D0985010

TEXTBOOK OF
Clinical Neurology

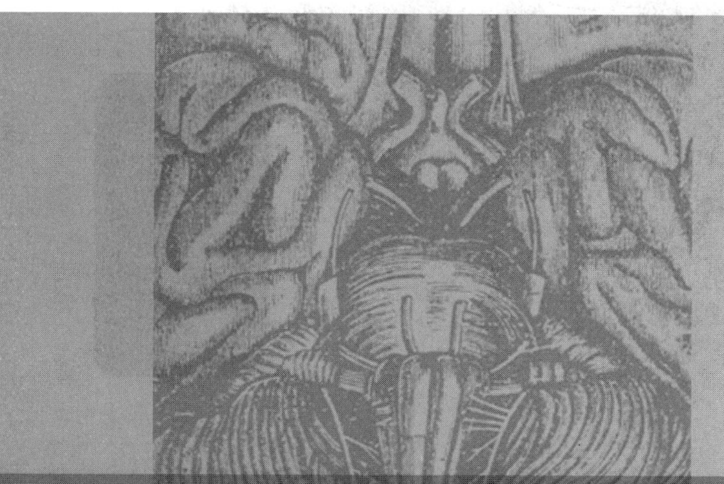

Second Edition

TEXTBOOK OF Clinical Neurology

CHRISTOPHER G. GOETZ, MD
Professor and Associate Chairman
Department of Neurological Sciences
Rush University
Rush-Presbyterian-St. Luke's Medical Center
Chicago, Illinois

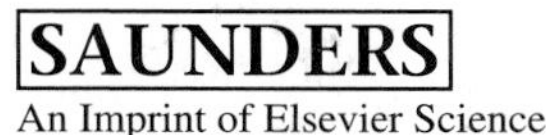

SAUNDERS
An Imprint of Elsevier Science

SAUNDERS
An Imprint of Elsevier Science

The Curtis Center
Independence Square West
Philadelphia, Pennsylvania 19106

TEXTBOOK OF CLINICAL NEUROLOGY
SECOND EDITION
ISBN 0–7216–3800–7

NOTICE

Neurology is an ever-changing field. Standard safety precautions must be followed, but as new research and clinical experience broaden our knowledge, changes in treatment and drug therapy may become necessary or appropriate. Readers are advised to check the most current product information provided by the manufacturer of each drug to be administered to verify the recommended dose, the method and duration of administration, and contraindications. It is the responsibility of the licensed prescriber, relying on experience and knowledge of the patient, to determine dosages and the best treatment for each individual patient. Neither the publisher nor the editor assumes any liability for any injury and/or damage to persons or property arising from this publication.

Previous edition copyrighted 1999

Library of Congress Cataloging-in-Publication Data

Textbook of clinical neurology/[edited by] Christopher G. Goetz.—2nd ed.
p. ; cm.
Includes bibliographical references and index.
ISBN 0–7216–3800–7
1. Nervous system—Diseases. 2. Neurology. I. Goetz, Christopher G.
[DNLM: 1. Nervous System. 2. Nervous System Diseases. WL 100 T3545 2003]
RC346. T446 2003
616.8—dc21

2002070829

Acquisitions Editor: Susan Pioli
Developmental Editor: Laurie Anello

Printed in the United States of America.

Last digit is the print number: 9 8 7 6 5 4 3 2 1

To my family,
Monica, Celine, Peter, and Elena Goetz,
and
To my colleague,
Eric J. Pappert, M.D.

Contents

Contributors

Michael J. Aminoff, M.D., D.Sc., F.R.C.P.
Professor of Neurology, School of Medicine, University of California; Attending Physician and Director, Clinical Neurophysiology Laboratories, University of California Medical Center, San Francisco, California
Electrophysiology

Russell Bartt, M.D.
Assistant Professor of Neurological Sciences, Rush Medical College; Attending Physician, Division of Neurology, Cook County Hospital, Chicago, Illinois
Autoimmune and Inflammatory Disorders

Anita L. Belman, M.D.
Professor of Neurology and Pediatrics, Department of Neurology, State University of New York at Stony Brook; Attending Neurologist, Stony Brook University Hospital Medical Center, Stony Brook, New York
Human Immunodeficiency Virus and Acquired Immunodeficiency Syndrome

Eduardo Benarroch, M.D., D.Sci.
Professor of Neurology, Consultant in Neurology, Mayo Clinic, Rochester, Minnesota
Autonomic Nervous System

Ramsis K. Benjamin, M.D., M.P.H.
Neuro-oncology Fellow, Department of Neurology, Massachusetts General Hospital; Neuro-oncology Clinical Fellow and Palliative Care Clinical Fellow, Departments of Neurology and Medicine, Massachusetts General Hospital, Boston, Massachusetts
Metastatic Neoplasms and Paraneoplastic Syndromes

Bruce O. Berg, M.D.
Professor Emeritus, Department of Neurology, University of California Medical Center, San Francisco, California
Chromosomal Abnormalities and Neurocutaneous Disorders

José Biller, M.D.
Professor and Chairman of Neurology, Indiana University School of Medicine; Chief of Services, Neurology, Indiana University Hospital, Indianapolis, Indiana
Neurovascular System

Thomas P. Bleck, M.D., F.C.C.M.
Louise Nerancy Eminent Scholar in Neurology and Professor of Neurology, Neurological Surgery, and Internal Medicine, University of Virginia; Director, Neuroscience Intensive Care Unit, University of Virginia, Charlottesville, Virginia
Levels of Consciousness and Attention

Bradley F. Boeve, M.D.
Assistant Professor of Neurology, Mayo Medical School, Consultant in Neurology, Division of Behavioral Neurology, Department of Neurology, Mayo Clinic, Rochester, Minnesota
The Degenerative Dementias

Karen I. Bolla, Ph.D.
Associate Professor of Neurology, Psychiatry and Behavioral Sciences, and Environmental Health, Johns Hopkins University School of Medicine and Bloomberg School of Public Health; Director of Neuropsychology, Johns Hopkins Bayview Medical Center, Baltimore, Maryland
Exogenous Acquired Metabolic Disorders of the Nervous System: Toxins and Illicit Drugs

Rebecca Brenden Bone, Ph.D.
Clinical Neuropsychologist, Division of Neurological Sciences, Department of Neurology, Rush-Presbyterian-St. Luke's Medical Center, Rush University, Chicago, Illinois
Neuropsychological Testing

Carsten G. Bönnemann, M.D.
Assistant Professor of Neurology and Pediatrics, University of Pennsylvania School of Medicine; Attending Neurologist, Department of Pediatrics, Children's Hospital of Philadelphia, Philadelphia, Pennsylvania
Developmental Structural Disorders

Derald E. Brackmann, M.D., F.A.C.S.
Clinical Professor of Otolaryngology and Head and Neck Surgery; Clinical Professor of Neurosurgery, University of Southern California School of Medicine; President, House Ear Clinic; Board of Directors, House Ear Institute, Los Angeles, California
Cranial Nerve VII: Facial Nerve

James B. Brewer, M.D., Ph.D.
Senior Resident, Department of Neurology, Johns Hopkins Medical Institute, Baltimore, Maryland
Memory

Paul Brown, M.D.
Senior Investigator, Laboratory for CNS Studies, National Institutes of Health, Bethesda, Maryland
Transmissible Spongiform Encephalopathy

Jean Lud Cadet, M.D.
Chief of Molecular Neuropsychiatry Section and Clinical Director, National Institute on Drug Abuse, National Institutes of Health, Baltimore, Maryland
Exogenous Acquired Metabolic Disorders of the Nervous System: Toxins and Illicit Drugs

Richard Camicioli, M.D., F.R.C.P.C.
Associate Professor of Medicine, University of Alberta; Attending Neurologist, Department of Medicine, University of Alberta Hospital and Glenrose Rehabilitation Hospital, Edmonton, Alberta, Canada
Gait and Balance

Mario Campero, M.D.
Assistant Professor, Department of Neurological Sciences, Faculty of Medicine, University of Chile, Santiago, Chile
Pain and Temperature

Louis R. Caplan, M.D.
Professor of Neurology, Harvard Medical School; Chief, Cerebrovascular Disease, Beth Israel Deaconess Medical Center, Boston, Massachusetts
Neurovascular Disorders

Richard J. Caselli, M.D.
Professor of Neurology, Mayo Medical School; Chairman, Division of Neurology, Mayo Clinic, Scottsdale, Arizona
The Degenerative Dementias

José Luis Castillo, M.D.
Associate Professor, Neurological Sciences, Faculty of Medicine, University of Chile; Neurologist, Clinical Neurophysiologist, Neurological Service, Hospital del Salvador, Santiago, Chile
Pain and Temperature

Gabriel Cea, M.D.
Assistant Professor of Neurology, Department of Neurology, University of Chile; Neurologist, Hospital del Salvador, National Health Service, Santiago, Chile
Pain and Temperature

Ronald D. Chervin, M.D., M.S.
Associate Professor, University of Michigan; Director, Sleep Disorders Center, University of Michigan, Ann Arbor, Michigan
Sleep Disorders

Chin-Sang Chung, M.D., Ph.D.
Professor, Department of Neurology, Sungkyunkwan University School of Medicine; Stroke Program Director, Department of Neurology, Samsung Medical Center, Seoul, Korea
Neurovascular Disorders

Cynthia L. Comella, M.D.
Associate Professor, Neurological Sciences, Rush University; Attending Neurologist, Rush-Presbyterian-St. Luke's Medical Center, Chicago, Illinois
Sleep and Wakefulness

Flavia B. Consens, M.D.
Clinical Assistant Professor, Department of Neurology, University of Michigan; Associate Director, Michael S. Aldrich Sleep Laboratory, University Hospital, University of Michigan, Ann Arbor, Michigan
Sleep Disorders

Peter B. Crino, M.D., Ph.D.
Assistant Professor, Department of Neurology, University of Pennsylvania, Philadelphia, Pennsylvania
The Trigeminal Nerve

Jeffrey L. Cummings, M.D.
Professor of Neurology, University of California, Los Angeles, California
Speech and Language

Asha Das, M.D.
Director, Medical Neuro-oncology, Department of Neurology, Cedars-Sinai Medical Center, Los Angeles, California
Metastatic Neoplasms and Paraneoplastic Syndromes

Cyrus K. Dastur
Medical Student, Drexel University College of Medicine; Department of Neuroradiology, Hahnemann University Hospital, Philadelphia, Pennsylvania
Neuroimaging

Hans Christoph Diener, M.D., Ph.D., F.A.H.A.
Chairman, Department of Neurology, University of Essen, Essen, Germany
Coordination and Ataxia

Richard L. Doty, Ph.D.
Professor, Department of Otorhinolaryngology: Head and Neck Surgery; Director, Smell and Taste Center, University of Pennsylvania, Philadelphia, Pennsylvania
Cranial Nerve I: Olfactory Nerve

Paul Richard Dyken, B.A., M.L.A., M.D.
Director, Institute for Research in Childhood Neurological Degenerative Diseases, Institute for Research in Childhood Neurodegenerative Diseases, Mobile, Alabama
Storage Diseases: Neuronal Ceroid-Lipofuscinoses, Lipidoses, Glycogenoses, and Leukodystrophies

Randolph W. Evans, M.D.
Clinical Associate Professor, Department of Neurology, University of Texas at Houston Medical School, Houston, Texas
Traumatic Disorders

Stanley Fahn, M.D.
H. Houston Merritt Professor of Neurology, Columbia University College of Physicians and Surgeons; Attending Neurologist, New York—Presbyterian Hospital, New York, New York
Hypokinesia and Hyperkinesia

Scott H. Faro, M.D.
Associate Professor of Radiological Sciences, Drexel University College of Medicine, Philadelphia, Pennsylvania
Neuroimaging

Mark A. Ferrante, M.D.
Director, EMG Laboratory, Bienville Orthopedic Associates, Biloxi, Mississippi; Clinical Associate Professor, Tulane University Medical Center, New Orleans, Louisiana
Body Fluid and Tissue Analysis; Endogenous Metabolic Disorders

Steven K. Feske, M.D.
Assistant Professor of Neurology, Harvard Medical School; Director, Stroke Division, Brigham and Women's Hospital, Boston, Massachusetts
Degenerative and Compressive Structural Disorders

Bruce L. Fetterman, M.D.
Clinical Assistant Professor, Otolaryngology, University of Tennessee, Memphis, Tennessee
Cranial Nerve VII: Facial Nerve

Nancy Foldvary-Schaefer, D.O.
Staff Neurologist, Section of Epilepsy and Sleep Disorders, Department of Neurology, Cleveland Clinic Foundation, Cleveland, Ohio
Epilepsy

Roy Freeman, M.D.
Associate Professor of Neurology, Department of Neurology, Harvard Medical School; Director, Autonomic and Peripheral Nerve Laboratory, Beth Israel Deaconess Medical Center, Boston, Massachusetts
Autonomic Nervous System

Joseph H. Friedman, M.D.
Professor and Chief, Section on Parkinson's Disease and Movement Disorders, Department of Clinical Neurosciences, Brown University Medical School; Chief, Division of Neurology, Memorial Hospital of Rhode Island, Pawtucket, Rhode Island
Mood, Emotion, and Thought

John D. E. Gabrieli, Ph.D.
Professor of Psychology, Stanford University, Stanford, California
Memory

Steven Galetta, M.D.
Van Meter Professor of Neurology, Department of Neurology, University of Pennsylvania Medical Center, Philadelphia, Pennsylvania
The Trigeminal Nerve

James Y. Garbern, M.D., Ph.D.
Associate Professor, Department of Neurology and Center for Molecular Medicine and Genetics, Wayne State University School of Medicine; Staff Neurologist, Harper University Hospital, Detroit, Michigan
Body Fluid and Tissue Analysis

Generoso G. Gascon, M.D.
Emeritus Professor, Clinical Neuroscience and Pediatrics, Brown University School of Medicine; Director, Division of Pediatric Neurology, Department of Neuroscience; Director, Department of Clinical Research, King Faisal Specialist Hospital and Research Center, Jeddah, Saudi Arabia
Aminoacidopathies and Organic Acidopathies, Mitochondrial Enzyme Defects, and Other Metabolic Errors

Jeffrey A. Golden, M.D.
Assistant Professor of Pathology, University of Pennsylvania School of Medicine; Associate Neuropathologist, Children's Hospital of Philadelphia, Philadelphia, Pennsylvania
Developmental Structural Disorders

Leslie J. Gonzalez-Rothi, Ph.D.
Professor of Neurology, University of Florida; Program Director, Brain Rehabilitation Research Center, VA Medical Center, Gainesville, Florida
Praxis

James Goodwin, M.D.
Associate Professor of Ophthalmology and Neurology, University of Illinois; Director, Neuro-ophthalmology Service, University of Illinois Eye and Ear Infirmary, Chicago, Illinois
Cranial Nerves III, IV, and VI: The Oculomotor System

Steven A. Greenberg, M.D.
Instructor, Department of Neurology, Harvard Medical School; Associate Neurologist, Department of Neurology, Brigham and Women's Hospital, Boston, Massachusetts
Degenerative and Compressive Structural Disorders

Robert C. Griggs, M.D.
Professor and Chairman, Department of Neurology, University of Rochester School of Medicine; Neurologist in Chief, Strong Memorial Hospital, Rochester, New York
Hereditary Nondegenerative Neuromuscular Disease

Timothy C. Hain, M.D.
Professor of Neurology, Otolaryngology, Physical Therapy, and Human Movement Sciences, Northwestern University; Director, Vestibular Laboratory, Chicago, Illinois
Cranial Nerve VIII: Vestibulocochlear System

John P. Hammerstad, M.D.
Professor Emeritus, Department of Neurology, Oregon Health and Sciences University, Portland, Oregon
Strength and Reflexes

Kenneth M. Heilman, M.D.
James E. Rooks Jr. Distinguished Professor of Neurology, University of Florida; Program Director, Shands Hospital at the University of Florida and the North Florida South Georgia Veteran Affairs Medical Center, Gainesville, Florida
Praxis

Wayne A. Hening, M.D., Ph.D.
Clinical Assistant Professor, Department of Neurology, University of Medicine and Dentistry of New Jersey, Robert Wood Johnson Medical School, New Brunswick, New Jersey
Sleep and Wakefulness

Neal Hermanowicz, M.D.
Associate Professor and Director, Movement Disorders Program, Vice Chair for Clinical Affairs, University of California, Irvine, and Phillip and Carol Traub Center for Parkinson's Disease, Irvine and Rancho Mirage, California
Cranial Nerves IX (Glossopharyngeal) and X (Vagus)

Beverly L. Hershey, M.D.
Clinical Assistant Professor, Department of Diagnostic Radiology, Thomas Jefferson University Hospital—Methodist Division, Philadelphia, Pennsylvania
Neuroimaging

Fred H. Hochberg, M.D.
Attending Neurologist, Department of Neurology, Massachusetts General Hospital, Boston, Massachusetts
Metastatic Neoplasms and Paraneoplastic Syndromes

Stacy S. Horn, D.O.
Assistant Clinical Professor, Department of Neurology, University of Pennsylvania; Pennsylvania Hospital, Philadelphia, Pennsylvania
Drug-Induced and Iatrogenic Neurological Disorders

Joseph Jankovic, M.D.
Professor of Neurology and Director of Parkinson's Disease Center and Movement Disorders, Baylor College of Medicine; Senior Attending Physician, Methodist Hospital, Houston, Texas
Movement Disorders

Todd J. Janus, M.D., Ph.D.
Assistant Professor, Neurological Sciences and Internal Medicine (Oncology), Rush Medical College, Chicago, Illinois
Primary Neurological Tumors

Horacio Kaufmann, M.D.
Associate Professor, Department of Neurology, Mount Sinai School of Medicine; Director, Neurology, Autonomic Disorders Research and Treatment Program, Mount Sinai School of Medicine, New York, New York
Autonomic Nervous System

Laurence J. Kinsella, M.D., F.A.C.P.
Associate Professor of Neurology, Saint Louis University; Chief, Division of Neurology and Neurophysiology, Tenet-Forest Park Hospital, Saint Louis, Missouri
Nutritional Deficiencies and Syndromes Associated with Alcoholism

Thomas Klockgether, M.D.
Professor and Chairman, Department of Neurology, University of Bonn; Head, Department of Neurology, University Hospital Bonn, Bonn, Germany
Ataxias

Robert A. Koenigsberg, D.O., F.A.O.C.R.
Professor of Radiology and Director of Neuroradiology, Department of Radiological Sciences, Drexel University College of Medicine, Philadelphia, Pennsylvania
Neuroimaging

Katie Kompoliti, M.D.
Assistant Professor of Neurological Sciences, Rush University; Adjunct Attending Physician, Neurological Sciences, Rush-Presbyterian-St. Luke's Medical Center, Rush University, Chicago, Illinois
Drug-Induced and Iatrogenic Neurological Disorders

William Kupsky, M.D.
Professor of Neurology, Psychiatry, and Behavioral Neuroscience, Clinical Neuroscience Center, Wayne State University School of Medicine, William Beaumont Hospital, Royal Oak, Michigan
Body Fluid and Tissue Analysis

Peter A. LeWitt, M.D., M.Med.Sc.
Professor of Neurology, Psychiatry, and Behavioral Neuroscience, Clinical Neuroscience Center, Wayne State University School of Medicine; William Beaumont Hospital, Royal Oak, Michigan
Body Fluid and Tissue Analysis

Grant T. Liu, M.D.
Associate Professor, Departments of Neurology and Ophthalmology, University of Pennsylvania School of Medicine; Neuro-ophthalmologist, Hospital of the University of Pennsylvania, Children's Hospital of Philadelphia, and the Scheie Eye Institute, Philadelphia, Pennsylvania
Cranial Nerve II and Afferent Visual Pathways

Elan D. Louis, M.D., M.S.
Assistant Professor of Neurology, Sergievsky Center, College of Physicians and Surgeons, Columbia University; Assistant Attending Neurologist, Columbia-Presbyterian Medical Center, New York, New York
Cranial Nerves XI (Spinal Accessory) and XII (Hypoglossal)

Betsy B. Love, M.D.
Volunteer Clinical Associate Professor, Department of Neurology, Indiana University College of Medicine, Indianapolis, Indiana
Neurovascular System

Paul Maertens, M.D.
Associate Professor of Neurology and Pediatrics, University of South Alabama, Mobile, Alabama
Storage Diseases: Neuronal Ceroid-Lipofuscinoses, Lipidoses, Glycogenoses, and Leukodystrophies

Mirjana Maletic-Savatic, M.D., Ph.D.
Assistant Professor of Neurology, State University of New York, Stony Brook, New York
Human Immunodeficiency Virus and Acquired Immunodeficiency Syndrome

Mario F. Mendez, M.D., Ph.D.
Professor of Neurology, University of California at Los Angeles; Director, Neurobehavior Unit, VA Greater Los Angeles Healthcare, Los Angeles, California
Speech and Language

Alan G. Micco, M.D., F.A.C.S.
Assistant Professor, Department of Otolaryngology and Head and Neck Surgery, Northwestern University Medical School, Chicago, Illinois
Cranial Nerve VIII: Vestibulocochlear System

Feroze B. Mohamed, Ph.D.
Assistant Professor, Department of Radiology, Drexel University College of Medicine, Philadelphia, Pennsylvania
Neuroimaging

Greg Morgan, M.D.
Neurology Associates, P.A., Austin, Texas
Proprioception, Touch, and Vibratory Sensation

Ziad S. Nasreddine, M.D., F.R.C.P.C.
Assistant Clinical Professor, Department of Neurology, Sherbrooke University and McGill University; Behaviorial Neurologist, Charles LeMoyne Hospital and Jewish General Hospital, Montreal, Quebec, Canada
Speech and Language

Barnett R. Nathan, M.D.
Assistant Professor, Departments of Neurology and Internal Medicine, University of Virginia, Charlottesville, Virginia
Cerebrospinal Fluid and Intracranial Pressure

Nancy J. Newman, M.D.
Professor and Leo Delle Jolley Professor, Departments of Ophthalmology, Neurology, and Neurological Surgery, Emory University School of Medicine; Director, Neuro-ophthalmology, Emory Eye Center, Atlanta, Georgia
Cranial Nerve II and Afferent Visual Pathways

John H. Noseworthy, M.D., F.R.C.P.C.
Professor and Chairman, Department of Neurology, Mayo Medical School, Clinic and Foundation, Rochester, Minnesota
Demyelinating Disorders of the Central Nervous System

John G. Nutt, M.D.
Professor of Neurology, Departments of Neurology, Physiology, and Pharmacology, Oregon Health and Science University and Portland VA Medical Center, Portland, Oregon
Gait and Balance

Pinar T. Ozand, M.D., Ph.D.
Chairman, Department of Genetics, and Senior Consultant, Medical Genetics, King Faisal Specialist Hospital and Research Center, Riyadh, Saudi Arabia
Aminoacidopathies and Organic Acidopathies, Mitochondrial Enzyme Defects, and Other Metabolic Errors

Istvan Pirko, M.D.
Neuroimmunology Fellow, Department of Neurology, Mayo Clinic, Rochester, Minnesota
Demyelinating Disorders of the Central Nervous System

Alison R. Preston, M.A.
Department of Psychology, Stanford University, Stanford, California
Memory

David E. Riley, M.D.
Associate Professor of Neurology, Case Western Reserve University School of Medicine; Director, Movement Disorders Center, University Hospitals of Cleveland, Cleveland, Ohio
Nutritional Deficiencies and Syndromes Associated with Alcoholism

Karen L. Roos, M.D.
John and Nancy Nelson Professor of Neurology, Department of Neurology, Indiana University School of Medicine, Indianapolis, Indiana
Viral Infections; Nonviral Infections

Michael Rose, B.Sc., M.D., F.R.C.P.
Honorary Senior Lecturer, Division of Neurosciences, Guy's, King's, and St. Thomas's School of Medicine, King's College, University of London; Consultant, Department of Neurology, King's College Hospital, London, United Kingdom
Hereditary Nondegenerative Neuromuscular Disease

Kathleen M. Shannon, M.D.
Associate Professor, Department of Neurological Sciences, Rush Medical College; Attending Physician, Department of Neurological Sciences, Rush-Presbyterian-St. Luke's Medical Center, Chicago, Illinois
Autoimmune and Inflammatory Disorders

Robert W. Shields, Jr., M.D.
Staff Neurologist, Cleveland Clinic Foundation, Cleveland, Ohio
Demyelinating Disorders of the Peripheral Nervous System

Nailah Siddique, R.N., M.S.N.
Clinical Nurse Specialist, Neuromuscular Disorders Program, Department of Neurology, Feinberg School of Medicine, Northwestern University, Chicago, Illinois
Degenerative Motor, Sensory, and Autonomic Disorders

Teepu Siddique, M.D.
Professor, Davee Department of Neurology and Clinical Neurosciences, Department of Cell and Molecular Biology; Abbott Laboratories Duane and Susan Burnham Research Professor; Director Neuromuscular Disorders Program, Feinberg School of Medicine, Northwestern University, Chicago, Illinois
Degenerative Motor, Sensory, and Autonomic Disorders

Todd L. Siegal, M.D.
Assistant Professor of Neuroradiology, Cooper Hospital, University Medical Center, Camden, New Jersey
Neuroimaging

Stephen D. Silberstein, M.D.
Professor, Department of Neurology, Jefferson Medical College, Thomas Jefferson University; Director, Jefferson Headache Center, Thomas Jefferson University Hospital, Philadelphia, Pennsylvania
Headache and Facial Pain

Glenn T. Stebbins, Ph.D.
Associate Professor, Department of Neurological Sciences, Rush-Presbyterian-St. Luke's Medical Center, Rush University, Chicago, Illinois
Neuropsychological Testing

Suzanne Stevens, M.D.
Assistant Professor, Departments of Psychology and Neurology, Rush-Presbyterian-St. Luke's Medical Center, Rush University, Chicago, Illinois
Sleep and Wakefulness

Robert Sufit, M.D.
Professor of Neurology, Feinberg School of Medicine, Northwestern University; Director, Neurologic Testing Center, Northwestern Memorial Hospital, Chicago, Illinois
Degenerative Motor, Sensory, and Autonomic Disorders

Margaret M. Swanberg, D.O.
Chief, Behavioral Neurology Section, Department of Neurology, Walter Reed Army Medical Center, Washington, D.C.
Speech and Language

Dagmar Timmann, M.D.
Associate Professor, Department of Neurology, University of Essen, Essen, Germany
Coordination and Ataxia

Fong Y. Tsai, M.D.
Professor and Chairman, Department of Radiological Sciences, University of California and Irvine Medical Center, Irvine, California
Neuroimaging

Chandan J. Vaidya, Ph.D.
Assistant Professor, Department of Psychology, Georgetown University, Washington, D.C.
Memory

Renato J. Verdugo, M.D., M.Sc.
Director, Department of Neurology, Faculty of Medicine, University of Chile, Santiago, Chile
Pain and Temperature

Arthur S. Walters, M.D.
New Jersey Neuroscience Institute at JFK Medical Center; Professor, Department of Neuroscience, Seton Hall University School of Graduate Medical Education; Clinical Professor of Neurology, University of Medicine and Dentistry of New Jersey—Robert Wood Johnson Medical School, New Brunswick, New Jersey
Sleep and Wakefulness

Robert T. Watson, M.D.
Professor, Department of Neurology, and Senior Associate Dean for Educational Affairs, Dean's Office, University of Florida College of Medicine, Gainesville, Florida
Praxis

Jack E. Wilberger, M.D., F.A.C.S.
Professor, Chairman, and Vice Dean of Neurosurgery, Drexel University College of Medicine, Allegheny General Hospital, Pittsburgh, Pennsylvania
Traumatic Disorders

Asa J. Wilbourn, M.D.
Clinical Professor of Neurology, Case Western Reserve School of Medicine; Director, EMG Laboratory, Cleveland Clinic, Cleveland, Ohio
Demyelinating Disorders of the Peripheral Nervous System

Elaine Wyllie, M.D.
Head, Section of Pediatric Epilepsy, Department of Neurology, Cleveland Clinic Foundation, Cleveland, Ohio
Epilepsy

William B. Young, M.D.
Assistant Professor of Neurology, Thomas Jefferson University; Attending, Department of Neurology, Thomas Jefferson Hospital, Philadelphia, Pennsylvania
Headache and Facial Pain

W. K. Alfred Yung, M.D.
Professor and Chairman, Department of Neuro-oncology, University of Texas M.D. Anderson Cancer Center, Houston, Texas
Primary Neurological Tumors

Preface

The first edition of *Textbook of Clinical Neurology*, published in 1999, was envisioned to answer an educational need not met by other textbooks. My original co-editor and I modeled the text after the three-part process used by clinical neurologists to diagnose and treat patients with neurological illnesses: establishing anatomical localization and definition of clinical syndromes based on the neurological examination and history (Part One), using diagnostic tools to clarify the syndromic diagnosis (Part Two), and explaining etiologies of neurological illnesses to establish the cause of neurological disorders (Part Three). In clinical practice, this three-step system is used in everyday diagnosis and treatment. In both the first and second editions, a clear and consistent format guides readers through this sequence.

Because neurological progress is an ongoing process that involves the rapid evolution of new information, I am pleased to offer readers this updated second edition, which applies reviewers' and colleagues' comments on the first edition to expand the information presented in the original chapters. This edition adds to the main elements of the original text a number of new features that make it unique among textbooks in the field. First, this multiauthor text incorporates the writings of internationally recognized experts in their respective fields of study. At the same time, however, firm, centralized editorial control ensures a homogeneous flow among the chapters and the parts. Second, each chapter includes not only a list of numbered references but also a list of Reviews and Selected Updates, which covers summaries and overviews as well as the latest published writings in clinical neurology. Third, to address the ongoing trend toward electronic education, every copy of the textbook includes a CD-ROM disk. The disk contains the complete text, as well as numerous videotape examples of disorders, interactive clinical exercises keyed to each chapter, and a search engine. To facilitate use of the CD-ROM, I have placed an icon in the margins of the printed text to indicate videotape entries.

A major administrative change in the second edition is the single editorship. Career and personal obligations prompted my colleague Eric Pappert to forgo his original co-editorship. As I have organized and completed this editorial project, however, I have remained cognizant that his intellectual rigor and high standards retain their imprint on this edition. Though removed from the cover and title page, his name appears in my dedication, and, in placing it there, I extend my hand to him in continued friendship.

The intent of the new and innovative approach to learning represented in this textbook is to capture the historically honored neurological method in its modern context. It is my aim for readers to move through the three parts of the book or the CD-ROM as they evaluate their patients, beginning with the anatomical syndromes, moving to the evaluation tools, and concluding with an etiology, always reviewing and previewing materials as in actual neurological practice. I have been pleased to see the first edition in wide use when I visit hospitals and universities. Rather than placed on a library shelf, the book is frequently left open on physicians' desks and put to active use on hospital units. I have seen residents carrying it during daily rounds and students working on the CD-ROM exercises. I have heard physicians discussing the many video cases as they relate to given patients in their practices. These are the markers of success that prompted me to take on the work of editing this new edition.

In addition to acknowledging the authors and the staff at Saunders, I extend my special thanks to Bernadette Gillard, whose editorial assistance, expertise, and careful attention to detail have made the preparation of this second edition of *Textbook of Clinical Neurology* a smooth process. The credits for the accompanying CD-ROM are provided in the opening panels of the program, but the expert work of both Steve Bick and Teresa Chmura on that project helped in the completion of the final corrections and details of the printed textbook as well.

I close this preface with two quotations borrowed from the first clinical neurologist of international proportion, the 19th-century physician Jean-Martin Charcot. The leitmotifs of his lectures have guided my career and retain their modernity in the 21st century. This second edition of *Textbook of Clinical Neurology* has been conceived and executed on the foundations of the teachings of this seminal neurologist:

Let us keep looking, in spite of everything. Let us keep searching. It is indeed the best method for finding, and perhaps, thanks to our efforts, the verdict we will give such an individual tomorrow will not be the same one we must give this patient today.

Let someone say of a doctor that he really knows his physiology or anatomy, that he is dynamic—these are not real compliments; but if you say he is an observer, a man who knows how to see, this is perhaps the greatest compliment one can receive.

—*Leçons du Mardi*, 1888

Christopher G. Goetz, M.D.
Chicago, Illinois

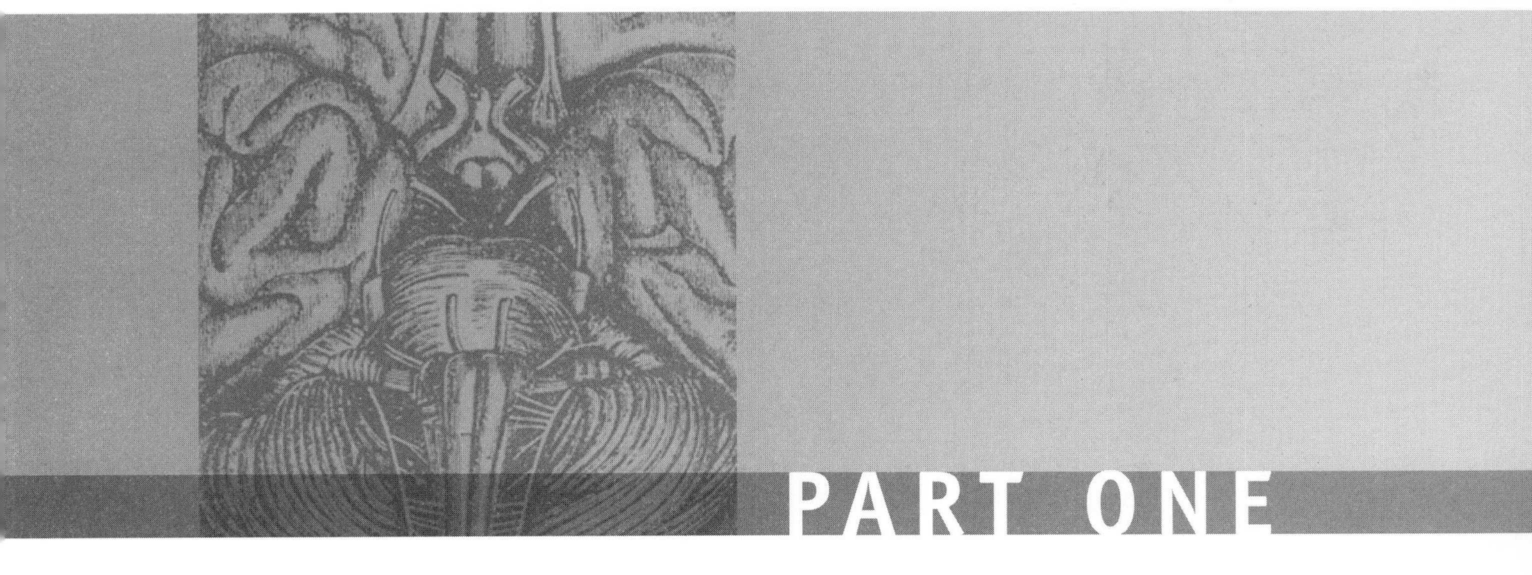

PART ONE

Neuroanatomical Localization and Syndromes

CHAPTER 1

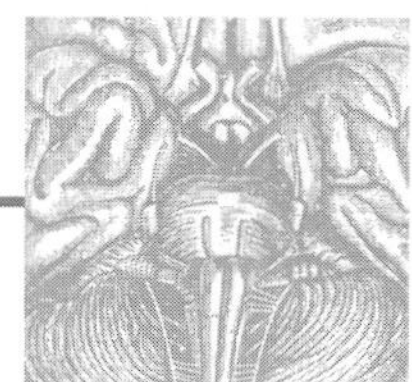

THOMAS P. BLECK

Levels of Consciousness and Attention

History and Definitions

Consciousness represents the core of our experience as human beings, and its alterations challenge our concepts of self and the meaning or value of life. For the physician, and especially the clinical neuroscientist, these alterations are among the greatest dilemmas, because the disorders that produce them often require swift diagnosis and management based primarily on the physical examination and most probable etiologies. The ancients, at least as far back as the Egyptians at the time of the Edwin Smith surgical papyrus, recognized that the brain was the seat of consciousness. However, the anatomical structures and physiological processes involved in awareness were not elucidated until the middle of the 20th century. The classic studies of Moruzzi and Magoun[1] established the importance of the midbrain reticular formation as the driving force of consciousness. McNealy and Plum[2] applied these concepts in their clinical observations, which were published in the 1960s, on patients with mass lesions. With some modifications by Ropper[3] in recent years, their discussion of the anatomy of lesions altering consciousness, as amplified in the classic text by Plum and Posner,[4] remains the foundation for analysis of the patient with altered consciousness. The other major source of insight into mechanisms of consciousness comes from the study of patients with epilepsy, particularly by Penfield and Jasper[5] and by Gloor.[6] The various theories used to explain loss of awareness during complex partial seizures and absence seizures have helped elucidate the interaction of the cortex and the reticular system.

For the purposes of this book, *consciousness* describes that set of neural processes that allow an individual to perceive, comprehend, and act on the internal and external environments. It is usually envisioned in two parts: *arousal* and *awareness*. Arousal describes the degree to which the individual appears to be able to interact with these environments; the contrast between waking and sleeping is a common example of two different states of arousal. In contrast, awareness reflects the depth and content of the aroused state. Awareness is dependent on arousal, because one who cannot be aroused appears to lack awareness. Awareness does not imply any specificity for the modality of stimulation. This stimulation may be external (e.g., auditory) or internal (e.g., thirst). *Attention* depends on awareness and implies the ability to respond to particular types of stimuli (modality-specific).[7]

Many terms that describe gradations of consciousness populate the clinical literature. *Stupor* refers to a condition in which the patient is less alert than usual but can be stimulated into responding. *Obtundation* describes a patient who appears to be asleep much of the time when not being stimulated. This eyes-closed state is not electroencephalographic (EEG) sleep, however. Stuporous or obtunded patients respond to noxious stimuli by attempting to deflect or avoid the stimulus. The *comatose* patient lies with eyes closed and does not make an attempt to avoid noxious stimuli. Such a person may display various forms of reflex *posturing* (defined later), but does not actively try to avoid the stimulus. After a period of coma, some patients may enter a *vegetative state*, in which the patient's eyes open and close, and the patient may appear to track objects about the room and may chew and swallow food placed in the mouth. However, the vegetative patient does not respond to auditory stimuli and does not appear to sense pain, hunger, or other stimuli. This is a state in which there is arousal but no awareness.

Delirium has been redefined in recent years by the psychiatric community through the *Diagnostic and Statistical Manual of Mental Disorders*. In this publication, delirium is defined as "a disturbance of consciousness that is accompanied by a change in cognition that cannot be better accounted for by a preexisting or evolving dementia. The disturbance develops over a short period of time, usually hours or days, and tends to fluctuate during the course of the day. There is evidence from the history, physical examination, or laboratory tests that the delirium is a direct physiological consequence of a general medical condition, substance intoxication or withdrawal, use of a medication, or toxin exposure, or a combination of these factors."[8]

Many other terms have been applied to gradations of consciousness but lack consistent definitions and usage. For this reason, one should eschew their employment and concentrate on clearly describing what the patient does spontaneously and in response to auditory, visual, and somatic stimulation. This discipline results in clearer communication among the clinicians caring for the patient.

Clinical History

Although the physician confronted with a patient whose alertness is reduced must be prepared to proceed without any external information, knowledge of the patient's history frequently provides important clues regarding the etiology of the problem and the initial approach to management. When an observer can provide the history of the present illness, immediate therapy for likely causes can be instituted. Even when only fragmentary information is available, such data allow the clinician to focus the evaluation more closely and, it is hoped, reach a diagnosis in a more timely fashion.

A history of trauma or underlying medical disease is important to establish, and a list of medications may suggest important intoxication or drug reactions. If the change in consciousness occurred suddenly, a cardiac or primary neurovascular event should be considered, whereas a subacute or slow decline in function may suggest other medical or metabolic causes. Any details on the immediate events surrounding the altered consciousness may help in isolating possible environmental factors, and knowledge of prior events of a similar nature leads the clinician to consider etiologies of a recurrent nature, like epilepsy. Particularly important information on associated medical or neurological signs that occurred just before the loss of consciousness, such as vomiting, altered speech or confusion, hemiparesis, or chest pains, are directly applicable to forming a list of possible diagnoses.

Anatomy of Consciousness and Attention

ANATOMY OF AROUSAL

Arousal requires the interplay of both the reticular formation and the cerebral hemispheres. The reticular components necessary for arousal reside in the midbrain and diencephalon; the pontine reticular formation is not necessary for arousal. The midbrain may be viewed as a driving center for the higher structures; loss of the midbrain reticular formation (MRF) produces a state in which the cortex appears to be waiting for the command or ability to function. This is manifested electroencephalographically as alpha coma, in which the resting electrical activity of the cortex appears relatively normal but cannot be altered by external or internal stimuli. This ascending midbrain reticular activating system extends upward into the hypothalamus to the thalamus. It receives collaterals from and is stimulated by every major somatic and sensory pathway directly or indirectly. Because of its many cellular components, this system is best regarded as a physiological rather than a precise anatomical entity. Nonetheless, at least three principle paths project out of the midbrain—one to the thalamic reticular nucleus and then to the cortex, one to the hypothalamus and then on to the basal forebrain and limbic system, and a third to the brain stem median raphe and locus caeruleus with consequent diffuse cortical projections.[9]

The precise mechanism of diencephalic involvement in arousal is uncertain. Information from the midbrain reticular formation passes to the thalamic reticular nucleus, through which these signals must pass in order to allow the cortex to function. The thalamic reticular nucleus acts predominantly to inhibit the cerebral cortex via outflow tracts that traverse numerous other thalamic nuclei. By increasing or decreasing thalamic inhibitory mechanisms on the cortex, the ascending reticular system from the midbrain provides a gating mechanism to enhance or diminish neuronal activation.[10] In patients with chronic subdural hematoma, diminished awareness appears to reflect a decrease in thalamic blood flow as a consequence of horizontal diencephalic shift.[11]

Disorders that distort the normal anatomical relationships of the midbrain, diencephalon, and cortex appear to impair arousal by interrupting the flow of information from the midbrain to the cortex. However, it is likely that the diencephalon plays a more active role in the control of arousal than simply that of a conduit. For example, in the prion disorder known as fatal familial insomnia (see Chapter 43), dysfunction of neurons in the anterior and ventral thalamic nuclei interfere with normal sleep-wake cycling to diminish or even completely prevent sleep.

Because of the diffuse anatomical substrate of arousal, little is known of the specific neurochemistry involved in the maintenance of arousal. It appears, however, that central acetylcholine and monoamine systems (noradrenaline and serotonin) have received the most attention. Cholinergic receptors exist at many levels of this system; antimuscarinic drugs often depress consciousness, and the centrally active cholinesterase inhibitor physostigmine reverses anticholinergic encephalopathy, both observations suggesting a direct role of the cholinergic system. Likewise, norepinephrine and serotonin are neurotransmitters in numerous areas of the brain stem reticular formation and may serve as direct or indirect chemical components of arousal pharmacology.[12]

Although older discussions of this material have stressed the role of downward shift of the midbrain in the production of coma, current concepts of pathological anatomy have been revised by the availability of computed tomography (CT) and magnetic resonance imaging (MRI). It is now clear that in patients with lateralized masses, the horizontal displacement of the diencephalon is more closely correlated with the degree of altered awareness than the vertical displacement. In patients with diffuse brain swelling, caudal vertical displacement of the diencephalon is important, but the actual mechanism of coma may relate more to elevated intracranial pressure (ICP), which compromises cerebral perfusion, than the actual movement. Terminally, both lateral masses and diffuse supratentorial brain swelling displace the brain stem caudally, separating it from the basilar artery (which remains fixed to the clivus).

Loss of function of both cerebral hemispheres interferes with normal arousal mechanisms. However, over days to weeks following a severe global cortical injury (e.g., hypoxia), the central nervous system appears to re-establish some degree of arousal. This is clinically apparent in the vegetative state, in which the patient manifests sleep-wake cycling. This condition appears to represent arousal without awareness, and is histopathologically characterized by loss of the cortex with preservation of brain stem and diencephalic reticular structures.

In summary, two primary types of lesions depress the level of arousal, either direct brain stem–diencephalic dysfunction involving the reticular formation and nuclei or bilateral cerebral dysfunction. Unilateral cortical lesions should not impair arousal function unless there is secondary compression or compromise of the other hemisphere or reticular structures, as sometimes occurs with herniation syndromes.

ANATOMY OF AWARENESS

Awareness implies that the individual is not only alert but is cognizant of self and surroundings. Interaction of the cerebral cortex and the reticular system is required for the individual to be aware. Analysis of patients in the vegetative state and the study of anencephalic infants provide a picture of reticular system function in the absence of the cerebral cortex. The opposite problem, that of understanding the function of the cortex in the absence of reticular system control, is difficult to study. First, almost all lesions damaging the midbrain or thalamic reticular structures also impair motor output, and second, although the cortex appears electroencephalographically to be idling, there is no electrical technique by which one can determine whether the cortex is aware. A few case reports suggest that olfactory stimulation (which does not require transit through the midbrain or thalamus to reach the cortex) may produce an EEG change, and patients in alpha coma due to a midbrain lesion will rarely alter this EEG pattern. These are the only suggestions that external stimuli can alter cortical function in the absence of reticular system driving. With current techniques, scientists are not able to examine whether the cortex of an individual with a reticular system lesion is able to perceive any internal state (e.g., hunger).

ANATOMY OF ATTENTION

Attention to specific aspects of the perceived universe depends on both awareness as a general property and on the specific anatomical structures that mediate the sensory phenomena involved. In order to attend to a particular stimulus, the pathways required for its perception must be functional (e.g., the visual system must carry information from the retina to the occipital cortex for visual attention to occur). Each primary sensory modality has one or more principal cortical regions that must function in order to attend to a stimulus (e.g., primary somatosensory cortex in the postcentral gyrus), but the presence of these areas alone is not sufficient for attention. Lesions affecting the more posterior portion of the nondominant parietal lobe, for example, produce extinction of the contralateral stimulus when stimuli are presented simultaneously on each side of the body. A lesion at the occipitoparietal junction produces a similar defect in visual perception of bilateral stimuli. With larger lesions, the patient appears to have increasingly more substantial deficits in awareness of the contralateral half of the universe, including the self.

Examination of Consciousness and Attention

DIRECTED NEUROLOGICAL EXAMINATION

Overview

The examination of the patient with altered consciousness begins by ensuring that the patient's vital signs and basic biochemistry are adequate to support brain function. It is essential to ensure that blood pressure, respiration, and oxygen saturation are adequate and that the patient is not hypoglycemic or thiamine deficient before proceeding with the examination outlined later. In many situations (e.g., emergency departments), naloxone is also administered at this point to reverse any putative effects of opiates. The empirical use of flumazenil to antagonize potential benzodiazepine intoxication as a routine measure is controversial because of the risk of provoking seizures or status epilepticus, especially in patients with mixed benzodiazepine and cyclic antidepressant overdoses.

The initial goals of the examination of the patient with apparent altered consciousness are first to determine whether the patient is conscious and then, in patients with altered awareness, to determine whether or not the reticular system is functional. Because altered awareness requires either reticular system dysfunction or bilateral hemispheric dysfunction, testing the structures immediately adjacent to the reticular system provides the major clues regarding the etiology of altered consciousness and thereby determines the direction of subsequent investigations. The major findings on examination and their expected anatomical correlates are presented in Table 1–1. These correlations are

TABLE 1–1. **Clinical Findings with Different Levels of Central Nervous System Dysfunction**

Dysfunction	Response to Noxious Stimuli	Pupils	Eye Movements	Breathing
Both cortices	Withdrawal	Small, reactive	Spontaneous conjugate horizontal movements; if none, cervico-ocular or vestibulo-ocular reflexes can be elicited	Posthyperventilation apnea or Cheyne-Stokes respiration
Thalamus	Decorticate posturing	Same as above, unless the optic tracts are also damaged	Same as above	Same as above
Midbrain	Decorticate or decerebrate posturing	Midposition, fixed to light	Loss of ability to adduct. Both eyes may be deviated laterally (wall-eyed) (CN III damaged)	Usually same as above; potential for central reflex hyperpnea
Pons	Decerebrate posturing	Usually small; may exhibit bilateral pinpoint pupils (especially with midline pontine hemorrhage); Horner's syndrome with lateral lesions	Loss of conjugate horizontal movements with retained vertical movements and accommodation. Often eyes are deviated medially (CN VII damage)	May exhibit central reflex hyperpnea, cluster (Biot's) breathing, or apneustic breathing
Medulla	Weak leg flexion (or none)	Usually small; Horner's syndrome with lateral lesions	Usually no effect on spontaneous eye movements; may interfere with reflex responses; rarely, nystagmus	Rarely, ataxic respiration; apnea if respiratory centers involved

with the level of *dysfunction*, which may involve a substantially larger portion of the nervous system than the degree of actual *damage*.[13]

The findings on these examinations are often summarized by use of the Glasgow Coma Scale.[14] Because the verbal response of intubated patients is difficult to assess, one either ignores it (assigning it a value of T, for intubated) or imputes a score based on the examiner's estimate of what the patient could do. Although the results of this evaluation are frequently presented as the sum of the values, this practice is of limited utility. This procedure is of value in indicating the severity of head injury, in which a total score of 3 to 8 indicates severe trauma, 9 to 13 moderate trauma, and 14 to 15 mild trauma. However, the real utility of the score is to provide a simple way of detecting changes in the examination over time, with good inter-rater reliability, in circumstances of global cerebral dysfunction (e.g., trauma, intoxication). The score has limited utility in patients with focal neurological dysfunction.

At all times in the initial examination of the patient with suspected impaired awareness, the examiner must recall that the patient may in fact be capable of sensing and remembering. Although noxious stimuli may be required for an adequate examination, the minimum necessary stimulation should be employed, and the examiner should always be cognizant of the need for explanation of procedures, especially potentially painful ones. This caveat should carry over from the first encounter with the patient throughout the course of treatment. Attempts to communicate the level of sedation in patients is particularly problematic. For patients who are intoxicated or therapeutically sedated, the scale proposed by Ramsay and colleagues is commonly used (Table 1–2).[15]

Assessment of Arousal

Observation of the Patient's Ambient State. A great deal can be learned by watching the patient before the formal examination. Is the patient lying still in bed when not stimulated (required for the diagnosis of coma), or does he or she exhibit spontaneous movements? Evaluation of the patient's spontaneous movements often yields information of localizing and lateralizing significance. An externally rotated leg in a comatose patient is frequently evidence of corticospinal tract dysfunction

TABLE 1–2. **Sedation Scale**

Level	Patient's State
1	Awake, anxious and agitated, or restless
2	Awake, cooperative, oriented, and tranquil
3	Awake but responds to commands only
4	Appears asleep (this is not true sleep) but responds brisky to a light glabellar tap or a loud auditory stimulus
5	Appears asleep, and responds only sluggishly to a light glabellar tap or a loud auditory stimulus
6	Appears asleep, with no response to stimuli

From Ramsay MA, Savage TM, Simpson BR, Goodwin R: Controlled sedation with alphaxalone-alphadolone. BMJ 1974;2:656–659.

due to a contralateral hemispheric lesion. Do the eyes open spontaneously, and are there other facial movements? Minor facial or extremity twitching is frequently the only physical finding in patients suffering from nonconvulsive status epilepticus. Is there evidence of trauma to the head or the rest of the body?

The examiner next asks the patient to follow verbal commands. Early in the examination, ask the patient to open the eyes and look up; this will detect patients with pontine lesions that prevent all other somatic motor output (the locked-in syndrome; see later). Such patients may appear comatose but are not, and care must be taken to recall that they are alert and cognizant, and have intact auditory and somatosensory systems despite their brain stem disorder.[16]

Pupillary Responses to Light. The parasympathetic reflex arc begins in the retina, traverses the base of the brain, runs through the midbrain, and returns to the pupil (see Chapters 8 and 9). Disorders altering pupillary constriction typically affect the midbrain or cranial nerve III. Compression of the superior colliculus (e.g., by a pineal region mass) interferes with input to the pretectal nuclei, resulting in pupils that are large (because the sympathetic system is not affected), unreactive to light, and sometimes displaying *hippus*. Lesions affecting the area of the Edinger-Westphal nucleus and the origins of cranial nerve III are the most important, because this area is adjacent to the superior pole of the midbrain reticular formation. Because the descending sympathetic efferent fibers also traverse this portion of the brain stem, dysfunction produces pupils that are midposition (4 to 6 mm in diameter), unreactive to light, and frequently slightly irregular. Such pupils are an ominous finding, usually indicating that coma is due to structural damage affecting the upper midbrain, and unless its etiology can be reversed quickly, the patient's coma is usually irreversible. Because the pupillary constrictor has a muscarinic, rather than a nicotinic, acetylcholine receptor, it is not affected by drugs given to block neuromuscular transmission. However, it is affected by systemic antimuscarinic drugs (e.g., atropine), so one must be cautious about interpreting the examination if such agents are being used.

Unilateral loss of pupillary constriction in the comatose patient may rarely indicate subarachnoid hemorrhage from an internal carotid aneurysm that compresses cranial nerve III at the origin of the posterior communicating artery. Much more commonly, such a finding indicates the presence of a mass lesion that has shifted the diencephalon laterally. Although older studies suggested that this finding arose from compression of the third cranial nerve by the herniating temporal lobe, the unilaterally dilated pupil appears to develop before actual movement of the medial temporal structures over the tentorial edge. Ropper's work demonstrates that unilateral pupillary dilation results from traction on cranial nerve III produced when the diencephalon, being pushed away from an expanding lateral mass, pulls the midbrain with it. Because cranial nerve III is tethered anteriorly at the cavernous sinus, the nerve ipsilateral to the mass is subjected to stretching and the pupil dilates. Early in the course of this process, therapies that decrease the degree of shift (e.g., administration of mannitol) can reverse the pupillary dilation.

The sympathetic pathways begin in the hypothalamus, descend through the brain stem and spinal cord to the first thoracic level, and then exit the central nervous system to traverse the face and reach the pupil. Most sedative drugs produce bilateral small pupils by antagonizing sympathetic outflow at the hypothalamic level; other agents, such as opiates, appear to have an additional effect of stimulating the parasympathetic system, resulting in very small (pinpoint) pupils. Lesions affecting the sympathetic system below the midbrain do not directly affect consciousness.

Conjugate Eye Movements. The position and movements of the eyes are observed, and certain easy-to-administer procedures are undertaken to evaluate the integrity of the cerebral hemisphere and brain stem. The neural pathways for the control of horizontal conjugate eye movements are outlined in Figure 1–1. Cortical control originates in the frontal gaze centers (Brodmann's area 8), and descending fibers controlling horizontal conjugate gaze cross the midline in the lower mid-

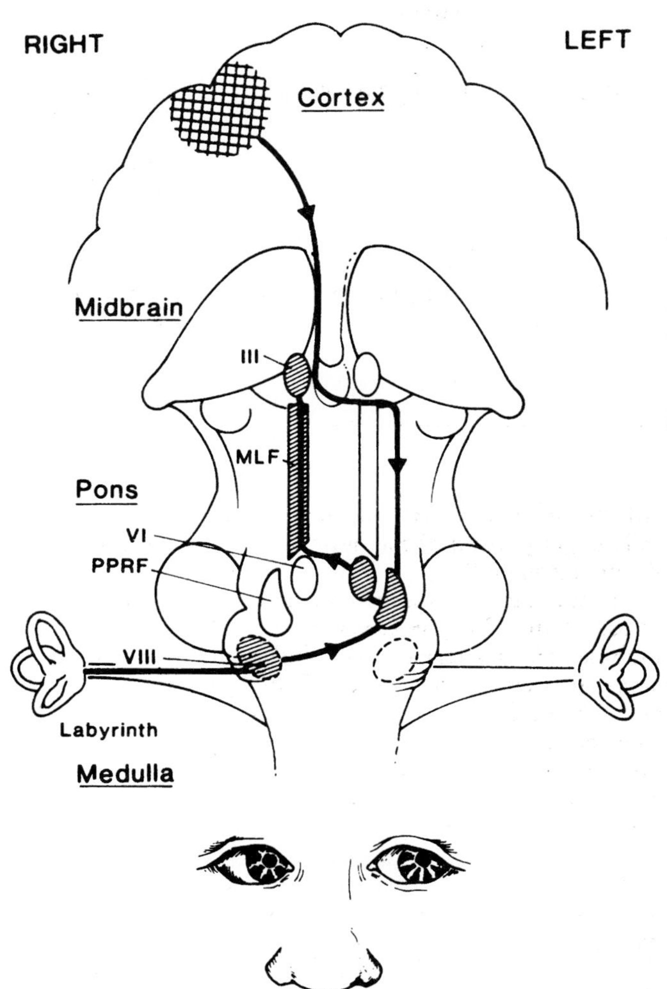

FIGURE 1–1. Conjugate vision pathways; nuclei and paths are shaded to include those important to left conjugate gaze: fibers from the right frontal cortex descend, cross the midline, and synapse in the left paramedian pontine reticular formation (PPRF). Fibers then travel to the nearby left cranial nerve VI nucleus (to move the left eye laterally) and then cross the midline to rise in the medial longitudinal fasciculus (MLF) to the right cranial nerve III nucleus (to move the right eye medially). In addition to the cortical influence on the left PPRF, there is vestibular influence. With cold water placed in the left external ear canal, the crossed pathway from the right vestibular nucleus to the left PPRF predominates and drives the eyes conjugately to the left. This procedure tests the integrity of the brain stem circuit that includes the vestibular nucleus, the PPRF, and cranial nerves III and VI and the MLF. If the eyes move to the side of cold water infusion, the brain stem from medulla to midbrain must be functioning. (From Weiner WJ and Goetz CG [eds]. Neurology for the Non-Neurologist, 3rd ed. Philadelphia, J.B. Lippincott Company, 1994.)

brain region and descend to the paramedian pontine reticular formation (PPRF) in the pons. The systems producing conjugate eye movements in the conscious and unconscious states vary slightly. Conscious horizontal conjugate eye movements depend on the PPRF for their coordination, whereas such movement in the unconscious patient appears to bypass this region and depend directly on the abducens nuclei for their coordination. Because these small structures are directly adjacent to each other and are caudal to the portion of the reticular formation necessary for consciousness, this distinction is not usually of consequence. The region of PPRF and adjacent neurons is thus the major area of confluence of pathways controlling horizontal eye movements. Neurons from the PPRF project to the nearby abducens nerve (cranial nerve VI) nucleus and thereby stimulate movements in the lateral rectus muscle of the eye ipsilateral to the PPRF and contralateral to the frontal gaze center. In addition, fibers from the abducens nerve nucleus cross the midline and ascend the median longitudinal fasciculus (MLF) to the medial rectus nucleus of the oculomotor nerve (cranial nerve III) in the midbrain. This activation stimulates adduction of the eye ipsilateral to the frontal gaze center, and conjugate gaze is thus completed. Because this system overlaps in space with the midbrain reticular formation, conjugate gaze examination is of vital importance in the comatose patient. In contrast to the pupillary constrictors, these muscles have nicotinic neuromuscular junctions and are therefore susceptible to neuromuscular junction blocking agents.

By following the pathways outlined in the figure, the consequences of lesions at various levels of the neuraxis can be deduced. Stimulation of fibers from the frontal gaze center of one cerebral hemisphere results in horizontal, conjugate eye movements to the contralateral side. If one frontal gaze center or its descending fiber tract is damaged, the eyes drift toward the involved cerebral hemisphere due to unopposed action of the remaining frontal gaze center. For example, a destructive lesion in the right cerebral hemisphere, involving descending motor fibers and frontal gaze fibers, causes a left hemiplegia, with head and eyes deviated to the right. In other words, the eyes appear to look at a destructive hemispheric lesion and look away from the resulting hemiplegia.

By contrast, a destructive left pontine lesion, for example, damages the left PPRF and surrounding region. The eyes, therefore, cannot move to the left and tend to deviate to the right. Because descending pyramidal tract fibers cross the midline in the medulla, damage to the pyramidal tract fibers in the pons on the left results in a right hemiplegia. Thus, the eyes appear to look away from a destructive pontine lesion but look toward the hemiplegia.

If the abducens nerve or nucleus is destroyed, there is a loss of abduction of the ipsilateral eye (cranial nerve VI palsy). With destruction of the tract of the medial longitudinal fasciculus, disconjugate gaze results, with loss of adduction of the ipsilateral eye (same side as the tract of the MLF). Abduction of the contralateral eye is preserved, but there is nystagmus in the awake patient. This type of disconjugate gaze abnormality is also termed internuclear ophthalmoplegia. The pathways for vertical eye movements are less well understood. Lower centers likely exist in the midbrain (pretectal and tectal) regions.

If a patient cannot follow verbal commands, two useful tests are employed to determine brain stem integrity. They activate the PPRF and subsequent pathways, not by cortical stimulation but rather by vestibular alterations. An oculocephalic or cervico-ocular (or doll's eyes) reflex is performed by turning the patient's head rapidly in the horizontal or vertical planes and by noting the movements or position of the eyes relative to the orbits. This test obviously should not be performed if a cervical neck fracture is suspected. If the pontine (horizontal) or midbrain (vertical) gaze centers are intact, the eyes should move in the orbits in the direction opposite to the rotating head. An abnormal response (no eye movement on moving the head) implies pontine or midbrain dysfunction and is characterized by no movement of the eyes relative to the orbits, or an asymmetry of movements.

Horizontal oculocephalic maneuvers are a relatively weak stimulus for horizontal eye movements. If a doll's eyes reflex is present, it is not necessary to continue with oculovestibular testing. If, however, the doll's eyes reflex is lacking, ice water calorics should be performed, because ice water is a stronger stimulus than oculocephalic maneuvers.

Oculovestibular responses (ice water calorics) are reflex eye movements in response to irrigation of the external ear canals with cold water. The head is raised to 30 degrees relative to the horizontal place, and the external canals are inspected for the presence of cerumen or a perforated tympanic membrane. Fifty to one hundred milliliters of cold water is instilled into the canal (waiting 5 minutes between each ear), and the resulting eye movements are noted. Ice water produces a downward current in the horizontal semicircular canal and decreases tonic vestibular output to the contralateral PPRF. Simplistically, one can think of this as an indirect means of stimulating the ipsilateral PPRF. Hence, after cold water instillation, there should be a slow, tonic, conjugate deviation of the eyes toward the irrigated ear if the brain stem is intact. In a comatose patient, there is a loss of the past-phase nystagmus, and only tonic deviation of the eyes is seen if appropriate pontine-midbrain areas are intact. Thus, if nystagmus is noted in a seemingly unconscious patient, the patient is not truly comatose.

Thus, a lack of oculovestibular responses suggests pontine-midbrain dysfunction. Ice water calorics can help differentiate between the conjugate gaze weakness or paralysis caused by either cortical (cerebral hemisphere) or brain stem (pontine) damage. Oculovestibular responses should not be altered in patients with only hemispheric pathology other than the loss of nystagmus.

Movement of the ipsilateral eye toward the irrigated ear but no movement of the contralateral eye suggests an abnormality of the contralateral MLF.

Although tradition dictates that the head be elevated 30 degrees (in order to place the horizontal semicircular canal in a vertical orientation, thereby maximizing the effect of gravity on endolymphatic movement), the superiority of this position over others has not been solidly demonstrated.

Breathing Patterns. Various respiratory patterns have localizing significance in the patient with altered consciousness. These patterns are recognizable by bedside observation. Before proceeding to detailed analysis of the respiratory pattern, the examiner should be certain that the upper airway is intact. If it is not, endotracheal intubation should be performed immediately unless the patient has an advance directive prohibiting this maneuver. The respiratory pattern can be easily assessed after intubation, recognizing the confounding effects of drugs given to facilitate the procedure and the increased work of breathing required by the smaller diameter of the new airway.

The respiratory pattern is determined by observation but should be interpreted in the light of arterial blood gas results. Tachypnea should be interpreted differently in patients who are hypoxic than in those who are normoxic. In the analysis of blood gas results, recall that the brain stem is primarily concerned with the maintenance of pH and PaO_2, not $PaCO_2$. Thus, compensation for a metabolic acidosis produces a pattern resembling central reflex hyperpnea, but the arterial blood gas analysis shows a pH below 7.35, which is indicative of a primary metabolic problem, such as diabetic ketoacidosis. The anatomical correlations of the major respiratory patterns are found in Table 1–1, and the patterns themselves are summarized in Table 1–3.

Motor Examination. The level of neurological dysfunction is often best defined by the motor examination. If the patient responds to noxious stimuli by any defensive maneuver, such as withdrawal from the stimulus, that patient is not truly comatose. Such a response may be seen in patients whose examinations otherwise suggest no cortical function, presumably because a noxious stimulus powerfully evokes an arousal response. Stereotyped posturing (spontaneous or induced) indicates that the cerebral cortices are no longer in command of the motor system.[17] The physiological levels of dysfunction are summarized in the motor component of the Glasgow Coma Scale (Table 1–4).

Experiments in animals led to the concepts of *decorticate* and *decerebrate* rigidity. These terms have produced endless confusion, and these states are perhaps better called by the labels used in the Glasgow Coma Scale: decorticate rigidity is abnormal flexion, and decerebrate rigidity is abnormal extension. Physiologically, these states reflect loss of higher motor control functions, either leaving the rubrospinal system in command (in flexor posturing) or ceding control to the vestibulospinal and reticulospinal systems (in extensor posturing). These postures do not mean that the higher control centers have been destroyed but indicate that they are not functioning. Patients

TABLE 1–3. **Respiratory Patterns in Patients with Alterations of Consciousness**

Pattern	Description	Localization	Comments
Posthyperventilation apnea	Apnea for more than 10 seconds after 5 deep breaths	Bilateral hemispheric dysfunction	Normally, the cerebral cortex triggers another breath within 10 seconds regardless of the $PaCO_2$
Cheyne-Stokes respiration	Rhythmic waxing and waning of respiratory amplitude	Bilateral hemispheric dysfunction	1. Periods of "apnea" are actually times when the respiratory amplitude is too low to measure, but the respiratory rhythm is unchanged 2. Congestive heart failure prolongs the reflex arc (blood leaving the lungs takes longer to reach the brain stem than is normal) and may produce this finding without any neurologic dysfunction
Central reflex hyperpnea (CRH) (formerly called central neurogenic hyperventilation)	Continuous deep breathing	Bilateral hemispheric (e.g., trauma), lower midbrain, upper pons, possibly medulla	When present in patients with brain stem lesions or subarachnoid hemorrhage, CRH is most commonly due to the hypoxia that accompanies neurogenic pulmonary edema. True central neurogenic hyperventilation is rare
Apneustic respiration	Prolonged inspiratory time ("inspiratory cramp")	Pons	Does not support adequate ventilation (true for all following patterns as well). Isolated lesions at these levels do not produce coma
Cluster (Biot's) breathing	Clusters of breaths punctuated by apnea	Lower pons	
Ataxic respiration	Infrequent, irregular breaths	Lower pons or upper medulla	
Ondine's curse	Failure of involuntary respiration with retained voluntary respiration	Medulla	
Apnea	No respiration	Medulla down to C4; peripheral nerve (e.g., acute inflammatory polyneuropathy), neuromuscular junction (e.g., myasthenia gravis), muscle	

TABLE 1–4. **Glasgow Coma Scale**

Item	Response	Score
Verbal response	Oriented	5
	Confused	4
	Inappropriate words	3
	Incomprehensible	2
	None	1
Eye opening	Spontaneous	4
	To speech	3
	To pain	2
	None	1
Motor	Obeys commands	6
	Localizes pain	5
	Withdraws	4
	Abnormal flexion	3
	Abnormal extension	2
	None	1

with lateral mass lesions may demonstrate flexor posturing on one side of the body and extensor posturing on the other (usually the side contralateral to the mass; see Chapter 15).

Assessment of Awareness

Although the comatose patient, by definition, does not manifest spontaneous eye opening (except in association with the vertical eye movements that may accompany a suppression-burst EEG pattern), the presence of spontaneous eye opening and even conjugate eye movements does indicate awareness; these findings are part of the vegetative state, in which the patient has arousal without awareness. Thus, testing for awareness must involve observation for the response to various stimuli and is not practically separable from testing for attention, because inattention to the stimuli chosen could be misinterpreted for unawareness (e.g., failure to respond to verbal commands on the part of a deaf patient). The patient who appears to be awake (i.e., aroused) but fails to attend to any stimuli (internal or external) is identified as lacking awareness.

Assessment of Attention

Tests of attention must include several modalities and be presented from both sides of the patient in order to avoid misinterpreting disorders of primary sensation or attention as disordered awareness. Typically, verbal, visual, and somatosensory stimuli are employed. Descriptions of the available tests for attention take up major portions of neuropsychology texts and are beyond the scope of this chapter. Only the basic principles commonly used in bedside screening of patients with impaired consciousness are discussed here.

Patients who are unable to respond to verbal commands (e.g., owing to receptive aphasia) may be able to direct themselves toward a voice or other sound (usually presented contralateral to the nondominant hemisphere). Assessing the response to visual stimuli may require passive eye opening (e.g., in patients with nondominant parietal lesions who have a transient apraxia of eyelid opening). Standardized tests of attention (e.g., the trailmaking test) are valuable in following patients over time, especially in assessing their response to therapy.

ASSOCIATED NEUROLOGICAL FINDINGS

Cerebral. The scope of potential physical findings related to lesions of the cerebral cortex in patients with altered awareness is itself the subject of several texts. Rather than attempting to perform specific tests of cortical function in these patients, one should concentrate on (1) using the neurological examination to identify lateralized lesions that may be affecting consciousness by shifting the diencephalon, and (2) detecting focal dysfunction that may be misinterpreted as altered consciousness (e.g., a patient with receptive aphasia who is misdiagnosed as confused or psychotic).

Cranial Nerves. In addition to the eye movements discussed earlier, the cranial nerve examination is crucial for the detection of brain stem lesions. Funduscopic examination may also provide a clue to the presence of elevated ICP. Conscious patients may exhibit nystagmus with a variety of intoxications. In anyone with a confusional state, detection of altered eye movements should prompt consideration of Wernicke's encephalopathy (see Chapter 40).

Motor/Reflexes/Cerebellar/Gait. Asterixis is a nonspecific sign of bilateral cortical dysfunction. Hemiparesis indicates a lesion of the upper motor neuron paths and may suggest either a contralateral cortical or paramedian brain stem lesion. Quadriplegia suggests a midline brain stem lesion. Signs of cerebellar dysfunction are unusual in patients with cerebellar infarcts or hemorrhages, which alter consciousness by producing brain stem compression or obstructive hydrocephalus. Finding cerebellar dysfunction or abnormal gait in a confused patient should raise the possibility of nutritional deficiencies (e.g., Wernicke's encephalopathy, vitamin B_{12} deficiency) or intoxications (see Chapters 39, 40, and 55).

Autonomic Nervous System. Autonomic instability can be both a cause and an effect of coma. In lesions affecting the descending sympathetic pathways from the hypothalamus to the brain stem, Horner's syndrome with a mildly constricted pupil ipsilateral to the lesion can be seen. Whereas diencephalic lesions are particularly associated with erratic changes in autonomic stability, the most common causes of coma with marked dysautonomia are intoxication and drug overdose (see Chapters 39 and 55).

Neurovascular. Because cardiac and vascular disease are commonly associated with coma, a thorough examination of these systems is essential. Arrhythmias, specifically atrial fibrillation, are associated with emboli that can shower the cortices and provoke multifocal bilateral cerebral dysfunction, leading to coma. The large vessels of the neck should be examined for evidence of carotid disease. The funduscopic examination likewise complements the neurovascular examination in detecting disease that affects central nervous system vasculature.

ASSOCIATED MEDICAL FINDINGS

Beyond measuring vital signs and detecting evidence of trauma, the general physical examination is most important for clues to systemic disorders that may alter consciousness. In the initial evaluation, detection of nuchal rigidity and skin lesions are the most important portions of the examination, because they may indicate the presence of bacterial meningitis (or, with nuchal rigidity, either subarachnoid hemorrhage or cerebellar tonsillar herniation). Other points of importance include evidence of hepatic disease, especially jaundice and signs of portal hypertension. An irregular cardiac rhythm raises the suspicion of systemic embolism, which may alter consciousness by producing a brain stem infarct or large bilateral cortical infarcts. Hematomas or purpura raise the possibility of platelet or coagulation disorders and may be associated with intracranial bleeding or conditions such as thrombotic thrombocytopenic purpura. Edema may reflect cardiac, hepatic, renal, or nutritional disorders.

Evaluation Guidelines

The use of neurodiagnostic studies in patients with altered consciousness with specific syndromes is outlined in Table 1–5.

Neuroimaging. Neuroimaging studies should be selected based on the patient's history and the initial examination. If a structural lesion is suspected, an emergent CT scan should be obtained to guide therapy. Patients with bilateral hemispheric dysfunction do not usually benefit from emergent CT scanning. Although MRI is almost always superior in quality to CT, the pulse sequences currently employed may not detect all cases of acute intracranial bleeding. CT scanning is usually faster and more readily available in emergent circumstances.[18] Positron-emission tomography may be useful in the study of vegetative patients but is not widely available.

Electrophysiology. An EEG is indicated in most patients with altered consciousness at some point in their evaluation, usually after a structural lesion has been excluded, because the history and examination are inadequate to detect many cases of nonconvulsive status epilepticus.[19] Patients in whom

TABLE 1–5. **Useful Studies in the Evaluation of Disorder of Level of Consciousness**

Syndrome	Neuroimaging	Electrophysiology	Fluid and Tissue Analysis	Neuropsychological Tests
Bilateral cortical dysfunction; confusion and delirium	Usually normal; may show atrophy; rarely bilateral chronic subdural hematoma or evidence of herpes simplex encephalitis; dural enhancement in meningitis, especially neoplastic meningitides	Diffuse slowing; often, frontally predominant intermittent rhythmic delta activity (FIRDA); in herpes simplex encephalitis, periodic lateralized epileptiform activity (PLEDS)	Blood or urine analyses may reveal etiology; CSF may show evidence of infection or neoplastic cells	In mild cases, difficulty with attention (e.g., trailmaking tests); in more severe cases, formal testing is not possible
Diencephalic dysfunction	Lesion(s) in or displacement of diencephalon; also displays mass displacing the diencephalon	Usually, diffuse slowing; rarely, FIRDA; in displacement syndromes, effect of the mass producing displacement (e.g., focal delta activity, loss of faster rhythms)	Usually not helpful	Usually not obtained
Midbrain dysfunction	Lesion(s) in the midbrain or displacing it	Usually, diffuse slowing; alpha coma; evoked response testing may demonstrate failure of conduction above the lesion	Rarely, platelet or coagulation abnormalities	Usually not performed
Pontine dysfunction	Lesion(s) producing syndrome; thrombosis of basilar artery	EEG: usually normal; evoked responses usually normal	Rarely, platelet or coagulation	Usually not performed abnormalities
Medullary dysfunction	Lesion(s) producing dysfunction	EEG: normal; brain stem auditory and somatosensory evoked responses may show conduction abnormalities	Rarely, platelet or coagulation abnormalities	Usually not performed
Herniation syndromes	Lesion(s) producing herniation; appearance of perimesencephalic cistern	Findings related to etiology	Findings related to etiology	Usually not performed
Locked-in syndrome	Infarction of basis pontis	EEG and evoked potential studies: normal	Findings related to etiology	Usually not performed
Death by brain criteria	Absence of intracranial blood flow above the foramen magnum	EEG: electrocerebral silence; evoked potential studies may show peripheral components (e.g., wave I of brain stem auditory evoked response) but no central conduction	Absence of hypnosedative drugs	Not done
Psychogenic unresponsiveness	Normal	Normal	Normal	Helpful after patient "awakens"

CSF, Cerebrospinal fluid; EEG, electroencephalogram; FIRDA, frontally predominant intermittent rhythmic delta activity; PLEDS, periodic lateralized epileptiform activity.

supratentorial structural lesions are present but are not adequate to explain the patient's state based on their location and size should also have an EEG performed.

Some EEG findings in patients with encephalopathy are characteristic; for example, frontally predominant rhythmic delta activity and triphasic waves are common in metabolic disorders. An alpha coma pattern indicates either a midbrain lesion, anoxia, or hypnosedative drug overdose. In the setting of a hypnosedative drug overdose, the patient has a good prognosis for recovery. An unexpectedly normal EEG, with alpha blocking on passive eye opening and normal sleep-wake cycling, should alert the physician to the likelihood of psychogenic unresponsiveness. The EEG may also provide clues to otherwise unexpected diagnoses, such as subacute spongiform encephalopathy, which may come to medical attention in the guise of an acute encephalopathy. Evoked response studies are of limited value in these patients, and although abnormalities may be present (see Table 1–5), these studies seldom contribute diagnostically or therapeutically useful data in this population.[20]

Body Fluid and Tissue Analysis. Although the concept of routine tests has fallen from favor in laboratory medicine circles because of pressure from third-party payors, the patient with unexplained bilateral hemispheric dysfunction should indeed have a battery of screening tests to allow the physician to detect treatable etiologies rapidly. At a minimum, these tests should include a complete blood count with differential, platelet estimate or count, prothrombin time, partial thromboplastin time, serum osmolality, and serum and urinary screening for drugs of abuse.

If oral drug ingestion is considered a possibility, gastric aspiration for analysis of the contents and removal of remaining unabsorbed drug is indicated. If the patient's airway protective reflexes are compromised, endotracheal intubation should be performed first. Induction of vomiting is no longer recommended in the emergency department because it may interfere with the use of activated charcoal to bind drugs. This substance may be used routinely unless acetaminophen ingestion is suspected, because it will interfere with the absorption of acetylcysteine as well.

Cerebrospinal Fluid. Cerebrospinal fluid analysis is crucial in some conditions that alter consciousness (e.g., suspected meningitis) and is irrelevant in others. Thus, the decision to perform a lumbar puncture is based on the entire clinical picture. If bacterial meningitis is suspected and the physician believes that an imaging study should precede the lumbar puncture in these patients, then appropriate antibiotic therapy should be started before the patient is sent for the imaging study. Pneumococcal and meningococcal meningitides may be so rapidly fatal that even a brief delay in instituting antibiotic treatment should not occur.

Subarachnoid hemorrhage, either as a single event or as a repeated phenomenon, can also be diagnosed by lumbar puncture. The pattern of red blood cells and various pigments helps in establishing whether a patient with a known subarachnoid hemorrhage and a new onset of depressed level of consciousness has re-bled or suffered another event like vasospasm.

In many instances of altered level of consciousness, ICP changes due to an intracranial mass lesion, ventricular obstruction, or other causes. As discussed in Chapter 26, ICP reflects the net effect of static and dynamic forces affecting the intracranial contents. In the clinical context of decreased intracranial compliance, relatively small changes in volume have the potential to effect dangerous changes in pressure when the ICP is already elevated. Therefore, sudden and nonlinear rises in pressure are particularly important to control through ICP monitoring. Whereas in the normal brain, the perfusion pressure (mean arterial pressure minus mean ICP) must drop below 40 mm Hg before cerebral blood flow is impaired, in the damaged brain, the determinate pressure is less clear. Furthermore, often pressure increases are not distributed evenly throughout the cranium, and compartmentalized, very high pressure areas may not be accurately recorded by ICP monitoring. These features are particularly problematic in the instance of focal lesions with risks of herniations.

Neuropsychological Tests. Although most focal cortical abnormalities should be detected by the bedside neurological examination, formal neuropsychological testing may be valuable for detecting focal neurological dysfunction in patients who are thought to have diffuse disorders. This may be especially valuable in patients who present with an acute encephalopathy but do not improve, or in whom subsequent information indicates that a more chronic dementing process may be present.

Clinical Syndromes

SYNCOPE

Syncope refers to rapid, transient loss of consciousness that is most commonly due to cardiovascular problems (e.g., arrhythmias) but that may also be a reflection of autonomic disturbances. These autonomic disturbances are frequently drug induced but may include such conditions as Shy-Drager syndrome. The other major differential diagnostic concern for the neurologist is a seizure presenting as loss of consciousness. The patient's history is essential in distinguishing conditions of inadequate cerebral blood flow from seizures.

Many patients with syncope of cardiac or autonomic origin have a brief tonic spasm when they lose consciousness, and a minority have a tonic-clonic seizure. This situation appears to be more common in children and young adults, and may be exacerbated if the patient is not allowed to become recumbent during the period of hypotension. The congenital syndromes of QT interval prolongation (e.g., Romano-Ward syndrome) are frequently misdiagnosed as a primary seizure disorder instead of a cardiac arrhythmia. Analyses of patients undergoing induced ventricular fibrillation as part of a cardiac electrophysiological study reveal a high incidence of seizures in this setting.[21] EEG should be reserved for cases in which there is a reason in the history or findings on examination to suspect seizures or in which the cardiac and autonomic evaluations have not yielded a diagnosis. Other than seizures or rare autonomic neuropathies, primary neurological disorders are extremely unlikely to cause syncope.

BILATERAL CORTICAL DYSFUNCTION

Confusion and delirium are common in hospitalized patients, especially the elderly. In this setting, drugs prescribed for the patient must be considered the first candidates for causing this state. Other common possibilities include nutritional disorders and withdrawal from alcohol or other hypnosedative agents. Even seemingly subtle changes in the patient's medication regimen, such as accidental discontinuation of a thyroid replacement medication, can lead to a metabolic encephalopathy with depressed consciousness. Patients in intensive care units (ICUs) are sometimes thought to develop delirium because of sleep deprivation, but this concept of ICU psychosis has come under attack in recent years, because almost all such patients have other reasons for acute confusion.

DIENCEPHALIC DYSFUNCTION

Disorders of the diencephalon may affect consciousness either directly, by interfering with reticular system function, or indirectly, by producing endocrine disorders. These conditions may develop slowly, as with anterior pituitary syndromes resulting in hypothyroidism or cortisol deficiency, or rapidly, as with osmoregulatory disorders. The lesions producing these problems may also affect the cerebral cortex, as in the case of neoplasms, and produce seizures or other focal neurological disorders. Patients with structural diencephalic lesions may have toxic downward eye deviation, small pupils, decorticate posturing, and Cheyne-Stokes respirations as an archetype, although varying combinations of signs may appear.

MIDBRAIN DYSFUNCTION

The classic midbrain syndrome associated with depressed consciousness involves midsized pupils, often unilateral cranial nerve III paresis with compensatory forced adduction (wall-eyes) and retractory nystagmoid movements. Decerebrate or decorticate posturing can occur, and a severe respiratory alkalosis can arise from central neurogenic hyperventilation. Rarely, patients with midbrain dysfunction can actually remain awake but have an altered state termed peduncular hallucinosis of Lhermitte. In this situation, the patient experiences intense visual hallucinations in a clear sensorium. These phenomena have been likened to dreams in an awake state, and disrupted brain stem pathways involved in sleep-wake physiology may be implicated in this remarkable syndrome.

PONTINE AND MEDULLARY DYSFUNCTION

Hemorrhage into the basis pontis frequently extends rostrally into the midbrain and appears to produce coma by interference with midbrain reticular function. This condition is associated with pinpoint pupils, presumably reflecting both parasympathetic irritation as well as sympathetic outflow disruption. Importantly, however, most patients presenting in coma with pinpoint pupils are suffering from an opiate overdose and not specific pontine dysfunction. Naloxone quickly reverses opiate pupillary changes but has no effect on pontine lesions. Patients with pontine lesions that cause coma from involvement of midbrain reticular dysfunction may also have a flaccid hemiparesis or paraparesis, irregular respirations termed apneustic, and a variety of extraocular palsies. These problems may include conjugate deviation of the eyes toward the hemiparetic body if the PPRF has a lesion, unilateral or bilateral cranial nerve VI palsies or an internuclear ophthalmoplegia if the MLF has a lesion. Cold caloric testing usually clarifies the ocular dysfunction.

Primary pontine lesions without midbrain involvement may mimic coma as the "locked-in" syndrome by interrupting almost all efferent pathways from the cerebral cortex. Infarction of the basis pontis disrupts the corticospinal tracts (producing tetraplegia), the PPRF and abducens nuclei (eliminating conjugate horizontal eye movements), and the facial nerves in their course around the abducens nuclei (resulting in complete facial paralysis). Because the MRF is spared, however, the patient is awake and alert; and because the sensory pathways have migrated to a posterior position in the pons, both the auditory and somatosensory systems are functional. The only voluntary motor act of which the patient is capable is conjugate vertical eye movements. When the patient is not actively moving the eyes, spontaneous vertical movements known as ocular bobbing may develop.

Although this condition was previously emphasized because of the possibility that a sentient patient would mistakenly be judged comatose, the advent of thrombolytic therapy for cerebrovascular diseases mandates that these patients be identified rapidly so that they may be considered for intravenous recombinant tissue plasminogen activator treatment. At present, studies of intra-arterial thrombolysis are in progress.

The locked-in state is occasionally mimicked by severe neuropathic disorders (e.g., acute inflammatory polyneuropathy, the Guillain-Barré syndrome) and other widespread peripheral disorders.

HERNIATION SYNDROMES

Herniation occurs when the brain is subjected to pressure gradients that cause portions of it to flow from one intracranial compartment to another. Although the brain has substantial elasticity, the arteries and veins responsible for its blood supply are relatively fixed in space, producing a risk that brain shifts will cause the moving portions to lose their blood supply. In the case of lateral herniation, the hernia itself may compress or distort vessels, similarly disrupting blood flow. Herniation also appears to produce dysfunction in important white matter pathways, such as those connecting the MRF to the thalamus, probably via geometrical distortion of the pathways themselves. Extracerebral structures, particularly cranial nerve III, are also susceptible to distortion when the brain shifts.

The classic herniation syndromes are well established in the clinical neurosciences; recent advances in imaging have changed some of our understanding of their pathological anatomy, but their clinical symptoms remain important.

Central Herniation Syndrome. Central herniation occurs when diffuse brain swelling (e.g., after trauma) or a centrally located mass causes the diencephalon to move caudally through the tentorial notch. Dysfunction of the reticular formation and cerebral hypoperfusion due to ICP elevation are the leading hypotheses explaining alteration of consciousness in this setting. Diencephalic dysfunction initially produces small reactive pupils because of loss of sympathetic output from the hypothalamus. At this stage, decorticate (flexor) posturing may be present spontaneously or is frequently elicited by noxious stimuli. As the midbrain begins to fail, the pupils enlarge to midposition, and posturing becomes decerebrate (extensor). Attempts to elicit horizontal eye movements may reveal failure of adduction with either cervico-ocular reflex (COR) or vestibulo-ocular reflex (VOR) testing; however, this is often only present briefly. Eventually, if the patient is breathing spontaneously, tidal volume decreases and the respiratory rhythm becomes irregular.

The initial cardiovascular response to diminished brain stem perfusion, regardless of etiology, is hypertension. In this setting, bradycardia is a reflex response to the systemic hypertension that is commonly seen in children but is less common in adults. There may be a tendency for bradycardia to occur more commonly in patients with posterior fossa masses, but this observation is confounded by the higher incidence of posterior fossa tumors in children. Respiratory disturbances, the third component of Cushing's triad, reflect the anatomical considerations discussed earlier and are not part of the same reflex system as the cardiovascular responses. In some clinical settings, such as head injury with diffuse brain swelling, spontaneous hyperventilation is commonly noted but its etiology remains obscure.

Lateral Mass Herniation (Uncal or Hippocampal Herniation) Syndrome. Although concepts of herniation due to an expanding lateral cerebral mass have changed in the past decade, there is a consistent sequence of physical findings that develops. The initial signs are usually those related to the mass itself (e.g., contralateral hemiparesis); as

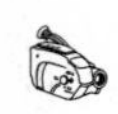

the diencephalon begins to shift away from the mass, consciousness begins to diminish, and an ipsilateral cranial nerve III palsy develops in about 85 percent of patients. When cranial nerve III is compressed against the tentorial notch, the pupillary fibers, located most peripherally in the nerve, are primarily damaged and the prominent sign is a large pupil. The remaining patients develop either simultaneous bilateral cranial nerve III palsies or, on occasion, an isolated contralateral cranial nerve III palsy. These findings presumably follow from the distortion of cranial nerve III anatomy described earlier, although the bilateral disturbance may also relate to midbrain ischemia as the brain stem begins to move away from the basilar artery. Imaging studies (CT or MRI) performed early in this process do not show transtentorial movement of the temporal lobe; this feature occurs later in the process, accounting for its implication as the cause of third nerve dysfunction in autopsy studies. Early in this process, the most common finding on imaging studies is an *enlargement* of the perimesencephalic cistern ipsilateral to the mass.

As lateral displacement of the midbrain continues, the contralateral corticospinal tract (in the cerebral peduncle) is compressed against the edge of the tentorium. This produces an *ipsilateral* hemiplegia, called the *Kernohan's notch* phenomenon. If the herniation process continues, the diencephalon and the ipsilateral temporal lobe may actually herniate downward through the tentorial notch. Because the uncus (containing the amygdala) and the hippocampus are the most medial portions of the temporal lobe, they are the first structures to cross the tentorial edge; this accounts for the older terms of *uncal* or *hippocampal* herniation. Movement of the more posterior aspects of the medial temporal lobe may compress the posterior cerebral artery (or arteries), producing ischemia in the medial temporal lobe and sometimes in the occipital lobe.

Subfalcine Herniation Syndrome. Herniation of the medial frontal structures (e.g., the cingulate gyrus) beneath the falx is commonly observed in patients with frontal lobe masses. Most of these patients present with signs related either to the mass itself or to the global increase in ICP that accompanies it. Rarely, this subfalcine herniation causes ischemia in the distribution of the anterior cerebral arteries.

Cerebellar Tonsillar Herniation Syndrome. Posterior fossa masses produce most of their findings by compression of the brain stem and cranial nerves, and by obstructive hydrocephalus. As the pressure gradient across the foramen magnum increases, however, the cerebellar tonsils may be pushed into, and eventually through, the foramen. This compresses the medulla and may produce apnea by inducing dysfunction in the medullary respiratory centers. Before losing consciousness, patients with cerebellar tonsillar herniation may complain of a stiff neck.

Upward Transtentorial Herniation Syndrome. Expanding posterior fossa masses usually herniate caudally because the obstructive hydrocephalus they produce prevents a pressure gradient across the tentorial opening. If these patients undergo ventriculostomy for relief of hydrocephalus, however, the possibility of upward herniation of the contents of posterior fossa into the diencephalic region exists. Many neurosurgeons prepare the patient for an emergent posterior fossa decompression just before performing the ventriculostomy in case this problem occurs.

PERSISTENT VEGETATIVE STATE

Following a severe brain insult, usually traumatic or anoxic, the comatose patient with a relatively intact brain stem usually begins to show the signs of the vegetative state discussed earlier.[22] Less commonly, the syndrome can be seen in the context of degenerative or severe developmental malformation disorders of the central nervous system. Approximately 10,000 to 25,000 adults and 6,000 to 10,000 children in the United States are diagnosed with this syndrome. Clinically, patients show no evidence of awareness of self or environment; no evidence of sustained, reproducible, purposeful behavioral response to stimuli; no evidence of language comprehension or expression; intermittent wakefulness; bowel and bladder incontinence; variably preserved cranial nerve and spinal reflexes; and sufficiently preserved hypothalamic and brain stem autonomic function to permit survival with medical and nursing care. The prognosis for further recovery to at least the level of ability to understand and follow commands varies with the mechanism of injury and with the age of the patient. In general, patients who remain in a vegetative state 3 months after an anoxic injury are expected to persist in that state indefinitely. Patients in a vegetative state at the time of hospital discharge after head trauma have an almost 50-percent likelihood of some further recovery over the next 12 months, and a small number regain consciousness between 12 and 36 months. However, the prognosis for functional recovery, in the form of returning to work or to school, is much worse. Although about one third of trauma patients younger than 30 years of age who awaken after prolonged vegetative state meet these goals, only some patients older than 30 years of age do so.

DEATH BY BRAIN CRITERIA

The ability to transplant organs successfully led to the need of criteria for brain death, and national and international definitions have been developed. Although the concept of brain death is embraced internationally, definitions vary considerably, without worldwide consensus on diagnostic criteria (Table 1–6).[23] Many now argue that current criteria are restrictive and should be expanded to include patients who have no reasonable chance of regaining consciousness.[24] If this change is to be made, a substantial shift in societal thinking about life and death may need to precede it. However, in North America, death by brain criteria is still considered to be irreversible loss of brain function, including that of the brain stem. The single exception to this rule appears to be in the area of osmolar control, and diabetes insipidus is not required for this diagnosis.

Many jurisdictions now permit organ recovery from patients immediately after cessation of cardiopulmonary function. This allows the families of patients who have been neurologically devastated but who are not dead to fulfill the patient's wish to donate organs. Although currently this technique is limited to renal and hepatic transplantation, it is evolving rapidly. This option requires careful forethought and planning, but can help a family gain some measure of peace in the face of an otherwise devastating loss.[25]

At present, most jurisdictions recognize the existence of death by brain criteria, but its precise definition varies with local practice. In general, the first stage in pronouncing death by brain criteria is a *permissive diagnosis*; that is, there must be a diagnosis adequate to explain death of the brain, including the brain stem. This need not be an etiological diagnosis; for example, a massive intracerebral hemorrhage qualifies as a permissive diagnosis, even if the etiology of the hemorrhage is unknown. This requirement helps exclude cases of hypnosedative overdose, in which the patient may appear dead but still recover. Importantly, this criterion does not require demonstration of an anatomical lesion, and a history of prolonged anoxia, for example, would suffice. One then proceeds to demonstrate that there is no detectable function above the level of the foramen magnum. Any sign of brain stem–mediated function, such as decerebrate posturing, eye movements, pupillary response to light, or coughing, negates the possibility of the diagnosis of death by current brain criteria. Brain stem testing includes an apnea challenge.[26]

Apnea testing involves observing the brain stem response to hypercapnia without producing hypoxemia. In order to prevent hypoxemia, a period (e.g., 20 minutes) of ventilation with 100 percent oxygen is required before starting the test. Although acidosis, rather than hypercapnia, is the real afferent trigger for ventilation, a $PaCO_2$ of 60 mm Hg (50 mm Hg in the United Kingdom) is usually the endpoint for this test. In order to reach this endpoint before hypoxemia supervenes, it is advisable to regulate ventilation during the period of preapneic oxygenation so that the $PaCO_2$ reaches 40 to 45 mm Hg before apnea begins. This period should also be used to ensure that the patient's core temperature is adequate (e.g., above 32° C), and that the results of assays for hypnosedative agents, if indicated, show that intoxication is not the cause of the patient's apparent lack of reflex responses.

Even though the patient has been adequately preoxygenated, some method of supplemental oxygen delivery is still necessary. This may be accomplished either by placing a suction catheter near the carina with a 10 L/min oxygen flow, or by using a continuous positive airway pressure (CPAP) circuit with 10 cm H_2O pressure. A CPAP circuit does not provide ventilation, so it does not interfere with observation for spontaneous respirations. Even with one of these methods employed, some patients with cardiorespiratory dysfunction may not tolerate the approximately 10 minutes of apnea necessary to raise the $PaCO_2$ to 60 mm Hg without becoming hypoxemic and hypotensive. In this circumstance, a confirmatory test may be necessary.

Apnea is then allowed under observation until the $PaCO_2$ reaches 60 mm Hg by arterial blood gas analysis.

TABLE 1–6. **Death by Brain Criteria in Several Countries**

	Law	Guideline	Apnea Test	Number of Physicians	Observation Time (hr)	Confirmatory Test
USA	P	P	PCO_2	2*	6	Optional
Canada	P	P	PCO_2	1	6	Optional
Mexico	P	P	A	A	24	Mandatory
Argentina	P	P	DVO	1	6	Mandatory
United Kingdom	P	P	PCO_2	2	6	Optional
France	P	P	PCO_2	1	A	Mandatory
Sweden	P	P	PCO_2	1	A	Mandatory
Israel	P	P	PCO_2	1	6 (24)†	Mandatory
China	A	A	A	A	A	Optional
Japan	P	P	PCO_2	1	A	Mandatory
Australia	P	P	PCO_2	2	2	Optional
New Zealand	A	P	PCO_2	2	2	Optional
India	P	P	DVO	4	A	Mandatory

*Based on data from 8 states.
†Observation time can be shortened or eliminated if one confirmatory test is positive for brain death.
P, Present law or guidelines; A, absent law or guidelines; PCO_2, target PCO_2 defined (50 or 60 mm Hg); DVO, disconnection from ventilator only.
Adapted from Wijdicks EFM: Brain death worldwide. Neurology 2002;58:20–25.

TABLE 1–7. **Selected Etiologies Associated with Changes in Level of Consciousness**

Etiological Category	Selected Specific Etiologies	Chapter
Structural Disorders		
Developmental	Hydrocephalus: obstructive or nonobstructive Neural tube defects Segmentation, cleavage defects Neuronal migration defects Posterior fossa abnormalities, Dandy-Walker, Chiari malformations	28
Degenerative and compressive	Paget's disease	29
Hereditary and Degenerative Disorders		
Storage diseases: Lipidoses, glycogen disorders, and leukoencephalopathies	Neuronal ceroid lipofuscinosis, especially NCL-2 Cerebrosidoses, especially type II Leukodystrophies, especially Canavan's disease (neonatal form) and Krabbe's disease	30
Amino/organic acidopathies, mitochondrial enzyme defects, and other metabolic errors	Aminoacidopathies, especially maple syrup urine disease, urea cycle disorders, propionic acidemia, methylmalonic acidemia Mitochondrial enzyme defects, especially Leigh's disease, Alper's disease, MERFF, MELAS, fatty acid oxidation disorders	31
Chromosomal abnormalities and neurocutaneous disorders	Conditions associated with generalized seizures, especially tuberous sclerosis and Sturge-Weber syndrome	32
The degenerative dementias	Alzheimer's disease (late) Pick's disease (late)	33
Movement disorders	Multiple system atrophy with syncope Huntington's disease (late)	34
Ataxias	Dandy-Walker syndrome Chiari malformations Multiple system atrophy with syncope	35
Degenerative motor, sensory, and autonomic disorders	Amyotrophic lateral sclerosis (late)	36
Acquired Metabolic and Nutritional Disorders		
Endogenous metabolic disorders	Electrolyte dysfunction, sodium, potassium, chloride, calcium Hormonal imbalances: especially thyroid, corticomineral steroids, and glucose metabolism	38
Exogenous acquired metabolic disorders of the nervous system: Toxins and illicit drugs	Solvents including methyl alcohol, ethylene glycol, carbon tetrachloride Organophosphates and organochlorides Illicit drugs, including cocaine, amphetamine analogs, and opioids	39
Nutritional deficiencies and syndromes associated with alcoholism	Alcohol stupor and withdrawal Vitamin deficiencies, including thiamine, B_{12}, folic acid, and biotin	40
Infectious Disorders		
Viral infections	All causes of viral meningitis and viral encephalitis	41
Nonviral infections	All organisms causing bacterial meningitis or encephalitis Abscesses with increased intracranial pressure	42
Transmissible spongiform encephalopathies	Kuru, Creutzfeldt-Jakob, Gerstmann-Straussler-Scheinker syndromes and fatal familial insomnia	43
HIV and AIDS	AIDS encephalopathy, AIDS dementia complex (late), dysautonomia from neuropathy or myelopathy, progressive multifocal leukoencephalopathy	44
Neurovascular Disorders	Unilateral strokes with secondary edema. Bilateral strokes or showering of emboli, brain stem strokes, subarachnoid hemorrhage	45
Neoplastic Disorders		
Primary neurological tumors	Unilateral tumors with secondary edema. Bilateral cerebral or primary brain stem tumors. Metabolic alterations, especially involving calcium	46
Metastatic neoplasms and paraneoplastic syndromes	Unilateral tumors with secondary edema. Bilateral cerebral or primary brain stem tumors. Metabolic alterations, especially involving calcium	47
Demyelinating Disorders		
Demyelinating disorders of the central nervous system	Multiple sclerosis (rare) Devic's disease	48
Demyelinating disorders of the peripheral nervous system	Guillain-Barré syndrome (with dysautonomia)	49

TABLE 1–7. **Selected Etiologies Associated with Changes in Level of Consciousness** *Continued*

Etiological Category	Selected Specific Etiologies	Chapter
Autoimmune and Inflammatory Disorders	Autoimmune cerebritis including giant cell arteritis, primary CNS arteritis, and hypersensitivity arteritis and autoimmune-induced dysautonomic states from peripheral nervous system involvement including polyarteritis and Wegener's granulomatosis. Systemic lupus erythematosus can affect either central or peripheral systems	50
Traumatic Disorders	Cortical contusion, epidural hematomas, subdural hematomas Traumatic hematomas, post-traumatic epilepsy	51
Epilepsy	All seizures associated with loss of consciousness, i.e., primary and secondary generalized seizures and all complex partial seizures with an alteration in consciousness	52
Headache and Facial Pain	Complicated migraine, basilar migraine	53
Sleep Disorders	Obstructive sleep apnea	54
Drug-Induced and Iatrogenic Neurological Disorders	Drugs associated with hypotension or seizures	55

AIDS, Acquired immunodeficiency syndrome; CNS, central nervous system; MELAS, mitochondrial myopathy, encephalopathy, lactic acidosis, and stroke-like episodes; MERFF, mitochondrial encephalopathy with ragged red fibers; NCL-2, neuronal ceroid lipofuscinosis type 2.

Although it may be possible to predict this point by following the trend in end-tidal CO_2 ($PetCO_2$) measurements, there is enough discrepancy between arterial blood $PaCO_2$ and $PetCO_2$ to indicate use of the arterial measurement. Visual observation is the standard method for detecting respiratory movement; this may be supplemented by airway pressure monitoring. Any respiratory movement negates the diagnosis of apnea. However, if the patient remains apneic despite a $PaCO_2$ of 60 mm Hg, the diagnosis of apnea is confirmed, and the patient, having met the other conditions cited as prerequisites, is declared dead by brain criteria.

If the patient is unable to tolerate the apnea test, or if some portion of the examination cannot be performed (e.g., trauma has rendered the face too swollen to examine the eyes), then a confirmatory test is necessary if the patient is to be diagnosed as dead. This is usually indicated only for potential organ donors, because there is no requirement that death be diagnosed in order to withdraw supportive measures, but at times may be helpful for the patient's family. Tests of cerebral perfusion (e.g., radionuclide angiography, conventional contrast angiography, or CT angiography) are usually employed to show that blood does not flow intracranially above the foramen magnum.[27] In some areas, transcranial Doppler blood flow velocity measurements are considered adequate for this purpose. Transorbital, transtemporal, and transforaminal approaches can be used.[28] Electrophysiological studies, such as EEG, have been used for this purpose but are prone to both false-positive (e.g., artifacts that cannot be distinguished from cerebral activity with certainty) and false-negative (due to hypothermia or hypnosedative drug intoxication) results (see Chapter 24, Fig. 24–4).

PSYCHOGENIC UNRESPONSIVENESS

This category includes patients who have a diagnosable psychiatric condition, such as catatonia or conversion disorder, and those who are malingering. The differential diagnosis of these conditions is beyond the scope of this chapter, but a few diagnostic points are important in order to raise the physician's suspicion of a psychogenic disorder. These conditions share two characteristics not seen in patients with neurological reasons for coma: First, they have the COR and VOR responses characteristic of awake patients and develop nystagmus and vomiting to cold caloric challenge. Second, their EEGs are not indicative of coma.

General Management Goals

Beyond the initial stabilization of the patient and the detection of conditions that require immediate specific treatment, the management of patients with altered consciousness is primarily supportive. The responsibility to protect patients from harm runs the gamut from keeping the confused ambulator from wandering away to endotracheal intubation and mechanical ventilation. Making an etiological diagnosis as rapidly as possible may permit specific treatment (Table 1–7).

Reviews and Selected Updates

American Academy of Neurology: Position paper on certain aspects of the care and management of the persistent vegetative state patient. Neurology 1989;39:125–126.

American Academy of Neurology: Position paper on certain aspects of the care and management of profoundly and irreversibly paralyzed patients with retained consciousness and cognition. Neurology 1993;43:222–223.

Bleck TP: Diagnosis and management of the comatose patient in the intensive care unit. *In*: Murray MJ, Coursin DB, Pearl RG, Prough DS (eds): Critical Care Medicine: Perioperative Management, 2nd ed. Philadelphia, Lippincott, Williams & Wilkins, 2002, pp.244–252.

Bleck TP, Smith MC, Pierre-Louis SJ, et al: Neurologic complications of critical medical illnesses. Crit Care Med 1993;21:98–103.

Bleck TP, Webb AR: The unconscious patient. *In* Webb AR, Shapiro MJ, Singer M, Suter P (eds): The Oxford Textbook of Critical Care. Oxford, Oxford University Press, 1999, pp 440–446.

Moruzzi G: The sleep-waking cycle. Rev Physiol 1972;64:1–165.

Quality Standards Subcommittee of the American Academy of Neurology: Practice parameters for determining brain death in adults. Neurology 1995;45:1012–1014.
Quality Standards Subcommittee of the American Academy of Neurology: Practice parameters: Assessment and management of patients in the persistent vegetative state. Neurology 1995;45:1015–1018.
Ropper AH: Lateral displacement of the brain and level of consciousness in patients with an acute hemispheral mass. N Engl J Med 1986;314:953–958.
Searle JR: Consciousness. Ann Rev Neurosci 2000;23:557–578.
Swash M, Beresford R: Brain death: Still unresolved issues worldwide. Neurology 2002;58:9–10.
Wijdicks EF: Neurological complications of critically ill patients. Anesth Analges 1996;83:411–419.
Young GB, Ropper AH, Bolton CF: Coma and Impaired Consciousness: A Clinical Perspective. New York, McGraw-Hill, 1997.

References

1. Moruzzi G, Magoun HW: Brain stem reticular formation and activation of the EEG. Electroencephalogr Clin Neurophysiol 1949;1:455–473.
2. McNealy DE, Plum F: Brain stem dysfunction with supratentorial mass lesions. Arch Neurol 1962;7:10–32.
3. Ropper AH: A preliminary MRI study of the geometry of brain displacement and level of consciousness with acute intracranial masses. Neurology 1989;39:622–627.
4. Plum F, Posner JB: The Diagnosis of Stupor and Coma. Philadelphia, F.A. Davis, 1980.
5. Penfield W, Jasper H: Epilepsy and the functional anatomy of the human brain. Boston, Little, Brown and Co, 1954.
6. Gloor P: Generalized cortico-reticular epilepsies. Some considerations on the pathophysiology of generalized bilaterally synchronous spike and wave discharge. Epilepsia 1968;9:249–263.
7. Devinsky O: Electrical and magnetic stimulation of the central nervous system. Historical overview. Adv Neurol 1993;63:1–16.
8. American Psychiatric Association: Diagnostic and Statistical Manual of Mental Disorders, 4th ed. Washington, DC, American Psychiatric Association, 1994, p 124.
9. Niedermeyer E: Consciousness: Function and definition. Clin Electroencephalogr 1994;25:86–93.
10. Yingling CD, Skinner JE: Regulation of unit activity in nucleus reticularis thalami by the mesencephalic reticular formation and the frontal granular cortex. Electroencephalogr Clin Neurophysiol 1975;39: 635–642.
11. Inao S, Kawai T, Kabeya R, et al: Relation between brain displacement and local cerebral blood flow in patients with chronic subdural haematoma. J Neurol Neurosurg Psychiatry 2001;71:741–746.
12. Moore RY, Bloom FE: Central catecholamine neuron systems: Anatomy and physiology of the norepinephrine and epinephrine systems. Ann Rev Neurosci 1979;2:113–168.
13. Samuels MA: The evaluation of comatose patients. Hosp Pract 1993;28:165–182.
14. Teasdale G, Jennett B: Assessment of coma and impaired consciousness. A practical scale. Lancet 1974;2:81–84.
15. Ramsay MA, Savage TM, Simpson BR, Goodwin R: Controlled sedation with alphaxalone-alphadolone. BMJ 1974;2:656–659.
16. Samuels MA: A practical approach to coma diagnosis in the unresponsive patient. Cleve Clin J Med 1992;59:257–261.
17. Christie JM, O'Lenic TD, Cane RD: Head turning in brain death. J Clin Anesth 1996;8:141–143.
18. Ishii K, Onuma T, Kinoshita T, et al: Brain death: MR and MR angiography. Am J Neuroradiol 1996;17:731–735.
19. Towne AR, Waterhouse EJ, Boggs JG, et al: Prevalence of nonconvulsive status epilepticus in comatose patients. Neurology 2000;54:340–345.
20. Markand ON: Brain stem auditory evoked potentials. J Clin Neurophysiol 1994;11:319–342.
21. Aminoff MJ, Scheinman MM, Griffin JC, et al: Electrocerebral accompaniments of syncope associated with malignant ventricular arrhythmias. Ann Intern Med 1988;108:791–796.
22. Multi-Society Task Force on PVS: Medical aspects of the persistent vegetative state. N Engl J Med 1994;330:1499–1508, 1572–1579.
23. Wijdicks EFM: Brain death worldwide. Neurology 2002;58:20–25.
24. Dobb GJ, Weekes JW: Clinical confirmation of brain death. Anaesth Intensive Care 1995;23:37–43.
25. Kimber RM, Metcalfe MS, White SA, Nicholson ML: Use of non-heart-beating donors in renal transplantation. Postgrad Med J 2001; 77:681–685.
26. Diringer MN: Early prediction of outcome from coma. Curr Opin Neurol Neurosurg 1992;5:826–830.
27. Dupas B, Gayet-Delacroix M, Villers D, Antonioli D, Veccherini MF, Soulillou JP: Diagnosis of brain death using two-phase spiral CT. Am J Neuroradiol 1998;19:641–647.
28. Lampl Y, Gilad R, Eschel Y, Boaz M, Rapoport A, Sadeh M: Diagnosing brain death using the transcranial Doppler with a transorbital approach. Arch Neurol 2002;59:58–60.

CHAPTER 2

SUZANNE STEVENS, CYNTHIA L. COMELLA,
ARTHUR S. WALTERS, and WAYNE A. HENING

Sleep and Wakefulness

History and Definitions

Sleep occupies approximately one third of the adult life. Although the FULL function of sleep is not understood, the inherent necessity for sleep is widely recognized and is present in almost all mammals. The notion that sleep is a time of rest and brain inactivity persisted until the 20th century, when electrophysiological techniques were applied to the study of sleep. Thereafter sleep was found to be a dynamic process, with the cyclical recurrence of different stages. The discovery of rapid eye movement (REM) sleep by Aserinsky and Kleitman in 1953[1] was a major advance in sleep research, stimulating physiological and clinical studies of sleep. Sleep is divided into two types: REM and non–rapid eye movement (NREM) sleep.[2]

REM sleep cycles on and off throughout the night. In a young adult, the first REM period occurs approximately 90 to 100 minutes after sleep onset, following an initial period of NREM sleep. The first REM period is on average the shortest of the night. Successive REM periods tend to be of progressively longer duration, with the longest REM period most often occurring in the early morning hours. In infancy, 50 to 80 percent of total sleep time consists of REM sleep. By age 2 years and through adulthood, the percentage of REM sleep falls to approximately 20 to 25 percent of total sleep time.

REM sleep is divided into tonic and phasic events, and has several characteristic features. The tonic REM events include (1) cortical desynchronization, with mixed frequency, fast activity on electroencephalography (EEG), similar to that observed in the waking state; (2) hippocampal synchronous theta activity that also occurs in waking; and (3) muscle atonia that is present in all but respiratory and ocular muscles, and is marked by a reduction in chin and limb electromyographic activity. The phasic components of REM sleep include the following features: (1) rapid eye movements, horizontal and vertical, occurring in bursts during REM; (2) muscle twitches punctuating the muscle atonia; (3) ponto-geniculo-occipital spikes (PGO) not observable on routine polysomnography (PSG); and (4) autonomic nervous system lability with fluctuations in respiratory rate, heart rate, and blood pressure.[3]

NREM sleep is divided into four stages: Stages 1 and 2 are considered light sleep. Stage 1 occupies 2 to 5 percent of sleep time and is marked by slow rolling eye movements; low-voltage, mixed-frequency EEG, and a low arousal threshold. Stage 2 makes up approximately 45 to 55 percent of total sleep time and is marked by the presence of K complexes and sleep spindles on EEG recordings. K complexes are composed of an initial negative sharp wave followed by a positive component. Sleep spindles are episodic, rhythmical complexes occurring with frequency of 7 to 14 cycles per second grouped in sequences lasting 1 to 2 seconds. Spindles can occur alone or can be superimposed on K complexes. Although spindles are a feature of Stage 2 sleep, they may also be present in Stage 3 and Stage 4 NREM sleep, and can even be found in REM sleep.

Stages 3 and 4 sleep are considered deep or slow-wave sleep (SWS). SWS is prominent in youth and diminishes in the elderly. SWS is present for approximately 10 to 20 percent of sleep time and predominates in the first part of the night. The arousal threshold is high in SWS. The EEG feature of SWS is the delta wave, a high-voltage (75 microvolts or more) wave pattern with a frequency range of 2Hz or slowes. Stage 3 sleep is defined as sleep consisting of 20 to 50 percent delta waves, and Stage 4 is defined as greater than 50 percent delta waves.[3, 4]

Clinical History

Obtaining a detailed clinical history is especially important when diagnosing a sleep disturbance because routine physical and neurological examinations during the waking hours are often not revealing. Information gathered from the history, such as age of onset, duration, and progression of the sleep complaint, often allow a general classification of the type of sleep disturbance. The International Classification of Sleep Disorders categorizes sleep disturbances as (1) dyssomnias or disorders that result in insomnia or excessive sleepiness; (2) parasomnias or disorders of arousal, partial arousal, or sleep stage transition; and (3) sleep disorders associated with medical or psychiatric disorders.[5] The dyssomnias include the intrinsic sleep disorders arising from bodily malfunctions, such as psychophysiological insomnia, obstructive and central sleep apnea, restless legs syndrome (RLS), and periodic limb movement disorder (PLMD). Examples of parasomnias include sleepwalking, sleep terrors, sleep talking, nightmares, REM sleep behavior disorder (RBD), bruxism, and enuresis. Sleep disorders associated with medical and psychiatric conditions include those secondary to mood disorders, alcoholism, neurological disorders such as parkinsonism and dementia, and gastroesophageal reflux.[6, 7]

Sleep complaints often involve three areas of sleep disturbance: (1) the perceived inability to obtain sufficient sleep (insomnia), (2) the presence of excessive sleepiness or fatigue during the day (excessive daytime somnolence [EDS]), and (3) the occurrence of unusual events during sleep (parasomnias) (see the section entitled Clinical Syndromes Involving the Anatomy of Sleep). The clinical history should investigate each of these areas because there is often overlap among them.

The first part of the interview examines the quantity and quality of sleep, including the hour of bedtime and final awakening, the latency from bedtime to onset of sleep, events that delay sleep onset, number and duration of nocturnal awakenings, activities during the night, and perceived sleep quality. Is there a variation in the timing of sleep from day to day? Those who work or attend school may sleep less during the week, then sleep much longer when their activites are not structured during the weekend.[8] Shift workers or those who work in the evening or at night may find it very difficult to obtain a consistent timing and duration of sleep. They may be always fighting the circadian clock, which keeps internal rhythms and levels of alertness set to a 24-hour cycle.[9] Patients with neurodegenerative diseases often have internal clocks that no longer function effectively. Sleep and wakefulness may occur haphazardly around the clock or may be reversed, with most sleep coming during the daylight hours.[10] Withdrawal from pharmacological agents, especially those that cause sedation, is another possible cause of sleep disruption.

A sleep diary is a useful adjunct to the patient history. The patient completes a sleep diary every day for a consecutive 14-day period. This daily record of the patient sleep cycle provides the clinician with an indication of the timing and quantity of sleep obtained. This method is particularly useful in diagnosing sleep phase shifts and timing of insomnia. Patients with delayed phase sleep may show an inability to fall asleep until late at night, with a corresponding late awakening. Likewise, patients with phase advanced sleep may fall asleep easily at an early hour but awaken early in the morning. In particular, sleep diaries allow for an assessment of spontaneous sleep patterns during weekends or vacation periods, when the necessity to accommodate a work or school schedule is not present. Actigraphy is a useful adjunct to a sleep diary. A wrist actigraph is worn by the patient for 2 weeks and continually records physical activity. Although it does not specifically record sleep, periods of quiescence suggesting sleep time, punctuated by periods of muscle activity, can be stored in the actigraph and later retrieved. In conjunction with a sleep diary, actigraphy is a powerful tool in estimating routine sleep patterns at home.[11]

The evaluation of sleep quality relies on the subjective perception of sleep. Several scales have been developed to assess overall sleep quality. Some of these scales have been validated.[12] The structured interview provides insight into several domains of sleep quality. How well does the patient sleep? Does the patient feel that sleep is troubled or insufficient? Good sleep satisfies several criteria: (1) it is sufficient—providing for adequate alertness and a feeling of vitality during the day; (2) it is efficient—easily initiated, continuously maintained, and not excessively prolonged; and (3) it is convenient—occurring during a period of time when the patient would not need or prefer to be awake, which is usually at night but may vary for those with other life demands, such as a nighttime job.

An evaluation of the presence and severity of daytime sleepiness is a vital part of the sleep interview. Patients whose sleep is significantly disrupted or fragmented,[13] or those who simply do not get enough sleep, may be sleepy during the daytime. Typically, EDS manifests as nodding off or napping during quiet, passive activities, such as reading, watching television, or listening to a lecture. In more severe cases, sleep may occur during active periods such as while eating, talking, or driving a motor vehicle. When EDS is severe, it can impair the quality of life and even lead to life-threatening situations, such as falling asleep while driving. In contrast to the EDS arising from nocturnal sleep disruption, narcoleptic patients may have attacks of sleep in which REM sleep occurs.

In determining whether or not there are unusual events during sleep, interview of the bed partner or family members who are able to observe the patient's sleep may be essential. A variety of abnormal events during sleep may impair sleep quality, cause patient discomfort, or interrupt the sleep of the bed partner. Snoring or gasping during sleep may be a sign of respiratory difficulties or sleep apnea. Unusual sleep-related movements can indicate the presence of or PLMD, nocturnal epilepsy, or RBD. Other behaviors may suggest the presence of sleep walking (somnambulism), sleep talking (somniloquy), tooth grinding (bruxism), or attacks of eating in a fuguelike state (nocturnal eating disorder).[5]

Events occurring before sleep onset may provide clues to the cause of insomnia. Good sleep hygiene, which can help sleep quality, involves consistent calming activities before sleep.[14] Poor sleep hygiene may interfere with the ability to sleep. Activities which may contribute to poor sleep hygiene include caffeine and nicotine intake, late-day napping, exercising immediately before bedtime, and using the bed to read, watch television, or work. Alcohol intake at bedtime may shorten sleep latency but often causes sleep fragmentation later in the night, with early morning awakening. Patients may report sensory phenomena in the legs or arms when they lie down to sleep. These sensations may be described as tingling, tightness, crawling sensations, or pain. These sensations may be severe enough to interfere with sleep onset and may be relieved only with movement of the limbs, or walking. This history suggests the diagnosis of RLS. PLMD is frequently associated with RLS and may cause disruption of sleep once sleep is obtained. A prominent jerk just at sleep onset that runs through most of the body, sometimes associated with a sensation or illusion of falling, is a hypnic jerk and is experienced by most people on occasion.[15]

Psychological states at the time of sleep onset are important to assess in patients with insomnia. Patients reporting excessive worries, ruminations over daytime problems, and anxiety may find that despite feeling sleepy, these intrusive thoughts cause alertness and prevent sleep onset. They may feel increased muscle tension. The duration and triggering factor for the insomnia is important to obtain. Patients experiencing transient insomnia related to particular life events may benefit from treatment strategies inappropriate for the patient with chronic, recurrent insomnia. Depression and anxiety are psychiatric disorders that are strongly associated with sleep disturbances. A psychiatric assessment may provide useful clues to the presence of these potentially treatable causes of insomnia.

Medical conditions may also interfere with normal sleep. Patients with rheumatoid arthritis may be awakened by pain. Patients with neuromuscular disease may awaken because of respiratory difficulty. Patients with Parkinson's disease may awaken because their medications have worn off and they are uncomfortable and unable to shift posture. Prostate disorders may lead to frequent awakenings to urinate during the night. The elderly may be at higher risk for frequent urination as a product of fragmented sleep.

Neuromuscular disorders, Parkinson's disease, multisystem atrophy, lung disease, obesity, acromegaly, or thyroid disease can all be associated with respiratory disturbances in sleep.[16] Different medical and neurological conditions, including iron deficiency, uremia, and peripheral neuropathy, are associated with RLS and PLMD.[17] Neurodegenerative disorders, such as Alzheimer's disease, may result in a breakdown of the circadian clock, which regulates the alternation of sleep and wakefulness. Tic disease may lead to parasomnias in children. Patients with Parkinson's disease, as well as those with neurodegenerative disease or brain stem strokes, may have RBD, in which dreams can be acted out with injurious consequences.[18]

A history of hallucinations either at sleep onset (hypnagogic) or on awakening from sleep (hypnopompic), sleep paralysis (the inability to voluntarily move on awakening), sleepiness during the day, and cataplexy (sudden loss of muscle tone during wakefulness) comprise the classic tetrad for narcolepsy. If present, they may indicate a diagnosis of narcolepsy, particularly if onset occurred during youth, adolescence, or young adulthood.[19] Not all narcoleptics have each of the symptoms in the tetrad.

Ingestion of medication is a particularly important part of the clinical history. There are many medications that cause drowsiness during the day or disrupted sleep at night. In severe cases, this disruption may lead to lethargy, confusion, or forgetfulness. Although sedative and hypnotic medications, particularly those with long half-lives, are usually recognized as a cause of daytime sleepiness, there are numerous additional agents that have a similar effect, including antihistamines, neuroleptic agents, antihypertensives, anticonvulsants, antiparkinsonian medications, antidepressants, analgesics, and muscle relaxants. Elderly patients, especially those with hepatic or renal insufficiency, may be particularly susceptible to medication side effects because a drug or its active metabolites may accumulate owing to impaired metabolism or excretion. Antiparkinsonian medications may cause vivid dreams and nightmares. The benzodiazepines and barbiturates may suppress SWS, decrease the amount of REM sleep, and exacerbate sleep apnea. With chronic use, these agents often lose their efficacy, and sudden discontinuation frequently causes rebound insomnia. Stimulants used for attention deficit disorder and in narcolepsy may cause insomnia. Dopamine-blocking agents including metoclopramide can aggravate RLS, whereas antidepressants, including tricyclic compounds and serotonin reuptake inhibitors, may activate PLMD.

A family history of sleep disturbance may suggest particular sleep disorders. In particular, RLS is familial and an autosomal dominant inheritance has been suggested by some pedigrees.[20] Narcolepsy and sleep apnea are other sleep disorders with genetic components. Genetic factors contribute to NREM parasomnias with most patients having a first-degree relative with a NREM parasomnia. The familial seizure disorder autosomal dominant frontal lobe epilepsy has been described.[21] Fatal familial insomnia is a rare disorder in which family history is helpful for a correct diagnosis, although diagnosis can be made with a determination of the nature of the prion protein.[22]

Anatomy of Normal Sleep

PHYSIOLOGICAL FUNCTION OF SLEEP

Sleep evolves during life and changes with maturation and aging. During infancy, 16 to 18 hours a day are spent sleeping, with sleep-wake states initially occurring every 3 to 4 hours. By 6 months of age, a more prolonged sleep period occurs during the night. REM sleep time occupies as much as 80 percent of sleep time in the newborn, with a steady decrease until only approximately 20 percent of sleep is REM in the adult. Sleep spindles appear at approximately 2 years of age. During adolescence, sleep requirement increases, and the sleep pattern is one of phase delay.[8] Because school schedules do not allow for late awakening, the most common cause of daytime sleepiness in this age group is insufficient sleep. In adulthood, the need for sleep is relatively constant. With aging, sleep tends to become more fragmented, and night sleep may decrease with a corresponding increase of daytime napping. With aging, the amount of SWS decreases. Although REM sleep time remains stable with aging, the pattern of REM sleep seen in the young adult with progressively longer REM periods is not observed in the elderly, who have REM sleep equally distributed over the course of the night.[23]

The function of sleep remains elusive.[24] Most sleep is NREM sleep, comprising 80 percent of total sleep time in the adult. The most critical part of NREM sleep occurs early at night, when most SWS occurs. SWS is the deepest, most difficult to interrupt, and most refreshing of the sleep stages. During recovery from sleep deprivation, SWS is the first to rebound.[25] The decline in the proportion of SWS with aging is possibly related to the overall deterioration of sleep, resulting in an increase in sleep complaints that characterize the older population. Third, for humans, primarily diurnal animals, sleep typically occurs at night. Whatever else sleep does, it likely reduces activity at the time when a diurnal, visually dependent animal cannot function effectively and thereby conserves resources. In evolution, the development of sleep as a block of reduced activity at night likely made that time available for other purposes. Functions that would be impaired by daylight activity could be shifted into the sleep period and integrated with the sleep state. As a result, many of the plausible functions of sleep may be adaptations to the reduced nocturnal activity that sleep ensures. Fourth, there may be no one single function of sleep but a group of different functions. As one summary statement to a recent publication of the proceedings of a conference on the function of sleep stated, "Research and speculation on the functions of sleep have yielded many viable possibilities."[26] Functions may vary in importance depending on the individual's age or activities, and none of these functions may be unique to sleep. The following section presents some of the plausible functions suggested for NREM sleep.

METABOLIC AND THERMOREGULATORY FUNCTIONS

Experiments with rats have suggested that during sleep deprivation, energy expenditure increases while temperature and weight drop until body systems begin to fail, beginning with the endocrine and immune systems.[27] These and other studies have led to the proposal that sleep conserves energy loss through thermoregulation, and when core body temperature decreases during sleep, heat loss to the environment is minimized. Confirmatory sleep deprivation studies have not been performed in humans, but humans naturally show lowered body temperature during sleep. A different interpretation of temperature changes begins during sleep with the observation that sleep in general and deeper NREM sleep in particular are increased when the body is heated;[28] therefore, sleep may allow the shedding of excess accumulated heat.[29] This approach emphasizes not the decreased rate of heat loss in sleep due to decreased core temperature but the reduced rate of heat production due to slowed metabolism. Sleep may be the prime period for anabolic activity. In primates, growth hormone, whose effects can be manifest at all ages in humans, is primarily secreted during the periods of deepest SWS early in the night.[30] In several studies of growth in children with growth disorders, total sleep correlated with rate of growth, suggesting that disrupted sleep could inhibit growth. In human males, the growth hormone secretion is positively associated with the amount of SWS.[31] Acute sleep loss has been associated with decreased glucose tolerance, lower thyrotropin concentrations, elevated evening cortisol levels, and increased activity of sympathetic nervous system activity.[32]

RESTORATIVE NEURAL FUNCTIONS

In the brain, there is evidence, although it is not yet conclusive, that overall RNA transcription and protein synthesis is most prominent during deep SWS. This activity may have particular importance for synaptic function. Even considering the alternation of SWS and REM sleep, when brain activity is often as high as during the waking state, it has been suggested that SWS allows for a recovery from so-called "activity debts." It has been hypothesized that the brain uses the materials produced and stored during SWS. The decline of cognitive function with sleep deprivation provides some evidence of these restorative or supportive functions of sleep. There is also some evidence that SWS responds to learning situations in animals and may play additional roles in consolidating memories.[33] Other possible related functions are a restoration of balance at the synaptic level. Neurons relatively quiescent during the waking period can be activated at night during both NREM and REM sleep, so that the entire network does not become imbalanced.[34] SWS may restore a functional balance of emotional states related to limbic system function.

Neuronal Circuits and Nuclei Underlying Sleep Rhythm

CIRCADIAN RHYTHMS

The timing and rhythmicity of the sleep-wake cycle is matched to the solar day-night cycle in humans. This rhythmical pattern is generated internally but is modified by environmental factors, in particular the light-dark cycle. The endogenous nature of the circadian rhythm is verified by the persistence of these rhythms when environmental conditions are held constant. For example, a human kept in isolation without access to a clock or a periodic light-dark cycle will maintain a regular sleep-wake cycle. According to Czeisler and colleagues, although the rhythm is maintained, the periodicity of the sleep-wake cycle under this free-running condition is approximately 24.2 hours. However, under the influence of the environmental light-dark cycle, this rhythm is entrained to the 24-hour solar day. The environmental cues that are able to entrain the internal clock mechanism are called *zeitgebers*. The most potent zeitgeber for sleep-wake rhythms in most organisms is light.

THE SUPRACHIASMATIC NUCLEUS

The anatomical structure serving as the internal circadian rhythm generator is the suprachiasmatic nucleus (SCN) of the anterior hypothalamus.[35,36] Lesions of the SCN in rodents abolish circadian rhythmicity, and disconnection of the SCN from the rest of the brain also results in a loss of circadian rhythms in the brain in spite of continued fluctuations within the SCN. Furthermore, in animals with ablations of the SCN, transplantation of fetal SCN tissue restores circadian rhythm.

Entrainment of these neurons occurs via the visual pathways linking photoreceptors of the retina to the SCN. There are two pathways: (1) a direct pathway called the retinohypothalamic tract (RHT) and (2) an indirect pathway called the geniculohypothalamic tract (GHT). Photoreceptors in the retina transduce light into nerve impulses and transmit information to ganglion cells, distributed over the entire retina. The ganglion cells contribute to the RHT, that travels through the optic nerve and optic chiasm. In the chiasm, two thirds of the axons cross and one third remain uncrossed. The RHT projects directly to the SCN. Collateral processes from the RHT continue in the optic tract to the lateral geniculate complex. From the lateral geniculate, the GHT projects to the SCN as the indirect pathway.

Efferent fibers from the SCN project to intrahypothalamic areas—encompassing the preoptic area, paraventricular nucleus, retrochiasmatic area, dorsomedial area, and extrahypothalamic sites, including the thalamus, basal forebrain, and periaqueductal gray. From these areas information is further relayed to the effector organs for particular biological rhythms.

In addition to controlling the circadian variability of the sleep-wake cycle, the SCN drives a similar circadian variability in locomotor activity, food intake, water intake, sexual behavior, core body temperature, and hormonal levels. Thus, cortisol is highest in the early morning hours between 4:00 to 8:00 AM, and thyroid-stimulating hormone increases just before sleep. Hormones both influence and are influenced by the circadian clock.

THE PINEAL GLAND AND MELATONIN

The pineal gland is a neuroendocrine gland that synthesizes and secretes melatonin (*N*-acetyl-5-methoxytryptamine).[37] The afferent input to the pineal gland is transmitted from the retinal photoreceptors through the SCN and sympathetic nervous system. The circadian rhythm of melatonin is controlled by the SCN but is strongly entrained by light. The two effects of light are, first, to regulate melatonin secretion in accordance with diurnal light-dark cycles and, second, to suppress melatonin if given in brief intense pulses. Melatonin secretion increases rather abruptly in the evening, about 2 hours before typical bedtime (dim light melatonin onset; DLMO), and then continues elevated during the night, reaching a peak level between 2:00 and 4:00 AM, then gradually falls during the latter part of the night, and is present at very low levels during the day. Exogenous melatonin has been used with some success to avoid jet lag and may be useful for treatment of phase-shifted sleep and sleep disturbance due to shift work. Melatonin is available through health food stores and has received strong public attention. However, at this time, there are no proven indications for melatonin.

NREM SLEEP

Sleep spindles usually arise from the gamma-aminobutyric acid (GABA)–ergic neurons in the reticular thalamic nucleus. These neurons have intrinsic oscillations with spontaneous slow depolarization on which rhythmical spikes are superimposed and serve as drivers for thalamocortical projection neurons. Dissection of the reticular thalamic region from the thalamocortical region or specific kainic acid lesions of reticular thalamic nuclei eliminates spindles. On scalp recordings, spindles occur maximally over the frontal and vertex areas. Depth electrode recordings in humans show that thalamic spindles are earlier and more frequent than those recorded on the scalp. Spindles occurring in the frontal leads may also originate in the supplementary cortex.[38]

The defining feature of Stages 3 and 4 sleep is the delta or slow wave. Thalamocortical cells are capable of generating delta waves, but other areas are involved as well, as shown by lesions of the anterior hypothalamus, preoptic region, and basal forebrain, all of which can abolish delta waves.

REM SLEEP

The anatomical substrates for the different components of REM sleep are as follows:

1. An important substrate is cortical desynchronization. The origin of the mixed frequency activity is the mesencephalic reticular formation. The reticular cells begin firing about 15 seconds before activation is manifest in the cortex, and their projections extend to the intralaminar nuclei of the thalamus with widespread projections to cortex.
2. Hippocampal theta activity is highly synchronous activity with a frequency of 5 to 10 Hz, which is generated in the dentate gyrus and medial entorhinal cortex. It involves the rostral pontine reticular formation in the area of the nucleus pontis oralis.
3. Muscle atonia, except for respiratory and ocular muscles, is a tonic event of REM sleep. Electrical stimulation studies have shown that muscle atonia occurs following activation of the medullary magnocellular reticular nucleus and the rostral nucleus pontis oralis. Muscle paralysis arises at the spinal cord level, from a centrally mediated hyperpolarization of the alpha motor neurons through the action of the inhibitory neurotransmitter glycine.
4. Muscle twitches are superimposed on the tonic muscle paralysis. The twitches arise from descending excitatory impulses, which transiently overcome motor neuron inhibition.
5. Rapid eye movements are another phasic event of REM sleep. Horizontal eye movements arise from burst neurons in the parabducens reticular formation in the pons, and vertical eye movements are associated with activation of the midbrain reticular formation. Positron emission tomography has shown that REM-related eye movements involve cortical areas similar to those used during wakefulness.
6. PGO activity is a phasic feature of REM sleep, generated in the pons and projected through the lateral geniculate body and other thalamic nuclei to the occipital cortex. PGO activity is of two types—type one occurs independent of eye movements, and type 2 occurs simultaneously with eye movements. PGO spike activity has been associated with fragmentary images or dreams.

7. Autonomic nervous system lability, with profound sympathetic activation and fluctuations in respirations, heart rate, and blood pressure, involves the parabrachial nuclei of pons. Other features of REM sleep include penile erections not associated with sexual stimulation or dream content and thermoregulatory suspension leading to a pseudopoikilothermic state. Additionally, there is an increase in cerebral metabolism and blood flow as compared with NREM sleep, particularly in the pons, thalamus and cingulate cortex.[39–41]

The regulation of REM sleep is primarily at the level of the brain stem, with REM-on and REM-off nuclei.[42] Although the putative trigger zone initiating REM sleep is not identified, the activity of brain stem areas during REM sleep has been studied, both electrically and pharmacologically. Brain stem nuclei with activity immediately preceding and persisting during REM sleep are the cholinergic cells in the dorsolateral tegmentum: the lateral dorsal tegmental (LDT) and the pedunculopontine tegmental (PPN) nuclei. These two nuclei comprise the main concentration of brain stem cholinergic neurons.[43] The projection areas of these nuclei include the basal ganglia; the limbic areas, including the preoptic area; the thalamic nuclei, including the lateral geniculate nuclei; and the cortex. The PPN plays a role in numerous feedback loops, involving locomotion and rhythmical functions, specifically control of sleep-wake cycles and generation of REM sleep. The cholinoceptive REM triggering zone located in the paramedian reticular formation receives input from LDT and PPN. Inhibition of these REM-on nuclei appears to arise from nearby REM-off cells, primarily the serotonergic neurons of the dorsal raphe and adrenergic neurons of the locus coeruleus.

The reciprocal-interaction model proposed by Hobson posits that control of REM sleep arises from anatomically distributed and neurochemically integrated populations of cells. This model is summarized by McCarley as involving four steps: (1) positive feedback of REM-on neurons through excitatory interconnections with reticular neurons; (2) excitation of REM-off neurons by REM-on neurons mediated through cholinergic pathways, although the reticular formation may actually be the origin of this process; (3) inhibition of REM-on neurons by REM-off neurons located in the dorsal raphe and locus coeruleus; and (4) inhibitory feedback of REM-off neurons through recurrent collateral or some other method of serotonin and norepinephrine feedback.[3]

The neuroanatomical areas involved in the generation of REM sleep have largely been identified through transections at different levels in the neuraxis. In transections separating the forebrain from the brain stem, REM sleep features are recorded caudal to the cut. These features include atonia, rapid eye movements, PGO spike bursts, and REM-like activation of the reticular formation. However, in this transection, thermoregulatory control is lost with an inverse relationship between temperture and amount of REM sleep. Transections between the locus coeruleus and the red nucleus, separating the pons from the midbrain, results in atonia, PGO spike bursts, rapid eye movements, and activation of the reticular formation in a rhythmical pattern caudal to the transection. Transections between the medulla and the pons result in a regular cycle of REM above the transection, with the exception of the generation of muscle atonia. Taken together, these experiments provide evidence that REM sleep is generated primarily in the pons.[39]

REM sleep is the form of sleep in which many dreams occur. When awakened during an episode of REM, the sleeper will report the contents of the dream approximately 85 percent of the time. The function of dreaming has remained elusive. Both physiological (related to memory and learning) and psychological roles have been proposed.[44]

Neurochemical Anatomy

Several primary neurotransmitters control circadian rhythm. SCN neurons are mostly GABAergic. The neurotransmitter released from the RHT is glutamate, affecting both *N*-methyl-D-aspartate (NMDA) and non-NMDA receptors in the SCN. The putative neurotransmitters of the indirect pathway, GHT, are GABA and neuropeptide Y. Cholinergic agonists like carbachol also have an effect on activity of the SCN, and their administration shifts the activity of the SCN in a manner similar to that of light exposure. Less pronounced effects on SCN activity have been described following clonidine, an alpha-2 receptor agonist. The SCN also receives nonentrainment afferents from serotonergic projections of the median and dorsal raphe nucleus of the midbrain and histaminergic projections from the posterior hypothalamic tuberomammillary neurons. Vasoactive intestinal polypeptide is a neurotransmitter in an efferent pathway from the SCN. The neurotransmitter from the SCN to the pineal is norepinephrine.[35]

The neurochemical constituents involved in the generation and maintenance of REM and NREM are listed in Table 2–1. Neurochemically, REM sleep is associated with an increase in cholinergic activity and a reduction in noradren-

TABLE 2–1. **Activity of Subpopulations of Cell Groups During Waking, Slow-Wave Sleep, and REM Sleep**

Nucleus	Primary Neurotransmitter	Waking Activity	Slow-Wave Sleep	REM Sleep
Pedunculopontine nucleus (PPN)	Acetylcholine	Increased	Decreased	Increased
Locus coeruleus	Norepinephrine	Increased	Increased	Decreased
Raphe nucleus	Serotonin	Increased	Increased	Decreased
Substantia nigra	Dopamine	Increased	Decreased	Increased

Reprinted from Garcia-Rill E: The pedunculopontine nucleus. Prog Neurobiol 1991;36:363–389, with permission of Elsevier Science.

ergic and serotonergic activity. In contrast, SWS is associated with increased serotonergic activity.[42–44]

HYPOCRETIN (OREXIN) SYSTEM

Hypocretin (orexin) is a brain neuropeptide contributing to the sleep-wake cycle and implicated in the etiology of narcolepsy. The function of this neuropeptide is thought to promote wakefulness and stimulate appetite. The cell bodies containing hypocretin are located in the dorsolateral hypothalamus and project to the locus coeruleus and numerous other areas of the brain including the cortex.[45] In animal models, alterations of the gene encoding hypocretin 2 receptors and preprohypocretin genes produce findings consistent with narcolepsy.[46, 47] In humans, reports of cerebrospinal fluid levels of hypocretin were markedly decreased in seven of nine narcoleptic patients but detected in normal amounts among the eight control subjects.[48] Human narcoleptic brains have been shown to have a dramatic reduction in the number of hypocretin neurons.[49] The hypocretin (orexin) system may offer further understanding of narcolepsy and offer a target for future treatment strategies.

Examination of the Patient with Sleep-Wake Cycle Complaints

NEUROLOGICAL EXAMINATION

Cerebral. The neurological examination focuses on the general state of alertness. Patients may appear sleepy or even nod off during the examination if EDS is severe. Cognitive and psychological functioning are assessed for evidence of dementia or depression, because both are associated with sleep pattern disruption. Excessive anxiety, fears, and concerns are frequent causes for insomnia, and clues to these problems may reveal themselves during cerebral assessments of memory, concentration, and attention.

Cranial Nerves. Cranial nerve lesions indicate brain stem pathology. Disorders of REM sleep, including narcolepsy and RBD, may reflect focal pathology in the pons, so specific attention to pontine cranial nerve function (trigeminal, abducens, facial, and vestibulocochlear) are essential. Bulbar dysfunction in the form of dysphagia, hoarseness, and dyspnea can occur in neuromuscular disorders and myopathies. In checking for the gag reflex, the upper airway can be examined, and a reddened palate and uvula are suggestive of snoring.

Motor/Reflexes/Cerebellar/Gait. Several disorders of the motor system are associated with sleep alterations. Strength should be examined, specifically the strength of the neck and respiratory muscles. Patients with myopathies, neuropathies, and neuromuscular junction disease can have significant chest wall weakness. In acute or chronic demyelinating polyneuropathy (Guillain-Barré syndrome), tendon reflexes are lost and there may be additional bulbar cranial nerve weakness. In patients with myasthenia gravis, initial inspiration and expiration volumes may be normal, but repeated testing demonstrates rapid fatigability and poor aeration. In multiple system atrophy, a diffuse degenerative condition with numerous areas of the nervous system affected, sleep complaints occur in the context of parkinsonism and signs of cerebellar dysfunction, such as dysmetria, ataxia, or tremors. Spinocerebellar atrophies are also associated with sleep disruption, and their motor signs are predominantly limb, trunk, and gait ataxia, along with sensory neuropathies. Whereas most movement disorders resolve during sleep, patients with tics may have significant sleep disruption from continuing tics, and patients with Parkinson's disease have difficulty going to sleep because of stiffness and shaking as well as further difficulty staying asleep. In addition, they have a frequent problem with vivid dreams and sleep fragmentation, and they may have RBD associated with injurious behaviors.

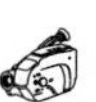

Sensory. A number of neuropathies are associated with sleep alterations, and hence the sensory examination, including both position and vibration testing for myelinated fiber function and pain and temperature testing for unmyelinated fiber function should be performed. RLS can be frequently exacerbated by neuropathy, and diabetes mellitus and spinocerebellar atrophies have characteristic neuropathic findings.

Autonomic Nervous System. The signs of central sleep apnea include the loss of respiratory airflow and the loss of respiratory muscle effort. The condition is thought to arise from alterations in the functioning of chemoreceptors monitoring hypoxic and hypercapnic influences on respiration. Patients should be examined for waking respiratory difficulties and cardiac functioning, in particular for congestive heart failure. Neuromuscular diseases likewise may predispose to episodes of sleep apnea, as can autonomic nervous system instability. Patients should be assessed for evidence of orthostatic hypotension and examined for those disorders with autonomic nervous system involvement, including multiple system atrophy, Guillain-Barré syndrome, and diabetes.

Neurovascular System. A general cardiac and vascular examination reveals signs of cardiac failure and blood pressure, specifically signs of pulmonary hypertension that is frequently associated with obstructive sleep apnea.

ASSOCIATED MEDICAL FINDINGS

The physical examination in a patient with a suspected sleep disorder focuses on several features. To assess for physical abnormalities associated with obstructive sleep apnea, particular attention is directed toward examination of height, weight, and blood pressure. Abnormalities of the upper airway, including nasal congestion, nasal polyps, deviated septum, enlarged tonsils, enlarged tongue, or low palate, can indicate possible contribution of these anatomical findings to airway obstruction. A reddened uvula and palate may be associated with loud snoring. Retrognathia and a small pharyngeal opening may also be seen in patients with sleep apnea.

Evaluation Guidelines

There are a variety of laboratory tests that directly or indirectly may apply to the evaluation of sleep and sleep disorders (Table 2–2).

TABLE 2–2. **Useful Studies for the Investigation of Sleep-Wake Cycle Disorders**

Syndrome	Neuroimaging	Electrophysiology	Fluid and Tissue Analysis	Neuropsychological Tests	Other Tests
Insomnia	Focal abnormality in post-traumatic, atrophy in degenerative diseases	PSG to indicate whether secondary to other sleep disorder EMG evidence of peripheral neuropathy in some patients with RLS	Metabolic or drug screening	Dementia, depression, anxiety, or other psychiatric disorder	Sleep diary for sleep patterns Forced immobilization test to assess for RLS
EDS	Focal abnormalities, brain stem abnormality in central sleep apnea	PSG assessing for nocturnal sleep disorder (sleep apnea, PLMD) Multiple sleep latency test with shortened latency with or without REM onset naps EMG showing neuromuscular disease	Arterial blood gas showing hypoxia, chronic carbon dioxide retention HLA blood typing Serological evidence of viral infection	Dementia, depression, anxiety, or other psychiatric disorder Reduced attention	Daytime sleepiness scales Sleep diary Oximetry Pulmonary function tests Cephalometry Pharyngeal examination
Parasomnia	Focal abnormality in brain stem area, thalamus, or hemisphere causing nocturnal seizure Brain stem/cerebellar atrophy consistent with multiple system atrophy	PSG with videotaping to show the behaviors and the stage of sleep during which they occur Electroencephalography for nocturnal seizures	Evidence of multiples sclerosis in CSF, prior viral infection	Dementia Psychological disturbances, post-traumatic stress disorder	None needed
Circadian disorders		Wrist actigraphy, PSG	None needed	Assessment for anxiety, depression	Sleep diary, employment history

CSF, Cerebrospinal fluid; EDS, excessive daytime somnolence; EMG, electromyography; HLA, human leukocyte antigen; PLMD, periodic limb movement disorder; PSG, polysomnography; REM, rapid eye movement, RLS, restless legs syndrome.

Neuroimaging. Neuroimaging is not usually necessary during the evaluation of a primary sleep disorder. If patients present with additional neurological symptoms and signs, or the clinical history is atypical, magnetic resonance imaging may be helpful.

Electrophysiology. Routine EEG may be indicated when a diagnosis of sleep-related seizures is suspected. Likewise, electromyography may provide valuable information if peripheral neuropathy is suspected associated with RLS, or if neuromuscular disorders are thought to be predisposing to sleep apnea. The standard test of sleep is overnight PSG. PSG is an overnight recording of sleep, monitoring EEG, eye movements, chin muscle tone, muscle activity of the limbs, electrocardiogram, respiratory effort, nasal airflow, and oxygen saturation. During polysomnography, a patient is closely monitored by a technician who is present throughout the night. Videotaping abnormal sleep behaviors is possible. PSG testing provides objective data concerning sleep latency, sleep efficiency, sleep staging, severity and type of sleep apnea, periodic limb movements, and parasomnias. PSG is of more limited usefulness in the evaluation of insomnia, unless insomnia arises from a primary sleep disorder, such as sleep apnea. The major drawback to PSG is the need to sleep in a controlled environment. For some patients, the strange surroundings reduce the ability to sleep normally, and obtaining an accurate sleep recording requires one night of adaptation before the actual recording night. Moreover, PSG is very labor intensive and expensive. Despite these drawbacks, PSG remains the most reliable test for certain sleep disturbances.

Body Fluid and Tissue Analysis. In patients with sleep apnea, obtaining a baseline arterial blood gas may be essential in guiding treatment. In patients with suspected narcolepsy, human leukocyte antigen blood typing may be descriptively interesting but does not confirm or eliminate a diagnosis. Obtaining other tests will depend on the individual case. Extensive fluid and tissue analysis is seldom necessary for most primary sleep disorders, but thyroid tests and drug screens should be obtained in most cases.

Neuropsychological Tests. Neuropsychological testing is useful for determining the presence and severity of cognitive impairment and mood disorders.

Other Tests. *Sleep diaries* allow a continuous subjective report of sleep. Patients are given a 2-week log, with each day divided into 30-minute or 60-minute intervals. Patients are instructed to fill out the log three to four times per day, indicating the time asleep for the previous 6- to 8-hour period. Patients can comment about their sense of alertness on awakening each morning and record unusual daytime or nighttime events. Sleep logs are inexpensive and convenient. Logs can provide valuable information about the circadian pattern of sleep and allow for an indefinite recording period. The drawback to sleep logs is the inaccuracy of self-report of sleep time and the inability to diagnose sleep disturbance. Sleep logs are a useful screening tool and can provide follow-up information for phase shifted sleep and insomnia.

Wrist actigraphy measures movement of the wrist and consists of a movement detector and memory storage. A wrist actigraph is approximately the size of a large watch and is worn continuously at home. When the recording period is complete, the stored movement data are transferred to a computer for analysis. Interpretation of actigraphic records assumes that movement is reduced during sleep compared with wakefulness. Patients who lie still but are awake for prolonged periods of time will have their sleep time overestimated. Similarly, patients with excessive movements during sleep may be considered to be awake and have an underestimate of sleep time. According to the American Sleep Disorders Association practice parameters, actigraphy serves as a useful adjunct to history, examination, and subjective sleep diary for the diagnosis and treatment of insomnia, circadian-rhythm disorders, and excessive sleepiness. However, actigraphy is not indicated for the routine diagnosis of any sleep disorder.[50]

The multiple sleep latency test (MSLT) consists of five 20-minute nap opportunities, with each nap separated by 2 hours. The patient lies down in a darkened room and is instructed to try to sleep. The time before any sleep is recorded for each nap, and the mean sleep latency for all five naps is then determined. Patients with a mean sleep latency of less than 5 minutes are considered to have pathological sleepiness; those with a mean sleep latency between 5 and 10 minutes are borderline, and those with a mean latency greater than 10 minutes are normal. During the naps, sleep is staged. If REM sleep occurs during two or more naps, the MSLT is consistent with a diagnosis of narcolepsy, provided other causes of sleep-onset rapid eye movements have been excluded. The interpretation of the MSLT test is more accurate if performed the day following overnight PSG. Sleep deprivation from the night before or drugs that suppress REM may yield deceptive results. The MSLT is indicated for assessment of narcolepsy, severity of EDS due to obstructive sleep apnea, other nocturnal sleep disturbances, and idiopathic hypersomnia.[51] Pupillometry measures the pupillary size. Pupils generally constrict and demonstrate instability when falling asleep. However, this is not used widely clinically as normative data is not available.

Ambulatory or portable sleep monitoring allows for recording of sleep in the patients home. It is less expensive than laboratory PSG and more convenient for patients. Portable monitors have been most often used for the assessment of sleep apnea. The limitations of portable monitoring include the variability in commercially available monitors. Recording channels may be limited, making a complete assessment of sleep problematic. There is no technician present in an unattended study to adjust for malfunctioning equipment or to reapply faulty or loose electrodes. According to the American Sleep Disorder Association's guidelines, portable monitoring is indicated only for patients who cannot be studied in the sleep laboratory or for follow-up studies when the diagnosis has already been established by standard PSG.[52]

Clinical Syndromes Involving the Anatomy of Sleep

This section discusses the sleep disorders as clinical syndromes (Table 2–3). See Chapter 54 for a discussion of the specific diagnoses and treatment of primary sleep disorders.

INSOMNIA

The insomnias encompass a number of different disorders predominantly by difficulty falling asleep or maintaining

TABLE 2–3. **Selected Etiologies of Disorders Affecting the Sleep-Wake Cycle**

Etiological Category	Specific Etiologies	Chapter
Developmental structural disorders	Enuresis from structural anomalies	28
Degenerative and compressive structural disorders	Obstructive sleep apnea, upper airway resistance syndrome	29
The degenerative dementias	Alzheimer's disease	33
Movement disorders	Parkinson's disease; multiple system atrophy; dopa-responsive dystonia; hyperkinetic movements: tics, chorea, dystonia, tremor, hemiballismus, hemifacial spasm, myoclonus of cortical origin	34
Degenerative motor, sensory, and autonomic disorders	Duchenne muscular dystrophy, myotonic dystrophy, limb girdle dystrophy, amyotrophic lateral sclerosis	36
Hereditary nondegenerative neuromuscular disease	Congential myopathies	37
	Kleine-Levin syndrome	38
Endogenous metabolic disorders	Thyroid disease	
Nutritional deficiencies and syndromes associated with alcoholism	Alcoholism	40
Transmissible spongiform encephalopathy	Fatal familial insomnia	43
Demyelinating disorders of the peripheral nervous system	Guillain-Barré syndrome	49
Autoimmune and inflammatory disorders	Rheumatoid arthritis, polymyositis, myasthenia gravis	50
Traumatic disorders	Post-traumatic hypersomnia	51
Epilepsy	Sleep epilepsy, nocturnal paroxysmal dystonia	52
Headache and facial pain	Sleep-related headaches	53
Sleep disorders	Narcolepsy, REM sleep behavior disorder, restless legs syndrome, periodic limb movement disorder, primary insomnia, sleepwalking, sleep talking, bruxism	54
Drug-induced and iatrogenic neurological disorders	Antidepressants; hypnotic-dependent sleep disorder, stimulant-dependent sleep disorder	55

consolidated sleep, or the problem of awakening early in the morning before adequate sleep is obtained. The definition of adequate sleep varies among individuals, with some perceiving 5 hours as sufficient and others feeling that 8 or 9 hours of undisturbed sleep is necessary to be rested and alert the following day. The history is crucial to determining the possible etiologies of insomnia.[53–56]

Sleep-onset insomnia refers to a prolonged latency from the time of going to bed until falling asleep. In psychophysiological insomnia, patients may complain of feelings of anxiety, tension, worry, or persistent reflections over the problems of the past or future as they lay in bed to sleep. In acute insomnia, there may be a precipitating event, such as the death or illness of a loved one, that is associated with the onset of insomnia. The pattern may become established over time, and the patient is left with a recurrent, persistent insomnia. In time, they may become apprehensive as they lie down to sleep, fearing that the struggle to obtain sleep will commence again. The greater the effort expended in trying to sleep, the more elusive sleep becomes. Watching the clock as each minute and hour passes only increases the sense of urgency, further confounding efforts to sleep. The bed may eventually be viewed as a battleground, and sleep is achieved more easily in a less typical environment.

Some patients report an inability to fall asleep quickly because of physical discomfort as they lie down. Patients with Parkinson's disease may observe stiffness and an inability to roll over in bed; patients with RLS may report unusual sensations of tightness, tension, creeping, or tingling in their calf muscles that is relieved only by movement; pain from arthritis, neuropathy, or muscle injury may be enhanced at night.

Patients with poor sleep hygiene may complain of sleep-onset insomnia. Late-day napping, caffeine and nicotine intake, exercising in the hours immediately before bed, or late night meals may all be factors contributing to insomnia. Using the bedroom and bed to work, read, eat, or watch television may also interfere with the ability to fall asleep.

Circadian rhythm disorders may also present as sleep-onset insomnia.[57] Patients with irregular sleep hours, such as shift workers or international travelers, are continuously fighting their inherent circadian rhythms. In particular, travel in an eastward direction may provoke an inability to sleep at the desired times in the new time zone. Adolescents are often phase delayed or so-called "night owls," preferring a later bedtime and awakening time. In some individuals, this pattern may carry over into adulthood, causing significant problems with maintaining an acceptable job schedule. These patients may be incorrectly diagnosed with sleep-onset insomnia rather than phase-delayed sleep.

Insomnia may arise secondary to neurological or psychological disorders.[58–60] Patients with dementia may have difficulty falling asleep at night. In some, there may even be a reversal of the normal day-night sleep cycle so that the patient is awake and wandering about throughout the night hours and napping intermittently during the day. Certain psychiatric disorders, such as major depression or bipolar disorder, may be the cause of insomnia. Particularly in the acute manic or hypomanic phase of bipolar illness, there may be significant problems with sleep onset. Schizophrenic patients may also report sleep-onset insomnia.

Many drugs may interfere with sleep.[61] Some agents, such as stimulants and antiparkinsonian drugs, may be directly associated with insomnia. Other drugs may cause insomnia when they are discontinued. In particular, the discontinuation of chronic sedative-hypnotic treatment may cause severe rebound insomnia. Establishing the pattern of medication intake and the association of medications with the onset of insomnia is vital to considering this factor as the cause of insomnia.

Sleep fragmentation refers to an inability to maintain sleep over the night with frequent nocturnal awakenings and variable ability to fall back to sleep. Sleep may be disturbed by a variety of causes. Alcohol intake before bed, while promoting sleep onset, often causes disruption of sleep toward the end of the night. Primary sleep disorders may disrupt nocturnal sleep. PLMD may cause a patient to awaken without being aware of the cause. Sleep apnea, likewise, may cause sleep fragmentation in a patient who reports that initial sleep latency is short. A patient with sleep apnea may awaken with choking, or a sense of being unable to breathe. PSG is usually necessary to diagnose these causes of insomnia.

Medical and neurological conditions, including nocturia, cardiac disease, rheumatoid arthritis, fibromyalgia, and neuromuscular diseases may also cause sleep fragmentation. Sleep fragmentation is commonly seen with neurodegenerative disorders.

Insomnia may also present as early-morning awakening. Patients with this type of insomnia complain that they wake up for no reason at an early hour in the morning and are not able to reinitiate sleep. This type of insomnia is often seen in patients with major depression and is a frequent complaint of the elderly. In phase-advanced sleep, the major sleep period occurs early so that bedtime and final awakening occur before the desired times.

EXCESSIVE DAYTIME SOMNOLENCE

EDS indicates the occurrence of abnormal sleepiness during the normal waking hours.[62] EDS may be associated with inadequate nocturnal sleep and can be a component to a primary sleep disorder.[63] EDS can also occur independently of insomnia. Primary sleep disorders, such as sleep apnea and PLMD, may disrupt nocturnal sleep, leading to sleep deprivation and EDS. Often, patients with these disorders have frequent arousals punctuating the night but are unaware of these brief events and focus only on their susceptibility to falling asleep during the day. When the condition is mild, inadvertent napping may occur only with sedentary activities during the normal nadirs in daytime alertness in the afternoon or evening. As EDS becomes more severe, patients may report nodding off during active periods, such as driving a car or when conversing. Narcolepsy is also characterized by a propensity to sleep during the day. Sometimes, these periods may present as microsleeps in which there is a sudden but momentary lapse of consciousness. During these short periods, automatic behaviors may occur and observers may not realize that the patient is asleep. Sleep attacks, the unexpected, cataclysmic onset of sleep, are also seen. Patients with narcolepsy may experience REM sleep and report the occurrence of dreams during these daytime naps. EDS may be the sole clinical manifestation of narcolepsy in some patients, occurring without associated cataplexy, hallucinations, or sleep paralysis.

EDS may also indicate primary hypersomnia.[64] Idiopathic hypersomnia is a neurological disorder characterized by nocturnal sleep that is prolonged but not refreshing and an insatiable sleep need. Daytime naps may be long and unsatisfactory. Patients may sleep for periods of up to 20 hours a day. PSG shows a relatively normal sleep architecture compared with the more fragmented sleep seen in narcolepsy. The multiple sleep latency test demonstrates pathological sleepiness, but REM sleep does not occur during the two or more naps. Hypersomnia may also be caused by medical conditions such as viral infections, especially mononucleosis and encephalitis, or hydrocephalus. It is usually necessary to obtain a PSG in order to distinguish among the disorders leading to the EDS syndrome.

PARASOMNIAS

Parasomnia refers to a group of disorders that involve the intrusion of unwanted events or acts into sleep. A feature of many of the parasomnias is the occurrence of abnormal muscle activation behaviors occur during sleep. These behaviors may be associated with REM or NREM sleep. NREM parasomnias typically occur during Stages 3 and 4 of NREM sleep, therefore usually occurring during the first third of the night. NREM parasomnias are largely considered disorders of arousal. Somnambulism or sleepwalking, sleep terrors, and confusional arousals are commonly occurring parasomnias during SWS. Usually, these disorders affect children and adolescents, and resolve during adulthood. However, these disorders may carry over into adulthood or arise as side effects of various medications. Sleepwalking may result in significant sleep-related injuries because patients may walk through windows or fall down stairs during their nocturnal wanderings.

Sleep complaints that occur during the transition from wakefulness to sleep often affect otherwise healthy individuals and include sleep starts, sleep talking, and rhythmical movement disorders such as head banging, body rocking, and head rolling. The hallmark of this group of disorders is their occurrence at sleep onset, with some also occurring during wakefulness.

The parasomnias associated with REM sleep include nightmares, sleep paralysis, and RBD.[18] REM-related parasomnias are more likely to occur later in the night, when REM sleep predominates. RBD usually affects older men, in contrast to the other REM- and NREM-related parasomnias. RBD may occur as an idiopathic disorder or be related to neurological disorders with pathology involving brain stem nuclei. RBD is considered a primary disorder of REM sleep that parallels oneiric activity in animals following selective lesions of the pontine nuclei controlling motor atonia. Patients with narcolepsy, another disorder of REM sleep, may also show features of RBD.

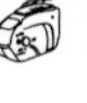

Sleep enuresis and bruxism are classified as parasomnias but are distinguished by their lack of complex-associated behaviors.

Additional sleep-related behavior disorders that may be confused with those described earlier include paroxysmal nocturnal dystonia and nocturnal epilepsy. These disorders appear as paroxysmal, stereotyped behaviors with sudden onset and resolution reflecting abnormal cortical activity rather than alterations in brain stem centers controlling REM sleep, or most commonly arising from NREM sleep.

CIRCADIAN RHYTHM DISORDERS

This group of disorders involves a disruption of the inherent circadian pattern of wakefulness and sleep.[40] Jet lag arises from transmeridian flights of long duration, usually through at least three time zones, and reflects the adaptation necessary to reset the internal rhythm to the day-night cycle of the destination. Jet lag is enhanced by the sleep deprivation that usually occurs before a prolonged trip, loss of sleep, and altered conditions during flight. Depending on the distance traveled, recovery may take 7 days or more, especially for eastward travel.

In contrast, shift workers are required to change their major sleep period without the reinforcement of external light-dark cycles and in the absence of social patterns that conform to their new sleep schedule. Following a single change in shift, 2 weeks may be needed for readjustment. However, often shift workers are required to change their schedules every 2 to 4 weeks, and frequently are progressively changed from night to afternoons to morning shifts. Thus, they may have a chronic desynchronization with their circadian clock.

Finally, there are so-called "natural night owls" and "morning larks" who are most comfortable with their major sleep period either later or earlier than can accommodate socially acceptable daytime activities, such as work or school.

Reviews and Selected Updates

Chokroverty S: Diagnosis and treatment of sleep disorders caused by co-morbid disease. Neurology 2000;54:S8–S15.

Czeisler CA, Duffy JF, Shanahan TL, et al: Stability, precision, and near-24-hour period of the human circadian pacemaker. Science 1999;284:2177–2181.

Dijk D-J, Edgar DM: Circadian and homeostatic control of wakefulness and sleep. *In* Turek FW, Zee PC (eds): Neurobiology of Sleep and Circadian Rhythms (series: Lung Biology in Health and Disease). New York, Marcel-Dekker, I, 1999, pp 111–147.

Kryger MH, Roth T, Dement WC: Principles and Practice of Sleep Medicine, 3rd ed. Philadelphia, WB Saunders, 2000.

Mahowald MW: Diagnostic testing. Sleep disorders. Neurol Clin 1996;14:183–200. Roth T, Roehrs T: Sleep organization and regulation. Neurology 2000;54(5 Suppl 1):S2–S7.

Silber MH: Sleep disorders. Neurol Clin 2001;19:173–186.

References

1. Aserinsky E, Kleitman N: Regularly occurring periods of eye motility and concomitant phenomena during sleep. Science 1953;118:273–274.
2. Carskadon MA, Dement WC: Normal human sleep: An overview. *In* Kryger MH, Roth T, Dement WC (eds): Principles and Practice of Sleep Medicine, 3nd ed. London, WB Saunders 2000, pp 15–25.
3. McCarley RW: Neurophysiology of sleep: Basic mechanisms underlying control of wakefulness and sleep. *In* Chokroverty S (ed): Sleep Disorders Medicine, 2nd ed. Boston, Butterworth-Heinemann 1999, pp 21–50.
4. Rechtschaffen A, Kales AA: A Manual of Standardized Terminology, Techniques and Scoring System for Sleep Stages of Human Subjects. Los Angeles, UCLA Brain Information Service/Brain Research Institute, 1968.
5. American Sleep Disorders Association: The International Classification of Sleep Disorders, revised: Diagnostic and Coding Manual. Rochester, Minnesota, American Sleep Disorders Association, 1997.
6. Chokroverty S: An approach to a patient with sleep complaints. *In* Chokroverty S (ed): Sleep Disorders Medicine, 2nd ed. Boston, Butterworth-Heinemann, 1999, pp 277–285.
7. Aldrich MS: Approach to the patient with disordered sleep. *In* Kryger MH, Roth T, Dement WC (eds): Principles and Practice of Sleep Medicine, 3rd ed. Philadelphia, WB Saunders, 2000, pp 521–525.
8. Carskadon MA: Patterns of sleep and sleepiness in adolescents. Pediatrician 1990;17:5–12.
9. Czeisler CA, Moore-Ede MC, Coleman RM: Rotating shift work schedules that disrupt sleep are improved by applying circadian principles. Science 1982;217:460–463.
10. Allen SR, Seiler WO, Stahelin HB, et al: 72-hour polygraphic and behavioral recordings of wakefulness and sleep in a hospital geriatric unit: Comparison between demented and non-demented patients. Sleep 1987;10:143–159.
11. Sadeh A, Hauri PJ, Kripke DF, Lavie P: The role of actigraphy in the evaluation of sleep disorders. Sleep 1995;18:288–302.
12. Buysse DJ, Reynolds CF, Monk TH, et al: The Pittsburgh sleep quality index: A new instrument for psychiatric practice and research. Psychiatry Res 1989;28:193–213.
13. Carskadon MA, Brown ED, Dement WC: Sleep fragmentation in the elderly: Relationship to daytime sleep tendency. Neurobiol Aging 1982;3:321–327.
14. Zarcone VP: Sleep hygiene. *In* Kryger MH, Roth T, Dement WC (eds): Principles and Practice of Sleep Medicine, 3rd ed. Philadelphia, WB Saunders, 2000, pp 657–661.
15. Oswald I: Sudden bodily jerks on falling asleep. Brain 1959;82:92–103.
16. Chokroverty S: Sleep, breathing, and neurological disorders. *In* Chokroverty S (ed): Sleep Disorders Medicine 2nd ed. Boston, Butterworth-Heinemann, 1999, pp 509–571.
17. Trenkwalder C, Walters AS, Hening WA: Periodic limb movements and restless legs syndrome. Neurol Clin 1996;14:629–650.
18. Olson EJ, Boeve BF, et al: Rapid eye movement sleep behaviour disorder: Demographic, clinical and laboratory findings in 93 cases. Brain 2000;123:331–339.
19. Overeem S, Mignot E, van Dijk JG, Lammers GJ: Narcolepsy: Clinical features, new pathologic insights, and future perspectives. J Clin Neurology 2001;18:78–105.
20. Ondo W, Jankovic J: Restless legs syndrome: Clinicoetiologic correlates. Neurology 1996;47:1435–1441.
21. Scheffer IE: Autosomal dominant nocturnal frontal lobe epilepsy. Epilepsia 2000;41:1059–1060.
22. Collins S, McLean CA, Masters CL: Gerstmann-Straussler-Scheinker syndrome, fatal familial insomnia, and kuru: A review of these less common human transmissible spongiform encephalopathies. J Clin Neuroscience 2001;8:387–397.
23. Bliwise DL: Sleep in normal aging and dementia. Sleep 1993;16:40–81.
24. Horne J: Why we sleep: The functions of sleep in humans and other mammals. New York, Oxford University Press, 1988.
25. Borbly AA, Baumann F, Brandeis D, et al: Sleep deprivation effects on sleep stages and EEG power density in man. Electroenceph Clin Neurophysiol 1981;51:483–493.
26. Moorcroft WH: Comments on the symposium and an attempt at synthesis. Behav Brain Res 1995;69:207–210.
27. Rechtschaffen A, Bergmann BM: Sleep deprivation in the rat by the disk-over-water method. Behav Brain Res 1995;69:55–63.
28. Horne JA, Reid AJ: Night-time sleep EEG changes following body heating in a warm bath. Electroencephalogr Clin Neurophysiol 1985; 60:154–157.
29. McGinty D, Szymusiak R: Keeping cool: A hypothesis about the mechanisms and functions of slow wave sleep. Trends Neurosci 1990; 13:480–487.
30. Finkelstein JW, Roffwarg HP, Boyar RM, et al: Age related change in twenty-four hour spontaneous secretion of growth hormone. J Clin Endocrinol Metab 1972;35:665–670.
31. Van Cauter E, Leproult R, Plat L: Age-related changes in slow wave sleep and REM sleep and relationship with growth hormone and cortisol levels in healthy men. JAMA 2000;284:861–868.
32. Spiegel K, Leproult R, Van Cauter E: .Impact of sleep debt on metabolic and endocrine function. Lancet 1999;354:1435–1439.
33. Giuditta A, Ambrosini MV, Montagnese P, et al: The sequential hypothesis of the function of sleep. Behav Brain Res 1995;69:157–166.
34. Krueger JM, Obál F Jr, Kapás L, Fang J: Brain organization and sleep function. Behav Brain Res 1995;69:177–185.
35. Miller JD, Morin LP, Schwartz WJ, Moore RY: New insights into the mammalian circadian clock. Sleep 1996;19:641–667.
36. Murphy PJ, Campbell SS: Physiology of the circadian system in animals and humans. J Clin Neurophysiol 1996;13:2–16.
37. Brzezinski A: Melatonin in humans. N Engl J Med 1997;336:186–195.
38. Jankel WR, Niedermeyer E: Sleep spindles. J Clin Neurophysiol 1985;2:1–35.
39. Siegel JM: Brainstem mechanisms generating REM sleep. *In* Kryger MH, Roth T, Dement WC (eds): Principles and Practice of Sleep Medicine, 2nd ed. Philadelphia, WB Saunders, 1994, pp 125–144.
40. Culebras A: Update on disorders of sleep and the sleep-wake cycle. Psychiatric Clin North Am 1992;15:467–489.
41. Jones BE: Paradoxical sleep and its chemical structural substrates in the brain. Neuroscience 1991;40:637–656.
42. Hobson JA, Lydic R, Baghdoyan HA: Evolving concepts of sleep cycle generation: From brain centers to neuronal populations. Behav Brain Sci 1986;9:371–448.

43. Garcia-Rill E: The pedunculopontine nucleus. Prog Neurobiol 1991;36:363–389.
44. Cartwright RD: Dreams and their meaning. *In* Kryger MH, Roth T, Dement WC (eds): Principles and Practice of Sleep Medicine. London, WB Saunders, 1994, pp 400–406.
45. Peyron C, Tighe DK, van den Pol AN, et al: Neurons containing hypocretin (orexin) project to multiple neuronal systems. J Neuroscience 1998;18:9996–10015.
46. Lin L, Faraco J, Li R, et al: The sleep disorder canine narcolepsy is caused by a mutation in the hypocretin (orexin) receptor 2 gene. Cell 1999;98:365–376.
47. Chemelli RM, Willie JR, Sinton CM: Narcolepsy in orexin knockout mice: Molecular genetics of sleep regulation. Cell 1999;98:409–412.
48. Nishino S, Ripley B, Overeem S, et al: Hypocretin (orexin) deficiency in human narcolepsy. Lancet 2000;355:39–40.
49. Thannickal TC, Moore RY, Nienhuis R, et al: Reduced number of hypocretin neurons in human narcolepsy. Neuron 2000;27:469–474.
50. American Sleep Disorders Association Report: Practice parameters for the use of actigraphy in the clinical assessment of sleep disorders. Sleep 1995;18:285–287.
51. American Sleep Disorders Association: The clinical use of the multiple sleep latency test. Sleep 1992;15:268–276.
52. Standards of Practice Committee of the American Sleep Disorders Association: Practice Parameters for the use of portable recording in the assessment of obstructive sleep apnea. Sleep 1994;17:372–377.
53. Hauri P: Case Studies in Insomnia. New York, Plenum Medical Book Company, 1991.
54. Alberto J, Silva CE, Chase M, et al: Special report from a symposium held by the World Health Organization and the World Federation of Sleep Research Societies: An overview of insomnias and related disorders-recognition, epidemiology and rational management. Sleep 1996; 19:412–416.
55. Edinger JD, Fins AI, Goeke JM, et al: The empirical identification of insomnia subtypes: A cluster analytic approach. Sleep 1996;19:398–411.
56. Spielman AJ, Nunes J, Glovinsky PB: Insomnia. Neurol Clin 1996;14:513–543.
57. Regestein QR, Monk TH: Delayed sleep phase syndrome: A review of its clinical aspects. Am J Psychiatry 1995;152:602–608.
58. Thase ME, Kupfer DJ, Ulrich RF: Electroencephalographic sleep in psychotic depression. Arch Gen Psychiatry 1986;43:886–893.
59. Hudson JI, Lipinski JF, Frandenburg FR, et al: Electroencephalographic sleep in mania. Arch Gen Psychiatry 1988;45:267–273.
60. Gierz M, Campbell SS, Giullin JC: Sleep disturbances in various nonaffective psychiatric disorders. Psychiatric Clin North Am 1987; 10:565–581.
61. Novak M, Shapiro CM: Drug-induced sleep disturbances. Focus on nonpsychotropic medications. Drug Saf 1997;16:133–149.
62. Lavie P: The touch of Morpheus: Pre-20th century accounts of sleepy patients. Neurology 1991;41:1841–1844.
63. Guilleminault C: Disorders of excessive sleepiness. Ann Clin Res 1985;17:209–219.
64. Guilleminault C, Pelayo R: Idiopathic central nervous system hypersomnia. *In* Kryger MH, Roth T, Dement WC (eds): Principles and Practice of Sleep Medicine, 3rd ed. Philadelphia, WB Saunders, 2000, pp 687–692.

CHAPTER 3

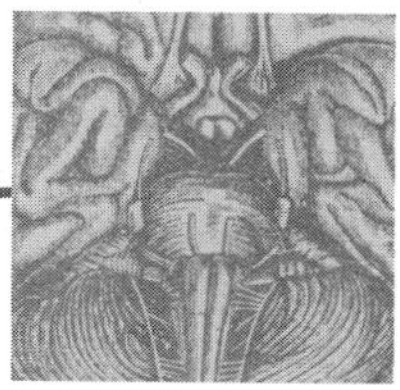

JOSEPH H. FRIEDMAN

Mood, Emotion, and Thought

History and Definitions

Mood is the term used to describe a sustained internal emotion and is to be distinguished from affect, which is more fluid, possibly changing from moment to moment.[1] The spectrum of moods is enormous, and each different mood is colored in a multitude of gradations and shades. The most obvious moods are sadness, joy, grief, and anger. The presence of one mood, of course, does not preclude the simultaneous presence of another. Sadness and anger, even opposite moods such as happiness and sadness, frequently coexist. *Affect* generally refers to the external expression of emotional content and may coincide or be at odds with a patient's mood. The terms *mood congruent* and *mood incongruent* are used to describe these forms of emotional or affective expressions. Two basic mood abnormalities, depression and mania, are recognized, and these occur on a continuum from normal to the clearly pathological. While minor symptoms may be an extension of normal sadness or elation, more severe symptoms are associated with discrete syndromes (affective disorders) that appear to differ qualitatively from normal processes. *Depression* is defined as a morbid sadness, dejection, or melancholy, whereas *mania* is a disordered mental state of extreme excitement. Both have accompanying emotional and cognitive and motoric features.

Emotional experience connotes the whole range of human feelings, including anxiety, fear, apathy, euphoria, depression, sadness, anger, and grief, as well as how the person experiences these various feelings, which are not mutually exclusive. Thus, most individuals constantly experience a wide variety of feelings of variable intensities that vary over time. *Emotional expression*, or affect, may be mood congruent, accurately reflecting the person's inner state, or incongruent, when the subject appears to be very happy or sad but in fact feels quite the opposite. Emotional expression has an enormous range, which is obviously wider in some people than in others. This range may be normal, expanded, or *restricted*, allowing little chance for either happy or sad emotions to be displayed. When expansive, emotional expression is amplified at both ends of the mood spectrum. *Flattened* affect is a lack of emotional display, and *labile* affect is an emotional state that changes rapidly and is out of proportion to changes in the situation. It is important to note that emotional experience and emotional expression are quite different. One can appear to be emotionally detached and have little concern or interest in the situation, when in fact one is greatly moved. Such a discordance between apparent and true emotion may be highly adaptive in some situations and cultures and not at all pathological.

Other terms involved in disorders of emotion and mood include *apathy*, which is a lack of feeling or indifference.[2] *Abulia* is a general behavioral slowing and lowered activity that may be associated with an inability or refusal to speak. *Akinetic mutism* is defined as a condition in which the patient appears awake and may follow the examiner with his or her eyes but lacks spontaneous motor and verbal responses. *Anxiety* is an uncomfortable and unjustified sense of apprehension that may be diffuse and unfocused and is often accompanied by physiological symptoms. An *anxiety disorder* connotes significant distress and dysfunction due to the anxiety. *Fear* can also produce the symptoms of anxiety, but, in contrast to anxiety, its cause is obvious and understandable.

Thought is in many ways unrelated to mood or emotions. Thought is evaluated in terms of the "process" or mechanics of thinking and also in terms of the content. In schizophrenia, one deals with "loosened" thought processes. *Psychosis* is a broad term defined variably in different places, but generally it implies a severe mental illness characterized by a loss of contact with reality leading to severe impairments in personal and social functioning. Psychosis is distinguished from delirium, in which there is an impairment of consciousness associated with an organic cause. Distinguishing these two syndromes may be difficult but is extremely important. Delirium usually has a more abrupt onset and a course that fluctuates more widely and more quickly than psychosis. Delirious patients are usually disoriented with significant attentional problems.

Hallucinations, hallucinosis, illusions, and delusions are terms that are frequently misused, leading to incorrect diagnoses, particularly by nonpsychiatrists. *Hallucinations* are false sensations that arise without a stimulus. Visual hallucinations appear real and are seen clearly in the light. They may be unformed like geometric shapes, or formed, simulating people, animals, or objects. Auditory hallucinations are sounds, such as voices or music, that are indistinguishable from real sounds. *Hallucinosis* refers to the presence of hallucinations in an otherwise normal mental state, without confusion, disorientation, or psychosis. Generally, hallucinations are experienced as real, whereas in hallucinosis the sensations are quickly interpreted as false. Hallucinations occur in every sensory realm, so that smells, taste, tactile sensations, and so on, may all occur. *Illusion* refers to an altered or misperceived sensation that is transformed, such as perceiving a lamp as a person. *Delusion* refers to a false and irrational belief that is unalterable by rational discourse. Typical delusions may include grandiosity, in which the patient believes he or she has great powers, or paranoia, in which the patient believes he or she is being followed. Hallucinations and delusions occur in a wide variety of psychoses including manic-depression and organic states.

Hallucinations and delusions are considered *positive symptoms*, meaning that they are extra or additional features superimposed upon normal behavior. This concept was pioneered by Hughlings Jackson, who considered positive symptoms a "release" phenomenon, in which inhibitory control is lost.[3] Other positive symptoms include bizarre behavior, pressured speech, and thought disorder. In contrast, *negative symptoms* refer to loss of affect, diminished thought, anhedonia (diminished interest and enjoyment), and diminished attention. Jackson attributed negative symptoms to a loss of neurons leading to a direct loss of function.[3]

Obsessive thoughts are unwanted and bothersome recurrent ideas, images, and impulses that intrude upon a patient and cannot be pushed out of consciousness. A *compulsion* is an irresistible need to perform an activity. Obsessions and compulsions usually go together. *Rituals* are a sequence of stereotyped behaviors that must be performed and often have a symbolic meaning.

Clinical History

The basic structure of the history and examination for a mood, emotion, or thought disorder is no different from that used for any medical or neurological problem. The only variation lies in how the history is obtained and how the patient answers questions and relays the clinical information. The process of response may therefore be even more important than the content of the historical details themselves. Another difference is that historical data, in a patient with a disorder of mood, emotion, or thought, often need corroboration or explication by third parties. The examiner should also obtain information about the premorbid state of the patient, including his or her development and environment, as important background on which to view the patient's current state. Personality changes are crucial indicators of mood and should be sought from family members. Progressive irritability or social withdrawal may be markers of depression, whereas new gregariousness and socializing may reflect a "decline" into mania. Finally, the time frame of the behavioral changes determines whether the event is acute, subacute, or chronic.

The presence of certain features typical of mood, emotion, or thought disorders must be pursued in a manner similar to that used for historical evaluation for any neurological or medical condition. Important details are evaluated so that pertinent positive and negative elements of the history supporting a diagnosis can be supplied. The clinician should know the symptoms of the illnesses considered in the differential diagnosis so that he or she can be sure that all pertinent questions have been asked. The history for a person with an affective illness must take into account both the mood state itself and the multiple somatic manifestations of mood disorders. Important questions about both depression and mania must be asked.

Depression is often associated with vegetative symptoms including disturbances of sleep and appetite, and loss of interest or pleasure in almost everything. Depressed people may state that they sleep excessively or insufficiently. They may note a loss of appetite or weight, or eat excessively. Because most depressed people lose energy and develop easy and excessive fatigue, these symptoms should be inquired about. Although some depressed patients become agitated, as if they were manic, most generally do not apply this energy in useful, purposeful activities. Patients may note that their thinking ability and attention span are reduced and that their decision-making capability has plummeted. The patient may exhibit low self-esteem and feelings of guilt and may be absorbed by thoughts of death. The depressed mood may not be perceived by the patient or even by associates and may be manifested only by irritability. A sexual history is important because sexual drive may be markedly decreased as well.

Special care must be taken in the particular situation of a potentially suicidal patient, and the topic should be addressed forthrightly. Depressed patients should always be questioned about their potential for suicide. A history of suicide attempts, a family history of suicide, a suicide note, and a history of impulsive behavior are all significant risk factors.

When mania is encountered, the patient or family may note that the patient's need for sleep has declined and that the sleep schedule has changed dramatically. There may be a history of going without sleep for a few days and impaired judgment. This impaired judgment may have led to the undertaking of huge projects based on an inflated belief in one's own power to control the outcome. The history may include details about money because large amounts may have been spent. Excessive or inappropriate sexual activity is also common.

When a patient has apathy or abulia, there is a near complete loss of feeling, initiative, movement, and thought. Very little historical information can be obtained directly from the patient, and the physician will have to rely on other family members or caretakers. In contrast, patients with anxiety and anxiety disorders often describe feelings of tension, irritability, or apprehension and may be mildly distractible during the interview. The presence of concomitant autonomic symptoms should be inquired about, including palpitations, diarrhea, cold clammy extremities, sweating, urinary frequency, insomnia, fatigue, and trembling.

Patients with psychotic disorders have a history of a grossly impaired sense of reality, often coupled with emotional disabilities. The violence-prone patient must be assessed in a safe situation, and the potential for violence should be openly acknowledged. Questions should be asked about previous episodes and the reason for the current violent outburst or threat. The interview situation must be stable and under control, with security personnel present, if necessary. During the interview, the patient may talk and act in a bizarre fashion, demonstrate delusions, or have illusions and hallucinations. During the conversation, the interviewer should note disturbances of both thought form and content. Abnormalities of thought include a loosening of associations with tangential topics of conversation. The flow of thoughts does not follow the usual orderly sequence that leads from one idea to another. Rather, it takes peculiar leaps that are difficult for listeners to follow both because the sequence is idiosyncratic and because the expressed thoughts may appear unrelated to the preceding thoughts. In addition, the content of thoughts may be bizarre. The patient may disrupt the flow of thoughts by including irrelevant information. New words, or neologisms, may be used that have no meaning. Disturbances of thought content, or delusions, may be bizarre, persecutory, or of grandeur. The patient may state that he or she believes he or she can control events through telepathy or may be convinced that there are "meanings" behind events and people's actions directed toward him or her.

Illusions are typically visual but may also be auditory or tactile. With visual illusions, the patient or family may note that the person may look at an object or person and see something other than what is actually there. The examiner should give specific examples, such as looking at a coat hanging in the closet or a light pole or lamp and perceiving a person, or looking at a bush and perceiving an animal. Similar examples involving sounds and tactile stimulation should be inquired about. Hallucinations should also be inquired about, and all sensory modalities should be investigated. Hallucinations may be unformed shapes or colors or formed images of people, animals, and objects. The images may be familiar or unfamiliar and may include relatives or friends who are living or dead, children, babies, or lilliputian figures. Threatening or frightening hallucinations may also occur and should be inquired about. The nature of the hallucinations may be relatively stereotypic for individual disorders. All primary nondementing psychotic disorders that include hallucinations feature auditory rather than visual hallucinations. These are mood congruent, meaning that the content reflects the emotional state of the patient. Drug-induced hallucinations are generally visual and are often without emotional content. It should also be noted that sensory deprivation, blindness in particular, may produce non-emotion-laden hallucinations in the impaired sensory modality. Visual hallucinations are also common in Lewy body dementia.

In the investigation of obsessive-compulsive behavior, the examiner should ask whether the patient experiences repeated images or ideas that are intrusive. Patients may note that these thoughts are unwanted, distressing, and occasionally frightening or violent, and that they are powerless to stop them. The examiner should ask whether the patient ruminates endlessly on certain thoughts such as whether the patient locked the door or performed other activities. The existence of rituals or compulsions should be sought. Patients should be asked if they must count, touch, or clean something to ward off unwanted happenings or to satisfy an obsession. These activities may consume a patient's whole day, rendering him or her unable to complete any necessary task.

Patients with impulse dyscontrol or aggression may not offer any complaints, yet family members may relate a detailed account. The spouse or relatives may note the patient's impulsiveness in everyday activities and an inability to resist performing inappropriate activities both at home and in public. The clinician should inquire about the use of both inappropriate words and physical actions. Additionally, family members should be asked about the presence of sudden outbursts or episodes of rage involving destructive behavior to property, abusive actions involving others, or self-mutilation. The patient's emotional response to his acts of destruction or aggression and his memory of the events may be very helpful in making a diagnosis.

In all settings of disorders of mood, emotion, and thought, a complete drug history is essential to uncover possible organic precipitants of behavioral changes. A medical and neurological review of systems is also crucial. Various medical conditions such as infections and endocrinopathies may present with disorders of mood, emotion, and thought, and other physical findings associated with these disorders may be helpful in arriving at the correct diagnosis. Neurologically, patients should be asked whether they have experienced asymmetrical weakness, numbness, memory problems, dysgeusia, or seizure activity, which may indicate a structural, metabolic, or infectious cause of the presentation. Finally, a family history provides important diagnostic information, since certain mental illnesses, including affective disorders, tend to be hereditary.

Anatomy of Mood, Emotion, and Thought

The neuroanatomic structures related to human mood, emotion, and thought function are complex, and research in this area is still under development. The association of various brain regions with particular functions is based primarily on studies of lesions and, more recently, on functional neuroimaging. Although generalizations based on these isolated cases are somewhat precarious, extended observations based on series of cases are somewhat more reliable. Additionally, although the findings of animal studies are highly reproducible, they do not necessarily apply to human behavior.[4] Early experiments on dogs and other animals demonstrated that decortication produced rage behavior when the animal was presented with previously nonthreatening stimuli. Later work in cats showed the importance of an intact diencephalon (thalamus and hypothalamus) in eliciting this response. If these lower structures were also damaged, strong emotional displays were not elicited. Other experiments on the hypothalamus of the cat demonstrated that when certain areas were stimulated, marked behavioral alterations were produced, including not only behavioral displays but also concomitant physiological changes appropriate to the behavior. For example, the cat displayed piloerection and hissing and baring of teeth with associated elevations of blood pressure, heart rate, and respiration.

Primary alterations in mood, emotion, and thought in humans have also been associated with abnormalities in certain regions of the brain and have primarily focused on the "limbic system" and on the temporal lobe and the frontal lobes.

LIMBIC SYSTEM

The term limbic lobe was coined by Broca in 1878 to describe a series of structures that envelop the brain stem. The word limbic is derived from limbus, meaning border in Latin,[5] and the limbic system encompasses the amygdala, hippocampus, septum, cingulate gyrus, cingulate cortex, hypothalamus, epithalamus, anterior thalamus, mammillary bodies, and fornix. The limbic system has rich connections throughout the brain, particularly with the primary sensory cortices, including the rhinencephalon for smell, the autonomic nervous system via the hypothalamus, and memory areas. The medial tip of the subthalamic nucleus may be included in the limbic system as well. Electrical stimulation of this nucleus for the treatment of Parkinson's disease has, on rare occasion, produced a joyous mood with nonpathological laughter. Early reports on strokes in the subthalamic nucleus described both hemiballismus and emotional changes.[6] Papez, in 1937, was the first to use clinical information obtained from patients with brain tumors in support of his proposed limbic mechanism of emotion and memory. Since that time, others have reported a correlation of abnormalities of this region with disorders of emotion, mood, and thought.

Starkstein and colleagues studied 11 patients with manic syndromes associated with brain injuries and demonstrated that secondary mania correlated with the presence of either anterior subcortical atrophy or a focal lesion of a limbic or limbic-connected region of the right hemisphere.[7] Follow-up studies of additional patients along with analysis of other cases of secondary mania from the literature indicated that the causative brain lesions were located mainly in limbic and limbic-related areas that have connections with the frontal lobes.[8, 9] More recently, positron-emission tomography (PET) studies performed on subjects experiencing transient sadness with recall of unhappy memories showed bilateral activation of paralimbic structures, whereas happy memories were associated with a widespread reduction in cortical cerebral blood flow.

Mega and colleagues[10] describe two main divisions of the limbic system, an orbitofrontal amygdala division involved in emotional associations and appetites, and a hippocampal cingulate division serving mnemonic and attentional activities.

The limbic system has also been implicated in such thought disorders as schizophrenia. In one study reporting magnetic resonance imaging (MRI) and cerebral blood flow studies in twins who were discordant for schizophrenia, the hippocampal area of nearly all affected individuals was smaller. Additionally, a number of well-controlled observations of postmortem brain samples of schizophrenics revealed a decrease in the size of the region including the amygdala, the hippocampus, and the parahippocampal gyrus.

Amygdala

The amygdala, a core part of the limbic system, has been the focus of particular research attention in the evaluation of mood and emotion. This structure, named for its almond shape, sits medially in the anterior temporal lobe above the hippocampal formation. It consists of two main nuclear regions and about a dozen individual nuclei, each with distinct cytological and histochemical features. The amygdala is in contact with the tail of the caudate nucleus, but it is dissimilar from this region from both structural and evolutionary viewpoints. Afferent inputs to the amygdala are varied and include projections from the olfactory cortex, hypothalamus, and thalamus. The two major efferent projections from the amygdala are the stria terminalis and the ventral amygdalofugal pathway. The former supplies the hypothalamus, the nucleus accumbens, and the bed nucleus of the stria terminalis. The latter projects to the hypothalamus, dorsal medial nucleus of the thalamus, and the cingulate gyrus. The amygdala also projects in a reciprocal fashion to brain stem nuclei involved in the autonomic changes that accompany fear and stress-related responses. Projections to somatosensory cortex and most of the temporal lobe have also been demonstrated.

The connections between the amygdala and the hypothalamus and visceral brain stem nuclei explain the complex physiological responses that occur with mood changes in general, specifically fear and the "fight or flight" response. Stimulation experiments in animals produce a variety of autonomic responses. The most common response is an accelerated respiratory rate with shallow breathing associated with increases or decreases in blood pressure and pulse. Gastric motility may increase or decrease, and urination as well as defecation may be induced. Piloerection, pupillary changes, salivation, and altered body temperature may also occur. These autonomic changes may result from sympathetic or parasympathetic systems. The amygdala is additionally implicated in modulation of the hypothalamic control over food intake. Lesions of the basolateral nucleus of the amygdala or bilateral destruction of the amygdala induces hyperphagia. Stimulation of the basolateral nucleus causes decreased appetite and arrest of feeding behavior.

In 1939, Kluver and Bucy described primates with bilateral anterior temporal lobectomies, including removal of the uncus, amygdala, and part of the hippocampus.[11] These animals became tame, and they lost the responses of fear and aggression. They mouthed all objects, regardless of how familiar or inappropriate, and they ate everything, including nonfood items. Sexual behavior increased dramatically for appropriate and inappropriate targets, and self-stimulation also occurred. A visual agnosia combined with an inability to screen out unimportant visual stimuli caused the animals to react to all stimuli in their visual field. Subsequent studies revealed that damage to the amygdala was the most important source of these behaviors. These data suggest that the amygdala gives sensory stimuli affective and motivational significance. In other experimental models, aggression has been provoked by stimulation of the amygdala, hypothalamus, and fornix and inhibited by stimulation of the frontal lobes.

Amygdala damage in humans usually occurs in patients undergoing elective surgery for controlling epilepsy, and in such cases these regions are presumed to be abnormal before ablation. Decreased aggression, increased placidity, or no emotional changes result.[12] In one case of amygdalectomy, the patient lost the ability to interpret facial emotions as well as the emotions conveyed by the nonverbal aspects of speech. In contrast, amygdala stimulation in humans has produced fear, confusion, amnesia, and altered awareness.

Temporal Lobe

Emotional attributes have also been associated with temporal lobe abnormalities in humans, even when the nature, localization, and extent of the abnormalities have been unknown. Most of these data involve epileptics with known seizure foci of the temporal lobe. Researchers have posited that patients with temporal lobe epilepsy who have not undergone surgery may have a "temporal lobe personality." In such studies, patients with right temporal lobe abnormalities have been thought to be more introspective and "obsessive," and those with left temporal lobe defects have been said to be extroverted and often concerned with "personal destiny."[13] Additional features perceived to be more common in temporal lobe epileptics than in normal controls include emotionality (more intense and sustained emotional response), euphoria, sadness, anger, guilt, hypermoralism, religiosity, hypergraphia, and passivity. These studies have been criticized on methodological grounds but suggest that emotionality, mood, and thought processes involve temporal lobe function albeit in complicated and still poorly understood ways.

Various reviews and long-term follow-up studies of patients with epilepsy who have undergone temporal lobectomies have led to several conclusions about the temporal lobe and psychotic behavior. Most reports suggest that when psychosis is present preoperatively, no improvement is demonstrated following the operation. In fact, psychosis may actually develop postoperatively, especially when the surgery involves the right temporal lobe. Postoperative depression and both early and late suicide are also reported as possible complications of temporal lobectomy. Improvement, however, may occur in other behaviors, particularly excessive aggression, irritability, and social misconduct.

FRONTAL CORTEX

Mood, emotions, and thought also involve structures outside the limbic system, and the frontal lobes in particular have a major role. The famous 1868 case of Phineas Gage, in which the subject survived an explosion in which a metal bar 3 cm wide by 1 meter long went through his left frontal lobe but then demonstrated a marked alteration in personality, clearly indicated the importance of the frontal lobe in behavior.

"The frontal lobes serve as the 'senior executive' of the brain and personality, acting to process, integrate, inhibit, assimilate, and remember perceptions and impulses received from the limbic system, striatum, and neocortical sensory receiving areas."[14] The frontal cortex of interest can be divided into three major domains: precentral, prefrontal, and limbic. The precentral cortex is composed primarily of the motor strip and premotor cortex. Further anterior is the prefrontal cortex, which is the largest region of the frontal lobe and includes the anterior pole. The prefrontal cortex may be further divided into mesial, dorsal, and orbital parts. The orbitofrontal region of the cortex is one of the main limbic efferent channels to the hypothalamic-hypophysial complex and the visceral motor system. The prefrontal cortex has connections with the association, premotor, and limbic cortices as well as with the amygdala, hippocampus, and dorsomedial thalamic nuclei. Although the prefrontal cortex projects to the striatum, it does not receive reciprocal fibers from this structure. Lichter and Cummings have proposed three major circuits connecting the frontal lobes with the subcortical structures, providing a framework for understanding the role of the frontal lobes in behavioral disorders. Based on analyses of lesions, the dorsolateral prefrontal-subcortical circuit appears to be involved with executive function (see Chapter 5). This type of function includes the process of supervising other brain functions related to developing and implementing a plan. The orbitofrontal-subcortical circuit is necessary for social behaviors and inhibition of inappropriate activities, and lesions of this area have been associated with obsessive-compulsive disorders. Finally, the medial frontal-subcortical circuit is involved with motivation; consequently, lesions of this region have been associated with apathy syndromes.

Lesions of the frontal lobe may cause different behavioral syndromes depending on their location and size. Bilateral disturbances of the frontal lobes, particularly slowly developing abnormalities such as tumors, can cause significant intellectual and affective decline that simulates the signs of Alzheimer's disease or other dementing disorders. Bilateral ventromedial frontal lobe damage produces inappropriate, uncontrolled histrionic displays of affect, with laughing or crying fits that are not precipitated by obvious stimuli and are unrelated to the subject's mood.[14] More commonly, frontal lobe lesions in humans cause a dulling or shallowness of response or a lability of mood, classically termed witzelsucht. This term refers to the inappropriate jocularity and facetiousness seen with such disorders. The humor is quite changeable, and the affect may be labile. There is a loss of pleasure but no depressed affect, as seen in patients with affective disorders. Increased volatility, especially in patients with orbital lesions, has led to hypotheses that dysfunction of the frontal-orbital cortex may be involved in mania, especially when the right hemisphere is involved.

Other focal lesions of the frontal cortex have also been associated with mood and emotion abnormalities. In a selected group of right-handed patients with a single stroke lesion in either the right or left hemisphere and no previous psychiatric history, Robinson and associates found that the severity of depression in these patients was significantly increased in those with left anterior lesions as opposed to any other location.[15] Additionally, the severity of depression correlated significantly with the proximity of the lesion to the frontal pole in the left anterior group. Patients with a right hemisphere lesion showed the reverse. Lesion analysis in post-stroke patients indicates that lesions of the left cortico-striato-pallido-thalamic-cortical circuits are most involved in depression unrelated to severity of the neurologic deficit.[16] These findings suggest that the location of the intrahemisphere lesion is in some way related to mood disorders in stroke patients, and the neuroanatomy of the biogenic amine-containing pathways in the cortex might explain the graded effect.

In the presence of frontal lobe dysfunction, patients are often impulsive and have little insight into their difficulties. They are also characterized by a lack of originality and creativity, an inability to focus attention, recent memory problems, and a tendency to display inappropriate emotional reactions (disinhibitions).[14, 16]

Investigations of patients with thought disorders such as schizophrenia have also consistently shown frontal lobe dysfunction. Morphological and imaging studies in these patients have shown other abnormalities including ventricular enlargement with atrophy involving the amygdala, parahippocampal gyrus, and superior temporal gyrus.[17] Single-photon emission computed tomography (SPECT) and PET have further revealed the presence of low metabolic rates in medial frontal regions[18] and in the dorsolateral prefrontal cortex.[19] MRI has revealed portions of the brain involved when patients are hallucinating during their scan.

SUBCORTICAL STRUCTURES

Mood and affective changes are seen in patients with subcortical dementia syndromes resulting from a disconnection between the frontal lobes and the basal ganglia. Behavior has been investigated in patients with certain specific disorders including Parkinson's disease, progressive supranuclear palsy (PSP), and Huntington's disease.[20] In each, the pathology has been located primarily in the basal ganglia, and all patients have had associated disorders of affect and cognition. Patients with Parkinson's disease or PSP are often depressed or apathetic and may develop delusions and hallucinations with drug therapy. These patients, particularly those with PSP, may demonstrate a pathological affect known as pseudobulbar affect, whereby they intermittently exhibit primary emotional displays in response to trivial stimuli. This situation is also seen in any condition causing bilateral lesions involving the bulbar regions of the neocortical motor system or its descending connections. Patients with Huntington's disease also become depressed, impulsive, and often psychotic. The clinicopathological correlation is complicated by the fact that our understanding of the pathology of each of these disorders is still incomplete, and cortex is not spared in these disorders. Other investigators have shown that secondary mania is associated with subcortical lesions of the white matter of the right frontal lobe, the right anterior limb of the internal capsule, and the right head of the caudate.

Recently, investigators have become interested in the role of the cerebellum in nonmotor function, including mood and executive function.[21] A syndrome of mutism and behavioral disturbances has been reported in some children after cerebellar resections, and several case reports have described "cortical type" behavioral disturbances resulting from purely cerebellar lesions.[22]

PHARMACOLOGICAL NEUROANATOMY

A number of neurotransmitters, specifically the catecholamines (norepinephrine and dopamine) and serotonin, are closely related to mood, emotion, and thought disorders.[23] Catecholamines are formed in brain, chromaffin cells, sympathetic nerves, and sympathetic ganglia from tyrosine, their amino acid precursor (Fig. 3–1). Tyrosine is taken up from the bloodstream and concentrated within the brain and other sympathetically innervated tissue via active transport. In the brain, tyrosine undergoes a series of chemical transformations, resulting in the formation of norepinephrine and dopamine. The conversion of tyrosine to dihydroxyphenylalanine (dopa), the first and rate-limiting step in this process, is controlled by tyrosine hydroxylase. This enzyme is stereospecific and requires molecular O_2, Fe^{2+}, and tetrahydropteridine as cofactors. The second enzyme involved in catecholamine biosynthesis is dopa decarboxylase, which requires pyridoxal phosphate (vitamin B_6) as a cofactor and converts dopa to dopamine. Dopamine-beta-hydroxylase utilizes molecular oxygen in the presence of ascorbic acid to convert dopamine to norepinephrine. In the adrenal medulla, norepinephrine can be further *N*-methylated by the enzyme phenylethanolamine-*N*-methyl transferase, forming epinephrine. Although it is largely restricted to the adrenal medulla, low levels of this enzyme have been noted in the mammalian brain.

The degree of sympathetic activity does not influence endogenous levels of norepinephrine. Studies have demonstrated that accelerated norepinephrine biosynthesis secondary to enhanced sympathetic activity is due to an increase in the activity of existing tyrosine hydroxylase and is not the result of increased enzyme synthesis. Tyrosine hydroxylase is inhibited by catechols and catecholamines, presumably within the neuron. When increased impulse flow causes more transmitter to be released and metabolized, the levels of intraneuronal norepinephrine are reduced, resulting in increased activity of tyrosine hydroxylase. More recently, several experiments have demonstrated that electrical stimulation of both central and peripheral catecholamine neurons results in an allosteric activation of tyrosine hydroxylase that persists following termination of the stimulation. This suggests that short-term mechanisms in addition to depletion of catecholamines are operative in altering tyrosine hydroxylase

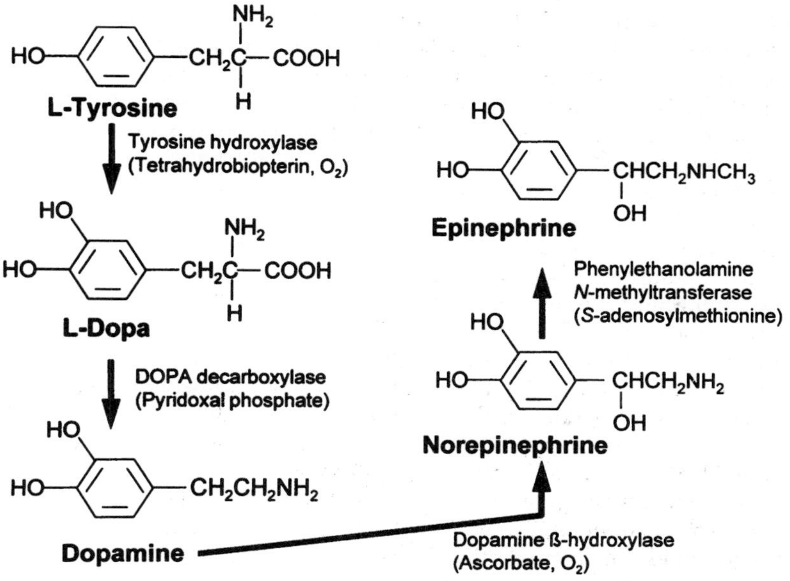

FIGURE 3–1. Catecholamine biosynthetic pathway. (Reproduced with permission from Siegel GJ, Agranoff BW, Albers RW, Molinoff PB: Basic Neurochemistry, 5th ed. New York, Raven Press, 1994.)

activity during increased neuronal activity. After prolonged increases in activity of catecholaminergic neurons, tyrosine hydroxylase formation is induced; however, this process appears to be nonspecific and also results in increased levels of dopamine-beta-hydroxylase levels.

Most norepinephrine is located within highly specialized subcellular particles, or granules, in sympathetic nerve endings of the central nervous system (CNS). Adenosine triphosphate likewise is contained in the granules. These vesicles serve as a depot for dopamine and oxidize this transmitter to norepinephrine. By storing the transmitters, the vesicles retard their diffusion out of the neuron and protect them from destruction by intraneuronal monoamine oxidase (MAO). The release of catecholamines can be influenced by direct local action at nerve terminals by catecholamines themselves as well as by prostaglandins, vasoactive amines, angiotensin II, acetylcholine, and polypeptides. Beta-2-adrenoceptors are believed to facilitate the release of norepinephrine, possibly by stimulation of adenylate cyclase, which leads to increased levels of cyclic adenosine monophosphate, followed by rises in intracellular Ca^{2+} concentrations.

The major enzymes involved in the metabolic degradation of catecholamines are MAO and catechol-O-methyl transferase (COMT) (Fig. 3–2). Monoamine oxidase converts catecholamines to their corresponding aldehydes, which are then rapidly metabolized, generally through oxidation by

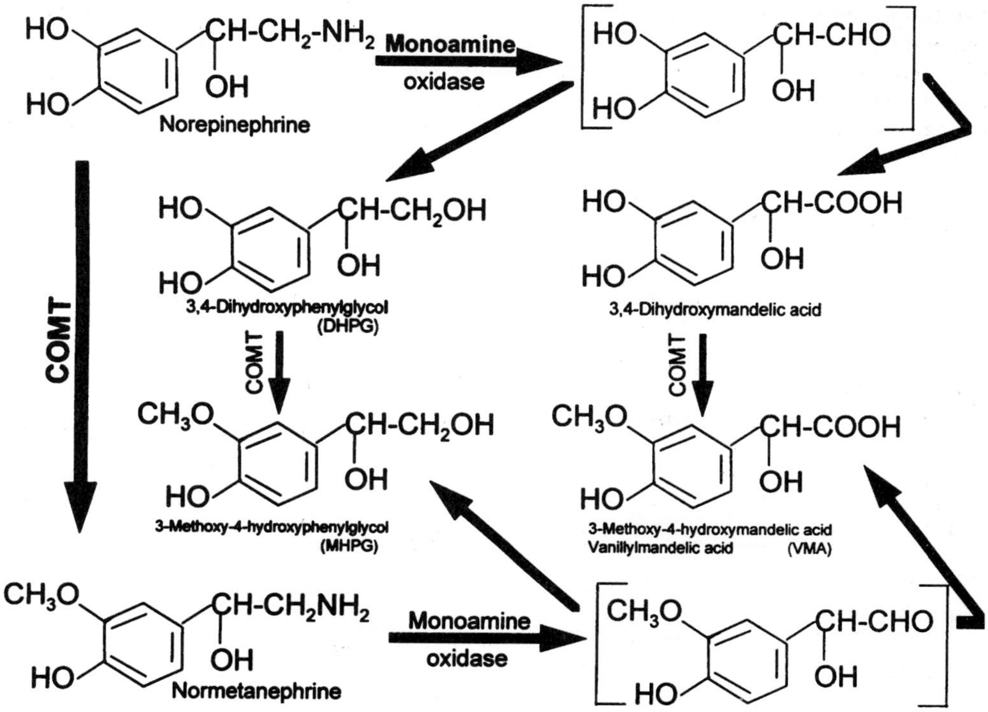

FIGURE 3–2. Degradative pathways of norepinephrine. COMT, Catechol-*O*-methyl transferase. (Reproduced with permission from Siegel GJ, Agranoff BW, Albers RW, Molinoff PB: Basic Neurochemistry, 5th ed. New York, Raven Press, 1994.)

aldehyde dehydrogenase to the corresponding acid. Monoamine oxidase is predominantly located in the outer membrane of mitochondria with possible microsomal localization. Extraneuronal MAO exists; however, it is predominantly an intraneuronal enzyme. In the human brain, at least two forms of MAO, type A and type B, have been identified. Certain agents have been shown to specifically inhibit these enzymes, including clorgyline, a specific type A inhibitor, and deprenyl, a selective type B inhibitor.

The second enzyme, COMT, is thought to be predominantly extraneuronal and requires S-adenosyl methionine and Mg^{2+} to become active. In peripheral sympathetic neurons, the aldehyde intermediate produced by MAO can be oxidized to the corresponding acid or reduced to glycols. Oxidation usually exceeds reduction, and vanillylmandelic acid is the major metabolite of norepinephrine and is detectable in the urine. In the CNS, reduction of the intermediate aldehyde formed by MAO predominates, and the major metabolite of norepinephrine found is 3-methoxy-4-hydroxy-phenethyleneglycol. Dopamine is metabolized to dihydroxyphenylacetic acid (DOPAC) through intraneuronal MAO following reuptake (Fig. 3–3). When released, dopamine is also metabolized to homovanillic acid (HVA) through the actions of COMT and then MAO. In humans, the major dopaminergic brain metabolite is HVA, and accumulation of this metabolite in the brain or cerebrospinal fluid can be used as an index of functional activity of this transmitter system. There are lesser amounts of DOPAC and 3-methoxytyramine in human brain tissue. Catecholamines released by neurons are subsequently taken up via a saturable membrane transport process that is dependent on temperature and requires energy. This process is also sodium dependent and can be blocked by the inhibition of Na^+/K^+-activated ATPase.

The largest group of norepinephrine neurons in the CNS is in the locus coeruleus, a compact bilateral cluster of approximately 12,000 large neurons in the caudal pontine central gray matter. Fibers from these cells form three major ascending noradrenergic tracts, including the central gray dorsal longitudinal fasciculus, the central tegmental, and the ventral tegmental-medial forebrain bundle tracts. These fibers innervate all cortices, specific thalamic and hypothalamic nuclei, and the olfactory bulb. A fourth tract ascends to innervate the cerebellar cortex, while the fifth fascicle descends into the mesencephalon and spinal cord; although they are largely ipsilateral, approximately one quarter of these fibers cross in some animals.

These central norepinephrine neurons have been thought to be involved in many neurophysiological functions, including learning, memory, sleep-wake cycle regulation, anxiety, and nociception, as well as in affective psychoses. In the catecholaminergic theory of affective disorders, it is hypothesized that depression may be related to a deficiency of catecholamine at important CNS receptors, whereas mania is associated with an excess catecholaminergic state. This hypothesis originally resulted from the observation that MAO inhibitors produced mood elevation, and, in contrast, drugs that depleted brain amines such as reserpine could produce depression. Furthermore, agents such as MAO inhibitors, tricyclic antidepressants, and stimulants that are effective in treating depression interact with brain catecholamine receptors and increase the availability of monoamines. More recent studies have shown that long-term treatment with some of these agents affects receptor numbers and causes physiological and behavioral changes in sensitivity to monoamine agents. Furthermore, there is a decrease in the number and sensitivity of postsynaptic beta-adrenergic receptors and an increase in sensitivity of central alpha-adrenergic receptors.

The CNS dopaminergic system is complex, and a proposed schema divides the anatomy into three systems including ultra-short, intermediate-length, and long-length systems.[23] The ultra-short systems encompass the interplexiform amacrine and periglomerular olfactory dopamine cells, which are unrelated to mood, emotion, or thought processes. The intermediate-length systems include the tuberohypophysial (connecting the arcuate and periventricular nuclei to the intermediate lobe of the pituitary and median eminence), the incertohypothalamic neurons (linking the dorsal-posterior hypothalamus with the dorsal anterior hypothalamus–lateral septal nuclei), and the medullary periventricular dopamine group (in the area of the dorsal motor nucleus, nucleus tractus solitarius, and periaqueductal gray). The long-length system connects the ventral tegmental and substantia nigra with the caudate-putamen (nigrostriatal) and limbic cortex–limbic

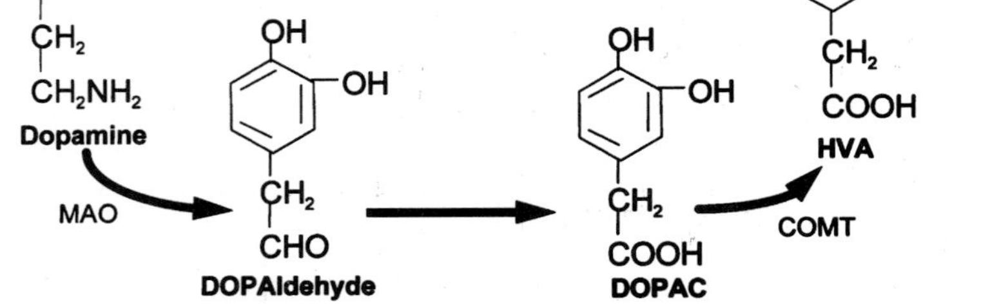

FIGURE 3–3. Major metabolites of dopamine. MAO, Monoamine oxidase; COMT, catechol-*O*-methyl transferase; HVA, homovanillic acid; DOPAC, 3,4-dihydroxyphenylacetic acid. (Reproduced with permission from Siegel GJ, Agranoff BW, Albers RW, Molinoff PB: Basic Neurochemistry, 5th ed. New York, Raven Press, 1994.)

system (mesocortical-mesolimbic). This long-length system is important in motor control and in mood, emotion, and thought processes.

Although dopamine synthesis and transmitter dynamics are shared by all dopamine cells, their physiology, pharmacology, and regulatory properties vary with location. Early investigations suggested that there were two broad classes of dopamine receptors (D_1 and D_2 classes); however, recently multiple additional subtypes have been identified (two D_1 and four D_2 classes). The D_1 receptors mediate dopamine-stimulated increases of adenylate cyclase and phosphoinositide turnover and are located in the striatum, nucleus accumbens, olfactory tubercle, and striatum. One D_1 receptor subtype, D_5, has a pharmacological profile that is similar to that of D_1 and stimulates adenylate cyclase activity, but it displays a higher affinity for dopamine and is located primarily in the limbic system. The D_2 receptors mediate the inhibition of adenylate cyclase and modulate phosphoinositide metabolism, as well as inhibiting the entry of Ca^{2+} through voltage-sensitive channels and enhancing K^+ conductance in the dopaminergic neuron. These receptors are located in the striatum, nucleus accumbens, retina, substantia nigra, ventral tegmental area, and pituitary gland. The D_3 receptor, a D_2 subtype, is found in highest levels in the limbic brain structures. Another D_2 subtype, the D_4 class, resembles the D_2 and D_3 receptors pharmacologically but has a higher affinity for clozapine, the atypical antipsychotic, and is found in the amygdala, hippocampus, and hypothalamus. Drugs that have dopaminergic effects may act via dopamine receptor–mediated effects as well as by non-receptor-mediated effects on presynaptic function and by effects that are mediated indirectly by interaction with other neurotransmitter systems that subsequently affect dopamine neurons.

Abnormalities in dopaminergic homeostasis have been implicated in patients with psychotic disorders, particularly schizophrenia. These theories suggest that such abnormalities of thought result from too much dopaminergic activity. This hypothesis evolved from the observation that, except for clozapine, the efficacy and potency of antipsychotics are correlated with the ability to antagonize the D_2 receptor. Additionally, amphetamines and other drugs that increase dopaminergic activity are able to produce psychotic behavior. Whether the cause of psychosis is related to excessive dopamine release or hypersensitivity of the dopamine receptors is unclear, as is which dopaminergic systems or receptors are involved. Furthermore, there is at present no direct experimental evidence that excessive dopamine-dependent neuronal activity or elevated dopamine levels at central synapses occur in schizophrenics. Although a significant elevation in HVA levels in the cerebrospinal fluid (CSF) of patients taking antipsychotic medications has been demonstrated, no differences in HVA levels in brain or CSF in normal subjects and unmedicated schizophrenics have been found. Other neurotransmitters may also be involved in psychosis, including norepinephrine, serotonin, and some amino acids. Glutamate, the most ubiquitous excitatory neurotransmitter in the CNS has become a recent focus of attention as well.[24] How these various systems interact is a matter of continued speculation.

Brain serotonin makes up only about 2 percent of the body's serotonin, much more being present in platelets, mast cells, and enterochromaffin cells. In the brain, serotonin is synthesized by the uptake of tryptophan, which is then hydroxylated by tryptophan hydroxylase to form 5-hydroxytryptophan (5-HTP). This enzyme requires molecular oxygen, reduced pteridine, and a sulfhydryl-stabilizing substance. This first enzyme is the rate-limiting step. When synthesized, 5-HTP is then decarboxylated to serotonin via amino acid decarboxylase. Serotonin is deaminated by MAO, producing 5-hydroxyindoleacetaldehyde, which can be further oxidized to 5-hydroxyindoleacetic acid (5-HIAA) or reduced to 5-hydroxytryptophol.

Serotonin synthesis apparently is not influenced by the concentration of 5-HT itself. This has been demonstrated by the fact that when 5-HT catabolism is blocked, brain serotonin concentration increases to three times that of controls. Furthermore, when 5-HIAA efflux is blocked, levels of this metabolite continue to rise linearly. These findings suggest that the rate of initial synthesis may be limited only by the availability of substrate and cofactors, or by other mechanisms. Serotonin-containing cells are concentrated in the pineal gland but are also found in discrete groups of cells in the midline regions of the pons and midbrain. The caudal cells project to the spinal cord and brain stem, while the rostral cell groups project to the limbic forebrain system, thalamus, neostriatum, and cerebellum. Raphe neurons receive dopaminergic input from the substantia nigra and the ventral tegmental area, norepinephrine input from the locus coeruleus, and other afferents from the hypothalamus, thalamus, and limbic forebrain. In the past decade, extensive pharmacological laboratory work has identified numerous serotonergic subsystems, including $5\text{-HT}_{1A\text{-}F}$, $5\text{-HT}_{2A\text{-}C}$, 5-HT_3, 5-HT_4, $5\text{-HT}_{5A\text{-}B}$, and 5-HT_7. More recently, specific receptor antagonists have also been developed that allow more refined pharmacological and neurochemical analysis of behaviors that relate to serotonin.

A wide array of homeostatic functions has been suggested for the serotonergic systems, including sleep-wake cycles. Alterations in serotonergic function have also been suggested in patients with certain psychiatric conditions such as affective illness, aggressive states, and schizophrenia. Low levels of serotonin in brain have been associated with depression and suicide, and drugs that enhance serotonin activity act as antidepressants. The selective serotonin reuptake inhibitors (SSRIs) have become the mainstay of antidepressant treatment in the United States, and drugs that block 5-HT_2 and dopamine D_2 receptors have proven more effective antipsychotics than the neuroleptic class of antipsychotics.[25]

Examination of Mood, Emotion, and Thought

DIRECTED NEUROLOGICAL EXAMINATION

The directed neurological examination should begin with a mental status evaluation, which includes a psychiatric assessment. This part of the examination actually begins during the history and may be expanded in a more formal fashion. The mental status examination should include assessments of level of alertness, orientation, and attention.

Stupor may be organic in origin or psychiatric. Hypervigilant states may develop with delirium tremens as well as with drug overdoses, such as amphetamine, phencyclidine, and cocaine, or with paranoid states in general. A fluctuating level of consciousness is more likely to be associated with an organic cause, and the presence of stupor will interfere with the remaining aspects of the cognitive examination. Sudden alterations in behavior, especially behavior with automatisms, may also suggest a seizure disorder; seizures of frontal lobe origin may be extremely bizarre, and sudden behavioral changes are often mistaken for psychogenic displays.

To assess mood, one must ask how the patient feels, yet the affect is also directly displayed. The patient may appear sad and tearful or ebullient and inappropriately expansive. The way the patient is dressed and presents herself or himself is important but is often overlooked. A slovenly appearance in a recently high-performing individual is a cause for concern, even if the subject scores well on tests of memory and the simple routine tasks demanded in an office cognitive examination. The way questions are answered is a significant aspect of the emotional evaluation. The examiner should notice whether the patient volunteers information or conceals it. Additionally, it should be noted whether questions are answered in a normal time frame or if there are delays that require several prompts to obtain an answer. Furthermore, the answers may be incomplete or minimally helpful, and the prosody of the speech may convey emotions or the lack of them.

The presence of a thought disorder will be conveyed during conversation and is independent of mood. When taking the history and examining patients, the clinician should look for "loose associations of thought" and the practice of skipping illogically from one idea to another seemingly unrelated idea. It should be observed whether a word with two meanings is used correctly the first time and then used incorrectly to develop an unrelated thought. A formal language examination may be helpful in distinguishing a thought disorder from an aphasia. But when the speech disorder is profound, the difference may be difficult to discern. There are certain features of psychotic speech that may be helpful and should be sought. Clanging, the use of similar sounding words together regardless of their meaning, is never present in aphasia, whereas dysarthria is not a feature of psychosis. Naming should not be impaired in thought disorder but is usually affected in aphasias. The examiner should note that many patients with thought disorders are either noncompliant and refuse to answer or may seem to purposefully misname things, requiring interpretation of the incorrect answers. Writing specimens of a psychotic subject should be obtained; they may be agrammatical or may contain neologisms, simulating aphasia. As in patients with some aphasias, the content of the speech of a patient with a thought disorder may be empty, and often, after a few minutes of monologue, the examiner may have no idea what information was conveyed. Thought-disordered speech may also be pressured and may be highly distractible. The clinician should note any figures of speech that may contain unusual allusions and references to bizarre or macabre things.

The examiner should also ask whether the patient is hearing or seeing things that aren't there and assess whether these hallucinations are interfering with complete cooperation. Delusions should be probed but not countered. Since the delusion is an irrational belief, argument over its logic is fruitless, but the examiner should not agree with it. Depending on the situation, either an explanation that the belief is a delusion but appears real to the patient can be given, or the clinician can simply take note of it and pass on to other subjects. In the case of drug-induced psychosis in Parkinson's disease, the most common delusion is of spousal infidelity, a problem that is often not shared with the neurologist owing to embarrassment by both the patient and the spouse. In this situation and occasionally in others, specific delusions should be asked about.

ASSOCIATED NEUROLOGICAL FINDINGS

Cranial Nerves. The cranial nerve examination is important for determining symmetry in general. Asymmetrical findings indicate a pathological process. The eye examination is the most important part of the cranial nerve examination. Gaze impersistence, an inability to maintain conjugate deviation of the eyes, may be seen in a frontal lesion. Small pupils may suggest narcotic use. Anticholinergic overdose may cause large pupils. A left-sided field cut or cortical blindness may be associated with a mass or infarct and in addition will be associated with a denial of illness. A bitemporal field cut indicates a chiasmal lesion, which can occur in a patient with a pituitary tumor in the presence of emotional abnormalities. A superior quadrantanopia may accompany temporal lobe tumors or other disorders. Fundi can reveal papilledema or emboli, pointing to systemic disease. Foster Kennedy syndrome, associated with a frontal meningioma, may present with behavioral changes, ipsilateral optic atrophy, and contralateral papilledema. Smell should also be tested in patients with behavioral abnormalities because it may be abnormal when orbital-frontal pathology is present.

Motor/Reflexes/Cerebellar/Gait. The motor examination may reveal several signs relevant to the assessment of mood and thought. Any abnormality such as a hemiparesis indicates an organic disorder. The finding of myoclonus or asterixis generally indicates a metabolic or toxic disorder and occurs only rarely with focal lesions. Tremor at rest is seen with neuroleptic drug use or Parkinson's disease, and these should be considered. Rigidity and akinesia should also be assessed; they may accompany catatonia, neuroleptic use, or any parkinsonian syndrome. Catatonic akinesia may include waxy flexibility and abnormal sustained postures including one limb being stretched out for extended periods. Adventitious movements such as chorea may be seen and usually indicate tardive dyskinesia following chronic exposure to dopamine-blocking drugs. Alternative explanations include dyskinesias in the presence of psychosis in Parkinson's disease, Huntington's disease, Sydenham's chorea, or systemic lupus erythematosus. Stereotypic movements such as clapping, tapping, and rubbing may suggest autism or mental retardation or may be seen with schizophrenia. Deep tendon reflexes may be accentuated during stress or anxiety. A few beats of clonus at the ankles may be acceptable in these settings. Babinski's sign, asymmetrical reflexes, or spastic tone should always suggest an organic process. "Frontal release" or "primitive" reflexes may occur as a normal finding, but these are commonly seen in patients with disorders of frontal lobe deterioration. The grasp reflex is normal in young children only and is always pathological in adults. Hoffman's sign and the palmomental reflex are common in the normal elderly, and their appearance can be interpreted as abnormal only if multiple frontal release signs are present or if their appearance is asymmetrical.

Sensory. The sensory examination is the most subjective part of the evaluation and can be difficult to interpret. The presence of a sensory abnormality triggers the same differential diagnosis as that used for a mentally normal person. It is important to test vibratory and position sensations in a patient with a mood or thought disorder. A sensory neuropathy should lead the clinician to assess nutritional problems (vitamin B_{12} deficiency), infections (human immunodeficiency virus [HIV] and syphilis), hypothyroidism, or malignancy. The gait should also be checked. An obviously factitious gait may cast doubt on the organicity of an unexplained mood, emotion, or thought abnormality encountered during other parts of the examination. However, gait ataxia and mood disorders may occur in the context of alcoholism and multiple sclerosis, and more rarely with hypothyroidism. Isolated right parietal signs such as extinction on double simultaneous stimulation or agrapesthesia may be the only physical findings associated with a confusional state induced by a right parietal infarct or tumor.

Autonomic Nervous System. The clinician should look for evidence of autonomic hyperactivity including the presence of palpitations, cold clammy extremities, sweating, sighing, trembling, or hypervigilance, which can be indicative of anxiety disorders, anxiety associated with neurological diseases, or drug withdrawal syndromes.

Neurovascular. The neurovascular examination is rarely helpful in patients with mood, emotion, or thought disorders.

ASSOCIATED MEDICAL FINDINGS

Assessment of vital signs, preferably performed prior to administration of medications, is very important. Fever should always be construed as a sign of organic disease and should trigger consideration of a spinal tap. In a patient taking a neuroleptic, fever may accompany the neuroleptic malignant syndrome and may warrant consideration of this diagnosis. The lethal catatonia syndrome is a disorder that mimics the neuroleptic malignant syndrome except for the lack of drug use. Once the vital signs are known, the general physical examination should be performed with the aim of identifying contributory factors to a behavior disorder. The general appearance may reveal obesity or cachexia. Central obesity and hirsutism suggest endocrine derangements, whereas hair loss may indicate lupus, thyroid disease, or simply an unrelated skin condition. Weight loss may be evident by excessive skin folds or a cachectic appearance and may accompany depressive syndromes. Baggy clothes, indicative of weight loss, may be supportive evidence. Changes in skin color may suggest endocrine disorders or a neurocutaneous syndrome. Evaluation of the head may reveal evidence of trauma or gingival hyperplasia, indicative most likely of chronic phenytoin use or proptosis from hypothyroidism. Heart auscultation may reveal murmurs of valvular disease. Both lupus and rheumatic fever may affect the heart valves and can cause a variety of neuropsychiatric syndromes. Subacute bacterial endocarditis, a chronic illness, may present with an abnormal mental state such as depression and mild dementia. Tachycardia may be observed in patients with anxiety and manic disorders. Abdominal examination may reveal evidence of liver disease. The extremities should be evaluated for intravenous track marks, the stigmata of the drug abuser.

Evaluation Guidelines (Table 3–1)

The tests that should be performed on patients with mood, emotion, or thought disorders depend on the clinical situation. Patients who present for the first time are obviously to be evaluated differently from patients who were once fully evaluated but have suffered a relapse. Which tests are ordered is considered best left to the examining physician. A recent psychiatric text[1] leaves the choice of tests up to the physician and avoids any blanket recommendation for imaging of the brain or other tests. This is analogous to the National Institutes of Health criteria for diagnosing Alzheimer's disease, which do not include brain imaging. Patients with long histories, although perhaps never fully evaluated with modern techniques, may not require testing because the natural course of alternative diagnoses may preclude their consideration (e.g., in a 65-year-old with a 40-year history of schizophrenia, a frontal lobe tumor is not the cause of the behavioral disorder).

Neuroimaging. Most American psychiatrists suggest that a psychotic patient should have at least one brain MRI and possibly an electroencephalogram to not miss the rare patient with a structural or physiological abnormality. An MRI study is more sensitive than a computed tomography (CT) scan primarily because it reveals white matter disease with far greater sensitivity. The usefulness of these studies is questionable in "routine" disorders of mood, emotion, and thought, but in atypical cases, those of late onset, or when focal neurological signs are present, an imaging study is imperative. In general, imaging is done to look for evidence of masses or infarcts for which CT is adequate. Lesions causing such changes are usually large or multiple, and CT is satisfactory and much less costly than MRI. In patients who have had a prior brain imaging study for a behavioral disorder, repeat studies are unlikely to shed further light on a potential organic cause.

SPECT studies have been available for several years using the hexamethylpropylenamine-oxime ligand to visualize brain metabolism, yet they have little diagnostic value for individual patients. In the future, as more ligands are developed, the prospect of depicting neurotransmitter or receptor densities throughout the brain is high. PET scans provide information about metabolism (glucose utilization), neurotransmitters, or receptors. Although several abnormalities have been found in a variety of disorders of mood, emotion, and thought, none occur with sufficient specificity to be diagnostic.

Electrophysiology. Electroencephalography (EEG) is helpful in the evaluation of seizure disorders and metabolic encephalopathy and, to a lesser extent, for documentation of regional physiological malfunctions. In patients with psychosis, the EEG should be normal, whereas metabolic disorders can cause disorganization and generalized slowing. The EEG can reveal physiological abnormalities that may not be reflected on structural imaging studies. Old trauma, a postictal state, or migraine headache may be associated with behavioral abnormalities and may cause focal EEG findings when

TABLE 3–1. **Useful Studies in the Evaluation of Patients with Disorders of Mood, Emotion, and Thought**

Syndrome	Neuroimaging	Electrophysiology	Fluid and Tissue Analysis	Neuropsychological Tests
Affective Disorder Syndromes				
Depression	Brain MRI/CT: Hydrocephalus	Not applicable	CBC, chemistries, TFTs, VDRL, toxicology, vitamin B_{12}, ESR, adrenal studies	California Verbal Learning, Wechsler Memory Scale, Controlled Oral Word Fluency, Beck Depression Inventory, Hamilton Depression Rating Scale, Geriatric Depression Rating Scale
Mania	Brain MRI/CT: Epilepsy, Huntington's disease, CNS neoplasm, trauma, stroke, encephalitis	EEG: Mania associated with epilepsy	CBC, chemistries, TFTs, VDRL, toxicology, heavy metal screen, vitamin B_{12}, ESR, adrenal studies, porphyria studies, genetic studies, evaluation	Minnesota Multiphasic Personality Inventory-2 (MMPI-2)
Psychotic Syndromes	Brain MRI/CT: Epilepsy, CNS neoplasms, stroke, trauma, carbon monoxide poisoning, hydrocephalus, encephalitis, Wernicke-Korsakoff syndrome	EEG: Psychosis associated with temporal lobe epilepsy	CBC, chemistries, TFTs, VDRL, toxicology, heavy metal screen, vitamin B_{12}, ESR, adrenal studies, CSF evaluation, HIV, ceruloplasmin, porphyria studies	Brief psychiatric rating scale; scale for assessment of positive symptoms; scale for assessment of negative symptoms
Apathy Syndromes	Brain MRI/CT: CNS neoplasms, stroke, trauma	EEG: Encephalopathy	Toxicology screen	Frontal Lobe Personality Scale
Anxiety Syndromes	Brain MRI/CT: Post-trauma, stroke, encephalitis, multiple sclerosis	EEG: Aura preceding seizures	CBC, chemistries, TFTs, VDRL, toxicology, vitamin B_{12}, adrenal studies, urinary metanephrines, ESR	State train anxiety inventory; anxiety disorders interview schedule
Obsessive-Compulsive Syndromes	Brain MRI/CT: Post-trauma	EEG: Temporal lobe epilepsy	Not applicable	Yale-Brown Obsessive-Compulsive Scale
Impulse Dyscontrol Syndromes	Brain MRI/CT: Degenerative disorders, CNS tumors, trauma, encephalitis	Sleep-deprived EEG with nasopharyngeal electrodes	CBC, chemistries, adrenal studies, TFTs, CSF evaluation, toxicology	Luria Complex Motor Tasks (go–no go); Wisconsin Card Sorting Test, California Verbal Learning Test; Behavioral Dyscontrol Scale; EXIT; MMPI-2; Frontal Lobe Personality Scale
Altered Sexuality Syndromes	Brain MRI/CT: Encephalitis, CNS tumors, hypothalamic lesions, trauma	EEG: Temporal lobe epilepsy	Prolactin, follicle-stimulating and luteinizing hormone levels, testosterone, estradiol, urine cortisol	MMPI-2

CBC, Complete blood count; TFTs, thyroid function tests; VDRL, venereal disease research laboratory test; CSF, cerebrospinal fluid; EEG, electroencephalography; MRI, magnetic resonance imaging; CT, computed tomography; ESR, erythrocyte sedimentation rate; HIV, human immunodeficiency virus; EXIT, executive interview.

the MRI is normal. Rarely, disorders of emotion, mood, or thought with "subclinical seizures" or complex partial status epilepticus may be diagnosed only with EEG. The use of evoked responses in neuropsychiatric disorders remains a research tool except when organic explanations such as multiple sclerosis are being actively considered.

Body Fluid and Tissue Analysis. "Routine" blood tests to assess for metabolic disorders are required for all patients with behavioral abnormalities. Sodium, glucose, creatinine, blood urea nitrogen, calcium, liver function tests, and thyroid hormone levels are mandatory. Depending on the situation, other blood studies such as serum ammonia, ceruloplasmin, porphobilinogen, drug levels, pregnancy tests, prolactin and other hormones, toxicology screens, vasculitic studies, and HIV and syphilis serologic tests may be appropriate. Gastric lavage is useful in patients with suspected drug ingestion and possibly when one is looking for blood as a source of hepatic encephalopathy. Genetic testing can be done when Huntington's disease is considered likely. Because of the putative biological nature of many depressions, certain research-related tests have been developed, including the dexamethasone suppression test, measurement of urinary 3-methoxy-4-hydroxyphenylglycol, and the thyrotropin-releasing hormone stimulation test. Unfortunately, these studies are not useful in routine clinical practice. A drug screen for amphetamines and other psychoactive medications should be included in the evaluation of patients with appropriate clinical presentations.

Cerebrospinal Fluid. Cerebrospinal fluid must be examined when meningitis (infectious or carcinomatous) and encephalitis are being considered. Cell counts are elevated in patients with infectious or malignant meningitis. There is a polymorphonuclear predominance with bacterial etiologies and a mononuclear predominance with viral, fungal, or malignant causes. There is also an elevated protein and low (bacterial) and normal to low (viral or fungal) glucose levels. Special stains, cultures, and immunofixation studies should be obtained when indicated. A high-volume tap for cytological examination should also be pursued when carcinomatous meningitis is being considered in the presence of a known or suspected malignancy. A single large-volume tap may be negative, and multiple lumbar punctures may be required to effectively document or rule out the possibility of this diagnosis.

Neuropsychological Tests. Neuropsychological testing can be extremely helpful in the diagnosis, prognosis, and treatment of patients with disorders of mood, emotion, and thought and is especially useful for distinguishing "organic" dementia from nonorganic disorders such as the pseudodementia of depression, or malingering. These tests may also help to identify and localize organic syndromes, contribute to the identification of borderline psychotic states, and provide baseline data on the patient's general and specific function. A large number of neuropsychological tests are available, and the tester must choose the appropriate studies. The Wechsler Adult Intelligence Scale provides three separate IQ scores, and various subtests can provide clues to the presence of disorders of attention and thought (see Chapter 27). The Minnesota Multiphasic Personality Inventory can produce a general description of the patient's personality characteristics, but it is not useful diagnostically. Other tests that may at times be useful in the evaluation of patients with mood, emotion, and thought disorders include the Bender-Gestalt, Rorschach, thematic aperception, and draw-a-person tests (see Chapter 27).

Clinical Syndromes (Table 3–2)

AFFECTIVE DISORDER SYNDROMES

Major depression has a lifetime prevalence of about 15 percent and is about 15 times as common as bipolar disorder (manic-depressive disorder). Major depression is about twice as common in women as in men in all countries and cultures and does not vary in occurrence among different races. It may occur at any age, but the majority of cases occur in adulthood. Studies suggest a genetic predisposition based on twin

TABLE 3–2. **Selected Etiologies Associated with Disorders of Mood, Emotion, and Thought**

Etiological Category	Selected Specific Etiologies	Chapter
Hereditodegenerative Disorders		
Storage diseases: lipidoses, glycogen disorders, and leukoencephalopathies	Cerebral lipidoses—psychotic features Metachromatic leukodystrophy—psychotic features	30
Amino/organic acidopathies, mitochondrial enzyme defects, and other metabolic errors	Homocystinuria—psychotic features Acute intermittent porphyria—psychotic features, depression	31
Degenerative dementias	Diffuse Lewy body disease—psychotic features, dyscontrol syndromes Alzheimer's disease—psychotic features, depression, dyscontrol syndromes	33
Movement disorders	Parkinson's disease—depression, anxiety, apathy Progressive supranuclear palsy—depression, anxiety, apathy Wilson's disease—psychotic or manic features, depression, anxiety Huntington's disease—psychotic or manic features, anxiety, dyscontrol syndromes, depression Tourette's syndrome—anxiety, obsessive-compulsive syndrome	34
Degenerative motor, sensory, and autonomic disorders	Fabry's disease—psychotic features	36

Table continued on following page

TABLE 3–2. **Selected Etiologies Associated with Disorders of Mood, Emotion, and Thought** *Continued*

Etiological Category	Selected Specific Etiologies	Chapter
Acquired Metabolic and Nutritional Disorders		
Endogenous metabolic disorders	Adrenal, parathyroid, thyroid dysfunction (hypo and hyper)—depression, manic features, anxiety, dyscontrol syndromes Cardiovascular disease, pulmonary insufficiency, anemia, hypoglycemia, pheochromocytoma—anxiety	38
Exogenous acquired metabolic disorders of the nervous system: toxins and illicit drugs	Carbon monoxide poisoning—psychotic features Heavy metals—psychotic features, anxiety Amphetamine, hallucinogens, belladonna alkaloids, barbiturate withdrawal, cocaine, phencyclidine—psychotic features, dyscontrol syndromes	39
Nutritional deficiencies and syndromes associated with alcoholism	Vitamin B_{12} deficiency—psychotic features, depression, anxiety Wernicke-Korsakoff syndrome—psychotic features Pellagra—psychotic features, anxiety Alcohol—psychotic and manic features Alcohol withdrawal—anxiety	40
Infectious Disorders		
Viral infections	Encephalitis—psychotic or manic features, anxiety, dyscontrol syndromes, altered sexuality Epstein-Barr virus—depression Postencephalitic—obsessive-compulsive syndrome	41
Nonviral infections	Neurosyphilis—psychotic or manic features, anxiety Tuberculosis—depression	42
Transmissible spongiform encephalopathy	Creutzfeldt-Jakob disease—psychotic features	43
HIV and AIDS	Depression Manic features	44
Neurovascular Disorders	Stroke involving temporal/frontal lobe—psychotic or manic features, anxiety, apathy Stroke involving right parietal lobe—depression, apathy	45
Neoplastic Disorders		
Primary neurological tumors	Cerebral glioma—psychotic and manic features, depression, anxiety, dyscontrol syndromes Parasagittal/orbital ridge meningioma—apathy and dyscontrol syndromes Hypothalamic/temporal lobe tumors—altered sexuality syndromes	46
Metastatic neoplasms and paraneoplastic syndromes	Cerebral metastasis—psychotic features, depression, mania, anxiety, dyscontrol syndromes, apathy	47
Demyelinating Disorders		
Demyelinating disorders of the central nervous system	Multiple sclerosis—manic features, depression, anxiety	48
Traumatic Disorders	Head trauma—depression, psychotic or manic features, apathy syndromes, anxiety, obsessive-compulsive syndrome, apathy	50
Autoimmune and Inflammatory Disorders	Systemic lupus erythematosus—psychotic features, anxiety Rheumatoid arthritis, temporal arteritis, polyarteritis nodosa—anxiety	51
Epilepsy	Temporal lobe epilepsy—psychotic or manic features, anxiety (aura), dyscontrol syndromes, altered sexuality syndromes	52
Headache and Facial Pain Sleep Disorders	Migraine—manic features, anxiety Sleep apnea, narcolepsy—depression	53 54
Drug-Induced and Iatrogenic Neurological Disorders	Ibuprofen, ampicillin, streptomycin, tetracycline, beta-blockers, vincristine, azathioprine, amantadine, cimetidine, prednisone, dopaminergics—depression Amphetamines, baclofen, isoniazid, dopaminergics, opiates, cimetidine, captopril—manic features Caffeine (and withdrawal), penicillin, sulfonamides, sympathomimetics, amphetamines—anxiety Barbiturates, amphetamines—dyscontrol syndromes Dopaminergics, amantadine—altered sexuality syndromes	55

studies and studies of adoptees but point to a complex interaction with the environment. The *Diagnostic and Statistical Manual of Mental Disorders*, 4th edition (DSM-IV) criteria for this diagnosis require either that the patient have a depressed mood or that the patient have a sustained loss of interest and pleasure. Some depressed patients have a depressed affect or become withdrawn or irritable but do not admit to or complain of feelings of sadness. Almost all, however, complain of reduced energy and easy fatigability, and most have weight disturbances. Their clinical presentation can vary, however, from profound retardation and withdrawal to an irritable, unrelieved agitation. Other symptoms include a loss of interest in activities, diminished emotional bonds, preoccupation with death, guilt, and a sense of worthlessness. The patient may have somatic complaints with memory impairment, fatigability, insomnia, anorexia or hyperrexia, weight loss or gain, and impaired libido. A thought disorder may be present with delusions, but hallucinations are uncommon. Most patients have two or more attacks, and some have clear periods between episodes. Most attacks gradually build over a period of a week to a month, and if untreated may last from 3 to 8 months. Diagnosis and treatment of depression are believed to be grossly inadequate. The World Health Organization ranked depression fourth among all disorders in importance. It is a common cause of disability of equal significance in the United States to heart disease, diabetes, and hypertension.

Major depression is to be distinguished from a lower intensity and more prolonged depressive state known as dysthymia. Major depression is associated with psychotic features such as delusions or hallucinations in about 15 percent of cases.

The diagnosis of depression in patients with neurological disease is often overlooked. This may occur because the depression is overshadowed by the primary disorder or by the belief that the affect is appropriate to the condition. And, in fact, it can be difficult to distinguish appropriate grieving from depression. In parkinsonian disorders, many of the features of depression—psychomotor retardation, depressed facial expression, soft noninflected speech—are also features of the neurological disorder itself.

The differential diagnosis of depression includes primary psychiatric syndromes other than major depression such as behaviors associated with schizophrenia, generalized anxiety disorder, and obsessive-compulsive neuroses. Medical and neurological disorders either associated with or mimicking depression include malignancy, infections, medications (steroids, reserpine, benzodiazepines, anticholinesterases), endocrinological dysfunction (Cushing's disease, hypothyroidism, apathetic hyperthyroidism, diabetes), pernicious anemia, and electrolyte and nutritional disorders (inappropriate secretion of antidiuretic hormone, hyponatremia, hypokalemia, hypercalcemia). Depression is also associated with multiple sclerosis, Parkinson's disease, head trauma, stroke (particularly of the left frontal lobe), and Huntington's disease. Interictal changes in temporal lobe epilepsy may mimic depression, particularly with right-sided epileptic foci. Patients with diencephalic and temporal region tumors may also present with depressive symptoms. Equally important, depressive signs and symptoms may be incorrectly diagnosed as dementia, especially in the elderly population, where depression induces a pseudodementia.

In patients with bipolar disorder, mania that is severe enough to compromise functioning must be present in addition to depression. The lifetime risk for developing bipolar disorder is 0.6 to 1.0 percent. While the type of inheritance is uncertain, there is a strong genetic influence. These manic periods usually develop over a few days and may be associated with hallucinations and delusions. The attacks are usually separated in time by months or years, but there may be more rapid cycling in a minority of patients. Symptoms consistent with mania include euphoria, emotional lability, irritability, an increased amount of energy, a marked decrease in time spent sleeping, and a demanding and egocentric demeanor. The patient may be loud and have word rhyming or pressured speech with a flight of ideas. He or she may demonstrate poor judgment, disorganization, and agitation, possibly accompanied by paranoia, delusions, or hallucinations.

The differential diagnosis of bipolar disorder includes other psychiatric syndromes including schizophrenia and personality disorders. Medical and neurological conditions that may be associated with mania or may be mistaken for bipolar disorder include CNS masses, infections (neurosyphilis, encephalitis), and hyperthyroidism. Steroids, cocaine, amphetamines, hallucinogens, baclofen, dopamine agonists methylphenidate, and levodopa may all cause symptoms consistent with mania. Other neurological disorders that may include mania as part of their presentation include multiple sclerosis, head trauma, stroke, temporal lobe epilepsy, and Wilson's disease.

PSEUDOBULBAR PALSY

Patients with pseudobulbar palsy demonstrate pathological laughing, crying, and grimacing, often following little or no stimulation. Spastic weakness of the lower cranial nerve muscles (cranial nerves V, VII, and IX through XII) may be noticed on examination with accompanying dysarthria. This syndrome may be seen in patients with upper motor neuron dysfunction including those with amyotrophic lateral sclerosis, multiple sclerosis, or bilateral cerebral infarction. Patients with PSP, Parkinson's disease, and other parkinsonian syndromes may have pseudobulbar palsy in addition to more classic signs and symptoms. Mutism associated with pseudobulbar symptoms has also been reported after the resection of posterior fossa tumors in children.[21] Most therapies are ineffective; however, trials of agents that modulate biogenic amines such as levodopa, amantadine, amitriptyline, and fluoxetine may ameliorate the paroxysms of abnormal affective behavior.

PSYCHOTIC SYNDROMES

Psychosis does not describe a specific diagnosis and may be seen in patients with both primary psychiatric disease and drug intoxication and in the presence of certain medical and neurological conditions. Psychotic patients have alterations in the normal processes of thought that result in an impaired sense of reality, which may be linked to emotional and cognitive abnormalities. The patient with psychosis may talk and act in a bizarre fashion and demonstrate hallucinations. The hallucinations may occur in one or more sensory modalities including tactile (the sensation of bugs crawling on the skin), auditory (threatening, critical, or insulting voices), and visual (lilliputian figures or animals). Additionally, delusions in the presence of full wakefulness may occur. These may be

of Parkinson's disease and PSP and can be difficult to distinguish from depression. Bilateral cingulate lesions can produce akinetic mutism and abulia, but these lesions are not necessarily symmetrical, and one can be cortical while the other is subcortical. Abulia can cause mutism and is characterized by a general slowing of behavior and lowered activity. Patients with abulia show little spontaneous motor or speech activity and may at times fail to respond for minutes or at all to questions or commands. If they occur at all, the responses are slow and apathetic. Akinetic mutism refers to a syndrome of variable severity caused by lesions of both medial frontal lobes causing decreased motivation, sometimes to a degree mimicking catatonia, with complete failure to initiate activity or to respond, even to painful stimuli. These patients may respond intermittently to noxious stimuli and may be doubly incontinent. All of these signs are related to supplementary motor area damage and can be seen with lesions anywhere in the ascending dopaminergic pathways. In these settings, primitive reflexes such as sucking and rooting may also emerge, but if the motor cortex is unaffected, the remainder of the examination may be unremarkable.

ANXIETY AND OBSESSIVE-COMPULSIVE DISORDER SYNDROMES

Anxiety is an extremely common occurrence that affects everyone at some time and is characterized by an unpleasant and unjustified sense of fear that is usually associated with autonomic symptoms including hypervigilance, palpitations, sweating, lightheadedness, hyperventilation, diarrhea, and urinary frequency as well as fatigue and insomnia. Anxiety is thought to be mediated through the limbic system, particularly the cingulate gyrus and the septal-hippocampal pathway, as well as the frontal and temporal cortex. Based on animal data, the amygdala is believed to be the mediator of the stress response causing the sympathetic response to fear. Lesions of the amygdala prevent such a response in animals. The term *anxiety disorder* is used to denote significant distress and dysfunction resulting from anxiety. There are several subsyndromes of anxiety. Generalized anxiety is probably the one most commonly encountered in neurological practice. Panic attacks may precipitate neurological consultation to exclude other paroxysmal disorders. It should be noted that the lactate infusion test will precipitate panic attacks in two thirds of subjects. Post-traumatic stress disorders may also be associated with episodic behavioral changes that bring a patient to neurological attention. Agoraphobia and other phobias are also subsumed under the umbrella term of anxiety. Chronic, moderately severe anxiety tends to run in families and may be associated with other anxiety disorders or depression. The differential diagnosis of anxiety states includes other psychiatric conditions such as anxious depression as well as schizophrenia, which may present as a panic attack with disordered thinking. Uncomplicated anxiety may be a common problem in patients who abuse alcohol and hypnotic-sedatives, amphetamines, and caffeine. Other medical conditions that may be associated with anxiety include hypoglycemia, hyperthyroidism, and pheochromocytoma. As an organic disorder, anxiety is not intrinsically part of any neurological disease, although it is commonly seen with Gilles de la Tourette's syndrome, Parkinson's disease, and various headache syndromes.

Patients with obsessive-compulsive disorders have intruding unwanted thoughts that are distressful and recurrent ideas, images, and impulses that cannot be pushed out of consciousness. The patient may ruminate on these thoughts endlessly, impairing his or her ability to function. Most of these individuals develop rituals and compulsions that are performed to ward off an unwanted occurrence or to fulfill an obsession. Anxiety may be associated with the obsessions, and the performance of certain rituals may temporarily relieve this anxiety. The cause of this condition is unknown, but abnormalities in CNS serotonergic neurons have been implicated. Various studies and reports suggest that the frontotemporal lobes, cingulum, and basal ganglia may play a role in the generation of this behavior. Obsessive-compulsive disorder occurs in approximately 2 percent of the population and is more common in first-degree relatives of afflicted patients. Typically, this disorder begins in the third decade of life and is usually chronic with few remissions. This abnormal behavior may occur in the presence of depression or may be associated with certain neurological disorders including postencephalitic parkinsonism and Gilles de la Tourette's syndrome.

IMPULSE DYSCONTROL AND AGGRESSION SYNDROMES

The impulse dyscontrol and aggression syndrome consists of an inability to resist an impulse to perform a harmful act; the impulse is accompanied by a buildup of tension needing to be released, and is followed by a feeling of satisfaction or relief when the act is committed.[27] This in turn is followed by either relief, remorse, or a sense of justification for the act. Impulse dyscontrol and aggression can occur in neurologically normal individuals, but this behavior becomes pathological when carrying out the impulse consistently harms the subject or others. These behaviors may occur in patients with psychiatric disorders and global or localized brain dysfunction. These disorders overlap with obsessive-compulsive disorders, personality disorders, and mood disorders.

A number of other neuropsychiatric conditions may be associated with aggression. In patients with psychotic disorders, such as those mentioned earlier, aggressiveness may be a component. This type of behavior may also be seen with manic episodes and usually arises from delusional beliefs. A primary psychiatric disorder known as intermittent explosive disorder is characterized by discrete episodes of unrestrained violence that result in serious assaultive acts or destruction of property. The degree of aggressiveness is grossly out of proportion to any precipitating psychosocial stressors, occurs in a person with a clear consciousness, and is not accounted for by another mental disorder or the direct effects of a substance or any medical or neurological condition. Although the etiology of this disorder is unknown, investigations have suggested that disordered limbic system function with decreases in serotonergic transmission may play an important role.

Aggression may occur in patients with other medical or neurological conditions, producing global brain dysfunction. With a reduced level of consciousness and altered sleep-wake cycles, patients with delirium (due to electrolyte derangements, infection, drugs, or postsurgical or postictal conditions) may experience transitory ill-formed delusions and misperceptions leading to aggression. Encephalitis secondary to herpes simplex virus can become manifest with aggressiveness and may be associated with memory difficulties, irritability, distractibility, apathy, and restlessness. An unusual syndrome associated with aggressive behavior is REM behavior disorder. Patients with this act out their aggressive dreams, which occur during REM sleep, causing harm to themselves or their bedmate. Most of these patients have this in association with a parkinsonian condition, usually idiopathic Parkinson's disease. Childhood attention-deficit disorder, although it becomes manifest generally with attentional impairment, may be associated with destructive behavior when it is severe. Self-mutilation in association with aggression is a prominent feature of both the Lesch-Nyhan and the Prader-Willi syndromes, and may be seen in any condition that causes mental retardation. Finally, aggression in the context of a general personality change may be seen in patients with global neurodegenerative disorders such as Alzheimer's disease and Huntington's disease. When more prominent frontal lobe involvement is present, as occurs in the frontal lobe dementias, explosive outbursts of rage may be seen.

Focal frontal lobe dysfunction in the presence of head injury, tumors, or stroke may lead to disinhibited behavior and a need to do things on the spur of the moment. Disinhibited behaviors accompanied by a lack of restraint of antisocial impulses but without aggression can occur in patients with orbitofrontal damage. Aggressive impulses in the form of rage in response to trivial irritations may arise in patients with dorsolateral prefrontal damage. Limbic system dysfunction, particularly with involvement of the ventromedial hypothalamus or amygdala, in which the affective significance of stimuli may be altered, may also be associated with rage and violent behavior. This condition typically occurs in patients with amnesia, hyperphagia, and other evidence of hypothalamic dysfunction and is usually associated with neoplastic invasion. Occasionally, impulsive behavior, aggressiveness, or just inappropriate behavior is ascribed to seizures of temporal lobe onset, but complex behaviors involving directed interactions with other individuals is rarely of convulsive origin. Drugs often are at the root of aggressive behavior, and doses that precipitate aggressiveness can be highly variable among individuals. For example, some patients become pathologically aggressive on very small amounts of alcohol.

ALTERED SEXUALITY SYNDROMES

Altered sexuality may take many forms. The loss of libido is the most common form and can present as inhibited excitement or orgasm. Hypoactive sexual desire may be due to a number of psychiatric, medical, and neurological disorders. Typically, the cause is functional and the condition occurs in the presence of anxiety or depression. Hyposexuality associated with hypergraphia, hyper-religiosity, irritability, and elation comprise the main features of the Gastaut-Geschwind syndrome. This syndrome has been described as an interictal syndrome in patients with epilepsy of temporal lobe origin. These patients may also demonstrate "viscosity," which refers to a stickiness of thought processes and an interpersonal adhesiveness, and circumstantiality, which is manifest as a difficulty in terminating conversations.

A vigorous sexual drive can be a normal variant of human sexuality, but when it interferes with normal activities of living or is pursued at inappropriate times and with unwilling partners, it is considered pathological. Historically, hypersexuality was described as part of the Kluver-Bucy syndrome in association with loss of anxiety, diminished aggression, hypermetamorphosis, visual agnosia, and hyperorality. This syndrome is rare in humans but has occurred as a result of encephalitis.[28] Lesions of the hypothalamus are the most likely to create sexual disinterest, but medial temporal lobe damage may produce the same result. Frontal lobe lesions often create disinhibited behavior that may or may not be associated with a change in libido. Hypersexuality may also occur in individuals with Parkinson's disease or other parkinsonian patients treated with dopaminergic agents including levodopa, dopamine agonists, and amantadine.

General Management Goals

AFFECTIVE DISORDER SYNDROMES

When secondary causes have been sufficiently evaluated, treatment of depression can be initiated. Treatment may include psychological therapies (supportive psychotherapy and behavior therapy) as well as pharmacological agents. Nearly 80 percent of patients with major and most chronic minor depressions respond to drug therapy, including tricyclic antidepressants, specific SSRIs, and MAO inhibitors. Electroconvulsive therapy may be necessary if medications fail or their use is not tolerated, if immediate therapy is indicated, or in some patients with psychotic depressions.

When manic symptoms are mild (hypomania), the patient may be followed as an outpatient with home supervision by family members. These patients may benefit by a short course of an antipsychotic drug. If they are manic, patients require hospitalization and may require acute antipsychotic therapy in combination with a benzodiazepine. These medications should be tapered and discontinued when the initial phase of the manic episode has subsided and the effects of more definitive therapy using lithium carbonate, carbamazepine, or valproic acid have been established. Lithium, while effective in the long term, takes time to have an effect so that acute intervention with these other medications may be required. It must be noted that some antidepressants used for treatment for depression in patients with bipolar affective disorder may trigger a manic spell in some patients. The anticonvulsant lamotrigine has been shown to be an effective antidepressant in bipolar disorder.

PSYCHOTIC SYNDROMES

Antipsychotics can be used in patients with acute psychoses while a specific etiology is being sought (Table 3–4). Most of the antipsychotics are sedating but act specifically on the psychosis and are not simply tranquilizers. All such drugs act preferentially on the positive symptoms but may also improve the negative symptoms of schizophrenia as well. The older antipsychotics were all neuroleptics, having dopamine receptor blocing properties that induced a wide variety of movement disorders. The newer agents, classified as "atypical antipsychotics," generally have a better effect on negative symptoms than the neuroleptics as well as a considerably more benign extrapyramidal side effect profile. Long-term follow-up for tardive dyskinesia syndromes is still necessary, however.

TABLE 3–4. **Common Antipsychotic Drugs and Doses**

Generic (Trade) Names	Dosage Form and Range: Oral	Dosage Form and Range: Parenteral (IM)
Phenothiazines		
Chlorpromazine (Thorazine)	200–800 mg/day	25–50 mg/dose
Fluphenazine (Prolixin)		
Hydrochloride	2–20 mg/day	None
Enanthate/decanoate	None	1.25–2.5 mg every 1–4 weeks
Trifluoperazine hydrochloride	5–20 mg/day	1–20 mg/dose
Thioxanthenes		
Thiothixene hydrochloride (Navane)	5–30 mg/day	2–4 mg/dose
Butyrophenone		
Haloperidol (Haldol)		
Hydrochloride	2–20 mg/day	2–5 mg/dose
Decanoate	None	25–250 mg every 2–4 weeks
Atypical Antipsychotics		
Clozapine (Clozaril)	6.25–900 mg/day	None
Risperidone (Risperdal)	2–8 mg/day	None
Olanzapine (Zyprexa)	10–15 mg/day	None
Quetiapine (Seroquel)	25–800 mg/day	None

Unfortunately, none of these agents are available as parenteral preparations; thus, for the acutely agitated noncompliant patient, parenteral preparations of traditional neuroleptics are required, sometimes in combination with benzodiazepines. A poorly understood observation has been that haloperidol, administered intravenously, is relatively free of extrapyramidal side effects, whereas the intramuscular and oral preparations have a high propensity to induce a variety of problems.

ANXIETY AND OBSESSIVE-COMPULSIVE DISORDER SYNDROMES

The drug treatment available for anxiety disorders is quite good. Although few drugs have been adequately tested in long-term trials of generalized anxiety, benzodiazepines are successful in about 70 percent of cases. There are no data to support one drug as more effective than the others, and the sedative side effects usually resolve without loss of efficacy. Buspirone is mildly less effective. Antidepressants may also be helpful. Although beta- blockers are helpful with the secondary autonomic symptoms of anxiety, they are not very helpful in treating the anxiety itself. Panic disorder is responsive to antidepressants (SSRIs, tricyclics and tetracyclics, MAO inhibitors, and the atypical antidepressants) as well as high-dose benzodiazepines (but not buspirone). Obsessive-compulsive disorder is generally treated with an SSRI or clomipramine, occasionally with a neuroleptic added for refractory patients.

IMPULSE DYSCONTROL AND AGGRESSION SYNDROMES

Aggressiveness is a common management issue for clinicians of various specialties and may be a primary reason for referral. While aggression is not a specific diagnosis and its etiology should be sought, many of these conditions are not directly treatable, and symptomatic therapy is indicated. A wide assortment of medications in various pharmacological classes have been studied for patients with aggression, primarily in open-label fashion, and none have been found uniformly helpful. In practice, the neuroleptics are the most widely used agents (see Table 3–2). Benzodiazepines are useful for short-term control of aggression, but long-term treatment with these agents should be avoided because of the possibility of paradoxical disinhibition and tolerance necessitating dose escalation. Lithium has been shown to be helpful in the reduction of “psychotic excitement,” not only in manic patients but also in those with aggression related to other conditions. Similarly, carbamazepine has been used to stabilize mood and may aid in the treatment of aggressive behaviors. Other agents that may be useful, alone or in combination, include the beta-blockers, clonidine, buspirone, and the SSRIs.[29] A new class of drugs, termed the serenics, was specifically developed for the treatment of destructive behaviors in humans. However, one such agent, eltoprazine hydrochloride, failed to show any significant effect when it was studied in patients with either Gilles de la Tourette’s syndrome or epilepsy with aggressive behaviors.

Reviews and Selected Updates

Dubois B, Slachevsky A, Litvan I, Pillon B: A frontal assessment battery at bedside. Neurology 2000;55:1621–1626.

Gold JM, Harvey PD: Cognitive deficits in schizophrenia. Psychiatr Clin North Am 1993;16:295–311.

Kotter R, Meyer N: The limbic system: A review of its empirical foundation. Behavioural Br Res 1992;52:105–127.

Lamberty GJ, Bieliauskas LA: Distinguishing between depression and dementia in the elderly: A review of neuropsychological findings. Arch Clin Neuropsychol 1993;8:149–170.

Lichter DG, Cummings JL (eds): Frontal-Subcortical Circuits in Psychiatric and Neurological Disorders. New York, The Guilford Press, 2001.

Salloway S, Malloy P, Cummings J (eds): The neuropsychiatry of limbic and subcortical disorders. J Neuropsychiatry Clin Neurosci 1997;9:313–510.

Shenton ME, Dickey CC, Frumin M, McCarley RW: A review of MRI findings in schizophrenia. Schizophr Res 2001;49:1–52.

Soares JC, Mann JJ: The functional neuroanatomy of mood disorders. J Psychiatr Res 1997;31:393–432.

Stielman KI: Disinhibition syndromes, secondary mania and bipolar disorder in old age. J Affect Disord 1997;46:175–182.

Tamminga CA, Frost DO: Changing concepts in the neurochemistry of schizophrenia. Am J Psychiatry 2001;158:1365–1366.

References

1. Sadock BJ, Sadock VA (eds): Kaplan and Sadock's Comprehensive Textbook of Psychiatry, 7th ed. Philadelphia, Lippincott, Williams and Wilkins, 2000.
2. Levy ML, Cummings JL, Fairbanks LA, et al: Apathy is not depression. J Neuropsychiatry Clin Neurosci 1998;10:314–319.
3. Andreason NC, Arndt S, Alliger R, et al: Symptoms of schizophrenia. Methods, meanings, and mechanisms. Arch Gen Psychiatry 1995;52: 341–351.
4. Aggleton JP: The contribution of the amygdala to normal and abnormal emotional states. Trends Neurosci 1993;16:328–333.
5. Kolb B, Whishlaw IQ: Fundamentals of Human Neuropsychology, 4th ed. New York, WH Freeman, 1995.
6. Krack P, Kumar R, Ardouin C, et al: Mirthful laughter induced by subthalamic nucleus stimulation. Mov Disord 2001;16:867–875.
7. Starkstein SE, Pearlson GD, Boston J, Robinson RG: Mania after brain injury: A controlled study of causative factors. Arch Neurol 1987;44:1069–1073.
8. Starkstein SE, Boston JD, Robinson RG: Mechanisms of mania after brain injury. 12 case reports and review of the literature. J Nerv Ment Dis 1988;176:87–100.
9. Starkstein SE, Mayber HS, Berthier JL, et al: Mania after brain injury: Neuroradiological and metabolic findings. Biol Psychiatry 1991;29:149–158.
10. Mega MS, Cummings JL, Salloway S, Malloy P: The limbic system: An anatomic, phylogenetic and clinical perspective. J Neuropsychiatry Clin Neurosci 1997;9:315–330.
11. Kluver H, Bucy PC: Preliminary analysis of functions of the temporal lobes in monkeys. Arch Neurol Psychiat 1939;42:979–1000.
12. Aggleton JP: The functional effects of amygdala lesions in humans: A comparison with findings from monkeys. *In* Aggleton JP (ed): The Amygdala: Neurobiological Aspects of Emotion, Memory and Mental Dysfunction. New York, Wiley-Liss, 1992, pp 485–503.
13. Bear DM, Fedio P: Quantitative analysis of interictal behavior in temporal lobe epilepsy. Arch Neurol 1977;34:454–467.
14. Joseph R: Frontal lobe psychopathology: Mania, depression, confabulation, catatonia, perseveration, obsessive compulsions and schizophrenia. Psychiatry 1999;62:138–172.
15. Robinson RG, Kubos KL, Starr LB, et al: Mood disorders in stroke patients: Importance of location of lesion. Brain 1984;107:81–93.
16. Beblo T, Wallesch C-W, Hermann M: The crucial role of frontostriatal circuits for depressive disorders in the postacute stage after stroke. Neuropsychiatr, Neuropsychol Behav Neurol 1999;12:236–246.
17. Shenton ME, Kikinis R, Jolesz FA, et al: Abnormalities of the left temporal lobe and thought disorder in schizophrenia. N Engl J Med 1992;327:604–612.
18. Siegel BV Jr, Buchsbaum MS, Bunney WE Jr, et al: Cortical-striatal-thalamic circuits and brain glucose metabolic activity in 70 unmedicated male schizophrenic patients. Am J Psychiatry 1993;150:1325–1336.
19. Lewis DA: Neural circuitry of the prefrontal cortex in schizophrenia. Arch Gen Psychiatry 1995;52:269–273.
20. Lauterbach EC, Cummings JL, Duffy J, et al: Neuropsychiatric correlates and treatment of lenticulostriate diseases: A review of the literature and overview of research opportunities in Huntington's, Wilson's and Fahr's diseases. J Neuropsychiatry Clin Neurosci 1998;10:249–266.
21. Akshoomoff NA, Courchesne E: A new role for the cerebellum in cognitive operations. Behav Neurosci 1992;106:731–738.
22. Pollack IF, Polinko P, Albright AL, et al: Mutism and pseudobulbar symptoms after resection of posterior fossa tumors in children: Incidence and pathophysiology. Neurosurgery 1995;37:885–893.
23. Cooper JR, Bloom FE, Roth RH: The Biochemical Basis of Neuropharmacology, 7th ed. New York, Oxford University Press, 1996.
24. Goff DC, Coyle JT: The emerging role of glutamate in the pathophysiology and treatment of schizophrenia. Am J Psychiatry 2001;158:1367–1377.
25. Hardman JG, Limbird LE (eds): Goodman and Gilman's The Pharmacological Basis of Therapeutics, 10th ed. New York, McGraw-Hill, 2001.
26. Kirkpatrick B, Buchanan RW, Ross DE, Carpenter WT Jr: A separate disease within the syndrome of schizophrenia. Arch Gen Psychiatry 2001;58:165–171.
27. Davidson RJ, Putnam KM, Larson CL: Dysfunction in the neural circuitry of emotion regulation: A possible prelude to violence. Science 2000;289:591–594.
28. Marlowe WBE, Mancall EL, Thomas JJ: Complete Kluver-Bucy syndrome in man. Cortex 1975;11:53–59.
29. Ryan JM: Pharmacologic approach to aggression in neuropsychiatric disorders. Semin Clin Neuropsychiatry 2000;5:238–249.

CHAPTER 4

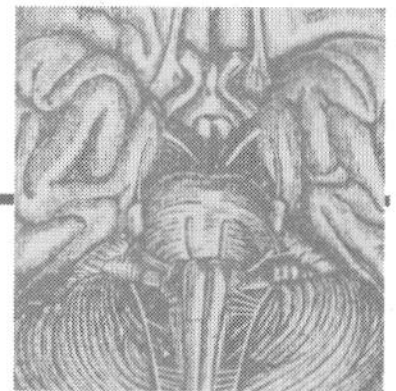

KENNETH M. HEILMAN, ROBERT T. WATSON,
and LESLIE J. GONZALEZ-ROTHI

Praxis

History and Definitions

Apraxia is a term that is applied to a diverse set of syndromes. However, this discussion will focus predominantly on limb apraxia. This term is defined as an inability to correctly perform learned skilled movements with the arms in the absence of primary sensory or motor impairments. To be classified as an apraxia, a patient's inability to perform learned movements cannot be caused by weakness, ataxia, seizures, or the superimposition of involuntary movements such as tremor, dystonia, chorea, ballismus, athetosis, or myoclonus. Patients with severe cognitive, memory, motivational, and attention disorders may also have difficulty in performing skilled acts without being apraxic. Whereas the presence of these disorders does not preclude the presence of apraxia, before apraxia is diagnosed, the clinician should be certain that these behavioral disorders do not fully account for the patient's inability to perform skilled acts.

There are several types of limb apraxia that are defined by both the nature of the errors made by patients and the means by which these errors are elicited on the neurological examination (Table 4–1). Liepmann was the first to systematically study limb apraxia around the turn of the century. His

TABLE 4–1. **Apraxias and the Types of Errors Committed to Commands**

Apraxia Type	Errors to Command: Postural	Errors to Command: Orientation	Discrimination: Movement	Comprehension	Imitation	Series	Mechanical Knowledge
Ideomotor							
Anterior	+++	+++	0	0	++	0	0
Posterior	+++	+++	+++	+++	++	0	0
Conduction	0	0	0	0	+++	0	0
Disassociation	+++	+++	0	0	0	0	0
Ideational	0	0	0	0	0	+++	0
Conceptual	0	0	0	0	0	0	+++

thorough and insightful description of an Imperial Counselor who had suffered a stroke and demonstrated "mixed aphasia and post-stroke dementia" provided the fundamental basis for models of apraxia. Liepmann discussed three types of apraxia: melokinetic (or limb-kinetic), ideomotor, and ideational. Limb-kinetic apraxia has since been considered an elemental motor disorder rather than a disorder of learned skilled movements and will not be further discussed in this chapter. Since Liepmann's initial descriptions, three other forms of apraxia, designated disassociation apraxia, conduction apraxia, and conceptual apraxia, have also been described and are included here.

Clinical History

While some patients complain of a loss of ability to perform skilled movements, most do not recognize their disability or complain about it. The activities to be inquired about include the use of common bathroom tools such as toothbrushes, razors, combs, and brushes. Furthermore, the clinician should ask whether the patient can prepare his or her own meals and use typical kitchen utensils including forks, knives, spoons, and other ancillary household equipment. Because the apraxia associated with hemispheric injury such as strokes and trauma is often associated with a hemiparesis, patients with these disorders who attempt to perform skilled acts with the nonpreferred arm during daily activities state that they are impaired. Although patients may attribute the difficulty to a premorbid clumsiness of the nonpreferred arm, this potential error in interpretation of the clinical history should not be committed by the physician.

Patients with hemispheric strokes may be anosognosic for the apraxia and state that they are able to use their nonpreferred hand correctly although they are clearly apraxic.[1] Additionally, many caretakers of chronically impaired individuals may find it easier to anticipate the patient's needs and perform mechanical tasks for them rather than await failures. It is, therefore, important to ask the caregiver about the presence of any impaired skills in the patient's activities of daily living. Since apraxia is most commonly seen in patients with strokes or Alzheimer's disease, special attention should be paid to obtaining the important elements of a history of praxis when the patient interview suggests these neurological disorders. Apraxia may, however, be seen in patients with many other diseases of the central nervous system including trauma and can be the presenting sign in those with corticobasal degeneration or primary progressive apraxia.

Anatomy of Praxis

Much of what we know about the anatomical basis of praxis (the ability to perform voluntary skilled movements) comes from the observations of patients with discrete cerebral lesions who have lost these abilities. To perform learned skilled movements, several types of knowledge are required. One must know how to move the limb through space (spatial trajectory) and how fast to move it. To successfully interact with the environment, a conceptual knowledge of praxis is also needed, such as what action is associated with a tool.

Liepmann and Maas[2] were the first to attempt to localize where this movement spatial temporal knowledge is stored. They described a patient with a right hemiparesis who was unable to correctly pantomime to command with his left arm. This patient had lesions of both the pons and the corpus callosum. Because this patient had a right hemiparesis, his right hand could not be tested. Since the work of Broca, it has been known that the left hemisphere in right-handed individuals is dominant for language. Liepmann and Maas could have attributed their patient's inability to pantomime with his left arm to a disconnection between the language and motor areas (i.e., the left hemisphere that mediates comprehension of the verbal command could not influence the right hemisphere's motor areas, which are responsible for controlling the left arm). However, this patient also could not imitate gestures or correctly use actual tools or objects. Therefore, a language-motor disconnection could not account for these findings. Liepmann and Maas posited that the left hemisphere of right-handed individuals contains movement formulas and that the callosal lesion in this patient disconnected these movement formulas from the right hemisphere's motor areas.

Geschwind and Kaplan[3] and Gazzaniga and co-workers[4] also found that their patients with callosal disconnection could not correctly pantomime to command with their left arm, but unlike Liepmann and Maas' patient, their patients could imitate and correctly use actual tools and objects with the left hand. The preserved ability to imitate and use actual tools and objects suggests that the inability to gesture to command, in these patients with callosal lesions, was induced by a language-motor disconnection rather than by a movement formula–motor disconnection. In addition, a disconnection between movement formula and motor areas should produce spatial and temporal errors, but many of the errors made by Liepmann and Maas' patient appeared to be content errors.

Watson and Heilman,[5] however, described a patient with an infarction limited to the body of the corpus callosum. This patient had no weakness in her right hand and performed all tasks flawlessly with her right hand. Yet, as Leipmann might have predicted, this patient could not correctly pantomime to command, imitate, or use actual tools with her left hand. Immediately after this patient's cerebral infarction, she made content errors, but subsequently she made primarily spatial and temporal errors. Her performance indicated that not only language but also movement representations were stored in her left hemisphere, and her callosal lesion disconnected these representations from the right hemisphere. In Watson and Heilman's patient, there appeared to be two types of representations that were stored in the left hemisphere: spatial-temporal movement representations (also called visual kinesthetic engrams) and conceptual knowledge about the relationship between tools and the actions required to use these tools.

Heilman and colleagues[6] and Rothi and associates[7] proposed that the movement representations (visual kinesthetic movement engrams), first posited by Liepmann, were stored in the left parietal lobe of right-handed individuals, and that destruction of the left parietal lobe should induce not only a production deficit (apraxia) but also a gesture comprehension-discrimination disorder. Apraxia induced by lesions of the premotor cortex, the pathways that connect premotor areas to motor areas, and the pathways that connect the parietal lobe with the premotor areas, may also cause production deficits. In these situations, patients make spatial and temporal errors, but, unlike parietal lesions, these lesions do not induce gesture comprehension and discrimination disorders. When patients with anterior and posterior lesions were tested, it was found that while both groups of patients were apraxic, the patients with a damaged parietal lobe had comprehension and discrimination disturbances, but those without parietal lesions did not.

As discussed fully in Chapter 15, the final common pathway that allows the muscles to move joints involves motor nerves that originate from the spinal cord. These spinal motor nerves are activated by corticospinal neurons, and the corticospinal tract is influenced by the premotor areas. In addition to direct connections with the spinal cord, the premotor area projects to the primary motor cortex. For each specific skilled movement, there is a set of spatial loci that must be traversed in a specific temporal pattern. It is proposed that movement formulas represented in the inferior parietal lobe are stored in a three-dimensional supramodal code. For the corticospinal neurons to properly activate the motor nerves, the stored spatial-temporal knowledge has to be transformed into a motor program.

The medial premotor cortex including the supplementary motor area (SMA) appears to play an important role in mediating skilled movements. Whereas electrical stimulation of the primary motor cortex induces simple movements, SMA stimulation induces complex movements that may include the entire forelimb. SMA receives projections from parietal neurons and projects to motor neurons. SMA neurons discharge before neurons in the primary motor cortex. Studies of cerebral blood flow, an indicator of cerebral metabolism and synaptic activity, have revealed that single repetitive movements increase activation of the contralateral primary motor cortex, but complex movements increase flow in the contralateral motor cortex and bilaterally in the SMA. When subjects remain still and think about making complex movements, blood flow is increased to the SMA but not to the primary motor cortex. Watson and colleagues[8] reported several patients with left-sided medial frontal lesions that included the SMA who made spatial and temporal errors when they attempted to perform learned skilled movements.

The convexity premotor cortex also receives projections from the parietal lobes as well as from the medial premotor cortex, and, like the medial premotor cortex, the convexity premotor cortex also projects to the primary motor area. Many skilled movements require that multiple joints be moved simultaneously. For example, when using a knife to cut a slice of bread, on the forward thrust, the shoulder must be flexed and adducted while the elbow is extended. On the backward thrust, the arm must be extended at the shoulder while the shoulder is abducted and the forearm is extended at the elbow. Lesions in the convexity premotor cortex impair multiple joint coordination. Unlike patients with parietal lesions, patients with convexity and medial premotor lesions could both comprehend and discriminate between well-performed and incorrectly performed pantomimes, demonstrating that their spatial-temporal movement representations were intact but could not be implemented.

It has been suggested that apraxia might be due to deep subcortical lesions including lesions of the basal ganglia or thalamus. Pramstaller and Marsden[9] reviewed 82 cases of "subcortical" apraxias that were studied by either neuroimaging modalities or neuropathological means. They concluded that isolated damage to the basal ganglia (putamen, caudate, and globus pallidus) does not induce apraxia. However, they noted that small lesions of the thalamus can sometimes cause apraxia, yet the exact role of the thalamus in higher-order motor control and apraxia remains to be determined.

Examination of Praxis

DIRECTED NEUROLOGICAL EXAMINATION

Because the diagnosis of apraxia is in part a diagnosis of exclusion, the clinician must perform a general neurological examination to determine whether the abnormal motor performance can be completely accounted for by nonapraxic motor, sensory, or cognitive disorders. Although the presence of elemental motor defects does not prohibit or preclude praxis testing, the examiner must interpret the results of praxis testing in light of the knowledge gained from the neurological examination.

When possible, both the right and left arms and hands should be tested. When one arm is weak or has another motor disorder that would interfere with testing, the nonparetic limb should be tested. Testing of praxis involves selectively varying input as well as varying task demands. If possible, the same items should be used for all subtests. First, patients should be requested to pantomime to verbal command (e.g., "Show me how you would use a bread knife to cut a slice of bread"). Both transitive gestures (i.e., using a tool and instrument) and intransitive gestures (i.e., communicative gestures such as waving good-bye) should be tested. The clinician should instruct the patient not to use the body part as the tool but instead pantomime the use of the tool. In addition, patients should be asked to imitate the examiner performing both meaningful and meaningless gestures. Independent of the results of the pantomime-to-command and imitation tests, patients should also be allowed to see and hold actual tools or objects and to demonstrate how to use the tool or object while they are seeing and holding these implements. In addition to having patients pantomime to verbal command, the examiner may also want to show them pictures of tools or objects for pantomime. The examiner should also allow patients to view real tools or the objects that tools work on (e.g., nails) and, without allowing them to hold the tool or object, ask them to pantomime the action associated with the tool or object. It may be valuable to see whether the patient can name or recognize transitive and intransitive pantomimes made by the examiner and can discriminate between well-and poorly performed pantomimes. Patients should also be asked to perform a task that requires several sequential motor acts (e.g., making a sandwich). Lastly, the examiner may want to determine whether the patient can match tools with the objects on which they operate (e.g., given a partially driven nail, will he select a hammer?) and whether a patient can develop tools to solve mechanical problems.

The types of errors made by patients with apraxia often define the nature of the praxis defect. Therefore, it is important to categorize errors, which can be done using a scoring system that classifies praxis errors into either content or production errors. Content errors include semantically related productions (pantomiming playing a trumpet rather than a

TABLE 4–2. **Types of Production and Content Errors Seen in Patients with Apraxia**

Error Type	Description	Example
Production Errors		
Spatial		
Postural	Use a body part as tool	Pantomiming the use of scissors, patients use fingers as blades
Orientation	Fail to orient forelimbs to an imaginary target	Pantomiming cutting a piece of paper in half with scissors, patients orient scissors laterally or not in consistent plane
Movement	Incorrect joint movement	Pantomiming the use of a screwdriver, patients rotate the arm at the shoulder and fix the elbow
Timing	Increased latency and incorrect speed	Absence of smooth sinusoidal speeds of movement when cutting with a knife
Content Errors		
Tool-object action knowledge	Lack of knowledge of the type of actions associated with tools, utensils, or objects	When pantomiming or using a screwdriver, the patient pantomimes a hammering movement or uses a screwdriver as a hammer
Tool-object association knowledge	Lack of knowledge of the association of a specific tool with a specific object	When shown a partially driven nail, the patient may select a screwdriver instead of a hammer from an array of tools
Mechanical knowledge	Lack of knowledge of overall mechanics of the use of tools	When attempting to drive a nail with no hammer available, the patient selects a screwdriver rather than a heavier tool (pliers)

trombone) and unrelated responses (e.g., making hammering movements rather than those associated with a trombone). Production errors include assuming the wrong posture, moving the incorrect joints, improperly coordinating multijoint movements, assuming an incorrect orientation, and making timing errors (Table 4–2). Each gesture produced by the patient may contain one or more praxis errors (see Rothi and colleagues[10] and Poizner and associates[11]).

ASSOCIATED NEUROLOGICAL FINDINGS

Because the diagnosis of apraxia is one of exclusion, a thorough neurological examination is indicated to rule out abnormalities of skilled motor movements that result from abnormalities of attention, language, primary visual disturbances, muscle weakness, ataxia, or disorders of primary sensory function (touch, proprioception). If any of these are present, the diagnosis of apraxia may be difficult to substantiate.

Cerebral. Since patients with apraxia commonly have other neurobehavioral dysfunction, a thorough neuropsychological examination is indicated, including an evaluation of directed attention and language function. Patients with left-sided parietal lesions of the supramarginal and angular gyri may have dyscalculia, finger agnosia, left-right disorientation, and agraphia (Gerstmann's syndrome). Additionally, patients may have alexia, aphasia, and constructional apraxia. Neglect for right-sided stimuli may occur but is uncommon. Patients with degenerative causes of apraxia, such as Alzheimer's disease, may also demonstrate memory loss, aphasia, and agnosia. Individuals with corticobasal degeneration may demonstrate frontal-subcortical dysfunction as well.

Cranial Nerves. Since patients with apraxia may have associated visual abnormalities due to involvement of the visual radiations in the parietal lobes, a bedside evaluation of the visual fields should be completed. Patients may demonstrate homonymous hemianopias or quadrantanopias. Visual pursuit and optokinetic nystagmus should be checked using a hand-held strip at the bedside because ipsilateral tracking abnormalities may be seen in patients with parietal lobe lesions. Occasionally, patients with apraxia related to more frontal lesions may demonstrate a conjugate gaze deviation.

Motor/Reflexes/Cerebellar/Gait. Patients with frontal lobe lesions associated with apraxia may have contralateral hemiparesis due to involvement of the motor cortex. Crural weakness without involvement of the arm and face suggests involvement of the medial frontal lobe; when acute, this suggests infarction in the territory of the anterior cerebral artery. These patients may also show evidence of callosal disconnection (see later discussion). Brachial-facial weakness suggests involvement of the distribution of the middle cerebral artery. Evaluation of tone and evaluation for the presence of abnormalities of movement is also important. Patients with apraxia as part of corticobasal degeneration may have rigidity, bradykinesia, and tremor or myoclonus.

Sensory. Cortical sensory loss including impaired two-point discrimination, agraphesthesia, and astereognosis indicates involvement of the parietal cortex and can occur in patients with apraxia due to vascular causes as well as in those with corticobasal degeneration.

Autonomic Nervous System. Disturbances of the autonomic nervous system generally do not occur in patients with apraxia.

Neurovascular. The patient's neck should be auscultated for the presence of vascular bruits because the presence of significant bilateral bruits is a risk factor for stroke that can cause apraxia in association with other neurological findings.

Evaluation Guidelines

Abnormalities of praxis are assessed by clinical history and the bedside neurological examination. Complementary investigations, such as neuroimaging, electrophysiology, fluid and tissue analysis, and neuropsychological testing, can contribute to the etiological diagnosis.

Neuroimaging. Neuroimaging can be very useful in localizing and identifying the various disorders that present with praxis abnormalities. While the clinical history and examination are most helpful in distinguishing apraxia due to an acute process such as stroke from a more chronic process such as the degenerative disorders, magnetic resonance imaging (MRI) and computed tomography (CT) are useful in differentiating the causes of stroke (hemorrhage, ischemia) and in ruling out central nervous system malignancies. Additionally, these imaging studies (particularly MRI) may show the areas of cortical atrophy in patients with degenerative disorders. Unilateral, predominantly parietal, atrophy suggests corticobasal degeneration, whereas bilateral temporoparietal atrophy is associated with Alzheimer's disease. Single-photon emission computed tomography (SPECT) may be useful in demonstrating decreased cortical activity when obvious atrophy is not observed. Positron-emission tomography (PET), utilizing oxygen metabolism and 18F-dopa uptake, can demonstrate asymmetrical hypometabolism in the posterior frontal, inferior parietal, and lateral temporal cortex, striatum, and thalamus in patients with corticobasal degeneration, whereas patients with Alzheimer's disease generally show hypometabolism of the parietotemporal and frontal association area, which may be asymmetrical or symmetrical, but striatal metabolism is preserved.

Electrophysiology. Electroencephalography is one measure of cortical function, and the finding of asymmetrical or symmetrical slowing may aid in the localization of pathology in patients with apraxia. Electromyography and nerve conduction studies are generally of little use in the evaluation of patientswith apraxia.

Cerebrospinal Fluid and Tissue Analysis. Cerebrospinal fluid (CSF) analysis is generally not helpful in differentiating the causes of apraxia, demonstrating at most nonspecific findings in patients with stroke or degenerative disorders. Brain biopsy, while potentially diagnostic in patients with apraxia associated with Alzheimer's disease or corticobasal degeneration, is indicated only in atypical cases or when the history and examination suggest other potentially treatable etiologies.

Neuropsychological Tests. In addition to bedside testing of praxis function, additional neuropsychological tests may be useful in differentiating early degenerative disorders such as Alzheimer's disease, corticobasal degeneration, or Pick's disease (see Chapter 33).

Clinical Syndromes (Table 4–3)

IDEOMOTOR APRAXIA

Ideomotor apraxia (IMA) is characterized by an impairment in the selection, sequencing, and spatial orientation of movements involved in gestures, including emblems and pantomimes. Two forms of ideomotor apraxia can be identified. A posterior form can be induced by left parietal cortex (angular or supramarginal gyrus) lesions, while an anterior form can occur following lesions anterior to the supramarginal gyrus that disconnect the visual kinesthetic motor engrams from the premotor and motor areas. Patients with posterior IMA have difficulty performing in response to command and imitation and do not discriminate well between poorly and well-performed acts. Patients with the anterior type of IMA also perform poorly to command or imitation but can comprehend and discriminate pantomimes (see Table 4–1).

When performing skilled acts, patients with IMA make primarily *spatial and temporal production errors* (see Table 4–2). Spatial errors can be divided into postural (or internal configuration), spatial orientation, and spatial movement subtypes. *Postural errors* are seen in patients with apraxia when they are asked to pantomime a skilled motor task and use a body part as a tool rather than acting as if they were using the particular implement.[12] For example, when certain patients with IMA are asked to pantomime the use of a pair of scissors, they may use their fingers for the blades. Although many normal subjects can make similar errors, it is important to instruct the patient specifically not to use a body part as a tool. Unlike normal subjects, patients with IMA continue to use their body parts as tools despite these instructions.[13]

TABLE 4–3. **Selected Etiologies Associated with Disorders of Praxis**

Etiological Category	Selected Specific Etiologies	Chapter
Hereditodegenerative Disorders		
Degenerative dementias	Alzheimer's disease	33
	Pick's disease	
	Corticobasal ganglionic degeneration	
Movement disorders	Corticobasal ganglionic degeneration	34
Neurovascular Disorders	Ischemic/hemorrhagic infarction	45
	Arteriovenous malformation	
Neoplastic Disorders		
Primary neurological tumors	Astrocytoma/glioblastoma/oligodendroglioma/meningioma	46
Metastatic neoplasms and paraneoplastic syndromes	Metastatic disease	47
Traumatic Disorders	Blunt or penetrating CNS trauma	51

Also unlike normal subjects, who, when asked to use a tool, orient that tool to an imaginary target of the tool's action, patients with IMA often fail to orient their forelimbs to the imaginary target. These are errors of *spatial orientation*. As an example, when asked to pantomime cutting a piece of paper with scissors, rather than keeping the scissors oriented in the sagittal plane, IMA patients may either orient the scissors laterally,[10] or they may not maintain any consistent plane.

When patients with IMA attempt to make a learned skilled movement, they often make the correct core movement (e.g., twisting, pounding, cutting), but their limb moves through space incorrectly.[10, 11] These *spatial movement errors* are caused by incorrect joint movements. Apraxic patients often stabilize a joint that they should be moving and move joints that should not be moving. For example, when pantomiming the use of a screwdriver, the patient with IMA may rotate his arm at the shoulder and fix his elbow. Shoulder rotation moves the hand in arcs when the hand should be rotating on a fixed axis. When multiple joint movements must be coordinated, the patient with apraxia may be unable to coordinate these actions to achieve the desired spatial trajectory. For example, when asked to pantomime slicing bread with a knife, both the shoulder and elbow joints must be alternately flexed and extended. However, when the shoulder flexes, the elbow should extend. When the joint movements are not well coordinated, patients may make primarily chopping or stabbing movements.

Patients with IMA may also make *timing errors*, including long delays before initiating a movement and brief multiple stops (stuttering movements), especially when changing direction.[13] In addition, when normal subjects make a curved movement, they reduce the speed of the movement, and when they move in a straight line, they increase the speed. Patients with IMA, however, do not demonstrate a smooth sinusoidal hand speed when performing cyclical movements such as cutting with a knife.

CONDUCTION APRAXIA

Patients with conduction apraxia show a greater impairment when imitating movements than when pantomiming to command. Because this constellation of signs is similar to those of the conduction aphasic who repeats poorly, Ochipa and colleagues termed this disorder conduction apraxia.[14] Patients with conduction apraxia can comprehend examiners' pantomimes and gestures but cannot perform the movements themselves. We, therefore, believe that patients' visual systems can access the movement representations (praxicons) and that these activated movement representations can activate semantics. It is possible that decoding a gesture requires accessing different movement representations than does programming an action. Therefore, according to Rothi and her co-workers, there may be two different stores of movement representations, an input praxicon and an output praxicon.[15] In the verbal domain, a disconnection of the hypothetical input and output lexicons induces conduction aphasia, and in the praxis domain, a disconnection between the input and output praxicons could induce conduction apraxia. Whereas the lesions that induce conduction aphasia are usually in the supramarginal gyrus or Wernicke's area, the lesions that induce conduction apraxia are unknown.

DISASSOCIATION APRAXIA

Patients with verbal disassociation apraxia cannot gesture normally to command but perform well with imitation and actual tools and objects. Heilman[16] described patients who, when asked to pantomime to command, looked at their hand but would not perform any recognizable action. Unlike the patients with ideomotor and conduction apraxia described previously, their ability to imitate motions and use objects was flawless. De Renzi and colleagues[17] also reported such patients as well as others who had a similar defect in other modalities. Others have reported patients with a disassociation apraxia of only the left hand following a callosal lesion.[3, 4] Whereas language in these patients was mediated by the left hemisphere, we posit that movement representations may have been bilaterally represented. Therefore, their callosal abnormalities induced a disassociation apraxia of only the left hand because the verbal command could not get access to the right hemisphere movement representations. Although the patient with callosal disassociation apraxia is not able to correctly carry out skilled learned movements of the left arm on command, these patients can imitate and use actual tools and objects with the left hand because these tasks do not require verbal mediation, and the movement representations stored in the right hemisphere can be activated by visual input.

Right-handed patients in whom both language and movement formulas are represented in the left hemisphere may show a combination of disassociation and ideomotor apraxia in the presence of callosal lesions.[5] When asked to pantomime with their left hands, patients may look at them and perform no recognizable movement (disassociation apraxia), but when imitating or using actual tools and objects, they may make the same spatial and temporal errors seen in patients with ideomotor apraxia.

Left-handed individuals may demonstrate an ideomotor apraxia without aphasia from a right hemisphere lesion. These left-handed individuals are apraxic because their movement representations were stored in the right hemisphere and were destroyed by the lesion.[18, 19] These left-handed persons are not aphasic because language is mediated by the left hemisphere (as is the case in the majority of left-handed people). If these left-handed individuals had a callosal lesion, they might have demonstrated a disassociation apraxia of the left arm and an ideomotor apraxia of the right arm.

The disassociation apraxia described by Heilman[16] from left hemispheric lesions was incorrectly termed "ideational apraxia." These patients and those of De Renzi and associates[17] probably had an intrahemispheric language-movement formula, visual-movement formula, or somesthetic-movement formula disassociation. The locations of the lesions that cause these intrahemispheric disassociation apraxia are not known.

IDEATIONAL APRAXIA

Patients with ideational apraxia are unable to carry out an ideational plan or a series of acts in the proper sequence.[20, 21] When performing a task that requires a series of acts, these patients have difficulty in sequencing the acts properly. For example, when writing and sending a letter, the patient with ideational apraxia may seal the envelope before inserting the letter. Unfortunately, the use of the term ideational apraxia has been confusing, since it has been used erroneously to label other disorders,[22, 23] including those involving disassociation apraxias[16] and conceptual apraxias. Many patients who demonstrate ideational apraxia have bilateral frontal and parietal dysfunction such as that seen with degenerative dementias including Pick's disease.

CONCEPTUAL APRAXIA

Whereas patients with ideomotor apraxia make production errors (e.g., spatial and temporal errors), patients with conceptual apraxia make *content and tool selection errors*. These patients may not recall the type of actions associated with specific tools, utensils, or objects (*tool-object action knowledge*) and therefore make content errors.[24, 25] For example, when asked to demonstrate the use of a screwdriver, either pantomiming or using the tool, the patient who has lost tool-object action knowledge may pantomime a hammering movement or use the screwdriver as if it were a hammer. Although this type of error may occur in the presence of an object agnosia, Ochipa and colleagues[25] reported a patient who could name tools and therefore was not agnosic but often used them inappropriately.

Patients with conceptual apraxia may be unable to recall which specific tool is associated with a specific object (*tool-object association knowledge*). For example, when shown a partially driven nail, they may select a screwdriver rather than a hammer from an array of tools. This conceptual defect may also be found in the verbal domain such that when an actual tool is shown to a patient, he or she may be able to name it (e.g., hammer), but when he is asked to name or point to a tool when its function is described, he cannot. These patients may also be unable to describe the functions of tools.

Patients with conceptual apraxia may also have impaired *mechanical knowledge*. For example, if they are attempting to drive a nail into a piece of wood and there is no hammer available, they may select a screwdriver rather than a wrench or pliers (which are hard, heavy, and good for pounding).[26] Mechanical knowledge is also important for tool development, and patients with conceptual apraxia may also be unable to correctly develop tools from available materials. Conceptual apraxia is perhaps most commonly seen in the degenerative dementia of the Alzheimer type,[26] but is also seen with hemispheric dysfunction.[27]

General Management Goals

The performance of learned motor tasks involves the ability to complete many of the activities of daily living including personal hygiene and meal preparation. As a result, the presence of apraxic deficits can result in the loss of independence for many patients. While physical rehabilitation may improve other associated neurological deficits following head trauma or stroke, the presence of apraxia can make occupational rehabilitation difficult because the patient will have difficulty in performing these skilled tasks. Recently, specific training programs have shown some promise in the rehabilitation of limb apraxia.[28] The clinician must inform patients and caregivers that apraxic patients should avoid participating in activities in which they may injure themselves or others. Occupational therapy and counseling may be useful for the patient and caregiver to teach various compensatory strategies. There is no pharmacological therapy that has been shown to be useful in treating apraxia.

Reviews and Selected Updates

Basso A, Faglioni P, Luzzatti C: Methods in neuroanatomical research and experimental study of limb apraxia. *In* Roy EA (ed): Neuropsychological Studies of Apraxia and Related Disorders. Amsterdam, North-Holland, 1985, pp 179–202.

De Renzi E: Methods of limb apraxia examination and their bearing on the interpretation of the disorder. *In* Roy EA (ed): Neuropsychological Studies of Apraxia and Related Disorders. Amsterdam, North-Holland, 1985, pp 45–64.

Heilman KM, Rothi LJG: Apraxia. *In* Heilman KM, Valenstein E (eds): Clinical Neuropsychology. New York, Oxford University Press, 1993, pp 141–163.

Roy EA (ed): Neuropsychological Studies of Apraxia and Related Disorders. Amsterdam, North-Holland, 1985.

References

1. Rothi LJG, Mack L, Heilman KM: Unawareness of apraxic errors. Neurology 1990;40:202.
2. Liepmann H, Mass O: Fall von linksseitiger Agraphie und Apraxie bei rechsseitiger Lahmung. Z Psychol Neurol 1907;10:214–227.
3. Geschwind N, Kaplan E: A human cerebral disconnection syndrome. Neurology 1962;12:675–685.
4. Gazzaniga M, Bogen J, Sperry R: Dyspraxia following diversion of the cerebral commissures. Arch Neurol 1967;16:606–612.
5. Watson RT, Heilman KM: Callosal apraxia. Brain 1983;106:391–403.
6. Heilman KM, Rothi LJ, Valenstein E: Two forms of ideomotor apraxia. Neurology 1982;32:342–346.
7. Rothi LJG, Heilman KM, Watson RT: Pantomime comprehension and ideomotor apraxia. J Neurol Neurosurg Psychiatry 1985;48:207–210.
8. Watson RT, Fleet WS, Rothi LJG, Heilman KM: Apraxia and the supplementary motor area. Arch Neurol 1986;43:787–792.
9. Pramstaller PP, Marsden CD: The basal ganglia and apraxia. Brain 1996;119:319–340.
10. Rothi LJG, Mack L, Verfaellie M, et al: Ideomotor apraxia: Error pattern analysis. Aphasiology 1988;2:381–387.
11. Poizner H, Mack L, Verfaellie M, et al: Three dimensional computer graphic analysis of apraxia. Brain 1990;113:85–101.
12. Goodglass H, Kaplan E: Disturbance of gesture and pantomime in aphasia. Brain 1963;86:703–720.
13. Raymer AM, Maher LM, Foundas A, et al: The significance of body part as tool errors in limb apraxia. J Int Neuropsychol Soc 1996;2:27.
14. Ochipa C, Rothi LJG, Heilman KM: Conduction apraxia. J Clin Exp Neuropsychol 1990;12:89.
15. Rothi LJG, Ochipa C, Heilman KM: A cognitive neuropsychological model of limb praxis. Cognitive Neuropsychol 1991;8:443–458.
16. Heilman KM: Ideational apraxia—a re-definition. Brain 1973;96:861–864.
17. De Renzi E, Faglioni P, Sorgato P: Modality-specific and supramodal mechanisms of apraxia. Brain 1982;105:301–312.
18. Heilman KM, Coyle JM, Gonyea EF, Geschwind N: Apraxia and agraphia in a left-hander. Brain 1973;96:21–28.
19. Valenstein E, Heilman KM: Apraxic agraphia with neglect induced paragraphia. Arch Neurol 1979;36:506–508.
20. Marcuse H: Apraktiscke Symotome bein linem Fall von seniler Demenz. Zentralbl Mervheik Psychiatr 1904;27:737–751.
21. Pick A: Sudien über motorische Apraxia und ihre Mahestenhende Erscheinungen. Leipzig, Deuticke, 1905.
22. De Renzi E, Pieczuro A, Vignolo L: Ideational apraxia: A quantitative study. Neuropsychologia 1968;6:41–52.
23. Zangwell OL: L'apraxie ideatorie. Nerve Neurol 1960;106:595–603.
24. De Renzi E, Lucchelli F: Ideational apraxia. Brain 1988;113:1173–1188.
25. Ochipa C, Rothi LJG, Heilman KM: Ideational apraxia: A deficit in tool selection and use. Ann Neurol 1989;25:190–193.
26. Ochipa C, Rothi LJG, Heilman KM: Conceptual apraxia in Alzheimer's disease. Brain 1992;114:2593–2603.
27. Heilman KM, Maher LM, Greenwald ML, Rothi LJG: Conceptual apraxia from lateralized lesions. Neurology 1997;49:457–464.
28. Smania N, Girardi F, Domenicali C, Lora E, Aglioti S: The rehabilitation of limb apraxia: A study of left brain damaged patients. Arch Phys Med Rehabil 2000;81:379–388.

CHAPTER 5

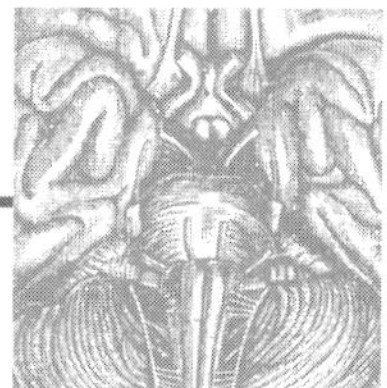

JOHN D. E. GABRIELI, ALISON R. PRESTON,
JAMES B. BREWER, and CHANDAN J. VAIDYA

Memory

History and Definitions

TYPES OF MEMORY

Memory in health and disease has been the focus of medical studies throughout history. In the first century, Pliny the Elder described a man who fell off a roof and afterward could not remember his mother, neighbors, and friends. Galen (130–200) placed emphasis on the ventricles as the anatomical key to mental processing, a view advocated by Nemesius of Syria, Posidonius of Byzantium, and several other early religious leaders whose views influenced medical thought. The perceived role of the ventricles declined during the Renaissance, and Thomas Willis entertained the idea that the cerebellum and brain stem controlled memory. Later, such figures as David Harley (1705–1757) and Charles Bonnet viewed memory in terms of vibration waves that oscillated in the brain. Scientific measurement of memory began in the late 1800s with Ebbinghaus' monograph and turned the study of memory away from philosophers and toward experimentalists. Studies of dementia, brain atrophy and memory decline, and trauma in relation to amnesia were conducted by several neurological luminaries, including Samuel Wilks, Jean Esquirol, and Alois Alzheimer. Linkage of memory with emotional elements was presented by James Papez, whose anatomical studies form much of the basis of modern knowledge of memory circuitry.

Memory is the recording, retention, and retrieval of knowledge. It accounts for all knowledge gained from experience—facts that are known, events that are remembered, and skills that are gained and applied. Memory is not a unitary faculty but rather an ensemble of various forms of learning that differ in their uses, their operating characteristics, and the neural networks that mediate their processing. A *memory system* may be defined as a particular neural network that mediates a specific form of mnemonic processing. Neurological or psychiatric diseases result in characteristic mnemonic deficits that reflect which memory systems are injured by a particular disease.

In regard to memory, several distinctions should be made between aspects of memory that are useful from the clinical perspective and those that are useful from the neuroscience perspective. One such distinction is between *declarative* and *nondeclarative* forms of memory.[1] Declarative memory corresponds to the everyday sense of memory and is responsible for the learning and remembrance of new events, facts, and materials. Thus, it encompasses both episodic memories (remembrance of personal experiences that took place at a particular place and time) and semantic memories (knowledge of generic information, such as the meaning of a word).[2] It is the form of memory people use to recollect facts and events consciously and intentionally and is therefore also referred to as *explicit* memory.

Nondeclarative memory refers to the many forms of memory that are not retrieved explicitly or intentionally but reflexively or incidentally. Remembering how to swim or ride a bicycle belong in this category. Nondeclarative forms of memory do not depend on the psychological processes or brain regions that are vital for declarative memory. These forms of memory guide current behavior on the basis of past experiences unrelated to any conscious awareness of those experiences and therefore are referred to as *implicit* memory. Implicit forms of memory include perceptual, motor, and cognitive *skill learning* (sometimes referred to as procedural memory), which is the increased accuracy, speed, or skill acquired for a given task during multiple training sessions in the absence of conscious awareness; classic and other sorts of *conditioning*, in which repeated pairing of an unconditioned stimulus, such as a tone, with an unconditioned response, such as salivation at the sight of food, leads to a conditioned response (salivation) when the tone is presented in the absence of the evoking stimulus (food); and *repetition priming*, which is the facilitated processing of a stimulus, such as a word or picture, due to prior exposure to that stimulus.

Temporal properties also distinguish one form of memory from another. *Immediate memory* refers to the recall of information without delay, either immediately after presentation or after uninterrupted rehearsal. Immediate memory is characterized by sharply limited capacities for how much and how long information can be remembered. For example, most people can remember no more than seven random digits and only as long as they rehearse the digits. Immediate memory often has perceptual characteristics. For example, errors in immediate memory for words are more likely to reflect word sounds than word meanings. *Working memory* is a multicomponent psychological system that mediates the temporary processing and storage of internal representations that guide and control action. Information is held in working memory only as long as it is useful for solving a problem at hand.

Long-term memory refers to permanent and large stores of episodic and semantic memories. Long-term memories are not, however, passively stored records of experience. Rather, they are constantly used to interpret new experiences. That ongoing use can alter the original memory (retrograde interference) and yield inaccurate memories (false or distorted memories). Long-term memory is often organized by meaning (semantics) or gist rather than by perceptual characteristics of experience. For example, people remember the content of a sentence they have read far better than the specific order of words or the font in which the sentence was seen. Similarly, people remember a set of related words (e.g., fruits) better than a set of unrelated words. It is common, however, to believe falsely that a particular fruit was in the set of words when it was not actually presented.

The relation between short-term and long-term memory is often misunderstood, in part because of various meanings of the term short-term memory. Sometimes the term short-term memory is used to refer to attention. An individual who cannot repeat back even a single digit or word is better described as having a deficit in attention than a deficit in any sort of memory. A second use of short-term memory is to refer to a memory mechanism that supports remembrance of information after a delay of seconds or minutes and without rehearsal. There is, however, no evidence of any anatomical memory system that has a temporal span between immediate and long term. There is, instead, constant and rapid loss of long-term memory for most events and facts. Therefore, memory of information after a brief delay of seconds or minutes will be superior to memory after a longer delay, but this difference reflects the dynamics of long-term memory and not the existence of any particular short-term memory store. It is often thought that information must go through short-term memory in order to reach long-term memory. This is correct if short-term memory refers to attention because people do not remember that which they do not notice. Surprisingly, this notion is incorrect if short-term memory refers to immediate memory. Patients with severe immediate memory deficits show minimal long-term memory deficits. This finding indicates that information from the environment enters immediate-memory and long-term memory stores in parallel rather than serially.

There is also a relation between working and long-term memory that is apparent on strategic memory tasks. Strategic memory tasks require manipulation of long-term memories rather than the mere retrieval of those memories. The mere retrieval of memories, for example, is sufficient to support performance on a recognition test in which an individual is asked to differentiate items that were seen earlier from those that were not. In contrast, an individual must initiate and use a strategy when asked to recall what items were seen or in what order the items were seen. For these strategic memory tasks, individuals must use a plan to "work with" long-term memories in order to solve a memory problem.

COGNITION AND MEMORY

Cognition refers to the mental processes of knowing, including high-level perception, language, and reasoning. Cognitive processes may be dichotomized as crystallized or fluid.[3] Crystallized processes involve the application of well-established knowledge and well-practiced routines, such as vocabulary knowledge. Fluid processes are invoked when a problem must be solved with a novel, flexible strategy, such as reasoning. Fluid processes are far more dependent on working memory capacity than crystallized processes are. Some factors influence cognitive functions in a global fashion. Education, for example, typically augments many cognitive abilities. There is, however, considerable evidence that various forms of cognition reflect psychologically and neurally distinct processes. For example, spatial and verbal cognition depend mostly on processes that are psychologically distinct and mediated by different brain regions.

Cognition has multiple relations with memory. Impaired cognition in a particular knowledge domain is usually correlated with both declarative and nondeclarative memory impairments in that domain. A patient with aphasia, for example, is likely to have impaired declarative and nondeclarative memory for words. Declarative memory, however, can be greatly impaired without affecting cognition except insofar as cognition depends on the acquisition of new declarative memories. Thus, individuals who cannot form new declarative memories can perform very well on many demanding tests of cognition. The same individuals, however, can fail relatively undemanding tests of cognition if they involve the explicit learning of new information.

Specific impairments in working memory can lead to broad difficulties in cognition because reduced working memory capacity limits the expression or use of acquired information in situations that require fluid thinking.

DISORDERS OF MEMORY

A disorder of declarative memory is defined as *amnesia*. A pure amnesia refers to a relatively circumscribed disorder of declarative memory that cannot be accounted for by non-mnemonic deficits such as attention, perception, language, or motivation. *Anterograde amnesia* refers to the inability to acquire new declarative memories. *Retrograde amnesia* refers to the loss of memories acquired prior to the onset of the amnesia. Retrograde amnesias are described as flat when they extend back uniformly through an individual's life. More often, however, retrograde amnesias are temporally graded, being most severe or limited to a time period preceding the onset of the amnesia, and less severe or absent for more remote experiences.[4] The gradient may reflect the time when the memory was acquired or the strength of the original memory. Depending on the size and location of lesions, amnesias can vary considerably in anterograde and retrograde scope and severity.

Dementia may be defined as a chronic and substantial decline in two or more areas of cognition. In addition to memory impairment, at least one of the following must occur: aphasia, agnosia, or a disturbance of executive function (see Chapter 33). The cognitive deficits must reflect a decline from the person's former function and must be sufficiently severe to cause impairment in occupational or social activities of daily living. Dementia differs from delirium because it is neither acute in onset nor a diffuse confusional state that affects all realms of function. It differs from amnesia in that dementia is not circumscribed to a declarative memory disorder. Dementia, however, can greatly affect memory ability in primary and secondary ways. Dementia can include a primary memory disability when declarative memory is one of the areas of decline. Indeed, many definitions of Alzheimer's disease, the most common dementing disorder, require that declarative memory be one of the areas of decline. Dementias can also affect memory ability in a secondary way when the multiple cognitive deficits impede memory performance. A dementia featuring a severe attentional disorder, for example, impedes many aspects of memory performance. For similar reasons, mental retardation, confusional states, inattention, or motivational difficulties such as depression all have broad and substantial secondary effects on memory performance.

Memory is also affected by nondisease influences such as aging. Older people in their sixties and seventies typically perform less well on standard measures of memory than younger people in their twenties and thirties.[5] This decline is sometimes referred to as *age-associated memory impairment*. Age-associated changes in the absence of overt disease, however, vary considerably for different kinds of cognition and memory. They are more severe for fluid than for crystallized aspects of cognition; indeed, crystallized cognition is often minimally affected. Working memory capacity appears to decline constantly across the life span; therefore, aging affects strategic memory far more than nonstrategic declarative memory performance. Semantic memory appears to be affected only in very old age. There are few, if any, age-associated changes in some forms of nondeclarative memory, such as repetition priming,[6] and there are severe declines in other forms of nondeclarative memory, such as conditioning.[7] Longitudinal studies provide evidence that age-associated memory impairment is accounted for partly by individuals who are in a preclinical form of Alzheimer's disease. It is unclear at present whether age-associated memory impairments reflect only preclinical forms of age-related diseases or whether age-related reductions in memory occur that are independent of disease processes.

Clinical History

Patients with memory deficits are, by definition, limited in their ability to provide information about their history, and this limitation is especially salient for patients who may be demented. Therefore, obtaining a clinical history from a patient complaining of memory disorders usually requires considerable cooperation from the patient's family or caregivers. In many cases, they are the ones who can most accurately recite the patient's problems. This fact introduces a challenge to the interpersonal skills of the examining physician because the patient must retain a feeling of central importance during the interview even though much information about the patient must come from these collateral sources.

The physician, after introductions, can elicit a general history that may be directed if the patient begins to go off-track. As the patient begins to tell the history of the present illness, the physician should be appraising the patient for a general view of affect and cognitive function, and for salient aspects of the patient's personality, educational background, and state of health. Information about the temporal onset and progression of memory impairment is useful in focusing the differential diagnosis. An acute onset of decline to a chronic level of memory dysfunction suggests a stroke or anoxic episode. An abrupt onset with a stepwise progression raises a suspicion of a vascular-based memory problem such as multi-infarct dementia. An insidious, slowly progressive, chronic decline shifts attention to the possibility of alcohol-related dementia or Alzheimer's disease. A more rapid progression of memory dysfunction over weeks to months may point to a depression-related memory loss or, especially if seizures are present also, to primary or metastatic tumors or encephalitis.

Family history should include the age and state of health or age at death and cause of death of at least the siblings, parents, grandparents, aunts, and uncles. Neurological disease in any relatives or the possibility of consanguinity should be pursued as a lead to uncovering a genetic etiology.

Occupational and intellectual achievements of the past should be elicited. A discordance between poor language or judgment relative to superior occupational and intellectual achievements in the past suggests causes that are not consonant with more pure amnesias. Further, high levels of premorbid functioning may mask the severity of current problems because such individuals can effectively compensate for memory loss. Paradoxically, individuals with high levels of premorbid functioning may be most sensitive to and concerned about memory disturbances, and they may interpret such age-associated disturbances as harbingers of Alzheimer's disease.

The past and current medical history should be thorough because memory disorders have a wide range of primary and secondary causes. Information about alcohol, drug, and dietary habits should be obtained. Substantial alcohol consumption, which should be quantified, may lead to memory dysfunction through Wernicke-Korsakoff psychosis or hepatorenal encephalopathy. A detailed drug history should be obtained because many medications directly or indirectly (e.g., via lethargy) reduce memory performance. Commonly used prescription and nonprescription drugs that may interfere with memory and cognition include analgesic, antihypertensive, anticholinergic, psychotropic, and sedative medications.

A history of surgery, trauma, or head injury should be pursued for the possibility of cerebral anoxia or direct trauma to the brain structures. Onset and progression of seizures and headaches should be clarified to direct suspicions of tumors, aneurysms, encephalitis, or epilepsy. A cancer history should raise a suspicion of metastases to the brain or paraneoplastic disorders, and known hypertension, stroke, or transient ischemic attacks point to a vascular cause of a memory disorder.

A history of depression is particularly notable because memory loss is often seen during depressive episodes, in which anxiety, guilt, and delusions are also present. For this reason, it is useful to assess the mood of the patient and make note of any insomnia or fatigue. A primary memory disorder, however, can affect a patient's mood, sleep, work, family relations, and daily activities. Personality changes, usually reported by the family, should be pursued to determine whether they are an incidental finding, a consequence of the memory dysfunction, or a clue to the underlying etiology, such as depression or frontal lobe tumors.

Finally, social and legal issues may have to be considered, especially when the findings are inconsistent across time or do not agree with the signs of an organic disorder. Stressful family situations may color the complaints of the patient or family. Legal motivations are salient in cases of insurance claims or conservatorships.

Anatomy of Memory (Table 5–1)

PAPEZ CIRCUIT

It is well recognized that the ability to recall and engender memories is intimately linked to the emotional makeup of such memories. Furthermore, several clinical conditions show combined deficits in these domains, suggesting a direct anatomical or physiological interaction of functions. In 1937, the neuroanatomist Papez published a study describing an anatomical circuit that involved a number of central nervous system nuclei and pathways that are important in aspects of memory and emotion. Familiarity with this Papez circuit allows clinicians to think systematically about the overall anatomical foundation of memory and to analyze which elements are involved in different aspects of memory function. The concept of a circuit is particularly important in dealing with memory, since lesions anywhere along the pathway may interrupt memory function, although the coloration of the deficit may be particularly influenced by the specific nuclei or path that is damaged (Fig. 5–1).

The circuit is schematically diagrammed in Figure 5–1*A*, and the anatomical nuclei and pathways are identified in the sagittal brain section shown in Figure 5–1*B*. The pathway is circular and provides continual reintegration of information. The two prominent cortical areas are the cingulate cortex and the hippocampus of the temporal lobe. Diffuse cortical impulses travel into the hippocampus, traverse the midline fornix pathway to the mammillary bodies of the hypothalamus, and continue to the anterior and dorsal thalamus. From these regions, information projects to the midline cingulate cortex, which finally projects diffusely to cortical regions.

ANATOMY OF DECLARATIVE MEMORY

A broad convergence of human and animal research indicates that declarative memory depends on an interaction between domain-specific neocortical regions and domain-

TABLE 5–1. **Clinico-anatomical Correlations of Memory Disorders**

Anatomical Site of Damage	Memory Finding	Other Neurological and Medical Findings
Frontal lobe	Lateralized deficits in working memory. Right spatial defects, left verbal defects, impaired recall with spared recognition	Personality change Perseveration Chorea, dystonia Bradykinesia, tremor, rigidity
Basal forebrain	Domain-independent declarative memory deficits	
Ventromedial cortex	Frontal lobe–type declarative memory deficits	Upper visual field defects
Hippocampus and parahippocampal cortex	Bilateral lesions yield global amnesia, unilateral lesions show lateralization of deficits—left: verbal deficits; right: spatial deficits	Myoclonus Depressed level of consciousness Cortical blindness Autonomations
Fornix	Global amnesia	
Mammillary bodies	Declarative memory deficits	Confabulation, ataxia, nystagmus, signs of alcohol withdrawal
Dorsal and medial dorsal nucleus thalamus	Declarative memory deficits	Confabulation
Anterior thalamus	Declarative memory deficits	
Lateral temporal cortex	Deficits in autobiographical memory	

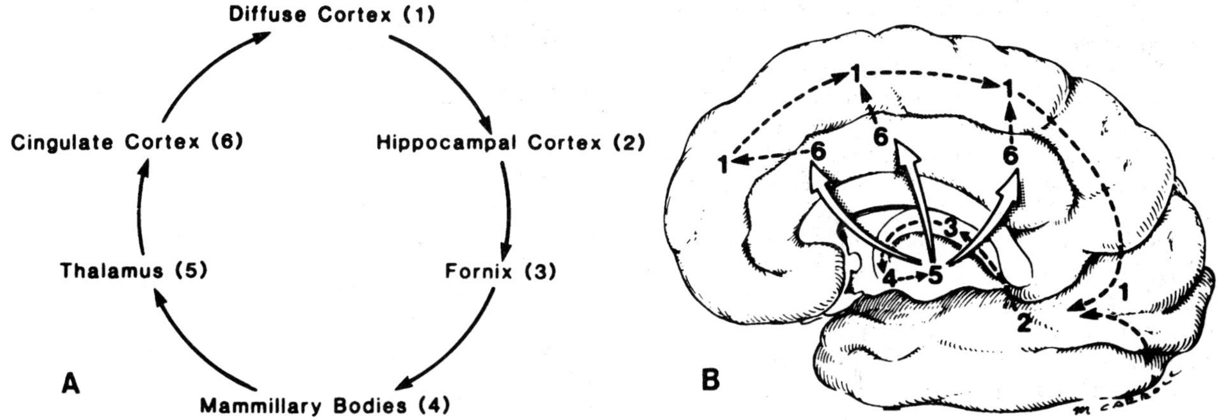

FIGURE 5–1. Papez circuit that integrates cortical and subcortical structures involved in memory or emotion. (From Goetz CG, Wilson RS: Behavioral Neurology. *In* Weiner WJ, Goetz CG [eds]: Neurology for the Non-Neurologist. Philadelphia, JB Lippincott, 1994, pp 184–194.)

independent medial-temporal, diencephalic, and basal forebrain regions.[1] Long-term memories are thought to be stored in the neocortex, the neocortical location reflecting the content of the memory. For example, knowledge about the visual appearance of a tool may be stored separately, perhaps near the visual neocortex, from knowledge about its use, which may be stored in areas that include the premotor regions.[8] Thus, relevant aspects of incoming information may be processed by domain-specific neocortical regions, and memory retrieval may involve reactivation of these regions, reflecting the retrieval of information stored in these domain-specific neocortical structures. For example, different brain regions involved in visual or auditory processing of an experience may be reactivated when that experience is remembered.[9–11] Memory of an event or fact, therefore, may be widely distributed in the neocortex with specific perceptual, conceptual, and emotional features of an event stored in specialized neocortical regions. The hippocampal complex has reciprocal connections with higher-order association cortices, and it is hypothesized that the hippocampal complex somehow binds or relates multiple features about an event or fact across physically disparate neocortical regions. Information processed in visual cortex, such as a person's face, and information processed in auditory cortex, such as a person's name, would elicit different patterns of activity in the hippocampal formation when experienced in isolation. However, when learned in association with one another, a face and a name may evoke a different pattern of activity from unassociated faces and names, suggesting that the hippocampal formation is important for combining distinct, domain-specific features of an experience.[12] Over time, the features somehow become consolidated and no longer require the hippocampal complex for binding. It is thought that temporally limited retrograde amnesia reflects the disruption of consolidation processes.

Damage to a neocortical region results in both the loss of previously acquired memory or knowledge stored in that area and an inability to acquire new memories involving that kind of knowledge. For example, patients with left temporal lesions lose specific knowledge about the names of animals, tools, or people, depending on the location of the lesion.[13] Thus, neocortical damage is thought to result in domain-specific memory deficits in which the loss of old memories and the inability to gain new memories reflect the kind of knowledge represented in that neocortical region.

In contrast, damage to medial temporal lobe, diencephalic, and basal forebrain regions yield widespread, or domain-independent, declarative memory deficits. Global amnesia can arise from damage to any one of these regions, even if the other regions remain intact. Bilateral damage to these regions can yield a global amnesia that affects all domains of declarative memory. Unilateral left- or right-sided lesions typically result in material-specific memory dysfunctions for, respectively, verbal or nonverbal information. An important exception to this rule occurs in patients with long-standing unilateral injury, such as that seen sometimes in epilepsy. In such cases, the relatively spared contralateral brain region may become critical for verbal and nonverbal memory functions.

The medial temporal region includes a number of interconnected but anatomically distinct structures: the amygdala, the hippocampal region that includes the cornu ammonis (CA) fields, dentate gyrus, and subiculum; the entorhinal cortex; the perirhinal cortex; and the parahippocampal cortex. Research with animals and humans indicates that these structures all have their own specialized roles in memory. It is now thought that the amygdala is not critical for most aspects of declarative memory. Rather, the amygdala appears to play a specific role in the emotional modulation of memories; its role in fear conditioning is especially well documented.[14] Focal damage to the CA1 region of the hippocampus is sufficient to result in a clinically substantial declarative memory deficit.[15] More widespread damage to the entorhinal, perirhinal, and parahippocampal regions (Fig. 5–2) results in increasingly devastating memory deficits.[16] In addition, the fornix constitutes the major subcortical output pathway of the hippocampal region. Damage to the fornix can produce global amnesia.[17] The specific mnemonic roles of medial temporal lobe regions critical for declarative memory ability have not yet been well characterized in humans. Functional neuroimaging and electrophysiological recordings in humans, however, have suggested that the formation of new declarative memories involves distinct, serially organized subprocesses associated with the parahippocampal cortex, the rhinal cortices, and the hippocampal formation.[18–20] Further, subicular and

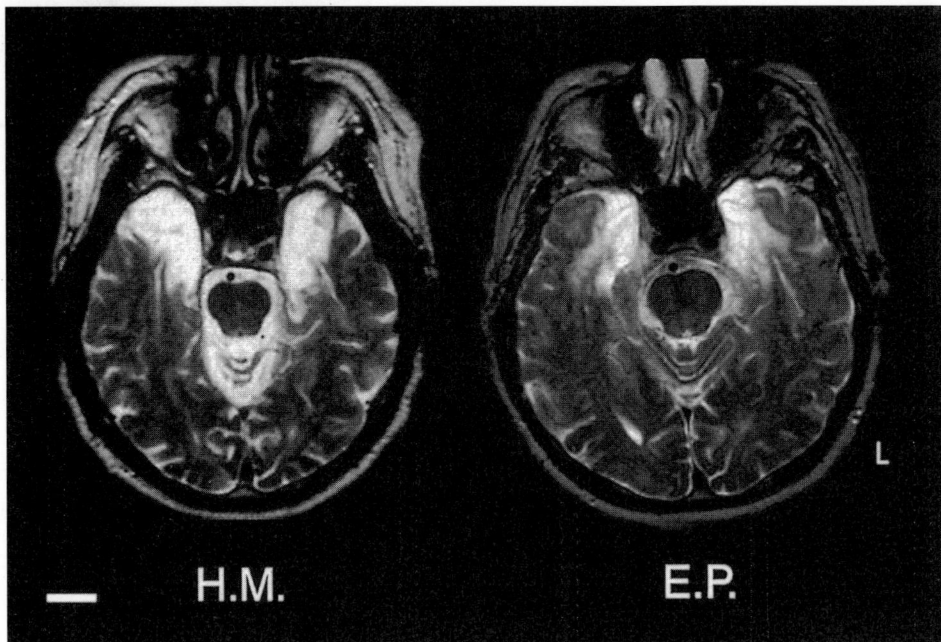

FIGURE 5–2. T2-weighted axial MRIs at the level of the temporal lobes of two patients with severe and selective global amnesias: H.M. *(left)* and E.P. *(right)*. Regions with brighter intensity indicate damaged tissue. Both patients sustained extensive medial temporal lobe damage, including hippocampal, entorhinal, perirhinal, and parahippocampal regions. Images are oriented such that the left side of the brain is on the right side of the image. The scale bar, 2 cm, applies to both images. (Reprinted from Stefanacci L, Buffalo EA, Schmolck H, et al: Profound amnesia after damage to the medial temporal lobe: A neuroanatomical and neuropsychological profile of patient E.P. J Neurosci 2000; 20(14): 7024–7036, copyright 2000 by the Society for Neuroscience.)

entorhinal areas appear to participate in the retrieval of recently[21] or more remotely[22] learned information.

Diencephalic regions linked to declarative memory include the dorsomedial and anterior nuclei of the thalamus, the mammillary bodies, the mammillothalamic fiber tract connecting the medial hippocampal complex to the anterior thalamic nuclei, and the ventroamygdalofugal fiber tract connecting the amygdala to the dorsomedial nuclei. The precise roles of these structures are not well specified, in part because damage tends to co-occur in multiple structures. For example, the mammillary bodies and dorsomedial nuclei are both greatly affected in alcoholic Korsakoff's amnesia. Acute thalamic lesions producing amnesia often injure both the dorsomedial nucleus and the surrounding mammillothalamic and ventroamygdalofugal tracts. The preponderance of the evidence favors a critical role for the dorsomedial nucleus of the thalamus and, perhaps, the surrounding fibers of the mammillothalamic tract.[23] The importance of the mammillary bodies is less certain. Lesions there sometimes appear to account for declarative memory deficits in patients[24] but do not produce the long-lasting memory impairments seen in monkeys that have sustained medial temporal or dorsomedial thalamic lesions. Declarative memory failure after diencephalic lesions appears to be quite similar to that seen after medial-temporal lesions, although additional nonmnemonic deficits may result from diencephalic lesions.

The basal forebrain is composed of midline structures, including the septal nuclei, diagonal band of Broca, and substantia innominata. These regions provide the largest input of acetylcholine, the neurotransmitter most directly implicated as critical for declarative memory, to the hippocampus and many neocortical areas. The basal forebrain also supplies to the cerebral cortex other neurotransmitters that contribute to the modulation of memory, including dopamine, norepinephrine, and serotonin. An extensive lesion to the basal forebrain yields a severe declarative memory impairment.[25] Partial damage to this and adjacent ventromedial frontal cortex often occurs after ruptures of anterior communicating artery aneurysms, which often lead to mild but persistent anterograde amnesia.[26]

There is increasing evidence of a correlation between the severity of anterograde amnesia and the extent of retrograde amnesia. Further, the severity of both anterograde and retrograde amnesia appear to correlate with the extent of medial-temporal injury.[15] Some patients with mild anterograde amnesias, however, show a surprising loss of personal memories concerning major life events or family members.[27] These patients typically have sustained damage to the more lateral temporal neocortex, which may store long-term autobiographical memory representations. These patients fail to exhibit the temporally graded retrograde amnesia characteristic of patients with lesions restricted to medial-temporal areas.

ANATOMY OF NONDECLARATIVE MEMORY

Whereas declarative memory depends on the integrity of a limited number of brain regions, nondeclarative memory encompasses all other forms of memory mediated by all other brain regions. In this sense, nondeclarative memory may be described as more diffuse in its neural representation. Each specific form of nondeclarative memory, however, is closely linked to specific brain structures and regions.

Immediate memory stores appear to be located in posterior neocortical regions, the location reflecting the modality (auditory or visual) and material (verbal or nonverbal) of the briefly retained information. For immediate auditory memory, left and right temporal-parietal cortices, respectively, mediate auditory verbal and nonverbal material. For immediate visual memory, left and right occipitoparietal cortices, respectively, mediate immediate verbal and nonverbal material. Thus, a reduced ability to immediately recall aurally presented digit strings occurs in patients with left temporal-parietal lesions.

Working memory processes that support selective aspects of declarative memory have been linked to the dorsolateral frontal cortex and to basal ganglia and cerebellar areas that are directly or indirectly linked to the dorsolateral frontal cortex. The prevailing view is that there are discrete dorsolateral frontal areas that direct the rehearsal of the immediate memory stores. Thus, keeping a spatial location in mind may involve a right frontal area that directs the maintenance of that information in a right parietal area, whereas keeping a word in mind may involve a left frontal area that directs the maintenance of that information in a left temporal or parietal area.[28] Specific basal ganglia and cerebellar areas appear to support the working memory capacity of particular frontal regions.

Implicit memory processes appear to depend on the same brain regions that mediate performance in any given domain. By this view, implicit memory reflects adaptive plasticity within neural systems that occurs in the course of the support by those systems of particular forms of behavior. Thus, motor-skill learning has been linked to pyramidal, extrapyramidal, and cerebellar motor systems.[29] Interestingly, perceptual and cognitive skill learning has also been linked to the same action systems, with some evidence indicating that they may reflect adjacent but separable frontostriatal and frontocerebellar circuits. Perceptual repetition priming has been linked to modality-specific neocortices (e.g., visual priming with visual cortex)[30] and conceptual repetition priming has been linked to polymodal linguistic neocortical regions in the left frontal and left temporoparietal areas.[31]

Classic conditioning has been well characterized as being dependent on the dentate and interpositus nuclei of the cerebellum in animals, and such conditioning depends on the same cerebellar structures in humans.[32] More complicated conditioning paradigms appear to require, in addition, medial-temporal regions.[33]

MEMORY-RELATED ANATOMICAL CHANGES

Memories are presumably formed by experience-induced changes in the operating characteristics of single cells, local circuits, and large-scale systems. Little is known directly about how these changes occur in the human brain. A great deal is known about some memory-related phenomena at cellular levels in in vitro and invertebrate models, such as the marine snail *Aplysia*. These findings offer suggestions about the cellular bases of human memories.

Aplysia withdraw their gills when stimulated with a brief jet of seawater. Repeated stimulation, however, leads to habituation such that the gills are no longer withdrawn. Habituation has been linked to decreasing presynaptic transmitter release. In other conditions, repeated stimulation can lead to sensitization. For example, a strong noxious stimulation, such as an electrical shock, can intensify a subsequent withdrawal response to a touch. Sensitization involves an increase of transmitter release from a facilitating interneuron.[34]

Long-term, but not short-term, memory processes require messenger RNA and protein synthesis.[35] These findings indicate that there are genes and proteins that guide long-term memories that are not invoked in short-term memories. These long-term changes may involve structural changes in presynaptic neurons. Long-term habituation may involve a pruning of presynaptic terminals, whereas sensitization may involve a proliferation of presynaptic terminals.[36] A strong candidate for a cellular basis of mammalian learning is long-term potentiation (LTP). A neuron becomes potentiated (i.e., increasingly responsive to new input of the same type) for minutes, days, or weeks when it is bombarded with brief but rapid series of stimulations. The fact that simultaneous stimulation of different synapses, or cooperativity, is required for LTP makes it a promising mechanism for associative learning at the level of a single cell. Cooperativity and other sources of evidence indicate that the postsynaptic neuron triggers LTP. LTP-induced changes in postsynaptic neurons are known to increase the concentration of calcium in dendrites, which activates a cascade of protein phosphorylation leading to changes in synaptic properties. LTP has been extensively studied in hippocampal synapses, in which *N*-methyl-D-aspartate glutamate receptors are of critical importance for the establishment, but not the maintenance, of LTP. There is evidence of similar mechanisms in the amygdala, cerebellum, and cerebral cortex. LTP in different brain regions exhibits different rates of development and stability, suggesting the involvement of multiple cellular mechanisms.

Another source of plasticity does not involve changes between existing synaptic connections but the formation of new neurons. Neurogenesis has been observed in the dentate gyrus of the hippocampus throughout the lives of many species,[37–39] including humans.[40] Not all newly generated hippocampal neurons survive, but hippocampal-dependent memory tasks can enhance the survival of these neurons, whereas hippocampal-independent memory tasks provide no such benefit.[41] In addition, these new neurons may be functionally important for memory formation in hippocampal-dependent memory tasks because a reduction in the number of such neurons impairs learning in such tasks.[42]

MEMORY-RELATED CHEMICAL CHANGES

The specific roles of different neurotransmitters in memory are just beginning to be appreciated. The cholinergic system appears to be critical for the acquisition of long-term declarative memories. In healthy subjects, cholinergic antagonists such as scopolamine impair declarative memory performance, whereas agonists such as physostigmine facilitate such performance.[43] Some nondeclarative forms of memory, however, are not affected by scopolamine. Cholinergic function decreases somewhat with age and greatly in patients with Alzheimer's disease,[44] and these changes may contribute importantly to corresponding reductions in declarative memory ability.

The catecholamines appear to have an important role in working memory. Dopaminergic function is decreased in patients with Parkinson's disease, who have reduced working memory capacity. There is some evidence that dopamine agonists can improve working memory capacity in patients with Parkinson's disease[45] and in healthy subjects.[46]

Examination of Memory

DIRECTED NEUROLOGICAL EXAMINATION

The first goal of the neurological examination of memory is to ascertain that memory impairment is not secondary either to a specific perceptual, motor, or cognitive disability or to a broad impairment of mental status. This goal can be accomplished by performing a mental status assessment and brief bedside tests of orientation, receptive and expressive language, and visual constructional abilities. Confusional states can be evaluated both informally, while the patient tells his or her history, by noting confusion or incoherence in thinking, anxiety level, and inconsistencies and inaccuracies about dates and symptoms, and formally by asking about the present day, date, place, and year. Further memory assessment should be undertaken only if a patient's level and content of consciousness and attention are determined to be unimpaired. One widely used standardized mental status test is the mini mental status examination.[47]

The second goal of the directed neurological examination is to characterize the nature of a primary memory problem by the use of brief tests of immediate, long-term, and remote memory. Tests of immediate memory require the patient to repeat exactly a series of random digits; normal adults can repeat 5 to 7 digits. Such tests assess the ability to attend to events adequately and to encode information. Immediate memory is relatively spared in patients with even the most severe amnesias and moderate dementias. Failure to immediately repeat 5 digits in the order presented suggests a problem in attention or orientation. The rare exceptions include patients with specific immediate memory deficits who may be differentiated from inattentive patients by virtue of their intact immediate memory in another modality (e.g., when shown 5 digits visually).

Tests of long-term memory (often referred to as short-term memory in standard neurological usage) require the patient to remember and later recall (e.g., after 3 minutes) three items of information (e.g., words or objects). It is useful to warn the patient that memory will be tested for the information and to have the patient immediately repeat the words or name the objects to rule out attentional, perceptual, and linguistic bases for any later memory failure. It is important that the delay between the study and the test be filled with activity such as counting before the patient is asked to recall the words or objects. Otherwise, a patient may quietly rehearse the words, and the test no longer measures long-term memory. In patients with expressive aphasia, demands on speech production may be bypassed by having the patient select the test object from a set of objects. Such tests assess the ability to learn new material and evaluate the possibility of anterograde amnesia.

Tests of remote memory used to evaluate the possibility of retrograde amnesia (often referred to as long-term memory in standard neurological usage) require patients to recall past personal, geographic, or historical facts (e.g., the names of the last six presidents).

ASSOCIATED NEUROLOGICAL FINDINGS

Cerebral. The presence of accompanying cortical signs other than memory loss helps to localize the anatomical basis of an amnestic syndrome. Accompanying dyspraxia, aphasia, or agnosia indicates that the cortex is involved in the pathological process. An assessment of affect is also important, because depression can produce a picture of seeming dementia (pseudodementia). Emotional lability or poor voluntary control over emotional expression (pseudobulbar affect) can occur in patients with conditions that affect both cortices or with progressive supranuclear palsy.

Cranial Nerves. In the context of compromised cognition, cranial nerve abnormalities are valuable in elucidating the underlying location and cause. Increased intracranial pressure is suggested by papilledema and cranial nerve VI paresis, and progressive supranuclear palsy often produces distinctive defects in volitional conjugate vertical gaze. A variety of extraocular muscle pareses and nystagmus may accompany Wernicke-Korsakoff syndrome, and visual field defects of a homonymous hemianopia pattern suggest the presence of deep lesions of the white matter pathways, which are seen in patients with thalamic and temporal lobe disorders. Multiple cranial nerve deficits are seen in patients with chronic meningitis.

Motor/Reflexes/Cerebellar/Gait. Chorea and dystonia suggest the possibility of Huntington's disease. Bradykinesia, tremor, rigidity, and postural reflex impairment are seen in Parkinson's disease, and myoclonus typifies postanoxia syndromes and spongiform encephalopathies, among other conditions. Primitive reflexes such as snout, plantar extension, and palmomental reflexes, such as rooting responses, suggest the presence of bilateral cortical, subcortical, or brain stem disease. Ataxia and other cerebellar signs may occur in patients with Wernicke-Korsakoff syndrome. Asymmetrical reflexes and mixed areas of weakness (e.g., a slight facial paresis on one side and a mild weakness of a leg or arm on the other side) suggest multiple strokes, often subcortical in location.

Sensory. Primary sensory function is difficult to test in patients with memory or cognitive impairment because they are often inattentive and inconsistent in their responses. If primary sensation is normal and a deficit in higher cortical sensory processing is present, such as astereognosis, extinction, or neglect, a cortical disorder should be suspected. Preferential vibration and position sensory loss in combination with memory problems may suggest vitamin B_{12} deficiency, whereas severe, painful crises and loss of pin and temperature sensation are more typical of syphilitic illness.

Autonomic Nervous System. In patients with diffuse sympathetic hyperactivity that can occur in the presence of hypothalamic lesions, bilaterally dilated pupils can occur, along with cardiac dysrhythmias and blood pressure instability.

Neurovascular. In the context of possible strokes, the neck vessels should be examined, and evidence of orthostatic hypotension should be sought.

ASSOCIATED MEDICAL FINDINGS

Impaired memory and cognitive functioning are characteristic of drug intoxication or withdrawal as well as of several systemic diseases such as vitamin deficiencies, endocrine disorders, chronic infections, and carcinomas. A general physical examination, therefore, is necessary to identify the precipitating cause. Typically, in disorders of memory such as dementia and amnesic syndromes, the patient does not appear to be acutely ill unless a systemic disorder is also present.

The general physical examination may reveal reversible memory disturbances, the most common causes of which are intracranial masses, normal pressure hydrocephalus, thyroid dysfunction, and vitamin B_{12} deficiency. Examination of the patient's general appearance, vital signs, skin and mucous membranes, head, neck, chest, and abdomen should reveal clinical signs that will aid in the differential diagnoses of dementia and amnesic syndromes. Fever, tachycardia, hypertension or hypotension, sweating, hypothermia, and impaired level of consciousness should suggest a systemic disease, anticholinergic intoxication, or withdrawal from ethanol or sedative drugs rather than an isolated memory disorder. Jaundice suggests hepatic disease; glossitis, intestinal problems, and yellowish skin suggest a vitamin B_{12} deficiency; hot, dry skin is often characteristic of anticholinergic drug intoxication. Hypothermia, hypotension, bradycardia, coarse dry skin, brittle hair, and subcutaneous edema are characteristic of hypothyroidism. Recent trauma to the head may be evidenced by scalp lacerations or contusions and pain. Positive Kernig's and Brudzinski's signs are found in cases of meningitis and subarachnoid hemorrhage.

Evaluation Guidelines (Table 5–2)

Neuroimaging. Neuroimaging techniques provide valuable information in the assessment of extent of structural and functional brain abnormalities in a patient. These data can be used to target further assessment of a patient's memory complaint. Gross structural abnormalities are often adequately revealed by computed tomography, but more refined volumetric assessment of the deep cortical structures such as the hippocampal formation and amygdala are better visualized by magnetic resonance imaging (MRI). Lesions that can be detected include space-occupying masses like tumors or abscesses and diffuse or focal degenerative illnesses involving the cortex and subcortical regions. Whereas diffuse atrophy typifies Alzheimer's disease, prominent frontal or parietal lobe atrophy is characteristic of Pick's disease. Contrast infusion studies highlight the abnormalities seen in vascular disorders and hence may help in leading the clinician to the proper etiological diagnosis.

Other functional neuroimaging techniques, such as positron-emission tomography and single photon emission computed tomography, assess global metabolic patterns and are useful in assessing the diffuse neuronal loss that occurs in degenerative diseases. For instance, in patients with dementias marked by memory loss, such as Alzheimer's disease, hypometabolism occurs primarily bilaterally in the temporal-parietal regions with relative sparing of the posterior cortices.[48] In contrast, in dementias marked by relative sparing of memory, such as Pick's disease, hypometabolism occurs primarily in the bilateral frontal cortices.[49] These techniques, plus, more recently, functional MRI, offer great potential for clinical application in the diagnosis and assessment of memory disorders. In their current state of development, however, they remain predominantly research tools because their specificity and sensitivity to specific diseases of memory are not yet sufficient for diagnostic purposes. They may, however, be useful when a patient's pattern of memory loss and sparing is difficult to comprehend and structural imaging reveals no lesions. In these cases, atypical functioning of a particular brain region may provide useful information.

Electrophysiology. Electroencephalography (EEG) is used routinely to detect the gross locus and nature of seizure activity in patients with epilepsy, although an abnormal EEG may result from any number of conditions, including tumors, abscesses, and subdural hematomas. Memory problems are mainly associated with medial temporal lobe epilepsy, and the nature of memory deficits varies with the epileptogenic hemisphere. EEG data are of limited value in indexing a memory deficit because often other areas of the epileptogenic hemisphere or the nonepileptogenic hemisphere may appropriate the memory functions normally subserved by the epileptic tissue. Consequently, the patient may present with very mild or no memory deficits. EEG data are valuable in the diagnosis of sleep disorders that can result in memory problems. In many dementing processes, the EEG shows a diffuse and nonspecific slowing that may be most predominant in the temporal regions. Distinctive processes, such as periodic 1- to 2-cycle-per-second slow-wave triphasic spike activity or a burst suppression pattern, may suggest dementing illnesses such as spongiform encephalopathies.

Body Fluid and Tissue Analysis. Memory impairment may occur secondarily to conditions such as drug and alcohol intoxication or withdrawal and to systemic diseases such as vitamin deficiencies, endocrine disorders (specifically thyroid disease), chronic infections, or carcinomas. These are often treatable conditions diagnosed by analysis of tissue (by biopsy) or fluids (by tests of blood and urine). When a treatable condition is found, further evaluation of memory need not be performed unless the memory impairment persists or becomes worse after the underlying disease has been treated. Some tests, such as the sedimentation rate, are nonspecific but lead the investigator toward other tests that may properly document a condition such as vasculitis or cerebritis. Choice of the biopsy site depends on the diagnosis being actively entertained—for example, amyloidosis is often diagnosed by rectal biopsy, whereas temporal arteritis is diagnosed by examination of the temporal artery itself. In patients with memory problems in whom management or treatment depends directly on a specific diagnosis, a brain biopsy should be considered. Instances include primary cerebral vasculitis, spongiform encephalopathies, tumors that require specific treatment, or likely infections, abscesses, or cysts.

Genetic testing is a new and growing potential source of evaluative information. In some cases (e.g., Huntington's disease), it is part of a standard diagnosis, but in other cases it is optional. In patients with Alzheimer's disease, atypical

TABLE 5–2. **Various Causes of Dementia**

Alzheimer's disease
Multi-infarct dementia
Alcoholic dementia
Intracranial tumors
Normal pressure hydrocephalus
Chronic drug intoxication
Metabolic states
Vitamin B_{12} deficiency, thyroid disease
Infectious illnesses
Spongiform encephalopathy, chronic meningitis, neurosyphilis, AIDS
Other neurological disorders
Parkinson's disease, progressive supranuclear palsy, Huntington's disease

early-onset cases may be screened for specific mutations on chromosomes 1, 14, and 21. More typical cases of Alzheimer's disease have been linked to apolipoprotein E4 alleles, but this linkage is probabilistic.[50] Because such genetic testing cannot definitively determine the diagnosis of Alzheimer's disease, drawbacks to such screening are salient. One drawback is that the appropriate diagnosis of dementia or Alzheimer's disease could be overly influenced by genetic information. A second drawback concerns the complex and controversial ethical issues involved in deciding whether this information should be available to the patient, family members, or insurers when the information does not define a disease. For these reasons, it is reasonable to suggest that apolipoprotein E testing is not yet appropriate for clinical use.

Cerebrospinal Fluid. Once a space-occupying lesion has been excluded, cerebrospinal fluid (CSF) may be obtained for analysis of treatable causes of memory problems. Infection, in the form of a chronic meningitis, is suggested by the presence of white blood cells and in patients with tertiary syphilis, inflammatory cells and positive serological tests (CSF, Venereal Disease Research Laboratories test) are diagnostic.

Neuropsychological Tests. One of the most important goals of neuropsychological testing is to determine whether the patient has a "pure" memory deficit or whether the deficit is due to a defect in some general cognitive function. Thus, neuropsychological testing should be comprehensive enough to identify the patient's strengths as well as weaknesses. The most widely used standard battery of tests of anterograde memory is the Wechsler Memory Scale (WMS)—Revised,[51] which includes a variety of subtests that assess verbal and nonverbal immediate and delayed memory and attention span. The battery yields five indices (verbal, visual, general memory, attention-concentration, and delayed recall). The criteria for a diagnosis of amnesia are considered a normal attention-concentration score but an impaired delayed recall score. Although the test is widely used, a major limitation is that it does not discriminate well between moderate and severe forms of amnesia. The WMS-R measures free recall and cued recall but not recognition memory, and therefore, both moderately and severely impaired patients often perform at the same low level. Further, it may not discriminate well between different types of memory disorders, such as that following frontal lobe lesions, which results in a selective memory impairment on recall tests, and that following temporal lobe lesions, which results in a global memory impairment on both recall and recognition tests.

A memory battery that does incorporate both recall and recognition measures is the California Verbal Learning Test (CVLT).[52] A strength of the CVLT is that it assesses the processes driving subjects' performance such as organizing strategies and sources of interference. Assessment of visuospatial memory, however, is not included. A widely used test of visuospatial memory is the Rey-Osterrieth Complex Figure Test,[53] which includes assessment of copying and of immediate and delayed recall. It is laborious to score but allows assessment of the perceptual strategies patients use or fail to use. Patients with left-hemisphere lesions often cannot remember internal details, whereas those with right-hemisphere lesions often cannot remember the general configuration.

Retrograde amnesia is more difficult to assess because it is culturally, geographically, and temporally specific to an individual. Further, it is difficult to ascertain what a person knew years ago. There are a few standardized tests in this area, including the Boston Retrograde Amnesia Battery,[54] which assesses the extent of the temporal gradient of a person's retrograde amnesia by incorporating pictures of famous people at different ages; a temporal gradient will be revealed if the amnesic patient recognizes the person at a young but not older age. These instruments are useful for documenting major losses of knowledge but have limited value in assessing subtle or very temporally limited (e.g., days, weeks, or months) retrograde amnesias.

Memory disorders are sometimes simulated by patients, particularly when amnesia would result in financial or legal gain. In such cases, neuropsychological testing can be helpful in distinguishing real from feigned memory loss. Often patients feigning amnesia mimic psychogenic amnesia, as shown in movies and on television, and report a total retrograde amnesia without any anterograde amnesia. Such a condition has not been documented in patients with verifiable lesions, although it may occur legitimately in a psychiatric form. It is worthwhile to note that psychogenic retrograde amnesias are highly selective in terms of what is forgotten. Patients may forget their identity and personal history, but they often remember public events. This is exactly the opposite of lesion-induced retrograde amnesia in which patients remember their identity and forget personal and public experiences on the basis of temporal factors. One approach to distinguishing real from feigned anterograde memory loss is to administer easy multiple choice recognition tests in which pseudoamnesic patients may perform less well than chance if they systematically avoid selecting the correct response. Another approach is the use of implicit memory tests that yield normal results in amnesic patients. Malingering subjects often perform poorly on these tests. Unaware of the findings that amnesic patients perform at normal levels, malingering subjects purposefully avoid using information presented earlier (Colorado Malingering Tests).[55]

Clinical Syndromes of Memory Dysfunction (Table 5–3)

DEMENTIA

Dementia refers to the loss of multiple acquired cognitive and emotional abilities sufficient to interfere with daily activities. It is defined by a behavioral syndrome and not by etiology or lesion location. Its onset is often insidious and its course is often progressive. Dementia is an age-associated syndrome that has a prevalence of 1 percent at age 60 and doubles every 5 years, becoming 30 to 50 percent by age 85.[56] More than 50 diseases may produce dementia, but Alzheimer's disease is thought to account for about 70 percent of dementia cases.[57] The second main cause is multi-infarct or vascular dementia; it may account for 10 to 20 percent of dementias. Other causes of dementia, including treatable causes, are rare. Although they account for relatively smaller percentages of dementias, some neurological diseases inevitably (e.g., Huntington's disease) or frequently (e.g., Parkinson's disease) result in dementia. For diseases that are age associated, such as Parkinson's disease, it is diffi-

TABLE 5-3. **Selected Etiologies Associated with Memory Disorders**

Etiological Category	Specific Etiologies	Chapter
Structural Disorders		
Developmental disorders	Compensated hydrocephalus	28
Hereditary and Degenerative Disorders		
Chromosomal abnormalities and neurocutaneous disorders	Consanguinity	32
Degenerative dementias	Alzheimer's disease, Pick's disease	33
Movement disorders	Parkinson's disease, Huntington's disease	34
Acquired Metabolic and Nutritional Disorders		
Endogenous metabolic disorders	Hepatic encephalopathy, hypothyroidism, anoxia	38
Exogenous acquired metabolic disorders:	Anticholinergic intoxication	39
Toxins and illicit drugs	Lead intoxication	
Nutritional deficiencies and syndromes associated with alcoholism	Korsakoff's psychosis	40
	Alcoholic withdrawal	
Infectious Disorders		
Viral infections	Herpes simplex encephalitis	41
Nonviral infections	Bacterial encephalitis	42
	Cerebral abscess, bacterial meningitis	
Transmissible spongiform encephalopathies	Creutzfeldt-Jakob disease	43
HIV and AIDS	AIDS dementia complex	44
Neurovascular Disorders	Multi-infarct dementia	45
	Posterior cerebral artery occlusion	
Neoplastic Disorders		
Primary neurological tumors	Primary tumor (especially those involving the medial temporal lobe, fornix, or thalamus)	46
Metastatic neoplasms and paraneoplastic syndromes	Metastatic melanoma, paraneoplastic syndrome	47
Demyelinating Disorders		
Demyelinating disorders of the central nervous system	Multiple sclerosis, subcortical arteriosclerotic encephalopathy (Binswanger's disease)	48
Traumatic Disorders	Traumatic head injury	51
Epilepsy	Medial temporal lobe epilepsy	52
Sleep Disorders	Insomnia, sleep apnea	54
Drug-Induced and Iatrogenic Neurological Disorders	Surgical lobectomy to treat medial temporal lobe epilepsy	55
	Electroconvulsive treatment	
	Medications: analgesic, antihypertensive, anticholinergic, psychotropic, sedative	

cult to know whether dementia reflects that disease per se or comorbid Alzheimer's disease.

Dementia, unlike pure amnesia, has a virtually unlimited range of specific presentations that depend on which particular abilities are compromised. Disabilities may occur in memory, language, spatial perception, cognition, attention, high-level motor control, emotion, and motivation. The breadth and diversity of presentation require the exclusion of other bases for widespread cognitive failure, including diminished arousal or wakefulness or an acute confusional state (e.g., drug intoxication). More circumscribed deficits, such as an aphasia or amnesia, must also be excluded. As discussed later for amnesia, focal damage to mental abilities like language or memory may appear superficially as a widespread disorder of cognition. For example, an aphasic individual could appear to fail in many areas of thought if he or she cannot adequately understand or respond to questions.

In patients with Alzheimer's disease, an impairment of declarative memory is typically the first sign. This is often manifested as forgetfulness in daily tasks, with appointments missed and possessions misplaced. The gradual progression of declarative memory failure is often noted when an individual fails to accomplish a habitual task, such as maintaining a checkbook, following a recipe, or following a route home. It may be noticed better by family members than by the patient, who is losing the very memory and other intellectual abilities needed to discern a decline in mental performance.

Two factors may obscure the declarative memory deficit. First, a mild degree of declarative memory difficulty is common in aging. Second, well-established knowledge and habits may continue to guide behavior and mask a declarative memory deficit for recent experiences and novel information. Remote memories appear intact relative to recent memories, but careful testing usually reveals a temporally extensive retrograde amnesia.[58]

A second cortical dementing illness is Pick's disease, or lobar cerebral atrophy.[59] The clinical picture is similar to that seen with Alzheimer's disease, although neuroimaging studies may reveal a preferential atrophic process in the frontal or parietal lobes. In some cases, the memory problems and dementia occur in the context of deficits that suggest the preferential lobar involvement: Personality changes, aphasia, and disinhibition typify Pick's disease patients with frontal lobe involvement, and apraxias are the prominent feature in those with parietal lesions.[60] In many patients with Pick's disease, however, the deficits appear to be more global, and the patients are not specifically separable clinically from subjects with Alzheimer's disease.

In the later stages of Alzheimer's disease, the cognitive deficits become more pronounced and pervasive.[61] The language deficit is severe in all aspects of production and comprehension. Patients lose their arithmetic skills. Spatial disorientation extends to simple everyday tasks such as dress. Patients forget how to use common objects and tools. Florid psychiatric symptoms occur, including delusions and visual hallucinations.[62] Parkinsonian motor signs become more apparent and lead to problems in locomotion. Finally, the patient lies in bed and must be fed and bathed. This progression occurs over a course of 5 or more years and often consists of alternating precipitous declines and plateaus of little apparent change.[63]

CORTICAL VERSUS SUBCORTICAL DEMENTING SYNDROMES

A distinction has been noted between the cortical dementia typically seen in Alzheimer's or Pick's disease and the subcortical dementia typified by Huntington's and Parkinson's disease but noted also in progressive supranuclear palsy, multiple sclerosis, Wilson's disease, and human immunodeficiency virus infection.[64] Dementia seen in diseases with primarily subcortical neuropathology features slowed movement (bradykinesia) and thought (bradyphrenia); disproportionate problems in the efficient use of memory; poor planning, judgment, and reasoning; and often affective changes.

The distinction is not absolute because most of these diseases are not limited to either cortical or subcortical regions, and therefore many patients exhibit elements of both kinds of dementia. Most of the differences between cortical and subcortical dementia are matters of degree and proportion rather than strict dichotomies. These characteristic differences in the patterns of dementias may be more distinct in the early, mild stages; the distinctions are less clear in later stages.

When measured formally, impairments in speed of mental processing, working memory, reasoning, and strategic memory (e.g., recall) are evident in nondemented patients with striatal diseases, including patients with early Parkinson's disease.[65] These deficits are highly intercorrelated, suggesting that they reflect a family of interacting memory processes mediated by frontostriatal neural circuits. In nondemented patients, these deficits may be circumscribed, and the patients perform normally on tests of immediate memory, semantic memory, nonstrategic declarative memory (recognition), and language. When dementia develops in a patient with a subcortical disease, problems in speed of mental processing, working memory, reasoning, and strategic memory then become disproportionately severe relative to other problems in language or memory. The disproportionate deficit in strategic memory may be contrasted with the more proportionate and global declarative memory deficits (e.g., recall and recognition) seen in persons with Alzheimer's disease or amnesia. In addition, demented patients with Parkinson's or Huntington's disease often have deficits in procedural forms of memory, motoric and nonmotoric, that remain intact in patients with Alzheimer's disease and amnesia. Thus, disproportionate impairments in speed of mental processing, working memory, reasoning, strategic memory, and procedural memory may reflect disproportionate damage to the frontostriatal regions in diseases that initially affect those brain regions.

AMNESIA

Amnesia refers to a relatively circumscribed deficit in declarative memory that cannot be accounted for by impairments in attention, language, motivation, reasoning, or other nonmnemonic abilities. It is defined by a behavioral syndrome and not by etiology or lesion location. The severity of the deficit can vary considerably, but at a minimum it interferes with daily activities and quality of life. The purity of the deficit also varies because many patients have some degree of other cognitive difficulties as well. To the extent that those difficulties are mild and do not account for the memory deficit, a patient may be classified as amnesic. Otherwise, a patient may be better classified as demented, with memory being one of multiple deficits. The amnesia is described as global if it extends to both verbal and nonverbal information. The amnesic patient performs well on tests of attention, reasoning, and general information as long as the tests do not make demands on declarative memory.

Patients with pure amnesia have a pervasive impairment on tests of declarative memory. The anterograde amnesia extends to memory for all sorts of materials and events in all modalities. It is apparent in both easy and difficult tests of memory. The severity of amnesia varies considerably, however, so that a mildly amnesic patient could perform well on easy tests of memory. Because judgment is preserved in amnesic patients, they are usually aware of having a memory problem. They may, however, underestimate the severity of the problem because they are aware only of memory difficulties at the present moment and cannot remember the sorts of memory failures they experienced earlier.

Amnesic patients perform normally on tests of immediate memory, classic conditioning, skill learning (motoric, perceptual, and cognitive), and perceptual and conceptual repetition priming.[1] Declarative memory, however, is often invoked by tests that are not ostensibly memory tests. Many complex tests of cognition require some degree of declarative memory, if only to remember the instructions for the test. Other tests confound anterograde amnesia with general knowledge. For example, a patient who became amnesic in 1985 would not know the current president of the United States and other sorts of widely known information about events since 1985. For the same reason, a purely amnesic patient could even fail to answer some questions used to probe orientation, such as where the patient is at present. The amnesic patient would not remember the name or address of a hospital or medical building and would not know the day, month, or year because all of these facts are learned via declarative memory. For these reasons, intelligent amnesic patients may earn a poor score on a standard dementia rating scale. Pure amnesia is quite rare, so routine application of assessment measures may be misleading.

Amnesia by definition features an anterograde amnesia, and a retrograde loss of memories is frequently but variably present. The retrograde amnesia is typically temporally graded, with more recent memories being most vulnerable to amnesia and remote memories most likely to be spared. In general, the severity of anterograde and retrograde amnesias are correlated. If a lesion extends laterally from medial temporal lobe areas, it may injure temporal lobe regions that normally represent autobiographical knowledge. Such a lesion would exacerbate the retrograde amnesia and lead to a more extensive loss of acquired memories, even important ones from remote time periods.

Amnesic syndromes can occur in isolation or can be accompanied by other neurological signs. In patients with the Wernicke-Korsakoff syndrome (see Chapter 40), which is often associated with thiamine deficiency but also with head trauma, epilepsy, and anoxia, amnesia may develop in the context of ataxia and extraocular muscle pareses. An overall confusional state may be seen early in such cases, but the enduring learning and memory deficit is the most distinctive mental aberration of this syndrome. In such cases, the anatomical lesion should be sought in the diencephalon, medial temporal lobes, mammillary bodies, and connecting pathways of these regions regardless of etiology.

PSEUDODEMENTIA

The term *pseudodementia* refers generically to treatable disorders that mimic dementia. The most common is depression. Depression and dementia can both lead to reduced motivation, impaired concentration, and mental slowing. Consequently, both diseases can lead to widespread cognitive and memory dysfunctions. Formal testing has shown that purely depressed patients perform better on declarative memory tests than genuinely demented patients, but this difference may be difficult to determine in particular patients. Because depression, with or without the co-occurrence of dementia, is treatable, it should be considered in any diagnostic evaluation. Some instruments, such as the Geriatric Depression Scale, may be useful in diagnosing depression in elderly individuals.

TRANSIENT GLOBAL AMNESIA

Transient global amnesia is a relatively rare syndrome characterized by a sudden onset of severe anterograde amnesia and confusion that often includes repetitive questioning. Patients are often disoriented in regard to time and place but usually not personal identity. The confusion may simply reflect a response to the amnesia (e.g., if an amnesic patient asks what is wrong with his or her memory or what the date is, he will forget any answer provided within moments). The absence of such overt confusion and repetitive questioning in chronic amnesia patients may reflect an eventual accommodation of the patient to the amnesic state. Transient global amnesia typically lasts for hours, although its duration may range from minutes to days. Retrograde amnesia is also common, although its severity varies much more than that of anterograde amnesia. Retrograde amnesia is usually extensive and is temporally graded. As the anterograde amnesia gradually resolves, the temporal extent of the retrograde amnesia appears to shrink. After recovery, the patient retains an amnesia for the period of the transient global amnesia and often for a few hours preceding it.[66] Transient global amnesia is often associated with atherosclerotic disease, especially ischemia in the posterior circulation, but seizure activity and migraine attacks have also been posited as a mechanism in some cases. In patients with this syndrome, an EEG may show abnormalities, although in most cases the findings are nonspecific. Attacks recur in less than 25 percent of patients, and fewer than 5 percent have more than three. The frequency of seizures or subsequent strokes is no different from that in a comparable age-matched population. No special treatment is indicated for these unusual cases of transient but traumatic memory impairment.

General Management Goals

The first goal is to diagnose any treatable memory problems. These include cases in which the problem is secondary to a treatable illness, such as depression or a systemic disease. Memory problems arising from medications may be treated by discontinuing any unneeded medications or considering alternative medications for needed treatments.

For untreatable causes of memory disorders, the main goal is to establish a framework for the care of patients who are or will be unable to take care of themselves. Informing the patient involves judgment about what information is useful to the patient. On the one hand, it is desirable to have the patient feel that he or she is at the center of the management goals. On the other hand, patients with severe memory disorders remember little of what is told to them, and discussions may produce distress for the patient with no benefit.

A primary consideration is the safety and security of the patient. Patients with dementia or pure amnesia have a limited ability to take care of themselves. Patients should be protected, therefore, from taking actions that may cause injury to themselves and others and for which they can no longer be held responsible. If a patient is still working, a plan for retirement should be initiated. A plan for the daily supervision of the patient should be developed that takes into account the present mental status of the patient and the resources of the family. It is usually advantageous, when possible, for the patient to sustain habits of daily activities in a familiar environment because these habits rely on abilities that are the last to decline. Supervision of the patient must be considered in terms of medical care, diet, medications, and daily activities. A common and difficult problem is determining when certain activities, particularly driving, become potentially dangerous. Legal issues, such as conservatorships, often arise at some stage of the disease. The nature of these issues varies a great deal between patients with chronic amnesia, in which the patient's judgment may remain intact, and those with dementia, in which judgment typically declines considerably. In both cases, however, patients cannot be responsible for or take care of themselves. For those with progressive diseases, however, hospitalization is inevitable.

Information given to family members is critical in several respects. First, they have to understand what the patients can and cannot do for themselves. This is important not only for practical reasons, but also because uninformed family members may misinterpret the actions of a memory-impaired patient as reflecting poor motivation or judgment. Therefore, family members must have as clear a picture as possible about the patient's abilities and disabilities.

Important information includes whether the memory impairment is chronic and whether it is likely to improve or become worse. It is useful for family members to understand whether the memory disorder is global or limited. It is also important for them to understand how pervasive a declarative memory disorder can be because few people appreciate how memory constantly supports the activities of daily living, including the taking of medications, preparing or eating meals, paying bills, and so on. Often, patients and family members are surprised by the contrast between anterograde amnesia and relative preservation of memory for remote periods. The severity and purity of the memory disorder dictate whether the patient can provide some degree of compensation in daily life. For example, patients with mild or moderate amnesias and without other major cognitive deficits can use notes or computers, especially small portable computers, to keep a useful record of goals and appointments. Even in these cases, however, frequent supervision is needed because important information may be ignored. Patients with severe amnesia or substantial additional cognitive deficits often cannot use such external memory devices effectively because they cannot even remember to use the devices.

It is also helpful to remind family members that memory-disordered patients retain many of their intellectual and emotional capacities and therefore need to have an active, regular schedule. Even patients with substantial memory or cognitive problems can slowly adapt to a regular, well-structured schedule. It is good to maintain a relatively normal sleep-wake cycle that ensures a good rest at night. This may require efforts to keep the patient awake during the day. Medications may be required to sustain a healthy sleep-wake cycle. Conversely, unexpected events can be exceptionally distressing to patients who cannot cope with novel circumstances.

In many respects, the diagnosis of dementia or chronic amnesia is as devastating to family members as to the patients. Family members face a long and difficult personal path in terms of emotional, financial, and often legal issues. This burden falls on the very shoulders of those who must now take exceptional responsibility for the care of their spouse, parent, or sibling. It is not uncommon for them to have strong feelings of denial, guilt, or blame. These feelings may not only affect the family members, but also compromise the supervision of the patient. It is important to monitor the mental health of family members and to encourage the use of appropriate resources, including social services and support groups.

Finally, medical care for the memory-disordered patient must be maintained. For example, a number of diseases that lead to memory disorders also lead to seizures that must be treated. Medical supervision is challenging because amnesic patients are often unable to provide any useful history, and demented patients may be unable to answer even simple questions about their present condition.

Reviews and Selected Updates

Alexander MP, Stuss DT: Disorders of frontal lobe functioning. Semin Neurol 2000;20:427–437.

Baddeley AD, Wilson BA, Watts FN: Memory Disorders. New York, Wiley & Sons, 1995.

Bennett MR, Hacker PM: Perception and memory in neuroscience: A conceptual analysis. Prog Neurobiol 2001;65:499–543.

Connor L: Memory in old age: Patterns of decline and preservation. Semin Speech Lang 2001;22:117–125.

Duke LM, Kaszniak AW: Executive control functions in degenerative dementias: A comparative review. Neuropsychol Rev 2000;10:75–99.

Duncan J, Owen AM: Common regions of the human frontal lobe recruited by diverse cognitive demands. Trends Neurosci 2000;23:475–483.

Ellis KA, Nathan PJ: The pharmacology of human working memory. Int J Neuropsychopharmacol 2001;4:299–313.

Gabrieli JDE: Differential effects of aging and age-related neurological diseases on memory subsystems of the human brain. *In* Boller F, Grafman J (eds): Handbook of Neuropsychology. Amsterdam, Elsevier/ North Holland, 1991.

Gabrieli JDE: Memory systems analyses of mneumonic disorders in aging and age-related diseases. Proc Natl Acad Sci USA 1996;93:13534–13540.

Geldmacher DS, Whitehouse PJ: Evaluation of dementia. N Engl J Med 1996;335:330–336.

Giovanello KS, Verfaellie M: Memory systems of the brain: A cognitive neuropsychological analysis. Semin Speech Lang 2001;22:107–116.

Langley LK, Madden DJ: Functional neuroimaging of memory: Implication for cognitive aging. Microsc Res Tech 2000;51:75–84.

Sorra KE, Harris KM: Overview of the structure, composition, function, development, and plasticity of hippocampal dendritic spines. Hippocampus 2000;10:501–511.

Spiers HJ, Maguire EA, Burgess N: Hippocampal amnesia. Neurocase 2001;7:357–382.

Squire LR: Memory and the hippocampus: A synthesis from findings with rats, monkeys, and humans. Psychol Rev 1992;99:195–231.

Tuokko HA, Frerichs RJ, Kristjansson B: Cognitive impairment, no dementia: Concepts and issues. Int Psychogeriatr 2001;13:183–202.

Verfaellie M, O'Connor M: A neuropsychological analysis of memory and amnesia. Semin Neurol 2001;20:455–462.

References

1. Cohen NJ, Squire LR: Preserved learning and retention of pattern-analyzing skill in amnesia: Dissociation of knowing how and knowing that. Science 1980;210:207–210.
2. Gabrieli JDE, Cohen NJ, Corkin S: The impaired learning of semantic knowledge following bilateral medial temporal-lobe resection. Brain Cog 1988;7:525–539.
3. Cattell RB: Theory of fluid and crystallized intelligence: A critical experiment. J Educ Psych 1963;54:1–22.
4. Butters N, Cermak LS: A case study of the forgetting of autobiographical knowledge: Implications for the study of retrograde amnesia. *In* Ruben D (ed): Autobiographical Memory. Cambridge, Cambridge University Press, 1986.
5. Salthouse TA: Adult Cognition: An Experimental Psychology of Human Aging. New York, Springer-Verlag, 1982.
6. Monti LA, Gabrieli JDE, Reminger SL, et al: Differential effects of aging and Alzheimer's disease upon conceptual implicit and explicit memory. Neuropsychology 1996;10:101–112.
7. Woodruff-Pak DS: Aging and classical conditioning: Parallel studies in rabbits and humans. Neurobiology 1988;9:511–522.
8. Martin A, Haxby J, Lalonde FM, et al: Discrete cortical regions associated with knowledge of color and knowledge of action. Science 1995;270:102–105.
9. Nyberg L, Habib R, McIntosh AR, Tulving E: Reactivation of encoding-related brain activity during memory retrieval. PNAS USA 2000;97: 11120–11124.
10. Vaidya CJ, Zhao M, Desmond JE, Gabrieli JDE: Evidence for cortical encoding specificity in episodic memory: Memory-induced re-activation of picture processing areas. Neuropsychologia 2002;40:2136–2143.
11. Wheeler ME, Petersen SE, Buckner RL: Memory's echo: Vivid remembering reactivates sensory-specific cortex. PNAS USA 2000; 97:11125–11129.
12. Small SA, Nava AS, Perera GM, DeLaPaz R, Mayeux R, Stern Y: Circuit mechanisms underlying memory encoding and retrieval in the long axis of the hippocampal formation. Nature Neurosci 2001;4:442–449.
13. Damasio H, Grabowski TJ, Tranel D, et al: A neural basis for lexical retrieval. Nature 1996;380:499–505.
14. Bechara A, Tranel D, Damasio H, et al: Double dissociation of conditioning and declarative knowledge relative to the amygdala and hippocampus in humans. Science 1995;269:1115–1118.

15. Rempel-Clower NL, Zola SM, Squire LR, et al: Three cases of enduring memory impairment after bilateral damage limited to the hippocampal formation. J Neurosci 1996;16:5233–5255.
16. Stefanacci L, Buffalo EA, Schmolck H, et al: Profound amnesia after damage to the medial temporal lobe: A neuroanatomical and neuropsychological profile of patient E.P. J Neurosci 2000;20(14):7024–7036.
17. Gaffan D, Gaffan EA: Amnesia in man following transection of the fornix: A review. Brain 1991;114:2611–2618.
18. Brewer JB, Zhao Z, Desmond JE, Glover GH, Gabrieli JD: Making memories: Brain activity that predicts how well visual experience will be remembered. Science 1998;281:1185–1187.
19. Fernandez G, Effern A, Grunwald T, et al: Real-time tracking of memory formation in the human rhinal cortex and hippocampus. Science 1999;285:1582–1585.
20. Wagner AD, Schacter DL, Rotte M, et al: Building memories: Remembering and forgetting of verbal experiences as predicted by brain activity. Science 1998;281:1188–1191.
21. Gabrieli JD, Brewer JB, Desmond JE, Glover GH: Separate neural bases of two fundamental memory processes in the human medial temporal lobe. Science 1997;276:264–266.
22. Haist F, Bowden Gore J, Mao H: Consolidation of human memory over decades revealed by functional magnetic resonance imaging. Nature Neuroscience 2001;4:1139–1145.
23. Von Cramon DY, Hebel N, Schuri U: A contribution to the anatomical basis of thalamic amnesia. Brain 1985;108:993–1008.
24. Dusoir H, Kapur N, Byrnes DP, et al: The role of diencephalic pathology in human memory disorder. Brain 1990;113:1695–1706.
25. Damasio AR, Graff-Radford NR, Eslinger PJ, et al: Amnesia following basal forebrain lesions. Arch Neurol 1985;42:263–271.
26. Irle E, Wowra B, Kunert HJ, et al: Memory disturbances following anterior communicating artery rupture. Ann Neurol 1992;31:473–480.
27. Kapur N, Ellison D, Smith MP, et al: Focal retrograde amnesia following bilateral temporal lobe pathology: A neuropsychological and magnetic resonance study. Brain 1992;115:73–85.
28. Smith E, Jonides J, Koeppe RA: Dissociating verbal and spatial working memory using PET. Cerebral Cortex 1996;6:11–20.
29. Heindel WC, Salmon DP, Shults CW, et al: Neuropsychological evidence for multiple implicit memory systems: A comparison of Alzheimer's, Huntington's, and Parkinson's disease patients. J Neurosci 1989;9:582–587.
30. Gabrieli JDE, Fleischman DA, Keane MM, et al: Double dissociation between memory systems underlying explicit and implicit memory in the human brain. Psychol Sci 1995;6:76–82.
31. Gabrieli JDE, Desmond JE, Demb JB, et al: Functional magnetic resonance imaging of semantic memory processes in the frontal lobes. Psychol Sci 1996;7:278–283.
32. Daum I, Schugens MM, Ackerman H, et al: Classical conditioning after cerebellar lesions in humans. Behav Neurosci 1993;107:748–756.
33. Daum I, Channon S, Polkey CE, et al: Classical conditioning after temporal lobe lesions in man: Impairment in conditional discrimination. Behav Neurosci 1991;105:396–408.
34. Kandel ER, Schwartz JH: Molecular biology of learning: Modulation of transmitter release. Science 1982;218:433–443.
35. Davis HP, Squire LR: Protein synthesis and memory: A review. Psychol Bull 1984;96:518–559.
36. Bailey CH, Chen MC: Morphological basis of long-term habituation and sensitization in Aplysia. Science 1983;220:91–93.
37. Gould E, McEwen BS, Tanapat P, Galea LA, Fuchs E: Neurogenesis in the dentate gyrus of the adult tree shrew is regulated by psychosocial stress and NMDA receptor activation. J Neurosci 1997;17:2492–2498.
38. Gould E, Tanapat P, McEwen BS, Flugge G, Fuchs E: Proliferation of granule cell precursors in the dentate gyrus of adult monkeys is diminished by stress. PNAS USA 1998;95:3168–3171.
39. Kempermann G, Kuhn HG, Gage FH: More hippocampal neurons in adult mice living in an enriched environment. Nature 1997;386:493–495.
40. Eriksson PS, Perfilieva E, Bjork-Eriksson T, Alborn AM, Nordborg C, Peterson DA, Gage FH: Neurogenesis in the adult human hippocampus. Nature Medicine 1998;4:1313–1317.
41. Gould E, Beylin A, Tanapat P, Reeves A, Shors TJ: Learning enhances adult neurogenesis in the hippocampal formation. Nature Neurosci 1999;2:260–265.
42. Shors TJ, Miesegaes G, Beylin A, Zhao M, Rydel T, Gould E: Neurogenesis in the adult is involved in the formation of trace memories. Nature 2001;410:372–376.
43. Polster MR: Drug-induced amnesia: Implications for cognitive neuropsychological investigations of memory. Psychol Bull 1993; 114:477–493.
44. Bartus RT, Dean RL, Beer B, et al: The cholinergic hypothesis of geriatric memory dysfunction. Science 1982;217:408–417.
45. Cooper JA, Sagar HJ, Doherty SM, et al: Different effects of dopaminergic and anticholinergic therapies on cognitive and motor function in Parkinson's disease. Brain 1992;115:1701–1725.
46. Luciana M, Depue RA, Arbisi P, et al: Facilitation of working memory in humans by a D2 dopamine receptor. J Cog Neurosci 1992;4:58–68.
47. Folstein MF, Folstein SE, McHugh PR: "Mini-mental state": A practical method for grading the cognitive state of patients for the clinician. J Psychiatr Res 1975;12:189–198.
48. Damasio AR, Van Hoesen GW, Hyman BT: Reflections on the selectivity of neuropathological changes in Alzheimer's disease. *In* Schwartz M (ed): Modular Deficits in Alzheimer-type Dementia. Cambridge, MIT Press, 1990, pp 226–238.
49. Hodges JR: Pick's disease. *In* Burns A, Levy R (eds): Dementia. London, Chapman & Hall, 1993, pp 62–80.
50. Roses AD: Apolipoprotein E genotyping in the differential diagnosis, not prediction, of Alzheimer's disease. Ann Neurol 1995;38:6–14.
51. Wechsler D: Wechsler Memory Scale—Revised Manual. San Antonio, The Psychological Corporation, 1987.
52. Delis DC, Kramer JH, Kaplan E, et al: CVLT: California Verbal Learning Test. San Antonio, The Psychological Corporation, 1987.
53. Rey A: L'examen psychologique dans les cas d'encephalopathie traumatique. Arch Psychol 1941;28:286–340.
54. Albert ML: Alexia. *In* Heilman KM, Valenstein E (eds): Clinical Neuropsychology. New York, Oxford University Press, 1979, pp 172–191.
55. Davis HP, Bajszar GM, Squire LR: Colorado Neuropsychology Tests. Colorado Springs, Colorado Neuropsychology Tests, 1994.
56. Evans DA, Funkenstein HH, Albert MS, et al: Prevalence of Alzheimer's disease in a community population of older persons. J Am Med Assoc 1989;262:2551–2556.
57. Mayeux R, Foster NL, Rossor M, et al: The clinical evaluation of patients with dementia. *In* Whitehouse PJ (ed): Dementia, Vol. 40. Philadelphia, F.A. Davis, 1993, pp 92–129.
58. Albert MS, Butters N, Brandt J: Patterns of remote memory in amnesic and demented patients. Arch Neurol 1981;38:495–500.
59. Parasuraman R, Haxby JV: Attention and brain function in Alzheimer's disease: A review. Neuropsychology 1993;7:242–272.
60. Solomon PR, Brett M, Groccia-Ellison ME, et al: Classical conditioning in patients with Alzheimer's disease: A multiday study. Psychol Aging 1995;10:248–254.
61. Keane MM, Gabrieli JDE, Fennema AC, et al: Evidence for a dissociation between perceptual and conceptual priming in Alzheimer's disease. Behav Neurosci 1991;105:326–342.
62. Gabrieli JDE, Corkin S, Mickel SF, et al: Intact acquisition and long-term retention of mirror-tracing skill in Alzheimer's disease and in global amnesia. Behav Neurosci 1993;107:899–910.
63. Arnold SE, Hyman BT, Flory J, et al: The topographical and neuroanatomical distribution of neurofibrillary tangles and neuritic plaques in the cerebral cortex of patients with Alzheimer's disease. Cerebral Cortex 1991;1:103–116.
64. Cummings JL, Benson DF: Subcortical dementia: Review of an emerging concept. Arch Neurol 1984;41:874–879.
65. Gabrieli JDE, Singh J, Stebbins GT, et al: Reduced working-memory span in Parkinson's disease: Evidence for the role of a fronto-striatal system in working and strategic memory. Neuropsychology 1996;10: 322–332.
66. Hodges JR, Salmon DP, Butters N: The nature of the naming deficit in Alzheimer's and Huntington's disease. Brain 1991;114:1547–1558.

CHAPTER 6

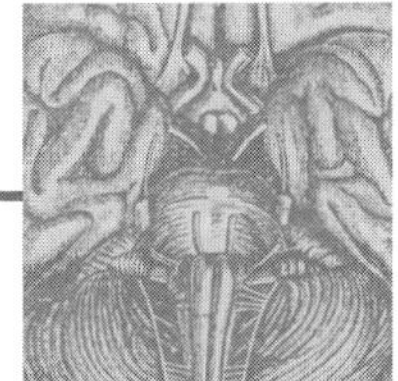

MARGARET M. SWANBERG, ZIAD S. NASREDDINE,
MARIO F. MENDEZ, and JEFFREY L. CUMMINGS

Speech and Language

History and Definitions

A wide variety of language disorders were described for many centuries before the modern interest in aphasia. The formal delineation of aphasia as presently recognized dates from 1861. In the early 19th century, similarly to other brain functions, language was considered to be subserved by a specific area in the brain. Opponents of this localization approach considered mental function to be a product of the entire brain working as a unit. In 1861, Paul Broca presented to the French Society of Anthropology the case of a patient who became speechless and then died. Postmortem studies revealed a large frontal lesion supporting the localization viewpoint. After this case, multiple clinicopathological studies were reported, confirming Broca's finding and lateralizing language function to the left hemisphere. In 1874, Karl Wernicke distinguished two types of aphasia, motor and sensory, which were clinically and anatomopathologically separable. He also postulated the existence of a conduction aphasia based on a diagrammatic scheme linking the sensory and motor components of language. Technological advancements, including neuroimaging techniques and more standardized aphasia batteries, have helped considerably in assessing patients with language disorders and in elucidating the intricate subsystems subserving language function.

Speech is the ability to vocalize by coordinating the muscles controlling the vocal apparatus. It is the mechanical aspect of oral communication. Speech disorders are termed dysarthria, a disturbance in articulation, or dysphonia, a disturbance in vocalization or phonation. Patients with dysarthria or dysphonia retain their language ability despite their speech disturbance.

Language refers to symbolic communication. It is the ability to converse, comprehend, repeat, read, and write. Language ability depends on central processing for either comprehension or formulation for expressing the sounds and symbols of prepositional communication. Language disorders are termed aphasias and involve language disturbances in comprehension, production, or both.

This chapter reviews clinical syndromes of both speech and language disorders. An overview of anatomy and physiology of speech and language is a first step toward understanding the pathophysiology underlying these disorders. Examination of speech and language disorders is emphasized and forms the basis for diagnosis, lesion localization, and treatment.

Clinical History

Clinical history is critical for speech and language assessment. Information from relatives, friends, or witnesses is often necessary owing to the patient's decreased ability to communicate. History taking should include the following components.

Temporal development of symptoms provides valuable information on the underlying pathophysiological process. An acute impairment of speech output indicates a possible underlying vascular, infectious, inflammatory, or traumatic pathology. A chronic and progressive course of symptoms is more suspicious for a degenerative or neoplastic process.

Description of the symptom is important in characterizing and differentiating speech and language disorders. Difficulty in articulation or vocalization implies a speech disorder, whereas the inability to find words, comprehend, read, or write is indicative of a language disorder. Differentiation of speech and language disorders has important localizing value for the underlying pathology within the nervous system and helps distinguish among different etiological processes.

Associated features should be sought. The presence of other neurological symptoms may help in localization of the pathological process or in discovering the cause of the disorder. For example, a patient who complains of progressive headaches, decreased level of consciousness, and weakness in the right upper extremity associated with language difficulties most likely has a left frontal expanding, neoplastic lesion.

Handedness should always be assessed. The left hemisphere is the dominant hemisphere for language for almost all right-handed adults and for many left-handed adults. This information has crucial significance for localization of the underlying disturbance.

Associated intercurrent or past medical illnesses are important clues to the underlying etiology of speech and language disorders. Vascular risk factors such as hypertension, diabetes, or evidence of atherosclerotic disease, including previous strokes or myocardial infarctions and smoking, should be assessed. A history of infection, trauma, alcohol or drug abuse, and malignancy also may be important.

Past psychiatric history should be reviewed. Psychiatric conditions such as schizophrenia, bipolar illness, and conversion disorders may present with speech and language symptoms closely mimicking a neurological syndrome.

Other important components of clinical history include *developmental and educational background and family history*. It is crucial to know the patient's previous language abilities including reading, writing, and the presence of a known developmental delay. This information may help distinguish a developmental disorder from an acquired disorder.

Anatomy of Speech and Language

ANATOMY OF SPEECH (NORMAL PHONATION AND ARTICULATION)

Normal speech involves a highly coordinated sequence of contractions of the respiratory musculature, larynx, pharynx, tongue, and lips. These muscles are innervated by the facial, vagal, hypoglossal (reviewed in Chapters 11, 13, and 14), and phrenic nerves. The nuclei of these nerves are controlled by the motor cortices through the corticobulbar tracts. Coordination of the movements of the articulatory structures requires simultaneous and coordinated activation of these cranial nerves, not only by direct cortical motor activation but also by indirect involvement of the basal ganglia and cerebellum. The basal ganglia and the cerebellum also are important participants in producing the prosodic aspects of speech, including pitch or frequency, stress or the differential emphasis placed on syllables, and rhythm or timing.

Thus, pathology affecting speech could be located at several sites within the motor systems. Speech is impaired when any of the following structures are damaged or dysfunctional: motor cortex and its outflow tracts, cerebellum, basal ganglia, brain stem, peripheral portions of cranial nerves controlling the speech apparatus, and target speech musculature, including facial muscles, pharynx, palate, tongue, vocal cords, diaphragm, and intercostal muscles.

ANATOMY OF LANGUAGE

Overview

Language processes are lateralized to the left hemisphere. This has been determined through anatomoclinical correlation in patients with language disturbances and associated brain pathology. It also has been demonstrated by electrical stimulation and seizure activity in the left hemisphere, as well as injection of sodium amytal in the left internal carotid, all causing language disturbances and speech arrest. Increased cerebral blood flow to the left hemisphere during language processing also confirms this lateralized brain function. There are anatomical differences between the left and right hemispheres. The planum temporale, the region on the superior surface of the temporal lobe posterior to Heschl's gyrus and extending to the posterior end of the sylvian fissure, is slightly larger on the left, which is consistent with Wernicke's area.[1] Computed tomography (CT) has shown the left occipital lobe to be longer than the right.

Approximately 90 percent of the general population are right-handed.[2] They prefer using their right hand for most motor activities, especially skillful tasks. Approximately 99 percent of right-handed individuals have language functions in the left hemisphere. There is a tendency for left-handed and ambidextrous individuals to have varying degrees of bilateral representation of language and visuospatial functions.[3] Left-handers are more likely to become aphasic because of the bilateral representation, but their aphasia tends to be milder and more brief than that of right-handers.[4] Specific cortical areas in the left hemisphere subserve distinct language functions. For example, the production or comprehension of a word requires serial and parallel processing of information through cortical and possibly subcortical circuits (Fig. 6–1).

Speech Comprehension and Production

Speech comprehension and production are complex processes. Words first reach the peripheral auditory apparatus, which transforms the mechanical input from the tympanic membrane into electrical impulses that travel to the brain stem cochlear nucleus, then to the medial geniculate nucleus of the thalamus via the trapezoid body and lateral lemniscus, finally reaching the primary auditory cortex (Heschl's gyrus) in the superior temporal gyrus. The auditory language content undergoes preliminary decoding in the auditory association

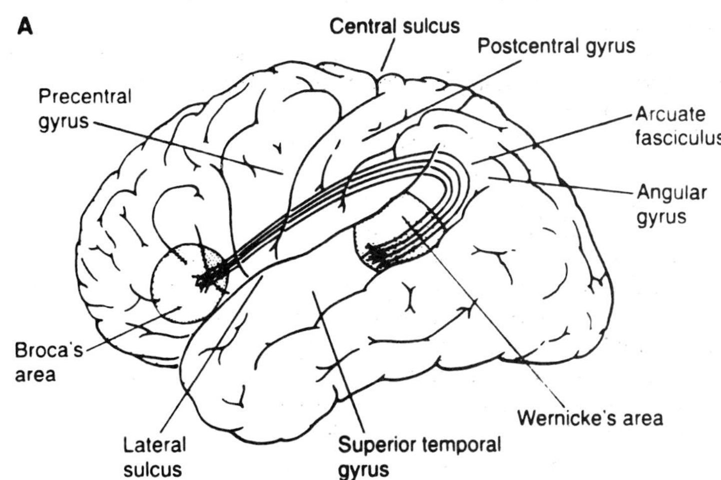

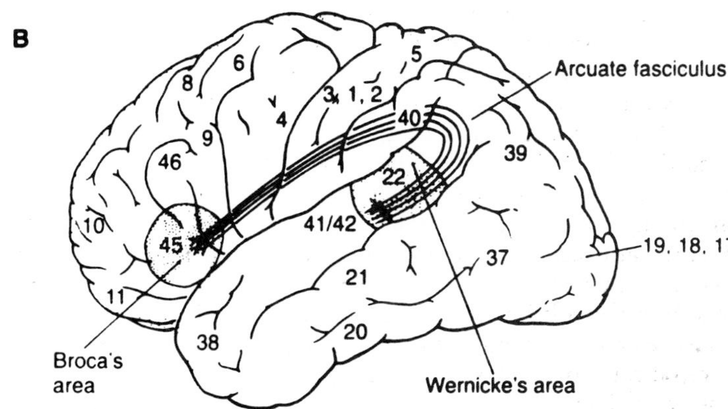

FIGURE 6–1. Primary language areas of the brain. (From Mayeux R: Disorders of language: The aphasias. *In* Kandel ER, Schwartz JH (eds): Principles of Neural Science, 3rd ed. New York, Elsevier, 1991.)

cortex, Wernicke's area (Brodmann's area 22) located in the posterior third of the left superior temporal gyrus (see Fig. 6–1). The sounds undergo further processing in the heteromodal association cortex, the angular gyrus, to provide the semantics (the meaning) and relate it to other incoming words, other sensory modalities, and past experiences. If the words are to be repeated, the auditory information is transmitted forward to Broca's area without necessarily passing through the angular gyrus. Information travels from Wernicke's area to the motor association cortex, Broca's area (Brodmann's area 44, 45 located in the posterior part of the inferior left frontal convolution), through the arcuate fasciculus, a band of white matter deep to the supramarginal gyrus connecting both language areas. Broca's area initiates a motor plan that is transmitted to the primary motor cortex (Brodmann's area 4) to pronounce the words. The motor cortex, in coordination with the supplementary motor area, basal ganglia, and cerebellum, sends corticobulbar fibers to implement speech sounds. (Figure 6–2 illustrates the four principal areas involved in comprehension of spoken language.)

Reading and Writing

Reading depends on visual stimuli (written words) reaching the primary visual cortex (Brodmann's area 17). The visual stimuli are then transmitted from the primary visual cortex, to the visual association cortex, or unimodal association cortex. The word stimuli are further processed in the heteromodal association cortex, the angular gyrus, for semantic meaning and integration with other sensory modalities

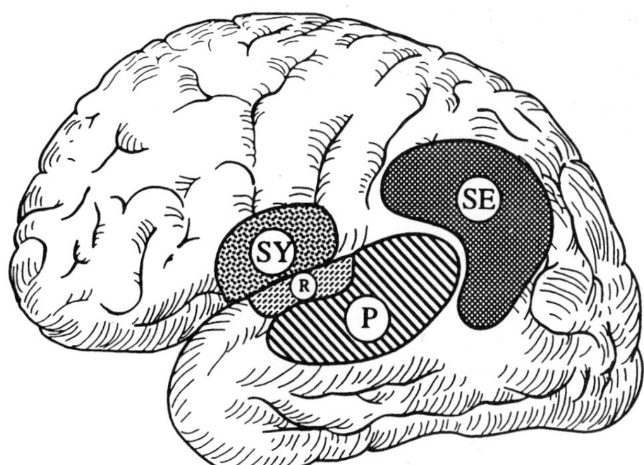

FIGURE 6–2. Artist's rendition of the four areas involved in comprehension of spoken language. R = receptive area (Heschl's gyrus); P = perceptive area (auditory association cortex); SE = semantic interpretation area (angular gyrus); SY = syntactical interpretation area (Broca's area). (From Benson DF, Ardila A: Aphasia: A Clinical Perspective. New York, Oxford University Press, 1996.)

and past experiences. If the words are to be read aloud, the information is transmitted forward from the visual association cortex to Broca's area through the arcuate fasciculus, without necessarily passing through the angular gyrus. From Broca's area, they are spoken using the same circuits as described earlier. A clinically pertinent fact is that visual information from the right visual cortex must travel through the posterior part of the corpus callosum to be further processed and read in the language regions of the left hemisphere.

Writing requires the transfer of language information to the motor association cortex superior to Broca's area and then to motor neurons in the primary motor cortex (Brodmann's area 4), projecting to the arm and hand. Writing to dictation involves the transfer of auditory information from Wernicke's area to the anterior motor areas; copying written material involves transfer of information from visual association cortex to the anterior motor areas for execution. Visuospatial input is also important in the orientation of written language.

ANATOMY OF THE AFFECTIVE ELEMENTS OF SPEECH AND LANGUAGE

The dominance of the right hemisphere in the processing of affective prosody is supported by numerous lesion studies,[5–7] and more recently by functional imaging data.[8] The ability to convey emotional meaning in speech, facial expressions, and gestures are functions of the right inferior frontal lobe (pars opercularis). The perception of affective components of communication is considered a function of more posterior areas in the right hemisphere.

LIMBIC AND SUBCORTICAL STRUCTURES PARTICIPATING IN LANGUAGE PROCESSING

In addition to the known left hemisphere cortical functions in language processing, other structures, including the insula, striatum, thalamus, and subcortical white matter, are involved in language function. The striatum is involved in speech output and prosody; the thalamus is important for cortical arousal and language comprehension. The subcortical white matter interconnects language areas.

Examination of Speech and Language

DIRECTED NEUROLOGICAL EXAMINATION

Speech. The examination of speech includes the assessment of speech volume, rate, articulation, prosody, and initiation.[9, 10] Each component of speech can be affected differently in various disorders. The examiner should assess speech through spontaneous conversation or by having the patient read a standardized passage to elicit a wide range of sounds including labials (sounds dependent on the lips), linguals (sounds dependent on the tongue), dentals (sounds requiring placing the tongue behind the front teeth), and gutturals (sounds depending on laryngeal control).

Speech volume may be increased with auditory perceptual problems. Reduced volume (hypophonia) is seen in extrapyramidal motor disorders and in peripheral disorders such as vocal cord paresis.

The *rate of speech* may be increased in Parkinson's disease, in which patients speak rapidly, and in patients with Wernicke's aphasia, who have pressured speech. In general, nonfluent aphasics speak slowly.

Articulation defect is a sign of motor impairment. Dysarthric speech often results in stereotyped speech errors, that is, repeating the same errors when trying to produce certain sounds. This helps distinguish dysarthric speech from paraphasic speech, in which substituted letters occur in a variable pattern.

Prosody evaluation includes assessment of the spontaneous inflection, prosodic matching of sentence structure (declarative sentence, questions, boundaries between clauses), assessment of affective intent, and assessment of pragmatic intent (humor, declarative, sarcastic, defensive). Speech inflection and prosodic matching of sentence structure are mediated by the left hemisphere, whereas affective intent is mediated by right hemisphere and basal ganglia functions.

Timing of speech initiation is related to supplementary motor area function and its outflow.[11, 12]

Laryngeal phonation, or breathiness, and resonance, or nasality, are two other qualities of speech that aid in localization. They are seen most often in patients with upper motor neuron lesions and spastic speech.

Language. The six main parts of the language examination can be performed at the patient's bedside. These parts include (1) expressive speech, (2) comprehension of spoken language, (3) repetition, (4) naming, (5) reading, and (6) writing.[13–15] The examiner can classify most aphasic syndromes after evaluating spontaneous speech, repetition, and comprehension (Fig. 6–3).

Expressive Speech. The evaluation of aphasia traditionally begins by observing the spontaneous or conversational speech of the patient. Aphasic verbal output is either nonfluent or fluent. Normal English output is 100 to 150 words per minute.[16] Nonfluent aphasic output is sparse (under 50 words per minute), produced with considerable effort, poorly articulated, of short phrase length (often only a single word), and dysprosodic (abnormal rhythm) and features a preferential use of substantive meaningful words with a relative absence of functor words (prepositions, articles, adverbs). Fluent aphasic output in contrast features many words, easily produced, with normal phrase length and prosodic quality but often omitting semantically significant words. Fluent aphasia, when severe, may sound empty and devoid of content. In addition, paraphasic errors (substitution of phrases or words) are often abundant in fluent aphasic output. Nonfluent aphasic output is associated with pathology involving the anterior left hemisphere,[17, 18] and fluent aphasia results from pathology posterior to the fissure of Rolando.

Comprehension of Spoken Language. Comprehension can be assessed in many ways;[19] four examples of clinical evaluations of comprehension include (1) *conversation*—engaging the patient in ordinary conversation probes the patient's ability to understand questions and commands; (2) *commands*—a series of single or multistep commands, such as asking the patient to pick up a piece of paper, fold it in two, and place it on a bedside stand; (3) *yes and no answers*—require only elementary motor function and can be used to assess various comprehension levels (e.g., are the lights on in

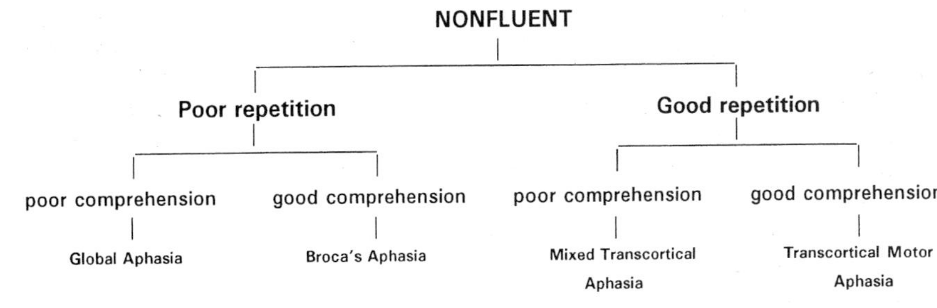

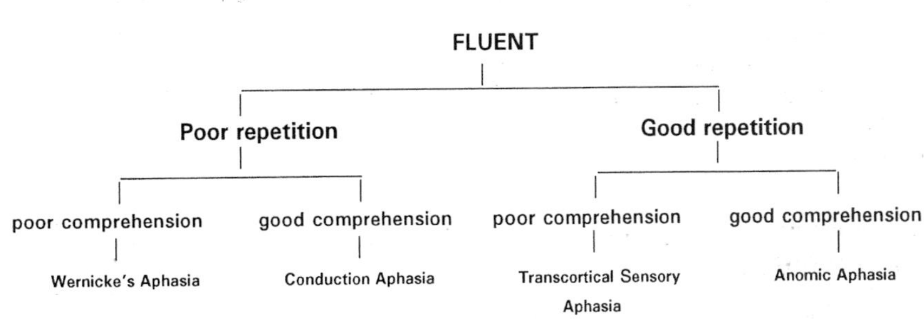

FIGURE 6–3. Algorithm for demonstration of aphasia syndromes.

this room?); and (4) *pointing*—requires a limited motor response (patients can be asked to point to the window, the door, and the ceiling; the patients are asked to point to these places in a specific sequence, and more difficult tasks also can be given [e.g., point to the source of illumination in this room]).

Despite all of these methods, comprehension remains difficult to assess. Patients may derive significant meaning from nonverbal cues (e.g., tone of voice, facial or arm gesture) and may lead the clinician to underestimate the comprehension deficit. Apraxia and other motor disorders may cause a failure to perform, leading to an overestimation of the deficits. Perseverative answers may further complicate comprehension assessment.

Comprehension is compromised by dysfunction of the heteromodal association cortex or Wernicke's area of the left hemisphere.

Repetition. The examiner tests repetition by requesting that the patient repeat digits, words, and sentences. A phrase like "no ifs, ands, or buts" poses special difficulty.[14] Aphasics with impaired repetition have pathology that involves the perisylvian region. In contrast, a strong, often mandatory tendency to repeat (echolalia) suggests an extrasylvian locus of pathology, often involving the vascular borderzone areas.

Naming. Disturbances in confrontational naming are the least specific language abnormalities. Naming is disturbed in most aphasic patients. Testing should evaluate the patient's ability to name objects (both high and low frequency), body parts, colors, and geometrical figures. If the patient fails, the examiner provides a phonemic cue (such as pronouncing the initial phoneme of the word) or a semantic cue (such as "You write with a ___."). Anomia is generally not a reliable localizing abnormality;[20] it occurs with lesions of the angular gyrus, posterior inferior temporal cortex, and temporal pole on the left but may occur in concert with other lesions.

Reading. The examination tests both reading aloud and reading for comprehension. In some cases, the two abilities are dissociated.

Writing. Writing is nearly always disturbed in aphasic patients. Writing provides a further sample of expressive language and permits evaluation of spelling, syntax, visuospatial layout, and mechanics. The examiner assesses writing to dictation and to command (e.g., describe your job), as well as copying.

ASSOCIATED NEUROLOGICAL FINDINGS

Cerebral. Many portions of the neurological examination are of considerable value in helping localize lesions associated with speech and language disorders.

When speech alterations are due to bilateral involvement of corticobulbar tracts, affective changes may be evident in which the patient expresses emotional incontinence (spasmodic crying and laughing). This is part of the pseudobulbar syndrome, which is described in the next section.

Language disturbances can be associated with other types of cognitive dysfunction, such as impaired memory, abstraction, visuospatial function, and praxis, as well as changes in personality (decreased inhibition), irritability, apathy, and agitation, which may indicate the presence of widespread dysfunction such as that encountered in degenerative dementing diseases. Evaluation for apraxia (which is defined as failure to carry out a maneuver on command, excluding any primary motor, sensory, or comprehension disorder) is important because ideomotor apraxia is often associated with nonfluent aphasias and conduction aphasia.

Cranial Nerves. Speech disorders are associated with lower motor neuron pathology including abnormalities of the neuromuscular junction. Therefore, it is important to search for any weakness, atrophy, and fasciculation in the facial musculature, the tongue, and the palate. Other cranial nerve function must be assessed; ptosis, ophthalmoplegia, and fatigability should be observed and tested. The gag reflex should be examined because it may be depressed in dysarthria of the lower motor neuron type and increased in dysarthria of the upper motor neuron type. A masked or unexpressive face and decreased blinking may be clues to the presence of an extrapyramidal cause of dysarthria.

Right homonymous hemianopia or quadrantanopia is helpful in localizing the site of pathology associated with language disorders. Anterior aphasias have little or no involvement of the visual fields compared with more posterior aphasic syndromes. The cranial nerves should also be assessed for the presence of a central type of facial muscle weakness on the right side. Occasionally, patients with acute onset of anterior aphasia have a conjugate gaze deviation to the left (see Chapter 1).

Motor/Reflexes/Cerebellar/Gait. Speech abnormalities in the presence of a significant spastic paralysis involving the entire side of the body suggest a deep-lying lesion involving the contralateral internal capsule. This type of lesion typically gives rise to spastic speech. When weakness is bilateral or unilateral but is associated with cranial nerve deficits on the opposite side, a brain stem lesion is suspected. Dysarthria associated with this type of insult is either flaccid or spastic, depending on the involvement of either the motor nuclei controlling the speech apparatus or their supranuclear pathways. Upper motor neuron signs including spasticity and hyper-reflexia should be sought as well as lower motor neuron signs including atrophy, fasciculation, and hyporeflexia and areflexia. These signs are helpful in distinguishing lesions producing spastic dysarthria from those causing flaccid dysarthria. Bradykinesia, rigidity, resting tremor, chorea, and dystonia are all signs suggestive of extrapyramidal disease and are usually associated with hypokinetic or hyperkinetic dysarthrias.

Cerebellar findings include ataxia, dysmetria on finger-to-nose and heel-to-shin testing as well as gaze-evoked nystagmus, dysmetric saccades, and rebound nystagmus. These findings are often associated with ataxic dysarthria.

Weakness involving only one limb with or without facial weakness is most suggestive of cortical pathology. Brachiofacial involvement suggests infarction of the territory of the middle cerebral artery and is usually associated with perisylvian aphasias; crural weakness without involvement of the arm and face suggests infarction in the territory of the anterior cerebral artery and is usually associated with transcortical motor aphasia. Greater weakness of proximal musculature in contrast to distal musculature is suggestive of involvement in the borderzone vascular areas and can be associated with extrasylvian aphasias (transcortical aphasias). Testing for ideomotor apraxia is helpful to localize pathology further within the left hemisphere. Language disturbances are not usually associated with cerebellar disease.

Sensory. Intact perception of light touch and proprioception with impaired sensation of pain and temperature occurring in an alternate pattern affecting one side of the face and the opposite side of the body helps localize pathology to the lateral brain stem or thalamus. Brain stem lesions could also affect lower cranial nerves such as cranial nerves IX, X, and XII and create a flaccid dysarthria.

Cortical sensory loss (astereognosia, impaired two-point discrimination, agraphesthesia) indicates involvement of the parietal cortex and can be associated with more posterior aphasia-producing lesions. Pseudothalamic pain that begins months after the onset of the sensory abnormality is seen after lesions affecting the white matter just deep to the supramarginal gyrus and can be associated with conduction aphasia.[13]

Neurovascular. The presence of significant bilateral vascular bruits on neurovascular examination is an important risk factor for stroke. Stroke patients could present with spastic dysarthria or pseudobulbar palsy secondary to single or multiple cerebral infarcts, respectively.

As for speech disorders, abnormal neurovascular examination suggests the presence of cerebrovascular disease. Multiple language disturbances and syndromes are caused by strokes. Transcortical aphasia occurs following borderzone infarction in patients with severe carotid stenosis during a hypotensive episode.

Evaluation Guidelines (Table 6–1)

Speech and language disturbances are assessed by clinical history, bedside speech and language assessment, and neurological examination. Complementary investigations, such as neuroimaging, electrophysiology, fluid and tissue analysis, neuropsychological testing, and other tests, help confirm the clinical diagnosis.

Neuroimaging. Several techniques are extremely helpful for localizing and identifying various types of pathologies underlying a speech or language disturbance. With the advent of CT and magnetic resonance imaging, the improved visualization of subcortical structures has implicated these regions in a growing number of speech and language disorders. Investigators have used positron-emission tomography and single-photon emission computed tomography to investigate aphasia and the anatomy of language. The studies have largely confirmed lesion-derived conclusions about the anatomy of language described earlier.[21]

Electrophysiology. Electroencephalography measures one parameter of brain function and can help in the localization of pathology. Repetitive magnetic stimulation has been used to localize lesions within the language-dominant hemisphere.[22] Electromyography and nerve conduction studies could assist in the diagnosis of peripheral causes of speech disorders, including motor neuron disease, and disorders of the neuromuscular junction.

Cerebrospinal Fluid. Lumbar puncture, blood and urine analysis, as well as more invasive procedures such as brain biopsy may be performed to confirm a diagnosis and help in the treatment of the underlying pathology, particularly in patients with inflammatory or infectious disorders.

Neuropsychological Tests. Numerous tests provide valuable information about cognitive function, particularly in patients suspected of having a degenerative disease underlying their language disturbance. Severe aphasia makes it impossible to perform meaningful neuropsychological assessment.

Other Tests. Of additional value, laryngoscopy (direct and indirect) and diaphragmatic fluoroscopy can be helpful in the diagnosis of peripheral causes of speech disorder affecting the larynx and diaphragm, respectively.

TABLE 6–1. **Useful Studies in the Evaluation of Speech and Language Disorders**

Disorder	Neuroimaging	Electrophysiology	Fluid and Tissue Analysis	Neuropsychological Tests	Other Tests
Dysphonia					
Muscle paralysis or fatigability	Mass lesion compressing cranial nerve X or on the vocal cords	Abnormal decrement of CMAP with repetitive stimulation in myasthenia gravis. Single-fiber EMG showing jitter in NMJ defects	Carcinoma of the vocal cords, carcinomatous meningitis	Normal language and cognitive function	Vocal cord pathology visualized by direct or indirect laryngoscopy
Dysarthria					
Spastic dysarthria	Multiple subcortical white matter disease	Prolonged sensory and visual evoked potentials in multiple sclerosis	Oligoclonal bands in CSF in multiple sclerosis	Pseudobulbar affect, psychomotor slowing, retrieval memory deficit	
Flaccid dysarthria	Brain stem lesion, atrophy, or normal	Fibrillation, fasciculation, and neurogenic recruitment on EMG testing, prolonged latencies	Increased protein in CSF with Guillain-Barré syndrome, carcinomatous meningitis	Normal language and cognitive function	
Ataxia dysarthria	Atrophy of cerebellum, stroke or cerebellar tumor	Decreased CMAP, SNAP in axonal polyneuropathy secondary to alcohol. CMAP potentiation with Eaton-Lambert syndrome	Increased CSF protein, anti-Purkinje cell antibodies, vitamin E deficiency	Normal language	Prolonged latencies of evoked potentials in multiple sclerosis
Extrapyramidal dysarthria	Stroke in basal ganglia, atrophy of the caudate			Mild cognitive decline, psychomotor slowing	
Aphasia					
Perisylvian aphasia	Stroke, tumor, abscess in perisylvian area	Slowing over the fronto-parieto-temporal region on EEG	Increased cholesterol, anticardiolipid antibodies	Decreased verbal memory	Holter and echocardiogram to rule out embolic causes of stroke, chest x-ray study
Extrasylvian aphasia (transcortical)	Stroke in borderzone vascular territory	Slowing over the left hemisphere on EEG			Doppler study of the carotids to rule out occlusion
Subcortical	Stroke in striatocapsular region or thalamus			Psychomotor slowing and possible decreased verbal memory	
Nonlocalizing (anomic)	Generalized atrophy or left hemisphere lesion	Slowing over the temporal lobes over the left hemisphere on EEG	Plaques and tangles or spongiform changes on brain biopsy	Prominent cognitive deficits: visuospatial, praxis, memory	Apolipoprotein E

Table continued on following page

TABLE 6–1. **Useful Studies in the Evaluation of Speech and Language Disorders** *Continued*

Disorder	Neuroimaging	Electrophysiology	Fluid and Tissue Analysis	Neuropsychological Tests	Other Tests
Other Disorders					
Alexia without agraphia	Left occipital infarct involving the splenum of the corpus callosum	EEG slowing over the left occipital cortex			
Alexia with agraphia	Generalized atrophy or focal infarct in left parietotemporal junction	Left centrotemporal slowing on EEG		Associated Gerstmann's syndrome plus anomia constitutes the angular gyrus syndrome	
Reiterative speech	Borderzone vascular infarct or generalized atrophy	Left hemisphere slowing on EEG	Plaques and tangles or spongiform changes on brain biopsy	Multiple cognitive deficits when there is underlying degenerative disorder	
Delirium	Usually normal or generalized atrophy	Abnormal chemistry panel, urine culture, positive hemoculture, abnormal liver or renal function		Multiple cognitive deficits	
Psychiatric disease	Normal	Normal	Normal	Bizarre thought content, flight of ideas, grandiosity, word salad	

CMAP, Compound muscle action potential; CSF, cerebrospinal fluid; EEG, electroencephalogram; EMG, electromyogram; NMJ, neuromuscular junction; SNAP, sensory nerve action potential.

TABLE 6–2. Speech Disorders

Dysphonia
Vocal cord muscle paralysis or fatigability
Spasmodic dysphonia

Dysarthria
Upper motor neuron (spastic dysarthria)
Lower motor neuron (flaccid dysarthria)
Cerebellar (ataxic dysarthria)
Extrapyramidal (hypo- or hyperkinetic dysarthria)
Mixed dysarthria

Speech-Related Disorders
Phonic tics and vocalization
Reiterative speech
Echolalia
Palilalia
Stuttering
Logoclonia

Clinical Syndromes

A discussion of speech disorders, including dysphonias, dysarthrias, and speech-related disorders is followed by a discussion of language disorders, including aphasias, alexias, and agraphias, and language-related disorders. Tables 6–2 and 6–3 outline the classification of speech and language disorders. This classification is meant to help in localizing various clinical syndromes according to current information regarding anatomoclinical correlations. Some entities could be classified in several subcategories, but they have been categorized under the most probable anatomical localization. Future research will help refine the classification. Three major speech disturbances are recognized: dysphonias, dysarthrias, and other speech-related disturbances.[23]

TABLE 6–3. Language Disorders

Aphasias
Perisylvian
  Broca's
  Wernicke's
  Conduction
  Global
Extrasylvian
Transcortical motor and supplementary motor area
  Transcortical sensory
  Transcortical mixed
Subcortical
  Thalamic, striatal, white matter
Nonlocalizing
  Anomic

Alexias and Agraphias

Language-Related Disorders
Aphemia
Pure word deafness
Others
  Delirium
  Psychiatric disorders
  Right hemisphere disorders
  Dementing diseases

DYSPHONIA

Dysphonia is the inability or reduced ability to vocalize due to a disorder of the larynx or its innervation. Dysphonic patients have a breathy sound resulting from abnormal apposition of the vocal cords.

Vocal Cord Dysfunction or Paralysis

Laryngitis is the most common cause of decreased voice volume, but laryngeal hypophonia may result from other causes such as damage to the superior laryngeal nerve, nodules or polyps of the larynx or vocal cords, or carcinoma involving the larynx. Muscle paralysis or fatigability can produce hypophonia, which is produced after excessive speaking. When a patient presents with variable hypophonia and/or dysarthria, a disorder of the neuromuscular junction should be sought. Dysphonia should lead to an investigation of laryngeal disease, either primary or secondary to an abnormality of innervation.

Spasmodic Dysphonia

Spasmodic dysphonia is a segmental dystonia and is usually nonprogressive. This unusual syndrome occurs in middle-aged or elderly individuals. Spasmodic dysphonia involves dystonic spasms of the laryngeal muscles. In the most common form, the adductor type, the voice will be strained, high-pitched, and commonly punctuated by repetitive brief interruptions of speech. Singing, whispering, or changing the voice's pitch may sometimes help lessen the spasms. Less commonly, the voice has a whispering, breathy quality, due to abduction spasms of the vocal cords.

DYSARTHRIA

Dysarthria is the inability or reduced ability to form or produce understandable speech due to lack of motor control over peripheral speech organs. Defects in articulation may be subdivided into several types: flaccid, spastic, ataxic, hypo/hyperkinetic, and mixed.

Flaccid Dysarthria

Flaccid dysarthria is also called lower motor neuron dysarthria or bulbar paralysis. This is due to disease affecting motor neurons in the medulla and lower pons or their intramedullary or peripheral extensions. Speech becomes slurred and progressively less distinct. There is special difficulty in the enunciation of vibrative letters such as "R"; lingual and labial consonants may become impossible with advancing paralysis. Speech has a nasal quality with bilateral paralysis of the palate as may be seen with diphtheria and poliomyelitis and in progressive bulbar palsy. The voice may have a raspy quality because of vocal cord paralysis. Facial diplegia as in Guillain-Barré syndrome affects the lips and impairs enunciation of labial consonants (B, M, P). Neurological examination may reveal atrophy and fasciculations of the tongue and weakness of the palate and the facial muscles. When a history of variable

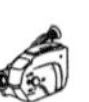

dysarthria or dysphonia, with prominent fatigability is elicited, a neuromuscular junction disorder such as myasthenia gravis should be considered.

Spastic Dysarthria

Spastic dysarthria is also called upper motor neuron dysarthria. It is a motor speech problem characterized by a harsh, low-pitched, slow, monotonous verbal output that sounds strained or strangled. This is the speech that characterizes pseudobulbar palsy (bilateral involvement of corticobulbar tracts) and, to a lesser degree, may be present following significant unilateral upper motor neuron disturbance. Spastic dysarthria may occur with nonfluent aphasia, particularly Broca's aphasia.

Mutism

Mutism is the total loss of speech. Several diseases and various sites of pathology can produce mutism. Peripheral disorders such as laryngitis or vocal cord paralysis occasionally can cause a mute state. Patients with aphemia (described later), global aphasia, transcortical motor aphasia, and aphasia with subcortical lesions frequently present with mutism. Persistent mutism is associated with bihemispheric involvement, particularly of the frontal lobes.[24, 25] Tissue destruction or dysfunction affecting the upper brain stem or the frontal cingulate/supplementary area bilaterally, can interfere with the initiation of both behavior and verbal output. When it is severe, this state is called akinetic mutism.[26] Mutism can also be of psychogenic origin.

Ataxic Dysarthria

Ataxic dysarthria is manifested by slowness of speech, altered rhythm, irregular breakdowns, and improper stress, producing an uneven, jumpy, and unpredictable output. Coordination of speech and of respiration is disturbed. There may not be enough breath to utter certain words or syllables, and others are expressed with greater strength than intended (explosive speech). This speech disorder is most commonly encountered with acute and chronic cerebellar disease.

Scanning speech is part of Charcot's triad (ataxia, nystagmus, scanning speech), which is historically considered to be pathognomonic for multiple sclerosis, but it is more common with head injuries. Scanning speech is characterized as a slow, deliberate, segmented, and monotonous output, presented as individual words or major segments of words. The output retains both grammatical and semantic competence, and articulation remains relatively normal. It is the prosodic quality, particularly of the rhythm and inflection, that are disrupted. The lesions producing this disorder are located at the level of the decussation of the brachium conjunctivum in the mesencephalon affecting crossed efferent cerebellar pathways and motor fibers in the cerebral peduncles, which lie in close proximity.[27] Although scanning speech is easily misinterpreted as a nonfluent aphasia, careful evaluation reveals that there is no true language impairment.

Hypokinetic and Hyperkinetic Dysarthria

Extrapyramidal disease is often associated with either hypokinetic or hyperkinetic dysarthria. Hypokinetic dysarthria occurs in Parkinson's disease and other rigid types of extrapyramidal disorders. This speech abnormality is characterized by rapid utterances, slurring of words, and decrescendo volume at the ends of sentences. The voice is low-pitched and monotonous, lacking both inflection and volume (hypokinetic and hypophonic). In advanced states, only whispering is possible. Festinations of speech with increasing rapidity as the sentence is uttered may occur.

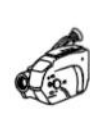

Two varieties of speech disorders can be classified as hyperkinetic. The first, *choreiform dysarthria*, features prolonged phoneme and sentence segments, intermixed with silences and showing variable, often improper, stress (phoneme inflections). This gives speech a bursting quality. This speech output occurs in choreiform disorders such as Huntington's disease and in myoclonic disorders. The second type, *dystonic dysarthria*, produces a slower speaking rate, with prolongation of the individual phonemes and segments and with abnormal, unexpected appearances of stress or of silence. Dystonic dysarthria occurs in dystonia musculorum deformans. Spastic dysphonia is one type of dystonic dysarthria.

Mixed Dysarthrias

In clinical practice, a mixed dysarthria syndrome that has characteristics of several types of motor speech disorders is commonly seen. Several classic neurological disorders, such as multiple sclerosis, Wilson's disease, and advanced amyotrophic lateral sclerosis, produce several variations of dysarthria concurrently including spastic, flaccid, ataxic, and hypokinetic and hyperkinetic dysarthrias.

SPEECH-RELATED DISORDERS

Miscellaneous speech-related disturbances not classified as dysarthrias or dysphonias include phonic tics, vocalizations, coprolalia, and reiterative speech disorders.

Phonic Tics and Vocalizations

Phonic tics are either simple or complex vocal tics. Simple vocal tics are similar in character to motor tics and are expressed as inarticulate noises and sounds (throat clearing, grunts, coughs, shouts, snorts, word accentuation). Complex vocal tics include articulate words, phrases, or sentences such as echolalia (involuntary repetition of the last sound, word, phrase, or sentence of another person) or coprolalia (involuntary utterance of socially unacceptable or obscene words, phrases, or sentences). Phonic tics, including various involuntary vocalizations and coprolalia, occur most often in Gilles de la Tourette syndrome. Degenerative diseases of the nervous system (e.g., neuroacanthocytosis, Huntington's disease), as well as use of neuroleptic medication and acquired brain injuries, also have been associated with tic disorder.

Reiterative Speech Disturbances (Table 6–4)

Echolalia. This syndrome is a nearly mandatory tendency to repeat what has just been said by the examiner. Fully developed echolalia encompasses entire phrases and sentences. The echoed phrase may be the only output the patient can offer. In other cases, the echoed phrase may be followed by a run of jargon output, with the patient appar-

TABLE 6–4. **Disorders Commonly Presenting with Reiterative Speech**

Echolalia
Transcortical sensory aphasia
Mixed transcortical aphasia
Gilles de la Tourette syndrome
Autism
Frontotemporal dementia
Huntington's disease
Neuroacanthocytosis
Palilalia
Parkinson's disease
Schizophrenia
Thalamic infarction
Alzheimer's disease
Idiopathic calcification of basal ganglia
Progressive supranuclear palsy
Stutter
Parkinson's disease
Huntington's disease
Progressive supranuclear palsy
Left cortical infarction
Left subcortical infarction
Logoclonia
Alzheimer's disease (late stages)
General paresis

ently unaware of what he or she is saying.[13] Most patients with echolalia show the completion phenomenon; thus, if started on a phrase that is not completed, "red, white, and . . . ," the correct word is supplied by the patient automatically. Echolalia is most often encountered in patients with transcortical aphasias, notably transcortical sensory and mixed transcortical aphasias. Echolalia is also encountered in many degenerative brain diseases.[28, 29]

Palilalia. This rare speech disorder is characterized by involuntary repetition of words and phrases during verbal output. In most instances, palilalia and aphasia are separate disorders, but palilalia has been reported with both anterior and posterior aphasias. Basal ganglia involvement has been suggested as the cause of some cases of palilalia. Palilalia can be seen in untreated schizophrenic patients, in paramedian thalamic damage, in the later stages of degenerative brain diseases such as Alzheimer's disease,[28, 29] and during electrical stimulation of left hemisphere sites.

Stutter. Many patients have a tendency to repeatedly iterate an uttered sound. It is common particularly among boys. Stutter can appear following brain damage in an individual who had not stuttered previously.[30]

The most common stutter is developmental stuttering, which is characterized by the involuntary repetition of the first syllable of a word. Initiation of the word is followed either by a machine gun–like repetition (stutter) or the presentation of the syllable followed by a prolonged silence (stammer). Both situations are accompanied by physical and emotional discomfort (stress). The patient with a newly acquired stutter produces repetitions and prolongations that are not restricted to the initial syllable. The patient does not exhibit evidence of anxiety associated with the difficult performance. Studies suggest that acquired stutter most often occurs with bilateral brain dysfunction. No focal neuroanatomical site or sites have been associated with acquired stuttering. The co-occurrence of acquired stutter and aphasia has been reported.

Logoclonia. This condition, in which a tendency to repeat the final syllable of a word occurs, often indicates bilateral brain dysfunction. Logoclonia is reported in later stages of dementia.[29]

APHASIAS

Language disorders affect the ability to comprehend and express spoken or written language, or both. Aphasias are the most classic syndromes and are presented first; disorders of written language, including alexias and agraphias as well as other related language disorders, are discussed in the next section.

The clinical characteristics of aphasia syndromes are summarized in Table 6–5.

Perisylvian Syndromes

Perisylvian syndromes include classic aphasic syndromes occurring with lesions along the left Sylvian fissure. They include Broca's, Wernicke's, and conduction aphasia

TABLE 6–5. **Language Disorders: Clinical Characteristics**

Type of Aphasia	Verbal Output	Paraphasia	Repetition	Comprehension	Naming	Reading (Aloud/ Comprehension)	Writing
Broca's	Nonfluent	Rare	Poor	Good	Poor	Poor/good	Poor
Wernicke's	Fluent	Common	Poor	Poor	Poor	Poor/poor	Poor
Conduction	Fluent	Common	Good	Good	Poor	Poor/good	Poor
Global	Nonfluent	Common	Poor	Poor	Poor	Poor/poor	Poor
Transcortical motor	Nonfluent	Rare	Good	Good	Poor	Poor/good	Poor
Transcortical sensory	Fluent	Common	Good	Poor	Poor	Poor/poor	Poor
Mixed transcortical	Nonfluent	Rare	Good	Poor	Poor	Poor/poor	Poor
Anomic	Fluent	Rare	Good	Good	Poor	Variable	Variable
Subcortical	Fluent or nonfluent	Good	Variable	Poor	Common	Variable	Variable

syndromes. Subtypes of Broca's and Wernicke's aphasia are described (Fig. 6–4).

Broca's Aphasia. In 1861, Paul Broca described an aphasic syndrome and correlated it with underlying pathology.[31] Broca's aphasia has since been called by several names. For instance, the same findings have been called expressive aphasia, anterior aphasia, and motor aphasia. The term Broca's aphasia is still the most universally recognized for this syndrome, and a specified anatomical localization has been widely accepted.

Verbal output in Broca's aphasia, which is assessed through conversational speech, is markedly reduced, often to fewer than 10 words per minute. The central feature of Broca's aphasia is a nonfluent verbal output[32]; it is sparse, poorly articulated, and produced with considerable effort. The quality of speech is markedly dysprosodic, lacking melody and rhythm. Sentences are very short, and most responses by a nonfluent aphasic are limited to single word sentences or telegraphic speech.[13] Even though very few words are produced by the nonfluent aphasic, the output often conveys significant information and may be well inflected. There is near absence of syntactical words (prepositions, articles, adverbs). The words produced are usually nouns, action verbs, or descriptive adjectives. This alteration of normal grammatical sentence structure is called agrammatism.[33]

Other language characteristics are less dramatic. The comprehension of spoken language is always significantly better than verbal output. Most patients with Broca's aphasia have some degree of comprehension defect; most often it is a difficulty understanding syntactical structures. The disturbance involves diminished comprehension of the same terms that the patients omit from their verbal expressions, and they have difficulty with relational words such as up and down, and inside and outside. Repetition of spoken language is abnormal. Confrontation naming is invariably poor. Patients often accept prompting well and improve in pronunciation or initiating articulation. This finding is characteristic of Broca's aphasia, even though it can be found in other types of aphasia. Reading out loud is very difficult for Broca's aphasia patients. Reading comprehension may be somewhat disturbed, but it is comparatively well preserved. Writing is abnormal, affecting both writing to command or copying written material. The letters are oversized, and multiple misspellings are common.

Neurological examination shows some degree of right-sided weakness in the majority of patients (over 80 percent) with a variable degree of severity. The weakness usually has a brachiofacial distribution. Hyperactive reflexes are frequently present on the involved side. Ideomotor apraxia, an inability to carry out on command a task that can be done spontaneously, frequently involves the nonparalyzed left hand of patients with Broca's aphasia.[13]

Sensory loss is not consistent. If a severe hemisensory loss is present at the onset but clears rapidly, a unilateral inattention syndrome is suggested rather than a true sensory defect.[34] Often, a conjugate ocular deviation to the left will be present initially. A visual field defect is uncommon and, if it is present, suggests more posterior neuroanatomical involvement.

The site of pathology in Broca's aphasia has been localized to the left posteroinferior frontal lobe, Brodmann's area 44, or simply Broca's area. Patients with the classic syndrome of Broca's aphasia often have associated deep-extending pathology involving the insula, basal ganglia, and periventricular white matter (Fig. 6–5).[15, 21, 35, 36] Various types of pathology, including trauma, tumor, infection, abcess, and others, can produce Broca's aphasia. The most common cause is cerebral vascular disease. Occlusion of one or several branches of the middle cerebral artery feeding the inferior frontal region is the most common cause of Broca's aphasia.

Broca's aphasia that rapidly improves is associated with lesions involving the frontal operculum but not extending deeply. These patients have a different clinical picture, and the condition has been called little Broca's aphasia or aphemia.[15] They may be left with a "breathy" voice or a

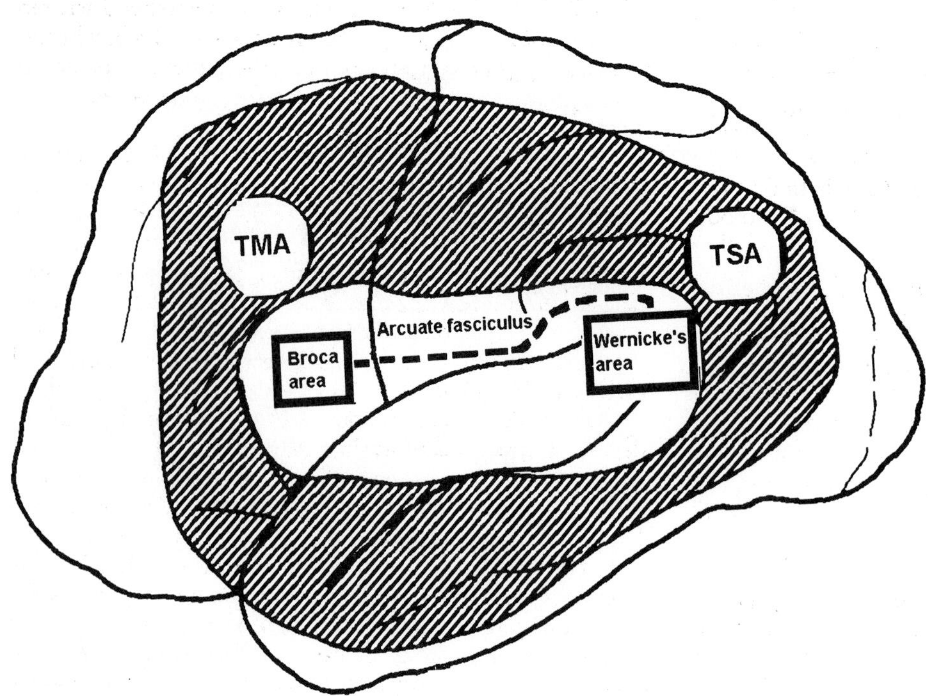

FIGURE 6–4. Lateral view of the left hemisphere indicating presylvian area (central clear region), and extrasylvian areas or borderzone area (cross-hatched region). TMA = region where a lesion may result in transcortical motor aphasia; TSA = region where a lesion may result in transcortical sensory aphasia.

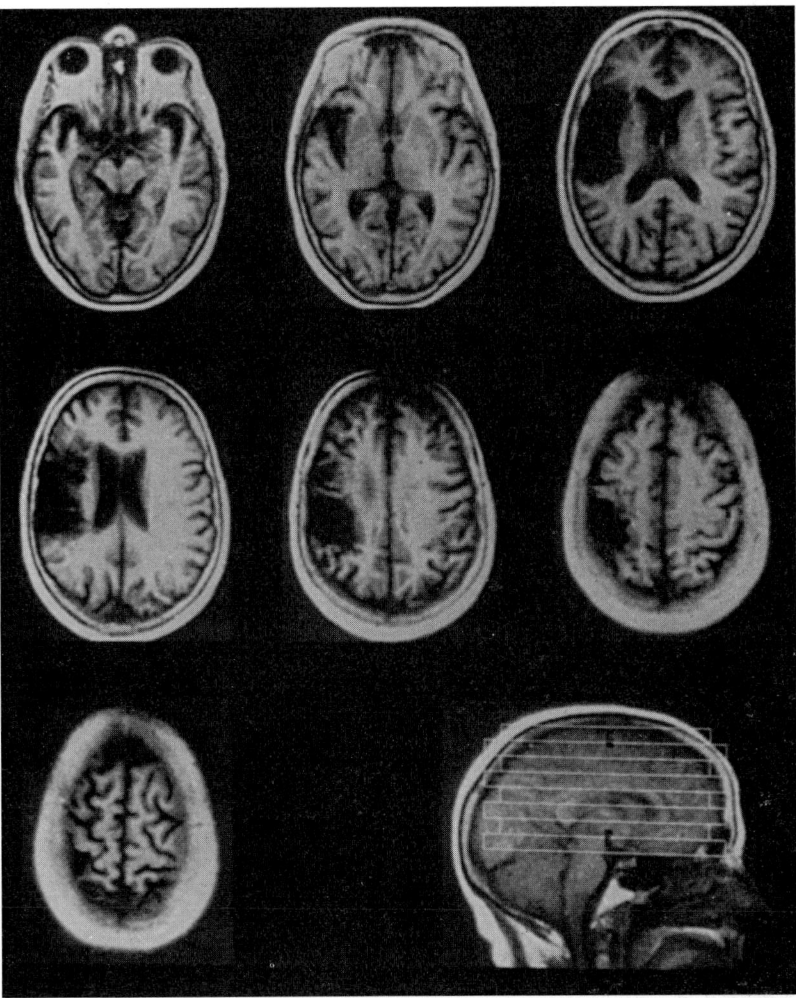

FIGURE 6–5. MRI of the brain showing a large, deep infarct involving Broca's area, the internal capsule, and the basal ganglia. (From Damasio H, Damasio AR: Lesion Analysis in Neuropsychology. New York, Oxford University Press, 1989.)

speech disorder that sounds like the accent of a non-native speaker (foreign accent syndrome).

Wernicke's Aphasia. In 1874, Karl Wernicke described a language impairment that was characterized by fluent verbal output and impaired comprehension. Essentially identical aphasia syndromes have also been called sensory aphasia or receptive aphasia.

Verbal output in Wernicke's aphasia is either normal or increased, sometimes over 200 words per minute.[16] Speech production demands little or no effort, and articulation is normal. Sentences are of normal length with normal prosody. However, sentences are devoid of meaningful words, so that almost no information is conveyed, an output that can be called empty speech; paraphasia is common.[13] Paraphasia may be literal when a syllable is substituted within a word (phonemic substitution) or semantic (also termed verbal paraphasia) when a word is substituted. Words can also be substituted by meaningless, nonsense words (neologisms). "Jargon aphasia" is a severe form of Wernicke's aphasia with rapid verbal output, abundant paraphasic substitutions, and incomprehensible verbalization. When patients have an increased output and speak incessantly, this is called logorrhea or pressured speech, an aphasic output nearly diagnostic of Wernicke's aphasia.

Comprehension of spoken language is disturbed in Wernicke's aphasia. The severity of the comprehension deficit is variable. Patients can sometimes understand a few words and even short sentences. Comprehension ability may decrease with testing, a phenomenon called fatigue or jamming. Two varieties of comprehension defect are described.[37] In one variety, the ability to comprehend spoken language is considerably worse than the ability to comprehend written language (the patient is predominantly word deaf), whereas in the other the opposite is true (the patient is predominantly word blind). Classic Wernicke's aphasia features a combination of the two.[19]

Other aspects of language are disturbed. Repetition of spoken language is invariably abnormal. Naming is often abnormal, and grossly paraphasic responses can be produced during confrontational naming. Reading out loud as well as reading comprehension are abnormal. Writing is also abnormal in Wernicke's aphasia. The output consists of well-formed letters combined in a meaningless manner. Correctly produced words may be scattered among the unintelligible combinations.

Neurological examination is often unrevealing. Some degree of cortical sensory loss may be present. A superior quadrantanopia suggesting involvement of the temporal radiation of the geniculocalcarine tract is often the only neurological deficit associated with Wernicke's aphasia. The absence of associated neurological deficits may lead to the erroneous diagnosis of psychosis or schizophrenia, particularly in younger patients, or dementia in older patients.

The pathology in most cases of Wernicke's aphasia is localized in the auditory association cortex of the posterosuperior portion of the first temporal gyrus of the left temporal lobe. When word deafness is predominant over word blindness, pathology tends to be deeper in the first temporal gyrus, involving Heschl's gyrus or its connections. Predominance of word blindness suggests greater involvement of the contiguous parietal cortex (primarily the angular gyrus). Pure word deafness is discussed in the next section. A variety of pathological entities are known to produce Wernicke's aphasia, including vascular events and tumors or abscesses of the temporal lobe.

The outcome and recovery of Wernicke's aphasia is less favorable than Broca's aphasia. With improvement, some ability to recognize spoken words appears. With continued improvement, the patient may be able to understand auditory material if it is presented slowly.[38] Recovery may be delayed by associated behavioral problems; most of the patients, however, are unaware of their deficit, making rehabilitation efforts difficult, and paranoid ideation is common.[13]

Conduction Aphasia. Conduction aphasia occurs in up to 15 percent of admissions of patients with aphasia in some reports.[37, 39] The defining feature of conduction aphasia is the repetition difficulty. Verbal output in conduction aphasia is fluent and paraphasic, but the amount of output is less than Wernicke's aphasia. Articulation is excellent, and comprehension of spoken language is intact. In contrast, the repetition of numbers or the naming of colors may be contaminated with phonemic paraphasias. Confrontational naming is also disturbed mainly because of paraphasic errors. Reading out loud may be similarily compromised; in contrast, reading silently for comprehension is intact. The ability to write is invariably disturbed to some extent. Most often, syllables and letters are substituted or misspelled or misplaced. Often, conduction aphasia is not diagnosed at the onset but develops in the recovery phase from Wernicke's aphasia. With further improvement, patients remain anomic.

The neurological examination often shows no abnormalities, but variable motor or sensory findings and ideomotor apraxia may be present. A pseudothalamic pain syndrome may develop in the recovery phase. Visual fields may show variable deficits reflecting involvement of different sites neighboring the locus of pathology underlying conduction aphasia.[13]

The site of pathology in conduction aphasia involves the left hemisphere arcuate fasciculus, most often deep to the supramarginal gyrus. This may produce a separation of the sensory and motor language areas, as originally suggested by Wernicke.[40, 41] Cases with features of conduction aphasia have been described with lesions outside this area, notably in the left supramarginal gyrus and left temporal gyrus.[37, 39] The most common cause of conduction aphasia is occlusion of a portion of the angular branch of the middle cerebral artery.

Global Aphasia. In global aphasia, all language functions are seriously impaired. The verbal output is always limited but not to a state of mutism. Single words or syllables can sometimes be produced, and occasionally, verbal output is limited to strings of a single syllable.[13] Some cases can produce highly automatic, overlearned phrases such as "How are you?" Comprehension is often better than verbal output but is also seriously disturbed. Repetition, naming, reading, and writing are all compromised. Neurological examination often shows hemiplegia, visual field loss, and sensory abnormalities. In some patients, the condition evolves from global aphasia to the other aphasia syndromes. Patients who do not make a rapid recovery soon after onset have a poor prognosis. The pathology may involve a large part of the left hemisphere, often in the distribution of the middle cerebral artery. Rare cases are reported, however, with a global aphasia but few associated neurological deficits. In those cases, small, strategically placed lesions involve Broca's and Wernicke's areas simultaneously.[42] Strokes are probably the most common cause, but a tumor, trauma, an infection, a gunshot wound, and other causes can all lead to severe global aphasia.

Extrasylvian Aphasias

In extrasylvian aphasias, pathology is localized outside the regions immediately bordering the sylvian fissure (see Fig. 6–4). There are three recognized aphasic syndromes in this category: transcortical motor, transcortical sensory, and mixed transcortical aphasias.

Transcortical Motor Aphasia. Transcortical motor aphasia resembles Broca's aphasia, but the patients are able to repeat. The term transcortical aphasia was suggested by Wernicke in 1881 and Lichtheim in 1885. It was also termed anterior isolation syndrome by Benson and Geschwind.[43] Verbal output is described as nonfluent and dysarthric, as in Broca's aphasia. But patients with transcortical motor aphasia have a stronger tendency to stutter, and output is often agrammatical and is produced with considerable effort. Comprehension of spoken language is normal. Sometimes the presence of associated apraxia might falsely suggest that the patient does not comprehend when asked to point to room objects or carry out commands. Repetition is usually good to excellent. Confrontational naming is often disturbed, and prompting with contextual cues or phonemic cues helps these patients considerably. Reading out loud produces poorly articulated speech. Comprehension of written language is intact and usually better than in patients with Broca's aphasia. Writing ability is always defective. It is often clumsily written with large letters, poor spelling, and agrammatical output. Most often, transcortical motor aphasia is seen in the recovery phase from Broca's aphasia. Patients with transcortical motor aphasia usually have variable recovery.

Neurological examination usually reveals right hemiplegia. Apraxia is very common, and conjugate ocular deviation is occasionally seen. Sensory loss and visual field loss do not occur.

Transcortical motor aphasia is not a frequent entity. Cases occur with lesions in the anterior watershed area or with occlusion of the left anterior cerebral artery. In some cases, pathology is located in the left frontal or prefrontal regions of the dominant hemisphere anterior or superior to Broca's area.[21] It is suggested that transcortical motor aphasia is the result of a separation of the pathways that connect the supplementary motor area with Broca's area.[44] Other patients have lesions of the left medial frontal region.

A variant of transcortical motor aphasia has been termed *supplementary motor area aphasia.* This syndrome is basically identical to transcortical motor aphasia but is produced by damage to the dominant hemisphere medial frontal structures, notably the cingulate cortex and supplementary motor area. Following initial mutism, patients with this disturbance develop a slow hypophonic output that improves considerably with repetition. In comparison with transcortical motor aphasia, patients with supplementary motor area aphasia have a characteristic neurological disturbance with weakness of the right lower extremity and shoulder but relatively normal strength in the arm and face. A similar pattern of sensory disturbance may or may not be present.[11] This syndrome is not common and occurs most often after occlusion of the dominant hemisphere anterior cerebral artery.

Transcortical Sensory Aphasia. Transcortical sensory aphasia is a distinct entity that features fluent output that is often contaminated by considerable paraphasia, including both neologistic and semantic substitutions. Comprehension of spoken language is severely disturbed. In striking contrast, repetition is intact. The patient is often echolalic, repeating most of the examiner's utterances with apparent unawareness of what is said. Naming is disturbed. Reading out loud may be preserved but is usually contaminated with paraphasic errors. Reading comprehension is defective. Writing is also abnormal.

Sensory abnormalities usually of the cortical type are found as well as a visual field defect. Occasionally, patients with transcortical sensory aphasia have a normal neurological examination and are misdiagnosed as schizophrenic.

The pathology underlying this syndrome is often located in the parietal and temporal areas, posterior to the perisylvian region. Occlusion of the left internal carotid with a subsequent posterior borderzone infarction frequently underlies transcortical sensory aphasia. Tumors in the parietotemporo-occipital junction area, as well as trauma, intracerebral hematoma,[45] and degenerative disorders such as Alzheimer's disease[46] are other reported causes.

Transcortical sensory aphasia may also follow the resolution of Wernicke's aphasia. The prognosis is usually guarded.

Mixed Transcortical Aphasia. Mixed transcortical aphasia, or isolation aphasia, is equivalent to global aphasia with preserved repetition.[47] Patients with this syndrome do not speak unless spoken to and their verbal output is almost entirely limited to what has been offered by the examiner, a true echolalia.[13] Patients may embellish the output in the form of the completion phenomenon or spontaneous correction of grammatical errors deliberately produced by the examiner. Thus, if told the beginning of a common phrase, the patient may not only repeat what has been said but continue the phrase to completion. Comprehension of spoken language is severely disturbed. The ability to repeat, although well preserved compared with all other language features, remains limited and is often below normal. The number of words in a sentence that can be repeated is often limited to three or four. Naming, reading out loud, reading for comprehension, and writing are severely compromised. When a response is elicited, it is often contaminated with paraphasias. Neurological examination reveals variable motor, sensory, and visual field deficits.

The pathology underlying mixed transcortical aphasia is most often located in both the anterior and posterior vascular borderzone cortical areas of the left hemisphere. Although borderzone pathology is rare in its pure form, individuals with acute left internal carotid occlusion or the residuals of severe cerebral edema or prolonged hypoxia may show the mixed transcortical language pattern. The course of this syndrome is one of improvement to a stable state of often severe language disability. The syndrome has been reported with unusual frequency in Creutzfeldt-Jakob disease.

Subcortical Aphasia

With the advent of brain imaging, language disorders that previously were difficult to characterize were found to have pathology affecting subcortical structures, particularly the basal ganglia and the thalamus.[48] Considerable variation is seen in the clinical picture depending on the specific subcortical structures involved, but several general characteristics help define the entity. First, there is typically an acute onset with mutism, recovering slowly to a hypophonic, slow, and poorly articulated output. Other language features vary depending on the site of subcortical pathology.

Aphasia has been reported following lesions in several different subcortical structures. Electrical stimulation and functional imaging studies have increased awareness of the role of these structures in language processing.[49, 50] Left thalamic lesions involving predominantly ventrolateral nuclei or anterior nuclei produce a mildly nonfluent aphasia with frequent paraphasias, impaired naming, logorrhea, and relatively preserved repetition and comprehension.[51] Hypertensive hemorrhage and ischemic lesions, particularly those involving the tuberthalamic artery, are the main causative etiologies. Basal ganglia lesions involving the striatum and internal capsule produce features of Wernicke's aphasia with dysarthria, hypophonia, and variable performance on repetition.[52, 53] These lesions resemble either a transcortical motor or sensory aphasia with the exception of the frequency of paraphasias and dysarthria. Except in rare cases and those involving large areas extending beyond the basal ganglia, recovery is significant.[19, 51–53]

Several theories have been proposed to explain the role of subcortical structures in the various forms of language impairment; these include cortical dysfunction secondary to mass effect and compression from blood in the thalamic/basal ganglia regions and dysfunction related to diaschisis. Another theory suggests a disconnection syndrome between cortical language areas and subcortical structures, proposing that there are "language loops" comparable to the cognitive loops involving subcortical structures and the frontal cortex. Subcortical mechanisms may impact the attentional and selective engagement properties of the thalamus. Subcortical structures may serve as a gating mechanism to control input and output and play a role in the ability of the thalamus to activate the specific regions of cortex required to carry out language functions.[50, 51, 54]

Nonlocalizing Aphasic Syndromes

Anomic Aphasia. Anomic aphasia is also known as amnestic aphasia and nominal aphasia. Anomia is a very frequent finding in aphasia to the extent that it is considered imprudent to suggest a diagnosis of aphasia in its absence.[13] Anomic aphasia refers to those aphasic syndromes in which the principal deficit is in confrontational naming. Although spontaneous speech is fluent and easily produced, there is an emptiness, which results from a lack of substantive words, with substitution of many nonspecific words that fail to communicate an idea satisfactorily. This vague output is called empty speech. Most often, excessive word-finding pauses typify the anomic output. If the description demands a substantive word that cannot be produced, another description may be tried. This rapidly produces a circuitous output called circumlocution.

Other language aspects are more intact. Comprehension is relatively well preserved. Reading and writing may be entirely normal, but not infrequently, there is abnormality in both. When anomia occurs by itself, it may result from pathology almost anywhere in the left hemisphere area and can even be seen in some cases of right hemisphere lesions.[13, 19] There is a fairly common syndrome in which anomic aphasia is associated with alexia plus Gerstmann's syndrome (agraphia, right-left disorientation, acalculia, and finger agnosia). In this syndrome, the pathology is localized in the left angular gyrus.[13, 14] Anomia is often the residual of more severe aphasic syndromes and remains the complaint of many well-recovered aphasics. Anomia also is seen in degenerative disorders such as Alzheimer's disease.

ALEXIAS AND AGRAPHIAS

Alexia Without Agraphia

Alexia without agraphia was first described by Dejerine in 1892 in a patient who suddenly lost the ability to read but had no other language disturbance. The only neurological finding of significance was a right homonymous hemianopia. Although the patient was unable to read except for some individual letters, he could write adequately. In patients with this syndrome, the patient can write but cannot read his or her own written output. If the letters of a word are read aloud, the patient can often put them together so that the word can be deciphered. The patient often has verbal alexia, which refers to an inability to read words (also called word blindness) but not literal alexia (letter blindness), retaining the ability to read letters. The patient with alexia without agraphia can recognize individual letters when they are drawn in the palm or palpated from embossed blocks. Patients with this syndrome do not lose the ability to see verbal stimuli, but visual information has lost access to the language area. Patients with this disorder also have greater difficulty in copying written material than in producing words to dictation. They can spell words out loud without difficulty. Many patients have disturbed color naming as well as a mild degree of anomia. Some have difficulty in reading numbers and others suffer from true acalculia.

The causative lesion is nearly always a stroke in the territory of the left posterior cerebral artery, with infarction of the medial occipital lobe, the medial temporal lobe, and the splenium of the corpus callosum. Dejerine suggested a disconnection between the intact right visual cortex and the left hemisphere areas mediating language, particularly the angular gyrus. Geschwind repopularized this disconnection theory.[55]

As a separate but closely related entity, Greenblatt[56] has described a syndrome that he named subangular alexia. Patients with this disorder have alexia without agraphia but with hemianopia. The structural pathology in these cases involves the white matter deep in the dominant parietal cortex, undercutting the angular gyrus.

Alexia with Agraphia

In 1891, Dejerine also described a syndrome of alexia with agraphia in a patient who suffered a cerebral vascular accident. The ability to read both letters and words is impaired, and thereis equal difficulty in comprehension of numbers and musical notation. Cues are of little help. Thus, tracing the letter with the finger does not aid in identification, and the patient with this type of alexia cannot decipher a word when it is spelled aloud for him. The writing disturbance is usually of equal severity. The ability to copy written material is far better than the ability to produce it on command. This syndrome may be considered an acquired illiteracy, in which a previously educated patient is rendered unable to read and write.

This disorder often overlaps with Wernicke's aphasia. In those cases, the patients often have a paraphasic output, impaired naming, and poor repetition, as well as disturbed written comprehension (word blindness) more than auditory comprehension (word deafness). Associated findings include right hemianopia or superior quadrantanopia, elements of Gerstmann's syndrome, and right-sided sensory loss. Most often, there is partial recovery, permitting only limited reading comprehension.

The most common locus of pathology in this syndrome is situated in the parietotemporal junction of the left hemisphere, particularly in the angular gyrus.

The association of alexia with agraphia in Gerstmann's syndrome and anomia has been called the angular gyrus syndrome, and the combined disorder almost invariably indicates a left hemisphere inferior parietal location of the causative pathology.[57]

Frontal Alexia

A number of features of frontal alexia are sufficiently distinctive to allow differentiation from the other varieties of alexia.[15] Most patients with the disorder can read, both aloud and for comprehension, but only isolated words from a given sentence are uttered; the recognized words are almost exclusively substantives. If relational words such as adjectives and prepositional phrases are the determining language structures, the patient may completely misinterpret the sentence. Nonfluent aphasia is often associated with frontal alexia. The site of pathology in frontal alexia involves the same locus as Broca's aphasia.

Other types of alexias have been described, including hemialexia following posterior corpus callosum section, unilateral paralexia, a manifestation of unilateral inattention, and other variants.[57]

Agraphia

Agraphia may be defined as a loss or impairment of the ability to produce written language, caused by brain dysfunction. Almost without exception, every individual with aphasia shows at least some degree of agraphia, and tests of writing ability can be used as a screening device to detect the presence of aphasia. Caution is necessary, however, because agraphia accompanies many disturbances other than aphasia.[13] Abnormalities of constructional skills, visuospatial discrimination, and disturbances of motor skills, such as ataxia, rigidity, spasticity, chorea, myoclonus, and tremor, cause major alterations in the quality of graphic output.

Three variations of agraphia are outlined.[13] *Left frontal (anterior) agraphia* is seen in patients with Broca's aphasia, and their written output parallels their verbal output. Words and letters are large and messy with poor spelling, and sentences are devoid of grammatical words (agrammatism). *Left parietotemporal (posterior) agraphia* is seen in patients with posterior aphasias, and written output parallels their spoken output. Literal and verbal paragraphias as well as empty writing are present. *Visuospatial agraphia* is most commonly associated with posterior right hemisphere defects causing constructional disturbance. The script is well formed, but there is a tendency for the written line to slant upward and for the left margin to be larger and increasing in size with subsequent lines.

LANGUAGE-RELATED DISORDERS

Aphemia

Aphemia was the term originally used by Broca to describe all language disturbances, but he later accepted the term aphasia promoted by Trousseau (1864). Bastian (1887) used aphemia to denote a specific syndrome described here; others have termed the same language abnormality pure motor aphasia, cortical anarthria, or apraxia of speech.

Aphemia traditionally is described as a disorder presenting with mutism but preserved ability to communicate using written language. More recent descriptions include patients with impaired writing abilities characterized by omission of prepositions and numerous spelling errors. When verbalization returns, the output is hypophonic, slow, and poorly articulated so as to be almost incomprehensible. Comprehension of spoken language is intact. Although both repetition and naming are severely disturbed because they demand vocalization, patients can comprehend written language and are able to write without difficulty. Primary laryngeal pathology should be ruled out.

Neurological examination reveals a transient right hemiplegia or hemiparesis without other neurological signs except for an often associated buccofacial apraxia. Patients have difficulty performing on command acts such as whistling, sucking, blowing, and winking. In contrast, they have no trouble performing limb activities such as imitating the use of a comb or a toothbrush, waving goodbye, and saluting.

In aphemia, the communication disturbance involves verbal output and is a speech problem rather than an impairment of language. There is often an overlap, however, between aphemia and the anterior aphasia syndromes. An aphemia-like state appears in some patients who have recovered from Broca's aphasia. Some investigators have even considered aphemia to be a minor subtype of Broca's aphasia, also called little Broca's aphasia.

However, aphemia differs from true Broca's aphasia because of the absence of agrammatism in the spoken and written output. Most often, aphemia improves to useful language output, but a dysprosodic speech quality remains, producing a so-called foreign accent syndrome, a disorder of rhythm, inflection, and articulation, suggesting that the patient is not a native speaker of the language. The pathology is located in or immediately inferior to Broca's area in the dominant hemisphere (see Fig. 6–5).[11]

Pure Word Deafness

Pure word deafness is a rare prelanguage syndrome in which only reception of spoken language is involved. Individuals with pure word deafness do not understand spoken language and cannot repeat. However, they are able to hear and identify adequately nonverbal sounds such as a whistle, a telephone ring, and a dog bark. Their reading is intact, and they often carry with them a writing tablet for others to use.[19]

There are two known loci of pathology. Some patients have a single lesion deep in the dominant superior temporal region affecting the primary auditory cortex or the pathways to it from the medial geniculate nucleus. More commonly, there is bilateral pathology involving the midportion of the superior temporal gyrus of both hemispheres. Wernicke's area (left auditory association cortex) is not involved.

Some cases of pure word deafness have associated paraphasic output and mild written language comprehension deficits. These cases should be classified as Wernicke's aphasias with predominant word deafness and relatively less word blindness (reading comprehension).

Pure word deafness is not a disturbance of language ability. Delivery of the auditory signal to the area mediating language interpretation is defective, which is a sensory transmission problem rather than a language disturbance. Pure word deafness resembles deafness more than aphasia. It has also been called auditory verbal agnosia.[58] Although pure word deafness is rare in isolation, it may be associated with posterior aphasic disorders.

Delirium

Delirium with fluctuating consciousness and disturbed thought content is associated with variable language difficulties with or without structural brain pathology. Patients often have impaired attention and do poorly on tasks such as digit span and mental control. Language disturbances can be the presenting feature of delirium, particularly in patients with decreased attention and concentration. Associated features may include agitation, hallucinations, confusion, and myoclonus.

Psychiatric Disorders

Psychiatric disorders can occasionally mimic classic language syndromes. Schizophrenics often present with verbal output described as word salad, containing bizarre words and sentences. Written output parallels the content of verbal output. These patients have no other language disturbances and are usually readily distinguished from Wernicke's or other posterior aphasias. Manic patients often present with logorrheic output, pressured speech, and grandiose content, but no other language disturbances are encountered that distinguish them from other classic aphasia syndromes.

Right Hemisphere Disorders

Right hemisphere disorders can affect language function, most commonly in left-handed individuals. Rarely, right-handed patients become aphasic after strokes in the right hemisphere, a phenomenon called crossed aphasia in dextrals. Even in right-handed people with typical left hemisphere dominance for language, subtle alterations in language function occur after right hemisphere damage. The right hemisphere has been considered the dominant hemipshere for the expression and detection of emotion in language, gestures, and

TABLE 6–6. **Clinico-anatomical Correlations of Speech and Language Disorders**

Anatomical Site of Damage	Speech or Language Syndrome	Other Neurological and Medical Findings	Common Etiologies	Comments
(L) Posterior inferior frontal lobe	Broca's aphasia	Brachiofacial weakness	Stroke, trauma, tumor, infection	Initial (L) conjugate gaze deviation
(L) Posterior superior temporal gyrus	Wernicke's aphasia	Visual field deficit	Stroke, temporal lobe abscess	
(L) Posterior sylvian region	Conduction aphasia	Cortical sensory deficit pseudothalamic pain	Stroke	Associated ideomotor apraxia
(L) Sylvian region	Global aphasia	Hemianopia, hemiplegia	Stroke, tumor, trauma, infection	
(L) Dorsolateral frontal cortex	Transcortical motor aphasia	Buccofacial apraxia, hemiparesis is occasional	Anterior borderzone vascular infarction	
(L) Temporoparieto-occipital junction	Transcortical sensory aphasia	Critical sensory deficit Visual field deficit	Posterior borderzone vascular infarction Degenerative disease	Echolalia is common
(L) Hemisphere, vascular border-zone areas	Mixed transcortical aphasia	Variable motor, sensory, and visual field deficits	Borderzone infarctions, anoxia, carbon monoxide poisoning	Echolalia very common
(L) Thalamus, striatum white matter	Subcortical aphasia	Hemiplegia/sensory loss	Stroke, ischemic and hemorrhagic	No visual field or cortical sensory loss
Unilateral or bilateral corticobulbar tracts	Spastic dysarthria	Unilateral or bilateral hyper-reflexia or spasticity	Stroke, demyelinating and degenerative disease	
Cerebellum	Ataxic dysarthria	Dysmetria, nystagmus, ataxia	Stroke, degenerative, toxic disorder; tumor	
Lower motor neuron, brain stem, or peripheral nerves	Flaccid dysarthria	Atrophy, fasciculation, decreased gag	Motor neuron disease, stroke, carcinomatous meningitis	Risk of aspiration pneumonia
Basal ganglia	Hypokinetic/ hyperkinetic dysarthria	Parkinsonism, dystonia, chorea	Degenerative disease, Parkinson's disease, Huntington's disease, stroke	
Vocal cords or their innervation	Dysphonia	Fatigability, ptosis	Laryngitis, vocal cord paralysis, myasthenia	May be a sign of laryngeal carcinoma

TABLE 6–7. **Selected Etiologies of Speech and Language Disorders**

Etiological Category	Selected Specific Etiologies	Chapter
Structural Disorders		
Developmental	Arnold-Chiari malformations	28
Hereditary and Degenerative Disorders		
Storage diseases: Lipidoses, glycogen disorders, and leukoencephalopathies	Adrenoleukodystrophy, Krabbe's disease, metachromatic leukodystrophy	30
The degenerative dementias	Alzheimer's disease, frontotemporal degeneration, Parkinson's disease, Huntington's disease	33
Movement disroders	Hallervorden-Spatz disease, Wilson's disease, progressive supranuclear palsy, Parkinson's disease, multiple system atrophy, Huntington's disease	34
Ataxias	Friedreich's ataxia, abetalipoproteinemia	35
Degenerative motor, sensory, and autonomic disorders	Amyotrophic lateral sclerosis	36
Hereditary nondegenerative neuromuscular disease	Myopathies	37
Acquired Metabolic and Nutritional Disorders		
Endogenous metabolic disorders	Hypothyroidism	38
Exogenous acquired metabolic disorders of the nervous system: Toxins and illicit drugs	Cocaine	39

TABLE 6–7. **Selected Etiologies of Speech and Language Disorders** *Continued*

Etiological Category	Selected Specific Etiologies	Chapter
Nutritional deficiencies and syndromes associated with alcoholism	Alcoholic cerebellar degeneration Vitamin E deficiency	40
Infectious Disorders		
Viral infections	Herpetic encephalitis	41
Nonviral infections	Toxoplasmosis or bacterial abscess of the temporal lobe	42
Transmissible spongiform encephalopathies	Creutzfeldt-Jakob disease, Gerstmann-Straussler syndrome	43
HIV and AIDS	Lymphoma, toxoplasmosis, AIDS dementia complex	44
Neurovascular Disorders	Vascular dementia; embolic, thrombotic, and hemorrhagic stroke	45
Neoplastic Disorders		
Primary neurological tumors	Glioblastoma, meningioma, astrocytoma	46
Metastatic neoplasms and paraneoplastic syndromes	Metastasis from lung, breast, melanoma, paraneoplastic cerebellar degeneration	47
Demyelinating Disorders		
Demyelinating disorders of the central nervous system	Multiple sclerosis, progressive multifocal leukoencephalopathy	48
Demyelinating disorders of the peripheral nervous system	Guillain-Barré syndrome	49
Autoimmune and Inflammatory Disorders	Myasthenia gravis	50
Traumatic Disorders	Contusion, subdural hematoma	51
Epilepsy	Frontal lobe epilepsy	52
Headache and Facial Pain	Migraine with aura	53
Sleep Disorders	Hypoxemia and hypotension with sleep apnea	54
Drug-Induced and Iatrogenic Neurological Disorders	Anterior cerebral infarction following aneurysm clipping	55

AIDS, Acquired immunodeficiency syndrome; HIV, human immunodeficiency virus.

faces, although a critical review of the literature has questioned these assumptions.[59, 60] Localization of emotional comprehension and emotional repetition have been less well characterized than comparable left hemisphere language functions. The inability to express affect in speech (affective motor aprosodia) has repeatedly been shown to result from lesions in the right frontal opercular region.[61] This syndrome is characterized by flat, robotic speech with loss of normal melody and emotional intonation. Affected patients also lack variability in the spacing of words and syllables to imply meaning. They rely more on semantic information to convey emotions. Frequently, this syndrome is interpreted as depression; however, patients deny the feeling or experience of being depressed. In addition, receptive amusia and other disorders of music appreciation are related disturbances predominantly associated with right hemisphere lesions.

Tables 6–6 and 6–7 summarize clinico-anatomical correlations and major etiological categories of speech and language disorders.

General Management Goals

Language and speech are basic for human existence, and their loss is often catastrophic. Most patients lose their ability to communicate in a sudden and unexpected way. In addition to the loss of language itself, patients may lose their employment, social position, recreational opportunities, and many other stabilizing factors of personal existence.[15] The prognosis of any speech and language disorder depends on many factors, including etiology, lesion site, severity, profile of aphasic deficits, age at onset, individual (crossed aphasics), or group characteristics (left-handedness).

Most clinicians agree that speech therapy may be helpful and begin treatment as soon as possible, but delays in treatment are not detrimental and are warranted until the patient is neurologically stable.[62] Therapy should be goal driven, not simply to maximize or optimize language function. The therapist should identify limiting factors, establish treatment plans for the treatable factors, and specify both the expected outcome and specific duration of treatment.

Treatment should also address complications of speech and language disorders. Depression is associated with left hemisphere injury, particularly in the deep frontal regions, and is associated with Broca's aphasia, global aphasia, or subcortical aphasia with anterior extension.[63, 64] Treatment of depression includes support and encouragement, concentration on domains in which the patient succeeds, and antidepressant medication. Paranoid and agitated behavior is occasionally observed in patients with posterior aphasic syndromes, particularly those with Wernicke's aphasia and pure word deafness;[65] management consists of antipsychotic drugs in low doses. Finally, patients with associated bulbar or pseudobulbar palsy are at increased risk for aspiration and secondary lung infection and should be monitored closely and considered for percutaneous gastric feeding tube.

Patients with aphasia are often assumed to be incompetent because of their reduced communication ability; the inability to communicate through verbal or written language, however, does not preclude aphasic patients from nonverbal communication, thinking, and expressing opinions. Even severely aphasic patients can live semi-independently and develop new interests and goals.

Reviews and Selected Updates

Bastian HC: On different kinds of aphasia. Brit Med 1887;2:931–936, 985–990.

Benson DF: Aphasia, Alexia, and Agraphia. New York, Churchill Livingstone, 1979.

Benson DF, Ardila A: Aphasia: A Clinical Perspective. New York, Oxford University Press, 1996.

Darley FL, Aronson EE, Brown JR: Motor Speech Disorders. Philadelphia, WB Saunders, 1975.

Dejerine J: Contribution à l'étude anatomo-pathologique et clinique des différentes variétés de cécité verbale. Mem Soc Biol 1892;4:61–90.

Demonet JF, Thierry G: Language and brain: What is up? What is coming up? J Clin Exp Neuropsych 2001;23:49–73.

Kertesz A: Aphasia. *In* Vinken PJ, Bruyn GW, Klawans HL (eds): Handbook of Clinical Neurology, Vol 45, Clinical Neuropsychology. Amsterdam, Elsevier, 1985.

Lecours AR, Lhermitte F, Bryans B: Aphasiology. London, Bailliere-Tindall, 1983.

Metter EJ: Speech Disorders. New York, Spectrum Publications, 1985.

Price CJ: The anatomy of language: Contributions from functional neuroimaging. J Anat 2000;197:335–359.

Saffran EM: Aphasia and the relationship of language and brain. Sem Neurol 2000;20:409–419.

Trousseau A: De l'aphasia. Gaz Hôp (Paris) 1864;37:13, 25, 37, 49.

References

1. Geschwind N, Quadfasel F, Segarra J: Isolation of the speech area. Neuropsychologia 1968;6:327–340.
2. Coren S, Porac C: Fifty centuries of right-handedness: The historical record. Science 1977;198:631–632.
3. Devinsky O: Behavioral Neurology. 100 maxims in neurology series, Vol I. Edward Arnold, 1992, pp 88–90.
4. Brown JW, Hecaen H: Lateralization and language representation. Neurology 1976;26:183–189.
5. Heilman KM, Bowers D, Speedie L, et al: Comprehension of affective and nonaffective prosody. Neurology 1984;34:917–923.
6. Starkstein SE, Federoff JP, Price TR, et al: Neuropsychological and neuroradiologic correlates of emotional prosody comprehension. Neurology 1994;44:515–522.
7. Schmitt JJ, Hartje W, Willmes K: Hemispheric asymmetry in the recognition of emotional attitude conveyed by facial expression, prosody, and propositional speech. Cortex 1997;33:65–81.
8. Buchanan TW, Lutz K, Mirzazde S, et al: Recognition of emotional prosody and verbal components of spoken language: An fMRI study. Cognitive Brain Research 2000;9:227–238.
9. Blumstein SE: Approaches to speech production deficits in aphasia. *In* Boller F, Grafman J (eds): Handbook of Neuropsychology, Vol I. Amsterdam, Elsevier, 1988, pp 349–365.
10. Darley FL, Aronson A, Brown J: Motor Speech Disorders. Philadelphia, WB Saunders, 1975.
11. Alexander MP, Benson DF, Stuss DT: Frontal lobes and language. Brain Lang 1989;37:656.
12. Gelmers HJ: Non-paralytic motor disturbances and speech disorders. The role of the supplementary motor area. J Neurol Neurosurg Psychiatry 1983;46:1052.
13. Benson DF: Aphasia, Alexia, and Agraphia. New York, Churchill Livingstone, 1979.
14. Benson DF, Geschwind N: The aphasias and related disturbances. *In* Baker NB, Baker LH (eds): Clinical Neurology. Philadelphia, J.B. Lippincott, 1988, Chapter 10, pp 1–34.
15. Benson DF, Ardila A: Aphasia: A Clinical Perspective. New York, Oxford Univesity Press, 1996.
16. Howes D, Geschwind N: Quantitative studies of aphasic language. *In* Mck Rioch D, Weinstein EA (eds): Disorders of Communication. Proceedings of the Association for Research in Nervous and Mental Disease, Vol XLII. Baltimore, Williams & Wilkins, 1964, pp 229–244.
17. Benson DF: Fluency in aphasia: Correlation with radioactive scan localization. Cortex 1967;3:373–394.
18. Wagenaar E, Snow C, Prins R: Spontaneous speech of aphasic patients: A psycholinguistic analysis. Brain Lang 1975;2:281–303.
19. Benson DF: Aphasia. *In* Heilman KM, Valenstein E (eds): Clinical Neuropsychology. New York, Oxford University Press, 1993, pp 17–36.
20. Benson DF, Geschwind N: The aphasias and related disturbances. *In* Baker AB, Joynt RJ (eds): Clinical Neurology, Vol I. Philadelphia, Harper & Row, 1985, Chapter 10, pp 1–32.
21. Alexander MP, Benson DF: The aphasias and related disturbances. *In* Joynt RJ (ed): Clinical Neurology, Vol I. Philadelphia, J.B. Lippincott, 1991, Chapter 10, pp 1–58.
22. Passarelli D, Santangello M, Rizzi R, et al: Rapid Rate Transcranial Magnetic Stimulation and Hemispheric Language Dominance: Usefulness and Safety in Epilepsy. Neurology, Vol I. Philadelphia, J.B. Lippincott, 1991.
23. Metter EJ: Speech Disorders. New York, Spectrum Publications, 1985.
24. Cappa SF, Guidotti M, Papagno C, Vignolo LA: Speechlessness with occasional vocalizations after bilateral opercular lesions: A case study. Aphasiology 1987;1:35–39.
25. Pineda D, Ardila A: Lasting mutism associated with buccofacial apraxia. Aphasiology 1992;6:285–292.
26. Plum F, Posner JB: Stupor and Coma, 3rd ed. Philadelphia, F.A. Davis, 1982.
27. Kremer M, Russell WR, Smyth GE: A mid-brain syndrome following head injury. J Neurol Neurosurg Psychiatry 1947;10:49–60.
28. Cummings JL, Benson DF, Hill MA, Read S: Aphasia in dementia of the Alzheimer type. Neurology 1985;35:394–397.
29. Cummings JL, Benson DF: Speech and language alterations in dementia syndromes. *In* Ardila A, Ostrosky F (eds): Brain Organization of Language and Cognitive Processes. New York, Plenum, 1989, pp 107–120.
30. Rosenfield DB, Nudelman HB: Stuttering. *In* Adelman G (ed): Encyclopedia of Neuroscience, Vol II. Boston, Birkhauser, 1987, pp 1149–1150.
31. Broca P, Perte de la Parole: Ramollissement chronique et destruction partielle du lobe anterieur gauche du cerveau. Bulletin, Societe d'Anthropologie (Paris) 1861;2:235–238.
32. Wernicke C: The symptom of complex aphasia. *In* Church ED (ed): Modern Clinical Medicine: Diseases of the Nervous System. New York, Appleton-Century-Crofts, 1908, pp 265–324.
33. Goodglass H, Berko J: Agrammatism and inflectional morphology in English. J Speech Hearing Res 1960;3:257–267.
34. Heilman KM: Neglect and related syndromes. *In* Heilman KM, Valenstein E (eds): Clinical Neuropsychology. New York, Oxford University Press, 1993, pp 279–337.
35. Damasio H: Cerebral localization of the aphasias. *In* Sarno MT (ed): Acquired Aphasia. New York, Academic Press, 1991, pp 45–73.
36. Kertesz A: Aphasia. *In* Vinken PJ, Bruyn GW, Klawans HL (eds): Handbook of Clinical Neurology, Vol 45, Clinical Neuropsychology. Amsterdam, Elsevier, 1985, pp 287–331.
37. Hecaen H, Albert ML: Human Neuropsychology. New York, John Wiley & Sons, 1978.
38. Albert ML, Bear D: Time to understand. A case study of world deafness with reference to the role of time in auditory comprehension. Brain 1974;97:383–394.
39. Benson DF, Sheremata WA, Bouchard R, et al: Conduction aphasia. Arch Neurol 1973;28:339–346.
40. Damasio H, Damasio A: The anatomical basis of conduction aphasia. Brain 1980;103:337–350.
41. Mendez MF, Benson DF: Atypical conduction aphasia: A disconnection syndrome. Arch Neurol 1985;42:886–891.
42. Legatt AD, Rubin MJ, Kaplan LR, et al: Global aphasia without hemiparesis: Multiple etiologies. Neurology 1987;37:201–205.
43. Benson DF, Geschwind N: The aphasias and related disturbances. *In* Baker AB, Baker LH (eds): Clinical Neurology, Vol I. New York, Harper & Row, 1971, Chapter 8, pp 1–24.
44. Freedman M, Alexander MP, Naeser MA: The anatomical basis of transcortical motor aphasia. Neurology 1984;34:409–417.

45. Kertesz A, Sheppard A, MacKenzie R: Localization in transcortical sensory aphasia. Arch Neurol 1982;39:475–478.
46. Murdoch BE, Chenery HJ, Wilks V, Boyle RS: Language disorders in dementia of the Alzheimer type. Brain Lang 1987;31:122–137.
47. Geschwind N, Quadfasel F, Segarra J: Isolation of the speech area. Neuropsychologia 1968;6:327–340.
48. Damasio AR, Damasio H, Rizzo M, et al: Aphasia with nonhemorrhagic lesions in the basal ganglia and internal capsule. Arch Neurol 1982;39:15–20.
49. Metz-Lutz M, Namer IJ, Gounot D, et al: Language functional neuroimaging changes following focal left thalamic infarction. Neuroreport 2000;11:2907–2912.
50. Johnson MD, Ojemann GA: The role of the human thalamus in language and memory: Evidence from electrophysical studies. Brain Cog 2000;42:218–230.
51. Karussis D, Leker RR, Abramsky O: Cognitive dysfunction following thalamic stroke: A study of 16 cases and review of the literature. J Neurol Sci 2000;172:25–29.
52. Chung C, Caplan LR, Yamamoto Y, et al: Striatocapsular haemorrhage. Brain 2000;123:1850–1862.
53. Kumral E, Evyapan D, Balkir K: Acute caudate vascular lesions. Stroke 1999;30:100–108.
54. Crosson B: Subcortical mechanisms in language: Lexical-semantic mechanisms and the thalamus. Brain Cog 1999;40:414–438.
55. Geschwind N: Disconnection syndromes in animals and man. Brain 1965;88:237–294, 585–644.
56. Greenblatt SH: Subangular alexia without agraphia or hemianopia. Brain Lang 1976;3:229–245.
57. Friedman R, Ween JE, Martin AL: Alexia. *In* Heilman KM, Valenstein E (eds): Clinical Neuropsychology. New York, Oxford University Press, 1993, Chapter 3.
58. Schneider A, Benson DF, Alexander DN, Schnider-Klaus A: Nonverbal environmental sound recognition after unilateral hemispheric stroke. Brain 1994;117:281–287.
59. Van Lancker D, Breitenstein C: Emotional dysprosody and similar dysfunctions. *In* Bogousslavsky J, Cummings JL (eds): Behavior and Mood Disorders in Focal Brain Lesions. Cambridge, Cambridge University Press, 2000, pp 327–368.
60. Schirmer A, Alter K, Kotz SA, Friederici AD: Lateralization of prosody during language production: A lesion study. Brain Lang 2000;76:1–17.
61. Pell MD: The temporal organization of affective and non-affective speech in patients with right-hemisphere infarcts. Cortex 1999;35:455–477.
62. Basso A: Therapy of aphasia. *In* Boller F, Grafman J (eds): Handbook of Neuropsychology, Vol 2. Amsterdam, Elsevier, 1989, pp 67–82.
63. Robinson RG, Chait RM: Emotional correlates of structural brain injury with particular emphasis on post-stroke mood disorders. Crit Rev Clin Neurobiol 1985;4:285–318.
64. Starkstein SE, Robinson RG: Depression in cerebrovascular disease. *In* Starkstein SE, Robinson RG (eds): Depression in Neurological Disease. Baltimore, Johns Hopkins University Press, 1993, pp 28–49.
65. Benson DF: Psychiatric problems in aphasia. *In* Sarno MT, Boov O (eds): Aphasia: Assessment and Treatment. New York, Masson, 1980, pp 192–201.

CHAPTER 7

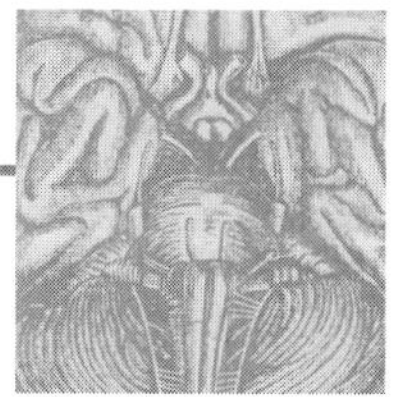

RICHARD L. DOTY

Cranial Nerve I: Olfactory Nerve

Definitions

Cranial nerve I (CN I) constitutes the primary receptor cells for the sense of smell. This nerve monitors the intake of airborne agents into the human respiratory system and largely determines, along with the sense of taste, the flavor and palatability of foods and beverages. In addition to purveying esthetic pleasures, CN I warns of spoiled foods, leaking natural gas, polluted air, and smoke and mediates elements of basic communication (e.g., mother-infant interactions). Of particular interest to the neurologist is the fact that alterations in the ability to smell are among the first, if not the first, signs of Alzheimer's disease and idiopathic Parkinson's disease.

Olfactory dysfunction can affect a patient's safety, nutritional status, and quality of life. Among 750 consecutive patients presenting to the University of Pennsylvania Smell and Taste Center with mainly olfactory problems, 68 percent experienced an altered quality of life, 46 percent reported changes in appetite or body weight, and 56 percent noted adverse influences on daily living or psychological well-being.[1] Many anosmics report increased use of sugar and seasonings to compensate for their olfactory disorder, a situation detrimental to persons with diabetes and salt-sensitive hypertension. In experimental settings, older persons with diminished smell function ingest foods that younger persons find distasteful, implying that such individuals are at considerable risk for food poisoning. It is well documented that a disproportionate number of elderly persons die from accidental gas poisoning, which is due, in large part, to their decreased ability to smell.

Most patients presenting with decreased "taste" function actually have decreased smell function. The perception of decreased ability to "taste" during deglutition is usually due to a loss of flavor sensations derived from retronasal stimulation of the olfactory receptors rather than to a loss of taste bud–mediated sensations per se. Thus, such flavors as coffee, chocolate, vanilla, strawberry, pizza, licorice, steak sauce, root beer, and cola disappear when CN I is markedly damaged, leaving intact only sweet, sour, salty, bitter, and umami (monosodium glutamate–like) sensations. Whole-mouth taste function is much more resilient to pathological or trauma-related alterations than is olfactory function, in large part because the taste buds have redundant innervation from several cranial nerves (i.e., CN VII, IX, and X).

The nomenclature for olfactory dysfunction is straightforward. *Anosmia* refers to a loss of ability to smell, whereas *hyposmia* or *microsmia* refers to diminished ability to smell. *Dysosmia* is distorted or perverted smell perception, such as when a rose smells more like garbage than a rose (*parosmia, cacosmia*) or when a "medicine-like" smell is present in the absence of odor stimulation following head trauma (*phantosmia*). *General* or *total anosmia* implies inability to smell all odorants on both sides of the nose. *Partial anosmia* implies an inability to smell certain odorants. In some cases, partial anosmia is indicative of a decreased sensitivity to a broad spectrum of odorants (*general hyposmia*), with the decrement exceeding the absolute threshold for only some odorants. *Specific anosmia*, the inability to smell one or a few odorants in the presence of an otherwise normal sense of smell, is rarely a reason for medical consultation. *Hyperosmia* is a rare condition of abnormally acute smell function. This occurs, for example, in some epileptic patients prior to the onset of ictal activity.

Olfactory dysfunction can be either *bilateral* or *unilateral* (sometimes termed *binasal* or *uninasal*). Thus, if a person has anosmia on the left side of the nose but not the right, the condition is described as unilateral left anosmia. Anosmia that is present on both sides of the nose is termed bilateral anosmia or, as noted previously, total anosmia.

Occasionally, complaints of dysosmia reflect foul odors that are produced either within the nasal cavity (e.g., as a result of infections within the nose) or within the body proper (e.g., as a result of altered metabolism). In the latter case, bad odors may come from saliva, exhaled breath, skin secretions, or urine. Although the basis of a number of such problems has nothing to do with alterations in any element of the olfactory pathway, the term dysosmia is still appropriate for describing the complaint, but not the clinical syndrome. Examples are trimethylaminuria (fish odor syndrome), in which a metabolic defect results in excretion of fish-like smelling amines, and cat's odor syndrome, a childhood neurological disorder associated with a defect in the enzyme β-methyl-crotonyl-CoA carboxylase.

Clinical History

A patient's description of the nature and onset of the chemosensory problem is an essential element of the clinical history, as is an historical assessment of the patient's general health, including endocrinological state, hospital admissions, surgical interventions, radiological treatments, and medications received for other conditions. The use of thyroid agents and drugs that affect cell turnover (e.g., chemotherapeutic drugs) may be of etiological significance. Retarded or delayed puberty in association with anosmia (with or without midline craniofacial abnormalities, deafness, and renal anomalies) suggests the possibility of Kallmann's syndrome. Importantly, associated events such as viral or bacterial respiratory infections, head trauma, exposure to toxic fumes, systemic diseases, and signs of early parkinsonism or central tumors are critical for arriving at an etiological diagnosis, which is possible in the majority of cases. Information related to exposure to environmental chemicals and signs of seizure activity (e.g., automatisms, occurrence of blackouts, déjà vu, etc.) should be sought, particularly in patients in whom heightened sensitivity is a symptom. Attention to the possibility of renal disease as well as liver disease is crucial, given reports of alterations of olfactory function in patients with cirrhosis of the liver, acute viral hepatitis, or renal dysfunction. Decreased olfactory function has been observed in some persons with human immunodeficiency virus infection.

In patients complaining of anosmia or hyposmia, it is useful to ask whether smell function is diminished or completely lost, localized to the right or left nostril, or both, and whether the dysfunction is for all odorants or only a few. Patients with loss due to nasal sinus disease are more likely to experience a gradual loss of function than those who have loss due to a prior upper respiratory infection or to head trauma.[1] Some patients report temporary recovery of function in circumstances in which nasal patency is increased, such as on warm days or during exercise, showering, or treatment with corticosteroids; this implies a problem with intranasal airway blockage (as in allergic rhinitis) rather than a sensorineural problem.

The smoking history should be explored in light of evidence that the ability to smell decreases as a function of cumulative smoking dose and that cessation of smoking can result in improvement in olfactory function over time.[2] A history of allergy should be sought, as should a history of current or past nasal or paranasal sinus infections. Inquiry should be made about nasal or paranasal sinus operations or other treatments such as the use of topical intranasal medications. Importantly, the association of nasal obstruction, headache, facial pain, postnasal discharge, purulent or clear rhinorrhea, ear symptoms, and throat symptoms should be sought with specific questioning. The order in which the symptoms appeared and regressed is at times helpful. The duration of the problem is important in relation to the possibility of spontaneous recovery, which is generally assumed to be unlikely after 6 months if damage to the olfactory epithelium has occurred.

The patient should be asked about olfactory distortions and whether they seem to be bilateral or are confined to one or the other nasal chamber. In various stages of olfactory epithelial degeneration or regeneration, a dysosmia—usually foul—is often present that may or may not require an inhaled stimulus for elicitation. Dysosmias are sometimes associated with certain mental disorders, including epilepsy, psychosis, schizophrenia, and depression-related syndromes such as the olfactory reference syndrome.[3] In some cases, aura-like dysosmic phenomena may occur without any evidence of seizure activity. Fortunately, most olfactory perversions are temporary, although long-standing cases have been reported.

Exploring a patient's complaint of taste loss is essential because it usually reflects an olfactory disorder. It is useful to have the patient differentiate between the loss of perception of flavors of food or beverages and the loss of perception of sweet, sour, bitter, and salty stimuli. The physician can ask whether the patient is able to perceive saltiness in potato chips, sourness in lemonade, or sweetness in sugar on cereal to arrive at this differentiation. A patient with anosmia may be able to taste the sweetness of an apple or a pear but is unable to distinguish between their flavors.

Anatomy of Cranial Nerve I (Table 7–1)

SENSORY RECEPTORS AND PRIMARY NEURONS

Cranial nerve I is the collection of approximately 6 million bipolar receptor cells whose cell bodies, dendrites, and initial axon segments are located within the olfactory neuroepithelium and whose axons project through the cribriform plate of the ethmoid bone to the anterior cranial fossa

TABLE 7–1. **Clinico-anatomical Correlation of Disorders of the Olfactory Nerve**

Anatomical Site of Damage	Typical CN I Finding	Other Neurological and Medical Findings	Common Etiologies
Sensory receptors and primary neuron	Hyposmia or anosmia Dysosmia Can be unilateral	With trauma, rare nasal leaks of CSF	Head trauma Upper respiratory infections Nasal or sinus disease Toxic exposure
Secondary neurons Olfactory bulb cells Anterior olfactory nucleus Medial and lateral striae	Hyposmia or anosmia Dysosmia Can be unilateral	Foster Kennedy syndrome Disinhibition, change in personality Gait dyspraxia, disinhibition, change in personality	Meningioma Neurodegenerative diseases (Alzheimer's disease, Parkinson's disease, Huntington's disease) Frontal lobe tumors Pituitary tumors Aneurysms
Medial dorsal nucleus of thalamus	Decreased odor identification Normal or increased odor thresholds*	Signs of Wernicke-Korsakoff syndrome: ataxia, extraocular paresis, nystagmus, memory problems including confabulations	Wernicke-Korsakoff syndrome Infarctions
Primary and secondary olfactory cortex	Decreased odor identification Normal or increased odor thresholds*	Lip smacking, automatisms during seizures Dementia, memory loss Tremor, bradykinesia Chorea, dementia Contralateral weakness, aphasia, homonymous quadrant visual field defects	Epilepsy Neurodegenerative disorders Alzheimer's disease Parkinson's disease Huntington's disease Tumors or infarcts

*Because of bilateral cortical and subcortical representation of olfactory function, unilateral lesions at this level generally do not cause clinically meaningful olfactory dysfunction.

(Fig. 7–1).[4] The olfactory neuroepithelium is a pseudostratified columnar epithelium supported by a highly vascularized lamina propria and is situated on the cribriform plate as well as on segments of the superior septum and both the superior and middle turbinates. Each bipolar receptor cell sends 3 to 50 cilia (which lack dynein arms and commonly have a 9 + 2 microtubule arrangement) from its dendritic knob into the overlying mucus. The cilia, which can radiate across the epithelial surface for over 30 μm, contain the receptor sites where odorants bind and provide a relatively large area for such binding. Assuming 6 million bipolar receptor cells, each containing 20 cilia 30 μm long and with an average diameter of 0.5 μm, the surface area of the cilia proves to be nearly 9 square inches.

In addition to bipolar receptor cells, the olfactory epithelium contains several other major cell types (see Fig. 7–1). The sustentacular or supporting cells, whose apical ends have microvilli that extend into the olfactory mucus, span the distance from the epithelial surface to the basal laminae and function to (1) mechanically isolate the bipolar receptor cells from one another, (2) secrete mucopolysaccarides, (3) transport molecules across the epithelium, and (4) detoxify and degrade odorants.[5] Some of the basal cells, located near the basement membrane, serve as precursors for the generation of other cell types within the neuroepithelium. The duct cells of Bowman's glands line passages through which most of the olfactory mucus is secreted, whereas the microvillar cells, located at the surface of the epithelium, send tufts of microvilli into the nasal mucus. The function of these flask-shaped cells is unknown. However, they number about 600,000 in humans.[4, 6]

The constituent bipolar neurons of CN I are unique in three respects. First, their apical processes are more or less directly exposed to the external environment. Second, unlike nearly all other neuronal cells, they have the propensity to regenerate from basal cells after being damaged; indeed, some of these cells die and replenish themselves at regular intervals, although others are more long-lived.[7] Third, each of these cells serves as both a receptor cell and as a first-order neuron, projecting an axon directly from the nasal cavity into the brain without an intervening synapse. Unlike the other major cell types of the epithelium, these cells have relatively little xenobiotic-metabolizing capacity[8] and are a primary route of invasion into the central nervous system of toxic agents and viruses. Indeed, it is believed that the majority of neurovirulent viruses first enter the CNS through this pathway.

Within the lamina propria, the unmyelinated and unbranched axons of the olfactory receptor cells coalesce into bundles of approximately 200 axons, each surrounded by ensheathing or Schwann cell mesoaxons. Axons within these bundles are in direct contact with one another and may interact metabolically and electrically.[9] These bundles in turn combine with other bundles to form the olfactory fila, which traverse the cribriform plate of the ethmoid bone through 50 or so foramina. The fila, on exiting from the cribriform plate, form a dense layer of axons on the surface of the olfactory bulb. From here, the receptor cell axons branch and

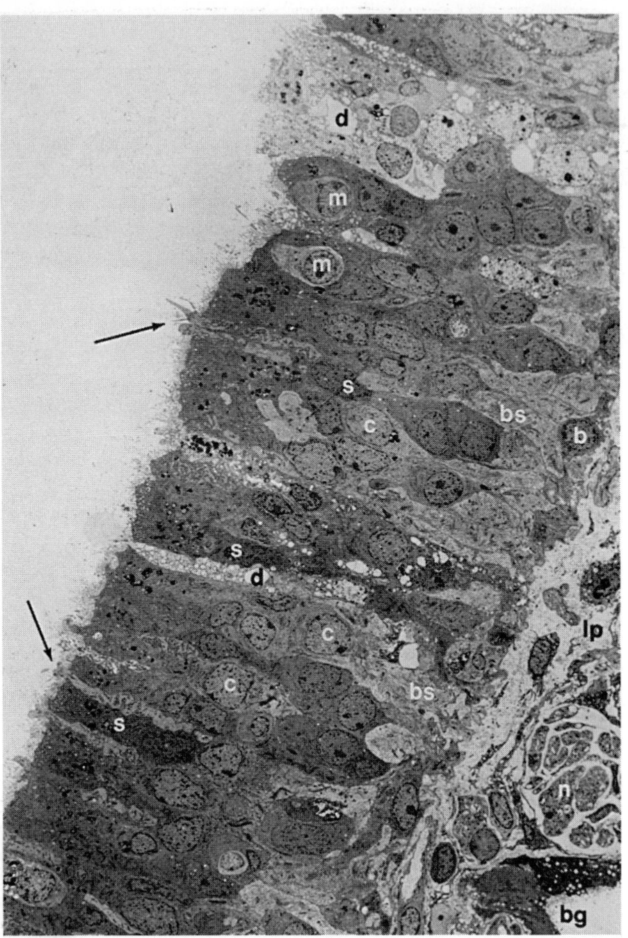

FIGURE 7–1. Low-power electron micrograph (×1000) of a longitudinal section through a biopsy of human olfactory mucosa taken from the nasal septum. Four cell types are indicated: ciliated olfactory receptor cells (c), microvillar cells (m), supporting cells (s), and basal cells (b). The arrows point to ciliated olfactory knobs of bipolar receptor cells; d indicates degenerating cells; bs, the base of supporting cells; lp, the lamina propria; n, a nerve bundle; and bg, a Bowman's gland. (From Moran DT, Rowley JC III, Jafek BW, et al: The fine structure of the olfactory mucosa in man. J Neurocytol 1982;11:721–746.)

synapse with second-order neurons within the glomeruli of the bulb.

SECONDARY SENSORY NEURONS: OLFACTORY BULB AND PROJECTIONS

The olfactory bulbs are complex ovoid structures located on the ventral surface of each frontal lobe dorsal to the cribriform plate.[10] Each bulb is composed of a number of types of cells, including neurons, afferent and efferent nerve fibers, microglia, astrocytes, and blood vessels, all surrounded by a thin layer of pia-arachnoid cells.[11] The cellular elements of the bulb are arranged in six concentric layers: the olfactory nerve layer (ONL), the glomerular layer (GL), the external plexiform layer (EPL), the mitral cell layer (MCL), the internal plexiform layer (IPL), and the granule cell layer (GCL). The GCL is the largest of these layers, making up about half the volume of the entire bulb. The anterior olfactory nucleus (AON) lies within the core of the posterior olfactory bulb and extends through the olfactory tract to the rostral part of the olfactory peduncle near the anterior perforated substance. This structure, which is considered to be an element of the primary olfactory cortex, contains pyramidal cells whose dendrites receive synapses from mitral and tufted cells as well as from the contralateral AON (via the anterior commissure [AC]) and numerous central brain structures. The axons of its pyramidal cells project to ipsilateral bulb neurons (mainly granule cells) as well as to the contralateral AON, bulb, or rostral olfactory cortex via the AC. Although termed a nucleus, the AON has a cortical structure with subdivisions based on cellular architecture and connectional patterns.[11]

The first synapse of a CN I bipolar neuron occurs in the olfactory bulb's *glomerulus*, a defining feature of both vertebrate and invertebrate olfactory systems (Fig. 7–2). The olfactory bulb of nonelderly humans has thousands of these 50- to 200-μm structures, arranged in single or double layers within the GL. With age, the number and integrity of the glomeruli greatly decrease, so that they are nearly absent in persons over the age of 80 years.[12] The development and maintenance of the glomeruli depend on trophic influences exerted by the receptor cells. Synapses between axons of the olfactory receptor cells and dendrites of second-order neurons occur within these structures. A given receptor cell projects to only one glomerulus, and a given glomerulus appears to receive most of its input from a restricted region of the epithelium.

The main afferent second-order neurons are termed mitral and tufted cells (see Fig. 7–2). The apical dendrites of these cells are influenced not only by the olfactory nerve terminals, but also by interneurons and centrifugal fibers, most of which are GABAergic or dopaminergic.[11]

CENTRAL CONNECTIONS

The olfactory tract, which contains both afferent and efferent fibers, is relatively flat posteriorly and becomes the olfactory trigone just rostral to the anterior perforated substance (so named because of the many small holes for blood vessels found throughout this region). At the edges of the trigone, the tract divides into the medial and lateral olfactory striae.

The axons of the mitral and tufted cells arise from the caudolateral part of the olfactory bulb and form the olfactory tract at the surface of the olfactory peduncle. According to Price,[12] the consensus of studies performed during the last two decades is that there is no medial olfactory tract in mammals. Thus, all mitral and tufted cell axons leave the olfactory bulb via the lateral olfactory tract to synapse on structures collectively termed the primary olfactory cortex. These structures are (1) the anterior olfactory nucleus, (2) the olfactory tubercle (poorly developed in humans), (3) the piriform cortex, (4) the anterior cortical nucleus of the amygdala, (5) the periamygdaloid complex, and (6) the rostral entorhinal cortex.[12] The components of the olfactory cortex have rich (and reciprocal) relations with a number of higher brain structures. For example, the entorhinal cortex supplies afferent fibers along the entire length of the hippocampus, including the dentate gyrus. Indeed, because of these connections, the olfactory system has the most direct access of all sensory systems to the hippocampus.[11] It is generally believed that the olfactory system is unique among sensory systems in sending fibers

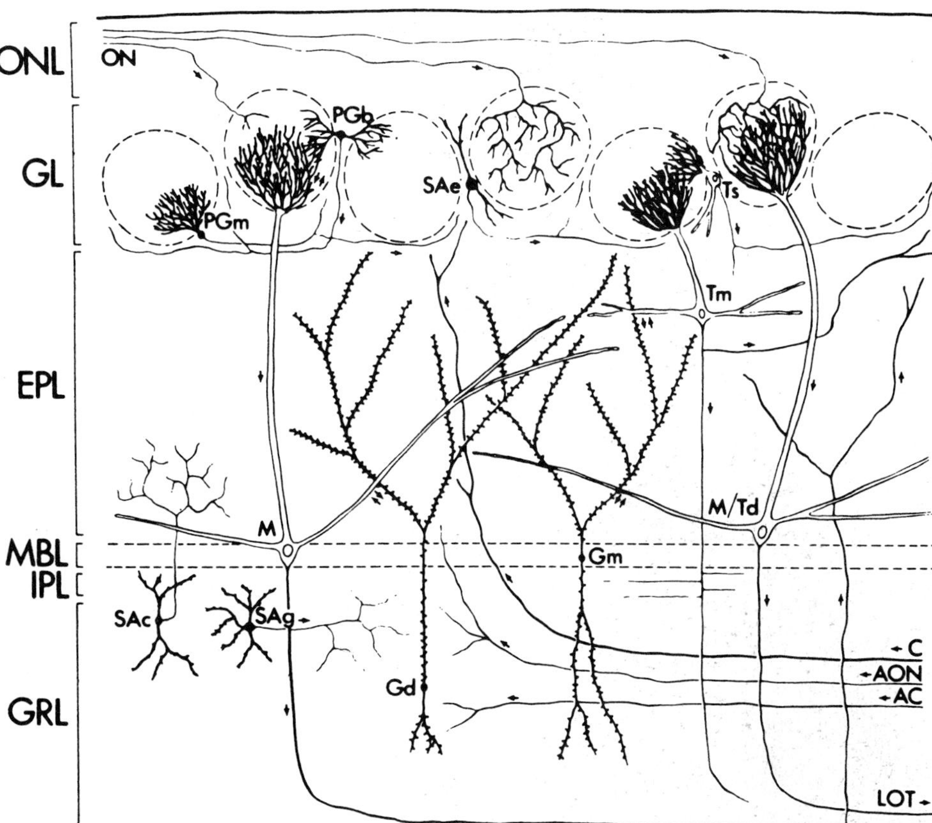

FIGURE 7–2. Diagram of major layers and types of olfactory bulb neurons in the mammalian olfactory bulb, as based on Golgi stained material. Main layers are indicated on left as follows: ONL, olfactory nerve layer; GL, glomerular layer; EPL, external plexiform layer; MBL, mitral body layer; IPL, internal plexiform layer; GRL, granule cell layer; ON, olfactory nerves; PGb, periglomerular cells with biglomerular dendrites; PGm, periglomerular cell with monoglomerular dendrites; SAe, short-axon cell with extraglomerular dendrites; M, mitral cell; M/Td, displaced mitral or deep tufted cell; Tm, middle tufted cell; Ts, superficial tufted cell; Gm, granule cell with cell body in mitral cell layer; Gd, granule cell with cell body in deep layers; SAc, short-axon cell of Cajal; SAg, short-axon cell of Golgi; C, centrifugal fibers; AON, fibers from the anterior olfactory nucleus; AC, fibers from anterior commissure; LOT, lateral olfactory tract. (From Shepherd GM: Synaptic organization of the mammalian olfactory bulb. Physiol Rev 1972; 52:864–917. Used with permission.)

directly to cortical regions without synapsing in the thalamus. Extensive interactions occur between the cells comprising the superficial and deeper laminae of each component of the olfactory cortex, as well as among the components themselves.[11]

In humans, it appears that most of the projections of the mitral and tufted cells extend to the more rostral elements of the primary olfactory cortex. It is presently believed that specific sites within the bulb do not preferentially communicate with specific sites within the primary olfactory cortex; that is, no obvious point-to-point topography exists.[11] Thus, small areas of the bulb can project to large areas of the olfactory cortex and vice versa.[12] Among the brain regions that exhibit reciprocal connections with the olfactory cortex are the orbitofrontal cortex, the dorsomedial and submedial thalamic nuclei, the lateral hypothalamus, the amygdala, and the hippocampus.[12] A major pathway from the olfactory cortex to the orbitofrontal cortex, is via the mediodorsal nucleus of the thalamus.

NEUROCHEMICAL OLFACTORY TRANSDUCTION PROCESSES

Peripheral olfactory transduction occurs in several stages: first, odorants move from the air phase of the nasal cavity into the aqueous phase of the olfactory mucus; second, odorants (most of which are hydrophobic) diffuse or are transported through this aqueous phase to the proteinaceous olfactory receptors; third, odorants bind to the receptors; fourth, action potentials are generated within the receptor neurons as a result of such binding; and fifth, integration of information occurs at higher levels, such as within the glomeruli of the olfactory bulb. Although some odorants stimulate nerve endings from CN V and perhaps other cranial nerves distributed in the nasal mucosa, nasal pharynx, or oral cavity, these involve primarily somatosensory sensations of the "common chemical sense," such as warmth or coolness, pungency, and irritation.

There is evidence that small water-soluble proteins, termed odorant-binding proteins, assist the movement of some hydrophobic, lipid-soluble molecules through the mucus to the receptor proteins of the olfactory cilia.[13] Such assistance may be selective, and at least some of these proteins may serve to inactivate odorant molecules or filter the number of such molecules reaching the receptors. For example, some odor-induced signals appear to be rapidly abolished by detoxification or biotransformation enzymes within the mucus.[14]

After reaching the cilia, odorants bind to receptor sites located on their surface. Different models of ligand-receptor interactions have been proposed, although little is known about the specific nature of the odorant-receptor interactions. There is evidence, however, that G-proteins play an important role in olfactory transduction. G-proteins have been identified in olfactory receptor cells,[15] and adenylate cyclase, an enzyme that is usually coupled to a G-protein, is highly active in olfactory cilia.[16] The activity of this enzyme in cilia is increased in the presence of guanosine triphosphate by a number of odorant ligands.[17] Interestingly, a positive correlation exists between an odorant's ability to activate adenyl cyclase activity in a frog ciliary preparation and both its perceived odor intensity to humans and the magnitude of the electro-olfactogram, a summated neural response produced in frog epithelia. This implies that a functional relation exists between the amount of adenyl cyclase activated and the intensity of odor perception.[18]

Recent studies indicate that there is marked genetic diversity in olfactory receptors. Buck and Axel,[19] in a pioneering study, identified a large multigene family that appears to code for odorant receptor proteins with seven transmembrane domains on rat olfactory sensory neurons. Subsequent studies have identified homologous gene families in a range of vertebrate forms, including humans.[20] As noted in a review by Sullivan and colleagues,[21] current estimates place the size of the olfactory receptor gene family in mammals at 500 to 1000 genes. This suggests that the basis of the ability of mammals to smell thousands of odorants derives from a wide range of ligand specificities.

It has long been known, mainly from single cell electrophysiological recordings, that individual olfactory receptor cells respond to a wide variety of odorants, leading earlier workers to label olfactory receptor cells "generalists." However, on closer scrutiny, it has become evident that such cells do not respond exactly to the same sets of stimuli, which allows for the possibility of cross-neuron coding. Recent research, incorporating gene probes from in situ hybridization studies, has provided three new pieces of information about the distribution of receptors on olfactory receptor cells and the relationship of such cells to higher-order structures.[21] First, most rodent olfactory receptor genes are expressed in only about 0.1 percent of the population of olfactory sensory neurons, in accordance with the hypothesis that each sensory neuron expresses only one or at most a few receptor genes. Second, neurons expressing the same gene do not clump together within the olfactory epithelium but seem to be randomly distributed within the epithelium in "spatial zones," across which different sets of olfactory receptor genes are expressed.[22] For example, in the mouse, four such zones, formed as a series of strips extending along the anterior-posterior axis of the nasal cavity, have been identified. Neurons that recognize the same odors (i.e., express the same olfactory receptor genes) are more or less confined to the same zone. Third, axons of neurons that express the same odorant receptor tend to converge on a small number of glomeruli within the olfactory bulb, suggesting that each glomerulus may be dedicated to only one or a very small number of receptor types, receiving input from only receptor cells expressing that receptor type. As noted by Sullivan and colleagues,[21] "a stereotyped and highly organized map of sensory information exists in the bulb, in which information provided by different ORs (odorant receptors) is mapped into discrete sites. As a single odorant can activate many glomeruli and a single glomerulus responds to many odorants, this map may well be a map of individual structural determinants, or epitopes, each shared by many odorants and recognized by different ORs."

A number of odorants produce a dose-related increase in intracellular cyclical adenosine 3′,5′-monophosphate (cAMP) in olfactory receptor cells,[17] thereby triggering the opening of cAMP-gated cation channels.[23] Some odorants also activate cyclic guanosine monophosphate (cGMP), which appears to play a role in the modulation of the sensitivity of olfactory receptor neurons, such as during adaptation.[24]

Examination of Cranial Nerve I

DIRECTED NEUROLOGICAL EXAMINATION

Essential components of the directed physical examination include a neurological evaluation emphasizing the cranial nerves and orbital contents (to direct attention to lesions of the skull base), as well as a general evaluation of the ears, upper respiratory tract, and head and neck. Although much can be gained by evaluating the nose using anterior rhinoscopy, nasal endoscopy allows a more thorough assessment. With this procedure, the rhinologist can often directly visualize the olfactory neuroepithelium and establish whether airflow access to the epithelium is blocked. In the nasal examination, the nasal mucosa is evaluated for color, surface texture, swelling, inflammation, exudate, ulceration, epithelial metaplasia, erosion, and atrophy. Discovery of purulent rhinorrhea, especially its site of origin, is considered significant; if it is present throughout the nasal cavity, rhinitis is suggested. If rhinorrhea is present in the middle meatus, maxillary or anterior ethmoid sinusitis is possible, whereas if the frontal recess is involved, frontal sinusitis is implicated. Finally, if rhinorrhea originates from the superior meatus or sphenoethmoidal recess, posterior ethmoid or sphenoid sinusitis is likely. The presence of polyps, masses, adhesions of the turbinates to the septum, and marked septal deviations all have the potential to decrease airflow to the olfactory epithelium. Allergy is suggested if the mucous membrane is pale, usually as a result of edema within the lamina propria. Chronic or acute exposure to environmental or industrial pollutants is suggested by metaplasia within the epithelium, as well as by swelling, inflammation, exudate, erosion, or ulceration. Atrophy of the lamina propria is suggested by unusual spaciousness, dryness, and crusting, as seen in atrophic rhinitis or rhinitis medicamentosa.

Quantitative testing of olfactory function is essential to (1) establish the validity of a patient's complaint, (2) characterize the specific nature of the problem, (3) reliably monitor changes in function over time, including those resulting from medical interventions or treatments, (4) detect malingering, and (5) establish compensation for permanent disability. It should be noted that some patients who present with complaints of anosmia or hyposmia actually have normal function relative to their peers. Others can be unaware of their deficits. For example, approximately 90 percent of patients with idiopathic Parkinson's disease have a demonstrable olfactory loss, yet less than 15 percent are aware of the problem until they are tested objectively.

Historically, a popular means of assessing the ability to smell has been to ask a patient to sniff a few small vials containing odorants such as coffee or cinnamon and then report whether or not an odor is perceived. Unfortunately, this procedure is akin to testing vision by shining an intense light into the eye and asking whether or not it can be seen. This problem is not corrected by asking the patient to attempt to identify an odor, since, without cues, even normal subjects have difficulty in identifying some odors. Although most olfactory disorders can be detected by administering a wide variety of nominally distinct olfactory tests, including tests of odor detection, discrimination, identification, and memory, interpretation of the findings of such tests must be done conservatively. All such tests are influenced by damage to the olfactory membrane, making it dangerous to assume, in any given case, that poor performance on a specific type of test (e.g., odor memory) has anything to do with damage to the neural circuits underlying the name of the test (e.g., odor memory circuits). The fact that the reliability (and hence sensitivity) of a number of such tests is low or unknown adds further difficulty to attempts to establish differential function.

Because assessment of olfactory function often has both medical and legal consequences, accuracy in olfactory testing is essential. Anosmia or hyposmia is a common consequence of head injury and is frequently the only residual neurological impairment of a fall or motor vehicle accident. In the United States, disability compensation is provided under the 1963 amendment to the Workmen's Compensation Law when a diminution of future earning power is apparent, and the Veterans Administration awards a 10 percent whole-body disability for total anosmia. The *Guides to the Evaluation of Permanent Impairment* published by the American Medical Association provide another authoritative basis for disability compensation.[25] However, this document equates total anosmia and total ageusia (a condition that exists rarely, if ever) with a 3 percent impairment of the whole person, a figure that is far below the amount given in most legal settlements for anosmia alone and that many view as insufficient. In Great Britain, disability benefits for anosmia resulting from an injury are available under the National Insurance Act as well under private accident insurance policies. Occupation must be taken into account in disability issues because loss or decreased smell function is quite a different matter for persons in some occupations (e.g., chefs, plumbers, wine tasters, municipal gas workers) than in others (e.g., sanitation workers).

A number of practical clinical quantitative tests of olfactory function of known reliability are now commercially available. The most widely used of these tests is the University of Pennsylvania Smell Identification Test (UPSIT), also known as the Smell Identification Test™ (Sensonics, Inc., Haddon Heights, NJ).[26, 27] The UPSIT, which can be self-administered in 10 to 15 minutes by most patients in the waiting room and scored in less than a minute by nonmedical personnel, consists of four booklets containing 10 odorants apiece. The stimuli are embedded in 10- to 50-μm diameter microencapsulated crystals located on "scratch and sniff" strips near the bottom of each page. Above each strip is a multiple choice question with four response alternatives. The patient is required to choose an answer, even if none seems appropriate or no odor is perceived (i.e., the test is forced-choice). This helps to encourage the patient to carefully sample each stimulus and provides a means of detecting malingering; since chance performance is 10 out of 40, very low scores reflect avoidance, and hence recognition, of the correct answer. Norms based on the administration of this test to nearly 4000 people are provided, and an individual's percentile rank is established relative to persons of the same age and gender.[27] This test makes it possible to classify an individual's function, on an absolute basis, into one of six categories: normosmia, mild microsmia, moderate microsmia, severe microsmia, anosmia, and probable malingering. The reliability of this test is high (test-retest Pearson *r*s > 0.90).

Other commercially available olfactory tests include the three-item forced-choice microencapsulated Pocket Smell Test™ (which is only a brief screening test), the 12-item Brief Smell Identification Test™ (B-SIT),[28] the five-odorant T&T olfactometer threshold test,[29] and a squeeze bottle odor threshold test kit termed the Smell Threshold Test™ (STT).[30] With the exception of the Pocket Smell Test™, the test-retest reliability coefficients of these tests are around 0.70. Norms that take into account both age and gender are available only for the UPSIT, STT, and B-SIT, although the small number of items in the latter test allows neither differentiation between degrees of olfactory loss nor a means for determining malingering.

Although most cases of olfactory dysfunction are bilateral, in some instances unilateral testing is needed. To accurately assess olfaction unilaterally, the naris contralateral to the tested side should be occluded to prevent or minimize crossing of inhaled or exhaled air at the rear of the nasopharynx to the opposite side (so-called retronasal stimulation). An easy way of doing this is to seal the contralateral naris using a piece of Microfoam tape (3M Corporation, Minneapolis, MN) cut to fit its borders. The patient is instructed to sniff the stimulus normally and to exhale through the mouth.

ASSOCIATED NEUROLOGICAL FINDINGS

Cerebral. The neurologist should be alert to signs of dementia (e.g., inattention, memory dysfunction, apathy, disorientation) in patients presenting with olfactory dysfunction, since decreased ability to smell is among the first signs of Alzheimer's disease and is also seen in some patients with Huntington's chorea, multi-infarct dementia, and Pick's disease. Evidence of fainting spells or blackouts, disorientation, seizure activity, and mood change should be sought because both increases and decreases in olfactory function are found in patients with temporal lobe epilepsy. Olfactory loss, along with short-term memory problems and associated confabulation, may help to define vitamin B_1 deficiency and the Wernicke-Korsakoff syndrome. Cognitive alterations (e.g., mental slowing, confusion, depression, and hallucinations) may also signal the presence of pernicious anemia.

Cranial Nerves. Optic disk examination and documentation of increased intraocular or intracranial pressure (papilledema) should be obtained because tumors in the olfactory groove or sphenoid ridge (e.g., meningiomas) can cause the Foster Kennedy syndrome, which is composed of three clinical hallmarks—ipsilateral anosmia or hyposmia, ipsilateral optic atrophy, and contralateral papilledema. Although rare, visual disturbances are caused by some forms of sinusitis, which can also alter chemosensation. For example, optic neuropathy has been reported secondary to cocaine-induced osteolytic sinusitis.[31] Altered visual contrast sensitivity, color perception, and perception of the visual vertical may provide additional information about a more diffuse chemosensory disorder. Hearing problems may reflect viral or bacterial infections in the middle ear that alter taste function in the anterior tongue via chorda tympani nerve (CN VII) damage or inflammation, as well as more general nasal sinus infections that also influence olfaction. Specifically, patients with Korsakoff's syndrome have deficits not only in memory and olfactory function but also in color discrimination and several measures of auditory perception, including dichotic listening tasks. Pupillary reaction to light is also sluggish in patients with this syndrome, and horizontal nystagmus and ophthalmoplegia, usually involving the bilateral lateral recti in isolation or with other extraocular muscle palsies, are also commonly present.

Applying small drops of sweet, sour, bitter, and salty tasting stimuli (with water rinses between applications) to the fungiform papillae on the front of the tongue (which are innervated by the chorda tympani division of CN VII) and on the circumvallate papillae at the rear of the tongue (CN IX) can be useful in identifying regional deficits and damage to specific nerves involved in taste perception. Alternatively, determination of thresholds to electrical stimulation using commercially available electrogustometers can also be employed. Iatrogenic factors, such as tonsillectomy, can damage CN IX fibers and produce taste distortions, whereas alterations in CN VII function (i.e., the chorda tympani nerve) can be caused by middle ear infections. Local factors (e.g., dryness, inflammation, edema, atrophy, abnormal surface texture, leukoplakia, erythroplasia, exudate, erosion, and ulceration) can influence taste function through a variety of means (e.g., gastric reflux), as can poor oral health and the use of smokeless tobacco.[32]

Motor/Reflexes/Cerebellar/Gait. Attention to ataxia, apraxia for orolingual movements, oculomotor abnormalities, coordination problems, gait disturbances, tremor, bradykinesia, and rigidity is critical, since alterations in the ability to smell are present in some patients with Huntington's chorea and multiple sclerosis, and in approximately 90 percent of patients with early-stage Parkinson's disease. In Korsakoff's syndrome, ataxia of the trunk but not of the limbs is frequently present, as are signs of acute alcohol withdrawal (e.g., tremor, delirium, and tachycardia).

Sensory. Decreased position, vibratory, temperature, and pain appreciation occurs in several neuropathies associated with hyposmia. These include diabetes, the neuropathy of renal and hepatic failures, and a large variety of toxic neuropathies. In patients with pernicious anemia, the large myelinated central fibers carrying position and vibration senses are preferentially affected. In the context of hepatitis, the acquired immunodeficiency syndrome, and other virus-related illnesses, hyposmia can occur along with an ascending polyneuropathy of the Guillain-Barré type. In seizure patients with uncal or temporal lobe foci that induce dysosmic auras, altered sensations in a hemibody distribution can occur as part of the seizure or as a postictal transient sequela.

ASSOCIATED MEDICAL FINDINGS

Evidence of a fever or stiff neck may help to determine the presence of an ongoing infection, including very serious disorders such as meningitis, which can be associated with chemosensory dysfunction. Flamboyant signs or inconsistencies in the examination may signal psychogenic factors or a propensity for malingering. Signs of diabetes should be sought, since both olfactory and gustatory dysfunction may be altered in this disorder.

Evaluation Guidelines

Neuroimaging. The sensitivity of computed tomography (CT) to soft tissue disease and bony changes makes it ideal for the investigation of the sinonasal cavities. All of the nasal cavity, paranasal sinuses, hard palate, anterior skull base, orbits, and nasopharynx should be scanned and, if central causes of olfactory dysfunction are suspected, the brain as well. Coronal scans are particularly valuable for the assessment of the paranasal anatomy, namely, the anterior nasoethmoid (ostiomeatal) region (i.e., the maxillary sinus ostium, infundibulum, uncinate process, and middle meatus). To better identify vascular lesions, tumors, abscess cavities, and meningeal or parameningeal processes, intravenous contrast enhancement is frequently employed. Presently, high-resolution CT appears to be the most useful and cost-effective screening tool for the assessment of sinonasal tract inflammatory disorders.

Magnetic resonance imaging (MRI) is superior to CT in the discrimination of soft tissue but is less sensitive than CT to bony cortical abnormalities or landmarks. Thus, MRI is the technique of choice for the evaluation of the olfactory bulbs, olfactory tracts, and intracranial causes of olfactory dysfunction because they can be visualized rather clearly on coronal scans. MRI is also the method of choice for the evaluation of skull base invasion by sinonasal tumors. Gadolinium-enhanced scans are particularly valuable in detecting dural or leptomeningeal involvement at the skull base. The paramagnetic contrast agent gadolinium-DTPA has been widely used to enhance the margins of sinonasal tumors and to distinguish solidly enhancing tumors from rim-enhancing inflammatory processes.[33]

Electrophysiology. Outpatient testing for EEG activity in individuals with dysosmia may be enhanced by using electrodes placed in the nasopharyngeal region or over the lower temporal areas. Inpatient EEG monitoring is indicated if epileptic-like olfactory events occur frequently but cannot be discerned by outpatient testing procedures.

Although odor-evoked potentials can now be measured accurately in most patients, the stimulus presentation equipment is complex and is at present very expensive; thus, such testing is available in very few clinics. The major technical problem is that trains of well-defined odorant pulses, with steep-onset gradients, must be imbedded in a humidified airstream that is flowed through the nose in a manner that does not evoke somatosensory afferents. To date, only late near-field potentials have been recorded using this technique. When available, evoked potential olfactometry is useful in detecting malingering as well as for providing information about olfactory function that does not depend on verbal or other overt responses of the patient.

Body Fluid and Tissue Analysis. In patients in whom a clear cause is not found, a complete blood count may be indicated to better define whether infective, nutritional, or hematopoietic processes are involved. A nonspecific indication of an autoimmune or inflammatory process can be obtained from the erythrocyte sedimentation rate. Although frank zinc deficiency has the potential to alter olfactory function, there is no evidence that zinc treatment of persons without stark zinc deficiency influences any olfactory disorder. Indeed, a double-blind clinical trial using a cross-over design in which zinc was compared to placebo showed no advantage of zinc over placebo in the treatment of hyposmia or hypogeusia.[34] Since vitamin B_1 deficiency is clearly implicated in the Wernicke-Korsakoff syndrome, determination of the erythrocyte thiamine level is indicated in patients with a significant history of suspected or documented chronic alcohol abuse. Early reports that vitamin A therapy may be of value in some cases did not include controls, making the efficacy of this therapy enigmatic.

Neuropsychological Tests. Given the close association between olfactory loss and several forms of dementia, including Alzheimer's disease and multi-infarct dementia, neuropsychological testing may be indicated to better identify the presence of dementia (for details of the tests listed following, see reference 35). The Mini-Mental State Examination is a widely used brief screening instrument for dementia and can be used alone or as a component of examination protocols such as the Consortium to Establish a Registry for Alzheimer's Disease (CERAD) battery. More extensive assessment of dementia can be obtained using either the Mattis Dementia Rating Scale, the Blessed Dementia Scale, the Boston Naming Test, or the logical memory and visual reproduction subtests of the Wechsler Memory Scale—Revised (WMS-R). The WMS-R and the California Verbal Learning Test have proved useful in patients in whom schizophrenia is suspected.

Malingering can be detected or is strongly suspected when a person scores below chance level on the UPSIT. Further verification of malingering can be obtained by administering neuropsychological tests specifically designed for this purpose. Among those that are widely used are Rey's memory test (RMT), also known as Rey's 3 × 5 test and the Rey 15-item memory test. The rationale behind this test is that malingerers typically fail at a memory task that all but the most retarded or severely brain-damaged persons perform easily. Another widely used test, the Portland digit recognition test, incorporates, like the UPSIT, a forced-choice procedure to ascertain whether test performance falls below that expected on the basis of chance. Unfortunately, this test takes nearly an hour to administer and provides no other neuropsychological information. Abbreviated versions of this test, however, are available.

Other Tests. To document changes in cellular aspects of the olfactory neuroepithelium, olfactory biopsies can be performed. In this procedure, a small amount of olfactory neuroepithelial tissue is stripped from the nasal septum by the rhinologist using small forceps or a specialized instrument and subsequently analyzed histologically.[36, 37] This procedure must be performed by a surgeon who is experienced in the technique, and multiple biopsies are usually needed, given the considerable metaplasia of respiratory-like epithelium in the region of the olfactory neuroepithelium.

Clinical Syndromes (Table 7–2)

ANOSMIA AND HYPOSMIA

Loss or decreased olfactory function is estimated to be present in approximately 1 percent of the American population under the age of 60 and in more than half of the population over that age.[38] The causes of loss or decreased olfactory function are variable, and simply establishing the presence of olfactory loss per se provides little insight into the cause. Nearly two thirds of patients with chronic anosmia or hyposmia (i.e., those that are presumably permanent) are due to prior upper respiratory infections, head trauma, and nasal and paranasal sinus disease, and most reflect damage to the olfactory neuroepithelium.[1] Other causes include iatrogenic interventions (e.g., septoplasty, rhinoplasty, turbinectomy, radiation therapy), intranasal neoplasms (e.g., papillomas, hemangiomas, and ameloblastomas), intracranial tumors or lesions (e.g., Foster Kennedy syndrome, olfactory groove meningiomas, frontal lobe gliomas), epilepsy, psychiatric disorders, exposure to environmental chemicals, hypothyroidism, renal disease, and kidney disease. According to Finelli and Mair,[39] the single most egregious error of neurologists in dealing with olfactory disturbances is the failure to recognize the symptom of anosmia as the principal or sole feature of an olfactory groove meningioma. Five to 10 percent of head trauma patients have olfactory dysfunction, and the majority of these have anosmia.[40] Of particular interest to the neurologist is the observation that olfactory dysfunction may be the first sign of Alzheimer's disease and idiopathic Parkinson's disease.[33] Olfactory testing can be useful in differentiating between Alzheimer's disease and depression.[41] Patients with intractable epilepsy who are candidates for temporal lobe resection have a hyposmic condition prior to surgery. In most of these cases, the hyposmia is bilateral, although asymmetry in function can be present, the greatest decrement being observed on the side of the focal damage. Interestingly, after surgical removal of diseased tissue in the right hemisphere, some measures of olfactory function improve significantly on the left side of the nose.

In most patients with congenital anosmia, MRI reveals a lack of or marked hypoplasia of the olfactory bulbs and stalks bilaterally. For example, in a study of 25 patients with congenital anosmia from the University of Pennsylvania Smell and Taste Center, MRI revealed an absence or hypoplasia of olfactory bulbs and tracts in all instances.[42] Verification of a physical cause of this disability proved to be quite therapeutic for some of these individuals.

DYSOSMIA

Dysosmia (disordered smell perception) presents as either a distortion in the perceived quality of an odor (*parosmia, cacosmia*) or as the presence of a strange odor in the absence of actual odor stimulation (*phantosmia* or *olfactory hallucinations*). Most dysosmias reflect dynamic elements associated with degeneration (or, more rarely, regeneration) of the olfactory epithelium and remit over time. However, it is common for patients with anosmia to report that prior to the onset of anosmia they experienced a period of weeks or months when dysosmia was present. Extremely debilitating chronic dysosmias have been reported that have required surgical intervention, such as ablation of portions of the olfactory epithelium[43] or removal of the olfactory bulbs.[44] Most such cases present unilaterally. More commonly, dysosmias are part of the sequelae of events that occur after the olfactory nerve fibers have been partially damaged by upper respiratory infections, head trauma, nasal sinus disease, or other disorders. In the majority of these cases, marked smell loss does not accompany the dysosmic condition, implying that it requires a relatively intact sensory system for expression.

In rare instances, dysosmias reflect aura-like processes that are suggestive of central brain tumors or lesions, particularly lesions of the temporal lobe. In some cases, aura-like

TABLE 7–2. **Selected Etiologies Associated with Disorders of Cranial Nerve I**

Etiological Category	Selected Specific Etiologies	Chapter
Structural Disorders		
Developmental	Kallmann's syndrome	28
Degenerative and compressive	Schizophrenia	
	Usher's syndrome	29
Hereditary and Degenerative Disorders		
Amino/organic acidopathies, mitochondrial enzyme defects and other metabolic errors	Trimethylaminuria	31
Chromosomal abnormalities and neurocutaneous disorders	Down's syndrome	32
Degenerative dementias	Alzheimer's disease	33
	Pick's disease	
Movement disorders	Idiopathic Parkinson's disease	34
	Huntington's disease	
Degenerative motor, sensory, and autonomic disorders	Amyotrophic lateral sclerosis	36
Acquired Metabolic and Nutritional Disorders		
Endogenous metabolic disorders	Diabetes	38
	Hypothyroidism	
	Kidney disease	
	Liver disease	
Exogenous acquired metabolic disorders of the nervous system: Toxins and illicit drugs	Toxic chemical exposure	39
Nutritional deficiencies and syndromes associated with alcoholism	Wernicke-Korsakoff syndrome	40
	Cirrhosis	
Infectious Disorders		
Viral infections	Upper respiratory viral infection	41
	Acute viral hepatitis	
	Acute poliomyelitis (CNs XI, XII)	
Nonviral infections	Bacterial meningitis	43
	Neurosyphilis (CN XII)	
	Pneumonia	
HIV and AIDS	Human immunodeficiency virus (HIV)	44
Neurovascular Disorders	Stroke	45
Neoplastic Disorders		
Primary neurological tumors	Foster Kennedy syndrome	46
Metastatic neoplasms and paraneoplastic syndromes	Metastatic carcinoma	47
Demyelinating Disorders		
Demyelinating disorders of the central nervous system	Multiple sclerosis	48
Autoimmune and Inflammatory Disorders	Allergies	50
Traumatic Disorders	Head trauma	51
Epilepsy	Temporal lobe epilepsy	52
Drug-Induced and Iatrogenic Neurological Disorders	Rhinitis medicamentosa	55
	Nasal surgery	
	Medications (neuroleptics)	

dysosmias can be chronic or occur regularly without producing any evidence or any clear sign of seizure activity (although, as noted earlier in this chapter, inpatient EEGs may be needed to detect infrequent partial seizure episodes). A few psychiatric syndromes, like olfactory reference syndrome, are also associated with dysosmic episodes, as are metabolic disturbances such as trimethylaminuria.

HYPEROSMIA

Hyperosmia (heightened smell function) is a relatively rare condition, usually of idiopathic origin, in which quantitative olfactory testing reveals heightened performance (e.g., UPSIT scores of 40 and detection threshold values that are several orders of magnitude below those of normal subjects). Although untreated adrenal cortical insufficiency is reportedly accompanied by hyperosmia,[45] this work has not been replicated, and animal studies have shown no evidence of heightened odor detection performance following adrenalectomy.[46] Indeed, adrenalectomy reduces rather than enhances peripheral nerve responses to a number of types of sensory stimuli, including tastants.[47] There have been suggestions of hyperosmia in patients with syndromes such as multiple chemical sensitivity, but the limited data available fail to support this notion.[48] Hyperosmia occurs in some patients with epilepsy during the interictal period, although, as noted earlier, patients with long-term epilepsy and intractable seizure activity, such as candidates for temporal lobe resection, typically are hyposmic.

DISSOCIATED OLFACTORY FUNCTION SYNDROMES

Some types of olfactory tests (e.g., tests of odor identification and discrimination) may be altered by central brain lesions that have little or no influence on other types of olfactory tests (e.g., odor detection thresholds). Thus, a dissociation between elements of the olfactory perceptual process may occur. For example, H.M., the only patient on record to have undergone bilateral temporal lobe resection, is said to perform normally on tests of odor detection, suprathreshold intensity discrimination, and adaptation, but abnormally on tests of odor quality discrimination and identification.[49] In one study, resection of left temporal lobes, right or left frontal lobes, and the right frontotemporal region significantly depressed scores on the UPSIT but not on a detection threshold test.[50] As noted earlier, however, care must be taken in the interpretation of such test results, given the fact that some olfactory tests, most notably some olfactory threshold tests, are relatively unreliable and thus insensitive to subtle alterations in smell function.

General Management Goals

Patients with complaints of olfactory dysfunction, regardless of etiology or anatomical localization, should receive careful sensory and neurological testing to ensure accurate categorization of both their sensory problem and, ideally, its physiological basis. In patients in whom anosmia or hyposmia is caused by airway blockage, treatment to relieve the edema or physical obstruction can be undertaken with optimism. Examples of treatments that have restored such function include allergic management, topical and systemic corticosteroid therapies, antibiotic therapy, and various surgical interventions. In cases in which tumors are the cause of the problem, their removal with the goal in mind of maintaining the integrity of the olfactory pathways can sometimes restore olfactory function. For patients with dysosmia, a careful review and systematic cessation of drugs that are potentially associated with the dysfunction may be fruitful in some instances, although this process can take several months, depending on the mode of action of the drugs involved and the number of medications being taken by the patient. In rare cases of long-term chronic dysosmia severe enough to produce depression, weight loss, or nausea because of the perversion of food flavor, surgical intervention may be indicated. If the dysosmia is unilateral (detected by blocking the flow of air to one side of the nose or by anesthetizing the olfactory membrane unilaterally), unilateral surgical intervention may correct the problem while sparing olfactory function on the contralateral side. Of the surgical approaches, intranasal ablation or stripping of tissue from the olfactory epithelium on the affected side is more conservative and less invasive than removing the olfactory bulb or tract through a craniotomy. Should the dysosmia reappear after such surgery, additional intranasal ablations may be performed.

Treatment of patients with anosmia due to sensorineural problems is challenging. Although there are a few advocates of zinc and vitamin therapies, sound empirical evidence of their efficacy is lacking. In patients in whom olfactory loss has been present for a long period of time and can be attributed to neural damage within the olfactory neuroepithelium, prognosis is poor, and no treatment is possible. Nevertheless, simply providing such patients with accurate information about their disorder, establishing objectively the degree and nature of the deficit, and ruling out the possibility of a serious disorder as the cause of the problem can diminish anxiety and may be very therapeutic. Because half of elderly persons with permanent olfactory loss are at or above the fiftieth percentile of their norm group, these individuals can be informed that while their olfactory function is below what it used to be, they still are outperforming most of their peers. This knowledge is extremely therapeutic and helps them place the natural age-related loss of olfactory function in a broader perspective.

Reviews and Selected Updates

Doty RL: Olfaction. Annual Rev Psychol 2001;52:423–452.

Doty RL: Olfactory dysfunction in neurodegenerative disorders. *In* Getchell TV, Doty RL, Bartoshuk LM, Snow JB Jr (eds): Smell and Taste in Health and Disease. New York, Raven Press, 1991, pp 735–751.

Doty RL, Hastings LM: Neurotoxic exposure and olfactory impairment. *In* Bleecker ML (ed): Clinics in Occupational Environmental Medicine (Neurotoxicology). Philadelphia, WB Saunders, 2001;1:1–29.

Doty RL, Yousem DM, Pham LT: Olfactory dysfunction in patients with head trauma. Arch Neurol 1997;54:1131–1140.

Duncan HJ, Smith DV: Clinical disorders of olfaction: A review. *In* Doty RL (ed): Handbook of Olfaction and Gustation. New York, Marcel Dekker, 1995, pp 345–365.

Ferreyra-Moyano H, Barragan E: The olfactory system and Alzheimer's disease. Int J Neurosci 1989;49:157–197.

Mesholam RI, Moberg PJ, Mahr RN, Gur RE, Doty RL: Olfaction and dementia: A meta-analysis review of olfactory functioning in Alzheimer's and Parkinson's disease. Arch Neurol 1998;55:84–90.

Moberg PJ, Agrin R, Gur RE, Gur RC, Turetsky BI, Doty RL: Olfactory dysfunction in schizophrenia: A qualitative and quantitative review. Neuropsychopharmacol 1999;21:325–340.

West SE, Doty RL: Influence of epilepsy and temporal lobe resection on olfactory function. Epilepsia 1995;36:531–542.

References

1. Deems DA, Doty RL, Settle RG, et al: Smell and taste disorders. A study of 750 patients from the University of Pennsylvania Smell and Taste Center. Arch Otolaryngol Head Neck Surg 1991;117:519–528.
2. Frye RE, Schwartz B, Doty RL: Dose-related effects of cigarette smoking on olfactory function. JAMA 1990;263:1233–1236.
3. Pryse-Phillips W: An olfactory reference syndrome. Acta Psychiat (Scand) 1971;47:484–509.
4. Moran DT, Rowley JC III, Jafek BW, et al: The fine structure of the olfactory mucosa in man. J Neurocytol 1982;11:721–746.
5. Getchell TV, Margolis FL, Getchell ML: Perireceptor and receptor events in vertebrate olfaction. Prog Neurobiol 1985;23:317–345.
6. Rowley JC, Moran DT, Jafek BW: Peroxidase backfills suggest the mammalian olfactory epithelium contains a second morphologically distinct class of bipolar sensory neuron: The microvillar cell. Brain Res 1989;502:387–400.
7. Hinds JW, Hinds PL, McNelly NA: An autoradiographic study of the mouse olfactory epithelium: Evidence for long-lived receptors. Anat Rec 1984;210:375–383.
8. Lewis JL, Dahl AR: Olfactory mucosa: Composition, enzymatic localization, and metabolism. *In* Doty RL (ed): Handbook of Olfaction and Gustation. New York, Marcel Dekker, 1995, pp 33–52.
9. Gesteland RC: Speculations on receptor cells as analyzers and filters. Experientia 1986;42:287–291.

10. Kratskin IL: Functional anatomy, central connections, and neurochemistry of the mammalian olfactory bulb. *In* Doty RL (ed): Handbook of Olfaction and Gustation. New York, Marcel Dekker, 1995, pp 103–126.
11. Shipley M, Reyes P: Anatomy of the human olfactory bulb and central olfactory pathways. *In* Laing DG, Doty RL, Breipohl W (eds): The Human Sense of Smell. Berlin, Springer-Verlag, 1991, pp 29–60.
12. Price JL: Olfactory system. *In* Paxinos G (ed): The Human Nervous System. San Diego, Academic Press, 1990, pp 979–998.
13. Pevsner J, Reed RR, Feinstein PG, et al: Molecular cloning of odorant binding protein: Member of a ligand carrier family. Science 1988;241:336–339.
14. Lazard D, Zupko K, Poria Y, et al: Odorant signal termination by olfactory UDP-glucuronosyl transferase. Nature 1991;349:790–793.
15. Jones DT, Reed RR: G_{olf}: An olfactory neuron specific-G protein involved in odorant signal transduction. Science 1989;244:790–795.
16. Kurihara K, Koyama N: High activity of adenyl cyclase in olfactory and gustatory organs. Biochem Biophys Res Commun 1972;48:30–33.
17. Sklar PB, Anholt RRH, Snyder SH: The odorant-sensitive adenylate cyclase of olfactory receptor cells. J Biol Chem 1986;261:15538–15543.
18. Doty RL, Kreiss DS, Frye RE: Human odor intensity perception: Correlation with frog epithelial adenylate cyclase activity and transepithelial voltage response. Brain Res 1990;527:130–134.
19. Buck L, Axel R: A novel multigene family may encode odorant receptors: A molecular basis for odor recognition. Cell 1991;65:175–187.
20. Selble LA, Townsend-Nicholson A, Llsmaa TP, et al: Novel G protein-coupled receptors: A gene family of putative human olfactory receptor sequences. Brain Res 1991;13:159–163.
21. Sullivan SL, Ressler KJ, Buck LB: Spatial patterning and information coding in the olfactory system. Curr Opin Genet Devel 1995;5:516–523.
22. Vassar R, Ngal I, Axel R: Spatial segregation of odorant receptor expression in the mammalian olfactory epithelium. Cell 1993;74:309–318.
23. Nakamura T, Gold GH: A cyclic nucleotide-gated conductance in olfactory receptor cilia. Nature 1987;325:442–444.
24. Leinders-Zufall T, Shepherd GM, Zufall F: Modulation by cyclic GMP of the odour sensitivity of vertebrate olfactory receptor cells. Proc Roy Soc Lond B 1996;263:803–811.
25. Guides to the Evaluation of Permanent Impairment, 2nd ed. Chicago, American Medical Association, 1984.
26. Doty RL, Shaman P, Dann M: Development of the University of Pennsylvania Smell Identification Test: A standardized microencapsulated test of olfactory function. Physiol Behav 1984;32:489–502.
27. Doty RL: The Smell Identification Test™ Administration Manual, 3rd ed. Haddon Heights, NJ, Sensonics, 1995.
28. Doty RL, Marcus A, Lee WW: The development of the 12-item cross-cultural smell identification test (CC-SIT). Laryngoscope 1996;106:353–356.
29. Yoshida M: Correlation analysis of detection threshold data for "standard test" odors. Bull Facul Sci Eng Chuo Univ 1984;27:343–353.
30. Doty RL: The Smell Threshold Test™ Administration Manual. Haddon Heights, NJ, Sensonics, 2000.
31. Neuman NH, DiLoreto DA, Ho JT, et al: Bilateral optic neuropathy and osteolytic sinusitis. JAMA 1988;259:72–74.
32. Mela DJ: Smokeless tobacco and taste sensitivity. N Engl J Med 1987;316:1165–1166.
33. Doty RL, Kobal G: Current trends in the measurement of olfactory function. *In* Doty RL (ed): Handbook of Olfaction and Gustation. New York, Marcel Dekker, 1995, pp 191–225.
34. Henkin RI, Schechter PJ, Friedewald WT, et al: A double blind study of the effects of zinc sulfate on taste and smell dysfunction. Am J Med Sci 1976;272:285–299.
35. Lezak MD: Neuropsychological Assessment, 3rd ed. New York, Oxford University Press, 1995.
36. Lovell MA, Jafek BW, Moran DT, et al: Biopsy of human olfactory mucosa: An instrument and a technique. Arch Otolaryngol 1982;108:247–249.
37. Lanza DC, Moran DT, Doty RL, et al: Endoscopic human olfactory biopsy technique: A preliminary report. Laryngoscope 1993;103:815–819.
38. Doty RL, Shaman P, Applebaum SL, et al: Smell identification ability: Changes with age. Science 1984;226:1441–1443.
39. Finelli PF, Mair RG: Disturbances of taste and smell. *In* Bradley WG, Daroff RB, Fenichel GM, Marsden CD (eds): Neurology in Clinical Practice, Vol 1. Boston, Butterworth-Heinemann, 1991, pp 209–216.
40. Costanzo RM, DiNardo LJ: Head injury and olfaction. *In* Doty RL (ed): Handbook of Olfaction and Gustation. New York, Marcel Dekker, 1995, pp 493–502.
41. McCaffrey RJ, Duff K, Solomon GS: Olfactory dysfunction discriminates probable Alzheimer's dementia from major depression: A cross-validation and extension. J Neuropsychiatry Clin Neurosci 2000;12:29–33.
42. Yousem DM, Geckle RJ, Bilker W, et al: MR evaluation of patients with congenital hyposmia or anosmia. Am J Radiology 1996;166:439–443.
43. Leopold DA, Schwob JE, Youngentob SL, et al: Successful treatment of phantosmia with preservation of olfaction. Arch Otolaryngol Head Neck Surg 1991;117:1402–1406.
44. Kaufman MD, Lassiter KRL, Shenoy BV: Paroxysmal unilateral dysosmia: A cured patient. Ann Neurol 1988;24:450–451.
45. Henkin RI, Bartter FC: Studies on olfactory thresholds in normal man and in patients with adrenal cortical insufficiency: The role of adrenal cortical steroids and of serum sodium concentration. J Clin Invest 1966;45:1631–1639.
46. Doty RL, Risser JM, Brosvic GM: Influence of adrenalectomy on the odor detection performance of rats. Physiol Behav 1991;49:1273–1277.
47. Kosten T, Contreras RJ: Adrenalectomy reduces peripheral neural responses to gustatory stimuli in the rat. Behav Neurosci 1985;99:734–741.
48. Doty RL, Deems DA, Frye R, et al: Olfactory sensitivity, nasal resistance, and autonomic function in the multiple chemical sensitivities (MCS) syndrome. Arch Otolaryngol Head Neck Surg 1988;114:1422–1427.
49. Eichenbaum H, Morton TH, Potter H, et al: Selective olfactory deficits in case H.M. Brain 1983;106:459–472.
50. Jones-Gotman M, Zatorre RJ: Olfactory identification deficits in patients with focal cerebral excision. Neuropsychologia 1988;26:387–400.

Supported by Grants P01-DC-00161, R01-DC-04278, R01-DC-02974, and R01-AG-17496 from the National Institute on Deafness and Other Communication Disorders, National Institutes of Health.

CHAPTER 8

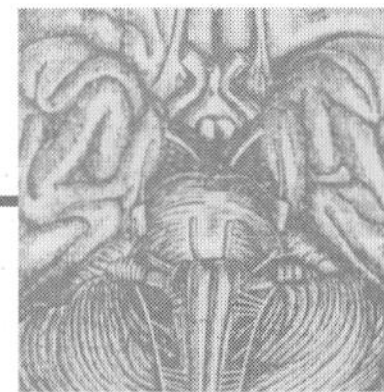

GRANT T. LIU and NANCY J. NEWMAN

Cranial Nerve II and Afferent Visual Pathways

History and Definitions

The afferent visual pathways encompass structures responsible for perceiving, relaying, and processing visual information: the eyes, optic nerves (cranial nerve II), chiasm, tracts, lateral geniculate nuclei, optic radiations, and striate cortex. In general, the visual abnormalities caused by lesions anterior to and including the chiasm cause acuity (clarity) loss, color deficits, and visual field defects (abnormal central or peripheral vision). From a neuro-ophthalmic standpoint, patients with unilateral retrochiasmal disturbances present primarily with visual field defects without acuity abnormalities. Higher-order processing, which is instrumental for interpreting visual images, occurs in extrastriate association cortex. Abnormalities in these areas cause, for instance, deficits in object recognition, color perception, and visual attention (neglect of visual stimuli in left or right hemifields).

This chapter reviews the neuroanatomical features of these structures and provides a systematic approach to the evaluation of clinical syndromes involving cranial nerve II, other parts of the afferent visual pathway, and higher cortical visual areas.

Clinical History

Common complaints encountered with visual loss include so-called negative phenomena such as blurry vision or gray vision. Patients with higher cortical disorders often have nonspecific complaints such as "I'm having trouble seeing" or "difficulty focusing." Patients with lesions of the afferent visual pathway may also complain of positive phenomena, such as flashing or colored lights (phosphenes or photopsias), jagged lines, or formed visual hallucinations (misperceptions of something that is not there). The level of visual image complexity of the positive phenomenon does not specify localization (see later).

The temporal profile of the visual loss suggests possible diagnoses, and its monocularity or binocularity helps in localization. As a general rule, acute or subacute visual deficits result from ischemic or inflammatory conditions or may be caused by a vitreous hemorrhage or retinal detachment. Chronic or progressive visual loss, in turn, may result from a compressive, infiltrative, or degenerative process. Cataracts, refractive error, open-angle glaucoma, and retinal disorders such as age-related macular degeneration or diabetic retinopathy also need to be considered when visual symptoms are insidious.

If a patient complains of monocular visual loss, a process in one eye or in the optic nerve should be considered. Painful monocular visual loss is characteristic of an inflammatory or demyelinating optic neuropathy. With binocular visual loss, a lesion of both eyes or optic nerves, or of the chiasm, tract, radiations, or occipital lobe should be investigated. Associated neurological deficits, such as motor or sensory abnormalities, also assist in localization and often indicate a hemispheric abnormality. Medical conditions should always be investigated in the review of systems. Hypertension and diabetes, for instance, predispose the patient to vascular disease, and a history of coronary artery disease should alert the examiner to the possibility of carotid artery insufficiency as well. Visual loss accompanied by endocrine symptoms, such as those consistent with hypopituitarism (e.g., amenorrhea, decreased libido, impotence) or pituitary hypersecretion (e.g., galactorrhea, acromegaly), suggests a process involving the chiasm.

Anatomy of Cranial Nerve II and Afferent Visual Pathways (Table 8–1)

OVERVIEW

Retinal ganglion cell axons carry visual information to the brain via the optic nerve, chiasm, and tract. A small portion subserves the pupillary light reflex by leaving the optic tract to reach the mesencephalon. Other axons synapse in the lateral geniculate body, which in turn sends projections via the optic radiations to reach striate cortex in the occipital lobe. Visual information undergoes higher-order processing in occipitotemporal, temporal, occipitoparietal, and parietal lobes.

EYES

The eyes are the primary sensory organs of the visual system. Before reaching the retina, light travels through the ocular media, consisting of the cornea, anterior chamber, lens, and vitreous. The size of the pupil, like the aperture of a camera, regulates the amount of light reaching the retina. The cornea and lens focus light rays to produce a clear image on the retina, and the ciliary muscle changes the lens shape to adjust for objects at different distances (accommodation).[1]

RETINA

Retinal processing of visual information occurs before its transmission through the optic nerve and remainder of the afferent visual pathway. The cone and rod photoreceptors first convert light (photons) to neuronal signals. The cones are located primarily in the middle of the retina, or *macula*, which is dedicated to central vision. The center of the macula, called the *fovea* centralis, is composed exclusively of cones. The rods occupy the retinal periphery. They subserve peripheral vision and are more useful in dim situations. Cones function best in bright light and are more important for color vision. Three types of cone photoreceptors are found, and each has a characteristic absorption spectra and responds best to blue, green, or red light. The perceived color of an object is based on the extent to which each of the three classes of cone photoreceptors is stimulated.[2]

The pigment molecules rhodopsin (in rods) and cone opsin (in cones) both contain 11-*cis*-retinal and are situated in the membrane of the outer segment of the photoreceptors. Light causes 11-*cis*-retinal to change to *trans*-retinal, and this process causes a conformational change in rhodopsin and cone opsin. The activated pigments stimulate transducin, which then activates cyclic guanosine monophosphate (cGMP) phosphodiesterase, which causes the breakdown of cGMP to 5′-GMP. Sodium channels, which are normally open in the dark, are then forced to close, resulting in hyperpolarization of the cell.[3] Photoreceptor signals are communicated to bipolar cells, then to the retinal ganglion cells, and these messages are modified by amacrine cells and horizontal cells (Fig. 8–1).[4]

The nasal retina receives visual information from the temporal field, and the temporal retina receives visual information from the nasal field. The superior and inferior halves of the retina have a similar crossed relationship with respect to lower and upper fields of vision. This type of parceling of visual information continues throughout the afferent visual pathway.

The majority of the blood supply of the eye travels via the ophthalmic artery, which is the first major intradural branch of the internal carotid artery, although there are external carotid anastomoses. The first major branch of the ophthalmic artery, the central retinal artery, pierces the dura of the optic nerve just behind the globe and travels within the nerve (Fig. 8–2). The central retinal artery then emerges at the disc surface where it typically branches into superior and inferior branches, each of which in turn divides into nasal and temporal branches to supply the four quadrants of the inner two thirds of the retina. The ophthalmic artery also gives rise to the long and short posterior ciliary arteries. The long posterior ciliary arteries pierce the sclera lateral to the optic nerve to supply the ciliary body and iris. The short posterior ciliary arteries enter the sclera near the optic nerve to supply the prelaminar portion of the optic nerve and outer one third of the retina. In some individuals, a cilioretinal artery, supplied by the choroidal circulation, may be seen at the temporal edge of the disc. The cilioretinal artery can provide an alternative blood supply to the papillomacular and macular regions in the event of a central retinal artery occlusion.[5]

OPTIC NERVE

The optic nerve has four major portions: intraocular, intraorbital, intracanalicular, and intracranial. The intraocular portion, the optic disc, consists of the unmyelinated

TABLE 8–1. **Clinico-anatomical Correlation of Disorders of Cranial Nerve II and Afferent Visual Pathways**

Anatomical Location	Visual Phenomena	Other Neurological and Medical Findings	Possible Etiologies
Retina	Transient monocular visual loss	Hollenhorst's plaque	Carotid disease, giant cell arteritis, migraine, vasospasm, cardiac emboli
	Acute monocular visual loss	Cherry-red spot, box-carring	Central retinal artery occlusion
	Subacute monocular visual loss	Retinal hemorrhage, cotton wool spots, dilated retinal veins	Central retinal vein occlusion
	Subacute monocular visual loss	Vitreous opacification	Vitreous hemorrhage
	Impaired visual acuity	Metamorphopsia	Central serous chorioretinopathy, macular degeneration
Optic nerve	Ipsilateral visual loss (decreased acuity, decreased color vision, central scotoma, altitudinal field defect)	Optic atrophy, optic disc swelling	Optic neuritis, ischemic optic neuropathy, compressive lesions
Optic chiasm	Bitemporal hemianopsia, decreased acuity and color vision	Optic atrophy	Pituitary adenoma, craniopharyngioma, optic glioma, meningioma, aneurysm
Optic tract	Contralateral incongruous homonymous hemianopia	Contralateral relative afferent pupillary defect, "bowtie" optic atrophy	Pituitary adenoma, craniopharyngioma, aneurysm
Optic radiations	Contralateral homonymous hemianopia	Preserved visual acuity, intact pupillary response, decreased OKN to side of lesion, sensory loss, hemiparesis	MCA stroke, temporal or parietal mass lesion
Occipital lobe	Contralateral congruous homonymous hemianopia (with or without macular sparing), quadrantic field defect, homonymous hemianopic central scotoma, cortical blindness (if bilateral)	Usually isolated deficits	PCA stroke, migraine, Alzheimer's, hypertensive encephalopathy
Association cortex	Cerebral hemiachromatopsia		Lingual and fusiform gyri lesion
	Alexia without agraphia		Left occipital lobe and splenium of corpus callosum lesion
	Visual agnosia, prosopagnosia		Bilateral medial occipitotemporal lesions
	Defective motion perception		Lateral occipitotemporal lesion (Brodmann area 39)
	Left hemifield visual neglect	Auditory and tactile neglect in left hemifield	Right parietal lesion
	Balint's syndrome (optic ataxia, simultanagnosia, ocular apraxia)		Bilateral occipitoparietal lesions
	Palinopsia		Temporo-occipital lesion(s)

OKN, Optokinetic nystagmus; MCA, middle cerebral artery; PCA, posterior cerebral artery.

retinal ganglion cell axons and astrocytes and is situated 3 to 4 mm nasal to the fovea. As the nerve exits the globe, it traverses the lamina cribrosa, which is a trabeculated meshwork of collagenous tissue. Just posterior to this, the optic nerve increases in diameter as it becomes myelinated by oligodendrocytes. At this point, the optic nerve is also invested with pia, arachnoid, and dura. The arachnoid extends to the sclera of the globe and contains cerebrospinal fluid (CSF) that is contiguous with that of the central nervous system. The dural covering fuses with the sclera around the optic nerve and more posteriorly blends into the periosteum of the optic canal.[5]

The intraorbital segment of the optic nerve is approximately 5 mm longer than the distance from the orbital apex to the posterior aspect of the globe. Within the orbital apex, the optic nerve is encased by the annulus of Zinn, which consists of the connective tissue origins of the superior, medial, lateral, and inferior rectus muscles. The nerve then passes through the optic foramen into the bony optic canal, which lies posteromedially in the sphenoid bone. The paired optic nerves course medially and rise at an angle of 45 degrees toward the chiasm. Intracranially, the optic nerves lie inferior to frontal lobes (gyrus recti) and anterior cerebral and anterior communicating arteries.[5]

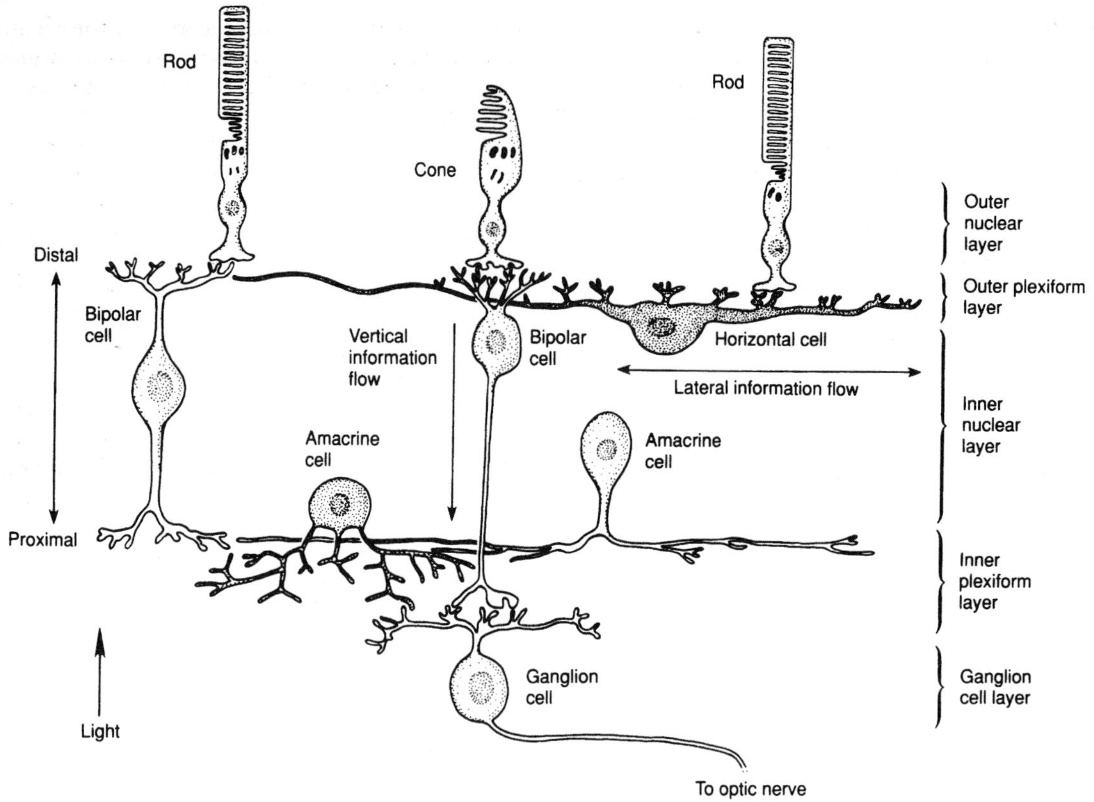

FIGURE 8–1. The three nuclear layers of the retina contain five major classes of cells: photoreceptors (rods and cones), bipolar cells, horizontal cells, amacrine cells, and ganglion cells. Photoreceptors, bipolar cells, and horizontal cells make synaptic connections with each other in the outer plexiform layer. The bipolar, amacrine, and ganglion cells make contact in the inner plexiform layer. Information flows vertically from photoreceptors to bipolar cells to ganglion cells and is modified by horizontal cells in the outer plexiform layer and amacrine cells in the inner plexiform layer. Output of visual information from the retina transported through the retinal ganglion cell axons (*bottom*). (From Tessier-Lavigne M: The retina and phototransduction. *In* Kandel ER, Schwartz JH, Jessell TM [eds]: Principles of Neural Science, 4th ed. New York, McGraw-Hill, 2000, p 515.)

The blood supply of the optic disc is derived from the arteriolar anastomotic circle of Zinn-Haller, which is supplied by the posterior ciliary arteries, the pial arteriole plexus, and the peripapillary choroid (see Fig. 8–2). Perforating branches of the ophthalmic artery supply the intraorbital segment of the optic nerve. The intracanalicular and intracranial portions of the optic nerve are supplied by a neurovascular network derived from the ophthalmic artery, internal carotid, anterior cerebral, and anterior communicating arteries. The central retinal artery does not directly supply the optic nerve.[5, 6]

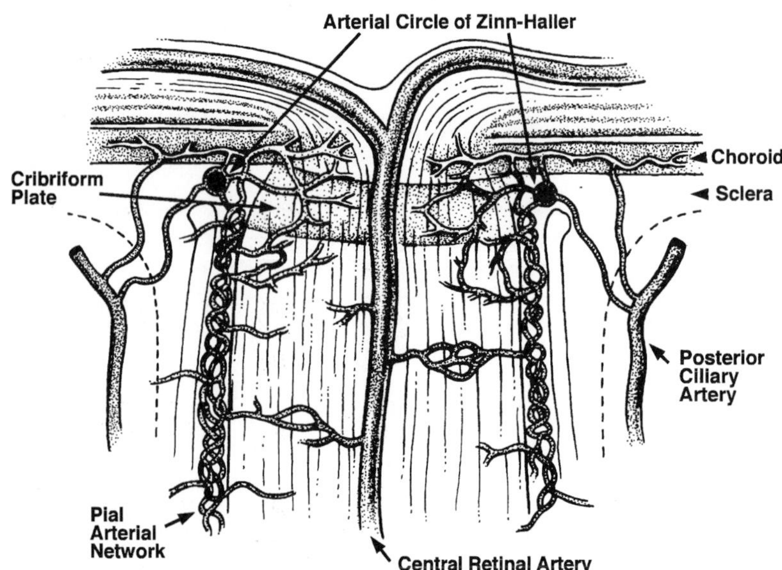

FIGURE 8–2. The blood supply of the optic nerve head is derived primarily from the arteriolar anastomotic circle of Zinn-Haller, which is supplied by the posterior ciliary arteries, the pial arteriole plexus, and the peripapillary choroid. (Redrawn from Hayreh SS: The central artery of the retina. Br J Ophthalmol 1963;47:655.)

OPTIC CHIASM

The optic nerves join at the optic chiasm, which lies in the suprasellar region, superior to the diaphragma sella, inferior to the third ventricle and hypothalamus, and just anterior to the infundibular stalk. The chiasm tilts forward at an angle of 45 degrees and most commonly lies directly above the pituitary fossa, although occasionally it may be prefixed or postfixed in position relative to the sella. Within the chiasm, fibers from the nasal retina cross, and the most ventral axons from the inferior nasal retina bend temporally through the contralateral optic nerve (Wilbrand's knee), whereas the fibers from temporal retina remain ipsilateral (Fig. 8–3). The existence of Wilbrand's knee has come into question.[7] The ratio of crossed to uncrossed fibers is 53 to 47 percent, respectively. The fibers transmitting visual information from the superior retina remain superior in the chiasm, whereas those from the inferior retina remain situated inferiorly. The papillomacular bundles lie superiorly and posteriorly within the chiasm.[1, 8]

Most of the fibers traveling through the optic chiasm are destined for the optic tracts and lateral geniculate bodies. Retinal projections may also exist from the posterior chiasm to the hypothalamus, specifically the suprachiasmatic nucleus or the supraoptic nucleus.[5] This pathway is thought to mediate the visual input responsible for diurnal variations of neuroendocrine systems. The chiasm's neuroanatomical locale in relation to surrounding vascular structures is important, given the potential aneurysms and subsequent visual field defects that they may produce. The carotid arteries ascend lateral to the optic chiasm, and the precommunicating segments of the anterior cerebral arteries lie superior to the chiasm.[6]

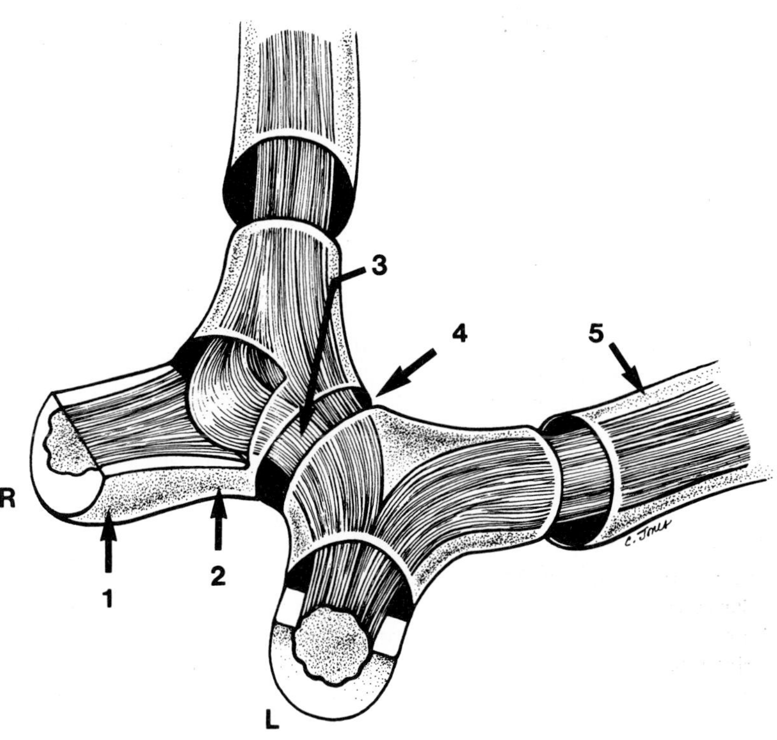

	Location	Left Eye	Right Eye	Comment
1	Right Optic Nerve			No light perception right eye
2	Junction of Right Optic Nerve and Chiasm			Junctional syndrome
3	Chiasm			Bitemporal hemianopsia (classic)
4	Posterior Chiasm			Central bitemporal hemianopic scotomas
5	Left Optic Tract			Incongruous right homonymous hemianopia

FIGURE 8–3. Optic chiasm: correlation of lesion site and field defect. (From Liu GT: Disorders of the eyes and eyelids. *In* Samuels MA, Feske S [eds]: The Office Practice of Neurology. New York, Churchill-Livingstone, 1996, p 46. Adapted from Hoyt WF, Luis O: The primate chiasm. Arch Ophthalmol 1963; 70:69–85. Copyright 1963, American Medical Association.)

The chiasm derives its blood supply from an inferior and superior anastomotic group of vessels.[9] The inferior group is made up of the superior hypophyseal arteries, which derive their blood supply from the internal carotid, posterior communicating, and posterior cerebral arteries. The superior group of vessels consists of precommunicating branches of the anterior cerebral arteries.[6]

OPTIC TRACT AND LATERAL GENICULATE BODY

The afferent visual fibers exit the chiasm posteriorly and diverge to form the left and right optic tracts, each of which is made up of ipsilateral temporal fibers and contralateral nasal fibers. The optic tracts sweep around and above the infundibulum, below the third ventricle, and superomedially to the uncal gyri. They then turn posterolaterally to the interpenduncular cistern, just ventral to the rostral midbrain and cerebral peduncles.

Most of the fibers synapse within the ipsilateral lateral geniculate nucleus; however, a few axons depart from the optic tract to complete the afferent limb of the pupillary light reflex. These fibers pass ventral to the medial geniculate nucleus; then they continue through the brachium of the superior colliculi before reaching the pretectal nuclei, where they synapse (Fig. 8–4). In turn, these nuclei connect bilaterally to the Edinger-Westphal nuclei in the oculomotor complex. Parasympathetic pupillary fibers leave the brain stem within cranial nerve III, then synapse in the ciliary ganglion in the orbit. Postganglionic fibers mediate pupillary constriction. Details regarding the Edinger-Westphal nuclei in oculomotor complex are contained in the chapter on cranial nerves III, IV, and VI (see Chapter 9).

The lateral geniculate nucleus (LGN), which is situated within the lateral recess of the choroidal fissure, above the ambient cistern, is considered part of the thalamus. Coronally, the LGN has six neuronal layers, and the input into each is monocular and retinotopically organized. Visual information from the ipsilateral eye synapses within laminae 2, 3, and 5, whereas that from the contralateral eye synapses within laminae 1, 4, and 6. Layers one and two contain large neurons (magnocellular LGN layers), whereas layers three through six contain smaller neurons (parvocellular LGN layers). Studies suggest the existence of at least two types of retinal ganglion cells (M and P, respectively) that project preferentially to each group, and that each layer may have distinct projections within the striate cortex as well. The medial horn of the LGN subserves the inferior visual field and the lateral horn subserves the superior visual field. The medial portion (hilum) subserves macular vision.

The blood supply of the optic tract is variable but typically comes from an anastomotic network made up of the anterior thalamic perforators (from the posterior cerebral artery) and the anterior choroidal artery (from the internal carotid artery). The LGN also has a rich anastomotic blood supply made up of the anterior and posterior choroidal arteries. The medial and lateral wedges of the LGN are supplied by the anterior choroidal artery, and the hilum (middle wedge) by the posterior choroidal artery. In about 50 percent of cases, small portions of the LGN receive blood from other small posterior cerebral artery (PCA) branches. Ischemic lesions to the posterior portion of the optic tract and the LGN are considered rare because of their rich anastomotic blood supply.[5,6]

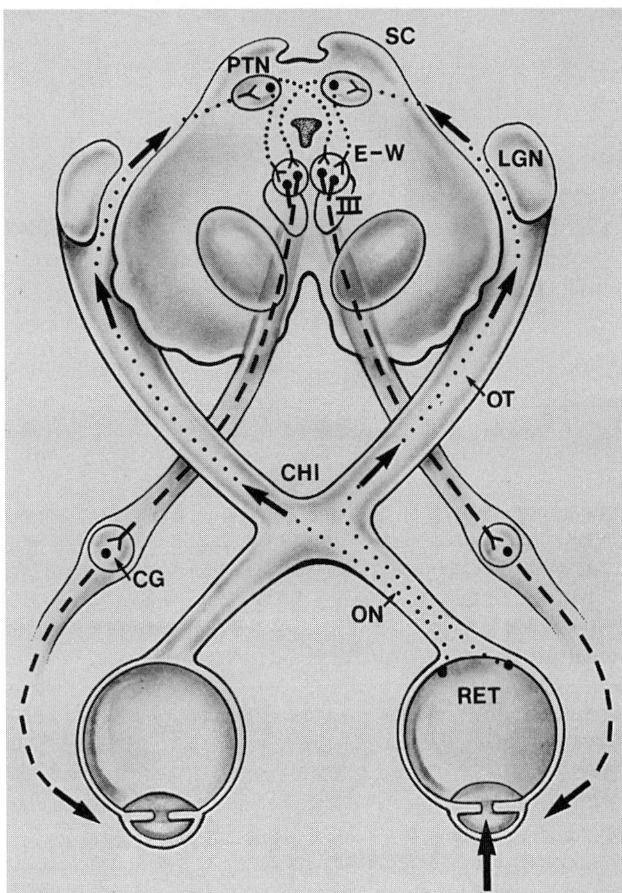

FIGURE 8–4. Pupillary light reflex–parasympathetic pathway. Light entering one eye (*straight black arrow, bottom right*) stimulates the retinal photoreceptors (RET), resulting in excitation of ganglion cells, whose axons travel within the optic nerve (ON), partially decussate in the chiasm (CHI), then leave the optic tract (OT) (before the lateral geniculate nucleus [LGN]) and pass through the brachium of the superior colliculus (SC) before synapsing at the mesencephalic pretectal nucleus (PTN). This structure connects bilaterally within the oculomotor nuclear complex at the Edinger-Westphal (E-W) nuclei, which issues parasympathetic fibers that travel within the third nerve (inferior division) and terminate at the ciliary ganglion (CG) in the orbit. Postsynaptic cells innervate the pupillary sphincter, resulting in miosis. Note light in one eye causes bilateral pupillary constriction. (From Liu GT: Disorders of the eyes and eyelids. *In* Samuels MA, Feske S [eds]: The Office Practice of Neurology. New York, Churchill Livingstone, 1996, p 61. Adapted from Slamovits TL, Glaser JS: The pupils and accommodation. *In* Glaser JS [ed]: Neuro-ophthalmology, 3rd ed. Philadelphia, Lippincott, Williams & Wilkins, 1999, p 528, with permission).

OPTIC RADIATIONS

The optic radiations (geniculocalcarine fibers) exit dorsally from the LGN, then spread into two major bundles. The group of fibers containing contralateral superior quadrant visual information (inferior fascicle) curves in an anteroinferior direction into the anterior pole of the temporal lobe, forming Meyer's loop. The superior fascicle lies deep within the parietal lobe and subserves visual information from the contralateral inferior quadrant. The temporal and parietal fascicles project in a retinotopic fashion to the lower and upper banks of calcarine cortex, respectively.

The temporal portion of the optic radiations receives its blood supply from the anterior choroidal artery and other middle cerebral artery (MCA) branches within the sylvian fissure, including the lenticulostriate and inferior temporo-occipital artery. The distal branches of the MCA, including the angular and posterior temporal arteries, supply the more superiorly situated parietal fascicles. The most posterior portions of the optic radiations, just before their entry into the occipital lobe, are supplied by the superior temporo-occipital sylvian artery branch of the MCA and the anterior temporal and calcarine arteries of the PCA.[5, 6]

STRIATE CORTEX

Brodmann area 17 (or V1, primary, calcarine, or striate cortex) is the end organ of the afferent visual system and is situated in the occipital lobe. The upper bank of striate cortex lies superior to the calcarine fissure, and the lower bank lies below the fissure. Other boundaries of striate cortex include the splenium of the corpus callosum anteriorly, interhemispheric fissure medially, and occipital pole posteriorly. Laterally, some striate cortex may be visible on the posterolateral outer surface of the occipital lobes.

Neuronal input arrives in a retinotopic fashion from fibers of the LGN and synapses within striate cortex, which is divided into six layers. The thick, light-colored layer IV is visible to the naked eye and has been termed the *striae of Gennari*. The parvocellular neurons synapse within the layer IV-C-beta, whereas the magnocellular cells synapse within layer IV-C-alpha.[10] Fibers from the medial aspect of the LGN, carrying information from the superior retina, project to the upper bank of the calcarine cortex, whereas those from the lateral aspect, carrying information from the inferior retina, project to the lower bank. The inferior visual fields are thus represented within the upper bank, and the superior visual fields are represented within the lower bank. Left and right visual fields are represented within right and left occipital lobes, respectively. Macular projections synapse in the occipital pole and occupy about one half the entire surface area of striate cortex. The occipital tip is devoted to foveal vision.

The majority of the blood supply to striate cortex derives from branches of the PCA: the calcarine artery, mostly, with lesser contributions from the posterior temporal and parieto-occipital arteries. In most cases, small penetrating branches from the calcarine artery supply both the upper and lower banks of calcarine cortex. In up to one third of cases, one major branch to each bank may be seen. At the occipital pole, there is an anastomosis between PCA vessels and the superior temporo-occipital sylvian artery from the MCA. This dual blood supply to the area responsible for central vision is one vascular explanation for macular sparing in the setting of PCA occlusion.

VISUAL ASSOCIATION AREAS

Extrastriate areas V2 and V3 surround V1 above and below the calcarine sulcus. Isolated and clinically apparent lesions of V2 and V3 are unusual, but a combined lesion of V2 and V3 restricted to the upper or lower bank typically is associated with a homonymous quadrantic visual field defect.[11]

Higher cortical processing of visual information occurs in visual association areas, which are divided anatomically and functionally into ventral and dorsal pathways. In general, the ventral stream (occipitotemporal) is more concerned with object recognition ("what") and represents the continuation of the parvocellular pathway.[10] Area V4, which is situated in the lingual and fusiform gyri, is responsible for color perception within the contralateral hemifield.[12] Bilateral mesial occipitotemporal regions are utilized in object and facial recognition.[13, 14] In contrast, the dorsal stream carries out functions related to spatial orientation (the "where" pathway) and is the extension of the magnocellular pathway.[10] The parietal lobe is devoted to directed attention. Evidence suggests that Brodmann area 39 (area V5), within the lateral occipitotemporal region, is analogous to monkey area MT and is important for motion perception.[15, 16]

Examination of Cranial Nerve II and Afferent Visual Pathways

DIRECTED NEUROLOGICAL EXAMINATION

Visual Acuity

Visual acuity is a measurement of the individual's capacity for visual discrimination of fine details of high contrast.[17] Best corrected visual acuity should be tested for each eye.[1] Distance vision is assessed with a standard Snellen chart and near vision with a hand-held card. If the patient does not bring corrective lenses for the examination, a pinhole can correct most refractive errors.

Acuity is most often recorded as, for example, 20/40, in which the numerator refers to the distance (in feet) from which the patient sees the letters and the denominator the distance from which a patient with normal vision sees the same letters. Visual acuity with the near card is often recorded using the standard Jaeger notation (J1, J3, etc.). If a patient is unable to read the largest Snellen letters (20/200 or 20/400), the acuity should be characterized by the ability to count fingers (CF) (and at what distance), detect hand motions (HM), or have light perception (LP). An eye that is blind has no light perception (NLP). Contrast sensitivity testing with sine-wave gratings is a useful adjunct in the evaluation of visual acuity. In younger preverbal patients, assessment of fixing and following in most instances is sufficient. When more accurate visual acuities are required, preferential looking tests (Teller's acuities) may be used.[18] These tests are based on the principle that a child would rather look at objects with a pattern stimulus (alternating black and white lines of specific widths) than at a homogeneous field. The smallest pattern that the child seems to prefer is an indicator of best visual acuity.

Visual acuity can be altered by macular, optic nerve, or chiasmal lesions. Disturbances that are posterior to the chiasm (retrochiasmal, i.e., tract, optic radiations, and occipital lobe) can affect visual acuity only if they are bilateral.

Color Perception

Color vision can be tested with standard pseudoisochromatic Ishihara or Hardy-Rand-Ritter plates, both of which contain numbers or geometrical shapes that the patient is asked to identify among different colored dots.[2] Qualitative inter-eye differences in color perception can be tested by comparing a red bottle top, for example, with each eye.

A patient with monocular "red desaturation" may state that with the affected eye the red bottle top appeared washed out, pink, or orange.

Color vision can be altered by macular, optic nerve, or chiasmal lesions. Retrochiasmal disturbances can produce abnormal color vision in the defective visual field. A lesion of the lingual and fusiform gyri can cause defective color vision in the contralateral hemifield.

Visual Field Testing

Testing the patient's visual fields can be accomplished at the bedside by finger confrontation methods in all four quadrants of each eye by asking the patient to "count my fingers" or "tell me when you first see my finger wiggling." In a patient who is aphasic, uncooperative, intubated, sedated, or very young, responses such as finger mimicry, pointing to targets presented, visual tracking, or reflex blink to visual threat allow for a gross assessment of visual field integrity. Color or subjective hand comparison is a useful adjunct to elicit defects respecting the vertical or horizontal meridians.[1] To test central or macular vision, an Amsler grid (similar to a piece of graph paper with a central fixation point) can be viewed by the patient. Patients may perceive abnormal areas on the grid that may correspond with visual field deficits.

Accurate documentation of visual fields requires kinetic testing with a tangent screen, Goldmann's perimeter, or automated threshold perimeter. The Goldmann's kinetic technique is useful when evaluating patients with significant neurological impairment, because it is shorter and involves interaction with the examiner. Threshold computerized perimetry of the central 30 degrees of vision is a more sensitive and reproducible test for patients with optic neuropathies and chiasmal disturbances. When visual fields are recorded, they are presented so that the right field is to the right and the left field to the left. The blind spot, corresponding to the optic nerve, is located approximately 15 degrees temporal to fixation and is recorded as an area without vision.[1]

The visual field can be altered by lesions anywhere in the afferent visual pathway, and the specific patterns in relationship to neuroanatomical structures are discussed in more detail later.

Higher Cortical Visual Function

It is often difficult to separate a dense left hemianopia from dense neglect in a patient with a large right parietal lesion. In instances when the deficits are more subtle, the examiner can screen for visual inattention by presenting visual stimuli, such as fingers, separately in each hemifield, then together on both sides of midline (double simultaneous visual stimulation). People with subtle visual inattention but intact fields see the stimulus when presented separately but not when shown simultaneously. Other bedside tests include letter cancellation, in which the patient is asked to find a specific letter or shape within a random array. Patients with left visual neglect may find the specified letter only when it appears on the right side of the page. When patients with left neglect are asked to bisect lines drawn randomly on a page, they may tend to "bisect" the lines to the right of their center.

In patients suspected of agnosias, informal tests of visual recognition can be performed at the bedside using common objects such as a pen, cup, or book. An inability to recognize faces (prosopagnosia) or interpret complex scenes (simultanagnosia) can be tested with magazine or newspaper photos and advertisements. Standardized facial and object recognition tasks are available during more formal neuropsychological testing.

Pupillary Examination

The size of each pupil can be measured in light and dark using the pupil scale found on most near-acuity cards. Pupillary light reactivity is tested with a bright light, such as a halogen transilluminator, while the patient fixes on a distant object (to avoid accommodation). While the light is shining in one eye, the ipsilateral pupillary light reflex, termed the *direct response*, and the contralateral, termed the *consensual response*, should be noted. Transient fluctuations in pupillary diameter are normal and are called *hippus*. The swinging flashlight test involves alternating a bright light equally at each eye to compare each pupil's reactivity to light. Because light from one eye will reach both Edinger-Westphal nuclei (see Fig. 8–4), normally both pupils react briskly when light is shone into just one eye, and the amount of constriction is the same regardless of which eye is stimulated.

If one eye has reduced vision owing to an optic neuropathy or large retinal process, light directed into that eye produces a relatively weaker pupillary response in both eyes (relative afferent pupillary defect [RAPD]) (Fig. 8–5).[1] Asymmetrical chiasmal disturbances may lead to an RAPD in the eye with worse acuity or greater field loss. Optic tract lesions can be associated with an RAPD in the contralateral eye, owing to interruption of the crossing nasal fibers, which outnumber the uncrossed temporal fibers. Because afferent pupillary fibers leave the afferent visual pathway before the geniculate, geniculocalcarine disorders are not associated with pupillary abnormalities.

Funduscopic Examination

The posterior pole of the eye can be viewed with a direct ophthalmoscope through an undilated pupil. Any media opacity due to corneal exposure, cataract, or vitritis, for instance, can create a hazy view. Posteriorly, the optic disc, retinal vasculature, macula, and peripapillary retina should be carefully examined (Fig. 8–6). Important details of the optic disc that should be noted include its color and contour and cup-to-disc ratio. The retinal vasculature should be evaluated in detail, with particular attention to the caliber of arteries and veins, branching patterns and, when suspected, possible emboli. The macula, best observed by asking the patient to look at the direct ophthalmoscope's light, is examined for evidence of degeneration, lipid deposition, detachment, edema, or change in pigment color. Thorough evaluation of the retinal periphery requires a pharmacologically dilated pupil and indirect ophthalmoscopy.

Optic disc swelling suggests an optic neuropathy or papilledema. Chronic optic nerve processes lead to disc atrophy. Macular disturbances are associated with central field loss and decrease in visual acuity. If large enough, other retinal abnormalities can also cause corresponding field loss. For instance, retinitis pigmentosa beginning peripherally causes field constriction, whereas an inferior branch retinal artery occlusion is associated with a superior altitudinal field defect.

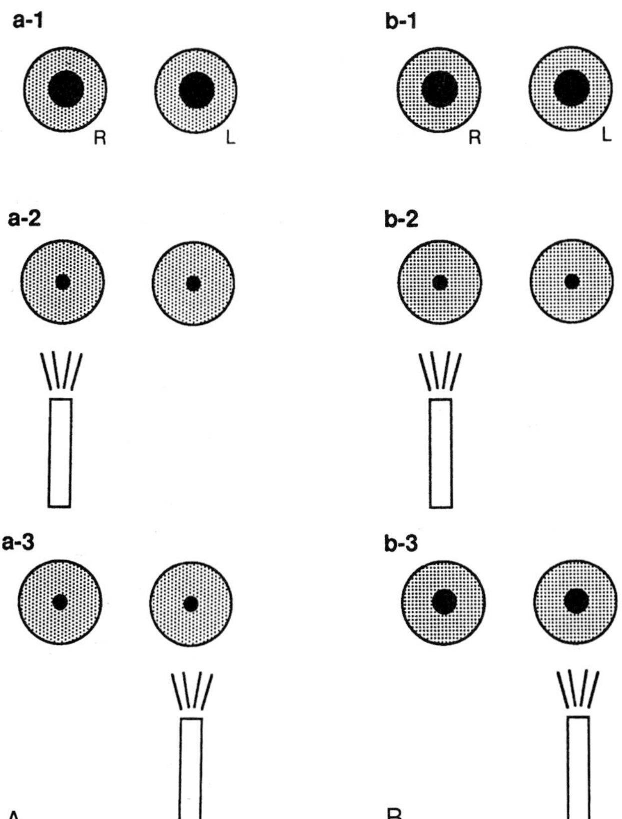

FIGURE 8–5. *A*, Normal swinging flashlight test, in which light directed in either eye elicits the same amount of pupillary constriction. *B*, Swinging flashlight test revealing a left relative afferent pupillary defect (L RAPD) in the hypothetical setting of visual loss in the left eye due to an optic neuropathy. Pupillary sizes are equal at rest in ambient lighting (b-1). Light stimulation of the good right eye results in brisk bilateral pupillary constriction (b-2). Light stimulation of the defective left eye produces comparatively weaker pupillary constriction, and both pupils dilate (b-3).

Ancillary Ophthalmological Techniques

The evaluation of patients with disorders of the afferent visual pathways often is enhanced by consultation with an ophthalmologist or neuro-ophthalmologist, who has ancillary ophthalmological equipment available. The most common cause of blurry vision is refractive error, and an ophthalmologist is the individual best equipped to make the required measurements. Applanation tonometry is a necessary screen for glaucoma. An exophthalmometer helps measure anterior protrusion of the eye, and it is indispensable when following proptosis, for example, in a patient with thyroid orbitopathy.

Slit lamp examination (biomicroscopy) uses what essentially is a horizontally mounted microscope and a special light source to visualize directly the cornea, anterior chamber, iris, vitreous, and posterior pole of the fundus (disc and macula, primarily). Indirect ophthalmoscopy, using a 20-diopter lens, allows more complete visualization of the posterior pole and peripheral retina. Both techniques follow pharmacological dilation of the pupil (usually 2.5 percent phenylephrine and 1 percent tropicamide topically), and each permits a stereoscopic view of the fundus, which is especially important when evaluating disc swelling, disc contour, cup-to-disc ratio, and macular edema. In addition, both slit lamp biomicroscopy and indirect ophthalmoscopy employ very bright light sources, allowing greater visualization of structures in the back of the eye when there is a media opacity such as a cataract.

ASSOCIATED NEUROLOGICAL FINDINGS

Cerebral. Hemianopias that result from lesions of the optic radiations are often associated with other "cortically based" neurological findings. Temporal lobe lesions may be accompanied by personality changes, complex partial seizures, memory deficits, fluent aphasia (if the dominant side is involved), or Klüver-Bucy syndrome (hypersexuality, placidity, hyperorality, visual and auditory agnosia, and apathy) with involvement of the anterior temporal lobes bilaterally. Conduction aphasia or Gerstmann's syndrome (finger agnosia, agraphia, acalculia, and right-left disorientation) suggests a dominant parietal lobe process. Left-sided neglect, topographic memory loss, constructional and dressing apraxias, in asssociation with a left hemianopia, suggest a nondominant parietal lesion. More parieto-occipital or occipitally based visual disturbances such as in Balint's

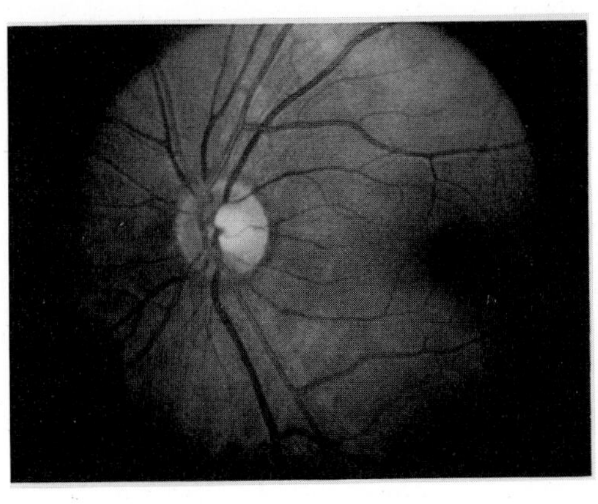

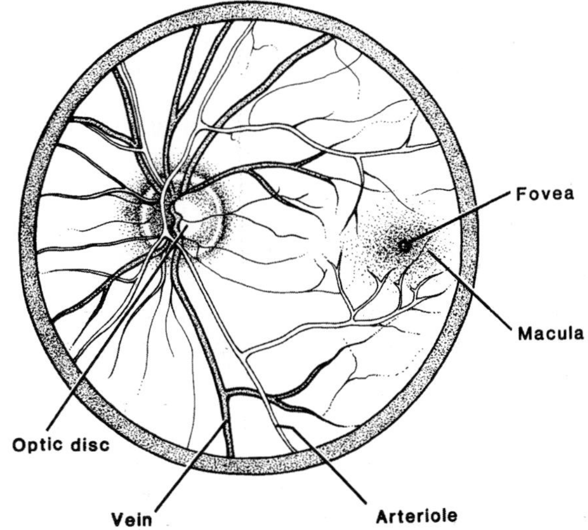

FIGURE 8–6. Photograph (*left*) of a normal left fundus. The corresponding illustration (*right*) identifies important structures. (From Liu GT: Disorders of the eyes and eyelids. *In* Samuels MA, Feske S [eds]: The Office Practice of Neurology. New York, Churchill Livingstone, 1996, p 41.)

syndrome or cortical blindness may accompany dementia in Creutzfeldt-Jakob disease, progressive multifocal leukoencephalopathy, or Alzheimer's disease.

Cranial Nerves. Lesions causing visual loss and ocular motility deficits frequently exhibit characteristic recognizable symptom complexes. For instance, orbital apex disturbances cause an optic neuropathy and cranial nerve III, IV, and VI dysfunction, as well as cranial nerve V distribution sensory loss, and oculosympathetic paresis. Suprasellar masses may compress the optic chiasm and, if large enough, can extend laterally to involve cranial nerves III, IV, VI, V1, and V2 within the cavernous sinus. In rare instances, seesaw nystagmus occurs in association with sellar lesions with bitemporal hemianopias. In this unique motility disturbance, one eye elevates and intorts while the other depresses and extorts, then the process reverses and repeats. Deep parietal lobe lesions can produce a homonymous hemianopia and poor tracking of objects moving toward the lesion. This effect results from involvement of the optic radiations and adjacent descending corticobulbar fibers from the parieto-occipitotemporal pursuit area.

In contrast, normal optokinetic responses can be expected in a hemianopia due to a lesion solely within the occipital lobe. Bilateral parietal lesions may cause abnormal initiation of voluntary eye movements, despite normal reflex saccades and pursuit (ocular motor apraxia), as seen in Balint's syndrome (see later). Hemianopias related to occipital lobe infarction may be associated with brain stem ocular motor dysfunction, if the etiology is vertebrobasilar occlusion. Patients with a hemianopia or neglect may have a gaze preference away from the visual deficit.

Patients with cerebellar disease and acquired nystagmus, particularly pendular, may complain of oscillopsia, the illusion of motion, and may suffer a reduction in visual acuity. Conversely, patients with bilateral visual loss involving the anterior visual pathways, especially if congenital or acquired in childhood, may develop nystagmus with jerk and pendular components.[19] Patients with severe visual loss of any type may also display a "searching" nystagmus in their attempt to localize objects without adequate visual feedback.

Patients with multiple sclerosis presenting with optic neuritis may have nystagmus or a unilateral or bilateral internuclear ophthalmoplegia, indicating previous white matter involvement in the posterior fossa.

Motor/Reflexes/Cerebellar/Gait. Hemispheric lesions may produce a homonymous field defect and ipsilateral hemiparesis when the optic radiations and motor strip or descending motor fibers are disrupted. A proximal posterior cerebral artery occlusion causes a similar clinical picture by leading to infarction of the cerebral peduncle in the midbrain and of the occipital lobe. Signs of cerebellar dysfunction such as nystagmus, truncal or appendicular ataxia, dysmetria, intention tremor, dysdiadochokinesia, or scanning speech together with a congruous homonymous hemianopia suggest vertebrobasilar occlusion. Patients with multiple sclerosis presenting with optic neuritis may have cerebellar signs indicating previous white matter involvement. Any process affecting both the afferent visual pathways and corticospinal tracts can cause visual loss and hyperreflexia. For instance, large hemispheric lesions can be expected to result in contralateral hemianopia and hyperreflexia. Conditions affecting central myelin (e.g., multiple sclerosis or acute disseminated encephalomyelitis) can cause optic or chiasmal neuropathy as well as spasticity and hyperreflexia. In central and peripheral dysmyelinating syndromes, there may be visual loss and hyporeflexia.

Sensory. A homonymous field defect in combination with ipsilateral sensory loss, astereognosis, decreased two-point discrimination, or graphesthesia suggests a parietal lesion. A process within the nondominant (usually right) parietal lobe can also produce a contralateral neglect syndrome or hemianopia, accompanied by contralateral sensory inattention. Pain, hemianesthesia, or choreoathetoid movements and an ipsilateral homonymous field deficit imply co-involvement of the thalamus and optic radiations.

Autonomic Nervous System. Autonomic system dysfunction, primarily because of pupillary and lacrimal disturbances, may lead to visual complaints. For instance, patients with pathological mydriasis due to parasympathetic dysfunction can suffer from photophobia or refractive error. The latter results from exposing spherical aberrations in the lens and cornea. Tonic pupils (Adie's pupils, for instance) are associated with accommodative insufficiency, and patients may complain of difficulty reading. Lacrimation abnormalities cause dry corneas, resulting in hazy views with irritative symptoms that are responsive to topical lubrication. Horner's syndrome (oculosympathetic dysfunction), by itself, should not cause visual abnormalities.

Neurovascular. Amaurosis fugax due to carotid stenosis may be associated with a carotid bruit, although that finding is notoriously unreliable. Cranial or ocular bruits may indicate an intracranial arteriovenous malformation or a carotid-cavernous fistula. In some instances of visual loss due to anterior ischemic optic neuropathy, underlying giant cell arteritis is suggested by tender, cord-like temporal arteries.

ASSOCIATED MEDICAL FINDINGS

A thorough but directed general examination of all patients can often provide important clues to neuro-ophthalmical diagnoses. It is impossible to list all the abnormalities one may find; however, some examples are reviewed.

Proptosis or periorbital fullness suggests an orbital process such as Graves' disease, orbital meningioma, or orbital pseudotumor. The patient's general appearance may suggest an underlying chromosomal, endocrinological, or metabolic disorder. For instance, disfiguring frontal bossing and enlargement of the mandible and hands are characteristic of acromegaly associated with a growth hormone–secreting pituitary adenoma. The heart rate, blood pressure, and carotid and cardiac examinations are important in any patient with a possible ischemic event. Patients with pseudotumor cerebri tend to be young females with obesity or a history of recent weight gain. Skin lesions such as erythema migrans (Lyme disease) or malar rash (systemic lupus erythematosus), and abnormal discolorations, such as café-au-lait spots and axillary freckling (neurofibromatosis), or hypopigmented ash-leaf spots (tuberous sclerosis) also may be helpful in guiding the evaluation of patients with visual disturbances.

Evaluation Guidelines (Table 8–2)

Neuroimaging. Most patients with suspected optic neuropathies should undergo neuroimaging to exclude a

TABLE 8–2. **Useful Studies in the Evaluation of Disorders of Cranial Nerve II and Afferent Visual Pathways**

Syndrome	Neuroimaging	Electrophysiology	Fluid and Tissue Analysis	Neuropsychological Tests	Other Tests
Retina	MRA: carotid occlusion, stenosis, or dissection	Abnormal electroretinogram if photoreceptors are affected	Elevated ESR in giant cell arteritis	N/A	Vascular occlusion on fluorescein angiography Thromboembolic source on cardiac echography, carotid ultrasound, or formal angiography
Optic nerve	MRI with gadolinium and fat saturation, coronal views: optic nerve enlargement or enhancement, or compressive mass lesion	Visual evoked potentials: decreased amplitude or increased latency	Elevated ESR in giant cell arteritis. CSF pleocytosis if inflammatory	N/A	N/A
Optic chiasm	MRI with gadolinium, thin coronal and sagittal cuts through sella: chiasmal enlargement or enhancement, or sellar compressive mass	N/A	CSF pleocytosis if inflammatory, endocrine studies showing evidence of hypopituitarism or hormone hypersecretion	N/A	N/A
Optic tract	MRI: compressive mass	N/A	N/A	N/A	N/A
Lateral geniculate body	MRI: infarction	N/A	N/A	N/A	N/A
Optic radiations	MRI: infarction or tumor MRA: carotid or MCA occlusion	N/A	N/A	Deficits in spatial ability and attention	Thromboembolic source on cardiac echography or carotid ultrasound
Occipital lobe	MRI: infarction or tumor MRA: posterior circulation occlusion	N/A	N/A	N/A	Thromboembolic source on cardiac echography
Higher cortical areas	MRI: infarction or tumor	N/A	N/A	Deficits in color perception or object or face recognition	Thromboembolic source on cardiac echography
Visual hallucinations	MRI: infarction or tumor	Epileptiform discharges on EEG if hallucinations are due to seizures	N/A	N/A	N/A
Other positive visual phenomena	MRI: infarction or tumor	Epileptiform discharges if positive phenomena are due to seizures	N/A	N/A	N/A

MRA, Magnetic resonance angiography; MRI, magnetic resonance imaging; ESR, erythrocyte sedimentation rate; EEG, electroencephalogram; CSF, cerebrospinal fluid; N/A, not applicable.

compressive or inflammatory process. The major exceptions are typical optic neuritis (although magnetic resonance imaging [MRI] scan may be appropriate to determine the prognosis for developing subsequent multiple sclerosis) or classic anterior ischemic optic neuropathy. Transient visual loss in the setting of migraine does not require neuroimaging when the historical features are characteristic and results of the neurological examination are normal. All patients with chiasmal and retrochiasmal patterns of visual loss should undergo imaging examination.

In general, MRI, with and without gadolinium, is the preferred technique for the evaluation of patients with suspected lesions of the afferent visual pathway.[20] In addition to the usual brain studies, some special instances require further neuroimaging. For instance, when an optic nerve process is suspected, MRI of the orbits with fat saturation and coronal views should be obtained. The chiasm is best imaged with additional thin cuts, coronal and sagittal, through the sellar area. Vascular disturbances, whether occlusive or aneurysmal, require MRI-angiography, and then in some instances, formal angiography. Computed tomography (CT) is helpful when fractures, bony erosion, or calcification is suspected, as in meningiomas or craniopharyngiomas.

Some experimental functional neuroimaging techniques may be helpful in cases when MRI or CT evaluation is inconclusive. Using positron-emission tomography or single-photon emission computed tomography techniques, hypoperfusion in visual association areas may be demonstrated in patients with visual agnosias, achromatopsia, and deficits in motion perception, for example. Functional MRI can highlight areas of cortical activation by detecting small changes in local blood flow.[21] Functional MRI technique may be more helpful for localization of normally functioning areas of brain, as in presurgical identification of cortical structures adjacent to brain tumors.[22]

Amaurosis fugax, central retinal artery occlusion, and ischemia in the middle and anterior cerebral artery distributions necessitate Doppler examination or MRI-angiography of the carotids. Echocardiography should be performed when a cardiac embolus or patent foramen ovale is suspected.

Electrophysiology. Other diagnostic tests used in combination with the clinical examination include electrophysiological testing such as an electroretinogram (ERG) or visual evoked potential (VEP). ERGs measure rod and cone photoreceptor function and help to distinguish the retinal degenerations and dystrophies. VEPs measure the cortical activity in response to flashes of light or checkerboard stimuli and, if abnormal, suggest a lesion of the afferent visual pathway. VEPs, when the result is normal, are particularly helpful in excluding organic lesions when functional visual loss is suspected. In addition, they can detect clinically silent lesions in the afferent visual pathway of patients with multiple sclerosis. VEPs should never take the place of the clinical examination and field testing, however, in the diagnosis or follow-up of patients with optic neuropathies or chiasmal disturbances. When cardiac source emboli are suspected, arrhythmias should be excluded by telemetry or Holter monitoring.

Body Fluid and Tissue Analysis. Blood studies are indicated when specific pathological processes are suspected. Vascular events may require evaluation of the erythrocyte sedimentation rate (ESR), rapid plasmin reagin, antinuclear antibody (ANA), and coagulation indices such as prothrombin time, partial thromboplastin time, and platelet count. The ESR, together with a C-reactive protein level, is especially important in transient or permanent visual loss in the elderly to rule out giant cell arteritis. In young individuals without an obvious risk factor for stroke, protein C, protein S, antithrombin III, Factor V Leiden mutation, antiphospholipid antibody, and anticardiolipin antibody levels should be obtained. A toxicology screen is necessary if drug use is suspected. Most intracranial mass lesions require either at least a brain biopsy if a primary neoplasm is suspected, or a metastatic evaluation if multiple metastases are more likely. In many cases of demyelinating disease, other autoimmune, inflammatory, and infectious disorders should be excluded by evaluating the ANA titer result, angiotensin-converting enzyme level, Lyme disease titer, and ESR, for instance.

When visual loss due to a sellar process is suspected, pituitary and hypothalamic function should be evaluated. The basic outpatient endocrinological panel should include serum prolactin, growth hormone (after a 75-g oral glucose load), insulin-like growth factor-I, adrenocorticotropic hormone, cortisol (serum morning sample or 24-hour urine free cortisol), thyroid-stimulating hormone, T_3, T_4, luteinizing hormone, follicle-stimulating hormone, estradiol, and testosterone level. Low values, and even normal ones in some instances, are consistent with hypopituitarism. High values imply pituitary hypersecretion by a pituitary adenoma.

Cerebrospinal Fluid. In some instances, CSF examination may aid in establishing the cause of visual loss. Inflammatory and infectious processes require CSF analysis (cell count, protein, glucose, Gram stain, and culture [bacterial, fungal, and viral when indicated]) when suspected. Carcinomatous or lymphomatous meningitis may require CSF cytology testing, including flow cytometry if available.

When pseudotumor cerebri is suspected in an individual with papilledema and normal neuroimaging results, a lumbar puncture is necessary to rule out meningitis, for example, and to document the CSF opening pressure. The lumbar puncture should be performed with the patient relaxed in a lateral decubitus position, with the head and spine at the same level and the neck and knees slightly flexed. To establish the diagnosis of pseudotumor cerebri, the CSF opening pressure should exceed 250 mm H_2O, which is the upper limit of normal for most obese and nonobese people.[23] Approximately 20 to 30 mL of CSF can be removed, although the optimal amount has not been studied. In suspected cases with a normal CSF opening pressure, monitoring for 1 hour with an epidural transducer or subarachnoid bolt may be considered,[24] but such a procedure is rarely done in clinical practice. The cell count and glucose levels should be normal, and the protein level normal or low.[25]

Lumbar punctures are not necessary in the evaluation of patients with typical isolated optic neuritis, because they rarely change the diagnosis and do not add to information garnered from an MRI in predicting the future development of multiple sclerosis.[26] The protein and glucose levels are usually normal, and only one third of patients have a pleocytosis that is between 6 to 27 white blood cells/mm^3 and rarely ever higher. Myelin basic protein can be detected in about one fifth of patients and IgG synthesis in about two fifths. Oligoclonal banding occurs in approximately half of these patients and is associated with the future development of clinically definite multiple sclerosis. Oligoclonal banding usually occurs in the presence of white matter lesions on MRI, however, which has been found to be highly correlated with the future evolution of multiple sclerosis. Therefore, oligoclonal banding adds little to the prognosis when neuroimaging, which is less invasive, has already been performed.[26]

Neuropsychological Testing. Neuropsychological assessment of higher cognitive functions can be used as an adjunct to the neuro-ophthalmic examination. By combining the disciplines of neurology and cognitive psychology, it is possible to analyze systematically the subcomponents of complex cognitive abilities or "information processing." The general functions that may be analyzed in detail include attention, speech and language, memory (short- and long-term, verbal and visual), visuospatial and perceptual functions (neglect, construction, praxia, and agnosia), and specific thought processes that include calculations, abstractions, judgment, and problem solving.[27]

Other Tests. Color stereo disc photographs aid frequently in the management of patients with optic disc swelling and pseudopapilledema due to disc drusen, for instance. Fluorescein angiography highlights the choroidal and retinal vasculature and involves intravenous injection of an aqueous fluorescein solution. Funduscopic pictures are taken before injection and at specific intervals after injection. This method detects vascular occlusion, abnormal retinal pigmentation or hemorrhages, and disturbances of the retinal pigmented epithelium. Truly swollen discs leak fluorescein, whereas, in general, discs with pseudopapilledema do not.

Clinical Syndromes (Table 8–3)

RETINA

Retina-related visual loss is usually painless and, in the acute setting, is almost always associated with some abnormality on funduscopic examination. Peripheral retinal disorders cause peripheral visual loss. Macular lesions tend to affect central vision and visual acuity. Symptoms of retinal degenerations include slowly progressive visual loss and poor night vision. Clues to underlying neurological disease may be provided by associated vascular, metabolic, hereditary, and degenerative retinal disorders.

Patients with transient monocular visual loss (amaurosis fugax) sometimes describe a descending "gray shade" that resolves after a few seconds or minutes.[28] A yellow cholesterol (Hollenhorst's) plaque may be seen at retinal vascular bifurcations, indicating an embolus from an atheromatous internal carotid artery or aortic arch. Emboli originating from calcific cardiac valves can produce similar symptoms but appear funduscopically as intra-arterial white plaques. Other causes of transient monocular visual loss include giant cell arteritis, retinal migraine, and vasospasm.

If the vascular obstruction persists, a completed central or branch retinal artery occlusion results. Typically the funduscopic examination reveals a normal optic disc, vessel attenuation, segmentation of the blood column ("box-carring" of arterial blood flow), retinal edema (pale and opaque), and a macular cherry-red spot. The latter results from the visible perfused choroid in the macular region, surrounded by opaque, infarcted ganglion cells, which are absent in the macula.

Painless monocular visual loss may also occur following a vitreous hemorrhage. Affected patients often report seeing large floaters in the affected eye, and blood within the vitreous impedes a complete fundus examination. These hemorrhages can result from neovascularization (e.g., diabetes) or acutely elevated intracranial pressure associated with a subarachnoid hemorrhage (Terson's syndrome).

Common causes of subacute monocular visual loss evolving over hours that involve the retina include retinal vein occlusions and retinal detachments. A patient with a central or branch retinal vein occlusion generally reports a painless loss of vision. Funduscopic examination reveals retinal hemorrhages; cotton wool spots; edema; and tortuous, dilated retinal veins. Peripheral visual loss may be reported, and decreased visual acuity suggests macular involvement or optic nerve ischemia. Retinal detachments are usually preceded by floaters and flashes of light (photopsias). If the macula becomes involved, the patient may experience acuity loss.

Central serous chorioretinopathy, which is characterized by elevation of the sensory retina with underlying serous fluid, affects the macula acutely. More insidious macular processes include age-related macular degeneration (exudative and nonexudative) and hereditary disorders such as Stargardt's disease.

Metabolic and energy disorders of neurological importance often produce characteristic retinal abnormalities that can cause progressive visual loss. These findings also provide important diagnostic clues, however. For instance, the presence of a macular cherry-red spot may suggest Tay-Sachs disease or sialidosis. Pigmentary retinal changes are often observed in Hallervorden-Spatz disease, neuronal ceroid lipofuscinosis, abetalipoproteinemia, mucopolysaccharidosis, or Refsum disease. Macular "salt and pepper" pigmentary retinopathy can be seen in patients with mitochondrial disorders such as MELAS syndrome (mitochondrial encephalomyopathy, lactic acidosis, and strokelike episodes), Kearns-Sayre syndrome, and chronic progressive external ophthalmoplegia.

OPTIC NERVE

Decreases in visual acuity and color vision, unilateral visual field loss, and an afferent pupillary defect suggest an optic neuropathy. Commonly associated field defects include arcuate, central, altitudinal scotomas, and constriction. The funduscopic examination may reveal an optic disc that is normal, swollen, or pale, depending on the etiology and temporal profile of the optic neuropathy. A glaucomatous disc has a normal rim, normal overall color, and an enlarged cup. Optic disc swelling, which is characterized by hyperemia, nerve fiber layer edema, venous congestion, obscuration of retinal vessels, and peripapillary hemorrhages, is indicative of active processes such as raised intracranial pressure or optic nerve inflammation, ischemia, or infiltration. Retrobulbar optic neuropathies by definition have no disc swelling because the pathology occurs more proximally, away from the optic nerve head. Optic disc pallor suggests an atrophic process and is seen at least to some degree in all chronic optic neuropathies when the damage has been present for weeks.

Although the most common optic neuropathy results from glaucoma (increased intraocular pressure), others associated with neurological disease include inflammatory, vascular,

TABLE 8–3. **Selected Etiologies Associated with Disorders of Cranial Nerve II and Afferent Visual Pathways**

Etiological Category	Specific Etiologies	Chapter
Structural Disorders		
Developmental structural disorders	Septo-optic dysplasia	28
Hereditodegenerative Disorders		
Storage diseases: lipidoses, glycogen disorders, and leukoencephalopathies	Adrenoleukodystrophy, Niemann-Pick disease, mucopolysaccharidoses	30
Amino/organic acidopathies, mitochondrial enzyme defects, and other metabolic errors	Cystinosis, Leber's hereditary optic neuropathy	31
Chromosomal abnormalities and neurocutaneous disorders	Optic pathway glioma in neurofibromatosis type-1	32
Degenerative dementias	Alzheimer's disease	33
Ataxias	Spinocerebellar degenerations	35
Acquired Metabolic and Nutritional Disorders		
Endogenous metabolic disorders	Diabetes	38
Exogenous acquired metabolic disorders of the nervous system, toxins and illicit drugs	Methanol	39
Nutritional deficiencies and syndromes associated with alcoholism	Nutritional amblyopia, B_{12} deficiency	40
Infectious Disorders		
Nonviral infections	Bacterial meningitis Lyme meningitis Tuberculous meningitis	42
Transmissible spongiform encephalopathy	Creutzfeldt-Jakob disease	43
HIV and AIDS	Progressive multifocal leukoencephalopathy	44
Neurovascular Disorders	Central retinal artery occlusion Ophthalmic artery occlusion Occipital or parietal lobe infarction	45
Neoplastic Disorders		
Primary neurological tumors	Optic pathway glioma Optic nerve meningioma Craniopharyngioma	46
Demyelinating Disorders		
Demyelinating disorders of the CNS	Optic neuritis/multiple sclerosis/Devic's	48
Autoimmune and Inflammatory Disorders	Giant cell arteritis Sarcoidosis Systemic lupus erythematosus	50
Traumatic Disorders	Traumatic optic neuropathy	51
Headache and Facial Pain	Migraine	53
Sleep Disorders	Narcolepsy	54
Drug-Induced and Iatrogenic Neurological Disorders	Functional visual loss Drugs Radiation	55

compressive, infectious, infiltrative, neoplastic, nutritional, toxic, congenital, and hereditary etiologies.

Patients with optic neuritis, which is an inflammatory optic neuropathy, present with acute monocular (usually) visual loss with pain exacerbated by eye movements. Two thirds of the cases are retrobulbar,[29] and visual loss results from inflammatory demyelination of the optic nerve. Most cases resolve spontaneously, but some patients continue to notice a transient loss of vision in the previously afflicted eye (Uhthoff's symptom) during periods of elevated body temperature during exercise or showering. Patients with optic neuritis who have multiple white matter lesions on MRI are at risk for developing multiple sclerosis.[30]

Some vascular etiologies of optic nerve dysfunction include ischemic optic neuropathy (nonarteritic or arteritic, secondary to giant cell arteritis), blood loss, and hypotension. Nonarteritic anterior ischemic optic neuropathy is an idiopathic, ischemic insult of the optic nerve head. Acute, painless visual loss (decreased acuity and an altitudinal defect, usually) and optic disc swelling characterize this disorder. The prognosis for visual recovery is relatively poor (in contrast to optic neuritis), and patients are typically older.[31] Presumed risk factors include a crowded, cupless optic disc; diabetes; and hypertension. Arteritic anterior ischemic optic neuropathy is associated with more severe visual loss,[32] and the disc swelling tends to be pallid.

The most common compressive lesions causing optic neuropathies are carotid-ophthalmic artery aneurysms and sellar masses (craniopharyngioma, meningioma, or pituitary adenoma/apoplexy). Primary neoplastic processes affecting the optic nerve include optic nerve gliomas (often associated with neurofibromatosis type 1), and optic nerve sheath meningiomas. Infiltrative processes (sarcoidosis, carcinomatous meningitis, leukemia, and lymphoma), nutritional deficiencies (cobalamin and thiamine deficiency), infections (syphilis), trauma, toxin exposures (ethambutol, methanol, and isoniazid), and congenital disc abnormalities (disc hypoplasia, congenital disc elevation, and optic nerve head drusen) may all cause optic neuropathies. The cause of tobacco/alcohol amblyopia, which appears classically as disc pallor and cecocentral scotomas, is unclear. The most common form of heredodegenerative optic neuropathy is the maternally inherited Leber's hereditary optic neuropathy.[33] Appearing in young males with severe, often sequential visual loss, this disorder is typically associated funduscopically with nonedematous disc elevation and peripapillary telangiectasias.

Pseudotumor cerebri (idiopathic intracranial hypertension) should be mentioned here because its major morbidity is visual loss related to optic nerve dysfunction. We dislike the term *benign intracranial hypertension* because the visual deficits can be severe and blinding. Patients should satisfy the following (modified Dandy's)[34] criteria: (1) signs and symptoms due to elevated intracranial pressure; (2) a normal result on neurological examination except for an abducens palsy; (3) modern neuroimaging excluding a mass lesion or other cause of elevated intracranial pressure; and (4) normal CSF parameters, except an elevated opening pressure (>250 mm H_2O). Patients are usually young obese females who may complain of headache, transient visual obscurations (seconds), pulsatile intracranial noises, or double vision. Almost uniformly, patients have papilledema; other causes of disc elevation, such as pseudopapilledema (optic nerve drusen or congenital nerve head elevation, for instance), should be excluded. Typically, visual acuity and color are preserved, but optic nerve-related visual field defects, which are best detected with computerized threshold perimetry, are present in over 90 percent of patients and include enlarged blind spots, generalized constriction, and inferior nasal field loss.

The combination of optic disc pallor and papilledema in the fellow eye is termed *Foster Kennedy syndrome*. Classically, the culprit lesion is a subfrontal mass, typically a meningioma, which compresses the ipsilateral optic nerve, causing disc atrophy. If the lesion is large enough to cause elevated intracranial pressure, papilledema results in the contralateral eye, but the ipsilateral optic nerve cannot swell because it is atrophic. Bilateral optic nerve compression is another possible mechanism.[35] Nontumor causes, resulting in the pseudo–Foster Kennedy syndrome, are actually more common. Examples include consecutive anterior ischemic optic neuropathy, characterized by new ischemic disc swelling in one eye accompanied by long-standing disc atrophy resulting from a previous event.

OPTIC CHIASM

A chiasmal process should be considered in patients with temporal field defects that respect the vertical meridian in either or both eyes, or in patients with visual loss of any type accompanied by an endocrinopathy. The most common field defect is a bitemporal hemianopsia, although the pattern of visual loss may vary depending both on the chiasm's position and the exact nature and location of the offending process (see Fig. 8–3). When a sellar mass is the cause, prefixed chiasms or more posteriorly situated lesions predispose to optic tract syndromes or central hemianopic scotomas. Postfixed chiasms or more anteriorly situated lesions are more likely to appear as an optic neuropathy or junctional scotoma with involvement of the ipsilateral optic nerve and Wilbrand's knee.

Patients with a bitemporal hemianopia are often without visual complaints unless visual acuity is abnormal, and such defects may not be apparent until the patient reads only the nasal half of the acuity chart. Some patients may complain of double vision because they may be unable to align the noncorresponding nasal fields of each eye (hemifield slide phenomenon). Asymmetrical lesions may produce an ipsilateral afferent pupillary defect, and color vision may be abnormal only in the defective field. Congenital or chronic processes may lead to optic atrophy, but rarely does a lesion compressing the optic chiasm lead to optic disc swelling without concomitant compression of the third ventricle. Rarely, patients present with asymmetrical shimmering nystagmus, torticollis, and head bobbing (mimicking spasmus nutans) or seesaw nystagmus.

Chiasmal syndromes are most commonly caused by sellar and suprasellar compressive masses. Such lesions are suggested by historical evidence of pituitary or hypothalamic dysfunction, and the differential diagnosis depends largely on the age of the patient. In the pediatric population, chiasmal-hypothalamic gliomas[36] and craniopharyngiomas[37] are most likely, whereas in middle-age to elderly patients, pituitary adenomas,[34] internal carotid aneurysms, craniopharyngiomas, and meningiomas should be considered. Compressive lesions usually produce insidious visual loss, and medical or surgical decompression may provide partial or complete visual recovery, especially in patients without evidence of optic atrophy. Rapid onset of visual loss and hypopituitarism suggests pituitary apoplexy.[38, 39] Rarely, chiasmal syndromes can be congenital as in septo-optic dysplasia (de Morsier's syndrome), characterized by hypoplasia of the optic nerves and chiasm, a hypoplastic or absent septum pellucidum, and pituitary ectopia.

OPTIC TRACT/LATERAL GENICULATE BODY

Complete lesions of both these structures cause dense contralateral homonymous hemianopias. Isolated syndromes involving these structures are rare. Incongruous homonymous hemianopias characterize partial optic tract and lateral geniculate body lesions (Fig. 8–7). A contralateral relative afferent pupillary defect can accompany an optic tract lesion; much rarer pupillary abnormalities include contralateral mydriasis (Behr's pupil) and hemianopic pupillary reactivity (Wernicke's pupil). Because of presynaptic interruption, patients may have bilateral optic atrophy with ipsilateral temporal pallor and contralateral "bowtie" or "band" atrophy. Visual acuity is normal in isolated tract lesions. Sellar and parasellar masses, especially craniopharyngiomas and aneurysms, commonly compress the optic tract. Isolated tract syndromes may also result from demyelination or rarely ischemia.

Although it is often difficult to distinguish clinically between lateral geniculate and tract syndromes, there are two unique exceptions owing to the geniculate's dual vascular

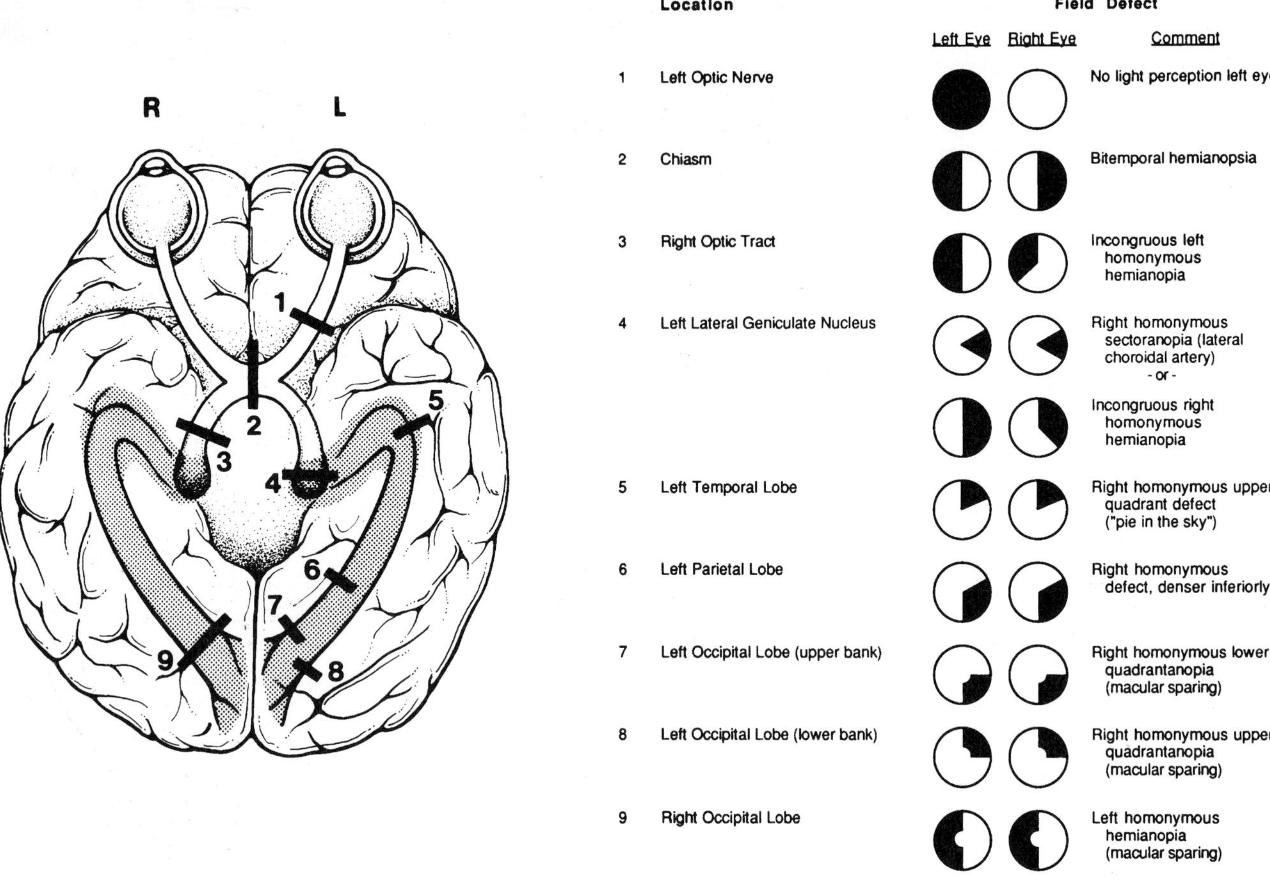

FIGURE 8–7. Visual pathways: correlation of lesion site and field defect, view of underside of the brain. Homonymous refers to a defect present in both eyes with the same laterality, whereas hemianopia refers to visual loss respecting the vertical meridian. Congruous fields are symmetrical in both eyes. Note that lesions of upper or lower occipital banks produce quadrantic defects, whereas lesions within temporal and parietal lobes cause field defects, which tend not to respect the horizontal meridian. (From Liu GT: Disorders of the eyes and eyelids. *In* Samuels MA, Feske S [eds]: The Office Practice of Neurology. New York, Churchill Livingstone, 1996, p 43. Adapted from Wurtz RH, Kandel ER: *In* Kandel ER, Schwartz JH, Jessell T [eds]: Principles of Neural Science, 4th ed. New York, McGraw-Hill, 2000, p 544.)

supply. A congruous homonymous horizontal wedge-shaped sectoranopia results from posterior choroidal artery infarction, whereas upper and lower homonymous sectoranopias result from anterior choroidal artery occlusion.

OPTIC RADIATIONS

An isolated lesion of Meyer's loop typically leads to a congruous or incongruous contralateral homonymous hemianopia denser superiorly (pie-in-the-sky defect), whereas lesions of the parietal lobe lead to defects more prominent inferiorly. In clinical practice, there is significant variation in these findings. Complete interruption of the optic radiations causes a dense homonymous hemianopia (Fig. 8–8A). Visual acuity is spared in unilateral lesions, but it can be impaired if bilateral lesions are present. Again, the pupillary responses are normal.

OCCIPITAL LOBE

Unilateral occipital lobe lesions, which are commonly due to vascular insults or primary and metastatic neoplastic lesions, cause a contralateral congruous homonymous hemianopia respecting the vertical meridian (Fig. 8–8A). Posterior cerebral artery infarction may produce a hemianopia with macular sparing (rather than macular splitting) (Fig. 8–8*B*), and this feature is specific to occipital lobe–related hemianopias. Proposed mechanisms include the dual vascular supply of the occipital poles, bilateral representation of the maculae, and test artifact due to poor central fixation by the patient. Posterior cerebral artery strokes may also spare the anterior striate cortex, the area that subserves temporal vision, thereby leading to homonymous hemianopias with preservation of the monocular temporal crescent (Fig. 8–8C).[40] This type of field defect is also highly suggestive of occipital lobe injury. Restricted lesions of the upper or lower banks of the calcarine cortex cause quadrantic field defects.

Bilateral upper or lower bank disturbances produce altitudinal hemianopias respecting the horizontal meridian. Homonymous hemianopic central scotomas are a telltale sign of a unilateral occipital lobe tip disturbance. Acuity is preserved with unilateral occipital lobe damage, but it can be impaired with bilateral geniculocalcarine lesions. Any level of visual acuity is possible with bilateral retrochiasmal lesions, but the acuities should be symmetrical unless there is superimposed anterior visual pathway disease.

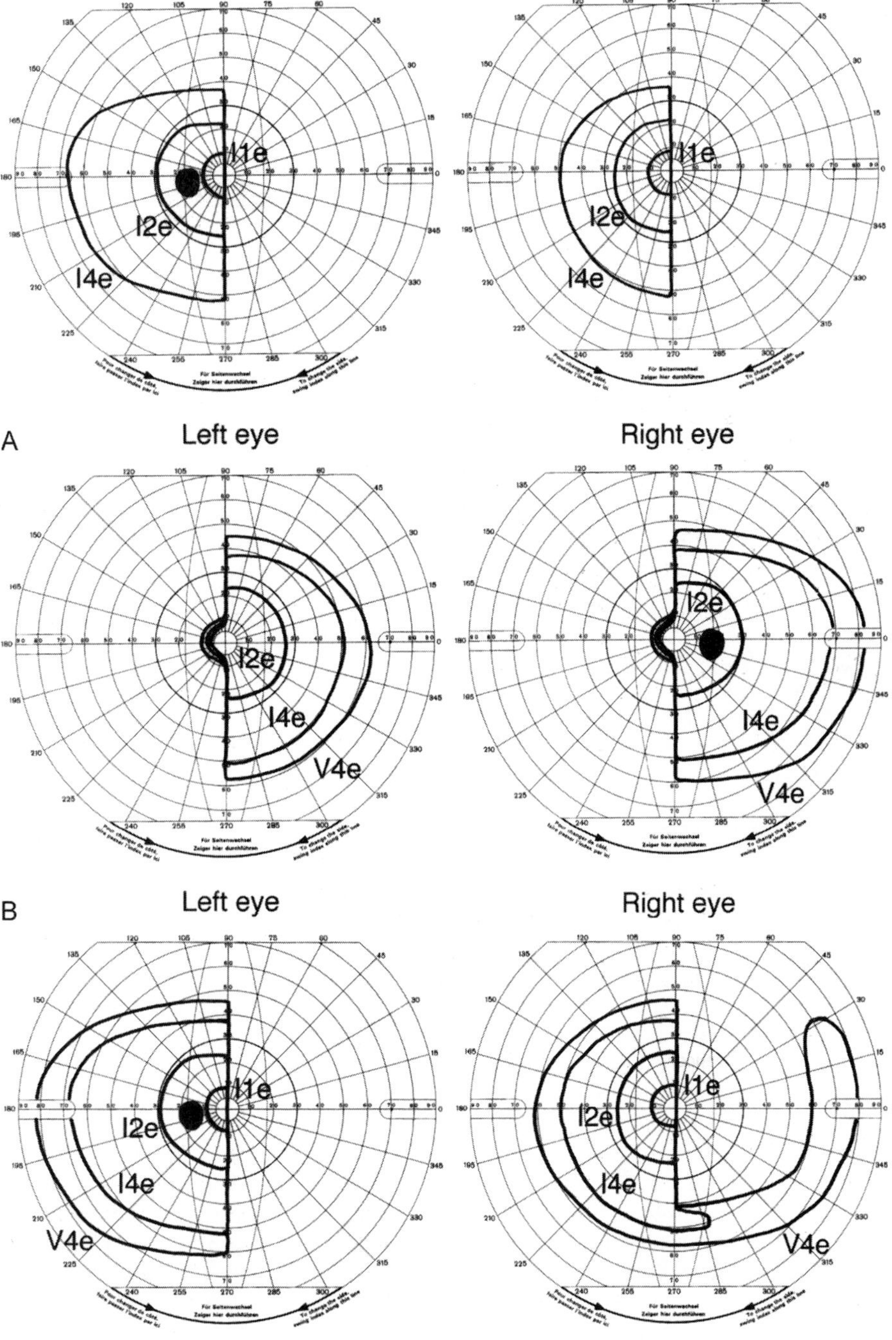

FIGURE 8–8. *A*, Complete, macular splitting right homonymous hemianopia due to a large left middle cerebral artery infarction. *B*, Macular sparing left homonymous hemianopia due to a right posterior cerebral artery stroke. *C*, Right homonymous hemianopia with sparing of the temporal crescent in the right eye. This resulted from a left posterior cerebral artery infarction which spared the anterior striate cortex on that side. (Reprinted with permission from Liu GT, Volpe NJ, Galetta SL. Neuro-ophthalmology: Diagnosis and Management. Philadelphia, WB Saunders, 2001, pp 307, 312, and 313.)

Hemianopias that are stroke-related are often isolated, unless a proximal posterior cerebral artery occlusion leads to a cranial nerve III palsy, ataxia, or ipsilateral hemiparesis from mesencephalic involvement, and memory or personality changes from mesial-temporal or thalamic involvement. A patient with a unilateral hemianopia due to occipital lobe infarction has a normal optokinetic response. In contrast, one with a hemianopia owing to an occipital lobe mass with edema extending into the parietal lobe may have an abnormal optokinetic response when the targets are drawn ipsilaterally to the lesion (Cogan's rule).

Cortical blindness, characterized by absent blink to threat and optokinetic responses, results from bilateral occipital lobe involvement. Clinically, patients with cortical blindness can be distinguished from those with pregeniculate lesions by the presence of intact pupillary light responses. Cortically blind patients may confabulate visual perceptions or deny their blindness (Anton's syndrome). Some of these patients have additional contributory cerebral lesions that alter recognition, memory, and behavior.

Unusual features observed following occipital lobe injury include unconscious vision in the blind hemifield (blindsight) and the recovery of motion perception (Riddoch's phenomenon). A "second," more primitive, retinal-tectal-pulvinal subcortical, extrastriate visual pathway has been proposed as a possible explanation. Polyopia (single objects appearing as several), palinopsia (persistence of visual images), and optic allesthesia (abnormal object orientation in space) are other unusual phenomena resulting from occipital, occipitoparietal, or occipitotemporal lesions.

Migrainous phenomena can involve the occipital lobes and manifest with transient hemianopic phenomena, with or without scintillations or phosphenes, followed by headache. Some patients experience only the visual prodrome without the headache (acephalgic migraine). In rare instances, a complicated migraine may lead to occipital lobe infarction and a fixed hemianopic defect.

In elderly patients, the differential diagnosis of occipital lobe dysfunction also includes Alzheimer's disease and hemorrhagic infarction due to amyloid angiopathy. Hypertensive encephalopathy or eclampsia can produce cortical blindness or transient hemianopias in patients of any age. Infectious causes include encephalitis, abscesses, progressive multifocal leukoencephalopathy, and Creutzfeldt-Jakob disease. In children, meningoencephalitis, adrenoleukodystrophy, and MELAS may be responsible for hemianopias. Ictal or postictal hemianopias are rare.

HIGHER CORTICAL LESIONS

Patients with lesions of visual association areas may have visual field defects if striate cortex is involved, but their visual complaints frequently cannot be explained by field loss alone. Further investigation often allows more accurate characterization of their symptoms.

Inferior occipital lobe dysfunction, involving the lingual and fusiform gyri, may result in a contralateral homonymous upper quadrantanopia and abnormal color vision in the contralateral hemifield (cerebral hemiachromatopsia). With left-sided lesions when the splenium of the corpus callosum or adjacent periventricular white matter is involved, alexia without agraphia (or pure alexia or "word blindness") may be observed. This represents a disconnection syndrome characterized by a right homonymous field defect and an inability to retrieve lexical visual information processed in the intact right occipital lobe.

Visual agnosia (the inability to recognize visual objects), in the absence of significant afferent visual pathway disruption, suggests bilateral medial occipitotemporal lesions disrupting the inferior longitudinal fasciculus, which is a white matter tract connecting striate cortex with the visual association areas of the temporal lobe. Prosopagnosia, a visual agnosia specific for faces, results from lesions to the fusiform face areas in the medial occipitotemporal regions. Defective motion perception is observed with lesions of Brodmann area 39 or lateral occipitotemporal cortex (area V5).[15]

Neglect or inattention to visual, tactile, or auditory stimuli in the left hemifield; dressing and constructional apraxia; and spatial disorientation suggest right hemispheric lesions. Neglect can occur without a hemianopia. Large parietal lesions frequently cause both, however, and in affected patients it may be difficult to separate dense visual neglect from field loss. The severity of neglect ranges from complete inattention to all stimuli in the left hemifield to subtle visual neglect of objects to the left only when stimuli are presented simultaneously on both sides of midline (double simultaneous stimulation).

Balint's syndrome is characterized by optic ataxia (a defect in reaching under visual guidance), simultanagnosia (an inability to recognize a whole picture despite the ability to perceive its parts), and ocular apraxia (a defect in voluntary eye movements). The symptom complex is caused by bilateral occipitoparietal lesions that are important for visual attention and foveal refixation. One or all elements may be present. Because the lesions commonly involve upper banks of occipital cortex, Balint's syndrome is commonly associated with inferior altitudinal field defects. Watershed infarctions are the usual cause, but Balint's syndrome may also be a prominent symptom of Alzheimer's disease or Creutzfeldt-Jakob disease.

VISUAL HALLUCINATIONS

These are visual images that the patient claims to see but that other observers do not. Visual hallucinations can be characterized as simple or unformed (e.g., dots, flashes, zigzags) versus complex or formed (actual objects or people). They may occur in patients with damage to the afferent visual pathways, sensory deprivation, migraine, seizures, brain stem lesions, drug toxicity or abuse, and psychiatric illnesses.[41]

Patients with visual loss due to a lesion anywhere within the afferent visual pathways may complain of hallucinations (positive visual phenomena) within the defective field.[42] This clinical scenario has been termed Charles Bonnet's syndrome. The complexity of the visual phenomenon is nonlocalizing. Patients may find these visual images pleasant or disturbing and may be embarrassed to volunteer their occurrence to their physician. Physiologically, they may represent visual phenomena released by lack of inhibitory input.[43] This mechanism may also explain visual hallucinations associated with severe sensory deprivation in prisoners of war.

Migraine visual aura may include positive phenomena such as stars, sparks, flashes, simple geometrical forms, enlarging scintillating scotomas, and fortification spectra.[44] Typically, auras develop over more than 4 minutes, last less than 1 hour, and precede or rarely accompany or follow the headache.[45] Uncommonly, the positive phenomena may persist in patients with or without "migrainous infarction."[46]

Epileptic visual hallucinations of occipital lobe origin may be very similar to migraine aura, and clinically the two disorders may be difficult to distinguish.[47] Secondary generalization, loss of consciousness, and ictal occipital discharges on electroencephalogram (EEG) may support a diagnosis of epilepsy, whereas transient visual loss, headache, and family history are more suggestive of migraine. Epileptiform discharges from other parts of the brain (the temporal lobe, for instance) may also produce positive visual phenomena. Other clinical features, however (autonomic, for example), are expected. In contrast to release hallucinations, the complexity of the visual phenomena may help localize the seizure focus. It is a useful generalization that occipital lobe seizures tend to be associated with simple visual hallucinations, whereas complex visual hallucinations are more likely the result of temporal lobe foci.

Peduncular hallucinations, consisting of vivid and life-like visual images of concrete objects, are rare sequelae of ventral midbrain injury. The hallucinations are frequently accompanied by sleep and cognitive disturbances. One clinicopathological study[48] suggested that their expression requires bilateral destruction of the medial substantia nigra pars reticulata.

Illicit drug use (cocaine, lysergic acid diethylamide [LSD], marijuana), medications (digoxin, anticholinergics, and dopaminergics), and parasympatholytic eye drops (atropine) may also be responsible for visual hallucinations. A psychotic psychiatric disorder is suggested when complex visual hallucinations are accompanied by occasional auditory hallucinations.[41] Normal people may experience both formed and unformed visual images on wakening (hypnopompic) or on going to sleep (hypnagogic). A number of degenerative neurological diseases (Parkinson's disease, progressive supranuclear palsy), in the setting of medication use (levodopa, dopamine agonists, monoamine oxidase inhibitors, and anticholinergics), can make visual hallucinations a common clinical disorder. Other disorders such as diffuse Lewy body disease may have visual hallucinations as a primary symptom as well.

OTHER POSITIVE VISUAL PHENOMENA

Phosphenes are flashes of light witnessed in patients with a blow to the eye, traction on the retina, optic nerve compression, or optic neuritis.[49] More complex positive visual phenomena include palinopsia (persistence of visual images), polyopia (multiple images), micropsia (shrunken images), macropsia (enlarged images), metamorphopsia (distortion of shape), and Alice-in-Wonderland syndrome (distortion of bodily image). All of these may occur during migraine aura. Metamorphopsia is a much more common complaint, however, among patients with macular disease. Palinopsia is more characteristically a symptom of occipitotemporal lobe damage.

FUNCTIONAL VISUAL LOSS

Nonphysiological or functional visual loss can be either subconscious (hysteria) or deliberate and willful (malingering). Commonly encountered neuro-ophthalmic complaints include visual impairment or complete loss of vision, visual field defects such as constricted fields, and monocular double vision. When confronted with a patient whose complaints and examination do not seem to correlate (subjective/objective mismatch) or whose visual deficit is nonphysiological, there are several clinical tools that help determine whether these findings are nonorganic.

The following clinical tests, when abnormal, are useful in a patient with suspected nonphysiological visual loss: (1) lack of a normal linear improvement of Snellen visual acuity with decreasing distance or increasing letter size (e.g., a patient who correctly identifies a 20/100 letter at 20 feet should equally identify a 20/50 letter at 10 feet); (2) presence of normal color vision and stereoacuity despite severely affected Snellen acuity; (3) normal menace or threat reflex, in which an approaching examiner's hand or bright light directed into the eye of interest causes a blink response; (4) presence of optokinetic nystagmus using an optokinetic nystagmus strip; (5) presence of fixation of a patient's eyes on his or her reflected image during the "swinging mirror" test; (6) suggestive Schmidt-Rimpler test result, which involves having the patient hold up his or her hand while instructed to look at it, which is a test of proprioception more so than vision. A patient with functional visual loss often looks everywhere but directly at the hand. Next, the patient is asked to touch the two index finger tips together, which, in nonorganic instances, may be performed improperly; and (7) normal EEG and psychogalvanic skin responses to light. With an intact afferent visual system, light shone into a normal eye causes a dampening of the posterior dominant alpha rhythm on EEG. The psychogalvanic skin reflex uses an electrode placed on the skin to measure the sympathetic response when a bright light is shone into the eye of interest. A normal response produces a deflection; no response is expected from the blind eye.[50] VEPs may also be helpful in this regard, although abnormal responses can be intentionally generated.

Monocular visual loss in the absence of a relative afferent pupillary defect or refractive error, media opacity, or retinal disorder suggests a nonorganic etiology. Tests that require binocularity (unbeknownst to the patient) can be extremely helpful in these cases. Perception of nine of nine stereo dots in the Titmus test requires 20/20 vision in both eyes.[51] During the Worth's four-dot test, the patient views red and green lights through a red glass over the right eye and a green one over the left. The right eye will see the red dots, and the left eye will see the green ones. It is impossible for an individual with one blind eye to see red and green dots simultaneously. In another maneuver, a prism is placed over the suspect eye while the patient reads the Snellen chart. Reading continues uninterrupted if the eye is blind. If vision is really normal in that eye, the patient pauses while refixating.[52] Perhaps the best stratagem is to fog the good eye secretively with a +10.00 diopter lens, then ask the patient to read the Snellen chart with both eyes. Any line read correctly must have been seen by the proported blind eye.

"Tunnel vision" is a classic nonphysiological visual field defect, and the patient usually complains of decreased peripheral vision.[53] Tangent screen testing reveals a lack of physiological expansion of the patient's perceived visual fields when the target size and distance from the screen are doubled. A patient's complaint of monocular hemianopia that upon formal visual field testing is present while testing the involved eye, absent while testing the unaffected eye, then present again when testing under binocular conditions is also nonphysiological. Although there are identifiable causes of monocular double vision, such as disturbances of the ocular media and some occipital lobe lesions, most are also considered nonphysiological, especially when they do not resolve with a pinhole.

General Management Goals

Some causes of visual loss, such as optic neuritis, tend to resolve spontaneously. Others due to compressive lesions and pituitary adenomas, for instance, have a good prognosis once the mass is removed surgically. Unfortunately, many of the vascular, hereditary, and degenerative causes of visual dysfunction have a poor prognosis for improvement.

Low vision aids may be helpful in some of these cases. In people with poor visual acuity, magnifiers can help them to read newspapers or other printed material. Closed circuit televisions, which enlarge written material without the distortion lenses may produce, are becoming popular for this purpose as well.

Patients with dense homonymous hemianopias can be offered prism therapy, but only a minority of them find it beneficial. A 30- to 45-diopter base-out Fresnel press-on prism is placed on the temporal half of an eyeglass ipsilateral to the hemianopia. This device projects images in the blind half of vision into the good half. The patients who like the prism therapy are those who use the prism to notice novel objects in their blind field; they then turn their head in that direction to use their good field to see the objects more clearly. Unfortunately, most individuals find this process too confusing and the result is suboptimal. It certainly does not improve their vision to the point at which they can drive. Base-out prism therapy should be attempted only in individuals who have normal mentation and in whom the hemianopia is isolated.

Experimental vestibular stimulation (by cold water, for instance) may have some efficacy in patients with visual neglect. We have no personal experience with this technique, however.

We have found that visual occupational therapy and rehabilitation is relatively unhelpful. Little proof exists that visual training after injury makes any difference in the speed or amount of visual recovery.

Reviews and Selected Updates

Glaser JS (ed): Neuro-ophthalmology, 3rd ed. Philadelphia, Lippincott, Williams & Wilkins, 1999.

Liu GT, Volpe NJ, Galetta SL: Neuro-ophthalmology: Diagnosis and Management. Philadelphia, WB Saunders, 2001.

Miller NR, Newman NJ (eds): Walsh and Hoyt's Clinical Neuro-ophthalmology, 4th ed. Baltimore, Williams & Wilkins, 1998.

References

1. Liu GT: Disorders of the eyes and eyelids. *In* Samuels MA, Feske S (eds): The Office Practice of Neurology. New York, Churchill Livingstone, 1996, p 40.
2. Hart WM: Acquired dyschromatopsias. Surv Ophthalmol 1987;32:10–31.
3. Tessier-Lavigne M: Visual processing by the retina. *In* Kandel ER, Schwartz JH, Jessell TM (eds): Principles of Neural Science, 4th ed. New York, McGraw-Hill, 2000, pp 507–522.
4. Dowling JE: The Retina. Cambridge, Belknap, 1987, pp 12–41.
5. Glaser JS, Sadun AA: Anatomy of the visual sensory system. *In* Glaser JS (ed): Neuro-ophthalmology. Philadelphia, Lippincott, Williams & Wilkins, 1999, pp 75–94.
6. Kupersmith MJ: Circulation of the eye, orbit, cranial nerves, and brain. *In* Neurovascular Neuro-ophthalmology. Berlin, Springer-Verlag, 1993, p 1.
7. Horton JC: Wilbrand's knee of the primate optic chiasm is an artefact of monocular enucleation. Trans Am Ophthalmol Soc 1997;95:579–609.
8. Newman NM: The visual afferent pathways. Anatomic considerations. *In* Neuro-ophthalmology: A Practical Text. Norwalk, CT, Appleton & Lange, 1992, p 3.
9. Bergland R: The arterial supply of the human optic chiasm. J Neurosurg 1969;31:327–334.
10. Zeki S: The P and M pathways and the "what and where" doctrine. *In* Zeki S (ed): A Vision of the Brain. Oxford, Blackwell Scientific, 1993, p 186.
11. Horton JC, Hoyt WF: Quadrantic visual field defects. A hallmark of lesions in extrastriate (V2/V3) cortex. Brain 1991;114:1703–1718.
12. McKeefry DJ, Zeki S: The position and topography of the human colour centre as revealed by functional magnetic resonance imaging. Brain 1997;120:2229–2242.
13. De Renzi E: Prosopagnosia. *In* Feinberg TE, Farah MJ (eds): Behavioral Neurology and Neuropsychology. New York, McGraw-Hill, 1997, pp 245–255.
14. Goldsmith Z, Liu GT: Facial recognition and prosopagnosia: Past and present concepts. Neuro-ophthalmology 2002;25:177–192.
15. Zeki S: Cerebral akinetopsia (visual motion blindness). A review. Brain 1991;114:811–824.
16. Tootell RB, Reppas JB, Kwong KK, et al: Functional analysis of human MT and related visual cortical areas using magnetic resonance imaging. J Neurosci 1995;15:3215–3230.
17. Frisen L: Visual acuity. *In* Clinical Tests of Vision. New York, Raven Press, 1990, pp 24–39.
18. Lamkin JC: Can this baby see? Estimation of visual acuity in the preverbal child. Int Ophthalmol Clin 1992;32:1–23.
19. Leigh RJ, Zee DS: The Neurology of Eye Movements, 3rd ed. New York, Oxford, 1999, p 442.
20. Pelak VS, Volpe NJ, Liu GT, Galetta SL: Neuroradiology in ophthalmology. Ophth Clin North Am 1998;11:339.
21. Liu GT, Fletcher DW, Bishop RJ, et al: Variability in visual cortex activation during prolonged functional magnetic resonance imaging. J Neuro-ophthalmol 1998;18:258–262.
22. Miki A, Liu GT, Modestino EJ, Bonhomme GR, Liu C-SJ, Dobre CM, Haselgrove JC: Functional magnetic resonance imaging of the visual system. Curr Opin Ophthalmol 2001;12:423–431.
23. Corbett JJ, Mehta MP: Cerebrospinal fluid pressure in normal obese subjects and patients with pseudotumor cerebri. Neurology 1983;33:1386–1388.
24. Radhakrishnan K, Ahlskog JE, Garrity JA, et al: Idiopathic intracranial hypertension. Mayo Clin Proc 1994;69:169–180.
25. Galetta SL, Liu GT, Volpe NJ: Neuro-ophthalmology. *In* Evans RW (ed): Diagnostic Testing in Neurology. Philadelphia, WB Saunders, 1999, pp 231–243.
26. Rolak LA, Beck RW, Paty DW, et al: Cerebrospinal fluid in acute optic neuritis: Experience of the optic neuritis treatment trial. Neurology 1996;46:368–372.
27. McCarthy RA, Warrington EK: Cognitive Neuropsychology. San Diego, Academic Press, 1990, p 1.
28. Gautier J-C: Amaurosis fugax [editorial]. N Engl J Med 1993;329:426–428.
29. Beck RW, Cleary PA, Anderson MM, et al: A randomized, controlled trial of corticosteroids in the treatment of acute optic neuritis. N Engl J Med 1992;326:581–588.
30. Optic Neuritis Study Group: The 5-year risk of MS after optic neuritis: Experience of the Optic Neuritis Treatment Trial. Neurology 1997;49:1404–1413.
31. The Ischemic Optic Neuropathy Decompression Trial Research Group: Optic nerve decompression surgery for nonarteritic ischemic optic neuropathy (NAION) is not effective and may be harmful. JAMA 1995;273:625–632.
32. Liu GT, Glaser JS, Schatz NJ, et al: Visual morbidity in giant cell arteritis: Clinical characteristics and prognosis for vision. Ophthalmology 1994;101:1779–1785.
33. Newman NJ: Leber's hereditary optic neuropathy: New genetic considerations. Arch Neurol 1993;50:540–548.
34. Smith JL: Whence pseudotumor cerebri? [editorial]. J Clin Neuro-ophthalmol 1985;5:55–56.
35. Watnick RL, Trobe JD: Bilateral optic nerve compression as a mechanism for the Foster Kennedy syndrome. Ophthalmology 1989; 96: 1793–1798.
36. Dutton JJ: Gliomas of the anterior visual pathways. Surv Ophthalmol 1994;38:427–452.
37. Repka MX, Miller NR, Miller M: Visual outcome after surgical removal of craniopharyngiomas. Ophthalmology 1989;96:195–199.
38. Cardoso ER, Peterson EW: Pituitary apoplexy: A review. Neurosurgery 1984;14:363–373.
39. Bills DC, Meyer FB, Laws ER, et al: A retrospective analysis of pituitary apoplexy. Neurosurgery 1993;33:602–608.
40. Lepore FE: The preserved temporal crescent: The clinical implications of an "endangered" finding. Neurology 2001;57:1918–1921.
41. Lessell S: Higher disorders of visual function: Positive phenomena. *In* Glaser JS, Smith JL (eds): Neuro-ophthalmology, Vol. 8. St. Louis, C.V. Mosby, 1975, p 27.
42. Lepore FE: Spontaneous visual phenomena with visual loss: 104 patients with lesions of the retinal and neural afferent pathways. Neurology 1990;40:444–447.
43. Cogan DG: Visual hallucinations as release phenomena. Arch Klin Exp Ophthalmol 1973;188:139–150.
44. Hupp SL, Kline LB, Corbett JJ: Visual disturbances of migraine. Surv Ophthalmol 1989;33:221–236.

45. Headache Classification Committee of the International Headache Society: Classification and diagnostic criteria for headache disorders, cranial neuralgias and facial pain. Cephalalgia 1988;8[suppl 7]:1–96.
46. Liu GT, Schatz NJ, Galetta SL, et al: Persistent positive visual phenomena in migraine. Neurology 1995;45:664–668.
47. Walker MC, Smith SJM, Sisodiya SM, et al: Case of simple partial status epilepticus in occipital lobe misdiagnosed as migraine: Clinical, electrophysiological, and magnetic resonance imaging characteristics. Epilepsia 1995;36:1233–1236.
48. McKee AC, Levine DN, Kowall NW, et al: Peduncular hallucinosis associated with isolated infarction of the substantia nigra pars reticulata. Ann Neurol 1990;27:500–504.
49. Gittinger JW, Miller NR, Keltner JL, et al: Sugarplum fairies. Visual hallucinations. Surv Ophthalmol 1982;27:42–48.
50. Miller BW: A review of practical tests for ocular malingering and hysteria. Surv Ophthalmol 1973;17:241–246.
51. Levy NS, Glick EB: Stereoscopic perception and Snellen visual acuity. Am J Ophthalmol 1974;78:722–724.
52. Kramer KK, La Piana FG, Appleton B: Ocular malingering and hysteria: Diagnosis and management. Surv Ophthalmol 1979;24:89–96.
53. Keane JR: Neuro-ophthalmic signs and symptoms of hysteria. Neurology 1982;32:757–762.

CHAPTER 9

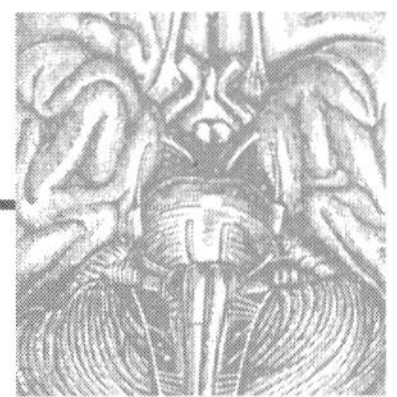

JAMES GOODWIN

Cranial Nerves III, IV, and VI: The Oculomotor System

History and Definitions

Cranial nerves III, IV, and VI and the muscles they innervate are involved in moving the eyes to allow inspection of visual objects. The act of positioning the image of an object on the retinal fovea, which is the locus of highest visual acuity and the psychological center of the visual field, is referred to as *fixation*. This is accomplished by activating combinations of extraocular muscles to achieve a specific angle of globe rotation in order to place the fovea in direct line with an image. *Fusion* denotes the primitive reflex action, organized within the central nervous system (CNS), in which the visual axes of the two eyes are made to converge on a single object of regard. This allows the same image in visual space to be focused simultaneously on the foveas of both eyes, and the image is perceived as a single object. The *visual axis* is an imaginary line connecting the fovea of the retina with the object of regard. It defines the direction of gaze and corresponds to the Y axis on Figure 9–1. *Strabismus* is present when there is deviation or misalignment of the visual axes.

There are nine cardinal positions of gaze, subdivided into primary, secondary, and tertiary positions. The primary position is straight ahead, and eccentric gaze develops when the two eyes deviate away from primary gaze. Secondary positions include straight up, straight down, straight in toward the nose, and straight out toward the temple. Tertiary positions are those away from the primary position with combined simultaneous horizontal and vertical deviation. These tertiary positions include elevation in adduction, elevation in abduction, depression in adduction, and depression in abduction. Abduction refers to movement of the eye toward the temple in the horizontal plane about a vertical axis, and adduction is the movement of the eye toward the nose in the horizontal plane about a vertical axis (Z axis, Fig. 9–1). Rotational movements relate to the eye's turning about an axis in the coronal or frontal plane of the globe. The axis may be vertical (horizontal rotation) or horizontal (vertical rotation) or oblique (oblique rotation) at any angle. *Torsional*

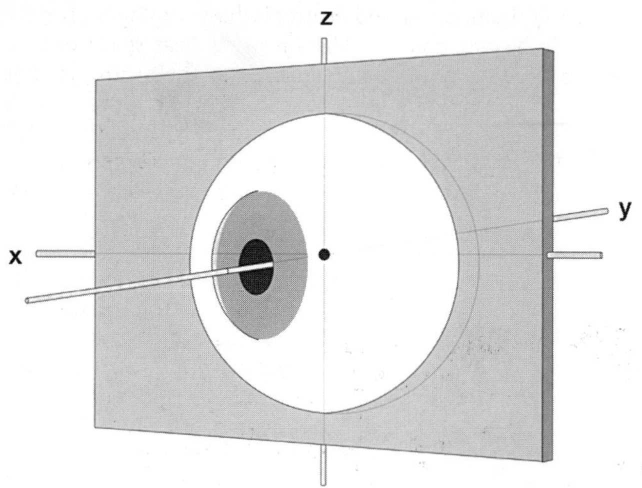

FIGURE 9–1. The axes of rotation of the eye. The Y axis corresponds to the line of sight when the eye is in the primary position looking straight ahead. (From Miller NR: Walsh and Hoyt's Clinical Neuro-ophthalmology, 4th ed, Vol 2. Baltimore, Williams & Wilkins, 1985.)

movements relate to an eye turning in the frontal plane about an anteroposterior axis through the center of rotation of the globe. The direction of torsion is specified by the movement of the 12 o'clock meridian of the limbus or corneal margin. *Intorsion* is defined as rotation of the point inward toward the nose or midline, and *extorsion* refers to rotation outward toward the temple. The rotation of both eyes in the same direction and at the same speed is known as *conjugate gaze*. This keeps the relative position of the visual axes constant (nearly parallel for distant objects, convergent for near objects). These conjugate movements of the two eyes are termed *versions* to distinguish them from *vergence movements*, in which the visual axes do not remain parallel but either converge or diverge.

Phoria denotes a latent eye deviation or deviation of the visual axes not present under conditions of binocular viewing. A phoria becomes manifest (becomes a tropia) when the image of the object of regard is made different in the two eyes such that the fusion mechanism cannot operate or operates inefficiently. *Tropia* is defined as deviation that is present with both eyes viewing, and hence is the condition that underlies diplopia. *Diplopia*, or double vision, is defined as seeing two separate images of the same object in visual space, with one of the images displaced from the other. Binocular diplopia results from the misalignment of the visual axes (the two eyes are looking in slightly different directions). This type is present only when the patient is viewing the object of regard simultaneously with both eyes and disappears when either eye is covered. *Polyopia*, or seeing three or more simultaneous images of a single object in visual space is categorically not a feature of binocular diplopia in humans. It is usually caused by an optical aberration in the refractive media of the eye, but a cerebral form also exists and is usually from lesions in the occipital-parietal lobes.

There are three systems of *conjugate* eye movement, including smooth pursuit, saccades, and the vestibulo-ocular reflex (VOR) that deviate the eyes in unison. Smooth pursuit eye movements stabilize on the fovea images of small objects moving in visual space. Saccades redirect the line of gaze to an object of interest, placing its image on the fovea. The VOR compensates for head movement, stabilizing gaze in space.

Clinical History

Because cranial nerves III, IV, and VI innervate the extraocular muscles that move the eyes, the striated muscles that elevate the upper eyelids, and the iris sphincters that constrict the pupils, several symptoms develop when damage occurs. In general, dysfunction of these nerves causes different combinations of binocular double vision from misalignment of the visual axes. Damage to cranial nerve III causes *ptosis* from weakness of the levator palpebrae muscle, as well as pupil mydriasis or dilatation from paresis of the iris sphincter muscle.

Altered function in the supranuclear control of the ocular motor system leads to conjugate gaze palsy or paresis in which the visual axes remain parallel or appropriately convergent on the object of regard. In these settings, the patient does not experience diplopia, because the two eyes simultaneously fail to achieve full movement in one or several directions from primary gaze. In some cases of conjugate gaze paresis, the eyes fail to deviate fully into the defective direction, and in other cases, the deficit is more subtle, so that the eyes deviate fully but move more slowly than they should or with an interrupted course. These dynamic alterations are generally without subjective symptoms and must be observed during the course of examination. Even patients with complete lack of gaze in a particular direction often have no complaints but automatically turn their head to compensate for the loss of eye deviation. The major exception to this principle is loss of downgaze, which generally creates much difficulty for the patient even when walking on a flat surface and especially in negotiating stairs and other uneven terrain. This is particularly irksome when coupled with the involuntary head and neck retraction or extension that often accompanies progressive supranuclear palsy (PSP) (see Chapter 34). Falling backward is common in PSP patients, and this problem should also be asked about specifically. A key symptom of pathological underactivity in the vestibulo-ocular reflex is *oscillopsia*, which is an illusory sense of movement of the visual environment as the head moves. This is a direct consequence of foveal image slippage engendered specifically by head movement, and the illusion ceases when the head is immobile. Vertigo, another common symptom of vestibular disorders, is often present when the head is still, although it is usually aggravated by head movement. Vertigo is a rotational illusion that is often accompanied by rhythmical oscillopsia as a consequence of nystagmus, in which case the rhythm is imposed by the regular fast phases of the nystagmus. The vertigo may be subjective, in which case patients feel as though they are rotating, or it may be objective, in which case they perceive that the environment is rotating.

The time course of the symptoms constitutes the best evidence for the etiology of the disorder and must be probed in detail. Diplopia is a markedly troublesome symptom, and it is either present or not, making its onset always acute. The angle of deviation between the eyes and the consequent distance between the two images may vary after onset, and this feature can be used to discern whether the course is stationary, progressive, or remitting. Symptoms from compressive cranial nerve lesions secondary to tumors and from degenerative conditions generally have a progressive course, whereas inflammatory diseases such as orbital inflammatory pseudotumor or Tolosa-Hunt syndrome (orbital and cavernous sinus inflammation, respectively) (see Chapter 53) often run either a course of remissions and exacerbations or a progressive course. Ischemic causes tend to produce a stationary course after acute onset.

Both ischemic and inflammatory disorders of cranial nerves III, IV, or VI tend to be associated with pain in the ipsilateral eye or orbit, sometimes with wide radiation to the brow, frontal, and temporal regions and downward into the cheek and even to the mandible. Malignant neoplasms may involve the cranial nerves III, IV, and VI anywhere along their courses, and pain can accompany the other features, especially when there is meningeal, bony, or dural infiltration. As with inflammatory diseases, the pain is usually centered on the ipsilateral orbit but may radiate widely. Not infrequently, intraorbital lesions, even malignant ones, can involve the cranial nerves without pain, possibly because they do not stretch or invade pain-sensitive structures, including muscle and particularly dura and periosteum. Absence of pain, therefore, should not in itself engender a false sense of security that the lesion causing the cranial neuropathy is benign.

A detailed characterization of the direction and circumstances of image separation is important in establishing which muscle or muscles, and hence, which cranial nerve or nerves, are involved. Horizontal diplopia arises from disorders affecting either the lateral rectus or medial rectus muscles. If the paretic muscle is one or both lateral rectus pair, the visual axes will be convergent (esotropia), and if the involved muscle is one or both medial recti, the visual axes will be divergent (exotropia). It is important to note that at minimal angles of binocular divergence, the patient often describes the visual experience as a blur rather than doubling of images. It is important to ask any patient with blurred vision if it clears on covering *either* eye, which will be the case for blur that is a result of minimal angle binocular diplopia. Blurring can be misconstrued for diminished acuity, but acuity is a function of cranial nerve II. Patients often cannot tell from the diplopia whether they have convergent or divergent eyes, because either condition produces horizontal image separation. Asking the patient when he or she covers the right eye whether the right or left image disappears can be helpful. If the eyes are exodeviated (divergent), the image to the left disappears. If the eyes are esodeviated (convergent), the image to the right disappears. A convenient way to remember the directions is to consider that *crossed* (X) diplopia results from eXodeviation (divergent visual axes, medial rectus weakness) and *homonymous*, or same side, diplopia results from esodeviation (convergent visual axes, lateral rectus weakness). The terms crossed and homonymous refer to the relation between the side of the eye covered and the relative position of the image that disappears—on the same (homonymous) or opposite (crossed) side. This same principle underlies diplopia testing and is considered in the examination section.

The visual axes are nearly parallel for viewing very distant objects. As the object of regard is brought progressively closer to the viewing subject, the person's visual axes must become more convergent to keep the images on both retinal foveas. Convergence is, therefore, a normal voluntary action in which the medial recti of both eyes are simultaneously activated and the resulting esodeviation is appropriate for near viewing. Because of this, patients with lateral rectus (cranial nerve VI) dysfunction and esotropia have diplopia only for relatively distant objects. All objects in near space can be fused by adding normal convergence to the esotropia that results from the muscle weakness. On the other hand, patients with exotropia do not have single vision at any distance. The presence or absence of fusion and single vision at some near point can be used to discern esotropia from exotropia.

Vertical image separation implies dysfunction of a vertically acting muscle in one or both eyes. These include the superior rectus and oblique and the inferior rectus and oblique muscles on either side. The details of image separation for vertical muscle imbalance must usually await examination using diplopia testing, but the patient may be able to supply some useful hints by way of history. Patients with a cranial nerve III dysfunction usually have mixed horizontal and vertical diplopia (oblique image separation) because several vertical muscles and the horizontally acting medial rectus muscle are commonly involved together. Also, these patients usually have some degree of upper eyelid ptosis, which is noticed by the patient on looking in the mirror. As ptosis becomes more severe, there is first restriction of the upper visual field and then loss of all vision when the pupil is completely covered. Asking the patient about upper field loss and total vision loss can help plot the time course of the ptosis. The most common neural cause of *isolated* vertical diplopia is cranial nerve IV dysfunction. The weak muscle is the superior oblique, which turns the eye down (depression) and does so most efficiently in adduction (horizontal deviation toward the nose). The image separation is widest in downgaze and looking to the side opposite the lesion, which brings the involved eye into adduction. If the patient can say that the vertical diplopia is wider looking down and widest looking down and to the left, then right superior oblique muscle weakness is most likely and vice versa. The diplopia is isolated in cranial nerve IV palsy because the nerve does not innervate any muscles other than the superior oblique and, in that respect, differs from cranial nerve III palsy, with its multiplicity of simultaneously involved muscles.

Patients with cranial nerve IV palsy often have torsional imbalance with excyclodeviation of the involved eye. Most patients automatically compensate by tilting and turning the head to minimize and sometimes eliminate diplopia. The resulting head position—tucked down, turned away, and tilted away—is characteristic and usually has been noticed as peculiar by others if not by the patient himself or herself. Patients often avoid diplopia altogether by using the compensatory head position. It can be useful to ask when people started saying things about the patient's head position, if it is unclear when the cranial nerve IV palsy really started. Also, it is useful to review family photographs from the patient's childhood and infancy. Head tilt in a childhood photo is good evidence of congenital cranial nerve IV palsy—a common condition that may present with the onset of diplopia later in life.

Oculomotor dysfunction may occur in the setting of any systemic disorder. One of the most common diseases to affect ocular motility is thyroid orbitopathy. The past history is particularly important because thyroid function studies are commonly normal when the patients present with orbital findings. A history of fatigue, weight change, skin alterations, heat intolerance, and other constitutional symptoms is thus important to elicit. A large contingent of patients who present with cranial mononeuropathies have a presumed ischemic etiology based on putative small vessel occlusive disease. These can usually present in persons older than 60 years of age, and many have other arteriosclerotic risk factors such as systemic hypertension or diabetes mellitus. A history of these disorders should be elicited by the interviewer. A full inquiry about multisystem signs and symptoms is essential to identify collagen vascular diseases such as periarteritis nodosa or systemic lupus erythematosus, which may be complicated by ischemic cranial mononeuropathy. Orbital inflammatory pseudotumor or Tolosa-Hunt syndrome may be caused by sarcoidosis, and the history should be probed for any of its many systemic manifestations including skin, muscle, joint, pulmonary, hepatic, or renal involvement. Myasthenia gravis frequently presents with ptosis and weakness of various extraocular muscles and may closely mimic cranial nerve lesions. This neuromuscular disorder (see Chapter 50) has the remarkable capacity to look like a pupil-sparing cranial nerve III palsy or, in a more limited case, internuclear ophthalmoplegia (INO) from a lesion along the medial longitudinal fasciculus (MLF) in the brain stem.[1] Myasthenia most frequently runs a remitting, exacerbating course with involvement of axial and appendicular muscle groups. It is important, therefore, to ask about past or concurrent weakness in the limbs, trouble swallowing, weak phonation, and trouble breathing. Finally, a full family history and review of all medications is necessary. Many commonly prescribed general medical and neurological drugs (carbamazepine, phenytoin) can be associated with diplopia, particularly at toxic levels.

Anatomy of Cranial Nerves III, IV, and VI (Table 9–1)

EXTRAOCULAR MUSCLES

Figure 9–2 represents a schematic diagram of the orbits viewed from above, with the eyes looking to the right. The superior rectus and superior oblique muscles are shown with their insertions on the top of the globes—the superior rectus muscle elevates the globe and the superior oblique muscle depresses the globe. The inferior rectus and oblique muscles insert at homologous sites on the bottom of the globe, and the horizontal vectors of pull are the same, except the inferior rectus muscle depresses the globe while the inferior oblique muscle elevates it. The adducted position of the left

TABLE 9–1. **Clinico-anatomical Correlation of Disorders of Cranial Nerves III, IV, and VI**

Anatomical Structure	Ocular Findings	Etiologies
Cranial Nerve III		
Nuclear	Bilateral ptosis and upgaze limitation; ipsilateral impairment of elevation, depression, adduction, and pupillary paralysis	Ischemia, central demyelinating disorders, neoplasm, inflammatory or infections (abscess) lesions
Fascicular	Ipsilateral limitation of ocular elevation, depression, adduction; ptosis; pupillary paralysis	Ischemia, central demyelinating disorders, neoplasm, and inflammatory or infectious (abscess) lesions
Subarachnoid	Ipsilateral limitation of ocular elevation, depression, adduction; ptosis; pupillary paralysis	Meningeal neoplastic, infectious, and inflammatory infiltrative disorders; aneurysm of the posterior communicating artery–internal carotid junction
Cavernous	Ipsilateral limitation of ocular elevation, depression, and adduction; ptosis; pupillary paralysis	Pituitary adenoma with lateral expansion, inflammatory (Tolosa-Hunt syndrome) and infection (aspergillosis), meningioma, giant carotid siphon aneurysm, pseudoaneurysm, carotid and dural branch to cavernous sinus fistulae, cavernous sinus thrombosis
Orbital	Ipsilateral limitation of ocular elevation, depression, and adduction; ptosis; pupillary paralysis	Orbital inflammatory pseudotumor, primary tumors (hemangioma, meningioma), metastatic tumors
Cranial Nerve IV		
Nuclear	Failure of the ipsilateral eye to depress fully in adduction; excyclodeviation; ipsilateral hyperdeviation (greatest in adduction and depression)	Ischemia, central demyelinating disorders, neoplasm, inflammatory or infectious (abscess) lesions
Fascicular	Failure of the ipsilateral eye to depress fully in adduction; excyclodeviation (torsion); ipsilateral hyperdeviation (greatest in adduction and depression)	Ischemia, central demyelinating disorders, neoplasm, inflammatory or infectious (abscess) lesions
Subarachnoid	Failure of both eyes to depress fully in adduction; excyclodeviation (torsion); ipsilateral hyperdeviation (greatest in adduction and depression)	Head trauma (downward/backward displacement of the brain stem with impaction of both cranial nerves IV) Ischemia, central demyelinating disorders, neoplasm, and inflammatory or infectious (abscess) lesions

TABLE 9–1. **Clinico-anatomical Correlation of Disorders of Cranial Nerves III, IV, and VI** *Continued*

Anatomical Structure	Ocular Findings	Etiologies
Cavernous	Failure of the ipsilateral eye to depress fully in adduction; excyclodeviation (torsion); ipsilateral hyperdeviation (greatest in adduction and depression)	Pituitary adenoma with lateral expansion, inflammatory (Tolosa-Hunt syndrome) and infectious (aspergillosis) lesions, meningioma, giant carotid siphon aneurysm, pseudoaneurysm, carotid and dural branch to cavernous sinus fistulae, cavernous sinus thrombosis
Orbital	Failure of the ipsilateral eye to depress fully in adduction; excyclodeviation (torsion); ipsilateral hyperdeviation (greatest in adduction and depression)	Orbital inflammatory pseudotumor, primary tumors (hemangioma, meningioma), metastatic tumors (lymphoma)
Cranial Nerve VI		
Nuclear	Conjugate gaze palsy ipsilateral to the lesion, plus failure of ipsilateral eye to abduct fully and esotropia	Ischemia, central demyelinating disorders, neoplasm, inflammatory or infectious (abscess) lesions
Fascicular	Failure of ipsilateral eye to abduct; esotropia greatest in gaze toward the lesion side	Ischemia, central demyelinating disorders, neoplasm, inflammatory or infectious (abscess) lesions
Subarachnoid	Failure of ipsilateral eye to abduct; esotropia greatest in gaze toward the affected side	Meningeal neoplastic, infectious, and inflammatory disorders; false-localizing cranial nerve VI palsy with elevated intracranial pressure
Cavernous	Failure of ipsilateral eye to abduct; esotropia greatest in gaze toward the lesion side	Pituitary adenoma with lateral expansion, inflammatory (Tolosa-Hunt syndrome) and infectious (aspergillosis) disorders, meningioma, giant carotid siphon aneurysm, pseudoaneurysm, carotid and dural branch to cavernous sinus fistulae, cavernous sinus thrombosis
Orbital	Failure of ipsilateral eye to abduct; esotropia greatest in gaze toward the affected side	Orbital inflammatory pseudotumor, primary tumors (hemangioma, meningioma), metastatic tumors (lymphoma)
Supranuclear Control		
Cortical	Long latency, hypometric contralateral saccades, increased frequency square wave jerks; low-gain (slow) ipsilateral smooth pursuit with catch-up (forward) saccades	Degenerative diseases, benign and malignant primary and metastatic neoplasms, focal infectious or inflammatory lesions, ischemic and hemorrhagic stroke
PPRF	Slow saccades, low-gain smooth pursuit with catch-up saccades, and conjugate gaze palsy all horizontal and ipsilateral	Benign and malignant primary and metastatic neoplasms, focal infectious or inflammatory lesions, ischemic and hemorrhagic stroke involving dorsal medial pons
Cerebellum	Gaze-evoked nystagmus with fast phases; ipsilateral, macro-square wave jerks, saccadic dysmetria, saccadic oscillations, macrosaccadic oscillations	Cerebellar degenerative diseases, benign and malignant primary and metastatic neoplasms, focal infectious or inflammatory lesions, ischemic and hemorrhagic stroke
Vestibular system	Vestibular (constant velocity slow-phase) nystagmus in plane of affected semicircular canal for peripheral lesions, pure upbeat for central lesions	Cerebellar degenerative diseases (flocculus and nodulus), benign and malignant primary and metastatic neoplasms, focal infectious or inflammatory lesions, ischemic and hemorrhagic stroke
MLF	Failure of ipsilateral eye to adduct during versions (conjugate gaze) to the side opposite the lesion; dissociated sustained or transient nystagmus of the abducting eye with fast phases away from lesion side	Multiple sclerosis, benign and malignant primary and metastatic neoplasms, focal infectious or inflammatory lesions, ischemic and hemorrhagic stroke
Gaze-holding system	Gaze-evoked nystagmus with fast phases ipsilateral	Cerebellar degenerative diseases (flocculus and nodulus), benign and malignant primary and metastatic neoplasms, focal infectious or inflammatory lesions, ischemic and hemorrhagic stroke

MLF, Medial longitudinal fasciculus; PPRF, paramedian pontine reticular formation.

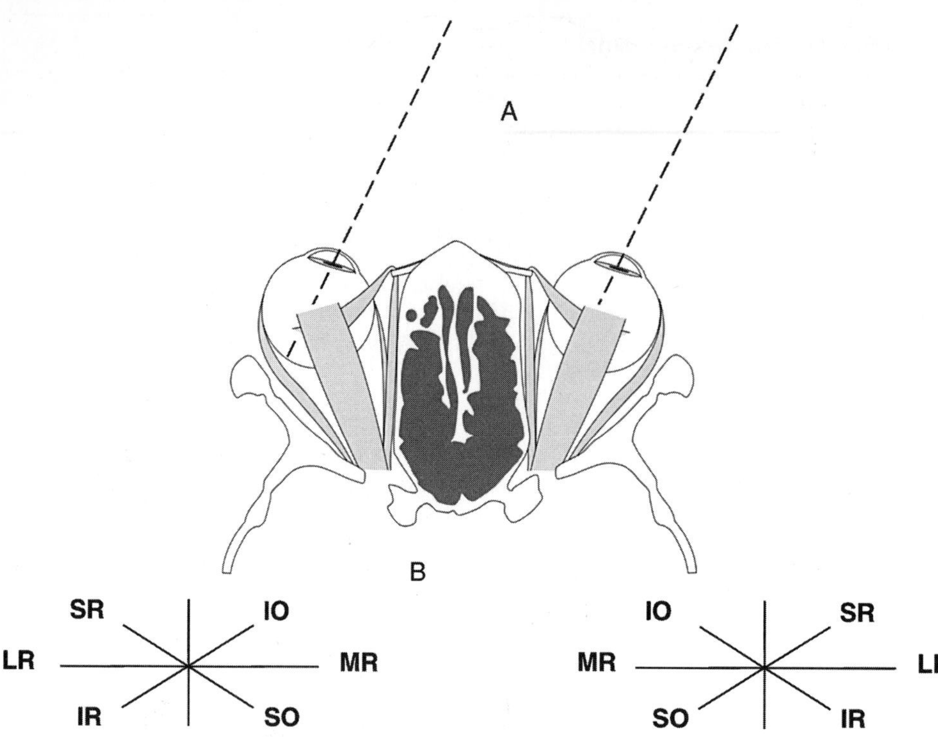

FIGURE 9–2. *A,* Axial section of the orbits viewed from above. The eyes are shown in conjugate right gaze, which places the right eye in the abducted position and the left eye in the adducted position. The superior oblique muscle is shown with its tendon passing through the trochlea or pulley on the anterior medial orbital rim. The rectus muscles are the primary elevators and depressors when the eye is in abduction, and the obliques perform this function with the eye in adduction. *B,* A diagram showing the position of maximum action of the extraocular muscles of the two eyes as viewed from in front of the patient. MR, medial rectus; LR, lateral rectus; SR, superior rectus; IR, inferior rectus; IO, inferior oblique; SO, superior oblique.

eye places the superior oblique in a position to depress the eye as a primary and direct action (see also Figure 9–2*B* and Table 9–2). The abducted position of the right eye puts the right superior rectus in position to elevate the right eye as a primary and direct action. The direction of pull of the left superior rectus muscle on the adducted left eye puts it in position to intort the eye as a primary and direct action (incyclodeviation or intorsion, rotation of the 12 o'clock meridian toward the nose or midline about the Z axis [see Fig. 9–1]). Similarly, the direction of pull of the right superior oblique muscle on the abducted right eye puts it in position to intort the right eye as its primary and direct action. More generally, the oblique muscles act as the pure depressor and elevator of the eye when it is in adduction, and the rectus muscles act as the pure depressor and elevator of the eye when it is in abduction. Conversely, the primary torsional action is carried out by the rectus muscles when the eye is in adduction and by the oblique muscles when the eye is in abduction. When the eyes are in primary position, the oblique and the rectus muscles both perform a mixture of vertical and torsional action. The action of the medial and lateral rectus muscles is simple relative to the vertical muscles. The medial rectus muscle adducts and the lateral rectus muscle abducts the eye.

The importance of these relationships lies in the fact that the binocular relative deviation is largest when the patient attempts to look into the direction of pull of the defective muscle. By determining the angles of deviation between the visual axes in all the cardinal positions of gaze, the weak muscle can be identified as the one that serves the cardinal position with the largest deviation.

TABLE 9–2. **Primary Actions of the Extraocular Muscles**

Muscle	Action	Optimum Position
Medial rectus	Adduction	
Lateral rectus	Abduction	
Superior rectus	Elevation	In abduction
Inferior rectus	Depression	In abduction
Superior oblique	Depression	In adduction
Inferior oblique	Elevation	In adduction

OCULOMOTOR NERVE (CRANIAL NERVE III)

Cranial nerve III innervates the medial rectus, superior rectus, inferior rectus, and inferior oblique muscles, along with the pupillary sphincter and the levator palpebrae that elevates the upper eyelid.

Cranial nerve III originates in a rostrocaudally elongated group of subnuclei clustered in the midbrain, just rostral to the level of the nucleus of cranial nerve IV. The architecture of this nuclear group has been the subject of intensive study over the years. The most widely accepted anatomical scheme is that of Warwick[2] and is represented in Figure 9–3. Warwick suspected that there is a subnucleus for each muscle and that these structures are in rostrocaudally elongated columns of cells. Axons from the more dorsally situated subnuclei pass through the middle and inferior columns of cells on their way to the point of exit from the ventral aspect of the midbrain near the cerebral peduncles. The nuclei for the inferior rectus, inferior oblique, and medial rectus muscles send axons only to the ipsilateral cranial nerve III. The caudal central subnucleus for the levator palpebrae is a midline structure and sends axons to both nerves. The Edinger-Westphal nucleus is also an unpaired midline nucleus situated rostral to the caudal central nucleus. Cells within this nucleus synapse in the ciliary ganglion in the inferior orbit. From this structure, postganglionic parasympathetic fibers innervate the pupillary sphincter muscle and the ciliary muscle that controls accommodation of the crystalline lens. Finally, the superior rectus subnucleus sends axons only to the contralateral third nerve trunk. These anatomical details lead to clinical rules by which one can determine whether a lesion is in the cranial nerve III nucleus or in the fascicular portion, which is more distal.

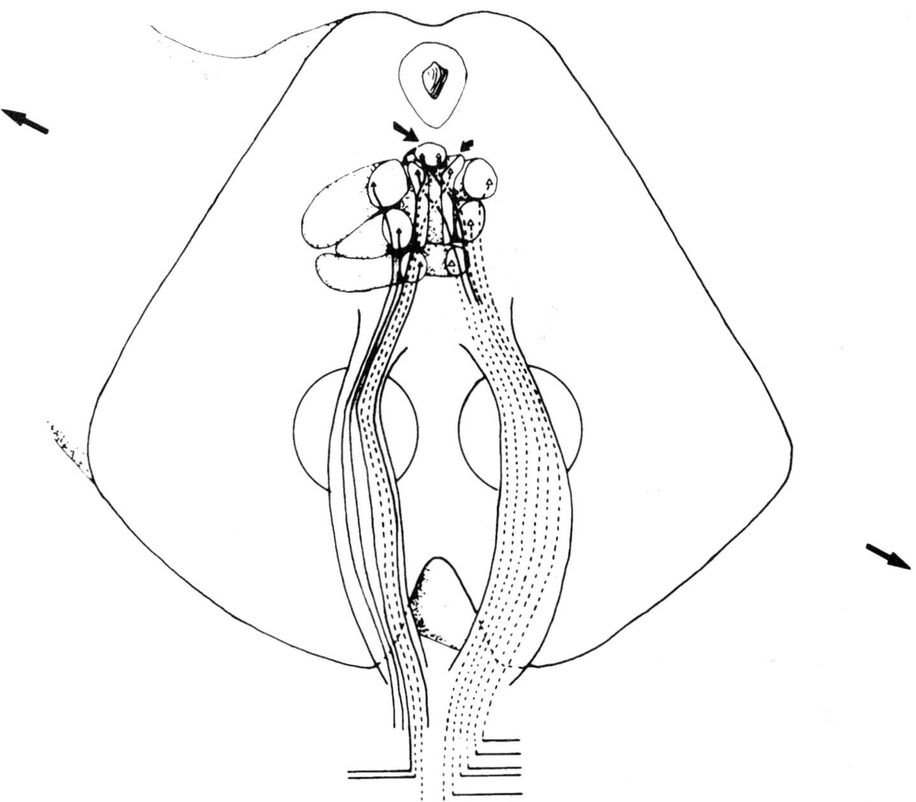

FIGURE 9–3. A cross section through the midbrain showing the cranial nerve III nuclear complex. The subnuclei extend in rostrocaudally oriented columns, as depicted in this three-dimensional representation modeled on Warwick's schemata. The letters superimposed on each nuclear group indicate the muscle innervated as follows: LP, levator palpebrae; SR, superior rectus; IR, inferior rectus; IO, inferior oblique; MR, medial rectus. A right nuclear cranial nerve III lesion is illustrated. Open triangles and dotted lines indicate lesioned neurons and their axons. Filled triangles and solid lines denote normal neurons and their axons. All of the outflow to the right cranial nerve III is lesioned. Crossed outflow from the right SR and LP subnuclei gives rise to paresis of contralateral eye elevation and ptosis. The left ptosis is partial because there is still ipsilateral (uncrossed) outflow from the left LP subnucleus to the left LP. The crossed pathway from left LP subnucleus to right LP is affected at the axonal level as the fibers course through the damaged right cranial nerve III complex (transition of solid lines to dotted); thus, right ptosis is complete. The contralateral elevator palsy and ptosis thus distinguish nuclear nerve palsy from fascicular palsy, in which the findings are limited to the ipsilateral eye. (From Goodwin JA: Eye signs in neurologic diagnosis. *In* Weiner WJ, Goetz CG: Neurology for the Non-neurologist, 3rd ed. Philadelphia, J.B. Lippincott, 1994, pp 298–348.)

Fascicular cranial nerve III involvement by intramedullary lesions can also be distinguished from extramedullary lesions by concomitant involvement of either the red nucleus (Claude's syndrome), cerebral peduncle (Weber's syndrome), or both (Benedikt's syndrome) (see Chapter 22).

Within the subarachnoid space, the nerve trunk is fed by branches of the posterior cerebral artery, superior cerebellar artery, and branches of the meningohypophysial trunk.[3] In the cavernous sinus, cranial nerve III runs superior to cranial nerve IV in the deep layer of the lateral wall of the cavernous sinus (Fig. 9–4). Cranial nerve III enters the orbit inferior to cranial nerve IV. Within the common tendon sheath of the extraocular muscles, the annulus of Zinn, cranial nerve III then divides into the superior and inferior rami (Fig. 9–5). The actual point of division varies among individuals and can occur within the cavernous sinus. The superior ramus of cranial nerve III innervates the superior rectus and levator palpebrae muscles, while the inferior ramus innervates the medial and inferior rectus muscles, inferior oblique muscle, and ciliary ganglion.

SYMPATHETIC INNERVATION OF THE PUPIL

In opposition to the pupillary constriction produced by cranial nerve III, the sympathetic system dilates the pupil. The dilator system functions by a reflex arc similar to the sphincter system. The afferent arm, however, is much less circumscribed than the light reflex. Afferent stimulation along pain and temperature pathways from the spinal cord generally causes pupillary dilatation that is abrupt in onset and lasts 20 to 60 seconds. More sustained dilatation often attends mental states involving fear, anxiety, or surprise. Because the sympathetic afferent pathways are anatomically ill defined, especially at rostral levels of the CNS, this discussion focuses on the efferent sympathetic pathways. Anatomical reports have shown sympathetic fiber degener-

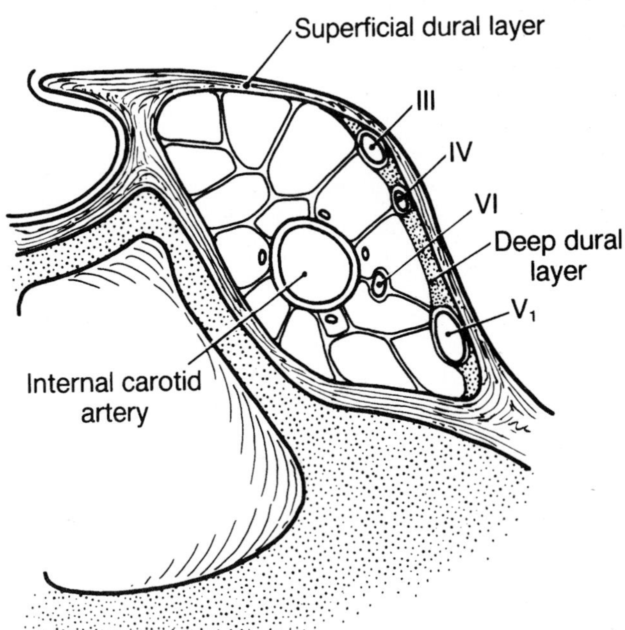

FIGURE 9–4. Diagram of the cavernous sinus. Oculomotor (III), trochlear (IV) (V_1), and ophthalmic division of the trigeminal and abducens cranial (VI) nerves are indicated. (From Miller NR: Walsh and Hoyt's Clinical Neuro-ophthalmology, 4th ed, Vol 2, Baltimore, Williams & Wilkins, 1985.)

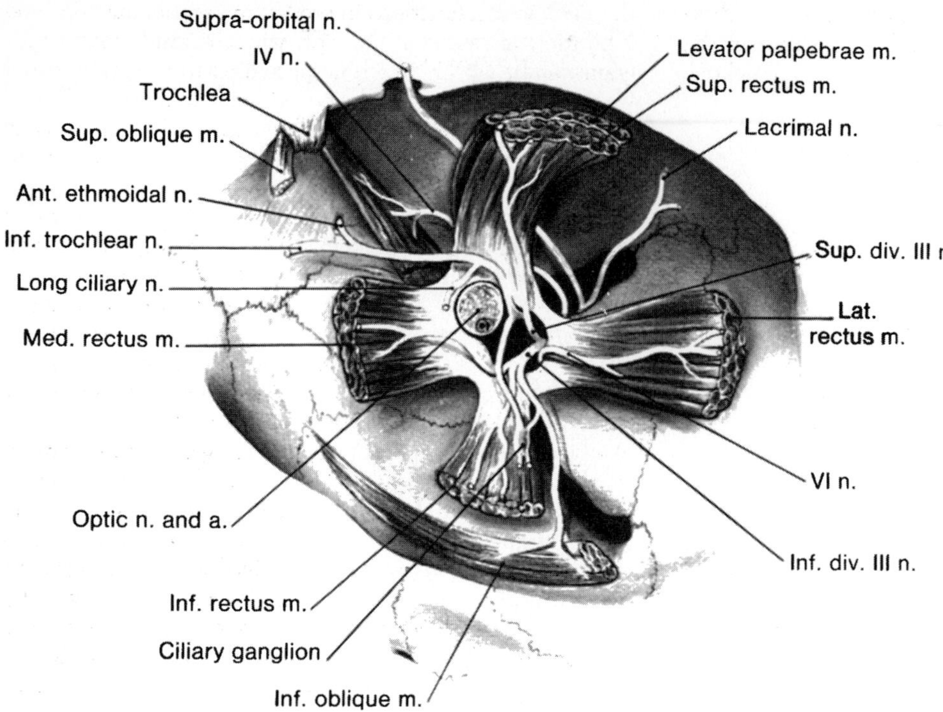

FIGURE 9–5. View of the posterior orbit showing the origins of the extraocular muscles and their relationships to the optic and ocular motor nerves. (Reproduced with permission from Miller NR: Walsh and Hoyt's Clinical Neuro-ophthalmology, 4th ed, Vol 2, Baltimore, Williams & Wilkins, 1985.)

ation in the upper brain stem after experimental lesions in the hypothalamus.[4] These studies document widely dispersed fiber tracts in the upper midbrain and diencephalon but none in the pons or medulla. The descending system is most likely a polysynaptic one, despite the clinical reference to "*the central neuron*" in the chain leading to the iris dilator. Clinical studies have documented that dorsolateral lesions throughout the brain stem often produce ocular sympathetic dysfunction ipsilaterally, whereas medial and ventral lesions do not. This is the basis for the widely accepted view that the polysynaptic central ocular sympathetic system is dorsolaterally disposed in the brain stem.

This pathway continues into the spinal cord to the C8 through T2 segmental levels, where the central fibers synapse with cells in the intermediolateral gray horns. This zone between C8 and T2 is commonly known as the *ciliospinal center of Budge and Waller*.[5] The central pathways through the cervical spinal cord are located very superficially (near the pia) in the lateral columns.[6] The preganglionic cells from the ciliospinal center send axons to the *paravertebral sympathetic ganglion chain* by way of the C8–T2 ventral roots. These preganglionic fibers travel upward in the sympathetic chain through the *stellate* (combined upper thoracic and lower cervical ganglion) and the *middle cervical* ganglions. They synapse with postganglionic cells in the *superior cervical* ganglion, which is usually found high in the neck, often under the angle of the mandible. This means that the common lesions that cause ocular sympathetic palsy (Horner's syndrome) interfere with preganglionic fibers as they course through the upper thorax and neck. Virtually all lesions producing postganglionic sympathetic dysfunction are intracranial and intraorbital, because the superior cervical ganglion is so near the base of the skull. The postganglionic axons at first travel in the adventitia of the carotid artery and those supplying vascular and sweat gland structures in the lower face travel with external carotid branches. The ocular sympathetics and those serving vasomotor and sudomotor function for the forehead travel with the internal carotid into the middle cranial fossa. A contingent of ocular sympathetic fibers takes a side path through the otic ganglion in the middle ear. This apparently explains the occasional occurrence of Horner's syndrome with middle ear infections. The main ocular sympathetic pathway, however, follows the carotid artery through its *siphon* region and then joins the *first division (ophthalmic) of the trigeminal nerve*, which carries it into the orbit. A sympathetic contingent passes through the parasympathetic ciliary ganglion, constituting the so-called sympathetic root of the ganglion, but no sympathetic synapses occur there. In the orbit, the ocular sympathetics innervate the iris dilator muscles together with small smooth muscles in the lids (Mueller's muscle), which contribute to upper lid elevation and lower lid depression.

TROCHLEAR NERVE (CRANIAL NERVE IV)

Cranial nerve IV is unique in that it exits from the brain stem dorsally and crosses to the other side before encircling the brain stem on the way to the cavernous sinus. This anatomy renders it particularly susceptible to trauma in which forces are brought to bear on the dorsal midbrain. This situation usually occurs in the setting of very severe head trauma in which the brain stem is forced downward and angulated backward by a sudden shift of supratentorial structures. The course of cranial nerve IV in the subarachnoid space is relatively protected from compressing lesions by the adjacent free edge of the tentorium. Within the cavernous sinus, cranial nerve IV can be found in the deep layer of the lateral wall inferior to cranial nerve III (see Fig. 9–4). Cranial nerve IV enters the orbit through the superior orbital fissure superior to cranial nerve III but outside the annulus of Zinn (see Fig. 9–5). It lies in the superior orbit, crosses over the superior rectus muscle, and innervates the superior oblique muscle.[7]

ABDUCENS NERVE (CRANIAL NERVE VI)

The abducens nucleus is medial and dorsal at the pontomedullary junction, separated from the floor of the fourth ventricle by the genu of the facial nerve. Within the abducens nucleus lateral rectus motor neurons intermix with internuclear neurons that send their axons across to the opposite MLF and then to the contralateral cranial nerve III. Axons of cranial nerve VI course almost directly ventral and exit from the pons near the midline. The axons emerge in the horizontal sulcus between the pons and medulla, lateral to the bundles of the corticospinal tract. Cranial nerve VI ascends underneath the pons in the prepontine cistern and enters Dorello's canal beneath Grüber's (petroclinoid) ligament. Within the cavernous sinus, the nerve is situated between the carotid artery medially and the ophthalmic branch of cranial nerve V. The large cells of the abducens nucleus innervate the lateral rectus muscle, while a small cell population innervates the contralateral medial rectus subnucleus of the oculomotor complex (cranial nerve III) via the MLF.

Supranuclear Control of Eye Movements

As with other motor anatomical systems, conjugate gaze has lower motor nuclei and an upper motor neuron control system.

The upper motor neuron supranuclear control resides bilaterally in the cerebral cortex and cerebellum, and the control networks that produce conjugate gaze functions are the saccade, pursuit, and vestibulo-ocular systems, each with a specific anatomical arrangement in the cerebral hemispheres, brain stem, and cerebellum. All of the supranuclear systems are concerned with *conjugate* eye movements, and destructive lesions in these systems cause conjugate deviation in the direction of the unopposed antagonist muscles. Dysconjugate eye movements indicate a disorder at or below (peripheral to) the nuclei of cranial nerves III, IV, and VI or in the pathways joining these nuclei.

ANATOMY OF THE SACCADE SYSTEM

Three important cortical areas are involved with saccade generation and include the frontal eye fields (FEF), the supplementary eye fields (SEF), and the parietal eye fields (PEF). Other zones of the association cortex that play a secondary, but important role in saccade generation are the prefrontal cortex (PFC) and posterior parietal cortex. The interrelationships of these structures are complex and are summarized with a clinical emphasis (Fig. 9–6).[8] The FEF is located in the lateral part of the precentral sulcus at the posterior end of the middle frontal gyrus. It is primarily involved with intentional conjugate visual exploration to the contralateral visual space and is active in the disengagement from fixation that must precede each refixation saccade. The FEF receives input from the PFC, which functions in prediction, spatial memory, and inhibition of saccades; the SEF, wherein reside motor programs; and the PEF, which is specialized to integrate spatial vectors and facilitate reflexive visual exploration.[9, 10] FEF output is directed to the superior colliculus (SC) and saccade generators (burst neurons) in the brain stem reticular formation.[11, 12]

The SEF is in the anterior part of the supplementary motor area in the posteromedial part of the superior frontal gyrus.[13, 14] It receives input from the PFC and from the posterior hemisphere,[9] and it projects to the FEF,[10] the SC, and the brain stem reticular formation.[15] The SEF functions to coordinate visual with other sensory and motor inputs to maintain eye position in space, despite head and body movement during and between successive saccades.[16–19] The PEF is situated in the superior part of the angular gyrus and supramarginal gyrus within Brodmann areas 39 and 40.[20, 21] Lesions of this area result in increased latency of reflexive, visually guided saccades[22] to the contralateral visual space, and this area has also been shown to be involved with disengagement from fixation as well as the triggering of reflexive visually guided saccades. The PEF seems more important in the reflexive exploration of the visual environment, while the FEF is more active with intentional (internally generated or willed) exploration.

The descending saccadic pathways most likely mimic those described in lower-order primates. In these animals, the frontal lobes project to the SC, which is then projected to the saccade generators in the pons (paramedian pontine reticular formation [PPRF]) for horizontal saccades and the midbrain for vertical saccades (see later). There are two parallel systems for the FEF and SEF. A subcortical circuit has also been demonstrated from the frontal cortex to the caudate nucleus and projects to the substantia nigra (pars reticularis) that sends inhibitory output to the SC, suppressing unnecessary saccades.

In a clinical example, a patient with an acute unilateral right-sided cerebral infarction resulting in left-sided limb weakness may maintain his or her eyes and head turned to the right. This patient's gaze may be brought to near the midposition, but attempts at saccades with the left gaze field are not possible. The doll's head maneuver does, however, bring the eyes past the midline to the left. In contrast, a patient with an acute unilateral right-sided pontine infarct will have left-sided limb weakness also, but gaze preference will be to the left with impaired rightward horizontal saccades. The doll's head maneuver will not bring the eyes past the midline.

ANATOMY OF THE PURSUIT SYSTEM

In contrast to the saccadic control, the conjugate pursuit system of each hemisphere controls binocular eye movements to the *ipsilateral* visual space.[23] Occipital visual areas (Brodmann areas 18 and 19) provide input on spatial vectors to the middle temporal (MT) and medial superior temporal (MST) cortexes. These areas are of primary importance in generating smooth conjugate pursuit eye movements.[24, 25] Efferents from MT and MST travel to the FEF, posterior parietal cortex, and brain stem reticular formation. Brain stem connections undergo a double decussation, resulting in each hemisphere's controlling ipsilateral smooth pursuit eye

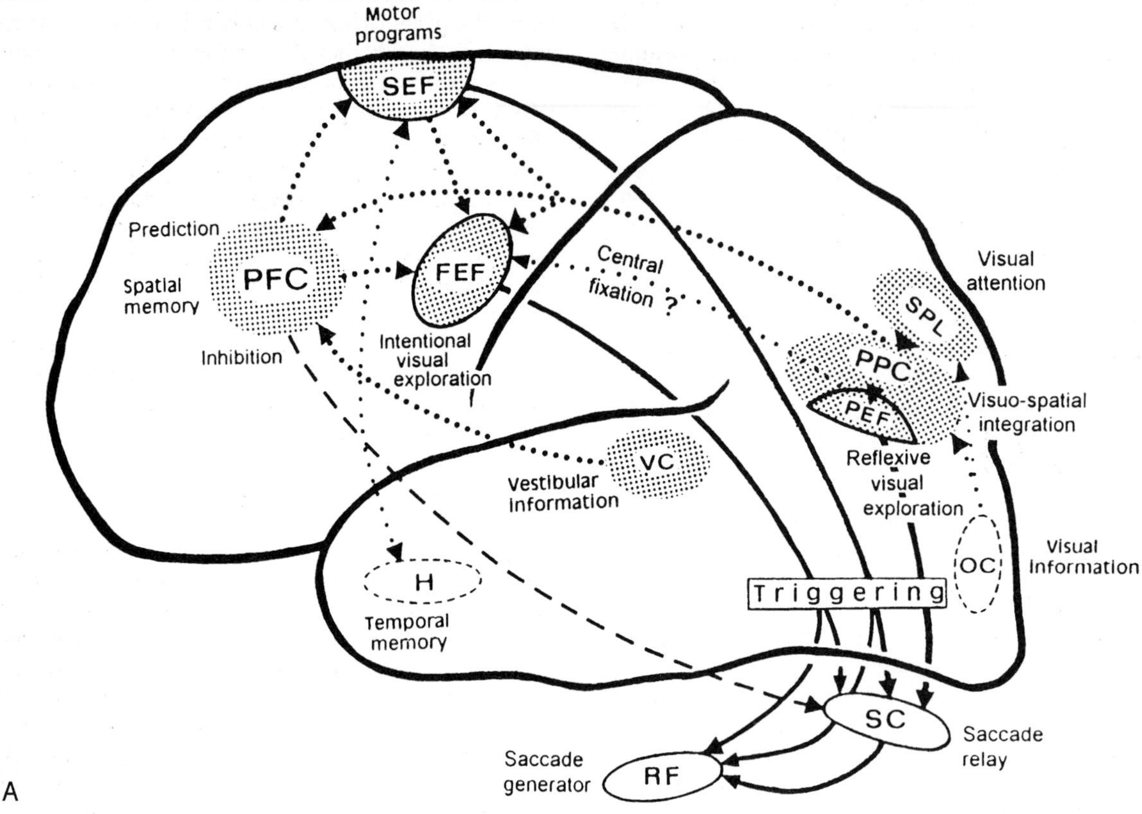

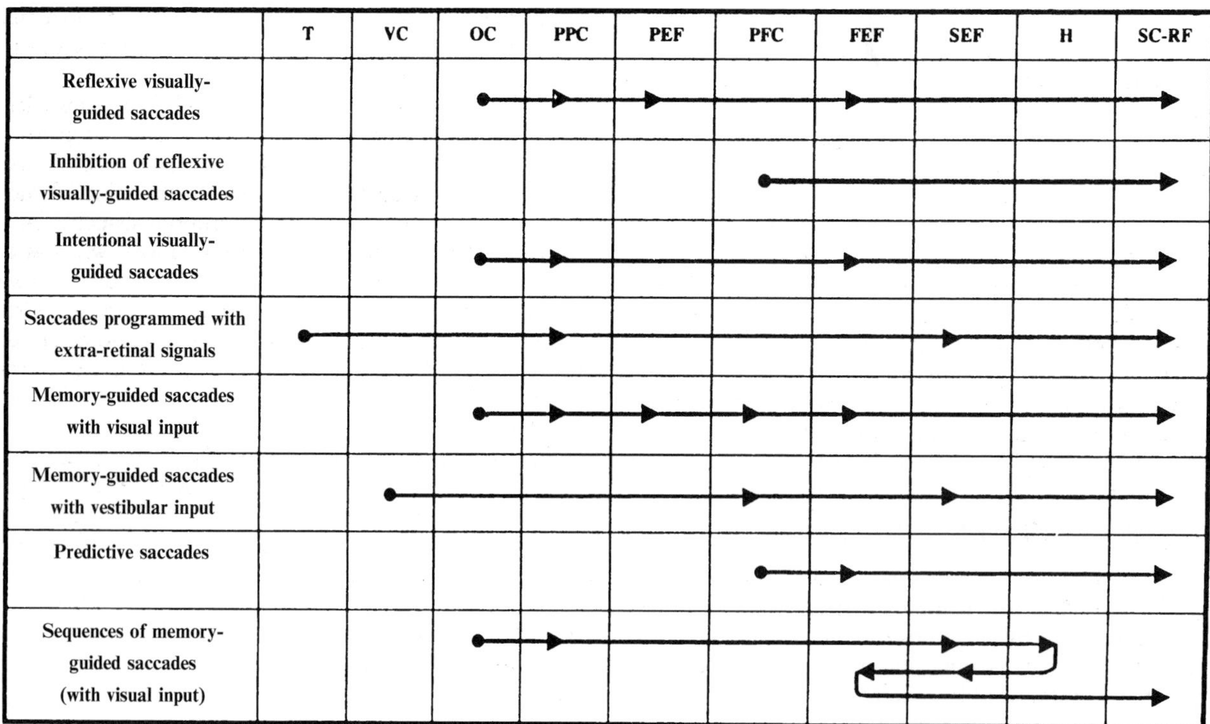

FIGURE 9–6. Hypothetical cortical pathways involved in saccade control. The cortical relays of saccade pathways are represented by arrowheads. FEF, frontal eye field; H, hippocampal formation; OC, occipital cortex; PEF, parietal eye field; PFC, prefrontal cortex (i.e., Brodmann area 46); PPC, posterior parietal cortex; SC and RF, superior colliculus and reticular formation; SEF, supplementary eye field; SPL, superior parietal lobule; T, thalamus; VC, vestibular cortex. (From Pierrot-Deseilligny C, Rivaud S, Gaymard B, et al: Cortical control of saccades. Ann Neurol 1995;557–567:37.)

movements.[26, 27] Selective lesions of MST bring about bilateral reduction of pursuit gain over the entire movement field, although this is most pronounced for ipsilateral pursuit.[28] Optokinetic nystagmus (OKN) gain is reduced by MST lesions.[29] Optokinetic nystagmus occurs when a series of vertical bars or a similar pattern is passed in front of the eyes. There is a slow following phase and a rapid jerk in the opposite direction.[30] Selective MT lesions produce impaired initiation of pursuit with motion in either direction in the contralateral hemifield of vision.[31]

Large cortical lesions, involving either frontal or parietal lobes, generally are associated with ipsilateral conjugate eye deviation that lasts a few days.[32] In these cases, forceful eye closure may be associated with conjugate eye deviation contralateral to the lesion.[33] Bilateral posterior cerebral hemisphere lesions lead to Balint's syndrome,[34] in which pursuit eye movements and OKN movements are defective in all directions and visually guided saccades have increased latency and diminished accuracy with relatively preserved intentional saccades. Involvement of angular gyrus and superior parietal cortex is thought to be responsible for the visual inattention that accompanies this syndrome. Optic ataxia refers to the inability of the patient to make accurate eye or limb movements under visual guidance. These patients also have a distinctive visual perceptual abnormality in which they cannot synthesize large visual figures that require multiple fixations to encompass. This is caused in part by the inability to make accurate saccades to the elements of the extended visual figure. This perceptual problem has been called amorphosynthesis or simultanagnosia by various authors.

Subcortical nuclei and pathways are undoubtedly important in generating smooth pursuit, although the result of focal lesions of these structures is uncertain. The thalamic pulvinar receives direct input from the retina and SC, and it projects to several cortical areas involved in the generation of eye movement. There is evidence that the pulvinar may function in visual suppression during saccades to eliminate perception of image motion as the eyes are traveling to a new fixation point. The pulvinar may also play a role in shifts in spatial attention and efference copy by which brain stem ocular motor structures provide feedback to cortical eye movement control systems about the moment-to-moment state of the eye movement. The internal medullary lamina of the thalamus receives input from brain stem nuclei, including the SC, vestibular nuclei, and nucleus prepositus hypoglossi, and provides reciprocal connections to the FEF, SEF, and PEF in the cerebral hemisphere. The clinical result of lesions involving the internal medullary lamina is uncertain. Such lesions may result in inaccuracy of memory-guided saccades, if another eye movement occurs between the saccade stimulus and the resulting saccade. Also, difficulties with disengaging fixation may occur, leading to increased saccade latency for visually guided saccades under certain stimulus circumstances.[35]

Thus, there is a fundamental distinction to be made between cerebral hemisphere and brain stem conjugate gaze control. At the cerebral level, the direction of the saccade control (contraversive) is opposite to the direction of the pursuit control (ipsiversive), while at the brain stem level both control ipsilateral movement. Clinical evidence demonstrates that pathways that control saccadic movements decussate caudal to the diencephalon but rostral to the pons, while the pursuit pathways either do not cross, or cross and recross. Patient studies suggest that hemisphere bidirectionality is preserved as far caudal as the thalamus and that the pursuit and saccade pathways both operate via the ipsilateral FEF outflow through the thalamus. Alternatively, the pursuit system may have pathways in the corona radiata separate from the saccade system outflow but funnel through the same region in the thalamus as the frontal system. The fact that some frontal lesions are associated with an ipsidirectional pursuit defect in conjunction with a contraversive saccade disorder supports the concept that the pursuit system outflow occurs via a common frontal–thalamic–brain stem pathway. However, the repeated observation of frontal lesions with isolated contralateral saccade disruption and normal pursuit weigh against a common pathway.

THE VESTIBULO-OCULAR SYSTEM

The vestibulo-ocular system maintains image stability on the fovea in the presence of head movement. The afferent arm of this reflex is initiated by acceleration receptors in the inner ear. The equivalent of mathematical integration is performed on the acceleration signal by the dynamic properties of the semicircular canal and cupula (see Chapter 12). The result of this integration is a signal proportional to head rotational velocity in space that is supplied to the vestibular nuclei by way of cranial nerve VIII. The information is then relayed to brain stem gaze centers, and slow eye movements with velocity equal to and direction opposite head rotation are generated. The arrangement of vestibular connections in the brain stem has been thoroughly reviewed.[36]

Because vertically acting rectus and oblique muscles exert mixed vertical and torsional rotations, the nystagmus resulting from vertical canal stimulation has mixed vectors and depends on the position of the eye in the orbit (abducted or adducted). The activation of the anterior semicircular canals produces upward and torsional slow phases, whereas activation of posterior canals induces downward and torsional movements. Each vestibular nucleus interacts with two motoneuron pools, one for each eye. Excitatory projections from vestibular nuclei cross the midline, but inhibitory connections do not. The pathways for upward and downward VORs differ.

Vestibular nuclei project to ocular motor neurons and to other nuclear groups that are important in various aspects of integrating the numerous inputs to eye movement. These include the nucleus prepositus hypoglossi and the nucleus of Roller, where integration of burst and step (holding) discharge patterns are assembled into a final oculomotor command. Outputs of the nucleus prepositus hypoglossi to burst cells initiate saccades and produce the fast phase of nystagmus.

INTERNUCLEAR OCULOMOTOR CONTROL: THE FINAL COMMON PATHWAY

Zones within the tegmental reticular formation in the brain stem serve to combine the various eye movement commands and to present an integrated set of final motor commands to the ocular motor nuclei. The PPRF refers to the zone surrounding cranial nerve VI nucleus on either side of midline in the pontine tegmentum. This area contains burst and pause cells that are important for horizontal saccade generation. The *rostral interstitial nucleus of the medial longitudinal fasciculus (riMLF)*, the *interstitial nucleus of Cajal (iC)*, the *nucleus of Darkschewitsch (nD)*, the *nucleus of the posterior commissure (nPC)*, and adjacent portions of the *mesencephalic reticular formation (MRF)* probably supply burst and pause commands for vertical saccades, and pass the final innervation pattern to the nuclei of cranial nerves III and IV. The integration of these systems has been reviewed extensively by Leigh and Zee.[37]

Commands for saccades and pursuit descend in the brain stem via supranuclear eye movement pathways outlined earlier. In addition, the vestibular nuclei in the medulla and the flocculi and noduli of the cerebellum provide vestibular inputs to both the horizontal eye movement system in the PPRF and to the vertical eye movement zones of the mesencephalic reticular formation, primarily the riMLF and iC. The final command signal for saccades and pursuit movements that descend on the ocular motor nuclei is a composite of inputs from a direct pathway and a pathway through the neuronal circuitry that performs a mathematical integration on the direct signal. This neural integration is probably a distributed function with components from the cerebellum (especially flocculus and paraflocculus), the nucleus prepositus hypoglossi, and the medial vestibular nucleus for horizontal gaze and the iC for vertical gaze. The PPRF was once thought to perform this function, but it has been established that lesions of this structure spare gaze holding, the primary function of the integrator for saccades.

Normal saccade velocity depends on normal function of *burst* neurons (velocity command) that provide the acceleration part of the movement. Without a proper burst, the resulting saccade is slow. The neural integrator produces a tonic *step* of innervation (position command) that is at just the right firing rate to sustain eye deviation at the endpoint of the saccade. When the neural integrator is leaky and produces a step innervation at too low a frequency of action potentials, the eyes reach the target accurately and with normal velocity on account of the burst. They then, however, drift back toward primary gaze, because the step or holding function is inadequate. After a certain amount of drift, a *position error* signal is generated calling for another saccade. This results in a repetitive cycle of saccades and back drifts that is called *gaze-evoked nystagmus* (see later).

When a novel visual stimulus calls for a saccadic refixation or when a command to look at a new fixation target is given, there is an obligate latent interval of between 100 and 200 milliseconds. This latent interval includes time for the visual stimulus in the peripheral field to travel along afferent pathways to the cerebral cortex, where the spatial coordinates of the object to be foveated are turned into motor commands or vectors having both direction and amplitude specifications. This computation of vectors and passage of the efferent commands to the brain stem requires additional time. It has also been postulated that the system works via intermittent data samples rather than continuous intake of afferent data. Thus, if a novel visual stimulus occurs just after a sample is taken, it will have to wait for the next sampling interval, perhaps 40 to 50 milliseconds later, before entry into the system. This could explain much of the latency variability observed for generation of individual saccades. The generation of saccades is a much more complex entity, however, and there is considerable controversy as to whether saccade vectors are calculated through intermittent or continuous sampling. It is also unclear whether saccade motor commands can be modified as the eyes are in motion during a saccade. Under ordinary circumstances, saccades behave as a *ballistic* movement—as with a thrown ball, the saccade trajectory is not modifiable after the movement begins. Under special test circumstances, however, it seems that some individuals are capable of modifying saccade trajectory in midflight. These special features of a few saccades in normals have not yet been adequately explained by existing models of brain stem circuitry.

Pursuit movements also depend on the combination of a velocity and position signal. When the direct innervation is not present, the eyes eventually attain the velocity of the stimulus, but the beginning acceleration to that velocity is slow. For pursuit commands, the direct pathway carries a step command, which is the velocity signal, and the neural integrator produces a ramp command that is the position signal. The slow eye movements of the vestibulo-ocular system also depend on a combined step-ramp signal for normal trajectory.

The organization of the vertical eye movement system is complex and incompletely understood at present. It appears that the riMLF contains primarily burst neurons that generate vertical saccades. Cells of iC, nD, nPC, and MRF carry the fully assembled burst-step firing pattern needed to perform saccades, pursuit, and vestibulo-ocular movements, as well as to hold the eyes in eccentric positions of gaze. Nuclei at the pontine and medullary levels are important in control of vertical eye movements. Bilateral lesions of the MLF, which carries complex ascending influences from vestibular nuclei and PPRF gaze centers, abolish vertical pursuit and VOR movements but spare saccades. Thus, the riMLF apparently has functional connections with the cerebral hemispheres independent of supranuclear pathways that operate via the PPRF. Although vertical saccades are spared with bilateral lesions of the ascending pathways, the eye position signal is abolished, and gaze paretic nystagmus occurs with upgaze and downgaze effort.

Efferents from the PPRF on one side connect with large motor cells in the ipsilateral cranial nerve VI nucleus for abduction of the ipsilateral eye and with small cells in the same nucleus, which, in turn, connect via the MLF with the opposite medial rectus subnucleus of cranial nerve III for adduction of the contralateral eye. Thus, a contraversive (opposite direction) saccade command from the right hemisphere descends to the left PPRF, then to the left abducens nucleus for abduction of the left eye and adduction of the right eye via the right MLF. This circuitry thereby produces conjugate gaze contralateral to the hemisphere issuing the command and ipsilateral to the activated PPRF. This network is illustrated schematically with participating brain stem and hemispheric pathways for conjugate leftward gaze (Fig. 9–7). Thus, the brain stem connections for ocular motility are arranged to provide *conjugate* gaze. Lesions affecting the internuclear gaze pathways distal to the PPRF, through the MLF, produce disconjugate gaze palsy such that only the abducting eye ipsilateral to the activated abducens nucleus has full deviation, often with dissociated or monocular nystagmus. The contralateral adducting eye moves either incompletely or

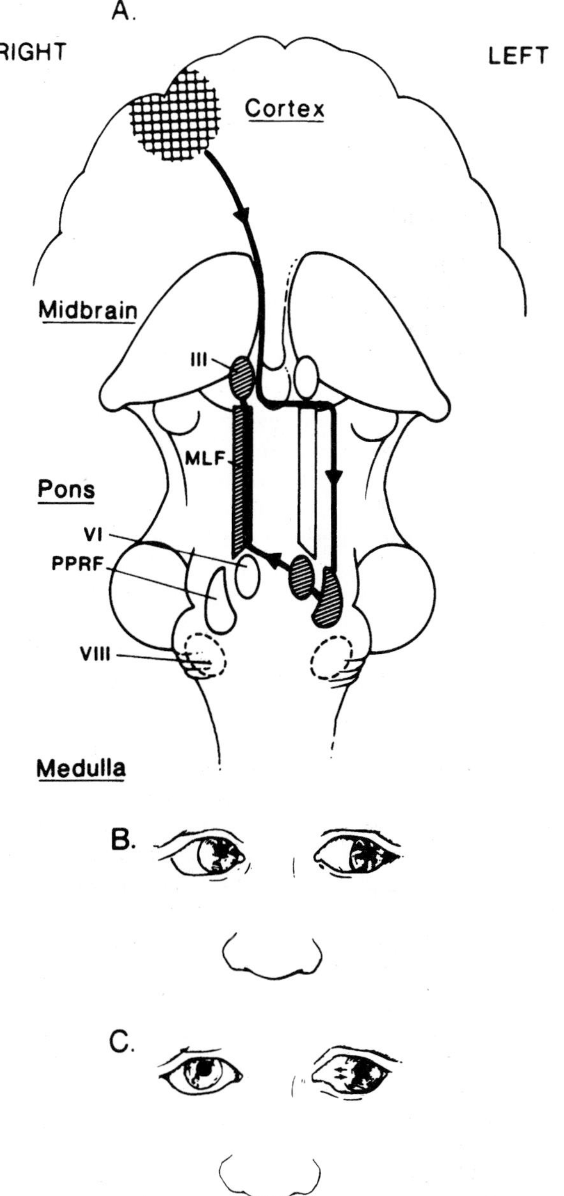

FIGURE 9–7. *A*, Semischematic diagram of the brain stem pathways and centers that serve horizontal conjugate gaze. Multisynaptic pathways from the right frontal cortex decussate in the midbrain and form synapses in the left pontine paramedian reticular formation (PPRF), which relays innervation to two cell populations within the nucleus of cranial nerve VI. The large cells in the nucleus send axons to the lateral rectus muscle to abduct the left eye. The small cell population gives rise to the pathway that decussates and ascends in the contralateral medial longitudinal fasciculus (MLF) and makes synaptic contact with cells of the medial rectus subnucleus of the cranial nerve III complex. This pathway gives rise to coordinated adduction of the right eye to complete the act of conjugate leftward gaze, as illustrated in *B*. A lesion in the MLF causes internuclear ophthalmoplegia, which is characterized by a failure of adduction of the ipsilateral eye during attempted conjugate gaze, as illustrated in *C*. The abducting eye often manifests dissociated or monocular nystagmus.(From Goodwin JA: Eye signs in neurologic diagnosis. *In* Weiner WJ, Goetz CG: Neurology for the Non-neurologist, 3rd ed. Philadelphia, J.B. Lippincott, 1994, pp 298–348.)

slowly. The eyes, however, remain *straight* with parallel visual axes when viewing objects at a distance in the primary position of gaze, which distinguishes INO from a cranial nerve III lesion or a primary defect of the medial rectus muscle, either of which causes divergence of the visual axes (exotropia) in primary gaze.

Examination of Cranial Nerves III, IV, and VI

DIRECTED NEUROLOGICAL EXAMINATION

The examination should begin during the clinical history, when there is the opportunity to observe the patient's head, eyes, and eyelids over an extended interval. During this period, it is important to notice general abnormalities of the globe or eyelid position or asymmetries of eye movement. Eyelid twitch and flutter may accompany eye movements in ocular myasthenia, and myasthenic involvement of the levator palpebrae may bring about progressive ptosis with sustained upgaze or even during sustained fixation near primary gaze. Thyroid orbitopathy characteristically includes a distinctive set of changes in the general appearance of the eyes, including lid puffiness, prominent extraocular muscle insertions, conjunctival edema (chemosis), conjunctival injection, forward displacement of one or both eyes (*proptosis*), *stare*, and *lid lag*. Each globe floats in orbital fat suspended within the orbit by ligamentous structures and by the extraocular muscles. The globe is free to rotate in all directions, but any rotation can be adequately described by measuring vectors, or components of the rotation in the vertical (X axis of rotation), horizontal (Z axis of rotation), and torsional (Y axis of rotation) planes. These three axes of rotation, which intersect at the hypothetical center of rotation of the globe, were defined by Fick and are depicted in Figure 9–1 in relation to Listing's plane. This plane is perpendicular to the visual axis (Y) with the eye in primary gaze, and any eye movement can be fully described by the rotation of the globe around a single axis in this plane.

In the subsequent sections, the examination of cranial nerves III (including the pupil—both parasympathetic and sympathetic components), IV, and VI, as well as the supranuclear control systems, are first presented. This is followed by a detailed approach to the examination of a patient with diplopia. In examining the function of these cranial nerves, patients should always be asked to look forward, maintaining the primary position, and then be instructed to look in all secondary and tertiary positions.

Examination of Cranial Nerve III and the Pupil

The patient with complete cranial nerve III dysfunction presents with abnormalities of all its extraocular muscles, including weakness of the levator palpebrae superioris, medial rectus, superior rectus, inferior rectus, and inferior oblique. As a result, the ipsilateral eye does not move fully into adduction, elevation, or depression, and there is upper eyelid ptosis. Looking forward, the patient's eye tends to deviate down and outward (exo) from residual tone in the superior oblique muscle (cranial nerve IV) and the lateral rectus muscle (cranial nerve VI). In attempted downgaze, there is intorsion of the globe produced by the normal action of the superior oblique muscle. This can best be observed by using conjunctival blood vessels as landmarks to visualize rotation of the globe about its anteroposterior (Y) axis. With intorsion, vessels nasal to the limbus move down while vessels on the temporal side of the cornea stay stationary or move up.

Partial or incomplete cranial nerve III dysfunction can result in weakness of one or a number of extraocular muscles. Thus, certain eye movements may be abnormal, corresponding to selected extraocular muscle dysfunction. This may occur when either the superior ramus (supplying the superior rectus and levator) or inferior ramus (supplying the medial and inferior recti, the inferior oblique, and ciliary ganglion) is affected in isolation. Dysfunction of the extraocular muscles that turn the eye as well as the levator palpebrae are together referred to as *external* ophthalmoplegia.

When assessing lid position, one must be careful of illusions created by asymmetrical skin folds, by altered position of the eye in the orbit (extraocular muscle palsies and strabismus), and even by anisocoria. The examiner uses all of these landmarks for assessing where the lid margin is expected to fall and whether its position is the same in the two eyes. Eyelid position and the relation of lid margins to landmarks such as skin folds is often asymmetrical for a variety of non-neurological reasons.

Cranial nerve III also innervates muscles within the eye, including the sphincter of the pupil and the ciliary muscle. With pupillary sphincter paralysis, the involved pupil is large and it reacts less to light stimulation of the retina than the contralateral pupil. The ciliary muscle exerts pull on radially oriented ligaments called zonules that attach around the perimeter of the crystalline lens. Ciliary muscle contraction induces slack in the zonules and allows the crystalline lens to assume a more spherical configuration, which shifts the focal plane of the eye to a nearer point in space—a process called accommodation. The neurological control of accommodation is obligatorily linked to that of convergence of the visual axes and that of pupillary meiosis (constriction). The three functions together serve the process of looking at near objects—convergence foveates the image in either eye, accommodation shifts the focal plane to that object, and meiosis increases the depth of focus for near vision. These three actions together are referred to as the *near triad.* Dysfunction of pupillary constriction and lenticular accommodation are referred to as *internal* ophthalmoplegia.

On examining the pupil, the clinician seeks evidence of either parasympathetic or sympathetic dysfunction by measuring pupil size in both bright and dim ambient illumination.

The ocular sympathetics innervate the radially oriented dilator smooth muscles in the iris, which are most active in dim light. The parasympathetic system via cranial nerve III innervates the pupillary sphincter muscle and is most active in bright light. In dim light, the pupillary sphincter muscle is reciprocally inhibited, and in bright light, the same is true of the dilator muscles. As a consequence, with parasympathetic lesions the anisocoria is greater in bright light (larger pupil abnormal) and with sympathetic lesions the anisocoria is greater in dim light (small pupil abnormal). For practical purposes, under clinical testing conditions, the pupillary reaction to light remains normal with ocular sympathetic dysfunction. The parasympathetic system determines the dynamic characteristics of the pupillary light reaction.

Abnormal lid position is best determined by measuring the distance between a central corneal light reflex and the upper and lower lid margins, respectively, and comparing these for symmetry between eyes. The light reflex, produced by shining a focused source of light on the eyes, does not move appreciably with variation in eye position. The distance from the light reflex to the upper and lower lid margins is called the margin-reflex distance (MRD). The distance to the upper lid is labeled MRD_1 and to the lower lid MRD_2. Both the MRD_1 and the MRD_2 are reduced on the side of an ocular sympathetic lesion, because Mueller's smooth muscle retracts both the upper and lower lids. Mueller's muscles work in opposition to the orbicularis oculi muscle (innervated by cranial nerve VII) (see Chapter 11) that encircles both lids and is the primary muscle of eye closure. In the setting of sympathetic dysfunction, the upper lid falls, whereas the lower lid rises with the nonfunctioning smooth muscle. An erroneous diagnosis of cranial nerve VII palsy can be made on the basis of apparent widening of one palpebral fissure (orbicularis oculi weakness) when the abnormality is a narrowed fissure on the other side secondary to an ocular sympathetic lesion. This error is more likely to occur if the normal range of facial asymmetry produces an apparent flattening of the nasolabial fold on the side of the wider palpebral fissure and if the pupillary meiosis is minimal or lacking in the ocular sympathetic palsy. Both the MRD_1 and the MRD_2 are larger on the side of a facial nerve palsy because the orbicularis is weak in both upper and lower lids. Pharmacological pupil testing for ocular sympathetic dysfunction can be a useful arbiter in this setting.

Cocaine (5- or 10-percent solution) can be used to diagnose the presence of Horner's syndrome, the clinical manifestation of ocular sympathetic dysfunction, including preganglionic and postganglionic types.[38] Within 40 minutes of the instillation of 1 drop of cocaine into each eye, relative anisocoria will increase if Horner's syndrome is present. This phenomenon occurs because cocaine blocks reuptake of the ambient norepinephrine released at the neuromuscular junctions of the iris sphincter. On the side of the lesion, there is less norepinephrine normally being released and, as a result, blocking reuptake results in less accumulated norepinephrine as compared with the normal side. Antihypertensive medications may prevent pupillary dilatation produced by cocaine and need to be considered when interpreting the results of this test. Hydroxyamphetamine (1-percent solution) can be used to distinguish between preganglionic (primary and secondary ocular sympathetic neurons) from postganglionic lesions. If this drug is used, testing should be delayed at least 24 to 48 hours after the use of cocaine solutions. When 1 drop of hydroxyamphetamine is instilled in the eyes, the suspected pupil will not dilate to the extent of the normal eye if a postganglionic (tertiary neuron) lesion is present. This results because hydroxyamphetamine causes the release of norepinephrine stored in the cytoplasmic vesicles in the postganglionic nerve terminals. If the tertiary, postganglionic neuron is intact, this drug will dilate the abnormal pupil as well as the normal side. If this occurs and a preganglionic lesion is thus suspected, further drug testing cannot delineate whether the neuronal abnormality is at the primary or secondary neuron (Fig. 9–8).

Examination of Cranial Nerve IV

Cranial nerve IV innervates the superior oblique muscle, which originates at the orbital apex and forms a tendon ante-

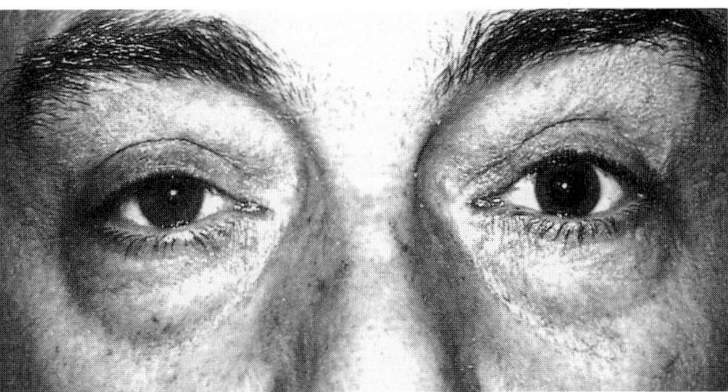

FIGURE 9–8. Positive para-hydroxyamphetamine test for postganglionic Horner's syndrome. The right (involved) pupil remains small while the left pupil has dilated after 1 percent para-hydroxyamphetamine is instilled into both eyes 30 minutes previously. There is mild right ptosis from disruption of ocular sympathetic innervation of Mueller's muscle.

riorly that passes through a pulley-like structure called the trochlea. The superior oblique muscle, therefore, originates functionally from the trochlea at the superior medial orbital rim and inserts on the top of the globe behind its equator. When the eye is in adduction, this muscle exerts a more or less direct downward pull and depresses the eye. When the eye is in abduction, the superior oblique muscle pulls the 12 o'clock meridian of the iris toward the nose, rotating the globe around an anteroposterior (Y) axis. This movement is called incyclodeviation (intorsion). When the eye is in the intermediate horizontal positions between adduction and abduction, the superior oblique exerts combined torsional and depressive actions. Weakness of the superior oblique muscle causes failure of depression of the globe that is maximal in adduction. This results in vertical diplopia, with the widest separation of images occurring in gaze away from the involved side (adduction) and down. Isolated superior oblique muscle weakness or cranial nerve IV palsy is more likely than cranial nerve III lesions to result in torsional imbalance. This is because only one of the vertically acting muscles is affected, leaving the other torting vertical muscles unopposed. Superior oblique weakness results in excyclodeviation (extorsion) of the involved eye. To compensate for this problem, the patient automatically tilts the head to the side opposite the palsy. Simultaneous incyclodeviation of the normal eye establishes parallelism and allows for torsional fusion of the images.

If the examiner tilts the head of a person with a right cranial nerve IV palsy to the right, even more intorsion than normal is required. The superior rectus is recruited in an effort to maximize the intorsional power. This results in further inappropriate elevation of the right eye, because the primary effect of superior rectus contraction is eye elevation. This is the basis for Bielschowsky's test for a cranial nerve IV palsy. The patient is directed to gaze straight ahead, and then the head is tilted to the right and to the left, making sure there is no vertical or horizontal eye rotation away from primary gaze. If the degree of elevation of the eye on the side of the cranial nerve IV palsy increases as the head is tilted toward the side of the palsied muscle, the test is positive. In addition to compensatory head tilt, the patient is likely to hold the head down to keep his or her eyes in upgaze and out of the field of maximum image separation. The compensatory triad is completed by turning the head away from the affected side to keep the involved eye relatively abducted.

Examination of Cranial Nerve VI

Cranial nerve VI innervates the lateral rectus muscle, which abducts the eye. With lesions of cranial nerve VI, the eyes are slightly crossed or convergent (esodeviated) in primary gaze. This is caused by the unopposed tone of the medial rectus, acting without the ipsilateral lateral rectus muscle. In gaze opposite the side of the palsy, the eyes are close to parallel, but as gaze is directed toward the side of the palsy, there is clear-cut failure of ipsilateral eye abduction and an increase in esotropia. In primary gaze, the involved eye may be used for target fixation, but this will result in deviation of the other eye. Which eye the patient chooses for fixation is a matter of habit that may not be disrupted by muscle paresis, even if the weakness is profound. The choice may also be influenced by visual acuity, and there is a strong tendency to fixate with the eye that has better vision. With acquired palsy of cranial nerve VI, the degree of esodeviation in primary gaze is usually different depending on the fixating eye. To observe primary versus secondary deviation, cover and then uncover each eye, observing the angle of the deviation just after the eye is uncovered. Primary deviation refers to the angle that results from fixation with the normal eye, and secondary deviation results from fixation with the paretic eye. Secondary deviation is larger because, in primary gaze, the eye with the weak muscle is struggling to abduct the eye even to the midposition against the tone of the medial rectus. For example, in the case of a right cranial nerve VI palsy, a great deal of rightward innervation is required by the right eye. According to Hering's law of equal innervation, the yoked medial rectus of the opposite (left) eye also receives this large amount of stimulation, and it adducts to a great degree, creating a large-angle esotropia. In contrast, when the nonparetic left eye is fixing, a standard quantity of rightward innervation is required, and a lesser deviation results from the failure of the right eye to abduct completely. On the examination, this difference between primary and secondary deviation is a good clinical clue to the presence of acquired nerve or muscle origin paretic deviation, as opposed to deviation caused by squint or childhood strabismus. In the latter disorder, the deviation remains the same regardless of the eye that is fixating.

Examination of the Supranuclear Control of Eye Movements

Saccade System. There is a growing body of literature showing that separate cortical zones are primarily involved in the generation of saccadic movements under different circumstances that can be tested individually.[8] *Intentional* saccades are internally generated by voluntary thought and the decision to act. *Reflexive* saccades are triggered by an external stimulus that the subject is instructed to look at when it occurs. This may be a visual or an auditory stimulus presented in the dark. *Goal-directed intentional saccades* have been further classified as *predictive* when they are made toward a repetitive stimulus that is presented at a predictable location, and as interval, or *memory-guided*, when they are made to a remembered location where the target is no longer present (could be auditory or visual). Also, *antisaccades* occur when the eye movement is in the direction opposite a saccade stimulus. Many of these conditions require elaborate stimulus presentation and eye movement recording systems, yet a bedside evaluation of some of these functions is possible.

The examiner can observe *spontaneous saccades*, which are internally triggered but not goal directed. These saccades can be observed throughout the history and examination by watching the patient produce these eye movements during speech or other motor activity.

In direct testing, the patient should first be given verbal directions to follow such as "look left" and "look down." This can be followed by *visually guided saccades*, which can be tested by asking the patient first to look at the examiner's nose and then to look at an object about 30 degrees to either side of midline. Appropriately placed objects are provided if the examiner holds his or her arms semiextended (elbows flexed about 90 degrees), with hands just a bit in front of his or her own facial plane. Patients should keep their heads stationary facing straight ahead during this type of testing to avoid introducing vestibulo-ocular components. Patients should be asked to refixate their gaze from the examiner's nose to one hand, then back to the nose. Reflexive, visually guided saccades are elicited in a slightly different manner. The examiner's hands should be extended in the same arrangement as noted earlier, but patients are instructed to refixate between the two hands, specifically when the examiner moves the fingers of one or the other hand. In this condition, the subject is waiting for a trigger signal that will result in a reflex eye movement.

The antisaccade task may also be completed at the bedside. In this maneuver, the patient is asked to look in the opposite direction to a novel visual target. The subject must suppress the natural tendency to make a saccade to a newly appearing visual stimulus. In all of these bedside studies, the examiner should observe the latency and accuracy of the eye movements, as well as whether multiple small saccades are necessary to complete the movement. Normal refixations (saccades) are smooth and accurate to verbally directed locations and between visual stimuli. Abnormalities include an increased latency to the generation of the eye movement and eye movements that fall short of the target (hypometric saccades) or overshoot the target (hypermetric saccades). Additionally, patients with hypometric saccades may produce multiple small saccades in order to generate the desired movement or may be unable to fully move their eyes to the extremes.

Optokinetic nystagmus may be useful in the evaluation of volitional (saccadic) gaze palsies when pursuit movements are normal. To obtain optokinetic responses, a striped drum, squares on a flag, or a tailor's tape with stripes can be used. The patient is asked to look at the apparatus or strip and count the lines as they pass. In normal individuals, as the stimulus passes in front of the patient, a slow phase of eye movements in the direction of the movement is followed by a rapid jerk in the opposite direction that repeats as long as the stimulus is present. In patients with a left frontal lesion, there may be an inability to volitionally make eye movements to the right, but slow-moving targets produce smooth pursuit to the right. Because rightward pursuit and saccades to the left are normal, when the OKN stimulus is rotated to the right, a normal OKN response occurs. Yet, with leftward targets, the fast phase to the right cannot be generated and a tonic deviation to the left occurs.

Pursuit System. Maintenance of a target on fovea with motion of the target in space is the task of the pursuit system. The goal of the pursuit system is to generate a smooth eye velocity that matches the velocity of a visual target. Testing this system requires that a stimulus be present, because patients cannot produce voluntary smooth eye movements in a stationary visual environment or in darkness. If the viewer's head remains stationary, the tracking of a moving target is achieved by matching the angular velocity of the eyes turning in the orbits to the angular velocity of the target moving across visual space. Smooth pursuit can be selectively tested by having the patient hold the head still while following the examiner's finger with the eyes. The finger movement must be slow and within the patient's visual field. The target must not be moved too rapidly, because the pursuit system in normal persons falls behind when the target velocities reach 40 to 50 degrees per second, producing saccadic pursuit. A target excursion that carries the patient's eyes from extreme right to extreme left gaze should take about 5 seconds. Normal pursuit is smooth with no inserted saccades. Pursuit is pathological if the normally smooth following eye movement is interrupted by a series of jerky movements in the direction of pursuit. The most frequently observed abnormality of pursuit is subnormal gain, in which the eyes fall progressively behind the target. The examiner cannot perceive the velocity of a patient's pursuit movements by inspection. Fortunately, the visual system does not tolerate the retinal position error that develops as the eyes fall behind the target, and an easily observed saccade is generated as soon as the eye is sufficiently far behind. These inserted catch-up saccades occur rhythmically, because it requires about the same amount of time to generate the needed position error throughout the course of the pursuit movement. This pursuit abnormality, best referred to as *low-gain pursuit with catch-up saccades*, has engendered various descriptive names including *saccadic pursuit*, and even *cogwheel pursuit* in patients with Parkinson's disease. This movement should not, however, be linked to the pathophysiology of parkinsonian cogwheeling. The saccadic pursuit of parkinsonism is simply the manifestation of low gain in the pursuit system. This does not differ from low-gain pursuit in other pathological conditions.

As with saccadic eye movements, optokinetic responses can be useful tools in evaluating pursuit defects, in that lesions affecting the deep parietal lobe cause an interruption in the descending occipitomesencephalic system for slow (pursuit) eye movements. Such lesions produce a homonymous hemianopia (contralateral) and an abnormal OKN when the targets are moved in the direction of the affected side; lesions only in the occipital or temporal lobes, although associated with a hemianopia, do not produce an abnormal OKN response (see later).

Vestibulo-ocular System. Zee has developed a practical approach to bedside or office examination of the vestibular system using simple tools.[36, 39] The sequence of tests is as follows:

1. Look for static imbalance (bias) between the two vestibular systems on either side of midline.
2. Look for dynamic imbalance using head movement and head position change.
3. Estimate the VOR gain.
4. Elicit vestibular nystagmus by rotating the patient.
5. Perform caloric testing.

Static imbalance is manifest as spontaneous nystagmus, the slow-phase velocity of which reflects the degree of imbalance between the tonic states of the vestibular system on the two sides. Spontaneous nystagmus may be present in primary gaze, although it is typical for vestibular nystagmus to emerge when fixation is suspended. This can be done by covering the eye or having the patient wear Frenzel's goggles with strong spherical convex lenses that eliminate the patient's ability to focus and fixate. Small amplitude nystagmus can be observed ophthalmoscopically by asking the patient to fixate with one eye while viewing the other eye's optic disc or other ocular fundus landmark. Slow-phase drift and rapid returns indicate the presence of nystagmus. On covering the fixating eye, the nystagmus typically increases in amplitude or may appear first. The direction of fundus motion is opposite the direction of visual axis movement. Spontaneous nystagmus should be assessed in the primary position, and in upward, downward, right, and left gaze, with estimation of the relative amplitude in the various gaze positions. It should also be noted whether the nystagmus is rhythmical and steady, as occurs in vestibular dysfunction, or variable in amplitude and frequency, changing with the degree of effort exerted while the patient attempts to maintain the eccentric gaze angle, as occurs with gaze-evoked nystagmus.

Dynamic imbalance is manifest as directional preponderance during vestibular stimulation, in which the VOR gain is greater in one direction than the other. This finding indicates differential sensitivity of vestibular mechanisms to oppositely directed labyrinthine inputs. To test for this, patients should be asked to shake their heads, first horizontally and then vertically, for 10 to 15 seconds in each direction. After each movement interval, the eyes are observed for nystagmus. After horizontal oscillation, the induced nystagmus slow phases are toward the lesion side, and after vertical oscillation, the induced *horizontal* nystagmus slow phases are opposite to the lesion side. These phenomena depend on the presence of a velocity-storage mechanism, which may be disrupted with severe lesions. In such cases, the nystagmus cannot be induced by head shaking. Also, other factors may lead to inverse directionality of the nystagmus. A single rapid head movement to either side can be used instead of prolonged shaking. The eyes should remain fixed on a stationary visual target, but if there is dynamic imbalance, the eye will be drawn off fixation and the observer will then see a small saccadic eye movement as the patient refixates. Paroxysmal positional vertigo is tested by hanging the head with position shifts. The patient is seated on an examination surface, so that when brought to supine position, the head hangs over the end of the surface. While in a sitting position, the head is turned to the right or left or is positioned straight ahead for each of a series of repetitions. The patient is then brought rapidly into a supine position with the head down 45 degrees from vertical and in one of the three turned positions. Transient nystagmus induced by these maneuvers is usually a sign of benign positional vertigo (see Chapter 12).

True *assessment of VOR gain* requires electronic eye movement testing, in which slow-phase velocity can be measured and compared with stimulus rotation velocity. A bedside test can be used in which the abnormal feature is reduced visual acuity during head motion. To perform this test, the patient is asked to read a near acuity card with the head stationary and during horizontal and then vertical sinusoidal head oscillations at a velocity of around 2 cycles per second. If the VOR gain is normal, the eye remains fixed on the optotypes and acuity does not change with head motion. With decreased gain, however, the eyes slip off fixation during head movement and acuity is worse, sometimes by several lines. Observing refixational saccades during head rotation is another sign of abnormal gain. When VOR gain is reduced, the movement of the saccades will be the opposite direction from the head movement, and if the gain is increased, the saccades occur in the same direction as the head movement.

Rotating the patient at a constant velocity in a swivel chair induces normal *vestibular nystagmus*. This maneuver is not practical for patient observation because the patient is moving relative to the examiner. After 45 seconds of constant rotation at a rate of about one turn every 3 seconds, the chair should be stopped and the patient's eyes observed for postrotational nystagmus. This is optimally performed through Frenzel's goggles, so the patient cannot suppress the nystagmus with visual fixation. Horizontal nystagmus can be induced by rotating the patient with the head upright, and vertical nystagmus is elicited by rotating with head tilted to one shoulder or the other. Rotation with the neck extended and head back normally induces torsional nystagmus.

Cold water caloric stimulation is another way to stimulate the various semicircular canals (see Chapter 1). In this setting also, the test is best performed with Frenzel's goggles.

Approach to Diplopia (Table 9–3)

The primary function of the extraocular muscle and the oculomotor system in general is to position the globes so that

TABLE 9–3. **Extraocular Muscles: Orbit and Gaze Positions Resulting in Maximal Deviation and Image Separation on Diplopia Testing**

Muscle	Deviation	Orbit Position with Maximum Deviation	Gaze Position with Maximum Deviation
Right medial rectus	Exotropia	Adduction	Left
Right lateral rectus	Esotropia	Abduction	Right
Right superior rectus	Left hypertropia	Elevation in abduction	Right, up
Right inferior rectus	Right hypertropia	Depression in abduction	Right, down
Right superior oblique	Right hypertropia	Depression in adduction	Left, down
Right inferior oblique	Left hypertropia	Elevation in adduction	Left, up
Left medial rectus	Exotropia	Adduction	Right
Left lateral rectus	Esotropia	Abduction	Left
Left superior rectus	Right hypertropia	Elevation in abduction	Left, up
Left inferior rectus	Left hypertropia	Depression in abduction	Left, down
Left superior oblique	Left hypertropia	Depression in adduction	Right, down
Left inferior oblique	Right hypertropia	Elevation in adduction	Right, up

the object of regard is seen as a single image in visual space regardless of the fact that it is viewed simultaneously by two eyes. Every point in visual space has a corresponding retinal location in either eye. The two points in the eyes that serve a single locus in visual space are called homologous retinal locations. Normally, the eyes are positioned such that all images fall on homologous retinal locations, and the subject sees a single fused image. Binocular diplopia results when the visual axes of the two eyes are divergent. In this state, the image of the object of regard is formed at nonhomologous points on the retinas of the two eyes. As a result, the object appears to be in two places simultaneously. The resulting diplopia can be analyzed by measuring the direction of separation and the distance between the two images, which is a direct measure of the angle at which the two visual axes diverge.

The apparent location of an object in visual space depends on where the image of that object is formed on the retina. The retinal fovea serves the center of the visual field or the perceptual sense of being straight ahead. Under normal conditions, the visual axes of the eyes are slightly convergent, and the image of the object of regard is formed on both foveas (F_1, F_2) (Fig. 9–9A). Using a red Maddox rod, the image of a point light source is turned into a red line that can be oriented either vertically or horizontally (Fig. 9–9*B–D* insets). The Maddox rod is an optical device that consists of a series of cylinders lying parallel to one another. A point of light viewed through a Maddox rod appears as a line perpendicular to the orientation of the cylinders (Fig. 9–10). The image line can be made to appear horizontal or vertical by reorienting the Maddox rod in front of the subject's eye. Retinal images formed on the nasal side of the fovea appear to be off center in the temporal visual field, whereas retinal images temporal to the fovea appear in the nasal field. Images formed on retinal sites above the fovea appear to be below the center, whereas images formed on the lower retina appear to be above the center.

Although each muscle has several vectors of force, a specific extraocular muscle turns the eye most efficiently in a single direction. Deviation of the eyes relative to one another is greatest when the patient attempts to look in the direction in which the weak muscle exerts its primary or maximal action. Using these basic principles, subjective and objective methods have been developed to analyze extraocular muscle imbalance. Subjective methods use the patient's own reported observations on the relative positions of images to measure image separation. Analysis of diplopia is aided if it can be established which image is being seen by which eye. The simplest method to perform this analysis is to place a colored glass over one eye and ask the patient where the colored image is relative to the white one as he or she views a point light source.

The Maddox rod has two advantages in diplopia testing as compared with the simple colored-glass test. First, mixed horizontal and vertical diplopia can be examined more accurately, because the patient can easily judge the vertical deviation by viewing a horizontal line and the horizontal deviation by viewing a vertical line. Second, because two dissimilar images (point of light and colored line) are viewed with the two eyes, the images are more completely dissociated and deviation is maximized. In contrast, when the patient views two differently colored but otherwise similar images, as with the colored-glass test, the fusion mechanism may not be entirely suspended and a deviation smaller than maximum might result.

Because some patients are unable or unwilling to give accurate subjective descriptions of their diplopia during the red glass or Maddox rod testing, the alternate cover and cover-uncover tests were devised as more objective tests for eye deviation (Table 9–4). Moving a cover (occluder) quickly back and forth from one eye to the other constitutes the *alternate cover* test. Because one eye remains covered at all times, there is no opportunity for the fusion reflex to operate. With this test, *latent* deviation (heterophoria) and *manifest* deviation (heterotropia, or strabismus) can be detected, but these conditions cannot be distinguished. In the cover tests, the examiner observes the resulting eye movements while moving the cover back and forth between eyes. The patient is instructed to maintain fixation on the object of regard. When the cover is shifted from one eye to the other, if the newly uncovered eye was deviated under cover, it will make a saccadic movement to attain fixation on the object of regard. The direction of these refixation movements indicates the direction in which the eye was deviated under cover. A movement toward the nose indicates that the eye was exodeviated (temporally), whereas an outward movement toward the temple indicates esodeviation (nasal deviation). If an eye moves upward when it is uncovered, it was deviated downward under cover and vice versa.

The *cover-uncover* test is useful in distinguishing heterotropia from heterophoria. Table 9–4 lists the movement of the two eyes as one eye is first covered and then uncovered in the three main conditions—orthophoria (no tendency to deviate, straight eyes with and without fusion), heterophoria (latent deviation, present only when fusion is suspended by cover), and heterotropia (manifest deviation, still present when fusion reflex is operational with both eyes uncovered). In using this table, one column (condition) should be considered at a time. Note that both the heterophorias and heterotropias are eye deviations relative to one another. In the heterophorias, the eye under the cover drifts into the deviated position relative to the other eye. When it is uncovered, the deviated eye makes a monocular movement to refixate. Patients with heterotropias commonly have a tendency for one eye to always be deviated when neither eye is covered. As an example, if a patient has exotropia with the right eye deviated, this occurs because the patient has chosen, usually unconsciously, to fixate with the left eye. This does not necessarily mean that the right eye has the weak muscle or muscles. If the left eye is covered, the patient can move the deviated right eye back to take up fixation, but because the refixation was a conjugate binocular movement, the patient's left eye is then deviated under the cover. On uncovering the left eye, the patient could subsequently maintain fixation with the right eye or make a conjugate binocular saccade to refixate with the left eye. A patient who is strongly left eye dominant or has better acuity with the left eye is likely to resume fixation with the left eye. A person who has no major visual dominance pattern or equal visual acuity with either eye may maintain fixation with the right eye. The cover tests are useful in patients with enough range of eye movement to make the various refixational movements. Even with nearly complete palsy of one or more muscles, it is still useful to measure angles of phoria in primary gaze as a measure of devi-

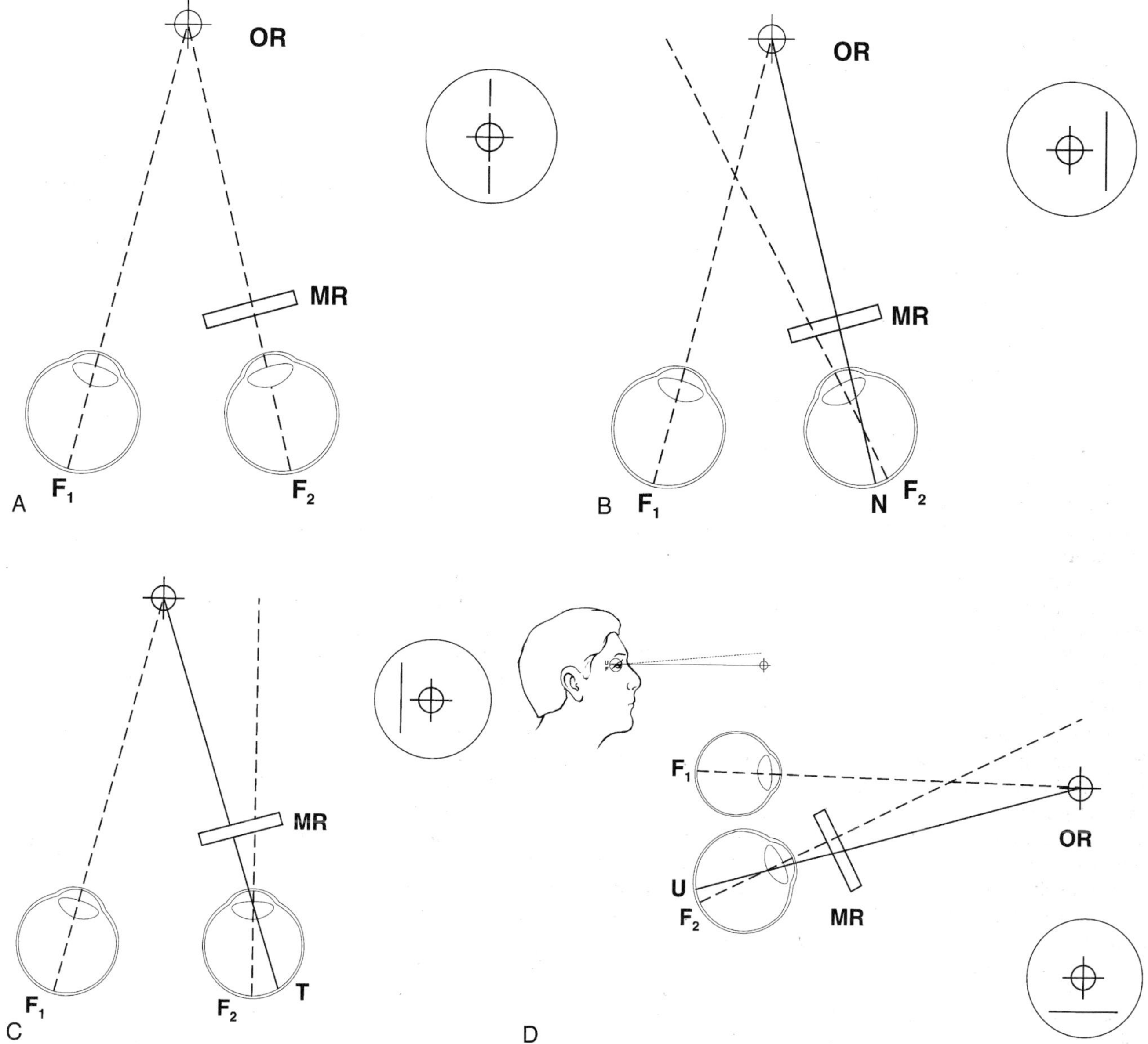

FIGURE 9–9. The two eyes in various deviated positions under conditions of Maddox rod testing. The inset at the right of each figure illustrates the relative positions of images of the object of regard (OR) seen with the left eye and of the line created by viewing through the Maddox rod (MR) with the right eye. In all cases, the Maddox rod is placed over the right eye (by convention) and that makes the right eye always the deviating eye because the patient is instructed to "look at the light" and he or she can see the light only with the left eye. *A*, Orthophoria—both eyes are foveating the images and the line (right eye image) runs through the light (left eye image). *B*, Esophoria—the eyes are converged, and the right eye image falls on nasal retina so the image in that eye (line) appears to be on the temporal (right) side of the light (left eye image). This is called homonymous diplopia because both the Maddox rod and the image from viewing through the rod are on the right (same) side. *C*, Exophoria—the eyes are divergent, and the image of the deviating right eye falls on temporal retina so the line (right eye image) appears displaced nasal to the light (left eye). This is called crossed diplopia because the image formed by the Maddox rod is on the left, with the rod over the right eye. *D*, Right hyperphoria—the right eye image falls on upper retina (above the fovea), and the right eye image (line) appears displaced below the light (left eye image).

ation tendency. This measurement can be followed over time for recovery or worsening.

ASSOCIATED NEUROLOGICAL FINDINGS

Cerebral. Cranial nerve III, IV, or VI neuropathies may be caused by meningeal infectious, inflammatory, and infiltrative lesions that may also affect cerebral function with impairment of consciousness or altered cognitive and language function. Because of its long intracranial course and its proximity to bony structures of the calvarium, isolated cranial nerve VI paresis can occur with large intracranial masses (false localizing signs of elevated intracranial pressure), especially involving the middle cranial fossa. Lesions in the pontine and midbrain reticular activating system can lead to impaired levels of consciousness, together with defective conjugate gaze and nystagmus.

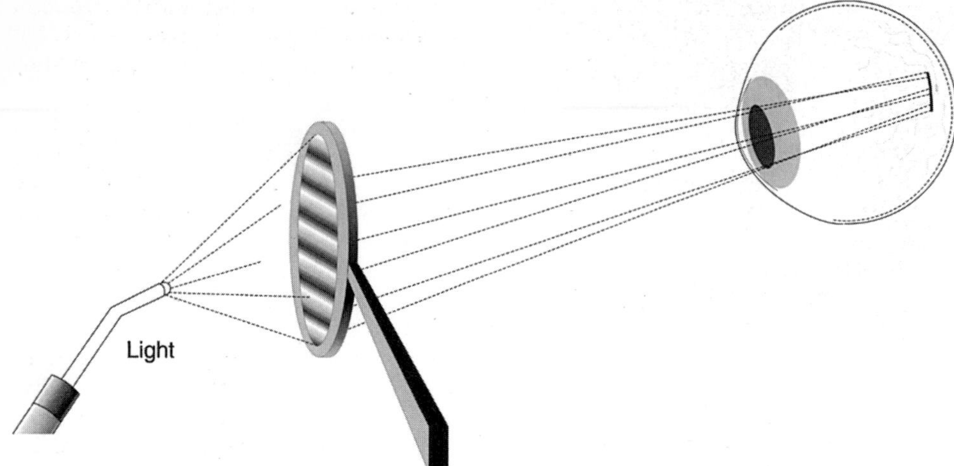

FIGURE 9–10. Diagram of a point light source viewed through a Maddox rod. The cylinders of the Maddox rod are oriented horizontally, and the image formed by the rod on the retina is a vertically oriented line or stripe.

Disorders of saccadic or pursuit movements may also be the direct result of cerebral pathology. Patients with pursuit abnormalities from parietal lobe lesions may have hemineglect or apraxia (nondominant) and language dysfunction or higher sensory dysfunction (dominant hemisphere). Abnormalities of saccades related to frontal lobe dysfunction may be accompanied by abulia, disinhibition, memory abnormalities, or apraxia. Patients with Wernicke's disease (see Chapter 40) may have ocular signs in the setting of disturbances in consciousness or mentation, including hallucinations, confusion, agitation, and anterograde amnesia. Abnormalities of saccadic or pursuit movements may also be accompanied by a homonymous hemianopia or quadrantanopia.

Cranial Nerves. Lesions in the cavernous sinus often involve the first two divisions of the trigeminal nerve as well as the oculomotor cranial nerves. Cranial nerve VI palsy with ipsilateral facial pain from trigeminal nerve dysfunction constitutes Gradenigo's syndrome of the petrous tip. It was commonly caused by spread of inflammation from adjacent mastoid air cells but has become infrequent in the antibiotic era. Tumors and even aneurysms in the same site can cause a similar presentation, so complete neuroradiological workup is in order. Optic neuritis may also coincide with disorders of cranial nerve III, IV, or VI in the setting of multiple sclerosis.

Motor/Reflexes/Cerebellar/Gait. Midbrain lesions involving the intramedullary fascicular portion of cranial nerve III can be associated with involvement of the cerebral peduncle with contralateral hemiparesis (Weber's syndrome), the red nucleus with ipsilateral tremor and chorea (Claude's syndrome), or ipsilateral cerebellar ataxia (Nothnagel's syndrome) (see Chapter 22). Raymond's syndrome of the pons consists of an ipsilateral cranial nerve VI paresis and contralateral hemiparesis, and when cranial nerve VII is also affected, the condition is termed Millard-Gubler syndrome. Because the cerebellum contributes to conjugate gaze mechanisms, lesions of the cerebellar pathways often cause abnormal conjugate gaze associated with unilateral or bilateral ataxia and tremor.

Parkinsonism or involuntary movements (chorea) in the setting of Parkinson's disease, Parkinson's plus syndromes, or Huntington's disease may be associated with abnormalities of saccadic eye movements (hypometria) or pursuit movements (cogwheel pursuit). Pyramidal signs may accompany INO with multiple sclerosis, and ataxia may be observed in patients with Wernicke's disease who often have nystagmus or cranial nerve VI palsy in addition. Finally, absent reflexes may be appreciated in conjunction with pupillary abnormalities in Adie's syndrome.

Sensory. An evaluation of the sensory system outside of that related to other cranial nerves is rarely helpful in the diagnosis of disorders of cranial nerves III, IV, and VI and their supranuclear control. Lesions in the brain stem tegmentum may cause syndromes involving cranial nerves III or VI

TABLE 9–4. **Movements of the Eyes During the Cover-Uncover Test**

Test Condition	Phoria	RE Tropia	LE Tropia
Cover RE	RE deviates under cover; LE maintains fixation	None: LE keeps fixation	LE takes up fixation: conjugate binocular shift but only RE observed
Uncover RE	RE monocular refixation movement; fusion re-established	None: LE keeps fixation	RE resumes fixation: conjugate binocular shift observed
Cover LE	LE deviates under cover; RE maintains fixation	RE takes up fixation: conjugate binocular shift but only RE observed	None: RE keeps fixation
Uncover LE	LE monocular refixation movement; fusion re-established	LE resumes fixation: conjugate binocular shift observed	None: RE keeps fixation

LE, Left eye; RE, right eye.

with contralateral hemihypesthesia, often in conjunction with lateralized cerebellar or pyramidal tract findings.

Autonomic Nervous System. Beyond testing the sympathetic and parasympathetic innervation related to the pupil, additional evaluation of the autonomic nervous system is rarely necessary.

Neurovascular. The neck and orbit should be auscultated for bruits. Carotid artery atheromas, particularly when complicated by hemorrhage or ulceration, as well as carotid artery dissection may be associated with ocular sympathetic dysfunction (Horner's syndrome).

ASSOCIATED MEDICAL FINDINGS

Because one of the most common causes of orbital infiltration is thyroid disease, patients with orbital signs such as proptosis, chemosis, and conjunctival injection together with abnormal ocular motility should be examined for goiter, pretibial myxedema, smooth moist skin, and loss of lateral eyebrows.[40] In thyroid disease, the extraocular muscles can develop edema, lymphocytic infiltration, and fibrosis, resulting in loss of elasticity more than loss of contractile strength. The diplopia that results from this restrictive feature is due to the tethering of the eye in an abnormal position by one or more shortened inelastic extraocular muscles.

Evaluation Guidelines (Table 9–5)

Neuroimaging. Lesions of cranial nerves III, IV, and VI may occur anywhere along the course of the nerves, from the nuclei in the brain stem to the orbits. The possibility of focal neoplastic or inflammatory lesions requires evaluation with neuroimaging. Magnetic resonance imaging (MRI) is more reliable than computed tomography (CT) for detecting brain stem, subarachnoid space, or cavernous sinus lesions. Proton density imaging best shows the MLF lesions in multiple sclerosis patients with internuclear ophthalmoplegia.[41]

MRI is also the best procedure for imaging the orbits when fat suppression (saturation) pulse sequences and gadolinium enhancement are used. Fat suppression renders the orbital fat dark so that any gadolinium enhancement (white) within the fat, muscles, or optic nerve can be reliably observed. Thin-section CT is still a potent imaging technique for supratentorial brain lesions and orbital study. It also is a cost-effective means to measure the extraocular muscle diameter and is a sensitive indicator of thyroid orbitopathy.

Saccular aneurysms remain a frequent and important cause of cranial nerve III palsy, and cerebral angiography should be used in evaluating cranial nerve III dysfunction because it is the only reliable way of finding such lesions. Because false-negative and false-positive results continue to be problematic, 1.5 Tesla magnetic resonance angiography (MRA) cannot yet be used in place of standard angiography. MRA using a 3-Tesla magnet may provide sufficient resolution to rule out posterior communicating artery aneurysm causing cranial nerve III palsy. False-positive MRA studies can lead the physician to interpret vascular loops as aneurysms, resulting in unnecessary surgical intervention. In a study of 142 patients comparing digital subtraction angiography (the gold standard for identifying aneurysms) with CT angiography and 3-dimensional time of flight MRA, the sensitivity for detection of aneurysms 5 mm or larger was 0.94 for CT angiography and 0.86 for MRA.[42] Particularly promising is multiplanar spiral CT angiography.[43]

Electrophysiology. Brain stem auditory evoked responses, somatosensory evoked responses, and pattern-reversal visually evoked responses are commonly used as indicators of demyelinating lesions, which can affect the conjugate gaze mechanisms and the individual cranial nerves as they course through the brain stem. There is no widely available electrophysiological method to examine the peripheral portions of cranial nerves III, IV, and VI.

Body Fluid and Tissue Analysis. Thyroid function testing is important to identify patients with thyroid orbitopathy, but it must be remembered that nearly half of patients have normal thyroid function at the time they present with orbital manifestations. Patients with lead and other heavy metal poisoning can present with elevated intracranial pressure and false-localizing cranial nerve VI palsy. Urine screen for heavy metals is an important adjunct to the workup of these patients.

Cerebrospinal Fluid. Cerebrospinal fluid (CSF) examination is often a critical part of investigation for dysfunction of cranial nerves III, IV, and VI because these nerves are often affected selectively in meningeal infections, as well as in inflammatory and neoplastic infiltrating disorders. In addition, patients with multiple sclerosis (see Chapter 48) may present a typical profile of CSF abnormalities, and patients with this disease often present with ocular motility disturbance from central lesions (gaze palsy, INO) and less frequently with ophthalmoplegia from plaques affecting the intramedullary portion of cranial nerves III, IV, or VI.

Neuropsychological Testing. There are no common specific indications for neuropsychological testing in patients with ocular motility disturbances, although altered pursuit or saccade dynamics may result from cerebral pathology that also affects higher cortical mental functions.

Clinical Syndromes (Table 9–6)

PUPILLARY SYNDROMES

Anisocoria

It is commonly written that 20 percent of the population has anisocoria of at least 0.4 mm in dim light, although published series cite highly variable percentages from 2 to 60 percent. The most common sort of variable anisocoria among healthy people has been called see saw anisocoria or simple central anisocoria. The mechanism is indeterminate; this benign condition may vary from one examination to the next or even reverse sides. Light stimulation of one or both eyes decreases the anisocoria, and the pupillary reactions to light, near, and psychosensory stimulation are all normal. A different sort of anisocoria among seemingly healthy normal people results when the consensual response is weaker than the direct response. This type of anisocoria is present only when either eye is stimulated individually with light and alternates sides because the illuminated pupil is always the smaller one. This characteristic may result from the selective dysfunction of the

TABLE 9–5. **Useful Studies in the Evaluation of Syndromes Involving Cranial Nerves III, IV, and VI**

Syndrome	Neuroimaging	Electrophysiology	Fluid and Tissue Analysis	Neuropsychological Tests	Other Tests
Anisocoria	MRI/CT brain and cervical spine; MRI: orbits with fat suppression and gadolinium	N/A	CSF analysis	N/A	Testing with pilocarpine, cocaine, hydroxyamphetamine; chest x-ray study
Adie's pupil	MRI: brain; orbits with fat suppression and gadolinium; CT: orbits	N/A	N/A	N/A	Testing with pilocarpine, cocaine, hydroxyamphetamine; chest x-ray study
Light-near dissociation	MRI brain: midbrain	EMG/NCV: peripheral neuropathy, Miller-Fisher variant of Guillain-Barré syndrome	CSF analysis, RPR, VDRL, fasting glucose	N/A	Testing with pilocarpine, cocaine, hydroxyamphetamine; chest x-ray study
Bilateral unreactive pupils	MRI brain: midbrain		CSF analysis	N/A	Testing with pilocarpine, cocaine, hydroxyamphetamine; chest x-ray study
Impaired smooth pursuit	MRI brain: parieto-occipital lobe, brain stem	N/A	HIV, drug screen, genetic studies (HD)	N/A	N/A
Impaired saccadic movements	MRI brain: frontal lobe, brain stem	N/A	TFTs, genetic studies (HD), HIV, immunoglobulins (AT), enzyme studies: Tay-Sachs' and Gaucher's diseases	N/A	Jejunal biopsy: Whipple's disease; bone marrow biopsy: Niemann-Pick
Gaze palsies	MRI brain: brain stem	N/A	CSF analysis	N/A	N/A
Skew deviation	MRI brain: brain stem	N/A	N/A	N/A	N/A
Ocular misalignment	MRI brain: brain stem, orbits	EMG/NCV: MG, botulism	CSF, muscle biopsy, fasting glucose	N/A	N/A
Nystagmus, central	MRI brain: brain stem	N/A	CSF analysis, drug screen, electrolytes	N/A	N/A
Ocular flutter/ opsoclonus	MRI brain: brain stem	N/A	CSF analysis, drug screen, antineuronal antibodies	N/A	Chest/ abdominal/pelvic CT
Monocular diplopia	MRI brain: occipital lobe (binocular)	N/A	N/A	N/A	Ophthalmological examination
Binocular diplopia	MRI brain: brain stem, orbits	EMG/NCV: MG, botulism	CSF analysis, drug screen, fasting glucose, muscle biopsy	N/A	N/A
Cavernous sinus syndrome	MRI brain (cavernous sinus, parasellar); MRA; cerebral angiography; orbital venography	N/A	CSF analysis	N/A	N/A
Orbital syndromes	MRI: orbits with fat suppression and gadolinium; CT: orbits	N/A	CSF analysis	N/A	N/A

AT, Ataxia-telangiectasia; CSF, cerebrospinal fluid; CT, computed tomography; EMG, electromyography; HD, Huntington's disease; HIV, human immunodeficiency virus; MG, myasthenia gravis; MRA, magnetic resonance angiography; MRI, magnetic resonance imaging; N/A, not applicable; NCV, nerve conduction velocity; TFTs, thyroid function tests.

TABLE 9–6. **Selected Etiologies Associated with Disorders of Cranial Nerves III, IV, and VI**

Etiological Category	Specific Etiologies	Chapter
Structural Disorders		
Developmental structural disorders	Arnold-Chiari malformation, cerebellar ectopias, basilar invagination	28
Hereditodegenerative Disorders		
Storage diseases: lipidoses, glycogen disorders, and leukoencephalopathies	Tay-Sachs', Gaucher's, Nieman-Pick C, and Pelizaeus-Merzbacher diseases	30
Amino/organic acidopathies, mitochondrial enzyme defects, and other metabolic errors	Maple syrup urine disease, nonketotic hyperglycinemia; Leigh's disease; mitochondrial myopathies	31
Chromosomal abnormalities and neurocutaneous disorders	Ataxia-telangiectasia	32
The degenerative dementias	Alzheimer's disease	33
Movement disorders	Parkinson's disease, progressive supranuclear palsy, Wilson's disease, Shy-Drager syndrome	34
Ataxias	Friedreich's ataxia, autosomal dominant cerebellar degeneration	35
Degenerative motor, sensory, and autonomic disorders	Parasympathetic dysautonomia, Shy-Drager syndrome, acute pandysautonomia	36
Acquired Metabolic and Nutritional Disorders		
Endogenous metabolic disorders	Diabetes, hypomagnesemia	38
Exogenous acquired metabolic disorders of the nervous system: toxins and illicit drugs	Botulism	39
Nutritional deficiencies and syndromes associated with alcoholism	Wernicke-Korsakoff syndrome, vitamin E deficiency	40
Infectious Disorders		
Viral infections	Brain stem encephalitis	41
Nonviral infections	Mucormycosis (diabetics), fungal meningitis	42
Neurovascular Disorders	Small vessel arteriosclerosis, berry aneurysm, artery dissection	45
Neoplastic Disorders		
Primary neurological tumors	Brain stem glioma, medial sphenoid ridge and parasellar meningioma; Pancoast's carcinoma (lung), lymph node metastases (cervical)	46
Metastatic neoplasms and paraneoplastic syndromes	Paraneoplastic brain stem encephalitis; meningeal carcinomatosis, neuroblastoma, ovarian carcinoma	47
Demyelinating Disorders		
Demyelinating disorders of the central nervous system	Multiple sclerosis	48
Autoimmune and Inflammatory Disorders	Systemic lupus erythematosus, periarteritis nodosa, vasculitis, myasthenia gravis	50
Traumatic Disorders	Blunt, penetrating head trauma	51
Epilepsy	Seizures (nystagmoid movements)	52
Headache and Facial Pain	Migraine, cluster headaches	53
Drug-Induced and Iatrogenic Neurological Disorders	Anticholinergics, phenytoin, carbamazepine, aminoglycosides	55

intercalated neuron that connects the midbrain pretectal nuclei and the Edinger-Westphal subnucleus of cranial nerve III. These and other normal pupillary phenomena, such as hippus (pupillary unrest) and early release after maximum light response, may confound detection of a relative afferent pupillary defect. Finally, it is important to note that with age, the pupils normally become smaller, and the average diameter of the pupils in darkness decreases at approximately 0.5 mm per decade after the second decade of life. Neurologically significant anisocoria occurs with lesions affecting parasympathetic components in cranial nerve III and with disorders of the ocular sympathetic system.

Ocular Parasympathetic Syndrome, Preganglionic. Lesions affecting cranial nerve III often cause anisocoria in which the pupil is larger in the affected eye and the degree of anisocoria (difference in size) is greater in bright than in dim light. The important causes of cranial nerve III lesions in this setting include intracranial aneurysms (typically those of the posterior communicating artery at its junction with the internal carotid artery)[44] and small vessel disease with resulting ischemic nerve lesions, such as that associated with diabetes. The pupillary sphincter is usually involved in the setting of an aneurysm or other extra-axial compression like temporal lobe herniation, because the pupillomotor fibers are arranged on the outside of the nerve. In contrast, pupillary function is most often spared when ischemic lesions of cranial nerve III are present.[45, 46] As a rule, the pupil is not solely affected in cranial nerve III lesions, because the autonomic component fibers are intimately associated with axons carrying motor innervation to the other muscles innervated by that nerve.

Ocular Parasympathetic Syndrome, Postganglionic (Adie's Pupil). Damage to the postganglionic parasympathetic pathways in the short posterior ciliary nerves produces the condition known as *tonic pupil*.[47, 48] This type of pupil is large and reacts very little to light when the stimulus is presented briefly but may contract slowly if the light stimulus is maintained for up to 30 to 40 seconds. Redilatation after the light is turned off is also very slow on the involved side. There is a greater pupillary constriction when the patient looks at a near object, and this difference is referred to as light-near dissociation. Tonic pupils are associated with patchy or generalized loss of deep tendon reflexes in Adie's syndrome.[49] This disorder is more common in women and is pathologically characterized by an idiopathic degeneration of spinal root and ciliary ganglia. It does not result in any clinically important sensory or motor defect apart from the are flexia. In Adie's tonic pupil, the axons of the postganglionic nerve degenerate one by one, producing paralysis of progressively more segments of the iris sphincter muscle.[50] Examination of the iris under magnification allows the examiner to perceive the segmental loss of constriction around the margin of the pupil in the early and intermediate stages of the disease. When a tonic pupil has been present for a period of time, all sectors become involved and, in general, the pupil becomes fixed at a small diameter.

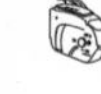

Ocular Sympathetic Syndromes. With ocular sympathetic lesions (Horner's or Claude Bernard's syndrome), the pathological pupil is the smaller one, and the anisocoria is greater in dim than in bright light. The light reflex is usually not perceptibly altered. This anisocoria is usually asymptomatic. Another finding in Horner's syndrome is mild ptosis of the upper eyelid from weakness of Mueller's smooth muscle in the lids. Less well recognized, however, is that weakness of Mueller's muscle in the lower lid also causes the lower lid to elevate. Upper lid ptosis and elevation of the lower lid together cause narrowing of the palpebral fissure. This contributes to an illusion that the involved eye is displaced backward in the orbit, which is the so-called apparent enophthalmos described with Horner's syndrome. A third component of Horner's syndrome involves sympathetic fibers serving the skin of the forehead just above the brow that travel with the nasociliary branch of the first (ophthalmic) division of the trigeminal nerve. With intracranial postganglionic sympathetic lesions, altered vasomotor tone and decreased sweating may be limited to a triangular patch of skin just above the brow extending to the midline. The sudomotor and vasomotor fibers to the skin of the lower face travel with branches of the external carotid artery after leaving the sympathetic paravertebral chain near the skull base and are spared with lesions rostral to this point of divergence.

The most important disorder that produces Horner's syndrome is malignancy involving the preganglionic sympathetic pathways in the neck or next to the apex of the lung. A minority of these preganglionic Horner's syndrome cases are secondary to trauma, usually resulting from penetrating neck wounds and root involvement in spinal injuries, and they should be obvious from the history and physical findings. In stellate ganglia anesthetic blocks, a transient Horner's syndrome predictably occurs because the preganglionic ocular sympathetic fibers go through this area. Inflammation, caused by suppurative infections and granulomatous diseases such as sarcoidosis or tuberculosis in cervical lymph nodes, is an occasional nonmalignant cause for preganglionic ocular sympathetic palsy. This etiology has become more prevalent in the AIDS era. Another important cause is carotid artery dissection, which presents with pain in the neck along with signs of ipsilateral cerebral hemisphere ischemia.

Postganglionic ocular sympathetic palsy is commonly associated with pain in the ipsilateral orbit and eye. In the early part of this century, a Norwegian ophthalmologist named Raeder reported this combination of pain, meiosis, and ptosis as a *paratrigeminal syndrome* with localizing value for mass lesions in the middle cranial fossa.[51] It is important to note that all four of his patients had, in addition to ocular sympathetic palsy, findings referable to the ipsilateral cranial nerves III through VI, either singly or in combination. During the past two decades, there has been growing awareness of patients with painful ocular sympathetic palsy without demonstrable middle fossa mass lesions. These patients often have histories of episodic retrobulbar and orbital pain that, in many cases, is typical of *cluster* or *histamine headache* (see Chapter 53).[52] The ocular sympathetic lesion occurs during a cluster of headaches and sometimes resolves spontaneously after the cluster has ended, although at times, it remains as a permanent sequel. This benign condition, considered a migraine variant, has been referred to as *Raeder's paratrigeminal syndrome, type II*, and to qualify for this diagnosis, patients must have no objective neurological deficits of cranial nerves III through VI. It has been speculated that in type II Raeder's syndrome, the postganglionic ocular sympathetic fibers are affected by edema in the wall of the carotid artery.

CNS (hypothalamus, brain, or spinal cord) lesions are an uncommon cause of Horner's syndrome and are almost always recognizable by the associated cranial nerve, cerebellar, motor, or sensory findings. A classic example is *Wallenberg's lateral medullary syndrome*, which is usually caused by occlusion of one vertebral artery with infarction in the distribution of the *posterior inferior cerebellar artery* (see Chapters 22 and 45). The attendant dorsolateral medullary lesion produces a syndrome that includes ocular sympathetic palsy along with facial numbness ipsilateral to the lesion, pain and temperature loss in the contralateral extremities, vertigo, dysphagia, and dysarthria.

Light-Near Dissociation

Light-near dissociation became a clinical sign relevant to etiological diagnosis when Argyll Robertson described it as a sign of neurosyphilis.[53, 54] The features of the Argyll Robertson pupil include (1) meiosis, (2) a normal afferent visual system (retina, optic nerve, chiasm, optic tract), and (3) failure of pupillary meiosis to light stimulation but normal pupillary constriction in response to accommodation and convergence with near viewing. In the original description, patients with this phenomenon had tabes dorsalis as well, and the pupil became an invaluable aid to the diagnosis of neurosyphilis. Light-near dissociation is not specific for neurosyphilis, however, and merely refers to the phenomenon in which the pupillary constriction in response to looking at near objects is greater than that in response to a bright light stimulus. The definition is imprecise because there is no way to quantify the degree of near effort that determines the amount of pupillary constrictor tone produced by the near stimulus. Many individuals make a poor effort when looking close up, and this may mask the presence of light-near dissociation.

Light-near dissociation may be due to input or output failure. Input failure occurs in bilateral prechiasmal lesions of the optic nerve or retina, chiasmal lesions, and bilateral optic tract lesions. As such, the examiner should establish whether the afferent visual system is functioning normally. If these conditions are present, the light reaction may be reduced and the near reaction left unaffected, creating a false light-near dissociation. Output failure can be the cause of Argyll Robertson pupil and occurs in the setting of diabetes mellitus, peripheral neuropathies, Adie's pupil (see earlier), and the Miller-Fisher variant of acute idiopathic demyelinating polyradiculopathy (see Chapter 49). Patients with midbrain compressive and ischemic lesions generally demonstrate large light-near dissociated pupils, in contrast to the classic description of Argyll Robertson, in which the pupils are small.[55] The mechanism of neurosyphilis-related Argyll Robertson pupil remains unknown.

Bilateral Unreactive Pupils

Failure of both pupils to react to both light and near stimuli has been described in cases of dorsal or rostral midbrain lesions, sometimes before the development of vertical gaze palsy or other ocular motility impairment.[55–59] An isolated unilateral (or bilateral) dilated, fixed pupil should also raise suspicion of pharmacological mydriasis. Patients or medical personnel may deliberately or inadvertently instill medications with parasympatholytic or anticholinergic activity into the eye. Pupils in this state will fail to constrict in the presence of pilocarpine (1 to 4 percent), whereas all fixed pupils from CNS or peripheral nervous system lesions become extremely meiotic in response to these concentrations of the drug.

OCULAR MISALIGNMENT SYNDROMES

Cranial Nerve III Palsy

Lesions of the oculomotor nerve can involve the nucleus in the midbrain, or nerve fascicles within the ventral midbrain, subarachnoid space, cavernous sinus, superior orbital fissure, or orbit. As an example, in the setting of an isolated right nuclear cranial nerve III lesion (see Fig. 9–7), there is complete disruption of the outflow of that nerve. Additionally, fibers from the *left* subnuclei for the superior rectus (contralateral outflow) and levator palpebrae (bilateral outflow) also are affected as they pass through the right-sided lesion. The combination of nuclear and fascicular damage results in partial bilateral ptosis and failure of elevation of both eyes. The ptosis contralateral to the lesion is usually incomplete because the levator receives some nondecussating neuronal fibers from the normal side of the caudal central nucleus. More ventral lesions in the brain stem only cause disruption of the fibers emerging from the ipsilateral cranial nerve III nucleus. The clinical characteristics of these *fascicular* cranial nerve III lesions are the same as those of any lesion distal to the nucleus, and only the functions of that ipsilateral nerve are affected. Localizing the lesion along the fascicular portion of the nerve depends on the presence of associated neurological features. Nuclear lesions are caused primarily by small infarcts secondary to occlusion of the medial penetrating vessels from the basilar artery (see Chapter 22),[60] or rarely by small hemorrhages. Other intramedullary lesions associated with cranial nerve III dysfunction include masses, including neoplastic (lymphoma, metastatic), inflammatory (sarcoidosis), and infectious (tuberculosis, fungal) etiologies.

Cranial nerve III palsy with concomitant involvement of other CNS structures leads to a constellation of findings that have been given various eponyms and usually are seen as stroke syndromes (see Chapter 22). Aneurysms of the posterior communicating artery are an important cause of cranial nerve III lesions from compression of the nerve outside the CNS. Compression can occur as the nerve passes near the vessel, at its junction with the supraclinoid portion of the internal carotid artery near the cavernous sinus.[44] Cranial nerve III palsy from an enlarging or bleeding saccular aneurysm of the posterior communicating artery is a neurological emergency, because the aneurysm is unstable and a fatal subarachnoid hemorrhage may occur. Clinical findings generally include cranial nerve III–innervated extraocular muscle dysfunction with pupillary sphincter paralysis. The latter dysfunction results from the compression of superficial parts of the nerve where the parasympathetic fibers are located.

In contrast, cranial nerve III lesions from diabetes or hypertension[45, 46] typically spare pupillary function. These disorders are associated with small vessel arteriosclerosis and affect deeper parts of the nerve. Involvement of the pupillary sphincter is more variable in inflammatory and neoplastic compressive disorders, but typically there is some degree of dysfunction. When attempting to determine whether a pupil-sparing cranial nerve III palsy is due to a medical or nonaneurysmal cause, knowledge of the degree of extraocular muscle dysfunction relative to the degree of internal ophthalmoplegia can be helpful.[44] A medical or ischemic cranial nerve III palsy is most likely when there is a total or near-total external ophthalmoplegia and complete or near-complete sparing of the pupillary sphincter. With incomplete external involvement, pupillary function is much less reliable as an indicator of whether the problem is caused by aneurysm or intrinsic ischemia.

Aberrant regeneration of fibers causes anomalous innervation of various muscles within the group that receives input from cranial nerve III when there has been axonal disruption and loss of continuity in the stromal channels that carry the axons within the nerve. Budding axons from the proximal segment of the damaged nerve gain access to the wrong stromal channels and grow into a muscle or muscles other than the one originally intended for that axon.

Typical clinical features of aberrant regeneration include elevation of the upper eyelid on depression (downward deviation) or adduction of the involved eye or segmental pupillary constriction with eye elevation, depression, or adduction.

This process of regrowth typically takes several months, and the clinical signs of aberrant regeneration are, therefore, not present in the early stages of the cranial nerve palsy. Cranial nerve III palsy from aneurysmal bleeding involves dissection of blood into the nerve with disruption of the axon channels, and this frequently sets the stage for late aberrant regeneration. On the other hand, ischemic cranial nerve III palsy less frequently leads to loss of continuity of the axon channels, and aberrant regeneration is an infrequent sequel.

Despite these general rules, aberrant regeneration has also been described following cranial nerve III palsy from trauma, compressive tumors, ophthalmoplegic migraine, basilar meningitis, ventral midbrain infection involving fascicles of cranial nerve III, and even following cranial nerve III palsy complicating diabetes.[61]

Cranial Nerve IV Palsy

In the setting of major head trauma, the dorsal midbrain and both fourth nerves are impacted in the notch of the tentorium cerebelli, and both nerves tend to be contused together. Because of bilateral injury to the ascending reticular formation, the patient is usually unconscious for a protracted period of time after the injury, following which there are complaints of vertical double vision. On examination, a relative elevation of the right eye (right hypertropia) in left gaze and relative elevation of the left eye (left hypertropia) in right gaze can be found. This reversal of vertical deviation indicates bilateral cranial nerve IV palsies. Unilateral cranial nerve IV palsy sometimes follows minor head trauma, and there is reason to believe that many of these cases represent decompensation of long-standing or congenital cranial nerve IV palsy that was not symptomatic. The mechanism of this occurrence is unclear, but it is important to ask patients with this disorder to bring in childhood photographs to search for head tilt that would indicate a congenital condition.

Cranial nerve IV palsies can also occur secondary to intraneuronal microvascular disease in elderly patients and are often associated with diabetes or long-standing hypertension, just as with ischemic cranial nerve III or VI palsies. The diplopia with ischemic cranial nerve IV involvement tends to improve over a period of several weeks or months following onset. Other causes of cranial nerve IV dysfunction include tumors in the region of the midbrain tectum and cavernous sinus, superior orbital fissure, and orbital disorders (see the section entitled Cavernous Sinus Syndrome).

Cranial Nerve VI Palsy

The abducens nucleus can be the site of a destructive lesion, particularly small vessel infarction or small focal hemorrhages. In these settings, ipsilateral paralysis of conjugate horizontal gaze results. In addition, peripheral cranial nerve VII palsy also occurs because the fascicles of nerve VII wrap over the superior aspect of the cranial nerve VI nucleus, forming a small bulge in the adjacent floor of the fourth ventricle (see Chapter 11). Nuclear cranial nerve VI lesions are also associated with more severely affected abduction of the ipsilateral eye than adduction of the contralateral eye, resulting in an esotropia and asymmetrical duction deficits. This phenomenon may be difficult to distinguish from a combined nuclear and fascicular lesion or separate lesions at the different sites. As with cranial nerves III and IV palsies, fascicular abducens nerve palsies can occur secondary to microvascular lesions in hypertensive and diabetic patients, in which case the abduction deficit tends to improve over a 3- to 6-month period. Conditions that can cause cranial nerve VI dysfunction include demyelination, neoplasia, inflammatory and infiltrating lesions of the cavernous sinuses, and leptomeninges (carcinomatous meningitis, chronic or acute infectious meningitis). Because of its long intracranial course along the bony ridges of the calvarium, cranial nerve VI is also susceptible to stretching and distortion more than other cranial nerves are. This phenomenon is characterized by failure of abduction in one or both eyes accompanying lesions remote from cranial nerve VI or the lateral rectus. This falsely localizing cranial nerve VI paresis occurs most commonly in the setting of raised intracranial pressure and as a transient phenomenon following lumbar puncture. This has been postulated to occur as a result of a transient shift of the brain stem secondary to changes in CSF pressure gradients. This unique susceptibility to small brain stem displacement is thought to result from the nerve's being fixed on one end at its emergence from the pons and at the other end, at Dorello's canal in the petrous tip.

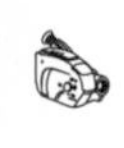

Internuclear Ophthalmoplegia (INO) and the Medial Longitudinal Fasciculus (MLF) Syndromes

Lesions affecting the MLF cause failure of the adducting eye to move, whereas the abducting eye deviates laterally to its full extent but has accompanying nystagmus during conjugate deviation. The medial rectus adducts without difficulty during convergence, distinguishing the paresis from a cranial nerve III or muscle lesion.

This striking pattern of disconjugate eye movements is referred to as *INO* because the lesion disconnects the nuclei of cranial nerves III and VI by causing failure of neural conduction in the internuclear pathway, the MLF. The peculiar monocular nystagmus can be either transitory (1 or 2 beats) or sustained. When the degree of dysfunction in the MLF is mild, the adducting eye may deviate fully but cannot attain the proper velocity during a saccadic refixation. In this case, there is a noticeable dissociation between the two eyes during the saccade, because the abducting eye completes the movement earlier than the adducting eye. To observe this phenomenon, it is necessary for the examiner to watch both of the patient's eyes simultaneously. This is best accomplished by looking at the bridge of the patient's nose from a distance of about 2 meters, so both of the patient's eyes can be clearly seen and differences can be appreciated in trajectory as the patient makes saccades to the right and left.

The clinical importance of diagnosing the MLF syndrome is its exquisite localizing value for lesions deep in the substance of the brain stem tegmentum. This general area in the brain stem contains the ascending reticular activating system, which is necessary for consciousness, along with several adjacent cranial nerve nuclei, and various ascending and descending sensory and cerebellar pathways. Therefore, the isolated occurrence of an MLF syndrome in an alert individual without other brain stem signs or symptoms suggests the presence of a highly discrete lesion. In the adult, this is caused by either small demyelinating plaques of multiple sclerosis, by small infarctions due to small vessel disease, and very occasionally can be encountered in the setting of head trauma. In children, the MLF syndrome can be the first sign of a brain stem glioma.

Differentiating between multiple sclerosis (see Chapter 48) and small vessel infarctions (see Chapters 22 and 45) can be problematic, because both tend to evolve acutely or subacutely and resolve over a period of days or weeks. Patients with multiple sclerosis are typically younger than 40 years old, whereas most individuals with infarctions are older than 60 years. Bilateral MLF lesions indicate multiple sclerosis, because a plaque may occur in the midline, whereas vascular lesions are often limited to one side by the margins of the vascular territory.

Patients with myasthenia gravis (see Chapter 50) can present with failure of adduction in one eye with dissociated nystagmus of the other eye. The dissociation between medical rectus function on lateral gaze compared with near convergence is, however, not typical of myasthenia gravis. Nonetheless, any patient presenting with the motility pattern that characterizes a pure MLF lesion, either unilateral or bilateral, without other signs suggestive of demyelinating or ischemic brain stem diseases, should have an edrophonium chloride (Tensilon) test as part of the workup (see Chapter 15).

In 1921, Lutz described a prenuclear (supranuclear) lesion causing failure of the ipsilateral eye to *abduct*, and he called this "posterior internuclear ophthalmoplegia" to distinguish it from the type of INO just described, which he called "anterior internuclear ophthalmoplegia." This can be distinguished clinically from a cranial nerve VI palsy by the lack of esotropia in the primary position of gaze just as in anterior internuclear ophthalmoplegia there is usually no exotropia in primary gaze. Involvement of the lower motor neurons in lesions of cranial nerves III or VI leads to reduced tone in the innervated muscle and deviation of the eye in primary gaze because of unopposed tone in the antagonist muscle. In these cases of internuclear or supranuclear lesions, the cranial nerve nucleus and its fascicles are normal. As a result, the resting tone of the innervated muscles remains normal, and the tonic imbalance between agonist and antagonist muscles that causes the deviation in primary gaze when the cranial nerve itself is involved is not present.

The existence of prenuclear abduction paresis has been controversial, but recently a series of 33 cases was published in which the lesion was localized rostral to the abducens nucleus using electrophysiological abnormalities in blink and masseter reflexes.[62] MRI and CT failed to identify these lesions in most cases, but the majority were thought to represent ischemic infarction and a few were thought to be multiple sclerosis plaques. The electrophysiological abnormalities were considered valid because they were ipsilateral to the symptoms and improved along with clinical improvement. All the cases had partial abduction palsy, and the patients did not have exotropia in primary gaze, consistent with the prenuclear location of the lesions. A suggested explanation of the observed findings was increased tone in the antagonistic medial rectus muscle, either from abnormal convergence or impaired medial rectus inhibition.

MONOCULAR DIPLOPIA

Monocular diplopia is generally a non-neurological condition in which images are split within the eye and fall on two places on the retina of that eye. This is commonly caused by irregularities in the refractive media of the eye, mostly in the crystalline lens (early cataract) or cornea. Deformity of the retina in or near the macula and fovea may also result in monocular diplopia. In these cases, two or more sets of photo receptors are activated simultaneously when the image should stimulate only one set. This type of diplopia persists when the opposite eye is covered. There is a cerebral form of mononuclear diplopia, usually resulting from lesions in the occipital-parietal lobes. It usually is present in both eyes together and singly (binocular monocular diplopia).

CAVERNOUS SINUS SYNDROME

Cranial nerves are often involved in lesions of the cavernous sinuses, including the third, the fourth, the sixth, and the first two divisions of the fifth. The most commonly encountered lesions in this area are inflammatory diseases of unknown etiology, aneurysms of the subclinoid internal carotid artery (siphon),[63] carotid artery and dural branch-cavernous sinus fistula,[64] and tumors. Meningiomas of the medial sphenoid ridge and pituitary tumors expanding laterally from the sella can also involve the cranial nerves within the cavernous sinuses.[65] A mucocele of the sphenoid and ethmoid sinuses can, on rare occasions, present this way as well.[66]

Granulomatous or primarily lymphocytic inflammation in the cavernous sinus and superior orbital fissure is known as the *Tolosa-Hunt syndrome*.[67, 68] It is manifest primarily by painful ophthalmoplegia and nearly always improves with steroid treatment. This relatively benign inflammatory disease must be distinguished, however, from other infiltrating lesions such as lymphomas, which may also respond transiently to steroid administration. An analysis of 108 patients with either benign lymphoid hyperplasia or malignant lymphoma revealed that there were no presenting or early clinical, laboratory, or tissue morphological features that reliably predicted the benign or malignant behavior of the lesion over the entire course of the illness.[69]

CONJUGATE GAZE PALSY SYNDROMES

Gaze palsies can be divided into disorders of vertical or horizontal gaze and further into nuclear or supranuclear lesions. Horizontal gaze palsies can be divided into impaired saccadic and pursuit eye movements.

Impaired Conjugate Saccadic Eye Movements

The saccade system generates very high velocity ballistic movements called saccades used primarily to examine the elements of a stationary but large or extended visual scene. An adult scans a scene in a highly organized way, extracting data from the highest informational areas but directing relatively few saccades to nonspecific or uninformative areas in the display. This efficient ocular scanning behavior develops progressively during infancy and can often be degraded in the presence of cerebral lesions, particularly those associated with dementia. This type of saccadic eye movement abnormality can be observed at the bedside examination, although quantitative characterization of saccadic behavior requires elaborate laboratory equipment. Where such facilities are available, saccadic eye movement *latency*, *velocity*, *metrics*, and *accuracy* can be measured. The average normal human takes about 200 milliseconds to generate a refixation eye movement or saccade to a new target presented in the visual periphery. A wide variation in the time required for each saccade exists, but the majority occur between 180 and 250 milliseconds.

Saccades have characteristic peak velocities that in normal persons bear a direct relationship to the size of the eye movement. Larger saccades are faster than smaller ones, but it is virtually impossible to perceive these subtle velocity variations by direct observation of the eyes in flight. Fortunately for diagnosis, pathology in the saccade system often slows refixational eye movements sufficiently that the movements are easily perceived as slow by direct inspection. Major reduction in saccade velocity generally indicates cerebellar or brain stem disorders, although minor slowing that usually requires electronic eye movement measurement to document can accompany cerebral hemisphere pathology, particularly if it involves the frontal lobes.

Another aspect of saccade abnormality is *dysmetria*, in which there is altered excursion amplitude—the eyes either fall short of their goal (*hypometric saccades*) or over shoot the target (*hypermetric saccades*). When saccades are hypometric, the eyes achieve the target by a series of small saccades, usually three or more. This gives the movement a jerky or ratchet-like quality that is easily observed. When counting the number of saccades necessary for the eyes to achieve a target 25 or 30 degrees to either side of center (*primary gaze*) in the examination, a normal patient often requires two and, occasionally, three saccades. A patient who consistently uses three or more saccades to make a 30-degree refixation can be considered abnormal. It is easier to be sure that saccade hypometria is significant if the number of saccades used for refixation to one side of primary gaze differs markedly from the number required to make an excursion of an equal distance to the other side. Overshoot, or *hypermetric*, saccades are also easily observed. Here, the eyes overshoot and attain the target via a series of decreasing amplitude reversals, each of which overshoots to a smaller degree than the preceding one. Each corrective saccade is separated from the last by the normal obligatory intersaccadic interval—around 200 milliseconds. This gives the movement a discontinuous quality as opposed to a smooth to-and-fro pendular appearance.

In the acute stages of vascular lesions—infarctions or hemorrhages—of one frontal lobe, the eyes are usually deviated tonically to the side of the lesion because of the suddenly unopposed tonic influence of the normal hemisphere. It can be deduced from this that the normal tone of a given hemisphere, and perhaps of the FEF specifically, brings about contralateral eye movements. This *contraversive* functional orientation is observed also in the disordered saccadic behavior that accompanies chronic frontal lobe lesions. In these cases, after the tonic eye deviation of the acute stage wears off and the patient is able to deviate the eyes fully in both directions, there remains a subtle disorder in which saccades directed away from the side of the lesion are *hypometric*. As an example, a patient with a right frontal lobe infarction has trouble looking volitionally to the left. During the first 4 or 5 days after the acute event, the patient's eyes may be strongly deviated to the right, sometimes along with forceful head and even torso deviation in the same direction. Gradually, the patient will be able to direct the gaze further to the left, and finally, full deviation is possible. An abnormally long latency period before initiating leftward eye movements during the acute stages may also be observed. This directional latency effect must be distinguished from bidirectional increased latency, which may represent altered mental function rather than a specific disorder of the saccade system.

In the chronic stages of this right hemispheric vascular lesion, leftward refixations may continue to evoke numerous hypometric saccades, whereas normometric single saccades are generated for rightward refixations. This contraversive organization is peculiar to the saccade system. The *pursuit* system operates in an *ipsiversive* mode, controlling eye movements toward the hemisphere that is active. This opposing functional orientation in the saccade and pursuit systems greatly enhances the diagnostic usefulness of eye signs related to these subsystems.

Impaired Smooth Pursuit Eye Movements

The pursuit system is highly susceptible to degraded function, and bidirectional low-gain pursuit may be a nonspecific abnormality in a variety of clinical settings in which the finding has no localizing value. Fatigue and the effects of many drugs bring about bidirectional symmetrical low-gain pursuit. Bidirectional low-gain pursuit is relatively common in the elderly and has little prognostic or localizing value. *Unidirectional low-gain pursuit*, however, is highly specific for a lesion of the horizontal gaze pathway on one side. Pursuit function in the cerebral hemisphere is *ipsiversive*, and unidirectional defective pursuit suggests a lesion of the parieto-occipital convexity on the side toward which pursuit demonstrates low gain. As an example, a right-sided posterior hemispheric lesion will cause low-gain pursuit with catch-up saccades rightward but will leave leftward pursuit unaffected. Large hemispheric lesions may involve both saccade and pursuit functions, in which case there are hypometric saccades in one direction (opposite the lesion) and low-gain pursuit in the other (toward the lesion). Low-gain pursuit can also be observed as part of the supranuclear conjugate gaze disorder that accompanies lesions of the rostral pons and midbrain, usually in conjunction with altered saccade parameters, but here, the saccades and pursuit are defective in the same direction.

Vertical Gaze Palsy

Vertical gaze palsy refers to the condition in which neither eye moves fully upward or downward. In contrast to horizontal gaze, there are no clinical disorders in which vertical gaze palsy is caused by cerebral hemisphere disease. Brain stem structures are thought to mediate vertical gaze through midbrain tectum and pretectal areas, and lesions in these regions commonly cause upward and downward gaze palsies in conjunction with other features. Aside from vertical gaze palsies, the common features include pupillary paralysis with unequal pupils (large or small), light-near dissociated pupils, convergence-retraction nystagmus, and variable degrees of ptosis or pathological lid retraction (Collier's sign). Retractory nystagmus is characterized by rhythmical backward movements of the globes into the orbits in a nystagmus-like cycle. In conjunction with globe retraction, there may be convergence movements of the two eyes with respect to one another. This constellation of symptoms constitute the *midbrain pretectal syndrome*, also referred to as the *periaqueductal gray matter syndrome* or *Parinaud's syndrome*.

This syndrome can result from mass lesions such as pinealomas compressing the midbrain pretectum as well as from intrinsic midbrain infarctions and/or hemorrhages. The syndrome is of localizing value but does not provide evidence for a specific etiology.

SKEW DEVIATION

Skew deviation refers to any acquired vertical binocular deviation that is caused by lesions affecting supranuclear input to the nuclei of cranial nerves III, IV, and VI rather than lesions affecting the cranial nerves themselves. These lesions are limited to the brain stem, but the location is highly variable and may occur at any level from midbrain to medulla. The vertical deviation may be comitant, such as with strabismus, or incomitant, sometimes mimicking cranial nerve IV lesions (deviation greater in downgaze and in adduction). Skew deviation is not specific for any etiology.

NYSTAGMUS SYNDROMES

Nystagmus is defined as a repetitive or cyclical ocular movement in which the slow phase of the motion is abnormal. Nystagmus can be further delineated by the specific movement of the eyes. Nystagmus characterized by repetitive cyclical bidirectional slow phases is termed *pendular nystagmus*, whereas *jerk nystagmus* has alternating slow and fast phases in which the fast phase is a normal saccade returning the visual axis to its original position. A feature common to all forms of nystagmus is that the eyes repeatedly return to the starting position of the cycle. There are three basic functional types of nystagmus: (1) unfettered, cyclical eye movement command generators; (2) tonic bias; and (3) inadequate holding power in eccentric gaze. The first and second types are characterized by abnormal positive influences on the conjugate gaze mechanisms. The third type results from a deficit of function in the gaze-holding mechanism and was originally termed gaze paretic nystagmus, but now gaze-evoked nystagmus is the preferred term.

The most frequent clinical example of the first type of mechanism is congenital nystagmus, in which the eyes are pulled off the object of regard by cyclical abnormal signals that enter the conjugate gaze–generating systems from an unknown site or sites. The return fast phase is a normal saccade bringing about re-foveation whence the cycle resumes. It has been proposed that the variation of slow-phase trajectory from one patient to the next with congenital nystagmus reflects various strategies employed by the CNS as a whole to maintain fixation or foveation. The variable visual acuity in these patients attests to the varied success of these strategies. Patients who keep foveation longer can achieve better levels of visual acuity.

The second mechanism, bias nystagmus, is most frequently encountered with vestibular system disorders and with lesions causing asymmetry of smooth pursuit conjugate gaze systems. The factor in common is that both the pursuit mechanism and the vestibular system are organized into two bilaterally symmetrical, tonically active systems in which the right and left sides oppose each other. Each system feeds commands into the horizontal and vertical gaze–generating systems, and in health, each side is equally active so there is no *net* driving force in any direction away from primary gaze. When disease affects one side more than the other, a net tonic drive or *bias* develops. The function of the vestibular system is to keep the visual axis on a fixed point in external visual space despite movement of the head in all planes (see Chapter 12). For instance, as the head rotates rightward at 10 degrees per second, an induced leftward eye movement at 10 degrees per second occurs, so that the external world remains fixed on the fovea. The VOR, however, does not supply the entire eye movement drive and works together with the pursuit system to optimize function.

Tonic vestibular system imbalance passes a tonic directional bias to the brain stem gaze centers, which causes the eyes to drift toward the side with less activity. The tonic influence of each side is contraversive, and a lesion creates underactivity of the ipsilateral system, with relative overactivity of the opposite system. The unopposed contraversive tone of the system opposite the lesion imposes eye drift toward the lesion side. This drift is checked by rhythmically occurring saccades in the opposite direction. The ensemble effect is rhythmical jerk-type nystagmus with slow-phase movements toward the side with the lesion and fast phases away from the lesion. This nystagmus is rhythmical because the slow-phase drift is constant velocity, determined by the degree of bias or imbalance between the two lateral vestibular subsystems, and the corrective saccades occur whenever a certain fixed amount of retinal position error between object of regard and fovea occurs.

The third mechanism, or gaze-evoked nystagmus, occurs when the patient is unable to maintain eye deviation away from primary gaze. When neural integration in the brain stem circuits is faulty, an inadequate step or position command results, and saccades made to eccentric gaze positions are followed by a backward drift of the eyes toward primary position. When a sufficiently large retinal error signal is generated (the object of regard is now on a peripheral retinal point), another saccade is generated to refixate the eccentric point. This results in a series of saccades and back drifts that constitute gaze-evoked nystagmus. This third type of nystagmus differs from vestibular and other bias forms of nystagmus in several ways. First, in gaze-evoked nystagmus, the velocity of the slow phase is determined by the difference between the oculomotor force being generated and the resisting forces that are tending to bring the eye back to primary position. These forces are largely contributed by elastic elements in the extraocular muscles and tendons and are greater when the eye is in a more eccentric position than when it is near primary gaze. This means that as the eyes drift back, the pulling force lessens as the elastic elements are less stretched, and the velocity of the slow phase declines exponentially. In vestibular nystagmus, on the other hand, the slow phase has constant velocity based on a fixed imbalance between the tonic forces of the two opposing vestibular systems. Second, gaze-evoked nystagmus depends on the continued effort of the subject to look in the direction of deficient holding power. As the urge to maintain the eccentric position wanes, the nystagmus slows down and may even stop with the eyes in a position close to primary gaze. Then if the subject is exhorted to look at the stimulus target, the nystagmus resumes. In general, vestibular nystagmus is faster than gaze-

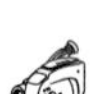

evoked nystagmus and keeps a fixed rate and rhythm. Third, gaze-evoked nystagmus is by definition not present in the primary position of gaze because it requires activation of a gaze shift. Vestibular nystagmus may be present in primary gaze if the intensity of the imbalance is great enough. Vestibular nystagmus is classified as first degree when it is present only with gaze in the direction of fast phase, second degree when it is present in primary gaze, and third degree when it is present in all positions of gaze.

OCULAR FLUTTER AND OPSOCLONUS

Abnormal repetitive eye movements in which the fast phase or saccades are abnormal include ocular flutter and opsoclonus. Opsoclonus is a continuous succession of multidirectional conjugate saccadic eye movements with no intersaccadic interval. In the acute stage, it is usually associated with violent ataxia and high-amplitude tremor of all limbs. As recovery occurs, some patients go through a phase in which there are spontaneous bursts of horizontal back-to-back saccades, again without an intersaccadic interval. In adults, opsoclonus usually results from brain stem encephalitis, either sporadic or as a remote effect of carcinoma. In infants and children, opsoclonus can be a remote manifestation of neuroblastoma. Ocular flutter comprises bursts of saccades in one plane, typically horizontal, during forward fixation. There are no intervals between saccades. Patients can manifest ocular flutter when developing or recovering from opsoclonus, and both disorders probably share pathophysiological mechanisms. Multiple sclerosis, hydrocephalus, head trauma, midbrain glioblastoma, thalamic hemorrhage, and sialidosis (cherry-red spot—myoclonus syndrome) have all been reported in association with ocular flutter.[70]

SUPERIOR OBLIQUE MYOKYMIA

Superior oblique myokymia refers to an aberration of superior oblique muscle innervation that causes episodic torsional oscillation of the involved eye. The patient experiences bursts of vertical and torsional oscillopsia and sometimes an increasing angle of vertical diplopia during a burst. Most cases are considered to be idiopathic, athough occasional cases caused by a tumor involving cranial nerve IV have been reported. A recent report documented probable cranial nerve IV compression by a small vascular branch causing superior oblique myokymia. Routine MRI was normal in this case, but the vascular structure in contact with cranial nerve IV ipsilateral to the symptoms was demonstrated using thin-slice (1.6 mm thick) MRI and "spoiled gradient recalled acquisition in the steady state" imaging. The authors suggested that vascular compression may bring about spontaneous discharges in trochlear axons similar to the mechanism thought to underlie hemifacial spasm when the facial nerve is compressed.[71]

ORBITAL SYNDROMES

In the orbit, cranial nerves III, IV, and VI and the extraocular muscles themselves can be involved by a nonspecific inflammatory disease with pathology identical to that in Tolosa-Hunt syndrome. Such orbital disease, called *orbital inflammatory pseudotumor* when the collagenous tissues and fat are primarily involved and *orbital myositis* when the extraocular muscles are primarily involved, frequently involves both the orbit and the anterior cavernous sinus through the superior orbital fissure.[72–74] The eye is painful and highly restricted in movement, usually in multiple directions. A condition with painful ophthalmoplegia reported as superior orbital fissure syndrome has no accompanying proptosis and has been most often ascribed to an inflammatory pachymeningitis from tuberculosis or syphilis, even when laboratory or pathological confirmation has been lacking.[75] Some cases have been thought to represent a sterile inflammatory reaction adjacent to infection in the paranasal sinuses.[76]

General Management Goals

Many of the disorders affecting cranial nerves III, IV, and VI are remitting, so management issues involve patient comfort. The most troublesome symptom in disorders of these cranial nerves is binocular diplopia that can be simply managed by having the patient patch one eye. Occluding one eye restricts the patient's visual field and results in a loss of depth perception. For this reason, driving is not recommended. Prism correction can be placed in the spectacle of one or both eyes to eliminate diplopia, at least for a range of eye positions near the primary position of gaze. Prisms bend light rays without altering the vergence of the rays. Corrective prisms are oriented to shift the image of the object of regard to the fovea of the deviating eye. An inexpensive plastic form of a prism can be applied to the patient's own glasses for short-term treatment. If the diplopia is going to be permanent or long lasting, then it is desirable to have the prism ground into the spectacle, because this is optically superior to the paste-on prism.

Reviews and Selected Updates

Barr D, Kupersmith M, Turbin R, Yang S, Iezzi R: Synkinesis following a diabetic third nerve palsy. Arch Ophthalmol 2000;118:132–134.

Hoyt WF, Keane JR: Superior oblique myokymia: Report and discussion on five cases of benign intermittent uniocular microtremor. Arch Ophthalmol 1970;84:461–467.

Leigh JR, Zee DS: The Neurology of Eye Movements, 2nd ed. Philadelphia, F.A. Davis Company, 1991.

Lutz A: Uber die bahnen der blickwendung und deren dissoziierung. (Nebst eines falles von ophthalmoplegia internuclearis anterior in verbindung mit dissoziierung der bogengange). Klin Monatsbl Augenheilkd 1923;70:213–235.

Miller NR: Walsh and Hoyt's Clinical Neuro-Ophthalmology, 4th ed, Vol 2. Baltimore, Williams & Wilkins, 1985.

Pierrot-Deseilligny C: Brainstem control of horizontal gaze: Effect of lesions. *In* Kennard C, Clifford-Rose F (eds): Physiologic Aspects of Clinical Neuro-Ophthalmology. London, Chapman and Hall, 1988.

Pierrot-Deseilligny C: Saccade and smooth-pursuit impairment after cerebral hemispheric lesions. Eur Neurol 1994;34:121–134.

Pierrot-Deseilligny C, Rivaud S, Gaymard B, et al: Cortical control of saccades. Ann Neurol 1995;37:557–567.

Sibony PA, Lessell S, Gittinger JW: Acquired oculomotor synkinesis. Surv Ophthalmol 1984;28:382–390.

References

1. Glaser JS: Myasthenic pseudo-internuclear ophthalmoplegia. Arch Ophthalmol 1966;75:363–366.
2. Warwick R: Representation of the extra-ocular muscles in the oculomotor nuclei of the monkey. J Comp Neurol 1953;98:449–503.

3. Asbury AK, Aldredge H, Hershberg R, Fisher CM: Oculomotor palsy in diabetes mellitus: A clinico-pathological study. Brain 1970;93:555–560.
4. Saper CB, Loewy AD, Swanson LW, Cowan WM: Direct hypothalamo-autonomic connections. Brain Res 1976;117:305–312.
5. Budge J, Waller A: Recherches sur la système nerveaux: Action de la partie cervicale du nerf grand sympathique et d'une portion de la moelle épinièresur la dilatation de la pupille. C R Acad Sci (Paris) 1851;33:370–374.
6. Kerr FWL, Brown JA: Pupillomotor pathways in the spinal cord. Arch Neurol 1964;10:262–270.
7. Sacks JG: Peripheral innervation of extraocular muscles. Am J Ophthalmol 1983;95:520–527.
8. Pierrot-Deseilligny C, Rivaud S, Gaymard B, et al: Cortical control of saccades. Ann Neurol 1995;37:557–567.
9. Cavada C, Goldman-Rakic PS: Posterior parietal cortex in the rhesus monkey. II. Evidence for segregated cortico-cortical networks linking sensory and limbic areas with the frontal lobe. J Comp Neurol 1989;287:393–445.
10. Schall JD, Morel A, Kaas JH: Topography of supplementary eye field afferents to frontal eye field in macaque: Implications for mapping between saccade coordinate systems. Vis Neurosci 1993;10:386–393.
11. Stanton GB, Goldberg MD, Bruce CJ: Frontal eye field efferent in the macaque monkey. J Comp Neurol 1988;271:473–506.
12. Seagraves MA: Activity of monkey frontal eye field neurons projecting to oculomotor regions of the pons. J Neurophysiol 1992;68:1967–1985.
13. Tehovnik EJ, Lee K: The dorsomedial frontal cortex of the rhesus monkey: Topographic representation of saccades evoked by electrical stimulation. Exp Brain Res 1993;96:430–442.
14. Tehovnik EJ, Lee KM, Schiller PH: Stimulation-evoked saccades from the dorsomedial frontal cortex of the rhesus monkey following lesions of the frontal eye fields and superior colliculus. Exp Brain Res 1994;98:179–190.
15. Shook BL, Schlag-Rey M, Schlag J: Primate supplementary eye field. I. Comparative aspects of mesencephalic and pontine connections. J Comp Neurol 1990;301:618–642.
16. Pierrot-Deseilligny C, Israel I, Berthoz A: Role of the different frontal lobe areas in the control of the horizontal component of memory-guided saccades in man. Exp Brain Res 1993;95:166–171.
17. Schlag J, Schlag-Rey M: Evidence for a supplementary eye field. J Neurophysiol 1987;57:179–200.
18. Heide W, Zimmermann E, Kompf D: Double-step saccades in patients with frontal or parietal lesions. Soc Neurosci Abstr 1993;19:427.
19. Muri RM, Roessler KM, Hess CW: Influence of transcranial magnetic stimulation on the execution of memorized sequences of saccades in man. Exp Brain Res 1994;101:521–524.
20. Pierrot-Deseilligny C, Rivaud S, Gaymard B, Agid Y: Cortical control of reflexive visually guided saccades in man. Brain 1991;114:1473–1485.
21. Anderson TJ, Jenkins IH, Brooks DJ: Cortical control of saccades and fixation in man: A PET study. Brain 1994;117:1073–1084.
22. Kompf D, Heide W: Saccades in parietal lesions. Neuro-ophthalmology 1994;14(suppl):535.
23. Pierrot-Deseilligny C: Saccade and smooth-pursuit impairment after cerebral hemispheric lesions. Eur Neurol 1994;34:121–134.
24. Dursteler MR, Wurtz RH: Pursuit and optokinetic deficits following chemical lesions of cortical areas MT and MST. J Neurophysiol 1988;60:940–965.
25. Komatsu H, Wurtz RH: Relation of cortical areas MT and MST to pursuit eye movements. I. Localization and visual properties of neurons. J Neurophysiol 1988;60:603.
26. Pierrot-Deseilligny C: Brainstem control of horizontal gaze: Effect of lesions. *In* Kennard C, Clifford-Rose F (eds): Physiologic Aspects of Clinical Neuro-Ophthalmology. London, Chapman and Hall, 1988, pp 209–223.
27. Sharpe JA, Morrow MJ, Johnston JL: Smooth pursuit: Anatomy, physiology and disorders. *In* Daroff R, Neetens A (eds): Neurological Organization of Ocular Movements. Berkeley, Kugler-Ghedini, 1990, pp 113–144.
28. Morrow MJ, Sharpe JA: Retinotopic and directional deficits of smooth pursuit initiation after posterior cerebral hemispheric lesions. Neurology 1993;43:595–603.
29. Kompf D: The significance of optokinetic nystagmus asymmetry in hemispheric lesions. Neuro-ophthalmology 1986;6:61–64.
30. Baloh RW, Yee RD, Honrubia V: Optokinetic nystagmus and parietal lobe lesions. Ann Neurol 1980;7:269–276.
31. Thurston SE, Leigh RJ, Crawford T, et al: Two distinct deficits of visual tracking caused by unilateral lesions of cerebral cortex in humans. Ann Neurol 1988;23:266–273.
32. Tijssen CC, Van Gisbergen JAM: Conjugate eye deviation after hemispheric stroke: A contralateral saccadic palsy? Neuro-ophthalmology 1993;13:107–118.
33. Sullivan HC, Kaminski HJ, Maas EF, et al: Lateral deviation of the eyes on forced lid closure in patients with cerebral lesions. Arch Neurol 1991;48:310–311.
34. Pierrot-Deseilligny C, Gray F, Brunet P: Infarcts of both inferior parietal lobules with impairment of visually guided eye movements, peripheral visual inattention and optic ataxia. Brain 1986;109:81–97.
35. Johnston JL, Sharpe JA, Morrow MJ: Spasm of fixation: A quantitative study. J Neurol Sci 1992;107:166–171.
36. Leigh RJ, Zee DS: The Neurology of Eye Movements, 2nd ed. Philadelphia, F.A. Davis Company, 1991, pp 15–78.
37. Leigh JR, Zee DS: The Neurology of Eye Movements, 2nd ed. Philadelphia, F.A. Davis Company, 1991, pp 198–205.
38. Thompson HS, Mensher JM: Adrenergic mydriasis of Horner's syndrome: Hydroxyamphetamine test for diagnosis of postganglionic defects. Am J Ophthalmol 1971;72:472–480.
39. Zee DS: The vestibulo-ocular reflex: Clinical concepts. *In* Zuber BL (ed): Models of Oculomotor Behavior and Control. Boca Raton, CRC Press, 1981, pp 257–278.
40. Dresner SC, Kennerdell JS: Dysthyroid orbitopathy. Neurology 1985;35:1628–1634.
41. Frohman EM, Zhang H, Kramer PD, et al: MRI characteristics of the MLF in MS patients with chronic internuclear ophthalmoparesis. Neurology 2001;57:762–768.
42. White PM, Teasdale EM, Wardlaw JM, Easton V: Intracranial aneurysms: CT angiography and MR angiography for detection: Prospective blinded comparison in a large patient cohort. Radiology 2001;219:739–749.
43. Hirai T, Korogi Y, Ono K, et al: Preoperative evaluation of intracranial aneurysms: Usefulness of intraarterial 3D CT angiography and conventional angiography with a combined unit—initial experience. Radiology 2001;220(2):499–505.
44. Trobe JD: Third nerve palsy and the pupil. Arch Ophthalmol 1988;106:601–602.
45. Rucker CW: Paralysis of the third, fourth and sixth cranial nerves. Am J Ophthalmol 1958;46:787–794.
46. Rush JA, Younge BR: Paralysis of cranial nerves III, IV, and VI: Cause and prognosis in 1,000 cases. Arch Ophthalmol 1981;99:76–79.
47. Harriman DGF, Garland H: The pathology of Adie's syndrome. Brain 1968;91:401–418.
48. Selhorst JB, Madge G, Ghatak N: The neuropathology of the Holmes-Adie syndrome. Ann Neurol 1984;16:138.
49. Adie WJ: Pseudo-Argyll Robertson pupils with absent tendon reflexes: Benign disorder simulating tabes dorsalis. BMJ 1931;1:928–930.
50. Thompson HS: Sector palsies of the iris sphincter in Adie's syndrome. *In* Thompson HS, Daroff R, Frisen L, et al (eds): Topics in Neuro-Ophthalmology. Baltimore, Williams & Wilkins, 1979, pp 113–115.
51. Raeder JG: Paratrigeminal paralysis of oculo-pupillary sympathetics. Brain 1924;47:149–158.
52. Grimson BS, Thompson HS: Raeder's syndrome: A clinical review. Surv Ophthalmol 1980;24:199–210.
53. Robertson DA: On an interesting series of eye symptoms in a case of spinal disease with remarks on the action of belladonna on the iris, etc. Edinburgh Med J 1869;14:696–708.
54. Robertson DA: Four cases of spinal miosis with remarks on the action of light on the pupil. Edinburgh Med J 1869;15:493.
55. Loewenfeld IE: The Argyll Robertson pupil, 1869–1969: A critical survey of the literature. Surv Ophthalmol 1969;14:199–299.
56. Loewenfeld IE: The Pupil: Anatomy, Physiology, and Clinical Applications. Detroit, Wayne State University Press, 1993, p 975.
57. Henkind P, Gottlieb MB: Bilateral internal ophthalmoplegia in a patient with sarcoidosis. Br J Ophthalmol 1973;57:792–796.
58. Freeman JW, Cox TA, Batnitzky S, et al: Craniopharyngioma simulating bilateral internal ophthalmoplegia. Arch Neurol 1980;37:176–177.
59. Seybold ME, Yoss RE, Hollenhorst RW, Moyer NJ: Pupillary abnormalities associated with tumors of the pineal region. Neurology 1971;21:232–237.
60. Kobayashi S, Mukuno K, Tazake Y, et al: Oculo-motor nerve nuclear complex syndrome. A case with clinico-pathological correlation. Neuro-ophthalmology 1986;6:55–59.

61. Messe SR, Shin RK, Liu GT, Galetta SL, Volpe NJ: Oculomotor synkinesis following a midbrain stroke. Neurology 2001;57:1106–1107.
62. Thomke F, Hopf HC: Abduction paresis with rostral pontine and/or mesencephalic lesions: Pseudoabducens palsy and its relation to the so-called posterior internuclear ophthalmoplegia of Lutz. BMC Neurol 2001;1:4.
63. Miller NR: Walsh and Hoyt's Clinical Neuro-Ophthalmology, 4th ed. Baltimore, Williams & Wilkins, 1985, pp 915–916.
64. Markwalder T, Meienberg O: Acute painful cavernous sinus syndrome in unruptured intracavernous aneurysms of the interal carotid artery. J Clin Neuro Ophthalmol 1983;3:31–35.
65. Keltner JL, Satterfield D, Dublin AB, Lee BCP: Dural and carotid cavernous sinus fistulas. Diagnosis, management, and complications. Ophthalmology 1987;94:1585–1600.
66. Leigh RJ, Zee DS: The Neurology of Eye Movements, 2nd ed. Philadelphia, F.A. Davis, 1991, pp 293–377.
67. Goodwin JA, Glaser JS: Chiasmal syndrome in sphenoid sinus mucocele. Ann Neurol 1978;4:440–444.
68. Tolosa E: Periarteritic lesions of carotid siphon with clinical features of a carotid infraclinoidal aneurysm. J Neurol Neurosurg Psychiatr 1954;17:300–302.
69. Hunt WE, Meagher JN, LeFever HE, Zeman W: Painful ophthalmoplegia: Its relation to indolent inflammation of the cavernous sinus. Neurology 1961;11:56–62.
70. Knowles DM, Jakobiec FA, McNally L, Burke JS: Lymphoid hyperplasia and malignant lymphoma occurring in the ocular adnexa (orbit, conjunctiva, and eyelids): A prospective multiparametric analysis of 108 cases during 1977 to 1987. Hum Pathol 1990;21:959–973.
71. Hashimoto M, Ohtsuka K, Hoyt WF: Vascular compression as a cause of superior oblique myokymia disclosed by thin-slice magnetic resonance imaging. Am J Ophthalmol 2001;131:676–677.
72. Bencherif B, Zouaoui A, Chedid G, et al: Intracranial extension of an idiopathic orbital inflammatory pseudotumor. Am J Neuroradiol 1993;14:181–184.
73. Clifton AG, Borgstein RL, Moseley IF, et al: Intracranial extension of orbital pseudotumour. Clin Radiol 1992;45:23–26.
74. Henderson JW: Inflammatory orbital tumors. *In* Henderson JW (ed): Orbital Tumors, 3rd ed. New York, Raven Press, 1994, pp 391–411.
75. Lakke JPWF: Superior orbital fissure syndrome: Report of a case caused by local pachymeningitis. Arch Neurol 1962;7:289–300.
76. Kretzschmar S, Jacot P: Des symptomes precoces et d'une etiologie souvent meconnue du syndrome de la fente sphenoidale. Schweiz Med Wschr 1939;69:1103–1107.

CHAPTER 10

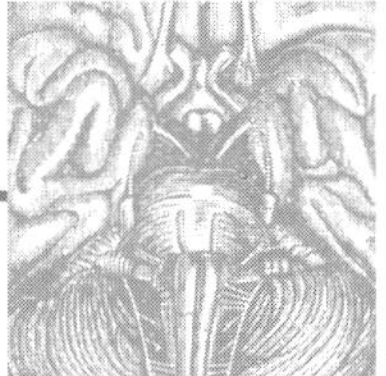

PETER B. CRINO and STEVEN GALETTA

The Trigeminal Nerve

History and Definitions

The trigeminal system contains both sensory and motor components and thus subserves and controls ipsilateral facial sensation and masticatory movements. The trigeminal sensory and motor nuclei extend in the brain stem from the pons to the upper cervical spinal cord. Pain, thermal, tactile, and kinesthetic sensory stimuli are received from the facial skin, oropharynx, nasal mucous membranes, sinuses, teeth, palate, dura, and masticatory muscles themselves. Motor fibers extend to the muscles of mastication as well as the tensor tympani and tensor veli palatini. Clinically, trigeminal dysfunction commonly is manifested as sensory changes such as paresthesias, dysesthesias, or anesthesia; paroxysmal or chronic pain; or difficulty chewing and swallowing. Traumatic, vascular, infectious, inflammatory, neoplastic, and demyelinating disorders can affect the trigeminal nerve at multiple points along the anatomical pathway from cortex, through the brain stem and trigeminal sensory ganglion, and out into peripheral trigeminal branches.

The first adequate clinical description of trigeminal neuralgia was made by Fothergill in 1773. Thereafter, Charles Bell (1829) demonstrated that the trigeminal nerve subserved sensation to the face. The trigeminal ganglion was excised in the late 19th century by Rose (1890), and the celebrated surgeon Horsley first sectioned cranial nerve V through an intradural middle fossa approach in 1891. Early 20th-century studies focused primarily on physiology, and more modern research has integrated neurochemistry, neuropharmacology, and microsurgical interventions in the treatment of trigeminal lesions.

Clinical History

When interviewing a patient with complaints referable to the trigeminal system, there are several key considerations to address. First is the nature of the patient's complaint (i.e., pain, sensory changes, sensory loss, or motor difficulty) because the characteristic clinical features are critical components of an appropriate neurological diagnosis. For example, lancinating excruciating pain suggests trigeminal neuralgia and is distinguished from the more tolerable yet disturbing paresthesias of trigeminal sensory neuropathy. Determination of whether the symptoms are intermittent, paroxysmal, or chronic and the temporal profile of symptom development (i.e., whether symptoms began in an acute, subacute, or indolent fashion) also provides diagnostic clues. Thus, sudden complaints of sensory loss, paresthesias, or motor dysfunction in the face are consistent with vascular, traumatic, or demyelinating processes, whereas similar complaints developing over weeks more often reflect neoplastic or inflammatory etiologies. Inquiries regarding a family history of neurological disorders that may run in families and have a possible genetic link, such as multiple sclerosis, stroke, brain tumor, or aneurysm, should be sought. Possible precipitating elements such as recent trauma, toxic exposures, illicit drug abuse, and all medication usage should be identified. It is also important to elicit other neurological symptoms such as autonomic, visual, ocular, or facial motor dysfunction, which may help to localize the lesion. Specifically, patients should be questioned regarding changes in facial sweating;

recurrent corneal irritation or abrasions; and difficulty blinking, swallowing, or speaking. Specific trigger points of facial pain suggest trigeminal neuralgia, and associated oropharyngeal or jaw pain may imply temporomandibular joint disease. It is imperative to identify past or concurrent medical or neurological disorders that may be related etiologically to a patient's complaints of trigeminal dysfunction. Specifically, a history of collagen vascular diseases, prior strokes, diabetes, neoplasms, granulomatous diseases, bleeding disorders, or recent and recurrent infections may prove helpful.

Anatomy of Cranial Nerve V (Table 10–1)

OVERVIEW

The trigeminal nerve is a mixed cranial nerve, and the afferent and efferent projections of cranial nerve V provide sensorimotor inputs and outputs to the face (see Table 10–1).[1] The multimodal sensory components (pain, temperature, position, and light touch) of the trigeminal system send projections via the thalamus to primary sensory cortices (Brodmann areas 3, 1, and 2). The three primary sensory nerves of the trigeminal system are named for the facial regions they innervate (e.g., ophthalmic [V1], maxillary [V2], and mandibular [V3]) (Fig. 10–1A). The unilateral cutaneous sensory distributions of these nerves overlap slightly in the facial midline, which has clinical relevance especially in assessing patients with nonorganic sensory loss (see later). In contrast, first order motor efferents originate in primary motor cortex (area 4) and project bilaterally to the pontine trigeminal motor nucleus. Axon collaterals extend to the thalamus and cerebellum. The motor projections innervate the muscles of mastication including the masseter, medial and lateral pterygoid, temporalis, mylohyoid, and anterior belly of the digastric muscles, as well as the tensors tympani and vela palatini. The motor portion of the trigeminal nerve runs with the mandibular (V3) sensory branch in the face.

MOTOR PORTION

Supranuclear Control and Upper Motor Neurons

Corticobulbar projections to the trigeminal motor nucleus (upper motor neurons) extend from facial regions of the precentral gyrus (first order neurons in primary and supplementary motor cortices, areas 4 and 6) via the corticobulbar tract

TABLE 10–1. **Clinico-anatomical Correlation of Localization of Lesions of CN V**

Anatomical Site of Damage	CN V Finding	Other Neurological and Medical Findings	Common Etiologies
Supranuclear			
Sensory cortex	Facial numbness, paresthesias	Neglect, apraxia, aphasia	Stroke, tumor, hemorrhage
Internal capsule	Hemifacial sensory loss	Hemiparesis of arm	Stroke, tumor, hemorrhage, MS
Corona radiata		Central 7th paresis	
VPM thalamus	Facial numbness, paresthesias, pain, cheiro-oral syndrome	Anornia, hemisensory deficit	Stroke, tumor, hemorrhage
Midbrain	Facial numbness, paresthesias, pain	Ophthalmoparesis	Stroke, MS, tumor, aneurysm
Nuclear			
Pons	Facial numbness, paresthesias, pain, trigeminal neuralgia, facial weakness	Ophthalmoparesis, CN VI, VII, VIII, Horner's syndrome	Stroke, tumor, hemorrhage, MS, syringobulbia, abscess, trauma
Medulla	Facial numbness, paresthesias, pain, trigeminal neuralgia	Ataxia, CN X, ophthalmoparesis, nystagmus, Horner's syndrome, Wallenberg's syndrome	Stroke, MS, tumor, aneurysm, abscess, vasculopathy
Preganglionic			
Cerebellopontine angle	Facial numbness	CN VII, VIII, headache, cerebellar dysergia	Neuroma, meningioma, meningitis (bacterial, TB, cancer), aneurysm, trauma
Middle cranial fossa			
Gasserian ganglion	Facial numbness, facial weakness	Gradenigo's syndrome, CN VI, VII	Tumor, infection, trauma
Skull base	Facial numbness, facial weakness	Headache, meningismus	Meningitis (bacterial, TB, cancer, sarcoid)
Trigeminal nerve branches V1			
Cavernous sinus	Facial numbness, pain	Headache, ophthalmoparesis, Horner's syndrome	Tumor, thrombosis, infection, trauma
Carotid–cavernous fistula	Facial numbness	Proptosis, bruit, ophthalmoparesis	Trauma
V2:Maxillary region	Facial numbness, numb cheek syndrome		Tumor, infarct, vasculopathy, trauma
V3:Mandibular region	Weakness of mastication, numb chin syndrome		Tumor, trauma, infarct

CN, Cranial nerve; VPM, ventroposteromedial; MS, multiple sclerosis; TB, tuberculosis.

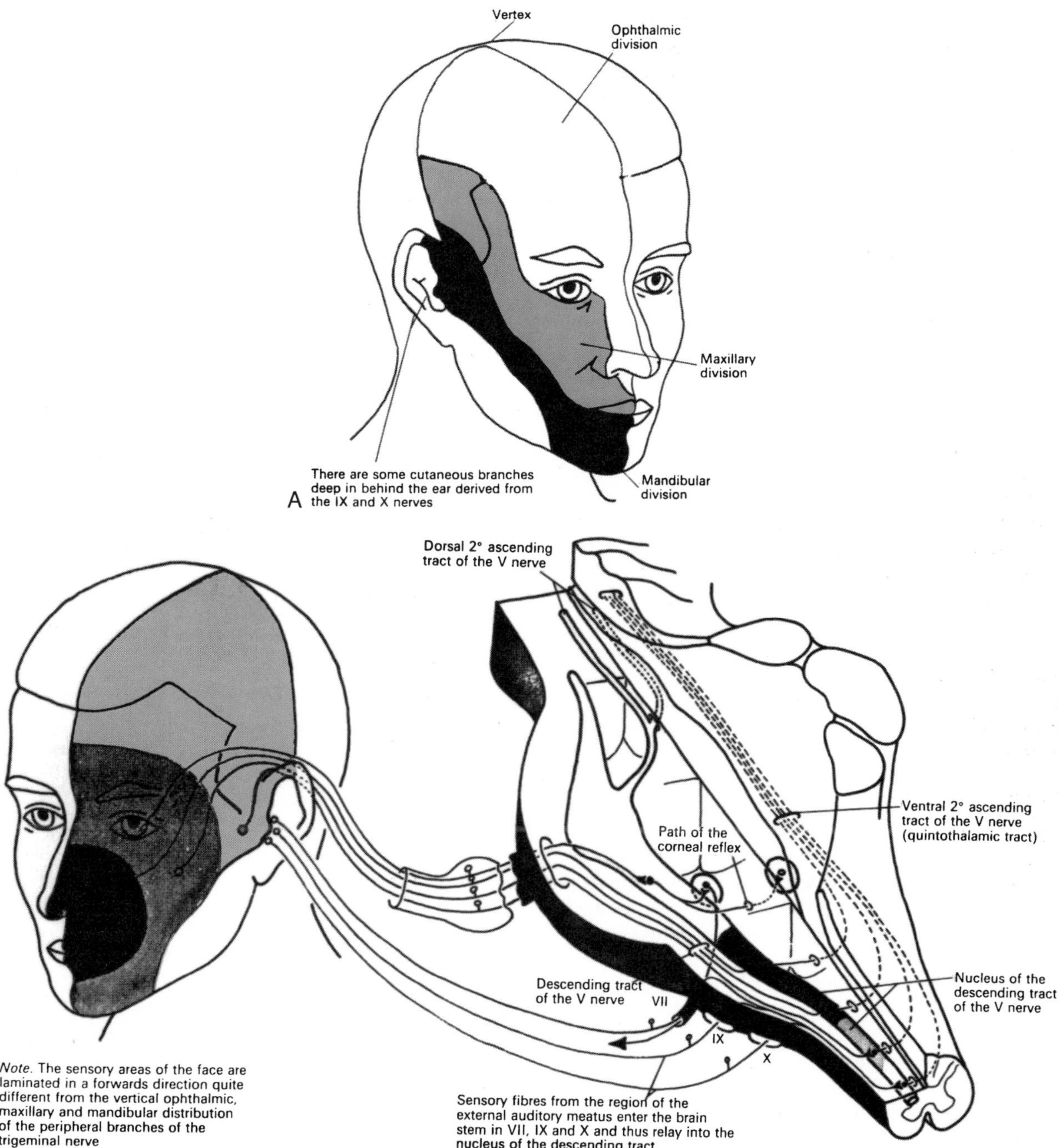

FIGURE 10–1. *A*, Cutaneous distribution and facial innervation of V1–V3. *B*, Anatomical relationship between cutaneous trigeminal fibers, the gasserian ganglion, and brain stem trigeminal nuclei and pathways. Note termination of afferent fibers via the descending (spinal) trigeminal tract into the spinal (descending) nucleus. The anterior innervation of the nose and mouth blends laterally with maxillary and preauricular innervation in a characteristic onion skin pattern. (From Patten JP: Neurological Differential Diagnosis: An Illustrated Approach, 2nd ed. Copyright © 1995 by Springer-Verlag, Berlin, Heidelberg. Used by permission of the publisher.)

to terminate directly on neurons within the pontine trigeminal motor nucleus or on adjacent pontine reticular interneurons, which project to motor nuclear cells.

Pontine Nucleus and Lower Motor Nucleus

The motor nucleus of cranial nerve V is located in the rostral pons medial to the principal sensory nucleus. The motor nucleus also receives fibers from the mesencephalic nucleus and mediates the efferent portion of the jaw jerk reflex. Motor trigeminal axons from the lower motor neurons project from the trigeminal motor nucleus to pass through the trigeminal sensory (gasserian or semilunar) ganglion (see later; Fig. 10–1*B*). Motor axons extend from the motor trigeminal nucleus in the pons and travel along the petrous portion of the temporal bone through Meckel's cave, which is a dural-lined cavity adjacent to the petrous apex housing the gasserian ganglion. Motor efferents pass through the gasserian ganglion, join sensory V3 fibers, and exit the skull base via the foramen ovale. Motor efferents in the face travel in association with sensory V3 fibers and reach the masticatory muscles via the medial and lateral pterygoid, deep temporal, masseteric, and mylohyoid nerves. These muscles serve to open (lateral pterygoids, digastric, and mylohyoid) and close (masseter, temporalis, and medial pterygoids) the jaw and provide medial and lateral jaw movements necessary for effective mastication. Small motor branches also extend to the tensor veli palatini and tensor tympani muscles. The tensor veli palatini in the posterior pharynx is active during swallowing and tenses the soft palate against the tongue. The tensor tympani is a small muscle in the middle ear recruited during continuous loud sound; it serves to draw the malleus and tympanic membrane toward the medial wall of the middle ear to dampen the vibrations of the tympanic membrane.

SENSORY PORTION

Receptors

Cutaneous receptors for the trigeminal nerve are primarily mechano-, thermo-, and nociceptive endings. These include pacinian corpuscles, free nerve endings, Merkel's discs, and Ruffini's endings. Although these are often associated with facial hairs, areas of particularly dense innervation include the lips, buccal and gingival surfaces, and the cornea. Some sensory nociceptive afferents are not myelinated, whereas others, and tactile and mechanical afferents, are heavily so. In addition, muscle spindles and Golgi tendon organs exist within facial muscles and extend via type Ia and Ib fibers to the pons.

First Order Neurons

Primary sensory neuron cell bodies for the afferent trigeminal fibers (V1–V3) are within the trigeminal (gasserian or semilunar) ganglion, which is embedded in the petrous portion of the temporal bone in the middle cranial fossa.[2, 3] In this area is Meckel's cave, a dural-lined cavity in the middle cranial fossa adjacent to the temporal lobe, which surrounds the gasserian ganglion and its branches as they exit into the petrous temporal bone. This region may be viewed by magnetic resonance imaging and is important clinically. A single large trigeminal sensorimotor root passes into the gasserian ganglion and then emits the three trigeminal divisions that exit the skull base via distinct foramina: V1 exits via the superior orbital foramen, V2 via the foramen rotundum, and V3 via the foramen ovale.

The ophthalmic division of the trigeminal nerve is entirely sensory (all modalities) and its branches innervate the orbit and eye (lacrimal and nasociliary branches); upper eyelid, forehead, and nose (frontal branches); nasal cavity; and nasal sinuses (nasociliary branches). V1 passes within the cavernous sinus where it lies inferolateral to the oculomotor, trochlear, and abducens nerves. From the cavernous sinus, V1 extends through the superior orbital fissure again in association with cranial nerves III, IV, and VI, before dividing into the lacrimal, frontal, and nasociliary nerves. Cutaneous fibers reach the skin via the supraorbital foramen along the ridge of the brow. V1 sensory afferents from the cornea provide afferents for the corneal reflex (see later). Smaller tentorial and dural branches innervate the tentorium cerebelli and dura mater.[4] Vasomotor fibers also branch from the trigeminal system (trigeminovascular innervation) to provide autonomic inputs to intracranial blood vessels. The majority of these fibers are believed to use calcitonin gene-related peptide, substance P,[5] and vasoactive intestinal peptide as transmitters.[6] Stimulation of the trigeminal ganglion in experimental animals and humans increases brain blood flow.[7, 8] Autonomic fibers to the lacrimal gland extend from the facial nerve and pterygopalatine ganglion to run with the lacrimal branch of V1, but they originate from the superior salivatory nucleus.

The maxillary division (V2) is also completely sensory; it innervates the skin of the cheek, nose, lower eyelid, upper lip, nasopharynx, soft and hard palate, maxillary sinus, and upper teeth. A small meningeal branch follows the middle meningeal artery and supplies the dura.[4] V2 fibers leave the gasserian ganglion, exit the foramen rotundum, and run inferiorly within the cavernous sinus. V2 axons pass through the pterygopalatine fossa, to exit the infraorbital foramen. These cutaneous branches include the zygomaticotemporal, zygomaticofacial, and infraorbital nerves, whereas branches innervating the nasopharynx and maxillary sinuses include the greater and lesser palatine nerves, nasopalatine nerve, and pharyngeal nerve. V2 innervation of the upper teeth, maxillary sinuses, and palate is via the anterior, middle, and posterior superior alveolar nerves, respectively. Autonomic fibers that originate from the facial nerve (superior salivatory) nuclei accompany V2 branches and comprise the superficial petrosal nerve. These fibers synapse within the pterygopalatine ganglion and provide parasympathetic input to the lacrimal, nasal, and palatine glands. Fibers of the superficial petrosal nerve unite with the deep petrosal nerve to form the nerve of the pterygoid canal. The deep petrosal nerve is a branch of the internal carotid plexus and carries postganglionic sympathetic fibers from the superior cervical ganglion to the lacrimal glands.

The mandibular division (V3) carries both sensory and motor fibers (see earlier) to the lower face. V3 axons leave the gasserian ganglion to exit the skull base via the foramen ovale. The fibers ramify through the deep face lateral to the medial pterygoid muscles and then divide into branches that provide sensation to the skin around the mandible, chin, and ear (lingual, auriculotemporal, and mental branches) and mucosa around the inner cheek (buccal branch), lower teeth (inferior alveolar nerves), and dura (meningeal branch). Parasympathetic fibers synapse within the otic and submandibular ganglia and project to the submandibular and parotid glands, respectively.

Proximal connections of the primary sensory neurons synapse in the brain stem in three sensory subnuclei that extend from the cervical spine to the pontomesencephalic junction. These include the spinal (descending) trigeminal tract and nucleus, the principal sensory nucleus, and the mesencephalic nucleus, each of which subserve a distinct trigeminal function. Sensory axons from V1- to V3-innervated regions of the face reach the trigeminal ganglion where cell bodies of these peripheral axons send central axons in a solitary sensory root into the midpons. Within the brain stem, these axon bundles bifurcate into fascicles that terminate rostrally in the principal sensory nucleus or caudally in the spinal trigeminal tract and nucleus.[9]

Fibers entering the spinal trigeminal tract pass caudally to the spinal nucleus in an inverted somatotopic organization (V1 ventrally, V2 medially, and V3 dorsally) and convey most of the nociceptive and cutaneous inputs mediated by the trigeminal system. The spinal trigeminal tract extends into the upper cervical spinal cord, and afferents synapse on immediately adjacent cells within the nucleus of the spinal trigeminal tract that lie medial to the tract for its entire length. The nucleus of the spinal trigeminal tract blends at its most rostral extent with the principal sensory nucleus (see later) and caudally with the substantia gelatinosa in the cervical spinal cord (see Chapters 19 and 20 on pain).

The spinal trigeminal nucleus may be divided cytoarchitecturally into a pars oralis, which receives sensory inputs from the oral and nasal regions, or the pars interpolaris and pars caudalis, which receive afferents from cutaneous portions of the face. Within the pars caudalis, four somatotopically organized laminae (I–IV) similar to the central gray area of the spinal cord parcel sensory inputs into pain and tactile stimuli. Two somatotopic homunculi for facial representation of pain are proposed within the spinal trigeminal nucleus. First, a rostrocaudal representation of facial innervation such that mandibular regions terminate more rostrally, followed by maxillary and ophthalmic regions more caudally extending into the cervical cord, has been proposed. This facial representation is distinct from the second homuncular pattern proposed, the so-called "onion skin" pattern, in which the mouth and nose (central regions) are represented rostrally in the brain stem, whereas the cheeks, eyes, and ears (more peripheral facial areas) are represented more caudally.

Impulses carrying tactile and pressure sense enter the midpons and extend rostrally to terminate in the principal trigeminal sensory nucleus. These inputs are somatotopically organized similar to the spinal trigeminal tract. Cells within the principal sensory nucleus have large receptive fields; they respond to various tactile and pressure stimuli applied to the skin, mucous membranes, palate, orbit, and teeth.

The third brain stem nucleus, the mesencephalic nucleus, is located dorsolaterally above the middle cerebellar peduncle near the pontomesencephalic junction and adjacent to the fourth ventricle. Afferent fibers to the mesencephalic nucleus travel within the motor root of the trigeminal nerve and convey primarily kinesthetic sensation from the teeth, oropharynx, and jaws. These afferents synapse on unipolar-shaped neurons. Stretch receptors in masticatory muscles send information regarding bite force to the mesencephalic nucleus and function as the afferent portion of the jaw jerk reflex (see later).

Second and Third Order Sensory Neurons

The second order sensory neurons located within the spinal trigeminal, main sensory, and mesencephalic nuclei send projections rostrally via the trigeminothalamic tract.[10, 11] Neurons within the pars oralis and caudalis of the spinal trigeminal nucleus and cell bodies from the mesencephalic and principal nuclei project medially into the pontine reticular formation, cross within the median raphe, and ascend contralaterally within the trigeminothalamic tract closely adjacent to the medial lemniscus.

Axons from the second order neurons terminate somatotopically within the venteroposteromedial nucleus (VPM) of the thalamus contralateral to their nucleus.[1, 10, 11] A smaller proportion of fibers terminate within the intralaminar nuclei. In contrast, a small fascicle of ipsilateral projections extend rostrally via the dorsal trigeminal tract to terminate in the VPM. Trigeminocerebellar fibers project bilaterally from the mesencephalic and motor trigeminal nuclei.

Third order thalamocortical projections from the VPM travel in the anterior limb of the internal capsule and terminate primarily in sensory cortical areas 3, 1, and 2.[10] Less dense projections reach the parietal lobule and the precentral gyrus. The presence of some sensory afferents in the cortical motor region explains why sensory abnormalities may be reported by patients with lesions affecting only the precentral gyrus.

Examination of the Trigeminal Nerve

DIRECTED NEUROLOGICAL EXAMINATION

Sensory Function of Cranial Nerve V

When assessing the trigeminal system, it is important to perform a directed and assiduous neurological examination because subtle alterations in function may provide clues to detect potentially serious neurological disease. Sensory and motor components should be tested separately, comparing right and left sides, and light touch, pin, and temperature sensation should be tested individually in V1 to V3. The cornea and sclera should be inspected for evidence of keratitis, which may be suggestive of diminished corneal (trigeminal) sensation or lacrimation, as well as the facial skin, oropharynx, teeth, gums, and nares for evidence of inflammatory, infectious, or neoplastic disorders. When considering trigeminal neuralgia or, less often, post-herpetic neuralgia, trigger points that elicit pain should be identified (see later). Localizing signs from involvement of the neuraxis in close proximity to the affected trigeminal region may be helpful. For example, other cranial neuropathies such as ocular motor dysfunction or facial weakness and Horner's syndrome may provide clues as to the lesion locus in combination with the trigeminal symptoms. In general, lesions that affect branches of V1 to V3 distal to the gasserian ganglion result in highly focal, circumscribed sensory loss within one division or subdivision of the trigeminal nerve. In contrast, pathological processes affecting the ganglion itself typically cause ipsilateral hemifacial sensory dysfunction. Lesions within the brain stem that affect the individual trigeminal nuclei may give a distinct picture of dissociated sensory loss in which pin, temperature, and light touch sensory modalities are differentially affected.

Sensory examination should assess pain, temperature, light touch, and vibration as well as checking the corneal and jaw jerk reflexes. Painful stimuli can reliably be delivered with a non-reusable pin applied evenly and gently to the skin (Fig. 10–2A through 10–2C). Two-point discrimination testing, especially on the lips, can be useful. Although temperature discrimination can best be assessed with glass tubes of hot or cold water, in clinical practice, touching the face with a tuning fork and asking if it feels cold is effective. Light touch can be tested with a cotton wisp or tissue paper stroked gently against the skin. Vibration may be assessed with a 125-Hz tuning fork held against the frontal bones, maxilla, and mandible.

It is important when performing a sensory examination to avoid suggesting or directing the patient into desired

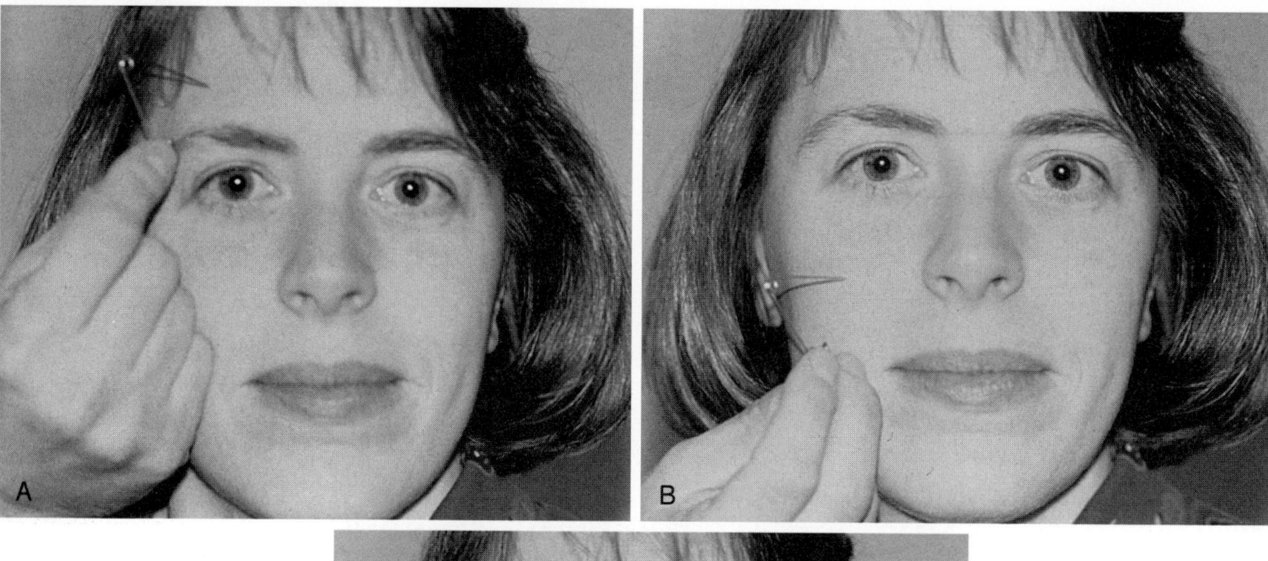

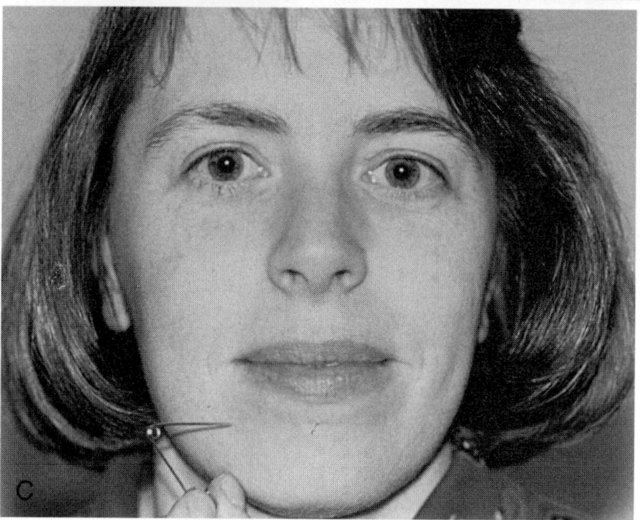

FIGURE 10–2. Sensory examination of the trigeminal nerve. Testing pain sensation in the cutaneous distribution of V1 (*A*), V2 (*B*), and V3 (*C*) by lightly touching the skin with a pin. Light touch and temperature modalities should also be assessed in the same distributions.

responses and to be vigilant for the malingering or hysterical patient. Thus, a conservative way to test sensation is to ask the patient to respond *yes* if present or *no* if not and then to determine a more subjective difference between the two responses. Comparisons should be made with the contralateral face. It is especially important to pay attention to upper cervical dermatomal distributions when assessing sensation along the angle of the jaw because there may be close overlap between sensory loss from a lesion affecting V3 and cervical spinal nerves of C2 to C3. Similarly, the distribution of the sensory fibers to the upper face and into the scalp merges near the vertex with fibers of the greater occipital nerve, which innervate the posterior scalp. The overlap in the midline of V1 to V3 cutaneous sensory fields is helpful in determining a malingering or hysterical patient. Thus, in patients complaining of hemifacial sensory loss, it is important to determine whether the pattern of loss abruptly stops at the midline or if there is a subtle gradation of loss proceeding from the affected to the normal side. In the former case, nonorganic causes should be suspected. By testing vibratory sensation on the frontal bone, malingering or hysterical patients can often be identified as those who report a difference in sensation despite the physiological impossibility of differences in vibratory sensation when essentially applying the tuning fork to the same albeit "right" or "left" bone. Similarly, loss of sensation on the forehead, which ends abruptly at the hairline, may suggest a nonorganic etiology, although facial sensory loss from leprosy affects facial cutaneous regions, which have a cooler temperature, but spares fibers at the hairline where the skin is warmer (personal communication, MJ Brown).

Motor Function of Cranial Nerve V

Evidence of trigeminal motor involvement such as muscle atrophy, spasm, or fasciculations; jaw deviation; difficulty chewing; and hyperacusis may be present. Atrophy of the temporalis is often easy to observe. To assess muscle bulk, the masseter may be pinched between the fingertips and the temporalis muscle should be palpated as the patient opens and closes the mouth (Fig. 10–3A). The strength of jaw opening (Fig. 10–3B), closure, and lateral deviation should be assessed because jaw closure is very strong and difficult to evaluate clinically, and subtle changes may not be easily detected.

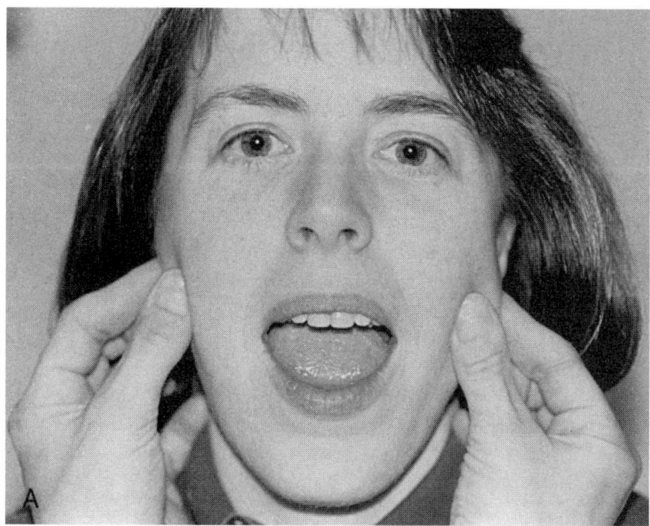

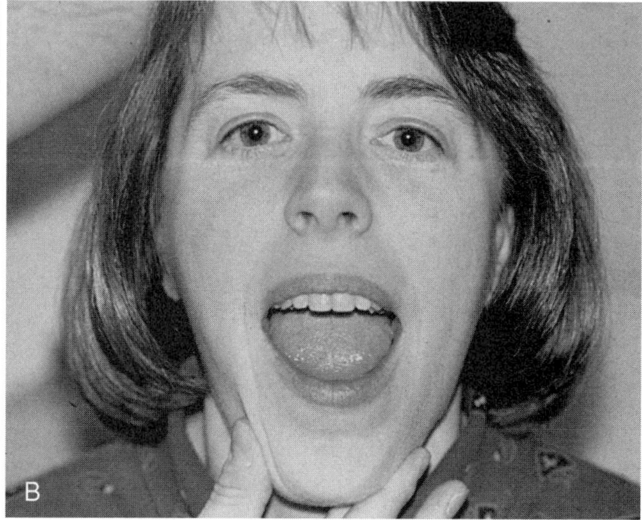

FIGURE 10–3. Motor examination of the trigeminal nerve. *A*, Palpation of the masseter muscles to assess muscle bulk, which may be diminished in lesions affecting the trigeminal motor nucleus or trigeminal nerve. *B*, Assessing strength of jaw opening is clinically easier than jaw closure.

If it is difficult for the patient to open the mouth against resistance, some degree of facial motor weakness is likely to be present. Weakness of the pterygoids resulting from nuclear or nerve lesions may produce ipsilateral jaw deviation (Fig. 10–3). Lower motor neuron processes involving the trigeminal motor nucleus such as motor neuron disease may produce fasciculations in association with muscle weakness and atrophy. One useful sign is the presence of masseteric spasm and contracture in association with ipsilateral hearing loss, facial numbness, diminished corneal reflex, and paretic facial muscles in patients with tumors infiltrating the dorsal pontine tegmentum.[12, 13]

Trigeminal Reflexes

The corneal reflex is a reliable measure of afferent trigeminal V1 and efferent facial nerve VII fibers (a V–VII reflex) and is present at infancy. Lightly touching the cornea with a tissue or cotton swab induces a rapid bilateral blink reflex (Fig. 10–4A). Touching the sclera or eyelashes, tapping the glabellar regions (glabellar blink reflex), presenting a light flash, or stimulating the supraorbital nerve induces a less rapid but still reliable response. Anatomically, afferent corneal V1 fibers may synapse within the spinal trigeminal nucleus as well as the main sensory nucleus. Short projection neurons project bilaterally to the facial nuclear neurons, which in turn project to the orbicularis oculi muscles. The latency of this response is between 25 and 72 msec and increases with advancing age. A brief latency difference exists between the stimulated and contralateral side of less than 6 msec. Extensive electrophysiological studies have characterized this reflex in great detail[14] in a number of neurological disorders. The corneal reflex may be slowed in various disorders affecting the trigeminal nerve, ganglion, or brain stem nuclei including posterior fossa and cerebellopontine angle tumors such as acoustic neuromas,

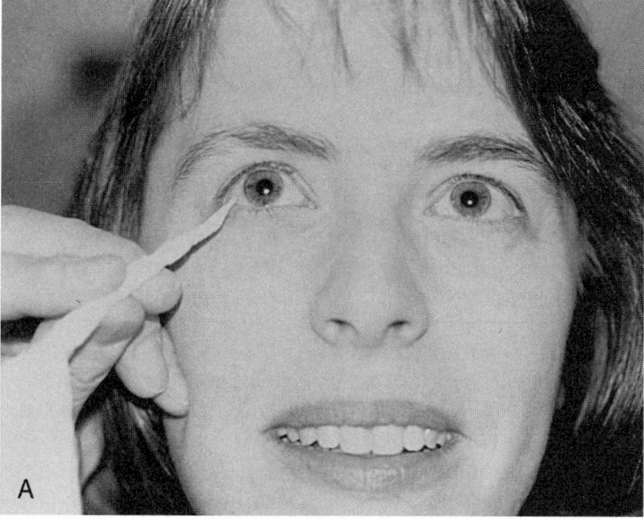

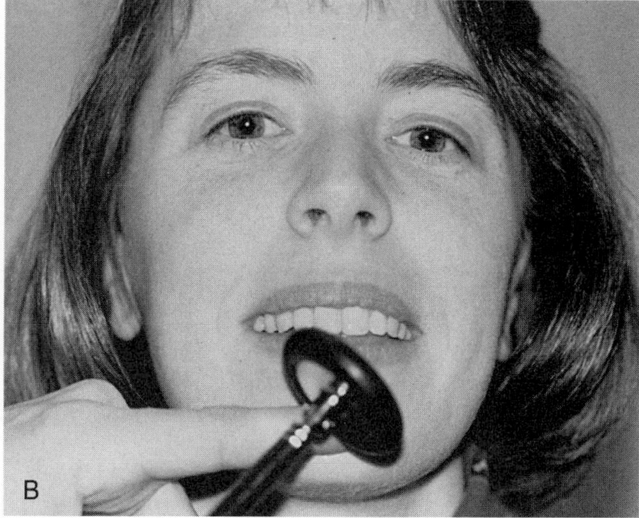

FIGURE 10–4. Trigeminal reflexes. *A*, The corneal reflex is elicited by lightly touching the cornea with a tissue or cotton swab. *B*, The jaw jerk reflex may be elicited by gently tapping a finger placed on the chin. Both of these reflexes may be brisk in supranuclear processes but diminished in nuclear or peripheral lesions.

multiple sclerosis, brain stem strokes (especially in Wallenberg's syndrome), and Parkinson's disease. Rarely, a delay in the corneal reflex has been reported ipsilateral to a hemispheric lesion.[15]

The jaw jerk reflex may indicate dysfunction of afferent sensory or efferent motor V3 fibers. Afferent axons for the jaw jerk reflex are from stretch receptors (muscle spindles) within the masseter, temporalis, and medial pterygoid muscles, which project centrally to the mesencephalic nucleus and induce a rapid, single jaw closure (jerk) mediated via motor trigeminal neurons that project back to these muscles. The jaw jerk is elicited by tapping the chin when the mouth is closed and the jaw relaxed (Fig. 10–4*B*). Other variations include tapping the thumb placed on the chin or a tongue blade placed on the lower teeth. Peripheral or brain stem nuclear processes that affect V3 neurons attenuate the jaw jerk reflex, whereas in lesions involving supranuclear trigeminal motor projections, exaggeration of the jaw jerk may be identified. Other trigeminal reflexes include the oculocardiac, corneomandibular, snout, and trigemino-abducens reflexes.[16]

ASSOCIATED NEUROLOGICAL FINDINGS

Cerebral. The presence of apraxia, hemispacial neglect, aphasia, or Gerstmann's syndrome in association with facial numbness is very helpful in identifying parietal lobe dysfunction in affected patients. Other important manifestations of parietal lobe dysfunction include a homonymous hemianopia (especially within the inferior quadrant); a cortical sensory syndrome in which astereognosis, diminished two-point discrimination, and agraphesthesia are features; and abolition of optokinetic nystagmus toward the side of the lesion.

Cranial Nerves. Ophthalmoparesis involving cranial nerves III, IV, or VI with trigeminal symptoms suggests cavernous sinus or superior orbital fissure pathology. If cranial nerves VI, VII, and/or VIII are involved (ophthalmoparesis, nystagmus, hearing changes), a petrous apex process such as Gradenigo's syndrome (see later) or lesion such as tumor within the lateral pons or cerebellopontine angle should be suspected. Similarly, detection of Horner's syndrome may indicate lateral brain stem or upper cervical spinal cord pathology.

Motor/Reflexes/Cerebellar/Gait. Hemiparesis can result from lesions within the postcentral gyrus and can overlap with sensory loss. Cerebellar abnormalities such as gait ataxia or nystagmus in association with facial numbness may point to a process within the cerebellopontine angle. Detection of Horner's syndrome alone or in combination with dysphasia and ataxia is consistent with a lesion in the lateral medullary region.

Sensory. Although the distribution of sensation on the lower face is via V3, the angle of the jaw is innervated by the C2 to C3 spinal nerves. Numbness or paresthesias in this region may reflect an intramedullary cervical cord process, but a psychogenic etiology should also be considered. "Crossed sensory" syndrome, wherein facial hypesthesia is central to body hypesthesia, indicates a brain stem lesion. Face and body hypesthesia on one side suggest a cortical, subcortical, or midbrain lesion.

Neurovascular. The detection of a bruit over the orbit is suggestive of a carotid–cavernous sinus fistula, especially in the setting of recent head trauma, and may be helpful in discerning trigeminal dysfunction from a cavernous sinus process. Other signs suggestive of carotid or systemic vascular disease increase the suspicion of stroke syndromes.

Evaluation Guidelines

In virtually every patient who presents with overt or subtle manifestations of trigeminal nerve dysfunction, some form of laboratory evaluation is indicated (Table 10–2). Careful and directed neurological examination dictates the most important tests to obtain.

Neuroimaging. Once a lesion has been reasonably localized to the cortex, white matter pathways, thalamus, or brain stem, neuroimaging is essential to support a definitive clinical diagnosis (for complete text, see reference 17). Although computed tomography (CT) scanning can provide useful information regarding bony change or intracranial hemorrhage, magnetic resonance imaging (MRI) renders high-resolution models of regions not readily visible by CT such as the brain stem. In addition, subtle abnormalities such as early multiple sclerosis plaques, small tumors, or infarcts can often be visualized with gadolinium-enhanced MR images. MRI with gadolinium is a very useful way to visualize Meckel's cave[18] and to detect enhancement within the trigeminal nerve roots or gasserian ganglion. MRI with fine sections through the orbits is useful in assessing an orbital mass lesion and pain referable to V1. Orbital CT may also be useful. MR angiography and CT may be utilized to identify compression of the trigeminal nerve by the superior cerebellar artery. CT is the method of choice to evaluate the petrous apex especially in disorders such as Gradenigo's syndrome.

Electrophysiology. Electroencephalography (EEG) may reveal focal slowing or epileptiform abnormalities such as sharp waves or spikes in patients with significant cortical or hemispheric lesions. Because tumors, infarctions, and hemorrhages may also cause seizures in addition to sensorimotor trigeminal dysfunction, EEG may be very useful. In addition, if symptoms described are paroxysmal or intermittent, focal seizures must be considered in the differential diagnosis. Brain stem auditory evoked potentials (BAEPs) may be useful in assessing the possibility of an intrinsic brain stem process as well as lesions within the adjacent cerebellopontine angle. For example, BAEPs may assist in identifying people with occult multiple sclerosis or small vessel brain stem strokes that may have subclinically affected pontine or medullary regions adjacent to the trigeminal nuclei.

Electrophysiological assessment of the corneal (blink) reflex latency can be reliably measured in an attempt to further localize a supranuclear, nuclear, or peripheral nerve process.[19] This electrically elicited response is similar to that tested at the bedside, and it allows measurement of the response latency after stimulating either the afferent trigeminal or efferent facial nerve components. The facial nerve can be stimulated directly at its exit near the mastoids and the direct response latency (contraction of the ipsilateral orbicularis oculi muscles) measured. For normal adults, this value is typically between 3.0 and 5.0 msec. In contrast, the afferent and efferent limbs of the blink reflex can be tested by stimulating the supraorbital nerve or tapping the glabellar regions and measuring response time to bilateral orbicularis contraction (normal values, approximately 30 msec; ipsilateral and contralateral latency differences less

TABLE 10–2. **Useful Studies in the Evaluation of the Trigeminal Nerve**

Syndrome	Neuroimaging	Electrophysiology	Fluid and Tissue Analysis	Neuropsychological Tests
Supranuclear	MRI with gadolinium for stroke, tumor, MS	EEG focal slowing or sharp waves	Increased protein, mild pleocytosis	Acalculia neglect
Nuclear lesions	MRI with gadolinium for stroke, tumor, MS	Abnormal BAEP, slowed blink reflex (V1)	Increased or normal protein, pleocytosis	NA
Preganglionic C-P angle	MRI with gadolinium for stroke, tumor, MS, meningitis, brain stem compression	Slowed blink reflex (V1)	Increased protein, pleocytosis, decreased glucose, abnormal cytology, positive CSF culture	NA
Gasserian ganglion	MRI with gadolinium for infection, tumor	Slowed blink reflex (V1)	Increased or normal protein, abnormal cytology, positive CSF culture	NA
Cavernous sinus	MRI with gadolinium for infection, thrombosis, aneurysm	Slowed blink reflex (V1)	CSF pleocytosis, low CSF glucose	NA
Peripheral CN V branches	Neuropathies	Slowed blink reflex (V1)	Increased or normal protein	NA
Trigeminal neuralgia	CN V root compression on MRI	No change	No change	NA

C-P, Cerebellopontine; MRI, magnetic resonance imaging; BAEP, brain stem auditory evoked potentials; NA, not applicable.

than 5 msec). Prolongation of the blink latency may be seen in compressive lesions of the trigeminal nerve, acoustic neuroma, Guillain-Barré syndrome, hereditary motor and sensory neuropathy type I, diabetes, and intrinsic brain stem processes. In contrast, clinical utility of trigeminal somatosensory evoked potentials is limited by technical problems of reliability and reproducibility.

Body Fluid and Tissue Analysis. Laboratory studies may reveal evidence of vasculopathies like systemic lupus erythematosus or Sjögren's syndrome. White blood count elevations may suggest infections, and eosinophilia may indicate fungal disease. Altered glucose tolerance is seen with diabetes mellitus. Vitamin levels may indicate deficiencies of thiamine, folate, vitamin B_{12}, pyridoxine, or vitamin A.

Cerebrospinal Fluid Evaluation. If infectious, neoplastic (especially meningeal carcinomatosis), or inflammatory (sarcoidosis) etiologies are suspected, cerebrospinal fluid (CSF) evaluation is warranted. CSF glucose level, protein level, differential white and red blood cell counts, and cytology tests are compulsory, whereas other studies to isolate mycobacterial, fungal, rickettsial, parasitic, and viral pathogens should be addressed on an individual basis. In the immunocompromised person (e.g., one with cancer, acquired immunodeficiency syndrome, and organ transplant), opportunistic pathogens causing infections such as cryptococcosis, candidiasis, mucormycosis, toxoplasmosis, and cytomegalovirus need to be seriously considered in the setting of any acute or subacute neurological presentation.

Clinical Syndromes

The trigeminal nerve may be involved in various neurological conditions, and, in most instances, the patient complains of sensory loss, paresthesias, pain, or difficulty eating (for complete review, see reference 16) (Table 10–3).

SUPRANUCLEAR SYNDROMES

Facial sensory loss may occur in the setting of lesions involving the trigeminothalamic pathways, corona radiata or internal capsule white matter projections from the VPM nucleus of the thalamus to primary sensory cortex, or within sensory cortex itself. Specific pathological processes affecting these pathways include ischemia, hemorrhage, neoplasm, and demyelinating diseases. All result in contralateral hemifacial and hemibody numbness. In seizures, facial tingling often occurs in association with hand numbness and suggests a lesion in the postcentral gyrus. In the cheiro-oral syndrome, ipsilateral numbness in the hand and at the corner of the mouth reflects an insult, typically vascular, at adjoining portions of the ventroposterolateral and VPM nuclei of the thalamus where the anatomical distributions of these regions are directly adjacent to one another. In contrast, a persistent deep, aching, poorly localized facial pain has been reported in patients with thalamic lesions including tumors, infarctions, and multiple sclerosis affecting the VPM nucleus. Often this syndrome is associated with small vessel infarctions of the thalamogeniculate artery.[20] The syndrome begins with transient facial hemisensory loss but then evolves into painful facial dysesthesias. Migraine headache may be misdiagnosed as trigeminal neuralgia, especially if pain is unilateral, although the duration of most headaches makes this distinction straightforward.

NUCLEAR (BRAIN STEM) SYNDROMES

Trauma, ischemic injury, and tumors may affect the trigeminal system within the brain stem. These syndromes

TABLE 10–3. **Selected Etiologies Associated with Trigeminal Nerve Disorders**

Etiological Category	Selected Specific Etiologies	Chapter
Structural Disorders		
Developmental	Brain stem vascular loop, syringobulbia	28
Degenerative and compressive	Paget's disease	29
Hereditary and Degenerative Disorders		
Chromosomal abnormalities and neurocutaneous disorders	Hereditary sensorimotor neuropathy 1 Neurofibromatosis (schwannoma)	32
Degenerative motor, sensory, and autonomic disorders	Amyotrophic lateral sclerosis	36
Acquired Metabolic and Nutritional Disorders		
Endogenous metabolic disorders	Diabetes	38
Exogenous disorders: Toxins and illicit drugs	Trichloroethylene, trichloroacetic acid	39
Nutritional deficiencies and syndromes associated with alcoholism	Thiamine, folate, B_{12}, pyridoxine, pantothenic acid, vitamin A deficiency	40
Infectious Disorders		
Viral infections	Herpes zoster, unknown	41
Nonviral infections	Bacterial, tuberculous meningitis, brain abscess, Gradenigo's syndrome, leprosy, cavernous sinus thrombosis	43
HIV and AIDS	Opportunistic infections, abscesses, herpes zoster	44
Neurovascular Disorders	Stroke, hemorrhage, aneurysm	45
Neoplastic Disorders		
Primary neurological tumors	Glial tumors, meningioma, schwannoma	46
Metastatic neoplasms and paraneoplastic syndromes	Lung, breast, lymphoma, carcinomatous meningitis	47
Demyelinating Disorders		
Demyelinating disorders of the central nervous system	Multiple sclerosis, acute demyelinating encephalomyelitis	48
Demyelinating disorders of the peripheral nervous system	Guillain-Barré syndrome, chronic inflammatory demyelinating polyneuropathy	49
Autoimmune and Inflammatory Disorders	Tolosa-Hunt syndrome, sarcoidosis, lupus, orbital pseudotumor	50
Traumatic Disorders	Carotid–cavernous fistula, cavernous sinus thrombosis, maxillary/mandibular injury	51
Epilepsy	Focal seizures	52
Headache and Facial Pain	Raeder's neuralgia, cluster headache	53
Drug-Induced and Iatrogenic Neurological Disorders	Orbital, facial, dental surgery	55

are characterized by sensory paresthesias, numbness, or pain in the distribution of the V1 to V3, along with combinations of cranial nerve palsies and distinct sensory and cerebellar system signs. Reflecting the lateral circumferential arterial supply to the lateral pons, ischemic lesions of the pontine tegmentum are often associated with dissociation of sensory modalities such that pain and temperature perception are dramatically diminished, whereas midline fiber tracts carrying light touch and deep pressure are spared. Pain similar to that of trigeminal neuralgia is rare. The lateral medullary or Wallenberg's syndrome[21] typically results from ischemic infarction of either the vertebral or posterior inferior cerebellar arteries, which provide vascular supply to the lateral medulla. Sensory loss may affect the entire ipsilateral face. Sensory loss results from damage to the spinal trigeminal tract, its nucleus, and rostral trigeminothalamic projections. Interestingly, some patients with Wallenberg's syndrome report facial pain or headache before neurological deficit.[22]

Persistent ipsilateral pain may be present in up to 50 percent of patients with a lateral medullary syndrome[21] typically in V1 or V2 distribution, which in some persists for months to years after the acute insult. The pattern of facial analgesia in patients with lateral medullary syndrome typically adheres to the cutaneous distribution of V1 to V3, although an onion-skin or radicular pattern of sensory loss has been described in which lesions affecting more rostral portions of the trigeminal sensory nuclei result in sensory loss in the nose and lips, whereas rostral and caudal lesions yield sensory loss in the cheeks and forehead (see Fig. 10–1). Associated neurological symptoms with Wallenberg's syndrome include ipsilateral Horner's syndrome, ataxia, and difficulty swallowing, with pain and temperature loss on the contralateral body (due to damage to the ascending spinothalamic tract). Lesions affecting the spinothalamic and spinal trigeminal tracts in the lateral medulla typically result in this crossed pattern of hemifacial and hemibody sensory loss (ipsilateral facial numbness with contralateral arm and leg numbness). Lesions involving more medial medullary regions result in unilateral facial and bodily sensory deficits contralateral to the lesion.[23] Medial medullary lesions presumably injure the crossed ventral trigeminothalamic tract.

Other pathological processes within the brain stem can produce trigeminal dysfunction. Tumors, hemorrhage (hypertensive, ruptured arteriovenous malformation), infarctions, demyelinating disease such as multiple sclerosis (Fig. 10–5), infections such as brain stem abscesses and brain stem encephalitis, and inflammatory conditions such as tuberculosis or sarcoidosis affecting the lateral pons or midbrain may result in ipsilateral or contralateral facial sensory loss, respectively, as well as severe paroxysmal hemifacial pain. Facial weakness, muscle atrophy, difficulty chewing, and diminished jaw jerk reflex may be identified in amyotrophic lateral sclerosis as well as other motor neuron disorders damaging the motor trigeminal nuclei. Traumatic or congenital syringobulbia can affect the sensory and motor portions of the trigeminal system within the midbrain, pons, or medulla.

PREGANGLIONIC SYNDROMES

Trigeminal nerve compression can occur in the area between the brain stem nuclei and the gasserian ganglion, specifically within the brain stem itself or in the cerebellopontine angle. Patients can present with reduced facial sensation in association with poor hearing, nystagmus, limb ataxia, facial weakness, and a diminished corneal reflex. Common lesions in this area include tumors[24] such as acoustic or trigeminal neuromas,[25] meningiomas, metastatic cancers, carcinomatous meningitis, and invasive nasopharyngeal carcinomas, inflammatory disorders such as sarcoidosis, or infectious processes such as mycobacterial (especially tuberculosis), fungal (candidal, histoplasmotic), parasitic, and bacterial organisms. Traumatic injury to this region may also result in sensory loss or motor deficits. Extensive brain stem and cerebellar signs may be evident from lesions in the cerebellopontine angle.

GASSERIAN GANGLION SYNDROMES

Numerous pathological processes occurring within the middle cranial fossa can result in trigeminal dysfunction by affecting the gasserian ganglion. In children, osteitis of the petrous apex following suppurative otitis media or mastoiditis, which leads to inflammation and infection affecting the trigeminal ganglion, may result in Gradenigo's syndrome. The syndrome is characterized by facial pain, headache, or sensory loss and a cranial nerve VI palsy, facial palsy (due to cranial nerve VII involvement), and deafness (due to cranial nerve VIII involvement). The pain is described as boring or throbbing, worse at night. Pain is aggravated by jaw or ear movement. It has been hypothesized that some of the dysesthetic sensation patients experience before or during episodes of Bell's palsy may reflect involvement of the trigeminal ganglion or nuclei in the brain stem.[26] A benign, self-limited trigeminal sensory neuropathy has been reported in children 7 to 21 days following a nonspecific febrile illness or upper respiratory infection.[27] Like other postinfectious cranial neuropathies involving the abducens, glossopharyngeal, or hypoglossal nerves, laboratory evaluations are normal or show only a mild CSF pleocytosis. Symptoms resolve usually within 1 to 2 months. It is unknown whether these postinfectious neuropathies result from peripheral nerve, ganglion, or brain stem pathology.

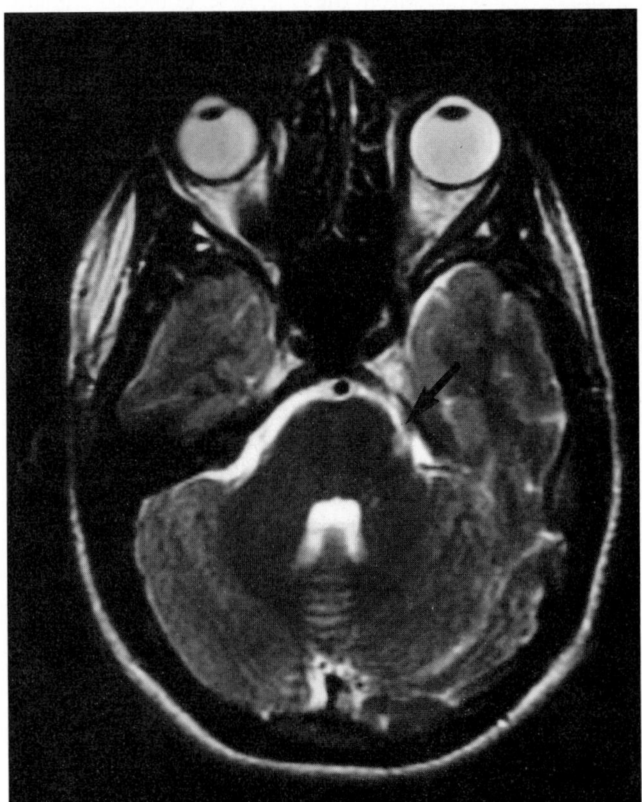

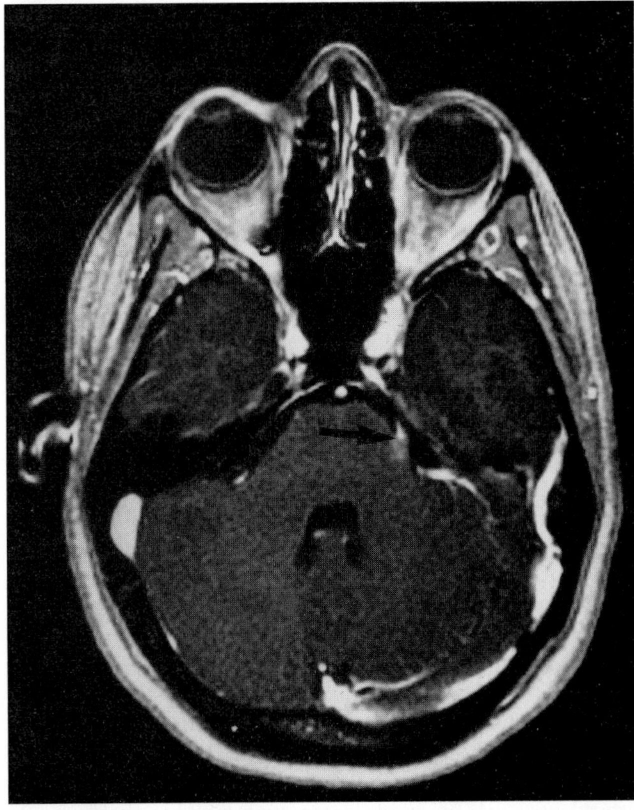

FIGURE 10–5. Axial MRI image from a patient with multiple sclerosis. *Left,* high signal abnormality along left trigeminal nerve course (*arrow*). *Right,* the nerve enhances after gadolinium injection (*arrow*).

Trigeminal sensory neuropathy may occur in association with connective tissue disorders such as mixed connective tissue disease, systemic sclerosis, Sjögren's syndrome, and systemic lupus erythematosus.[28, 29] Symptoms including facial dysesthesias, numbness, and loss of taste may be the presenting complaints.[30] In such cases, based on radiographical and electrophysiological testing, involvement of the gasserian ganglion is likely. Various infectious processes within the middle cranial fossa including syphilis, tuberculosis, and bacterial meningitis can affect the gasserian ganglion by inflammation, ischemia, or direct compression. Similarly, neoplasms in this region (meningiomas, schwannomas) can compress the ganglion within Meckel's cave.

SYNDROMES OF LESIONS INVOLVING PERIPHERAL BRANCHES OF CRANIAL NERVE V

Another disorder similar to both cluster headache and trigeminal neuralgia is Raeder's paratrigeminal neuralgia.[31] This syndrome is characterized by intense pain in the distribution of V1, lacrimation, conjunctival injection, rhinorrhea, and ipsilateral pupillary mydriasis (Horner's syndrome). This syndrome may be idiopathic or may result from pathology affecting the ipsilateral carotid artery or structures within the middle cranial fossa. In the idiopathic form, patients tend to be middle-aged or elderly males who develop a severe throbbing orbital or retro-orbital headache upon awakening. Additional signs such as lacrimation, conjunctival injection, and oculosympathetic dysfunction develop later. Therapy includes ergotamine tartrate, methysergide, and systemic corticosteroids. In both cluster headache and Raeder's syndrome, the pain in V1, duration of attacks, and associated features help distinguish the condition from trigeminal neuralgia. Raeder's paratrigeminal neuralgia may not actually represent a distinct clinical entity because those patients with an isolated Horner's syndrome likely have cluster headaches, whereas those with ocular motility impairment have a cavernous sinus process until proven otherwise. Furthermore, it is important to consider the possibility of a carotid dissection in a patient who presents with an isolated painful Horner's syndrome.

The skull base and exit points of V1 to V3 (i.e., at the superior orbital fissure, foramen ovale, or foramen rotundum) can be diseased and can result in focal sensory or sensorimotor trigeminal dysfunction. For example, acute or resolved bacterial, tuberculous, carcinomatous, or granulomatous (sarcoid) meningitis can result in inflammation, infiltration, or congestion of the basal meninges through which V1 to V3 nerve roots exit the skull. In Paget's disease, narrowing of the skull foramina can also lead to cranial (trigeminal) neuropathy. If V3 is affected, motor and sensory manifestations may be identified in one or more branches of the trigeminal system (Fig. 10–6).

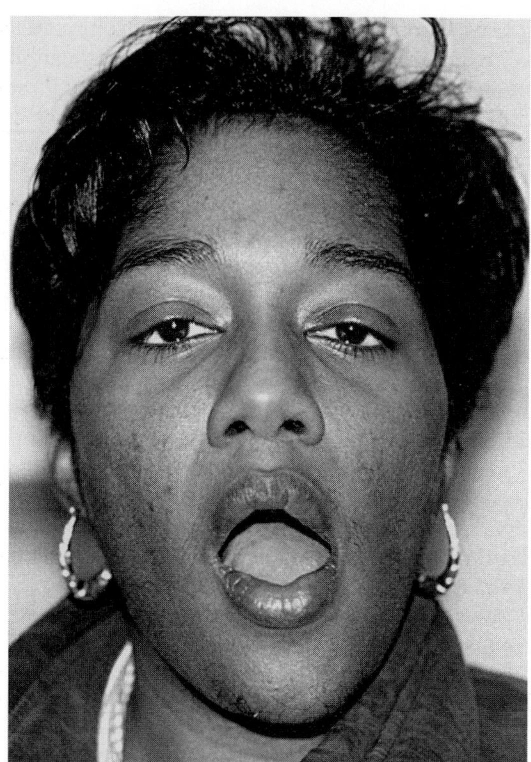

FIGURE 10–6. Left-sided trigeminal nerve involvement from sarcoid involving the skull base and meninges. Weakness of the pterygoids and masseters manifested as ipsilateral (leftward) jaw deviation and weakness of jaw opening.

Various pathological processes including tumors, aneurysms, infarctions, trauma, and infections can damage the ophthalmic division of the trigeminal nerve.[32] Superior orbital fissure involvement is characterized by numbness, paresthesias, or pain in the distribution of V1 and within the orbit, Horner's syndrome, and ophthalmoparesis. Involvement of the optic nerve suggests extension into the orbital apex. If, on funduscopic examination, there is evidence of venous congestion, cavernous sinus thrombosis is likely. Cavernous sinus thrombosis is almost always caused by spread of an infection from the face, nose, or mouth. Patients may initially complain of fever, malaise, and frontal headache, but they subsequently develop proptosis, ptosis, ophthalmoparesis, and vasocongestion. Initially the CSF test result may be normal, but findings characteristic of meningitis may occur if treatment is delayed. Mortality is linked to spread of bacteria to the meninges, which warrants early and intensive antibiotic therapy. In contrast, carotid–cavernous sinus arteriovenous fistulae may be congenital in children but in adults are more commonly the result of trauma. Carotid–cavernous sinus arteriovenous fistulae also occur in women during pregnancy or at childbirth. On examination, pulsating proptosis, conjunctival erythema, ophthalmoparesis, and a bruit over the globe may be found. Diagnosis by CT or angiography is usual, and treatment with neurosurgical or invasive radiological approaches is warranted.

In addition, there are several syndromes involving the peripheral trigeminal branches. Cluster headache appears as multiple attacks of severe head or facial pain and may be confused with trigeminal neuralgia.[33] Cluster headache typically occurs in middle-aged men and is more prominent at night. Attacks are of short duration; they occur in clusters that recur with variable frequency. Unlike trigeminal neuralgia, trigger points are not a characteristic feature. The associated symptoms of cluster headache such as lacrimation, conjunctival injection, sweating, ipsilateral nasal blockage, miosis, and ptosis are quite distinct from symptoms of trigeminal neuralgia. Studies have suggested, however, that disruption of normal autoregulatory trigeminovascular innervation may be responsible for cluster headache.[33]

Crescendo orbital pain or frontal headache can herald impending internal carotid artery occlusion presumably from irritation or ischemia to peripheral trigeminal branches. Similarly, a cluster of symptoms including facial, orbital, or neck pain or facial paresthesias in association with an ipsilateral Horner's syndrome may reflect dissection of the cervical portion of the internal carotid artery.[34] These symptoms may also be prodromal. Excruciating pain in the supraorbital headache in association with a pupil involving cranial nerve III palsy is almost pathognomonic for an intracranial (especially posterior communicating artery) aneurysm. Ipsilateral orbital or ocular pain has also been reported in association with posterior cerebral artery occlusion, which may reflect ischemic damage to regions of the tentorium adjacent to the occipital lobes that are innervated by V1.

Circumscribed facial paresthesias in V1 to V3 distributions have been identified in patients with diabetes mellitus, Guillain-Barré syndrome, hereditary sensory motor neuropathy I,[35] chronic inflammatory demyelinating polyneuropathy, nutritional deficiencies, and other peripheral neuropathological disorders. Vascular infarction of the nerve branches, for example, in vasculitis can also result in sensory loss. Compressive or infiltrative processes affecting any of the peripheral trigeminal branches result in focal, well-circumscribed sensory loss or paresthesias (see numb chin syndrome, later). Dental trauma and exposure to various toxic substances such as trichloroethylene and trichloroacetic acid can also result in circumscribed facial sensory loss or paresthesias in the trigeminal distribution.

The temporomandibular joint (TMJ) syndrome refers to recurrent pain in the region of the jaw, ear, occiput, and supraorbital regions, which is believed to result from degeneration or malocclusion of the TMJ. Erosion of the bony surfaces within the glenoid fossa may cause irritation of several adjacent nerves including the auriculotemporal and chorda tympani trigeminal nerves. Patients may report an increase in pain in the evening and pain referred to the oropharynx. Rarely, a sensation of hearing dullness or auricular congestion may be noted. The TMJ syndrome may result from local trauma, neoplastic invasion, ankylosis, or inflammation, although some cases reflect nonorganic or ill-defined joint pain syndromes. On examination, the TMJ may appear lax and may be painful to passive motion or palpation. Correction of an underlying malocclusion may be curative, but other measures include analgesics, jaw exercises, soft diet, and tricyclic antidepressants.[36]

The numb chin syndrome (mental neuropathy) often reflects a bony lesion affecting the mental foramen through which V3 passes to innervate the chin and mandible.[37, 38] Patients often report numbness or pain on one or both sides of the chin, which may extend to the lip or submandibular region. Frequent causes include granulomatous diseases such as histiocytosis X; primary bony malignancies such as osteosarcoma, fibrosarcoma, and plasmacytoma; and metastatic lesions from lung, breast, and prostate carcinoma[39] as well as lymphoma (especially Burkitt's lymphoma). Development of a numb chin in a patient with cancer in remission may indicate relapse. Nonmalignant etiologies include collagen vascular disorders, trauma, periodontal disease, benign bony cyst, focal idiopathic osteolysis (Gorham's disease),[40] and sickle cell disease. A variant of the numb chin syndrome is the numb cheek syndrome, which results from a bony lesion affecting the infraorbital foramen or the maxillary sinus and trigeminal branch V2.[41] On rare occasions, focal motor weakness affecting the masticatory muscles results from damage to motor branches of V3.

Evaluation of patients with focal sensory loss over the chin or malar region begins with a full, careful sensory examination to determine whether the sensory loss results from a distal or proximal trigeminal lesion. Specifically, mental neuropathy causes focal sensory loss over the lower lip and chin, whereas more proximal V3 dysfunction results in more widespread sensory disturbance and may be associated with dysfunction of other cranial nerves. Motor involvement is characterized by ipsilateral jaw deviation, flaccidity of the floor of the mouth, and wasting of the ipsilateral temporalis muscle. Weakness of the tensor tympani results in difficulty detecting low-pitched sounds. Careful examination of the oropharynx, dentition, and skin over the chin should also be performed because erythema and edema may be present over a focal bony lesion. Plain radiographs of the mandible may be very useful in establishing the diagnosis because they may be revealing in about 50 percent of cases. If the result is abnormal, bone scan and biopsy of the lesion itself may be indicated. A search for occult malignancy employing CT of the chest and abdomen, prostate-specific antigen (in men), and bone marrow biopsy may be necessary. If radiographs are normal, evaluation of the brain and cranial nerves by MRI (with contrast) and lumbar puncture for cytology is indicated because a brain stem lesion or carcinomatous meningitis may cause focal trigeminal dysfunction.

Corneal hypesthesia and orbital pain may result from local corneal dystrophies or reflect damage to branches of V1, which innervate these structures. Viral (herpetic) infections, diabetes, leprosy, and vitamin A deficiency can result in unilateral or bilateral corneal hypesthesia. In addition, the pain associated with anterior uveitis, acute angle-closure glaucoma, and optic neuritis is mediated through V1 orbital sensory fibers. Clinically, a diminished corneal reflex may be detected. In the orbit, inflammatory conditions such as cellulitis, pseudotumor, or neoplasms (lymphoma, metastatic tumors) may present as orbital pain in association with ophthalmoparesis. Trigeminal involvement in orbital pseudotumor is uncommon. Infections within the orbit including those from bacterial and fungal pathogens such as *Streptococcus* and *Mucor*, respectively, can also result in a painful ophthalmoplegia. The Tolosa-Hunt syndrome (painful ophthalmoplegia) is characterized by steady, unremitting retro- and supraorbital pain (in the cutaneous V1 distribution) in association with paresis of cranial nerves III, IV, and VI, and a diminished corneal reflex (for review, see reference 42). Sensory loss and pain in V2 distribution may also occur. Less frequently, the optic nerve and oculosympathetic fibers may be affected as well. Symptoms may persist for weeks to months. Pathologically, a low-grade, granulomatous, noninfectious, inflammatory process adjacent to the cavernous sinus or within the superior orbital fissure has been identified consisting of lymphocytes and plasma cells. The Tolosa-Hunt syndrome typically responds dramatically to systemic corticosteroids, although symptoms may recur over months to years. Spontaneous remissions have also been reported.

Other causes of decreased sensation within the globe and conjunctiva are orbital surgery or orbital trauma, which affect

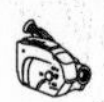

nasociliary and frontal branches of V1. In herpes zoster ophthalmicus (Fig. 10–7), inflammation and vesicular eruption involving all branches of V1 as well as small arterioles within the gasserian ganglion may result in excruciating, lancinating pain in the periorbital region.[43] Symptoms of herpes zoster ophthalmicus typically begin 2 to 3 days before the appearance of vesicles and may diminish after 2 to 3 weeks. Hypalgesia and paresthesias may be noted during and after lesions heal. Pain may persist after the rash is gone only to evolve into post-herpetic neuralgia. This syndrome consists of burning, lancinating, aching pain in the V1 territory often in association with paresthesias and hyperpathia. As in trigeminal neuralgia, trigger points can evoke pain in response to cutaneous stimuli.[44, 45]

Atypical facial pain can also reflect trigeminal branch disorders.[43, 46] Some patients experience persistent facial pain that is not confined to the distribution of V1 to V3 and that differs in character from classic trigeminal neuralgia. Many of these atypical facial pain syndromes, including Charlin's nasociliary neuralgia, Sluder's pterygopalatine ganglion syndrome, and Vail's vidian neuralgia, involve portions of the trigeminal nerve. They are also characterized by numerous autonomic symptoms such as lacrimation, conjunctival injection, altered sweating, salivation, facial flushing, and nasal congestion, which are believed to result from involvement of the autonomic ganglia (ciliary, pterygopalatine) in the face. These atypical facial neuralgias are additionally characterized by nondermatomal localization of pain; bilateral symptoms; continual instead of paroxysmal pain; lack of clear trigger zones; and deep, poorly localized pain.[46] Appropriate therapy for these debilitating and often refractory disorders is often unsatisfactory and has consisted of surgical ablation of peripheral pain fibers, peripheral or sympathetic nerve blockade, transcutaneous electrical stimulation, tricyclic antidepressants, and narcotic and nonnarcotic analgesics.

TRIGEMINAL NEURALGIA (TIC DOULOUREUX)

Painful neuralgia of the trigeminal nerve results in the clinical syndrome of tic douloureux or trigeminal neuralgia.[47] The paroxysmal disorder presents as excruciating, lancinating painful spasms affecting one or more divisions of cranial nerve V. Trigeminal neuralgia is unilateral and usually affects the second or third division of cranial nerve V (3rd > 2nd > 1st). In less than 5 percent of cases, V1 is affected, whereas V3 is affected in more than 70 percent of cases.[48] Rarely, pain may occur bilaterally, although simultaneous bilateral spasms are quite atypical. The pain occurs spontaneously as brief lightning-like spasms lasting seconds to minutes, or pain may be precipitated by cutaneous or auditory stimuli. In many instances, there is a demonstrable trigger point that can reproduce pain, and some patients may be unable to chew, eat, drink, shave, or brush their teeth for fear of triggering a spasm.[49] Paroxysms recur throughout the day and night. Between attacks, there are no symptoms, but the patient is usually anxious about having another attack. Objective sensory or motor deficits are not a feature, although a subjective report of hypesthesias over the face may be reported. Often there is a temporal summation of stimuli necessary to invoke a response. The pain is reported as lancinating, stabbing, searing, burning, or electrical, and the intensity is such that the patient often winces or grimaces in a tic-like fashion. Trigeminal neuralgia affects approximately 155 people per million population and has a slight female predominance (3:2). It is the most common neuralgia, and its incidence peaks in middle age. The age of onset is important, however, because the appearance of trigeminal neuralgia in a young patient should raise the suspicion of demyelinating disease such as multiple sclerosis[50, 51] or another structural brain stem disorder.[52–54]

Pathological analyses of trigeminal biopsy specimens taken during vascular decompression have described focal

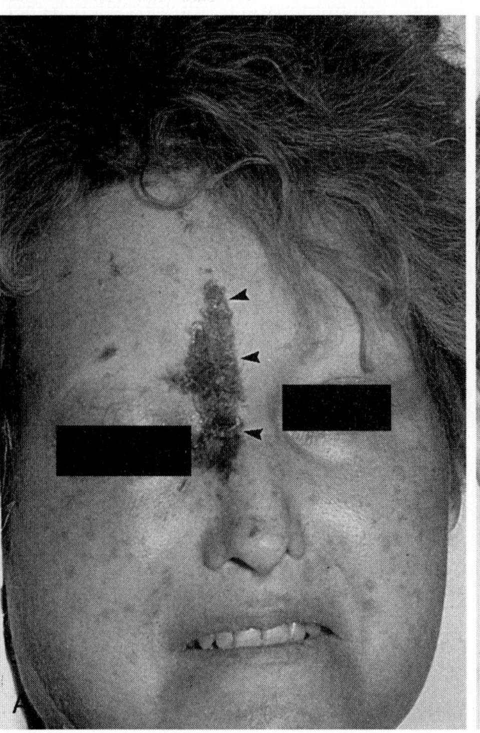

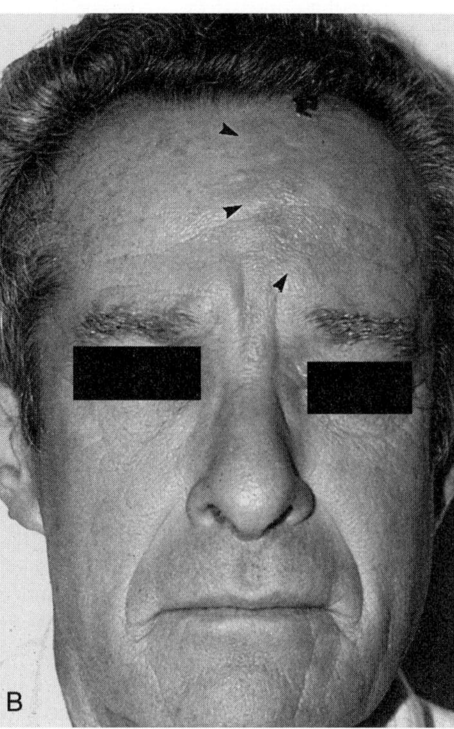

FIGURE 10–7. Acute (*A*) and resolving (*B*) herpes zoster (*arrows*). In *A*, there is selective involvement of the nasociliary branch of the trigeminal nerve.

demyelination but no inflammatory cells.[55–57] Abnormal ephaptic nonsynaptic neurotransmission between demyelinated trigeminal axons within the nerve root, ganglion, or spinal trigeminal nucleus may provide the physiological substrate for the paroxysmal pain characteristic of trigeminal neuralgia, especially if initiated by cutaneous stimuli.[58]

On physical examination, objective neurological deficits are not present. The patient, however, may appear emaciated if, for example, a trigger point is initiated during chewing, or males may appear disheveled if shaving induces a spasm. Laboratory study results are normal. Careful inspection and palpation of the teeth, gums, nares, nasal sinuses, palate, and pharynx should be performed because disease processes such as infections or inflammatory disorders in these regions can cause significant facial pain. MRI of patients with trigeminal neuralgia may be helpful in identifying other etiologies or associated disorders.

The diagnosis of tic douloureux can usually be made by history alone, but the disorder must be distinguished from other causes of facial pain syndromes such as glossopharyngeal neuralgia, which can be confused with tic douloureux that involves the third division of cranial nerve V. Herpes zoster or post-herpetic neuralgia may also provide some diagnostic confusion. Tumors or vascular lesions of the cerebellopontine angle[25] or within the trigeminal ganglion itself may induce pain similar to that of trigeminal neuralgia, although these disorders can be distinguished by findings of trigeminal sensory loss, atrophy of facial masticatory muscles, diminished corneal reflexes, and involvement of other adjacent brain stem structures that are not characteristic of trigeminal neuralgia. The nature of the pain in these cases is also distinct from that of trigeminal neuralgia in that it is often continuous and unremitting rather than episodic.[58]

General Management Goals

In approaching any patient with symptoms referable to the trigeminal system, it is necessary to localize the pathological process; identify associated symptoms; determine prognosis; and provide relief from pain, discomfort, and functional disability. Regardless of etiology, a detailed and directed neurological examination most often yields the correct anatomical localization.

Once determined that the likely etiology is, for example, within the brain, brain stem, or cranial vault, a rational first step is MRI of the brain with and without gadolinium contrast. Fine cuts may be obtained through the orbits, using fat saturation sequences to diminish intraorbital fat artifact. Similarly, dedicated coronal images may be taken to focus on the cavernous sinus. Recently, vascular compression of the trigeminal nerve in trigeminal neuralgia has been directly demonstrated by MRI and MR angiography.[59] Once appropriate neuroimaging has been performed, other diagnostic studies such as lumbar puncture may be indicated, especially if infectious or carcinomatous processes are suspected. Electrophysiological studies such as somatosensory evoked potentials may be somewhat helpful in peripheral trigeminal neuropathies. In either central or peripheral causes, neurosurgical consultation may be warranted, especially when there is compression of the trigeminal nerve roots or branches.

Prompt relief of the severe pain associated with this disorder must not be neglected. Both medical and surgical approaches should be considered when appropriate. Over the short term, nonsteroidal anti-inflammatory agents and narcotics may provide symptomatic relief. In patients with refractory neuropathic pain, treatment with tricyclic compounds such as amitriptyline, nortriptyline, or carbamazepine may be indicated. In patients with medically intractable facial pain, including tic douloureux, more invasive therapeutic approaches have been attempted. These strategies include peripheral glycerol injections,[60] stereotactic gamma knife radiosurgery,[61] percutaneous balloon compression of the trigeminal ganglion,[62] and even repetitive transcranial magnetic stimulation.[63]

Reviews and Selected Updates

Atlas S: Magnetic Resonance Imaging of the Brain and Spine. New York, Raven Press, 1991.

Brodal P: The trigeminal nerve. *In* The Central Nervous System. New York, Oxford, 1992, pp 328–331.

Gass A, Kitchen N, MacManus DG: Trigeminal neuralgia in patients with multiple sclerosis: Lesion localization with magnetic resonance imaging. Neurology 1997;49:1142–1144.

Maciewicz R, Scrivani S: Trigeminal neuralgia: Gamma radiosurgery may provide new options for treatment. Neurology 1997;48:565–566.

Miller N: Facial pain and neuralgia. *In* Miller NR (ed): Walsh and Hoyt's Clinical Neuro-Ophthalmology, 4th ed. Baltimore, Williams & Wilkins, 1988.

Rowland LP: Injury to cranial and peripheral nerves. *In* Rowland LP (ed): Merritt's Textbook of Neurology. Philadelphia, Lea and Febiger, 1989, pp 413–443.

References

1. Carpenter MB: Core Text of Neuroanatomy, 4th ed. Philadelphia, Williams & Wilkins, 1991, pp 176–182.
2. Burr HS, Robinson GB: An anatomical study of the gasserian ganglion, with particular reference to the nature and extent of Meckel's cave. Anat Rec 1925;29:269–282.
3. Gudmundsson K, Rhoton AL, Rushton JG: Detailed anatomy of the intracranial portion of the trigeminal nerve. J Neurosurg 1971;35:592–600.
4. Feindel W, Penfield W, McNaughton F: The tentorial nerves and localization of intracranial pain in man. Neurology 1960;10:555–563.
5. Liu-Chen L-Y, Gillespie SA, Norregaard TV, et al: Co-localization of retrogradely transported wheat germ agglutinin and the putative neurotransmitter substance P within trigeminal ganglion cells projecting to the cat middle cerebral artery. J Comp Neurol 1984;225:187–192.
6. Uddman R, Edvinnson L, Ekman R, et al: Innervation of the feline cerebral vasculature by nerve fibers containing calcitonin gene-related peptide: Trigeminal origin and co-existence with substance P. Neurosci Lett 1985;62:131–136.
7. Goadsby PJ, Edvinnson L: Release of vasoactive peptides in the extracerebral circulation of humans and the cat during activation of the trigeminovascular system. Ann Neurol 1988;23:193–196.
8. Tran-Dinh YR, Thurel C, Cunin G, et al: Cerebral vasodilation after the thermocoagulation of the trigeminal ganglion in humans. Neurosurgery 1992;31:658–662.
9. Torvick A: Afferent connections to the trigeminal sensory nuclei, the nucleus of the solitary tract, and adjacent structures: An experimental study in the rat. J Comp Neurol 1956;106:51–141.
10. Jones EG: The Thalamus. New York, Plenum Press, 1988.
11. Williams MN, Zahm DS, Jacquin MF: Differential foci and synaptic organization of the principle and spinal trigeminal projections to the thalamus in the rat. Eur J Neurosci 1994;6:429–453.
12. Radolsky I: Dorsal pontines tumor syndrome. Z Gesamte Neurol Psychiatry 1935;152:530–537.
13. Tensor RB, Corbett JJ: Myokymia and facial contraction in brain stem glioma. Arch Neurol 1974;30:425–427.
14. Kimura J, Rodnitzky RL, Van Allen MW: Electrodiagnostic study of the trigeminal nerve: Orbicularis oculi reflex and masseter reflex

in trigeminal neuralgia, paratrigeminal syndrome and other lesions of the trigeminal nerve. Neurology 1970;20:574–577.

15. Kimura J: Effects of hemispheral lesions on the contralateral blink reflex: A clinical study. Neurology 1974;24:168–174.
16. Miller N: Facial pain and neuralgia. *In* Walsh and Hoyt's Clinical Neuro-Ophthalmology, 4th ed. Baltimore, Williams & Wilkins, 1988.
17. Atlas S: Magnetic Resonance Imaging of the Brain and Spine. New York, Raven Press, 1991.
18. Rubenstein D, Stears RLG, Stears JC: Trigeminal nerve and ganglion in the Meckel cave: Appearance at CT and MR imaging. Radiology 1994;193:155–159.
19. Kimura J: Electrodiagnosis in Diseases of Nerve and Muscle: Principles and Practice, 2nd ed. Philadelphia, F.A. Davis, 1989.
20. Dejerine J, Roussy G: Le syndrome thalamique. Rev Neurol 1906;14:521–532.
21. Currier RD, Giles CL, DeJong RN: Some comments on Wallenberg's lateral medullary syndrome. Neurology 1961;11:778–791.
22. Hornsten G: Wallenberg's syndrome: Part I. General symptomatology with special reference to visual disturbances and imbalance. Acta Neurol Scand 1974;50:434–446.
23. Matsumoto S, Okuda B, Imai T, Kameyama M: A sensory level on the trunk in lower lateral brain stem lesions. Neurology 1988;38:1515–1519.
24. Posner JB: Cancer involving cranial and peripheral nerves. *In* Posner JB (ed): Neurologic Complications of Cancer. Philadelphia, F.A. Davis, 1995, pp 181–182.
25. Martini D, Har-El G, Johnson C: Trigeminal neurinoma. Ann Otol Rhinol Laryngol 1994;103:652–654.
26. Hanner P: Trigeminal dysfunction in patients with Bell's palsy. Acta Otolaryngol 1986;101:224–226.
27. Blau JN, Harris M, Kennett S: Trigeminal sensory neuropathy. N Engl J Med 1969;281:873–877.
28. Lecky BRF, Hughes RAC, Murray NMF: Trigeminal sensory neuropathy. Brain 1987;110:1463–1485.
29. Olney RK: AAEM minimonograph #38: Neuropathies in connective tissue disease. Muscle Nerve 1992;15:531–542.
30. Forster C, Brandt T, Hund E, et al: Trigeminal sensory neuropathy in connective tissue disease: Evidence for the site of the lesion. Neurology 1996;46:270–271.
31. Raeder JG: Paratrigeminal paralysis of oculo-pupillary sympathetic. Brain 1924;47:149–158.
32. Glaser J: Textbook of Clinical Neuro-Ophthalmology. Philadelphia, JB Lippincott, 1990.
33. Goadsby PJ, Edvinnson L: Human *in vivo* evidence for trigeminovascular activation in cluster headache. Brain 1994;117:427–434.
34. Fisher CM: The headache and pain of spontaneous carotid dissection. Headache 1981;22:60–65.
35. Coffey RJ, Fromm GH: Familial trigeminal neuralgia and Charcot-Marie-Tooth neuropathy. Surg Neurol 1991;35:49–53.
36. Reik L, Hale M: The temporomandibular joint pain-dysfunction syndrome: A frequent cause of headache. Headache 1981;21:151–156.
37. Massey EW, Moore J, Schold SC: Mental neuropathy. Neurology 1981;31:1277–1281.
38. Brazis PW, Vogler LB, Shaw KE: The numb cheek-lip lower lid syndrome. Neurology 1991;41:327–328.
39. Lossos A, Siegal T: Numb chin syndrome in cancer patients: Etiology, response to treatment, and prognostic significance. Neurology 1992;42:1181–1184.
40. Malter IM: Massive osteolysis of the mandible: Report of a case. J Am Dental Assoc 1972;85:148–150.
41. Campbell WW: The numb cheek syndrome: A sign of infraorbital neuropathy. Neurology 1986;36:421–423.
42. Kline LB: The Tolosa-Hunt syndrome. Surv Ophthalmol 1982;27:79–86.
43. Schott GD: Neurogenic facial pain. Trans Ophthalmol Soc 1980;100: 253–256.
44. Weller THE: Varicella and herpes zoster. N Engl J Med 1983;309: 1434–1440.
45. Olson ER, Ivy HB: Stellate block for trigeminal zoster. J Clin Neuro-Ophthal 1981;1:53–55.
46. White JC, Sweet WH: Pain and the Neurosurgeon. A Forty Year Experience. Springfield, IL, Charles C Thomas, 1969, pp 129–147.
47. Illingworth R: Trigeminal neuralgia: Surgical aspects. *In* Rose FC (ed): Handbook of Clinical Neurology. Amsterdam, Elsevier, 1986, pp 449–458.
48. Dandy WE: Concerning the cause of trigeminal neuralgia. Am J Surg 1934;24:447–455.
49. Roberts AM, Person P: Etiology and treatment of idiopathic trigeminal and atypical facial neuralgias. Oral Surg 1979;48:298–308.
50. Rushton JG, Olafson RA: Trigeminal neuralgia associated with multiple sclerosis. Arch Neurol 1965;13:383–386.
51. Olafson RA, Rushton JG, Sayre GP: Trigeminal neuralgia in a patient with multiple sclerosis: An autopsy report. J Neurosurg 1966;24:755–759.
52. Leibrock LG, Moore GF, Yetter M: Malpositioned endolymphatic shunt causing trigeminal neuralgia: Case report. Acta Neurochir 1994;126:192–194.
53. Janetta PJ: Arterial compression of the trigeminal nerve at the pons in patients with trigeminal neuralgia. J Neurosurg 1967;26:159–167.
54. Janetta PJ: Observations on the etiology of trigeminal neuralgia, hemifacial spasm, acoustic nerve dysfunction, and glossopharyngeal dysfunction: Definitive microsurgical treatment and results in 117 patients. Neurochirgica 1977;20:145–154.
55. Hamlyn PJ, King TT: Neurovascular compression in trigeminal neuralgia: A clinical and anatomic study. J Neurosurg 1992;76:948–954.
56. Hilton DA, Love S, Gradidge T, et al: Pathological findings associated with trigeminal neuralgia caused by vascular compression. Neurosurgery 1994;35(2):299–303.
57. Richards P, Shawdon H, Illingworth R: Operative findings on microsurgical exploration of the cerebellopontine angle in trigeminal neuralgia. J Neurol Neurosurg Psychiatry 1983;46:1098–1101.
58. Love S, Coakham HB: Trigeminal neuralgia: Pathology and pathogenesis. Brain 2001;124:2347–2360.
59. Bakshi R, Lerner A, Fritz JV, Sambuchi GD: Vascular compression in trigeminal neuralgia shown by magnetic resonance imaging and magnetic resonance angiography image registration. Arch Neurol 2001;58:1290–1291.
60. Erdem E, Alkan A: Peripheral glycerol injections in the treatment of idiopathic trigeminal neuralgia: Retrospective analysis of 157 cases. J Oral Maxillofac Surg 2001;59:1176–1180.
61. Friedman DP, Morales RE, Goldman HW: Role of enhanced MRI in the follow-up of patients with medically refractory trigeminal neuralgia undergoing stereotactic radiosurgery using the gamma knife: Initial experience. J Comput Assist Tomogr 2001;25:727–732.
62. Skirving DJ, Dan NG: A 20-year review of percutaneous balloon compression of the trigeminal ganglion. J Neurosurg 2001;94: 913–917.
63. Lefaucheur JP, Drouot X, Nguyen JP: Interventional neurophysiology for pain control: Duration of pain relief following repetitive transcranial magnetic stimulation of the motor cortex. Neurophysiol Clin 2001;31:247–252.

CHAPTER 11

DERALD E. BRACKMANN and BRUCE L. FETTERMAN

Cranial Nerve VII: Facial Nerve

History and Definitions

The first significant contribution to facial nerve anatomy was the description of its course through the temporal bone by Gabriel Fallopius in 1550. The British neurologist Sir Charles Bell made the next important discovery in 1829, when he described that the sensory innervation to the face was provided by cranial nerve V (CN V), whereas the motor function was supplied by cranial nerve VII (CN VII).[1] Over the years, much more has been learned about the anatomy and function of the facial nerve.

The facial nerve has a mixed function, primarily motor, but also sensory and parasympathetic. Consisting of approximately 10,000 fibers, CN VII has two segments, a skeletal motor root (contributing about 70 percent of the axons) and the nervus intermedius, which carries the sensory and autonomic fibers (the remaining 30 percent).[2] A lesion may involve the facial nerve anywhere along its course, and based on specific signs and symptoms, the location of the pathology can be deduced. A distinction can be made between central and peripheral facial weakness. Because of bilateral supranuclear innervation of the upper facial musculature, a central palsy spares forehead and brow motion. A peripheral palsy, however, involves both upper and lower facial muscles. In addition, with a central palsy, there may be preservation of emotional or involuntary facial motion, which is not seen with a peripheral paralysis.[3, 4]

The most common cause of facial nerve dysfunction is Bell's palsy, an idiopathic peripheral facial weakness. Named after Sir Charles Bell, Bell's palsy is a diagnosis of exclusion, applied only after other causes of facial paralysis are ruled out.

Clinical History

Many aspects of the patient's history help the clinician determine the anatomical site of lesion for a facial nerve disorder, as well as lead to the proper diagnosis. Some basic historical information to gather includes the following:

Temporal Presentation. Sudden onset suggests an inflammatory or vascular etiology (e.g., Bell's palsy or stroke), whereas a slowly progressive palsy suggests a neoplastic process, especially if there are episodes of facial twitching (e.g., facial nerve neuroma). The length of time with the paralysis and any spontaneous improvement should be noted, because Bell's palsy should improve within 6 months, whereas palsy caused by a tumor does not. In patients with a history of trauma or surgery, a palsy occurring immediately afterward suggests transection of the nerve (which requires prompt surgical evaluation), whereas a delayed onset usually implies edema of the nerve (which usually improves with time). If there are recurrent episodes of palsy on the same side, one should consider tumor as the etiology; however, if the recurrence is contralateral, one should consider Bell's palsy.

Extent of Involvement. It is important to assess the amount of facial palsy present initially, so that changes over time can be documented. The exact areas of weakness should be noted, because sparing of forehead motion or emotional facial expression suggests a central etiology, whereas palsy of both the upper and lower face suggests a peripheral lesion. If only one or two distal branches of the facial nerve are affected, possible etiologies include parotid gland tumors, facial surgery, or facial trauma. Bilateral involvement, called facial diplegia, can be found in Lyme disease, Möbius' syndrome, Bell's palsy, and Guillain-Barré syndrome (Table 11–1).[5, 6]

Precipitating Elements. Alcoholism, diabetes mellitus, autoimmune diseases, malignancy, hypertension, sarcoidosis, acute porphyria, hyperthyroidism, and pregnancy have been associated with facial palsy. In addition, many infectious diseases can cause CN VII palsy, such as tuberculosis, mononucleosis, poliomyelitis, syphilis, and human immunodeficiency virus. A recent ear infection, with or without otorrhea, is suspicious for an otological infection or cholesteatoma as the possible etiology. An upper respiratory infection commonly precedes Bell's palsy. Facial palsy has been seen after immunizations for polio and rabies and after exposure to toxins like arsenic, carbon monoxide, and ethylene glycol. A family history of facial nerve palsy is seen with Melkersson-Rosenthal syndrome and occasionally with Bell's palsy. Maternal infections (e.g., rubella), drugs used during pregnancy (e.g., thalidomide), and a difficult delivery, especially if forceps were used, have been associated with facial palsy at birth.[3]

Associated Features. A history of other neurological disorders or any evidence of neurological symptoms (e.g., headache, hemiplegia, loss of sensation, cranial nerve dysfunction, changes in balance or tendency to veer toward the same side) should be elicited, while seeking evidence of central pathology. In addition, it is imperative to check for signs and symptoms referable to the ear (e.g., otalgia, otorrhea, hypersensitivity to sound, hearing loss, tinnitus, or vertigo). To help localize the site of lesion, one should note whether other functions of CN VII are involved in patients with facial weakness (e.g., change in tearing, change in taste, reduced salivation). A history of vesicles in the ear, especially if there are CN VIII symptoms, suggests Ramsay Hunt syndrome. A history of tick bites and rash (erythema chronicum migrans) suggests Lyme disease. Facial swelling and fissuring of the tongue is seen with Melkersson-Rosenthal syndrome.[7]

TABLE 11–1. **Known Causes of Facial Diplegia[5, 6]**

	Cause
Congenital	Möbius' syndrome Thalidomide Absence of facial musculature
Infectious	Lyme disease Poliomyelitis Otitis media, acute or chronic (including cholesteatoma) Meningitis Encephalitis Syphilis Leprosy Malaria Tetanus Mononucleosis Herpes zoster Acquired immunodeficiency syndrome Botulism
Postinfectious	Guillain-Barré syndrome
Idiopathic	Bell's palsy Heerfordt's syndrome (sarcoidosis) Amyloidosis Melkersson-Rosenthal syndrome Stevens-Johnson syndrome
Hereditary	Osteopetrosis (Albers-Schonberg disease) Hyperostosis corticalis generalisata (Van Buchem's disease) Sclerostenosis Dystrophia myotonica Facioscapulohumeral dystrophy
Neoplastic	Meningeal tumors (leukemia, lymphoma) Extra-axial tumors (epidermoid cancer, ependymoma) Pontine glioma Neurofibromatosis 2
Metabolic	Diabetes mellitus Porphyria
Collagen diseases	Polyarteritis nodosa Temporal arteritis Systemic lupus erythematosus Sjögren's syndrome
Toxic	Ethylene glycol Wernicke-Korsakoff syndrome
Traumatic	Temporal bone fracture Facial lacerations Birth trauma
Iatrogenic	Arterial embolization Bilateral acoustic neuroma excision
Miscellaneous	Multiple sclerosis Parkinson's disease Pseudobulbar palsy Cerebrovascular accident Benign intracranial hypertension Miller Fisher syndrome Idiopathic cranial polyneuropathy Facial apraxia Myasthenia gravis

Anatomy of Cranial Nerve VII

(Table 11–2)

MOTOR DIVISION

The motor root contains myelinated special visceral efferent fibers for the muscles of facial expression (including the buccinator and the platysma), muscles of the external ear, stapedius, stylohyoid, and posterior belly of the digastric.

Upper Motor Neuron: Supranuclear Control

The cortical projections (corona radiata) originate from pyramidal neurons located in the lower third of the precentral gyrus of the frontal motor cortex. The cortical representation of the face, from uppermost cortex to lower, begins

TABLE 11–2. **Clinico-anatomical Correlation of Disorders of Cranial Nerve VII**

Anatomical Site of Damage	CN VII Finding	Other Neurological and Medical Findings	Common Etiologies	Comments
Motor cortex	Palsy of lower face (upper face spared); tone and emotional movements intact; tearing, salivation, taste intact	Hemiparesis (ipsilateral) Tongue weakness (ipsilateral) Frontal lobe signs	Vascular lesion of motor cortex or internal capsule on the side contralateral to the weakness	Facial weakness rarely seen as sole finding. Spasticity and hyperreflexia are found
Pontine nucleus	Facial palsy on same side as the lesion (upper and lower); tearing, salivation, taste intact	Hemiparesis (contralateral) Abducens palsy (ipsilateral)	Infarction (Millard-Gubler and Foville's syndromes), pontine glioma, multiple sclerosis, thalidomide toxicity, Möbius' syndrome	The lesion is below the facial decussation and above the corticospinal decussation. If congenital, may see anomalies of the ear or jaw
Cerebellopontine angle	Facial palsy on same side as the lesion (upper and lower); tearing, salivation, taste may be abnormal	Decreased hearing, increased tinnitus, vestibular impairment (CN VIII); facial numbness (CN V); ataxia, incoordination (cerebellum)	Acoustic neuroma, meningioma, facial nerve neuroma, cholesteatoma	CN VIII is usually involved, and its symptoms are usually the chief complaint, especially unilateral hearing loss. As lesions enlarge, other structures are involved
Internal auditory meatus (meatal segment)	Facial palsy on same side as the lesion (upper and lower); tearing, salivation, taste probably involved	Decreased hearing, increased tinnitus, vestibular impairment (CN VII)	Intracanalicular neuroma (acoustic or facial)	Signs and symptoms from CN VII and CN VIII only
Facial canal: labyrinthine segment	Facial palsy on same side as the lesion (upper and lower); tearing, salivation, taste probably involved	Decreased hearing, increased tinnitus, vestibular impairment (cochlea or vestibule involvement)	Bell's palsy, Ramsay Hunt syndrome, temporal bone fracture, hemangioma	When the facial canal is involved, the cochlea and/or the vestibular organs may be involved. Hearing loss can be conductive or sensorineural
Facial canal: tympanic segment	Facial palsy on same side as the lesion (upper and lower); salivation, taste probably involved (tearing spared)	Decreased hearing, increased tinnitus, vestibular impairment	Bell's palsy, otitis media, cholesteatoma, temporal bone fracture	If there was trauma, check for CSF otorrhea, blood in ear canal, Battle's sign, impaired consciousness
Facial canal: mastoid segment	Facial palsy on same side as the lesion (upper and lower); salivation, taste may be involved (tearing spared)	Decreased hearing, increased tinnitus, vestibular impairment	Bell's palsy, otitis media, cholesteatoma, glomus tumor	Lesions before the chorda tympani have impaired salivation and taste
Stylomastoid foramen	Facial palsy on same side as the lesion (upper and lower); tearing, salivation, taste not involved	Evidence of facial trauma, parotid or pharyngeal mass, uveitis	Facial laceration, fracture, or surgery; parotid tumors; sarcoidosis	Sparing of peripheral branches may be seen

CSF, Cerebrospinal fluid.

with the forehead, followed by the periorbital muscles, midface, and perioral muscles. Motor cortex for the tongue is next in line. These fibers join the corticobulbar tract and pass caudally within the posterior aspect of the internal capsule near its genu. When the fibers reach the midbrain, they join the medial third of the cerebral peduncle. Continuing through the basal portion of the pons with the pyramidal tract, most fibers cross in the caudal pons to reach the contralateral facial motor nucleus. Some fibers descend lower than the nucleus, cross to the other side, and then ascend to that side's nucleus (recurrent bundle of Dejerine). Other fibers, however, never decussate and synapse in the ipsilateral facial nucleus. The cortical fibers for the upper face (i.e., the frontalis, upper portion of the orbicularis oculi, and the corrugator superciliae) project to both the ipsilateral and contralateral facial nucleus. The supranuclear fibers for the lower facial muscles, however, travel only to the contralateral facial nucleus. This anatomical fact explains how unilateral supranuclear lesions characteristically spare the function of the upper face.

Emotional control of facial motion is provided by extrapyramidal input, which travels within the reticular formation from the frontal areas, thalamus, and globus pallidus to the facial motor nucleus. If a supranuclear lesion spares this input, emotional facial expressions (e.g., surprise or pain) are generally preserved despite facial palsy. Conversely, lesions of the midbrain or thalamus can cause contralateral palsy of emotional facial expressions with intact voluntary motion. In addition, lesions of the globus pallidus or its projections to the facial nucleus can cause facial bradykinesia. Despite the resulting masklike facies, some facial motion is detectable, originating from the cortical volitional and other extrapyramidal emotional pathways.[1, 4]

Pontine Nucleus

The motor nucleus of the facial nerve lies within the reticular formation of the lower third of the pons, bordered dorsally by the trigeminal nucleus and ventromedially by the superior olivary nucleus. Within the motor nucleus, four cell groups have been described that innervate specific muscles. The dorsomedial cell group sends fibers to the auricular and occipital muscles via the posterior auricular nerve. The ventromedial cell group gives rise to the cervical branch, which innervates the platysma. Fibers for the stapedius muscle and the temporal and zygomatic branches originate from the intermediate cell group. The lateral cell group contributes to the buccal and possibly to the mandibular branches. The exact cell group innervating the stylohyoid and posterior belly of the digastric is uncertain, but some feel that the origin may be the dorsal or accessory facial nucleus.[8, 9]

The special visceral efferent fibers emerge from the dorsal side of the facial motor nucleus and travel dorsomedially under the floor of the fourth ventricle. In this location, the fibers are called the *funiculus teres*, and the elevation of this bundle within the upper half of the floor of the ventricle creates the eminentia teres. The motor root fibers extend medially and cephalad toward the abducens nucleus. When the fibers reach the area below the medial part of the abducens nucleus, they turn laterally to cross the front of the abducens nucleus and continue to curve around its lateral border. After looping around the abducens nucleus, the fibers travel caudally between the medial border of the trigeminal nucleus and the lateral edge of the facial motor nucleus. The motor fibers exit the caudolateral border of the pons in the cerebellopontine angle medial to CN VIII. The medial-to-lateral loop around the abducens nucleus is called the *internal genu of the facial nerve* (Fig. 11–1). This anatomical relationship explains how certain disorders of facial nerve motor function can be associated with abducens palsy.[10, 11]

NERVUS INTERMEDIUS

Also called the nerve of Wrisberg, the nervus intermedius contains general visceral afferent, special visceral afferent, and general visceral efferent fibers that convey sensation from the posterior region of the external auditory canal and concha; taste from the anterior two thirds of the tongue; and secretomotor function for the lacrimal glands, submandibular and sublingual glands, and minor salivary glands in the nasal cavity, paranasal sinuses, and palate (Fig. 11–2). In the cerebellopontine angle, the nervus intermedius travels from the pons to the internal auditory meatus between the motor root and CN VIII. The geniculate ganglion, found within the temporal bone along the course of the facial nerve, contains the primary cell bodies of the special visceral afferent taste fibers and general somatic afferent sensory fibers. The preganglionic general visceral efferent fibers and special visceral

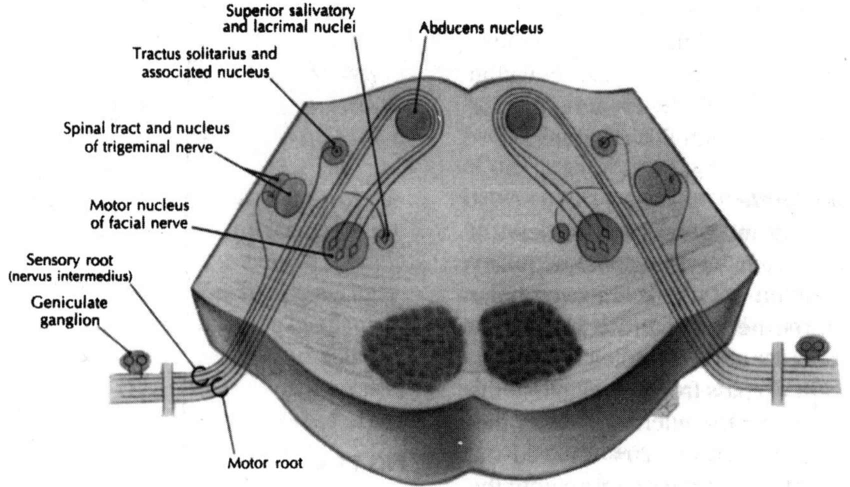

FIGURE 11–1. Facial nerve projections within the pons. (From LaRouere MJ, Lundy LB: Anatomy and physiology of the facial nerve. *In* Jackler RK, Brackmann DE [eds]: Neurotology. St. Louis, Mosby-Year Book, 1994, pp 1271–1281.)

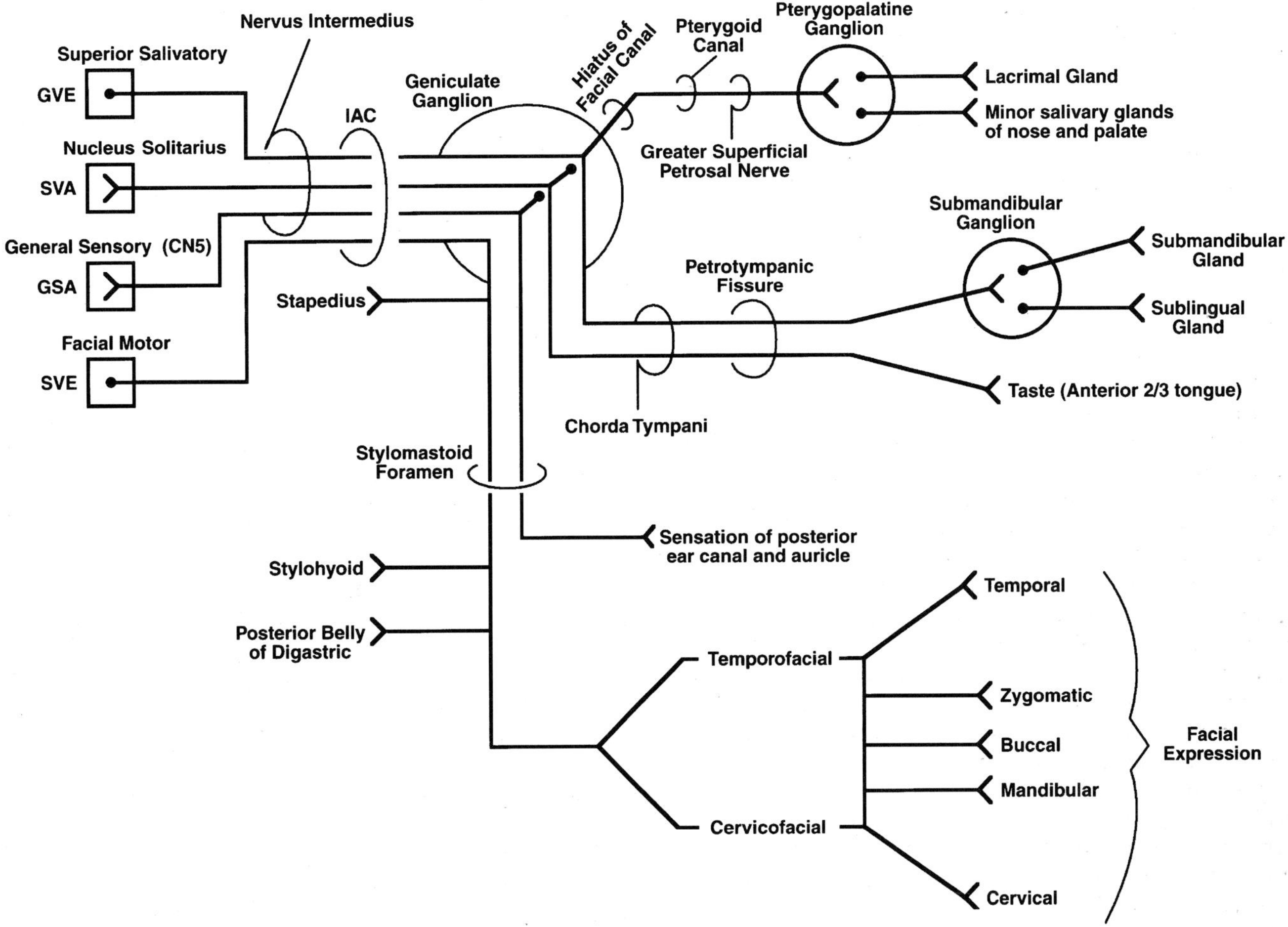

FIGURE 11–2. Diagram of facial nerve anatomy. GVE, General visceral efferent; SVA, special visceral afferent; GSA, general somatic afferent; SVE, special visceral efferent; IAC, internal auditory canal.

efferent fibers pass through the geniculate ganglion without synapsing. The chorda tympani and the greater superficial petrosal nerve are subdivisions of this nerve.

Sensory Nucleus

The general somatic afferent fibers from the posterior aspect of the external auditory canal, lateral pinna, and mastoid region (carried within the posterior auricular nerve) travel centrally in the nervus intermedius to the dorsal part of the primary sensory nucleus of CN V within the pons. Hypesthesia of the posterior external auditory canal has been found to be an early sign of tumors within the internal auditory canal (e.g., acoustic neuroma). It is speculated that sensory fibers are more susceptible to the effects of pressure than motor axons.[12, 13]

Parasympathetic Nucleus

The general visceral efferent fibers originate from the superior salivatory nucleus and the lacrimal nucleus in the dorsal pons and are carried distally within the nervus intermedius. After joining the motor root of the facial nerve, two main branches carry the parasympathetic fibers to their destination. At the geniculate ganglion, the greater superficial petrosal nerve branches at the hiatus of the facial canal and travels anteromedially through the middle fossa within the pterygoid canal. Contained within this nerve are preganglionic fibers destined for the lacrimal gland and the minor salivary glands of the nasal cavity, paranasal sinuses, and palate. The deep petrosal nerve, carrying postganglionic sympathetic fibers, joins the greater superficial petrosal nerve to form the nerve of the pterygoid canal (vidian nerve). At the pterygopalatine ganglion (found within the pterygopalatine fossa), the parasympathetic fibers synapse with postganglionic neurons, which continue toward their target organs.

The preganglionic fibers for the submandibular and sublingual salivary glands pass through the geniculate ganglion and then leave the mastoid segment of the facial nerve within the chorda tympani. The chorda tympani travels through the temporal bone within the canal of Huguier and enters the infratemporal fossa via the petrotympanic fissure, where it joins the lingual nerve (CN V). Within the submandibular ganglion, the parasympathetic fibers synapse with the postganglionic cells that innervate the submandibular and sublingual salivary glands.

Gustatory Nucleus

The special visceral afferent fibers from the taste buds of the anterior two thirds of the tongue (i.e., tongue anterior to the sulcus terminalis) also travel within the chorda tympani.

As stated earlier, the cell bodies for taste fibers are located within the geniculate ganglion. The gustatory afferent fibers are carried centrally by the nervus intermedius to cells in the rostral part of the nucleus of tractus solitarius in the medulla. Also synapsing within this nucleus are the taste fibers from other areas of the oral cavity, pharynx, and larynx carried by CN IX and CN X. Intermingling of these three cranial nerves occurs here.[10]

LOWER MOTOR NEURON: PERIPHERAL ROUTE OF CN VII

Cerebellopontine Angle

The intracranial segment (within the angle) measures about 23 to 24 mm long and 1 to 2 mm wide and runs obliquely (anteriorly and laterally) from the pontomedullary sulcus to the internal auditory canal.[14, 15] Both the motor root and the nervus intermedius emerge from the brain stem ventrolaterally near the posterior aspect of the pons, 9.5 to 14.5 mm from the midline and 0.5 to 2.0 mm medial to where CN VIII enters the brain stem. At times, the facial nerve axons pass through the transverse fibers of the middle cerebellar peduncle.[14] Within the subarachnoid space of the cerebellopontine angle, CN VII is joined by CN VIII, which travels lateral and slightly inferior to the facial nerve (Fig. 11–3). The nervus intermedius runs between CN VIII and the motor root of CN VII (hence its name). While in the cerebellopontine angle, the facial nerve has no epineurium and is covered only with pia mater. The trigeminal nerve is located anteriorly. The anterior inferior cerebellar artery is associated with the nerves and usually is found ventrally, between the nerves and the pons.[9]

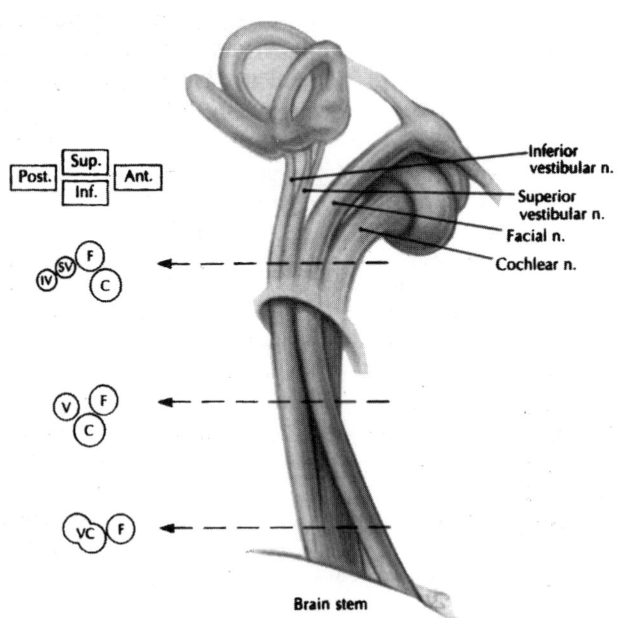

FIGURE 11–3. Relationship of the facial nerve to the cochlear and vestibular nerves from the cerebellopontine angle through the internal auditory canal. (From LaRouere MJ, Lundy LB: Anatomy and physiology of the facial nerve. *In* Jackler RK, Brackmann DE [eds]: Neurotology. St. Louis, Mosby–Year Book, 1994, pp 1271–1281.)

Internal Auditory Meatus of Temporal Bone

The meatal segment (within the internal auditory canal) is about 7 to 8 mm long. The nervus intermedius joins the motor root to form a common trunk that occupies the area nervi facialis, which lies within the anterosuperior segment of the meatus. The motor fibers are more anterior, whereas the nervus intermedius fibers remain posteriorly. At the lateral end of the meatus, a horizontal partition, the transverse or falciform crest, separates the facial from the cochlear nerve inferiorly. In addition, a vertical crest (Bill's bar) separates the facial from the superior vestibular nerve located posteriorly. The blood supply to this region is the labyrinthine artery, a branch of the anterior inferior cerebellar artery.

Facial Canal

Beginning at Bill's bar and ending at the stylomastoid foramen, this portion is comprised of three segments: (1) labyrinthine (3 to 4 mm long); (2) tympanic (12 to 13 mm long); and mastoid (15 to 20 mm long). The labyrinthine segment, which lies within the narrowest portion of the bony facial canal, extends from the anterosuperior region of the fundus to the geniculate ganglion. To reach the geniculate fossa, it passes between the ampulla of the superior semicircular canal and the cochlea and travels forward and downward. At the geniculate ganglion, the nerve turns 75 degrees posteriorly, thus creating the external genu. This marks the beginning of the tympanic segment. Exiting 90 degrees anteriorly from the geniculate is the first branch of CN VII, the greater superficial petrosal nerve.

The tympanic segment continues along the medial wall of the tympanic cavity, a few millimeters medial to the incus. It courses superior and posterior to the cochleariform process, along the upper edge of the oval window, and inferior to the lateral semicircular canal. At the origin of the stapedius tendon from the pyramidal process, the nerve turns 120 degrees, continuing inferiorly as the mastoid segment. The mastoid segment has two branches—the nerve to the stapedius and the chorda tympani. During its course through the mastoid along the posterior aspect of the external auditory canal, the nerve travels slightly posteriorly and usually passes lateral to the inferior aspect of the tympanic annulus. At times, however, the facial nerve may be lateral to the annulus during its entire descent, which puts the nerve at risk during mastoid surgery.[16, 17] The major blood supply for the facial nerve within the facial canal is the superficial petrosal branch of the middle meningeal artery (proximally) and the stylomastoid artery (distally).[18]

Stylomastoid Foramen

CN VII exits the temporal bone via the stylomastoid foramen, which is between the mastoid and styloid processes and deep to the posterior belly of the digastric. Almost immediately, the nerve enters the parotid gland. After traveling anteriorly about 2 cm within the parotid, the nerve divides at the posterior border of the ramus of the mandible into an upper temporofacial and a lower (and smaller) cervicofacial nerve. Classically, these divide again at the pes anserinus into the temporal, zygomatic, buccal, mandibular, and cervical branches. Many anastomoses exist between these branches, and many variations in the branching patterns have been described.[19] After emerging from the superior, anterior, and inferior margins of the parotid gland, these branches enter the deep surface of their target muscle. Ultimately, all the facial muscles are innervated by CN VII, except for the levator palpebrae superioris (CN III). The extratemporal portion of the facial nerve derives its blood supply from the stylomastoid, posterior auricular, superficial temporal, and transverse facial arteries.[18]

Examination of CN VII

DIRECTED NEUROLOGICAL EXAMINATION

Motor Evaluation

First, the clinician should observe the patient at rest for symmetry and the presence of any involuntary movements (e.g., fasciculations, tics). Signs of facial weakness include flattening of the nasolabial groove, slower blinking, and loss of facial wrinkles. Next, clinicians should check the amount of voluntary motion in each of the five peripheral branches by having the patient perform the following: (1) temporal—raise the eyebrows, wrinkle the brow; (2) zygomatic—close the eyes gently, and with maximal effort try to keep the eyes closed while the examiner attempts to open them; (3) buccal—smile, show teeth, puff out the cheeks; (4) mandibular—pout, purse the lips; (5) cervical— sneer. The clinician should determine if the patient exhibits Bell's phenomenon, which is an upward and outward rolling of the globe when eyelid closure is attempted. When there is incomplete closure, this phenomenon protects the cornea by placing it under the upper eyelid and moving it laterally. While testing the facial expressions, synkinesis should be sought, which is unintentional motion of a group of muscles when another group is voluntarily contracted (e.g., contraction of the eyelid during smiling). To differentiate a central palsy, clinicians should look for sparing of upper facial motion and for preservation of emotional facial expressions (e.g., surprise, pain). Both sides of the face should be examined closely to rule out bilateral involvement. A change in loudness perception suggests involvement of the nerve branch to the stapedius muscle. This hyperacusis can be confirmed subjectively by checking auditory function with finger rub or tuning forks and can be documented objectively by acoustic reflex testing during an audiometric evaluation.

Examiners must be careful not to confuse transferred contralateral motion with weak motion of the involved side. For example, the contralateral frontalis can create some wrinkles in the forehead of the involved side, and contralateral midfacial muscles can cause motion of the involved side. To prevent confusion, the examiner should cover the contralateral side to focus solely on the involved side before comparing the two sides. In addition, by holding the skin of the uninvolved side against the facial skeleton, midfacial motion from the contralateral side can be minimized. Likewise, examiners should not confuse active eye closure with the normal, gravity-assisted passive closure of the eyelids, which occurs after the levator palpebrae superioris is relaxed.[20]

Sensory Evaluation

The response to solutions of the four fundamental tastes (sweet—sucrose, sour—citric acid, salty—sodium chloride, and bitter—quinine sulfate) should be evaluated in the anterior two thirds of the tongue. The patient should be instructed not to eat or smoke for several hours before testing. Before test solutions are applied, the mouth is rinsed with distilled water. Then, using cotton swabs, a test solution is placed on the lateral, anterior tongue. The patient should be instructed to state whether the solution is sweet, sour, salty, bitter, unknown, or without taste. Between test solutions, the mouth should be swished with distilled water. Each side should be tested separately. To eliminate olfaction, patients should pinch their nose or hold their breath during the testing.

The somatic sensation of the posterolateral external ear canal and concha should be tested in the usual fashion (cotton wisp, pinprick, and other) and the results compared with the sensation of the surrounding areas and with the contralateral side.

Reflexes

Several reflexes related to facial nerve function can be tested, including the following: (1) corneal reflex—tactile stimulation of the cornea normally causes both eyes to blink simultaneously. The afferent limb is from CN V (ophthalmic division), whereas the efferent limb is from CN VII (motor root). Depending on the reflex patterns elicited, one can differentiate between a CN V or CN VII lesion. For example, if right-sided corneal stimulation does not cause both right and left eyelid closure, but left-sided stimulation does, there is a right CN V deficit. Similarly, if both right- and left-sided corneal stimulation cause the left eye to blink, but not the right, there is a right CN VII lesion. (2) Orbicularis oculi reflex—the examiner pulls the skin lateral to the lateral canthus with the thumb and index finger and then taps the thumb lightly with a reflex hammer, resulting in orbicularis oculi contraction. This stretch reflex shows hyporeflexia in peripheral palsy and hyperreflexia with central palsy. (3) Blink reflex—normally every 2 to 15 seconds there is spontaneous bilateral blinking. (4) Auditory palpebrae reflex—sudden, unexpected loud sound causes a single bilateral eyelid closure. Sudden bright lights also cause reflex eyelid closure. (5) Palmomental reflex—tapping or stroking of the palm causes contraction of the ipsilateral mentalis muscle. This pathological reflex is seen with pyramidal tract disease and helps diagnose a central palsy. Another reflex seen with central lesions is the snout reflex, in which tapping of the lips causes pursing of the lips. (6) Other reflexes associated with CN VII include the glabellar (tapping of the glabella causes both eyes to blink), supraorbital (tapping of the supraorbital ridge causes the ipsilateral eye to blink), nasolacrimal (irritative or painful nasal stimulation causes tearing), nasal (ipsilateral facial contraction after tickling of the nasal mucosa), and oculogyric-auricular (contraction of the auricular muscles after lateral gaze).[21]

Parasympathetic Evaluation

Infranuclear lesions can cause a reduction in ipsilateral tear production if they occur at, or proximal to, the geniculate ganglion. The Schirmer test provides a quantitative evaluation of tear production. Sterile strips of filter paper are folded into the shape of a hook and placed into each lower conjunctival fornix. After 5 minutes, the degree of wetting is measured and compared between sides. A unilateral reduction of more than 30 percent of the total amount of lacrimation of both eyes or bilateral tearing of less than 25 mm is considered significant. This test consists of an afferent limb (CN V) and an efferent limb (CN VII); however, unilateral corneal stimulation from the filter paper should cause bilateral, equal lacrimation. Therefore, because both eyes are tested simultaneously, a unilateral CN V lesion does not result in decreased tearing.[22, 23]

A lesion distal to the geniculate ganglion may result in excessive tear production. If there is corneal irritation resulting from poor eye closure, lacrimation may be increased. In addition, ectropion resulting from orbicularis oculi weakness and loss of facial tone disrupts the normal flow of tears. Instead of being circulated by blinking and cleared by the canaliculi (aided by the pumping action of the periorbital muscles), tears pool in the lower conjunctival sac and spill over the lower lid margin.[24]

ASSOCIATED NEUROLOGICAL FINDINGS

Cerebral. Cognitive function and abilities with language should be examined, as the clinician seeks impaired attention or concentration, slurred speech, dysarthria, or aphasia. Affect and emotions should be noted, looking for personality changes, apathy, inappropriate crying, or emotional outbursts. Memory should be assessed for deficits. Subfluent aphasia occurs in the context of a right central CN VII lesion, whereas cerebellar speech deficits may be found with peripheral disorders of CN VII, especially if the cerebellopontine angle is involved.

Cranial Nerves. The optic discs should be visualized for signs of increased intracranial pressure or stigmata of systemic conditions like hypertension or diabetes. Direct and consensual pupillary reflexes and extraocular movements, especially abduction of the globe (CN VI), should be evaluated. Facial sensation in the three divisions, as well as motor function of the muscles of mastication, should be checked to assess if CN V is also involved, as in a cerebellopontine lesion. Audition should be evaluated with tuning forks, looking for ipsilateral sensorineural or conductive hearing loss. If nystagmus is present, its direction and other characteristics should be documented. Unilateral vestibular weakness should be tested with the Mittelmeyer test (the patient marches in place with eyes closed and hands outstretched; there is a tendency to turn toward the side of vestibular weakness). Palatal sensation and movement, vocal cord motion, trapezial strength, and tongue function should be evaluated.

Motor/Reflexes/Cerebellar/Gait. Hemiparesis ipsilateral to the facial paralysis suggests a cortical or subcortical lesion, whereas contralateral hemiparesis suggests a pontine lesion near the facial motor nucleus. Reflexes should be checked for increased function, as is seen with a central nervous system lesion, or decreased function, as is seen in various neuropathies. The existence of flaccidity, atrophy, and fasciculations should be noted; these are indicative of a neuropathic process. Involuntary movements of the face in the form of synkinesis may suggest an old lesion with re-innervation. In patients with facial diplegia, ascending diffuse distal weakness with loss of reflexes suggests Guillain-Barré syndrome, whereas facial diplegia with diffuse proximal muscle weakness is seen more often in myopathies. When associated with facial weakness, the complex of ataxia, incoordination, and other signs of cerebellar disease suggest a brain stem or cerebellopontine angle lesion.

Sensory. A loss of sensation to pinprick, temperature, light touch, or vibration of the face or body (contralateral or ipsilateral) suggests lateral brain stem involvement or a cerebellopontine angle lesion. With ischemic damage from mid-pons to lower medulla, there is a loss of pain, temperature, and corneal reflex from the ipsilateral side of the face (descending tract of CN V), combined with pain and temperature loss from the contralateral side of the body (spinothalamic tract). Patients with lower brain stem lesions usually have intact proprioception and other signs of lateral medullary damage (Wallenberg's syndrome), whereas those with upper brain stem injury have impaired proprioception. In addition, those with upper pontine lesions have sensory loss from the contralateral side of the face and body.

Neurovascular. Because it is both a risk factor for and cause of intracranial vascular disorders, the presence of hypertension should be evaluated by both blood pressure determination and systemic examination (e.g., retinal vessel evaluation). Bruits and other evidence of carotid artery disease may point to thromboembolic disease as an etiology. A tender and enlarged temporal artery, especially with an elevated erythrocyte sedimentation rate, suggests temporal arteritis.

ASSOCIATED MEDICAL FINDINGS

The skin should be checked for rashes, lesions, or evidence of insect bites. The head and neck should be examined for masses, signs of trauma, or postoperative scars. The auricle and ear canal should be examined thoroughly for vesicles, ulcers, or other lesions. The tympanic membrane should be checked for perforation, drainage, or cholesteatoma. Infections, neoplasms, and evidence of prior otological surgery should be sought while examining the middle ear. The oral cavity and pharynx should be checked for masses, ulcerations, fissuring of the tongue, and other lesions. The parotid should always be palpated for tumors and inspected for inflammation. If nonsuppurative parotitis, uveitis, and mild fever are found, Heerfordt's disease, a variant of sarcoidosis, may be present. Endocrinological function should be evaluated, because diabetes insipidus or other evidence of pituitary dysfunction can signify neurosarcoidosis. If there is incomplete eyelid closure, the cornea should always be checked for ulceration or infection, because loss of vision from exposure keratitis can occur.

Evaluation Guidelines

Neuroimaging. Radiographical studies are helpful in determining the site of lesion and should be obtained whenever the etiology is unclear; when the paralysis is recurrent, progressive, or atypical; or if there was trauma (Table 11–3). If there is evidence of cerebellopontine angle or internal

TABLE 11–3. **Useful Tests in the Evaluation of Disorders of Cranial Nerve VII**

Syndrome	Neuroimaging	Electrophysiology	Fluid and Tissue Analysis	Neuropsychological Tests	Other Tests
Supranuclear facial paresis	MRI, CT for infarction, tumor	EEG: abnormal wave patterns in seizures	CSF: increased RBC	Mental status impairment	N/A
Nuclear lesions: Millard-Gubler and Foville's syndromes	MRI for infarction, tumor		CSF: increased RBC	N/A	N/A
Cerebellopontine angle lesion	MRI for tumor	ABR: delay in wave V or increased interaural difference	N/A	N/A	Audiogram: sensorineural hearing loss ENG: vestibular weakness
Facial canal lesion	MRI, CT for tumor, fractures, inflammation		N/A	N/A	Audiogram: sensorineural or conductive hearing loss; acoustic reflex: absent; electrogustometry: reduced; salivary flow: reduced; Schirmer's test: reduced
Stylomastoid foramen syndrome	MRI for tumor, fracture		N/A	N/A	
Hemifacial spasm	MRI for vascular loop compression		N/A	N/A	
Postparalytic movements and synkinesis		N/A	N/A	N/A	N/A
Myokymia	MRI for pontine tumor, MS plaques	EMG: spontaneous activity at 30–70 per second	CSF: elevated IgG and gamma globulin	N/A	N/A

MRI, Magnetic resonance imaging; CT, computed tomography; EEG, electroencephalogram; ABR, auditory brain stem response; CSF, cerebrospinal fluid; RBC, red blood cell; ENG, electronystagmography; MS, multiple sclerosis; EMG, electromyography; N/A, not applicable.

auditory canal pathology (e.g., facial weakness with ipsilateral sensorineural hearing loss, tinnitus, and/or vestibular abnormalities), magnetic resonance imaging (MRI) with gadolinium enhancement should be obtained. MRI can also demonstrate intracranial, temporal bone, base of skull, and facial soft tissue lesions. High-resolution computed tomography (CT) is useful in defining the bony anatomy of the facial canal. CT readily demonstrates fractures (face, mandible, temporal bone) and bony abnormalities (congenital anomalies, osteopetrosis). It helps differentiate between intratemporal facial nerve neuromas (smooth upward displacement of bone overlying the geniculate with expansion of the tympanic segment) and hemangiomas (irregular bony erosion around the geniculate). In addition, CT can show the extent of bone erosion with lesions like cholesteatoma, glomus tumors, carcinoma, and skull base osteomyelitis.[25]

Electrophysiology. Electroencephalography may help distinguish supranuclear causes of facial nerve dysfunction, especially in the instances of suspected epilepsy with a postseizure paresis, called *Todd's paresis*. Nerve conduction studies should be performed in patients with a unilateral complete paralysis. In testing the involved side, if the threshold is 3.5 mA greater than the contralateral ("normal") side, there is a poor prognosis for spontaneous recovery. This test, however, is not absolutely reliable, and even when there is complete transection of the facial nerve, it conducts impulses distal to the injury for up to 72 hours (until wallerian degeneration occurs).[23] Electroneurography can be used to determine the peak-to-peak amplitude of the evoked compound action potential of the involved side compared with the other side. Because the amplitude is considered proportional to the number of functioning motor fibers, if there is a 90 percent or greater reduction in the amplitude of the affected side (which represents more than 90 percent degeneration of the nerve), the prognosis is poor.

Muscle action potentials generated by voluntary and spontaneous activity can be measured through electromyography. By placing needles within the facial musculature, electrical silence can be seen in acute paralysis, severe muscle wasting, hypoplasia of the nerve or muscle, or normally innervated muscle in a resting state. Voluntary potentials are present with voluntary contraction. Polyphasic potentials appear during nerve regeneration from 4 to 6 weeks after onset of the paralysis. Fibrillation potentials represent degeneration of the motor nerve; they are usually seen 10 to 14 days after nerve injury. Electromyography is helpful in patients with long-standing facial paralysis and in infants with congenital facial paralysis, but it is not very useful with acute paralysis.

By using electrodes to record the blink reflex after percutaneous stimulation of the supraorbital nerve, a trigeminofacial reflex can be tested. Measuring conduction of the reflex arc between CN V (afferent) and CN VII (efferent) tests both central and peripheral segments of the facial nerve. Currently, the trigeminofacial reflex is the only direct test able to measure intracranial pathology of the facial nerve.[26]

Auditory brain stem response can be further used to evaluate brain stem anatomy when a retrocochlear or nuclear cause of facial nerve dysfunction is considered. Delay in the absolute latency of ipsilateral wave V or an interaural difference in wave V of more than 0.2 ms suggests retrocochlear involvement of CN VIII. This observation helps localize the etiology of facial palsy as within or proximal to the internal auditory canal (e.g., acoustic or facial nerve neuroma).

Body Fluid and Tissue Analysis. Basic tests to obtain include complete blood count with differential (for infectious mononucleosis, leukemia, inflammation), chemistry panel (for systemic diseases), fluorescent treponemal antibody titer (for syphilis), and erythrocyte sedimentation rate/antinuclear antibody test/rheumatoid factor (for collagen vascular disease). Depending on the clinical presentation, other tests may be helpful, including thyroid function tests, glucose tolerance test, angiotensin-converting enzyme levels (sarcoidosis), antibody titers (Lyme disease, Epstein-Barr virus, herpes zoster virus, human immunodeficiency virus), monospot test/heterophile antibody titers (mononucleosis), serum heavy metal/toxin levels (lead, arsenic, mercury, carbon monoxide), urine analysis (porphyria, diabetes, sarcoidosis), and stool analysis (*Clostridium botulinum* toxin). In patients with congenital facial nerve paralysis, one should consider testing for chromosomal abnormalities.[27]

Muscle biopsies are helpful in determining the existence of a mitochondrial myopathy. In addition, if a facial re-animation procedure is considered in patients with long-standing facial paralysis or in infants with congenital facial paralysis, facial muscle biopsy should be performed to determine whether viable muscle fibers are present. If the musculature has degenerated and has been replaced by fibrosis, any procedure attempting to bring only neural input to the area will fail.[23] In patients requiring a tissue diagnosis, biopsies of skin lesions, subcutaneous nodules, enlarged lymph nodes, or salivary gland tissue may reveal disorders such as sarcoidosis, parotid gland tumor, or vasculitis (e.g., temporal arteritis or periarteritis nodosa).

Cerebrospinal Fluid. If the possibility of central nervous system infection or malignancy exists, a lumbar puncture should be performed. After noting the opening pressure and qualities of the fluid, samples should be sent for cell count, chemistry levels, microbiological staining and culture, antigen titers, and cytology testing. Intracranial hypertension, meningitis (bacterial, fungal, mycobacterial, viral, carcinomatous, aseptic), and malignant processes such as metastasis (lung, breast, melanoma), leukemia, lymphoma, and other primary intracranial neoplastic processes can be detected. In addition, the diagnosis of other etiologies can be supported, like Guillain-Barré syndrome (increased protein level), multiple sclerosis (elevated IgG and gamma globulin levels), syphilis (positive serology result), and subarachnoid or intracerebral hemorrhage (red blood cells).

Other Tests. Audiometry should be performed in all patients with facial palsy. Because CN VII is intimately related to CN VIII in the cerebellopontine angle and internal auditory canal and because the facial canal courses by the cochlea and through the middle ear, many causes of palsy have an associated hearing loss. The type of loss (sensorineural versus conductive) as well as the extent (mild to profound) are essential factors for localization and planning of treatment. Another useful audiometrical test is the acoustic reflex test, which measures the contraction of the stapedius muscle in response to auditory stimuli. The result can localize the site of lesion as proximal or distal to the branch to the stapedius (mastoid segment of the facial nerve). Tests of vestibular function, like electronystagmography, may be helpful in differentiating central from peripheral lesions in patients who have accompanying vertigo.

By evaluating taste or salivation, the status of the chorda tympani nerve can be determined. Based on impairment, lesions can be localized as proximal or distal to this branch of the mastoid segment. For example, electrogustometry can measure the taste threshold in response to a small electric current applied to the anterior tongue. The current elicits a metallic or bitter taste, and by controlling the amount of current, the threshold for gustation can be obtained. An elevated threshold suggests involvement of the chorda tympani. Salivary flow can be analyzed by cannulating Wharton's duct. The salivary production is measured for 5 minutes, and a reduction of 25 percent between sides signifies chorda tympani involvement. In addition, salivary flow can be evaluated indirectly by checking the pH of the saliva, because the pH rises with increased salivation. A pH of 6.1 or less is considered to be significant for reduced flow.[2]

When certain systemic disorders are suspected to be the etiology of the facial palsy, chest radiography should be obtained. Based on characteristic radiographic findings, the diagnosis of sarcoidosis, tuberculosis, lymphoma, or lung cancer can be supported.

Clinical Syndromes (Table 11–4)

SYNDROMES OF PARESIS

Supranuclear Facial Paresis—Central Facial Palsy

In a central facial palsy, only the lower face is paralyzed, especially perioral musculature. Facial tone is intact (no atrophy), and there are no fasciculations. Despite loss of voluntary motion, emotional expression is preserved. With cortical lesions, hemiplegia of the same side as the facial palsy can be found, with upper extremity involvement more than lower. Lesions of the cortex or internal capsule on the side opposite the facial palsy cause the aforementioned symptom complex. If the dominant hemisphere is involved, aphasia may be present. With corticobulbar involvement of other cranial nerves, impairment of speech or swallowing may result. If the lesion is deeper (e.g., basal ganglia), volitional motion may be intact; however, the facial motor response to emotional stimuli is impaired. In acute supranuclear lesions, initially there

TABLE 11–4. **Selected Etiologies Associated with Disorders of Cranial Nerve VII**

Etiological Category	Selected Specific Etiologies	Chapter
Structural Disorders		
Developmental	Möbius' syndrome, absence of facial musculature	28
Degenerative and compressive	Osteopetrosis, sclerosteosis, hyperostosis corticalis generalisata, benign intracranial hypertension	29
Hereditary and Degenerative Disorders		
Amino/organic acidopathies, mitochondrial enzyme defects and other metabolic errors	Acute porphyria	31
Movement disorders	Hemifacial spasm, Parkinson's disease, Gilles de la Tourette's syndrome, facial dystonia Meige's disease or Brueghel's syndrome, facial contortion, bilateral	34
Degenerative motor, sensory, and autonomic disorders	Amyotrophic lateral sclerosis	36
Hereditary nondegenerative neuromuscular disease	Dystrophia myotonica	37
Acquired Metabolic and Nutritional Disorders		
Endogenous metabolic disorders	Diabetes mellitus, hyperthyroidism	38
Exogenous acquired metabolic disorders of the nervous system		
Toxins and illicit drugs	Thalidomide, carbon monoxide, ethylene glycol, arsenic	39
Nutritional deficiencies and syndromes associated with alcoholism	Wernicke-Korsakoff syndrome	40
Infectious Disorders		
Viral infections	Herpes zoster, herpes simplex, influenza, coxsackie, enterovirus, polio, mumps, mononucleosis	41
Nonviral infections	Otitis externa, otitis media, mastoiditis, syphilis, tuberculosis, leprosy, Lyme disease, cat scratch disease, mucormycosis, botulism, malaria	42
Neurovascular Disorders	Stroke, internal carotid artery aneurysm	45
Neoplastic Disorders		
Primary neurological tumors	Pontine glioma, neuroma (acoustic, facial), meningioma, hemangioma, cholesteatoma, glomus tumor	46
Metastatic neoplasms and paraneoplastic syndromes	Leukemia, lymphoma, myeloma, from salivary gland (adenoid cystic), skin (melanoma), breast, lung, kidney, head/neck	47
Demyelinating Disorders		
Demyelinating disorders of the central nervous system	Multiple sclerosis	48
Demyelinating disorders of the peripheral nervous system	Guillain-Barré syndrome	94
Autoimmune and Inflammatory Disorders	Bell's palsy, sarcoidosis, myasthenia gravis, Sjögren's syndrome, temporal arteritis, systemic lupus erythematosus, periarteritis nodosa	50
Traumatic Disorders	Facial laceration, face/mandible/temporal bone fracture, birth trauma, barotrauma, lightning	51
Epilepsy	Focal epilepsy, Ramsay Hunt syndrome	52
Headache and Facial Pain	Cerebellopontine angle lesion	53
Drug-Induced and Iatrogenic Neurological Disorders	Parotid or facial cosmetic surgery, otological or neurotological surgery, local anesthesia, arterial embolization	55

may be hyporeflexia, which over time is replaced with hyperreflexia.

Nuclear or Pontine Lesions

If the lesion is near the facial nucleus, an ipsilateral facial palsy is seen with a contralateral hemiplegia (corticospinal tract has not crossed yet). A concomitant deficit of CN VI may be seen because of the internal genu's relationship with the abducens nucleus. Two syndromes involving this region have been described.[4]

Millard-Gubler syndrome yields ipsilateral paralysis of CN VII, with contralateral hemiplegia of the extremities. The syndrome is usually caused by interruption of blood supply to the pons, with involvement of CN VII after its decussation and the corticospinal tract before its decussation.

Foville's syndrome is similar to Millard-Gubler syndrome, in that there is ipsilateral facial paralysis with contralateral hemiplegia; however, in addition, there is ipsilateral abducens palsy and paralysis of conjugate gaze due to concurrent involvement of the abducens nucleus.

Peripheral Nerve Lesions

Cerebellopontine Angle Syndrome. Pathology involving CN VII in this region often involves CN VIII (sensorineural hearing loss, tinnitus, vestibular weakness). Depending on the size and exact location of the lesion, other structures in this region can be affected, like the cerebellum (ataxia, incoordination) and CN V (reduced facial sensation, impaired corneal reflex). Common etiologies include acoustic neuromas and meningiomas.

Facial Canal Syndrome. The location of the lesion determines the actual deficit. In the labyrinthine segment, facial palsy is seen with ipsilateral hearing loss and vestibular weakness. In addition, hyperacusis and a decrease in tearing and in salivation with loss of taste can be detected. With lesions of the tympanic segment that are distal to the greater superficial petrosal nerve, all of the above may be found, except that lacrimation is intact. If the mastoid segment is involved, as with tympanic lesions, hearing and balance may be affected, and lacrimation is preserved. Whether the lesion is proximal to the nerve branch for the stapedius or to the chorda tympani determines whether there is hyperacusis, decreased salivation, or loss of gustation. Hemangiomas, neuromas, cholesteatomas, temporal bone fractures, and the inflammation causing Bell's palsy are some disorders of the facial canal that can cause facial palsy (see Fig. 11–4).

Stylomastoid Foramen Syndrome. A lesion after the nerve leaves the temporal bone results in only a lower motor neuron deficit of the mimetic muscles. Atrophy and fasciculations are found. Pathology of individual nerve branches can be seen with parotid tumors (e.g., adenoid cystic carcinoma), with facial or mandibular trauma, and after facial surgery (e.g., parotidectomy, face lift, and submandibular gland excision).

Idiopathic Facial Palsy. Despite a thorough workup, 60 to 75 percent of all cases of facial paralysis are of unknown etiology and are called Bell's palsy.[28] The annual incidence of

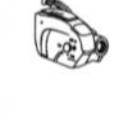

Bell's palsy is about 20 per 100,000, with an increasing incidence seen with increasing age. The male-to-female and left-to-right ratio is approximately equal. Seven to 9 percent have a history of prior facial palsy, and 4 to 9 percent have a positive family history for Bell's. High-risk patients include pregnant women and patients with diabetes mellitus or multiple sclerosis. Without treatment, improvement is noted within 3 weeks in 85 percent of patients, with the remainder showing improvement by 3 to 6 months. In addition, about 70 percent regain normal function, about 15 percent have some residual weakness, and the remainder have poor return of function. By 6 months, therefore, all patients with Bell's palsy should show some improvement, and thus none should have a persistent total facial paralysis.[29, 30]

Clinical characteristics of typical Bell's palsy include the following: peripheral CN VII dysfunction involving all distal branches; sudden onset with maximal facial weakness usually reached within several days; impaired result on acoustic reflex test in 90 percent; viral prodrome in 60 percent; numbness or pain of the ear, tongue, or face in 50 percent; chorda tympani nerve appears red in 40 percent; reduction in ipsilateral tearing or salivary flow in 10 percent; and spontaneous improvement within 6 months.[3]

Based on accumulated clinical and experimental evidence, the most commonly accepted cause of Bell's palsy is herpes simplex infection. Treatment, therefore, consists of acyclovir and steroids, which have been shown to hasten the recovery and to lessen the ultimate degree of dysfunction.[28, 31, 32] Adour and colleagues have shown that 92 percent of patients regain normal facial motion when given a 10-day course of acyclovir (400 mg by mouth 5 times daily) and prednisone (60 mg/day orally for 5 days, then tapered down by 10 mg/day for 5 days).[32] In addition to the specific treatment, all patients with weak eyelid closure should take general precautions to avoid ocular complications. Patients should use artificial tears throughout the day, ophthalmic ointment at night, and either an eye moisture chamber or taping closed of the affected eyelid during sleep.

Despite using acyclovir and prednisone, some patients never regain good facial function. This subset of patients with poor prognosis may benefit from surgical decompression of the entire infratemporal facial nerve. To determine which patients will have a poor return of function, electroneurography is used, and those showing more than 90 percent degeneration within 21 days have been found to benefit from surgical decompression.[33, 34] Decompression in this setting, however, is controversial.[31, 33] If surgery is offered, both a

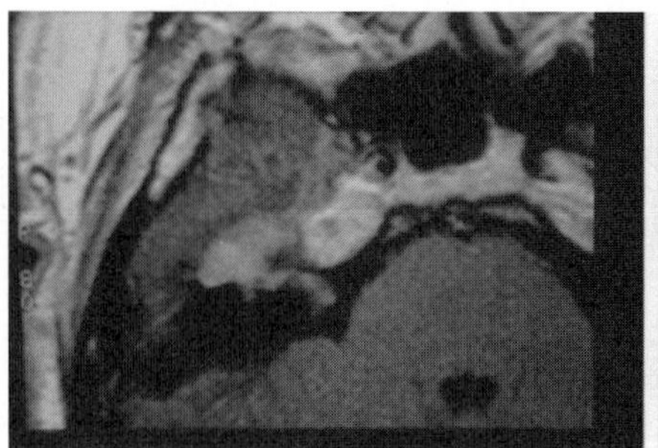

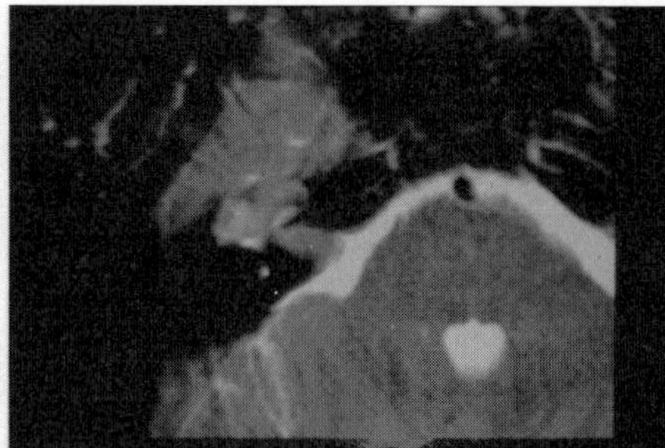

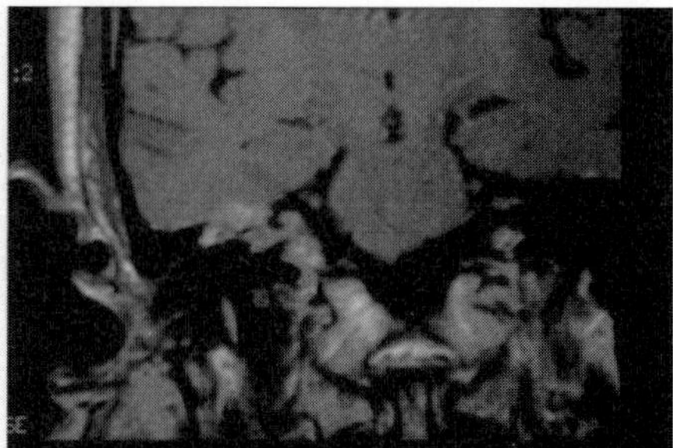

FIGURE 11–4. MRI of brain in a 52-year-old male with right facial twitching, right hearing loss, and headaches. A right-sided tumor of the facial nerve extending from the cerebellopontine angle to mastoid segment is shown. Facial nerve neuroma was suspected, and this was confirmed histologically after removal of the tumor via middle fossa craniotomy.

middle cranial fossa and a transmastoid approach are required. Because the presumed site of entrapment is the meatal foramen (beginning of the labyrinthine segment), middle fossa access is needed to decompress this region. The remainder of the infratemporal facial nerve can then be decompressed via the transmastoid approach.[33, 34]

SYNDROMES OF OVERACTIVATION

Hemifacial Spasm

This movement disorder is characterized by unilateral, involuntary, episodic tonic and clonic contraction of muscles innervated by CN VII. It usually begins as twitches around the eye and progresses to involve the remaining ipsilateral facial muscles, even during sleep. The spasms are painless, can be provoked by voluntary facial motion and emotional stress, and occur most often in middle-aged women. The exact etiology is unknown, but many believe that compression of the motor nerve root at the brain stem by a vascular loop causes focal demyelination and focal ectopic excitation. Impulses resulting from the chronic stimulation conduct centrifugally to the facial nerve nucleus, which causes hyperactivity of the nucleus with resultant bursts of hemifacial spasm.[35] The condition also has been seen after recovery from Bell's palsy and in certain patients with tumors adjacent to CN VII (e.g., parotid gland tumor, cerebellopontine angle meningioma, and acoustic schwannoma).[36] Hemifacial spasm must be differentiated from blepharospasm, which is an involuntary spasm involving both orbicularis oculi muscles.

Myokymia

This is a progressive, irregular fibrillation of individual facial muscle fibers. Usually, it begins in the frontalis and extends to involve all the ipsilateral facial muscles. Electromyographic findings include spontaneous activity of motor units at a rate of 30 to 70 per second. Common causes include pontine gliomas and multiple sclerosis.[4]

RE-INNERVATION SYNDROMES

Postparalytic Movements and Synkinesis

Synkinesis is unintentional motion of a group of muscles when another group is voluntarily contracted. It results from postparalytic re-innervation of different muscles by axons from the same motor neuron. An example is eyelid closure when the patient smiles.

Crocodile Tears

Also called Bogorad's syndrome, it is characterized by unilateral lacrimation during meals in patients with a history of facial palsy. After paralysis with neural degeneration, regenerating axons from the superior salivatory nucleus intended for the chorda tympani instead enter the greater superficial petrosal nerve. Rather than synapsing in the submandibular ganglion to regulate the sublingual and submandibular glands, these preganglionic parasympathetic fibers end up in the pterygopalatine ganglion. Therefore, during meals, the stimulus for increased salivation results in stimulation of the lacrimal gland, with a resultant increase in tearing.

Gustatory Sweating

Also known as Frey's syndrome, this results from anomalous re-innervation of sweat glands by axons intended for the parotid gland. Normally, sweat glands are innervated by postganglionic sympathetic fibers, which are unique in that they use acetylcholine as the transmitter (rather than norepinephrine). The parotid gland is innervated by postganglionic parasympathetic fibers also using acetylcholine as their transmitter to regulate salivary flow. After parotidectomy, the cholinergic fibers originally intended for the parotid gland end up innervating the sweat glands. While eating, stimuli that should cause an increase in salivation instead lead to facial sweating. Parotidectomy is the most common cause.

General Management Goals

General treatment for patients with facial palsy is concerned mainly with protection of the eye from exposure keratitis, especially when an ipsilateral CN V deficit exists. During the day, artificial tears should be used frequently to keep the eye moist. Sunglasses are worn outside. Areas with air contaminated by excessive particulate matter or noxious fumes (e.g., construction sites, textile factories) should be avoided. To protect the cornea while asleep, ophthalmic ointment is instilled. Then, either the eyelid is carefully taped shut or a moisture chamber is used. Other measures to protect the eye are room humidifiers, tape for lid support, and soft contact lenses. Any corneal abrasion or infection should be treated immediately to avoid possible visual complications. If there is deterioration in visual function, ophthalmology consultation is needed.

Specific treatments for facial palsy are aimed at the underlying etiology. Consultation with the appropriate specialist is necessary for facial palsy caused by tumors, cholesteatoma, skull base osteomyelitis, or middle ear infection. Infectious, metabolic, collagen vascular, or toxic causes should be corrected as required by the particular disease. Prompt surgical consultation is needed for patients with facial nerve paralysis after either blunt or penetrating trauma.[37]

For the patient with a permanent facial paralysis despite medical and surgical treatment, many surgical options are available to improve facial function and appearance. These include static sling procedures with fascia lata or alloplastic strips, dynamic procedures with temporalis or masseter transposition, hypoglossal–facial nerve anastomosis, cross-facial nerve grafting, free muscle grafts, and microvascular freenerve-muscle grafts.[38] In addition, the placement of gold weights or springs within the upper eyelid, canthoplasty, and lower lid shortening can help with eye closure. Associated procedures include brow or face lift, entropion or ectropion repair, and lip transposition.[39] In patients who are not surgical candidates or who refuse operative intervention, facial neuromuscular retraining is an alternative therapy that may help patients inhibit their synkinesis.[40]

Reviews and Selected Updates

Bauer CA, Coker NJ: Update on facial nerve disorders. Otolaryngol Clin North Am 1996;29:445–454.

Dew LA, Shelton C: Iatrogenic facial nerve injury: Prevalence and predisposing factors. Ear Nose Throat J 1996;75:724–729.

Graham MD, House WF (eds): Disorders of the Facial Nerve: Anatomy, Diagnosis, and Management. New York, Raven Press, 1982.

Grogan PM, Gronseth GS: Practice parameters: Steroids, acyclovir, and surgery for Bell's palsy (an evidence-based review): Report of the Quality Standards Subcommittee of the American Academy of Neurology. Neurology 2001;56:830–836.

House JW, Brackmann DE: Facial nerve grading system. Otolaryngol Head Neck Surg 1985;93(2):146–147.

May M, Schaitkin BM (eds): The Facial Nerve, 2nd ed. New York, Thieme Medical Publishers, 2000.

References

1. LaRouere MJ, Lundy LB: Anatomy and physiology of the facial nerve. *In* Jackler RK, Brackmann DE (eds): Neurotology. St. Louis, Mosby–Year Book, 1994, pp 1271–1281.
2. Hughes GB: Prognostic tests in acute facial palsy. Am J Otol 1989;10(4):304–311.
3. May M, Klein SR: Differential diagnosis of facial nerve palsy. Otolaryngol Clin North Am 1991;24(3):613–645.
4. Nelson JR: Facial paralysis of central nervous system origin. Otolaryngol Clin North Am 1974;7(2):411–424.
5. Teller DC, Murphy TP: Bilateral facial paralysis: A case presentation and literature review. J Otolaryngol 1992;21(1):44–47.
6. Keane JR: Bilateral seventh nerve palsy: Analysis of 43 cases and review of the literature. Neurology 1994;44:1198–1202.
7. Alioglu Z, Caylan R, Adanir M, Ozmenoglu M: Melkersson-Rosenthal syndrome: Report of three cases. Neurol Sci 2000;21(1):57–60.
8. Carpenter MB, Sutin J: The pons. *In* Carpenter MB, Sutin J: Human Neuroanatomy, 8th ed. Baltimore, Williams & Wilkins, 1983, pp 358–409.
9. Malone B, Maisel RH: Anatomy of the facial nerve. Am J Otol 1988;9(6):494–504.
10. Crosby EC, DeJonge BR: Experimental and clinical studies of the central connections and central relations of the facial nerve. Ann Otol Rhinol Laryngol 1963;72:735–755.
11. Gray H: The hindbrain. *In* Pick TP, Howden R (eds): Gray's Anatomy, 15th ed. New York, Bounty Books, 1977, pp 681–684.
12. Hitselberger WE, House WF: Acoustic neuroma diagnosis: External auditory canal hypesthesia as an early sign. Arch Otolaryngol 1966;83:218–221.
13. Folan-Curran J, Cooke FJ: Contribution of cranial nerve ganglia to innervation of the walls of the rat external acoustic meatus. J Peripher Nerv Syst 2001;6(1):28–32.
14. Lang J: Cerebellopontine angle, pons and internal auditory meatus. *In* Clinical Anatomy of the Posterior Cranial Fossa and Its Foramina. New York, Thieme Medical Publishers, 1991, pp 83–91.
15. Schuknecht HF: Anatomy: The facial nerve. *In* Pathology of the Ear, 2nd ed. Philadelphia, Lea & Febiger, 1993, pp 42–45.
16. Litton WB, Krause CJ, Cohen WN: The relationship of the facial canal to the annular sulcus. Laryngoscope 1969;79:1584–1604.
17. Proctor B: The anatomy of the facial nerve. Otolaryngol Clin North Am 1991;24(3):479–504.
18. Sataloff RT: Embryology of the facial nerve. *In* Embryology and Anomalies of the Facial Nerve and Their Surgical Implications. New York, Raven Press, 1991, pp 3–90.
19. Bernstein L, Nelson RH: Surgical anatomy of the extraparotid distribution of the facial nerve. Arch Otolaryngol 1984;110:177–183.
20. Jongkees LBW: Practical application of clinical tests for facial paralysis. Arch Otolaryngol 1973;97:220–223.
21. Kellman RM: Physiology and pathophysiology. Am J Otol 1989;10(1):62–67.
22. Cramer HB, Kartush JM: Testing facial nerve function. Otolaryngol Clin North Am 1991;24(3):555–570.
23. Dobie RA: Tests of facial nerve function. *In* Cummings CW, Fredrickson JM, Harker LA, et al (eds): Otolaryngology—Head and Neck Surgery, 2nd ed, Vol IV. St. Louis, Mosby–Year Book, 1993, pp 2718–2725.
24. May M, Hardin WB: Facial palsy: Interpretation of neurologic findings. Laryngoscope 1978;88:1352–1362.
25. Jager L, Reiser M: CT and MR imaging of the normal and pathologic conditions of the facial nerve. Eur J Radiol 2001;40(2):133–146.
26. Hughes GB: Prognostic tests in acute facial palsy. Am J Otol 1989;10(4):304–311.
27. Punal JE, Siebert MF, Angueira FB, Lorenzo AV, Castro-Gago M: Three new patients with congenital unilateral facial nerve palsy due to chromosome 22q11 deletion. J Child Neurol 2001;16(6):450–452.
28. Bauer CA, Coker NJ: Update on facial nerve disorders. Otolaryngol Clin North Am 1996;29(3):445–454.
29. Adour KK, Byl FM, Hilsinger RL, et al: The true nature of Bell's palsy: Analysis of 1,000 consecutive patients. Laryngoscope 1978;88:787–801.
30. Peitersen E: The natural history of Bell's palsy. Am J Otol 1982;4(2):107–111.
31. Adour KK: Medical management of idiopathic (Bell's) palsy. Otolaryngol Clin North Am 1991;24(3):663–673.
32. Adour KK, Ruboyianes JM, Von Doerstein PG, et al: Bell's palsy treatment with acyclovir and prednisone compared with prednisone alone: A double-blind, randomized, controlled trial. Ann Otol Rhinol Laryngol 1996;105(5):371–378.
33. Marsh MA, Coker NJ: Surgical decompression of idiopathic facial palsy. Otolaryngol Clin North Am 1991;24(3):675–689.
34. Gantz BJ, Rubinstein JT, Gidley P, Woodworth GG: Surgical management of Bell's palsy. Laryngoscope 1999;109:1177–1188.
35. Jannetta PJ, Abbasy M, Maroon JC, et al: Etiology and definitive microsurgical treatment of hemifacial spasm: Operative techniques and results in 47 patients. J Neurosurg 1977;47:321–328.
36. Galvez-Jimenez N, Hanson MR, Desai M: Unusual causes of hemifacial spasm. Semin Neurol 2001;21(1):75–83.
37. Bascom DA, Schaitkin BM, May M, Klein S: Facial nerve repair: A retrospective review. Facial Plast Surg 2000;16(4):309–313.
38. Conley J, Baker DC: The surgical treatment of extratemporal facial paralysis: An overview. Head Neck Surg 1978;1:12–23.
39. Papel ID: Rehabilitation of the paralyzed face. Otolaryngol Clin North Am 1991;24(3):727–738.
40. Diels HJ: Facial paralysis: Is there a role for a therapist? Facial Plast Surg 2000;16(4):361–364.

CHAPTER 12

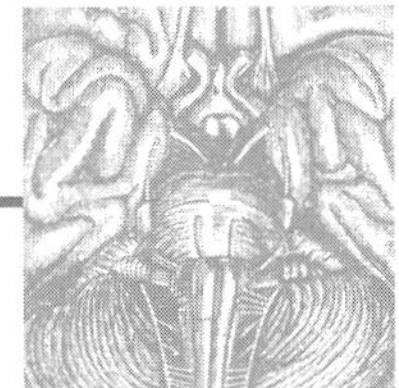

TIMOTHY C. HAIN and ALAN G. MICCO

Cranial Nerve VIII: Vestibulocochlear System

History and Definitions

Sound consists of sinusoidal waves of air pressure, and *hearing* is the perception of sound. The understanding of speech depends on the perception of complex, time-varying multifrequency sound. Hearing is possible when the pitch or frequency range of sound is between 20 and 20,000 cycles/sec (Hz) and when the sound is appropriately loud. The *loudness* of sound is measured in decibels. Clinically, such as during audiometry, decibels are expressed as units of hearing level, and are computed by the formula DB = 20 log P_{test}/P_{ref}, where P_{test} is the sound pressure level in question and P_{ref} is the sound pressure just barely audible by a group of young adults. *Tinnitus* is the false perception of a sound, or the perception of a sound that is not normally perceived, such as the pulse. A single sinusoidal tone corresponds to a ringing noise. Complex multifrequency sounds may be perceived as hissing, buzzing, roaring, or even as speech or music.

Hearing loss consists of a reduction, relative to normal standards, of the ability to perceive sound. Three subtypes are recognized: conductive, sensorineural, and central. In conductive hearing loss, mechanical transmission of sound into the sensory receptors in the cochlea is impaired. In sensorineural hearing loss, there is a loss of function in the sensory receptors in either the cochlea or the auditory nerve. In central hearing loss, there is a lesion in the brain stem or auditory cortex.

Vertigo is a false sensation of movement that is usually caused by disorders of the vestibular system, including the inner ear and/or parts of the central nervous system involved in processing of vestibular signals. Vertigo is often accompanied by imbalance as well as secondary symptoms such as nausea and fatigue. *Dizziness* is a less specific term often used by patients to indicate vertigo as well as a host of other symptoms such as giddiness or lightheadedness, confusion, and imbalance. The vestibular system senses movement by detecting angular velocity and linear acceleration. The semicircular canals are excellent detectors of angular (rotational) velocity. The otolith organs are detectors of linear acceleration that may be related to either movement of the head or changes in orientation to the earth's gravitational field.

The history of the vestibulocochlear system can be traced from the times of the ancient Greeks.[1] Plato theorized that "hearing is motion initiated by sound in the ears and ending in the region of the liver." Aristotle (384 BC–322 BC) outlined the concept of "inner ear" in the occiput of the skull as forming the basis of hearing. In 97 AD, Rufus of Ephesus described the auricular anatomy of the inner ear using the words *helix*, *antihelix*, and *tragus*, which are terms that are still in use today. Galen (130–200 AD) introduced the term *labyrinth* to describe the inner structure of the inner ear in temporal bone.

Vesalius (1564) named two of the ossicles, the malleus (drumstick or hammer) and incus (anvil). Eustachio (1510–1571) discovered the eustachian tube, which maintains equal pressure on both sides of the tympanic membrane. In 1850, Corti described the sensory epithelium of the cochlea, and the organ of Corti is his namesake. Rinne, in 1855, developed the use of tuning fork tests in the diagnosis of middle ear disease. Ménière, in 1861, described a disorder of increased pressure in the inner ear, a disease that now bears his name. Barr, in 1901, described the use of a ticking watch to quantify hearing loss. Barany received the Nobel Prize in 1909 for his work describing the caloric test. Fletcher, in 1923, described the electric audiometer. Bekesy received the Nobel Prize in the 1950s for his discovery of the traveling wave mechanism for the stimulation of the cochlea. In more recent years, the surgical specialty of neuro-otology has emerged, driven by availability of the operative microscope and the need for advanced training and subspecialization to surgically treat otosclerosis and acoustic neuromas.

Clinical History

Disorders of the vestibulocochlear system, namely dizziness and hearing disturbances, are common and have diverse causes. Accordingly, the history must be unusually thorough. To be adequate, the history should be all-encompassing or should follow a heuristic approach in which questions are dynamically selected as the interview progresses. In the all-encompassing approach, the examiner should first obtain a definition of symptoms. Does the patient complain of vertigo, a secondary symptom (such as nausea), a nonspecific symptom (giddiness or lightheadedness), or something unlikely to be caused by dysfunction of cranial nerve VIII (e.g., confusion or syncope)? With respect to hearing complaints, the clinician should ascertain whether one or both sides is affected, what types of sounds are poorly perceived (low-pitched, high-pitched, speech only, speech with background noise), whether there is an accompanying tinnitus (ringing, pulsatile, multifrequency sound such as roaring, auditory hallucinations), and whether there is otalgia or an abnormal sensation in the ear such as fullness. It is particularly important to inquire about coincident headaches, because migraine is a frequent source of vertigo.

Next, the physician should inquire about timing. Are symptoms constant or episodic? If episodic, how long do they last? Vertigo caused by benign paroxysmal positional vertigo (BPPV) usually lasts 10 seconds. Vertigo from attacks of Ménière's disease typically lasts 2 hours. Vestibular neuritis persists for weeks, and central vertigo may persist for years. The clinician should establish whether the various symptoms are related in time. This finding is particularly important for certain disorders that present as symptom complexes, such as the headache and dizziness of vertebrobasilar migraine or the typical quadrad of tinnitus, vertigo, aural fullness, and fluctuating hearing that typifies Ménière's disease.

All patients with vertigo should be queried regarding *triggering or exacerbating factors* (Table 12–1). In vertiginous patients, it is particularly important to inquire about positional triggers, because about 20 percent of all vertigo is caused by BPPV (see later).

A medication history should be taken because numerous medications can induce vertigo or impair hearing. Anticonvulsants, antihypertensives, and sedatives are common sources of dizziness and vertigo, and ototoxic medications (Table 12–2) may additionally be the source of hearing disturbances or ataxia. All current medications as well as previous exposure to ototoxins should be noted. In persons with hearing complaints, a history of noise exposure should also be obtained.

The *family history* is important to obtain, because there may be other family members who have migraine, seizures, Ménière's disease, oteosclerosis, or early-onset hearing loss. The *review of systems* should explore psychiatric problems (especially anxiety and panic), vascular risk factors, cancer, autoimmune disease, neurological problems (especially migraine, stroke, transient ischemic attack, seizures, multiple sclerosis), otological surgery, and general medical history (especially thyroid dysfunction, diabetes, and syphilis).

TABLE 12–1. **Triggering or Exacerbating Factors for Vertigo**

- Changes in position of the head or body
- Standing up
- Rapid head movements
- Walking in a dark room
- Loud noises
- Coughing, blowing the nose, sneezing, straining, or laughing
- Underwater diving, elevators, airplane travel
- Exercise
- Shopping malls, narrow or wide open spaces, grocery stores, escalators (visual sensitivity complex)
- Foods, not eating, salt, monosodium glutamate
- Alcohol
- Menstrual periods or hormonal manipulations
- Boat or car travel
- Anxiety or stress

TABLE 12–2. **Ototoxic Medications**

Antibiotics
Mainly vestibulotoxic
- Gentamicin
- Streptomycin
- Tobramycin

Mainly cochleotoxic
- Vancomycin
- Kanamycin
- Neomycin
- Amikacin

Diuretics (Mainly Cochleotoxic)
- Furosemide
- Bumetanide
- Ethacrynic acid

Quinine (Cochleotoxic)

Aspirin and Sodium Salicylate (Cochleotoxic, Reversible)

Chemotherapy (Mainly Mixed Toxicity)
- *Cis*-platinum (mainly cochleotoxic)
- Nitrogen mustard
- Actinomycin
- Bleomycin

TABLE 12–3. **Clinico-anatomical Correlations of Disorders of Cranial Nerve VIII—Auditory System**

Anatomical Location	Signs/Symptoms	Associated Neurological Findings
Cerebral cortex	Aphasia Auditory hallucinations	Normal hearing
Brain stem	Unilateral hearing loss Tinnitus Poor word recognition	Vestibular disorder
Cerebellopontine angle	Unilateral hearing loss Tinnitus Poor word discrimination	Vestibular disorder Facial weakness Facial numbness
Cochlear nerve	Unilateral hearing loss Tinnitus	Vestibular disorder
Cochlea	Hearing loss Tinnitus Hyperacusis	Facial weakness Aural fullness
Middle ear	Hearing loss Tinnitus	

Anatomy of the Vestibulocochlear System (Tables 12–3 and 12–4)

AUDITORY SYSTEM

Sound impinging on the ear is transmitted through a mechanical system including the tympanic membrane and ossicular chain, ending at the stapes. Sound energy is then converted into changes in neural firing, which is passed more centrally through a complex cross-connected network of neurons. This neural network can be considered as a series of four orders of neurons. First order neurons are derived from the auditory (spiral) ganglion; second order neurons are those in the neighborhood of the cochlear nuclei in the brain stem. Third order neurons are found at the level of the inferior colliculus, and fourth order neurons travel from the medial geniculate body in the thalamus to the auditory cortex. Considerably more detail about these pathways can be found in Webster and colleagues.[2]

TABLE 12–4. **Clinico-anatomical Correlations of Disorders of Cranial Nerve VIII—Vestibular System**

Anatomical Location	Signs/Symptoms	Associated Neurological Findings
Cerebral cortex	Quick spins	Confusion
Brain stem	Vertigo Ataxia	Nystagmus Weakness Numbness Dysarthria Diplopia
Cerebellopontine angle	Vertigo Ataxia	Nystagmus Hearing loss Facial weakness Facial numbness
Vestibular nerve	Quick spins Vertigo Ataxia	Nystagmus
Labyrinth	Vertigo Ataxia	Hearing symptoms Oscillopsia Pressure sensitivity

First Order Neuron

The vestibular and cochlear divisions of the inner ear are depicted in Figure 12–1A. Longitudinally (Fig. 12–1B), the labyrinth is composed of an outer compartment containing perilymph (similar to extracellular fluid) and an inner compartment containing endolymph (similar to intracellular fluid). The hair cells are embedded in the floor of the inner compartment, the basilar membrane. Two types of hair cells are in the cochlea, inner and outer. When sound is transmitted to the cochlea, oscillations are set up in the basilar membrane, and this stimulates the *inner hair cells*. Place-code mapping occurs between frequency of sounds to areas of the cochlea called a *tonotopic distribution*, which results in registration of higher frequencies at the base of the cochlea and lower frequencies at the apex.

The more numerous *outer hair cells* are motile and may help to dynamically tune the system. Appreciation of the motile nature of outer hair cells has led to a new test of hearing called *otacoustical emissions* or *OAEs* (see later). *Reissner's membrane* roofs the compartment containing the hair cells. In certain conditions in which endolymph pressure is increased (e.g., Ménière's disease), Reissner's membrane may bow out or rupture. The *spiral ganglion of the cochlea* is wrapped around the cochlea and receives output from the hair cells to create the *auditory nerve*, which runs with the vestibular nerve and facial nerve in the internal auditory canal. In addition to the afferent fibers in the vestibulocochlear nerve, there are also *efferent fibers*, which supply the outer hair cells.

Second Order Neuron

The cochlear nerve enters the brain stem at the pontomedullary junction, where it bifurcates and terminates in the two major subdivisions of the cochlear nucleus—the dorsal and ventral cochlear nuclei (Fig. 12–2). The most important outflow is to the *trapezoid body*, which contains fibers destined for the bilateral superior olivary nuclei in the brain stem. The *superior olive* is concerned with sound localization, based in interaural differences in sound timing and intensity. The superior olive is also an essential part of the stapedius reflex, which is a protective reflex in the middle ear. The simplest stapedius reflex arc involves the spiral ganglion neurons, the cochlear nucleus, superior olive, and facial nerve nucleus. Output from the superior olive joins crossed and uncrossed axons from the cochlear nucleus to form the *lateral lemniscus*. This pathway ascends to the inferior colliculus. Because the lateral lemniscus contains second order neurons from the cochlear nucleus and third and fourth order neurons from the superior olive, it contributes to three waves of the auditory brain stem response (described later). The tonotopic arrangement of the cochlea is maintained in the cochlear nucleus, lateral lemniscus, and reticular formation.

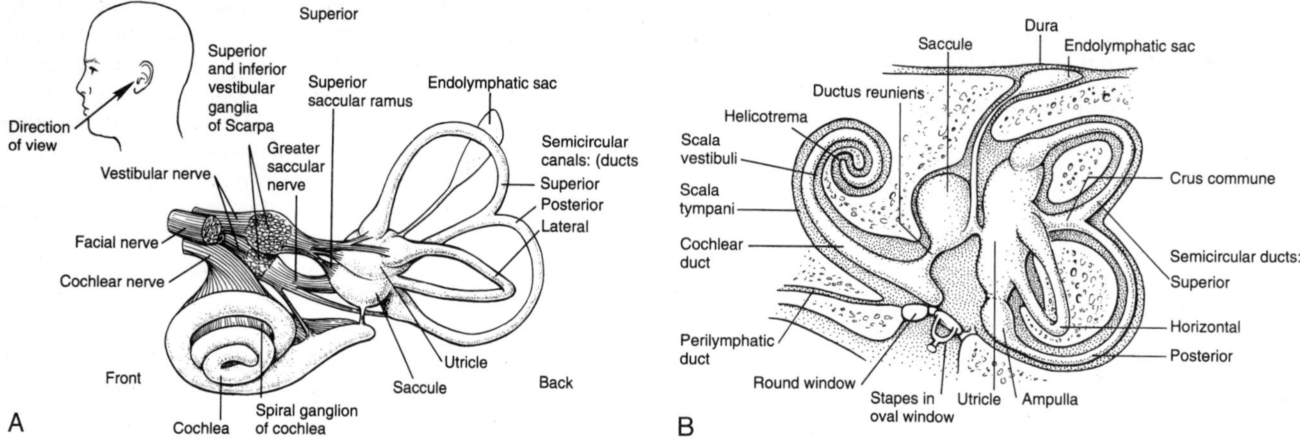

FIGURE 12–1. The cochlea (*A*) and vestibular labyrinth (*B*). (From Kandel ER, Schwartz JH, Jessell TM [eds]: Principles of Neural Science, 3rd ed. East Norwalk, CT, Appleton & Lange, 1991.)

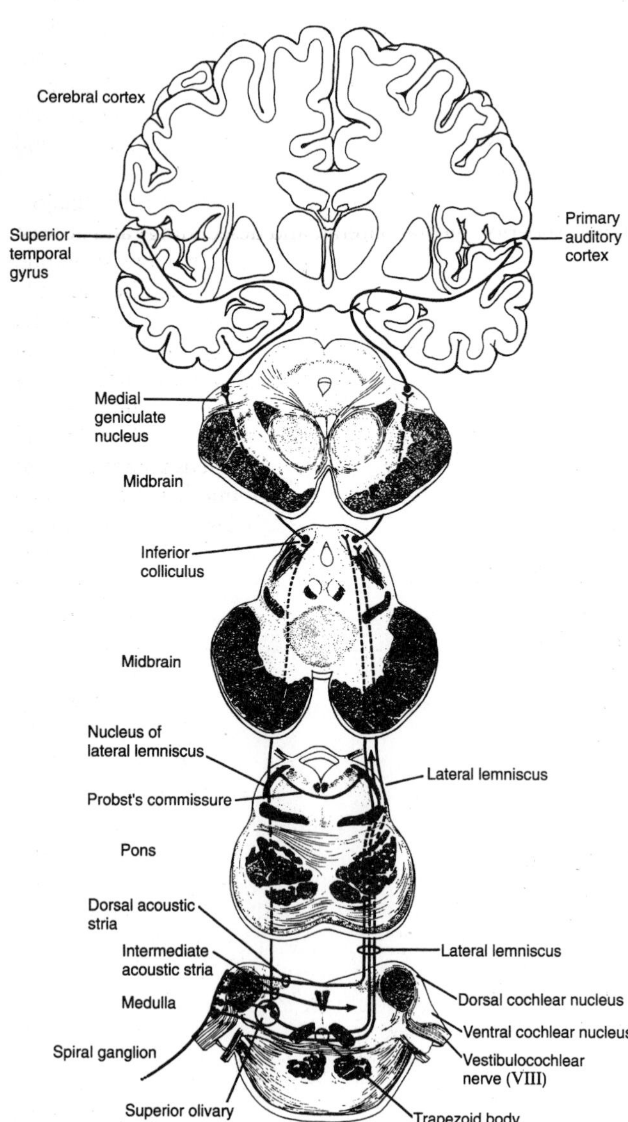

FIGURE 12–2. Central auditory pathways. (Reprinted with permission from Kandel ER, Schwartz JH, Jessell T: Principles of Neural Science, 3rd ed. East Norwalk, CT, Appleton & Lange, 1991, p 495.)

Because of the extensive crossing that occurs early in the central auditory circuitry, central auditory lesions usually do not cause monaural hearing loss.

Third Order Neuron

The inferior colliculus is a major integrating center for the auditory system and serves as a center for feedback pathways to the lower auditory system. Output from the inferior colliculus ascends to the medial geniculate body of the thalamus.

Fourth Order Neuron

The medial geniculate body is the major auditory nucleus of the thalamus. Parts of the medial geniculate are hypothesized to function in directing auditory attention. The medial geniculate body sends output to the primary auditory cortex, also known as the *transverse temporal gyri of Heschl* (Brodmann areas 41 and 42) and auditory association cortex (areas 22 and 52) (Fig. 12–3). The medial geniculate also sends output to the auditory motor cortex, which controls body responses to sound. The auditory cortex is divided into three areas, including a primary area (AI), a secondary area (AII), and a remote projection region (Ep). Investigators have varied in assigning area 42 to the primary or secondary auditory cortex. The ventral medial geniculate projects almost entirely to AI, whereas the surrounding auditory areas receive projections from the rest of the geniculate body. As with the lower auditory systems, tonotopic relationships are maintained.

VESTIBULAR SYSTEM

The peripheral vestibular system consists of a set of three-dimensional angular velocity transducers, the semicircular canals, and a set of three-dimensional linear acceleration transducers, the otoliths (utricle and saccule) (see Fig. 12–1).[3] These transducers are suspended by an assembly of membranes and connective tissue, the *membranous labyrinth,* within channels in the temporal bone, the *bony labyrinth.* Three important spatial arrangements characterize the semicircular canals. First, each canal within each labyrinth is *perpendicular* to the other canals, which is analogous to the spatial relationship between two walls and the floor of a rec-

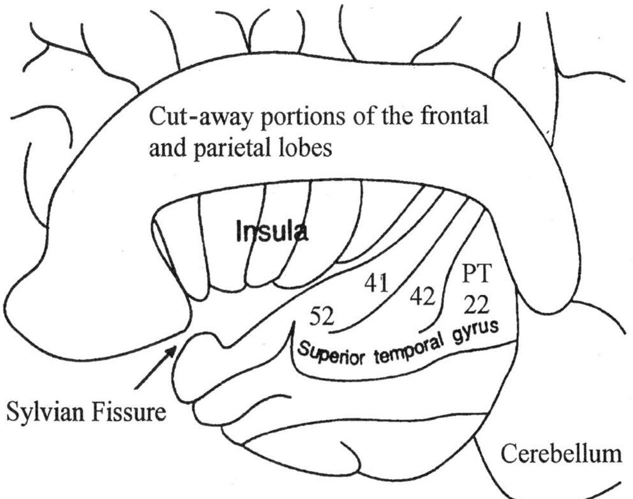

FIGURE 12–3. Cortical auditory areas. Portions of the frontal and parietal lobes have been cut away above the sylvian fissure to expose the insula and the superior temporal lobe. The number of Heschl's gyrus is variable. In this illustration, primary auditory cortex (41) is shown on the first transverse gyrus of Heschl, and area 42 is shown on the second transverse gyrus. PT, planum temporale. (Modified from Webster DB, Popper AN, Fay RF: The Mammalian Auditory Pathway: Neuroanatomy. New York, Springer-Verlag, 1992, p 17.)

tangular room. Second, the planes of the semicircular canals, between the labyrinths, conform very closely to each other. The six individual semicircular canals become three *co-planar* pairs: (1) right and left lateral; (2) left anterior and right posterior; and (3) left posterior and right anterior. Third, the planes of the canals are close to the planes of the extraocular muscles. This relationship allows relatively simple connections between sensory neurons related to individual canals and motor output neurons, which are related to individual ocular muscles.

The otoliths register linear acceleration, and they respond both to linear head motion and to static tilt with respect to the gravitational axis. The otolithic membranes contain calcium carbonate crystals called *otoconia*, and, therefore, they have substantially more mass than the surrounding structures. The increased mass of the otolithic membrane causes the maculae to be sensitive to gravity. In contrast, the cupulae of the semicircular canals have the same density as the surrounding endolymphatic fluid and are insensitive to gravity. Like the canals, the otoliths are arranged in a manner to enable them to respond to motion in all three dimensions. In an upright person, the saccule is vertical (parasagittal), whereas the utricle is horizontally oriented (near the plane of the lateral semicircular canals). In this posture, the saccule can sense linear acceleration in its plane, which includes the acceleration oriented along the occipitocaudal axis and linear motion along the anteroposterior axis. The utricle senses acceleration in its plane, which includes lateral accelerations along the interaural axis, as well as anteroposterior motion.

Vestibular Ganglion and Nerve

Vestibular nerve fibers are the afferent projections from the bipolar neurons of Scarpa's ganglion. The vestibular nerve transmits afferent signals from the labyrinths through the *internal auditory canal* (IAC). In addition to the vestibular nerve, the IAC also contains the cochlear nerve (hearing), the facial nerve, the nervus intermedius (a branch of the facial nerve), and the labyrinthine artery. The IAC travels through the petrous portion of the temporal bone to open into the posterior fossa at the level of the pons. The vestibular nerve enters the brain stem at the pontomedullary junction and contains two divisions, the superior and inferior vestibular nerves. The *superior vestibular nerve* innervates the utricle, as well as the superior and lateral canals. The *inferior vestibular nerve* innervates the posterior canal and the saccule. Because a common disorder of the vestibular nerve, vestibular neuritis, often spares the inferior division, clinical situations can arise where there is a partial injury to the vestibular nerve.[4]

Vestibular Nuclei

The primary vestibular afferents transmit information mainly to the vestibular nuclear complex and the cerebellum. The vestibular nuclear complex is the primary processor of vestibular input, and it implements direct, fast connections between incoming afferent information and motor output neurons. The cerebellum monitors vestibular performance and keeps it "calibrated." In both locations, vestibular sensory input is processed in association with somatosensory and visual sensory input.

The *vestibular nuclear complex* consists of four "major" nuclei (superior, medial, lateral, and descending) and at least seven "minor" nuclei (Fig. 12–4). It is a large structure, located primarily within the pons but also extending caudally into the medulla. The superior and medial vestibular nuclei are relays for the vestibulo-ocular reflex (VOR). The medial vestibular nucleus is also involved in vestibulospinal reflexes (VSR), and it coordinates head and eye movements that occur together. The lateral vestibular nucleus is the principal nucleus for the VSR. The descending nucleus is connected to all of the other nuclei and the cerebellum, but it has no primary outflow of its own. The vestibular nuclei are linked together via a system of *commissures*, which for the most part are mutually inhibitory. The commissures allow information to be shared between the two sides of the brain stem, and they implement the pairing of canals (discussed earlier).

In the vestibular nuclear complex, processing of the vestibular sensory input occurs concurrently with the processing of extravestibular sensory information (proprioceptive, visual, tactile, and auditory). Extensive connections between the vestibular nuclear complex, cerebellum, ocular motor nuclei, and brain stem reticular activating systems are required to formulate appropriate efferent signals to the VOR and VSR effector organs, the extraocular and skeletal muscles. The vestibular nucleus sends outflow to the oculomotor nuclei, spinal cord, cerebellum, and vestibular cortex.

Three major white matter pathways connect the vestibular nucleus to the anterior horn cells of the spinal cord. The *lateral vestibulospinal tract* originates from the ipsilateral lateral vestibular nucleus, which receives the majority of its input from the otoliths and the cerebellum. This pathway generates antigravity postural motor activity, primarily in the lower extremities, in response to the head position changes that occur with respect to gravity. The *medial vestibulospinal tract* originates from the contralateral medial,

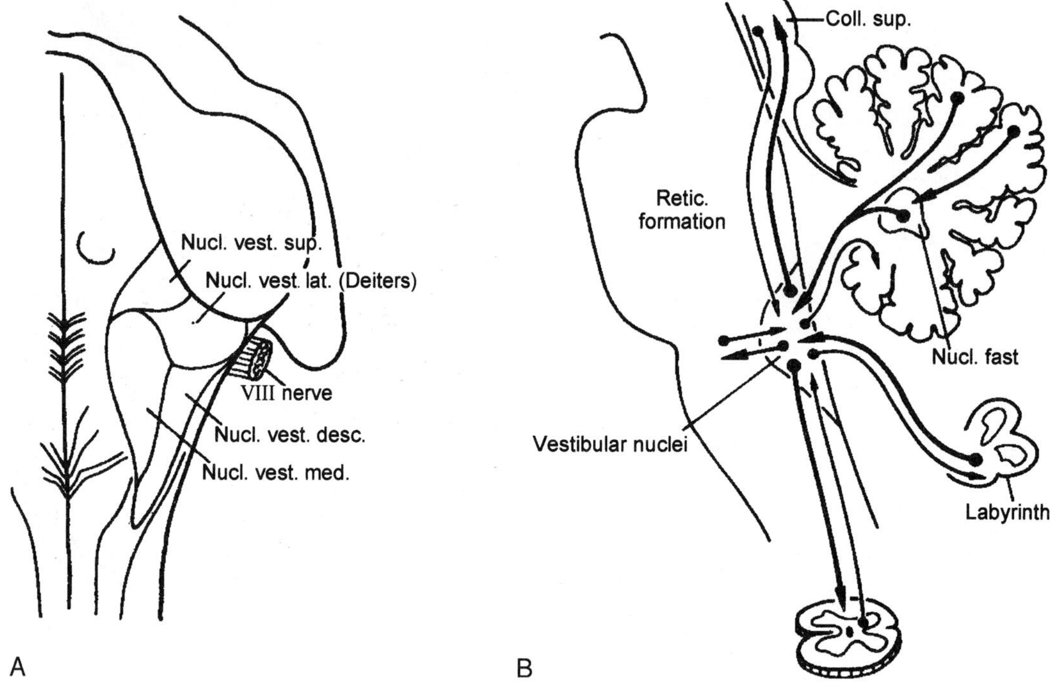

FIGURE 12–4. *A,* The four main vestibular nuclei in man as projected on the dorsal surface of the brain stem. *B,* A simplified diagram of the main connections of the vestibular nuclei. (From Brodal A: Neurological Anatomy in Relation to Clinical Medicine, 3rd ed. Copyright 1969, 1981 by Oxford University Press, Inc. Used by permission of Oxford University Press, Inc.)

superior, and descending vestibular nuclei; it mediates ongoing postural changes in response to semicircular canal sensory input (angular head motion). The medial vestibulospinal tract descends only through the cervical spinal cord in the medial longitudinal fasciculus; it activates cervical axial musculature.

The *reticulospinal tract* receives sensory input from all of the vestibular nuclei, as well as all of the other sensory and motor systems involved with maintaining balance. This projection has both crossed and uncrossed components, and it is very highly collateralized. As a result, its pathway through the entire extent of the spinal cord is poorly defined. The reticulospinal tract is probably involved in most balance reflex motor actions, including postural adjustments made to extravestibular sensory input (auditory, visual, and tactile stimuli).

The cerebellum is a major recipient of outflow from the vestibular nucleus complex, and it is also a major source of input to the vestibular nucleus itself. Most of the signal traffic is routed through the inferior cerebellar peduncle. The cerebellum is not required for vestibular reflexes, but when removed, vestibular reflexes become uncalibrated and ineffective. Originally, the *vestibulocerebellum* was defined as the portions of the cerebellum that received direct input from the primary vestibular afferents. It is now appreciated that most parts of the cerebellar vermis (midline) respond to vestibular stimulation. The cerebellar projections to the vestibular nuclear complex have an inhibitory influence on the vestibular nuclear complex. The *cerebellar flocculus* adjusts and maintains the gain of the VOR.[5] Lesions of the flocculus reduce the ability of experimental animals to adapt to disorders that reduce or increase the gain of the VOR. The cerebellar *nodulus* adjusts the duration of VOR responses; it is also involved with processing of otolith input.

VASCULAR ANATOMY

The arterial circulation of the inner ear (Fig. 12–5) is completely supplied by the *labyrinthine artery*. The labyrinthine artery has a variable origin. Most often it is a branch of the *anterior inferior cerebellar artery* (AICA), but occasionally, it is a direct branch of the basilar artery. As it enters the inner ear, it divides into the *anterior vestibular artery* and the *common cochlear artery*. The anterior vestibular artery supplies the vestibular nerve, most of the utricle, and the ampullae of the lateral and anterior semicircular canals. The common cochlear artery divides into a main branch, the *main cochlear artery*, and the *vestibulocochlear artery*. The main cochlear artery supplies the cochlea. The vestibulocochlear artery supplies part of the cochlea, ampulla of the posterior semicircular canal, and inferior part of the saccule. The labyrinth has no collateral anastomotic network and is highly susceptible to ischemia. Only 15 seconds of selective blood flow cessation is needed to abolish auditory nerve excitability.[6]

The *vertebral-basilar arterial system* provides the vascular supply for both the peripheral and central auditory vestibular system. The posterior inferior cerebellar arteries branch off the vertebral arteries. They supply the surface of the inferior portions of the cerebellar hemispheres, as well as the dorsolateral medulla, which includes the inferior aspects of the vestibular nuclear complex. The *basilar artery* is the principal artery of the pons. The basilar artery supplies central vestibular structures via *perforator branches*, which penetrate the medial pons; *short circumferential branches*, which supply the anterolateral aspect of the pons; and *long circumferential branches*, which supply the dorsolateral pons. The AICA supplies both the peripheral vestibular system, via the labyrinthine artery, as well as the ventrolateral cerebellum and the lateral tegmentum of the lower two thirds of the

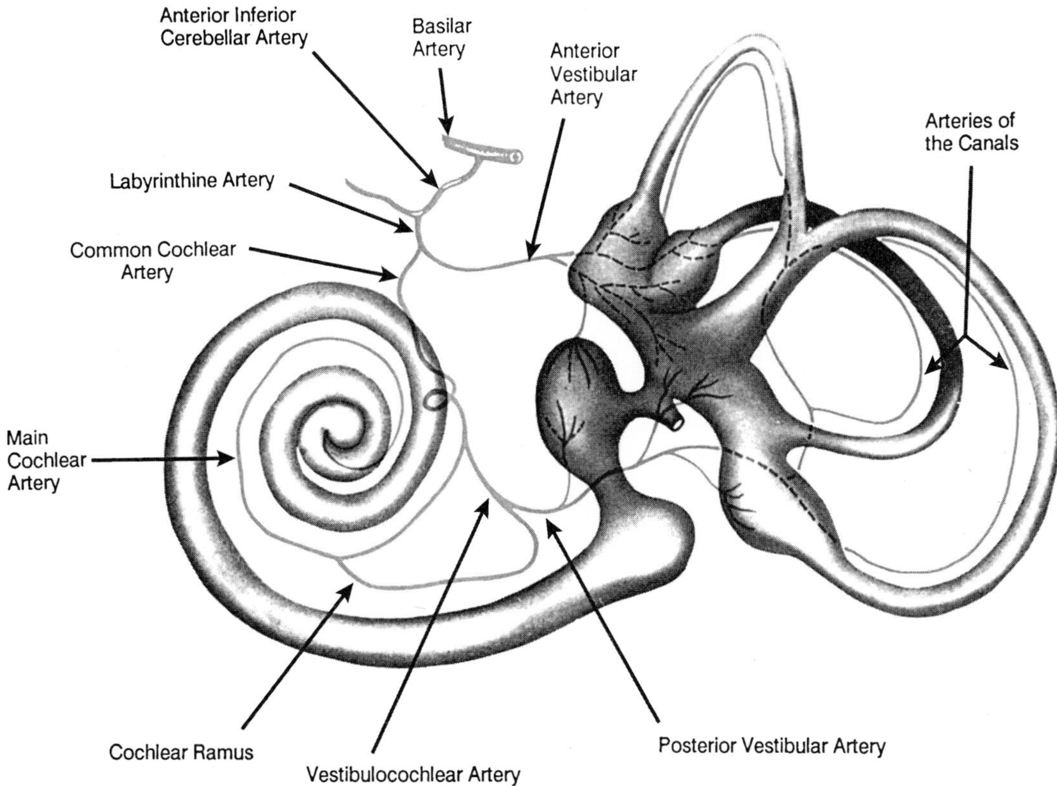

FIGURE 12–5. Arterial supply of the inner ear. (From Schuknecht HF: Pathology of the Ear. Philadelphia, Lea & Febiger, 1993, p 64.)

pons. Central auditory cortex is mainly supplied by the middle cerebral artery.

Examination of the Vestibulocochlear System

DIRECTED NEUROLOGICAL EXAMINATION

The "directed" or focused neurological examination for the assessment of cranial nerve VIII includes an evaluation of the external ear, hearing, and vestibular responses. The examination begins with an assessment of *gait and balance*.

Gait can often be observed as the patient walks into the examination room. The most useful test to quantify balance is the *eyes-closed tandem Romberg's* test. Low-normal performance consists of the ability to stand for 6 seconds, heel to toe, with eyes closed. Young adults should be able to perform this test for 30 seconds, but performance declines with age. It is helpful to develop a judgment as to how much ataxia is appropriate for a given degree of vestibular injury. Patients with *bilateral vestibular loss* are moderately ataxic—they make heavy use of vision and (with a narrow base) are unsteady when their eyes are closed. No patient with bilateral vestibular loss can stand in eyes-closed tandem Romberg's test position for 6 seconds. Patients with an additional superimposed posterior column position sense deficit, as well as patients with cerebellar dysfunction, are unsteady even with their eyes open. Patients with *chronic unilateral vestibular loss* show very little ataxia, and they can usually perform the eyes-closed tandem Romberg's test. The need to quantify ataxia does not come up in patients with recent unilateral vestibular imbalance, because these patients have a prominent nystagmus. Although numerous vestibulospinal tests have been described over the years, such as the Unterberger and Fukuda stepping test, the test results are not clinically useful because of variable performance in the normal population. In patients with head injury or in those in whom there are other reasons to suspect a central nervous system (CNS) origin of imbalance, basal ganglia function (pulsion/retropulsion tests) should also be performed.

The examination proceeds with an inspection of the external ear and ear canal looking for malformations, infections, masses, or asymmetry. Next, the tympanic membranes should be inspected for wax, perforation, otitis, or mass lesions. It is usually prudent to remove wax before embarking on more sophisticated diagnostic procedures. The tympanic membranes contribute about 20 db to the hearing level. Disorders such as perforation, scarring, fluid accumulation, or wax impaction can cause a conductive hearing loss. A normal tympanic membrane is translucent. Fluid behind the tympanic membrane imparts a straw color.

For *bedside hearing assessment*, Rinne's and Weber's tests can be used. In Weber's test, a vibrating 512-Hz tuning fork is placed on the patient's forehead. If the sound predominates in one ear, the patient may have either a conductive hearing loss in that ear or a contralateral sensorineural hearing loss. In Rinne's test, the base of a vibrating tuning fork is placed on the mastoid and then placed about an inch away from the ear. Sound is normally appreciated better through air than through bone. If sound is heard better through bone, it is likely that there is a conductive hearing loss. Other tuning fork tests include Bing's and Schwabach's tests. In Bing's test, the fork is struck and placed on the mastoid tip. The examiner alternately occludes the patient's ipsilateral external meatus. If the patient has normal hearing or a sensorineural loss, he or she notices a change in intensity with occlusion. If the patient has a conductive hearing loss, he or she notices no change. Schwabach's test is contingent on the examiner having normal hearing; the patient's hearing is compared with the examiner's. For bone conduction testing, if the patient stops hearing the sound before the examiner, this finding is consistent with a sensorineural loss. If the patient hears the sound longer than the examiner, it suggests a conductive hearing loss.

In current clinical practice, the wide availability of excellent audiometric testing allows a much briefer screening maneuver to be used with excellent results. The examiner's thumb and second finger are rubbed together at an arm's length from one of the patient's ears. Persons with normal hearing can perceive this sound at this distance. If the sound is not perceptible, this noise is brought closer and closer until it is heard, and the distance is recorded. This simple test identifies high-tone hearing loss, and an unexpected loss or asymmetrical findings may warrant formal audiogram studies or further investigations with the tuning fork maneuvers described earlier.

Spontaneous nystagmus is next assessed using Frenzel's goggles, which are illuminated, magnifying goggles worn by the patient. The goggles are placed on the patient, and over the next 10 to 15 seconds, the eyes are observed for the presence of spontaneous nystagmus. The typical nystagmus produced by inner ear dysfunction is a "jerk" nystagmus—the eyes slowly deviate off center and then there is a rapid jerk, which brings them back to the center position. Most other patterns of nystagmus (e.g., sinusoidal, gaze-evoked) are of central origin. If Frenzel's goggles are not available, clinicians can obtain similar information about nystagmus from the ophthalmoscopic examination, by monitoring the movement of the back of the eye. Because the back of the eye moves in the opposite direction to the front of the eye, for horizontal and vertical movements, the examiner must remember to invert the direction of the nystagmus when noting the direction of the fast phase. Furthermore, an attempt should be made to determine the effect of fixation on nystagmus. Nystagmus derived from the inner ear is increased by removal of fixation, whereas nystagmus of central origin is variably affected by fixation. Some types of central nystagmus, such as congenital nystagmus, may increase with fixation. Most forms of central nystagmus, however, decrease with fixation. Frenzel's goggles are an excellent means of removing fixation. In the ophthalmoscope test, fixation can also be removed by covering the opposite eye.

If there is little or no spontaneous nystagmus and if Frenzel's goggles are available, the *head-shake test* may be performed in an attempt to provoke a nystagmus. In this maneuver, the patient's eyes are closed and the head is moved in the horizontal plane, back and forth, for 20 cycles. A 45-degree excursion of the head to either side and a 2-cycle/second frequency should be used. Nystagmus lasting 5 seconds or more is indicative of an organic disorder of the ear or CNS and supports further detailed investigation.

All patients with vertigo should receive a *Dix-Hallpike positional test* (Fig. 12–6). The patient is first positioned on the examination table, so that when lying flat the head will extend over the end of the table. If Frenzel's goggles are available, they are used; however, the test may be adequately performed without them. The patient is moved backward rapidly to lie on the table in the head-hanging-down position. The eyes are observed for the development of nystagmus. If no dizziness or nystagmus is appreciated after 20 seconds, the patient is returned to the sitting position. The head is then repositioned 45 degrees to the right, and the patient is again brought down to the head-right supine position. After another 20 seconds, the patient is returned to the sitting position, and the procedure is repeated to the left (head-left). A burst of nystagmus, provoked by either the head-right or head-left position, should be sought. The nystagmus of classic BPPV beats upward and also has a rotatory component, such that the top part of the eye beats toward the down ear. The nystagmus typically has a latency of 2 to 5 seconds, lasts 5 to 60 seconds, and is followed by a downbeating nystagmus when the patient is placed upright in sitting position. A lateral-canal variant of BPPV occurs in which the eyes beat horizontally, the direction depending on head position. The "geotrophic" form beats toward the down ear. The "ageotrophic" form beats away from the down ear. Nystagmus that is sustained longer than 1 minute is unlikely to be BPPV.

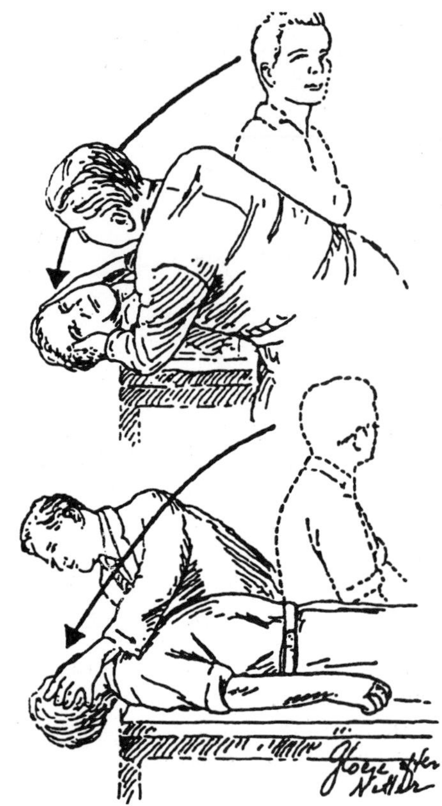

FIGURE 12–6. Dix-Hallpike maneuver. (From Baloh RW, Halmagyi GH [eds]: Disorders of the Vestibular System. New York, Oxford University Press, 1996, p 331.)

Although other positional tests can be used, they are of considerably less utility than the Dix-Hallpike test because of the relatively low incidence of causes of positional nystagmus other than BPPV. Central positional nystagmus such as a persistent downbeat or lateral beating nystagmus may be registered best by simple positional maneuvers wherein the head is supine rather than hyperextended, as in the Dix-Hallpike maneuver. Rarely, patients may develop nystagmus related to the position of their head on neck rather than with respect to gravity, and in these instances, maneuvers should be done wherein the trunk is rotated with respect to a stable head.

Maneuvers used in the *assessment of VOR gain* are aimed at documenting bilateral vestibular loss. They need not be done unless the patient has failed the eyes-closed tandem Romberg's test (see earlier). *The dynamic illegible* E test is the easiest and most sensitive of these tests. Using an eye chart located at least 10 feet away from the patient, visual acuity is recorded with the head still. Then, the examiner moves the patient's head horizontally at roughly 1 Hz, ±30 degrees, and visual acuity is again recorded. Normal individuals lose zero to two lines of acuity with head movement. Patients with partial to complete loss of vestibular function have a reduction of three to seven lines of acuity. The *ophthalmoscope test* is done when the dynamic illegible E test result is positive. The examiner focuses on the optic disc and then gently moves the head as described earlier. If the disc moves with the head, it confirms that the VOR gain is abnormal. This test is less sensitive than the illegible E test but is objective in nature. The *rapid doll's head test* can also be used when the illegible E test result is positive. The examiner stands in front of the patient, and the patient focuses on the examiner's nose. The examiner slowly rotates the patient's head to one side, roughly 30 degrees. Then, while asking the patient to continue to fixate, the head is rapidly rotated to the opposite mirror image position. In a normal subject, the eyes remain fixated on the examiner's nose throughout the entire procedure, moving equal and opposite to the head. In a patient with a poor VOR, such as in bilateral vestibular loss, a refixational eye movement is necessary after the head has stopped moving. This test can also sometimes detect unilateral vestibular lesions, because there may be a refixation saccade only when the head is rotated toward the bad side.

The *hyperventilation test* is most useful in patients with normal examinations up to this point. In this test, the patient breathes deeply and forcefully for 30 breaths at a rate of roughly one breath per second. Immediately after hyperventilation, the eyes are inspected for nystagmus with Frenzel's goggles, and the patient is asked if the procedure reproduced symptoms. A subjectively positive test result without nystagmus suggests the diagnosis of hyperventilation syndrome and is thought to be a sign of an anxiety disorder. Nystagmus induced by hyperventilation can occur in patients with tumors or irritation of cranial nerve VIII or in the setting of multiple sclerosis.

There are several additional tests performed in persons in whom a perilymph fistula or superior canal dehiscence is suspected. These patients will complain of pressure sensitivity or sound-induced vertigo. A loud noise, such as the Barany noise box, can be combined with Frenzel's goggles to document sound-induced vertigo. The Valsalva maneuver also may provoke nystagmus.

ASSOCIATED NEUROLOGICAL FINDINGS

Cerebral. Assessment of *cognitive function* does not often contribute to diagnosis of syndromes involving cranial nerve VIII. Unless there are specific issues suggested by history, this portion of the neurological examination can usually be omitted. The examination for aphasia should be undertaken if it appears that there is a discrepancy between the ability to detect sound versus the patient's ability to interpret sound. For example, an individual with cortical deafness may startle to a handclap but otherwise appears deaf.

Cranial Nerves. Other *cranial nerves* are rarely involved in processes that affect cranial nerve VIII. Corneal reflexes should be assessed when there are sensory complaints involving the face. Rarely, tumors of cranial nerve VIII grow larger than 3 cm and may compress cranial nerve V. Because cranial nerve VII travels with VIII in the IAC, the examiner should evaluate facial movement. Facial weakness is unusual even with large acoustical neuromas, however. In the brain stem, the nuclei of cranial nerves IX, X, and XI are close to that of VIII, and an assessment of the voice, palatal function, and gag may reveal unilateral weakness in certain patients. A careful oculomotor examination is crucial for detecting many subtypes of central vertigo.

Motor/Reflexes/Cerebellar/Gait. The motor examination should include assessment of power in the upper and lower extremities. The cerebellar examination should particularly focus on the assessment of upper extremity coordination. Reflexes should be checked, because asymmetry or a positive Babinski's sign may be a valuable clue to a brain stem disorder.

Sensory. When the history suggests a sensory disturbance, examination should be made of pinprick in the face and extremities. Position sense should be checked in all ataxic patients.

Autonomic Nervous System. The pupils should be also checked for Horner's syndrome (miosis, ptosis, and rarely anhydrosis), because the sympathetic system in the brain stem is at times affected with cranial nerve VIII dysfunction, particularly with vascular lesions (Wallenberg's syndrome). Blood pressure and pulse are taken with the patient standing, and if the blood pressure is low (110/70 or lower), it should be repeated with the patient lying flat. These procedures are intended to exclude orthostatic hypotension, which needs to be considered in patients with symptoms suggestive of postural vertigo or ataxia.

Neurovascular. The carotid and subclavian arteries are examined by auscultation in all patients with symptoms that suggest cranial nerve VIII dysfunction.

ASSOCIATED MEDICAL FINDINGS

The heart and the carotid and subclavian arteries should be auscultated. In patients with pulsatile tinnitus, the head should be auscultated for bruits. In patients with potential syncope who are younger than 70 years of age and have no carotid bruit, 10 seconds of carotid sinus massage may be undertaken. This is done with the patient in the sitting position, first on one side, then on the other, in an attempt to reproduce symptoms.

Evaluation Guidelines (Tables 12–5 and 12–6)

Numerous laboratory procedures are commonly used for evaluation of patients with vertigo and dizziness. For efficiency and cost, procedures should be selected according to specific symptom complexes present in the patient.

TABLE 12–5. **Useful Studies in the Evaluation of Disorders of Cranial Nerve VIII**

Syndrome	Neuroimaging	Electrophysiology	Fluid and Tissue Analysis	Neuropsychological Tests	Other Tests
Central hearing disorders	Temporal cortex lesion: MRI, CT	N/A	N/A	Abnormal	Poor word recognition on audiometry
Peripheral hearing loss	Usually normal MRI, CT	BAER ECOG	N/A	N/A	Audiogram abnormal
CPA syndrome	Lesion in CPA: MRI, CT	BAER	CSF	N/A	Audiogram abnormal
Central vertigo	Brain stem or cerebellum lesion: MRI, CT	BAER	CSF Blood	N/A	ENG Rotatory chair test
Peripheral vertigo: BPPV	Normal	Normal	N/A	N/A	ENG
Ménière's disease	Normal	BAER ECOG	N/A	N/A	Audiogram ENG
Vestibular neuritis	MRI may show enhancement of vestibular nerve	N/A	N/A	N/A	ENG
Bilateral vestibular loss	Normal	N/A	N/A	N/A	ENG Rotatory chair Audiogram

MRI, Magnetic resonance imaging; CT, computed tomography; MLR, middle latency response; BAER, brain stem auditory evoked responses; ECOG, electrocochleography; N/A, not applicable; ENG, electronystagmography.

Neuroimaging. Skull films, cervical spine films, computed tomography (CT) scans of the head, and CT scans of the sinuses are not routinely recommended in the evaluation of vertigo or hearing disturbances. Magnetic resonance imaging (MRI) of the head can be used to evaluate the structural integrity of the brain stem, cerebellum, periventricular white matter, cranial nerve VIII complexes, and sinuses. The T1 MRI with gadolinium contrast is the most useful study. MRI is not routinely needed to evaluate vertigo or hearing disturbance without accompanying neurological findings. Although the MRI may show enhancement of the vestibular nerve in vestibular neuritis, the expense of this study should be considered when attempting to document the existence of this self-limited condition. MRI with contrast is preferred to brain stem auditory evoked responses (BAER) testing, when acoustic neuroma is suspected, because it detects tumors at an earlier stage. CT of the temporal bone provides higher resolution than MRI and is preferred in the evaluation of lesions involving bone, particularly when otosclerosis or cholesteatoma is suspected. CT of the temporal bone is also crucial in detecting bony dehiscence of the superior semicircular canal, which is a cause of sound-induced vertigo.[7]

Electrophysiology. *Electroencephalography* has a low yield in most disorders related to cranial nerve VIII but is indicated when there is unexplained vertigo after head trauma or for the "quick spin" symptom complex. The BAER test, also known as *auditory brain stem response test*, assesses the auditory nerve and brain stem pathways. This test is usually ordered to rule out an acoustic neuroma, and this study has roughly 90 percent sensitivity. Because BAER results may be inaccurate in patients who have no high-frequency hearing, audiometry is recommended before BAER testing. The presence of abnormal BAER results is an indication for an MRI evaluation of the posterior fossa (T1-weighted image with contrast). For cost efficiency, BAERs need not be obtained if an MRI is planned, and the MRI is generally the preferred test in most instances. Electrocochleography (ECOG) is a variant of the BAER in which electrodes are placed on the eardrum to obtain better definition of the cochlear potential. ECOG is sometimes helpful to confirm a diagnosis of Ménière's disease.

Numerous more unusual electrophysiological tests can be used to infer the integrity of central auditory pathways. The middle latency response is generated by thalamocortical pathways. The "mismatch" response is a test of higher-order auditory discrimination. The role of these tests in clinical practice is uncertain.

Body Fluid and Tissue Analysis. *Blood tests* are triggered by specific symptom complexes, and there is no routine set of values obtained in every patient. Whereas thyroid dysfunction and vitamin B_{12} deficiency can be detected by appropriate diagnostic assays, chemistry panels, complete blood counts, glucose tolerance tests, and allergy tests need not be routinely ordered. Similarly, urine testing is rarely productive in disorders of cranial nerve VIII.

Cerebrospinal Fluid. Lumbar puncture has limited usefulness in disorders of cranial nerve VIII. Occasionally, it may be indicated in pursuit of the diagnosis of neurosyphilis, Lyme disease, multiple sclerosis, and meningeal carcinomatosis.

Neuropsychological Tests. Neuropsychological testing of speech and language may be helpful in patients in whom the diagnosis of a central hearing disturbance is being entertained. Otherwise, these procedures have limited usefulness in the evaluation of disorders of cranial nerve VIII. The

TABLE 12-6. Laboratory Procedures for Disorders Related to Cranial Nerve VIII

Test	Indication
Neuroimaging	
MRI of head	Central vertigo or hearing loss, abnormal BAER
MRA	TIA or CVA
CT scan of temporal bone	Suspect fistula, cholesteatoma, mastoiditis, congenital abnormality
Electrophysiology	
EEG	Post-traumatic vertigo Vertigo with disturbed consciousness
BAER	Asymmetrical hearing loss
MLR	Central hearing disturbance
Fluid and Tissue Analysis	
FTA	Hearing symptoms
Lyme titers	Tick bite with hearing symptoms or vertigo
Glycosylated hemoglobin	Ménière's symptom complex
ANA	Ménière's symptom complex
TSH	Ménière's symptom complex
Neuropsychological Testing	Central hearing disturbance Malingering
Audiological Testing	
Audiogram	Vertigo, hearing symptoms
ECOG	Secondary test for Ménière's and perilymphatic fistula
Otoacoustic emissions	Infant hearing screening
Vestibular Testing	
ENG	Vertigo
Rotatory chair	Bilateral vestibular loss Ototoxin exposure Secondary test to confirm abnormal ENG
Fistula test	Pressure sensitivity
Posturography	Malingering
Other Tests	
Ambulatory event monitoring	Syncope
Holter monitoring	Syncope
Tilt-table testing	Syncope

MRI, Magnetic resonance imaging; MRA, magnetic resonance angiography; CT, computed tomography; EEG, electroencephalogram; BAER, brain stem auditory evoked responses; MLR, middle latency response; FTA, fluorescent treponemal antibody; ANA, antinuclear antibody; TSH, thyroid stimulating hormone; ECOG, electrocochleography; ENG, electronystagmography; TIA, transient ischemic attack; CVA, cerebrovascular accident.

Minnesota Multiphasic Personality Inventory has some usefulness when the diagnosis of malingering is being considered. Neuropsychological testing may also be useful in determining how much anxiety is associated with the patient's symptom complex.

Other Tests. The audiogram is the single most useful test in the patient with a hearing disorder and/or vertigo. In hearing disorders, the audiogram is crucial in defining the degree and type of loss. In patients with vertigo, abnormalities in the audiogram usually narrow the differential diagnosis down to otological vertigo. Accompanying the audiogram is a battery of related measures. The *tympanogram* measures middle ear pressure, and tympanometry is helpful in identifying a perforated eardrum or middle ear infection. *Acoustic reflexes* measure the stapedius and tensor tympani reflex-generated eardrum movement in response to intense sound, and they can be helpful in corroborating particular types of hearing loss. Reflexes that are present at abnormally low levels suggest recruitment with a cochlear site of lesion. Reflexes that decay rapidly suggest a retrocochlear lesion.

The *word recognition score* (also called *speech discrimination*) measures the ability to repeat words presented at a comfortable loudness. Word recognition can be impaired by both auditory distortion and central abnormalities such as a nonfluent aphasia. Speech reception threshold measures the auditory threshold of hearing for words. It should be consistent with pure-tone hearing. When they are not consistent, a nonperipheral hearing disturbance is more likely.

The short-increment sensitivity index, alternate binaural loudness balance, and Bekesey's tests are no longer used in most clinical practices. Audiometry is particularly useful in the diagnosis of Ménière's disease. A fluctuating low-tone sensorineural hearing loss is typical of this condition (Fig. 12–7).

Otoacoustic emissions have become an added option to the hearing evaluation. A click is usually used to generate the response. The outer hair cells generate a sound in response to the stimulus, and this sound is captured by a microphone in the ear canal. The test has proven useful for infant hearing screening.

Four types of vestibular tests are selected according to the clinical situation. *Electronystagmography* (ENG) is the most useful, and it consists of a battery of procedures that can identify vestibular asymmetry (such as that caused by vestibular neuritis) and that document spontaneous or positional nystagmus (such as that caused by BPPV). Because of anatomical variability and technical difficulty, the ENG result can be misleading, most commonly suggesting an abnormality when none exists.

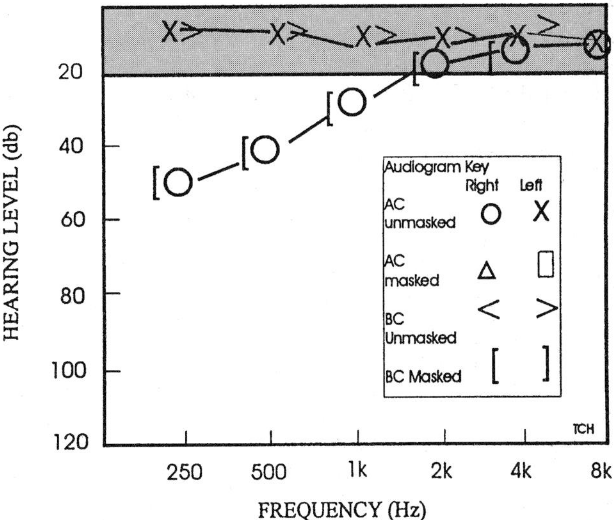

FIGURE 12–7. Audiogram depicting the low-tone sensorineural loss typical of Ménière's disease. The gray shaded area indicates the normal range. The left ear (*X marks*) is normal at all frequencies. The right ear (*circles*) has decreased hearing on both air and bone for lower frequencies.

An abnormal result that does not fit the clinical picture should be confirmed with *rotatory chair* testing. Rotatory chair testing measures vestibular function of both inner ears together and is also highly sensitive and specific for bilateral loss of vestibular function. Although rotatory chair testing does not establish the side of a unilateral vestibular lesion, there is a characteristic pattern of unilateral loss. For this reason it can also be helpful in corroborating an abnormal ENG. *Fistula testing* involves the recording of nystagmus induced by pressure in the external ear canal. Its sensitivity to a perilymph fistula is only 50 percent, but it is the only objective procedure that is available to substantiate a clinical suspicion of fistula. *Posturography* is an instrumented variant of the Romberg's test. Posturography can be helpful in quantifying imbalance. Additionally, it sometimes will detect malingering when the test demonstrates inconsistent patterns of balance.

Syncope is a common differential diagnosis in the evaluation of disorders of cranial nerve VIII; it is sometimes useful to check patients for arrhythmia or abnormal control of blood pressure. *Ambulatory event monitoring* or Holter monitoring is used to detect arrhythmia or sinus arrest. *Tilt-table testing* is sometimes advocated for the diagnosis of syncope. At present, however, there is a lack of data establishing a link between tilt-table test abnormalities and successful treatment outcomes, and thus the role of the tilt-table test in the evaluation of dizzy patients is presently unclear.

Clinical Syndromes (Table 12–7)

SYNDROMES PRIMARILY INVOLVING HEARING

Hearing loss is highly prevalent, especially in the older population, and three types are commonly encountered: conductive, sensorineural, and central hearing loss. In conductive hearing loss, sound is not transmitted into the inner ear. Diagnosis is ordinarily made via observation of an "air-bone gap" on audiometry, meaning that hearing is superior when sound is transmitted in such a way that it bypasses the middle ear ossicular chain. Causes include a buildup of ear wax, foreign body in the ear canal, otosclerosis, external or middle

TABLE 12–7. **Selected Etiologies Associated with Disorders of Cranial Nerve VIII**

Etiological Category	Specific Etiologies	Chapter
Structural Disorders		
Developmental structural disorders	Arnold-Chiari malformation Mondini malformation	28
Degenerative and compressive structural disorders	Paget's disease	
Hereditodegenerative Disorders		
Storage diseases: Lipidoses, glycogen disorders, and leukoencephalopathies	Hurler's, Hunter's, Sanfilippo's, Morquio's syndromes Krabbe's disease	29
Chromosomal anomalies and the neurocutaneous disorders	Waardenburg's, Usher's, Down's, Pendred's syndromes	32
Acquired Metabolic Disorders and Nutritional Disorders		
Endogenous metabolic disorders	Kernicterus	38
Nutritional deficiencies and syndromes associated with alcoholism	Wernicke's (central vertigo)	
Infectious Disorders		
Viral infections	Vestibular neuritis Herpes zoster oticus Cytomegalovirus (infants)	41
Nonviral infections	Chronic, acute otitis media (bacterial) Meningitis (bacterial, fungal) Syphilis	42
Neurovascular Disorders	AICA, PICA syndromes Subarachnoid hemorrhage	45
Neoplastic Disorders		
Primary neurological tumors	Acoustic neuroma Cholesteatoma	46
Demyelinating Disorders		
Demyelinating disorders of the central nervous system	Multiple sclerosis	48
Traumatic Disorders	Blunt head trauma	51
Epilepsy	Central vertigo	52
Headache and Facial Pain	Central vertigo (vertebrobasilar migraine)	53
Drug-Induced and Iatrogenic Neurological Disorders	Vestibular ototoxicity: aminoglycosides	55

AICA, Anterior inferior cerebellar artery; PICA, posterior inferior cerebellar artery.

ear infections, allergy with serous otitis, and perforation of the tympanic membrane. Characteristically, hearing aids work well for this population.

Sensorineural hearing loss is the most common type of hearing loss, occurring in 23 percent of the population older than 65 years of age. The term *sensorineural* is used to indicate that there is either a cochlear or a cranial nerve VIII lesion. The diagnosis of a sensorineural pattern hearing loss is made through audiometry, which shows a significant hearing loss without the air-bone gap characteristic of conductive hearing disturbances. Common causes include old age (when the hearing pattern is often somewhat confusingly called *presbycusis*), Ménière's disease, toxin exposures (such as to high-dose aspirin), and noise. Treatments are mainly aimed at preventing further damage. If the loss is minor, avoidance of noise and of ototoxic medications are appropriate "treatments." If the loss is significant, a hearing aid should be tried. Occasionally, persons with acquired deafness can be treated with a surgically implanted prosthesis that directly stimulates the spiral ganglion.

Central hearing loss is extremely rare compared with the sensorineural or conductive types. The diagnosis is usually not made by the pure-tone audiogram, which often yields a normal result. Rather, patients usually have an aphasia, which may be associated with disproportionally poor scores on the speech reception threshold tests or word recognition scores portions of the audiogram.

Pure word deafness is a rare subtype of central deafness. This disorder is defined as disturbed auditory comprehension without difficulties with visual comprehension. Patients characteristically have fluent verbal output, severe disturbance of spoken language comprehension and repetition, and no problems with reading or writing.[8] Nonverbal sounds are correctly identified. The lesion is classically postulated to be a disruption in connections between the dominant Heschl's transverse gyrus and the medial geniculate as well as callosal fibers from the opposite superior temporal region. Initially, it appears commonly as Wernicke's aphasia. With recovery, difficulties in auditory comprehension persist. Although usually caused by a stroke, pure word deafness can arise from other causes of focal cortical lesions such as tumors.

Auditory agnosia, another rare subset of central deafness, is typified by relatively normal pure-tone hearing on audiometry, but inability to interpret (recognize) nonverbal sounds such as the ringing of a telephone. Inability to interpret nonverbal sounds but preserved ability to interpret speech may be a result of a right hemisphere lesion alone.[8] Amusia is a particular type of auditory agnosia in which only the perception of music is impaired. Again, right-sided temporal lesions are thought to be the cause.

Cortical deafness is essentially the combination of word deafness and auditory agnosia. It is characterized by an inability to interpret either verbal or nonverbal sounds with preserved awareness of the occurrence of sound (for instance, by a startle reaction to a clap). In most instances, the cause is bilateral embolic strokes in the area of Heschl's gyri. Patients present with sudden deafness evolving later so that they can hear sounds but are unable to recognize their meaning. Relatively few cases of this disorder have been studied, and it is possible that bilateral lesions of the central auditory pathways, other than the speech cortex, can also result in these deficits.

Auditory hallucinations consist of an illusion of a complex sound such as music or speech. These hallucinations most commonly occur as a result of an injury to the superior temporal auditory association areas. Penfield discovered that stimulating this area induced an auditory sensation that seemed real to patients. Auditory hallucinations can also occur as a result of temporal lobe seizure.[9]

SYNDROMES PRIMARILY INVOLVING VESTIBULAR FUNCTION

Conditions that involve vestibular function can be separated into peripheral (otological vertigo) and central subgroups. Patients with these syndromes present clinically with a combination of vertigo and ataxia. Practically, there are far more cases of otological vertigo than central vertigo, and for this reason, in clinical practice, a detailed understanding of otological vertigo is essential.

Benign Paroxysmal Positional Vertigo

Benign paroxysmal positional vertigo (BPPV) is the cause of half of all cases of otological vertigo; it accounts for about 20 percent of all patients with vertigo. BPPV is diagnosed by the history of positional vertigo with a typical nystagmus pattern (a burst of upbeating/torsional nystagmus) on Dix-Hallpike positional testing. Symptoms are precipitated by movement or a position change of the head or body. Getting out of bed or rolling over in bed are the most common "problem" motions. A burst of nystagmus can often be provoked by placing the head in positions wherein the posterior canal is made vertical in space, and ENG testing may be helpful in documenting this condition. BPPV is usually a straightforward clinical diagnosis. Ordinarily there is no need to obtain neuroradiological tests, audiometric testing, or posturography.

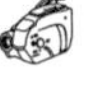

It is currently thought that BPPV is caused by the presence of free debris, possibly otoconia, within the semicircular canals, which is dislodged from the otolith organs by trauma, infection, or degeneration (Fig. 12–8). The otoconial debris can move about after changes in head position, causing vertigo and nystagmus when the debris tumbles through the semicircular canals. The duration of symptoms is brief, because dizziness occurs only while the debris shifts position. Physical treatments based on the manipulation of the head

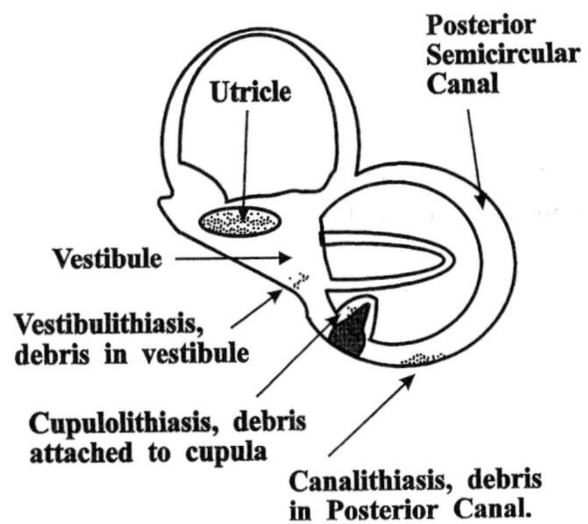

FIGURE 12–8. Debris hypothesis of benign paroxysmal positional vertigo. Otoconia displaced from the utricle gravitate to the most dependent parts of the inner ear.

are the most effective remedies for BPPV. These maneuvers reposition the otolithic debris to an insensitive location within the inner ear.[10]

Vestibular Neuritis and Other Unilateral Vestibulopathies

Vestibular neuritis is a self-limited otological condition. Patients present with vertigo, nausea, ataxia, and nystagmus. Most cases of vestibular neuritis are monophasic. Hearing is not impaired, and when there are similar symptoms with abnormal hearing, the syndrome is termed *labyrinthitis*. A strong nystagmus is seen acutely, and Frenzel's goggles are particularly useful in seeing these eye movements. Vestibular neuritis is thought to be caused by viral infections of the vestibular ganglion.

Similar symptoms may be seen with other etiologies. Ménière's disease is usually recognized by the episodic pattern (see later). Herpes simplex virus infection of the vestibular nerve is recognized by a combination of ear pain and the presence of vesicles on the external canal. Acoustic neuroma (discussed later) is recognized by a slower course and the occurrence of hearing loss. Vascular disorders such as a labyrinthine artery infarction are generally impossible to exclude, and their diagnosis is suggested by an identical symptom complex combined with vascular risk factors.

No laboratory testing is needed in straightforward cases. When a central disorder is suspected in the setting of multiple cerebrovascular risk factors or neurological diseases, however, further laboratory testing may be helpful to confirm the anatomical diagnosis. Electronystagmography testing often reveals a significantly decreased caloric response on one side as well as spontaneous nystagmus. Rotational testing is not necessary, but when obtained, it typically shows reduced gain and increased phase lead. Posturography is also not necessary, but results are typically abnormal, indicating that balance is impaired.

In vestibular neuritis, severe distress associated with constant vertigo, nausea, and malaise usually lasts 2 or 3 days, and less intense symptoms ordinarily persist for 1 or 2 weeks. The treatment strategy involves the use of vestibular suppressants and antiemetics (Tables 12–8 and 12–9). Roughly 10 percent of patients may take as long as 2 months for the condition to improve substantially. These patients usually have a significant fixed vestibular paresis combined with central dysfunction that slows their compensation. For example, patients with alcoholic cerebellar degeneration or persons of advanced age may recover much more slowly. Such patients often benefit from vestibular exercises.

Vestibular exercise instructions may be given to patients in the form of a handout.[11] These exercises are done three times daily, moving from the easier procedures to more difficult ones, as recovery ensues. Specialized physical therapy programs are also available in which individualized therapy can be offered and supervision provided, when appropriate. It should also be noted that numerous avocational activities serve well to promote vestibular compensation, and depending on the abilities and interests of patients, clinicians may prescribe golf, bowling, racquetball, bicycling, or even T'ai Chi.

Cerebellopontine Angle Syndrome

Acoustic neuromas and other tumors such as meningiomas, which can appear at the cerebellopontine angle, usually display asymmetrical sensorineural hearing loss. Usually, patients in the fifth or greater decade present with mild vertigo or ataxia, accompanied by a significant asymmetrical hearing loss. Generally, there are no other physical examination abnormalities, and facial and sixth nerve functions are ordinarily normal.

If the hearing loss is minor, an audiogram may be performed within 6 months. If hearing loss progressively worsens, an MRI scan with gadolinium should be pursued. If a

TABLE 12–8. **Vestibular Suppressants***

Drug	Dose	Adverse Reactions	Pharmacological Class and Precautions
Meclizine (Antivert, Bonine)	12.5–50 mg every 4–6 hours	Sedating, precautions in prostatic enlargement, glaucoma	Antihistamine Anticholinergic
Lorazepam (Ativan)	0.5 mg twice daily	Mildly sedating Drug dependency	Benzodiazepine
Clonazepam (Klonopin)	0.5 mg twice daily	Mildly sedating Drug dependency	Benzodiazepine
Scopolamine (Transderm-Scop)	1.5 mg patch every 3 days	Topical allergy with chronic use. Precautions in glaucoma, tachyarrhythmias, prostatic enlargement	Anticholinergic
Dimenhydrinate (Dramamine)	50 mg every 4–6 hours	Same as meclizine	Antihistamine Anticholinergic
Diazepam (Valium)	2–10 mg (1 dose) given acutely orally, intramuscularly, or intravenously	Sedating Respiratory depressant Drug dependency Precaution in glaucoma	Benzodiazepine

*Doses listed are used in adults. Drugs are arranged in order of preference.

TABLE 12-9. **Antiemetics**

Drug	Usual Dose*	Adverse Reactions	Pharmacological Class
Meclizine (Antivert, Bonine)	12.5–50 mg every 4–6 hours orally	Sedating Precautions in glaucoma, prostate enlargement	Antihistamine and anticholinergic
Metoclopramide (Reglan)	10 mg orally three times daily or 10 mg intramuscularly	Restlessness or drowsiness Extrapyramidal	Dopamine antagonist
Ondansetron (Zofran)	4–8 mg orally single dose	Headache	5-HT_3 antagonist
Prochlorperazine (Compazine)	5 mg or 10 mg intramuscularly or orally every 6–12 hours or 25 mg rectal every 12 hours	Sedating Extrapyramidal	Phenotniazine
Promethazine (Phenergan)	12.5 mg–25 mg orally every 6–8 hours or 12.5–25 mg rectal every 12 hours 12.5 mg intramuscularly every 6–8 hours	Sedating Extrapyramidal	Phenothiazine
Trimethobenzamide (Tigan)	250 mg orally three times daily or 200 mg intramuscularly three times daily	Sedating Extrapyramidal	Similar to phenothiazine
Thiethylperazine (Torecan)	10 mg orally, up to three times daily or 2 mL intramuscularly, up to three times daily	Sedating	Phenothiazine

*Doses listed are used in adults.

tumor is identified and is small, or the patient is reluctant to have surgery, the tumor may be followed with periodic evaluations. MRI should be repeated every year, or more frequently if there is a substantial change in hearing. In many instances, lesions remain stable over many years and surgery can be avoided. Gamma knife treatment is an emerging modality and may also be used when surgery is refused or when the patient is a poor surgical risk.

Ménière's Disease

Classic Ménière's disease presents as a quadrad of paroxysmal symptoms, including tinnitus, monaural fullness, fluctuating hearing, and episodic vertigo. This clinical picture is sometimes called the "hydrops" symptom complex, inferring that the mechanism is related to dilation and rupture of the endolymphatic compartment of the inner ear. The tinnitus is characteristically of two types. Between attacks, the tinnitus is characteristically a ringing noise (about 75 percent of the population has ringing tinnitus from time to time). During an attack, the tinnitus becomes a multifrequency noise such as a roar, hiss, or buzz. Patients also generally complain of monaural fullness, a sensation as if the ear were full of water, beginning a day or two before an attack. Hearing is normal at the onset of the condition, but with each attack a low-frequency sensorineural reduction in hearing appears (see Fig. 12–6), and then it usually resolves a day or two later. After many attacks, hearing begins to decline and involves the high frequencies. Ultimately, many individuals with Ménière's disease develop permanent sensorineural pattern deafness.

The clinical picture of Ménière's disease varies widely, with some patients developing deafness with their first attack and others retaining normal hearing after several decades of repeated attacks. Variants of Ménière's disease include a form that follows head injury (labyrinthine concussion or delayed endolymphatic hydrops) and a bilateral form attributed to autoantibodies or genetic predisposition.

The diagnosis of classic Ménière's disease can be made purely by history, but most commonly it is made by combining a history of episodic vertigo and hearing symptoms with audiometric documentation of a fluctuating low-tone sensorineural hearing loss. Electrocochleography may be useful in cases when the history is not classic. It is conventional practice to obtain several blood tests including fluorescent treponemal antibody, antinuclear antibody, complete blood count, and fasting blood glucose after diagnosing Ménière's disease to identify specific treatable causes.

In the treatment of Ménière's disease, vestibular suppressants and antiemetics are used in a way similar to that described for vestibular neuritis (see Tables 12–8 and 12–9). Because bouts generally last only 2 hours, acute treatment is usually episodic. Often patients can anticipate an attack and can start taking an antiemetic and/or vestibular suppressant before their full-blown symptoms occur. It is presently generally accepted that reduction of salt intake with a no-added-salt diet and daily use of a salt-wasting diuretic is helpful in reducing the number and intensity of spells over the long term.

Effective surgical treatment of Ménière's disease is based on procedures that destroy vestibular function. Three procedures are commonly used today, including labyrinthectomy, selective vestibular nerve section, and transtympanic gentamicin treatment. Gentamicin treatment is presently growing rapidly in popularity.

Central Vertigo

In neurological practice, central vertigo typically makes up only about 25 percent of diagnoses of patients presenting

TABLE 12–10. Common Causes of Central Vertigo

Stroke and TIA
Cerebellum
AICA distribution
PICA distribution
Vertebrobasilar migraine
Adult form
Childhood variant (benign paroxysmal vertigo of childhood)
Seizure (temporal lobe)
Multiple sclerosis, postinfectious demyelination
Arnold-Chiari malformation
Tumors of cranial nerve VIII, brain stem, or cerebellum
Paraneoplastic cerebellar degeneration
Wernicke's syndrome

TIA, Transient ischemic attack; AICA, anterior inferior cerebellar artery; PICA, posterior inferior cerebellar artery.

with vertigo, because otological vertigo and vertigo of unknown cause are much more frequent (Table 12–10). Stroke and transient ischemic attacks account for one third of cases of central vertigo. Vertigo attributed to vertebrobasilar migraine accounts for another 15 percent of cases. A large number of individual miscellaneous neurological disorders such as seizures, multiple sclerosis, and the Arnold-Chiari malformation make up the remainder.

General Management Goals

General pharmacological management of conditions affecting hearing is nearly nonexistent, in spite of many attempts over the years using vasoactive agents, steroids, and agents for allergy.[12] When a specific etiology is known, such as Ménière's disease, treatment directed at the cause may be used, but there is no effective pharmacological management of tinnitus or hearing loss.

Hearing aids are indicated when hearing loss is significant and "aidable," meaning that improvement in word recognition scores may be obtained with amplification. Hearing aids are expensive. They are often not covered by standard insurance policies, and there are considerable performance differences between basic and "deluxe" models. For these reasons, hearing aids should ideally be fit by an experienced audiologist who offers at least a 1-month tryout period.

For tinnitus, an assortment of medications may be empirically tried, including antidepressants, minor tranquilizers, and anticonvulsants. Hearing aids or "maskers" (devices that generate white noise) are helpful in a few patients.

With respect to symptomatic management of peripheral vestibular disorders (see Tables 12–4 and 12–5), vestibular suppressants and antiemetics are generally used. In patients with static and significant structural vestibular lesions, vestibular rehabilitation approaches, including vestibular exercises, are substituted. In patients with central vestibular disorders, treatment approaches are generally eclectic. Agents used in peripheral disorders are usually tried, followed by empirical trials of other medication groups, including benzodiazepines and anticonvulsants. Vestibular rehabilitation again may be quite useful in this group.

Certain medications should be used with caution in patients with disorders of cranial nerve VIII. A surprisingly large number of frankly ototoxic medications are in common clinical use (see Table 12–2). It is usually prudent to eliminate as many of these medications as possible in such patients. In addition, it is common practice to use potentially addictive medications, such as benzodiazepines, in the management of patients with vertigo or imbalance when other medications fail. Although these agents are indispensable in these settings, the doses should be kept low and patient use should be monitored.

Hearing protection is often indicated in patients with damage to cranial nerve VIII, and patients need to be explicitly warned to avoid loud noises and use hearing protection devices in excessively noisy environments.

Reviews and Selected Updates

Baloh RW, Foster CA, Yue Q, Nelson SF: Familial migraine with vertigo and essential tremor. Neurology 1996;46:458–460.

Baloh RW, Halmagyi GH (eds): Disorders of the Vestibular System. New York, Oxford University Press, 1996.

Brandt T: Phobic postural vertigo. Neurology 1996;46(6):1515–1519.

Fife TD, Tusa RJ, Furman JM, et al: Assessment: Vestibular testing techniques in adults and children: Report of the Therapeutics and Technology Assessment Subcommittee of the American Academy of Neurology. Neurology 2000;55:1431–1441.

Gomez CR, Cruz-Flores S, Malkoff MD, et al: Isolated vertigo as a manifestation of vertebrobasilar ischemia. Neurology 1996;47(1):94–97.

Lawden MC, Bronstein AM, Kennard C: Repetitive paroxysmal nystagmus and vertigo. Neurology 1995;45:276–280.

Rascol O, Hain TC, Brefel C, et al: Antivertigo medications and drug-induced vertigo. A pharmacological review. Drugs 1995;50(5):777–791.

Schuknecht HF: Pathology of the Ear. Philadelphia, Lea & Febiger, 1993.

Therapeutics and Technology Assessment Subcommittee: Assessment: Electronystagmography. Neurology 1996;46:1763–1766.

References

1. Peuder DJ: Practical otology. Philadelphia, JB Lippincott, 1992.
2. Webster DB, Popper AN, Fay RF (eds): The Mammalian Auditory Pathway: Neuroanatomy. New York, Springer-Verlag, 1992.
3. Anson BJ, Harper DG, Winck TR: The vestibular system. Anatomic considerations. Arch Otolaryngol 1967;85:497–514.
4. Goebel JA, O'Mara W, Gianoli G: Anatomic considerations in vestibular neuritis. Otol Neurotol 2001;22:512–518.
5. Lisberger SG, Miles FA, Zee DS: Signals used to compute errors in monkey vestibuloocular reflex: Possible role of the flocculus. J Neurophysiol 1984;52:1140–1153.
6. Perlman HB, Kimura RS, Fernandez C: Experiments on temporary obstruction of the internal auditory artery. Laryngoscope 1959;69:591.
7. Minor LB: Superior canal dehiscence syndrome. Am J Otol 2000;21:9–19.
8. Mesulam M: Principles of Behavioral Neurology. Philadelphia, F.A. Davis, 1985.
9. Weiser HG: Depth recorded limbic seizures and psychopathology. Neurosci Biobehav Rev 1983;7:427.
10. Epley JM: The canalith repositioning procedure: For treatment of benign paroxysmal positional vertigo. Otol Head Neck Surg 1992;107:399–404.
11. Hain TC: Episodic vertigo. *In* Rakel R (ed): Conn's Current Therapy. Philadelphia, WB Saunders, 1996, pp 869–874.
12. Ruckenstein MJ, Rutka JA, Hawke M: The treatment of Ménière's disease: Torok revisited. Laryngoscope 1991;101:211–218.

CHAPTER 13

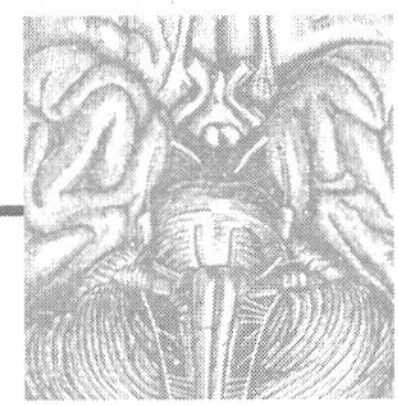

NEAL HERMANOWICZ

Cranial Nerves IX (Glossopharyngeal) and X (Vagus)

History and Definitions

The glossopharyngeal and vagus nerves have been described since antiquity. Galen of Pergamus (131–201 AD) included them in his descriptions of neuroanatomy, grouping together cranial nerves IX, X, and XI as a single nerve.[1] Centuries later, the anatomy of the glossopharyngeal and vagus nerves was elucidated in greater detail by the Prussian anatomist Samuel Thomas von Soemmering (1755–1830) in his treatise on the 12 cranial nerves. Although study of the glossopharyngeal nerve in isolation is impractical, the vagus nerve, with its numerous thoracic and abdominal visceral innervations, has long held the attention of physiologists, including the Russian Nobel Laureate Ivan Petrovich Pavlov (1849–1936), who, with E.O. Schumov-Simanovskaja, published in 1895 their prominent paper describing vagus nerve innervation for gastric secretion in dogs. The clinical consequences of pathology, particularly trauma and tumors, on the glossopharyngeal or vagus nerves have been described by a number of authors who have attached their names to syndromes of the lower cranial nerves, beginning with John Hughlings Jackson in 1883.

Cranial nerves IX and X, the glossopharyngeal and vagus nerves, respectively, have their nuclei in the medulla, and they serve motor, sensory, and autonomic functions. Both nerves are formed by the joining of rootlets that emerge from the lateral medulla in a groove formed between the olive and the inferior cerebellar peduncle. The two nerves travel closely in their proximal courses, both exiting the skull at the jugular foramen, and consequently they are typically affected together by intracranial pathology. The name of the glossopharyngeal nerve refers in Latin to its targets of function, *glosso* referring to tongue and *pharyngeal* to the beginning of the alimentary canal. The vagus nerve is aptly named as well, with its numerous afferent and efferent functions in the head, neck, chest, and abdomen; *vagus* is a Latin adjective meaning wandering or roving.

Both nerves have components of branchial motor fibers (special visceral efferent) providing innervation of striated muscle, visceral motor fibers (general visceral efferent) to secretory glands, and both visceral and general sensory functions (general visceral and general somatic afferent). Additionally, the glossopharyngeal nerve has special afferent fibers receiving taste sensation from the posterior third of the tongue. Together cranial nerves IX and X provide sensory and motor innervation of the larynx and pharynx, including the afferent and efferent limbs of the gag reflex, and exteroceptive information for these structures: the tongue, the auditory meatus and tympanic membrane, and parts of the ear. The glossopharyngeal nerve also provides afferent input from the baroreceptors of the carotid sinus and the chemoreceptors of the carotid body. The vagus nerve subserves esophageal peristalsis, heart rate and blood pressure modulation, gastric secretion, and bowel motility.

Clinical History

The primary clinical symptom of cranial nerve IX dysfunction is dysphagia or choking, and the most readily identified sign of vagal nerve damage is hoarseness. The clinical histories of patients with symptoms referable to the glossopharyngeal and vagus nerves necessarily reflect the location of the nerve dysfunction and the process producing it. Dependent upon these two factors, the temporal appearance of symptoms may vary widely, ranging, for example, from the acute onset of hoarseness and dysphagia due to brain stem infarction involving the vagus nerve nuclei to the insidious appearance of hoarseness without dysphagia produced by the encroachment of a pulmonary neoplasm on the intrathoracic recurrent laryngeal branch of the vagus nerve.

Intraparenchymal brain lesions of the medulla at the level of the glossopharyngeal and vagus nerves typically affect the nuclei of both, and possibly also of cranial nerve VIII, resulting in symptoms of vertigo, hoarseness of speech, and dysphagia. Because cranial nerves IX, X, and XI pass together through the jugular foramen at the base of the skull, a lesion at this location can cause added neck muscle weakness.[2] Rarely, throat pain occurs, specifically in the syndrome of idiopathic glossopharyngeal neuralgia, in which fleeting pain at the base of the tongue is sometimes triggered by chewing or swallowing. An intramedullary lesion of the vagal motor nucleus producing vocal cord weakness and hoarseness of speech likely also affects adjacent structures, such as the spinal tract and nucleus of cranial nerve V, the spinothalamic tract, and cerebellar fibers. Hence, associated symptoms include a crossed sensory disturbance (ipsilateral face and contralateral limbs) and ataxia. An ipsilateral Horner's syndrome may be present from involvement of descending sympathetic fibers, although the patient is unlikely to describe accompanying symptoms, because an intracranial but extramedullary lesion of the vagus nerve also involves cranial nerves IX and XI. The presence or absence of dysphagia, with hoarseness of speech, is an important clue to the localization of the lesion of the vagus nerve. Hoarse speech without dysphagia occurs when the lesion site of the vagus nerve is below the upper cervical levels where the pharyngeal branches exit. This lesion most commonly occurs at the level of the recurrent laryngeal nerve branch. Possible mechanisms include an expanding aneurysm or dissection of the thoracic aorta, mediastinal adenopathy, and pulmonary neoplasms.[3, 4]

Head, neck, or oral trauma and surgery of these structures may result in damage to cranial nerves IX and X. Head and neck injury may compromise both nerves at the jugular foramen.[5] Vocal cord paralysis is a recognized complication of neck surgery, including thyroidectomy and carotid endarterectomy.[6, 7] Both procedures may injure laryngeal branches of the vagus nerve by manipulation or transection. The recurrent laryngeal nerve is injured by thyroidectomy at a rate of approximately 7 percent, producing ipsilateral paralysis of all the laryngeal muscles except for the cricothyroid. This injury, often unrecognized at the time of surgery, may result in breathiness of speech and risk for aspiration. The prognosis for recovery is favorable.[6, 8]

Underlying medical conditions or their treatment may cause injury to the glossopharyngeal and vagus nerves. Patients with neoplasms that involve the head or neck, either primary tumors or metastases, may experience impaired swallowing as a consequence of nerve compression at the jugular foramen or other sites.[9] Infectious or inflammatory processes involving the central nervous system (CNS) at the level of the brain stem can produce cranial neuropathies. Although cranial nerves IX and X may be involved, they generally do not produce prominent symptoms or signs. Neurological manifestations of sarcoidosis typically involve cranial nerves, particularly the facial nerve, yet involvement of cranial nerves IX and X can occur in conjunction with facial weakness, and their function should be assessed.[10] Cranial nerves IX and X may also be damaged as a consequence of diabetes, syphilis, or alcoholism.[11, 12]

Patients may have respiratory complaints, because abnormalities of ventilatory drive by hypoxic stimulation can occur with involvement of carotid body chemoreceptor afferent fibers from the glossopharyngeal nerve.[13] Patients may also have symptoms of lightheadedness and orthostatic dizziness from involvement of baroreceptor afferent fibers from the carotid sinus.[14] The Guillain-Barré syndrome may have associated autonomic dysfunction resulting from demyelination of glossopharyngeal afferents from the carotid sinus and vagal fibers, producing instability of blood pressure and heart rhythm, and bowel motility disturbance such as ileus.[15, 16] A history of all medications and toxin exposures is important, because cranial nerve neuropathy due to exposure to known neurotoxins may involve the glossopharyngeal and vagus nerves. Patients undergoing cancer treatment with the chemotherapeutic agent vincristine may rapidly develop jaw pain due to peripheral injury of the glossopharyngeal nerve.[17]

Anatomy of Cranial Nerve IX (Table 13–1)

MOTOR FIBERS

Nucleus

The nucleus ambiguus runs in a rostral to caudal direction in the medulla and is located in the ventrolateral reticular formation, posterior to the inferior olivary nuclear complex and anteromedial to the spinal trigeminal nucleus (Fig. 13–1).[18, 19] The rostral portion of the nucleus ambiguus gives rise to special visceral efferent fibers of the glossopharyngeal nerve, which innervate the stylopharyngeus muscle. This muscle originates from the styloid process and descends between the internal and external carotid arteries to the upper wall of the pharynx. Contraction of the stylopharyngeus muscle aids in raising the larynx and elevating and expanding the pharynx during swallowing. The nucleus ambiguus is also the source of special visceral efferent fibers of cranial nerves X and XI, which together with cranial nerve IX innervate the muscles of the pharynx and larynx.

TABLE 13–1. **Clinico-anatomical Correlation of Disorders of Cranial Nerves IX and X**[2, 48, 49]

Anatomical Site of Damage	CN IX or X Finding	Other Neurological and Medical Findings	Common Etiologies	Comments
Intracranial, intra-or extramedullary at the level of the medulla, involving CN X, XI, and XII	Ipsilateral paralysis of the soft palate, pharynx, and larynx producing hoarseness and dysphagia	Ipsilatral weakness of the sternocleidomastoid and trapezius muscles, and atrophy and weakness of the ipsilateral tongue	Infarction, neoplasm	Jackson's syndrome
Nucleus ambiguus, CN XI nuclei and extramedullary fibers	Ipsilateral paralysis of the soft palate, pharynx, and larynx producing hoarseness and dysphagia	Ipsilateral weakness of the sternocleidomastoid and trapezius muscles	Infarction, neoplasm, idiopathic neuropathy	Schmidt's syndrome
Extramedullary fibers of CN X and XII	Ipsilateral paralysis of the soft palate, pharynx, and larynx producing hoarseness and dysphagia	Atrophy and weakness of the ipsilateral tongue	Trauma, neurofibroma of the CN X and XII nerves, parotid tumor	Tapia's syndrome
Jugular foramen involving CN IX, X, and XI	Ipsilateral paralysis of the soft palate, pharynx, and larynx producing hoarseness and dysphagia	Ipsilateral paralysis of the sternocleidomastoid and trapezius muscles	Trauma, neoplasm, jugular bulb thrombosis, internal carotid artery aneurysm	Vernet's syndrome
Retropharyngeal space, involving CN IX to XII	Ipsilateral paralysis of the soft palate, pharynx, and larynx producing hoarseness and dysphagia	Ipsilateral weakness of the sternocleidomastoid and trapezius muscles, and atrophy and weakness of the ipsilateral tongue	Neoplasm, trauma, internal carotid artery dissection, coiling of the internal carotid artery	Collet-Sicard syndrome
Retropharyngeal space, involving CN IX to XII, and cervical sympathetic fibers	Ipsilateral paralysis of the soft palate, pharynx, and larynx producing hoarseness and dysphagia	Ipsilateral weakness of the sternocleidomastoid and trapezius muscles, atrophy and weakness of the ipsilateral tongue, and ipsilateral Horner's syndrome	Cervical internal carotid artery dissection, lung apex neoplasm	Villaret's syndrome
Vagus nerve below higher cervical levels where branches to the pharynx exit	Ipsilateral paralysis of the larynx producing hoarseness without dysphagia		Neoplasm, trauma	
Lateral medulla	Ipsilateral vocal cord paralysis producing hoarseness, ipsilateral weakness of the palate and pharynx; the uvula will be drawn to the intact side, dysphagia	Ipsilateral pain around the eye, face, or ear, vertigo; nausea and vomiting; impaired pain and temperature sensation of the ipsilateral face and contralateral limbs; unsteady gait and ataxia of ipsilateral limbs	Thrombosis or dissection of the vertebral artery occluding the opening to the posterior inferior cerebellar artery	Wallenberg's syndrome (lateral medullary syndrome)

CN, Cranial nerve.

Upper Motor Neuron, Supranuclear Control

The nucleus ambiguus receives bilateral input primarily from the precentral gyrus of the cerebral cortex. These corticobulbar fibers travel through the internal capsule and brain stem in association with the corticospinal tract and terminate on reticular formation neurons, which transmit signals to the nucleus ambiguus.

Lower Motor Neuron, Peripheral Pathways

The motor fibers emerge from the medulla in a groove between the inferior cerebellar peduncle and the olive as part of the rootlets comprising the glossopharyngeal nerve. The nerve travels laterally through the posterior fossa and exits the skull through the jugular foramen together with cranial nerves X and XI. The fibers to the stylopharyngeus muscle travel downward in the neck deep to the styloid process and reach the muscle around its posterior margin.

SENSORY FIBERS

Sensory Organs and First Order Neurons

First order neurons for sensory functions of the glossopharyngeal nerve have their cell bodies located in either the superior or inferior glossopharyngeal ganglia, which are found at the jugular foramen. Taste from the posterior third of the

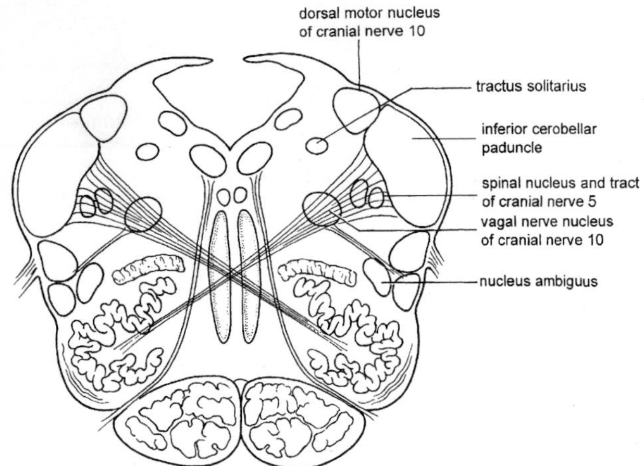

FIGURE 13–1. Cross section of the medulla. The ninth and tenth cranial nerve nuclei lie in the lateral portion of the medulla, in close juxtaposition with the eighth cranial nerve nucleus, the spinal nucleus of cranial nerve V, and the inferior cerebellar peduncles.

tongue is detected by chemical stimulation of cells within taste buds and then is conveyed by the special afferent fibers. The first order neuron for taste has its cell body located in the inferior glossopharyngeal ganglion. The central processes of these neurons project to the rostral nucleus solitarius. The specific means for detection of pain, temperature, and tactile sensation in areas served by the glossopharyngeal nerve are presumably similar to those elsewhere in the body. Pain, temperature, and tactile sensation from the posterior third of the tongue, upper pharynx, tonsils, skin behind the external ear, inner aspect of the tympanic membrane, and eustachian tube are conveyed by general somatic afferent fibers of the glossopharyngeal nerve. Cell bodies for these first order neurons lie in both the superior and inferior glossopharyngeal ganglia. The central processes of these neurons enter the medulla and descend in the spinal trigeminal tract and synapse within the caudal part of the spinal trigeminal nucleus.

Nuclear and Supranuclear Control

The axons of cells in the nucleus solitarius conveying taste from the posterior third of the tongue ascend and terminate at the ventral posterior nuclei of the thalamus. These neurons in turn project to the inferior third of the postcentral gyrus for taste perception. The secondary neuron cell bodies for pain, temperature, and tactile sensation are located in the spinal trigeminal nucleus. Their processes cross the midline in the medulla and ascend to terminate at the contralateral ventral posterior nucleus of the thalamus. From this point, the third order neurons project to the postcentral, sensory cortex region.

AUTONOMIC FIBERS

Nucleus

The inferior salivatory nucleus gives rise to general visceral efferent fibers that provide input for parotid gland secretion. The afferent limb for autonomic reflexive control of respiration and cardiac output is provided by general visceral afferent fibers of the glossopharyngeal nerve. These fibers convey impulses to the nucleus solitarius from chemoreceptors of the carotid body and baroreceptors from the carotid sinus regarding blood oxygen tension and blood pressure, respectively.

Supranuclear Control

The salivatory nucleus receives input from the hypothalamus. The output influencing parotid gland secretion may be modulated by emotional stimuli, such as fear causing dryness of mouth, or by sensory input, such as pleasant odors of food producing increased secretion (mouth watering).

Peripheral Pathways

The glossopharyngeal general visceral efferent fibers reach the otic ganglion, which lies below the foramen ovale. Postganglionic fibers from the otic ganglion then provide input to the parotid gland.

Anatomy of Cranial Nerve X

MOTOR FIBERS

Nucleus

The nucleus ambiguus is the origin of special visceral efferent fibers of the vagus nerve, which supply striated muscles of the tongue and larynx, and all of the striated muscles of the soft palate and the pharynx except for the tensor veli palatini and the stylopharyngeus (which are innervated by branches of cranial nerves V and IX, respectively) (see Table 13–1). The palatoglossus is the only tongue muscle supplied by the vagus nerve; the remainder are supplied by cranial nerve XII. The palatoglossus muscle originates in the soft palate and passes through the tongue in a transverse fashion. Together with the styloglossus muscle, it acts to elevate the posterior tongue.

Upper Motor Neuron, Supranuclear Control

The nucleus ambiguus receives input from motor areas of the cerebral cortex, particularly the precentral gyrus. The cortical input is bilateral and indirect. The corticobulbar fibers terminate first on adjacent reticular formation fibers, which in turn transmit signals to the nucleus ambiguus. The nucleus also receives sensory input from the larynx, pharynx, and airways, which mediate reflexive actions such as coughing, swallowing, and vomiting.

Lower Motor Neuron, Peripheral Pathways

The special visceral efferent fibers exit the skull through the jugular foramen with the vagus nerve and then divide into three major branches: the pharyngeal nerve, superior laryngeal nerve, and recurrent laryngeal nerve. The pharyngeal and superior laryngeal nerves branch from the vagus high in the neck. The recurrent laryngeal nerve branches at the base of the neck on the right and in the thorax on the left (Fig. 13–2). The pharyngeal nerve enters the pharynx and divides into the pharyngeal plexus to supply the muscles noted earlier. The superior laryngeal nerve descends and

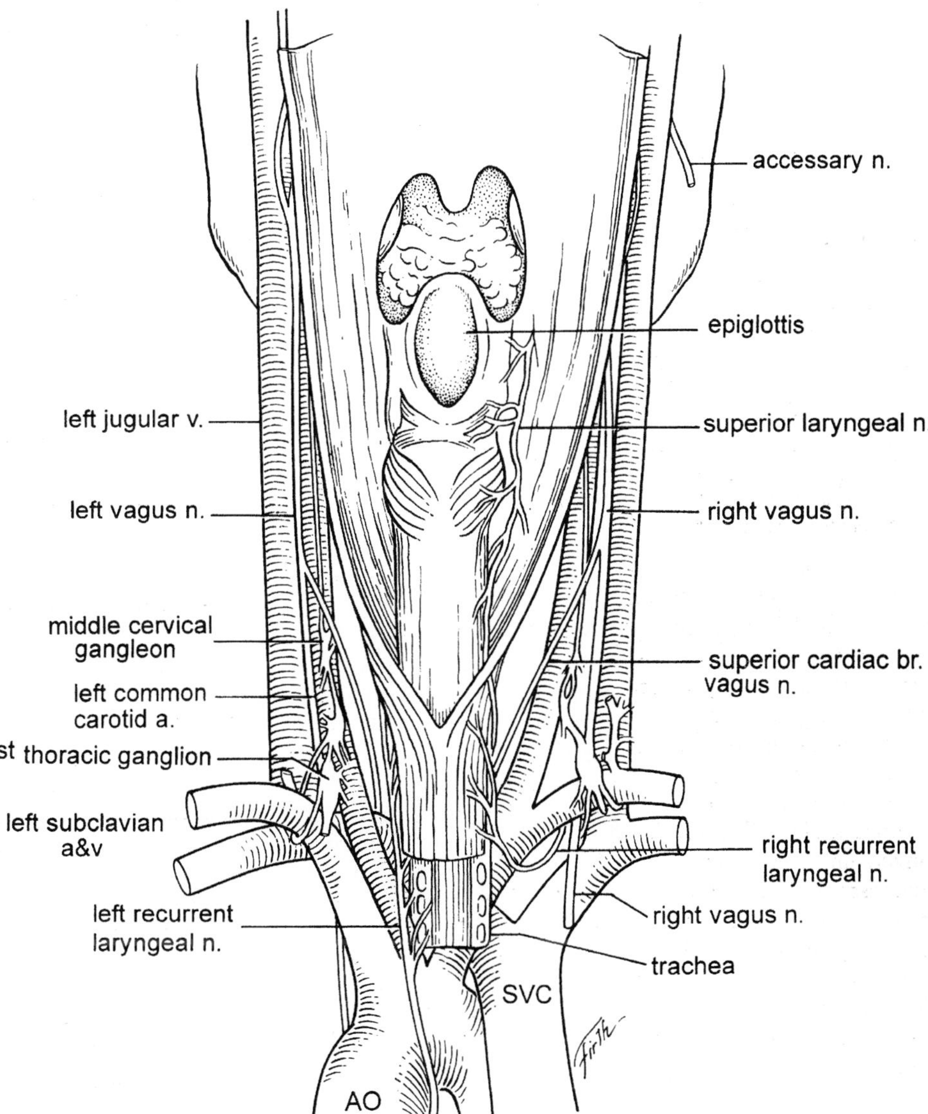

FIGURE 13–2. Diagram of the vagus nerve (cranial nerve X), specifically, its branch, the recurrent laryngeal nerve, and its relationship to the large vessels of the neck. The right and left nerves are not identical, and the recurrent laryngeal nerve branches at the base of the neck on the right and in the thorax on the left.

divides to reach the cricothyroid and the inferior constrictor muscles. The right and left recurrent laryngeal nerves take different paths to reach their destination, supplying all of the intrinsic muscles of the larynx except the cricothyroid. On the right, the recurrent laryngeal nerve descends anterior to the subclavian artery, loops posteriorly beneath it, and then turns upward again, running along the right side of the trachea to the larynx. The left recurrent laryngeal nerve passes under the aortic arch and travels upward in a groove between the left trachea and esophagus to the larynx.

SENSORY FIBERS

Sensory Organs and First Order Neurons

General somatic efferent fibers of the vagus nerve convey sensations of pain, temperature, and touch from the meninges of the posterior fossa, the back of the ear, the external auditory canal, the external tympanic membrane, the larynx, and the pharynx. Sensation from the vocal cords and the larynx below this level is carried by sensory fibers of the recurrent laryngeal nerve. Sensation above the vocal folds is conveyed by the internal laryngeal nerve, which is a branch of the superior laryngeal nerve. The cell bodies for sensation of the ear, external auditory meatus, and tympanic membrane are in the superior vagal ganglion (jugular ganglion); the remaining fibers have their cell bodies in the inferior vagal ganglion (nodose ganglion). Both the superior and inferior vagal ganglia are located on the proximal vagus nerve intracranially at the jugular fossa near the jugular foramen. The central processes of both ganglia enter the medulla and descend in the spinal trigeminal tract to the trigeminal nucleus.

Visceral afferent fibers of the vagus nerve carry visceral sensation from the intestines, stomach, esophagus, tongue, part of the pharynx, lungs, bronchi, trachea, and larynx. These fibers also convey signals from chemoreceptors detecting blood oxygen tension located in the aortic body and baroreceptors for blood pressure in the aortic arch. Cell bodies for all visceral afferent fibers are in the inferior vagal ganglion. Their central processes descend in the tractus solitarius in the medulla to reach the nucleus of the tractus solitarius.

Nuclear and Supranuclear Control

After reaching the spinal trigeminal nucleus, impulses for pain, temperature, and tactile sensation are carried by second order neuron fibers, crossing in the medulla, to the contralateral ventral posterior nucleus of the thalamus. The third order neurons in the thalamus project to the sensory cortex via the internal capsule. The nucleus of the tractus solitarius, along with the reticular formation and hypothalamus, has connections to the dorsal vagal motor nucleus for reflexive control of cardiac, respiratory, and gastrointestinal functions.

AUTONOMIC FIBERS

Nucleus

The dorsal vagal motor nucleus is the origin of the preganglionic, parasympathetic fibers (general visceral efferent) of the vagus nerve. This nucleus is a column of cells located in the floor of the fourth ventricle medial to the nucleus ambiguus. These parasympathetic fibers of the vagus control secretion of glands in the mucosa of the larynx, pharynx, gut from the esophagus to the colon at the splenic flexure, pancreas, liver, and lungs. Fibers to the stomach are responsible for acid secretion. Activation of the parasympathetic fibers to the heart results in slowing of the heart rate; such activation also produces a negative inotropic effect on heart muscle contraction. The vagus parasympathetic fibers also innervate smooth muscle of the airway and gut. These fibers carry signals to open the airway during breathing, to produce bronchoconstriction, and also to coordinate peristalsis of the esophagus and intestine.

Supranuclear Control

The dorsal motor nucleus of the vagus receives input from the hypothalamus, the nucleus of the tractus solitarius, the reticular formation, and the olfactory system.

Peripheral Pathways

The parasympathetic fibers affect numerous body functions in structures within the neck, thorax, and abdomen. They leave the cranium with the vagus nerve through the jugular foramen. These preganglionic fibers terminate near their target sites on ganglia associated with plexuses at several locations, including the esophagus, pharynx, lungs, heart, and intestines. The parasympathetic functions of the vagus nerve are addressed in the chapter on the autonomic nervous system.

Examination of Cranial Nerves IX and X

DIRECTED NEUROLOGICAL EXAMINATION

Cranial Nerve IX

The functions of the glossopharyngeal nerve overlap with those of other cranial nerves, making it difficult to test in isolation.

Motor. The sole skeletal muscle innervation of cranial nerve IX is the stylopharyngeus, which aids in elevation of the pharynx. The oral cavity should be inspected visually at rest to ascertain whether asymmetrical lowering of the pharynx is present. The pharynx is elevated also by the palatopharyngeus and salpingopharyngeus muscles, both of which derive their nerve supply from the vagus nerve. Lesions of the glossopharyngeal nerve therefore may not produce any noticeable clinical motor effect.

Autonomic. The activity of parotid gland salivary secretion through Stensen's duct reflects autonomic functioning of the glossopharyngeal nerve. The duct is located on the inside of the cheek opposite the crown of the second upper molar tooth. Secretion from the parotid glands should be symmetrical, although the amount of saliva normally produced may vary. This quantity may be tested by having the patient suck on a lemon wedge, or by injecting pilocarpine intravenously, and then assessing saliva volume from the duct. Reduced volume of one side suggests glossopharyngeal autonomic dysfunction on that side. Saliva volume measurements for this purpose are impractical and are virtually never done.

Sensory. The sensory function of the glossopharyngeal nerve most accessible to testing is general visceral sensation (tactile, pain, temperature) of the posterior and lateral aspects of the pharynx, and the posterior third of the tongue and the tonsils. Testing is done by touching the soft tip of a cotton applicator to either side of these areas and asking the patient about asymmetry of sensation. Tactile sensation in these areas also serves to trigger the gag, or pharyngeal, reflex. Testing taste sensation of the posterior third of the tongue cannot be done reliably in the clinic. Testing may be accomplished in a laboratory setting by stimulating this area of the tongue with an electrical current.

Reflexes. The gag, or pharyngeal, reflex is centered in the medulla and consists of the reflexive motor response of pharyngeal elevation and constriction with tongue retraction in response to sensory stimulation of the pharyngeal wall, posterior tongue, tonsils, or faucial pillars. This reflex is examined by touching the posterior pharynx with the soft tip of a cotton applicator and visually inspecting for elevation of the pharynx. Both sides of the pharynx should be examined for both the afferent and efferent limbs of the reflex by touching one side first and then the other, while watching for symmetry of pharyngeal movement. The normal reflex response varies, and it may be reduced in the elderly or in smokers. Asymmetry of the reflex is the feature most indicative of pathology.

Cranial Nerve X

Motor innervations of the vagus nerve to the soft palate, larynx, and pharynx are readily available for testing.

Motor. Inspection of the palate on phonation shows deviation of the uvula to the intact side with a unilateral vagus nerve lesion. The unaffected muscles contract normally, drawing the uvula upward and pulling it laterally away from the side of the lesion. A lesion involving the branches of the vagus nerve to the larynx produces vocal cord paresis on that side. The affected cord lies between abduction and adduction. The patient may demonstrate a mild hoarseness, or speech may be unaffected because of compensatory movement of the intact vocal cord. A lesion affecting innervation to the palate produces speech with a nasal quality. This quality is due to inability to close the nasal passage by palate elevation during phonation, allowing air to escape into and resonate within the nasal cavity. The patient may also have dysphagia due to involvement of pharyngeal muscles, with liquids escaping into the nasal cavity during swallow. Vocal cord function can be assessed by listening to the patient's speech to detect a hoarse or breathy voice with reduced volume. Cord function is best examined by visualization using indirect or direct laryngoscopy. Videostroboscopy recording using the fiberoptic direct laryngoscope may also be helpful to assess vocal cord movement.

Sensory. Sensory testing of the vagus nerve cannot be reliably accomplished in the routine neurological examination. Regions of the body that have vagus sensory innervation are either inaccessible or also have sensory input from cranial nerves V and IX.

Autonomic. The carotid sinus baroreceptors are innervated by the carotid sinus nerve branch of the glossopharyngeal nerve. Their stimulation results in heart rate reduction mediated by the vagus nerve. Testing the integrity of these fibers by carotid artery massage is not only impractical and unreliable but also is potentially dangerous. This maneuver may produce asystole or ventricular arrhythmia and should be done only where resuscitative means are immediately available, and not as part of a neurological examination. The vagus nerve is the efferent limb also of the oculocardiac reflex, where heart rate is decreased by pressure on the eyeball. The afferent impulses for this reflex are conveyed by the trigeminal nerve. The heart rate may slow slightly when the reflex is intact. Heart rate is influenced by numerous factors, however, and this reflex is not a reliable test for vagus nerve integrity. Testing of autonomic functions related to the vagus nerve is addressed in the chapter on the autonomic nervous system.

Reflexes. The vagus nerve participates in several reflexes, including coughing, swallowing, sneezing, yawning, and hiccups, but only the gag reflex lends itself to routine testing in the neurological examination. The gag reflex involves afferent fibers provided by the glossopharyngeal nerve (and, in some people, also the vagus nerve) and motor efferents to the pharynx, soft palate, and tongue from the vagus. The reflex is elicited by tactile stimulation of the walls of the pharynx or the posterior tongue. The reflex consists of symmetrical contraction and elevation of the pharynx and retraction of the tongue. This process is described earlier in the section on reflex testing of the glossopharyngeal nerve.

ASSOCIATED NEUROLOGICAL FINDINGS

Cerebral. Dysphagia and changes in speech similar to that which is produced by a lesion of the cranial nerves or their nuclei may occur with interruption of the corticobulbar fibers, which provide the brain stem nuclei with innervation from the frontal cerebral cortex. This condition is referred to as *pseudobulbar palsy*. The brain stem nuclei receive bilateral input; consequently, a unilateral lesion does not result in bulbar symptoms. Speech and swallowing disorders are due to bilateral injury of these pathways. The interruption may occur at any point from the cortex to the brain stem, but most commonly the interruption is due to ischemic injury.[20] Clinical findings indicative of cerebral lesions producing these pseudobulbar symptoms may include aphasia, sensory changes, or corticospinal tract findings such as limb spasticity, increased tendon and jaw jerk reflexes, and an extensor plantar response. Patients with pseudobulbar palsy also may have impaired emotional control with unprovoked laughter or crying, and emergence of primitive reflexes such as suck and snout.

Cranial Nerves. Lesions of the nuclei of cranial nerves IX or X usually affect adjacent brain stem structures, producing ipsilateral sensory disturbance of the face from involvement of the fibers of the descending tract and nucleus of cranial nerve V, vertigo from vestibular nuclei, contralateral limb sensory changes from the lateral spinothalamic, and ipsilateral limb ataxia caused by involvement of the inferior cerebellar peduncle. Cranial nerves IX and X travel closely together between the brain stem and the jugular foramen and consequently are rarely affected independently of one another in their intracranial locations. More peripherally, a lesion at the jugular foramen also affects the spinal accessory nerve, which passes through this opening with the glossopharyngeal and vagus nerves. In addition to disturbance of speech, swallow, and gag, the patient demonstrates weakness of the sternocleidomastoid and trapezius muscles. Cranial nerve XII may be involved together cranial nerves IX, X, and XI by trauma, infection, or neoplasm at the retroparotid space. A lesion of cranial nerve XII produces deviation of the tongue to the side of the lesion when the tongue is protruded.

Motor/Reflexes/Cerebellar/Gait. Changes in muscle tone can be indicative of neurological disease involving cranial nerves IX and X. Cerebral lesions causing pseudobulbar palsy with alteration of speech and dysphagia may be associated with limb spasticity due to corticospinal tract injury. Parkinsonism caused by various etiologies frequently is associated with difficulties in speech and swallowing. No specific lesions exist of the cranial nerves, but rather the subcortical control is affected bilaterally. Patients with progressive supranuclear palsy particularly have prominent difficulty with speech and dysphagia. In patients with suspected cranial nerve IX or X lesions, the presence of abnormal reflexes, such as an extensor plantar response, or the emergence of rudimentary reflexes like the suck or snout are indicators of CNS pathology. Disorders of the neuromuscular junction also produce dysarthria and dysphagia. Repetitive testing of ocular or limb muscle power may produce an inordinate amount of fatigue and weakness pointing to a diagnosis of myasthenia.

A brain stem lesion producing impairment of speech and swallow may also include ataxia of ipsilateral limbs and gait by injury to the inferior cerebellar peduncle that lies adjacent to the nuclei of nerves IX and X.

Sensory. Alteration of pain and temperature sensation of the ipsilateral face with sensory changes of contralateral limbs in association with dysphagia and dysarthric or hoarse speech indicate a brain stem lesion. Sensory changes of the limbs and face on the same side may be produced by a cerebral lesion that contributes to a pseudobulbar state.

Autonomic Nervous System. Disorders of vagal nerve autonomic function may result in symptoms relating to cardiopulmonary and gastrointestinal functions, none of which are testable in the neurological examination. These may be assessed by specialized tests such as the tilt-table cardiac examination or studies of gastrointestinal motility.

Neurovascular. The precise mechanism of neurally mediated syncope (vasovagal vasomotor syncope) remains undetermined. These fainting spells are often provoked by unpleasant sensory stimuli and are accompanied by bradycardia, peripheral vasodilation, and hypotension. Blockage of the vagally mediated bradycardia with atropine does not eliminate the vasodilation and hypotension or the syncope. Vascular function is not a means of assessing glossopharyngeal or vagal status in a setting other than a research environment.

Evaluation Guidelines (Table 13–2)

Neuroimaging. Lesions of the medulla such as infarction or neoplasm, or extramedullary, intracranial lesions, are better visualized by magnetic resonance imaging (MRI) than by computed tomography (CT). Some lesions that involve bone, especially the skull base, may be detected by CT or radiographs, the latter usually requiring the neurologist to request special views of the base of the skull. Imaging should be employed to assist in defining lesion type when the clinical examination indicates an intracranial process.

Electrophysiology. Disorders of speech and swallow suspected to be due to neuromuscular disorders such as motor neuron disease or myasthenia gravis may be evident on electrophysiological testing. Repetitive stimulation on nerve conduction studies and single fiber assessment of jitter may aid in the diagnosis of myasthenia. Electromyography (EMG) of the tongue or limb muscles may demonstrate denervation indicative of motor neuron disease. The location of a nerve lesion producing vocal cord paralysis may be established by EMG testing of the thyroarytenoid and cricothyroid laryngeal muscles.[21] Evidence of denervation restricted to the cricothyroid or thyroarytenoid muscle alone indicates neuropathy of the superior laryngeal or recurrent laryngeal nerves, respectively. Denervation of both muscles places the lesion proximally in the laryngeal nerve or the vagus. Laryngeal EMG has also been useful in discriminating laryngeal dystonia (spasmodic dysphonia) from voice tremor and other disorders producing speech problems.[22]

Body Fluid and Tissue Analysis. Occasionally, biopsy of tissue outside the CNS may be productive in establishing a diagnosis involving cranial nerves IX and X. Amyloid neuropathy involving the cranial nerves may be demonstrated on peripheral nerve biopsy. Sarcoidosis with basilar meningitis and cranial neuropathies may be evident on lung or lymph node biopsy.

Cerebrospinal Fluid and Intracranial Pressure. Lumbar puncture should be accomplished in cases of suspected CNS infectious or inflammatory disorders.

Neuropsychological Testing. Patients with pseudobulbar palsy may have findings of cognitive impairment on formal neuropsychological testing.

Other Tests. Patients with voice disorders should undergo careful otolaryngological evaluation of the neck and pharynx

TABLE 13–2. **Useful Tests in the Evaluation of Disorders of Cranial Nerves IX and X***

Syndrome	Neuroimaging	Electrophysiology	Fluid and Tissue Analysis	Neuropsychological Tests	Other Tests
Supranuclear lesions unilateral or bilateral	CT or MRI evidence of structural lesion, most commonly ischemic infarction of the frontal lobe	EEG may demonstrate nonspecific abnormalities	Not applicable	Evidence of cognitive impairment	None
Nuclear lesions: lateral medulla	MRI evidence of ischemic infarction. CT is not optimal imaging modality in this region. Angiographic evidence of impaired flow in the vertebral or basilar arteries	No findings	Not applicable	No abnormal findings	None
Proximal peripheral nerves: Cerebellopontine angle lesion	MRI or CT evidence of contrast enhancing mass lesion	Abnormal interwave separation (waves I–III, I–V) on brain stem auditory evoked potential	Not applicable	None	None
Middle peripheral nerve lesion at base of skull or nasopharynx	MRI or CT evidence of neoplasm or trauma	None	Not applicable	None	None
Far distal peripheral nerve lesions	MRI or CT evidence of neoplasm or trauma	Not applicable	Not applicable	None	None

*With cross-references to chapters on neuroimaging, electrodiagnostics, tissue analyses, neuropsychological testing, and other tests.
MRI, Magnetic resonance imaging; CT, computed tomography; EEG, electroencephalogram.

and visualization of the vocal cords by either indirect or direct laryngoscopy. Paresis of the left vocal cord may result from disease processes in the chest involving the recurrent laryngeal nerve, such as an expanding aortic aneurysm, mediastinal adenopathy, or lung neoplasm. Chest radiographs, and possibly CT, should be employed to evaluate patients with suspected thoracic disease. Intravenous administration of edrophonium (Tensilon test) may be helpful in diagnosis of suspected myasthenia gravis.

Clinical Syndromes (Table 13–3)

SUPRANUCLEAR LESIONS

Interruption of the corticobulbar tracts providing innervation of cranial nerve motor nuclei from the cerebral precentral motor cortex produces disturbances of speech, swallowing, chewing, and occasionally breathing known as *pseudobulbar palsy*. Patients with this disorder may also have emotional lability with exaggerated crying or laughter in response to minimal provocation. Because the nuclei of cranial nerve IX and X receive bilateral innervation, a unilateral lesion may be silent or may produce only mild symptoms. Supranuclear lesions are responsible for weakness of speech, chewing, and swallowing; the muscles do not also produce prominent atrophy because the lower motor neuron and its trophic effect on the muscle remain intact. Palate and gag reflexes remain intact, even heightened, and abnormal reflexes such as the snout and suck may be present, along with an increased jaw jerk reflex. Patients with pseudobulbar palsy may have dementia due to cerebral pathology involving bilateral frontal areas.

Acute onset of pseudobulbar palsy in one series of 13 patients was associated with infarction in the operculum, the internal capsule, or corona radiata or hemorrhage in lenticular nuclei.[23] Six of these patients had no prior history of stroke. Only one of these patients was described as having neuropsychological deficits, and all improved or recovered from the pseudobulbar symptoms within a few weeks.

Supranuclear innervation of speech is also derived from extrapyramidal pathways. Basal ganglia dysfunction is

TABLE 13–3. **Etiologies of Lesions of Cranial Nerves IX and X**

Etiological Category	Selected Specific Etiologies	Chapter
Structural Disorders		
Developmental	Immaturity of cervical vagus nerve fibers	28
Degenerative compressive	Paget's disease	29
Hereditary and Degenerative Disorders		
The degenerative dementias	Bifrontal pathology, especially Alzheimer's, Pick's disease	33
Movement disorders	Adductor spasmodic dysphonia Abductor spasmodic dysphonia Parkinsonism	34
Degenerative motor, sensory, and autonomic disorders	Amyotrophic lateral sclerosis	36
Acquired Metabolic and Nutritional Disorders		
Endogenous metabolic disorders	Neuropathy of glossopharyngeal afferent and vagus efferent fibers of circulatory reflexes, especially diabetes	38
Nutritional deficiencies and syndromes associated with alcoholism	Neuropathy of glossopharyngeal afferent and vagus efferent fibers of circulatory reflexes, poor nutrition, alcoholism	40
Infectious Disorders		
Nonviral infections	Syphilis	42
Neurovascular Disorders	Strokes with bifrontal pathology (pseudobulbar paresis) Lateral medullary syndrome, posterior fossa, arteriovenous malformation	45
Neoplastic Disorders		
Primary neurological tumors	Schwannoma	46
Metastatic neoplasms and paraneoplastic syndromes	Tumor to base of skull, nasopharynx, chest	47
Demyelinating Disorders of the Peripheral Nervous System	Guillain-Barré syndrome	49
Autoimmune and Inflammatory Disorders	Sarcoidosis Myasthenia gravis	50
Traumatic Disorders	Compromise of jugular foramen contents by basilar skull fracture	51
Epilepsy	Intractable epilepsy	52
Headache and Facial Pain	Glossopharyngeal neuralgia	53
Drug-Induced and Iatrogenic Neurological Disorders	Vincristine Injury of the recurrent laryngeal nerve by thyroidectomy	55

believed to be the source of focal dystonias involving the larynx causing adductor and abductor spasmodic dysphonia.[24] The former type is the far more common of the two. Involuntary adduction of the cords during phonation produces speech that has an interrupted, strangulated quality that is often effortful for the patient. In the less common abductor type of spasmodic dysphonia the patient has a breathy voice. As in other forms of focal dystonia, the patient may employ certain "tricks" to briefly overcome the dystonia, presumably by using other motor pathways to accomplish the desired movement. Some patients with spasmodic dysphonia may find their voice nearly normal when singing or shouting. These fluctuations of symptoms and ability to speak have in the past resulted in psychiatric diagnoses, leading to inappropriate and unproductive therapies and, when the correct diagnosis is established, a lingering resentment and hostility on the part of the patients toward physicians.

Symptomatic treatment of adductor dysphonia has been quite successful by injection of small amounts of botulinum toxin into the thyroarytenoid muscle of the larynx.[25–27] This technique is regarded by many as the treatment of choice for this disorder. Treatment of the abductor type of spasmodic dysphonia by botulinum toxin injection has been technically more difficult and has produced less satisfactory results, although some investigators have reported success targeting the posterior cricoarytenoid or the cricothyroid muscles.[28, 29]

Unilateral stimulation of the vagal nerve has been established as an effective means to treat medically refractory epilepsy.[30] Electrodes from an implantable pacemaker device are attached to the left vagus nerve in the neck and provide intermittent stimulation. The mechanism of reducing seizures is believed to involve activation of cortical and subcortical connections to the vagal nuclei. Patients receiving vagal nerve stimulation for treatment of epilepsy have been reported to experience improvement in daytime drowsiness and altered REM sleep patterns.[31] Further, vagal nerve stimulation is under investigation as a means to treat depression that has been inadequately responsive to medical management.[32]

NUCLEAR LESIONS

The lateral medullary syndrome, known also as Wallenberg's syndrome, is the prototype lesion involving the nuclei of cranial nerves IX and X. The syndrome results from infarction of the medulla by vertebral artery thrombosis or dissection that may also produce occlusion of the opening to the posterior inferior cerebellar artery.[33]

Presenting symptoms often include a stabbing pain in the eye, face, or ear ipsilateral to the side of infarction, presumably as a result of involvement of the nucleus of the descending tract of cranial nerve V. Vertigo or a sense of dysequilibrium occurs commonly because of injury of the vestibular nuclei. Nausea and vomiting are often accompanying symptoms, and they may also arise from vestibular nuclei involvement. Intractable hiccups are rarely caused by lesions of the medulla but may be present in lateral medullary infarction.[34, 35] Involvement of the nucleus ambiguus causes ipsilateral vocal cord paralysis and a hoarse voice, as well as ipsilateral weakness of the palate and pharynx. Palate elevation on phonation is asymmetrical, with the uvula drawn to the intact side, and the patient experiences dysphagia. Impaired sensation to pain and temperature occurs in a crossed fashion involving the ipsilateral face and contralateral limbs caused by involvement, respectively, of the descending tract of the cranial nerve V and the spinothalamic tract. Injury of spinocerebellar fibers and of the inferior cerebellar peduncle results in an unsteady gait and ataxia of the ipsilateral limbs. An ipsilateral Horner's syndrome occurs from involvement of the descending sympathetic fibers from the hypothalamus. Limb weakness, tendon reflex changes, and extensor plantar responses do not occur because the corticospinal fibers are ventrally located at this level of the medulla and are outside of the area of injury. Ipsilateral facial weakness may be present even though the infarction does not extend beyond the lateral medulla. The triad of Horner's syndrome, ipsilateral limb ataxia, and contralateral limb numbness reliably indicates lateral medullary infarction.[36]

Unless cerebellar infarction is also present, cranial CT often does not identify the infarction.[36, 37] Imaging by MRI is clearly superior to CT to visualize lesions in the medulla. The prognosis for recovery from a lateral medullary cerebrovascular accident is generally good, although in some cases, the infarction may potentially be fatal because of secondary edema and herniation or obstructive hydrocephalus and increased pressure in the posterior fossa. In this circumstance, emergency surgical intervention with ventricular drainage or decompressive craniotomy may be lifesaving.[38] The area of infarction may also be extended by propagation of clot into the basilar artery, or by vessel-to-vessel embolism from the vertebral artery to the basilar artery.[39]

PROXIMAL PERIPHERAL LESIONS

The glossopharyngeal and vagus nerves pass through the area of the cerebellopontine angle, formed by the junction of the pons, medulla, and cerebellum, before exiting the skull through the jugular foramen. In this area, both nerves may be compromised by an expanding mass lesion, most commonly a schwannoma originating from the vestibular portion of cranial nerve VIII within the internal auditory canal. The syndrome of a cerebellopontine angle tumor generally begins as tinnitus with hearing loss and dysequilibrium or frank vertigo, which may be episodic. As the tumor expands, cranial nerve V becomes involved, resulting in ipsilateral facial pain and numbness and loss of the corneal reflex. The cerebellum or cerebellar peduncles may become compressed, producing ataxia. Unilateral impingement on the vagus nerve causes mild hoarseness and asymmetrical elevation of the soft palate. Schwannoma arising from the glossopharyngeal nerve is a rare occurrence, but, interestingly, the presenting symptom of patients with this tumor is most commonly hearing loss.[40] This occurs because the mass emanating from the glossopharyngeal nerve is clinically silent until it has enlarged to the point that it is impinging on adjacent structures.

MIDDLE PERIPHERAL LESIONS

Lesions at the jugular foramen, retropharyngeal space, or other peripheral locations produce syndromes involving cranial nerves IX and X, and sometimes also cranial nerves XI and XII. The lesions may be due to various potential etiologies, including neoplasm, infection, and trauma. The syndromes are associated with the names of authors describing them and are listed in Table 13–1. The jugular foramen syndrome, also known as *Vernet's syndrome*, involves cranial nerves IX, X, and XI. The syndrome is comprised of weakness of the ipsilateral vocal cord, palate, and pharynx and the trapezius and sternocleidomastoid muscles. A lesion in the retropharyngeal space is responsible for Villaret's syndrome, which involves cranial nerves IX, X, XI, and XII and produces anesthesia of the palate, larynx, and pharynx; weakness of the trapezius and sternocleidomastoid muscles; atrophy and weakness of the tongue; and Horner's syndrome. This last feature is due to involvement of cervical sympathetic fibers.

FAR DISTAL PERIPHERAL LESIONS

Isolated lesions of either the glossopharyngeal or vagus nerves are unusual. As noted earlier, glossopharyngeal nerve abnormalities may be clinically undetectable unless adjacent structures are also involved. Perhaps the most common vagus nerve lesion is that involving the recurrent laryngeal nerve, resulting in ipsilateral vocal cord paresis and hoarseness of voice. The left nerve has a longer course, with its looped recurrence in the chest rather than in the neck, as on the right. The nerve passes around the aorta before returning rostrally to the larynx. The left recurrent laryngeal nerve may be compromised by an expanding aortic arch aneurysm or other intrathoracic processes, such as enlargement of the left atrium of the heart, pulmonary neoplasm, or mediastinal adenopathy. Both right and left superior or recurrent laryngeal nerves may be injured during the course of neck surgery such as thyroidectomy. Vocal cord paralysis has been described with vagal neuropathy attributed to diabetes or alcohol consumption and with vagal neuritis in association with herpes simplex and herpes zoster.[41, 42] Superior laryngeal branch neuralgia produces pain in the area of the thyroid cartilage radiating to the ear, and it is triggered by talking or swallowing. This is a rare disorder; treatment is with carbamazepine. Immaturity of the cervical vagus fibers may play a role in sudden infant death syndrome.[43]

GLOSSOPHARYNGEAL NEURALGIA

This is an uncommon disorder, occurring with an annual crude incidence of 0.7 per 100,000 population.[44] The pain of glossopharyngeal neuralgia is located at the base of the tongue, tonsils, ear, or angle of the jaw and is triggered by talking, swallowing, and coughing. Glossopharyngeal neuralgia produces symptoms similar in character to those of trigeminal neuralgia: brief, recurrent, stabbing pains lasting seconds to a couple of minutes. Of these two cranial nerve disorders, glossopharyngeal neuralgia is less common; the ratio of trigeminal to glossopharyngeal neuralgia is 5.9:1.[45] The attacks of glossopharyngeal neuralgia are comparatively more mild, and in contrast to trigeminal neuralgia, bilateral symptoms frequently occur.[44] The course tends to be relapsing and remitting.

Epidemiological data from a population in Minnesota found men and women equally affected with rates of incidence highest in the sixth through eighth decades.[44] Syncope is an unusual accompaniment of glossopharyngeal neuralgia.[46] Spontaneous discharges of the glossopharyngeal nerve to the medulla may cause bradycardia or even asystole by reflexive vagal nerve cardiac inhibitory output.[47] The syncopal episode is produced by this bradycardia together with hypotension caused by reduced sympathetic output. Clonic jerking mimicking seizure may accompany the syncopal spells, although electroencephalographic recording during spells has demonstrated slowing and suppression of activity rather than seizure activity.[48]

Glossopharyngeal neuralgia is divided into idiopathic and symptomatic forms, with the latter due to identifiable pathology such as oropharyngeal or neck carcinoma, a posterior fossa arteriovenous malformation, or multiple sclerosis.[49–52] Although results of the neurological examination are normal in idiopathic glossopharyngeal neuralgia, patients with symptoms of this disorder should have careful examination of the oral cavity and neck and brain imaging with attention to the posterior fossa to exclude underlying pathology. Treatment for the symptoms of glossopharyngeal neuralgia includes the medications used for trigeminal neuralgia, including carbamazepine, baclofen, phenytoin, or combinations of these.

Surgical treatment is an option for patients with symptoms refractory to medical therapy. Sectioning of the rootlets of the glossopharyngeal nerve effectively terminates symptoms but obviously sacrifices the nerve. Alternatively, microvascular decompression has also been successful in treating this disorder and spares the function of the glossopharyngeal nerve. This technique is based on the idea that the neuralgia is due, at least partly, to an adjacent blood vessel producing mechanical irritation to the glossopharyngeal nerve. In one series of 40 patients, the most common offending blood vessel was the posterior inferior cerebellar artery, followed by an artery and vein combination.[53] In this surgery, the glossopharyngeal nerve is identified along with the offending vessels and they are separated. A piece of Teflon felt may be placed between the nerve and an artery. Successful treatment of the neuralgia, by medical or surgical means, should also eliminate any associated syncopal episodes.

General Management Goals

During the initial evaluation of a patient with disorders attributable to cranial nerves IX and X, few specific precautions for management are indicated. Bilateral vagus nerve lesions, regardless of the pathological process, occlude the airway by opposition of the vocal cords in the midline. This condition is an emergency and requires endotracheal intubation to maintain airway patency. Patients with bradycardia or asystole due to increased vagal output are treated initially with atropine or cardiac pacing until the causative process is addressed. It should be kept in mind that the condition of patients with lateral medullary syndrome by infarction may be unstable. Clinical status may decline rapidly with life-threatening consequences by pressure effects in the posterior fossa or by extension of the area of infarction by propagation of clot or embolization from the vertebral artery into the basilar artery. Emergency neurosurgical intervention may be required to alleviate brain stem compression.

Reviews and Selected Updates

Ballotta E, DaGiau G, Renon L, et al: Cranial and cervical nerve injuries after carotid endarterectomy: A prospective study. Surgery 1999;125:85–91.

Berthoud HR, Neuhuber WL: Functional and chemical anatomy of the afferent vagal system. Auton Neurosci 2000;85:1–17.

Cooper E: Nicotinic acetylcholine receptors on vagal afferent neurons. Ann NY Acad Sci 2001;940:110–118.

Fallen EL, Kamath MV, Tougas G, Upton A: Afferent vagal modulation. Clinical studies of visceral sensory input. Auton Neurosci 2001;90:35–40.

Haerer AF: DeJong's The Neurologic Examination, 5th ed. Philadelphia, JB Lippincott, 1992, pp 227–242.

Harati Y: Anatomy of the spinal and peripheral autonomic nervous system. *In* Low PA (ed): Clinical Autonomic Disorders. Boston, Little, Brown 1993, pp 30–35.

Thomas PK, Mathias CJ: Diseases of the ninth, tenth, eleventh, and twelfth cranial nerves. *In* Dyck PJ, Thomas PK, Griffen JW, et al (eds): Peripheral Neuropathy, 3rd ed, Vol 2. Philadelphia, WB Saunders, 1993, pp 869–879.

Wilson-Pauwels L, Akesson EJ, Stewart PA: Cranial Nerves. Philadelphia, B.C. Decker, 1988, pp 113–137.

Zagon A: Does the vagus nerve mediate the sixth sense? Trends Neurosci 2001;24:671–673.

References

1. McHenry LC: Garrison's History of Neurology. Springfield, IL, Charles C Thomas, 1969, pp 19, 93.
2. Roger J, Bille J, Vigouroux RA: Multiple cranial nerve palsies. *In* Vinken PJ, Bruyn GW (eds): Handbook of Clinical Neurology, Vol 2. New York, John Wiley & Sons, 1969, p 99.
3. Khan IA, Wattanasauwan N, Ansari AW: Painless aortic dissection presenting as hoarseness of voice: Cardiovocal syndrome: Ortner's syndrome. Am J Emerg Med 1999;17:361–363.
4. Rafay MA: Tuberculous lymphadenopathy of superior mediastinum causing vocal cord paralysis. Ann Thorac Surg 2000;70:2142–2143.
5. Connolly B, Turner C, DeVine J, Gerlinger T: Jefferson fracture resulting in Collet-Sicard syndrome. Spine 2000;25:395–398.
6. Lo CY, Kwok KF, Yuen PW: A prospective evaluation of recurrent laryngeal nerve paralysis during thyroidectomy. Arch Surg 2000;135:204–207.
7. Maroulis J, Karkanevatos A, Papakostas K: Cranial nerve dysfunction following carotid endarterectomy. Int Angiol 2000;19:237–241.
8. Crumley RL: Laryngeal synkinesis revisited. Ann Otol Rhinol Laryngol 2000;109:365–371.
9. Sicenica T, Venkata Balaji G, Klein A, et al: Villaret's syndrome in a man with prostate carcinoma. Am J Med 2000;108:516–517.
10. Castroagudin JF, Gonzalez-Quintela A, Moldes J, et al: Acute reversible dysphagia and dysphonia as initial manifestations of sarcoidosis. Hepatogastroenterology 1999;46:2414–2418.
11. Berry H, Blair RL: Isolated vagus nerve palsy and vagal mononeuritis. Otolaryngology 1980;106:333–338.
12. Novak DJ, Victor M: The vagus and sympathetic nerves in alcoholic polyneuropathy. Arch Neurol 1974;30(4):273–284.
13. Evans RJC, Benson MK, Hughes DTD: Abnormal chemoreceptor response to hypoxia in patients with tabes dorsalis. BMJ 1971;1:530–531.
14. Sharpey-Schafer EP, Taylor PJ: Absent circulatory reflexes in diabetic neuritis. Lancet 1960;1:559–561.
15. Fagius J, Wallin GB: Microneurographic evidence of excessive sympathetic outflow in the Guillain-Barré syndrome. Brain 1983;106(3):589–600.
16. Camilleri M: Disorders of gastrointestinal motility in neurologic diseases. Mayo Clin Proc 1990;65(6):825–846.
17. McCarthy GM, Skillings JR: Jaw and other orofacial pain in patients receiving vincristine for the treatment of cancer. Oral Surg Oral Med Oral Pathol 1992;74:299–304.
18. Carpenter MB, Sutin J: Human Neuroanatomy, 8th ed. Baltimore, Williams & Wilkins, 1983, p 315.
19. Wilson-Pauwels L, Akesson EJ, Stewart PA: Cranial Nerves. Philadelphia, B.C. Decker, 1988, p 113.
20. Rondot P: Central motor disorders. *In* Vinken PJ, Bruyn GW (eds): Handbook of Clinical Neurology, Vol 1. New York, John Wiley & Sons, 1969, pp 198–221.
21. Simpson DM, Sternman D, Graves-Wright J, et al: Vocal cord paralysis: Clinical and electrophysiological features. Muscle Nerve 1993;16:952–957.
22. Blitzer A, Lovelace RE, Brin MF, et al: Electromyographic findings in focal laryngeal dystonia. Ann Otol Rhinol Laryngol 1985; 94:591–594.
23. Besson G, Bogousslavsky J, Regli F, et al: Acute pseudobulbar or suprabulbar palsy. Arch Neurol 1991;48:501–507.
24. Tolosa E, Pena J: Involuntary vocalizations in movement disorders. Adv Neurol 1988;49:343–363.
25. Whurr R, Lorch M, Fontana H, et al: The use of botulinum toxin in the treatment of adductor spasmodic dysphonia. J Neurol Neurosurg Psychiatry 1993;56:526–530.
26. Blitzer A, Brin MF, Stewart CF: Botulinum toxin management of spasmodic dysphonia (laryngeal dystonia): A 12-year experience in more than 900 patients. Laryngoscope 1998;108:1435–1441.
27. Bhattacharyya N, Tarsy D: Impact on quality of life of botulinum toxin treatments for spasmodic dysphonia and oromandibular dystonia. Arch Otolaryngol Head Neck Surg 2001;127:389–392.
28. Blitzer A, Brin MF, Stewart C, et al: Abductor laryngeal dystonia: A series treated with botulinum toxin. Laryngoscope 1992;102:163–167.
29. Bielamowicz S, Squire S, Bidus K, et al: Assessment of posterior cricoarytenoid botulinum toxin injections in patients with abductor spasmodic dysphonia. Ann Otol Rhinol Laryngol 2001;110:406–412.
30. DeGiorgio CM, Schachter SC, Handforth A, et al: Prospective long-term study of vagus nerve stimulation for the treatment of refractory seizures. Epilepsia 2000;41(9):1195–2000.
31. Malow BA, Edwards J, Marzec M, et al: Vagus nerve stimulation reduces daytime sleepiness in epilepsy patients. Neurology 2001;57(5):879–884.
32. Rush AJ, George MS, Sackeim HA, et al: Vagus nerve stimulation (VNS) for treatment-resistant depressions: A multicenter study. Biol Psychiatry 2000;47(4):273–275.
33. Hosoya T, Watanabe N, Yamaguchi K, et al: Intracranial vertebral artery dissection in Wallenberg syndrome. Am J Neuroradiol 1994;15(6):1161–1165.
34. Chang YY, Chen WH, Liu JS, et al: Intractable hiccup caused by medulla oblongata lesions. J Formosan Med Assoc 1993;92:926–928.
35. Kim JS: Sensory symptoms in ipsilateral limbs/body due to lateral medullary infarction. Neurology 2001;57(7):1230–1234.
36. Sacco RL, Freddo L, Bello JA, et al: Wallenberg's lateral medullary syndrome. Clinical-magnetic resonance imaging correlations. Arch Neurol 1993;50:609–614.
37. Kim JS, Lee JH, Suh DC, et al: Spectrum of lateral medullary syndrome. Correlation between clinical findings and magnetic resonance imaging in 33 subjects. Stroke 1994;25:1405–1410.
38. Jauss M, Krieger D, Hornig C, et al: Surgical and medical management of patients with massive cerebellar infarctions: Results of the German-Austrian Cerebellar Infarction Study. J Neurol 1999;246(7):628.
39. Fisher CM, Karnes W, Kubik C: Lateral medullary infarction: The pattern of vascular occlusion. J Neuropathol Exp Neurol 1961;20:323–325.
40. Sweasey TA, Edlestein SR, Hoff JT: Glossopharyngeal schwannoma: Review of five cases and the literature. Surg Neurol 1991;35:127–130.
41. Guo YP, McLeod JG, Baverstock J: Pathological changes in the vagus nerve in diabetes and chronic alcoholism. J Neurol Neurosurg Psychiatry 1987;50:1449–1454.
42. Tang SC, Jeng JS, Liu HM, et al: Isolated vagus nerve palsy probably associated with herpes simplex virus infection. Acta Neurol Scand 2001;104(3):174–177.
43. Becker LE, Zhang W: Vagal nerve complex in normal development and sudden infant death syndrome. Can J Neurol Sci 1996;23(1):24–33.
44. Katusic S, Williams DB, Beard CM, et al: Incidence and clinical features of glossopharyngeal neuralgia, Rochester, Minnesota, 1945–1984. Neuroepidemiology 1991;10:266–275.
45. Katusic S, Williams DB, Beard CM, et al: Epidemiology and clinical features of idiopathic trigeminal neuralgia and glossopharyngeal neuralgia: Similarities and differences, Rochester, Minnesota 1945–1984. Neuroepidemiology 1991;10:276–281.
46. Ferrante L, Artico M, Nardacci B, et al: Glossopharyngeal neuralgia with cardiac syncope [review]. Neurosurgery 1995;36:58–63.
47. Barbash GI, Keren G, Korczyn AD, et al: Mechanisms of syncope in glossopharyngeal neuralgia. Electroencephalogr Clin Neurophysiol 1986;63:231–235.
48. Lagerlund TD, Harper CM Jr, Sharbrough FW, et al: An electrographic study of glossopharyngeal neuralgia with syncope. Arch Neurol 1988;45:472–475.
49. Paterson AJ, Lamey PJ: Oropharyngeal squamous cell carcinoma presenting as glossopharyngeal neuralgia [letter]. Br J Oral Maxillofac Surg 1992;30:278–279.
50. Metheetrairut C, Brown DH: Glossopharyngeal neuralgia and syncope secondary to neck malignancy. J Otol 1993;22:18–20.
51. Galetta SL, Raps EC, Hurst RW, et al: Glossopharyngeal neuralgia from a posterior fossa arteriovenous malformation: Resolution following embolization. Neurology 1993;43:1854–1855.
52. Minagar A, Sheremata WA: Glossopharyngeal neuralgia and MS. Neurology 2000;54(6):1368–1370.
53. Resnick DK, Janetta PJ, Bissonette D, et al: Microvascular decompression for glossopharyngeal neuralgia. Neurosurgery 1995;36:64–68.

CHAPTER 14

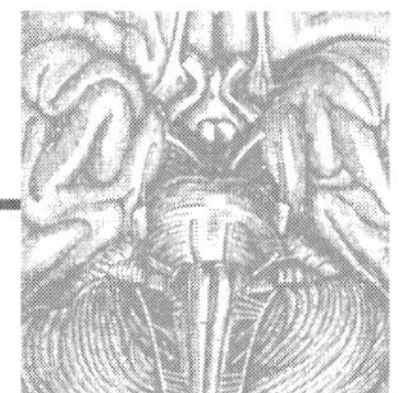

ELAN D. LOUIS

Cranial Nerves XI (Spinal Accessory) and XII (Hypoglossal)

History and Definitions

The assignment of numbers to the cranial nerves may be traced back to Galen (circa 130–201 AD) and perhaps even to Marinus of Tyre (circa 100 AD).[1] Galen recognized 11 of the 12 structures that we now designate as cranial nerves, lumping several of these together such that there were seven paired cranial nerves. Galen combined what we now know as cranial nerves IX through XI, calling these structures the sixth cranial nerve. In his system, the hypoglossal nerve was the seventh and final cranial nerve. The Galenic system for numbering the cranial nerves persisted for one and a half millennia.[1] It was still used by Andreas Vesalius, the Italian anatomist, in his text *De Fabrica* in 1543.[2, 3] Thomas Willis, the English physician and anatomist, numbered the cranial nerves at eight rather than seven. In his celebrated text of 1664, *Cerebri Anatome*,[4] he provided the first thorough description of the spinal accessory nerve. It is said that he used the word "accessory" because the nerve was accessory to the vagus nerve.[1, 2, 5] Samuel von Soemmering, the Prussian artist, inventor, paleontologist, and clinical investigator, has been credited with the first modern enumeration of the 12 cranial nerves in 1778.[1]

The spinal accessory nerve (cranial nerve [CN] XI) and hypoglossal nerve (CN XII) share a number of features. These nerves, along with cranial nerves IV and VI, are classically viewed as pure motor nerves, meaning that they subserve only motor functions, and they do not carry sensory or autonomic fibers.[6] A recent study of spinal accessory nerve samples, however, suggested that this nerve may carry sensory fibers as well.[7] Nuclei of the spinal accessory and hypoglossal nerves lie in the medulla, along with the nuclei of the glossopharyngeal (CN IX) and vagus nerves (CN X).[8]

This chapter focuses on those disturbances of the spinal accessory and hypoglossal nerves that result in weakness rather than overactivity of innervated muscles, because the latter is discussed in other chapters on involuntary movements (see Chapters 16 and 34).

Clinical History

Patients with dysfunction of structures innervated by CN XI or XII or their supranuclear input may present to the physician with various complaints. The more common complaints when CN XI is involved are difficulty rotating the head, complaint that the head "droops" forward, or complaint that the shoulders seem asymmetrical or misshapen. The more common complaints when CN XII is involved are slurred speech, garbled speech, speaking with "marbles in my mouth," difficulty chewing, complaints that "my tongue gets in the way," or difficulty swallowing. Occasionally, a patient

TABLE 14–1. Clinico-anatomical Correlation of Disorders of Cranial Nerves XI and XII

Anatomical Site of Damage	CN XI or XII Finding	Other Neurological and Medical Findings	Common Etiologies
Supranuclear (cerebral hemisphere)	Neck weakness, tongue deviation	Hemiparesis with spasticity and extensor plantar responses, pseudobulbar palsy, cognitive deficits, personality changes, urinary incontinence, gait apraxia, primitive reflexes (e.g., suck, snout, glabellar), paratonic rigidity (gegenhalten)	Stroke, brain tumor, multiple sclerosis, brain abscess
Supranuclear (pontine)	Dissociated weakness (ipsilateral SCM and contralateral trapezius), contralateral weakness with spasticity, and deviation of the eyes toward the weakness	Facial numbness (CN V), weakness of the palate (CN X), or autonomic dysfunction. Contralateral loss of pain and temperature in the body and ipsilateral loss of pain and temperature in the face	Stroke, multiple sclerosis, brain abscess, brain tumor
Nuclear	Bilateral lesions may result in diminished ability to rotate the neck, inability to protrude the tongue, slurred and indistinct speech, impaired swallowing, and possibly some respiratory difficulty. The medial medullary syndrome results in ipsilateral tongue weakness and contralateral weakness and impaired tactile and proprioceptive sense of the arm and leg	With vascular lesions, bilateral pyramidal signs and diminished vibration and position sensation can occur	Motor neuron disease, poliomyelitis, brain stem abscess, syringobulbia, strokes
Within the cranium or in the region of the foramen magnum	Neck and tongue weakness	Cranial nerve IX and X involvement (depressed gag, palatal paresis, and vocal cord paralysis)	Platybasia, Paget's disease, glomus tumors, acoustic neuromas, meningiomas, metastases to the skull base, syphilis, tubercular meningitis, sarcoidosis
Within the region of the jugular foramen	Vernet's syndrome (ipsilateral weakness of the SCM and trapezius)	Vernet's syndrome (ipsilateral loss of taste and depressed sensation over the posterior one third of the tongue, ipsilateral depressed gag reflex and palatal weakness, ipsilateral vocal cord paralysis, and ipsilateral weakness of the SCM and trapezius muscles)	Tumor, basal skull fracture
In the retroparotid or retropharyngeal spaces, and distal peripheral nerve lesions	Collet-Sicard syndrome (ipsilateral weakness of the SCM, trapezius, and tongue)	Collet-Sicard syndrome (same as Vernet's syndrome, with the addition of weakness of the ipsilateral tongue)	Surgical trauma, local infections, neck irradiation or local tumors

SCM, Sternocleidomastoid; CN, cranial nerve.

notices that the tongue is asymmetrical, appearing small and wrinkled on one side with protrusion. These complaints may be associated with neurological signs, including weakness of the sternocleidomastoid (SCM) and trapezius muscles (with or without atrophy), winging of the scapula, deviation and weakness of the tongue (with or without atrophy), dysarthria, and dysphagia.[9–12]

Patients may present with complaints of acute, subacute, and chronic onset. Acute presentations, characterized by the rapid onset of symptoms and signs, include the medial medullary syndrome (i.e., an acute cerebrovascular event involving the posterior circulation), basal skull fracture, shoulder trauma, and dislocation of upper cervical vertebra. Subacute presentations include lesions due to multiple sclerosis, brain stem abscesses, and tuberculous meningitis. Chronic presentations are typically seen in motor neuron disease, acoustic neuroma, meningioma, and other tumors of the central and peripheral nervous system.[11]

Dysfunction of cranial nerves XI and XII may be the result of various precipitating events or underlying etiologies, and several of these were alluded to earlier. These include trauma to the head, neck, or shoulder region (basal skull fracture, stab wound, or gunshot wound of the neck; dislocation of upper cervical vertebra; shoulder trauma), various infectious etiologies including bacterial (tuberculosis, brain abscess, syphilis) and viral (acute poliomyelitis), inflammatory or granulomatous processes (multiple sclerosis, Guillain-Barré syndrome, neurosarcoidosis), metabolic disorders (Paget's disease), structural disorders (platybasia, syringobulbia), exogenous toxins (botulism), acute cerebrovascular events (medial medullary syndrome), neoplasms (glomus cell tumor, neurofibroma, meningioma, acoustic neuroma, metastatic carcinoma), and iatrogenic events (radiation therapy involving the neck, neck surgery).[11, 13] Dysfunction also may be idiopathic.[14, 15]

Lesions of these cranial nerves may be accompanied by any of a large number of associated diseases, symptoms, or signs, including the several systemic illnesses (systemic sarcoidosis, tuberculosis, carcinoma, syphilis), other neurological disorders (multiple sclerosis, Guillain-Barré syndrome, motor neuron disease), and other associated symptoms and signs referable to involvement of regional anatomy, particularly long tracts passing through the brain stem (resulting in weakness with spasticity, dysautonomia, sensory disturbances, gait instability, and incoordination) and other cranial nerves (resulting in facial numbness, nystagmus, dysphagia).[11, 12]

Anatomy (Table 14–1)

CRANIAL NERVE XI

Nucleus

The spinal accessory nerve (CN XI) is classified as a special visceral efferent nerve because it innervates striated muscles that arise embryologically from the branchial arches.[6] CN XI consists of two distinct portions, the cranial (or accessory) portion and the spinal portion (Fig. 14–1).[8] These are sometimes referred to as the *ramus internus* and *ramus externus*, respectively,[12] each with distinctive embryological development.[16]

The cranial and spinal portions of CN XI arise from separate nuclei. The nucleus for the cranial portion of the nerve is the most caudal part of the nucleus ambiguus, which is the longitudinal column of cells that is dorsal to the inferior olivary nucleus in the medulla.[17] The nucleus ambiguus is composed of cells controlling several functions outside of the domain of CN XI: (1) motor neurons supplying the muscles of the soft palate, pharynx, and larynx; (2) preganglionic parasympathetic neurons involved with control of heart rate; and (3) afferent input from brain stem sensory nuclei, especially the nucleus of the spinal tract of the trigeminal nerve and the nucleus of the tractus solitarius. The nucleus for the spinal portion of CN XI is the accessory nucleus, which is a longitudinal column of cells in the anterior horn of the upper five cervical segments of the spinal cord.[8, 17] As is too often the case in the biological sciences, nomenclature is somewhat muddled, and it is important not to confuse (1) the *accessory nucleus* in the cervical spinal cord, which gives rise to the spinal portion of CN XI; and (2) the cranial or *accessory portion of CN XI*, arising from the nucleus ambiguus in the medulla.

Lower Motor Neuron, Peripheral Pathways

Cranial nerve XI fibers extend peripherally from two distinct nuclei: the caudal portion of the nucleus ambiguus in the medulla and the accessory nucleus in the cervical spinal cord. Fibers from the caudal portion of the nucleus ambiguus leave the brain stem caudal to the vagus nerve, as the cranial root of CN XI.[8, 17] Fibers from the accessory nucleus exit the cervical spinal cord as a series of rootlets. These unite to form a common trunk. They then ascend as the spinal root of CN XI, passing upward through the foramen magnum, and uniting with the cranial root of CN XI near the medulla. The united cranial and spinal roots of the accessory nerve exit

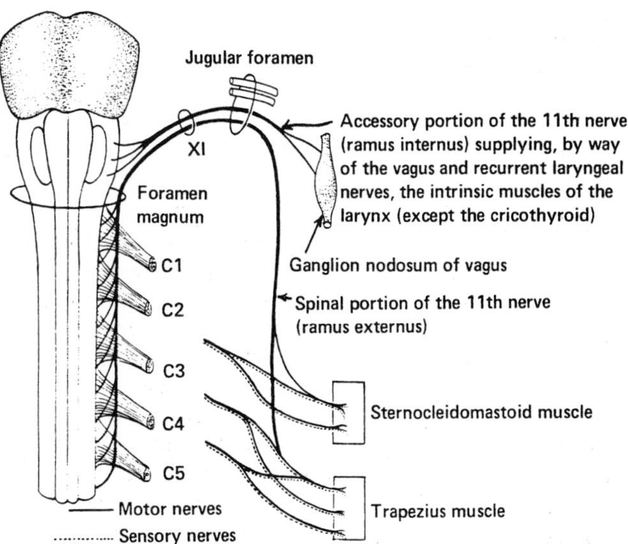

FIGURE 14–1. Schematic of the cranial and spinal portions of CN XI.

the cranium through the jugular foramen.[8, 13, 17, 18] At this point, the spinal accessory nerve lies within the same dural sheath as the vagus nerve, separated from it by a fold of arachnoid.[12]

After exiting the cranium through the jugular foramen, the spinal accessory nerve divides into two portions: (1) the fibers from the nucleus ambiguus join the vagus nerve to form the inferior laryngeal nerve; this nerve innervates the intrinsic muscles of the larynx; (2) the fibers from the accessory nucleus first innervate the SCM muscle and then innervate the three portions of the trapezius muscle.[19] The middle and lower portions of the trapezius muscle are innervated by cervical roots.[8, 17, 19, 20]

A number of connections exist between cranial nerve XI and other nerves. In particular, in the neck, cranial nerve XI unites at several points with the first through fourth cervical nerves.[12]

Some investigators have soundly suggested that the cranial portion of CN XI is actually no more than a mislabeled inferior branch of CN X.[10] First, the cranial portion of CN XI innervates the intrinsic muscles of the larynx rather than the SCM or trapezeii. Second, the cranial portion of CN XI only travels with the spinal portion for a short distance before joining CN X.[10] When the function of CN XI is assessed in the standard neurological examination, only the spinal portion is tested.[20]

Upper Motor Neuron, Supranuclear Control

The nature of the supranuclear input to each of the paired nuclei of cranial nerve XI is not well understood. It is generally believed that these nuclei receive bilateral supranuclear input, and that this input arises from the lower portion of the precentral gyrus. Although the input for the trapezius muscle is believed to be derived primarily from the contralateral hemisphere,[13] the input for the SCM is less well understood but is thought to be derived predominantly from the ipsilateral hemisphere.[21] Although a minority have argued that the supranuclear fibers for the SCM do not decussate, there is a body of evidence, from isolated case reports, that there is a double decussation.[13, 22–25] The precise location of these decussations is not entirely known, although the first decussation may occur in the subthalamic region, midbrain, or pons, and the second may occur in the medulla or cervical spinal cord below the level of the first cervical root.[21] Not surprisingly, the supranuclear input for the trapezius muscle travels separately in the brain stem from the supranuclear input for the SCM muscle, and there have been a number of reports of the pathological dissociation of the two.[26, 27]

The primary supranuclear input for the trapezius muscle is located ventrally in the brain stem and crosses the brain stem in either the midbrain or pons. The supranuclear input for the SCM muscle is located in the brain stem tegmentum, and it decussates twice. Some investigators have suggested that the sternal head of the SCM (responsible for rotation of the head in the contralateral direction) is innervated by the ipsilateral hemisphere, but the clavicular head of the SCM (responsible for tilting the head to the ipsilateral side) is innervated by the contralateral hemisphere.[28] Teleologically, this may be understood as an example of the concept that each cerebral hemisphere controls movement in the contralateral hemispace rather than just in contralateral muscle groups.[28]

CRANIAL NERVE XII

Nucleus

The hypoglossal nerve is classified as a general somatic efferent (GSE) nerve because it innervates striated muscle that arises embryologically from the somites.[6, 8] The nucleus of CN XII is located in the medulla, ventral to the floor of the fourth ventricle. The hypoglossal triangle, or trigonum hypoglossi, in the floor of the fourth ventricle serves as an external landmark for the rostral portion of the hypoglossal nucleus.[17] As with some of the other pure motor cranial nerves, the nucleus is situated medially in the brain stem, which is a result of embryological anatomical relationships. The hypoglossal nucleus, formed by a column of large cells, is approximately 1.8 cm in length. It transverses much of the length of the medulla.[8, 18] Numerous fibers cross the midline of the medulla to connect the paired hypoglossal nuclei.[12] Several discrete smaller nuclear groups surround the hypoglossal nucleus in the medulla, including the nucleus intercalatus, nucleus prepositus, and the nucleus of Roller.[8]

Lower Motor Neuron, Peripheral Pathways

Upon exiting the hypoglossal nucleus, the hypoglossal nerve travels ventrolaterally, passing through the medullary reticular formation, just lateral to the lateral margin of the medial longitudinal fasciculus and the medial lemniscus, and through the medial segments of the inferior olivary nucleus.[12] The nerve exits the ventral aspect of the medulla in the preolivary or ventrolateral sulcus, between the medullary pyramid and the inferior olive, and medial to cranial nerves IX, X, and XI.[6, 17] When the nerve exits the medulla, it is comprised of 10 to 15 separate rootlets on each side.[13] These rootlets coalesce to form two larger bundles, and these perforate the dura mater separately, uniting after their passage through it.[18]

The hypoglossal nerve exits the posterior fossa through the hypoglossal canal.[17] It descends in the neck close to the angle of the mandible. It passes beneath the internal carotid artery and the internal jugular vein, then travels forward between these two blood vessels and crosses the external carotid artery.[12] The branches of the hypoglossal nerve are the meningeal (sending branches to the dura mater in the posterior cranial fossa), descending (sending branches to the omohyoid, sternohyoid, and sternothyroid muscles), thyrohyoid (sending branches to the thyrohyoid muscle), and muscular (sending branches to the extrinsic and intrinsic muscles of the tongue) (Fig. 14–2).[17, 18] The extrinsic muscles of the tongue include the genioglossus, styloglossus, hyoglossus, and chondroglossus muscles, whereas the intrinsic muscles of the tongue include the superior and inferior longitudinales, transversus, and verticalis muscles.[12] The emphasis in the standard neurological examination, with regard to hypoglossal nerve function, is on the function of the extrinsic muscles of the tongue.[10, 12]

Upper Motor Neuron, Supranuclear Control

The supranuclear input for the hypoglossal nerve is better understood than that for the spinal accessory nerve.[29] As with the latter, the supranuclear input is derived from the lowest portion of the precentral gyrus.[10] The corticobulbar

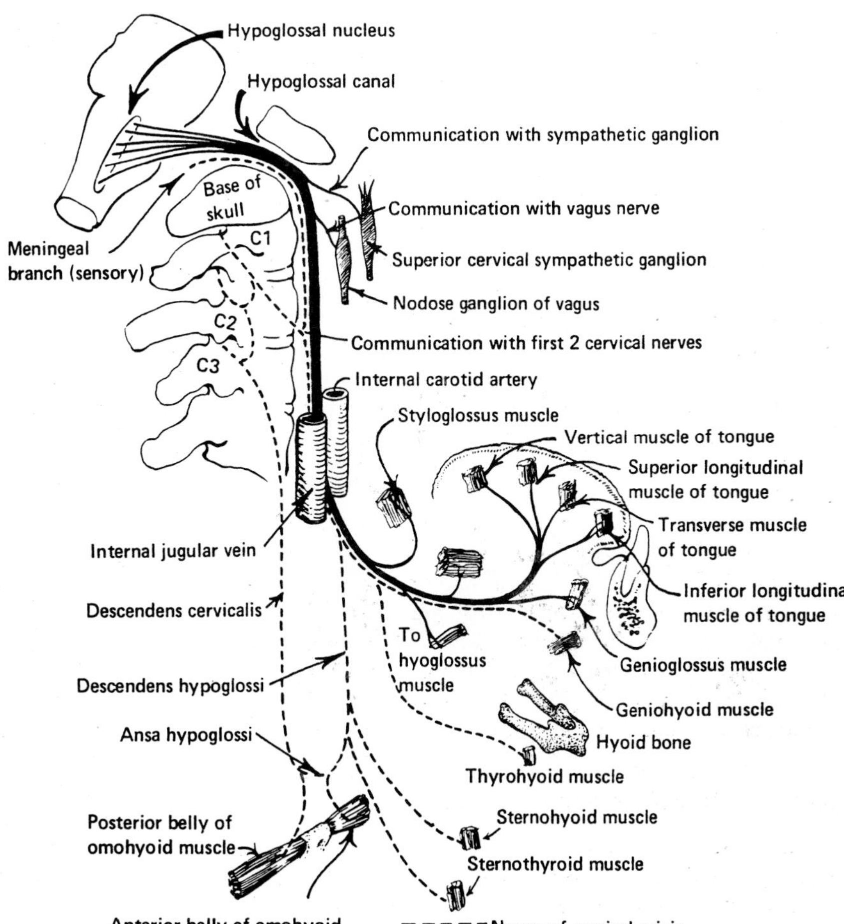

FIGURE 14–2. The origin and innervation of CN XII.

afferents, which travel by way of the genu of the internal capsule and the middle of the cerebral peduncle, are predominantly contralateral, although some are also ipsilateral.[10, 17] The supranuclear input for the genioglossus muscle may be strictly contralateral.[13, 26]

Examination of Cranial Nerves XI and XII

DIRECTED NEUROLOGICAL EXAMINATION

Cranial Nerve XI

The examination of CN XI consists of two parts: observation (at rest and during action) and palpation. Abnormal findings include atrophy; fasciculations; neck or shoulder deviation; and limitations in range, strength, or speed of motion.

Examiners should observe the neck and back while the patient is seated or standing, paying particular attention to the SCM muscle and the upper portion of the trapezius muscle. Atrophy or asymmetry should be noted. Fasciculations may be present with nuclear or lower motor neuron lesions. A unilateral paralysis of the SCM muscle causes little if any change in the position of the head while in the resting state. Bilateral paralysis may cause the neck to fall backward. Paralysis of the upper or middle portion of the trapezius muscle may alter the position of the scapula (Fig. 14–3). The upper part of the scapula may fall laterally away from the shoulder and vertebral column, and the interior part may be drawn inward.[9, 12]

The speed, strength, and range of motion should be assessed. The major action of the SCM muscle, through its sternal head, is to turn the head to the opposite side.[9, 28] Additionally, through its clavicular head, the SCM tilts the head to the ipsilateral side. To examine the right SCM muscle, the patient should turn the chin completely toward the left shoulder, and the examiner should attempt to overcome the movement. During this maneuver, it is important for the examiner to press against the patient's cheek rather than the mandible, because with the latter maneuver, one is testing not only the SCM but also the lateral pterygoid muscle (CN V) as well.[12] The SCM muscle is also involved in neck flexion, and when both SCM muscles act simultaneously, the result is to bring the head forward and downward. This movement may be tested by asking the patient to flex the neck while the examiner exerts firm pressure on the forehead.[12]

To assess the strength of the rostral portion of the trapezius muscle, the patient should elevate or shrug the shoulders and maintain this movement against resistance.[10] The rostral portion of the trapezius muscle also retracts the head and draws it to the ipsilateral side,[12] and this movement may be tested as well. The rostral and middle portions of the trapezius muscle normally stabilize the scapula, and a lesion of CN

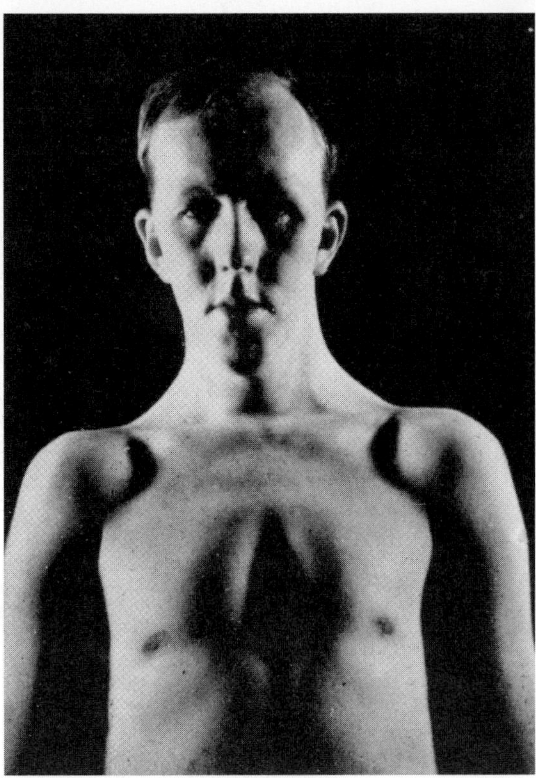

FIGURE 14–3. Bilateral atrophy of the sternocleidomastoid muscles.

XI may cause winging of this structure. This muscle action is tested by asking the patient to extend the arms forward and horizontally. CN XI lesions cause winging of the scapula, although to a milder degree than that seen with dysfunction of the serratus anterior muscle.[9]

The SCM and the trapezius muscles should be palpated for the presence of atrophy or hypertrophy. Proper palpation of the sternal head of the SCM muscle is aided by asking the patient to turn the head to the opposite side against resistance. When activated, the right SCM turns the chin to the left.[9, 20]

A unilateral hemispherical lesion does not usually cause marked deviation of the head, although some weakness may be present. In cortical or subcortical strokes, the head can deviate to the side of the lesion, away from the hemiparetic body, making rehabilitation efforts frustrating. Atrophy and fasciculations are not present in an upper motor neuron lesion.[12] Irritative cortical foci may result in seizures accompanied by forced deviation of the head to the contralateral side.[23] A unilateral supranuclear lesion in the upper brain stem may produce dissociated weakness, with ipsilateral weakness of the sternal head of the SCM and contralateral weakness of the trapezius.[12] Nuclear lesions of CN XI are rare. These lesions result in muscle weakness as well as atrophy and fasciculations. Unilateral nerve lesions produce weakness of the involved muscles as well as some deviation and possibly winging of the scapula. Bilateral nerve lesions result in diminished ability to rotate the neck, and the neck may fall either backward or forward, depending on whether the SCMs or trapezeii muscles are more involved. Because other cervical muscles such as the scaleni and splenii play a major role in neck deviation, flexion, and extension, a complete paralysis of neck muscles does not occur even with bilateral lesions of CN XI.[12]

Cranial Nerve XII

The examination of CN XII consists of three parts: observation, palpation, and percussion. The examiner should assess the tongue for atrophy; fasciculations; deviation; limitations in the range, strength, or speed of motion; and involuntary movements.

The tongue is observed as it rests in the mouth, with attention to atrophy, fasciculations, deviation, tremor, myoclonus, or chorea (see Chapter 34).[9] Atrophy, if present, may be particularly noticeable at the tip or borders of the tongue, resulting in a scalloped appearance with multiple small folds (Fig. 14–4).[10, 12] A fine rippling of the tongue due to incomplete relaxation should not be confused with fasciculations.[20] Even while the tongue is "resting" in the floor of the mouth, there is some activity of the styloglossus muscles. These muscles pull the tongue upward and backward. When there is a unilateral hypoglossal nerve lesion, the resting tongue may deviate slightly away from the side of the lesion because of unopposed action of the styloglossus muscles.[12]

The tongue should be observed during protrusion. The examiner should note atrophy, tremor, chorea, or deviation. The genioglossus muscle causes protrusion of the apex of the tongue. When there is a unilateral lesion of the hypoglossal nerve, the protruding tongue deviates toward the side of the lesion owing to the unopposed action of the normal genioglossus muscle.[9, 10] When there are complete bilateral nuclear or hypoglossal nerve lesions, the patient is unable to protrude the tongue at all. In general, when examining the protruding tongue for deviation, it is very important to choose appropriate landmarks.[9, 13] For example, if the lips are

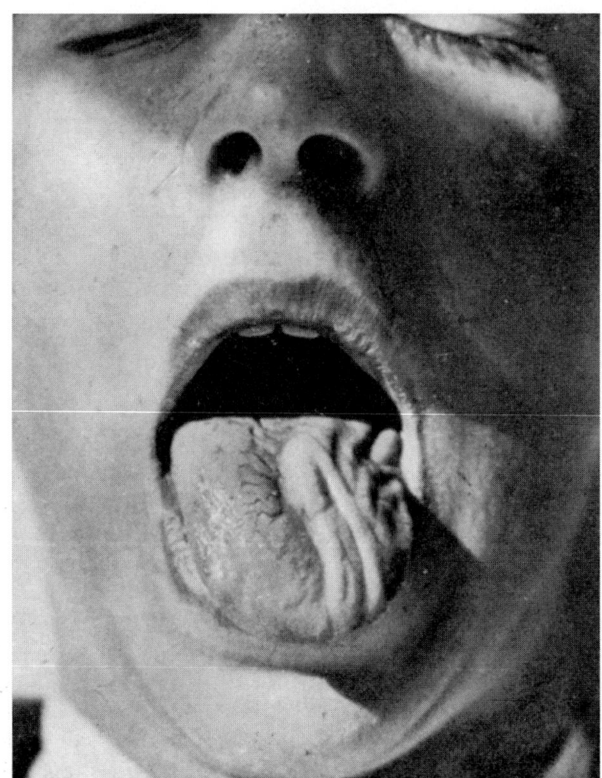

FIGURE 14–4. Lesion of the left hypoglossal nerve resulting in weakness and atrophy of the left half of the tongue.

used as a landmark, in the setting of unilateral facial weakness, the tongue may falsely appear to deviate toward the weak side. A more appropriate landmark in this and most other settings is the space between the two upper central incisors. This space should be aligned with the median raphe of the tongue.[9, 20]

The tongue is observed during movements other than protrusion. First, the speed and range of motion should be assessed by asking the patient to wiggle the tongue rapidly from side to side, and to point the tip upward and downward. Second, the strength of tongue motion should be assessed by asking the patient to press the tip of the tongue sideways against the inside of the cheek, while the examiner exerts opposing pressure by placing an index finger on the outer aspect of the cheek.[9] Third, speech, and particularly lingual sounds, should be assessed for the presence of dysarthria.

Palpation and percussion comprise the final aspects of the examination of the tongue. Palpation of the tongue between the examiner's thumb and index finger sometimes confirms the presence of atrophy.[10, 20] When a diagnosis of myotonia is being considered, the tongue should be tapped with a percussion hammer. A myotonic response is characterized by a contraction that is very slow to disappear.[9]

In a unilateral supranuclear lesion, the tongue may deviate toward the contralateral side; however, atrophy and fasciculations are not present. In a unilateral nuclear or hypoglossal nerve lesion, the tongue is atrophic on the ipsilateral side. On protrusion, it clearly deviates toward the side of the nuclear or nerve lesion.[10] In this setting, speech, swallowing, and respirations should be unaffected. If there are bilateral nuclear or nerve lesions, the tongue is diffusely atrophic, and the patient is unable to protrude the tongue at all. Additionally, articulation (especially lingual sounds) may be impaired, with slurred and indistinct speech. Swallowing and respiration may be impaired as the tongue falls back into the pharynx.[12] Fasciculations may be present either unilaterally or bilaterally in progressive disorders that involve the nucleus (e.g., amyotrophic lateral sclerosis or syringobulbia). Forced deviation of the tongue may be a manifestation of a seizure, and involuntary movements of the tongue may be a feature of myoclonus, or rarely Parkinson's disease (tremor), Huntington's disease (chorea), or tardive dyskinesia or tardive dystonia (oral-buccal-lingual movements).[12]

ASSOCIATED NEUROLOGICAL FINDINGS

Cerebral. With regard to CN XI or XII, bihemispherical lesions may result in significant weakness of the SCM, trapezeii, or extrinsic tongue muscles. Other features that confirm the presence of bihemispherical lesions are urinary incontinence, gait apraxia, pseudobulbar palsy (i.e., dysarthria, dysphagia, and emotional incontinence), cognitive deficits, and alterations in personality.

Cranial Nerves. Dysfunction of neck or tongue musculature may be the result of lesions in the brain stem affecting supranuclear, nuclear, or nerve fibers of CN XI or CN XII. Other features of a brain stem lesion are facial numbness (CN V), weakness of the palate (CN X), or autonomic dysfunction, indicating involvement of cranial nerve nuclei or sympathetic fibers in close proximity to the nuclei of CN XI or XII. Additionally, although supranuclear lesions may result in both head and eye deviation (due to connections between the accessory nucleus and the medial longitudinal fasciculus), a peripheral lesion of the spinal accessory nerve should not be accompanied by eye deviation.

Motor/Reflexes/Cerebellar/Gait. When examining a patient with a suspected lesion of CN XI or XII, it is important to perform a thorough motor examination. The examiner should note any primitive reflexes (e.g., suck, snout, glabellar) or paratonic rigidity (gegenhalten). These signs, along with pseudobulbar palsy, may be indicative of bilateral frontal lobe lesions. In addition, weakness in other ipsilateral muscles in the face, arm, or leg, accompanied by hypertonia, hyper-reflexia, or extensor plantar responses, is suggestive of an upper motor neuron lesion,[30] whereas weakness with atrophy, loss of reflexes, or fasciculations are signs of either a lower motor neuron lesion or neuronopathy. The supranuclear fibers for the sternal head of the SCM muscle probably decussate twice: once in the midbrain or pons and a second time in the medulla or cervical spinal cord.[23] Hence, a lesion in the right side of the pons may result in (1) left-sided weakness (involvement of corticospinal tract fibers before their decussation in the medulla) and (2) weakness of the left SCM muscle and deviation of the head to the left (i.e., the same side as the hemiparesis) because of involvement of the supranuclear input to the left SCM muscle after the first but before the second decussation. In contrast, a lesion in the right cerebral hemisphere or right internal capsule or high in the right midbrain, before the initial decussation of the supranuclear fibers to the SCM, may result in (1) left-sided weakness due to involvement of the corticospinal tract fibers before their decussation and (2) weakness of the right SCM muscle and deviation of the head to the right (i.e., the side opposite the hemiparesis).[13]

When dysfunction of CN XI or XII is present, it is also important to perform a thorough examination of coordination and gait. The presence of cerebellar signs ipsilateral to CN XI or XII deficits may be indicative of involvement of the inferior cerebellar peduncle, which is consistent with a lesion in the region of the medulla.

Sensory. The sensory examination is especially important in assessing brain stem dysfunction because of the distinctive pattern of findings seen only with damage to this structure. The nucleus ambiguus is situated just medial to the spinothalamic and trigeminothalamic tracts in the medulla. Contralateral loss of pain and temperature in the body and ipsilateral loss of pain and temperature in the face confirm a lesion in the medulla in the region of the nucleus ambiguus. The medial lemniscus is located in the medial medulla, ventral to the hypoglossal nucleus, and tongue weakness with simultaneous loss of position and vibratory sense implies a lesion in this area (i.e., Dejerine's syndrome or anterior spinal artery syndrome of the medulla).[8, 13]

Autonomic Nervous System. Lesions of the brain stem may sometimes involve autonomic pathways. An examination of the autonomic nervous system involves assessment of pulse rate, blood pressure in different positions (lying, seated, and standing), changes in skin color and texture, changes in hair and nails, decreased or excessive perspiration (e.g., anhidrosis in Horner's syndrome), and reflexes (e.g., pupillary, oculocardiac).

Neurovascular. Carotid dissection as well as brain stem stroke are etiologies of lower cranial nerve dysfunction, and the patency of the carotid artery may be preliminarily assessed at the bedside. Auscultation may reveal a bruit (i.e., partial occlusion). Palpation of the carotid pulse may reveal unilateral or even bilateral diminished pulsation, indicative of partial or complete occlusion of this blood vessel.

Evaluation Guidelines (Table 14–2)

The following tests may aid in the diagnosis of problems affecting cranial nerves XI and XII.

Neuroimaging. Various neuroimaging studies may be useful.[31–33] *Plain films of the skull* may provide diagnostic information in platybasia (flattening of the base of the skull so that the angle formed by an imaginary line connecting the anterior margin of the foramen magnum, the tuberculum sella, and the nasion is greater than 143 degrees), Paget's disease (areas of increased and decreased bone density, giving the bones a cotton-wool appearance), and basal skull fracture. *Head computed tomography* may be diagnostic in meningioma (homogeneous contrast-enhancing lesions with well-defined borders), acoustic neuroma (a well-defined uniformly enhancing tumor in the cerebellopontine angle, along with widening of the internal auditory canal), and skull fracture. *Head magnetic resonance imaging* is useful in the diagnosis of a multitude of lesions including syringobulbia (a syringobulbar cavity), multiple sclerosis (plaques), tuberculous or carcinomatous meningitis (meningeal enhancement), brain abscess (a thin rim of contrast enhancement that surrounds a central zone of low attenuation), medial medullary syndrome (infarction in the medial medulla), and metastatic cancer. *Doppler studies* or an *angiogram* may be useful with regard to the workup of the medial medullary syndrome resulting from vascular occlusion in the posterior circulation.

Electrophysiology. A number of electrophysiological studies may provide valuable diagnostic clues. *Electromyography* (EMG) with nerve conduction studies may be useful to diagnose Guillain-Barré syndrome (reduction in conduction velocity, slowing of F wave conduction velocity, nerve conduction block) and motor neuron disease (widespread fibrillations and positive sharp waves). *Evoked potentials* (visual, brain stem auditory, somatosensory) may be useful in the diagnosis of multiple sclerosis.

Cerebrospinal Fluid. Cerebrospinal fluid (CSF) analysis may aid in the diagnosis of lesions of CN XI and XII. Elevated CSF protein level is a feature of multiple sclerosis, neurosarcoidosis, tuberculous meningitis, and poliomyelitis. A low CSF glucose level may be present in tuberculous meningitis, carcinomatous meningitis, and neurosarcoidosis. CSF leukocytosis may be found in neurosarcoidosis and tuberculous meningitis. Albuminocytological dissociation (elevated CSF protein level in the relative absence of CSF leukocytosis) is a feature of Guillain-Barré syndrome. CSF oligoclonal bands are a feature of multiple sclerosis. Cytological examination of cellular material in the CSF may be diagnostic in carcinomatous meningitis. CSF cul-

TABLE 14–2. **Useful Studies in Evaluating Lesions of Cranial Nerves XI and XII**

Syndrome	Neuroimaging	Electrophysiology	Fluid and Tissue Analysis	Other Tests
Supranuclear lesions, unilateral or bilateral	Head MRI, CT	Evoked potentials	CSF	N/A
Supranuclear lesion in pons	Head MRI Head CT	Evoked potentials	CSF	N/A
Nuclear lesions	Head MRI	EMG/NCV	CSF	CBC, throat washings, stool or blood cultures (abscess, polio) Serum alkaline phosphatase Chest radiograph, PPD Serum angiotensin-converting enzyme, chest radiograph Serum VDRL
Lesion within the cranium or in the region of the foramen magnum	Plain skull film Head MRI Head CT	BAER, audiometry	CSF, lymph node biopsy	N/A
Lesions in the region of the jugular foramen	Head MRI Plain films of head, head CT	N/A	CSF	N/A
Lesions in the retroparotid or retropharyngeal spaces, and far distal peripheral nerve lesions	Neck MRI	N/A	N/A	N/A

MRI, Magnetic resonance imagery; CT, computed tomography; EMG/NCV, electromyogram/nerve conduction velocity; CSF, cerebrospinal fluid; CBC, complete blood count; BAER, brain stem auditory evoked response; PPD, purified protein derivative; VDRL, Venereal Disease Research Laboratory test; N/A, not applicable.

tures along with analysis of genetic material by polymerase chain reaction may be diagnostic in infections of the CSF. CSF pressure may be elevated in a number of processes including abscesses, neurosarcoidosis, and tuberculous meningitis.

Body Fluid and Tissue Analysis. Blood work may also be of diagnostic value (e.g., alkaline phosphatase levels in Paget's disease, angiotensin-converting enzyme levels in sarcoidosis, Venereal Disease Research Laboratory test in syphilis, viral cultures in poliomyelitis, genetic testing in neurofibromatosis). Purified protein derivative is helpful in diagnosing tuberculosis, as is lymph node biopsy in sarcoidosis.

Neuropsychological Tests. This technique has limited value in diagnosis of processes involving CN XI and XII.

Other Tests. Plain films of the chest are of diagnostic value in evaluating pulmonary disorders that extend beyond the pleura to involve CN XI, including tuberculosis, lung carcinoma, and pulmonary sarcoidosis.

Clinical Syndromes

SUPRANUCLEAR HEMISPHERICAL LESIONS
(Table 14–3)

The supranuclear input to CN XI and XII is not fully understood. Although input is thought to be bihemispheri-

TABLE 14–3. **Selected Etiologies Associated with Disorders of Cranial Nerve XI and Cranial Nerve XII**

Etiological Category	Specific Etiologies	Chapter
Structural Disorders		
Developmental	Platybasia (CN XII)	28
	Syringobulbia (CNs XI, XII)	
Degenerative and compressive	Paget's disease	29
Hereditary and Degenerative Disorders		
Chromosomal abnormalities and neurocutaneous disorders	Neurofibromatosis (CN XII)	32
Movement disorders	Dystonia (CNs XI, XII)	34
	Huntington's disease (CN XI)	
	Myoclonus (CN XII)	
Degenerative motor, sensory, and autonomic disorders	Amyotrophic lateral sclerosis (CNs XI, XII)	36
Acquired Metabolic and Nutritional Disorders		
Endogenous metabolic disorders	Paget's disease (CN XII)	38
Exogenous acquired metabolic disorders of the nervous system: Toxins and illicit drugs	Botulism (CN XII)	39
Infectious Disorders		
Viral infections	Acute poliomyelitis (CNs XI, XII)	41
Nonviral infections	Tubercular meningitis (CN XII)	42
	Neurosyphilis (CN XII)	
	Brain stem abscess (CN XII)	
Neurovascular Disorders	Medial medullary syndrome (CN XII)	45
	Dissecting carotid aneurysm (CN XII)	
	Cortical and subcortical vascular lesion (CN XI)	
	Lateral pontine lesion (CN XI)	
Neoplastic Disorders		
Primary neurological tumors	Glomus cell tumor (CN XII)	46
	Acoustic neuroma (CN XII)	
	Meningioma (posterior fossa) (CN XII)	
Metastatic neoplasms and paraneoplastic syndromes	Metastatic carcinoma (CN XII)	47
Demyelinating Disorders		
Demyelinating disorders of the central nervous system	Multiple sclerosis (CN XII)	48
Demyelinating disorders of the peripheral nervous system	Guillain-Barré syndrome (CN XII)	49
Autoimmune and Inflammatory Disorders	Neurosarcoidosis (CNs XI, XII)	50
Traumatic Disorders	Basal skull fracture (CNs XI, XII)	51
	Shoulder trauma (CN XI)	
	Gun shot wound (CN XII)	
	Stab wound (CN XII)	
	Dislocation of upper cervical vertebrae (CNs XI, XII)	
Epilepsy	Focal epilepsy (CN XI)	52
Drug-Induced and Iatrogenic Disorders	Neck irradiation (CNs XI, XII)	55
	Neck surgery (CNs XI, XII)	
	Medications (neuroleptics) (CNs XI, XII)	

cal in general, some muscles probably receive predominantly ipsilateral input (SCM), whereas others receive predominantly contralateral input (trapezius, genioglossus). A destructive unilateral supranuclear lesion (e.g., infarction, hemorrhage, tumor, multiple sclerosis, brain abscess) may result in some weakness of neck and tongue musculature so that the chin deviates toward the lesion. Atrophy and fasciculations are not present in an upper motor neuron lesion.[11, 12] An irritative unilateral supranuclear lesion (e.g., a seizure focus) may result in forced deviation of the head or tongue away from the lesion.[12]

PONTINE LESIONS

A unilateral lesion in the brain stem (e.g., stroke, multiple sclerosis, abscess, tumor) may produce dissociated weakness, with ipsilateral weakness of the SCM and contralateral weakness of the trapezius.[12] In addition, the supranuclear fibers for the SCM muscle probably decussate twice. A lesion in the right side of the pons may result in left-sided weakness (i.e., involvement of the corticospinal tract fibers before their decussation in the medulla) and possible deviation of the head to the left (i.e., involvement of supranuclear input to the left SCM muscle after the first but before the second decussation). Involvement of the paramedian pontine reticular formation may also result in deviation of the eyes toward the weakness.

NUCLEAR LESIONS AT THE LEVEL OF THE MEDULLA (CN XI AND XII) AND CERVICAL CORD (CN XI)

The nuclei of CN XI or XII may be involved in a number of disease processes including motor neuron disease, poliomyelitis, brain stem abscess, and syringobulbia.[34] In addition to muscle weakness, these lesions may result in atrophy and fasciculations. Bilateral involvement of these nuclei may result in diminished ability to rotate the neck, inability to protrude the tongue, slurred and indistinct speech, impaired swallowing, and possibly some respiratory difficulty. The medial medullary syndrome, which is caused by occlusion of the vertebral artery, results in paralysis and atrophy of the tongue on the side of the lesion (due to involvement of cranial nerve XII or its nucleus), weakness of the arm and leg on the side opposite the lesion (due to involvement of the pyramidal tracts before their decussation), and impaired tactile and proprioceptive sense of the side of the body opposite to the lesion (due to involvement of the medial lemniscus).[13, 35]

LESIONS WITHIN THE CRANIUM OR IN THE REGION OF THE *FORAMEN MAGNUM*

A large number of different pathological processes in this region may impinge on either cranial nerves XI or XII. Additionally, other cranial nerves in the posterior fossa may be involved (CN IX and X). Platybasia and Paget's disease, indirectly through their effects on the bony structures in this region, may impinge on these cranial nerves. Tumors, including glomus tumors, acoustic neuromas, meningiomas, and metastases to the skull base, may impinge on cranial nerves XI or XII. A number of infectious processes, including syphilis and tuberculosis,[36] may result in dysfunction of CN XI and XII. Combined dysfunction of CN IX through XII may result in neck and tongue weakness, depressed gag, palatal paresis, and vocal cord paralysis.

LESIONS WITHIN THE REGION OF THE *JUGULAR FORMAMEN*

These lesions may affect CN IX, X, and XI, which exit the skull through this foramen. The resultant syndrome, Vernet's syndrome, is characterized by the following features: ipsilateral loss of taste and depressed sensation over the posterior one third of the tongue, ipsilateral depressed gag reflex and palatal weakness, ipsilateral vocal cord paralysis, and ipsilateral weakness of the SCM and trapezius muscles.[11, 13, 37]

LESIONS IN THE RETROPAROTID OR RETROPHARYNGEAL SPACES AND DISTAL PERIPHERAL NERVE LESIONS

CN XI and XII may be affected by a number of distal peripheral nerve lesions resulting from surgical trauma,[38–44] local infections, stretch,[45, 46] neck irradiation,[47] or local tumors.[48–52] A dissecting carotid aneurysm may result in hypoglossal nerve palsy.[53] A self-limited idiopathic hypoglossal nerve palsy also has been reported.[54, 55] The resultant findings (i.e., weakness and atrophy) in peripheral nerve lesions have been described earlier. Occasionally, a lesion may affect CN IX through XII, with a resultant Collet-Sicard syndrome, characterized by the same features as Vernet's syndrome described earlier, with the addition of weakness of the ipsilateral tongue.[11, 13]

General Management Goals

Patients with dysfunction of either CN XI or CN XII may exhibit a number of problems with communication and swallowing, as well as difficulty resulting from weakness of the neck or trapezius muscle. Difficulty with swallowing may be amenable to swallowing therapy, including oral exercises and methods of postural facilitation. A soft mechanical diet with thickened liquids may decrease the likelihood of tracheal aspiration; however, a nasogastric tube or even a percutaneous gastrostomy device may be required.

Difficulty with articulation and communication may be amenable to speech therapy; however, augmentive and alternative communication devices may be required. Devices vary from the simple (e.g., boards with letters, words, or symbols) to the more complex (e.g., electronic communicators).

Weakness of the neck may be aided by a cervical orthotic device, and that, as well as weakness of the trapezius, may be aided by conventional physical therapy techniques such as range of motion and strengthening exercises, compensatory techniques, EMG feedback, and functional electrical stimulation.[56]

Reviews and Selected Updates

Ballotta E, DaGiau G, Renon L, et al: Cranial and cervical nerve injuries after carotid endarterectomy: A prospective study. Surgery 1999;125:85–91.

Brodal P: Cranial nerves: The hypoglossal nerve and the accessory nerve. In The Central Nervous System: Structure and Function, 2nd ed. New York, Oxford University Press, 1997, pp 451–453.

Keane JR: Twelfth-nerve palsy: Analysis of 100 cases. Arch Neurol 1996;53:561–567.

Sawczuk A, Mosier KM: Neural control of tongue movement with respect to respiration and swallowing. Crit Rev Oral Biol Med 2001;12:18–37.

Strauss WL, Howell AB: The spinal accessory nerve and its musculature. Q Rev Biol 1939;11:387.

Toyoda K, Imamura T, Saku Y, Oita J: Medial medullary infarction. Neurology 1996;47:1141–1147.

References

1. Rucker WC: History of the numbering of the cranial nerves. Mayo Clin Proc 1966;41:453–461.
2. Skinner HA: The Origin of Medical Terms. New York, Hafner Publishing, 1970.
3. Vesalius A: De Humani Corporis Fabrica Libri Septum. Basel, Ex oficina I. Oporini, 1543.
4. Willis T: Cerebri Anatome; Cui Accessit Nervorum Descriptio Et Usus, Studio Thomae Willis. Amstelodami, Casparum Commelinum, 1664.
5. Schmidt JE: Medical Discoveries. Who and When. Springfield IL, Charles C Thomas, 1959.
6. Martin JH: Neuroanatomy: Text and Atlas, 1st ed. New York, Elsevier, 1989.
7. Bremmer-Smith AT, Unwin AJ, Williams WW: Sensory pathways in the spinal accessory nerve. J Bone Joint Surg 1999;81:226–228.
8. Carpenter M: Core Text of Neuroanatomy, 4th ed. Baltimore, Williams & Wilkins, 1991.
9. Monrad-Krohn GH: The Clinical Examination of the Nervous System, 10th ed. New York, Paul B. Hoeber, 1955.
10. Mayo Clinic and Mayo Foundation: Clinical Examinations in Neurology, 5th ed. Philadelphia, WB Saunders, 1981.
11. Chusid JG: Correlative Neuroanatomy & Functional Neurology, 19th ed. Los Altos, CA, Lange Medical Publishers, 1985.
12. Haerer AF: DeJong's The Neurological Examination, 5th ed. Philadelphia, JB Lippincott, 1992.
13. Brazis PW, Masdeu JC, Biller H: Localization in Clinical Neurology, 2nd ed. Boston, Little, Brown, 1990.
14. Combarros O, Alvarez de Arcaya A, Berciano J: Isolated unilateral hypoglossal nerve palsy: Nine cases. J Neurol 1998;245:98–100.
15. Giuffrida S, Lo Bartolo ML, Nicoletti A, et al: Isolated, unilateral, reversible palsy of the hypoglossal nerve. Eur J Neurol 2000;7:347–349.
16. Skorzewska A, Bruska M, Wozniak W: The development of the spinal accessory nerve in human embryos during the 5th week (stages 14 and 15). Folia Morphol 1994;53:177–184.
17. Barr ML, Kiernan JA: The Human Nervous System: An Anatomical Viewpoint, 4th ed. Philadelphia, Harper & Row, 1983.
18. Gray H: Gray's Anatomy, 37th ed. New York, Churchill Livingstone, 1989.
19. Kierner AC, Zelenka I, Burian M: How do the cervical plexus and the spinal accessory nerve contribute to the innervation of the trapezius muscle? As seen from within using Sihler's stain. Arch Otolaryngo 2001;127:1230–1232.
20. DeMyer W: Technique of the Neurological Examination: A Programmed Text, 3rd ed. New York, McGraw-Hill, 1980.
21. DeToledo JC, Dow R: Sternomastoid function during hemispheric suppression by amytal: Insights into the inputs to the spinal accessory nerve nucleus. Mov Disord 1998;13:809–812.
22. Bender MB, Shanzer S, Wagman IH: On the physiologic decussation concerned with head turning. Confin Neurol 1964;24:169–181.
23. Geschwind N: Nature of the decussated innervation of the sternocleidomastoid muscle. Ann Neurol 1981;10:495.
24. Iannone AM, Gerber AM: Brown-Séquard syndrome with paralysis of head turning. Ann Neurol 1982;12:116.
25. Mastaglia FL, Knezevic W, Thompson PD: Weakness of head turning in hemiplegia: A quantitative study. J Neurol Neurosurg Psychiatry 1986;49:195–197.
26. Kuypers HGJM: Corticobulbar connections to the pons and lower brainstem in man: An anatomical study. Brain 1958;81:364–388.
27. Manion-Espaillat R, Ruff RL: Dissociated weakness of sternocleidomastoid and trapezius muscles with lesions in the CNS. Neurology 1988;38:796–797.
28. DeToledo J, Smith DB, Kramer RE, et al: Cortical innervation of the sternocleidomastoid in humans. Clinical and neurophysiological observations. Ann Neurol 1989;26:171.
29. Muellbacher W, Mamoli B: The course of the cortico-hypoglossal projections in the human brainstem: Functional testing using transcortical magnetic stimulation. Brain 1997;120:1909–1910.
30. Louis ED, King D, Sacco RL, et al: Upper motor neuron signs in acute stroke: Prevalence, interobserver reliability, and timing of initial examination. J Stroke Cerebrovasc Dis 1995;5:49–55.
31. Orbay T, Aykol S, Seckin Z, et al: Late hypoglossal nerve palsy following fracture of the occipital condyle. Surg Neurol 1989;31:402–404.
32. Yock DH: Imaging of CNS Disease, 2nd ed. St Louis, Mosby–YearBook, 1991.
33. Thompson EO, Smoker WR: Hypoglossal nerve palsy: A segmental approach. Radiographics 1994;14:939–958.
34. Atsumi T, Miyatake T: Morphometry of the degenerative process in the hypoglossal nerves in amyotrophic lateral sclerosis. Acta Neuropathol 1987;73:25–31.
35. Gan R, Noronha A: The medullary vascular syndromes revisited. J Neurol 1995;242:195–202.
36. Richards IM, White AM, O'Sullivan MM, et al: Unilateral palsy of the hypoglossal nerve in a patient with tuberculosis of the first cervical vertebra. J Rheumatol 1989;28:540–542.
37. Schweinfurth JM, Johnson JT, Weissman J: Jugular foramen syndrome as a complication of metastatic melanoma. Am J Otolaryngol 1993;14:168–174.
38. Morrell S, Roberson JR, Rooks MD: Accessory nerve palsy following thoracotomy. Clin Orthop 1989;238:237–240.
39. Marini SG, Rook JL, Green RF, et al: Spinal accessory nerve palsy: An unusual complication of coronary bypass. Arch Phys Med Rehabil 1991;72:247–249.
40. Sweeney PJ, Wilbourn AJ: Spinal accessory (11th) nerve palsy following carotid endarterectomy. Neurology 1992;42:674–675.
41. Davidson BJ, Kulkarny V, Delacure MD, et al: Posterior triangle metastases of squamous cell carcinoma of the upper aerodigestive tract. Am J Surg 1993;166:395–398.
42. Donner TR, Kline DG: Extracranial spinal accessory nerve injury. Neurosurgery 1993;32:907–910.
43. Nagai K, Sakuramoto C, Goto F: Unilateral hypoglossal nerve paralysis following the use of the laryngeal mask airway. Anaesthesia 1994;49:603–604.
44. Blackwell KE, Landman MD, Calcaterra TC: Spinal accessory nerve palsy: An unusual complication of rhytidectomy. Head Neck 1994;16:181–185.
45. Dellon AL, Campbell JN, Cornblath D: Stretch palsy of the spinal accessory nerve. Case report. J Neurosurg 1990;72:500–502.
46. Logigian EL, McInnes JM, Berger AR, et al: Stretch-induced spinal accessory nerve palsy. Muscle Nerve 1988;11:146–150.
47. Johnston EF, Hammond AJ, Cairncross JG: Bilateral hypoglossal palsies: A late complication of curative radiotherapy. Can J Neurol Sci 1989;16:198–199.
48. Chang KC, Huang JS, Liu KN, et al: Neurinoma of the spinal accessory nerve: Report of a case. J Formos Med Assoc 1990;89:593–597.
49. Sanghvi VD, Chandawarkar RY: Carotid body tumors. J Surg Oncol 1993;54:190–192.
50. Singh B, Shaha AR: Solitary malignant schwannoma invading the hypoglossal nerve. Ear Nose Throat J 1994;73:842–844, 847–849.
51. Okura A, Shigemori M, Abe T, et al: Hemiatrophy of the tongue due to hypoglossal schwannoma shown by MRI. Neuroradiology 1994;36:239–240.
52. Ortiz O, Reed L: Spinal accessory nerve schwannoma involving the jugular foramen. Am J Neuroradiol 1995;16:986–989.
53. Koch J, Klotz JM, Kahle G, et al: Unilateral caudal cranial nerve paralysis in extracranial carotid dissection [German]. Fortschr Neurol Psychiatry 1994;62:46–49.
54. Sugama S, Matsunaga T, Ito F, et al: Transient, unilateral, isolated hypoglossal nerve palsy. No To Hattatsu 1992;14:122–123.
55. Lee SS, Wang SJ, Fuh JL, et al: Transient unilateral hypoglossal nerve palsy: A case report. Clin Neurol Neurosurg 1994;96:148–151.
56. Laska T, Hannig K: Physical therapy for spinal accessory nerve injury complicated by adhesive capsulitis. Phys Ther 2001;81:936–944.

CHAPTER 15

JOHN P. HAMMERSTAD

Strength and Reflexes

History and Definitions

Recognition that paralysis resulted from injuries to the nervous system was described in the Hippocratic writings, but it was the work of three men—Galen of Pergamon (130–200 AD), Andreas Vesalius (1514–1564), and Thomas Willis (1621–1675)—that established the foundation of our current knowledge of the functional anatomy of weakness.[1] Galen, who was also physician to the Roman emperor Marcus Aurelius, was the first experimental physiologist. His vivisection studies on the brain established that cutting into the brain produced paralysis, but he gave undue attention to the ventricles as the source of the weakness rather than the substance of the hemispheres. Galen's experiments on the spinal cord were more definitive; he showed different levels of paralysis by sectioning different regions of the cord, including hemisections that caused paralysis on the same side of the body. Little more was added to our knowledge of the nervous system until the Renaissance anatomist Vesalius refined Galen's anatomical observations of the central nervous system and corrected Galen's misconceptions about the function of muscles and the anatomy of nerves. Galen thought that muscles were mere protective flesh for the tendons, which produced movement when excited by the animal spirits flowing from the ventricle through hollow nerves. Vesalius recognized that Galen's "flesh" was the "particular organ of motion and not merely the stuffing and support of the fibers." He also recognized that nerves were solid, not hollow, and when ligated, produced paralysis according to which nerve was divided.

The English physician Thomas Willis recognized that weakness could result from lesions at all levels of the nervous system and that the distribution of the paralysis was determined by the site of the lesion. Charles Bell (1774–1842) and Brown-Séquard (1817–1894) further refined our understanding of the functional anatomy of paralysis, and Robert Bentley Todd (1809–1860) described epileptic hemiplegia. In more modern times, John Hughlings Jackson contributed the concept of the hierarchical nature of the motor system, and Wilder Penfield refined the localization of motor function in the motor cortex by defining the now familiar motor homunculus by direct stimulation of the cortex in patients undergoing surgery for epilepsy.

Willis and Descartes introduced the notion of reflexes and reflex action, but until the latter half of the 19th century, tendon jerks and cutaneous reflexes were not appreciated as valuable aids in localizing lesions and diagnosing diseases of the nervous system. In his paper of 1875, Erb was the first to describe systematically the tendon reflexes and their exaggeration in patients with hemiplegia and paraplegia, although he acknowledged that his observations were not new to his neurological colleagues. Erb also described ankle clonus. A few years later, William Gowers noted that knee jerks were diminished or lost in diseases of the nerve roots or the muscle itself. Although the cutaneous flexor withdrawal reflex had already been described, Babinski pointed out in 1876 the diagnostic importance of the extensor response of the great toe when the sole of the foot is scratched. A few years later, the brilliant English experimental neurophysiologist, Sir Charles Sherrington, defined the nature of reflex arcs and the importance of reciprocal inhibition in his landmark book, *The Integrative Action of the Nervous System.*[2] Other late 19th century neurologists also contributed important observations to help localize and diagnose diseases causing weakness. Charcot described the atrophy and fasciculations of muscle in amyotrophic lateral sclerosis, and Duchenne described the features of muscular dystrophy, including pseudohypertrophy.

Degrees and location of muscular weakness and changes in muscle tone are described by more or less precise terms. Paralysis refers to a complete loss of voluntary movement, whereas paresis is a reduced but not complete abolition of voluntary movement. Palsy is an older term that has been used interchangeably with either paralysis or paresis; currently, its use is confined to historical diagnoses that have been retained in conventional use such as Bell's palsy and cerebral palsy. The distribution of the paralysis or paresis is modified by the prefixes mono (for involvement of one limb), para (for involvement of both legs), hemi (for the limbs on one side of the body), and quadra or tetra (for all four limbs). A brachial paresis (or paralysis) refers to a monoparesis of an arm, and crural refers to involvement of one leg.

Changes in muscle tone that are elicited by passive movements of the limbs are described by the following terms. *Flaccidity* is the absence of normal muscle tone, while *spasticity* and *rigidity* are abnormal increases in muscle tone. Spasticity differs from rigidity in that it selectively increases the tone in the flexor muscles of the arm and the extensors of the leg, whereas rigidity affects flexors and extensors equally. The *gegenhalten* (German "hold against") phenomenon is felt as an increase in tone but is the result of resistance with an equal and opposite force by the patient to the examiner's attempt to move the limb passively.

The terms *lower motor neuron* and *upper motor neuron* are often used to differentiate two basic types of weakness: the first, due to a lesion of the motor neuron in the anterior spinal gray matter and its axon coursing to the muscle through the spinal roots and peripheral nerves and the second, due to a lesion that interrupts the descending motor pathways from supraspinal neurons that converge on the lower motor neuron pool. These very useful terms in clinical neurology derive from the concept that pools of upper motor neurons exist in a hierarchical order in the brain stem and motor cortex and converge via several different pathways on the lower motor neuron pool consisting of alpha and gamma motor neurons.

The *neuromuscular junction* is the specialized anatomical connection between the motor nerve endings and the skeletal muscle. The muscles that convert the electrical impulse into the force that produces movement is striated muscle, which is often referred to as skeletal muscle; this muscle type contrasts with smooth muscle, which responds to activation of the autonomic nervous system.

The term *fatigability* is used in a general sense to describe the feeling of being tired and not being able to put out full effort. It is also used more precisely to define a change in force-generating capacity of the neuromuscular apparatus brought about by muscular activity. Normal fatigue results from intense muscular contraction. When one or more muscles used in a specific task become weaker and weaker with repetitive but normal use, the phenomenon is referred to as fatigability and implies dysfunction at the neuromuscular junction.

Finally, *weakness* should be differentiated from *dyspraxia* (see Chapter 4). Weakness is an inability to carry out a desired movement with normal force because of a reduction in strength of the muscles necessary to carry out the movement. In dyspraxia, strength is normal, and the inability to perform a movement results from a failure in the motor centers in the cortex that plan and provide the proper commands to execute the movement.

Clinical History

For disorders of strength, as for other disorders of the nervous system, the clinical history is primarily important in defining the location and cause of the disorder. The onset (sudden or insidious), rate of progression (gradual or rapid), and temporal profile (intermittent, step-wise, or stable and chronic) help narrow the diagnostic possibilities. Precipitating elements associated with onset of the disorder, such as trauma, exposure to toxins, recent infections, or travel, provide important clues. Because the molecular and genetic natures of more and more neurological disorders are being defined, it is most important to take a careful family history. Other medical illnesses and the medications taken for them may be important determinants of the cause. Lifestyle and habits, and drugs, both prescribed and illicit, including alcohol, vitamins, and special diets, are potential causes of weakness. Other neurological illnesses or features may also help in localizing the lesion and defining the cause of the weakness. For example, dementia or a speech and language disorder may localize the problem to the cortex; the distribution of numbness, pain, and other sensory symptoms helps to localize the lesion causing weakness. The phenomenon of fatigability typifies a lesion of the neuromuscular junction.

Anatomy of Strength and Reflexes

OVERVIEW OF VOLUNTARY MOTOR FUNCTION

The motor systems are responsible for initiating and coordinating all movements that are part of the normal and abnormal behavioral repertoires. The motor systems generate three general types of movements. *Reflex responses* are rapid, stereotyped involuntary movements elicited by a stimulus that requires a quick reaction at an involuntary level—for example, withdrawal of a bare foot that has touched a sharp or hot object. *Rhythmical movements* such as walking and running require a stereotyped sequence of muscle activation (see Chapter 18). *Voluntary movements* are the most complex.

They are goal-directed and initially require conscious direction. Through practice, skilled movements such as playing a piano become more automatic and require less conscious direction.

The three types of movements correlate with the overall organization of the motor system, which is *hierarchical* and contains three major components: local reflex networks in the spinal cord; motor integration areas of the brain stem; and motor integration areas of the cerebral cortex. The spinal cord contains the circuitry for the reflex responses and some rhythmical motor patterns, whereas the brain stem system contains circuits for more complex patterns of motor movements including rhythm generators. The cortex is the command center that plans and initiates movements and uses the reflex and patterned responses of the brain stem and spinal cord to generate the details of the movement.[3]

The motor systems do not function in isolation and require a constant flow of sensory information to produce the appropriate movement. The sensory system is also organized in a hierarchical fashion and provides appropriate sensory information to each level of the motor system. In addition to these three hierarchical levels, two other parts of the motor system regulate movement, the cerebellum (see Chapter 17) and the basal ganglia (see Chapter 16). The cerebellum improves the coordination and accuracy of movement by comparing sensory feedback from the periphery with the descending motor commands, and the basal ganglia receive inputs from both motor and sensory cortical regions and project principally to areas of the frontal cortex that are involved in motor planning.

In addition to this hierarchical organization, many pathways operate in *parallel* and can act independently to control motor output. Thus, higher centers can adjust the operation of different spinal circuits independently to produce combinations of movements required for complex tasks. For example, postural reflexes residing in the brain stem maintain the ballet dancer's body position and balance while the cortex initiates a reaching movement of the arms.

Ultimately, all of these descending hierarchical and parallel pathways converge on a set of motor neurons in the spinal cord that give rise to the motor nerves that innervate skeletal muscle and produce movement. These are the *lower motor neurons* of the ventral gray matter of the spinal cord. Sometimes they are referred to as the final common pathway. In contrast, the motor neurons that generate voluntary, rhythmical, and reflex responses are the *upper motor neurons*. Most of the control signals coming from the upper motor neuron do not act directly on the lower motor neuron but use networks of interposed neurons known as *interneurons*, or the internuncial pool of neurons. These neurons are very important in integrating the reflex and rhythmical patterns of movement. The final effector of movement, skeletal muscle, responds in two modes, tonic and phasic contractions. For example, muscles involved in posture contract tonically, whereas those involved in voluntary limb movements contract in a phasic pull and push of joints. Phasic movements require coordinated contractions of agonists and antagonists. In the sections that follow, these elements of the motor system are discussed in more detail, starting with the muscle and the neuromuscular junction and then proceeding with the lowest level of hierarchical organization, the spinal cord, and progressing through the brain stem to the cortex. The parallel processing of motor control is discussed for each of these levels.

MUSCLE

Skeletal muscle is the effector of all motor commands from the CNS. The degree of movement, or force, depends on the magnitude of neural excitation of skeletal muscle. Striated muscle is composed of bundles of *myofibers*, which are the multinucleated cells of muscle. Muscles are composed of two types of myofibers that are distinguished by their energy metabolism. *Type I* fibers correspond to the slow-contracting fibers that rely primarily on aerobic oxidative metabolism and are involved in more sustained contractions such as maintenance of posture. *Type IIA* fibers are fast-contracting but are also capable of sustained activity. These fibers are both aerobic and anaerobic; although oxidative enzymes are present, their activity is slightly less than that of type I fibers. *Type IIB* fibers are characterized by anaerobic or glycolytic metabolism and correspond to the fast-contracting fibers that are recruited for short periods of vigorous exercise.[4] The differences in the predominant metabolic enzymes used by these two types of muscle fibers can be readily seen by histochemical stains specific for the enzymes of either type.

Each myofiber contains many bundles of slender filaments called *myofibrils* (Fig. 15–1). Under the electron microscope, myofibrils are seen to contain dark bands alternating with light bands bisected by a narrow dark line called the Z line, which gives a regular striated appearance to the muscle. The segment from one Z line to another is called a *sarcomere*; this is the unit of contraction because it contains the contractile proteins responsible for transforming chemical energy into mechanical force. Each sarcomere consists of thick filaments, primarily composed of the protein *myosin*, and thin filaments, which contain *actin*. Actin interacts with myosin to produce contraction of the muscle. The thin filaments also contain regulatory proteins including tropomyosin and troponin.[5]

Two other ultrastructural elements are important in the process of contraction[4] (Fig. 15–2). The *transverse tubule* (T-tubule) is a specialized invagination of the plasma membrane of the myofiber, the sarcolemma. The T-tubule is responsible for propagation of the action potential into the interior of the myofiber in response to depolarization of the sarcolemma. The other important structure involved in contraction is the *sarcoplasmic reticulum*, which is a set of tubules and cisterns surrounding the myofibrils. The sarcoplasmic reticulum stores calcium, which is released or taken up again in the process of *excitation-contraction coupling* and relaxation. In response to neurally initiated depolarization of the sarcolemma, calcium is released from the sarcoplasmic reticulum. The sudden increase in calcium concentration changes the conformation of the regulatory proteins on the thin filament, allowing interaction between myosin and actin to form cross-bridges and contraction. Contraction is terminated by the reuptake of calcium into the sarcoplasmic reticulum. This active transport of calcium requires energy. If energy is not available to reduce the calcium accumulation in sarcoplasm, the actin and myosin cross-bridges persist and relaxation does not occur. When this occurs after death, it is known as rigor mortis.

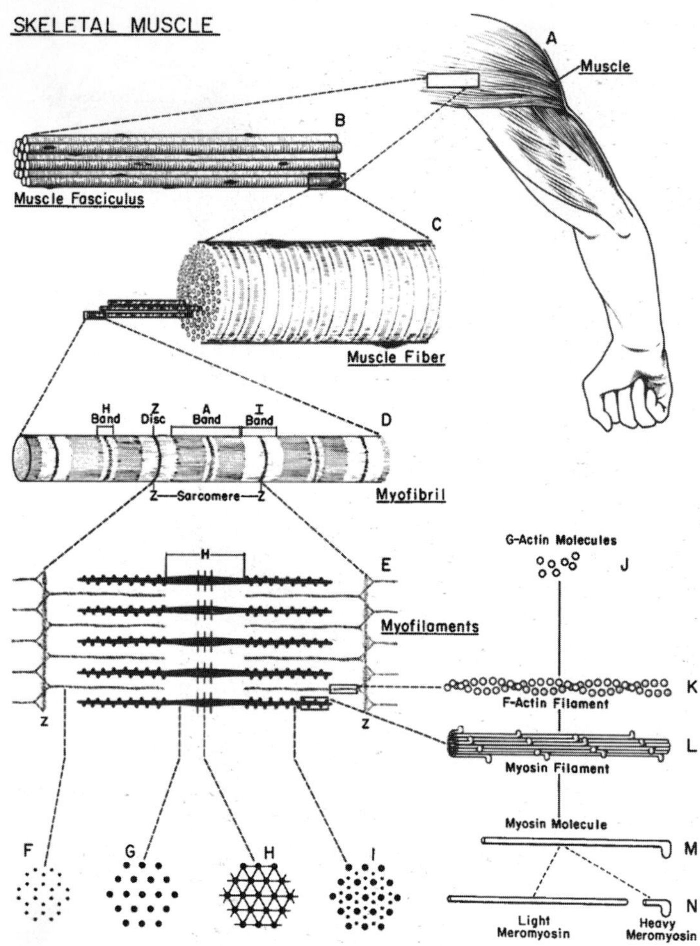

FIGURE 15–1. Histological and molecular structure of skeletal muscle. E represents a longitudinal section of a sarcomere showing the arrangement of the myofilaments actin (thin filaments) and myosin with projecting bridges (thick filaments). F, G, H, and I are cross sections through the sarcomere showing the arrangements of the thin and thick filaments at the sites indicated. (From Bloom W, Fawcett DW: A Textbook of Histology. Philadelphia, WB Saunders, 1968.)

A variety of metabolic disorders of muscle are possible if defects occur at any step in this orderly sequence of excitation-contraction coupling and relaxation. Disturbances in sodium channels in the sarcolemma membrane result in episodic weakness, giving rise to the disorder known as *periodic paralysis* (see Chapter 37). Muscle weakness can result from a shortage of fuel when defective glycolytic enzymes cannot convert glycogen to glucose (*glycogen storage diseases*) or when the machinery that converts glucose to energy is defective (*mitochondrial disorders*) (see Chapter 31). Defects in the uptake of calcium into the sarcoplasmic reticulum disrupt relaxation and also result in weakness (*myotonia, myotonic dystrophy*) (see Chapter 36).

All of these defects in the contraction and relaxation of muscle are genetic in origin. Recently, work in molecular genetics has shown that the muscular dystrophies, in particular *Duchenne's and Becker's dystrophies*, result from a defective gene that codes for a major structural protein in the sarcolemmal membrane known as *dystrophin* (see Chapter 36).[6] Immunohistochemical studies show that dystrophin is completely absent in Duchenne's dystrophy, whereas in Becker's dystrophy, the dystrophin protein is either smaller than normal or is present in low levels.

NEUROMUSCULAR JUNCTION

The transfer of information from the axon potentials of motor nerves to the muscle occurs at a specialized synapse, the neuromuscular junction. After entering muscle, the axon of a motor neuron divides into many thin branches or twigs. Each of these twigs makes contact with only one myofiber, approximately midway between its ends. At this motor endplate, the axonal twig divides further and forms a complex of approximately 50 boutons, each making synaptic contact with the muscle cell. The lower motor neuron uses *acetylcholine* as its chemical transmitter. When an action potential from the lower motor neuron reaches the neuromuscular junction, normally enough acetylcholine is released to produce a suprathreshold *excitatory endplate potential*, which produces a propagated *muscle action potential* and a twitch in the fiber innervated by that alpha motor neuron. This involves two major events, presynaptic release of the acetylcholine and interaction with the postsynaptic receptor.

In the presynaptic terminal, acetylcholine is synthesized from acetyl CoA and choline and is catalyzed by *choline acetyltransferase*. The acetylcholine is packaged in synaptic vesicles and is released into the synaptic cleft after a nerve action potential arrives by a process that requires calcium and is called *stimulus-secretion coupling*. The entry of calcium in the presynaptic terminal through voltage-gated channels triggers the fusion of the synaptic vesicles with the presynaptic cell membrane.[7] This fusion of the vesicular and plasma membrane opens the vesicle to the synaptic cleft, releasing its contents in a process known as *exocytosis*. Synapsin I, a phosphoprotein localized in vesicles, may

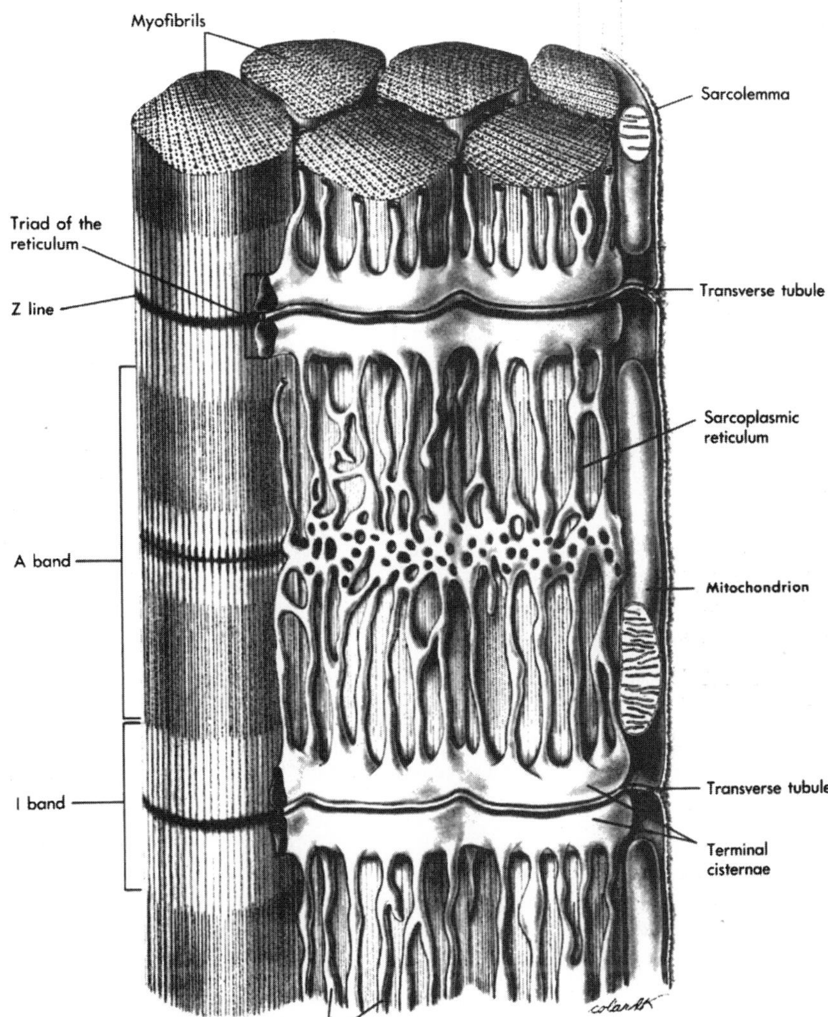

FIGURE 15–2. The transverse tubule system, showing the relationship of the sarcoplasmic reticulum and transverse tubular system to the myofibrils. (From Bloom W, Fawcett DW: A Textbook of Histology. Philadelphia, WB Saunders, 1970.)

mediate translocation of vesicles to the membrane. The subsequent steps involve a complex of proteins collectively referred to as SNARE proteins.[8] The clostridial neurotoxins, *botulinum toxin* and *tetanus toxin*, inhibit exocytosis by acting as proteases to cleave specific SNARE proteins at different sites, depending on the toxin and its serotype. There are seven botulinum toxin serotypes, two of which, types A and B, are used clinically to take advantage of their ability to inhibit release of acetylcholine at the neuromuscular junction to relieve muscle spasms in dystonia, spasticity, and related disorders. After acetylcholine has been released, the presynaptic membrane is pinocytotically recaptured, and the vesicles are remade and repleted with acetylcholine.[9] The acetylcholine binds to a receptor on the postsynaptic membrane. If sufficient acetylcholine is released, the postsynaptic membrane is depolarized, resulting in the *endplate potential*. The probability that an interaction will occur between the released acetylcholine and its receptor on the postsynaptic membrane is increased by concentration of the *cholinergic receptors* along postjunctional folds at the neuromuscular junction. The cholinergic receptor is of the *nicotinic type*. The action of acetylcholine is terminated by *acetylcholine esterase*, which catabolizes it into its two constituents, and the choline is recaptured for reuse by low-affinity transport in the nerve terminal.

LOWER MOTOR NEURON POOL

Contraction of skeletal muscle can occur only when a nervous impulse is conducted down the axons of the motor neuron. The motor neurons lie in the ventral horn of the spinal cord and are known as *lower motor neurons*. There are two types of motor neurons that provide a parallel system of innervation of the muscle. The larger *alpha motor neurons* innervate the extrafusal muscle fibers, and the smaller *gamma motor neurons* innervate the intrafusal muscle fibers of the *muscle spindle* (Fig. 15–3). The axons of the motor neurons leave the spinal cord through the ventral roots and continue into the ventral and dorsal branches (rami) of the spinal nerves. The dorsal rami innervate the paravertebral muscles of the neck and trunk, and the ventral rami innervate the rest of the trunk and the extremities. In the brain stem, the motor neurons in the cranial nerve motor nuclei send axons to innervate the muscles of the tongue, pharynx, larynx, palate, face, and extraocular muscles. Because signals to skeletal muscle from any part of the motor system rely on activation of the lower motor neuron pool, Sir Charles Sherrington coined the term *final common pathway* to describe the function of the lower motor neurons. The activation of different numbers and combinations of alpha motor neurons by other motor centers determines the force and

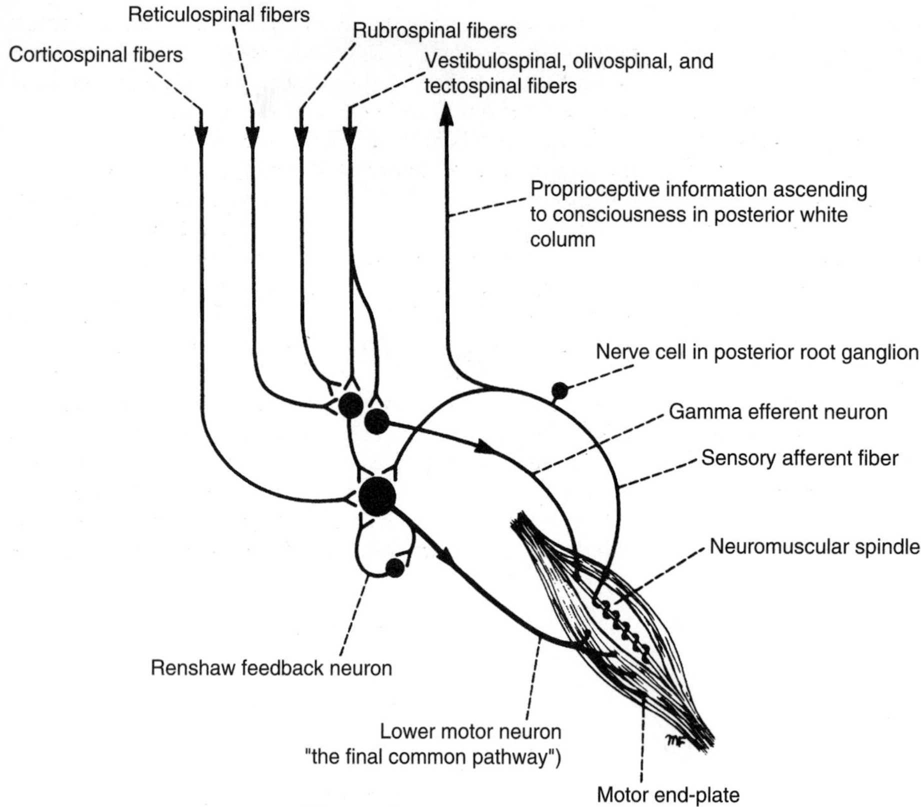

FIGURE 15–3. The parallel organization of the alpha and gamma lower motor neurons (black cell bodies). The alpha motor neurons innervate extrafusal skeletal muscle; the gamma motor neuron innervates the intrafusal muscle fibers to ensure proper sensory feedback from the muscle spindle. The activity of both motor neurons is modulated by multiple segmental and suprasegmental inputs. (From Snell RS: Clinical Neuroanatomy for Medical Students. Boston, Little, Brown & Co., Inc., 1987.)

speed of the resulting movement. The accuracy of a movement depends on sensory feedback. The parallel gamma motor neuron system provides a way for the motor system to ensure the accuracy of the sensory information it is receiving.

Alpha Motor Neuron

Nerve impulses generated by the alpha motor neuron cause contraction of extrafusal muscle fibers, resulting in the generation of force and movement. The axon of the alpha motor neuron divides into numerous branches when it enters the muscle, and each terminal branch makes synaptic contact with one muscle cell. The number of terminal branches and muscle cells innervated by an individual alpha motor neuron may vary greatly but generally corresponds to the size of the motor neuron. An alpha motor neuron and all the muscle cells innervated by it are called a *motor unit*, another term introduced by Sherrington. Therefore, all muscle cells innervated by that alpha motor neuron contract simultaneously when an *action potential* is generated by that motor neuron. The size of a motor unit may range from as few as 10 muscle cells innervated by one motor neuron to more than 1000. The smallest motor units are found in muscles that are used for delicate precise movements such as the extraocular muscles, the larynx, and the intrinsic muscles of the hand. The largest motor units are found in large powerful muscles involved in more forceful movements that require less precise control like the back and thigh muscles.[3]

The myofibers belonging to the same motor unit may be scattered throughout the muscle, but they are all of the same fiber type. Therefore, all of the myofibers in a given motor unit have the same characteristics with regard to maximal force, velocity of contraction, and endurance. Also, there is a correlation between the size of the motor units and the fiber type. The smallest motor units consist of type I fibers, whereas the largest ones consist of type IIB fibers.

The difference in fiber types amplifies the difference in the maximal force that can be generated by the large and small motor units. Therefore, in the largest motor units, where type II fibers predominate, not only are there more myofibers, but each one can also generate more force. Smaller motor units made up of type I fibers are found in muscles used for finely graded changes of force needed for more precise control.

The force of a muscle contraction can be increased in a graded manner by two means. One is a gradual increase in the number of alpha motor neurons activated, which results in the *recruitment* of more and more motor units and thus more myofibers. When a muscle contraction is initiated, the smallest, most fatigue-resistant, and slowest motor units are recruited first; as the force is increased, larger and faster-contracting motor units that are more susceptible to fatigue are recruited successively. This concept was demonstrated by Henneman and colleagues,[10] who referred to it as the "size" principle. They also described the relationship between the size of a motor unit (i.e., the number of myofibers innervated) and the size of its motor neuron. The smallest motor neurons are more excitable and thus are activated first. The largest motor neurons are not as easily excited but have the highest maximum firing frequencies and can generate the quickest forceful movements. Therefore, the *size principle* ensures selection of the motor units that are best suited for a particular kind of movement.

The other method of increasing the force of muscle contraction and movement is to increase the firing frequency of the alpha motor neurons already recruited, thereby increasing the force developed by each motor unit. A single action potential from a motor neuron produces only a very brief contraction of the myofiber, or twitch. If no other action potentials arrive within a tenth of a second, no movement is produced. However, if action potentials arrive at closer and closer intervals, the individual twitches become a sustained contraction. As the firing frequency of the motor neuron increases, the tension and force generated increase also; this is referred to as summation. The maximum muscle contraction at the maximum firing frequency is known as *fused tetanus*. Unfused tetanus occurs at submaximum firing frequencies.

Motor neurons are *somatotopically organized* in the ventral gray matter of the spinal cord. Within the ventral gray, the motor neurons are grouped in longitudinally oriented columns (Fig. 15–4). Each column contains the alpha and gamma motor neurons to one or a few functionally similar muscles. Generally, each column extends through more than one segment of the cord. Therefore, each muscle receives motor fibers through more than one ventral root and spinal nerve. This explains why destruction of one root or spinal nerve by a lumbar disc protrusion, for example, produces weakness but not complete paralysis of a muscle.

Another level of organization is seen in the distribution of the neurons supplying the axial muscles versus those supplying the extremities. The motor neurons innervating the paravertebral muscles are located most medially in the ventral gray, whereas those supplying the muscles of the extremities are located more laterally. This arrangement can be seen most dramatically on cross sections of segments of the cord that send fibers to the extremities; the ventral horn is much larger and extends more laterally in the cervical and lumbar enlargements. There is also a dorsal-ventral organization in which the motor neurons supplying the proximal muscles of the extremities lie more ventrally in the ventral gray than those supplying the distal muscles of the hand and foot.

The spinal cord is divided into *segments*, each giving rise to a dorsal and ventral root, which combine to form a spinal

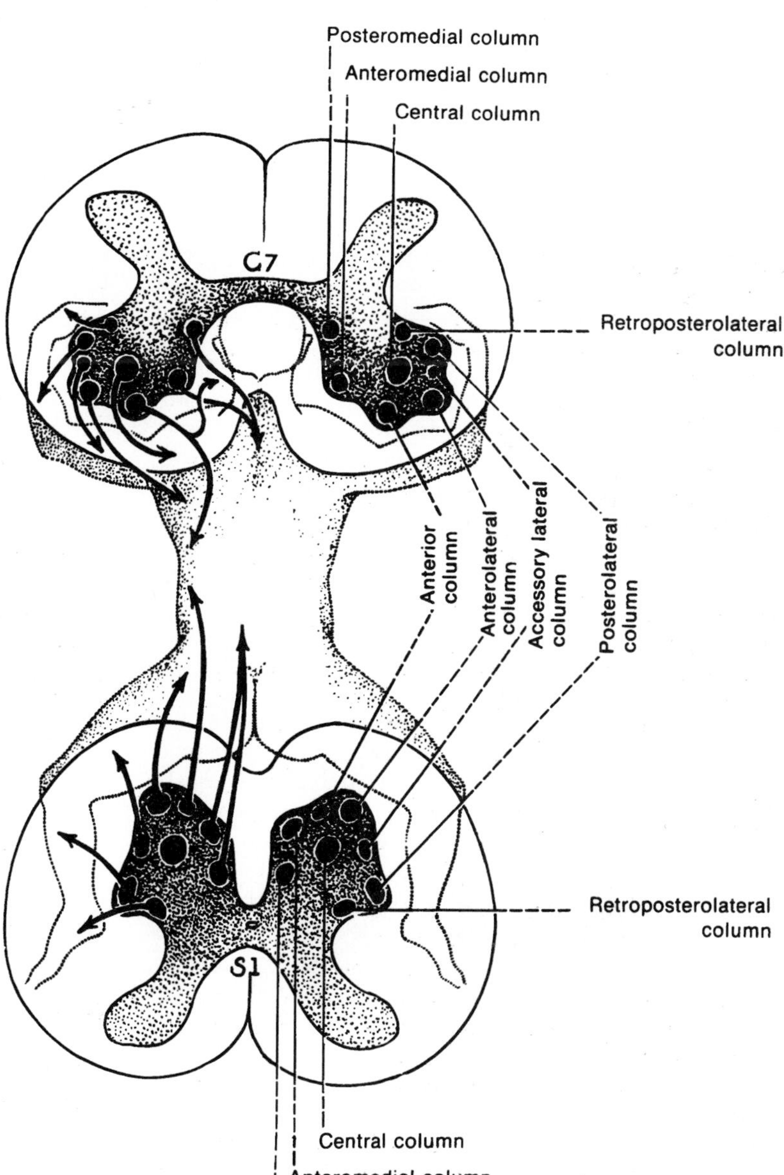

FIGURE 15–4. Functional organization of the lower motor neurons in the spinal cord. (From Bossy: Atlas of Neuroanatomy and Special Sense Organs. Philadelphia, WB Saunders, 1970.)

nerve. The axons of all the motor neurons located in one spinal segment leave the spinal cord through one ventral root and continue into the spinal nerves.

These spinal nerves conform to the embryological *myotomes*. This myotomal organization can still be seen in the rostral caudal distribution of innervation from the cervical and lumbar cord segments innervating the upper and lower extremities, respectively. The proximal muscles of the shoulder and hip girdle are innervated by the more rostral segments of the cervical cord (C5–C6) and the lumbar cord (L2–L4), whereas the intrinsic muscles of the hand and the more distal leg and foot muscles are innervated by the lowermost segments of the cervical (C8–T1) and lumbar (L5–S1) segments. There are the same number of thoracic (12), lumbar (5), and sacral (5) spinal roots as vertebral bodies. However, there are eight cervical spinal roots, whereas there are only seven cervical vertebral bodies. The first pair of cervical nerves exits from the vertebral column between the atlas and the skull. Each of the remaining cervical nerves from C2 to C7 leaves the spinal column *above* the vertebra of the corresponding number. Because there are eight pairs of cervical nerves and only seven cervical vertebrae, the eighth cervical nerve leaves the spinal column between C7 and T1. The first thoracic nerve and all the remaining spinal nerves pass out from the vertebral column *below* the vertebra of like number.

After leaving the spinal column, the cervical and lumbar nerves combine to form the brachial plexus and the lumbosacral plexus from which the peripheral nerves to the arm and leg are formed. As a result, motor axons from one spinal segment are distributed to several peripheral nerves. Looking at it from the standpoint of the muscle, each limb muscle receives motor axons from more than one spinal segment. As noted earlier, destruction of one spinal nerve therefore produces only a weakness rather than a paralysis of a muscle. Destruction of the peripheral nerve innervating the muscle, however, interrupts all of the motor innervation for that muscle, resulting in paralysis and atrophy of the muscle. Knowledge of the peripheral nerves, the spinal nerves contained in them, and the muscles innervated by them is crucial in localizing lesions in the subdivisions of the lower motor neuron, whether in the spinal nerve, plexus, or peripheral nerve. Diagrams of the important relationships are contained in Figures 15–5 to 15–7.

The cervical, brachial, and lumbosacral plexuses are formed by the anterior primary rami of the spinal nerve roots (the posterior rami innervate the paravertebral muscles). In the plexuses, the roots become reorganized into peripheral nerves, which then contain contributions from two or more spinal roots. Therefore, to accurately localize a lesion to a specific part of a plexus, one has to know the motor and sensory supply of all peripheral nerve components supplied by that division.

The *cervical plexus* is formed by the anterior primary rami of C1 through C4 behind the sternocleidomastoid and in front of the scalenus medius and levator scapulae muscles. The motor branches of the plexus supply the muscles of the neck. Injuries to the cervical plexus are infrequent, but any of its branches can be injured by penetrating wounds, surgery, or enlarged lymph nodes (see Fig. 15–6A). Involvement of the cervical plexus may also compromise the closely associated cranial nerves XI and XII. In patients with lesions of the cer-

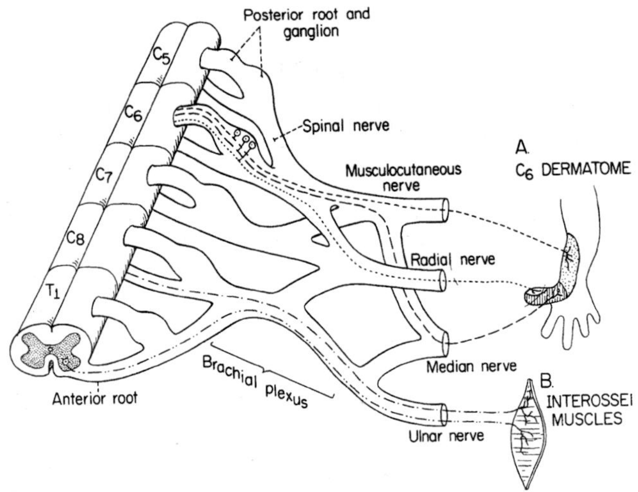

FIGURE 15–5. The axons of the lower motor neurons form the spinal roots, one for each spinal segment *(A)*. The spinal roots (containing both sensory and motor axons) recombine to form the brachial plexus *(B)*, from which the major peripheral nerves are formed (Adapted from Patton HD, Sundsten JW, Crill W, Swanson PD: Introduction to Basic Neurology. Philadelphia, WB Saunders, 1976.)

vical plexus, sensory symptoms in the form of head and neck dysesthesia and pain may predominate over motor signs.

Injuries are more common to the *brachial plexus*, which is formed from the anterior primary rami of C5 through T1. It extends from the spinal column to the axilla and is divided into five major components starting proximally and proceeding distally. The first components are the roots, which recombine to form trunks, and then divisions, cords, and finally branches. Figure 15–6 shows a diagram of the anatomy of the brachial plexus.

The *lumbosacral plexus* is derived from the anterior primary rami of the twelfth thoracic through the fourth sacral levels and is contained within the psoas major muscle. Although many more roots contribute to the lumbosacral plexus, it is somewhat simpler than the brachial plexus. Two major nerves, the femoral nerve and the sciatic nerve, are formed from the plexus (see Fig. 15–7).

Gamma Motor Neuron

Like the alpha motor neurons, the gamma motor neurons lie in the ventral horn of the spinal cord interspersed among the alpha motor neurons innervating the same muscle. Gamma motor neurons innervate the *intrafusal* muscle fibers of a specialized sensory organ, the *muscle spindle*.[11] The muscle spindle consists of a small bag of muscle fibers that lie in parallel with the extrafusal skeletal muscle fibers. Therefore, when the muscle lengthens or shortens, the intrafusal muscle spindle fibers are stretched or relaxed correspondingly. The intrafusal fibers are surrounded by sensory nerve endings that become 1a afferents to the dorsal root ganglion. When the intrafusal fibers are stretched as the muscle is lengthened, the sensory fibers are activated, providing sensory feedback about the degree of lengthening that has occurred. When the muscle contracts and shortens, the intrafusal spindle fibers also shorten. If this were a completely passive system, the intrafusal fibers would relax and the sensory endings would become silent, providing no helpful feedback information about the state of the

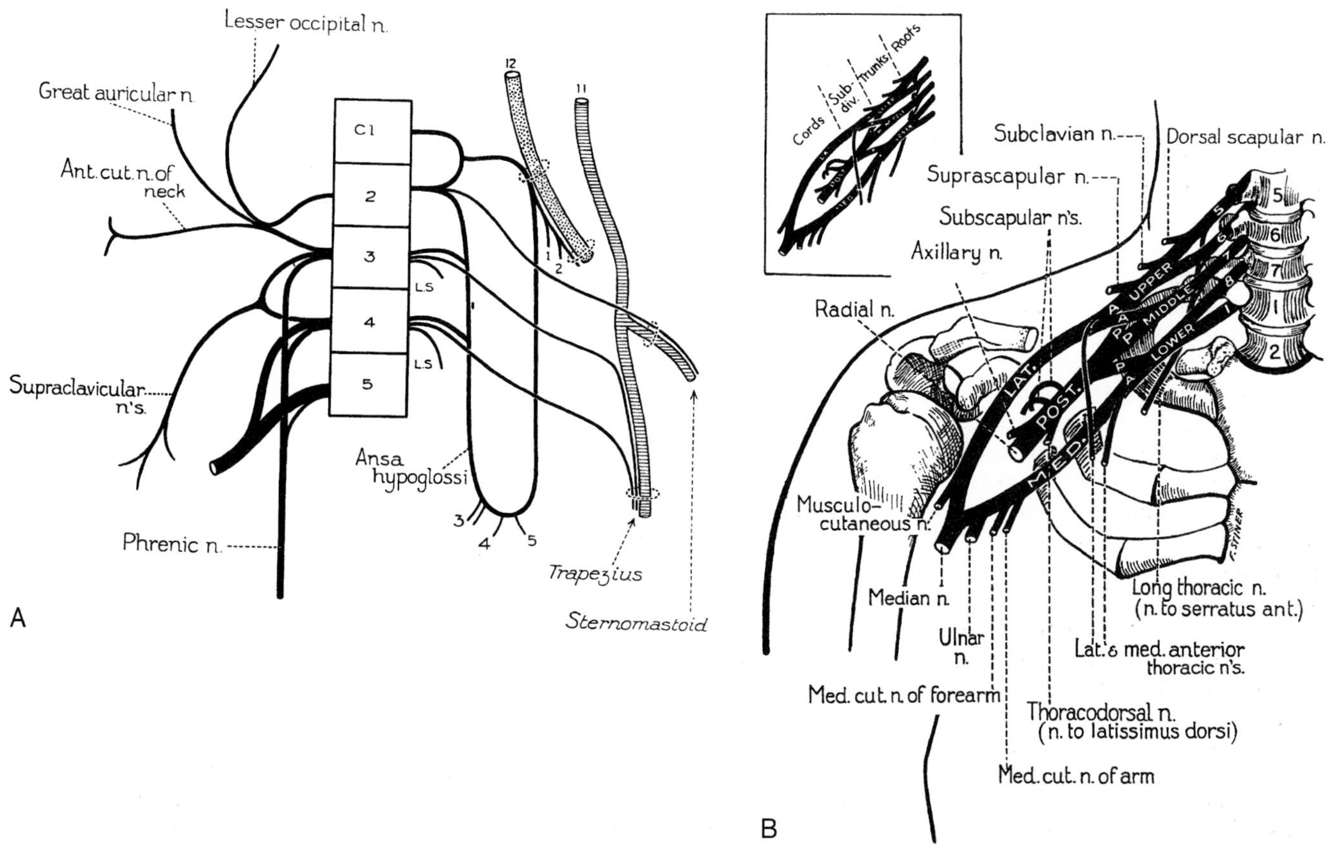

FIGURE 15–6. *A* and *B*, The organization of the brachial plexus. The spinal roots C5–T1 recombine to form trunks (upper, middle, and lower), divisions (anterior and posterior), and cords (lateral, posterior, and medial). (From Haymaker N, Woodhall B: Peripheral Nerve Injuries. Philadelphia, WB Saunders, 1953.)

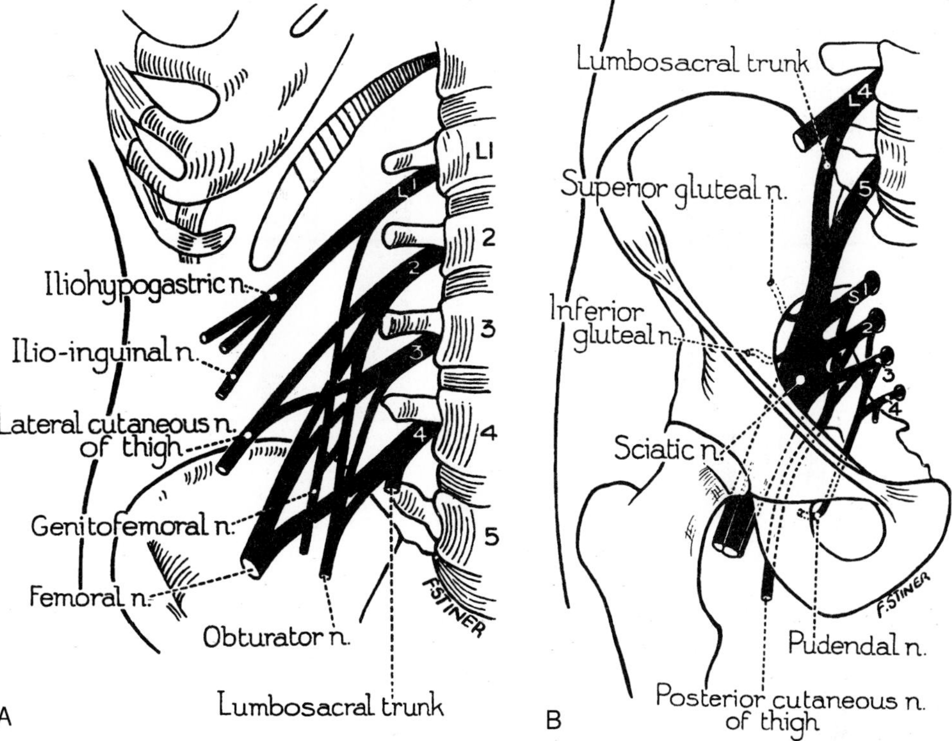

FIGURE 15–7. *A*, The lumbar plexus. *B*, The sacral plexus. The lumbosacral trunk is the connection between the lumbar and sacral plexus. (From Haymaker N, Woodhall B: Peripheral Nerve Injuries. Philadelphia, WB Saunders, 1953.)

muscle. To prevent this inefficient circumstance, gamma motor neurons are activated, maintaining tension in the intrafusal fibers to continue to provide precise sensory information.

This phenomenon can be observed experimentally if alpha motor neurons are excited in isolation. When the muscle contracts, there is a pause in volleys from the 1a afferent. When the gamma motor neuron is excited at the same time, the afferent volleys do not pause. This simultaneous activation of alpha and gamma motor neurons during muscle contraction is called *alpha-gamma co-activation*; it is an excellent example of sensory motor integration in the nervous system. By this means, innervation of the muscle spindle by an independent system of gamma motor neurons allows the central nervous system to adjust the sensitivity of the spindle and fine-tune the information it receives (Fig. 15–8).

Another sensory organ, the *Golgi tendon organ*, also conveys information about the state of the muscle. The Golgi tendon organs lie in the muscle tendon and, unlike the muscle spindle, are coupled in series with the extrafusal muscle fibers. Therefore, both passive stretch and active contraction of the muscle increase the tension of the tendon and activate the tendon organ receptor. In contrast to the activity of the muscle spindle, which depends on muscle length, the Golgi tendon organ conveys information about muscle tension. Together they convey precise information about the length, tension, velocity, and force of the muscle contraction, thus allowing greater precision of movement.[12]

Changes in muscle tone, defined as resistance to passive stretch of muscle, are an important feature of diseases of the motor system. At one time, an important component of normal resting muscle tone was thought to be the result of low-level background alpha-gamma co-activation. However, more recent studies in fully relaxed individuals indicate that the viscoelastic properties of muscle and tendons account for normal resting tone.[13] Common experience indicates that resting muscle tone can vary considerably depending on the state of relaxation of the muscle as well as its viscoelastic properties. Some studies have shown that the passive viscoelastic properties of muscle may contribute to increased tone in patients with chronic spasticity and rigidity, but the most important determinants of pathological alterations in tone are the result of alterations in stretch reflexes.

Alpha and Gamma Motor Neurons and Reflex Arcs

Reflex actions are the simplest form of coordinated movement. A reflex action is a stereotyped response to a specific sensory stimulus. The reflex elicited depends on the site of the stimulus, and the strength of the stimulus determines the amplitude of the response. Reflex responses are used by higher motor centers to generate more complex movements and behaviors. The neural circuitry responsible for reflex actions is present at different levels of the motor system, and disturbances in these reflexes are important for localizing lesions in the motor system. Some reflexes, especially spinal and brain stem reflexes, are normally observed or elicited only in the developing nervous system. As the nervous system and higher motor centers mature, these reflexes are suppressed, only to re-emerge if damage to the higher motor centers modulates the reflex. The unmasking of spinal reflexes in particular is a good example of the hierarchical organization of the motor system.

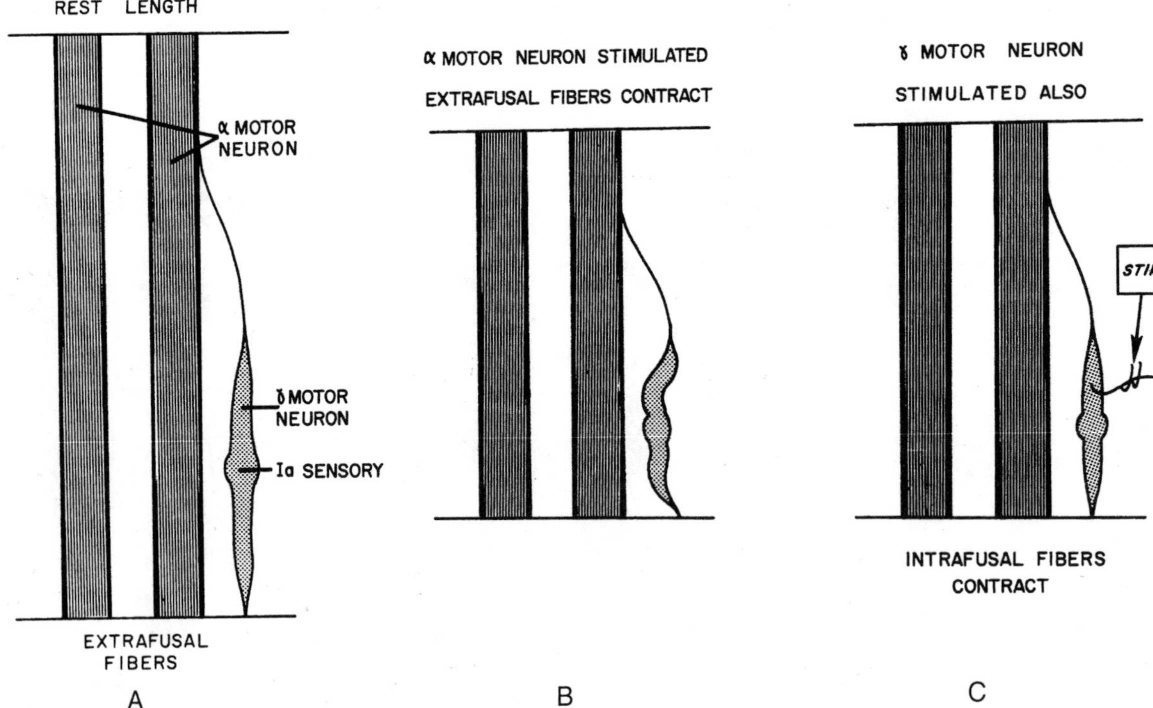

FIGURE 15–8. The effect of gamma activation on maintenance of tone in the muscle spindle. *A*, The extrafusal fibers innervated by the alpha motor neuron and the intrafusal muscle fibers of the muscle spindle innervated by the gamma motor neuron lie in parallel. *B*, Condition that would exist if the intrafusal fibers of the muscle spindle did not have a separate innervation to maintain tone when the alpha motor neuron fires causing contraction and shortening of the extrafusal skeletal muscle. *C*, Firing of the gamma motor neurons activates the muscle spindle to maintain normal tone and responsivity of the 1a afferent (alpha-gamma co-activation).

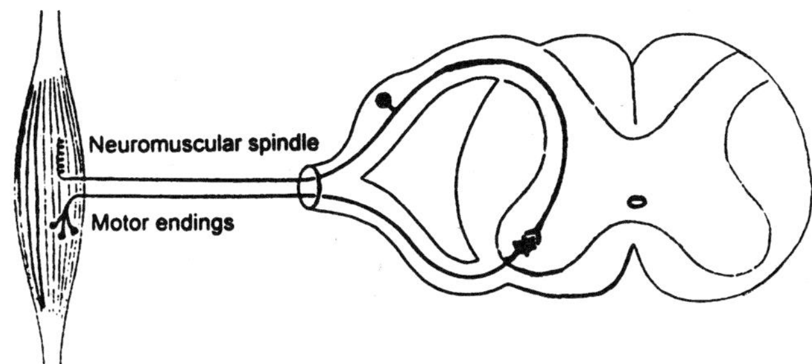

FIGURE 15–9. The two neuron monosynaptic phasic stretch reflex. A rapid stretch of a muscle increases the discharge rate of the 1a afferent fibers from the muscle spindle. The 1a afferent entering the spinal cord directly excites the alpha motor neuron, causing contraction of agonist muscles to oppose the lengthening. (From Gardner E: Fundamentals of Neurology. Philadelphia, WB Saunders, 1968.)

The *monosynaptic stretch reflex* is the simplest spinal reflex. As the name implies, the reflex muscle contraction is elicited by lengthening or stretching the muscle. To evoke this reflex, the muscle must be stretched rapidly, which produces a short phasic contraction. Thus, this reflex is termed a *phasic stretch reflex.*[14] In the human subject, sudden stretch is produced by tapping a tendon with a reflex hammer.

Sherrington demonstrated that this reflex could be eliminated by cutting either the dorsal or the ventral root, thus establishing that this reflex requires both sensory input from the muscle to the spinal cord and motor output from the motor neurons to the muscle.[2] The sensory receptor for the afferent limb of the reflex is the muscle spindle.[11] Sudden lengthening of the muscle by the tap on the tendon causes an increase in the discharge rate of type 1a nerve fibers from the muscle spindle. The 1a afferents entering the spinal cord excite motor neurons to both agonist and synergist muscles, causing contractions that oppose the lengthening (Fig. 15–9). Branches from the 1a afferents also excite interneurons that inhibit antagonist motor neurons, causing the antagonist muscles to relax. Thus, this reflex can be seen as a negative feedback loop that resists changes in muscle length. Note that although contraction of the agonist muscles results from a simple monosynaptic connection between the 1a afferent and the alpha motor neuron, relaxation of the antagonist muscles requires an *inhibitory interneuron* and a phenomenon called *reciprocal inhibition* (Fig. 15–10).

INTERNUNCIAL POOL

More complex reflexes use even more of these inhibitory interneurons, sometimes referred to as the *internuncial pool.*

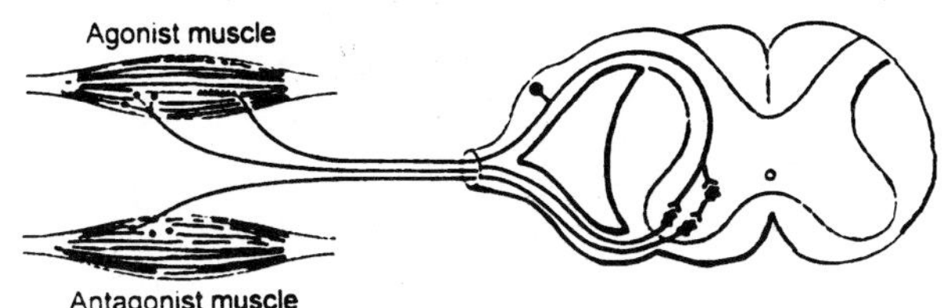

FIGURE 15–10. Reciprocal inhibition. When the agonist muscle is activated by the monosynaptic phasic stretch reflex, a branch from the 1a afferent of the muscle spindle also excites interneurons that inhibit the antagonist motor neurons causing relaxation of the opposing antagonist muscle. (From Gardner E: Fundamentals of Neurology. Philadelphia, WB Saunders, 1968.)

One of these inhibitory interneurons with a special action was described by Birdsie Renshaw and is known by his name.[15] The *Renshaw cell* receives a recurrent collateral, that is, a branch of the axon of the alpha motor neuron before it leaves the ventral horn (Fig. 15–11). The axons of the Renshaw cell contacts the alpha motor neuron. An action potential down the axon of the alpha motor neuron also excites the Renshaw cell through the recurrent collateral. The Renshaw cell in turn inhibits the same alpha motor neuron and other alpha motor neurons that innervate agonists. The Renshaw cell also inhibits the inhibitory interneuron mediating the reciprocal inhibition. In this way, the Renshaw cell shortens the reflex contraction of the agonist and, at the same time, shortens the reciprocal inhibition of the antagonist. Through this mechanism, the motor neurons can inhibit their own activity. This seems to be important in preventing alpha motor neurons from sending long trains of action potentials in response to a brief stimulus. The Renshaw cell and other internuncial neurons receive input from the higher motor centers, which can modulate the activity of these neurons and fine-tune the reflex movements. This means that the spinal reflexes provide the nervous system with elementary and automatic motor patterns that can be activated either by sensory stimuli or by descending signals from higher motor centers. Supraspinal input can therefore modify or suppress the expression of the reflex through the internuncial pool of inhibitory interneurons.

Clearly, most spinal reflexes are mediated by polysynaptic circuits that allow the reflex to be modified and the movement to be more finely coordinated. The most important of the *polysynaptic* spinal reflexes is the *flexor reflex* (Fig. 15–12). It is stimulated by a noxious *cutaneous stimulus* to the leg. The response is a withdrawal of the leg from the source of the painful stimulus. Teleologically, this reflex is important in

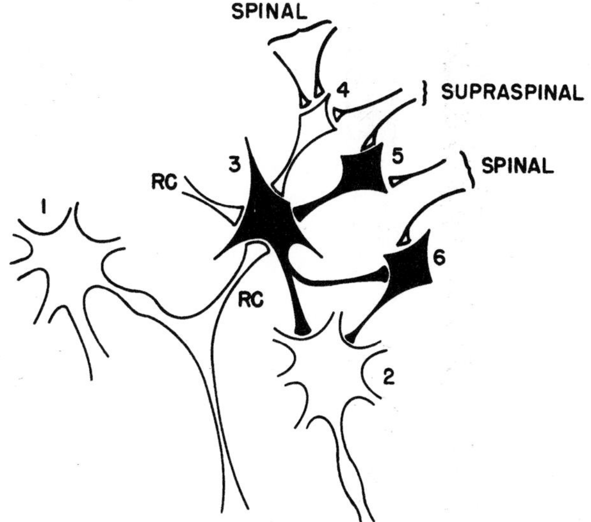

FIGURE 15–11. The internuncial pool of inhibitory interneurons. White cells and synapses are excitatory; the black cells are inhibitory. 1 and 2 are anterior horn cells; 3 is the Renshaw cell; 4, 5, and 6 are interneurons. Note the spinal and supraspinal inputs to the inhibitory interneurons. Note also the recurrent collateral from the alpha motor neuron contacting the Renshaw cell, which in turn makes contact with the anterior horn cell and sends a recurrent collateral to inhibit the inhibitory interneuron mediating reciprocal inhibition. (From Curtis BA, Jacobson S, Marcus EM: Introduction to the Neurosciences. Philadelphia, WB Saunders, 1972.)

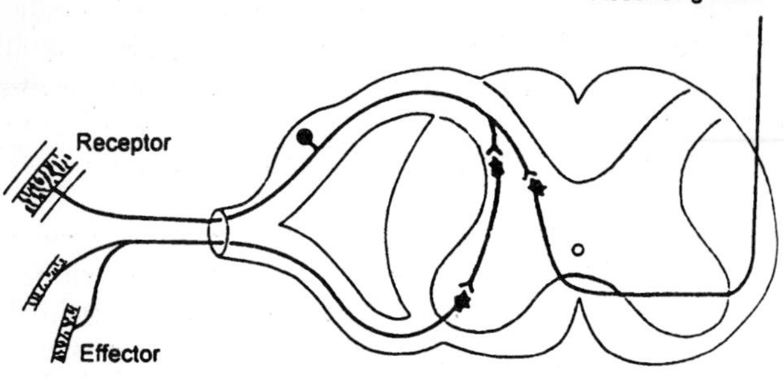

FIGURE 15–12. The polysynaptic flexor reflex. The impulses from a cutaneous receptor excite the alpha motor neuron to the effector muscles through an intermediate neuron. Additional impulses also reach the cerebral hemisphere by way of an ascending tract. (From Gardner E: Fundamentals of Neurology. Philadelphia, WB Saunders, 1968.)

preventing injury to the foot from stepping on a sharp or hot object. As with other reflexes, the strength of the response corresponds to the strength of the stimulus. In a normal individual, only a painful stimulus elicits the reflex. When descending motor pathways that suppress and modulate the reflex are damaged, a lighter, nonpainful stimulus may elicit the reflex. This was discovered by Babinski when he scratched the sole of the foot of a patient with central nervous system lesions. With the light nonpainful stimulus, the strength of the response parallels the extent to which the upper motor neuron lesion has allowed upregulation of the reflex. In a patient with a small hemispheral lesion, only a small fragment of the reflex may be elicited, that is, extension of the great toe, known as the *Babinski sign* (Fig. 15–13). With complete transection of the spinal cord, the entire withdrawal reflex with flexion at the hip, knee, and ankle may occur.

The sensory limb of this reflex arc is mediated by cutaneous receptors of fast-conducting 1a afferents that converge on the internuncial pool of inhibitory interneurons. While the motor neurons to the flexor muscles are excited, the extensor muscles are inhibited through reciprocal inhibition.

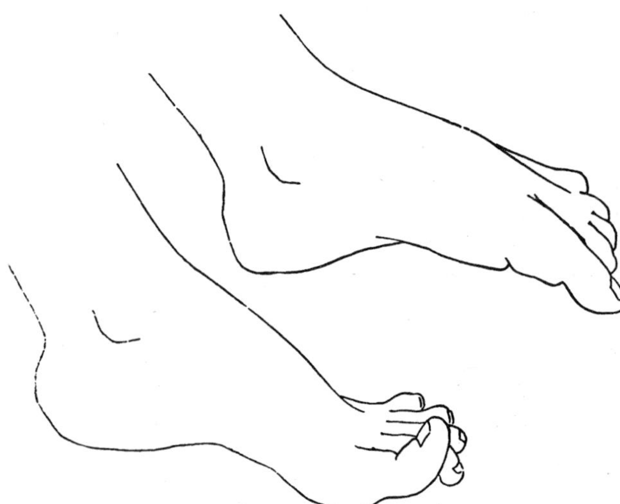

FIGURE 15–13. Babinski's sign. *Top*, The normal adult response to stimulation of the lateral plantar surface of the foot. *Bottom*, The normal infant and abnormal adult response. (From Gardner E: Fundamentals of Neurology. Philadelphia, WB Saunders, 1968.)

At the same time, motor neurons to the extensors of the contralateral leg are activated and the flexors are relaxed to compensate for the shift of weight to the contralateral leg while the ipsilateral leg is withdrawn from the painful stimulus. This *crossed extensor reflex* maintains postural support during withdrawal from a painful stimulus.

One can readily appreciate that the spinal circuits responsible for flexion withdrawal and crossed extension do more than mediate protective reflexes. They also serve to coordinate limb movements and voluntary movements. The interneurons in these pathways receive conversion inputs from different types of afferent fibers, not just pain fibers, as well as from descending pathways. Therefore, this convergence combines inputs from many different sensory sources including commands for voluntary movement through the descending pathway. This integration of sensory input is necessary for the regulation of precise movements because voluntary movements also produce excitation of cutaneous and joint receptors as well as muscle receptors.

Another cutaneous reflex of clinical significance is the *superficial abdominal reflex* (Fig. 15–14). This reflex is elicited by stroking the skin of the abdomen, which causes a reflex contraction of the abdominal muscles beneath the stimulus. Thus, stroking the upper abdomen causes contraction of the upper abdominal muscles, whereas stimulation of the lower abdomen causes contraction of the lower abdominal muscles. This relationship between the location of the stimulus and the muscles that contract is called a *local sign*. Other examples are contraction of the *cremasteric* muscles of the scrotum in response to stroking the skin of the inner thigh and the reflex contraction of the external anal sphincter when the perianal skin is stroked.

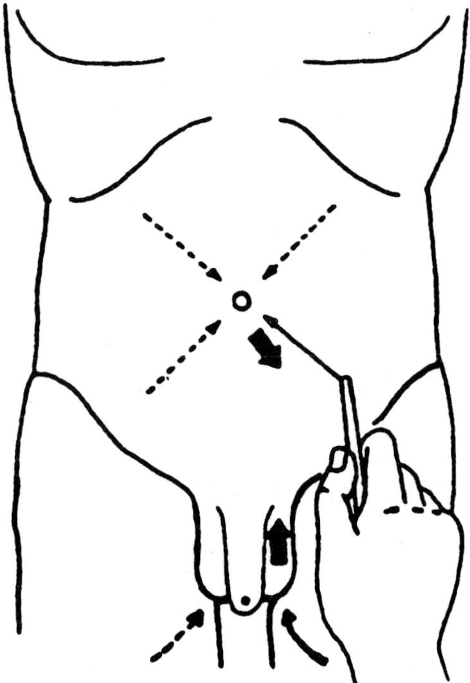

FIGURE 15–14. The superficial abdominal reflex. The examiner strokes the skin with a stick as diagrammed. Stroking the upper quadrant tests thoracic segments 7–9 and the lower quadrants for T10–T12.

The normal function of the short-latency phasic stretch reflex is hard to define. In a fully relaxed individual who can exert total voluntary control over the excitability of the motor neurons, the stretch reflex does not appear to contribute to muscle tone. However, when these descending influences are interrupted, the excitability of the motor neurons involved in the stretch reflex is enhanced. This can be seen in the alteration of muscle tone called *spasticity*.

The pathophysiology of spasticity may involve several mechanisms. Hyperexcitability of the alpha motor neurons from a primary intrinsic change in membrane properties may account for certain elements of spasticity, but most of the changes in lower motor neuron function are thought to be secondary to alterations in suprasegmental synaptic input. With regard to the 1a afferent pool, there are several types of suprasegmental inhibition that may be altered in spasticity. Presynaptic inhibition mediated by axo-axonic synapses on 1a terminals is reduced by suprasegmental disease, causing normal stimuli to 1a afferents to induce an exaggerated response. In addition, the 1a system on paired flexor and extensor muscles normally functions in a coordinated fashion to reduce the likelihood that antagonistic muscle groups will be co-activated during a muscle contraction. In the condition of spasticity, this type of 1a inhibition is lost, resulting in inefficient co-contractions that can compromise motor function. In addition, 1a inhibitory interneurons are also affected by descending excitatory pathways, and when these latter paths are damaged, the interneurons from flexors to extensors and from extensors to flexors are affected differently. In addition to the changes in the 1a system, nonreciprocal 1b inhibition is also reduced or even replaced by facilitation in spastic patients, suggesting that important physiological alterations occur in this system as well. In fundamental contrast to all of these mechanisms, recurrent inhibition via Renshaw cell activity is actually increased in patients with spinal cord lesions and spastic paresis. The specific descending pathways of influence are discussed subsequently.

In addition to the short-latency monosynaptic stretch reflex, a second reflex contraction of muscle occurs at a longer latency.This *long-latency stretch reflex* (sometimes referred to as the long-loop stretch reflex) is mediated by a polysynaptic reflex pathway and has different properties from the short-latency monosynaptic stretch reflex.[16] The strength of the long-latency reflex depends on whether the muscle is relaxed or active at the time of stretching and whether the subject is instructed to resist the stretch or to let go. The strength of the reflex may also change during learning of a motor task. Therefore, this reflex can adapt quite readily to voluntary descending control from the higher motor centers. This kind of control appears to be mediated through the internuncial pool of interneurons, which can regulate the excitability of the motor neurons and therefore the degree of muscle contraction.

The function of the long-latency stretch reflex is as hard to define as that of the short-latency reflex, but based on the elegant experiments of Marsden and associates,[17] it appears to compensate for changes in resistance during slow precision movements. In these experiments, while the subject flexed the thumb with a constant speed against a force of constant magnitude, the force was suddenly changed at unpredictable times. The change in compensatory force by the subject occurred at a latency that was faster than that of voluntary contraction and consistent with a polysynaptic long-latency reflex. The stretch reflex appeared to function to keep the sensitivity of the muscle spindles at a high level so that the slightest perturbations could be detected and the activity of the alpha motor neurons could be adjusted appropriately.

A disturbance in the long-latency stretch reflexes may be responsible for the characteristic increased muscle tone seen in patients with Parkinson's disease and known as *rigidity*. In contrast to spasticity, rigidity is felt as a constant resistance to stretch that occurs in both flexion and extension of a joint; it may be felt during passive stretching of muscles that are too slow to elicit the spastic catch.

Delwaide's studies on spinal interneuron activity provide the best explanation for the pathophysiology of rigidity.[18] The magnitude of rigidity correlates well with a reduction in short-latency autogenic 1b inhibition and simultaneous 1a interneuron facilitation. Activation of the descending reticulospinal tract from the nucleus reticularis gigantocellularis in experimental animals elicits this same pattern of 1b inhibition and 1a facilitation, suggesting that this system is involved in rigidity. Studies in monkeys who are rigid and parkinsonian due to exposure to the toxin 1-methyl-4-phenyl-1,2,3,6-tetrahydropyridine (MPTP) in fact show excessive activation of this pathway.

UPPER MOTOR NEURON POOL

There are many neurons in the cerebral cortex and brain stem that initiate and modify movement through their connections with the lower motor neurons in the anterior spinal gray. These projections also synapse on the internuncial pool of interneurons, which in turn make contact with the alpha and gamma motor neurons. These are known as the *upper motor neurons*. These supraspinal motor neurons in the cerebral cortex and brain stem are interconnected with each other and participate to various degrees in all automatic and voluntary movements. Descending tracts from the motor centers in the brain stem are primarily involved with posture and automatic movements, whereas the motor areas of the cerebral cortex are required for voluntary movement.

Corticospinal Tract

The corticospinal tract is composed of axons of *pyramidal neurons* located in lamina 5 of the cerebral cortex. Most of the axons of the corticospinal tract come from neurons in the precentral gyrus (Brodmann area 4),[19] although significant contributions come from many other areas of the cortex, especially premotor area 6 and supplementary motor area. This is the only motor tract that passes directly from the cerebral cortex to the spinal cord without making any intermediate synaptic connections. The cytoarchitecture of the primary motor area, supplementary motor area, and premotor cortex is distinct from that of the adjacent sensory and prefrontal regions. Layer 4, the major afferent layer for the sensory cortex, is absent in the motor areas, and hence these motor regions are often termed agranular.

Layer 5 in the primary motor cortex contains the distinctive giant pyramidal neurons known as *Betz cells*. The axons of these cells become the corticospinal or pyramidal tract and represent one of several descending influences on the motor neurons of the brain stem and spinal cord. The remaining cells mostly come from the supplementary motor and premotor cortex. Most of these axons terminate on interneurons in the internuncial pool of the ventral gray of the spinal cord. Axons that connect monosynaptically with the lower motor neurons are involved in control of the distal muscles of the extremities, especially the intrinsic muscles of the hand that control finger movements.[3] Upper motor neurons in the cerebral cortex also send axons to the motor nuclei of the cranial nerves and form the *corticobulbar tract*. The motor neurons in the primary motor area have a somatotopic organization. The *homunculus* was mapped by Penfield and colleagues[20] by electrically stimulating the surface of the cortex during epilepsy surgery in humans. Stimulation of most of the lateral surface of the primary motor area produced movement in the mouth, tongue, face, and hand muscles, which is consistent with the importance of fine voluntary control of these structures (Fig. 15–15A).

The axons of the corticospinal tract gather together, forming the corona radiata, and descend through the posterior limb of the *internal capsule* into the middle two thirds of the *cerebral peduncles of the midbrain*. In this descent, the fibers shift position, and those representing the face become most medial, while those of the legs become most lateral. The corticospinal fibers become less recognizable as a tract as they course through the ventral two thirds of the pons. They form bundles interspersed with a variety of other descending and crossing white matter tracts. When the fibers enter the medulla, they form a very discrete, easily recognizable bundle on the ventral aspect of the medulla known as the *pyramids*. Because it is such an easily recognizable bundle of nerve fibers, the corticospinal tract is often referred to as the *pyramidal tract*, although the pyramids also contain fibers other than those in the corticospinal system.[21] Half to three fourths of the fibers of the pyramidal tract originate in areas 4 and 6 anterior to the central sulcus, and the rest come from areas posterior to the central sulcus in the parietal lobe.

At the caudalmost level of the medulla, most of the corticospinal fibers cross the midline in the decussation of the cervical medullary junction and continue in the lateral funiculus of the spinal cord as the *lateral corticospinal tract*. A much smaller number of fibers continue uncrossed in the ventral

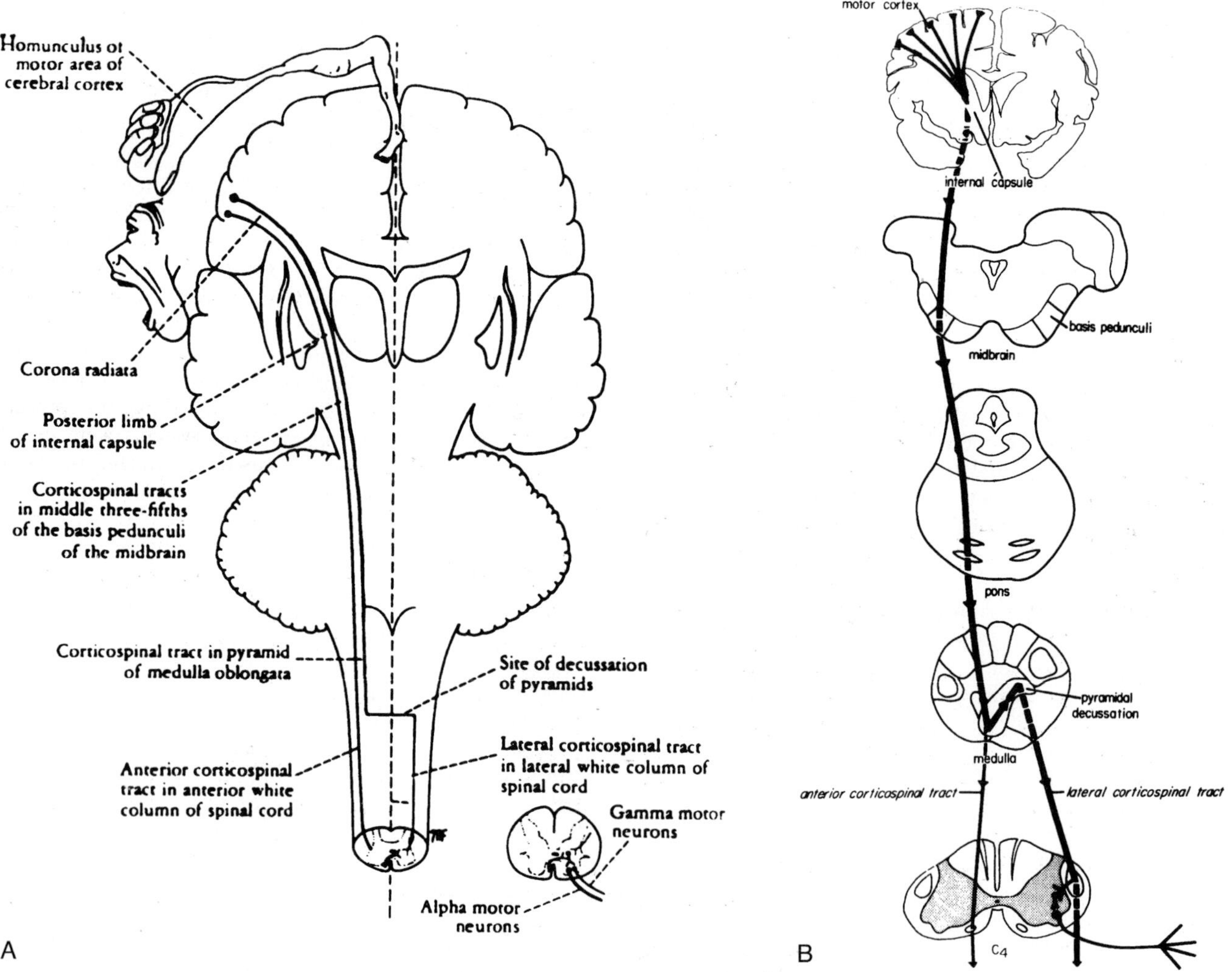

FIGURE 15–15. The corticospinal tract. *A*, The course of the corticospinal tract from primary motor cortex in Brodmann area 4 to the spinal cord. *B*, The fibers destined for the limbs decussate at the cervical medullary junction and become the lateral corticospinal tract. The fiber destined for axial musculature continues uncrossed in the anterior corticospinal tract. (From Snell RS: Clinical Neuroanatomy for Medical Students. Boston, Little, Brown & Co., Inc, 1987.)

funiculus as the *ventral corticospinal tract*. The lateral corticospinal axons terminate in internuncial pools and motor neurons involved in movement of the contralateral extremities, whereas the ventral corticospinal axons terminate in the medial and ventral portions of the anterior gray in which are found neurons innervating the paravertebral muscles involved in posture (see Fig. 15–15*B*). The corticospinal tracts and their relationship to other descending pathways in the spinal cord are shown in Figure 15–16.

Corticobulbar fibers destined for the motor nuclei of the cranial nerves leave the corticospinal tract in the brain stem. Muscles of the head, except for the lower facial muscles, receive both crossed and uncrossed corticobulbar fibers. Therefore, as a rule, in a patient with a lesion of the corticobulbar tract on one side, one seldom sees significant weakness of the jaw, tongue, pharynx, or larynx (Fig. 15–17).

Because the corticospinal tract extends from the cerebral cortex to the spinal cord, its considerable length makes it vulnerable to lesions at many different sites along its path. One of the most common lesions is ischemia resulting from occlusion of an artery. Therefore, it is helpful to know the vascular supply of the corticospinal tract as it courses through the brain and spinal cord (see Chapter 22).

Brain Stem Motor Tracts

Whereas the corticospinal tracts direct voluntary movements of the distal extremities, the brain stem motor tracts are responsible for the automatic reflexes involved in posture.[22] The one exception is the *rubrospinal tract*, which forms a *lateral pathway* that terminates in the same part of the ventral gray as the pyramidal tract and is involved in distal limb movements.[23] The *medial pathways* include the reticulospinal, vestibulospinal, and tectospinal tracts. The medial pathways travel in the ventral columns of the spinal white matter and terminate in medial ventral motor neurons innervating the axial and proximal limb muscles.

The *reticulospinal tract* originates from several nuclear groups in the reticular formation in the pons and medulla (Fig. 15–18). The reticulospinal system also receives input from a variety of other sources, including the cerebral cortex and the vestibular nuclei, and integrates this information in maintaining posture. Crude voluntary proximal movements of the extremities seen in monkeys with a pyramidal tract lesion probably result from the corticoreticular portion of the reticulospinal input.

The *vestibulospinal tracts* originate in the vestibular nuclei and convey information from the vestibular labyrinth (Fig. 15–19). The vestibulospinal tract has two parts. The largest is the lateral vestibulospinal tract, which originates in the lateral vestibular (Deiters') nucleus and reaches all levels of the spinal cord. Its input to both alpha and gamma motor neurons is excitatory and maintains contraction of antigravity muscles to maintain posture. The medial vestibulospinal tract reaches only the cervical and upper thoracic segments of the cord; it mediates reflex head movements in response to vestibular stimuli.

The *tectospinal tract* arises in the superior colliculus and is involved in coordination of head and eye movements.

The *rubrospinal tract* that forms the lateral pathway arises in the magnocellular portion of the *red nucleus* (Fig. 15–20). In the cat, it is an important pathway for controlling movements of the distal extremities, but in humans, it has become a vestigial pathway whose function has been taken over by the corticospinal tract.[23] Most of the red nucleus in the human, the parvicellular portion, contains smaller neurons whose major connections are with the cerebellum and inferior olive.

REFLEX INTEGRATION OF MOTOR PATHWAYS

Postural Reflexes

Because postural reflexes are difficult to study without special techniques[24] in normally functioning animals and humans, and because the pathways involved are intermingled with many other neural systems in the brain stem, postural reflex abnormalities are detected primarily in animals with large lesions of the brain stem. Experimentally, this was demonstrated most vividly when Sherrington transected the brain stem below the red nucleus in a cat. By interrupting the descending tracts from the cerebral cortex, the postural reflexes mediated by the brain stem systems were greatly exaggerated. This produced increased tone in the antigravity muscles, allowing the cat to be stood on all four legs. This is called *decerebrate rigidity*. Decerebrate rigidity with tonic extension of all four limbs is also seen in humans with lesions of the midbrain and upper pons.[25] In humans with brain stem lesions, the rigid extension of the limbs is not persistently

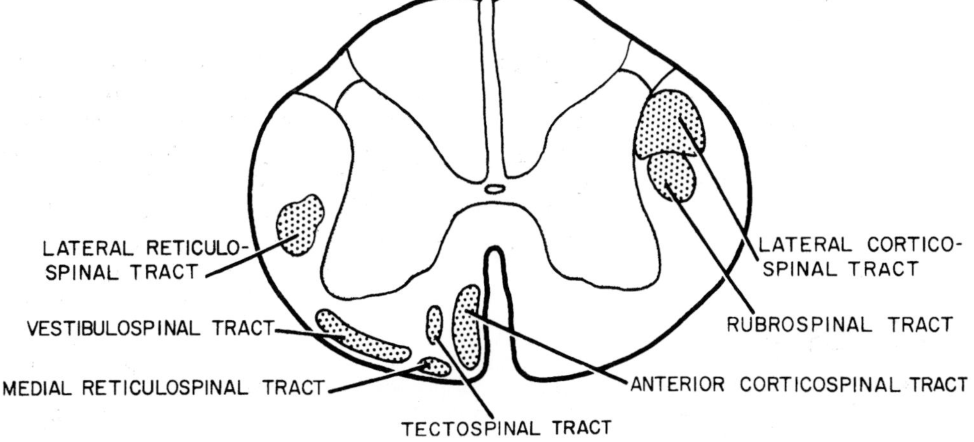

FIGURE 15–16. Several motor tracts of the spinal cord, showing the relationship between the lateral corticospinal tract and the others. (From Curtis BA, Jacobson S, Marcus EM: Introduction to the Neurosciences. Philadelphia, WB Saunders, 1972.)

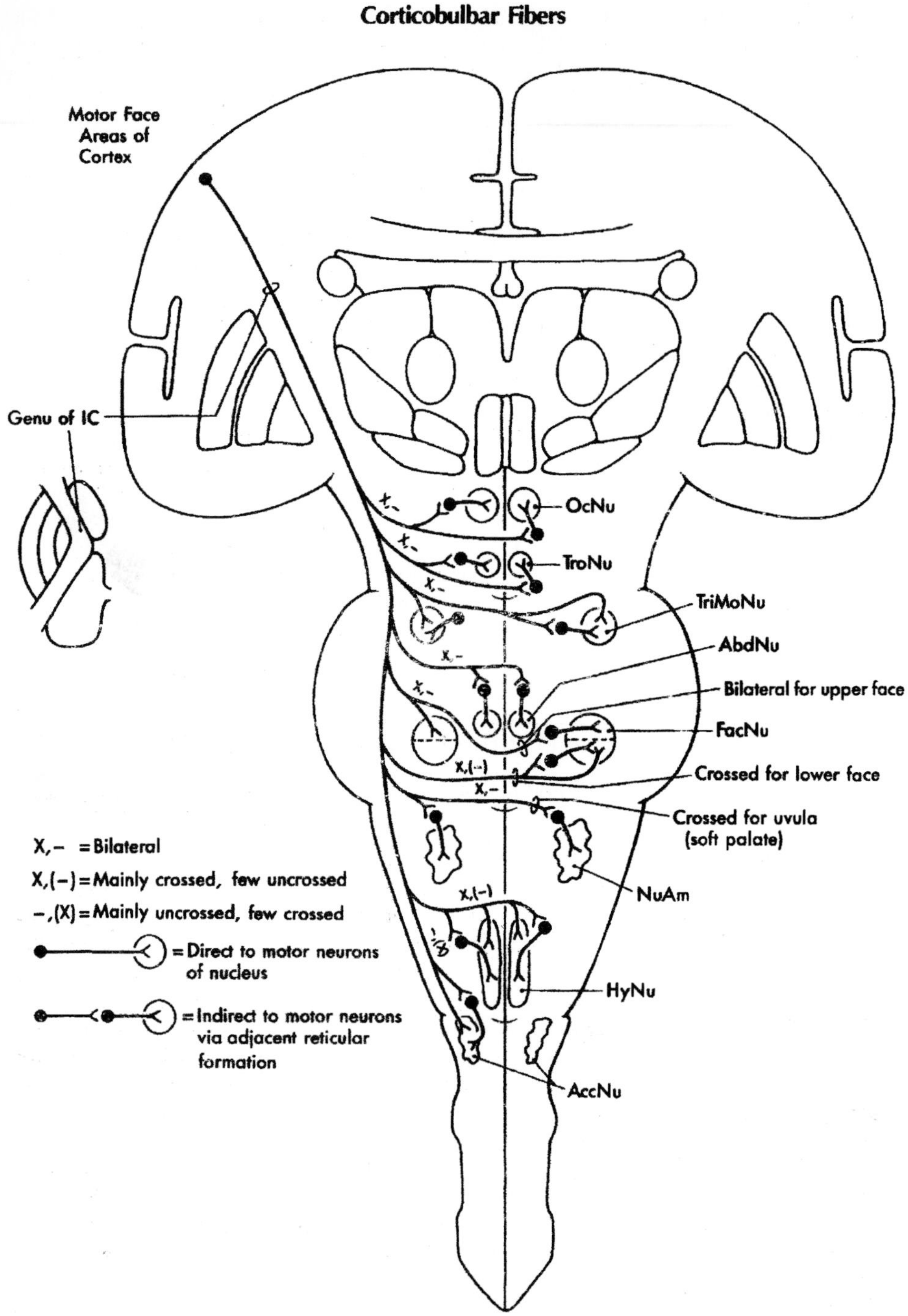

FIGURE 15–17. The corticobulbar tract. Note that the motor cortex of each hemisphere sends fibers to both the ipsilateral (uncrossed) and contralateral (crossed) cranial nerve nuclei, with the exception of the accessory nucleus and that part of the facial nerve nucleus that supplies the lower face. (From Haines DE: Neuroanatomy, 4th ed. Baltimore, Williams & Wilkins, 1995.)

maintained but may be paroxysmal, often in response to external stimuli, and is then referred to as *decerebrate posturing* (Fig. 15–21).

Decorticate rigidity is a posture in which the arms are flexed and adducted and the legs are extended due to lesions above the midbrain in the cerebral hemispheres. The posture is usually bilateral and is essentially the same as a bilateral spastic hemiplegia.

Tonic Neck Reflexes

Reflex changes in muscle tone and posture, especially in the extremities when the relationship of the head to the body is changed, are known as neck reflexes. Neck reflexes are not usually seen in normally functioning humans and animals. Stimulation of the labyrinths (labyrinthine reflexes) produces effects on muscle tone and posture that are exactly the opposite of the neck reflexes, thereby holding these in balance in the normal individual. However, in decerebrate animals, human infants, and children with cerebral palsy, the neck reflexes may be unmasked and can be demonstrated by turning the head from side to side. For example, when the head is rotated to the right, an increase in extensor tone occurs in the ipsilateral extremities and an increase in flexor tone is seen in the contralateral extremities, producing the so-called fencer's posture.

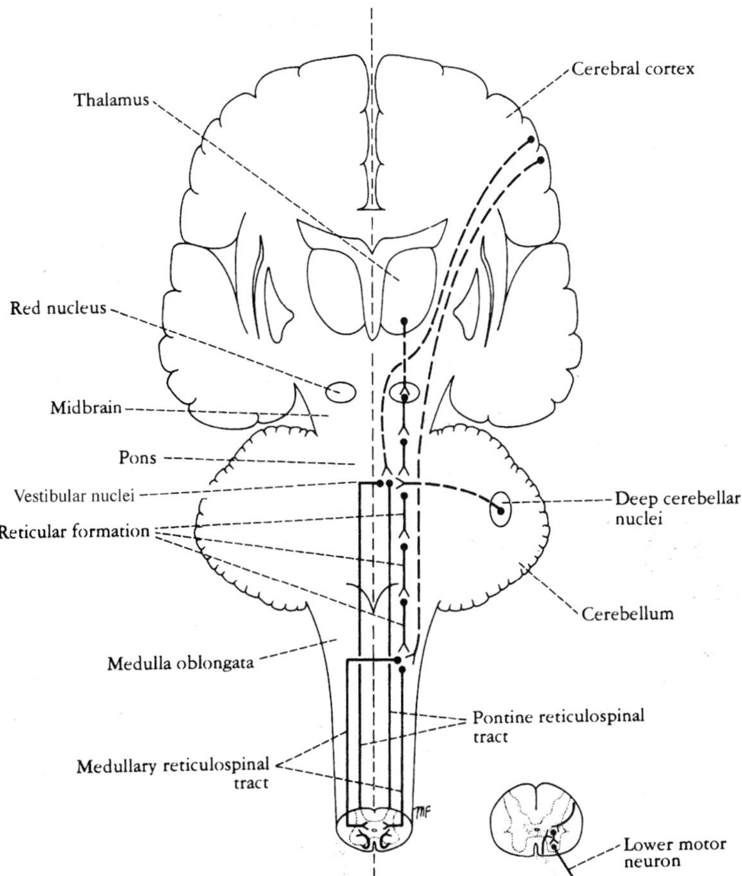

FIGURE 15–18. The reticulospinal tracts. Note the multiple inputs including cerebral cortex and vestibular nuclei. (From Snell RS: Clinical Neuroanatomy for Medical Students. Boston, Little, Brown & Co., Inc., 1987.)

Locomotor Reflexes

Pattern generators for locomotion reside in these brain stem systems. Pattern generators for locomotion also exist at a spinal level, although in humans the brain stem generators are more important. Locomotion is examined in more detail in Chapter 18.

PHARMACOLOGY OF THE MOTOR SYSTEM

The lower motor neuron uses *acetylcholine* as its neurotransmitter. The internuncial pool of neurons in the spinal cord are all inhibitory neurons that use the amino acid neurotransmitters *gamma-aminobutyric acid (GABA)* and *glycine*. Whereas glutamate is the most important excitatory neurotransmitter in the brain as well as the motor system, GABA is the most widely distributed and major chemical neurotransmitter used in the inhibitory systems. Some output neurons in the basal ganglia and cerebellum use GABA as their transmitter, but most GABA is contained and utilized by local circuit inhibitory interneurons including the internuncial pool in the spinal cord. GABA is synthesized from glutamate by the enzyme *glutamic acid decarboxylase* (GAD) and is catabolized by the enzyme *GABA-transaminase* (GABA-t). Drugs that inhibit GABA-t such as some newly developed antiepileptic drugs increase the concentrations of GABA and inhibitory tone. Drugs can also act as agonists at GABA receptors. Clinically useful drugs such as the benzodiazepines and baclofen presumably reduce spasticity by stimulating GABA receptors at inhibitory synapses in the spinal cord.[26] The drugs picrotoxin and bicuculline block GABA receptors, thereby producing excessive excitation and leading to tetanic muscle spasms or convulsions. *Glycine* is the principal neurotransmitter of the Renshaw cell. Strychnine is a specific antagonist at the glycine receptor. In small doses *strychnine* has been used as part of herbal or homeopathic preparations as an "energizer." In higher concentrations it causes convulsions by blocking normal inhibitory feedback on the motor neurons. Tetanus toxin unleashes unrestrained motor neuron activity by blocking the exocytic release of glycine and GABA.

The motor neurons of the cerebral cortex use *glutamate* as their transmitter. This includes all motor outputs from the cerebral cortex including the corticospinal and corticobulbar tracts as well as inputs to the rubrospinal and tectospinal systems. Aspartate has also been proposed as a neurotransmitter at some of the synapses, including those involved in inhibitory feedback on motor neurons, but evidence favoring it is much less compelling than that concerning glutamate.

Examination of Strength and Reflexes

DIRECTED NEUROLOGICAL EXAMINATION

Assessment of Muscle Bulk

The patient should be in a state of sufficient undress for the physician to be able to appreciate his or her general bodily habitus and especially the muscle bulk of the extremities.

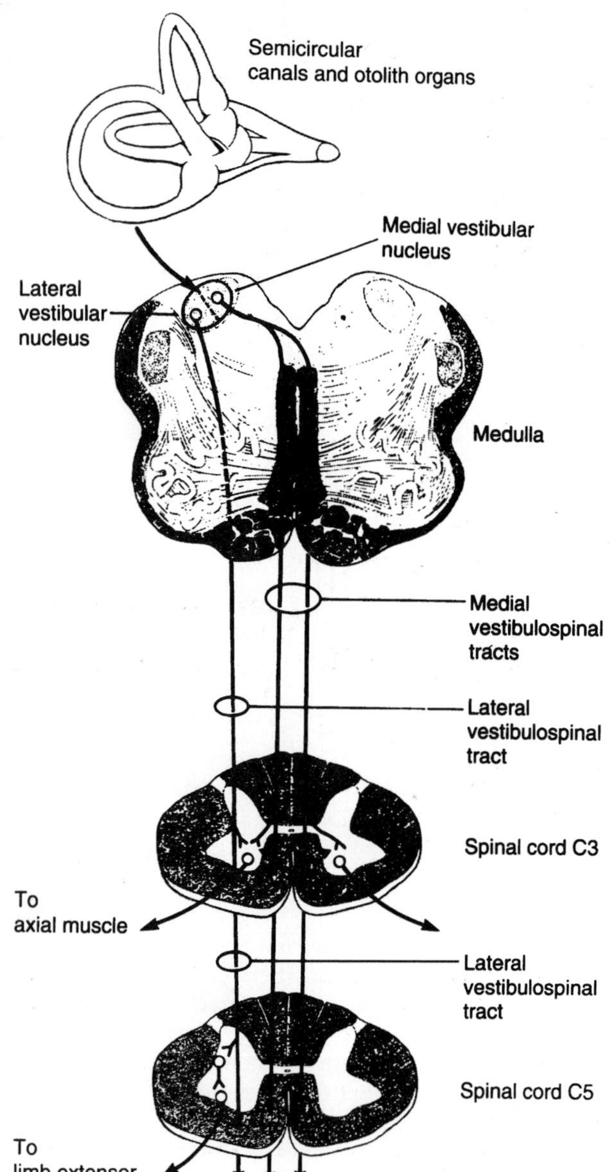

FIGURE 15–19. The vestibulospinal tract. The inputs from the lateral vestibulospinal tract to the alpha and gamma motor neurons excite antigravity axial muscles. The medial vestibulospinal tract terminates in the cervical and upper thoracic segments to mediate reflex head movements in response to vestibular stimuli. (From Kandel ER, Schwartz JH, Jessell TM: Principles of Neural Science. Norwalk, CT, Appleton & Lange, 1991.)

Before actual testing of muscle strength begins, simple observation may disclose asymmetries in muscle bulk of the extremities or more focal atrophy of specific muscles or muscle groups. The upper extremities should be inspected in both the pronated and supinated positions, which is especially important to appreciate differences in the extensor and flexor compartments of the forearm. The lower extremities should be observed from the front and the back while the patient is standing.

If a significant asymmetry or focal atrophy is apparent, the bulk of the muscle groups in the arm, forearm, thigh, and leg can be measured objectively by measuring the girth and comparing sides. The point at which the circumference is to be measured is marked with a ballpoint pen, usually at the point of greatest estimated girth. To find the same site on the opposite limb, the distance to the closest bony landmark is measured, and that measurement is used on the opposite limb to obtain precise symmetrical measurements. Muscle bulk is usually greater in the dominant limb; a difference of 1.0 cm is accepted as within the range of normal in the leg and thigh, and 0.5 cm is acceptable in the forearm and arm.

In most cases, a significant difference indicates hypotrophy of the smaller side. However, in some cases, the difference may be the result of an unusual hypertrophy or pseudohypertrophy in patients with muscular dystrophy. Pseudohypertrophy in a patient with muscular dystrophy is generally symmetrical and most commonly involves the calves. Therefore, any disparity in muscle bulk between the upper and lower extremities should also be sought. During the inspection of muscle bulk, one should also look for fasciculations. The ease with which fasciculations may be seen depends on how much subcutaneous tissue is present. In thin elderly men with suspected amyotrophic lateral sclerosis, the shoulder girdle and pectoral muscles are often a good place to look for fasciculations. In patients with more subcutaneous adipose tissue, the first dorsal interosseous muscle of the hand is better. Forcible contraction or percussion of the muscle may increase the frequency of the fasciculations.

Fasciculations are a feature of disorders of the anterior horn cell or root compression. Therefore, fasciculations are often viewed as an ominous sign. They need not be because they are commonly experienced as a benign phenomenon in the absence of any disorder of the motor neuron or spinal nerve roots.[27] Fasciculations of a benign nature can generally be distinguished from fasciculations secondary to lower motor neuron disease by several features. They have a predilection for males and for certain muscle groups, especially the calves and thighs. When they occur in the arm muscles, they tend to be seen as a repetitive twitch in the same muscle fascicle as opposed to the random nonstereotyped twitches of many parts of the muscle seen in patients with anterior horn cell disease. Benign fasciculations in the calves are more difficult to distinguish clinically because they may be frequent and multiple and have a more malignant appearance. However, there is no associated weakness or atrophy of the affected muscles with benign fasciculations. Electrophysiologically, a benign fasciculation appears like a normal motor unit; there are no other features of denervation in the muscle. A malignant fasciculation in a patient with motor neuron disease is more complex and has a longer duration and a higher amplitude.[28] The predilection toward benign fasciculations in males tends to be familial and increases progressively with age.

Assessment of Tone

Muscle tone is assessed by asking the patient to relax completely while the examiner moves each joint through the full range of flexion and extension. Patients vary in their ability to relax. Generally, it is easier for them to relax the lower extremities in the sitting position, whereas the upper limbs can be examined in either the sitting or lying position. Some patients, especially mildly demented elderly people, find it difficult not to voluntarily help move the limb in the desired direction. In a completely relaxed patient, no resistance should be felt at the wrist and elbow, and minimal resistance at the shoulder, knee, and ankle. It is very important to compare sides because a minimal but pathological increase in

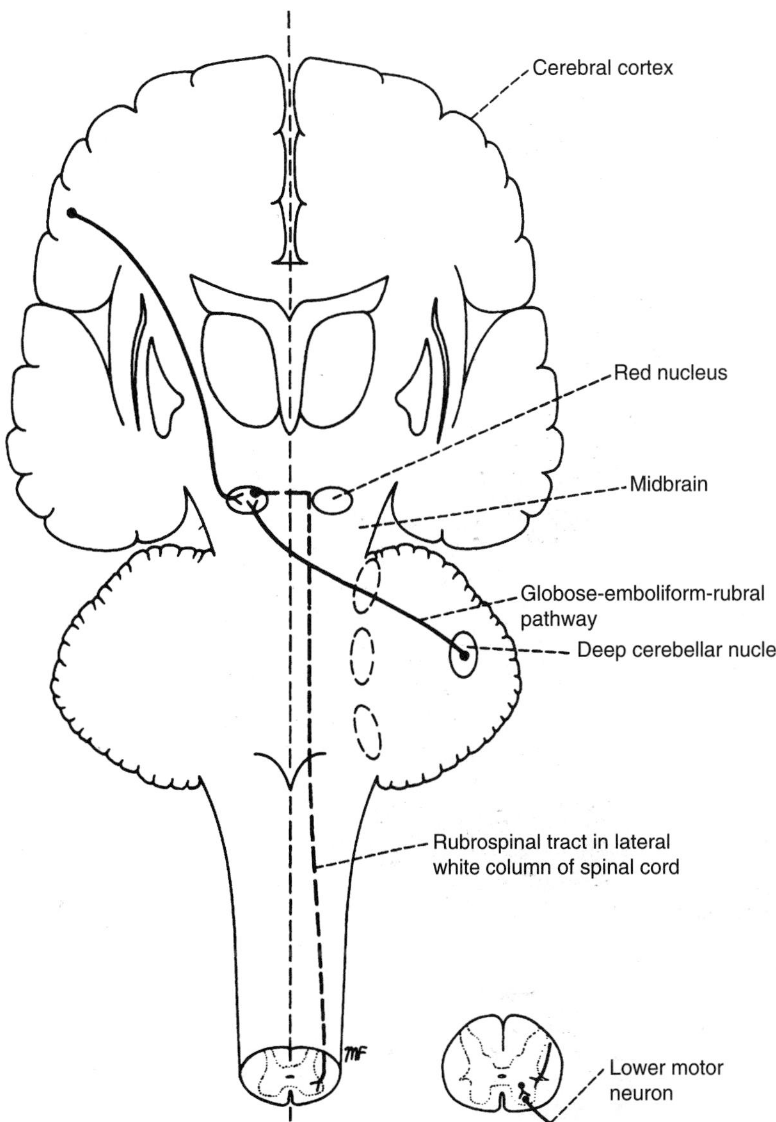

FIGURE 15–20. The rubrospinal tract. (From Snell RS: Clinical Neuroanatomy for Medical Students. Boston, Little, Brown & Co., Inc., 1987.)

tone may initially be considered normal until one compares it with the normal side. The degree of relaxation varies from patient to patient, and any change from normal is necessarily somewhat subjective. In assessing tone, it is also important to recognize that patients with non-neurological disease, specifically pain or bone or joint abnormalities, may demonstrate resistance to passive movement, thus confounding the examination.

Flaccidity, in particular, may be difficult to judge.[29] Certain maneuvers may be helpful in showing a difference from one

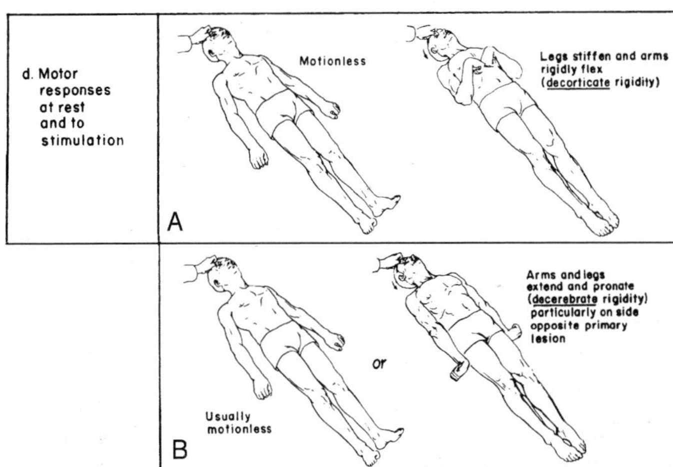

FIGURE 15–21. Decorticate *(A)* and decerebrate *(B)* posturing. (From Plum F, Posner JB: Diagnosis of Stupor and Coma. Philadelphia, F.A. Davis, 1980.)

side to the other. For example, flexion of the wrist can be compared by noting the distance the thumb can be brought to the flexor aspect of the forearm. Another maneuver is to shake the forearm and observe the floppiness of the movements of the hand at the wrist, or, with the arms raised overhead, compare the degree of flexion or limpness of the wrist on each side. The lower extremities can be tested by rapidly flexing the thigh after instructing the patient to let the leg flop. The sudden flexion of the thigh raises the knee. In a patient with normal tone, the heel may come off the bed slightly and transiently and then drag along the sheet as the thigh is flexed. The heel of the flaccid leg will be dragged across the bed from the very beginning, while the spastic leg will jerk upward and the heel may never fall back to the bed.

In assessing *hypertonus*, one must differentiate between spasticity and rigidity. In *spasticity*, the distribution of increased tone is very specific for the upper and lower extremities. The flexors of the arm (primarily the biceps) and the extensors and adductors of the leg display a greater increase in tone. This can be vividly seen in the classic hemiplegic posture in which the arm is flexed at the elbow and wrist and adducted against the chest while the leg is stiffly extended and the foot is inverted and flexed in a plantar direction. One can see spasticity in the adductors of the leg in the tendency of the hemiplegic leg to "scissor" over the good leg; this scissoring is most easily seen in a patient with spastic paraplegia. When the patient is lying down, the increase in tone in the adductors of the thigh can be felt by rapidly rotating the thigh back and forth to detect the increase in tone when the thigh is rotated externally.

The difference in tone in the flexors of the arm and the extensors of the leg can also give rise to the *spastic catch*, or the clasped knife phenomenon. This is a manifestation of the heightened stretch reflex that occurs in patients with lesions of the upper motor neuron pathways. By rapidly flexing and extending the elbow or knee, a sudden stretch is put on the muscle by lengthening it. The reflex contraction resists this lengthening and is sometimes referred to as the *lengthening reaction*. It is felt as a catch or interruption in the velocity of extension at the elbow or flexion at the knee. It is important to extend the elbow or flex the knee rapidly because the rate of stretch is important in eliciting the maximum response. The muscle spindles are maximally activated with a rapid stretch. Even with a very rapid stretch, a free interval occurs at the start of the movement, followed by the resistance. As the muscle is lengthened further, the resistance gives way, a process that has been compared to opening the blade of a clasped knife.

In contrast to spasticity, *rigidity* involves an equal increase in tone in the flexors and extensors. The increase in tone is felt throughout the range of movement, and has been compared to bending a lead pipe. As the rigidity increases, it becomes more difficult to rapidly flex and extend the joint. In fact, it may be easier to feel the rigidity with slower movements. It is important, however, to flex and extend the joint repetitively because the rigidity may gradually build up in intensity with repeated motion. Often the rigidity is not felt as a continuous smooth change, as implied by the terms plastic or lead pipe. Instead, a rapid and rhythmical succession of catches and releases occurs that has been compared to a lever jumping from one cog to another in the turning of a cog wheel, hence the term cog wheel rigidity. The physiological explanation for cog wheeling and rigidity is still being debated; current evidence favors a disturbance in the long-loop stretch reflex (see earlier discussion of muscle tone in the section, Gamma Motor Neuron). It is important to note that the phenomenon of cog wheeling can occur in patients with *essential or familial tremor* in the presence of normal tone and may be confused with parkinsonism. In these instances, the clinician feels the alternate activation of the flexors and extensors that produce the tremor, but does not feel the hypertonicity.

The *gegenhalten phenomenon* is not a true increase in muscle tone but a pseudovoluntary resistance by the patient against any passive movement of the limb. Each attempt at moving the limb by the examiner is met with an equal and opposing force. This can give rise to the appearance of increased tone. It is involuntary to the extent that the patient has great difficulty in voluntarily suppressing the urge to resist. Gegenhalten is usually associated with diffuse cerebral disease and dementia.

Assessment of Strength

The strength of a movement can be measured according to certain criteria; the most commonly used scale is that devised by the Medical Research Council[30] (Table 15–1). The grade assigned to the muscle is the maximum force generated by an effort to move the involved body area. Judgment of the presence of mild weakness depends on making appropriate comparisons, one arm versus the other, or the arms versus the legs, or extension versus flexion. The examiner should always look for patterns of weakness and compare the weak limb or muscle against the normal one in the same individual. Of course, if the weakness is generalized, judgment must be based on an estimate of the power normally generated by the age and bulk of the muscle.

More objective measurements can be made with the use of specially designed instruments to measure force. The only one widely used in clinical practice measures grip strength. Recently an electronic strain-gauge that measures maximum isometric force has also been used in clinical research trials for the treatment of amyotrophic lateral sclerosis.[31] Some degree of objective measurement can also be obtained through formal assessment by a specially trained physical therapist. These semiquantitative methods (semiquantitative because they require the full cooperation of the patient being examined) are not primarily used for diagnostic purposes but

TABLE 15–1. **The Medical Research Council Rating of Muscle Strength**

Scale	Muscle Strength
0	No contraction
1	Flicker or trace of contraction
2	Active movement, with gravity eliminated
3	Active movement against gravity
4	Active movement against gravity and resistance
5	Normal power

From Medical Research Council: Aids to the Examination of the Peripheral Nervous System. Memorandum No. 45. London, Crown Publishing, 1976.

rather for measuring changes that occur over time in response to some disease or treatment.

The most important purpose of strength testing is to discover whether there is a particular pattern of weakness that can be used to localize the lesion. Is it a hemiparesis, suggesting a hemispheric lesion; a paraparesis, which is consistent with a spinal cord lesion; or a proximal pattern of weakness compatible with a myopathic process versus a distal pattern that is consistent with neuropathy? (Table 15–2)

Even more important than tests of the strength of individual movements are tests of the ability of the patient to perform functional movements that bring out more subtle deficits escaping detection when muscle strength is tested against resistance. For example, a very subtle weakness of the leg may be noticed if the patient has some difficulty in hopping in one place. Because the leg and thigh muscles are so powerful, the patient's ability to walk, hop on either foot, and walk on the heels and toes is important. A mild upper motor neuron weakness may be betrayed by a slight circumduction or external rotation of the leg or even by an occasional scuffing of the sole against the floor. One may be able to differentiate an L5 from an S1 radiculopathy due to a herniated disc

TABLE 15–2. Patterns of Weakness That Aid in Localization

Distribution of Weakness, UMN or LMN Signs	Location of Lesion
Limbs and lower face on same side (spastic hemiparesis, UMN)	Contralateral cerebral hemisphere
All four limbs (spastic tetraparesis, UMN), speech (spastic dysarthria), swallowing with hyperactive jaw and facial jerks (pseudobulbar palsy, UMN)	Bilateral cerebral hemispheres
Hemiparesis (UMN) plus cranial nerve signs (LMN)	Brain stem
Tetraparesis (UMN) plus cranial nerve signs (LMN)	Brain stem
All four limbs (spastic tetraparesis, UMN)	Mid-or upper cervical cord
Lower limbs (UMN) and hands (LMN)	Low cervical cord
Lower limbs (spastic paraparesis, UMN)	Thoracic spinal cord Bilateral, medial motor cortex
All limbs, proximal > distal (LMN)	Muscle (myopathy or dystrophy)
Legs, distal > proximal (LMN)	Nerve (polyneuropathy)
Ocular muscles, eyelids, jaw, face, pharynx, tongue (LMN)	Neuromuscular junction (NMJ)
Jaw, face, pharynx, tongue; sparing ocular muscles, eyelids (UMN and LMN)	Motor neuron disease
Specific muscle groups in one limb (LMN)	Nerve root, plexus or peripheral nerve

UMN, Upper motor neuron; LMN, lower motor neuron.

if weakness of dorsiflexion of the foot reduces the ability to walk on the heels (L5 lesion), whereas a weakness of the gastrocnemius diminishes the ability to rise on the toes (S1 lesion). Walking may demonstrate a decrease in arm swing that is consistent with an upper motor neuron or basal ganglia lesion of one hemisphere.

A variety of functional tests of the upper extremities can be used to bring out subtle weakness or spasticity. Probably the most widely used test in the one in which the patient is asked to extend the arms in the fully supinated position while keeping the eyes closed. A mildly paretic arm gradually becomes pronated and sometimes flexed and drifts downward, showing the "*pronator drift*." Other tests not as well validated by widespread use are the digiti quinti minimi sign (hyperabduction of the outstretched fifth finger on the paretic side) and the forearm rotator sign (the patient rotates the forearms around each other; the paretic arm tends to stay fixed while the good arm rotates around it). Because paretic muscles move more slowly with reduced amplitude, some repetitive tasks, such as finger tapping or the forearm rotator test, are used to look for asymmetrical movements. However, interpretation of these tests may be more difficult because it may be hard to differentiate an abnormality from the bradykinesia of Parkinson's disease or even from problems with coordination secondary to cerebellar disease.

Because walking requires not just strength but the interplay of all the motor and sensory systems that are necessary for balance and the execution of motor programs, it is one of the most important parts of the neurological examination. A normal gait excludes a wide variety of neurological disorders (see Chapter 18). Abnormal gait patterns may provide powerful clues to the localization of a lesion. Upper motor neuron weakness is generally accompanied by spasticity, which produces a gait with a stiff jerky quality. The classic example of a lower motor neuron weakness is the steppage gait typical of a motor neuropathy in which weakness of dorsiflexion of the feet requires the patient to lift the legs higher to prevent the toes from scuffing the pavement. This appearance is accompanied by an excessive slapping of the forefoot against the floor. It may occur unilaterally in a patient with a pressure palsy of the peroneal nerve. The incomplete dorsiflexion of the foot combined with the slapping of the forefoot on the ground gives rise to the appearance of the "drop foot." The foot may also be inverted because of the unopposed action of the posterior tibial muscle. However, one must be careful to differentiate this condition from dystonia of the foot, which commonly produces a posture of flexion and inversion of the foot. The ability to dorsiflex the foot should be carefully examined in such patients; in patients with dystonia it will be normal, whereas in those with a peroneal palsy it will not.

A characteristic gait and posture are apparent in patients with myopathic weakness, in which the proximal muscles are much weaker than the distal ones. The weakness of the lumbar paraspinal muscles results in a hyperlordosis, and failure of the myopathic girdle muscles to fix the pelvis on one side when the other leg is being advanced gives rise to a ducklike waddling appearance. When a proximal myopathic weakness is suspected, other important functional tests include tests of the ability to rise from a squat or out of a chair, or to step up onto a stool or chair. Another helpful test in children with suspected muscular dystrophy is rising from a supine to a standing position. They cannot simply sit up and then push themselves to a standing position because truncal and hip girdle weakness prevents it. Instead, they roll to a prone position, push themselves up on all fours, and then quickly grab their thighs and walk up the thighs to a standing position (*Gower's sign*).

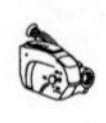

Fatigability

Normal fatigue associated with intense muscular contraction is accompanied by a reduction in the motor-unit firing rate, which is thought to be the result of a reduction in the excitatory drive to the motor neurons, which is a central mechanism.[32] The phenomenon of fatigability with normal levels of muscle activity is a specific characteristic of disorders of the neuromuscular junction and is accompanied by a decrement in amplitude, not frequency, of the muscle action potential. This phenomenon is demonstrated most easily with electrophysiological techniques in the clinical neurophysiology laboratory. However, there are methods for bedside testing of the ability to produce a repetitive forceful movement or tonic muscle contraction. Jolly devised a grip ergometer connected to a smoke drum that could demonstrate the classic decrement in force produced by each attempt by the patient to produce a maximum grip. The *Jolly test* has subsequently been modified, depending on the availability of material at the bedside and the ingenuity of the examiner. One readily available method is to inflate a blood pressure cuff, which the patient can grip and squeeze repetitively. The height of the excursions of the mercury manometer can be readily monitored, and the decrement in pressure produced by each squeeze is readily appreciated.

Such methods of quantitating fatigability are especially important when one is assessing the patient's response to the acetylcholinesterase inhibitor *edrophonium chloride* (Tensilon) as a test for myasthenia gravis. For example, one may test how many squats can be performed before and after the injection of Tensilon. The muscles or movements to be tested depend to a great extent on the patient's symptoms, but whenever possible, a movement should be chosen that can be quantitated as accurately as possible. Another quantifiable method is the length of time a posture can be held. For example, if the patient complains of ptosis or double vision, the length of time the patient can maintain upward vision before ptosis or diplopia occurs can be estimated. Another is the length of time a patient can hold the arms out before they fall below a horizontal 90 degrees. Sometimes the fatigability of the muscles involved in myasthenia gravis cannot be readily quantified. For example, weakness of the face has to be judged on a more subjective basis. Usually, the weakness is bilateral and symmetrical, and milder examples may escape notice until after Tensilon clearly produces a change in facial movements and expression. Reading a standard passage can help in measuring the time it takes for the speech to become mushy and dysarthric.

The Tensilon test is performed by giving incremental intravenous injections of 10 mg (1 mL) of the drug. A test dose of 2 mg (0.2 mL) is given first to monitor the heart rate (preferably with electrocardiography) to avoid bradycardia and vasodepressor syncope, which occasionally occur with higher doses. If this dose is tolerated and no definite improvement in strength occurs, another 3 to 4 mg is given. If there is still no response, the final 4 to 5 mg is given.

TABLE 15–3. **Scale for Amplitude of Tendon Reflexes**

Scale	Tendon Reflex Amplitude
0	Absent with reinforcement
1	Present but decreased in amplitude and velocity from the normal range and elicited with reinforcement
2	Normal amplitude and velocity without reinforcement
3	Increased in amplitude and/or velocity with spread to adjacent site
4	Increased in amplitude and/or velocity with spread to adjacent site and duplication of the jerk or clonus

Assessment of Reflexes

Tendon jerks are conventionally graded on a scale of zero to 4, with zero representing absent jerks and 4 representing hyperactivity with clonus. A commonly used scale with accompanying definitions is shown in Table 15–3. Superficial cutaneous reflexes are noted as present or absent. Tendon reflexes are elicited with a percussion hammer, of which many types are available. The two most commonly used are the hammer developed at the National Hospital for Nervous Diseases at Queen Square in London, and the tomahawk-shaped hammer used most often by American neurologists. The "Queen Square" hammer comes in a variety of sizes. The mallet should have sufficient weight and the handle should be long enough to easily create enough momentum to produce a sharp but nonpainful tap on the desired tendon. The sites at which the tendon reflexes are most commonly tested are listed in Table 15–4, which notes the myotome level of innervation involved in the reflex arc.

Finger flexor jerks may be obtained in two different ways. The more common method is the one described by Hoffman. The middle finger is held between the second and third fingers of the examiner and the distal phalanx is flicked downward by the examiner's thumb. A positive *Hoffman sign* is a reflex flexion of the fingers, most easily seen in the thumb. A more reliable way of obtaining this flexion reflex of the fingers was described by *Trömner*. The examiner lays the fingers of the patient's hand on his own and taps his own fingers. The sudden stretch on all of the patient's fingers elicits a more reliable response, which is a reflex flexion of the fingers that can be felt by the examiner and also observed in the thumb as in the Hoffman sign. Like the tendon jerk, the reflex is most apt to be obtained in patients with hyperactive reflexes. However, the reflexes need not be pathologically

TABLE 15–4. **Myotomal Innervation of Tendon Reflexes**

Reflex	Spinal Segment	Peripheral Nerve
Biceps jerk	C5–C6	Musculocutaneous
Brachioradialis	C5–C6	Radial
Triceps jerk	C6–C7	Radial
Flexor finger jerk	C7–C8	Median and ulnar
Knee jerk	L2–L4	Femoral
Ankle jerk	L5, S1–S2	Sciatic

hyperactive because this reflex can be seen in normal individuals. The reflex has clinical significance when it is asymmetrical and confirms a suspected asymmetry in the tendon jerks. The presence of a Hoffman sign by itself is not necessarily pathological and must be interpreted in the context of other tendon jerks and other signs of an upper motor neuron lesion such as ankle clonus and a Babinski's sign.

Reflex clonus, the repetitive contraction of a muscle or muscle group, is also obtained by putting a sudden stretch on a muscle. It is most commonly and easily elicited at the ankle. The Achilles tendon is stretched by rapidly dorsiflexing the foot and holding it in the dorsiflexed position. This can be done with the patient in either a sitting or lying position but is generally obtained most reliably in the supine position with the examiner holding the leg flexed at the knee and rapidly dorsiflexing the foot with an upward and outward motion. In the sitting position, it may be more readily elicited using a combination of a tap on the tendon with the hammer followed by holding the foot in a dorsiflexed position. In a patient with fully developed ankle clonus, repetitive plantar flexion of the foot can be maintained virtually indefinitely as long as an upward pressure is maintained on the foot. Patellar (quadriceps) clonus can be obtained by producing a quick forcible downward displacement of the patella, which puts a stretch on the patellar or quadriceps tendon. In patients with severe spasticity, one may also obtain clonus in the fingers, elicited by the Hoffman or Trömner maneuver, or in the jaw by tapping it with a hammer. Occasionally, one to two beats of clonus can be obtained at the ankle in normal individuals with naturally brisk reflexes. Generally speaking, however, clonus cannot be obtained at any site in the normal individual. The severity of clonus parallels the severity of spasticity and hyper-reflexia.

The presence of the flexor reflex in the form of extension or dorsiflexion of the great toe (i.e., the sign described by Babinski) is referred to in many ways. Some report it as the presence or absence of the *Babinski's sign* (see Fig. 15–13). To avoid confusion, some prefer to describe the response of the great toe to stimulation of the plantar surface of the outer sole. Thus, the plantar (or toe) response is described as flexor or extensor. Another colloquial way to refer to the presence of a Babinski sign is to describe it as an "up going toe." The preference of the author is to refer to it as a flexor or extensor plantar response.

The extensor plantar response is most reliably obtained with the method of stimulation described by Babinski. Others have described additional methods of stimulation that also produce the extensor toe response.[33] This reflects an expansion of the reflexogenous zone or receptive field when the upper motor neuron lesion is more complete and/or mature, especially in patients with spinal cord lesions. The most commonly used alternative to the Babinski method is the Chaddock maneuver, which consists of rubbing the lateral surface of the foot with the edge of a tongue blade or key from the heel to the little toe. The Oppenheim maneuver involves applying heavy pressure with the thumb and forefinger to the anterior surface of the tibia and stroking downward from the infrapatellar region toward the ankle. Bing obtained the extensor toe response by pricking the dorsum of the foot or great toe with a pin, and Gordon obtained it by squeezing the calf muscles. These other maneuvers are mainly useful in the patient who is very ticklish in whom it is difficult to differentiate spontaneous withdrawal from reflex responses. Another sign of upper motor neuron disease is the crossed adductor reflex.

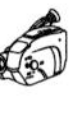

Diffuse cerebral disease can unmask reflexes normally present only in the infant. These are generally referred to as *primitive reflexes*. They are sometimes referred to as frontal release signs because they are most commonly seen in demented individuals with frontal lobe disease. The *snout reflex* is a component of the suck reflex in which there is a puckering movement of the lips in response to pressure or light tapping on the lips. The facial jerks are usually increased in this situation, and it may not be possible to differentiate between the two. The most convincing demonstration that this is a primitive reflex occurs when stroking the cheek elicits the same response it would in an infant or if visual presentation of an object moving toward the mouth produces the response ("visual suck"). The *grasp reflex* may also be unilateral or asymmetrical and reflects unilateral or asymmetrical frontal lobe disease. It is elicited by diverting the patient's attention and casually stroking the palm of the hand with two or three fingers. If the reflex is present, the examiner's fingers will be grasped with increasing force; the harder the examiner tries to extricate his fingers, the harder the patient grips. Patients may literally be lifted off the bed and the fingers pried open only with great difficulty after the examiner has put the arm back in a resting position. The *palmomental reflex* is obtained by scratching the palm of the hand and observing the reflex contraction of the mentalis muscle of the chin. This reflex is seen more often in demented individuals but may also be seen in normals and is too unreliable to be used as a diagnostic sign of dementia.

Stretch reflexes can also be obtained by putting a sudden stretch on muscles that lack a tendon. This is done by directly tapping the muscle with the aid of the examiner's fingers and the reflex hammer. The two best examples are the facial jerk and the jaw jerk. To obtain the *facial jerk*, the examiner first stretches the skin of the patient's nasolabial fold with the index and middle finger of one hand and then taps these fingers with the reflex hammer, producing a reflex contraction in the underlying facial muscles. A reflex contraction in the muscles of mastication, the *jaw jerk*, is more easily obtained by simply tapping the point of the chin with the reflex hammer. Usually, the examiner's fingers are put on the point of the chin and interposed between the blow of the hammer and the patient's chin.

As in the detection of weakness, it is the pattern of changes in the reflexes that is sought as an aid in localization. For upper motor neuron lesions, the distribution of hyperreflexia is the most valuable aid. The most common pattern is one of asymmetry between the sides because of a lesion in one cerebral hemisphere. The presence of symmetrical hyperreflexia, spasticity, clonus, and Babinski's signs indicates an interruption of the corticospinal tracts bilaterally, which could be a result of bilateral hemispheral disease or a brain stem or spinal cord lesion. The differentiation between these possible sites can usually be determined by associated signs (Table 15–5). If the disease is hemispheral, the corticobulbar tracts are also interrupted, producing a pseudobulbar palsy with spastic dysarthria, dysphagia, and increased facial and jaw jerks. Other signs of diffuse cerebral dysfunction may also be present such as dementia. If the lesion is in the brain stem, bilateral corticospinal dysfunction is often associated with

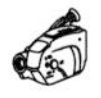

TABLE 15–5. **Clinico-anatomical Correlations for Disorders Affecting Strength and Reflexes**

Anatomical Site of Damage	Strength and Reflex Findings	Other Neurological and Medical Findings	Common Etiologies	Comments
Upper Motor Neuron Syndromes				
Pyramidal lesions				
Cortex and subcortex	Contralateral hemiparesis, hyper-reflexia, spasticity, Babinski's sign	*Cortex:* Left: aphasia, apraxia Right: constructional apraxia Homonymous hemianopia on paretic side *Subcortex:* No aphasia or sensory loss	Stroke, neoplasm	If parietal sensory cortex is affected, primary sensory modalities are reduced but not lost Integration of sensory information is affected, causing graphesthesia, extinction of sensory stimuli, and astereognosis
Brain stem	Large bilateral lesion: tetraparesis, bilateral hyper-reflexia, Babinski's sign Small lesions: contralateral hemiparesis, hyper-reflexia, Babinski's sign	Coma, decerebrate posturing Ipsilateral cranial nerve palsy	Stroke, trauma	Basis pontis lesions cause "locked in" syndrome: tetraparesis with paralysis of horizontal eye movements and jaw, face, and bulbar muscles, but consciousness and vertical eye movements and blinking are preserved
Spinal cord	Tetraparesis or paraparesis, bilateral hyper-reflexia, Babinski's sign, normal jaw jerk	Sensory level, no cranial nerve signs	Trauma, multiple sclerosis	See Table 15–13 for other spinal cord syndromes
Diffuse excitation of internuncial pool	Weakness of ocular, facial, or bulbar muscles (cephalic tetanus), diffuse hyper-reflexia	Rigidity, tetanic seizures	Tetanus, stiff-person syndrome	
Lower Motor Neuron Syndromes				
Progressive spinal atrophy syndrome	Progressive weakness, muscular atrophy, loss of tendon reflexes	No sensory symptoms or loss	Genetic	Classification based on hereditary pattern, age of onset, rate of progression and muscles affected—e.g., generalized infantile-onset lethal form: Werdnig-Hoffman disease; proximal childhood onset: Wohlfart-Kugelberg-Welander disease
Radiculopathy	Weakness of individual or combinations of muscles in one limb, reduction or loss of reflexes in myotomal pattern	Dermatomal sensory loss	Herniated intervertebral disc	

Plexopathy	Weakness and loss of tendon reflexes of muscles supplied by more than one spinal or peripheral nerve	Pain and sensory change in distribution of more than one spinal or peripheral nerve	Autoimmune, inflammatory, trauma, tumor	
Peripheral neuropathy, mononeuropathy	Weakness of muscles supplied by single peripheral nerve	Sensory change in distribution of single peripheral nerve	Entrapment, trauma, diabetes mellitus	See Table 15–11 for most common examples
Polyneuropathy	Symmetrical weakness and loss of tendon reflexes, distal before proximal; legs before arms	Symmetrical distal sensory loss; legs before arms	Diabetes mellitus, alcoholism, uremia	
Combined Upper and Lower Syndromes				
Motor neuron disease	Weakness, atrophy, and fasciculations of jaw, facial, bulbar, and limb muscles, hyper-reflexia	No sensory abnormalities; no weakness of eyelids or ocular muscles	Amyotrophic lateral sclerosis (ALS)	Tendon reflexes are especially quick and "snappy." Despite hyper-reflexia, Babinski's signs may not be present early in the disease
Myelopathy	Weakness, atrophy, fasciculations, loss of reflex at level of lesion (cervical cord); weakness, hyper-reflexia below level of lesion; bilateral Babinski's signs	Sensory loss below level of lesion	Multiple sclerosis, trauma	See Table 15–13 for various myelopathic syndromes
Neuromuscular Junction Syndromes				
Neuromuscular junction	Weakness of ocular, jaw, facial, and bulbar muscles and limbs; normal reflexes	No sensory abnormalities, fatigability (MG)	Autoimmune (MG); exogenous toxin (botulism)	Note that myasthenia gravis commonly affects ocular muscles (diplopia) and eyelids (ptosis), whereas ALS does not
Presynaptic cholinergic cell	Limb weakness, dysphagia, loss of knee jerks	Dry mouth, loss of taste, impotence	Association with neoplasia (paraneoplastic syndrome)	Autoantibodies against calcium channel
Myopathic Syndromes				
Muscle	Bilateral symmetrical, proximal weakness; reflexes are retained until weakness is severe	Skin rash (dermatomyositis)	Autoimmune or inflammatory (polymyositis); muscular dystrophy	

MG, Myasthenia gravis.

disturbances of consciousness or cranial nerve dysfunction. A cervical cord lesion produces hyper-reflexia and spasticity in the limbs with normal function in the cranial muscles and a normal jaw jerk. In the presence of diffuse hyper-reflexia of the tendon jerks, normal cerebral function and normal speech increase the probability that the lesion is at the level of the cervical cord. A normal jaw jerk therefore is helpful in confirming the localization. If the reflexes are normal in the upper extremities but abnormal in the lower extremities, the lesion is at the thoracic cord level. In contrast to exaggerated tendon reflexes in the presence of an upper motor neuron lesion, the superficial abdominal reflexes are absent. These reflexes also may be helpful in localizing lesions to the midthoracic cord if they are present in the upper quadrants and absent in the lower.

Lower motor neuron lesions are accompanied by a reduction or loss of both the tendon jerks and the superficial cutaneous reflexes. Once again, the distribution of the absent reflexes can define the localization of the lesion. For example, loss of one ankle jerk indicates a lesion of the S1 nerve root. A symmetrical absence of ankle jerks and a reduction in knee jerks indicate a neuropathy. A mild reduction in knee jerks with normal ankle jerks suggests a myopathy. Absence of cremasteric and anal reflexes reflects disease of the lumbosacral cord or roots.

Other Observations

Comparison of the contraction of the upper and lower abdominal muscles yields another sign that is valuable in localizing thoracic cord lesions. This comparison is made by palpating the muscles while the patient lifts the head off the pillow, causing contraction over the abdominal muscles. In a patient with a mid-to lower thoracic cord lesion, the upper abdominal muscles may contract while the lower ones remain flaccid. This maneuver may also result in an upward movement of the umbilicus, as noted by Lord Beevor, for whom this sign is named.

The presence of *atrophy* and *fasciculations* is further evidence of a lower motor neuron lesion. A focal or segmental distribution suggests a root lesion. Fasciculations are seldom seen with peripheral nerve lesions; therefore, atrophy without fasciculations is more compatible with a peripheral nerve lesion. If fasciculations are confined to the upper extremities, it is very important to check the tongue. Atrophy and fasciculations of the tongue suggest the presence of diffuse lower neuron disease, that is, amyotrophic lateral sclerosis, whereas atrophy and fasciculations confined to the arms, especially the intrinsic muscles of the hands, could indicate cervical cord pathology such as a tumor, spondylitic myelopathy, or syringomyelia.

Myotonia, which is impaired relaxation of muscle from its contracted state, can be demonstrated in two ways. The first is direct percussion of the muscle. In the normal muscle, the tap produces such a brief contraction and relaxation to the normal resting state that it is not seen. In a myotonic muscle, the contraction remains as a dimple for a few seconds before the contraction subsides. In a smaller muscle such as the thenar eminence, the contraction is strong enough to produce adduction of the thumb. Impaired relaxation can also be readily demonstrated after a forceful grip; the patient with myotonia has marked difficulty in relaxing and opening the fingers. Myotonia in the eyelids can be demonstrated by asking the patient to look upward and then rapidly look down; this produces a pronounced lid lag. The impaired relaxation of muscle in patients with myotonia is the result of impaired uptake of calcium by the sarcoplasmic reticulum.

Mirror movements are most often seen in children with cerebral palsy or as a rare inherited disorder. These movements are most readily demonstrated by asking the patient to produce a rapid alternating movement of the hand; when he does so, it will be mirrored by the same movement in the opposite hand. This phenomenon is also sometimes referred to as *synkinesis*.

Though the level of the patient's relaxation (or nervousness) can sometimes influence the state of the tendon reflexes, both the tendon and the superficial reflexes are the only truly objective attributes of the neurological examination, since the patient cannot voluntarily alter them in most cases. A sophisticated patient may be able to fake a Babinski sign, but an experienced observer can usually detect the fakery, which occurs very rarely. In contrast, estimation of muscle strength depends on the patient's cooperation and effort. Therefore, it is possible for the patient to voluntarily change the level of effort, thus producing the impression of weakness. It is important to recognize when the patient is not putting out a full effort or is intentionally trying to deceive the examiner for whatever reason.

The most common pattern of feigned weakness is a sudden collapse of the limb after an initial, often normal effort. It may be a phasic ratchet-like collapse as the muscle is tested, most commonly the biceps. Another pattern is seen when the arm is in the abducted position. When the arm is pushed downward, the patient bends his trunk to that side, giving the impression that his arm is being pushed downward when in fact the relationship with the trunk remains the same. If the adventitious nature of the weakness is not obvious, one can usually bring it out by testing the muscle strength rapidly and simultaneously in the arms starting at the shoulders and proceeding distally as rapidly as possible so the patient does not have time to think about what his response should be. As a result, the good side may collapse in unison with the bad side after an initial symmetrical effort. This is usually most easily demonstrated when testing abduction of the fingers.

With the patient lying supine, one can judge the effort put forth in the lower extremities by placing one hand between the heel and the examining table while testing the ability of the patient to raise the other leg off the table. With full effort, the heel on the table is forced downward to support the raising of the opposite leg. When full effort is used to raise the good leg, one can feel the normal downward pressure of the "weak" leg. When the weak leg is supposed to be raised, one may feel very little if any pressure under the leg with presumably normal strength, indicating that the patient is not trying to raise the weak leg. In fact, the pressure under the heel of the good leg may decrease. When this pattern of effort is present, it is referred to as a *Hoover's sign*.

It is important to identify *psychogenic paralysis* of a limb or a paraplegia, and certain observations and tests are helpful in revealing the true nature of such a weakness. A paralyzed arm that is held limply at the side will flail back and forth when the patient's shoulders are shaken back and forth. If, instead, the arm is observed to remain tightly held against the body, it has normal strength and tone. Hysterical paraplegia may be suspected by the ease with which the patient is able to roll over and move in bed and can be confirmed by the presence of normal reflexes. If the patient can walk, he exhibits behavior that indicates that he is markedly exaggerating the effort to take a step and in the process displays extraordinary strength and coordination.

ASSOCIATED NEUROLOGICAL FINDINGS

(See Table 15–5)

In addition to patterns of weakness and reflex changes, clinical findings in other neural systems will confirm or further help in localizing the source of the weakness.

Cerebral. A command center for conjugate gaze is located in each frontal lobe. When one is damaged, the unopposed action of the other causes deviation of the eyes to the side of the lesion and away from the hemiplegia. The motor cortex is very close to Broca's area, and a nonfluent or Broca's aphasia often accompanies a right hemiplegia of cortical origin. The sensory cortex is across the Rolandic fissure, and a cortical sensory loss often accompanies hemiplegia. Lesions in the hemispheral visual pathways will result in a contralateral homonomous hemianopia.

Cranial Nerves. Cranial nerve dysfunction and the pattern of involvement define the brain stem as the source of the lesion causing the weakness. Since the pyramidal tract is a midline structure in the brain stem, midline damage causes weakness and hyper-reflexia, usually bilaterally, and affects cranial nerves III and IV (midbrain), VI and VII (pons), and XII (medulla).

Cerebellar/Gait. Brain stem lesions causing weakness also commonly affect connections with the cerebellum, producing ataxia and dyssynergia. These components of cerebellar motor dysfunction may be difficult to see depending on the severity of the weakness. Proximal weakness can produce wavering when the patient puts a finger to the nose, which is very reminiscent of a cerebellar intention tremor. In this situation, one must examine the patient's coordination in finger and hand movements. One helpful test is repetitive tapping of the forefinger against the flexor crease of the thumb. Pyramidal and extrapyramidal lesions slow the rate of movement, but accuracy in hitting the target is unaffected, whereas in patients with cerebellar disease, the rate may be normal, but the accuracy is impaired and the rhythm of tapping is erratic. Rapid alternating movements of the hands are slow and regular in pyramidal and extrapyramidal disease; in cerebellar disease, the rate and rhythm are irregular and clumsy.

Walking is one of the most important tests in differentiating upper from lower motor lesions causing weakness. The spasticity caused by an upper motor neuron lesion can be seen in the very stiff jerky movements of the legs. Spasticity of the adductor muscles produces scissoring (i.e., a tendency for the legs to cross over one another from one step to the next). If the upper motor lesion is unilateral, the spastic leg is often circumducted with the leg extended at the knee while the arm is held in a flexed posture, that is, the typical hemiplegic posture. Distal weakness due to a lower motor neuron lesion produces floppy feet that slap on the floor and must be lifted high to prevent the toe from dragging and tripping the patient. Weakness of the hip girdle, most often seen in patients with myopathies, results in weakness of fixation of the pelvis and a waddling ducklike walk. Often the gait is widened to increase stability because otherwise the gait is made more unstable by the hip girdle weakness.

Sensory. The presence or absence of sensory symptoms and signs and the pattern and type of sensory change are very helpful in confirming which level of the motor system is involved in producing weakness. A relatively mild hemisensory loss affecting touch and proprioception more than pain and accompanied by impairment of stereognosis, graphesthesia, and two-point discrimination is characteristic of a lesion in the contralateral sensory cortex. A change in touch and pain sensation in the ipsilateral face and contralateral body is characteristic of a unilateral lateral medullary lesion (Wallenberg's syndrome). Spinal cord lesions often affect sensation on both sides of the body; the upper level of the sensory loss, especially in regard to pain and temperature, helps to define the level of the lesion. When half the cord is damaged, a pattern of loss of proprioception and vibration ipsilateral to the lesion and contralateral loss of pain and temperature sensation is characteristic of the Brown-Séquard syndrome. Central cord lesions produce a suspended sensory loss affecting pain and temperature sensation with sparing of the sacral dermatomes, and vibration and proprioception (see Chapters 19 and 20). Lesions of the conus medullaris or cauda equina produce loss of sensation in the perineum. Careful mapping of a more localized area of sensory loss in a limb can differentiate a dermatomal pattern of loss consistent with a spinal root lesion from a peripheral nerve distribution. An absence of sensory symptoms or signs indicates that the weakness results from disease in the motor neurons, muscle, or neuromuscular junction.

Autonomic Nervous System. At the bedside, some aspects of the autonomic nervous system can be tested. The most easily appreciated lesion is an impairment of sympathetic innervation to the cranial structures producing ipsilateral ptosis, miosis, and anhidrosis of the face (Horner's syndrome). Horner's syndrome may result from lesions of the descending sympathetic fibers in the brain stem and spinal cord in which the pattern of weakness, the presence or absence of cranial nerve signs, and sensory changes are more important in localizing the lesion. The presence of Horner's syndrome is more helpful in localization of a lesion when a spinal root or brachial plexus lesion is suspected. The preganglionic sympathetic fibers leave the spinal cord with the C8 and T1 spinal roots, which become the lower trunk of the brachial plexus. Therefore, lesions of the C8 or T1 nerve roots (e.g., herniated disc) or lower trunk of the brachial plexus (e.g., apical lung tumor) may be associated with Horner's syndrome. The postganglionic sympathetic fibers course along the carotid arteries into the cranium. Occasionally an occlusion of the common carotid artery produces an ipsilateral Horner's syndrome along with a contralateral hemiparesis.

The parasympathetic pupillomotor fibers from the Edinger-Westphal nucleus in the third nerve nuclear complex of the midbrain is impaired with lesions of the third nerve nucleus or nerve, which result in a paralysis of the pupillary sphincter, producing pupillary dilatation. Attention to autonomic function, especially sweating, can be helpful in defining the level of acute transverse spinal cord lesions. A loss of sweating occurs below the level of the lesion. Sometimes this can be appreciated by lightly rubbing the dorsal surface of the forefinger along the skin, starting below the expected level of the lesion and stroking upward; the finger slides easily over the smooth dry skin below the lesion but sticks momentarily as it meets the normal moist skin at the upper border of the lesion.

Orthostatic hypotension is sometimes described by the patient as weakness rather than as a presyncopal lightheaded fainting sensation. Diffuse autonomic dysfunction with orthostatic hypotension is a feature of multiple system atrophy (olivopontocerebellar atrophy and Shy-Drager syndrome). Orthostatic blood pressures are checked after 3 minutes in a recumbent posture and again after 3 minutes of standing. The pulse rates are also taken in the supine and standing positions. In patients with autonomic dysfunction, the pulse rate does not rise to compensate for the fall in blood pressure, whereas in those with hypovolemic orthostasis, a significant compensatory increase in pulse rate is seen.

Neurovascular. The neck vessels should be examined in patients in whom strokes are suspected. Evidence of small vessel disease in the form of poor pulses or trophic skin changes may suggest diabetes or vasculopathic causes of weakness.

ASSOCIATED MEDICAL FINDINGS

Examination of other organ systems is most useful in finding clues that may establish the cause of the weakness. Examination of the skeletal system can help to confirm localization of the lesion in certain circumstances. For example, the presence of a scoliosis may increase suspicion of a thoracic cord lesion. An asymmetry in the length or size of the limbs on one side suggests a deficit in growth during development that is compatible with a congenital hemispheral motor lesion.

Examination of the skin may disclose the café-au-lait spots or axillary freckling of neurofibromatosis, a hairy patch or dimple over the lumbar spine at the site of a tethered cord, or inflammatory skin changes compatible with dermatomyositis. If a stroke or transient ischemic attack is suspected, it is especially important to examine the heart for murmurs and arrhythmias and the carotid arteries for a bruit or pulse deficit. Inflammation or deformities of the joints may also limit the ability of the patient to exert full strength and give a false sense of weakness. The optic fundi should be examined for the presence of papilledema and lesions of the retina and macula that may be seen in patients with metabolic, developmental, or inflammatory diseases.

Evaluation Guidelines (Table 15–6)

A wide variety of tests are now available to the neurological clinician. The workup must be tailored to the situation and guided by a careful analysis of the neurological examination and history. The findings on the neurological examination localize the lesion to the nervous system and to the area where the attention should be focused. They also narrow the possible causes of the disorder. The list of possible causes is narrowed further by the history, which gives the clinician the temporal profile of the disease process.

Neuroimaging. Neuroimaging has become a powerful tool in confirming the localization of lesions. Magnetic resonance imaging (MRI) is the most powerful imaging tool available, but in some cases, computed tomography (CT) is equally effective (e.g., in some tumors) or better (e.g., bony abnormalities, hemorrhage) in visualizing the lesion. Because it has a much higher resolution and is not subject to artifact from neighboring bony structures, MRI is the test of choice for imaging the posterior fossa. MRI is also the tool of choice for visualizing the spinal canal except in circumstances (e.g., cervical spondylosis, vascular malformations) when myelography with CT may be superior for identifying the extent of the root or cord involvement. Conventional radiographs of the spinal column may be indicated when infectious, neoplastic, degenerative, or developmental disorders of bone are suspected.

Electrophysiology. Electromyography and measurement of nerve conduction velocities can be crucial in identifying, localizing, and determining the extent and severity of disorders in the lower motor neuron unit. The electromyographer still needs guidance from the history and neurological examination to tailor his evaluation to the appropriate region and choose the proper test to gain accurate and confirmatory observations most efficiently. With these tools, it is possible to differentiate an anterior horn cell disorder from a lesion of the spinal root or nerve or to differentiate disorders of the neuromuscular junction from primary muscle disease.

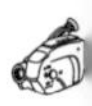

Body Fluid and Tissue Analysis. Examination of the cerebrospinal fluid (CSF) via a lumbar puncture has been one of the standbys in neurological diagnosis. Because it is virtually identical in composition to the extracellular fluid, changes in the chemical or cellular composition of CSF can reflect a variety of diseases. Analysis of the CSF is most useful in diagnosing subarachnoid hemorrhages or infections and inflammatory disorders that produce an excess of white cells or changes in immunoglobulin.

Tests for specific bacterial and fungal antigens are now available for diagnosing the more common bacterial (e.g., influenza, pneumococcal, meningococcal) or fungal (e.g., cryptococcal) meningitides. Polymerase chain reaction tests for certain viruses are now available. It is no longer necessary to perform a brain biopsy to diagnose herpes simplex encephalitis.

Immunohistochemical techniques have made muscle biopsy even more useful in diagnosing any disorder affecting muscle including mitochondriopathies. Nerve biopsies are usually less informative and are generally useful only in patients with inflammatory disorders affecting the nerves or their blood supply, or in those with amyloidosis for detecting the deposition of amyloid.

Except as a tool for making a diagnosis of a tumor or abscess, brain biopsy is used sparingly to diagnose rare encephalitides (e.g., Creutzfeldt-Jakob disease) or vasculopathies (e.g., granulomatous angiitis).

Neuropsychological Tests. If cerebral lesions are suspected, neuropsychological testing may identify evidence of a single, multifocal, or diffuse process. Special tests for aphasia, apraxia, and spacial orientation identify and lateralize cortical lesions.

TABLE 15–6. **Useful Studies for the Evaluation of Disorders of Muscle Strength and Reflexes**

Syndrome	Neuroimaging	Electrophysiology	Fluid and Tissue Analysis	Neuropsychological Tests
Upper Motor Neuron Syndromes				
Pyramidal lesions				
Cortex and subcortex	MRI or CT of brain: lesion contralateral to hemiparesis	N/A	CSF pressure	Lateralized right or left hemisphere dysfunction Left: tests of language, praxis Right: tests of construction, spatial orientation
Brain stem	MRI: local lesion	N/A	N/A	N/A
Spinal cord	MRI or CT myelography: extrinsic versus intrinsic lesion	Somatosensory evoked potentials (SSEP): delayed conduction with median or tibial nerve stimulation	CSF: protein, glucose, IgG, WBC, RBC	N/A
Decerebrate and decorticate posturing	MRI or CT scan: lesion in midbrain (decerebrate); bilateral hemisphere (decorticate)	N/A	N/A	N/A
Diffuse excitation of internuncial pool	N/A	EMG: continuous motor potentials	Blood and CSF: GABA, GAD autoantibodies (stiff-person syndrome)	N/A
Lower Motor Neuron Syndromes				
Progressive spinal atrophy syndrome	MRI: atrophy of spinal cord (late stages)	EMG: denervation-fibrillations, fasciculations, positive sharp waves, giant MUAPs	Muscle biopsy: grouped atrophy Blood: DNA analysis	N/A
Radiculopathy	MRI or CT myelography: compression of nerve root by disc or bony spur	EMG: denervation potentials in muscles supplied by affected root	Blood: FBS	N/A
Plexopathy	MRI: infiltrating mass	EMG: denervation of muscles supplied by multiple roots	Blood: FBS, ESR, SR, ANA, SPEP	N/A
Peripheral neuropathy				
Mononeuropathy	N/A	EMG/NCV: abnormal nerve conduction of affected nerve results in denervation of muscle supplied by that nerve	Nerve biopsy: inflammation, demyelination Blood: ESR, ANA, SPEP, FBS	N/A
Polyneuropathy	N/A	EMG/NCV: abnormalities of all nerves; legs affected before arms	CSF: protein Nerve biopsy: inflammation, demyelination, amyloid Blood: ESR, ANA, SPEP, FBS, B_{12}, T4/TSH, anti-nerve antibodies	N/A

Table continued on following page

TABLE 15–6. **Useful Studies for the Evaluation of Disorders of Muscle Strength and Reflexes** *Continued*

Syndrome	Neuroimaging	Electrophysiology	Fluid and Tissue Analysis	Neuropsychological Tests
Combined Upper and Lower Syndromes				
Motor neuron disease	MRI: cervical cord may be atrophic	EMG: denervation with giant MUAPs, normal NCV	Muscle biopsy: grouped atrophy Blood: CK normal to mildly elevated	N/A
Myelopathy	MRI, CT myelography	Somatosensory evoked potentials Visual evoked potentials (if multiple sclerosis is suspected)	CSF: protein, IgG, oligoclonal bands, inflammatory cells Blood: VDRL, B_{12}, long chain fatty acids	N/A
Spinal shock	MRI, CT myelography	N/A	N/A	N/A
Neuromuscular Junction Syndromes				
Myasthenia and botulism	Chest CT	EMG: decremental response to repetitive nerve stimulation	Blood: acetylcholine receptor antibodies Botulinum toxin	N/A
Eaton-Lambert syndrome	Chest x-ray, mammography, pelvic ultrasound	EMG: incremental response to repetitive nerve stimulation	Blood: striated muscle antibodies	N/A
Myopathic Syndromes				
Myopathy	N/A	EMG: small-amplitude polyphasic MUAPs	Skin/muscle biopsy: inflammation, mitochondrial abnormalities, necrosis and fibrosis, histochemical analysis Blood: CK, ESR	N/A

MRI, Magnetic resonance imaging; CT, computed tomography; EMG, electromyography; CSF, cerebrospinal fluid; WBC, white blood count; RBC, red blood count; GABA, gamma-aminobutyric acid; GAD, glutamic acid decarboxylase; DNA, deoxyribonucleic acid; NCV, nerve conduction velocity; MUAP, motor unit action potential; FBS, fasting blood sugar; SR, sedimentation rate; ANA, antinuclear antibodies; SPEP, serum protein electrophoresis; ESR,erythrocyte sedimentation rate; B_{12}, vitamin B_{12}; T4/TSH, thyroxine/thyroid-stimulating hormone; VDRL, Venereal Disease Research Laboratory; CK, creatine kinase; IgG, immunoglobulin G; N/A, not applicable.

Other Tests. Edrophonium chloride (Tensilon), a short-acting cholinesterase inhibitor, is used in the diagnosis of myasthenia gravis (Tensilon test). As explained earlier in the discussion of fatigability, a symptomatic muscle that is most amenable to semiquantitative testing is chosen for the measurement of fatigability before and after the intravenous injection of edrophonium. This test is sometimes done in conjunction with injection of a saline placebo. However, because muscarinic as well as nicotinic receptors are stimulated by the accumulation of acetylcholine in the synaptic cleft, this test is difficult to perform in a blinded fashion because intestinal cramping and muscle fasciculations in the eyelids are generally produced by the edrophonium. The muscarinic effects may also cause a bradycardia that is sufficiently severe to induce fainting, and rarely asystole occurs in what appears to be an idiosyncratic reaction. Therefore, a small test dose of 0.2 mL is given first to assess for an idiosyncratic reaction before the remaining 0.8 mL is given. The effects are short lasting but are long enough to assess strength in the muscles chosen for testing. A positive test (i.e., a significant improvement in muscle strength) is consistent with myasthenia gravis.

A forearm ischemia test is used to diagnose disorders of energy production in muscle. This test is especially useful in patients with deficiencies of enzymes that break down and utilize glycogen. The prototypical disorder that can be diagnosed by this test is McArdle's disease, or alpha-phosphorylase deficiency. Normally, in the presence of ischemia, muscle can shift to anaerobic glycolysis to satisfy its energy needs. In alpha-phosphorylase deficiency, glycogen cannot be used, and the muscle becomes weak and then develops an electrically silent cramp identical to that seen in rigor mortis. More sophisticated tests of oxygen utilization and energy production by muscle can be done in a human performance laboratory. Magnetic resonance spectroscopy is becoming more widely available for analyzing the level and distribution of high-energy phosphate compounds.

Physical therapists trained in evaluating the strength of individual muscles can be very helpful in systematically and semiquantitatively assessing and documenting changes in muscle strength over time. Pulmonary function tests are used to assess the presence and degree of weakness in the respiratory muscles in patients with disorders of the neuromuscular junction or acute inflammatory demyelinating polyneuropathy (Guillain-Barré syndrome).

Clinical Syndromes (Table 15–7)

UPPER MOTOR NEURON SYNDROMES

The upper motor neuron syndrome is marked by weakness, spasticity, hyperactivity of the tendon reflexes, and the presence of the flexor reflex (Babinski's sign). This pattern of motor disturbance occurs when there is an interruption of the descending projections from the motor neurons in the cerebral cortex and brain stem that modulate excitation of the internuncial pool of inhibitory interneurons and the alpha and gamma motor neurons. The net effect is a reduction of inhibitory influences and an increase in excitatory tone, producing exaggeration of the muscle stretch reflexes (hyperreflexia), increased muscle tone (spasticity), weakness, and disinhibition of the flexor reflex (Babinski's sign). Several clinical syndromes affect the upper motor neurons.

The upper motor neuron syndrome is primarily a reflection of interruption of the corticospinal (pyramidal) tract. Because the corticospinal tract extends from the cerebral cortex to the lumbosacral spinal cord, the pattern of weakness and associated reflex abnormalities depends on the site of the lesion along the considerable length of this pathway. Because there are two halves to the brain and consequently two corticospinal tracts, the pattern also depends on which side is affected or whether both sides are affected. Also, the clinical signs on the affected side depend on whether the lesion is above or below the decussation of the tracts in the cervical medullary junction. A unilateral lesion of the cerebral motor cortex will affect the other side of the body. Depending on the size of the lesion, it might affect only one limb or even a part of one limb. For example, a small stroke in the arm area could produce a brachial monoplegia. Because the leg area is on the medial side of the hemisphere at the apex of the motor strip, the leg areas from each hemisphere face each other in the interhemispheric fissure. Therefore, a *parasagittal lesion* in the interhemispheric fissure could affect both legs and produce a syndrome of paraparesis, simulating a spinal cord lesion. This is most commonly produced by a parasagittal meningioma (Table 15–8).

Hemiparesis most commonly results from a lesion in the contralateral cerebral cortex. Depending on its location in the hemisphere and the side affected, other associated signs can further localize the lesion (Table 15–9). Because of the considerable length of the corticospinal tract, hemiparesis can also result from lesions anywhere along its path (see Table 15–9). Because the axons from the motor neurons gather together in the posterior limb of the internal capsule (Fig. 15–22), a lesion in this location may be very small and still cause a complete hemiparesis (face, arm, body, and leg). Weakness that affects the entire side of the body equally without associated sensory signs (or aphasia if the lesion is in the left hemisphere) has been referred to by Fisher, in a clever redundancy, as a "*pure motor hemiplegia*."[34] Less commonly, small strokes (lacunar infarcts) can produce more focal weakness depending on the region of the internal capsule involved. Weakness in the face and arm can produce the *dysarthria-clumsy hand syndrome*.[35]

Lesions of the corticospinal tract as it traverses the brain stem also affect other structures in the brain stem, producing recognizable syndromes depending on the location and size of the lesion. Unilateral lesions of the pyramidal tract in the cerebral peduncle of the midbrain may involve the neighboring third nerve, red nucleus, or superior cerebellar peduncle (brachium conjunctivum). Lesions in this area are generally lacunar infarcts in hypertensive individuals that result from occlusion of small paramedian arteries supplying these structures. As the pyramidal tract enters the pons, the fibers become intermingled with other ascending and descending tracts in the basis pontis. It is still possible for lacunar infarctions to involve the pyramidal tracts primarily, producing a pure motor hemiparesis with or without facial involvement that is similar to the syndrome resulting from a lacunar infarct in the posterior limb of the internal capsule. The corticobulbar and corticopontocerebellar fibers are also present,

TABLE 15–7. **Selected Etiologies of Conditions That Affect Strength and Reflexes**

Etiological Category	Specific Etiologies	Chapter
Structural Disorders		
Developmental	Hydrocephalus; neural tube defects; segmentation, cleavage, and midline defects; neuronal migration defects	28
Degenerative and compressive	Degenerative disc disease; cervical spondylosis; ankylosing spondylitis; fibrous dysplasia; Paget's disease of bone; compressive neuropathies	29
Hereditary and Degenerative Disorders		
Storage disease: Lipidoses, glycogen disorders, and leukoencephalopathies	Gangliosidoses; sphingomyelinoses; cerebrosidoses; mucopolysaccharidoses; mucolipidoses; glycogen storage diseases; leukodystrophies	30
Amino/organic acidopathies, mitochondrial enzyme defects, and other metabolic errors	Maple syrup urine disease (MSUD); urea cycle disorders (UCD); propionic acidemia (Pa); methylmalonic acidemia (MMA); deficiency of phenylalanine hydroxylase (Pah); homocystinuria; glutaricaciduria type 1; subacute necrotizing encephalomyelopathy; Alper's disease; myoclonic epilepsy and ragged red fibers; mitochondrial encephalopathy, lactic acidosis, and stroke-like episodes; fatty acid oxidation disorders; Hartnup's disease; Menkes' disease; porphyrias	31
Chromosomal abnormalities and neurocutaneous disorders	Neurofibromatosis; tuberous sclerosis	32
The degenerative dementias	Progressive aphasia; progressive frontal lobe/frontotemporal syndrome; progressive perceptual motor syndrome; ALS-dementia complex; multiple system atrophy	33
Movement disorders	Multiple system atrophy; stiff-person syndrome	34
Ataxias	Friedreich's ataxia; congenital ataxias; autosomal dominant cerebellar ataxia	35
Degenerative motor, sensory, and autonomic disorders	Amyotrophic lateral sclerosis; spinal muscular atrophy; hereditary spastic paraplegias; dystrophinopathies; limb girdle muscular dystrophies; fascioscapulohumeral muscular dystrophy; scapuloperoneal syndrome; myotonic dystrophy; oculopharyngeal muscular dystrophy; Emery-Dreifuss muscular dystrophy; distal myopathies; hereditary sensory and motor neuropathies; hereditary sensory and autonomic neuropathies; Shy-Drager syndrome	36
Hereditary nondegenerative neuromuscular disease	Channelopathies; congenital myopathies; malignant hyperthermia; Brody's disease; congenital myasthenias; familial amyloid polyneuropathy; giant axonal neuropathy; Isaac's disease	37
Acquired Metabolic and Nutritional Disorders		
Endogenous metabolic disorders	Hypocalcemia; hypercalcemia; hyperthyroidism; hypothyroidism; diabetes	38
Exogenous acquired metabolic disorders of the nervous system: Toxins and illicit drugs	Arsenic; inorganic lead; manganese; inorganic mercury; organic mercury; organophosphate insecticides; organochlorine insecticides; snake and spider venoms; tick paralysis; chickpea (lathyrism); diphtheria; tetanus; botulism; cocaine; amphetamine analogs	39
Nutritional deficiencies and syndromes associated with alcoholism	Thiamine; niacin/nicotinic acid; cobalamin (vitamin B_{12}); pyridoxine (vitamin B_6); Strachan's syndrome; postgastroplasty polyneuropathy; Marchiafava-Bignami disease; alcoholic myopathy; alcoholic neuropathy	40
Infectious Disorders		
Viral infections	Meningitis; encephalitis; neuritis; myelitis	41

Nonviral infections	Acute bacterial meningitis; recurrent bacterial meningitis; abscess (bacterial, fungal, paracytic); intracranial thrombophlebitis; subdural empyema (bacterial, fungal, paracytic); extradural abscess (cranial and spinal epidural); myelitis (Lyme disease); neuritis (Lyme disease); syphilitic; dorsal root ganglion disease; cyst formation (echinococcus); myopathy (parasites); tick paralysis	42
Transmissible spongiform encephalopathies	Sporadic disease; familial disease; iatrogenic disease	43
HIV and AIDS	HIV-related neuropathies; HIV-related myopathy; progressive HIV-related encephalopathy; HIV-associated neoplasms; opportunistic infections; cerebrovascular complications	44
Neurovascular Disorders	Ischemic stroke; hemorrhagic stroke; subarachnoid hemorrhage; arteriovenous malformations; subdural hematomas; epidural hematomas; spinal cord strokes	45
Neoplastic Disorders		
Primary neurological tumors	Parasagittal meningioma; infiltrative CNS tumor	46
Metastatic neoplasms and paraneoplastic syndromes	Intraparenchymal metastasis; meningeal and ventricular metastases; spinal metastases; peripheral nerve metastases; paraneoplastic encephalomyelopathies; paraneoplastic motor neuron diseases; paraneoplastic neuromuscular junction and muscle disorders; paraneoplastic peripheral neuropathies	47
Demyelinating Disorders		
Demyelinating disorders of the central nervous system	Multiple sclerosis; neuromyelitis opica; isolated inflammatory demyelinating CNS syndromes; acute disseminated encephalomyelitis	48
Demyelinating disorders of the peripheral nervous system	Acute inflammatory demyelinating polyradiculoneuropathy; chronic inflammatory demyelinating polyradiculoneuropathy; monoclonal gammopathies of undetermined significance; neuropathy with multiple myeloma; neuropathy with osteosclerotic myeloma; motor neuropathy with multifocal conduction block	49
Autoimmune and Inflammatory Disorders	Inflammatory vasculopathies; rheumatoid arthritis; systemic lupus erythematosus; progressive systemic sclerosis; myasthenia gravis; dermatomyositis/polymyositis; eosinophilic myositis; inclusion body myositis; Sjögren's disease; Behçet's disease; Mollaret's syndrome; sarcoid	50
Traumatic Disorders	Acute head injury; spinal cord injury; whiplash injuries; trauma-induced brachial and lumbosacral plexopathies; mountain sickness; decompression sickness; lightning and electrical injuries	51
Epilepsy	Todd's paresis; epilepsies related to CNS lesions	52
Headache and Facial Pain	Complicated (hemiplegic) migraine	53
Sleep Disorders	Narcolepsy	54
Drug-Induced and Iatrogenic Disorders	Anesthetics; cholinesterase inhibitors; penicillins; aminoglycosides; sulfonamides; isoniazid; rifampin; ethambutol; amphotericin B; chloroquine; alkylating agents; methotrexate; vinca alkaloids; cisplatin; thiamine; pyridoxine; penicillamine; clofibrate; lovastatin and pravastatin; coronary artery bypass graft; cardiac catheterization; percutaneous transluminal coronary angioplasty; radiation damage; vaccinations	55

HNP, Herniated nucleus pulposis; AIDS, acquired immunodeficiency syndrome; CMV, cytomegalovirus; IC/MCA, internal carotid/middle cerebral artery; AIDP, acute inflammatory demyelinating polyneuropathy.

TABLE 15–8. **Anatomical Localization of Paraparesis**

Location of Lesion	Pattern of Weakness, Reflexes, and Associated Signs
Bilateral medial hemispheres (leg area motor cortex)	Spastic paraparesis with no sensory level
Thoracic	Paraparesis with hyper-reflexia of legs, normal reflexes in arms; thoracic sensory level
Lumbar	Paraparesis, loss of reflexes, double incontinence with flaccid bladder and sphincters

and a lacunar infarction in the basis pontis, especially one at the junction of the upper third and lower two thirds, may result in a *dysarthria-clumsy hand syndrome* that is similar to the clinical presentation of a lacune in the genu of the internal capsule. Another lacunar infarct syndrome is a homolateral ataxia and hemiparesis, which is more severe in the lower extremity. This also may be associated with dysarthria, nystagmus, and paresthesia from a lesion in the contralateral pons. Lesions (usually strokes) that include the pontine tegmentum produce a characteristic syndrome composed of an ipsilateral cranial nerve palsy and a contralateral hemiparesis (see Table 15–9). These uncommon clinical syndromes are described in more detail in Chapter 45.

TABLE 15–9. **Anatomical Localization of Hemiparesis**

Location of Lesion	Characteristics of Hemiparesis and Associated Signs
Cerebral cortex	Contralateral arm is affected more than leg or face; sometimes tongue (deviates to weak side) Left hemisphere: aphasia, apraxia Right hemisphere: inattention to left half of body, visual space; constructional apraxia Homonymous hemianopia on weak side Decreased graphesthesia, extinction of sensory stimuli
Internal capsule	Contralateral arm equal to leg; face may be spared No sensory loss or aphasia
Brain stem	Contralateral arm equal to leg plus ipsilateral cranial nerve palsy
Midbrain	Third nerve palsy (Weber syndrome)
Pons	Sixth and seventh nerve palsies (peripheral); ipsilateral conjugate gaze palsy possible (Foville's syndrome)
Medulla	Twelfth nerve palsy
Cervical spinal cord (hemicord)	Ipsilateral weakness of arm and leg, sparing face; ipsilateral loss of proprioception and vibration Contralateral loss of pain and temperature (Brown-Séquard syndrome)

Bilateral lesions of the basis pontis (infarction, hemorrhage, central pontine myelinolysis) produce the "*locked-in syndrome*" (Table 15–10). The patient is quadraparetic due to bilateral corticospinal tract involvement and aphonic due to involvement of the corticobulbar fibers to the lower cranial nerves, and occasionally his horizontal eye movements are impaired owing to bilateral involvement of the fascicle of the sixth cranial nerve as it exits the pons. Because the patient cannot move or speak, he may initially appear to be in a coma. However, because the tegmentum of the pons is spared, the reticular formation is intact, and the patient is awake. Vertical eye movements and blinking are still intact, and the patient is able to communicate via eye blinks.

Hemorrhages in the pons that produce tetraplegia owing to destruction of the basis pontis usually also affect the dorsal tegmentum, producing sudden coma, pinpoint pupils, ophthalmoplegia, hyperthermia, and progression to death. A more restricted hemorrhage may occur in the lateral tegmentum of the pontomesencephalic junction, producing a more restricted syndrome that includes small reactive pupils with the smaller pupil ipsilateral to the lesion, ipsilateral conjugate palsy due to involvement of the paramedian pontine reticular formation, ipsilateral ataxia due to involvement of cerebellar connections, and contralateral hemiparesis and hemisensory deficits. Occasionally, the ocular motor abnormality is an ipsilateral skew deviation or internuclear ophthalmoplegia caused by involvement of the medial longitudinal fasciculus.

Although we often refer to the corticospinal tract as the pyramidal tract and to weakness from a lesion as a pyramidal weakness, weakness resulting from lesions of the pyramids in the medulla is very seldom seen. The medullary pyramids are supplied by the paramedian arteries branching off the vertebral artery and, more inferiorly, from the interior spinal artery. Occlusion of these arteries can produce infarction of the ipsilateral pyramid, medial lemniscus, and hypoglossal nerve and nucleus, producing a contralateral hemiplegia with sparing of the face and ipsilateral paresis and atrophy of the tongue. Occasionally, there is a contralateral loss of position of vibratory sensation due to involvement of the medial lemniscus. Because the more dorsolateral spinothalamic tract is unaffected, pain and temperature sensation are spared. However, infarction of the medulla occurs much more commonly in the vascular supply of the lateral medulla, producing the *Wallenberg* or *lateral medullary syndrome*, which spares the pyramids (see Chapters 13, 14, 22, and 45).

Developmental malformations of the brain stem such as the Chiari malformations or tumors in the foramen magnum at the cervical medullary junction more commonly produce weakness by involvement of the medullary pyramids and the upper cervical cord at the place where they decussate into the corticospinal tracts of the lateral and ventral funiculi of the spinal cord. A spastic tetraparesis (generally the legs are more involved than the arms) occurs in varying combinations with weakness of the tongue and pharynx, nystagmus (due to involvement of the inferior cerebellar peduncle), and facial hypalgesia (due to involvement of the descending tract of the trigeminal nerve) (see Table 15–10). A syringomyelic syndrome occurs if central cavitation of the cord is present. This characteristically produces a loss of pain and temperature sensation over the shoulders and a lower motor neuron syndrome of the upper extremities with weakness, atrophy,

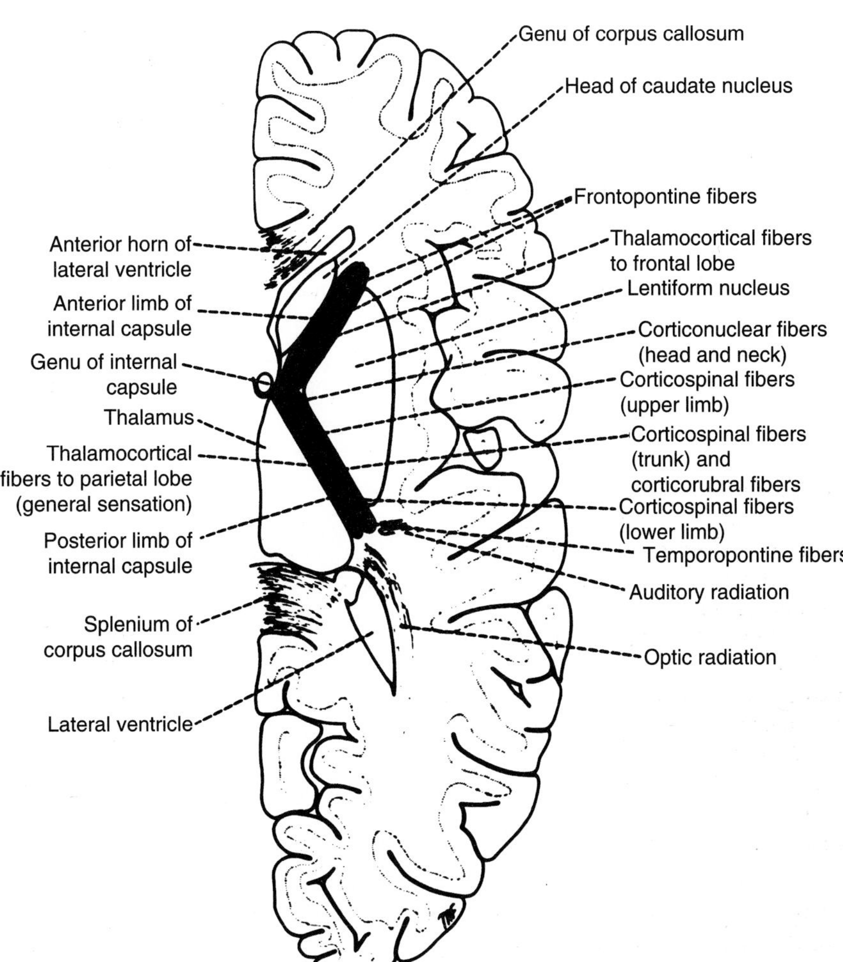

FIGURE 15–22. Cross section of the cortex showing the internal capsule and its fiber arrangements. (From Snell RS: Clinical Neuroanatomy for Medical Students. Boston, Little, Brown Co., Inc., 1987.)

TABLE 15–10. **Anatomical Localization of Tetraparesis**

Location of Lesion	Pattern of Weakness, Reflexes, and Associated Signs
Bilateral cerebral hemispheres	Tetraparesis, spastic dysarthria, dysphagia with hyper-reactive jaw and facial jerks (pseudobulbar palsy), decorticate posturing (large acute lesions)
Midbrain	Tetraparesis, coma, mid-size poorly reactive pupils, decerebrate posturing
Basis pontis	"Locked-in" syndrome; tetraparesis, paralysis of horizontal eye movements, jaw, face, pharynx, and tongue muscles; preservation of eye blink, vertical eye movements, consciousness
Cervicomedullary junction	Tetraparesis with or without weakness of pharynx and tongue
High cervical	Tetraparesis, no cranial nerve palsies, normal jaw and facial jerks
Midcervical	Tetraparesis with preservation of shoulder movements

fasciculations, and loss of reflex. The distribution of the weakness and loss of reflex depends on which segments of the cervical spinal cord are involved.

The characteristic pattern of weakness seen in patients with upper motor neuron lesions of the spinal cord is weakness combined with appropriate reflex changes on both sides of the body with no signs of cerebral, cortical, or brain stem dysfunction. The level of the lesion is defined by whether the arms are involved (cervical cord) or just the legs (thoracic cord). More exact definition of the level of the lesion is made by noting the distribution of lower motor neuron involvement if the lesion is in the cervical cord or by noting the sensory level resulting from involvement of the ascending sensory tracts with lesions in either the thoracic or cervical cord. These characteristic clinical syndromes are described in more detail in the later section on combined upper and lower motor neuron lesions (see Table 15–7).

SYNDROME OF DIFFUSE EXCITATION OF INTERNUNCIAL POOL

When the inhibitory tone in gamma motor neurons provided by the inhibitory interneuron in the internuncial pool is removed, the spontaneous excitability of the lower motor neurons is unleashed. This phenomenon of unrestrained excitation of contraction of the skeletal muscles is known as *tetanus*. In the most common generalized form of tetanus, all skeletal muscle, both agonists and antagonists as well as diaphragm, paravertebral, and respiratory muscles, contract uncontrollably in paroxysms of painful muscle spasms (tetanic seizures) (see Table 15–5). In the absence of any inhibitory check, any environmental stimuli increase the intensity of the paroxysms, preventing coordinated respiratory movements. Tetanus may remain localized to the area of the wound (local, or cephalic, tetanus if wound is of the face or head). Tetanus is produced by impairment of function of the neurotransmitters employed by the inhibitory interneurons (i.e., GABA and glycine). Tetanus toxin blocks glycine receptors. Antibodies against glutamic acid decarboxylase (GAD), the GABA-synthesizing enzyme, are produced by certain cancers and diabetes mellitus, resulting in the *stiff-person syndrome*[36] (see Chapter 34).

LOWER MOTOR NEURON SYNDROMES

Diseases of the lower motor neuron may affect the cell body itself in the anterior spinal gray or its axon as it leaves the spinal cord in the spinal root and becomes a peripheral nerve. Signs of disease of the lower motor neuron include muscular weakness, atrophy, fasciculations, and loss of tendon reflexes.

Progressive Spinal Muscular Atrophy Syndromes

There may be selective degeneration of the anterior horn cells of the spinal cord or brain stem or both. This results in a progressive weakness and wasting of muscle and loss of tendon reflexes. The upper motor neuron is not affected. The spinal muscular atrophies are genetic diseases of childhood and adolescence and, less commonly, adulthood. Regardless of whether they are recessive or dominant, the defect is linked to the same region on chromosome 5. In addition to patterns of heredity, clinical classifications are based on age of onset, rate of progression, and the muscles affected.[37] The infantile-onset form (*Werdnig-Hoffman disease*) is the most severe (lethal) form and is recessive. The later-onset, more benign forms are more likely to be dominant. The variety that affects the proximal musculature and simulates muscular dystrophy is known as the *Wohlfart-Kugelberg-Welander syndrome*. The distal musculature is preferentially affected in various combinations with the ocular and bulbar muscles in *Kennedy's syndrome*.

Lower motor neuron disorders that are restricted to certain cranial nerve nuclei or combinations are much less common. The *Möbius syndrome*, which affects the sixth and seventh cranial nerves, appears to be a failure of development of the motor neurons and presents as a congenital disorder. The progressive bulbar palsy of *Fazio-Londe* is a rare fatal disease that affects all motor nuclei of the brain stem.

Radiculopathy Syndromes

Lesions of the spinal nerves and roots produce weakness, atrophy, and sometimes fasciculations in the muscles innervated by the affected root or, in some cases, multiple roots. Localization of the specific nerve root affected by the lesion requires a knowledge of each group of muscles supplied by a single anterior spinal root (*myotome*) and each cutaneous area supplied by the posterior spinal root (*dermatome*). Differentiation of these syndromes from peripheral nerve or plexus lesions thus depends on the distribution of the motor and sensory signs and whether the signs conform to those produced by a particular myotome or dermatome. Root lesions may interrupt the afferent or efferent arc of the phasic stretch reflex and thus affect tendon jerks. Thus, a reduction or loss of a reflex is very helpful in localizing the root involved. Table 15–4 correlates the reflex in the cervical or lumbosacral root subserving that reflex.

The spinal nerve roots may be injured directly by trauma or compressed by lesions such as tumors or herniated discs. The most common radiculopathies affect the fifth and sixth cervical roots and the fifth lumbar and first sacral roots, since those are the roots most often compressed by herniated discs. Because muscles are innervated by more than one spinal nerve root, it may be difficult to differentiate a C5 from a C6 or a C6 from a C7 root injury. For example, a C6 root lesion may depress either the biceps or triceps reflex. Differentiating a C5 from a C7 root lesion is easier because the C5 lesion reduces the biceps jerk, whereas the C7 reduces the triceps. The same muscles are also the weakest. Therefore, one must also use the distribution of pain and sensory loss as a guide to supplement the motor signs and provide a pattern of motor and sensory change that can be assigned to one spinal segment.

In the lower extremity, the differentiation of an L5 from an S1 root lesion is most readily made by watching the patient walk on the heels and toes. Weakness of dorsiflexion (difficulty in walking on the heels) is usually due to an L5 root lesion, reflecting the fact that the anterior tibial muscle receives its major innervation from that segment. Difficulty in walking on the toes due to weakness of the gastrocnemius muscles reflects the fact that its major innervation is provided by the S1 root. The ankle jerk may be affected by either lesion but is more often abolished by the S1 root lesion.

Plexopathy Syndromes

Plexopathies are more difficult to recognize and localize than lesions of the spinal roots or peripheral nerves because the anatomy of the plexuses is so complex (see Figs. 15–6 and 15–7). Brachial plexopathies present with a variety of clinical syndromes that depend on the part of the plexus involved. Trauma is the most frequent cause of damage, which usually results from a traction, compression, or stretch injury of the plexus. The most common syndromes are summarized in Table 15–11. The brachial plexus is also subject to injury from radiation or malignancies, compression by tumors in lymph nodes or the apex of the lung, or immunologic attack (*"brachial neuritis"* or *Parsonage-Turner syndrome*). The best clue to the presence of a brachial plexopathy is a motor and sensory deficit that involves more than one spinal or peripheral nerve. The motor signs (weakness, atrophy, and loss of tendon jerk) are much more prominent than the sensory changes, which are often patchy and incomplete. Diffuse aching pain, sometimes quite severe, is often present.

Lesions of the brachial plexus most commonly affect the upper and lower trunks. The upper trunk of the plexus is affected most commonly, giving rise to paralysis and atrophy in muscles supplied by the C5–C6 roots that comprise the upper trunk (*Erb-Duchenne type*). This upper trunk palsy is most often due to traumatic hyperextension of the head and shoulder but can be due to direct pressure caused by carrying

TABLE 15–11. **Examples of Plexopathies Causing Weakness**

Plexopathy	Pattern of Weakness	Causes
Brachial		
Upper trunk (C5–C6)	"Porter's tip position"; biceps, brachioradialis jerks reduced or absent	Pressure on shoulder ("knapsack palsy"); brachial neuritis
Lower trunk (C8–T1)	Wrist and finger flexion, intrinsic hand muscles	Trauma, Pancoast's tumor of lung
Lumbosacral		
Lumbar segments (T12–L4)	Flexion, adduction, and eversion of thigh; absent knee jerk	Tumor, surgical trauma
Sacral segments (L5–S3)	Hip extension, abduction and internal rotation of thigh, flexion of leg and all movements of foot ("flail foot"); absent ankle jerk	Tumor, surgical trauma
Entire Plexus	Incomplete weakness of various muscles	Diabetes mellitus, idiopathic plexitis

heavy objects (knapsack palsy). The upper trunk is the part of the plexus most commonly affected by an idiopathic inflammatory neuritis (Parsonage-Turner syndrome). The *lower brachial plexopathy (Dejerine-Klumpke type)* is usually the result of trauma to the lower trunk of the plexus, which contains the eighth cervical and first thoracic roots. It is the plexus lesion most often associated with an infiltrating tumor from the apex of the lung (Pancoast tumor). Because the sympathetic fibers destined for the superior cervical ganglion exit the spinal cord with the first thoracic root, *Horner's syndrome* (ptosis, miosis, and anhidrosis) may result; if present, it can be a helpful confirmatory sign.

Like lesions of the brachial plexus, a lumbosacral plexopathy is recognized by deficits in the distribution of multiple spinal and peripheral nerves in the lower extremity (see Table 15–11). Also like the brachial plexus, the lumbosacral plexus is affected by idiopathic inflammatory neuritis, radiation, and infiltrating neoplasms. It is less likely to be injured by trauma than the brachial plexus, but pelvic hematomas in the psoas muscle resulting from anticoagulation and surgical trauma are more common. Lesions of the lumbar segments produce weakness of all movements of the thigh with reduction or loss of the patellar tendon jerk. Lesions of the sacral portion of the plexus result in a weakness of the foot and flexion of the knee with reduction or loss of the ankle jerk. Because most of the motor output of the lumbar portion of the plexus is contained in the femoral nerve and the output of the sacral portion is found in the sciatic nerve, it may be difficult to distinguish lumbosacral plexus lesions from lesions of their respective major peripheral nerves. To distinguish a lumbar plexus lesion from a femoral neuropathy, a diligent search should be made for weakness of the adductor muscles innervated by the obturator nerve or of sensory loss in the inguinal region or over the genitalia, which are outside the distribution of the femoral nerve. Weakness of abduction and internal rotation of the thigh and of hip extension, or sensory loss on the posterior thigh in the distribution of the posterior femoral cutaneous nerve, helps to distinguish a lesion of the sacral plexus from a sciatic palsy, which lacks these signs.

Peripheral Neuropathy and Mononeuropathy Syndromes

Interruption of the motor fibers in a motor or mixed nerve leads to weakness or paralysis and atrophy of the muscles innervated by that nerve. Fasciculations are less likely to occur in peripheral nerve lesions than in root or anterior horn cell lesions. Table 15–12 lists the peripheral nerves most often affected by lesions, the muscles they supply, and any

TABLE 15–12. **Examples of Common Neuropathies Causing Weakness**

Neuropathy	Patterns of Muscle Weakness and Reflex Changes	Common Causes
Long thoracic nerve (C5–C7)	Winged scapula (serratus anterior)	Pressure on shoulder, weight lifting
Axillary nerve (C5–C6)	Abduction of arm (deltoid)	Dislocated shoulder, brachial neuritis
Musculocutaneous nerve (C5–C7)	Flexion of forearm (biceps), biceps jerk	Infarction due to vasculopathy (DM, PAN)
Median nerve (C5–T1)	Abduction (abductor pollicis brevis, opponens pollicis) and opposition of thumb	Entrapment—pronator or carpal tunnel syndrome
Ulnar nerve (C7–T1)	Intrinsic muscles of hand except those innervated by median nerve; "claw hand"	Pressure at elbow, entrapment in cubital tunnel
Radial nerve (C5–C8)	Extensors of wrist and fingers, "wrist drop" triceps, triceps jerk (if compressed in axilla)	Pressure in axilla ("crutch palsy") or spiral groove of humerus ("Saturday night palsy")
Femoral nerve (L2–L4)	Flexion of thigh, leg extension (psoas, quadriceps), knee jerk	Surgical trauma, DM
Common peroneal nerve (L4–L5)	Dorsiflexors and everters of foot	Pressure palsy at fibular head

DM, Diabetes mellitus; PAN, polyarteritis nodosa.

stretch reflex subserved by that nerve. Because a muscle is generally served by only one peripheral nerve, the weakness and wasting in that muscle are generally easier to detect than in a root lesion because the same muscle is generally served by two or more myotomes. The localization is confirmed by the pattern of sensory loss, which in most cases differs from the segmental dermatomal loss secondary to a root lesion. Lesions of a single peripheral nerve are most commonly due to entrapment, trauma, or infarction of the nerve secondary to diabetes or an inflammatory vasculitis. When a single peripheral nerve is damaged, it is termed a *mononeuropathy*. *Mononeuropathy multiplex* refers to involvement of several major named nerves in more than one limb. This condition most often occurs in systemic diseases such as autoimmune vasculitis, especially polyarteritis nodosa and diabetes mellitus.[38]

In *polyneuropathy*, the essential feature is impairment of function of many peripheral nerves simultaneously, causing symmetrical loss of function starting in the distal extremities. The legs are almost always affected before the arms. Hyporeflexia or areflexia often precedes any overt motor or sensory symptoms. The ankle jerks are affected first and then the knee jerks before any change occurs in the reflexes of the arms.

Polyneuropathies may be mainly sensory, mixed motor and sensory, or primarily motor. The motor component begins as weakness and atrophy in the intrinsic muscles of the feet; atrophy of the extensor digitorum brevis is often the first helpful clue. If the motor impairment progresses, the leg muscles are affected next, producing weakness of dorsiflexion and plantar flexion of the foot. Only then may the intrinsic muscles of the hand be affected. Generally, the more proximal muscle groups are not affected unless a rapidly progressive disorder is present such as an *acute inflammatory demyelinating polyneuropathy (AIDP, Guillain-Barré syndrome)* or another neuropathy mimicking AIDP such as porphyria and acquired immunodeficiency syndrome. The common distal symmetrical and slowly progressive polyneuropathies are most often due to systemic disorders, especially diabetes mellitus, alcoholism, and uremia.

COMBINED UPPER AND LOWER MOTOR NEURON SYNDROMES

Motor Neuron Syndromes

Motor neuron disease refers to a group of disorders in which selective degeneration of both upper and lower motor neurons occurs.[39] *Amyotrophic lateral sclerosis* (ALS, Lou Gehrig's disease) is the prototypical motor neuron disease. Several varieties or subtypes are recognized based on the sites at which the motor neurons are first and most prominently involved. The spinal form most commonly affects the lumbosacral segments first, producing weakness, atrophy, and fasciculations in one leg as the initial manifestations. At the same time, the upper motor neurons are generally affected, so instead of loss of reflexes to accompany the atrophy and fasciculations, hyper-reflexia occurs, producing the characteristic combination of upper and lower motor neuron involvement. Onset of disease in the brain stem affects the lower cranial nerve nuclei, producing a *progressive bulbar palsy*. Lower motor neuron degeneration becomes evident by weakness, atrophy, and fasciculations of the tongue and weakness of voluntary palatal movement, while upper motor neuron involvement is shown by the very brisk gag reflex and jaw jerk. The otolaryngologist is often the first consultant asked to see the patient because a nasal voice and dysphagia are present. Occasionally, the upper motor neurons are selectively affected at the onset, producing a slowly progressive spastic tetraparesis and pseudobulbar palsy (primary lateral sclerosis). Often, an EMG can record the fibrillations, positive sharp waves, and giant action potentials typical of lower motor neuron involvement before the signs become clinically manifest. Regardless of the mode of onset, the disorder eventually involves the motor neurons of the entire neuraxis.

From a diagnostic standpoint, it is most important to differentiate ALS from potentially treatable lesions in the cervical canal that compress the nerve roots and spinal cord, producing a characteristic syndrome of lower motor neuron signs in the hands and upper motor neuron signs in the legs. Imaging of the cervical spine is important to rule out *cervical spondylosis* or tumor. ALS is confirmed by electromyographic demonstration of denervation in a combination of facial or bulbar muscles and lower extremities.

Paralytic poliomyelitis is now rare in the vaccinated western world. The neurotrophic polio virus attacks nerve cells in the hypothalamus, thalamus, brain stem, reticular formation, vestibular nuclei, and nuclei of the cerebellum, but the major hallmark of the disease is destruction of the lower motor neurons in the motor nuclei of the brain stem and anterior horn of the spinal cord. The severity and distribution of the bulbar and spinal paralysis is quite variable. The most common bulbar symptoms are weakness of the face, larynx, and pharynx. Spinal paralysis is more common than bulbar paralysis. Weakness develops rapidly, usually attaining its maximum severity in 48 hours, and is accompanied by coarse fasciculations. The tendon jerks may be hyperactive during the acute phase but then diminish and eventually are lost as the weakness of the limb muscles progresses. Limb weakness is often asymmetrical and patchy. Muscle atrophy is generally appreciated within 3 to 4 weeks of the paralysis and is permanent. In addition to the disability produced by the weakness and atrophy, progression of muscle weakness may occur many years after the acute paralytic illness (post-polio syndrome).

Myelopathic Syndromes

The *transverse myelopathy* syndrome interrupts the ascending tracts from below the level of the lesion and all descending tracts from above this level. Therefore, all motor and sensory function below the level of the spinal cord injury is lost. Trauma is the most frequent cause of complete loss of function at the site of the injury. In practice, many lesions are incomplete, although there is evidence of involvement of the entire cross-sectional extent of the cord. Demyelinating and inflammatory processes account for most examples of incomplete lesions and are often referred to as *transverse myelitis*. All sensory modalities are lost below the level of the lesion. There is often a zone of disagreeable dysesthesia at the uppermost border of the sensory loss. Radicular pain is common at the level of the lesion. If an infectious or neoplastic process is present in the epidural space (epidural abscess) or in the vertebrae (metastatic cancer), localized vertebral pain may be elicited by percussion of the spinous processes.

The pathological processes that produce transverse myelopathy are often acute and initially produce a flaccid areflexic paralysis known as spinal shock (Table 15–13). Within days, the motor syndrome becomes characteristic of an upper motor neuron paralysis with hyper-reflexia and bilateral extensor plantar responses. At the level of the lesion, segmental lower motor neuron signs may persist owing to injury to the anterior horns or the ventral roots. The lower motor neuron signs are a reliable indicator of the level of the spinal cord injury. They may be quite obvious in the cervical level but can be subtle and hard to detect at the thoracic cord level.

Marked disturbances in autonomic function can occur below the level of the lesion. Loss of sweating and trophic skin changes occur, as well as loss of temperature control and vasomotor instability, which can result in sudden changes in body temperature and blood pressure, including hypertensive crises. Initially, after an acute lesion, the bladder is atonic, and the anal sphincter is flaccid. Later they become spastic, leading to involuntary evacuation of the bladder and bowels.

The *Brown-Séquard syndrome* produces a characteristic combination of motor and sensory signs below the level of the lesion. Interruption of the descending corticospinal tract produces an ipsilateral spastic weakness. Also, ipsilateral loss of proprioception below the level of the lesion results from interruption of the ascending fibers in the posterior columns.

TABLE 15–13. **Myelopathies or Spinal Cord Syndromes**

Location of Lesion	Characteristic Signs
Complete transection (transverse)	Complete loss of motor and sensory function below level of lesion (tetraplegia or paraplegia) Acute: flaccid, areflexia (spinal shock) Chronic: spasticity, hyper-reflexia, Babinski's signs, spastic bladder
Hemisection (Brown-Séquard syndrome)	Ipsilateral hemiplegia or monoplegia, ipsilateral loss of vibration, proprioception Contralateral loss of pain and temperature below level of lesion
Central	"Suspended" sensory loss: "cape" sensory loss over shoulders from cervical lesion most common Loss of pain and temperature, sparing of vibration and proprioception ("dissociated" sensory loss) Weakness, atrophy, fasciculations, loss of reflex in extremity of affected segment (usually arm or cervical)
Anterior (anterior spinal artery syndrome)	Loss of motor function below level of lesion, flaccid tetraplegia or paraplegia. Loss of pain and temperature sensation below level of lesion with preservation of vibration, proprioception. Loss of bladder and bowel control
Caudal (conus medullaris)	Hypotonic bladder and rectal sphincters. Pain and loss of sensation in saddle distribution in perineum

Loss of pain and temperature sensation occurs contralateral to the hemisection because the crossed spinothalamic tract is interrupted. The sensory level that is responsive to pain and temperature is usually located one or two segments below the level of the lesion. When the Brown-Séquard syndrome results from an extramedullary lesion, there may be segmental lower motor neuron and sensory signs at the level of the lesion due to damage to the roots and anterior horn cells, and these signs are the most reliable indication of the level of the lesion. This syndrome is most apparent in patients with traumatic hemisections of the spinal cord (e.g., due to a stab wound). Other causes are extramedullary tumors or abscesses and, less commonly, intrinsic lesions, especially vasculitis (as in systemic lupus erythematosus). The full-blown hemisection syndrome is not commonly encountered (see Table 15–13).

The *central cord* syndrome is most often caused by *syringomyelia* and intramedullary cord tumors. The pathological process starts centrally and proceeds centrifugally, producing motor and sensory signs that evolve characteristically for this syndrome. Characteristically, the syndrome presents as a combination of segmental loss of pain and temperature sensation and lower motor neuron signs. This pattern occurs because the crossing fibers of the spinothalamic tract conveying pain and temperature sensation are initially compromised but posterior column sensation is preserved (*disassociated sensory loss*). Because only the decussating spinothalamic tract fibers are affected, the loss of pain and temperature is bilateral but affects only those segments of the spinal cord involved in the pathological cavitation or by the tumor, thus producing a *suspended sensory loss* with normal sensation above and below the lesion. In patients with syringomyelia, this pattern characteristically begins in the upper cervical segments, producing a loss of pain and temperature over the shoulders in a cape distribution. The syringomyelia or tumor usually invades the anterior horns early, producing the segmental lower motor neuron syndrome with weakness, wasting, and loss of reflex. As the lesion expands centrifugally, it may compromise the lateral corticospinal tracts, producing an upper motor neuron syndrome below the level of the lesion and loss of proprioception and vibratory sensation below the level of the lesion as it extends into the posterior columns (see Table 15–13).

When the anterior horns are affected in the cervical cord, wasting occurs first in one hand and then in the other. At the thoracic level, the disease affects the lower motor neurons innervating the paraspinal musculature, resulting in a scoliosis. Finally, if the lesion extends into the spinothalamic tracts themselves, pain and temperature sensation below the level of the lesion may be lost. Because the spinothalamic tracts are arranged in a laminated pattern with the sacral segments in the most lateral and ventral position, the sacral dermatomes are often preserved (*sacral sparing*).

The *anterior spinal artery* syndrome produces a distinctive combination of motor and sensory signs. Circulation to approximately the ventral two thirds of the spinal cord is supplied by the anterior spinal artery. Occlusion of the anterior spinal artery thus produces infarction in the ventral and most of the lateral funiculi, which include the anterior horns and the lateral corticospinal and spinothalamic tracts. Infarction leads to a subacute onset of a flaccid paralysis below the level of the lesion with loss of pain and temperature sensation below the level of the lesion. Position sense, vibration, and light touch are spared because the dorsal column supplied by the posterior spinal arteries is preserved. Infarction of the spinal cord usually occurs at borderzones between the major arterial systems supplying the spinal cord. These watersheds are at the T1–T4 and L1 spinal cord levels.

NEUROMUSCULAR JUNCTION SYNDROMES

Myasthenia Gravis

The defect in neuromuscular transmission in myasthenia gravis (see Chapter 50) produces a pure muscular weakness without the atrophy, fasciculations, or reflex changes seen in motor neuron disease.[40] Myasthenia gravis also causes a pattern of weakness in the ocular and cranial muscles that is different from that seen in amyotrophic lateral sclerosis. A weakness of the extraocular muscles and eyelids producing diplopia and ptosis is common in patients with myasthenia gravis but rare in those with amyotrophic lateral sclerosis (see Table 15–2). Facial weakness is also common in myasthenia gravis, and the combination of ptosis and weakness of eye closure may be duplicated only by an acute inflammatory demyelinating polyneuropathy (Guillain-Barré syndrome), which has a very different temporal profile.

The other characteristic feature of myasthenia gravis is *fatigability*. The myasthenic muscle rapidly weakens with continued or repetitive use. The physiological counterpart is the *decremental* response to repetitive stimulation of a peripheral nerve. Rest can temporarily restore the muscle to almost normal strength, but diplopia and ptosis return as the patient uses the eyes. The nasal voice and mushy dysarthric speech resumes as he speaks, and difficulty with chewing and swallowing occurs as he eats. Limb and postural muscles are generally less affected.[41]

Myasthenic Syndrome (Eaton-Lambert Syndrome)

Although weakness reminiscent of myasthenia gravis is the presenting complaint in most people with Eaton-Lambert syndrome,[42] the phenomenon of fatigability is less prominent, and the distribution of weakness, which affects the limbs and spares the extraocular muscles and eyelids, is also different. Pharyngeal weakness with dysphagia is the only weakness of the cranial musculature regularly encountered. Also in contrast to myasthenia gravis, autonomic dysfunction and reflex changes develop. Dry mouth and perversion of taste are common. Knee jerks are often reduced or absent.[43]

Occasionally, patients with the Eaton-Lambert myasthenic, syndrome describe a warming-up phenomenon, which is the opposite of fatigability; as a muscle is used repetitively, it may gain in strength, although with continued use fatigability returns. The clinical warming-up phenomenon correlates with an *incremental* increase in the amplitude of the muscle action potential with repetitive stimulation. The initial low amplitude of the muscle action potential occurs because an antibody blocks a calcium channel, slowing the entry of calcium into the presynaptic terminal to initiate vesicular release of acetylcholine.[44] Because it is only a partial blockade, however, enough calcium eventually enters with repetitive depolarizations to allow the amplitude of response to increase and strength to improve, at least temporarily.[45] In many but not all cases, the antibody against the calcium channel is generated by a cancer; thus, the Eaton-Lambert myasthenic syndrome is often a paraneoplastic disorder.[46]

Other Disorders of the Neuromuscular Junction

Botulism produces a rapidly developing paralysis. Because it usually affects the ocular and cranial musculature first, and the weakness develops so rapidly, botulism can be confused with a brain stem stroke or encephalitis. It rapidly becomes generalized to include all skeletal musculature and then may be mistaken for AIDP (Table 15–14). In typical cases, these conditions can be distinguished from each other by the fact that botulism starts in the ocular and cranial musculature and produces a descending paralysis, whereas AIDP starts as a weakness in the legs and produces an ascending paralysis that eventually includes the cranial musculature. This rule applies very well to botulism, which almost invariably begins in the ocular and cranial musculature, but may be violated by

TABLE 15–14. **"Acute" Generalized Weakness**

Location of Lesion	Differentiating Features	Causes
Midbrain	Coma, mid-size poorly reactive pupils, decorticate/ decerebrate posturing, hyper-reflexia, bilateral Babinski's signs	Stroke, trauma, tentorial herniation secondary to mass lesion
Basis pontis	Conscious; paralysis of horizontal eye movements and of jaw, face, pharynx, and tongue with preservation of vertical eye movements, eye blink; UMN spastic tetraparesis ("locked-in" syndrome)	Stroke
Spinal cord (spinal shock)	Flaccid paraplegia (tetraplegia), sensory loss below level of lesion with absent tendon reflexes but with extensor plantar responses; hypotonic bladder and sphincters	Trauma, infarction, metastatic tumor, transverse myelitis
Polyradicular neuropathy	Limb weakness (legs before arms), areflexia, absent or flexor toe response, minimal distal sensory loss without a sensory level	Acute inflammatory demyelinating polyneuropathy, tick paralysis, poliomyelitis
Neuromuscular junction	Ocular (including loss of pupillary light reflex) and pharyngeal weakness followed by generalized weakness without sensory loss and preservation of consciousness	Botulism, organophosphates

AIDP, which sometimes begins in the cranial musculature and descends. However, the early loss of pupillary reflexes in botulism and the predilection of AIDP for the facial and lower cranial nerves can clearly distinguish the two disorders. Weakness resulting from botulism is prolonged, lasting months, because the toxin permanently impairs the presynaptic release of acetylcholine from the terminals to which the toxin is bound. Neuromuscular transmission and strength return only after the nerve terminals sprout new endings.

MYOPATHIC SYNDROMES

In general, diseases of muscle (myopathies) are recognized by the characteristic pattern of proximal shoulder and hip girdle weakness with relative preservation of distal strength (see Table 15–2). Myopathic syndromes also differ from symmetrical polyneuropathies in their effect on reflexes. In contrast to polyneuropathies in which the distal reflexes are lost early, in myopathies, the reflexes are reduced in proportion to the degree of weakness; only with severe weakness in the end stages of a myopathy are the reflexes lost (see Table 15–5). Myopathies can be further differentiated from neuropathies by the lack of any sensory abnormalities. Atrophy of muscle may occur in myopathies but develops very slowly over the course of several years, whereas in motor neuron disease it develops much more rapidly. Also, no fasciculations are seen in myopathies. In certain muscular dystrophies, especially *Duchenne's muscular dystrophy*, pseudohypertrophy of the calf and deltoid muscles may occur owing to infiltration of the muscle by fat. The patient with myopathy often has a typical facial expression with ptosis, open mouth, and facial immobility.

As is often the case in medicine, there are exceptions to these general rules. The distal muscles may be weaker than the proximal muscles (e.g., *myotonic dystrophy*, *inclusion body myositis*), or a motor neuron disorder may affect the proximal musculature more than the distal, mimicking a myopathy (*Kugelberg-Welander syndrome*). Some myopathies affect the cranial and ocular muscles rather than limb muscles, as in, for example, the *chronic progressive external ophthalmoplegia* (CPEO) syndrome. The abnormal eye movements can be differentiated from those in myasthenia gravis; in CPEO, eye movements are restricted symmetrically and diplopia is not a complaint, whereas in myasthenia gravis double vision is a common symptom.

If special attention is given to the distribution of muscle weakness, the age and sex of the patient, and the family history, the likely diagnosis can often be determined. Some myopathies are congenital and have a different prognosis from rapidly progressive myopathies of childhood onset in boys that are usually dystrophinopathies. Dominantly inherited dystrophies have a later onset and a more benign course and have a rather uniform pattern of involvement (e.g., fascioscapulohumeral dystrophy). Mitochondrial myopathies preferentially affect the ocular and cranial musculature and are often accompanied by dysfunction in other organ systems. Inflammatory and infectious myopathies generally affect older individuals. The exception is dermatomyositis, which may occur at any age but is accompanied by characteristic skin changes.

SYNDROME OF "ACUTE" GENERALIZED WEAKNESS

Occasionally the pace of a disease is so rapid that by the time the patient is seen in the hospital the weakness has become generalized. The history of the mode of onset and the early course of the disease may not be available or may be confused by inaccurate observations. Therefore, accurate formulation of the problem depends on the examination and on localization of the level of the motor system that is damaged and is producing the weakness (see Table 15–14). The first step in the differentiation is to determine whether the patient is in a coma. The "locked-in" patient with a basis pontis lesion may initially appear comatose because he cannot move or speak and has lost the ability to make horizontal eye movements. However, the ability to blink and make vertical eye movements is preserved, and one should attempt to establish a communication code using eye blinks. In severe cases of botulism and AIDP, even ocular movements may be totally paralyzed, but no decorticate or decerebrate posturing is present nor any hyper-reflexia, and there are no Babinski's signs to indicate the presence of an intrinsic brain stem lesion.

Another potential source of confusion is the differentiation of AIDP without cranial neuropathy from an acute transferase myelopathy with spinal shock. Interruption of the descending motor tracts due to an acute transection of the spinal cord not only produces a paralysis below the level of the lesion but also causes a loss of all reflex activity. Tendon reflexes are lost, and initially there is no Babinski's sign. However, Babinski's signs generally appear within a matter of hours to a few days at most, helping to differentiate between the two. Also, in patients with acute transverse myelopathy, there is a well-defined sensory level, whereas in those with AIDP there is minimal if any sensory loss, which is generally distal with no sensory level.

EPISODIC WEAKNESS SYNDROME

There are a number of unusual syndromes in which weakness is intermittent or fleeting. These are listed in Table 15–15. Because of the phenomenon of fatigability and recovery after rest, the patient with myasthenia gravis may complain of episodic weakness. Myasthenia gravis is seldom confused with these other disorders because of the features mentioned earlier and the predilection of the weakness for the ocular and cranial muscles. An episodic hemiparesis is more apt to lead to confusion. The most common cause of this is *transient ischemic attack*, but the potential for confusion is greater with *partial motor seizures* or *hemiplegic migraine*. These entities can be differentiated clinically by paying careful attention to the mode of onset and the course of the weakness. Transient ischemic attack, produces an abrupt and simultaneous onset of weakness in all the muscles that will be affected during the attack. A partial motor seizure may become manifest as an inhibition of motor function, producing a stepwise progression of weakness from one body part to the next ("march") over many seconds to a few minutes as the wave of excitation or inhibition spreads along the cortical motor strip. The more common clonic jerking of the limbs may be followed by a postictal weakness (*Todd's paresis*) that lasts minutes to hours. The weakness of hemiplegic migraine takes even longer to develop than the inhibitory

TABLE 15–15. **Episodic Weakness—Differential Diagnosis**

Disorders	Key Features	Diagnostic Tests
Common		
Transient ischemic attack	All symptoms begin at once	Carotid ultrasound
Less Common		
Partial motor seizure with Todd's paresis	Gradual "march" of symptoms in several seconds to a few minutes	EEG
Hemiplegic migraine	Gradual development over several minutes; family history	
Myasthenia gravis	Fatigability, recovery with rest; predilection for ocular and cranial muscles	Tensilon test, repetitive stimulation test
Hysteria	Normal reflexes	
Cataplexy	Triggered by emotion; association with other features of narcolepsy; episodes very brief	Sleep study
Sleep paralysis	Narcolepsy; terminated by touch	Sleep study
Drop attacks	Sudden loss of postural tone without loss of consciousness	MRI, magnetic resonance angiography (MRA), x-ray of cervical spine with flexion-extension, EEG
Rare		
Periodic Paralysis	**Familial**	**Serum K+**
Hypokalemic	Nocturnal occurrence; lasts hours to days	Carbohydrate load after exercise
Hyperkalemic with myotonia	Myotonia induced by exposure to cold	KCl load
Hyperkalemic without myotonia	More frequent; provoked by rest after exercise	
Normokalemic	More severe and prolonged than hyperkalemic	KCl load

seizure, usually requiring several minutes to reach its completion.

Psychogenic paralysis can usually be readily diagnosed by the normal state of the reflexes and the nonanatomical distribution of sensory loss. When they are distracted or think they are unobserved, patients with this form of paralysis can usually be observed to move or use the affected body part in a way that should not be possible. The *cataleptic attack* is sudden and brief and is usually triggered by emotion. The history reveals other features of the *narcolepsy* syndrome. Another feature of narcolepsy is *sleep paralysis*. The attack generally occurs when the patient is beginning to arouse and awaken early in the morning. As the patient becomes aware of his surroundings, it is apparent that he is paralyzed and cannot move or talk, although respiration is unaffected. This attack can be aborted by an external stimulus, usually touch; sometimes the patient himself can abort the paralysis by imagining a touch. This phenomenon differentiates the attack of sleep paralysis from periodic paralysis (see later discussion). An attack of sleep paralysis may also be accompanied by frightening hallucinations (*hypnogogic hallucinations*).

The term *drop attack* refers to sudden falling spells without warning, loss of consciousness, or postictal symptoms. These attacks are very brief and are presumed to result from a sudden loss of muscular strength due to dysfunction of the corticospinal tracts at the level of the pyramidal tracts in the medulla or the high cervical cord. The attacks may result from brief ischemia to this region as in a vertebrobasilar ischemic attack or transient compression by excessive movement of the odontoid in a patient with an unstable atlantoaxial articulation. The ligament holding the odontoid in place may be destroyed by rheumatoid arthritis or trauma, and certain movements of the head, especially extension, can cause the odontoid to transiently compress the cervicomedullary junction. Similar attacks of tetraparesis can also occur in the chronic cerebellar tonsillar herniation characteristic of the *Chiari malformation* or in patients with severe congenital cervical spinal stenosis during Valsalva maneuvers or after falls. In the latter examples of mechanical compression, the weakness is generally more prolonged than it is in the classic drop attack, in which the person is immediately able to get to his or her feet after hitting the ground. There is also a syndrome of idiopathic drop attacks in elderly women that has a benign prognosis.

By definition, drop attacks occur without loss of consciousness, but in practice it may be difficult to differentiate these from akinetic seizures or certain varieties of syncope in which the loss of consciousness is so brief that it is difficult for the patient to decide whether he lost consciousness or not. One must probe very carefully to elicit a history of a brief warning to identify syncope or obtain an EEG to rule out an akinetic seizure.

The most interesting and rare disorders causing episodic weakness are the *periodic paralyses*, which are associated with genetic disorders of the potassium and sodium channels. In the great majority of cases these disorders are familial and autosomal dominant. Currently, they are classified according to the level of serum potassium during the attack (see Table 15–15). During an attack variable weakness of the limbs occurs, and usually the legs are affected before the arms. Then the weakness may progress to affect the trunk muscles, but the diaphragm, sphincters, and cranial and ocular musculature are generally spared. The attack usually evolves over minutes to several hours and may last a few hours if the attack is mild or several days if it is severe. These forms of paralysis can also be distinguished from each other by the factors that provoke an attack of weakness, the duration and severity of the attacks, and the presence of myotonia.

General Management Goals

TREATMENT OF WEAKNESS

The occupational therapist and physical therapist can offer help that is of paramount importance in the rehabilitation of the patient with weakness. Strengthening and stretching exercises maintain the weak muscles in maximum tone and keep the joints from developing contractures, which further limit movement. The patient can be trained to use adaptive movements to facilitate function and to use canes and walkers, assessing which ones produce the maximum benefit. Splints and braces can be used to stabilize the joints.

TREATMENT OF SPASTICITY

A number of options are now available for the treatment of spasticity that interferes with gait or produces uncomfortable spasms such as the flexor spasms typical of spinal cord lesions. It must be emphasized, however, that spasticity may be helpful in compensating for weakness, especially in gait. Over zealous treatment of spasticity may in fact cause a decrement in function, particularly gait, especially when drugs with systemic effects are used. The development of botulinum toxin injections now offers the option of targeting muscles to avoid the deleterious effects of drugs on helpful spasticity.

Drugs with systemic effects are now used primarily in patients who are confined to a wheelchair or bed. These drugs facilitate relaxation of muscles, allowing easier transfers from bed to chair and faciliating hygiene as well as alleviating painful flexor spasms. The drugs used are baclofen, diazepam, and tizanidine.

Injections of botulinum toxin into spastic leg adductors can facilitate nursing care;[47] injections into the arm muscles can relieve painful spasms.[48] Injections of botulinum toxin into specific muscles also can be used in ambulatory patients to facilitate normal gait patterns while preserving spasticity in muscles that are necessary for walking. Injections into the gastrocnemius-soleus muscle can facilitate a conversion from toe walking to plantigrade foot placement. Botulinum toxin injections are useful when a dynamic spasticity is present but very little, if any, permanent contracture. If a fixed contracture has developed, it may be necessary to release the contracted tendons surgically. These procedures are most commonly done to release the Achilles, adductor, and hamstring tendons.

Reviews and Selected Updates

Brodal P: Motor Systems. The central nervous system: Structure and function. New York, Oxford, 1992, pp 199–284.

Carpenter RH: Sensorimotor processing: Charting the frontier. Curr Biol 1997;7:348–351.

Corcos DM: Movement deficits caused by hyperexcitable stretch reflexes in spastic humans. Brain 1986;109:1043–1058.

Georgopoulos A: Current issues in directional motor control. Trends Neurosci 1995;18:506–510.

Johnson EA: Clostridial toxins as therapeutic agents: Benefits of nature's most toxic proteins. Ann Rev Microbiol 1999;53:551–575.

Leigh PN, Swash M: Motor Neuron Disease. Basel, Springer-Verlag, 1995.

Litvan I, Mangone CA, Werden W, Bueri JA: Reliability of the NINDS myotatic reflex scale. Neurology 1996;47:969–972.

Matthews PBC: The human stretch reflex and the motor cortex. Trends Neurosci 1991;14:87–91.

References

1. Spillane JD: The Doctrine of the Nerves. Oxford, Oxford University Press, 1981.
2. Sherrington C: The Integrative Action of the Nervous System, 2nd ed. New Haven, Yale University Press, 1947.
3. Evarts E, Wise SP: The Motor System in Neurobiology. Amsterdam, Elsevier, 1985.
4. Kakulas BA, Adams RD: Diseases of Muscle: Pathological Foundations of Clinical Myology, 4th ed. Philadelphia, Harper & Row, 1985, pp 130–131.
5. Peachey LD: Skeletal muscle. *In* Brooks VB (ed): Handbook of Physiology. Baltimore, Williams & Wilkins, 1983.
6. Hoffman EP: Genotype/phenotype correlations in Duchenne/Becker muscular dystrophy. *In* Partridge TA (ed): Molecular and Cell Biology of Muscular Dystrophy. London, Chapman & Hall, 1993, pp 12–36.
7. Protti DA, Reisin R, Mackinley TA, Uchitel OD: Calcium channel blockers and transmitter release at the normal human neuromuscular junction. Neurology 1996;46:1391–1396.
8. Xu T, Binz T, Niemann H, Neher E: Multiple kinetic components of exocytosis distinguished by neurotoxin sensitivity. Nature Neurosci 1998;1:192–200.
9. John R, Sudhof TC: Synaptic vesicles and exocytosis. Ann Rev Neurosci 1994;17:219–246.
10. Henneman E, Clamann HP, Gillies JD, Skinner RD: Rank order of motoneurons within a pool: Law of combination. J Neurophysiol 1974;37:1338–1349.
11. Mathews PBC: Evolving views on the internal operation and functional role of the muscle spindle. J Physiol 1981;320:1–30.
12. Houck JC, Crago PE, Rymer WZ: Functional properties of the Golgi's tendon organs. *In* Desmedt JE (ed): Spinal and Supraspinal Mechanisms of Voluntary Motor Control and Locomotion. Progress in Clinical Neurophysiology, Vol 8. Basel, Karger, 1980, pp 33–43.
13. Basmajian JV: Muscles Alive. Their Functions Revealed by Electromyography, 5th ed. Baltimore, Williams & Wilkins, 1985.
14. Berardelli A, Hallett M, Kaufman C, et al: Stretch reflexes of triceps surae in normal man. J Neurol Neurosurg Psychiatry 1982;45:513–525.
15. Renshaw B: Activity in the simplest spinal reflex pathways. J Neurophysiol 1940;3:373–387.
16. Marsden CD, Rothwell JC, Day BL: Long-latency automatic responses to muscle stretch in man: Origin and function. *In* Desmedt JE (ed): Motor Control Mechanisms in Health and Disease. New York, Raven Press, 1983, pp 509–539.
17. Marsden CD, Merton PA, Morton HB: Stretch reflex and servo-action in a variety of human muscles. J Physiol 1976;259:531–560.
18. Delwaide PJ, Pepin JL, Maertens de Noordhout A: Short-latency autogenic inhibition in patients with Parkinsonian rigidity. Ann Neurol 1991;30:83–89.
19. Jane JA, Yashon D, DeMeyer W, Bucy PC: The contribution of the precentral gyrus to the pyramidal tract of man. J Neurosurg 1967;26:244–248.
20. Penfield W, Rasmussen T: The Cerebral Cortex of Man: A Clinical Study of Localization of Function. New York, Macmillan, 1950.
21. Davidoff RA: The Pyramidal Tract. Neurology 1990;40:332–339.
22. Patton HD: Reflex regulation of movement and posture. *In* Rush TC, Patton HD (eds): Physiology and Biophysics, 19th ed. Philadelphia, WB Saunders, 1965, pp 181–206.
23. Kennedy PR: Corticospinal, rubrospinal and rubro-olivary projections: A unifying hypothesis. Trends Neurosci 1990;13:474–478.
24. Nashner LM: Adaptation of human movement to altered environments. Trends Neurosci 1982;5:358–361.
25. Plum F, Posner JB: The Diagnosis of Stupor and Coma, 3rd ed. Philadelphia, F.A. Davis, 1980.
26. Davidoff RA: Antispasticity drugs: Mechanisms of action. Ann Neurol 1985;17:107–116.
27. Blexrud MD, Windebank AJ, Daube JR: Long-term follow-up of 121 patients with benign fasciculations. Ann Neurol 1993;34:622–625.
28. Eisen A, Stewart H: Not-so-benign fasciculation. Ann Neurol 1994;35:375–376.
29. Van der Meche FGA, Van Gijn J: Hypotonia: An erroneous clinical concept? Brain 1986;109:1169–1178.
30. Medical Research Council: Aids to the Investigation of Peripheral Nerve Injuries, Memorandum No. 45. London, Crown Publishing, 1976.
31. Andres PL, Hedlund W, Finison L, et al: Quantitative motor assessment in amyotrophic lateral sclerosis. Neurology 1986;36:937–941.

32. Fuglevand AJ: Neural aspects of fatigue. Neuroscientist 1996;2:203–206.
33. DeJong RN: The Neurologic Examination, 4th ed. Hagerstown, MD, Harper & Row, 1979, p 456.
34. Fisher CM, Curry HB: Pure motor hemiplegia of vascular origin. Arch Neurol 1965;13:30–33.
35. Fisher CM: A lacunar stroke: The dysarthria-clumsy hand syndrome. Neurology 1967;17:614–617.
36. Grimaldi LME, Martino G, Braghi S, et al: Heterogeneity of autoantibodies in Stiff-Man Syndrome. Ann Neurol 1993;34:57–64.
37. Russman BS, Iannacone ST, Buncher CR, et al: Spinal muscular atrophy: New thoughts on the pathogenesis and classification scheme. J Child Neurol 1992;7:347–353.
38. Dyck PJ, Dyck PJB, Grant IA, Fealey RD: Ten steps in characterizing and diagnosing patients with peripheral neuropathy. Neurology 1996;47:10–17.
39. Tandan R: Clinical features and differential diagnosis of classical motor neuron disease. *In* Williams AC (ed): Motor Neuron Disease. New York, Chapman & Hall, 1994, pp 3–27.
40. Drachman DB: Myasthenia gravis: Immuno-biology of a receptor disorder. Trends Neurosci 1983;6:446–451.
41. Pachner AR: Myasthenia gravis. Immunol Allergy Clin North Am 1988;8:277–293.
42. Eaton LM, Lambert EH: Electromyography and electric stimulation of nerves in diseases of the motor unit: Observations of the myasthenic syndrome associated with malignant tumors. JAMA 1957;163: 1117–1124.
43. Engel AG: Myasthenia gravis and myasthenic syndromes. Ann Neurol 1996;16:519–534.
44. Kim YI, Neher E: IgG from patients with Lambert-Eaton syndrome blocks voltage-dependent calcium channels. Science 1988;239:405–408.
45. Sanders DB: Lambert-Eaton myasthenia syndrome: Clinical diagnosis, immune-mediated mechanism and update on therapies. Ann Neurol 1995;37:563–573.
46. Lennon VA, Kryzer JJ, Griesmann MS, et al: Calcium-channel antibodies in the Lambert-Eaton syndrome and other paraneoplastic syndromes. N Engl J Med 1995;332:1467–1474.
47. Snow BJ, Tsui JK, Bhatt MH, et al: Treatment of spasticity with botulinum toxin: A double-blind study. Ann Neurol 1990;28:512–515.
48. Grazko MA, Polo KB, Jabbari B: Botulinum toxin A for spasticity, muscle spasms, and rigidity. Neurology 1995;45:712–717.

CHAPTER 16

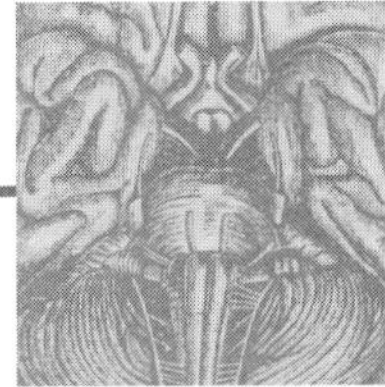

STANLEY FAHN

Hypokinesia and Hyperkinesia

History and Definitions

In an attempt to distinguish the class of motor disturbances resulting from lesions of the basal ganglia, Kinnier Wilson coined the term extrapyramidal in his famous 1912 article[1] describing hepatolenticular degeneration, now known as Wilson's disease. This term was widely adopted thereafter and continues to be used today. The *extrapyramidal system* refers to the basal ganglia with their anatomical connections, and *extrapyramidal disorders* are hypokinetic and hyperkinetic states that ensue from lesions in these anatomical sites. Unfortunately, these terminologies are not absolutely accurate, and extrapyramidal is more a functional concept than a purely anatomical one. There are many other motor pathways that are anatomically extrapyramidal and yet not necessarily related to the basal ganglia, including cerebellar, reticulospinal, vestibulospinal, and rubrospinal pathways. Furthermore, most outflow from the basal ganglia goes to the cerebral cortex via the thalamus and eventually influences the pyramidal system. In fact, a lesion of the pyramidal system that results in paralysis will eliminate the abnormal movements that originate from a basal gangliar disturbance. Another problem with the term extrapyramidal is the different ways it is used, creating ambiguity and possible misunderstanding. Although Wilson conceived of the term to refer to all types of hypokinetic and hyperkinetic disorders, psychiatrists today usually use the term extrapyramidal side effects to represent only drug-induced parkinsonism.

At present, the term movement disorder largely replaces the older term extrapyramidal disease because it is more descriptive and accurate. Almost all movement disorders stem from disturbances in the basal ganglia or their connections, but there are important exceptions. Myoclonus is one major example of a movement disorder of brain stem, cortical, or spinal cord origin, and conditions such as painful legs/moving toes and the so-called jumpy stump syndrome emerge from injuries to the peripheral nervous system.

Movement disorders are clinically characterized by hypokinesia or hyperkinesia, and sometimes both. Hypokinesia technically means decreased amplitude of movement, but it is used also to represent bradykinesia (decreased speed of movement) and akinesia (absence of movement). The important element in hypokinesias is paucity of movement in the absence of weakness or paralysis. Hypokinesia is the hallmark of parkinsonism, a term that broadens hypokinesia when it is associated with tremor, rigidity, or balance problems. Hyperkinesia means excessive movement and generally refers to a wide variety of abnormal *involuntary* movements or dyskinesias. Occasionally some syndromes have a combination of hypokinetic and hyperkinetic components, such as the rare syndrome of rapid-onset dystonia-parkinsonism.[2] Hyperkinetic voluntary movements, which are common in attention deficit disorders and some psychiatric disorders such as mania, are not generally considered as hyperkinesias in this context. The listing of the various

TABLE 16–1. **List of Movement Disorders**

Hypokinesia (Parkinsonism)	Poverty of movement in speed or amplitude, synonymous with akinesia and bradykinesia
Pure parkinsonism	Akinesia or rest tremor associated with rigidity and/or postural reflex deficits
Parkinsonism-plus	Parkinsonism occurring in association with other signs, such as vertical gaze paresis, hypotension and dysautonomia, apraxias
Hyperkinesias	Involuntary movements that occur spontaneously or during activity, synonymous with dyskinesias
Akathitic movements	Stereotypic movements (usually legs) that occur in response to internal restless feelings
Athetosis	Twisting contorsion, a form of dystonia, usually associated with birth injury or cerebrovascular accidents
Ballismus	Violent chorea, involving large muscle groups
Chorea	Involuntary rapid and irregular movements
Dystonia	Twisting, sustained posture
Hemifacial spasm	Unilateral facial contractions
Hyperekplexia	Enhanced and pathological startle response
Myoclonus	Shocklike jerks, focal or generalized
Stereotypy	Repetitive movement, simple or complex
Tics	Stereotypy that typically involves face, neck, and vocal apparatus more than other body parts
Tremor	To-and-fro oscillation around a joint

hypokinesias and hyperkinesias along with definitions of each are presented in Table 16–1.

Important characteristics used to describe and classify hyperkinesias include regularity, velocity and duration, and anatomical distribution. In terms of regularity, tremors are generally rhythmical to-and-fro movements; likewise, tics and stereotypies are repetitive movements that are highly predictable in quality, although intermittent in frequency. In contrast, chorea is best characterized by rapid movements flowing irregularly from one body part to another without a predictable pattern. In terms of velocity and duration, rapid movements include myoclonus, chorea, ballismus, clonic tics, and some tremors. Slow movements are dystonic or athetotic, showing a sustained contraction of muscles, often with a twisting component. Finally, several hyperkinesias have a propensity to involve certain body regions; for example, akathitic movements almost always affect the legs, and tics tend to be most prominent in the face, eyes, and neck. Dystonic movements occur in all body regions but are particularly common in the neck muscles (torticollis).

Clinical History

There are several symptoms that are suggestive of hypokinesia. Patients report difficulty getting out of chairs, especially car seats and sofas; trouble turning over in bed; and an overall reduced speed of activities of daily living. Patients and families might interpret slowness as a sign of old age or early arthritis and not suspect a neurological disorder. Some patients may misinterpret hypokinesia as weakness. Slowness and fatigue, although they are particularly prominent in hypokinesia, can be features of depression, catatonia, or hypothyroidism.

Trouble starting and stopping can also be seen with hypokinesia. Parkinsonian patients may complain of start-hesitation or freezing[3] during turning, when they are trying to reach a target, or when they are passing through a doorway. Difficulty stopping is the complaint of patients who have festination as part of hypokinesia, and these patients have a tendency to build up speed as they walk, even to the point of running. They cannot stop until coming to a barrier, such as a wall. The mechanism is considered to be a combination of the loss of postural reflexes and the flexed posture, which brings the center of gravity in front of the feet.

Falling is an important historical feature of movement disorders, and all adults who fall without ready explanation should be evaluated neurologically. In parkinsonian disorders, patients eventually develop loss of postural reflexes, which can lead to poor balance and falling. This problem is particularly apparent to patients with freezing. Falling occurs in other movement disorders as well, especially in patients with Huntington's disease, in whom loss of postural reflexes occurs in association with a stuttering, dancing gait. Truncal ataxia due to cerebellar or proprioceptive impairment may cause a wide-based staggering stance and gait, which patients interpret as "walking like a drunk."

Falling is also a common feature of hyperekplexia or excessive startle syndrome. In this disorder, often inherited with a defect in the gene for the glycine receptor,[4] a sudden noise or threat can trigger the patient to lose muscle tone and then fall. In this disorder, the patient has an exaggerated startle reflex,[5] which can be measured electrophysiologically. If patients have a delayed reaction to sudden noise or threat, a psychogenic problem should be considered.[6, 7]

Another cause of falling is positive and negative myoclonus. The positive myoclonic jerk can result in a patient being thrown off balance. Negative myoclonus, especially of the thigh muscles when the patient is standing or walking, produces a bouncing stance, and the sudden inhibitions of the muscles lead to a fall. Posthypoxic myoclonus is the most common cause of this type of negative myoclonus,[8] and in these cases, patients complain of sudden body jerks that cause them to lose balance control without warning.

Not knowing what to call the various forms of hyperkinesias, patients may use terms such as muscle jerks and shaking movements to describe their disorder. Only the examination can definitively differentiate the type of dyskinesia, but the history can suggest the most likely categories. Sudden muscle jerks are usually myoclonus or tics. Rhythmical movements are usually tremors, rhythmical (segmental) myoclonus, or the repetitive movements of tardive dyskinesia, such as oral-lingual-buccal dyskinesias, body rocking, and marching in place. In dystonia, movements may occur or increase with volitional activity such as writing, pouring liquids, buttoning, and walking. The timing of abnormal movements is important to document, especially with tremors. Parkinsonian tremor occurs while the affected body part is at rest, such as the hands lying quietly in the patient's lap. Postural tremor, associated with many noradrenergic drugs, hyperthyroidism, or essential tremor, is seen when the limb is maintained against gravity and is usually made worse during activity; it typically worsens with handwriting, and the patient often complains of large, sloppy handwriting. Cerebellar endpoint kinetic tremor is seen when the patient's limb attempts to reach a target; this type of tremor causes extreme sloppiness, spilling, and soiling of clothes.

In most movement disorders, the onset of symptoms is insidious, although frequently patients date them to an incident such as a frightening event or trauma. An exception to this rule is hemiballismus, which often is sudden in onset and related to a cerebrovascular accident involving the subthalamic nucleus.

Sudden movement induces some special forms of dyskinesia. A history of intermittent attacks of dyskinesias that arise just as a person stands up or starts to run immediately raises the suspicion of a paroxysmal dyskinesia,[9] such as paroxysmal kinesigenic dyskinesia. In addition to sudden movement, startle or hyperventilation can also be the precipitating factor.[9] Prolonged exercise can induce attacks of hyperkinesia as well and leads to the diagnosis of paroxysmal exertional dyskinesia.[10] Other types of paroxysmal dyskinesias are more commonly induced by fatigue, stress, or ingestion of caffeine and alcohol. Paroxysmal nonkinesigenic dyskinesias, however, especially those without a family history, are often psychogenic in etiology.[11] Most psychogenic movement disorders are continual rather than intermittent and can present as any type of hyperkinesia[6] and even hypokinesia[12] and gait disorders. There are many historical clues to suspect the psychogenic etiology of a movement disorder,[6] including their frequent distractability, inconsistency of signs, and abrupt, strokelike onset.[13]

Medication exposure requires a special place in the clinical history of a movement disorder. The most important drugs that induce movement disorders are those that are dopamine D_2-receptor antagonists, the so-called dopamine receptor blocking agents. These drugs can cause acute dystonic reactions, acute akathisia, drug-induced parkinsonism, neuroleptic malignant syndrome, and the tardive dyskinesia syndromes. The last entity presents a wide variety of dyskinesias,[14] which are characterized by their frequent persistence even after drug withdrawal. Drugs, and certain endocrine compounds such as thyroxine, epinephrine, and insulin that alter noradrenergic tone, can exaggerate physiological tremor. Anticonvulsants can induce chorea, and valproate may even induce hypokinesia. Cocaine can induce chorea,[15] tics,[16] and opsoclonus-myoclonus.[17]

Although movement disorders are primary motor conditions, a number of sensory phenomena can occur. Painful muscle cramps are most often due to neuromuscular disease[18] but can occur with severe rigidity or stiff-person syndrome.[19] Dystonia can sometimes be painful, particularly drug-induced forms. Painful foot cramping due to dystonic spasms can be an early sign of parkinsonism.[20] Also in parkinsonism,[21] as well as in tardive syndromes,[22] pain may be focal in the oral and genital areas and have a burning quality or numbness and itching. In patients with akathisia, a movement disorder associated with a primary subjective restlessness, patients frequently describe a vague but intense discomfort in their body with an urge to move about, and which is relieved by movement.

In addition to these historical elements, a careful medical and family history is important in evaluating hypokinesia and hyperkinesia. The medical history should include an evaluation of all body systems, including the mind, because dementia, psychosis, depression, and various personality traits such as attention deficit disorder and hyperactivity, and obsessive-compulsive disorder can help in diagnosis and co-morbidity analyses. Several primary movement disorders are hereditary, and therefore the creation of a family tree focusing on the type of movement disorder the patient has along with other neurological and psychiatric disorders may prove pivotal to the final neurological diagnosis.

Anatomy of the Basal Ganglia

The basal ganglia are a group of subcortical nuclei, most of which are located in proximity to the thalamus and hypothalamus. These regions and their white matter pathways connect to the cortex and indirectly to descending pyramidal and other spinal cord pathways that modulate motor and cognitive programs (Figs. 16–1 and 16–2). There is no dedicated basal ganglia–spinal tract, and the so-called final common pathway for basal gangliar motor function involves the corticospinal pyramidal tract and the lower motor neuron (see Chapter 15). Although they are highly complex, these anatomical connections have been schematized in block diagrams in order to test specific hypotheses related to hypokinesia and hyperkinesia (Fig. 16–3). The specific nuclei of primary focus are the caudate nucleus and putamen, collectively known as the striatum; the globus pallidus (both internal and external segments, termed GP_i and GP_e); the subthalamic nucleus; and the substantia nigra (pars compacta and pars reticulata).

BASAL GANGLIAR CONNECTIONS

Anatomical discussions of the basal ganglia usually consider structures in afferent and efferent relationship with the striatum. The caudate and putamen complex contains several different neuronal types, the most abundant population being the medium spiny neuron which uses gamma-aminobutyric acid (GABA) as its neurotransmitter. This neuron sends its axonal projection out of the striatum and also has several recurrent axon collaterals that are distributed primarily within its own intrastriatal dendritic field. In addition, the striatum contains numerous large cholinergic interneurons, known as large aspiny neurons, as well as somatostatin-rich cells that contain nitric oxide synthase for production of the neuromodulator nitric oxide.[23]

Cortical and thalamic afferents to the caudate and putamen are somatotopically organized and excitatory, using glutamate as their neurotransmitter.[24] The brain stem input is primarily from the pars compacta substantia nigra (SNc), a dopaminergic pathway. The substantia nigra is a melanin-rich structure located dorsal to the pyramidal tracts (crus cerebri) in the midbrain. These dopaminergic nigrostriatal fibers have both an excitatory and an inhibitory effect on target (GABA-containing) neurons in the striatum. There are two distinct efferent pathways from the striatum that ultimately reach the internal segment of the globus pallidus

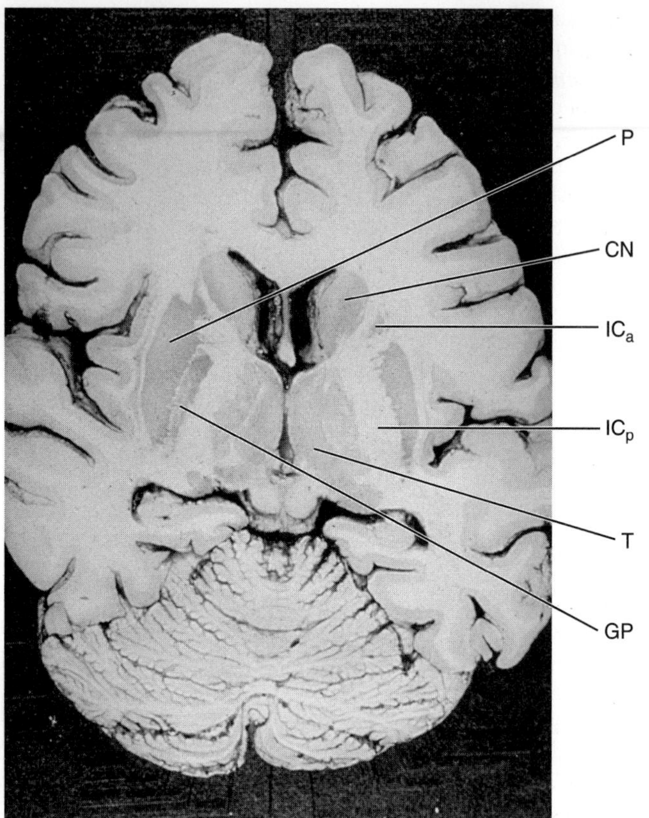

FIGURE 16–1. Transverse section of a human brain with basal ganglia identified. CN = caudate nucleus, P = putamen, GP = globus pallidus, T = thalamus, IC_a = internal capsule anterior limb, IC_p = internal capsule posterior limb.

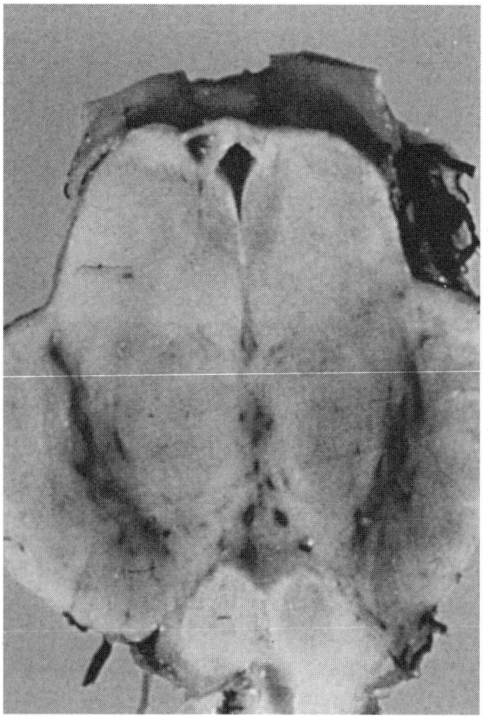

FIGURE 16–2. Cross section of a human midbrain with the black band of dark melanin-rich substantia nigra (SN) and the pyramidal tract that lies anteriorally.

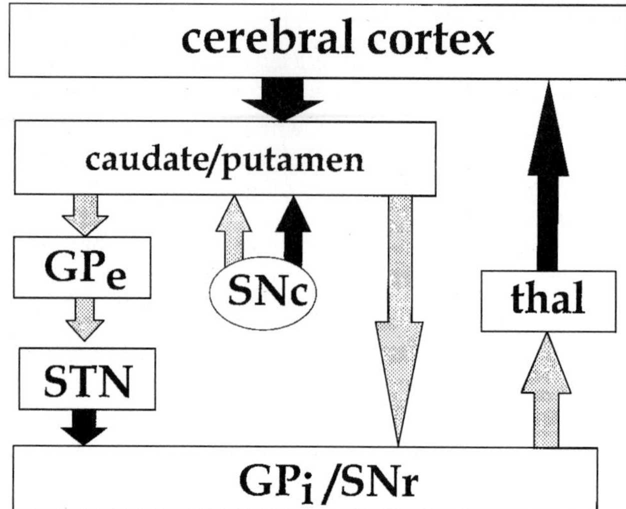

FIGURE 16–3. Schema of anatomical nuclei and pathways involving the basal ganglia. Black arrows represent excitation, and speckled arrows represent inhibition. Note the two primary pathways that leave the striatum—the "direct" pathway that flows monosynaptically to the GP_i and the "indirect" pathway that has intermediate synapses in the GP_e and the subthalamic nucleus. GP_i = globus pallidus internal segment; GP_e = globus pallidus external segment; STN = subthalamic nucleus; SNr = pars reticularis of the substantia nigra; SNc = pars compacta of the substantia nigra; thal = thalamus.

(GP_i) and the pars reticulata of the substantia nigra (SNr). They are conveniently named the direct and the indirect pathways. The effect of the D_1 dopamine receptors on medium spiny neurons in the direct pathway is excitatory. Because the direct pathway's monosynaptic GABA efferents from the striatum to the GP_i and SNr are inhibitory, the net effect of dopamine (and D_1 receptors) via the direct pathway is to inhibit the GP_i and SNr. The indirect pathway from the striatum reaches the same destination, but sends GABA efferents first to the GP_e, which then sends GABA efferents to the subthalamic nucleus. The effect of the D_2 dopamine receptors on medium spiny neurons in the indirect pathway is inhibitory. The glutaminergic efferents from the subthalamus to the GP_i and SNr are excitatory. The net effect of the subthalamic nucleus on the GP_i and SNr via the indirect pathway is also inhibitory. It has three inhibitory fibers followed by an excitatory one. But the final excitatory pathway in the indirect pathway is inhibited because of the three sequential inhibitory pathways reaching the subthalamic nucleus (see Fig. 16–3). Thus, the ultimate effect of dopamine from the subthalamic nucleus, whether via the direct or indirect pathways, is to inhibit GP_i and SNr neurons.[25]

Efferent pathways directed beyond the basal ganglia to the thalamus and cortex emanate primarily from the GP_i and pars reticulata of the substantia nigra. This influence is a tonic inhibitory one via GABAergic cells that project to the ventral anterior and ventral lateral thalamic nuclei and, to a lesser extent, to other thalamic regions, as well as the brain stem. The various influences on GP_i provide phasic modulation of the tonic inhibition on the thalamus. The final part of this loop involves the thalamocortical projections, which are excitatory, probably using glutamate as the neurotransmitter, and synapse in the motor, supplementary motor, and premotor cortices.[26]

INTRASTRIATAL STRUCTURE

Within the striatum, there is a large neuronal matrix compartment, comprising approximately 80 percent of the striatum, and a smaller compartment interdigitated with the matrix and known as striosomes or patches. Both the matrix and striasomal neurons receive inputs from dopamine cells coming from the pars compacta of the substantia nigra. Both cell types send efferent projections to the GP_e, and these cells all contain enkephalin. In contrast, however, the matrix population also sends efferents to the substantia nigra pars reticulata and the GP_i, whereas the striasomal cells project in large part back to the pars compacta. These projection cells contain substance P and dynorphin.[27]

ADDITIONAL BRAIN STEM–CORTICAL LOOPS

A series of anatomical loops have been identified that are involved in the genesis of myoclonus, presumably through transmission of aberrant electrical discharges. A cortical loop has been proposed involving diffuse areas of the cortex, but predominantly the sensorimotor area, the pyramidal tract, medial lemniscus, and thalamus, with return fibers to the cortex. Complementing and interacting with the cortical loop is the spino-bulbar-spinal reflex, which primarily involves the brain stem reticular formation. Sensory impulses entering the spinal cord ascend bilaterally within the spinoreticular pathway, project to the nucleus reticularis gigantocellularis of the medial medullary reticular formation, descend within the reticulospinal tract, and eventually terminate on interneurons at various spinal cord levels influencing alpha motor neurons. In several instances of myoclonus, involvement of nuclei and pathways involving the cerebellum has also been identified. Specifically, the network connecting the red nucleus, dentate nucleus, and the inferior olivary nucleus (triangle of Guillain and Mollaret) has been directly implicated as playing a role in rhythmical palatal myoclonus. In other clinical settings, myoclonus can be associated with damage to the dentate nucleus, superior cerebellar peduncles, and the spinocerebellar pathways, with preservation of the red nucleus and olives. Finally, a spino-spinal loop with involvement of the flexor reflex afferents has been implicated in the generation of rhythmical myoclonus that occurs in a spinal segmental distribution. In contrast, repetitive, nonrhythmical jerks resulting in flexion at the trunk, hips, knees, and neck may be produced by abnormal electrical activity generated within the cord and transmitted via the propriospinal system, so-called propriospinal myoclonus.

NEUROTRANSMITTERS

Although neurotransmitters relate to all neuroanatomical discussions, they are of particular interest in relation to the basal ganglia and their function. Much of the basic understanding of neurotransmitters in clinical medicine came from studies of human basal gangliar disorders, and most medical specialists in this area of neurology have a sound foundation in neurochemistry and neuropharmacology. Additional material related to neurotransmitters was reviewed in the discussion of Mood, Emotion, and Thought (see Chapter 3). A neurotransmitter is an endogenous chemical that relays information from one neuron to another through synaptic release and receptor activation. To qualify as a neurotransmitter, five classic criteria must be demonstrated: (1) presence within neurons, (2) synthetic pathways with identified enzymes, (3) release mechanisms from the neuron into the synapse, (4) metabolic pathways to effect the removal of the chemical, and (5) mimicry of neuronal activity by iatrogenic application of the neurochemical. Few chemicals accepted as neurotransmitters actually fulfill all criteria within the central nervous system.

Dopamine

This simple catecholamine is synthesized in four major central nervous system pathways, and the most important and most widely understood involves the nigrostriatal pathway of the basal ganglia. The synthetic pathway for dopamine is tyrosine—1→dopa—2→dopamine. The rate-limiting enzyme is tyrosine hydroxylase (enzyme 1), and the second synthesizing step involves aromatic amino acid decarboxylase (enzyme 2). Once dopamine is produced in the nigral cell, it is transported along the axon to the striatal terminals, where it is released from vesicles into the synaptic cleft. There are receptors for dopamine on the striatal cells (postsynaptic receptors) as well as presynaptic or autoreceptors on the nigral axon. Depolarization of the autoreceptor raises the resting potential of the presynaptic neuron and makes the neuron easier to depolarize; on the other hand, the gradient between resting potential and action potential has been reduced, so that the end result is a decreased release of dopamine. This important mechanism provides for self-regulation of dopamine function. Activation of the postsynaptic receptors by dopamine can lead to depolarization or hyperpolarization, depending on the receptor site. An important concept for all neurotransmitters, including dopamine, is that the final result, hyperpolarization or depolarization, is dependent on both the transmitter and its receptor. The concept of an inhibitory transmitter should be abandoned for the more accurate concept of an inhibitory interaction between neurotransmitter and receptor.

Dopamine activity can be increased by four mechanisms: (1) increased synthesis, (2) increased release, (3) prolongation of neurotransmitter activity, and (4) direct receptor stimulation. Synthesis of the neurotransmitter can be increased by giving dopa because it is the product beyond the rate-limiting enzyme and there is ordinarily an abundant amount of aromatic amino acid decarboxylase in the central nervous system. When dopa is combined with a peripherally active decarboxylase inhibitor, more dopa is delivered across the blood-brain barrier and can be used to synthesize central dopamine. Increased release can be effected by drugs such as cocaine, amphetamine, and methylphenidate, all forcing release of presynaptic catecholamines. The normal metabolism of dopamine involves reuptake of dopamine into the presynaptic cell, with subsequent metabolism by two enzymes, monoamine oxidase (MAO) and catechol O-methyltransferase (COMT). Prolongation of dopamine activity can be effected by blocking reuptake or altering enzyme activity. Amantadine and possibly some tricyclic antidepressant medications operate on the dopaminergic system through blockade of reuptake. MAO inhibitors and COMT inhibitors for human use also increase dopaminergic activity. Finally, direct activation of the dopamine receptors on the striatal cell can be induced by agonists like bromocriptine, pergolide, and other drugs. Importantly, orally administered dopamine itself has no place in altering the central nervous system dopamine levels, because, being a positively charged molecule, it cannot cross the blood-brain barrier.

Dopamine function can be antagonized by three basic mechanisms: (1) decreased synthesis, (2) decreased release, and (3) blockade of dopamine receptors. Alpha-methyl paratyrosine inhibits the synthesis of dopamine by blocking the rate-limiting enzyme tyrosine hydroxylase. Because this is also the rate-limiting enzyme for the synthesis of norepinephrine, the use of this drug has widespread effects on the autonomic nervous system. Vesicular packaging of dopamine for proper release is blocked by reserpine and tetrabenazine, which are very potent dopamine antagonists. However, these drugs are nonspecific and also inhibit vesicular storage of norepinephrine and serotonin. Finally, receptor blockade occurs with phenothiazine neuroleptics or haloperidol. These drugs are relatively specific for the dopaminergic system but are not specific to any one dopaminergic pathway. Hence, when one tries to block dopamine function in one region, one may also block dopaminergic function in other basal gangliar and nonbasal gangliar systems. Dopaminergic pathways include the nigrostriatal, mesolimbic, mesocortical, and hypothalamic circuit involving prolactin. Many of the side effects of these potent drugs can be explained by these overlap effects.

Dopamine receptors fall into two major categories, those associated with (D_1 group) or independent of (D_2 group) adenyl cyclase. The D_1 group includes receptor types D_1 and D_5, and the D_2 group includes D_2, D_3, and D_4. In relationship to the striatum and its double dopaminergic input from the substantia nigra, the direct pathway involves the D_1 receptors and the indirect pathway involves D_2 systems.

Acetylcholine

Acetylcholine is synthesized from dietary choline, and acetyl coenzyme A by the enzyme choline acetyltransferase (CAT). There are two types of cholinergic receptors in basal gangliar structures, nicotinic and muscarinic. The cholinergic interneurons within the striatum are primarily muscarinic, but nicotinic receptors also populate the striatum as well as other basal gangliar nuclei. Because CAT is the rate-limiting enzyme, its function cannot easily be increased. Hence, augmentation of presynaptic acetylcholine has remained largely an unrealized dream for neuropharmacologists. The normal metabolism of acetylcholine takes place within the cholinergic synapse by the extracellular enzyme acetylcholinesterase. The centrally active acetylcholinesterase inhibitor physostigmine increases the available acetylcholine at central cholinergic receptors and increases cholinergic activity transiently. Its use in clinical medicine is limited by its short duration of action, its usual parenteral use, and its peripheral side effects. Newer centrally acting cholinesterase inhibitors that can be administered orally have been developed. These include donepezil, rivastigmine, and galantamine, all of which are marketed for impaired memory. Cholinergic receptor antagonists have been available for the muscarinic population since the 19th century. Originally called belladonna alkaloids, they block the muscarinic receptors of the pupil as well as the central nervous system and hence were used in the past by women who wanted large pupils as a sign of beauty. Antimuscarinic drugs are used to treat parkinsonism and dystonia. These agents can impair short-term memory.

Gamma-Aminobutyric Acid

Unlike acetylcholine and dopamine, GABA is a tiny amino acid that serves both as a neurotransmitter and as an intermediate metabolite in the normal function of cells. GABA is synthesized from glutamate, another amino acid neurotransmitter, by way of the vitamin B_6–dependent enzyme, glutamate decarboxylase. The presence of this enzyme has helped investigators in deducing whether GABA is present in a cell as a neurotransmitter or as a metabolite in other cell functions. The metabolism of GABA can proceed by two paths, via GABA transaminase or via the Krebs cycle.

GABAergic cells have a dense representation within the basal ganglia. Striatal GABAergic cells co-exist with either substance P or enkephalins and send axons to the substantia nigra pars compacta and reticulata, and to the external and internal globus pallidi. The pathways from the external globus pallidus to the subthalamic nucleus and from the internal globus pallidus to the thalamus also use GABA. In all known systems, GABA appears to interact with its receptor systems to inhibit or hyperpolarize.

Glutamate

This amino acid has high depolarization potential in many neuronal populations. Like GABA, it is an intermediate in cellular metabolism, so the presence of glutamate in a cell does not necessarily suggest neurological activity. As a neurotransmitter, however, glutamate functions with its receptors in an excitatory or depolarizing system at primary afferent nerve endings, the granule cells of the cerebellum, the dentate gyrus, and the corticostriatal and subthalamopallidal pathways important to basal gangliar function. The differentiation between glutamate-containing and aspartate-containing neurons is difficult with present technology. Glutamate activates receptors sensitive to either N-methyl-D-aspartate (NMDA), kainate, or quisqualate (non-NMDA).

Norepinephrine

This catecholamine neurotransmitter has its main cell populations in the hypothalamus, the lateral tegmentum, and the locus ceruleus. It is synthesized from dopamine, and therefore shares the same enzymes, including the rate-limiting tyrosine hydroxylase. Norepinephrine, however, has a unique enzyme associated with its synthesis called dopamine β-hydroxylase that transforms dopamine into norepinephrine. The presence of this unique enzyme is the primary way that noradrenergic cells are identified in the central nervous system. Norepinephrine is released from vesicles and activates two primary receptor systems, α and β. Like dopamine, norepinephrine is removed from the synapse by active reuptake into the presynaptic cell and then is metabolized by two enzymes, MAO and COMT. The final metabolic product of norepinephrine is 3-methoxy-4-hydroxymandelic acid (vanillylmandelic acid), although another metabolite, 3-methoxy-4-hydroxyphenyleneglycol, is often followed as the preferred marker of central nervous system norepinephrine metabolism. The noradrenergic system is more fully discussed in Chapter 3.

Serotonin

This indolamine neurotransmitter has its main cell bodies in the dorsal raphe nucleus of the brain stem as well as the spinal cord, hippocampus, and cerebellum. In parallel to dopamine, it is synthesized by a two-step process, first with a rate-limiting enzyme and then a general enzyme. The first step takes tryptophan to 5-hydroxytryptophan (5-HTP) with the rate-limiting enzyme, tryptophan hydroxylase. The second step takes this intermediate to serotonin (5-hydroxytryptamine, or 5-HT) by aromatic amino acid decarboxylase, which is the same enzyme involved in dopamine synthesis. There are several types of serotonin receptors spread throughout the brain, and they are classified by their location, enzymatic linkage, and propensity for various ligands. Serotonin is metabolized like the catecholamines, by active reuptake into the presynaptic cell and then metabolism by MAO (see also Chapter 3).

BASAL GANGLIAR INTERACTIONS WITH THE CEREBELLUM

Besides the basal ganglia, the cerebellum also has profound influences on motor function. Major cerebellar outflow paths converge on the ventral anterior and ventral lateral nuclei of the thalamus, and hence, these nuclei serve as a coordination center for the basal ganglia and cerebellar inputs to the cortex. Similar to the basal ganglia, the cerebellum influences the pyramidal system primarily through thalamocortical projections, and when cerebellar lesions occur, patients are poorly coordinated but are not weak. The cerebellar system, however, functions differently from the basal ganglia in that it has its own direct afferent paths from the entire cortex, as well as the spinal cord. The cerebellum appears to be important for rapid corrections of gross motor movements, whereas the basal ganglia affect more complex motor controls. As such, the prototype of a cerebellar lesion is sloppy execution (dyssernergia) of simple motor tasks and terminal tremor, but without the superimposition of other abnormal involuntary movements (see Chapter 17).

ANATOMICAL AND PHYSIOLOGICAL HYPOTHESES FOR HYPOKINESIA AND HYPERKINESIA

Based on these data, models of hypokinetic and hyperkinetic disorders have been proposed and examined in animals as well as in humans. In monkeys treated with the toxin *N*-methyl-4-phenyl-1,2,3,6-tetrahydropyridine, profound hypokinesia develops, and pathologically, there is highly focused damage of the pars compacta substantia nigra (Fig. 16–4). Physiologically, as predicted by a resultant enhancement of the indirect pathway and a diminished influence of the direct pathway, the degenerated pars compacta and the associated loss of striatal dopamine lead to increases in the neuronal discharge of the subthalamic nucleus and tonic discharges from the GP_i. The resultant enhanced inhibition of the thalamus reduces cortical activation and correlates with reduced volitional movement in these experimental animals. In concert, there appears to be an altered phasic responsiveness by the GP_i to proprioceptive stimuli. Numbers of responding cells increase, and the receptive field becomes less specific, with loss of directional effects and responses from multiple joints. It has been suggested that such changes account for rigidity and for altered timing and coordination of volitional movements in hypokinesia. Direct lesioning or high-frequency stimulation of the subthalamic nucleus, GP_i, and thalamus can relieve hypokinesia (see Chapter 34).

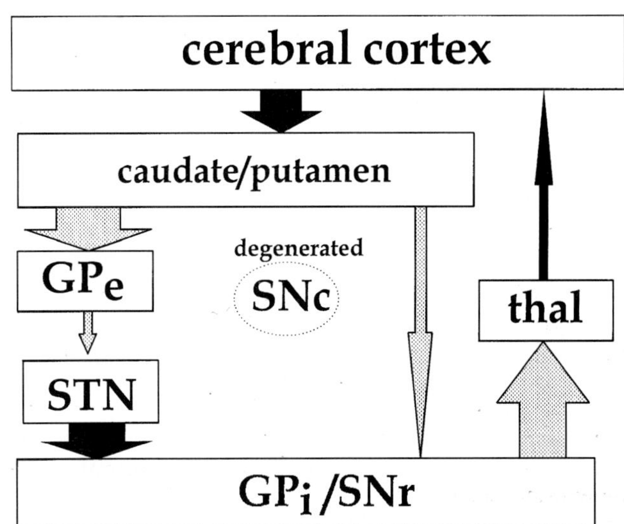

FIGURE 16–4. Schema of hypokinesia, with reduced input from SNc, enhanced activation of the excitatory subthalamopallidal fibers in the indirect pathway and reduced function of the direct pathway. Output from the GP_i is enhanced with more inhibition at the level of the thalamus and less activation of the cortex. Abbreviations: see Figure 16–3.

The same anatomophysiopharmacological model has been applied to hyperkinesia as well, with the disorder Huntington's disease serving as the prototype (Fig. 16–5). In this case, the primary driving aberration involves the indirect striatal pathway with selective loss of the GABA-enkephalin–containing cells projecting from the striatum to the GP_e. Resultant overactivation of GP_e excessively inhibits the subthalamic nucleus; the thalamus is no longer inhibited, with resultant overexcitation of cortical signals and hyperkinesia. Evidence that this model is sound for at least some forms of hyperkinesia includes the known pathological

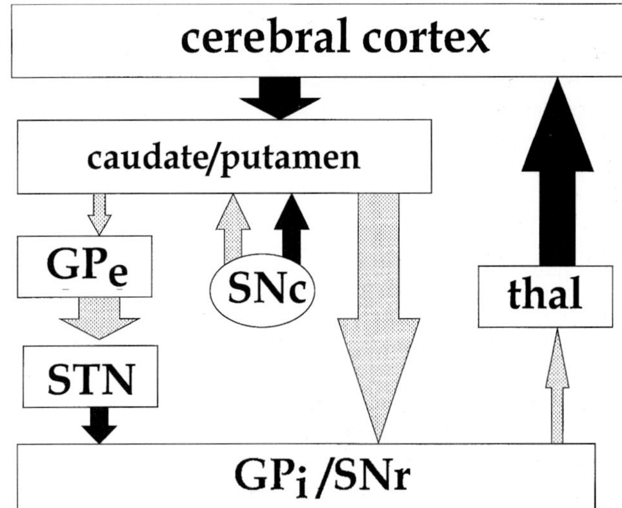

FIGURE 16–5. Schema of hyperkinesia, diminished activation of the excitatory subthalamopallidal fibers in the indirect pathway, and enhanced function of the direct pathway. Output from the GP_i is decreased with less inhibition at the level of the thalamus and more motor activation of the cortex. Abbreviations: see Figure 16–3.

changes in Huntington's disease, the cessation of hyperkinetic drug-induced dyskinesias in Parkinson's disease patients after lesions of the GP_i, and the well-documented induction of ballistic hyperkinesias after destruction of the subthalamic nucleus. However, the large variety of dyskinesias is not explained by this model at the present time.

Examination of Hypokinesia and Hyperkinesia (Table 16–2)

DIRECTED NEUROLOGICAL EXAMINATION

In assessing hypokinesia or hyperkinesia, the directed neurological examination aims to categorize the disorder phenomenologically and to detect the activities that maximize abnormal movements. With this information and support from appropriate diagnostic tests (see Part Two), the diagnosis of a movement disorder by specific name and etiology can be determined (see Chapter 34). In assessing hypokinesia or hyperkinesia, three primary testing paradigms are used: (1) rest, (2) maintenance of a static posture, and (3) volitional activity. Tone is determined at rest, with attention to changes with posture or activity. A final task that is requisite to any evaluation of hypokinesia or hyperkinesia is walking, because this activity integrates several functions, and specific patterns of gait dysfunction are particularly helpful in characterizing a movement disorder.

Patient at Rest

The patient needs to be observed sitting quietly in a comfortable position; occasionally, it is necessary to observe the patient lying supine. In assessing the rest position, be certain that the extremities are fully relaxed and supported so that the patient is not holding a posture. When engaged in conversation, most individuals have spontaneous gestures of their hands, often cross one leg over the other, and smile when chatting. In hypokinetic disorders, there is a paucity of

TABLE 16–2. **Clinico-anatomical Correlation of Disorders Associated with Hypokinesia and Hyperkinesia**

Hypokinetic or Hyperkinetic Finding	Common Anatomical or Neurochemical Lesion	Other Neurological and Medical Findings	Selected Common Etiologies
Hypokinesia			
Parkinsonism—pure	Degeneration of substantia nigra	None	Parkinson's disease
	Blockade of striatal dopamine receptors	If drug induced, may have chorea or dystonia in addition to parkinsonism	Drugs: usually neuroleptics
Parkinsonism-plus	Multifocal or diffuse neuronal degeneration with or without degeneration of substantia nigra	Progressive supranuclear palsy: vertical gaze paresis Multiple system atrophy: hypotension, dysautonomia, and impotency	Primary neurodegenerative condition
Hyperkinesias			
Tremors	Postural and action tremor: heightened activity of central noradrenergic systems	If hyperthyroid, will have anxiety, increased sweating; proptosis	Hyperthyroidism Prescription drugs Illicit drugs Essential tremor
	Cerebellar kinetic tremor: white matter lesions in cerebellum or brain stem	May have other signs of white matter central nervous system illness, Lhermitte's sign, optic atrophy, pyramidal signs	Multiple sclerosis Vascular disease
Chorea	Striatal degeneration	Dementia	Huntington's disease
	Striatal dopaminergic hypersensitivity	Psychotic behavior or depression	Tardive dyskinesia
Ballismus	Subthalamic nucleus lesions	Weakness	Vascular disease
Tics and sterotypies	Dopaminergic hypersensitivity—site unknown	Attention deficit disorder, obsessive-compulsive behaviors	Gilles de la Tourette syndrome
		Mental retardation	Rett syndrome, Angelman's syndrome Down syndrome
Dystonia	Putamen lesions, pallidal lesions, or no specific lesion	Usually no other signs Tremor and chorea	Idiopathic torsion dystonia Neuroleptic tardive dyskinesia
Athetosis	Globus pallidal lesion Thalamic lesion	Weakness	Cerebrovascular accident
Myoclonus	Cortex, brain stem, or spinal cord	Epilepsy Palatal myoclonus	Cortical myoclonus Reticular myoclonus Segmental myoclonus
Hemifacial spasm	Cranial nerve VII or no specific lesion	Mild weakness of facial muscles	Usually idiopathic, can have compressive lesions

movement, including lack of normal gesturing and spontaneous movements. The face is hypomimetic, with lack of expression, and there is reduced rate of blinking. Rest tremor, if present, is elicited when the hands and feet are completely relaxed.

In hyperkinesias, key information is obtained by observing the patient at rest in complete repose without talking. Relaxing these patients and finding the best rest position can be a challenge. It is important to recognize that a sitting position is one of rest for the extremities, but one of activation for the trunk. In dystonia, in which movements are often absent during rest and activate with a maintained posture, the examiner must be particularly vigilant to correctly identify postures that are resting and active. As such, in truncal dystonia, a kyphotic posture may be present when the patient is sitting erect or standing in seeming repose, because the trunk muscles are activated in these positions. To test for resolution or diminution in the rest posture, these patients must lie supine or prone. Likewise, neck hyperkinesias must be studied with great care to achieve a rest position. Cervical dystonia may be prominent with the patient quietly sitting, but in fact, the neck muscles are very active in the sitting posture and the rest position for the neck requires head support, such as the patient resting the back of the head against a wall or high-backed chair.

Many other hyperkinesias are present at rest, such as athetosis, ballismus, chorea, moving digits, myokymia, and tics. Patients with akathisia resist sitting quietly because the urge to move increases, and even when instructed to remain still, they persist with movements such as caressing the scalp, crossing and uncrossing the legs, spontaneously standing up, and even moaning. Involuntary vocalizations that occur in tic disorders or gasping choreic sounds may be audible when the patient is sitting comfortably, and voluntary phonic sensory tricks, used by dystonic patients to break sustained contractions of the eyelids, jaw, or pharynx, occur frequently when the patient is sitting quietly.

Importantly, tics are highly influenced by environment, and patients are usually able to suppress their tics at least partially in the presence of the observer. Encouraging them to sit in a restful position in a quiet room, especially in isolation with a video camera running, may permit an observer to appreciate a wide variety of tics, both motor and phonic, that otherwise would not be documented in the neurological examination.

If myoclonus or a heightened startle reflex is suspected, the investigator should suddenly clap the hands or drop a book on the floor to surprise the patient. Such a maneuver should be performed with the patient sitting and not standing, because patients can have both positive jerks and negative myoclonus, the latter associated with loss of postural tone and falling.

Maintenance of a Posture

Postural tremor is maximized when the patient assumes and attempts to maintain a posture. In the case of a patient with hand tremor, there may be no tremor at rest, but when the hands are outstretched, a fine or coarse tremor develops. Patients with myoclonus may extend their arms well and maintain them for several seconds, when suddenly a lightning-like jerk displaces their shoulder or upper arm. These myoclonic jerks may be so brisk as to cause the patient to drop objects or fling them. With postural tremors, during the finger-to-nose test, finger oscillations will be seen as the patient moves from the finger to the nose, but at each endpoint, the tremor abates and the subject effectively hits the target without dyssynergia. During handwriting, as the hand assumes the writing posture, tremor occurs and a large, shaky signature develops. Dystonic patients also develop tremor often when they are forced to maintain a posture that activates their dystonia. This dystonic tremor is believed to be the patient's own compensatory movement to overcome the dystonia. Therefore, the tremor can usually be maximized in the position that opposes the natural dystonic contraction and minimized or even aborted completely in the position of natural dystonic deformity. One of the clinical hallmarks of chorea is termed motor impersistence, and patients are unable to maintain a posture without the superimposition of the random choreic movements. The tongue darts involuntarily back into the mouth when the subject tries to maintain it protruded, and when the subject tries to grip the examiner's hand or finger with steady pressure, there is uncontrolled squeezing and release (milk-maid grip).

Execution of Tasks

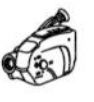

Many tasks are interrupted by hypokinesia and hyperkinesia, and the structured neurological examination of the motor system usually includes a series of simple maneuvers of high yield. Finger tapping is slow and cramped in hypokinesia, and sloppy and overridden with additional movements in chorea or cerebellar dyssynergia. The same task may precipitate a spasm of contorted hand posture in a dystonic. Likewise, foot tapping brings out the same features in the lower extremities. Handwriting is useful to evaluate because bradykinesia causes a small and cramped parkinsonian script (micrographia); action tremor causes a large, tremulous signature; and dystonia induces irregular script and often the patient will need to adjust the pen several times because of painful spasms or involuntary dystonic movements. The finger-to-nose task helps distinguish postural tremor from kinetic or endpoint tremor, which is usually associated with cerebellar ataxia (see Chapter 17). In postural tremor, the tremor is seen through the trajectory movement but the patient's finger stabilizes at the endpoint (either the examiner's finger or the patient's nose). The kinetic tremor actually augments at the endpoint.

Speech is another particularly valuable task to evaluate, because it allows the examiner to detect dysarthria, hypophonia, and language disorders and also presents an opportunity as a window of intelligence. Talking is a common motor act that induces overflow dystonic or choreic movements elsewhere in the body and can bring out action dystonia of the tongue, face, or jaw muscles. In many patients with blepharospasm as a form of dystonia, the forced eyelid closure may be relieved by talking or humming.

Movement disorders of all types can affect the production and clarity of speech. In the hypokinetic disorders, decreased amplitude of speech (hypophonia) and lack of inflection (aprosody) are most common. Hypophonia can become so severe that the voice may be restricted to a bare whisper. Other speech abnormalities can also occur in parkinsonism, such as palilalia. In parkinsonism, palilalia is the repetition of the first syllables of words; in patients with Gilles de la

Tourette syndrome, palilalia is manifested by a repetition of phrases (also called palilogia). Patients with Parkinson's disease can also have transient speech arrests in the middle of talking due to the freezing phenomenon. They can also have tachyphemia, which is very rapid speech with no pausing between syllables; the words run together and the listener cannot easily distinguish them. Myoclonus can interrupt speech. Lingual dystonia results in impaired, indistinct speech because the tongue does not move normally. Some patients with oromandibular dystonia or blepharospasm may make sounds to break the dystonic contractions; these are basically sensory tricks.

In addition to palilalia, patients with Gilles de la Tourette syndrome may have echolalia (repeating phrases of others) or coprolalia (uttering obscenities or fragments of obscene words), as well as a variety of vocal tics representing words, sounds, coughs, sniffs, or throat clearing. In addition, they may make sudden increased amplitude of their speech, and they can have speech blocks, which are interruptions of the patient's conversation that occur during a sequence of motor tics.

Voice tremor is usually a manifestation of vocal cord tremor and sometimes vocal cord adductor dystonia. Occasionally, voice tremor is the result of pronounced neck tremor. Tardive dyskinesia of respiratory muscles can also produce a lack of smoothness of speech.

Speech apraxia can be seen in apractic syndromes, including corticobasal degeneration. Speech is often hesitant in this disorder, as it is in progressive supranuclear palsy.

Movement disorders by themselves do not regularly cause language difficulties unless some other neurological disorder is present, such as dementia. Importantly, although speech is a relevant aspect of disability in hypokinesia and hyperkinesia, the clinician must also consider upper motor neuron, lower motor neuron, and cerebellar disorders in evaluating speech (see Chapter 6).

Tone

Tone represents the resistance to passive movement of a joint. Unlike spasticity, which is characteristic of upper motor neuron disease (see Chapter 15), rigidity, the hallmark of hypokinesia, is increased tone of both flexor and extensor muscles. Often, in parkinsonism, there is a cogwheeling character to the hypertonicity (cogwheel rigidity). Dystonic patients also have increased tone when the dystonia is active, although the tone in uninvolved groups is generally normal. In chorea, the tone is often reduced (hypotonia) and the excess movements take on a puppet-like quality as they flow from one body part to another. In patients with tics, the tone is normal.

Walking

As discussed in greater detail in Chapter 18, gait integrates numerous neuroanatomical systems, including pyramidal, extrapyramidal, cerebellar, visual, vestibular, and cognitive. In hypokinesia, the patient has a hunched, flexed posture, and the arms do not swing well during walking. The steps are small, and often the patient walks on the toes (marche à petits pas). If the body is flexed forward, there may be a propulsive running gait (festination) as the patient attempts to avoid falling forward. Alternatively, the patient may fall backward, especially when pivoting. In hyperkinesias, a variety of abnormalities are seen. In chorea, there is a lilting, stuttering, dance-like quality of walking, often accompanied by hypotonic limbs that move too freely with superimposed random choreic hand or arm movements. In dystonia, walking brings out the spasms, so the patient may begin normally but, after several seconds or minutes, develop inversion of the foot, hyperextension of the large toe, and cramps. Tics may abate during walking or occur during pauses. After assessing walking, the clinician must test for postural reflexes by standing behind the patient and giving a brisk pull on the shoulders (pull test). Patients should be warned and instructed to resist this postural threat, but in several movement disorders, they will take several steps backward or even fall. The examiner must be prepared to catch the patient.

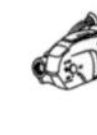

ASSOCIATED NEUROLOGICAL FINDINGS

Cerebrum. Because the basal ganglia circuits include the cortex and because the caudate nucleus is particularly involved with cognition, the cerebral examination can have important contributory findings in patients with hypokinesia or hyperkinesia. Bedside screening tests of dementia and depression are very useful, and an assessment of aphasia and apraxia indicates likely cortical lesions.

Cranial Nerves. Most cranial nerve functions are retained in hypokinesia and hyperkinesia. Ocular saccades can be slowed in Huntington's disease, and vertical conjugate gaze paresis should specifically suggest hypokinetic disorders like progressive supranuclear palsy. The facial nerve (cranial nerve VII) may be affected in patients with hemifacial spasm, and the patient may have a mildly flattened nasolabial fold at rest. Tongue protrusion and movements can reveal bradykinesia as a sign of parkinsonism, tremor as a sign of parkinsonism or other cause of tremor, and macroglossia as a sign of tardive dyskinesia. Independent of speech assessment (see earlier), the palate should be examined for the possibility of palatal myoclonus.

Motor/Reflexes/Cerebellar/Gait. Most of the pertinent motor findings in hypokinesia and hyperkinesia are discussed in the section entitled Directed Neurological Examination. In almost all instances, strength is preserved and deep tendon reflexes are normal.

Sensory System. Although patients may complain of pain or altered sensations in hypokinesia and hyperkinesia, the systematic sensory examination of pain or temperature and position or vibration senses is generally normal. In cases of the hypokinetic disorder corticobasal degeneration, cortical sensory loss and graphanesthesia may occur. In the condition painful legs/moving toes, which often is preceded by peripheral nervous system damage, the sensory examination shows signs suggestive of neuropathy or radiculopathy (see Chapters 19 and 20).

Autonomic Nervous System. Several movement disorders are accompanied by dysautonomia, and furthermore, many of the drug treatments for hypokinetic and hyperkinetic disorders affect autonomic nervous function. Orthostatic hypotension in the face of hypokinesia, rigidity, and gait abnormalities suggests multiple system atrophy. In patients with this condition, the normal tachycardia that develops on standing does not regularly occur and patients may actually lose consciousness in the first few minutes on standing (see Chapters 21 and 34).

Neurovascular. Most cases of movement disorders do not have a vascular etiology, but abnormal vascular findings on examination can suggest very specific syndromes. Small vessel disease in the brain can be a cause of a lower body parkinsonism with a shuffling gait, so-called vascular parkinsonism. Chorea can result from systemic lupus erythematosus; flushed skin and vascular evidence of hyperviscosity suggests polycythemia, associated with chorea and ballismus; and vascular neck disease or evidence of cardiac embolic sources raises the possibility of multifocal strokes that can lead to parkinsonism or hyperkinesias.

DIRECTED GENERAL EXAMINATION

The general medical examination provides useful diagnostic information in patients with hypokinesia and hyperkinesia. The skin examination in patients with Parkinson's disease shows seborrhea, scaly skin, and often patches of excessive dryness. Increased salivation and drooling are typical. The eyes should be examined in patients with movement disorders to detect the presence of Kayser-Fleischer rings from copper deposits in the cornea (Wilson's disease), and proptosis and lid-lag suggests hyperthyroidism, which is frequently associated with chorea or postural tremors.

Evaluation Guidelines (Table 16–3)

Neuroimaging. Many of the primary neurodegenerative movement disorders, whether hypokinetic or hyperkinetic, show no abnormalities on magnetic resonance imaging (MRI) or computed tomography (CT) scans other than mild to moderate cerebral atrophy. However, in Huntington's disease and in neuroacanthocytosis, two conditions associated with chorea, there may be focal atrophy of the caudate nucleus, leading to the appearance of enlarged lateral ventricles, without a comparable increase in size of the temporal horns. Similarly, in multiple system atrophy of the olivopontocerebellar type, localized atrophy of the pons and cerebellum may be prominent. In cases of hypokinesia, the MRI scan shows increased signal intensity in the outer rim of the putamen on T2-weighted images in multiple system atrophy. There is decreased T2 signal from excessive iron deposition in the globus pallidus in Hallervorden-Spatz syndrome and in a new entity, neuroferritinopathy, in which dystonia is a clinical feature.[28] MRI and CT scans are particularly useful in disclosing secondary causes of movement disorders. Cerebrovascular accidents, abscesses, and tumors can be identified, as well as calcium deposition that may suggest parathyroid disease, old hemorrhage, or infections. Hypokinesia caused by carbon monoxide intoxication likewise has a characteristic pattern of cystic degeneration of the globus pallidus. Other neuroimaging techniques may prove useful in particular situations, such as single photon emission computed tomography scanning in corticobasal degeneration, in which focal parietal lobe hypoactivity can sometimes be detected. Positron-emission tomography scanning with the use of selective ligands is used extensively in research centers to monitor patients with hypokinesia and hyperkinesia, but it is not used in a regular clinical setting (see Chapters 23 and 34).

Electrophysiology. Electroencephalography (EEG) is useful in studying any intermittent movement disorder, but the recording obtained must include episodes of the patient's movements in order to determine if there is a cortical event that occurs simultaneously. Cases of paroxysmal dyskinesias can sometimes be associated with epileptiform discharges in the contralateral frontal cortical region, and although they may not be detected in a standard EEG, double-density electrodes may provide the phase-reversal indicative of a seizure. In myoclonic disorders, the EEG is important for documentation of a possible associated cortical event at the time of the myoclonic jerk detected by electromyography (EMG). Sensory evoked potentials and specialized computerized back-averaging techniques can be used with simultaneous EMG to clarify the brain stem or cortical origins. Tremors can be characterized with accelerometer recordings applied over agonist and antagonist muscle groups. In the evaluation of dystonic patients who will receive injections of botulinum toxin (see Chapter 34), the muscles maximally involved in the spasms can be identified with EMG needle recordings at the time of the injection. A variety of research electrophysiological tests are used for the study of movement disorders and their quantification, but these tests are largely restricted to specialty centers.

Fluid and Tissue Analysis. Few blood and urine tests are of primary interest in the characterization of movement disorders. Basic electrolytes, complete blood count, liver function tests, and thyroid function tests are standard tests that can be helpful screens. In cases of dystonia or tremor in which the specific condition known as Wilson's disease is considered, 24-hour urine levels of copper excretion and serum ceruloplasmin levels are useful. In specific cases, blood ammonia levels, coagulation profiles, or blood viscosity can be analyzed. In cases of chorea, unusual tics, or dystonic movement, fresh blood smear analysis for acanthocytes can be diagnostic. Childhood aminoacidopathies or other metabolic disorders with hypokinesia or hyperkinesias are diagnosed with specialized tests for enzyme levels or storage compounds found in blood, urine, or various biopsy tissues (see Chapters 30 and 31). For a growing number of genetic illnesses with movement disorders that include Huntington's disease, generalized torsion dystonia, spinocerebellar degenerations, and dentatorubral-pallidoluysian atrophy, genetic tests can be diagnostic. In cases of acute onset of disorders, a toxicology screen is essential.

Cerebrospinal Fluid (CSF). Whereas alterations in various neurochemical metabolites such as homovanillic acid (dopamine) and 5-hydroxyindolacetic acid (serotonin) are of research interest in various movement disorders, their levels are neither diagnostic nor useful specifically in dealing with disease progression. CSF drainage over several days may have diagnostic value in normal pressure hydrocephalus, and a beneficial result may have predictive value in a subsequent ventriculoperitoneal shunt.

Neuropsychological Tests. These tests help document cognitive and affective dysfunction that can be useful in determining diagnoses like Huntington's disease, Alzheimer's disease, and diffuse Lewy body disease, and also in guiding potential decisions regarding medical therapy. For example, when movement disorders are associated with depression or

TABLE 16–3. **Useful Studies in the Evaluation of Hypokinesia and Hyperkinesia Syndromes**

Syndrome	Neuroimaging	Electrophysiology	Fluid and Tissue Analysis	Neuropsychological Tests
Hypokinesia				
Pure parkinsonism	In Parkinson's disease, MRI and CT are normal; PET scans of F-dopa can show decreased uptake	Usually not used. Can study tremor with accelerometer	Copper, ceruloplasmin, and thyroid	Can detect depression, dementia
Parkinsonism-plus syndromes	In multiple system atrophy, putamen can have hyperdensity in T2-weighted images; SPECT scans can show decreased activity in frontal parietal lobe	Rectal EMG may be useful in multiple system atrophy	In multiple system atrophy catecholamines can be studied	Can detect evidence of dyspraxia, aphasia, cortical or subcortical dementia patterns
Hyperkinesia				
Postural tremor	Normal	Tremor can be studied with accelerometer	Thyroid, drug levels especially lithium, amphetamines, and tricyclic antidepressants	Not usually useful
Action-endpoint tremor	May show cerebellar white matter lesions	Evoked potentials may show evidence of widespread white matter disease as in multiple sclerosis	Lithium level; CSF can be studied for multiple sclerosis	Not usually useful. Pseudobulbar affect can be seen with multiple sclerosis
Chorea, choreoathetosis, and ballismus	In Huntington's disease, there is reduced volume of caudate nucleus Generalized cerebral atrophy	Not usually useful	Acanthocytes by fresh red blood smear, thyroid, drug levels of anticonvulsants Genetic testing for Huntington's disease	Dementia can be detected, along with impulsive behavior and depression
Tics and stereotypies	Normal	Not usually useful	None used	Attention deficit disorder and obsessive-compulsive behaviors are frequent problems in tic patients
Dystonia	Normal, can have lesion in putamen in some forms of secondary dystonia	Not usually useful except EMG is often used to guide botulinum toxin injections for therapy	Blood test now can identify gene in idiopathic torsion dystonia	Depression and pain can be important contributors to disability
Akathisia	Normal	Not useful	Not useful	Patients can be psychotic, depressed, and anxious
Myoclonus	Usually normal; in postanoxic mycolonus, there may be diffuse cortical and subcortical damage	EEG helps detect seizures; also can show diffuse slow wave activity in encephalopathies; in research centers, back-averaging techniques can study origin of myoclonus	Electrolytes, calcium, magnesium, thyroid function for metabolic causes of myoclonus	Dementia, difficulties concentrating

CSF, Cerebrospinal fluid; CT, computed tomography; EMG, electromyography; F-dopa, fluorodopa; MRI, magnetic resonance imaging; PET, positron-emission tomography; SPECT, single photon emission computed tomography; EEG, electroencephalography.

dementia, drugs that are associated with side effects such as depression, confusion, or psychosis need to be avoided or used in reduced doses. Some movement disorders commonly co-exist with specific types of behavioral patterns, for example, Gilles de la Tourette syndrome and attention deficit disorder or obsessive-compulsive disorder, and neuropsychological evaluations complement the neurological examination in identifying such combinations.

Clinical Syndromes

HYPOKINESIA SYNDROMES (Table 16–4)

The term hypokinetic syndrome is synonymous with parkinsonism. In addition to slowness, parkinsonism, as a clinical syndrome of multiple etiologies, is manifested by combinations of several cardinal symptoms and signs (Table 16–5). At least two of the cardinal features should be present before the syndromic diagnosis of parkinsonism is made, with one of them being hypokinesia or tremor at rest. Parkinsonism can occur in isolation without other neurological signs, or can occur as part of a larger neurological syndrome, termed descriptively Parkinson-plus syndromes. The specific diagnosis depends on details of the clinical history, physical examination, and laboratory findings (see Chapter 34).

Parkinsonism

Primary parkinsonism, or Parkinson's disease, is the most common type of parkinsonism encountered by the neurologist, but drug-induced parkinsonism is probably far more prevalent. Dopamine receptor antagonists, which are usually prescribed for psychotic behavior but occasionally for gastrointestinal disturbances, are the likely causative agents. In these forms of primary and secondary parkinsonism, the

TABLE 16–4. **Selected Etiologies Associated with Hypokinesia and Hyperkinesia Syndromes**

Etiological Category	Specific Etiologies	Chapter
Structural Disorders		
Developmental	Hemiatrophy-hemiparkinsonism	28
	Hydrocephalus causing gait dysfunction that resembles parkinsonism	
	Pseudodystonia can occur in syringomyelia and Arnold-Chiari malformations	
Degenerative and compressive	Pseudodystonia from atlantoaxial subluxation	29
Hereditary and Degenerative Disorders		
Storage diseases: Lipidoses, glycogenoses, and leukodystrophies	Neuronal ceroid-lipofuscinosis especially type 1, 4, 6, GM_1-gangliosidosis type III, GM_2 gangliosidosis, sphingomyelinosis type C	30
Amino/organic acidopathies, mitochondrial enzyme defects, and other metabolic errors	Mitochondrial disorders, Leigh's disease, glutaricacidemia, methylmalonicacidemia, homocystinuria, Hartnup's disease, Lesch-Nyhan syndrome	31
Chromosomal abnormalities and neurocutaneous disorders	Fragile-X syndrome, Rett syndrome, Down syndrome, tuberous sclerosis	32
Degenerative dementias	Huntington's disease, Alzheimer's disease, Pick's disease	33
Movement disorders	Parkinson's disease, progressive supranuclear palsy, multiple system atrophy, Huntington's disease, Gilles de la Tourette syndrome, essential myoclonus, dystonia, hemifacial spasms	34
Ataxias	Spinocerebellar ataxias	35
Degenerative motor, sensory, and autonomic disorders	ALS-Parkinson-dementia complex of Guam	36
	Tremors in Charcot-Marie-Tooth and Roussy-Levy diseases	
Hereditary nondegenerative neuromuscular disease	Neuromyotonias can appear as pseudodystonias	37
Acquired Metabolic and Nutritional Disorders		
Endogenous metabolic disorders	Hyperthyroidism, hypothyroidism, hypoparathyroidism, hyperparathyroidism, diabetes, hypoglycemia, hyperestrogen states including pregnancy	38
Exogenous acquired metabolic disorders of the nervous system: Toxins and illicit drugs	Lead, mercury, manganese, methyl alcohol, toluene, trichlorethane, carbon tetrachloride, carbon monoxide, MPTP, cocaine, amphetamine derivatives	39
Nutritional deficiencies and syndromes associated with alcoholism	Alcohol, thiamine deficiency, vitamin B_{12} deficiency	40
Infectious Disorders		
Viral infections	Influenza (encephalitis lethargica)	41
Nonviral infections	Abscess, encephalitis, vasculitis (Sydenham's chorea)	42
Transmissible spongiform encephalopathies	Creutzfeldt-Jakob disease, kuru	43
HIV and AIDS	AIDS encephalopathy, opportunistic infections and abscesses	44

Table continued on following page

TABLE 16–4. **Selected Etiologies Associated with Hypokinesia and Hyperkinesia Syndromes** *Continued*

Etiological Category	Specific Etiologies	Chapter
Neurovascular Disorders	Cerebrovascular accidents, AVMs	45
Neoplastic Disorders		
Primary neurological tumors	Primary tumors affecting basal ganglia or white matter connecting pathways	46
Metastatic neoplasms and paraneoplastic syndromes	Metastatic tumors affecting basal ganglia or white matter connecting pathways; stiff-person syndrome as perineoplastic syndrome	47
Demyelinating Disorders		
Demyelinating disorders of the central nervous system	Multiple sclerosis (especially paroxysmal dyskinesias and cerebellar tremor)	48
Demyelinating disorders of the peripheral nervous system	Distal chorea can develop in patients with peripheral neuropathy	49
Autoimmune and Inflammatory Disorders	Sydenham's chorea, systemic lupus erythematosus, chorea, stiff-person syndrome	50
Traumatic Disorders	Dystonia, pugilist encephalopathy causing parkinsonism-plus, stump dyskinesia, painful legs/moving toes	51
Epilepsy	Epilepsia-related paroxysmal dyskinesias. Tremor can be a sign of epilepsia partialis continua. Myoclonus can be part of the myoclonic epilepsies	52
Sleep Disorders	REM-behavioral disorder, restless legs	54
Drug-Induced and Iatrogenic Neurological Disorders	Anticonvulsants, lithium, tricyclic antidepressants, phenothiazine antipsychotics, narcotics, methotrexate, metoclopramide, oral contraceptive	55

AIDS, Acquired immunodeficiency syndrome; ALS, amyotrophic lateral sclerosis; AVM, arteriovenous malformation; HIV, human immunodeficiency virus; MPTP, 1-methyl-4-phenyl-1,2,3,6 tetrahydropyridine.

syndrome usually occurs in isolation, without other neurological signs. Hypokinesia is manifested cranially by masked facies (hypomimia), decreased blinking, soft speech with loss of inflection (aprosody), and drooling of saliva due to decreased spontaneous swallowing. In the arms, there is slowness in shrugging the shoulder and raising the arm, loss of spontaneous movement such as gesturing, smallness and slowness of handwriting (micrographia), and difficulty with hand dexterity for shaving, brushing teeth, and putting on make-up. In the legs, there is a short-stepped, shuffling gait with slowed foot movements, and in the trunk, there is difficulty arising from a chair, getting out of automobiles, and turning in bed. Bradykinesia thus encompasses a loss of automatic movements as well as slowness in initiating movement on command and reduction in amplitude of the voluntary movement. The latter can be observed as decrementing amplitude with repetitive finger tapping or foot tapping. The ability to carrying out two activities simultaneously is affected,[29] and this difficulty may represent bradykinesia as well.[30]

TABLE 16–5. **Cardinal Features of Parkinsonism**

Tremor at rest
Rigidity
Bradykinesia/hypokinesia
Flexed posture of neck, trunk, and limbs
Loss of postural reflexes
Freezing

Rigidity is another cardinal feature of parkinsonism. Rigidity is usually manifested by a ratchet-like tension in the range of motion, so-called cogwheel rigidity. As the disease advances, the patient begins to assume a flexed posture, particularly of the elbows, knees, thorax, and neck. Eventually, the flexion can become extreme. The patient begins to walk with the arms flexed at the elbows and the forearms placed in front of the body, and with decreased arm swing. With the knees slightly flexed, the patient tends to shuffle the feet, which stay close to the ground and are not lifted up as high as in normals; there is loss of heel strike, which would normally occur when the foot moving forward is placed onto the ground.

Loss of postural reflexes occurs later in the disease. The patient has difficulty righting himself after being pulled off balance. A simple test for the righting reflex is for the examiner to stand behind the patient and give a firm tug on the patient's shoulders toward the examiner, warning the patient in advance that he or she should try to maintain balance by taking a step backward. Normally, a person can recover in one step. A mild loss of postural reflexes can be detected if the patient requires several steps to recover balance. A moderate loss is manifested by a greater degree of retropulsion. With a more severe loss, the patient would fall if not caught by the examiner, who must always be prepared for such a possibility. With a marked loss of postural reflexes, a patient cannot withstand a gentle tug on the shoulders or cannot stand unassisted without falling. In order to avoid having the patient fall to the ground, it is wise to have a wall behind the examiner, particularly if the patient is a large, bulky individual.

A combination of loss of postural reflexes with stooped posture can lead to festination, whereby the patient walks faster and faster, trying to catch up with his or her center of gravity to prevent falling.

The freezing phenomenon[31] usually begins with start-hesitation; that is, the feet take short, sticking, shuffling steps before the patient can begin walking. With progression, the feet seem to become glued to the ground when the patient needs to walk through a crowded space (e.g., a revolving door) or when trying to move a fixed distance in a short period of time (e.g., crossing the street at the green light or entering an elevator before the door closes). Often, patients develop destination-freezing, that is, stopping before reaching the final destination. For example, the patient may stop too soon when reaching a chair in which to sit down. With further progression, sudden transient freezing can occur when the patient is walking in an open space or when he perceives an obstacle in his walking path.

When faced with a patient with parkinsonism, the major differential diagnoses include primary Parkinson's disease and drug exposure to agents such as dopamine receptor blockers (antipsychotics, some antinausea medications, and metoclopramide), dopamine-depleting drugs (alpha-methyldopa, reserpine, and tetrabenazine), and some illicit drugs. Cerebrovascular accidents, infections, toxins, and other neurodegenerative diseases usually cause parkinsonism in the context of additional neurological signs (see later).

Parkinsonism-Plus Syndromes

The same constellation of features can occur in patients who have additional signs of neurodegenerative lesions, and these syndromes are termed Parkinson-plus. This heterogenous group of disorders has a large variety of supplementary signs, but some diagnoses have particularly typical ones: supranuclear vertical gaze paresis is typical of progressive supranuclear palsy; apraxias and cortical sensory loss are typical of corticobasal degeneration; and dysautonomia, ataxia, and endpoint kinetic tremors are typical of multiple system atrophy. There is considerable overlap among these syndromes and, in early stages, with primary parkinsonism. In defining a patient with a hypokinetic syndrome, these additional signs must be systematically evaluated in order to differentiate to the maximal degree possible Parkinson's disease from Parkinsonism-plus syndromes (see Chapter 34). Secondary causes of parkinsonism, such as trauma, cerebrovascular accidents, and infection, can also cause parkinsonism plus other neurological features, but usually these patients lack the particular constellation of signs distinctive of the neurodegenerative disorders.

HYPERKINESIA SYNDROMES (see Table 16–4)

Tremors

Tremor is an oscillating movement affecting one or more body parts, such as the limbs, neck, tongue, chin, or vocal cords. It is usually rhythmical and regular. Tremor can be due to alternate or simultaneous contractions of agonists and antagonists. The rate, location, amplitude, and constancy varies, depending on the specific type of tremor and its severity. It is helpful to determine whether or not the tremor is present at rest (with the patient sitting or lying in repose), with posture-holding (with the arms extending in front of the body), with action (such as writing), or with intention maneuvers (such as bringing the finger to touch the nose). Etiologies and treatment differ according to these types.  Postural tremors are seen in familial tremor, in hyperthyroidism, and with some prescribed medications including lithium carbonate, tricyclic antidepressants, and theophylline. Action and intention tremors are discussed in the chapter on ataxia (Chapter 35), and other tremors are examined in the chapter on movement disorders (Chapter 34).

Chorea, Choreoathetosis, and Ballismus

Chorea refers to involuntary, irregular, purposeless, nonrhythmical, abrupt, rapid, unsustained movements that flow from one body part to another. Although many neurologists erroneously label almost all nonrhythmical, rapid involuntary movements as choreic, many in fact are not. Nonchoreic rapid movements can be tics, myoclonus, and dystonia. The prototypical choreic movements are those seen in Huntington's disease, in which the brief and rapid movements are irregular and occur randomly as a function of time.

When choreic movements are infrequent, they appear as isolated, small amplitude, brief movements, somewhat slower than myoclonus but sometimes difficult to distinguish from it. When chorea is more pronounced, the movements occur almost continually, presenting as a pattern of involuntary movements flowing from one site to another on the body.

Random choreic movements can be partially suppressed, and the patient with this type of chorea can often hide some of the movements by incorporating them into semipurposeful movements, known as parakinesia. Random chorea is usually accompanied by the inability to maintain a sustained contraction, often medically termed motor impersistence. A common symptom of motor impersistence is the dropping of objects. Motor impersistence is detected by examining for an inability to keep the tongue protruded and by the presence of milk-maid grips due to an inability to keep the fist in a sustained tight grip.

Athetosis refers to slow, writhing, continuous movements. These movements are more commonly appendicular but can also involve axial musculature, including the neck, the face, and the tongue. When athetosis is not present in certain body parts at rest, it can often be brought out by having the patient carry out voluntary motor activity elsewhere on the body. This phenomenon is known as overflow. For example, speaking can induce increased athetosis in the limbs, neck, trunk, face, and tongue. The speed of these involuntary movements can sometimes be faster and blend with those of chorea, and the term choreoathetosis is used. Sometimes athetosis is associated with sustained contractions, producing abnormal posturing. In this regard, athetosis blends with dystonia.

Athetosis most commonly occurs as a result of injury to the basal ganglia in the neonatal period or during infancy. When athetosis occurs in infants, the movements are slow and twisting; it should be considered a form of dystonia. In adults, athetosis is usually unaccompanied by posturing and its speed approaches that of chorea. This form of choreoathetosis can be considered a form of chorea.

Ballismus refers to very large amplitude choreic movements. Because of the speed of choreic movements, these large-amplitude excursions of the limbs are expressed by flinging and flailing movements when they involve proximal musculature. Ballismus is most frequently unilateral, and this form is referred to as hemiballismus. This disorder is usually the result of a lesion of the contralateral subthalamic nucleus or multiple small infarcts (lacunes) in the contralateral striatum. In rare instances, ballismus occurs bilaterally (biballismus) due to bilateral lacunes in the basal ganglia. Like chorea, ballismus sometimes occurs as a result of overdosage of levodopa.

Tics and Stereotypies

Tics can be divided into abnormal movements (motor tics), abnormal sounds (vocal tics), and combinations of the two. When motor and vocal tics are present and are of childhood onset and chronic duration, the designation of Gilles de la Tourette syndrome is commonly applied. Motor and vocal tics can be simple or complex and burst forth for brief moments from a background of normal motor activity.[32] Thus, they are paroxysmal in occurrence unless they are so severe as to be continual. Simple motor tics may be impossible to distinguish from a myoclonic or choreic jerk; basically, they are abrupt, sudden, single, isolated movements. Examples include a shoulder shrug, head jerk, dart of the eyes, and twitch of the nose. Most of the time, simple tics are repetitive, such as a run of eye blinking. When multiple simple tics occur in a sequence that is repeated over and over, the tics change from simple to complex. It is reasonable to view simple tics as formes frustes of complex tics. Even when tics are simple jerks, more complex forms of tics may also be present, allowing one to establish the diagnosis by associated tics. Tics frequently vary in severity over time and can have remissions and exacerbations.

Complex motor tics are very distinct, consisting of coordinated patterns of sequential movements that can appear in different parts of the body and are not necessarily identical from occurrence to occurrence in the same body part. Examples of complex tics include such acts as touching the nose, touching other people, head shaking with shoulder shrugging, kicking of legs, and jumping. Obscene gesturing (copropraxia) is another example.

Tics are usually preceded by an uncomfortable feeling that is relieved by carrying out the movement. Unless they are very severe, tics can be suppressed voluntarily for various periods of time. But when they are suppressed, inner tension builds up and is only relieved by an increased burst of more tics.

In addition to being as rapid as myoclonic jerks, tics can also be sustained contractions, resembling dystonic movements. The complex sequential pattern of muscular contractions in dystonic tics makes the diagnosis obvious in most cases. Moreover, torsion dystonia is a continual hyperkinesia, whereas tics are paroxysmal bursts of varying duration.

Involuntary ocular movements can be an important feature for differentiation of tics from other dyskinesias. Whether a brief jerk of the eyes or more sustained eye deviation, ocular movements can occur as a manifestation of tics. Very few other dyskinesias involve ocular movements. The exceptions are (1) opsoclonus (dancing eyes), which is a form of myoclonus; (2) ocular myoclonus (rhythmical vertical oscillations at a rate of 2 Hz) that often accompanies palatal myoclonus; and (3) oculogyric spasms (a sustained deviation of the eyes, thus a dystonia) associated with dopamine receptor blocking drugs or as a consequence of encephalitis lethargica.

Vocal tics can range from simple throat-clearing sounds or grunts to verbalizations and the utterance of obscenities (coprolalia). Sniffing can also be a phonic tic, involving nasal passages rather than the vocal apparatus. Like motor tics, phonic tics can also be divided into simple and complex tics. Throat-clearing and sniffing represent simple phonic tics, whereas barking and verbalizations are considered complex phonic tics.

Involuntary phonations occur in only a few other neurological disorders besides tics. These include the moaning in akathisia and in parkinsonism from levodopa toxicity, the brief sounds in oromandibular dystonia and Huntington's disease, and the sniffing and spitting occasionally encountered in Huntington's disease.

Stereotypy refers to simple or complex movements that repeat themselves continually and identically. There may be long periods of minutes between movements,[33] or they may be very frequent. When they occur at irregular intervals, stereotypies may not always be easily distinguished from motor tics, compulsions, gestures, and mannerisms. In their classic monograph on tics, Meige and Feindel[34] distinguished between motor tics and stereotypies by describing tics as acts that are impelling but not impossible to resist, whereas stereotypies, although illogical, are without an irresistible urge. The odd, complex movements seen in patients with schizophrenia, mental retardation, and autism are considered to be those of stereotypy. Involuntary movements that are continuous (uninterrupted) and repeat themselves over and over again unceasingly are a continuous stereotypy. This pattern is the hallmark of abnormal movements in patients with classic tardive dyskinesia due to neuroleptic drugs (see Chapter 55).

Dystonia

Dystonia refers to twisting movements that are sustained at their peak, are frequently repetitive, and often progress to prolonged abnormal postures. Agonist and antagonist muscles contract simultaneously to cause dystonic movements. The speed of the movement varies widely from slow (athetotic dystonia) to shocklike (myoclonic dystonia). When the contractions are very brief (i.e., less than a second), they are referred to as dystonic spasms or myoclonic dystonia. When they are sustained for several seconds, they are called dystonic movements. And when they last minutes to hours, they are known as dystonic postures. When they are present for weeks or longer, the postures could lead to permanent fixed contractures.

In primary dystonia, the movements typically occur when the affected body part is carrying out a voluntary action (action dystonia) and are not present when that body part is at rest. With progression of the disorder, dystonic movements can appear at distal sites when other parts of the body are voluntarily moving (overflow), such as occurs also in athetosis; with further progression, dystonic movements become present when the body is at rest. Even at this stage, dystonic movements are usually made more severe with voluntary activity. Whereas idiopathic dystonia often begins as action dystonia and may persist as the kinetic (clonic) form, symptomatic dystonia often begins as fixed postures (tonic form).

When a single body part is affected, the condition is referred to as focal dystonia. Common forms of focal dystonia are spasmodic torticollis (cervical dystonia), blepharospasm (upper facial dystonia), and writer's cramp (hand dystonia). Involvement of two or more contiguous regions of the body is referred to as segmental dystonia. Generalized dystonia indicates involvement of one or both legs, the trunk, and some other part of the body.

Although classic torsion dystonia may appear in the beginning stages only as an action dystonia, it usually progresses to manifest as continual contractions. In contrast to this continual type of classic torsion dystonia, a variant of dystonia also exists in which the movements are sudden in onset and transient, known as paroxysmal dyskinesias. Besides occurring in hereditary forms, dystonia is a component of a number of other neurodegenerative disorders (Wilson's disease, Hallervorden-Spatz disease) and several metabolic disorders. Additionally, perinatal cerebral injury, encephalitis, strokes, tumors, and trauma have been implicated as causes of dystonia (see Chapter 34). Among other disorders to be differentiated from dystonia are tonic tics (also called dystonic tics), which also appear as sustained contractions.

Akathisia

Akathisia (from the Greek, meaning unable to sit still) refers to a feeling of inner restlessness, which is relieved by moving about. The typical akathitic patient, when sitting, may stroke the scalp, cross and uncross the legs, rock the trunk, squirm in the chair, and get out of the chair often to pace back and forth, and even make noises such as moaning. The characteristic feature is that akathitic movements are complex movements and usually stereotypic; the other major disorders showing complex movements are tics, compulsions, and mannerisms. Carrying out these motor acts brings relief from akathisia. If a specific body part is affected, it may give a sensation of burning or pain, which, again, is relieved by moving that body part. A somewhat common expression of akathisia is the vocalization of continual moaning or groaning. Akathitic movements and vocalizations can be transiently suppressed by the patient if he or she is asked to do so.

The most common cause of akathisia is iatrogenic. It is a frequent complication of drugs that block dopamine receptors, such as the antipsychotic drugs. It can occur when drug therapy is initiated (acute akathisia) or after chronic treatment (tardive akathisia). Acute akathisia is eliminated on withdrawal of the medication. Tardive akathisia is associated with the syndrome of tardive dyskinesia and is usually made worse on sudden discontinuation of the medication. The exact mechanism of akathisia is not known, but heightened dopaminergic activity or supersensitive dopaminergic receptors, possibly in the limbic system, may be involved (see Chapter 55).

Tardive akathisia commonly accompanies tardive dyskinesia and, like tardive dyskinesia, is aggravated by discontinuing the neuroleptic agent; it is usually relieved by increasing the dose of the offending drug, which masks the movement disorder. When they are associated with tardive dyskinesia, the akathitic movements can be rhythmical, such as body rocking or marching in place. In this situation, it is difficult to be certain whether such rhythmic movements are due to akathisia or tardive dyskinesia.

Myoclonus

Myoclonus refers to motor jerks that are sudden, brief, shocklike involuntary movements caused by muscular contractions (positive myoclonus) or inhibitions (negative myoclonus). The most common form of negative myoclonus is asterixis, which is commonly seen accompanying various metabolic encephalopathies. In asterixis, the brief flapping of the limbs is due to transient inhibition of the muscles that maintain posture of those extremities.

Myoclonus can appear as irregular jerks, rhythmical jerks (such as palatal myoclonus and ocular myoclonus, with a rate of approximately 2 Hz), or oscillatory jerks that occur in a burst and then fade. Rhythmical myoclonus is typically due to a structural lesion of the brain stem or spinal cord (segmental myoclonus), but not all cases of segmental myoclonus are rhythmical. Myoclonic jerks occurring in different body parts are often synchronized, a feature that may be specific for myoclonus. The jerks can often be triggered by sudden stimuli such as sound, light, visual threat, or movement. Myoclonus has a relationship to seizures in that both seem to be the result of hyperexcitable neurons.

Cortical reflex myoclonus usually presents as a focal myoclonus and is triggered by active or passive muscle movements of the affected body part. It is associated with high-amplitude somatosensory evoked potentials and with cortical spikes observed by computerized back-averaging, which is time-locked to the stimulus. Reticular reflex myoclonus is more often generalized or spreads along the body away from the source in a timed-related sequential fashion.

The fact that rhythmical myoclonic jerks of one body part are synchronized with contractions elsewhere is a strong argument for categorizing such movements as myoclonus and not as tremor. Furthermore, oculopalatal myoclonus persists during sleep. As a general rule, all movement disorders except myoclonus disappear during sleep.

Often, myoclonic jerks appear with the body at rest, but action myoclonus, in which myoclonic jerks appear when the affected body part is in voluntary activity, also occurs. Action or intention myoclonus is more often encountered after cerebral hypoxia and with certain degenerative disorders, such as the Ramsay Hunt syndrome. Usually, action myoclonus is more disabling than rest myoclonus.

Hemifacial Spasms

Hemifacial spasm, as the name indicates, refers to unilateral facial muscle contractions. Generally, these spasms are continual, although there are periods of quiescence. Often the movements can be brought out by having the patient forcefully contract the facial muscles; then when the patient relaxes, the involuntary movements often appear. The disorder is believed to involve the facial nerve, and sometimes it is due to compression of the nerve by a blood vessel.[35] As the name implies, hemifacial spasm involves only one side of the face. It usually affects both upper and lower parts of the face, but patients are commonly more concerned about closure of the eyelid than of the contractions of the cheek or at the corner of the mouth. It can be easily distinguished from blepharospasm, because blepharospasm involves the face bilaterally and often the dystonic contractions spread to contiguous structures, such as oromandibular and nuchal muscles. Blepharospasm is rarely due to unilateral dystonia. In such a circumstance, it would be difficult clinically to distinguish it from hemifacial spasm. EMG may be of assistance because hemifacial spasm may be associated with some facial nerve denervation and ephaptic transmission may be detected. The contractions in both hemifacial spasm and blepharospasm are intermittent but tend to be sustained when they appear.

General Management Goals

Management of hypokinesia and immobility includes medical and physical therapies. Whereas the specific drug or surgical intervention depends on the etiology and the type of hypokinesia, all forms may benefit from careful attention to proper support tools in the home and walking aids. Sometimes a visit to the home by a physical or occupational therapist is useful for an assessment of needs. Because freezing episodes can be precipitated by low-lying objects and crowded conditions, many families remove all unnecessary furnishings from the patient's walking area. Visual cues like striped lines on the floor may also help patients with prominent freezing to overcome the blockage and encourage the initiation of movement. The patient who falls may need to wear knee, elbow, and hip padding. If the patient is highly immobilized, venous status and pulmonary emboli are risks, especially if the patient remains in bed.

The hyperkinetic patient likewise may need protective clothing if he bumps himself from flinging movements. Braces and splints should generally be avoided, because the movements persist and the braced extremity or trunk will be injured. Attention to weight and nutrition is important in hyperkinetic patients because hyperkinetic patients may be hypermetabolic and use unexpectedly high calories and fluids. If swallowing is affected by either hypokinesia or hyperkinesia, attention must be directed to proper nutrition, and some patients with advanced diseases require feeding tubes.

Reviews and Selected Updates

Beal MF: Energetics in the pathogenesis of neurodegenerative diseases. Trends Neurosci 2000;23:298–304.

Bhatia KP, Griggs RC, Ptacek LJ: Episodic movement disorders as channelopathies. Mov Disord 2000;15:429–433.

Bolam JP, Hanley JJ, Booth PAC, Bevan MD: Synaptic organisation of the basal ganglia. J Anat 2000;196:527–542.

Brooks DJ: Imaging basal ganglia function. J Anat 2000;196:543–554.

Camargo EE: Brain SPECT in neurology and psychiatry. J Nucl Med 2001;42:611–623.

Crossman AR: Functional anatomy of movement disorders. J Anat 2000;196:519–525.

Deuschl G, Raethjen J, Lindemann M, Krack P: The pathophysiology of tremor. Muscle Nerve 2001;24:716–735.

Eidelberg D, Edwards C: Functional brain imaging of movement disorders. Neurol Res 2000;22:305–312.

Filion M: Physiologic basis of dyskinesia. Ann Neurol 2000;47(Suppl 1): S35–S41.

Galvin JE, Lee VMY, Trojanowski JQ: Synucleinopathies—Clinical and pathological implications. Arch Neurol 2001;58:186–190.

Greenamyre JT: Glutamatergic influences on the basal ganglia. Clin Neuropharmacol 2001;24:65–70.

Nakano K, Kayahara T, Tsutsumi T, Ushiro H: Neural circuits and functional organization of the striatum. J Neurol 2000;247:1–15.

Obeso JA, Olanow CW, Nutt JG (eds): Basal ganglia, Parkinson's disease and levodopa therapy. Trends Neurosci 2000;23(Suppl):S1–S126.

Sudarsky L: Gait disorders: Prevalence, morbidity, and etiology. Adv Neurol 2001;87:111–117.

Vitek JL, Giroux M: Physiology of hypokinetic and hyperkinetic movement disorders: Model for dyskinesia. Ann Neurol 2000;47(Suppl 1):S131–S140.

References

1. Wilson SAK: Progressive lenticular degeneration: A familial nervous system disease associated with cirrhosis of the liver. Brain 1912;34:295–509.
2. Pittock SJ, Joyce C, O'Keane V, et al: Rapid-onset dystonia-parkinsonism—A clinical and genetic analysis of a new kindred. Neurology 2000;55:991–995.
3. Fahn S: The freezing phenomenon in parkinsonism. Adv Neurol 1995;67:53–63.
4. Shiang R, Ryan SG, Zhu YZ, et al: Mutations in the 1 subunit of the inhibitory glycine receptor cause the dominant neurologic disorder, hyperekplexia. Nat Genet 1993;5:351–358.
5. Matsumoto J, Hallett M: Startle syndromes. *In* Marsden CD, Fahn S (eds): Movement Disorders 3. Oxford, Butterworth-Heinemann, 1994, pp 418–433.
6. Fahn S: Psychogenic movement disorders. *In* Marsden CD, Fahn S (eds): Movement Disorders 3. Oxford, Butterworth-Heinemann, 1994, pp 359–372.
7. Thompson PD, Colebatch JG, Brown P, et al: Voluntary stimulus-sensitive jerks and jumps mimicking myoclonus or pathological startle syndromes. Mov Disord 1992;7:257–262.
8. Lance JW, Adams RD: The syndrome of intention or action myoclonus as a sequel to hypoxic encephalopathy. Brain 1963;86:111–136.
9. Fahn S: The paroxysmal dyskinesias. *In* Marsden CD, Fahn S (eds): Movement Disorders 3. Oxford, Butterworth-Heinemann, 1994, pp 310–345.
10. Demirkiran M, Jankovic J: Paroxysmal dyskinesias: Clinical features and classification. Ann Neurol 1995;38:571–579.
11. Bressman SB, Fahn S, Burke RE: Paroxysmal non-kinesigenic dystonia. Adv Neurol 1988;50:403–413.
12. Lang AE, Koller WC, Fahn S: Psychogenic parkinsonism. Arch Neurol 1995;52:802–810.
13. Koller W, Lang A, Vetere-Overfield B, et al: Psychogenic tremors. Neurology 1989;39:1094–1099.
14. Fahn S: The tardive dyskinesias. *In* Matthews WB, Glaser GH (eds): Recent Advances in Clinical Neurology, Vol 4. Edinburgh, Churchill Livingstone, 1984, pp 229–260.
15. Daras M, Koppel BS, Atos-Radzion E: Cocaine-induced choreoathetoid movements (crack dancing). Neurology 1994;44:751–752.
16. Pascual-Leone A, Dhuna A: Cocaine-associated multifocal tics. Neurology 1990;40:999–1000.
17. Scharf D: Opsoclonus-myoclonus following the intranasal usage of cocaine. J Neurol Neurosurg Psychiatry 1989;52:1447–1448.
18. Rowland LP: Cramps, spasms, and muscle stiffness. Rev Neurol (Paris) 1985;141:261–273.
19. Thompson PD: Stiff people. *In* Marsden CD, Fahn S (eds): Movement Disorders 3. Oxford, Butterworth-Heinemann, 1994, pp 373–405.
20. Melamed E: Early-morning dystonia: A late side effect of long-term levodopa therapy in Parkinson's disease. Arch Neurol 1979;36:308–310.
21. Ford B, Louis ED, Greene P, Fahn S: Oral and genital pain syndromes in Parkinson's disease. Mov Disord 1996;11:421–426.
22. Ford B, Greene P, Fahn S: Oral and genital tardive pain syndromes. Neurology 1994;44:2115–2119.
23. Dawson VL, Dawson TM, London ED, et al: Nitric oxide mediates glutamate neurotoxicity in primary cortical cultures. Proc Natl Acad Sci USA 1991;88:6368–6371.
24. Alexander GE, Crutcher MD: Functional architecture of basal ganglia circuits: Neural substrates of parallel processing. Trends Neurosci 1990;13:266–271.

25. Parent A: Extrinsic connections of the basal ganglia. Trends Neurosci 1990;13:254–258.
26. Ilinsky IA, Jouandet ML, Goldman-Rakic PS: Organization of the nigrothalamocortical system in the Rhesus monkey. J Comp Neurol 1985;236:315–330.
27. Young AB, Penney JB Jr: Biochemical and functional organization of the basal ganglia. *In* Jankovic J, Tolosa E (eds): Parkinson's Disease and Movement Disorders, 3rd ed. Baltimore, Williams & Wilkins, 1998, pp 1–13.
28. Curtis ARJ, Fey C, Morris CM, et al: Mutation in the gene encoding ferritin light polypeptide causes dominant adult-onset basal ganglia disease. Nat Genet 2001;28:345–349.
29. Schwab RS, Chafetz ME, Walker S: Control of two simultaneous voluntary motor acts in normals and in parkinsonism. Arch Neurol Psychiatry 1954;72:591–598.
30. Fahn S: Akinesia. *In* Berardelli A, Benecke R, Manfredi M, Marsden CD (eds): Motor Disturbances II. London, Academic Press, 1990, pp 141–150.
31. Fahn S: The freezing phenomenon in parkinsonism. Adv Neurol 1995;67:53–63.
32. Fahn S: Motor and vocal tics. *In* Kurlan R (ed): Handbook of Tourette's Syndrome and Related Tic and Behavioral Disorders. New York, Marcel Dekker, 1993, pp 3–16.
33. Tan A, Salgado M, Fahn S: The characterization and outcome of stereotypic movements in nonautistic children. Mov Disord 1997;12:47–52.
34. Meige H, Feindel E: Tics and Their Treatment. Translated from the French by Wilson SAK. London, Appleton, 1907.
35. Jannetta PJ: Surgical approach to hemifacial spasm: Microvascular decompression. *In* Marsden CD, Fahn S (eds): Movement Disorders. London, Butterworth Scientific, 1982, pp 330–333.

CHAPTER 17

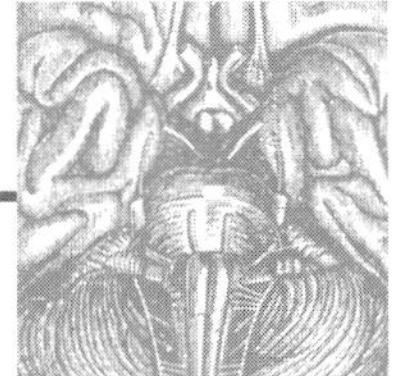

DAGMAR TIMMANN and HANS CHRISTOPH DIENER

Coordination and Ataxia

History and Definitions

The work of the French/Polish neurologist, Babinski, and the English neurologist, Holmes, have been most influentual on the development of concepts and terminology of cerebellar disease utilized by modern clinical neurologists.[1, 2, 3]

The cardinal sign of cerebellar disease is ataxia [Greek, a (negative article) + taxi (order)]. The term *ataxia* is used to denote disturbances of coordinated muscle activity (= incoordination).[4] Cerebellar ataxia is defined as lack of accuracy or coordination of movement that is not due to paresis, alteration in tone, sensory loss, or the presence of involuntary movements.[5]

Cerebellar ataxia relates to motor dysfunctions of the limbs, trunk, eyes, and bulbar musculature. *Ataxia of gait* refers to incoordination of walking that might be so severe that the patient cannot walk (*abasia*). Postural ataxia refers to *ataxia of stance* and *sitting*, and includes *truncal ataxia*. The patient may be unable to sit or stand without support (*astasia*). *Limb ataxia* refers to incoordination of limb movements and ataxia of speech to cerebellar *dysarthria*.

Cerebellar ataxia embraces all abnormal motor phenomena related to cerebellar dysfunction. Different terms are commonly used to describe different aspects of ataxia. *Dysmetria* refers to disturbance of the trajectory or placement of a body part during active movement, both in range and direction. *Hypometria* refers to a movement undershooting its target, and *hypermetria* indicates a movement in which the limb overshoots its goal. *Bradyteleokinesia* describes terminal slowing before reaching the target. *Decomposition of movement* refers to errors in the sequence and speed of the component parts of a movement (i.e., a breakdown of a multijoint movement into its constituent parts). Movements previously fluid and accurate become erratic and jerky. *Asynergia* and *dyssynergia* are commonly used as synonyms to denote decomposition of movement. *Dysdiadochokinesis* refers to decomposition of alternating or fine repetitive movements. Deficits appear in the rate of alternation as well as the completeness of the sequence.

Cerebellar disease results in *postural* and *limb tremor*. There may be a rhythmic tremor of the body that can evolve into a severe *titubation*. Limb tremor occurs as a kinetic and, to a lesser extent, static tremor. *Kinetic tremor* occurs as an oscillatory movement when the subject initiates a movement of the limb or during the course of moving the limb. The tremor becomes more prominent as the moving limb approaches a target. It has commonly been described as *intention tremor*, but the term kinetic tremor better describes the clinical appearance. *Static tremor* develops if the patient attempts to maintain a limb in a fixed position. Usually the position can be sustained steadily for several seconds, but then the limb develops a rhythmical oscillation generated at the proximal limb muscles.

A variety of eye movement abnormalities are seen in cerebellar disease. Gaze-evoked *nystagmus* is a common finding. Other frequent abnormalities are impairment of smooth pursuit and saccadic (*ocular dysmetria*) eye movements, inability to suppress the vestibulo-ocular reflex (VOR) by fixation, and abnormalities of optokinetic nystagmus.

Hypotonia, hyporeflexia, and *asthenia* were described as typical symptoms of acute cerebellar lesions by Holmes.[3] Hypotonia refers to a decrease in the resistance to passive movements of the limbs, associated with *pendular tendon reflexes,* typified by the lower leg swinging back and forth several times after the knee tendon is tapped with the reflex hammer.

Clinical History

The following aspects of the clinical history should be considered: mode of inheritance, age at disease onset, progression rate, accompanying symptoms, and exposure to toxins.

A positive family history suggests a form of inherited ataxia. Different ataxic disorders start in infancy, childhood, or adulthood. Patients and relatives should be asked about delayed motor milestones or poor athletic performance at school. The course of the disease might be of acute (over minutes or hours) or subacute (over days or weeks) onset, nonprogressive from birth, and episodic or slowly progressive (over months or years). Congenital ataxias are frequently nonprogressive after birth.[6] The acute onset of severe headache in association with ataxia suggests a diagnosis of cerebellar hematoma or ischemia. A recent history of trauma, such as a fall on the back of the head, suggests hematoma or craniocerebral injury. Subacute onset is found in viral cerebellitis, multiple sclerosis, paraneoplastic cerebellar syndromes, posterior fossa tumors or abscesses, spongiform encephalopathies, and alcoholic cerebellar degeneration. Episodic ataxia in adults might be caused by drug ingestions, multiple sclerosis, transient vertebrobasilar ischemic attacks, foramen magnum compression, intermittent obstruction of the ventricular system, and dominantly inherited periodic ataxia. In children and young adults, a metabolic disorder should be expected. Chronic progressive ataxia suggests an inherited or idiopathic degenerative ataxia.

Patients should be asked if symptoms are worse in the dark. Ataxia largely due to sensory loss is typically enhanced by lack of visual feedback. Facial droop, vertigo, hearing loss, numbness, or diplopia associated with ataxia suggests a disorder in the brain stem. The history of previous subacute monocular visual loss suggests a diagnosis of multiple sclerosis. Some degenerative ataxias are associated with gradual visual loss. Occipital headache and projectile vomiting in conjunction with ataxia are associated with raised intracranial pressure in the presence of a posterior fossa lesion. Headache and vomiting are commonly worse on coughing, bending, and walking and in the morning. Incontinence associated with dementia and gait ataxia suggests normal pressure hydrocephalus. Postural hypotension and extrapyramidal signs are associated with multiple system atrophy. Skeletal abnormalities like scoliosis and pes cavus, as well as diabetes and cardiac symptoms, are associated with Friedreich's ataxia. Repeated infections are associated with ataxia telangiectasia.

Patients should be asked whether they are receiving antiepileptic agents (phenytoin), cytotoxic drugs (fluorouracil, cytarabine), or lithium. They should be questioned on excessive or frequent alcohol consumption, and whether they have been exposed to any toxins (heavy metals, solvents). Ataxia can be associated with intestinal disease (sprue, vitamin E deficiency), metabolic disorders (hypothyroidism), or physical stress (heat stroke).

Anatomy of Coordination (Tables 17–1 and 17–2)

OVERVIEW

The cerebellum occupies most of the posterior cranial fossa. It is separated from the cerebral hemispheres by the tentorium cerebelli and overlies the brain stem. The cerebellum consists of two large hemispheres and a midline structure, the vermis. Midline structures are involved in the control of motor execution, balance, and eye movements, and the lateral parts of the hemispheres are involved in motor planning. Lesions of the midline structures result in disturbances of stance, gait, and ocular movements, whereas lesions of the cerebellar hemispheres primarily affect limb movements.[7]

Several classifications have been used to subdivide the cerebellum based on anatomical, phylogenetic, and functional (i.e., termination of cerebellar afferents and efferents) findings. Anatomically, the cerebellum is subdivided into three major components, the flocculonodular, anterior, and posterior lobes, the latter two forming the corpus cerebelli. The anterior lobe is separated from the posterior lobe by the primary fissure, and the flocculonodular lobe is separated from the posterior lobe by the posterolateral fissure. The three lobes are subdivided into several lobules. The terminology used to identify the lobules is not uniform and is often contradictory. Several nomenclature systems use individual names. For example, the cerebellar tonsil is the most caudal lobule of the hemispherical part of the posterior lobe (Fig. 17–1). Larsell has introduced a numbering system, which consists of Roman numerals in the vermis and the prefix H in the hemispheres. A modified version of the Larsell terminology has recently been proposed by Schmahmann and co-workers.[8]

The terms archicerebellum, paleocerebellum, and neocerebellum originate from phylogenetic and embryological studies. The neocerebellum refers to the youngest and the archicerebellum to the oldest parts of the cerebellum. The neocerebellum corresponds to the cerebellar hemispheres and the middle part of the vermis. The paleocerebellum consists of anterior and posterior parts of the vermis (except the nodulus), and the archicerebellum corresponds to the flocculonodular lobe.

The terms vestibulocerebellum, spinocerebellum, and pontocerebellum originate from termination sides of cerebellar *afferent* projections. These subdivisions match well with the subdivisions based on phylogenetic studies. The flocculonodular lobe (archicerebellum) and adjoining parts of the

TABLE 17–1. **Cerebellar Systems: Anatomy and Clinical Correlations**

Origin of Afferent Input	Afferent Cerebellar Peduncle	Projection Area of Cerebellar Cortex (Where Afferents Synpase on Purkinje Cells)	Cerebellar Nucleus (Where Purkinje Cell Axons Terminate)	Efferent Cerebellar Peduncle	Efferent Destination	Function	Syndrome* (Which Results When System Is Diseased)
Vestibular nerve and nuclei	Inferior *Restiform body*	Flocculonodular lobe; adjoining caudal vermis	Fastigial; direct projections to vestibular nuclei	Inferior	Vestibular nuclei	Balance and eye movements	Truncal ataxia: cannot sit up without falling over; oculomotor signs
Vestibulocerebellum		***Archicerebellum***	***Medial Zone***				
Dorsal spinocerebellar tract	Inferior *Restiform body*	Anterior lobe (rostral vermis; intermediate cerebellum); caudal vermis	Fastigial: interposed (emboliform and globose)	Superior (to opposite red nucleus)	Interposed: rubralspinal tract; fastigial: vestibular nuclei	Ongoing execution of movement; gait	Anterior lobe syndrome: difficulty walking with little incoordination of other tasks
Ventral spinocerebellar tract	Superior *Brachium conjunctivum*						
Spinocerebellum		***Paleocerebellum***	***Medial, Intermediate Zone***				
Contralateral hemisphere	Middle *Brachium pontis*	Cerebellar hemispheres and middle part of vermis	Dentate	Superior (to opposite red nucleus)	Rubral-thalamic tract (going back up to cortex where the afferents originated)	Motor planning: coordination of arms and legs	Poor limb coordination
Corticoponto-cerebellum		***Neocerebellum***	***Lateral Zone***				

* Unilateral lesions in the cerebellum cause ipsilateral limb ataxia because the major output pathway of the cerebellum is crossed and disturbs the action of the corticospinal and rubrospinal tracts, which are also crossed.

TABLE 17–2. **Clinco-anatomical Correlation of Coordination Disorders**

Anatomical Location	Cerebellar Signs/Symptoms	Associated Neurological Findings
Rostral Vermis (So-Called Anterior Lobe)	Ataxia of stance and gait Anteroposterior body sway (3 Hz) Romberg positive Infrequent: dysarthria, nystagmus	Alcoholic cerebellar degeneration: Peripheral neuropathy
Caudal Vermis (Including Flocculonodular Lobe)	Truncal, postural and gait ataxia Omnidirectional body sway (1 Hz) Romberg negative Tendency to fall Saccadic slow pursuit, nystagmus Inability to suppress Vestibulo-ocular reflex	Acute, focal lesions: Headache Vomiting Change in consciousness
Cerebellar Hemisphere	Ipsilateral limb ataxia: Hypotonia Decomposition of movement Dysdiadochokinesis Kinetic tremor Past-pointing Deviation of gait Dysarthria	Acute, focal lesions: Headache Vomiting Change in consciousness
Pancerebellum	Truncal and bilateral limb ataxia Ataxia of gait and stance Dysarthria Oculomotor disturbances	Heredoataxias: Pyramidal signs Extrapyramidal signs Peripheral neuropathy Cranial neuropathy Dementia
Posterior Inferior Cerebellar Artery	Ipsilateral limb ataxia Nystagmus	Vertigo, headache Nausea, vomiting Ipsilateral Horner's syndrome, V, IX, X nerve palsy Contralateral impaired body pain and temperature sensation
Anterior Inferior Cerebellar Artery	Ipsilateral limb ataxia Nystagmus (Dysarthria)	Nausea, vomiting Vertigo Tinnitus Ipsilateral Horner's syndrome, deafness, facial paralysis, impaired facial pain and temperature sensation Contralateral impaired body pain and temperature sensation
Superior Cerebellar Artery	Ipsilateral limb ataxia Dysarthria Nystagmus Gait ataxia	Nausea, vomiting Headache Ipsilateral Horner's syndrome Contralateral loss of facial and body pain and temperature sensation Contralateral IV nerve palsy

caudal vermis have been named vestibulocerebellum because of heavily projecting vestibular afferents; the anterior and posterior parts of the vermis (paleocerebellum) and paravermal parts of the cerebellar hemispheres were called spinocerebellum because of their spinal afferents; and the cerebellar hemispheres (neocerebellum) were called cerebrocerebellum or pontocerebellum based on their main input from the cerebellar cortex, synaptically interrupted in the pontine nuclei (Fig. 17–2).

On the basis of the *efferent* projections from the cerebellar cortex to the cerebellar nuclei, Jansen and Brodal,[9] and later Chambers and Sprague,[10] suggested a subdivision into three longitudinal (= sagittal) zones: a medial zone (vermis) projecting to the fastigial nucleus, an intermediate (paravermal part of cerebellar hemisphere) zone projecting to the interposed nuclei (itself composed of two nuclei, the globose and emboliform), and a lateral (lateral part of cerebellar hemisphere) zone projecting to the dentate nucleus. Voogd[11] showed that the longitudinal subdivision was more detailed by using a special method to stain myelin. He found seven longitudinal zones termed A and B (medial zone), C1–C3 (intermediate zone), and D1 and D2 (lateral zone). Hawkes

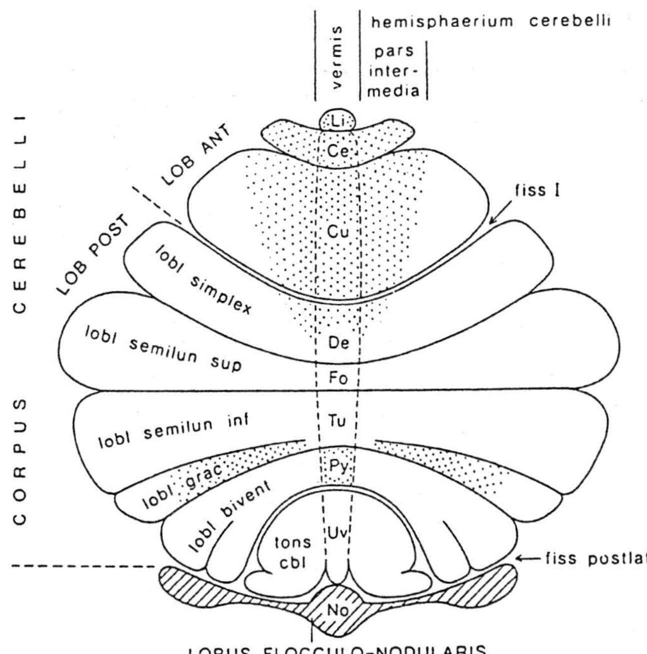

FIGURE 17–1. The cerebellar cortex, unfolded into one plane, showing the fields of termination of cerebellar afferent projections (= mossy fiber system): pontocerebellar fibers (*open contours*), spinocerebellar fibers (*dotted areas*) and vestibulocerebellar fibers (*hatched areas*). LOB POST = Posterior lobe; LOB ANT = anterior lobe; lobl simplex = lobulus simplex; lobl semilun sup = superior semilunar lobule; lobl semilun inf = inferior semilunar lobule; lobl grac = gracile lobule; lobl bivent = biventer lobule; tons cbl = cerebellar tonsil; fiss I = primary fissure; fiss postlat = posterolateral fissure; Li = lingula; Ce = central lobe; Cu = culmen; De = declive; Fo = folium vermis; Tu = tuber vermis; Py = pyramis; No = nodulus; Uv = uvula. (With permission from Nieuwenhuys R, Voogd J, van Huijzen C: The Human Central Nervous System. A Synopsis and Atlas. Berlin, Springer, 1988, p 162.)

and colleagues[12] described at least 32 parasagittal cerebellar compartments as defined by using molecular markers, so-called zebrins.

Two inverted somatotopic maps have been charted for the cerebellar cortex. The leg is represented anteriorly within the anterior lobe, with the arm and face represented successively more posteriorly. In the posterior lobe, the arrangement is the reverse, with the face represented anteriorly (Fig. 17–3).[13, 14]

The cerebellum is connected with the brain stem by afferent and efferent fibers passing through three pairs of tracts, called the inferior, middle, and superior cerebellar peduncle (or restiform body, brachium pontis, and brachium conjunctivum). The middle cerebellar peduncle contains only afferent fibers. In the inferior peduncle, most fibers are afferent, whereas in the superior cerebellar peduncle, most fibers are efferent.

CEREBELLAR AFFERENTS

The cerebellar cortex receives afferent input from most parts of the peripheral (proprioceptive, cutaneous, vestibular, and visual, except olfactory) and central nervous system. The afferent fibers reach the cerebellar cortex through the three cerebellar peduncles. Vestibular afferents reach the cerebellum by the inferior cerebellar peduncle, innervating primarily the flocculonodular lobe. Spinocerebellar afferents reach the cerebellum by the inferior cerebellar peduncle (dorsal spinocerebellar tract) and the superior cerebellar peduncle (ventral spinocerebellar tract), innervating primarily the anterior lobe of the cerebellum and the caudal vermis. Corticopontine projections reach the cerebellum by the middle cerebellar peduncle projecting to the contralateral cerebellar hemispheres.

The afferent fibers consist of mossy fibers, climbing fibers, and monoaminergic fibers. The two most important types of excitatory cerebellar afferents, mossy and climbing fibers,

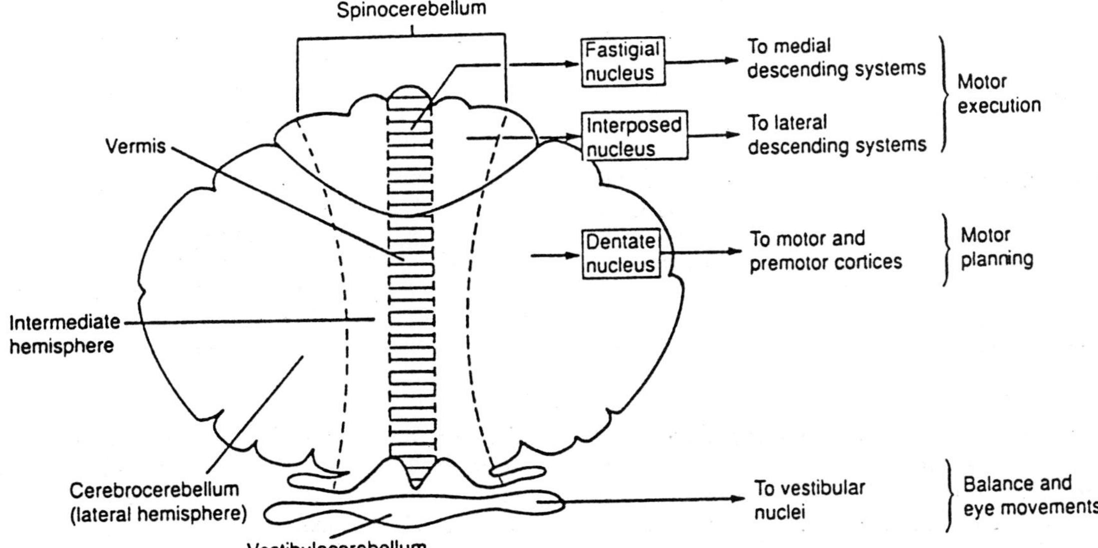

FIGURE 17–2. The cerebellum has three functional components based on different inputs—the vestibulocerebellum, the spinocerebellum, and the cerebrocerebellum or pontocerebellum—and based on different outputs, a medial zone (≅ vermis) projecting to the fastigial nucleus, an intermediate (≅ paravermal parts of hemispheres) zone projecting to the interposed nucleus, and a lateral zone (≅ lateral part of hemisphere) projecting to the dentate nucleus. The main efferents from the flocculonodular lobe project directly to the vestibular nuclei. (From Ghez C: The cerebellum. *In* Kandel ER, Schwartz JH, Jessell TM (eds): Principles of Neural Science, 3rd ed. Norwalk, Appleton & Lange, 1991, Fig. 41–7, p 633.)

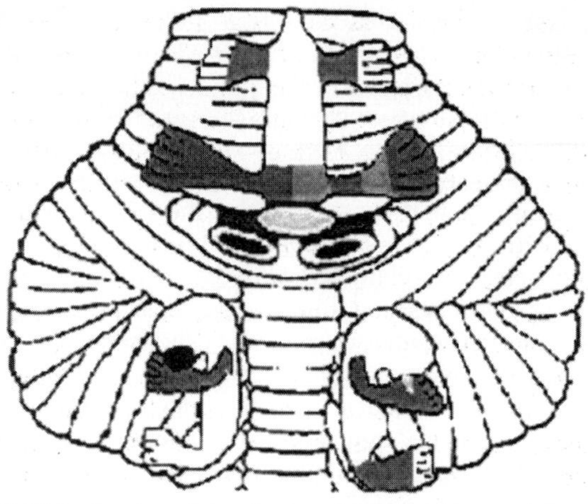

FIGURE 17–3. Somatotopic localization of the cerebellar cortex. Display of the cerebellar homunculi based on animal experiments by Snider and Eldred (1951)[14]; superimposed are areas of fMRI activations as revealed by a human sensorimotor mapping study.[13] (Adapted from Grodd et al: Sensorimotor mapping of the human cerebellum: fMRI evidence of somatotopic organization. Human Brain Mapping 2001;13:55–73; Fig. 7c, p 68. Copyright © John Wiley & Sons. This material is used by permission of Wiley-Liss, Inc., a subsidiary of John Wiley & Sons, Inc.)

have been defined based on how the fibers end in the cerebellar cortex. Mossy fiber terminals are characterized by their mosslike appearance on histological examination, whereas climbing fibers climb in a characteristic way along the cell body and dendrites of the Purkinje cell. Each mossy fiber terminates on numerous granular cells, and each of these contacts many Purkinje cells. Climbing fibers directly contact Purkinje cells with each Purkinje cell receiving branches from only one climbing fiber. Climbing fibers originate solely from the inferior olive in the brain stem.[15] Mossy fibers form the major cerebellar input. They originate from different brain stem nuclei (e.g., pontine, vestibular, trigeminal, and reticular nuclei) and neurons in the spinal cord.[16]

Besides the vestibular system, the spinocerebellar tracts send mossy fibers directly to the cerebellum. From the trunk and legs, the dorsal and ventral spinocerebellar tracts enter the cerebellum through the ipsilateral inferior and contralateral superior cerebellar peduncle, respectively. From the arms and neck, the cuneocerebellar tract enters the cerebellum through the ipsilateral inferior cerebellar peduncle. Many afferent pathways have additional relay stations (pontine nuclei, inferior olives) before they enter the cerebellum. The pontine nuclei represent the most important relay for corticocerebellar pathways. From the pontine nuclei, corticopontine projections enter the cerebellum mainly through the contralateral middle cerebellar peduncle. The pontine nuclei convey afferents mainly from cerebral motor areas including the primary motor cortex, somatosensory cortex, supplementary motor and premotor areas, and the posterior parietal lobes. The inferior olives receive afferents mainly from the spinal cord and also from several other cortical and brain stem areas. From the inferior olive, climbing fibers enter the cerebellum through the contralateral inferior cerebellar peduncle. Mossy and climbing fiber spinocerebellar afferents end mostly in the spinocerebellum of the same side. Some pass uncrossed; other fibers cross twice. The primary destination of afferent fibers is the Purkinje cell located in the Purkinje cell layer of each lobe of the cerebellar cortex. Collaterals are sent to the deep cerebellar nuclei.

CEREBELLAR NUCLEI

The cerebellar cortex of the vermis and the intermediate and lateral parts of each hemisphere are connected to different deep cerebellar nuclei. Each half of the cerebellum contains four distinct nuclei. The vermis projects to the fastigial nucleus, the intermediate part of the cerebellar hemisphere to the emboliform and globose nuclei, and the lateral part of the hemisphere to the dentate nucleus (see Figs. 17–2 and 17–4). The fastigial nucleus is located most medially, followed by the globose and emboliform nucleus and, most laterally, the dentate nucleus. The emboliform and globose nuclei in humans resemble the anterior and posterior interposed nuclei in animals.

CEREBELLAR EFFERENTS

The Purkinje cells form the principal projections from the cerebellar cortex to the deep cerebellar nuclei. The Purkinje cells of the vestibulocerebellum project directly to the vestibular nuclei in the brain stem, which are functionally analogous to the cerebellar nuclei, and indirectly via efferents from the fastigial nuclei.

The cerebellar nuclei transmit the main output of the cerebellum. The efferent fibers from the cerebellum are distributed to several parts of the central nervous system (see Fig. 17–4). Cerebellar output is directed essentially to the ipsilateral brain stem where subsequent crossing of the midline often occurs. Most of the efferents leave the cerebellum via the superior cerebellar peduncle and a few via the inferior cerebellar peduncle. Efferent cerebellar pathways descend to the brain stem and spinal cord or ascend to the cerebral cortex.

Efferents from the fastigial nuclei (medial zone) project to the vestibular nuclei and the reticular formation via the inferior cerebellar peduncle. Brain stem and spinal cord motor neurons can be influenced through the vestibulospinal and reticulospinal tracts. Efferents from the globose and emboliform nuclei (intermediate zone) project both to the contralateral thalamus and the red nucleus and leave the cerebellum primarily in the superior cerebellar peduncle. Output fibers from the dentate nuclei (lateral zone) end in the contralateral thalamus (primarily in ventral lateral thalamic nucleus) and some in the contralateral red nucleus. The main efferent output from the red nucleus goes to the spinal cord (rubrospinal tract). The main projection from the thalamus goes to the primary motor cortex. In addition, projections are sent to premotor and prefrontal ("cognitive") areas of the contralateral frontal cortex.[17] In unilateral cerebellar lesions, symptoms of limb ataxia occur ipsilaterally because the major parts of both the cerebellar efferents and the motor tracts (corticospinal and rubrospinal tracts) cross within the brain stem (double-crossing).

INTERNAL STRUCTURE

The cerebellar cortex is a uniform structure. It is divided into three distinct layers, the molecular layer, the Purkinje cell layer, and the granular layer. The cerebellar cortex contains five types of neurons: (1) the Purkinje, (2) granule, (3) Golgi, (4) stellate, and (5) basket cell. The molecular layer is the outermost layer and contains primarily the axons of the granule

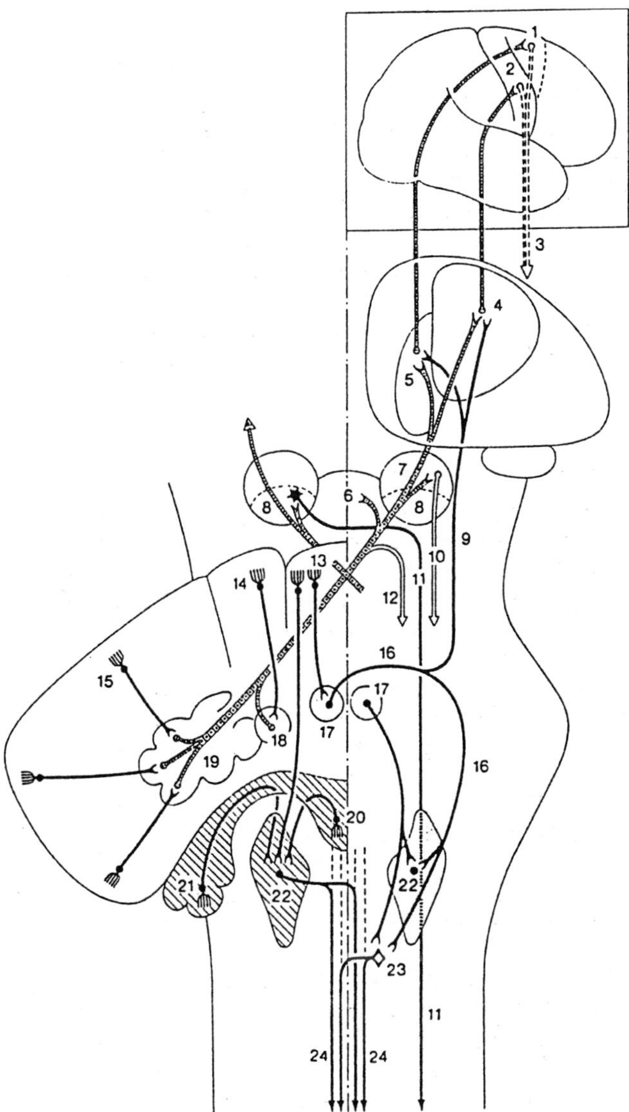

FIGURE 17–4. The efferent connections of the cerebellum. 1, Premotor cortex. 2, Motor cortex. 3, Pyramidal tract. 4, Ventral lateral thalamic nucleus. 5, Ventral anterior thalamic nucleus. 6, Griseum centralis mesencephali. 7, Red nucleus (parvocellular part). 8, Red nucleus (magnocellular part). 9, Uncinate cerebellar fasciculus (ascending ramus). 10, Central tegmental tract. 11, Rubrospinal tract. 12, Superior cerebellar peduncle. 13, Vermis. 14, Intermediate part of cerebellar hemisphere. 15, Cerebellar hemisphere. 16, Uncinate cerebellar fasciculus. 17, Fastigial nucleus. 18, Interposed nucleus. 19, Dentate nucleus. 20, Nodulus (flocculonodular lobe). 21, Flocculus (flocculonodular lobe). 22, Vestibular nuclei. 23, Reticular formation. 24, Medial longitudinal fasciculus. (From Nieuwenhuys R, Voogd J, van Huijzen C: The Human Central Nervous System. A Synopsis and Atlas. Berlin, Springer, 1988, p 166.)

cells, termed parallel fibers, as well as dendrites of the Purkinje and Golgi cells, climbing fibers, and two types of interneurons (stellate and basket cells). The large pear-shaped cell bodies of the Purkinje cells are aligned side by side in a single layer, known as the Purkinje cell layer. The extensive dendritic tree of the Purkinje cell extends into the molecular layer in a single plane. The granular layer is the innermost layer and contains primarily densely packed, small granule cells as well as a few larger interneurons (Golgi cells).

The mossy fiber afferents terminate in the granular cell layer. Mossy fiber contacts with dendrites of the granule and Golgi cell are known as cerebellar glomeruli. The mossy fibers alter the activity of the Purkinje cell via the parallel fibers, which are the axons of the granule cells. Each Purkinje cell receives inputs from numerous granule cells, and each granule cell collects inputs from several mossy fibers. The climbing fibers connect directly with the dendrites of the Purkinje cell. Each Purkinje cell receives input from a single climbing fiber, and one climbing fiber contacts 1 to 10 Purkinje cells.

The Purkinje cell is the only output neuron of the cerebellar cortex. Purkinje cells have an inhibitory action on the cerebellar nuclear neurons. Both mossy and climbing fiber afferents have an excitatory action on the Purkinje cell. The excitatory input is modulated by inhibitory interneurons (stellate and basket cells in the molecular layer, and Golgi cells in the granular layer).

Oscarsson[18] proposed that the cerebellar cortex consists of numerous structural-functional units with distinct efferent and climbing fiber afferent connections, known as *microzones*. Ito[19] introduced the concept of *corticonuclear microcomplexes*. He defined a microcomplex as a cortical microzone and an associated group of nuclear cells that regulates a single function of motor control.

PHARMACOLOGY OF THE CEREBELLUM

Ito[19] discovered that all Purkinje cells are inhibitory and use the inhibitory amino acid gamma-aminobutyric acid (GABA) as their neurotransmitter. Granule cells are excitatory and use the excitatory amino acid glutamate as their neurotransmitter. The inhibitory interneurons (stellate, basket, and Golgi cells) use the inhibitory amino acid GABA as their neurotransmitter. The efferent fibers from the cerebellar nuclei are generally thought to be excitatory, and glutamate is a likely candidate. The neurotransmitters of the excitatory mossy and climbing fibers are thought to include the excitatory amino acids glutamate and aspartate. Monoaminergic fibers originate in different afferent systems and are distributed equally throughout the cerebellum. The origin of most noradrenergic fibers lies within the locus coeruleus, of serotoninergic afferents within many dorsal raphe nuclei, and of histaminergic fibers within the hypothalamus. The cerebellum has a low content of identified neuropeptides (e.g., calcitonin gene–related peptide and corticotropin-releasing factor), which are of unknown functional importance.[20]

VASCULAR ANATOMY OF THE CEREBELLUM

The blood supply of the cerebellum is provided by the vertebrobasilar arterial system. The three major branches are the posterior inferior cerebellar artery (PICA), the anterior inferior cerebellar artery (AICA), and the superior cerebellar artery (SCA). The PICA usually arises from the vertebral artery, the AICA from the basilar artery, and the SCA from the basilar artery before its bifurcation into the posterior cerebral arteries. Variations in the size and distribution of these vessels are frequent, and all major branches are highly anastomotic. All cerebellar arteries supply cerebellar as well as brain stem structures. Therefore, vascular disorders frequently damage the cerebellum and brain stem together.

Branches of the PICA supply the inferior aspect of the cerebellar hemispheres and inferior vermis extending up to the horizontal fissure. Whether the PICA supplies the dentate nucleus is debated and it probably supplies the fastigial nucleus as well. The PICA sometimes supplies the lateral medullary area and usually part of the dorsal medullary area. Branches of the AICA supply the flocculus, adjacent lobules of the inferior and anterior cerebellum, and the middle cerebellar peduncles. The AICA supplies the lower third of the lateral pontine territory in most cases, its middle third frequently, and in a few individuals the superior part of the lateral region of the medulla. The labyrinthine artery, which supplies the inner ear, arises frequently from the AICA. The SCA supplies the superior parts of the cerebellum down to the horizontal fissure. It supplies all deep cerebellar nuclei and most of the cerebellar white matter. The SCA supplies the dorsolaterotegmental area of the upper pons (Fig. 17–5).[21, 22]

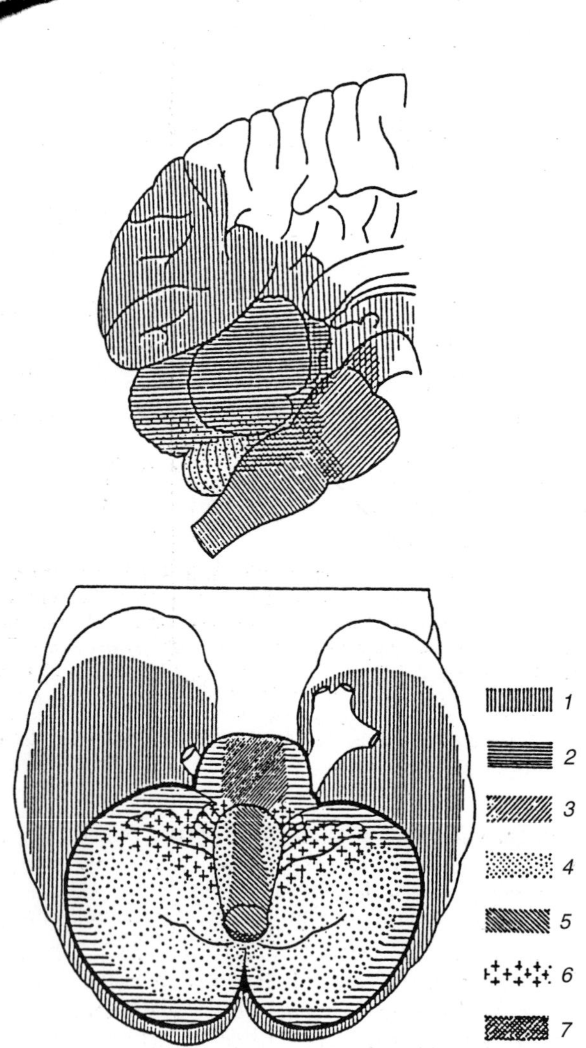

FIGURE 17–5. Vascular anatomy of the cerebellum. (*Top*: lateral view; *bottom*: ventral view.) 1, Posterior cerebral artery. 2, Superior cerebellar artery (SCA). 3, Basilar artery. 4, Posterior inferior cerebellar artery (PICA). 5, Anterior spinal artery, vertebral artery. 6, Anterior inferior cerebellar artery (AICA). 7, Posterior spinal artery. (Adapted from Gänshirt H: Zerebrale Zirkulationsstörunjem. *In* Hopf HC, Poeck K, Schliack H (eds). Neurologie in Klinik und Praxis. Stuttgart, Thieme, 1983; Fig. 9 b and c, p 2.9.)

Examination of Coordination and Ataxia

DIRECTED NEUROLOGICAL EXAMINATION

Clinical signs and symptoms were comprehensively described and summarized by Holmes,[3] Goldstein,[23] and later by Dow and Moruzzi,[24] Gilman and associates,[25] and Harding.[26] Different rating scales have been proposed to score the severity of cerebellar ataxia.[27]

Posture and Gait

Evaluation of posture and gait is critical in cerebellar disorders. Ataxia of gait might be the only abnormal sign in certain cases of cerebellar degeneration. Walking capacities are observed during a 10-meter test including a half turn. Patients with cerebellar disorders walk with a wide-based, staggering gait and consequently take a zigzag course, making it seem as if they were intoxicated by alcohol. Steps are short, unequal in length, and irregular. The legs often are lifted too high and brought down with undue force. The arms do not swing synchronously with the movement of the opposite leg. Velocity of gait is reduced. Gait ataxia might be visible only when the patient walks on tandem, backwards, or without visual feedback. However, cerebellar ataxia may be so severe that the patient cannot walk (abasia). Supporting a severely ataxic patient, the examination of gait reveals decomposition of truncal and leg movements, with the legs preceding while the trunk remains behind. Symptoms are more prominent during sudden changes of direction, for example, turning or stopping suddenly, or rising quickly from a chair. A tendency to fall or deviate to one side suggests a unilateral cerebellar lesion on the same side. Patients may compensate by shortening their steps and shuffling (i.e., keeping both feet on the ground simultaneously).

Standing and sitting capacities are observed. The stance usually is on a broad base, with the feet several inches apart. In the mildest form, patients have difficulties standing with their feet together, in tandem position, or on one foot. However, the patient may be unable to sit or stand without support (astasia), with a tendency to fall backward or toward the side of the lesion. There may be a rhythmical tremor of the body, appearing usually as a rocking of the trunk forward and backward, from side to side, or in a rotatory movement that can evolve into a severe titubation. Romberg's sign might be present or absent in cerebellar disorders, depending on the site of the lesion. Lesions of the anterior lobe lead to anteroposterior body sway with a frequency of about 3 Hz. This form of postural tremor is provoked by eye closure (presence of Romberg's sign). Patients rarely fall because the body tremor is opposite in phase in head, trunk, and legs, resulting in a minimal shift of the center of gravity. Lesions of the lower vermis cause omnidirectional postural tremor of head and trunk, with frequency components below 1 Hz. This kind of postural tremor is not enhanced by eye closure (Romberg's sign is not present).[28]

Voluntary Motor Acts

Upper Limb Ataxia. Limb ataxia is generally more marked in upper limbs than in lower limbs, in complex movements than in simple movements, and in fast movements than in slow movements. Several aspects of upper limb ataxia might be observed using the finger-nose test. Patients are asked to move an arm from an outstretched horizontal position to touch the tip of the nose or to alternatively touch the examiner's finger and the patient's own nose. Visual control is required. Initiation of movement is delayed (Fig. 17–6A). The arm often first flexes and then swings about until the finger reaches the nose. Thus, the arm movement is decomposed in time into its constituent parts (decomposition of movement).[29] Defective postural stabilization of the limb and trunk might be present during the arm movement, with increased sway of proximal arm muscles and movement of the trunk in the opposite direction. The movement path of the finger is erratic and jerky, and the nose is rarely touched at once (dysmetria; Fig. 17–6B). Subjects more frequently overshoot the target (hypermetria) and rarely stop the movement too soon (hypometria). Errors in initiation, direction, and range become more prominent when a change of direction is required. The patient is instructed to follow with the finger the abruptly initiated horizontal arm movements of the examiner as fast as possible (finger-chase test). Kinetic cerebellar tremor occurs as an oscillatory movement that becomes more prominent as the moving limb approaches a target (see Fig. 17–6B). Tremor on action is a prominent symptom in diseases involving the dentate nucleus or superior cerebellar peduncle. Kinetic tremor is greatest when patients use visual cues to guide the movement. Past-pointing is examined in Barany's pointing test. The patient is asked to hold both arms extended horizontally in front. The examiner's forefinger touches the patient's extended forefinger. The patient is asked to bring the arm downward and up again (or upward and down again) to reach the examiner's finger. After a few practice trials with preserved vision, the patient is asked to close the eyes. In addition to overshooting its target (dysmetria), the forefinger of the affected limb deviates almost constantly outward, away from the examiner's finger position.

The ability to execute rapidly alternating movements is tested by raising the forearm vertically and making alternating movements of the hand or by patting with one hand, rapidly alternating between palm up and palm down. In cerebellar subjects, movements are irregular (dysdiadochokinesis) and slow (bradydiadochokinesis) (Fig. 17–6C). Slowness at the turning points could result from delays in movement initiation or dysmetria, or both, at the end of the movement.

Impaired execution of fine finger movements is tested by bringing each finger of one hand separately in succession to the tip of the thumb. All fingers tend to flex simultaneously, and the ability of the thumb to keep a correct posture is impaired. Investigating a variety of more complex tasks, like buttoning or handling objects, may demonstrate disturbance of activities of everyday life. Prehension involves moving the hand to an object, a coincident shaping of the hand in anticipation of the object, and a final closing of the fingers to formulate the grasp. Cerebellar subjects open their fingers excessively wide in anticipation of the object and close their fingers with undue force to grasp the object (signe de la préhension). Writing is often affected. Maintaining a low isometric force between thumb and index finger, for example, when holding a pen while writing, is impaired. The pencil is held incorrectly and is pressed too firmly on the paper. Writing becomes labored and slow. The letters are irregular in size and enlarged (megalographia).

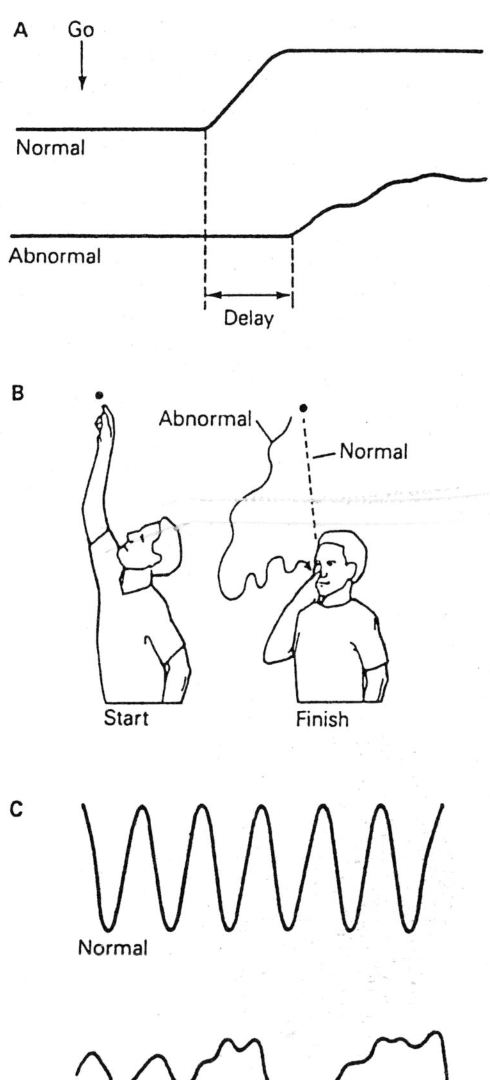

FIGURE 17–6. Typical defects in upper limb ataxia. *A,* Initiation of movement is delayed. *B,* Dysmetria (inaccuracy in range and direction) and kinetic tremor. *C,* Dysdiadochokinesis, an irregular pattern of alternating movements, can be seen in the abnormal position trace. (From Ghez C: The cerebellum. *In* Kandel ER, Schwartz JH, Jessell TM (eds). Principles of Neural Science, 3rd ed. Norwalk, Appleton & Lange, 1991; Fig. 41–16, p 643. Adapted from Thach WT, Montgomery EB: Motor system. *In* Pearlman AL, Collins RC (eds): Neurobiology of Disease, 3rd ed. New York, Oxford University Press, 1990, pp 168–196.)

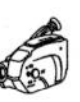

Lower Limb Ataxia. The disturbances of lower limb ataxia are usually less severe compared with disturbances of gait. Several aspects of lower limb ataxia might be observed using the heel-to-shin test. The test is performed in the supine position, and the head is tilted so that visual control is possible. The patient is asked to raise one leg, place that heel on the knee, and then slide the heel down the anterior surface of the leg toward the ankle. On reaching the ankle joint, the leg is again raised in the air to a height of approximately 40 cm, and the action is repeated. Similar to upper limb ataxia, initiation of movement is delayed. The thigh might be bent on the trunk before the knee is adequately flexed, or the knee might flex first (decomposition of movement). The movement path of the heel is erratic and jerky, and the knee is rarely touched at once (dysmetria). Kinetic tremor is specifically observed when the patient holds the heel on the knee for a few seconds before sliding down the anterior tibial surface. Another example of decomposition of trunk and leg movements has been described by Babinski:[1] In attempting to sit up from the supine position by flexion of the trunk, the heel of the affected side often rises from the bed.

Speech

Fluency and clarity of speech are tested by asking the patient to repeat several times a standard phrase, for instance, "A mischievous spectacle in Czechoslovakia," and by syllable repetition tasks.

Articulation, phonation, and respiration are disturbed. Subsequently, the melodic aspects of the speech become abnormal (dysprosody). Comprehension and expression of meanings via words remain intact. Patients show reduced articulatory precision resulting in slurred pronunciation of consonants ("imprecise consonants") and vowels ("disturbed vowels"). Articulatory deficits frequently are present inconsistently, giving rise to the perception of "irregular articulatory breakdowns." The speech tempo is slowed either in connected speech or syllable repetition tasks. There may be increased separation of syllables with excess and equal stress ("scanning speech"). Phonation may be monotonous with rough (hoarse) voice quality. Fluctuation of pitch and loudness and voice tremor may be present. Cerebellar speech often becomes more elaborated.[30, 31]

Oculomotor System

A variety of eye movement abnormalities are seen in cerebellar disease, particularly in midline cerebellar lesions. Gaze-evoked nystagmus is a common finding, with the slow phase of the nystagmus being toward the primary eye position. The subject is asked to look laterally at the finger of the examiner. The movements assessed are mainly horizontal, but they may be oblique, rotatory, or vertical. It may be associated with slow- and fast-phase reversal on return to the primary position (rebound nystagmus). Rebound nystagmus appears to be specific for cerebellar lesions. Downbeat or upbeat nystagmus and sustained horizontal nystagmus may also be present.

Another frequent abnormality is impairment of smooth pursuit eye movements, which are slower than normal and cause the patient to make catch-up saccades in an attempt to keep the moving target near the fovea (saccadic pursuit or jerkiness of smooth pursuit). The subject is asked to follow the slow lateral finger movement of the examiner. Dysmetria of saccades are examined using the following procedure: The two index fingers of the examiner are placed in each temporal visual field of the patient, whose eyes are in the primary position. The patient is then asked to look laterally at the finger on the right and on the left, and the average overshoot or undershoot is estimated. On attempted fixation, the eyes may overshoot the target and then may oscillate through several cycles until precise fixation is attained (ocular dysmetria). Square wave jerks (Gegenrucken) refer to inappropriate saccades disrupting fixation, which are immediately followed by a corrective saccade.

An inability to suppress the VOR and abnormalities of optokinetic nystagmus are frequently found. The ability to suppress VOR is tested by asking the patient to elevate the arms in front of him and fixate one thumb while slowly rotating the upper body. Normal subjects can maintain fixation.

Cerebellar and brain stem disorders, particularly those associated with paraneoplastic etiologies, have been associated with ocular flutter and opsoclonus. Ocular flutter refers to brief bursts of spontaneously and conjugated oscillations of the eyes in the horizontal direction. Opsoclonus is the term of description given when the eyes oscillate in a variety of directions (syn. "dancing eye movements," "ataxic conjugate eye movements").

Other Cerebellar Signs

Patients with chronic cerebellar lesions usually have normal muscle tone and normal tendon reflexes. Hypotonia refers to a decrease in the resistance to passive movements of the limbs in acute cerebellar damage, which usually disappears within a few days or weeks. As a result of hypotonia, Holmes[3] described an increased swinging of the affected limbs in rapid passive movements. Furthermore, when the forearms are held vertically in a patient with a unilateral lesion, the affected wrist flexes more than the unaffected one. Also, if the arms are held outstretched and gently tapped, the affected arm moves in wider excursions. In patients with acute cerebellar lesions due to hypotonia, tendon reflexes have been described as being less brisk, with the involved limb continuing to swing inertly like a pendulum (pendular reflexes).

The rebound phenomenon can be used to examine the inability to stop an ongoing movement. Excessive rebound is tested by pulling forcefully on the patient's forearm while the patient flexes the elbow. When the forearm is unexpectedly released, the hand of the affected side flies unchecked to the patient's shoulder (Stewart-Holmes sign).

Recent studies suggest that the cerebellum may play a role in selected aspects of cognition, including temporal processing, frontal lobe function, higher-order speech, and visuospatial processing. In patients with cerebellar lesions, detailed neuropsychological testing may reveal deficits in cognitive planning (e.g., tower of Hanoi), verbal fluency, and word generation tasks. Agrammatism and mutism have been reported as well. However, presenting symptoms are almost always motor, and unless more extensive damage or degeneration occurs beyond the cerebellum, cerebellar disorders are not associated with general intellectual impairment, such as dementia.[32]

ASSOCIATED NEUROLOGICAL FINDINGS

Pure cerebellar syndromes are rare. Cerebellar symptoms are frequently associated with brain stem dysfunction because of the cerebellum's close proximity to the brain stem. Vascular disorders frequently damage the cerebellum and brain stem together because all cerebellar arteries supply cerebellar as well as brain stem structures. Degenerative cerebellar disorders are frequently accompanied by pyramidal and extrapyramidal symptoms. Cerebellar symptoms might be mimicked by frontal lobe lesions.

Cerebral. Frontal signs include motor abnormalities, impairment of cognitive function, and changes in personality. There are important anatomical connections between the contralateral frontal lobe and ipsilateral cerebellum. Therefore, frontal lobe disorders might cause cerebellar-like symptoms with walking difficulties and clumsiness. However, frontal lobe tumors commonly start with mental symptoms. Cognitive dysfunction accompanies some degenerative ataxic disorders. Incontinence associated with dementia and gait ataxia suggests normal pressure hydrocephalus.

Cranial Nerves. The history of previous subacute monocular visual loss suggests a diagnosis of multiple sclerosis. Some degenerative ataxias are associated with gradual visual loss due to retinitis pigmentosa. Diplopia, facial numbness, facial droop, vertigo, or hearing loss resulting from associated cranial neuropathies (cranial nerves III, IV, V, VI, VII, and VIII) associated with ataxia suggests a disorder in the brain stem. Tumors of the cerebellopontine angle, such as acoustical neurinomas, are frequently associated with nerve palsies of cranial nerves V, VII, and VIII.

Motor/Reflexes/Gait. A slight loss of muscular power and increased fatigability of muscles may occur with acute cerebellar disorders. However, paresis associated with increased muscular tone, hyper-reflexia, and extensor plantar reflexes (Babinski's sign) suggest an additional involvement of upper motor neurons (corticospinal or pyramidal syndrome). Paresis accompanied with atrophy, hypotonia, and loss of tendon reflexes (areflexia) suggests the involvement of the lower motor neuron and is usually associated with polyneuropathy (e.g., in Friedreich's ataxia). Several demyelinating neuropathies may give rise to prominent tremor and sensory ataxia, which might be confused with cerebellar ataxia, such as the demyelinating type of hereditary motor and sensory neuropathy, chronic inflammatory and paraproteinemic neuropathies, and Refsum's disease. In these cases, ataxia is improved by visual feedback. The Miller-Fisher variant of Guillain-Barré syndrome may present with cerebellar ataxia of subacute onset, usually associated with areflexia, ophthalmoplegia, and facial weakness.

Rigidity, akinesia, and static tremor suggest parkinsonism and are associated with multiple system atrophy. Abnormal involuntary movements might occur in cerebellar disorders. Powerful but brief involuntary movements at the beginning of the movement are due to intention myoclonus, not tremor, and occur in diseases involving the dentate nucleus or the superior cerebellar peduncle. Palatal tremor occurs in lesions of the inferior olive in the brain stem or dentato-olivary pathway. Hemiballismus and chorea are associated with basal ganglia disorders.

Sensory. Pure cerebellar lesions do not cause disturbances in sensation. Hemianesthesia involving one side of the body suggests an additional lesion of the contralateral parietal lobe. Crossed sensory disturbances with a loss of pain on one side of the face and on the opposite side of the body are common in patients with a brain stem lesion. Symmetrical sensory impairment over the feet, legs, and hands associated with reflex loss and various degrees of paresis suggests peripheral neuropathy. Peripheral neuropathies are frequently associated with degenerative cerebellar disorders.

Autonomic Nervous System. Horner's syndrome (miosis, ptosis, and retraction of the eyeball) and ipsilateral dysautonomia (increased skin temperature due to vasomotor paralysis and anhidrosis due to impaired sudomotor function) associated with cerebellar ataxia suggest an additional brain stem lesion. Postural hypotension, bladder dysfunction, and erectile dysfunction are associated with multiple system atrophy. Urgency of micturition is common in multiple sclerosis and might be present in degenerative ataxic disorders.

Neurovascular. Fundal examination may disclose diabetic, hypertensive, or atherosclerotic retinal changes. Auscultation of the mastoid may reveal a bruit in a patient with stenosis of a vertebrobasilar artery or vascular malformation. A carotid or subclavian bruit might be heard in a patient with symptomatic artherosclerotic disease of the vertebrobasilar arteries. A reduced radial pulse and blood pressure suggests subclavian stenosis and might be associated with subclavian steal syndrome.

ASSOCIATED MEDICAL FINDINGS

Skeletal abnormalities like kyphoscoliosis and pes cavus, as well as diabetes and cardiac symptoms, are associated with Friedreich's ataxia. Cold intolerance, dry skin, and hair loss indicate hypothyroidism. Pulmonary and gynecological examination might show signs of bronchial or ovarian carcinoma, respectively. Cervical adenopathy might reveal Hodgkin's disease. Subacute, reversible ataxia associated with pyrexia suggests viral cerebellitis. Repeated bronchopulmonary infections suggest ataxia-telangiectasia. Examination of the cardiovascular system might disclose a structural cardiac lesion or rhythm disturbances, which indicate a possible cardiac cause of emboli.

Evaluation Guidelines (Table 17–3)

The first step in the diagnosis of ataxia is to distinguish between focal cerebellar disease (hemorrhage, ischemia, neoplasms, abscess, or parasitic infections) and nonfocal lesions. This distinction is achieved by the use of imaging methods. Further diagnostic testing should be guided by considering the mode of inheritance, age at disease onset, progression rate, and accompanying symptoms. Some disorders have a highly characteristic clinical phenotype, and the expected diagnosis can be confirmed by a specific laboratory test (see Chapter 35).

Neuroimaging. Immediate computed tomography (CT) scanning or magnetic resonance imaging (MRI) has to be performed in the setting of acute and subacute cerebellar ataxia. Posterior fossa lesions carry the risk of increased intracranial pressure and death because of the cerebellar tonsils moving downward and compressing the brain stem within the foramen magnum. Angiography of the vertebrobasilar vascular system should be performed if the diagnosis of an aneurysm, vascular malformation, or basilar artery thrombosis is suspected based on the findings of the CT or MRI scan.

Compared with CT scanning, MRI offers an increased capacity for demonstrating cerebellar (and brain stem) lesions because of a lack of bone artifact, high resolution, and the capability of imaging different planes. MRI demonstrates cerebellar atrophy as well as spinal and brain stem involvement in degenerative cerebellar disorders. In addition, MRI

TABLE 17–3. **Useful Studies in the Evaluation of Coordination Disorders**

Syndrome	Neuroimaging	Electrophysiology	Fluid and Tissue Analysis	Neuropsychological Tests	Other Tests
Truncal, gait, and stance ataxia (absence of Romberg's sign)	CT or MRI: brain	Posturography, ENG	CSF	N/A	N/A
Stance and gait ataxia (presence of Romberg's sign)	CT or MRI: brain	Posturography	Blood count, gamma-glutamyl transpeptidase, thiamine, liver enzymes	N/A	
Unilateral limb ataxia	CT or MRI: brain cerebral angiography	N/A	CSF	N/A	Carotid echogram
Truncal, stance, gait, and bilateral limb ataxia	CT or MRI: brain	Posturography ENG. Extracerebellar involvement: VEP, SSEP, AEP, MEP, NCVs, EEG	CSF, genetic testing, cholestanol, alpha-fetoprotein, immunoglobulins, lipids, vitamin E, VLCFA, ACTH (in males), lactate, pyruvate, muscle biopsy, ceruloplasmin, thyroxine, anti-gliadin, anti-myosin, anti-GAD, Phytanic acid. *To exclude malignancy:* urinary catecholamine levels, anti-Purkinje cell antibodies, bone marrow biopsy. Associated with mental retardation: hexosaminidase, arylsulfatase A, galactocerebrosidase	N/A	Friedreich's ataxia: electrocardiogram, echocardiogram. *To exclude malignancy:* chest x-ray, pelvic imaging, mammogram
Cerebellar speech	CT or MRI: brain	N/A	CSF	N/A	Carotid echogram
Paroxysmal ataxia	CT or MRI: brain	ENG	*Infancy and early childhood:* blood ammonia, pyruvate, lactate, amino acids, urinary amino acids. *Adult onset:* CSF	N/A	N/A
Cerebellar oculomotor signs	CT or MRI: brain	ENG	CSF	N/A	N/A

ACTH, Adrenocorticotropic hormone; AEP, auditory evoked potentials; CSF, cerebrospinal fluid; CT, computed tomography; ENG, electronystagmography; MEP, magnetic evoked potentials; MRI, magnetic resonance imaging; N/A, not applicable; NCVs, nerve conduction velocity studies; SSEP, somatosensory evoked potentials; VEP, visual evoked potentials; VLCFA, very long-chain fatty acids; anti-GAD, glutamate decarboxylase antibodies.

is much more sensitive to white matter lesions, particularly demyelination. Therefore, MRI should be performed when multiple sclerosis is suspected.

Electrophysiology. Electrophysiological tests are applied to confirm extracerebellar lesions. Nerve conduction studies are performed when lesions of the peripheral nervous system are expected. Evoked potentials show lesions of the visual (visual evoked potentials), auditory (auditory evoked potentials), and somatosensory (somatosensory evoked potentials) systems. Involvement of the corticospinal tract is demonstrated using magnetic evoked potentials. Demonstration of prolonged latencies of multimodal evoked potentials is helpful in the diagnosis of multiple sclerosis.

Electronystagmography is a useful laboratory tool to confirm and quantify cerebellar oculomotor disorders. Posturography is applied to quantify ataxia of stance and may distinguish spinocerebellar, vestibulocerebellar, and spinal ataxias. Lesions of the anterior lobe lead to anteroposterior body sway with a frequency of about 3 Hz. Lesions of the lower vermis cause omnidirectional postural tremor of head and trunk with frequency components below 1 Hz. Spinal ataxia leads to predominantly lateral body sway.[28]

Electroencephalography should be performed in cases with associated epilepsy.

Body Fluid and Tissue Analysis. Genetic testing will confirm a suspected diagnosis of Friedreich's ataxia (early disease onset, areflexia, dysarthria, posterior column signs). Diabetes mellitus should be excluded in Friedreich's ataxia. Alpha-fetoprotein is increased and immunoglobulins are decreased in ataxia telangiectasia. In the presence of xanthomas, cholestanol should be analyzed to confirm cerebrotendinous xanthomatosis.

Genetic testing is available for an increasing number of inherited ataxias, particularly for autosomal dominant cerebellar ataxias after the age of 20 years.[33] To date, direct DNA testing is available for spinocerebellar ataxia (SCA) types 1, 2, 3, 6, 7, 8, 10, 12, and 17 and dentatorubral-pallidoluysian atrophy (DRPLA). Dominant ataxia and retinal degeneration is always associated with the SCA7 mutation (see Chapter 35).

In early-onset (< 25 years) recessive and sporadic disease and in adult-onset sporadic ataxia, metabolic disorders should be excluded. Lipids (abetalipoproteinemia), vitamin E (abetalipoproteinemia, ataxia with isolated vitamin E deficiency), very long-chain fatty acids, adrenocorticotropic hormone (adrenoleukodystrophy, X-chromosomal inheritance), lactate and pyruvate (mitochondriopathies), phytanic acid (Refsum's disease), ceruloplasmin (Wilson's disease), and thyroxine (hypothyroidism) should be analyzed. A muscle biopsy should be performed in cases of suspected mitochondrial myopathy. Inflammatory (viral infections) and immune-mediated disorders (antigliadin and antiendomysium antibodies [sprue]) should be excluded. Antibodies against glutamic acid decarboxylase disorders can also be assayed.

Poisoning or drug intoxication has to be excluded. Anemia, macrocytosis, and raised gamma-glutamyltranspeptidase suggest alcoholic cerebellar degeneration. Serum anti-Purkinje cell antibodies (anti-Yo, anti-Hu, and anti-Ri) are useful in the diagnosis of paraneoplastic cerebellar degeneration. In children, neuroblastoma may be associated with paraneoplastic cerebellar degeneration leading to opsoclonus. Urinary catecholamine levels are increased (see Chapter 47).

Investigations of early-onset, chronic progressive ataxia commonly associated with multiple system involvement should include arylsulfatase A (metachromatic leukodystrophy), galactocerebrosidase (globose cell leukodystrophy [Krabbe's disease]), and hexosaminidase (GM2-gangliosidosis). Ultrastructural analysis of lymphocytes and skin should be considered (neuronal ceroid lipofuscinosis). Intermittent ataxia associated with mental retardation and onset in infancy or early childhood suggest a metabolic disorder (e.g., urea cycle deficiences, aminoacidurias, and disorders of lactate metabolism). Screening investigations include blood ammonia, amino acids, urinary amino acids, pyruvate, and lactate (see Chapter 31).

In the presence of myoclonus, tissue biopsies can be helpful: skin, muscle, and liver for Lafora disease; muscle for myoclonic epilepsy with ragged red fibers (MERFF); and lymphocytes or skin for neuronal ceroid lipofuscinosis. In suspected sialidosis type 1, sialo-oligosaccharides in urine and neuraminidase activity in white blood cells should be analyzed.

In the presence of retinal degeneration, vitamin E (abetalipoproteinemia, ataxia with isolated vitamin E deficiency), lipid electrophoresis (abetalipoproteinemia), and phytanic acid (Refsum's disease) should be analyzed. Analysis of skin and lymphocytes may reveal neuronal ceroid lipofuscinosis. Retinal-macular cherry-red spot is associated with sialidosis type 1 and macular degeneration with SCA7.

Cerebrospinal Fluid. Lumbar puncture and examination of the cerebrospinal fluid (CSF) are applied when inflammatory or infectious disorders are expected. Pleocytosis, increased total protein content, and oligoclonal bands are found in patients with multiple sclerosis, viral cerebellitis, and paraneoplastic cerebellar disorders. In addition, cerebrospinal fluid anti-Purkinje cell antibodies (anti-Yo, anti-Hu, and anti-Ri) are useful in the diagnosis of paraneoplastic cerebellar degeneration. Lactate in CSF is increased in mitochondrial disease.

Neuropsychological Tests. Degenerative forms of ataxia, which are frequently associated with extracerebellar lesions, might present with dementia. Neuropsychological testing is useful to confirm and quantify existing cognitive deficits. In pure cerebellar disorders, detailed neuropsychological testing may reveal minor abnormalities such as frontal lobe or higher-speech dysfunction.

Other Tests. In subacute-onset ataxia, a thoracic x-ray study and pelvic imaging are required to exclude malignancies (small cell lung cancer, ovarian or breast cancer, or Hodgkin's disease) causing paraneoplastic cerebellar degeneration. Abdominal and thoracic CT scan as well as bronchoscopy might be required. An electrocardiogram and echocardiogram should be performed in Friedreich's ataxia, because of frequent associated heart disease.

Schellong test and urodynamic testing are performed to confirm autonomic dysfunction suggestive of multiple system atrophy.

Clinical Syndromes (see Tables 17–3 and 17–4)

Three syndromes of cerebellar dysfunction are commonly distinguished on purely clinical grounds. Symptoms that are

TABLE 17–4. **Selected Etiologies Associated with Disorders of Coordination**

Etiological Category	Selected Etiologies	Chapter
Structural Disorders		
Developmental structural disorders	Pontocerebellar and granule cell hypoplasia Joubert's syndrome, Gillespie's syndrome, Dandy-Walker malformation, malformations	28
Hereditary and Degenerative Disorders		
Storage diseases: Lipidoses, glycogen disorders, and leukoencephalopathies	Abetalipoproteinemia, hypobetalipoproteinemia (Bassen-Kornzweig disease), Refsum's disease, cerebrotendinous xanthomatosis, GM_2 gangliosidoses (Tay-Sachs disease), Niemann-Pick disease, cholestanolosis, metachromatic leukodystrophy, ceroid lipofuscinosis, sialidosis, arylsulfatase C deficiency	30
Amino/organic acidopathies, mitochondrial enzyme defects, and other metabolic errors	Ornithine-transcarbamylase deficiency, arginosuccinase deficiency, arginase deficiency, hyperornithinemia, Hartnup's disease, maple syrup urine disease, isovalericacidemia, gamma-glutamylcysteine synthetase deficiency, Leigh's syndrome, multiple biotin-dependent carboxylase deficiencies, pyruvate dehydrogenase deficiency, mitochondrial myopathy	31
Chromosomal abnormalities and neurocutaneous disorders	Von Hippel-Lindau disease Ataxia-telangiectasia	32
Movement disorders	Multiple system atrophy: striatonigral degeneration, olivopontocerebellar atrophy, Shy-Drager syndrome Wilson's disease	34
Ataxias	**Autosomal Recessive** Friedreich's ataxia Infantile-onset spinocerebellar ataxia (IOSCA) Autosomal recessive spastic ataxia (Charlevoix-Saguenay) Early-onset cerebellar ataxia (EOCA): with retained reflexes with hypogonadism (Holmes' ataxia) with deafness with optic atrophy and mental retardation (Behr syndrome) with cataract and mental retardation (Marinesco-Sjögren syndrome) with pigmentary retinopathy (Hallgren syndrome) with extrapyramidal features with myoclonus (Ramsay-Hunt syndrome) **Autosomal Dominant** ADCA type I: SCA1, SCA2, SCA3 (Machado-Joseph disease), SCA4, SCA8, SCA12, SCA13, SCA17 ADCA type II: SCA7 ADCA type III: SCA5, SCA6, SCA10, SCA14, SCA15, SCA16 Dentatorubral-pallidoluysian atrophy (DRPLA) Episodic ataxia type 1 Episodic ataxia type 2 X-linked recessive spinocerebellar ataxia	35
Acquired Metabolic and Nutritional Disorders		
Exogenous acquired metabolic disorders of the nervous system: Toxins and illicit drugs	Heavy metals (mercury, thallium), solvents (toluene)	39
Nutritional deficiencies and syndromes associated with alcoholism	Alcoholic cerebellar degeneration (thiamine deficiency), vitamin E deficiency	40
Infectious Disorders		
Viral infections	Chronic panencephalitis of congenital rubella, subacute sclerosing panencephalitis, varicella, measles, rubella, echo, coxsackie A/B, polio, Epstein-Barr, herpes simplex, postinfectious disseminated encephalomyelitis, mumps, cytomegalie virus	41
Nonviral infections	Legionella pneumoniae, mycoplasma pneumoniae, toxoplasmosis, Lyme disease, Plasmodium falciparum, cysticercosis, tuberculosis	42
Transmissible spongiform encephalopathy	Creutzfeldt-Jakob disease, Gerstmann-Sträussler disease	43
Neurovascular Disorders	Hemorrhage, ischemia	45

TABLE 17-4. **Selected Etiologies Associated with Disorders of Coordination** *Continued*

Etiological Category	Selected Etiologies	Chapter
Neoplastic Disorders		
Primary neurological tumors	Astrocytoma, medulloblastoma, cerebellopontine angle tumors (acoustic neurinoma, mengioma)	46
Metastatic neoplasms and paraneoplastic syndromes	Metastases: lung > melanoma > breast > gynecological > gastrointestinal > lymphoma Paraneoplastic: In adults: lung, ovary, breast, lymphoma In children: neuroblastoma	47
Demyelinating Disorders		
Demyelinating disorders of the central nervous system	Multiple sclerosis	48
Demyelinating disorders of the peripheral nervous system	Miller-Fisher variant of GBS	49
Traumatic Disorders	Gunshot injuries, falls, traffic accidents, heat stroke	51
Epilepsy	Minor epileptic status Lafora disease SCA10, SCA17 Mitochondriopathes	52
Headache and Facial Pain	Migraine (e.g., SCA6)	53
Drug-Induced and Iatrogenic Neurological Disorders	Phenytoin, lithium, 5-fluorouracil, cytosine arabinoside	55

ADCA, Autosomal dominant cerebellar ataxia; GBS, Guillain-Barré syndrome; SCA, spinocerebellar ataxia.

the result of disease of the flocculonodular lobe induce the archicerebellar or flocculonodular syndrome. Damage to the anterior lobe of the corpus cerebelli or, perhaps more properly, to the medial part of the corpus cerebelli causes the paleocerebellar or anterior lobe syndrome. Lesions of the lateral parts of the corpus cerebelli, which in man are chiefly the posterior part of the cerebellar hemispheres, induce the neocerebellar syndrome.

It has already been noted by Dow and Moruzzi in 1958[24] that, although the corpus cerebelli can be subdivided morphologically into an anterior and posterior lobe, there is considerable evidence that a division into medial, intermediate, and lateral parts may be of greater physiological significance. The clinical description of the paleocerebellar syndrome results chiefly from dysfunction of the medial parts of the cerebellum. The clinical description of the neocerebellar syndrome results chiefly from damage to the posterior lobe but may actually result from damage to the lateral and intermediate parts of the anterior lobe as well. Damage of those parts of the posterior lobe that project to the fastigial nucleus does not likely cause the neocerebellar syndrome.

In spite of the three prototypic descriptions, cerebellar syndromes in practice often reflect more than one of the functionally different subdivisions of the cerebellum. Furthermore, there is no difference between the symptoms of ataxia that results from lesions of afferent and efferent cerebellar pathways (e.g., of cerebellar peduncles or within the brain stem) and those that result from the cerebellum itself.

In addition, pure cerebellar syndromes are rare. Cerebellar symptoms are frequently accompanied by brain stem symptoms. Cerebellar disorders involve the medulla and pons early either directly or indirectly by pressure or obliteration of vessels. Pressure effects are common in the posterior fossa, where expansion is anatomically limited.

A remarkable degree of compensation occurs in lesions of the cerebellum, which are particularly marked in children and slowly progressive disorders.

TRUNCAL, GAIT, AND STANCE ATAXIA (ABSENCE OF ROMBERG'S SIGN)

Lesions of the flocculonodular lobe and adjoining parts of the caudal vermis (so-called archicerebellar or flocculonodular syndrome) mainly due to tumors or hemorrhage cause postural ataxia of head and trunk during sitting, standing, and walking. Patients frequently fall while sitting. The classic example is medulloblastoma, which occurs most often in the cerebellum in children between 5 and 10 years of age. Cerebellar symptoms are first limited to unsteadiness of gait and stance. In patients with such lesions, visual stabilization of posture, as evaluated by comparing sway with eyes closed and sway with eyes open, is impaired (absence of Romberg's sign). Severe postural sway is present with eyes open and is essentially unchanged with eyes closed. Coordinated movements of the upper and lower limbs (tested when the patient is lying in bed) are relatively preserved. Saccadic slow pursuit, nystagmus, and an inability to suppress the VOR are frequently present.

STANCE AND GAIT ATAXIA (PRESENCE OF ROMBERG'S SIGN)

Damage to the spino- or paleocerebellar parts of the anterior lobe (so-called anterior lobe or paleocerebellar syndrome) is characterized by an ataxia of stance and gait, with

varying degrees of instability of the trunk and ataxia of legs. The arms are affected to a much lesser extent, and nystagmus and dysarthria are infrequent signs. The classic example is alcoholic cerebellar degeneration. Lesions of the anterior lobe lead to anteroposterior body sway with a frequency of about 3 Hz. Visual stabilization of posture is relatively preserved and the tremor is provoked by eye closure (presence of Romberg's sign). Patients rarely fall because the body tremor is opposite in phase in head, trunk, and legs, resulting in a minimal shift of the center of gravity.

UNILATERAL LIMB ATAXIA

Holmes fully described symptoms of the lateral parts of the posterior lobe in his classic studies of injuries of the cerebellum. In unilateral lesions, the symptoms occur on the side of the lesion. Diseases of the cerebellar hemisphere (so-called neocerebellar or pontocerebellar syndrome) due to hemorrhage, infarction, or neoplasms are associated with severe disturbances of limb movements, including hypotonia in acute lesions, dysmetria, decomposition of movement (asynergia), dysdiadochokinesis, and, if the dentate nucleus is involved, kinetic tremor. Past-pointing and deviation of gait to the affected side are associated symptoms.

TRUNCAL, GAIT, STANCE, AND BILATERAL LIMB ATAXIA

Symmetrical involvement of both hemispheres and vermis produces bilateral limb ataxia and ataxia of stance and gait, as happens in most forms of cerebellar degeneration. Dysarthria and oculomotor disturbances are also frequently present. Extracerebellar signs are often associated, such as pyramidal and extrapyramidal signs, ophthalmoplegia, and peripheral neuropathy.

PAROXYSMAL ATAXIA

Paroxysmal ataxia with onset in infancy or early childhood is usually associated with mental retardation.[6] A metabolic disorder should be expected. Episodic ataxia in adults might be caused by drug ingestion, multiple sclerosis, transient vertebrobasilar ischemic attack, foramen magnum compression, intermittent obstruction of the ventricular system, and dominantly inherited periodic ataxia.

Autosomal dominant forms of paroxysmal cerebellar ataxia are characterized by ataxia attacks of gait and stance, dysarthria, vertigo, and nystagmus. In episodic ataxia type 1, attacks last for a few seconds or minutes, and patients present with interictal facial myokymia. In episodic ataxia type 2, attacks last for a few hours to several weeks. In most patients, there are mild neurological signs between attacks, such as gaze-evoked down-and-out nystagmus and mild gait ataxia. Rarely, paroxysmal cerebellar ataxia type 2 is associated with progressing and disabling permanent cerebellar deficits (see Chapter 35).[34]

CEREBELLAR SPEECH

Hemispherical disorders are associated with cerebellar dysarthria more frequently than are vermal lesions. The paramedian regions of the superior cerebellar hemispheres are most relevant for the development of cerebellar dysarthria.[35,36] Left hemispherical cerebellar lesions appear to be more frequently associated with cerebellar dysarthria than right hemispherical or vermal lesions. Cerebellar dysarthria is frequently present in degenerative forms of cerebellar ataxias and multiple sclerosis. Cerebellar hemorrhage, infarcts (in particular of the SCA), tumors, and trauma may all cause cerebellar speech.

CEREBELLAR OCULOMOTOR SIGNS

Three principal syndromes of cerebellar oculomotor disorders can be identified: (1) the syndrome of the dorsal vermis and underlying fastigial vermis, (2) the syndrome of the flocculus and paraflocculus, and (3) the syndrome of the nodulus.[37] Lesions of the dorsal vermis and fastigial nucleus cause saccadic dysmetria and mild deficits of smooth pursuit. Lesions of the nodulus are accompanied with prolongation of vestibular responses, positional nystagmus, and periodic alternating nystagmus, which is a spontaneous horizontal nystagmus that changes direction every few minutes. Lesions of the flocculus and paraflocculus cause impaired smooth pursuit; gaze-evoked, rebound, and downbeat nystagmus; impaired optokinetic nystagmus; impaired VOR suppression; and disability to adjust the gain of the VOR. Other cerebellar oculomotor signs cannot be localized to specific cerebellar regions at present, such as square-wave jerks, upbeat nystagmus, and pendular oscillations. These three syndromes are frequently found in patients with degenerative forms of cerebellar ataxia. Cerebellar hemorrhage, tumors, and infarcts may all cause cerebellar eye signs by direct involvement of midline cerebellar structures. Medulloblastomas involving the nodulus and uvula are frequently associated with positional nystagmus. Downbeat nystagmus is frequently associated with paraneoplastic cerebellar ataxia.

The intermediate (interposed nucleus) and lateral cerebellum (dentate nucleus) appear to be involved also in oculomotor control. Their exact role, however, is currently unknown.

General Management Goals

Acquired ataxias need to be treated according to the primary disorder. However, ataxia is often associated with progressive degenerative disease, and it is rarely possible to influence the underlying cause. Only a few forms of inherited ataxias can be treated effectively, such as episodic ataxias using acetazolamide. In most cases, no pharmacological treatment is known. The pharmacological trials using various drugs—GABA agonists (baclofen, sodium valproate), choline chloride, lecithin, physostigmine, gamma-vinyl gamma-aminobutyric acid, thyrotropin-releasing hormone, 5-hydroxytryptophan, buspirone, amantadine, and a combination of sulfamethoxazole and trimethoprim—have been disappointing. Other drugs, such as vitamin E, idebenone, or coenzyme Q10 in Friedreich's ataxia, are still being investigated in clinical trials. Physical therapy is the most important treatment of disorders of coordination and ataxia. Dyssynergia might be reduced by placing additional weight on an ataxic limb to increase inertia. Genetic testing is available in an increasing number of hereditary cerebellar ataxias.[38] However, genetic counseling has to be carefully approached because hereditary cerebellar ataxias are not treatable. Genetic counseling should agree with the guidelines for predictive and prenatal DNA analysis published by the International Huntington's Association and the World Federation of Neurologists. Drugs such as lithium and phenytoin, which are associated with cerebellar dysfunction, should be avoided. Additional neurological symptoms, like spasticity, and physical signs, like diabetes, heart disease, and skeletal deformity, are treated in a common fashion.

Reviews and Selected Updates

Brodal P: The Central Nervous System. Structure and Function, 2nd ed. New York, Oxford University Press, 1998.

Holmes G: The cerebellum of man. Brain 1939;62:1–30.

Klockgether T (ed): Handbook of Ataxia Disorders. New York, Basel, Marcel Dekker, 2000.

Manto M-U, Pandolfo M (eds): The Cerebellum and Its Disorders. Cambridge, Cambridge University Press, 2001.

Thach WT: What is the role of the cerebellum in motor learning and cognition? Trends Cogn Sci 1998;2:331–337.

Voogd J, Glickstein M: The anatomy of the cerebellum. Trends Neurosci 1998;21:370–375.

References

1. Babinski J: De l'asynergie cérbélleuse. Rev Neurol 1899;7:806–816.
2. Babinski J: Sur le role du cervelet dans les actes volitonnels nécessitant une succession rapide de mouvements: Diadococinésie. Rev Neurol 1902;10:1013–1015.
3. Holmes G: The symptoms of acute cerebellar injuries due to gunshot injuries. Brain 1917;40:461–535.
4. Anthoney TR: Neuroanatomy and the neurologic exam. A thesaurus of synonyms, similar-sounding, non-synonyms and terms of variable meaning. Boca Raton, FL, CRC Press, 1994.
5. DeJong RN: The Neurological Examination, 4th ed. Hagerstown, MD, Harper & Row, 1979.
6. Harding AE: Clinical features and classification of inherited ataxias. *In* Harding AE, Deufel T (eds): Advances in Neurology. New York, Raven Press, 1993, pp 1–14.
7. Dichgans J, Diener HC: Clinical evidence of functional compartmentalization of the cerebellum. *In* Bloedel JR, Dichgans J, Precht W (eds): Cerebellar Functions. Berlin, Springer, 1985, pp 126–147.
8. Schmahmann JD, Doyon J, Toga AW, Petrides M, Evans AC: MRI Atlas of the Human Cerebellum. San Diego, Academic Press, 2000.
9. Jansen J, Brodal A: Experimental studies on the intrinsic fibers of the cerebellum. II. The corticonuclear projection. J Comp Neurol 1940;73:267–321.
10. Chambers WW, Sprague JM: Functional localization in the cerebellum. I. Organization in longitudinal cortico-nuclear zones and their contribution to the control of posture, both extrapyramidal and pyramidal. J Comp Neurol 1955;103:105–129.
11. Voogd J: The importance of fiber connections in the comparative anatomy of the mammalian cerebellum. *In* Llinas R (ed): Neurobiology of Cerebellar Evolution and Development. Chicago, American Medical Association, 1969, pp 493–514.
12. Hawkes R, Brochu G, Dore L, et al: Zebrins: Molecular markers of compartmentation in the cerebellum. *In* Llinas R, Sotelo C (eds): The Cerebellum Revisited. New York, Springer-Verlag, 1992, pp 22–55.
13. Grodd W, Hülsmann E, Lotze M, Wildgruber D, Erb M: Sensorimotor mapping of the human cerebellum: fMRI evidence of somatotopic organization. Hum Brain Map 2001;13:55–73.
14. Snider RS, Eldred E: Cerebro-cerebellar relationships in the monkey. J Neurophysiol 1951;15:27–40.
15. Szentagothai J, Rajkovits K: Über den Ursprung der Kletterfasern des Kleinhirns. Z Anat Entwicklungsgesch 1959;121:130–141.
16. Bloedel JR, Courville J: A review of cerebellar afferents system. *In* VB Brooks (ed): Handbook of Physiology. Bethesda, MD, American Physiological Society, 1982, pp 735–830.
17. Middleton FA, Strick PL: Anatomical evidence for cerebellar and basal ganglia involvement in higher cognitive function. Science 1994;266:458–461.
18. Oscarsson O: Functional units of the cerebellum—sagittal zones and microzones. Trends Neurosci 1979;2:143–145.
19. Ito M: The Cerebellum and Neural Control. New York, Raven Press, 1984.
20. Oertel WH: Neurotransmitters in the cerebellum: Scientific aspects and clinical relevance. *In* Harding AE, Deufel T (eds): Advances in Neurology. Inherited Ataxias, Vol 61. New York: Raven Press, 1993, pp 33–75.
21. Tatu L, Moulin T, Bogousslavsky J, Duvernoy H: Arterial territories of human brain: Brain stem and cerebellum. Neurology 1996;47:1125–1135.
22. Amarenco P, Hauw J-J, Caplan LR: Cerebellar infarctions. *In* Lechtenberg R (ed): Handbook of Cerebellar Diseases. New York, Marcel Dekker, 1993, pp 251–290.
23. Goldstein K: Das Kleinhirn. *In* Bethe A, von Bergmann G, Embden G, Ellinger A (eds): Handbuch der Normalen und Pathologischen Physiologie, Vol 10. Berlin, Springer, 1927, pp 222–317.
24. Dow RS, Moruzzi G: The Physiology and Pathology of the Cerebellum. Minneapolis, University of Minnesota Press, 1958.
25. Gilman S, Bloedel J, Lechtenberg R: Disorders of the Cerebellum. Philadelphia, F.A. Davis Company, 1981.
26. Harding AE: Ataxic disorders. *In* Bradley WG, Daroff RB, Fenichel GM, Marsden CG (eds): Neurology in Clinical Practice. Boston, Butterworth-Heinemann, 1991, pp 337–346.
27. Trouillas P, Takayanagi T, Hallett M, et al: International Cooperative Rating Scale for pharmacological assessment of the cerebellar syndrome. The Ataxia Neuropharmacology Committee of the World Federation of Neurology. J Neurol Sci 1997;145:205–11.
28. Diener HC, Dichgans J: Pathophysiology of cerebellar ataxia. Mov Disord 1992;7:95–109.
29. Bastian AJ, Martin TA, Keating JG, Thach WT: Cerebellar ataxia: Abnormal control of interaction torques across multiple joints. J Neurophysiol 1996;76:492–509.
30. Brown JR, Darley FL, Aronson AE: Ataxic dysarthria. Int J Neurol 1970;7:302–318.
31. Ziegler W, Wessel K: Speech timing in ataxic disorders: Sentence production and rapid repetitive articulation. Neurology 1996;47:208–214.
32. Schmahmann JD (ed): The Cerebellum and Cognition. Int Rev Neurobiol 1997;Vol. 41.
33. Klockgether T: Recent advances in degenerative ataxias. Curr Opin Neurol 2000;13:451–455.
34. Griggs RC, Nutt JG: Episodic ataxias as channelopathies. Ann Neurol 1995;37:285–287.
35. Lechtenberg R, Gilman S: Speech disorders in cerebellar disease. Ann Neurol 1978;3:285–290.
36. Ackermann H, Vogel M, Petersen D, et al: Speech deficits in ischemic cerebellar lesions. J Neurol 1992;239:223–227.
37. Robinson FR, Fuchs AF: The role of the cerebellum in voluntary eye movements. Ann Rev Neurosci 2001;24:981–1001.
38. Tan EK, Ashizawa T: Genetic testing in spinocerebellar ataxias: Defining a clinical role. Arch Neurol 2001;58:191–195.

CHAPTER 18

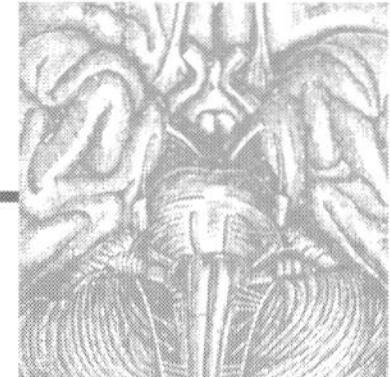

RICHARD CAMICIOLI and JOHN G. NUTT

Gait and Balance

History and Definitions

Walking is a product of three interrelated nervous system functions: locomotion, balance, and adaptation. Locomotion comprises the stereotyped patterns of muscle activation (synergies) of limbs and trunk that produce repetitive stepping. The nervous system must be able both to initiate and arrest stepping and to alter stepping patterns for turns, different speeds, and different support surfaces. Balance or equilibrium synergies include a number of postural responses that enable an individual to arise and remain erect during standing and locomotion. Standing is an active process (static postural response) in which the sway of the body is kept within the limits of the base of support provided by the feet. Anticipatory postural responses are changes in postural muscle groups that precede voluntary movements made to offset disturbances in balance that would result from the voluntary movement. For example, paraspinal and leg muscle activation precedes voluntary movements of the arm in a standing person to protect the person's upright stability. Anticipatory postural responses are feed-forward responses. They anticipate the perturbation of balance caused by the voluntary action. Reactive postural responses are feedback responses. They protect against unexpected external perturbations and are triggered by sensory cues indicating that the body is outside the limits of stability.

Adaptation refers to the adjustment of locomotor and balance synergies to the constraints produced by the environment, the body, and the ongoing voluntary activities. The gait pattern of normal individuals at any point in time depends on the person's perception of the environment, the condition of the body (clothes, shoes, disease), and the individual's personal goals. In addition to locomotor and balance synergies, a secure gait depends on the following: (1) information about the environment and the position of the body in the environment as relayed by proprioceptive, vestibular, and visual pathways; (2) ability to interpret and integrate the afferent information; (3) ability to produce force through the bones, joints, and muscles; (4) ability to modulate force for optimum performance; and (5) ability to select and adapt locomotor and balance synergies to the environmental requirements and the individual's capabilities.

Clinical History

Gait and balance difficulties generally present as complaints of slow or unsteady walking and of falls. Questions about the speed of walking, the length of the steps taken, the width between the feet, and any difficulties experienced with initiating walking provide clues to the gait disorder. Additionally, the ability to turn and a tendency to trip or bump into things or appear drunk are important clues.

The environment or conditions in which the person finds it difficult to walk also offer clues to the gait pattern and guide the physical examination. The clinician should specifically inquire about difficulties in turning over in bed, getting in or out of a car, and arising from a chair because these can be indicators of imbalance.

Falls require a detailed history because they are unlikely to be observed during the examination. Several recent falls that are clearly remembered by the patient or a family member should be explored in detail. Details of the exact location and activity of the patient when the fall occurred may indicate environmental or patient-related precipitants. Had the patient just arisen from a lying or sitting position, suggesting orthostatic hypotension? Or did the feet "get tangled" while turning around, suggesting incoordination? Did the patient trip, suggesting weakness of the dorsiflexors of the ankle, increased tone characteristic of spasticity, or the shuffling of parkinsonism? Was there lightheadedness, vertigo, or loss of consciousness, suggesting orthostatic hypotension, a labyrinthine disorder, or syncope? How exactly did the patient fall? Crumpling (breaking at the knees) suggests a loss of consciousness (syncope, seizure) or of strength (transient ischemic attack). Falling backward like a log is particularly common in patients with extrapyramidal disorders. Was falling related in any way to meals, suggesting postprandial hypotension, or to drug intake, suggesting drug-induced hypotension or impairment of attention and coordination?

In other aspects of the history, the physician should probe for evidence of proprioceptive, vestibular, and visual disturbances and for signs of pain or deformity of the bones and joints that could affect gait. The relationship of falls to the environment may give clues to neurologic impairment. For example, increased instability under poor lighting conditions or uneven surfaces may suggest impairment of sensory input or processing. Weakness sufficient to disturb balance and gait is generally recognized by the patient. Proximal weakness may be qualified by asking if the patient has difficulty reaching for items above their head level, rising from a chair, or going up stairs. Slowness and clumsiness in other motor activities and dysarthria may offer clues to cerebellar and extrapyramidal disorders. Urinary urgency and incontinence are common in multi-infarct states and normal pressure hydrocephalus. The history may suggest that the patient exhibits impaired judgment or attention span that might contribute to falls. If cognitive impairment is suspected an informant other than the patient should be interviewed for elaboration of the circumstances surrounding falls and to assess for the presence of cognitive or functional impairment.

The mode of onset of gait difficulties gives clues to the disease process producing them. Sudden onset suggests vascular disease; gradual onset suggests a degenerative disorder. The medication history is also very important because some drugs can affect the sensory-motor systems, thereby causing balance and gait disturbances. Examples of such drugs include the benzodiazepines, which affect the vestibular system; phenytoin, which affects the cerebellum; and neuroleptics, which involve the basal ganglia. Falls are associated with sedative-hypnotics, which may affect attention and judgment, and with drugs that produce orthostatic hypotension.

Anatomy of Gait and Balance (Table 18–1)

Normal gait and posture depend on the normal function of various structures along the entire neuroaxis. This includes the cortical, subcortical, and spinal cord regions as well as the final common pathway of motor neurons, the neuromuscular junctions and the muscles they innervate. The anatomy and neurological examination of the motor, sensory, cerebellar, and basal gangliar components of normal gait and posture are addressed in specific chapters. This chapter integrates the function of those regions with the important spinal, subcortical, and cortical structures involved in gait and posture.

SPINAL CORD

Locomotor synergies are present in the spinal cord. Spinally transected vertebrates, including humans, can

TABLE 18–1. **Clinico-anatomical Correlation of Disorders of Gait and Balance**

Anatomical Location	Gait Abnormalities	Associated Findings
Cerebral Cortex	Freezing Disequilibrium Falls	Dementia Grasp reflex Hyperreflexia Urinary urgency and incontinence
Brain Stem	Disequilibrium Astasia	Eye movement and pupillary abnormalities Hyperreflexia
Basal Ganglia	Freezing Hypokinetic gait Hyperkinetic gait Astasia	Rigidity, tremor Bradykinesia Chorea and dystonia
Cerebellum	Ataxia	Dysmetric limbs Dysmetric eye movements
Vestibular System	Ataxia	Nystagmus Difficulty with tandem walk
Spinal Cord	Spastic gait Sensory ataxia	Sensory level/loss Increased tone (may be posturally dependent) Increased DTRs Babinski's sign
Peripheral Nerve	Foot drop Sensory ataxia	Reduced or absent DTRs Peripheral weakness Peripheral sensory loss
Muscle/ Neuromuscular Junction	Waddle	Hip and shoulder girdle weakness

DTRs, Deep tendon reflexes.

produce coordinated stepping movements without any input from supraspinal neural structures. The spinal networks that produce patterned muscle activation, termed central pattern generators, are distributed throughout the spinal cord. The rhythmical muscle activation that is a part of coordinated stepping can be generated from even a few isolated segments of the hemitransected spinal cord. The central pattern generator has been deduced to consist of excitatory and inhibitory interneurons using glycine, glutamate, and acetylcholine as neurotransmitters. Interneurons and collaterals connect the ipsilateral and contralateral central pattern generators to produce reciprocal movements of the limbs. Propriospinal neurons connect different levels to produce coordination between the hind limbs and axial muscles and the arms or front legs. The pattern of central pattern generator activation can determine the speed of locomotion and the direction of locomotion (forward or backward). The output of the central pattern generator is the motoneuron. Coordinated, sequential activation of the limbs and axial muscles involved in stepping is produced by the rhythmical excitation and inhibition of the motoneurons of various muscles.

Input to central pattern generators includes local sensory input and descending input from the brain stem via the reticulospinal pathways. Locomotion in spinal animals or fictive locomotion (rhythmical firing of motor neurons innervating limbs in the isolated spinal cord in vitro) can be induced by brain stem stimulation, sensory input, treatment with monoamine precursors or agonists (e.g., L-dopa, clonidine) in vivo, and treatment with excitatory amino acids in vitro. Spinal locomotion can be modified by sensory input and level of electrical or chemical stimulation. For example, progression from a slow walk to a trot to a gallop can be induced by increasing the speed of the treadmill on which the animal stands or by increasing the amount of electrical excitation of brain stem locomotor regions. In the isolated spinal cord, central pattern generators are adaptable to a limited degree based on peripheral sensory input. The limb that encounters an obstacle is reflexively lifted higher to clear the obstacle. However, the locomotor pattern is stereotyped and does not anticipate environmental constraints on locomotion or the needs of the animal. Nor does the spinal cord have the balance synergies that are essential for successful locomotion. The important point is that the actual programming of the muscle activation required for gait is present at the spinal level. Higher centers initiate gait and adapt it to individual needs. For straightforward walking, the higher centers need not specify the individual muscle activations necessary to produce locomotion but instead activate the central pattern generators.[1, 2] This arrangement does not preclude supraspinal control of individual muscles during locomotion when precise foot placement is necessary.[3]

BRAIN STEM

The brain stem has three important functions in balance and locomotion: (1) setting the activity of the spinal central pattern generators to determine the initiation and speed of locomotion; (2) setting postural tone; and (3) modulating the force generated by the muscles activated by the central pattern generators.

Control of the spinal cord central pattern generators is exerted by the subthalamic and midbrain locomotor regions and relayed to the spinal cord by the reticulospinal tracts. The subthalamic locomotor region is defined physiologically as an area in the posterior lateral hypothalamus from which locomotion can be evoked by stimulation in the decerebrate animal (an animal whose brain stem has been transected just below the thalamus). The subthalamic locomotor region is not in the subthalamic nucleus but is medial and dorsal to it. This region is not associated with any particular cell group, and stimulation of it may excite axons passing through the area. A cat with an intact thalamus and basal ganglia but with the cortex removed walks continuously in a nondirected manner, termed obstinate progression. This behavior has been interpreted as disinhibition of the subthalamic locomotor region or of the influences that pass through the area. Stimulation of the subthalamic locomotor region in an intact cat induces locomotion and searching behavior.[4]

The midbrain locomotor region is also defined physiologically but appears to overlap at least partially the pedunculopontine nucleus. This fact is important because the pedunculopontine nucleus receives a major input from the basal ganglia and from the sensorimotor and limbic cortex.[5] This area may represent one way in which the cortex and basal ganglia affect the initiation of locomotion.[6] Progressive increases in electrical stimulation of the midbrain locomotor region of decerebrate monkeys induce stepping first in the contralateral limb, then in both limbs, and finally in a gallop. The midbrain locomotor region can also be stimulated by injections of gamma-aminobutyric acid (GABA) antagonists that are thought to disinhibit the midbrain locomotor region from tonic GABAergic input from the basal ganglia. Stimulation of the midbrain locomotor region in the neurologically intact cat induces locomotion that appears to be initiated to avoid a painful or frightening stimulus.[4, 6, 7]

Output of the locomotor regions descends by way of the medullary reticulospinal tract, which arises from the ventral medial reticularis gigantocellularis and magnocellularis nuclei. This tract traverses the ventral medial spinal cord, and lesions of the tract prevent locomotion and impair balance.[7, 8]

The role of the brain stem in postural control is evident by the postural responses that can be elicited in decerebrate animals. Vestibular, neck, and righting reflexes are present in decerebrate animals that have an intact brain stem.[9] Stimulation in the dorsal tegmental fields of the pons causes an intact cat to cease walking and reduces postural tone, so that the cat sits and then lies down. Conversely, more inferior stimulation in the ventral tegmental fields of the pons increases postural tone and induces locomotion, so that a supine cat rises and then begins to walk. These stimulation sites indicate that postural and locomotor responses may be mediated, at least partially, by the same brain stem structures.[4] In humans, lesions in the medial tegmental region of the rostral pons cause unstable walking with truncal ataxia, whereas lesions in the base (anterior portion) of the pons lead to limb ataxia and hemiparesis without truncal ataxia.[10]

Brain stem systems do not simply turn on the spinal central pattern generators, as is done experimentally by electrical stimulation of the locomotor regions. Recordings from brain stem reticulospinal neurons that activate the spinal central pattern generators as well as from vestibulospinal and rubrospinal neurons demonstrate that activity in these pathways is phase-locked to the step cycle. This phasic activity is largely abolished if the cerebellum is ablated. The phasic activity in these descending tracts does not determine the frequency of stepping but enhances its force and rhythmicity.[3, 11] The tectospinal tract influences the posture of the head and neck and its orientation to visual targets. This tract arises from the superior colliculus, a structure that receives a major input from the substantia nigra pars reticulata, hence providing another connection between the basal ganglia and the postural and locomotor systems.

CEREBELLUM

The cerebellum is not considered to be the origin of postural or locomotor responses because total ablation of the cerebellum does not abolish these responses. The cerebellum, however, refines the force and timing of locomotor and postural responses. Thus, the execution of these responses in an animal with cerebellar ablation is uncoordinated and dysmetric.[12] The cerebellum receives information about each step cycle through the spinocerebellar pathways (see Chapter 17). Many Purkinje cells fire in synchrony with various parts of the step cycle. The cerebellum partially exerts its influence on locomotion by affecting the activity of the reticulospinal, vestibulospinal, and rubrospinal pathways, which are phasically active during stepping and contribute to coordinated rhythmic stepping. Rhythmical firing in these descending bulbospinal pathways is largely abolished by cerebellar ablation.[3] The cerebellar projections to the thalamus and thence to the frontal cortex may also affect gait and balance, although this possibility has not been explored. Stimulation of the Hook bundle in the cerebellum in decerebrate cats has been shown to induce locomotion, suggesting that a cerebellar locomotor region exists.[13]

BASAL GANGLIA

The basal ganglia may have direct input to the brain stem nuclei controlling posture and balance via the pedunculopontine nucleus (midbrain locomotor region) and the superior colliculus (tectospinal tract).[6] The majority of the basal ganglia output is directed back to the frontal cortex, and this influence is presumably responsible for the hallmarks of disease of the basal ganglia, hypokinesia and hyperkinesia (see Chapter 16). The execution of locomotor and postural responses, like other movements, may also be hypokinetic (parkinsonian) or hyperkinetic (choreic, dystonic).

CORTEX

The cortex is completely unnecessary for routine walking in the cat, as evidenced by the performance of decorticate cats (animals in which the cortex has been removed but the basal ganglia and thalamus are left intact). However, the cat with frontal cortex or medullary pyramid lesions cannot perform stepping that requires precise placement of the feet, for example, walking on the rungs of a horizontal ladder. This indicates that "skilled walking" requires input from the motor cortex. The motor cortex has neurons that fire in phase with stepping and, therefore, like the reticulospinal, vestibulospinal, and rubrospinal systems, probably facilitates precise stepping. Stimulation of the medullary pyramid can reset the step cycle. This indicates that the corticospinal tract can affect the central pattern generators and may have a role in initiating and modifying the locomotor pattern produced by the central pattern generators.[3] The sensorimotor cortex also has connections to the midbrain locomotor region and may affect the central pattern generators through this link. Stimulation of the motor cortex can induce discrete movements of a limb, preceded by the appropriate anticipatory postural responses, indicating that the cortex has a role in anticipatory postural responses. Lesions of the frontal cortex may also affect anticipatory reflexes.[14]

Other anatomical areas are undoubtedly important in balance and locomotion. The areas reviewed here are responsible for the proper mechanical execution of balance and locomotion in a relatively stereotyped fashion. They do not explain the adaptation of gait to the individual's goals, the perception of the environmental dangers to balance and upright position, and the development of appropriate strategies to cope with environmental hazards. It is important to realize that the posture and gait observed in an individual are a product of the more or less hard-wired locomotor and postural responses modified by the individual at conscious and subconscious levels to adapt these responses to his or her needs. Posture and gait patterns are not fixed and stereotyped neurological signs as are deep tendon reflexes.

Examination of Gait and Posture

DIRECTED NEUROLOGICAL EXAMINATION

In examining a patient with complaints regarding gait and balance, sitting balance is first evaluated. If an inability to sit upright is found, profound imbalance or weakness is suggested. The examiner should check to see whether titubation (rhythmical tremor or shaking of the trunk and head) is present, suggesting cerebellar disease, or whether there is a tendency to lean progressively in one direction, suggesting hemiparesis or basal ganglia disease. To make sitting balance more challenging and to bring out subtle abnormalities, the clinician should ask the subject to sit on the examining table with the arms and legs not touching any support surface.

Next, the ability to arise from a chair should be tested. This maneuver tests the patient's strength and anticipatory postural responses. The physician should check to see whether the patient can arise and if he or she can organize rising appropriately (brings the feet under the body, leans forward, and uses the arms to push). If the patient is unable to rise without pushing himself off the chair, proximal muscle weakness or impaired central recruitment of force is suggested, as in Parkinson's disease or pyramidal tract lesions (e.g., myelopathy).

Standing unaided, which tests static balance, should then be evaluated. The examiner should determine whether the patient can stand without assistance or whether titubation or excessive sway is present, indicating cerebellar disease. The distance between the feet should be noted, because feet placed wide apart suggest problems with lateral stability (seen in patients with cerebellar disease, multi-infarct state, or proprioceptive loss). Furthermore, the presence of any discrepancy between standing with the eyes open and with the eyes closed (Romberg's sign) should be determined because this finding may indicate defective proprioception. Balancing on one foot is a more stringent test of static balance. Healthy individuals, younger than age 80 years, should generally be able to manage this task for 10 seconds with their eyes open or closed. Individuals older than 80 years of age may not be able to stand on one foot for 10 seconds with their eyes closed, reflecting impaired proprioception or central processing of sensory input.[15]

Finally, the gait should be examined. Gait initiation reveals the integrity of locomotor synergies. Abnormalities that should be sought include delays of seconds (freezing) and delays with a series of small steps (start hesitation) on the initiation of gait. These are common signs of frontal lobe, subcortical white matter, and basal ganglia lesions. Once gait has started, the examiner should check to see whether the maintenance of stepping is disturbed by passage through narrow spaces, distractions, or turns. Reduction of gait speed and stride length are nonspecific indicators of gait and balance disturbances. Speed slows and steps shorten in most disorders of gait and balance in which patients perceive postural insecurity.[16] Healthy people adapt the same gait pattern on slippery surfaces. Occasionally, gait is not slowed in proportion to postural instability, for example, in those with progressive supranuclear palsy, indicating difficulties with perception, attention, or judgment. The distance between the feet while walking (gait base) is an indicator of lateral stability. Typically, the base narrows as a patient changes from standing to walking. As with the standing base, a widened base during walking generally indicates sensory, cerebellar, or frontal lobe dysfunction. Head movements during walking may offer a clue to vestibular function. Patients with diminished or absent vestibular function often try to minimize head movements while walking, giving them a stiff appearance. Asking the patient with a vestibular disorder to rotate the head while walking causes the gait to become ataxic.

The cadence of gait is important because it is an indicator of motor coordination. Steps should be regular and symmetrical. In certain disorders, they may be dysmetric, choreic, dystonic, parkinsonian, hemiparetic, or spastic, thereby disturbing the normal free movements of stepping and altering gait cadence. Both cerebellar ataxia and subcortical white matter disease lead to increased variability in step length and timing.[17] Observation of arm swing can identify a variety of motor function problems. Involuntary movements often appear in the arms during walking, particularly dystonia, chorea, and rest tremor. Unilaterally decreased arm swing is common in early parkinsonism and mild hemiparesis. Decreased arm swing does not always have a neurological explanation because musculoskeletal disorders can induce changes as well.

Turning or pivoting while walking is more posturally demanding than walking straight ahead, and abnormalities may emerge during turning that are inapparent during straight walking. Widening of the base only during turns or taking an extra one or two short steps during turning to maintain balance may be the earliest sign of cerebellar ataxia. "En bloc" turns (in which the head, torso, and legs turn together as a rigid unit rather than in sequence beginning with rotation of the head and followed in turn by the shoulders and then the hips and legs) suggest parkinsonism or caution. With more severe imbalance, en bloc turns are associated with slow, small steps, and the patient may freeze during turning in the so-called turn hesitation that is very typical of patients with parkinsonism and frontal lobe gaits. Gait velocity and step length may be improved in patients with Parkinson's disease when "OFF" (after withdrawal of medications) by having them walk with the assistance of visual cues, such as horizontal stripes placed on the ground, suggesting that external cueing may activate alternative cortical pathways to initiate and maintain locomotion. This improvement is not evident in normal pressure hydrocephalus.[18]

Tandem walking tests lateral stability and should be observed because it is a sensitive indicator of cerebellar and vestibular dysfunction. Finally, the process of pushing the patient to the side and pulling him backward (with the examiner maintaining a position to keep the patient from falling) tests reactive postural responses. These responses may be deficient in patients with basal ganglia disease or frontal or subcortical lesions.

ASSOCIATED NEUROLOGICAL FINDINGS

Cerebral. In the mental status examination, the physician may detect abnormalities of cognition and attention that may cause falls owing to a lack of insight, inability to interpret and adapt to the environment, or inattention to environmental dangers. Dementia is common in patients with multi-infarct state and normal pressure hydrocephalus, which may be associated with gait disturbances.

Cranial Nerves. The cranial nerve examination may reveal signs of sensory or motor dysfunction that could affect gait. Decreased visual acuity, visual field deficits, or visual neglect may cause a patient to adopt a cautious gait pattern and may contribute to falls. Likewise, extraocular muscle dysfunction causing diplopia and gaze palsies may distort and reduce visual information, thereby causing falls. Selective paresis of voluntary downgaze is a common sign in patients with progressive supranuclear palsy, a disorder that often presents with unexplained falls. Nystagmus is a marker of vestibular, cerebellar, and brain stem pathology that may disturb balance synergies. Dysarthria is a sensitive indicator of cerebellar, basal ganglia, and corticobulbar dysfunction.

Motor/Reflexes/Cerebellar/Gait. In the motor examination, the clinician should search for weakness, particularly in the legs and hips, that may affect walking. Changes in tone may indicate corticospinal tract involvement (spasticity), parkinsonism (rigidity), and diffuse cortical dysfunction with dementia (gegenhalten or paranoia. Involuntary movements may suggest basal ganglia disease (chorea, dystonia, and rest tremor) or other cortical disease (myoclonus).

COORDINATION. Coordination is often abnormal in patients with gait and balance problems. Finger-to-nose and heel-to-shin testing examines cerebellar function. Rapid alternating movements may be rapid but sloppy or dysmetric, indicating cerebellar dysfunction. It is important to recognize that gait ataxia need not be associated with limb ataxia. This dissociation may be seen in midline cerebella diseases or brain stem lesions. Rapid alternating movements may also be slow and hypometric, indicating parkinsonism, or slow and clumsy, indicating corticospinal tract disturbances. Finally, disorganized alternating movements may suggest apraxia and along with motor perseveration may indicate parietal, subcortical, or frontal dysfunction. Abnormalities of repetitive finger tapping and handwriting are common in disorders that affect the cerebellum, basal ganglia, and cortical sensorimotor areas.

REFLEXES. Deep tendon reflexes are important in differentiating various causes of weakness and altered tone that might influence posture and gait. Hyperreflexia is common in patients with corticospinal tract disorders; hyporeflexia is common in those with peripheral nerve diseases that produce weakness and proprioceptive sensory loss. The presence of Babinski's sign indicates corticospinal tract dysfunction.

Sensory. Sensory testing that emphasizes proprioception in the toes, ankles, and knees is particularly important for balance and walking, but may be insensitive to peripheral nerve dysfunction. Evidence of abnormal pin-prick, light touch, or vibration sense are more sensitive indicators of peripheral neuropathy and may offer clues to sensory dysfunction that might contribute to impaired balance.

Autonomic Nervous System. Orthostatic hypotension may cause falls. It is important to recognize that the presence of orthostatic hypotension may vary during the day; it is most prominent after meals and after taking some medications. Therefore, the absence of orthostatic changes in blood pressure in the clinic does not exclude orthostatic hypotension as a cause of falls.

Neurovascular. Auscultation and palpation of the carotid and other superficial cranial vessels may suggest a vascular cause of gait dysfunction. Poor distal pulses are associated with atherosclerotic vascular disease and embolic disease. Retinal vessels also offer clues to the presence of systemic vascular disease.

ASSOCIATED MEDICAL FINDINGS

If falls cannot be explained by neurological abnormalities, cardiac syncope must be considered, and the cardiac examination may be informative. The spine, joints, and limbs should be inspected for abnormalities or pain that might affect walking.

Evaluation Guidelines (Table 18–2)

Laboratory evaluation of patients with gait and balance abnormalities is largely determined by the findings derived from the history and physical examination that point to dysfunction in specific neural structures, and these tests are covered in other chapters. For example, a gait disturbance associated with proprioceptive sensory loss should trigger a workup for peripheral neuropathy or spinal cord (posterior column) disease depending on the accompanying signs. General guidelines pertaining specifically to gait and balance disturbances are indicated here.

Neuroimaging. Magnetic resonance imaging (MRI) of the head is indicated for patients in whom the cause of a gait disturbance is not apparent from the history and neurological examination or in whom start hesitation or disequilibrium is evident. Hydrocephalus, frontal lesions, subcortical gray and white matter lesions, and brain stem lesions may be found that were not suspected from the history or physical examination. Computed tomography of the head reveals less information about white matter and subcortical structures but excludes hydrocephalus, frontal lesions, and large subcortical abnormalities. It does not exclude lesions or malformations of the foramen magnum, which are best assessed by MRI. Incident high signal changes on MRI are associated with the development of gait impairment in the elderly.[19] The presence of spasticity and posterior column signs will direct imaging toward the spine, particularly the cervical region, if no explanation is apparent from brain imaging.

Electrophysiology. Nerve conduction velocities and electromyography are useful in differentiating muscle, nerve, and motoneuron causes of weakness. Brain stem and visual evoked responses may help in assessing pathology in the brain stem and visual pathways. Electroencephalography may help in detecting encephalopathy as a cause of inattention and falls and, combined with a Holter monitor, may be useful in patients with unexplained crumpling falls (collapsing) to exclude seizures or cardiogenic syncope.

Body Fluid and Tissue Analysis. Pernicious anemia sometimes causes gait disorders that are out of proportion to the peripheral neuropathy or myelopathy that is present. Testing for vitamin B_{12} is indicated for patients with no obvious cause of their gait and balance difficulties; borderline cases might reveal an elevated methylmalonic acid or homocysteine level. Analysis for autoantibodies may be indicated in patients with neuropathy. A urine drug screening test may reveal drug use that explains ataxia or inattention and falls. Although some hereditary spinocerebellar ataxias can be diagnosed by genetic testing, it is important to bear in mind that many cases that are familial have negative genetic testing, and some gene-positive cases have a negative family history.

Cerebrospinal Fluid. Large-volume lumbar spinal taps (30 to 50 ml of cerebrospinal fluid removed) sometimes cause a transient improvement in gait, cognitive functioning, and urinary continence in patients with normal pressure hydrocephalus.[20] The sensitivity and accuracy of this test are not known.

Other Tests. Electronystagmography and rotational tests are used to examine peripheral labyrinthine and central vestibular function. Posturography is used to examine a standing patient's ability to maintain balance as proprioceptive and visual sensory information is reduced or distorted. Posturography can also be used to differentiate the contributions of the visual, vestibular, and proprioceptive systems to a patient's balance. Gait analysis, which measures gait speed, cadence, foot clearance, single support time (when one foot is in the swing phase of stepping), and double support time (when both feet are in contact with the ground), and the trajectories of limbs, is rarely indicated for the diagnosis of gait disturbances. It generally quantifies the observations of an astute clinician. For intermittent gait abnormalities, videotapes made by the family of the patient during times of difficulty may be very informative. Pulse and blood pressure recordings obtained at home in relation to falls may also yield helpful clues. Finally, a visit by an experienced physical therapist or occupational therapist to the home of a patient with unexplained falls may reveal environmental causes of falls.

Clinical Syndromes (Table 18–3)

Because gait and balance disturbances are common manifestations of functional disturbances of many parts of the

TABLE 18–2. **Useful Studies in the Evaluation of Disorders of Gait and Balance**

Syndrome	Neuroimaging	Electrophysiology	Fluid and Tissue Analysis	Neuropsychological Tests	Other Tests
Synergies					
Freezing	CT or MRI: Frontal or subcortical white matter lesions; multiple lacunes; hydrocephalus	N/A	N/A	Cognitive impairment	N/A
Frontal disequilibrium	CT or MRI: Frontal or subcortical white matter lesions; multiple lacunes; hydrocephalus	N/A	Large volume CSF tap	Cognitive impairment	N/A
Frontal gait	CT or MRI: Frontal or subcortical white matter lesions; multiple lacunes; hydrocephalus	N/A	N/A	Cognitive impairment	N/A
Sensory Abnormalities					
Proprioceptive	MRI: Spinal cord posterior column lesion	Slowed NCV Decreased sensory action potential	VDRL, FTA-ABS, HIV, vitamin B_{12}, methylmalonic acid, homocysteine, SSEP, UPEP, ENA (e.g., anti-Ro, La) CSF: protein, glucose, IgG index, oligoclonal bands		
Vestibular	MRI: Brain stem or labyrinth and cranial nerve VIII lesions	Abnormal ENG BAER	Glucose, thyroid studies, FTA-ABS, CBC, vasculitic work-up		Vascular studies
Visual	CT or MRI: Visual pathways or orbital lesions	VER	Glucose, thyroid studies		Slit-lamp examination Perimetry tensilon test
Perception/orientation					
Thalamic/putaminal and midbrain astasia	MRI: Lesions in thalamus, putamen, midbrain	N/A	N/A	N/A	N/A
Progressive supranuclear palsy	MRI: Atrophy of midbrain	N/A	N/A	Cognitive impairment	N/A
Force					
Bones, joints, ligaments	N/A	N/A	RA factor, ESR, ANA	N/A	N/A
Waddling	N/A	EMG: Myopathic changes	CK, ESR, thyroid studies, muscle biopsy	N/A	N/A
Foot drop	MRI: Stenosis of lumbosacral canal and foramina	NCV: Slowed conduction EMG: Denervation	Glucose, nerve biopsy	N/A	N/A

Table continued on following page

TABLE 18–2 **Useful Studies in the Evaluation of Disorders of Gait and Balance** *Continued*

Syndrome	Neuroimaging	Electrophysiology	Fluid and Tissue Analysis	Neuropsychological Tests	Other Tests
Force Scaling					
Hemiplegic or paraplegic gait	CT or MRI: Brain or spinal cord lesions	SSEP	Vitamin B_{12}, methylmalonic acid, homocysteine, ACE CSF: IgG, WBC	N/A	N/A
Cerebellar ataxia	MRI: Brain stem and cerebellar lesions	N/A	Thyroid studies Toxicology screen CSF: IgG, cells, Anti-Purkinje cell Ab, vitamin E, genetic tests for SCA, acanthocytes, anti-gliadin antibody, transglutaminase antibody	N/A	N/A
Parkinsonian gait	CT or MRI: Hypointense putamen in MSA	N/A		N/A	N/A
Choreic gait	MRI: Putaminal lesions; atrophy of striatum	N/A	Copper, ceruloplasmin HD gene test Acanthocytes Anticardiolipin Ab, ASO	Cognitive impairment	N/A
Dystonic gait	CT or MRI: Putaminal or thalamic lesions	N/A	Copper, ceruloplasmin, liver biopsy	N/A	Slit-lamp examination
Adaptation					
Cautious	N/A	N/A	N/A	N/A	N/A
Dementia	CT or MRI: Cortical atrophy; other cortical lesions	N/A	Thyroid studies, CBC, electrolytes, Vitamin B_{12}, glucose	Memory, distractibility, cognitive impairment	N/A
Attention and balance	CT or MRI: Cortical atrophy	EEG: Slowing	Metabolic screen, drug screen	Inattention	N/A
Post-fall	N/A	N/A	N/A	Anxiety	N/A
Psychogenic	N/A	N/A	N/A	Hysterical traits, suggestibility, depression	N/A

CT, Computed tomography; MRI, magnetic resonance imaging; EMG, electromyography; ESR, erythrocyte sedimentation rate; NCV, nerve conduction velocity; VER, visual evoked responses; VDRL, venereal disease research laboratories; CSF, cerebrospinal fluid; HIV, human immunodeficiency virus; CK, creatine kinase; ANA, antinuclear antibody; WBC, white blood cells; SSEP, somatosensory evoked potentials; HD, Huntington's disease; EEG, electroencephalography; BAER, brain stem auditory evoked response; Ab, antibody; MSA, multiple system atrophy; ENG, electronystagmography; N/A, not applicable; ENA, extractable nuclear antigen; ASO, antistreptolysin-O antibody; CBC, complete blood count; ACE, angiotensin converting enzyme.

TABLE 18–3. **Selected Etiologies Associated with Disorders of Gait and Balance**

Etiological Category	Selected Etiologies	Chapter
Structural Disorders		
Developmental structural disorders	Chiari malformation with hydrocephalus	
	Normal pressure hydrocephalus	28
Degenerative and compressive structural disorders	Degenerative disc disease	29
Hereditary and Degenerative Disorders		
Storage diseases: Lipidoses, glycogen disorders, and leukoencephalopathies	Adrenoleukodystrophy	
	Metachromatic leukodystrophy	
	Krabbe's disease	
	Pelizaeus-Merzbacher disease	30
Amino/organic acidopathies, mitochondrial enzyme defects, and other metabolic errors	GTP cyclohydrolase mutations (dopa-responsive dystonia)	31
Chromosomal abnormalities and neurocutaneous disorders	Neurofibromatosis type II	
	Ataxia-telangiectasia	32
Degenerative dementias	Alzheimer's disease	
	Frontotemporal dementia	33
Movement disorders	Huntington's disease	
	Parkinson's disease	
	Progressive supranuclear palsy	
	Multiple system atrophy	
	Corticobasal degeneration	34
Ataxias	Autosomal dominant spinocerebellar ataxias	
	Friedrich's ataxia (Ar)	
	Refsum's disease (Ar)	
	Episodic ataxias	35
	Vitamin E deficiency	
Degenerative motor, sensory, and autonomic disorders	Amyotrophic lateral sclerosis	
	Duchenne muscular dystrophy	
	Hereditary sensory motor neuropathies	
	Hereditary spastic paraparesis	36
Hereditary nondegenerative neuromuscular disease	Congenital myopathies	37
Myelopathies		
Acquired Metabolic and Nutritional Disorders		
Endogenous metabolic disorders	Thyroid myopathy	
	Diabetic neuropathy	38
Exogenous acquired metabolic disorders of the nervous system: toxins and illicit drugs	Lathyrism	39
Nutritional deficiencies and syndromes associated with alcoholism	Thiamine deficiency	
	Vitamin B_{12} deficiency	40
Infectious Disorders		
Viral infections	HTLV-I infection, labyrinthitis	41
Nonviral infections	Syphilis	
	Lyme disease	
	Chronic meningitis	42
Transmissible spongiform encephalopathy	Creutzfeldt-Jakob disease	43
HIV and AIDS	Vacuolar myelopathy	44
Neurovascular disorders		
	Binswanger's disease, infarction, hemorrhage, vascular malformation (brain, spinal)	45
Neoplastic Disorders		
Primary neurological tumors	Butterfly glioma, midsaggital mengioma	46
Metastatic neoplasms and paraneoplastic syndromes	Any metastasis to brain, brain stem, spinal cord	
	Paraneoplastic cerebellar degeneration	47
Demyelinating Disorders		
Demyelinating disorders of the central nervous system	Multiple sclerosis	48
Demyelinating disorders of the peripheral nervous system	Guillian-Barré syndrome	
	Chronic inflammatory demyelinating polyneuropathy	49

Table continued on following page

TABLE 18–3 **Selected Etiologies Associated with Disorders of Gait and Balance** *Continued*

Etiological Category	Selected Etiologies	Chapter
Autoimmune and Inflammatory Disorders	Myasthenia gravis, systemic lupus erythematosis, sarcoidosis, vasculitis, Sjörgen's syndrome, antiphospholipid antibody syndrome	50
Traumatic Disorders	Dementia pugilistica	51
Drug-Induced and Iatrogenic Neurological Disorders	Neuroleptics, sedative-hypnotics, anticonvulsant toxicity	55

HIV, Human immunodeficiency virus; AIDS, acquired immunodeficiency virus; GTP, guanosine triphosphate; HTLV-I, human t-cell lymphotrophic virus type 1.

nervous system, alterations in gait are important physical signs in diagnosing dysfunction of these structures. Diseases affecting the proprioceptive, vestibular, or visual sensory systems commonly produce an unsteady or ataxic gait. Weakness produced by muscle and motor nerve diseases alters locomotion in characteristic patterns. Upper motor neuron disorders cause weakness and spasticity, which typically become evident during locomotion. Basal ganglia disorders produce distinctive hypokinetic and hyperkinetic gaits. Cerebellar dysfunction causes ataxia. However, many gait and balance disorders seen in the clinic are not readily explained by disturbances of a single neural structure.

As described earlier in the section on anatomy, some of the basic circuitry governing locomotion and balance is known. However, many clinical abnormalities of gait and posture are not due to disturbances of this basic circuitry but to the individual's adaptation (or failure of adaptation) of normal or slightly abnormal balance and gait synergies to day-to-day living. The neuroanatomical basis of this higher level of control and adaptation of balance and gait is less well understood. For this reason, gait and balance syndromes are arranged by systems rather than anatomically; they include disorders of (1) locomotor and balance synergies, (2) primary sensory function, (3) perception/orientation, (4) force production, (5) force scaling, and (6) adaptation/cognition/attention.

DYSSYNERGY/SYNERGY SYNDROMES

Although *locomotor synergies*, the basic patterns of muscle contraction and relaxation that produce coordinated rhythmic stepping, exist in the spinal cord, dyssynergies resulting from discrete spinal lesions are not commonly recognized clinically. This is partly because spinal lesions that would disrupt the central pattern generators would probably affect the motor neurons, producing weakness or paralysis, and would also disrupt the ascending and descending tracts, producing other neurological dysfunctions. However, release of locomotor synergies can be seen in patients with damage to the central nervous system. Automatic or spinal stepping can be elicited in humans with clinically complete cervical or thoracic cord transection by having the patients partially supported on a moving treadmill.[21] Automatic stepping, probably due to stimulation of the brain stem locomotor regions, also occasionally occurs in patients with brain stem lesions and with coma, such as occurs with central herniation.[22]

Freezing gait, or difficulty in initiating and maintaining locomotion, may represent an interruption of automatic access to the brain stem locomotor regions or spinal central pattern generators. The feet of a patient with freezing seem to stick to the floor, and the patient may be at a loss as to how to start walking. This gait pattern has been given the graphic term gait ignition failure. Its milder form is termed start hesitation because a hesitation of several seconds ensues before the patient can begin to walk. When gait is finally initiated, it may begin with small steps that increase in length, sometimes to normal length, a phenomenon termed slipping clutch gait. Turns are accomplished with slow, small steps and sometimes freezing, termed turn hesitation. Any distraction that interrupts the patient's concentration on walking, such as being asked a question or passing through a narrow opening, may precipitate freezing. Freezing may be overcome by tricks that convert walking from an automatic act of moving from one place to another to a cortically directed process of voluntary movements of the legs and feet. Thus, patients may initiate gait by focusing on stepping on a particular spot on the floor, pretending to kick something, or stepping over an object. A plausible but unproved interpretation of these clinical observations is that locomotion in patients with freezing is achieved by cortically directing the individual movements of the limbs until stepping is initiated; then the more automatic stepping generated from the brain stem locomotor regions and spinal central pattern generators can function, but always under the constant surveillance of the cortex. Distraction in these patients brings locomotion to a halt by interfering with the necessary cortical supervision of walking.

Freezing is most commonly seen in patients with Parkinson's disease as the disease advances (see Chapters 16 and 34).[23] However, frontal cortex and deep white matter lesions sometimes produce freezing with little or no imbalance and with no other parkinsonian signs. Further localization to specific frontal regions or to specific cortical bulbar tracts has not been possible, to date. Patients with these frontal and subcortical lesions may have marked freezing, but once under way they have an almost normal or completely normal stride. Arm swing is frequently preserved, which helps to differentiate isolated gait ignition failure from the freezing characteristic of parkinsonism. The base may be normal, as in parkinsonism, but often is widened, which is atypical of parkinsonism. There may be an exaggerated side-to-side sway of the trunk in an attempt to raise the feet off the floor, another feature not found in parkinsonism. Nevertheless, this freezing gait resembles the more common parkinsonian freezing gait pattern so closely that it is often referred to as lower half parkinsonism.[24, 25]

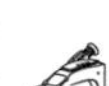

Balance or *equilibrium synergies* organized in the brain stem are highly stereotyped and are not context sensitive. In day-to-day living, balance synergies are adapted to the environment, body position in space, previous experience, and expectation by the higher centers. Decerebrate and decorticate posturing and tonic neck reflexes are reflex brain stem postural synergies that are released by extensive cortical and subcortical lesions (see Chapters 1 and 15). Abnormal posturing (fencer's position) may also be produced by mesial frontal lobe stimulation or epileptic discharges.

Frontal disequilibrium may be seen in patients with lesions of the frontal lobes or deep white matter. This gait abnormality is associated with an imbalance that may represent loss of access to balance synergies, inappropriate selection of synergies, or release of inappropriate brain stem synergies. Hydrocephalus, frontal infarcts, multiple lacunar infarcts in deep white matter, and frontal masses can produce frontal disequilibrium, a profound disturbance of balance that may preclude standing.[24, 26, 27] Patients with frontal disequilibrium have difficulty in rising to stand. This is due to patients not bringing their feet under themselves as they try to rise. In addition, they may not even place both feet on the ground. Helped to an erect position, they cannot stand independently because they do not bring their weight over their feet. Many hyperextend the trunk and push backward in seeming disregard for their support base. Stepping may be bizarre with crossing of the legs and no coordination between the trunk and the legs. This clinical phenomenon was first described by Bruns in 1892 and is sometimes termed Bruns' ataxia or frontal ataxia. It is important to recognize that this form of ataxia is different from that produced by cerebellar lesions, which result in problems with scaling and timing of steps. Frontal disequilibrium is also sometimes termed apraxia of gait; however, this term seems inappropriate because gait is limited by balance, not by locomotor difficulties.[28]

Frontal gait is a combination of imbalance (that does not preclude locomotion), small steps, and freezing. It is more common than the two extremes described previously, frontal disequilibrium and isolated gait ignition failure. Frequently, but not always, the base is widened.[28] The frontal gait pattern has also been referred to as marche à petits pas. Frontal disequilibrium and frontal gait disorders are often accompanied by other frontal lobe signs such as grasp reflexes, dementia, pseudobulbar palsy, and urinary urgency and incontinence.

SENSORY GAIT SYNDROMES

The adaptation of spinal and brain stem synergies to an individual's goals and limitations (i.e., context) requires a knowledge of the relations of the body segments to each other, the situation of the body in space and the gravitational field, and the presence of environmental hazards and aids to balance and locomotion. This information is largely derived from the somatosensory, vestibular, and visual senses. Generally, one sensory system is adequate to orient a person and permit normal balance and gait. Balance and gait difficulties arise if environmental information is inadequate because of reduced sensory input or if a mismatch between the sensory information provided by the three sensory systems occurs because the environmental clues are ambiguous or the information is distorted by diseased sensory systems.

Sensory ataxia arises from a proprioceptive sensory loss in the lower extremities and may be produced by diseases affecting large myelinated peripheral nerves, dorsal roots, or posterior columns. The gait disorder is often first recognized when the patient is suddenly deprived of vision, such as occurs when walking into a dark room or closing the eyes to wash the face. At this mild stage, the only abnormalities detectable on examination may be a slight unsteadiness when the person stands with the feet together and the eyes closed (Romberg's sign), walks with the eyes closed, walks backward, or makes sudden turns. Patients may adapt to mild sensory abnormalities by walking more slowly or taking smaller steps. With more severe sensory loss, the patient shows increased sway when standing and walks with a widened base and irregular steps. The feet may be raised too high, thrown too far forward, and brought down too quickly. At this stage, the gait resembles that of a person with cerebellar ataxia. The patient's eyes are focused on the feet and the ground immediately in front of them. Diverting the eyes away from the feet may cause the patient to fall. Reactive or protective postural responses as induced by the pull test may be delayed because proprioceptive input to signal movement of the center of mass relative to the base of support is absent. A cane may aid in walking, perhaps through proprioceptive cues appreciated in the hands. With severe proprioceptive sensory loss, the patient may not be able to stand unaided, even though strength is retained. Neurological examination reveals a profound loss of position sense at the toes and ankles and generally also at the knees and hips in patients with ataxia on the basis of proprioceptive sensory loss. Other aspects of the neurological examination help in differentiating the peripheral nerve and spinal cord posterior column origin of the sensory loss.

Vestibular ataxia is seen in patients with vestibular dysfunction; its severity depends on the speed with which dysfunction develops, the extent of the lesion, and the degree of compensation. The person with longstanding complete loss of vestibular function, for example from aminoglycoside antibiotics, may appear completely normal under most circumstances. The effects of the vestibular deficit may emerge only when the person is in an environment in which vision and proprioceptive clues are reduced or deceptive. Subtle signs in these patients include an en bloc appearance, which restricts the movement of the head during walking. Ataxia may be elicited in these patients by asking them to rotate the head from side to side while walking. The ability to balance on one foot or to walk in tandem with the eyes open or closed may also be impaired.[29]

Vestibular function that is present but distorted causes more difficulty with balance and gait. Patients are very dependent on visual information, but their deficient vestibulo-ocular reflexes make it difficult for them to differentiate between self and environmental movement. For example, such patients find it difficult to walk on a busy city sidewalk because of the surrounding movement of pedestrians and vehicular traffic. These patients generally describe unsteadiness, but not vertigo. The gait may be characterized by staggering and veering in response to erroneous perceived self-motion. Acute vestibular lesions are generally associated with vertigo and produce prominent difficulties with gait and balance. The sudden onset of vertigo may be associated with an inability to walk or even to stand.

Historical features suggestive of vestibular disorders include the following: (1) spontaneous vertigo; (2) vertigo induced by movement, Valsalva maneuvers, noise, exercise, and heat; (3) visual blurring induced by head and body movements; and (4) disequilibrium induced by body movements and movements in the surrounding environment. Findings on examination that suggest vestibular dysfunction include spontaneous or positional nystagmus, en bloc gait (particularly minimizing head movement), ataxia with head movement, and difficulty in balancing on one foot or on a compliant surface that reduces sensory input (e.g., thick foam) with the eyes closed.[30]

Visual ataxia is unsteadiness caused by visual deficits. Under normal circumstances, humans are very dependent on vision for balance; foveal vision appears to be most important, but peripheral vision also contributes to balance. Disturbances in visual acuity or visual fields increase body sway and predispose the person to falls. People adjusting to new bifocals may feel unsteady or even fall. Vision may also be affected by abnormalities of eye movements. Limitation of eye movements, particularly downward movement, or an imbalance between the extraocular muscles, producing diplopia, can cause balance difficulties and falls.[31]

Multisensory disequilibrium occurs with deficits in multiple sensory systems. No single deficit is sufficient to cause a problem, but the sum causes difficulties in orientation in space.[32]

HIGHER SENSORY PROCESSING SYNDROMES

Patients may have normal sensory input from the proprioceptive, vestibular, and visual systems but be unable to integrate and interpret the information because of abnormalities in higher sensory processing.[33] Failure of sensory integration may be related to distortion of the spatial maps known to exist in the parietal cortex, putamen, ventral premotor cortex, superior colliculus, and frontal eye fields.[34] Faulty interpretation of the position of the body segments to each other and the position of the body in space may elicit inappropriate balance and gait synergies.

Thalamic, *midbrain*, and *putaminal astasia* may represent abnormalities of orientation. Posterolateral thalamic lesions impair an individual's ability to judge verticality and may be associated with postural instability. Infarcts and hemorrhages in the midbrain tegmentum, dorsal thalamic nuclei, and putamen produce striking problems with balance. Patients with these lesions have adequate strength, primary sensation, and coordination but cannot stand without drifting and falling to the side or backward unless corrective efforts are made. In patients with lesions of the thalamus, this clinical picture has been referred to as thalamic astasia,[35] and similar clinical presentations have been described in patients with midbrain[36] and putaminal[37] vascular lesions. Abnormalities of eye movements (vertical gaze palsies, skewed eye position, and counter-rotation) may offer clinical clues to mischief in these subcortical regions, but more often brain imaging establishes the diagnosis.

Progressive supranuclear palsy (PSP) may be another example of disorientation caused by degeneration in the subcortical regions, particularly the midbrain tectum. Patients with PSP often present with unexplained falls, an essentially normal straight ahead gait, and minimal extrapyramidal signs. The disequilibrium appears when the subject turns while walking or is pulled backward or pushed from the side (lateral instability). The patient often falls with apparently no protective responses. This presentation differs from that of idiopathic Parkinson's disease, in which imbalance appears later in the course of the disease and is generally accompanied by the classical parkinsonian gait. Other findings on examination that confirm this diagnosis are decreased or absent downgaze and pseudobulbar palsy (see Chapter 34). PSP generally progresses to an inability to stand unaided.[38]

Lesions in the *posterior parietal cortex* are known to produce neglect and spatial disorientation.[33] The effect on balance and gait is not well documented, but it is easy to imagine that lesions in these areas could impair gait and balance. "Pusher syndrome," in which patients tend to lean towards a parietal lesion (away from hemiparesis), has been described, highlighting the importance of the cortex in maintaining upright posture.[39]

MOTOR FORCE DISORDERS

The musculoskeletal system is required to execute the locomotor and balance synergies. Skeletal, joint, muscle, motor nerve, and motor neuron disorders may preclude ambulation or force the nervous system to adopt unique strategies to carry out ambulation.

Articular, bone, and *connective tissue disorders* of the trunk and lower extremities may alter gait because of mechanical restraints or pain. However, the extent to which a person can adapt ambulation to the presence of bony deformities and artificial limbs is remarkable if the central nervous system is undamaged. The compensated gait pattern may be bizarre but provides mobility. A slow and careful gait in which movement of some joints (particularly the hips and knees) is restricted to reduce pain is referred to as an antalgic or arthritic gait. The examination should reveal pain and limitation of movement at the affected joints.

Muscular dystrophies, *myositis*, and *myopathies* generally affect the proximal muscles more than the distal muscles and cause weakness of the trunk and pelvic girdle. Weakness of the medial glutei prohibits fixation of the pelvis on the support leg during walking. To prevent the pelvis from tilting toward the swing leg, the trunk flexes laterally, toward the support leg. The successive movements of the trunk from side to side during walking produce a characteristic waddling gait. Examination demonstrates rather profound weakness in the hips if the gait disturbance is due to weakness.

Peripheral motor neuropathies typically affect the distal muscles and produce weakness at the ankle, particularly dorsiflexion of the ankle. If the ankle does not dorsiflex sufficiently, hip flexion must be increased to raise the leg so that the toe will not catch on the support surface. This produces a steppage gait or foot drop. Foot drop causes patients to trip frequently because the toe does not clear some minor obstacle on the ground. Distal weakness and reflex abnormalities are present on examination.

FORCE SCALING DISORDERS

Disorders of the cerebellum, basal ganglia, and corticospinal tracts do not eliminate balance and gait synergies but they disrupt their execution. These synergies are apparently inappropriately scaled—that is, they are too big or too small or are distorted by other involuntary movements. Postural disturbance is often considered a key component of *parkinsonism*. Patients with advanced disease may appear to have absolutely no response to a push or a pull, toppling over like a log if not caught. However, muscle electromyographic activity recorded from postural muscles generally shows that such patients have appropriate reactive postural responses at normal latencies. The problem is that the postural response is hypometric and generates insufficient force to produce an effective and timely correction. Thus, some of the postural abnormalities seen in parkinsonism appear to be related to the same physiological abnormalities that cause bradykinesia (an inability to energize the muscles quickly and forcefully).

A very typical progression of gait abnormalities occurs in patients with parkinsonism. Initially, the only abnormality is reduced arm swing, generally unilaterally because the disease commonly begins unilaterally. Subsequently, the steps become shorter, and the speed of walking slows. The trunk is flexed (simian posture). Turns become slower, and the head, neck, and trunk move together as a rigid unit, the en bloc turn. Later, the patient may find it difficult to start to walk, and the feet remain apparently stuck to the floor (start hesitation). Once gait is underway, it looks much more normal (although the flexed posture and reduced arm swing remain) as long as the patient walks straight ahead in an open area. Turns may again cause the feet to "stick" to the floor and may be accomplished by making small shuffling steps (turn hesitation). Walking may become slower or stop completely when the patient passes through a narrow space such as a doorway or is distracted (freezing). Because the feet slow or stop and the trunk may be leaning forward in anticipation of moving forward, hesitation and freezing at starts and turns may cause falls forward onto the knees or outstretched arms. Some patients may attempt to compensate by taking multiple small rapid steps (propulsion). Postural instability can be brought out by pulling the patient backward, causing the individual to take multiple steps backward (retropulsion) or at times fall backward without a postural response. Eventually, walking may become impossible without assistance because of the freezing and hypometric protective postural responses. Throughout this deterioration of the parkinsonian gait, the base remains narrow. If a wide base is present in a patient with other signs of parkinsonism, the clinician must consider other syndromes such as multiple system atrophy, spinocerebellar atrophies, and multi-infarct gait disorders.

Choreic gaits are largely normal locomotor and balance synergies distorted by involuntary movements. In patients with moderately severe chorea, the involuntary movements of the legs cause a characteristic gait pattern. The trajectory of the leg and the position of the foot when it makes contact with the ground vary from step to step. Choreic movements may flex and extend the trunk and otherwise interrupt the smooth forward progression of the gait. The consequence is an erratic, jerky gait pattern marked by hesitations in some steps, variable length of steps, and variable contact with the ground, so that the patient may rise on the toes for one step and then land on the side of the foot or the heel next. This produces a stuttering or dancing gait that has been likened to a puppet on a string. With severe chorea, gait may be precluded by the superimposed involuntary movements.

Dystonic gaits are characterized by involuntary, sustained, twisting movements of the limbs and trunk that affect locomotion. Initially, dystonia tends to occur only when the patient is engaged in specific activities (action dystonia). For example, dystonic spasms may affect a leg when the person walks forward but not backward. This characteristic of the gait is often incorrectly interpreted as suggesting hysteria. Dystonic posturing of the arms is often brought out by asking the patient to walk on the toes or heels. With time, dystonic postures may be present at rest. Dystonia may remain restricted to one group of muscles or one limb, or it may be generalized. The gait pattern reflects the distribution of dystonic spasms. Because childhood-onset dystonia often begins in a leg, abnormalities of walking or running (described as a limp by parents) are the first signs of the disorder.

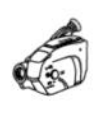

Cerebellar disorders appear to produce hypermetric anticipatory and reactive postural responses and dysmetric limb movements that have impaired timing and force. The basic synergies for balance and gait are not deranged. That is, the cerebellum modifies the execution of the synergies that are generated elsewhere in the nervous system. Mild cerebellar gait ataxia shows up as impaired ability to tandem walk and the need for an extra balancing step or two on quick turns. With increasing cerebellar dysfunction, the base widens, and the stepping cadence becomes more irregular. The response to a push is often an overreaction, but the protective response is an appropriate synergy, inappropriately scaled. Severe cerebellar dysfunction may preclude standing and walking because of the marked dysmetria of the postural responses and stepping.

Cerebellar gait ataxia is often described as three distinct syndromes. Lesions of the flocculonodular lobe (vestibulocerebellum) produce clinical abnormalities resembling those produced by vestibular lesions. There is marked disequilibrium with falling in any direction. There may be a truncal tremor when the patient is sitting or standing (titubation). Medulloblastomas are frequently associated with this syndrome. Lesions of the anterior vermis (spinocerebellum) produce a wide-based gait with a slow and irregular cadence and superimposed lurching. The patient may have few or no other signs of ataxia except when standing and walking. Alcoholic cerebellar degeneration primarily affects the anterior vermis and produces the same picture.[40] Lesions of the lateral cerebellar lobes (frontocerebellum) produce ataxia of limb movements and consequently an ataxic gait. Infarcts, hemorrhages, and tumors are common causes of this syndrome. These syndromes are not reliable indicators of the anatomical location of cerebellar pathology.[41] In clinical practice, a cerebellar ataxic gait with no other prominent cerebellar signs is attributed to midline cerebellar dysfunction. A cerebellar ataxic gait with limb ataxia, dysarthria, and ocular dysmetria is attributed to involvement of the lateral cerebellar lobes.

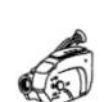

Spastic hemiparetic and *paraparetic gaits* result from disruption of the corticospinal tracts and produce unilateral or bilateral weakness and spasticity. The patterns of automatic postural responses, anticipatory responses, and gait are basically preserved, although less force (scaling deficit), delays in distal muscle activation, and co-contraction are present. If there is adequate strength, spasticity rarely prohibits ambulation, although it may make gait precarious.

The movements of the affected leg or legs are slow, stiff, and effortful. Most of the forward movement of the spastic leg comes from the hip. Because of the weakness of the

dorsiflexors of the ankle and the increased (spastic) tone in the leg, the leg moves as a rigid pillar in a semicircle during the swing phase (circumduction) to prevent catching the toe. The toe often scrapes along the floor and may catch on small irregularities, causing falls. The toes of the shoes are scuffed and worn out of proportion to the remainder of the sole of the shoe. The person with a spastic gait, like the patient with peripheral neuropathy and foot drop, is trying to overcome the weakness of dorsiflexion of the ankle, but the stiffness of the leg prevents the spastic patient from adopting the steppage gait and requires circumduction of the leg to accomplish the swing phase (bringing the leg forward for a step). The legs may even cross the midline at the end of the swing phase because of the increased tone in the adductors of the thigh, producing the scissoring gait typical of severe spasticity. There may be a marked discrepancy between the signs of spasticity elicited when the patient is supine (hyperreflexia, spastic catch in the legs, Babinski's signs) and the degree of spasticity apparent when the patient walks.

SYNDROMES OF IMPAIRED ADAPTATION AND DEPLOYMENT STRATEGIES

The individual must be able to adapt synergies to the environment and situation. Much of this process occurs at a subconscious level and operates through the frontal lobe and possibly the basal ganglia. In addition, some adaptation takes place at a conscious level and is dependent on attention, learning, and insight, functions that are associated with frontal lobe function. A normal person's gait changes appropriately depending on whether the surface is flat, rough and uneven, or slippery (such as ice) and on the kind of footwear being worn (shoes, thongs, skis, stilts). Likewise, postural synergies are adapted to the situation. The postural response to a perturbation felt when standing at the end of a low diving board depends on whether the pool is filled with water and how the person is attired. Thus, equilibrium and gait are adapted to the situation through awareness of the body and the environment as well as through the use of insight, judgment, and past experience.

The cortex is not necessary for ordinary walking in laboratory animals such as cats. It is necessary for *skilled walking*, for example, when the cat must place its feet precisely such as when walking on the rungs of a horizontal ladder. Similarly, in humans, the frontal motor areas are presumed to be involved in precise locomotion such as walking on uneven surfaces, avoiding obstacles on the ground, and dancing.

The *cautious gait*, often inappropriately referred to as a *senile gait*, is characterized by slower, shorter steps and en bloc turns. It is not a pathological gait pattern but is a more conservative balance and gait pattern, the proper response to perceived postural insecurity in the anterior-posterior direction. A normal person assumes a cautious gait pattern on an icy surface. Older individuals assume a cautious gait pattern when they perceive that their balance or their ability to regain their balance is impaired. Widening of the base of support is an appropriate response to uncertainty about when and where the feet will make contact with the support surface and the risk of falls laterally. Just as a normal person widens the base of support on a pitching ship deck, an older individual with a cerebellar, vestibular, or somatosensory disorder widens his or her base.[28]

Although dementia is not associated with a particular gait pattern, many epidemiological studies of falls in the elderly identify dementia as one risk factor for falls.[42, 43] Patients with Alzheimer's disease (AD) have normal cadence, but are slower, with decreased stride length, compared with age-matched elderly. People with AD have increased susceptibility to distractors, which might increase their risk for falls.[44] Some falls appear to be due to poor insight; the patient attempts to do things that are not reasonable for his or her physical capabilities and environmental situation. Demented patients do not attend to their environment. It is probable that if dementia is combined with any problems with balance and gait, the chances of falls are markedly increased because the patient will be unable to adapt to the disabilities. In conclusion, demented patients may have normal balance synergies but cannot use them effectively because of their impaired attention and insight and an inability to profit from experience. The converse is also true. Some patients with severely compromised balance and gait synergies never fall because of their insight and carefulness.

Although balance and gait are thought of as "subconscious" functions, it has been demonstrated that attentional demands are needed to maintain balance and locomotion. As the difficulty of balancing or walking increases, as is common in the elderly, more attention is required.[45, 46] Attentional demands are increased by using a walker.[47] Thus, inattention or distraction may impede balance and walking. The increased risk of falling associated with psychotropic drug use[42] may be related to the drug's effects on attention and not solely to alterations in sensory-motor function. Patients with unexplained falls may be encephalopathic from medical illnesses as well as drugs.[48]

The *post-fall syndrome* consists of a sudden inability to walk without the support of objects or the assistance of another person; it occurs after a fall, and there is no evidence of a neurological or orthopedic abnormality that explains the inability to walk.[49, 50] With assistance, many of these patients can learn to walk normally. This inability to walk appears to be due to excessive fear—a perceived insecurity of balance that does not match the person's physical capacity. It might be termed an overcautious gait.

Psychogenic gait disorders can take many forms, including hemiparetic and paraparetic disorders, ataxic disorders, trembling, buckling of knees, and dystonic abnormalities. Features that suggest psychogenic gait disorders include (1) variability in gait from time to time, particularly with suggestion or distraction; (2) excessive slowness and hesitation in walking; (3) tandem walking with much arm waving and swing foot wavering combined with prolonged periods of balancing on the stance foot; (4) bizarre gait patterns with no explanatory neurological findings; and (5) other historical and neurological signs suggesting a psychogenic disorder.[51] Neurological disorders that are sometimes improperly labeled as psychogenic are (1) dystonia, because the postures may be strange and may be present only during certain specific tasks (e.g., during walking but not running); (2) thalamic astasia, because of the striking evidence of disequilibrium combined with a lack of other neurological signs; and (3) frontal gait disorders, because of balance and gait dysfunction without other neurological signs in the presence of personality changes.

TABLE 18–4. Etiological Classification of Gait Disorders in Descending Order of Prevalence from a Gait Disorders Clinic

Myelopathy
Sensory deficits
Multiple infarcts
Unknown causes
Parkinsonism
Hydrocephalus
Cerebellar disorders
Miscellaneous disorders
Psychogenic
Toxic/metabolic

General Management Goals

Although characterizing gait impairment (Table 18–4) and instituting a specific treatment plan based on a precise diagnosis is important, general measures should always be considered in patients who present with gait disorders or falls. The first management goal is patient safety, and a number of nonspecific strategies can be used to achieve this goal. Since falls are dangerous, their prevention must be of paramount concern. Stabilizing walking aids such as walkers, canes, and other support aids may be useful in weak or unstable patients, but the patients must be specifically trained to use these objects correctly. Some patients, especially those with a gait marked by freezing, may find such aids of more hazard than benefit. Padded clothing, knee pads, and elbow guards may also be used. Physical therapists are often particularly skilled in advising on the use of medical ambulation aids.

The next management goal is to identify the neural dysfunction that contributes to the patient's gait and balance difficulties. A differential list of diseases that should be investigated in the search for treatable pathologies can be developed and a prognosis established. Characterization of balance and gait disorders in terms of systems dysfunction will help to identify correctable problems such as decreased visual acuity that is amenable to refraction or cataract removal, weakness that is amenable to bracing, and so on. It is important to recognize that balance and gait disorders may have multifactorial causes[52] and that there need not be a unique cause for the patient's difficulties. An attempt to correct all potential contributors to gait and balance problems is worthwhile.[53, 54]

When these goals have been accomplished, physical therapy programs for strengthening and improved balance can be refined.[55] Further evaluation and experimentation with various assistive devices may be useful, and therapists can instruct the patient and family how to best use these. The occupational therapist can evaluate the home for safety and may suggest the use of grab bars, new lighting, floor coverings, a different furniture arrangement, and so forth to prevent falls.[54]

Reviews and Selected Updates

Bronstein AM, Brandt T, Woollacott MH (eds): Clinical Disorders of Balance, Posture, and Gait. London, Arnold, 1996.

Burleigh-Jacobs A, Horak FB, Nutt JG, Obeso JA: Step initiation in Parkinson's disease: Influence of levodopa and external triggers. Mov Disord 1997;12:206–215.

Capaday C: The special nature of human walking and its neural control. Trends in Neurosci 2002; 25:370–376.

Masdeu JC, Sudarsky L, Wolfson L (eds): Gait Disorders of Aging: Falls and Therapeutic Strategies. Philadelphia, Lippincott, Williams and Wilkins, 1997.

Report of the Therapeutics and Technology Assessment subcommittee of the American Academy of Neurology: Posturography. Neurology 1993; 43:1261–1264.

Ruzicka E, Hallett M, Jankovic J (eds): Advances in Neurology, Volume 87: Gait Disorders. Philadelphia, Lippincott, Williams & Wilkins, 2001.

References

1. Grillner S, Wallen P: Central pattern generators for locomotion with special reference to vertebrates. Annu Rev Neurosci 1985;8:233–261.
2. Grillner S, Deliagina T, Ekeberg O, et al: Neural networks that co-ordinate locomotion and body orientation in lamprey. Trends Neurosci 1995;18:270–279.
3. Armstrong DM: Supraspinal control of locomotion. J Physiol 1988;405:1–37.
4. Mori S, Sakamoto T, Ohta Y, et al: Site-specific postural and locomotor changes evoked in awake, freely moving intact cats by stimulating the brainstem. Brain Res 1989;505:66–74.
5. Pahapill PA, Lozano AM: The pedunculopontine nucleus and Parkinson's disease. Brain 2000;123:1767–1783.
6. Garcia-Rill E: The basal ganglia and the locomotor regions. Brain Res Rev 1986;11:47–63.
7. Eidelberg E, Walden JG, Nguyen LH: Locomotor control in Macaque monkeys. Brain 1981;104:647–663.
8. Lawrence DG, Kuypers HGJM: The functional organization of the motor system in the monkey II. The effects of lesions of descending brainstem pathways. Brain 1968;91:15–36.
9. Magnus R: Physiology of posture. Lancet 1926;2:531–536, 585–588.
10. Mitoma H, Hayashi R, Yanagisawa N, Tsukagoshi H: Disturbances in patients with pontine medial tegmental lesions. Arch Neurol 2000;57:1048–1057.
11. Mori S: Contribution of postural muscle tone to full expression of posture and locomotor movements: Multi-faceted analyses of its setting brainstem-spinal cord mechanisms in the cat. Jpn J Physiol 1989;39:785–809.
12. Rademaker GGJ: The Physiology of Standing (Das Stehen). Minneapolis, University of Minnesota Press, 1980.
13. Mori S, Matsui T, Kuze B, et al: Stimulation of a restricted region in the midline cerebellar white matter evokes coordinated quadrupedal locomotion in the decerebrate cat. J Neurophysiol 1999;82:290–300.
14. Massion J: Movement, posture, and equilibrium: Interaction and coordination. Prog Neurobiol 1992;38:35–56.
15. Camicioli R, Panzer VP, Kaye J: Balance in the healthy elderly: Posturography and clinical assessment. Arch Neurol 1997;54:976–981.
16. Elble RJ, Hughes L, Higgins C: The syndrome of senile gait. J Neurol 1992;239:71–75.
17. Ebersbach G, Sojer M, Wissel J, et al: Comparative analysis of gait in Parkinson's disease, cerebellar ataxia and subcortical arteriosclerotic encephalopathy. Brain 1999;122:1349–1355.
18. Stoltze H, Kuhtze-Buschbeck JP, Johnk K, Illert M, Deuschl G: Comparative analysis of gait disorder of normal pressure hydrocephalus and Parkinson's disease. J Neurol Neurosurg Psychiatry 2001;70:289–297.
19. Whitman GT, Tang T, Lin A, Baloh RW: A prospective study of cerebral white matter abnormalities in older people with gait dysfunction. Neurology 2001;57:990–994.
20. Wikkelso C, Andersson H, Blomstrand C, Lindqvist G: The clinical effect of lumbar puncture in normal pressure hydrocephalus. J Neurol Neurosurg Psychiatry 1982;45:64–69.
21. Dietz V, Colombo G, Jensen L: Locomotor activity in spinal man. Lancet 1994;344:1260–1263.
22. Hanna JP, Frank JI: Automatic stepping in the pontomedullary stage of central herniation. Neurology 1995;45:985–986.
23. Giladi N, McDermott MP, Przedborski S, et al. and the Parkinson Study Group: Freezing of gait in PD: Prospective assessment in the DATATOP cohort. Neurology 2001;56:1712–1721.
24. Thompson PD, Marsden CD: Gait disorder of subcortical arteriosclerotic encephalopathy: Binswanger's disease. Mov Disord 1987;2:1–8.
25. Yanagisawa N, Ueno E, Takami M: Frozen gait of Parkinson's disease and vascular parkinsonism—A study with floor reaction forces and EMG. *In* Shimamura M, Grillner S, Edgerton VR (eds): Neurobiological Basis of

Human Locomotion. Tokyo, Japanese Scientific Society Press, 1991, pp 291–304.

26. Adams RD, Fisher CM, Hakim S, et al: Symptomatic occult hydrocephalus with "normal" cerebrospinal fluid pressure: A treatable syndrome. N Engl J Med 1965;273:117–126.
27. Meyer JS, Barron DW: Apraxia of gait: A clinicophysiological study. Brain 1960;83:261–284.
28. Nutt JG, Marsden CD, Thompson PD: Human walking and higher level gait disorders, particularly in the elderly. Neurology 1993;43:268–279.
29. Shumway-Cook A, Horak FB: Rehabilitation strategies for patients with vestibular deficits. Neurol Clinics North Am 1990;8:441–457.
30. Horak FB, Shupert CL: Role of the vestibular system in postural control. *In* Herdman SJ, Whitney SL, Borello-France DF (eds): Vestibular Rehabilitation. Philadelphia, F.A. Davis, 1994, pp 22–46.
31. Paulus WM, Straube A, Brandt T: Visual stabilization of posture: Physiological stimulus characteristics and clinical aspects. Brain 1984;107:1143–1163.
32. Drachman DA, Hart CW: An approach to the dizzy patient. Neurology 1972;22:323–330.
33. Karnath H: Subjective body orientation in neglect and the interactive contribution of neck muscle proprioception and vestibular stimulation. Brain 1994;117:1001–1012.
34. Gross CG, Graziano MSA: Multiple representations of space in the brain. Neuroscientist 1995;1:43–50.
35. Masdeu JC, Gorelick PB: Thalamic astasia: Inability to stand after unilateral thalamic lesions. Ann Neurol 1988;23:596–603.
36. Felice KJ, Keilson GR, Schwartz WJ: Rubral gait ataxia. Neurology 1990;40:1004–1005.
37. Labadie EL, Awerbuch GI, Hamilton RH, Rapesak SZ: Falling and postural deficits due to acute unilateral basal ganglia lesions. Arch Neurol 1989;45:492–496.
38. Litvan I, Mangone CA, McKee A, et al: Natural history of progressive supranuclear palsy (Steele-Richardson-Olszewski syndrome) and clinical predictors of survival: A clinicopathological study. J Neurol Neurosurg Psychiatry 1996;60:615–620.
39. Karnath H-O, Ferber S, Dichgans J: The origin of contraversive pushing: Evidence for a second graviceptive system in humans. Neurology 2000;55:1298–1304.
40. Victor M, Adams RD, Mancall EL: A restricted form of cerebellar cortical degeneration occurring in alcoholic patients. Arch Neurol 1959;1:579–688.
41. Gilman S, Bloedel JR, Lechtenberg R: Disorders of the Cerebellum. Philadelphia, F.A. Davis, 1981.
42. Tinetti ME, Speechley M, Ginter SF: Risk factors for falls among elderly persons living in the community. N Engl J Med 1988;319:1701–1707.
43. Salgado R, Lord SR, Packer J, Ehrlich F: Factors associated with falling in elderly hospital patients. Gerontology 1994;40:325–331.
44. Camicioli R, Howieson D, Lehman S, Kaye J: Talking while walking: The effect of a dual task in aging and Alzheimer's disease. Neurology 1997;48:955–988.
45. Teasdale N, Bard K, LaRue J, Fleury M: Cognitive demands of posture control. Exper Aging Res 1993;19:1–13.
46. Lajoie Y, Teasdale N, Bard C, Fleury M: Attentional demands for static and dynamic equilibrium. Exp Brain Res 1993;97:139–144.
47. Wright DL, Kemp TL: The dual-task methodology and assessing the attentional demands of ambulation with walking devices. Phys Ther 1992;72:306–315.
48. Sudarsky L: Geriatrics: Gait disorders in the elderly. N Engl J Med 1990;322:1441–1446.
49. Marks I: Space "phobia" a pseudo-agaraphobic syndrome. J Neurol Neurosurg Psychiatry 1981;44:387–391.
50. Murphy J, Isaacs B: The post-fall syndrome: A study of 36 elderly patients. Gerontology 1982;82:265–270.
51. Lempert T, Brandt T, Dieterich M, Huppert D: How to identify psychogenic disorders of stance and gait. J Neurol 1991;238:140–146.
52. Duncan PW, Chandler J, Studenski S, et al: How do physiological components of balance affect mobility in elderly men? Arch Phys Med Rehabil 1993;74:1343–1349.
53. Tinetti ME, Speechley M: Prevention of falls among the elderly. N Engl J Med 1989;320:1055–1059.
54. Tinetti ME, Baker DI, McAvay G, et al: A multifactorial intervention to reduce the risk of falling among elderly people living in the community. N Engl J Med 1994;331:821–827.
55. Province MA, Hadley EC, Hornbrook MC, et al: The effects of exercise on falls in elderly patients: A preplanned meta-analysis of the FICSIT trials. JAMA 1995;273:1341–1347.

CHAPTER 19

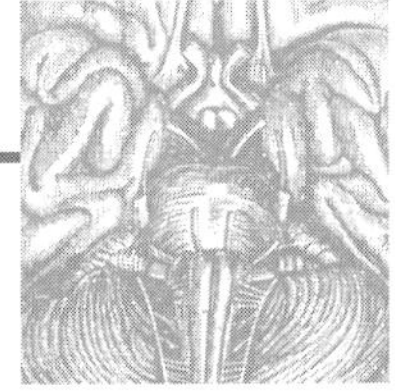

GREGORY W. MORGAN

Proprioception, Touch, and Vibratory Sensation

History and Definitions

The direct relation of somatic sensation to the nervous system was first put forth by Herophilus of Chalcedon in the third century BC. Through careful dissections, he identified nerves as structures directly connected to the brain and spinal cord and attributed sensation and motor function to them.[1] The concept of the subdivision of somatic sensation into modalities was solidified by the specificity theory of Müller, who proposed that the stimulation of certain primary afferent fibers yielded a specific modality of sensation and that these specific nerve fibers were tuned to respond to only certain stimuli.[2]

The specificity theory's greatest challenge came from the experimental findings of Lele and Weddell, who noted that free nerve endings in the cornea produced sensations of more than one modality.[3] Subsequently, many subtypes of mechanoreceptors were shown to respond to various types of stimuli.[4] However, the elegant intraneural microstimulation studies of Ochoa and Torebjörk have demonstrated that an elementary sensation can be reliably elicited by stimulation of a single mechanoreceptive unit.[5] Most likely, modality specificity exists at the most fundamental levels of the sensory unit at threshold levels of stimulation, but suprathreshold levels of stimulation activate receptors nonspecifically.

Because the sensory modalities of proprioception, vibration, and touch share neurophysiology, clinical concurrence, and some anatomy beyond the level of the mechanoreceptors, these sensations are considered together.

Proprioception is any postural, positional, or kinetic information provided to the central nervous system by sensory receptors in muscles, tendons, joints, or skin; *touch* is the sensory modality concerned with the ability to perceive superficial, non-noxious stimulation of the skin; and *vibration*, which is sometimes referred to as *pallesthesia*, is the ability to perceive sinusoidal rhythmic stimulation on both a superficial and deep level.

Alterations in sensation are often spoken of in terms of hyperesthesia, hypesthesia, and paresthesia. *Hyperesthesia* is an exaggeration of any sensory modality response. Hyperesthesia is distinct from *hyperpilaphesie*, which represents augmentation of tactile faculties in response to other sensory deprivation (e.g., touch in the blind). *Hypesthesia* represents a diminution of any sensory modality; however, it is most frequently used in the discussion of painful and tactile stimulation. *Paresthesia* reflects a perversion of sensation, producing a perception that is abnormal in character (e.g., tingling on tactile stimulation) or abnormal sensations that an individual experiences in the absence of stimulation, including feelings of tingling, burning, prickling, crawling, and so on. Paresthesia has also been applied in a general sense to refer to sensations of a purely subjective nature.[6]

Clinical History

Sensory complaints can be subdivided into positive and negative phenomena. Negative phenomena, hypesthesia or hypalgesia, reflect a loss of sensation on stimulation. Positive phenomena are represented by hyperesthesia and paresthesia. Examples include pain perceived with light stimulation of the skin or a sensation of ants crawling on the skin in the absence of any external stimulation. Negative phenomena generally reflect failure along sensory channels secondary to either conduction block or fiber loss at any site along the sensory axis. Paresthesia or spontaneous pain, however, is most likely due to neural hyperactivity generated ectopically from damaged fibers.[7]

A number of descriptors may be used by the patient to indicate a sensory loss: numbness, dead weight, prickling, tingling, "pins and needles," aching, tightness, creeping, itching, and burning. It is important to clarify the symptoms with the patient. Such terms as *numbness* may be used when actually the patient is experiencing weakness or, conversely, the patient is referring to an extremity feeling weak or heavy when indeed there is diminished sensation.

Several historical factors are critical in determining the etiology of a patient's sensory complaints. Chief among these is the distribution of the perceived sensory loss. Localization is the foundation for generating an accurate and complete list of conceivable causes. Some examples of the distribution of sensory loss and typical localizations are listed in Table 19–1. The patient should also be asked to describe the temporal presentation, clinical course (static, progressive, stepwise, relapsing/remitting), duration, and severity of symptoms. Any precipitating or provocative factors for the sensory complaints should be noted.

Abnormalities of touch sensation are likely readily recognized by the patient, whereas impairment of vibration is generally not noted by patients because this sensory inflow is not a part of the daily conscious experience. Proprioceptive loss is most likely recognized by the patient as a lack of coordination in the limbs or impairment in gait. An early sign of proprioceptive loss may be unmasked by asking if the patient has difficulty walking or reaching for objects in the dark.

It is important to determine if there are any associated neurological deficits to aid in localization and determination of etiology, such as motor deficits, cranial neuropathies, language deficits, sensory neglect, deep tendon reflex changes, limb or gait ataxia, or autonomic dysfunction.

TABLE 19–1. **The Pattern of Sensory Loss Seen in Lesions Throughout the Sensory Axis**

Distribution of Sensory Loss	Clinical Diagnosis
Single nerve	Mononeuropathy
Multiple peripheral nerves in a single arm	Infraclavicular brachial plexopathy
Single nerve root	Radiculopathy
Multiple spinal roots in a single arm	Supraclavicular brachial plexopathy
Multiple spinal roots in a single leg	Lumbrosacral plexopathy
Symmetrical distal extremities	
Legs > arms	Polyneuropathy (e.g., diabetes)
Arms > legs	Polyneuropathy (e.g., vitamin B_{12} deficiency)
Symmetrical proximal extremities	Polyneuropathy (e.g., Tangier disease)
Multifocal peripheral nerve distribution	Mononeuritis multiplex
Multifocal partial nerve distribution	Subcortical white matter (e.g., multiple sclerosis)
Distinct sensory level	Spinal cord lesion
With sacral sparing	Extrinsic cord compression or central cord lesion
Saddle distribution	Conus medullaris or cauda equina
Incomplete hemibody	Brain stem
Hemibody	Thalamic lesion
Face and arm sparing leg	Sensory cortex or superficial subcortical white matter

The presence of any familial history of sensory complaints or conditions causing sensory dysfunction must be investigated. In particular, a determination of the pattern of inheritance of a peripheral neuropathy may greatly aid in making a diagnosis.

Underlying medical conditions that may predispose the patient to disease of the sensory axis must be explored, with careful attention to past medical illnesses, trauma, toxin exposure, and medications. Patients may present with sensory complaints as their only recognizable manifestation of toxin exposure. Toxic neuropathies secondary to medications or environmental exposure are seldom purely sensory neuropathies; however, Table 19–2 lists some medications that may cause a predominantly sensory neuropathy. Although the sensory complaints associated with a toxic neuropathy may vary, pathologically there may be a predilection for involvement of a certain fiber type population. Almost all predominantly sensory toxic neuropathies due to medications are axonopathic rather than myelinopathic.

Anatomy of Proprioception, Touch, and Vibratory Senses (Table 19–3)

RECEPTORS

Sensation begins most distally with the transduction of mechanical stimulation by mechanoreceptors in the dermis, epidermis, muscles, and joints. To stimulate the axon

TABLE 19-2. **Medications Causing Predominantly Sensory Neuropathies Along with the Fiber Type Preferentially Affected as Seen on Pathologic Specimens**

Medication	Fiber Type Preferentially Affected Pathologically
Almitrine	Large greater than small
Chloramphenicol	Small greater than large
Cisplatin	All fibers
Dideoxycytidine (ddC)	All fibers
Disulfiram	All fibers
Metronidazole	All fibers
Misonidazole	All fibers
Phenytoin	Large greater than small
Pyridoxine	All fibers
Taxol	All fibers
Thalidomide	Small greater than large
Vincristine	Small greater than large

associated with a mechanoreceptor, the stimulus must first pass through intervening tissues. This process is referred to as *stimulus accession*. This is followed by *stimulus transduction*, in which the stimulus energy is transformed into electrical energy by depolarization of the axon terminal in proportion to the amount of mechanical energy applied. The amplitude of the mechanical stimulus determines the frequency at which the action potentials are initiated.[8] This temporal summation of afferent impulses is preserved throughout the afferent course and is decoded centrally as subjective stimulus sensation magnitude. Increasing the intensity of a mechanical stimulus not only increases the firing frequency of the discharging mechanoreceptor, but also recruits more sensory units. The intrinsic properties of the mechanoreceptors, however, determine how sustained the impulse activity is when stimulated.[9] Rapid adaptation of a mechanoreceptor indicates that the unit is firing only as long as the stimulus is moving. Slow adaptation indicates that the unit also fires when the stimulus is held constant.[10]

Four subtypes of mechanoreceptors that have large fiber afferent nerves associated with them have been identified: (1) Meissner's end organ (RA) with rapid adaptation, a distinct receptor field border, and small receptive field size; (2) paciniform end organ (PC) with rapid adaptation, obscure field borders, and large field size; (3) Merkel's end organ (SA I) with slow adaptation, distinct field borders, and a small receptive field; and (4) Ruffini's end organ (SA II) with slow adaptation, obscure field borders, and large field size.[11]

TABLE 19-3. **Clinico-anatomical Correlation of Lesions Involving Proprioception and Vibration Sensations**

Anatomical Site of Damage	Sensory Findings	Other Neurological and Medical Findings
Sensory receptors	Local diminution of all modalities	Edema or inflammation of skin
Primary neuron	Distal to proximal gradient loss of all modalities	Distal weakness and atrophy of lower extremity muscles, areflexia
Peripheral nerve		
Sensory root ganglion	Vibration and proprioceptive loss greater than pain and temperature in distal extremities; arms and legs equally affected; limb ataxia	Areflexia; may have xerophthalmia, xerostomia, arthritis, rash, or pulmonary mass lesion
Dorsal columns and other spinal tracts	Proprioceptive and vibratory loss generally in bilateral lower extremities	Pupillary abnormalities, areflexia, ataxia in lower extremities
Secondary neurons	Selective loss of vibration and proprioception, in lower extremities for gracilis and in upper extremities for cuneatus	Cranial nerve deficit in lower brain stem
Nucleus cuneatus and gracilis		
Medial lemniscus	Loss of proprioception, vibration, and discriminative touch on the contralateral half of the body usually in an incomplete distribution	Cranial nerve palsy; the particular nerve involved is important in localizing at what level the medial lemniscus is lesioned as it courses through the length of the brain stem
Tertiary neurons	Loss or decrease of all modalities on entire contralateral half of body, frequently accompanied by spontaneous pain	May be associated thalamic aphasia, memory deficit, or rubral tremor
Ventroposterolateral and ventroposteromedial nuclei		
Internal capsule	Loss of all modalities or combinations of selective loss of pain and temperature or vibration, proprioception, and discriminative modalities. Distribution is near complete or incomplete hemibody contralateral to the lesion; associated hemiparesthesia may be noted	
Sensory cortex	Mild and often transient loss of pain, temperature, and vibration; more severe and sustained loss of proprioception and discriminative touch. There is variability in distribution and severity from moment to moment. Distal extremities are affected more severely than proximal extremities, and extremities are affected more than the trunk. Unilateral face and arm or leg alone may be affected	Neglect, aphasia, extinction on double simultaneous stimulation

Any given mechanoreceptor may respond to various types of mechanical energy; however, most are particularly sensitive to one form of stimulation. This selectivity tends to be greatest at or near threshold levels of stimulation, that is, activation of the smallest number of sensory units necessary for stimulus perception.[12]

It has been demonstrated, from intraneural microstimulation of a single myelinated fiber associated with a mechanoreceptor, that elementary sensations can be perceived and sensory quality, magnitude, and localization can be resolved at a cognitive level.[5] Microstimulation of a single RA unit produces a sensation of intermittent tapping or fluttering. These receptors are related to texture discrimination in glabrous skin such as the fingertips.[13] Microstimulation of a PC receptor produces a sensation of vibration or tickle. Microstimulation of an SA I receptor produces a sensation of pressure,[5] and these receptors appear to be critical in resolving the spatial structures of objects or surfaces.[13, 14] Microstimulation of SA II receptors evokes no sensation when stimulated in isolation; however, they are excited by skin stretching and joint movement.[15] The Ia afferents that represent the primary endings of muscle spindles also produce no sensation when stimulated in isolation.[16]

FIRST-ORDER NEURON

Beyond the mechanoreceptors, the sensory impulses are propagated centrally by a population of afferent nerve fibers. The cross-sectional diameter, degree of myelination, and conduction velocity of peripheral nerve fibers are useful categories that relate directly to the modality subserved by certain mechanoreceptors and nerve fiber populations. The accepted composition of the sensory nerve compound action potential includes Aαβ myelinated fibers (30–72 m/sec); Aδ lightly myelinated fibers (4–30 m/sec); and C unmyelinated fibers (0.4–2 m/sec).[17] There is an association between activity in a fiber population and the sensation perceived: Aαβ fibers convey light touch, proprioception, vibratory, and discriminative sensations (large fiber modalities); Aδ fibers convey sensation of pinprick and coldness; and C fibers convey the sensation of dull aching and warmth. These latter two groups reflect the small fiber modalities discussed in Chapter 20 on pain and temperature sensation.

In the case of the largest myelinated fibers, conduction block due to demyelination or conduction failure due to axonal damage can lead to impaired sensory impulse transmission centrally and thus a corresponding sensory deficit in these large fiber modalities. Uniform conduction slowing per se does not seem to have a clinical correlate. In patients with hereditary sensorimotor neuropathy type I, conduction velocities can approach 10 to 15 m/sec in the largest fiber population (normal for lower extremities is 40 m/sec and in upper extremities it is 50 m/sec) with few sensory symptoms. However, if there is an unequal slowing of conduction of select fibers within the Aαβ population (differential slowing), it is likely to interfere with clinical tests that depend on the delivery of synchronized bursts of impulses such as vibratory sensation.[18]

These peripheral nerve fibers of the first-order neurons have their associated soma in the dorsal root ganglia (DRG). The separation of modalities that originated in the peripheral mechanoreceptors appears to be preserved in the DRG anatomically, with the most rapidly conducting peripheral fibers associated with a subpopulation of large clear cells within the DRG.[12] On a neurophysiological level, membrane properties of DRG cells are correlated with the specific peripheral mechanoreceptor type and peripheral nerve fiber conduction velocity.[19] The DRG neurons are T-shaped structures, with the afferent sensory axons coming from the peripheral nerve and separate axonal projections that transmit the impulse centrally to the spinal cord through the dorsal roots.

Within the dorsal roots, the various sensory fibers are intermingled. However, as the fibers enter the spinal cord, the large myelinated fibers assume a more medial position. The more lateral aspect of the bundle is composed of thinly myelinated and unmyelinated fibers that ascend three to six segments and descend four to five segments before synapsing within the spinal cord gray matter of the dorsal horn. The spinal cord gray matter is described in terms of laminae, the separate areas being denoted cytoarchitectonically. These laminae often represent separate nuclei with distinctive functions. Lamina IV plays a role in light touch, and lamina VI receives afferents from group I muscle afferents, for example. Most of the fibers that enter the dorsal columns of the spinal cord do so without synapsing in the dorsal horn. The dorsal columns generally represent direct projections from the DRG neurons to the nuclei gracilis and cuneatus within the brain stem. However, some of the primary afferents coursing in the dorsal columns send projections to the propriospinal neurons in the dorsal horn and some axons of second-order neurons from the dorsal horn course in the dorsal columns and terminate on dorsal column nuclei.

The classical view is that the impulses ascending in the fibers of the dorsal columns mediate sensations of touch, deep pressure, vibration, proprioception, and sensory discrimination. The fibers in the dorsal columns are steadily pushed in a medial direction as they course rostrally. The fibers entering at more rostral levels intrude themselves between the ascending fibers and the dorsal horn. The medial portion is referred to as the funiculus gracilis and is composed of fibers from caudal to and including the lowest six thoracic levels, and the lateral portion is referred to as the funiculus cuneatus and is composed of the upper six thoracic segments and cervical segments.[20] The funiculus cuneatus occupies most of the ventral aspect of the dorsal columns, abutting the commissure from the second to the sixth cervical cord segments. At C3 it occupies all of the ventral aspect. There is a topographical representation within the dorsal columns by submodality such that discriminative touch is most superficial (dorsal), vibration is represented most deeply (ventral), and proprioception is intermediate.[21]

SECOND-ORDER NEURON

The dorsal column fibers terminate in the nucleus gracilis and cuneatus at the level of the medulla. Again, the nucleus gracilis is medial to the cuneatus and each nucleus subserves the same body region, as represented in its respective funiculus. In these nuclei, the primary afferent fibers synapse and the second-order sensory afferents send projections more rostrally through the medial lemniscus after the fibers decussate as the internal arcuate fibers in the medulla. The somatotopic organization is preserved throughout the course of the medial lemniscus. The medial lemniscus remains medial in the medulla and pons, sweeping more laterally at the level of the midbrain.

THIRD-ORDER NEURON

The fibers of the medial lemniscus terminate in the ventroposterolateral (VPL) nucleus of the thalamus. This pathway is organized somatotopically such that the fibers from the nucleus gracilis end most laterally within the VPL nucleus and those from the nucleus cuneatus end in the larger, medial part of the VPL nucleus. The VPL nucleus is the origin of the third-order sensory afferent neuron that sends projections to somatosensory cortex (Fig. 19–1).

Primary somatosensory cortex consists of the postcentral gyrus and its medial extension into the paracentral lobule (Brodmann areas 1, 2, and 3). There is somatotopic organization such that the amount of tissue within the primary sensory cortex that represents a particular region of the body is related to the importance of that region in somatic sensation and not to its absolute size. For example, the thumb has a much greater area of cortical representation than does the proximal arm. In the region of the postcentral gyrus, the calf and the foot are represented on the medial surface of the hemisphere and then laterally follow the foci for the thigh, abdomen, thorax, shoulder, arm, forearm, hand, fingers, and face. The foci for the bladder, rectum, and genitalia are located on the lowest aspect of the medial surface of the hemisphere (Fig. 19–2).

With regard to the subdivision of cortical regions by modality, Powell and Mountcastle have shown in monkey cortex that over 90 percent of the neurons in area 2 are related to receptors of the deep tissues of the body such as the joints, in area 3 most of the cells are activated by cutaneous stimuli, and area 1 has an intermediate position in terms of the modality specificity of its neurons.[22]

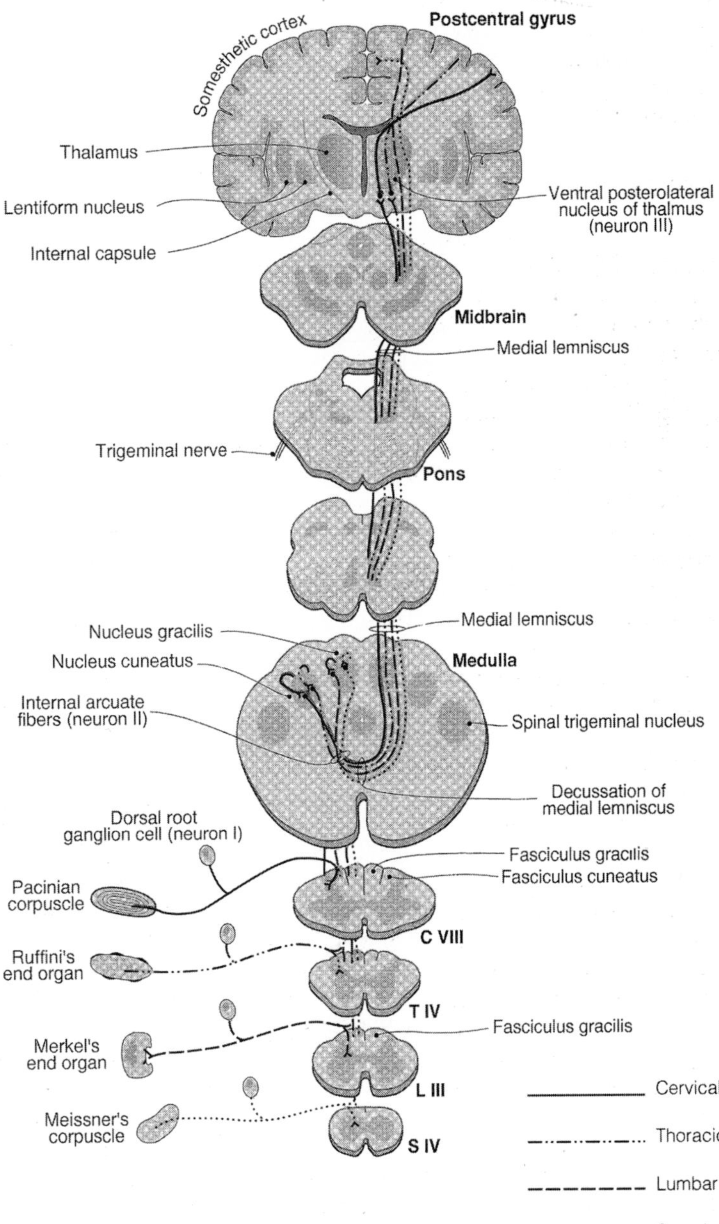

FIGURE 19–1. The formation and course of the posterior columns in the spinal cord and the medial lemniscus in the brain stem. The posterior columns are formed from uncrossed ascending and descending branches of spinal ganglion cells. Ascending fibers in the fasciculi gracilis and cuneatus synapse on cells of the nucleus gracilis and cuneatus. Fibers forming the medial lemniscus arise from cells of the nuclei gracilis and cuneatus, cross in the lower medulla, and ascend to the thalamus. Impulses mediated by this pathway include proprioceptive, vibratory, and discriminative touch. Spinal ganglia and afferent fibers entering the spinal cord at different levels are coded as in legend. (Modified from Carpenter MB: Human Neuroanatomy. Baltimore, Williams & Wilkins, 1983.)

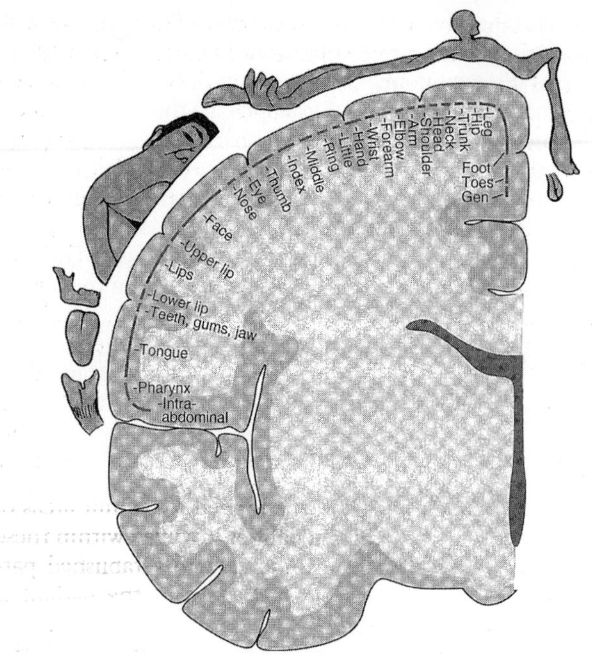

FIGURE 19–2. Sensory homunculus. This diagram shows the relative size and distribution of the parts of the cerebral cortex from which sensations localized to different parts of the body can be elicited on electrical stimulation in man. (From Penfield W, Rasmussen T: The Cerebral Cortex of Man. New York, Simon and Schuster, 1950.)

Adjacent to primary sensory cortex are smaller cortical zones that receive input from primary somatosensory cortex referred to as secondary sensory areas. Although contralateral representation of the body predominates, there is some bilateral representation within these areas.

SPINOCEREBELLAR PATHWAYS

A second type of sensory information enters the spinal cord through the dorsal columns. These fibers generally carry spinocerebellar impulses that terminate in various regions of the cerebellum and thus do not reach a level of conscious sensation.

The dorsal spino-olivary tract ascends within the dorsal columns, synapses in the cuneatus and gracilis nuclei, and then relays impulses to the contralateral accessory olivary nucleus. These fibers arise in the spinal cord and are activated by cutaneous and group Ib receptor afferents. The function of these fibers is largely spinocerebellar. There are fibers traveling in the anterior funiculi that have a similar termination and are referred to as the anterospino-olivary tract.

The dorsal spinocerebellar tract (DSCT) arises from neurons in the dorsal nucleus of Clarke from the T1 to L2 levels. The principal afferent fibers to Clarke's nucleus are collaterals of primary afferent fibers that are observed to descend directly from the dorsal columns. These cells have afferent peripheral inputs from muscle spindles, Golgi tendon organs, and touch and pressure receptors. The fibers enter the cerebellum through the inferior cerebellar peduncle in the medulla and terminate on the ipsilateral vermis. These impulses are utilized in the fine coordination of posture and movement of individual limb muscles.

The ventral spinocerebellar tract arises from cells in the dorsal horn and ascends largely contralaterally in the lateral funiculus of the cord ventral to the dorsal spinocerebellar tract. The fibers come from levels below the midthoracic cord. These fibers enter the cerebellum through the superior cerebellar peduncle.

The cuneocerebellar tract (CCT) is the forelimb equivalent of the DSCT. It consists of two separate components: one exteroceptive, which is activated by cutaneous afferents and higher threshold muscle afferents, and one proprioceptive, which is activated by group I muscle afferents. The CCT terminates ipsilaterally in lobule V of the anterior lobe of the cerebellum.[23]

DISCRIMINATIVE TOUCH, VIBRATION, AND CONSCIOUS SENSE OF JOINT/MUSCLE MOVEMENT

There are three elements of proprioception with separate peripheral receptor representation: (1) the perception of limb movement is mediated by muscle spindle receptors, cutaneous mechanoreceptors, and joint receptors; (2) the perception of limb position is mediated by muscle spindle receptors and cutaneous mechanoreceptors; and (3) the perception of force of muscular contraction is mediated by corollary discharges and tendon organ receptors.[24] Specific mechanoreceptors that have been implicated in proprioception include SA II cutaneous afferents that respond to planar stretch of the skin and muscle spindle endings that respond to muscle stretch. Neither of these receptors evokes a coherent sensation when stimulated in isolation. This suggests that spatial summation among various receptors is critical for the perception of position sense.[16]

Proprioception is transmitted through heavily myelinated nerve fibers. The cell body of the first-order neuron is in the DRG and goes without synapsing into the ipsilateral funiculus gracilis or cuneatus to synapse in the nucleus gracilis or cuneatus within the medulla. As these fibers travel in the dorsal columns they are topographically localized between the fibers transmitting vibration and those transmitting discriminative touch in the intermediate region of the dorsal columns. The second-order neurons are located within the gracilis and cuneatus nuclei. The third-order neurons are located in the VPL nucleus of the thalamus following the course of the dorsal column nuclei to the somatosensory cortex, as previously mentioned. The sensory cortex gets very precise information on the position and movements of the joints.

Pacinian corpuscles (PC) are the mechanoreceptors responsible for the sensory transduction of vibratory sensation. These receptors are excited by very rapid changes in tissue distortion such as that produced by sinusoidal vibration.[12] When the skin is locally anesthetized by cocaine, there is a many-fold elevation in threshold for frequencies in the range of 5 to 40 Hz, whereas that for higher frequencies is scarcely unchanged. This suggests that the perception of vibration depends on two separate primary afferents: one innervating the skin and the other innervating the deep tissues.[11] Detection of vibration of the frequency range of 5 to 40 Hz probably depends more on RA transduction, whereas PC units account for detection at higher frequencies of vibration.[25] As stimulus intensity is increased, PC fibers may initially discharge irregularly or at some submultiple of the stimulus frequency. With slight increments, however, the point of phase locking between stimulus and firing of afferent nerve fiber is quickly reached.[8]

Vibratory stimuli are transmitted through large myelinated, group Aβ fibers through the dorsal columns to the somatosensory cortex. Like proprioceptive fibers, the first-order neurons are in the DRG, second-order neurons in the cuneatus and gracilis nuclei, and third-order neurons in the VPL nucleus of the thalamus. With regard to the cortical representation of vibratory sensation, many years ago Holmes stated that the "appreciation of vibration is possible through the thalamus alone."[26] Although the thalamus may play a significant role in the appreciation of vibratory sensation, Mountcastle has clearly demonstrated activity in cortical neurons in response to vibratory stimulation and has localized the function of frequency discrimination to a cortical level.[27]

Discriminative or complex touch includes two-point discrimination, touch localization, direction of movement of an object drawn on the skin, stereognosis, and graphesthesia. The finest levels of surface structure are transduced by RA and PC afferent fibers.[28] It is most probable that these complex sensations result from a simultaneous stimulation of several types of receptors. The nerve fibers transmitting discriminative modalities have their first-order neuron origin in the DRG. These fibers enter the DRG through myelinated fibers in the medial division of the dorsal root. They follow an identical course to that of proprioceptive fibers to the somatosensory cortex by means of the dorsal columns. Within the dorsal columns these fibers occupy the most posterior region.[29]

LIGHT TOUCH AND PRESSURE

The mechanoreceptors associated with light touch include the RA and SA I. The sensory nerve fibers are large and myelinated. The central course of the fibers subserving tactile sensation is more diffuse than that of the other large fiber modalities with fibers coursing in both the anterior spinothalamic tract and the dorsal columns. It has long been recognized that a morbid process confined to the dorsal column will give no clear-cut loss of simple tactile sensibility. Conditions are similar for lesions affecting the anterolateral sensory tracts. It appears that if one of the two systems subserving touch sensibility is damaged, the reduction is so mild that it is of no practical clinical relevance.[20]

Tactile sensory nerve fibers have their first-order neurons in the DRG and enter the spinal cord through the medial division of the dorsal root. These fibers are largely thought to traverse the medial strand of the dorsal roots and enter the dorsal columns ascending to the contralateral thalamus (see previous discussion of course of dorsal columns). Other fibers bifurcate into ascending and descending fibers that synapse within a few segments in the dorsal horn and laminae I, IV, V, and some of VI and VII. Some of these second-order neurons decussate in the anterior commissure and ascend in the contralateral anterior spinothalamic tract to the VPL nucleus of the thalamus. Within the thalamus the tactile sensory fibers are placed slightly caudad to those conveying pain. These third-order neurons then ascend to somatosensory cortex. The organization of this modality at the cortical level is not well understood.

Pressure is related to tactile sense but involves the perception of pressure sensations other than light touch from subcutaneous structures. It is closely related to proprioception and is mediated through the dorsal columns.

Examination of the Position, Touch, and Vibratory Sensory Systems

DIRECTED NEUROLOGICAL EXAMINATION

The sensory examination is performed to delimit areas of abnormal sensation and the modalities involved within these limits and to compare these findings with established patterns of abnormal sensation. To ensure that the patient is attentive and cooperative, the examiner may need to interrupt the examination and complete it at a later time if the patient becomes fatigued or inattentive. The importance of the abnormal findings on the sensory examination are greatly enhanced by reproducibility, and it may be necessary to reexamine affected areas to verify initial findings.

In the patient who is without subjective sensory complaints, a quick survey of the body is all that is necessary, keeping in mind the distribution of the major sensory peripheral nerve and segmental root distributions (Figs. 19–3 through 19–5) and verifying that sensation perception is symmetrical. If there are specific sensory complaints or if abnormalities are found on the survey examination, a focused examination should be carried out to determine the exact distribution and the modalities impaired.

Some areas of the body are physiologically more sensitive to touch, and caution should be used in declaring an abutting area hypesthetic when only a minor difference in sensation occurs in these border zones. These areas include the antecubital fossa, supraclavicular fossa, and neck. An additional potential pitfall in misinterpreting a normal sensory examination is that as one passes from one skin area to an adjacent area supplied by a much higher spinal segment, it is normal for the patient to sense a sudden increase in the stimulus at the point of the segmental border. An example is seen on the chest where dermatomes C4 and T2 abut.[30] Some physical factors that may contribute to anesthesia on the sensory examination include areas of thicker skin, such as the elbow, or regions covered by calluses.

Some helpful landmarks and anatomical considerations to keep in mind when performing the sensory examination are in the following list:

C1 has no supply to the skin.
The interaural line is the border between the areas supplied by the ophthalmic division of the trigeminal nerve and the C2 segment.
C5–C6 supply the radial side of the arm, forearm, and hand.
C8–T1 supply the ulnar side of the forearm and hand.
T3 supplies the axilla.
T4 supplies the nipple region.
T8 supplies the rib margin.

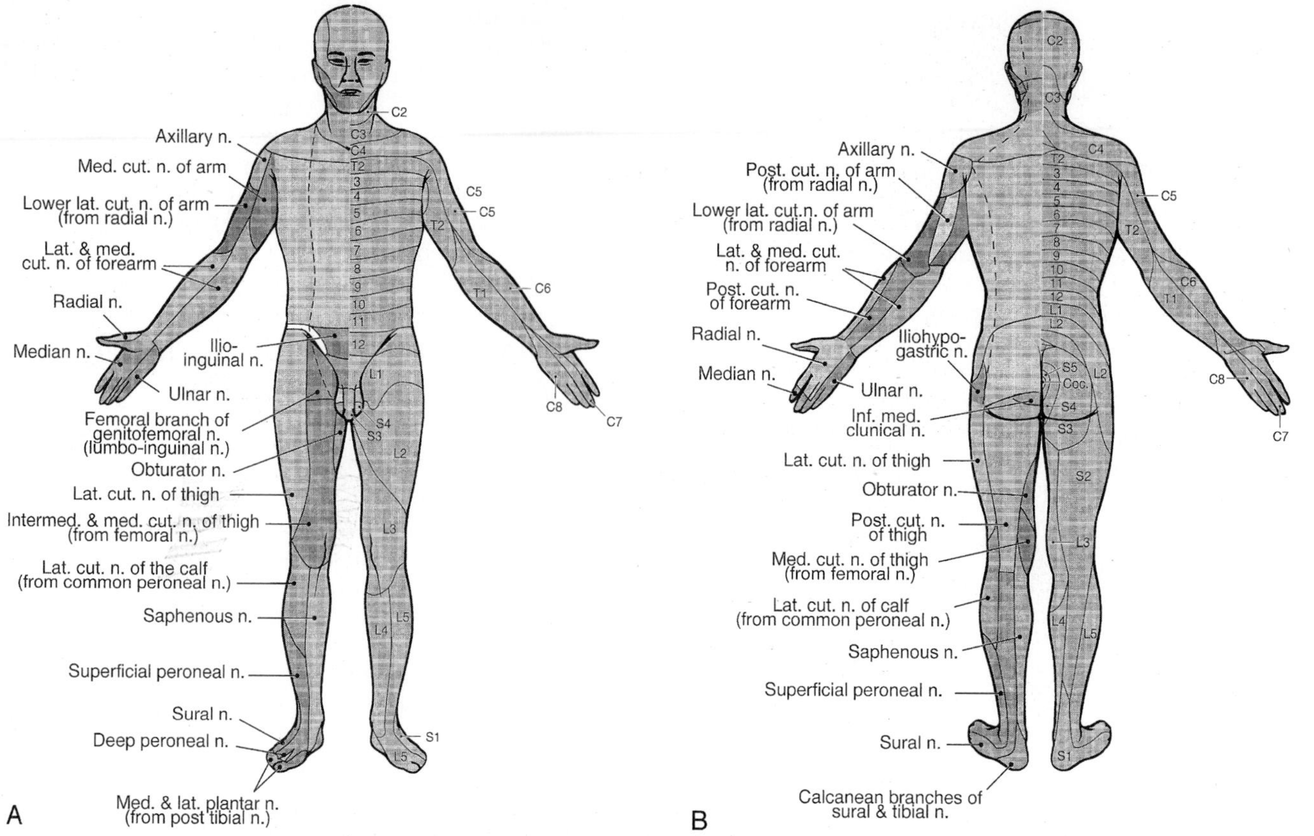

FIGURE 19–3. *A*, Anterior view. The right side of the body depicts the cutaneous fields of the peripheral nerves. The unlabeled areas on the thorax are innervated by the cutaneous branches of the anterior primary rami. The left side of the body depicts the segmental (dermatomal) innervation of the skin. *B*, Posterior view. The right side of the body depicts the segmental (dermatomal) innervation of the skin. The left side of the body depicts the cutaneous fields of the peripheral nerves. The unlabeled area on the left back is innervated by the cutaneous branches of the posterior primary rami. (*A* and *B*, modified from Haymaker W, Woodhall B: Peripheral Nerve Injuries. Philadelphia, WB Saunders, 1953.)

T10 supplies the umbilicus.
T12–L1 supply the groin.
L5 supplies the dorsum of the foot, lateral leg, and great toe.
S1 supplies the small toe, sole of the foot, and the posterior thigh and leg.
S4–S5 supply the perineal region concentric to the coccyx and not the anus.

When a region of hypesthesia has been identified, either subjectively by the patient or on the survey examination, the most reliable method of defining the hypesthetic zone is to proceed from the hypesthetic area to areas of reportedly normal sensation. It is more typical for there to be a gradient of loss at the borders of the hypesthetic region rather than abrupt change at the segmental, peripheral nerve, or midline borders. This is due to some overlap of innervation in the border regions from adjacent peripheral nerves and segmental innervation.

In performing the sensory examination the observer can assess *threshold sensation*, which measures a single nerve fiber innervating a receptor or group of receptor cells, or *innervation density*, which measures multiple overlapping peripheral receptive fields.[31] In peripheral nerve disease, threshold changes tend to be more sensitive for identifying an abnormality. Examples are cutaneous pressure threshold for the slowly adapting mechanoreceptor population and cutaneous vibratory threshold for the rapidly adapting mechanoreceptor population. Once nerve fibers have degenerated there is a decrease in innervation density that is measured by two-point discrimination.[32]

Proprioception. Proprioception, or position sense, can be assessed in a number of ways:

1. With the patient's eyes closed, place his or her hand in a particular position, remove it, and ask the patient to resume the position. Alternatively, have the patient try to imitate the assumed position with the other hand. Poor performance on this exercise could also be related to a motor deficit or higher cortical dysfunction.
2. With the patient's eyes closed, hold the sides of one of his or her digits between your thumb and finger so that no uneven pressure above or below the digit reveals the direction of movement and then move the articulation up or down. The patient should identify the direction of passive movement, and the threshold for accurate detection is noted by the examiner. The normal threshold for passive movement of an articulation is 5 to 10 degrees in the interphalangeal joint of the index finger and 1 degree at the shoulder.[33] It is important to clearly identify the directions of movements of the joint with exaggerated excursion before testing so that the results are not falsified by miscommunication.
3. Have the patient hold his hand outstretched. Look for wavering of a hand or pseudoathetoid movements.

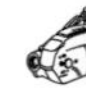

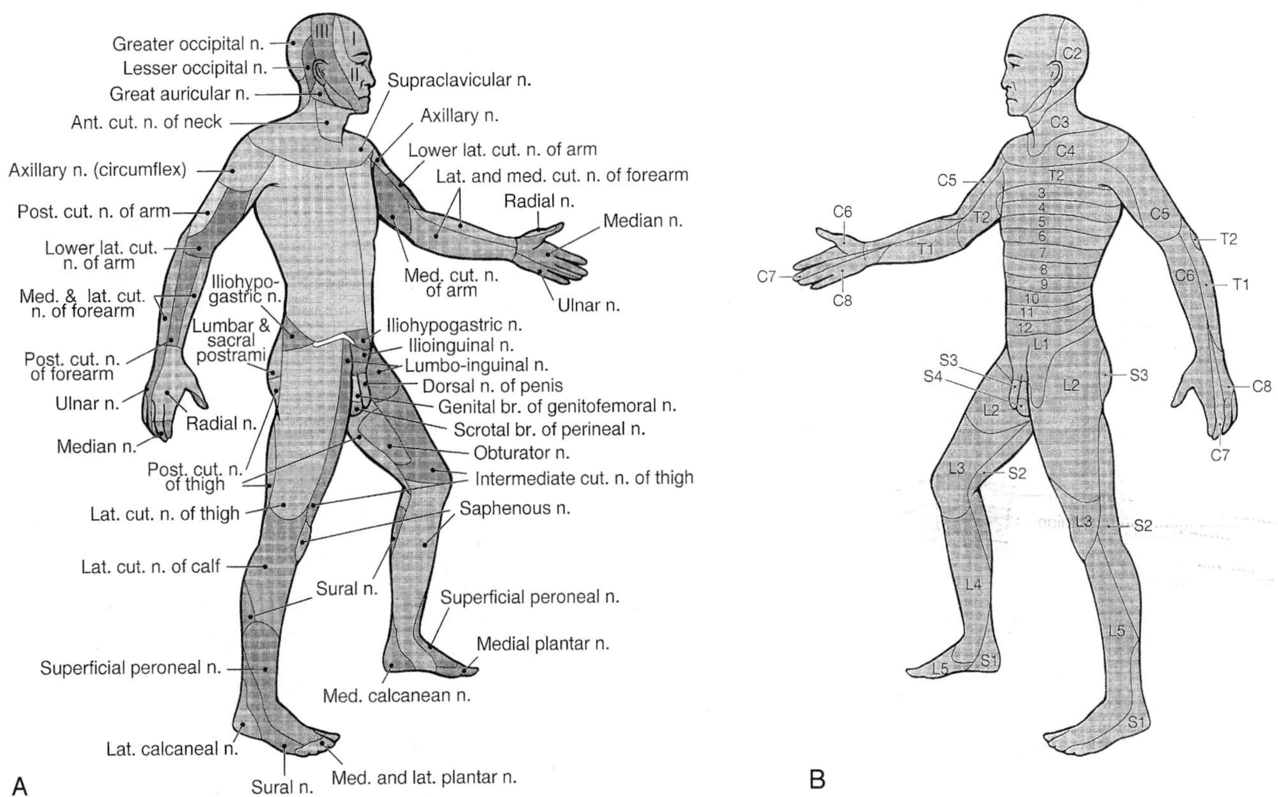

FIGURE 19–4. Side view. *A*, A side view of the cutaneous fields of the peripheral nerves. *B*, A side view of the dermatomes. (Both figures modified from Haymaker W, Woodhall B: Peripheral Nerve Injuries. Philadelphia, WB Saunders, 1953.)

4. Ask the patient to place his or her forefinger accurately on the tip of the nose and his or her heel accurately on a knee.
5. Romberg testing. The Romberg sign is present when the patient is able to stand with the feet together while the eyes are open but sways or falls when the eyes are closed.

Pathologically, with minimal impairment of proprioception there is first loss of the sense of position of the digits, then of the sense of motion. As the process becomes more extensive, loss of recognition for an entire extremity or even at times for the entire body develops.

Vibration. The testing of vibration is an important part of the sensory examination because it is often the first sensation to disappear in nerve injury. The acknowledgment of vibration as a discrete modality is attributed to Weber in 1842.[34] It was Rumpf who introduced the tuning fork to clinical medicine,[35] and the clinical studies of Symms and Williamson secured vibratory sensation assessment as a part of the routine bedside examination.[36, 37]

Vibration is generally assessed with a 128- or 256-Hz tuning fork. The tuning fork is struck against a hard surface with sufficient force to cause the prongs to touch each other and emit a sound. It is applied with a pressure equal only to the weight of the apparatus over an area with a paucity of subcutaneous tissue, such as the anterior tibial area in the leg or the malleoli. The tuning fork is allowed to run down by itself, and the patient is asked to indicate when he or she can no longer feel it. The examiner should make sure the patient is not listening to the humming sound generated but is in fact attending to the vibratory sensation. The examiner should also note the duration of perceived vibration and quickly move the tuning fork to the identical spot on the contralateral limb without striking it again. It is normal to perceive 3 to 5 additional seconds of vibration after such a transference. Areas that can be tested include the great toe, anterosuperior iliac crest, sacrum, spinous process of the vertebrae, sternum, clavicle, styloid processes of the ulna or radius, and finger joints. It is best to apply the tuning fork to an affected site first and then to the same, contralateral, nonaffected site for comparison. An average duration can be quantitated over four to five trials.

The threshold for vibratory perception is lower in the arms than in the legs,[38] with distal sites being more sensitive than proximal ones. In the order of most sensitive to least sensitive areas to vibratory threshold perception are palm; pad of the finger; dorsum of the finger; dorsum of the hand; dorsum of the great toe; sternum and malleolus; lip, tongue, forehead, mastoid, and patella; forearm; and sacrum.[38] Thibault lists normal values of duration of vibratory perception as 19.21 seconds for the index fingerpads and 13.36 seconds for the ankle.[39] Vibratory thresholds are increased in the legs but not the arms in patients older than 50. The degree of the impairment increases with age.[40]

Touch. General tactile sensation is tested by the use of a light stimulus such as a wisp of cotton, feather, tissue, or fingertip. The stimulus should be so light that no pressure on subcutaneous tissues is produced. An allowance for decreased

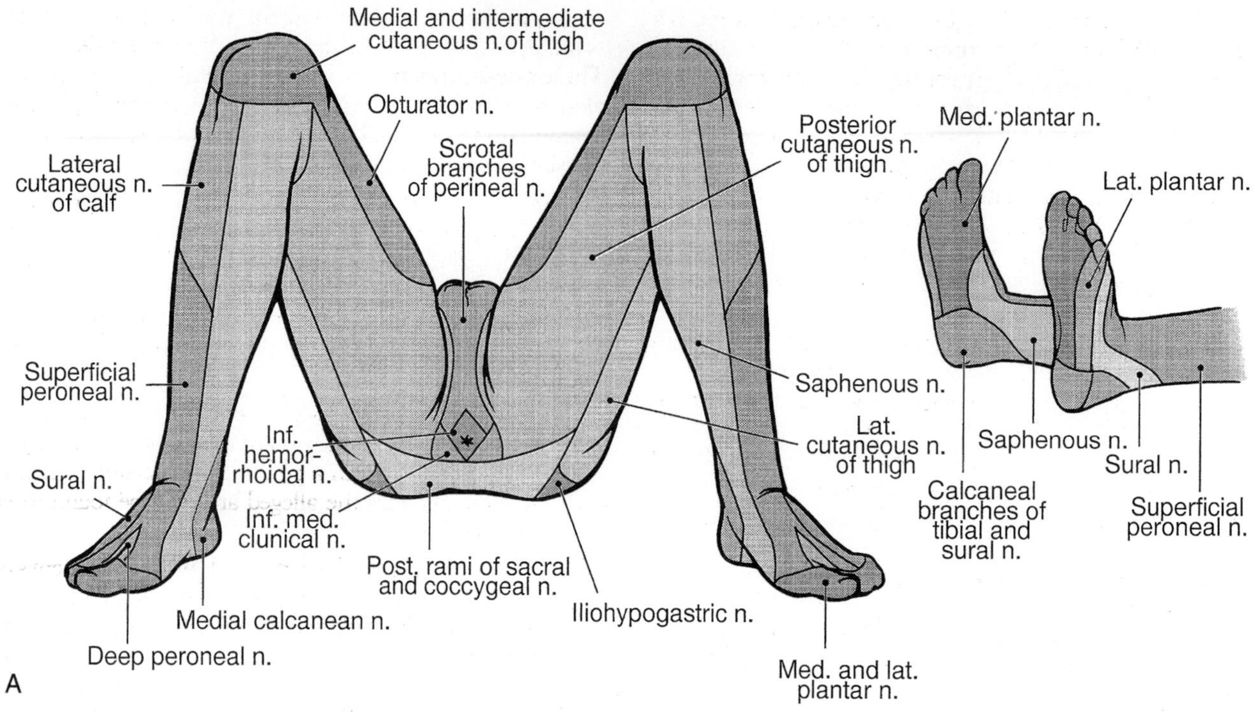

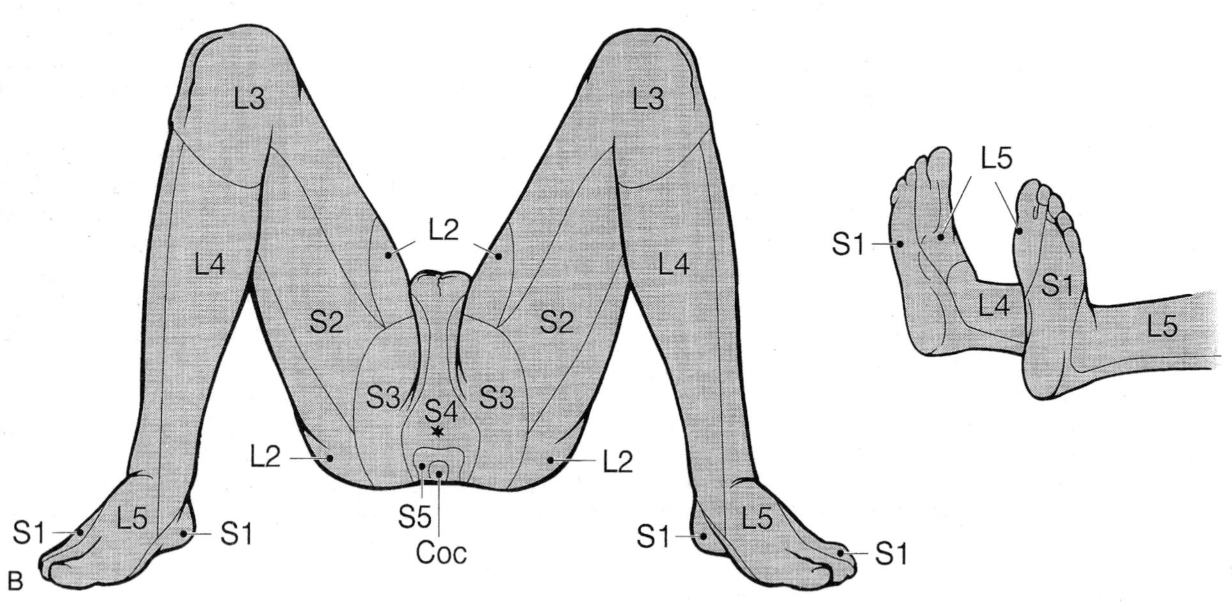

FIGURE 19–5. Perineum and limbs. *A*, Cutaneous fields of the peripheral nerves of the perineum and limbs. *B*, Segmental (dermatomal) innervation of the skin of the perineum and limbs. (Modified from Haymaker W, Woodhall B: Peripheral Nerve Injuries. Philadelphia, WB Saunders, 1953.)

perception should be made for the thicker skin on the palms and soles. The tips of the tongue, lips, genitalia, and fingertips are the most sensitive areas. The upper arms, buttocks, and trunk are much less sensitive. The examination should be conducted with the patient's eyes closed, and the patient is instructed to inform the examiner when the stimulus was perceived. For milder degrees of impairment of light touch, a relative difference from side to side or abutting regions should be investigated.

A systematic approach to the assessment of the threshold of light touch is provided by the Semmes-Weinstein nylon monofilaments. The thickness of these monofilaments is standardized, creating a specific level of force at the point at which the nylon monofilament bends after contact with the skin. There are 20 graduated nylon filaments calibrated in terms of the logarithm of 10 times the force in milligrams required to buckle the filament. Established normal values have been published.[41, 42]

Tactile thresholds are increased in the elderly.[43] In normal persons, distal sites tend to have lower thresholds than proximal ones. In decreasing order of sensitivity are thumbs, palms, plantar surface of foot, and proximal arm.

Two-Point Discrimination. Two-point discrimination is a function of slowly adaptive peripheral mechanoreceptors and a measurement of innervation density. It is best carried out with a two-pronged instrument with blunt ends because sharp pointed objects will tend to stimulate pain fibers rather than touch. Localization is most accurate on the palmar surfaces of the fingers, especially the thumb and index finger. On the fingers it should be possible to discriminate two points separated by less than 5 mm; however, on the dorsum of the foot a distance as great as 5 cm as the lowest level of discrimination may be normal.

Testing of Higher Cortical Function. Other discriminative modalities include graphesthesia, stereognosis, topesthesia, baresthesia, and double simultaneous stimulation. In the presence of normal tactile sensation, abnormalities in these discriminative modalities generally reflect a disorder of cortical sensation. In fact, however, graphesthesia and stereognosis may be impaired by lesions in the dorsal columns and rostrally.

Graphesthesia is tested by tracing a number or letter or figure on the surface of the skin. Test areas include the palm, anterior forearm, thigh, and lower leg. The clearest figures for interpretation tend to be 8, 4, and 5, whereas 6, 9, and 3 tend to be the most difficult.

Stereognosis depends on the sense of light touch and position. It is tested by placing an object in a patient's hand and having him or her identify it with eyes closed. The patient can manipulate the object freely in the hand but should not use the contralateral hand at the same time. If the patient is unable to identify the object, comparison with the contralateral hand should be made. Most studies of normal subjects indicate that familiar objects can be named within 5 seconds of contact.[44] Baresthesia can be assessed in a similar fashion by placing two objects of different weight in sequence in the patient's hand and having him or her identify which is heavier.

Double simultaneous stimulation is tested with the patient's eyes closed, alternating patterns of touch of one limb and then two limbs simultaneously that are contralateral to each other. The patient must identify where he or she is touched. Extinction of a hemibody field is identified such that touch on the affected side is always recognized when done in isolation; however, when the nonaffected side and the affected side are stimulated simultaneously, the affected side is not recognized. This is generally associated with lesions affecting the contralateral parietal lobe.

Stimulus localization or topesthesia can be examined either by asking the patient to touch with his or her finger where the examiner has touched or by asking the patient to state where he or she has been touched. The latter method eliminates joint position sense as a factor.

Examination in Suspected Psychogenic Sensory Loss. The sensory examination is subjective by nature, and it can be very difficult to delineate those patients who have factitious, feigned, or nonphysiological sensory findings. A number of clues and approaches can be utilized in the sensory examination if a nonorganic cause of the sensory complaints is suspected, including skin that is hyperesthetic for one sensationand anesthetic for another; anesthesia exactly to the midline; absolute loss of all cutaneous sensation; midline change for the sense of vibration over bony areas; and inapparent hyperesthesia when the patient is distracted.

A number of methods can be used during the sensory examination to assess for possible psychogenic sensory loss. These assessments are best applied in patients who are clearly alert and cooperative and in whom the standard sensory examination has raised a high degree of suspicion for nonphysiological sensory impairment:

1. Have the patient close his or her eyes and respond "yes" when he or she believes that a stimulus has been applied and "no" when he or she does not feel that a stimulus was applied. Occasionally, a patient with a nonorganic sensory complaint will be identified such that the timing of the answer "no" exactly coincides with each stimulus contact.
2. With the patient's eyes covered, find out by the aid of a light stimulus the alleged anesthetic area and mark the boundaries of it with a pen. If this procedure is repeated at short intervals the alleged area will be found to vary considerably.
3. The zig-zag test can be performed. With the patient's eyes covered, the border of an hypesthetic or anesthetic zone is marked. The observer starts again at the periphery of the limb and works upward with the stimulus in a zig-zag fashion. In the patient with a nonorganic sensory loss, the limit may have shifted downward and repeated tests will continue to bring it lower. The patient is led to feel a greater distance has been covered in a straight line reference. If an altered sensation depends on a genuine lesion of the sensory axis, the sense of localization is not called on and such a migration of the border of the hypesthetic zone is not seen.[45]
4. With the patient's eyes covered, the examiner draws figures of different shapes on the patient's skin. The figures are initially drawn such that part of the outline falls within the alleged anesthetic area and part without. The patient with nonorganic sensory loss may correctly identify the figure even when a critical portion of the figure necessary for identification is drawn within the alleged anesthetic area.
5. With the patient's eyes covered, cross his or her hands behind the back with the palms facing forward and then proceed to test his or her sensibility. In the patient with nonorganic sensory loss the observer may see bending of the alleged insensible finger as it is touched or hesitation in responding to the stimulus.[45]

ASSOCIATED NEUROLOGICAL FINDINGS

Cerebral. There are some potential distortions of body image that may accompany sensory loss helping to localize the sensory deficit to the cerebral cortex. Examples are *anosodiaphora*, which is a lack of concern over a profound loss of sensation or other neurological deficit; *anosognosia*, which reflects a lack of awareness of a profound sensory or neurological deficit; and *asomatognosia*, which represents loss of awareness of one half of the body. Additionally, the patient may manifest sensory neglect with a lack of orienting responses to unilateral stimuli. An aphasia and an increased susceptibility to distracting stimuli manifested as lack of attention or poor concentration are also signs localizing an accompanying sensory deficit to the cerebral cortex.

Thalamic sensory deficits may be associated with unilateral hyperpathia.

Cranial Nerves. As the medial lemniscal fibers course through the brain stem they may be lesioned at any level. The level can be identified by an associated cranial nerve deficit (e.g., cranial nerve III in the midbrain or cranial nerve VII in the caudal pons). Patterns of multifocal sensory loss in the face, extremities, and trunk may represent multiple sclerosis. It is essential in such circumstances to look for typical findings of an internuclear ophthalmoplegia or an afferent pupillary defect on cranial nerve examination that might suggest remote or concurrent optic neuritis or a demyelinating plaque in the brain stem.

Bilateral facial weakness in a lower motor pattern may accompany mild distal extremity sensory loss in acute inflammatory demyelinating polyradiculoneuropathy.

Motor/Reflexes/Cerebellar/Gait. Motor power can be assessed and the distribution of any weakness found noted, such as the distal symmetrical weakness of peripheral neuropathy, which aids in localization of the deficit found on sensory examination. The examiner should look for atrophy of muscles and fasciculations that might suggest a peripheral nervous system process. Muscle tone should be assessed. Deep tendon reflexes are extremely important in the assessment of patients with sensory complaints because they are frequently abnormal in the patient with a lesion in the sensory axis. One should look for the antalgic gait of a painful limb, such as in lumbosacral radiculopathy, or the slapping gait associated with a proprioceptive deficit. Ataxia or pseudoathetosis of the extremities may be associated with a proprioceptive loss in the affected limb.

Autonomic Nervous System. The autonomic nervous system can be evaluated in a noninvasive manner at the bedside with the following assessments: blood pressure and heart rate response to standing, isometric exercise, heart rate variation with respiration, Valsalva ratio, and plasma norepinephrine levels with standing.[46]

Neurovascular. The size, character, and quality of heart sounds and gallop rhythms should be estimated. One should look for the stigmata of cardiogenic embolization: Osler nodes, Janeway lesions, and Roth spots are examples. The pulse is noted for 1 minute in a search for irregularities. The femoral artery, carotid artery, supraclavicular artery, and orbit are auscultated for evidence of bruits. The distal lower extremities are examined for color changes and ulceration characteristic of venous insufficiency.

ASSOCIATED MEDICAL FINDINGS

A good general medical examination of all systems is necessary to aid in generating a differential diagnosis for conditions affecting the sensory axis and can also aid in localization. Diseases commonly associated with peripheral nervous system dysfunction include cancer, diabetes mellitus, the acquired immunodeficiency syndrome, connective tissue disorders, alcohol abuse, uremia, myxedema, and paraproteinemias.

Evaluation Guidelines (Table 19–4)

Neuroimaging. Plain radiographs may be helpful with peripheral localized nerve injury, such as identifying a humeral dislocation in the setting of an infraclavicular brachial plexopathy. Cervical spine or lumbar spine radiographs are useful in radicular complaints, and a chest radiograph is needed to evaluate lower trunk plexopathy of the brachial plexus to look for a cervical rib or an upper lobe structural lesion.

If the clinical pattern of sensory loss suggests a brain stem or hemispheric lesion, neuroimaging of the brain with magnetic resonance imaging (MRI) or computed tomography is indicated. MRI or myelography may be indicated based on sensory loss that localizes to the spinal column (e.g., myelopathy or radiculopathy). Also, if a lesion localizes to either the lumbar or brachial plexuses, an MRI of these regions should be obtained, especially if the patient has a history of cancer.

In a suspected sensory loss of hemispheric origin, focal cerebral blood flow studies with SPECT scanning may be helpful in localizing a focal structural lesion or impairment of circulation.

Electrophysiology. The most important supplement to the history and physical examination in the patient with possible peripheral nervous system disease is an electrodiagnostic examination consisting of nerve conduction studies and electromyography. The sensory nerve conduction studies directly assess the large fiber peripheral sensory nervous system distal to the dorsal root ganglion. This examination is useful in localization of mononeuropathies, generalized peripheral neuropathies, and plexopathies. Although the needle electrode examination assesses only motor axon involvement, it can be helpful in localizing sensory complaints in the spinal nerve root proximal to the region assessed by the standard sensory nerve conduction studies.

Somatosensory evoked potentials allow assessment of sensory impulse conduction along the entire sensory axis from peripheral nerve to sensory cortex. They have their greatest application in lesions proximal to the dorsal root ganglion. In the upper extremity the median nerve is the most frequent site of stimulation; in the lower extremity it is the tibial nerve. This test is useful in patients with multiple sclerosis, brain stem structural lesions, Friedreich's ataxia, spinal cord injury, plexopathy, or radiculopathy. The brain stem auditory evoked response may be useful in identifying a subclinical focus of demyelination in multiple sclerosis, a brain stem structural lesion, or Friedreich's ataxia.

Body Fluid and Tissue Analysis. In a patient with peripheral neuropathy a serological workup including a complete blood cell count, antinuclear antibody, erythrocyte sedimentation rate, rheumatoid factor, glucose level, vitamin B_{12} level, thyroid function tests, test for human immunodeficiency virus, blood urea nitrogen determination, phosphate level, cholesterol level, triglyceride level, cryoglobulin level, serum protein electrophoresis, porphobilinogen/epsilon-aminolevulinic acid value, urine heavy metal level, and vitamin E level covers the majority of identifiable causes.

Specifically for a pure sensory neuropathy, an abbreviated serological evaluation with complete blood cell count, chemistry panel, vitamin B_{12} level determination, erythrocyte sedimentation rate, anti-SSA and anti-SSB tests for Sjögren's syndrome, and anti-Hu antibody test for paraneoplastic sensory neuropathy is sufficient, owing to the limited differential diagnosis.

Cerebrospinal Fluid. A lumbar puncture can be helpful when multiple sclerosis, myelitis, meningitis, acute inflammatory demyelinating polyneuropathy, and certain other peripheral neuropathies are suggested. Attention should be paid to the white blood cell count, protein value, IgG synthesis rate, IgG index, and oligoclonal banding.

TABLE 19–4. **Useful Studies in the Evaluation of Disorders of Touch and Vibration Sensations**

Syndrome	Neuroimaging	Electrophysiology	Fluid and Tissue Analysis	Other Tests
Primary sensory neuropathy	Normal	Low-amplitude sensory response; prolonged distal latency or slow conduction velocity confined to the single sensory nerve involved	Normal	Plain radiograph may demonstrate fracture locally
Diffuse sensory polyneuropathy	Normal	Generalized low-amplitude sensory responses on nerve conduction studies	Elevated ESR, anti-Hu antibody, anti-ssA, anti-ssB HIV, low vitamin B_{12}	Lip biopsy positive for Sjögren's syndrome
Dorsal root ganglia: tabes dorsalis	Normal	Abnormal tibial sensory evoked potential	Positive RPR, FTA, mild lymphocytic pleocytosis in cerebrospinal fluid with elevated protein level	
Radiculopathy	Nerve root compression due to osteophyte, herniated disc, or other structural lesion	Normal sensory nerve conductions; may have low-amplitude CMAP and denervation of NEE if there is motor root involvement; abnormal sensory evoked potential	Normal	
Plexopathy	Mass compressing plexus such as tumor or hematoma	Low amplitude sensory and motor nerve conduction responses in involved nerves; Mykoymic potentials on NEE in radiation plexopathy		Chest radiograph shows cervical rib or apical lung lesion
Spinal cord lesion: posterior column	Structural lesion involving posterior column: infarction, spondylitic changes, tumor, epidural hematoma	Abnormal tibial sensory evoked potential	Elevated cerebrospinal fluid protein, IgG index, positive oligoclonal bands	
Combination of spinal cord and peripheral nerve lesions: vitamin B_{12} deficiency	Normal	Abnormal sensory evoked potential Cord level on NEE Normal sensory conductions	Low vitamin B_{12}, megaloblastic anemia	
Psychogenic sensory loss	Normal	Normal	Normal	

ESR, Erythrocyte sedimentation rate; HIV, human immunodeficiency virus; AIDS, acquired immunodeficiency syndrome; RPR, rapid plasma reagin test; FTA, fluorescent treponemal antibody test; CMAP, compound muscle action potential; NEE, needle electrode examination.

Other Tests. Lip biopsy for high clinical suspicion of Sjögren's syndrome and nerve biopsy for progressive neuropathy of unclear etiology or suspected vasculitis may be done. A punch biopsy of the skin to determine intraepidermal nerve fiber density is a useful diagnostic test in patients with suspected sensory polyneuropathy and normal nerve conduction studies and electromyography.[47] This procedure carries a lower morbidity than peripheral nerve biopsy and allows a direct analysis of the small caliber C and A delta nerve fibers that innervate the skin.[48] This technique shows a distinction between sensory neuropathy and sensory ganglionopathies. In the former, there is a greater degree of loss of intraepidermal nerve fiber loss distally. In the latter, there is a non-length-dependent degeneration of somatic unmyelinated fibers.[49]

Clinical Syndromes (Table 19–5)

The sensory examination aims to establish the sensory modality involved, the intensity of involvement, and the anatomical distribution of the sensory change. In combination, these patterns isolate the likely neurological location of disease and later suggest etiology.

In lesions of the peripheral nervous system the sensory loss tends to be intense, with fixed, clearly defined zones. With central nervous system sensory deficits the boundaries are vague and the deficit is more mild as compared with peripheral processes. There may be considerable variation in both the distribution of and intensity of this type of sensory deficit.

TABLE 19–5. **Etiology of Disorders Affecting Position and Vibration Senses**

Etiological Category	Specific Etiologies	Chapter
Structural Disorders		
Developmental	Tethered spinal cord	28
Degenerative and compressive	Herniated disc	29
Hereditary and Degenerative Disorders		
Storage diseases: lipidoses, glycogen disorders, and leukoencephalopathies	Tangier disease	30
Amino/organic acidopathies	Hereditary tyrosinemia	31
Chromosomal abnormalities and neurocutaneous disorders	Neurofibromatosis with foramen magnum tumor or neurofibrom	32
Movement disorders	Parkinson's disease	34
Ataxias	Friedreich's ataxia	35
Degenerative motor, sensory, and autonomic disorders	Hereditary spastic paraplegia	36
Hereditary nondegenerative neuromuscular disease	Hereditary sensory autonomic neuropathy I	37
Acquired Metabolic and Nutritional Disorders		
Endogenous metabolic disorders	Hypothyroid neuropathy	38
Exogenous acquired metabolic disorders of the nervous system: toxins and illicit drugs	Pyridoxine toxic neuropathy	39
Nutritional deficiencies and syndromes associated with alcoholism	Vitamin B_{12}—subacute combined degeneration	40
Infectious Disorders		
Viral infections	Herpes zoster "shingles"	41
Nonviral infections	Acute disseminated encephalomyelitis	42
Human immunodeficiency virus infection and acquired immunodeficiency syndrome	Distal sensorimotor peripheral neuropathy Mononeuritis multiplex	44
Neurovasular Disorders	Parietal stroke Abdominal aortic dissection	45
Neoplastic Disorders		
Primary neurological tumors	Neurofibroma	46
Metastatic neoplasms and paraneoplastic syndromes	Brachial plexopathy—usually lower trunk Sensory ganglionitis	47
Demyelinating Disorders		
Demyelinating disorders of the central nervous system	Multiple sclerosis	48
Demyelinating disorders of the peripheral nervous system	Chronic inflammatory demyelinating polyradiculoneuropathy	49
Autoimmune and Inflammatory Disorders	Sensory neuronopathy associated with Sjögren's syndrome	50
Traumatic Disorders	Infraclavicular brachial plexopathy from humeral dislocation	51
Epilepsy	Parietal lobe irritative focus with focal sensory seizure	52
Headache and Facial Pain	Migraine with sensory aura	53
Drug-Induced and Iatrogenic Neurological Disorders	Radiation plexitis Postanesthesia brachial plexopathy	55

MECHANORECEPTOR DYSFUNCTION

Non-neural factors including dermatitis, keratosis, cutaneous inflammation, and edema may compromise sensation either through limiting stimulus accession to the mechanoreceptor or through mechanoreceptor decay. The pattern of the sensory deficit will correspond to the distribution of the local cutaneous process.

PRIMARY SENSORY NEUROPATHY: PURE SENSORY DISTAL NERVE LESIONS

Primary sensory neuropathies reflect a focal mononeuropathy of a nerve that carries only sensory fibers. Some examples include the following (see also Figs. 19–3 and 19–4):

- Meralgia paresthetica with involvement of the lateral femoral cutaneous nerve
- Gonalgia paresthetica due to entrapment of the infrapatellar saphenous nerve
- Cheiralgia paresthetica due to entrapment of the superficial branch of the radial nerve
- Medial antebrachial cutaneous neuropathy
- Dorsal ulnar neuropathy
- Sural neuropathy

DIFFUSE SENSORY POLYNEUROPATHY

In generalized peripheral neuropathy the sensory loss is length dependent such that it begins symmetrically at the most distal aspect of the lower extremities and ascends proximally. Generally the distal upper extremities will begin to show involvement when the sensory deficit in the lower extremity has ascended to the level of the proximal calf. In the most severe stage of peripheral neuropathy only a midline strip over the posterior trunk and neck and the peripheral aspects of the face have sustained sensation.[50] Examples of causes of diffuse sensory neuropathy include a dysproteinemic state (IgM monoclonal gammopathies with antimyelin-associated glycoprotein), amyloidosis (generally small fiber), hereditary, diabetes mellitus, uremia, hypothyroidism, immunological (scleroderma, sarcoid), and toxins. A generalized peripheral neuropathy can show selective involvement of certain fiber types such as large myelinated fibers. In these circumstances there will be a dissociated sensory loss with a deficit of vibration and proprioception while sparing pain and temperature on sensory examination. Examples of these conditions include Friedreich's ataxia, Charcot-Marie-Tooth disease, uremia, and Guillain-Barré syndrome.

There are more unusual length-dependent generalized symmetrical proximal neuropathies such that the shortest peripheral nerves are selectively involved. This results in sparing of sensation at the distal aspects of the extremities. This pattern may be seen in the neuropathy associated with Tangier disease, in acute intermittent porphyria, and in a unique familial sensorimotor neuropathy.[51]

PLEXOPATHY

Sensory loss due to a lesion of the brachial plexus will appear in the distribution of two or more peripheral nerves if the lesion is infraclavicular and in the distribution of multiple cervical dermatomes if the lesion is supraclavicular. All sensory modalities may be involved.

In radiation-induced plexopathy, 77 percent of patients have upper trunk involvement predominantly that generally occurs 3 months to 26 years after irradiation of the chest. It is quite characteristic to find myokymia on the needle electrode examination in these patients.[52] Metastatic plexopathy has a predilection for the lower trunk, possibly owing to its proximity to the axillary lymph nodes. Pain is a predominant and early symptom in metastatic plexopathy.

Other causes of brachial plexopathy include traction, obstetrical paralysis, surgical injury, neuralgic amyotrophy, true neurogenic thoracic outlet syndrome, and trauma.

In the lumbar region, a pattern of weakness, loss of reflexes, and sensory disturbance is found that cannot be localized to a single lumbosacral root or peripheral nerve. Pain is a prominent early manifestation when secondary to neoplasm. The differential diagnosis includes idiopathic plexitis, vasculitis, diabetic polyradiculopathy, infection (e.g., with herpes zoster or *Schistosoma japonicum*), hereditary liability to pressure palsies, hemorrhage, trauma, obstetrical complications, and tumor irradiation.

DORSAL ROOT: RADICULOPATHY

Radiculopathy is generally associated with back or neck pain radiating into an extremity. The pain is poorly localizing for nerve root level but typical in the fact that it is radiating. There will generally be a loss of all modalities of sensation in a dermatomal distribution, a corresponding weakness in a myotomal distribution (i.e., with ventral root involvement as well), and segmental hyporeflexia. The most common cause is a herniated disc or osteophyte compressing on a nerve root. A structural lesion such as a neurofibroma or a metastatic focus must also be taken into consideration as possible causes.

DORSAL ROOT GANGLION/DORSAL HORN LESIONS: TABES DORSALIS

Generalized sensory neuropathies should be distinguished from subacute sensory neuronopathies, which are characterized by pain, paresthesia, and numbness in the limbs. The latter demonstrate a marked loss of proprioception and vibration, ataxia, and areflexia in an entire limb with a loss of pain and temperature to a lesser degree. The sensory loss may be more pronounced in the upper extremities than the lower extremities; therefore, it is not strictly length dependent, distinguishing it from a polyneuropathy. Other clinical features distinguishing sensory neuronopathy from sensory polyneuropathy are listed in Table 19–6. The differential diagnosis is Sjögren's syndrome, paraneoplastic origin, hereditary disease, cisplatin toxicity, vitamin B_6 toxicity, and idiopathic disease. The lesion is at the level of the dorsal root ganglion.

Dorsal root ganglion and dorsal horn lesions tend to have very similar anatomical patterns of sensory loss to radiculopathies; however, dorsal horn lesions are more likely to have dissociated loss as the dorsal root fibers separate into the medial (large myelinated) and lateral (thinly myelinated and unmyelinated) bundles as they enter the dorsal horn.

Tabes dorsalis is characterized by diminished proprioception and vibration in the legs, sensory ataxia of gait, areflexia, and aching/lancinating pains in the legs. Additionally, there may be autonomic disturbances, including bladder atony, pupillary abnormalities, and impotence. Generally there is preservation of touch, pain, and temperature sensation. Distal weakness and atrophy may be a late manifestation of tabes dorsalis attributed to extension of syphilitic process to the anterior horn cell. Pathologically, tabes dorsalis is concentrated in the dorsal roots, dorsal funiculi, and posterior columns of the lumbosacral and lower thoracic spinal cord. The dorsal root ganglion is rarely affected.

SPINAL CORD: MYELOPATHY

Generally with transverse lesions of the spinal cord, there is a demonstrable sensory level with bilateral loss of all modalities of sensation below a definite level. With involvement of the dorsal columns there is loss of proprioception,

TABLE 19-6. **Clinical Features Helpful in Distinguishing Sensory Neuronopathy from Axon Loss Sensory Polyneuropathy**

Severe proprioceptive loss
Severe sensory ataxia
Sensory deficits that are not strictly length dependent (i.e., hands may be more impaired than feet)
Asymmetrical sensory deficits
Skin punch biopsy shows equal amounts of intraepidermal nerve fiber loss at distal and proximal sites of biopsy

discriminative modalities, and vibration within a couple of levels caudad to the lesion site. With smaller lesions it is possible to selectively involve certain dorsal column modalities owing to the topographical distribution of the various modalities: fibers carrying discriminative touch are most posterior, vibratory fibers are most anterior, and proprioceptive fibers are intermediate within the dorsal funiculi. There will be no significant loss of light touch; however, pressure sensation may be impaired. Examples are a metastatic lesion to the spinal cord, cord infarction, and multiple sclerosis plaque.

In the patient with a pattern sparing sensation in the sacral dermatomes, an extrinsic cord compression or central cord lesion is suggested at the level of the upper border of the sensory deficit. Sensory loss confined to the sacral dermatomes, a so-called saddle lesion, localizes the lesion to the conus medullaris or cauda equina. There will be involvement of all modalities; however, if there is preservation of touch, the lesion is more likely to be in the conus medullaris.

Central cord lesions and anterior spinal artery syndrome are discussed in Chapter 20. Brown-Séquard syndrome is discussed in Chapter 15.

COMBINATION OF SPINAL CORD AND PERIPHERAL NERVE LESIONS: SUBACUTE COMBINED DEGENERATION

Subacute combined degeneration is characterized by mild distal weakness in the lower limbs associated with increased patellar reflexes, absent ankle reflexes, bilateral Babinski responses, unsteady gait, and positive Romberg sign. Vibration and proprioception are impaired. Vitamin B_{12} deficiency is implicated as the cause. This is a disease of posterior and lateral columns of the spinal cord with associated sensorimotor peripheral neuropathy.

BRAIN STEM LESIONS

A unilateral lesion of the medial lemniscus, usually vascular in origin, is followed by an impairment or loss of vibration, proprioception, and reduced or abolished sense of discriminative touch on the contralateral half of the body if the lesion is situated above the crossing of the fibers in the medulla. Owing to the segmental arrangement of the fibers in the long ascending tracts, there frequently will not be a complete unilateral sensory or motor impairment. Circumscribed areas of sensory loss are not rare, and the regions presenting sensory impairment are only distinctly outlined.[20] Because of the medial placement of the medial lemniscus, the midline cranial nerves or medial longitudinal funiculus are affected, causing ocular paresis that helps to define the level of the brain stem involved.

THALAMIC LESIONS

A lesion in the thalamus causes a loss or a decrease of all modalities of sensation on the half of the body contralateral to the lesion. Very small lesions such as lacunes strategically placed in the thalamus may cause tract-specific sensory deficits confined to a variable pattern of modalities. In thalamic disorders, sensations evoked by peripheral stimulation may outlast the stimulus for a longer period of time than is normally the case.[26]

SENSORY CORTICAL LESIONS

Acutely, in pure cortical lesions, all modalities are affected; however, the modalities of deep sensation (proprioception and discriminative touch) tend to be involved more than the superficial sensory modalities. Vibratory sensation is the exception. Head noted that vibratory sensation was consistently diminished with lesions of the sensory cortex albeitmildly as compared with peripheral lesions.[53] With time, pain, touch, and temperature tend to return. The sense of discriminative touch is usually permanently and severely impaired.

There is generally unilateral loss of these modalities. When the loss is over one entire half of the body with cortical lesions the limbs are almost invariably more involved than the face or trunk. This is partly because in the limbs loss of spatial perception is usually the most prominent feature, whereas the face and trunk are poorly endowed with sensibility of this quality.

As the lesion becomes more superficial it would have to be increasingly large to affect all the diverging fibers. Superficial lesions, therefore, tend to affect one localized area only. The sensory disturbances are usually more marked in the distal than in the proximal segments of the limbs, probably owing to wider representation in the cortex.

Responses are characteristically variable from moment to moment. There is not a definite or sharp border, as the sensory loss generally fades away gradually into the region of normal sensibility. The different parts of the body do not regain their sensibility at the same rate. The face regains it fastest, especially the oral region, then the larynx and anogenital region. The distal parts of the extremities have restitution that is far from complete. Patients with cortical lesions may also experience sensory phenomena like the inability to recognize their own limbs, or alien hand syndrome.

SENSORY SYNDROMES ASSOCIATED WITH PSYCHOGENIC SENSORY LOSS

A psychogenic sensory loss should be suspected in patients with sensory loss that demonstrates hyperesthesia for one modality in a given area and anesthesia for another in the same area, absolute loss of all cutaneous sensation, hyperesthesia that resolves with mild distraction, and sensory levels that correspond to the patient's body image rather than organic sensory levels. The examiner should look for abrupt midline changes, vibration asymmetry over a fixed bone that spans the midline, vibration asymmetry at a fixed midline point as the tuning fork is pivoted from one side to the other, and marked variation with repeated examination. The validity of determining a psychogenic sensory loss with these factors has been debated.[54, 55]

General Management Goals

Regardless of the cause of the sensory loss in the patient with an insensate extremity, it is important to increase the patient's awareness of potential injuries. For example, the patient should be instructed (1) not to use the insensate hand when cooking or smoking; (2) not to place the insensate extremity in hot water; and (3) not to type on a manual typewriter or play a piano/guitar to avoid trauma to the hands.

In the patient with a functional impairment secondary to sensory loss, a rehabilitative process should be instituted. The objectives of sensory re-education are to improve the perception of sensory information arising from receptors in the hand and to improve motor skills. It is important for the patient to integrate the involved limb into normal movement patterns as early as possible.

The principle of sensory re-education focuses on allowing the patient to learn to make sense of unfamiliar somatic sensations through repeatedly matching them to vision and at the same time developing tactics of perception in the form of purposeful exploratory movements of the hand. One method illustrating the latter is to have patients attempt to differentiate objects from a background medium such as sand, rice, or beans. To re-educate moving touch perception, the patient can be asked to repeatedly discriminate between a square nut and a hexagonal one, each of which is rolled across the finger. Constant touch can be rehabilitated by having the patient discriminate between large and small nuts. As discrimination improves, smaller objects are used to increase the difficulty.[56]

Reviews and Selected Updates

Chien HF, Tseng TJ, Lin WM, Yang CC, Chang YC, Chen RC, Hsieh S: Quantitative pathology of cutaneous nerve terminal degeneration in the human skin. Acta Neuropathol 2001;102(5):455–461.

Horak FB: Postural ataxia related to somatosensory loss. Adv Neurol 2001;87:173–182.

Jortner BS: Mechanisms of toxic injury in the peripheral nervous system: Neuropathologic considerations. Toxicol Pathol 2000;28(1):54–69.

McDonald WI: Physiological consequences of demyelination. *In* Sumner A (ed): The Physiology of Peripheral Nerve Disease. Philadelphia, WB Saunders, 1980, pp 265–286.

Ochoa JL: Positive sensory symptoms in neuropathy: Mechanisms and aspects of treatment. *In* Asbury AK, Thomas PK (eds): Peripheral Nerve Disorders, Vol 2. Oxford, Butterworth Heinemann, 1995, pp 44–58.

Olesen LL, Jensen TS: Prevention and management of drug-induced peripheral neuropathy. Drug Safety 1991;6:302–314.

Reid V, Cros D: Proximal sensory neuropathies of the leg. Neurol Clin 1999 Aug;17(3):655–667.

Reinhardt F, Wetzel T, Vetten S, Radespiel-Troger M, Hilz MJ, Heuss D, Neundorfer B: Peripheral neuropathy in chronic venous insufficiency. Muscle Nerve 2000;23(6):883–887.

Thomas PK, Griffin JW: Neuropathies predominantly affecting sensory or motor function. *In* Asbury AK, Thomas PK (eds): Peripheral Nerve Disorders, Vol 2. Oxford, Butterworth Heinemann, 1995, pp 59–94.

References

1. Rufus Ephesius. De anatomia partium hominis 71–75. *In* Von Staden H: Herophilus. Cambridge, Cambridge University Press, 1989, pp 200–201.
2. Müller J: Handbuch der Physiologie des Menschen, Vol 2. Coblenz, J Hölscher, 1841, pp 249–503.
3. Lele PP, Weddell G: The relationship between neurohistology and corneal sensibility. Brain 1956;79:119–154.
4. Bishop GH: My life among the axons. Ann Rev Physiol 1965;27:1–18.
5. Ochoa J, Torebjörk E: Sensations evoked by intraneural microstimulation of single mechanoreceptor units innervating the human hand. J Physiol 1983;342:633.
6. Gowers WR: A Manual of Diseases of the Nervous System, Vol 1. London, J and A Churchill, 1886.
7. Ochoa JL, Torebjörk HE: Paresthesiae from ectopic impulse generation in human sensory nerves. Brain 1980;103:835–853.
8. Mountcastle VB, Talbot WH: A neural base for the sensation of flutter-vibration. Science 1967;155:597–600.
9. Lindblom U, Ochoa J: Somatosensory function and dysfunction. *In* Asbury AK, McKhann GM, McDonald WI (eds): Diseases of the Nervous System: Clinical Neurobiology, 2nd ed. Philadelphia, WB Saunders, 1992, pp 213–228.
10. Vallbo ÅAB, Olsson KÅA, Westberg K-G, et al: Microstimulation of single tactile afferents from the human hand. Brain 1984;107: 727–749.
11. Vallbo ÅAB, Johansson RS: The tactile sensory innervation of the glabrous skin of the human hand. *In* Gordon G (ed): Active Touch: The Mechanisms of Recognition of Objects by Manipulation, A Multi-Disciplinary Approach. Oxford, Pergamon, 1978, pp 29–54.
12. Birder LA, Perl ER: Cutaneous sensory receptors. J Clin Neurophysiol 1994;11:534–552.
13. Johnson KO, Hsaio SS: Neural mechanisms of tactual form and texture perception. Annu Rev Neurosci 1992;15:227–250.
14. LaMotte RH, Srinivasan MA: Tactile discrimination of shape: Responses of slowly adapting mechanoreceptive afferents to a step stroked across the finger pad. J Neurosci 1987;214:1655–1671.
15. Macefield G, Gandevia SC, Burke D: Perceptual responses to microstimulation of single afferents innervating joints, muscles, and skin of the human hand. J Physiol 1990;429:113–129.
16. Burke D, Gandevia SC, McKeon B: The afferent volleys responsible for spinal proprioceptive reflexes in man. J Physiol 1983;339:535.
17. Burgess PR, Perl ER: Cutaneous mechanoreceptors and nociceptors. *In* Iggo A (ed): Handbook of Sensory Physiology, Vol 2. Berlin, Springer-Verlag, 1973, pp 29–78.
18. Gilliatt RW, Willison RG: Peripheral nerve conductions in diabetic neuropathy. J Neurol Neurosurg Psychiatry 1962;25:11–18.
19. Koerber HR, Druzinsky RE, Mendell LM: Properties of somata of spinal dorsal root ganglion cells differ according to peripheral receptor innervated. J Neurophysiol 1988;60:1584–1596.
20. Brodal A: Neurological Anatomy in Relation to Clinical Medicine, 3rd ed. Oxford, Oxford University Press, 1981, pp 46–147.
21. Ross RT: Dissociated loss of vibration, joint position and discriminatory tactile senses in disease of spinal cord and brain. Can J Neurol Sci 1991;18:312–319.
22. Powell TPS, Mountcastle VB: Some aspects of the functional organization of the postcentral gyrus of the monkey: A correlation of findings obtained in a single unit analysis with cytoarchitecture. Bull Johns Hopkins Hosp 1959;105:133–162.
23. Erkerot CF, Larson B: Differential termination of the exteroceptive and proprioceptive components of the cuneocerebellar tract. Brain Res 1972;36:420–424.
24. Jones LA: The perception of force and weight: Theory and research. Psychol Bull 1986;100:29–42.
25. Talbot WH, Darian-Smith I, Kornhuber HH, et al: The sense of flutter-vibration: Comparison of the human capacity with response patterns of mechanoreceptive afferents from the monkey hand. J Neurophysiol 1968;31:301–334.
26. Holmes G: Disorders of sensation produced by cortical lesions. Brain 1927;50:413–427.
27. Mountcastle VB, Talbot WH, Sakata H, et al: Cortical neuronal mechanisms in flutter-vibration studies in unanesthetized monkeys: Neuronal periodicity and frequency discrimination. J Neurophysiol 1969;32:452–484.
28. Jones LA: Peripheral mechanisms of touch and proprioception. Can J Physiol Pharmacol 1994;72:484–487.
29. Schneider RC, Khan EA, Crosby EC, et al (eds): Correlative Neurosurgery, 3rd ed. Springfield, IL, Charles C Thomas, 1982, p 1022.
30. Bickerstaff ER (ed): Neurological Examination in Clinical Practice, 3rd ed. Oxford, Blackwell Scientific Publications, 1973.
31. Gelberman RH, Szabo RM, Williamson RV, et al: Sensibility testing in peripheral nerve compression syndromes. J Bone Joint Surg 1983;6:632–638.
32. Dellon AL: Clinical use of vibratory stimuli to evaluate peripheral nerve injury and compression neuropathy. Plast Reconstr Surg 1980;65:466–476.
33. Cohen LA: Analysis of position sense in human shoulder. J Neurophysiol 1957;21:550–568.
34. Weber EH: Tastsinn und Gemeingefühl. *In* Wagner R (ed): Handwörterbuch der Physiologie. Brunswick F Vieweg u Sohn, 1842,

p 401. Reprinted in Ostwald W: Klassiker der Exacten Wissenschaften. Leipsig, W. Englemann, 1905.
35. Rumpf J: Ueber einen Fall von Syringomyelie nebst Beitragen zur Untersuchung der Sensibilitat. Neurol Zentralbl 1889;8:185.
36. Symms JLM: A method of stimulating the vibratory sensation, with some notes on its application in diseases of the peripheral and central nervous system. Lancet 1918;1:217.
37. Williamson RT: Vibration sensation in disease of the central nervous system. Am J Med Sci 1922;164:715–727.
38. Cosh JA: Studies on the nature of vibration sense. Clin Sci 1953;12:131–151.
39. Thibault A, Forget R, Lambert J: Evaluation of cutaneous and proprioceptive sensation in children: A reliability study. Dev Med Child Neurol 1994;36:796–812.
40. Pearson GH: Effect of age on vibratory sensibility. Arch Neurol Psychiatry 1928;20:482–496.
41. Bell-Krotoski JA: Light touch-deep pressure testing using Semmes-Weinstein monofilaments. *In* Hunter JM, Schneider LW, Mackin EJ, et al (eds): Rehabilitation of the Hand: Surgery and Therapy. St. Louis, C. V. Mosby, 1990, pp 585–593.
42. Omar GE: Sensibility testing. *In* Omer GE, Spinner M (eds): Management of Peripheral Nerve Injuries. Philadelphia, WB Saunders, 1980, pp 3–15.
43. Tornbury JM, Mistretta CM: Tactile sensitivity as a function of age. J Gerontol 1981;36:34–39.
44. Dannenbaum RM, Jones LA: The assessment and treatment of patients who have sensory loss following cortical lesions. J Hand Ther 1993;6:130–138.
45. Jones AB, Llewellyn LJ: Malingering or the Simulation of Disease. London, William Heinemann, 1917.
46. McLeod JG, Turk RR: Disorders of the autonomic nervous system: II. Investigation and treatment. Ann Neurol 1987;21:519.
47. McArthur JC, Stocks EA, Hauer P, Cornblath DR, Griffin JW: Epidermal nerve fiber density: Normative reference range and diagnostic efficiency. Arch Neurol 1998;55(12):1513–1520.
48. Barohn RJ: Intraepidermal nerve fiber assessment: A new window on peripheral neuropathy. Arch Neurol 1998;55(12):1505–1506.
49. Lauria G, Sghirlanzoni A, Lombardi R, Pareyson D: Epidermal nerve fiber density in sensory ganglionopathies: Clinical and neurophysiologic correlations. Muscle Nerve 2001;24(8):1034–1039.
50. Thomas PK, Ochoa J: Clinical features and differential diagnosis. *In* Dyck PJ, Thomas PK (eds): Peripheral Neuropathy, 3rd ed. Philadelphia, WB Saunders, 1993, pp 749–774.
51. Sabin TD: Classification of peripheral neuropathy: The long and short of it. Muscle Nerve 1986;9:711.
52. Chad DA, Recht LD: Neuromuscular complications of systemic cancer. Neurol Clin 1991;9:901–918.
53. Head H: Sensation and the cerebral cortex. Brain 1918;41:58–201.
54. Gould R, Miller BL, Goldberg MA, et al: The validity of hysterical signs and symptoms. J Nerv Ment Dis 1986;174:593–597.
55. Rolak L: Psychogenic sensory loss. J Nerv Ment Dis 1988;176:686–687.
56. Schatt AH: Hand rehabilitation. *In* DeLisa JA, Ganz BM (eds): Rehabilitation Medicine, 2nd ed. Philadelphia, JB Lippincott, 1993, pp 1191–1205.

CHAPTER 20

RENATO J. VERDUGO, JOSÉ G. CEA, MARIO CAMPERO, and JOSÉ LUIS CASTILLO

Pain and Temperature

History and Definitions

The theory of the specificity of sensation, proposed at the end of the last century, maintains that a separate anatomical pathway conveys each type of sensation. This theory has been repeatedly questioned. Sir Henry Head postulated the existence of two sets of sensory inputs to the central nervous system (CNS), the epicritic and the protopathic inputs. Epicritic sensation allowed discrimination of touch, temperature, and pain, whereas protopathic sensation was a poorly localized, unpleasant, and long-lasting sensation. This protopathic sensation was physiologically inhibited in the CNS by the epicritic system. Head based his conclusions on careful observations of the recovery of sensation after experimental division of his own cutaneous nerves. Later, Trotter and Davies dismissed the theory of epicritic and protopathic sensations after performing equally careful experiments on themselves, maintaining that Head's findings could all be attributed to activity in the regenerating nerve fibers. The debate continues about whether sensation, particularly pain, is the result of a pattern of activity in the afferent sensory pathways or of activity in separate specific channels.

Pain is the consequence of stimulation of pain-sensitive structures and is often an early sign of disease or tissue damage. When pain is the result of physiological activity in the normal pain receptors, and there is no primary dysfunction of the nervous system, it is called nociceptive pain. Nociceptive pain may indicate a disorder in any other system or organ, and its diagnosis and treatment involve different medical specialties. Pain resulting from the dysfunction of the central or peripheral nervous system is called neuropathic pain,[1] and its treatment usually involves the neurological team. Neuropathic pain actually involves different kinds of pain and reflects several different pathophysiological mechanisms (see later discussion).

Clinical History

Sensory dysfunction involves two types of symptoms: "negative" and "positive" sensory phenomena.[2] A negative sensory phenomenon is an expression of a deficit of sensory function such as loss of warm or cold sensation or hypalgesia. However, patients rarely recognize these deficits, and because of the protective role of nociceptors, such deficits frequently lead to painless, repetitive traumatic lesions such as those occurring in the hands among patients with syringomyelia or in the feet of diabetics.

A positive sensory phenomenon is an expression of an abnormally increased function of the sensory system such as paresthesias or neuropathic pain. Neuropathic pain may be spontaneous or stimulus-induced.[2] Spontaneous neuropathic pain has certain attributes that must be explored separately: quality, intensity, and distribution. Spontaneous pain may have a burning quality, usually referred to the skin, when it is the expression of discharges of the peripheral C-nociceptors.[3] Such pain may be sharp when it is caused by excitation of small myelinated A-delta nociceptive cutaneous afferents.[2] Electric-like shooting pains, radiating to a limb segment or the face, are usually the result of the generation of ectopic impulses in the nociceptive pathways.[4] Unmyelinated C-fiber muscle afferents responsive to noxious mechanical and chemical stimuli have been described in the awake human being. Activity in this type of afferent is perceived as a cramp-like sensation.[5]

In evaluating pain, it is useful to rate its intensity using verbal or visual analogue scales to record changes over time or with response to treatment. A frequently used scale rates pain between 0 and 10, 0 being no pain and 10 being "the worst pain one can imagine." The distribution of pain helps to localize the site of the lesion; for example, radicular, nerve, plexus, and central pains have a more or less stereotyped distribution (see later discussion).

Stimulus-induced neuropathic pain is traditionally divided into allodynia (pain induced by a stimulus that is normally not painful) and hyperalgesia (increased pain produced by a stimulus that normally causes pain). In clinical practice, hyperalgesia and allodynia always coexist, and in this text the term hyperalgesia is used to refer to both. Hyperalgesia is usually elicited by mechanical and thermal stimuli. Mechanical hyperalgesia has been divided into dynamic and static subtypes.[6] Dynamic mechanical hyperalgesia is the unpleasant sensation induced by light stroking of the skin; static mechanical hyperalgesia is pain induced by sustained light pressure of the symptomatic area. Selective blockade of myelinated fibers abolishes dynamic mechanical hyperalgesia without affecting static hyperalgesia. In thermal hyperalgesias, a thermal stimulus, either cold or heat, is perceived as abnormally painful.[7]

Spontaneous pain and hyperalgesia may be influenced by several factors, especially temperature. For example, heat may increase burning pain owing to the sensitization of C-nociceptors, whereas cold may relieve it. On the other hand, cold increases spontaneous burning pain in patients with selective loss of small myelinated fibers.[7] Patients with neuropathic pain often volunteer information about autonomic symptoms such as sweating and trophic alterations. An increase in temperature may be an expression of vasomotor sympathetic denervation or neurogenic inflammation.[8] A decrease in temperature may be the result of a reflex increase in sympathetic vasomotor tone in response to pain or the development of sympathetic denervation supersensitivity.

Neuropathic pain is usually chronic or recurrent, as in diabetic polyneuropathy or in the recurrent attacks of lancinating root pain. An exception is the acute burning pain characteristic of herpes zoster.

Anatomy of Pain and Temperature Sensation

RECEPTORS AND FIRST ORDER NEURONS

Pain and temperature are sensations mediated at a primary afferent level by fibers of a smaller diameter than those mediating touch, vibration, and position sense. Cold sensation is mediated by small myelinated fibers (A-delta fibers) and possibly by unmyelinated afferents;[9] warm sensation is mediated by unmyelinated warm specific C fibers, and pain is mediated by small myelinated A-delta nociceptors and unmyelinated C, nociceptors.[2] In animals, the cold receptors are located within the superficial layers of the skin, whereas the warm receptors are found deeper. The characteristics of cold and warm receptors in humans are not well understood.

The anatomical and functional aspects of cutaneous pain afferents have been studied in detail. The skin, subcutaneous tissues, muscles, and joints are sensitive to a variety of potentially harmful mechanical, thermal, and chemical stimuli. Numerous free nerve endings are responsible for conveying sensory information that is decoded as pain in the central nervous system. Although the ultrastructural characteristics of pain receptors (nociceptors) are not well known, classically two types have been characterized in the human skin according to their receptor-response features: those associated with unmyelinated C fibers and those associated with small myelinated A-delta fibers.[2]

The glabrous and hairy skin is richly innervated by nociceptors with unmyelinated C fibers. These are known as C-polymodal nociceptors (CPNs) because they respond to a variety of noxious stimuli (i.e., mechanical, thermal, and chemical stimuli). A single CPN innervates an area of skin approximately 1 cm square, usually in a single continuous receptive field. These nociceptors have thresholds that are well below the level at which actual tissue damage occurs. CPNs respond to capsaicin, the active substance of hot pepper, and other chemical stimuli such as acid pH and bradykinin. These CPNs also respond to temperatures below 15° C.[10]

A-delta nociceptors have been described in detail in the skin of subhuman primates, but their features have been studied less thoroughly in humans. In humans they seem to respond mainly to mechanical stimulation. A-delta nociceptors display a smaller, usually punctiform, receptive field and have higher mechanical and heat thresholds than CPNs.

A third type of cutaneous nociceptor composed of unmyelinated C fibers has been recently described. These nociceptors are activated only during inflammation. In the absence of inflammatory changes, they do not respond even to very high noxious stimulation.[11] These afferents have been also described as mechano- and heat-insensitive (MiHi), and different populations of MiHi afferents possibly mediate hyperalgesia and itch.[12, 13]

The sensations evoked by activation of A-delta and C nociceptors are different. Excitation of cutaneous CPNs evokes a pure burning sensation, as demonstrated during selective microneurographic stimulation of CPNs[3] and during selective blockade of myelinated fibers during compression ischemia.[14] A-delta nociceptors evoke sharp pain that is projected to a punctiform area.

In addition to their role in pain sensation, CPNs are involved in neurogenic inflammation. Excitation of CPNs determines release of algogenic substances from nociceptive terminals in the skin, causing local vasodilatation and thus reddening of the skin. This flare reaction spreads some centimeters around the site of stimulation through an axonal reflex that depends on a network of fine dermal afferent fibers, originally described as a nocifensor system.[8] Denervation of the skin impairs the flare reaction.

It is classically stated that after experimental injury, an area of flare appears around the site of the injury and the area of hyperalgesia widens. Hyperalgesia occurring at the site of injury is defined as primary hyperalgesia and is a characteristic response to heat and mechanical stimuli.[15] Hyperalgesia that occurs in a wider area of undamaged surrounding skin is defined as secondary hyperalgesia. It is also classically stated that secondary hyperalgesia extending beyond the area of flare is elicited only by mechanical stimulation. It has long been accepted that primary hyperalgesia is the consequence of sensitization of CPNs at the site of the injury, whereas secondary hyperalgesia is due to plastic changes in the CNS.[16] The latter theory is supported by the fact that sensitized CPNs have not been regularly found in areas of secondary hyperalgesia, and plastic changes in dorsal horn neurons take place after peripheral injuries. Nevertheless, it is possible that secondary hyperalgesia relies also on peripheral mechanisms as originally proposed by Lewis.[8] In fact, heat hyperalgesia is also present in the area of secondary mechanical hyperalgesia when heat pain is tested with suprathreshold stimuli; furthermore, the area of flare is wider than that traditionally considered to match the area of both mechanical and heat hyperalgesia.[17] Finally, MiHi nociceptors develop heat and mechanical sensitivity in areas of secondary hyperalgesia.[18]

SECOND ORDER NEURONS (Fig. 20–1)

Both A-delta and C-primary nociceptive afferents have their cell bodies in the dorsal root ganglion and synapse centrally with second order neurons located in the dorsal horns. However, before contacting second order neurons in the spinal cord, the axons of these afferents divide into descending and ascending branches that run a few segments in the tract of Lissauer, giving off collaterals to the superficial layers of the dorsal horn. At least three types of neurons are distributed in the superficial layers of the dorsal horn in cats and subhuman primates. These are (1) nociceptive-specific neurons, (2) wide dynamic range (WDR) neurons, and (3) inhibitory and excitatory interneurons.[19] Nociceptive-specific neurons, located mainly in lamina I of Rexed, receive inputs mainly from primary nociceptive afferents. These neurons project into the contralateral spinothalamic tract, and their activity is modulated by local interneurons. WDR neurons, although responding more vigorously to inputs from nociceptive afferents, also discharge in response to nonnoxious stimuli. They are mostly located in lamina V, although some of them are also found in laminae I and II. It has been proposed that in humans these neurons also project into the contralateral spinothalamic tract.[20]

Neurophysiological experiments in animals have shown that sensitization and expansion of the receptive fields of second order neurons occur following massive input from primary nociceptive afferents induced by a peripheral tissue injury. This finding has led to the hypothesis that, after a peripheral injury, input from low-threshold mechanoreceptors evokes pain rather than tactile sensation, and this pain may spread beyond anatomical peripheral boundaries. However, the behavioral consequences in animals and the clinical expression in humans of these changes are far from clear.[21]

Nociceptive-specific and WDR neurons project mainly through the spinothalamic tract (STT), the most prominent ascending nociceptive pathway in the spinal cord. The axons from lamina I are located dorsolateral to the axons from lamina V in the STT in some mammals. In humans, anterolateral chordotomies largely abolish pain sensitivity, and electrical stimulation of the STT elicits pain.[22] Second order nociceptive neurons also project to higher regions through the spinoreticular, spinomesencephalic, and spinocervical tracts, and some project into the posterior columns.[19] The spinomesencephalic and spinocervical tracts project to the reticular formation, the thalamus, and the periaqueductal gray nuclei.

THIRD ORDER NEURONS

Projections of nociceptive ascending neurons of the dorsal horn end in the ventral posterior nuclei of the thalamus, mainly the ventral posterior lateral (VPL) nucleus. This nucleus receives input from neurons in lamina I and V and projects to the primary somatosensory cortex.[20] The ventral posterior medial nucleus receives input from second order nociceptive neurons in the trigeminal nuclei. Additionally, the intralaminar nuclei, which have complex receptive fields, receive input from the deep dorsal horn laminae and the reticular formation of the brain stem. This thalamic region is probably concerned with arousal rather than with pain sensation itself. On leaving the dorsal horn, these axons sweep anteriorly in the spinal cord, cross the midline, and ascend to the VPL nucleus of the thalamus. The tract is laminated in that the sacral fibers are most lateral, followed in turn by the lumbar, thoracic, and cervical fibers.

In the primary somatosensory cortex, two main types of neurons have been described. One group, which receives inputs from the VPL thalamus, displays a small, contralateral receptive field. The other group comprises neurons that have wide receptive fields, usually bilateral; they probably receive inputs from the medial thalamic nuclei. Just as in the other sensory modalities, there is probably a simultaneous process for distributing noxious information to the different cortical areas.[20]

The facial sensations of pain and temperature are carried by cranial nerve V (see Chapter 10) and ascend separately to the thalamus.

The thalamocortical projections and the primary sensory cortex in the parietal lobe have a homuncular sensory pattern,

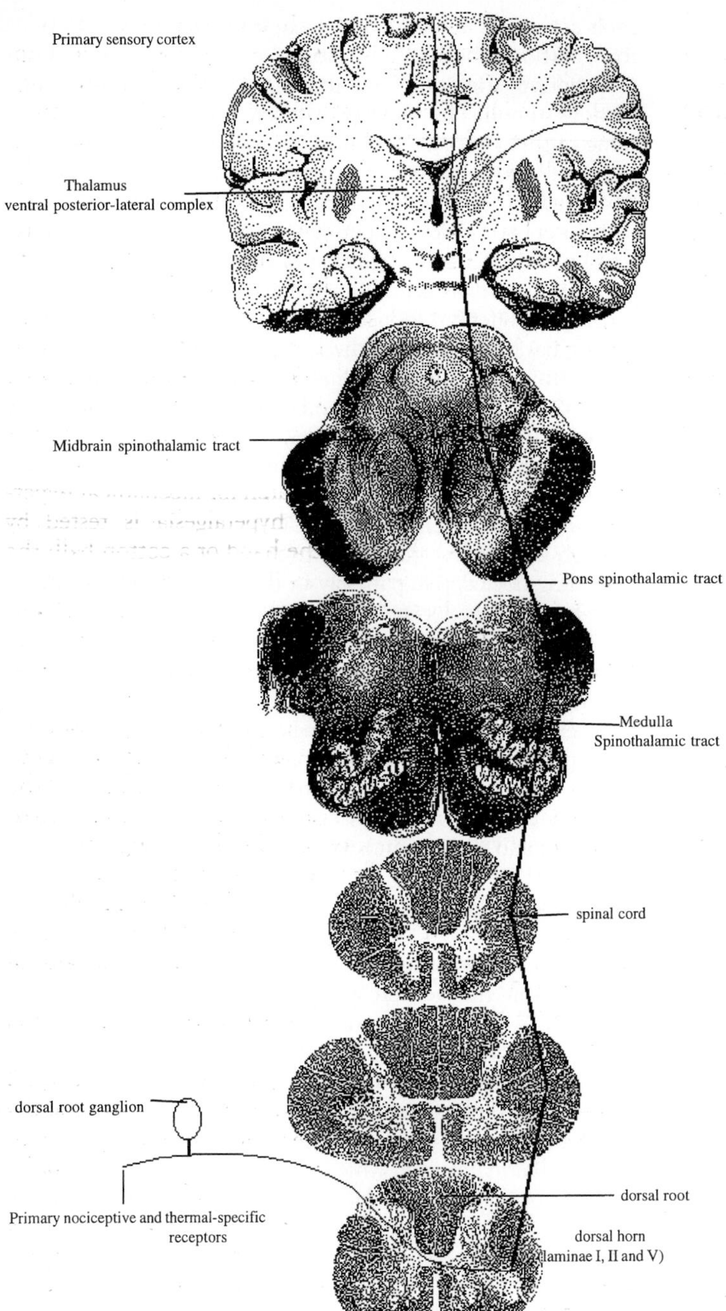

FIGURE 20–1. Pain and temperature pathway. Primary nociceptive and thermospecific afferents with their cell body in the dorsal root ganglia. These afferents send their central projection to the superficial laminae of the dorsal horns (laminae I to IV). Second order neurons project mainly into the contralateral spinothalamic tract ascending through the lateral brain stem to the ventral posterior lateral and to the anterior and intralaminar thalamic nuclei. These third order afferent neurons project into the primary sensory cortex.

in which the projections for the face are closest to the sylvian fissure, those for the hand and arm are above, and those for the leg lie near the central sulcus. In the thalamocortical projections and the cortex, all sensory modalities coalesce (see Chapter 19).

PAIN CONTROL MECHANISMS IN THE CENTRAL NERVOUS SYSTEM

Electrical stimulation of the periaqueductal gray matter reduces the perception of pain by suppressing the activity in the ascending nociceptive pathways. Descending pathways terminating in nociceptive neurons in the spinal cord carry out this modulation. Neurons in the periaqueductal and periventricular gray matter send excitatory connections to the serotoninergic raphe magnus and gigantocellularis nuclei and pass through the posterior columns to inhibit nociceptive second order neurons in the superficial dorsal horns directly. The nuclei also activate enkephalin interneurons. Enkephalin interneurons presynaptically inhibit the input from the primary nociceptive afferents.

Local circuits in the dorsal horn are essential for processing nociceptive input and modulating ascending and descending nociceptive pathways. Primary C-nociceptive fibers act on second order dorsal horn neurons through the release of substance P and glutamate; the former acts on neurokinin receptors and the latter on N-methyl-D aspartate receptors. These receptors are important in the long-term sensitization of dorsal horn neurons that is possibly involved in neuropathic pain. Descending noradrenergic and serotoninergic pathways contact dendrites of the spinothalamic tract neurons as well as enkephalin-containing inhibitory neurons in the superficial dorsal horn. Enkephalin-containing dorsal horn interneurons inhibit the release of glutamate and substance P from primary nociceptive neurons. These interneurons also suppress nociceptive input postsynaptically on spinothalamic tract neurons.

Opiates seem to exert an analgesic effect at the same sites where analgesia is produced by electrical stimulation. The mesencephalic periaqueductal gray matter and the rostral ventral medulla are extremely sensitive to morphine. Mu receptors are found mainly in the mesencephalic periaqueductal gray matter and in the superficial dorsal horn together with enkephalin-containing neurons. The activity of the descending pathways that control nociceptive inputs is thought to be excitatory on inhibitory morphine-sensitive interneurons. Recent observations indicate that in addition to their central action, opiates modulate primary nociceptive afferents at a receptor level.[22]

GATE CONTROL THEORY

Sir Henry Head was the first to propose that activity in large-caliber afferent fibers may modulate activity in the pain pathway. In 1959, based on observations in patients with postherpetic neuralgia, Noordenbos[23] proposed that after a nerve lesion affecting mainly myelinated nerves occurred, disinhibition of second order neurons in the dorsal horns followed, resulting in hyperalgesia. Later, Melzack and Wall[24] proposed the gate control theory of pain, which suggested that activity in low-threshold mechanoreceptors inhibited the discharges in second order nociceptive afferents through an inhibitory interneuron. This theory is supported by the observation that pain is relieved by transcutaneous electrical nerve stimulation (TENS), which may stimulate predominantly large-caliber afferent fibers. However, the specific effect of TENS remains to be proved.

The gate control theory of pain contrasts with more recent results of neurophysiological experiments showing sensitization and expansion of receptive areas of WDR neurons following a transient nociceptive input to the spinal cord. These plastic changes would allow input from low-threshold mechanoreceptors to excite second order neurons, signaling pain.[21] Recent re-evaluations of the TENS unit cast doubt on its conclusive utility[25] and suggest that its beneficial effect may be largely attributed to placebo effects.[26]

Examination of Pain and Temperature Sensory Systems (Table 20–1)

DIRECTED NEUROLOGICAL EXAMINATION

In a patient complaining of pain with neuropathic characteristics, the neurological evaluation is a fundamental step that has two goals: first, to establish the presence or absence of a neurological lesion, and second, to determine the relationship between the neurological lesion found and the symptoms of the patient.

A full sensory examination is necessary in any patient with sensory symptoms. This is not an easy task and requires the full attention and cooperation of the patient. Since cold, warm, and pain sensations are mediated by different systems, the indemnity of one of them does not imply normality of the others. Cold and warm sensations can be examined at the bedside using tubes filled with cold or hot water. As each stimulus is gently applied to a body area, the patient should respond as soon as he or she feels the temperature stimulus by identifying its quality. A correct response that requires several seconds to be sensed may indicate slowed conduction along pain pathways. Pain is usually evaluated by disposable pinprick testing. Comparing a patient's response to a sharp and a dull stimulus monitors the integrity of this system; again, both the rapidity and the accuracy of the response must be assessed. The neurological evaluation must also include a search for mechanical hyperalgesias. Dynamic mechanical hyperalgesia is tested by lightly rubbing the skin with the hand or a cotton ball; the patient with a lesion feels an unpleasant burning sensation. To test for static mechanical hyperalgesia, a fixed mechanical stimulus such as a mild pinch is applied to the skin; the patient with a sensory abnormality describes an intense sharp or burning pain.

In the neurological examination, the clinician must consider the distribution of negative and positive sensory manifestations. A peripheral polyneuropathy affecting the small-caliber afferent fibers causes warm and cold hypesthesia and hypalgesia in a typical distal stocking and glove distribution. The areas of mechanical and cold or hot hyperalgesias may initially be distal, but as the pathological process becomes worse and the most distal parts become denervated, hyperalgesia is only found more proximally in the extremity.

In patients with lesions of a peripheral root or nerve trunk, negative and positive sensory manifestations are usually confined to the anatomical territory of the nerve or root affected. Occasionally, the area of hyperalgesia may expand beyond the relevant anatomical territory. This phenomenon has been explained by the plastic changes occurring in second order sensory neurons,[21] but, as discussed earlier, the clinical expressions of these plastic changes are unknown. When a peripheral nerve lesion causes the painful syndrome, expansion of the area of hyperalgesia beyond its anatomical boundaries seldom occurs.[27]

In patients with central disorders, the distribution of positive and negative sensory manifestations also helps to localize the lesion. With syringomyelia, a typical bilateral segmental distribution of pain and temperature sensory loss occurs in the cervical segments because of the central cord involvement of the crossing second order neuronal axons. In patients with brain stem lesions, there may be a loss of pinprick and thermal sensations on the ipsilateral side of the face and the contralateral side of the body. In those with thalamic lesions, the sensory manifestations involve the entire contralateral half of the body; although they are often vaguely localized, they can be intensely uncomfortable. Hemispheric lesions are more prominent on the face and upper extremity or on the lower extremity alone, depending on whether the damage involves the convexity or the medial aspect of the hemispheres.

TABLE 20–1. **Clinico-anatomical Correlation of Disorders of Pain and Temperature Sensations**

Anatomical Site of Damage	Sensory Findings	Other Neurological and Medical Findings	Common Etiologies	Comments
Sensory Receptors	Hypesthesia to cold and warm and hypoalgesia	Changes in skin color, edema, hypo- or hyperthermia	Traumatic or surgical scars	
Primary Neuron				
Peripheral nerve	Hypesthesia to cold and warm or mechanical hyperalgesia in stocking and glove or dermatomal distribution	Redness of skin, hyperthermia, swelling Pale discoloration of skin, coldness Distal muscle weakness and atrophy, diminished tendon reflexes	Diabetic polyneuropathy, traumatic and entrapment neuropathies, plexopathies	Examination of responses to cold, warmth, and pain is the most useful tool for localizing a painful nerve lesion
Sensory root ganglion	Asymmetrical numbness, tingling, and lancinating pains. Loss of position sense	Pupillary abnormalities, areflexia	Neoplasia, Sjögren's syndrome, monoclonal gammopathy	
Secondary Neurons				
Internal arcuate	Suspended loss of pain and temperature sensations. Less impairment of touch, vibration, and position senses	Distal muscle atrophy and areflexia in upper extremities; trophic changes in the hands	Syringomyelia, central spinal cord tumors	Clinical presentation may be asymmetrical
Lateral ST tract	Contralateral loss of cold, warm, and pain sensations. Sometimes spontaneous pain and mechanical hyperalgesia. Ipsilateral loss of joint position and vibration senses	Ipsilateral pyramidal syndrome, Horner's syndrome, cerebellar signs	Lateral compression of spine (Brown-Séquard syndrome), lateral infarction of medulla (Wallenberg's syndrome)	"Classic" traumatic hemisection of the spine is rare
Tertiary Neurons				
VPL, VPM	Contralateral hypesthesia for all sensory modalities. Lancinating spontaneous pain	Contralateral pyramidal syndrome, homonymous hemianopia	Thalamic hemorrhage or infarction	
Internal capsule	Contralateral sensory loss	May present with pure sensory loss or with contralateral pyramidal syndrome	Deep small infarction	
Sensory cortex	Hemisensory loss is greater in lower or upper extremity	Neglect, aphasia	Large vessel infarct, tumors	

VPL, Ventral posterior lateral nucleus: VPM, ventral posterior medial nucleus; ST, spinothalamic.

ASSOCIATED NEUROLOGICAL FINDINGS

Cerebral. Contralateral sensory neglect, sometimes associated with sensory loss, is a feature of cortical lesions affecting the right hemisphere. In patients with thalamic lesions, tactile, vibration, and position senses are also lost in the contralateral side of the body, frequently associated with hemianopsia and motor hemiparesis. Contralateral sensory neglect is difficult to evaluate in patients with thalamic lesions owing to the prominent sensory loss. It has been traditionally stated that thalamic pain is particularly distressing, although this statement may be applicable to any chronic neuropathic pain syndrome.

Cranial Nerves. Lesions affecting the lateral spinothalamic tract in the pons may involve the ipsilateral cranial nerves V and VII. In the medulla, the lateral spinothalamic tract is close to cranial nerves IX and X, the descending trigeminal nucleus, the sympathetic pathway, and the cerebellum. Vascular lesions involving these structures cause the classic Wallenberg syndrome.

Motor/Reflexes/Cerebellar/Gait. Hemispheric lesions may cause contralateral hemiparesis in addition to hemisensory impairment. Brain stem lesions cause contralateral limb weakness with cranial nerve involvement ipsilateral to the lesion. Syringomyelia characteristically involves the anterior horn cells, causing muscle weakness and atrophy in the hands. With peripheral neuropathy, distal weakness occurs and is usually of greater magnitude in the lower extremities.

When the thick myelinated afferent fibers in the periphery or dorsal columns are involved, an ataxic sensory gait may be seen. In lumbar radicular pain syndrome, the patient assumes an antalgic posture with the knee of the affected side in partial flexion and the back bent toward or away from the painful side.

Autonomic Nervous System. Sweating may be disturbed in patients with several neuropathic pain disorders. When the autonomic fibers are spared, sweating is usually increased because of the greater activity of the sympathetic fibers. At the same time, the affected limb may be cold because of the increased sympathetic tone. It must be kept in mind that coldness may also be an expression of increased vasoconstriction due to sympathetic denervation supersensitivity. Warmth and redness of the painful parts may be an expression of sympathetic denervation (before the development of supersensitivity) or antidromic discharge of C nociceptors causing neurogenic inflammation. Orthostatic hypotension, resting tachycardia, and impairment of reflex tachycardia to hypotension are signs of autonomic dysfunction that are easily assessed at the bedside.

Neurovascular. Painful neuropathies, especially in diabetics, may be associated with evidence of small vessel disease in the form of poor distal pulses and retinal vessel abnormalities. In patients with sudden onset of pain syndromes in a stroke-like distribution, the neurovascular examination may reveal large vessel abnormalities and differences in the carotid pulses on palpation.

ASSOCIATED MEDICAL FINDINGS

Trophic changes are common in neuropathies involving small-caliber afferents such as diabetic polyneuropathy. These include loss of hair and skin atrophy to deep ulcers in the feet. Visceral enlargements may be found in patients with neuropathies associated with alcohol, neoplasm, polyneuropathy, organomegaly, endocrinopathy, monoclonal protein and skin changes (POEMS), and amyloidosis. Patients with vasculitic neuropathies may have skin petechiae, respiratory symptoms, and signs and evidence of hepatic or renal involvement.

Evaluation Guidelines (Table 20–2)

Neuroimaging. Magnetic resonance imaging (MRI) is a useful procedure for investigating morphological changes in the peripheral nerve trunks and plexus. It is useful in the evaluation of traumatic lesions, tumors of the peripheral nerves, and adjacent tissues involving the nerves or plexus. MRI is also the most useful imaging test for the evaluation of structural disorders of the spinal cord and roots. Computed tomography is a complementary test used to evaluate bone changes in the spine. Radiographs of the spine are limited to the study of bone and joint lesions.

Electrophysiology. Several neurophysiological tests are used to evaluate disorders of the central or peripheral nervous system affecting pain and temperature sensations. Nerve conduction studies and needle electromyography allow for precise localization and characterization of a peripheral nerve lesion disclosing an axonal or demyelinating disorder. It must be stressed that conventional electrophysiological studies evaluate the function of motor and large-caliber afferent fibers, leaving unexplored the function of small-caliber afferents involved in pain and temperature sensation. Furthermore, conventional electrophysiological studies are unable to explore the pathophysiological substrate of positive sensory phenomena, even those involving large-caliber afferents such as cutaneous paresthesias. Therefore, a normal nerve conduction study does not necessarily rule out a peripheral nerve lesion as the cause of the pain. Conversely, an abnormal study does not necessarily imply that an identified peripheral nerve lesion is the cause of painful symptoms.

Microneurography is the process of recording the electrical activity of nerve fibers using an intraneural microelectrode. This is an electrophysiological way of exploring small- and large-caliber afferent fibers including the pathophysiological substrate of positive sensory phenomena. The procedure is time consuming and has a high incidence of false-negative results. It is mainly an experimental procedure and is not used in routine clinical studies.

A test commonly used for the routine clinical evaluation of small-caliber afferent pathways is the Quantitative Somatosensory Thermotest (QST).[28] A ramp of ascending or descending stimulating temperature, operating on the Peltier principle, is applied to the skin of the patient through a thermostimulator. It is a psychophysical test in which the patient signals his or her threshold for cold, warmth, cold pain, and heat pain sensations. The threshold for cold sensation is the result of activity of A-delta small myelinated channels specific for cold sensation; the threshold for warm sensation is the expression of function of unmyelinated warm-specific C channels, and cold pain and heat pain sensations are the result of activity of unmyelinated CPNs.[28]

TABLE 20–2. **Useful Studies in the Evaluation of Disorders of Pain and Temperature Sensations**

Syndrome	Neuroimaging	Electrophysiology	Fluid and Tissue Analysis	Neuropsychological Tests	Other Tests
Primary Sensory Neuropathy	Normal	Low-amplitude sensory responses, cold and warm hypesthesia in QST, mild reduction of motor nerve conduction velocity	Nerve biopsy shows axonal loss predominantly of unmyelinated fibers	Normal	
Mononeuropathy	Normal	Impaired motor and sensory nerve conduction across site of lesion, signs of denervation in muscles innervated by nerve affected	Depending on severity of entrapment, focal demyelination and axonal loss occurs, predominantly of large myelinated fibers	Normal	
Diffuse Sensory Polyneuropathy	Normal	Low-amplitude sensory nerve action potentials, hypesthesia to cold and warm sensations in QST	Elevated ESR, glycosylated hemoglobin E, abnormal glucose tolerance test, HIV	Normal	
Multisystem Degeneration	Normal	Normal	Normal	Dementia in some patients	Abnormal ECG
Dorsal Root Ganglia	Normal	Low-amplitude sensory nerve action potentials, normal motor studies, abnormal somatosensory evoked potentials	Monoclonal gammopathies, loss of myelinated fibers in sural nerve biopsy	Normal	Lip biopsy for Sjögren's syndrome
Radiculopathy	MRI of the spine may show disk herniation or osteophyte compression of root	Normal sensory conduction study, low-amplitude CMAP and signs of denervation in needle EMG Thermal hypesthesia in the dermatome in QST, abnormal somatosensory evoked potentials	Normal	Normal	
Plexopathy	Mass compression or infiltration of plexus	Sensory and motor nerve conduction abnormalities Denervation in needle EMG, thermal hypesthesia and possibly thermal hyperalgesia in QST	Elevated ESR		Fracture of pelvis in traumatic injury of sacral plexus; chest x-ray shows apical lung lesions or cervical rib
Syringomyelia	MRI: central spinal cord cavity, extension to medulla Associated Arnold-Chiari malformation	Denervation in affected segments	Normal	Normal	

QST, Quantitative Somatosensory Thermotest; ESR, erythrocyte sedimentation rate; HIV, human immunodeficiency virus; ECG, electrocardiography; AIDS, acquired immunodeficiency syndrome; MRI, magnetic resonance imaging; CMAP, compound muscle action potentials; EMG, electromyography.

The thresholds determined by QST are the result of activity of the whole afferent pathways involved in thermal sensations in the peripheral and central nervous systems, and therefore an abnormal pattern does not have a precise localizing diagnostic value. Nevertheless, certain abnormal patterns are characteristic of some clinical syndromes. A peripheral neuropathy typically produces warm hypesthesia first; as the disease progresses, cold hypesthesia may develop. This pattern occurs because warm sensation depends more on the number of stimulated fibers than cold sensation.[28] In patients with myelopathy without peripheral nerve involvement, pure cold hypesthesia may typically occur.[29, 30] QST may also disclose cold or heat hyperalgesia, showing the presence of abnormally low pain thresholds induced by low or high temperature. Cold or heat hyperalgesias are often present with cold or warm hypesthesias.

Patients with nerve lesions may also have changes in skin temperature[31] that can be measured by thermography. This modality, however, lacks convincing sensitivity and specificity for the diagnosis of the presence of a nerve lesion. The symptomatic area may be hyperthermic or hypothermic. Hyperthermia may be an expression of cutaneous vasodilatation secondary to sympathetic denervation or, alternatively, an expression of antidromically induced vasodilatation by discharges in C nociceptors.[8, 32] Hypothermia is an expression of either a physiological increase in sympathetic vasoconstrictor tone in response to pain or increased vasoconstriction due to sympathetic denervation supersensitivity.[32]

The American Academy of Neurology Therapeutics and Technology Assessment Subcommittee has made specific recommendations for the use of thermography in neurological practice. This report concluded that infrared thermography may provide information about altered cutaneous temperatures and may be useful in characterizing reflex sympathetic dystrophy, focal autonomic neuropathies, and focal nerve injuries. It is not reliably useful for evaluating neck and back pain, radiculopathy, musculoskeletal pain, or entrapment neuropathy.[33]

Electrophysiological study of the central somatosensory pathways is done classically through somatosensory evoked potentials by electrical stimulation of the peripheral nerves. This method explores only the large-caliber afferent lemniscal pathway. The recent development of the carbon dioxide laser somatosensory evoked potentials may allow exploration of the small-caliber spinothalamic pathway.

Body Fluid and Tissue Analysis. Fluid, nerve, and muscle biopsies have diagnostic value in inflammatory, neoplastic, deposit (amyloid), and some toxic peripheral neuropathies. Electron microscopy is essential for the morphological evaluation of unmyelinated fibers.

Cerebrospinal Fluid. Neoplastic infiltration of nerve roots may cause an increased cerebrospinal fluid cell count and protein content. Neoplastic cells may also appear.

Clinical Syndromes (see Tables 20–1 and 20–3)

SENSITIZATION OF C-POLYMODAL NOCICEPTORS
(Figs. 20–2 and 20–3)

This syndrome, described by Ochoa,[32] is characterized by burning pain and mechanical hyperalgesia that is increased by heat and relieved by cold. The skin is red and hyperthermic due to neurogenic inflammation. QST shows heat hyperalgesia, frequently combined with warm hypesthesia. The presence of sensitized C nociceptors has been described in a few patients.[34] Similar manifestations can be induced experimentally in normal subjects after injection of capsaicin. CPN sensitization can be seen in many of the conditions described subsequently.

TRIPLE COLD SYNDROME

In the triple cold syndrome there is burning pain that is increased by cold and relieved by heat. The skin is cold and pale because of vasoconstriction due to sympathetic denervation supersensitivity. QST shows cold hypesthesia combined with cold hyperalgesia and a paradoxical hot burning sensation. A lesion composed of small myelinated fibers with relative sparing of unmyelinated fibers has been described in these patients.[35] A similar QST pattern is seen in normal subjects during selective blockade of myelinated fibers. It has been proposed that cold hyperalgesia is due to central release of a C-nociceptive input, which is normally inhibited by cold-specific A-delta fibers.

The triple cold syndrome can be seen in any of the disorders described later, and occasionally, particularly in the elderly, it presents without apparent cause.

PRIMARY SENSORY NEUROPATHY

Primary sensory neuropathies are rare hereditary conditions. Four main types have been described: dominantly inherited sensory neuropathy (hereditary sensory and autonomic neuropathy [HSAN] type I in Dyck's classification,[36] recessively inherited sensory neuropathy or Riley-Day syndrome [HSAN type II], familial dysautonomia [HSAN type III]), and congenital sensory neuropathy with anhidrosis [HSAN type IV]; see Chapter 36).

HSAN type I begins in the second decade of life with impairment mainly of pain and temperature sensations. Spontaneous pain and mutilating acropathy are common. Autonomic symptoms, such as loss of distal sweating and bladder dysfunction, may be present but are not characteristic. As the disease worsens, other sensory modalities are affected, and mild distal muscle wasting and weakness develop. Histological studies have shown that axonal loss occurs, predominantly involving unmyelinated fibers. Motor conduction velocity is usually normal, and sensory action potentials are reduced or absent. There may be distal denervation signs on electromyography (EMG).

HSAN type II is usually present from birth and affects all sensory modalities. There may be autonomic involvement and mild distal muscle weakness. Motor conduction velocity is slightly reduced, and sensory action potentials are absent. EMG may show signs of denervation.

Familial dysautonomia (HSAN type III) is an autosomal recessive disorder most often described in Jews; it is characterized by autonomic disturbances from birth. Absent tendon reflexes and failure to respond to pain are also present. Histologically, severe and moderate losses of unmyelinated and small myelinated axons occur, respectively. The amplitude of sensory action potentials is severely reduced.

In congenital sensory neuropathy with anhidrosis (HSAN type IV), a selective loss of small myelinated axons occurs with an almost complete absence of unmyelinated fibers.

TABLE 20–3. **Selected Etiologies Associated with Disorders of Pain and Temperature Sensation**

Etiological Category	Specific Etiologies	Chapter
Structural Disorders		
Developmental structural disorders	Syringomyelia	28
Degenerative and compressive structural disorders	Herniated disk/radiculopathy, entrapment mononeuropathies	29
Hereditary and Degenerative Disorders		
Storage diseases: Lipidoses, glycogen disorders, and leukoencephalopathies	Adrenomyeloneuropathy Tangier's disease Refsum's disease	30
Amino/organic acidopathies, mitochondrial enzyme defects, and other metabolic errors	Tyrosinosis	31
Chromosomal abnormalities and neurocutaneous disorders	Neurofibromatosis	32
Degenerative dementias	Homocystinuria (deficiency of cobalamin coenzyme synthesis)	33
Movement disorders	Neuroacanthosis	34
Ataxias	Friedreich's ataxia Late-onset cerebellar ataxia	35
Degenerative motor, sensory, and autonomic disorders	Hereditary sensory and autonomic neuropathy (HSAN I–IV), hereditary spastic paraplegia	36
Hereditary nondegenerative neuromuscular disease	Familial amyloid neuropathy	37
Acquired Metabolic and Nutritional Disorders		
Endogenous metabolic disorders	Diabetic polyneuropathy	38
Exogenous acquired metabolic disorders of the nervous system: Toxins and illicit drugs	Arsenic, mercury, platinum *N*-hexane	39
Nutritional deficiencies and syndromes associated with alcoholism	Subacute combined degeneration	40
Infectious Disorders		
Viral infections	Herpes zoster radiculopathy	41
Nonviral infections	Syphilis	42
HIV and AIDS	Mononeuritis multiplex Distal polyneuropathy	44
Neurovascular Disorders	Central post-stroke pain syndromes Anterior spinal artery infarct	45
Neoplastic Disorders		
Primary neurological tumors	Ependymoma	46
Metastatic neoplasms and paraneoplastic syndromes	Extradural cord compression Gangliomas	47
Demyelinating Disorders		
Demyelinating disorders of the central nervous system	Multiple sclerosis	48
Demyelinating disorders of peripheral nervous system	Guillain-Barré and CIDP, POEMS	49
Autoimmune and Inflammatory Disorders	Sjögren's ganglionopathy Mononeuritis multiplex in polyarteritis nodosa	50
Traumatic Disorders	Spinal injuries Brachial plexus and root avulsion Traumatic mononeuropathies	51
Epilepsy	Focal sensory	52
Drug-Induced and Iatrogenic Neurological Disorders	Radiation plexopathies Disulfiram-induced polyneuropathies	55

HIV, Human immunodeficiency virus: AIDS, acquired immunodeficiency syndrome: POEMS, polyneuropathy, organomegaly, endocrinopathy, monoclonal protein, and skin changes: CIDP, chronic inflammatory demyelinating polyneuropathy.

MONONEUROPATHY

A mononeuropathy is a lesion of one nerve by a local process, usually compression or, less frequently, trauma or a vascular cause. Clinical examination typically demonstrates negative and positive sensory phenomena restricted to the territory of the nerve involved. Compression of a nerve affects the myelinated fibers first. Nerve conduction studies may be particularly useful in the detection of additional, more widespread disease of the nerves that predisposes to local lesions, as seen in diabetes (see Chapters 29 and 38).

Entrapment of the median nerve at the carpal tunnel is one of the most common forms of mononeuropathy. Classic

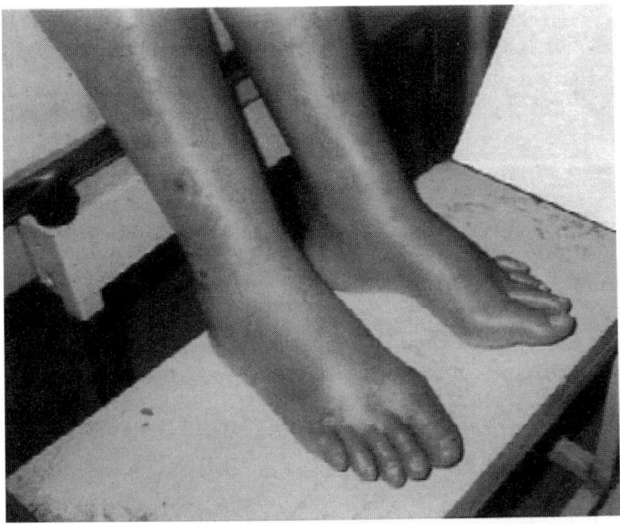

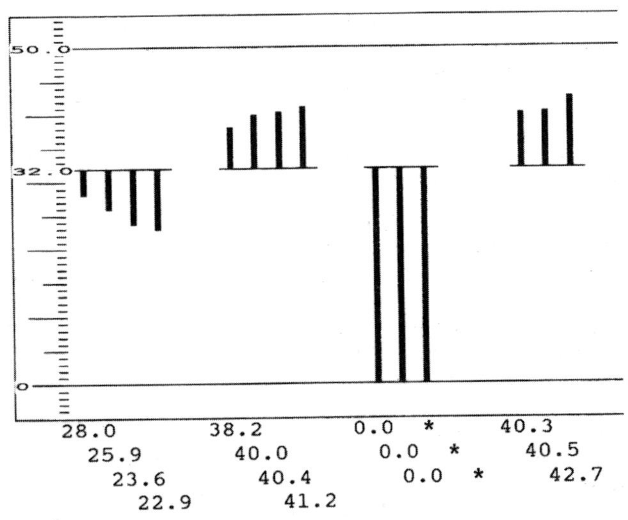

FIGURE 20–2. Typical aspects of the syndrome of sensitization of C-polymodal nociceptors. Left, red and hot skin in stocking distribution in a case of painful polyneuropathy. Right, typical QST pattern. Each vertical line represents the thermal threshold signaled by the patient in the following order: cold and warm sensation and cold and heat pain. Note the combination of warm hypoesthesia (the first four lines up, which correspond to warm sensation, are abnormally high) with heat hyperalgesia (the last four lines up, which correspond to heat pain, are abnormally low).

symptoms include nocturnal paresthesias in the thumb, index, and middle fingers. Numbness, tingling, and burning pain in the median nerve distribution can be present and sometimes awakens the patient from sleep. Pain can be referred to proximal segments up to the shoulder. Hypesthesia to light touch and an increased two-point discrimination threshold in fingers innervated by the median nerve are common findings. Frequently, the sensation in the thenar eminence is not affected because the palmar cutaneous nerve emerges from the median nerve before the carpal tunnel. Mechanical hyperalgesia is sometimes present in the same territory. The presence of atrophy of the thenar eminence and weakness of the intrinsic muscles of the hand innervated by the median nerve depend on the duration of the entrapment. Although it is asymmetrical, the condition is frequently bilateral, the dominant side used for writing being affected more severely. Sensory conduction velocity across the wrist is delayed in more than 90 percent of patients. In most patients, a reduction in motor conduction velocity across the wrist is also present. Several predisposing factors exist: pregnancy, diabetes mellitus, rheumatoid arthritis, hypothyroidism, amyloidosis, gout, acromegaly, and fractures of the wrist. Surgical treatment is recommended if there is sensory loss, muscle weakness, atrophy of the thenar eminence, or severe EMG changes.

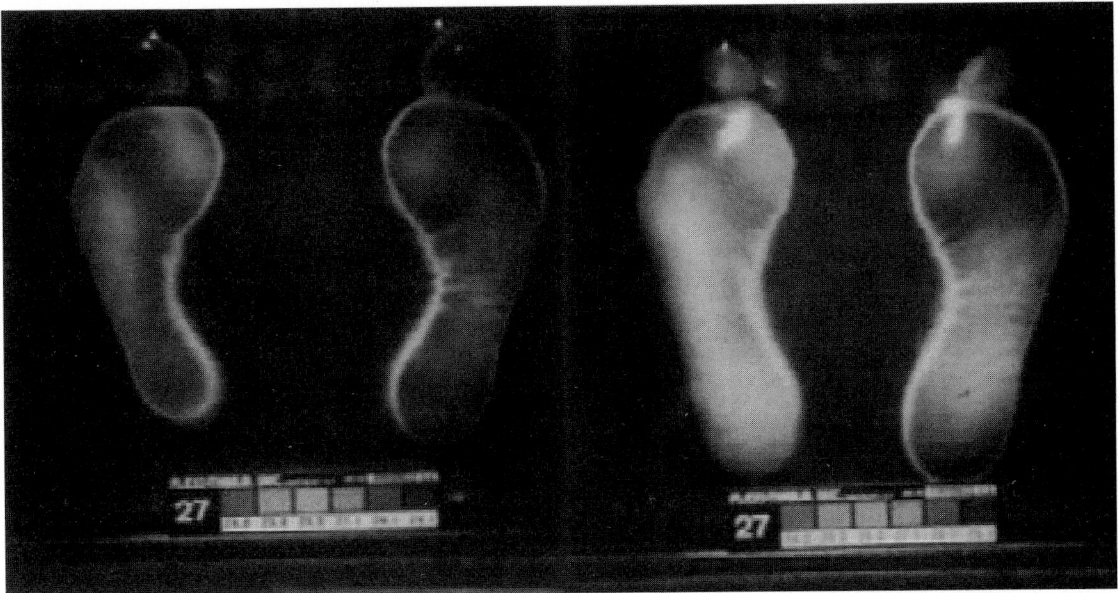

FIGURE 20–3. Thermographic recordings of syndrome of sensitization of C-polymodal nociceptors. Thermographic recording of both feet before (*left*) and after (*right*) immersion of hands in cold water. Note lowering of temperature of the feet in response to immersion of hands in cold water, indicating the presence of sympathetic vasomotor reflex activity.

Meralgia paresthetica is a pure sensory entrapment neuropathy. The lateral femoral cutaneous nerve derives from the second and third lumbar roots within the psoas muscle and runs to the anterior superior iliac spine; it then passes medial to the spine beneath the inguinal ligament, and as it runs down, it divides into anterior and posterior divisions. This nerve is frequently compressed in this course through the inguinal ligament, for example, in pregnancy, in obese patients, or even by a tight belt or corset. It can also be involved in patients with a psoas hematoma or a fracture of the anterior portions of the ilium. Numbness, painful burning, and itching in the lateral aspect of the thigh are the main complaints. Examination reveals hypesthesia to touch and pinprick or dysesthesia in the same area. The diagnosis is made mainly on clinical grounds and can be confirmed by the absence (in 58 percent of cases) or delay latency (17 percent of cases) of the sensory nerve potential of the lateral femoral cutaneous nerve. Underlying diabetes should be excluded. In patients with compression at the inguinal ligament, symptomatic treatment of the pain, weight reduction, and avoidance of tight garments are indicated. In refractory cases neurolysis may be considered.

DIFFUSE SENSORY POLYNEUROPATHY

In polyneuropathies the peripheral nervous system is involved diffusely, and the symptoms and signs are more or less symmetrical, predominantly distal, and of gradual onset. Some exceptions to this distal distribution are seen in those with lead neuropathy, familial amyloidosis type 2, adult-onset Tangier's disease, and occasionally porphyria. Usually all types of fibers are involved, and most neuropathies cause sensory, motor, and autonomic manifestations. Muscle weakness is more prominent in patients with inflammatory demyelinating neuropathy, hereditary motor sensory neuropathy, and porphyria. Sensory deficits are more common in those with diabetic polyneuropathy, carcinoma, Sjögren's syndrome, acquired immunodeficiency syndrome, or inherited conditions. Orthostatic hypotension and other autonomic dysfunctions are usually associated with diabetes, Guillain-Barré syndrome, amyloidosis, porphyria, and sensory inherited neuropathies. Positive sensory phenomena such as pain, paresthesias, and hyperalgesia are also common manifestations of polyneuropathy involving large- and small-caliber afferent fibers. The sensitization of nociceptors and the triple cold syndromes described previously are rare examples of positive sensory phenomena in patients with polyneuropathy, particularly painful diabetic polyneuropathy.

DORSAL ROOT GANGLION SYNDROMES

Sensory ganglionitis is usually acute or subacute and is characterized by rapidly progressive sensory symptoms including sensory ataxia. Frequently, asymmetrical numbness, tingling, and lancinating pains are present in different body segments including the face. These varied symptoms were originally described in patients with tabes dorsalis, arsenic poisoning, and diphtheria. Signs such as pupillary abnormalities, areflexia, and loss of position sense are common. Sensory ganglionitis has also been associated with neoplasias, monoclonal gammopathies, and Sjögren's syndrome. Sural nerve biopsy shows a loss of large myelinated fibers. Inflammatory changes and degeneration or loss of neurons have been found in the dorsal root ganglion in most cases. Reduced or absent sensory nerve action potentials and normal EMG recordings are characteristic features.

RADICULOPATHY

Pain due to root compression is generally accompanied by dermatomal sensory loss, muscle weakness, and decreased or absent tendon reflexes. One of the most common causes of radiculopathy is disk herniation. Compression of the nerve roots by a lateral disk herniation is frequent in the lumbar spine because the posterior vertebral ligament is weaker at the sides than in the center at this level. Because the meningeal sheath follows the roots, radiculopathies can also be caused by leptomeningitis and meningeal carcinomatosis.

Root avulsions occur in the cervical region but are rare in the lower segments. Because epineural and perineural sheaths are absent at the origins of the nerve roots, avulsions occur at this site in stretching accidents.

Herpes zoster radiculopathy is an interesting root lesion characterized by burning pain and skin eruption in a dermatomal distribution. During the acute attack, there is an inflammatory reaction that excites the nociceptors within the nervi nervorum, producing the burning pain that precedes and accompanies the skin eruption. In some patients, the burning pain and mechanical hyperalgesia persist for more than 2 months after the skin lesions have healed (post-herpetic neuralgia). Persistence of the sensitization of nociceptors is a possible mechanism,[37] but a central mechanism has also been proposed based on changes of sensitivity within the area of post-herpetic neuralgia.[38]

PLEXOPATHY

Patients with plexopathies show different patterns of motor and sensory loss, depending on which portion of the plexus is affected. In the upper extremity, plexopathies involving the entire plexus produce weakness and sensory loss from C5–T1. The patient loses all sensation in the whole arm and the ability to make movements. In patients with upper trunk lesions, abduction of the arm and flexion of the forearm are impaired because of C5–C6 sensory loss and decreased biceps and brachioradialis tendon reflexes. Lower trunk lesions cause weakness of the intrinsic muscles of the hand and wrist flexors with sensory loss over the two medial fingers and the medial aspect of the hand and arm. By definition, these are lesions distal to the dorsal rami and dorsal ganglion, so no fibrillations occur in the paraspinal muscles, and there is reduction in amplitude of the sensory nerve action potentials of the nerve involved.

In the lower extremity, plexopathies can affect the lumbar or sacral plexus or both. Lumbar plexopathies (L2–L4) affect hip flexion, extension of the knee, and thigh adduction and present sensory loss in the anteromedial aspect of the thigh and impaired knee reflexes. Sacral plexopathies (L5–S1) affect extension and abduction of the hip, knee flexion, and flexion and dorsiflexion of the foot, and there is sensory impairment in the posterior aspect of the thigh, anterolateral and posterior aspects of the leg, and dorsolateral and plantar surfaces of the foot; the ankle jerk may be decreased or absent. Again, EMG studies are fundamental in localizing the lesion because multiple root lesions may present similar clinical pictures.

Several principles must be kept in mind regarding lesions of the plexus. Stretching and contusion are the main mechanisms of traumatic lesions of the brachial plexus, whereas pelvic fractures and hip surgery are common traumatic causes of lumbosacral lesions. Neoplastic plexopathies are characteristically painful; in the brachial plexus, more than 70 percent involve the lower trunk and are mainly due to axillary lymph node infiltration.[39] In the lumbosacral plexus, neoplastic plexopathies are produced by direct infiltration; the distribution is 31 percent and 51 percent for the lumbar and sacral trunks, respectively.[40] Painless and progressive weakness is the hallmark of radiation plexopathies, which typically occur in the upper trunk of the brachial plexus and in the lower part of the lumbosacral plexus, where they are usually bilateral but asymmetrical.

CENTRAL SPINAL CORD SYNDROME: SYRINGOMYELIA

Syringomyelia is a cavitating disorder of the central spinal cord and is usually located in the lower cervical and upper thoracic segments. A bilateral, frequently asymmetrical, segmental sensory loss of pain and temperature sensations is a common finding. Chronic pain in the impaired segments is an important complaint in about one third of patients. Initially, only the pain and temperature fibers are damaged when they cross the midline, but as the syrinx size increases, the dorsal columns are also affected. Anterior expansion produces segmental areflexia, muscle weakness, and atrophy. The intrinsic muscles of the hand are often affected. The corticospinal pathway can be involved in the later stages. Lower brain stem symptoms and signs can appear when the cavity expands into the medulla oblongata or even into the pons. Cranial nerves IX through XII may be involved, usually asymmetrically. Pain and thermal hypesthesia in the face may occur in the onion skin pattern characteristic of nuclear involvement of the trigeminal nerve. Central nystagmus may also be present.

Spinal trauma, possibly through an intraspinal hematoma, may also cause syringomyelia.[41] Alternatively, a flexion-extension injury mechanism and cord ischemia due to hypotension may also produce a central spinal cord syndrome. The differential diagnosis includes intramedullary tumors. MRI is the most useful method of diagnosis of these pathological processes.

CAUDA EQUINA VERSUS *CONUS MEDULLARIS* SYNDROME (Table 20–4)

Radicular pain is a frequent presentation of the cauda equina syndrome, usually in association with radicular sensory loss (saddle anesthesia), asymmetrical paraplegia with loss of the tendon reflexes, muscle atrophy, and bladder dysfunction. The principal causes of this syndrome are tumors, lumbar spinal stenosis, ruptured lumbar disk, arachnoiditis, and spinal fracture. When the conus medullaris is impaired, radicular pain is less prominent. The principal and early disturbances are urinary retention and constipation. In addition, there may be loss of pinprick sensation in the perianal region, impotence, and sometimes muscle weakness of the lower limb.[42]

TABLE 20–4. **Differences Between Cauda Equina and Conus Lesions**

	Cauda Equina	Conus
Pain	Severe radicular pain	Back pain, less severe radicular pain
Hypesthesia	Radicular sensory loss (saddle hypesthesia)	Usually restricted to perianal region
Motor deficits	Asymmetrical areflexic paraplegia	Distal paresis of lower limbs
Sphincters	Urinary retention	Urinary retention plus atonic anal sphincter
Sexual dysfunction	Sometimes impotence	Impotence frequent

COMBINED RADICULAR AND MYELOPATHY SYNDROMES

Cervical spondylosis is probably the most frequent cause of myelopathy. Degenerative changes of the spine, especially in the lower cervical vertebrae, may initially cause local pain that can involve not only the site of the lesion but also the paravertebral areas and sometimes the shoulder or hips. Radicular burning or shooting pain radiating to the sensory distribution of the root in the neck, shoulder, and upper extremity may also be the initial symptom. This pain may have an acute onset or may evolve over weeks, months, or even years. A third but less frequent kind of pain is a diffuse burning pain in the back and lower limbs that may appear several months after the spinal cord injury and is associated with lesions in the spinothalamic pathway. Another frequent symptom is cutaneous paresthesias, which follow more precisely the root pattern distribution. C5 and C6 roots are most frequently damaged. In patients with compression of the spinal cord, it is possible to find spasticity and Babinski's sign in the lower extremities associated with a reduction in the vibration and position senses. Pain and thermal sensations are usually spared.

SPINAL CORD HEMISECTION

Spinal cord hemisection, also known as Brown-Séquard syndrome, is characterized by contralateral loss of pain and temperature below the site of the lesion due to damage of the spinothalamic pathway, and also ipsilateral loss of position sense and pyramidal syndrome due to lesions of the dorsal columns and the corticospinal tract (see also Chapters 15 and 19). At the level of injury there is an area of spontaneous pain and hyperalgesia in a dermatomal distribution.

TRANSVERSE MYELOPATHY

Transverse myelitis is an inflammatory disease of the spinal cord that may be due to postinfection mechanisms or a direct effect of the infection, or may be idiopathic. The clinical features include ascending paresthesias, back pain, weakness of the lower limbs, and urinary retention associated with bilateral loss of superficial and deep sensation below the lesion (see also Chapters 15 and 19). The presence of a sensory loss level, usually in the trunk, differentiates transverse myelopathy from an acute polyneuropathy.

Spinal cord trauma usually affects the most mobile regions of the vertebral column, the cervical column and the union between the thoracic and lumbar segments. When the spinal cord is completely severed, all movements, sensations, and reflex activities are lost below the level of the lesion; this is the so-called spinal shock. This state can last for weeks to months, and then an increased reflex activity develops. Many patients describe paresthesias or a dull or burning pain below the level of the spinal cord lesion that can be very distressing. Beric and colleagues[43] have noted that in patients who have sustained cervical or thoracic spinal cord injury, pain may develop if another occult lesion develops in the conus or cauda equina. A selective deafferentation of the spinothalamic pathway with preservation of the function of the dorsal columns has also been postulated as the cause of post-traumatic pain.[44] Burning dysesthesia has also been described after complete spinal cord transection; it is attributed to abnormal discharge of the thalamic neurons.[45]

Spinal cord ischemia, usually as a result of a complication of spontaneous aortic dissection, is a rare cause of transverse myelopathy. A complete spinal cord transection or an anterior spinal artery syndrome can be produced. Patients usually present with severe pain in the trunk and sometimes the lower limbs, together with paraplegia and sensory loss. Hemorrhage into the spinal cord is also infrequent; it is caused by vascular malformations and bleeding diseases. Vascular malformations usually cause both ischemic and hemorrhagic lesions.

ANTERIOR SPINAL ARTERY SYNDROME

When the anterior spinal artery is obstructed, the anterior portion of the spinal cord, including both the lateral spinal thalamic tracts and the corticospinal tracts bilaterally, is infarcted. The resulting syndrome comprises paraplegia or quadriplegia of sudden onset and loss of pinprick and temperature sensation below the lesion. Position and vibratory senses are normal because the posterior spinal arteries supply the dorsal columns.

CENTRAL POST-STROKE SYNDROME (THALAMIC PAIN SYNDROME)

Dejerine and Roussy reported in 1906 the development of lancinating pain in the contralateral half of the body following a thalamic stroke. Today the disorder is called central post-stroke pain (CPSP) because it is not restricted to thalamic lesions. It has been associated with lesions in the hemispheres, particularly the parietal lobule, the brain stem, and even the cerebellum.[46, 47] Andersen and colleagues[42] reported that 8 percent of stroke patients have CPSP. In addition to pain, patients complain of mechanical and thermal, particularly cold, hyperalgesia.

All patients with CPSP seem to have a lesion in the spinothalamic pathway; pain is not an obligatory consequence of this lesion because many patients have loss of temperature and pain sensations without pain. As described for spinal cord disorders, preservation of touch, vibration, and proprioception has been reported in many patients.[47, 48] In patients with pain after parietal lesions, a disruption of the interconnections between the cauda insula and the opercular region of the parietal cortex and the thalamus has been suggested.[49] Pain is severe and is usually resistant to all kinds of treatment. Amitriptyline can reduce the pain in some patients with CPSP, probably because of inhibition of noradrenaline and serotonin reuptake. Drugs that act on the excitatory amino acids and the gamma-aminobutyric acid–ergic systems are also being tested.

BRAIN STEM PAIN LOSS SYNDROMES

In patients with lateral pontine and medullary lesions, usually vascular in origin, loss of pain and temperature sensations on the contralateral side of the body and the ipsilateral side of the face occurs, along with poor coordination of the ipsilateral extremities due to dysfunction of the cerebellar peduncle (see also Chapters 22 and 45). Other laterally placed cranial nerves are damaged, as are the descending sympathetic fibers.

CORTICAL PAIN SYNDROME

A number of unusual cortical lesions involving the parietal and parieto-occipital lobes can affect the patient's ability to react to pain. In these instances, usually dissociation occurs between the primary pain sensation and the emotive and motor withdrawal responses implicit in the normal pain reaction. Pain asymbolia is a condition wherein the patient recognizes pain and can distinguish it from touch and other sensations but does not recognize discomfort and makes no effort to avoid painful stimuli. Typically, the patient can identify a pin pricking him but reports that it does not hurt. Associated with this condition may be a global disregard for other forms of danger, along with a sensory aphasia, impairment of spatial orientation, and the presence of right-left confusion, including a fully developed Gerstmann syndrome. Most anatomical correlations link this syndrome with the dominant parietal lobe. Pain hemiagnosia, usually described in lesions of the right parietal lobe, is associated with a left hemiplegia and left hypersensitive sensory reaction to even light touch. In this case, there is a heightened emotive reaction to pain, and the patient groans and becomes inappropriately distressed at mild tactile stimuli. Despite this overreaction, however, the patient cannot identify exactly where the pain is and makes no effort to push the examiner away or protect the affected extremity.

In asymbolia for pain, patients have no evidence of a primary sensory deficit but lack appropriate motor and emotional responses to painful stimuli. Unilateral neglect and disorders of the body schema are often associated findings. The syndrome has been described after different lesions, mostly vascular, of the dominant inferior parietal lobe, frontoparietal cortex, somatosensory area, parietal operculum, and the adjacent insular cortex on either hemisphere. An interruption of connections between the sensory cortices and the limbic system has been suggested as the cause of this syndrome.[50]

Unilateral neglect may be a manifestation of injury to the right hemisphere. Attention is impaired, and the patient is unable to recognize or explore stimuli located within the left hemispace.

INSENSITIVITY TO PAIN

Thrush[51] first reported four siblings with painless injuries and bone fractures due to insensitivity to pain, but since that time, no clear cause of this clinical syndrome has been found. In the original description, no demonstrable lesion was found in the central and peripheral sensory pathways, but recently Larner and associates[52] re-evaluated two of the patients described by Thrush and found a sensory and autonomic neuropathy; they recommended a prolonged follow-up and sequential nerve biopsies to clarify this diagnosis. Familial cases occur, and a genetic factor is likely. Five subgroups of patients with congenital insensitivity to pain and temperature have been described:[53] congenital analgesia with minimal or no demonstrable lesion in the central or peripheral nervous system, congenital analgesia with anhidrosis, congenital analgesia in dizygote twins, congenital sensory neuropathy, and familial dysautonomia (see Chapter 36).

SENSORY SYSTEMS ASSOCIATED WITH PSYCHOGENIC SENSORY LOSS

Conversion reactions, Münchausen's syndrome, and malingering can present with sensory abnormalities. These conditions are often related to anxiety and depression and may be reinforced by the attention of the family. Criteria listed in the fourth edition of the *Diagnostic and Statistical Manual of Mental Disorders* (DSM-IV) include a temporal relationship with relevant psychological stressors and an "unconscious" motivation for the symptoms. One of the most frequent psychogenic sensory losses encountered is pinprick hemihypesthesia with a very clear limit at the midline or including loss of hearing and vision on the same side. If one limb is hypesthetic or anesthetic, all sensory modalities are impaired in a uniform way. These contradictory findings may help in making a correct diagnosis. However, an organic disease such as multiple sclerosis must be ruled out through a careful evaluation including clinical and laboratory tests. Pain with neuropathic characteristics is also a frequent expression of predominantly psychogenic disorders.[27]

CAUSALGIA

Causalgia means burning pain. It was first described in wounded soldiers in the American Civil War. At present, post-injury pain syndromes have been divided into complex regional pain syndrome type I (reflex sympathetic dystrophy) and complex regional pain syndrome type II (causalgia[1]). Reflex sympathetic dystrophy develops without evidence of nerve injury, whereas a traumatic nerve lesion causes causalgia. Historically, the sympathetic nervous system has been involved in the pathogenesis of both conditions,[54] leading to the concept of sympathetically maintained pain. However, later experience with placebo-controlled sympathetic blocks has questioned this concept.[55] Actually, causalgia and reflex sympathetic dystrophy are nonspecific terms that can be applied to different unrelated painful neuropathic disorders.

General Management Goals (Table 20–5)

General management of these patients includes pharmacological and nonpharmacological aspects. The first step in the management of a patient with neuropathic pain should be to give the patient a careful explanation of the cause or origin of the pain.

Tricyclic antidepressants have an important place in the management of neuropathic pain,[56] particularly ongoing burning pain such as that seen in diabetic polyneuropathy. Several clinical controlled trials have suggested that these drugs have good analgesic efficacy in several pain syndromes such as painful polyneuropathy and post-herpetic neuralgia. In addition to reducing ongoing burning pain, tricyclic antidepressants may also reduce brief lancinating pains and cutaneous hyperalgesia. Their analgesic effect is not related to their antidepressant activity, and they do not reduce the pain threshold in normal skin. Their analgesic effect seems to be related to the blockade of serotonin and norepinephrine (NE) reuptake. However, although mixed reuptake blockers such as amitriptyline and imipramine and selective NE reuptake blockers such as desipramine have proved useful, selective serotonin reuptake blockers such as paroxetine are not consistently useful. Citalopram may, however, have some beneficial effect.

Anticonvulsants are useful for relieving lancinating pain resulting from ectopic impulse generation at peripheral and central levels. As with the local anesthetics, the mechanism of action of anticonvulsants seems to be related to the membrane-stabilizing effect of these drugs. Phenytoin and carbamazepine are the anticonvulsants most used. Gabapentine has also been useful in diabetic painful neuropathy and post-herpetic neuralgia.[57] Lamotrigine has a partial beneficial effect.[58]

Topical local anesthetic preparations that can penetrate the skin are another treatment alternative for neuropathic pain. EMLA cream (eutectic mixture of local anesthetics), a mixture of 2.5 percent lidocaine and 2.5 percent prilocaine, as well as preparations of tetracaine in liposomes (phospholipid membrane vesicles designed to penetrate the stratum corneum) and other local anesthetic preparations have been extensively used in patients with post-herpetic neuralgia. The mechanism of action may be related to the inhibition of entry of sodium into the cell. Regenerating nerve endings develop dense concentrations of sodium channels, and here local anesthetics may exert a strong analgesic action. Unfortunately, as for other therapies, only a few controlled trials testing the use of local anesthetics for neuropathic pain have been conducted.

At the present time, there are no controlled trials that show a beneficial effect of long-term opioid therapy in patients with nonmalignant pain. In the short term, some clinical trials have challenged the conventional belief that these drugs have no role in treating these afflictions. Nevertheless, the published literature shows striking disparities, which may reveal differences in the groups of patients selected, the drugs tested, or the specific cause of the pain.[59] More controlled clinical trials are necessary to establish the role of opioids in the treatment of neuropathic pain. At present, they should be restricted to very selective cases.

As a consequence of the recent observations that NMDA receptors may be involved in the sensitization of WDR neurons and the increase in glutamate activity in different central nuclei in animal models of chronic pain, NMDA-receptor antagonists have become the objects of substantial investigations of the management of neuropathic pain. The main drawback of NMDA-receptor antagonists is their

TABLE 20–5. **Pharmacological Agents Used to Treat Neurological Pain Syndromes**

Drug Class	Antidepressants	Anticonvulsants	Opioids	NMDA-Receptor Antagonists	Capsaicin	Topical Local Anesthetics
Prototype Drug	Amitriptyline	Carbamazepine	Codeine	Ketamine	Capsaicin	EMLA
Usual Route and Dose	Oral use 12.5–150 mg	Oral use 200–800 mg tid	Oral use 30–60 mg daily	Intravenous intrathecal or oral less often	Topical use 0.025–0.1 mg strength	Topical use bid
New Drugs	Citalopram	Gabapentin Lamotrigine Topiramate				
Anatomical Area of Activity	Periaqueductal gray	Central or peripheral nervous system	Periaqueductal gray, dorsal horns of spinal cord, peripheral nociceptors(?)	Spinal cord second order neurons	C-nociceptor peripheral fibers	C-nociceptor peripheral fibers
Mechanism of Action	Blockade of serotonin and norepinephrine reuptake	Membrane-stabilizing effect	Mu opioid receptor agonist	Noncompetitive NMDA-receptor antagonist	Depletion of substance P in peripheral receptors	Inhibition of sodium entry into cells
Diabetic Neuropathy						
Generally used?	Yes, tricyclics	Yes, carbamazepine (CBZ) and gabapentin (G)	No	Yes	Yes, capsaicin	No
NNT	3	2.3 (CBZ); 3.8 (G)		Unknown	5.9	
CI	(2.4–4.4)	(1.5–3.8) (CBZ); (2.4–8.7) (G)		Unknown	3.8–13.0	

Post-herpetic Neuralgia						
Generally used?	Yes, tricyclics	Yes, gabapentin	No	No	Yes, capsaicin	No
NNT	Unknown	3.8		Unknown	5.3	
CI	Unknown	(2.4–8.7)		Unknown	(2.3–∞)	
Central Post-stroke Pain						
Generally used?	Yes, tricyclics	Yes, carbamazepine	No	Yes	No	No
NNT	1.7	3.4		Unknown		
CI	Unknown	Unknown		Unknown		
Traumatic Neuropathy						
Generally used?	No	Yes	No	No	No	Yes
NNT	Unknown	Unknown				Unknown
CI	Unknown	Unknown				Unknown
Side Effects	Dry mouth, tremor, sedation, constipation, increased appetite, cardiovascular signs with high doses	Nausea, drowsiness, visual disturbances, blood disorders, Steven-Johnson syndrome	Constipation, drowsiness, nausea	Diplopia, nystagmus, dream-like states, nightmares	Unbearable induction pain, local skin irritation	Local dermatitis

NNT, Number needed to treat, i.e., number of patients that have to be treated to obtain relief of pain by at least 50% of basal intensity in one patient; CI, confidence interval; NMDA, *N*-methyl-D-aspartate; EMLA, eutectic mixture of local anesthetics.

mental side effects. Ketamine, used for years as an anesthetic, might reduce pain in humans if used in subanesthetic doses. Results with dextrorphan, an opioid traditionally considered devoid of analgesic effects, are contradictory.

Capsaicin is the active substance extracted from hot pepper; after long-term application to the skin it produces hypalgesia. This effect is probably due to depletion of substance P. Capsaicin preparations have been reported to relieve pain in about one third of patients with painful diabetic neuropathy and post-herpetic neuralgia. This effect has been reported with concentrations of 0.025, 0.075, and 0.1 percent. Topical capsaicin has not been extensively used in clinical practice because of the intense burning pain and the increased mechanical hyperalgesia it produces during the first weeks of application before relief of pain occurs.

Topical anti-inflammatory agents such as aspirin, indomethacin, diclofenac, and benzydamine have been used in pain associated with trauma and inflammation. Their analgesic effects are probably due to desensitization of the nociceptors through blockade of receptors of inflammatory mediator, stabilization of neuronal membranes, and inhibition of prostaglandin synthesis. Nevertheless, clinical trials are still inconclusive.

TENS is traditionally used to obtain relief from different types of pain, but its specific effect against placebo is still the subject of debate.[25, 26]

Sympathetic blocks of different kinds have been traditionally used in the belief that the sympathetic system maintains pain. Nevertheless, this therapy has been recently challenged on the basis of placebo-controlled trials.[60]

Reviews and Selected Updates

Bowsher D: Pain syndromes and their treatment. Curr Opin Neurol Neurosurg 1993;6(2):257–263.

Galer BS, Jensen MP: Development and preliminary validation of a pain measure specific to neuropathic pain: The neuropathic pain scale. Neurology 1997;48:322–339.

Kost RG, Straus SE: Postherpetic neuralgia—pathogenesis, treatment, and prevention. N Engl J Med 1996;335:32–42.

Nasreddine ZS, Saver JL: Pain after thalamic stroke. Neurology 1997;48:1196–1199.

Ochoa JL: Pain mechanisms in neuropathy. Curr Opin Neurol 1994;7:407–414.

Ochoa JL, Verdugo RJ: Reflex sympathetic dystrophy. A common clinical avenue for somatoform expression. Neurol Clin 1995;13:351–363.

Rowbotham MC: Chronic pain: From theory to practical management. Neurology 1995;45:S5–S10.

References

1. Merskey H, Bogduk N (eds): Classification of Chronic Pain. Description of Chronic Pain Syndromes and Definition of Pain Terms, 2nd ed. Seattle, IASP Press, 1994.
2. Lindblom U, Ochoa JL: Somatosensory function and dysfunction. *In* Asbury AK, McKhann GM, McDonald WI (eds): Disease of the Nervous System, 2nd ed. Philadelphia, Ardmore Medical Books (WB Saunders), 1993, pp 213–228.
3. Ochoa JL, Torebjörk HE: Sensations evoked by intraneural microstimulation of C nociceptor fibers in human skin nerves. J Physiol 1989;415:583–599.
4. Nordin M, Nystrom B, Wallin V, Hagbarth KE: Ectopic sensory discharges and paresthesias in patients with disorders of peripheral nerves, dorsal roots and dorsal columns. Pain 1984;20:231–245.
5. Simone DA, Marchettini P, Caputi G, Ochoa JL: Identification of muscle afferents subserving sensation of deep pain in humans. J Neurophysiol 1994;72:883–889.
6. Ochoa JL, Yarnitsky D: Mechanical hyperalgesias in neuropathic pain patients: Dynamic and static subtypes. Ann Neurol 1993;33:465–472.
7. Ochoa JL: Thermal hyperalgesia as a clinical symptom. *In* Willis W (ed): The Second Bristol Myers Squibb Symposium on Pain Research. Hyperalgesia and Allodynia. New York, Raven Press, 1992, pp 151–165.
8. Lewis T: Pain. New York, Macmillan, 1942.
9. Campero M, Serra J, Bostock H, Ochoa JL: Slowly conducting afferents activated by innocuous low temperature in human. J Physiol 2001;535:855–865.
10. Campero M, Serra J, Ochoa JL: C-Polymodal nociceptors activated by noxious low temperature in human skin. J Physiol 1996;497:565–572.
11. Meyer RA, Davis KD, Cohen RH, et al: Mechanically insensitive afferents (MIAs) in cutaneous nerves of monkeys. Brain Res 1991;561:252–261.
12. Weidner C, Schmelz M, Schmidt R, et al: Functional attributes discriminating mechano-insensitive and mechano- responsive C nociceptors in human skin. J Neurosci 1999;19:10184–10190.
13. Schmelz M, Schmidt R, Bickel A, Handwerker HO, Torebjork HE: Specific C-receptors for itch in human skin. J Neurosci 1997;17: 8003–8008.
14. Torebjörk HE, Hallin RG: Perceptual changes accompanying controlled preferential blocking of A and C fibre responses in intact human skin nerves. Exp Brain Res 1973;16:321–332.
15. Hardy JD, Wolff HG, Goodell H: The nature of cutaneous hyperalgesia. *In* Pain Sensations and Reactions. Baltimore, Williams & Wilkins, 1952, pp 173–215.
16. LaMotte RH, Shain CN, Simone DA: Neurogenic hyperalgesia: Psychophysical studies of underlying mechanisms. J Neurophysiol 1991;66:190–211.
17. Serra J, Campero M, Ochoa JL: Mechanisms of neurogenic flare in human skin. J Neurol 1994;241(Suppl):S34.
18. Serra J, Campero M, Ochoa JL: Sensitization of "silent" C-nociceptors in areas of secondary hyperalgesia (SH) in humans (abstract). Neurology 1995;45:S47.
19. Jessel TM, Kelly DD: Pain and analgesia. *In* Kandel ER, Schwartz JH, Hessell TM (eds): Principles of Neural Sciences. Norwalk, CT, Appleton and Lange, 1991, pp 385–399.
20. Mayer DJ, Price DD, Becker DP: Neurophysiological characterization of the anterolateral spinal cord neurons contributing to pain perception in man. Pain 1975;1:51–58.
21. Dubner R: Neuronal plasticity and pain following peripheral tissue inflammation or nerve injury. *In* Bond MR, Charlton JE, Woolf CJ (eds): Proceedings of the Sixth World Congress on Pain. Amsterdam, Elsevier Science Publishers, 1991, pp 263–276.
22. Stein C: Peripheral mechanisms of opioid analgesia. Anesth Analg 1993;76:182–191.
23. Noordenbos W: Pain. Amsterdam, Elsevier Science Publishers, 1959.
24. Melzack R, Wall PD: Pain mechanisms: A new theory. Science 1965;150:971–978.
25. Milne S, Welch V, Brosseau L, et al: Transcutaneous electrical nerve stimulation (TENS) for chronic low back pain. [Systematic Review] Cochrane Back Review Group. Cochrane Database of Systematic Reviews. Issue 4, 2001.
26. Carroll D, Moore RA, McQuay HJ, et al: Transcutaneous electrical nerve stimulation (TENS) for chronic pain. [Systematic Review] Cochrane Pain, Palliative Care and Supportive Care Group. Cochrane Database of Systematic Reviews. Issue 4, 2001.
27. Ochoa JL, Verdugo RJ, Campero M: Pathophysiological spectrum of organic and psychogenic disorders in neuropathic pain patients fitting the description of causalgia or reflex sympathetic dystrophy. *In* Gebhart GF, Hammond DL, Jensen TS (eds): Proceedings of the Seventh World Congress on Pain. Seattle, IASP Press, 1994, pp 483–494.
28. Verdugo RJ, Ochoa JL: Quantitative somatosensory thermotest. A key method for functional evaluation of small calibre afferent channels. Brain 1992;115:893–913.
29. Castillo JL, Cea JG, Verdugo RJ, Cartier L: Sensory dysfunction in HTLV-I associated myelopathy/tropical spastic paraparesis. A comprehensive neurophysiological study. Eur Neurol 1999;42:17–22.
30. Castillo JL, Cea JG, Cartier L, Verdugo RJ: HTLV-I seronegative idiopathic progressive spastic paraparesis: Clinical and neurophysiological study of the sensory features. Rev Med Chil 2001;129:735–741.
31. Verdugo RJ, Ochoa JL: Use and misuse of conventional electrodiagnosis, quantitative sensory testing, thermography, and nerve blocks in the evaluation of painful neuropathic syndromes. Muscle Nerve 1993;16:1056–1062.

32. Ochoa JL: The newly recognized painful ABC syndrome: Thermographic aspects. Thermology 1986;2:65–107.
33. American Academy of Neurology: Therapeutics and Technology Assessment Subcommittee. Assessment of thermography in neurologic practice. Neurology 1990;40:523–525.
34. Cline MA, Ochoa JL, Torebjörk HE: Chronic hyperalgesia and skin warning caused by sensitized C nociceptors. Brain 1989;112:621–647.
35. Ochoa JL, Yarnitsky D: The triple cold ("CCC") syndrome: Cold hyperalgesia, cold hypoesthesia and cold skin in peripheral nerve disease. Brain 1994;117:185–197.
36. Dyck PJ: Neuronal atrophy and degeneration predominantly affecting peripheral sensory and autonomic neurons. *In* Dyck PJ, Thomas PK, Lambert EH, Bunge R (eds): Peripheral Neuropathy. Philadelphia, WB Saunders, 1984, pp 1557–1599.
37. Bennett GJ: Hypotheses on the pathogenesis of herpes zoster-associated pain. Ann Neurol 1994;35(Suppl):S38–S41.
38. Nurmikko T: Sensory dysfunction in postherpetic neuralgia. *In* Boivie J, Hansson P, Lindblom U (eds): Touch, Temperature and Pain in Health and Disease: Mechanisms and Assessment. Progress in Pain Research and Management, Vol. 3. Seattle, IASP Press, 1994, pp 133–141.
39. Kori SH, Foley KM, Posner JB: Brachial plexus lesions in patients with cancer: 100 cases. Neurology 1981;31:45–50.
40. Jaeckle KA, Young DF, Foley KM: The natural history of lumbosacral plexopathy in cancer. Neurology 1985;35:8–15.
41. Nashold BS: Paraplegia and pain. *In* Nashold BS Jr, Ovelmen-Levitt J (eds): Deafferentation Pain Syndromes: Pathophysiology and Treatment. New York, Raven Press, 1991, pp 301–319.
42. Archibald DJ, McGrath PJ, Ritvo PG, et al: Pain prevalence, severity and impact in a clinic sample of multiple sclerosis patients. Pain 1994;58:89–93.
43. Beric A, Dimitrijevic MR, Light JK: Pain in spinal cord injury with occult caudal lesions. Eur J Pain 1992;13:1–7.
44. Beric A, Dimitrijevic MR, Lindblom U: Central dysesthesia syndrome in spinal cord injury patients. Pain 1988;34:109–116.
45. Lenz FA, Tasker RR, Dostrovsky JO, et al: Abnormal single-unit activity recorded in the somatosensory thalamus of a quadriplegic patient with central pain. Pain 1987;31:225–236.
46. Boivie J, Leijon G, Johansson I: Central post-stroke pain—a study of the mechanisms through analyses of the sensory abnormalities. Pain 1989;37:173–185.
47. Vestergaard K, Nielsen J, Andersen G, et al: Sensory abnormalities in consecutive, unselected patients with central post-stroke pain. Pain 1994;61:177–186.
48. Andersen G, Vestergaard K, Ingeman-Nielsen M, Jensen TS: Incidence of central post stroke pain. Pain 1995;61:187–193.
49. Schmahmann JD, Leifer D: Parietal pseudothalamic pain syndrome. Arch Neurol 1992;49:1032–1037.
50. Berthier M, Starkstein S, Leiguarda R: Asymbolia for pain: A sensory-limbic disconnection syndrome. Ann Neurol 1988;24:41–49.
51. Thrush DC: Autonomic dysfunction in four patients with congenital insensitivity to pain. Brain 1973;96:591–600.
52. Larner AJ, Moss J, Rossi ML, Anderson M: Congenital insensitivity to pain: A 20 year follow up. J Neurol Neurosurg Psychiatry 1994;57:973–974.
53. Moffie D: Congenital insensitivity to pain. *In* Vinken PJ, Bruyn GW, Klawans HL, Mathews WB (eds): Neuropathies, Vol. 51. Handbook of Clinical Neurology. Amsterdam, Elsevier Science, 1987, pp 563–568.
54. Ochoa JL, Verdugo RJ: Reflex sympathetic dystrophy. Definitions and history of the ideas. A critical review of human studies. *In* Low PA (ed): The evaluation and management of clinical autonomic disorders. Boston, Little, Brown, 1993, pp 473–492.
55. Verdugo RJ, Ochoa JL: "Sympathetically maintained pain." I. Phentolamine sympathetic block questions the concept. Neurology 1994;44:1003–1010.
56. Max MB: Antidepressants as analgesics. *In* HL Fields, JC Liebeskind (eds): Pharmacological Approaches to the Treatment of Chronic Pain: Management, Vol.1. Seattle, IASP Press, 1994, pp 229–246.
57. Backonja MM: Anticonvulsants (antineuropathics) for neuropathic pain syndromes. Clin J Pain 2000;16:S67–S72.
58. Eisenberg E, Lurie Y, Braker C, Daoud D, Ishay A: Lamotrigine reduces painful diabetic neuropathy. A randomized, controlled study. Neurology 2001;57:505–509.
59. Portenoy RK: Opioid therapy for chronic nonmalignant pain: Current status. *In* HL Fields, JC Liebeskind (eds): Pharmacological Approaches to the Treatment of Chronic Pain: New Concepts and Critical Issues. Progress in Pain Research and Management, Vol. 1. Seattle, IASP Press, 1994, pp 247–288.
60. Kingery WS: A critical review of controlled clinical trials for peripheral neuropathic pain and complex regional pain syndromes. Pain 1997;73:123–139.

CHAPTER 21

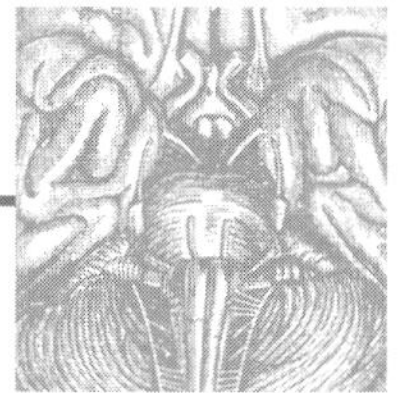

EDUARDO BENARROCH, ROY FREEMAN, and HORACIO KAUFMANN

Autonomic Nervous System

History and Definitions

The early concepts of the autonomic nervous system date back to the Roman period, during which Galen described the sympathetic chain ganglion and the rami communicantes. Although he hypothesized that this chain originated in the brain and provided sensory function, he thought that the numerous interconnections allowed the spirits to travel between the various organs, maintaining a physiological "sympathy." Much later, in the 17th century, Bartholomeo Eustachio investigated the ganglionated nerves but did not contribute further to our understanding of this system. While still believing that this chain descended from the brain, Thomas Willis (1664) placed its origin in the posterior fossa and associated it with involuntary or automatic motion—specifically, with the motion of the heart and respiration. François Pourfour du Petit noted that pupil size and the amount of secretions from the eye were altered when the cervical sympathetic nerves were cut and cast doubt on the sensory function of the sympathetic chain. In 1732, Winslow introduced the term sympathetic nerve, describing great, middle, and small components. In the 19th century, a flurry of research on the autonomic nervous system resulted in Walter Gaskell concluding that this system was actually composed of two subsystems. At the turn of the century, the terms preganglionic, postganglionic, and autonomic were first used by John Newport Langley, who theorized that this system contained both peripheral and central components. During this century, further refinements in our understanding of the autonomic nervous system were contributed by Thomas Elliott, Walter Dixon, and Otto Loewi, among others.

In discussing the autonomic nervous system and disorders related to it, a number of common terms require definition. Orthostatic hypotension (Greek, *orthos*: straight; *statikos*: causing to stand) refers to decreases of 20 mm Hg in systolic blood pressure and 10 mm Hg in diastolic pressure after standing. Syncope (Greek, *synkope*: cessation, pause), which can occur in the presence of autonomic dysfunction, is characterized by a loss of consciousness and postural tone due to a reversible reduction in blood flow to the reticular activating system in the brain stem. When both the sympathetic and parasympathetic neurotransmissions fail, the condition is typically termed a pandysautonomia. When only acetylcholine neurotransmission fails, the term cholinergic dysautonomia is used, whereas the term adrenergic dysautonomia is used to describe isolated failure of noradrenergic neurotransmission.

Clinical History

The presenting symptoms of patients with autonomic failure are extremely varied because the autonomic nervous system (ANS) controls the visceral processes involving the cardiovascular system, gastrointestinal system, urinary bladder, and sexual function as well as thermoregulation. Defective autonomic innervation of blood vessels can cause orthostatic hypotension, and with the subsequent reduction in blood flow to the brain, a variety of symptoms can develop. Typically, patients complain of visual disturbances (e.g., blurring, tunneling, or darkening of vision), sensations such as dizziness, lightheadedness, giddiness, and feeling faint, as well as a dull neck and shoulder ache (so-called coathanger pain). When orthostatic hypotension is pronounced and cerebral blood flow decreases below a critical level (approximately 25 mL/min/100 g), syncope occurs.

Orthostatic symptoms may be worse in the morning because nocturnal hypertension results in renal sodium and water loss and intravascular volume depletion.[1] Patients may also note that the symptoms of orthostatic hypotension are worse after eating, after standing still for a period of time, or following exercise or exposure to a warm environment such as a hot shower. All these circumstances divert blood from the central circulation (to the splanchnic area postprandially, to the skin following a hot shower, and to the lower part of the body while standing still) and thus reduce venous return to the heart.

Patients with gastrointestinal autonomic dysfunction have a variety of symptoms resulting from abnormal motility of the stomach and gut. The examiner should inquire about the presence of constipation, diarrhea, nausea, postprandial vomiting, bloating, belching, loss of appetite, and early satiety. Urinary bladder symptoms associated with autonomic dysfunction include hesitancy, poor stream production, increased intervals between micturition, and a sense of inadequate bladder emptying. Patients may also report symptoms associated with urinary retention and overflow incontinence. Male patients may additionally complain of impotence, which often is the earliest symptom of generalized autonomic failure. Sympathetically mediated ejaculatory failure may be an early complaint that precedes erectile failure.

Other characteristic symptoms of autonomic failure are caused by deficient thermoregulatory sweating. Initially, patients may notice reduced sweating only by the presence of dry socks and a lack of skin moisture. When abnormalities are severe, the patient may develop heat intolerance, flushing, or even heat-stroke symptoms.

Pure autonomic failure with no other neurological deficits is rare. More often, autonomic failure occurs in combination with other neurological disorders such as Parkinson's disease and multiple system atrophy (see Chapter 34). In these patients, it is important for the examiner to inquire about abnormalities in gait, changes in facial expression, the presence of dysarthria, difficulty in swallowing, and balance problems. Autonomic failure also occurs in patients with some peripheral neuropathies, such as those associated with diabetes and amyloidosis. Symptoms related to these disorders (e.g., limb weakness and sensory deficits) should also be sought. Because autonomic failure may be caused by lesions at different levels of the nervous system, a history of secondary trauma, cerebrovascular disease, tumors, infections, or demyelinating diseases should be established. Additionally, because the most frequent type of autonomic dysfunction encountered in medical practice is pharmacological, a thorough review of medication use, especially antihypertensives and psychotropic drugs, should be undertaken.

Some conditions may be confused with autonomic failure, including neurally mediated syncope, which is referred to as vasovagal, vasodepressor, or reflex syncope. This condition is caused by a paroxysmal reversal of the normal pattern of autonomic activation that maintains blood pressure in the standing position; these patients do not have autonomic failure. A detailed history is important to differentiate this disorder. In contrast to patients with chronic autonomic failure in whom syncope appears as a gradual fading of vision and loss of awareness, patients with neurally mediated syncope often have signs and symptoms of autonomic overactivity such as diaphoresis and nausea prior to the event. This distinction and the episodic nature of neurally mediated syncope should be part of a thorough clinical history.

Anatomy of the Autonomic Nervous System

The term autonomic (autonomous, self-governing) nervous system was introduced to describe "the system of nerves which controls the unstriated tissue, the cardiac muscle and the glandular tissue of mammals."[2] Originally, the term applied only to neurons with axons outside the central nervous system (CNS). More recently, the discovery that discrete neuronal groups in the brain stem, diencephalon, and cerebral cortex are involved in the control of autonomic function has broadened the definition of the ANS to include not only peripheral afferent and efferent pathways but also a complex network of neurons within the CNS.

The cell bodies of afferent autonomic (visceral) neurons are in the dorsal root ganglia of the spinal or cranial nerves and travel in both sympathetic and parasympathetic nerves toward the CNS (Fig. 21–1). The autonomic CNS neurons are located at many levels from the cerebral cortex to the spinal cord. Efferent autonomic pathways are organized in two major outflows: the sympathetic and parasympathetic. Finally, the enteric nervous system, which is considered a separate and independent division of the autonomic nervous system, is located in the walls of the gut.

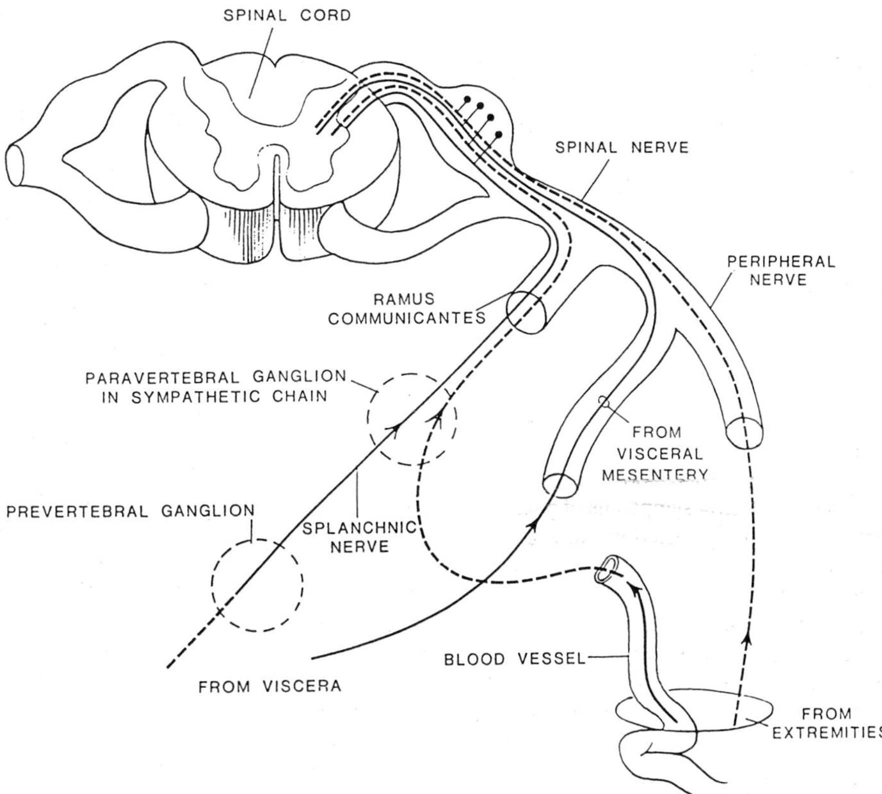

FIGURE 21–1. Organization of visceral and somatic afferents in the spinal cord. (Reproduced from Westmoreland BF, et al: Medical Neurosciences: An Approach to Anatomy, Pathology, and Physiology by Systems and Levels, 3rd ed. Boston, Little, Brown, 1994. By permission of Mayo Foundation.)

CENTRAL AUTONOMIC NETWORK

The ANS, like the somatic nervous system, is organized in segmental levels. Neurons in the cerebral cortex, basal forebrain, hypothalamus, midbrain, pons, and medulla participate in autonomic control. Autonomic neurons are reciprocally interconnected by neurochemically complex pathways and constitute a functional unit referred to as the central autonomic network (CAN).[3,4] The CAN integrates visceral, humoral, and environmental information to produce coordinated autonomic, neuroendocrine, and behavioral responses to external or internal stimuli. Within the CAN, there is segmental and regional specialization for the control of autonomic functions. A coordinated response is generated through interconnections among the amygdala and the neocortex, basal forebrain, ventral striatum, hypothalamus, and autonomic and somatic motor nuclei of the brain stem.[3–5]

Cerebral Cortex and Amygdala

The insular and medial prefrontal cortices (paralimbic areas) and nuclei of the amygdala are the higher centers involved in the processing of visceral information and the initiation of integrated autonomic responses. The insular cortex is the primary viscerosensory cortex and receives viscerotopically organized sensory information from visceral and arterial chemoreceptors and baroreceptors. Functional studies show activation of the human insular cortex in response to maneuvers that activate cardiovascular afferents.[6] The insula and the anterior cingulate cortices area activated by nociceptive inputs and initiate autonomic responses associated with affective behavior.[7] The amygdala receives exteroceptive and interoceptive information and provides it with emotional significance. The central nucleus of the amygdala projects to the hypothalamus, periaqueductal gray, and autonomic nuclei of the brain stem to integrate autonomic, endocrine, and motor responses to emotionally relevant stimuli.[8]

Hypothalamus

The hypothalamus integrates the autonomic and endocrine responses that are critical for homeostasis. It is functionally divided into three longitudinal zones: a *periventricular zone* involved in circadian rhythms and endocrine responses; a *medial zone* involved in the control of sexual function, osmoregulation, and thermoregulation; and a *lateral zone* involved in behavioral arousal (Fig. 21–2).[9] All three zones project to the autonomic nuclei of the brain stem and spinal cord.

The paraventricular hypothalamic nucleus is the site of integrated autonomic and neuroendocrine responses to stress. It contains different subpopulations of "effector" neurons including magnocellular neurons that secrete vasopressin, parvicellular neurons that produce corticotrophic-releasing hormone and other regulatory hormones that control pituitary function, and neurons that innervate all brain stem and spinal autonomic nuclei.[10] The medial preoptic nucleus contains thermosensitive neurons that initiate autonomic, endocrine, and motor responses. Warm-sensitive neurons, excited by an increase in core temperature, initiate responses such as skin vasodilatation, sweating, and slow-wave sleep, which lead to heat loss. Cold-sensitive neurons initiate vasoconstriction and shivering. In humans, these thermoregulatory sudomotor and vasomotor pathways descend in the equatorial plane of the lateral column of the spinal cord.

The lateral hypothalamic area participates in arousal, motivated motor behavior, and autonomic control. Some

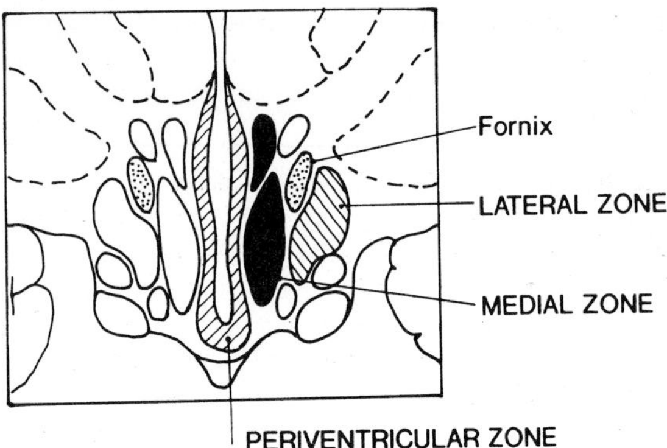

Hypothalamic Area

Zone	Function
Periventricular	Autonomic
	Circadian rhythms
	Neuroendocrine
Medial	Homeostasis
	Reproduction
Lateral	Arousal
	Motivated behavior

FIGURE 21–2. Subdivisions of the hypothalamus. (Reproduced from Westmoreland BF, et al: Medical Neurosciences: An Approach to Anatomy, Pathology, and Physiology by Systems and Levels, 3rd ed. Boston, Little, Brown, 1994. By permission of Mayo Foundation.)

neurons of this region synthesize orexin/hypocretin and project to cholinergic and monoaminergic regions of the brain stem regulating rapid-eye-movement sleep. Dysfunction of this system has been implicated in the mechanism of narcolepsy.[11] These lateral hypothalamic neurons, as well as neurons in the ventromedial hypothalamus, including the arcuate nucleus, are the targets of leptin, a hormone secreted from adipose tissue in response to food intake. Leptin directly activates neurons of the arcuate nuclei to inhibit food intake and simultaneously inactivates neurons of the lateral hypothalamus that ordinarily increase food intake.[12] The hypothalamic autonomic pathways descend predominantly ipsilaterally in the dorsomedial and ventrolateral tegmentum of the brain stem.

Periaqueductal Gray Matter

The periaqueductal gray matter (PAG) of the midbrain is the site of integrated autonomic, behavioral, and antinociceptive stress responses. It is organized into separate columns that control specific patterns of response to stress.[13] The lateral PAG mediates sympathoexcitation, opioid-independent analgesia, and motor responses consistent with the fight-or-flight reaction. The ventrolateral PAG produces sympathoinhibition, opioid-dependent analgesia, and motor inhibition. The PAG constitutes a critical relay station for the micturition reflex (see later discussion on Bladder).

Brain Stem

Neurons in the medulla are critical for the control of cardiovascular, respiratory, and gastrointestinal functions. The medullary nucleus of the solitary tract (NTS) is the first relay station for the arterial baroreceptors and chemoreceptors, as well as cardiopulmonary and gastrointestinal afferents.[3] The NTS integrates multiple autonomic reflexes and projects to other central autonomic regions. Neurons in the reticular formation of the ventrolateral medulla are arranged in distinct groups that maintain cardiomotor, vasomotor, and respiratory functions. Neurons in the rostral ventrolateral medulla project directly to sympathetic preganglionic neurons and maintain basal arterial blood pressure, while neurons in the ventral medulla are critical for respiratory rhythmogenesis. The nucleus ambiguus provides parasympathetic innervation to the heart.[14,15]

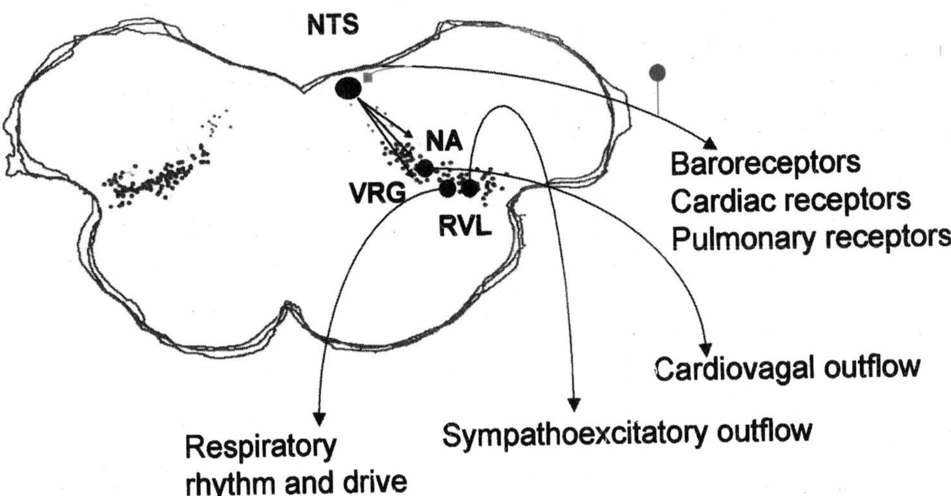

FIGURE 21–3. Basic circuitry of the medullary cardiorespiratory reflexes. Inputs from baroreceptors, cardiac receptors, chemoreceptors, and pulmonary receptors reach the central nervous system via branches of the glossopharyngeal (CN IX) and vagus (CN X) nerves. These afferents synapse on specific neuronal groups of the nucleus tractus solitarius (NTS), which is the first relay station for the cardiorespiratory reflexes. Neurons of the NTS project to the nucleus ambiguus (NA) and dorsal vagal nucleus, which provide vagal outputs to the heart and respiratory systems; to neurons of the ventral respiratory group (VRG) involved in generation of respiratory rhythm and control of spinal respiratory motor neurons; and to neurons of the rostral ventrolateral medulla (RVL), which provide sympathoexcitatory inputs to the preganglionic neurons of the spinal cord.

These ventromedullary vasomotor, cardiomotor, and respiratory neurons form a network that is coordinated via interneurons of the medullary reticular formation.[14] Together with the NTS, this network is involved not only in the generation of respiratory and cardiovascular rhythms but also in complex motor patterns such as vomiting, swallowing, sneezing, and coughing. The descending reticulospinal pathways for the automatic control of breathing and blood pressure, as well as those for sweating and micturition, run in the ventral half of the white matter of the lateral columns of the spinal cord (Fig. 21–3).

EFFERENT AUTONOMIC PATHWAYS

The autonomic output to effector organs consists of a two-neuron pathway with one synapse in the peripheral autonomic ganglia. The central neuron is called preganglionic, and the ganglionic neuron is called (illogically) postganglionic. Sympathetic preganglionic neurons are located in the intermediolateral cell column of the gray matter of the spinal cord at all thoracic and high lumbar levels (T1–L3) (thoracolumbar outflow) (Fig. 21–4A). Parasympathetic preganglionic neurons are located both in the brain stem and at the sacral (S2–S4) level of the spinal cord (craniosacral outflow) (Fig. 21–4*B*). Sympathetic and parasympathetic preganglionic axons emerge from the brain stem or spinal cord as small myelinated fibers, but postganglionic sympathetic and parasympathetic axons to the peripheral effector organs are unmyelinated.

Sympathetic Outflow

Preganglionic sympathetic neurons are organized into different functional units that control blood flow to the skin and muscles, secretion of sweat glands, skin hair follicles, systemic blood flow, as well as the function of viscera. Preganglionic sympathetic neurons receive direct descending excitatory input from the paraventricular and lateral nuclei of the hypothalamus as well as the ventromedial and ventrolateral medulla. These pathways coordinate selective rather than massive patterns of sympathetic discharge by innervating different specific subsets of preganglionic sympathetic neurons. Selectivity is further refined by the release of different neurotransmitters.[16]

Preganglionic sympathetic axons exit through the ventral roots and pass through the white rami of the corresponding spinal nerve toward paravertebral or prevertebral ganglia (see following paragraphs). These axons have a segmental organization, but their distribution does not follow the dermatomal pattern of somatic nerves. Segments T1–T3 innervate the head and neck, T3–T6 the upper extremities and thoracic viscera, T7–T11 the abdominal viscera, and T12–L2 the lower extremities and pelvic and perineal organs.

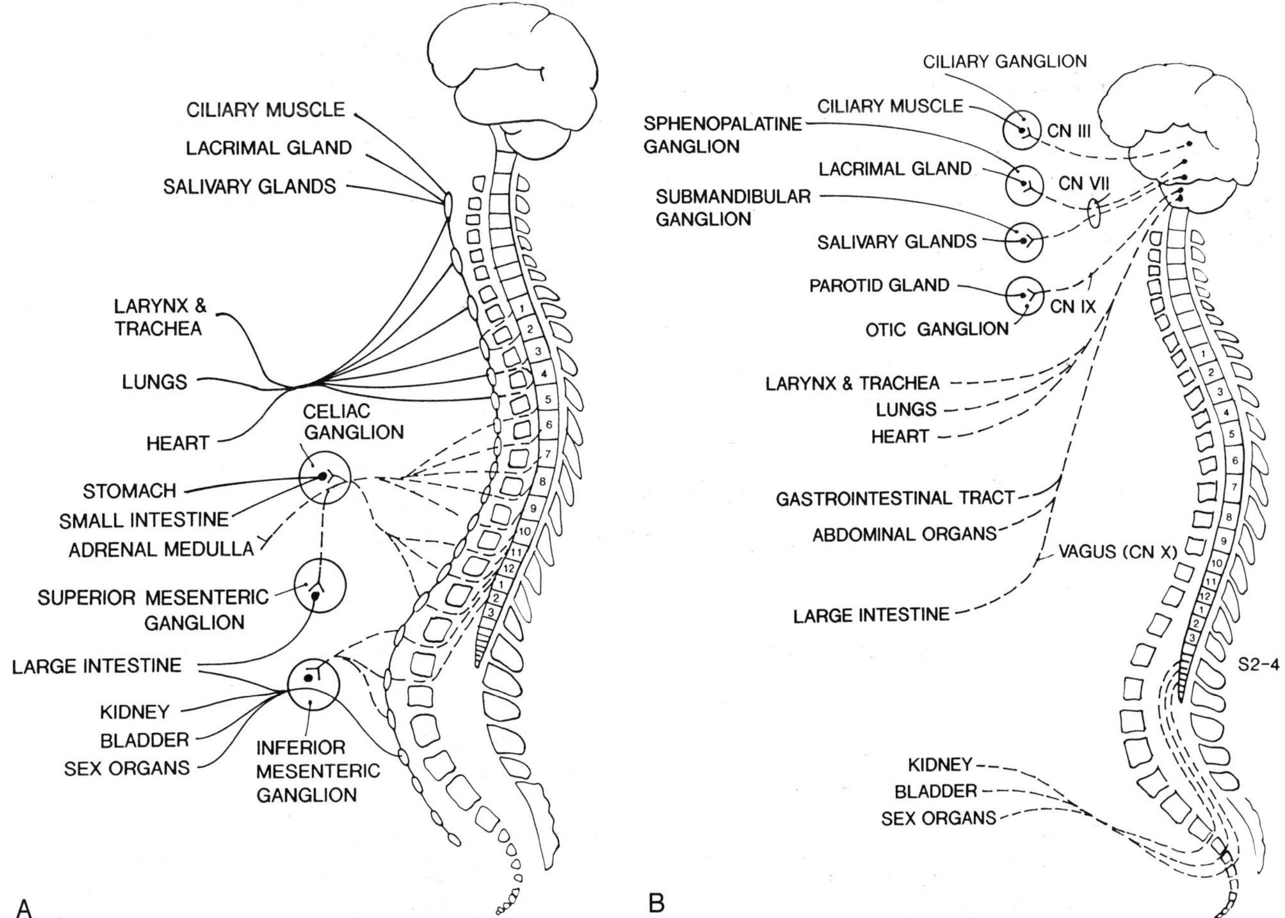

FIGURE 21–4. Sympathetic (*A*) and parasympathetic (*B*) divisions of the autonomic nervous system: efferent systems. (Modified from Noback C, Demarest R: The Human Nervous System. Basic Principles of Neurobiology. New York, McGraw Hill, 1981, p 228.)

Sympathetic ganglia are organized into two anatomical and functionally distinct groups: paravertebral and prevertebral ganglia. At the paravertebral ganglia (located at the sides of the spinal cord), preganglionic fibers may synapse on a postganglionic neuron at the same level or branch and run rostrally or caudally to synapse on a large number of postganglionic neurons at different levels. Preganglionic fibers also pass through the paravertebral ganglia without synapsing to form the splanchnic nerves that innervate the prevertebral ganglia (located anterior to the spinal cord) or the adrenal medulla.

The paravertebral ganglia provide long unmyelinated axons to all sympathetically innervated tissues and organs except those in the abdomen, pelvis, and perineum. The superior cervical ganglion (T1–T2) provides pupilodilator and sudomotor fibers to the face. The stellate ganglion (T2–T6) innervates the upper limb through branches of the brachial plexus, and the lumbar sympathetic ganglia (T9–L1) innervate the lower limb through branches of the lumbosacral plexus. The postganglionic sympathetic fibers join the peripheral somatic nerve via the gray rami communicantes, and thus their distribution is similar to that of the corresponding somatic nerve. Sympathetic fibers in somatic nerves provide vasomotor, sudomotor, and pilomotor innervation to the extremities and trunk. The lower cervical and upper thoracic ganglia innervate the heart via the cardiac plexus and the tracheobronchial tree via the pulmonary plexus.

The prevertebral ganglia innervate the abdominal, pelvic, and perineal organs. Preganglionic fibers from T5–T12 levels are carried by the thoracic splanchnic nerves, which pierce the diaphragm and enter the abdomen to synapse on the celiac and superior mesenteric ganglia. These form the celiac plexus, which innervates all abdominal viscera except the descending colon. Sympathetic activation produces splanchnic vasoconstriction, inhibition of secretion and motility of the gut, as well as secretion of epinephrine, renin, and glucagon. Preganglionic axons from L1–L3 levels, carried by the lumbar splanchnic nerves, synapse on the inferior mesenteric ganglion. The postganglionic axons innervate the descending colon, rectum, bladder, and genitalia via the hypogastric plexus. Sympathetic nerves inhibit muscle contractility of the bladder and bowel, thus allowing storage of urine and feces. These postganglionic neurons also produce the contraction of the vas deferens that is necessary for ejaculation.[17]

Parasympathetic Outflow

The cranial parasympathetic neurons are located in the general visceral efferent column of the midbrain, pons, and medulla. Their preganglionic axons travel in cranial nerves III, VII, IX, and X (see Chapters 9, 11, and 13). Parasympathetic outputs carried via cranial nerve III produce pupillary constriction and accommodation of the lens. Output carried via cranial nerves VII and IX stimulates lacrimal and salivary secretion. The vagus nerve (cranial nerve X) provides the most widespread brain stem parasympathetic output. Vagal preganglionic neurons are located in the dorsal motor nucleus, which controls respiratory and abdominal viscera, and in the region of the nucleus ambiguus, which innervates the heart. The vagus provides inputs to parasympathetic ganglia located in or near the target organs, and its main effects are cardioinhibitory, visceromotor, and secretomotor.

The sacral preganglionic parasympathetic neurons are located in the intermediolateral cell column at the S2–S4 levels of the spinal cord. Their axons pass through the ventral roots to the pelvic splanchnic nerves (nervi erigentes), which join the inferior hypogastric (pelvic) plexus. The sacral parasympathetic system is critical for defecation, micturition, and erection.[17]

Efferent Autonomic Neurotransmitters

Acetylcholine is the neurotransmitter of the sympathetic and parasympathetic preganglionic neurons. Acetylcholine produces fast excitation of ganglion neurons via nicotinic receptors. The main postganglionic sympathetic neurotransmitter is norepinephrine, which acts through alpha- and beta-adrenergic receptors. The sympathetic innervation of the sweat glands is mediated by acetylcholine, acting via muscarinic receptors. The main postganglionic parasympathetic neurotransmitter is acetylcholine, which acts through different subtypes of muscarinic receptors. Postganglionic sympathetic terminals to the heart and smooth muscles also release adenosine triphosphate and neuropeptide Y, whereas postganglionic parasympathetic terminals may release vasoactive intestinal polypeptide or nitric oxide.

Alpha-adrenergic receptors mediate sympathetically induced pupillary dilatation (mydriasis), vasoconstriction, and contraction of the vas deferens and bladder and rectal internal sphincters. Beta receptors mediate cardiac stimulation, vasodilation, bronchodilatation, relaxation of the bladder, and endocrine-metabolic effects. Muscarinic receptors mediate pupil constriction (miosis), salivary and lacrimal secretion, cardiac inhibition, bronchoconstriction, stimulation of motility and secretion in the gastrointestinal tract, evacuation of the bladder and rectum, and erection.

AFFERENT AUTONOMIC PATHWAYS

Visceral afferents transmit conscious sensations (e.g., gut distention, cardiac ischemia) and unconscious visceral sensations (e.g., blood pressure, chemical composition of the blood). Their most important function is to initiate autonomic reflexes at the local, ganglion, spinal, and supraspinal levels.[18] Visceral receptors are innervated by small myelinated and unmyelinated fibers that have cell bodies in the dorsal root ganglia of the spinal or cranial nerves. Spinal visceral afferents are carried by thoracolumbar sympathetic and sacral parasympathetic nerve trunks. In the spinal cord, they branch extensively and synapse on viscerosomatic neurons in the dorsal horn and intermediate gray matter. These neurons receive convergent visceral and somatic inputs and are the substrate for referred pain (i.e., visceral pain referred to overlying or nearby somatic structures). Visceral sensation is carried primarily by the spinothalamic and spinoreticular pathways, which transmit visceral pain and sexual sensations. The dorsal columns may relay sensations related to micturition, defecation, and gastric distention. Viscerosensory inputs, after a relay in the thalamic nuclei, project to the insula and other cortical autonomic areas.[18]

Brain stem visceral afferents are carried by the vagus and glossopharyngeal nerves and have their cell bodies in the nodose and petrosal ganglia, respectively. Vagal afferents carry information from aortic, cardiac, pulmonary, and gastrointestinal receptors. Glossopharyngeal afferents carry signals from baroreceptors and chemoreceptors in the carotid sinus. These vagal and glossopharyngeal afferents synapse on neurons of the NTS. Taste and general visceral afferent information from the NTS is relayed, either directly or via the parabrachial nucleus, to the ventroposteromedial nucleus of the thalamus, which in turn projects to the insular cortex. Brain stem visceral afferents are important in complex automatic motor acts such as swallowing, vomiting, and coughing.

AUTONOMIC INNERVATION OF SPECIFIC ORGANS

Cardiovascular System

The heart receives parasympathetic and sympathetic innervation. The cell bodies of the parasympathetic preganglionic neurons innervating the heart are located in the medulla (nucleus ambiguus and dorsal motor nucleus of the vagus).[15]

The axons of these neurons, which are part of the vagus nerve, join the cardiac neural plexus after entering the thorax to synapse with neurons in the intracardiac ganglia. From these ganglia, short postganglionic parasympathetic neurons emerge to innervate the myocardial tissue. Vagal innervation is particularly abundant in the nodes and the atrioventricular conduction system.

The heart draws its sympathetic innervation from neurons in the intermediolateral columns of the spinal cord at the T1–T4 levels. Axons of these neurons synapse in superior, middle, and inferior (stellate) cervical ganglia, which are the origin of postganglionic sympathetic neurons that reach the heart in a mixed neural plexus along with preganglionic parasympathetic neurons. Sympathetic axons innervate the sinoatrial and atrioventricular nodes, the conduction system, and myocardial muscle fibers, most prominently in the ventricles. The arteries and veins of the systemic circulation are innervated primarily by the sympathetic system.

Postganglionic parasympathetic neurons release acetylcholine, which activates muscarinic receptors in the heart, causing a decrease in heart rate as well as reductions in the conduction, excitability, and contractility of myocardial cells. Postganglionic sympathetic axons release norepinephrine, which, primarily via beta-adrenergic receptors, increases heart rate and the conduction, excitability, and contractility of the myocardium. Cardiac vagal neurons are activated through the baroreflex (see later discussion) when arterial pressure increases and are inhibited during inspiration. Because acetylcholine acts quickly and is rapidly inactivated by cholinesterase, the vagus controls heart rate on a beat-to-beat basis.

Sympathetic outflow to the arteries, arterioles, and veins of the peripheral circulation produces vasoconstriction by activating alpha-adrenergic receptors. The presence of vasodilator cholinergic sympathetic fibers to skeletal muscle in humans is debatable. Sympathetic vasoconstrictor outflow to the blood vessels of skeletal muscle is strongly modulated by the baroreflex (see later discussion) and is important for buffering acute changes in arterial pressure. Splanchnic vasoconstriction produced by sympathetic activation is critical for the maintenance of arterial pressure in the upright posture. Loss of splanchnic vasomotor outflow is the main mechanism causing orthostatic hypotension in autonomic failure.

Autonomic outflow to the heart and blood vessels is controlled on a moment-to-moment basis by a variety of reflexes, which are initiated by arterial baroreceptors and chemoreceptors and by several types of cardiac receptors. Of these reflexes, the one that has been best studied is the arterial baroreflex, which is a classic negative feedback mechanism that buffers fluctuations in arterial blood pressure. Afferent fibers in the vagus and glossopharyngeal nerves with cell bodies in the nodose and petrosal ganglia are sensitive to pressure or mechanical distention (i.e., baroreceptors). These neurons have arborizations that are distributed in the adventitial layer of the carotid sinus and the aortic arch, and their first synapse occurs in the NTS. Impulses from the NTS modify the activity of cardiac vagal motor neurons in the nucleus ambiguus and neurons in the ventrolateral medulla that control sympathetic outflow. When arterial pressure increases, afferent baroreceptor discharge in the NTS increases. This results in a rapid increase in cardiovagal efferent activity, which slows the heart, and in inhibition of sympathetic vasoconstrictor outflow, which causes vasodilatation. Conversely, when blood pressure falls, for example when standing up, baroreceptors are "unloaded," and their afferent discharge to the NTS decreases. This results in reflex sympathetic excitation and parasympathetic inhibition, which cause vasoconstriction and tachycardia.

Cardiovascular reflexes also control the release of vasopressin from the supraoptic and paraventricular hypothalamic nuclei. These neurons are tonically inhibited by baroreceptor input, and therefore a fall in arterial pressure elicits an increase in vasopressin release.[19]

Skin

Sympathetic innervation of the skin plays an important role in thermoregulation and the expression of emotional states. The sympathetic outflow to the skin includes cholinergic neurons innervating sweat glands (sudomotor neurons) and adrenergic neurons innervating blood vessels and hair follicles (vasoconstrictor and pilomotor neurons). Cutaneous vasomotor activity and sweating in the face is controlled by the T2–T3 segments of the spinal cord via the superior cervical ganglion. Postganglionic axons accompany branches of the internal carotid (for innervation of the forehead) and external carotid arteries (innervating the rest of the face) and follow branches of the trigeminal nerve. Sympathetic outflow produces vasoconstriction in the ears and lips but predominantly vasodilatation in the rest of the face. Fibers from the stellate ganglion (which receives innervation from T2–T6 preganglionic neurons) innervate the arm via branches of the brachial plexus. The lumbar sympathetic ganglia (which receive innervation from T9–L1 preganglionic neurons) innervate the lower limb via branches of the lumbosacral plexus. The trunk is innervated by the intercostal nerves.

Exposure to cold produces skin vasoconstriction (pallor) and piloerection (goose flesh) via alpha-adrenergic mechanisms; conversely, a warm environment elicits vasodilatation (redness, flushing) and sweating via muscarinic receptors. During certain emotional states (fear, anxiety) and hemodynamic stimuli (severe fall in arterial pressure), both vasoconstrictor and sudomotor outputs are activated simultaneously, producing a cold, clammy skin ("cold sweat").

Gastrointestinal Tract

The dorsal nucleus of the vagus innervates the entire gastrointestinal tract with the exception of the proximal esophagus and the distal colon and rectum. The vagus produces increases in propulsive motility, relaxation of sphincters, and secretions of the exocrine and endocrine glands of the stomach, intestine, pancreas, and liver. Sympathetic outflow to the gastrointestinal tract, which arises from preganglionic neurons at the T1–L1 segments of the spinal cord and relays, via the splanchnic nerves, in the celiac and mesenteric ganglia, is involved in reflexes that decrease gut motility. Extrinsic vagal and sympathetic influences are relayed and integrated at the level of the enteric nervous system, located in the wall of the gut.

Bladder

The function of the bladder, rectum, and sexual organs is controlled by three outflows: sacral parasympathetic, lumbar sympathetic, and somatic. Control of the bladder serves as a paradigm for innervation of the other pelvic organs. The sacral parasympathetic (S2–S4) output to the bladder is carried via the pelvic nerves and is mediated by muscarinic cholinergic receptors. These parasympathetic nerves promote bladder emptying (micturition) through activation of the detrusor muscle and relaxation of the bladder neck. The lumbar sympathetic (T11–L2) output is carried via the hypogastric nerves. The sympathetic nerves produce relaxation of the detrusor muscle by way of beta receptors and contraction of the bladder neck by way of alpha receptors, thus favoring storage of urine. The sacral somatomotor output, which arises from motor neurons of the nucleus of Onuf (S2–S4) and is carried by the pudendal nerve, stimulates contraction of the external sphincter via nicotinic cholinergic receptors. Activation of these somatomotor nerves promotes storage of urine.[17]

In normal individuals, micturition involves a spino-ponto-spinal reflex that is initiated by bladder tension receptors and integrated in pontine micturition centers. This reflex coordinates the simultaneous activation of sacral parasympathetic autonomic neurons and inhibition of somatic sphincter motor neurons, thus allowing synergistic bladder contraction and sphincter relaxation during micturition.[17]

Interruption of the sacral parasympathetic outflow in patients with lesions of the conus or cauda equina results in a hypotonic areflexic bladder. In patients with spinal cord lesions, the suprasegmental pathway is interrupted, and micturition occurs through segmental spinospinal sacral reflexes, which are triggered by perineal or nociceptive stimulation. In this condition, bladder and sphincter contractions are not well coordinated, resulting in detrusor-sphincter dyssynergia. Cortical inputs are responsible for voluntary control of initiation and interruption of micturition. Lesions involving the medial aspects of the frontal lobes, including the anterior cingulate and paracentral gyri, result in involuntary but coordinated micturition, referred to as uninhibited bladder.

Other Organs

Autonomic innervation of the pupil (see Chapter 9) and the lacrimal and salivary glands (see Chapters 11 and 13) is reviewed in the chapters discussing the specific cranial nerves controlling these structures.

Examination of the Autonomic Nervous System

DIRECTED NEUROLOGICAL EXAMINATION

The directed bedside neurological examination includes clinical observation and pharmacological testing with adrenergic and cholinergic agonists. Pharmacological tests can detect a decrease or increase in response of the effector organs due to denervation supersensitivity. Denervation supersensitivity is a manifestation of postganglionic, as opposed to preganglionic, neuronal autonomic failure.[20]

Skin

The examiner may recognize sudomotor failure by noting a dryness of the skin and a lack of resistance to gentle stroking with the fingerpads or to a tuning fork run over the skin. Sudomotor failure may take the form of an isolated generalized anhidrosis or a diffuse autonomic failure with other associated findings. A search should be made for localized increases in or absence of sweating and for asymmetrical patterns of skin temperature or color. In patients with disturbances of autonomic innervation of the face, the physician may note gustatory sweating, flushing, and facial anhidrosis. Acral vasomotor changes that may be observed include acrocyanosis, pallor, mottling, livedo reticularis, or erythema.[21] Skin temperature changes can be assessed by palpation. Other findings to be noted include atrophic skin changes, alopecia, hypertrichosis, nail thickening, skin decoloration or deformation, and Charcot's joints. Allodynia and hyperalgesia are components of a complex regional pain syndrome that in some cases may involve sympathetic mechanisms.

A bedside intradermal injection of pilocarpine can be used to assess the sweat glands; a supersensitive response to diluted pilocarpine indicates the presence of postganglionic sympathetic sudomotor denervation. Intradermal injection of histamine produces a "triple response" (erythema, flare, and wheal) through an axon reflex mediated by nociceptive C-afferent fibers. Loss of the histamine flare indicates severe loss or absence of nociceptive C axons, as in patients with familial dysautonomia or peripheral neuropathies affecting the sympathetic nerves.

Cardiovascular Reflexes

To assess cardiovascular autonomic function, blood pressure and heart rate should be measured while the patient is supine and after he or she has been standing for at least 3 minutes. In normal conditions, there is a 5- to 20-mm Hg drop in systolic blood pressure on changing from the supine to the standing position with no change or only a slight rise in diastolic pressure; heart rate increases 5 to 25 beats per minute[22] (see later section, Evaluation Guidelines).

Orthostatic hypotension is defined as a reproducible fall of more than 20 mm Hg in systolic pressure or of more than 10 mm Hg in diastolic pressure within 3 minutes of adopting the erect position.[23] In patients with severe orthostatic intolerance, it is useful to monitor the length of time the patient can stand in place before he or she experiences symptoms. Severe orthostatic hypotension results in a "standing time" of less than 30 seconds. If orthostatic hypotension is not apparent, it is useful to ask the patient to squat several times and then repeat the blood pressure measurement. The presence of orthostatic hypotension without reflex tachycardia is evidence of sympathetic and cardiovagal failure. If a reflex tachycardia is present, hypovolemia should be excluded. However, the presence of tachycardia does not exclude an autonomic cause of orthostatic hypotension. An increase in heart rate of more than 30 beats per minute above the basal rate or more than 120 beats per minute on adopting the erect position, if associated with symptoms, is characteristic of the postural tachycardia syndrome. This syndrome is a heterogeneous disorder that has multiple possible causes.[24]

Bladder

Clinical evaluation of bladder function includes assessment of the ability to control initiation or interruption of micturition voluntarily and the integrity of the bladder and perianal sensation. Reflexes that are integrated at the level of the conus medullaris and are mediated by sensory and motor roots in the cauda equina should also be checked. The bulbocavernosus and anal reflexes are somatic reflexes that are integrated at the S2–S4 levels, and the scrotal and internal anal reflexes are autonomic reflexes that are integrated at the S2–S4 and T12–L2 levels, respectively. Palpation and percussion of the bladder can identify the presence of abnormal bladder distention. Measurement of post-void residual urine after catheterization is used to assess residual urinary volume.

Pupil

Examination of the pupil is fully reviewed in the chapter on evaluation of cranial nerve III (Chapter 9).

Lacrimal Glands

Reduced or absent tearing occurs with lesions that affect the parasympathetic innervation of these glands (see Chapter 11). Schirmer's test is a means of quantifying lacrimal gland secretion; it consists of application of a standard sterile filter paper strip over the lower eyelid border. The standard minimum for tear production is a length of wetness of this strip of 15 mm after 5 minutes.

ASSOCIATED NEUROLOGICAL FINDINGS

Cerebral. Assessment of mental status, particularly the function of the frontal lobe, is important because it allows detection of abnormalities involving memory or the higher cognitive processes, which may be associated with incontinence due to uninhibited neurogenic bladder.

Cranial Nerves. Examination of the optic and oculomotor nerves allows for the localization of lesions that produce asymmetrical pupils or absent pupillary responses to light. Because the pupilloconstrictor fibers are located peripherally in the oculomotor nerve, compressive (extrinsic) lesions such as aneurysms or an uncal herniation elicit unilateral mydriasis before extraocular motor paralysis. Intrinsic (vascular) lesions, such as the neuropathy resulting from diabetes, affect the central fascicles of the nerve and produce a "pupil-sparing" oculomotor palsy. There are some exceptions to this classic distinction. Examination of the function of the trochlear and abducens nerves and of facial sensation in the ophthalmic and maxillary distribution of the trigeminal nerve helps to localize lesions at the level of the cavernous sinus and orbit. A facial nerve palsy may be associated with absence of lacrimation. Nystagmus, vertigo, and paralysis of the glossopharyngeal, vagus, and spinal accessory cranial nerves may occur in patients with lateral medullary infarctions that produce ipsilateral Horner's syndrome. These features, which suggest lower brain stem dysfunction, may also accompany syringobulbia, which is associated with orthostatic hypotension, and Arnold-Chiari malformations, which produce syncope.[25] In patients with symmetrical polyneuropathies such as Guillain-Barré syndrome, facial diplegia and other cranial nerve pareses can occur, especially in patients with the Miller-Fisher variant, which is often associated with autonomic instability.

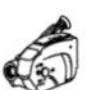

Motor/Reflexes/Cerebellar/Gait. Autonomic dysfunction is a frequent accompaniment of central and peripheral motor syndromes. Muscle weakness in the distribution of a peripheral nerve or root may accompany hyperhidrosis or vasomotor changes resulting from nerve injury. Distal symmetrical motor weakness with loss of the deep tendon reflexes indicates a large-fiber peripheral polyneuropathy that can be seen in patients with peripheral demyelinating diseases such as Guillain-Barré syndrome and in those with certain toxic or drug reactions to agents such as vincristine. Proximal muscle weakness and areflexia occur in patients with prejunctional neuromuscular transmission defects that occur with cholinergic autonomic failure, such as botulism[26] and the Lambert-Eaton myasthenic syndrome.

Spastic paraparesis is frequently found in patients with neurogenic bladder and detrusor-sphincter dyssynergia (e.g., as in multiple sclerosis). Areflexia in the lower extremities, which is associated with loss of the anal and bulbocavernosus reflexes, indicates a lesion of the cauda equina that produces hypotonic bladder, bowel hypomotility, and sphincter incontinence. Extrapyramidal, pyramidal, cerebellar, and autonomic deficits in varying combinations are characteristic of multiple system atrophy (i.e., the Shy-Drager syndrome), a neurodegenerative disorder of unknown etiology. Autonomic failure may also accompany Parkinson's disease with its associated resting tremor, bradykinesia, rigidity, and postural reflex impairment.

Sensory. Distal, symmetrical loss of sensation to pinprick and temperature is typical of the small-fiber peripheral neuropathies associated with diffuse autonomic failure (e.g., diabetes, amyloidosis). Insensitivity to pain occurs in patients with some hereditary sensory and autonomic neuropathies, including familial dysautonomia (Riley-Day syndrome). Loss of the vibration and joint position sense occurs in paraneoplastic sensory ganglioneuronopathies and Sjögren's syndrome—both of which are commonly associated with autonomic failure. Hypesthesia and allodynia in a limb, associated with vasomotor and sudomotor changes, occur in patients with damage to a peripheral nerve (causalgia) or the poorly understood reflex sympathetic dystrophy.

ASSOCIATED MEDICAL FINDINGS

Skin examination may reveal angiokeratomas in the trunk and lower limbs in patients with Fabry's disease, and the tongue may be enlarged in those with amyloidosis. Absence of fungiform papillae may also be demonstrated in children with familial dysautonomia (Riley-Day syndrome).

Evaluation Guidelines (Table 21–1)

Neuroimaging. Magnetic resonance imaging (MRI) is useful for the evaluation of patients with focal or organ-specific autonomic syndromes. It can detect lesions that involve the frontal lobes (e.g., hydrocephalus) or the cervical, thoracic, or lumbar spine, producing different types of neurogenic bladder. It is also indicated for the detection of hypothalamic lesions, lateral medullary infarctions, syringomyelia, or lesions in the cavernous sinus that produce Horner's syndrome. MRI of the neck is required when a diagnosis of paragangliomas arising from the carotid body or the vagus nerve is considered in patients with severe baroreflex failure. MRI of the abdomen can localize pheochromocytomas arising from chromaffin cells in the adrenal medulla or elsewhere in the abdomen, and imaging of the neck, chest, and pelvis should be used when pheochromocytomas are considered.

Neuroimaging has a low yield in the evaluation of patients with generalized autonomic failure, although it may show atrophy of the basal ganglia, pons, or cerebellum in patients with multiple system atrophy. In these patients, areas of hypointensity in T2-weighted MRI images of the posterolateral putamen have been reported.

Electrophysiology. Electromyography (EMG) and nerve conduction velocities (NCVs) are useful in evaluating patients with peripheral neuropathy. However, the studies may be normal in conditions that selectively affect small nerve fibers. Small-fiber function may be assessed using quantitative sensory testing to determine the sensory threshold for heat and cold sensation; these sensory modalities are mediated by the C-and A-delta nerve fibers. This technique measures the intensity of a stimulus necessary to evoke a specific sensation. EMG and NCVs are used to evaluate peripheral nerve injuries that may result in focal autonomic abnormalities. NCV studies may also be used to identify the cause of the predominantly cholinergic autonomic abnormalities that accompany the prejunctional disorders of neuromuscular transmission (e.g., botulism, the Lambert-Eaton myasthenic syndrome, and the autonomic abnormalities that accompany paraneoplastic sensory ganglioneuronopathy). Finally, EMG of the external anal sphincter may show denervation in patients with lesions of the conus or cauda equina and in patients with multiple system atrophy.

Electrodermal activity is generated by the sweat glands and overlying epidermis and mediated by supraspinal sites that include the orbitofrontal cortex, the posterior hypothalamus, the dorsal thalamus, and the ventrolateral reticular formation. This response, which occurs spontaneously and can be evoked by stimuli such as respiration, startling, mental stress, and electrical stimuli, is referred to as the sympathetic skin response or peripheral autonomic surface potential. The sympathetic skin response is used in some EMG laboratories to assess sudomotor function. It consists of a slow change in the electrical potential of the skin of the palms and feet that depends on sweat production and is evoked reflexively by unexpected noise, deep inspiration, and electrical stimuli. Absence of the sympathetic skin response occurs in patients with autonomic failure, but it has limited specificity and no localizing value.

Microneurographic recordings of activity in sympathetic fibers innervating muscle and skin allow direct assessment of sympathetic vasoconstrictor and skin sudomotor outflows, respectively. However, because this technique is laborious and invasive and requires considerable expertise as well as a very cooperative patient, it remains only a research tool.

Electroencephalography may show epileptiform activity in the temporolimbic areas, which may be associated with syncope or other paroxysmal autonomic phenomena. Sleep polysomnograms in patients with multiple system atrophy may allow the physician to make a diagnosis of sleep apnea.

Body Fluid and Tissue Analysis. Blood tests useful in the evaluation of patients with autonomic failure include blood glucose and glycosylated hemoglobin (diabetes), protein immunoelectrophoresis and genetic tests for the transthyretin variant (amyloidosis), vitamin B_{12} (pernicious anemia), erythrocyte sedimentation rate, antinuclear antibody (connective tissue diseases), extractable nuclear antigen (Sjögren's disease), antineuronal nuclear (anti-Hu) antibody (paraneoplasia), human immunodeficiency virus serology and, in selected cases, porphyrins (acute intermittent porphyria) or alpha-galactosidase (Fabry's disease). Some patients with acute or subacute autonomic neuropathy have antibodies against the $\alpha 3$ subunit of the ganglionic nicotinic acetylcholine receptor.[27]

Measurements of plasma cortisol in the morning and evening and, as previously mentioned, plasma catecholamines in the supine and standing positions may be helpful in the evaluation of patients with orthostatic hypotension.

Cerebrospinal Fluid. Cerebrospinal fluid examination may show albuminocytological dissociation with an elevated protein concentration and no pleocytosis in patients with Guillain-Barré syndrome and other acute pandysautonomias. Abdominal fat aspirate, rectal biopsy, or sural nerve biopsy should be considered in patients in whom amyloid neuropathy or Fabry's disease is suspected, and salivary or lacrimal gland biopsy should be done in patients in whom Sjögren's syndrome is suspected.

SPECIAL AUTONOMIC FUNCTION TESTING

Many laboratory tests are used to diagnose autonomic disorders, quantify autonomic function, and evaluate the efficacy of treatment. Disorders for which autonomic testing provides useful information include those involving generalized autonomic failure such as the Shy-Drager syndrome, Parkinson's disease, and pure autonomic failure; suspected distal small-fiber and other peripheral neuropathies; orthostatic intolerance of uncertain etiology; syncope; localized autonomic disorders; unexplained autonomic symptoms or

TABLE 21–1. **Useful Studies in the Evaluation of Disorders of the Autonomic Nervous System**

Syndrome	Neuroimaging	Electrophysiology	Fluid and Tissue Analysis	Neuropsychological Tests	Other Tests
Pandysautonomia					
Preganglionic disorders (multiple system atrophy)	MRI brain: decreased putaminal signal intensity on T2-weighted images	EMG of anal sphincter: large motor units	Supine NE normal; no increase with standing	N/A	Cardiovagal and adrenergic innervation tests abnormal; TST abnormal
Autonomic ganglionic and postganglionic disorders	N/A	NCV/EMG: Abnormal in peripheral neuropathies with motor/sensory involvement	Supine plasma NE low; no increase with standing ANNA: paraneoplastic syndromes	N/A	Cardiovagal and adrenergic innervation tests abnormal; TST abnormal Rectal biopsy: amyloidosis
Pure Cholinergic Dysautonomia	N/A	EMG abnormal in botulism and LEMS	Normal plasma NE Antibodies to voltage-gated calcium channels: LEMS	N/A	GI motility studies
Pure Adrenergic Dysautonomia	N/A	N/A	Very low plasma NE	N/A	Test of adrenergic innervation abnormal; TST normal
Focal Disorders					
Telencephalic	MRI brain	EEG monitoring for limbic seizures	N/A	Temporal lobe dysfunction	N/A
Diencephalic	MRI brain	N/A	Endocrinological tests for hypothalamic dysfunction Elevated creatinine kinase	Memory Cognition	N/A
Brain stem	MRI brain	N/A	CSF abnormalities in MS	N/A	N/A
Spinal cord	MRI spinal cord	N/A	CSF abnormalities in MS	N/A	Bladder EMG or cystometrogram

MRI, Magnetic resonance imaging; EMG, electromyography; NCV, nerve conduction velocity; LEMS, Lambert-Eaton myasthenic syndrome; ANNA, antineuronal nuclear antibody (anti-Hu); NE, norepinephrine; TST, thermoregulatory sweat test; CSF, cerebrospinal fluid; MS, multiple selerosis.

signs; and complex regional pain syndromes. The blood pressure and heart rate response to active standing, the passive head-up tilt test, and the Valsalva maneuver are the most commonly performed noninvasive tests used to assess reflex circulatory control.

Evaluation of Cardiac Vagal Innervation

Heart Rate Response to Deep Breathing. Normally, heart rate varies from beat to beat, primarily due to changes in vagal activity. The most noticeable variation is that which is synchronous with the respiratory cycle (respiratory sinus arrhythmia). Heart rate increases during inspiration and decreases during expiration. The heart rate response to deep breathing is maximal at around six deep breaths per minute. Laboratory measures of heart rate variability include the peak-to-trough amplitude during a single breath, the standard deviation of the electrocardiogram R-R intervals during 1 minute, and other statistical measures such as the mean square successive difference, the expiratory-inspiratory ratio (E/I ratio), and the mean circular resultant.[28, 29] The subject's age and the rate and depth of respiration influence heart rate variation in response to deep breathing. When these variables are taken into account, the maximum heart rate variation in response to deep breathing is the best noninvasive test for the assessment of cardiac vagal innervation.[28, 29]

Heart Rate Response to Valsalva Maneuver. The Valsalva maneuver is typically performed by blowing through a mouthpiece connected to a mercury manometer for 15 or 20 seconds. The mercury column of the manometer is maintained at 40 mm. The normal cardiovascular response to a Valsalva maneuver has four phases (Fig. 21–5). Phase 1 consists of a transient rise in arterial pressure and an associated decrease in heart rate. In phase 2, during the expiratory phase of the maneuver, there is a gradual fall in blood pressure followed by a recovery. An increase in heart rate accompanies this phase. Phase 3 consists of a sudden brief fall in blood pressure with an accompanying increase in heart rate that occurs with the cessation of straining. In phase 4 there is an increase in blood pressure above the resting value (the "overshoot") that is accompanied by a bradycardia. Phases 1 and 3 most likely reflect mechanical factors, while phases 2 and 4 are a consequence of sympathetic, vagal, and baroreflex interactions. The Valsalva ratio (i.e., the ratio between the tachycardia occurring during the maneuver and the postmaneuver bradycardia) provides an index of cardiac vagal function.[30]

Heart Rate Response to Postural Change (The "30:15 Ratio"). The heart rate changes that occur during the first 30 seconds of standing result mostly from modification of cardiovagal activity and are blocked by atropine (Fig. 21–6). Heart rate increases sharply on standing, peaking at about 12 seconds (about the fifteenth beat). It then becomes progressively slower until about 20 seconds after standing (so that the thirtieth R-R interval is usually the longest), and then it gradually rises again. This transient relative bradycardia is due to reflex activation of efferent cardiac vagal fibers. These changes are reflected by the 30:15 ratio, which is calculated by dividing the longest R-R interval around the thirtieth beat by the shortest R-R interval around the fifteenth beat ($RR_{max\ 30}/RR_{min\ 15}$ ratio). In subjects with abnormal cardiovagal function, the bradycardia is reduced or absent.[31–33]

Other tests of cardiovagal function include the *carotid sinus massage*, the *cold face test* (which assesses the trigeminovagal reflex), the *atropine test*,[22] and *power spectral analysis*, which detects high-frequency oscillations of heart rate.[34]

Evaluation of Cardiovascular Sympathetic Innervation

Cardiovascular Response to Postural Change. Measurement of changes in blood pressure and heart rate induced by passive tilt or active standing is the most useful test of sympathetic function. During upright tilt to 60 degrees or more, normal subjects undergo a transient reduction in systolic, diastolic, and mean blood pressure, followed by a recovery within 1 minute. The heart rate also increases by 10 to 20 beats per minute. Patients with adrenergic failure have a marked reduction in systolic, diastolic, and pulse pressure with no recovery, and they have an inadequate compensatory tachycardia.[22, 35]

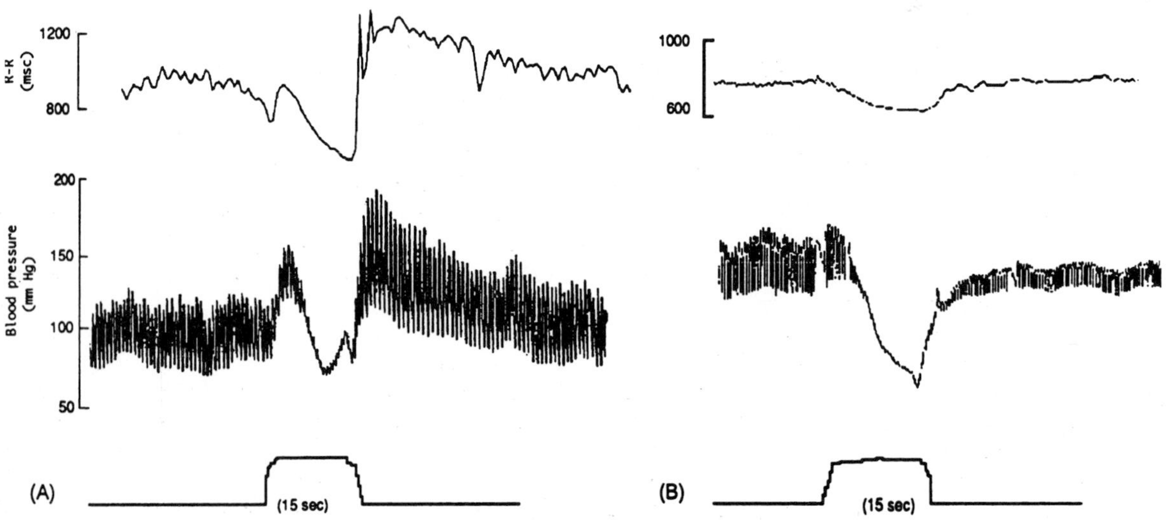

FIGURE 21–5. Valsalva maneuver induced changes in R-R intervals and blood pressure by Finapress recording in (*A*) a normal subject and (*B*) a patient with autonomic failure. (Reproduced with permission by Korczyn A: Handbook of Autonomic Nervous System Dysfunction. New York, Marcel Dekker, Inc, 1996.)

A) 36 y.o. male with autonomic failure

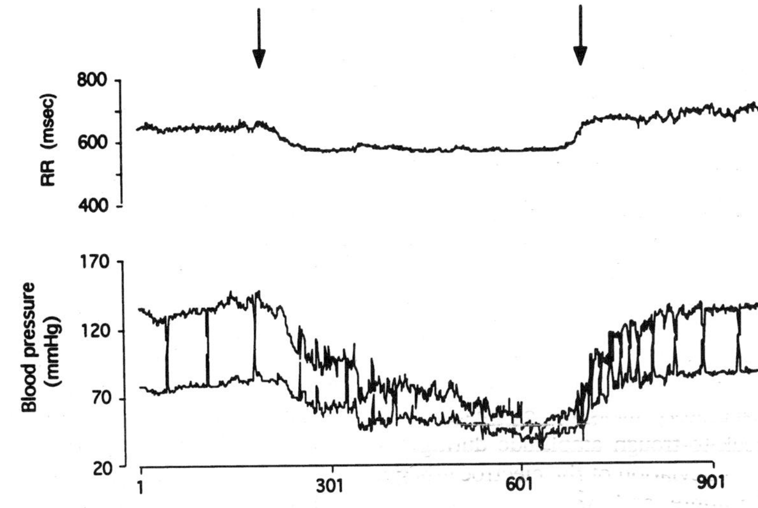

B) 28 y.o. male with neurally mediated syncope

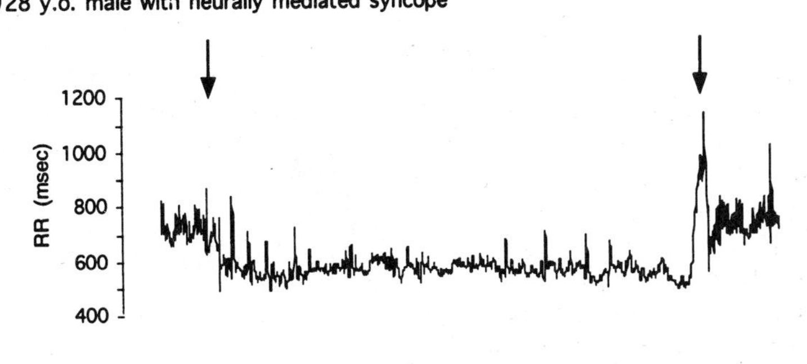

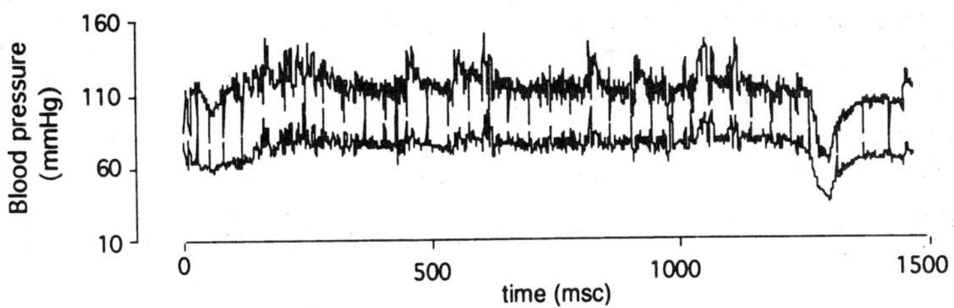

FIGURE 21–6. Posturally induced changes in continuous R-R intervals and blood pressure by Finapress recordings in (*A*) a subject with primary autonomic failure and (*B*) a subject with neurally mediated syncope. The initial arrow denotes when the head is tilted up, and the latter arrow denotes when the head is tilted down after syncope has been induced. (Reproduced with permission from Robertson D, Low P, Polinsky R, et al: Primer on the Autonomic Nervous System. San Diego, Academic Press, 1995.)

Blood Pressure Response to Valsalva Maneuver. Beat-to-beat recordings of the blood pressure during a Valsalva maneuver may be used to measure cardiac adrenergic function. Sympathetic failure is characterized by a profound decrease of blood pressure in phase 2 and an absence of the blood pressure "overshoot" in phase 4 of the Valsalva maneuver.[30]

Other Tests. Other tests used to assess sympathetic cardiovascular outflow include the hemodynamic response to physical or emotional perturbations such as immersion of a hand in cold water for 1 minute (*cold pressor test*), isometric exercise (e.g., the *sustained handgrip* maneuver), or emotional stress (e.g., *mental arithmetic*). In normal subjects, these maneuvers produce increases in diastolic pressure of more than 15 mm Hg and in heart rate of more than 10 beats per minute.[22] The *venoarteriolar reflex* is an axon reflex mediated by sympathetic C fibers. This reflex is provoked by distention of the veins of a dependent limb that produces local arteriolar constriction; the reflex can be detected by a decrease in skin blood flow.[22]

In research laboratories, other techniques used to evaluate autonomic circulatory control include the application of lower body negative pressure, which pools blood in the lower part of the body and elicits autonomic responses similar to those induced by standing up. The neck chamber device can also be used. This device modifies carotid artery transmural pressure and allows assessment of the carotid sinus baroreflexes. Finally, changes in heart rate in response to pressor or depressor drugs can be evaluated.[22]

Plasma Catecholamines. Circulating norepinephrine (NE) originates primarily in the sympathetic nerves innervating the blood vessels of muscles. Plasma NE constitutes approximately 10 percent of NE released into the synaptic cleft that escapes neuronal reuptake and "spills over" into the bloodstream. Patients with postganglionic autonomic disorders, such as pure autonomic failure or diabetic neuropathy,

TABLE 21–2. **Differentiation of Preganglionic Versus Postganglionic Disorders**

	Preganglionic	Postganglionic
Pandysautonomia	Multiple system atrophy	Pure autonomic failure Small-fiber neuropathy
Plasma norepinephrine	Normal	Reduced
Norepinephrine response to standing	Abolished	Abolished
Norepinephrine response to edrophonium	Normal	Impaired
Blood pressure response to tyramine	Increased	No increase
Blood pressure response to norepinephrine	Increased, with normal threshold	Decreased threshold (denervation supersensitivity)
Vasopressin response to standing	Impaired	Normal or exaggerated
Thermoregulatory sweat responses	Impaired	Impaired
Cholinergic sudomotor axon reflex	Normal	Impaired
Horner's syndrome		
Pupil response to phenylephrine	Dilated	No response
Pupil response to diluted alpha-agonist	No response	Dilated (supersensitivity)
Adie's pupil		Constricts with diluted muscarinic agonist (denervation supersensitivity)

frequently have reduced plasma NE levels at rest in the supine position. In normal subjects, plasma NE levels double with the assumption of the upright posture. In contrast, this response is absent in patients with both pre- and postganglionic sympathetic failure.[35] Determination of plasma and urinary levels of NE metabolites, such as dihydroxyphenylglycol (DHPG) and normetanephrine, may also be useful for separating preganglionic from postganglionic causes of autonomic failure (Table 21–2).[36] In patients who lack dopamine beta hydroxylase, the enzyme that converts dopamine to NE, NE in plasma is virtually undetectable, whereas dopamine is high and increases further with maneuvers that increase sympathetic neural discharge.[37]

Norepinephrine levels can be measured following an infusion of edrophonium, a cholinomimetic agent. This agent induces the release of NE by stimulating the sympathetic ganglia. NE levels can also be measured following the infusion of tyramine, an indirect sympathomimetic agent, which releases NE from sympathetic terminals. The pressor response to an infusion of NE and other alpha-adrenergic agonists may be used to assess denervation supersensitivity and baroreflex function.

These pharmacological tests have been used to differentiate preganglionic from postganglionic causes of sympathetic failure. Postganglionic autonomic failure is characterized by decreased NE release and lack of a pressor response to edrophonium and tyramine. There is also a decreased threshold for the pressor effects of NE and other adrenergic agonists consistent with denervation hypersensitivity.[20]

Evaluation of Sympathetic Cholinergic (Sudomotor) Innervation

Testing of the eccrine sweat glands can localize the site of sympathetic nervous system dysfunction in patients with autonomic failure. Thermoregulatory sweat testing is used to evaluate both the central and peripheral sympathetic efferents, including the hypothalamus, the cervical and thoracic spinal cord, the peripheral autonomic nerves, and the sweat glands. This test, however, does not differentiate between preganglionic and postganglionic causes of anhidrosis. Postganglionic sudomotor function can be determined by measuring the sweat output after iontophoresis or intradermal injection of cholinergic agonists such as pilocarpine, nicotine, or methacholine. These agents either stimulate the sweat glands directly or affect a neighboring population of sweat glands via an axonal reflex. The site of a lesion can be established if the thermoregulatory sweat test is combined with a test measuring postganglionic sudomotor function. For example, an abnormal result of a thermoregulatory sweat test combined with normal postganglionic function indicates a preganglionic cause of anhidrosis. On the other hand, an abnormal thermoregulatory sweat test result in a patient with abnormal postganglionic function indicates a postganglionic cause of anhidrosis. Skin potential recordings that measure skin conductance, skin resistance, or the sympathetic skin potential provide an alternative measure of sudomotor function. The following tests of sudomotor function may be performed.

Thermoregulatory Sweat Test. Thermoregulatory sweating is tested by raising the body temperature with an external heating source. This test evaluates the distribution of sweating by measuring the change in color of an indicator powder such as iodine with starch, quinizarin, or alizarin-red in response to a rise in core body temperature.[38]

Quantitative Sudomotor Axon Reflex Test. The quantitative sudomotor axon reflex test (QSART) provides a quantitative measure of postganglionic sudomotor function. The sudomotor response measured by the QSART is mediated by an "axon reflex" carried by unmyelinated postganglionic sympathetic cholinergic sudomotor fibers. This axon reflex can be elicited by iontophoresis of a cholinergic agonist.[39, 40]

Sweat Imprint. A sweat imprint is formed by the secretion of active sweat glands into a plastic or silicone mold in response to iontophoresis of a cholinergic agonist. This test can be used to determine sweat gland density, sweat droplet size, and sweat volume per unit of area.

Clinical Syndromes Involving the Autonomic Nervous System (Table 21–3)

Clinical syndromes involving ANS dysfunction may be divided into those involving diffuse autonomic failure and pure cholinergic or adrenergic disorders (Table 21–4).

TABLE 21–3. **Selected Etiologies Associated with Disorders of the Autonomic Nervous System**

Etiological Category	Selected Etiologies	Chapter
Structural Disorders		
Developmental structural disorders	Arnold-Chiari malformation	28
	Syringomyelia	
	Normal pressure hydrocephalus	
Hereditary and Degenerative Disorders		
Movement disorders	Multiple system atrophy	34
Degenerative motor, sensory, and autonomic disorders	Riley-Day syndrome	36
	Pure autonomic failure	
Hereditary nondegenerative neuromuscular disease	Amyloidosis	37
Acquired Metabolic and Nutritional Disorders		
Endogenous metabolic disorders	Diabetes	38
Nutritional deficiencies and syndromes associated with alcoholism	Wernicke's encephalopathy/thiamine deficiency	40
Infectious Disorders		
Viral infections	Poliomyelitis	41
Transmissible spongiform encephalopathy	Fatal familial insomnia	43
HIV and AIDS	HIV-associated neuropathy	44
	HIV-related Guillain-Barré syndrome	
Neurovascular Disorders	Vertebrobasilar ischemia	45
Neoplastic Disorders		
Primary neurological tumors	Brain stem glioma	46
Demyelinating Disorders		
Demyelinating disorders of the central nervous system	Multiple sclerosis with bladder dysfunction	48
Demyelinating disorders of the peripheral nervous system	Guillain-Barré syndrome	49
Autoimmune and Inflammatory Disorders	Lambert-Eaton myasthenic syndrome	50
Traumatic Disorders	Spinal cord: blunt or penetrating trauma	51
Epilepsy	Temporal/limbic seizures	52
Headache and Facial Pain	Cluster headaches	53
Drug-Induced and Iatrogenic Neurological Disorders	Drugs: chemotherapeutic agents (vincristine)	55

AIDS, Acquired immunodeficiency syndrome: HIV, human immunodeficiency virus.

DIFFUSE AUTONOMIC FAILURE (PANDYSAUTONOMIA)

Central (Preganglionic) Disorders

Multiple System Atrophy. Multiple system atrophy (MSA, Shy-Drager syndrome) is a degenerative disorder of the CNS that affects the extrapyramidal, cerebellar, and autonomic neurons (see Chapter 34). Autonomic dysfunction in patients with MSA is due to the loss of preganglionic neurons in the brain stem and spinal cord. Patients with MSA typically present with diffuse autonomic failure and parkinsonian, cerebellar, or pyramidal deficits in different combinations.[41] Autonomic features include orthostatic intolerance, erectile dysfunction in males, bowel hypomotility, urinary incontinence due to denervation of the external urinary sphincter, and respiratory disturbances (sleep apnea and laryngeal stridor). There is usually a poor response to levodopa.[42] Pathologically, cell loss and gliosis in striatonigral, olivopontocerebellar, and autonomic neurons are evident, and intracytoplasmic oligodendroglial and neuronal inclusions are frequently present.

Parkinson's Disease. Autonomic dysfunction in patients with Parkinson's disease (see Chapter 34) is rarely as severe as that seen in patients with MSA. Autonomic failure frequently occurs late in the course of the illness and is often associated with levodopa and dopamine agonist therapy. In patients with Parkinson's disease, Lewy bodies are found not only in central but also in peripheral neurons, suggesting that autonomic dysfunction in this disorder may be caused by both preganglionic and postganglionic neuronal dysfunction.

Autonomic Ganglionic and Postganglionic Disorders

Pure Autonomic Failure. Pure autonomic failure (PAF) is an idiopathic, sporadic, degenerative disorder of the autonomic nervous system of adult onset.[43] Unlike MSA and Parkinson's disease, PAF has no motor manifestations. In patients with PAF, intracytoplasmic eosinophilic inclusion bodies with the histologic appearance of Lewy bodies, similar to those found in Parkinson's disease, are identified in neurons of the substantia nigra, locus ceruleus, thoracolumbar and sacral spinal cord, as well as sympathetic ganglia and postganglionic nerves.[44] The disorder is slowly progressive and has a better prognosis than MSA (see Table 21–2).

Autonomic Peripheral Neuropathies and Neuropathies. Acute autonomic neuropathies with prominent sympathetic

TABLE 21–4. **Autonomic Nervous System Syndromes**

Diffuse Autonomic Failure (Pandysautonomia)
Preganglionic autonomic failure—central neurodegenerative diseases
Multiple system atrophy (Shy-Drager syndrome)
Parkinson's disease with autonomic failure
Ganglionic and postganglionic disorders—peripheral neurodegenerative disorders
Pure autonomic failure
Peripheral neuropathies and neuronopathies with autonomic failure
Acute and subacute (preganglionic and postganglionic)
Acute pandysautonomia
Guillain-Barré syndrome
Paraneoplastic pandysautonomia
Others (porphyria, toxins, drugs)
Chronic small-fiber (postganglionic) neuropathies
Diabetes
Amyloidosis
Hereditary (familial dysautonomia, Fabry's disease)
Subacute or chronic sensory and autonomic ganglionopathies
Paraneoplastic
Sjögren's syndrome
Other peripheral neuropathies
Infections (human immunodeficiency virus)
Connective tissue disease (systemic lupus erythematosus)
Metabolic-nutritional (alcohol, uremia, vitamin B_{12} deficiency)
Pure Cholinergic or Adrenergic Disorders
Cholinergic dysautonomias
Associated with neuromuscular transmission defect
Botulism (acute)
Lambert-Eaton myasthenic syndrome (chronic)
Not associated with neuromuscular transmission defect
Acute cholinergic dysautonomia
Chronic idiopathic anhidrosis
Adie's syndrome
Chagas disease
Adrenergic dysautonomias
Pure adrenergic neuropathy
Dopamine–beta-hydroxylase deficiency

and parasympathetic involvement (i.e., acute pandysautonomia) occur in isolation or accompany the Guillain-Barré syndrome and acute paraneoplastic neuropathies. The protein level in the cerebrospinal fluid may be elevated, and the autonomic features may respond to intravenous immunoglobulin. Paraneoplastic dysautonomia may occur in association with carcinoma of the lung, pancreatic carcinoma, Hodgkin's disease, testicular cancer, and other neoplasms. Paraneoplastic gastrointestinal dysfunction with constipation and intestinal pseudo-obstruction has been reported in patients with small-cell carcinoma of the lung and elevated titers of anti-Hu antibodies. Acute autonomic dysfunction may also be a feature of porphyria and of the neuropathies due to drugs (e.g., vincristine, taxol, cisplatin) and toxins (e.g., thallium, acrylamide).[45]

Dysautonomia is a prominent feature of some chronic neuropathies affecting small-diameter unmyelinated fibers. Diabetes mellitus is the most common cause of autonomic neuropathy in the developed world. Typical features of diabetic autonomic neuropathy are orthostatic intolerance, impotence, voiding difficulties, gastroparesis, constipation alternating with diarrhea, and gustatory sweating. Patients with primary or familial amyloid neuropathy typically present with distal sensory symptoms, although the autonomic manifestations may be the presenting feature (see Chapter 37). Sensory neuronopathy with autonomic failure may be a paraneoplastic phenomenon that may be associated with Sjögren's syndrome (see Chapter 50) or may be idiopathic.[45]

Hereditary sensory and autonomic neuropathies (HSANs) are characterized by prominent sensory loss and dysautonomia. Autonomic manifestations are mild in patients with HSAN type I and II but prominent in those with HSAN type III (Riley-Day syndrome, familial dysautonomia) (see Chapter 36). Familial dysautonomia is an autosomal recessive disorder that is seen primarily in Ashkenazi Jewish children. Its clinical features include insensitivity to pain and temperature, absence of tears, hypoactive corneal and tendon reflexes, and absence of fungiform papillae of the tongue. Patients with familial dysautonomia have poor suck and feeding responses, esophageal reflux with vomiting and aspiration, uncoordinated swallowing, episodic hyperhidrosis, vasomotor instability, postural hypotension, hypertensive crises, supersensitivity to cholinergic and adrenergic agents, and absent histamine flare.[27] HSAN types IV and V, characterized by congenital insensitivity to pain and anhidrosis, have been linked to different mutations of the trkA gene encoding for the nerve growth factor receptor.[46]

Fabry's disease is an X-linked recessive disorder caused by a deficiency of alpha-galactosidase A (see Chapter 30). Its manifestations include painful distal peripheral neuropathy; a truncal reddish-purple macular papular rash; angiectases of the skin, conjunctiva, nail bed, and oral mucosa; progressive renal disease; corneal opacities; and cerebrovascular accidents. The autonomic manifestations include hypohidrosis or anhidrosis, reduced saliva and tear formation, impaired histamine flare, and gastrointestinal dysmotility.[45]

PURE CHOLINERGIC OR ADRENERGIC DISORDERS

Cholinergic Dysautonomias. Acute or chronic cholinergic dysautonomias may occur in isolation or in patients with impaired neuromuscular transmission. In the Lambert-Eaton myasthenic syndrome (see Chapter 50) and in botulism (see Chapter 39), acetylcholine release from motor as well as autonomic neurons fails. Thus, neuromuscular and autonomic cholinergic neurotransmission is impaired, and muscle weakness, reflex loss, and autonomic failure result.[26]

Chronic disorders that affect cholinergic function without neuromuscular impairment include Adie's syndrome, chronic idiopathic anhidrosis, Ross's syndrome (a combination of Adie's pupils and segmental anhidrosis), and Chagas' disease, a disease caused by *Trypanosoma cruzi* that affects the neurons of the parasympathetic ganglion and produces megaesophagus, megacolon, and cardiomyopathy (see Chapter 42).

Pure Adrenergic Neuropathy. Dopamine–beta-hydroxylase deficiency is a hereditary disease characterized by an inability to convert dopamine (DA) to NE. This disorder is characterized by severe orthostatic hypotension accompanied by ptosis, ejaculatory failure, nocturia, nasal congestion, and hyperextensible joints. Typically, the serum NE/DA ratio is 0.1 (normal 10).[37]

AUTONOMIC DYSFUNCTION SECONDARY TO FOCAL CENTRAL NERVOUS SYSTEM DISEASE

The autonomic nervous system syndrome may also be classified anatomically into telencephalic, diencephalic, brain stem, and spinal cord disorders (Table 21–5).

Telencephalon Syndromes. Temporolimbic seizures may induce changes in heart rate, heart rhythm, and blood pressure. Cardiovascular manifestations of seizures include sinus tachycardia or bradyarrhythmias (including sinus arrest) with syncope. Seizure-induced ventricular tachycardia and fibrillation have been implicated in sudden death. Other autonomic manifestations of seizures include flushing, pallor, shivering, sweating, symmetrical or unilateral piloerection, visceral sensations, vomiting (ictus emeticus), and respiratory changes.[4, 47] Ischemic damage to the insula has been associated with cardiac arrhythmias and contralateral hyperhidrosis. When the cingulate and paracentral cortices are involved, urinary incontinence may occur because of uninhibited bladder contractions.

Diencephalon Syndromes. Disorders affecting the hypothalamus may produce disturbances of thermoregulation, osmotic balance, endocrine function, and state of alertness.[4] Chronic expanding lesions such as tumors or granulomas cause hypothermia, whereas acute lesions may cause hypothermia or hyperthermia. Wernicke's encephalopathy should be suspected in alcoholic and other malnourished patients presenting with unexplained hypothermia, particularly in the presence of disturbances of consciousness and oculomotor function.[4] Episodic hyperhidrosis with hypothermia may occur with no apparent cause,[48] as a manifestation of agenesis of the corpus callosum and neighboring regions of the basal forebrain,[49] or during paroxysms of autonomic hyperactivity.

TABLE 21–5. Level-Specific Central Autonomic Nervous System Disorders

Telencephalon	Stroke
	Temporolimbic seizures
Diencephalon	Wernicke's syndrome
	Episodic hyperhidrosis with hypothermia
	Paroxysmal autonomic hyperactivity
	Fatal familial insomnia
	Iatrogenic
	Neuroleptic malignant syndrome
	Serotonin syndrome
Brain stem	Tumors
	Vertebrobasilar disease
	Syringobulbia
	Arnold-Chiari type I malformation
	Inflammation (multiple sclerosis, poliomyelitis)
Spinal cord	Trauma
	Syringomyelia
	Multiple sclerosis
	Tetanus
	Stiff-person syndrome

Although such paroxysmal autonomic hyperactivity in patients with brain tumors and other diseases of the diencephalon has been referred to as diencephalic seizures, this term is a misnomer. The electroencephalogram shows no ictal activity, and the episodes are refractory to antiepileptic drugs. Paroxysmal autonomic hyperactivity was first described in patients with tumors situated in the region of the third ventricle that caused hydrocephalus and abrupt increases in intracranial pressure. The majority of cases, however, are due to severe closed head injuries marked by episodic increases in intracranial pressure and acute hydrocephalus following subarachnoid hemorrhage.[4]

Sympathetic hyperactivity also occurs in a transmissible spongiform encephalopathy characterized by severe atrophy of the anteroventral and dorsomedial nuclei of the thalamus. This autosomal dominant prion disease presents with disruption of endocrine circadian rhythms, motor dysfunction, and progressive intractable insomnia—thus its name, familial fatal insomnia (see Chapter 43).[50]

Brain Stem Syndromes. Cerebrovascular disease is the most common cause of dysautonomia associated with brain stem dysfunction. Transient ischemic attacks in the basilar artery territory may present with paroxysmal hypertension before any focal neurological deficit becomes apparent. Lateral medullary infarction (Wallenberg's syndrome) produces Horner's syndrome and, occasionally, more severe autonomic abnormalities such as profound bradycardia, supine hypotension, or central hypoventilation.[4]

Other brain stem disorders associated with autonomic dysfunction include tumors, syringobulbia, Arnold-Chiari malformation type 1, multiple sclerosis, and poliomyelitis. Brain stem tumors may present with intractable vomiting, orthostatic hypotension, or paroxysmal hypertension. Syringobulbia may produce Horner's syndrome, orthostatic hypotension, cardiovagal dysfunction, lability of arterial pressure, and central hypoventilation.[25] Syncope, sleep apnea, and cardiorespiratory arrest have been reported in association with the Arnold-Chiari malformation type 1. Less common manifestations of brain stem dysfunction include hypertension due to involvement of the medullary reticular formation in poliomyelitis (see Chapter 41); autonomic hyperactivity, most likely due to disinhibition of preganglionic sympathetic and parasympathetic neurons in tetanus (see Chapter 39); and fulminant neurogenic pulmonary edema due to demyelination of the area surrounding the NTS in patients with multiple sclerosis (see Chapter 48).[4]

Spinal Cord Syndromes. Traumatic spinal cord injury, particularly injury above the T5 level, is associated with severe and disabling cardiovascular, gastrointestinal, bladder, and sexual dysfunction. These patients have both supine and orthostatic hypotension and are at risk of developing bradycardia and cardiac arrest during tracheal suction or other maneuvers that activate the vagovagal reflexes. Vasopressin and the renin-angiotensin-aldosterone system have an enhanced role in maintenance of orthostatic arterial pressure in patients with spinal cord lesions. Lack of vasomotor and sudomotor thermoregulatory responses below the level of the lesion may lead to severe hypothermia or hyperthermia in response to changes in environmental temperature. Acute spinal injury or spinal shock produces a paralytic atonic bladder. The pattern of dysfunction seen in the chronic stages of disease, however, depends on the level of the lesion. Lesions above the sacral parasympathetic nucleus produce spastic bladder, commonly with detrusor-sphincter dyssynergia, whereas lesions of the conus medullaris produce a flaccid, areflexic bladder.

In patients with chronic tetraplegia with lesions at or above the T5 level, stimulation of the skin, muscle, or viscera innervated by segments below the lesion may result in a massive reflex activation of sympathetic and sacral parasympathetic outflows, referred to as autonomic dysreflexia.[51] Stimuli that trigger autonomic dysreflexia arise primarily from the bladder, bowel, or skin. Vasodilation above the level of the lesion produces flushing of the face, chest, and upper arms and congestion of the nasopharyngeal mucosa. There may be excessive sweating above the anesthetic dermatome, piloerection, pallor in the abdomen and lower extremities, and pupillary dilatation. Severe hypertension is a prominent feature of autonomic dysreflexia and can result in hypertensive encephalopathy or intracranial, subarachnoid, or retinal hemorrhage. The combined parasympathetic and sympathetic stimulation may cause potentially dangerous supraventricular and ventricular arrhythmias.

Multiple sclerosis (MS) may affect autonomic pathways at the level of the spinal cord, brain stem, or diencephalon. Bladder, bowel, and sexual dysfunction are prominent autonomic manifestations of MS. The pathophysiological basis of the bladder dysfunction seen in patients with MS is detrusor hyper-reflexia and detrusor-sphincter dyssynergy. Subclinical abnormalities in cardiovascular sympathetic and parasympathetic function and abnormal thermoregulatory sweating detected by testing in the autonomic laboratory are common in patients with MS.

Syringomyelia produces partial interruption of sympathetic output pathways in the intermediolateral cell columns. Its autonomic manifestations include Horner's syndrome, sudomotor and vasomotor dysfunction, and trophic changes in the limbs, especially the hands.

Tetanus and the stiff-person syndrome may be associated with sympathetic hyperactivity due to lack of synaptic inhibition of preganglionic autonomic neurons. This results in hyperpyrexia, sweating, tachycardia, hypertension, tachypnea, and pupillary dilatation, usually associated with the muscle spasms.

TOPOGRAPHIC OR ORGAN-SPECIFIC DISORDERS
(Table 21–6)

Pupils

Argyll Robertson Pupils. Argyll Robertson pupils are irregular and smaller than normal in darkness and demonstrate lack of the pupillary light reflex with preserved pupillary constriction during accommodation and convergence for near objects. These features, as in patients with large pupils with light-near dissociation, usually indicate a lesion in the rostral midbrain at the level of the posterior commissure.

Adie's Pupil. These tonic pupils are large and irregular in shape, poorly reactive to light, and indicate a lesion of the ciliary ganglion or short ciliary nerves. On slit-lamp evaluation, regional palsies of the iris sphincter are visible. These pupils have a hypersensitive constrictor response to administration of diluted muscarinic agonists, such as a 2.5 percent solution of methylcholine chloride or a 0.1 percent solution of pilocarpine. Adie's pupils are tonic pupils associated with reduced or absent tendon reflexes.

TABLE 21–6. **Topographic or Organ-Restricted Autonomic Disorders**

Disorders of the Pupil
Affecting parasympathetic outflow
Third nerve lesion
Argyll Robertson pupil
Adie's pupil
Affecting sympathetic outflow
Horner's syndrome
Pourfour du Petit syndrome
Facial Hyperhidrosis and Flushing
Gustatory sweating
Harlequin syndrome
Cluster headache
Vasomotor and Sudomotor Disorders of the Limb
Vasomotor disorders
Raynaud's phenomenon
Acrocyanosis
Livedo reticularis
Erythromelalgia
Essential hyperhidrosis
Complex neuropathic pain syndromes
Painful distal peripheral neuropathy
Nerve trauma (causalgia)
Undetermined and multifactorial: Complex regional pain syndrome
Reflex sympathetic dystrophy
Neurogenic Bladder
Spastic bladder with or without detrusor-sphincter dyssynergia
Flaccid bladder
Gastrointestinal Dysmotility
Pseudo-obstruction
Sexual Dysfunction
Erectile dysfunction
Ejaculation dysfunction

Horner's Syndrome. A unilateral small pupil is commonly due to underactivity of the ipsilateral sympathetic pathways. Miosis is commonly associated with ptosis (lid droop) due to sympathetic denervation of the tarsal muscle and facial anhidrosis (loss of sweating). This combination is known as Horner's syndrome. Oculosympathetic paralysis occurs ipsilaterally owing to (1) central lesions involving the hypothalamospinal pathways at the dorsolateral brain stem tegmentum (e.g., a lateral medullary infarct); (2) preganglionic lesions (e.g., compression of the sympathetic chain by a tumor in the apex of the lung); or (3) postganglionic lesions at the level of the internal carotid plexus (e.g., lesions of the cavernous sinus). Postganglionic Horner's syndrome does not result in facial anhidrosis because pupilodilator and sudomotor axons follow separate paths along branches of the internal and external carotid arteries, respectively.

Local instillation of drugs that affect sympathetic neurotransmission in the pupil helps to localize the lesion causing oculosympathetic paralysis. Cocaine hydrochloride (5 to 10 percent), which prevents NE reuptake, will not dilate a pupil that is miotic because of a lesion anywhere in the sympathetic pathway. The responsible lesion can be further localized by hydroxyamphetamine hydrobromide (Paredrine 1 percent), which is an indirect sympathomimetic agent that releases norepinephrine from the synaptic terminals, thus eliciting pupillary dilatation in patients with preganglionic but not postganglionic Horner's syndrome. Phenylephrine hydrochloride (Neo-Synephrine) is a direct alpha-agonist that in a low concentration (1 percent) dilates the pupil only in patients with a postganglionic Horner's syndrome associated with denervation hypersensitivity of the pupil.

Facial Hyperhidrosis and Flushing

Facial flushing may result from the release of tonic sympathetic vasoconstriction, active sympathetic vasodilatation, increased parasympathetic activity via the greater petrosal nerve, and the release of vasoactive peptides. Gustatory sweating and flushing occur in the following conditions: idiopathic hemifacial hyperhidrosis associated with hypertrophy of the sweat glands; following bilateral cervicothoracic sympathectomy with reinnervation of the superior sympathetic ganglion by preganglionic sympathetic fibers destined for the sweat glands; after local damage to the autonomic fibers traveling with the peripheral branches of the trigeminal nerve (e.g., in parotid or submaxillary gland surgery or V3 zoster) with reinnervation of sweat glands and blood vessels by parasympathetic vasodilator fibers destined for the salivary glands; and accompanying peripheral neuropathies, most frequently diabetes mellitus.[52]

Sympathetic failure may produce loss of sweating and flushing as manifestations of Horner's syndrome. In contrast, the Porfour du Petit syndrome consists of a dilated pupil with flushing and hyperhidrosis due to sympathetic hyperactivity. This syndrome is seen in patients with sympathetic nervous system lesions, frequently following injuries of the neck that damage the sympathetic plexus around the carotid artery. The harlequin syndrome consists of a sudden onset of flushing and sweating on one side of the face. This disorder may be due to lesions in the contralateral central or peripheral sympathetic nervous system pathways. Attacks of cluster headache may be accompanied by ipsilateral signs of parasympathetic hyperactivity (lacrimation and nasal discharge), sympathetic overactivity (forehead sweating), and ocular sympathetic paralysis (miosis and ptosis). The mechanisms producing these phenomena have no widely accepted explanation. Changes in both the sympathetic and the trigeminovascular pathways may be responsible for the autonomic features that accompany migraine and cluster headaches.[52]

Vasomotor and Sudomotor Disorders of the Limbs

Hyperhidrosis may be generalized or localized. Localized hyperhidrosis is rare and may occur with injury to the spinal cord (e.g., in syringomyelia), peripheral nerves (e.g., with partial median or sciatic nerve injury), or eccrine sweat glands. Perilesional hyperhidrosis may surround an anhidrotic region produced by a lesion of the sympathetic ganglia or rami. The axillary eccrine sweat glands are activated by thermal stimuli, whereas the palmar and plantar glands are activated by emotional stimuli. Primary or essential hyperhidrosis affects the axillary, palmar, and plantar regions and may be familial. Available medical treatments, including systemic anticholinergics and beta-blockers and topical agents such as aluminum antiperspirants and tap water iontophoresis, are largely ineffective. Surgical sympathectomy significantly reduces sweating but has frequent side effects, including pneumothorax, Horner's syndrome, and compensatory sweating in other areas of the body. Recently, intradermal injections of botulinum toxin type A, which blocks the release of acetylcholine during nerve stimulation, have been reported to reduce excessive sweating in patients with primary palmar hyperhidrosis.[53] Generalized hyperhidrosis may be secondary to infections, malignancies, or neuroendocrine disorders (e.g., pheochromocytoma, thyrotoxicosis, acromegaly, carcinoid, anxiety, hypotension, hypoglycemia, and cholinergic agents).[52]

Vasomotor disorders in the limbs include Raynaud's phenomenon, acrocyanosis, livedo reticularis, vasomotor paralysis, and erythromelalgia. Raynaud's phenomenon is the episodic, bilateral, symmetrical change in skin color (pallor, followed by cyanosis and terminating in rubor after rewarming) that is provoked by cold or emotional stimuli. This response is due to episodic closure of the digital arteries. There is, however, no consistent evidence of exaggerated sympathetic outflow to the skin. Raynaud's phenomenon may be associated with connective tissue disease (e.g., scleroderma, rheumatoid arthritis, psoriasis), occupational trauma (such as the use of pneumatic hammers or chain saws producing vibration), the thoracic outlet syndrome, the carpal tunnel syndrome, or certain drugs (e.g., beta-blockers, ergot alkaloids, methysergide, vinblastine, bleomycin, amphetamines, bromocriptine, and cyclosporine).[52]

Acrocyanosis is a symmetrical distal blue discoloration, usually occurring below the wrists and ankles, that is due to arteriolar constriction and is aggravated by cold. In contrast, livedo reticularis is a vasomotor disorder that affects the extremities and the trunk and is due to vasospasm with obstruction of the perpendicular arterioles or stasis of blood in the superficial veins. It may be a benign disorder or may be associated with vasculitis, antiphospholipid antibodies (Sneddon's syndrome), connective tissue disease, hyperviscosity syndrome, thrombocythemia, and drugs (e.g., amantadine, quinine, and quinidine).[52]

Vasomotor paralysis may be seen in patients with lesions of the sympathetic pathways at the level of the spinal cord, preganglionic nerves, ganglia, or postganglionic nerves. Examples include surgical sympathectomy (e.g., for treatment of selective cases of hyperhidrosis, Raynaud's phenomenon, and reflex sympathetic dystrophy), trauma (e.g., carpal tunnel syndrome, ulnar nerve lesions), and tumor infiltration (e.g., Pancoast's tumor, malignant retroperitoneal disease).

Erythromelalgia is a painful acral erythematous condition that occurs with cutaneous warming and is associated with an intense burning sensation. It may occur in patients with small-fiber neuropathies. The mechanism may be activation of neurogenic flare by a polymodal C-nociceptor axon and release of vasodilator and algogenic neuropeptides such as substance P.[21]

Regional Pain Syndromes

Reflex sympathetic dystrophy (chronic regional pain syndrome type 1) is a pain syndrome defined as a continuous burning pain, hyperpathia (exaggerated response to painful stimuli), and allodynia (perception of an innocuous stimulus as painful) in a portion of an extremity. This disorder is associated with signs of sympathetic hypoactivity or hyperactivity and usually follows minor trauma that does not involve major nerves. Causalgia (chronic regional pain syndrome type 2) is a similar syndrome that occurs after partial injury of a nerve or one of its major branches. Vasomotor and sudomotor instability, manifestations of sympathetic hyperactivity or hypoactivity, are commonly seen. Reflex sympathetic dystrophy is not a single pathological entity, but different central, peripheral, and psychogenic mechanisms may coexist in a particular case. Sympathetic blockade may be of benefit.[21]

Neurogenic Bladder

Disturbances at different levels of the bladder control system result in the development of neurogenic bladder. Neurogenic bladders can be subdivided into two types: the reflex or upper motor neuron type, and the nonreflex or lower motor neuron type. The terms reflex and nonreflex denote the presence or absence, respectively, of bulbocavernosus and anal reflexes. The reflex type of neurogenic bladder includes the uninhibited bladder associated with lesions of the medial frontal region that results in urinary incontinence but not urinary retention because the detrusor-sphincter synergy is preserved. The automatic bladder results from lesions of the spinal cord that interrupt the pathway from the pontine micturition centers. An automatic bladder is associated with urgency, frequency, incontinence, and urinary retention that is due to detrusor-sphincter dyssynergia. The lower motor neuron type of neurogenic bladder, such as that occurring with lesions of the cauda equina or peripheral nerves, is characterized by incomplete bladder emptying, urinary retention, and overflow incontinence.[13]

General Management Goals

ORTHOSTATIC HYPOTENSION

Management of orthostatic hypotension requires patient education to avoid factors that precipitate a fall in blood pressure. Patients should be made aware of the hypotensive effects of certain drugs, large meals, environmental temperature increases, and physical activities. Other instructions include institution of a high-fiber diet to lessen straining resulting from constipation and the use of physical maneuvers that help to increase postural tolerance. These maneuvers include crossing the legs, lowering the head in a stooped position, bending forward, and placing a foot on a chair or squatting. Some patients may be helped by sleeping with the head of the bed elevated 15 to 30 cm (the reverse Trendelenburg position) to avoid supine hypertension and decrease nocturnal natriuresis and volume depletion. This maneuver alone may reduce postural hypotension in the morning. To reduce postprandial hypotension, patients should eat smaller, low-carbohydrate meals more frequently and drink strong coffee. Finally, custom-fitted elasticized garments (a Jobst or Barton-Carey leotard) may reduce venous pooling in the legs.

Pharmacological interventions are directed toward increasing intravascular volume and peripheral vascular resistance without markedly increasing supine hypertension. Volume expansion can be achieved by ensuring adequate hydration (2 to 2.5 L of fluid per day) and increasing sodium intake (150 to 250 mEq, or 10 to 20 g).

Fludrocortisone is the drug most frequently used for the treatment of orthostatic hypotension in patients with autonomic failure. Even at low doses, it expands blood volume by its mineralocorticoid action. The initial dose is 0.1 mg po qd; this is increased slowly in 0.1-mg increments at 1- to 2- week intervals. Few patients require more than 0.4 mg. Side effects include volume expansion, congestive heart failure, supine hypertension, and hypokalemia.

The next line of therapy entails the use of vasoconstricting sympathomimetic agents. Several types are available. Indirect sympathomimetic drugs, such as ephedrine and methylphenidate (Ritalin), release NE both centrally and peripherally and therefore may produce tachycardia, anxiety, and tremor. Direct alpha-agonists, such as phenylephrine, may be helpful but have erratic gastrointestinal absorption, a short duration of action, and an increased risk of supersensitive hypertensive responses and tachyphylaxis; phenylpropanolamine, previously frequently used to treat this disorder, increases the risk of intracerebral hemorrhage, particularly in women.[54] Midodrine, a pro-drug metabolized in the liver to desglymidrodrine, is a potent alpha-1 adrenergic agonist that acts on both the arteries and the veins. This agent is well absorbed following oral administration and does not cross the blood-brain barrier.[55] All sympathomimetic agents may produce supine hypertension and should not be used at night.

Dihydroxyphenylserine is a synthetic amino acid that is decarboxylated by L-amino acid decarboxylase to norepinephrine, thus bypassing the dopamine–beta-hydroxylase step of catecholamine synthesis. It is therefore the agent of choice for the treatment of hypotension in patients with inherited dopamine–beta-hydroxylase deficiency. Its efficacy in more common forms of autonomic failure is currently under investigation.

Recombinant epoietin alfa (25 to 75 U/kg sc two or three times weekly) corrects the mild anemia frequently seen in patients with severe autonomic failure and may increase blood pressure and orthostatic tolerance.[56] Other agents that may be of benefit in the treatment of orthostatic hypotension include ergotamine tartrate, dihydroergotamine, monoamine oxidase inhibitors, yohimbine, and nonsteroidal anti-inflammatory agents. It is unclear whether any of these agents is effective.

Severe supine hypertension, particularly at night, is a troublesome feature of this disorder that may be prevented by sleeping in the reverse Trendelenburg position, avoiding vasoconstrictor drugs in late afternoon, and eating a small carbohydrate-rich snack or drinking alcohol before bedtime. If needed, a short-acting vasodilator agent (e.g., nifedipine 10 mg po) may also be used at night.

NEUROGENIC BLADDER

Detrusor Hyper-reflexia Without Outlet Obstruction. In patients with detrusor hyper-reflexia without outlet obstruction, the treatment most frequently given is an anticholinergic drug such as oxybutynin, tolterodine, propantheline, or dyclomine. Timed voiding and moderate fluid restriction are helpful in reducing frequency, urgency, and urge incontinence.

DDAVP may also be useful in patients with significant incontinence and nocturia. In patients with severe spasticity, both intrathecal baclofen infusion and dorsal rhizotomy may be effective. Augmentation cystoplasty has a place in the treatment of patients with MS and refractory detrusor hyper-reflexia.

Detrusor Hyper-reflexia with Outlet Obstruction. Treatment of patients with detrusor hyper-reflexia and detrusor-sphincter dyssynergia is more difficult, and these patients are at higher risk of sustaining upper urinary tract damage. Alpha-1 antagonists such as phenoxybenzamine or prazosin may decrease bladder-outlet sphincter tone. Dantrolene, baclofen, or benzodiazepines may reduce the tone of the striated external sphincter. The most useful method is the combined use of anticholinergics and intermittent self-catheterization. Surgical external sphincterotomy or diversion procedures are treatments of last resort.

Detrusor Areflexia or Poor Bladder Contractility. Bethanechol hydrochloride is a muscarinic agonist that has a relatively selective action on the urinary bladder and may be effective in treating patients with chronic detrusor atony or hypotonia. Other options include the use of adrenergic antagonists, prostaglandins, and narcotic antagonists, but their efficacy is unproved. The simplest and most effective form of management in patients with hypotonic bladder and detrusor areflexia is intermittent self-catheterization. Patients who are unable to perform intermittent self-catheterization because of motor difficulties may require an indwelling catheter or suprapubic diversion. Women may benefit from using the Credé maneuver. In patients with conus or cauda equina lesions, alpha-adrenergic agonists (e.g., ephedrine or phenylpropanolamine) may be used to increase bladder outlet resistance.

SEXUAL DYSFUNCTION

Treatment of organic impotence includes treatment of secondary psychological problems and reducing or eliminating aggravating factors such as poor sleep, chronic pain, malnutrition, alcohol use, and some medications. Yohimbine can be used orally to increase penile arterial vasodilatation and enhance relaxation of the cavernous trabeculae. Direct injection of papaverine (direct smooth muscle relaxant), phentolamine, or prostaglandin E1 into the corpora cavernosa may be effective but poses the risks of priapism and scarring of the tunica albuginea. Sildenafil is now the drug of choice in the treatment of male erectile dysfunction of various etiologies. By inhibiting phosphodiesterase type 5, the enzyme within the corpus cavernosum responsible for breakdown of cyclic guanidine monophosphate (cGMP), sildenafil increases vasodilatation and enhances penile erection. Nitric oxide is the principal neurochemical for penile erection. Within the trabecular myocyte (corpus cavernosum), nitric oxide activates a soluble guanylyl cyclase that elevates intracellular levels of cGMP. This, in turn, stimulates the activities of cGMP-dependent protein kinases, which then phosphorylate certain proteins and ion channels, resulting in smooth muscle relaxation (and erection). During the return to the flaccid state, cGMP is hydrolyzed to GMP by the highly specific cGMP-binding phosphodiesterase type 5 (PDE5). Sildenafil is a specific PDE5 inhibitor that prevents the hydrolysis of cGMP, thereby augmenting penile smooth muscle relaxation and erection. A vacuum device may also be used to enhance corporal filling.[57]

GASTROINTESTINAL DYSMOTILITY

The principles of management of any gastrointestinal motility disorder include restoration of hydration and nutrition by the oral, enteral, or parenteral route; suppression of bacterial overgrowth; use of prokinetic agents or stimulant laxatives; and resection of localized disease.

Bowel Hypomotility. The first line of treatment of bowel hypomotility is to increase dietary fiber as well as water intake and exercise. Psyllium or methylcellulose with a concomitant increase in fluid intake may be used to further increase stool bulk. Some caution is required in diabetic patients, in whom high fiber may pose a risk of distention, cramping, and potential bezoar formation in the presence of gastroparesis. If these measures are ineffective, stool softeners (e.g., docusate sodium) or lubricants (e.g., mineral oil) together with an osmotic agent (e.g., milk of magnesia or lactulose) may be used. Glycerine suppositories or sodium phosphate enemas promote fluid retention in the rectum and thus stimulate evacuation. Contact cathartics such as diphenylmetane derivatives (e.g., phenolphthalein, bisacodyl) or anthraquinones (e.g., senna and cascara) should be used sparingly because these agents may damage the myenteric plexus, producing a "cathartic bowel."

This regimen can be used in conjunction with the prokinetic agents, which include the following: metoclopramide, which has antiemetic effects due to blockade of central dopaminergic D2 receptors and indirect prokinetic effects through cholinergic mechanisms; domperidone, a peripheral D2 receptor antagonist; cisapride, which increases the release of acetylcholine from neurons of the myenteric plexus but has been associated with an increase in ventricular tachyarrhytmias and is no longer generally available; erythromycin, which mimics the prokinetic actions of motilin, a gastrointestinal polypeptide; and misoprostol, a synthetic prostaglandin E1 analogue. Patients who do not respond to medical therapy may require colonic surgery.

Bowel Hypermotility. Diarrhea may result from bacterial overgrowth in patients with intestinal hypomotility. A trial with tetracycline or metronidazole is generally conducted in patients with unexplained chronic diarrhea, particularly if steatorrhea is present. Prokinetic agents may paradoxically improve diarrhea in this situation. If these measures fail, synthetic opioid agonists such as loperamide or diphenoxylate can be used. Opioid agonists decrease peristalsis and increase rectal sphincter tone. Clonidine, an alpha-2 agonist, has been used to treat diarrhea associated with diabetic dysautonomia.

Idiopathic fecal incontinence may be associated with delayed conduction in the pudendal nerves and denervation changes in the sphincter muscles. High-fiber bulking agents may be beneficial because semi-formed stools are easier to control than liquid feces. Fecal disimpaction is indicated in some patients. Daily tap water enemas aid in clearing the residue from the rectum between evacuations and may improve continence. Biofeedback may be successful in some cases. Patients who undergo surgical sphincter repair may gain some continence for solid stool, although the presence of pudendal neuropathy is associated with a poor outcome. Other surgical treatments include colostomy, artificial anal sphincters, and creation of a neosphincter with muscle grafts.

Reviews and Selected Updates

Benarroch EE, Chang FL: Central autonomic disorders. J Neurophysiol 1993;10:39.

Blottner D: Nitric oxide and fibroblast growth factor in autonomic nervous system: Short- and long-term messengers in autonomic pathway and target-organ control. Prog Neurobiol 1997;51:423–438.

Kaufmann H: Neurally mediated syncope and syncope due to autonomic failure: Differences and similarities. J Clin Neurophysiol 1997;14:183–196.

Morrison SF: Differential control of sympathetic outflow. Am J Physiol Regul Integr Comp Physiol 2001;281:R683–R698.

Shields RW: Functional anatomy of the autonomic nervous system. J Neurophysiol 1993;10:2–13.

Therapeutics and Technology Assessment Subcommittee: Assessment: Neurological evaluation of male sexual dysfunction. Neurology 1995;45:2287–2292.

van Lieshout JJ, Wieling W, Karemaker JM: Neural circulatory control in vasovagal syncope. Pacing Clin Electrophysiol 1997;20:753–763.

References

1. Kaufmann H, Oribe E, Pierotti AR, et al: Atrial natriuretic factor in human autonomic failure. Neurology 1990;40:1115–1119.
2. Langley JN: The autonomic nervous system. Brain 1903;26:1–26.
3. Loewy AD: Central autonomic pathways. *In* Loewy AD, Spyer KM (eds): Central Regulation of Autonomic Functions. New York, Oxford University Press, 1990, pp 88–103.
4. Benarroch EE: The central autonomic network: Functional organization, dysfunction, and perspective. Mayo Clin Proc 1993;68:988–1001.
5. Loewy AD: Forebrain nuclei involved in autonomic control. Prog Brain Res 1991;87:253–268.
6. King AB, Menon RS, Hachinski V, Cechetto DF: Human forebrain activation by visceral stimuli. J Comp Neurol 1999;413:572–582.
7. Verberne AJ, Owens NC: Cortical modulation of the cardiovascular system. Prog Neurobiol 1998;54:149–168.
8. Ledoux JE: Emotions and the amygdala. *In* Aggleton JP (ed): Neurobiological Aspects of Emotion, Memory, and Mental Dysfunction. New York, Wiley-Liss, 1992, pp 339–351.
9. Saper C: Hypothalamus. *In* Paxinos G (ed): The Human Nervous System. New York, Academy Press, 1990, pp 389–413.
10. Swanson LW: Biochemical switching in hypothalamic circuits mediating responses to stress. Prog Brain Res 1991;87:181–200.
11. Kilduff TS, Peyron C: The hypocretin/orexin ligand-receptor system: Implications for sleep and sleep disorders. Trends Neurosci 2000;23:359–365
12. Elmquist JK, Elias CF, Saper CB: From lesions to leptin: Hypothalamic control of food intake and body weight. Neuron 1999;22:221–232.
13. Bandler R, Shipley MT: Columnar organization in the midbrain periaqueductal gray: Modules for emotional expression? [published erratum appears in Trends Neurosci 1994;17(11):445—see comments]. Trends Neurosci 1994;17:379–389.
14. Guyenet PG: Role of the ventral medulla oblongata in blood pressure regulation. *In* Leowy AD, Spyer KM (eds): Central Regulation of Autonomic Functions. New York, Oxford University Press, 1990, pp 145–167.
15. Spyer KM: Annual Review Prize Lecture: Central nervous mechanisms contributing to cardiovascular control. J Physiol 1994;474:1–19.
16. Janig W: Spinal cord reflex organization of sympathetic systems. Prog Brain Res 1996;107:43–77.
17. de Groat WC, Booth AM: Autonomic systems to the urinary bladder and sexual organs. *In* Dyck PJ, Thomas PK (eds): Peripheral Neuropathy, 3rd ed. Philadelphia, WB Saunders, 1993, pp 198–207.
18. Cervero F, Foreman RD: Sensory innervation of the viscera. *In* Loewy A, Spyer KM (eds): Central Regulation of Autonomic Function. New York, Oxford University Press, 1990, pp 103–125.
19. Kaufmann H, Oribe E, Miller M, et al: Hypotension-induced vasopressin release distinguishes between pure autonomic failure and multiple system atrophy with autonomic failure. Neurology 1992;42:590–593.
20. Polinsky RJ, Kopin IJ, Ebert MH, Weise V: Pharmacologic distinction of different orthostatic hypotension syndromes. Neurology 1981;31:1–7.
21. Freeman R, Dover JS: Autonomic neurodermatology (Part I): Erythromelalgia, reflex sympathetic dystrophy, and livedo reticularis. Semin Neurol 1992;12:385–393.
22. Kaufmann H: Investigation of autonomic cardiovascular dysfunction. *In* Korczyn AD (ed): Handbook of Autonomic Nervous System Dysfunction. New York, Marcel Dekker, 1995, pp 427–468.
23. The Consensus Committee of the American Autonomic Society and the American Academy of Neurology: Consensus statement on the definition of orthostatic hypotension, pure autonomic failure, and multiple system atrophy. Neurology 1996;46:1470.
24. Low PA, Opfer-Gehrking TL, Textor SC, et al: Postural tachycardia syndrome (POTS). Neurology 1995;45:S19–S25.
25. Nogues MA, Newman PK, Male VJ, Foster JB: Cardiovascular reflexes in syringomyelia. Brain 1982;105:835–849.
26. Jenzer G, Mumenthaler M, Ludin HP, Robert F: Autonomic dysfunction in botulism B: A clinical report. Neurology 1975;25:150–153.
27. Vernino S, Low PA, Fealey RD, et al: Autoantibodies to ganglionic acetylcholine receptors in autoimmune autonomic neuropathies. N Engl J Med 2000;343:847–855.
28. Eckberg DL: Human sinus arrhythmia as an index of vagal cardiac outflow. J Appl Physiol 1983;54:961–966.
29. Ewing DJ, Borsey DQ, Bellavere F, Clarke BF: Cardiac autonomic neuropathy in diabetes: Comparison of measures of R-R interval variation. Diabetologia 1981;21:18–24.
30. Benarroch EE, Opfer Gehrking TL, Low PA: Use of the photoplethysmographic technique to analyze the Valsalva maneuver in normal man. Muscle Nerve 1991;14:1165–1172.
31. Ewing DJ, Campbell IW, Murray A, et al: Immediate heart-rate response to standing: Simple test for autonomic neuropathy in diabetes. BMJ 1978;1:145–147.
32. Borst C, Wieling W, van Brederode JF, et al: Mechanisms of initial heart rate response to postural change. Am J Physiol 1982;243:H676–H681.
33. Freeman R: Heart rate variability—the time domain. *In* Low PA (ed): Management of Clinical Autonomic Disorders. Boston, Little, Brown and Company, 1997, pp 297–308.
34. Freeman R, Saul JP, Roberts MS, et al: Spectral analysis of heart rate in diabetic autonomic neuropathy. A comparison with standard tests of autonomic function. Arch Neurol 1991;48:185–190.
35. Ziegler MG, Lake CR, Kopin IJ: The sympathetic nervous system defect in primary orthostatic hypotension. N Engl J Med 1977;296:293–297.
36. Goldstein DS, Polinsky RJ, Garty M, et al: Patterns of plasma levels of catechols in neurogenic orthostatic hypotension. Ann Neurol 1989;26:558–563.
37. Robertson D, Goldberg MR, Onrot J, et al: Isolated failure of autonomic noradrenergic neurotransmission. Evidence for impaired beta-hydroxylation of dopamine. N Engl J Med 1986;314:1494–1497.
38. Fealey RD, Low PA, Thomas JE: Thermoregulatory sweating abnormalities in diabetes mellitus. Mayo Clin Proc 1989;64:617–628.
39. Low PA, Caskey PE, Tuck RR, et al: Quantitative sudomotor axon reflex test in normal and neuropathic subjects. Ann Neurol 1983;14:573–580.
40. Vallbo AB, Hagbarth KE, Torebjörk HE, Wallin BG: Somatosensory, proprioceptive, and sympathetic activity in human peripheral nerves. Physiol Rev 1979;59:919–957.
41. Bannister R, Oppenheimer DR: Degenerative diseases of the nervous system associated with autonomic failure. Brain 1972;95:457–474.
42. Kaufmann H: Multiple system atrophy. Curr Opin Neurol 1998;11:351–355.
43. Bradbury S, Eggelston C: Postural hypotension: Report of 3 cases. Am Heart J 1925;1:73–86.
44. Hague K, Lento S, Morgello S, Caro S, Kaufmann H: The distribution of Lewy bodies in pure autonomic failure: Autopsy findings and review of the literature. Acta Neuropathologica 1997;94:192–196.
45. McLeod JG, Tuck RR: Disorders of the autonomic nervous system: Part 1. Pathophysiology and clinical features. Ann Neurol 1987;21:419–430.
46. Houlden H, King RHM, Hashemi-Nejad A, et al: A novel TRK A (NRTK1) mutation associated with hereditary sensory and autonomic neuropathy type V. Ann Neurol 2001;49:521–525.
47. Freeman R, Schachter SC: Autonomic epilepsy. Semin Neurol 1995;15:158–166.
48. Kloos RT: Spontaneous periodic hypothermia. Medicine (Baltimore) 1995;74:268–280.
49. Klein CJ, Silber MH, Halliwill JR, et al: Basal forebrain malformation with hyperhidrosis and hypothermia: A variant of Shapiro's syndrome. Neurology 2001;56:254–256.
50. Montagna P, Cortelli P, Gambetti P, Lugaresi E: Fatal familial insomnia: Sleep, neuroendocrine and vegetative alterations. Adv Neuroimmunol 1995;5:13–21.
51. Mathias CJ, Frankel HL: Autonomic disturbances in spinal cord lesions. *In* Bannister R, Mathias CJ (eds): Autonomic Failure. New York, Oxford University Press, 1992, pp 839–881.

52. Freeman R, Waldorf HA, Dover JS: Autonomic neurodermatology (Part II): Disorders of sweating and flushing. Semin Neurol 1992;12:394–407.
53. Saadia D, Voustianiouk A, Wang AK, Kaufmann H: Botulinum toxin type A in primary palmar hyperhidrosis: Randomized, single-blind, two-dose study. Neurology 2001;57:2095–2099.
54. Kernan WN, Viscoli CM, Brass LM, et al: Phenylpropanolamine and the risk of hemorrhagic stroke. N Engl J Med 2000;343:1826–1832.
55. Kaufmann H, Brannan T, Krakoff L, et al: Treatment of orthostatic hypotension due to autonomic failure with a peripheral alpha-adrenergic agonist (midodrine). Neurology 1988;38:951–956.
56. Perera R, Isola L, Kaufmann H: Effect of recombinant erythropoietin on anemia and orthostatic hypotension in primary autonomic failure. Clin Auton Res 1995;5:211–213.
57. Lue TF: Erectile dysfunction. N Engl J Med 2000;342:1802–1813.

CHAPTER 22

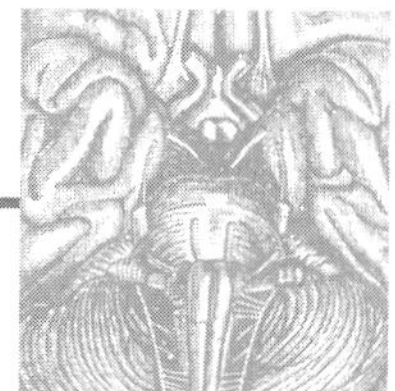

BETSY B. LOVE and JOSÉ BILLER

Neurovascular System

History and Definitions

The modern study of neurovascular function owes much of its success to important, early contributors to the field. Some of the earliest drawings of the cerebral circulation were done in the 1500s by Andreas Vesalius.[1] Gabriel Fallopius provided a detailed description of the cerebral vasculature, including a description of what was later called the circle of Willis.[1] Thomas Willis was the first to describe the function of the circle that bears his name.[1] Vascular anatomy was transformed into physiology through the work of William Harvey in the early 1600s.[1] The most important early advances in the study of "apoplexy" were a result of meticulous studies of the cerebral blood vessels of patients with apoplexy by Johann Jakob Wepfer.[2] The actual demonstration that the paralysis was on the side opposite the brain lesion in "apoplexy" was through the work of Domenico Mistichelli, and François Bayle was among the first to relate atherosclerosis in cerebral arteries to "apoplexy."[2]

A transient ischemic attack (TIA) is an episode of focal, nonconvulsive neurological dysfunction caused by a reversible interference of the blood supply to an area of the retina or brain that lasts less than 24 hours, and often lasts less than 30 minutes. The episodes are sudden and often are unprovoked. They reach a maximum intensity almost immediately. The duration of a TIA was determined on an arbitrary basis. Subsequent studies have revealed that the typical carotid distribution TIA lasts less than 10 to 20 minutes.[3, 4]

A completed (established) stroke is the preferred term to describe an acute episode of focal brain ischemia that lasts longer than 24 hours. Most completed strokes reach a maximal neurological deficit within an hour of onset. Older terms that have been used in the past include apoplexy (literally meaning "struck with violence" or "being thunderstruck") and cerebrovascular accident. Both of these older terms imply a random, unpredictable, or uncertain nature to these events, which often is not the case.

Stroke in evolution or progressive stroke describes a temporal profile in which the neurological deficit occurs in a stepwise or progressive pattern. In the carotid artery distribution, there is usually little likelihood of progression after 24 hours. In the vertebrobasilar distribution, progression may continue for up to 72 hours.[5] There are numerous causes to consider (Table 22–1) when there is "progression" of an ischemic event.

Stroke may be divided into ischemic infarctions, which may be bland or hemorrhagic, and hemorrhages, including intracerebral hemorrhages and subarachnoid hemorrhages. Ischemic infarctions can be due to intrinsic vascular occlusion (thrombus) or an occlusion from intravascular material that originates elsewhere, such as heart or other vessels (embolism).

Common focal sites of cerebrovascular atherosclerosis include the proximal common carotid artery, the origin of the internal carotid artery, the carotid siphon, and the proximal middle cerebral and vertebral arteries. The aortic arch has been recognized as a source for atheroembolism.

Small arteries are also susceptible to atherosclerotic changes. Examples of these small arteries would be the lenticulostriate arteries, thalamoperforating arteries, the basilar paramedian penetrating arteries, and the medullary arteries. These arteries supply the deep cerebral white matter. The most frequent sites of lacunar infarcts are the putamen, basis pontis, thalamus, posterior limb of the internal capsule, and caudate nucleus. They may also occur in the anterior limb of the internal capsule, subcortical cerebral white matter, and cerebellar white matter.

Overall, embolism accounts for between 15 and 30 percent of strokes.[6–8] Emboli that cause brain ischemia may arise from the heart, the aorta, the venous system in combination with a transcardiac defect, or from other intracerebral or extracerebral arteries (artery-to-artery embolism).

Diffuse perfusion deficits may lead to brain ischemia and may occur with severe hypotensive crises due to sepsis, anaphylaxis, acute blood loss, pharmacological alterations, cardiac surgery, and other acute medical crises. These situations may lead to infarctions, typically in the border zone regions (watershed areas) between the anterior, middle, and posterior cerebral arteries.

Hemorrhages may be subarachnoid, intraparenchymal, or a combination of both. Intraparenchymal hemorrhages are the result of bleeding from an arterial source directly into the brain. Subarachnoid hemorrhages are the result of bleeding into the subarachnoid spaces.

Another distinction needs to be made between hematomas within the brain parenchyma, which are referred to as intracerebral, and those outside the brain parenchyma, which are referred to as extracerebral. Examples of extracerebral hematomas are subdural and epidural hematomas.

TABLE 22–1. **Causes of Neurological Worsening After an Ischemic Event**

Thrombus propagation
Occlusion of a stenotic artery due to thrombus
Recurrent embolism
Hemorrhagic transformation
Failure of collateral blood supply
Hypoperfusion due to systemic hypotension
Hypovolemia or decreased cardiac output
Hypoxia
Cerebral edema
Herniation
Seizures
Medication effects
Medical conditions such as pneumonia, pulmonary embolus, myocardial ischemia, congestive heart failure, electrolyte disturbances, or urosepsis

Clinical History

One of the first questions to address in the history is whether the problem involves neurovascular dysfunction. The clinical hallmark of many forms of neurovascular dysfunction is an acute focal change in neurological status. Therefore, an event that has an indistinct onset or course may not involve the neurovascular system. There are two exceptions to consider. One is the indistinct time of onset of symptoms in an individual who awakens with the neurological dysfunction. The other is a stuttering or waxing or waning course that can be seen in some patients with cerebral arterial thrombosis. In most instances of neurovascular dysfunction, the neurological deficit is maximum from its onset, with the involved body parts being simultaneously affected. The diagnosis of neurovascular dysfunction is weakened if there is a series of events in which neurological deficits accumulate, or if there is a march of symptoms from one area to another. Focal seizures can usually be differentiated by obtaining a history of associated involuntary motor activity and a march of symptoms. A gradual onset of symptoms with accumulation of deficits over time would suggest the possibility of a space-occupying lesion. It would be distinctly unusual for neurovascular dysfunction to present with positive neurological phenomena such as visual hallucinations or scintillating visual symptoms. Fleeting positive visual phenomenon would be more consistent with migraine. Isolated vertigo may be more consistent with a labyrinthine disorder. Hypoglycemia should be considered in the diabetic patient with transient paresis or aphasia, particularly if there is associated altered consciousness or confusion.

Specific details need to be sought in the history to adequately evaluate the possible underlying type and mechanism of neurovascular dysfunction. It is important to review any cerebrovascular risk factors with the patient, including a history of cardiac disorders, hypertension, hematological abnormalities, hyperlipidemia, diabetes, tobacco use, alcohol or drug use, migraine, oral contraceptive use, and a personal history or family history of TIA or stroke. Information should be obtained about use of medications such as oral anticoagulants or antiplatelet agents and the use of illicit drugs. Patients may have other medical illnesses associated with stroke, including connective tissue diseases, malignancies, and hypercoaguable states. Rarely, a preceding or concurrent infection may predispose to stroke. A history of recent trauma should be sought in patients with symptoms of carotid or vertebral dissection. A history of posterior circulation symptoms with arm exercise may suggest a subclavian steal syndrome.

It is often difficult to differentiate an ischemic infarction from a hemorrhage. Some historical features that suggest a hemorrhage would be an altered level of consciousness or a seizure at the onset, vomiting, or a severe headache. However, onset headaches can also be present in 17 percent of patients with ischemic infarction.[9] A carotid dissection may present with pain involving the neck, ipsilateral head, or the periorbital region.

While it is difficult to distinguish cardiogenic stroke from other causes based on the neurological profile, historical features that may suggest a cardioembolic cause are an abrupt onset with a maximum deficit at the onset, a history of infarctions in more than one vascular territory, or systemic emboli to the limbs or other organs.

Patients noting monocular visual loss or having complaints of a speech disorder suggestive of aphasia most likely have carotid distribution ischemia. Complaints of binocular visual loss, vertigo, balance difficulties, gait instability, bilateral or alternating weakness or altered sensation, swallowing difficulties, or diplopia suggest ischemia in the vertebrobasilar distribution. Etiologies other than vertebrobasilar ischemia should be considered with isolated vertigo, diplopia, or dysarthria. Localization of the neurovascular dysfunction to the cortical or subcortical region may be possible based on historical features. Patients with complaints of any degree of altered consciousness may have cortical or combined subcortical and cortical ischemia. Loss of vision in one field or forced eye deviation usually implies a cortical or combined cortical and subcortical localization. A history of weakness or sensory loss affecting the face, arm, and leg equally usually implies a subcortical or brain stem localization. Complaints of severe dysarthria are often indicative of a subcortical or combined cortical and subcortical infarction.

Anatomy of the Neurovascular System

EXTRACRANIAL ARTERIAL SYSTEM

Heart, Aorta, Common Carotid, Subclavian, Innominate Arteries

The ascending aorta arises from the left ventricle. The aortic arch gives rise to several important branches. The first branch of the aorta is normally the innominate artery, which is also referred to as the brachiocephalic trunk. Shortly after its origin, the innominate artery divides into the right subclavian and right common carotid arteries. The right vertebral artery arises from the right subclavian artery, courses posteromedially, and then enters the foramen transversarium of C6. The right common carotid artery bifurcates into the internal and external carotid arteries in the midcervical region, usually at C3 or C4, about 3 cm below the angle of the mandible. However, the bifurcation may be as rostral as C1 or as caudal as T2.

The next branch of the aorta is the left common carotid artery, which bifurcates into the internal and external carotid arteries at the same level as the right common carotid artery (Fig. 22–1). The last branch of the aortic arch is the left subclavian artery. The left vertebral artery is the first branch of the left subclavian artery. This branch usually arises from the superior portion of the artery and then courses cephalad to enter the foramen transversarium of C6.

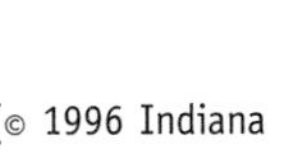

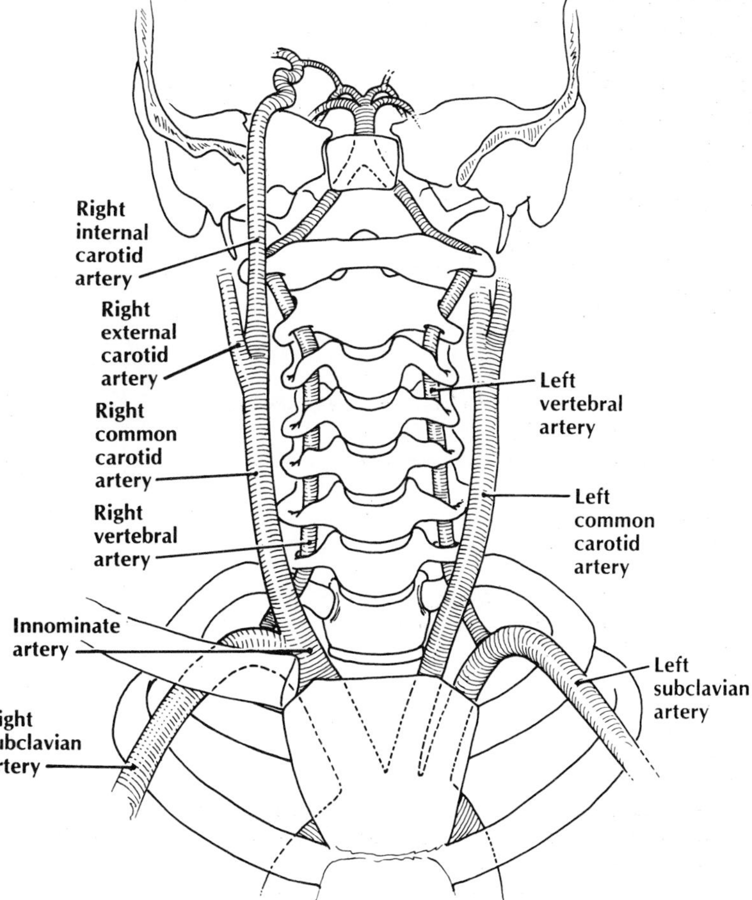

FIGURE 22–1. Branches of the aortic arch. (© 1996 Indiana University Medical Illustration Dept.)

It is reported that the left vertebral artery is as large as or larger in caliber than the right vertebral artery in approximately 75 percent of cases.[10]

External Carotid Artery and Branches

The external carotid artery arises from the common carotid artery in the midcervical region. The proximal portion of this artery lies anteromedial to the internal carotid artery, but as it ascends, it courses posteromedially to supply structures of the face. The external carotid artery has nine major branches (Fig. 22–2). Several of these branches, particularly the maxillary artery and its branches, the ascending pharyngeal artery, and the facial artery, can be important sources of collateral blood flow in the event of internal carotid artery occlusion. The order in which these branches arise and the selected important structures they supply are as follows:

1. Superior thyroid artery, which supplies the larynx and portions of the thyroid.
2. Ascending pharyngeal artery, which supplies portions of the meninges, middle ear, lower cranial nerves, and the upper cervical nerves.
3. Lingual artery, which supplies the tongue and pharynx.
4. Facial artery, which supplies the face, palate, and pharynx.
5. Occipital artery, which supplies musculocutaneous structures of the scalp and neck.
6. Posterior auricular artery, which supplies the scalp, tympanic cavity, pinna, and the parotid gland.
7. Maxillary artery, which is the larger terminal branch that has three major portions, each with its own branches. The most important branches to remember are the middle meningeal artery, which can be lacerated in head trauma and produce an epidural hematoma, and the anterior deep temporal artery, which can be a source of collateral blood flow through the ophthalmic artery when the internal carotid artery is occluded.
8. Transverse facial artery, which with the facial artery supplies the buccal area.
9. Superficial temporal artery, which is the smaller terminal branch that supplies the anterior two thirds of the scalp and portions of the face.

Vertebral Extracranial Portion and Anterior Spinal Artery

The vertebral artery is divided into four segments.[11] The first or V1 segment is the portion from its origin at the subclavian artery to its entry into the costotransverse foramen of C6 or C5. The second or V2 segment travels between C6 and C2, entirely within the transverse foramina. The third or V3 segment takes a tortuous course between C2 to the suboccipital triangle between the atlas and the occiput, where it is covered by the atlanto-occipital membrane. The fourth or V4 segment is the intracranial portion, after it has pierced the dura mater to enter the foramen magnum to join the opposite vertebral artery at the medullopontine level.

The anterior spinal artery is formed by the anastomosis of the two branches of the vertebral arteries. This artery extends from the olivary nucleus to the conus medullaris and supplies the ventral surface of the medulla and the anterior two thirds of the spinal cord.

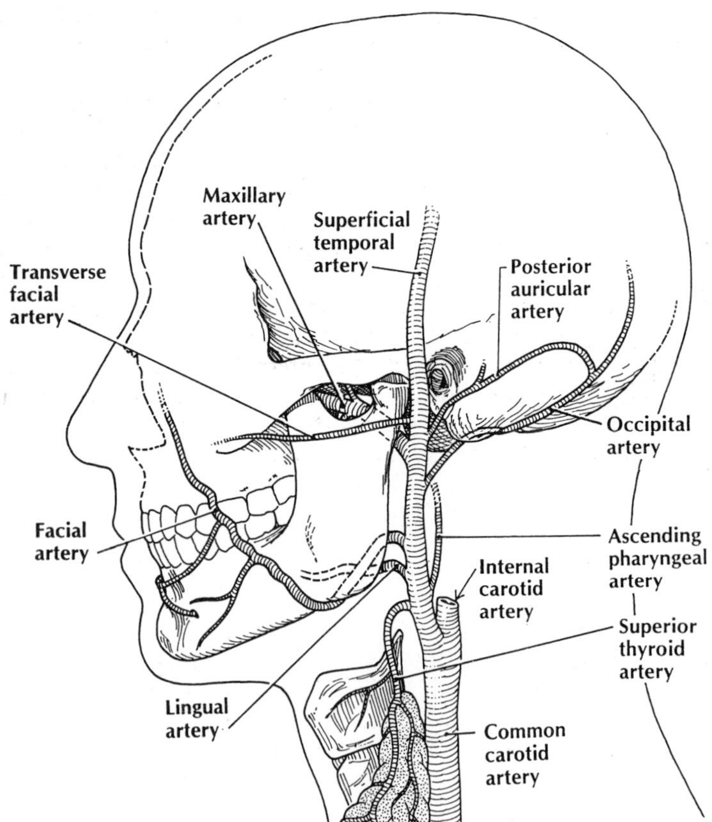

FIGURE 22–2. Major branches of the external carotid artery. (© 1996 Indiana University Medical Illustration Dept.)

INTRACRANIAL ARTERIAL SYSTEM: CIRCLE OF WILLIS

Internal Carotid Artery and Branches (Ophthalmic and Anterior Choroidal)

The internal carotid artery (ICA) can be conceptually divided into three main segments: cervical, petrosal, and intracranial. The cervical portion extends from the carotid bifurcation to the base of the skull. This segment has no branches. The petrosal segment begins after the artery enters the base of the skull and travels through the carotid canal in the petrous portion of the temporal bone. The artery then crosses the foramen lacerum and enters the cavernous sinus. The intracranial portion begins distal to the petrosal segment and proximal to the anterior clinoid process. At this point, the presellar and juxtasellar portions of the ICA are distinguished. The juxtasellar portions lies within the cavernous sinus and is closely associated with cranial nerves III, IV, VI, and the ophthalmic and maxillary divisions of cranial nerve V. Meningohypophyseal branches arise from the presellar and juxtasellar portions to supply the meninges and the posterior lobe of the hypophysis. The ICA pierces the dura mater medial to the anterior clinoid process to become supraclinoid.

The first major branch of the ICA, the ophthalmic artery, arises at the level of the anterior clinoid process (Fig. 22–3). After initially running intracranially, this artery traverses the optic canal and then goes to the orbit. The most important of the ocular branches is the central retinal artery. Numerous anastomotic channels between the internal and external carotid arteries ultimately involve the ophthalmic artery.

After giving rise to the ophthalmic artery, the ICA gives rise to the posterior communicating artery (PCoA) and then the anterior choroidal artery (AChA). The AChA has a proximal or cisternal segment that courses posteromedially below the optic tract and medial to the uncus of the temporal lobe. The artery then turns laterally and passes through the crural cistern and around the cerebral peduncle to enter the choroidal fissure of the temporal lobe.[12] The distal or plexal segment of the AChA starts at the choroidal fissure and goes posteriorly in a cleft of the temporal horn. The AChA may terminate near the lateral geniculate body or extend around the pulvinar of the thalamus.[12] There is a rich anastomotic relationship between the AChA and the lateral posterior choroidal, posterior communicating, and posterior cerebral arteries. Therefore, the regions supplied by the AChA and its branches can be extensive, but also variable. Possible regions supplied by this artery include the choroid plexus of the temporal horn, the amygdaloid nucleus, the piriform cortex and uncus of the temporal lobe, the hippocampus and dentate gyri, the lateral geniculate body, the optic tract and the origin of the optic radiations, the genu and inferior and medial parts of the posterior limb of the internal capsule, the medial globus pallidus, tail of the caudate nucleus, and the upper brain stem. After giving off the AChA, the ICA bifurcates to form the anterior cerebral and middle cerebral arteries (see Figs. 22–3 and 22–4).

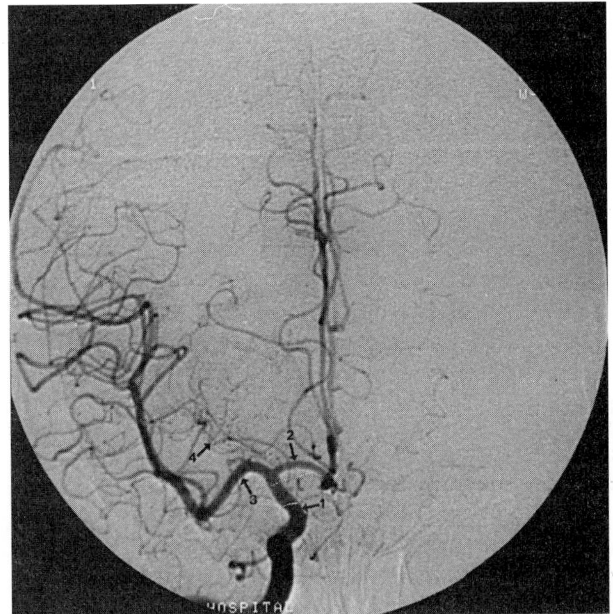

FIGURE 22–4. AP internal carotid artery arteriogram, arterial phase. 1, Internal carotid artery. 2, Anterior cerebral artery. 3, Middle cerebral artery. 4, Medial lenticulostriate arteries. (Courtesy of Karen S. Caldemeyer, M.D.)

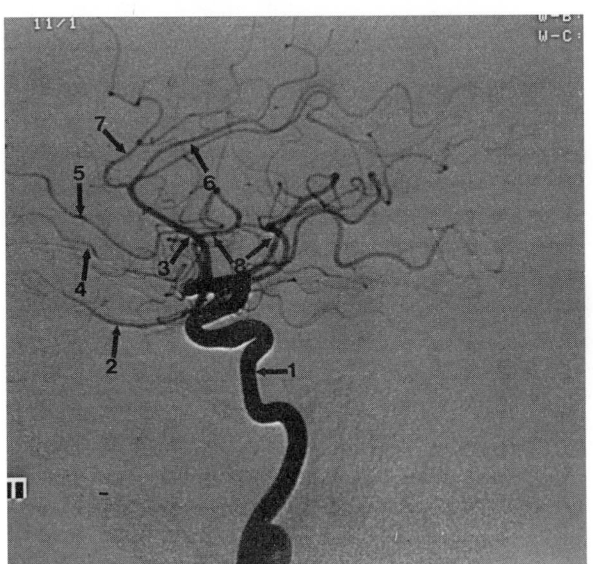

FIGURE 22–3. Lateral internal carotid artery angiogram, arterial phase. 1, Internal carotid artery. 2, Ophthalmic artery. 3, Anterior cerebral artery. 4, Orbitofrontal branch. 5, Frontopolar branch. 6, Callosomarginal branch. 7, Pericallosal branch. 8, Middle cerebral artery branches. (Courtesy of Karen S. Caldemeyer, M.D.)

Circle of Willis

The circle of Willis is an arterial anastomosis at the base of the brain that connects the internal carotid and vertebrobasilar arterial systems. The circle surrounds the ventral surface of the diencephalon adjacent to the optic nerves and tracts. The anterior portion of the circle of Willis consists of the two internal carotid arteries, the anterior cerebral arteries, and the anterior communicating artery. The posterior portion of the circle consists of the proximal portions of the posterior cerebral arteries and the two posterior communicating arteries.

Anterior Cerebral and Anterior Communicating Artery

The anterior cerebral artery (ACA) arises below the anterior perforated substance and runs anteromedially to the interhemispheric fissure, where it joins the opposite ACA by way of the anterior communicating artery (ACoA). The ACA supplies the medial surface of the cerebrum and the upper border of the frontal and parietal lobes.[13]

The ACA is often divided into A1 and A2 segments. The A1 segment is the horizontal, proximal portion that extends from the origin of the ACA to its union with the contralateral ACA by way of the ACoA. The A2 segment is the portion of the ACA that is distal to the ACoA. It runs superiorly into the interhemispheric fissure, coursing around the genu of the corpus callosum. It has an important relationship anatomically to two other midline structures, lying above the optic chiasm and the pituitary gland.

The ACA gives rise to medial lenticulostriate, pericallosal, and hemispheric branches (see Fig. 22–4). The medial lenticulostriate branches include basal branches, which supply the dorsal aspect of the optic chiasm and hypothalamus, and the medial striate artery (recurrent artery of Heubner), which supplies the anteroinferior limb of the internal capsule and the anterior aspects of the putamen and caudate nuclei. The callosal branches arise from the pericallosal artery, which is that portion of the ACA distal to the ACoA. Some reserve the term pericallosal artery for the segment beyond the origin of the callosomarginal artery. The ACA and the pericallosal arteries also supply the septum pellucidum and the fornix. The hemispheric branches supply the medial surface of the hemisphere and include the orbitofrontal, frontopolar, internal frontal (anterior, middle, and posterior), paracentral, and internal parietal (superior and inferior) branches.

Middle Cerebral Artery and Its Branches

The middle cerebral artery (MCA), the largest branch of the ICA, arises below the medial part of the anterior perforated substance. It supplies most of the lateral surface of the cerebral hemisphere, including the lateral frontal, parietal and temporal lobes, insula, claustrum, and extreme capsule.[14]

The MCA is divided into proximal, sylvian, and distal segments. The posterior-superior aspect of the proximal segment gives rise to the lenticulostriate arteries that supply the corona radiata, external capsule, claustrum, putamen, part of the globus pallidus, body of the caudate nucleus, and superior portion of the anterior and posterior limbs of the internal capsule. Other branches that may arise from the horizontal segment are the orbitofrontal and the anterior temporal arteries, but there are many variations. The sylvian segment includes all of the branches on the insula of Reil and in the sylvian fissure. After the takeoff of the anterior temporal artery, the main trunk of the MCA usually bifurcates into two branches: a superior and inferior division. Less common patterns include a trifurcation into superior, middle, and inferior divisions and a ramification pattern into four or more trunks. One branch gives rise to the anterior or proximal group of arteries, and the other branch gives rise to the posterior or distal group. The anterior group includes the orbitofrontal, precentral, central, and anterior parietal arteries. The posterior group includes the posterior parietal, posterior temporal, and the angular or terminal arteries.

Posterior Communicating Artery

The PCoA arises from the posteromedial aspect of the intracranial ICA and runs caudally and medially, above the oculomotor nerve to join the posterior cerebral artery. The two PCoAs from each side provide a connection between the carotid and vertebrobasilar systems. The PCoAs supply the anterior and medial portions of the thalamus, and the walls of the third ventricle.

Posterior Cerebral Artery and Branches

The posterior cerebral arteries (PCAs) usually arise as the terminal bifurcation of the basilar artery ventral to the midbrain (Fig. 22–5). Approximately 15 to 22 percent of people have a fetal (embryonic) origin of the PCA from the ICA.[15, 16] The PCA supplies the occipital lobes, inferomedial portions of the temporal lobes, midbrain, thalamus, and deep structures including the choroid plexus and ependyma of the third and lateral ventricles. The first branches are the small thalamoperforating arteries that penetrate and supply the midbrain, thalamus, and lateral geniculate body. The next branches are the medial and lateral posterior choroidal arteries that supply the posterior portion of the thalamus and the choroid plexus. An anterior division of the PCA gives rise to the inferior temporal arteries (hippocampal, anterior, middle, posterior, and common temporal arteries) that supply the

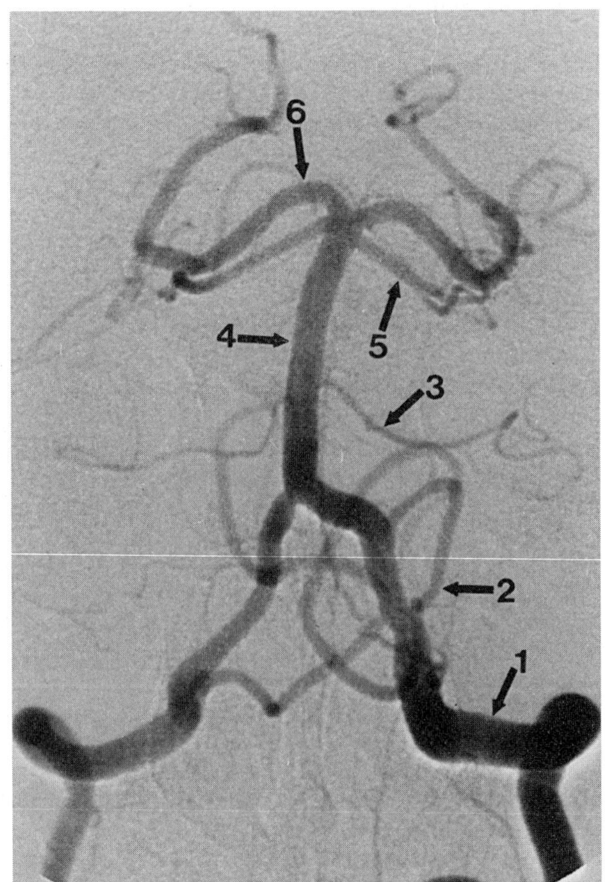

FIGURE 22–5. AP vertebral angiogram. 1, Vertebral artery. 2, Posterior inferior cerebellar artery. 3, Anterior inferior cerebellar artery. 4, Basilar artery. 5, Superior cerebellar artery. 6, Posterior cerebral artery. (Courtesy of Karen S. Caldemeyer, M.D.)

inferior portions of the temporal lobes. A posterior division includes the two terminal branches of the PCA; the parieto-occipital artery, which supplies part of the cuneus and precuneus, the superior occipital gyrus, and occasionally, the precentral and superior parietal lobule; and the calcarine artery, which supplies the visual cortex, inferior cuneus, and part of the lingual gyrus. The splenial arteries may arise directly from the PCA or from the parieto-occipital artery.

VERTEBRAL SYSTEM

Vertebral Arteries

The vertebral arteries (VAs) normally arise as the first branches of the subclavian artery (see Fig. 22–1). They course superiorly and medially to enter the transverse foramen of C6. The VAs course vertically through the transverse foramen of C3-C6 and then turn superolaterally to pass through the C2 foramen. After the arteries pass through the foramen of the atlas, they curve around the atlanto-occipital joint and lie in a horizontal groove along the posterior arch of C1. The VAs then curve cephalad to enter the skull through the foramen magnum.

Basilar Artery

The basilar artery is formed by the union of the two vertebral arteries, which takes place at the lower border of the ventral pons (see Fig. 22–5). It continues superiorly to terminate in the interpeduncular cistern by dividing into the PCAs. The branches of the basilar artery can be divided into paramedian arteries, short circumferential arteries, and long circumferential arteries. The paramedian vessels are four to six in number, and they penetrate into the pontine parenchyma to supply the medial basal pons. The short circumferential arteries enter the brachium pontis to supply the ventrolateral basis pontis. The long circumferential arteries include the superior cerebellar artery (SCA), anterior inferior cerebellar artery (AICA), and the internal auditory artery.

Long Circumferential Arteries (PICA, AICA, SCA)

The arterial supply to the cerebellum includes the posterior inferior cerebellar artery (PICA), the AICA, and the SCA. The PICA is the largest branch of the vertebral artery (see Figs. 22–5 and 22–6). The PICA encircles the medulla to supply the lateral medulla. The distal portion of PICA then bifurcates into a medial trunk that supplies the vermis and the adjacent cerebellar hemisphere and a lateral trunk that supplies the cortical surface of the tonsil and cerebellar hemisphere.

The AICA most often arises directly from the basilar artery (see Figs. 22–5 and 22–6). Rarely, it may arise from the vertebral artery. In its normal course, it runs across the pons, enters the cerebellopontine angle cistern, and then forms a tight loop before running over the cerebellum. AICA supplies the lateral tegmentum of the lower two thirds of the pons and the ventrolateral cerebellum. The internal auditory artery arises from AICA to supply the auditory and facial nerves.

The SCA arises from the basilar artery near its terminal bifurcation (see Figs. 22–5 and 22–6). It courses posterolaterally in the perimesencephalic cistern to circle the brain stem in the region between the pons and the mesencephalon. The SCA supplies the superolateral cerebellar hemispheres, the superior cerebellar peduncle, the dentate nucleus, and part of the middle cerebellar peduncle.

VASCULAR SUPPLY TO THE SPINAL CORD

Extraspinal System (Extramedullary Arteries)

The anterior spinal artery arises from the anastomosis of two branches from the intracranial vertebral arteries. It travels in the anterior sulcus of the spinal cord and extends from the level of the olivary nucleus to the conus medullaris. It supplies the ventral surface of the medulla and the anterior two thirds of the spinal cord. The artery is continuous in the upper cervical region. However, in the segments inferior

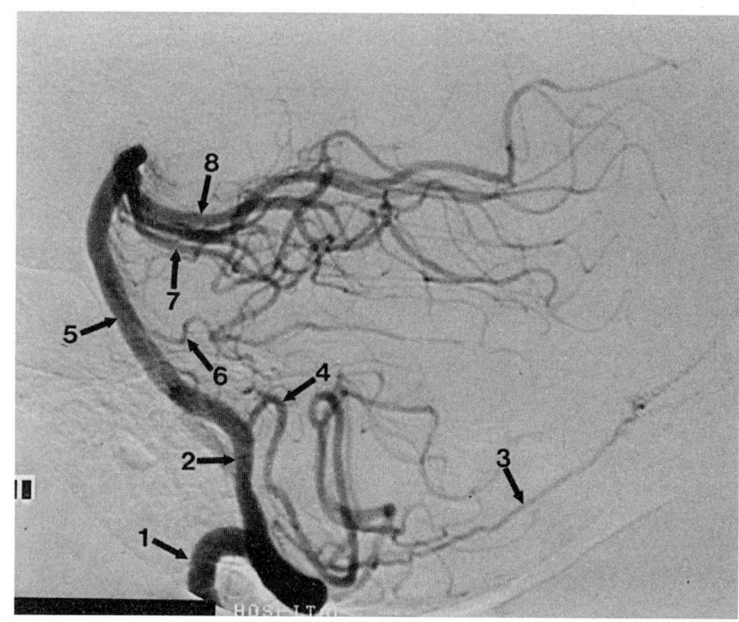

FIGURE 22–6. Lateral vertebral. 1, V-3 segment of the vertebral artery. 2, V-4 segment of the vertebral artery. 3, Posterior meningeal artery. 4, Posterior inferior cerebellar artery. 5, Basilar artery. 6, Anterior inferior cerebellar artery. 7, Superior cerebellar artery. 8, Posterior cerebral artery. (Courtesy of Karen S. Caldemeyer, M.D.)

to the upper cervical region, it consists of anastomosing branches from the anterior radicular arteries.

The two posterior spinal arteries most commonly arise from the vertebral arteries. However, in some instances, they arise from the PICA. There are contributions from numerous posterior radicular arteries that form an anastomotic network on the posterior surface of the spinal cord.[17] These arteries supply the posterior one third of the spinal cord. The anterior and posterior spinal arteries join in an anastomotic loop at the conus medullaris.[18]

The different regions of the spinal cord receive an unevenly distributed blood supply. The upper cervicothoracic region between C1 and T2 is richly vascularized by the anterior spinal artery in the most superior segments, and radicular arteries in the lower cervical and upper thoracic segments. The artery of the cervical enlargement is the most important of these radicular arteries. There are a number of radiculomedullary arteries that feed the posterior spinal arteries. The intermediate or midthoracic portion of the cord between T3 and T8 is poorly vascularized by intercostal arteries. There is a single radiculomedullary artery between T6 and T8. There are a limited number of segmental feeders to the posterior spinal arteries. In the lower or thoracolumbosacral region, there is again a rich vascular supply through the radiculomedullary branches of the intercostal and lumbar arteries. One important artery is the great anterior radicular artery of Adamkiewicz (artery of the lumbar enlargement). There are numerous posterior radicular arteries at this level. An understanding of these variations is important in spinal cord vascular syndromes, particularly with hypoperfusion of the spinal cord due to hypotension.

Intraspinal System (Intramedullary Arteries)

Branches of the anterior and posterior spinal arteries form a vascular plexus or peripheral vasocorona that encircles the cord. There are also sulcal arteries arising from the anterior spinal system that travel in the anterior median fissure of the cord and then branch and penetrate the cord. There are fewer sulcal arteries in the midthoracic region, which may contribute to the susceptibility of this region to ischemia. The branches of this plexus supply a major portion of the white matter and the dorsal horns of the gray matter. The arterial supply of the gray matter is richer than that of the white matter. The gray matter, except the dorsal horns, is supplied by the largest branches of the anterior spinal artery called the sulcocommissural arteries. The dorsal horns and the funiculi are supplied by paired posterior spinal arteries, posterior medullary feeders, and perforating pial branches.

ARTERIAL STRUCTURE

Arteries are classified into three categories based on their size and histological features. The large or elastic arteries, such as the aorta and its major branches, have three layers: the tunica intima, the tunica media, and the tunica adventitia. In large arteries, the intima is a smooth layer of thin endothelial cells on a basement membrane, the media is the muscular layer that is rich in elastic tissue, and the adventitia is a layer of connective tissue with elastic fibers, nerve fibers, and the vasa vasorum. With aging, the elastic fibers of the media in large vessels become less resilient. This causes less expansion with blood pressure elevations and predisposes to tortuosity. The medium or muscular arteries also consist of three layers. The distinguishing features of muscular arteries are the internal elastic lamina that forms the outer limit of the intima and the external elastic membrane that forms the outer layer of the media and is more defined than in large arteries. The adventitial layer in muscular arteries contains more nerves than this layer in large vessels due to their role in autonomic control. Arteriosclerosis and atheromatosis are most characteristic of the large and medium-sized vessels. Medial calcific sclerosis can affect medium-sized arteries. Finally, small arteries are characterized by a progressive loss of the three layers such that arterioles have no identifiable layers. The extracranial cerebral arteries have the usual structure of elastic or muscular arteries. However, intracranial arteries differ because they have no external elastic lamina and there is no vasa vasorum.[19]

BLOOD-BRAIN BARRIER

The microcirculation of the brain is unique because of the blood-brain barrier (BBB). This barrier to free metabolic exchange keeps a homeostatic environment around neurons. There are actually two parts to the BBB, including the BBB itself and the blood–cerebrospinal fluid (CSF) barrier.[20] The BBB consists of capillary endothelial cells that are joined at tight junctions devoid of fenestrae. There is very little pinocytosis occurring, and passage of substances depends on their affinity for lipids and the presence of carrier proteins. The blood-CSF barrier consists of the periventricular region, including the choroid plexus, median eminence, and the area postrema. In these locations, there is active pinocytosis that allows small molecules into the subependymal interstitial space. Cerebral edema occurs when there is an increase in water content in the brain. Cerebral infarctions, hemorrhages, and contusions cause vasogenic edema as a result of leakage of water and plasma directly into the central nervous system due to damaged capillary endothelial cells that have lost their BBB function.

VENOUS SUPPLY

The venous system of the head and neck is extensive. Emphasis is made here only to those vessels that are relevant to cerebrovascular syndromes (Fig. 22–7).

The blood from the brain is drained by the cerebral veins, which empty into dural sinuses that are primarily drained by the internal jugular veins. The extracranial draining veins of the neck consist of the external jugular vein, the internal jugular vein, and the vertebral vein.

The venous drainage of the brain and meninges can be divided into the diploic veins, the meningeal veins, the dural sinuses, and the cerebral veins. The diploic veins run between the tables of bone of the skull to drain the diploë. These vessels communicate extensively with the extracranial venous system, the meningeal veins, and the dural sinuses. The meningeal veins are epidural vessels that supply drainage for the falx cerebri, the tentorium, and the cranial dura mater. The major dural sinuses include the superior and inferior sagittal sinuses, the cavernous and intracavernous sinuses, the superior and inferior petrosal sinuses, the occipital sinus, and the straight, transverse, and sigmoid sinuses.[21]

The dural sinuses that are most often affected by thrombosis are the superior sagittal sinus (SSS), the lateral sinuses (LS), and the cavernous sinuses (CS). The SSS originates

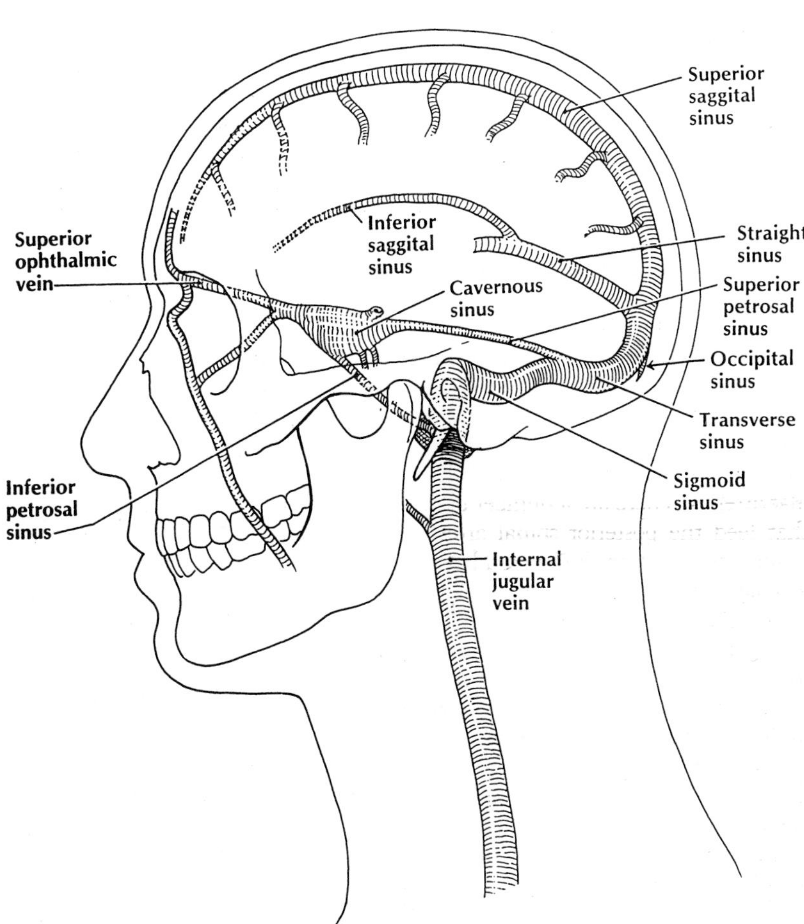

FIGURE 22–7. Major veins of the cerebral venous system. (© 1996 Indiana University Medical Illustration Dept.)

near the crista galli where it communicates with the facial and nasal veins.[21] It courses posteriorly in the midline along the falx cerebri, and then courses backward toward the occipital protuberance, where it joins the lateral and straight sinuses to form the torcular Herophili. The SSS drains a major portion of the cortex. Due to its connection with the diploic veins that drain the scalp through the emissary veins, the SSS can be affected by infections or contusions of the face and scalp.

The LS course from the torcular Herophili to the jugular bulbs. They have a transverse portion that lies in the attached border of the tentorium and a sigmoid portion that runs on the mastoid process. Due to the latter anatomical configuration, this sinus can be affected by mastoiditis and otitis media. The drainage territory of the LS includes the cerebellum, brain stem, and the posterior portion of the cerebral hemisphere.

The CS are paired venous structures that lie next to the sphenoid bone. There are several important structures that lie in the region of the CS, including cranial nerves (CNs) III, IV, V_1, and V_2 in the lateral wall, and CN VI and the carotid artery with its sympathetic plexus in the central portion of the sinus. The CS drain blood from the orbits and the anterior portion of the base of the brain. They drain via the superior and inferior petrosal sinuses into the internal jugular veins.

The three important groups of veins that drain blood from the brain are the superficial cerebral veins, the deep cerebral veins, and the veins of the posterior fossa. The superficial cerebral veins lie along the cortical sulci. These vessels drain the cerebral cortex and portions of the white matter. The frontal, parietal, and occipital cortical veins drain into the SSS, while the middle cerebral veins drain into the LS. The middle cerebral veins run along the sylvian fissure to drain the opercular region. These veins are unique because they have no muscular layers or valves, which enables them to dilate and reverse the direction of blood flow if a sinus into which they drain is occluded. The deep cerebral veins, including the internal cerebral and basal veins, drain blood from the deep white matter of the cerebral hemispheres and the basal ganglia. These veins join to form the great vein of Galen, which subsequently drains into the straight sinus. The veins of the posterior fossa are divided into three major systems. The superior group drains into the galenic system. The anterior group drains the anterior cerebellum, pons, and medulla. The posterior group drains into the torcular Herophili and adjacent dural sinuses. They supply the cerebellar tonsils and the posteroinferior cerebellar hemispheres.

Examination of the Neurovascular System

DIRECTED NEUROLOGICAL EXAMINATION

The carotid artery should be palpated gently for the presence and the intensity of the impulse. The artery should be auscultated for a bruit. However, a bruit is not always indicative of carotid artery stenosis. In addition, the absence of a bruit does not rule out carotid stenosis. A vertebral artery bruit can be auscultated over the posterior upper cervical region. The temporal region, the orbits, and the mastoid region are good locations to auscultate cranial bruits, as in the case of arteriovenous malformations or aneurysms. Attention should be paid to the scalp, looking for prominence, or tenderness of the superficial temporal artery that may be seen with temporal arteritis. Bounding pulsation of the superficial temporal or the supraorbital arteries may be seen with internal carotid occlusive disease owing to increased collateral flow through the external carotid artery. Necrosis of the scalp can be seen with temporal arteritis.

Attention should be paid to the ocular globe, looking for scleral injection, dilated ocular and orbital vessels, pulsating exophthalmos, chemosis, or ophthalmoplegia that can be seen with carotid-cavernous fistulas. A dilated funduscopic examination can demonstrate the ocular manifestations of carotid vascular disease, including hypoperfusion or venous stasis retinopathy, anterior ischemic optic neuropathy, retinal infarctions, and rubeosis iridis. There may be evidence of microemboli such as bright orange-yellow, refractile, or Hollenhorst plaques; white platelet–fibrin intra-arterial plugs; or gray-white nonrefractile calcific emboli.

A careful auscultation of the heart should focus on the detection of structural lesions or rhythm disturbances. The aorta and peripheral pulses should be palpated and auscultated to provide clues to underlying peripheral atherosclerosis.

ASSOCIATED NEUROLOGICAL FINDINGS

Cerebral. Patients with ischemic stroke or intracerebral hemorrhage may have a number of varied cortical deficits (Table 22–2). Patients should be evaluated for disturbances in attention, emotion, memory, language, and speech. Examination of higher cortical functions may be difficult acutely, but serial examinations are often helpful to detect the type and extent of cognitive disturbances.

A basic mental status examination should be performed, evaluating orientation, object recall, calculations, reading, writing, and comprehension. Patients should be examined for disturbances in spatial relationships including anosognosia, spatial disorientation, hemispacial neglect, constructional apraxia, and other apraxias that are seen with nondominant hemisphere lesions. Finger agnosia and right-left disorientation are seen with dominant hemispheric lesions. The typical deficits seen with the various stroke syndromes are detailed in Table 22–2.

Detailed classification of aphasia subtypes is helpful in localizing the area of stroke. There are typical findings with regard to fluency, comprehension, repetition, and naming with lesions in different locations (see Chapter 6).

Cranial Nerves. Visual acuity should be checked with correction to evaluate for a decrement that can be seen with retinal vascular lesions. A dilated funduscopic examination may show evidence of retinal emboli. Visual fields examination may show a homonymous hemianopia that can be seen with MCA or PCA territory stroke or with PCA occlusion secondary to basilar artery disease. Bilateral homonymous hemianopia results in cortical blindness and is most often due to simultaneous or successive PCA occlusions.

Vertical eye movements are impaired with midbrain infarctions. Examination of CN III may disclose an oculomotor paresis that can be seen with the midbrain syndromes, an aneurysm at the junction of the internal carotid and posterior communicating arteries, an aneurysm of the ICA in the cavernous sinus, or with uncal herniation. Horizontal eye movements are impaired with pontine infarctions. CN IV may be affected with midbrain infarction or hemorrhage. CN VI may be affected by pontine infarction or hemorrhage, carotid aneurysms or carotid-cavernous fistulas within the cavernous sinus, or compressive lesions within the prepontine cistern such as with fusiform basilar artery aneurysms. Pupillary responses may be helpful in localization of the vascular lesion. Pinpoint pupils that are reactive are seen with pontine tegmental lesions. Fascicular or peripheral III nerve lesions seen with compression due to aneurysms and herniation produce an ipsilateral dilated and unresponsive pupil. Lesions in the midbrain tegmentum produce midposition, irregular, and corectopic pupils (noncentered). Lesions in the midbrain tectum produce midposition and unreactive pupils, often with spontaneous hippus.

Horner's syndrome (ptosis, miosis, and anhidrosis) may be seen with disruption of the descending oculosympathetic system in lateral medullary infarctions (Wallenberg's syndrome), infarctions in the territories of the superior cerebellar or anterior inferior cerebellar arteries, or mesencephalic hemorrhages. Cervical carotid dissection or occlusion can be associated with postganglionic Horner's syndrome.

An internuclear ophthalmoplegia (INO), characterized by adduction weakness on the side of the medial longitudinal fasciculus lesion and monocular nystagmus of the abducting eye, can be seen with brain stem infarctions. The INO may be unilateral or bilateral.

CN IV may be affected with midbrain infarction or hemorrhage. CN V may be affected with vascular disease of the pons or medulla or in the cavernous sinus. Dysfunction of CN VII can be manifested as a central facial palsy due to supranuclear corticobulbar lesions that cause a contralateral paresis of the lower portion of the face, with relative sparing of upper facial function. This type of involvement is commonly seen with cortical or subcortical cerebral hemorrhage or ischemia. A peripheral type facial nerve palsy with paralysis of the upper and lower facial muscles can be seen with pontine lesions.

Acute hearing loss can occur with AICA infarctions. Vascular lesions of the auditory cortex do not lead to complete deafness, even if the lesions are bilateral. Pure word deafness can occur with unilateral or bilateral temporal lesions affecting Heschl's gyri. Due to the binaural representation of the ascending auditory tracts above the level of the cochlear nuclei, lesions of the brain stem involving the auditory pathways do not cause deafness.

Dysfunction of CN IX and X with vascular lesions is manifested by dysphagia and an altered gag response. Bilateral supranuclear corticobulbar lesions, as can occur with bilateral infarctions, can result in severe dysphagia as well as other pseudobulbar signs. Lateral medullary infarctions affect CN IX and X function due to involvement of the nucleus ambiguus and cause hoarseness, hiccups, dysphagia, and paralysis of the pharynx, palate, and vocal cords.

Lesions of CN XII can be assessed by observing the tongue at rest and with protrusion. With supranuclear lesions due to infarction or hemorrhage, the tongue will deviate toward the

TABLE 22–2. **Clinico-anatomical Correlation of Disorders of Neurovascular Function**

Anatomical Site of Damage	Neurovascular	Cerebral	Cranial Nerves	Motor/Reflexes/Cerebellar/Gait	Sensory	Autonomic Nervous System
Diffuse Ischemia: Hypoperfusion						
Cerebral	Usually normal	Confusion, somnolence	Lower altitudinal defect; saccade/pursuit defects	Bibrachial weakness	Bibrachial sensory loss	Orthostatic hypotension
Spinal cord	Usually normal	Normal	Normal	Paralysis below lesion	Sensory loss below lesion	Orthostatic hypotension, bladder/bowel incontinence
Extracranial steal syndrome	Decreased radial pulse in affected arm	Normal	Transient CN dysfunction	Transient uni- or bilateral quadriparesis	Transient sensory loss, body not face	Decreased blood pressure in affected arm
TIA						
Carotid	Carotid bruit, decreased carotid pulse, atherosclerosis	Transient aphasia and dysarthria	Ipsilateral amaurosis fugax, contralateral HH	Transient contralateral weakness or clumsiness	Transient bilateral sensory loss	Cardiac arrhythmia, hypertension
Vertebrobasilar	Vertebral or basilar bruit	Normal	Transient CN findings–diplopia, dysarthria	Transient bilateral weakness or clumsiness	Transient bilateral sensory loss	Cardiac arrhythmia, hypertension
Focal CVA—Carotid System						
Carotid	Carotid pulse diminished or absent	Depressed consciousness, global aphasia	Retinal emboli, contralateral HH, conjugate eye deviation	Weakness contralateral face, arm, leg	Contralateral hemisensory loss face, arm, leg	Cardiac arrhythmia, hypertension
Middle cerebral	Possible bruit mid/upper cervical area	Aphasia (left), apraxia (right)	Contralateral HH	Weakness contralateral face, arm greater than leg	Contralateral hemisensory loss face, arm, greater than leg	Cardiac arrhythmia, hypertension
Anterior cerebral	Possible bruit mid/upper cervical area	Emotional lability, aphasia (left), apraxia (right)	Conjugate eye deviation	Weakness contralateral leg more weak than face, arm	Contralateral hemisensory loss, leg more involved than face and arm	Cardiac arrhythmia, hypertension
Anterior choroidal	Possible cervical bruit, atherosclerosis	Affect changes, hemineglect	Contralateral HH	Weakness contralateral face, arm, leg	Contralateral hemisensory loss face, arm, leg	Cardiac arrhythmia, hypertension
Small vessel (lacunar infarction)	Usually normal	Dementia (multiple lacunar strokes)	Usually normal (except for CN VII)	Paralysis, if present, usually involves face, arm, leg	Sensory loss, if present involves face, arm, leg	Hypertension

Table continued on following page

TABLE 22–2 **Clinico-anatomical Correlation of Disorders of Neurovascular Function** *Continued*

Anatomical Site of Damage	Neurovascular	Cerebral	Cranial Nerves	Motor/Refelexes/ Cerebellar/Gait	Sensory	Autonomic Nervous System
Focal CVA—Vertebrobasilar System						
Posterior inferior cerebellar	Possible vertebral bruit	Normal	Ipsilateral weak palate, Horner's syndrome, decreased p/t ipsilateral face	Ipsilateral limb ataxia	Decreased p/t contralateral body	Cardiac arrhythmia, hypertension
Anterior inferior cerebellar	Normal	Normal	Ipsilateral deafness, ipsilateral facial weakness, decreased sensation ipsilateral face	Ipsilateral limb ataxia	Decreased p/t contralateral body	Cardiac arrhythmia, hypertension
Superior cerebellar	Normal	Normal	Nystagmus, ipsilateral deafness, diplopia (CN IV)	Ipsilateral limb ataxia	Decreased all sensory modalities contralateral body	Cardiac arrhythmia, hypertension
Posterior cerebral	Possible vertebral bruit	Visual agnosia, visual neglect, dyslexia	Contralateral HH, cortical blindness, Balint's syndrome	Usually normal, possible chorea or ballism	Normal unless thalamic pain	Cardiac arrhythmia, hypertension
Medial midbrain basilar	Usually normal	Normal	Internuclear ophthalmoplegia, CN III paresis	Contralateral body weakness, ataxia	Normal	Cardiac arrhythmia, hypertension
Medial pontine basilar	Usually normal	Normal	Internuclear ophthalmoplegia, CN6 paresis or conjugate eye deviation to side of lesion	Contralateral body weakness, bilateral lesions cause quadraparesis and "locked-in" syndrome	Normal, may have decreased position and vibration contralateral body	Cardiac arrhythmia, hypertension
Medial medullary	Usually normal	Normal	CN XII: dysarthria, may have upbeat nystagmus	Contralateral body weakness, ataxia	Decreased position and vibration contralateral body	Cardiac arrhythmia, hypertension
Transient global amnesia	Normal	Loss of memory for recent events, cannot learn new information	Normal	Normal	Normal	Normal

Hemorrhage						
Subarachnoid	Possible cranial bruits	Variable depressed level of consciousness	CN III paresis if internal carotid posterior communicating artery aneurysm Fundus: subhyaloid hemorrhages	Normal, unless intraparenchymal extension or secondary vasospasm	Normal, unless intraparenchymal extension or secondary vasospasm	Hypertension, cardiac arrhythmia
Intracranial hematoma	Possible cranial bruits	Depressed level of consciousness	Depends on location: brain stem-CN findings prominent; cortical/subcortical-HH; thalamic-conjugate downward deviation	Hemi- or quadriplegia	Cannot assess well if comatose. If thalamus or parietal lobe affected, hemisensory loss contralateral	Hypertension
Extracranial hematoma	Normal	Normal or depressed level of consciousness	Normal, possible CN VI palsy from increased intracranial pressure	Varying degree of hemiparesis	Varying degree of hemisensory loss	Normal or Cushing's triad if increased intracranial pressure
Vascular Anomalies						
Intracranial steal	Cranial bruits	May have cognitive deficits	Transient visual deficits	Transient hemiparesis	Transient hemisensory deficits	Normal
Vessel dissection	Diminished carotid, superficial temporal, or supraorbital pulses	Normal unless infarction occurs	CN XII lesions, other CN (II, III, V, XI) may be involved; Horner's syndrome	Variable hemiparesis	Variable hemisensory loss	
Vascular fistula	Orbital bruit, ocular pulsation	Normal	Variable visual loss and restriction of eye movements and chemosis	Normal	Normal	Normal
Spinal Cord Ischemia						
Anterior spinal artery	Aortic pulsation or aortic dissection	Normal	Normal	Flaccid paraplegia or quadriplegia below lesion	Loss of pain and temperature below lesion	Hypotension
Posterior spinal artery	Normal	Normal	Normal	Loss of reflexes below lesion	Loss of position and vibration below lesion	Hypotension

HH, Homonymous hemianopia; p/t, pain/temperature sensation

side of the hemiplegia. This nerve can also be affected in its intramedullary course due to infarction or hemorrhage. The medial medullary syndrome can cause paresis of the tongue with the tongue protruding away from the hemiplegia.

Motor/Reflexes/Cerebellar/Gait. The motor deficits with cerebrovascular disease can vary from a mild limb drift to hemiplegia. The different clinical syndromes have different patterns of motor deficits, and the extent of weakness varies (see Table 22–2). The presence of bilateral or crossed weakness may suggest vertebrobasilar circulation ischemia, particularly in the presence of other signs of vertebrobasilar ischemia. Weakness of the face and arm more than the leg usually indicates MCA ischemia. Involvement of the face, arm, and leg equally can be seen with capsular or pontine ischemia. Prominent weakness of the leg may be seen with ACA ischemia. In spinal cord vascular lesions, there is paralysis below the level of the lesion if the anterior spinal artery is involved.

It is also important to evaluate tone, since hypotonia may be seen with cerebellar lesions and varying degrees of hypertonicity can be seen with cerebral infarcts or hemorrhages or with brain stem compression. Paratonia (gegenhalten phenomenon) is present often with frontal infarction or hemorrhage.

Asymmetry of the muscle stretch reflexes or a unilateral extensor toe sign or Hoffman response may be the only indication of corticospinal tract dysfunction. There may be "primitive" reflexes, such as a grasp or snout reflex with extensive frontal lesions.

Ataxia or dystaxia of the limbs, trunk, or gait is seen with cerebellar lesions. The gait may be wide based with impaired tandem gait. Asynergia, dysdiadochokinesia, and dysmetria may be present. The presence of truncal ataxia and titubation suggests a lesion in the midline cerebellum.

Sensory. Tactile sensory loss may be seen with many of the stroke syndromes (see Table 22–2). Patients can be tested for graphesthesia and stereognosis. Lesions of the postcentral gyrus in the parietal lobe can cause contralateral sensory loss with astereognosis, impaired position sense, and impaired tactile sensation greater than to pain, temperature, and vibration. There may be extinction to double simultaneous tactile stimulation. Hemisensory deficits can occur with thalamic infarctions in the territory of the thalamogeniculate arteries that supply the somatosensory nuclei. There are crossed sensory findings with lateral medullary infarctions.

In spinal cord vascular lesions, there is loss of pain and temperature sensation below the level of the infarction if the anterior spinal artery is involved. Loss of position, vibration, and light touch sensation below the level of the lesion is seen with infarction of the posterior spinal artery.

Autonomic Nervous System. Other autonomic testing is usually normal with disturbance of neurovascular function. With the anterior spinal artery syndrome, there is loss of bowel, bladder, and sexual function due to dysfunction of autonomic pathways.

Orthostatic blood pressure and pulse will provide information on ambient autonomic function and reflex response to gravitational changes. In cases in which vascular abnormalities in the neck are suspected (e.g., subclavian steal syndrome), left versus right blood pressure and pulse comparisons are useful.

Evaluation Guidelines

The goals of the diagnostic evaluation are to establish the diagnosis of ischemic or hemorrhagic cerebrovascular disease as a cause of the patient's symptoms and to determine the underlying cause of the event. Early diagnosis and management in the first few hours after stroke are critical. Since proper management begins with an accurate diagnosis, it is paramount to differentiate between cerebral infarction and hemorrhage. The tests that may assist with diagnosis are detailed in Table 22–3. There are a number of potential etiologies of cerebral infarction and hemorrhage that need to be considered (Tables 22–3 and 22–4; see Chapter 45).

Neuroimaging. In all patients with suspected ischemic stroke, an unenhanced computed tomogram (CT) of the brain is the first test to differentiate between infarction and hemorrhage. In addition, other disorders that mimic acute cerebrovascular disease must be excluded, including tumors, abscesses, and subdural hematomas. Intravenous contrast-enhanced CT is needed only when these diagnoses are a consideration. Thin CT cuts through the posterior fossa should be done if posterior fossa pathology is suspected. Magnetic resonance imaging (MRI) is superior to CT in cerebral ischemia, particularly in the evaluation of ischemic areas in the posterior fossa. Diffusion-weighted MRI can detect areas of cerebral ischemia within minutes after the onset of stroke.

In patients with suspected intracerebral hemorrhage, CT is the most effective initial test to accurately identify the location, site, direction of extension, and type of an acute intracerebral hemorrhage. The presence and degree of hydrocephalus, ventricular shift or compression, and edema can be assessed. While MRI is not often used acutely, it becomes an important diagnostic tool later for identifying whether vascular malformations or tumors are present.

Carotid Doppler ultrasonography is used as a noninvasive means of evaluating for stenosis or occlusion of the common and proximal portions of the internal and external carotid arteries. Transcranial Doppler ultrasound is a technique that allows identification of alteration in direction or velocity of flow in the basal intracranial arteries. This test can be helpful in subarachnoid hemorrhage to evaluate for vasospasm.

Angiography is indicated in patients who are possible candidates for carotid endarterectomy with moderate to severe carotid artery stenosis on noninvasive testing or in patients with suspected vasculitis, arterial dissection, or with suspicion of other intracranial vasculopathies. Cerebral angiography plays an important role in the evaluation of selected patients with intracerebral hemorrhage. Angiography is of importance when there is reason to suspect an aneurysm, arteriovenous malformation (AVM), vasculitis, or moyamoya disease. Angiography is performed in patients who have an atypical location for hypertensive hemorrhage or in the young patient without hypertension.

In patients with spinal cord ischemia, a spinal MRI may show an area of infarction or hemorrhage or a vascular malformation.

Body Fluid and Tissue Analysis. A basic workup that should be performed in all patients with ischemic stroke includes a complete blood count with differential and platelet count, erythrocyte sedimentation rate, prothrombin time with International Normalized Ratio (INR), activated

TABLE 22–3. **Useful Tests in the Evaluation of Disorders of Neurovascular Function**

Syndrome	Neuroimaging: MRI/CT	Electrophysiology	Fluid and Tissue Analysis	Neuropsychological Tests	Other Tests
Ischemia					
Diffuse hypoperfusion					
Cerebral	Uni- or bilateral infarcts in "watershed" areas	EEG: diffuse slowing	NA	Depressed LOC	None
Spinal cord	Infarct in thoracic "watershed" areas	SSEP delay	NA	Normal	None
Extracranial steal syndrome	Normal unless infarct occurs	EEG usually normal	NA	NA	None
TIA					
Focal ischemia					
Large vessel	Infarct in involved region	Polymorphic delta waves over region	Lab tests*	Variable depending on site	Chest x-ray, ECG, NV tests†
Small vessel (lacunae)	Small infarcts subcortex and brainstem	Normal	Lab tests*	Variable depending on site	Chest x-ray, ECG, NV tests†
Hemorrhage					
Subarachnoid	Blood subarachnoid space, MR angiogram may visualize aneurysm	Varying degrees of diffuse slowing	CSF: RBCs/xanthochromia	Depressed LOC dependent on extent of bleeding, hydrocephalus, and vasospasm	Cerebral angiography to show aneurysm
Intracranial hematoma	Intraparenchymal blood	EEG: polymorphic slow waves over region	Decreased CSF cystatin C (cerebral amyloid angiopathy)	Variable depressed LOC depending on site	Biopsy of hematoma site may reveal tumor cells or cerebral amyloid angiopathy
Extracranial hematomas	Extradural or subdural defects	EEG: attenuated background over hematoma	NA	Variable degrees of depressed consciousness	Cerebral angiogram: avascular mass
Vascular Anomalies					
Intracranial steals	MRI/CT: vascular mass	EEG: slow waves in contralateral hemisphere	Normal	Variable cognitive effects depending on site of AVM	AVM on cerebral angiogram
Vessel dissection	Cerebral or brain stem infarct	EEG: polymorphic slow waves over ipsilateral hemisphere	Normal	Aphasia in carotid dissection	Dissection seen on angiogram
Fistula	MRI/CT: dilated vascular structure, esp. cavernous sinus	Normal	NA	Normal	Cerebral or MR angiogram; dilated vascular channels
Spinal cord ischemia	MRI: infarction of cord	SSEP: normal (anterior spinal artery) or prolonged (posterior spinal artery)	NA	NA	Spine x-rays, aortic ultrasound, TEE, angiography useful in aortic dissection

*Lab tests = standard battery of tests of neurovascular evaluation; includes CBC with differential, platelet count, ESR, PT, PTT, plasma glucose, BUN, creatinine, lipid analysis, luetic serology, urinalysis. More detailed testing for hematological abnormalities are added as indicated.

†NV tests = noninvasive diagnostic procedures are carotid and vertebral duplex, 2-D echocardiography, or TEE. These are useful in evaluating a cerebrovascular lesion. Cerebral angiography is invasive and therefore used only in selected instances.

MRI, Magnetic resonance imaging; CT, computed tomography scan; EEG, electroencephalography; LOC, level of consciousness; SSEP, somatosensory evoked potentials; AVM, arteriovenous malformation; NA, not applicable; TEE, transesophageal echocardiography.

TABLE 22–4. **Selected Etiologies Associated with Neurovascular Disorders**

Etiological Category	Selected Specific Etiologies	Chapter
Structural Disorders		
Developmental structural disorders	Saccular aneurysms Arteriovenous malformations	28
Hereditary and Degenerative Disorders		
Storage diseases: Lipidoses, glycogen disorders, and leukodystrophies	Fabry's disease	30
Amino/organic acidopathies, mitochondrial enzyme defects, and other metabolic errors	MELAS Menke's disease	31
Chromosomal abnormalities and neurocutaneous disorders	Rendu-Osler-Weber, Ehlers-Danlos type IV	32
Movement disorders	Sydenham's chorea	34
Hereditary nondegenerative neuromuscular disease	Inherited disease producing accelerated atherosclerosis Inherited nonatherosclerotic vasculopathies	37
Acquired Metabolic and Nutritional Disorders		
Endogenous metabolic disorders	Acquired prothrombotic states	38
Exogenous acquired metabolic disorders of the nervous system: Toxins and illicit drugs	Heroin, cocaine, phencyclidine, phenylpropanolamine, amphetamines, methanol intoxication	39
Nutritional deficiencies and syndromes associated with alcoholism	Binge alcohol intoxication	40
Infectious Disorders		
Viral infections	Herpes zoster arteritis	41
Nonviral infections	Meningovascular syphilis, meningitis (bacterial, tuberculosis), fungal infections, sarcoidosis	42
HIV and AIDS	Bleeding diatheses, opportunistic infection	44
Neurovascular Disorders	Arterial hypertension Atherosclerotic vasculopathy Embolic cardiac diseases, valvular heart disease, arrhythmias, intracardiac defects, cyanotic congenital heart disease, atrial myxoma, infective endocarditis Hemoglobinopathies Vascular anomalies (e.g., aneurysms, AVMs) Nonatherosclerotic vasculopathies Cerebral venous thrombosis	45
Neoplastic Disorders		
Primary neurological tumors	Intracranial hemorrhage into tumor	46
Metastatic neoplasms and paraneoplastic syndromes	Paraproteinemias, intracranial hemorrhage	47
Autoimmune and Inflammatory Disorders	Temporal arteritis Takayasu's arteritis Wegener's granulomatosis Polyarteritis nodosa Behçet's disease Buerger's disease	50
Traumatic Disorders	Arterial dissection Extracerebral hemorrhage	51
Headache and Facial Pain	Migraine	53
Drug-Induced and Iatrogenic Disorders	Oral contraceptives MAO inhibitors Radiation vasculopathy Anticoagulants/thrombolytics Stroke associated with surgery	55

partial thromboplastin time, plasma glucose level, blood urea nitrogen, serum creatinine, lipid analysis, luetic serology, and urinalysis (see Table 22–3).

A basic evaluation that should be performed in all patients with intracerebral hemorrhage includes a complete blood count with differential and platelet count, prothrombin time with partial thromboplastin time, erythrocyte sedimentation rate, plasma glucose, serum alkaline phosphatase, serum aspartate aminotransferase, serum calcium, blood urea nitrogen, serum creatinine, and urinalysis. Additional paraclinical evaluation is listed in Table 22–3.

Cerebrospinal Fluid. There is almost no indication for a lumbar puncture in patients suspected of having ischemic stroke or intracerebral hemorrhage. Rarely, patients suspected of having infection as a cause of stroke may need CSF analysis. In patients with intracerebral hemorrhage or a large hemispheric stroke, a lumbar puncture can be dangerous because of sudden intracranial compartmental shifts with resultant herniation. Patients with suspected subarachnoid hemorrhage with a CT scan that does not reveal hemorrhage should undergo a lumbar puncture. There is no need to perform a lumbar puncture if the CT scan shows subarachnoid blood.

Neuropsychological Tests. Depression occurs in 30 to 50 percent of stroke patients within 2 years of the initial event.[22] Poststroke depression produces physical, emotional, and cognitive symptomatology and may have a major impact on the recovery of these patients. Approximately 40 to 50 percent will display depressive symptomatology in the first month after stroke. About half of the patients meet criteria for major depression. The other half have minor depressive symptoms. A particularly interesting finding, not corroborated by all investigators, has been that depression is most common with strokes involving the frontal lobe and head of the caudate nucleus, particularly with lesions close to the frontal pole. Depression is more common with lesions affecting the left dorsolateral frontal lobe in comparison with the right frontal pole. One possible explanation for this neuroanatomical correlation is that such lesions may interrupt noradrenergic and serotoninergic pathways. Poststroke depression responds to tricyclic antidepressants and selective serotonin reuptake inhibitors. Persuading patients to comply with treatment requires a detailed explanation of the potential unwanted effects of the medications. The selection of the antidepressant is based on the side effect profile of the medication and the clinical characteristics of the patient.

Other neuropsychiatric problems that can occur after stroke include mania, anxiety, bipolar affective disorders, and psychosis. Another problem that can develop is a pseudobulbar affect or emotional incontinence that may be due to bilateral infarctions. These patients often respond to nortriptyline.[22]

Other Tests. Other tests that should be performed in all patients with ischemic stroke include chest roentgenography and electrocardiography. Cardiac investigations to determine whether emboli have a cardiac source are advised in selected circumstances. Two-dimensional echocardiography in older patients with ischemic stroke is often limited to those with clinical clues of heart disease. Two-dimensional echocardiography should be considered in all patients younger than 45 years with otherwise unexplained ischemic stroke. Transesophageal echocardiography should be used in selected individuals, particularly for the evaluation of mitral and aortic prosthetic valves or vegetations, or whenever there is a need for better visualization of the left atrial appendage or interatrial septum, or when a right-to-left shunt or debris from atherosclerosis of the aortic arch is suspected.

Clinical Syndromes

There are a number of syndromes that result from ischemia or hemorrhage involving the central nervous system. Table 22–2 details typical clinical features, while Table 22–3 details tests that assist in the diagnosis of the syndromes. Causes of stroke are discussed in Chapter 45.

DIFFUSE HYPOPERFUSION SYNDROMES (CEREBRAL AND SPINAL CORD)

As discussed in the section on arterial anatomy, the midthoracic spinal cord is a border zone or watershed area that is susceptible to ischemia due to the unequal blood supply in this region. In situations of systemic hypoperfusion, there can be a spinal cord infarction. Conditions such as an aortic dissection can also cause a global decrease in spinal cord perfusion that results in gray matter infarction with relative sparing of the white matter tracts.

There can be border zone or watershed infarctions in the brain between the major arterial circulations. These conditions may occur with severe hypotension or in association with cardiac surgery. There are several described syndromes.[23]

If there is ischemia in the border zone territory of the anterior, middle, and posterior cerebral arteries, there may be bilateral parieto-occipital infarcts. There can be a variety of visual defects, including lower altitudinal visual field defects, optic ataxia, cortical blindness, disorders of ocular pursuit, and abnormalities in judging size, distance, and movement. If there is ischemia between the territories of the anterior and middle cerebral arteries bilaterally, a syndrome of bibrachial sensorimotor impairment can occur. Initially, there is weakness of the entire upper limbs, but later the weakness may be confined to the forearms and hands. Saccadic eye movements may be impaired due to involvement of the frontal eye fields. In ischemia to the border zone regions between the middle and posterior cerebral arteries, there can be bilateral parietotemporal infarctions. Patients have cortical blindness initially that may improve. However, there are a number of defects in higher cortical function, including dyslexia, dysgraphia, dyscalculia, and memory defects, that persist.

EXTRACRANIAL STEAL SYNDROMES FROM DISEASE OF THE AORTIC BRANCHES

Occlusive disease in the subclavian arteries or the innominate artery can give rise to extracranial steal syndromes. The most defined syndrome is the subclavian steal syndrome. In this condition, occlusive disease in the proximal subclavian artery can lead to a siphoning of blood away from the brain by a reversal of flow down the vertebral artery on the affected side to the ischemic limb. The pulse and blood pressure are diminished in the affected limb. The symptoms may include headache, vertebrobasilar ischemia, and limb claudication, often precipitated by exercise. A bruit may be heard over the subclavian artery. The limb may become cyanotic if it is held above the level of the heart. It should be noted that a majority of persons with subclavian steal detected by noninvasive techniques have no neurological symptoms.[24]

TRANSIENT ISCHEMIC ATTACKS (TIAs)

A TIA is a transient episode of focal neurological or retinal dysfunction secondary to impaired blood supply in a vascular territory. Clinical signs typical of TIAs in the carotid and vertebrobasilar territories are outlined in Table 22–2. It should be noted that transient vertigo, diplopia, dysarthria, or dysphagia in isolation is insufficient to establish a diagnosis of vertebrobasilar TIAs. In addition, isolated drop attacks in which the patient falls to the ground, maintains consciousness, and then arises without a deficit are seldom due to vertebrobasilar ischemia. The annual risk of stroke after a TIA is 3 to 4 percent per year. However, the risk of a subsequent stroke is at least three times greater for individuals who have had a TIA than in those individuals who have not had a TIA.[25]

Amaurosis fugax may be described as a sudden onset of a "fog," "haze," "scum," "curtain," "shade," "blur," "cloud," or "mist." A curtain or shade pattern with the loss of vision moving superiorly to inferiorly is described only by 15 to 20 percent of patients.[26, 27] Less commonly, there can be a concentric visual loss presumed to be due to marginal perfusion causing diminished blood flow to the retina. The visual loss is sudden in onset, often brief in duration, and painless in nature. The length of visual loss is usually 1 to 5 minutes and rarely lasts more than 30 minutes. Positive phenomena such as scintillation, fortification spectra, or flashing lights are rarely indicative of amaurosis fugax. After an episode of amaurosis fugax, the vision is usually fully restored, although some patients may have permanent visual loss due to a retinal infarction (see Table 22–2).[27]

In amaurosis fugax, it is key to evaluate for ICA stenosis with a carotid duplex ultrasound and to exclude temporal arteritis or a cardiac abnormality as a cause.

CAROTID SYSTEM STROKE SYNDROMES

Internal Carotid Artery Occlusion

Occlusion of the ICA can produce symptoms and signs of infarction in either the ACA or MCA territories (or both) as described below. PCA territory infarctions can be seen with ICA occlusion if a fetal origin of the PCA is present. The sole feature that distinguishes the MCA syndrome from a carotid artery syndrome is the presence of amaurosis fugax.[28, 29] Infarctions are often large, involving multiple lobes. Cerebral edema may be a life-threatening concern. The carotid pulse may be absent ipsilaterally. Horner's syndrome may be present due to oculosympathetic involvement along the carotid artery.

Middle Cerebral Artery Syndrome

An MCA infarction is one of the most common manifestations of cerebrovascular disease (Fig. 22–8). The clinical picture with an MCA infarction is varied and depends upon whether the site of the occlusion is in the stem, the superior division, the inferior division, or the lenticulostriate branches and whether there is good collateral blood flow.

When the stem of the MCA is occluded, there is usually a resultant large infarction with contralateral hemiplegia, conjugate eye deviation toward the side of the infarct, hemianesthesia, and homonymous hemianopia. There is associated global aphasia if the dominant hemisphere is involved and hemineglect with nondominant hemispheral lesions. The difference between an upper division MCA infarction and a MCA stem lesion is that the hemiparesis usually affects the face and arm more than the leg with upper division infarction. Broca's aphasia is more common in upper division infarcts due to preferential involvement of the anterior branches of the upper division in occlusions. With lower division MCA syndromes, a Wernicke type aphasia is seen

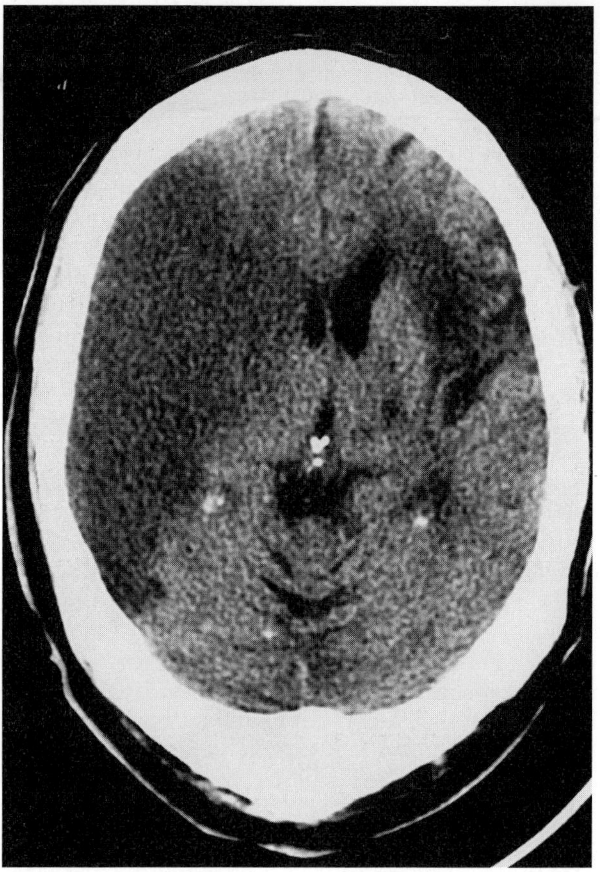

FIGURE 22–8. CT of a large acute right middle cerebral artery territory infarction. (Courtesy of Karen S. Caldemeyer, M.D.)

with dominant hemisphere infarction and behavioral disturbances are seen with nondominant infarction. A homonymous hemianopia may be present. A lenticulostriate branch occlusion may cause a lacunar infarction with involvement of the internal capsule producing a syndrome of pure motor hemiparesis. These described syndromes are variable and are dependent on the presence of collaterals and whether edema is present.[30–32]

Alexia with agraphia may occur with left angular gyrus involvement. Gerstmann's syndrome, which consists of finger agnosia, acalculia, right-left disorientation, and agraphia, may be seen with dominant hemisphere parietal lesions. The perisylvian aphasias seen with dominant hemispheral infarctions may be of the Broca, Wernicke, conduction, or global type, depending on the site and extent of involvement. Anosognosia most commonly is associated with right hemispheric strokes. Nondominant infarction may cause inattention, neglect, denial, apraxia, impaired prosody, and rarely acute confusion and agitated delirium.[33] A contralateral homonymous hemianopia or contralateral inferior quadrantanopia can occur with infarctions in either hemisphere.

Anterior Cerebral Artery Syndrome

ACA territory infarctions are uncommon. They can be seen in patients with vasospasm after subarachnoid hemorrhage due to ACA or ACoA aneurysms. Excluding these causes, the percentage of acute cerebral infarcts that are in the ACA territory is less than 3 percent.[34–36] The characteristics of ACA infarction vary according to the site of involvement and the extent of collateral blood flow.[37] Contralateral weakness involving primarily the lower extremity and, to a lesser extent, the arm is characteristic of infarction in the territory of the hemispheric branches of the ACA (see Table 22–2). Other characteristics include abulia, akinetic mutism (with bilateral mesiofrontal damage), impaired memory or emotional disturbances, transcortical motor aphasia (with dominant hemispheric lesions), deviation of the head and eyes toward the lesion, paratonia (gegenhalten), discriminative and proprioceptive sensory loss (primarily in the lower extremity), and sphincter incontinence (see Table 22–2).

An anterior disconnection syndrome with left arm apraxia due to involvement of the anterior corpus callosum can be seen. Pericallosal branch involvement can cause apraxia, agraphia, and tactile anomia of the left hand. Infarction of the basal branches of the ACA can cause memory disorders, anxiety, and agitation.

Infarction in the territory of the medial lenticulostriate artery (artery of Heubner) causes more pronounced weakness of the face and arm without sensory loss due to this artery's supply of portions of the anterior limb of the internal capsule.

Anterior Choroidal Artery Syndrome

The AChA syndrome is often characterized by hemiparesis as a result of involvement of the posterior limb of the internal capsule, hemisensory loss due to involvement of the posterolateral nucleus of the thalamus or thalamocortical fibers, and hemianopia secondary to involvement of the lateral geniculate body or the geniculocalcarine tract[38, 39] (see Table 22–2). The visual field defect that is seen with AChA infarcts is characterized by a homonymous defect in the superior and inferior visual fields that spares the horizontal meridian.[40] In a small number of patients, there may be left spatial hemineglect with right hemispheric infarctions and a mild language disorder with left hemispheric infarctions.[39, 41] With bilateral infarctions in the AChA territory, there can be pseudobulbar mutism and a variety of other features including facial diplegia, hemiparesis, hemisensory loss, lethargy, neglect, and affect changes.[42]

LACUNAR STROKE SYNDROMES

While there are over twenty described lacunar syndromes, the four that have been best described will be addressed here. These syndromes have been described with ischemic lacunar infarctions as well as with discrete hemorrhages.[43]

Pure motor hemiparesis is characterized by a unilateral motor deficit involving the face, the arm and, to a lesser extent, the leg. There may be a mild dysarthria. There is no associated aphasia, apraxia, or agnosia. In addition, there is no sensory, visual, or higher cortical dysfunction. This syndrome may be secondary to a lacunar infarction in the posterior limb of the internal capsule, corona radiata, basis pontis, cerebral peduncle, or the medullary pyramid.[44] However, an ischemic cortical lesion may also cause a pure motor hemiparesis.[43]

Pure sensory stroke (pure hemisensory or paresthetic stroke) is characterized by unilateral numbness, paresthesias, and a hemisensory deficit involving the face, arm, trunk, and leg. Subjective complaints may be out of proportion to objective findings. Lacunae in the ventroposterolateral nucleus of the thalamus may cause this syndrome. However, pure sensory stroke can also be due to ischemic infarctions in the corona radiata or in the parietal cortex.[43]

Ataxic hemiparesis (homolateral ataxia and crural paresis) is characterized by weakness that is more prominent in the lower extremity in association with ipsilateral arm and leg incoordination. Involvement of the face is uncommon. Dysarthria is usually not present. There may be an extensor plantar response. Lacunae in the posterior limb of the internal capsule, basis pontis, red nucleus, or in the thalamocapsular region can cause this syndrome.[43, 45]

The dysarthria–clumsy hand syndrome is characterized by supranuclear facial weakness, tongue deviation, dysphagia, dysarthria, impaired fine motor control of the hand, and an extensor plantar response. There is no sensory deficit. Lacunae in the basis pontis, at the junction of the upper one third and lower two thirds of the pons, or in the genu of the internal capsule may cause this syndrome.[43]

VERTEBROBASILAR STROKE SYNDROMES

The circumferential vessels perfuse the lateral brain stem, and the perforant vessels directly from the large basilar or vertebral arteries perfuse the midline structures. While obstruction of the circumferential arteries gives rise to standard syndromes, there is great variability in the perforant vessels, and therefore several syndromes are described. As a rule, midline syndromes affect the pyramidal system, consciousness, and midline cranial nerves (extraocular muscles), whereas lateral syndromes affect the cerebellum, sensation, and the lateral cranial nerves. There are additional overlap syndromes when vessels perfuse areas in between.

Posterior Inferior Cerebellar Artery Syndrome

The areas of the cerebellum supplied by the PICA are variable. There are several different patterns of PICA territory cerebellar infarctions. Typical clinical findings are detailed in Table 22–2. If the medial branch territory is affected, involving the vermis and vestibulocerebellum, the clinical findings include prominent vertigo, ataxia, and nystagmus. If the lateral cerebellar hemisphere is involved, patients can have vertigo, gait ataxia, limb dysmetria and ataxia, nausea, vomiting, conjugate or dysconjugate gaze palsies, miosis, and dysarthria. If the infarction is large, there may be altered consciousness or confusion. Hydrocephalus or herniation may develop. There is also a syndrome of combined dorsolateral medullary and cerebellar infarction that may be due to a vertebral artery occlusion or a medial PICA occlusion.[46] While a PICA occlusion can be the cause of Wallenberg's (lateral medullary) syndrome, this syndrome is more often due to an intracranial vertebral artery occlusion (Fig. 22–9).[47]

Anterior Inferior Cerebellar Artery Syndrome

The AICA syndrome causes a ventral cerebellar infarction that has a characteristic clinical picture[48, 49] (see Table 22–2). The signs and symptoms that are seen include vertigo, nausea, vomiting, and nystagmus due to involvement of the vestibular nuclei. There may be ipsilateral facial hypalgesia

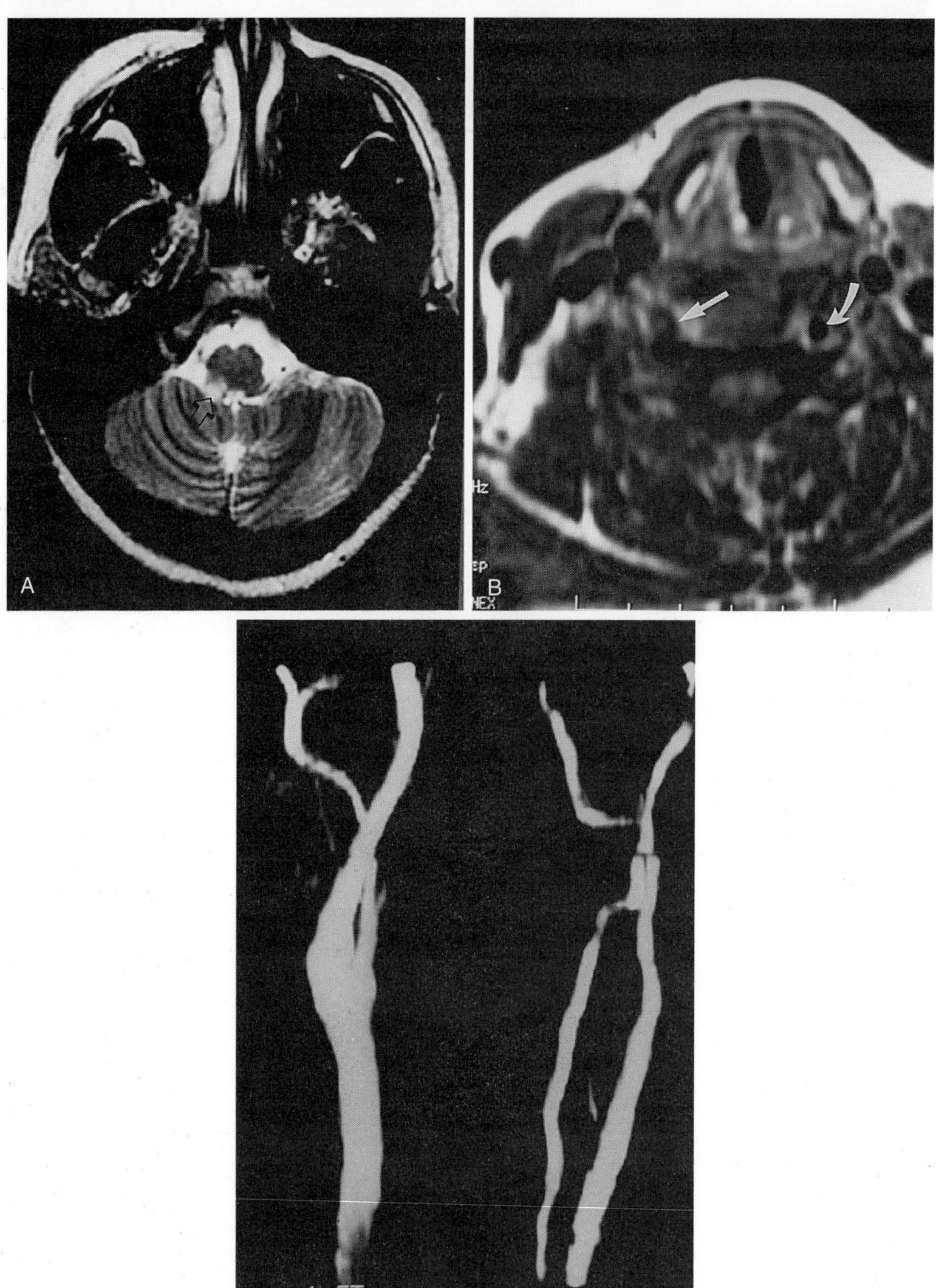

FIGURE 22–9. Forty-seven-year-old man involved in motor vehicle accident presenting with lateral medullary syndrome due to a vertebral artery dissection. *A,* T2-weighted image shows hyperintensity in the right posterior lateral medulla (*arrow*). *B,* Axial T1-weighted image shows lack of flow void in the right vertebral artery (*straight arrow*). Notice the normal flow void in the left vertebral artery (*curved arrow*). *C,* Time of flight magnetic resonance arteriogram shows no flow in the right vertebral artery. (Courtesy of Karen S. Caldemeyer, M.D.)

and thermoanesthesia and corneal hypesthesia due to involvement of the trigeminal spinal nucleus and tract. There is ipsilateral deafness and facial paralysis due to involvement of the lateral pontomedullary tegmentum. Ipsilateral Horner's syndrome is present due to compromise of the descending oculosympathetic fibers. There is contralateral trunk and extremity hypalgesia and thermoanesthesia due to involvement of the lateral spinothalamic tract.

Finally, there is ipsilateral ataxia and asynergia due to involvement of the cerebellar peduncle and cerebellum.

Superior Cerebellary Artery Syndrome

Infarction in the territory of the SCA produces a dorsal cerebellar syndrome that may also involve the lateral superior pons[50] (see Table 22–2). Vertigo may be present, although it is less common with SCA infarcts than with the other cerebellar syndromes. Nystagmus is present due to involvement of the medial longitudinal fasciculus and the cerebellar pathways. Ipsilateral Horner's syndrome is seen due to involvement of the descending sympathetic tract. Ipsilateral ataxia and asynergia and gait ataxia are noted due to involvement of the superior cerebellar peduncle, brachium pontis, the superior cerebellar hemisphere, and the dentate nucleus. There is an intention tremor due to involvement of the dentate nucleus and superior cerebellar peduncle. Choreiform dyskinesias may be present ipsilaterally. Contralaterally, there is hearing loss due to lateral lemniscus disruption and trunk and extremity hypalgesia and thermoanesthesia due to spinothalamic tract involvement. A contralateral fourth nerve palsy may be present due to involvement of the midbrain tectum. The diagnostic findings are detailed in Table 22–3.

Midline Basilar Artery Syndromes: Midbrain

It should be emphasized that there is great variability in the arterial blood supply to the brain stem. The syndromes that are described may be oversimplified, and several variations are possible.

Weber's Syndrome. Weber's syndrome (ventral cranial nerve III fascicular syndrome) is due to infarction in the distribution of the penetrating branches of the PCA affecting the cerebral peduncle, especially medially with damage to the fascicle of CN III and the pyramidal fibers. The resultant clinical findings are contralateral hemiplegia of the face, arm, and leg due to corticospinal and corticobulbar tract involvement and ipsilateral oculomotor paresis, including a dilated pupil. A slight variation of this syndrome is the midbrain syndrome of Foville, in which the supranuclear fibers for horizontal gaze are interrupted in the medial peduncle, causing a conjugate gaze palsy to the opposite side.

Benedikt's Syndrome. Benedikt's syndrome is caused by a lesion affecting the mesencephalic tegmentum in its ventral portion, with involvement of the red nucleus, brachium conjunctivum, and the fascicle of CN III. This syndrome is due to infarction in the distribution of the penetrating branches of the PCA to the midbrain. The clinical manifestations are ipsilateral oculomotor paresis, usually with pupillary dilation and contralateral involuntary movements, including intention tremor, hemiathetosis, and hemichorea.

Claude's Syndrome. Claude's syndrome is caused by lesions that are more dorsally placed in the midbrain tegmentum than with Benedikt's syndrome. There is injury to the dorsal red nucleus that results in more prominent cerebellar signs without the involuntary movements. There is oculomotor paresis.

Nothnagel's Syndrome. Nothnagel's syndrome is characterized by an ipsilateral oculomotor palsy with contralateral cerebellar ataxia. Infarctions in the distribution of the penetrating branches of the PCA to the midbrain are the cause of this syndrome.

Parinaud's Syndrome. Parinaud's (dorsal rostral midbrain) syndrome can result from infarctions in the midbrain territory of the PCA penetrating branches. This syndrome is characterized by supranuclear paralysis of eye elevation, defective convergence, convergence-retraction nystagmus, light-near dissociation, lid retraction (Collier's sign), and skew deviation.

Top of the Basilar Syndrome. Top of the basilar syndrome is due to infarction of the midbrain, thalamus, and portions of the temporal and occipital lobes.[51, 52] It is due to occlusive vascular disease, often embolic in nature, of the rostral basilar artery. The signs that may be present include the following:

1. Behavioral abnormalities, including somnolence, peduncular hallucinosis (see Chapter 8), memory disturbances, and agitated delirium.
2. Ocular findings, including unilateral or bilateral paralysis of upward or downward gaze, disordered convergence, pseudoabducens palsy, convergence-retraction nystagmus, abnormalities of abduction, Collier's sign (elevation and retraction of the upper eyelids), skew deviation, and oscillatory eye movements. Visual defects that may be present include hemianopia, cortical blindness, and Balint's syndrome (see Chapter 8).
3. Pupillary abnormalities, including small and reactive pupils, large or midposition and fixed pupils, corectopia, and occasionally oval pupils.
4. Motor and sensory deficits.

Midline Vertebrobasilar Syndromes: Pons

While there are many named pontine syndromes, the most beneficial categorization is based on neuroanatomical divisions.

Locked-in Syndrome. Locked-in syndrome (de-efferented state) is the result of bilateral ventral pontine lesions that produce quadriplegia, aphonia, and impairment of the horizontal eye movements in some patients. Wakefulness is maintained due to sparing of the reticular formation. Patients can move their eyes vertically and can blink because the supranuclear ocular motor pathways lie more dorsally (see Chapter 1). In some patients, there is a "herald" hemiparesis that makes the lesion appear to be cortical in nature. However, within a few hours, there is progression to bilateral hemiplegia and CN findings associated with the locked-in syndrome.[53]

Medial Inferior Pontine Syndrome. This syndrome is due to occlusion of a paramedian branch of the basilar artery. There is ipsilateral paralysis of conjugate gaze to the side of the lesion, abducens palsy, nystagmus, and ataxia. Contralateral to the lesion, there is hemibody impairment of tactile and proprioceptive sensation and paralysis of the face, arm, and leg.

Medial Midpontine Syndrome. Medial midpontine syndrome is due to ischemia of the medial midpontine region from occlusion of the paramedian branch of the midbasilar artery. It can lead to ipsilateral limb ataxia. Contralateral to the lesion, there is eye deviation and paralysis of the face, arm, and leg. While there are predominant motor symptoms, there can be variable impaired touch and proprioception.

Lateral and Combined Vertebrobasilar Syndromes

Lateral Midpontine Syndrome. Occlusion of the paramedian branch of the midbasilar artery can lead to ipsilateral impaired sensory and motor function of the trigeminal nerve with limb ataxia.

Total Unilateral Inferior Pontine Syndrome. An occlusion of the AICA can lead in some circumstances to a combination of the symptoms and signs seen with the lateral and medial pontine syndromes.

Lateral Pontomedullary Syndrome. This syndrome can be seen with occlusion of the vertebral artery. The manifestations seen are a combination of the medial and lateral inferior pontine syndromes.

Lateral Medullary Syndrome (Wallenberg's Syndrome). The lateral medullary syndrome is most often due to occlusion of the vertebral artery. Less commonly, it is due to occlusion of the PICA. This syndrome produces an ipsilateral Horner syndrome; loss of pain and temperature sensation of the face; weakness of the palate, pharynx, and vocal cords; and cerebellar ataxia. Contralateral to the lesion, there is hemibody loss of pain and temperature sensation.

Total Unilateral Medullary Syndrome. Occlusion of the vertebral artery can lead to a combination of medial and lateral medullary syndromes.

Midline Vertebrobasilar Syndrome: Medulla

Medial Medullary Syndrome. This syndrome is less common than the lateral medullary syndrome. It may be due to occlusion of the vertebral artery, a branch of the vertebral artery, or the lower basilar artery. The findings with this syndrome include an ipsilateral lower motor neuron paralysis of the tongue and contralateral paralysis of the arm and leg. In addition, there is contralateral hemibody loss of tactile, vibratory, and position sense.

Thalamic Infarction

The main arterial supply to the thalamus arises from the PCoAs and the perimesencephalic segment of the PCA. Localization of the arterial territory responsible for a thalamic infarction often can be determined from clinical findings. Thalamic infarctions typically involve one of the four major vascular regions: posterolateral, anterior, paramedian, and dorsal.

Posterolateral thalamic infarctions result from occlusion of the thalamogeniculate branches arising from the P2 segment of the PCA. Three common clinical syndromes may occur: pure sensory stroke, sensorimotor stroke, and the thalamic syndrome of Dejerine-Roussy. Findings in Dejerine-Roussy syndrome contralateral to the involved thalamus may include hemianesthesia, transient slight hemiparesis, hemiataxia, choreoathetoid movements, athetoid posture, paroxysmal pain, and homonymous hemianopia (often due to simultaneous medial occipital infarction).

Anterior thalamic infarction results from occlusion of the polar or tuberothalamic artery. Findings may include predominant neurobehavorial disturbances such as abulia, apathy, disorientation, lack of insight, and personality changes. There may also be facial paresis for emotional movement, contralateral hemiparesis and visual field defects, dysphagia with left-sided lesions, and hemineglect and impaired visuospatial processing with right-sided lesions.

Infarctions in the territory of the paramedian artery may also involve the paramedian region of the midbrain. Occlusion of the top of the basilar artery can cause this syndrome. Findings may include transient loss of consciousness or somnolence, behavioral changes, recent memory loss with anterograde and retrograde components, disorders of vertical gaze and convergence, contralateral hemiataxia, asterixis or motor weakness, and delayed action tremor in the contralateral limbs.

Dorsal thalamic infarction results from occlusion of the posterior choroidal arteries. These infarctions are characterized by the presence of homonymous hemianopia or homonymous horizontal sectoranopia. There may also be an asymmetrical optokinetic response and hemibody (face and arm) hypesthesia. Involvement of the pulvinar may account for thalamic aphasia.

Posterior Cerebral Artery Syndrome

The signs and symptoms seen with PCA territory infarctions are variable, depending on the site of the occlusion and the availability of collateral blood flow. Unilateral infarctions in the distribution of the hemispheral branches of the PCA may produce a contralateral homonymous hemianopia. This is due to infarction of the striate cortex, the optic radiations, or the lateral geniculate body. There is partial or complete macular sparing if the infarction does not reach the occipital pole. The visual field defect may be limited to a quadrantanopia. A superior quadrantanopia is caused by infarction of the striate cortex inferior to the calcarine fissure or the inferior optic radiations in the temporo-occipital lobes. An inferior quadrantanopia is the result of an infarction of the striate cortex superior to the calcarine fissure or the superior optic radiations in the parieto-occipital lobes (see Chapter 8).

There may be more complex visual changes, including formed or unformed visual hallucinations ("release hallucinations"), visual and color agnosias, and prosopagnosia (agnosia for familiar faces).[54] Finally, there can be some alteration of sensation with PCA hemispheral infarctions, including paresthesias and altered position, pain, and temperature sensations.

Infarction in the distribution of the callosal branches of the PCA involving the left occipital region and the splenium of the corpus callosum produces alexia without agraphia.[55] In this syndrome, patients can write, speak, and spell normally. However, they are unable to read words and sentences. Naming of letters and numbers may be intact. However, there can be inability to name colors, objects, and photographs.[56] Right hemispheric PCA territory infarctions may cause contralateral visual field neglect. Amnesia may be present with PCA infarctions that involve the left medial temporal lobe or when there are bilateral mesiotemporal infarctions. In addition, an agitated delirium may occur with bilateral penetrating mesiotemporal infarctions. Large infarctions of the left posterior temporal artery territory may produce an anomic or transcortical sensory aphasia (see Chapter 6).[57]

Infarctions in the distribution of the penetrating branches of the PCA to the thalamus can cause aphasia if the left pulvinar is involved, akinetic mutism, global amnesia, and/or Dejerine-Roussy syndrome. In the latter syndrome, the patient has contralateral sensory loss to all modalities, severe dysesthesias on the involved side (thalamic pain), vasomotor disturbances, transient contralateral hemiparesis, and choreoathetoid or ballistic movements. There are also a number of syndromes that can result from infarctions in the distribution of the penetrating branches of the PCA to the midbrain that were previously discussed with the midbrain syndromes. Bilateral infarctions in the distribution of the hemispheric branches of the PCAs may cause bilateral homonymous hemianopia. With bilateral occipital or occipitoparietal infarctions, one can have cortical blindness, often with denial or unawareness of blindness (Anton's syndrome). Another syndrome—Balint's syndrome—may be seen with bilateral occipital or parieto-occipital infarctions. The characteristics of this syndrome include optic ataxia, psychic paralysis of fixation with inability to look to the peripheral field, and disturbance of visual attention.

Transient Global Amnesia Syndrome

Transient global amnesia (TGA) is an episode of total amnesia that lasts little more than 24 hours. Patients classically ask many questions repeatedly. During the episode, there are no visual, motor, sensory, or brain stem abnormalities. After the episode, the individual has no recall for the events during the period of TGA, but there are no other cognitive residuals. The mechanism of TGA is not known. Theories advanced suggest either medial temporal lobe seizure activity or a vascular phenomenon, such as PCA territory ischemia involving the medial temporal lobes bilaterally. There seems to be an association with strenuous exertion, sexual intercourse, and emotional stress.[58]

SPINAL CORD STROKE SYNDROMES

Anterior Spinal Artery Syndrome

The anterior spinal artery syndrome is characterized by an abrupt onset of flaccid paraplegia or tetraplegia below the level of the lesion due to bilateral corticospinal tract damage. There is thermoanesthesia and analgesia below the level of the lesion due to compromise of the spinothalamic tracts bilaterally. Position, vibration, and light touch are spared due to preservation of the dorsal columns, which are supplied by the posterior spinal arteries. Bowel and bladder function is impaired. There may be associated radicular or "girdle" pain.

These infarctions most commonly occur in the "watershed" areas or boundary zones where the distal branches of the major arterial systems of the cord anastomose, between the T1 and T4 segments and at the L1 segment. Common etiologies of arterial spinal cord infarction are detailed in Table 22–3.

Posterior Spinal Artery Syndrome

The posterior spinal artery syndrome is uncommon, probably due to the presence of numerous posterior radicular arteries and the reversal of flow that is possible at the conus medullaris if there is compromise of the artery of Adamkiewicz. The characteristics of this syndrome are loss of proprioception and vibration sense below the level of the lesion and loss of segmental reflexes. The common etiologies are listed in Table 22–3.

SUBARACHNOID HEMORRHAGE SYNDROME

Aneurysmal subarachnoid hemorrhage (SAH) syndrome accounts for 6 to 8 percent of all strokes, affecting approximately 28,000 individuals each year in the United States. The most common cause of spontaneous SAH is a ruptured intracranial saccular aneurysm (Fig. 22–10). In addition, SAH may be due to many other causes that are outlined in Tables 22–3 and 22–4.

The clinical presentation of SAH is usually an abrupt onset of a severe headache, photophobia, nausea, vomiting,

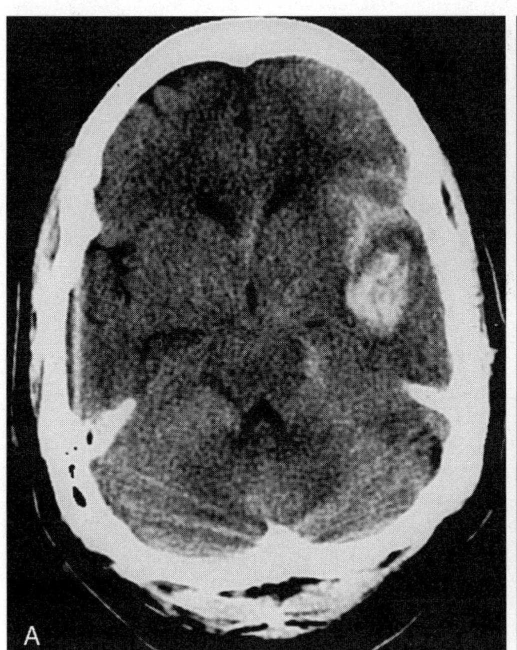

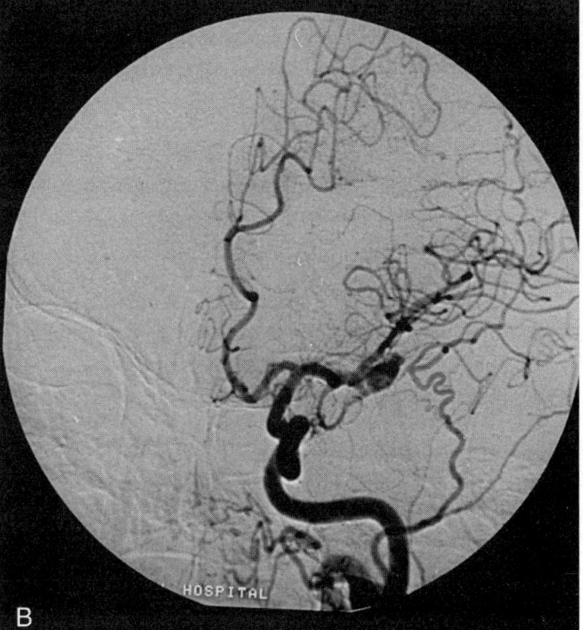

FIGURE 22–10. *A,* Nonenhanced axial CT shows subarachnoid hemorrhage in the left sylvian fissure and adjacent intraparenchymal hemorrhage in the temporal lobe. *B,* AP left common carotid arteriogram shows a lobulated left middle cerebral artery trifurcation aneurysm. (Courtesy of Karen S. Caldemeyer, M.D.)

meningismus and, often, unconsciousness and other neurological deficits (see Table 22–2). In some instances, a premonitory headache, representing a sentinel bleed, may occur days to weeks before the presenting hemorrhage. Misdiagnosis of SAH occurs in up to 25 percent of cases.[59] A ruptured aneurysm should be suspected in patients complaining of "sudden onset of the worst headache of my life," later onset of migraine headache with no family history of migraine, a change in the headache pattern in a known migraineur, severe localized and persistent headache, and severe "vascular" headaches that are refractory to conventional therapy.

Neurological signs are detailed in Table 22–2. Meningismus with nuchal rigidity and Kernig's sign is present in two thirds of patients. A dilated ophthalmologic examination may show papilledema or hemorrhages (see Table 22–2). Ptosis or diplopia due to oculomotor nerve palsy can be seen with internal carotid–posterior communicating artery aneurysms, distal basilar aneurysm, or uncal herniation. Other neurological findings depend on the location of the aneurysm.

Clinical deterioration after SAH may be due to multiple causes, including seizures, electrolyte disturbances such as hyponatremia, cerebral vasospasm, rebleeding, hydrocephalus, and development of medical complications such as pneumonia, hypotension, electrolyte abnormalities, and cardiac arrhythmias. Diagnosis and treatment of these disorders are detailed in Part 3.

SYNDROMES OF EXTRACRANIAL HEMATOMAS

Subdural Hematoma

Subdural hematomas can be acute, subacute, or chronic. Acute subdural hematomas occur within 24 to 48 hours after an injury. They can be secondary to arterial or venous bleeding into the subdural space. The usual cause is a blow to the head by falling or being struck. The neurological symptoms depend on the area of the brain involved. There can be rapidly evolving focal signs that produce aphasia, memory disturbances, hemiparesis and hemisensory deficits, and altered consciousness. Signs of increased intracranial pressure may be present. Diagnosis is made by CT scan. Chronic subdural hematomas present at weeks to months after the injury. Patients presenting with this type of hematoma include the elderly with cerebral atrophy, patients with epilepsy, patients with alcohol dependence, and persons with coagulation defects. These hematomas may become quite large without producing symptoms. The neurological findings may vary from no or minimal deficit, to focal neurological symptoms that may be transient or progressive. In some, there may be florid symptoms of increased intracranial pressure with headaches, nausea, vomiting, and papilledema. There may be accompanying seizures. Diagnosis of a chronic subdural hematoma may require a CT scan without and with contrast due to the possibility of isodensity of the hematoma with the surrounding brain at some point in its evolution (see Chapter 23).

Epidural Hematoma

The most important type of epidural hematoma to be acquainted with is the acute epidural hematoma usually due to arterial bleeding from damage to the middle meningeal artery. Patients with this condition may have a history of trauma with a lucid interval followed by rapid development of focal neurological signs and deterioration in consciousness. The deterioration is due to high-pressure arterial bleeding with increased intracranial pressure. Like subdural hematomas, epidural hematomas can present subacutely or chronically, with the same time frame and similar symptoms. A CT scan classically shows a lens-shaped density that does not follow sulcal margins (Fig. 22–11). Skull x-rays may show an associated skull fracture. Prompt diagnosis is important

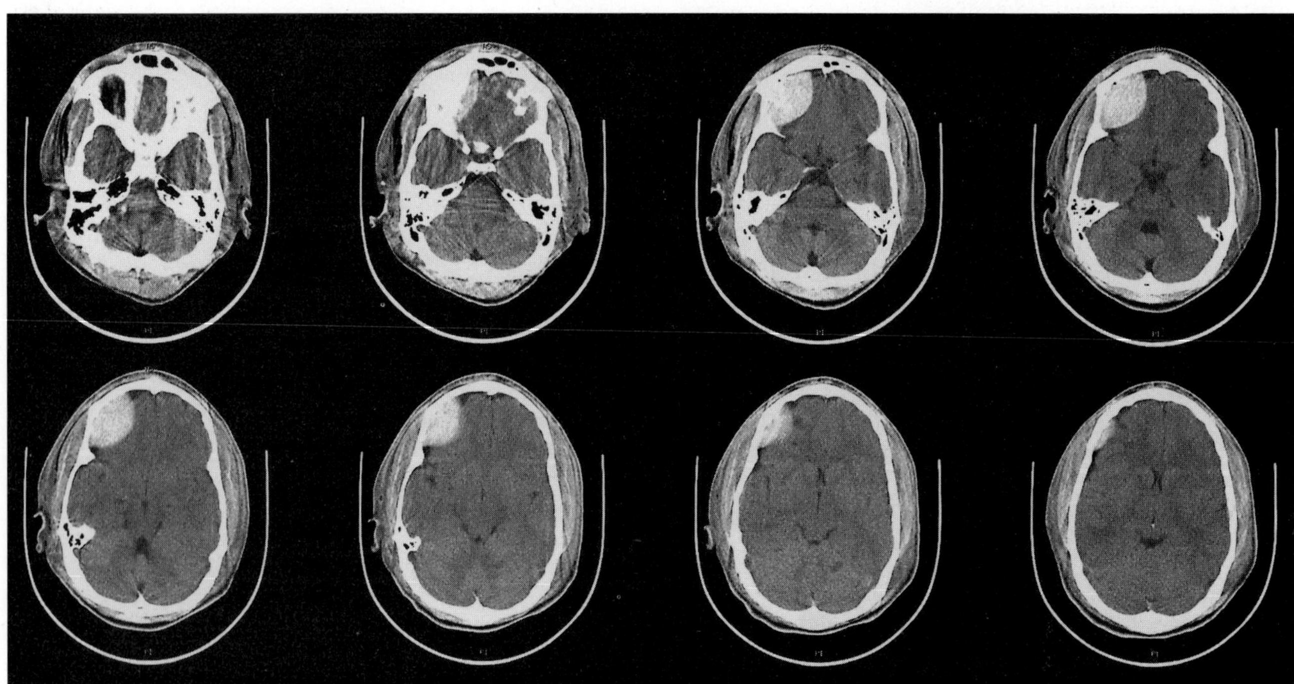

FIGURE 22–11. Nonenhanced axial CT shows a lens-shaped frontal density consistent with an acute epidural hematoma.

because a craniotomy with evacuation of the clot is often needed.

INTRACRANIAL STEAL SYNDROMES

In some patients with AVMs that are large and are fed by both deep and superficial vessels, there has been some anecdotal clinical support for intracerebral steal. The theory is that the presence of low-resistance shunt vessels compromises blood and nutrient flow to adjacent areas of the brain supplied by the same blood vessels, causing transient or permanent damage to neurons.[60] The clinical reports, although limited in number, report that these patients with AVMs have a variety of focal neurological deficits, cognitive deficits, visual deficits, and seizures that recover after the AVM is excised. In most patients, the neurological deficits are confined to the area of the brain supplied by the AVM. However, there have been reports of electroencephalogram abnormalities in the hemisphere contralateral to the AVM and lower cerebral blood flow in the contralateral hemisphere that may support relative areas of ischemia.[61] More documentation of this syndrome in large numbers of patients is needed.

VASCULAR DISSECTION SYNDROMES

Dissections of arteries develop when there is blood extravasated within the medial or subintimal layers of the arterial wall with resultant compromise of the arterial lumen and development of a pseudoaneurysm. Vascular dissections can be associated with blunt trauma, penetrating trauma, or even trivial trauma. There are a number of associated conditions, including fibromuscular dysplasia, Marfan's syndrome, Ehlers-Danlos type IV syndrome, atherosclerosis, pronounced vessel tortuosity, moyamoya, cystic medial degeneration, pharyngeal infections, alpha$_1$-antitrypsin deficiency, and luetic arteritis. However, dissections may occur spontaneously. Cervicocephalic arterial dissections may present with ischemic stroke due to arterial occlusion or secondary embolization. The vessel that is most commonly involved is the extracranial carotid artery between C2 and the base of the skull. The vertebrobasilar system, intracranial carotid, and middle cerebral arteries are less frequently involved.[62] The patients may present with symptoms of transient retinal ischemia, hemispheric or posterior fossa ischemia, cerebral infarction, or subarachnoid hemorrhage. Pain along the forehead, eye, face, or neck may be present with carotid dissections. Vertebral dissections can cause pain in the occiput and neck. Other associated symptoms may include Horner's syndrome, audible bruits, and pulsatile tinnitus. Other cranial nerves that may be involved include CN II, III, V, VII, VIII, IX, X, XI, and XII.[63] Diagnosis requires a high level of clinical suspicion that is confirmed with typical arteriographic signs (see Chapters 45 and 50).

CAROTID-CAVERNOUS FISTULA

A carotid-cavernous fistula is an abnormal communication between the carotid artery and the veins of the cavernous sinus, creating a high-pressure, high-flow system. There is often a history of trauma. Patients may present with an audible bruit and progressive pulsatile proptosis with chemosis, restricted eye movement, and progressive visual loss in late stages (see Table 22–2). The diagnosis is made by cerebral angiography, but a CT scan with contrast, MRI, or magnetic resonance angiography may show the lesion (see Table 22–3 and Chapter 23).

CEREBRAL VENOUS THROMBOSIS

Intracranial venous occlusive disease is significantly less common than arterial disease. The symptoms can be nonspecific. The symptoms that are present depend upon the venous structure that is affected, the extent and rapidity of thrombosis, and the extent of venous collaterals. Common symptoms include headache, nausea, vomiting, altered consciousness, and seizures. Examination may show papilledema, meningismus, and subtle focal neurological deficits (see Table 22–2). Possible findings on CT and MRI are presented in Table 22–3. Diagnosis may be made with magnetic resonance venography or conventional or digital intravenous angiography (Fig. 22–12).

SYNDROMES OF INTRACEREBRAL HEMORRHAGE

There are general features of the clinical syndrome of intracerebral hemorrhage that may help to characterize it. Historical features include a presentation that is maximum at the onset in one third of patients and gradual with smooth progression over 30 minutes in two thirds of patients. Interestingly, most hemorrhages occur during activity rather than during sleep.[64, 65]

A headache is present in approximately one half of patients. Nausea and vomiting are present in over 50 percent of patients. The level of consciousness may be variable. Seizures rarely occur at the onset. There is usually no history of any prodromal attacks. There is often a history of arterial hypertension. On examination, meningeal irritation can be seen if the bleeding extends to the subarachnoid space. Retinal hemorrhages may be present on funduscopic examination (see Table 22–2). There are a number of potential etiologies of intracerebral hemorrhage (see Table 22–3).

The various forms of intracerebral hemorrhage have distinctive clinical presentations that are dependent on the location, size, direction of spread, and the rate of development of the bleeding[64] (see Table 22–2). The results of testing are detailed in Table 22–3.

Putaminal Hemorrhage

A putaminal hemorrhage is the most common form of intracranial hemorrhage because the putamen is the most common site involved with hypertensive intracranial hemorrhage. Hemorrhages in this location may be confined to the putamen, or they may enlarge to involve the internal capsule, corona radiata, centrum semiovale, temporal lobe, or intraventricular system. The classic presentation with putaminal hemorrhages that are large involves rapidly progressing contralateral hemiparesis or hemiplegia with less severe contralateral hemisensory loss.[66] Rarely, with a small hematoma, there can be a pure motor hemiparesis.[67] There is a conjugate horizontal gaze palsy, with the eyes conjugately deviated toward the side of the hematoma. Homonymous hemianopia is present. A dominant hemisphere putaminal hemorrhage produces associated global aphasia, while a nondominant lesion results in hemi-inattention with apractagnosia, left

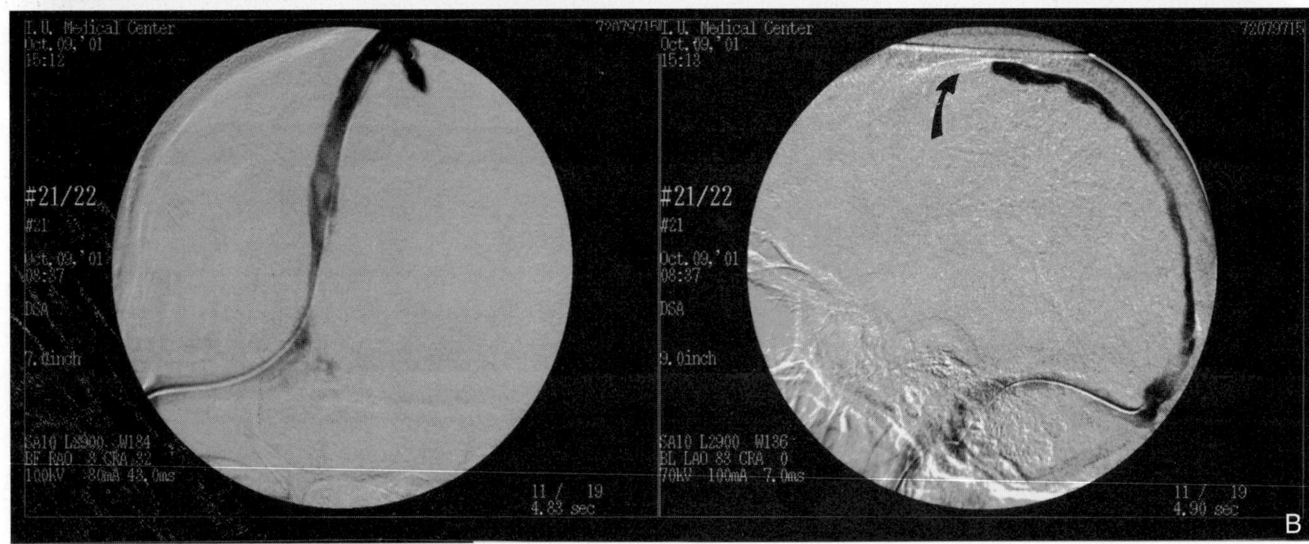

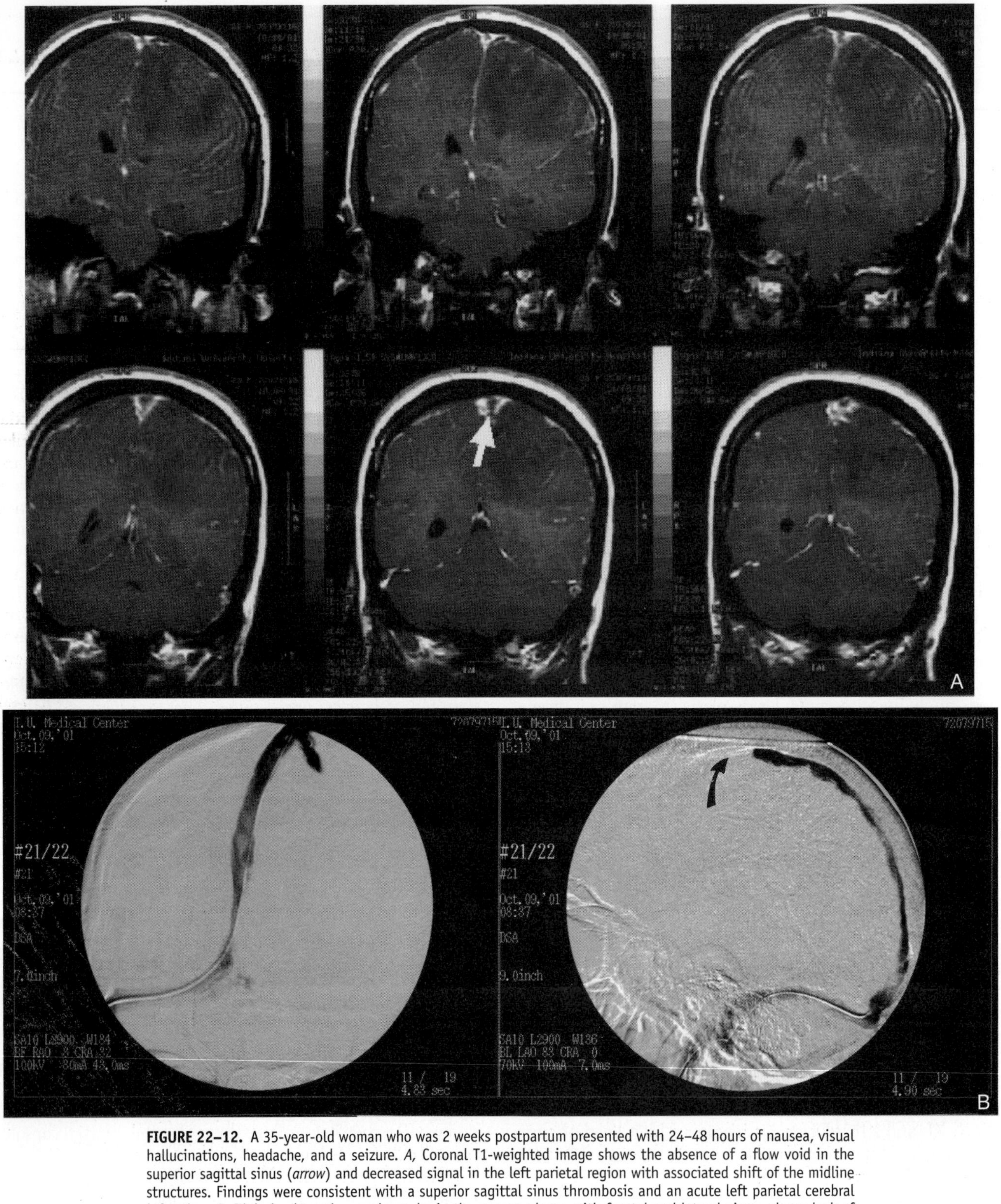

FIGURE 22–12. A 35-year-old woman who was 2 weeks postpartum presented with 24–48 hours of nausea, visual hallucinations, headache, and a seizure. *A,* Coronal T1-weighted image shows the absence of a flow void in the superior sagittal sinus (*arrow*) and decreased signal in the left parietal region with associated shift of the midline structures. Findings were consistent with a superior sagittal sinus thrombosis and an acute left parietal cerebral infarction. *B,* Digital subtraction angiography in the venous phase, with frontal and lateral views, shows lack of filling of the superior sagittal sinus consistent with superior sagittal sinus occlusion (*curved arrow*).

visual neglect, and constructional apraxia.[68] Occasionally, patients with a nondominant putaminal hemorrhage have allesthesia, in which a noxious stimulus on the side of the hemisensory disturbance is perceived on the opposite normal side in the corresponding area.[69] Pupillary size is normal unless there is associated uncal herniation.

Lobar Hemorrhage

This type of hemorrhage refers to bleeding occurring within the subcortical white matter. Underlying structural lesions are more common than arterial hypertension as a cause. The clinical presentation can resemble that of an embolic cerebral infarction. There are characteristic findings with hemorrhages in different locations.[70] With frontal lobe hemorrhages, characteristic findings are abulia, contralateral hemiparesis, and a conjugate gaze palsy toward the side of the hemorrhage. Parietal lobe hemorrhages may cause contralateral hemisensory loss, neglect of the contralateral visual field, mild hemiparesis, and occasionally a hemianopia or anosognosia. A temporal lobe hemorrhage may present with variable degrees of visual field deficit, or occasionally agitated delirium. With dominant temporal lobe hemorrhages, there can be a Wernicke aphasia. If there is an extension into the dominant parietal lobe, there can be conduction or global aphasia. A hemorrhage in the occipital lobe may cause a contralateral homonymous hemianopia and ipsilateral orbital pain.[70, 71]

Thalamic Hemorrhage

The usual cause of thalamic hemorrhages is hypertension. However, an underlying structural lesion such as a vascular malformation or tumor is another consideration. Thalamic hemorrhages may be confined to the thalamus or may extend laterally to involve the internal capsule, inferomedially to compress the subthalamus and midbrain, or medially to involve the third ventricle. Classic signs of a thalamic hemorrhage include a hemisensory deficit with a lesser degree of hemiparesis. Ocular findings may include convergence-retraction nystagmus, impairment of vertical gaze, pupillary light-near dissociation, downward-inward deviation of the eyes (depression-convergence syndrome), unilateral or bilateral pseudo–sixth nerve paresis, skew deviation and conjugate gaze palsy to the side of the lesion ("wrong-way eyes"), and a conjugate horizontal gaze palsy. If the hemorrhage is located in the posterior thalamus, there can be distinctive features.[72]

Pontine Hemorrhage

The signs and symptoms of pontine hematomas depend on size, location, and presence or absence of ventricular involvement or hydrocephalus. Primary pontine hematomas usually are symmetrically placed at the junction of the basis pontis and tegmentum. Large pontine hematomas cause coma, decerebrate rigidity, quadriparesis, centrally positioned eyes with absent oculocephalic and oculovestibular reflexes, and pinpoint reactive pupils. Ocular bobbing, characterized by rapid conjugate downward movements of the eyes followed by a slow upward drive to primary position, may be present. Hyperthermia and respiratory abnormalities may be present. Partial damage to the lateral basis pontis may cause pure motor hemiparesis. Lateral pontine tegmentum hemorrhage may cause ipsilateral conjugate gaze paresis, ipsilateral internuclear ophthalmoplegia, the "one-and-a-half" syndrome, and ocular bobbing (see Chapter 9). Lateral tegmental hemorrhages may cause ipsilateral hemiataxia with contralateral hemiparesis and hemisensory deficits.

Cerebellar Hemorrhage

The signs present with cerebellar hematomas depend on their location and size and whether there is associated brain stem compression or hydrocephalus. The most common location for a cerebellar hemorrhage is in the region of the dentate nucleus. The vermis is less frequently involved. The most frequently observed findings are truncal or limb ataxia, ipsilateral gaze palsy, and small reactive pupils. Other ocular findings may include skew deviation, gaze-paretic nystagmus, or ocular bobbing. Other cranial nerve findings may include ipsilateral peripheral facial weakness and ipsilateral absence of the corneal reflex. Dysarthria is often present.

TABLE 22–5. **Vascular Dementias**
Multi-infarct dementia
Strategically placed infarcts
Binswanger disease (subacute arteriosclerotic encephalopathy)
Cerebral amyloid angiopathies
CADASIL (cerebral autosomal dominant arteriopathy with subcortical infarcts and leukoencephalopathy)
Dementia linked to hypoperfusion
Neoplastic angioendotheliosis
Hemorrhagic lesions causing dementia
Subacute diencephalic angio-encephalopathy
Cortical micro-infarction (granular cortical atrophy)
Other (mixed-Alzheimer's disease-Vascular Dementia, etc.)

Caudate Hemorrhage

Caudate hemorrhages can cause headache, nausea, vomiting, meningismus, confusion, and decreased short-term memory.[73] Findings that are variably present include a transient contralateral conjugate gaze paresis, contralateral hemiparesis, transient hemisensory deficits and, rarely, ipsilateral Horner's syndrome.

Vascular Dementia Syndrome

Vascular dementia is the second most common cause of dementia in the United States and Western Europe, and the most frequent cause of dementia in Japan, Russia, and other Eastern countries. It is defined as a global decline in intellectual functioning, without a change in the level of consciousness, that is produced by cerebrovascular disease. A number of conditions are classified under the category of vascular dementia (Table 22–5). The pathological substrates that can produce vascular dementia are extensive. Any lesion in the brain rostral to the upper brain stem can potentially affect cognition. Cerebrovascular disease can affect cognition by destroying the neural components (cortical areas) of the networks or their connections (white matter and subcortical relay centers).[74] The size and location of the region affected by cerebrovascular disease is important in delineating the clinical manifestations. The diagnostic criteria for vascular dementia are listed in Table 22–6.[75]

General Management Goals

Rapid diagnosis of stroke and initiation of treatment are important to maximize recovery and to prevent recurrence of stroke (see Chapter 45). Patients with an acute stroke should be admitted to the hospital for emergency evaluation and treatment, preferably in a stroke unit or intensive care unit

TABLE 22-6. DSM-IV Diagnostic Criteria for Vascular Dementia

A. The development of multiple cognitive deficits manifested by both
   1. memory impairment (impaired ability to learn new information or to recall previously learned information)
   2. one (or more) of the following cognitive disturbances:
      a. aphasia
      b. apraxia
      c. agnosia
      d. disturbance in executive functioning
B. The cognitive deficits in criteria A1 and A2 each cause significant impairment in social or occupational functioning and represent a significant decline from a previous level of functioning
C. Focal neurological signs and symptoms
D. The deficits do not occur exclusively during the course of a delirium

where close medical and nursing observation is available. A multidisciplinary approach with referral to specialists with expertise in stroke is beneficial. Care should focus not only on the treatment of the stroke, but also on the prevention of complications.

Patients should be thoroughly investigated in an attempt to determine the likely etiology of the stroke. Appropriate therapy should be instituted to reduce the likelihood of a recurrent stroke. Choices for therapy that are available include fibrinolytic agents; antiplatelet therapies such as aspirin, clopidogrel, ticlopidine, or aspirin in combination with modified-release dipyridamole; anticoagulation with heparin acutely followed by warfarin (usually reserved for a cardiac etiology of stroke); and carotid endarterectomy (in appropriate situations). The choice of treatment needs to be made on a case-by-case basis and is influenced by a number of variables. The most important factors are the time interval from stroke, the severity of the neurological impairments, the results of the baseline brain imaging studies, and the cause of the stroke.[76]

In the patient with an intracranial hemorrhage, hemostatic defects should be sought and corrected, if present. Offending drugs such as warfarin, heparin, and thrombolytic therapy should be stopped and, in appropriate situations when there is an antidote, reversed immediately. Neurosurgical consultation and intervention may be indicated in patients with large cerebellar infarctions; large, nondominant hemispheric ischemic infarctions with deterioration and herniation; and in selected patients with accessible, large lobar hemorrhages, when there is a progressive course. Patients with cerebellar hemorrhages should have an immediate neurosurgical consultation. Further guidelines for specific therapy are detailed in Part 3 (see Chapter 45).

Frequent neurological checks are vital to early recognition of neurological changes associated with herniation, recurrent or progressive stroke, recurrent hemorrhage or vasospasm in the patient with subarachnoid hemorrhage, and seizures. Cerebral edema with resultant herniation is the leading cause of death in the first week after an ischemic or hemorrhagic stroke.[77] Cerebral edema caused by ischemia overlaps both cytotoxic and vasogenic forms.

In patients with stroke, the blood pressure should be monitored frequently or even continuously for the first 48 to 72 hours. It is not unusual for the blood pressure to be transiently elevated after a stroke. Within a few days, the blood pressure may return to prestroke levels. Whether transient elevations should be treated is controversial.[78, 79] It is important not to overtreat the blood pressure and cause hypotension. The most important objective is to maintain adequate cerebral blood flow in the presence of impaired autoregulation.

Cardiac monitoring is recommended for the first 24 to 48 hours after stroke due to the high frequency of cardiac dysfunction associated with stroke. In approximately 3 percent of cases, concomitant cerebral and myocardial ischemia can occur. A variety of cardiac arrhythmias can occur after ischemic or hemorrhagic stroke and subarachnoid hemorrhage (SAH), including tall P waves, longer or shorter PR and QT intervals, ST-segment elevation or depression, peaked or inverted T waves, U waves, sinus bradycardia, wandering atrial pacemaker, paroxysmal atrial pacemaker, nodal bradycardia, AV block, premature atrial or ventricular contractions, atrial fibrillation and flutter, and AV dissociation. These abnormalities have generally been attributed to increased circulating levels of catecholamines. If ischemic electrocardiographic changes occur, serial creatine kinase and lactate dehydrogenase isoenzymes are indicated. Ventricular wall motion abnormalities have been demonstrated by echocardiography in patients with aneurysmal SAH. Patients with SAH often have microscopic changes consistent with subendocardial necrosis at post mortem.

Prevention of pulmonary complications is necessary in the bedridden patient or in the patient with impaired oropharyngeal function. Management of the airway and maintenance of adequate oxygenation and ventilation should be accomplished immediately. Ventilatory assistance is indicated if there are signs of respiratory depression, a Glasgow Coma Scale of less than or equal to 8, or raised intracranial pressure and herniation. Pneumonia is the most common cause of non-neurological death in the first 2 to 4 weeks after a stroke.[80] The mortality rate from pneumonia is as high as 15 to 25 percent. It is important to place a temporary enteral feeding tube if there is evidence of oropharyngeal dysfunction to avoid aspiration. Good pulmonary toilet is needed, including chest physical therapy, frequent turning, and volumetrics.

Lower extremity deep venous thrombosis (DVT) in the hemiparetic limb is a common occurrence if DVT prophylaxis is not initiated. If there are no contraindications, low-dose subcutaneous unfractionated heparin or low-molecular-weight heparin should be instituted. If heparin is contraindicated, as in the patient with intracranial hemorrhage, intermittent pneumatic compression stockings are recommended.

The patient's nutritional status and fluid requirements should be assessed. Patients with a large ischemic stroke may need fluid restriction during the first few days. In patients with intracranial hemorrhage, one should try to maintain euvolemia. In patients with SAH, strict fluid restrictions should be avoided due to the possible risk of increasing cerebral ischemia in patients developing vasospasm. The patient's swallowing function should be assessed before intake of fluid or food is initiated. Patients who have significant oropharyngeal dysfunction will require parenteral or tube feeding.

Indwelling catheters should be placed only if absolutely necessary and should be removed at the earliest possible time to avoid urosepsis. The chronic use of an indwelling catheter should be limited to patients with incontinence or urinary retention that is refractory to other treatments.

The development of pressure sores occurs in approximately 15 percent of patients after a stroke.[81] Steps to avoid this complication include frequent inspection of the skin, routine skin cleansing, frequent turning, use of special mattresses and protective dressings, maintaining adequate nutritional status, and trying to improve the patient's mobility as soon as possible after stroke.

One of the most common causes of injury to the patient with a stroke is falling. Assessments of the risk for falling should be made at regular intervals during the acute hospitalization. Measures should be instituted to minimize the risk of falls. Rehabilitation plays an important role in recovery in patients who are good candidates for intensive therapies.

Mortality is highest within the first 30 days after stroke and remains elevated to different degrees depending on the presenting stroke syndrome, stroke subtype, and other comorbidities.[82] The risk for recurrent stroke is greatest within the first 30 days. Only about half of those surviving a stroke are independent 6 months after a stroke, and the quality of life is decreased.[82]

Reviews and Selected Updates

Bassetti C, Bogousslavsky J, Mattle H: Medial medullary syndrome. Neurology 1997;48:882–890.

Biller J, Feinberg WM, Castaldo JE, et al: Guidelines for carotid endarterectomy: A statement for healthcare professionals from a Special Writing Group of the Stroke Council, American Heart Association. Circulation 1998; 97:501–509.

Chen J, Simon R: Ischemic tolerance in the brain. Neurology 1997;48:306.

Hornig CR, Bauer T, Carmen S, et al: Hemorrhagic transformation in cardioembolic cerebral infarction. Stroke 1993;24(3):465.

Shah MV, Biller J: Medical and surgical management of intracerebral hemorrhage. Semin Neurol 1998; 18:513–519.

Tatu L, Moulin T, Bogousslavsky J: Arterial territories of human brain. Neurology 1996;47:1125–1135.

References

1. Bell BA: Early study of cerebral circulation and measurement of cerebral blood flow. *In* Wood JH (ed): Cerebral Blood Flow. New York, McGraw-Hill, 1987, pp 3–16.
2. Fields WS, Lemak NA: A history of stroke: Its recognition and treatment. New York, Oxford University Press, 1989, pp 3–148.
3. Pessin MS, Duncan GW, Mohr JP, Poskanzer DC: Clinical and angiographic features of carotid transient ischemic attacks. N Engl J Med 1977;296(7):358–362.
4. Toole JF, et al: Transient ischemic attacks. A prospective study of 225 patients. Neurology 1978;28(8):746–753.
5. Millikan CH, McDowell FH: Treatment of progressive stroke. Prog Cerebrovasc Dis Stroke 1981;12(4):397–409.
6. Bogousslavsky J, Cachin C, Regli F, et al: Cardiac sources of embolism and cerebral infarction—clinical consequences and vascular concomitants: The Laussane Stroke Registry. Neurology (NY) 1991;41(6):855–859.
7. Foulkes MA, Wolf PA, Price TR, et al: The Stroke Data Bank: Design, methods, and baseline characteristics. Stroke 1988;19(5):547–554.
8. Kunitz SC, Gross DR, Heyman A, et al: The pilot stroke data bank: Definition, design, data. Stroke 1984;15(4):740–746.
9. Gorelick PB, Hier DB, Caplan LR, Langenberg P: Headache in acute cerebrovascular disease. Neurology 1986;36(11):1445–1450.
10. Osborn AG: Aortic arch and its branches. *In* Introduction to Cerebral Angiography. Philadelphia, Harper & Row, 1980, pp 35–45.
11. Krayenbuhl H, Yasargil M: Radiological anatomy and topography of the cerebral arteries. *In* Vinken P, Bruyn G (eds): Handbook of Clinical Neurology, Vol. 2. Amsterdam, North-Holland Publications, 1972, pp 65–84.
12. Osborn AG: The anterior choroidal artery. *In* Introduction to Cerebral Angiography. Philadelphia, Harper & Row, 1980, pp 74–82.
13. Berman SA, Hayman LA, Hinck VC: Correlation of CT cerebral vascular territories with function: I. Anterior cerebral artery. Am J Roentgenol 1980;135(2):253–257.
14. Ring BA: Middle cerebral artery: Anatomical and radiographic study. Acta Radiol 1982;57:289–293.
15. Alpers BJ, Berry RG, Paddison RM: Anatomical studies of the circle of Willis in normal brain. Arch Neurol Psychiatry 1959;81:409–417.
16. Saeki N, Rhoton AL Jr: Microsurgical anatomy of the upper basilar artery and the posterior circle of Willis. J Neurosurg 1977;46(5):563–578.
17. Shoenen J: Clinical anatomy of the spinal cord. Neurol Clin 1991;9(3):503–510.
18. Hughes JT: Vascular disorders. *In* Pathology of the Spinal Cord, 2nd ed. Philadelphia, WB Saunders, 1978, pp 61–90.
19. Barnett HJM: Delayed cerebral ischemic episodes distal to occlusion of major cerebral arteries. Neurology (NY) 1978;28:769–774.
20. Pardridge WM, Oldendorf WH, Cancilla P, Frank HJL: Blood-brain barrier: Interface between internal medicine and the brain. Ann Intern Med 1986;105:82–95.
21. Osborn, Anne G: Veins of the head and neck. *In* Introduction to Cerebral Angiography. Philadelphia, Harper & Row, 1980, pp 110–118.
22. Robinson RG, Parrikh MR, Lipsey JR, et al: Pathological laughing and crying following stroke: Validation of a measurement scale and a double blind treatment study. Am J Psychiatry 1993;150:286–290.
23. Howard R, Trend P, Russell RWR: Clinical features of cerebral arterial border zones after periods of reduced cerebral blood flow. Arch Neurol 1987;44:934–940.
24. Hennerici M, Klemm C, Rautenberg W: The subclavian steal phenomenon: A common vascular disorder with rare neurologic deficits. Neurology (NY) 1988;38:669–673.
25. Davis PH, Dambrosia JM, Schoeberg BS, et al: Risk factors for ischemic strokes: A prospective study in Rochester, Minnesota. Ann Neurol 1987;22:319–327.
26. Gautier JC: Clinical presentation and differential diagnosis of amaurosis fugax. *In* Bernstein EF (ed): Amaurosis Fugax. New York, Springer-Verlag, 1990, pp 74–78.
27. Marshall J, Meadows S: The natural history of amaurosis fugax. Brain 1968;91:419–434.
28. Fisher CM: Occlusion of the internal carotid artery. Arch Neurol Psychiatry 1951;69:346–355.
29. Pessin MS, Hinton RC, Davis KR, et al: Mechanisms of acute carotid stroke. Ann Neurol 1979;6:245–252.
30. Waddington MM, Ring AB: Syndromes of occlusions of middle cerebral artery branches. Angiographic and clinical correlation. Brain 1968;91:685–696.
31. Boller F: Strokes and behavior disorders of higher cortical functions following cerebral disease. Disorders of language and related function. Stroke 1981;12(4):532–534.
32. Mesulam MM, Waxman SG, Geschwind N, Sabin TD: Acute confusional states with right middle cerebral artery infarction. J Neurol Neurosurg Psychiatry 1976;39:84–89.
33. Mori E, Yamadori A: Acute confusional state and acute agitated delirum: Occurrence after infarction in the right middle cerebral artery territory. Arch Neurol 1987;44:1139–1143.
34. Bougousslavsky J, Regli F: Anterior cerebral artery territory infarction in the Lausanne Stroke Registry: Clinical and etiological patterns. Arch Neurol 1990;47:144–148.
35. Gacs G, Fox AJ, Barnett HJM, Viñuela F: Occurrence and mechanism of occlusion of the anterior cerebral artery. Stroke 1983;14: 952–959.
36. Kazui S, Sawada T, Kuriyama Y, et al: A clinical study of patients with cerebral infarction localized in the territory of the anterior cerebral artery. Jpn J Stroke 1987;9:317–319.
37. Critchley M: Anterior cerebral artery and its syndromes. Brain 1930;53:120–138.
38. Bruno A, Graff-Radford NR, Biller J, Adams HP: Anterior choroidal artery territory infarction: A small vessel disease. Stroke 1989;20:1591–1592.
39. Decroix JP, Graveleau P, Massan N, Cambier J: Infarction in the territory of the anterior choroidal artery: Clinical and computerized tomographic study of 16 cases. Brain 1986;109:1071–1085.
40. Helgason C, Caplan LR, Goodwin J, Hedges T: Anterior choroidal artery territory infarction: Report of cases and review. Arch Neurol 1986;43:681–686.

41. Bogousslavsky J, Miklossy J, Regli F, et al: Subcortical neglect: Neuropsychological, SPECT, and neuropathological correlation with anterior choroidal artery territory infarction. Ann Neurol 1988;23:448–452.
42. Helgason C, Wilbur A, Weiss A, et al: Acute pseudobulbar mutism due to discrete bilateral capsular infarction in the territory of the anterior choroidal artery. Brain 1988;111:507–524.
43. Kappelle LJ, van Gijn J: Lacunar infarcts. Clin Neurol Neurosurg 1986;88:3–17.
44. Chokroverty S, Rubino FA, Haller C: Pure motor hemiplegia due to pyramidal infarction. Arch Neurol 1965;13:30–32.
45. Helweg-Larsen S, Larsson H, Henrikson O, Sorenson PS: Ataxic hemiparesis: Three different locations studied by MRI. Neurology 1988;38:1322–1324.
46. Amerenco P, Hauw JJ, Henin D, et al: Les infarctus du territoire de l'artère cérébelleuse postéro-inférieure: Ètude clinico-pathologique de 28 cas. Rev Neurol 1989;145:277–279.
47. Fisher CM, Karnes W, Kubik C: Lateral medullary infarction: The pattern of vascular occlusion. J Neuropathol Exp Neurol 1961;20:323–333.
48. Adams R: Occlusion of the anterior inferior cerebellar artery. Arch Neurol 1943;49:765–774.
49. Syper AW, Alvord EC: Cerebellar infarction: A clinicopathological study. Arch Neurol 1975;32:357–359.
50. Kase CS, White JL, Joslyn JN, et al: Cerebellar infarction in the superior cerebellar artery distribution. Neurology 1985;35:705–711.
51. Caplan LR: Top of the basilar syndrome. Neurology 1980;30:72–79.
52. Mehler MF: The rostral basilar artery syndrome. Diagnosis, etiology, prognosis. Neurology 1989;39:9–16.
53. Fisher CM: "The herald hemiparesis" of basilar artery occlusion. Arch Neurol 1988;45:1301–1303.
54. Blust JCM, Behrens MM: "Release hallucinations" as the major symptom of posterior cerebral artery occlusion. A report of 2 cases. Ann Neurol 1977;2:432–436.
55. Damasio AR, Damasio H: The anatomic basis of pure alexia. Neurology 1983;33:1573–1583.
56. Derenzi E, Zambolin A, Crisi G: The pattern of neuropsychological impairment associated with left posterior cerebral artery territory. Brain 1987;110:1099–1116.
57. Kertesz A, Shepard A, MacKenzie R: Localization in transcortical sensory aphasia. Arch Neurol 1982;39:475–478.
58. Miller JW, Petersen RC, Metter EJ, et al: Transient global amnesia: Clinical characteristics and prognosis. Neurology 1987;37:733–737.
59. Kassell NF, Kongable GL, Torner JC, et al: Delay in referral of patients with ruptured aneurysms to neurosurgical attention. Stroke 1985;16:587–590.
60. Wade JPH, Hachinski V: Cerebral steal: Robbery or maldistribution. *In* Wood JH (ed): Cerebral Blood Flow: Physiologic and Clinical Aspects. New York, McGraw-Hill, 1987, pp 467–480.
61. Hachinski V, Norris JW, Cooper PW, Marshall J: Symptomatic intracranial steal. Arch Neurol 1977;34:149–153.
62. Biller J, Hintgen WL, Adams HP Jr, et al: Cervicocephalic arterial dissections: A ten-year experience. Arch Neurol 1986;43:1234–1238.
63. Mokri B, Silbert PL, Schievink WI, Piepgras DG: Cranial nerve palsy in spontaneous dissection of the extracranial internal carotid artery. Neurology 1996;46:356–359.
64. Fisher CM: Clinical syndromes in cerebral hemorrhage. *In* WS Fields (ed): Pathogenesis and Treatment of Cerebrovascular Disease. Springfield, IL, Charles C Thomas, 1961, pp 318–332.
65. Fisher CM: Pathological observations in hypertensive cerebral hemorrhage. J Neuropathol Exp Neurol 1971;30:536–550.
66. Hier DB, Davis KR, Richardson EP, Mohr JP: Hypertensive putaminal hemorrhage. Ann Neurol 1977;1:152–159.
67. Tapia JF, Kase CS, Sawyer RH, Mohr JP: Hypertensive putaminal hemorrhage presenting as pure motor hemiparesis. Stroke 1983;14:505–506.
68. Ojemann RG, Mohr JP: Hypertensive brain hemorrhage. Clin Neurosurg 1976;23:220–244.
69. Kawamura M, Hirayama K, Shinohara T, et al: Alloaesthesia. Brain 1987;110:225–236.
70. Ropper AH, Davis KR: Lobar cerebral hemorrhages. Acute clinical syndromes in 26 cases. Ann Neurol 1980;8:141–147.
71. Kase CS, Williams JP, Wyatt DA, Mohr JP: Lobar intracerebral hematomas: Clinical and CT analysis of 22 cases. Neurology 1982;32:1146–1150.
72. Hirose G, Kosoegawa H, Saeki M, et al: The syndrome of posterior thalamic hemorrhage. Neurology 1985;35:998–1002.
73. Stein RW, Kase CS, Hier DB, et al: Caudate hemorrhage. Neurology 1984;34:1549–1554.
74. Martinez-Lage P, Hacinski V: Multiple-infarct dementia. *In* Barnett HJM, Mohr JP, Stein BM, Yatsu FM (eds): Stroke Pathophysiology, Diagnosis and Management, 3rd ed. Philadelphia, Churchill Livingstone, 1998, pp 875–894.
75. American Psychiatric Association: Diagnostic and Statistical Manual of Mental Disorders, 4th ed. Washington, American Psychiatric Association, 1994.
76. Adams HP Jr: Treatment of acute ischemic stroke: selecting the right treatment for the right patient. Eur Neurol 2001;45:61–66.
77. Silver FL, Norris JW, Lewis AJ, Hachinski V: Early mortality following stroke: A prospective review. Stroke 1984;15:492–496.
78. Hayashi M, Kobayashi H, Kawano H, et al: Treatment of systemic hypertension and intracranial hypertension in cases of brain hemorrhage. Stroke 1988;19:314–321.
79. Adams HP Jr, Brott TG, Crowell RM, et al (eds): Guidelines for the management of patients with acute ischemic stroke. Stroke 1994;25:1901–1914.
80. Bounds JV, Wiebers DO, Whisnant JP, et al: Mechanisms and timing of deaths from cerebral infarction. Stroke 1981;12:474–477.
81. Roth EJ: Medical complications encountered in stroke rehabilitation. Phys Med Rehabil Clin North Am 1991;2(3):563–567.
82. Sacco RL, Wolf PA, Gorelick PB: Risk factors and their management for stroke prevention: Outlook for 1999 and beyond. Neurology 1999;53:S15–S24.

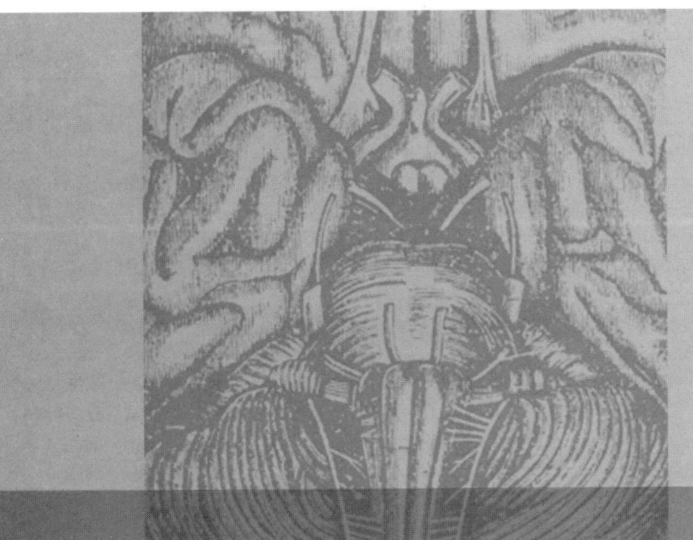

PART TWO

Neurodiagnostic Tools

CHAPTER 23

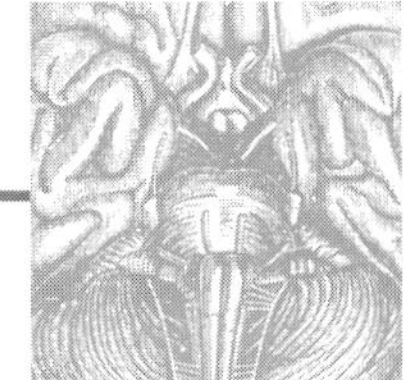

ROBERT A. KOENIGSBERG, SCOTT H. FARO, BEVERLY L. HERSHEY, TODD L. SIEGAL, FEROZE B. MOHAMED, CYRUS K. DASTUR, and FONG Y. TSAI

Neuroimaging

Imaging of the nervous system encompasses a wide variety of modalities that have undergone rapid evolution in the past few decades. Although still employed, plain film analysis of the skull and spine is not routine in the initial investigation of patients with neurological signs and symptoms. Computed tomography (CT), developed in the 1970s, remains a common radiographic technique, particularly for the acutely traumatized patient. Magnetic resonance imaging (MRI), which came into widespread clinical usage in the 1980s, has supplanted CT for evaluation of many suspected pathological processes of the brain and spine. Depending on availability, MRI is often the initial study ordered, particularly in an outpatient setting. MRI continues to be a rapidly evolving field, encompassing techniques such as magnetic resonance angiography (MRA) and spectroscopy. Myelography, introduced in the early 1900s, has been replaced to varying degrees by MRI, owing to the noninvasive nature of the latter. Myelography is still regarded as useful in visualizing the intradural nerve roots and is performed in selected cases, particularly when MRI is contraindicated. Throughout the century, myelography has evolved into a much safer examination, owing to development of contrast agents with dramatically reduced neurotoxicity. Angiography, introduced in 1927, remains the gold standard for evaluation of neurovascular disease. Interventional neuroradiology, also known as endovascular surgical neuroradiology, a field that has evolved in the past two decades, offers patients therapy through catheter-based angiographic techniques. Ultrasonography is most useful for evaluating the neonatal brain and spine and

TABLE 23–1. **Neuroimaging Applications in Diagnosis and Therapy**

Technique	Diffuse or Multifocal Cerebral	Focal Cerebral	Subcortical	Brain Stem	Spinal Cord
Plain film	Neoplasm Metabolic Congenital	Neoplasm	Not useful	Not useful	Trauma Neoplasm Degenerative
CT	Hemorrhage Calcification Infarct Neoplasm Inflammation Vascular	Hemorrhage Calcification Infarct Neoplasm Inflammation Vascular	Hemorrhage Calcification Infarct Neoplasm Inflammation Vascular	Hemorrhage Calcification Infarct Neoplasm Inflammation Vascular	Hemorrhage Calcification Neoplasm Inflammation
MR	Neoplasm Inflammation Hemorrhage Vascular White matter disease Congenital Infarct	Neoplasm Inflammation Hemorrhage Vascular White matter disease Congenital Infarct	Neoplasm Inflammation Hemorrhage Vascular White matter disease Infarct	Neoplasm Inflammatory Hemorrhage Vascular White matter disease Infarct	Neoplasm Inflammatory Hemorrhage Vascular White matter disease Infarct
Myelography	Not useful	Not useful	Not useful	Not useful	Degenerative Neoplasm Hematoma Inflammatory Vascular Congenital
Angiography	Mass effect Vasculopathy Atherosclerosis	AVM tumor Aneurysm Atherosclerosis	AVM tumor Aneurysm Atherosclerosis	AVM tumor Aneurysm Atherosclerosis	AVM
Ultrasonography	Hemorrhage (Neonatal) Congenital Neoplasm Infection Vascular	Hemorrhage (Neonatal) Congenital Neoplasm Infection Vascular	Hemorrhage (Neonatal) Congenital Neoplasm	Congenital Neoplasm	Congenital Neoplasm
PET-SPECT	Vascular Neoplasm Infection Degenerative Trauma	Vascular Neoplasm Infection Degenerative Trauma	Vascular Neoplasm Infection Degenerative Trauma	Not useful	Not useful

AVM, Arteriovenous malformation.

extracranial vascular disease. Transcranial Doppler studies are useful in selected patients for assessing intracranial vascular disease. Ultrasonography has also been used in the operative setting. Positron-emission tomography and single photon emission computed tomography are nuclear medicine techniques that offer physiological information (Table 23–1).*[VGC1]

*Individual subsection authors: Plain Film Analysis, Todd L. Siegal; Computed Tomography, Beverly L. Hershey; Magnetic Resonance Imaging, Scott H. Faro, Robert A. Koenigsberg, and Cyrus K. Dastur; Functional Magnetic Resonance Imaging, Feroze B. Mohamed, Scott H. Faro, and Robert A. Koenigsberg; Cerebrospinal Fluid Flow—Phase Contrast Imaging, Scott H. Faro and Feroze B. Mohamed; Magnetic Resonance Imaging of the Spine, Scott H. Faro and Robert A. Koenigsberg; Magnetic Resonance Angiography, Scott H. Faro and Feroze B. Mohamed; Magnetic Resonance Venography, Cyrus K. Dastur, Robert A. Koenigsberg, Scott H. Faro, Feroze B. Mohamed, and Fong Y. Tsai; Myelography, Todd L. Siegal; Neuroangiography, Robert A. Koenigsberg and Scott H. Faro; Ultrasonography, Robert A. Koenigsberg; Positron-Emission Tomography and Single Photon Emission Computed Tomography, Scott H. Faro and Robert A. Koenigsberg.

Plain Film Analysis

BASIC PRINCIPLES AND TECHNIQUES

Standard views of the skull are the posteroanterior (PA), lateral, anteroposterior (AP), half-axial (Towne), and base. The PA view demonstrates the frontal and ethmoidal sinuses, frontal bones, nasal cavity, superior orbital rims, and mandible. The frontal, parietal, temporal, and occipital bones; the sella turcica; the orbital roofs; the mastoid region; and the lateral aspect of the facial bones are demonstrated on the lateral view. The Towne view shows the zygomatic arches, the foramen magnum, the occipital bone, and the mastoid region. The base view demonstrates the basal structures of the skull. To evaluate the facial bones and sinuses, the occipitomental (Waters) view is often used. CT imaging, though, has largely supplanted the use of plain films, particularly in the evaluation of the "specialty regions" (i.e., the paranasal sinuses, orbits, temporal bones, and sella).

Conventional radiographic examination of the spine plays a critical role in the initial evaluation of the trauma patient. Because the cervical cord is prone to damage from unnecessary manipulation, the initial radiographic examination is usually limited to two or three projections that provide the optimal amount of clinically pertinent information. Plain film examination of the spine is also an invaluable tool in the screening of patients for degenerative, inflammatory, and neoplastic conditions and serves as an excellent imaging modality by alerting the physician to the presence and degree of abnormalities. Of all the spine examinations involving radiation, plain film radiography gives the lowest dose, averaging 0.2 rad to the ovaries for a four-view lumbar examination. The testicular dose is 10 to 50 percent of the ovarian dose.

NORMAL FINDINGS

The skull varies considerably in shape and consists of a superior portion, the vault, and an inferior portion, the base. Along the base lie the orbits, sella turcica, and the temporal bones. The skull bones are composed of outer and inner tables of compact bone separated by the diploic space containing bone marrow. The inner table contains grooves for vascular structures such as the middle meningeal artery branches, and care should be taken not to confuse these for linear fractures. Pacchionian depressions house arachnoid granulations that are related to venous lacunae communicating with the superior sagittal sinus. From the midline they commonly extend 2.5 to 3.0 cm, and any inner table depression beyond that distance should be considered suspicious, possibly an inner table erosion secondary to a neoplasm.[1] Beyond age 3, the cranial sutures appear similar to those of adults, and portions undergo actual closure at variable ages. Normal intracranial calcifications involve the dura, pineal gland, habenular commissure, choroid plexus, arachnoid granulations, and basal ganglia. The latter can be seen in hypothyroidism and pseudohypothyroidism but are most often physiological.

For the spine, the lateral view is the single most useful projection because it can demonstrate most post-traumatic lesions of the cervical spine.[2] The lateral projection clearly demonstrates the vertebral bodies, apophyseal joints, anterior arch of the atlas, atlanto-odontoid distance, odontoid process, spinous processes, and disc spaces. A mandatory requirement is the demonstration of the C7 vertebral body. The four smooth contour lines of the normal cervical spine are apparent on the lateral view and should be evaluated to exclude interruption or angulation. The lines include the anterior and posterior vertebral lines, the spinolaminar line (defines the posterior margin of the spinal canal), and the posterior spinous line. Evaluation of the prevertebral soft tissues can also be performed because the retropharyngeal and retrotracheal spaces are adequately demonstrated and may be pathologically widened in traumatic or nontraumatic conditions.

The anterior projection demonstrates the C3 to C7 vertebral bodies, intervertebral disc spaces, lateral masses, uncinate processes, uncovertebral (Luschka) joints, and the spinous processes that, superimposed upon the bodies, resemble teardrops. To provide adequate visualization of C1 and C2, a variant of the AP projection is often obtained, termed the *open-mouth* or *odontoid view*. The atlanto-occipital and atlantoaxial joints, odontoid process, and lateral masses of C1 and C2 are effectively demonstrated.

The oblique view of the cervical spine demonstrates the neural foramina and facet alignment. Neural canal stenosis typically occurs secondary to degenerative spur formation arising from the uncinate processes anteriorly or from the respective facet joints posteriorly. Pathological foraminal widening can be associated with neurofibromas as seen in cases of neurofibromatosis. Rarely, vascular masses of the spine, particularly those associated with the vertebral artery, can be expansile and mimic benign neural tumors. In cases of spine trauma, the oblique view can be helpful in delineating fracture dislocations of the articular processes, particularly in cases of perched or jumped facet injuries. The oblique view of the lumbar spine is the single most useful view in evaluating for suspected spondylolytic defects through the pars interarticularis.

TYPES OF DETECTABLE ABNORMALITIES

With the advent and marked success of both CT and MRI, the clinical utility of skull and spine radiography has declined. However, it remains useful in the detection and diagnosis of fractures, abnormal calcifications, developmental anomalies, and osteolytic or osteoblastic disorders. Degenerative spinal conditions and osteophytic changes are still commonly evaluated with spine films.

NEUROLOGICAL APPLICATIONS IN DIAGNOSIS AND TREATMENT

Generalized Diseases

Metabolic and Systemic Diseases. Renal osteodystrophy, hyperparathyroidism, and acromegaly represent some of the metabolic and endocrine disturbances that the skull responds to. However, the importance of radiographic findings has decreased with the routine laboratory determination of certain diseases. The skull characteristically demonstrates mottling of the vault, manifesting a "salt and pepper" appearance. Occasionally, cystlike lesions, or brown tumors, may occur. The findings in renal osteodystrophy are identical to those of primary hyperparathyroidism. Findings in acromegaly include thickening of the calvarium and expansion of the supraorbital ridge and frontal sinus, but the clinical manifestations and hormonal assay are more sensitive and objective determinations of disease severity.

Cranial Diseases

Neoplasms and Destructive Lesions. Skull radiography remains valuable in the evaluation of destructive lesions and metabolic abnormalities. By far the most common neoplastic involvement of the skull is secondary to metastasis or invasion from adjacent neoplasm. Metastatic carcinoma, multiple myeloma, and lymphoma usually present as lucent or lytic lesions and represent the most common malignancies affecting the calvarium. Breast carcinoma commonly manifests as large and variable-sized lucencies. In males, prostate carcinoma is the most common cause of osteoblastic metastasis. There is little to differentiate osteomyelitis from neoplasm radiographically, but, fortunately, osteomyelitis of the calvarium is rare in North America and many other parts of the world.

Structural and Developmental Abnormalities. Several acquired abnormalities can be demonstrated by plain films. Fibrous dysplasia classically features sclerosis, lucency, and thinning and bulging of the inner table. This entity can be confused with Paget's disease but is encountered in a younger age group and often ceases to grow at about the third decade of life. The classic calvarial presentation of eosinophilic granuloma is that of a sharply circumscribed lucency involving the diploë and inner and outer tables, similar in appearance to that of a destructive lesion. Indeed, the differential considerations are metastatic neoplasm, infection, and recent surgical repair. Hemangiomas of the calvarium usually have an unmistakable "Aunt Minnie" appearance on plain film. These lesions are typically discrete, predominantly lucent areas with a reticular or "spoke wheel" trabecular bony configuration. Further, a prominent diploic vascular channel is frequently identified entering the lesion; this may represent an enlarged draining venous channel. The initial or lytic phase of Paget's disease results in areas of sharply demarcated lucency termed *osteoporosis circumscripta*. Subsequent stages demonstrate enlarged, coarsened trabeculae; thickening of the cortex; and nonhomogeneous patchy densities referred to as a "cotton wool" appearance. Paget's disease can be confused with other entities, but the patient's age, blood chemistry, and involvement of other bones aid in the formulation of an appropriate differential diagnosis.

Developmental alterations can also be demonstrated on radiographic examination of the skull. Sutural abnormalities such as premature closure (craniosynostosis) or widening (from increased intracranial pressure seen in aqueductal atresia and Dandy-Walker syndrome) can be identified. Decreased size of one half of the cranium along with the compensatory, ipsilateral skull thickening are key findings in the Dyke-Davidoff syndrome of cerebral hemiatrophy secondary to intrauterine and perinatal internal carotid artery infarction. Childhood anemias and sickle cell disease classically demonstrate generalized skull thickness or density. Decreased thickness and density can be seen in osteogenesis imperfecta. Defects in bone can occur with cranial myelomeningoceles, dermal sinuses, and epidermoids.

Trauma. Skull radiography is generally not indicated for cranial trauma because many patients with a skull fracture have no neurological sequelae and many with severe intracranial abnormalities have no associated skull fractures. Patients with significant cranial injury or post-traumatic neurological symptoms should be evaluated by CT. There are two situations in which the skull fracture itself poses a clinical threat. The depressed fracture and fracture associated with a penetrating injury are of great concern. However, the symptoms associated with such injuries will invariably direct the clinician to use CT for evaluation. Plain films are valuable in demonstrating facial fractures, which often occur in recognizable patterns. Cortical disruption and displacement of osseous fragments represent direct signs of fracture. Indirect signs include paranasal sinus opacification or air-fluid levels, orbital emphysema, and soft tissue prominence. One side of the facial skeleton should always be compared with the other, and asymmetrical radiodensities should be regarded as suspicious findings.

Spinal Diseases

Spinal Fractures and Post-Traumatic Spinal Destabilization. Most unstable of all cervical spine injuries, the flexion teardrop fracture can be identified on the lateral view.[3] This fracture, characterized by anterior avulsion of a teardrop-shaped fragment by disruption of the anterior longitudinal ligament as well as fracture of the posterior elements and posterior displacement of the involved vertebrae, should be distinguished from the stable extension teardrop fracture. Although also demonstrating an anteriorly displaced fragment, this injury shows no subluxation, and the spinolaminar and posterior vertebral lines are preserved. The lateral view can also effectively demonstrate unilateral or bilateral locked facets (unstable), dens fractures (type 2 unstable), the stable clay-shoveler (fracture of the C6/C7 spinous process), and simple wedge fractures.

Symmetrical and bilateral fractures involving the anterior and posterior arches of C1 characterize the unstable Jefferson fracture, best demonstrated on the open-mouth odontoid view. Odontoid fractures, with emphasis being placed on transverse fracture through the base (type 2, unstable), can often be diagnosed on this view even though detail of an injury is often lacking. The AP view affords identification of fractures involving the bodies of C3 through C7 as well as abnormalities of the intervertebral disc spaces and uncovertebral joints.

Familiarization with the radiological findings that indicate instability is imperative in evaluation of the trauma patient.[4] These findings include displacement of the vertebrae, disruption of the posterior vertebral body line, and widening of the apophyseal joints. Widening and elongation of the vertebral canal with evidence of increased interpedicular distance also indicates instability. The single presence of any of these findings represents enough radiological proof to assume instability. The same principles for determining the stability of a cervical spine injury apply to those of the thoracolumbar spine.

The AP and lateral views compose the standard radiographic projections for evaluating traumatic thoracic spine injuries. For lumbar spine evaluation, AP, lateral (including a view of L5 through S1), and oblique views are traditionally obtained. By using the same general principles mentioned earlier, burst fractures, fracture/dislocations, and distraction fractures can be identified. The Chance, or "seat-belt" fracture, is an injury at the thoracolumbar junction that can be stable or unstable, depending on the extent and severity. Fracture/dislocations are notoriously unstable.

Degenerative and Inflammatory Bone Disease. Osteoarthritis, degenerative disc disease, spondylosis deformans, and diffuse idiopathic skeletal hyperostosis represent degenerative conditions that involve the spine and will frequently co-exist in the same patient. The anatomical site of degenerative change determines the type of degenerative disease.[5]

Degenerative changes involving the synovial joints (atlantoaxial, costovertebral, apophyseal, and sacroiliac) produce osteoarthritis of these structures. The defining radiological features are identical to other synovial joints and include joint space narrowing, subchondral sclerosis and cyst formation, and osteophyte formation. The mid- and lower cervical and lumbar spine frequently demonstrate apophyseal joint degenerative changes. Involvement of the apophyseal joints often discloses gas within the joint, termed the *vacuum phenomenon*. This is virtually pathognomonic for an advanced degenerative process. Oblique views can be valuable in demonstrating posterior osteophytes, which may encroach on the neural canal sac. Frequently, however, CT is required to demonstrate such findings.

Degenerative disc disease is secondary to degenerative changes within the intervertebral disc and may also manifest the "vacuum phenomenon" in long-standing degenerated discs.[6] Disc space narrowing and marginal osteophytosis of the adjacent vertebral bodies are also prominent features of this entity. Degenerative spondylolisthesis can be seen in patients with degenerative disc disease and apophyseal joint arthritis (Fig. 23–1).

Abnormalities of the annulus fibrosis can promote anterior and anterolateral disc herniation leading to the formation of anterior and lateral osteophytes, a process termed *spondylosis deformans*. Indeed, the primary radiological feature of this entity is extensive osteophytosis, and, unlike degenerative disc disease, the disc spaces are relatively well preserved.

Diffuse idiopathic skeletal hyperostosis demonstrates extensive osteophytosis without significant sclerosis or intervertebral disc space narrowing. Flowing ossification is characteristically seen along the anterior aspect of the vertebral bodies, stretching across the disc space. The findings are secondary to ossification involving the ligaments, entheses, and fibrous articulations. The radiological characteristics are best demonstrated on the lateral view.

The offending bacterial organism of the infectious spondylitis can be varied, with staphylococci, streptococci, *Escherichia coli*, *Proteus*, and *Pseudomonas* being the most common. Bacterial spread is usually by the hematogenous route, being common in immunocompromised individuals and intravenous drug abusers, but it may also be iatrogenic, occurring after spinal surgery, lumbar puncture, or complicating diagnostic discography. The most common location is the lumbar region, and the lesion is detected on plain radiographs by loss of disc space stature along with rarefaction of the adjacent endplates. If untreated, significant vertebral body involvement may lead to collapse of the vertebral body, resulting in wedge deformities, focal kyphosis, and/or scoliosis. The inflammatory process may extend beyond the confines of the vertebral body into the paraspinal soft tissues or posteriorly into the epidural space of the central canal with abscess formation and thecal sac compression. CT and MRI allow excellent visualization of the extent of these inflammatory processes, which cannot be adequately assessed with plain film radiography.

The most common location for spinal tuberculosis is the lower thoracic and upper lumbar regions. The granulomatous process usually begins in the anterior third of the vertebral bodies and spreads along the spinal axis beneath the paraspinal ligaments. The intervertebral disc space in tuberculous spondylitis remains relatively intact for a longer period of time than in pyogenic infections. In untreated chronic cases of spinal tuberculosis, paraspinal, paravertebral, and

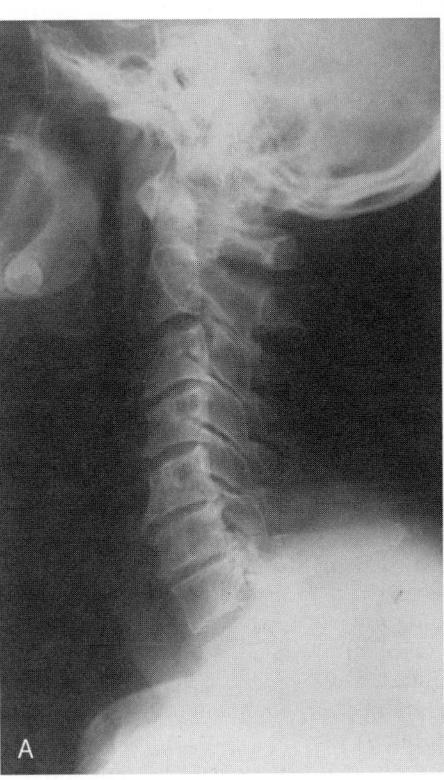

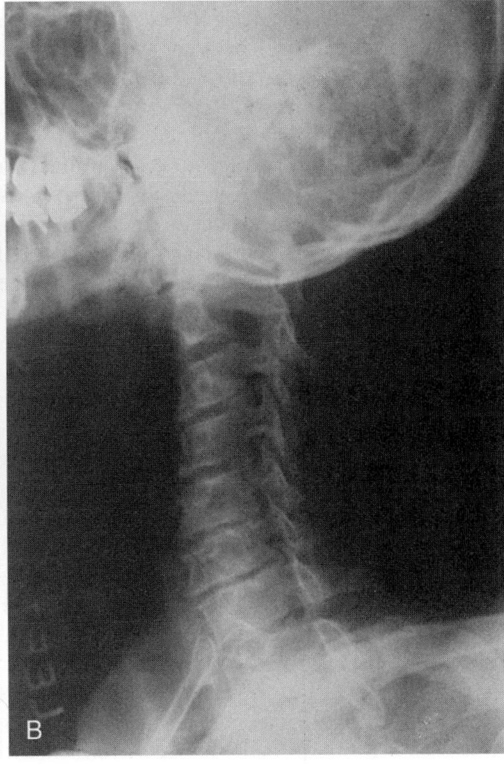

FIGURE 23–1. Cervical spondylosis. *A*, Lateral x-ray of cervical spine demonstrates chronic degenerative disc disease from C3–C4 through C6–C7 with varying degrees of disc space narrowing and associated endplate spur formation at each level. *B*, Right anterior oblique x-ray of cervical spine demonstrates multilevel neural canal stenosis from C3–C4 through C6–C7 secondary to chronic degenerative spur formation arising from the uncinate processes.

psoas abscesses frequently occur. The psoas abscess may calcify.

Neoplasms. By far the most common extradural malignancy of the spine is the metastatic lesion. Although breast and prostate cancer are known for their osteoblastic or sclerotic lesions, most metastases are osteolytic. Spine metastases can involve all vertebral levels but most commonly affect the lower thoracic and lumbar spine.

The most common plain film finding is pedicle destruction, even though in adults the initial site of involvement is typically the vertebral body. Pathological compression fractures, multiple lytic vertebral body lesions, and paraspinous soft tissue masses are other common expressions of metastatic neoplasms. A discriminating eye can sometimes detect an indistinct posterior vertebral body margin, a clue to epidural metastatic disease. MRI, however, is a highly sensitive imaging study that can portray epidural and paraspinous soft tissue involvement as well as cord compression. Breast, lung, and prostate cancer are commonly associated with epidural spinal cord compression. Other common adult metastatic primary lesions include renal cell carcinoma, melanoma, lymphoma, multiple myeloma, and sarcoma.

Computed Tomography

BASIC PRINCIPLES AND TECHNIQUES

The advent of computed tomography was one of the most exciting developments in the history of neuroimaging. For the first time, direct visualization of the brain became possible. Although MRI has surpassed CT in displaying neuroanatomy and pathology, CT remains a mainstay for several reasons. Wider availability and lower costs of CT are considerations in today's managed care environment. CT is easier to perform in the setting of acute trauma and in the ventilated patient. Owing to the speed with which CT images can be obtained, high-quality studies are more feasible in the patient unable to cooperate for examination. Patients with implanted devices such as cardiac pacemakers, spinal stimulators, aneurysm clips, and other surgical implants, as well as patients harboring ferromagnetic foreign bodies, are not MRI candidates.[7] Disadvantages of CT include the potential need for iodinated contrast material to visualize vessels and many intracranial pathological processes, artifacts related to beam hardening (which particularly limits evaluation of posterior fossa structures) or the presence of metallic foreign bodies, and difficulty in obtaining imaging planes other than the axial. The latter particularly limits evaluation of the spine.

CT is a technique in which a tightly collimated x-ray beam is directed through the patient. The patient is placed in the CT gantry, and the x-ray beam travels in a circular path around the patient. Detectors 180 degrees opposite the beam measure x-ray attenuation, or removal of the photons from the beam. The x-ray beam is collimated in a range from 1 to 10 mm, depending on the size of the structure being examined. The patient is moved by the same increment as the slice thickness for contiguous images of the area of interest. The signal from the radiation detector must be digitized by means of an analogue-to-digital converter so that the image can be constructed using a computer algorithm. Images are reconstructed by convention; air is seen as black and bone as white. Air is the tissue with the least attenuation of x-rays and on the Hounsfield scale (named after Godfrey N. Hounsfield, the inventor of CT) is arbitrarily designated as −1000. Bone, the greatest attenuator, is designated as +1000, with water as 0. Table 23–2 lists the approximate Hounsfield units for anatomical tissues encountered on head CT, in order from dark to bright. Resolution of small structures is a function of pixel size, determined by field of view (typically 23 cm for a routine head) and matrix size (typically 512).[8]

A recent technological advance is the development of helical CT, which requires a new system or updated hardware and software to perform. Helical CT differs from conventional CT in that the patient is moved continuously through the x-ray beam, dramatically shortening scanning times. There is some loss of resolution with this technique as scanning times decrease, such that in routine brain imaging, helical scanning is not employed. Helical scanning is useful when a rapid collection of data is necessary, such as in the traumatized or uncooperative patient. Helical scanning has made CT angiography possible, because rapid collection of images is needed after a bolus of contrast medium is injected.[9] The latest advance in CT imaging is the coupling of helical technology with multislice imaging, allowing for extremely rapid and detailed simultaneous multislice acquisitions.

The typical radiation dose for a head CT is 40 to 60 milligray (mGy). There are a number of factors influencing dose, such as voltage (kVp), current (mA), scan time (seconds), field of view, rotation angle, filtration, collimation and section thickness, and spacing. The dose distribution also depends on the size, shape, tissue density, and elemental composition of the patient.[10]

Morbidity of CT is mainly that of reactions to intravenous contrast medium administration. Today, nonionic contrast medium is available with significant reduction in the number and severity of adverse reactions. Lower cost has allowed CT use to become more routine. Patient conditions in which only nonionic contrast medium should be administered include prior reaction to iodinated contrast medium, asthma, multiple allergies, cardiac disease, and pulmonary hypertension.[11]

Patients with allergic histories can also be given a steroid pretreatment consisting of prednisone, 50 mg, orally 13, 7, and 1 hour before dye injection with diphenhydramine (Benadryl),

TABLE 23–2. **Appearances of Tissues on Computed Tomography**

Tissue	Hounsfield Unit	Gray Scale
Air	−1000	Black (↓↓↓)
Fat	−100	Black (↓↓)
Cerebrospinal fluid	0	Black (↓)
Brain	30	Gray (−)
Extravasated blood	100	White (↑↑)
Contrast medium enhancement	100	White (↑↑)
Bone	1000	White (↑↑↑)

↓↓↓, Marked hypoattenuation; ↓↓, moderate hypoattenuation; ↓, mild hypoattenuation; −, isoattenuation (to brain); ↑↑, moderate hyperattenuation; ↑↑↑, marked hyperattenuation.

50 mg, 1 hour before if desired.[12] In this patient population, it is preferable to avoid contrast medium–enhanced CT if at all possible, with MRI providing an excellent alternative. If MRI is contraindicated, and the patient has a history of laryngospasm or hypotension with previous use of contrast medium, an anesthesiologist should be present during the contrast medium administration. Acute renal failure is an absolute contraindication to the administration of contrast medium. Renal insufficiency should be regarded as a relative contraindication, and again MRI is recommended as the study of choice. Patients on dialysis can be imaged safely with contrast medium, preferably with dialysis planned soon after the study.

CT can be used to guide stereotactic brain biopsy, a technique that is especially helpful for tissue diagnosis of small or deep-seated lesions. Stereotactic radiation therapy, stereotactic craniotomy, brachytherapy, and management of brain stem lesions can also be planned from CT images. For most stereotactic procedures, the patient is placed in a device such as a Brown-Robert-Wells head ring. CT scanning is performed, and the lesion of interest is targeted using the head ring as an external reference. A computer transforms the two-dimensional coordinates of rods fixed in the head ring and the targeted lesion into three-dimensional space so that the trajectory of the biopsy needle can be planned.[13] Frameless stereotactic techniques have also been developed.

The standard head CT is performed with the gantry angled parallel to the orbitomental line obtaining images in the axial plane. Five-millimeter sections are obtained through the posterior fossa to ensure adequate visualization of the fourth ventricle with 10-mm sections through the supratentorial space. Thinner sections (1–3 mm) are employed for detailed examination of small anatomical regions such as the temporal bone, sella, orbits, and paranasal sinuses. Direct coronal imaging is essential for evaluation of these structures and may be used to visualize lesions in the tentorial region or at the vertex. Coronal imaging requires repositioning the patient in the gantry with the neck hyperextended either supine or prone. Gantry angulation can help reduce the degree of cervical extension but often is insufficient alone for direct coronal imaging. Patients with cervical spine disease, airway obstruction, or obesity also may not be able to tolerate positioning for coronal imaging, and intubated patients cannot be placed in this position.

Filming of head CT images is done at narrow windows (60–80 HU) to accentuate the minor difference in Hounsfield units between white and gray matter, with white matter being slightly lower in attenuation. In cases of trauma, metastatic disease, bone infection, or neoplasm, bone windows (2000–4000 HU) should be obtained to evaluate for fracture, bone destruction, or hyperostosis associated with meningiomas. Bone windows are also useful in detection of intracranial air and can separate air and fat density. At these windows, the brain is not seen. A bone algorithm, a computer reconstruction technique, can also be employed and is particularly useful in evaluating small or thin bones, such as the ossicles in the middle ear, the facial bones, and skull base. Acquisitions in bone algorithm alone give detailed bone information, but the images cannot be filmed at brain windows as they will be unsatisfactory. Subdural windows (150–200 HU) are necessary to identify acute subdural hematomas, which blend in with the calvarium on routine brain images (Fig. 23–2).

NORMAL FINDINGS

A normal unenhanced head CT scan shows midline position of the third and fourth ventricles and the septum pellucidum/fornix positioned between the lateral ventricles. The bodies of the lateral ventricles need not be symmetrical. Mild differences in the sizes of the frontal, temporal, and occipital horns are common. There should be density discrimination between the white matter (centrum semiovale, corona radiata, internal capsule, and brachium pontis) and gray matter. No focal white matter low densities should be seen in young or middle-age patients. Patients older than the age of 65 may

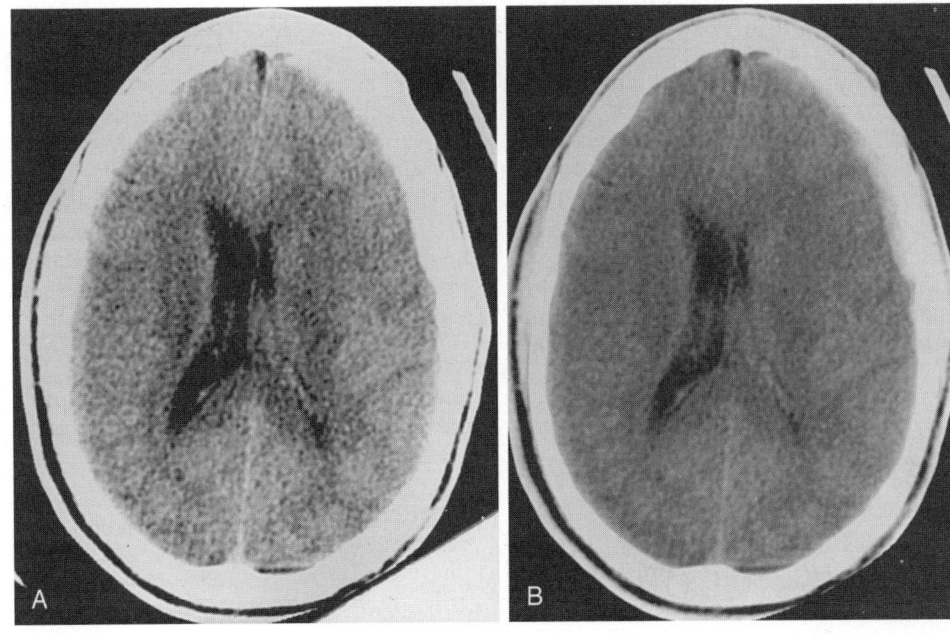

FIGURE 23–2. Twenty-three-year-old man status post motor vehicle accident. *A,* An acute frontal subdural hematoma causes compression of the left lateral ventricle, but it is difficult to see at routine brain windows (60). *B,* At subdural windows (150), the hematoma is identified subjacent to the calvarium.

show mild periventricular hypodensities as part of the normal aging process. Ventricular and subarachnoid space size is variable between individuals. In general, the ventricles and subarachnoid spaces are small in younger patients and increase in size with increasing age. In an older patient, the ventricles should not be dilated out of proportion to the subarachnoid space size.

Normally calcified structures are the pineal gland and the glomus of the choroid plexus in the trigone of the lateral ventricle. Calcification may be seen throughout the choroid plexus, including the temporal horns and the outlets of the fourth ventricle. Occasionally, the habenula (directly anterior to the pineal gland) may show calcification. The arteries of older patients are not uncommonly calcified. Calcification of the globus pallidus can be physiological and becomes more prominent with advancing age. Calcification in dural structures, including the walls of venous sinuses, is seen as a normal variant. Excessive calcifications of vascular or dural structures may indicate an underlying pathological process.

Arteries and veins show normal enhancement owing to the higher attenuation of blood containing iodinated contrast material. Lack of a blood-brain barrier and the tight junctions between endothelial cells allow enhancement of the dural structures (falx and tentorium) and pituitary gland. The choroid plexus in the ventricular system usually shows mild to moderate enhancement owing to its vascular nature. This enhancement can be prominent in the outlets of the fourth ventricle, simulating a vascular lesion.

In evaluation of spine CT, the intervertebral disc is seen as having a higher density than that of the contents of the spinal canal. The spinal canal has relatively low attenuation owing to the presence of cerebrospinal fluid (CSF), particularly in the lumbar region. The nerve roots of the cauda equina may be visualized in the posterior portion of the thecal sac. Roots in the cervical and thoracic subarachnoid space cannot be visualized unless intrathecal contrast medium is present. The intervertebral foramina contain mostly fat, which outlines the dorsal root ganglion and is best appreciated in the lumbar region. In the cervical region, soft tissue density of the nerve root is seen in the inferior neural foramen, whereas in the lumbar spine the root is seen in the superior aspect of the foramen. The osseous structures should be smooth with no encroachment upon the central canal, neural foramina, or lateral recesses. Linear lucencies representing veins may be seen in the vertebral bodies and are corticated, distinguishing them from fracture lines. The basivertebral venous plexus exits the vertebral body midway between the superior and inferior endplates and has a dorsal calcified cap that should not be mistaken for an osteophyte. The ligamenta flava are visualized particularly well in the lumbar spine but should not indent the thecal sac.[14]

TYPES OF DETECTABLE ABNORMALITIES

Computed Tomography Without Contrast Medium Enhancement

CT is an excellent study to evaluate for acute intracranial hemorrhage, particularly in the subarachnoid space (Fig. 23–3). Acute hemorrhage is detected as high attenuation owing to clot retraction with separation of the high-density erythrocytes from lower-density plasma. Unclotted, active bleeding may be detected in either epidural or subdural hemorrhages as a relative lucency, commonly referred to as the "swirl sign."

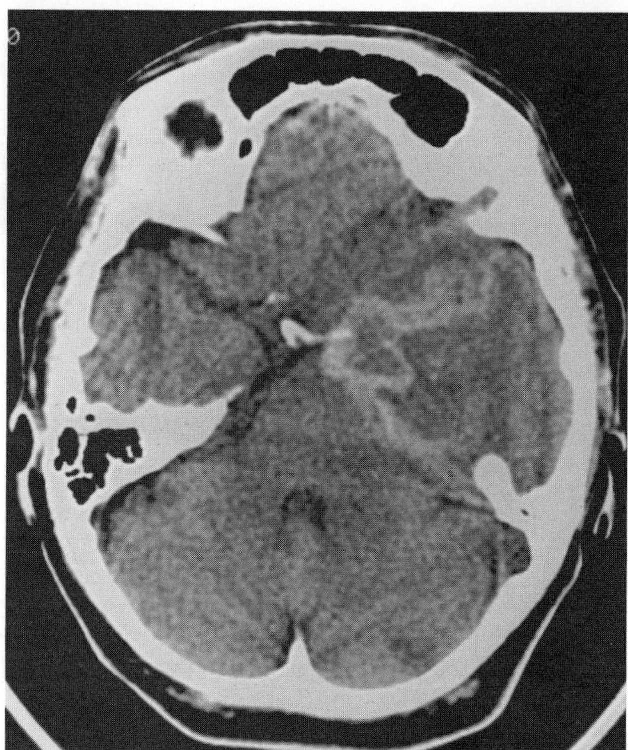

FIGURE 23–3. Middle-aged woman presenting with what she reported as the worst headache of her life and third nerve palsy. Acute subarachnoid hemorrhage is present in left-sided basal cisterns secondary to rupture of a posterior communicating artery aneurysm. Central lucency represents the aneurysm.

Edema is identified as low attenuation owing to the presence of increased water content. Cytotoxic edema associated with infarct or diffuse anoxia is seen as low density in the gray matter, representing abnormal accumulation of intracellular water (Fig. 23–4). Vasogenic edema is the abnormal accumulation of extracellular water in the white matter, seen as "fingers" or "fronds" of low attenuation following white matter tracts.

CT is valuable in detecting mass effect including subfalcine, descending transtentorial (uncal), ascending transtentorial, and transsphenoidal herniations (see Chapter 1). Cerebellar tonsillar herniation is infrequently detected and can be missed secondary to beam hardening artifact at the level of the foramen magnum.

Evaluation of ventricular size can be done by CT. Enlargement of the temporal horns out of proportion to the lateral ventricular bodies is helpful in recognizing early hydrocephalus. Hydrocephalus with marked dilatation of the ventricles and relative effacement of sulci is typical of more advanced cases. CT can be helpful to follow ventricular size after shunting.

CT is very useful for detecting intracranial calcifications, such as those seen in congenital infections, vascular lesions, metabolic disease, and neurocutaneous disorders. The location and distribution of calcifications is key in differentiating

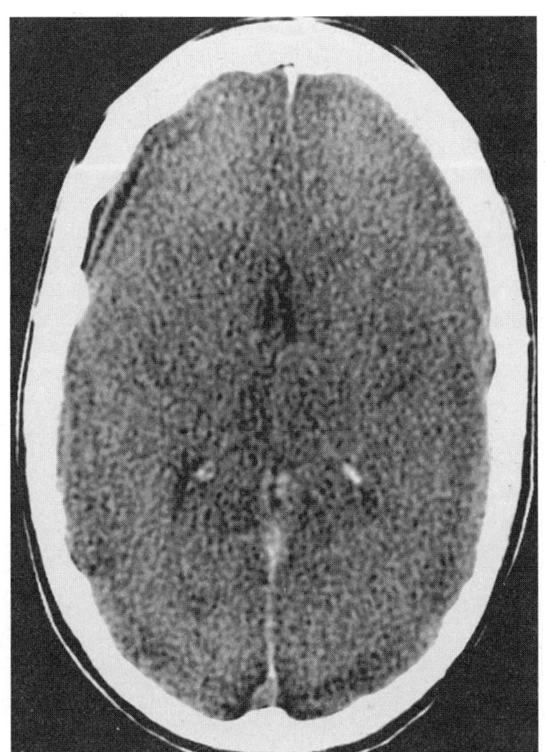

FIGURE 23–4. Thirty-four-year-old woman status post cardiorespiratory arrest and resuscitation. CT shows severe diffuse cerebral (cytotoxic) edema with loss of white-gray matter differentiation and compression of ventricles and subarachnoid spaces secondary to anoxia.

these various causes. The identification of calcification in a neoplasm aids in differential diagnosis.

Although congenital brain malformations can be seen on CT, MRI is the modality of choice owing to direct multiplanar imaging with visualization of structures such as the corpus callosum and improved sensitivity for migrational abnormalities. CT is complementary in the evaluation of encephaloceles and meningomyeloceles in regard to identifying bone defects.

CT is preferred for evaluating acute fractures of the calvarium, skull base, and spine. Fractures are identified as lucencies without sclerotic margins. These features aid in differentiating fractures from vascular grooves or sutures. In the spine, CT can uniquely demonstrate bone impingement on the central canal, implying possible spinal cord injury. Epidural hematomas are occasionally but not consistently identified in the spine (Fig. 23–5). Again, the spinal cord is typically not directly visualized without the use of intrathecal contrast medium.

CT and MRI provide complementary information about neoplasms of the vertebrae, particularly in the case of spine hemangioma (Fig. 23–6). Infection of the spine is better evaluated by MRI, although CT can provide very useful information regarding bone destruction and paravertebral soft tissue involvement.

Many pathological processes of the extracranial head and neck can be identified by CT. High-resolution thin-section CT is the test of choice for evaluation of the paranasal sinuses and middle ear structures owing to its exquisite bone detail highlighted by air. CT affords better evaluation of the paranasal sinuses, although the intracranial extent of neoplasm or infection is best evaluated by MRI. CT and MRI can both be used for the evaluation of the orbits, with the orbital fat providing excellent contrast for the optic nerve and extraocular muscles with either technique. CT provides information about calcification, which may be seen in tumors, drusen, and vascular lesions.

Computed Tomography with Contrast Medium Enhancement

In general, it is preferable to perform neuroimaging with MRI than to perform CT with contrast medium enhancement.

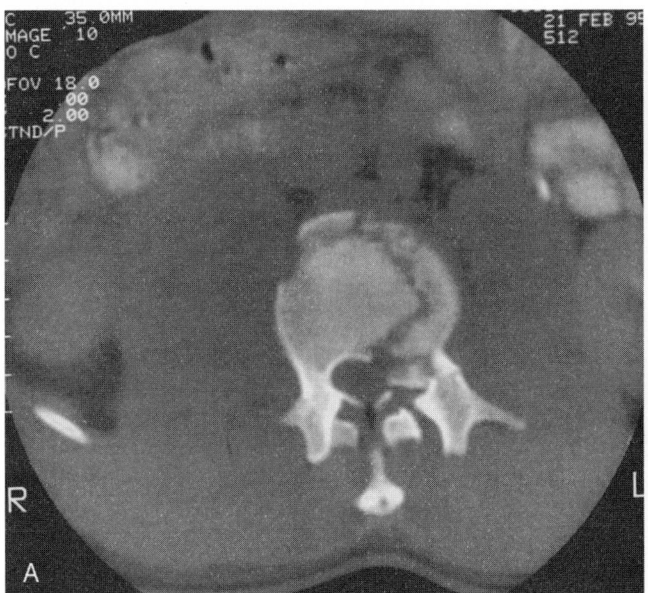

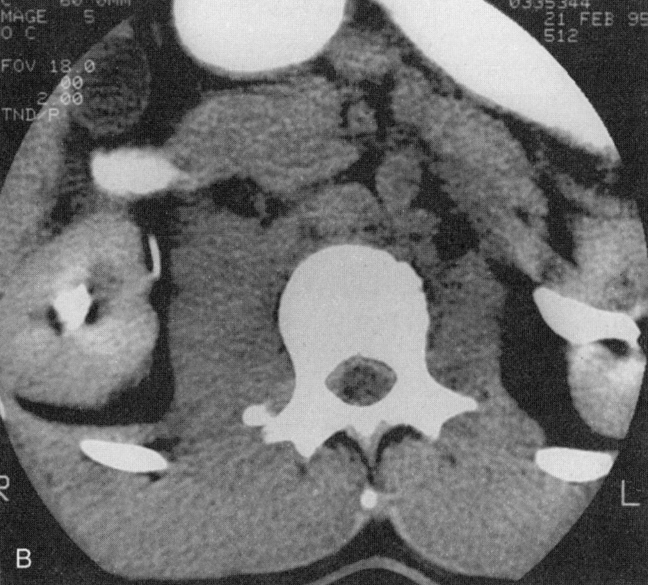

FIGURE 23–5. Twenty-three-year-old man status post motor vehicle accident. *A,* Bone windows from a lumbar CT reveal a burst fracture of L2. *B,* Soft tissue window demonstrates an anterior epidural hematoma at the L1 level.

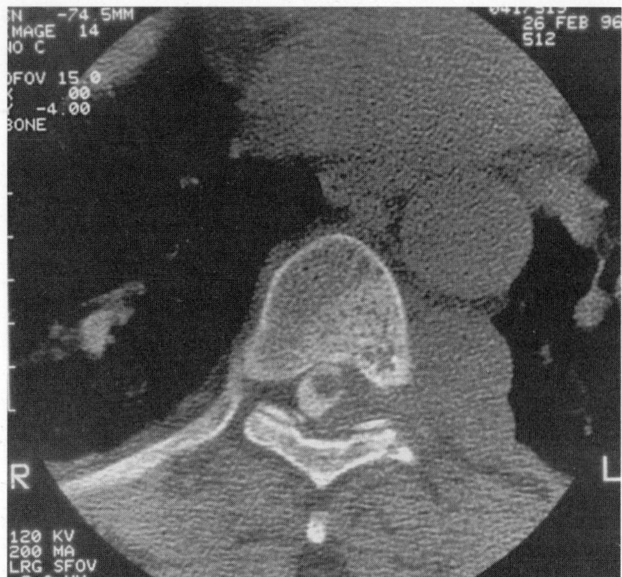

FIGURE 23–6. Fifty-five-year-old man with asymptomatic mass lesion identified on chest x-ray. CT myelogram reveals hyperdense spiculated lesion of the T7 vertebral body with soft tissue components in the paraspinal and epidural space consistent with hemangioma.

MRI is more sensitive to subtle changes in tissue signal and is superior to CT in initial as well as follow-up evaluation of enhancing lesions such as neoplasms, infection, and vascular lesions. MRI affords evaluation of masses in multiple planes and is especially useful in surgical or stereotactic irradiation planning. Meningeal disease is better evaluated by MRI and can be missed on CT owing to volume averaging with the skull coupled with the normal bright enhancement of the meninges.

Contrast medium–enhanced CT is useful in patients who cannot undergo MRI and when MRI is not readily available. Contrast medium aids in the detection of intracranial lesions that may otherwise be poorly delineated or invisible on unenhanced CT. Patterns of enhancement can be helpful in differential diagnosis of intracranial masses.

CT is not as sensitive in the detection of white matter and neurodegenerative disorders as MRI and should not be used as the primary imaging modality. If MRI is contraindicated, CT may identify white matter lesions secondary to demyelination or dysmyelination, and contrast medium enhancement is occasionally useful in differential diagnosis.

NEUROLOGICAL APPLICATIONS IN DIAGNOSIS AND TREATMENT

CT is useful in detecting structural abnormalities causing multifocal, focal, or subcortical cerebral dysfunction. Evaluation of the brain stem is generally limited to the midbrain and upper pons. CT has limited usefulness in the evaluation of the spinal cord and nerve roots. CT is not useful in the evaluation of neuromuscular disease.

Cranial Diseases

Intra-axial Disorders. CT can often identify lesions responsible for cerebral dysfunction and is ordered in the acutely ill neurological patient with a history of trauma, stroke, "worst headache" of life, anticoagulation or bleeding diathesis, or seizure. In any case of suspected acute intracranial hemorrhage, intravenous contrast medium should not be immediately administered because contrast medium enhancement and acute extravascular blood have similar attenuation characteristics. Likewise, evaluation for infarction should be performed without contrast medium enhancement to exclude hemorrhage and also because subacute infarction may show mild enhancement such that it is indistinguishable from normal cortex. Where available, perfusion CT imaging can be obtained in acute stroke patients to access the extent of ischemic brain. Typical unenhanced scans performed within the first 24 hours of clinical symptomatology of infarct may not reveal any detectable abnormality. Early signs of middle cerebral artery infarct include hyperdensity of the artery (thrombus, embolus), loss of differentiation of insular cortex (insular ribbon sign), and obscuration of the lentiform nuclei from adjacent capsular white matter structures due to edema, as well as effacement of the sylvian fissure and sulci. Should urgent angiography be necessary in acutely ill patients, caution should be taken when interpreting CT imaging studies performed over the next 24 hours because residual intravascular contrast can be present, particularly in patients with renal insufficiency or failure.

Differential diagnosis of enhancing lesions includes primary brain neoplasm, metastasis, abscess, infarct, demyelinating disease, resolving hematoma, and vascular malformation. Abscesses, metastases, and high-grade primary neoplasms incite prominent vasogenic edema, whereas other enhancing lesions usually show less edema. Demyelinating disease shows ring or solid enhancement in the acute stage, commonly in a periventricular location. Resolving hematomas show ring enhancement 1 to 2 weeks after hemorrhage at the margin of the hematoma bed. Arteriovenous malformations demonstrate enlargement of feeding arteries and draining veins with central dense enhancement representing the "nidus." Cavernous angiomas show enhancement in a solid pattern and are often hyperdense without contrast medium owing to calcification. CT can detect venous angiomas utilizing contrast medium due to lack of any quantifying features other than the enhancing aberrant vein.

Intracranial calcifications are seen in a variety of disease processes. Arteriovenous malformations, aneurysms, and cavernous angiomas all may contain calcifications. Of the neurocutaneous disorders, tuberous sclerosis and Sturge-Weber syndrome show characteristic patterns. Patients with tuberous sclerosis demonstrate calcifications that are mainly periventricular in location (Fig. 23–7). Patients with Sturge-Weber syndrome show a gyriform pattern of calcification seen in the posterior temporal, parietal, and occipital cortex. Patients with neurofibromatosis may also demonstrate parenchymal calcifications in the basal ganglia and elsewhere. Excessive basal ganglia calcifications are seen in many metabolic disorders usually related to calcium metabolism. Neoplasms that calcify include gliomas (particularly oligodendrogliomas), meningiomas (Fig. 23–8), ependymomas, craniopharyngiomas, and choroid plexus papillomas. The most common acquired intracranial infection to demonstrate intracranial calcification is cysticercosis.

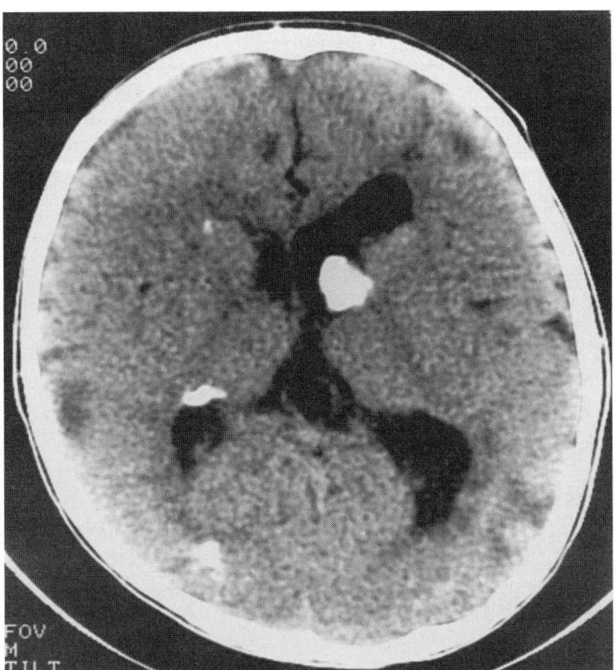

FIGURE 23–7. One-year-old male with tuberous sclerosis. CT without contrast reveals periventricular calcifications, the largest at the left foramen of Monro.

CT plays a complementary role to MRI in evaluation of patients with cranial nerve palsies. CT excels in evaluation of the bony skull base and can detect pathological processes such as tumor, infection, and primary bone lesions as they encroach upon, enlarge, or destroy foramina. Because all the cranial nerves have a close relationship to the skull base, bone detail thin-section scanning should be obtained in all patients with these palsies. Of the cranial nerves, only the optic nerve can be directly visualized by CT. Patients with monocular visual loss may demonstrate enhancement and/or enlargement of the optic nerve.

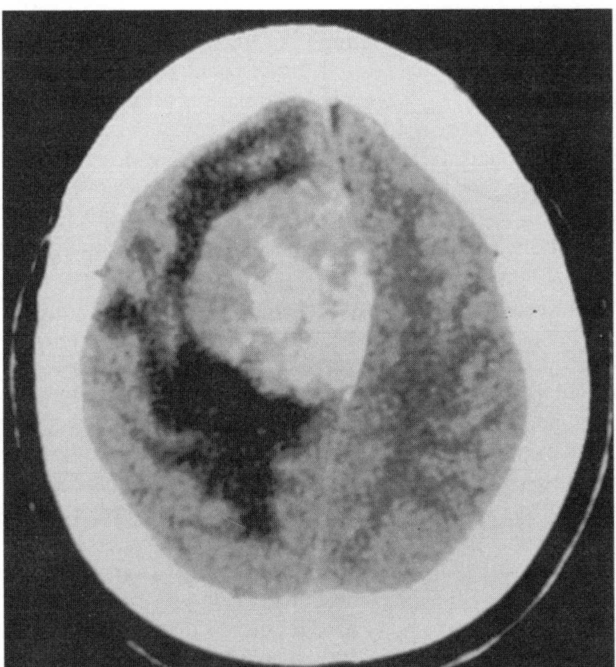

FIGURE 23–8. Sixty-year-old woman with right parasagittal meningioma. Without contrast, the lesion is hyperdense and contains calcifications. Low-density white matter represents vasogenic edema.

Spinal Disease

MRI is generally the test of choice for evaluating upper or lower motor neuron disease localized to the spinal cord, spinal roots, or plexi. In particular, CT should not be used as a primary imaging modality in suspected spinal cord compression because soft tissue lesions such as abscesses, hematomas, and sometimes disc herniations may be missed. CT serves a complementary role in defining bone lesions causing spinal cord compression once the level of interest has been identified by MRI or myelography, predominantly if MRI is contraindicated. Metastatic disease, discogenic disease with osteophyte formation and calcification of disc material/ligaments, infection, and primary bone tumors or metabolic lesions are examples of pathological processes in which CT can add or supplement information to MRI. CT can visualize nerve roots surrounded by low-attenuation fat particularly in the lumbar neural foramen and is useful in evaluating bone encroachment on the neural foramina from endplate osteophyte formation, facet degeneration, or uncinate process osteophytes of the cervical spine. CT myelography can visualize nerve roots and the spinal cord in the thecal sac and is particularly useful in the patient who cannot undergo MRI.

Magnetic Resonance Imaging

BASIC PRINCIPLES AND TECHNIQUES

Gorter is given credit for the origin of the concept of nuclear magnetic resonance (NMR) in 1936.[15] Work was continued by Purcell and Block in the mid-1940s with their Nobel Prize–winning discovery of the magnetic resonance phenomenon. Experimentation was limited to very small quantities of materials that were contained within a vacuum chamber. In the late 1960s, Jackson reported NMR experiments on animal tissues. Damadian, in 1972, was the first to describe whole-body NMR for medical diagnosis. Shortly after, in 1973, Lauterbur theorized using magnetic field gradients to create a position-dependent NMR signal. The first MR images of detailed human anatomy were produced by Aberdeen in 1976. The widespread clinical use of MRI began approximately in 1980 and continues to grow at an exponential pace.

NMR is the science that forms the basis for MRI. Abundant water molecules within the human body contain hydrogen protons that act as microscopic magnets. When the human body is placed into a static main magnetic field, approximately 50 percent of the magnets align parallel to this main magnetic field. The remainder align in an antiparallel fashion. These magnets cancel each other out, although approximately one in a million bar magnets is not canceled out and creates the basis of a tiny magnetic net vector. These microscopic magnets form the basis of the intrinsic signal that is used to generate clinical images.

These net magnetic vectors align with the axis of the main magnet and rotate at a specific frequency known as the Larmor frequency. A second type of magnetic field known as gradient fields is used to augment the main magnetic field and allow for anatomical localization of the specific spinning protons. Finally, there is a third type of magnetic field known as a resonance frequency field and referred to as a radiofrequency (RF) pulse. This RF pulse is a very low amplitude that oscillates near the Larmor frequency (63.87 MHz for a 1.5-Tesla [T] MR image). When the RF pulse is applied, the spinning protons become excited and flip their orientation to a predetermined flip angle, which is usually 90 degrees for a spin-echo technique. When the RF field is turned off, these excited spinning protons convert to a relaxed state, releasing energy. This energy can be measured with head, body, or surface coils and forms the basis for image formation.

The intrinsic high tissue contrast medium for MRI is one of the major strengths of this modality. Whereas CT uses differences in x-ray attenuation coefficients of two adjacent tissues, the MR signal is intrinsic and is generated by changing the proton spins in response to an external RF pulse. The different macromolecular characteristics of the intercellular and extracellular protons within the water molecules determine the intrinsic MR signal that is displayed for diagnostic interpretation. The macromolecular spin magnetization returns to its equilibrium state through a process defined by two relatively independent relaxation times, referred to as T1 and T2.

After a 90-degree RF pulse the proton magnetization net vector rotates from the axis of the main magnet (z axis, longitudinal magnetization) to the transverse plane (x and y axes, transverse magnetization). When the RF pulse ends, the longitudinal magnetization recovers toward 100 percent in an exponential manner. The time it takes for the proton to recover 63 percent of its longitudinal magnetization is referred to as *T1* or *spin-lattice relaxation*. In a similar fashion, when the RF pulse ends, the transverse magnetization is 100 percent and decays toward zero. The time it takes the proton to lose 63 percent of its transverse magnetization is termed *T2* or *spin-spin relaxation time*. The energy signal formed during this decay process is referred to as free induction decay. This signal is intrinsically weak. It is enhanced by the addition of a second 180-degree RF pulse, which follows the first 90-degree RF pulse. This second RF pulse refocuses the protons and creates a spin-echo signal. The time from the 90-degree pulse to the spin-echo signal is termed the *TE*. This process is repeated, and the repetition time between the 90-degree pulses is called *TR*.

Images can be created that have relative T1 weighting (T1W) or T2 weighting (T2W) by varying the TR and TE. A T1-weighted image has a TR less than 1000 msec and a TE less than 50 msec. A T2-weighted image has a TR greater than 2000 msec and a TE greater than 60 msec. An intermediate so-called proton density weighing has a TR greater than 2000 msec and a TE less than 40 msec.

NORMAL FINDINGS

There are basic MR signal patterns of normal tissues in the brain. These patterns are shown in Table 23–3.

TABLE 23–3. **Magnetic Resonance Findings**

	T1	T2
Fat	↑↑	↓
Bone	↓↓	↓↓
Gray matter	–	–
White matter	↑	↓
Cerebrospinal fluid	↓	↑↑

Signal is relative to gray matter that is intermediate in signal intensity on T1W and T2W images.

–, Intermediate signal intensity; ↑, small increase; ↑ ↑, bright; ↓, small decrease; ↓ ↓, dark.

TYPES OF DETECTABLE ABNORMALITIES

The MR signal characteristics of a lesion on T1- and T2-weighted sequences enable the differential diagnosis of any particular brain abnormality to be narrowed. A summary of signal characteristics is shown in Table 23–4. There are specific and nonspecific patterns of MR signal regarding normal and abnormal tissues. The most specific patterns are seen with respect to CSF, fat, bone, and stages of intracranial hemorrhage.

CSF has decreased signal on T1-weighted images, intermediate signal on proton density, and increased signal on T2-weighted images. When evaluating a cystic lesion, one must determine if the lesion follows CSF signal characteristics on all pulse sequences. If the lesion does not, it is considered atypical. Lesions that follow CSF signal typically represent arachnoid cysts or dilated CSF spaces as seen in Virchow-Robin spaces or secondary to encephalomalacia. Complicated fluid may show increased signal on both T1- and T2-weighted sequences. These abnormalities suggest the presence of proteinaceous or complex hemorrhagic fluid and may harbor malignancy.

Fat has increased signal on T1-weighted images and decreased signal on T2-weighted images. Lesions that follow this pattern most commonly represent fat, as seen in congenital lipomas and teratogenic tumors. Confirmation of a fatty lesion can be obtained with a fat saturation RF pulse sequence.

Each stage of hemoglobin molecular breakdown has its own peculiar imaging signature based on the MR signal. That is, the stages of hemorrhage, whether acute, subacute, or chronic, generate unique changes that are uniquely shown only by MRI. These signals range from nearly isointense to hypointense signal as seen in acute hemorrhages to increased signal seen on both T1- and T2-weighted images observed in late subacute or chronic hemorrhages.[16, 17] The identification of hemosiderin typifies chronic cerebral hemorrhage. The signal patterns of brain hemorrhage are summarized in Table 23–5.

MR signal patterns are recognizable with common diseases such as cerebral edema, neoplasm, abscess, infarcts, or demyelinating processes. These entities demonstrate a nonspecific pattern of decreased signal on T1-weighted images and increased signal on proton density and T2-weighted images. Therefore, to obtain a differential diagnosis with a high degree of accuracy, this information is linked with

TABLE 23-4. **Signal Characteristics of the T1W and T2W Images***

T1W		T2W	
Fat Intracellular methemoglobin Extracellular methemoglobin Complex proteins Complex calcifications Entry slice Flow in vessels Slow flow in vessels Melanin Contrast medium enhancement	↑ signal	Extracellular methemoglobin Cerebrospinal fluid Edema Neoplasms Abscess Demyelination Dysmyelination Acute to subacute infarcts	↑ signal
Cerebrospinal fluid Bone Ligaments Air Calcifications Deoxyhemoglobin Hemosiderin Flow void in vessels Acute to subacute infarcts	↓ signal	Bone Ligaments Air Calcifications Deoxyhemoglobin Intracellular methemoglobin Hemosiderin Flow void in vessels Fat	↓ signal

*In relation to gray matter.

anatomical location, morphology, and a degree of contrast medium enhancement. These, with good clinical history, all help in arriving at a correct differential diagnosis.

NEUROLOGICAL APPLICATIONS IN DIAGNOSIS AND TREATMENT

In general, owing to high tissue contrast between tissues and multiplanar imaging, MRI is the study of choice to evaluate all lesions in the brain and spine. CT, however, is more sensitive than MRI for the evaluation of calcifications, subtle fractures, and remains pivotal in the diagnosis of acute subarachnoid hemorrhage. Additionally, MRI cannot be performed in patients who have intraorbital foreign bodies, pacemakers, or non-MRI-compatible implants, such as artificial heart valves, vascular clips, cochlear implants, or ventilators. When approaching a lesion that is seen on an MRI of the brain, the specific location of this lesion must be identified. If one begins superficially and moves inward toward the deeper spaces of the brain, the first important space is the extracalvarial soft tissues, consisting of skin, muscle, and facial structures. The bony calvarium is next composed of the outer table, bone marrow within the diploic space, and inner table. The next space to consider is the extra-axial leptomeningeal structures, which include the epidural, subdural, and subarachnoid spaces. The layer beneath the subarachnoid space is the pia mater, which is closely adherent to the gray matter cortical ribbon. Deep to the pial layer lie the intra-axial structures. These structures include the cortical gray matter, the underlying white matter, the deeper basal ganglionic structures, and the brain stem as well as the ventricular system. On routine MRI of the brain there are additional structures to examine, which include the orbits, the paranasal sinuses, temporal bone, and skull base.

Calvarial-Related Lesions

Bone abnormalities include primary and secondary masses. Metastatic lesions and rare primary tumors such as osteogenic sarcomas or giant cell tumors can affect the calvarium. Additional secondary neoplastic processes that can involve the diploic (marrow) space include leukemia and lymphoma. Benign neoplastic processes include neurofibroma in a patient with neurofibromatosis (type I), soft tissue fibromas, and dermoid and epidermoid tumors. These can affect the skull, resulting in bony deformities, or can directly

TABLE 23-5. **Magnetic Resonance Signal Change of Hemorrhage**

	Acute (6 hours–3 days)	Early Subacute (day 3 to day 7)	Late Subacute (1 week to 1 month)	Chronic (months to years)
T1W	↓	↑	↑	↑
T2W	↓↓	↓	↑	↑
Pathophysiology	Deoxyhemoglobin	Intracellular methemoglobin.	Extracellular methemoglobin	Extracellular methemoglobin and hemosiderin ring*

*After slow reabsorption of the extracellular methemoglobin, only decreased signal hemosiderin persists.

involve the calvarium. Hemangiomas can be seen as enhancing, expansile masses originating within the diploic space.

Inflammatory lesions within the extracalvarial soft tissues typically include benign processes such as sebaceous cysts or cellulitis. Primary calvarial inflammatory lesions include osteomyelitis or an infected postoperative bone flap.

Bony lesions and congenital fibro-osseous lesions such as fibrous dysplasia or Paget's disease are common calvarial abnormalities. A common bone marrow disorder is conversion from fatty marrow to hematopoietic marrow in patients with anemia. Primary loss of normal hematopoietic elements with conversion to dense fibrous matrix can be seen in myelofibrosis.

Cranial Diseases

Extra-axial Space Lesions. Congenital tumors of epidermal and mesodermal origin that arise from the skull base and cerebellopontine angle are typically epidermoid tumors. These tumors are usually eccentric and are locally invasive. Congenital tumors that contain all three embryonic layers are termed dermoid tumors. These tumors tend to occur in the midline at the skull base and within the suprasellar cistern. More aggressive neoplasms to consider include ependymomas, which arise from ependymal cells most commonly within the fourth ventricle or cerebellopontine angle. Secondary neoplastic involvement of the pachymeninges include lymphoma, metastasis from lung or breast, or possibly an adenocarcinoma from an unknown primary tumor. These lesions may present as a single metastatic focus or can result in diffuse carcinomatosis.[18]

The most common dural-based tumor is the meningioma, which represents a primary neoplasm of the dura (Fig. 23–9). These tumors commonly involve the dural convexities, but may also involve the falx, cerebellar tentorium, and skull base. Rarely, these tumors present as intraventricular masses or masses involving the foramen magnum. Meningiomas typically enhance densely with contrast material and can display a signature "dural tail" representing contiguous involvement of the dura beyond seemingly defined tumor margins.

Inflammatory processes such as epidural empyema from an adjacent sinus infection may occur. Subdural effusions have been described in children with systemic *Haemophilus influenzae* infections. The most common inflammatory process to consider is a meningitis, which may be of viral, fungal, or bacterial origin.

An important pattern of abnormality is diffuse pachymeningeal thickening with homogeneous enhancement following an intravenous injection of contrast agent (gadolinium). The differential diagnosis includes carcinomatosis, sarcoidosis, meningitis, or a more recently described entity referred to as central CSF hypotensive pachymeningitis.[19] The exact cause of this last entity is not well understood, but it is believed to be related to either a CSF leak or an abnormal CSF metabolic process.[16] One of the more common extra-axial lesions is a post-traumatic epidural or subdural hematoma.[20] These lesions are occasionally imaged primarily by MR, but more frequently are imaged as an adjunct to CT scanning. MRI can be helpful in clarifying the involved extra-axial space and its secondary effects, as well as evaluating the hemorrhage age or chronicity. Lesions within the subarachnoid space that follow CSF signal on all pulse sequences and demonstrate mass effect represent congenital or post-traumatic (acquired) arachnoid cysts.

Intra-axial Space Lesions. Small focal lesions at the gray matter/white matter junction, which demonstrate mass effect, surrounding edema, and contrast medium enhancement, most commonly represent metastatic lesions. Large enhancing masslike lesions that involve both the gray matter and white matter and that do not follow a wedgelike distribution typically represent primary brain gliomas. Low-grade (I, II) gliomas typically do not enhance, whereas higher-grade gliomas (III, IV) usually do. A low-grade neoplastic process must also be considered if there is a focal, nonenhancing enlargement of the gray matter cortex that continues to have mass effect over a 3- to 4-week interval. This lack of change will help differentiate a low-grade glioma from a cortical infarct.

Peripheral cortical inflammatory processes secondary to meningitis may lead to cerebritis or consequently, a focal

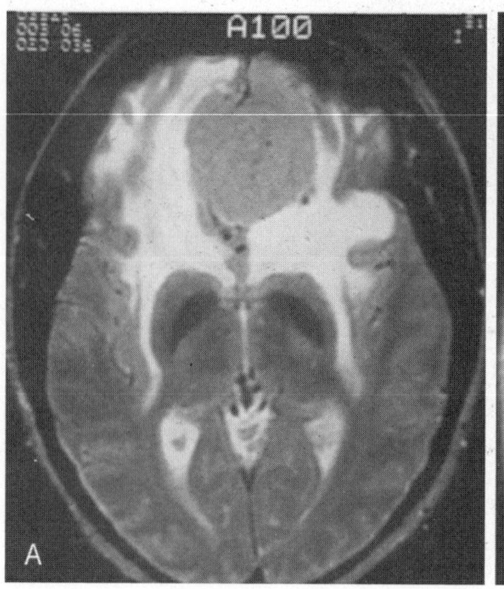

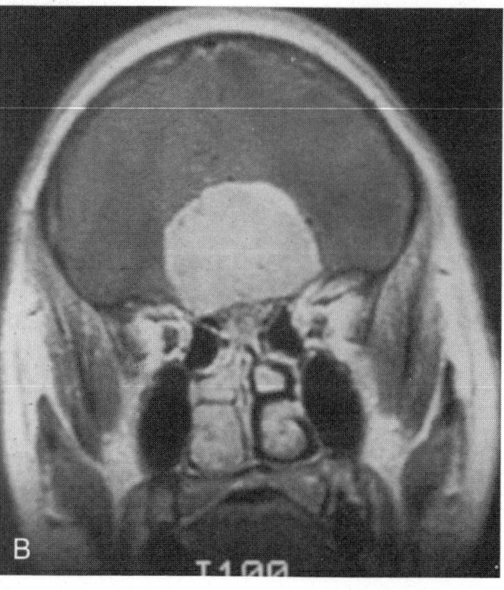

FIGURE 23–9. Olfactory groove meningioma. *A,* Axial T2-weighted image shows a mass attached to the anterior falx (dural extension). Note relative low signal on T2-weighted image and surrounding signal edema. *B,* Coronal T1-weighted image after contrast shows homogeneous enhancement of the dural-based extra-axial mass.

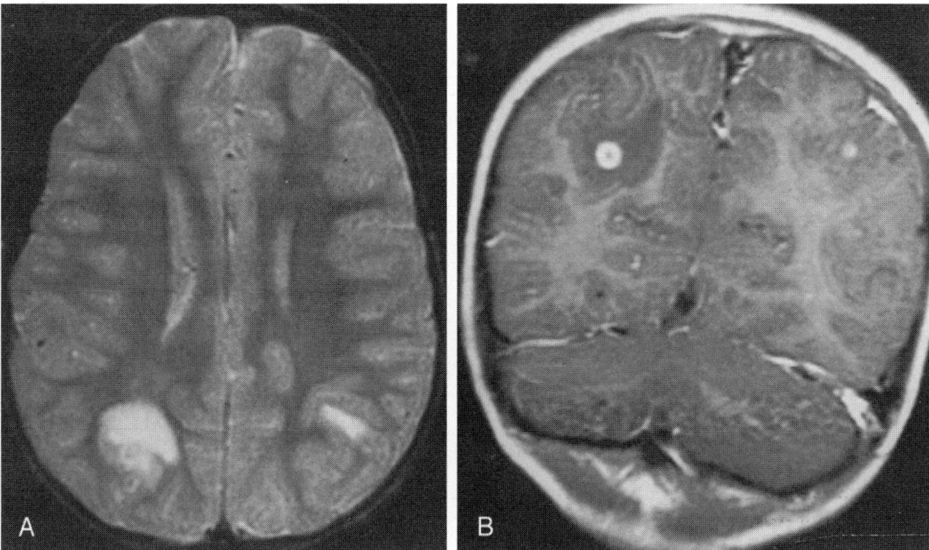

FIGURE 23–10. Cysticercosis. *A,* Axial T2-weighted image shows two parietal lobe lesions with up signal. *B,* Coronal T1-weighted image after contrast shows small ring-enhancing lesions.

abscess. Viral inflammatory processes of the cortex and subcortical white matter may occur and are most commonly secondary to a herpesvirus infection. Multifocal enhancing lesions in the gray matter/white matter junction, brain stem, and cerebellum may represent multifocal abscesses in the appropriate clinical setting (Fig. 23–10).

A wedge-shaped lesion that involves both white and gray matter and follows a vascular distribution usually represents an infarction from cerebrovascular disease. Acute infarctions may become evident on routine T2W spin-echo images within 12 to 24 hours of onset. The most sensitive pulse sequence is a water diffusion coefficient weighted technique.[21] This pulse sequence can detect an infarct within the first few minutes of onset. MR perfusion imaging can further be helpful in differentiating a devascularized brain territory (Fig. 23–11), and an appropriate mismatch between diffusion and perfusion imaging can help guide appropriate neurointervention. Peripheral vascular venous occlusions of the superior sagittal sinus or adjacent cortical draining veins may lead to a cortical or a cortical/subcortical venous infarction.

Lesions that primarily involve the white matter are most commonly secondary to small vessel occlusive disease or a demyelinating process. Small rounded infarctions less than 1 cm within the deep white matter, basal ganglion, cerebellum, or brain stem in an adult older than 50 years of age most commonly represent lacunar infarctions. Also in this population, tiny lesions within the periventricular white matter are usually secondary to small vessel ischemic disease. Demyelinating lesions secondary to multiple sclerosis may mimic this appearance but typically are present in younger adults. Lesions of multiple sclerosis may present as early as the second decade as rounded or ovoid lesions in the periventricular deep white matter. Ovoid lesions that are perpendicular to the long axis of the body of the lateral ventricles represent demyelination within perivascular spaces termed *Dawson's fingers*. Additional lesions can present in the corpus callosum, brain stem, and spinal cord. In children younger than the age of 10, periventricular white matter lesions and basal ganglionic, brain stem, or cerebellar lesions may represent an acute disseminated encephalomyelitis, typically secondary to a postviral or postvaccine autoimmune process (Fig. 23–12).

Multiple sclerosis and acute disseminated encephalomyelitis are the most common acquired leukoencephalopathies. Another leukoencephalopathy to consider is human immunodeficiency virus encephalopathy, which is a diffuse process.

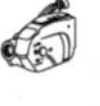

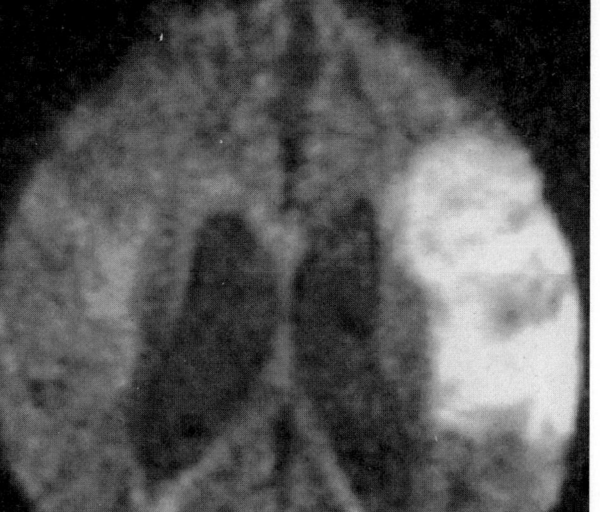

FIGURE 23–11. DWI demonstrating abnormal decreased signal in the left middle cerebral artery distribution.

Multifocal lesions with minimal mass effect and no abnormal contrast medium enhancement in an immunocompromised patient may represent progressive multifocal leukoencephalopathy. Postradiation and/or postchemotherapeutic leukoencephalopathy should be considered. There are a wide variety of congenital dysmyelinating disorders, the most common of which are metachromatic leukodystrophy, adrenoleukodystrophy, and Canavan's disease. All of these dysmyelinating diseases represent congenital enzymatic defects.

Within the deeper basal ganglionic structures, brain stem, or cerebellum, the most common lesions are focal infarctions and demyelination. Much less common lesions include focal encephalitis or gliomas. Focal mass lesions within the brain stem or cerebellum may occur within an older adult and most commonly represent metastasis. A primarily cystic lesion with an enhancing mural nodule within the cerebellum in a child represents a pilocystic astrocytoma. In a young adult, a similar-appearing lesion most likely represents a hemangioblastoma, which may be a manifestation of von Hippel-Lindau disease. A focal expansile lesion within the brain stem most commonly in the pons in a young child typically represents a brain stem glioma (Fig. 23–13). In a child, the primary differential diagnosis for a posterior fossa mass includes, in decreasing frequency, a primitive neuroectodermal tumor (medulloblastoma), brain stem glioma, cerebellar pilocystic astrocytoma, and ependymoma.

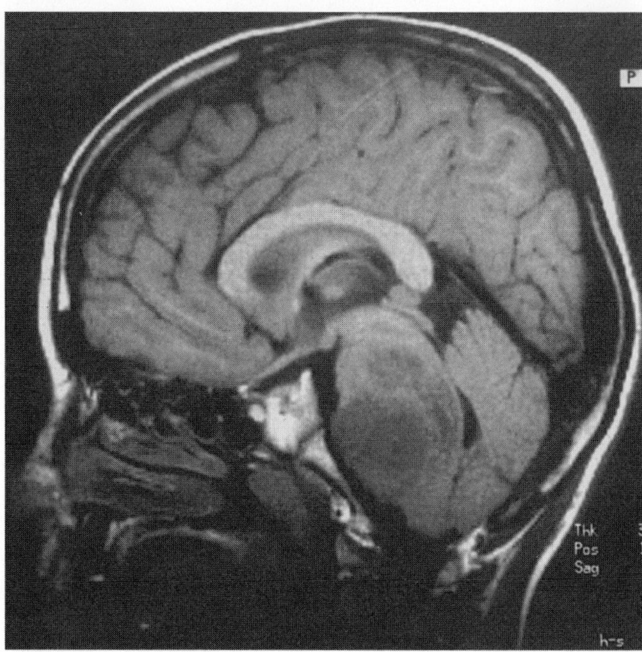

FIGURE 23–13. Brain stem glioma. Midline sagittal T1-weighted image shows a focal enlargement of the pons with decreased signal.

Vascular malformations are most commonly found within the intra-axial space, although they may be present solely within an extra-axial space. These lesions represent a spectrum from benign cavernous angiomas, which have a low bleeding potential, to arteriovenous malformations that carry a bleeding potential of 2 to 4 percent per year.[17] Cavernous angiomas have characteristic appearances of lobulated blood-filled channels with a rim of hemosiderin. Arteriovenous malformations have serpiginous tangles of flow voids with adjacent feeding arteries and draining veins. Dural malformations may be difficult to detect by MRI alone due to an inherent lack of brain parenchymal involvement.[22]

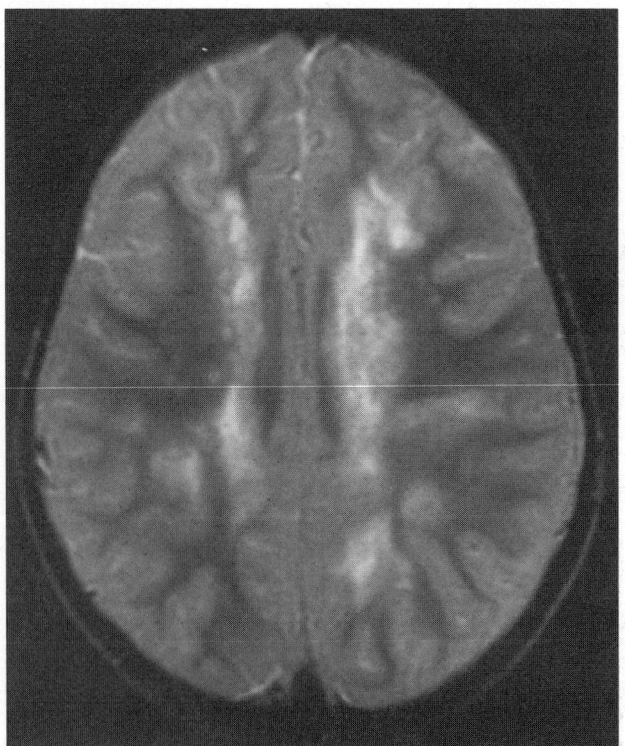

FIGURE 23–12. Acute disseminated encephalomyelitis. Axial T2-weighted image shows multiple white matter lesions.

Primary neoplasms, although uncommon, do occur. These tumors include choroid plexus papilloma or carcinoma; central neurocytomas, which are characteristically attached to the septum pellucidum (Fig. 23–14); interventricular meningiomas; and ependymomas. Colloid cysts typically originate within the region of the roof of the anterior portion of the third ventricle and typically are usually benign. Occasionally, these cysts may cause acute hydrocephalus and rarely death in a young adult from brain herniation.

Functional Magnetic Resonance Imaging

Functional magnetic resonance imaging (fMRI), based on blood oxygenation level–dependent (BOLD) imaging[23] of the brain, provides functional data of cerebral activation during any given task (e.g., motor, visual, cognitive). This method allows for a quantitative nonclinical method for assessing changes in cerebral function as related to cerebral activities (i.e., performance of physical or cognitive tasks). The BOLD fMRI technique allows for detection of minute changes in cerebral oxygenation. In fMRI, examining the signal intensity differences in an imaging voxel between the presence and absence of a stimulus identifies areas that are

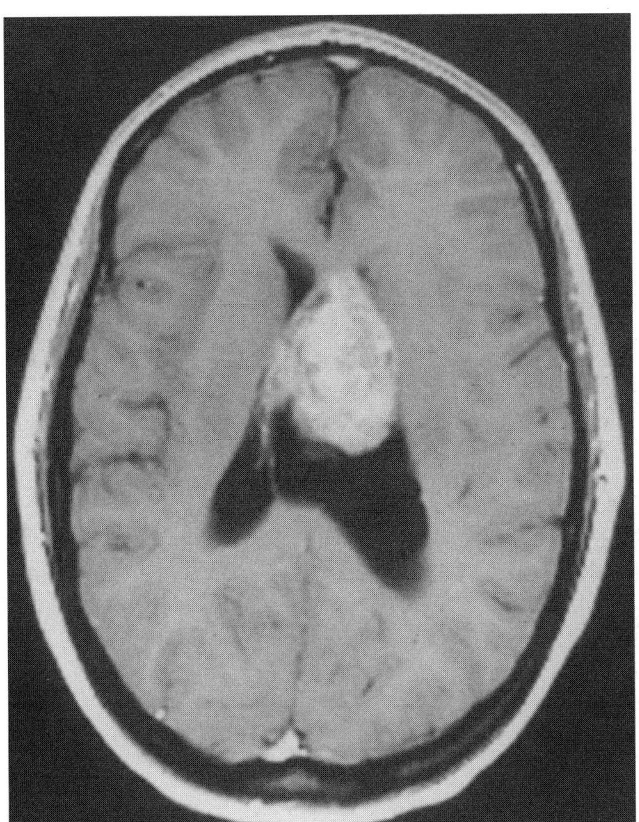

FIGURE 23–14. Central neurocytoma. Axial post-contrast T1-weighted image shows a heterogeneously enhancing, rounded intraventricular mass within the anterior portion of the lateral ventricle.

receiving increased blood flow, which is used as a marker for increased functional activity. This methodology has been widely used and has shown promising results for fMRI studies of various pathways of the brain, including the language, memory, and visual pathways (Fig. 23–15).

Cerebrospinal Fluid Flow—Phase-Contrast Imaging

Physiological CSF flow information can be obtained using a proton phase–sensitive (phase contrast, PC) technique. Moving tissue such as CSF causes shifting of the phase of the spinning protons. The phase shifting can be measured and qualitative direction of flow and quantitative flow velocity can be measured using a PC technique. CSF flow is a dynamic process that moves in a to-and-fro motion. The flow of CSF through the aqueduct of Sylvius, basal cisterns, and foramen magnum normally changes direction two to three times per second with a net slow flow in the superior to inferior direction. Cardiac gating can be performed with the PC technique, and flow information can be determined at selected intervals during the cardiac cycle. This flow information can be displayed in a cine loop, demonstrating the temporal and spatial changes of CSF flow. There are several clinical indications for CSF flow–PC imaging, which include characterizing partial versus complete aqueductal stenosis; determining the patency of an internal ventriculostomy (endoscopic osteotomy in the floor of the third ventricle to bypass an aqueductal obstruction); characterizing increased CSF velocity in normal pressure hydrocephalus; and characterizing the CSF flow around the basal cisterns and cervicomedullary junction in Chiari I malformation.

Magnetic Resonance Imaging of the Spine

Since the mid-1980s, MRI of the spine has attained acceptance as the premier modality in the evaluation of spine diseases. MRI is eloquent in the evaluation of both

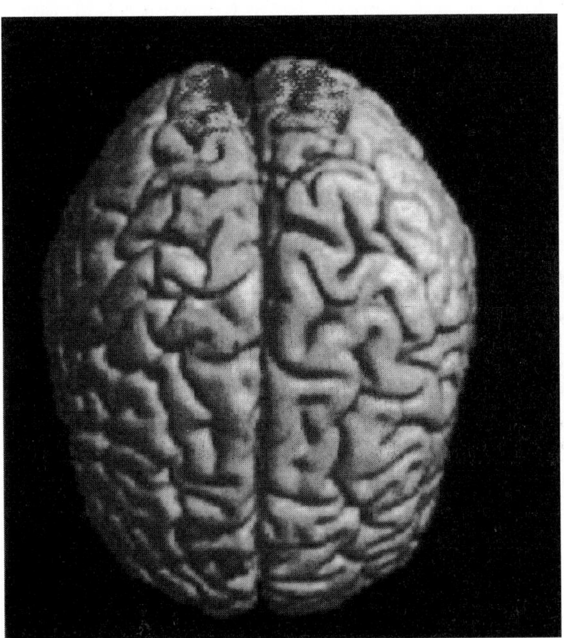

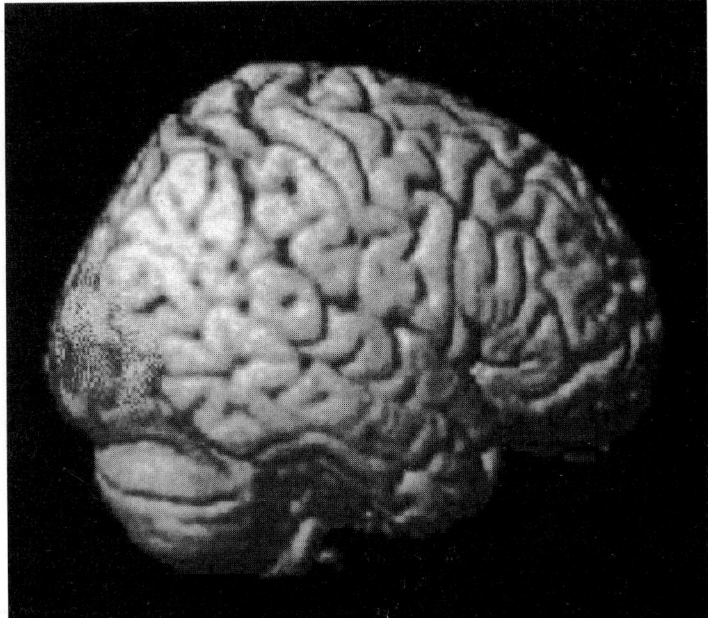

FIGURE 23–15. Frontal and lateral 3D fMRI rendering of functional activity in the occipital lobe secondary to a visual stimulus.

benign and malignant spinal processes and is further unique in its inherent noninvasive ability to image the spinal cord and surrounding structures. Structures such as CSF, dura, and adjacent ligaments are routinely seen and evaluated. The utility of spine MRI can be discussed in terms of the three classic categories of spine disease: extradural, intradural-extramedullary, and intramedullary processes.

A frequent cause of epidural disease is intervertebral disc pathology. MRI can uniquely image the intervertebral disc directly, without the use of contrast material. Disc integrity can be assessed in terms of degeneration, abnormal disc bulges, or herniations. High-resolution T2-weighted images of the disc can diagnose annular and circumferential tears that previously required injection of contrast material (i.e., CT discography). Any effect on spinal contents, either the spinal cord or existing nerves in the cervical and thoracic regions, or nerve impingement on either the cauda equina or existing nerve roots in the lumbar region can be assessed. Additionally, inherent signal aberrations within the intervertebral discs can also be analyzed for primary intrinsic disc abnormalities such as infectious discitis and associated vertebral osteomyelitis.

Although MRI is inherently poor for showing dense, cortical bone, it is extremely useful in the evaluation of infiltrative bone marrow diseases. Both degenerative and malignant bone marrow changes can be detected and categorized based on MR signal patterns. Benign processes such as post-traumatic bone edema, fatty bone marrow infiltration, or benign neoplasms such as primary vertebral hemangiomas can be readily distinguished from carcinomatous changes (i.e., vertebral plasmacytoma or frank metastatic disease with or without vertebral destruction or paravertebral soft tissue involvement). MRI is also useful in the analysis of degenerative spondylosis and complications of spondyloarthropathies as well as in the evaluation of benign or malignant spinal canal or foraminal stenosis. MRI is pivotal in the emergency evaluation of post-traumatic spinal cord compression.

Infrequently, intradural extramedullary masses present for evaluation. In the cervical and thoracic regions, meningiomas, neuromas, and arachnoid cysts predominate, whereas, in the lumbar spine, schwannomas, ependymomas or, rarely, intradural disc herniations are more common. Occasionally, intradural extramedullary metastases are encountered that may stud the spinal cord and meninges with metastatic deposits.

MRI is uniquely sensitive in detecting the presence of intramedullary spinal cord diseases. Common primary intramedullary neoplasms that can be elucidated include astrocytoma, ependymoma, and spinal cord hemangioblastoma. Contrast medium–enhanced MRI can help differentiate spinal cord edema, as seen in these entities, from the primary tumoral masses. Other causes of abnormal signal within the spinal cord include inflammatory or demyelinating diseases such as acute disseminating encephalomyelitis, transverse myelitis, and multiple sclerosis. The evaluation of spinal cord edema secondary to trauma, either from chronic discogenic disease or in situations of acute complex fracture injuries, is essential, particularly in national trauma centers.

Magnetic Resonance Angiography

BASIC PRINCIPLES AND TECHNIQUES

MRI techniques have been developed to image the flowing blood. Magnetic resonance angiography (MRA) and venography (MRV) are used to study the flow in various vessels and have proved to be robust in routine clinical examination of vascular diseases. In this section the basic underlying principles of MRA and the major clinical uses are discussed.

There are two major MRA techniques that are used in MRI that exploit either the longitudinal spin magnetization or transverse spin magnetization of the protons in blood to visualize flowing blood. They are the time-of-flight (TOF) technique, which utilizes the inflow-outflow of the moving spins within the selected imaging volume to image the blood flow, and the phase-contrast technique, which utilizes the flow-induced phase variations of the MRA signal caused by the motion of the blood. These MRA techniques by convention depict the blood flow as bright in contrast to the dark surrounding stationary tissues. The MRA data are post-processed with a maximum intensity projection (MIP) algorithm and may be displayed in multiple angiographic projections and angulations.

NORMAL FINDINGS

The TOF method uses the longitudinal magnetization, such that the blood flowing into the selected volume during the RF excitation period is fully relaxed, whereas the magnetization from the stationary tissue is saturated, and hence the signal from the blood is brighter compared with that of the stationary tissue. This phenomenon was first described in a nonimaging context by Singer.[24] After RF excitation, the longitudinal magnetization recovers exponentially with time constraint T1 and is typically much longer than with T2W. In a volume of stationary tissue and flowing blood, during every TR interval, the magnetization recovers incompletely throughout the volume, acquiring T1W that suppresses particularly the signals with longer T1. This is referred to as saturation. The degree of T1W depends on the solution of the Bloch equation, which is a function of TR, T1, and the excitation flip angle $\propto$. Usually a TR of 30 to 100 msec and flip angles of 10 to 60 degrees are used. These imaging parameters can be optimized for maximum suppression of the stationary tissues and better flow visualization.

In TOF imaging, faster flow through a vessel lumen running perpendicularly through the slice partially or completely exits the slice in the interval between the 90- and 180-degree excitation pulses.[25] Consequently, the 180-degree pulse fails to invert the nuclei, and the signal is diminished. However, with slow flow, washout of the spins between the 90-degree and the 180-degree pulses is minimal. The previously excited outgoing slice is replaced during the TR interval by the inflow of fully magnetized spins from outside the volume, giving a brighter signal than the one acquired from stationary tissue. This phenomenon is generally referred to as entry phenomenon or flow-related enhancement. Furthermore, the heavy T1W associated with these short TR sequences suppresses stationary tissue, an important contributor to the contrast between the stationary and the flowing signal. Therefore, the TOF method primarily uses these flow-related enhancement phenomena to image the blood vessels.

Two major techniques exist in TOF MRA: two-dimensional TOF (2D TOF) and three-dimensional TOF (3D TOF) imaging techniques. Two-dimensional TOF is advantageous because of its sensitivity to slow flow rates, minimal saturation effects for normal flow velocities, and short acquisition times (5 to 7 minutes). Although widely used, the technique has a few limitations. The appearance of the moving blood varies when the imaging plane is not perpendicular to the slice select direction. Owing to the in-plane flow, the blood vessels that run parallel to the imaging plane experience multiple RF pulses and eventually become saturated. Hence, the portion of the vessel traversing the imaging plane may exhibit some reduction in signal intensity and appear artifactually narrowed or even discontinued. Preliminary work with 2D TOF and magnetization transfer (MT) in the carotid artery bifurcation has shown an improved signal-to-noise ratio (SNR) and greater sharpness of vessel margins.[26] The 3D TOF MRA technique offers a wide number of advantages over its 2D counterpart. The 3D volume acquisition techniques offer superior SNR and high spatial resolution and are sensitive to fast and intermediate flow. The other major advantage of this technique is that the acquisition can be made in thin slices, thereby reducing voxel size and hence decreasing intravoxel dephasing of the moving blood. The use of surface coil along with small imaging voxels has been shown to significantly improve SNR and vessel conspicuity in normal and diseased carotid arteries.[27] Three-dimensional TOF is relatively insensitive to slow flow and is effective only for relatively small 3D volumes, because blood is saturated by multiple RF pulses while traversing the slab. Recently, MRA using 3D TOF with MT has been widely used in routine clinical imaging of the circle of Willis owing to their excellent stationary tissue suppression capabilities.[28] Preliminary work with 3D TOF acquired with dual 20- and 60-degree flip angles demonstrates improved SNR and vessel definition.[29] Contrast-enhanced 3D TOF imaging has further enhanced detail to near angiographic quality.

In contrast to TOF, the phase-contrast angiography technique uses the flow-induced phase variations of the MRA signal caused by the motion of the blood. These phase shifts induced by blood flow can be selectively modulated using bipolar flow-encoding gradients, and, therefore, images of flow can be generated. With this strategy, two sets of data are acquired under identical conditions, except that the polarity of the bipolar flow-encoding gradients is alternated during data acquisition. This modulates the velocity-induced phase shift for spins having macroscopic motion (flowing blood) and has no effect on stationary spins. MRA projections are created by subtraction of one data set from another, remove the signal from stationary tissues, and retain the signal from the flow. Moreover, the phase shift of the image can also be used to obtain a phase map of the image. This phase map is usually displayed in gray scale and indicates the regions where flow has occurred.

The two most popular methods that are currently used image the slab volume either with sequential time-averaged 2D slices[30] or with simultaneous acquisition of 3D volume slabs[31] and are generally referred to as 2D or 3D phase-contrast angiography. The 2D phase-contrast angiograms, like 2D TOF, are obtained as sequential individual slices. In 3D phase-contrast MRA the data are collected in three dimensions. This has several advantages over the 2D phase-contrast technique, such as isotropic voxels, reduction in phase variations, and flexibility in cross-sectional presentation of the feature of interest. However, the overall imaging time is much higher as compared with the 2D technique. In the past few years, cine phase-contrast MRA, a variant of 2D phase-contrast MRA in which cardiac gating is used to generate images at different points within the cardiac cycle, has become widely used. This method has been used to analyze temporal flow of blood in carotid arteries in the neck[32] and flow of CSF in the brain.[33]

NEUROLOGICAL APPLICATIONS IN DIAGNOSIS AND TREATMENT

Extracranial Disease

Carotid Bifurcation Lesions. One of the primary uses of MRA is the evaluation of the lesions in the carotid artery bifurcation. Atherosclerotic lesions within the carotid bulb and proximal internal carotid artery are major factors contributing to the development of cerebrovascular ischemia. The appropriate treatment of patients with asymptomatic and symptomatic carotid stenosis remains controversial. The North American Symptomatic Carotid Endarterectomy Trial[34] and the European Carotid Surgery Trial[35] demonstrated that patients with transient ischemic attacks or nondisabling stroke ipsilateral to a carotid stenosis of 70 percent or more have been found to have a significant incidence of further strokes. In a group of patients with asymptomatic carotid stenosis of 50 percent or more, Hobson and associates and the Veterans Affairs Cooperative Study Group showed that carotid endarterectomy reduced the overall incidence of ipsilateral neurological events in this population.[36] Although the exact degree of carotid stenosis that would affect patient management (i.e., medical or surgical) has not been definitely determined, these studies have set the current trends. Noninvasive techniques that accurately measure the degree of carotid stenosis will continue to be a very important part in the workup of these patients. Figure 23–16 shows an example of an MRA of a complex stenosis.

Atherosclerotic disease is most prevalent at arterial bifurcations and usually involves the carotid bulb of the internal carotid artery. The development of plaque and stenosis at the carotid bulb is believed to be related to the anatomy of the carotid bifurcation and associated complex hemodynamic forces that cause microscopic intimal injury and subsequent initiation of the atherosclerotic cascade. The complex flow (vortices, separation of flow streams, and slow flow) within the carotid bifurcation is well demonstrated using computer simulation based on images obtained by digital subtraction angiography (DSA) and MRA.[24]

Complex flow is one of the major causes of intravoxel dephasing, which leads to signal loss in MRA. An example of MRA signal loss distal to a carotid stenosis is shown in Figure 23–17. Comparison is made with DSA and computer simulation of temporal blood in this vessel. DSA remains the gold standard to characterize carotid bifurcation disease; however, numerous investigations have shown that noninvasive MRA has the potential to replace DSA as a screening test and obviate the need for diagnostic carotid angiography.[37, 38]

Intracranial Disease

Lesions in the Circle of Willis. The primary uses of circle of Willis MRA are to screen for the presence of unruptured aneurysms that came to medical attention due to incidental discovery by MRI and to assess for the presence of intracranial atherosclerotic disease. The use of MRA as a noninvasive screening test to identify congenital berry aneurysms before rupture in groups at risk (e.g., adult polycystic kidney disease, family history of aneurysm) would also be desirable. Several studies have shown that the sensitivity of MRA to detect congenital aneurysms 5 mm or greater is approximately 90 percent.[39–41] Figure 23–18 shows an aneurysm detected with MRA. Aneurysms smaller than 5 mm do rupture, although the incidence is reduced. MRA is considered an accurate noninvasive screening test for patients at risk for aneurysms. Conventional DSA, however, remains the gold standard for preoperative planning as well as for the assessment of ruptured aneurysms resulting in subarachnoid hemorrhage. Nevertheless, MRA frequently may have a complementary role in the assessment of patients suffering subarachnoid hemorrhage when DSA is inconclusive.

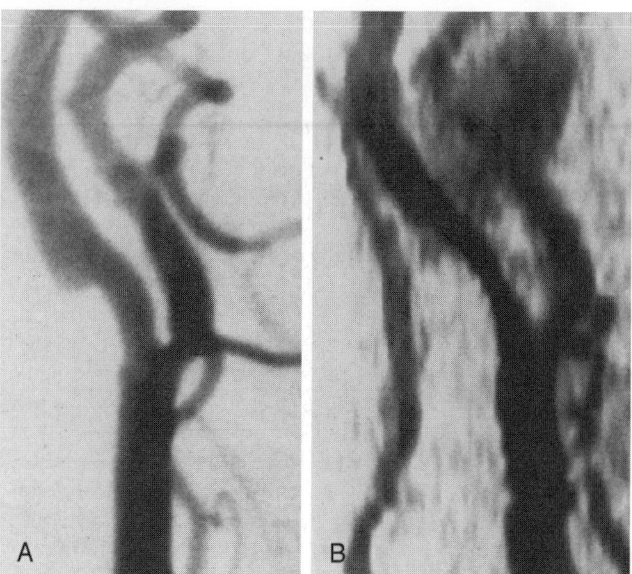

FIGURE 23–17. Carotid bifurcation of patient with atherosclerotic disease. *A,* Selected digital subtraction arteriogram of carotid artery bifurcation showing a mild to moderate (approximately 33 percent) stenosis in the proximal internal carotid artery. *B,* Axial two-dimensional TOF (surface coil) shows a smooth, approximately 50 percent stenosis in the proximal internal carotid artery. Exaggeration of the degree and length of stenosis is present. For color simulation of vascular flow pattern in the carotid bifurcation in this patient during the acceleration phase of systole, see the CD-ROM. (From Faro SH, Vinitski S, Ortega HV, et al: Carotid magnetic resonance angiography: Improved image quality with dual 3-inch surface coils. Neuroradiology 1996;38:403–408.)

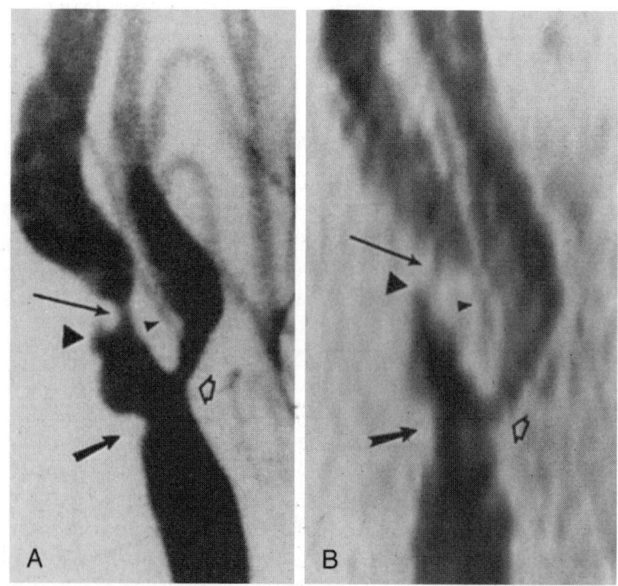

FIGURE 23–16. Carotid bifurcation of a patient with arteriosclerosis. *A,* Digital subtraction arteriogram shows mild stenosis in proximal carotid bulb *(short arrow)*, moderate to marked stenosis in external carotid artery *(open arrow)*, and marked stenosis (approximately 85 percent) in distal bulb/proximal internal carotid artery *(long, thin arrow)*. Contrast medium collection probably represents ulceration *(large arrowhead)*. Ascending pharyngeal artery *(small arrowhead)*. *B,* Axial two-dimensional TOF (surface coil). Accurate demonstration of moderate to marked stenosis in external carotid artery *(open arrow)*. Small elongation of mild stenosis in proximal bulb *(arrow)*. Slight exaggeration of marked stenosis (to approximately 90 percent) in distal bulb/proximal internal carotid artery *(long, thin arrow)*. Signal is lost within the proximal portion of this stenosis. Ulceration *(large arrowhead)* and ascending pharyngeal artery *(small arrowhead)* are identified. (From Faro SH, Vinitski S, Ortega HV, et al: Carotid magnetic resonance angiography: Improved image quality with dual 3-inch surface coils. Neuroradiology 1996;38:403–408.)

Other Applications. Vascular malformations, either pial (intramedullary) or dural (extramedullary), may be detected with MRA. Serpiginous flow patterns and voids, either within or extrinsic to the spinal cord, can suggest specific diagnoses. Even the presence of unexplained spinal cord edema may suggest angiodysgenic myelomalacia (Foix-Alajouanine syndrome) in the presence of an underlying vascular malformation. Intravenous contrast medium administration in MRI of the spine further aids in the delineation of spinal cord tumors and has proved helpful in the evaluation of the postoperative spine, particularly in the differentiation between nonenhancing recurrent disc herniation from enhancing postoperative scar.

Magnetic Resonance Venography

The MR method to examine the cerebral venous system including the dural sinuses is MRV. A 2D TOF technique is used, which has the advantage of increased sensitivity to slower-flowing vessels and generally a larger region of coverage in comparison to 3D TOF techniques. Two-dimensional TOF is a slice-by-slice technique, and flow-

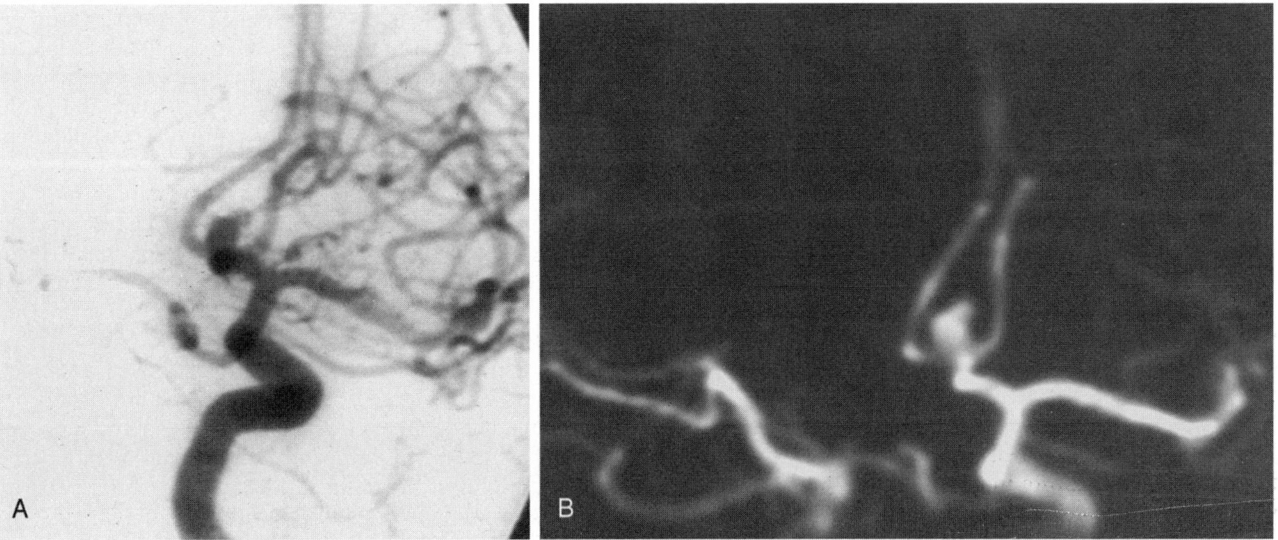

FIGURE 23–18. *A,* DSA image shows a well-defined 5- to 6-mm anterior communicating artery aneurysm with distal tip. *B,* Three-dimensional TOF MRA accurately shows the aneurysm.

related signal is maximized when a flowing vessel is perpendicular to the imaging slice. Patients are primarily scanned in the coronal plane using a slice thickness of 1.5 to 2 mm. Coronal imaging maximizes flow in the superior sagittal sinus (SSS) and transverse sinuses. Decreased flow may occur in the distal SSS due to in-plane dephasing artifact (flowing vessel is parallel to the imaging slice). An additional axial 2D TOF MRV through the region of the distal SSS may be used to decrease dephasing artifact. Note that the transverse sinus may be congenitally small (most commonly the left) and may mimic a thrombosed vessel. Examination of the raw data prior to the MIP postprocessing will demonstrate the congenitally attenuated vessel. Patients with the diagnosis of thrombosis of the SSS or transverse sinuses can be assessed and followed with serial MRV studies (Fig. 23–19).

Myelography

BASIC PRINCIPLES AND TECHNIQUES

The beginning of myelography has its "roots" in the early 1900s when subarachnoid injections of air were performed to localize spinal cord tumors. This technique of pneumomyelography was eventually supplanted by the subarachnoid injection of an iodized poppy seed oil, Lipiodol, the myelographic medium of choice during the 1930s. Lipiodol had its disadvantages, including a very high viscosity, its immiscibility with CSF (thereby making it difficult to perform satisfactory diagnostic studies as well as remove on completion of the study), and its irritating nature to the leptomeninges. In 1940, Pantopaque was introduced. This oil-based contrast agent was less viscid and less irritating to the leptomeninges

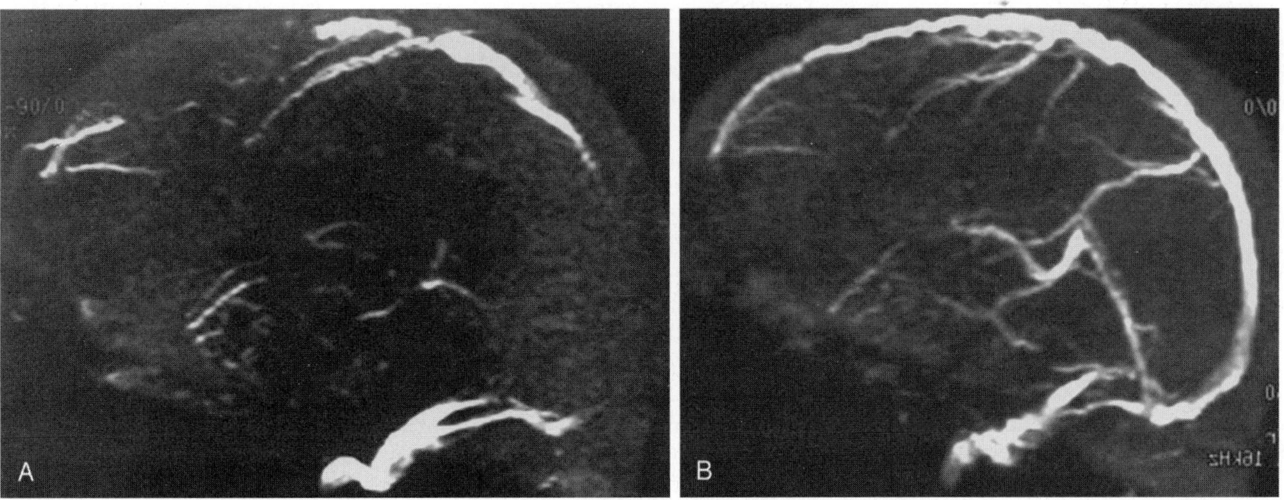

FIGURE 23–19. *A,* MRV shows loss of flow-related signal in the proximal and distal and straight sinuses (SS) and superior sagittal sinus (SSS) in a patient with dehydration and dural sinus thrombosis. *B,* Follow-up MRV showed reconstitution of the SSS and SS.

than Lipiodol. Its lower specific gravity allowed it to flow more freely in the subarachnoid space with fewer tendencies to form large irregular globules; accordingly, removal on completion of the study was easier to perform than its predecessor. Pantopaque soon became the contrast medium of choice in the United States until the late 1970s, although it was still far from being an ideal subarachnoid contrast agent. Its relative immiscibility in CSF resulted in its inability to enter nerve root sleeves, thereby making it difficult to evaluate far posterolateral disc abnormalities. A 20-gauge spinal needle or larger was required during Pantopaque insertion and removal, and the use of this relatively large-sized needle commonly resulted in spinal headaches from CSF leakage at the puncture site. Furthermore, Pantopaque was still difficult to remove in entirety after completion of the study. When left behind, Pantopaque was absorbed slowly at the rate of approximately 1 mL/yr and could further produce local changes of arachnoiditis.

In the early 1930s, experimental studies were carried out with Abrodil, a water-soluble organic iodine compound widely used in the Scandinavian countries for lumbar myelography. Abrodil never achieved popularity in the United States as a result of its marked hypertonicity in comparison to CSF, which produced significant irritation to the leptomeninges and neural elements. Water-soluble myelography was revitalized in the United States during the early 1970s with the introduction of Conray and Dimer-X, salts of iodinated acids. These compounds, like Abrodil, caused significant neurotoxic effects, including meningeal and radicular irritation, as a result of their hypertonicity.

As a result of ongoing investigations, metrizamide was marketed as a synthetic nonionic water-soluble contrast medium that had a much lower osmolality than the salts of iodinated acids. This contrast agent provided safe examination of the entire spinal column without significant neurotoxicity.

Within recent years, in an attempt to further reduce the incidence of serious side effects, other nonionic water-soluble contrast agents, such as Isovue and Omnipaque, have been synthesized and are now in wide use. In many institutions, iopamidol (Isovue) is used for subarachnoid injections. In the concentration used for lumbar myelography (200 mg iodine/mL), iopamidol is only mildly hyperosmolar when compared with CSF (413 vs. 301 mOsm/kg H_2O) and has dramatically fewer neurotoxic side effects than the salts of iodinated acids. Iopamidol is rapidly excreted in the kidneys with undetectable plasma levels at 48 hours in the absence of renal dysfunction. The most common adverse reactions are headache, nausea, vomiting, and transient worsening of neck, back, or leg symptomatology. Hypotensive collapse and shock are rare, with only isolated reports being found in the literature. The usual recommended adult dose range for iopamidol when performing myelographic procedures is 2000 to 3000 mg iodine. This is equivalent to 10 to 15 mL Isovue-M200, which is used for lumbar myelography, and to 10 mL maximum Isovue-M300, which is used for cervical myelography. Modern myelographic studies are approached via lumbar injection of contrast material, and virtually all patients have a postmyelogram CT evaluation to supplement the conventional diagnostic myelographic imaging procedure.

Before a myelogram is performed, certain information should be obtained from all patients. In those individuals with a prior history of dye allergy, bronchial asthma, hay fever, and food allergies, premedication with corticosteroids and antihistamines is indicated to prevent or minimize possible allergic reactions. Patients should also be well hydrated before and after the myelographic procedure. Dehydration may contribute to acute renal failure in patients with a history of diabetes, advanced vascular disease, or pre-existing renal disease. Knowledge as to current prescription and nonprescription medications as well as underlying disease states is extremely important. Specifically, elective studies should not be performed on patients who are receiving oral or intravenous anticoagulants, and the use of aspirin should be discontinued for approximately 48 hours before the myelographic procedure. Drugs that lower the seizure threshold such as monoamine oxidase inhibitors, tricyclic antidepressants, and central nervous system stimulants should be withheld for 48 hours before and after the myelographic procedure. Prior to myelography, serum creatinine, blood urea nitrogen, and coagulation profile including prothrombin time, partial thromboplastin time, and platelet counts may be obtained to access procedure risk, particularly in the elderly population.

During lumbar myelography, a 22-gauge spinal needle is inserted either in the midline between the spinous processes or slightly off midline through the rhomboid fossa at the level of L2–L3, or L3–L4. This puncture site is preferred over the L4–L5 and L5–S1 levels because of the higher incidence of herniated discs and spinal stenosis at these lower levels. Alternatively, if premyelography imaging studies or certain clinical information is available, the puncture site can be performed at these lower lumbar levels when significant disease is known to exist at the level of L2–L3. The lumbar injection should be performed slowly over a period of 1 to 2 minutes to avoid excessive mixing with CSF and subsequent loss of contrast medium as well as premature cephalad dispersion.

In most instances, cervical myelography can be adequately performed by means of a lumbar puncture with subsequent fluoroscopic guidance of a more concentrated dose of contrast medium into the cervical region by gravity. Alternatively, a lateral C1–C2 puncture can be performed with the needle placement in the posterior third of the spinal canal between the C1–C2 neural arches. At all costs, intracranial entry of a bolus of contrast medium should be avoided because this could possibly lead to acute neurotoxic effects.

Meticulous radiographic technique is essential to obtain quality diagnostic examinations. Low voltage (KVp) with optimal milliampere-seconds (mas) maximizes contrast detail. Air gaps should also be eliminated to reduce scatter and increase edge sharpness. In both the lumbar and the cervical regions, AP, lateral, shallow, and steep oblique views should be obtained with the addition of AP and lateral views of the conus during lumbar myelography. For thoracic myelography, AP and lateral views are routinely filmed.

Postmyelography CT of abnormal lumbar disc levels should be performed in the prone position. Imaging can be deferred for up to 4 hours to reduce the degree of contrast within the desired area to be studied. Before obtaining the postmyelogram CT scan, the patient should be helped to roll over several times to thoroughly mix the contrast medium and avoid pooling in dependent portions of the spinal canal.

Routine postprocedure orders include keeping the patient's head elevated 30 to 45 degrees for 12 to 24 hours with close neurological monitoring. Oral fluids should be encouraged and diet prescribed as tolerated. All movements should be monitored by hospital personnel and performed slowly with the patient's head maintained in an upright position.

NORMAL FINDINGS

Routinely, with either cervical or lumbar myelography, there is symmetrical filling of the nerve root sleeves without evidence of nerve root displacement or nerve root sleeve truncation. The size and direction of the spinal roots vary at different levels. The largest roots are the lower lumbar and upper sacral roots, which innervate the lower extremities. Accordingly, the roots of the lower four cervical and first thoracic nerves are also large, owing to their upper extremity innervation. The upper cervical and remaining thoracic nerve roots are rather small in comparison, and the lower sacral and coccygeal nerve roots are the smallest. Discrepancies in length and direction of spinal nerve roots are secondary to the spinal cord being much shorter than the vertebral canal. In the cervical region, the relatively short nerve root traverses the lower portion of its respective neural canal in a horizontal direction. The thoracic nerve roots are directed obliquely downward, with the length and degree of obliquity increasing from the upper to the lower thoracic levels. Because the spinal cord ends at approximately L1, the lumbar, sacral, and coccygeal nerve roots descend in a nearly parallel course, with the length of the roots increasing successively from above downward. This group of nerve roots below the level of termination of the cord is termed the *cauda equina*. The thecal sac should have a smooth contour without evidence of narrowing or mass effect from extradural abnormalities. There should be smooth tapering of the distal thecal sac at a variable distance below the L5–S1 disc space to a smooth "pencil point" appearance. The silhouette of the cervical and thoracic cord as well as the appearance and position of the conus should be closely scrutinized for intramedullary expansile lesions.

TYPES OF DETECTABLE ABNORMALITIES

The use of water-soluble intrathecal contrast medium has markedly decreased over the past 10 to 15 years with the introduction of CT and, more recently, MRI. Before these more advanced imaging tools, water-soluble myelography was the gold standard in evaluating patients with back pain and had the ability to evaluate spinal stenosis, disc bulges and herniations, other extradural impressions on the thecal sac, spinal cord enlargement, and various inflammatory conditions. However, intrathecal contrast medium enhancement still lacked sensitivity in evaluating lateral disc herniations and specificity in determining the exact cause for extradural impressions on the thecal sac and cord enlargement. With the use of CT and MRI, it is now possible to further define the factors contributing to spinal stenosis and to offer a much more exact and detailed differential diagnosis for the etiology of intramedullary lesions. With this added preciseness has come the general acceptance of these imaging modalities over myelography by other physicians not formally trained in radiological sciences.

Certain situations still warrant the use of water-soluble myelography. In extremely obese patients, in whom image resolution is significantly degraded on both CT and MRI studies, myelography in conjunction with postmyelography CT of abnormal levels still plays an important role in the diagnosis of spinal disease. Likewise, in patients with marked claustrophobia, in patients in whom MRI is contraindicated (e.g., those patients with intracerebral aneurysm clips, pacemakers, transcutaneous electrical nerve stimulation units, orbital metallic foreign bodies), or in patients with postoperative metallic internal fixation devices, myelography and postmyelography CT remain the imaging studies of choice. In our experience, myelography, in conjunction with postmyelography CT, is as sensitive in the evaluation of subtle cases of arachnoiditis as MRI.

NEUROLOGICAL APPLICATIONS IN DIAGNOSIS AND TREATMENT

Extradural Spinal Lesions

The most common disorder seen while performing myelography is the extradural defect. Ventral extradural defects at the level of the disc space are caused by a variety of conditions, including disc bulges, disc herniations, posterior endplate spur formation, epidural hematomas, inflammatory processes, and epidural tumor, with or without associated adjacent bone involvement. Anterolateral extradural defects at the level of the disc space are routinely caused by posterolateral disc herniations, which will also result in nerve root displacement or nerve root sleeve truncation and the classic double-density sign seen on a lateral radiograph with the patient in the prone position (Fig. 23–20). Posterior and posterolateral extradural defects at or near the level of the disc space are usually the result of chronic degenerative changes of the posterior elements, including hypertrophic facet disease, ligamentum flavum hypertrophy, and the occasional synovial cyst arising from a markedly degenerated facet joint. Less common causes include metastatic disease to the posterior elements in association with a posterior epidural tumor component. An anterior or anterolateral extradural defect not limited to the disc space level could be the result of a migrated free disc fragment, epidural hematoma, inflammatory process, or metastasis. Far lateral disc herniations within the lateral aspect of the neural canal that extend beyond filling of the nerve root sleeve are radiographically silent on myelography. Similarly, a significant percentage of disc bulges and herniations at the L5–S1 level are nondescript using conventional myelography owing to the rather prominent anterior epidural space at this level that allows for posterior extension of disc material without associated thecal sac compression or nerve root displacement.

Intramedullary Spinal Lesions

Intramedullary lesions causing enlargement of the spinal cord or conus with concomitant narrowing of the adjacent subarachnoid space include primary cord neoplasms such as ependymomas, astrocytomas, and hemangioblastomas;

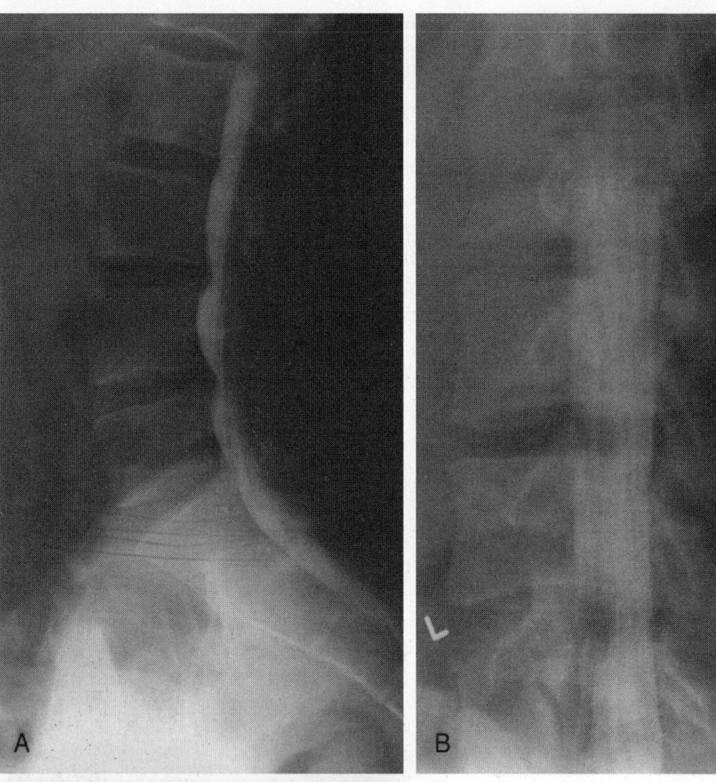

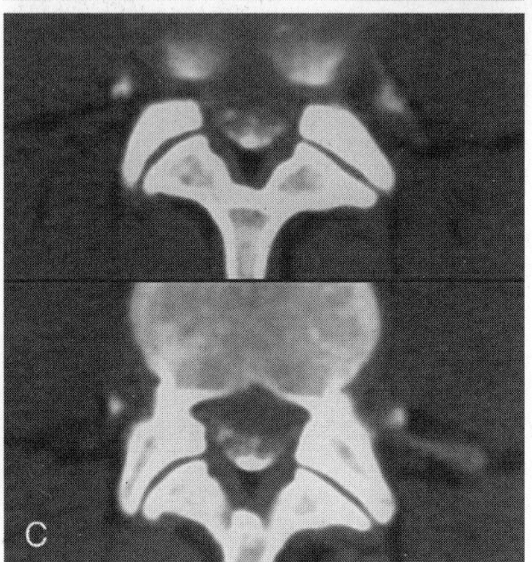

FIGURE 23–20. *A,* Prone cross-table lateral view of lumbar myelogram. Prominent ventral impressions upon the contrast column are present at L3–L4 and L4–L5. Much milder ventral impressions are seen at L2–L3 and L5–S1. A so-called double-density sign consistent with an eccentric posterior disc herniation is present at L3–L4 and L4–L5. *B,* Prone left anterior oblique view of lumbar myelogram. Left-sided filling defects are present at L3–4 and L4–L5 secondary to eccentric posterior disc herniations at both levels. *C,* Axial CT scans at and just below L3–L4 disc space demonstrate moderate-sized broad-based central and left-sided posterior disc herniation extending into left lateral recess. This eccentric posterior disc herniation would account for the double-density sign seen in *A.*

metastases; inflammatory conditions such as sarcoidosis and abscess formation; cord hematomas and infarcts; vascular malformations; and congenital lipomas, dermoids, and epidermoids. Although these groups of lesions will most certainly cause widening of the silhouette of the cord or conus, the intrinsic pathology and extent of these intramedullary lesions are far better imaged with MRI.

Intradural Extramedullary Spinal Lesions

Intradural extramedullary lesions such as meningiomas and the majority of neurofibromas can be adequately studied with myelography followed by CT. Whereas the intrinsic characteristics of these lesions is best evaluated with MRI, myelography and postmyelography CT still play an important role in the presurgical evaluation of these lesions. Subtle cases of arachnoiditis or the determination of the level of a dural tear in a postoperative pseudomeningocele is as adequately visualized with myelography and postmyelography CT as with MRI (Fig. 23–21). Myelography and postmyelography CT are excellent diagnostic tools in evaluating patients with brachial plexus traction injuries presenting with nerve root sleeve tears and nerve root avulsion injuries. The communication of intradural and extradural arachnoid cysts, sacral cysts, and Tarlov cysts with the subarachnoid space can be accurately evaluated with myelography and postmyelography CT.

Neuroangiography

BASIC PRINCIPLES AND TECHNIQUES

Diagnostic neuroangiography is the study of the central nervous blood vessels and related cervicocerebral vasculature using radiographs obtained during the simultaneous injection

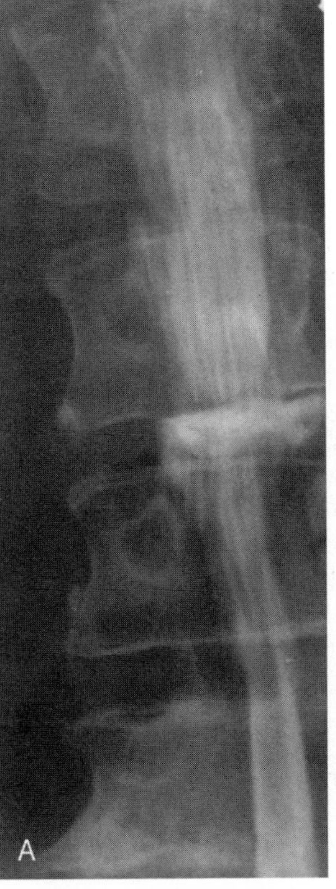

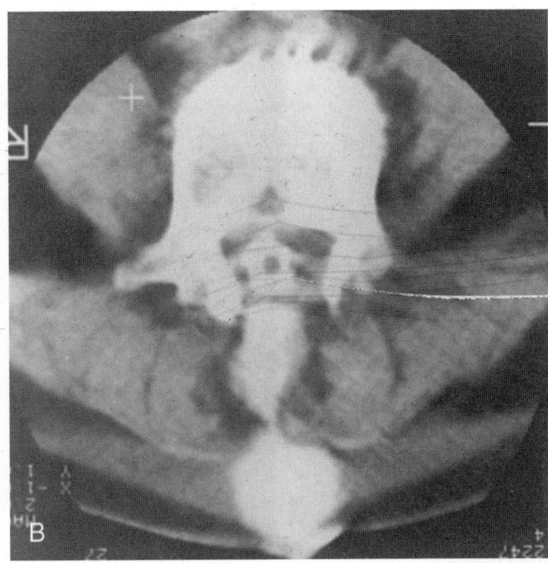

FIGURE 23–21. Adhesive arachnoiditis. *A,* Anteroposterior view of lumbar myelogram. The thecal sac below the level of the L2–L3 disc space is narrowed and featureless with central clumping of distal nerve roots giving the appearance of a pseudocord. Note absence of posterior elements at L3 and L4 secondary to prior decompressive laminectomy surgery. A small amount of contrast has inadvertently been injected into L2–L3 disc space during lumbar puncture. *B,* Postmyelogram CT scan through the L3–L4 disc space. Central clumping of lumbosacral nerve roots with "pseudocord" appearance is once again noted. Large bilobed pseudomeningocele protruding through laminectomy defect into deep and superficial soft tissues represents postoperative complication secondary to dural tear with continued CSF leak.

of intravascular contrast media. Cerebral angiography was first introduced by Moniz in 1927 and remains today, a vital tool in the neuroradiological evaluation of cerebrovascular diseases. Although neuroangiography had been historically used to evaluate many types of central nervous system diseases, CT and MRI have largely supplanted diagnostic angiography in the primary evaluation of central nervous system diseases.[42] Further, state-of-the-art CT and MRI offer advanced vascular imaging capabilities, yielding excellent "angiographic" types of information. Nevertheless, diagnostic neuroangiography continues to remain the gold standard in the evaluation of vascular diseases related to the head, neck, and spine, and further provides a platform for neurointerventional procedures.

The goal of neuroangiography is to define and outline the cerebral vasculature, both for diagnostic and potentially therapeutic purposes. Typical cerebral angiography is performed using the femoral arterial approach to gain access to the cerebrovascular arterial tree. Alternatively, in selected cases, the axillary, brachial, or direct cervical approaches may be used as necessary. After access, nonselective catheterization of the aortic arch or selective catheterizations of the cervical arteries (specifically, the carotid or vertebral arteries) can be performed. Contrast medium is injected through the catheter with simultaneous radiographic filming of appropriate vascular territories such that diagnostic images of the cerebral vasculature are obtained. Current microcatheter technology also permits superselective angiographic analysis of smaller branch vessels of the brain, for both diagnosis and management of intracranial diseases.

Conventional film-screen technology in modern cerebral angiography has largely been replaced by digital subtraction technology. State-of-the-art digital suites now image with a 1024^2 matrix resolution, providing exquisite vascular detail. In addition, digital angiography allows rapid image acquisition, instantaneous review, and pixel shifting capabilities, providing vascular resolution unsurpassed by conventional filming. For these reasons, conventional film-screen angiography is rapidly becoming outmoded, and most new, dedicated neuroangiographic suites are now constructed solely with digital angiographic capabilities.

NORMAL FINDINGS

Neuroangiography is used today primarily as a diagnostic modality in the evaluation of patients with vascular diseases of the central nervous system. Typical four-vessel cerebral angiography includes selective catheterizations of both internal carotid and vertebral arteries with angiographic filming in the AP, lateral, or oblique planes as needed. Additionally, imaging of the aortic arch as well as the cervical carotid and vertebral arteries may be necessary in the evaluation of many patients suffering cerebrovascular disease. Angiographic filming is acquired during the arterial, capillary, and venous phases, because each phase reveals important vascular information. For example, the arterial phase is critical in the evaluation of entities such as cerebral aneurysms, cervical or intracranial arterial stenosis, or arterial occlusions. In contrast, the capillary and venous phases may reveal important data regarding vascular malformations, tumor neovascularity, venous stenoses, or venous thrombi. The measurement of the intracranial transit time of contrast material may further provide insight regarding focal or diffuse central nervous system abnormalities. Therefore, all phases of the angiographic study can provide important information regarding the overall health of the central nervous system. Yet, angiography maintains flexibility in that studies may be tailored to answer specific clinical questions.

Risks of neuroangiography are generally related to the complexity of the angiographic procedure, with an estimated 1 percent overall incidence of neurological deficit and a 0.5 percent incidence of persistent deficit.[43] Risks include local bleeding or arterial injuries secondary to vascular access. The intra-arterial positioning of an angiographic catheter within the arterial tree carries a risk of injury to the intimal lining of the arterial wall, particularly in patients with pre-existing atherosclerosis. This, coupled with the intra-arterial injection of contrast media, presents a risk of arterial dissection or stroke due to distal embolization. Lastly, there are potential risks associated with the use of iodinated contrast material, including allergic reactions and systemic organ effects such as renal damage. In preparing to study a patient with an allergic history, the current recommendation is 50 mg of prednisone orally 13, 7, and 1 hour prior to the procedure. Diphenhydramine 50 mg orally may also be administered 1 hour prior to the procedure.

TYPES OF DETECTABLE ABNORMALITIES

Angiography may be useful in detecting vascular lesions causing focal or bilateral cerebral dysfunctions, subcortical dysfunctions, or brain stem or spinal cord abnormalities. Abnormal size and contour of the appropriate vessel lumen, abnormal distribution of vessels, and abnormal sequences of vascularization (early or late) can be seen. Additionally, displacement of vessels by extrinsic lesions can be detected along with endovascularization from tumors. In the section that follows, angiography is discussed in relationship to diagnosis and management of patients with ischemic brain disease, intracranial aneurysms, vascular malformations, and neoplasms. Although intracranial masses and their mass effects classically distort the cerebral vasculature, the primary diagnosis of intracranial masses has shifted to CT and MRI and is not addressed in this section. Angiography is not currently useful in the evaluation of peripheral nervous system or neuromuscular diseases.

NEUROLOGICAL APPLICATIONS IN DIAGNOSIS AND TREATMENT

Cranial Lesions

Ischemic Cerebrovascular Disease. Diagnostic angiography in ischemic brain disease allows evaluation of the cerebral circulation from the aortic arch level to the terminal intracranial vessels.[44] This provides a thorough evaluation for vascular lesions potentially causing stroke. Lesions most commonly diagnosed are atherosclerotic in origin. However, stenosis may be secondary to other entities, such as fibromuscular dysplasia, dissection, intimal hyperplasia, or radiation-induced vasculopathy. Cerebral angiography is also useful in evaluating patients with suspected vasculopathies. Angiography can uniquely identify abnormal regions of arterial narrowing or beading as seen in extracranial or intracranial arteritis (Fig. 23–22).

A primary goal in cerebrovascular disease therapy is stroke prevention. Hemodynamically significant stenosis carries an increased stroke risk, particularly when involving the carotid artery. Angiography remains key in detecting both extracranial and intracranial disease and allows precise characterization of inner plaque contour, including assessment of ulceration and stenosis measurement.

Traditionally, surgical treatments such as carotid endarterectomy have been the treatment of choice in the correction of cervical or intracranial stenosis.[45] A growing literature now supports the use of endovascular techniques as an alternative in controlling cerebrovascular disease.[46] The use of stent-

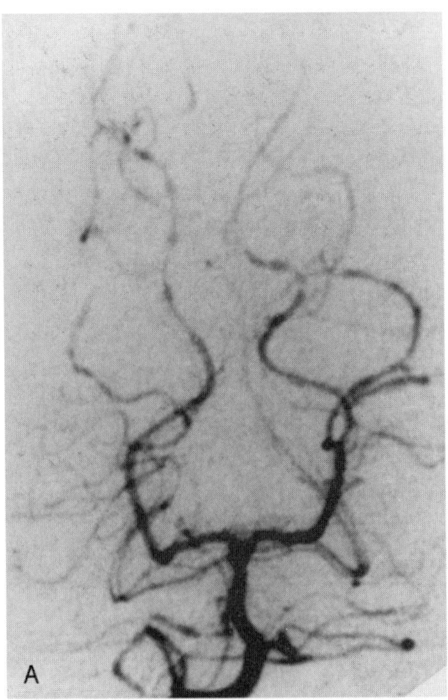

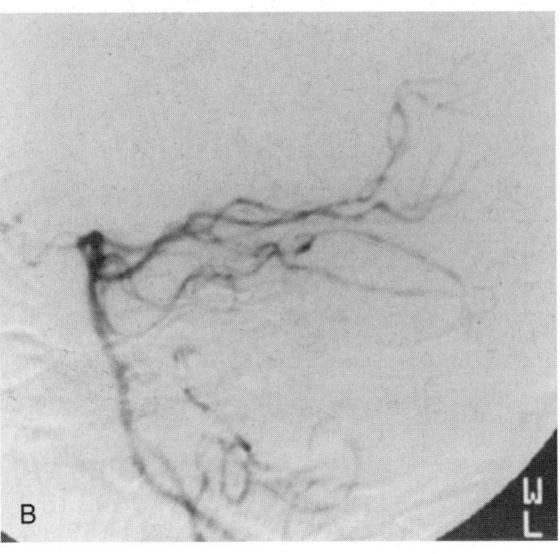

FIGURE 23–22. Arteritis. *A,* Anteroposterior right vertebral angiogram demonstrating diffuse beading of the posterior cerebral arteries. *B,* Lateral view.

supported percutaneous transluminal angioplasty (PTA) in the treatment of subclavian, vertebral, or even carotid territory stenosis is growing.[47] Advancing stent technology has further added to the success of cervical carotid PTA. Cervical carotid PTA trials are ongoing at this time, many of which include the use of distal embolization protection devices (i.e., umbrellas and balloons) (Fig. 23–23). These techniques will undoubtedly challenge carotid endarterectomy as the treatment method of choice for cervical carotid stenosis.[48–52] Further, intracranial PTA is now technically feasible in both the carotid and vertebral territories. Combination therapy may also be considered for tandem lesions.

Stroke literature now supports prompt neurointervention with thrombolytics in patients who generally present with major cerebral arterial occlusive disease within 6 hours of acute neurological symptoms. In these cases, angiography precisely localizes sites of arterial occlusion and accesses collateral vasculature. Microcatheter delivery of thrombolytic agents directly into the occlusive thrombus can potentially re-establish normal arterial flow. This treatment has the potential to avert an impending stroke or significantly reduce the overall extent of cerebral infarction.

Brain infarction or hemorrhage occasionally may result secondary to venous occlusive disease. CT or MRI ordinarily establishes the identification of venous thrombus. Angiography or cerebral venography may be necessary when the diagnosis is obscure. Angiography can demonstrate absence of flow within a dural sinus or identify intraluminal filling defects. When necessary, a thrombosed dural sinus can be treated with direct microcatheter delivery of thrombolytics, balloon angioplasty, or thrombectomy devices, resulting in clot lysis. The treatment goal here is to reduce vascular congestion and re-establish normal venous outflow.

Aneurysms and Vascular Malformations. Cerebral angiography remains the gold standard in the evaluation of patients suffering from subarachnoid hemorrhage. A complete angiographic evaluation of all cerebral arteries, particularly the circle of Willis bifurcations, is mandatory (Fig. 23–24A). Generally, in cases of suspected brain aneurysm, all cerebral vessels are studied because of the frequency of multiple aneurysms. Standard four-vessel angiography detects aneurysms in 85 percent of patients who present with subarachnoid hemorrhage. If initial angiography is negative, repeat angiography is generally indicated in 10 to 14 days, increasing aneurysm detection rate by approximately 5 percent. Many neurosurgical centers favor prompt neurosurgical or endovascular intervention in cases of acute subarachnoid hemorrhage. This is in an effort to eliminate the incidence of aneurysm rebleeding and sudden death. In addition to standard neurosurgical clipping, various detachable coil devices are now approved for intracranial aneurysm therapy in the United States, offering an endovascular alternative for treatment of intracranial aneurysms[53] (Fig. 23–24B).

Cerebral angiography is pivotal in the evaluation of central nervous system vascular malformations, particularly arteriovenous malformations (AVM). Although MRI is highly sensitive in detecting central nervous system malformations, precise vascular mapping of AVM remains essential. Angiography uniquely shows detailed information regarding the angioarchitecture of AVM (i.e., feeding arteries, nidus, and draining veins) (Fig. 23–25). Also, additional risk for AVM rupture, such as associated feeding arterial pedicle aneurysms or venous stenosis, can be identified. Treatment options such as surgical resection, endovascular embolization, radiotherapy, or combination remain dependent on precise angiographic characterization.

Neoplasm. The assessment of neovascularity may be warranted in the evaluation of selected intracranial tumors, particularly when surgical resection is planned. Embolization procedures in these types of cases are not intended to be cur-

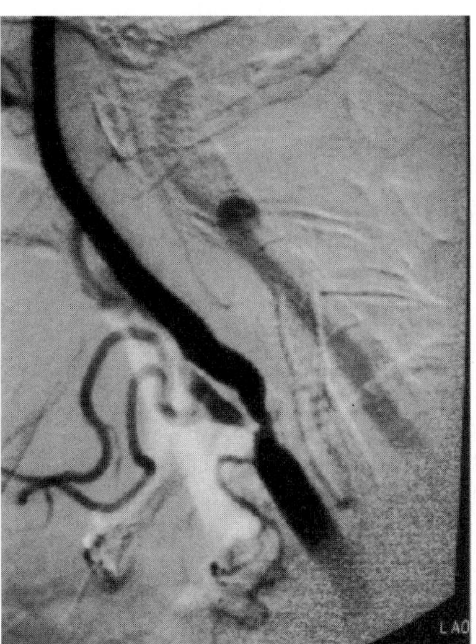

A

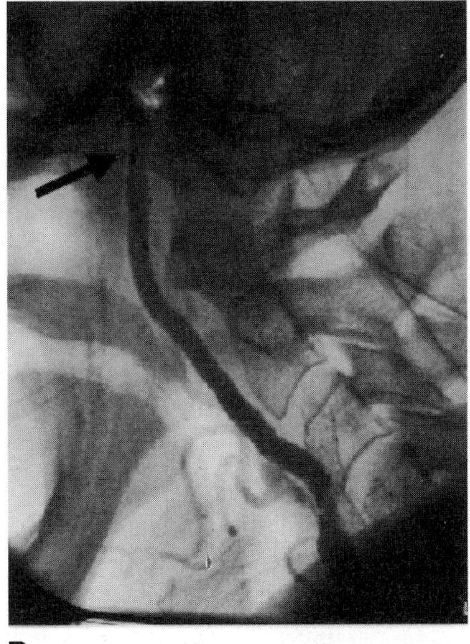
B

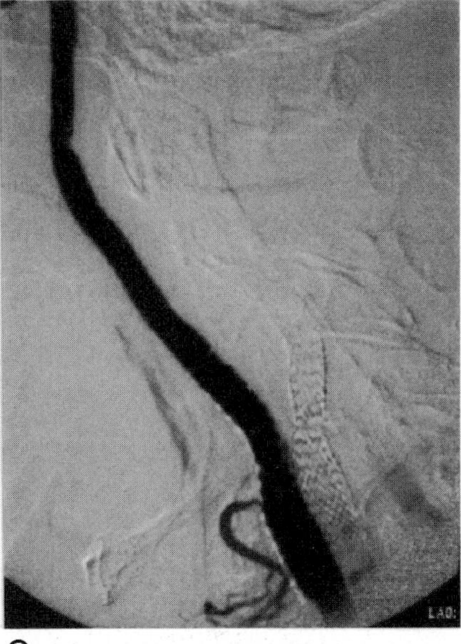

C

FIGURE 23–23. Carotid stent. *A,* Right common carotid arteriogram demonstrating high-grade internal carotid stenosis at the level of the cervical bifurcation. *B,* Introduction of filter wire providing distal protection. *C,* Post-stent supported angioplasty. No residual internal carotid artery stenosis remains.

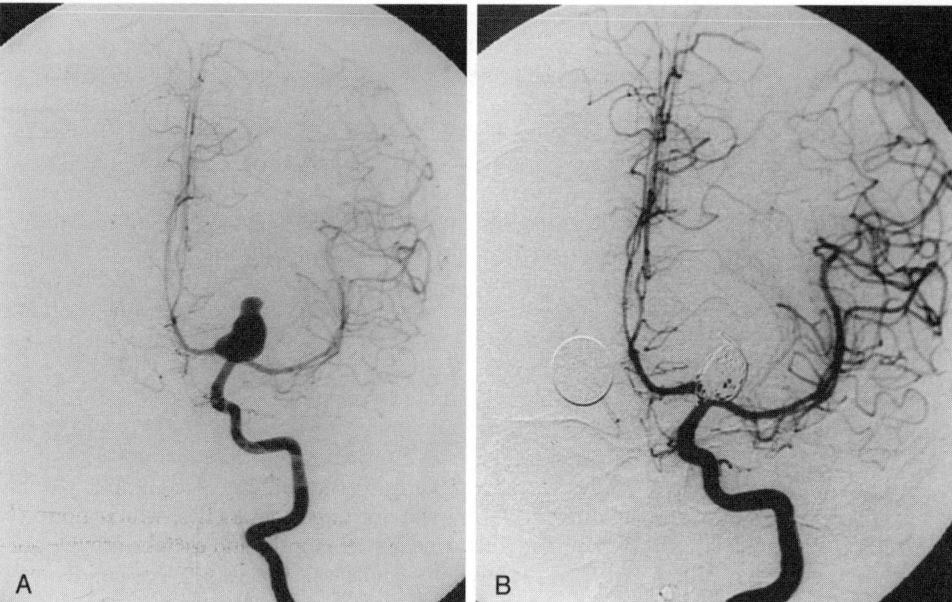

FIGURE 23–24. Aneurysm. *A,* Left internal carotid arteriogram demonstrating giant, lobulated internal carotid bifurcation aneurysm. *B,* Appearance following successful GDC coiling.

ative. Rather, embolization is used to reduce blood loss at surgery and help lower overall perioperative surgical morbidity. Intracranially, embolization is most commonly applied to bulky extra-axial tumors such as meningiomas to facilitate surgical resection. Cervical angiography and embolization may be helpful in managing the abnormal vascularity associated with head and neck tumors. These techniques can be useful in patients with paragangliomas of the head and neck, metastatic nodal disease from thyroid or kidney, and Castleman's disease. In these types of cases, the angiographic tumor blush can be quite intense and presurgical embolization can be very helpful.

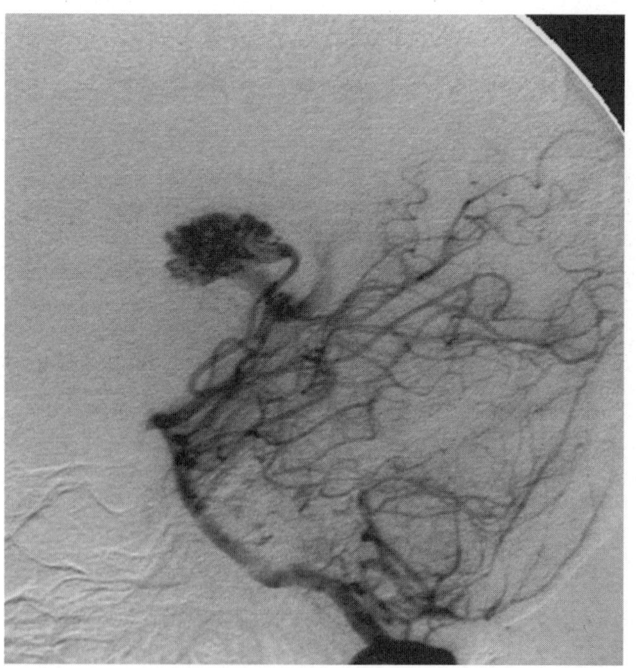

FIGURE 23–25. Vertebral angiogram demonstrating a deep left hemispheric arteriovenous malformation fed by the posterior choroidal artery with deep venous drainage.

Spinal Vascular Lesions

Spinal angiography remains key in the analysis of vascular disorders of the spine. Vascular malformations of the spinal cord lead to serious spinal cord morbidity and paralysis. The treatment plan frequently depends on angiographic delineation of these malformations. Angiography delineates the intramedullary or extramedullary location of the AVM nidus, the feeding arteries including their relationship to the artery of Adamkiewicz, and venous drainage (Fig. 23–26).

Neovascularity secondary to spinal cord tumors can be demonstrated angiographically, providing complementary information to CT and MRI. In selected cases, spinal embolization can also be a useful adjunct.[54] For example, vertebral hemangiomas, aneurysmal bone cysts, giant cell tumors, or metastatic disease of the spine can demonstrate intense vertebral neovascularity. Preoperative embolization can be valuable to attaining a successful surgical resection.

Ultrasonography

Diagnostic ultrasonography (US) uses sound waves above the audible level to generate diagnostic medical images. US operates on the principles of sound propagation; therefore, the patient is not exposed to ionizing radiation. US has various imaging applications, with specific uses in neurological disorders. It is readily available in hospitals or outpatient imaging facilities, and it typically is less costly than other, comparable diagnostic imaging modalities. Routinely, images are obtained in real time, within a gray scale format. US uses a variety of transducers, which are available for different applications. Diagnostic US can be coupled with Doppler devices, with or without color, allowing flow measurements in vascular structures, such as commonly employed for carotid artery studies.

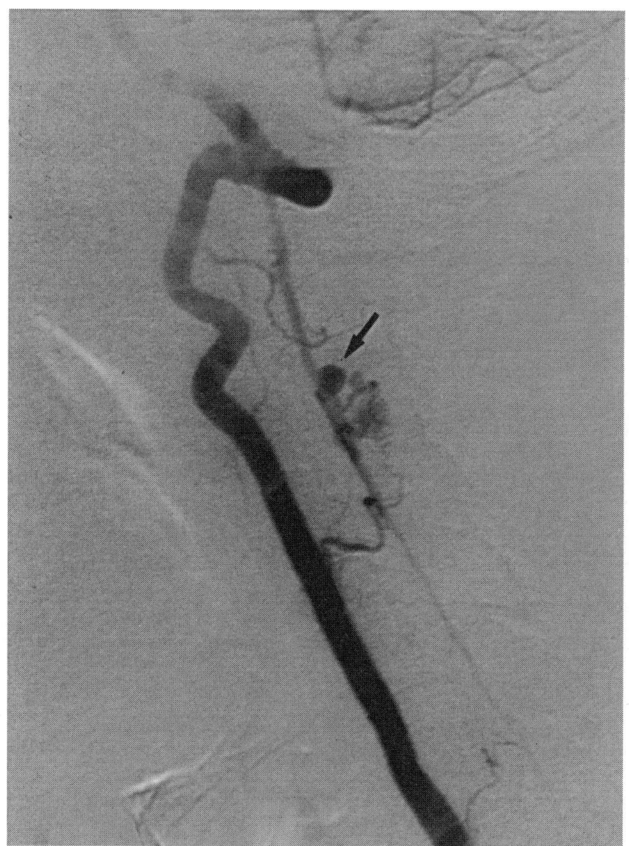

FIGURE 23–26. Right vertebral angiogram demonstrating a spinal arteriovenous malformation fed chiefly by a vertebral muscular branch vessel. An aneurysm is present on the arterial feeder *(arrow)*.

BASIC PRINCIPLES AND TECHNIQUES

Ultrasonography depends on the presence of sonographic "windows," which allow sound wave propagation and detection of echo signals. These signals form the basic sonographic units for image generation. Therefore, as a general rule, US is indicated when visualization of the target object is not blocked by intervening bone or air, such as calvarium or bowel gas. This limitation does not completely negate the use of US in the evaluation of adult brain disorders, as discussed later. The usefulness of US as an imaging tool in pediatrics is particularly appealing owing to its inherent lack of ionizing radiation.

Carotid US consists of gray scale imaging to assess location and extent of plaque and Doppler to measure flow velocities and degree of stenosis. Color may be added to the Doppler to improve visualization of the flow lumen and optimize the Doppler angle.[55] The term *carotid duplex*, currently in vogue, represents the union of these entities.[56, 57] Measurements of peak systolic velocity and end-diastolic velocity are made in the distal common carotid artery, carotid bulb, and cervical internal carotid artery. Color information enhances the ability of carotid duplex in the identification of maximal flow velocity points and further is useful in allowing precise transducer placement in patients when high-flow jets are encountered.[58]

The bony calvarium severely inhibits sound propagation, which has limited the ability of US to directly image the brain in adults. However, research led to the development of transducers capable of measuring intracranial flow velocities of key vascular structures despite the presence of intervening bone. This technology resulted in the development of transcranial Doppler (TCD), the study of the intracranial arteries using the spectral analysis of blood flow velocity. The technique generally employs a 2-MHz pulsed Doppler transducer. Vessel identification is based on the cranial window utilized, transducer position, and depth of sample volume. The direction and velocity of blood flow is recorded, noting the relationship to the terminal internal carotid and response to common carotid artery compression.[59, 60] Unfortunately, TCD may be limited by the thickness of the calvarium, which simply may not allow the measurement of intracranial Doppler signals.

NORMAL FINDINGS

Direct brain imaging in the pediatric age group is possible owing to the presence of large fontanelles, which normally remain open until age 6 to 9 months and thereby provide adequate windows to extensively image the brain. Routine imaging consists of a series of coronal and sagittal images typically obtained through the anterior fontanelle. Additional views can be obtained through other windows as necessary. Details regarding cerebrum and cerebellum are routinely seen and include views of the cerebral hemispheres, the deep ganglionic structures, thalami, ventricles, and posterior fossa.

Carotid imaging is typically performed with either a 5- or 7-MHz linear array transducer maintaining a duplex Doppler angle between 30 and 60 degrees and a sample size of 2 to 4 mm. Transverse and longitudinal images of the cervical carotid artery are routinely obtained that provide anatomical detail regarding the cervical carotid bifurcations. Normal flow velocities in the carotid arteries range between 60 and 100 cm/sec. The cervical vertebral arteries can also be evaluated, but this examination is inherently limited owing to the bony spine. The goal of vertebral artery US is to identify stenotic or occlusive disease or retrograde flow such as seen in subclavian steal syndrome. Representative images can be obtained with Doppler waveforms recording the presence and direction of flow.

TYPES OF DETECTABLE ABNORMALITIES

In infants and very young children, brain structures can be visualized and congenital anomalies thereby detected. Differences in transduction by tissue, fluid, and blood permit a differentiation of hydrocephalus, cysts, and hemorrhage. Various tumors and vascular disorders, especially vascular malformations, can also be detected with US. In newborns up to 6 months of age, spinal cord lesions can also be detected with US because the posterior elements are membranous rather than bony. In adults, US is used primarily for evaluation of vascular lesions of the head and neck, specifically, stenosis, obstruction, and dissection.

NEUROLOGICAL APPLICATIONS IN DIAGNOSIS AND TREATMENT

Cranial Lesions

Intracranial Hemorrhage and Premature Infants. Due to advances in neonatology, increasing numbers of infants are evaluated for neurological disorders secondary to prematurity. This coupled with primary neurological diseases has led to wide use of US as a leading diagnostic imaging tool in the neurological evaluation of children.[61] Regions of the brain hemorrhage can be readily diagnosed and graded, typically on a scale of 1 to 4 (Table 23–6). Hemorrhages can range in size from a small, solitary petechial hemorrhage to multiple large parenchymal hemorrhages with associated ventricular changes. Noninvasive follow-up imaging of these hemorrhages can be repeated as necessary without concern for radiation exposure. Small, germinal matrix hemorrhages, common in premature infants, carry the best long-term neurological prognosis (Fig. 23–27). In contrast, intraventricular hemorrhages may be seen in premature infants, representing a higher-grade hemorrhage. Larger parenchymal hemorrhages represent the more severe spectrum of premature brain injury and typically result in long-term neurological deficits. Hydrocephalus may complicate brain hemorrhage, which can be readily diagnosed and followed with US.

Congenital and Acquired Neonatal Disorders. US can provide useful information regarding other intracranial pediatric abnormalities, particularly in the newborn period. For example, congenital abnormalities such as Chiari malformations, agenesis of the corpus callosum, anencephaly, aqueductal stenosis, holoprosencephaly, and encephaloceles can be evaluated. Congenital pediatric neoplasms that occur in the first year of life such as choroid plexus papilloma and carcinoma, gliomas, primitive neuroectodermal tumors, and vascular disorders (e.g., the vein of Galen malformation) can be elucidated. Infectious diseases of the brain may result in abnormal intracranial fluid collections, complicating meningitis or encephalitis. US can be useful in providing guidance for needle aspirations of these collections.

Limitations of US include decreased detection rates of convexity lesions, such as extra-axial hemorrhages or masses (i.e., subarachnoid hemorrhage). Periventricular leukomalacia or the effects of perinatal asphyxia can be imaged but can also be challenging to recognize. As necessary, US information can be supplemented by other imaging tests, such as CT or MRI, to improve detection of conditions not recognized by US.

Intracranial Vascular Lesions

The indications for TCD continue to evolve but primarily focus on stroke prevention. TCD is useful in inferring the presence of intracranial stenosis or occlusions of major intracranial arteries and may further document routes of collateral circulation. One important role for TCD is for screening and follow-up of intracranial vasospasm complicating subarachnoid hemorrhage. Vasospasm typically peaks on days 3 through 7 after subarachnoid hemorrhage. TCD is useful in screening these patients for the onset of vasospasm, before clinical symptomatology (Fig. 23–28). This allows for early treatment planning, before the patient becomes symptomatic. TCD can be useful intraoperatively, for example, providing continuous intraoperative recording of the middle cerebral artery during carotid endarterectomy and, therefore, can help identify patients needing an indwelling shunt. Other developing indications of TCD include screening patients for intracranial stenosis that complicates sickle cell disease, identification of flow disturbances in migraine, and identification of AVM. In the latter instance, the nidus of AVM can be analyzed showing routes of supply and drainage and may further show flow reductions in AVMs after interventions. Lastly, TCD may be useful in accessing venous diseases such as sagittal sinus thrombosis and may play a future role in brain death determination.

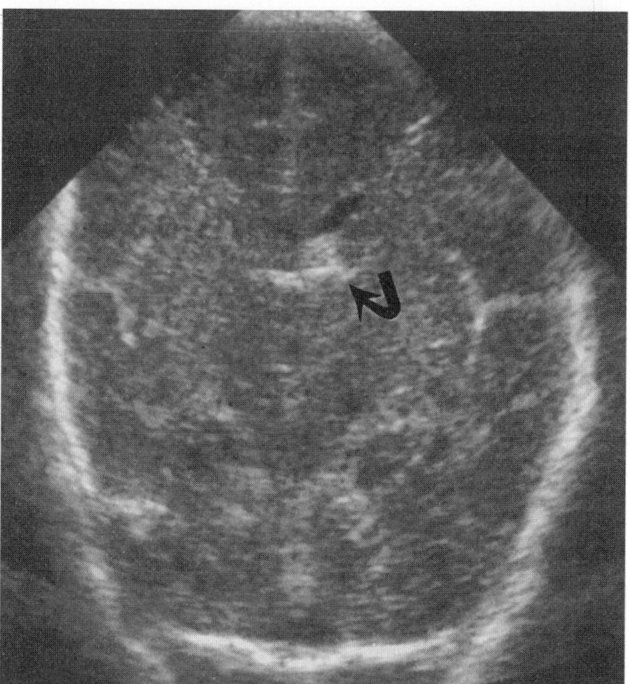

FIGURE 23–27. Cranial ultrasound of infant demonstrating left germinal matrix hemorrhage *(arrow)*.

TABLE 23–6. Grades of Intracranial Hemorrhage

Grade	Description
I	Subependymal hemorrhage into one or both germinal matrices
II	Germinal matrix hemorrhage with intraventricular extension, no hydrocephalus
III	Germinal matrix hemorrhage with intraventricular extension and hydrocephalus
IV	Germinal matrix hemorrhage with intraparenchymal extension

Vascular Lesions in the Neck

The prevalence of stroke in the United States has led to development of screening modalities aimed toward recognition and correction of stroke risk factors. Increasingly, atherosclerotic disease involving the cervical carotid and vertebral arteries is recognized for its inherent risk in stroke. The Asymptomatic Carotid Atherosclerosis Study demonstrated benefit in ipsilateral stroke reduction with carotid endarterectomy for patients with asymptomatic stenoses of extracranial carotid artery greater than or equal to 60 percent.[62] The North American Symptomatic Carotid Endarterectomy Trial demonstrated strong benefit with carotid endarterectomy in sympto-

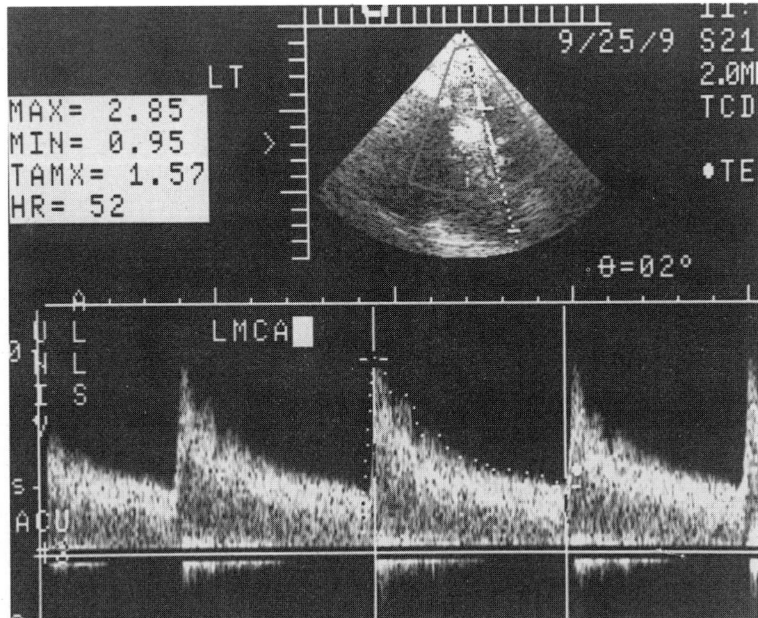

FIGURE 23–28. Transcranial Doppler image of left middle cerebral artery showing elevated flow velocities in the left middle cerebral artery status post subarachnoid hemorrhage consistent with vasospasm.

matic patients with ipsilateral carotid stenosis greater than or equal to 70 percent.[63] Therefore, because the majority of strokes are currently believed to be embolic in etiology, carotid screening becomes justified. The presence of significant stenosis of the carotid bifurcation is now generally accepted as an indication for intervention in both asymptomatic and symptomatic patients.

US of the cervical vasculature has several key advantages compared with other imaging modalities as a screening study.[64–66] These include patient comfort, lack of procedure risk, and high sensitivity and specificity in detecting cervical stenosis. Information regarding surface contour and internal characteristics of plaque can be routinely obtained. US limitations include operator dependency and possible error, field of view limitations (thorax inferiorly and the mandible superiorly), technical problems related to vessel tortuosity, and kinking, dense calcifications, and the potential to miss a trickle of blood in cases of high-grade, 99 percent stenosis. The latter in particular continues to justify the need for additional imaging studies in cases of suspected complete carotid occlusion and in cases in which information beyond the US field of view is needed. Indications for cervical US include evaluation of cervical bruit, transient ischemic attack, and stroke. Figure 23–29 demonstrates an example of a severe cervical carotid bifurcation plaque with angiographic correlation. US is also useful in following progression of atherosclerosis in cases of known plaque or in detecting other cervical pathologies, such as arterial dissection (Fig. 23–30).

At many institutions, carotid stenosis is graded based on a sliding scale developed by Bluth.[67] Mild carotid stenosis results in broadening of the normal ultrasonic spectral waveform with mild elevation of peak systolic velocity (PSV) due to turbulent flow from small plaques. In contrast, higher degrees of stenosis result in higher flow velocities, which can be seen in both systole and diastole. Generally, PSV greater than 130 cm/sec indicates moderate stenosis whereas PSV greater than 250 cm/sec indicates severe stenosis. Systolic and diastolic ratios between the stenotic internal carotid artery and the common carotid artery are also calculated and, if increased, may further indicate regions of carotid narrowing. Ratio analysis can aid in identifying false-positive and false-negative results in conditions such as systemic hypertension. Routinely, all high-flow jets are also recorded. A point can be reached in which flow velocities can diminish. These areas can further define abnormal regions of critical carotid stenosis.

Pediatric Spinal Lesions

Imaging of spinal abnormalities is useful in children up to 3 to 6 months of age as the posterior elements are membranous not bony. Beyond this age, these elements calcify and generally US would then need to be complemented with another imaging modality. Early evaluation and differentiation of neural tube defects, such as lipomas, meningoceles, myelomeningoceles, and tethered spinal cord, is possible. US can evaluate the subcutaneous structures and allow for recognition of abnormal spinal canal development, including spinal cord abnormalities. Even in older children, the presence of abnormal skull dimples, pores, or hair tufts can be evaluated for underlying spinal dysraphism. Rarely, US can be useful in evaluating spinal neoplasm or syrinx development.

Positron-Emission Tomography and Single Photon Emission Computed Tomography

BASIC PRINCIPLES AND TECHNIQUES

Kuhl and Edwards pioneered the original work of radionucleotide emission tomography in 1963.[68] This research demonstrated the initial use of radionucleotide tracers to

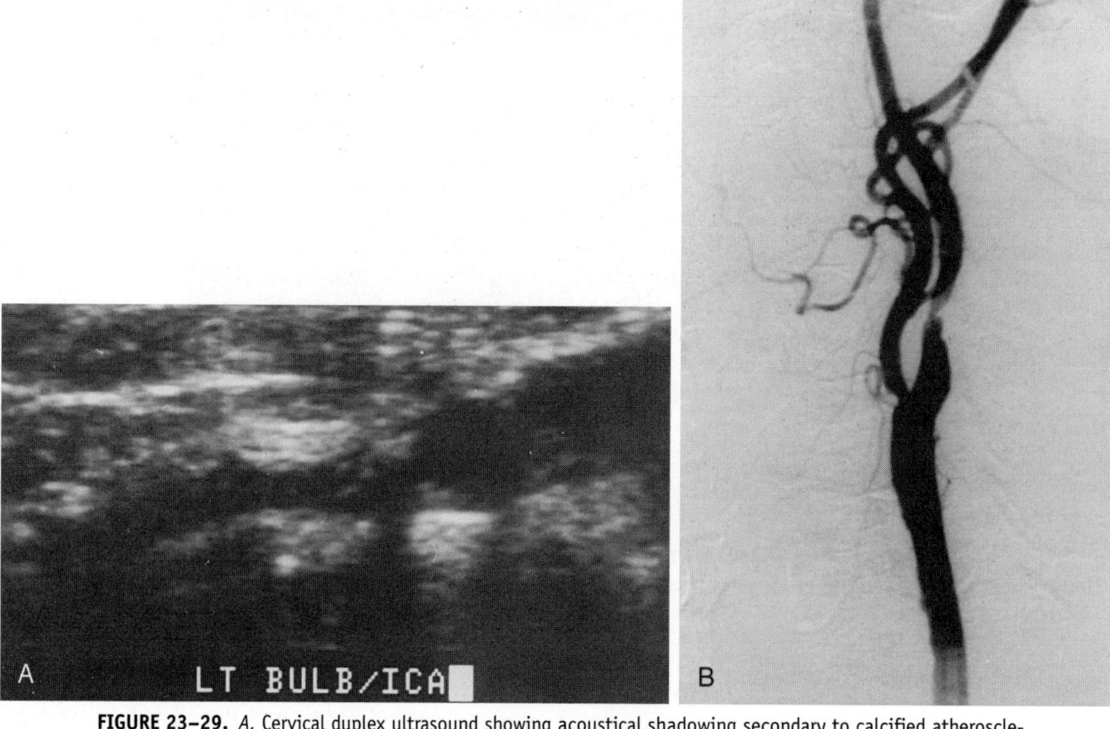

FIGURE 23–29. *A,* Cervical duplex ultrasound showing acoustical shadowing secondary to calcified atherosclerotic plaque. *B,* Corresponding carotid angiogram confirming stenosis.

create axial reconstructed images. It became apparent that the relative low resolution of this technique was a limitation as research began to focus on the functional imaging capabilities of this technique. Early work with CT in the early 1970s demonstrated the correlation between focal lesions in the brain and lesions demonstrated by radionucleotide emission tomography. Single photon emission computed tomography (SPECT) imaging uses radionucleotides that release gamma radiation. Gamma cameras detect the radiation released in 360 degrees and create multiplanar re-formations. In the

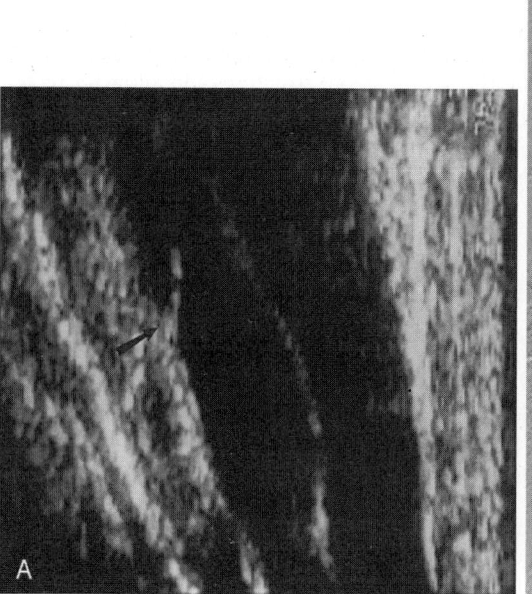

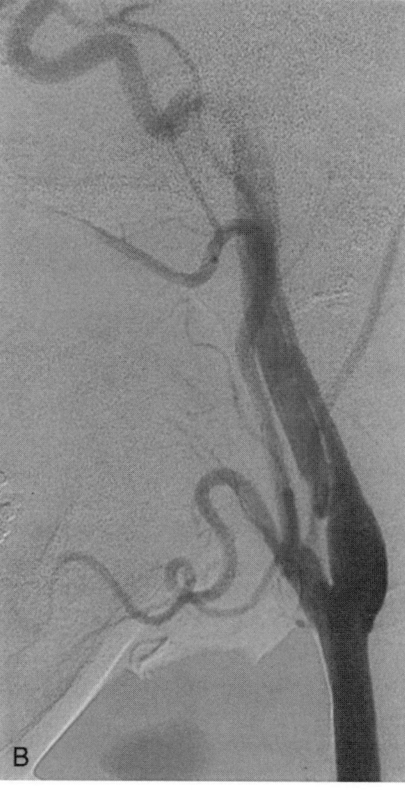

FIGURE 23–30. *A,* Ultrasound of right internal carotid demonstrating flap consistent with arterial dissection *(arrow). B,* Diagnostic right internal carotid angiogram confirming arterial dissection.

early 1980s iodine-based radionucleotides were initially used to determine symmetrical brain function. The uptake and distribution of such radionucleotides within the brain is believed to be proportional to blood flow.[69] Major breakthroughs occurred in the late 1980s with the introduction of technetium-99m–labeled compounds, the most common of which was hexamethylpropylene amineoxime (HMPAO).

A second major technique that investigates functional and, to a lesser degree, anatomical details within the brain is positron-emission tomography (PET). This procedure uses positron-emitting radionucleotides. This is in distinction to SPECT imaging, which uses gamma emitters. Positron-emitting particles decay by releasing two annihilation radiation particles into opposite directions that are separated by 180 degrees. Data is postprocessed and reformatted into multiple planes. Sokoloff, in 1977, described the use of the radionucleotide ^{14}C-deoxyglucose.[70] This was a major advancement in functional imaging of the brain that enabled the measurement of glucose uptake and metabolism. Shortly after, the most commonly used PET agent, ^{18}F-deoxyglucose (FDG), was introduced. The development of ligands associated with specific neurochemical receptors or other proteins has broadened the use of PET and SPECT to include a growing number of degenerative or biochemical disorders.

NORMAL FINDINGS

Radionucleotides are evenly distributed into the brain parenchyma for both PET and SPECT scanning. The calvarium and ventricles represent photopenic regions. The brain images can be displayed in axial, coronal, or sagittal projections. Under normal conditions, when a subject performs a motor, language, visual, or other sensory task, ^{18}F-deoxyglucose PET scans will identify increased glucose metabolism in the involved cortical region.

TYPES OF DETECTABLE ABNORMALITIES

SPECT and PET imaging have showed comparable detection of diseased states. In chronic pathological states, the cerebral blood flow demonstrated by SPECT correlates to abnormal metabolic activity that is shown by PET imaging. Unfortunately, PET imaging requires cyclotron-produced nucleotides. This, as well as cost, has limited PET to major research facilities. SPECT imaging is more accessible owing to recent advances in stability of radionucleotides and in computer technology. These factors have led to a significant increase in the resolution of the SPECT images. Both PET and SPECT can detect generalized hypometabolism in anoxia, degenerative disease, trauma, and aging or a focal hypometabolism. Hypermetabolism due to increased blood flow can be imaged as seen in tumors, infections, or seizure foci. In degenerative illnesses with neurotransmitter defects (e.g., Parkinson's disease and Huntington's disease), focal deficits can be detected, although these applications remain largely in the research realm.

NEUROLOGICAL APPLICATIONS IN DIAGNOSIS AND TREATMENT

Cerebrovascular Disease

Cerebrovascular disease is the third leading cause of death in the United States. The ability to rapidly diagnose acute stroke has both therapeutic and prognostic value. Acute intra-arterial thrombolysis of a recently formed thrombus is a new pioneering procedure that may significantly decrease the morbidity and mortality of cerebrovascular disease. PET is able to demonstrate a rise in regional oxygen extraction fraction indicating an evolving stroke. These changes are often demonstrated earlier and show more extensive tissue damage than what is predicted by CT or MRI. However, work with diffusion-weighted MRI suggests that this may be the most sensitive imaging study for acute stroke.[71] In patients with reversible ischemic injury there is a decrease in regional cerebral blood flow that is termed *misery perfusion*. These patients would have a false-positive PET and SPECT scan. Areas of chronic infarction generally demonstrate decreased regional cerebral blood flow and oxygen and glucose metabolism. SPECT imaging can identify areas of decreased blood flow in patients with acute infarcts not detectable by CT.

A diagnostic test to identify high-risk patients who would benefit from surgical intervention of an arteriosclerotic lesion within the carotid bifurcation can also be of great value. A pharmacological stress test with acetazolamide, which causes cerebrovascular dilatation and increased regional cerebral blood flow, has been investigated.[72] Others have investigated the prognostic value of the ratio of regional cerebral blood flow to regional cerebral blood volume.[73] The regional cerebral blood volume can be determined with technetium-99m–labeled red blood cells. As the regional cerebral blood flow decreases, the regional cerebral blood volume increases to maintain perfusion. This procedure has been described as an indicator of cerebral perfusion reserve, thus defining a patient's risk for infarction. SPECT and PET have also demonstrated "luxury perfusion," which represents the areas of subacute stroke that receive increased blood flow in relation to the non-affected brain. This is most likely due to an increase in an aerobic metabolism in the region of infarction. SPECT has also demonstrated hypoperfusion of the contralateral cerebellum in patients with cortical strokes termed *crossed cerebellar diaschisis*. This is believed to be secondary to disruption of the corticopontine tracts uniquely seen by SPECT.

Brain Tumors

The majority of tumor investigation imaging has been with PET. FDG is the primary positron emitter used today. In general, high-grade neoplasms demonstrate increased metabolism whereas low-grade neoplasms demonstrate relatively decreased activity. There has been high correlation between metabolic activity determined by PET and histological grade of the neoplasm.[74] One of the many uses of PET scanning is to distinguish tumor recurrence from radiation necrosis. Focal areas of decreased metabolic activity help diagnose areas of radiation necrosis, whereas tumor recurrence shows increased metabolic activity. PET remains one of the most sensitive tests to differentiate between these two entities.

SPECT has a more limited role in the evaluation of brain tumors. Some enthusiasm has been displayed with the use of SPECT to differentiate a lymphoma from toxoplasmosis in immunocompromised patients. Imaging with thallium-labeled gamma emitters demonstrates increased activity within lymphomas and decreased activity within toxoplasmosis[75] (Fig. 23–31).

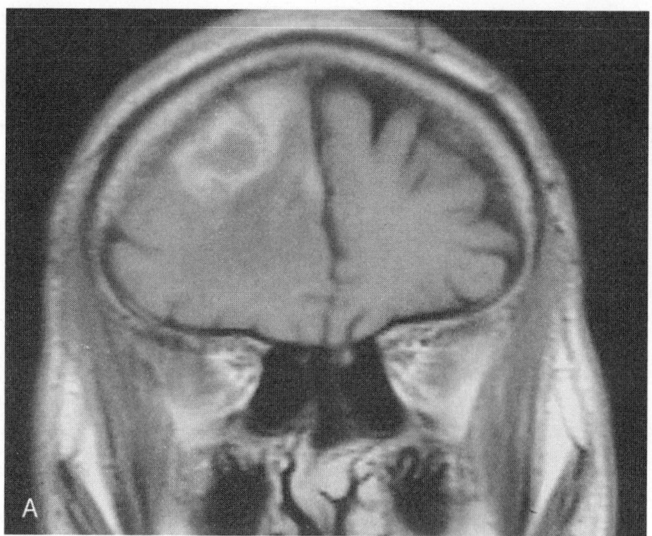

FIGURE 23–31. A 30-year-old HIV-positive male presents with mental status changes. *A,* MR (post-contrast T1W image) demonstrates a focal masslike lesion with ring enhancement within the right frontoparietal area. The primary differential diagnosis is between lymphoma and toxoplasmosis. *B,* Thallium SPECT scan shows abnormal increased uptake representing a primary CNS lymphoma.

Dementia

Within the past decade there has been much excitement about the use of PET and SPECT to evaluate dementia. Alzheimer's disease is the most common cause of dementia in the United States. There have been numerous studies that have described decreased regional glucose metabolism in healthy older subjects within the frontal, parietal, and temporal lobe regions.[76] Current PET normalizes regional values using internal standards such as the cerebellum or calcarine fissure region. Characteristic patterns of decreased regional glucose metabolism within the parietal and temporal lobes have been described in patients with Alzheimer's disease.[77] In these patients there is relative preservation of the calcarine fissure region, sensory motor region, cerebellum, and basal ganglion region. Decreased metabolic rates for oxygen have also been reported in the same regions that demonstrate areas of decreased glucose metabolism in patients with Alzheimer's disease.[78] Patients with progressive Parkinson's 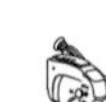 disease have a similar pattern to that seen in patients with Alzheimer's disease. Multiple-infarct dementia occurs after multiple lacunar infarctions. PET can therefore demonstrate the corresponding multifocal regions of decreased glucose metabolism[79] that typify the focal lesions demonstrated by CT or MRI. Significant decreases in glucose metabolism within the frontal and temporal lobes have been described in patients with Pick's disease, which can be detected by PET.[80] Patients with Huntington's chorea, a disorder of the extrapyramidal system, have shown a decrease in glucose metabolism within the caudate nuclei.[81] These findings may present before atrophy of the caudate nuclei is demonstrated by CT or MRI.

Decreased regional cerebral blood flow demonstrated with SPECT has shown a similar pattern of decreased glucose metabolism in comparison to PET. Most investigators believe that SPECT is a test of equal sensitivity to characterize dementia.

Cerebral Trauma

In severe head trauma there is a strong association between a diffuse axonal injury and decreased brain metabolism. It has been demonstrated that diffuse and focal areas of decreased metabolism can recover over time. Correlations have been found between post-traumatic decreases in glucose metabolism identified by PET and decreased regional cerebral blood flow identified with SPECT. Focal lesions identified on CT demonstrate a larger area of abnormal regional cerebral blood flow by SPECT.[82] A goal of SPECT research in head trauma has been to use this method to characterize prognosis of focal lesions as well as cases of more widespread diffuse axonal injury.

Seizure Disorders

SPECT and PET have been investigated as complementary noninvasive studies for localization of seizure foci. CT, MRI, and electroencephalography (EEG) are the primary noninvasive methods used to localize an epileptic focus but do not always identify a lesion. These patients may require invasive placement of depth electrodes to definitively elucidate a seizure focus. SPECT has been helpful in demonstrating regional decreased cerebral blood flow within a seizure focus between seizures and increased regional cerebral blood flow ictally. PET studies have also shown decreased metabolism between seizures within a seizure focus and increased metabolic activity ictally. In both SPECT and PET, up to approximately 80 percent of patients who demonstrated a focal EEG abnormality also demonstrated an associated perfusion or metabolic activity defect within the same region.[83] The rapid availability of cyclotron-produced nucleotides is, again, a limiting factor for the use of PET for the ictal stage.[84] HMPAO is the SPECT radionucleotide of choice. This tracer is taken up by the brain during the first vascular pass and does not redistribute after the first few minutes. Imaging can then be obtained up to 3 to 4 hours after the seizure ictus. There is an additional increased sensitivity if an ictal SPECT scan can be obtained. Research suggests that a more stable SPECT imaging agent, ethyl cystinate dimer, which is chemically more stable than HMPAO, has the potential to become the radionucleotide of choice.

Degenerative Disorders: Parkinson's Disease and Huntington's Disease

PET can use a number of ligands other than glucose, and these applications are of particular interest in neurological disorders involving neurotransmitter abnormalities. Parkinson's disease and Huntington's disease are the prototypical examples (see Chapter 34) of such conditions, but dystonias and other movement disorders have also been studied with PET.[85] To study the activity of the nigrostriatal dopaminergic system, fluorodopa (a derivative of levodopa) is typically used. Receptor agonists can be used to study postsynaptic function of the same system. Whereas these ligand "probes" remain research tools at the present time, increasing experience may lead to their use in regular clinical neurological practice. In animal models of Parkinson's disease, there is a good correlation between fluorodopa uptake and striatal dopamine content. An even higher correlation exists between uptake and the number of dopamine cells in the substantia nigra zona compacta, an area specifically affected by Parkinson's disease. In patients with severe clinical disability from Parkinson's, fluorodopa scans show lower uptake than those of patients with mild disease. Possible future applications include its potential use in patients with tremors in whom the diagnosis of Parkinson's disease is clinically unclear. Such scans may also prove useful in monitoring the success of such therapies as tissue transplants. In Huntington's disease, most PET attention has focused on its putative utility in preclinical detection and the monitoring of clinical disease progression.

Reviews and Selected Updates

American Academy of Neurology: Assessment: Positron emission tomography. Neurology 1991;41:163–167.

American Academy of Neurology: Performance/interpretation qualifications: Computed tomography. In AAN Practice Handbook. American Academy of Neurology, St. Paul, MN, 1991, pp 27–28.

American Academy of Neurology: Performance/interpretation qualifications: Positron emission tomography imaging. *In* AAN Practice Handbook. American Academy of Neurology, St. Paul, MN, 1989, pp 81–82.

American Academy of Neurology: SPECT and neurosonology qualifications approved. Neurology 1991;41:13A.

American Academy of Neurology: Training guidelines for MRI imaging. Neurology 1988;38:21A.

Cook GJ, Maisey MN: The current status of clinical PET imaging. Clin Radiol 1996;51:603–613.

Kuikka JT, Belliveau JW, Hari R: Future of functional brain imaging. Eur J Nucl Med 1996;23:737–740.

Le Bihan D: Functional MRI of the brain: Principles, applications and limitations. J Neuroradiol 1996;23:1–5.

Longworth C, Honey G, Sharma T: Science, medicine, and the future: Functional magnetic resonance imaging in neuropsychiatry. BMJ 1999; 319:1551–1554.

Pritchard JW, Cummings JL: The insistent call from functional MRI. Neurology 1997;48:797–800.

Sawle GV: Imaging the head: Functional imaging. J Neurol Neurosurg Psychiatry 1995;59:454.

Spencer SS, Theodore WH, Berkovic SF: Clinical applications: MRI, SPECT, and PET. Magn Reson Imaging 1995;13:1119–1124.

References

1. Taveras J: Anatomy and examination of the skull. *In* Taveras J, Ferrucci J (eds): Radiology, rev ed. Vol. 3. Philadelphia, JB Lippincott, 1991, pp 1–9.
2. Greenspan A: Orthopedic Radiology, 2nd ed. New York, Gower Medical Publishing, 1992, pp 12.1–12.19.
3. Rogers LF: Radiology of Skeletal Trauma, 2nd ed. Vol. 1. New York, Churchill Livingstone, 1992, pp 301–579.
4. Harris JH, Edeiken-Monroe B: The Radiology of Acute Cervical Spine Trauma, 2nd ed. Baltimore, Williams & Wilkins, 1987, pp 65–91.
5. Resnick D, Niwayama G: Degenerative disease of the spine. *In* Resnick D (ed): Diagnosis of Bone and Joint Disorders, 3rd ed. Vol. 3. Philadelphia, WB Saunders, 1995, pp 1372–1454.
6. Nizard RS, Cardinne L, Bizot P, Witvoet J: Radiologic assessment of lumbar intervertebral instability and degenerative spondylolisthesis. Radiol Clin North Am 2001;39:55–71.
7. Shellock F: Pocket Guide to MR Procedures and Metallic Objects. Philadelphia, Lippincott-Raven, 1996.
8. Villafana T: Physics and instrumentation: CT and MRI. *In* Lee SH, Rao KCVG (eds): Cranial Computed Tomography and MRI, 2nd ed. New York, McGraw-Hill, 1987, pp 1–70.
9. Schwartz RD: Helical (spiral) CT in neuroradiologic diagnosis. Radiol Clin North Am 1995;33:981–995.
10. Rothenberg LN, Pentlow KS: Radiation dose in CT. Radiographics 1992;12:1225–1243.
11. Greenberger PA, Patterson R: The prevention of immediate generalized reactions to radiocontrast media in high risk patients. J Allergy Clin Immunol 1991;87:867–872.
12. Mafee MF: The eye and orbit. *In* Som PJ, Curtin HD (eds): Head and Neck Imaging, 3rd ed. St. Louis: Mosby–Year Book, 1996, pp 1059–1129.
13. Heilbrun MP, Brockmeyer D, Sunderland P: Stereotactic surgery for mass lesions of the cranial vault. *In* Apuzzo MLJ (ed): Brain Surgery. New York: Churchill Livingstone, 1993, pp 390–405.
14. Johnson BA, Tanenbaum LN: Contemporary spinal CT applications. Neuroimaging Clin N Am 1998;8:559–575.
15. Gorter CJ: Paramagnetic Relaxation. Amsterdam, Elsevier, 1947.
16. Atlas S: Magnetic Resonance Imaging of the Brain and Spine. Lippincott, Williams, & Wilkins, Philadelphia, 2001.
17. Gomori JM, Grossman RI, Goldberg HI, et al: Intracranial hematomas: Imaging by high field MR. Radiology 1985;157:87–93.
18. Hoffman JM: New advances in brain tumor imaging. Curr Opin Oncol 2001;13:148–153.
19. Hochman MS, Naidich TP, Kobetz SA, Fernandez-Maitin A: Spontaneous intracranial hypotension with pachymeningeal enhancement on MRI. Neurology 1992;42:1628–1630.
20. Gomori JM, Grossman RI: Mechanisms responsible for the MR appearance and evaluation of intracranial hemorrhage. Radiographics 1988;8:427–440.
21. vanGelderen P, de Vleeschouwer MH, Des Pres D, et al: Water diffusion and acute stroke. Magn Reson Med 1994;31:154.
22. Calamante F, Thomas DL, Pell GS, Wiersma J, Turner R: Measuring cerebral blood flow using magnetic resonance imaging techniques. J Cereb Blood Flow Metab 1999;19:701–735.
23. Ogawa S, Tank DW, Menon R, et al: Intrinsic signal changes accompanying sensory stimulation: Functional brain mapping with magnetic resonance imaging. Proc Natl Acad Sci 1992;89:5951–5955.
24. Singer JP: Blood flow rates by nuclear magnetic resonance measurements. Science 1959;130:1652.
25. Wherli FW, Shimakawa A, Gullberg GT, et al: Time-of-flight MR flow imaging: Selective saturation recovery with gradient refocussing. Radiology 1986;160:781.
26. Faro SH, Haselgrove JC, Wang Z, et al: Carotid MR angiography: Optimization with magnetization transfer. Radiology 1993;189(P): 243.
27. Faro SH, Vinitski S, Ortega HV, et al: Carotid magnetic resonance angiography: Improved image quality with dual 3-inch surface coils. Neuroradiology 1996;38:403–408.
28. Wolff SD, Balaban RS: Magnetization transfer contrast (MTC) and tissue water proton relaxation in vivo. Magn Reson Med 1989; 10:135.

29. Faro SH, Mohamed FB, Vinitski S, Ahmed KY: High resolution multiple flip angle (MFA) 3D time of flight MR angiography: A new technique to study the carotid bifurcation. Radiology 1994;193(P):266.
30. Dumolin CL, Hart HR: Magnetic resonance angiography. Radiology 1986;161:717.
31. Dumolin CL, Souza SP, Walker MF, et al: Three dimensional phase contrast angiography. Magn Reson Med 1989;9:130.
32. Faro SH, Ortega HV, Mohamed FB, et al: Temporal signal loss in the normal carotid bifurcation: Analysis with gated 2D phase contrast MR angiography and computer modelling. Proceedings of the 34th annual meeting of the American Society of Neuroradiology, Seattle, WA, 1996, pp 246–247.
33. Henry-Feugeas MC, Idy-Peretti I, Blanchet B, et al: Temporal and spatial assessment of normal cerebrospinal fluid dynamics with MR imaging. Magn Reson Imaging 1993;11:1107.
34. NASCET Collaborators: Beneficial effect of carotid endarterectomy in symptomatic patients with high-grade stenosis. N Engl J Med 1991;325:445–453.
35. Vanninen R, Manninen H, Koivisto K, et al: Carotid stenosis by digital subtraction angiography: Reproducibility of the European Carotid Surgery Trial and the North American Symptomatic Carotid Endarterectomy Trial measurement methods and visual interpretation. AJNR 1994;15:1635–1641.
36. Hobson RW II, Weiss DG, Fields WS, et al, and Veterans Affairs Cooperative Study Group: Efficacy of carotid endarterectomy for asymptomatic carotid stenosis. N Engl J Med 1993;328:221–227.
37. Blatter DD, Bahr AL, Parker DL, et al: Cervical carotid MR angiography with multiple overlapping thin-slab acquisition: Comparison with conventional angiography. AJR 1993;161:1269–1277.
38. Masaryk AM, Ross JS, DiCello MC, et al: 3DFT MR angiography of the carotid bifurcation: Potential and limitations as a screening examination. Radiology 1991;179:797–784.
39. Huston J, Nichols DA, Luetmer PH, et al: Blinded prospective evaluation of sensitivity of MR angiography to known intracranial aneurysms: Importance of aneurysm size. AJNR 1994;15:1607–1614.
40. Korogi Y, Takahashi M, Mabuchi N, et al: Intracranial aneurysms: Diagnostic accuracy of three-dimensional, Fourier transform time-of-flight MR angiography. Radiology 1994;193:181–186.
41. Ronkainen A, Puranen MI, Hernesniemi JA: Intracranial aneurysms: MR angiographic screening in 400 asymptomatic individuals with increased familial risk. Radiology 1995;195:35–40.
42. Osborn AG: Technical aspects of cerebral angiography. *In* Diagnostic Cerebral Angiography. Philadelphia, Lippincott, Williams & Wilkins, 1999, pp 421–445.
43. Heiserman JE, Dean BL, Hodak JA, et al: Neurologic complications of cerebral angiography. Am J Neuroradiol 1995;15:1401–1407.
44. Wolpert SM, Caplan LR: Current role of cerebral angiography in the diagnosis of cerebrovascular diseases. AJR 1992;159:191–197.
45. Higashida RT, Halbach VV, Tsai FY, et al: Interventional neurovascular techniques for cerebral revascularization in the treatment of stroke. AJR 1994;163:793–800.
46. Mathias K, Jager H, Hennings S, Gissler HM: Endoluminal treatment of internal carotid artery stenosis. World J Surg 2001;25:328–334.
47. Vitek JJ, Roubin GS, New G, Al-Mubarek N, Iyer SS: Carotid angioplasty with stenting in post-carotid endarterectomy restenosis. J Invasive Cardiol 2001;13:123–125.
48. Hobson RW, Goldstein JE, Jamil Z, et al: Carotid restenosis: Operative and endovascular management. J Vasc Surg 1999;29:228–235.
49. Phatouros CC, Higashida RT, Malek AM, et al: Carotid artery stent placement for atherosclerotic disease: Rationale, technique, and current status. Radiology 2000;217:26–41.
50. Al-Mubarak N, Roubin GS, Vitek JJ: Systematic comparison of the early outcome of angioplasty and endarterectomy for symptomatic carotid artery disease. Stroke 2000;31:3079–3083.
51. Roubin GS, New G, Iyer SS, et al: Immediate and late clinical outcomes of carotid artery stenting in patients with symptomatic and asymptomatic carotid artery stenosis: A 5-year prospective analysis. Circulation 2001;103:532–537.
52. Chastain HD, Campbell MS, Iyer S, et al: Extracranial vertebral artery stent placement: In-hospital and follow-up results. J Neurosurg 1999;91:547–552.
53. Guglielmi G, Vinuela F: Intracranial aneurysms. Guglielmi electrothrombotic coils. Neurosurg Clin North Am 1994;5:427–435.
54. Merland JJ, Reizine D, Laurent A, et al: Embolization of spinal cord vascular lesions. *In* Vinuela F, et al (eds): Interventional Neuroradiology: Endovascular Therapy of the Central Nervous System. New York, Raven Press, 1992, pp 153–165.
55. Carsten CG III, Elmore JR, Franklin DP, et al: Use of limited color-flow duplex for a carotid screening project. Am J Surg 1999;178:173–176.
56. Huston J III, James EM, Brown RD Jr, et al: Redefined duplex ultrasonographic criteria for diagnosis of carotid artery stenosis. Mayo Clin Proc 2000;75:1113–1140.
57. Fox AJ: Comparisons between carotid duplex sonography and cerebral angiography in assessing the degree of carotid stenosis. AJNR 2000;21:618–619.
58. Dix J, Skrocki J: Evaluation of carotid stenosis. AJNR 2000;21:639–642.
59. Lupetin AR, Davis DA, Beckman I, Dash N: Transcranial Doppler sonography: I. Principles, technique and normal appearances. Radiographics 1995;15:179–191.
60. Lupetin AR, Davis DA, Beckman I, Dash N: Transcranial Doppler sonography: II. Evaluation of intracranial and extracranial abnormalities and procedural monitoring. Radiographics 1995;15:193–209.
61. Harlow C, Hay TC, Rumack CM: The pediatric brain. *In* Rumack CM, Wilson SR, Charboneau JW (eds): Diagnostic Ultrasound. St. Louis, Mosby–Year Book, 1991, pp 1009–1044.
62. Executive Committee of the Asymptomatic Carotid Atherosclerosis Study: Endarterectomy for asymptomatic carotid artery stenosis. JAMA 1995;273:1421–1428.
63. North American Symptomatic Carotid Endarterectomy Trial (NASCET) Collaborators: Beneficial effect of carotid endarterectomy in symptomatic patients with high-grade carotid stenosis. N Engl J Med 1991;325:445–453.
64. Kurtz AB, Middleton WD: Vascular system. *In* Thrall JH (ed): Ultrasound: The Requisites. St. Louis, Mosby–Year Book, 1996, pp 464–487.
65. Zweibel WJ: Duplex sonography of the cerebral arteries: Efficacy, limitations, and indications. AJR 1992;158:29–36.
66. Robinson ML: Duplex sonography of the carotid arteries. Semin Roentgenol 1992;27:17–27.
67. Bluth EI, Stavros AT, Marich KW, et al: Carotid duplex sonography: A multicenter recommendation for standardized imaging and Doppler criteria. Radiographics 1988;8:487–506.
68. Kuhl DE, Edwards RQ: Image separation of radioisotope scanning. Radiology 1963;80:653–662.
69. Kuhl DE, Barrio JR, Huang S-C, et al: Quantifying local cerebral blood flow by N-isopropyl-*p*-^{123}I-iodoamphetamine (IMP) tomography. J Nucl Med 1982;23:196–203.
70. Sokoloff L, Reivich M, Kennedy C, et al: The (^{14}C) deoxyglucose method for the measurement of local cerebral glucose utilization: Theory, procedure and normal values in the conscious and anesthetized albino rat. J Neurochem 1977;28:897–916.
71. Siewart B, Patel MR, Warach S: Stroke and ischemia. MRI Clin North Am 1995;3:529–540.
72. Sullivan HG, Kingsbury TB IV, Morgan ME, et al: The rCBF response to Diamox in normal subjects and cerebrovascular disease patients. J Neurosurg 1987;67:525–534.
73. Baron JC, Frackowiak RSJ, Herholz K: Use of PET methods for measurement of cerebral energy metabolism and hemodynamics in cerebrovascular disease. J Cereb Blood Flow Metab 1989;9:723–742.
74. DiChiro G: Positron emission tomography using [^{18}F] fluorodeoxyglucose in brain tumors: A powerful diagnostic and prognostic tool. Invest Radiol 1986;22:360–371.
75. Ruiz A, Ganz WI, Donovan Post J, et al: Use of thallium-201 brain SPECT to differentiate cerebral lymphoma from *Toxoplasma* encephalitis in AIDS patients. AJNR 1994;15:1885–1894.
76. Yoshii F, Barker WW, Chang JY, et al: Sensitivity of cerebral glucose metabolism to age, gender, brain volume, brain atrophy, and cerebrovascular risk factors. J Cereb Blood Flow Metab 1988;8:654–661.
77. Duara R, Grady C, Haxby J, et al: Positron emission tomography in Alzheimer's disease. Neurology 1986;36:879–887.
78. Frackowiak RSJ, Pozzilli C, Legg NJ, et al: Regional cerebral oxygen supply and utilization in dementia: A clinical and physiological study with oxygen-15 and positron tomography. Brain 1981;104:753–778.
79. Benson F, Kuhl DE, Hawkins ME, et al: The fluorodeoxyglucose ^{123}F scan in Alzheimer's disease and multiinfarct dementia. Arch Neurol 1983;40:711–714.
80. Kamo H, McGeer R, Harrop R, et al: Positron emission tomography and histopathology in Pick's disease. Neurology 1987;37:439–445.
81. Hayden MR, Martin WRW, Stoessl AJ, et al: Positron emission tomography in the early diagnosis of Huntington's disease. Neurology 1986;36:888–894.

82. Abdel-Dayem HM, Sadek SA, Kouris K: Changes in cerebral perfusion after acute head injury: Comparison of CT with Tc-99m HM-PAO SPECT. Radiology 1987;165:221–226.
83. Rowe CC, Berkovic SF, Sia STB, et al: Localization of epileptic foci with postictal single photon emission computed tomography. Ann Neurol 1989;26:660–668.
84. Lee JS, Lee DS, Kim SK: Localization of epileptogenic zones in F-18 FDG brain PET of patients with temporal lobe epilepsy using artificial neural network. IEEE Trans Med Imaging 2000;19:347–355.
85. Ilgin N: Functional imaging of neurotransmitter systems in movement disorders. QJ Nucl Med 1998;42:179–192.

CHAPTER 24

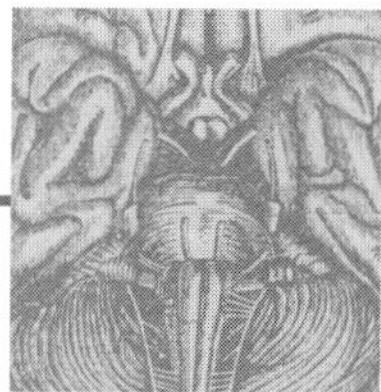

MICHAEL J. AMINOFF

Electrophysiology

Electroencephalography

BASIC PRINCIPLES AND TECHNIQUE

Electroencephalography is a noninvasive technique in which the electrical activity of the brain is recorded from the scalp to evaluate the function of the brain. It is thus complementary, rather than an alternative, to neuroimaging techniques. The differences in voltage between electrodes placed in different regions of the scalp are recorded and amplified. The polarity, frequency, amplitude, distribution, and changes with time of this activity are then studied to determine whether the findings are normal or abnormal and whether they suggest any particular type of underlying pathological process.

Electrodes are placed on the scalp based on standardized, internationally agreed locations (the 10–20 system).[1] The potential difference between pairs of scalp electrodes (bipolar derivation) or between individual scalp electrodes and a common reference point such as the linked ears (referential derivation) is then recorded as the electroencephalogram (EEG) on moving paper or viewed on the screen of an oscilloscope. Recordings are made simultaneously from pairs of electrodes in an organized sequence or pattern termed a *montage*, which is generally either longitudinal or transverse in orientation.[2] In longitudinal montages, recordings are made from electrodes in a sagittal plane; in bipolar derivations, recordings are between linked pairs of electrodes, whereas in referential derivations, the recordings are between each electrode and the reference point. In transverse montages, recordings are made from electrodes in a straight coronal plane. The recordings are then displayed in anterior-to-posterior or left-to-right sequences.

For recording purposes, the input from each pair of electrodes (or from active and reference electrodes) is connected to the two inputs of a differential amplifier in such a way that the input from the active electrode is connected to input one and from the reference electrode (or, with bipolar recordings, from the more posterior or right-sided electrode) to input two. The recording arrangement is such that an upward deflection indicates either increased negativity at the electrode connected to input one or increased positivity at input two.

In recording the EEG, an attempt is generally made to activate abnormalities by hyperventilation for about 3 minutes, and also by photic stimulation at flash rates up to 20 Hz. Other common activating procedures include sleep during the recording procedure and sleep deprivation on the night before the examination.[2]

It is sometimes necessary to monitor the EEG for several days in patients with episodic behavioral disturbances to record during some of the episodes and determine whether they have electrocerebral accompaniments such as occur with epileptic seizures. This can either be undertaken in a long-term video EEG monitoring unit in the hospital or, in some instances, by recording the EEG with an ambulatory cassette EEG system. The latter approach can be undertaken in the home setting and does not require continuous supervision by specialized personnel. Tapes last for 24 hours and can generally be reviewed in less than 1 hour.[3]

The traditional method of EEG interpretation depends on visual analysis, which is subjective and very time intensive. Quantitative or automated (computerized) techniques for analysis are being developed but are not yet in widespread use for routine purposes.

It is important to distinguish between cerebral activity and artifactual discharges of biological or nonbiological origin. Bioelectric artifacts include ocular, cardiac, respiratory, movement, muscle, and sweat artifacts. These various artifacts have characteristic appearances that facilitate their recognition. Artifacts may also arise from the equipment or electrodes and especially from variation in electrode impedance. Other artifacts may arise from the environment in which the recording is made, such as from other electrical equipment, intravenous infusion lines, and static electricity generated by nylon clothing.

The electrocerebral activity recorded from the scalp consists not of action potentials but of the summated synaptic potentials from large numbers of cortical neurons. It thus reflects the summated excitatory and inhibitory postsynaptic cortical potentials. This activity is markedly attenuated by the skull and scalp and is therefore considerably greater when recorded from the cortical surface.

NORMAL EEG ACTIVITY

The cerebral activity recorded at electroencephalography is generally rhythmic; that is, it consists of regularly recurring waveforms of similar duration and morphology. It is widely believed that the rhythmicity is imposed on the cerebral cortex by a thalamic pacemaker.[4]

Activity recorded in the human EEG is characterized by its frequency. In normal adults, a posteriorly predominant 8- to 12-Hz rhythm is present and is attenuated by eye opening; this is designated the alpha rhythm (Fig. 24–1). Faster-frequency activity, or beta activity, is also present to a variable extent, has a generalized distribution, and is enhanced by certain medications such as benzodiazepines. Activity slower than 8 Hz is designated as theta (4 to 7 Hz) or delta (less than 4 Hz) activity. Such slow activity is a normal feature of certain stages of sleep but is generally not present in awake alert adults.

ABNORMAL EEG ACTIVITY

The pathophysiology of abnormal EEG activity is multifactorial and difficult to clarify. Increased excitability of the cerebral cortex probably accounts for cortical spike activity. More generalized spike-wave bursts probably depend on thalamocortical projections. The delta activity recorded under certain pathological circumstances probably reflects lesions involving predominantly the cerebral white matter. When subcortical nuclei are involved, either alone or in association with pathology affecting the cerebral cortex itself, paroxysmal slow activity is seen and may include spike discharges.[5]

Slow activity sometimes occurs with a localized distribution and varies in rhythm, rate, and amplitude with time. Such a focal polymorphic slow-wave disturbance, when present continuously, suggests an underlying structural lesion involving the cerebral white matter (Fig. 24–2) but provides no clue as to its nature. Transient polymorphic slow-wave activity is suggestive of either migraine or a postictal state after a partial (focal) seizure.

Intermittent rhythmical slow activity may occur with a frontal emphasis in adults or an occipital emphasis in children and is a nonspecific finding that has been described in a variety of settings, including metabolic disturbances, hydrocephalus, and diencephalic lesions.

A diffusely slowed record during wakefulness is nonspecifically abnormal but is seen most commonly in patients with diffuse encephalopathic processes such as a metabolic disturbance or encephalitic disorder (Fig. 24–3). It may also reflect long-standing diffuse cerebral dysfunction such as occurs in patients with a perinatal static encephalopathy.

Focal attenuation of EEG activity reflects destructive disease of the cerebral cortex, whereas more diffuse attenuation may result from severe encephalopathic processes and occurs also in certain degenerative disorders such as Huntington's disease. Electrocerebral silence or inactivity, in recordings made under conditions to enhance the presence of any underlying low-voltage EEG activity, is suggestive of neocortical brain death but may also occur in patients who are hypothermic or have taken an overdose of drugs that depress the central nervous system (CNS) (Fig. 24–4).[6] In some instances, the EEG consists of bursts of mixed-frequency activity occurring on a relatively quiescent background. This so-called burst-suppression pattern may occur with any severe encephalopathy, such as after severe cerebral anoxia or after head trauma, after overdose of CNS depressant drugs, and with anesthesia.

Epileptiform discharges consist of abnormal paroxysmal events containing sharp waves or spike discharges, at least in part. A spike discharge is a potential having a sharp contour and a duration of less than 80 msec, whereas a sharp wave has

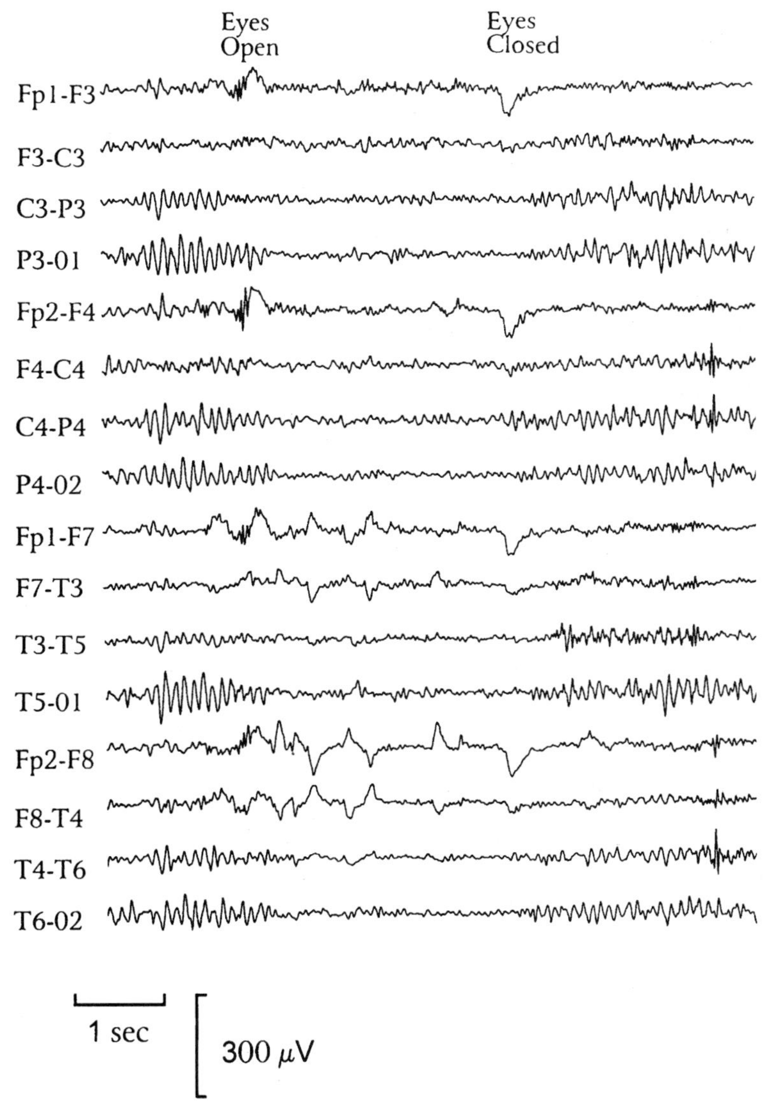

FIGURE 24–1. A posteriorly predominant 9-Hz alpha rhythm is present when the eyes are closed and is attenuated by eye opening in the EEG of this normal subject. Electrode placements in this and succeeding figures are as follows: Fp, frontopolar; F, frontal; C, central; P, parietal; O, occipital; T, temporal; A, earlobe; Sp, sphenoid. Right-sided placements are indicated by even numbers, left-sided placements by odd numbers, and midline placements by Z.

a duration of between 80 and 200 msec. They may occur without any clinical correlates or significance but are found interictally with a greater incidence than normal in patients with epilepsy.

Periodic lateralized epileptiform discharges are lateralized epileptiform discharges that occur with a regular periodicity. They occur in association with acute hemispheric pathology such as an infarct or rapidly expanding tumor,[7, 8] typically in obtunded patients with a focal neurological deficit and often recurrent seizures, and are commonly replaced after several weeks by a continuous polymorphic slow-wave disturbance.

Repetitive complexes consisting of slow waves, sharp activity, or both occur with a regular periodicity and generalized distribution in various disorders. Such periodic complexes are especially characteristic of certain infective disorders of the brain but may also occur after severe cerebral anoxia, head injury, or generalized seizures; with deep anesthesia; and in cerebral lipidosis.

Certain EEG patterns are worthy of mention because they are frequently regarded as abnormal when, in fact, they are simply normal variants of no pathological significance. Such patterns include 14- and 6-Hz positive spikes, small sharp spikes (sometimes referred to as benign epileptiform transients of sleep), wicket spikes, 6-Hz spike-wave activity, and rhythmical temporal bursts of sharpened theta activity, all of which occur most commonly during drowsiness or light sleep.[2]

CLINICAL USES OF THE EEG

The EEG is useful in the evaluation of patients with several types of neurological disorders, including seizures, encephalopathy, and focal cerebral abnormalities. It also provides an ancillary aid to the diagnosis of brain death and may suggest certain specific neurological diagnoses when characteristic EEG findings are recorded in patients with clinical disorders of uncertain nature.

Epilepsy

The EEG is important in the evaluation of patients with known or suspected epilepsy. The interictal occurrence of epileptiform activity in a patient with an episodic behavioral disorder that may represent seizure activity increases markedly the probability of epilepsy.[9] In patients with epilepsy, the EEG

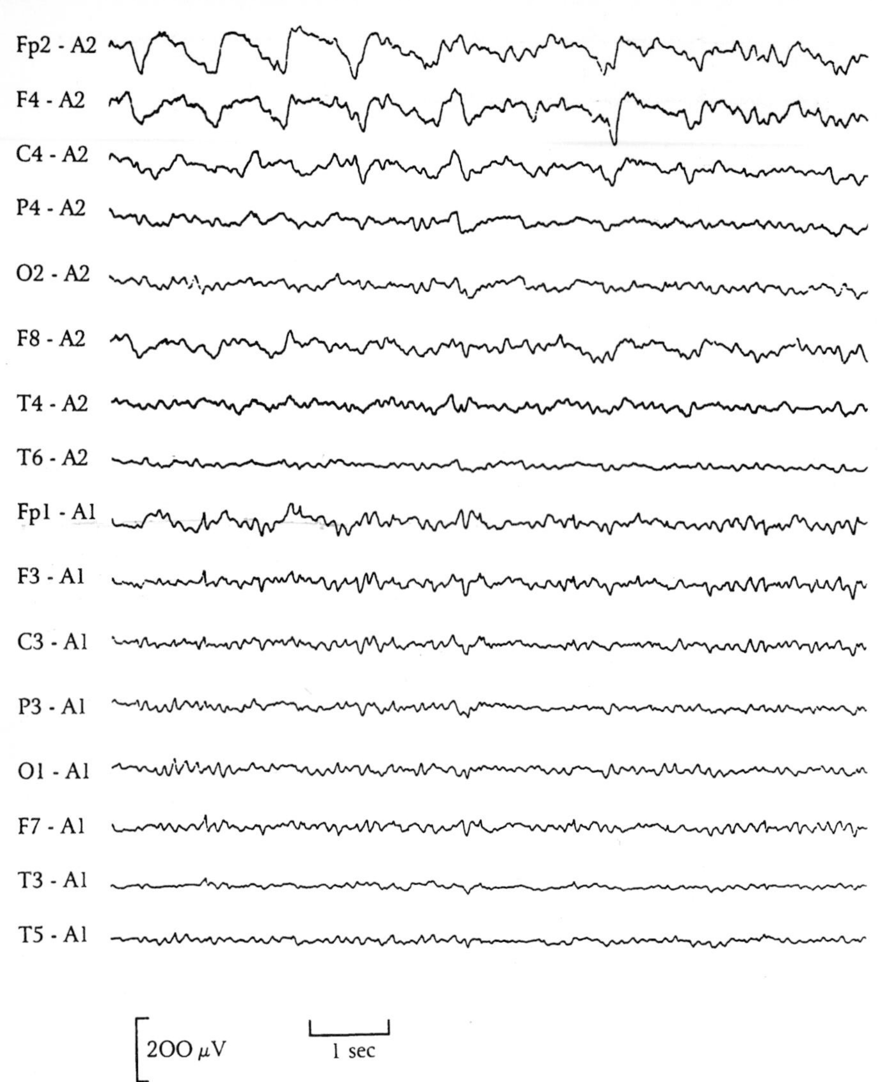

FIGURE 24–2. EEG showing a focal polymorphic slow-wave disturbance in a patient with a right frontal glioma.

findings help to classify the seizure disorder, often permitting a distinction between seizure types when this cannot be made clinically. For example, the EEG findings permit typical absence seizures to be distinguished from complex partial seizures and generalized seizures to be distinguished from partial seizures having rapid secondary generalization (Fig. 24–5). Such findings therefore suggest the appropriate anticonvulsant drug for treating individual patients and provide a guide to prognosis. A guide to prognosis is also provided by the background EEG activity—a slowed background implies a poorer prognosis than otherwise. In addition, a normal background activity EEG permits certain epileptic syndromes with

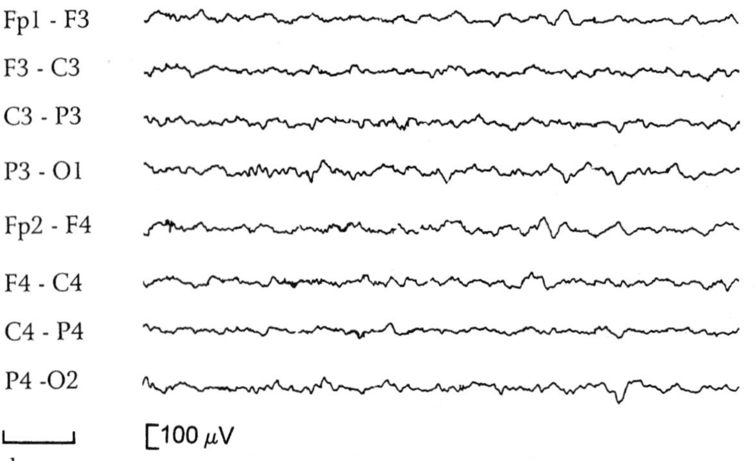

FIGURE 24–3. Diffusely slowed EEG in an obtunded patient with a metabolic encephalopathy.

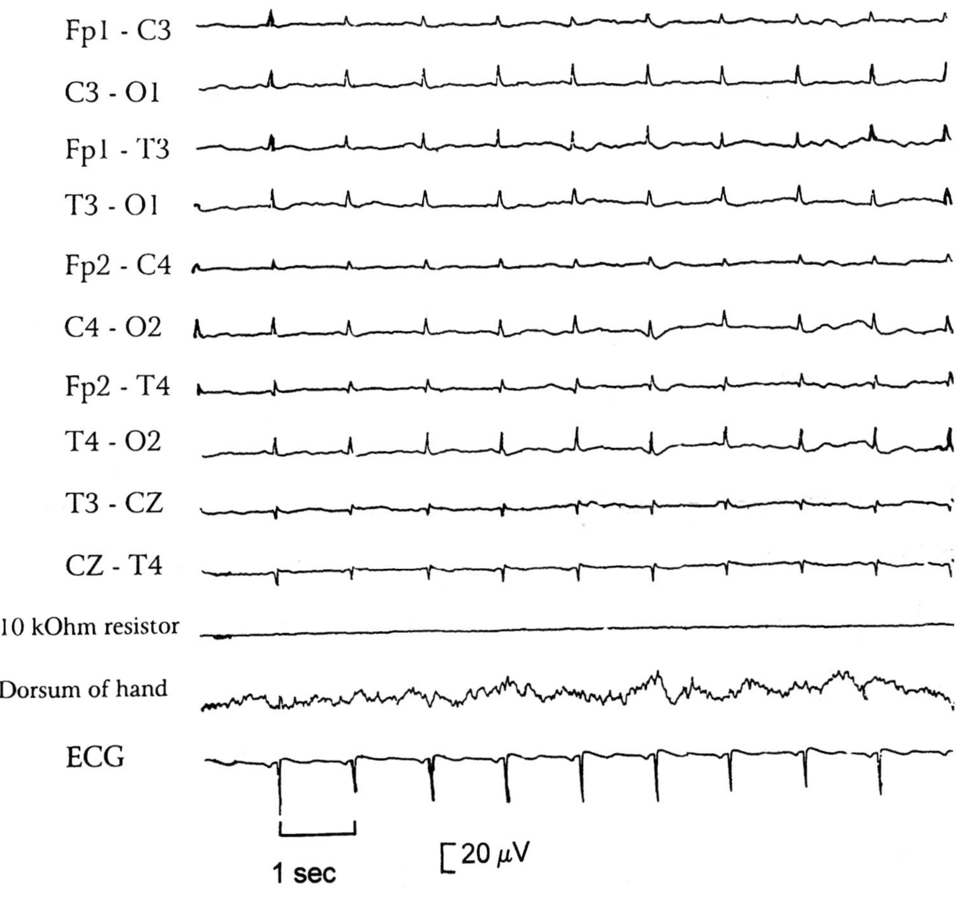

FIGURE 24–4. Electrocerebral silence in the EEG of a brain-dead patient following attempted resuscitation after cardiopulmonary arrest.

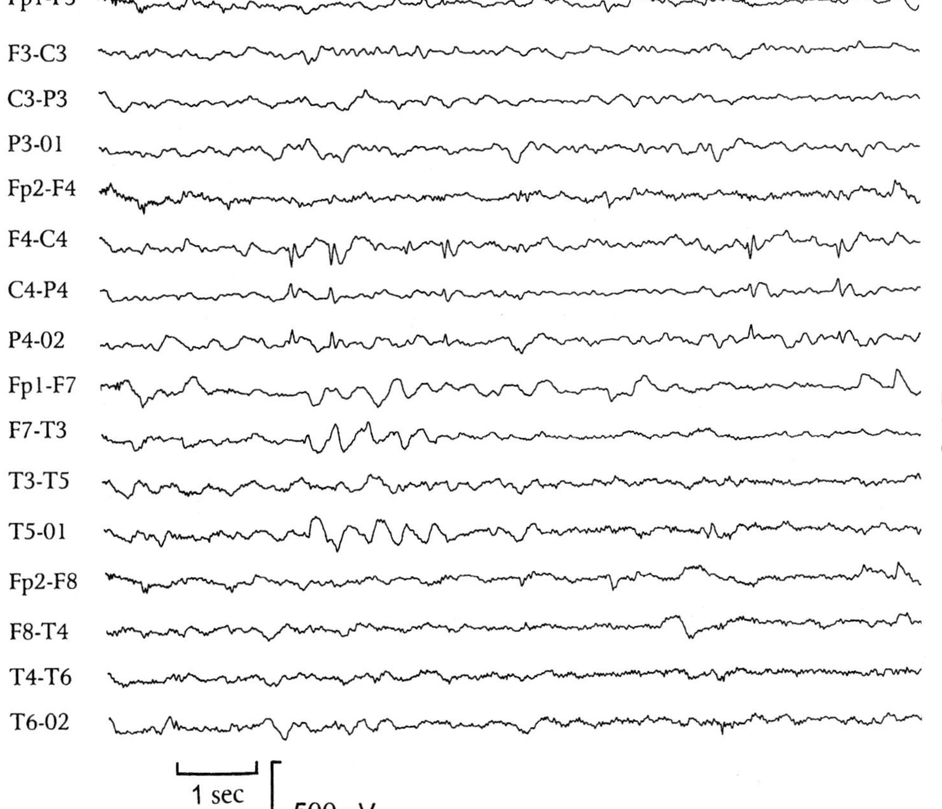

FIGURE 24–5. EEG in a woman with complex partial seizures, showing focal spike discharges in the right central region.

specific prognostic implications to be recognized. For example, benign rolandic epilepsy of childhood has a characteristic interictal EEG pattern (rolandic spikes) and a good prognosis, whereas anterior temporal spike discharges are typically associated with complex partial seizures and imply a poorer outcome.

When surgery is under consideration for the treatment of medically intractable seizures, the EEG has a major role in localizing seizure foci, provided that actual seizures can be recorded. This generally requires admission to a hospital, where the EEG can be recorded continually while patients are video-monitored.

The interictal EEG findings may suggest certain characteristic seizure disorders. *Hypsarrhythmia* refers to a pattern characterized by high-voltage, irregular slow activity with superimposed multifocal spike discharges. It is typically found in children with infantile spasms, although some children with infantile spasms do not have this EEG pattern and it is sometimes found in patients without infantile spasms.[10] Generalized spike-wave activity suggests primary generalized epilepsy when it occurs interictally at 3 Hz and is bilaterally symmetrical and bisynchronous (Fig. 24–6) and Lennox-Gastaut syndrome when it is at 1 to 2 Hz and irregular in frequency and morphology. Polyspike-wave activity occurs with myoclonic epilepsy, including juvenile myoclonic epilepsy of Janz.

The ictal EEG recorded during a tonic-clonic convulsion is always abnormal, but the findings may be obscured by muscle and movement artifact. A transient attenuation of ongoing electrocerebral activity or the development of low-voltage fast activity heralds the onset of the seizure (Fig. 24–7), followed by the appearance of rhythmic, repetitive activity at about 10 Hz that gradually becomes intermixed with increasing amounts of slow activity until the record is characterized by spike-wave activity as the tonic phase of the seizure is succeeded by the clonic phase. This is followed in turn by a transient attenuation of the background EEG and then by irregular slow activity before the EEG reverts to its preictal appearance. During tonic seizures, the EEG shows generalized, repetitive spike activity or an attenuation of the ongoing background activity. During a typical absence attack, by contrast, the EEG is characterized by 3-Hz spike-wave activity, and during myoclonic seizures, it is characterized by polyspike-wave activity at 4 to 5 Hz. The EEG may show no ictal accompaniments during simple partial seizures, and this should not be taken to imply that the seizures are nonorganic in origin. In other patients with such seizures and in those with complex partial seizures, the EEG shows rhythmic, organized, localized discharges (Fig. 24–8) with or without spike activity that may become more generalized as the seizure proceeds and may be followed postictally by a transient flattening of the traces and then by polymorphic slow activity with a localized or generalized distribution.

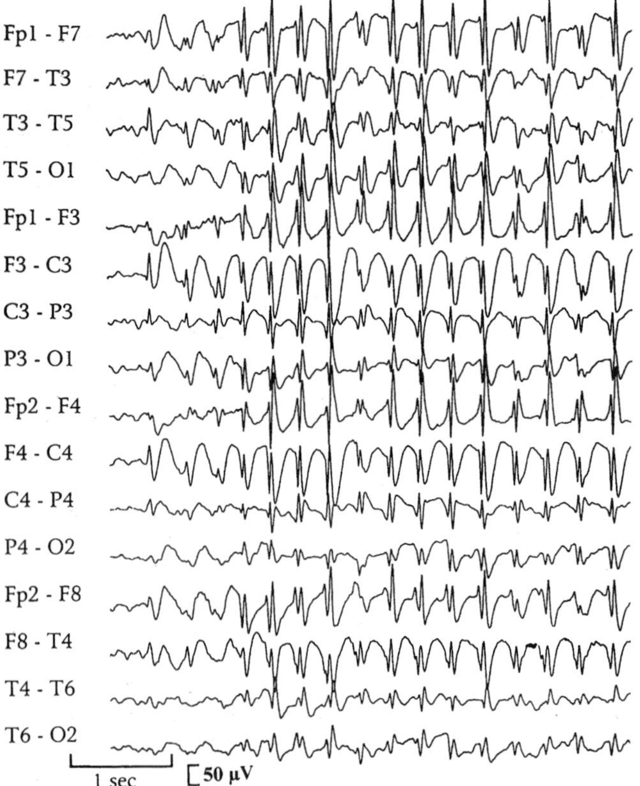

FIGURE 24–6. Burst of generalized 3- to 4-Hz spike-wave activity occurring interictally in a patient with primary generalized epilepsy.

During tonic-clonic (major motor or grand mal) status epilepticus the EEG shows repeated electrographic seizures. The EEG is not required for diagnostic purposes, however, except when patients have been paralyzed pharmacologically to facilitate management; when coma has been induced to control refractory status, the EEG has an important role in monitoring the level of anesthesia. In patients with nonconvulsive status epilepticus, the basis for the abnormal mental status can only be recognized by the EEG finding of continuous, generalized spike-wave activity (so-called spike-wave stupor) or repeated partial seizures. This underscores the importance of obtaining an EEG in any patient with a change in mental status of uncertain basis.

Focal Cerebral Pathology

With the advent of new imaging techniques, the role of the EEG in screening patients for suspected focal intracranial pathological processes has declined, except in developing countries. In fact, however, the EEG detects disturbances of function whereas imaging procedures detect structural abnormalities, so that the two approaches are complementary, not alternatives. EEG abnormalities are sometimes generalized in patients with focal intracranial pathology, detracting from the value of the technique in localizing the lesion but emphasizing its importance in reflecting the extent of functional impairment. Thus, generalized slowing of the EEG commonly reflects a disturbance in the level of consciousness. Even when focal abnormalities are present, they generally provide no indication as to the nature of the underlying pathology. They typically consist of a localized slow-wave disturbance (see Fig. 24–2) or an attenuation of background electrocerebral activity, sometimes accompanied by focal spikes or sharp waves.

Abnormal States of Consciousness

The EEG is an important means of investigating patients with a disturbance of consciousness. It may suggest the cause of the abnormal mental state, helps to determine the depth of coma, and provides a guide to prognosis. Moreover, the

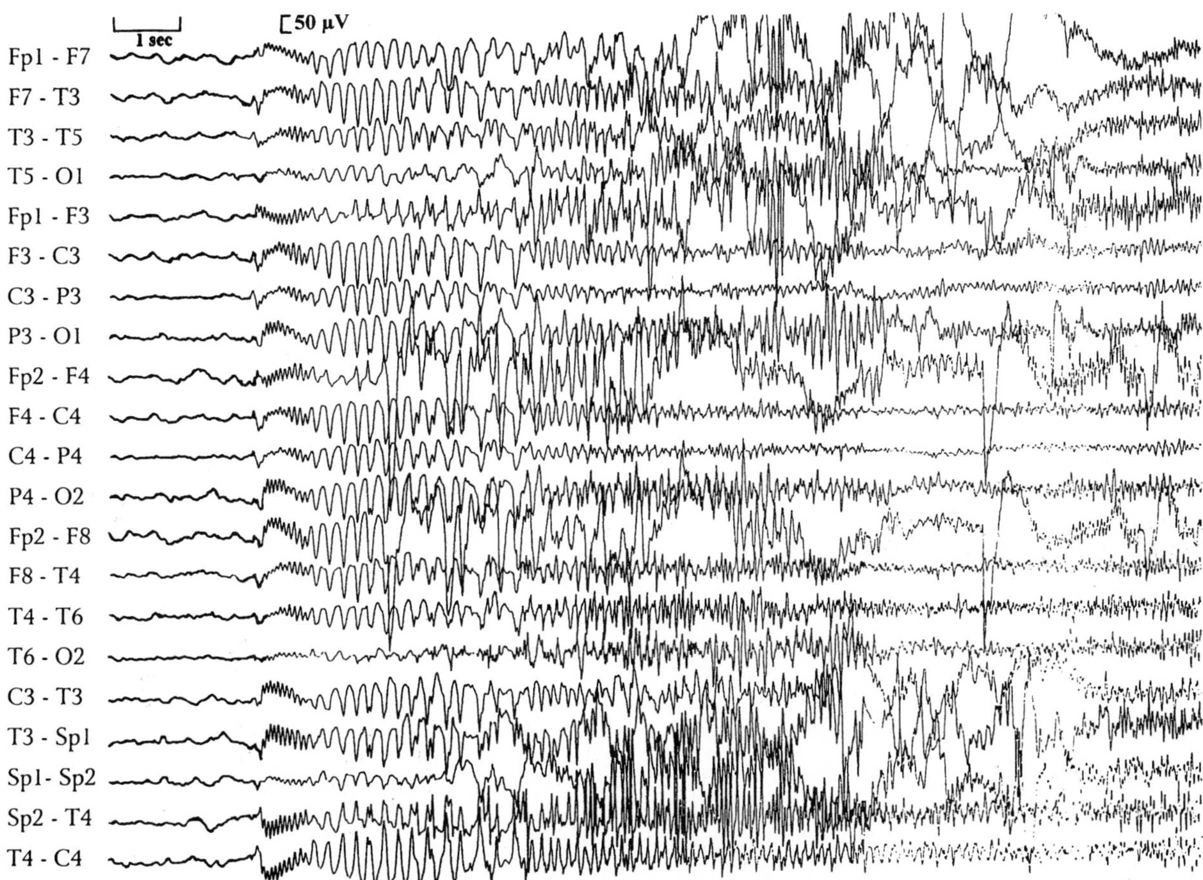

FIGURE 24–7. EEG recorded at the onset of a generalized clonic-tonic-clonic seizure, showing the development of bisynchronous low-voltage generalized fast activity that then becomes intermixed with increasing amounts of slow activity as the seizure continues.

EEG is an important means of distinguishing between unconscious states and neurological disorders simulating unconsciousness, such as the locked-in syndrome, in which the EEG is normal or shows only minor nonspecific changes.

In patients with a disturbance of consciousness due to diffuse cerebral dysfunction, the EEG typically showed generalized slowing (see Fig. 24–3) without focal or lateralizing features. In some metabolic encephalopathies, triphasic waves are conspicuous, but these are a nonspecific finding. When epileptiform discharges or electrographic seizures are found in the EEG, they suggest that a postictal state or status epilepticus is responsible for the obtundation.

In coma after head injury, the EEG is likely to be diffusely slowed but focal abnormalities (slowing, spike discharges, or an attenuation of activity) may be superimposed. These localized abnormalities may relate to hematoma or cerebral contusion, ischemia, or edema.

Alpha-pattern coma designates coma associated with alpha-frequency activity in the EEG. The alpha-frequency activity is usually widespread in distribution and nonreactive to external stimuli. It is found most commonly after a cardiac or cardiorespiratory arrest and also occurs after pontine strokes and occasionally with a drug overdose. Alpha-pattern coma was originally thought to imply a poor prognosis, but the outlook relates more to the cause of the coma than to the presence of alpha-frequency activity in the EEG.[11, 12]

In some comatose patients the EEG shows a burst-suppression pattern, indicating a severe encephalopathic process such as an anoxic encephalopathy. The finding of electrocerebral silence indicates that irreversible brain damage and neocortical brain death have occurred. A similar finding may also relate to hypothermia or the presence of CNS depressant drugs, however, and these conditions must always be excluded before prognostic implications are ascribed to the EEG changes.

Other Applications

In patients with encephalitis or meningoencephalitis, the EEG typically shows diffuse slowing without any specific features. Characteristic abnormalities are, however, found in certain infectious disorders of the brain. In herpes simplex encephalitis, periodic lateralized complexes may occur over one or both temporal regions, usually repeating once every 1 to 4 seconds (Fig. 24–9).[13] These discharges may take up to 2 weeks to develop, and their absence does not exclude the diagnosis. Their presence provides strong support for it, however, and their bilateral occurrence implies a poorer prognosis for survival than otherwise. In subacute sclerosing panencephalitis, generalized periodic complexes are seen, often lasting for up to 3 seconds and with an interval 3 to 15 seconds between complexes. A similar pattern is sometimes observed in patients who have taken phencyclidine.[14] In Creutzfeldt-Jakob disease (Fig. 24–10), periodic complexes are typically triphasic in configuration and occur at a rate of approximately 1 Hz. Their occurrence in patients with a rapidly progressive dementia strongly supports the diagnosis.[15, 16]

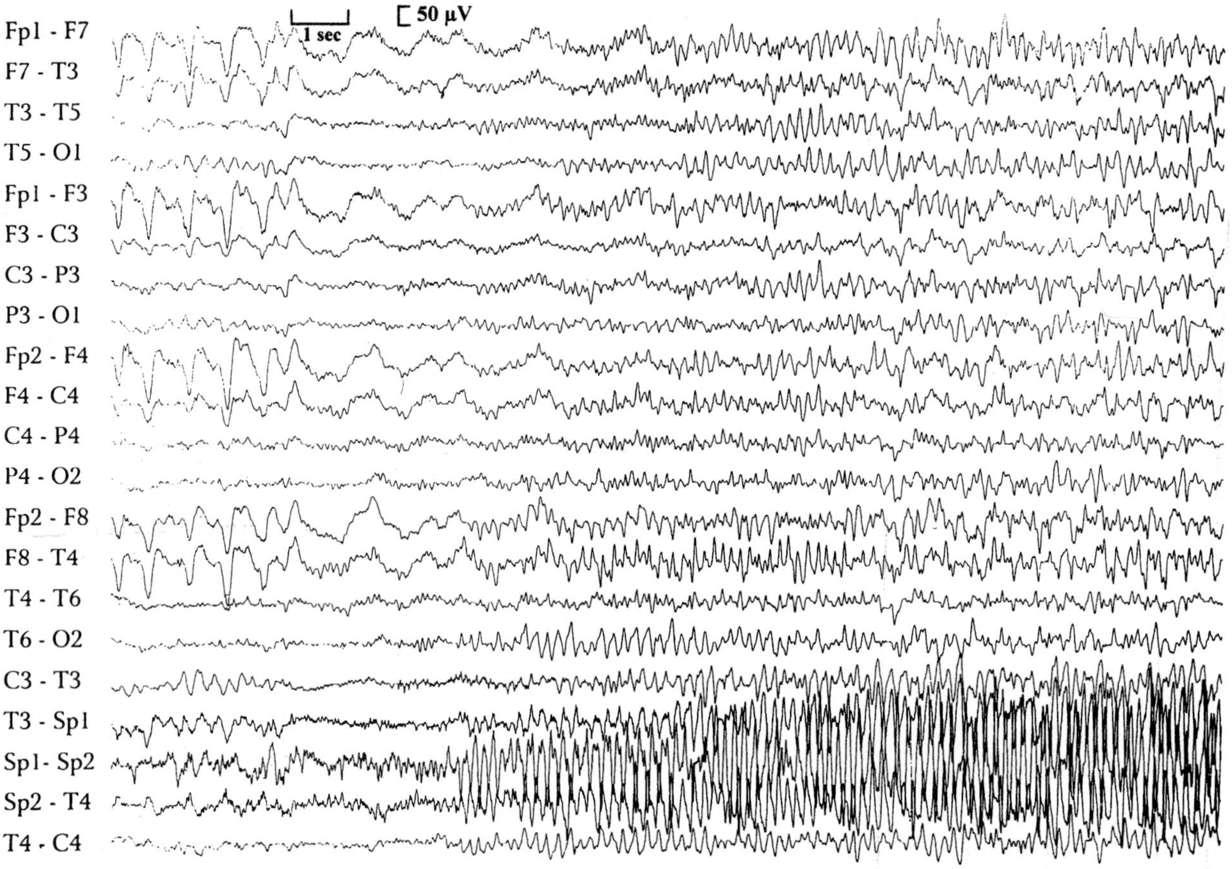

FIGURE 24–8. Repetitive focal spike activity arising in the right anteromesial temporal region (right sphenoidal electrode at Sp2) at the onset of a complex partial seizure in a patient with epilepsy

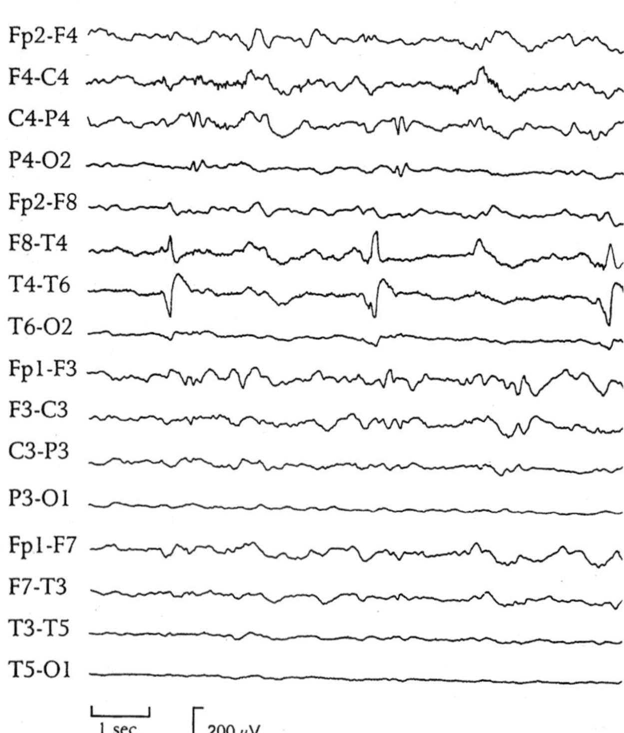

FIGURE 24–9. Repetitive complexes occurring in the right temporal region of a child with herpes simplex encephalitis.

The EEG findings are of little relevance to the diagnosis of migraine. They are usually normal, but focal or generalized slow activity may be found, especially during or immediately after migrainous attacks. Epileptiform transients are also encountered in some patients.

Abnormalities may be found in demented patients and consist usually of a nonspecific loss of the alpha rhythm and the presence of excessive slow activity. Focal slowing may also occur, especially in Alzheimer's disease. A normal EEG in no way excludes a diagnosis of dementia, but a diffusely abnormal record supports a diagnosis of dementia as opposed to pseudodementia. The EEG findings may suggest the cause of the dementia, such as in Creutzfeldt-Jakob disease or subacute sclerosing panencephalitis, or when a focal structural lesion is present.

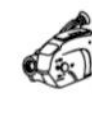

The EEG findings after head trauma reflect the severity of injury and level of consciousness. They do not improve the ability to predict which patients are likely to develop posttraumatic epilepsy.

Polysomnography

BASIC PRINCIPLES AND TECHNIQUE

Disorders of sleep are common and often respond well to treatment. Polysomnography is important in diagnosing and characterizing such disorders. It involves recording the EEG

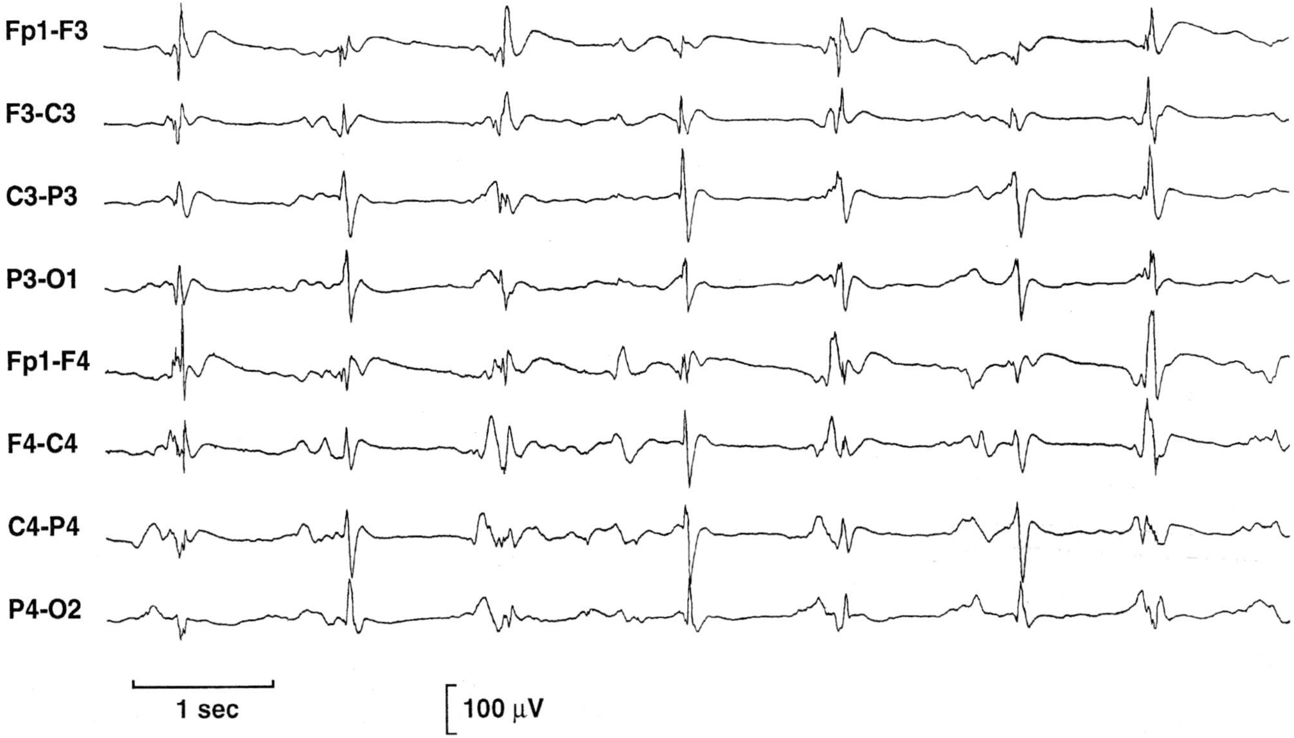

FIGURE 24–10. EEG of a patient with Creutzfeldt-Jakob disease showing periodic complexes that often have a triphasic configuration.

on two or a few channels to characterize the stage of sleep while recordings are also made of eye movements, mentalis muscle activity (chin EMG), electrocardiogram, respiration, and oxygen saturation. Respiratory movements are recorded by measurement of air flow through the nasal passages and the mouth using thermistors and by recording thoraco-abdominal excursions with surface electrodes. Oxygen saturation is measured using an ear oximeter. A microphone can be taped to the face to record snoring.

NORMAL POLYSOMNOGRAPHIC FINDINGS

The EEG shows a characteristic sequence of events during sleep. During drowsiness (Stage 1 sleep) the alpha rhythm is attenuated and the background consists of mixed frequencies. Rolling eye movements are characteristic. During Stage 2 sleep, the background EEG consists of diffuse theta and slower activity superimposed on which are vertex sharp waves, sleep spindles (bursts of 12- to 14-Hz activity that occur bilaterally in the central regions), and K-complexes (high-voltage slow-wave complexes). During slow-wave (Stages 3 and 4) sleep, high-voltage theta and slower activity is present, with activity at 2 Hz or less being present for up to 50 percent of the time in Stage 3 sleep and for more than this in Stage 4 sleep. Tonic activity is present in the mentalis muscle during these stages of sleep. During rapid-eye-movement (REM) sleep, the EEG resembles that of Stage 1 sleep, but rapid eye movements occur in all directions and tonic muscle activity is either absent or markedly reduced.

Sleep goes through these various stages sequentially from Stage 1 to Stage 4 and then back to Stage 2 over about 90 minutes, following which REM sleep occurs. Such sleep cycles usually occur about three or four times each night, with the amount of REM sleep increasing in later cycles.

ABNORMAL FINDINGS AND CLINICAL USES OF POLYSOMNOGRAPHY

Polysomnography is important in the investigation of patients with excessive daytime somnolence, disorders of initiating and maintaining sleep, disorders of the sleep-wake cycle, and disorders associated with certain sleep stages (parasomnias).

It is important in confirming the existence of insomnia and characterizing its nature by determining, for example, whether it is associated with nocturnal myoclonus or periodic leg movements. Some patients complain of insomnia but, in fact, have a normal amount of sleep. Patients with complaints of excessive daytime somnolence may have sleep apnea, which can be diagnosed by polysomnography. Apnea is defined in this context as the cessation of air flow at the mouth and nostrils for at least 10 seconds, whereas hypopnea refers to a reduction in respiratory air flow to one third of its basal value, with an associated reduction of abdominal and thoracic respiratory movements and a decline in oxygen saturation. The number of respiratory irregularities per hour of sleep can be calculated by dividing the number of apneic and hypopneic episodes by the total sleep time in minutes and multiplying the result by 60. A value of 5 or less is regarded as within the normal range.[17] Polysomnography further indicates whether sleep apnea syndrome relates to a central disturbance, an obstructive disturbance in the oropharynx (Fig. 24–11), or a mixed disorder. Sleep apnea is dangerous because various cardiac abnormalities may occur during the apneic episodes, sometimes resulting in death. Polysomnography permits the severity of the syndrome and the presence of cardiac

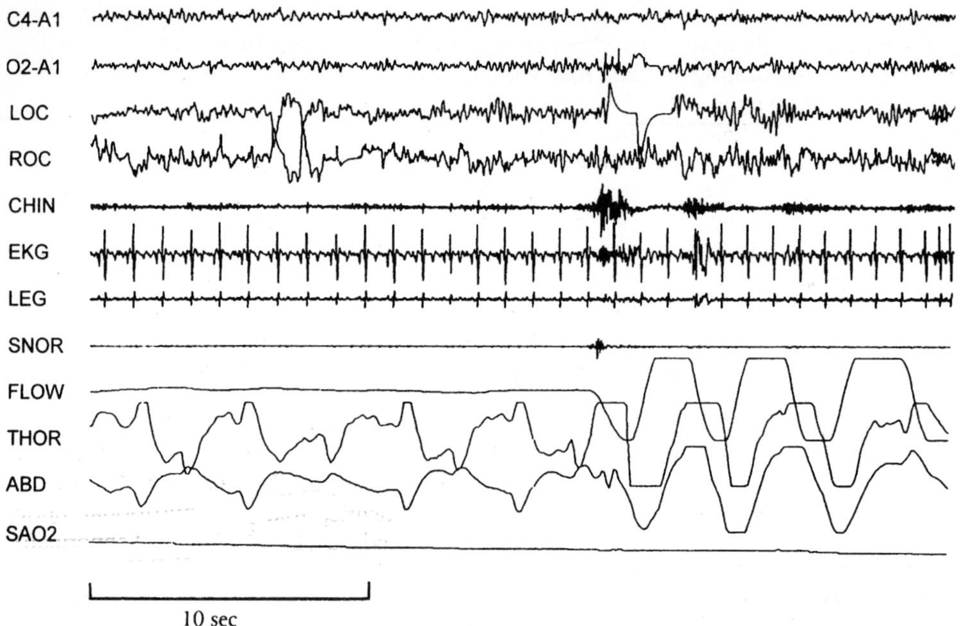

FIGURE 24–11. Polysomnogram of a patient with obstructive sleep apnea. An obstructive apneic episode is seen during REM sleep and is characterized by cessation of air flow associated with oxygen desaturation, accompanied by attempted respiratory movements of the thoracic and abdominal musculature.

abnormalities to be determined, thereby indicating the need for prompt therapeutic intervention.

Another important cause of excessive daytime sleepiness is narcolepsy, which is diagnosed by the multiple sleep latency test. This quantifies the time required to fall asleep and allows the recognition of abnormally short latencies for going into REM sleep.[18, 19] Patients are monitored for five periods of 20 minutes at intervals of 2 hours, during which they are allowed to fall asleep; between these periods, they are kept awake and alert. A mean daily score of less than 5 minutes indicates a pathological level of daytime sleepiness. The number of sleep-onset REM periods (with REM sleep occurring within 15 minutes of sleep onset) is determined. Normally, REM sleep does not occur during these periods; two sleep-onset REM episodes strongly support a diagnosis of narcolepsy. The sensitivity and specificity of the test, however, are not clearly defined.[20]

Certain complex behavioral disorders may disrupt sleep. These parasomnias are best characterized also by polysomnography. They tend to occur particularly during slow-wave sleep, and precise diagnosis facilitates appropriate treatment. In other patients, seizures may occur during sleep and these can be recognized by the study. Further discussion of sleep disorders is provided in Chapter 54.

Overview of Evoked Potentials

Stimulation of certain sensory systems leads to the generation of cerebral potentials that can be recorded over the scalp with surface electrodes. The latency and morphology of these evoked potentials depend on the eliciting stimulus. Evoked potentials are generally of low voltage and are intermixed with background EEG activity. For this reason, they are not easily seen without computer averaging of a number of responses so that signals that are time locked to the stimulus are enhanced, whereas other electrocerebral activity is averaged out.

Evoked potential recordings provide a means of detecting lesions in the afferent pathways under study. They assess the functional integrity of these pathways, whereas imaging techniques such as magnetic resonance imaging evaluate their anatomical basis. Thus, evoked potential studies sometimes reveal abnormalities missed by magnetic resonance imaging, and vice versa. The findings may be important for diagnostic purposes, in following the course of certain neurological disorders, or for determining the extent of pathological involvement.[21] In patients with known pathological processes involving the CNS, evoked potential studies help to detect and localize lesions. Subclinical abnormalities may be detected in a variety of disorders, and multifocal abnormalities occur not only in multiple sclerosis but also in a variety of different settings. The electrophysiological findings must therefore be interpreted in the clinical context in which they are obtained. Evoked potential studies are also helpful in the evaluation of ill-defined complaints to categorize more precisely the functional integrity of any afferent pathways that may be responsible for the symptoms in question.[21]

The clinical utility of the various evoked potential studies in widespread use depends on the context in which they are obtained. Although some investigators have attempted to localize lesions on the basis of the electrophysiological findings, precise localization by this approach may not be possible. The generators of many of the recorded components are not known with confidence, and some components may have multiple generators.

Evoked potentials have been used to monitor neural structures at risk during surgical procedures, such as correction of scoliosis, in an attempt to minimize or prevent neurological damage. When an evoked potential abnormality occurs during the surgical procedure, it is hoped that alteration or reversal of the procedure may prevent or minimize damage. However, the utility of intraoperative monitoring is not well established in most circumstances. Moreover, even if an electrophysiological change occurs intraoperatively, it sometimes remains unclear whether this simply predicts an adverse outcome rather than actually permitting that outcome to be prevented if the surgical technique is modified. Nevertheless, in limited contexts, it is clear that intraoperative monitoring is beneficial. During posterior fossa surgery, for example, recordings of brain stem auditory evoked potentials are helpful in monitoring the status of the eighth cranial nerve to prevent its damage, and stimulation of the seventh cranial nerve aids in identifying this nerve and ensuring its functional continuity. Similarly, somatosensory evoked potential studies to monitor spinal cord function seem to reduce the morbidity associated with the surgical correction of scoliosis.

Visual Evoked Potentials

BASIC PRINCIPLES AND TECHNIQUE

Monocular stimulation generates a cerebral response that is best recorded over the occipital region. Either a flash or a pattern that occurs without change in background luminance can be used to elicit the response. Responses to approximately 100 stimuli are generally averaged to obtain robust and unambiguous potentials. For pattern stimulation, the seated subject looks at the center of a television screen on which is displayed a checkerboard pattern of white and black squares. The pattern reverses at about 1 Hz so that the white squares become black, and vice versa, without change in total luminance. The size of the checks is usually between 15 and 50 minutes of arc at the subject's eye, and the entire pattern should subtend at least 10 degrees of visual angle. Pattern-reversal stimuli generate robust responses and have a higher yield of abnormalities than flash stimuli. Small checks (15 to 30 minutes) preferentially activate the macular region and are the most widely used stimulus.

NORMAL VEP FINDINGS

The typical visual evoked potential (VEP) elicited by a pattern-reversal stimulus is a negative-positive-negative complex that is recorded maximally in the midoccipital region with reference to either the midfrontal region or the linked ears.[22] The positivity is the most conspicuous and consistent of these potentials and has a latency to its peak of approximately 100 msec (Fig. 24–12). It is therefore called the P100 response, and it is to this component that attention is directed.

In analyzing the VEP, the latency of the P100 response is measured after stimulation of each eye and then the interocular difference in latency is determined. These values are compared with normal values obtained using an identical stimulation and recording technique. This is important because certain physical attributes of the stimulus (such as its contrast or the check size) normally influence the response latency. The amplitude of the response and the latency of the preceding and succeeding negativities (the N75 and N145, respectively) are of uncertain clinical utility, but absence of the P100 is abnormal.

ABNORMAL FINDINGS AND CLINICAL USES OF THE VEP

Visual evoked potentials are useful in evaluating the function of the anterior visual pathways. They are not useful in evaluating lesions posterior to the optic chiasm.

In patients with an acute optic or retrobulbar neuritis, the P100 response is initially lost; with time, it recovers and is then found to have a markedly prolonged latency that generally persists indefinitely (see Fig. 24–12),[23, 24] even if apparently complete clinical recovery occurs. The VEP is therefore an important means of evaluating patients with suspected optic neuritis and may be delayed even when magnetic resonance imaging of the optic nerve is normal.[24] Abnormalities may relate to either recent or long-standing pathological processes. The VEP may be abnormal in patients without a past history of optic neuritis, thereby providing evidence of subclinical involvement of the optic nerve. For this reason, it is useful to record the VEP in such patients when multiple sclerosis is a diagnostic possibility.[25]

Other disorders may also lead to VEP abnormalities. In particular, ocular pathology (e.g., refractive error, inability to focus on the pattern stimulus, or glaucoma) may be responsible. Compressive, ischemic, toxic, or nutritional optic neuropathies may also produce VEP changes, and abnormalities occur in Leber's hereditary optic atrophy.[26, 27] Compressive lesions of the optic nerve typically lead to VEPs that are markedly abnormal in shape as well as delayed in latency;[28] in ischemic or toxic neuropathies, the response is usually markedly attenuated in amplitude without being delayed significantly.[26] The findings, however, have always to be interpreted in the clinical context in which they were obtained.

The VEP findings are of little help in the evaluation of lesions posterior to the optic chiasm. It has been suggested that VEPs can be used to evaluate the visual fields, but the approach is time consuming, requires the close cooperation and attention of patients, and is no better or even less sensitive than standard tests of perimetry.[29, 30] In patients with cortical blindness, the VEP may be normal or abnormal—the presence of a normal response should therefore not lead, in itself, to a diagnosis of nonorganic visual loss.[31]

The pattern-elicited VEP can be used to measure refractive error or detect amblyopia in preverbal children who are unable to cooperate for behavioral testing.[32] For refractive purposes, the VEP is recorded while different lenses are placed in front of the eye to determine the lens with which the VEP to small (15 minute) checks is of largest amplitude

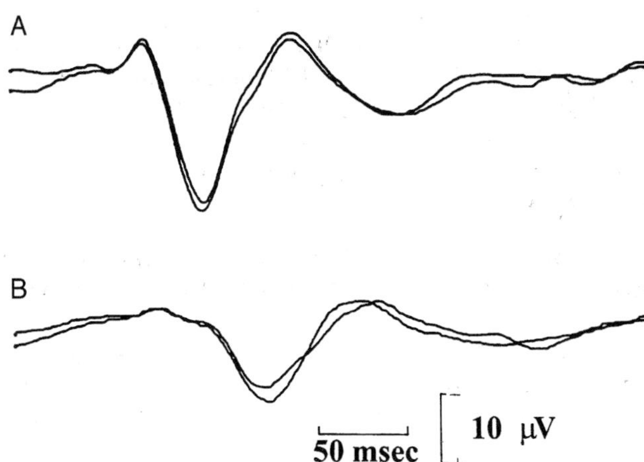

FIGURE 24–12. Visual evoked potential elicited by 50-minute checks and recorded between the midoccipital and midfrontal regions with monocular stimulation in a normal subject (*A*), and a patient with a past history of optic neuritis (*B*). Two trials are superimposed to show the replicability of the findings. The P100 response in *B* is prolonged to 146 msec.

and shortest latency; this lens will be the optimal one for the patient. By an analogous approach, the interocular difference in size of the VEP elicited by small checks is important as a means of detecting unilateral amblyopia at an early age, when recovery may still be possible.

Brain Stem Auditory Evoked Potentials

BASIC PRINCIPLES AND TECHNIQUE

Potentials generated in the auditory nerve and in different regions of the auditory pathways in the brain stem can be recorded at the vertex of the head after auditory stimulation.[33] These brain stem auditory evoked potentials (BAEPs) occur within 10 msec of the stimulus, which for clinical purposes is a monaural click. This is usually set at approximately 65 dB above the patient's hearing threshold and is delivered through earphones while the opposite ear is masked by white (i.e., mixed-frequency) noise. The attention of the subject is not required. Because the BAEP is of very low voltage, between 1000 and 2000 responses are generally recorded so that the BAEP can be extracted by averaging from the background noise.

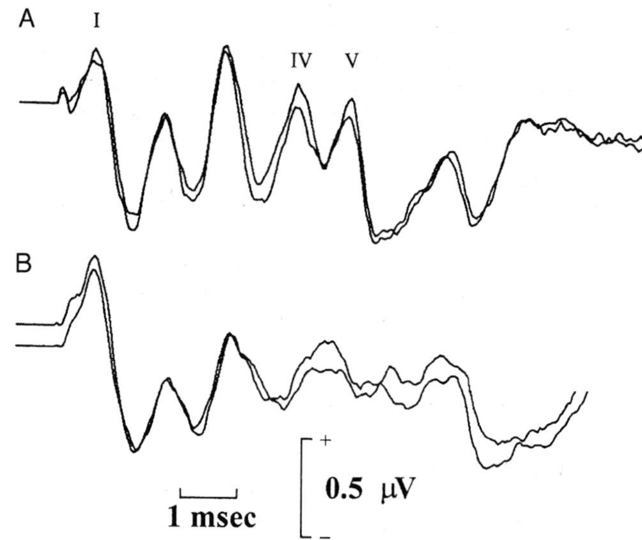

FIGURE 24–13. Brain stem auditory potential elicited by monaural stimulation at 75 dBSL and recorded with an ipsilateral mastoid reference in a normal subject (*A*), and a patient with a structural lesion involving the upper pons (*B*). Two trials are superimposed to show the replicability of the findings. It can be seen that waves IV and V are markedly attenuated in the response recorded in *B*.

NORMAL BAEP FINDINGS

The BAEP consists of a series of up to seven components (identified by Roman numerals) that occur within 10 msec of the click stimulus and are generated in different regions of the peripheral and central auditory pathways. Wave I and the early part of wave II represent the auditory nerve action potential. Wave III probably arises in the region of the superior olive, whereas waves IV and V arise in the midbrain and inferior colliculus. Waves VI and VII are of uncertain origin and, because of their inconsistency in normal subjects, are of little clinical utility.

The most consistent components are waves I, III, and V, and it is to these that attention is directed when BAEPs are evaluated for clinical purposes. The absolute latency of these components, the intervals between them (the so-called interpeak latencies), and the amplitude of wave V relative to wave I are assessed. Interside differences in interpeak latency are also measured and may reveal minor abnormalities. Figure 24–13 illustrates a normal response.

ABNORMAL FINDINGS AND CLINICAL USES OF THE BAEP

The BAEP is an important means of evaluating function of the eighth cranial nerve and the central auditory pathways in the brain stem.

In infants, young children, and adults who are unable to cooperate for behavioral testing, BAEPs can be used to evaluate hearing.[34] The wave V component of the response is generated by auditory stimuli that are too weak to generate other components. As a screening test of hearing, then, the electrophysiological threshold for eliciting wave V is determined. An impairment of auditory acuity is suggested if a stimulus intensity greater than 40 dB is required. BAEPs provide a sensitive screening test for acoustic neuromas or other lesions in the cerebellopontine angle involving the eighth cranial nerve. Indeed, the BAEP findings may be abnormal at a time when imaging studies show no definite abnormality.

The BAEP is also useful in assessing the integrity of the brain stem (see Fig. 24–13). Although the auditory pathways have a bilateral course, a unilaterally abnormal BAEP nevertheless suggests an ipsilateral, structural brain stem lesion. The presence of normal BAEPs in comatose patients suggests either that the coma is due to bihemispheric disease or that it relates to metabolic or toxic factors; abnormal BAEPs in this context imply brain stem pathology and a poorer prognosis than otherwise. When coma is due to brain stem pathology, the BAEP findings help in localizing the lesion: alteration of wave V suggests midbrain dysfunction, and alteration of waves I to III indicates a lesion in the lower brain stem.[35] In patients with brain death, the BAEP should be absent apart from wave I and the early part of wave II, which are generated peripherally. In many patients with suspected brain death, however, all BAEP components, including wave I, are absent, and it is then not possible to exclude other causes (such as technical factors or deafness) for the absent response.[36]

BAEPs have been used to detect subclinical brain stem pathology in patients with suspected multiple sclerosis.[37, 38] However, the yield in this circumstance is less than with the visual or somatosensory evoked potentials, possibly because the auditory pathway is relatively short or is more likely to be spared.

Somatosensory Evoked Potentials

BASIC PRINCIPLES AND TECHNIQUE

Stimulation of a mixed nerve or its sensory branch leads to a response that can be recorded from the nerve more proximally or distally (the sensory nerve action potential), as well as over the spine and scalp. The scalp response is small and obscured by the ongoing EEG, and for this reason it is often necessary to average up to 2000 responses after stimulation of a nerve in the arm or 4000 responses with stimulation of a nerve in the leg, depending on the amount of background noise, to obtain well-defined responses.

The somatosensory evoked potential (SEP) depends on the functional integrity of the fast-conducting large-diameter group IA muscle afferent fibers and group II cutaneous afferent fibers and on the posterior columns of the cord, although some fibers may follow a different, extralemniscal pathway. It is elicited for clinical purposes by an electrical stimulus that is sufficient to produce a slight muscle twitch when a mixed nerve is stimulated or to generate a sensory nerve action potential that is about 50 percent of maximum. It is generally well tolerated, even when applied with a repetition rate of about 3 or 5 Hz. SEPs can also be elicited by cutaneous nerve or dermatomal stimulation, but the role of these approaches, especially in the evaluation of suspected radiculopathies, is uncertain. SEPs are best recorded with surface electrodes. Over the scalp, either a bipolar derivation (both recording electrodes placed on the scalp) or a referential derivation (involving a noncephalic reference electrode) may be used.

NORMAL SEP FINDINGS

SEP components are defined by polarity and latency. With stimulation of a nerve in the arm, recording between the contralateral "hand area" of scalp and contralateral Erb's point, that is, in a referential derivation, demonstrates a P9 potential that reflects activity at or just beyond the brachial plexus. A P13–P14 potential reflects postsynaptic activity in the medial lemniscus, and an N20 component is generated in the primary somatosensory cortex (Fig. 24–14). A variety of other potentials may also be detected but are clinically less helpful and are not discussed further. With stimulation of the tibial nerve at the ankle, a P38 response is recorded over the scalp in the midline and represents activation of the

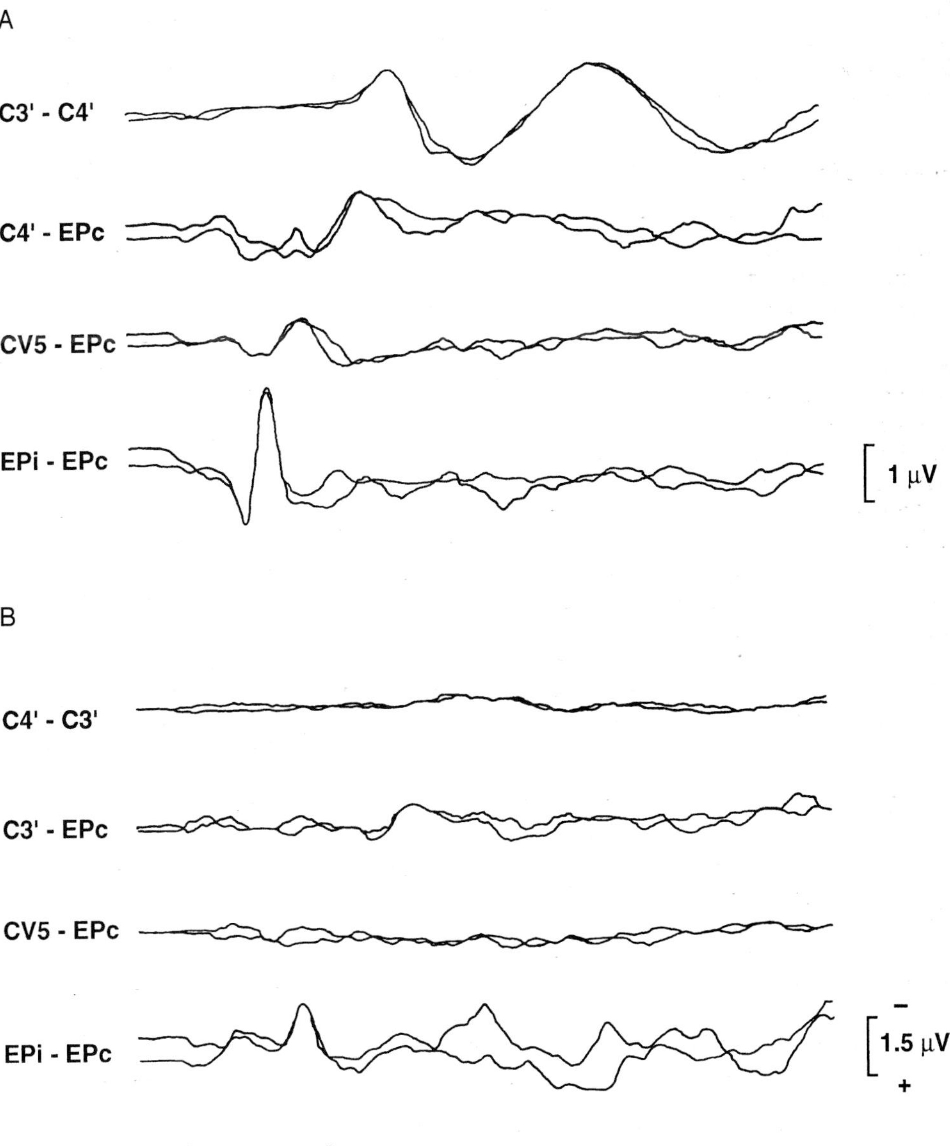

FIGURE 24–14. Median-elicited somatosensory evoked potential elicited in *A*, a normal subject by right-sided stimulation, and *B*, a patient with multiple sclerosis by left-sided stimulation. Two trials are superimposed to show the replicability of the findings. In the responses recorded in the patient, an Erb's point potential is present but responses over the cervical spine and scalp are absent. EP, Erb's point; CV5, 5th cervical spine; i, ipsilateral; c, contralateral; other abbreviations as in earlier illustrations.

primary somatosensory cortex (Fig. 24–15). Recordings over the cervical spine after stimulation of the nerve in the arm reveals an N13/P13, whereas stimulation of a leg nerve elicits a negative peak over the cauda equina and lumbar spine.

The presence or absence of these obligate components of the response and their latency and interpeak latency are recorded. Amplitude measurements may also be made, but abnormalities should not be based solely on amplitude criteria, except when an obligate response is absent. The absolute latency of individual components, but not the interpeak latency, varies with limb length.

As with the BAEP, it has generally been assumed that different components of the SEP reflect sequential activation of neural generators. However, potentials can be generated by a change in the physical characteristic of the volume conductor as, for example, when an impulse passes from the arm to the axilla.[39, 40]

ABNORMAL FINDINGS AND CLINICAL USES OF THE SEP

Somatosensory evoked potentials are helpful in detecting and localizing lesions of the somatosensory pathways within the CNS but provide no indication about the nature of the underlying pathological processes. They are of little value in evaluating the peripheral nervous system, except when there is concern about the functional integrity of nerves that are not easily accessible for conventional nerve conduction studies.[41] SEPs have been used to evaluate patients with suspected radiculopathies. Abnormalities would not be expected in the SEP obtained by a stimulation of a polysegmental nerve trunk in patients with isolated root lesions, and cutaneous nerve or dermatomal stimulation has given conflicting results and should therefore be regarded as investigational.[42]

In patients with multiple sclerosis, SEP abnormalities may indicate the presence of subclinical lesions, thereby helping to establish the diagnosis.[43] The presence of such abnormalities may also suggest that vague sensory complaints have an organic basis when this is hard to determine clinically. The SEP is abnormal in about 80 percent of patients with multiple sclerosis (see Figs. 24–14 and 24–15), but SEP abnormalities are found in only about 30 percent of patients when this is merely a diagnostic possibility. The yield is greater in SEPs elicited by stimulation of a nerve in the legs than the arms and is more likely when there are pyramidal signs in the stimulated limb or legs.[44] The most common abnormality found in patients with multiple sclerosis is loss or marked attenuation of the cervical response after stimulation of the median or ulnar nerve, and there may be an increase in central conduction time.[45] Subclinical SEP abnormalities may also indicate sensory involvement in patients with hereditary spinocerebellar degenerations, hereditary spastic paraplegia, AIDS, and a deficiency of vitamin B_{12} or vitamin E, and are therefore not pathognomonic of multiple sclerosis.[43, 46]

SEPs may indicate involvement of the central somatosensory pathways by other disorders at the spinal, brain stem, or thalamic levels. In patients with unilateral lesions of the cerebral hemisphere, the SEPs are often normal unless there is a clinical sensory disturbance, when they may be lost or markedly attenuated.

The SEP has been used to provide a prognostic guide in comatose patients.[36, 43, 47–49] In particular, loss bilaterally of the N20 response after stimulation of the median nerve is commonly associated with a fatal outcome or development of a persistent vegetative state. In patients with unilateral loss of the N20, the outcome is more variable; with bilaterally preserved N20 responses, approximately 50 percent of comatose patients regain useful function, 25 percent remain in a vegetative state, and the remainder die. Based on several other studies, it seems reasonable to conclude that patients with absent cortical SEPs bilaterally are unlikely to recover cognition, but the presence of normal SEPs does not predict that useful recovery will necessarily follow. The bilateral absence of all responses later than the N13–N14 response is supportive of brain death, when this is diagnosed by clinical criteria.[36]

After spinal injury, the SEP findings vary over the scalp after stimulation of a leg nerve, depending on the timing of the examination and the severity of the lesion. The absence of any cortical response in the acute stage after cord injury should not be taken to imply that the lesion is complete or that recovery will fail to occur. Preserved responses or their early return, however, indicate a better prognosis, although the degree of functional recovery varies.

SEPs have been used intraoperatively to monitor cord function, but it is not clear how useful they are in this con-

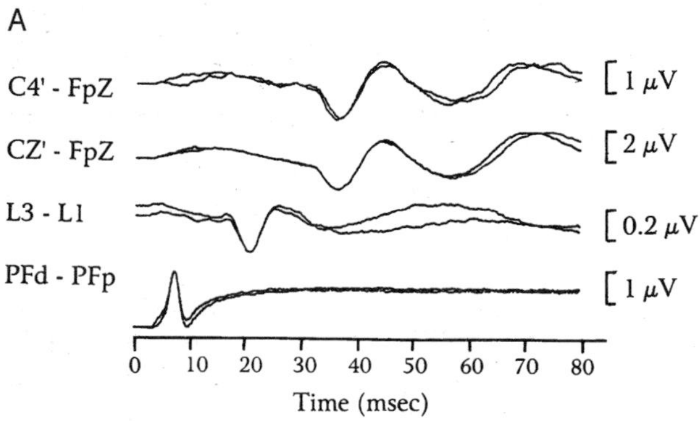

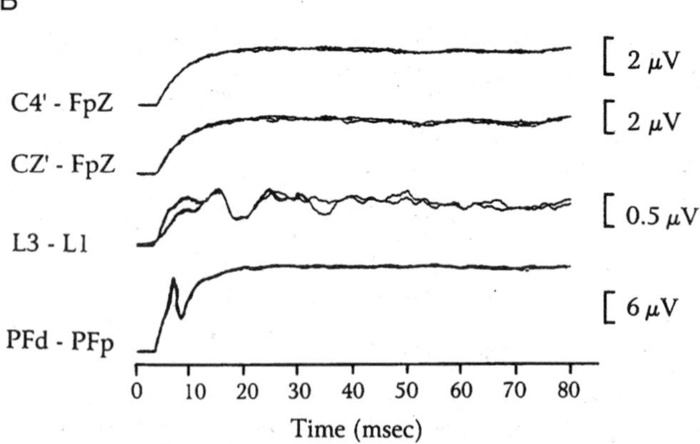

FIGURE 24–15. Responses recorded over the popliteal fossa, and over the spine and scalp to stimulation of the left tibial nerve at the ankle. Two trials are superimposed to show the replicability of the findings. *A* shows the finding in a normal subject, and *B* shows the response in a patient with multiple sclerosis. No response is present over the scalp in the patient. PF, popliteal fossa; L1, first lumbar spine; L3, third lumbar spine; d, distal; p, proximal; other abbreviations as in earlier illustrations.

text. Recent work suggests that this approach is helpful in reducing the morbidity of scoliosis surgery.

Motor Evoked Potentials

Magnetic stimulation of the brain and spine elicits so-called motor evoked potentials (MEPs). This technique is usually well tolerated by patients and poses no immediate safety hazards. The latency of the motor responses can be measured, and central conduction time can be estimated by comparing the latency of the responses elicited by cerebral and spinal stimulation. Abnormalities have been described in patients with a variety of central disorders including multiple sclerosis, amyotrophic lateral sclerosis, stroke, and certain degenerative disorders.[50] The clinical utility of these techniques, however, is unclear and at the present time the magnetic stimulation of central structures is regarded as investigational in the United States.

Electromyography

BASIC PRINCIPLES AND TECHNIQUE

Electrical activity can be recorded by a needle electrode placed within muscle. The potentials are amplified, displayed on an oscilloscope screen, and fed through a loudspeaker so they can be monitored by ear. Several different types of needle electrodes are in common use, but the most popular is the concentric needle electrode. This consists of a fine silver or platinum wire, insulated except at its tip, that is contained within a pointed steel shaft; the potential difference between the outer shaft and inner wire is recorded.

The electrical activity recorded from muscle, that is, the electromyogram (EMG), provides a guide to the pathological site in patients with disease of the motor units. Pathological processes can be localized to the neural, muscle, or junctional components of the motor units. In neuropathic diseases, the pattern of affected muscles also permits a lesion to be localized to the spinal cord, nerve roots, limb plexuses, or peripheral nerves. The EMG findings are not, however, pathognomonic of specific diseases and do not in themselves provide a definitive diagnosis.

NORMAL EMG ACTIVITY

When a needle electrode is inserted into a muscle, a brief burst of activity occurs for 2 to 3 seconds or less. Once this insertion activity has settled, spontaneous activity is not present in normal muscle except in the endplate region, where endplate "noise" can be recorded and corresponds to the nonpropagated miniature endplate potentials generated by the spontaneous release of acetylcholine at the neuromuscular junctions.

When slight voluntary contraction is initiated, a few of the motor units within the muscle are activated and initially fire irregularly and at a low rate. With increasing effort, they fire more rapidly; and, at a certain firing rate, additional units are recruited. With further effort, so many units are active that individual potentials cannot clearly be distinguished, leading to a complete "interference pattern" on the trace of the oscilloscope (Fig. 24–16).

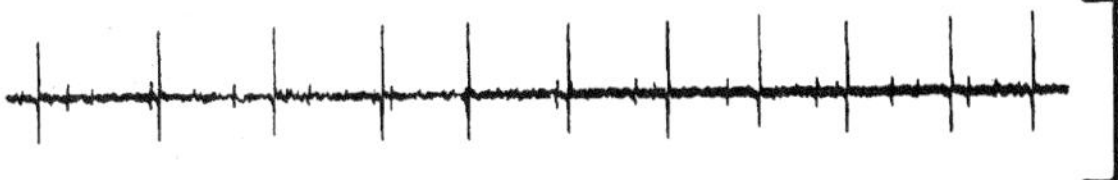

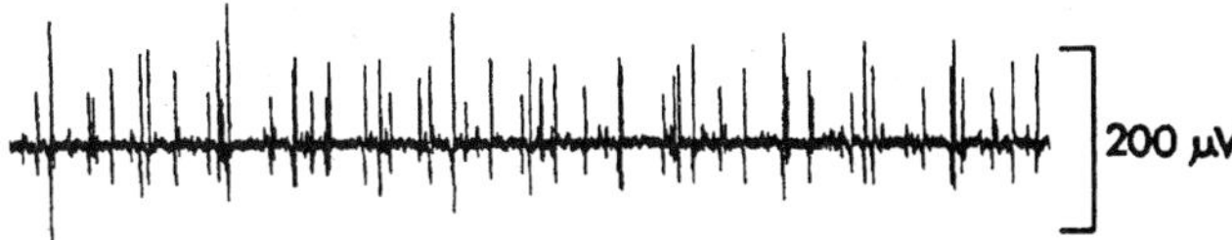

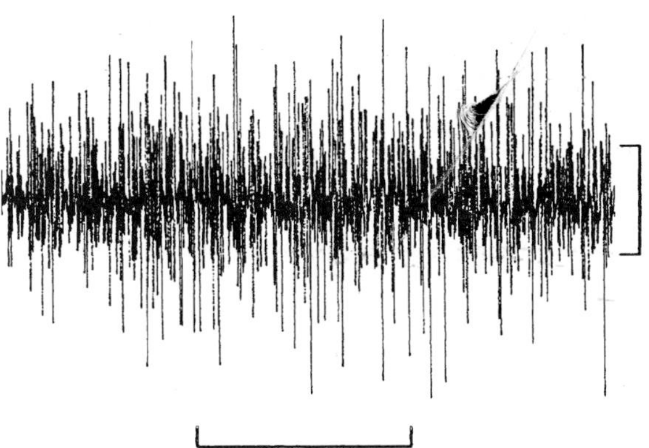

FIGURE 24–16. Motor unit activity during increasing voluntary effort. The number of units activated increases with the force of contraction, and eventually (bottom trace) individual potentials can no longer be recognized. In accordance with conventions, an upward deflection in this and subsequent figures indicates that the active electrode is negative with respect to the reference one. (From Aminoff MJ: Electromyography in Clinical Practice, 3rd ed. New York, Churchill Livingstone, 1998.)

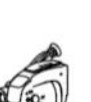

Individual motor unit action potentials are usually biphasic or triphasic in configuration, but up to 10 to 15 percent are polyphasic, that is, they have five or more phases. They normally have a duration of between 2 and 15 msec and an amplitude of between 300 μV and 3 mV (Fig. 24–17).

ABNORMAL EMG ACTIVITY

Insertion activity is increased in neuropathic and certain myopathic or myotonic disorders and in myositis. Abnormal spontaneous activity is present in various neuromuscular diseases. *Fibrillation potentials* (Fig. 24–18) are biphasic or triphasic discharges with a positive onset except in the endplate region; they have an amplitude of about 300 μV, have a duration of up to 5 msec, fire up to 20 times per second, and represent action potentials generated in single muscle fibers. They usually fire rhythmically, and this probably reflects oscillations of the resting membrane potential of skeletal muscle fibers.[51] *Positive sharp waves* (Fig. 24–19) may be found in association with them and consist of an initial positive deflection followed by a slow deflection in the negative direction. Although similar in size to fibrillation potentials, they often last for 10 msec or more and may discharge at rates up to 100 per second. Fibrillation potentials and positive sharp waves are found in conditions with increased muscle fiber irritability. They occur in denervated muscle but may not appear for 3 to 4 weeks after an acute neuropathic lesion.

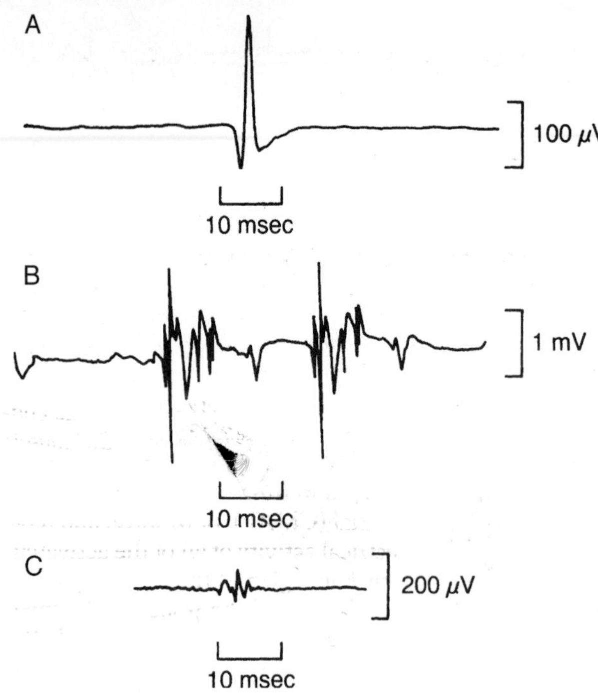

FIGURE 24–17. Motor unit action potentials. *A*, Normal potential. *B*, Long-duration polyphasic potential (shown twice). *C*, Short-duration, low-amplitude, polyphasic potential. (From Aminoff MJ: Electromyography in Clinical Practice, 3rd ed. New York, Churchill Livingstone, 1998.)

They are also found in patients with inflammatory disorders of muscle, occasionally in patients with muscular dystrophies, after muscle trauma, in patients with certain metabolic disorders (such as acid maltase deficiency), and in association with botulism.

In patients with chronic partial denervation, as well as with certain of the muscular dystrophies or inflammatory disorders of muscle, *complex repetitive discharges* are found. These have a high discharge frequency, but their amplitude and frequency remain constant (Fig. 24–20). They appear to arise in the muscle itself and are probably initiated by a fibrillating muscle fiber that then depolarizes adjacent fibers by ephaptic transmission.[52] By contrast, in the *myotonic discharges* (Fig. 24–21) that characterize certain myotonic disorders with delayed relaxation after voluntary contraction, high-frequency trains of action potentials occur spontaneously, wax and wane in amplitude and frequency, and relate to a disorder of the muscle fiber membrane.

Fasciculation potentials have the dimensions of motor unit action potentials (see later) and represent the spontaneous activation of all the muscle fibers in individual units. They produce a sudden dull thump over the loudspeaker. They are found most often with disease of the anterior horn cells but may also occur with other neuropathic disorders, occasionally with certain myopathic disorders (as in thyrotoxicosis), and sometimes as an isolated phenomenon without pathological significance. Studies in patients with diverse lower motor neuron lesions have revealed that they may arise at multiple sites along motor axons or the cell bodies of diseased motor neurons,[53] but in most instances they originate at the distal extremity of the axon.[54] Myokymic discharges, in which motor unit action potentials discharge spontaneously in characteristic patterns, are discussed following.

The motor unit action potentials may show characteristic abnormalities in various diseases of the motor units. In *myopathies*, the number of muscle fibers in individual motor units is reduced. In consequence, the mean duration and amplitude of the motor unit action potentials is reduced (see Fig. 24–17) and the incidence of polyphasic potentials is increased. Moreover, because the individual units generate less tension than normal, an increased number is recruited for any given degree of voluntary activity. By contrast, in *neuropathic disorders*, the number of motor units—but not their content of muscle fibers—is reduced; indeed, if denervated muscle fibers have been re-innervated by sprouting from the axon terminals of surviving units, the number of fibers per unit may actually be increased. In consequence, motor unit action potentials may be longer in duration and larger in amplitude than normal, with an increased incidence of polyphasic potentials, indicating that re-innervation has occurred (see Fig. 24–17).

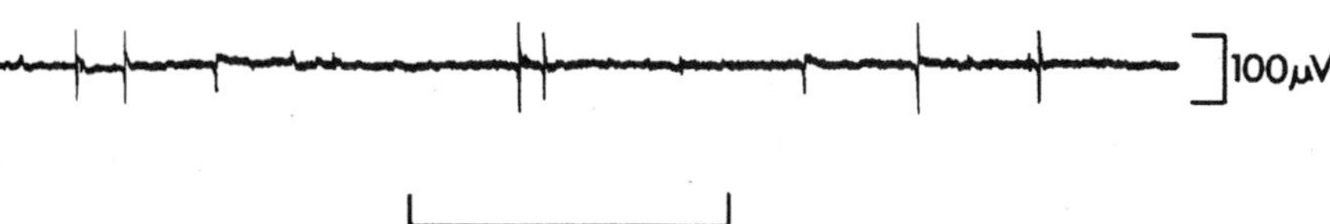

FIGURE 24–18. Fibrillation potentials recorded in partially denervated muscle. (From Aminoff MJ: Electromyography in Clinical Practice, 3rd ed. New York, Churchill Livingstone, 1998.)

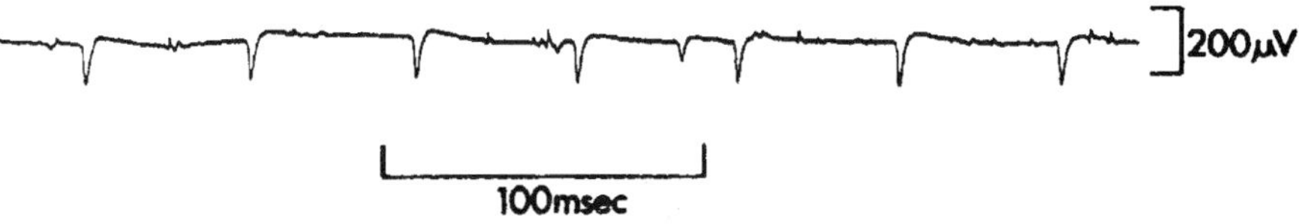

FIGURE 24-19. Positive sharp waves recorded in partially denervated muscle. (From Aminoff MJ: Electromyography in Clinical Practice, 3rd ed. New York, Churchill Livingstone, 1998.)

During mild voluntary activity, there is an increase in the rates at which individual units begin firing and at which they fire before additional units are recruited; and during maximal effort the interference pattern is reduced.

In disorders with *abnormal neuromuscular transmission*, such as myasthenia gravis, motor unit action potentials vary in amplitude and area during continued activity and, in addition, there is an excess of small, short-duration potentials in affected muscle. The variability of the potentials reflects the reduced safety factor for neuromuscular transmission, as a consequence of which there is variation in the number of muscle fibers firing with each discharge of the unit. Single-fiber electromyography is a technique in which action potentials are recorded from two or more muscle fibers belonging to the same motor unit by means of a special electrode, and the temporal variability (or jitter) between the two action potentials at consecutive discharges is measured.[55] This jitter reflects variation in neuromuscular transmission time in the two motor endplates involved. An increased jitter is therefore to be expected in patients with diseases of neuromuscular transmission, and impulse blocking may also occur.

Myokymic discharges consist of a spontaneously occurring grouped pattern of firing of motor units; double, triple, or multiple discharges occur, followed by a period of silence and then by another grouped discharge. They may occur in patients with radiation-induced plexopathy or myelopathy and occasionally with chronic radiculopathies or entrapment neuropathies, Guillain-Barré syndrome, multiple sclerosis, or gold intoxication; they may also be found in facial muscles in patients with brain stem gliomas.[56, 57]

Nerve Conduction Studies

BASIC PRINCIPLES AND TECHNIQUE

Needle electromyography is generally performed in conjunction with nerve conduction studies, which may be undertaken to determine the functional integrity of the peripheral nerves. For motor conduction studies, the nerve is stimulated at two or more points along its course while the electrical response is recorded of one of the muscles supplied by it. Electrical stimuli are preferred and must be of sufficient intensity to excite all of the fibers in the nerve. The muscle response is recorded by surface or subcutaneous needle electrodes, with the active electrode being placed over the endplate region and the reference electrode over the muscle tendon. The response recorded in this way is called the compound muscle action potential (CMAP), or M wave, and represents the sum of the electrical activity of all of the activated muscle fibers within the pickup region of the recording electrode. The shape, size, and latency of the response obtained by stimulating the nerve at different sites is compared. By measuring the distance between stimulation sites and the difference in latency of the responses elicited by stimulation at these sites, the conduction velocity can be determined for the fastest conducting fibers along the intervening segments of the nerve (Fig. 24–22). In the arms, the normal range of maximal motor conduction velocity is between 50 and 70 m/sec, while in the legs the corresponding velocities are between 40 and 60 m/sec.

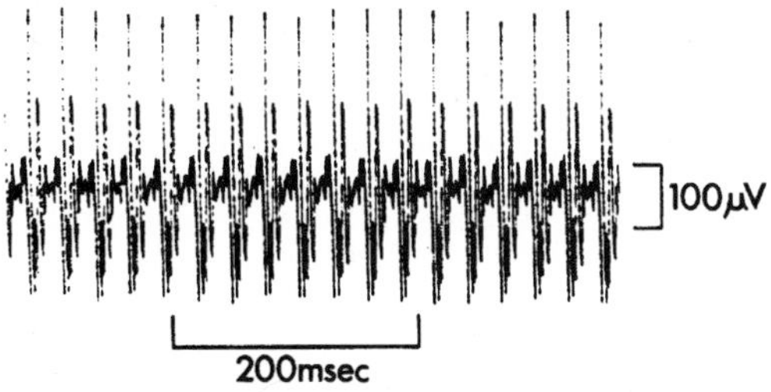

FIGURE 24-20. Spontaneous, high-frequency repetitive discharge of action potentials in a partially denervated muscle. (From Aminoff MJ: Electromyography in Clinical Practice, 3rd ed. New York, Churchill Livingstone, 1998.)

Sensory nerve conduction studies involve stimulating a sensory nerve either orthodromically or antidromically and recording the response at another point along the course of that same nerve. The calculated conduction velocity is the same, but the response is larger with antidromic stimulation. Responses can also be recorded from a purely sensory nerve after stimulation of the parent nerve trunk from which it originates, or vice versa.

In patients with *focal conduction block* involving an individual nerve, the CMAP elicited by stimulating the nerve above the site of the lesion is reduced in amplitude compared with more distal stimulation and, in severe cases, is completely lost. Sensory nerve action potentials are also small or unrecordable when the lesion is located between stimulation and recording sites. With focal *conduction slowing* (but not block), the size of the CMAP is reduced as the distance increases between the stimulating and recording electrodes. Motor and sensory conduction velocities are slowed across the region of the nerve encompassing the lesion, and sensory nerve action potentials may be markedly attenuated or unrecordable because of dispersion. *Axon-loss lesions* are characterized by an attenuated muscle response, by reduced or absent sensory nerve action potentials, and by electromyographic signs of denervation in the affected muscle. Motor or sensory conduction velocity is normal or reduced only minimally, when it can be recorded.

CLINICAL USES OF NERVE CONDUCTION STUDIES

Motor conduction studies are helpful in indicating that weakness is due to pathology of the peripheral nerves rather than other parts of the motor unit. Sensory conduction

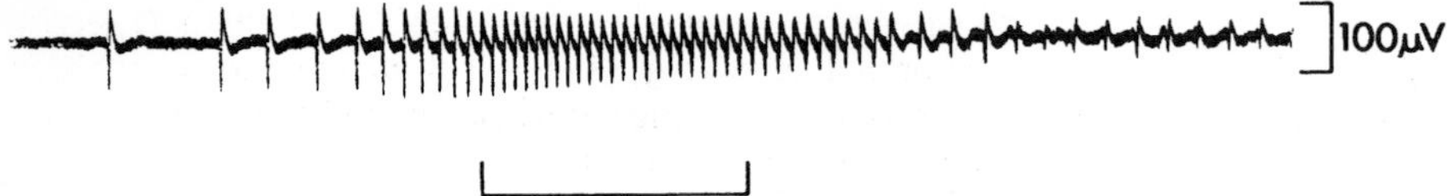

FIGURE 24–21. A myotonic discharge evoked by electrode movement. (From Aminoff MJ: Electromyography in Clinical Practice, 3rd ed. New York, Churchill Livingstone, 1998.)

studies may indicate that sensory symptoms are due to an impairment of peripheral nerve function or, when normal, to a lesion proximal to the dorsal root ganglia. Motor and sensory conduction studies are important in determining the presence and extent of a peripheral neuropathy, distinguishing between a polyneuropathy and mononeuropathy multiplex, recognizing the selective involvement of motor or sensory fibers, and following the course of peripheral nerve disease. The nature of the abnormalities found on motor or sensory conduction studies may suggest the type of underlying pathology and, in particular, whether this is primarily axonal loss or segmental demyelination.[58] Nerve conduction studies are also important as a means of recognizing subclinical polyneuropathies and in detecting and localizing a focal lesion involving individual nerves.

Focal nerve lesions may result from injury or compression at sites of entrapment of the nerve by neighboring anatomical structures. Common entrapment neuropathies include compression of the median nerve at the wrist (carpal tunnel syndrome); the ulnar nerve at the elbow, cubital tunnel, or Guyon's canal; and the peroneal nerve at the head of the fibula. Electrophysiological studies are very important in localizing the lesion in such disorders and also in excluding the possibility of a subclinical polyneuropathy manifest primarily by the entrapment neuropathy. The findings depend on the duration and severity of nerve damage, the rapidity of its evolution, and the underlying disorder.[59]

F-Response and H-Reflex Studies

BASIC PRINCIPLES AND TECHNIQUE

F responses are evoked from muscle as the result of antidromic activation of motor neurons by a peripheral electrical stimulus. The stimulus should be of greater intensity than is required to elicit a maximal CMAP and may not always elicit an F response. F responses are small (usually less than 5 percent) compared with the CMAP (Fig. 24–23), and their latency and amplitude vary considerably even when the stimulating and recording arrangements remain constant, presumably because different anterior horn cells are activated antidromically. Various parameters of F waves can be measured, but the most popular is the minimum latency of 10 or more responses.

The H reflex, named after Hoffmann who first described it, can be recorded easily only from the gastrocnemius-soleus muscle in the legs and the flexor carpi radialis muscle in the forearm in response to stimulation of the nerve to these muscles. The stimulus required to elicit the response is lower in intensity than is necessary to elicit CMAPs of maximal size (Fig. 24–23). The afferent pathway subserving the H reflex consists of spindle afferent (a) fibers, and the efferent arc is via the alpha motor axons. The H reflex is not easily obtained from other muscles except in infants or patients with pyramidal lesions, limiting its clinical utility.

NORMAL FINDINGS

The latency of the H reflex or F response depends on a subject's height or limb length, and normal values must therefore be obtained with this in mind to permit appropriate evaluation of the results from patients. It may also be helpful to compare interside differences in latency of the responses in individual patients; for H and F responses from the soleus muscle, or the F responses from the intrinsic hand muscles, this is normally less than 2 msec.[60]

ABNORMAL FINDINGS AND CLINICAL USES OF F-RESPONSE AND H-REFLEX STUDIES

F-response and H-reflex studies are sometimes useful in the evaluation of patients with peripheral neuropathies, particularly when the pathological process is so proximal that

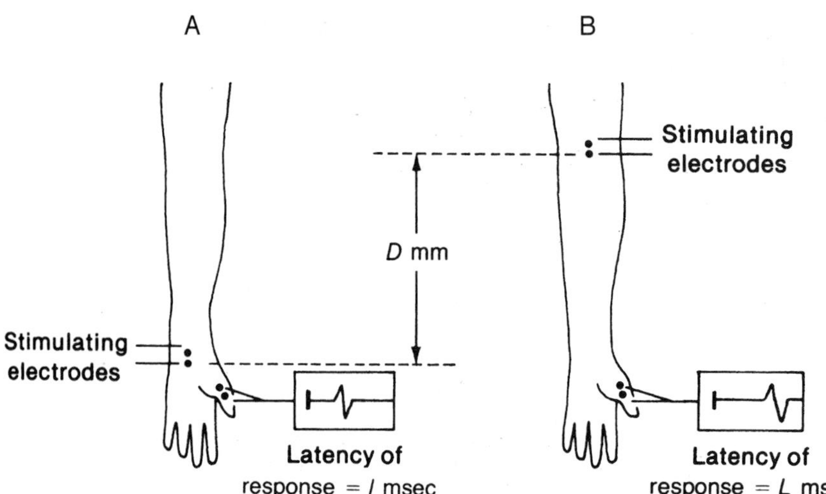

FIGURE 24–22. Arrangement for measuring motor conduction velocity in the forearm segment of the median nerve. The nerve is stimulated distally *(A)* and proximally *(B)*, and the evoked potentials are recorded from the abductor pollicis brevis muscle. (Ground electrode not shown.) Maximal motor conduction velocity (m/sec) between the proximal and distal sites of stimulation is calculated by dividing the distance between these sites by the difference in latency of the responses. (From Aminoff MJ: Electromyography in Clinical Practice, 3rd ed. New York, Churchill Livingstone, 1998.)

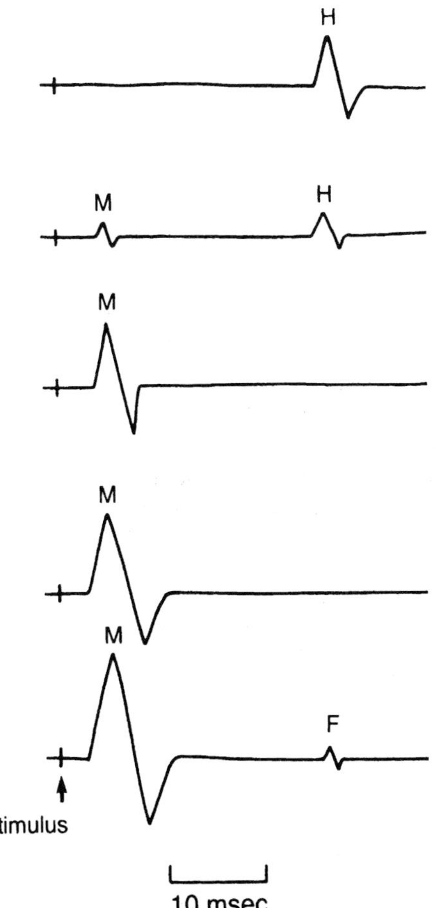

FIGURE 24–23. Diagrammatic representation of the relationship between the direct (M) response, F response, and H reflex, and the intensity of the eliciting stimulus. With low-intensity stimulation of the tibial nerve, an H reflex is elicited from the soleus muscle. As the intensity of stimulation increases, the H reflex declines and a small M wave is seen. With a higher stimulus intensity, the H reflex disappears and the M wave increases in size until it is maximal. Following the maximal M wave, a small F response is sometimes seen. (From Aminoff MJ: Electromyography in Clinical Practice, 3rd ed. New York, Churchill Livingstone, 1998.)

conventional nerve conduction studies fail to reveal any abnormalities. A prolongation of the minimum F-response latency may occur in patients having polyneuropathies with involvement of motor fibers, sometimes when conventional nerve conduction studies are normal. Abnormalities are sometimes encountered with radiculopathies, but these patients generally have abnormalities on needle electromyography so that the added F-response abnormality does not influence management. H-reflex abnormalities (lost or delayed responses) may also be found in patients with polyneuropathies or with a lesion anywhere along the pathways subserving the reflex.

Blink Reflex

BASIC PRINCIPLES AND TECHNIQUE

The blink reflex is a polysynaptic reflex that is most conveniently recorded from surface electrodes placed over the orbicularis oculi muscle after electrical stimulation of the supraorbital nerve (Fig. 24–24). The afferent arc of the reflex is subserved by the trigeminal nerve, and the efferent arc is subserved by the facial nerve.

NORMAL FINDINGS

The response is characterized by a short-latency (approximately 10 msec) ipsilateral response that is designated R1, followed by a more asynchronous, bilateral response having a latency of 28 to 30 msec that is designated R2 (Fig. 24–25).

ABNORMAL FINDINGS AND CLINICAL USES OF THE BLINK REFLEX

The blink reflex may be helpful in revealing the presence of a subtle trigeminal or facial nerve lesion. Ipsilateral trigeminal nerve lesions lead to responses that are either lost or have a prolonged latency bilaterally. A unilateral facial nerve lesion, by contrast, leads to a delayed or absent response on the affected side regardless of which side is stimulated.

The blink reflex may be abnormal with polyneuropathies, thereby indicating the extent of the disorder. Abnormalities may also occur with tumors in the cerebellopontine angle involving either or both nerves or the brain stem and with brain stem lesions involving the central pathways subserving the reflex, such as in multiple sclerosis, sometimes in the absence of clinical evidence of brain stem involvement.

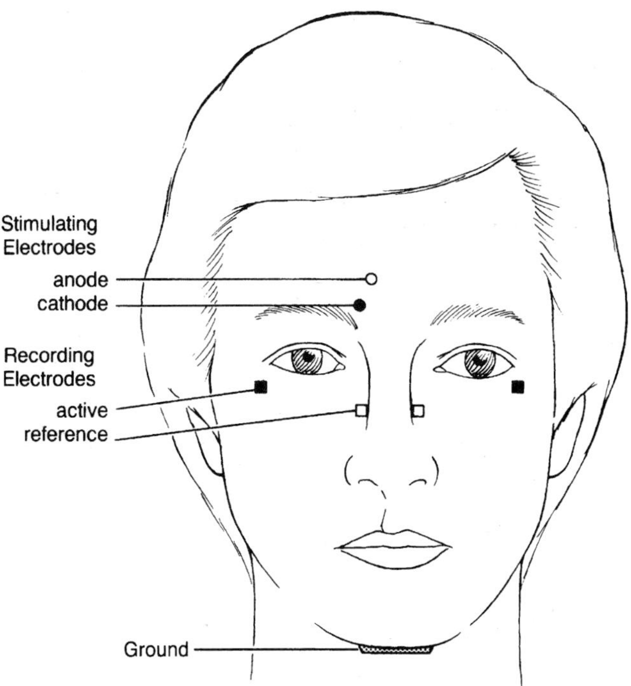

FIGURE 24–24. Arrangements for eliciting the blink reflex. (From Aminoff MJ: Electromyography in Clinical Practice, 3rd ed. New York, Churchill Livingstone, 1998.)

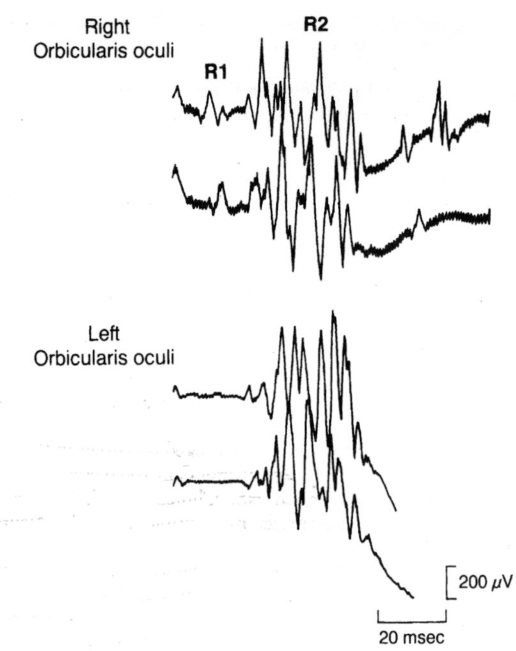

FIGURE 24–25. The blink reflex elicited by electrical stimulation of the right supraorbital nerve in a normal adult. Two separate responses are shown. The R1 component of the response is present only on the side that is stimulated, whereas R2 is present bilaterally. (From Aminoff MJ: Electromyography in Clinical Practice, 3rd ed. New York, Churchill Livingstone, 1998.)

Repetitive Nerve Stimulation

BASIC PRINCIPLES AND TECHNIQUE

Electrophysiological techniques are important in the evaluation of neuromuscular transmission. The amount of acetylcholine released by a nerve impulse—and thus the size of the endplate potential—is influenced by preceding activity in the junctional region. This normally is of little consequence, because the amount of acetylcholine released far exceeds that required to generate endplate potentials above the threshold for activating muscle fiber action potentials. Reduction in this safety factor, however, may alter the number of muscle fibers activated by an impulse and thus the size of the CMAP elicited by a supramaximal stimulus to the motor nerve. The size of the electrical response evoked in muscle by two or more supramaximal stimuli, or by a single stimulus applied after a 30-second period of maximal voluntary activity or tetanic stimulation, therefore reflects the efficacy of neuromuscular transmission.

NORMAL FINDINGS

There is normally no change in size of the responses to paired or repetitive shocks delivered to the motor nerve at rates of up to 10 Hz or in the response to single shocks delivered before and after maximum voluntary activity or tetanic stimulation.

ABNORMAL FINDINGS AND CLINICAL USES OF REPETITIVE NERVE STIMULATION

Repetitive nerve stimulation is a useful technique for evaluating neuromuscular transmission. In diseases in which such transmission is impaired, the muscle response to repetitive nerve stimulation may show abnormal alterations in size or area. In myasthenia gravis, a progressive decrement in the response may occur with repetitive stimulation (especially at 2 to 3 Hz), or an initial decrement may be followed by a leveling off of the response at a reduced size. Abnormalities are more likely to be found in proximal rather than distal limb muscles and in facial rather than limb muscles. Normal findings do not exclude the diagnosis. By contrast, in patients with Lambert-Eaton myasthenic syndrome or botulism, the response to a single stimulus is abnormally small and stimulation at a slow rate leads to a further reduction in response size; with rapid rates of stimulation, a progressive increase in size of the response occurs.

Reviews and Selected Updates

Aminoff MJ: Electrodiagnosis in Clinical Neurology, 4th ed. New York, Churchill Livingstone, 1999.

Aminoff MJ: Electromyography in Clinical Practice, 3rd ed. New York, Churchill Livingstone, 1998.

Brown WF, Bolton CF, Aminoff MJ (eds): Neuromuscular Function and Disease: Basic, Clinical, and Electrodiagnostic Aspects. Philadelphia, WB Saunders, 2002.

Chiappa KH (ed): Evoked Potentials in Clinical Medicine, 3rd ed. New York, Lippincott-Raven, 1997.

Gronseth GS, Ashman EJ: Practice parameter: The usefulness of evoked potentials in identifying clinically silent lesions in patients with suspected multiple sclerosis (an evidence-based review). Report of the Quality Standards Subcommittee of the American Academy of Neurology. Neurology 2000;54:1720–1725.

Jablecki CK, Andary MT, Floeter MK, et al: Practice parameter: Electrodiagnostic studies in carpal tunnel syndrome. Report of the American Association of Electrodiagnostic Medicine, American Academy of Neurology, and the American Academy of Physical Medicine and Rehabilitation. Neurology 2002;58:1589–1592.

Kimura J: Electrodiagnosis in Diseases of Nerve and Muscle: Principles and Practice, 3rd ed. New York, Oxford University Press, 2001.

References

1. Jasper HH: Report of the Committee on Methods of Clinical Examination in Electroencephalography. Electroencephalogr Clin Neurophysiol 1958;10:370–375.
2. Aminoff MJ: Electroencephalography: General principles and clinical applications. *In* Aminoff MJ (ed): Electrodiagnosis in Clinical Neurology, 4th ed. New York, Churchill Livingstone 1999, pp 37–80.
3. Ebersole JS: Ambulatory electroencephalographic monitoring. *In* Aminoff MJ (ed): Electrodiagnosis in Clinical Neurology, 4th ed. New York, Churchill Livingstone, 1999, pp 151–168.
4. Steriade M, Gloor P, Llinas RR, et al: Basic mechanisms of cerebral rhythmic activities. Electroencephalogr Clin Neurophysiol 1990;76:481–508.
5. Gloor P, Kalabay O, Giard N: The electroencephalogram in diffuse encephalopathies: Electroencephalographic correlates of grey and white matter lesions. Brain 1968;91:779–802.
6. American Electroencephalographic Society: Minimum technical standards for EEG recording in suspected cerebral death. J Clin Neurophysiol 1994;11:10–13.
7. Chatrian GE, Shaw CM, Leffman H: The significance of periodic lateralized epileptiform discharges in EEG: An electrographic, clinical and pathological study. Electroencephalogr Clin Neurophysiol 1964;17:177–193.
8. Markand ON, Daly DD: Pseudoperiodic lateralized paroxysmal discharges in electroencephalogram. Neurology 1971;21:975–981.
9. Goodin DS, Aminoff MJ: Does the interictal EEG have a role in the diagnosis of epilepsy? Lancet 1984;1:837–839.
10. Hahn JS, Tharp BR: Neonatal and pediatric electroencephalography. *In* Aminoff MJ (ed): Electrodiagnosis in Clinical Neurology, 4th ed. New York, Churchill Livingstone, 1999, pp 81–127.
11. Iragui VJ, McCutchen CB: Physiologic and prognostic significance of "alpha coma." J Neurol Neurosurg Psychiatry 1983;46:632–638.
12. Sorensen K, Thomassen A, Wernberg M: Prognostic significance of alpha frequency EEG rhythm in coma after cardiac arrest. J Neurol Neurosurg Psychiatry 1978;41:840–842.

13. Upton A, Gumpert J: Electroencephalography in diagnosis of herpes-simplex encephalitis. Lancet 1970;1:650–652.
14. Fariello RG, Black JA: Pseudoperiodic bilateral EEG paroxysms in a case of phencyclidine intoxication. J Clin Psychiatry 1978;39:579–581.
15. Chiofalo N, Fuentes A, Galvez S: Serial EEG findings in 27 cases of Creutzfeldt-Jakob disease. Arch Neurol 1980;37:143–145.
16. Levy SR, Chiappa KH, Burke CJ, et al: Early evolution and incidence of electroencephalographic abnormalities in Creutzfeldt-Jakob disease. J Clin Neurophysiol 1986;3:1–21.
17. Guilleminault C, Anagnos A: Polysomnographic evaluation of sleep disorders. *In* Aminoff MJ (ed): Electrodiagnosis in Clinical Neurology, 4th ed. New York, Churchill Livingstone, 1999, pp 631–653.
18. Carskadon MA, Dement WC: The multiple sleep latency test: What does it measure? Sleep 1986;5:S67–S72.
19. Carskadon MA, Dement WC, Mitler MM, et al: Guidelines for the multiple sleep latency test (MSLT): A standard measure of sleepiness. Sleep 1986;9:519–524.
20. Van den Hoed J, Kraemer H, Guilleminault C, et al: Disorders of excessive daytime somnolence: Polygraphic and clinical data for 100 patients. Sleep 1981;4:23–37.
21. Aminoff MJ: Evoked potential studies in neurological diagnosis and management. Ann Neurol 1990;28:706–710.
22. American Electroencephalographic Society: Guidelines on evoked potentials. J Clin Neurophysiol 1994;11:40–73.
23. Halliday AM, McDonald WI, Mushin J: Delayed visual evoked response in optic neuritis. Lancet 1972;1:982–985.
24. Miller DH, Newton MR, van der Poel JC, et al: Magnetic resonance imaging of the optic nerve in optic neuritis. Neurology 1988;38:175–179.
25. Bottcher J, Trojaborg W: Follow-up of patients with suspected multiple sclerosis: A clinical and electrophysiological study. J Neurol Neurosurg Psychiatry 1982;45:809–814.
26. Celesia GG: Visual evoked potentials in clinical neurology. *In* Aminoff MJ (ed): Electrodiagnosis in Clinical Neurology, 4th ed. New York, Churchill Livingstone, 1999, pp 421–438.
27. Aminoff MJ, Goodin DS: Visual evoked potentials. J Clin Neurophysiol 1994;11:493–499.
28. Groswasser Z, Kriss A, Halliday AM, et al: Pattern- and flash-evoked potentials in the assessment and management of optic nerve gliomas. J Neurol Neurosurg Psychiatry 1985;48:1125–1134.
29. Maitland CG, Aminoff MJ, Kennard C, et al: Evoked potentials in the evaluation of visual field defects due to chiasmal or retrochiasmal lesions. Neurology 1982;32:986–991.
30. Celesia GG, Meredith JT, Pluff K: Perimetry, visual evoked potentials and visual evoked spectrum array in homonymous hemianopsia. Electroencephalogr Clin Neurophysiol 1983;56:16–30.
31. Celesia GG, Bushnell D, Toleikis SC, et al: Cortical blindness and residual vision: Is the "second" visual system in humans capable of more than rudimentary visual perception? Neurology 1991;41:862–869.
32. Birch EE: Visual evoked potentials in infants and children. *In* Aminoff MJ (ed): Electrodiagnosis in Clinical Neurology, 4th ed. New York, Churchill Livingstone, 1999, pp 439–449.
33. Jewett DL, Williston JS: Auditory-evoked far fields averaged from the scalp of humans. Brain 1971;94:681–696.
34. Picton TW, Taylor MJ, Durieux-Smith A: Brainstem auditory evoked potentials in infants and children. *In* Aminoff MJ (ed): Electrodiagnosis in Clinical Neurology, 4th ed. New York, Churchill Livingstone, 1999, pp 485–511.
35. Uziel A, Benezech J: Auditory brain-stem responses in comatose patients: Relationship with brain-stem reflexes and levels of coma. Electroencephalogr Clin Neurophysiol 1978;45:515–524.
36. Goldie WD, Chiappa KH, Young RR, et al: Brainstem auditory and short-latency somatosensory evoked responses in brain death. Neurology 1981;31:248–256.
37. Stockard JJ, Stockard JE, Sharbrough FW: Detection and localization of occult lesions with brainstem auditory responses. Mayo Clin Proc 1977;52:761–769.
38. Chiappa KH: Use of evoked potentials for diagnosis of multiple sclerosis. Neurol Clin 1988;6:861–880.
39. Kimura J, Mitsudome A, Yamada T, et al: Stationary peaks from a moving source in far-field recording. Electroencephalogr Clin Neurophysiol 1984;58:351–361.
40. Kimura J, Mitsudome A, Beck DO, et al: Field distribution of antidromically activated digital nerve potentials: Model for far-field recording. Neurology 1983;33:1164–1169.
41. Aminoff MJ: Use of somatosensory evoked potentials to evaluate the peripheral nervous system. J Clin Neurophysiol 1987;4:135–144.
42. Aminoff MJ: Segmentally specific somatosensory evoked potentials. Neurol Clin 1991;9:663–669.
43. Aminoff MJ: The use of somatosensory evoked potentials in the evaluation of the central nervous system. Neurol Clin 188;6:809–823.
44. Davis SL, Aminoff JJ, Panitch HS: Clinical correlations of serial somatosensory evoked potentials in multiple sclerosis. Neurology 1985;35:359–365.
45. Eisen A, Stewart J, Nudleman K, et al: Short-latency somatosensory responses in multiple sclerosis. Neurology 1979;29:827–834.
46. Aminoff MJ, Eisen A: Somatosensory evoked potentials. *In* Aminoff MJ (ed): Electrodiagnosis in Clinical Neurology, 4th ed. New York, Churchill Livingstone, 1999, pp 513–536.
47. Greenberg RP, Becker DP, Miller JD, et al. Evaluation of brain function in severe human head trauma with multimodality evoked potentials: II. Localization of brain dysfunction and correlation with post-traumatic neurological conditions. J Neurosurg 1977;47:163–177.
48. Hume AL, Cant BR: Central somatosensory conduction after head injury. Ann Neurol 1981;10:411–419.
49. Brunko E, Zegers de Beyl D: Prognostic value of early cortical somatosensory evoked potentials after resuscitation from cardiac arrest. Electroencephalogr Clin Neurophysiol 1987;66:15–24.
50. Murray NMF: Motor evoked potentials. *In* Aminoff MJ (ed): Electrodiagnosis in Clinical Neurology, 4th ed. New York, Churchill Livingstone, 1999, pp 549–568.
51. Thesleff S, Ward MR: Studies on the mechanism of fibrillation potentials in denervated muscle. J Physiol 1975;244:313–323.
52. Stalberg E, Trontelj JV: Abnormal discharges generated within the motor unit as observed with single-fiber electromyography. *In* Culp WJ, Ochoa J (eds): Abnormal Nerves and Muscles as Impulse Generators. New York, Oxford University Press, 1982, pp 443–474.
53. Roth G: The origin of fasciculations. Ann Neurol 1982;12:542–547.
54. Landau WH: The essential mechanism in myotonia: An electromyographic study. Neurology 1952;2:369–388.
55. Stalberg E, Trontelj J: Single Fiber Electromyography, 2nd ed. New York, Raven Press, 1994.
56. Albers JW, Allen AA, Bastron JA, et al: Limb myokymia. Muscle Nerve 1981;4:494–504.
57. Radu EW, Skorpil V, Kaeser HE: Facial myokymia. Eur Neurol 1975;13:499–512.
58. Thomas PK: The morphological basis for alterations in nerve conduction in peripheral neuropathy. Proc R Soc Med 1971;64:295–298.
59. Stewart JD: Focal Peripheral Neuropathies, 3rd ed. Philadelphia, Lippincott, Williams & Wilkins, 2000.
60. Fisher MA: H-reflex and F-response studies. *In* Aminoff MJ (ed): Electrodiagnosis in Clinical Neurology, 4th ed. New York, Churchill Livingstone, 1999, pp 323–336.

CHAPTER 25

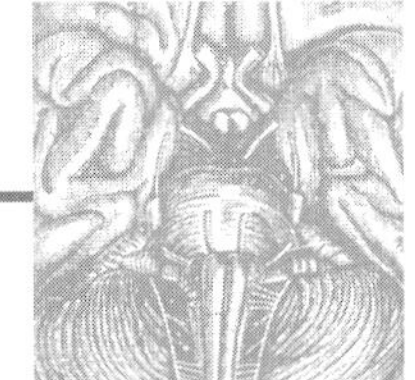

PETER A. LEWITT, JAMES Y. GARBERN,
MARK A. FERRANTE, and WILLIAM KUPSKY

Body Fluid and Tissue Analysis

For the variety of applications it offers, clinical laboratory testing for neurological disease has undergone revolutionary change in recent years. Diagnostic capabilities for metabolic diseases, for rapid detection of infection, and for determining genetic risk factors are only a few examples of recent developments in testing capabilities. Results from the clinical laboratory are the only way to evaluate for certain neurological disorders. Laboratory tests have become an expensive part of the medical enterprise, but often they can provide the most cost-effective means for answering diagnostic questions.

Abnormalities detected by laboratory testing are not always attributable to a particular neurological disorder. Clinicians sometimes need to apply a process of decision-tree logic to derive useful information from laboratory results. Another limit of abnormal test results is that they do not always point to the mechanism of disease. The latter point was well known to a 19th-century founder of clinical laboratory medicine, Claude Bernard, who made the analogy that "as familiar as we might become with the structure of a mill, there is still much to learn before we would know the craft of a miller." The imprint of disease on the tissues and fluid compartments of the body provides an important but sometimes imperfect tool for solving clinical problems and guiding therapy. False-positive and false-negative findings, other sources of artifactual results, multimodal distributions of normal values, and the constant evolution of new information all are reasons that clinicians need to maintain a broad base of knowledge concerning laboratory medicine.

Certain screening laboratory studies, including complete blood counts, electrolytes, and tests of renal and hepatic function, are commonly used in the evaluation of many neurological conditions. Other studies such as drug and toxicological screens (see Chapter 39) as well as nutritional (see Chapter 40), coagulation (see Chapter 45), immunological (see Chapter 50), and enzymatic studies (see Chapters 30 and 31) may be useful in specific clinical settings and are covered in their respective chapters in Part Three of this textbook. This chapter focuses on the proper use of genetic studies and primary neurological tissue (muscle, nerve, and brain) in the diagnosis of neurological disease.

Genetic Studies

The pace of discovery of genes responsible for hereditary neurological diseases has been escalating over recent years. The sheer number of genetically defined disorders already is too large to permit comprehensive coverage of the molecular diagnosis of these disorders in a single chapter. In addition, there will be no doubt that some of the information presented here will be superseded or rendered obsolete as scientific advances occur. Rather, the necessary background information to understand key concepts and discoveries will be presented, along with some general guidelines to enable the reader to select the most efficient and beneficial approach (which may be to refer the patient to a geneticist) to the diagnosis and counseling of a patient suspected of having a genetic neurological condition.

In order to fully appreciate the current findings and to rationally approach the investigation of a patient suspected of having a genetic disorder, it is essential to understand some basic principles of genetics and molecular biology.

THE HUMAN GENOME

All biological activities depend directly or indirectly on the proteins that lie within cells. The totality of genetic information for an organism is referred to as the genome. The human genome is divided among 23 pairs of chromosomes; females have two X chromosomes and 22 pairs of autosomes (nonsex chromosomes) and males have an X and a Y chromosome in addition to the 22 pairs of autosomes. Genetic information is contained in the linear sequence of nucleotides, or bases, in deoxyribonucleic acid (DNA). Each chromosome is a single enormous molecule of linear DNA associated with a complex assortment of proteins that play structural and regulatory as well as enzymatic roles during DNA replication and gene expression. The autosomes are numbered according to their sizes and contain over 200 million bases in chromosome 1 to about 50 million bases in chromosome 22.

It is estimated that there are some 50,000 to 100,000 genes in the human genome. They range in size from about 100 bases for genes for structural ribonucleic acids (RNAs) to about 2.5 million bases for the largest known gene, dystrophin. Gene expression is the sequence of processes from messenger RNA (mRNA) synthesis, or transcription, to protein synthesis, or translation. Gene transcription is a complex process and begins with the regulated initiation of transcription from a transcription initiation site. This initiation process is of fundamental importance and is mediated by proteins termed transcription factors. A primary transcript is synthesized down the length of the entire gene from the 5′ to the 3′ end. The information in most genes is broken up into discontinuous pieces termed *exons*, which are separated by *introns*, or intervening sequences. These introns are removed from the primary transcript through splicing. Most spliced products then have a string of adenosine bases added to their 3′ ends. This spliced and polyadenylated product is the mRNA, which is then transported to the cytoplasm of the cell and serves as a template for the synthesis of protein.

An individual gene, therefore, is the composite not only of the sequences that code for protein, but also the introns, the transcribed but not translated regions at the 5′ and at the 3′ ends of the mRNA, and sequences that regulate the transcription initiation, termination, and splicing processes. Regulatory sequences can flank the transcription initiation and termination sites or even lie within introns or exons (Fig. 25–1).

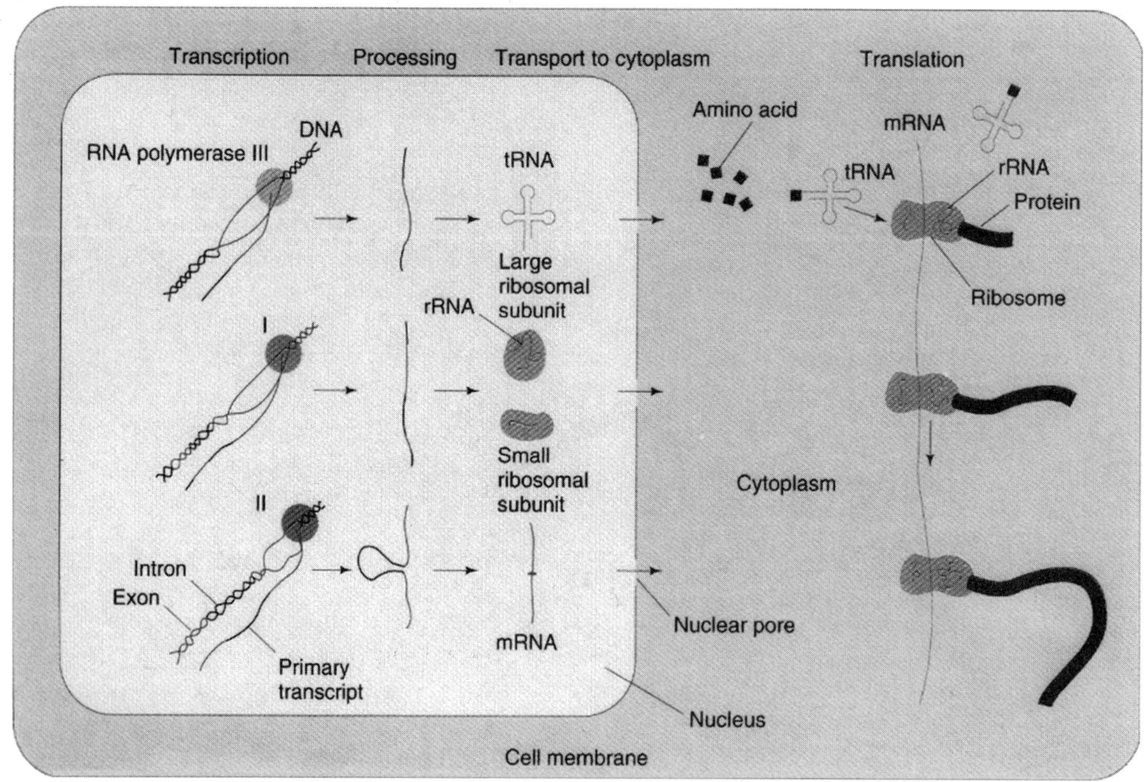

FIGURE 25–1. Eukaryotic gene expression. The initial step in gene expression is the transcription of the primary RNA transcript. The intervening regions, or introns, that separate the exons that contain the protein coding regions are removed from the primary transcript by splicing. The spliced transcript is modified at its 5′ and 3′ ends (not shown), and the mature mRNA is then transported out of the nucleus and into the cytoplasm, where it serves as the template for translation, the process of decoding the RNA sequence into protein using the ribosomes and transfer RNA (tRNA) molecules that both "read" the genetic code words, or codons, and provide a single amino acid that is added to the growing polypeptide chain. (Adapted from Griffiths AJF, Miller JH, Suzuki DT, Lewontin RC, Gelbart, WM: An Introduction to Genetic Analysis 6.0. New York, W.H. Freeman, 1996.)

The sequence of bases in an mRNA encodes the amino acid sequence of the protein for a gene. Nucleotide information is interpreted in groups of three bases, termed codons. With four nucleotide bases, there are 64 possible codons. Four codons are particularly important. AUG encodes methionine, which is always the first amino acid of the primary translation product (which may be cleaved to make a mature protein product). The codons UAG, UGA, and UAA are stop codons. Mutations that cause disease can be as subtle as the substitution of one nucleotide base for another. The consequences of point mutations demonstrate the great variety of effects that result from an alteration in a gene and illustrate most of the key problems that result from mutations. The results of such a mutation depend critically on the location of the mutation within the gene as well as on the particular bases that are involved. If the mutation lies within the coding region (also known as the open reading frame), the result could be the substitution of one amino acid for another. Some point mutations result in no change of the amino acid and are termed *silent mutations*. Other protein coding region mutations can result in the conversion of an amino acid encoding codon into a termination or stop codon. A mutation affecting an initiation codon would prevent translation initiation unless another AUG codon was present elsewhere. Point mutations can occur outside of the coding region. Consequences include obliteration or creation of splice sites, destruction or creation of transcription initiation or termination sites, or of regulatory sites.

Mutations can also result from deletions or insertions, that range in size from one to thousands of nucleotides. When an insertion or deletion lying within the coding region for a protein involves a number of bases that is not a multiple of 3, then the coding frame is disrupted, resulting in a protein sequence that diverges from the normal sequence from that point on, unless a second mutation restores the proper reading frame.

A recently recognized but important category of mutations, properly considered a subtype of insertion, is the trinucleotide repeat expansion mutations (Table 25–1). These mutations are characterized by an elongation of a gene region characterized by repeats of a three-nucleotide sequence. The precise sequence varies among these disorders as does the scale of expansions. There are some general distinctions that can be drawn, however, to characterize all these repeat expansion mutations. When the trinucleotide, or triplet, repeat unit lies outside of the coding region, the expansions can reach a very large size. The mutations that cause fragile-X mental retardation syndrome (FMRI) are expansions of a region involving the trinucleotide CCG that lies in the 5′ untranslated but transcribed portion of the gene. Normally, there are about 5 to 50 CCG repeats in this region, but affected individuals can have hundreds or even thousands of such repeats. Expansions of over several hundred triplet

TABLE 25–1. Trinucleotide Repeat Disorders

Disorder	Gene	Chromosome	Repeat Unit	Normal Repeat Number (range/ pathological range)	Other Mutations
Huntington's disease	Huntingtin	4p16.3	CAG	15–20/39–~100	
X-linked spinal and bulbar atrophy	Androgen receptor	Xq11	CAG	15–20/40–~100	
SCA I	Ataxin-1 (ATX1)	6p23	CAG	–6–36/39–83	
SCA II	Ataxin-2 (ATX2)	12q24	CAG	15–31/34–400	
Machado-Joseph/ SCA III	MJD	14q24.3	CAG	12–40/55–86	
SCA VI	CACNL1A4	19p13	CAG	4–16/20–33	Other mutations cause episodic ataxia or hemiplegic migraine
SCA7	Ataxin-7	3p21.1–p12	CAG	4–19/37–>300	
SCA8	Ataxin-8	13q21	CTA/CTG	15–50/80–250	Some with very large repeats do *not* have ataxia
SCA10	Ataxin-10	22q13	ATTCT	10–22/800–4500	
SCA12	Protein phosphatase 2A	5q31	CAG	6–26/66–78	
SCA17	TATA binding protein	6q27	CAG	30	
DRPLA	DRPLA	12p13	CAG	3–36/49–~88	
Myotonic dystrophy	Myotonin	19q13.2	CTG	5–27/50–thousands	
Fragile-X	FMR-1	Xq28.3	CCG	6–54, premutation 56–200/~200–thousands	ILE367ASN,1BP DEL, ACT125CT, FS159TEACT125CT, FS159TER,IVS1, G-T, –1 AND G-A, +1
Friedreich ataxia	Frataxin	9q	GAA	7–38/66 –~1700	Intron 17; other point mutations can cause Friedreich ataxia

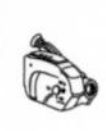

repeats have been found in patients with myotonic dystrophy (Steinert's disease), where the repeat unit CTG is normally present in 5 to 27 copies and lies in the 3′ untranslated region of the myotonin gene. The Friedreich ataxia triplet repeat mutation is due to expansion of a GAA repeat that has a normal length of 7 to 22 repeats and that lies in the seventeenth intron of a gene believed to be a phosphoinositol kinase gene. Patients can have several hundred copies of the triplet. Interestingly, point mutations in the FMRI and Friedreich ataxia genes can also cause mental retardation and Friedreich ataxia, respectively.

The other type of triplet repeat mutations involves repeats of the nucleotide bases CAG, which encode the amino acid glutamine, and lie within the coding domains of their respective genes. Not only is the repeat unit the same for these disorders, but also the scale of the repeat expansion is also quite similar: The length of the normal repeat is approximately 20, whereas affected individuals have 40 or more repeats. To date, all of the mutations of this type described are of special importance to neurologists, as the major syndromes affect the brain, spinal cord, or muscles.

Mutations affecting mitochondrial DNA cause a wide variety of clinical neuromuscular syndromes and can affect any part of the central and peripheral nervous systems, the muscles, and other organs. Mutations may arise sporadically, such that there is no family history of disease, or may be transmitted via maternal inheritance with up to 100 percent of a mother's offspring receiving the genetic defect. This unique phenomenon arises because all mitochondria are inherited from the ovum. Another special feature of mitochondrial inheritance arises from the fact that mixtures of normal and abnormal mitochondria can exist not only within a single cell, but also in different tissues. *Homoplasmy* refers to the state of having uniformly normal or abnormal mitochondria in a tissue, while *heteroplasmy* refers to the state of having a mixture of normal and abnormal mitochondria in a tissue. Typically over 90 percent of the mitochondria need to be abnormal before abnormal clinical symptoms and signs are apparent. It is important to recognize that some disorders, such as Kearns-Sayre syndrome (KSS), may cause abnormal mitochondria to develop in some tissues, such as ocular muscles, but not in others, such as peripheral blood leukocytes. In such a situation (which is common in the case of KSS), molecular testing for the deletions of the mitochondrial genome may not be detected in blood samples but may be present in other tissues, such as muscle.

TESTING METHODS (Table 25–2)

High-Resolution Karyotype

The lowest resolution genetic test is the karyotype analysis. In this test, a sample of cells (e.g., blood leukocytes or amniotic fluid cells) are grown in tissue culture medium in the presence of mitotic inhibitors that arrest cells at metaphase. The cells are then "squashed" to spread the chromosomes on the microscope slide. The chromosomes can then be stained to reveal a pattern of bands along the length of the chromosome arms. This form of testing is able to assess whether the cells have the normal number of chromosomes and can determine whether interchanges of chromosome arms between chromosomes (i.e., translocations) have occurred. Depending on their size, this analytic method can also detect some deletions or duplications of chromosomal regions. A typical high-resolution test can detect deletions of approximately 10 million base pairs or more. Smaller deletions or duplications (submicroscopic deletions) will not be seen, such as the duplication found in most patients with Charcot-Marie-Tooth disease IA (CMTIA) (Fig. 25–2).

Fluorescent in situ Hybridization (FISH)

FISH analysis is a useful method for determining deletions or duplications of specific chromosomal regions. The technique involves staining chromosomes by hybridization with a nucleic acid probe that has been covalently labeled with a fluorescent molecule that can be visualized with a conventional fluorescence microscope. Typical probes range from a few thousand bases to tens of thousands of bases in length. In addition to staining chromosomal spreads prepared as described previously for conventional karyotype analysis, the method can also be used to stain chromosomes in interphase, or nonmitotic, cells, which has the advantage that the DNA is not tightly wound into densely packed chromatin, so that relatively closely spaced fluorescent markers can be resolved microscopically. Examples of this technique include detection of the 1.5 million base duplication in CMTIA, and detection of the submicroscopic deletions responsible for the Smith-Magenis, or for the Prader-Willi/Angelman syndromes. This method is very valuable in basic research as a straightforward method for localizing genes to specific chromosomal regions.

Single Gene Mutation Screening

Mutation detection specificity and sensitivity concerns apply to molecular diagnostic testing as well as to conventional biochemical testing. It is important to understand the nature(s) of mutations that are known to occur in a gene in question as well as to understand the range of potential mutations that can occur for any gene. The type or types of mutations that can cause a genetic disease determine how comprehensive or sensitive a screening test is. The trinucleotide repeat disorders represent a group of genetic diseases that can be screened easily and with great sensitivity, because the mutations are of a single type and occur in a single region of respective genes. On the other hand, disorders such as X-linked Charcot-Marie-Tooth disease (Connexin 32 gene) or myotonia congenita (skeletal muscle chloride channel) are more difficult to screen, since different families affected by the disease will often have unique, or private, mutations such as single base changes or small insertions or deletions. With large genes, the molecular detection of mutations can be quite daunting, to the point that, while technically feasible, particularly with relatively rare disorders, there may not be commercial laboratories willing to develop screening tests. By virtue of the natures of their mutations, however, some genetic disorders can be detected by relatively convenient tests even when they are caused by private mutations. Although the dystrophin gene, responsible for Duchenne and Becker muscular dystrophies, is an extremely large gene with many exons, mutations tend to be fairly sizable (tens or hun-

TABLE 25–2. **Molecular Testing Methods**

Method	Disease Examples	Limitations of Testing	Comments
Karyotype	Complex phenotypes (contiguous gene syndromes, aneuploidies, [e.g., Down's syndrome]); balanced translocation	Will not detect chromosomal anomalies smaller than approximately 5 megabases; may miss small balanced translocations	
FISH	Pelizaeus-Merzbacher disease (PMD), Charcot-Marie-Tooth disease 1A	Will not detect point mutations	May need to use point mutation testing (e.g., ASO, direct sequencing) if negative
Allele-specific oligonucleotide	Canavan disease, cystic fibrosis, factor V Leiden, MELAS, MERRF, NARP	Examines only the more common point mutations; will not detect any other mutations	May need to perform SSCP or direct sequencing if negative; will not detect large gene duplications/deletions
Trinucleotide repeat expansion	HD, SCA1, 2, 3, 6, 7, 8, 10, 12, 17, FRDA, muscular dystrophy, DRPLA, FMR	Will miss other mutations, e.g., episodic ataxia-2, FRDA caused by point mutations in the frataxin gene; may not detect large expansions	May need to do Southern blot if only single allele (repeat length) is detected, which can appear to be the case with huge expansions; will not detect large deletions or duplications
PCR/RFLP	PMD; many other diseases	Will miss mutations outside of region(s) amplified by PCR	
Direct sequencing	Numerous	Will miss large duplications/deletions; will miss mutations in regions not amplified in the PCR (e.g., intronic mutations, regulatory region mutations); may not be able to reliably distinguish pathological mutations from polymorphisms	Labor and time intensive; expensive
SSCP; heteroduplex analysis	PMD; others	Will miss large deletions/duplications, mutations outside of PCR-amplified region(s)	Often used as sceening test; may miss up to 20 percent of point mutations within the amplified region(s)
Linkage	Neurofibromatosis, Duchenne muscular dystrophy, many others	Laborious; requires multiple family members, including normal as well as affected individuals	Appropriate for diseases where gene has not yet been identified but has been localized to a particular chromosomal region; can be used for nondisclosing linkage analysis, e.g., determining whether a child of a clinically normal parent is at risk for developing HD, but where the parent does not wish to find out if she/he definitely has inherited HD
PCR/gel electrophoresis	Duchenne muscular dystrophy	Will miss point mutations and mutations outside of PCR-amplified segment(s)	Most appropriate for conditions resulting frequently from intragenic deletions; may detect duplications/deletions
Premature protein truncation	Neurofibromatosis I	Will miss missense and other small mutations, duplications	Depends on RNA expression of the gene; useful when significant proportion of mutations result in frameshift or nonsense changes; will not detect about 30 to 40 percent of NFI mutations; may not be reliable for prenatal testing

ASO, Allele-specific oligonucleotide; DRPLA, dentatorubropallidolysian atrophy; FISH, fluorescent in situ hibridization; HD, Huntington's disease; NFI, neurofibromatosis I; PCR, polymerase chain reaction; RFLP, restriction fragment legth polymerization; SSCP, single-strand confirmation polymorphism

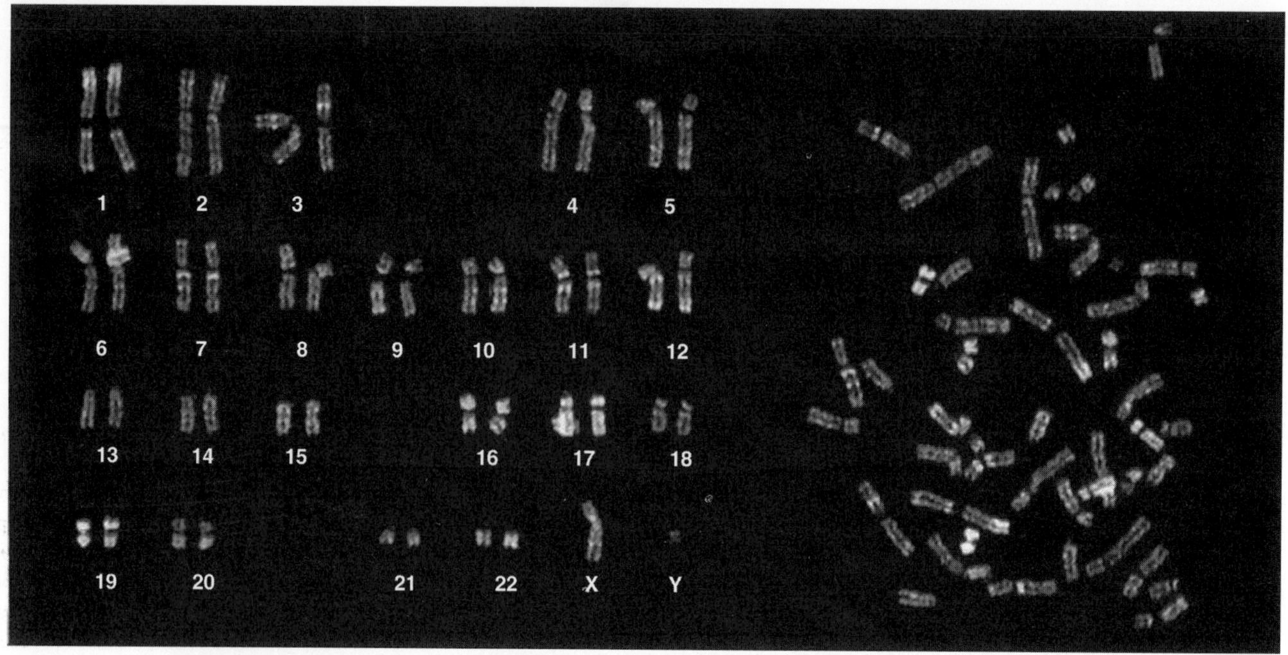

FIGURE 25–2. Flurorescent in situ hybridization (FISH) of metaphase chromosomes. The right side of the photomicrograph shows the original distribution of chromosomes from a single cell whose nucleus has been ruptured to release the chromosomes, which are stained with a red fluorescent probe to a gene on chromosome 11. The images of the chromosomes on the right side of the figure have been excised and organized on the left side of the figure to easily examine each pair of chromosomes from this karyotypically normal male. (Adapted from Griffiths AJF, Miller JH, Suzuki DT, Lewontin RC, Gelbart WM: An Introduction to Genetic Analysis 6.0. New York, W.H. Freeman, 1996.)

dreds of bases) deletions in most cases. Because particular gene regions are "hot spots" for these deletions, polymerase chain reaction (PCR) simultaneous amplification (so-called multiplex PCR) of the dystrophin gene regions that are most often deleted can detect mutations in about 75 percent of cases. Neurofibromatosis I (NFI) is another example of a genetic disorder affecting a large gene caused by many private mutations. The majority of mutations lead to premature termination of protein synthesis of the neurofibromin protein. Because the neurofibromin gene is expressed in white blood cells, the premature protein truncation test can screen leukocyte RNA for the neurofibromin mRNA that can be specifically amplified and then used as a template for in vitro protein synthesis. After electrophoresis of the neurofibromin generated synthetically and detection by antibody on Western blot, mutations can be reliably inferred if the immunoreactive neurofibromin is a smaller size than the normal protein. The premature protein truncation assay is now commercially available and is reported to detect mutations in the NFI gene in about 70 percent of individuals who fulfill the clinical criteria for NFI. When mutations are not found in a clinically affected individual, mutation detection then becomes more problematic. Currently there is no commercial laboratory that offers testing for mutations in the remaining 30 percent of NFI individuals. When the clinical situation merits an intensive search for mutations in a gene, it is hoped that future advances in genetic screening and sequencing technology will facilitate mutation identification.

A description of some of the most common techniques in current use illuminate the available dimensions of molecular biological diagnostics.

Polymerase Chain Amplification

Polymerase chain amplification is a critical technique that is central to many detection tests. Even though it does not enable direct mutation detection in all cases, it enables the generation of large amounts of DNA for testing applications. Routine PCR is limited to the amplification of specific small (up to several hundred base pairs in length) regions of a single gene that are bracketed by a pair of opposing DNA primers that define the origins and directions of DNA synthesis of a target gene (Fig. 25–3).

Because each strand of the double helix can be used as a template for DNA synthesis, for each repetitive cycle of DNA denaturation, primer annealing, and DNA synthesis, there is a doubling in the number of amplified DNA regions. Thus, a several billionfold amplification of a gene region is readily achievable from even a minute amount of DNA. As mentioned, PCR is the basis for detecting trinucleotide repeat expansion mutations and for detecting deletions of the dystrophin gene. PCR is also used to amplify segments of a gene suspected of having a mutation. The PCR products are then used in a variety of assays that can screen for mutations.

Single-Strand Conformation Polymorphism (SSCP) Analysis

This modification of PCR technology has the capability of detecting single base mutations and is a very valuable means of screening for small mutations. PCR products, generally a few hundred bases in length, when denatured and subjected to electrophoresis will usually show measurable differences in electrophoretic migration, due to the differences in confor-

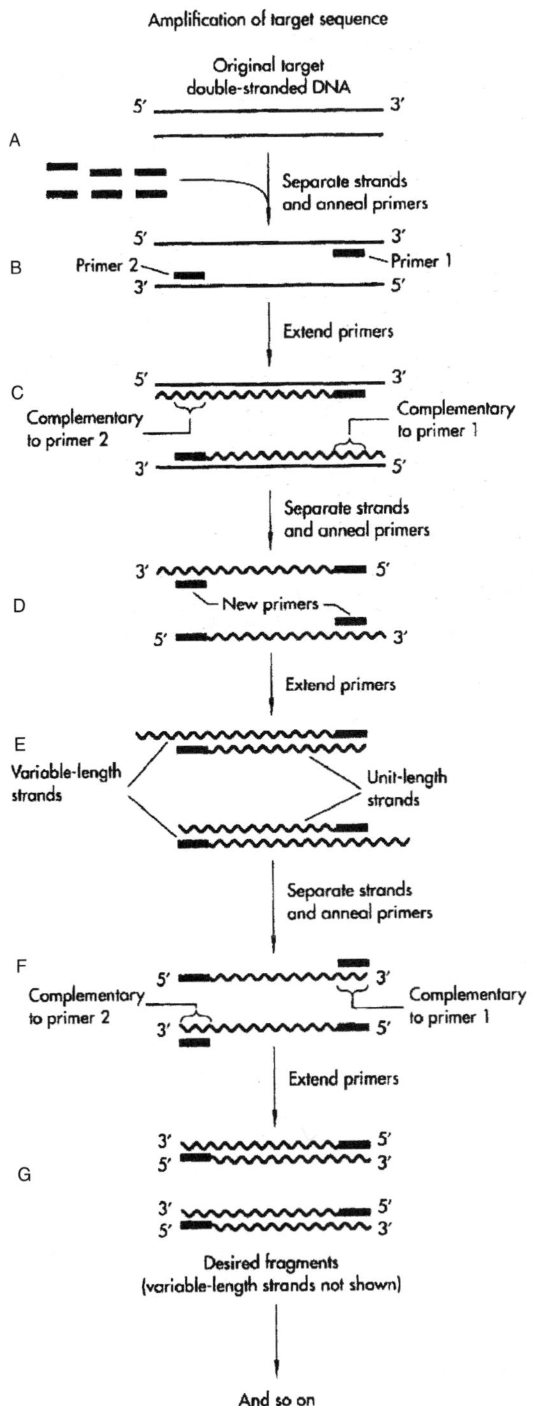

FIGURE 25–3. Polymerase chain reaction. Short, synthetic, single-stranded DNA primers that hybridize to opposing strands of the target DNA are typically spaced a few hundred to a few thousand bases apart *(A)* and are allowed to anneal to thermally denatured DNA *(B)*. *C,* DNA polymerase, typically isolated from thermophilic bacteria, is allowed to synthesize the complementary DNA, beginning from the primer. *D,* The newly synthesized DNA products are thermally denatured, then cooled to allow the primers to anneal again, and the DNA polymerase reaction again allowed to proceed. Step D is repeated, typically about 30 times, to exponentially amplify the product strands, which after round 3 of the reaction preferentially amplifies the short double-stranded DNA product whose termini are defined by the two primers. A typical 30-cycle PCR theoretically can amplify a single DNA molecule over 200 million times. (Adapted from Griffiths AJF, Miller JH, Suzuki DT, Lewontin RC, Gelbart WM: An Introduction to Genetic Analysis 6.0. New York, W.H. Freeman, 1996.)

mation of the dissociated single strands of DNA. Mutations in a gene may further alter the electrophoretic migration of dissociated DNA strands which have been PCR amplified. This is the basis of SSCP analysis. SSCP when properly designed can detect about 80 percent or even more of point mutations (mutations as small as a single base difference) within the region amplified. If needed for precise definition of the mutation, direct sequencing of the PCR product can be done.

Allele-Specific Oligonucleotide (ASO) Hybridization

This method is primarily used to detect specific point mutations. Certain diseases are caused by a common mutation that recurs spontaneously or by an inherited mutation that is responsible for most occurrences of the disease. An example of the former is achondroplasia, which is acquired by spontaneous mutation of the fibroblast growth factor receptor 3 gene. For unknown reasons, a specific base substitution occurs spontaneously in this disorder. An example of a disorder with a specific point mutation in most affected individuals is sickle cell anemia, where individuals with the affected allele inherited it from a common ancestor. With properly designed oligonucleotides, single-stranded DNA probes of about 20 bases in length, it is possible to detect specifically either the normal or mutant gene variant by hybridization of the probes to PCR-amplified DNA segments.

Direct Gene Sequencing

The definitive method for point mutation detection is to sequence the gene directly. For large genes such as the NFI gene or the dystrophin gene, such a direct screen would be impractical with current technology. For some genes, however, this technique is the method of choice. For example, the entire prion protein gene coding region conveniently lies within a single exon that can be amplified by PCR with a single pair of primers. Current methods can now readily scan the entire coding sequence of the gene in cases of suspected hereditary prion mutations. Other genes, such as the proteolipid protein gene that is mutated in Pelizaeus-Merzbacher disease, with relatively short and few exons, are also amenable to direct sequencing for mutation screening.

Southern Blot Hybridization

There are several neurogenetic syndromes that are caused by increased or decreased numbers of otherwise normal genes. CMTIA and Pelizaeus-Merzbacher disease are most often caused by duplications of the peripheral myelin protein-22 (PMP22) and proteolipid protein genes, respectively. Hereditary neuropathy with predisposition to pressure palsies is due to a loss of one copy of the PMP22 gene. These alterations in gene number or dosage had actually been overlooked previously. The most straightforward method of detecting these changes is to examine the signal intensities of the altered gene region compared to the level of a gene region lying outside the duplicated or deleted region. These differences can be overlooked unless specifically sought. The originally used method relied on the standard Southern blot technique (named after its inventor). For this technique, genomic DNA, usually isolated from peripheral leukocytes, is digested with an appropriate restriction endonuclease, subjected to electrophoresis through agarose gels, and transferred to nylon membranes for hybridization to labeled gene probes. For dosage analysis, a gene probe that spans the junction of the normal and dose-altered genomic region is hybridized to the filter. If a restriction enzyme site exists that separates the normal from altered copy number regions, then the probe will hybridize to a normal level to a DNA restriction fragment in the normal copy region. If the copy number for the gene is increased or decreased, the signal intensity will be altered (Fig. 25–4).

Restriction Fragment Length Polymorphism (RFLP) Analysis

By chance, mutations that alter the sequence of a gene may create or abolish a sequence cleavable by bacterial proteins called restriction endonucleases. These enzymes cut double-stranded DNA wherever a specific short, usually 4 to 10 base, sequence occurs. The discovery of these enzymes was key to the advances in recombinant DNA technology and modern molecular analysis. When a restriction site is created or abolished, the pattern of DNA fragments generated by the appropriate enzyme is also changed. Because restriction analysis is technically easy to perform, it is a preferred method when informative (Fig. 25–5).

Methods of gene hunting that rely on RFLP analysis take advantage not only of restriction site variation within the gene itself, but also site variations that lie outside but nearby the gene in question. For example, prior to the discovery of the Huntington's disease (HD) gene, RFLP analysis was the mainstay of genetic diagnosis of presymptomatic individuals. Nearby restriction site variations outside the HD gene could be used to mark the abnormal chromosome with high (over 95%) reliability, even though these restriction site polymorphisms were not the cause of the disease.

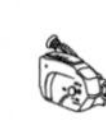

LIMITATIONS OF TESTING

It is important to recognize that the sensitivity of genetic testing varies from one clinical condition to the next, and that it is important to apply testing in the appropriate context. The molecular test for HD is very sensitive and specific, but there are other clinical conditions that can present not only with adult onset chorea, but also may even have an autosomal dominant pattern of inheritance. For example, spinocerebellar ataxia I and dentatorubropallidoluysian atrophy have autosomal dominant patterns of inheritance but are caused by triplet repeat expansions of unique genes distinct from huntingtin, the gene affected in HD. Therefore a negative HD test only has value in an asymptomatic person if the genetic test is positive in a clinically affected blood relative. The diagnosis of NFI is best established clinically, because the search for gene mutations is currently too laborious to be practical in most cases. The premature protein truncation test is the most sensitive molecular test for this disease but only detects abnormalities in about 70 percent of cases.

In cases where the gene product, generally a protein, is well characterized functionally, it is usually more effective to screen for abnormalities by functional testing. For example, the lysosomal storage diseases are caused by defective enzymes that can be assayed directly. Thus, the most effective screening test is a direct assay of enzyme function or of substrates or breakdown products of the enzyme in question in a specimen such as serum, urine, or, in certain circumstances, cells, such as fibroblasts obtained by skin biopsy. The category of mitochondrial diseases presents special complicating factors in making a diagnosis, because the diseases due to mtDNA mutations are not reflected in the genomic DNA and the proportion of mutant mitochondria can vary tremendously from tissue to tissue. For example, the blood leukocyte mitochondrial assays may be normal in patients with KSS, necessitating muscle biopsy in many cases to find the DNA deletions that make the diagnosis.

As the number of testable genetic conditions grows, it is anticipated that the approach to diagnostic evaluation will become more complicated and more expensive. For the inherited ataxias alone, there are at least 20 different disease-causing genes. For the most part, these disorders cannot be reliably distinguished solely through clinical history and evaluation, and genetic testing is the only reliable method to differentiate them. Guidelines for rational and cost-efficient testing will need to be developed, perhaps by developing panels of tests for the most common genetic causes, and secondary panels for the rarer causes. Geographic and ethnic factors, as well as clinical features, when appropriate, may help narrow the number and sequence of tests that need be done to establish the diagnosis.

Although genetic testing may be somewhat expensive, once a diagnosis is established, no further testing is needed, and testing for other affected relatives can be focused with precision. Furthermore, genetic diagnosis is essential for rational family planning using prenatal and preimplantation genetic testing. In the future, molecularly confirmed diagnoses will be essential to identify those individuals who are appropriate for disease-specific treatments for these disorders.

Ethics of Testing

Particularly for genetic testing, where molecular test results not only provide diagnostic information, but can also predict the onset of disease in many cases, it is important to advise patient on potential implications of genetic information in regard to their economic and social well-being, their own health, and that of relatives. Adverse genetic risk information potentially could affect an individual's employment and insurance status. Confidentiality must be maintained according to the patient's wishes in virtually all situations.

Need for Counseling

It is very important to ensure that counseling be included as part of a program of genetic testing. The diagnostic and therapeutic team should include a geneticist and genetic counselor to provide understandable information to the patient and family, thereby enabling them to comprehend maximally the direct and more subtle implications of genetic disease. Especially for presymptomatic and prenatal testing for hereditary diseases, it is often necessary to have several counseling sessions in order for the patient to decide on which avenue to proceed. In many cases, and not just limited to presymptomatic testing for HD, psychological evaluations and counseling should be an integral part of the testing

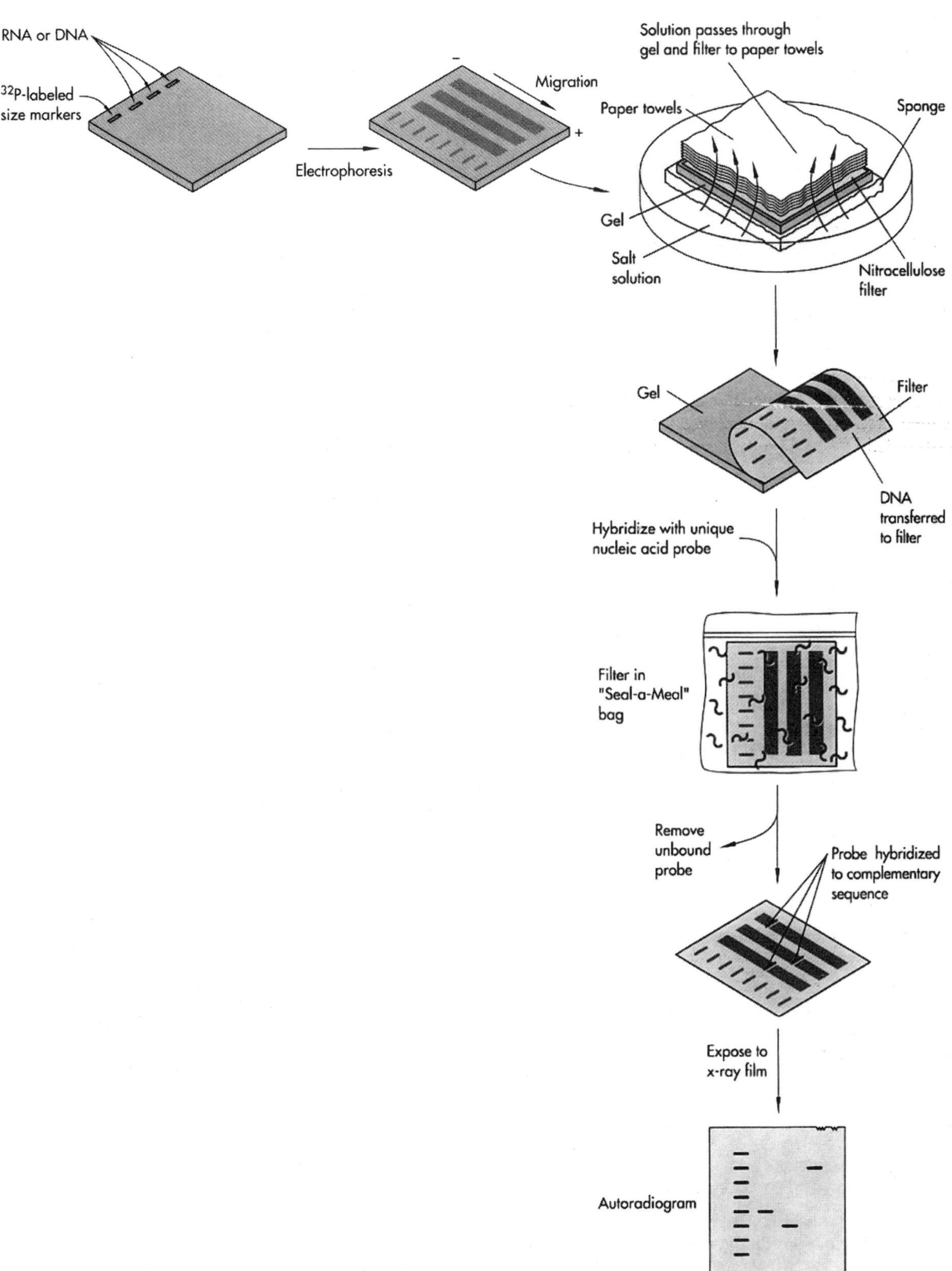

FIGURE 25–4. Southern blot. DNA fragments, typically after a restriction digest or after PCR, are electrophoretically separated on agarose gels, which sieve the fragments according to size (smaller fragments migrate more quickly). The DNA fragments are transferred, in this case by capillary transfer, to a sheet of nitrocellulose (nylon is also used) under conditions that also denature the DNA into single-stranded molecules that can be recognized by appropriate complementary probes. The nitrocellulose filter is then hybridized with a labeled (usually radioactively tagged) single-stranded probe that sticks to the specific target. The hybridized filter is then exposed to x-ray film and the signals revealed by developing the film. (Adapted from Griffiths AJF, Miller JH, Suzuki DT, Lewontin RC, Gelbart WM: An Introduction to Genetic Analysis 6.0. New York, W.H. Freeman, 1996.)

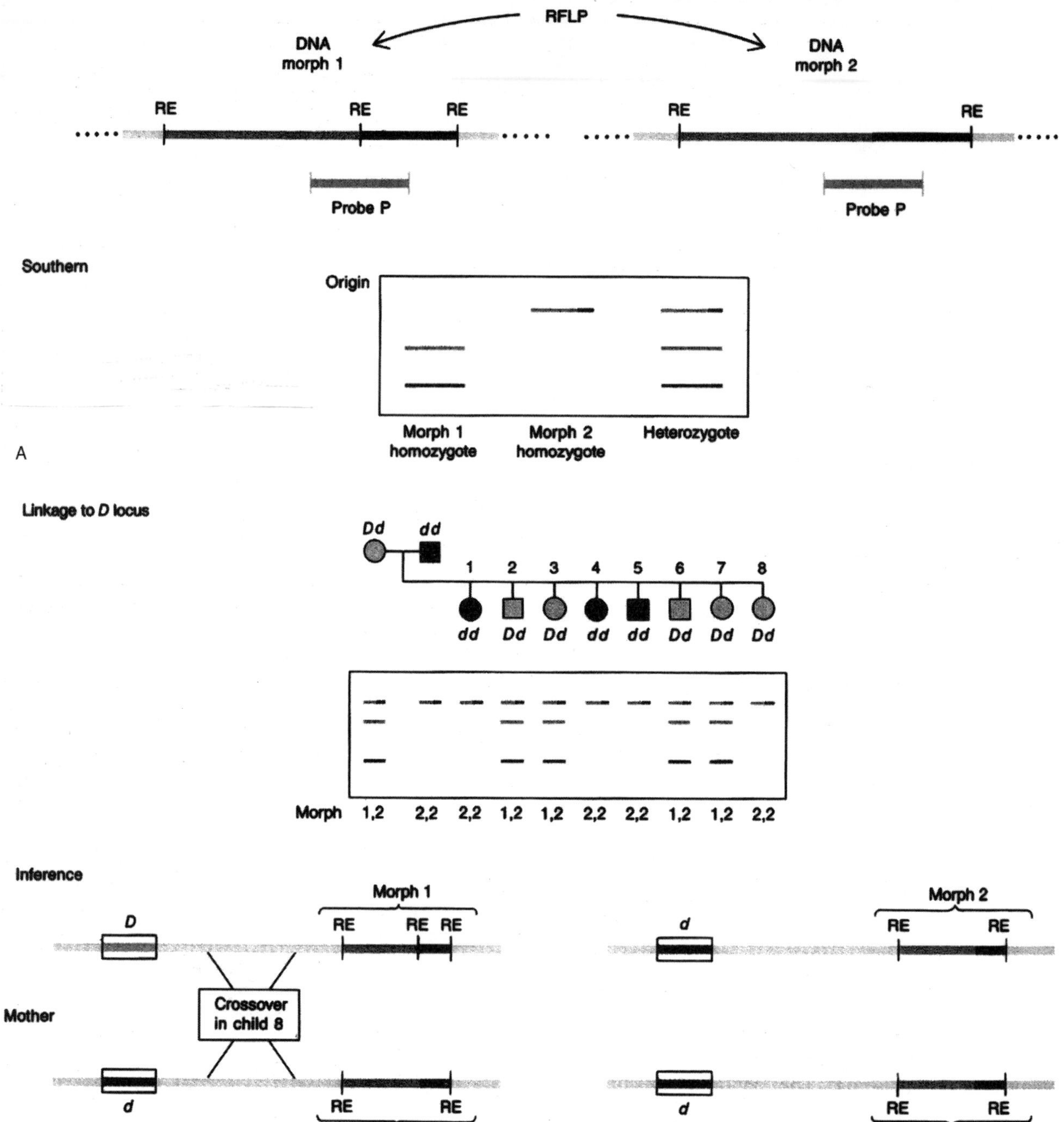

FIGURE 25–5. *A,* Detection of a restriction fragment length polymorphism (RFLP). A probe *(P)* hybridizes to a genomic region that straddles a region that contains a polymorphic restriction endonuclease site (the middle one on "morph 1"). The morph 1 region is digested into two fragments of different size that both hybridize to the probe, whereas the morph 2 region is digested such that only a single fragment (whose size happens to be the sum of the sizes of the two fragments in morph 1) is detected. The lower part of the figure is a Southern blot of an agarose gel showing the patterns of hybridization that result. *B,* Inheritance of an RFLP in a hypothetical family with an autosomal dominant disease (gene symbolized as "D," with normal allele indicated as "d"). Note that the polymorphic restriction site is near but not within the d gene. On most of the chromosomes with the mutant D gene, there is an extra restriction endonuclease site (RE, as in *A),* so that most of the affected family members have a pattern of three bands, a large band corresponding to the normal allele, and the two smaller bands resulting from the additional restriction site. Individual 8, however, although affected, has the restriction pattern of a normal person due to a recombination, schematized in the lower part of the figure. Such "recombinants" are extremely useful in mapping the location of, and eventually finding, new disease genes. (Adapted from Griffiths AJF, Miller JH, Suzuki DT, Lewontin RC, Gelbart, WM: An Introduction to Genetic Analysis 6.0. New York, W.H. Freeman, 1996.)

TABLE 25–3. **Useful Web Sites for Genetics and Genetic Testing**

Web Site	URL	Comments
Online Mendelian Inheritance in Man	*http://www.ncbi.nlm.nih.gov/entrez/query.fcgi?db=OMIM*	The most comprehensive database of human inherited disease; page also includes many links to other genetics and genomics resources
Genetests	*http://www.geneclinics.org*	Web site developed primarily for geneticists with clinical reviews of inherited diseases and links to laboratories offering genetic testing
Human Gene Mutation Database	*http://archive.uwcm.ac.uk/uwcm/mg/hgmd0.html*	Comprehensive repository for disease-causing mutations
Athena Diagnostics	*http://www.athenadiagnostics.com*	Commercial site that specializes in testing for neurogenetic disorders; owns licenses for some tests, e.g., Charcot-Marie-Tooth 1A.

process before, during, and after molecular test results are disclosed (Table 25–3).

Muscle Enzymes and Biopsy

FOREARM EXERCISE TESTING

Muscle fibers develop tension and shorten, thereby producing movement. These processes, including contraction and relaxation, are coordinated by the nervous system and are energy-requiring. Skeletal muscle meets its energy demands by converting chemical energy into mechanical energy. One feature unique to skeletal muscle compared with other tissues is the energy requirement difference between its resting and fully active states, a value that can approach two to three orders of magnitude.[1] When the metabolic energy demands of active muscle cannot be met by the available energy sources, muscle fatigue and dysfunction occur. In such settings, when abnormalities of muscle biochemistry are responsible for the decreased energy supply, the term *metabolic myopathies* is applied. For diagnostic purposes, these disorders can be divided into two groups: (1) exercise-induced (dynamic) myopathies, in which symptoms such as weakness, cramping, myalgias, and stiffness appear during exercise; and (2) stable, or slowly progressive (static), myopathies (Tables 25–4 and 25–5).[2] Muscle energy metabolism may be assessed through exercise testing. The results of these studies may refine the differential diagnosis and reduce the cost of the microscopic analysis. Additionally, when the microscopic evaluation is unrevealing, provocative exercise testing may confirm the presence of a metabolic defect. Common types of exercise testing include forearm (grip) exercise that primarily provides information about the integrity of glycolytic metabolism; incremental bicycle ergometry that yields information about the integrity of aerobic metabolism; and ^{31}P magnetic resonance spectroscopy that provides information about the intracellular metabolites of energy metabolism (i.e., adenosine triphosphate [ATP], inorganic phosphate, and phosphocreatine). Because exercise testing is an important part of the investigation of muscle disease, particularly with disorders of skeletal muscle energy metabolism, it is essential that physicians understand skeletal muscle energy metabolism.

Skeletal Muscle Energy Metabolism

Although muscle contraction is ATP-consuming, the ATP content of a contracting muscle changes little during a sustained contraction. Interestingly, muscle ATP stores are incapable of sustaining a muscle contraction for more than a single second. Phosphocreatine, a high-energy compound with an intramuscular concentration approximately four- to fivefold that of ATP, permits rapid ATP regeneration through the rephosphorylation of adenosine diphosphate (ADP). This reaction is catalyzed by creatine kinase, an enzyme

TABLE 25–4. **Metabolic Defects That Produce Exercise-Induced Muscle Symptoms**

- Disorders of carbohydrate metabolism
  - Myophosphorylase deficiency (McArdle's disease; type V glycogenosis)
  - Phosphofructokinase deficiency (Tarui's disease; type VII glycogenosis)
  - Phosphoglycerate kinase deficiency (type IX glycogenosis)
  - Phosphoglycerate mutase deficiency (type X glycogenosis)
  - Lactate dehydrogenase deficiency
  - Phosphorylase b kinase deficiency
- Disorders of lipid metabolism
  - Carnitine palmitoyl transferase deficiency
  - Long-chain acyl-coenzyme A dehydrogenase deficiency
  - Short-chain 3-hydroxyacyl-coenzyme A dehydrogenase deficiency
- Defects of the respiratory chain
  - Defects of complex I, complex III, and complex IV
  - Coenzyme Q10 deficiency
- Others
  - Myoadenylate deaminase deficiency
  - X-linked myopathy with abnormal dystrophin
  - Idiopathic

Modified from Rifai Z, Griggs RC: Metabolic myopathies. *In* Samuels MA, Feske S, Mesulam MM, et al (eds): Office Practice of Neurology. New York, Churchill Livingstone, 1996, pp 600–604.

TABLE 25–5. **Metabolic Defects That Produce Static Muscle Weakness**

Disorders of carbohydrate metabolism
Acid maltase deficiency (type II glycogenosis)
Debrancher enzyme deficiency (type III glycogenosis)
Brancher enzyme deficiency (type IV glycogenosis)
Phosphorylase b kinase deficiency
Phosphofructokinase deficiency
Myophosphorylase deficiency
Disorders of lipid metabolism
Muscle carnitine deficiency
Systemic carnitine deficiency
Mitochondrial myopathies

Modified from Rifai Z, Griggs RC: Metabolic myopathies. *In* Samuels MA, Feske S, Mesulam MM, et al (eds): Office Practice of Neurology. New York, Churchill Livingstone, 1996, pp 600–604.

found in large quantities in skeletal muscle tissue. Nevertheless, this anaerobic energy source is depleted in less than a minute, and even when combined, these two sources of readily available energy are incapable of maintaining high-intensity exercise. For this reason, skeletal muscle tissue must rely on other energy sources when sustained exertion is necessary.

In the nonfasting individual, the energy requirements of skeletal muscle are met by the metabolism of either carbohydrate (e.g., glycogen, glucose) or lipid (e.g., free fatty acids). The principal source of carbohydrate for skeletal muscle metabolism is intracellular glycogen, which is formed from blood glucose, via glycogenesis, and stored within the myocyte. When energy is required, glycogen is hydrolyzed to glucose (glycogenolysis) and then to pyruvate (glycolysis). In addition to pyruvate, glycolysis also generates ATP and nicotinamide adenine dinucleotide hydrogen (NADH) (reduced form of nicotinamide adenine dinucleotide [NAD^+]). Under aerobic conditions, pyruvate is subsequently metabolized to acetyl-CoA. The latter compound enters the Krebs' (tricarboxylic acid) cycle, yielding further molecules of ATP and NADH, as well as flavin adenine dinucleotide hydrogen ($FADH_2$). The reducing equivalents generated by glycolysis and the Krebs' cycle (i.e., the NADH and $FADH_2$) enter the electron transport system, a chain of enzymes located on the inner mitochondrial membrane, and are oxidized. The energy released from their oxidation is used to drive the phosphorylation of ADP to ATP. The maximum derivable energy from the aerobic metabolism of one molecule of glucose is 38 molecules of ATP. Conversely, under anaerobic conditions, because pyruvate is converted to lactate and the generated reducing equivalents cannot be metabolized by the electron transport system, only four molecules of ATP are generated from one molecule of glucose. Hence, the metabolism of carbohydrate is much more energy-efficient in the presence of oxygen (i.e., aerobic metabolism) than in its absence (i.e., anaerobic metabolism). The skeletal muscle fatigue (i.e., the inability to maintain high-intensity exertion for more than several minutes) associated with anaerobic glycolysis results from end-product accumulation (ADP, inorganic phosphorus, hydrogen ion), not from a lack of oxygen.[1] Although blood glucose can be used directly, most carbohydrate energy is derived from glycogen. Unlike carbohydrate storage, which is primarily intramuscular, lipid storage is primarily extramuscular. For this reason, the primary source of lipids during skeletal muscle metabolism is plasma free fatty acids; the lipid present within the myocyte contributes to a much lesser extent. Since the rate of free fatty acid mobilization is slow, the contribution of lipid metabolism during initial energy generation is limited. In addition, although carbohydrate can undergo both aerobic and anaerobic metabolism, lipid can only be metabolized aerobically and consequently cannot be utilized during anaerobic conditions.

As expected, the exact ratio of carbohydrate and lipid utilized for muscle energy metabolism, a topic recently summarized in an editorial by Layzer,[3] reflects many variables, including the intensity of exertion and its duration, the blood concentration of free fatty acids and oxygen, the amount of blood flow to the muscle, the muscle glycogen concentration, and the muscle's capacity for oxidative metabolism. At rest and during light exercise, skeletal muscle tissue metabolism is aerobic, and consequently it aerobically metabolizes free fatty acids for its energy. As the degree of intensity increases, the supply of lipid-derived energy becomes unable to keep pace with the energy requirement. For this reason, a greater proportion of energy must be contributed by carbohydrate. In general, enough glycogen is available to work intensively for 3 to 4 hours.[4] Should effort continue after the glycogen supply is depleted, the slower rate of lipid metabolism immediately diminishes the magnitude of the ongoing effort. At maximum intensity (e.g., sprinting at full speed), skeletal muscle energy is supplied through anaerobic glycolysis. Initially, the readily available energy substrates are exhausted (i.e., ATP and phosphocreatine), and aerobic glycolysis begins. Although simultaneous changes enhance oxidative metabolism (i.e., increased blood flow to muscle, increased oxygen uptake), they are insufficient to meet the energy demands of maximum exertion. Thus, anaerobic glycolysis occurs and pyruvate is converted to lactate. As lactate accumulates, oxygen debt increases, a term that refers to the additional oxygen required, during recovery, to oxidize the accumulated lactate. Again, this level of exertion can be maintained only for several minutes.[5] Through aerobic exercise training, athletes enhance their muscles' capacity for oxidative (aerobic) metabolism. Thus, during submaximal efforts, the blend of substrate used contains a greater percentage of lipid and, for this reason, less glycogen. As a result, the glycogen supply lasts longer, as does the individual's endurance.

Technique

Forearm exercise testing can be performed in a number of ways. Traditionally, the patient was asked to repetitively squeeze a handheld ergometer while a blood pressure cuff was maintained above systolic pressure. The blood pressure cuff, by inducing ischemia, ensures that oxidative phosphorylation cannot occur. A simple technique for evaluating lactate production in response to ischemic forearm exercise was described by Munsat in 1970.[6] In that report, rested and fasting individuals squeezed a handheld ergometer, with a workload of 4 to 7 kg-m, at 60 Hz for 1 minute. (Alternative methods are to sustain 1.5-second contractions that are separated by 0.5-second rest periods for 1 full minute[7] or squeezing a hand dynamometer to 50 percent of maximum grip strength until exhaustion—usually about 10 minutes.[2]) Although the serum lactate concentrations vary significantly among the studied individuals (the standard deviation approximated 60 percent of the mean), their *relative change* (rather than their absolute change) is fairly constant for a given individual. The serum lactate concentration peaks within 5 minutes (within 3 minutes for 90 percent of the tested individuals) of work cessation at a value that is three- to fivefold greater than the initial resting value. Because ischemic work induces pain, it is fortunate that the best correlation between the degree of serum lactate rise and the total work performed occurs when the exercise period is limited to 1 minute, a period of ischemic exercise that most individuals can tolerate. The relationship of forearm work and lactate production without ischemia was also evaluated and appears to produce comparable results, provided the workload exceeds 6 to 7 kg-m. In other words, the work intensity must be sufficiently strenuous to exceed the individual's aerobic threshold, thereby inducing anaerobic energy metabolism. This technique avoids the use of blood pressure cuff–induced ischemia, which may be hazardous to patients with glycolytic defects (may cause severe muscle necrosis).[2, 7]

Regardless of the technique used, the anaerobic condition blocks oxidative phosphorylation, thereby ensuring dependence on anaerobic glycolysis. Pre-exercise and postexercise (1, 2, 4, 6, and 10 minutes) venous lactate and ammonia levels are determined from venous blood samples collected from a catheter placed in an antecubital vein proximal to the deep veins of the forearm (e.g., the median vein). A three-way stopcock can be connected; blood samples are obtained from the side port and a slow infusion of normal saline maintains catheter patency. Normally, the lactate value rises three- to fivefold (resting level is ~1 mmol/L) within 1 to 2 minutes, whereas the ammonia value rises two- to tenfold within 2 to 5 minutes of exercise.[1, 2, 5] In the presence of a metabolic disorder, however, different metabolite patterns may be observed: With a *defect in glycolysis*, ammonia elevation occurs, but lactate elevation is diminished or does not occur. With *myoadenylate deaminase deficiency*, lactate elevation occurs, but elevation of ammonia does not. In the setting of *mitochondrial disorders*, lactate elevation is excessive, and with *poor effort*, neither lactate nor ammonia concentrations increase. As expected, with *disorders of lipid metabolism*, the metabolite profile is normal. Although the major source of blood lactate is muscle, the blood lactate concentration rises with anxiety, hyperventilation, muscular activity, and food intake, and, therefore, the patient should be relaxed, still, and in a fasting state.[6]

MUSCLE BIOPSY

The decision to proceed with a muscle biopsy is made after a thorough medical and neurological history, examination, laboratory evaluation, and electromyogram (EMG) study, thereby permitting the formulation of a preliminary diagnosis and, hence, dictating the studies required of the muscle biopsy specimen. The history characterizes the weakness (e.g., its rate of onset, distribution, time course, precipitants [e.g., exercise-induced], associated symptoms, and family pedigree). The clinical examination quantifies the weakness and identifies any associated features (e.g., myotonia). The laboratory assessment (e.g., serum creatine kinase, urine myoglobin) screens for abnormalities of the blood and urine and EMG provide information typically not obtainable in other ways, including (1) the identification of a disorder other than a myopathy (e.g., motor neuron disease, neuromuscular junction defect), thereby avoiding an unnecessary muscle biopsy; (2) further characterization of the myopathy (e.g., its distribution, its associated electrical features [e.g., fibrillation potentials]), thereby further defining the diagnostic possibilities; and (3) the identification of the best muscle for biopsy. As expected, the information obtained from the muscle biopsy specimen is related to the underlying disorder, as well as its severity and rate of progression. When the patient is free of muscle weakness, the muscle biopsy is unlikely to show any significant changes. Other important variables influencing the yield of the muscle biopsy include (1) the particular muscle biopsied; (2) the way in which the muscle biopsy specimen is processed; and (3) the particular studies performed on the specimen. Consequently, this subsection includes a discussion of these important variables. Most important, however, it is necessary for the clinician, the person performing the biopsy, the pathologist, and, when indicated, the referring pathology laboratory to carefully plan their approach to the evaluation of the muscle specimen.

Muscle Selection and Technique

Myopathic processes do not affect all skeletal muscles equally. Therefore, a risk of sampling error among muscle biopsy specimens is always present. For this reason, it is paramount to select the muscle that will most likely yield the desired information. Important clinical and electrodiagnostic data to consider in making this determination include (1) the degree of involvement of the muscle; (2) the rapidity of onset of the disease process; (3) the muscle's history; (4) the pathological familiarity of the muscle; (5) the accessibility of the muscle; and (6) the EMG examination findings. A clinically unaffected muscle should be avoided, because it may not be involved pathologically. A severely affected muscle is also avoided, since it may only show end-stage features (e.g., atrophy, fat, and fibrosis) rather than the distinguishing features of a specific disorder. Although a moderately affected muscle should be sought in patients with a slowly progressive disorder, a more severely affected muscle may provide the greatest diagnostic yield in individuals with acute disorder. The chosen muscle additionally should neither be involved with another disease process (e.g., radiculopathy) nor have suffered a recent (i.e., within 1 month) injection or needle electrode examination (i.e., EMG). The needle electrode examination should generally be performed on only one side of the body (and this should be clearly labeled in the chart) and is used to help in the identification of a muscle meeting sampling criteria so that the homologous muscle in the contralateral extremity may be sampled.

In general, the most frequently biopsied upper extremity muscles are the deltoid and biceps brachii, and the most frequently biopsied lower extremity muscles are one of the quadriceps (e.g., vastus lateralis) because the range of normal for these muscles is well defined. Although the gastrocnemius is frequently cited as a useful muscle, it should be avoided because of its type 1 muscle fiber predominance, its greater susceptibility to random pathological changes, and its pennate nature.[7] The problem with pennate muscles (i.e., muscles in which the tendon insertion extends throughout the muscle) is that inadvertent sampling near the myotendinous junction can occur. This region tends to have more central nucleation, muscle fiber size variability, and split muscle fibers. As expected, the muscle chosen must be easily accessible.

The technique of muscle biopsy is usually not difficult in the hands of an experienced individual. The skin and subcutaneous tissues are anesthetized (e.g., 2 percent Xylocaine [lidocaine]), while carefully avoiding muscle infiltration. A small incision is then placed in the belly region (i.e., away from the myotendinous junction) along the long axis of the muscle and is extended only to the fascia. In most cases, three specimens are collected: (1) an unclamped specimen for histochemistry (the most important piece); (2) a clamped specimen for electron microscopy; and (3) a clamped specimen for histopathology. A fourth specimen can be obtained and frozen in the event further studies are deemed necessary.

The *specimen for histochemistry* should be 2 to 3 cm in length and about as round as a pencil. It should be handled gently by its ends using tweezers and placed in a cool, normal saline-moistened piece of gauze to prevent drying out (soaked gauze may interfere with freezing and produce artifacts). The gauze-wrapped muscle specimen is then placed in a screw-cap vial for later freezing. The specimen should be rapidly transported to the pathology laboratory; otherwise it may lose its enzymatic activity. Many techniques exist for the preparation of the frozen specimen. Typically, it is gently immersed in a Pyrex beaker containing 2 inches of liquid nitrogen–cooled isopentane (−140° to −155° C), frozen for roughly 30 seconds, and then removed and immediately placed in a previously cooled specimen container (e.g., another screw-cap vial). When the specimen is sent to an outside reference laboratory, the specimen container should be placed in an insulated shipping container filled with dry ice.

The *specimen for electron microscopy* can be slightly smaller and should be gently raised (e.g., with Metzenbaum scissors) just high enough to permit the placement of a muscle clamp. The clamp is then locked and the muscle specimen cut just *outside* the clamped sites. Clamping helps avoid contraction artifact. A less cumbersome technique involves the suturing of the muscle tissue specimen (e.g., with 3-0 silk) to a piece of tongue depressor before excising it (i.e., it is sutured in situ). Once removed, the muscle specimen is then placed in a 4 percent buffered glutaraldehyde fixative (or Karnovsky's fixative).

The *specimen for histopathology* is obtained similar to that for electron microscopy, with the exception that it is fixed in formalin. The fixed specimens should be shipped separately from the frozen specimen. It is important to include the patient's name, the sampled muscle, the procurement time, and a brief note detailing the clinical presentation and workup findings to date, as well as a list of pending studies. Importantly, when specialized studies are planned (e.g., mitochondrial DNA studies), larger tissue specimens may be necessary. For this reason, the reference laboratory should be contacted before performing the muscle biopsy so that the required amount of tissue is procured.

The indications for an open biopsy, as opposed to a needle biopsy, are unsettled. There are two major advantages of open biopsies—a larger specimen can be obtained and the specimen can be fixed at its in situ length, thereby preventing contraction artifact. The two major advantages of a needle biopsy are the limited scarring and the ability to sample multiple sites (in either the same or different muscles) in a single session. Disadvantages of this technique include the smaller specimen size and greater orientation difficulty. In general, the experience of the person performing the biopsy and the expertise of the laboratory personnel dictate which technique is utilized.

Diagnostic Staining Methods

Overview. A brief overview of pertinent neuromuscular anatomy and physiology, including muscle fiber types, is a necessary preface to a discussion of the various stains and reactions. Skeletal muscles are composed of muscle fibers and connective tissue elements termed endomysium, perimysium, and epimysium. Epimysium surrounds the muscle belly and also lies between fascicles. Fascicles are surrounded by perimysium and are composed of groups of muscle fibers that are individually surrounded by endomysium. Small arteries, arterioles, veins, and nerve twigs are contained within the perimysium. Unlike the epimysium, which may contain adipose tissue, the perimysium of adults is usually devoid of adipocytes. Muscle fibers are cylindrical, polygonal (in adult cross sections), multinucleated syncytia derived from myoblast fusion. The muscle cytoplasm is termed sarcoplasm, and the muscle membrane is termed sarcolemma. Muscle nuclei (roughly five per fiber in cross section) are located just below the sarcolemma (up to 3 percent may be more centrally placed). Satellite cells are located subjacent to the sarcolemma and are covered by the basement membrane, which surrounds the entire muscle fiber. These function as a reserve cell population (discussed later). Each muscle fiber contains hundreds of myofibrils that are composed of repeating subunits, termed sarcomeres, containing the contractile elements (e.g., actin, myosin). Tubular extensions of the sarcolemma, termed T-tubules, extend transversely into the muscle fiber between the myofibrils. These structures permit the passage of electrical activity into the depths of the muscle fiber, thereby ensuring a maximal contraction. A second intermyofibrillar system of tubules is the sarcoplasmic reticulum, which is oriented parallel to the myofibrils (i.e., perpendicular to the T-tubules). The ends of these tubules are dilated into cisternae. The T-tubules are surrounded on both sides by the terminal cisternae of the sarcoplasmic reticulum. The nearness of these structures permits the electrical activity traversing the T-tubules to induce calcium release from the sarcoplasmic reticulum, thereby initiating muscle contraction. These tubular structures, as well as the aqueous sarcoplasm and mitochondria, are collectively termed the intermyofibrillar network.

There are two major types of muscle fibers, type 1 and type 2, each with different histochemical and physiological properties that give them specificity for certain activities. Type 1 fibers contain more oxidative enzymes, mitochondria, capillaries, and myoglobin and are hence best suited for aerobic metabolism and nonfatiguing activities (e.g., standing still). Type 2 fibers contain fewer mitochondria, and more abundant glycogen and glycolytic enzymes and are best suited for anaerobic metabolism and, consequently, those activities requiring maximal energy outputs (e.g., bench-pressing). Type 2 fibers are further subdivided into types 2A, 2B, and

2C. The type 2A fibers are more oxidative in nature than the type 2B fibers; type 2C fibers are present in fetal muscle, as well as regenerating muscle. Individual human skeletal muscles are composed of both muscle fiber types. The functional unit of movement is the motor unit, which consists of all the muscle fibers innervated by the same lower motor neuron. Its size, like that of the muscle fiber (discussed later), is dependent on the particular muscle. Although different types of muscle fibers compose an individual human skeletal muscle, the muscle fibers of a given motor unit are all identical in type (since this determination is made by the innervating lower motor neuron). The muscle fibers of a given motor unit normally are randomly distributed among the muscle fibers of other motor units. Although the relative abundance of fiber types among different muscles varies, the proportion of muscle fiber types observed in adults is as follows: type 1 (30 to 40%), type 2A (20 to 30%), and type 2B (40 to 50%); thus, there are roughly twice as many type 2 fibers as type 1 fibers, whereas in children, the ratio of type 1 fibers to type 2 fibers is nearly equal.[8] Type 1 fiber predominance is present when more than 55 percent of the fibers are type 1, whereas type 2 fiber predominance occurs when more than 80 percent of the muscle fibers are type 2.[9] The mean diameter of powerful muscles is 85 to 90 microns, as opposed to weaker, more distal muscles that have a mean diameter of 20 microns.[9] The muscle fiber type also influences diameter. In general, the diameter of type 1 fibers is less than or equal to that of type 2 fibers. Regarding gender, male type 1 fibers are equal to those of females, whereas male type 2 fibers are larger than those of females, a reflection of hormonal influences.[9]

Frozen Specimen. This, the most important specimen, is utilized for a variety of histochemical stains and reactions, some of which are listed in Table 25–6. The hematoxylin and eosin stain is useful for characterizing the general morphology (e.g., myocytes, nuclei, connective tissue, blood vessels, nerves) of the skeletal muscle specimen. The hematoxylin component identifies cell nuclei, and hence nuclear position, and muscle cross-striations; the eosin portion counterstains the cytoplasm reddish pink. Connective tissue appears darker with eosin staining. The modified Gomori trichrome stain stains nuclei and mitochondria red and myocytes blue-green. This stain is useful in identifying ragged-red fibers. The periodic acid–Schiff stain causes glycogen to appear purple. This stain readily identifies glycogen storage disorders, as well as capillaries. Oil red O stains lipid orange. Its utility, like that of the Sudan black stain, is in the identification of lipid storage disorders. Nicotinamide adenine dinucleotide dehydrogenase-tetrazolium reductase (NADH-TR) is an oxidative enzyme reaction that, like other reactions of this type, reflects the concentration of mitochondria within myocytes. This reaction colors myocytes purple-gray. By highlighting the sarcoplasmic reticulum, T-tubules, and mitochondria (i.e., the intermyofibrillar network), this reaction causes the sarcoplasm to take on a granular appearance. Although oxidative enzyme reactions differentiate the different muscle fiber types (i.e., type 1 > 2A > 2B), these reactions should not be used for fiber typing since atrophied type 2 fibers appear darker (i.e., appear like type 1 fibers). Succinate dehydrogenase, a Krebs' cycle enzyme, selectively stains mitochondria, as does cytochrome-c oxidase, a respiratory chain enzyme. Thus, unlike NADH-TR, the tubular elements are not highlighted. These two reactions can be used to determine whether intermyofibrillar aggregates are mitochondrial or tubular elements. The myofibrillar ATPase reaction is the most accurate method of muscle fiber typing.[9] The color characteristics are determined by the preincubation pH. In short, acidic pHs (e.g., 4.3, 4.6) cause type 1 fibers to appear darker than type 2 fibers, whereas alkaline pHs (e.g., 9.4) cause the type 2 fibers to appear darker. When preincubated at pH 4.3, the type 2A and 2B fibers are lighter than the type 2C fibers, which are intermediate in intensity; at pH 4.6, the type 2A fibers are lighter than the type 2B and 2C fibers, which are intermediate in intensity. Thus, preincubation at pH 4.3 permits the 2C fibers to manifest. Acid phosphatase, a lysosomal enzyme, facilitates the identification of degeneration (since necrotic fibers have increased lysosome content), inflammatory cells, and lysosomal storage disorders (e.g., acid maltase deficiency). Acid phosphatase is stained red, whereas the background is green. The alkaline phosphatase reaction stains regenerating fibers black, as well as normal capillary basement membranes; the background is yellow. Nonspecific esterase highlights endplates, lysosomes, and macrophages. It also identifies recently (i.e., within 6 months) denervated muscle fibers. The denervation-induced atrophy causes these fibers to appear smaller and darker. Sulfonated alcian blue stains amyloid "sea foam" green; it stains mast cells red. The alkaline Congo red stain causes amyloid to appear red, and, when viewed under polarized light, an apple green birefringence is observed.

TABLE 25–6. Selected Stains and Reactions and Their Usefulness in Evaluating Skeletal Muscle

Stains	
Hematoxylin and eosin	Hematoxylin: nuclei, cross-striations (purple) Eosin: cytoplasm (red), connective tissue (darker red)
Modified Gomori trichrome	Nuclei, mitochondria, T-tubules, sarcoplasmic reticulum (red); myocytes (blue-green)
Periodic acid–Schiff	Glycogen (purple; type 1 >2; glycogen storage disorders)
Oil red O	Lipid (orange; type 1 >2; lipid storage disorders)
Reactions	
NADH-TR	T-tubules, sarcoplasmic reticulum, mitochondria Type 1 (dark); type 2A (intermediate); type 2B (light)
Succinate dehydrogenase	Krebs' cycle enzyme; selectively stains for mitochondria
Cytochrome-c oxidase	Respiratory chain enzyme (orange-brown; type 1 >2)
ATPase (pH 4.3)	Type 1 (dark); type 2 (light)
ATPase (pH 4.6)	Type 1 (dark); type 2A (light); type 2B (intermediate)
ATPase (pH 9.4)	Type 1 (light); type 2 (dark)
Acid phosphatase	Degeneration (stains red; background fir green)
Alkaline phosphatase	Regeneration (stains black; background yellow)
Nonspecific esterase	Acetylcholinesterase (yellow-red; type 1 >2)

These stains and reactions, on transverse section, permit the shape, diameter, and intermyofibrillar pattern of the myocyte, as well as the arrangement and proportion of muscle fiber types, to be determined. Adult muscle fibers appear polygonal, and their cross-sectional diameters vary, depending on the specific skeletal muscle (discussed earlier). Within a given section, they are somewhat uniform. The intermyofibrillar pattern is best demonstrated with the histochemical reactions for oxidative enzymes and should appear uniform. Two examples of the histopathological features that disrupt the intermyofibrillar network include target fibers and central cores. Since the muscle fiber types of different motor units are interspersed, normal muscle shows a checkerboard pattern of light and dark fibers. This same reaction permits the recognition of fiber type disproportion and those disorders confined predominantly to one muscle fiber type (e.g., atrophy, cytoarchitectural abnormalities). When atrophy is identified, it should be further characterized as to muscle fiber type involved. When atrophy is due to a chronic denervating disease, the checkerboard pattern of type 1 and type 2 fibers is altered by collateral sprout-related reinnervation. Thus, the adjacent atrophied myocytes are of the same histochemical fiber type. Conversely, when atrophy is due to disuse, the checkerboard arrangement of muscle fiber types is maintained because collateral sprouting does not occur. Certain cytoarchitectural abnormalities are more pronounced in one muscle fiber type (Table 25–7).

Target fibers are a cardinal feature of neurogenic disorders and are composed of three "rings": (1) a central light-staining ring; (2) an intermediate dark-staining ring; and (3) a peripheral normal-staining ring. They are most predominant among type 1 muscle fibers. With central core disease, the NADH-TR reaction produces central unreactive zones, termed central cores, among affected myocytes. Thus, these structures are composed of two rings: a central ring of absent staining surrounded by a normally staining periphery. Again, type 1 fibers are mainly affected. Rod bodies (nemaline myopathy), which originate from Z disc material, appear reddish purple in the modified Gomori trichrome stain. Because a small number of muscle fibers in muscular dystrophy and polymyositis have been noted to contain these structures,[9] a diagnosis of nemaline myopathy requires the presence of numerous rod bodies in many muscle fibers. As previously noted, the modified Gomori trichrome stain is also useful in the identification of mitochondria and the tubular system of muscle. This stain readily identifies subsarcolemmal collections of mitochondria, termed ragged-red fibers, as well as sarcoplasmic reticulum–derived collections, termed tubular aggregates. Both of these abnormalities stain red. Because tubular aggregates are also highlighted by the NADH-TR reaction, but not by the succinate dehydrogenase reaction, they are easily differentiated from mitochondrial aggregates. Although these structures are frequently seen with hyperkalemic periodic paralysis, they are not diagnostically specific for this condition. Rimmed vacuoles have blue margins with hematoxylin and eosin and red margins with the modified Gomori trichrome stain. They are seen in association with inclusion body myopathy, oculopharyngeal muscular dystrophy, distal myopathy, and denervated muscle.

TABLE 25–7. Preferential Fiber Type Involvement

Preferential Atrophy

Type 1 fibers: Myotonic dystrophy (prominent), nemaline myopathy, centronuclear myopathy, congenital fiber type disproportion

Type 2 (especially 2B) fibers: Disuse, corticosteroid excess (exogenous, endogenous)*

Cytoarchitectural Abnormalities

Type 1 fibers: Target fibers, central cores (central core disease), rod bodies (nemaline myopathy), mitochondrial abnormalities

Type 2 fibers: Tubular aggregates

*Type 2 fiber atrophy, especially if limited to type 2B fibers, is a nonspecific finding most frequently indicating disuse.

Regarding the two other specimens, the glutaraldehyde-fixed specimen is embedded in plastic for electron microscopy (discussed later), whereas the formalin-fixed specimen is embedded in paraffin for light microscopy. Paraffin sections, which are routinely stained with hematoxylin and eosin (viewed in polarized light) and trichrome (viewed in bright field optics), can serve several purposes.[10] Longitudinally oriented sections permit the identification of cross-striation loss, inflammatory infiltrates, and blood vessel wall changes and can also serve as backup material.

Specialized Studies. Immunocytochemical techniques utilize commercially prepared antibodies to identify absent or abnormal proteins (e.g., dystrophin, laminin, complement cascade components) and to characterize cell types (e.g., lymphocyte subclasses), among other functions. For example, antibodies against dystrophin can confirm the diagnosis of Duchenne muscular dystrophy when blood tests are uninformative; antibodies against cell markers can demonstrate immune deposits distinctive of dermatomyositis; and antibodies against the membrane attack complex can identify cells targeted for destruction by the immune system. Enzyme histochemistry permits the biochemical analysis of muscle homogenates for specific enzymes (e.g., phosphofructokinase), and electron microscopy is available when ultrastructural examination of the tissue specimen (e.g., diagnosis of congenital myopathies, inclusion body myopathy, mitochondrial inclusions, tubular aggregates) is required.

Moreover, some histopathological changes are pathognomonic of a particular disorder. In general, the more specialized the study, the more likely its results will have pathognomonic significance (e.g., immunocytochemical studies [dystrophin], electron microscopy [inclusion body myopathy, congenital myopathies with pathognomonic ultrastructural features], and enzyme histochemistry studies for specific enzymes). In addition, certain morphological features, such as atrophy, are indicative of an underlying muscle disorder. For example, perifascicular atrophy, in which the muscle fibers near the edges of the fascicle are atrophied, is the hallmark of dermatomyositis, whereas panfascicular atrophy is indicative of Werdnig-Hoffmann disease.

Myopathic and Neurogenic Changes

The histopathological features observed in skeletal muscle biopsies can be subdivided into two pathological processes—those due to interruption of innervation (i.e., neuropathic changes) and those due to dysfunction of the muscle fiber itself (i.e., myopathic changes). Because nerve and muscle pathophysiologies dictate the observed changes, a brief overview of this topic initiates this subsection. As previously discussed, the functional unit of movement is the motor unit. This structure consists of a single lower motor neuron, its peripherally directed axon, and all of the muscle fibers it innervates. With lower motor neuron and motor axon disorders, because the affected axons undergo wallerian degeneration, the muscle fibers of an entire motor unit are denervated. Denervated muscle fibers undergo several changes, including downregulation of contractile element synthesis and contractile element resorption, both of which permit their survival, albeit in an atrophied state. If these muscle fibers are not reinnervated within approximately 20 months, they will be replaced by connective tissue. With incomplete nerve lesions, the uninvolved motor axons can sprout collaterals to the denervated muscle fibers, thereby "adopting" them. This process increases the number of muscle fibers innervated by the adopting lower motor neuron. With myopathic disorders, random muscle fiber loss occurs, rather than loss of whole motor unit territories. However, collateral sprouting may still occur with a myopathy. When a portion of a muscle fiber is degenerated (i.e., segmental necrosis), the muscle fiber functions as two separate fibers, the portion with the motor endplate (i.e., the innervated fiber) and the portion without it (i.e., the denervated fiber). Because the regenerative capacity of muscle is considerable, the denervated portion can be adopted by collateral sprouting. Also, precursor cells (satellite cells) proliferate and fuse with each other to regenerate the destroyed portion of the muscle. Muscle fibers that are not reinnervated undergo degeneration, a process associated with extensive collagen deposition and fatty infiltration.

Histological Features Associated with Neuropathic Processes. Histological features associated with neuropathic processes include angular atrophic fibers, group atrophy, fiber type grouping, target fibers, nuclear bags, and the presence of minimal interstitial fibrosis.[8] Of these features, the most typical attribute is atrophy, a process resulting in the appearance of small angulated (in cross section) muscle fibers, not selective for fiber types, scattered throughout the specimen. The atrophy also causes the intensity of staining to increase; thus, the denervated fibers appear darker (e.g., nonspecific esterase). Normally, the intermixing of muscle fiber types produces a random checkerboard pattern when skeletal muscle tissue is stained using fiber type-specific techniques. Because collateral sprouting increases the number of muscle fibers innervated by the adopting lower motor neurons and, as previously discussed, converts them to its own histochemical type, fiber type grouping occurs. For this reason the normal checkerboard staining pattern of muscle fibers diminishes. As denervation continues, assuming reinnervation keeps pace, larger and larger groups of contiguous fibers of the same histochemical type are observed (the sine qua non of reinnervation). Atrophy of these groups produces grouped atrophy, the hallmark of chronic denervation. The extreme version of grouped atrophy is panfascicular atrophy, a feature indicative of Werdnig-Hoffmann disease. Fiber type grouping must be distinguished from fiber type predominance (discussed earlier).

Histological Features Associated with Myopathic Processes. Primary disorders of muscle may affect solely the sarcolemma, a single region (segment) of the muscle fiber, or the entire muscle fiber. Thus, the histological features observed vary with the particular myopathic process. Features considered to be indicative of a myopathic process include rounded fibers, central nucleation, muscle fiber size variability, fiber splitting, segmental necrosis, muscle fiber necrosis (degeneration), cellular inflammation, myophagocytosis, regeneration (i.e., basophilic fibers), an increase in connective tissue elements, and structural abnormalities (e.g., vacuoles [glycogen, lipid], ragged-red fibers [mitochondrial myopathies], granulomas [sarcoid], and microorganisms [toxoplasmosis, trichinosis], as well as those structural changes associated with various congenital myopathies [e.g., rod bodies, central cores]).[8] Centrally located nuclei may be observed in up to 3 percent of normal muscle tissue specimens, but when present in a higher percentage, this indicates an underlying myopathy. This finding is especially prominent in the muscle fibers of patients with myotonic dystrophy (see Chapter 36). In fact, when internal nuclei appear in most of the muscle fibers of the sample, this diagnosis is strongly implicated. However, when a *single* central or paracentral nucleus appears in essentially every myocyte, the diagnosis of centronuclear myopathy is indicated. The combination of atrophy and hypertrophy contributes to the wide variability of muscle fiber size. Because muscle fiber splitting normally occurs near myotendinous junctions, muscle biopsies from this region may appear myopathic, and, consequently, sampling in this region is discouraged. When viewed in cross section, connective tissue septae, often with adjacent nuclei, are seen traversing the affected (i.e., split) muscle fibers. When muscle fiber necrosis destroys only a portion of the myocyte, the term *segmental necrosis* is applied. In this situation, proliferating satellite cells may regenerate the destroyed segment, thereby reinnervating the portion lacking a motor endplate. Features of regeneration include basophilic sarcoplasm (due to the rich ribonucleic acid content) and large nuclei with prominent nucleoli. However, when reinnervation occurs by collateral sprouting, small foci of fiber type grouping may be observed. Hence, small patches of fiber type grouping should not be considered synonymous with a neuropathic process. Inflammatory cell collections may have a perivascular distribution (e.g., collagen vascular disorder, dermatomyositis) or be most pronounced intracellularly (e.g., facioscapulohumeral dystrophy). With dystrophic myopathies, the thin connective tissue layers separating individual muscle fibers thicken and the muscle fibers may undergo considerable fibrosis. Regarding disease tempo, muscle fiber necrosis, basophilia, and myophagocytosis are features typical of an active myopathic process, whereas muscle fiber splitting is more characteristic of a chronic myopathy.[11]

Nerve Tissue

Biopsy of the peripheral nerve has somewhat limited use. It is generally performed in suspected neuromuscular diseases in order to aid in the distinction between segmental demyelination and axonal degeneration, particularly when the clinical evaluation, laboratory studies, and electrophysiological examinations are nondiagnostic or contradictory. Nerve biopsy may also be useful in the diagnosis of a number of specific disorders with characteristic findings that may involve a peripheral nerve such as amyloidosis, vasculitis, sarcoidosis, and some neoplasms.[12] Diagnostic nerve biopsy is generally restricted to a relatively expendable sensory nerve such as the sural, although portions of peripheral motor nerve twigs may be available for examination as part of muscle biopsy. Because of the limited amount of nervous system tissue available for examination and the relatively limited repertoire of pathological findings, peripheral nerve biopsy has a high chance of being noninformative unless the procedure is performed to answer a specific question in the context of the other clinical and electrophysiological findings.

NERVE SELECTION AND TECHNIQUES

Biopsy of peripheral nerve is usually completed either as a full-thickness nerve biopsy (i.e., a complete transection of the nerve to remove a segment) or as a fascicular biopsy (i.e., a longitudinal dissection of the nerve to remove segments of only one or several fascicles), sparing at least a portion of the nerve. Full-thickness nerve biopsy is considered technically easier to perform and is preferable when the pathological evaluation should include both nerve fibers and surrounding connective tissue and vascular structures. Fascicular nerve biopsy usually produces a smaller deficit and is favored when larger nerves are biopsied.

The choice of peripheral nerve biopsy site is limited by the potential deficits arising from nerve transection. The most common sites are the sural nerve or the superficial peroneal nerve, both subcutaneous sensory nerves in the lower extremity. In occasional cases, the superficial radial nerve in the upper extremity or the greater auricular nerve is also sampled. As noted earlier, concomitant biopsy of skeletal muscle to include small intramuscular nerve twigs may supplement the examination of the peripheral nervous system. Peripheral nerve biopsy may also be combined with skin biopsy, removing an ellipse of overlying skin, when morphological or tissue culture examination of skin is desired for diagnosis of metabolic or degenerative disease.

The sample amount is varied and should be judged, on the one hand, by the amount of tissue needed for the proposed studies and, on the other hand, by the fact that deficits arising from transection of the nerve during biopsy will not necessarily be increased by removing the extra centimeter or two that transforms a nondiagnostic biopsy into a useful diagnostic tool. For most purposes, a 2- to 3-cm segment of full-thickness nerve or fascicles is adequate to provide tissue for standard light and electron microscopic examination, including preparation of teased nerve fibers and frozen section.

TESTING METHODS

The usual morphological techniques for examination of peripheral nerve include standard light microscopy and electron microscopy, supplemented by morphometric studies, examination of teased nerve fibers, and examination of frozen sections when special studies such as immunohistochemistry are needed (Table 25–8).[13] For light and electron microscopy and teased nerve studies, specimens are usually fixed in glutaraldehyde solution. Cross sections are standard and useful for morphometric studies. Longitudinal sections are also useful for demonstrating some pathological findings, including focal processes such as vasculitis that may be irregularly distributed along the length of the nerve and missed in a given cross section. For light microscopic examination, resin-embedded sections stained with dyes such as toluidine blue give good morphological resolution. The same tissues can be subsequently processed for electron microscopy. Formalin-fixed or glutaraldehyde-fixed paraffin-embedded tissues and frozen sections give less resolution but generally permit examination of larger expanses of tissue and may be useful for some special stains, including some immunohistochemical procedures. Teased nerve fiber preparations, involving the dissection of single nerve fibers from fascicles of fixed nerve, are used for examination of sequential internodes of myelin along the fiber and are essential for proper assessment of various conditions involving axonal degeneration, regeneration, segmental demyelination, and remyelination. Morphometric procedures allow for the scoring of abnormalities.

TABLE 25–8. **Morphological Examination of Peripheral Nerve**

Technique	Fixation	Use
Routine light microscopy	Formalin, paraffin	Survey (vasculitis, amyloidosis)
	Glutaraldehyde, paraffin, or resin	Survey
Frozen specimen light microscopy	None	Special stains (immunohistochemistry, metachromasia)
Teased nerve examination	Glutaraldehyde, osmium	Myelin internodes
Electron microscopy	Glutaraldehyde, osmium, resin	Fine structure

Brain and Meningeal Tissue

In the earlier part of this century, diagnostic brain biopsy was often considered a technique of last resort. The development of improved imaging techniques such as computed tomography (CT) and magnetic resonance imaging (MRI) now permits a high degree of definition of lesions, including both anatomical localization and pathological characteristics. Concomitant developments in neurosurgical techniques, including stereotactic or computer-guided neurosurgery, microsurgical techniques, and intraoperative neurosurgery such as electrocorticography, now permit access to brain tissue with relatively little morbidity, even in vulnerable areas such as motor cortex, the diencephalon, and the brain stem.[14–16]

Diagnostic biopsy of a brain lesion, possibly followed by resection, is now essential in the diagnosis and management of most primary brain tumors and often plays a role in the management of metastatic disease as well. Diagnostic brain biopsy may also play a role in the management of other mass lesions of a non-neoplastic nature, such as distinguishing between reactive and neoplastic mass lesions. Diagnostic brain biopsy currently also has a more limited use in certain forms of infectious, degenerative, or metabolic diseases that affect the brain. In some of these disease categories, the need to sample brain tissue has been lessened because of the development of improved imaging studies and other ancillary diagnostic techniques. Recent rapid developments in genetics and molecular diagnosis may further supplant the need to obtain central nervous tissues in some circumstances but may also create as yet unforeseen needs for brain tissue. In addition, brain tissue resection is part of the management of some forms of chronic intractable epilepsy.

Despite the improvements in neurosurgical and other clinical practice, removal of nonregenerating brain tissue is still accompanied by risk of permanent neurological deficit. Additional risks of intraoperative complications such as hemorrhage, cerebral infarction, or infection and of postoperative complications such as scarring with formation of an epileptic focus must also be considered. The decision to remove brain tissue must be balanced between the attendant risks and the utility of a tissue diagnosis.[17]

TISSUE SELECTION AND TECHNIQUES

Diagnostic brain biopsy is usually performed as stereotactic biopsy or open craniotomy.[16] Stereotactic brain biopsy, using CT or MRI guidance, is usually completed by the aspiration of tissue through a needle inserted into the area of the lesion. Although this technique is particularly useful in cases in which the lesion is small, deep-seated, or located in a sensitive area such as the motor cortex or deep nuclei, the amount of tissue removed is small and may hinder diagnosis. The procurement of multiple biopsies along the needle trajectory, however, may provide a more complete picture of the pathological process. For accessible lesions, open craniotomy permits the intraoperative assessment of pathological processes by direct observation and may be performed when biopsy and resection are contemplated. This procedure may also be considered when maintenance of the anatomic relationship of the biopsy specimen is desired. Stereotactic localization techniques can also be applied to open craniotomy procedures and are sometimes useful in planning and monitoring resections.

The choice of biopsy site depends on the suspected diagnosis.[18] In the setting of a structural or mass lesion (brain tumor), whether neoplastic or non-neoplastic, tissue from the area of imaging abnormality is the obvious choice, although the pathological lesion and the imaged lesion may not be equivalent. Infiltrating gliomas, for example, may extend well beyond the area of contrast enhancement seen on imaging studies, and occasional lesions that appear discrete on imaging studies such as MRI may be remarkably ill-defined and elusive in the operating room or in the pathology laboratory. In the case of a mass lesion, the amount and pattern of sampling should also be guided by the suspected diagnosis. The amount of tissue sufficient for diagnosis cannot be predicted and often depends on the nature of the disease process. A few cells from a cerebrospinal fluid or needle aspiration of tissue may be sufficient in the diagnosis of metastatic carcinoma or lymphoma, whereas even postmortem examination of the entire brain may be inadequate to establish a precise diagnosis in some degenerative or metabolic diseases.[19, 20] Direct communication between the clinician and the pathologist prior to the surgical procedure is the best method of ensuring that tissue sampling is appropriate.

Intraoperative evaluation of tissue samples by frozen section or other preparation has several roles. Frozen sections may provide a specific diagnosis in some cases, but in many situations a definitive diagnosis can be made only after evaluation of all tissue specimens and with adjunctive studies. Frozen sections are sometimes used to guide resection of a mass lesion. In many cases, particularly in primary biopsies of undefined lesions, frozen section is most useful in the assessment of whether the tissue sample appears adequate to answer the clinical question. It also is useful in the selection and processing of the tissue for other pertinent studies, even if a precise diagnosis cannot be rendered intraoperatively.[21]

In the case of large tumors, abscesses, or other reactive lesions, the abnormal brain region may be heterogeneous. Sampling of central areas of complete tissue necrosis in tumors or abscesses may not yield diagnostic tissue. The relationship of the lesioned tissue to the adjacent brain is often important in assessing the nature of the pathological process, for example, demonstrating the infiltrating border in gliomas, the presence of residual or recurrent tumor in radiation necrosis, or the boundary between demyelinated or necrotic brain and normal brain. Microorganisms are often present at the expanding edge of infectious lesions but absent in the necrotic center. Stereotactic biopsy offers the advantage of obtaining multiple samples along a single needle trajectory and is useful in evaluating heterogeneous lesions such as gliomas, in which different areas of the tumor may show different degrees of malignancy, as well as in reactive lesions.

Intraoperative monitoring of brain function by techniques such as electrocorticography is useful in guiding sampling or resections in sensitive areas such as the motor strip. These techniques are also essential in mapping epileptic foci and can be used in conjunction with conventional imaging studies and special studies such as positron-emission tomography.

In the absence of a mass lesion or defined area on imaging studies, noneloquent areas of the cerebrum are generally selected. The type of tissue sampled (e.g., gray or white brain matter, leptomeninges) should also be guided by the suspected diagnosis. The most useful specimen should be large enough to allow for the proper orientation by the pathologist and to be divided into pieces adequate for special studies (see later). For degenerative or metabolic diseases, infectious diseases (viral encephalitis), and diffuse disorders (cerebral vasculitides), a wedge of brain tissue consisting of cerebral cortex, overlying leptomeninges, and underlying white matter provides the most useful tissue sample and should be large enough to provide material for ancillary studies (e.g., biochemical analysis, electron microscopy).

TESTING METHODS

Morphological techniques include cytological studies (the evaluation of individual cells in fluids) and histological studies (the evaluation of cells in their tissue context). The latter involve light microscopy with routine and special stains, electron microscopy, histochemistry, and immunohistochemistry. Typical methods of fixation and staining for each technique are summarized in Table 25–9. Ancillary studies that supplement the armamentarium of morphological techniques

TABLE 25–9. **Diagnostic Brain Biopsies: Common Tissue Techniques**

Evaluation	Biopsy Technique	Fixative	Staining
Cytological	Imprint/touch Smear/squash	Alcohol	Rapid hematoxylin and eosin, Diff-Quik, Papanicolaou
Routine histological	Frozen section Paraffin section	Alcohol Formalin, B5	Rapid hematoxylin and eosin, metachrome B, special staining
Special histological: histochemistry, immunohistochemistry	Frozen section Frozen or paraffin	None Variable	Enzymes, biochemical reactions Monoclonal or polyclonal antibodies
Electron microscopy	Thick section Thin section	Glutaraldehyde/OsO_4	Toluidine blue Lead citrate/uranyl acetate

include microbiology (e.g., bacterial, viral, fungal cultures), cytogenetics (e.g., karyotype analysis), molecular genetics (e.g., polymerized chain reaction), and biochemical analyses.

The choice of morphological and ancillary techniques depends on the nature of the lesion and the available material. Although most pathological diagnoses are made on sections of formalin-fixed paraffin-embedded tissues stained with hematoxylin and eosin or a comparable general tissue stain, some diagnoses require other stains to be used on the paraffin-embedded tissues or even other methods of tissue handling and fixation (freezing, glutaraldehyde fixation, and plastic embedding for electron microscopy; submission of unfixed tissues in special handling media for cytogenetic or microbiological studies). Before fixation, tissue should be divided and processed appropriately for these studies. Consideration of the expected diagnosis, obtained from the preoperative workup or from intraoperative frozen section, is essential in the planning and optimal handling of the diagnostic brain biopsy. Familiarity with a particular institution's manual of laboratory procedures that list recommendations for handling tissues for specific tests and communication with the neurosurgeon and pathologist in advance of the biopsy procedure are necessary to avoid inappropriate handling of valuable specimens.

SPECIFIC INDICATIONS

Categories of central nervous system (CNS) disease amenable to diagnosis by brain biopsy or mimicking types of disease normally presenting as neurosurgical conditions are summarized in Table 25–10. This disorder can be grouped into conditions that present with mass lesions, focal or multifocal nonmass lesion abnormalities, and diffuse abnormalities. Mass lesions include most neoplasms and neoplastic or non-neoplastic cysts, some forms of infection (abscesses, cerebritis, tuberculomas, some encephalitides), specific vascular disorders (hemorrhages, early infarcts), malformations or developmental lesions (hamartomas, some migrational abnormalities), and a variety of miscellaneous conditions (e.g., sarcoidosis, acute multiple sclerosis, and adrenoleukodystrophy). Conditions that produce imaging study abnormalities that are not necessarily mass lesions include some neoplasms (infiltrating gliomas, gliomatosis, lymphomas), cerebrovascular disorders (vasculitides, vasculopathies), infections (viral encephalitis, progressive multifocal leukoencephalopathy, CNS syphilis), degenerative diseases (Creutzfeldt-Jakob disease, and other dementias), inflammatory and immunological disorders (acute disseminated encephalomyelitis, limbic encephalitis, Rasmussen's encephalitis), developmental and malformative disorders (cortical migrational disorders and dysplasias), toxic and metabolic disorders (leukodystrophies, central pontine myelinolysis, mitochondrial encephalopathies), and some forms of epilepsy (mesial temporal sclerosis, malformations). Finally, some conditions show either no imaging study abnormalities or show only atrophy without focal findings, for example, degenerative diseases (Alzheimer's disease, Parkinson's disease), toxic and metabolic diseases (hepatic encephalopathy, many storage diseases), and most cases of idiopathic epilepsy.

Mass Lesions (Table 25–11)

Tumors. The differential diagnosis of a mass lesion presumed to be neoplastic can be limited by considering the age of the patient and the location of the tumor. Table 25–12 lists examples of tumors encountered in certain nervous system locations in the pediatric and adult age groups. Diagnostic biopsy is usually directed toward the mass lesion. As noted

TABLE 25–10. **Brain and Meningeal Biopsy Diagnoses**

Category	Examples
Neoplasms	Gliomas, metastatic tumors, CNS lymphoma
Infections (inflammatory)	HIV encephalitis, opportunistic infections (toxoplasma, cytomegalovirus, herpes simplex, *Cryptococcus*), bacterial abscess, cysticercosis, tuberculosis, sarcoidosis
Degenerative diseases	Creutzfeldt-Jakob disease, Alzheimer's disease, Pick's disease
Vascular diseases	Vasculitis, amyloid angiopathy, vascular malformations, CADASIL
Epilepsy	Mesial temporal sclerosis, dysplasias and malformations, Rasmussen's encephalitis
Metabolic diseases	Leukodystrophies, storage diseases, mitochondrial diseases

CNS, Central nervous system; HIV, human immunodeficiency virus.

TABLE 25-11. **Differential Diagnosis of Space-Occupying Central Nervous System Lesions**

Neoplasms	Intra-axial: gliomas, metastatic tumors, lymphoma Extra-axial: meningiomas, nerve sheath tumors
Infections	Abscesses (bacterial, fungal, parasitic), granulomas (tuberculosis, sarcoidosis), necrotizing lesions (toxoplasma, some focal viral encephalitides)
Cerebrovascular	Hemorrhages, acute infarctions
Demyelinating	Acute multiple sclerosis, adrenoleukodystrophy
Cysts	Metastatic neoplasms, primary neoplasms (gliomas), primary developmental disorders (arachnoid, neuroepithelial, colloid, enterogenous)

earlier, the possibilities of tissue heterogeneity and central necrosis should be taken into account by adequate sampling of different areas, including the interface between tumor and adjacent brain. A preliminary intraoperative assessment by frozen section is useful to gauge the adequacy of the specimen for diagnosis and to predict how tissues should be handled for ancillary studies. Neoplasms that may present without evidence of a mass lesion and mimic other forms of neurological disease include neoplasms disseminated in the subarachnoid space (metastatic carcinoma, glioma, lymphoma), infiltrating gliomas (low-grade astrocytomas, oligodendrogliomas, or gliomatosis cerebri), and some forms of mixed neuronal and glial neoplasms (dysembryoplastic neuroepithelial tumor) and lymphomas. Non-neoplastic mass lesions such as infections can be suspected on intraoperative frozen section evaluation, and appropriate ancillary studies can be done.

Radiation Necrosis. Following therapeutic radiation therapy for intracerebral neoplasms, the distinction between recurrent neoplasm and radiation necrosis is often difficult. Diagnostic brain biopsy is often useful in demonstrating residual or recurrent neoplasm and may show the coagulative tissue necrosis and vasculopathic changes characteristic of radiation necrosis in adjacent brain parenchyma, with or without evident tumor. Diagnostic brain biopsy can be performed as part of the therapeutic removal of necrotic tissue as well.

Non-neoplastic Cysts. Diagnostic biopsy of a cyst wall can be performed as part of cyst fenestration or drainage and may be useful in distinguishing between neoplastic and non-neoplastic cystic mass lesions.

Infections. Infectious diseases of the CNS are diagnosed by a variety of means, including assessment of clinical history, standard laboratory studies, serological and microbiological evaluation of blood and cerebrospinal fluid, and imaging studies. Diagnostic brain biopsy plays a limited role in this setting. In the case of mass lesions or focal brain lesions, diagnostic brain biopsy may be useful in distinguishing between neoplasms and infections. Diagnostic brain biopsy evaluated by morphological and microbiological studies (including molecular biological techniques) may also be useful in identifying an organism that has failed to be diagnosed by blood or cerebrospinal fluid studies. Diagnostic brain biopsy is also performed when a suspected infectious lesion fails to respond to a trial of antimicrobial therapy. Diagnostic brain biopsy is also performed in some patients with human immunodeficiency virus (HIV) infection and certain CNS complications. The spectrum of possible infectious complications in these patients is large and varied. Common CNS infections include toxoplasma cerebritis, cryptococcal and other fungal infections of the meninges or brain parenchyma, herpes simplex and cytomegalovirus encephalitis, and progressive multifocal leukoencephalopathy (JC virus). Although these infections often present with characteristic clinical and imaging features, a considerable overlap among these infections and primary CNS lymphoma can occur. In HIV patients who fail a trial of antimicrobial agents for a suspected infection, diagnostic brain biopsy may also be useful.

Degenerative Diseases

Many degenerative diseases are characterized by neuronal loss and gliosis in various brain structures without distinctive features. Diagnosis by brain biopsy remains inconclusive in many cases. In patients with a rapidly progressive dementia, a distinction can be made between Creutzfeldt-Jakob disease and degenerative disorders by the presence of spongiform changes or

TABLE 25-12. **Differential Diagnosis of Neoplastic Central Nervous System Tumors**

Age	Cerebral Hemispheres	Diencephalon	Posterior Fossa	Cerebral Meninges	Spinal Cord
Adulthood	Astrocytoma, glioblastoma, oligodendroglioma, metastatic tumor, lymphoma	Astrocytoma, glioblastoma, colloid cyst, pituitary adenoma	Metastatic tumor, hemangioblastoma	Meningioma, CN VIII schwannoma, metastatic carcinoma, lymphoma	Meningioma, nerve sheath tumors, astrocytoma, ependymoma
Childhood	Astrocytoma, ependymoma, choroid plexus tumor, primitive neuroectodermal tumor	Germ cell tumors, craniopharyngioma	Medulloblastoma, ependymoma, cerebellar pilocytic astrocytomas, brain stem astrocytoma, choroid plexus tumor	Leukemia, lymphoma	Nerve sheath tumors, astrocytoma

CN, Cranial nerve.

prion proteins in the former. In addition, the demonstration of senile plaques and neurofibrillary tangles in a random biopsy of cerebral cortex, while suggestive of Alzheimer's disease, does not exclude the possibility of other forms of neurodegenerative disease or the presence of other concomitant disease. Because of the variability of distribution of the pathological changes in most degenerative disorders, random biopsies may be nondiagnostic. For adequate evaluation, a piece of cerebral cortex with overlying leptomeninges and underlying white matter that can be oriented is desirable. Tissue should be considered potentially infectious, and precautions for Creutzfeldt-Jakob disease should be taken according to local institutional guidelines. The tissue should be fixed and reserved for possible electron microscopy or other studies.

Vascular Diseases (Table 25–13)

Surgical resection of tissue is occasionally performed in the setting of cerebrovascular disease. Diagnostic brain or meningeal tissue biopsy is usually performed when CNS vasculitis is suspected. Resection of brain tissue is usually performed for the diagnosis and treatment of vascular malformations. Symptomatic treatment of acute cerebrovascular diseases, usually hemorrhages and traumatic lesions, by evacuation of hematoma with removal of damaged brain tissue, may provide histological evidence of specific etiologies such as amyloid angiopathy, hypertensive vasculopathy, or cerebral autosomal dominant arteriopathy with subcortical infarcts and leukoencephalopathy (CADASIL). CADASIL can be diagnosed in some cases by ultrastructural examination of small blood vessels on skin punch biopsy. Some cases of cerebrovascular disease, such as infarcts, present as mass lesions and may be clinically mistaken for neoplasms.

TABLE 25–13. Tissue Diagnoses in Cerebrovascular Disease

Vasculitis	Primary CNS vasculitis, CNS involvement in systemic vasculitis, infectious vasculitis
Vascular malformations	Arteriovenous malformation, cavernous angioma, venous angioma
Vasculopathies and diseases presenting as intracranial hemorrhages	Amyloid angiopathy, hypertensive vasculopathy, vasculitis, primary or metastatic neoplasms, infections
Cerebrovascular diseases mimicking mass lesions	Recent infarction

Metabolic Diseases

Diagnosis of metabolic and storage disorders by brain biopsy has been superseded in many conditions by biochemical and molecular genetic analysis of more readily obtainable non-CNS cells and tissues. In cases in which metabolic or storage disease involving the CNS is suspected but no metabolic defect can be identified by other means, random biopsy of cerebral cortex and white matter may provide either positive or useful negative information. Reserved frozen or properly fixed tissues may prove useful later when subsequent clinical clues or testing techniques become available.

Epilepsy

Some patients with intractable epilepsy may benefit from surgical resection of brain tissue (see Chapter 52). In patients with complex partial seizures originating in the temporal lobe, temporal lobectomy with partial hippocampectomy may be beneficial. Examination of medial temporal lobe structures may disclose evidence of neuronal loss and gliosis in the hippocampus, amygdala, or adjacent gray matter structures (mesial temporal sclerosis). In occasional cases, other pathological findings (neoplasm, vascular malformation, cicatrix) may account for an epileptogenic focus. In some patients with intractable epilepsy with focal abnormalities demonstrated by electrophysiological, conventional neuroimaging modalities, or physiological imaging modalities such as positron-emission tomography scanning, removal of the focus is indicated. Pathological findings may include cortical migrational abnormalities, dysplasias, vascular malformations, glial scars, neoplasms, or focal infections. More widespread resections such as lobectomy or even hemispherectomy are occasionally performed with patients with established neurological deficits and more extensive malformations or with progressive lesions such as Rasmussen's encephalitis. Despite the finding of a focal lesion on one or more studies, no specific pathology is found in a large percentage of cases.

Reviews and Selected Updates

Engel AG: The muscle biopsy. *In* Engel AG, Franzini-Armstrong C (eds): Myology, 2nd ed. New York, McGraw-Hill, 1994, pp 822–831.

Fatallah-Skaykh HM: Fiction, reality, and molecular neurology. Arch Neurol 2000;57:63–64.

Fischbach FT: Blood Studies. A Manual of Laboratory and Diagnostic Tests, 5th ed. Philadelphia, Lippincott-Raven, 1996, pp 147–252.

Genetics Testing Task Force of the American Academy of Neurology: Practice parameter: Genetic testing alert. Neurology 1996;47:1343–1344.

Haller RG, Bertocci LA: Exercise evaluation of metabolic myopathies. *In* Engel AG, Franzini-Armstrong C (eds): Myology, 2nd ed. New York, McGraw-Hill, 1994, pp 807–821.

MacMillan JC, Harper PS: Clinical genetics in neurological disease. J Neuro Neurosurg Psychiatry 1994;57:7–15.

Rosenberg RN, Prusiner SB, DiMauro S, et al (eds): The Molecular and Genetic Basis of Neurological Disease. Boston, Butterworth-Heinemann, 1993.

References

1. Haller RG, Bertocci LA: Exercise evaluation of metabolic myopathies. *In* Engel AG, Franzini-Armstrong C (eds): Myology, 2nd ed. New York, McGraw-Hill, 1994, pp 807–821.
2. Rifai Z, Griggs RC: Metabolic myopathies. *In* Samuels MA, Feske S, Mesulam MM, et al (eds): Office Practice of Neurology. New York, Churchill Livingstone, 1996, pp 600–604.
3. Layzer RB: How muscles use fuel. N Engl J Med 1991;324:411–412.
4. Sudarsky L: Muscle. *In* Sudarsky L (ed): Pathophysiology of the Nervous System. Boston, Little, Brown, 1990, pp 25–47.
5. Martin A, Haller RG, Barohn R: Metabolic myopathies. Curr Opin Rheumatol 1994;6:552–558.
6. Munsat TL: A standardized forearm ischemic exercise test. Neurology 1970;20:1171–1178.
7. Griggs RC, Mendell JR, Miller RG (eds): Evaluation and Treatment of Myopathies. Philadelphia, F.A. Davis, 1995.
8. Prayson RA: Skeletal muscle pathology. Neuropathology review course. Cleveland Clinic Foundation, Cleveland, 1994, pp 50–63.
9. Heffner RR Jr: Neuromuscular disease. 32nd Annual Neuropathology Review Course. Armed Forces Institute of Pathology, San Antonio, 1994, pp 1–30.

10. Engel AG: The muscle biopsy. *In* Engel AG, Franzini-Armstrong C (eds): Myology, 2nd ed. New York, McGraw-Hill, 1994, pp 822–831.
11. Brooke MH, Cwik VE: Disorders of skeletal muscle. *In* Bradley WG, Daroff RB, Fenichel GM, et al (eds): Neurology in Clinical Practice, 2nd ed. Boston, Butterworth-Heinemann, 1996, pp 2003–2047.
12. Hauw JJ, Eymard B: Muscle and nerve biopsies. *In* Mohr JP, Gautier JC (eds): Guide to Clinical Neurology. New York, Churchill Livingstone, 1995, pp 91–118.
13. Vital C, Vallat JM (eds): Ultrastructural Study of the Human Diseased Peripheral Nerve, 2nd ed. New York, Elsevier, 1987, pp 1–22 and passim.
14. McKeever PE, Blaivas M, Nelson JS: Tumors: Applications of light microscopic methods. *In* Garcia JH (ed): Neuropathology: The Diagnostic Approach. St. Louis, Mosby, 1997, pp 31–38.
15. Esiri MM: Oppenheimer's Diagnostic Neuropathology: A Practical Manual, 2nd ed. Oxford, Blackwell Scientific, 1996.
16. Chandrasoma PT, Apuzzo MLJ: Stereotactic Brain Biopsy. New York, Igaku-Shoin, 1989, pp 65–73.
17. Gautier JC, Mohr JP: Autopsy and brain biopsy. *In* Mohr JP, Gautier JC (eds): Guide to Clinical Neurology. New York, Churchill Livingstone, 1995, pp 85–90.
18. Burger PC, Scheithauer BW, Vogel FS: Surgical Pathology of the Nervous System and Its Coverings, 4th ed. New York, Churchill Livingstone, 2002.
19. Stanley MW: Cerebrospinal fluid cytology. *In* Garcia JH (ed): Neuropathology: The Diagnostic Approach. St. Louis, Mosby, 1997, pp 1–30.
20. Bigner SH: Cerebrospinal fluid. *In* Bigner DD, McLendon RE, Bruner JM (eds): Russell and Rubenstein's Pathology of Tumors on the Nervous System, 6th ed. New York, Oxford University Press, 1998.
21. Goebel HH: Neurodegenerative diseases: Biopsy in children. *In* Garcia JH (ed): Neuropathology: The Diagnostic Approach. St. Louis, Mosby, 1997, pp 581–636.

CHAPTER 26

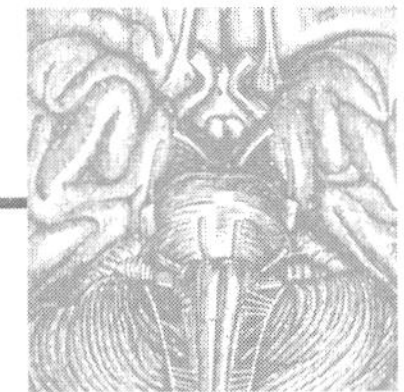

BARNETT R. NATHAN

Cerebrospinal Fluid and Intracranial Pressure

History

The cerebrospinal fluid (CSF) has served as an aid to the diagnosis and treatment of a variety of central nervous system (CNS) disorders for more than 100 years. In 1891, Quinke first developed the technique of spinal puncture and introduced it into clinical practice.[1] He was the first to use a needle with a stylet, to measure opening and closing pressures, and to pioneer the measurement of CSF glucose, protein, and cell counts. Much of the CSF literature in the early part of the 20th century dealt with changes related to bacterial meningitis and neurosyphilis.[2]

The notion that elevated intracranial pressure (ICP) can occur began in 1783 when Alexander Monroe posited that the skull is a closed container and its contents are nearly incomprehensible. These concepts were expanded in 1824 by George Kellie, who proposed that the volume of the blood within the brain was constant. In 1846, Burrows suggested that the volume of blood within the brain could only change in a reciprocal manner with the CSF and brain parenchyma. This concept formed the foundation of the Monroe-Kellie hypothesis, and modern theories of pressure-volume relationships still refer to this hypothesis. Early anatomists hypothesized that the choroid plexus was the source of CSF because of its location within the ventricles. This hypothesis was substantiated by Dandy and Blackfan[3] and then by Harvey Cushing,[4] who observed oozing of fluid from the choroid plexus during neurosurgery. Later, Ames provided definitive proof that the majority of intraventricular CSF was produced by the choroid plexus.[5, 6]

Cerebrospinal Fluid and the Ventricular System

ANATOMY

The choroid plexus produces the majority of the CSF in addition to smaller amounts secreted by the ependyma and the perivascular spaces. The choroid plexus is derived embryologically from the neural epithelium and is composed of two layers, including a specialized ependymal cell layer composed of the epithelial lining of the ventricular system and a highly vascularized pia mater layer. This bilayered structure, known as the choroidal epithelium, is folded into microvilli and forms a brush border on which cilia are present on the apical surfaces of some of these cells (Fig. 26–1). The choroidal epithelium with accompanying blood vessels and interstitial connective tissue collectively form the choroid plexus.

The choroidal epithelium shares many characteristics with the blood-brain barrier. The concept of a blood-brain barrier was first considered in the 19th century when Paul Ehrlich injected dye into the blood of animals and noted that all the organs except the brain were stained. Later, in 1913, Edwin Goldmann injected dye into the CSF compartment and found that the brain was stained but no dye appeared in the blood. From these findings, the hypothesis that the brain was separated from blood and that the brain capillaries provide this barrier was proposed. When electron microscopy became available, it was revealed that capillary endothelial cells rest on a basement membrane and form a tube joined by continuous tight junctions with the merging of the outer

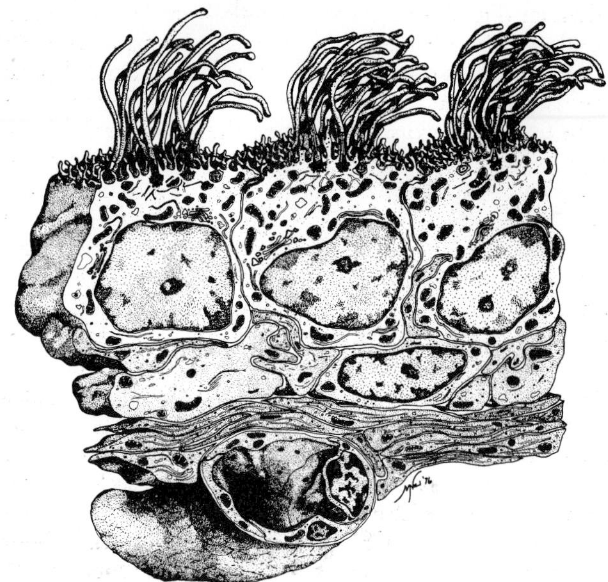

FIGURE 26–1. Diagram of choroidal epithelium demonstrating the ependymal microvilli and cilia forming a brush border into the ventricular lumen. (From Page RB, Leure-dePree AE: Ependymal alterations in hydrocephalus. *In* Wood JH [ed]: Neurobiology of Cerebrospinal Fluid. New York, Plenum Press, 1983, p 802.)

leaflets of two adjoining cells. This barrier is involved in protecting the brain from substances in the blood, selectively transporting desired blood constituents, and metabolizing or modifying substances transported between compartments.

The properties of brain endothelial cells that differentiate them from systemic capillaries include complex tight junctions between individual capillary endothelial cells, which provide a high electrical resistance. These junctions are formed through the merging of the outer leaflets of two adjoining cells. Second, little bulk flow of molecules occurs through these cells because of the paucity of pinocytotic vesicles and fenestrae. These two features protect the brain from various neurotoxic agents that may be present in the blood. Only substances that can cross biological membranes owing to their lipophilic character may diffuse unrestricted across the blood-brain barrier. Specific carrier systems, however, do exist in the brain endothelial cells and allow for the controlled exchange of substances between the system blood and the nervous system. These include facilitated diffusion in the case of the glucose transporter and adenosine triphosphate (ATP)–dependent active transport mechanisms. Third, in addition to the endothelial cells, pericytes, perivascular microglia, and astrocytes contribute to the barrier. Pericytes are contractile adventitial cells and serve as the counterpart to the smooth muscle of large systemic vessels. Whereas evidence exists to suggest that these cells are necessary for the growth and integrity of the capillary endothelial cells and cellular transport, their exact function is unknown. Perivascular microglial cells are derived from bone marrow and most likely migrate to the brain. In proximity to the capillary endothelial cells, these microglial cells most likely serve as phagocytes. Finally, astrocytic endfeet are also closely associated with capillary endothelial cells and are separated from the cell plasma membrane by only the basal lamina. The astrocytes and their associated processes may be involved in the induction of the blood-brain barrier.

The choroid plexus is found in the walls of the lateral ventricles, and this structure is continuous with choroid plexus in the roof of the third ventricle. Additionally, the fourth ventricle contains a T-shaped choroid plexus that projects into the cavity from the roof. Whereas the choroid plexus of the lateral ventricles receives its arterial supply from the anterior and posterior choroidal arteries, the third ventricular choroid plexus is supplied by branches of the posterior cerebral artery. The posterior inferior cerebellar artery supplies the choroid plexus of the fourth ventricle.

After the CSF is secreted by the choroid plexus, it circulates throughout the ventricular system and the subarachnoid space that surrounds the brain and spinal cord (Fig. 26–2). The anatomy of the ventricular system allows for movement of CSF in and around all the major structures of the brain. The lateral ventricles are located within the cerebral hemispheres and communicate with the third ventricle via the foramina of Monroe. The third ventricle lies caudal to the lateral ventricles and is a midline structure within the diencephalon. At its caudal end, the third ventricle is connected by the aqueduct of Sylvius to the fourth ventricle, which is situated between the brain stem and cerebellum. Cerebrospinal fluid then flows into the basal cisterns and subarachnoid space by the lateral foramina of Luschka and the medial foramen of Magendie. From these cisterns, the CSF flows throughout the subarachnoid space and over the hemispheric convexities and around the spinal cord.

CSF is reabsorbed into the venous system by numerous microscopic arachnoid villi and larger but less common arachnoid granulations. The granulations have a collagenous

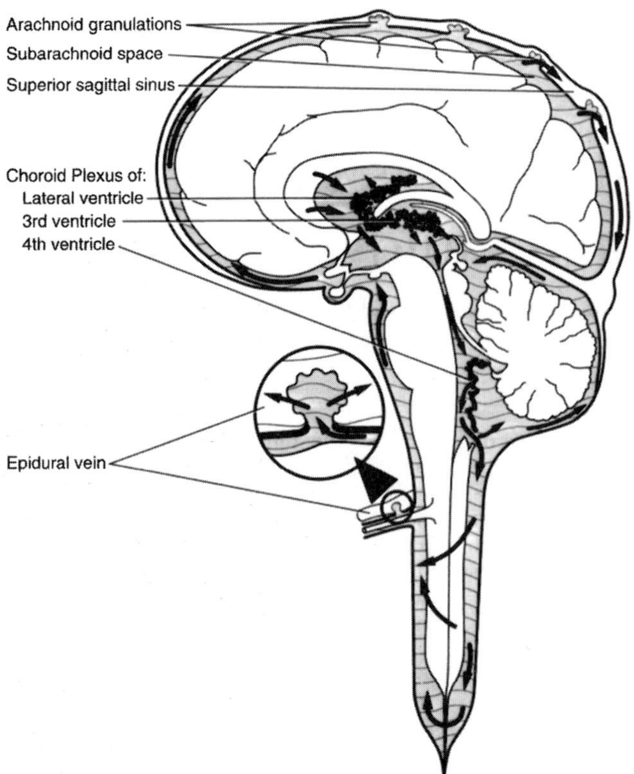

FIGURE 26–2. The ventricular system. This diagram demonstrates the flow of cerebrospinal fluid from the choroid plexus to the arachnoid villi. (From Fishman RA: Cerebrospinal fluid in diseases of the nervous system. *In* Fishman RA [ed]: Cerebrospinal Fluid in Diseases of the Nervous System, 2nd ed. Philadelphia, WB Saunders, 1992, p 8.)

trabecular core with associated channels and a cap of arachnoid cells on the apex. Villi and granulations represent outpouchings of the arachnoid membrane that penetrate gaps in the dura and protrude within the venous sinuses (Fig. 26–3). Arachnoid villi are also present at various levels of the spinal cord and surrounding spinal nerve roots.

PHYSIOLOGY

Secretion and Absorption

It is estimated that the average adult ventricular system and subarachnoid space contain between 90 and 150 mL of CSF with nearly 80 percent being present in the ventricles. The production of CSF occurs at a rate of about 500 mL/day (20 mL/hour), and the entire amount of CSF is replenished five times a day. The secretion of CSF by the choroid plexus is linked to the hydrostatic pressure within the plexus capillaries that moves water and electrolytes into the interstitial space and subsequently into the choroidal epithelium (Fig. 26–4).[7] Water and ions are then transferred into the ventricular cavity by either traversing the tight apical junctions or the plasma membrane of the apical villus. Because the secretion of CSF is associated with the transport of sodium, ion pumps are involved in this transfer, and the movement of sodium is linked to the membrane-bound enzyme sodium-potassium–activated ATPase that has been identified on the brush border and intercellular clefts.[8] In addition to the sodium-potassium ion exchange at the apical surface, basolateral sodium-hydrogen antiports and apical and basal chloride-bicarbonate antiports are also present in the choroidal epithelium (Fig. 26–5). Typically, a net secretion of sodium, chloride, and bicarbonate occurs from the plasma to the CSF, yet ion exchanges can occur in either direction and depend on the relative levels of various ions in the cells and the CSF.

The exact mechanisms regulating the action of these ion pumps and the permeability of the choroidal epithelium is incompletely understood, yet a strong correlation exists between the rate of sodium exchange and the rate of spinal fluid formation.[9] The rate of sodium exchange is, in turn, partially regulated by the permeability of bicarbonate, and the enzyme carbonic anhydrase is important in this relationship. This enzyme is present in the cytosol of the choroidal epithelium and catalyzes the formation of carbonic acid from water and carbon dioxide.[10, 11] Carbonic acid then freely dissociates to bicarbonate and a hydrogen ion that are available to participate in their respective ion pumps. Investigators have demonstrated that a carbonic anhydrase inhibitor such as acetazolamide can reduce CSF sodium exchange by 50 to 100 percent[10] and can reduce CSF production significantly.[11] Other factors may influence the rate of CSF formation (Table 26–1), although most findings are based on animal studies and the results cannot necessarily be extended to human physiology.

Because CSF production is in equilibrium with absorption, approximately 0.35 mL of CSF are absorbed every minute. This rate is the bulk flow of fluid and does not represent the absorption of individual constituents such as ions and proteins. These latter CSF components are exchanged at individual rates that depend on the rate of fluid absorption, the degree of active transport of the solute from the CSF, and the amount of solute diffusion into the parenchyma of the brain and brain capillaries.[7] The process in which fluid and

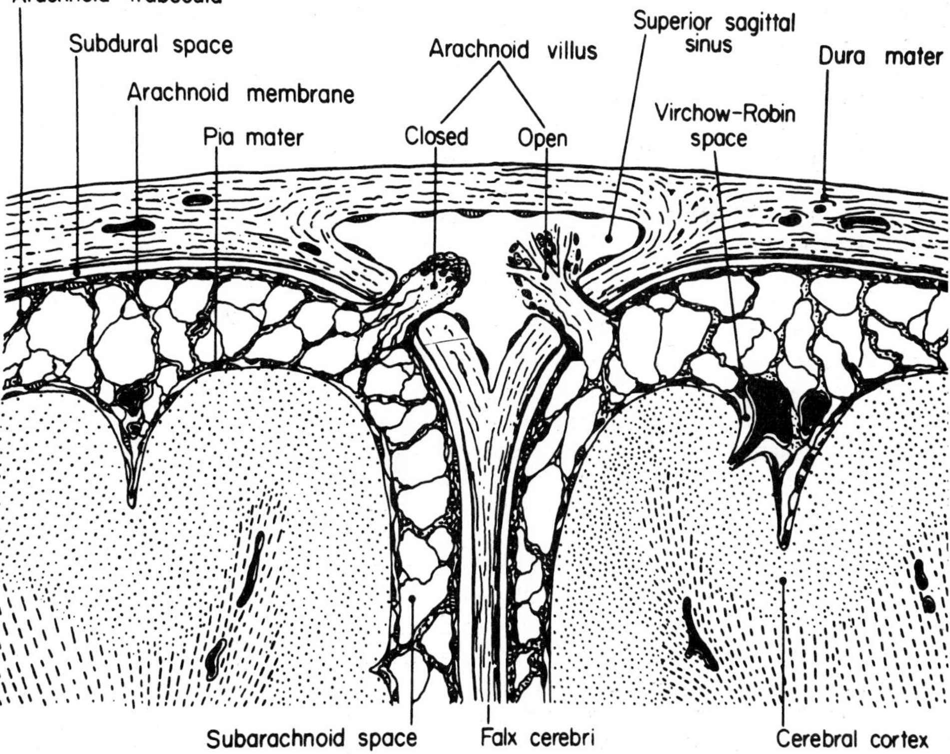

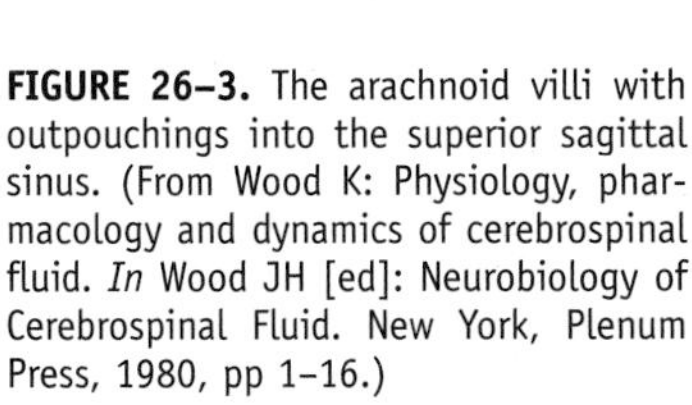
FIGURE 26–3. The arachnoid villi with outpouchings into the superior sagittal sinus. (From Wood K: Physiology, pharmacology and dynamics of cerebrospinal fluid. *In* Wood JH [ed]: Neurobiology of Cerebrospinal Fluid. New York, Plenum Press, 1980, pp 1–16.)

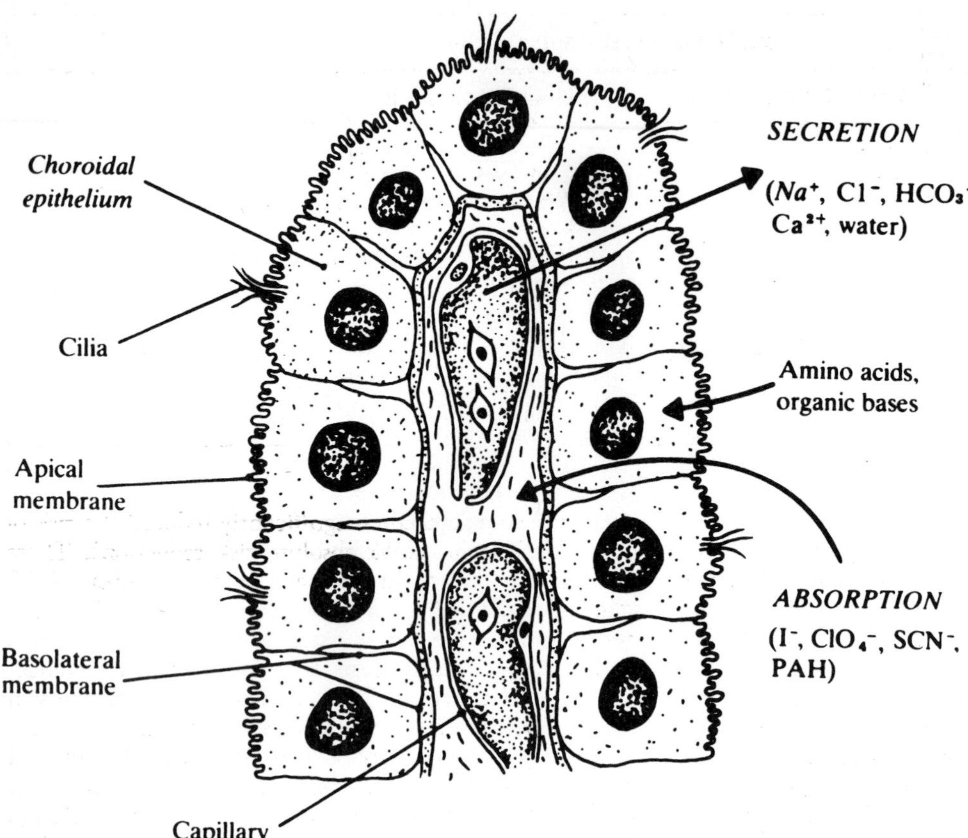

FIGURE 26–4. Diagrammatic representation of the choroid plexus with respect to the relationship of a variety of ions and small molecules. (From Wright EM: Transport processes in the formation of the cerebrospinal fluid. Rev Physiol Biochem Pharmacol 1978;83:1–34.)

other molecules move across the villi and granulations to enter the venous system is not entirely understood, but possible mechanisms include direct flow through a tubular system,[12] the use of giant vacuoles,[13] pinocytosis, and extracellular transport.[14]

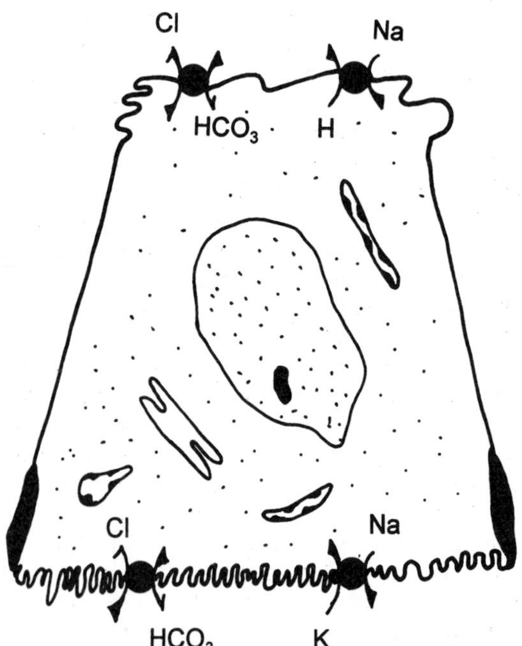

FIGURE 26–5. Demonstration of the sodium/hydrogen ion, sodium/potassium, and chloride/bicarbonate pumps in a choroid epithelium cell. (Modified from Johansen CE, Parandoosh Z, Smith OR: Cl = HCO_3 exchange in choroid plexus: Analysis by the DMO method for cell pH. Am J Physiol 1985;249:478.)

Composition

In addition to the major ions, CSF contains oxygen, sugars (e.g., glucose, fructose, polyols), lactate, proteins (e.g., albumin, globulins), amino acids, urea, ammonia, creatinine, lipids, neurotransmitters and their metabolites, hormones (e.g., insulin, gastrin), and vitamins. Whereas the regulation of many CSF constituents is unknown, some are transported into the CSF by facilitated diffusion using a proteolipid carrier (e.g., glucose). In general, CSF glucose concentration is about 60 percent of the serum. CSF concentrations of sodium, chloride, and magnesium are the same or greater than those in the serum; however, potassium, calcium, and glucose concentrations are lower (Table 26–2).

Acquisition

The technique of the lumbar puncture (LP), or spinal tap, was first developed by Quinke in 1891 and has likely changed little since that time. Before performing an LP to obtain CSF, a patient's coagulation profile should be checked. If the results of these studies demonstrate a thrombocytopenic (platelet count less than 20,000/μL) or a prolonged prothrombin time or partial thromboplastin time, these abnormalities should be corrected before the LP.[15] In adults, the LP is best performed with the patient in the lateral decubitus position with the head and spine parallel to the floor. This positioning is particularly important for the accurate measurement of the opening and closing pressures. After positioning the patient, certain landmarks should be palpated, beginning with the iliac crest. An imaginary line that runs between the crests will intersect approximately the L3–L4 interspace. Once this area is

TABLE 26–1. **Factors That May Influence the Formation of Cerebrospinal Fluid**

Agent	Effect on CSF Production	Presumed Mechanism
Cholera toxin	Increases	Stimulates adenosine monophosphate
Alpha-adrenergic drugs	Increases	Stimulates adenylate cyclase
Hyperosmolality	Decreases	Alteration in ionic concentrations
Hypothermia	Decreases	Unknown
Furosemide	Decreases	Inhibition of the sodium-potassium-chloride co-transport system
Dopamine (D1) antagonists	Decreases	Unknown
Vasopressin	Decreases	Reduces choroidal blood flow
Atrial natriuretic hormone	Decreases	Modulates cyclic GMP activity
Acetazolamide	Decreases	Inhibition of carbonic anhydrase
Ouabain	Decreases	Inhibition of sodium-potassium ATPase

located, the spinal processes of L3 and L4 should be palpated and between them the interspace may be felt. This procedure is easily accomplished in thin patients but may be difficult in obese or edematous individuals.

When the landmarks are located, the patient should pull the knees into the chest and assume the so-called fetal position. This maneuver helps widen the vertebral interspace. The clinician should appropriately prepare the skin surface using a sterilizing agent and then place the sterile draping. One to two percent lidocaine should be injected intradermally and then is infiltrated into the deeper tissues. Once the patient is anesthetized, a spinal needle with a stylet should be inserted into the skin toward the interspace. Some debate exists as to the optimum gauge of spinal needle that should be used. Although fewer post-LP headaches occur when finer-gauge needles are used,[16] it is more difficult to remove CSF and accurately measure pressures. A 20- or 22-gauge needle is generally used. In order to reduce the risk of post-LP headache, the needle should be advanced with the bevel parallel to the long axis of the spine,[17] which will prevent the transection of the fibers of the longitudinal ligament. Instead, this technique causes the separation of these fibers. Alternatively, an atraumatic needle may be used. A randomized, controlled trial of atraumatic versus standard needles demonstrated that the use of atrauamtic needles significantly reduced the risk of post-LP headache (25% absolute risk reduction). There was, however, a slight increase in the number of LP attempts when using an atraumatic needle.[18] When the needle reaches the longitudinal ligament, there will be a slight increase in resistance, yet with continued advancement a sudden decrease in the amount of resistance will occur. When this is felt, the needle has passed through the longitudinal ligament and has entered the subarachnoid space (Fig. 26–6). At this point, the removal of the stylet results in the flow of CSF. If no fluid flows, the stylet should be replaced and the needle should be rotated 90 degrees so that the bevel is oriented cephalad. The needle may need to be further adjusted or reinserted if the CSF fails to flow from the needle. Each time the needle is reinserted, the stylet should be replaced.

TABLE 26–2. **Normal Cerebrospinal Fluid Constituents**

Substance	Plasma	CSF
Sodium (mEq/L)	140.0	144.0
Potassium (mm/L)	4.6	2.9
Magnesium (mEq/L)	1.6	2.2
Calcium (mg/dL)	8.9	4.6
Chloride (mEq/L)	99.0	113.0
Bicarbonate (mm/L)	26.8	23.3
Inorganic phosphate (mg/dL)	4.7	3.4
Protein (g/dL)	6.8	0.028 (28 mg/dL)
Glucose (mg/dL)	110.0	50 to 80
Osmolality	0.3	0.29
pH	7.4	7.3
pCO_2 (mm Hg)	41.1	50.5

Adapted from Wood K: Physiology, pharmacology and dynamics of cerebrospinal fluid. *In* Wood JH (ed): Neurobiology of Cerebrospinal Fluid, Vol. 1. New York, Plenum Press, 1980, p 87.

When the CSF begins to flow, a manometer may be attached to the hub of the spinal needle, which allows the CSF to flow into the manometer tube. This maneuver should be done immediately in order to avoid spuriously low opening pressure readings. Often some fluid has already been removed. The CSF should be allowed to rise into the tube until a steady state is reached. Coughing, talking, or performing the Valsalva maneuver can falsely elevate the pressure reading. It may also be helpful to allow the patient to come out of the fetal position to reduce the amount of intra-abdominal pressure, which may affect opening pressure measurements. A normal opening pressure ranges from 10 to 20 cm H_2O (approximately equivalent to 5 to 15 mm Hg). Following the measurement of the opening pressure, the CSF can be collected for analysis.

When acquiring the CSF, the clinician should number the tubes and maintain this order during the CSF collection. After the CSF fluid is collected, the manometer should be reconnected and a closing pressure should be measured. This value is usually less than the opening pressure; however, the range of closing pressure values depends on the amount of CSF removed. A low opening pressure may indicate a CSF leak or a spinal subarachnoid obstruction, which does not allow for communication of the lumbar space with the cranium. Disorders that elevate the opening pressure (greater than 20 cm H_2O) are numerous, including mass-occupying lesions and diffuse cerebral inflammatory or toxic processes. The closing pressure is used to assess the pressure reduction after an LP, particularly in cases of therapeutic lumbar puncture.

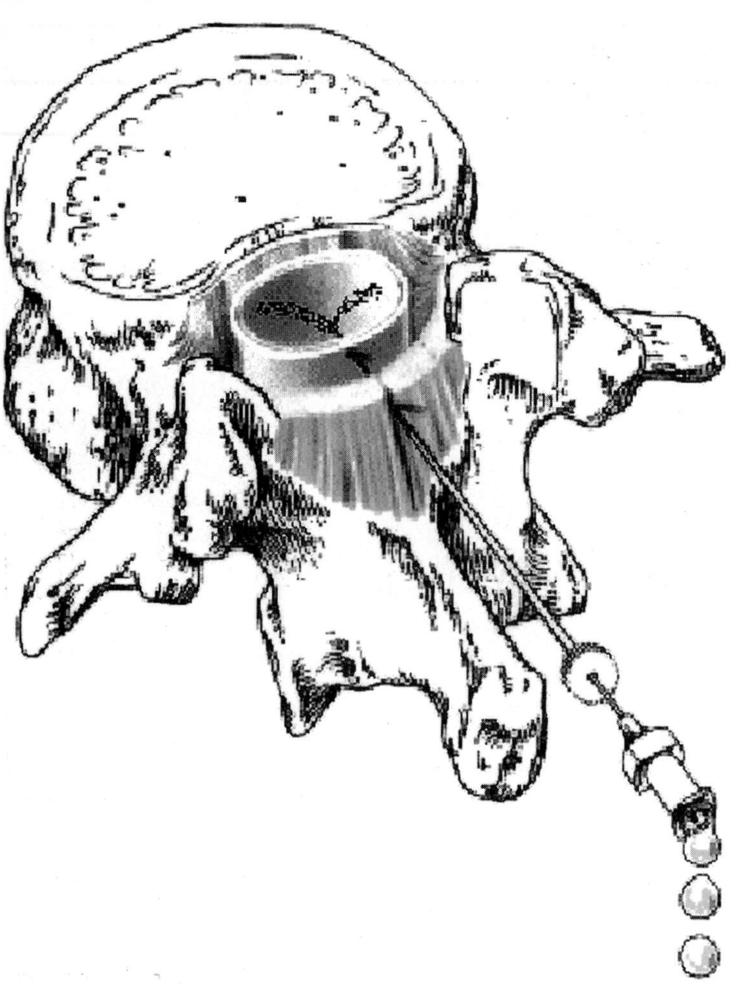

FIGURE 26–6. Diagram demonstrating the passage of the spinal needle through the fibers of the longitudinal ligament and into the subarachnoid space. (Available from: *http://www.emergemedical.com.au/Products/Images/Eldor%20Spinal%20Needles.pdf.*)

Before withdrawing the spinal needle, the stylet should not be reinserted, to lessen the likelihood of contamination. It is not necessary for the patient to lie supine for any specific amount of time after the LP, because controlled studies have clearly demonstrated that position does not reduce the risk of a post-LP headache.[19]

The LP may also be performed in the sitting position, or CSF may be collected with cisternal or lateral cervical punctures under fluoroscopic guidance. The advantages of performing the LP in a sitting position are threefold: (1) the midline is much easier to determine; (2) some patients find that tightly flexing the hips while sitting is more comfortable than the fetal position; and (3) gravity can assist the flow of the CSF in cases of low CSF pressures. This technique is essentially the same as that of the lateral decubitus position, but the patient is upright. The patient should be asked to sit on the edge of the bed or examination table and lean forward as far as possible. This position is best accomplished with the patient leaning forward on a table that is slightly higher than the bed. With the physician standing behind the patient, the iliac crests are palpated, and at the intersection of these structures and in the midline lies the L3–L4 interspace. This area is prepped, draped, and anesthetized similarly to the earlier description. Again, the needle is inserted with the bevel facing laterally so as not to tear the fibers of the longitudinal ligament. The angle of insertion is upward in this position, toward the umbilicus. In this position, neither opening or closing pressures can be accurately determined. In order to obtain the pressure readings, the patient may be moved to the lateral decubitus position once the spinal needle is in the subarachnoid space.

Other than the L3–L4 interspace, several other lumbar levels may be used to perform the LP including L4–L5 and L5–S1. More rostral levels should not be attempted because spinal cord trauma may occur. If anatomical restrictions exist such as occurs in severe spinal spondylosis, previous spinal surgery with fusion, or morbid obesity, and impedes the acquisition of CSF levels, an attempt should be made to obtain CSF under fluoroscopic guidance. If this procedure is unsuccessful, CSF may be obtained through a cisternal or lateral cervical puncture. These procedures should be performed by an experienced clinician under radiographical guidance. A cisternal puncture is performed by placing the spinal needle in the cisterna magna and carries the risk of brain stem or upper cervical cord damage. A lateral cervical puncture involves the insertion of the spinal needle in the C1–C2 interspace from a posterolateral approach and also has the risk of damage to the cervical cord.

When an asymmetrical CNS process or an increase in ICP is suspected, a computed tomography (CT) or magnetic resonance imaging scan should be obtained prior to an LP. If a mass lesion is found, the LP should be delayed. On the other hand, diffuse cerebral processes that predictably elevate the opening pressure, such as pseudotumor cerebri[20] and some

TABLE 26-3. **Etiologies of Increased CSF Protein in 4157 Patients**

			Increased				Range		
Diagnosis	**Total**	**Normal, 45 mg/dL or Less**	**Slightly, 45 to 75 mg/dL**	**Moderately, 75 to 100 mg/dL**	**Greatly, 100 to 500 mg/dL**	**Very Greatly, 500 to 3600 mg/dL**	**High (mg/dL)**	**Low (mg/dL)**	**Average**
Purulent meningitis	157	3	7	12	100	35	2220	21	418
Tuberculous meningitis	253	2	30	37	172	12	1142	25	200
Poliomyelitis	158	74	44	16	24	0	366	12	70
Neurosyphilis	890	412	258	102	117	1	4200	15	68
Brain tumor	182	56	45	22	57	2	1920	15	115
Cord tumor	36	5	4	3	14	10	3600	40	425
Brain abscess	33	9	15	3	6	0	288	16	69
Aseptic meningitis	81	37	20	7	17	0	400	11	77
Multiple sclerosis	151	102	36	9	4	0	133	13	42
Polyneuritis	211	107	33	17	44	10	1430	15	74
Epilepsy (idiopathic)	793	710	80	2	1	0	200	7	31
Cerebral thrombosis	300	199	78	13	10	0	267	17	46
Cerebral hemorrhage*	247	34	41	32	95	45	2110	19	57
Uremia	53	31	13	8	1	0	143	19	57
Myxedema	51	12	28	3	8	0	242	30	71
Cerebral trauma†	474	255	84	43	73	19	1820	10	100
Acute alcoholism	87	80	5	2	0	0	88	13	32
Total	4157	2128	821	331	743	134			

*Results on fluids removed at first lumbar puncture are used in most instances.
†Increase of protein usually due to presence of admixed serum.
From Fishman RA: Cerebrospinal fluid in diseases of the nervous system. *In* Fishman RA (ed): Cerebrospinal Fluid in Diseases of the Nervous System, 2nd ed. Philadelphia, WB Saunders, 1992, p 431.

forms of encephalitis or meningitis,[21] may be benefited by frequent LPs to lower ICP.

Whereas LP is considered a standard, safe diagnostic intervention, headache is a common sequel, occurring in approximately 30 percent of cases. In the American Academy of Neurology practice guidelines, the following factors were identified to reduce the risk of post-LP headaches: (1) small needle sizes, (2) assurance that bevel direction is parallel to dural fibers, and (3) replacement of the stylet before the needle is withdrawn. There was no established evidence that recumbency after the procedure or increased fluid intake influenced the frequency or severity of post-LP headache.

NORMAL AND PATHOLOGICAL FINDINGS (see Tables 26–2, 26–3, and 26–4)

The general appearance of CSF is clear and colorless, because it is more than 99 percent water. Color of CSF is observed only in pathological circumstances. Whereas the term xanthochromia means yellow color, it has been used for the presence of other colors as well. Because of this practice, the actual color of the CSF should be stated and a gradation of its magnitude (from 1+ to 4+) should be noted. A yellowish tinge can be found with any cause of a markedly increased protein (greater than 200 mg percent). A yellow or pink color is found when hemoglobin has been released into the CSF from prior bleeding and sufficient time has passed for its breakdown to bilirubin and other pigments. Oxyhemoglobin is red but becomes pink or yellow when diluted. The concentration of oxyhemoglobin is maximal within the first 36 hours and disappears by 14 days. Bilirubin is yellow and is first detected in the CSF 10 hours after subarachnoid bleeding. Its concentration is maximal at 2 days and may persist for up to a month. Other causes for coloration of CSF include an elevated systemic bilirubin from liver disease; a brownish or gray coloration in the presence of CNS melanoma; and a greenish tinge related to leukemic meningeal infiltration.

Fluid that is obviously blood tinged or bloody indicates a traumatic tap or the presence of a subarachnoid hemorrhage. In traumatic taps, the CSF usually clears as sequential amounts are collected and is unlikely to have a pink- or yellow-tinged supernatant. The CSF may occasionally clot if the ratio of blood to CSF is high. Bloody CSF from subarachnoid hemorrhage does not clear with sequentially collected tubes and may demonstrate xanthochromia if the bleeding occurred over 2 to 4 hours before the LP. If the CSF is acquired over 12 hours after the onset of subarachnoid hemorrhage, virtually all patients' CSF will demonstrate xanthochromia.[22]

Whenever the viscosity of CSF is increased, the most likely explanation is a marked increase of protein content. If sufficient fibrin is present, the free flow of CSF can be impaired and spontaneous clotting of the CSF can occur (Froin's syndrome). Turbidity detected in CSF when a collection tube is twirled in the beam of a bright light is indicative of the presence of at least 200 or more leukocytes per microliter. Turbidity may also be caused by the presence of microscopic fat globules that have traveled to the brain as

Text continued on page 522

TABLE 26–4. **Selected Disorders and Associated CSF Studies**

Domain	Disorder	Useful CSF Studies	Expected Results	Comments
		Cerebral Dysfunction		
Infectious	Meningitis (purulent)	pr, gl, cell cts, gs, cx, op	↑ pr, ↓ gl, ↑ CSF PMNs, + gs and cx, + bacterial ag's, ↑ op ↑ LA	+ cryptococcal ag and india ink in cryptococcal meningitis Mononuclear cells possible in partially rx'd bacterial meningitis
	Meningitis (aseptic)	pr, gl, cell cts	↑ pr, nl gl, ↑ CSF WBC (10 to 1000 mononuc cells/mm^3)	PMNs possible in early aseptic meningitis
	Encephalitis	pr, gl, cell cts, gs, cx	mildly ↑ pr (50 to 100 mg/dL), nl gl, ↑ CSF WBC 50 to 100/mm^3 (mononuc) ↑ RBC/xanthochromia, + CSF PCR	Herpes simplex encephalitis
	HIV encephalopathy	pr, gl, cell cts	mildly ↑ pr, nl gl, nl or few WBC	
	Neurosyphilis (acute)	VDRL, pr, gl	↑ pr (>45 mg/dL), ↑ WBC (5 to 500 mononuc/mm^3), + VDRL	CSF parameters may be normal
	Neuroborreliosis	pr, gl, cell cts, OCB, ab's	↑ pr (~100 mg/dL), nl or ↓ gl, ↑ WBC (~100 mononuc/mm^3), + OCB, + Lyme ab's	CSF normalizes in stage III
	Tuberculous meningitis	pr, gl, cell cts, op, acid-fast stain, cx	↑ pr (100 to 200 mg/dL), ↓ gl (<45 mg/dL), ↑ WBC (25 to 100 mononuc/mm^3), ↑ op	May be spinal block; stain and culture require large amts. of CSF
	Abscess	Not recommended		May be dangerous to perform LP in the face of abscess; risk of herniation or ventricular rupture
	Creutzfeldt-Jakob	pr, gl, cell cts	Normal	14-3-3 protein in CSF (not readily available)
	Progressive multifocal leukoencephalopathy	JC virus PCR	+ JC virus PCR	CSF o/w normal
	Cysticercosis	pr, gl, cell cts, op	↑ pr, ↓ gl, ↑ WBC (mixed w/eosinophilia), ↑ op	CSF eosinophils constitute 20 to 75 percent
Cerebrovascular	Stroke	pr, cell cts	mildly ↑ pr and WBC	Not routinely performed; ↑ LDH, AST and CK-BB in cortical CVA
	Subarachnoid hemorrhage	pr, gl, cell cts, color	↑ ↑ pr, ↓ gl, ↑ ↑ RBC, ↑ WBC, xanth	pr can be normal or significantly ↑, gl can be normal or slightly ↓
	Venous thrombosis	cell cts, op	↑ RBC, ↑ op	WBC may be ↑ if 2° to septic thrombosis
	Anoxic brain			Not routinely performed; CK-BB, NSE, MBP may be useful

Dementia	Alzheimer's disease	pr, gl, cell cts	normal parameters	Abnormal CSF helps r/o AD
Degenerative	Huntington's disease	pr, gl, cell cts	normal	Abnormal CSF helps r/o Huntington's disease
	Wilson's disease	pr, gl, cell cts	normal	Abnormal CSF helps r/o Wilson's disease
Neoplastic	Meningeal carcinomatosis	pr, gl, cell cts, cyt, op	↑ pr (24 to 1200 mg/dL), ↓ gl, ↑ WBC (PMN), + cyt, mildly ↑ op	Large volumes of CSF and multiple LPs increase cytology yield
	Craniopharyngioma	cell cts	↑ WBC (mononuc)	A cause of chronic chemical meningitis
Metabolic	Hepatic encephalopathy	pr, color	↑ pr possible xanth	Not routinely performed; op may be ↑; CSF glutamine ↑
	Uremic encephalopathy	pr, cell cts, urea	mildly ↑ pr and WBC, ↑ urea,	Not routinely performed
	Myxedema coma	pr	↑ pr (100 to 300 mg/dL)	
	Mitochondrial encephalopathies	pyruvate, lactate	↑ pyruvate, lactate	MELAS
Demyelinating	Multiple sclerosis	pr, gl, cell cts, OCB, MBP, IgG index	↑ pr, mildly ↑ WBC, nl gl, + OCB, + MBP, ↑ IgG index	Abnormal CSF in 90 percent of cases; pr and cell cts nl in 2/3
	Acute disseminated encephalomyelitis	pr, gl, cell cts, OCB	mildly ↑ pr and WBC, nl gl, + OCB	OCBs may disappear after resolution
Autoimmune	Sarcoid	pr, gl, cell cts	↑ pr (50 to 200 mg/dL), mildly ↓ gl (30 to 40 mg/dL), ↑ WBC (10 to 100 mononuc/mm^3)	ACE ↑ in 50 percent, but not specific
	Behçet's disease	pr, cell cts	↑ pr, ↑ WBC (mixed response) 10 to 200 cell/mm^2	CSF results quite varied
	Angiitis	pr, gl, cell cts, op	↑ pr, ↓ gl, ↑ WBC (mononuc), ↑ op	Abnormal CSF in 80 to 90 percent
Other disorders	Normal pressure hydrocephalus	Diagnostic high volume LP, op	Gait and mental status improvement after LP, nl op	High volume LP (40 to 50 cc of CSF)
	Pseudotumor cerebri	pr, cell cts, op	↓ pr, nl cell cts, ↑ op (250 to 600 mm H_2O)	CSF removal may be therapeutic in some cases
	Migraine	See comments		Little available data. May have ↑ pr and cell cts in severe complicated migraine
	Generalized seizure	pr, cell cts	nl ↑ pr, mild ↑ WBC	Postictal
	Reye's syndrome	pr, gl, cell cts, op	pr and gl nl, <10 cell/mm^2; ↑ op	

Table continued on following page

TABLE 26–4. **Selected Disorders and Associated CSF Studies** *Continued*

Domain	Disorder	Useful CSF Studies	Expected Results	Comments
		Cranial Nerve Dysfunction		
	Miller-Fisher variant of GBS	See GBS	See GBS/comments	Pr more commonly nl than in GBS
	Optic neuritis	pr, cell cts, OCB	Mild ↑ pr (45 to 60 mg/dL), 50 percent with mild ↑ WBC (mononuc), + OCB	+ OCB increase risk of MS
	Lyme disease	cell cts	Mild ↑ WBC (mononuc)	
	Bell's palsy	pr, gl, cell cts	nl CSF	Abnormal CSF helps r/o Bell's palsy
	Trigeminal neuralgia			Not routinely performed; may have ↑ substance P and ↓ monoamines
	Kearns-Sayre syndrome	pr	↑ pr (70 to 400 mg/dL)	
		Motor Dysfunction		
CNS	Parkinson's disease			Not routinely performed. Abnormal CSF helps r/o Parkinson's disease
	Huntington's disease	See above		Abnormal CSF helps r/o Huntington's disease
	Wilson's disease	See above		Abnormal CSF helps r/o Wilson's disease
	Neurosyphilis (paretic)	VDRL, pr, cell cts,	+ + VDRL, pr: 50 to 100 mg/dL, cell cts: 25 to 75 leukocytes/mm^2	CSF abnormalities increase with duration of disease
	HTLV-1	pr, gl, IgG, OCB	mild ↑ pr, nl gl, ↑ IgG, + OCB	Serum + HTLV-1 ag
	Poliomyelitis	pr, gl, cell cts	mild ↑ pr (50 to 200 mg/dL), nl gl, mild ↑ CSF WBC (mononuc)	CSF WBC ↓ with time
	Spinal cord tumor	pr, gl, cell cts, cytology	may be ↑ ↑ pr, nl gl, ↑ WBC (mononuc), + cyt	Froin's syndrome (spinal cord block) may sig ↑
	Tetanus	pr, gl, cell cts	↑ pr (90 to 150 mg/dL), nl gl, nl cell cts	Care must be taken not to induce tetany. Normal cell cts differentiate from meningitis
	Stiffman's syndrome	pr, cell cts, IgG, OCB	nl pr, nl cell cts, ↑ IgG, ? + OCB	

Motor Neuron	ALS	pr, cell cts	mild ↑ pr and cell cts	Nondiagnostic
	Guillain-Barré (GBS)	pr, cell cts	↑ pr, nl cell cts	Pr peaks between 1 and 3 wks. Cell cts >5 should prompt search for another cause
Nerve	Brachial plexopathy	pr, cell cts	mild ↑ pr (50 to 60 mg/dL), nl cell cts	
	Chronic inflammatory demyelinating polyradiculopathy (CIDP)	pr, gl, cell cts	↑ pr (100 to 200 mg/dL), nl gl, mild ↑ WBC (5 to 50 cell/mm^3)	Similar to GBS; pr elevation correlates with severity; + WBC in 10 percent
	Inherited neuropathy	pr, gl, cell cts	mod ↑ pr (50 to 200 mg/dL), nl cell cts	
Muscle	Myopathy or myositis			Not routinely performed
		Cerebellar Dysfunction		
Cerebellitis	pr, gl, cell cts	pr, gl, cell cts	mildly ↑ pr, nl gl, cell cts usually <100/mm^2 (mononuc)	Usually secondary to varicella- zoster
	Paraneoplastic cerebellar disease	pr, cell cts, abs	mild ↑ pr, mild ↑ WBC (8 to 20 cells/mm^3) + anti-Yo or anti-Hu ab	Anti-Yo in ovarian, uterine, or breast CA. Anti-Hu seen in lung CA
		Sensory Dysfunction		
Neuropathy	Diabetic	pr, gl, cell cts	↑ pr (50 to 400 mg/dL), nl cell cts, ↑ gl (secondary diabetes)	
	CIDP	See above		
	Inherited neuropathies	See above		
	Neurosyphilis (tabes dorsalis)	VDRL, pr, gl, cell cts	3/4 w/+ VDRL, CSF freq o/w WNL	CSF may resemble paretic form, but parameters improve w/progression

abs, Antibodies; ACE, angiotensin-converting enzyme; AD, Alzheimer's dementia; ag, antigen; AST, aspartate aminotransferase; bact, bacteria; CA, cancer; cell cts, cell counts; cerebrovasc, cerebrovascular; CK-BB, creatinine kinase BB isoenzyme; CSF, cerebrospinal fluid; CVA, cerebrovascular accident (stroke); cyt, cytology; degen, degenerative; gl, glucose; gs, Gram stain; LA, lactic acid; LDH, lactate dehydrogenase; MBP, myelin basic protein; mononuc, mononuclear cells; nl, normal; NPH, normal pressure hydrocephalus; NSE, neuron-specific-enolase; OCB, oligoclonal bands; OP, opening; o/w, otherwise; pr, protein; r/o, rule out; rx'd, treated; sig, significantly; VDRL, venereal disease research laboratory test; wks, weeks; WNL, within normal limits; xanth, xanthochromia.

emboli. The presence of erythrocytes will impart turbidity up to a concentration of 400 cells/μL, above which there will be pink coloration from their hemoglobin content.

Six common CSF studies include the cell count and differential, Gram stain and culture, blood glucose, and protein concentrations and direct observation for color and character.

Cell Counts

CSF cell counts (red blood cell [RBC] count and white blood cell [WBC] count) with differentials should be performed on every specimen. Typically, the CSF contains no RBC/μL and 0 to 1 WBC/μL. Cook and Brooks[23] reported that the normal CSF WBC in 11 patients was 0.826 + 0.733 cells/μL with differentials of approximately 66 percent lymphocytes, 33 percent monocytes, and 1 percent polymorphonuclear cells. Fishman has also noted that the normal CSF should contain no more than five lymphocytes or mononuclear cells per microliter, and counts greater than 6 cells/μL are abnormal. A traumatic LP causes elevations of RBCs and WBCs, but these elevations are differentiated from subarachnoid hemorrhage because the former elevations are high in the first tube but clear in the later tubes. To determine whether an elevated CSF WBC is due to blood from a traumatic tap or other causes, an expected ratio can be used. If the elevated WBC is due to blood in the CSF, 1 WBC/μL for every 700 RBC/μL is found. If the WBC exceeds this ratio, its origin must be accounted for from other etiologies such as infection or inflammation.

Glucose

As noted in Table 26–2, the CSF glucose concentration is normally 60 percent of the plasma glucose concentration, and under nonpathological conditions, this ratio changes proportionately in response to a rising or falling plasma glucose event with a 4-hour lag time. This linear ratio of CSF to plasma glucose concentration decreases as the plasma glucose exceeds 500 mg/dL. The reason for this decrease is unclear, but it may reflect the saturation of the carrier-mediated transport of glucose at high plasma concentrations.[7] As a result, it is important to obtain a concomitant serum glucose level at the time of the CSF sample. Although an elevated CSF glucose level (hyperglycorrachia) results from an elevated plasma glucose level, a decreased CSF glucose concentration (hypoglycorrachia) may be due to a variety of causes including hypoglycemia. The other etiologies include bacterial meningitis[24, 25] (including typical bacteria, tuberculosis, and neurosyphilis), fungal meningitis, certain viral meningitides (mumps),[26] subarachnoid hemorrhage,[27] carcinomatosis meningitis, chemical meningitis, and meningitis resulting from parasitic organisms (cysticercosis, trichinosis, amebiasis). If 0.4 is used as the lower limit of the normal CSF to serum glucose ratio, values below 0.4 have a sensitivity of 80 to 91 percent and a specificity of 96 to 98 percent for bacterial meningitis versus aseptic meningitis (inflammatory cells without evidence of a common bacterial pathogen).[28, 29] The CSF glucose value often returns to normal before other CSF determinations (such as protein or lactate), and some investigators have suggested serial determinations to guide treatment decisions.[25] The CSF glucose level may take several weeks to return to normal despite the normalization of the protein concentration and cell count.[30]

Protein

The majority of CSF protein is derived from the serum, and the CSF to serum albumin ratio is approximately 1:200. This ratio implies that the entry rate of protein from the serum to the CSF is approximately 200 times less than its exit rate.[7] The CSF protein concentration varies at different levels of the neuroaxis and generally increases from the cephalad to caudal levels. Elevation in lumbar CSF protein is a nonspecific but sensitive indicator of CNS disease.[7] Table 26–2 illustrates the various disorders that can cause an elevation in the CSF protein level.[23] A very high CSF protein concentration (greater than 500 mg/dL) is an infrequent finding but can occur with bacterial meningitis, subarachnoid hemorrhage, or spinal-subarachnoid block. When a significant amount of blood is present in the CSF (e.g., subarachnoid hemorrhage), a correction for the total protein concentration should be calculated. The presence of 1000 RBCs in the CSF results in the increase of protein by 1 mg/dL. A spinal-subarachnoid block can cause Froin's syndrome and is usually the result of a spinal cord tumor and can cause very significant elevations in CSF protein (greater than 1000 mg/dL).[23] Protein concentrations of 100 mg/dL or greater have sensitivity and specificity for bacterial meningitis of 82 and 98 percent, respectively, as compared with aseptic meningitis,[31] and if the concentration is 200 mg/dL, the sensitivity is 86 percent and the specificity is 100 percent.[28] A lower than normal CSF protein level may occur in young children (6 months to 2 years of age), in patients with pseudotumor cerebri, and in patients with unintended loss of CSF from frequent LPs, a lumbar drain, or a lumbar dural CSF leak.

Certain proteins arise within the intrathecal compartment. Among these are immunoglobulins produced by CNS lymphocytes, transthyretin (produced by choroid plexus), and various structural proteins found in brain tissue (including glial fibrillary acidic, tau, and myelin basic proteins). The last group of proteins and transthyretin are found only in trace amounts, whereas immunoglobulins comprise a substantial fraction of normal CSF (5 to 12 percent). Electrophoretic techniques can be used to define the gammaglobulins as a heterogeneous group of proteins. Because serum IgG comprises nearly 20 percent of the total serum protein, a variety of formulas have been used to correct the CSF IgG level for the contribution derived from the blood in order to determine the CNS (Fig. 26–7). Contamination of the CSF with blood may significantly elevate the IgG index and the IgG synthesis rate.

The electrophoretic separation of CSF proteins can be accomplished through the use of agarose gel and by the staining of the bands that are produced. Within the gamma

$$\text{IgG index} = \frac{\text{Immunoglobulins}_{\text{CSF}}/\text{immunoglobulins}_{\text{Serum}}}{\text{Albumin}_{\text{CSF}}/\text{albumin}_{\text{Serum}}}$$

FIGURE 26–7. Formula for the determination of cerebrospinal fluid immunoglobulin. (From Fishman RA: Cerebrospinal fluid in diseases of the nervous system. *In* Fishman RA [ed]: Cerebrospinal Fluid in Diseases of the Nervous System, 2nd ed. Philadelphia, WB Saunders, 1992, p 431.)

region, three patterns of bands may be observed including one clone (monoclonal), many clones (polyclonal), and a few bands (three to five bands, or oligoclonal bands).[7] Each band represents a homogeneous protein that is secreted by a single clone of plasma cells.

Oligoclonal bands (OCBs) are present in the CSF when three to five bands are seen on gel electrophoresis. This finding implies that a single clonal population of plasma cells is responsible for each band. More than one OCB rarely occurs in normal CSF. A serum sample should also be obtained simultaneously with the acquisition of the CSF to determine whether the OCBs are unique to the CSF. Oligoclonal bands are present in 83 to 94 percent of patients with multiple sclerosis, 100 percent of patients with subacute sclerosing panencephalitis, 25 to 50 percent of patients with other inflammatory CNS disorders (CNS lupus, neurosarcoidosis, cysticercosis, Behçet's and viral, fungal, and bacterial infections), as well as most with some brain tumors and Guillain-Barré syndrome. Because OCBs are present in such varied conditions, their presence offers little to a specific diagnosis.

Gram Staining

Examining the CSF with Gram stain is useful to diagnose bacterial meningitis.[24] A Ziehl-Neelsen acid-fast stain should also be performed if tuberculous meningitis is a diagnostic possibility. CSF cultures should be done in the setting in which an infectious process is suspected. Bacteria that commonly cause meningitis are routinely cultured on standard preparations. *Mycobacterium* can also be cultured, yet several weeks (or more) may be required to grow these organisms. Viral cultures may be ordered; however, the yield is generally low. Fungal cultures should be performed in clinical settings of suspected chronic meningitis.

Specialized Tests

In addition to these routine studies, various specialized tests may also be useful in specific clinical settings.

The measurement of the CSF acid-base status is not normally part of the routine evaluation of this body fluid. In experimental studies, normal subjects have a CSF pH that is slightly lower than the pH of arterial blood and a pCO_2 that is higher. In contrast, bicarbonate levels are generally equal. Comparisons between CSF obtained through cisternal and lumbar punctures reveal that the pH is typically lower and pCO_2 higher in lumbar CSF. Again, bicarbonate levels are not significantly different. The variations between the cisternal and lumbar CSF samples may reflect differences in rates of local metabolism relative to clearance rates,[32] and the clinical measurement of the lumbar CSF pH may be an unreliable indicator of the metabolic state of the CNS.

Because the concentration of CSF lactate is dependent on CNS glycolysis,[33] the measurement of this agent may be helpful in the diagnosis of bacterial meningitis. This concentration of lactate increases proportionally to the number of inflammatory cells in the CSF.[34] A lactate concentration of 4.2 mmol/L accurately predicted 24 out of 25 cases of bacterial meningitis, whereas no patients with presumed viral meningitis had a lactate level that exceeded this value. Unlike the glucose concentration, CSF lactate levels typically remain elevated for a significant time after appropriate therapy is initiated.[25] This finding may be helpful in the diagnosis of bacterial meningitis when antibiotics had been given before the acquisition of CSF. Increased lactate may also result from a cerebral hemorrhage, malignant hypertension, hepatic encephalopathy, diabetes mellitus, and hypoglycemic coma.[35]

Perhaps an even better marker for bacterial meningitis is the measurement of CSF concentrations of C-reactive protein (CRP). In a meta-analysis of studies published from 1981 through 1995, Gerdes and colleagues analyzed 24 studies examining the use of CSF concentrations of CRP for the diagnosis of bacterial meningitis.[36] These studies were heterogeneous in design, with some involving children only, some adults and children, and some adults only, some using quantitative and some qualitative measures of CRP. Although most of these studies were small, some enrolled large numbers of patients (250–478) and most compared patients with bacterial versus viral meningitis. Gerdes and colleagues found that the sensitivity ranged from 18 to 100 percent and the specificity ranged from 75 to 100 percent. In spite of these wide-ranging values and varying methods, the odds ratio was quite high at 241 (95% CI:59–980) for diagnosing bacterial meningitis.

The measurement of CSF glutamine can be a helpful test in diagnosing patients with confusion in the setting of hepatic encephalopathy. Glutamine is formed by the combination of ammonia, which is toxic to the CNS, and alpha-ketoglutarate in the brain. This process helps protect the CNS from the effects of ammonia. Normally, the CSF concentration of ammonia is less than one half of arterial levels, but may increase dramatically in patients with hepatic failure.[7] Although a correlation exists between increased levels of ammonia and glutamine and the severity of encephalopathy, technical difficulties exist that hamper the ability to use these indices in acute settings.[7]

Various biogenic amines (and their metabolites) may be measured within the CSF, including dopamine (homovanillic acid [HVA]), serotonin (5-hydroxyindoleacetic acid [5-HIAA]), and norepinephrine (3-methoxy-4-hydroxyphenylglycol [MHPG]). Significant ventricular to lumbar gradients exist for HVA and 5-HIAA, although MHPG levels are nearly equivalent. Decreased lumbar CSF levels of HVA and 5-HIAA have been reported in patients with parkinsonism and Alzheimer's disease. Whereas decreased HVA levels have also been documented in the ventricular CSF of patients with dystonia, cerebral palsy, multiple sclerosis, and posthypoxic states, no significant differences in 5-HIAA levels are apparent. Biogenic amine levels have also been studied in psychiatric patients, and whereas normal HVA levels are present in the lumbar CSF of patients with schizophrenia, decreased 5-HIAA concentrations are present in depressed subjects. Increased lumbar CSF MHPG levels have been identified in patients with cerebral infarction and hemorrhage. Animal studies further reveal that changes in biogenic amine levels in the CSF parallel CNS changes; however, delays in the clearance of these metabolites from the CSF complicate the interpretation of the values obtained. Because of these physiological constraints and the nonspecific nature of changes in biogenic amine levels, their measurement remains a research tool and has little clinical applicability.

Tumor cells can also be found in the CSF and occur in association with neoplasms of the brain or meninges. The cytopathological identification of these cells requires the acquisition of large volumes of CSF (more than 20 mL) and the sample should be brought immediately to the laboratory to minimize cell lysis and morphological changes. Serial LPs may be necessary to obtain positive cytological results. In a study of the usefulness of CSF cytology and autopsy, Glass and co-workers reported that 26 percent of patients with metastatic brain tumors had positive CSF cytology.[37] In another study, the cytological examination of the CSF identified metastatic involvement of the meninges in 70 percent of cases.[38] The detection of other CSF markers may be useful for the diagnosis of primary or metastatic malignancies including astroprotein (glioblastoma), carcinoembryonic antigen (carcinomas), beta-2-microglobin (lymphoblastic leukemia and lymphoma), alpha-fetoprotein (germ cell tumors), chorionic gonadotropin (choriocarcinoma and testicular tumors), and ferritin (carcinomas).[39]

Finally, it is possible to measure a wide variety of enzymes in the CSF, although few are clinically important and most are not routinely obtained. An elevated lactate dehydrogenase (LDH) may occur in bacterial meningitis[40] and cortical versus lacunar strokes.[41] Elevated levels of CSF creatinine kinase-BB are also present in a wide variety of conditions that cause parenchymal damage. Lysozyme levels are increased in processes similar to those previously mentioned, whereas adenosine deaminase elevations can occur in tuberculous meningitis.[38]

Intracranial Pressure

BASIC PRINCIPLES

Intracranial hypertension may result from a wide variety of surgical and medical conditions. The association between elevated ICP and the potential for devastating brain stem herniation has been recognized for centuries. Because the skull is essentially a closed container, its contents have only limited compressibility. The intracranial contents are composed of three compartments: (1) the brain and interstitial fluid, which comprise approximately 80 percent of the intracranial space; (2) intravascular blood, which accounts for 10 percent of intracranial space; and (3) the CSF (in the ventricles and subarachnoid space), which comprises the final 10 percent. In order to maintain physiological ICP, an increase in volume of one compartment must lead to a compensatory decrease in the volume of another compartment. As an example, diffuse cerebral edema causes an increase in the parenchymal and interstitial compartment that necessitates a compensatory decrease in the amount of blood or CSF (or both) in the intracranial space. Similarly, an increase in the CSF compartment (hydrocephalus) must lead to a decrease in the parenchymal or blood compartments.

The body is able to regulate and modify the diameter of brain arterial vasculature to maintain a relatively constant

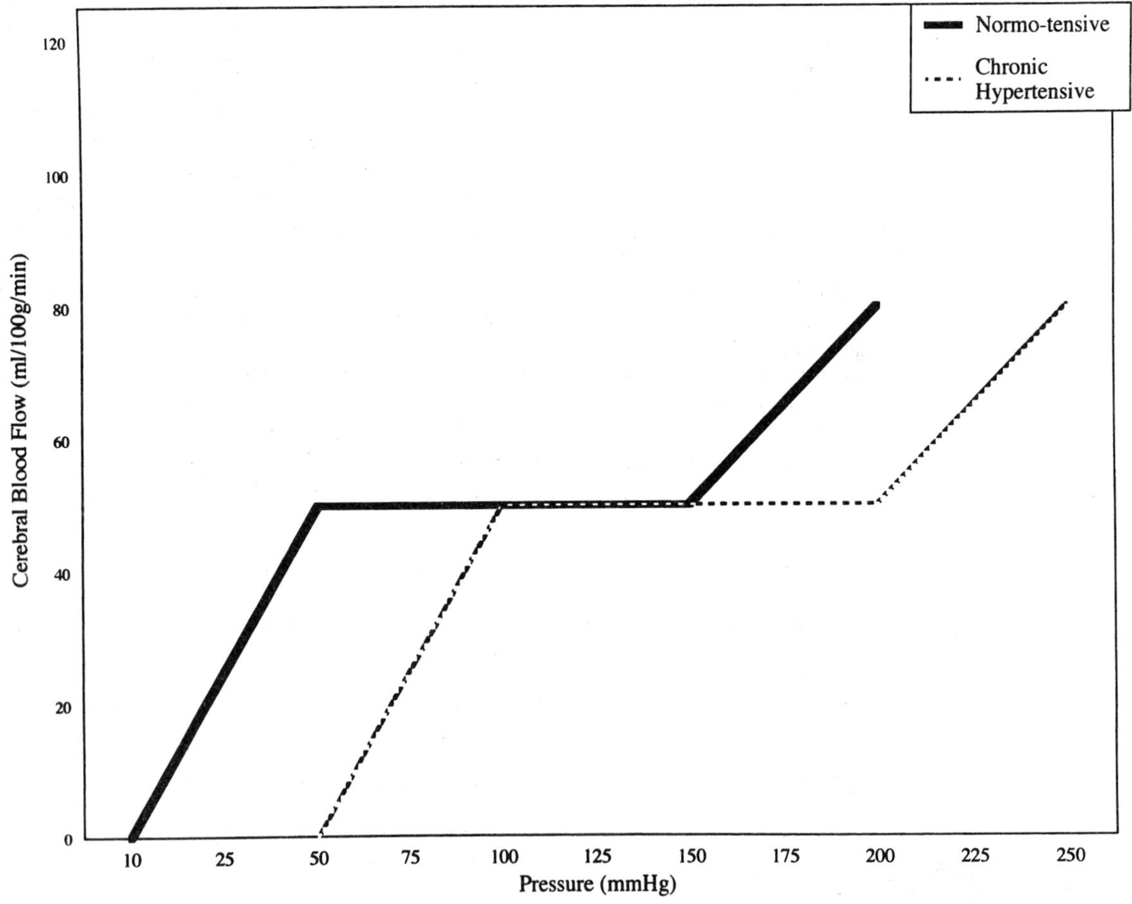

FIGURE 26–8. This graph illustrates the approximate mean arterial pressures in which the brain is able to autoregulate blood flow (flat portion of graph). The hashed line illustrates the shift to the right in a person with chronic hypertension.

TABLE 26–5. **Causes of Increased Intracranial Pressure**

Space-Occupying Lesions
Intracerebral hemorrhage
Epidural hemorrhage
Subdural hemorrhage
Tumor
Abscess

Diffuse Cerebral Edema
Meningitis
Encephalitis
Hepatic encephalopathy
  Reye's syndrome
  Acute liver failure
Electrolyte shifts
  Dialysis
Hypertensive encephalopathy
Postanoxic brain injury
Lead encephalopathy
Uncompensated hypercarbia
Head trauma
  Diffuse axonal injury

Hydrocephalus
Subarachnoid hemorrhage
Meningitis
Aqueductal stenosis
Idiopathic

Miscellaneous
Pseudotumor cerebri
Craniosynostosis
Venous sinus thrombosis

amount of blood flow over a range of systemic blood pressures that vary among patients (Fig. 26–8). This regulatory mechanism, termed autoregulation, allows the brain to regulate the flow of blood to meet its metabolic needs. Under normal conditions, the cerebral blood flow ranges between 50 and 60 mL per 100 g brain per minute (approximately 700 to 850 mL blood/min for the whole brain)[7] and accounts for about 20 percent of the total cardiac output. In patients with chronic hypertension, the graph is shifted to the right (see Fig. 26–8). The cerebral vasculature is innervated by cholinergic-, noradrenergic-, and neuropeptide-containing neurons; however, it is unlikely that these neurotransmitters contribute significantly to autoregulation, although they certainly contribute to cerebral blood flow. The control of autoregulation more likely arises from the intrinsic sensitivity of the vascular smooth muscle cells to tension across the vessel wall. Additionally, hydrogen ions also have effects on the vessels, and increases in their concentration result in dilatation. The precise role of the mechanisms involved in cerebral vasculature autoregulation under all conditions remains unclear.

Many of the diseases or syndromes that increase ICP do so by causing cerebral edema (Table 26–5). The pathophysiology of cerebral edema is based on one (or more) of three causes (Table 26–6). In vasogenic edema, an increase in capillary permeability occurs through the widening of tight junctions and increases in pinocytotic vesicles at the level of the blood-brain barrier. Because a disruption of the blood-brain barrier occurs with this disorder, magnetic resonance imaging and computed tomography studies administered with contrast typically demonstrate brain parenchymal enhancement. In cytotoxic edema, a swelling of the neurons, glia, and endothelial cells of the brain is present. Cytotoxic edema occurs in the setting of a decreased energy supply to brain cells (i.e., hypoxia) or osmotic disequilibrium (i.e., dialysis disequilibrium). The third type of cerebral edema occurs with hydrocephalus and results in an increase in interstitial fluid in the periventricular region. Through this mechanism, hydrocephalus raises ICP by increasing CSF volume and causing periventricular cerebral edema.

ICP MONITORING

Recording the ICP was initially performed through LPs in the 1890s by Quinke. Although the opening pressure is routinely measured at the time spinal taps are performed, this technique is not appropriate for long-term ICP monitoring.

Because clinical signs of elevated ICP, such as the Cushing response (systemic hypertension, bradycardia, and irregular respirations),[42] are usually a late finding and may never even occur,[43] it is important to directly measure ICP with an invasive device in appropriate settings. Furthermore, because increases in ICP may result in a decrease in cerebral perfusion pressure (CPP) if autoregulation fails, early intervention can be hastened by the direct measurement of ICP. Normal ICP ranges from approximately 10 to 20 cm H_2O (or about 5 to 15 mm Hg). CPP is calculated by subtracting the ICP from the mean arterial pressure (MAP) (CPP = MAP − ICP). Cerebral vasculature autoregulation cannot maintain appropriate cerebral blood flow and perfusion at CPP levels below 50 mm Hg. Long-term ICP monitoring was initiated in the

TABLE 26–6. **Types of Cerebral Edema**

	Vasogenic	Cytotoxic	Hydrocephalus
Pathogenesis	Increased capillary permeability	Cellular swelling	Increased intraventricular fluid
Location	White matter	Gray and white matter	Ventricular, periventricular white matter
Edema fluid	Plasma filtrate	Intracellular H_2O and sodium	Cerebrospinal fluid
Extracellular fluid volume	Increased	Decreased	Increased
Syndromes	Tumor, abscess, infarction, hemorrhage, lead encephalopathy, ischemia, meningitis	Hypoxia, ↓ osmolality, ischemia, meningitis, Reye's syndrome	Communicating and noncommunicating hydrocephalus

Adapted from Fishman RA: Cerebrospinal Fluid in Diseases of the Nervous System. Philadelphia, WB Saunders, 1992.

1950s and 1960s with the introduction of ventricular catheterization. This procedure involves insertion of a sterile catheter into the lateral ventricle that is guided by either skull-based landmarks or through stereotactic placement. Once within the ventricle, CSF may be drained and the ICP can be monitored. The latter may be completed by either direct visualization of the height of the CSF column generated outside the body or through its measurement by an external transducer. Possible complications of the ventricular catheter include subdural, epidural, or intracerebral hematomas and infection. A risk of so-called upward herniation exists if an infratentorial mass is present and CSF is quickly removed from the supratentorial lateral ventricles. Other systems for the measurement of ICP do not involve direct entry into the ventricles. Collectively, these devices are termed intracranial bolts, although this is a misnomer, and historically, they consist of hollow screws that are inserted through the skull and extend into the subarachnoid space. After the placement of these devices, tubing filled with sterile saline is attached to the bolt and a pressure monitor. True bolts are rarely used today, yet multiple systems are available that may use a hollow screw-like device. These devices usually use a pressure transducer or a fiber-optic cable inserted through the hollow bolt that directly measures the pressure within the subdural or subarachnoid space or in the brain parenchyma. Compared with the ventriculostomy, the risk of hemorrhage and ventriculitis is lower with this procedure.

After the ICP monitoring device is inserted, a waveform may be generated. Because the ICP varies with both respirations and the cardiac cycle, positive deflections of 2 to 10 mm H_2O can be observed in a patient who is not receiving positive-pressure ventilation immediately after systole and during exhalation. Maneuvers to test the function of the ICP monitor include asking patients to increase their intrathoracic pressure (by using the Valsalva technique), which causes an increase in the ICP. Alternatively, a modified Queckenstedt test may be performed in which the jugular veins are lightly compressed. Because this maneuver causes a decrease in the venous drainage from the brain, an increase in the ICP occurs, and if the intracranial compliance is low, this is rapidly observed. Neither of these tests should be performed in patients with critically elevated ICP. In these patients, evidence for plateau waves (acute elevations in ICP [600 to 1300 mm H_2O] that last 5 to 20 minutes and then return to baseline) may be present. These waves may represent an autoregulatory response to insufficient cerebral blood flow (secondary to elevated ICP) that produces vasodilatation, an increased cerebral blood flow, and, in turn, further elevations of the ICP.[44] Because of the presumed underlying pathophysiology, the presence of plateau waves suggests a poor prognosis.

The clinical conditions for performing ICP monitoring or ventricular drainage are limited. In severe head trauma with diffuse intracerebral edema, ICP monitoring may aid in guiding therapeutic interventions; however, no randomized, controlled studies exist to determine if ICP monitoring affects long-term outcome. Other conditions that may require ICP monitoring to guide interventions include large intracranial hemorrhages or strokes, encephalitis or bacterial meningitis, acute and fulminant hepatic encephalopathy, intracranial tumors, and Reye's syndrome. In patients with normal pressure hydrocephalus, transient elevations in ICP (similar to plateau waves) may be present during rapid-eye-movement sleep, and documentation of these waves may aid in determining which patients could improve with shunting.

TREATMENT OF INCREASED INTRACRANIAL PRESSURE

The treatment of increased ICP involves a few standard procedures (Table 26–7). Perhaps the easiest method for decreasing ICP is proper positioning of the patient and the avoidance of situations that can increase intrathoracic pressure. Placing the patient in an upright (or close to upright) position will lower ICP by promoting an increase in venous flow and will avoid compression of the jugular veins. Additionally, if high pressures associated with positive-pressure ventilation are managed, increases in ICP can be reduced. The administration of intravenous mannitol or hyperventilation can quickly lower ICP in most patients, yet both procedures have possible adverse side effects and are not long lasting. Mannitol treatment may lead to dehydration or electrolyte imbalance as a result of its potent osmotic diuretic effect. The beneficial effects of hyperventilation are short lived because the body quickly compensates for the induced respiratory alkalosis by producing a metabolic acidosis. Theoretically, overhyperventilation may also lead to significant vasoconstriction with associated cerebral ischemia. Corticosteroids are best used to treat increased ICP in the setting of vasogenic edema (see Table 26–5) such as occurs with brain tumors or abscesses and have little value in the setting of a patient with a stroke or head trauma. The management of blood pressure is also important in patients with an elevated ICP, because although lowering the systemic

TABLE 26–7. **Treatment Options for Elevated Intracranial Pressure**

Treatment	Dose	Advantages	Limitations
Hypocarbia by hyperventilation	pCO_2 25 to 33 mm Hg RR 10 to 16/min	Immediate onset, well tolerated	Hypotension, barotrauma, duration usually hours or less
Osmotic	Mannitol 0.5 to 1 g/kg	Rapid onset, titratable, predictable	Hypotension, hypokalemia, duration hours or days
Barbiturates	Pentobarbital 1.5 mg/kg	Mutes BP and respiratory fluctuations	Hypotension, fixed pupils (small), duration days
Hemicraniectomy	Timing critical	Large sustained ICP reduction	Surgical risk, tissue herniation through wound

RR, Respiratory rate.

blood pressure can lower ICP, it may also lower CPP. Beta-blockers or mixed beta- and alpha-blockers provide the best antihypertensive effects without causing significant cerebral vasodilatation that can lead to elevated ICP. Finally, in rare cases of hydrocephalus, direct drainage of CSF by ventriculostomy may be extremely useful.

NORMAL-PRESSURE HYDROCEPHALUS (NPH)

Pathogenesis and Pathophysiology. NPH is the result of an imbalance between production and resorption of the CSF, usually around the brain convexities. Whereas there is full communication between the ventricles and the subarachnoid space (communicating hydrocephalus), the communication between the subarachnoid space and the arachnoid villi and granulations is not intact, so fluid is not transferred efficiently to the superior sagittal sinus. Subarachnoid hemorrhage, meningitis, head trauma, and elevated levels of CSF protein all cause thickening of the arachnoid or obstruction of the subarachnoid space. A relatively large number of patients do not have an identifiable cause for hydrocephalus, and, pathophysiologically, their lesion best fits with reduced resorption of CSF, based on studies of increased resistance to CSF outflow.[45] Less frequently, intracranial tumors, stenosis of the aqueduct of Sylvius, and arachnoid cysts (causes mainly discussed in the previous section) can cause NPH due to obstruction within the ventricular system, and normal pressure is maintained as a result of apparent compensations.

In spite of its name, it appears that intracranial pressure in NPH is not always normal. Physiological experiments suggest that a transient elevation of pressure may increase ventricular size and a new fluid balance is reached with normal pressure but with a higher force, based on Pascal's law of pressure in fluids. Other mechanisms may include abnormal ventricular distensibility, increased CSF pulse amplitude, and increased transmantle pressure gradients between the intraventricular and subdural spaces that lead to expansion of the ventricles.

Epidemiology and Risk Factors. NPH has its highest prevalence in the late middle-aged and elderly groups, and is rare in patients younger than 60 years of age. On the other hand, neonates, infants, children, adolescents, and young adults can develop primary or secondary NPH. It accounts for 5 percent of patients with dementia in the older age group, but its prevalence in the general population is unknown.

Clinical Findings and Associated Disorders. The triad of progressive dementia, gait disturbance, and urinary incontinence was originally described by Adams and colleagues.[46] In most instances, gait disturbance is the first sign, followed by dementia, and, later, urinary dysfunction. The gait is slow, unsteady, and wide-based. Steps are usually short, and patients have difficulty picking their feet off the ground to ambulate (so-called magnetic gait). Turning is difficult and takes several steps. On examination, there is bradykinesia, and the legs may be spastic with increased reflexes. Patients may have difficulty in handwriting and dressing, and may appear to be mildly parkinsonian, but their tremor, if present, is usually postural, not resting. One particular feature is the discrepancy between leg function during walking and simulated walking when sitting. Patients can usually move their legs well and imitate walking while in a chair, but they become awkward and severely impaired as soon as they attempt to walk. This dyspraxia for gait eliminates a pyramidal lesion.

Cognitive decline is clinically multidimensioned and involves impaired attention, poor memory, and poor executive function.[47] Apathy and bradyphrenia are common, whereas aphasia and upper extremity limb dyspraxia are uncommon.

Neuroanatomically, the gait dysfunction and urinary impairment are believed to relate to the stretched fibers innervating the legs and sphincters that project through the vicinity of the frontal horns of the ventricular system. Compromised microcirculation due to increased intraparenchymal pressure may contribute to the cognitive impairment. Positron-emission tomography (PET) data suggest that glucose utilization defects are widespread in NPH and involve subcortical and cortical regions.

Evaluation and Differential Diagnosis. Because the clinical picture of NPH is not specific, especially in the younger patient, several diagnostic tests play a crucial diagnostic role. CT or MRI scans are important to establish the presence of hydrocephalus. The diagnosis of NPH is supported when the anterior ventricular horns measure greater than 30 percent of the diameter of the cranial cavity and the inferior horns are wider than 2 mm. On T2-weighted MRI, increased signal in the periventricular areas occurs due to presumed transependymal exudation of CSF. Other findings can suggest alternate diagnoses: for example, a normal-sized fourth ventricle with dilated third and lateral ventricles usually indicates aqueductal stenosis.

Clinically, dementing illnesses of all types must be differentiated from NPH (see Chapter 33). Alzheimer's disease is not associated with marked gait dysfunction, and a patient with multi-infarct dementia or Binswanger's disease may have a similar clinical presentation to a patient with NPH but has MRI signs of multiple strokes. In younger patients, in whom the classic clinical triad may not be met, the differential diagnosis is wider.

A lumbar puncture usually reveals normal CSF pressure. Furthermore, removal of 20 to 50 mL of CSF may cause clinical improvement in cognitive and gait dysfunction supporting the diagnosis of NPH. Intermittent pressure B-waves detected by intracranial monitoring devices suggest decreased brain compliance and NPH. Radioisotope cisternography is used most often but is not particularly specific. Whereas in normal subjects isotope injected intrathecally can be seen around the brain convexity within 48 hours, reflux into the ventricles and stasis beyond 48 hours are often seen with NPH. However, this finding has relatively low predictive accuracy in the diagnosis of NPH and the response to therapy by shunting procedures.[48]

Management and Prognosis. The primary treatment is large-volume lumbar puncture and eventual ventricular shunting. However, selection of patients for shunting is controversial; most reports agree that dementia of less than 2 years' duration and typical gait and urinary dysfunction should be considered for shunting as long as there is no evidence for a multi-infarct state on MRI scans. Medical management can include acetazolamide or digoxin to decrease CSF production. The rate of complications of CSF-diverting procedures is approximately 30 percent, with 5 percent being serious with long-term sequelae.[49] Subdural hematomas, intracranial infections, stroke, and failure of the shunt are the major complications. The proportion of patients who experience long-term benefit from this treatment range from 25 to 80 percent.

Syndromes of Altered CSF Dynamics. Several syndromes occur when the normal production or flow of CSF is altered. Those syndromes related to obstruction of the ventricular system, either the foramen leaving the lateral ventricles or the third or fourth ventricle cause "obstructive hydrocephalus" discussed primarily in Chapter 1 because altered level of consciousness is the usual overriding symptom. Another condition, normal pressure hydrocephalus, as a syndrome, is discussed in this chapter and further details are available in various Chapters in Part III dealing with specific etiologies associated with this clinical picture.

Reviews and Selected Updates

Evans RE, Armon C, Frohman EM, Goodin DS, Therapeutics and Technology Assessment Subcommittee of the American Academy of Neurology: Prevention of post-lumbar puncture headaches. Neurology 2000;55:909–914.

Fishman RA: Cerebrospinal Fluid in Diseases of the Nervous System, 2nd ed. Philadelphia, WB Saunders, 1992.

Greenlee JE: Approach to diagnosis of meningitis. Cerebrospinal fluid evaluation. Infect Dis Clin North Am 1990;4:583–598.

Hartman A, Stingele R, Schnitzer M: General treatment strategies for elevated intracerebral pressure. *In* Hacke W (ed): Neurocritical Care. Berlin, Springer-Verlag, 1994, pp 101–115.

Quality Standards Subcommitte of the American Academy of Neurology: Practice Parameter: Lumbar puncture. American Academy of Neurology, 1992, pp 149–155.

Roos KL, Bonnin JM: Acute bacterial meningitis. *In* Bleck TP (ed): Nervous System and Eye Infections. Philadelphia, Churchill Livingstone, 1995, pp 1.1–1.12.

Ropper AH, Rockoff MA: Physiology and clinical aspects of raised intracranial pressure. *In* Ropper AH (ed): Neurological and Neurosurgical Intensive Care. New York, Raven Press, 1993.

Wood K: Physiology, pharmacology and dynamics of cerebrospinal fluid. *In* Wood JH (ed): Neurobiology of Cerebrospinal Fluid. New York, Plenum Press, 1980, pp 1–16.

References

1. Haymaker W, Baer K: The Founders of Neurology. Springfield, IL, Charles C Thomas, 1953, pp 356–359.
2. Levinson A: Cerebrospinal Fluid in Health and Disease. St. Louis, C.V. Mosby, 1929.
3. Dandy WE, Blackfan KD: Internal hydrocephalus. An experimental, clinical and pathological study. Am J Dis Child 1914;8:406–482.
4. Cushing H: Studies on cerebrospinal fluid. J Med Res 1914;31:1–19.
5. Ames A, Sakanoue M, Endo S: Na, K, Ca, Mg and Cl concentrations in the choroid plexus fluid and the cisternal fluid compared to plasma ultrafiltrate. J Neurophysiol 1964;27:672–681.
6. Ames A, Higashi K, Nesbitt FB: Relation of potassium concentration in the choroid plexus to that of plasma. J Physiol 1965;181:506–515.
7. Fishman RA: Cerebrospinal Fluid in Diseases of the Nervous System. Philadelphia, WB Saunders, 1992.
8. Wright EM: Transport processes in the formation of the cerebrospinal fluid. Rev Biochem Pharmacol 1978;83:1–34.
9. Davson H, Segal M: Physiology of Cerebrospinal Fluid and Blood Brain Barriers. Boca Raton, CRC Press, 1996, pp 264–268.
10. Davson H, Luck C: The effect of acetazolamide on the chemical composition of the aqueous humor and cerebrospinal fluid of some mammalian species and the rate of turnover of 24Na in these fluids. J Physiol (London) 1957;209:131–153.
11. Tschirgi R, Frost RW, Taylor JL: Inhibition of cerebrospinal fluid formation by a carbonic anhydrase inhibitor, 2-acetylamino-1, 3, 4-thiodiazole-5-sulfonamide (Diamox). Proc Soc Exp Biol Med 1954;87:373–376.
12. Welch K, Pollay M: The spinal arachnoid villi of the monkeys *Cercopithecus aethiops sabaeus* and *Macaca irus*. Anat Rec 1963;145:43–48.
13. Tripathi BS, Tripathi RC: Vacuolar transcellular channels as a drainage pathway for cerebrospinal fluid. J Physiol (London) 1974;239:195–206.
14. Butler AB, Mann JD, Maffeo CJ, et al: Mechanism of cerebrospinal fluid absorption in the normal and pathologically altered arachnoid villi. *In* Wood JH (ed): Neurobiology of Cerebrospinal Fluid. Vol. 2. New York, Plenum Press, 1983, pp 707–726.
15. Edelson RN: Spinal subdural hematomas complicating lumbar puncture: Occurrence in thrombocytopenic patients. Arch Neurol 1974;31:134–137.
16. Tourtellotte WW, Henderson WG, Tucker RP, et al: A randomized, double blind clinical trial comparing 22 versus 26 gauge needle in the production of post-lumbar puncture headache in normal individuals. Headache 1972;12:73–78.
17. Thomas SR, Jamieson DR, Muir KW: Randomised controlled trial of atraumatic versus standard needles for diagnostic lumbar puncture. BMJ 2000;321:986–990.
18. Lybecker H, Moller JT, May O, Nielson HK: Incidence and prediction of post-dural puncture headache. A prospective study of 1021 spinal anesthesias. Anesth Analg 1990;70:389–394.
19. Dieterich M, Brandt T: Is obligatory bedrest after lumbar puncture obsolete? Eur Arch Psychiatr Neurol Sci 1985;235:71–75.
20. Greer M: Management of benign intracranial hypertension (pseudotumor cerebri). Clin Neurosurg 1968;15:161–174.
21. van Gemert HM, Vermeulen M: Treatment of impaired consciousness with lumbar punctures in a patient with cryptococcal meningitis and AIDS. Clin Neurol Neurosurg 1991;93(3):257–258.
22. Vermeulen M, Hasan D, Blijenberg B, et al: Xanthochromia after subarachnoid haemorrhage needs no revisitation. J Neurol Neurosurg Psychiatry 1989;52:826–828.
23. Cook JD, Brooks BR: Lymphocyte subpopulations in human cerebrospinal fluid. *In* Wood JH (ed): Neurobiology of Cerebrospinal Fluid. Vol. 1. New York, Plenum Press, 1980, pp 507–523.
24. Tugwell P, Greenwood BM, Warrell DA: Pneumococcal meningitis: A clinical and laboratory study. Quar J Med 1976;45:583–601.
25. Bonadio WA: The cerebrospinal fluid: Physiologic aspects and alterations associated with bacterial meningitis. Pediatr Infect Dis J 1992;11:423–32.
26. Wilfert CM: Mumps meningoencephalitis with low cerebrospinal fluid glucose, prolonged pleocytosis and elevation of protein. N Engl J Med 1969;280:855–859.
27. Sambrook MA, Hutchison EC, Aber GM: Metabolic studies in subarachnoid hemorrhage and strokes. II. Serial changes in cerebrospinal fluid and plasma urea electrolytes and osmolarity. Brain 1973;96:191–202.
28. Genton B, Berger JP: Cerebrospinal fluid lactate in 78 cases of adult bacterial meningitis. Intensive Care Med 1990;16:196–200.
29. Donald PR, Malan HC, van derWalt A: Simultaneous determination of cerebrospinal fluid glucose and serum glucose concentrations in the diagnosis of bacterial meningitis. J Pediatr 1983;103:413–415.
30. Swartz MN, Dodge PR: Bacterial meningitis—a review of selected aspects. I. General clinical features, special problems and unusual meningeal reactions mimicking bacterial meningitis. N Engl J Med 1965;272:957–959.
31. Donald PR, Malan C: Cerebrospinal fluid lactate and lactate dehydrogenase activity in the rapid diagnosis of bacterial meningitis. S Afr Med J 1986;69:39–42.
32. Plum F, Price RW: Acid-base balance of cisternal and lumbar cerebrospinal fluid. N Engl J Med 1973;289:1346–1350.
33. Posner JB, Plum F: Independence of blood and cerebrospinal fluid lactate. Arch Neurol 1967;16:492–496.
34. Kolmel HW, von Maravic M: Correlation of lactic acid level, cell count and cytology in cerebrospinal fluid of patients with bacterial and non-bacterial meningitis. Acta Neurol Scand 1988;78:6–9.
35. Yao H, Sadoshima S, Nishimura Y, et al: Cerebrospinal fluid lactate in patients with diabetes mellitus and hypoglycemic coma. J Neurol Neurosurg Psychiatry 1989;52:372–375.
36. Gerdes LU, Jorgensen PE, Nexo E, Wang P: C-reactive protein and bacterial meningitis: A meta-analysis. Scand J Clin Lab Invest 1998;58:383–393.
37. Glass JP, Melamed M, Chernik NC, Posner JB: Malignant cells in the cerebrospinal fluid (CSF): The meaning of a positive CSF cytology. Neurology 1979;29:1369–1375.
38. Position Paper, Health and Public Policy Committee and American College of Physicians: The diagnostic spinal tap. Ann Intern Med 1986;104:880–885.
39. Knight JA: Advances in the analysis of cerebrospinal fluid. Ann Clin Lab Sci 1997;27(2):93–104.
40. Knight JA, Dudek SM, Haymond RE: Early (chemical) diagnosis of bacterial meningitis: Cerebrospinal fluid glucose, lactate and lactate dehydrogenase compared. Clin Chem 1981;27:1431–1434.
41. Donnan GA, Zapf P, Doyle AE: CSF enzymes in lacunar and cortical strokes. Stroke 1983;14:266–269.

42. Cushing H: Concerning a definite regulatory mechanism of the vasomotor center which controls blood pressure during cerebral compression. Johns Hopkins Hosp Bull 1901;12:290–292.
43. Marshall LF, Smith RW, Shapiro HM: The influence of diurnal rhythms in patients with intracranial hypertension: Implications for management. Neurosurgery 1978;50:100–102.
44. Rosner MJ, Becker DP: Origin and evolution of plateau waves. Experimental observations and a theoretical model. J Neurosurg 1961;50:312–324.
45. Kosteljanetz M: CSF dynamics and pressure-volume relationships in communicating hydrocephalus. J Neurosurg 1986;64:45–52.
46. Adams RD, Fisher CM, Hakim S, et al: Symptomatic occult hydrocephalus with "normal" cerebrospinal fluid pressure: A treatable syndrome. N Engl J Med 1965;273:117–126.
47. DeMol J: Neuropsychological symptomatology in normal pressure hydrocephalus. Schweitz Arch Neurol Psychiatr 1986;33–45.
48. Vanneste J, Augustjin P, Davies GAG, et al: Normal pressure hydrocephalus. Is cisternography still useful in selecting patients for a shunt? Arch Neurol 1992;49:366–370.
49. Vanneste J, Augustjin P, Dirven C, et al: Shunting normal-pressure hydrocephalus: Do the benefits outweigh the risk? A multicenter study and literature review. Neurology 1992;42:54–59.

CHAPTER 27

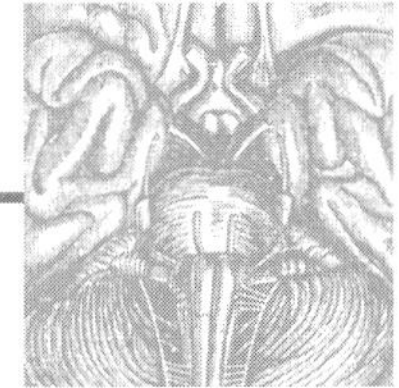

REBECCA BRENDEN BONE and GLENN T. STEBBINS

Neuropsychological Testing

History and Definitions

Neuropsychology is the subspecialty of psychology that studies brain–behavior relationships. Neuropsychology is a diverse field that includes experimental neuropsychology, the study of brain–behavior relationships in nonhumans; cognitive neuropsychology, the study of normal cognition in humans; behavioral neuropsychology, the blending of behavioral theory and neuropsychological principles; and clinical neuropsychology, the study of brain–behavior relationships in humans. When a physician requests neuropsychological testing for a patient, a clinical neuropsychologist will likely provide the assessment.

In most states, clinical neuropsychologists are licensed as clinical psychologists and have specialized training (both pre- and postdoctoral) in neuropsychology. The major role of clinical neuropsychologists is the assessment of cognitive function in individuals with known or suspected brain damage. Cognitive functions may be conceptualized as those processes by which an individual perceives both external and internal stimuli; selects pertinent stimuli and inhibits nonpertinent stimuli; records, retains, and recalls information; forms associations between stimuli and manipulates information in the pursuit of a goal; and outputs information through the expression of overt behavior. Clinical neuropsychology is based on the premise that assessments of these overt behaviors provide information about the functional integrity of the central nervous system.

The development of the science of neuropsychology is found in the works of Gall,[1] Broca,[2] James,[3] Watson,[4] Lashley,[5] Goldstein,[6] Halstead,[7] and Luria.[8] Early theories of the relationship between neurological functioning and cognition proposed independent modules of function, demonstrated most clearly by the phrenologist Gall. According to this theory, specific brain regions, reflected by bumps on the skull, were associated with specific behavior. With the advances in localization of function, in part owing to patient case studies, Broca refined our understanding of language processing, specifically within the realm of expressive language functions. James' and Watson's contributions to the principles of psychology in general, and neuropsychology specifically, led to an increased sensitivity to the need for empirical data to support theories of cognitive function, and the application of the scientific method to psychological studies. The work of Lashley and Goldstein led to a better understanding of the relationship between brain localization and behavior in neurologically healthy and neurologically damaged individuals. Halstead and Luria, through differing methods, clearly demonstrated that the assessment of overt behaviors could be used to identify brain damage with accuracy.

Although current understanding of the relationship between neuroanatomical structures and behavior rejects the skull-based tenets of phrenology, discovery of the neuroanatomical substrates of cognitive function remains a major goal of neuropsychology. It is hypothesized that cognitive function depends on both localized areas of specific functions as well as recursive connections between multiple brain areas that contribute, in toto, to cognition. In order to understand such a complex system, neuropsychology is a composite field of study integrating various disciplines including psychology, neurology, clinical neurosciences, psychiatry, statistics, and physiology.

The role of clinical neuropsychology is to elucidate the effects of brain damage on behavior, and to be able to account for the influences of other factors such as genetic, developmental, emotional, and experiential contributions on cognitive functioning. In order to accomplish this goal, neuropsychologists assess patients' cognitive function using behavioral tests. Two main approaches to neuropsychological assessment are typically used by clinicians: the quantitative approach, typified by standardized assessment techniques and comparison of individual performance measures against normative expectations, and the qualitative approach typified by in-depth analysis of individual performance characteristics using relatively standardized measures to elicit pathognomonic signs. Although these two approaches developed semi-independently, current practices in clinical neuropsychology incorporate aspects of both.[9] Not only do neuropsychologists use both quantitative and qualitative approaches to testing, they also test cognitive function in a multidimensional manner. For example, the assessment of verbal memory, a form of cognition, may be assessed by simply asking patients to remember a list of words. This approach to testing is inadequate by itself, however, because verbal memory is more complex than simply remembering lists of words. Therefore, assessment of verbal memory entails testing memory for lists of words, pairs of words, sentences, and short stories, using both immediate recall, delayed recall, and recognition paradigms. Such an assessment strategy provides enough data to analyze fully specific deficits in cognitive abilities that may be shared by multiple processes and allows for a finer discrimination of abilities and impairments.

The complexity and depth of knowledge about brain–behavior relationships are reflected in the vast number of volumes devoted to their description. This chapter provides an overview of adult clinical neuropsychology with the aim of assisting practitioners in the use and interpretation of neuropsychological data.

Overview of Testing

PURPOSES OF NEUROPSYCHOLOGICAL EXAMINATION

With the advent of modern structural imaging techniques such as computed axial tomographic (CAT) imaging, and magnetic resonance imaging (MRI), and even newer functional imaging techniques such as positron emission tomography (PET) and functional magnetic resonance imaging (fMRI), the use of neuropsychological assessments to identify the location and type of CNS lesion has waned.[6–8] However, because they identify and quantify both cognitive strengths and deficits, neuropsychological assessments are widely used in current neurological practice.[9] Indeed, the Therapeutics and Technology Assessment Subcommittee of the American Academy of Neurology rated neuropsychological assessments as an established adjunct to neurological examinations.[10]

Traditionally, neuropsychological assessment can be thought of as either diagnostic or descriptive. With regard to diagnostics, neuropsychological testing is commonly used to diagnose a variety of difficulties or pathologies. For example, neuropsychologists are often asked to diagnose conditions such as mental retardation, specific learning disabilities, mild cognitive impairment, or dementia. Clinical neuropsychologists are also frequently referred patients in which there is a question of differential diagnosis. In such cases, the neuropsychological testing is tailored to rule out one of two possible diagnoses, or to differentiate psychiatric from neurological difficulties. For example, depression and disorders of memory can share common clinical features: problems with attention and concentration, short-term memory difficulties, or deficits in working memory and processing speed. Thus, determining what specific brain functions are compromised, as well as which cognitive functions are intact, can help differentiate between two disorders. Separating which difficulties are attributable to a major depressive episode from those which are attributable to a true memory impairment or dementia is useful not only for diagnostic purposes, but is also critical for the implementation of appropriate treatment options and long-term prognosis.

Neuropsychological testing can also be used for descriptive purposes. Examination questions that are descriptive in nature inquire into the specific characteristics of the patient's condition, and the test battery is tailored to answer questions concerning relative cognitive strengths and weaknesses of a particular patient. The value of the test battery depends upon two psychometric characteristics: sensitivity and specificity. While the sensitivity of a test refers to the probability of correctly classifying an individual as abnormal who is performing abnormally with regard to a specific function or functions, the specificity of a test is the probability of classifying a normally functioning person as normal. In general, it is essential to know the specificity of a given test score cut-off, and to acquire as much information as possible about that cut-off's resulting sensitivity to various types of disorders. For example, the Mini-Mental Status Examination uses a cut-off of 24 out of 30 as a marker for impairment. This cut-off appears to be sensitive and specific with regard to cognitive dysfunction in aging populations. Once baseline data has been established for a patient, repeated testing sessions can then be used to document deterioration or improvement of cognition and the relative rates of change between functions for the individual patient.

Referrals generally fall into the diagnostic or descriptive category, although the referral source may not be specifically asked questions pertaining to specific diagnoses or inquire about the descriptive nature of a patient's deficits. Most referrals for neuropsychological assessments, however, are generally made within one of five specific domains: patient care, rehabilitation, educational planning, forensic issues, and treatment outcome analyses.

Patient Care

The largest number of referrals for neuropsychological assessments involve issues of patient care. Neuropsychological examinations are particularly informative for conditions in which neuroimaging results and other laboratory findings are not informative. For example, testing is often requested to assess the CNS effects of toxic exposure, mild head injury, dementing conditions, and in differentiating psychiatric conditions from neurological illnesses. Neuropsychological data can provide valuable information for the identification of these processes as well as the extent of resultant CNS damage.

Neuropsychological examinations may also be used to characterize the patient's current levels of cognitive and emotional functioning in association with a known or suspected CNS process. Often these data are used to monitor changes in the patient's neuropsychological status across repeated examinations,[11] so the effect of various treatment interventions on cognitive abilities can be assessed. Additionally, since neuropsychological assessments provide detailed information on both intact and impaired abilities, these assessments are useful for providing medical staff and family caregivers information on the patient's strengths as well as deficits. This information is particularly helpful in coordinating efforts to help the patient and family adjust to a given condition and make appropriate plans.

A newer application of neuropsychological examinations to neurological care is the use of screening examinations. In contrast to a full neuropsychological examination, which typically requires from 3 to 12 hours of testing, screening examinations usually require less than 1 hour. A typical screening examination tests functioning in attention, orientation, short-term and long-term memory, expressive and receptive language abilities, abstract reasoning, and intelligence. Although these shorter examinations do not give the depth of information that a full neuropsychological examination provides, they still offer basic information on the integrity of each of these abilities.[12] The data from screening examinations are particularly helpful in identifying patients in need of full examinations.

Another purpose of neuropsychological assessment in patient care situations is to assist in the differentiation of psychiatric from neurological illnesses. Often a patient presents with a neurological complaint that does not clearly follow accepted pathophysiological principles. The presentation may be as obvious as functional blindness, but can be as subtle as memory loss owing to severe depression. Neuropsychologists are able to use their training in clinical psychology as well as their knowledge of neurological systems to aid in identifying these conditions.

Rehabilitation

With the increase in cognitive rehabilitative programs for patients with CNS damage, neuropsychologists help to identify patients who can benefit from such efforts, document cognitive abilities in need of rehabilitation, provide goals for therapy, develop individual rehabilitation plans, and track the efficacy of rehabilitative interventions. Neuropsychological assessments are particularly well-suited to address these issues and are a cost-effective addition to rehabilitative efforts.[13]

Educational Planning

As with other psychological assessments, neuropsychological assessments can provide important information for educational planning, especially for children. Documentation of basic intellectual abilities helps determine appropriate classroom placement (e.g., enriched environment, special education) for school-age children. Such tests also aid in the identification of children with severe intellectual deficits, such as mental retardation. Differences between intellectual ability and academic achievement are used in the identification of specific learning disabilities. In neurological conditions such as Gilles de la Tourette's syndrome, neuropsychological assessments can be an integral component to individual educational plans by identifying strengths and weaknesses in academic abilities, as well as indicating comorbid conditions like attention deficit disorder, hyperactivity, and obsessive-compulsive behaviors.

Forensic Issues

Neuropsychological assessments are used to document the presence and extent of cognitive impairments following accidents or injury. Levels of present functioning can be compared with estimates of pre-morbid functioning to assign a monetary value to present and future lost abilities.

Treatment Outcomes Research

Neuropsychologists are trained in research designs and methods. With this knowledge they are able to assist in the design, implementation, and analysis of clinical research projects. They are often asked to apply their knowledge of cognitive assessment to suggest outcome measures, which may include standard neuropsychological tests or experimental measures. One example of this is quality of life measures, which are the increasing focus of clinical drug trials and neurosurgical interventions in neurological illness.

INTEGRATION WITH NEUROLOGICAL EXAMINATION

Neuropsychological assessments are ancillary to the typical neurological examination, and establish better precision of the type and extent of cognitive and behavioral deficits found on bedside testing. To accomplish this goal, neuropsychological tests need to be standardized, valid and reliable, and need to make meaningful comparisons of patient-derived data to normative performance.

Standardization of neuropsychological testing procedures allows for the comparison of performance across time and across individuals. Because the interpretation of neuropsychological tests requires consistent assessment methods, neuropsychological tests are standardized to testing environment, presentation of instructions, presentation of testing stimuli, seeking clarification of response from the patient, scoring procedures, and interpretative methods. Standard testing methods provide all patients with an equal opportunity to perform the required task.

Another important aspect to neuropsychological assessment is the use of reliable and valid tests. Reliability refers to the degree to which a given test score represents differences in the behavior of interest as opposed to error. Reliability measures include the degree to which a test provides consistent scores across different time points (test-retest reliability); the degree to which a test provides consistent scores across different examiners (inter-rater reliability); the degree to which the test is internally consistent (split-half reliability); and the degree to which a test provides consistent score across alternate forms of the test (alternate-form reliability).[14] A valid test is one that measures what it is purported to measure. This aspect of test development and utilization depends upon many factors. Validity measures include the degree to which the items of the test cover the relevant domain of interest but not other domains (content validity); the degree to which the test agrees with either a gold standard of the domain of interest or another test designed to measure the same domain (concurrent validity); the degree to which a test does *not* agree with another test designed to measure a different domain (discriminant validity); and the degree to which a test measures the theoretical construct under study (e.g., intelligence) (construct validity).

The relationship between reliability and validity is statistically constrained. Validity scores cannot exceed the square of reliability scores. Thus, a test can be highly reliable but invalid, but a test can never be valid and unreliable. One way to increase reliability of a given test is the use of the preceding standardized testing methods. If the manner in which a test is administered varies across examiners or across testing sessions, extraneous error is introduced, which lowers reliability and validity.

The ability to make meaningful comparisons of an individual patient's performance to normative expectations is constrained by how test performance is interpreted. Neuropsychological assessments are usually requested to identify and quantify some form of cognitive impairment. Thus, neuropsychological tests are designed to assess deficits in performance.[15] In order to assess impairments, there must be some knowledge of normal expectancies of performance. Thus, testing results must have a referent for comparison, either individual comparisons or normative comparison groups.

Individual comparisons of test performance are the most obvious method for identification of deficits. In individual comparisons previous data from a patient are used to compare with present performance. Thus, if a patient demonstrated above-average performance on a test of verbal memory prior to developing herpes simplex encephalitis, but performed at the below-average range of performance on the same test following the illness, one could conclude that a decline in verbal memory had occurred. In reality such a situation rarely occurs because neuropsychological data are usually not available from the period prior to disease or trauma. Even when such data are available there are other possible explanations for the decline in performance. If for any reason the scoring on the first or second exam is incorrect, scores are artificially inflated or minimized. Again, standardization of testing methods and concerted efforts to eliminate testing bias help to reduce this occurrence.

A second referent for neuropsychological test performance interpretation is the population-based comparison. This method is most frequently used in neuropsychological assessment and involves the comparison of individual patients' test scores to *norms* that detail performance on the measure of interest by a standardization sample. A relative ranking of the individual's score can then be determined according to the performance of the normative sample. A norm is constructed by sampling a large number of individuals, called the standardization sample, on the measure of interest. The standardization sample should be representative of the population of interest. Thus, if one wishes to develop norms for adult performance on a measure of general intelligence, the standardization sample must include individuals from all relevant age ranges, gender distributions, and educational strata. The norms provided for the Wechsler Adult Intelligence Scale–Third Edition (WAIS-III)[16] are an example of such a procedure and the norms of WAIS-III performance are reflective of this population.

Random sampling is required for the development of most norms, because a random sample, stratified for pertinent variables, is one of the assumptions of a normal distribution. Sampling theory states that large, random samples of test scores will approach a normal distribution as the sample size approaches infinity. The characteristics of a normal distribution are particularly well-suited to norm development (Fig. 27–1). In a normal distribution the measures of central tendency (mean, median, mode) are unitary and the dispersion of scores (standard deviation) on either side of mean is symmetrical. The shape of a normal distribution has been called a bell-shape curve because it peaks in the middle and trails off as you approach either tail. The characteristics of a normal distribution allow the ranking of average performance. Approximately 68 percent of all cases (or WAIS-III scores in our example) fall within one standard deviation of the mean, and approximately 95 percent of all cases fall within two standard deviations of the mean. This characteristic allows for a meaningful comparison of an individual's score to the standardization sample. Therefore, one can express an individual's performance in terms of standard deviations away from the mean of the standardization sample; z-scores, which represent the individual's score minus the mean of the standardization sample divided by the standard deviation of the standardization sample; or a percentile ranking based on the standardization sample. In most neuropsychological assessments, one of these methods for ranking an individual's performance will be reported.

Comparison of an individual's performance to these norms then provides a meaningful yardstick to identify strengths and weaknesses. If someone is performing above the mean of the standardization sample, that performance is above average for the population. Such a comparison scheme is very helpful in tracking patients' abilities and disabilities. It does, however, raise the question of whether lower than average performance really equals impaired performance. Since the standardization sample assumes normal distributional properties, the probability of occurrence of any score can be calculated. In most clinical neuropsychological assessments, performance is defined as impaired when the probability of obtaining a score that low or lower in the standardization sample is less than 5 percent. This corresponds to the standard level of significance used in most statistical analyses.

Because the standardization sample is used to interpret individual test performance, an important consideration in all neuropsychological assessments is the adequacy of the sample. Even with well-normed tests such as the WAIS-R, care needs to be exercised when comparing specific individuals with the standardization sample. For example, the standardization sample for the WAIS-III has adequate representation of individuals up to the age of 89, but does not provide any normative information for individuals over the age

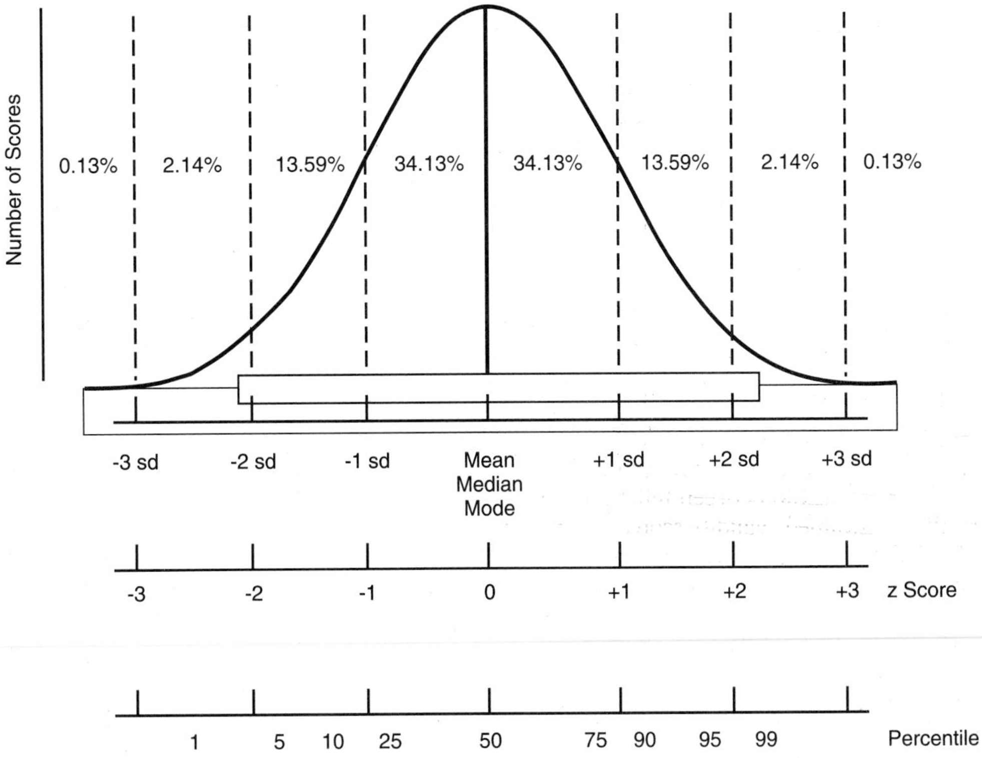

FIGURE 27–1. The normal distribution is approached when many scores of a given test are collected from a random sample. This distribution is symmetrically shaped with common measures of central tendency (mean, median, mode) and equal variance on either side. The percentages of cases falling within each standard deviation are presented between the dashed lines. The ranking of any single score may be represented by standard deviation units, z score units, or percentile ranking. sd, standard deviation.

of 89. Thus, if the performance on a 92-year-old patient on the WAIS-III is compared with this standardization sample the results may not truly reflect the performance of all 92-year-old persons.

Many other tests used in neuropsychological assessments have much more limited standardization samples, and as such may be subject to erroneous interpretations. The interpretation of many neuropsychological tests is based on standardization samples of less than 100 scores. Heaton and colleagues[17] have attempted to generate better norms for many commonly used neuropsychological tests. Their efforts have surely led to improved interpretative methods. However, even this effort suffers from a lack of generalizability to the populations of interest. This is because the standardization samples they used were not randomly selected but rather were composed of volunteers from limited geographic regions. Therefore, it is important for the consumer of neuropsychological assessment results to be aware of how the interpretations are made and the norms used in those interpretations.

HIERARCHY OF TESTING FUNCTIONS

A given cognitive function is usually composed of multiple discrete functions. Memory performance is affected not only by the ability to recognize and recall stimuli but also by the ability to perceive, process, and store those stimuli, and, finally, to reproduce them in an observable fashion. Most neuropsychologists approach patient assessment using a general hierarchy of functions involved in cognition.

The primary components of this hierarchy are the perception of stimuli, ability to attend to the stimuli, and the ability to generate some form of response. In consideration of these issues, one of the first cognitive functions to be tested in almost all examination formats is level of consciousness (see Chapter 1). If a patient is comatose there is little need to conduct neuropsychological testing. Testing of sensory systems (usually visual, auditory, tactile, and proprioceptive) is also conducted to ensure adequate stimuli processing. Finally, in order to assess a patient, a competent effector system that enables a response must be present. Therefore, testing of basic motor, vocal, and praxis abilities is conducted. If deficits are noted in any of these basic abilities, the neuropsychologist uses that information in the interpretation of other cognitive tests to increase or decrease confidence in those results. Once these three levels of abilities have been tested, testing of higher cognitive functions (e.g., intelligence, reasoning, language) can begin.

TESTING BATTERIES VERSUS INDIVIDUALIZED TESTING

There are two basic approaches to testing methods in neuropsychological assessments: the use of comprehensive testing batteries or the use of individualized testing. Each approach has its strengths and weaknesses, and most neuropsychologists use a combination of these two approaches to capitalize on the strengths and minimize the weaknesses.

The Battery Approach

Neuropsychological testing batteries provide a structured approach to the assessment of cognitive function. Although there are many neuropsychological testing batteries, two batteries are most commonly used: the Halstead-Reitan Battery[18] and the Luria-Nebraska Neuropsychological Battery.[19] The Halstead-Reitan Battery is a collection of tests that Halstead found to discriminate normal individuals from patients with organic brain disease. The core of the Halstead-Reitan Battery includes six tests developed by the authors (measuring abstract reasoning, tactile performance, tactile/visual–spatial memory, rhythm perception and memory, speech–sound perception, and primary motor speed) and seven tests developed by other individuals (measuring intelligence, psychomotor speed, sequencing abilities, language function, sensory function, grip strength, and personality functioning). The entire battery requires at least 6 hours for administration, not including scoring and interpretation, so testing often requires multiple visits. The original standardization sample for the development of the Halstead-Reitan Battery norms was inadequate; new norms have been generated using a larger and perhaps more representative standardization sample.[17] The Halstead-Reitan Battery appears to be adequate in discriminating brain-damaged individuals from neurologically healthy individuals, but is not sensitive to mild cognitive impairment or to precise localization. Despite these limitations, the Halstead-Reitan Battery is the most commonly used neuropsychological assessment battery.

The Luria-Nebraska Neuropsychological Battery[19] developed out of the extensive investigations of behavioral neurology conducted by the Russian neurologist Luria and the work of Christensen,[20] who brought Luria's theories and methods of neuropsychological testing to America. The battery uses selected Luria test items that best discriminate brain-damaged patients from neurologically healthy individuals. It consists of 269 individual items that are scored on a zero (no impairment) to 2 (impairment) scale. The test items are simple and complex commands and problems, such as motor commands and arithmetic. The 269 items are composed of 11 clinical/ability scales measuring motor abilities, rhythm sense and reproduction, tactile abilities, visual abilities, receptive speech, expressive speech, writing, reading, arithmetic abilities, memory function, and intelligence. Three additional scales provide information as to the presence of pathognomonic signs, left hemisphere damage, and right hemisphere damage. Administration of the Luria-Nebraska Neuropsychological Battery is approximately 2 to 3 hours (substantially less than the Halstead-Reitan Battery).

Although authors of the Luria-Nebraska Neuropsychological Battery have published numerous articles in support of its reliability and validity, other investigators have not been able to replicate these results.[21] The inadequate validity and reliability of the Luria-Nebraska Neuropsychological Battery are owing primarily to the lack of any theoretical model used in its development. Whereas the strength of Luria's original work was his ability to generate hypotheses about brain-behavior relationships and methods to tests these hypotheses, the developers of the Luria-Nebraska Neuropsychological Battery were unable to emulate this strength.

Individualized Testing Approach

The main advantage to the battery approach is that it allows for the collection of massive amounts of information on the status of cognitive functioning in a highly standardized manner. This advantage is contrasted with numerous disadvantages: the time required for a complete assessment is often excessive and fatigues the patient; the batteries often include assessment measures that are not necessary for a given patient, and, conversely, the batteries do not provide comprehensive assessments of all cognitive functions. By recognizing these limitations, most neuropsychologists use an individualized approach to testing.

An individualized approach allows the neuropsychologist to use pertinent information to guide test selection. For example, if neuropsychological assessment is requested for a patient with diagnosed Alzheimer's disease, the neuropsychologist knows that trying to complete a Halstead-Reitan Battery would not only be unfair to the patient but would also provide little useful information. Instead, the examiner may choose to use a number of shorter tests with lower performance ranges to allow for extremely low scores. Using this approach, the neuropsychologist chooses tests (either from existing batteries or tests designed to assess specific deficits) that assess cognitive functions relevant to a given patient. Thus, examination time is shortened, and the specificity of the testing results is increased. Inevitably, however, the selection of tests introduces a certain bias, and some domains of good or bad function may be missed.

Neuropsychologists have a vast array of tests from which to choose when using the individualized approach. Over 700 tests of cognitive functioning are available, assessing such complex functions as intelligence and such basic functions as primary motor speed. Although a detailed description of all of these neuropsychological tests is well beyond the scope of this chapter, the next section provides a brief description of the most commonly used tests and their role in assessing specific cognitive domains. This review is limited to the most commonly used tests in neuropsychological assessments of adults.

Neuropsychological Tests

ORIENTATION, ATTENTION, AND VIGILANCE

Impairments in orientation, attention, and vigilance are common sequelae to brain damage, and regardless of the localization of brain pathology, these abilities are often compromised. When a patient is disoriented and unable to attend to ongoing events, there is usually severe pathology. In addition, inability to attend to ongoing stimuli makes the interpretation of neuropsychological tests of higher cognitive functions, such as intelligence or memory, difficult. Therefore, the assessment of orientation, attention, and vigilance is an integral part of all neuropsychological assessments and usually is performed first.

Orientation Tests: Personal, Temporal, and Spatial

Standard bedside mental status examinations always assess orientation to person, time, and place. Usually this information is gathered from interviewing the patient in an open manner, and is not part of a standardized test. Many tests of cognitive function include questions assessing orientation, although they may not provide selective scores for orientation. Specific tests with orientation questions, or tests designed to assess orientation, are listed here.

Mini-Mental State Examination (MMSE).[22] The MMSE includes questions that assess orientation to time ("What is today's date?" "Month?" "Day of the week?"

"Year?") and orientation to place ("Where are you now?" "What state are you in?" "County?" "City?" "What is the name of this place?"). Each item is scored as pass or fail. Although the orientation section of the MMSE does not provide a separate score, a failure of two or more items is reflective of impaired performance.

Wechsler Memory Scale–Third Edition (WAIS-III).[23] Although the majority of this test's items assess memory function, there is a subtest, Information and Orientation, that assesses orientation to person, place, or time. Failure of two or more items is considered impaired.

Temporal Orientation Test (TOT).[24] The TOT is designed to assess specifically orientation to time. The questions include knowledge of current hour and minutes, date, day of the week, month, and year. Errors are assigned negative scores depending on the amount of disorientation. The error score is subtracted from 100 and any score less than 95 is reflective of impaired performance.

Money Road Map Test (MRMT).[25] The MRMT assesses the ability of the patient to identify left and right directions at different orientations. The patient views a map on which the examiner traces a route. At each turn, the patient has to identify whether the examiner made a left or right turn. In order to perform this test correctly, patients must be able to reorient mentally to the perspective of the examiner and to different orientations of the route. If a patient makes more than 10 errors (out of 32 turns) his or her performance is considered impaired.

Finger Localization Test.[26] This test of personal orientation requires the patient to identify which finger has been stimulated by the examiner under visual guidance, and in the absence of visual input. A variant of this test is found in the Halstead-Reitan Battery, which assigns numbers to each finger of each hand, and requires the patient to identify which hand and which finger number has been stimulated in the absence of visual input.

Left-Right Orientation Test.[27] This test of left-right orientation requires the patient to display lateralized body parts (e.g., "show me your left hand"), identify laterality of the examiner's body (e.g., "point to my left hand"), and touch lateralized body parts of the examiner (e.g., "touch my left hand"). In order to perform this task correctly, the patient must be able to reverse personal orientation when confronted with identifying laterality of the examiner. The normative data for this test are very limited, but a cut-off score of four errors is suggestive of impaired left-right orientation.

Mental Status Tests

Mental status tests are used to assess overall level of cognitive functioning. These tests are brief to administer and not very comprehensive. They tend to include a few questions on orientation, attention, memory, language, and sometimes praxis. Although mental status testing provides basic information on the integrity of most cognitive functions, the tests tend to lack sensitivity to detect mild cognitive impairment. In addition, most tests of mental status do not have normative data, so the effects of various demographic variables (e.g., age, gender, education) are unknown. Despite these limitations, the tests provide useful information, and some form of mental status testing should be a part of all neuropsychological assessments.

Mini-Mental State Examination (MMSE).[22] In addition to the preceding orientation questions, the MMSE includes items assessing registration of information, recall of three words, attention and sequencing abilities (serial sevens, or spell world backward), naming, repetition, following spoken commands, writing, and copying. The test provides a general summary of cognitive function, but does not assess any cognitive domain in depth. The maximum score for the MMSE is 30, and a cut-off score of 24 is considered to indicate impaired performance.

Although the MMSE is the most commonly used mental status test, it has a number of problems. First, one must accept the basic limitation of any screening exam. Since the test has a limited number of questions, adequate testing of cognitive function is not possible. Practically, however, the MMSE score is used as an indicator of intact or impaired performance. The cut-off score of 24 is associated with relatively high false-negative rates (test indicates absence of impairment when impairment is present) and relatively high false-positive rates (test indicates impairment when no impairment is present). Additionally, MMSE score is affected by education, race, and gender. Despite these limitations, the MMSE provides a "quick-and-dirty" assessment of overall cognitive function, and in most contexts a score of 22 or lower is considered an accurate mark of clinically significant cognitive impairment.

Mental Status Questionnaire (MSQ).[28] The MSQ is composed of items assessing orientation to time and place and ability to name the current and past presidents of the United States. The maximum score of the MSQ is 10 errors, and individuals making more than 2 errors are considered moderately impaired. This cut-off score suffers from the same limitations as the MMSE.

Short-Portable Mental Status Questionnaire (SPMSQ).[29] The advantage of the SPMSQ over the MMSE and MSQ is that normative data have been gathered to aid in interpreting performance. This represents a major advantage to the SPMSQ. However, the test still suffers from problems with false-positives and false-negatives (particularly in patients with mild cognitive impairment).

Tests of Attention and Vigilance

Testing attention involves assessment of the ability to attend to stimuli, the ability to focus attention on selected stimuli, and ability to inhibit attention to inappropriate stimuli. Tests of vigilance also require the active updating of information in an ongoing display requiring attention. All of these abilities are essential to intact cognitive function. Information on attention and vigilance should be reported in all neuropsychological assessments.

Simple Reaction Time (SRT). SRT tasks require the patient to respond, as quickly as possible, to a stimulus. The time the patient takes to respond (RT) is usually measured in milliseconds. Slowed RT is one of the most sensitive measures of impaired cognitive functioning, but individual data are difficult to interpret owing to the large inter- and intrapatient variability.

Choice Reaction Time (CRT). There are many measures of CRT, but all follow a basic paradigm: the patient is required to respond to one stimulus but to not respond to another. An example of this is the Continuous Performance Test, in which the patient is asked to respond, as quickly as possible, to a rare stimulus that is embedded in a stream of ongoing similar stimuli. These tests assess the patient's ability to maintain attention and vigilance for the target stimulus and the ability to inhibit responses to the nontarget stimuli. Individual differences are difficult to interpret owing to large inter- and intrapatient variability.

Span Tests. Tests of span capacity are a more standard form of assessing attention and vigilance than reaction time measures. In addition to assessing attention, span tests also require some form of short-term memory. However, forward span tests (see following discussion) are thought to be more reflective of attentional abilities. When backward span (repeating a sequence heard in the reverse order of presentation) is used, different cognitive processes are required, including working (or short-term) memory, so that the test is no longer a pure measure of attention.

The most commonly used span measures are the Digit Span tests from the WAIS-III and the Wechsler Memory Scale-Third Edition (WMS-III).[23] In these tests, patients listen to random sequences of numbers presented in increasing length, and immediately repeat each sequence. Two trials at each span length are presented, and maximum span is the number of digits the patient can correctly repeat on at least one trial. Average performance on this measure is considered to be between five and nine digits.[30] Another type of span test is the Letter-Number Sequencing subtest of the WAIS-III and WMS-III. Similar to the Digit Span subtest, the Letter-Number Sequencing subtest requires the patient to repeat back a sequence of letters and numbers. However, during this subtest, the patient must now manipulate the letters and numbers by first repeating back all the numbers in numerical order, and then all the letters in alphabetical order. Both digit and letter span are measures of verbal ability. A nonverbal span measure is the Corsi Block Test.[31] In this test the patient is presented with an array of nine blocks arranged in a random order. The examiner touches blocks in sequences of increasing length. The patient is required to reproduce the sequence at each length. As in the digit span test, two trials are given at each sequence length and maximum span is the number of blocks the patient taps in the correct order on at least one trial. Average performance on this test is similar to digit span. The Spatial Span subtest of the WMS-III is an equivalent test to the Corsi Block Test, and has good standardization and normative data.

Attention/Concentration Subtests of the WMS-III. Two subtests of the WMS-III (discussed following) that assess attention and concentration are the Letter-Number Sequencing subtest and the Spatial Span subtest. Together these subtests form the composite measure of Working Memory. One major advantage to the use of these measures is that they have good normative information (see WMS-III description later) and can be converted to age-adjusted standard scores with a mean of 100 and a standard score of 15. The use of these standard scores allows for comparisons across many different neuropsychological tests (e.g., WAIS-III).

Paced Auditory Serial Addition Test (PASAT).[32] The PASAT is a test requiring attention and vigilance. In this test, the patient listens to a tape recording of digits presented one at a time. The task for the patient is to add each number to the one immediately preceding it. For example, the recording might present the numbers 1, 7, 5, 4. The patient adds the first two numbers (1 + 7) and responds with the number 8. The patient then adds the second two numbers (7 + 5) and responds with the number 12. The patient then adds the third two numbers (5 + 4) and responds with the number 9. This continues for a total of 61 numbers presented in a random order. The test can be given at different rates of presentation ranging from a slow rate of one number every 2.4 seconds to the fastest rate of one number every 1.2 seconds. This test assesses attention and vigilance because the patient is required to not only attend to the relevant stimuli (numbers) but also be vigilant to changes in the ongoing presentation. This is an extremely sensitive measure of vigilance. However, the test also involves working or short-term memory because the patient must "hold" in short-term memory the preceding number while formulating a response. Although this is a sensitive test, the norms for interpretation are limited.

Digit Symbol.[16] This subtest of the WAIS-III presents the patient with a row of numbers one through nine, each paired with nonsense symbols (e.g., inverted T). Below this key are empty boxes with numbers above each box. The patient is required to transcribe the symbol corresponding to the number above the box as quickly as possible. This measure requires focused attention and switching behavior between the key and the target boxes. One advantage of this test is the extensive WAIS-III norms available on performance expectations. This test also requires motoric speed and may not be appropriate for patients with marked motor impairment. A variant of this test is available that requires a verbal response only, thus decreasing motoric demands.[33]

Symbol Search.[16] This subtest of the WAIS-III presents the patient with two target symbols (nonsense symbols) and an array of additional symbols (nonsense symbols). The patient is required to respond yes if the array of additional symbols contains one or more of the target symbols, and respond no if the array of additional symbols does not contain one or more of the target symbols. Again, one advantage of this test is the extensive WAIS-III norms available on performance expectations. This test also requires motoric speed, and thus, should not be used with patients who have motor impairments.

Trail Making Test.[34] There are two forms to this test: Trail Making Tests A and B. Trail Making Test A provides an assessment of complex attention. This test requires the patient to connect randomly positioned numbered circles in numeric order as quickly as possible. Form B presents the patient with numbered circles and circles with letters. The patient is required to connect the circles in numeric and alphabetic order as quickly as possible, alternating between numbers and letters. Both Forms A and B require focused attention for successful performance. In addition, Form B requires the patient to switch cognitive sets between numbers and letters. Both forms of the Trail Making Test are highly dependent upon motoric speed, and may not be appropriate for patients with marked motor impairment (e.g., Parkinson's disease).

Cancellation Tests. Another useful test of attention and vigilance is that which requires the patient to seek a selected stimulus out of a background of similar stimuli. One such measure is the Letter Cancellation Test[35] where the patient is required to cancel selected letters, designs, or words from a background of nontarget letters, designs, or words. Another cancellation test is the Visual Search and Attention Test

(VSAT).[36] Here, the patient is required to cancel out either a letter or symbol of varying colors. Because cancellation tasks are timed measures requiring motoric responses, they may not be appropriate for patients who have marked motor impairment.

Clinical Situations for Testing Orientation, Attention, and Vigilance

Neuropsychological data on orientation, attention, and vigilance abilities are useful in defining dysfunction in all levels of neurological functioning. Such tests are particularly useful in cases of toxic and metabolic abnormalities (see Chapters 38 and 39), which affect level of consciousness (see Chapter 1), sleep/wake cycles (see Chapter 2), and memory functioning (see Chapter 5). In addition, attentional testing is essential for patients who evidence neglect or dyspraxia (see Chapter 4). Useful information on patients with psychiatric presentations is also provided when attention is assessed (see Chapters 1 and 3). When requesting neuropsychological assessment of orientation, attention, and vigilance, it is important to request testing on all aspects of attention and vigilance including simple attention, focused attention, and set-shifting.

INTELLECTUAL ABILITIES

Intelligence is considered to be the culmination of cognitive abilities. The testing of intelligence involves assessments of attention, reasoning, memory, language, perception, and construction. Intelligence tests should provide an overview of cognitive function integrity. Most tests of intelligence do not adequately assess all cognitive abilities, however.

Intelligence Quotients

These tests are the current gold standard in intelligence testing and include the WAIS–III.[16, 36, 37] Each Wechsler test is used for different age ranges: the WPPSI-R test is for ages 3 years to 7 years and 3 months; the WISC-III test is for ages 6 years to 16 years 11 months; and the WAIS-III test is for ages 16 years to 74 years 11 months. Because the different Wechsler tests are similar in construction, interpretation, and psychometric concerns (standardization, norms, reliability), only the WAIS-III will be discussed.

In keeping with the idea that intelligence is the culmination of cognitive function, the WAIS-III is composed of different subtests, each assessing different cognitive functions (Table 27–1). Because of this composition, the various subtests are listed under different subheadings in this chapter. In addition, since the WAIS-III assesses many different cognitive functions, it is often the framework for neuropsychological assessment, and provides an overview of the integrity of cognitive abilities. Results for subtest performance often guide further (and more extensive) testing of selected functions.

The WAIS-III provides three summary measures: Verbal IQ, Performance IQ, and Full Scale IQ. The IQ score repre-

TABLE 27–1. **Subtests of the Wechsler Adult Intelligence Scale–Third Edition and Cognitive Functions They Assess**

Verbal Scales (Verbal IQ)	**Cognitive Function Assessed**
Vocabulary	Vocabulary knowledge Semantic memory
Similarities	Reasoning, problem solving, concept formation Executive function
Arithmetic	Attention/concentration Executive function Processing speed Calculations
Digit Span	Attention/concentration Short-term memory
Information	General fund of information
Comprehension	Reasoning, problem solving, concept formation Executive function
Performance Scales (Performance IQ)	
Picture Completion	Reasoning, Problem solving, concept formation Executive function
Digit Symbol	Attention/concentration Executive function (sequencing) Motor function Processing speed
Block Design	Construction Praxis Spatial reasoning Motor function Processing speed
Matrix Reasoning	Visual-Spatial processing Abstract reasoning
Picture Arrangement	Reasoning, problem solving, concept formation Executive function (sequencing)

sents an age-adjusted scaling of an individual's intellectual performance. This provides a standard measure that can be compared across individual patients or within a given patient over chronological age. Due to the extensive norms for the WAIS-III (see preceding discussion) these measures may be generalized to the population of the United States. The Wechsler tests have been translated into many different languages, and adequate norms exist for most of these modifications. The characteristics of the standardization sample of IQ scores (Verbal, Performance, and Full Scale) are a mean performance of 100, with a standard deviation of 15. In addition, individual subtest performance can be converted to standard scores with associated variability. Thus, the clinician is able to classify individual performance for both summary IQ measures and individual subtest performance against these values and provide a relative ranking of performance.

The summary IQ scores are extremely useful in educational settings. Although these scores are useful, care needs to be exercised in their use. Because IQ scores represent the culmination of cognitive abilities, they are extremely susceptible to brain damage.[15] The presence of a potentially reversible impairment in one of the basic elements of cognitive function (e.g., attention/vigilance) will provide artificially low IQ performance. Therefore, IQ scores need to be interpreted in the context of a complete neuropsychological examination.

One particularly difficult issue in intellectual performance is the diagnosis of profound intellectual impairments, or mental retardation. First, this diagnosis has major consequences for an individual. Once assigned with the label of mental retardate, educational and occupational opportunities are limited. The individual is guided away from mainstream educational settings and provided with specialized training. Second, there are no universally accepted diagnostic criteria for mental retardation. The usual criterion is IQ performance greater than two standard deviations below the mean (e.g., an IQ score of less than 70 on the WAIS-III). Because the performance level for mental retardation is so low, however, statistical reliability of the standardization sample is also low. As seen in Figure 27–1, as the scores decrease (or increase) toward the tail of the distribution, the number of sample scores drops dramatically. The representativeness of cases at these extreme levels is limited and hence it is problematic to generalize the results to the population of interest. Because of these issues, it is incumbent on the examiner to base the diagnosis of mental retardation on multiple assessments of intellectual performance and not on a single measure.

The use of IQ scores in neuropsychological assessments is limited to providing a basic measure of cognitive functional integrity. Comparison of Verbal IQ performance to Performance IQ performance has been suggested to provide an assessment of dominant (verbal) and nondominant (performance) hemispheric function. Actuarial studies of this Verbal IQ/Performance IQ comparison, however, have not supported its use in this capacity.[38] Verbal IQ measures do provide some indication of dominant hemispheric integrity, but Performance IQ measures do not reliably indicate nondominant hemispheric integrity. This lack of reliability is due to basic differences between verbal and performance measures. Whereas most subscales comprising Verbal IQ are not timed, all Performance IQ subscales are. This difference adversely affects the Performance IQ scores of individuals with compromised motor and cognitive speed (e.g., patients with basal ganglia damage). In addition, there are basic differences in sensitivity to brain damage between verbal and performance subscales. The subtests of Verbal IQ tend to require overlearned abilities such as vocabulary knowledge and general information. These abilities are, in general, less affected by brain damage. The subtests of Performance IQ tend to require novel abilities, such as reproducing visual patterns using colored blocks. These abilities are, in general, more affected by brain damage. This difference between overlearned and novel abilities is evident in aging, and reflected in the performance of the standardization sample.

In contrast to the use of summary IQ scores for neuropsychological assessment, the analysis of subscale performance is very useful. As shown in Table 27–1, each subscale assesses specific (and overlapping) cognitive abilities. The pattern of performance on the subtests can provide useful information in forming hypotheses as to possible impairment in various cognitive abilities. These hypotheses can then be tested with additional, more focused, assessments. The use of subscale performance patterns has resulted in various interpretative methods for specific neuropsychological use.

Premorbid Estimates of Intellectual Function

In order to provide useful information on general cognitive functioning, current measures of intelligence need to be compared with premorbid level of functioning. Because neuropsychological testing results are typically not available for the period prior to neurologic trauma, neuropsychologists are forced to estimate premorbid abilities.[39] There are three basic approaches to estimation of premorbid intellectual functioning: estimates derived from life-history variables believed to be correlated with measures of cognitive functioning (e.g., years of education); measures of best current cognitive functioning, or "present abilities," which are used to estimate a minimum level of premorbid functioning; and comparison of an individual's test results to population-based estimates of normal performance (norm-based comparisons as discussed previously). Each of these approaches has associated error that needs to be considered in the interpretation of neuropsychological testing data.

The first method, estimates based on life-history variables, offers a potential wealth of information that is thought to be related to the cognitive performance. Estimates derived from life-history variables may include basic demographic information such as age, education, and gender but may also include information from developmental history, medical history, occupational history, and academic history. The application of these data to an estimate of premorbid functioning can be accomplished in either qualitative or quantitative methods. The qualitative approach allows the examiner to form a "best-guess" of premorbid functioning.[39] For example, the estimated premorbid functioning for an individual with a normal developmental history, outstanding academic history, a college degree, and an occupational attainment of CEO of a major corporation would be higher than an individual with a normal developmental history, poor academic history, a high school diploma, and an occupational attainment of sales clerk. Although this information may be helpful, it does not provide an actual estimate of premorbid functioning.

The quantitative approach to the use of life-history information typically uses demographic information such as age, education, and gender to provide an estimate of the range of premorbid test scores for a given individual.[40, 41] This approach is useful because specific ranges of test scores may be generated to be compared with current scores, but typically does not take full advantage of nonquantifiable information such as developmental and medical history.

The second method of estimating premorbid cognitive abilities, the "present abilities" approach, uses current test scores to provide a lower-bound estimate of prior functioning. The theory underlying this approach is that neurological damage does not affect all cognitive abilities equally and that an individual's highest test score on current testing is most likely to reflect intact performance. Therefore, that highest test score can be used to provide an estimate of overall premorbid cognitive functioning. For example, if an individual is scoring at the below average range of performance on tests of verbal memory, verbal comprehension, and verbal fluency but is performing at the average range on a test of visual-spatial skills and nonverbal reasoning, the examiner may assume that the individual was performing at least at the average range on all measures. Of course, this estimate is only meant to provide an interpretative guide, as other explanations for a given pattern of intact and impaired performance are possible.

A more standardized method than the "present abilities" approach for estimating premorbid IQ is found in tests such as the National Adult Reading Test (NART)[42] and its variants. These tests rely on current performance of reading ability or vocabulary knowledge to estimate premorbid abilities. Both reading ability (particularly reading of phonically irregular words such as *debt*) and vocabulary knowledge tend to be less affected by brain damage than other cognitive abilities. By using these abilities to estimate premorbid IQ, the examiner is able to get an estimate of a lower-bound to previous IQ.[43]

All of these approaches to premorbid IQ estimation are subject to many caveats. First, the range of scores provided by the quantitative approaches is limited. With these measures, it is not possible to get very high or very low IQ estimates. Second, these approaches overestimate low IQ performance and underestimate high IQ performance. Third, each approach is associated with differing levels of statistical error, usually measured as the standard error of estimate. For example, the quantitative approaches have standard errors ranging between 7 and 16 points. Since the standard deviation of IQ is 15 points, these estimates can at best provide a range of possible scores equal to or greater than one standard deviation. Therefore, extreme care needs to be applied to the use of these estimates. Most neuropsychologists will use a combination of quantitative and qualitative approaches to the estimation of premorbid IQ.

Other Intelligence Tests

The Wechsler scales are not the only method for the assessment of intellectual abilities. Due to space limitations we cannot list all tests of intelligence. However, other tests of intellectual abilities tend to follow two different assessment methods: tests of verbal abilities and tests of nonverbal abstraction. The first method, testing of verbal abilities, is represented by tests such as the Peabody Picture Vocabulary Test–Revised (discussed in the section on Perception and Construction Abilities), in which patients are asked to choose which of four pictures best identifies a spoken word. This method is based on the high correlation between vocabulary knowledge and IQ.[44] The second method, tests of nonverbal abstraction, is represented by the Raven's Progressive Matrices Test (discussed in the section on Reasoning and Problem Solving Through Concept Formation), in which patients must abstract general principles and rules from patterns. This method tends to correlate well with the Full Scale IQ from the Wechsler scales.

Tests of Academic Achievement

Tests of academic achievement typically assess standard academic skills such as reading, writing, arithmetic skills, and spelling. The scores derived from these measures provide important information on neuropsychological and educational abilities. They allow comparisons of an individual patient's educational development to normative expectations. They also help identify specific areas in need of remediation. Finally, academic achievement tests provide important information in the diagnosing of specific learning disabilities. The presence of learning disabilities is suggested when there is a large discrepancy between measures of intellectual ability and measures of academic achievement. Additional testing is required to formally assign a diagnosis of learning disabilities. The most commonly used tests of academic achievement are the Peabody Individual Achievement Test-Revised (PIAT-R)[45] and the Wide Range Achievement Test–Third Edition (WRAT-III).[46] Both of these tests assess reading, arithmetic, and spelling. The PIAT-R has additional scales assessing the patient's fund of general information and reading recognition. Both tests provide information as to an individual patient's academic achievement in terms of grade level, standard score, and standing.

Clinical Situations for Tests of Intellectual Abilities

Intellectual assessment is very important for patients presenting with impairments of higher cognitive functioning such as memory, language, and reasoning. Because these higher cognitive functions are highly correlated with intelligence, intelligence assessment allows the examiner to interpret scores of memory, language, and reasoning performance in light of basic intellectual abilities. Intellectual assessments are not particularly helpful in patients with disturbances in level of consciousness (see Chapter 1), disrupted sleep/wake cycles (see Chapter 2), or neglect and dyspraxia (see Chapter 4). Additionally, the comparison of intellectual abilities and academic achievement is helpful in identifying patients who may have learning disabilities. In children with developmental or neurodegenerative disorders affecting the cortex or subcortex (see Chapters 28, 33, and 34) and those with chromosome alterations, enzyme defects, or storage abnormalities (see Chapters 30–32), these assessments help in tailoring educational efforts and expectations. When intelligence testing is requested, the referring physician should ask for a reporting of subscale performance as well as summary IQ scores.

REASONING AND PROBLEM SOLVING THROUGH CONCEPT FORMATION

Reasoning and problem solving are highly related to intellectual functioning. Similar to intellectual function, these abilities tend to be impaired following damage to the CNS. Specific location of injury appears to be less important to reasoning impairments, as does the presence of CNS disturbance. Impairments in reasoning and problem solving result in difficulties in all areas of daily functioning. Patients may not be able to form generalizations from a given situation and interpret events concretely. Tests of reasoning and conceptualization usually assess verbal or nonverbal abilities.

Tests of Verbal Reasoning and Concept Formation

Comprehension.[16] This subtest of the WAIS-III is a test of verbal conceptualization. Patients are required to answer questions or interpret proverbs that require problem solving (e.g., "What does 'a rolling stone gathers no moss' mean?"). Scoring is based on partial credit on most items for concrete responses and full credit on responses reflecting abstraction of general principles. One advantage of this test is the extensive WAIS-III norms available on performance expectations.

Similarities.[16] This subtest of the WAIS-III requires the patient to identify the common elements between seemingly uncommon stimuli. The test begins with simple problems (e.g., "How are an orange and banana alike?"), and progress to more difficult problems (e.g., "How are praise and punishment alike?"). Scoring awards full credit for complete abstractions, partial credit for concrete responses, and no credit for incorrect responses. One advantage of this test is the extensive normative data from the WAIS-III standardization sample.

Arithmetic.[16] This subtest of the WAIS-III presents the patient with progressively more difficult arithmetic word problems. The test is timed so the patient must attempt to complete each problem as quickly as possible. In addition, bonus points are given for some of the difficult problems when the patient responds very quickly. Since this test is a subtest of the WAIS-III, it benefits from extensive normative data.

Tests of Nonverbal Reasoning and Concept Formation

Category Test.[18] The Category Test is part of the Halstead-Reitan Battery and tests visual concept formation. In this test, patients see slides with four stimuli and are required to identify the concept presented on each slide. The principle remains the same in each of six different sets of slides, but changes between sets. A final set of slides presents pictures viewed in previous sets as a test of memory for the solution. This test can be very frustrating for patient and examiner alike, but is one of the more sensitive measures in the Halstead-Reitan Battery.

Raven's Progressive Matrices.[47] These tests (Colored Progressive Matrices, Standard Progressive Matrices, and Advanced Progressive Matrices) measure visual concept formation and problem solving. Patients are presented with multiple designs that are linked by a common conceptual pattern. The final design is missing, and the patient must choose which of six to eight alternative final designs is correct. The range of abilities this test assesses is very large, from the concrete to extremely abstract. Extensive normative data are available for British norms, and adequate norms are available for U.S. norms.

Wisconsin Card Sorting Test (WCST).[48] This test of visual concept formation adds cognitive set-shifting to concept formation. Patients are presented with four "target" cards with simple colored designs that can be sorted by three concepts. The patients match probe cards with identical colored design to the target cards according to whatever concept they generate. The only feedback to the patient after each trial is whether his or her response is correct. The order of sorting concept is fixed, but unbeknownst to the patient, changes after a set number of correct responses. Thus, patients must be able to switch the concept they were using for the previous trials.

Clinical Situations for Tests of Reasoning and Problem Solving Through Concept Formation

Because reasoning and problem-solving abilities are closely associated with intellectual functioning, testing should be requested in those situations that require intelligence testing.

VERBAL FUNCTION

Disturbances in language function are one of the most noticeable impairments in cognitive abilities. They can be the result of generalized cognitive deterioration, as in dementing conditions (see Chapter 33), or confusional states (see Chapters 38–40 and 55). Likewise, they may be due to specific lesions, as in transcortical aphasia (see Chapter 6) or psychiatric conditions (see Chapter 3), as in psychotic word salad or neologisms. Most assessments of verbal function include testing of expressive abilities (spontaneous speech, naming, repetition of words and phrases, writing) and receptive abilities (comprehension of speech, comprehension of written material).

Aphasia Batteries (see Chapter 6)

Boston Diagnostic Aphasia Examination (BDAE).[49] This battery is a comprehensive assessment of verbal function. It provides information on 12 areas of language abilities using 34 subscales. Assessments include verbal comprehension, written comprehension, writing to dictation, naming, articulation, spontaneous speech, repetition, reading, following simple and complex commands, speech fluency, and prosody. The test provides an overall severity rating score and a profile of subtest performance. This test is very useful in providing a comprehensive assessment of verbal function, but because of the number of items, testing time is quite long. Therefore, this battery is mostly used for specific diagnosis and rehabilitative planning of aphasic patients. Because of scoring and normative information, separate subtests can be given independently for a more focused (and shorter) examination of specific areas of verbal function.

Multilingual Aphasia Examination (MAE).[50] This test is similar to the BDAE in that it provides a comprehensive assessment of language function. The administration time is shorter, however. MAE tests were taken from the Neurosensory Center Comprehensive Examination for Aphasia. An advantage to the MAE is that alternate forms are provided, so repeated testing can be conducted without contamination of practice effects. Subtests of the MAE can also be given independently of the complete battery.

Neurosensory Center Comprehensive Examination for Aphasia (NCCEA).[51] This battery provides detailed assessments of reading, writing, articulation, visual abilities, and tactile abilities. The battery has 20 subtests measuring visual naming, description of use of objects, tactile naming, digit repetition forward and backward, sentence construction, identification of objects, oral reading for single words and sentences, visual naming of objects, written naming of objects, writing to dictation, writing from copy, and articulation. In addition, four "control tests" are provided. These tests are given if the patient makes errors on the tactile naming, visual naming, or reading tests. Extensive norms are provided for each subtest, so they may be used independently. Administration time is usually under 2 hours, which makes this battery practical in everyday clinical use.

Aphasia Screening Tests

Because most aphasia batteries require extensive time for administration, screening measures have been developed. These screening tests have variable reliability, sensitivity, and specificity to language impairments.

Aphasia Screening Test.[18] This test is part of the Halstead-Reitan Battery and is composed of 32 items testing reading, articulation, spelling, repetition, naming, calculations, and construction. Administration time is brief (approximately 15 to 30 minutes). Each ability is tested with one or two items, so the range of abilities is not great. In addition, studies of the diagnostic utility of this test have been disappointing.[52]

Token Test.[53] This test is extremely sensitive to impairments in verbal functions. It does not provide specific information as to type of verbal disturbance, however. The patient is presented with tokens of different shapes (i.e., circles, squares, triangles), sizes, and colors. The patient is required to perform certain acts with the tokens, such as point to selected tokens, touch them, pick them up, and place one token on top of another. Administration and scoring are very simple and the testing time is brief (approximately 15 minutes). Because this test requires comprehension of detailed information, it is sensitive to patients with disturbances of attention and vigilance. This test is particularly useful in identifying the presence of verbal function disturbances and whether additional, more detailed testing is required.

Individual Tests of Verbal Skills

The most commonly used individual tests of verbal skills come from the previously discussed batteries. Because of the common use of these individual tests, a few are presented following:

Naming Test.[50] This test comes from the MAE. Patients are required to name common and uncommon objects depicted in line drawings.

Boston Naming Test.[54] This naming test is not part of any battery, but is often added to the BDAE. Patients are required to name 60 objects depicted in line drawings. The objects range from simple and common objects such as a tree to complex and uncommon objects such as an abacus. If a patient is unable to name an object, he or she is given a phonemic cue and a semantic cue.

Controlled Oral Word Association Test.[50] This test measures verbal fluency and comes from the MAE. Patients are required to generate as many words as possible, as quickly as possible, to a given letter. Proper nouns, numbers, and the plural form of a produced word are not allowed. The patient is given three 1-minute trials using three different letters. A variant of this test also requires the patient to generate exemplars from different categories (e.g., four-legged animals, things found in a grocery store, parts of a building).

Sentence Repetition.[50] This test is part of the MAE and requires the patient to repeat spoken sentences. The first item is simple, composed of three syllables, and the last item is complex, composed of 24 syllables. In addition to testing repetition, this test assesses verbal memory.

Clinical Situations for Tests of Verbal Function

Assessment of language function is necessary for all neuropsychological examinations. Not only do these tests provide information about verbal function, they also assess basic skills needed to complete other neuropsychological tests. Usually, requests for administration of aphasia batteries are limited to patients with documented verbal impairments. Screening tests or individual tests of naming, comprehension, verbal fluency, repetition, reading, and writing should be requested for all referrals. In the assessment of patients with vascular disease (see Chapters 22 and 45), cortical developmental (see Chapter 28), or degenerative processes (see Chapters 31–35), language testing can help in identifying deficits and tracking verbal decline or improvement.

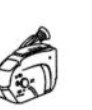

MEMORY (see Chapters 5 and 33)

The ability to record, retain, and reproduce information constitutes memory functioning. Memory is not a unitary phenomenon, however. There are different forms of memory (Table 27–2) including memory requiring awareness (explicit memory) as well as memory that occurs in the absence of awareness (implicit memory; see Chapter 5). All standard clinical assessments of memory test explicit memory. Even within explicit memory there are different forms. Semantic

TABLE 27–2. **Wechsler Memory Scale–Third Edition, Primary and Optional Indexes**

Primary Indexes	Optional Indexes
Auditory Presentation	**Auditory Presentation**
Logical Memory I and II	Information and Orientation
Verbal Paired Associates I and II	World Lists I and II
	Mental Control
Letter-Number Sequencing	Digit Span
Visual Presentation	**Visual Presentation**
Faces I and II	Visual Reproduction I and II
Family Pictures I and II	
Spatial Span	

memory represents the ability to learn information about the world in general. Episodic memory represents memories that are tied to specific episodes. For example, the knowledge that a bicycle has two wheels, pedals, a seat, and handlebars represents semantic memory; it is not possible to identify when this information was acquired. The memory of the first time one rode a bicycle is an example of episodic memory; the events surrounding that first ride are part of the memory trace. Most clinical neuropsychological tests of memory test a combination of semantic and episodic explicit memory. There are many different memory tests, both batteries and tests of single abilities.

Wechsler Memory Scale–Third Edition (WMS-III).[23] The WMS-III is a memory assessment battery composed of 17 subtests (Table 27–3). The 17 subtests include

1. Information/Orientation—assessing general personal information and orientation to person, place, and time;
2. Logical Memory I—assessing recall of orally presented stories;
3. Faces I—assessing ability to recognize visually presented target faces from distracter faces;
4. Verbal Paired Associates I—assessing recall memory for orally presented word pairs that have been previously learned;
5. Family Pictures I—assessing recall of visually presented family scenes involving four family members;
6. Word Lists I—assessing recall of an orally presented list of words;
7. Visual Reproduction—assessing ability to reproduce difficult-to-verbalize designs after a brief exposure;
8. Letter–Number Sequencing—assessing ability to manipulate and recall letters and numbers;
9. Spatial Span—assessing ability to reproduce increasingly longer spatially separated sequences of forward and backward taps on blocks;
10. Mental Control—assessing speeded performance for reciting the alphabet, counting forward and backward, days of the week forward and backward, months of the year forward and backward, counting by 6s while stating days of the week in order;
11. Digit Span—assessing forward and backward digit span;
12. Logical Memory II—assessing ability to recall information from the stories in Logical Memory I after a 30-minute delay, as well as assessing recognition of information from stories;
13. Faces II—assessing ability to recognize visually presented target faces from Faces I after a 30-minute delay;
14. Verbal Paired Associates II—assessing ability to recall associations from Verbal Paired Associates I after a 30-minute delay, as well as assessing recognition of word pairs;
15. Family Pictures II—assessing recall of visually presented family scenes from Family Pictures I;
16. Word Lists II—assessing recall of the orally presented list of words from Word List I after a 30-minute delay;
17. Visual Reproduction II—assessing ability to recall the designs presented in Visual Reproduction I after a 30-minute delay, as well as specific sub-subtests to assess recognition of correct figures from nontarget figures, copying of figures to assess visual perception abilities, and a subtest to analyze discrimination abilities.

Ten of these subtests contribute to eight indices, namely the Auditory Immediate Index (Logical Memory I and Verbal Paired Associates I), Visual Immediate Index (Faces I and Family Pictures I), Immediate Memory Index (Logical Memory I, Verbal Paired Associates I, Faces I, and Family Pictures I), Auditory Delayed Index (Logical Memory II and Verbal Paired Associates II), Visual Delayed Index (Faces II and Family Pictures II), Auditory Recognition Delayed Index (Logical Memory II Recognition and Verbal Paired

TABLE 27–3. **Subtests of the Wechsler Memory Scale–Third Edition That Form the Primary Indexes and the Memory Functions They Assess**

Indexes and Subtests	Cognitive Function Assessed
Auditory Immediate Index	
Logical Memory I	Verbal long-term memory Verbal learning
Verbal Paired Associates I	Verbal long-term memory Verbal learning
Visual Immediate Index	
Faces I	Nonverbal long-term memory Nonverbal learning
Family Pictures I	Nonverbal long-term memory Nonverbal learning
Immediate Memory Index	
Logical Memory I	
Verbal Paired Associates I	
Faces I	
Family Pictures I	
Auditory Delayed Index	
Logical Memory II	Verbal delayed memory Verbal learning
Verbal Paired Associates II	Verbal delayed memory Verbal learning
Visual Delayed Index	
Faces II	Nonverbal delayed memory Nonverbal learning
Family Pictures II	Nonverbal delayed memory Nonverbal learning
Auditory Recognition Delayed Index	
Logical Memory II Recognition	Recognition of verbal information
Verbal Paired Associates II Recognition	Recognition of verbal information
General Memory	
Logical Memory II	
Verbal Paired Associates II	
Faces II	
Family Pictures II	
Working Memory	
Letter–Number Sequencing	Auditory processing Attention/concentration Executive function
Spatial Span	Visual–Spatial processing Attention/concentration Executive function

Associates II Recognition), General Memory Index (Logical Memory II, Verbal Paired Associates II, Faces II, and Family Pictures II), and Working Memory Index (Letter-Number Sequencing and Spatial Span). The standardization sample for the WMS-III follows the same method as that used in the WAIS-III (although with a smaller standardization sample size), so good normative data are provided for each subtest as well as the index scores.

Rey Auditory Verbal Learning Test (RAVLT).[55] This test of verbal memory presents the patient with multiple trials of learning a list of 10 words. Following each presentation of the study list, the patient is asked to recall as many words as possible. Following the fifth repetition of this study list, a new study list is introduced followed by a recall trial. Following this recall, the patient is asked to recall as many of the words from the first list as possible. Finally, a recognition test is given if delayed recall is defective. This test provides information on immediate verbal memory, rate of learning, occurrence of retroactive and proactive interference, delayed recall, and recognition.

California Verbal Learning Test (CVLT).[56] This variant of the RAVLT increases the number of words on each list to 16 and uses words belonging to one of four categories of "shopping list" items. The testing procedure is also modified to provide a cued recall where the categories are provided to the patient to aid recall.

Rey-Osterrieth Complex Figure.[57] In this nonverbal test of memory, patients are presented with a difficult-to-verbalize complex line drawing. They are first asked to copy the figure, with no mention of being required to remember the design for later recall. After a brief delay (approximately 3 minutes) the patient is asked to reproduce the design. Delayed memory is tested again in 30 minutes. One potential difficulty with this test is that most of the elements that make up the complex design can be assigned a verbal label (e.g., a square on top of a triangle with a flag on top), so some verbal memory contamination can occur. This difficulty is common to most nonverbal tests of cognitive abilities.

Clinical Situations for Memory Tests

Because memory is a basic ability of higher cognitive function, some assessment of memory ability should be conducted for most patients. Memory assessment is particularly important for patients with suspected dementing illnesses (see Chapter 33), toxic and metabolic conditions (see Chapters 38, 39, and 55), and possible depression (see Chapter 3). When requesting memory assessment, information on form of memory tested should be provided.

PERCEPTION AND CONSTRUCTION ABILITIES

The ability to perceive stimuli is one of the basic requirements for the assessment of cognitive function. Therefore, tests of visual, auditory, and tactile perception are common in neuropsychological assessments. Certain alterations in perception, such as neglect, are diagnostically informative.

Visual Perception and Construction

Tests of visual perception typically assess color perception, object recognition, visual organizational abilities, visual scanning, and differentiation of figure from ground. Most neuropsychological assessments will assess color perception informally. The Color Vision Screening Inventory[58] is occasionally used by examiners, however. This test provides a screening measure of color blindness.

Peabody Picture Vocabulary Test–Revised.[59] This test is discussed in the section on Tests of Verbal Function; it can be used to assess ability to visually recognize objects.

Benton Facial Recognition Test.[60] This test of visual object recognition uses faces as stimuli. Patients are presented with a target face on one page and six faces on the adjacent page. One of the six faces matches the target face. The test progresses in difficulty from easy (a duplicate of the target face is presented in the six faces) to hard (the matching face differs from the target face in orientation and lighting). Since both the target and matching face are seen together, memory requirements are minimized.

Judgment of Line Orientation (JLO).[61] This test assesses ability to match lines of different orientation to target lines. Difficulty increases on this test by varying the length of the matching lines. Since both target and matching lines are seen together, memory requirements are minimized.

Hooper Visual Organization Test (HVOT).[62] This test presents the patient with 30 easily recognized objects that have been decomposed into parts and randomized. The patient is required to identify each object. Successful performance on this test requires the patient to mentally reorganize the decomposed images into the complete shape. There have been a number of normative studies of performance on the HVOT, but none is fully adequate.

Picture Arrangement.[16] This subtest of the WAIS-III requires the patient to rearrange a series of pictures that, when placed in the correct order, tell a story. One advantage of this test is the extensive normative data generated for the WAIS-III.

Letter Cancellation Test.[35] This visual scanning test is discussed in the section on Tests of Attention and Vigilance. When systematic errors occur on this test, such that the patient completes only one side of the page, the possibility of visual neglect is raised.

Line Bisection Test.[63] This test presents the patient with lines drawn in different locations on a page. The patient is required to draw a perpendicular line through the lines on the page. Visual scanning is required to locate all the lines on the page. As with the cancellation tests, if systematic errors occur, where the patient does not bisect the line on one side of the page, the possibility of visual neglect is raised.

Embedded Figures Test.[64] This test differentiates figure from ground and consists of 16 line drawings of figures on one page, and a complex figure that contains the target figure and overlapping figures. The patient is required to trace the target figure in the complex figure. Scoring is on a pass-fail basis, with extra credit given for fast performance.

Rey-Osterrieth Complex Figure.[57] This test of visual construction is discussed in the section on Memory. Information on visual construction can be found from performance on the copy portion of this test.

Clock Drawing Test.[65] This test of visual construction in which the patient is required to draw a clock with all the numbers and "set" the clock at 20 minutes to four o'clock. Clock drawing has been a part of bedside mental status testing for a long time, but scoring had been somewhat arbitrary. The addition of explicit scoring criteria has improved interpretation.

Developmental Test of Visual-Motor Integration (VMI).[66] This visual construction test was originally developed for the assessment of children. It is also useful in assessing adult visual constructional abilities, however. The patient is required to copy 24 geometric designs ranging from simple (a single line) to complex. Adequate norms for children exist for this test, and its range of performance can be extended to adults.

Three-Dimensional Block Construction.[67] This test assesses constructional abilities in three dimensions. Patients are presented with 29 blocks of different shapes in a prearranged order. A model is shown to the patient, who is told to use some or all of the blocks to re-create the model. In all, three models are presented to the patient. A maximum of 5 minutes is allowed to complete each model. Adequate norms exist for this test.

Auditory Perception

Auditory perception is tested for acuity, perception of organized sounds, and rhythms.

Sensory Examination.[18] This test is part of the Halstead-Reitan Battery and assesses auditory perception to single and simultaneous stimulations. The examiner stands behind the patient and gently rubs two fingers together next to each ear. This tests auditory perceptual problems in each ear, and also the presence of extinction to double-simultaneous stimulation.

Speech–Sound Perception Test.[18] This test is part of the Halstead-Reitan Battery. Patients listen to 60 nonsense syllables on a tape and must choose among four options of printed versions of the sounds. One problem with this test is that individuals who have high-frequency hearing loss tend to perform poorly.

Seashore Rhythm Test.[18] This test is part of the Halstead-Reitan Battery. Patients listen to two sets of tape-recorded rhythms and are required to judge whether the rhythms are the same or different. The test includes easy items with a few beats and complex items with many beats. Because the patient must remember the first rhythm and must attend rapidly to changing stimuli, this test also measures memory and attention.

Tactile Abilities

Testing of tactile abilities in most neuropsychological assessments is limited to the hands. This information is particularly important for assessing the effects of tactile deficits on test performance.

Sensory Examination.[18] This test is part of the Halstead-Reitan Battery. The tactile ability assessment includes Fingertip Number Writing, where the examiner traces a number on each finger and asks the patient to report the number without visual guidance, and Tactile Finger Recognition (discussed in the section on Tests of Attention and Vigilance), where the patient must identify which finger has been touched by the examiner without visual guidance.

Face–Hand Test.[18, 68] This is a test of single and simultaneous stimuli on either side of the patient's hand, face, or both. Information from this test is helpful in identifying the presence of tactile inattention.

Tactile Form Perception.[69] This test requires the patient to recognize geometric forms placed in one hand hidden from view, and identify a drawing of the object in a multiple-choice format. Adequate norms are provided for this test. A variant of this test is found in the Halstead-Reitan Battery, which uses three-dimensional forms and requests verbal responses as opposed to multiple-choice responses.

Clinical Situations for Tests of Perception and Construction Abilities

Assessment of perception and construction abilities is very important, not only to aid in diagnosis of inattention (neglect) and constructional apraxia, but also to assess the competency of basic skills required for adequate testing. Most of the tests presented also can assess attention and vigilance. Testing is appropriate for all patients except perhaps for those with alterations in level of consciousness (see Chapter 1), or dementia (see Chapter 33).

EXECUTIVE FUNCTION AND MOTOR PERFORMANCE

Executive Function

Traditionally, executive functions have been ascribed to the frontal lobes. They involve the ability to assess ongoing stimuli for relevance to specific goals, the formation of goals, planning action to achieve goals, ability to evaluate plans for efficacy, and executing plans. According to this description, executive functions involve many processes associated with reasoning and intellectual performance. Indeed, the Digit Symbol subtest of the WAIS-R (discussed in the section on Tests of Attention and Vigilance), Category Test, Wisconsin Card Sorting Test, Raven's Progressive Matrices (all discussed in the section on Tests of Reasoning and Problem Solving Through Concept Formation), Rey-Osterrieth Complex Figure (discussed in the section on Memory), and tests of visual scanning (discussed in the section on Perception and Construction Abilities) can all be used to assess executive function. Following is a list of a few additional tests.

Porteus Mazes.[70] This test of planning requires the patient to trace a path through progressive difficult mazes without entering any blind alleys. Scoring is based on number of errors (entering a blind alley) and on time to complete the mazes. Both of these measures have been found to be sensitive to patients with frontal-lobe damage.

Design Fluency.[71] This test of mental flexibility requires the patient to create as many designs as possible that are not objects or shapes in 5 minutes. Next, the patient is required to make as many designs as possible using only four lines (straight or curved) in 4 minutes. Adequate norms exist for this test.

Stroop Word–Color Interference Test.[72] This test of inhibition has three trials. The first trial requires the patient to read the color names printed in black ink as quickly as possible. On the second trial, the patient is required to name the color of colored dots as quickly as possible. The third trial requires the patient to name the color of ink of color name words. The color name does not match the color of the ink. Forty-five seconds are allowed for completion of each trial. Scores for each trial indicate the number of correct responses. An interference score can be generated that quantifies the patient's ability to inhibit the inappropriate response of reading the color name as opposed to the color of ink used to print the name in the third trial.

Motor Performance Tests

Assessment of motor performance is particularly helpful in identifying integrity of each hemisphere and subtle motor performance. Tests of motor performance include simple motor speed, strength, and complex motor/dexterity abilities.

Finger Tapping Test.[73] This is a test of primary motor speed of the index finger of each hand. Patients tap a finger as quickly as possible for five consecutive 10-second trials. Because fatigue may affect performance, a rest period is given between each trial. Large differences between left and right finger speed may reflect lateralized hemispheric dysfunction. Adequate norms are available for this test.

Hand Dynamometer.[18] This test measures grip strength in each hand. Patients are given three trials with each hand, the first considered practice. Large differences between left and right grip strength may reflect lateralized hemispheric dysfunction. Adequate norms are available for this test.

Purdue Pegboard Test.[74] This test of finger dexterity requires patients to place pegs in vertically arranged holes. They perform the task using each hand separately and then using both hands. Each trial last 30 seconds. Large differences between left and right performance in comparison to performance using both hands may reflect lateralized hemispheric dysfunction. Adequate norms are available for this test.

Clinical Situations for Tests of Executive Function and Motor Performance

Assessment of executive function is very important for patients presenting with impairments of higher cognitive functioning such as memory, language, and reasoning. Because these higher-cognitive functions are highly correlated with planning, inhibition of inappropriate responses, and goal execution, executive function assessment also aids the examiner in interpretation of tests assessing memory, language, intelligence, and reasoning performance. Assessment of executive function is also helpful in patients with disturbances in level of consciousness (see Chapter 1), disrupted sleep/wake cycles (see Chapter 2), and neglect and dyspraxia (see Chapter 4).

EMOTIONAL FUNCTIONING

Most assessments of emotional functioning are conducted during the interview with the patient. This information can be gathered in a standardized or nonstandardized format. Tests of emotional functioning ought to be used to generate hypotheses as to the presence of dysfunction with follow-up of these hypotheses occurring during the interview (see Chapter 3). There are two general formats to tests of emotional functioning: objective tests and projective tests. Only objective tests will be presented in this section.

Minnesota Multiphasic Personality Inventory-2 (MMPI-2).[75] This self-report test is an objective measure of personality function composed of 567 true-false questions. The questions were chosen based on their ability to differentiate emotionally impaired individuals from nonimpaired individuals. The MMPI-2 has 10 clinical scales and 4 validity scales. Profiles of the clinical scales can suggest the presence of many different emotional disorders, ranging from mild depression to psychotic conditions. This test has acceptable norms, although the standardization sample was limited in racial diversity. Care needs to be exercised in the interpretation of the MMPI-2 when applied to patients with brain damage, because many of the symptoms elicited by MMPI-2 questions are common to neurological patients.

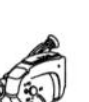

Beck Depression Inventory.[76] This objective self-report measure assesses the presence of depressive symptoms experienced by the patient within the past week. It is composed of 21 questions. Each question is scored on a 4-point scale ranging from no impairment (0) to severe impairment (3). The maximum score is 63; a cut-off score indicative of mild depressive symptoms is greater than 10 and for severe depressive symptoms is greater than 30. One problem with the use of the Beck Depression Inventory with brain-damaged patients is that many of the items reflect somatic concerns and social changes associated with neurologic damage.

Geriatric Depression Scale.[77] This objective self-report measure of depression was designed for use in elderly patients. The test consists of 30 yes or no questions. A cut-off score of 13 is recommended as an indication of depression.

Clinical Situations for Tests of Emotional Functioning

The assessment of emotional functioning is important for three reasons. First, emotional disturbance often follows or accompanies CNS damage. Examples include cerebrovascular disease (see Chapters 22 and 45), neurodegenerative disorders (see Chapters 33–36), and metabolic, nutritional and drug-induced encephalopathies (see Chapters 38–40 and 55). Not only do patients face adjustments to physical function, they also often must make social adjustments that can affect emotional functioning. Second, emotional disturbances can affect cognitive functioning. Although the diagnosis of pseudodementia, or dementia related to depression, does not appear to be real dementia, severe depression can cause impairments in attention, vigilance, and motivation, which may affect performance on memory tests. Third, assessment of emotional functioning is required to differentiate functional from neurological disorders.

Practical Issues

In order to serve the patient best, neuropsychological assessments need to be a cooperative effort between the neuropsychologist and the referring neurologist. The neurologist needs to be as specific as possible when formulating the referral questions. Any pertinent patient information, such as current and past medical status, current medications, brief description on the history of the present illness, and a brief review of physical and neurologic examination results should also be provided. This information helps guide the neuropsychologist in the selection of testing materials and approach to the patient. If testing is to be conducted in the hospital, the patient's schedule needs to include blocks of time when no other clinical tests are scheduled (e.g., radiology, discharge planning) so that the patient may be tested without interruptions and when maximally alert and attentive. The neuropsychologist needs to communicate with the neurologist before testing to discuss the assessment plan, including which cognitive abilities will be tested, the approximate length of testing, and when the neurologist can expect the written report. After the assessment is completed, but before submitting the written report, the neuropsychologist generally contacts the neurologist to provide preliminary feedback. The written report, delivered shortly thereafter, should be brief but complete, including a listing of the tests administered, some form of score report, usually a percentile or standard score for each test, a summary of the findings, and an interpretation of these findings. The brevity of the report depends on the nature of the referral and the questions the neurologist has posed.

Reviews and Selected Updates

Connolly JF, D'Arcy RC: Innovation in neuropsychological assessment using event-related brain potentials. Int J Psychophysiol 2000;37:31–47.

Filipek PA, Accardo PJ, Ashwal S, et al: Practice parameter: screening and diagnosis of autism: report of the Quality Standards Subcommittee of the American Academy of Neurology and the Child Neurology Society. Neurology 2000;55:468–479.

Gioia GA, Isquith PK, Guy SC, Kenworthy L: Behavior rating inventory of executive function. Neuropsychol Dev Cogn Sect C Child Neuropsychol 2000;6:235–238.

Jones BL, Eberle JA: Learning disabilities: diagnostic considerations from an educational perspective. Semin Clin Neuropsychiatry 2000;5:157–163.

Kolb B, Whishaw IQ: Fundamentals of Human Neuropsychology, 3rd ed. New York, W.H. Freeman, 1990.

Lezak MD: Neuropsychological Assessment, 3rd ed. New York, Oxford University Press, 1995.

McCaffrey RJ, Williams AD, Fisher JM, Laing LC: The Practice of Forensic Neuropsychology: Meeting Challenges in the Courtroom. New York, Plenum Press, 1997.

Shuren JE, Grafman J: The neurology of reasoning. Arch Neurol 2002;59:916–919.

Spreen O, Strauss E: A Compendium of Neuropsychological Tests. Administration, Norms, and Commentary. New York, Oxford University Press, 1991.

Taylor MJ, Heaton RK: Sensitivity and specificity of WAIS-III/WMS-III demographically corrected factor scores in neuropsychological assessment. J Int Neuropsychol Soc 2001;7:867–874.

Verfaellie M, O'Connor M: A neuropsychological analysis of memory and amnesia. Semin Neurol 2000;20:455–462.

Zigmond MJ, Bloom FE, Landis SC, et al: Fundamental Neuroscience. San Diego, Academic Press, 1997.

References

1. Spurzheim JG: Phrenology. Philadelphia, Lippincott, 1908.
2. Berker EA, Berker AH, Smith A: Translation of Broca's 1865 report. Arch Neurol 1986;43:1065–1072.
3. James W: The Principles of Psychology. New York, Dover, 1890.
4. Watson JB: Behaviorism, rev. ed. New York, Norton, 1930.
5. Lashley KS: Brain Mechanisms and Intelligence: A Quantitative Study of Injuries to the Brain. Chicago, University of Chicago Press, 1929.
6. Goldstein K: The Organism. New York, American Book, 1939.
7. Halstead WC: Brain and Intelligence. Chicago, University of Chicago Press, 1947.
8. Luria AR: Higher Cortical Functions in Man. New York, Basic Books, 1966.
9. Kaplan E: A process approach to neuropsychological assessment. *In* Boll T, Bryant BK (eds): Clinical Neuropsychology and Brain Function: Research, Measurement, and Practice. Washington, American Psychological Association, 1988, pp 14–38.
10. Therapeutics and Technology Assessment Subcommittee of the American Academy of Neurology: Assessment: neuropsychological testing of adults. Considerations for neurologists. Arch Neurol 1996;47:592–599.
11. Costa L: Clinical neuropsychology: prospects and problems. Clinical Neuropsychologist 1988;2:3–11.
12. Stordant M: Longitudinal studies of aging and age-associated dementias. *In* Boller F, Grafman J (eds): Handbook of Neuropsychology, Vol 4. Amsterdam, Elsevier, 1990, pp 32–39.
13. Kaszniak AW, Bortz JJ: Issues in evaluating the cost-effectiveness of neuropsychological assessments in rehabilitation settings. *In* Glueckauf RL, Sechrest LB, Bond GR, McDonel EC (eds): Improving Assessment in Rehabilitation and Health. Thousand Oaks, CA, Sage, 1993, pp 176–195.
14. Anastasi A: Psychological Testing. New York, Macmillan, 1982.
15. Russell EW: The psychometric foundation of clinical neuropsychology. *In* Filskov SB, Boll TJ (eds): Handbook of Clinical Neuropsychology, Vol 2. New York, John Wiley, 1986, pp 45–80.
16. Wechsler D: WAIS-R Manual. New York, Psychological Corp., 1981.
17. Heaton RK, Grant I, Matthews CG: Comprehensive Norms for an Expanded Halstead-Reitan Battery: Demographic Corrections, Research Findings, and Clinical Applications. Odessa, TX, Psychological Assessment Resources, 1991.
18. Reitan RM, Wolfson D: The Halstead-Reitan Neuropsychological Test Battery: Theory and Clinical Interpretation. Tucson, AZ, Neuropsychology Press, 1985.
19. Golden CJ, Purisch AD, Hammeke TA: Luria-Nebraska Neuropsychological Battery: Forms I and II. Los Angeles, Western Psychological Services, 1985.
20. Christensen AL: Luria's Neuropsychological Investigation, 2nd ed. Copenhagen, Munksgaard, 1979.
21. Spiers PA: Have they come to praise Luria or to bury him? The Luria-Nebraska Battery controversy. J Consult Clin Psychol 1981;49:331–341.
22. Folstein MF, Folstein SE, McHugh PR: Mini-mental state: a practical method for grading the cognitive state of outpatients for the clinician. J Psychiatr Res 1975;12:189–198.
23. Wechsler D: Wechsler Memory Scale–Revised. New York, Psychological Corp., 1987.
24. Benton AL, Van Allen MW, Fogel ML: Temporal orientation in cerebral disease. J Nerv Ment Dis 1964;139:110–119.
25. Money J: A Standardized Road Map Test of Directional Sense. Manual. San Rafael, CA, Academic Therapy Publishers, 1976.
26. Benton AL: Right-Left Discrimination and Finger Localization. New York, Hoeber-Harper, 1959.
27. Benton AL, Hamsher K, Varney NR, Spreen O: Contributions to Neuropsychological Assessment. New York, Oxford University Press, 1983.
28. Kahn RL, Miller NE: Assessment of altered brain function in the aged. *In* Stordant M, Siegler I, Ellis M (eds): The Clinical Psychology of Aging. New York, Plenum Press, 1978, pp 43–70.
29. Pfeiffer E: SPMSQ: Short Portable Mental Status Questionnaire. J Am Geriatr Soc 1975;23:433–441.
30. Miller GA: The magical number seven, plus or minus two: some limits on our capacity for processing information. Psych Rev 1956;63:81–97.
31. Milner B: Interhemispheric differences in the localization of psychological processes in man. Brit Med Bul 1979;27:272–277.
32. Gronwall DMA: Paced Auditory Serial Addition Task: a measure of recovery from concussion. Precept Mot Skills 1977;44:367–373.
33. Smith A: Sumbol Digit Modalities Test (SDMT). Manual (revised). Los Angeles, Western Psychological Services, 1982.
34. Army Individual Test Battery. Manual of Directions and Scoring. Washington, DC, War Department, Adjutant General's Office, 1944.
35. Talland GA, Schwab RS: Performance with multiple sets in Parkinson's disease. Neuropsychologia 1964;2:45–53.
36. Wechsler D: Wechsler Intelligence Scale for Children, 3rd ed. San Antonio, TX, Psychological Corp., 1991.
37. Wechsler D: Manual for the Wechsler Preschool and Primary Scale of Intelligence. New York, Psychological Corp., 1967.
38. Larrabee GJ: Another look at VIQ-PIQ scores and unilateral brain damage. Int J Neurosci 1986;29:141–148.
39. Wilson RS, Stebbins GT: Interpreting the findings: Estimating premorbid ability and preexisting neuropsychological deficits. *In* Doerr HO, Carlin A (eds): Forensic Neuropsychology. New York, Guilford Press, 1991, pp 89–98.
40. Wilson RS, Rosenbaum G, Brown G: The problem of premorbid intelligence in neuropsychological assessment. J Clin Neuropsych 1979;1:49–54.

41. Barona A, Reynolds CR, Chastain R: A demographically based index of premorbid intelligence for the WAIS-R. J Consult Clinical Psychol 1984;52:885–887.
42. Nelson HE: The National Adult Reading Test (NART): Test Manual. Windsor, UK, NFER-Nelson, 1982.
43. Stebbins GT, Wilson RS, Gilley DW, et al: Use of the National Adult Reading Test to estimate premorbid IQ in dementia. Clin Neuropsychol 1990;4:18–24.
44. Matarazzo JD: Wechsler's Measurement and Appraisal of Adult Intelligence, 5th ed. Baltimore, Williams & Wilkins, 1972.
45. Markwardt FC: The Peabody Individual Achievement Test–Revised. Circle Pines, MN, American Guidance Service, 1989.
46. Jastak JF, Wilkinson GS: Wide Range Achievement Test–Revised. Wilmington, DE, Jastak Assessment Systems, 1984.
47. Raven JC, Court JH, Raven J: Manual for Raven's Progressive Matrices. London, H.K. Lewis, 1976.
48. Heaton RK: Wisconsin Card Sorting Test. Manual. Odessa, TX, Psychological Assessment Resources, 1981.
49. Goodglass H, Kaplan E: The Assessment of Aphasia and Related Disorders, 2nd ed. Philadelphia, Lea and Febiger, 1987.
50. Benton AL, Hamsher K: Multilingual Aphasia Examination. Iowa City, IA, AJA Associates, 1989.
51. Spreen O, Benton AL: Neurosensory Center Comprehensive Examination for Aphasia. Victoria, BC, University of Victoria Neuropsychology Laboratory, 1977.
52. Snow WG: Standardization of test administration and scoring criteria: Some shortcomings of current practice with the Halstead-Reitan Test Battery. Clin Neuropsychol 1987;1:250–262.
53. De Renzi E, Vignolo L: The Token Test: a sensitive test to detect receptive disturbances in aphasics. Brain 1962;85:665–678.
54. Kaplan EF, Goodglass H, Weintraub S: The Boston Naming Test, 2nd ed. Philadelphia, Lea and Febiger, 1983.
55. Rey A: L'examen clinique en psychologie. Paris, FR, Press Universaire de France, 1964.
56. Delis DC, Kramer JH, Kaplan E, Ober BA: California Verbal Learning Test: Adult Version. San Antonio, TX, Psychological Corp., 1987.
57. Osterrieth PA: Le test de copie d'une figure complex: Contribution a l'etude de la perception et de la memoire. Archives de Psychologie 1944;30:286–356.
58. Coren S, Hakstian A: Color vision screen without the use of technical equipment: Scale development and cross validation. Precept Psychophys 1988;43:115–120.
59. Dunn LM, Dunn LM: Peabody Picture Vocabulary Test-Revised. Manual. Circle Pines, MN, American Guidance Service, 1981.
60. Benton AL, Van Allen MW: Impairment in facial recognition in patients with cerebral disease. Cortex 1968;4:344–358.
61. Benton AL, Hannay HJ, Varney NR: Visual perception of line direction in patients with unilateral brain disease. Neurol 1975;25:907–910.
62. Hooper HE: The Hooper Visual Organization Test. Manual. Beverly Hills, CA, Western Psychological Services, 1958.
63. Schenkenberg T, Bradford DC, Ajax ET: Line bisection and unilateral visual neglect in patients with neurologic impairment. Neurol 1989;30:509–517.
64. Spreen O, Benton AL: Embedded Figures Test. Victoria, BC, University of Victoria, 1969.
65. Strub RL, Black FW: The Mental Status Examination in Neurology. Philadelphia, F.A. Davis, 1977.
66. Beery KE: Developmental Test of Visual-Motor Integration. Administration and Scoring Manual. Chicago, Follett Publishers, 1967.
67. Benton AL: Visuoperceptive, visuospatial, and visuoconstructive disorders. *In* Heilman KM, Valenstein E (eds): Clinical Neuropsychology. New York, Oxford University Press, 1979.
68. Bender MB, Fink M, Green M: Patterns in perception on simultaneous tests of face and hand. Arch Neurol Psychiat 1951;66:355–362.
69. Weinstein S: Functional cerebral hemispheric asymmetry. *In* Kinsbourne M (ed): Asymmetrical Function of the Brain. Cambridge, Cambridge University Press, 1978, pp 17–48.
70. Porteus SD: Porteus Maze Test. Fifty Years Application. New York, Psychological Corp., 1965.
71. Jones-Gotman M, Milner B: Design fluency: The invention of nonsense drawings after focal cortical lesions. Neuropsychologia 1977;15:653–674.
72. Stroop JR: Studies of interference in serial verbal reactions. J Exp Psychol 1935;18:643–662.
73. Spreen O, Strauss E: A Compendium of Neuropsychological Tests. Administration, Norms, and Commentary. New York, Oxford University Press, 1991.
74. Purdue Research Foundation: Purdue Pegboard Test. Lafayette, Indiana, Lafayette Instrument, no date.
75. Butcher JN, Dahlstrom WG, Graham JR, et al: MMPI-2: Minnesota Multiphasic Personality Inventory-2. Manual for Administration and Scoring. Minneapolis, University of Minnesota Press, 1989.
76. Beck AT: Beck Depression Inventory. San Antonio, Psychological Corp., 1987.
77. Yesavage J, Brink TL: Development and validation of a geriatric depression scale: a preliminary report. J Psychiatr Res 1983;17:37–49.

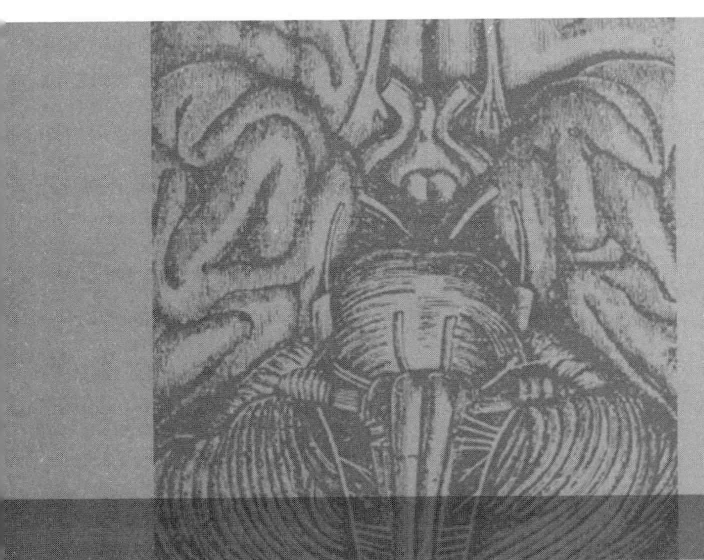

PART THREE

Etiological Categories of Neurological Diseases

CHAPTER 28

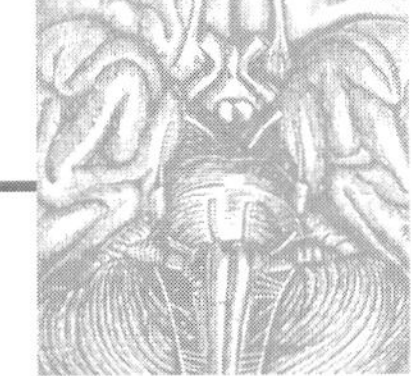

JEFFREY A. GOLDEN and CARSTEN G. BÖNNEMANN

Developmental Structural Disorders

This chapter reviews the major structural malformations and associated problems related to the central nervous system (CNS) and surrounding structures. Hydrocephalus, although not a specific structural disorder, is discussed in the first section because of the importance and frequency with which hydrocephalus occurs in many of the disorders that follow in the chapter. Furthermore, the evaluation and diagnosis of hydrocephalus plays a pivotal role in clinical management of many malformations. Following hydrocephalus, disorders of development are discussed according to the approximate developmental timing of the pathogenesis. Because the developmental timing for many disorders is not known or is only speculative, disorders have also been grouped into major categories.

Hydrocephalus

Hydrocephalus is one of the most common manifestations of developmental disorders. A fundamental understanding of the principles, evaluation, and management of congenital and neonatal hydrocephalus is essential for physicians involved in the care of infants with developmental structural disorders of the CNS. Hydrocephalus, in the strictest definition, denotes an increased volume of cerebrospinal fluid (CSF) within the skull, most frequently in the ventricles. Unfortunately the use of various definitions in a wide variety of clinical presentations and pathological abnormalities has resulted in confusion surrounding the definition and meaning of the term *hydrocephalus*. In this chapter, hydrocephalus is defined as an increase in the volume of CSF within the ventricular system independent of the actual head circumference. Entities such as "normal pressure hydrocephalus" will not be discussed as they are generally not considered malformations and occur mainly in an adult population.

Pathogenesis and Pathophysiology. In contrast with normal CSF physiology discussed in Chapter 26, hydrocephalus is the result of a disturbance in normal CSF fluid dynamics. Two terms frequently used when discussing hydrocephalus are obstructive (noncommunicating) and nonobstructive (communicating) hydrocephalus. These terms were first coined by Harvey Cushing to describe the results of injection of air (pneumoencephalography) into the subarachnoid space or dye into the ventricles. If the air was found to move into the ventricles or the dye out to the subarachnoid space, the cause of the hydrocephalus was considered nonobstructive. If no communication between the spaces was found, the cause of the hydrocephalus was considered obstructive. These terms were used to help define the pathophysiological mechanisms underlying the hydrocephalus. While conceptually appealing, Adams and Victor[1] challenged the value of this distinction, pointing out that increased pressure leading to hydrocephalus is virtually always a result of blockage,[2] whether along the pathway of CSF flow or at the site of resorption. Overproduction of CSF, as reported in rare cases of choroid plexus papillomas, is not likely to represent a common, if even plausible, cause of hydrocephalus. Thus, the entities included in this section, with the exception of the destructive lesions, will be discussed, when known, in reference to where the blockage occurs (Table 28–1).

Hydrocephalus associated with congenital malformations and disruptions often is associated with flattened gyri and reduced sulci. If hydrocephalus develops in utero, the cerebral hemispheres may show an abnormal gyral pattern characterized by multiple complex small gyri. This abnormal gyration has been called microgyria, polygyria, or stenogyria. It is important to distinguish this gyral abnormality from polymicrogyria (see later discussion). The primary basis for distinction relies on the abnormal cortical lamination in polymicrogyria and the normal cortical cytoarchitecture in hydrocephalus related to gyral abnormalities. Although a six-layer neocortex is recognized in polygyria, neuronal populations may be significantly reduced. It is equally important to remember that true polymicrogyria and hydrocephalus may coexist in certain malformations.

When hydrocephalus occurs as a function of increasing intracranial CSF fluid volume, intracranial pressure will begin to increase as well. In an attempt to relieve the increased intracranial pressure the head circumference will begin increasing by widening of the sutures. Although the cranial sutures have begun fusion by 2 years of age, they can often be "split" open if the intracranial pressure rises prior to the age of complete skull ossification (8 to 10 years). At the same time the fontanelles, if still open, will become tense and bulging. The majority of conditions that are discussed in this chapter result in hydrocephalus prior to fusion of the cranial sutures; thus, an enlarging head occurs concurrently with the hydrocephalus.

Clinical Features and Associated Disorders. Signs and symptoms of postnatal hydrocephalus depend on the expandability of the skull. As outlined earlier, prior to fusion of the sutures the skull is able to expand, resulting in an enlarged head circumference and tense fontanelles. In addition to the finding of a tense or bulging fontanelle, the separation of sutures can give rise to the so-called "cracked pot" sound on percussion of the skull. The scalp veins may be prominent, especially frontally. The absolute head circumference measured at only one time point cannot be used as a strict diagnostic guide; instead, it is important to follow the trajectory of the head circumference plot over a brief period of time. Any upward crossing of percentiles over a few weeks is potentially relevant and requires urgent investigation. Clinical signs and symptoms may be minimal or completely absent.[3] When present, irritability, frequent crying, unexplained vomiting (especially in the morning), and persistent or increasing headaches may all signal hydrocephalus. Alternatively, as a result of chronically increased intracranial pressure there may be developmental delay, disinterest in the environment with a "dull" affect, endocrine dysfunction, unsteady gait, and increased tone in the legs.[4] In the newborn period bradyarrhythmia and apneic spells may be the only clinical sign of overt hydrocephalus.

Ophthalmological signs often occur early and are important to recognize. Disturbances of extraocular movements include a supranuclear upgaze paresis, giving rise to the "setting sun phenomenon" in infants. In this condition, the eyes appear driven downwards and the white of the sclera is seen above the iris. This phenomenon is probably related to aqueductal distention with compression of periaqueductal structures, or by pressure on the quadrigeminal plate by a dilated third ventricular subpineal recess. Unilateral or bilateral abducens and/or trochlear paresis can also occur. Swelling of the optic nerve head (papilledema) occurs in hydrocephalus before closure of the sutures only with very rapidly progres-

TABLE 28–1. **Overview of the Differential Diagnosis of Congenital Hydrocephalus**

Etiology	Specific Causes*	Mechanism of Hydrocephalus
Tumors	Most types, benign and malignant	Blockage of CSF pathway
Malformations	Many	
	Chiari II	Unknown
	Dandy-Walker	Unknown
	Aqueductal anomalies	Obstruction of CSF flow at the level of the cerebral aqueduct
	Forking/stenosis	
	X-linked hydrocephalus	
Infectious/post-infectious	Abscess	Obstruction by a mass lesion
	Meningitis/ventriculitis	Obstruction of CSF resorption and/or obstruction due to fusion of ventricular wall
	Congenital infections	
	CMV	Adhesions and fusion of ventricular wall
	Toxoplasmosis	Ex vacuo and/or mass lesion
Vascular/hemorrhagic	Vascular malformation	Mass lesion of post-hemorrhage
	Post-hemorrhagic	
	Germinal matrix origin	Intraventricular blood obstructs CSF flow
	Choroid plexus origin	
Destructive	Hydranecephaly	Ex vacuo
Secondary	Porencephaly	Ex vacuo
	Perinatal leukomalacia	Ex vacuo

*The entities listed are only a partial list and are not meant to reflect a complete differential diagnosis.

sive hydrocephalus. On the other hand, chronic and long-standing hydrocephalus can lead to optic atrophy, resulting in papilledema no longer being apparent. In neonatal hydrocephalus stretching of the optic radiations and cortices can also result in a picture of cortical blindness. Another unusual neurological manifestation of hydrocephalus is the so called "bobble-head-doll" syndrome, in which the patient shows rhythmical to-and-fro movements of the head in the upright position. It is related to obstructive lesions in and around the aqueduct as well as to cystic lesions of the third ventricle, but its pathophysiology is unknown.

Long-standing untreated hydrocephalus has been associated with a neuropsychological profile referred to as the "cocktail-party syndrome."[5] Characteristic manifestations include a fluent and profuse speech that lacks content and is pragmatically deficient. Chronic hydrocephalus may also result in precocious puberty. Earlier detection, primarily as a result of improved imaging of the central nervous system, along with advances in treatment and management have resulted in these manifestations of chronic hydrocephalus being relatively rare.

The special case, a hereditary form of hydrocephalus, occurs in familial aqueductal stenosis, most frequently inherited as an X-linked trait. Mutations in the gene for L1-CAM, a neuronal surface glycoprotein implicated in migration and fasciculation of neuronal cells,[6] have been identified in one subtype (linked to chromosome Xq28). How mutations in this molecule lead to aqueductal stenosis is unclear. The condition should be considered in diagnosing both infants and children with hydrocephalus because, in the case of Xq28-linked familial aqueductal stenosis, in about 50 percent of affected males, mental retardation, spastic paraparesis, and adducted thumbs may not become apparent until later in life.

Differential Diagnosis. Hydrocephalus does not necessarily mean an enlarged head, although an enlarged or enlarging head often is the presenting feature. The converse is also not necessarily true; an enlarged head (macrocephaly) is not equivalent to hydrocephalus. Several metabolic disorders, hamartomatos, and other genetic conditions can be associated with macrocephaly independent of hydrocephalus.[7] If the brain itself is enlarged without a significant component of hydrocephalus, the term megalencephaly is appropriately applied. Examples include neurofibromatosis type I, several of the overgrowth syndromes such as Sotos syndrome, Alexander's disease, metabolic disorders such as Canavan's disease, several of the gangliosidoses, and glutaricaciduria type I. Malformations and disruptions with enlarged ventricles but without CSF flow obstruction have to be differentiated by careful imaging. Holoprosencephaly and hydranencephaly provide examples. In the newborn, congenital infections, especially toxoplasmosis, must be considered as well as the possibility of preceding intracerebral hemorrhage potentially causing aqueductal stenosis as well as diminished CSF absorption. Space-occupying lesions around the midbrain, tectum, and pineal region must also be excluded by appropriate imaging studies.

Evaluation. The diagnosis of hydrocephalus relies on the application of neuroimaging techniques combined with the clinical features outlined in the beginning of this section.[8] Plain radiographs of the skull may show an irregular, shallow scalloping of the inner bone table. Although hydrocephalus will be obvious on computed tomography (CT) or cranial ultrasound, precise anatomical definition of the blockage level is best investigated by magnetic resonance imaging (MRI). Assessment of the cerebral aqueduct in the sagittal plane, including evaluation of a flow void through the aqueduct, is also possible via this technique. On CT or MRI, CSF driven transependymally into the periventricular white matter may be apparent as low attenuation on CT or high signal on T2-weighted MRI sequences.

Evaluation must take into account whether the cranial sutures are open or closed. The ventricular size with an expandable skull versus a fixed volume skull can be dramatically different even with an equal increase in intraventricular pressure. In the case of open sutures, even moderate rises of pressure can expand the ventricles enormously and the surrounding brain may appear compressed to a thin band. A dramatic reconstitution of the cerebral mantle may be seen after shunting, sometimes with reversion of some pre-existing neurological deficits, in particular impaired visual function. On the other hand, in the fixed volume skull, even enormously elevated intraventricular pressures may give rise to only moderate expansion of ventricular size, especially with "communicating" hydrocephalus. "Arrested" or inactive hydrocephalus with apparently normal pressure measurements may pose a special problem for management decisions, as spotcheck measurements of CSF pressure by lumbar puncture may not accurately reflect chronic CSF dynamics. Longer, continuous monitoring of intracranial pressure using a subdural or epidural device has been advocated for such cases. These investigations are not without risk for the patient and are not universally recommended. Meticulous attention to clinical details in order to decide whether the hydrocephalus is symptomatic should guide treatment decisions.

Early prenatal detection of hydrocephalus is possible, but it should be kept in mind that hydrocephalus may develop only after 16 to 18 weeks gestation. Of paramount importance is the detection of additional CNS and extracerebral malformations, as these may heavily influence the prognosis and management decisions.

Management and Prognosis. Shunting of the CSF from the ventricles is the mainstay of therapy for hydrocephalus.[9] The predominant shunt systems currently in use are ventriculoperitoneal shunting (VP) devices with pressure-controlled valves placed under the scalp close to the burr hole. The major complications associated with VP shunt treatment involve mechanical problems, shunt-related infections, and functional problems. Signs of increased intracranial pressure with headache, lethargy, and vomiting will be apparent in most of the situations in which shunting is impaired. Functional overshunting can also occur, albeit less frequently. Headache again is the most common clinical symptom, but in contrast to the headache associated with increased intracranial pressure, headache resulting from overshunting tends to be relieved in the recumbent position. Shunt infections are a serious complication and are most often caused by *Staphylococcus aureus*. Unexplained fever, which can sometimes be low-grade, and chronic or frank meningitis usually is the presenting feature. Treatment is with penicillinase-resistant antibiotics, but culturing the pathogen for determination of drug susceptibility should be attempted in all cases. Replacement of all hardware is frequently necessary. Abdominal complications of VP-shunting include peritonitis, perforation of an abdominal organ, peritoneal cysts, and the development of hydroceles in boys. Seizures, especially during the first year after shunting, occur in approximately 5.5 percent of patients. The incidence of developing seizures declines after the first year. In the Xq28-linked familial aqueductal stenosis VP-shunting is indicated as well. Importantly, the development of mental retardation and spastic paraparesis appears to be independent from the ventricular dilatation per se and does not improve with the treatment.

Under certain circumstances such as neonatal posthemorrhagic hydrocephalus, in which some patients may show resolution of the hydrocephalus without more permanent intervention, temporizing measures may be useful. Daily lumbar punctures removing substantial amounts of CSF have been used, but this treatment still requires more systematic clinical evaluation. Pharmacological intervention consists of a combination of high-dose acetazolamide with furosemide, which can reduce CSF production considerably. Careful monitoring for the development of nephrocalcinosis (particularly problematic in premature infants treated with this combination of drugs) and electrolyte imbalances is essential. The management of neonatal posthemorrhagic hydrocephalus is rather complex and beyond the scope of this chapter.[10]

The detection of a fetal ventriculomegaly by ultrasound has created a new problem in the management of hydrocephalus that requires insight into the natural history of fetal ventriculomegaly.[11, 12] The prognosis is strongly influenced by the co-existence of major neural and extraneural abnormalities. In one large series,[12] 50 percent of detected cases died in utero or the pregnancy was electively terminated, mainly because of the detection of major additional anomalies. Of the remaining 50 percent only a small percentage of cases were found to develop progressive ventriculomegaly in utero on follow-up investigations. These infants were shunted immediately after delivery and had relatively good outcomes. In an even smaller percentage, the ventriculomegaly resolved, also with a favorable outcome. Of the majority that were stable in utero, a little more than half remained stable postnatally and their ultimate prognosis was dependent on the presence of additional associated anomalies and malfunctions. The other group developed postnatal progression of the hydrocephalus requiring shunting. The outcome was good in the infants without additional anomalies. This pattern also holds true for hydrocephalus detected at birth.[13] Given the importance of additional anomalies for the ultimate prognosis, once fetal ventriculomegaly is identified, a complete workup should be conducted at an experienced center. Currently no definite benefit to intrauterine shunting has been demonstrated.

Neural Tube Defects

Defects in formation of the neural tube account for 0.001 to 1 percent of all human malformations, depending on the reference population, making this group of disorders among the most common major malformations. Neural tube closure defects are also among the oldest recorded malformations. For example, a mummy from ancient Egypt, investigated by Etienne Geoffroy Saint-Hilaire, was determined to have anencephaly. A curious observation in the 16th century of a child with a froglike head and face, now believed to represent anencephaly, was born to a woman who had a frog placed on her hand during a febrile illness and represents the first indication that neural tube closure defects may result from environmental factors.[14] This example of "maternal impression," a theory widely postulated for many centuries as the cause of some congenital anomalies, including the "Elephant Man," is noteworthy because of the now recognized association of maternal hyperthermia and neural tube closure defects.[15]

Pathogenesis and Pathophysiology. The prevailing theory on the pathogenesis of neural tube defects is that they result from a failure of the neural folds to come together to form the neural tube as opposed to splaying open of a closed neural tube. Experimental models and studies in humans have supported this contention. Although monoallelic disorders are occasionally associated with neural tube closure defects,[16] most data implicate a multifactorial etiology for the occurrence of neural tube closure defects. Neural tube closure defects are common in animals, including mice, in which mutant strains have been invaluable in identifying many genes important for neural tube closure. Strain differences in the susceptibility to neural tube closure defects have been recognized, consistent with the multifactorial model. Similarly, environmental factors have been identified that result in neural tube closure defects. Recent data also indicate that at least in the cranial region, neural tube closure occurs not in a single continuous closure, but at multiple sites and in a coordinated pattern. Each defined site may be under the control of different genes and be susceptible to different environmental factors (Fig. 28–1).[17, 18]

Given that several of the known environmental risk factors can be controlled, it is important to appreciate the embryonic timing of neural tube closure and therefore the gestational age at which these defects are believed to arise. Closure of the neural folds begins on approximately day 20 after fertilization and is complete by approximately day 28. This is approximately 1 to 2 weeks beyond the time a women is expecting her normal menstrual cycle. Thus, during this critical time of development for the nervous system, a woman is frequently still unaware that she is pregnant. As a result, preventive measures have to be already in place before conception.

Epidemiology and Risk Factors. The past decades have witnessed an overall decline in the incidence of neural tube closure defects, although the etiology for this decline remains elusive. Epidemiological and experimental investigations into potential environmental risk factors, particularly in Wales and Ireland, have failed to identify an obvious single source. Several environmental factors have been linked to neural tube closure defects including maternal diabetes, maternal hyperthermia, and some anticonvulsants (valproic acid and carbamazepine in particular)[19]; however, the elimination of some of these minor risk factors is not sufficient to explain the overall declining incidence.[20] Recently, vitamin supplementation, particularly folate, has been linked to a reduced risk for having a second child with a neural tube closure defect.[21, 22] Preliminary data indicate that similar supplementation may also reduce the risk for all mothers.[23] The mechanisms by which vitamin supplementation prevents neural tube closure defects are poorly understood.

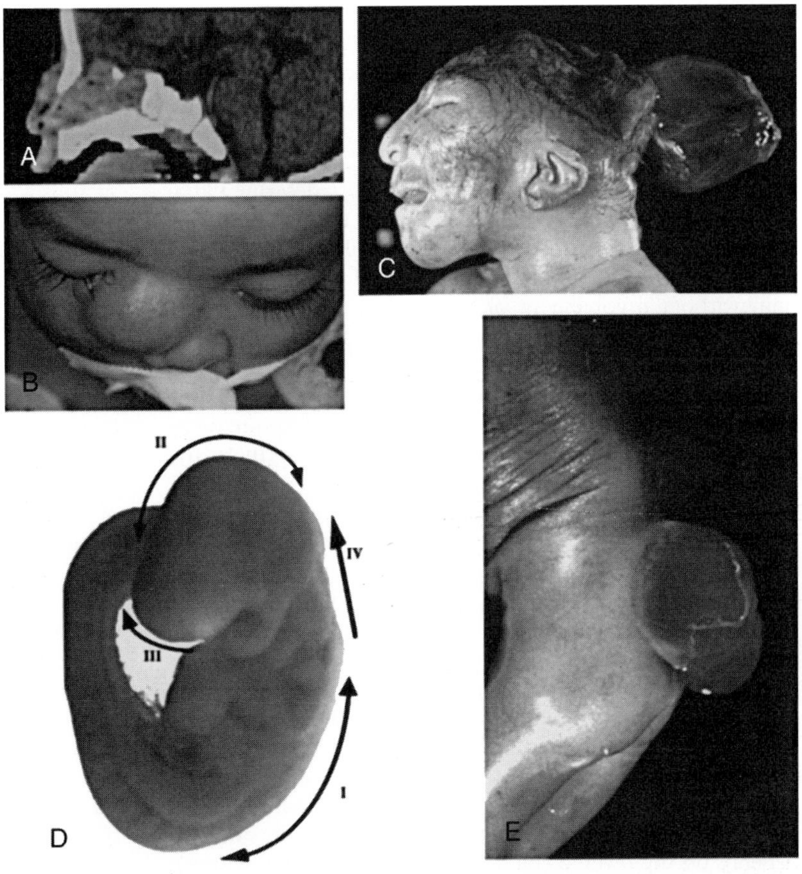

FIGURE 28–1. Neural tube closure defects located at multiple sites along the neuroaxis. A CT scan *(A)* and clinical photograph *(B)* of a patient with a frontal (nasal glioma) encephalocele. *C,* An encephalocele/anencephaly isolated to the occipital region. *D,* This case showed an open defect at the top of the encephalocele with extensive loss of neural tissue, placing this case in the category of anencephaly. *E,* A lumbosacral myelomeningocele with an intact membrane over the defect that involved the spinal cord. A model of neural tube closure defects. Defects in closures III, IV, and I may account for the examples shown in *A* and *B* and *C* and *E,* respectively. (From Golden J, Chernoff G: Intermittent pattern of neural tube closure in two strains of mice. Teratology 1993;47:73-80.)

As alluded to already, it is likely that many factors play roles in the causation of neural tube closure defects, and the actual etiology is more often than not multifactorial. Genetic factors certainly play an important role in at least conferring a predisposition to having a child with a neural tube closure defect. These genetic and environmental factors are likely to act synergistically to increase a women's risk for having a child with a neural tube closure defect.

Clinical Features and Associated Disorders. Neural tube defects can be divided into cranial and caudal, although occasional cases may involve both (e.g., encephalocele in conjunction with myelomeningocele). The terminology of a neural tube closure defect often provides a description of the type and location of the defect. *Anencephaly* in the strict sense means absence of the head, however, the term practically refers to an absence of the brain and the calvarium covering the brain. Although some cases have partial sparing of supratentorial or more commonly infratentorial structures, the vast majority of cases show a complete absence of most of the brain. The anterior pituitary, eyes and lower brain stem are usually spared. Although the tissue fated to become the brain is present in the embryo, it is generally believed that direct contact between the neural epithelium and the amniotic fluid leads to degeneration of the former. The remaining tissue covering the basal cranium is a highly vascular and friable membrane referred to as the *area cerebrovasculosa. Rachischisis* refers to cases of anencephaly with a contiguous spinal defect involving at least the cervical spine region and extending for varying degrees down the spinal column. In the majority of cases there is associated polyhydramnious and a significant proportion are stillborn. Infants born alive do not survive, and their neurological function is primarily limited to brain stem and spinal reflexes. Seizures, at times resembling infantile spasms, have been observed in some infants.

Encephaloceles and cranial meningoceles are distinguished from anencephaly by the former having an epidermal covering over the cranial neural tube closure defects. Both entities are associated with a defect in the skull with protrusion of the leptomeninges alone in the case of a meningocele, and leptomeninges and underlying brain in encephalocele. The size of an encephalocele can vary from a barely visible bulge to those larger than the infant's head. Occasionally, no clear bony defect or attachment to the underlying brain can be identified, particularly with lesions located in the inferior frontonasal region. This form of a frontal encephalocele is sometimes called a "nasal glioma," although the term is misleading because there is no neoplasm. These lesions may not be immediately obvious on external examination and may present as intranasal masses, pharyngeal obstruction, or with recurrent meningitis. Hypertelorism, median cleft lip, or hypothalamic dysfunction can also be associated. The location of an encephalocele can be helpful in the diagnosis of specific syndromes. For example, the Meckel-Gruber and Walker-Warburg syndromes are frequently associated with occipital encephaloceles; anterior encephaloceles are found more commonly in Roberts' syndrome and as isolated malformations more commonly in Southeast Asia. Parietal encephaloceles are less common. The extent of the cortex "herniated" into the cele correlates with the neurological deficits. Malformed cortex within or adjacent to the cele, in addition, can give rise to seizures.

Neural tube closure defects involving the spinal cord can involve the meninges alone (meningocele) or the meninges and underlying spinal cord (myelomeningocele). Most caudal neural tube closure defects occur in the lumbar region, followed by the lumbosacral region, but can also be located in cervical, thoracic, or sacral regions. The terms *spina bifida occulta* and *spina bifida cystica* are also used to describe variations of these defects. These terms refer to the bony changes of the vertebral column. Spina bifida occulta is defined as a defect in the posterior bony components of the vertebral column without involvement of the cord or meninges. These defects are often found incidentally on radiographic studies or are picked up because of a subtle clinical finding such as a tuft of hair or a cutaneous angioma or lipoma in the midline of the back marking the location of the defect. On rare occasions a sinus tract may communicate from the skin to the underlying dura.

The clinical presentation is largely dependent on level and content of the defect. Pure meningoceles without involvement of the spinal cord may be largely asymptomatic. Neurological disability is greatest in patients with myelomeningoceles. Infants with defects at or above L2 are more likely to have skeletal deformities, including kyphosis and scoliosis, dislocated hips, and clubfeet (see later discussion). The degree of motor paresis is dependent on the level of the neural tube closure defect and is discussed in more detail under Management and Prognosis. Involvement of the kidneys, urinary tract, and bladder with various forms of incontinence and reflux is very common and similarly depends on the level of the lesion (see following discussion).

Several disorders frequently included in the spectrum of spinal neural tube defects are tethered cords, spinal lipomas, and sacral teratomas, although these entities do not arise as a result of a failed neural tube closure. Nonetheless, spinal dysraphisms are occasionally associated with these lesions. The etiological relationship between these disorders remains unclear. Tethering of the cord can present late and insidiously with progressive gait disturbances, atrophy of various muscle groups or the entire limb, loss of reflexes, loss of sensation in particular in the sacral dermatomes, and sphincter disturbances.[24] The gait abnormality results from weakness and lower extremity spasticity. Pain in the gluteal, perianal, and other pelvic areas as well as the limbs associated with cramping can occur in particular with later presentation. Early and seemingly fixed deformities as well as sudden and dramatic deteriorations can also be seen. Deteriorations may occur in particular during periods of rapid growth. Partial duplication of the spinal cord, diastatomyelia, can give rise to a similar picture, although the symptoms are often more strictly unilateral.

Myelomeningoceles, particularly those arising in the lumbosacral regions, are frequently associated with other defects along the neuroaxis and the surrounding mesoderm. The cranial bones may show regional thinning resulting in radiographic and transilluminative lucencies. These defects, also known as Lückenschädel, are present in far greater than 50 percent of term children with myelomeningoceles, but are rarely diagnosed after 2 years of age. Although these bony lucencies frequently occur in patients with myelomeningoceles, especially in the additional presence of hydrocephalus, they are not specific for this disorder and may be found incidentally or in association with hydrocephalus only. The base of the skull is also abnormally flattened (platybasia) in most patients with myelomeningoceles, resulting in a shallow angle between the clinoid process and the foramen magnum.

The cerebral hemispheres can show malformations that are not clearly linked to the neural tube defect. The associated anomalies range from those that are found infrequently, such as agenesis of the corpus callosum, polymicrogyria, and pachygyria, to frequent findings such as an enlarged massa intermedia. Probably the most common finding associated with myelomeningocele is the Chiari II malformation, also referred to by some authors as Arnold-Chiari malformation. This hindbrain malformation is present in greater than 95 percent of children with myelomeningoceles. Although a broad spectrum of findings are part of the Chiari II malformation,[25] the change found in virtually all cases includes displacement of the cerebellar vermis (and to a lesser extent the inferior lateral cerebellar hemispheres) over the dorsal aspect of the cervical spinal cord (Fig. 28–2) within the upper vertebral column. The fourth ventricle, pons, and medulla are similarly elongated and partially located within in the spinal canal. The lower medulla may be kinked. Forking of the aqueduct, aqueductal stenosis, and/or aqueductal atresia may be present. Less common findings include fusion (beaking) of the inferior tectum and anomalies of cranial nerve nuclei. Hydrocephalus is a common complication of myelomeningoceles, and may manifest pre- or postnatally. The etiology of the hydrocephalus is not always clear, although the aqueductal changes could account for some of the cases. Clinically, the Chiari II malformation may present with lower brain stem and cranial nerve dysfunction. Dysphagia leading to feeding difficulties, drooling, nasal regurgitation, strider, vocal cord paralysis, and life-threatening apnea spells may all occur. Cyanotic episodes are ominous, carrying a considerable risk of mortality. Nystagmus, retrocollis, and opisthotonus can also be seen. Later presentation of the Chiari II malformation may include additional loss of head control, newly arising weakness in the arms, and increasing spasticity leading to quadriparesis.

In addition to dysraphism, other malformations may be concurrently found in the spinal cord.[25] The two most frequent abnormalities of the spinal cord are hydromyelia (dilations of the central canal) and syringomelia (a glial lined cavity within the parenchyma of the spinal cord). They may occur in isolation or may be found together (hydrosyringomyelia). These disorders may be localized to a short segment of the spinal cord or extend along great distances. It is also important to recognize that these conditions are not specific to dysraphisms and can even occur post-traumatically. Partial (diastematomyelia) and complete (diplomyelia) duplications of the spinal cord are occasionally present in association with myelomeningocele. These potentially associated anomalies are not specific for dysraphisms of the spinal cord, and each may be found in isolation or with other CNS malformations.

Differential Diagnosis. The diagnosis of a neural tube defect usually is quite obvious, except in rare cases of small or hidden encephaloceles and with *forme fruste* lesions such as dural sinus tracts. In some cases of aplasia cutis congenita, there may be bony skull defects without cystic outpouching of components of the CNS, making the diagnosis of a neural tube defect diffficult. Tumors such as caudal lipomas, teratomas, and dermoids may occasionally mimic a neural tube

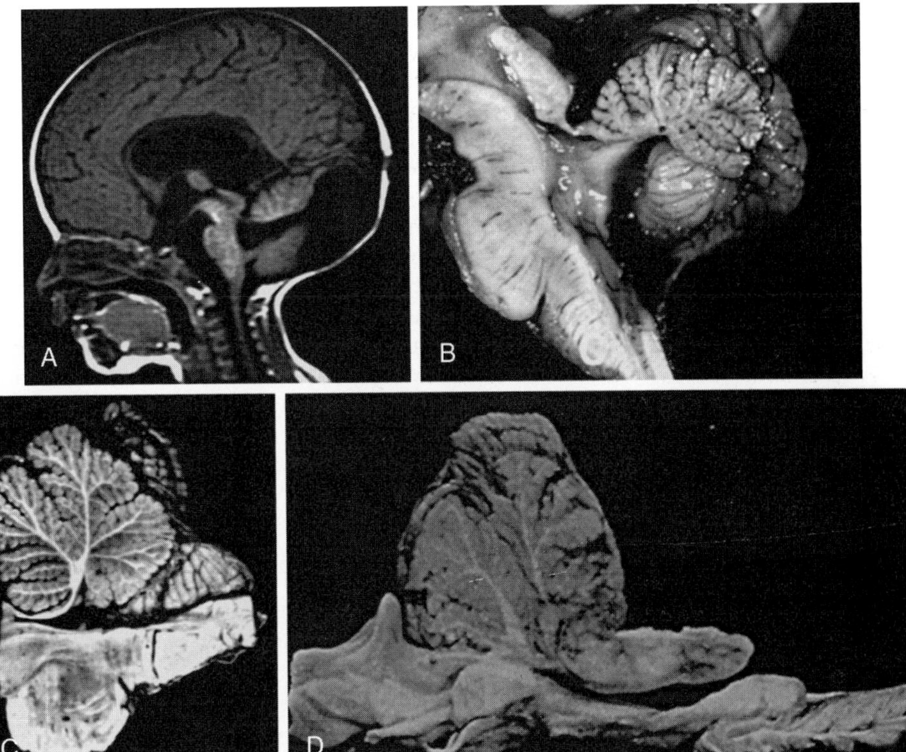

FIGURE 28–2. Examples of several posterior fossa anomalies. A midsagittal MRI (*A*) and photograph of a brain (*B*) with Dandy-Walker malformations. The cerebellar vermis is rotated anteriorly and there is a cystlike dilation of the fourth ventricle. *C*, A Chiari I malformation is characterized by a tongue of cerebellar tonsils extending over the cervical spinal cord. The cerebellar vermis is intact and shows no displacement. *D*, The Chiari II malformation is characterized by the cerebellar vermis extending as a tongue of tissue into the cervical spinal canal. The inferior vermis is white, corresponding to the extreme gliosis usually seen in this disorder. Note the beaking of the inferior tectum, the elongated and distorted pons and medulla, with the kinking of the lower medulla.

closure defect. The amniotic band sequence can also disrupt the neural folds and/or cranium, resulting in a defect resembling a neural tube closure defect.[21] Disruptions due to the amniotic band sequence are often easily distinguished from neural tube closure defects by the asymmetry, the presence of facial clefts, and the presence of extremity amputations. The signs and symptoms of tethering of the cord and related anomalies have to be differentiated from other progressive spinal cord diseases, including tumors, multiple sclerosis, spinal cord infarction, and progressive spastic paraparesis.

Evaluation. The diagnosis of anencephaly is readily made on examination of the affected infant. The evaluation of children with less dramatic neural tube defects is more complex. Occipital encephaloceles may be part of a syndrome with important genetic and prognostic implications. For example, the Meckel-Gruber syndrome and the Walker-Warburg syndrome, both mentioned previously, are autosomal recessive disorders with a poor prognosis. A special case is the frontonasal encephalocele. Clear rhinorrhea from CSF leakage following the removal of a nasal "polyp" requires immediate evaluation with imaging and prophylactic antibiotic treatment instituted before surgical repair. A complete endocrine evaluation is particularly important in sphenoidal encephaloceles. In general, careful imaging, preferably using both MRI and CT scanning with bone windows, is important for the evaluation of encephaloceles to outline their content and anatomical relationships for treatment planning.

In the evaluation of the infant with spinal dysraphism, particularly the lumbosacral forms, it is important to be aware of the commonly associated Chiari II malformation as well as of the possibility of coexisting hydrocephalus. Myelomeningoceles outside of the lumbosacral region have a less consistent association with hydrocephalus.

It is currently recommended that every child with myelomeningoceles be screened for the presence of hydrocephalus with at least transfontanelle ultrasound, because the development of signs and symptoms may be delayed. Careful morphological and functional urological assessment is of major importance in children with myelomeningoceles. Only in very low lesions at S3 will there be a flaccid, and therefore relatively easy to manage, bladder. Higher lesions are often associated with incoordination of the detrusor and external urethral sphincter.

Management and Prognosis. In anencephaly the prognosis for survival without maximal support for an affected infant is extremely poor, and a significant proportion of infants are stillborn. Because survival of live-born infants can be prolonged with the assistance of life support systems, anencephalic infants are potential organ donors, but purposeful life prolongation for this use is controversial.

The management for dysraphic disorders begins with the planning of an atraumatic delivery. The avoidance of labor by prelabor cesarean section significantly improves neurological outcome in children with myelomeningoceles.[26] Larger encephaloceles are also managed in this fashion. Decisions concerning the surgical management in the encephaloceles are dependent on the clinical context in which the encephalocele occurs, including the identification of syndromes and other associations important for prognosis and genetic counseling (see Van Allen and colleagues[17] for a more complete list of associations and syndromes). Most encephaloceles are sporadic, however, so that prognosis and management are solely based on the extent of the individual defect. Generally, surgical excision and closure are recommended, even if there are significant associated malformations; the goal of surgery in these cases may be simply to improve caregiving for the affected infant. More urgent surgery may be indicated in the case of CSF leaks to prevent meningitis. The prognosis and neurological outcome are significantly better in anterior encephaloceles as opposed to parietal and occipital lesions, particularly those involving the posterior fossa contents (see later discussion of Chiari III). Frequently a sporadic encephalocele, frontal or occipital, can be surgically managed with fairly good outcome.

The surgical treatment of spinal dysraphism in most centers is now directed at closing all but the prognostically worst cases. Although early treatment is preferable, there are no strong data supporting improved outcome from emergency closure. Timely closure does, however, reduce the rate of infectious complications. A planned operation within the first 24 to 48 hours after delivery currently is the standard of treatment, although some delay of the closure under antibiotic coverage does not seem to adversely affect outcome. Concurrent shunting of co-existing hydrocephalus is often necessary and advisable even for what might appear to be "arrested" ventriculomegaly. Prevention of meningitis or ventriculitis is extremely important, because the outcome for cognitive development is inversely related to the occurrence of such complications. Therefore antibiotic prophylaxis is used before and around the time of surgery, in particular with open defects. A new surgical intervention that has shown significant initial promise is fetal surgery to close the defect, although further studies are required to determine which patients are the best candidates and to assess the safety and long-term outcome of this intervention.

Surgical management of the Chiari malformation itself may become necessary when prominent brain stem signs persist despite adequate treatment of the hydrocephalus.[27] In these selected cases decompression via suboccipital craniectomy and cervical laminectomy can be beneficial. Urological management plays a prominent role in the care of these children.[28] It is very important to avoid secondary dilatation of the proximal urinary system creating the potential for chronic pyelonephritis and renal damage. Urological complications continue to be a leading cause of morbidity in children with myelomeningocele. Various conservative (intermittent catheterization, anticholinergic medication) and surgical regimens for bladder management may be appropriate.[29] Rectal incontinence can often be successfully managed with conservative treatment such as very regulated and scheduled emptying of the bowel. Several late complications of myelomeningoceles can arise. Scoliosis, especially with lesions at or above L2, and traction on the cord, may result from the defect alone. Postsurgical complications include spinal cord infarction, compression of the cord by subarachnoid cysts, and inclusion cysts arising from trapped skin appendages.

The distribution of weakness and deficits on examination is an important predictor for later ambulation. Involvement above the L3 level in general creates motor deficits that preclude ambulation; lesions below S1 usually allow for unaided ambulation. If the deficit level falls between S1 and L3, a number of assisting devices may be useful for ambulation.[30]

Tethering of the cord may be found as a late complication after meningomyelocele repair,[31] but may also occur as a "primary" abnormality (see previous discussion). In all cases surgical untethering of the cord is recommended. The associated pain responds best to surgical treatment, and ambulation and bladder function may improve as well. However, sphincter dysfunction often remains a permanent problem even after complete release. Given the potential for rapid deterioration with incomplete neurological recovery, even prophylactic surgery in an otherwise asymptomatic child seems advisable.

Primary prevention of neural tube defects currently focuses on dietary folate replacement around the time of conception. Such a supplementation has been shown to not only reduce the risk for the birth of a second affected child, but may also be effective in reducing the primary incidence of neural tube defects. Given the early timing of the failure of neural tube closure, supplementation may be too late when an unplanned pregnancy is noted. The question of general diet fortification with folate is still being debated.[32]

Prenatal detection of neural tube defects has become routine through screening programs using serum and amniotic chemistry and prenatal ultrasound. Elevated serum or amniotic fluid alpha-fetoprotein (AFP) and elevated acetylcholinesterase in the amniotic fluid are found in almost all open neural tube defects. The peak of sensitivity for maternal serum AFP levels lies somewhat later than the amniotic fluid determination and is optimal at 16 to 18 weeks' gestation. Before that time, the levels may be normal despite the presence of a neural tube closure defect. The specificity of this test is much lower so careful follow-up testing needs to be done after the determination of an elevated value. This surveillance commonly includes a high-level fetal ultrasonography and often amniocentesis to measure AFP and acetylcholinesterase in the amniotic fluid. This determination is highly sensitive for open neural tube closure defects, but not always completely specific, since there are other causes for elevated AFP in the amniotic fluid. AFP levels combined with acetylcholinesterase analysis in the amniotic fluid approaches a sensitivity of 100 percent with much improved specificity. In addition, fetal ultrasonography can provide an additional level of confidence with very high sensitivity in experienced hands at even 14 to 16 weeks' gestation. Indirect signs such as the lemon sign, referring to a symmetrical bifrontal narrowing of the skull, and cerebellar abnormalities are helpful in addition to the often-difficult direct demonstration of the defect. Fetal ultrasonography can also assist in dating of the pregnancy, an important factor in the calculation of the AFP values, as the normal and abnormal ranges are dependent on the gestational age of the fetus.

Segmentation, Cleavage, and Midline Defects

The group of disorders discussed in this section are believed to arise from a defect in midline development. The result is a failure of midline structures, like the corpus callosum, to form. Included are also abnormalities in the separation of the neural tube into two hemispheres. This later defect is believed to result in holoprosencephaly and the related disorders that will be discussed.

Pathogenesis and Pathophysiology. Completion of neural tube closure is followed by segmentation in the anterior-posterior axis. Although these segments were originally defined morphologically, recent data have demonstrated a coordinated expression of a variety of developmentally regulated genes, mostly members of transcription factor families such as the homeobox genes. In more general terms these data have suggested that the segmental organization of the nervous system is established through a combinatorial regional expression and regulation of specific developmental genes.[33, 34] These segments form the progenitors to all structures recognized in the adult nervous system. Holoprosencephaly is now believed to arise from a defect in this early dorsal-ventral patterning of the rostral neural tube midline.[38] In addition to the anterior-posterior organization of the nervous system, bilateral symmetry arises in the cerebral hemispheres. At approximately 5 to 6 weeks post-fertilization the prosencephalon, the most rostral segment of the nervous system, shows differential growth as two distinct hemispheres. The most anterior point of the neural tube, the lamina terminalis, is the location from which the major crossing fibers between the cerebral hemisphere will arise. Both the anterior commissure and the corpus callosum have their anlagen in the lamina terminalis. From there the corpus callosum grows back over the top of the third ventricle to form its genu, body, and splenium. Failure of the prosencephalon to grow into two symmetrical hemispheres and defects in the region of the lamina terminalis are believed to give rise to the class of defects commonly referred to as cleavage defects or midline defects.

Epidemiology and Risk Factors. Among the midline defects, holoprosencephaly is the best characterized and studied, and this section will focus primarily on this disorder as a model of a segmentation defect. Holoprosencephaly is a relatively rare malformation of the CNS, frequently associated with specific craniofacial anomalies including midline facial clefts, cyclopia, and nasal anomalies. The incidence in liveborn children with normal chromosomes has been estimated to be approximately 0.48 to 0.88 per 10,000.[35, 36] In contrast, the rate among human aborted fetuses was estimated at 40 per 10,000, indicating a high rate of fetal loss.[37]

Several environmental/maternal factors have been associated with the holoprosencephaly sequence. In humans, the best recognized association is with maternal diabetes. Maternal ethanol consumption has also been anecdotally associated and is supported by experimental studies.[38] Excluding those cases of holoprosencephaly resulting from exposure to a teratogen, it is likely that the majority of remaining cases will have a recognizable genetic etiology. Furthermore, it is possible that even those cases associated with a teratogenic exposure occur against the background of a genetic predisposition, similar to the risk of a chronically alcoholic woman having a child with the fetal alcohol syndrome.

Because the holoprosencephaly sequence can occur in the setting of other well-recognized syndromes, the evaluation of a fetus, infant, or child with holoprosencephaly must include a complete investigation for other systemic anomalies. It has been estimated that up to 25 percent of patients with holoprosencephaly have a recognizable syndrome.[35, 36] Syndromes that may show holoprosencephaly as a feature include pseudotrisomy 13, Smith-Lemli-Opitz, Pallister-Hall, Meckel, velocardiofacial, Genoa, Lambotte, Martin, and Steinfeld syndromes.[38] As will be discussed in the following sections, the Smith-Lemli-Opitz syndrome, due to a defect in cholesterol biosynthesis[39] at the level of 3ß-hydroxy-steroid-Δ^7-reductase, is of particular interest because it also has a link to a specific signaling pathway involving the human sonic hedgehog homolog (SHH) molecule. Affected patients have severe hypocholesterolemia, and cholesterol is required for normal SHH signaling.

In addition to these recognized syndromes, a number of nonrandom chromosomal abnormalities have been found in patients with holoprosencephaly. Chromosomal anomalies have been reported in 24 to 45 percent of live-born infants,[35, 36] the most common of which is trisomy 13. This has been estimated to account for greater than 50 percent of the chromosomal abnormalities in patients with cytogenetic abnormalities, and up to 70 percent of children with trisomy 13 have holoprosencephaly. In addition to trisomy 13, several other chromosomal anomalies have been identified in patients with holoprosencephaly.[38]

Based on nonrandom cytogenetic rearrangements, at least 12 chromosomal regions on 11 chromosomes may contain genes that may play a role in the pathogenesis of holoprosencephaly. Four of these loci have been designated *HPE1* (21q22.3), *HPE2* (2p21), *HPE3* (7q36), and *HPE4* (18p).[40] Since that time, *SHH* was found to map within the minimal critical region for *HPE3* and mutations identified. Confirmation that *SHH* plays a role in the pathogenesis of holoprosencephaly has come from mice that are homozygous mutant for the *SHH* gene and show a holoprosencephaly-like sequence.[41] Other genes that have been identified to date in holoprosencephaly include *TGIF, ZIC2, and PTC.*[42] Other genes are likely to also be identified.

Clinical Features and Associated Disorders. Holoprosencephaly is frequently divided into subtypes according to the extent of cerebral hemisphere involvement, although these distinctions are probably artificial. The most commonly used classification scheme defines three subtypes: alobar, semilobar and lobar holoprosencephaly.[43] Alobar holoprosencephaly is the most severe of these (Fig. 28–3A). The brain shows no evidence of a midsagittal fissure. The corpus callosum is absent and the olfactory bulbs and tracts are almost always absent as well. Varying degrees of fusion of the basal ganglia and thalamus are present. This form of holoprosencephaly is most frequently associated with severe facial malformations (see later discussion). Semilobar holoprosencephaly is characterized by an incomplete fusion of the cerebral hemispheres (Fig. 28–3B). The occipital and parietal lobes tend to be more or less separated, whereas the frontal lobes show varying degrees of fusion. Again, the corpus callosum is absent in all cases and the olfactory bulbs and tracts absent in most. The basal ganglia and thalamus are variably involved but at least partially fused in all cases. In lobar holoprosencephaly a midline fissure is present over the entire dorsal aspect of the brain; however, in at least the medio-orbital region of the frontal lobe there is fusion across the midline. The olfactory bulbs and tracts are again absent in the vast majority of cases, as is the corpus callosum. The posterior fossa contents are usually unremarkable in holoprosencephaly. Only in the most severe cases of alobar holoprosencephaly can anomalous development of the cerebellum occasionally be seen. On the other hand, absence of the corticospinal tracts is a common finding and is believed to be the consequence of the severe malformation of the cerebral cortex with subsequent failure of formation of proper motor projections. A spectrum of quite distinctive facial dysmorphisms can be part of the holoprosencephalic malformation sequence. These facial abnormalities are expressions of the underlying profound disturbance of midline development, affecting prechordal mesoderm important in facial development as well. The facial phenotypes can be ranked in

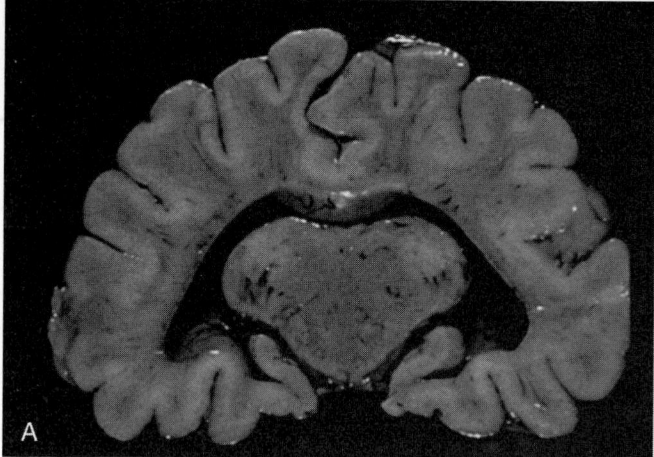

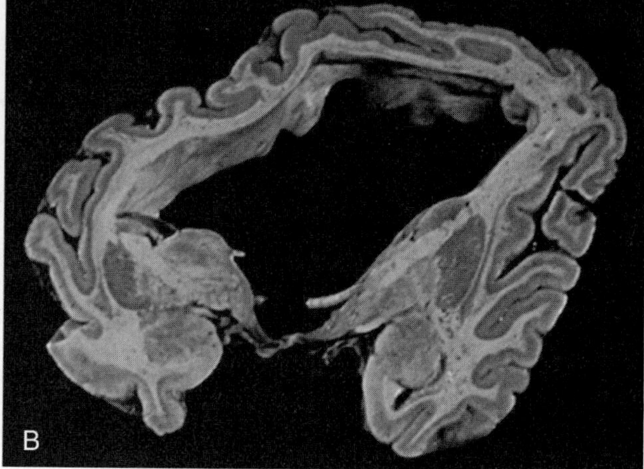

FIGURE 28–3. Semilobar and alobar holoprosencephaly. *A,* In semilobar and lobar holoprosencephaly there is an apparent midline sagittal (interhemispheric) fissure (coronal section of brain). However, coronal sections reveal the cerebral cortex to be continuous across the midline. Furthermore, no corpus callosum is present. The thalamus is abnormally shaped with marked midline fusion. *B,* Alobar holoprosencephaly has no indication of a midline fissure on coronal sections or when viewing the brain dorsally. Again there is no evidence of a corpus callosum, only subcortical white matter across the midline.

descending order of their severity: (1) cyclopia (the eye and orbits are fused or in various states of incomplete separation, agnathia may also be present); (2) ethmocephaly (instead of a nose, a proboscis is present and often located above the incompletely separated, or severely hypoteloric, eyes): (3) cebocephaly (the nose is between and below the hypoteloric eyes, but there is only a single blindly ending nostril): (4) premaxillary agenesis or aplasia of the primary palate, associated with hypotelorism and often midline cleft lip and palate: (5) milder facial dysmorphism with hypotelorism, flat base of the nose, and milder midline or bilateral clefting: (6) minimal forms such as single central incisor. While it is generally true in the holoprosencephaly spectrum that the face predicts the brain,[44] exceptions do occur. In general, the severe facial dysmorphisms of cyclopia, cyclopia with agnathia, ethmocephaly, cebocephaly, and severe hypotelorism with agenesis of the primary palate and a median cleft lip and palate usually go along with the severe alobar form of holoprosencephaly. The correlation of severity of the facial appearance and brain morphology is less pronounced at the mild end of the spectrum of facial phenotypes. Although the full-fledged facial phenotypes seem to be always associated with holoprosencephaly, cases of for example agnathia (but without cyclopia) or central cleft lip and palate, have been seen in patients with a morphologically normal-appearing brain and also with brains that have malformations distinct from the holoprosencephaly sequence. The reverse correlation, namely that a holoprosencephalic brain necessarily goes along with an abnormal brain, is less strict, as a normal face can be seen even in severe holoprosencephaly. Distinct genetic causes for holoprosencephaly with a normal face are emerging (e.g., ZIC 2 mutations). Thus, the brain does not necessarily predict the face.

The clinical presentation of holoprosencephaly is very much dependent on the degree of CNS involvement. Infants with severe alobar forms often die shortly after birth. Survivors frequently present with severe mental retardation, seizures with infantile spasms early on, severe motor impairments, poikolothermia, and endocrine insufficiencies. In the milder forms of holoprosencephaly, longer survival with various degrees of psychomotor retardation is possible. Endocrine dysfunction may become apparent, with diabetes insipidus and growth hormone deficiency often reported. It should be re-emphasized that only the "classical" facial phenotypes are predictive of the severe alobar holoprosencephaly with its associated very poor prognosis; a number of partial facial phenotypes, such as midline cleft lip or midface hypoplasia, are not necessarily associated with the most severe malformations in the spectrum.[17]

In families with autosomal dominant holoprosencephaly, carriers of the gene with minimal expression of the defect (e.g., hypotelorism or a single central incisor) can be neurologically normal. There may be considerable variability of expression within a given family, with severely involved cases occurring alongside milder ones. Autosomal recessive holoprosencephaly has been reported as well and in some families is associated with heart and limb defects.

Evaluation. Most cases of holoprosencephaly occur sporadically, but may also be a feature of one of several malformation sequences or syndromes.[17] Therefore, part of the clinical evaluation of a patient with holoprosencephaly must include a careful workup for additional malformations, since this information may provide the diagnosis of a specific syndrome with potentially far-reaching genetic implications. Because of the associations with some deletion/microdeletion syndromes, high-resolution karyotype analysis (+/–FISH analysis) (see Chapter 25) with special emphasis on chromosomes 2p21, 3p, 7q36, 13q, 18p11.3, and 21q22.3 is recommended in all cases of holoprosencephaly. Specific gene mutation analysis is also warranted for *SHH*, *TGIF*, *PTC*, and/or *SIX3* in selected cases. If the affected proband is not available, chromosome analysis in the parents is important to rule out a carrier status for a balanced translocation. Possible misdiagnoses in the severe forms of alobar holoprosencephaly include hydranencephaly, hydrocephalus, and large, expanded interhemispheric cysts that sometimes are associated with agenesis of the corpus callosum. Expanded large posterior third ventricular cysts can be mistaken for semilobar holoprosencephaly. Bridging of cerebral cortex across the midline deep in the interhemispheric fissure can be missed in very mild cases of lobar holoprosencephaly and is best evaluated on coronal T1-weighted MRI. The prenatal diagnosis of holoprosencephaly is largely based on ultrasound examination. A first trimester diagnosis is possible based on ultrasound findings of a lack of a midline echo indicative of a monoventricle, cyclopia or marked hypotelorism, a flattened profile of the nose, and microcephaly. Transvaginal ultrasound enhances the visibility of these findings, especially early in gestation. Prenatal diagnosis by ultrasound of mild forms such as lobar holoprosencephaly may be impossible.

Management and Prognosis. The management of a patient with holoprosencephaly depends on the extent of clinical involvement, and focuses predominately on seizure control (see Chapter 52). The prognosis for all live-born children with severe forms of holoprosencephaly is extremely poor. The rare cases associated with true hydrocephalus due to CSF flow obstruction need to be differentiated from verticulomegaly as a feature of the malformation itself, and treated with VP shunting. Prognosis similarly parallels the ability to control the seizures. Mental retardation may be mild in the least severely affected individuals, but is almost always profound in the more severely affected individuals. In cases of holoprosencephaly with less complete CNS involvement, surgical correction of the craniofacial malformations, such as cleft lip and/or palate, may be appropriate. Endocrine dysfunctions respond to hormone replacement therapy.

Other Segmentation and Cleavage Disorders

Septo-optic dysplasia is pathologically defined as absence of the septum pellucidum in combination with hypoplastic optic nerves. This clinical constellation of symptoms and signs has also been referred to as De Morsier syndrome. Other abnormalities are variably reported, suggesting considerable heterogeneity underlying this phenotype. Clinically there is optic nerve hypoplasia resulting in visual impairment, endocrine abnormalities resulting from hypothalamic-pituitary insufficiency, and not infrequently seizures, especially in cases where there has been disruption of cortical development as well. The degree of visual impairment can vary from blindness leading to the development of amaurotic nystagmoid eye-movements a few months after birth, to normal vision in a few cases. The endocrine insufficiencies can cause symptomatic hypoglycemias, diabetes insipidus, and later growth hormone deficiency may become apparent. These can and should be treated by standard endocrine replacement protocols. Although retardation of cognitive development occurs, especially in patients with obvious concomitant cortical anomalies, a number of cases with normal cognitive development are on record. Most cases of septo-optic dysplasia have been sporadic; however, there are two observations in siblings and in cousins suggesting the existence of a form with autosomal recessive inheritance. It is an important consideration in the differential diagnosis in children presenting with optic hypoplasia.[45]

Agenesis of the corpus callosum can be found as an isolated malformation or in association with other malformations.[17] A growing number of inborn errors of metabolism also include agenesis of the corpus callosum as part of their clinical spectrum. In complete absence of the corpus callosum the cingulate gyrus is altogether absent and sulci are found radiating down the medial aspect of the brain from the dorsal surface to the high riding roof of the third ventricle (Fig. 28–4). Coronal sections or images often reveal slightly dilated ventricles with an irregular "batwing" contour. A white matter tract, known as the bundle of Probst, can frequently be found running in the anterior-posterior direction just above the

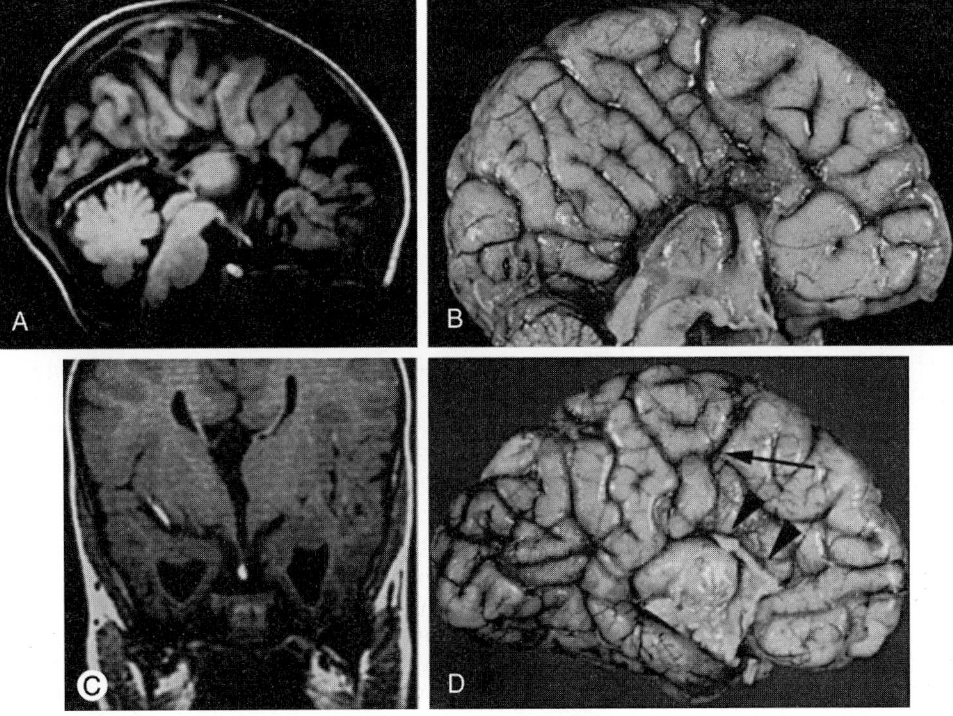

FIGURE 28–4. Partial and complete agenesis of the corpus callosum. *A,* Midsagittal MRI of a patient with complete agenesis of the corpus callosum. The medial gyri are seen radiating to the third ventricle. *B,* Midsaggital section of the brain from a patient with complete agenesis of the corpus callosum. A comparison of *A* and *B* shows remarkably similar findings. *C,* Coronal MRI of another patient with agenesis of the corpus callosum. The lateral ventricles show the classic batwing form, and dilation is seen in the temporal horns of the lateral ventricles and the third ventricle. *D,* Midsagittal section of a brain with partial agenesis of the corpus callosum. The partial corpus callosum present *(arrowheads)* extends from the lamina terminalis posteriorly. The cingulate (partially obscured by the arrowheads) extends the length of the corpus callosum. A sulcus *(arrow)* extends from the dorsal surface of the brain to the third ventricle only, posterior to the formed corpus callosum.

lateral ventricle where the fibers of the corpus callosum would normally collect into the commissure. Partial agenesis is recognized by the absence to variable degrees of the posterior corpus callosum with sparing of the rostrum and genu. In cases of partial agenesis of the corpus callosum the cingulate gyrus is present only to the extent that the corpus callosum exists. The anterior commissure, also derived from the lamina terminalis, is absent in cases of complete agenesis of the corpus callosum, but is usually spared in cases of partial agenesis of the corpus callosum.

Isolated agenesis of the corpus callosum is sometimes discovered incidentally either on imaging studies that were obtained for other reasons or at autopsy. In isolation, the abnormality can be clinically largely silent and deficits may only be discovered on careful neuropsychological assessment. Findings resembling disconnection syndromes have been described in some patients, however, this is by no means a constant feature and in the majority of patients this cannot be demonstrated. Patients with agenesis of the corpus callosum have a higher incidence of seizures and mental retardation, partially reflecting the slightly higher incidence of telencephalic migrational abnormalities also seen in these patients. It should be noted however, that patients with mental retardation and/or seizures are also more likely to have CNS imaging that skews the ascertainment of clinicopathological correlations in agenesis of the corpus callosum towards more affected individuals.

Because it can be assumed that the clinical manifestations of agenesis of the corpus callosum most often depend on the associated CNS anomalies rather than on the lack of the corpus callosum itself, careful assessment for such associated malformations is mandatory. Although agenesis of the corpus callosum can be diagnosed on a CT scan (high-riding third ventricle, parallel configuration of the lateral ventricles, and colpocephaly), MRI is far superior in diagnosing associated structural abnormalities such as disturbances of neuronal migration. Partial agenesis of the corpus callosum is also seen very clearly on sagittal MRI. Midline cysts not associated with agenesis of the corpus callosum, holoprosencephaly as well as extreme hydrocephalus with thinning or disruption but without agenesis of the corpus callosum, need to be considered in the differential diagnosis. In secondary disruption of the corpus callosum, associated developmental features such as lack of the cingulate gyrus and presence of a bundle of Probst are not found. The potential diagnosis of an underlying metabolic disorder (e.g., nonketotic hyperglycinemia, infantile lactic acidosis associated with pyruvate carboxylase or PDH deficiency, Smith-Lemlie-Opitz syndrome, and Zellweger syndrome) has to be considered, depending on the clinical context. In patients with additional malformations of the brain and/or extraneural structures, a karyotype should be performed as well. A special problem is posed by the prenatal detection of absence of the corpus callosum on ultrasound. The presence of additional abnormalities and an abnormal karyotype is a poor prognostic indicator for developmental outcome, whereas outcome can be favorable if the agenesis of the corpus callosum is a truely isolated malformation.[46] However, subtle associated brain malformations can be impossible to detect on prenatal ultrasound.

Arrhinencephaly, or absence of the olfactory bulbs and tracts, is also considered in the midline defects although the pathogenesis may be quite distinct. Arrhinencephaly can be found as an isolated malformation or in conjunction with a variety of malformation syndromes. Clinically, bilateral arrhinencephaly manifests as anosmia. Although arrhinencephaly is frequently included in the midline dysplasias and can represent a mild manifestation within the holoprosencephaly spectrum, it would be incorrect to conclude that every isolated case of arrhinencephaly belongs with this spectrum. Quite likely, arrhinencephaly can result from a number of independent mechanisms. One example of a non-holoprosencephaly-sequence syndrome associated with arrhinencephaly is Kallmann syndrome. This syndrome is characterized by a combination of arrhinencephaly resulting in anosmia with hypogonadotropc hypogonadism, resulting from gonadotropin-releasing hormone (GnRH) deficiency.[47] Other neurological features may be associated. The syndrome can be inherited in an autosomal dominant, recessive, or X-linked recessive pattern. The gene for the X-linked form has been identified. It shares homology with neural-cell adhesion molecules, and the developmental defect has been linked to the failure of GnRH producing neurons to reach the hypothalamus.[47]

Neuronal Migration Defects

Pathogenesis and Pathophysiology. Anomalous cerebral cortical development is generally characterized as a cortical migrational abnormality, although an actual defect in migration has only been conclusively demonstrated for a relatively few disorders. Recently Rorke[48] has hypothesized a variety of factors that must be considered in the pathogenesis of cortical migrational abnormalities. Among the various components of development, cellular proliferation, cell death, postmigrational intracortical growth and development, and extracellular matrix abnormalities can each be implicated as a possible pathogenetic mechanism.

The human cerebral cortical malformations classified as disorders of neuronal migration include the lissencephaly/pachygyria/subcortical band heterotopia spectrum, periventricular nodular heterotopia, and polymicrogyria. The lissencephalies and periventricular nodular heterotopia clearly represent cell migration defects. However, other malformations, such as polymicrogyria, have pathogeneses yet to be elucidated. Because the classification relies more on pathogenic mechanisms than on clinical grounds, these divisions are presented in this section.

LISSENCEPHALY

Lissencephaly was derived from the Greek words "lissos" (smooth) and "encephalos" (brain), and describes the smooth appearance of an agyric brain. Microscopic examination of the cerebral cortex is variable, but the normal six-layer cytoarchitecture is absent in all cases. Lissencephaly has become the paradigm of a neuronal migration disorder.

Classical Lissencephaly (Type I)

Classical lissencephaly, also known as type I lissencephaly in the pathology literature, is a malformation where the surface of the brain is completely, or nearly completely, devoid of gyri and sulci (Fig. 28–5). Macroscopically the malforma-

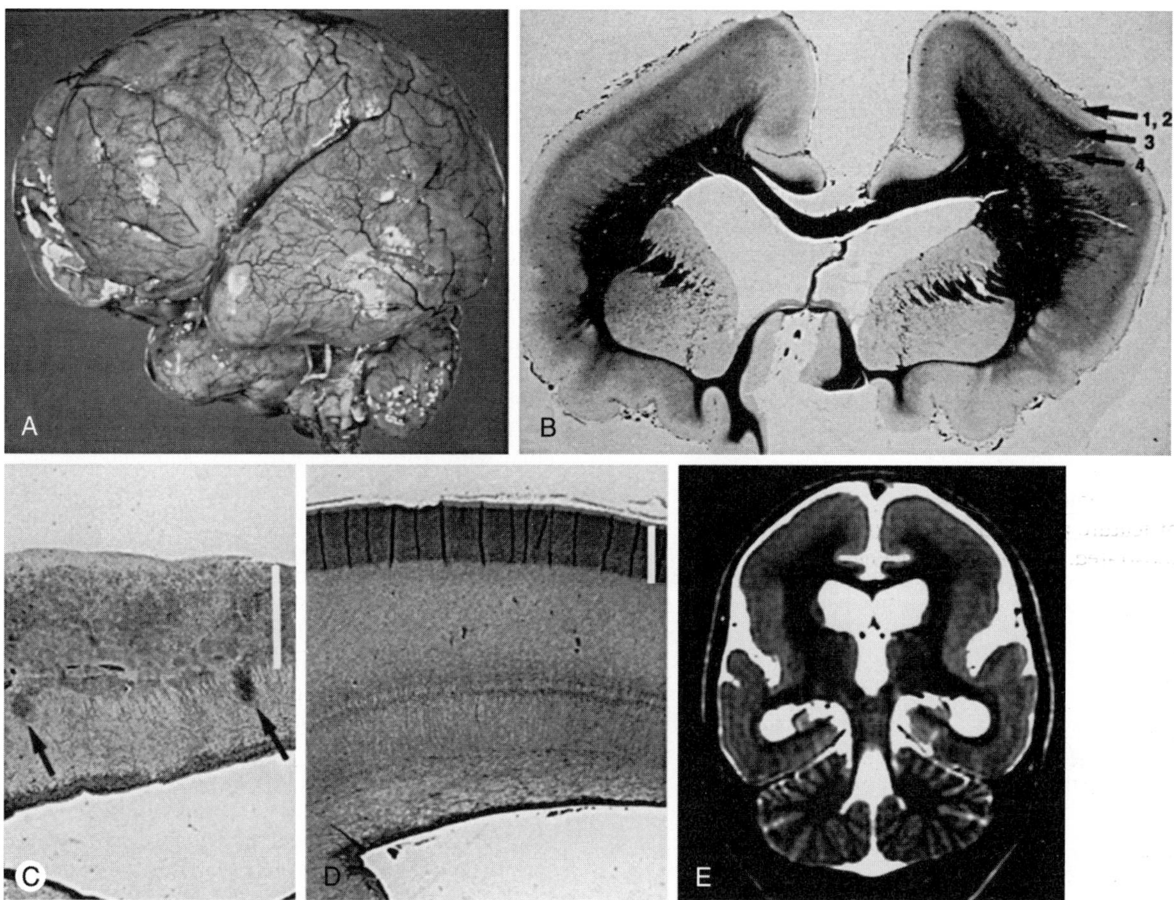

FIGURE 28–5. Lissencephaly type I and type II. *A,* A brain from an 8-month-old infant with Walker-Warburg syndrome demonstrating type II lissencephaly. Note the smooth surface of the brain, slight irregularities of the cortical surface can best be appreciated in areas of light reflection on the specimen. *B,* A coronal section stained for myelin that demonstrates the four layers of type I lissencephaly (e.g., the Miller-Dieker syndrome): *1* corresponds to the molecular layer, *2* is a cellular layer with mostly large neurons, *3* is a layer containing myelinated fibers, and *4* is a broad heterogeneous cell-rich layer. Note that the cortical plate takes up more than half of the total thickness of the cerebral mantle. *C,* A histological section through the cerebral mantle of a 20-week gestational age fetus with Walker-Warburg syndrome. One half of the thickness of this section is taken up by the totally disorganized cortical plates *(white bar).* In addition there are subcortical heterotopias pointed out by the arrows. *D,* Age-matched control. Here the cortical plate *(white bar)* takes up only a fraction of the whole thickness of the mantle. *E,* iA T2-weighted coronal MR image of type I lissencephaly.

tion spectrum ranges from agyria and pachygyria to subcortical band heterotopia with a relatively normal gyral pattern.[49] Histologically classical lissencephaly reveals a four-layered cortex replacing the normal 6-layered ribbon.[49] The outermost layer is the molecular layer (layer 1), layer 2 is a band of pyramidal neurons, layer 3 is composed of myelinated fibers and fewer neurons. This layer can be seen by neuroimaging. Finally, layer 4 is composed of a broad band of disorganized neurons. The white matter occasionally contains grey matter heterotopia. Anomalies of the inferior olivary nucleus, cerebellum, and the corticospinal tracts may also be present.

Classical lissencephaly due to deletions or mutations of the *LIS1* gene on chromosome 17p13.3 is found in the *Miller-Dieker Syndrome* (MDS) and isolated lissencephaly sequence (ILS). MDS is a contiguous gene syndrome and is due to deletions of chromosome 17p13.3 involving the *LIS1* gene and presumably other specific genes at this chromosomal locus. Patients have distinct facial features and may have other associated congenital anomalies, such as omphaloceles or cardiac anomalies. In contrast, ILS is associated with small deletions or intragenic mutations of *LIS1*.

Patients with MDS usually have lissencephaly at the severe end of the spectrum with complete agyria. In ILS the cortical malformation ranges between agyria and pachygyria. The cortical malformation with a *LIS1* abnormality is more severe posteriorly,[50] whereas patients with lissencephaly and *DCX* mutations show a more severe involvement of the frontal lobes (see later discussion). The overall severity of the lissencephaly in ILS appears to be related to the type and location of the mutation.

Mutations in the *DCX* gene located on the X chromosome are associated with subcortical laminar heterotopia, also known as "double cortex," in females.[51, 52] The assumed mechanism for this anomaly is explained by the normal and random X-inactivation that occurs in females. When the chromosome carrying the mutated copy of *DCX* is inactivated, that cell will presumably behave like a normal cell and migrate to the cortical plate. In contrast, if the chromosome with the normal copy of *DCX* is inactivated, only the mutant allele will be expressed. Thus, two populations of cells exist in the ventricular zone. Those cells expressing the mutant allele become localized in the white matter forming a band of heterotopic neurons, whereas the cells expressing the normal copy migrate to form the cortical plate in the normal location. Males with *DCX* usually have classical lissencephaly, but have also presented with subcortical laminar heterotropia. Both the type of mutation and somatic mosaicism have been associated with this milder phenotype in males. In pedigrees, where females have subcortical laminar heterotopia and males lissencephaly, a *DCX* mutation has so far always been identified. In females with sporadic subcortical laminar heterotopia the figures vary, but in those with bilateral diffuse bands, or thin frontal bands only, the mutation rate appears to be high.

Other Lissencephaly Syndromes

Several other syndromes with lissencephaly as a component have been identified (see *http://www.geneclinics.org*). The best characterized of these is lissencephaly with cerebellar hypoplasia. Recently linkage to *RELN* was found in two consanguineous pedigrees. The similarity of the brain defects to those seen in the Reeler mouse made this a suitable candidate gene. Further studies identified distinct *RELN* splicing mutations in each family.[53] To date the pathology of the lissencephaly and cerebellar hypoplasia has not been reported in a patient with a known *RELN* mutation. However, this does suggest that other genes in the *RELN* pathway are good candidates for lissencephaly with cerebellar hypoplasia and related disorders. Additional variants of lissencephaly have been identified radiographically and pathologically; the genetic bases for these have not yet been delineated.

Cobblestone Lissencephaly

Cobblestone lissencephaly, also known as type II lissencephaly in the pathology literature, is also referred to as "cobblestone cortex." It occurs in a group of disorders associated with congenital muscular dystrophy and eye abnormalities. The Walker-Warburg syndrome, muscle-eye-brain disease, and Fukuyama congenital muscular dystrophy are entities within this group and appear to be autosomal recessive. In contrast to classical lissencephaly where there is a slowing or delay in cell migration, the pathogenesis of cobblestone lissencephaly is believed to be an overmigration. Disruption of the pial-glial limitans results in cells migrating past the cortical plate proper and into the leptomeninges, forming a rind of neurons admixed with the leptomeninges over the surface of the brain (see Fig. 28–5). Agenesis of the corpus collosum, hindbrain deformities, cerebellar dysplasia, and Dandy-Walker malformation are also frequently associated with the Walker-Warburg syndrome. Neuroimaging can identify these cerebral malformations, as well as pachygyria and polymicrogyria, white matter abnormalities, hydrocephalus, and posterior cephaloceles.[54]

Walker-Warburg syndrome is the most severe of these disorders. The eye abnormalities include microphthalmia, cataracts, glaucoma and retinal dysplasia. A congenital muscular dystrophy is also a constant finding. Prognosis is usually poor with death within the first few years of life. The surface of the brain shows smooth and nodular areas, appearing like a cobblestone street. In cross-section, the cortical band is thickened but not to the same extent as in classical lissencephaly. The six-layer cerebral cortex is replaced with two broad bands of neurons. The outer band is a disorganized collection of neurons, glia, collagen bundles and blood vessels. The inner layer is a disorganized collection of neurons thought to be the remnant of the true cortical plate. The pial-glial limitans appears disrupted at multiple points and can usually be found between these two disorganized layers of gray matter.

Muscle-eye-brain disease of Santavouri, most commonly reported in the Finnish population, is generally milder than Walker-Warburg syndrome, with a longer survival. Eye abnormalities can be similar to Walker-Warburg syndrome, with myopia being the most consistent feature. It is also associated with a muscular dystrophy. Muscle-eye-brain disease has been linked to 1p32-34 and the gene identified as an enzyme involved in Golgi-based O-linked glycosylation (protein O-mannose beta-1,2-N-acetylglucosaminyltransferase.[55] One of the proteins normally glycosylated by this enzyme could be alpha dystroglycan, an extracellular matrix receptor expressed both in skeletal muscle and in the CNS.

Fukuyama congenital muscular dystrophy is another disorder with some features that resemble Walker-Warburg syndrome and muscle-eye-brain disease; however, the involvement of the eye and brain is less severe, compared to Walker-Warburg syndrome in particular. Patients show psychomotor deficits and progressive loss of muscle function. Linkage to chromosome 9q31 was established; subsequently a novel gene was identified encoding the protein now named *fukutin*.[56] *Fukutin* also appears to have a role as a glycosyltransferase, so that the defects in CNS development and in muscle must be related to faulty glycosylation of specific muscle and brain proteins such as alpha dystroglycan. Fukuyama congenital muscular dystrophy is extremely rare outside of Japan. Interestingly, an ancient 3′UTR retrotransposon insertion, yielding reduced but intact mRNA expression, has been identified as the molecular basis for many of the Japanese cases.[56] Others within Japan and elsewhere have a point mutation affecting the coding region.

PERIVENTRICULAR NODULAR HETEROTOPIA

Heterotopia are ectopic collections of neurons. The pathogenesis of heterotopia located in the cerebral white matter is believed to be a failure of neurons to migrate to the cortical plate. They may occur as single lesions adjacent to the ventricle or in the more superficial white matter. In some cases, there are multiple nodules lining the ventricles. This latter entity is known as periventricular nodular heterotopia (PVNH). Microscopic examination shows that many neurons remain in the ventricular zone and accumulate as nodules lining the ventricular surface.

Studies of families with women who have PVNH associated with epilepsy and pregnancy loss consistent with lethality in males pointed towards a PVNH locus on the X chromosome. Linkage was found to Xq28 in a number of families, and subsequently mutations in the gene coding for the actin crosslinking protein filamin 1 or filamin A (*FLN1*), were identified in patients with PVNH.[57] The majority of patients with *FLN1* mutations have diffuse continuous heterotopia around the lateral ventricles, but the cortex appears

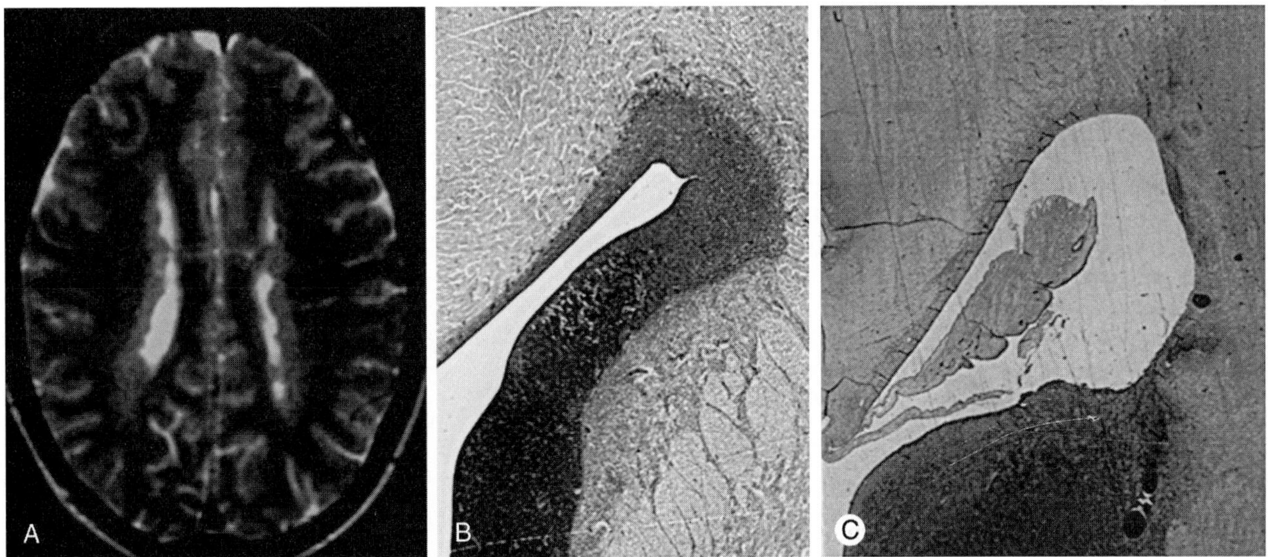

FIGURE 28–6. Periventricular nodular heterotopia. *A,* MRI from a patient with extensive periventricular heterotopia. The heterotopia are the same signal intensity as the cerebral cortex and scallop the margin of the ventricular surface. Histological sections from a normal fetus at 20 weeks' gestation *(B)* and from a similar age fetus with periventricular heterotopia *(C)*. The germinal tissue normal present around the angle of the lateral ventricle is replaced by several nodules of maturing gray matter (heterotopia). (*A,* Courtesy of Dr. C. Walsh.)

relatively normal. One of the mechanisms explaining the phenotype of PVNH in females is random X-inactivation resulting in two populations of neurons, those expressing the mutant allele, which presumably reside in the periventricular region as heterotopia and those that express the normal allele and migrate out to the cortical plate.

Single or multiple heterotopia are collections of disorganized grey matter in inappropriate locations (Fig. 28–6). Heterotopia in the cerebral hemispheres, other than the subcortical band heterotopia and bilateral periventricular heterotopia described previously, can take on one of many patterns. They may occur as focal, isolated anomalies found incidentally upon imaging or at autopsy, or they may have clinical manifestations as described following. Occasionally an isolated heterotopian or multifocal cerebral heterotopia is associated with an overlying cortical malformation. In addition to white matter heterotopia, glial and neuroglial heterotopia are often found in the leptomeninges overlying a cortical anomaly or around the base of the brain. The displaced tissue can form a radiographically and grossly identifiable plaque over the surface of the brain.

POLYMICROGYRIA AND OTHER DISORDERS OF CORTICAL DEVELOPMENT

Polymicrogyria is frequently recognized as a fine stubbling on the surface of the brain (described as "Moroccan leather" in appearance). By MRI and gross examination of brain sections, the cerebral cortex shows a complex set of small gyri that appear fused to each other. Microscopic examination confirms the gross impression, highlighting the small complex gyri and fusion of layer 1. Controversy exists as to whether polymicrogyria is a malformation or a disruption of development. The answer is likely that both mechanisms are involved in different forms of polymicrogyria. Given that polymicrogyria is almost always present at the margins of disruptions such as porencephaly and in the setting of malformation such as Zellweger's syndrome and triploidy, the conclusion often drawn is that polymicrogyria has multiple pathogeneses. Although there are certain microscopic differences depending on whether the polymicrogyria is caused by disruption or malformation, there still exists some overlap in the microscopic features of polymicrogyria regardless of the presumed pathogenesis. Unlike lissencephaly/pachygyria, the border between polymicrogyria and normal cortex is quite distinct and layer 6 in adjacent normal cortex and the deepest layers of the malformed polymicrogyric cortex are contiguous (Fig. 28–7). Based on the pathological features of polymicrogyria, the timing is later in neocortical development, generally believed to arise from defects occurring between 17 to 18 weeks' and 24 to 26 weeks' gestation.

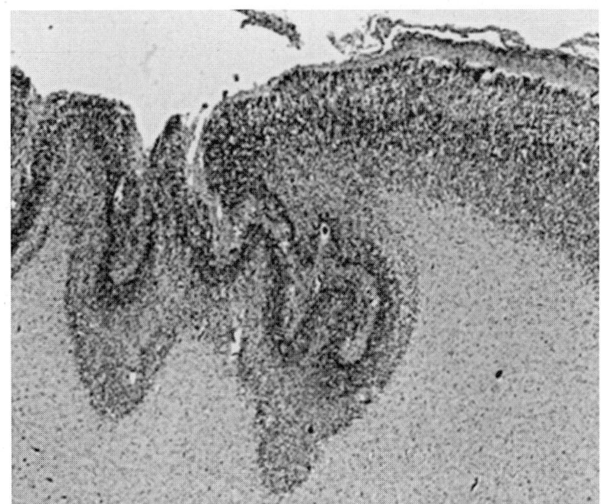

FIGURE 28–7. Polymicrogyria. The border of polymicrogyria and normal cortex. The border is extremely well delineated. The polymicrogyria is characterized by fusion of layer 1, continuity of layer 4, and extensive undulating folds of cerebral cortex.

Focal cortical dysplasias or cortical migrational anomalies are another group of anomalies of cerebral cortical development that are being recognized with increasing frequency (Fig. 28–8). The increasing practice of surgery in the management of intractable seizures has resulted in the recognition of a variety of cortical malformations in a significant number of cases. Although polymicrogyria and pachygyria have been seen in many cases, the most frequent anomaly has been labeled focal cortical dysplasia. This disorder is characterized by a disruption in the lamination pattern and maloriented neurons in inappropriate layers including layer 1 and in the cerebral white matter.[58] The pathogenesis remains unknown.

Epidemiology and Risk Factors. The incidence of neuronal migrational abnormalities disorders is unknown. Most of the cortical migrational disorders, particularly the diffuse ones, show a variety of inheritance patterns.[54] Other cases show no clear inheritance and appear to be sporadic. A variety of enviromental risk factors have been associated with the development of neuronal migrational disorders, including retinoic acids, methylmercury, and radiation. In utero infections, particularly viral, are also known to result in cortical migrational abnormalities. The pathogenesis for viral-induced migrational disorders remains unknown, although a destructive process is speculated to underlie the defect.

Clinical Features and Associated Disorders. The most striking clinical context in which type I lissencephaly is seen is the Miller-Dieker syndrome. Classical facial features include bitemporal hollowing, a rather short nose with a broad bridge and upturned nares, long and thin upper lip, small chin, and mildly low-set and posteriorly rotated ears. Although this constellation is referred to as the Miller-Dieker facial dysmorphism, the findings can be rather subtle. Most individuals with type I lissencephaly present in the neonatal period with marked hypotonia. Later, a spastic quadriparesis will dominate the picture. Seizures are a constant part of the clinical picture; they can start as neonatal seizures, but more commonly present as infantile spasms with myoclonic and tonic seizures, that later lead into a Lennox-Gastaut syndrome with the additional occurrence of atonic seizures. The electroencephalogram (EEG) typically shows fast α- and β-activity admixed with high-amplitude slow activity. Mental and psychomotor retardation are usually profound. Cardiac anomalies occur in 20 to 25 percent, and there can be genital anomalies in about 70 percent of males.

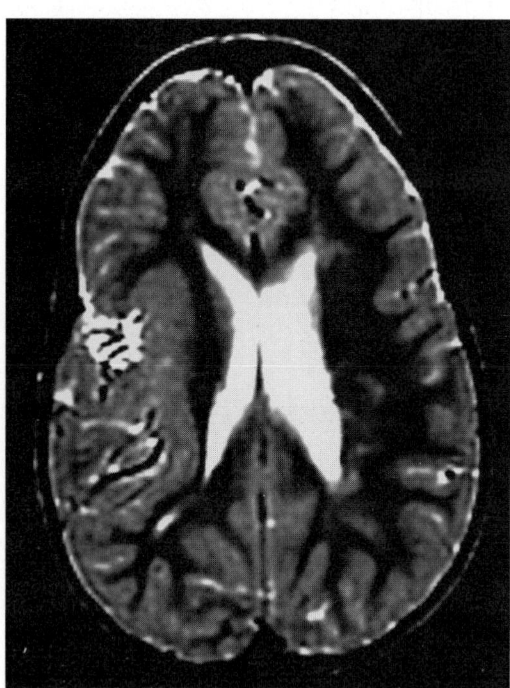

FIGURE 28–8. Focal cortical dysplasia. A horizontal MRI from a patient with focal cortical dysplasia. The left hemisphere shows a normal cortical ribbon; however, in the left hemisphere posterior frontal lobe, the cortical ribbon is abnormally thickened and the sulcal pattern is lost. The underlying white matter may be slightly thin.

Type II lissencephaly occurs in a group of disorders associated with congenital muscular dystrophy, often involving the eyes as well. The Walker-Warburg syndrome, muscle-eye-brain disease, and Fukuyama muscular dystrophy are entities within this group. Walker-Warburg syndrome is the most severe of these disorders with a high proportion of neonatal lethality. The brain malformation often is complex with associated hydrocephalus, cerebellar hypoplasia (and occasionally Dandy-Walker malformation), and sometimes an occipital encephalocele. Clinically Walker-Warburg syndrome is characterized by profound hypotonia in the neonatal period due to the combined muscle and CNS involvement. The eyes can be affected in a number of ways, most frequently by retinal dysplasia, although anterior chamber malformations, cataracts, choroidal colobomata, optic nerve hypoplasia, and microphthalmia can all occur. Serum CK levels are elevated. Arthrogryposis may be present, and additional contractures may develop later. This condition is inherited in an autosomal recessive fashion and no gene or genetic localization has, as yet, been defined.

Muscle-eye-brain disease of Santavouri has many features that resemble Walker-Warburg syndrome. The disorder is most prevalent in Finland[59] but clearly also occurs outside of that country. This condition also presents at birth or during the first few months of life with hypotonia and weakness. Serum CK levels are consistently elevated after 1 year of age and often earlier. Subsequent psychomotor development is markedly delayed; however, many patients will acquire the ability to stand and walk. Mental retardation and seizures are common. The EEG is usually abnormal and progressively so after about 6 to 7 years of age. Most patients show a progressive motor deterioration, confounded by increasing spasticity and contractures by 5 years of age. The eye abnormalities consist of high myopia, retinal degeneration, and optic atrophy. Congenital glaucoma and juvenile cataracts may also be present. The visual evoked potentials tend to be progressively delayed and of abnormally high amplitude with an abolished ERG at the same time. Neuroimaging often reveals less severe, but comparable findings of muscle-eye-brain disease to Walker-Warburg syndrome. Hydrocephalus is seen frequently, and patchy white matter involvement can be seen on T2-weighted MRI.

Fukuyama congenital muscular dystrophy is the second most common muscular dystrophy in Japan[60]; only Duchenne muscular dystrophy is identified more frequently. It appears to be extremely rare outside of Japan. In contrast to muscle-eye-brain disease and Walker-Warburg syndrome, eye involvement is generally less frequent and less severe. Patients show considerable psychomotor retardation and progressive muscular weakness and contractures. Seizures occur in about 50 percent of cases. When present, ocular findings include myopia and optic atrophy. MRI of the brain demonstrates the areas of pachygyria as well as polymicrogyria. Areas of abnormal T2 signal on MRI can be seen in the white matter. The cerebellum is only mildly affected and hydrocephalus is rare.

Polymicrogyria has a less heterogenous clinical presentation than lissencephaly. For all practical purposes, the different forms of polymicrogyria, independent of their syndromic or etiological context, present with seizures and potentially also mental retardation, depending on the extent of the abnormality. The various syndromic associations of polymicrogyria are discussed later under Differential Diagnosis.

Heterotopia can be sporadic, inherited in a simple Mendelian trait, or be part of a more complex syndrome. When in isolation, the main presenting feature is seizures of various kinds, but they are by no means obligatory. Onset of the seizures can be from childhood (most commonly) to adulthood. Focal, multifocal, and generalized seizures can occur, with infantile spasms and the Lennox-Gastaut syndrome seen at the severe end of that spectrum. Other neurological problems such as motor impairments and mental retardation may coexist. The risk for these additional manifestations is lowest when the abnormality is localized to the periventricular region, higher in the white matter heterotopia, and highest in the diffuse subcortical band heterotopia. However, even in the latter condition quite normal psychomotor development can be seen, although infrequently.

The initial presentation of cortical dysplasia is most commonly the onset of various types of seizures. With this presentation there are no clear signs or symptoms that would predict a cortical dysplasia versus another cortical lesion. The age of seizure onset tends to be in childhood, but can be delayed into adulthood or can be as early as infancy.[61] When presenting in infancy, the clinical picture can vary from clearly focal appearing seizures to infantile spasm with relatively minimal or no focal clinical or EEG features. Later, the seizures may also include tonic seizures as well as drop attacks. Onset during the first few days of life as an early infantile epileptic encephalopathy has also been described.[62] EEG findings can be quite variable.[61, 63]

Differential Diagnosis. Among the conditions with lissencephaly type I, the Miller-Dieker phenotype is distinguished from ILS, by the lack of distinctive facial features in the latter. However, some degree of bitemporal hollowing and a small chin may be seen in ILS as well. Furthermore, FISH analysis has demonstrated microdeletions in a significant number of ILS cases.[64] However, other probes appear to distinguish the two entities, suggesting a difference in the physical extent of the deletions. Whether the obvious contiguous gene hypothesis, involving the loss of multiple adjacent genes, accounts for the additional anomalies in the Miller-Dieker syndrome awaits the discovery and analysis of the lissencephaly gene. Other cases of ILS could possibly result from mutations in other genes.

The differential diagnosis of the lissencephaly II syndromes can be quite difficult at times. These difficulties are reflected in the many essentially synonymous designations of these syndromes, including the muscle-eye-brain syndrome, HARD+/–E (*h*ydrocephalus, *a*gyria, *r*etinal *d*ysplasia, +/–*e*ncephalocele), and CODM (congenital ocular dysplasia/muscular dystrophy) syndromes. Although there is no difference in principle between Walker-Warburg syndrome and muscle-eye-brain disease beyond the degree of severity, this does not automatically prove that they are allelic variants at the same gene locus. With the identification of the muscle-eye-brain disease gene it is now clear that the two are genetically distinct. Fukuyama muscular dystrophy, despite many similar features, usually does not include the severe eye and brain anomalies found in the Walker-Warburg syndrome.

Many other syndromes and associations may show variable forms of lissencephaly, pachygyria and polymicrogyria as features, and many cases are not easily classified into any particular syndrome (Table 28–2).[65] Discussions of these rare disorders has recently been reviewed.[54] A number of metabolic conditions can also be associated with pachygyria/lissencephaly. The most frequent syndrome to show such an association (along with polymicrogyria) is the Zellweger syndrome.[66] This is a disorder of peroxisomal biogenesis that is characterized by marked neonatal hypotonia, facial dysmorphism, wide-open fontanelles, and renal and hepatic abnormalities. Neonatal adrenoleukodystrophy and bifunctional enzyme deficiency are also peroxisomal disorders that may show migrational abnormalities. Glutaricaciduria type II, pyruvate dehydrogenase deficiency, nonketotic hyperglycenamia, and sulfite oxidase deficiency/molybdenium cofactor deficiency are examples of other metabolic disorders that occasionally include cortical dysplasia as one of the manifesting features.

The differential diagnosis of conditions with polymicrogyria is extensive,[54] reflecting the nonspecific nature of the malformation. In addition to the lissencephaly II conditions discussed already, Aicardi, Neu Laxova, Zellweger, and Smith-Lemlie-Opitz syndromes could be mentioned as monogenic conditions. Polymicrogyria can also occur with a variety of chromosomal abnormalities. As outlined previously, disruptive and destructive disorders can have polymicrogyria associated with them. The most common association is with congenital cytomegalovirus (CMV), and the timing of this is probably similar to the disruptions of porencephaly and hydranencephaly. In fact, both of these disorders have been reported with congenital CMV infection as well as other congenital infections. Extensively fused polymicrogyria can be difficult to differentiate from pachygyria on imaging.

Periventricular as well as subcortical band heterotopia can occur as X-linked inherited conditions, mapping to different

TABLE 28–2. **Summary of Syndromes with Cortical Malformations***

Disorder	Cerebrum	Cerebellum	Hydrocephalus	Eye	Muscle	Other
MDS	A	–	–	–	–	–
ILS	A	–	–	–	–	–
WWS	A,P,E	DWS	+	+	+	+
MEB	A,P,E	DWS	+	+	+	–
Fukuyama	A,P	–	+/–	+/–	+	–
NL	A,P	+	–	+	–	+
Zellweger's	A,P	+	–	–	–	+
NRS	A	+	–	–	–	–

*Not a Complete List.

A, Agyria; DWS, Dandy-Walker malformation; E, encephalocele; ILS, isolated lissencephaly sequence; MDS, Miller-Dieker syndrome: MEB, muscle-eye-brain disease; NL, Neu-Laxova syndrome; NRS, Norman Roberts syndrome; P, pachygyria; WWS, Walker-Warburg syndrome.

regions on the X chromosome.[67] In familial band heterotopia, affected females present with the heterotopia and often seizures, whereas affected males show a more severe brain malformation, including lissencephaly. This may be due to random X-inactivation in females preventing full expression of the defect, and also raises the possibility that a spectrum of developmental disturbances, from focal heterotopia to lissencephaly, exists with a common pathogenesis.[64, 68, 69] In familial periventricular heterotopia affected male family members also have a more severe malformation and clinical phenotype than affected female siblings.[69] Again, a number of syndromes include neuronal heterotopia with some regularity. For example, in Aicardi syndrome heterotopia are as constant a feature as agenesis or hypoplasia of the corpus callosum. Retinal lacunae, cerebellar abnormalities, and hemivertebrae may also be found in this syndrome. Aicardi syndrome is probably an X-linked dominant male lethal condition, so that only girls are affected clinically. The presentation includes severe early seizures (infantile spasms) and profound psychomotor retardation. The list of metabolic conditions associated with polymicrogyria includes the peroxisomal disorders as well as Smith-Lemlie-Opitz syndrome, an inborn error of cholesterol metabolism diagnosed by demonstrating an elevated level of plasma 7-dehydrocholesterol.

Polymicrogyria and focal cortical dysplasia can be difficult to differentiate because of the similar clinical presentation with seizures. Imaging is the mainstay of diagnosis (see later discussion). The so-called "benign focal epilepsies of childhood" are important to differentiate from "fixed" cortical malformations, because the prognosis and management are different.

Evaluation. The diagnosis of the Miller-Dieker syndrome and also the isolated lissencephaly sequence is based on the finding of a smooth brain surface with widely open sylvian fissures on neuroimaging studies, an appearance that has been referred to as the figure 8 sign. The broad cortex in relation to the extremely narrow white matter can be seen on MRI. Cytogenetically visible deletions of the critical chromosomal region 17p13.3 are seen in about two thirds of clinically convincing cases.[64] More than 90 percent of cases show loss of this critical region when FISH analysis is employed.

Cobblestone (type II) lissencephaly has an appreciably different MRI appearance, with a grey to white matter ratio of 1:1. As for all of the other disorders of neuronal migration, careful evaluation of the morphology of the cortex by MRI is essential. In cases of cobblestone lissencephaly/pachygyria, especially in the presence of associated CNS malformations or abnormalities of the eyes, the group of congenital muscular dystrophies with eye and brain involvement has to be considered. Determination of serum CK levels and muscle biopsy may become necessary. Once the diagnosis of a congenital muscular dystrophy with structural brain abnormalities has been made, the differential diagnosis between the individual conditions should follow the preceding considerations. Prenatal diagnosis of the Walker-Warburg syndrome by ultrasound is possible, though not always easy. The posterior fossa anomalies and demonstration of retinal detachment are helpful.

The workup for focal cortical abnormalities of migration also relies heavily on extremely high-quality MRI, as some of these lesions can be very hard to detect. Clinical suspicion must remain high and hints, such as delayed myelination in a cortical region, may be valuable in defining the location of the abnormality. The value of functional imaging techniques such as positron-emission tomography, single-photon emission computed tomography, and perfusion-diffusion MRI at this point cannot be generalized. These techniques are under active development. Several special MRI techniques, such as 3D surface rendering, are being evaluated for this purpose and also appear quite promising. At a minimum, high-resolution imaging with thin cuts and optimal grey to white matter resolution for the age of the patient is essential. On EEG, focal very high amplitude rhythmical activity is quite characteristic of cortical dysplasias; however, it is recorded in less than half of the cases. Other EEG patterns, such as focal abnormal fast activity, have no particularly predictive value for a focal dysplasia. At times the surface EEG can be quite normal or appear to show primary generalized spike and wave discharges. An additional important diagnostic problem is the question whether the underlying lesion is unifocal or multifocal. Multifocal discharges on the EEG do not necessarily mean multifocality of the dysplasias, though they certainly can. Conversely, electrographic evidence for only one focus does not exclude the existence of additional foci. Long-term videotelemetry monitoring may be helpful in evaluating these questions. In cases where seizures are resistant to medical management and there is a high degree of suspicion for a focal cortical abnormality but lack of noninvasive evidence, intraoperative electrophysiology may prove useful. Guided by this approach, resected pathological material will often show features of cortical dysplasia.

Management and Prognosis. In general, the prognosis for patients with Miller-Dieker syndrome and the Walker-Warburg syndrome is very poor and many patients do not survive infancy. Very little psychomotor development if any takes place. Insertion of a gastric tube may be necessary to provide adequate nutrition, prevent aspiration, and facilitate care. Treatment of the frequently prominent seizures follows general guidelines. Whereas most cases have poor outcome, milder cases are on record for both syndromes.

In the congenital muscular dystrophies with structural brain abnormalities the brain malformation may require surgical intervention for the hydrocephalus or sometimes for the encephalocele in the Walker-Warburg syndrome. If the hydrocephalus is due to aqueductal stenosis and a Dandy-Walker anomaly is present, shunting of both the lateral ventricles and the posterior fossa cyst may become necessary. The prognosis is better in muscle-eye-brain disease, and although patients often acquire the ability to walk, there may be secondary deterioration because of increasing spasticity. In this condition, the ophthalmological management becomes very important: high myopia, cataracts, glaucoma, and retinal detachment may all require intervention.

Because the resulting epileptic syndrome in disorders of neuronal migration is frequently medically intractable, surgical extirpation of the lesion is often desirable, and earlier surgical intervention may improve the overall developmental prognosis by preventing the development of an epileptic encephalopathy. For an isolated focus of polymicrogyria or cortical dysplasia presenting with intractable seizures, extirpation can be a curative option; however, multifocality is not an automatic contraindication against the surgery, because extirpation of a major focus may result in overall improvement of seizure control. The presurgical and intraoperative evaluation is essential for success of the surgery and is dealt with in detail by Wyllie.[70] For isolated epileptogenic heterotopias, surgical excision also is an option, whereas the drop attacks that can be seen in the diffuse bilateral band heterotopias may respond to callosotomy.[71]

OTHER DISORDERS OF NEURONAL MIGRATION AND CORTICAL FORMATION

Ulegyria is another distinct cortical anomaly. It is best characterized as a fusion of layer 1 at the depths of sulci with relative sparing of the crests of the gyri. The fusion is frequently associated with gliosis in the cortex, neuronal loss, and obliteration of the cortical lamination. The scarring at the depth of a sulcus and sparing at the surface of the brain results in a mushroom appearance when the gyrus is viewed on cross section. These lesions have very well-defined borders and discrete islands of preserved neurons within the lesion. The histology and location, frequently in an arterial zone, has led to the contention that ulegyria arises late in gestation or in early neonatal life as a vascular injury to the immature cortex, possibly related to a hypoperfusion. Ulegyria may be clinically silent or cause seizures similar to polymicrogyria discussed previously.

Megalencephaly, or an enlarged brain volume, can be sporadic, autosomal dominant, autosomal recessive, or part of a recognized syndrome or disease (Table 28–3).[7] In generalized megalencephaly, a diffuse broadening of the cerebral gyri, an increased white matter and grey matter volume, and frequently normal sized ventricles occur. The brain is usually microscopically normal, although several reports have suggested an increased cell volume. In the familial megalencephaly with autosomal dominant inheritance, the majority of cases are neurologically normal. Hydrocephalus and extracerebral fluid collections have to be ruled out by imaging in all cases.

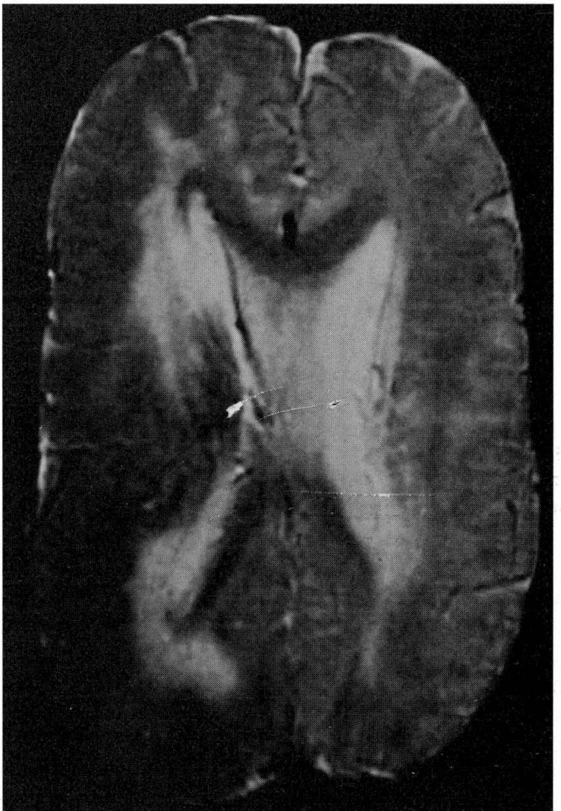

FIGURE 28–9. Hemimegalencephaly. A horizontal T2-weighted MRI demonstrates the moderately larger right hemisphere compared to the left. The cerebral cortex is poorly defined on the right side and the T2 imaging highlights the abnormal signal intensity of the cerebral white matter on the same side.

TABLE 28–3. **Selected Conditions Presenting with Megalencephaly/Hemimegalencephaly**

Isolated Familial Megalencephaly
Autosomal dominant
Autosomal recessive

Syndromes of Parenchymal Overgrowth
Neurocutaneous syndromes
- Neurofibromatosis I
- Tuberous sclerosis
- Proteus syndrome
- Klippel-Trenaunay-Weber
- Riley-Smith syndrome
- Shapiro-Shelman syndrome
- Linear sebaceus nevus syndrome

Generalized overgrowth syndromes
- Sotos syndrome
- Ruvalcaba-Myhre-Smith syndrome
- Beckwith-Wiedemann syndrome
- Weaver syndrome
- Bannayan-Zonana syndrome

Metabolic Disorders
Alexander disease
Canavan disease (N-acetyl asparto acylase deficiency)
GM_1 and GM_2 gangliosidosis
Glutaricaciduria type 1

Other Associations
Achondroplasia
Agenesis of the corpus callosum

Hemimegalencephaly (Fig. 28–9) may occur in isolation or be associated with a specific syndrome, the most widely recognized of which are the Beckwith-Wiedemann syndrome and the linear sebaceus nevus syndrome. The abnormally large cerebral hemisphere shows regions of broad and fused gyri. Cross sections of the hemispheres reveal regions of thickened cerebral cortex and frequently heterotopia in the cerebral white matter. Microscopically the hemisphere shows marked disorganization with regions resembling pachygyria. In other regions the neurons of the malformed cortex are abnormally spaced and disorganized in orientation. The clinical presentation of hemimegalencephaly is quite variable.[72] One clue to the possible existence of hemimegalencephaly is the identification of body asymmetries, especially of the skull and face, or the recognition of other features of a syndrome associated with hemihypertorphy. Most patients with hemihypertrophy present during the first year of life with frequent, focal seizures or infantile spasms. Some infants show asymmetries of motor development that can be subtle or present as frank hemiparesis. The EEG is variable, showing a fast rhythmic pattern in the alpha to beta range, burst-suppression patterns, spike-wave, and/or repetitive triphasic complexes. Some authors assign a poor prognosis to repetitive triphasic complexes. Mental retardation is frequently associated with hemimegalencephaly and appears to be primarily correlated with the severity of the epilepsy. Patients with normal development and intelligence and/or well-controlled partial seizures have been reported. The association of hemimegalencephaly with Wilms' tumor of the kidney is important to recognize. Given the difficulties of medical seizure control in the majority of cases and the adverse effects that ongoing seizures potentially have for developmental outcome, early modified hemispherectomy has been repeatedly advocated and successfully performed in these children.[73]

Microcephaly is defined by the head circumference being two standard deviations below that predicted by the body size. This definition does not provide any indication of the nature of the brain abnormality. The etiology of microcephaly is complex (Table 28–4) and includes conditions that restrict brain growth (such as the craniosynostosis), destroy formed brain substance before completion of brain growth (e.g., hypoxic-ischemic insults and some infections), or intrinsically impair brain growth. The latter can be the result of a metabolic insult (exogenous or inborn) or a defect within the developmental process of brain formation itself (as is assumed to be the case in the "primary" genetic microcephalies, the chromosome breakage syndromes, and the majority of syndromes associated with microcephaly). It should be kept in mind that a small head circumference at birth does not rule out metabolic conditions, nor does a normal head circumference at birth rule out primary genetic causes of microcephaly. Microcephaly is a manifestation of many syndromes and is very common in syndromes that have mental retardation and cortical migration abnormalities as a component. Jones[21] compiled 39 syndromes with microcephaly as a frequent component and an additional 21 syndromes associated occasionally with microcephaly. One hundred and seventy six syndromes have been reported with at least one case of documented microcephaly.[17] Patients who appear to have a "primary" form of significant microcephaly, meaning not associated with other malformative features, are sometimes referred to as having microcephalia vera. This heterogeneous condition (autosomal recessive and X-linked forms have been identified) shows a striking reduction of head circumference up to 5 standard deviations below the mean. There is no facial dysmorphism associated. These individuals are severely mentally retarded, have no recognizable speech, but are often described as having a relatively preserved personality. Although these patients often have a somewhat lumbering gait, there is a paucity of other neurological findings. Skull films at birth show the sutures to be present. The brains are usually quite small, less than 300 g (normal, 1200 to 1500 g), and show a primitive gyral pattern. The cortex is thickened and disorganized without clear lamination. Isolated microcephaly can also be transmitted as an autosomal dominant trait. In this condition the degree of microcephaly usually is not as pronounced, and intelligence is relatively preserved. Given the preponderance of genetic conditions presenting with isoloated microcephaly, Tolmie and colleagues[74] calculated an empirical recurrence risk of 19 percent after a single affected proband.

TABLE 28–4. **Various Conditions Associated with Microcephaly**

Primary Small Brain Size
Nongenetic insults (pre-, peri-, postnatal)
- Infectious
- Vascular disruption, hypoxic-ischemic insult
- Irradiation
- Toxins and teratogens
- Malnutrition
- Metabolic
- Trauma (including shaken baby)

Genetic conditions
- Chromosomal disorders (e.g., trisomy 21, trisomy 13, 5p- [cri du chat] syndrome)
- Metabolic and degenerative conditions with onset before completion of brain growth (e.g., PKU, Smith Lemlie-Opitz syndrome, infantile neuronal ceroid lipofuscinosis)
- Chromosomal instability and premature aging disorders (e.g., Bloom syndrome, Cockayne syndrome, Nijmegen breakage syndrome)
- Monogenic or sporadic "syndromic" disorders (e.g., Cornelia de Lange syndrome, Meckel syndrome, Rubinstein-Taybi syndrome; also microcephalia vera and microcephaly "plus")

Restriction of Brain Growth
Disorders of bone and cartilage
- Nongenetic (endocrinopathies)
- Genetic (craniosynostosis, skeletal dysplasias)

External restriction of skull growth in utero

Posterior Fossa Anomalies

Pathogenesis and Pathophysiology. The development of the brain stem and cerebellum has been extensively investigated at the anatomic, cellular, and molecular levels.[42] The cerebellum is entirely derived from the rhombic lip, a dorsal ridge of the developing neural tube located at the junction between the midbrain and hindbrain (rhombencephalon). Proliferation and migration at the rhombic lip results in caudal growth of the cerebellar anlagen, resulting in the cerebellum forming the roof of the fourth ventricle. Complete aplasia of the cerebellum is an extremely rare condition and most cases are believed to represent secondary disruptions of normal development, primarily on a vascular basis. Cerebellar hypoplasia on the other hand is more common and diverse in its etiology.

In the 1890s Chiari described a group of malformations of the posterior fossa, each characterized by a displacement of the cerebellum.[75] *Chiari II* malformations, also known as the Arnold-Chiari malformation, have been described previously in this chapter (see Neural Tube Defects). *Chiari I* malformations are distinguished from Chiari II malformations by the displacement of the cerebellar tonsils (as opposed to the vermis in cases of the Chiari II malformation) over the cervical spinal cord (see Fig. 28–2). The Chiari I malformation is occasionally equated with herniation syndromes involving pressure coning and necrosis of the cerebellar tonsils. These two entities, however, should remain distinct, the Chiari I representing a malformation with resultant cerebellar displacement and the other entity the result of increased pressure within the posterior fossa. Occasionally hydromelia or syringomyelia may be associated with the Chiari I malformation, as with the Chiari II malformation; however, myelomeningoceles are not associated with Chiari I malformations.

The rare *Chiari III malformation* represents a displacement of the cerebellum into an occipital encephalocele. Occipital encephaloceles can involve either the occipital lobes of the cerebral hemispheres or the posterior fossa elements. As mentioned previously, encephaloceles involving the posterior fossa elements, and the cerebellum in particular, frequently carry a poor prognosis.

The *Dandy-Walker malformation*, by the strictest definition, includes a cystlike dilation of the fourth ventricle, an anteriorly rotated cerebellar vermis that is partially or completely absent, and an enlarged posterior fossa with an elevated tentorial insertion.[76] The Dandy-Walker malformation is not a true cyst of the fourth ventricle, but a cystlike dilation of the ventricle resulting from the abnormally anteriorly rotated vermis and an extended posterior medullary vellum.

Joubert's syndrome is due to absence or partial absence of the cerebellar vermis, but this syndrome can be distinguished neuropathologically from the Dandy-Walker malformation by the absence of a cystically dilated fourth ventricle. Relatively few brains clinically diagnosed as Joubert's syndrome have been pathologically studied. One problem related to understanding the pathological findings in this syndrome is the lack of a clearly defined clinical spectrum. Patients described as having Joubert syndrome have shown a wide spectrum of clinical findings (see later discussion), including variation among different families, suggesting possibly more than one etiology and clearly demonstrating genetic heterogeneity.

Möbius' syndrome involves focal deficits primarily involving cranial nerves VI and VII and can be unilateral or bilateral. Although disagreements exist as to the precise definition of this syndrome, the presence of bilateral deficits of both cranial nerves VI and VII justify the designation. Whether unilateral deficits involving one or multiple cranial nerves should be included as cases of Möbius' syndrome remains controversial. Although very few cases have been studied pathologically, most data agree that destructive lesions, frequently assumed to be vascular in origin, are the basis for most cases of Möbius' syndrome. Whether congenital absence of cranial nerve nuclei exists as a distinct entity is unknown.

Several clinical syndromes are believed to result from a "miswiring" in the nervous system that is from the establishment of aberrant neural connections resulting from failure of certain connections to form or be maintained. Duane's syndrome is discussed later. Another example of this phenomenon is the *Marcus Gunn phenomenon*, in which patients present with a jaw-winking and elevation or drooping eyelids provoked by sucking in the infant, smiling, swallowing, or speaking. Usually this phenomenon becomes less pronounced with age. This syndrome is believed to result from misdirected neuronal connections between cranial nerves III, V, and other cranial nerves.

Epidemiology and Risk Factors. Given the diverse group of anomalies that afflict the posterior fossa, it is impossible to give a concise estimate for the incidence or prevalence of this group of disorders. Some of the anomalies are found in almost constant association with other malformations. For example, the Chiari II malformation (discussed with myelomeningoceles) is almost uniformly associated with lumbosacral neural tube closure defects and thus the incidence parallels the incidence of myelomeningoceles. Other anomalies, like the Dandy-Walker malformation, may be found either as an isolated malformation, in conjunction with other malformations (e.g., cardiovascular), or as part of a syndrome (e.g., Meckel-Gruber syndrome, Walker-Warburg syndrome). Risk factors also vary depending on the malformation in question. Möbius' syndrome, for example, is found more frequently among children born with congenital heart malformations than in isolation. Dandy-Walker malformations have been associated with maternal retinoic acid exposure and warfarin exposure. A complete discussion of the risk factors and associated syndromes involving the posterior fossa has recently been compiled.[17]

Clinical Features and Associated Disorders. *Cerebellar hypoplasia* and *aplasia* may present with any combination of hypotonia, motor delays, cognitive delays, ataxia and head/truncal titubations, irregularities of speech rhythm, and nystagmus. However, clinically asymptomatic cases of cerebellar hypoplasia or even aplasia are well documented in the older literature.

The *Dandy-Walker malformation* is clinically quite heterogeneous. In addition to cerebellar features, some cases exhibit other CNS abnormalities such as agenesis of the corpus callosum, brain stem anomalies, and migrational abnormalities that will have bearing on the clinical picture. Mental retardation is also variable and frequently correlates with the presence of associated anomalies. Patients without associated anomalies may have relatively normal intelligence and development.[77] The evaluation of an individual with the Dandy-Walker malformation therefore requires a careful search for such associated abnormalities. Ataxia and brain stem dysfunction are often the presenting features and are believed to result from local pressure effects on the brain stem and cerebellum. Due to pressure fluctuations in the posterior fossa, these symptoms can occur intermittently. Presentation can be as late as in adulthood with headache and progressive neurological deterioration. Although hydrocephalus is often included in the definition of the Dandy-Walker malformation, it is often not present at birth, and may develop and present in the first year of life or later. Although occasionally a clear etiology for the hydrocephalus, such as aqueductal stenosis, is identified, in most cases there is no clear obstruction of CSF flow. Lack of patency of the foramen of Magendie and the foramina of Lushka, once considered the pathogenesis of the malformation, is rare and unlikely to be the etiology of the hydrocephalus in most cases.

Joubert syndrome usually presents with abnormalities of respiratory rate control in infancy (in particular episodic tachypnea, but also respiratory pauses), rhythmic tongue protrusion, abnormal eye movements, ataxia, and mental retardation.[78, 79] Structural eye abnormalities such as chorioretinal colobomata have been described. The degree of developmental delay can be quite variable and is not uniformly as severe as initially thought.

Chiari I malformation has a clinical spectrum that has broadened in recent years with the increasing use of MRI, the imaging modality of choice for the diagnosis of this condition. As opposed to the Chiari II malformation (see previous discussion of neural tube closure defects), the Chiari I malformation usually becomes symptomatic in teenage to early adult years, although the initial presentation can also be in an infant or older adult. The initial complaint is often neck pain, at times presenting with torticollis or retrocollis. If cervical spinal cord syringomyelia co-exists, symmetrical, asymmetrical, or even totally unilateral arm pain can be the initial complaint. Neurological symptoms and signs also are dependent on the neural structures involved. Predominant impairment of the brain stem and cerebellar tonsils by either compression at the level of the foramen magnum or by extension of the syrinx into the brain stem (syringobulbia) can lead to a variety of brain stem and cerebellar signs. In the very young age group, sleep apnea, stridor, and feeding difficulties may be the presenting symptoms. Eye movement abnormalities are relatively common. Oscillopsia is reported by the patient, and a variety of forms of nystagmus can be seen on examination. Downbeating nystagmus, especially when accentuated by lateral downgaze, should alert the examiner to a potential problem at the craniocervical/pontomedullary junction. Torsional nystagmus may also be present, especially in the presence of syringomyelia/syringobulbia. Lower cranial nerve impairment can lead to dysphagia and aspiration, which may first present as late as the eighth decade. When complicated by syringobulbia, asymmetrical cranial nerve involvement up to cranial nerve V may be present. Imbalance and vertigo with truncal ataxia may indicate impairment of the vestibulo- and spinocerebellar systems. With the coexistence of syringohydromyelia this clinical picture becomes even more complicated. Forty to 75 percent of cases of Chiari I have an associated syringomyelia, depending on the series and method of ascertainment.[80] When the patient is presenting with symptoms referable to the spinal cord, syringomyelia can be demonstrated in over 90 percent of cases. The most common location of maximal expansion is C4 to C6, though the cavity can expand up and down the entire cord. The cavity often is centrally or slightly asymmetrically located, thus first impairing crossing fibers in the anterior spinal commissure. Since these fibers carry sensory information for predominantly pain and temperature, and the posterior columns can be relatively spared, a dissociated sensory loss may result; thus pain and temperature sensation may be disturbed in a capelike distribution over the shoulders and down the arms, while light touch and joint position remain relatively unaffected. Compromise of the anterior horn cells may result in patchy weakness, amyotrophy, and loss of reflexes in the arms. These findings are often asymmetrical or even unilateral. With expansion of the cavity additional symptoms, including long tract signs and symptoms, can become apparent. Another important manifestation of syringomyelia, especially in childhood, is progressive scoliosis, sometimes the earliest sign of a syringomyelia. Skeletal anomalies of the skull base can be associated with the Chiari I malformation as well, most frequently basilar impression (see later discussion). Other skeletal anomalies of the craniocervical junction associated with the Chiari I malformation include the Klippel-Feil anomaly and atlanto-occipital assimilation.

In contrast to these predominantly cerebellar syndromes, other conditions have more clinical signs of brain stem dysfunction. In the broadest clinical definition *Möbius' syndrome* refers to a combination of bilateral symmetrical and asymmetrical facial weakness associated with abnormalities of horizontal gaze, most often deficiencies of abduction. Other cranial nerve functions can be impaired as well, especially IX, XII, V, and occasionally III. The impairment of lower cranial nerves can lead to early feeding difficulties, problems with swallowing, and atrophy of the tongue that is frequently unilateral. Neurosensory deafness may also be associated. A variety of somatic anomalies may be present in patients with Möbius' syndrome.[81] At least 50 percent of cases have limb anomalies. Thirty percent have talipes deficiencies, and 20 percent exhibit hypoplasia of digits, transverse terminal defects, or syndactyly. The Poland anomaly (absence of the pectoral muscle with or without radial ray abnormality of the upper extremities) and the Klippel-Feil anomaly can also be associated. Concurrent congenital heart disease, urinary tract anomalies, and hypogonadism/hypogenitalism are less frequent. Mild mental retardation is reported in 10 to 15 percent of patients with Möbius' syndrome; however, psychomotor development can also be slowed because of communication and social interaction problems that may result from the cranial nerve palsies. Most cases of Möbius' syndrome appear to occur sporadically, and may in some cases indicate a disruptive sequence. The association with Poland anomaly is sometimes referred to as Poland-Möbius' syndrome and may be familial.

Another syndrome involving cranial nerve nuclei is *Duane's syndrome*. This syndrome consists primarily of limited abduction with widening of the palpebral fissure on attempted abduction and globe retraction on the affected side on attempted adduction. It is due to deficient abducens innervation to the lateral rectus with compensatory innervation by cranial nerve III. Again, most of the described cases have been sporadic; however, familial occurences have been seen in the context of a number of anomalies such as limb anomalies, eye anomalies and deafness.[81] The combination of Duane anomaly, Klippel-Feil anomaly, and perceptive deafness has been referred to as Wildervanck (cervico-oculo-acoustic) syndrome. It is of uncertain inheritance. *Marcus-Gunn* (jaw-winking) *syndrome* consists of unilateral ptosis, with elevation of the ptotic lid to a position higher than the opposite side upon opening of the mouth, especially with deviation of the mouth to the opposite side. This is often first noted in the infant while sucking. There are a few families with a suggestion of a dominant mode of inheritance with incomplete penetrance.

Differential Diagnosis. Cases of congenital cerebellar hypoplasia have been reported as autosomal recessive and probably also with X-linked inheritance.[82] Cerebellar hypoplasia and pontocerebellar hypoplasia have been associated with a number of other syndromes.[82] Together these findings indicate that cerebellar hypoplasia is genetically heterogeneous. A recently recognized group of metabolic disorders of protein glycosylation can also present with a picture of neonatal olivo-ponto-cerebellar atrophy.[83] Prenatal cytomegalovirus infection also needs to be investigated in infants with congenital cerebellar hypoplasia or aplasia, especially in cases with co-existing deafness and retinopathy.

Because the *Dandy-Walker malformation* may be part of a considerable number of syndromes,[17] evaluation of the internal organs, particularly the heart and kidneys, as well as a skeletal and muscular assessment[84] is essential once a Dandy-Walker malformation is recognized. Differential diagnostic considerations have to include conditions that can cause cyst-like expansions in the posterior fossa. These include arachnoid cysts, mega cisterna magna, and cystic tumors. MRI is the imaging modality of choice given the problems of visualizing the posterior fossa by CT scanning. True cysts, such as arachnoid or ependymal cysts, in the posterior fossa may mimic a Dandy-Walker malformation; however, in contrast with the enlarged fourth ventricle associated with Dandy-Walker malformations, the fourth ventricle is compressed in the presence of a true cyst.

In Joubert's syndrome there is no cystic dilatation in the posterior fossa, so that the cerebellar hemispheres are seen to lie closely opposed without an intervening vermis. A similar cerebellar picture of agenesis of the cerebellar vermis without a posterior fossa cyst has been seen in several other syndromes, including the oro-facio-digital syndrome type VI of Papp-Varadi, as well as other syndromes with vermal hypoplasia/agenesis.[84] Patients with oro-facio-digital syndrome type VI of Papp-Varadi often have an unusual V-shaped partially duplicated metacarpal on hand x-rays, and sometimes hamartomatous nodules under the tongue can be found. An unequivocal distinction between these syndromes is not always possible.

The differential diagnosis in the Chiari I malformation with syringomyelia is broad given the protean range of the possible clinical symptoms. Multiple sclerosis, spinal muscular atrophy, amyotrophic lateral sclerosis, spinocerebellar ataxias, mononeuropathy multiplex, cervical disc and degenerative disease, and a variety of other disorders of the spinal cord and cerebellum can all be confused with the condition on clinical grounds. Imaging will resolve the majority of these differential diagnostic points. The situation can be more difficult in patients with prominent neurological symptoms but only borderline abnormal findings on imaging. Alternative diagnoses have to be considered seriously in that scenario. A cavity in the spinal cord can also have a traumatic (hematomyelia), inflammatory (necrotizing myelopathy), metabolic (Leigh disease), or neoplastic (astrocytoma and ependymoma) basis. Of the neurocutaneous disorders neurofibromatosis I and von Hippel-Lindau disease can be associated with a syrinx. Demonstration of a flow void within the cavity by MRI can be helpful to demonstrate continuity with the CSF spaces.

Möbius' syndrome must be differentiated from neuromuscular diseases with a prominent component of facial weakness, especially those with involvement of the extraocular muscles. In boys, centronuclear myopathy in particular should be considered because of the congenital presentation in the X-linked form. Mitochondrial myopathies, myasthenic syndromes and, in cases with only facial involvement, myotonic dystrophy and facio-scapulohumeral dystrophy as well as some of the structural congenital myopathies need to be considered. In cases with an unclear history of symptom onset, a multitude of acquired causes for multiple cranial nerve palsies has to considered. These causes include trauma to the skull base and cranial nerves; infection of the meninges, skull base, and cavernous sinus; inflammation of the nerves, brain stem, or cavernous sinus; tumors of the skull base; and meningeal neoplastic spread.

Differentiation between Möbius' and Duane's syndromes should be possible in most cases given the sparing of the face and lower cranial nerve nuclei in the latter. Duane's syndrome itself needs to be differentiated from other causes of abducens palsy in childhood, where the elaborate co-innervation phenomena of Duane's syndrome are usually not seen. More bizarre associated eye movement abnormalities can be seen in Duane's syndrome and may confuse the picture. The globe retraction can sometimes be difficult to appreciate, especially in infants.

Evaluation. Imaging for posterior fossa malformations is best done with MRI. The relationship between the cerebellar vermis and fourth ventricle and cisterna magna needs particular attention. Diagnosis of cerebellar and/or pontine hypoplasias can be difficult in mild cases and strictly speaking requires age-matched controls for comparison. As mentioned before, for any unusual posterior fossa anomaly, screening for additional malformations may lead to a syndrome diagnosis. Ultrasound of the heart and internal organs, a skeletal x-ray survey, and an ophthalmological evaluation are recommended. In cases of young patients with Joubert's syndrome an overnight sleep study may alert to respiratory irregularities and apnea spells. In cases of hydrocephalus associated with the Dandy-Walker malformation, evaluation should follow the guidelines outlined in the section on hydrocephalus.

Diagnosis of the Chiari I malformation as well as of syringomyelia relies on clinical suspicion as well as on adequate imaging. The imaging modality of choice is (as previously mentioned) MRI, especially sagittal images. The now routine inclusion of these images in any MRI study of the head has led to the discovery of a number of asymptomatic Chiari I malformations and asymptomatic cases of syringomyelia. It has also become apparent that the clinical picture is broader and more varied than the classical clinical syndromes described. The question frequently arises about the significance of low-lying tonsils that are discovered incidentally on a cranial MRI examination. The tonsils normally retract upward with age so their location must be interpreted in an age dependent context. The cut-off in the first 10 years of life appears to be 6 mm below the level of the foramen magnum, from 10 to 30 years it would be 5 mm, and after that 4 mm. Herniations greater than 12 mm are almost invariably symptomatic, on the other hand, about 30 percent of individuals with significant displacements of 5 to 10 mm are asymptomatic.[85] Similarly, syrinx cavities can be quite large with minimal clinical symptoms.

Patients with the different brain stem syndromes need to be evaluated in an effort to rule out disorders that may mimic these syndromes (see Differential Diagnosis) and also to define the extent of the abnormalities and establish the presence of any associated malformations. In Möbius' syndrome this may require (in addition to a careful neurological and ophthalmological examination) brain stem auditory evoked responses; CK determination; imaging of the brain, posterior fossa, and skull base by MRI; a skeletal radiographic survey, and echocardiography.

Management and Prognosis. Treatment of the Chiari I complex consists mainly of decompressing the structures trapped in the foramen magnum. Surgical approaches for pediatric[86] and adult[87] patients are comparable. Most often a suboccipital craniectomy, with or without dural patch grafting, and cervical laminectomies are performed, but anterior approaches may become necessary in selected cases to achieve satisfactory decompression. Occasionally, very large syrinx cavities require drainage by fenestration or shunting into the subarachnoid space. In general, the decompressive surgery at the foramen magnum is the more successful of the two,[87] and co-existing syrinx cavities may even shrink or resolve postoperatively without further intervention. Signs and symptoms referable to brain stem compression respond better to surgery then symptoms related to the spinal cord, even when syrinx decompression is included in the operation. Major pre-existing sensory or motor deficits are poor prognosticators for functional recovery.[86]

Treatment of the Dandy-Walker malformation is also surgical by shunting of the hydrocephalus and the dilated fourth ventricle via a double ventriculo- and cysto-peritoneal shunt.[88] This intervention may allow for normal mental development in the absence of additional CNS malformations.

The respiratory abnormalities associated with Joubert's syndrome usually improve after infancy. If significant and life-threatening apnea periods occur, home ventilation may be utilized successfully during the initial high-risk period. In case of severe feeding difficulties the placement of a gastric tube may be appropriate. Psychomotor retardation is not as uniformly severe as initially thought, and efforts to ensure best possible cognitive development should be undertaken.

Although disabilities resulting from the Möbius' syndrome can initially be very significant, including feeding difficulties and language problems, these tend to improve with time. Therefore, temporary placement of a feeding tube may be indicated in severe cases. The facial immobility can cause a significant social handicap and needs to be addressed in the management plan for such patients.

Abnormalities of the Skull and Spine

CRANIOSYNOSTOSIS

Pathogenesis and Pathophysiology. Craniosynostosis refers to the premature fusion of one or more of the cranial sutures. The premature fusion of cranial sutures results in abnormal and often asymmetrical growth of the cranium with resulting effects on both the underlying brain and the outward appearance of the head. There may be nonprogressive hydrocephalus in patients with craniosynostosis. Intracranial pressure may be elevated with or without hydrocephalus, especially when the absolute intracranial volume is increased (as can be the case in sagittal synostosis). Significant advances in understanding the pathogenesis of craniosynostosis are based on the recognition that mutations in members of a family of genes segregate with craniosynostosis and syndromes with craniosynostosis as one of the features. Point mutations in the fibroblast growth factor receptors (FGFR) were first recognized in the *FGFR2* gene in Crouzon's syndrome and subsequently also in Apert's, Jackson-Weiss', and Pfeiffer's syndromes. Mutations in *FGFR1* are found in Pfeiffer's syndrome. These findings have clearly linked these genes to the development of craniosynostosis.[89] Many of these syndromes have overlapping defects in other parts of the musculoskeletal system and other organ systems that are likely to result from the pleotropic expression of the FGFRs. Mapping of the mutations in the FGFRs has shown that mutations in different parts of these receptors, including the intracellular, the extracellular, and the transmembrane domains, account for some of the variation in clinical expression. Why mutations in different regions of these genes have such unique phenotypes is currently speculative. Some of the mutations render the receptor constitutively active, explaining the dominant inheritance. Several syndromes associated with a dwarfed stature can also result from mutations in an FGFR. Specifically thanatophoric dysplasia and achondroplasia/hypochondroplasia result from mutations in *FGFR3*.[89] Some cases of thanatophoric dysplasia include a cloverleaf skull, a severe form of craniosynostosis (see later discussion). It is already clear that other genes are also involved in the development of craniosynostosis.[90] For example, mutations in the homeobox gene *MSX2* have been linked to the Boston type of craniosynostosis,[91] but appear to be rare. In addition to these now molecularly characterized syndromes, there are many cases of craniosynostosis that are of unknown etiology and others arise from apparently nongenetic causes, such as the amniotic rupture sequence.

Clinical Features and Associated Disorders. In 1988, Cohen[92] reviewed all the syndromes with craniosynostosis as one of the features recognized up to that date. He found 64 described syndromes; over the subsequent years many more have been added. About 80 to 90 percent of all cases of craniosynostosis are sporadic and not part of a recognized syndrome. The sagittal suture is most often affected, leading to an elongated appearance of the skull with a normal face. This skull shape is referred to as scaphocephaly or dolichocephaly. Girls are affected slightly more often than boys and there are usually no neurological deficits associated with this craniosynostosis. Although the biparietal diameter is low, the actual head circumference is usually above the 95th percentile, so that the actual intracranial volume is normal or even increased. Impairment of brain growth usually does not occur, although the intracranial pressure may be elevated in some cases. Premature closure of the lambdoid sutures can occur in an asymmetrical fashion (plagiocephaly) or symmetrically (brachycephaly) (Fig. 28–10). Both conditions occur

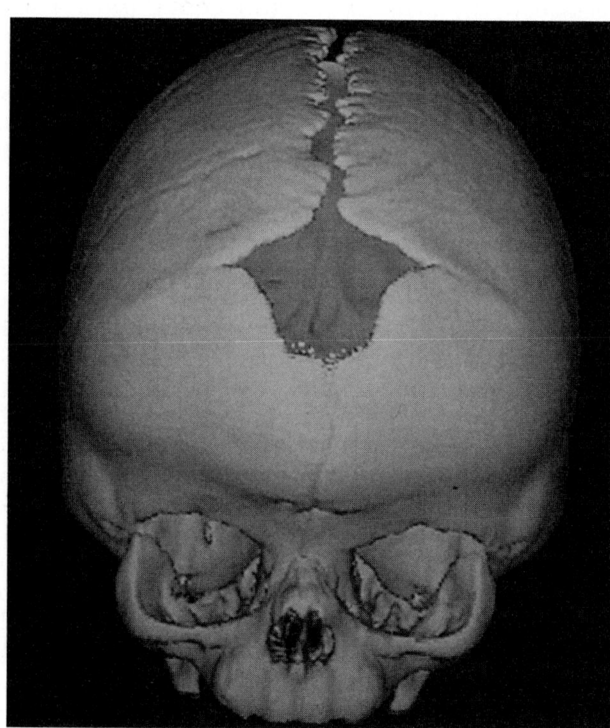

FIGURE 28–10. Craniosynostosis. A three-dimensional reconstruction of MRI from a patient with Apert syndrome. The coronal sutures are prematurely closed and the saggital suture is abnormally wide.

more commonly in boys. Brachycephaly, in particular, has a higher incidence of neurological complications and mental retardation. Optic atrophy with resulting visual impairment can be caused by traction of the chiasm and optic nerves due to upward displacement of the chiasm in the foreshortened skull. Increased intracranial pressure may also develop in premature synostosis of the coronal sutures and lead to optic atrophy as well as to more diffuse neurological damage. The incidence of mental retardation in brachycephaly remains high even in cases after surgical correction of increased intracranial pressure. Metopic craniosynostosis is rather rare and often occurs in a syndromic context such as the Opitz trigonocephaly syndrome (C syndrome) or in conjunction with holoprosencephaly. Asymmetrical closure of the lambdoid suture leads to another form of plagiocephaly. These single suture synostoses can be very mild phenotypically. A particularly severe situation can result from the combined closure of the coronal and sagittal sutures (oxycephaly). Here microcephaly and crowding of the intracranial content may result. In the most severe form, the sagittal, coronal, and lambdoid sutures are affected, resulting in the cloverleaf, or trilobed, skull (Kleeblattschädel). Patients with the cloverleaf skull anomaly show a bulging forehead, proptotic eyes, and severe neurological impairment.

Syndromic craniosynostosis only accounts for about 15 percent of cases of craniosynostosis. The two most common conditions are Crouzon and Apert syndrome, which account for about two thirds of syndromic craniosynostosis cases. In Crouzon syndrome synostosis of the coronal, sagittal, and lambdoid sutures are the most common. Ocular proptosis resulting from shallow orbits is a constant feature. Visual impairment occurs in about half of the patients.[93] Traction and compression in the optic canals leads to optic atrophy in 22 percent of cases and legal blindness in 7 percent.[94] Conductive hearing loss is quite common and occurs in about 55 percent of patients.[94] Headaches are a concern in about one third of the patients, and seizures have been reported in up to 12 percent of patients.[94] Mental deficiency is rare. This disorder follows autosomal dominant transmission. Apert syndrome (acrocephalosyndactyly) is an autosomal dominant disorder characterized by coronal synostosis in conjunction with a malformed and short cranial base resulting in a short and high skull (brachyturricephaly) and hand anomaliles. Platybasia is often associated. In infancy there is a wide and gaping defect in the region of the sagittal and metopic sutures. Again visual impairment is common.[93] Optic atrophy and conductive hearing loss can also occur in Apert syndrome. As opposed to Crouzon syndrome, mental deficiency is common in this condition; in one series half of the patients had an IQ below 70.[95] However, normal or above average intelligence can certainly be seen. The structure of the CNS can be affected in a number of ways; the most frequent includes agenesis or hypoplasia of the corpus callosum, migrational anomalies, and gyral abnormalities. Ventriculomegaly does not necessarily mean hydrocephalus, which is rather uncommon in Apert syndrome. Hand anomalies in Apert syndrome consist of fused middle fingers involving at least digits 2, 3, and 4. For most of the more severe craniofacial syndromes with craniosynostosis upper airway obstruction can become a problem relevant for management.[96]

Differential Diagnosis. Craniosynostosis is a defining feature of many syndromes.[17] Metabolic conditions that can lead to a premature fusion of cranial sutures include hyperthyroidism, hypercalcemia, and hypophosphatasia. Asymmetries of the skull are also seen in other conditions without craniosynostosis such as hemimegalencephaly, hemiatrophy, and unilateral destructive lesions of the brain that result in a marked size difference between the two cerebral hemispheres. The amniotic band rupture sequence can also give dramatic alterations in skull shape. A small head per se does not mean premature closure of the sutures, but retarded brain growth as a primary abnormality has to be considered. Earlier closure of the sutures can be seen under these circumstances and this constellation would not be considered a craniosynostosis. Severe constraint in utero can have the same effect. A number of other position-dependent asymmetries of skull shape can be seen, especially in hypotonic infants or infants with other external restrictions of skull growth. Finally, there exists a long list of syndromes that include unusual skull configurations not based on premature fusion of cranial sutures.

Evaluation and Management. Although skull films were traditionally the modality of choice for the evaluation of craniosynostosis, CT with 3-D reconstructions are now the method of choice for the evaluation of the cranial skeleton and planning of management. The goal of evaluation should not only be the delineation of the various anatomical abnormalities, but also an attempt at a specific diagnosis in a given case of craniosynostosis. This may include the clinical recognition of a syndrome; direct mutation analysis of selected FGFR genes may be appropriate in selected cases.

Treatment for the craniosynostosis is surgical and involves excision of the fused suture and separation of the bony margins by an implanted matrix. Good results can usually be obtained,[97] especially when surgery is performed before 6 months of age. Given that the intracranial pressure can be elevated with single suture synostosis, the indication for repair has moved away from purely cosmetic indications. For the Kleeblattschädel deformity, early subtotal craniectomy is the only reasonable attempt at correction, although the severity of the overall condition may prohibit invasive treatment. The acrocephalosyndactyly syndromes may require surgical approaches to the associated hand malformations, in particular polydactyly and syndactyly. Careful attention needs to be paid to vision and hearing in craniosynostosis patients. Hearing aids may be necessary for adequate communication and language development. Shunting for hydrocephalus is rarely necessary.

OTHER DISORDERS OF THE SKULL AND SPINE

Dwarfism

Although dwarfism is primarily a defect of the musculoskeletal system, central and periphereal nervous system manifestations are encountered in a variety of these disorders associated with short stature, most of which are beyond the scope of this chapter. The most frequent neurological manifestations are a result of impingement of the nervous system as a result of narrowing of bony foramina. For example, in some dwarfism syndromes, such as achondroplasia, narrowing of the foramen magnum can obstruct CSF flow and result in hydrocephalus. In achondroplasia the development of clinical symptoms usually requires a narrowing of the foramen magnum to under –3 to 4 SD (standard deviations are available in radiology texts). *Thanatophoric dysplasia*, due to mutations in the same genes as achondroplasia (see preceding discussion), has a unique neuropathology of the brain[98] with deep radial fissures arranged as spokes on a wheel distorting the temporal lobes (Fig. 28–11). Microsopically the temporal lobes, particularly medially, are disorganized, often showing polymicrogyria. Polymicrogyria may also occur outside the temporal lobes.

The diagnosis of thanatophoric dysplasia is important for management decisions and for the purpose of genetic counseling. Clinically there are short limbs, a narrow thorax with short ribs, a short spine with flat vertebral bodies, and large-appearing cranium with flat nasal bridge. There are two subtypes: the more common type I with bowed bones but no cloverleaf skull, and a second form (type 2) with straight bones but with a complex craniosynostosis giving rise to the cloverleaf skull. Hydrocephalus is common with the type II form. Both forms are associated with mutations in *FGFR3*.

Achondroplasia can be associated with a number of neurological complications.[99] Stenosis at the level of the foramen magnum can cause a high cervical or lower medullary myelopathy. In case of the latter apneic spells or respiratory insufficiency can result; the former can give rise to long tract symptomatology including frank quadriparesis. Stenosis of the spinal canal with myelopathy and/or radiculopathy can occur at any level. Careful assessment for lower extremity hyper-reflexia, clonus, and Babinski signs is important for the early recognition of a myelopathy. Surgical decompression may become necessary in these cases. The development of hydrocephalus in achondroplasia is possible due to stenosis at the level of the foramen magnum, though this is not very common. A milder degree of hydrocephalus has been postulated to be due to impaired CSF resorption because of diminished venous return from the cranial compartment. A degree of macrocephaly, however, is part of the "normal" clinical manifestations of achondroplasia and does not automatically imply hydrocephalus. Thus, head circumference measurements should be compared with head circumference charts specifically corrected for achondroplasia. The numerous skeletal dysplasias, many of which have secondary neurological complications, are beyond the scope of this chapter (see McKusick[100] for complete discussions).

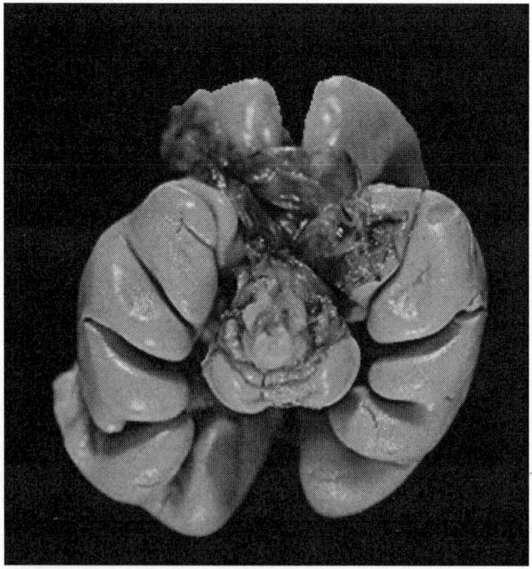

FIGURE 28–11. Thanatophoric dysplasia. A ventral view of the brain from a 20-week fetus with thanatophoric dysplasia. Radially oriented, deep fissures in the medial temporal lobe replace the normal smooth surface at this age and are pathopneumonic for this disorder.

Skull Base and Neck Deformities

Malformations and deformities of the skull base can be part of a number of conditions. Included among these are craniosynostosis syndromes (short and steep cranial base), neurofibromatosis 1 (aplasia of the sphenoid wing), Chiari type I and II (platybasia, flat cranial base), osteogenesis imperfecta (basilar impression, invaginated cranial base), and Hajdu-Cheney syndrome (basilar impression), as well as others. They can also occur in isolation or in a familial context. Other conditions such as Paget's disease, rickets, rheumatoid arthritis, and hypoparathyroidism have to be considered in the differential diagnosis. Nuchal pain and vertigo may be early and nonspecific complaints. If present, downbeating nystagmus in primary position accentuated by gaze position down and out may provide a diagnostic clue for pathology at the craniocervical junction. The neurological syndrome of basilar impression, including platybasia and the more extreme convexobasia, can begin insidiously with increasing spasticity in the lower extremities, ataxic gait, and loss of proprioception also in the upper extremities. In addition, lower cranial nerve function, including dysphagia, may become impaired late in the course.[101] The neck may be short and cervical motility impaired, and there may be nuchal pain in addition causing neck stiffness and torticollis at presentation. Symptoms and signs of associated conditions such as the Chiari malformations and syringomyelia can complicate the picture. Sagittal CT reconstruction plus sagittal MRI is the optimal imaging modality combination to confirm the diagnosis and delineate the bony abnormalities. Surgical decompression at the foramen magnum is the treatment of choice, occasionally requiring additional laminectomies of C2 and C3 with cervico-occipital fusion. Platybasia (defined as the angle between planes of the anterior cranial fossa and the clivus being greater than 140 degrees) in isolation is generally asymptomatic.

Congenital fusion of the cervical vertebrae is known as the *Klippel-Feil anomaly*. Presumably this reflects a failure of segmentation rather than a secondary fusion. This anomaly can be part of a number of syndromes (such as Turner's, Noonan's, and Wildervanck's syndromes), but can also occur sporadically or be inherited in isolation as an autosomal dominant or autosomal recessive trait. The fusion of vertebrae can extend beyond the cervical spine, but most commonly is restricted to levels C2 and C3 or C5 and C6. Clinically there is a short neck, low posterior hairline, and limitation of neck movements, in particular rotation and bending to the sides. Atlanto-occipital anomalies are frequently associated with the Klippel-Feil anomaly and one of the major reason for associated morbidity. Kyphosis and scoliosis are often associated, as is spina bifida occulta in some cases.[102] Many patients also have a variety of genitourinary anomalies, including unilateral renal agenesis.[102] Hearing impairment can be seen in about 20 percent. Other skeletal malformations such as the Sprengel deformity can be associated. The main neurological complications result from craniocervical instability with the possibilty of spinal cord compromise. It has also been noted that patients with the Klippel-Feil anomaly may have mirror movements on neurological examination,[103] but the reason for this observation is not clear.

Occipitalization of the atlas, or assimilation of the atlas, refers to the fusion of the anterior arch and ring of C1 with the foramen magnum. A Chiari type 1 malformation, Klippel-Feil anomaly, achondroplasia, and syringomyelia may be associated. Atlanto-axial instability (atlas-dens interval greater than 3 mm) can occur in rheumatoid arthritis but also in a number of genetic conditions and syndromes, most notably Down's syndrome. It is recommended to screen trisomy 21 patients at 5 and 10 years for atlanto-axial instability and if present restrict potentially harmful physical activities.

Reviews and Selected Updates

Barkovich AJ, Kuzniecky RI, Jackson GD, Guerrini R, Dobyns WB: Classification system for malformations of cortical development. Neurology 2001;57:2168–2178.

Caviness VS Jr, Takahashi T, Nowakowski RS: Neocortical malformation as consequence of nonadaptive regulation of neuronogenetic sequence. Ment Retard Dev Disabil Res Rev 2000;6:22–33.

Cornette L, Verpoorten C, Lagae L, Plets C, Van Calenbergh F, Casaer P: losed spinal dysraphism: A review on diagnosis and treatment in infancy. Europ J Paediatr Neurol 1998;2:179–185.

Gleeson JG: Classical lissencephaly and double cortex (subcortical band heterotopia): *LIS1* and *doublecortin*. Curr Opin Neurol 2000;13:121–126.

Kinsman SL, Plawner LL, Hahn JS: Holoprosencephaly: Recent advances and new insights. Curr Opin Neurol 2000;13:127–132.

MacCollin M, Kwiatkowski: Molecular genetic aspects of the phakomatoses: tuberous sclerosis complex and neurofibromatosis 1. Curr Opin Neurol 2001;14:163–170.

Mochida GH, Walsh CA: Molecular genetics of human microcephaly. Curr Opin Neurol 2001;14:151–156.

Muenke M, Cohen MM Jr: Genetic approaches to understanding brain development: Holoprosencephaly as a model. Ment Retard Dev Disabil Res Rev 2000;6:15–21.

Pasqualetti M, Rijli FM: Homeobox gene mutations and brain stem development disorders: Learning from knockout mice. Curr Opin Neurol 2001;14:177–184.

Pomeroy SL, Kim JY: Biology and pathobiology of neuronal development. Ment Retard Dev Disabil Res Rev 2000;6:41–46.

Walsh CA: Genetics of neuronal migration in the cerebral cortex. Ment Retard Dev Disabil Res Rev 2000;l6:34–40.

References

1. Adams R, Victor M: Principals of Neurology, 5th ed. New York, McGraw-Hill, 1993.
2. Russell D: Observations on the pathology of hydrocephalus. Medical Research Council Special Report Series No. 265: Her Majesty's Stationery Office, London, 1949.
3. Kirkpatrick M, Engleman H, Minns RA: Symptoms and signs of progressive hydrocephalus. Arch Dis Child 1989;64:124–128.
4. Di Rocco C, Caldarelli M, Ceddia A: "Occult" hydrocephalus in children [see comments]. Childs Nerv Syst 1989;5:71–75.
5. Hagberg B, Sjorgen I: The chronic brain syndrome of infantile hydrocephalus. A follow-up study of 63 spontaneously arrested cases. Am J Dis Child 1966;112:189–196.
6. Jouet M, Rosenthal A, Armstrong G, et al: X-linked spastic paraplegia (SPG1), MASA syndrome and X-linked hydrocephalus result from mutations in the L1 gene. Nat Genet 1994;7:402–407.
7. De Myer W: Megalencephaly: Types, clinical syndromes and management. Pediatr Neurol 1986;2.
8. Barkovich AJ, Kjos BO: Nonlissencephalic cortical dysplasias: Correlation of imaging findings with clinical deficits [see comments]. AJNR 1992;13:95–103.
9. Kanev PM, Park TS: The treatment of hydrocephalus. Neurosurg Clin North Am 1993;4:611–619.
10. Volpe J: Neurology of the Newborn, 3rd ed. Philadelphia, WB Saunders, 1994.
11. Hudgins RJ, Edwards MS, Goldstein R, et al: Natural history of fetal ventriculomegaly. Pediatrics 1988;82:692–697.
12. Rosseau GL, McCullough DC, Joseph AL: Current prognosis in fetal ventriculomegaly. J Neurosurg 1992;77:551–555.
13. Fernell E, Uvebrant P, von Wendt L: Overt hydrocephalus at birth—origin and outcome. Childs Nerv Syst 1987;3:350–353.
14. Warkany J: Congenital Malformations. Notes and Comments. Chicago, Year Book Medical, 1971.
15. Clarren S, Smith D, Harvey M, Ward R: Hyperthermia: A prospective evaluation of a possible teratogenic agent in man. J Pediatr 1979;95:81–83.
16. Jones K: Smith's Recognizable Patterns of Human Malformations, 5th ed. Philadelphia, WB Saunders, 1996.
17. Van Allen MI, Kalousek DK, Chernoff GF, et al: Evidence for multisite closure of the neural tube in humans. Am J Med Genet 1993;47:723–743.
18. Golden J, Chernoff G: Multiple sites of anterior neural tube closure in humans: Evidence from anterior neural tube defects (anencephaly). Pediatrics 1995;95:506–510.
19. Holmes L: Spina bifida: Anticonvulsants and other maternal influences. *In* Bock G, Marsh J (eds): Neural Tube Defects. London, John Wiley and Sons, 1994, pp 232–244.
20. Stevenson R, Hall J, Goodman R: Human Malformations and Related Anomalies. New York, Oxford University Press, 1993.
21. MRC Vitamin Study Research Group: Prevention of neural tube defects: Results of the Medical Research Council Vitamin Study. Lancet 1991;338:131–137.
22. Kirke PN, Daly LE, Elwood JH: A randomised trial of low dose folic acid to prevent neural tube defects. The Irish Vitamin Study Group. Arch Dis Child 1992;67:1442–1446.
23. Czeizel AE, Dudas I: Prevention of the first occurrence of neural-tube defects by periconceptional vitamin supplementation. N Engl J Med 1992;327:1832–1835.
24. Schmidt DM, Robinson B, Jones DA: The tethered spinal cord. Etiology and clinical manifestations. Orthop Rev 1990;19:870–876.
25. Gilbert J, Jones K, Rorke L, Chernoff G, James H: Central nervous system anomalies associated with meningomyelocele, hydrocephalus, and the Arnold-Chiari malformation: Reappraisal of theories regarding the pathogenesis of posterior neural tube closure defects. Neurosurgery 1986;18:559–564.
26. Luthy DA, Wardinsky T, Shurtleff DB, et al: Cesarean section before the onset of labor and subsequent motor function in infants with meningomyelocele diagnosed antenatally [see comments]. N Engl J Med 1991;324:662–666.
27. Rauzzino M, Oakes WJ: Chiari II malformation and syringomyelia. Neurosurg Clin North Am 1995;6:293–309.
28. Hernandez RD, Hurwitz RS, Foote JE, Zimmern PE, Leach GE: Nonsurgical management of threatened upper urinary tracts and incontinence in children with myelomeningocele. J Urol 1994;152: 1582–1585.
29. Khair B, Azmy A, Carachi R, Fyfe A, Drainer I: Continent urinary diversion using Mitrofanoff principle in children with neurogenic bladder. Eur J Pediatr Surg 1993;3:8–9.
30. Samuelsson L, Skoog M: Ambulation in patients with myelomeningocele: A multivariate statistical analysis. J Pediatr Orthop 1988;8:569–575.
31. Herman JM, McLone DG, Storrs BB, Dauser RC: Analysis of 153 patients with myelomeningocele or spinal lipoma reoperated upon for a tethered cord. Presentation, management and outcome. Pediatr Neurosurg 1993;19:243–249.
32. Wald N: Folic acid and neural tube defects: The current evidence and implications for prevention. *In* Bock G, Marsh J (eds): Neural Tube Defects. London, John Wiley and Sons, 1994, pp 192–211.
33. Puelles L, Rubenstein J: Expression patterns of homeobox and other putative regulatory genes in the embryonic mouse forebrain suggest a neuromeric organization. TrendsNeurosci 1993;16:472–479.
34. Lumsden A, Keynes R: Segmental patterns of neuronal development in the chick hindbrain. Nature 1989;337:424–428.
35. Croen LA, Shaw GM, Lammer EJ: Holoprosencephaly: Epidemiologic and clinical characteristics of a California population. Am J Med Genet 1996;64:465–472.
36. Olsen CL, Hughes JP, Youngblood LG, Sharpe-Stimac M: Epidemiology of holoprosencephaly and phenotypic characteristics of affected children: New York State, 1984–1989. Am J Med Genet 1997;73:217–226.
37. Matsunaga E, Shiota K: Holoprosencephaly in human embryos: Epidemiologic studies of 150 cases. Teratology 1977;16:261–272.

38. Golden JA: Holoprosencephaly: a defect in brain patterning. J Neuropathol Exp Neurol 1998;57:991–999.
39. Kelley RL, Roessler E, Hennekam RC, et al: Holoprosencephaly in RSH/Smith-Lemli-Opitz syndrome: Does abnormal cholesterol metabolism affect the function of Sonic Hedgehog? Am J Med Genet 1996;66:478–484.
40. Ming JE, Muenke M: Holoprosencephaly: From Homer to Hedgehog. Clin Genet 1998;53:155–163.
41. Chiang C, Litingtung Y, Lee E, et al: Cyclopia and defective axial patterning in mice lacking Sonic hedgehog gene function. Nature 1996;383:407–413.
42. Wallis DE, Muenke M: Molecular mechanisms of holoprosencephaly. Mol Genet Metab 1999;68:126–138.
43. Friede R: Developmental Neuropathology, 2nd ed. Berlin, Springer-Verlag, 1989.
44. DeMyer W, Zeman W, Palmer C: The face predicts the brain: Diagnostic significance of median facial anomalies from holoprosencephaly (arhinencephaly). Pediatrics 1964;34:711–718.
45. Brodsky MC, Glasier CM: Optic nerve hypoplasia. Clinical significance of associated central nervous system abnormalities on magnetic resonance imaging [published erratum appears in Arch Ophthalmol 1993; 111:491]. Arch Ophthalmol 1993;111:66–74.
46. Gupta JK, Lilford RJ: Assessment and management of fetal agenesis of the corpus callosum. Prenat Diagn 1995;15:301–312.
47. Rugarli EI, Ballabio A: Kallmann syndrome. From genetics to neurobiology. JAMA 1993;270:2713–2716.
48. Rorke L: A perspective: The role of disordered genetic control of neurogenesis in the pathogenesis of migration disorders. J Neuropath Exp Neurol 1994;53:105–117.
49. Pilz D, Stoodley N, Golden JA: Neuronal migration, cerebral cortical development, and cerebral cortical anomalies. J Neuropathol Exp Neurol 2002;61:1–11.
50. Pilz DT, Matsumoto N, Minnerath S, et al: LIS1 and XLIS (DCX) mutations cause most classical lissencephaly, but different patterns of malformation. Hum Mol Genet 1998;7:2029–2037.
51. des Portes V, Pinard JM, Billuart P, et al: A novel CNS gene required for neuronal migration and involved in X-linked subcortical laminar heterotopia and lissencephaly syndrome. Cell 1998;92:51–61.
52. Gleeson JG, Allen KM, Fox JW, et al: Doublecortin, a brain-specific gene mutated in human X-linked lissencephaly and double cortex syndrome, encodes a putative signaling protein. Cell 1998;92:63–72.
53. Hong SE, Shugart YY, Huang DT, et al: Autosomal recessive lissencephaly with cerebellar hypoplasia is associated with human RELN mutations. Nature Genetics 2000;26:93–96.
54. Norman M, McGillivray B, Kalousek D, Hill A, Poskitt K: Congenital Malformations of the Brain: Pathological, Embryological, Clinical, Radiolological and Genetic Aspects. New York, Oxford University Press, 1995.
55. Yoshida A, Kobayashi K, Manya H, et al: Muscular dystrophy and neuronal migration disorder caused by mutations in a glycosyltransferase, POMGnT1. Dev Cell 2001;1:717–724.
56. Kobayashi K, Nakahori Y, Miyake M, et al: An ancient retrotransposal insertion causes Fukuyama-type congenital muscular dystrophy. Nature 1998;394:388–392.
57. Fox JW, Lamperti ED, Eksioglu YZ, et al: Mutations in filamin 1 prevent migration of cerebral cortical neurons in human periventricular heterotopia. Neuron 1998;21:1315–1325.
58. Mischel P, Nguyen L, Vinters H: Cerebral cortical dysplasia associated with pediatric epilepsy. Review of neuropathologic features and proposal for a grading system. J Neuropath Exp Neurol 1995;54:137–153.
59. Santavuori P, Somer H, Sainio K, et al: Muscle-eye-brain disease (MEB). Brain Dev 1989;11:147–153.
60. Fukuyama Y, Osawa M, Suzuki H: Congenital progressive muscular dystrophy of the Fukuyama type: Clinical, genetic and pathological considerations. Brain Dev 1981;3:1–29.
61. Aicardi J: The place of neuronal migration abnormalities in child neurology. Can J Neurol Sci 1994;21:185–193.
62. Pedespan JM, Loiseau H, Vital A, Marchal C, Fontan D, Rougier A: Surgical treatment of an early epileptic encephalopathy with suppression-bursts and focal cortical dysplasia. Epilepsia 1995;36:37–40.
63. Quirk JA, Kendall B, Kingsley DP, Boyd SG, Pitt MC: EEG features of cortical dysplasia in children. Neuropediatrics 1993;24:193–199.
64. Dobyns WB, Truwit CL: Lissencephaly and other malformations of cortical development: 1995 update. Neuropediatrics 1995;26:132–147.
65. Aicardi J: The agyria-pachygyria complex: A spectrum of cortical malformations. Brain Dev 1991;13:1–8.
66. Volpe JJ, Adams RD: Cerebro-hepato-renal syndrome of Zellweger. An inherited disorder of neuronal migration. Acta Neuropathol 1972;20:175–198.
67. Huttenlocher PR, Taravath S, Mojtahedi S: Periventricular heterotopia and epilepsy. Neurology 1994; 44:51–55.
68. Eksioglu Y, Scheffer I, Cardenas P, et al: Periventricular heterotopia: An X-linked dominant epilepsy locus causing aberrant cerebral cortical development. Neuron 1996;16:77–87.
69. Dobyns WB, Andermann E, Andermann F, et al: X-linked malformations of neuronal migration. Neurology 1996;47:331–339.
70. Wyllie E: The Treatment of Epilepsy: Principles and Practice. Philadelphia/London, Lea & Febiger, 1993.
71. Palmini A, Andermann F, Aicardi J, et al: Diffuse cortical dysplasia, or the "double cortex" syndrome: The clinical and epileptic spectrum in 10 patients. Neurology 1991;41:1656–1662.
72. Barkovich AJ, Chuang SH: Unilateral megalencephaly: Correlation of MR imaging and pathologic characteristics. AJNR 1990;11:523–531.
73. Vigevano F, Di Rocco C: Effectiveness of hemispherectomy in hemimegalencephaly with intractable seizures. Neuropediatrics 1990;21:222–223.
74. Tolmie JL, McNay M, Stephenson JB, Doyle D, Connor JM: Microcephaly: Genetic counselling and antenatal diagnosis after the birth of an affected child. Am J Med Genet 1987;27:583–594.
75. Chiari H: Veränderungen des Kleinhirns, des Pons und der Medulla oblongata in Folge von Congenitalerhydrocephalie des Grosshirns. Denkschrift Akad Wiss Wien 1896;63:71–116.
76. Brown J: The Dandy-Walker malformation. *In* Vinken PJ, Bruyn GW (eds): The Handbook of Clinical Neurology, Vol 30. Amsterdam, Elsevier, 1977.
77. Golden J, Rorke L, Bruce D: Dandy-Walker syndrome and associated anomalies. Pediatr Neurosci 1987;13:38–44.
78. Joubert M, Eisenring JJ, Andermann F: Familial dysgenesis of the vermis: A syndrome of hyperventilation, abnormal eye movements and retardation. Neurology 1968;18:302–303.
79. Boltshauser E, Isler W: Joubert syndrome: Episodic hyperpnea, abnormal eye movements, retardation and ataxia, associated with dysplasia of the cerebellar vermis. Neuropadiatrie 1977;8:57–66.
80. Menezes AH: Chiari I malformations and hydromyelia—complications. Pediatr Neurosurg 1991;17:146–154.
81. Engle EC: The genetics of strabismus: Duane, Moebius, and fibrosis syndromes. *In* Traboulsi EI (ed): Genetic diseases of the eye. New York, Oxford University Press, 1999.
82. Barth PG: Pontocerebellar hypoplasias. An overview of a group of inherited neurodegenerative disorders with fetal onset. Brain Dev 1993;15:411–422.
83. Jensen PR, Hansen FJ, Skovby F: Cerebellar hypoplasia in children with the carbohydrate-deficient glycoprotein syndrome. Neuroradiology 1995;37:328–330.
84. Bordarier C, Aicardi J: Dandy-Walker syndrome and agenesis of the cerebellar vermis: Diagnostic problems and genetic counselling. Dev Med Child Neurol 1990;32:285–294.
85. Elster AD, Chen MY: Chiari I malformations: Clinical and radiologic reappraisal. Radiology 1992;183:347–353.
86. Nagib MG: An approach to symptomatic children (ages 4–14 years) with Chiari type I malformation. Pediatr Neurosurg 1994;21:31–35.
87. Bindal AK, Dunsker SB, Tew JM Jr: Chiari I malformation: Classification and management. Neurosurgery 1995;37:1069–1074.
88. Osenbach RK, Menezes AH: Diagnosis and management of the Dandy-Walker malformation: 30 years of experience. Pediatr Neurosurg 1992;18:179–189.
89. Muenke M, Schell U: Fibroblast-growth-factor receptor mutations in human skeletal disorders. Trends Genet 1995;11:308–313.
90. Winter RM: Recent molecular advances in dysmorphology. Hum Mol Genet 1995;4:1699–1704.
91. Jabs EW, Muller U, Li X, et al: A mutation in the homeodomain of the human MSX2 gene in a family affected with autosomal dominant craniosynostosis. Cell 1993;75:443–450.
92. Cohen MM Jr: Craniosynostosis update 1987. Am J Med Genet 1988; 4(Suppl):99–148.
93. Hertle RW, Quinn GE, Minguini N, Katowitz JA: Visual loss in patients with craniofacial synostosis. J Pediatr Ophthalmol Strabismus 1991; 28:344–349.
94. Kreiborg S: Crouzon syndrome. A clinical and roentgencephalometric study. Scand J Plast Reconstruct Surg 1981;18(Suppl):1–198.
95. Patton MA, Goodship J, Hayward R, Lansdown R: Intellectual development in Apert's syndrome: A long term follow up of 29 patients. J Med Genet 1988;25:164–167.

96. Moore MH: Upper airway obstruction in the syndromal craniosynostoses. Br J Plast Surg 1993;46:355–362.
97. Vander Kolk CA: Craniofacial surgery. Clin Plast Surg 1994;21:4.
98. Wongmontkolrit T, Bush M, Roessmann U: Neuropathological findings in thanatophoric dysplasia. Arch Pathol Lab Med 1984;107:132–135.
99. Hecht JT, Butler IJ: Neurologic morbidity associated with achondroplasia. J Child Neurol 1990;5:84–97.
100. McKusick V: Mendelian Inheritance in Man. Catalogs of Human Genes and Genetic Disorders, 11th ed. Baltimore, Johns Hopkins University Press, 1994.
101. Aicardi J: Diseases of the Nervous System in Childhood. London, Mac Keith Press, 1992.
102. Van Kerckhoven MF, Fabry G: The Klippel-Feil syndrome: A constellation of deformities. Acta Orthop Belg 1989;55:107–118.
103. Gunderson CH, Solitare GB: Mirror movements in patients with the Klippel-Feil syndrome. Neuropathologic observations. Arch Neurol 1968;18:675–679.

CHAPTER 29

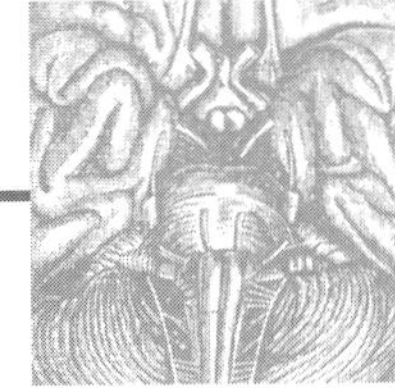

STEVEN K. FESKE and STEVEN A. GREENBERG

Degenerative and Compressive Structural Disorders

History and Definitions

A variety of neurological disorders result from abnormalities of bones, ligaments, muscles, and other mesenchymal tissue that compress the nervous system. In many instances the result is a focal disorder of nervous system function such as a mononeuropathy, a root syndrome, or the compression of intracranial contents by abnormalities of the skull. Much of our clinical knowledge of the peripheral system is derived from these kinds of lesions—for instance, the dermatomal map, which every student of the nervous system carries in his or her black bag, is in part derived from the study of patients with a herniated disc and root compression. Much of the standard neurological examination of the sensory system is derived from studies carried out by Henry Head 80 years ago in patients (including himself) who had lesions of individual peripheral nerves.

Degenerative Structural Disorders

DEGENERATIVE DISC DISEASE

Pathogenesis and Pathophysiology. The vertebral disc is composed of the inner gelatinous nucleus pulposus and the surrounding annulus fibrosus. Vertebral disc herniation refers to rupture of the annulus with displacement of the central nucleus. In youth, the disc is highly elastic. With the passage of time, the direct vascular supply to the vertebrae and discs decreases, and they undergo the accumulated effects of axial loading. The resulting decreases in water content, oxygen content, and metabolic efficiency lead to a disc that is more compressible, less elastic, and more prone to tear and rupture. Disc rupture and herniation can cause pain by several mechanisms. The periosteum of the bony spine, the ligaments, the outer fibrous annulus of the vertebral discs, and the dura are all innervated by nociceptive afferents from the spinal nerves. A ruptured or torn fibrous disc may generate local pain owing to mechanical stress on these pain-sensitive structures. Also, the exposed disc material has a direct toxic effect and elicits a local inflammatory response, both of which may promote increased pain sensitivity. In addition to these local effects, the mass of the herniated disc material may compress the spinal roots by protruding into the lateral recess or the neural foramen, or it may protrude into the spinal canal, compressing the spinal cord in the cervical or thoracic region or the cauda equina in the lumbosacral region. Details of the mechanisms by which compression causes neurological dysfunction are complex and probably include mechanical alteration of axonal membranes, impaired axonal flow, and ischemia due to compromise of the microcirculation with resultant edema and eventual demyelination. Finally, regional muscle spasm may accompany other effects, adding to the pain and disability.

The accumulation of degenerative lesions in the spine may compromise the area of the central canal available to the spinal cord in the cervical region or to the cauda equina in the lumbosacral region enough to cause symptomatic spinal stenosis with or without discrete disc herniation. Most commonly, these lesions include degenerative discs that bulge posteriorly, a hypertrophied ligamentum flavum that bulges anteriorly, and hypertrophied facet joints that crowd into the bony canal posterolaterally (Fig. 29–1). Less common lesions may contribute to the problem, hastening significant stenosis: congenitally short pedicles, spondylolisthesis without spondylolysis, or abnormal angulation of the bony spine.

Epidemiology and Risk Factors. Vertebral disc degenerative changes are a universal accompaniment of aging. Teenagers rarely develop symptomatic disc herniation. The peak incidence of symptoms occurs between the ages of 30 and 50. Patients often describe the onset of low back pain, usually remittent and without specific features in their twenties, perhaps after identifiable trauma, and the onset of more specific symptoms that leads to the diagnosis of disc herniation is often not preceded by further trauma. Probably the accumulation of degenerative changes to the annulus and the preservation of the expansile gelatinous nucleus, overlapping with a period of life when job and sports-related activities increase the amount of mechanical stress on the body, account for this peak in the incidence of disease. The incidence then falls off in the older population, probably due to the lack of mobility of the desiccated disc and the relative lack of physical activity. Women and men are affected approximately equally.

There is a tendency toward disc herniation in some families, such as those with congenital spinal anomalies, including fused and malformed vertebrae and lumbar spinal stenosis due to short pedicles. Patients with increased weight and tall stature are at increased risk for this condition. Also, acquired spinal disorders, such as common degenerative arthritis and ankylosing spondylitis, predispose to disc degeneration. Various behaviors that increase risk include sedentary occupations, physical inactivity, motor vehicle use, vibration, and smoking. In younger women, pregnancy and delivery are associated with lumbosacral herniation, and new symptoms

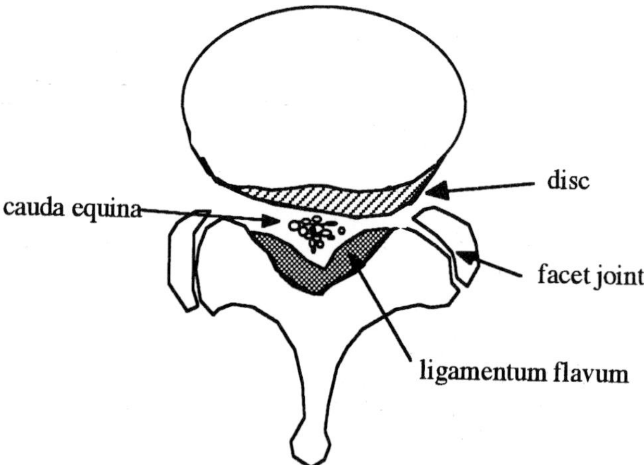

FIGURE 29–1. Lumbosacral spinal stenosis. L4 vertebra in cross section. Posterior bulging of the intervertebral disc, hypertrophy of degenerated facet joints, and hypertrophy of the ligamentum flavum crowd into the central canal to cause lumbar spinal stenosis.

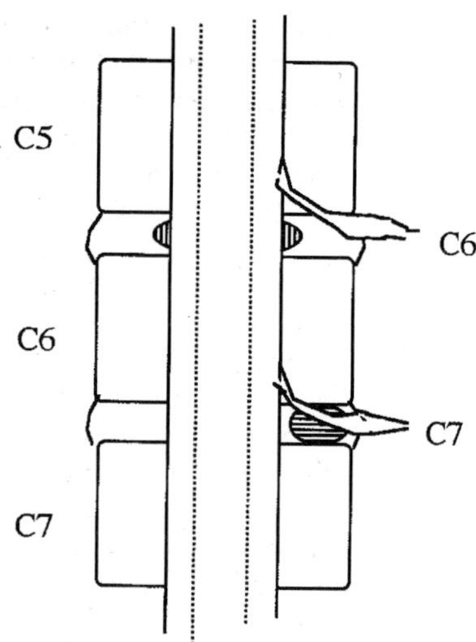

FIGURE 29–2. Cervical disc herniation. At the cervical levels, roots emerge from the spinal cord near their level of exit. Each root emerges above its corresponding vertebra, with C8 emerging between C7 and T1. Posterolateral herniation at this level causes compression of the exiting root *(horizontal hatching)*. Hence, C6–C7 herniation causes C7 compression, and so on. A large central herniation in this region can compress the spinal cord and cause a cervical myelopathy *(vertical hatching)*.

of cervical disc herniation may occur in part because of the bending and lifting involved in child rearing.

Clinical Features and Associated Disorders. The most common site of disc herniation in the cervical region is the C6–C7 level, followed by C5–C6, C7–T1, and C4–C5. Patients typically develop some local pain in the neck that radiates to the shoulders or the interscapular region. In the most common lateral herniations, radicular symptoms ensue. These symptoms include pain in the shoulder and arm, which may follow a dermatomal pattern but more typically is deep and aching and only roughly corresponds to the involved dermatome. At the cervical levels, the roots emerge laterally to exit through the neural foramina *above* the correspondingly numbered vertebral bodies. Because the spinal cord and bony vertebral levels are roughly aligned in the neck, the level of herniation corresponds to the level of root irritation. Hence, C6–C7 herniation affects the C7 root (Fig. 29–2). Pain may be exacerbated by coughing or straining. Numbness is more likely to supply reliable localizing information than pain. Compression of the C6 root typically causes numbness in the thumb and index finger, and compression of the C7 root typically involves the index and middle fingers. When compression is severe, myotomal weakness, reflex loss, and, with time, fasciculations and atrophy may ensue. With C6 compression, the biceps, brachioradialis, pronator teres, and radial wrist extensors may be weak, and the brachioradialis and biceps reflexes may be diminished or lost. With C7 weakness, the wrist and finger extensors and the triceps are typically weak. The triceps reflex may also be diminished or lost. With C8 compression, there is often interscapular pain and pain in the medial aspect of the arm and hand with weakness of the hand intrinsic muscles. The finger flexor reflex may be lost. Lesions above C6 are less common and are associated with correspondingly more proximal sensory symptoms and weakness. Lesions of the C5 root may cause shoulder pain and pain and numbness in the lateral aspect of the upper arm. Many muscles can be used to test the C5 root, including the infraspinatus, supraspinatus, deltoid, biceps, and supinator. Lesions above this level may cause neck pain and sensory loss in the neck, supraclavicular area (C3), and acromioclavicular area (C4) of the shoulder. Lesions involving the spinal cord or roots above C4 may paralyze the diaphragm and cause respiratory compromise (Table 29–1).

In the lumbosacral region, the most common site of herniation is the L5–S1 level, followed by the L4–L5 level and then higher levels. Symptoms of lumbosacral herniation often follow lifting or twisting injuries, or they may result from accumulated low-level trauma. Pain typically occurs in the parasacral area and radiates to the buttocks. Below C8, the roots exit through the neural foramina *below* the correspondingly numbered vertebral bodies. In patients with the most common posterolateral herniation, dermatomal radicular pain typically occurs at the level below the emerging root, which usually escapes entrapment above the protruding disc. Hence, L5–S1 herniation affects the S1 root (Fig. 29–3). With posterolateral L5–S1 herniations and S1 root entrapment, the pain radiates to the posterior aspect of the thigh and, especially when the root is stretched, into the posterolateral lower leg, lateral heel, and sole. This pattern can be demonstrated by straight-leg raising, in which the smaller the angle of elevation required to elicit pain, the greater the suggestion that root compression is responsible.[1] Characteristic pain on elevation of the opposite leg may be even stronger evidence of root compression.[2] Some patients with symptoms that are exacerbated by root traction avoid full weight bearing on the heel of the involved side, standing with the knee flexed and the heel off the floor. When pain is less severe, symptoms may be elicited by having the patient walk on the heels. Numbness is felt in the posterolateral leg, lateral aspect of the heel, and the sole of the foot. The gastrocnemius and hamstrings may be weak, and the ankle jerk may be diminished or lost. More lateral herniation of the L5–S1 disc or herniation of the L4–L5 disc may entrap the L5 root. Here the pain may be similar, with adjustment of the findings to fit the L5 dermatome and myotome. Numbness is most marked on the dorsum of the foot. Weak muscles include the foot elevators (tibialis anterior group), everters (peronei), and invertors (tibialis posterior), and the toe extensors (extensor hallucis longus). Herniations at higher levels in the lumbosacral region cause pain and deficits that correspond to the roots involved (Table 29–2).

In addition to these radicular syndromes, patients with central herniations in the cervical or thoracic region may develop pain and acute myelopathic symptoms with spasticity and quadriparesis or paraparesis, sensory loss at or below the segmental dermatome of the lesion, hyperactive reflexes, and Babinski's signs. Soon after an acute lesion develops, the reflexes may diminish because of spinal shock. Patients with lumbosacral central herniation may develop acute compression of the cauda equina. This causes radicular pain, paresthesias, and sensory loss referable to multiple bilateral roots, bilateral leg weakness, and loss of the lower extremity reflexes. Bowel and bladder dysfunction may occur early. When subtle, this dysfunction may be limited to asymptomatic bladder retention noted only on postvoid catheterization. When dysfunction is more severe, there may be perianal and perineal sensory loss, loss of anal tone and reflexes (the reflex anal sphincter constriction due to perianal skin stimulation or anal wink and the bulbocavernosus reflex), and fecal and urinary retention and incontinence.

Degenerative herniations in the thoracic region are uncommon, and symptoms and findings at these levels should raise a suspicion of other underlying lesions, such as tumor or abscess. Disc herniations at this level may cause radiating dermatomal pain resulting from root compression; more frequently, they progress to spinal cord compression.

The symptom most suggestive of lumbar spinal stenosis is neurogenic claudication. Low back pain radiates to the buttocks and thighs and may extend more distally along the lumbosacral dermatomes. This pain is brought on by walking. Unlike vascular claudication, rest in the upright position does not relieve the pain, but rest while seated or forward bending, such as leaning on a shopping cart, may provide relief. Pain is exacerbated by spinal extension, such as downhill walking. When spinal stenosis is severe, patients bend forward while walking. Symptoms and signs may be either mechanical, due to bone, ligament, and joint involvement,

TABLE 29–1. **Cervical Radiculopathies**

Root	Muscle Weakness	Action	Location of Pain	Reflex Change
C5	Deltoid	Shoulder abduction (15–90°)	Lateral shoulder	Biceps
	Biceps	Elbow flexion	Lateral upper arm	
	Supraspinatus	Shoulder abduction (0–15°)	Lateral epicondyle	
	Infraspinatus	Humerus external rotation		
C6	Brachioradialis (5,6)	Elbow flexion in semipronation	Posterior shoulder, lateral forearm	Brachioradialis
	Pronator teres (6,7)	Pronation	Thumb and index finger	
	ECR (6,7)	Radial wrist extension		
C7	Triceps (6,7,8)	Elbow extension	Posterior shoulder	Triceps
	ECR (6,7)	Radial wrist extension	Medial forearm	
	ED (7,8)	Finger extension	Index and middle fingers	
C8	Flexor pollicus longus	Thumb flexion	Interscapular medial forearm	Finger flexors
	FDS, FDP	Finger flexion	Little finger	
T1	Interossei	Finger abduction	Medial forearm	None
	Abductor digiti minimi	Little finger abduction	Medial epicondyle	

ECR, Extensor carpi radialis; ED, extensor digitorum; FDS, flexor digitorum superficialis; FDP, flexor digitorum profundus. Actual motor innervation is multisegmental. Most of the myotomal overlap is disregarded here to emphasize clinically useful localization.

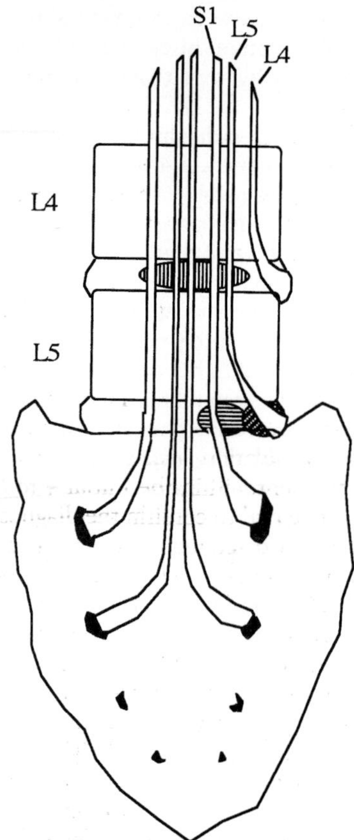

FIGURE 29–3. Lumbosacral disc herniation. The most common posterolateral herniation compresses the nerve root traveling downward to emerge one level below the level of the exiting root. Hence, L5–S1 herniation most commonly compresses the descending S1 root *(horizontal hatching)*. More lateral herniation may compress the root exiting at the level of herniation *(diagonal hatching)*. A large central herniation may compress multiple bilateral descending roots of the cauda equina *(vertical hatching)*.

or radicular, due to compromise of the lateral recesses or neural foramina.

Proximal compression resulting from root entrapment may increase the vulnerability of nerves to dysfunction due to distal entrapment. This double crush phenomenon is presumed to be a result of disturbed axoplasmic flow and disrupted architecture of the neurofilaments. Therefore, when surgical repair of a distal entrapment fails to provide the expected relief, a contributing radiculopathy resulting from degenerative disc disease should be considered.

Differential Diagnosis. Disc herniations must be differentiated from other causes of acute and chronic neck, back, and extremity pain; radiculopathy; and myelopathy. Malignant and benign tumors affecting the spine; infection; epidural hematoma; various arthritides, including rheumatoid arthritis, ankylosing spondylitis, and Reiter's syndrome; and other spondyloarthropathies may present with similar early symptoms and signs. Various anomalies, such as conjoined spinal roots and multiple roots emerging through a single foramen, may also be confused with disc disease. Degenerative arthritis of the spine can cause symptoms by many mechanisms, including disc herniation, and the various lesions that are causing symptoms in a particular person should be differentiated as clearly as possible to allow directed therapy.

Evaluation. A careful history and physical examination are critical in the evaluation of disc herniation. It has been well established with all imaging modalities that asymptomatic patients have a high incidence of anatomical lesions. To detect clinically relevant illness properly, it is therefore essential to establish the closest possible clinical correlation of the symptoms and signs with the anatomical findings of the various imaging studies. The initial history should screen for problems that raise a suspicion of severe underlying disease. All patients should be questioned about trauma, cancer, infections, recent fever, and the use of anticoagulant medications. The underlying family history and risk factors for

TABLE 29–2. **Lumbosacral Radiculopathies**

Root	Muscle Weakness	Action	Location of Pain	Reflex Change
L1	Iliopsoas (sometimes but mainly L2,3)	Hip flexion (mainly 2,3)	Inguinal crease	None
L2	Iliopsoas (2,3)	Hip flexion	Anterior and lateral thigh	Cremasteric
L3	Adductor group	Hip adduction	Medial thigh and knee	Knee
	Quadriceps	Knee extension		
L4	Quadriceps	Knee extension	Medial lower leg	Knee
	Tibialis anterior	Foot dorsiflexion	Medial malleolus	
L5	EHL, EHB	Great toe extension	Anterolateral lower leg	Tibialis posterior
	EDL, EDB	Toe extension	Dorsum of foot	Internal hamstrings
	Tibialis anterior	Foot dorsiflexion		
	Peroneii	Foot eversion		
	Tibialis posterior	Foot inversion		
	Gluteus medius	Hip abduction		
	Internal hamstrings	Knee flexion		
S1	Biceps femoris	Knee flexion	Lateral heel	Ankle
	Gastrocnemius soleus	Foot plantar flexion	Sole of foot	
	FDB	Toe flexion		
	Gluteus maximus	Hip extension		

EHL, Extensor hallucis longus; EHB, extensor hallucis brevis; EDL, extensor digitorum longus; EDB, extensor digitortum brevis. Actual motor innervation is multisegmental. Most of the myotomal overlap is disregarded here to emphasize clinically useful localization.

tumor, infection, hematoma, and various disorders that predispose to disc disease should be sought. The physical examination, likewise, is undertaken to seek evidence of other severe underlying disease and to localize and classify the pain and any deficits as mechanical, radicular, or myelopathic. It is most important to immediately establish the presence of major deficits that demand rapid diagnosis and treatment. These include the cauda equina or conus syndrome, acute or progressive myelopathy, and severe radicular motor deficits. If, on the other hand, the findings are consistent with a ruptured disc and either no deficit or a mild to moderate one, it is reasonable to temporize before pursuing a workup to evaluate the cause thoroughly. If plain radiographs of the affected area reveal no evidence of unexpected lesions, conservative therapy for disc herniation may be tried before further imaging is performed. This approach is justified by the good prognosis for spontaneous recovery of patients with acute radiculopathy with mild to moderate deficits. When the clinical examination leaves doubt about the localization of the lesion, electromyography (EMG) can supplement the diagnosis of radiculopathies and suggest other localizations, such as plexopathies and neuropathies. EMG is more sensitive if it is delayed until at least 10 to 14 days after the onset of a new deficit.

The tests available for imaging include plain radiographs, computed tomography (CT), myelography with or without CT, and magnetic resonance imaging (MRI). X-ray studies can be used to screen for unexpected infection, tumor, or deformity of the bony spine. Radiographs cannot show the neural tissues or the disc itself, but loss of disc space height and other degenerative changes may provide some indirect diagnostic information. Interpretation of plain radiographs must be tempered by an awareness of the high frequency of degenerative findings in asymptomatic populations. Plain radiographs taken under conditions of flexion and extension can also be used to assess spinal stability. Myelography is invasive, indirect, and nonspecific; however, it retains certain advantages in the era of MRI. It can visualize the entire length of the spine and best defines the root sleeves. Although myelography alone cannot distinguish between osteophytes and a herniated disc compromising a foramen, when combined with CT, it provides the best visualization of lateral pathology and small osteophytes. It is now most commonly used to answer specific questions that remain after the MRI examination. CT is superior to MRI in distinguishing soft tissue from bone. MRI has emerged as the preferred imaging choice in most cases. It demonstrates bone and soft tissues directly, easily allows multiplanar visualization, and is suited to the visualization of multiple levels. The high contrast of epidural fat and the cerebrospinal fluid (CSF)-filled thecal sac allows accurate assessment of subtle compression in most cases.

Lumbar spinal stenosis is evaluated by CT or MRI. MRI best demonstrates the relationship of the bony and neural structures. CT best demonstrates lateral recess stenosis. Although the dimensions of the bony canal can be used as guidelines, diagnosis must ultimately be based on the correlation of stenosis with the clinical findings. The transverse interfacet dimension should be greater than 16 mm. A dimension of less than 10 mm indicates severe stenosis. An anteroposterior dimension of less than 12 mm suggests stenosis; however, this finding is less sensitive in patients with symptomatic disease. A lateral recess of 3 mm or less suggests stenosis.

Management. The crucial initial step in management of patients with disc herniation syndrome is to identify those lesions that merit further evaluation and immediate therapy. In the remaining cases, the good prognosis for early recovery justifies a trial of conservative therapy before definitive imaging is done. Conservative therapy includes rest in a position of comfort followed by early remobilization, gentle exercises, and analgesics for pain as needed. Nonsteroidal anti-inflammatory agents probably provide little relief in most cases. For severe pain, judicious time-limited use of narcotics should be considered. Oral and epidural corticosteroids can be helpful. Many other modalities are available, but there are few reliable data about their effectiveness in populations: medical and physical measures (e.g., ice, heat, massage, and ultrasound) that address secondary muscle spasm, transcutaneous electrical nerve stimulation, acupuncture, exercise, and traction.[3] If improvement within the initial 4 to 6 weeks is not satisfactory, it is helpful to confirm the diagnosis by imaging. This may provide a diagnosis of an unsuspected condition, localization for epidural steroid injection, or information about suitability for eventual surgery.

Clear indications for surgery include the presence of acute myelopathy, cauda equina syndrome, severe or progressive motor deficits, and intractable pain. When conservative measures fail to provide a satisfactory response within 6 to 12 weeks, surgery should also be considered. Studies comparing the outcome of surgical therapy with conservative care suggest that early recovery occurs more often with surgery. Although the benefits of surgery are lost with prolonged follow-up periods, it is important to point out that in an often cited study, patients in the conservative therapy group who had not responded to this therapy received surgery.[4] Newer microsurgical techniques allow shorter hospitalization and rehabilitation periods but have not been shown to improve long-term outcome. The success rate of chymopapain chemonucleolysis has not reached that of surgery in most hands, and this treatment carries significant risks. Percutaneous nucleotomy has also been disappointing and should not be pursued given the current level of experience.

For patients with lumbar spinal stenosis, initial therapy is symptomatic, with analgesics, pain-modulating medications, and physical and occupational therapy. When significant disability and pain remain despite conservative measures, referral for surgical decompression should be considered.

Prognosis and Future Perspectives. The prognosis for the relief of pain and a full functional recovery is good. With bed rest alone, Weber found that 70 percent of patients experienced decreased pain and improved function within 4 weeks, and 60 percent had returned to work.[5] Seventy percent were functionally unrestricted at 1 year. With selective surgery, 90 percent of patients should have a good functional recovery within a year. Patients with psychosocial problems tend to do worse with either therapy, but those with appropriate indications respond better to surgery. Sensory dysfunction does not recover as fully as motor function, and a large proportion of patients retain some sensory deficits. Patients in whom relapse occurs should be re-evaluated for new lesions that are potentially addressable by surgery; however, the success rate of surgery declines with follow-up procedures, and a significant proportion of patients with disc herniation experience relapse with chronic low back pain.

Research into the mediators and biomechanics of pain may further elucidate the mechanisms of pain in disc disease and provide other conservative therapies. Improved imaging techniques may further refine the selection of patients for surgery. It is hoped that improved surgical selection and further refinements in surgical technique may continue to improve outcome and shorten the period of disability.

CERVICAL SPONDYLOSIS

Pathogenesis and Pathophysiology. Degenerative changes of the spine universally accompany aging, and the accumulation of such degenerative changes in the cervical spine constitutes cervical spondylosis. These spondylotic changes become clinically important when they cause pain or neurological dysfunction. Aging leads to desiccation and shrinkage of the intervertebral discs. The resultant loss of vertebral height narrows the intervertebral foramina. The weakening of the containing fibrous annulus allows bulging of the desiccated discs, which may then form transverse bars that protrude posteriorly, compromising the spinal canal. Their protrusion more laterally into the foramina may further compromise this space. Osteophytes and hypertrophic osteoarthritic changes of the facet and uncovertebral joints may further impinge on the spinal canal and foramina. Hypertrophy of the ligamentum flavum, which runs longitudinally along the posterior wall of the spinal canal, may compromise this space even more (Fig. 29–4). Intuition suggests that compression of the cervical spinal cord and nerve roots by the stenosis of the spinal canal and foramina is responsible for the myelopathy and radiculopathies characteristic of cervical spondylosis. However, a finer understanding of the pathogenesis of this disorder has been elusive. Proposed explanations of the neurological deficit include (1) direct compression by stenosis adequate to compromise the cord and roots, (2) rubbing of the spinal cord and roots on protruding skeletal structures that may not themselves be severely compressive, and (3) arterial or venous compromise. All of these factors may play a role. Pathological study shows the presence of distorted and flattened spinal cords that correspond to spondylotic bars. Demyelination of the lateral columns occurs at the stenotic site and caudally and of the posterior columns rostrally. This demyelination corresponds to the sites of rubbing: anteriorly and inferiorly with neck flexion and posteriorly and superiorly with extension. In the central gray matter ischemic changes with neuronal loss are seen. Sometimes syringomyelia can be found. Root sleeves may be thickened and rootlets adherent.

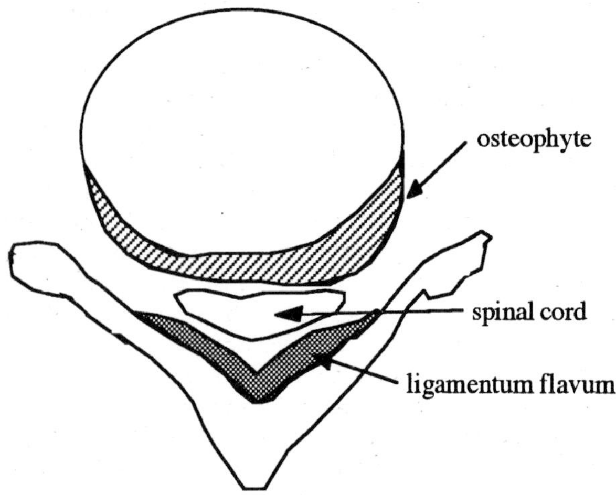

FIGURE 29–4. Cervical spondylosis. C5 vertebra in cross section. Posterior osteophytes of the vertebral endplate and hypertophy of the ligamentum flavum compromise the cervical spinal canal and cause flattening of the spinal cord.

Epidemiology and Risk Factors. The major risk factor for cervical spondylosis is aging. Although trauma may contribute, there is usually no history of significant trauma. Screening of asymptomatic patients shows a high frequency of spondylotic changes that increases with advancing age. By age 59, 70 percent of women and 85 percent of men have changes on radiographs, and by age 70, the number increases to 93 percent of women and 97 percent of men.[6] Up to 75 percent of these patients have abnormal neurological findings by age 65, but fewer have symptoms of spondylosis.[7] Heavy labor and especially occupations that expose the patient to vibration probably increase the risk of spondylosis.

Clinical Features and Associated Disorders. The major clinical features are the symptoms and signs referable to cervical myelopathy and radiculopathy. Patients may complain of neck pain and pain radiating into the arms. There may be weakness of the legs and sensory loss, especially of position sense. The weakness or sensory loss may be discovered when an elderly patient presents for gait problems or falls rather than after a direct complaint. Bowel and bladder dysfunction are uncommon complaints accompanying advanced cervical myelopathy. Most commonly, the onset of symptoms is insidious; however, occasionally an elderly patient with spondylosis presents with catastrophic onset of quadriparesis or paraparesis after a fall.

Typically, there is some limitation of neck mobility. Examination of the cranial nerves should be normal, although the jaw jerk may be increased in some cases. Weakness is common in the lower extremities, especially in the iliopsoas, hamstrings, and extensors of the feet and toes. Tone in the lower extremities is spastic, and Babinski's sign may be present. Sensory loss to light touch, vibration, and joint position is sometimes found. The major deficits in lower extremity function are determined by the degree of myelopathy. Findings in the upper extremities vary depending on the level of central canal stenosis and the degree of cervical root involvement. Patients may have mild weakness with brisk reflexes. When roots are compromised, especially in the lower cervical myotomes, atrophy, weakness, and fasciculations may be found, at times mimicking the signs of amyotrophic lateral sclerosis. Sensory loss in the upper extremities may also be seen, following a simple radicular pattern or, more commonly, a patchy distribution, presumably due to multiple root and cord involvement.

The main associated features are those of disorders that compromise the cervical spine and predispose to osteoarthritis. These include prior trauma, prior disc herniation, various congenital anomalies of the cervical spine, and underlying systemic arthritic disorders.

Differential Diagnosis. The issue of differential diagnosis is particularly important when one is dealing with a condition that is commonly present as an asymptomatic radiological finding. When a patient presents with a combination of radicular signs and symptoms accompanied by cervical myelopathy, the diagnosis of spondylotic disease is not difficult. However, this clinical presentation is not common, and most patients have either myelopathy resulting from central protrusions or radiculopathy resulting from lateral protrusions, but not both. The differential diagnosis must therefore cover conditions that cause pure myelopathy, motor neuron disease, and combined myelopathy and radicular or neuropathic lesions.

The syndrome of slowly progressive spastic weakness of the extremities, worse in the lower than in the upper extremities, may be produced by a variety of pathological causes. Some of these are listed here along with clues that may help to distinguish them from spondylotic myelopathy.

MULTIPLE SCLEROSIS (see Chapter 48). Age of onset, gender, and types of neurological findings do not reliably distinguish chronic spinal multiple sclerosis. Early onset of bladder symptoms, visual complaints, and mental status changes should be sought. Cranial MRI may demonstrate periventricular bright lesions on T2-weighted images in the majority of patients with multiple sclerosis. Visual evoked responses and oligoclonal bands in the CSF, if abnormal, are helpful.

AMYOTROPHIC LATERAL SCLEROSIS (see Chapter 36). In most patients with amyotrophic lateral sclerosis, lower motor neuron signs are evident from the beginning, but spasticity predominates in a few. The finding of atrophy of muscle and increased reflexes in the same myotome strongly suggests amyotrophic lateral sclerosis. Bulbar symptoms or signs should be carefully sought on examination and should be evaluated with EMG. The sensory loss from radicular or long tract involvement, common in cervical spondylosis, should be absent. In one recent series, 5 percent of patients with amyotrophic lateral sclerosis underwent a cervical laminectomy in the hope of arresting progressive spasticity, emphasizing how commonly the two conditions co-exist.

PRIMARY LATERAL SCLEROSIS A few patients with a slowly progressive, purely spastic condition are found to have a degenerative disease allied to amyotrophic lateral sclerosis, but without lower motor neuron features.

SUBACUTE COMBINED DEGENERATION OF THE SPINAL CORD (see Chapter 40). Vitamin B_{12} deficiency should never be overlooked. A low serum B_{12} level, hypersegmented polymorphonuclear leukocytes, and macrocytic anemia are some of the abnormalities found in early cases. The lesions of vitamin B_{12} deficiency begin in the cervical or thoracic cord, and deficits are often primarily sensory, which is quite uncommon in patients with cervical spondylosis.

DURAL ARTERIOVENOUS FISTULA Several decades ago it was believed that spinal arteriovenous malformations presented either as subarachnoid hemorrhage or as the lumbar syndrome of painful cauda equina deficit. It is now known that small arteriovenous fistulas in the spinal dura can cause myelopathy with either a stepwise progression or abrupt onset. Most malformations are seen on MRI or myelography; however, some require selective angiography of the segmental arteries that supply the cord for definitive diagnosis.

MYELOPATHY ASSOCIATED WITH AIDS (see Chapter 44). A subacute vacuolar change in the spinal cord may develop in patients with human immunodeficiency virus infection, usually in those with frank acquired immunodeficiency syndrome (AIDS) and a history of multiple opportunistic infections. Most patients are younger than the average patient with spondylosis. The clinical findings often emphasize an ascending sensory disorder.

HTLV-I MYELOPATHY (see Chapter 41). A slowly progressive spastic paraparesis with early bladder involvement in a patient from a region endemic for human T-cell leukemia-lymphoma virus (HTLV)-I infection should prompt suspicion of this infectious cause. Patients typically have milder spasticity of the upper extremities. Diagnosis can be made by identifying the presence of antibodies to HTLV-I in serum.

FAMILIAL SPASTIC PARAPLEGIA These patients can be recognized by their family history of progressive leg weakness and gait difficulty among several relatives. The most common inheritance pattern is autosomal dominant linked to mutations in the spastin gene on chromosome 2p. However, other autosomal dominant, autosomal recessive, and X-linked types also occur. Laboratory testing for mutations in the spastin gene is now available.

SYRINGOMYELIA. Cervical syringomyelia may occur in isolation or in association with the Chiari malformation, trauma, or tumor. Patients typically have lower motor neuron signs in the upper extremities due to involvement of the central gray matter and upper motor neuron signs in the upper and lower extremities due to involvement of the descending corticospinal tracts. The segmental loss of spinothalamic modalities of sensation and the neuropathic quality of the accompanying neck, back, and extremity pain as well as the context of an associated underlying problem suggest the diagnosis. MRI demonstrates the syrinx.

COMPRESSIVE LESIONS AT THE CRANIOCERVICAL JUNCTION. The Chiari malformation may cause myelopathy, vertigo, and ataxia. There may be an associated syringomyelia. Basilar impression due to instability of the atlanto-occipital joint or atlantoaxial instability, as in rheumatoid arthritis, may cause slowly progressive myelopathy. These lesions often occur in the context of spondylotic lesions, and it is very important to clarify the source of progressive findings. Certain tumors, such as meningiomas and schwannomas, at the craniocervical junction may also mimic the signs of cervical spondylosis. Often the history suggests a loss of function on one side followed by progression of signs to all four extremities. Downbeating nystagmus suggests the localization. Imaging high enough to demonstrate the craniocervical junction is crucial before cervical myelopathy is attributed to spondylotic lesions.

Evaluation. Evaluation begins with a careful history and examination. This is especially important because of the known high rate of radiological spondylotic abnormalities in asymptomatic populations. It is very important to establish the best possible correlations between the clinical findings and the imaging abnormalities. Available imaging modalities include plain radiographs, CT myelography, and MRI. Plain films can show many of the degenerative changes of bony elements; however, they do not reveal the relationship of these to the neural structures. Simple flexion and extension films performed with care can also demonstrate spinal instabilities that are not apparent on MRI or CT myelography. MRI is the easiest noninvasive means of diagnosis. MRI can demonstrate the dimensions of the spinal canal and foramina and distortion of the spinal cord and roots caused by the impingement of bony structures. Gadolinium enhancement can demonstrate the presence of various alternative lesions that may be under consideration. CT myelography can be used to answer any questions that remain after MRI. The myelogram may fail to show complete block even when significant spondylotic myelopathy is present.

Management. Conservative management of cervical spondylosis includes immobilization with a cervical collar and the use of non-narcotic, nonsteroidal medications for pain. The symptoms and signs in most patients stabilize with this therapy; that is, the myelopathy does not progress, and in some patients it improves. Yet controlled studies evaluating the benefit of immobilization are limited.[8] When radicular pain is the major problem demanding further intervention, epidural steroid injections can be effective. We refer patients for neurosurgical evaluation and surgical therapy when their myelopathy progresses despite these conservative measures, after careful consideration of other diagnostic possibilities as listed earlier. There has been no documentation of long-term benefit from surgery, although many series have shown evidence of benefit in the short term.[8] Posterior decompressive laminectomy is the procedure that has the longest history. However, unless it is performed over many levels, it will not relieve multilevel compression. Wide decompression performed over a number of segments may be complicated in later years by a swan neck deformity owing to the loss of posterior supporting elements. The anterior approach with interbody fusion is especially suitable for patients with single level nerve root compression. Its benefits for cord compression are less well defined. When radicular symptoms are due to bony osteophytes, foraminotomy may relieve the symptoms and signs of root compression. Although the benefit of surgery has not been systematically validated, and many patients improve spontaneously or with immobilization by a collar, clinical experience with individual cases suggests that selected patients do benefit and show marked improvement shortly after decompressive surgery.

Prognosis and Future Perspectives. The natural history of cervical spondylosis is not known. Although the course of the disease is progressive and most patients have chronic symptoms, the large majority remain stable for many years and do not require surgical intervention.

MRI has greatly advanced the precision of diagnosis while sparing most patients the discomfort and risk of myelography. Future advances in imaging may further facilitate diagnosis. Rowland has pointed out our great lack of knowledge of the natural history of cervical spondylosis as well as the need for controlled trials to demonstrate the effects of surgery and clarify surgical indications.[9] Such studies, if they are done, will require a cooperative effort and careful definition of clinically relevant questions.

ANKYLOSING SPONDYLITIS

Ankylosing spondylitis (AS) is one of the group of seronegative forms of arthritis, which also includes Reiter's syndrome and psoriatic arthritis. There is a close association with the HLA-B27 type, and the disease is more than three times more common in men than in women. In many patients, the disease seems to progress slowly for years, primarily with back pain, and then stabilizes without much disability. In some cases the disease progresses to total spinal fusion, producing a typical bamboo spine on x-ray. In all patients, the presence of sacroiliac joint disease on radiographs is required to make the diagnosis. There are two major neurological complications of AS: a cauda equina syndrome of unclear etiology and several types of cervical spinal cord compression due to dislocation or deformity.

Ankylosing spondylitis is less common in black populations and in people of Japanese ancestry, in parallel with the lower expression of HLA-B27 in these groups. There is a considerable familial incidence of AS. Approximately 20 percent of patients with AS have joint disease in the peripheral joints, not in the vertebral column or pelvis, and it is in this group that the neurological complications seem to be most frequent.

Patients with the cauda equina syndrome of AS have a gradual and relatively symmetrical loss of function in the L5, S1, and S2 roots.[10] Both motor and sensory fibers are affected. Foot drop, weakness of plantar flexion, and perianal sensory loss are typical. Nearly all patients develop bladder and bowel incontinence. The cervical spine disorder most often associated with AS is instability at the craniocervical junction because of ligamentous laxity at the level of the odontoid process.[11] Some patients have stepwise subluxation of the cervical spine, resembling that seen in seropositive rheumatoid arthritis. In either case, myelopathy may develop, often with significant sensory loss in the hands, as well as quadriparesis. As in rheumatoid arthritic disease, there may be marked instability of the cervical spine or craniocervical junction with much local pain, sudden changes in neurological symptoms with postural change, and eventual requirement for surgical fusion. Patients with AS may have uveitis or cardiac disease. Fractures of the fully or partially fused spine, especially if osteopenia exists, are common.

The cauda equina syndrome can be confused with lumbar disc disease, but the distinguishing features of the former are symmetry and early loss of bladder function. The craniocervical instability of AS produces a myelopathy that may be insidious and difficult to distinguish from general weakness, myopathy, nerve entrapment, or generalized neuropathy.

The diagnosis should be confirmed radiologically; there are specific criteria for the diagnosis of AS.[12] Cauda equina syndrome is accompanied by a distinctive radiological change, consisting of a wide patulous distention of the subarachnoid space in the sacral region, often with erosion of the overlying sacral bone. The cause of this distended space is unknown, nor is it clear how this distention contributes to nerve root dysfunction.[13] CSF examination does not suggest arachnoiditis. The cervical spine should be fully visualized by MRI, and the position of the odontoid should be carefully noted. In rheumatoid arthritis patients, asymptomatic widening of the space between the odontoid and the arch of C1 (normally 3 mm or less) is observed. In AS, unrecognized fracture, odontoid dislocation, or atlantoaxial dislocation can occur.

Unfortunately, no specific therapy is available for patients with the cauda equina syndrome. A scattering of case reports indicate that some authors have attempted decompression of the thecal sac. Decompressive laminectomy is of no value. Fractures or cervical dislocations may require fusion.

Compressive Structural Disorders

FIBROUS DYSPLASIA

Pathogenesis and Pathophysiology. Our understanding of the pathogenesis of fibrous dysplasia has advanced greatly in recent years. Investigators have identified a missense point mutation of the gene that codes for the alpha subunit of the G-protein, Gsα, in affected bone and other tissues in patients with fibrous dysplasia and the McCune-Albright syndrome (polyostotic fibrous dysplasia, café au lait spots, and precocious puberty in females).[14] The absence of this mutation in nonaffected tissues in patients with the disease suggests that a somatic mutation occurs early in embryogenesis to create a genetic mosaic. The mutated Gsα proteins activate adenylate cyclase and increase signaling through the cyclic adenosine monophosphate (cAMP)–protein kinase A pathway.[15] Recent work suggests that the resultant phosphorylation of transcription factors enhances transcription of the proto-oncogenes c-*fos* and c-*jun* and translation of their proteins in affected tissues.[16, 17] These findings surely represent only part of the molecular story, and it is likely that enhanced production of other oncoproteins is yet to be discovered.[18]

These molecular changes result in a gain of function that probably underlies the bony and endocrinological lesions characteristic of fibrous dysplasia. The functional result is a disorder of lamellar bone remodeling and repair. The pathological result is a replacement of normal bone and marrow elements by a vascular fibrous tissue composed of whorls of proliferating fibroblasts with haphazardly arranged trabeculae of metaplastic bone and fluid-filled cystic areas lined by multinucleated giant cells. The appearance is similar to that of osteitis fibrosa cystica due to hyperparathyroidism but is distinguished by the absence of osteoblasts. The abnormal bone originates from the medullary cavity and grows outward, thinning the bony cortex.[19] The high prevalence in puberty, the accelerated expansion of lesions during pregnancy, and the association with precocious puberty in females in the McCune-Albright syndrome[20, 21] suggest a hormonal influence that is, so far, poorly understood. Estrogen and progesterone receptors have been identified in affected bone.[22] Patients with fibrous dysplasia have an accelerated turnover of bone, and many have elevated serum alkaline phosphatase levels, reflecting increased osteoblastic activity. Those with extensive disease also have elevated urinary hydroxyproline, reflecting increased turnover of collagen, a measure of the activity of osteoclasts. Serum calcium and inorganic phosphorus remain normal, reflecting compensatory increases in bone formation and resorption. Fibrous dysplasia is generally considered to occur sporadically. Sassin and Rosenberg found no positive family histories among 50 cases with cranial fibrous dysplasia.[19] This result is consistent with the current hypothesis that the disorder results from a somatic mutation early in embryological development.

Epidemiology and Risk Factors. The age of onset is variable, but the disorder most commonly presents in childhood, especially during the period of most rapid bone growth. However, in one series of 50 patients with fibrous dysplasia of the skull, over half came to medical attention after age 18. There is no difference in incidence based on race or sex for the most typical forms.[19] However, the McCune-Albright syndrome occurs more frequently in females. As noted earlier, the bony lesions may expand at an accelerated rate during pregnancy.

Clinical Features and Associated Disorders. About 70 percent of patients have the monostotic form involving a single bone. The remainder have the disseminated polyostotic form, which is often predominantly unilateral. Sites of involvement vary, the ribs and long bones being the most common sites. The skull is involved in about 50 percent of polyostotic cases and in 10 to 27 percent of monostotic cases.[19] Most of the clinical manifestations that prompt neurological evaluation are due to skull involvement. Table 29–3 shows the frequency of skull bone involvement found in a series of 50 patients.[19] A more recent series found the ethmoids to be most commonly involved.[23] Lesions causing complications may be overrepresented in these series, since they are more likely to be referred for specialty care. Patients may present with a variety of focal neurological findings secondary to the compressive effects of the involved bone (Fig. 29–5). Visual impairment followed by hearing loss and tinnitus are the most common presenting neurological complaints. Although various other cranial neuropathies may occur as a result of the compressive effects of involved bone, these are rare enough that none were seen in two large studies of cases involving the skull.[19, 24] Optic nerve compression

TABLE 29–3. **Frequency of Skull Bone Involvement by Fibrous Dysplasia**

Bone	Number of Cases (N = 50)
Frontal	28
Sphenoid	24
Frontal + sphenoid	18
Optic canal involved	10 (3 bilateral)
Temporal	8
Parietal	6
Occipital	2

Adapted from Sassin JF, Rosenberg RN: Neurological complications of fibrous dysplasia of the skull. Arch Neurol 1968;18:363–369.

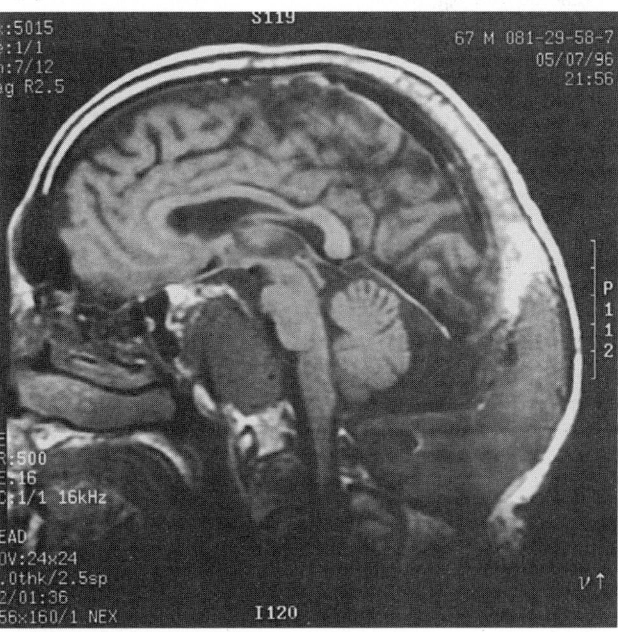

FIGURE 29–5. Fibrous dysplasia. Sagittal T1-weighted MRI scan of the head. Fibrous tissue is seen replacing bone of the occiput and skull base. This patient presented with acute hoarseness that was presumed to be due to compression of the accessory nerve in the skull base.

with visual symptoms is common when the frontal and sphenoid bones are involved. A proptotic and downward displaced eye is often seen when these bones are involved and should prompt questions about visual symptoms and a radiological evaluation of the optic canal. Patients with stenosis of the optic canal may complain of decreased acuity or blurring of vision, scintillating scotoma, flashing light, or graying of vision when pressure is applied to the globe. Optic atrophy may be seen on funduscopic examination. The visual symptoms may be slowly progressive, and they have often been present for some time when the patient presents. Patients may also have progressive facial asymmetry and deformity resulting from facial nerve involvement. Patients with hearing deficits typically have conductive loss due to stenosis of the external canal and middle ear by the involved temporal bone. A nonthrobbing headache may be a common complaint as well. Sassin and Rosenberg's patients also had an increased incidence of seizures (6 of 50), confirming the findings of prior reports.[19] The reason for this association is not known.

Fibrous dysplasia has been associated with various other disorders. Cutaneous pigmentation occurs in over 50 percent of those with the polyostotic form. The McCune-Albright syndrome consists of polyostotic fibrous dysplasia, usually largely unilateral, with café au lait spots and various forms of endocrine hyperfunction, especially precocious puberty in females.[20, 21] Rarely, other endocrine abnormalities, including hyperthyroidism, acromegaly, Cushing's syndrome, hyperparathyroidism, and diabetes mellitus, may occur. Some patients may have a progressive diffuse facial deformity called leontiasis ossea; however, this facies may be caused by other disorders as well, including Paget's disease and craniometaphyseal dysplasia.[24] Malignant transformation to sarcoma occurs in about 0.5 percent of patients with fibrous dysplasia and 4 percent of those with the McCune-Albright syndrome.[25] This tumor is rare in the skull.[24]

Differential Diagnosis. Fibrous dysplasia must be differentiated from benign and malignant neoplasms, including meningioma with adjacent hyperostosis, sarcomas or fibromas replacing bone, bone cysts, and various orbital masses, including eosinophilic granuloma, Hand-Schüller-Christian disease, and orbital pseudotumor.[24, 26] In addition, other metabolic diseases of bone must be considered, including Paget's disease, hyperparathyroidism, hyperostosis frontalis interna, osteopetrosis, and craniometaphyseal dysplasia (Pyle's disease). In general, age of onset, other clinical features, and radiological features easily distinguish these disorders. Rarely, the cranial hyperostosis found in hematological disorders causing bone marrow hyperplasia or cyanotic heart disease may cause confusion.

Evaluation. Evaluation should seek to distinguish fibrous dysplasia from other tumors or metabolic diseases and to assess the presence of deficits that require follow-up or surgical intervention. Plain x-ray films, CT, and MRI can distinguish fibrous dysplasia from tumors and characterize other metabolic disorders. Meningioma with adjacent hyperostosis is distinguishable on CT and MRI by its typical enhancement and its extension into the cranial cavity. Fibrous dysplasia expands into the outer table, leaving the inner table and cranial contents undisturbed.[24] Imaging dedicated to the optic foramina should be done when the frontal and sphenoid bones are involved. Skeletal survey and increased uptake on bone scintiscanning can identify asymptomatic areas of involvement. Serum alkaline phosphatase levels are often elevated, but serum calcium and inorganic phosphorus are normal, helping to differentiate hyperparathyroidism. When following patients with frontal and sphenoid involvement who have not had surgery, photographs of the head, quantitation of proptosis, documentation of acuity and visual fields, and funduscopic examinations for optic atrophy should be performed along with radiological views of the optic canal. These parameters may then be followed every 3 to 6 months until it is clearly established that no progressive visual loss has occurred. The onset of pain, increasing alkaline phosphatase levels, rapid growth, or invasion into cortical bone should raise a suspicion of possible malignant transformation. Biopsy may be needed to distinguish progression of fibrous dysplasia from malignant transformation.

Management. Because of a lack of medical therapies, treatment has been primarily surgical. Recently bisphosphonates and bisphosphonates in combination with surgery have been shown to relieve bone pain, to prevent fractures, to lower the levels of markers of disease activity, and to decrease disability.[27–29] When visual symptoms are present in patients with a small or diminishing optic canal, surgical decompression by unroofing the optic canal can in most cases arrest progression. Such treatment rarely leads to significant return of function; therefore, patients at risk for visual loss must be closely followed. The lesions are highly vascular, and intraoperative bleeding and intrabony hematomas may complicate surgery. Radiotherapy is contraindicated because it greatly increases the risk of malignant transformation. Because lesions may progress more rapidly during pregnancy, careful follow-up, especially for visual symptoms, must be maintained. Decisions about surgery during pregnancy should be based on the neurological status of the patient.

Prognosis and Future Perspectives. The course in most cases is benign. Leeds and colleagues followed 15 patients for 6 to 39 years and found that radiological progression was slight or equivocal in all except two patients.[24] Although the lesions become less active after skeletal maturation, progression does not necessarily stop with bone growth, and the lesions may reactivate during maturity. The increased understanding of this disease and the development of bisphosphonates have now provided a promising new medical therapy for patients with significant symptoms. Recent success in elaborating the molecular mechanisms of intracellular signaling and their alterations in fibrous dysplasia and other diseases has opened a rich field in which our understanding of the pathogenesis of fibrous dysplasia can be deepened. The elaboration of this work is likely to clarify the endocrinological manifestations of fibrous dysplasia and to lead to further refinements in therapy.

PAGET'S DISEASE

Pathogenesis and Pathophysiology. Paget's disease (osteitis deformans) is a metabolic bone disease of unknown etiology characterized by increased osteoclast size and activity that results in resorption of bone followed by reactive new bone formation. This process produces areas of bone resorption with new bone laid down in an abnormally dense mosaic pattern. The osteoclasts in affected bone contain nuclear and cytoplasmic viruslike inclusions and paramyxoviral transcripts, and evidence has been presented of an association with various paramyxoviruses, including measles virus, respiratory syncytial virus, and canine distemper virus. However, the role that viral infection may play in the pathogenesis remains unclear. It has been speculated that the disorder represents the late effect of viral infection on osteoclasts or their precursors and that affected osteoclasts tend to form multinucleated syncytia, which have increased resorptive activity. Normal osteoblasts may then be stimulated by the primary pathological osteolytic disorder. Although recent studies have suggested susceptibility loci on chromosomes 6p and 18q in some families, subsequent studies have confirmed the genetic heterogeneity of Paget's disease and the infrequency of linkage to these loci.[30–32]

Epidemiology and Risk Factors. Paget's disease is the second most common metabolic bone disease in the elderly population, after osteoporosis. It is most common in patients of northern European ancestry and is uncommon among Asians and Africans. Males predominate slightly. The prevalence in the elderly population of the United States is 1 to 3 percent, with 0.1 to 0.2 percent of patients having significant symptoms.[33] The risk is increased in relatives of those affected, but pedigrees do not support direct inheritance.

Clinical Features and Associated Disorders. The disease typically begins in middle age or later and varies from limited asymptomatic involvement of a single or few sites to widespread symptomatic disease. The femur, pelvis, and spine are most commonly affected, although any bone may be involved. Skull involvement is also common. The most typical presenting symptoms are focal progressive bone pain, deformity due to expansion of bone, and structural failure such as vertebral compression fracture or bowing of weight-bearing long bones. Enlarging hat size due to progressive skull expansion is a classic symptom. Other typical facial changes include enlarged and coarsened orbits and prognathism. Patients may also notice focal increases in skin temperature due to increased blood flow at affected sites. The most common neurological symptoms are headache, deafness, and problems resulting from spinal disease. The cause of the deafness is unclear. Both auditory nerve compression and involvement of the middle ear ossicles have been suggested as mechanisms; however, autopsy studies have not borne out either hypothesis.[33, 34] The main mechanisms presumed to cause neurological symptoms are compression of neural and vascular structures by overgrowth of bone into limited spaces, traction on neural structures displaced by bony deformity, and possibly a vascular steal phenomenon resulting from the local high blood flow demand of pagetic bone (Table 29–4). Involvement of the skull may cause basilar impression with consequent problems, including headache, ataxia, hydrocephalus, myelopathy, or cranial neuropathies. Patients may develop intradiscal lesions with spinal stenosis and, rarely, extramedullary hematopoiesis. These lesions may cause back pain or may progress to cause spinal cord and nerve root compression. Yet compressive symptoms due to spinal disease are uncommon, and when they occur in patients with Paget's disease, the possibility of sarcomatous degeneration should be considered. High-output heart failure due to the highly vascular shunts is rare.

From 1 to 5.5 percent of patients with Paget's disease develop osteogenic sarcoma.[35] Other tumors, such as giant cell tumor of bone, are less common. The pagetic osteogenic sarcoma is osteolytic, and pathological fracture is the most common presentation. Malignant degeneration should also be suspected when a rapid increase in pain or growth is noted or when compressive spinal findings emerge. About 5 percent of patients have hyperparathyroidism, but the mechanism of this association is not known. A complex array of vitamin D–related disorders may also accompany Paget's disease.

Differential Diagnosis and Evaluation. The differential diagnosis includes primary and metastatic bony tumors, especially prostate cancer, and other metabolic bone disorders that produce lytic lesions and hyperostosis. Degenerative arthritis may cause confusion, especially when one is trying to determine the source of symptoms when the two diseases co-exist.

Plain radiographs of affected bones are still the primary means of diagnosis. The bones are expanded, often with thickening of the cortex. There may be a peripheral edge of lytic fronts and a small intracortical lytic area. It is common

TABLE 29–4. **Neurological Complications of Paget's Disease of Bone**

Deficit/Localization	Proposed Mechanisms of Injury
Hearing Loss	
Conductive	Involvement of middle ear ossicles
Sensorineural	Compression/traction of auditory nerve
Spinal Cord and Root Involvement	Compression of central canal and foramina
Radiculopathy (esp. lumbosacral)	Compression, traction
Myelopathy (esp. thoracic)	Compression, vascular compromise (possible steal)
Cranial Nerve and Brain Stem	
Olfactory nerve	Sphenoid thickening compromising lamina cribosa
Optic nerve	Optic canal stenosis, orbital compression, possible vascular steal
Ocular motor nerves	Superior orbital fissure stenosis, possible vascular steal
Trigeminal nerve	Foraminal compression, possible vascular steal
Facial nerve	Facial canal stenosis, possible vascular steal
Lower cranial nerves, brain stem, cerebellum	Foraminal stenosis, basilar impression, platybasia, and vertebral artery compression within the foramina transversaria

Major cateogories are listed in order of decreasing relative frequency. Among cranial nerve deficits, those of the lower cranial nerves are most common.

to find lytic lesions predominating in the skull. The most striking feature is typically osteosclerosis, which may have a fluffy appearance. The sclerosis is often intermixed with lytic disease. Uniformly sclerotic ivory vertebrae may be seen. Radionuclide scanning demonstrates greatly increased uptake and is the most sensitive test to establish the extent of involvement. CT can be used to distinguish osteolytic lesions missed on plain radiographs and can identify soft tissue masses (Fig. 29–6). In this regard, it may be an important adjunct in the differentiation of benign lesions from tumor. The urinary hydroxyproline-creatinine ratio is elevated, reflecting increased bone resorption. Greatly elevated bone alkaline phosphatase levels reflect increased osteoblastic activity and are characteristic. The relative elevations of these values reflect the predominance of either lytic (early) or blastic (late) disease. Serum calcium is usually normal unless some other factor, such as immobilization, tips the balance in favor of resorption and hypercalcemia. Inorganic phosphorus is normal or slightly elevated. When malignant degeneration is suspected, as in a patient with a pathological fracture, early biopsy should be pursued.

Management. The management of Paget's disease has changed in recent years. Both bisphosphonate and calcitonin attack the underlying metabolic disorder by inhibiting bone resorption. Newer bisphosphonate derivatives offer advantages that have made them emerge as the favored therapy, yet both bisphosphonate and calcitonin are still used to prevent the development of long-term complications. Etidronate, the first bisphosphonate available, provides definite benefit by inhibiting osteoclast activity. However, it interferes with the normal mineralization of new bone. The newer bisphosphonates, such as pamidronate and alendronate, are similarly effective without impairing mineralization at effective doses.[36] These agents may be given in short courses intravenously, and alendronate can be given chronically by mouth. The urinary hydroxyproline level begins to fall within days of an intravenous dose, and the serum alkaline phosphatase declines later and more gradually. These substances remain in bone for a long time and may promote prolonged remissions. Subcutaneous or nasally administered calcitonins also inhibit osteoclasts. Symptomatic relief follows; however, the effect is short-lived, and the agents must be continued to maintain this effect. A loss of effect during therapy may be due to the formation of neutralizing antibodies, which occurs in about one fourth of those treated, or to the downregulation of calcitonin receptors.[37] The cytotoxic plicamycin used for hypercalcemia of malignancy causes a rapid improvement but is more toxic than the bisphosphonates or calcitonins. Gallium nitrate has antiosteoclastic activity, but data on its clinical use do not yet support its use outside of controlled trials. The goals of treatment are to normalize metabolism as evidenced by biochemical markers and to relieve symptoms. Most patients obtain relief from bone pain. Reversal of neurological deficits and stabilization—and rarely improvement—of hearing often follows therapy. There has been radiological evidence of healing of osteolytic lesions. Patients who develop compressive spinal cord syndromes unresponsive to medical therapy require surgical intervention. Malignant lesions should be treated aggressively with radical resection for best results. Chemotherapy has not yet been shown to be effective. Early detection is currently the only available way to improve survival. Patients require life-long surveillance for tumor recurrence. With the currently available array of effective therapies for Paget's disease, it is most important that patients be properly referred for expert care.

Prognosis and Future Perspectives. Many patients remain asymptomatic. Newer drug therapies can now address bone pain and other rarer symptoms and may offer long-term remission. However, as noted previously, prevention or early detection of neurological deficits is essential to avoid loss of function, since therapy is more likely to arrest than to reverse them. The prognosis after malignant degeneration has occurred, however, remains poor, with only about 10 percent of patients surviving 5 years.[38] Research in Paget's disease has produced advances in the understanding of the possible underlying etiology, genetic associations, the metabolic processes that promote the disorder, and the application of several new therapies. Further clarification of the viral hypothesis, elaboration of genetic associations, development of improved diagnostic metabolic markers, and refinement of management with antiosteoclastic agents are expected in the future.

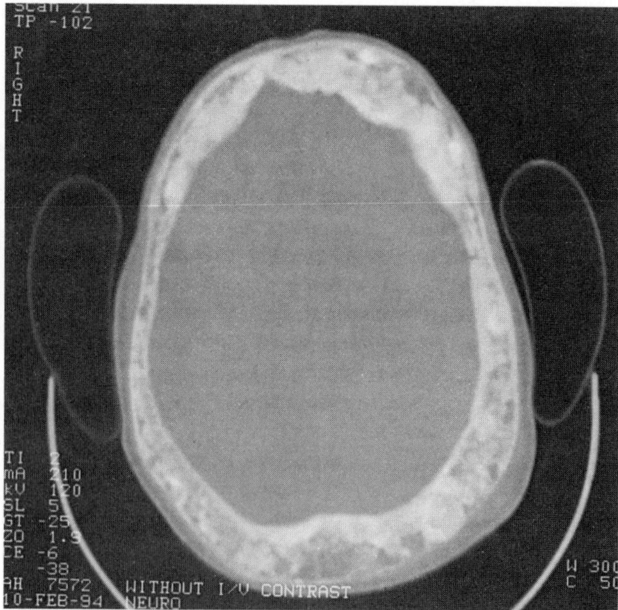

FIGURE 29–6. Paget's disease of bone. Head CT bone windows show thickening of the bony calvarium with osteosclerotic and lytic lesions.

OTHER COMPRESSIVE DISORDERS

Numerous other less common structural disorders are occasionally associated with compressive neurological signs and symptoms, including hyperostosis frontalis interna, anomalies of the craniocervical junction, congenital and acquired abnormalities of the spinal cord, generalized skeletal abnormalities, and such miscellaneous disorders as arachnoid diverticula. The clinical signs and symptoms of these disorders are summarized in Table 29–5.

COMPRESSIVE NEUROPATHIES

Compressive neuropathies should be distinguished from focal neuropathies. Although all compressive neuropathies are focal, not all focal neuropathies are due to compression. Other focal neuropathies may be ischemic, inflammatory, neoplastic, or idiopathic. Furthermore, compressive neuropathies

TABLE 29–5. **Other Structural Disorders and Associated Neurological Syndromes**

Disorder	Neurological Syndrome
Hyperostosis frontalis interna	Headache
Anomalies of the craniocervical junction region	
Basilar impression	Brain stem, cerebellar, and cranial nerve compression
Chiari malformation	Brain stem, cerebellar, and cranial nerve compression
Atlantoaxial subluxation (e.g., congenital, rheumatoid arthritis, Down's syndrome)	Cord/lower brain stem compression
Congenital and acquired abnormalities of the spinal cord	
Klippel-Feil syndrome	Cord and root compression
Scoliosis	Cord and root compression
Kyphosis	Cord and root compression
Generalized skeletal abnormalities	
Achondroplasia	Spinal stenosis, disc disease, basilar impression
Mucopolysaccharidoses	Cord and root compression, basilar impression
Down's syndrome	Atlantoaxial subluxation, basilar impression
Osteoporosis	Cord and root compression
Osteopetrosis	Brain stem and cord compression
Osteomalacia	Cord and root compression, basilar impression
Osteitis fibrosa cystica (hyperparathyroidsim)	Basilar impression
Osteogenesis imperfecta	Basilar impression
Miscellaneous disorders	
Arachnoid diverticula	Cord and root compression

are not synonymous with entrapment neuropathies. Prolonged but self-limited compression, such as may occur during anesthesia or other periods of unconsciousness, may result in a focal compressive neuropathy but without entrapment. The common sites of nerve entrapment are listed in Table 29–6.

Compressive Disorders of the Median Nerve

Carpal Tunnel Syndrome

PATHOGENESIS AND PATHOPHYSIOLOGY. The carpal tunnel is formed by the transverse carpal ligament anteriorly and the bones of the wrist posteriorly, laterally, and medially. The median nerve and finger flexor tendons pass through the tunnel so that narrowing of the space or inflammation of the tendon synovial sheaths (tenosynovitis) may result in compression of the median nerve. Studies with recording wicks placed in the canal show that flexion or extension elevates the canal pressure, and it is clear clinically that such wrist deviation typically worsens symptoms.[39] Although nonspecific tenosynovitis is the most common cause of rising canal pressure, other causes may be relevant: amyloidosis may infiltrate the tendon sheaths, rheumatoid arthritis may cause synovial tissue to invade the canal, or hypothyroidism may cause tissue edema.

TABLE 29–6. **Clinical and Electrodiagnostic Features of Common Nerve Entrapment Syndromes**

Nerve	Location	Sensory	Motor	Electrodiagnostic
Median	Wrist	D1–lateral D4	Thumb abduction and opposition	Reduced amplitude SNAP Prolongation of distal sensory and motor latencies
Ulnar	Elbow	Ulnar: Palmar medial D4–D5 + medial palm DUC: Dorsal medial D4–D5 + palm	Finger abduction (dorsal IO); finger adduction (palmar IO)	Reduced amplitude ulnar-D5 and DUC SNAPs Slowing of across-elbow motor segment Needle EMG abnormalities in FDI and FCU
Peroneal	Fibular head	Lateral calf from knee to ankle; dorsum of foot to web space D1–D2	Foot dorsiflexion (TA) and eversion (PL)	Reduced amplitude superficial peroneal SNAP Slowing of across-fibular head motor segment EMG abnormalities in TA, PL, but not TP, GM
Lat. cut. N. of thigh	Inguinal ligament	Lateral thigh	None	Normal

SNAP, Sensory nerve action potential; DUC, dorsal ulnar cutaneous nerve; IO, interossei muscles; FDI, first dorsal interosseous; FCU, flexor carpi ulnaris; TA, tibialis anterior; PL, peroneus longus; TP, tibialis posterior; GM, gluteus medius.

CLINICAL FEATURES. The median nerve may be compressed at the wrist within the carpal tunnel, resulting in the carpal tunnel syndrome (CTS). The principal symptom of CTS is a sensation of nocturnal paresthesias in the hand. The patient often awakens and feels the need to shake out the hand. Symptoms when unilateral are typically in the dominant hand, unless there is a history of a predisposing factor such as a wrist fracture or rheumatoid arthritis affecting the nondominant hand. With increased severity, there may be intermittent pins and needles paresthesias in the hands during particular activities such as driving a car or even continuous numbness in several fingertips. When continuous sensory symptoms are present, the clinical finding of a sensory disturbance splitting the fourth digit is helpful in defining a median nerve lesion. Weakness of thumb abduction perpendicular to the palm (abductor pollicis brevis, APB) is occasionally present, but in most patients, the physical examination is normal. Signs of mechanical irritability of a nerve, when elicited properly, are helpful. In particular, induction of tingling or brief electrical sensations in the tips of any of the second through fourth digits with tapping of the wrist over the median nerve (Tinel's sign) is highly suggestive of CTS. The production of wrist pain alone with this maneuver or other vague sensory symptoms should not be interpreted as evidence of nerve compression.

ELECTROPHYSIOLOGICAL ASPECTS. Electrophysiological studies (EMG and nerve conduction studies) may be extremely helpful in establishing the diagnosis. Considerable uncertainty remains, however, about the cut-off points of "normal" values because differing definitions of the gold standard for normal function have been applied in numerous studies. For example, some studies have used circular reasoning, defining the normal population clinically and then excluding initially chosen normal subjects after performing nerve conduction studies and obtaining "abnormal" values.[40, 41]

Nonetheless, consensus does exist that sensory studies are more sensitive than motor studies for detection of CTS and that performance of any of three sensory comparison studies is more sensitive than more routine sensory tests.[42] A reasonable approach to electrophysiological diagnosis is to start with performance of median-second digit and ulnar-fifth digit antidromic sensory studies. If these studies are normal, a more sensitive comparison study such as the median-ulnar mixed palmar interlatency difference can be performed.[43] Median-APB motor studies are also typically performed. The wide range of normal values for all of these studies creates problems of interpretation in some cases.[44–47] The value of needle EMG studies when nerve conduction studies are diagnostic for CTS has been debated.[48, 49] There are electrophysiological severity grading scales that depend on needle EMG results, but because these scales are not clearly of value in determining management, the additional discomfort to the patient is usually a significant deterrent.[50]

TREATMENT. Many patients with CTS are managed successfully by conservative means. Use of a wrist splint at night and during the day for particular activities, such as long periods of driving, should be advocated. The splint should hold the wrist in a relatively neutral position. Prolonged or continuous wrist splinting may lead to reduced range of motion and should be discouraged.

The role of steroid injections for treatment is controversial.[51–53] It is clear that injections into the carpal tunnel may damage the median nerve; short- or long-term benefit superior to sham treatment or the use of wrist splints has not been established. Some authors have advocated injections proximal to the carpal tunnel as an effective treatment, yet this approach has not been compared to conservative therapy with wrist splints or no intervention.[54]

Patients who have persistent symptoms following conservative management should be considered for surgical treatment. The results of surgery release are generally excellent. Forty percent of patients are asymptomatic following surgery, and another 40 percent have only trivial residual symptoms. Postoperative long-lasting incisional pain, slight weakness of the wrist, and neurological worsening have been found in 10 percent of patients in surgical outcome studies.[55] Several procedures for endoscopic carpal tunnel release have been introduced. Overall, these seem to have efficacy that is about equal to that achieved with standard release procedures.[56]

Compression of the Median Nerve at Sites Other Than the Wrist. Median neuropathies may occur in the axilla from crutches, subclavian or axillary artery aneurysms, or hematomas. In the upper arm, compression during deep sleep or unconsciousness may occur. At the elbow, supracondylar spurs and ligaments are rare causes of compression.

Many patients with forearm pain receive a diagnosis of pronator teres syndrome. This syndrome has been variously defined. A "true" pronator teres syndrome resulting in compression of the median nerve by the pronator teres muscle is extremely rare, with very few well-documented cases published in the literature.[57]

Compressive Disorders of the Ulnar Nerve

Ulnar Neuropathies at the Elbow

PATHOGENESIS AND PATHOPHYSIOLOGY. The ulnar nerve may be compressed at the region of the elbow, either at the condylar groove or the cubital tunnel. Though the terms "tardy ulnar neuropathy" and "cubital tunnel syndrome"[58] have been used to refer to all ulnar neuropathies at the elbow, they should be reserved for much more specific syndromes. Habitual elbow leaning and prolonged elbow flexion, particularly during sleep, are the most likely causes of ulnar compressive neuropathy. Alterations in elbow anatomy, such as old fractures or the deformities of rheumatoid arthritis, may predispose to the development of ulnar neuropathy. The postoperative occurrence of ulnar neuropathy is common, particularly after coronary artery bypass. Diabetes mellitus is a frequent predisposing factor.

CLINICAL FEATURES. The most common symptoms are numbness and paresthesias in the medial hand. When there is significant motor involvement, difficulty with fine movements such as turning a key or buttoning may occur. Pain is of little localizing value when present, though symptoms of focal mechanical irritability, as with all compression neuropathies, are much more specific.

The sensory examination is important, particularly in cases of early disease, in which sensory abnormalities may be the only findings. Involvement of the dorsal ulnar cutaneous and ulnar sensory territories results in a sensory disturbance that includes the dorsal and ventral medial hand up to the level of the wrist, the medial aspect of the fourth digit, and all of the fifth digit. Sparing of the dorsum of the hand may suggest an ulnar neuropathy at the wrist, though the selective fascicular involvement of the nerve when compressed at the elbow makes this sign unreliable. Clinical evaluation should include a careful study of the pattern of weakness. Ulnar neuropathy causes weakness of adduction of all fingers and abduction of the second through fourth digits. Involvement of flexor digitorum profundus may result in weakness of flexion of the terminal phalanx of the fourth and fifth digits, and wrist flexion, particularly medially, may be weak from involvement of the flexor carpi ulnaris.

With lesions of the ulnar nerve above and at the elbow, there can be atrophy and flattening of the hypothenar eminence and interossei. The hand may demonstrate a "claw-hand" deformity (*main en griffe*), with the fifth, the fourth, and, to a lesser degree, the third fingers hyperextended at the metacarpophalangeal joints and flexed at the interphalangeal joints. The hyperextension at the metacarpophalangeal joints results from paralysis of the interossei and ulnar lumbricals and causes the unopposed action of the long finger extensors. The flexion at the interphalangeal joints is due to tension from the long finger flexors. Ulnar paresis or paralysis also affects extension at the interphalangeal joints of the second to fifth fingers, adduction and abduction of the second to fifth fingers, and abduction and opposition of the fifth finger. Froment's prehensile thumb sign (*signe du journal*) may be present as a result of adductor pollicis weakness. This sign occurs when a sheet of paper, grasped between the thumb and index finger by the patient, is pulled away; to retain the paper, the patient with ulnar neuropathy extends the proximal phalanx of the thumb and flexes the distal phalanx.

ELECTROPHYSIOLOGICAL ASPECTS. The electrophysiological evaluation should focus on the amplitudes of the ulnar-fifth digit and dorsal ulnar cutaneous sensory nerve action potentials (SNAPs), including comparison to the contralateral side, and the ulnar-ADM (abductor digiti minimi) and ulnar-FDI (first dorsal interosseus) across elbow motor conduction velocities, including short-segment incremental ("inching") studies. Needle EMG studies of ADM, FDI, and flexor carpi ulnaris are also helpful. A common finding is reduction in the amplitudes of the SNAPs without localizing across elbow slowing, resulting in a nonlocalizing ulnar neuropathy by electrophysiological criteria.

TREATMENT. Conservative management, consisting of avoiding elbow pressure and prolonged flexion, is effective in most patients.[58] The decision to recommend surgical treatment is almost always made with great reluctance, as clinical experience with the benefits of surgical approaches is often discouraging. Three surgical procedures are performed. *Cubital tunnel decompression* is limited to sectioning of the flexor carpi ulnaris aponeurosis. *Anterior transposition* of the nerve involves sectioning of the aponeurosis followed by mobilization of the nerve out of the condylar groove with placement either subcutaneously or submuscularly. *Medial epicondylectomy* removes the bony prominence against which the ulnar nerve abuts and variously "stretches" the aponeurosis.

Compression of the Ulnar Nerve at Sites Other Than the Elbow. The ulnar nerve is occasionally compressed at the wrist or in the palm and rarely in the upper arm or axilla. In the palm, repeated external pressure rather than ongoing structural compression is usually the cause, though ganglionic cysts in the hand and at the wrist are an important cause to recognize. Because of the detailed pattern of branching of the distal ulnar nerve, several distinct clinical syndromes may occur, including variously palmar ulnar sensory loss (without dorsal ulnar cutaneous involvement) and weakness of hypothenar, other nonhypothenar ulnar innervated hand muscles, or both. Electrophysiological studies may be of significant value in distinguishing these cases from ulnar neuropathy at the elbow.

Compressive Disorders of the Radial Nerve

In distinct contrast to the well-defined chronic structurally compressive causes of median and ulnar neuropathies, chronic compressive neuropathies of the radial nerve are rare. Subacute or acute compression is much more common. This may be caused by crutches in the axilla, by compression against the shaft of the humerus during deep sleep or unconsciousness ("Saturday night palsy"), or by fractures of the humerus. One chronic syndrome may occur, affecting the superficial radial nerve, a purely sensory branch that is vulnerable to compression near the wrist from a bracelet or wrist watch. The clinical features of the largely acute syndromes are straightforward and are understood from the anatomy of the radial nerve. Weakness of wrist and finger extension are the most obvious clinical features. Involvement of the brachioradialis, as determined by its bulk when contracted, is important in localization to the upper arm when the triceps is spared. Apparent weakness of finger abduction with severe finger extensor weakness should not be interpreted as ulnar nerve involvement; the inability to extend the fingers results in considerable loss of mechanical advantage for abduction. Sensory loss is typically in the territory of the superficial radial nerve in the dorsal web space.

There is a radial tunnel located beneath the extensor carpi radialis, 3 to 4 cm distal to the lateral epicondyle, and the "radial tunnel syndrome" has been variously used to refer to a syndrome of compression of the posterior interosseous nerve (PIN), the distal pure motor branch of the radial nerve, in its course through the supinator muscle. The existence of a compressive syndrome of the PIN is uncertain. At best, it is extremely rare. When the "radial tunnel syndrome" is limited to refractory forearm pain and tenderness, terms such as "resistant tennis elbow" seem more applicable. Attributing pain to compression of the PIN without demonstrable weakness or electrophysiological findings is usually a mistake and should be avoided.

Compression of the Medial Cord or Lower Trunk of the Brachial Plexus: Thoracic Outlet Syndrome

Clinical Features. It is important to distinguish true neurogenic thoracic outlet syndrome (TOS) from other syndromes labeled thoracic outlet syndrome, often as an explanation for chronic pain.[59] True neurogenic TOS is rare and has a highly characteristic presentation. It results from compression of the medial cord or lower trunk of the brachial plexus due to a rudimentary cervical rib or aberrant band between the transverse process of the C7 vertebra and the sternum or first or second rib.

Gradually progressive weakness and wasting of median and, to a lesser extent, ulnar innervated hand muscles with medial forearm and ulnar hand sensory disturbance is the hallmark presentation of this disorder. This pattern of involvement is so distinctive that little else besides a medial cord or lower trunk plexus lesion can cause it. A T1 root lesion or intramedullary cord lesion, such as a syrinx, might produce a similar picture; the presence of a Horner's syndrome should alert one to these localizations.

Evaluation. Nerve conduction studies and EMG are valuable in the evaluation of this disorder. The electrodiagnostic findings are distinctive. Reduction in amplitudes of the ulnar, dorsal ulnar cutaneous, and medial antebrachial cutaneous sensory nerve action potentials distinguish this disorder from intraspinal (T1 root or cord) causes. Reduction in amplitudes of median-APB and, to a lesser extent, ulnar-ADM compound muscle action potentials and needle EMG abnormalities in these muscles but not median innervated middle trunk and lateral cord muscles (pronator teres and flexor carpi radialis) are characteristic.

Radiological studies are also crucial in the evaluation of this disorder. Plain cervical spine films may demonstrate a rudimentary cervical rib (Fig. 29–7). These ribs may also be seen on chest AP lordotic views, though less well. MRIs of the neck and plexus characteristically do not show the ribs and may be falsely reassuring. However, they may be of value in excluding other causes, such as neoplastic invasion of the medial cord of the plexus.

Treatment. The treatment of true neurogenic thoracic outlet syndrome requires surgical removal of the rib or aberrant band. Surgical exploration may be indicated in a typical case without a radiologically verified rib or ligamentous band.

Compressive Disorders of the Lower Extremities

With the exception of the common peroneal nerve at the fibular head and the lateral femoral cutaneous nerve of the thigh at the inguinal ligament, chronic compressive neuropathies of the lower extremities are rare. Acute compressive syndromes as with the upper extremity, however, may occur. Acute major trauma, deep hemorrhage, tumor, surgical complications, and ganglionic cysts account for most of these. Some postoperative focal neuropathies are caused by stretch injuries to nerves.

Common Peroneal Neuropathy at the Fibular Head

CLINICAL FEATURES. Acute compression of the common peroneal nerve at the fibular head results from its vulnerable fixed position against the fibula. Similar to many acute compressive syndromes, vulnerable positioning during deep sleep or prolonged unconsciousness with the legs crossed or flexed at the knees is the most common cause. Chronic compression from habitual leg crossing is also common. Loss of eversion of the foot, if the superficial division is involved, or of dorsiflexion of the toes and ankle, if the deep division is involved, or of both may occur. Sensory loss is much more apparent with lesions of the superficial division. The sensory loss involves the lateral calf, the lateral malleolus, the dorsum of the foot, and the medial three or four toes up to the inter-

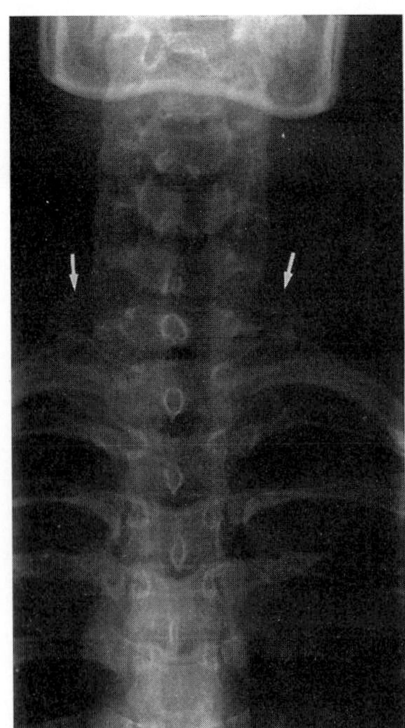

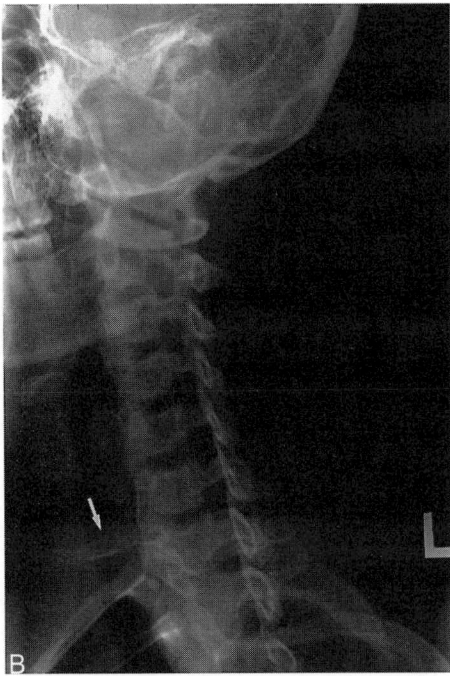

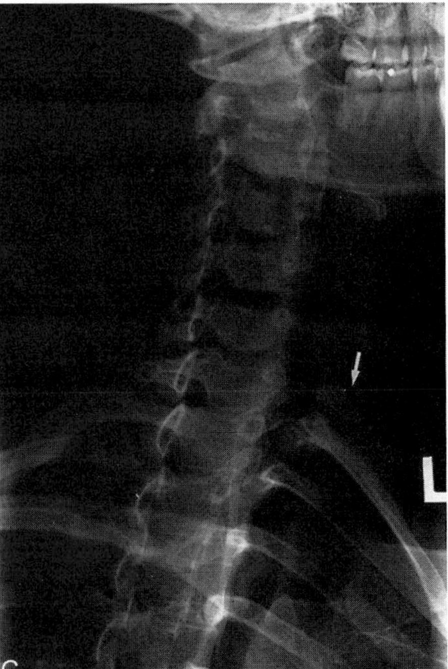

FIGURE 29–7. A 23-year-old woman with true neurogenic thoracic outlet syndrome secondary to cervical ribs. She complained of 10 years of right hand, forearm, and finger flexor cramps and 3 years of progressive right hand weakness and numbness of medial hand and forearm. Examination showed thenar greater than hypothenar weakness and wasting. Electrodiagnostic studies demonstrated absent ulnar and medial antebrachial cutaneous sensory nerve action potentials and absent median to abductor pollicis brevis compound motor action potential (CMAP), with normal amplitude for ulnar to abductor digiti minimi CMAP. *A,* AP cervical spine view demonstrating bilateral cervical ribs. *B* and *C,* Oblique views demonstrating articulating ribs *(arrows).*

phalangeal joint. With lesions of the deep division, the sensory loss is smaller and involves the small area between the first and second toes and the web space and the adjacent portion of the dorsum of the foot. In common acute compressive peroneal lesions, pain is not a typical complaint, and there are few or no sensory symptoms. With compression from ganglionic cysts or other masses, patients may experience radiating pain and slowly progressive motor and sensory disturbances.

ELECTROPHYSIOLOGICAL ASPECTS. Electrophysiological evaluation of the peroneal nerve can be extremely helpful in establishing a diagnosis of peroneal neuropathy at the fibular head. The superficial peroneal sensory nerve action potential may or may not be reduced, depending on whether there is just focal demyelination at the fibular head or axonal degeneration. The peroneal-EDB (extensor digitorum brevis) and peroneal-TA (tibialis anterior) motor studies may demonstrate a focal segment across the fibular head with conduction block or slowing. Needle EMG studies may show abnormalities in tibialis anterior and peroneus longus, but not other L5 muscles such as tibialis posterior, hamstrings, or gluteus medius.

Compression of the Lateral Cutaneous Nerve of the Thigh. Lateral cutaneous neuropathy of the thigh, also referred to as meralgia paresthetica, is also a common focal neuropathy in the legs. This purely sensory nerve arises directly from the lumbar plexus at the fusion of the dorsal divisions of the ventral primary rami of L2 and L3. The nerve has a variable course at the inguinal ligament, where it may pierce the ligament or pass above or below it. Although compression by the inguinal ligament is rarely documented, it is widely believed that entrapment or angulation at the inguinal ligament is the cause of neuropathy in most patients with this syndrome.

Pain and parethesias, often burning or stinging in the lateral thigh, are the typical symptoms. There is no weakness or alteration in the knee reflex. Electrodiagnostic studies are only helpful if a femoral neuropathy is suspected, because they are typically normal in meralgia paresthetica. The natural history is often of spontaneous improvement, though some patients do have long-lasting symptoms, and surgical procedures are quite effective.[60]

Other Compressive Disorders of the Lower Extremities. There are other uncommon compressive neuropathies of the lower extremities. The distal portions of the tibial and peroneal nerves in particular may be affected by chronic external trauma. Two syndromes that are rare at best deserve discussion: the piriformis syndrome and the tarsal tunnel syndrome.

The piriformis syndrome is often invoked to explain buttock pain of unknown cause; the implication is that compression of the proximal sciatic nerve as it passes under the piriformis muscle is the cause. Documentation in the literature of cases with clinical and electrodiagnostic findings of a sciatic neuropathy is extremely rare, and in an extensive survey, only two cases came close to meeting rigid criteria.[61] It has been suggested that, analogous to the situation with thoracic outlet syndrome, the diagnosis of true neurogenic piriformis syndrome be reserved for such extremely rare cases.

Similarly, the tarsal tunnel syndrome, consisting of pain in the ankle with or without paresthesias in the sole of the foot, has been attributed to compression of the distal tibial nerve as it passes through the tarsal tunnel at the ankle. Although referrals for tarsal tunnel syndrome are common in electrodiagnostic laboratories, convincing cases clinically or electrophysiologically are extremely rare.

Reviews and Selected Updates

American Academy of Neurology, American Association of Electrodiagnostic Medicine, and American Academy of Physical Medicine and Rehabilitation: Practice parameter for electrodiagnostic studies in carpal tunnel syndrome (summary statement). Neurology 1993;43:2404–2405.

American Academy of Neurology Quality Standards Subcommittee: Practice parameters: Carpal tunnel syndrome. AAN Practice Handbook 1992, pp 131–136.

American Academy of Neurology Quality Standards Subcommittee: Practice parameters: Magnetic resonance imaging in the evaluation of low back syndrome (summary statement). Neurology 1994;44:767–770.

Chen J-R, Rhee RSC, Wallach S, et al: Neurologic disturbances in Paget's disease of bone: Response to calcitonin. Neurology 1979;29:448–457.

Dawson DM: Entrapment neuropathies of the upper extremity. N Engl J Med 1993;329:2013–2018.

Jablecki CK, Andary MT, Floeter MK, et al: Practice parameters: Electrodiagnostic Medicine, American Academy of Neurology 2002; 58:1589–1592.

Rosenbaum RB, Ochoa JL: Carpal Tunnel Syndrome and Other Disorders of the Median Nerve. Boston, Butterworth-Heinemann, 1993.

Rowland LP: Surgical treatment of cervical spondylotic myelopathy: Time for a controlled trial. Neurology 1992;42:5–13.

Stewart JD: Focal Peripheral Neuropathies, 3rd ed. New York, Elsevier, 2001.

Weber H: Spine update: The natural history of disc herniation and the influence of intervention. Spine 1994;19:2234–2238.

References

1. Troup JDG: Straight-leg raising (SLR) and the qualifying tests for increased root tension: Their predictive value after back and sciatic pain. Spine 1981;6:526–527.
2. Scham SM, Taylor TKF: Tension signs in lumbar disc prolapse. Clin Orthop 1971;75:195–204.
3. Deyo RA, Loeser JD, Bigos SJ: Herniated lumbar intervertebral disk. Ann Intern Med 1990;112:598–603.
4. Weber H: Lumbar disc herniation: A controlled, prospective study with ten years of observation. Spine 1983;8:131–140.
5. Weber H: Spine update: The natural history of disc herniation and the influence of intervention. Spine 1994;19:2234–2238.
6. Irvine DH, Foster JB, Newell DJ, Klukvin RN: Prevalence of cervical spondylosis in a general practice. Lancet 1965;2:1089–1092.
7. Pallis C, Jones AM, Spillane JD: Cervical spondylosis. Incidence and implications. Brain 1954;77:274–289.
8. Fouyas IP, Statham PF, Sandercock PA, Lynch C: Surgery for cervical radiculomyelopathy (Cochrane Review). Cochrane Database Syst Rev 2001;3:CD001466.
9. Rowland LP: Surgical treatment of cervical spondylotic myelopathy: Time for a controlled trial. Neurology 1992;42:5–13.
10. Bartleson JD, Cohen MD, Harrington TM, et al: Cauda equina syndrome secondary to longstanding ankylosing spondylitis. Ann Neurol 1983;14:662–669.
11. Fox MW, Onofrio BM, Kilgore JE: Neurological complications of ankylosing spondylitis. J Neurosurg 1993;78:871–878.
12. Suarez-Almazor ME, Russell AS: Anterior atlantoaxial subluxation with spondyloarthropathies: Association with peripheral disease. J Rheumatol 1988;15:973–975.
13. Confavreux C, Larbre JP, Lejeune E, et al: Cerebrospinal fluid dynamics in the tardive cauda equina syndrome of ankylosing spondylitis. Ann Neurol 1991;29:221–223.
14. Bianco P, Riminucci M, Majolagbe A, et al: Mutations of the GNAS1 gene, stromal cell dysfunction, and osteomalacic changes in non-McCune-Albright fibrous dysplasia of bone. J Bone Miner Res 2000;15:120–128.

15. Weinstein LS, Shenker A, Gejman PV, et al: Activating mutations of the stimulatory G-protein in the McCune-Albright syndrome. N Engl J Med 1991;325:1688–1695.
16. Candeliere GA, Glorieus FH, Prud'homme J, St. Arnaud R: Increased expression of the *c-fos* proto-oncogene in bone from patients with fibrous dysplasia. N Engl J Med 1995;332:1546–1551.
17. Sakamoto A, Oda Y, Iwamoto Y, Tsuneyoshi M: A comparative study of fibrous dysplasia and osteofibrous dysplasia with regard to expressions of *c-fos* and *c-jun* products and bone matrix proteins: A clinicopathologic review and immunohistochemical study of *c-fos*, *c-jun*, type 1 collagen, osteonectin, osteopontin, and osteocalcin. Hum Pathol 1999;30:1418–1426.
18. Sassone-Corsi P: Signaling pathways and *c-fos* transcription response—Links to inherited diseases. N Engl J Med 1995;332:1576–1577.
19. Sassin JF, Rosenberg RN: Neurological complications of fibrous dysplasia of the skull. Arch Neurol 1968;18:363–369.
20. McCune DJ, Bruch H: Osteodystrophia fibrosa: Report of a case in which the condition was combined with precocious puberty, pathologic pigmentation of the skin and hyperthyroidism, with a review of the literature. Am J Dis Child 1937;54:806–848.
21. Albright F, Butler AM, Hampton AO, Smith P: Syndrome characterized by osteitis fibrosa disseminata, areas of pigmentation and endocrine dysfunction with precocious puberty in females: Report of five cases. N Engl J Med 1937;216:727–746.
22. Kaplan FS, Fallon MD, Boden SD, et al: Estrogen receptors in bone in a patient with polyostotic fibrous dysplasia (McCune-Albright syndrome). N Engl J Med 1988;319:421–425.
23. Lustig R, Holliday MJ, McCarthy EF, Nager GT: Fibrous dysplasia involving the skull base and temporal bone. Arch Otolaryngol Head Neck Surg 2001;127:1239–1247.
24. Leeds N, Seaman WB: Fibrous dysplasia of the skull and its differential diagnosis: A clinical and roentgenographic study of 46 cases. Radiology 1962;78:570–582.
25. Yabut SM Jr, Kenan S, Sissons HA, Lewis MM: Malignant transformation of fibrous dysplasia: A case report and review of the literature. Clin Orthop 1988;228:281–288.
26. Stompro BE, Wolf P, Haghighi P: Fibrous dysplasia of bone. Am Fam Physician 1989;39:179–184.
27. Lala R, Matarazzo P, Bertelloni S, et al: Pamidronate treatment of bone fibrous dysplasia in nine children with McCune-Albright syndrome. Acta Paediatr 2000;89:188–193.
28. Zacharin M, O'Sullivan M: Intravenous pamidronate treatment of polyostotic fibrous dysplasia associated with the McCune-Albright syndrome. J Pediatr 2000;137:403–409.
29. O'Sullivan M, Zacharin M: Intramedullary rodding with bisphosphonate treatment of polyostotic fibrous dysplasia associated with the McCune-Albright syndrome. J Pediatr Orthop 2002;22: 255–260.
30. Nance MA, Nuttall FQ, Econs MJ, et al: Heterogeneity in Paget's disease of the bone. Am J Med Genet 2000;92:303–307.
31. Hocking L, Slee F, Haslam SI, et al: Familial Paget's disease of bone: Patterns of inheritance and frequency of linkage to chromosome 18q. Bone 2000;26:577–580.
32. Good D, Busfield F, Duffy D, et al: Familial Paget's disease of bone: Nonlinkage of the PDB1 and PDB2 loci on chromosomes 6p and 18q in a large pedigree. J Bone Miner Res 2001;16:33–38.
33. Bone HG, Kleerekoper M: Clinical review 39: Paget's disease of bone. J Clin Endocrinol Metab 1992;75:1179–1182.
34. Schuknecht HF: Myths in neuro-otology. Am J Otol 1992;13:124–126.
35. Hadjipavlou A, Lander P, Srolovitz H, Enker IP: Malignant transformation in Paget disease of bone. Cancer 1992;70:2802–2808.
36. Delmas PD, Meunier PJ: Drug therapy: The management of Paget's disease of bone. N Engl J Med 1997;336:558–566.
37. Singer FR, Fredericks RS, Minkin C: Salmon calcitonin therapy for Paget's disease of bone: The problem of acquired clinical resistance. Arthritis Rheum 1980;23:1148.
38. Frassica FJ, Sim FH, Frassica DA, Wold LE: Survival and management considerations in postirradiation osteosarcoma and Paget's osteosarcoma. Clin Orthop 1991;270:120–127.
39. Gelberman RH, Hergenroeder PT, Hargens AR, et al: The carpal tunnel syndrome: A study of carpal canal pressures. J Bone Joint Surg 1981;63A:380–383.
40. Mills KR: Orthodromic sensory action potentials from palmar stimulation in the diagnosis of carpal tunnel syndrome. J Neurol Neurosurg Psychiatry 1985;48:250–255.
41. Sander HW, Quinto C, Saadeh PB, Chokroverty S: Median and ulnar palm-wrist studies. Clin Neurophysiol 1999;110:1462–1465.
42. American Association of Electrodiagnostic Medicine: Literature review of the usefulness of nerve conduction studies and electromyography for the evaluation of patients with carpal tunnel syndrome. Muscle Nerve 1999;22(Suppl 8):S145–S167.
43. Uncini A, Di Muzio A, Awad J, et al: Sensitivity of three median-to-ulnar comparative tests in diagnosis of mild carpal tunnel syndrome. Muscle Nerve 1993;16:1366–1373.
44. Salerno DF, Franzblau A, Werner RA, et al: Median and ulnar nerve conduction studies among workers: Normative values. Muscle Nerve 1998;21:999–1005.
45. Salerno DF, Werner RA, Albers JW, et al: Reliability of nerve conduction studies among active workers. Muscle Nerve 1999;22:1372–1379.
46. Hennessey WJ, Falco FJ, Braddom RL: Median and ulnar nerve conduction studies: Normative data for young adults. Arch Phys Med Rehabil 1994;75:259–264.
47. Redmond MD, Rivner MHL: False positive electrodiagnostic tests in carpal tunnel syndrome. Muscle Nerve 1988;11:511–518.
48. Gnatz S: Needle EMG is important. Muscle Nerve 1999;22:282–283.
49. Conway RR: Needle EMG is often unnecessary. Muscle Nerve 1999;22:283–285.
50. Bland JD: A neurophysiological grading scale for carpal tunnel syndrome. Muscle Nerve 2000; 23:1280–1283.
51. Davies T: Injection with methylprednisolone for carpal tunnel syndrome. Study is needed to determine best treatment for this syndrome. BMJ 2000;320:646.
52. Hayward AC: Injections with methylprednisolone for carpal tunnel syndrome. Study does not show long term benefits of injection for the syndrome. BMJ 2000;320:646.
53. Wong SM, Hui AC, Tang A, et al: Local vs systemic corticosteroids in the treatment of carpal tunnel syndrome. Neurology 2001; 56:1565–1567.
54. Dammers JW, Veering MM, Vermeulen M: Injection with methylprednisolone proximal to the carpal tunnel: Randomized double blind trial. BMJ 1999;319:884–886.
55. Cseuz KA, Thomas JE, Lambert EH, et al: Long term results of operation for carpal tunnel syndrome. Mayo Clin Proc 1966;41:232–241.
56. Brown RA, Gelberman RH, Seiler JG, et al: Carpal tunnel release. A prospective randomized assessment of open and endoscopic methods. Am J Bone Joint Surg 1993;75:1265–1275.
57. Morris HH, Peters BH: Pronator syndrome: Clinical and electrophysiological features in seven cases. J Neurol Neurosurg Psych 1976;39:461–464.
58. Dellon AL, Hament W, Gittlesohn A: Non-operative management of cubital tunnel syndrome: An 8-year prospective study. Neurology 1993; 43:1673–1677.
59. Cuetter AC, Bartoszek DM: The thoracic outlet syndrome: Controversies, overdiagnosis, overtreatment, and recommendations for treatment. Muscle Nerve 1989;12:410–419.
60. Williams PH, Trzil KP: Management of meralgia paresthetica. J Neurosurg 1991;74:76–80.
61. Stewart JD: Focal Peripheral Neuropathies, 3rd ed. New York, Elsevier, 2001.

CHAPTER 30

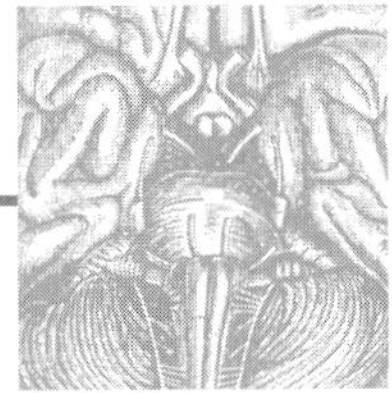

PAUL MAERTENS and PAUL RICHARD DYKEN

Storage Diseases: Neuronal Ceroid-Lipofuscinoses, Lipidoses, Glycogenoses, and Leukodystrophies

The storage diseases are characterized by pathological reactions that lead to the intracellular accumulation of abnormal material in the nervous system. They include disorders that may affect the entire nervous system, or primarily the gray or white matter. Most, but not all, are pediatric conditions, but adult variants are being recognized. Although there are many systemic manifestations of these illnesses, this discussion deals primarily with the neurological aspects of these diseases.

Neuronal Ceroid-Lipofuscinoses

Neuronal ceroid-lipofuscinoses (NCLs) are a group of lysosomal storage diseases characterized by neurological symptoms and the accumulation of autofluorescent waxy lipopigments within the lysosomes of neurons and other cells. The conglomerate term neuronal ceroid-lipofuscinoses was coined by Zeman and Dyken in 1969 to emphasize the neurological involvement, clinically and pathologically.[1] The disorders are linked to a number of celebrated names in neurological history, including Batten, Jansky, Bielschowsky, Santavuori, and Kuf, each of whom described clinical variants of these multidimensional disorders. In 1998, a classification of eight forms of NCLs was developed to consolidate earlier clinical and genetic descriptions[2] (Table 30–1).

Pathogenesis and Pathophysiology. In the NCLs, waxy lipopigments, composed of ceroid and lipofuscin, accumulate in neurons and non-neuronal tissue. The ceroid composition

TABLE 30–1. **Neuronal Ceroid-Lipofuscinoses**

Type	Name	Enzyme Deficiency	Prominent Cytosome	Storage	Genetics	Age of Onset	Major Signs
NCL 1	Santavuori's (acute infantile)	PPT1	GROD	SAP	1p32(AR)	3 to 18 months	Fulminating psychomotor deterioration, seizures
NCL 2	Bielschowsky's (acute late infantile)	TPP1	CV	Subunit c	11p15(AR)	2 to 4 years	Seizures followed by acute decline in motor and mental functions with vegetative state in 2 years
NCL 3	Batten's (juvenile chronic form)	Battenin	FP	Subunit c	16p12(AR)	4 to 12 years	Blindness, seizures, dementia; mixed pyramidal and extrapyramidal signs
NCL 4	Kuf's (adult)	Not known	GROD, FP, RL	Subunit c	AR or AD	Adult	Chronic motor, cerebellar, or extrapyramidal signs and mental deterioration, seizures
NCL 5	Finnish variant (childhood)	407 amino acids protein	CV, RL, FP	Subunit c	13q22(AR)	4 to 7 years	Blindness, dementia, seizures
NCL 6	Lake's (late infantile)	Linclin	CV, RL, FP	Subunit c	15q21–23(AR)	2 to 8 years	Blindness, seizures, chronic myoclonus
NCL 7	Turkish variant (late infantile)	Not known	FP, CV, RL	Subunit c	AR	1 to 6 years	Seizures, followed by psychomotor decline
NCL 8	Northern epilepsy (juvenile)	Lysosomal membrane protein	RL, CV	Subunit c	8p23(AR)	5 to 10 years	Seizures, mental deterioration, motor impairment

TPP1, Tripeptidyl peptidase 1; PPT1, palmitoyl protein thioesterase 1; FP, fingerprint profile; CL, curvilinear profile; GROD, granular osmiophilic deposits; RL, rectilinear profile; AR, autosomal recessive; AD, autosomal dominant; Subunit c, subunit c of ATP synthase; SAP, saposins A and D.

of inclusion bodies varies in different forms of NCL. "Subunit c" of mitochondrial adenosine triphosphate (ATP) synthase accumulates in all forms of NCL, except for the infantile form, or Santavuori's disease (NCL 1), in which sphingolipid activator proteins, saposins A and D, accumulate.[3] In addition to proteins, storage materiel includes lipids, metals, and dolichyl pyrophosphoryl oligosaccharides. All subsequent symptoms are based on this accumulation, with resultant cellular dysfunction and death in differently maturing groups of neurons of the cerebral cortex and retina. It has been speculated that cellular death is apoptotic.[4] A combination of metabolic and mechanical factors also lead to the dysfunctional state. The lipopigments accumulate first in the larger neurons and tend to cluster around the axonal hillock. Inert lipopigments and debris progressively accumulate in an area rich in inhibitory synapses. Thereafter, the waxy pigments gradually spread to other parts of the neuron, ultimately involving the rest of the cell body while sparing the dendritic tree. Progressive swelling of the neuron occurs, followed by cellular death, subsequent disruption of the cell membranes, extracellular extrusion of debris, and its accumulation within scavenger cells. By this time, smaller neurons are involved as well as glia, endothelium, and fibrocytes. Lipopigments accumulate to a mild extent in almost all cells of the body, including lymphocytes, eccrine cells, fibroblasts, endothelial cells, ganglion cells of the rectum, and conjunctival cells. This observation permits detection of the "diagnostic" cytosomes without the need for brain biopsy. It must be emphasized, however, that the absence of such material in non-neuronal sites does not exclude the diagnosis, and the presence of similar osmophilic bodies does not establish it.

The slow process of waxy pigment accumulation first in the axonal hillock may account for the epileptogenesis that is often present, particularly in the late infantile (NCL 2), the classic juvenile (NCL 3), and the juvenile Northern epilepsy (NCL 8) forms. It is speculated that classic seizures are precipitated by an overriding glutaminergic state caused by cancellation of the inhibitory influences at the axonal hillock. Hyperglutaminergic states may also lead to more rapid loss of other neurological functions.

All NCLs are autosomal recessive except for the rare families with the adult autosomal dominant form of Kuf's disease, as first described by Boehme in 1971. It is notable that the proposed gene defects are different for the different forms of the disorder (see Table 30–1). The infantile form (NCL 1) results from a lysosomal palmitoyl-protein thioesterase 1 (*PPT1*) deficiency due to mutations of the *PPT1* gene on chromosome 1q32. Bielschowsky's disease (NCL 2) results from a lysosomal tripeptidyl peptidase 1 (*TPP1*) deficiency due to mutations in the *TPP1* gene on chromosome 11p15. In the classic juvenile form (NCL 3), a genetic defect exists in chromosome 16p12. The genes of the childhood Finnish (NCL 5) and early juvenile (NCL 6) forms are carried on chromosomes 13p31–32 and 15q21–23, respectively. The proteins encoded by these last three genes are proteins of predicted transmembrane topology. The gene of the juvenile Northern epilepsy (NCL 8) form has been mapped on chromosome 8p23.[5] The loci for the two adult forms, NCL 4 and the NCL 7, are not known.

Epidemiology and Risk Factors. These genetic diseases are probably present in all ethnic and racial groups around the world. One series in the United States found that NCL 3 was the most common form, followed by NCLs 2, 1, 7, 4, and 6 (see Table 30–1), in that order. These data agree with experiences in Germany, Britain, the Netherlands, and Sweden. In Poland, on the other hand, the late infantile (NCL 2) form is encountered more frequently. This may possibly hold true for the other Eastern European countries as well. In Finland, the more common type is the acute infantile Santavuori form. It is so common there and so rare elsewhere that it is often called the Finnish form. In Saudi Arabia, the vast majority of NCL patients suffer from a form that is relatively uncommon in the United States, the early juvenile NCL 6. All the families with NCL 7 are from Turkey.

Clinical Features and Associated Disorders. The rapidly progressive infantile form or Santavuori's disease (NCL 1) has its onset within the first year of life, after a symptom-free period between birth and 3 months of age. Then a sudden and dramatic psychomotor collapse occurs with loss of neurological and visual functions. The collapse may or may not be associated with drug-refractory seizures or severe myoclonus. After the age of 2 years, a brownish discoloration of the macula, retinal degeneration, and optical atrophy develop. Death occurs between 8 and 13 years of age. Variants mimicking late infantile and juvenile NCL have been described.

In the acute late infantile form or Bielschowsky's disease (NCL 2), on average, the first symptom seldom appears after 4 years of age. The condition's hallmark is a seizure disorder that begins precipitously, progresses rapidly, and ultimately becomes refractory to all anticonvulsant medications. The initial seizures are usually described as drop attacks, myoclonic, partial, or generalized seizures, although nearly all types of seizures often occur within a short period of time. In this rapidly developing disorder, severe intellectual and mental deterioration is seen. The child becomes nonambulatory, usually before the age of 6 years. During this time, vision is progressively lost, yet because of the general loss of neurological function, such an isolated sign is often not recognized. Compared to patients with the juvenile form, a characteristic retinopathy occurs with striking retinal artery attenuation, patches of retinal atrophy, and symmetrical macular granular degeneration.

In the classic juvenile chronic form (NCL 3) or Batten's disease, neurological dysfunction occurs at disease onset, usually between the ages of 5 and 15 years.[6] Whereas patients may be referred initially to an ophthalmologist or psychiatrist, by age 10, the patient is most often referred to a neurologist. The obvious behavioral symptoms have progressed from a learning deficiency to frank dementia. Likewise, visual dysfunction has usually progressed to blindness. There is a slow and steady progression of neurological symptoms. Three stages of clinical deterioration occur. The first phase involves visual and behavioral disturbances, and the middle phase consists of seizures and motor dysfunction related to a mixture of pyramidal and extrapyramidal symptoms. In the terminal phase, the preceding symptoms worsen, and there may be changes in affect and motor signs including myoclonus. The three phases are steadily progressive and form an overall monophasic illness that distinguishes NCL 3 from the other disorders described in this chapter.

As a general rule, phase one lasts from 6 months to 5 years, phase two from 2 to 10 years, and phase three from 1 to 10 years. This pattern results in a life expectancy that ranges from 3 to 25 years after the initial visual-neurological symptoms are noted. The course of disability is generally directly proportional to control of the seizures. Once seizures become refractory and frequent, the course proceeds rapidly downhill to a vegetative state.

Kuf's adult form of NCL (NCL 4) has two major clinical presentations.[7] Type A begins with late-onset progressive myoclonic epilepsy and subsequent subacute loss of mental functions but relative preservation of motor skills. Type B is marked by predominant motor dysfunction. This dysfunction may become manifest as pure cerebellar ataxia or progressive rigidity. NCL 4 is not associated with retinal changes.

The childhood form or "Finnish" variant (NCL 5) presents with visuomotor problems and/or behavior problems between 4 and 7 years of age. Mental deterioration often precedes the onset of retinal degeneration, seizures, and myoclonus.

The late infantile "Gypsy" variant form or Lake's disease (NCL 6) has clinical features that overlap those of the late infantile and juvenile forms. There may be fewer retinal abnormalities than in NCL 2 or NCL 3, but other features characteristic of both the juvenile and late infantile forms are seen. Onset occurs between 18 months and 8 years of age, and the course is subacute compared to the chronic juvenile and acute late infantile forms of the disease.

The "Turkish" late infantile variant (NCL 7) has a phenotype similar to Bielschowsky's disease. The juvenile "Northern epilepsy" form of NCL is characterized by onset of epilepsy (generalized tonic-clonic, complex partial seizures) between 5 and 10 years of age. Mental regression is slow. Retinal degeneration is never observed. Dysarthria and incoordination become severe in adulthood.

Differential Diagnosis. The most important step in the differential diagnosis is to identify the order of the characteristic symptoms, taking into account the fact that the retinal picture may be of greatest importance. This evaluation separates the retinal NCLs (NCL 1, 2, 3, 5, 6, and 7) from the nonretinal NCLs (NCL 4 and 8). The differential diagnosis for the group includes all neurodegenerative diseases characterized by epilepsy, blindness, motor failure, and dementia, including the gangliosidoses and sphingomyelinoses.

Evaluation. A battery of laboratory tests is important in the workup of NCL patients. Neuroimaging studies show abnormalities characteristic of the type and stage of disease and demonstrate that most NCLs are ultimately atrophic poliodystrophies involving the cerebral cortex. Certain unique types such as the spinocerebellar form show selective involvement of the cerebellum in which autofluorescent storage material accumulates in Purkinje cells.[8] In NCL patients with epilepsy, electroencephalography (EEG) shows epileptogenic patterns. Electroretinograms are decreased or absent in patients with the retinal NCL types. Particularly in NCL 2, exaggerated evoked potential responses are seen, especially following tactile or somatosensory stimulation. Evoked potential exaggeration also occurs in some other NCLs.

Clinical and histopathological evaluations are essential to make the specific diagnoses. Ultrastructural cellular cytosome alterations are seen on electron microscopy in extracerebral tissue such as ganglion cells in the rectal submucosa, in eccrine cells and fibrocytes of the skin, in endothelial cells in vessels, in lymphocytes in the peripheral blood, and in conjunctival cells. Extracerebral evaluation may not be entirely infallible. Many current diagnostic problems stem from confusion about the cytosomes themselves. Osmophilic inclusions occur frequently as an artifact of tissue preparation for electron microscopy and do not always represent the diagnostic inclusion of the NCL. Four suggestive cytosomes are important, and two of these are diagnostic (see Table 30–1). The osmophilic fingerprint cytosomes (FP) are highly characteristic as lymphocytic inclusions in NCL 3. FP without membrane-bound vacuole are seen in biopsy samples of NCL 4, 5, 6, and 7. The second diagnostic osmophilic cytosome is the curvilinear body (CV), which characterizes NCL 2. Some atypical CVs are seen in NCL 5, 6, 7, and 8. The third important ultrastructural cytosomes are the "granular osmophilic deposits" (GROD), which are the dominant cytosomes in NCL 1, but can be seen in association with other inclusions in NCL 4. The fourth inclusion is the rectilinear body (RL). RL is seen in association with other inclusions in NCL 4, 5, 6, 7, and 8. The least diagnostic cytosome is the classic lipofuscin body.

A large proportion of the storage material involved in NCL consists of the mitochondrial protein called subunit *c*. This material is found in very high quantities in NCL 2 but is also seen in increased amounts in other NCLs except NCL 1. The most direct and precise means of confirming the diagnosis of NCL 1 is based on the enzyme assay of *PPT1*.[9]

Management. Bone marrow transplant and embryonic stem cell transplant may be beneficial in some patients. Symptomatic treatment, particularly proper anticonvulsant therapy, is important in all NCL disorders. Sodium valproate has been used with success. Antioxidants may improve the symptoms in some cases, and trials of these medications have been undertaken in patients with NCLs 1, 2, 3, and 6. It has been suggested that long-term antioxidant treatment and vitamin E may delay loss of intellectual and motor function and may be helpful in seizure control as well. Extrapyramidal symptoms such as dystonia and myoclonus are treated symptomatically, and behavioral modification techniques may be useful, particularly in the chronic forms. If the symptomatology is of long standing, palliation of the symptoms may be extremely useful in supporting a long and often useful life for the patient. School placement and modified educational programs are important in patients with the chronic forms of disease.

Lipidoses

GANGLIOSIDOSES

As a group, the gangliosidoses (Table 30–2) are autosomal recessive lysosomal storage disorders characterized biochemically by accumulation of gangliosides, molecules composed of ceramide and a sialic acid (an oligosaccharide containing *N*-acetyl neuraminic acid). Blocks at various intermediate steps of ganglioside catabolism cause accumulation of specific gangliosides GM_1, GM_2, and GM_3 in nervous system and other tissues. GM_1-gangliosides accumulate when beta-galactosidase, a component of the lysosomal multienzyme complex (LMC), is deficient. This LMC contains beta-galactosidase, sialidase, *N*-acetylgalactosamine-6-sulfate sulfatase, and the lysosomal carboxypeptidase (cathepsin A). LMC is involved

TABLE 30–2. **Gangliosidoses**

Type	Name	Enzyme Defect	Storage Product	Genetics	Age of Onset	Primary Clinical Features
GM_1-gangliosidosis type I	Infantile form	Beta-galactosidase	GM_1	Autosomal recessive	Birth	Cherry-red spot in 50 percent, edematous face, hepatosplenomegaly, seizures, mental and motor retardation
GM_1-gangliosidosis type II	Late infantile form	Beta-galactosidase	GM_1	Autosomal recessive	6 to 18 months	As above, but slower in evolution
GM_1-gangliosidosis type III	Adult form	Beta-galactosidase	GM_1	Autosomal recessive	Adult	Prominent extrapyramidal signs without hepatosplenomegaly
Beta-galactosidosis		Beta-galactosidase and sialidase	GM_1	Autosomal recessive	Variable	Same as GM_1-gangliosidosis
GM_2-gangliosidosis type I	Tay-Sachs: infantile form	Hexosaminidase A	GM_2	Autosomal recessive	Infants	Hyperexcitability, blindness, cherry-red spot
GM_2-gangliosidosis type II	Juvenile form	Hexosaminidase A	GM_2	Autosomal recessive	5 years	Seizures, dementia, pyramidal and extrapyramidal motor signs
GM_2-gangliosidosis type III	Adult form	Hexosaminidase A	GM_2	Autosomal recessive	Adult or adolescence	Variable pictures, including myelopathic, motor neuron, or extrapyramidal signs
GM_2-gangliosidosis: Activator factor abnormality		Partial hexosaminidase A deficiency due to activator factor dysfunction	GM_2	Autosomal recessive	Childhood	Similar presentation to Tay-Sachs disease
GM_2-gangliosidosis	Sandhoff's disease	Hexosaminidase A and B	Globoside and GM_2 ganglioside	Autosomal recessive	Infants	Clinically similar to Tay-Sachs but with hepatosplenomegaly
GM_3-gangliosidosis	Hematoside sphingolipo-dystrophy	*N*-acetylgalactos-aminyl transferase	GM_3 (hematoside)	Autosomal recessive	Infants	Respiratory difficulties, seizures, with delayed motor and mental retardation

in catabolism of glycolipids, glycoproteins, and mucopolysaccharides. GM_1-gangliosidosis and Morquio's type B disease are caused by mutations in the beta-galactosidase gene on chromosome 3p21.[10] Galactosialidosis is caused by mutations in the cathepsin A gene on chromosome 20q13 and results in a beta-galactosidase and sialidase deficiency.[11] *N*-acetylgalactosamine-6-sulfate sulfatase deficiency causes Morquio's type A disease (see mucopolysaccharidoses). Sialidase deficiency leads to sialidosis (see mucolipidoses). GM_2-gangliosides accumulate when the activity of hexosaminidase A, a heteropolymer of alpha and beta polypeptides, is deficient or when the GM_2 glycoprotein activator is deficient. GM_2-gangliosidoses with hexosaminidase A deficiency can result from mutations in either the alpha subunit on chromosome 15q23 (type I GM_2-gangliosidosis)[12] or the beta subunit on chromosome 5 (type II GM_2-gangliosidosis or Sandhoff's disease).[12] GM_2-gangliosidosis with partial or no hexosaminidase A deficiency results from mutations in the GM_2 glycoprotein activator gene on chromosome 5q32–33 (type III GM_2-gangliosidosis).[13] GM_3-gangliosides accumulation results from *N*-acetylgalactosaminyl transferase deficiency, an enzyme important in the synthesis of GM_1 and GM_2 from GM_3. In all forms, the ganglion cells in the submucosal enteric plexus contain characteristic lysosomal inclusions with various membranous and vesicular profiles.

Pathogenesis and Pathophysiology. All the gangliosidoses are characterized by storage of abnormal gangliosides in neurons and other parts of the nervous system (see Table 30–2). In all of the gangliosidoses, there is a dramatic accumulation of lipid that distends the neuronal cell body; the resulting mechanical factors interfere with metabolic function and ultimately destroy the cell. Different neuronal populations are involved and produce different symptoms. The storage is primarily neuronal and tends to occur mainly in the large neurons of the polioencephalon. The weight and volume of the affected brain increase markedly during the second year of life; it can often weigh well over twice the normal amount for age and sex. Thereafter, cystic degeneration of the remaining cortex and subcortex occurs. The neuropathological process is not limited to the brain, and motor neurons of the anterior horn cells of the spinal cord are also affected. Pathological examination of these disorders reveals distorted and ballooned neurons. Fusiform swelling of the axons, termed torpedoes, occurs, and astrocytic proliferation is seen. White matter degeneration occurs secondary to the neuronal dysfunction and cell death. Electron microscopic studies show the gangliosides usually tightly packed within the individual cells. In most gangliosidoses, these cytosomes, or membranous cytoplasmic bodies, are osmophilic and often take on a loosely "whorled" form.

Epidemiology and Risk Factors. These exclusively autosomal recessive genetic disorders are globally distributed. Because intermarriage among relatives increases gene frequency, there are often pockets of these diseases in certain sequestered populations. Thus, type I GM_2-gangliosidosis, or Tay-Sachs disease, has a high frequency among Ashkenazi Jews. Although this disease was once considered rare in black populations, it has been recently noted to occur in the southern United States in areas with a history of consanguinity.[14] In Saudi Arabia, which has high consanguinity and reproduction rates, there is also a high gene frequency of the GM_2-gangliosidosis known as Sandhoff's disease.[15]

Clinical Features and Associated Disorders. GM_1-gangliosidoses, designated generalized gangliosidosis by Norman and colleagues in 1959,[16] affect the brain and organs outside the central nervous system.[17] Keratan sulfate, a mucopolysaccharide, is the major storage material in the liver, while GM_1 ganglioside accumulates in nerve cells. Urine mucopolysaccharides are usually normal. Galactose-containing oligosaccharides are excreted in urine,[18] and bone marrow biopsy may show foamy histiocytes. There are clinical similarities between children with these diseases and those with mucolipidoses. In *type I GM_1-gangliosidosis (infantile form)*, the onset of symptoms is at birth or shortly after. Nonpitting edema of the face and extremities produces a dull, heavy-appearing facies with frontal bossing, depressed nasal ridge, low-set ears, and large maxilla. The gums and tongue may be large. Ocular signs include a cherry-red spot in about 50 percent of such patients, but corneal clouding is unusual. Macrocephaly may be noted. Hepatosplenomegaly is frequently prominent. Intellectual and motor developments are retarded from birth, and children eat poorly, gain weight slowly, and are generally weak and incoordinated. Joints tend to be enlarged, and the long bones are wide in the center and tapered at the ends; kyphoscoliosis and breaking of vertebrae are usual. Myotactic hyper-reflexia, hypertonus, and flexion contractures occur. Seizures usually occur late in the disease, and affected children, blind, deaf, and in respiratory failure associated with infection, die by the age of 2 years. A subgroup of patients with infantile GM_1-gangliosidosis present with a cardiomyopathy resembling Pompe's disease.

Type II GM_1-gangliosidosis (late infantile form) follows a more prolonged course and shows a less precipitous decline in activity. There is no visceral storage or bone involvement. Vision is preserved. Onset of symptoms occurs between 6 and 18 months. Incoordination, spasticity, mental impairment, and seizures are progressive. The affected patients may appear normal through the first years of life. Death occurs before 10 years of age.

Type III GM_1-gangliosidosis (adult type) is characterized by a slowly progressive course with predominant extrapyramidal signs of dystonia and postural reflex impairment. Rigidity is common, and speech disturbances and increased muscle tone are frequent additional features. Neuronal ganglioside storage occurs in the basal ganglion,[19] and, in contrast to the infantile, no visceral or skeletal changes occur. Magnetic resonance imaging (MRI) demonstrates symmetrical high-intensity lesions in the putamen on T2-weighted images. It has been suggested that the putaminal lesions may be primarily responsible for the dystonia.[20] Intellectual deterioration is always present, usually in association with incoordination, spasticity, myoclonus, and seizures. Survival is prolonged.

Galactosialidosis affects the neurons and organs outside of the nervous system. Gangliosides are stored in the nervous system while sialyloligosaccharides and sialoglycoproteins are stored in other tissues. Urine mucopolysaccharides are normal. Sialyloligosaccharides are found in the urine[18] and bone marrow biopsy may show foamy histiocytes. Vacuolated lymphocytes are frequently found in the blood smear. Three clinical phenotypes are recognized. *Type 1 (infantile)* resembles GM_1-gangliosidosis, except for milder seizures and corneal clouding as additional findings in 50 percent of patients. Cherry-red spots are noted in half of the patients. *Type 2 (juvenile)* is characterized by the triad myoclonus, ataxia, and angiokeratoma. Mental deterioration and visceromegaly are not features of this disorder. Visual impairment results from corneal clouding and cherry-red spots.[11]

GM_2-gangliosidoses affect primarily the nervous system where GM_2-gangliosides are stored. Visceromegaly and bone dysplasia are not a feature, except for Sandhoff's disease. Urine mucopolysaccharides are normal, except in Sandhoff's disease. Oligosaccharides are not found in the urine, and bone marrow contains no storage cells. Vacuolated lymphocytes are not in the blood smear. The clinical features of all three types of GM_2-gangliosidoses are essentially identical with progressive dementia and cherry-red spots as cardinal features. The symptoms in Tay-Sachs disease (infantile form) are uniform in type and timing of development. The first clinical manifestations occur within 6 months of birth, yet the infant appears normal for the first 3 months. Initially, excessive hyperexcitability and irritability develop, and infants have a heightened startle reflex to noises and tactile stimuli. Hypotonia and a delay in motor and mental development are characteristic. During the first 6 months of life, the child's visual acuity is usually deficient and continues to deteriorate to the point of blindness by 1 year of age. The early blindness is thought to be retinal in origin, since the GM_2-ganglioside storage lesion is within the ganglion cells of the macula, and normal pupillary responses persist. The macular cherry-red spot, appearing in all cases within the first 3 months of life, is highly characteristic, although it tends to disappear late in the disease owing to total retinal atrophy. The color of the macula has little pathophysiological significance compared to the milky, whitish halo found around the macular region.[10] This finding is a result of the buildup of opaque gangliosides. Because of this macular lesion, the baby has fixation defects and searching conjugate eye movements. At times, the extreme hyperexcitability and reactivity suggest frank seizure activity. If seizures occur, they are of a myoclonic character that closely resembles infantile spasms (see Chapter 52). The progression of symptoms continues through the second and sometimes third year of life, and most children die before the age of 4. Megalocephaly is predominant even in the terminal stages.

A *juvenile variant of type II GM_2-gangliosidosis* follows a much different course. These children first become ill after 5 years of age, and death occurs within 10 years following a course of seizures; progressive dementia; and cerebellar, pyramidal, extrapyramidal, and spinal dysfunction as well as optic atrophy.[21] This form of the disease may present as a progressive pure form of dystonia and dementia that begins before 5 years of age. Later in life these patients have a hypokinetic-rigid syndrome. These cases differ from the classic form of GM_2-gangliosidosis in the regional preferences of the storage process.[22] MRI shows mild to moderate brain atrophy.

Adult-onset type III GM_2-gangliosidosis has been reported with a number of phenotypic patterns, and the clinical picture may vary within families. Adults between 16 and 28 years of age, who have had very mild symptoms in childhood, develop pronounced motor symptomatology. In some patients, spinocerebellar degeneration is predominant.[23] These individuals do not have seizures, funduscopic abnormalities, or dementia. Other adult patients may show predominant extrapyramidal abnormalities with dystonia and choreoathetosis.[24] Some cases resemble juvenile spinal atrophy,[25] and others have a pure psychosis without cognitive decline.[26] A burning dysesthesia may be the presenting complaint.[27]

Patients with Sandhoff's disease have clinical symptoms that are similar to those characteristic of Tay-Sachs disease, with hyperacusis, decreased vision, a cherry-red macular spot, decerebrate rigidity, and megalocephaly. In addition, hepatosplenomegaly is seen, and the tubular epithelial cells of the kidneys are filled with sphingolipids. Cardiomyopathy and mitral insufficiency may be present, and death usually occurs between 2 and 4 years of age.[28] There are some variants of Sandhoff's disease, including a juvenile form in which patients are normal until 5 years of age, when they develop a progressive cerebellar ataxia, slurred speech, intellectual deterioration, and progressive hyper-reflexia and hypertonia. Funduscopic examination may be normal.

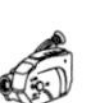

A few cases have been reported of infants with severe neurological and systemic problems that have been traced to excessive accumulation of *GM_3-ganglioside (hematoside)* in tissues[29] without GM_1 or GM_2. In these cases, there is a decrease in the enzyme N-acetylgalactososaminyl transferase, which is important in the synthesis of GM_1 and GM_2 from GM_3. These infants have pronounced respiratory difficulties in the first weeks of life, when generalized seizures become prominent. Poor motor and mental development is typical, and dysplastic features such as an enlarged tongue, high-arched palate, inguinal hernia, and loose skin are found. The hands and feet are broad, and there is marked hirsutism. Generalized muscle hypotonia, poor responses, and diminished reflexes develop, but the optic fundi are normal, and the liver and spleen are minimally enlarged. Because of dysphagia and difficulty in feeding, death usually occurs within the first few months of life. On autopsy, spongy degeneration in the brain stem and diencephalon is evident, and intracytoplasmic bodies are seen in astrocytes.

Differential Diagnosis. The other group of degenerative disorders that should be considered in the differential diagnosis is the cerebroretinal syndromes. In patients with some variant forms, such as the neuronal ceroid-lipofuscinoses, primary movement disorders and spinocerebellar degeneration must be considered.

Evaluation. The electroretinographical abnormalities and delayed or absent visual evoked responses suggest a retinal involvement. Urine oligosaccharides are abnormal in GM_1-gangliosidosis and galactosialidosis. Urine mucopolysaccharides are abnormal in Sandhoff's disease. No biochemical marker is found in other GM_2-gangliosidoses. Definite diagnosis requires testing of specific enzymes. In GM_2-gangliosidosis, false-positive results are seen in patients treated with oral steroids or pregnant patients. Pseudodeficiency has also been reported in a non-Jewish patient; the diagnosis can be confirmed by DNA testing.[28] False-negative results are due to specific mutations in the hexosaminidase gene[30] or to GM_2 glycoprotein activator gene deficiencies. Identification of storage material in rectal biopsy may be helpful in such cases. Special testing is warranted for populations at particular risk. Since approximately 80 percent of patients with Tay-Sachs disease are of Jewish ancestry, massive population screening studies of white blood cell enzymes to detect the carrier state have been successful. Amniotic fluid removed early in pregnancy and chorionic villi may also be studied to determine whether the Tay-Sachs disorder is present. Several pitfalls should be avoided in diagnosing patients with gangliosidosis. For example, there is often confusion between Sandhoff's disease and Tay-Sachs disease because of similar clinical and biochemical results. DNA testing, coupled with enzyme analysis, provides a good level of sensitivity and specificity.

Management, Prognosis, and Future Perspectives. Definitive treatment is not available for patients with most of the gangliosidoses, but some experimental approaches may be effective. Enzyme replacement therapy with multiple laminar lyposomes coated with human IgG has not been effective.[21] Bone marrow transplantation is being used, but the attendant risks of radiation to the brain and chronic immunosuppressive therapy are worrisome. Palliative therapies are helpful. The prognosis remains dismal. Future research with enzyme replacement, inhibitors, and activators; identification of new enzyme activators; and genetic counseling are all indicated.

SPHINGOMYELINOSES

As a group, the sphingomyelinoses are lysosomal storage disorders of autosomal recessive inheritance characterized biochemically by the accumulation of sphingomyelin, a molecule containing a ceramide, a phosphoric acid ester, and choline.

There are at least four types of sphingomyelinoses or Niemann-Pick's disease (types A, B, C, and D), all of which are neurodegenerative disorders except type B (Table 30–3). A prominent visceromegaly is the rule, except for some patients with late-onset type C and D diseases. A rapid deterioration is more frequent in patients with early-onset disease. In contrast, late-onset cases are characterized by a slow progression. Approximately 50 percent of affected patients belong in the type A group, characterized by severe neurological symptoms. Type A and B diseases result from molecular defects in the acid sphingomyelinase (ASM). The ASM gene is mapped to chromosome 11p. Type A and type B diseases are caused by allelic point mutations and deletions within the ASM gene. Type C disease results from molecular defects in either NPC1 protein, a lysosomal permease belonging to one of the superfamilies of efflux pumps, or in the HE1 protein, a protein that interacts with NPC1.[31, 32] The NPC1 gene has been identified and maps to chromosome 18q11. The HE1 gene maps to chromosome 14q24. Niemann-Pick's disease type C results from mutations in the NPC1 gene (NPC1) or in the HE1 gene (NPC2). Niemann-Pick's disease type D is an allelic variant of NPC1.[33]

Type A disease, or infantile form, is marked by failure to thrive, hypotonia, and hepatosplenomegaly. A macular cherry-red spot is noted in 50 percent of patients. Eye movements are normal. Seizures are common. Developmental regression with loss of reactivity to the environment is relentless. Recurrent infection is often a major problem, and death occurs before 5 years of age.

In some cases, peripheral nervous system involvement is detected with slow nerve conduction velocities. In such patients, type C disease can be classified into four major groups according to the onset of neurological symptoms (i.e., early infantile, late infantile, juvenile, and adult). In the early infantile form, cholestasis and biliary atresia are associated with a rapid neurological deterioration. In the late infantile form, the patients usually seem normal until 2 years of age, when psychomotor deterioration with ataxia, dysarthria, and drooling develop. Most patients belong to the juvenile form, also known as dystonic juvenile lipidosis. These patients may present with behavioral and motor difficulties. They often develop dystonia with selectively swollen cells in the basal ganglia. Dystonia starts distally and gradually becomes generalized. Features of supranuclear vertical gaze palsy are noted when the patient is asked to look down. Degeneration of the macula may be associated with a cherry-red spot. In the adult form, cognitive and psychiatric disturbances (psychosis, catatonia) may be prominent. Vertical supranuclear palsy leads to difficulties negotiating stairs. Visceromegaly is mild when present, and many patients never develop this problem.

Type D, or Nova Scotia variant, however, is characterized by early onset of hepatosplenomegaly and neurological difficulties similar to those seen in type C beginning between the second and the fourth year of life. The clinical course is protracted with survival into adulthood.[34] In patients with Niemann-Pick's disease, foamy histiocytes can be found in the bone marrow and spleen, and hepatic cells show small clusters of histiocytes that resemble sea-blue histiocytes.[35] No unusual characteristics mark the plasma lipoprotein profile.

Most histological information has been obtained from studies of the infantile or type A form. Very often, the central nervous system of these patients is gliotic, small, and atrophic. The gray matter shows necrotic changes with large neurons that are distended and ballooned with apparent storage of sphingomyelin. In some patients, there are extensive abnormalities in the spinal cord, midbrain, and cerebellum. The white matter is rarely affected. Changes in retinal cells similar to those in the brain are seen. Biochemical assay of membranous cytoplasmic bodies reveals large amounts of sphingomyelin and cholesterol.

The differential diagnosis rests with the other storage diseases. In patients with type A (with hepatosplenomegaly) and type C (with vertical supranuclear palsy), most confusion in diagnosis involves the cerebrosidoses. Dystonia with intellectual deterioration has been reported in NPC1, juvenile-onset metachromatic leukodystrophy, and the late-onset gangliosidoses. Diagnosis is suspected on identifying excessive amounts of sphingomyelin and the foamy cells. The definite diagnosis is made by measuring sphingomyelinase activity or by linkage analysis and sequence analysis of the mutated genes. Antenatal diagnosis of types A and B disease can be made. Of the various therapy approaches, hematopoietic stem cell–mediated gene therapy and exogenous recombinant protein replacement have attracted the most interest.

CEREBROSIDOSES

Cerebrosidoses are autosomal recessive diseases characterized by lysosomal storage of cerebroside, a molecule composed of ceramide and hexose. Lipid-laden macrophages, Gaucher's cells, are found in most tissues. Gaucher's cells have an excentric nucleus and a wrinkled tissue paper cytoplasm. In the vast majority, the enzyme glucocerebrosidase (glucosylceramide beta-glucosidase) is deficient. The abnormal gene is located on chromosome 1q21. Rare cases are caused by a deficiency of Saponin C, a heat-stable cofactor required for normal catalytic function of glucocerebrosidase (see metachromatic leukodystrophy). There are three forms of cerebrosidosis, or Gaucher's disease: type I (adult), type II

TABLE 30–3. **Sphingomyelinoses (Niemann-Pick's Disease) and Cerebrosidoses (Gaucher's Disease)**

Type	Name	Enzyme Defect	Storage Product	Genetics	Age of Onset	Primary Clinical Features
Sphingomyelinoses						
Type A	Classic Niemann-Pick's disease	Sphingomyelinase	Sphingomyelin	Autosomal recessive: prenatal detection available	Infants	Hepatosplenomegaly, Niemann-Pick cells in bone marrow Prominent neurological findings, motor and mental retardation, cherry-red spot in 50 percent
Type B	Non-neurological variant	Sphingomyelinase	Sphingomyelin	Autosomal recessive: prenatal detection available	Chronic progressive	No neurological signs and massive hepatosplenomegaly
Type C	Childhood or adult	NPC1 protein or HE1 protein	Sphingomyelin and cholesterol	Autosomal recessive	2 to 4 years chronic and progressive or adult onset	Hepatosplenomegaly variably present; Niemann-Pick cells in bone marrow Prominent neurological findings, especially dystonia
Type D	Nova Scotian variant	NPC1 protein	Sphingomyelin and cholesterol	Autosomal recessive	2 to 4 years chronic and progressive	Clinically similar to type C. Most neurological signs may be secondary to hepatosplenopathy
Cerebrosidoses						
Type I	Classic Gaucher's disease, chronic, non-neuropathic form	Glucose cerebrosidase	Glucose cerebroside	Autosomal recessive	Adults	Chronic disease involving viscera and blood-forming tissues, non-neurological
Type II	Infantile or neurological Gaucher's disease	Glucose cerebrosidase	Glucose cerebroside	Autosomal recessive	Infants	Prominent neurological signs with early opisthotonos, severe mental and motor retardation and death by age 2 years
Type III	Juvenile	Glucose cerebrosidase	Glucose cerebroside	Autosomal recessive	Juveniles	Variable hepatosplenomegaly and moderate neurological signs of motor and mental retardation

(infantile), and type III (juvenile) (see Table 30–3). Gaucher's disease is the most frequently reported of the lysosomal storage diseases and is particularly frequent among Ashkenazi Jews.[21]

Type I disease, so-named because it was first described by Gaucher, is the chronic, non-neuropathic form.[36] This form is usually found in adults and is a predominantly chronic disease involving the viscera (splenomegaly, hypersplenism) and blood-forming tissues (bone crisis). Type II, on the other hand, is an acute neuropathic disease found in infants. It is almost always apparent by 6 months of age but may present as early as the newborn period, frequently with hyperextension or opisthotonic posturing of the head. The posturing is believed to be due to Gaucher's cells in the meninges at the base of the brain. Affected babies have early strabismus or heterotropia, generalized hypertonia, and difficulty in swallowing, a fairly consistent neurological clinical triad. Ichthyosis is the presenting symptom in some patients. Profound psychomotor retardation develops, and laryngospasm, myoclonus, bulbar impairment, supranuclear vertical and horizontal gaze palsy, and seizures may be evident. Brain MRI may be normal or show hydrocephalus. Rapidly progressive central nervous system (CNS) deterioration occurs combined with splenomegaly. Some children have relatively mild systemic symptoms. Most patients with this form of cerebrosidosis die by the age of 2 years. The course of disease is similar in many respects to the fulminating course of type A sphingomyelinosis. The infantile neuronal form of Gaucher's disease does not have a proclivity toward Jewish ancestry. Type III cerebrosidosis is a subacute neuronopathic disease, most often found in juveniles and associated with variable neurological and systemic features. Most patients present in childhood with refractory seizures and mental decline. These patients may also have myoclonus, and the diagnosis should be considered in children with the progressive myoclonic epilepsies (see Chapter 52). In other children, ataxia and/or dystonia are the presenting symptoms. Horizontal supranuclear gaze palsy is a predominant sign. Death may occur between the second and fourth decade. Although this classification of Gaucher's disease into three entities is accepted, exceptions to it do occur,[37] such as a rare non-neuronopathic form occurring in early infancy and a neuronopathic form with supranuclear gaze palsy and parkinsonism seen in adults.[38]

Full clinical assessment of neuropathic cases includes a careful neurological examination, eye movement examination, a detailed funduscopic examination, a family history, neuropsychometric and neurophysiological evaluations, and brain imaging. Bone marrow aspirate can be used to identify Gaucher's cells. Definite diagnosis is made by enzyme analysis. The finding of sulfatides in the urine of a patient with type II disease should suggest a prosaposin deficiency.

Intravenous enzyme replacement therapy is available using recombinantly produced glucocerebrosidase. This therapy improves the neurological outcome in neuronopathic cases.[39]

MUCOPOLYSACCHARIDOSES

Mucopolysaccharides (Table 30–4) are constituents of connective tissue composed of alternating units of polymerized hexuronic acids and hexose amines. As a group, mucopolysaccharidoses are characterized by somatic dysplasia, slowly deteriorating mentation and motor control, storage of mucopolysaccharide within cellular lysosomes, and urinary excretion of glycosaminoglycans (heparin sulfate, dermatan sulfate, or related compounds). It is generally agreed that the causative defect in the mucopolysaccharidoses (MPS) involves lysosomal hydrolysis. Because of faulty breakdown of glycosaminoglycans, these products are stored within the lysosomes, distending the lysosome and the cell body. Mucopolysaccharides represent the major component of the lysosomal storage material, particularly in fibroblasts. In lymphocytes, storage vacuoles have been called Reilly bodies. Because the brain is also a prime storage site, mental retardation is a prominent feature of all MPS. There are 13 subclasses of MPS (see Table 30–4).[40]

The mucopolysaccharidoses are inherited as autosomal recessive diseases, with the exception of Hunter's syndrome, which is sex-linked. The global frequency of the varieties of MPS has not been clearly established. Population studies in the Netherlands indicated that Sanfilippo's syndrome type A is the most common form, with an estimated frequency of 1:24,000 in that population.[41] In British Columbia, the incidence of Hunter's syndrome was estimated at 1:78,000,[42] but in Israel its frequency may be higher. Sanfilippo's syndrome type B is seen particularly often in Greece,[42] and in the Cayman Islands a high frequency of Sanfilippo's syndrome type A has been found, with an estimated carrier frequency of 1:10.

As a group, these diseases are marked by striking somatic dysplasia, slowly deteriorating neurological and systemic symptoms, storage of mucopolysaccharides in the lysosomes, and excretion of mucopolysaccharides in the urine (see Table 30–4). Although each type has a specific enzyme deficit, the similar spectrum of clinical manifestations in all MPS disorders makes biochemical differentiation essential.

Mucopolysaccharidoses I are caused by an alpha-iduronidase deficiency. This enzyme is required for the hydrolysis of alpha-iduronic acid from the terminal end of dermatan and heparan sulfate. The gene has been assigned to 4p16.3. Three clinical syndromes result from this defect. For many reasons, Hurler's disease (type 1) has become the prototypical MPS. Patients who have this syndrome in early infancy may appear reasonably normal, but by 6 months of age it is obvious that a severe disorder is present. The abnormal facial appearance is one of the first signs noted, and hepatosplenomegaly and umbilical and inguinal hernias are soon detected. Affected infants may have chronic rhinorrhea associated with frequent colds, recurrent airway infections, and otitis media. When children with Hurler's disease attempt to sit, a characteristic kyphoscoliosis is often observed, which progresses with time. Ultimately, a frank gibbus deformity, one of the earliest described clinical features of the disease, develops. Vision is often impaired in Hurler's disease because of corneal clouding. Although the infant with Hurler's disease may develop some sitting and walking skills as well as early language skills, these are soon lost. Severe mental retardation becomes apparent, and patients are usually bedridden before the end of the juvenile period. Patients with Hurler-Scheie's disease (type 2) have severe joint involvement, short stature, small thoraces, hepatosplenomegaly, coarse facial features, and corneal clouding. They may have near-normal mental abilities. The small thorax and cardiac involvement in this dis-

TABLE 30–4. **Mucopolysaccharidoses and Mucolipidoses**

Type	Name	Enzyme Defect	Storage Product	Genetics	Age of Onset	Primary Clinical Features
Mucopolysaccharidoses (MPS)						
1	Hurler's (MPS I)	α-L-iduronidase	Heparan sulfate (HS) and dermatan sulfate (DS)	Autosomal recessive	Birth or by 6 months	Abnormal facial appearance, hepatosplenomegaly, kyphoscoliosis, corneal clouding, mental retardation
2	Hurler-Scheie's MPS V/I	α-L-iduronidase	Heparan sulfate (HS) and dermatan sulfate (DS)	Autosomal recessive	First year	Severe joint involvement, coarse facial features, hepatosplenomegaly, corneal clouding, but near-normal mentation
3	Scheie's (MPS V)	α-L-iduronidase	Heparan sulfate (HS) and dermatan sulfate (DS)	Autosomal recessive	First year	Normal stature and less severe neurological deficits than in types 1 and 2
4	Hunter's (MPS II)	Iduronate 2-sulfatase	Heparan sulfate (HS) and dermatan suflate (DS)	X-linked	First year	Similar to Hurler, but without corneal clouding
5, 6, 7, 8	Sanfilippo's A, B, C, D (MPS III)	A: Heparan sulfatase B : *N*-acetyl-glucosaminidase C : *N*-acetyl-CoA-acetyl-transferase D: *N*-acetyl-α, D-glucosamine-6-sulfatase	A: Heparan sulfate B : Heparan sulfate C: Heparan sulfate D: Heparan sulfate	Autosomal recessive	First year	Hepatosplenomegaly and facial coarseness less than in Hunter and Hurler. Mental and motor retardation, death by age 10. Among the subgroups, C is the mildest. In all subgroups, patients excrete heparan sulfate
9, 10	Morquio's A, B (MPS IV)	A: Acetyl-galactosamine-6-sulfatase B : β-galactosidase	Keratan sulfate and chondroitoin sulfate Keratan sulfate	Autosomal recessive	First year	Skeletal dysplasia with compressive neurological signs (severe in A, mild in B). No or little mental retardation. Corneal clouding 50% and organomegaly less prominent compared to other MPS. Survival to middle age

Table continued on following page

TABLE 30–4 **Mucopolysaccharidoses and Mucolipidoses** *Continued*

Type	Name	Enzyme Defect	Storage Product	Genetics	Age of Onset	Primary Clinical Features
11	Maroteaux-Lamy (MPS VI)	Arylsulfatase B	Dermatan sulfate	Autosomal recessive	First year	Growth retardation, coarse features, myelopathy
12	Sly's (MPS VII)	β-glucuronidase	Dermatan sulfate and heparan sulfate	Autosomal recessive	First year through childhood	Hepatosplenomegaly, psychomotor retardation, coarse features
13	Multiple sulfatase deficiency	Arylsulfatase A, B, and C	Dermatan sulfate and heparan sulfate	Autosomal recessive	First year	Variable signs, including mental retardation and coarse facial features
Mucolipidoses (ML)						
1	Sialidosis type 1 (ML I)	Neuraminidase (sialidase)	Oligosaccharide, glycolipids	Autosomal recessive	Adolescence	Cherry-red spot, myoclonic seizures, painful neuropathy, mildly coarse facial features
2	Sialidosis type 2 (ML I)	Neuraminidase (sialidase)	Oligosaccharide, glycolipids	Autosomal recessive	Infants	More severe than sialidosis. Facial and somatic dysmorphism, progressive mental retardation
3	I-cell disease (ML II)	*N*-acetylglucosamylphosphotransferase	Oligosaccharide, glycolipids	Autosomal recessive	Infants	Severe disease. Facial and somatic dysmorphism, progressive severe mental retardation, hepatosplenomegaly. Death often by age 10
4	Pseudo-Hurler's (ML III)	*N*-acetylglucosamine–1-phosphotransferase	Oligosaccharide, glycolipids	Autosomal recessive	Childhood	Mild in comparison to I-cell. Corneal clouding. Survival to adulthood
5	Berman's mucolipidosis (ML IV)	Mucolipin I	Oligosaccharide, glycolipids	Autosomal recessive	Childhood	Most patients of Ashkenazi Jewish extraction

ease often reflect mitral valve insufficiency. Scheie's syndrome (type 3) usually occurs in individuals of normal size, and their neurological deficits are less severe than those seen in patients with types 1 and 2 disease. These patients have only mild hepatosplenomegaly with marked coarseness of the facial features or severe mental retardation. Dysostosis multiplex or bony involvement is also mild, although a common feature is carpal tunnel symptomatology. It is rare for neurological problems to be severe enough to cause early complaints. Generally, ocular involvement, specifically corneal clouding or retinal abnormalities suggesting degeneration, lead to suspicions of an MPS disorder. In most instances, the diagnosis is not made before the age of 10 years, and frequently it is not recognized until age 20 or later.

Mucopolysaccharidoses II are caused by iduronosulfatase deficiency. The gene maps on Xq28. Two types of Hunter's syndrome have been suggested, one with predominant mental retardation and one not associated with retardation. Children with Hunter's syndrome may have a facial appearance similar to that characteristic of Hurler's syndrome, but the cornea is not clouded in Hunter's disease. In fact, corneal findings are the most important features distinguishing Hunter's from Hurler's disease. Patients with Hunter's syndrome often have a macular skin rash over the arms, shoulders, and thighs that may change in character. Urinary excretion of heparan and dermatan sulfate is similar in Hunter's and Hurler's diseases.

The four forms of *mucopolysaccharidoses III* or Sanfilippo's syndrome (MPS III, types 5–8) are caused by four enzyme defects: heparan sulfatase (or sulfamidase) (type A), *N*-acetylglutaminidase (type B), acetyl-CoA *N* acetyltransferase (type C), and *N*-acetylglucosamine-6-sulfatase (type D). Type A is caused by sulfamidase gene mutations on chromosome 17q25.3.[43] Type B is caused by *N*-acetyl-CoA *N*-acetyltransferase gene mutations on chromosome 17q21.1.[44] Type D is caused by *N*-acetylglucosamine-6-sulfatase mutations on 12q14.[45] Clinical symptoms usually start after 2 years of apparently normal development and include hyperactivity, aggressive behavior, delayed speech, sleep disturbances, coarse hair, hirsutism, and diarrhea. There are only mild somatic manifestations such as short stature, slight coarsening of facial features, and mild contractures. Hepatomegaly, when present, only appears late in the course of the illness. Mental deterioration is progressive and motor impairment soon leads to loss of ambulation. Myoclonus appears late in the course of the illness. These children are bedridden in the second decade, and death usually occurs by the midteens. Patients with type D disease have a later onset, an attenuated phenotype with normal stature, hyperactivity, mental retardation, a slower progression, and prolonged survival. Sanfilippo's syndrome is a classic example of a neurodegenerative disease with a monophasic downhill course.

Mucopolysaccharidosis IV is caused by the deficiency of two enzymes, components of the lysosomal multienzyme complex (LMC): type A is caused by *N*-acetylgalactosamine-6-sulfate sulfatase deficiency and type B is caused by beta-galactosidase deficiency. Mutations in the *N*-acetylgalactosamine-6-sulfate sulfatase gene on chromosome 16q24.3 cause type A disease, and mutations in the beta-galactosidase gene on chromosome 3p21[10] cause type B disease. In 1929, Morquio[46] described a syndrome characterized by severe skeletal dysplasia. Clinically, the severe classic syndrome (type A) can be differentiated from mild variant (type B). In both forms, mental symptomatology is absent or only mildly present. Neurological symptoms may result from compression of the spinal cord or medulla. The skeletal changes include joint laxity, shortness of stature, pectus carinatum, shortened vertebrae, genu valgum, pes planus, and enlarged joints. The neck is short, and the odontoid process in the cervical region is often underdeveloped, accounting for the atlantoaxial subluxation seen.[47] There are no cherry-red spots. Corneal clouding is present in 50 percent of cases, and hepatomegaly is less prominent than in other forms of mucopolysaccharidosis. Cardiac involvement may include aortic regurgitation. Patients usually survive until middle age.

These disorders are most easily confused with the mucolipidoses and the GM_1-gangliosidoses because of the associated facial and somatic progressive dysmorphisms. Full general and neurological assessments are necessary, and even with a full family history, these recessive diseases may not be fully expressed in an immediate family constellation. Important laboratory evaluations include identification of mucopolysaccharides in the urine and assays for enzyme defects in leukocytes and cultured fibroblasts (see Table 30–4).

Bone marrow transplant appears to slow down neurological deterioration. Symptomatic palliative therapies are available, but these are slowly progressive diseases, and life expectancy is limited.

MUCOLIPIDOSES

The mucolipidoses (MLs) are a group of autosomal recessive lysosomal storage diseases characterized biochemically by accumulation in tissues and brain of glycolipids and glycoproteins. Each of the five types of mucolipidoses may be confused phenotypically with the mucopolysaccharidoses (see Table 30–4). However, in all mucolipidoses, urine mucopolysaccharides are normal, differentiating them readily from mucopolysaccharidoses. There is no specific race or ethnic predilection except for the ML type 4.

Mucolipidosis type 1 (or sialidosis) is caused by a sialidase (neuraminidase) deficiency. Sialidase is a component of the LMC (see GM_1-gangliosidosis). Sialidosis is caused by several mutations in the sialidase gene on chromosome 6p.[21] Bone marrow aspirates contain foamy histiocytes and vacuolated lymphocytes. Urine mucopolysaccharides are normal. Oligosaccharides and glycoproteins are found in the urine. Sialidosis may have two phenotypes. *Sialidosis type 1 or nondysmorphic type* is also known as the *cherry-red spot-myoclonus syndrome*.[48] Patients present in the second decade with a progressive visual impairment, myoclonus, and gait abnormalities. Once visual pathology is evident, including night blindness or loss of color vision, the disease becomes progressive.[48] A cherry-red spot is uniformly present and lens opacities occur frequently. Myoclonus is typically generalized and triggered by startle, auditory stimuli, smoking, and menstruation. Intellectual deterioration may be a late occurrence. Painful neuropathy, delayed nerve conduction velocity, generalized convulsive seizures, ataxia, and dysostosis multiplex ensue. Facies may be coarse but to a lesser extent than in the mucopolysaccharidoses.

In *sialidosis type 2 or dysmorphic type*, the onset of symptoms always occurs early in life. Babies may be born with hydrops fetalis. The somatic and facial features are invariably coarse. Dysostosis multiplex, periosteal cloaking, and hepatosplenomegaly dominate, and contractures of major bony articulations, inguinal hernias, and mild hepatosplenomegaly are common findings. Angiokeratoma corporis diffusum may be prominent. Neurological impairment is slowly progressive and is marked by dementia and other signs such as ataxia, hypotonia, reduced muscle mass, and cherry-red spots.

Mucolipidosis type 2 and 3 are caused by a *N*-acetylglucosaminyl phosphotransferase, resulting in a deficient targeting and phosphorylation of the mannose in newly synthesized glycoprotein acid hydrolases. The gene for this enzyme has been designated GNPTA and maps to 4q21–q23.[49] Assaying lysosomal enzymes in plasma shows increased activity of lysosomal enzymes. Bone marrow aspirates contain vacuolated plasma cells and lymphocytes. Vacuoles are also seen in fibroblasts. *Mucolipidosis type 2* or I-cell disease presents in the neonatal area with coarse facies reminiscent of Hurler's disease, hepatosplenomegaly, umbilical hernias, kyphoscoliosis, and lumbar gibbus. Mild forms of dysostosis multiplex are seen, but these are much less severe than those seen in patients with Hurler's disease. The thorax is usually small, joint movement is restricted, and the tongue is large, often with gingival hyperplasia. Corneal haziness is common, and cardiac involvement includes cardiomegaly and aortic insufficiency. Both intellectual and motor retardation become obvious in the first months of life. These children are severely ill and frequently die in the first decade of life from cardiopulmonary failure.

Mucolipidosis type 3 or pseudo-Hurler's disease is a milder form characterized by a later clinical onset, usually in childhood, and some may live into adulthood but are mentally retarded. Linear growth is severely affected, corneal clouding and aortic regurgitation are common, and older patients show joint stiffness. Facial coarseness is minimal.

Mucolipidosis type 4 is caused by a defect in mucolipin 1, a membrane protein involved in endocytosis and showing homology to a group of calcium channels of the TRP/TRPL family. Mutations in the MCOLN1 gene on chromosome 19p13.3–p13.2 are responsible for mucolipin 1 deficiency.[50] Fibroblasts are similar to those seen in I-cell disease. Patients with ML type 4 lack dysmorphic features, hepatosplenomegaly, and bony changes. Visual impairment and severe corneal clouding appear in the first year of life. Myopathy and psychomotor retardation are profound.

The MLs are most easily confused with the mucopolysaccharidoses. They are biochemically distinguishable by the lack of the mucopolysacchariduria characteristic of the MPS. There are some clinical and biochemical similarities with the GM_1-gangliosidoses. Detailed and skilled clinical evaluation of systemic as well as neurological factors is essential in addition to assays for lysosomal enzymes and mucopolysaccharides in the urine. No specific therapy is available.

Glycogenoses

Pathogenesis and Pathophysiology. The glycogenoses or glycogen storage diseases are disorders in which glycogen accumulates within a number of tissues. These diseases are named for the specific enzyme deficiency that occurs in the glycogen metabolic pathway (Table 30–5), and their ordering follows the enzymatic steps involved in glycogen synthesis and catabolism.[51, 52] Most enzymes are cytosolic except for the lysosomal acid alpha-glucosidase. If the deficient enzyme is expressed predominantly in the liver, hypoglycemia usually accompanies the clinical signs. If the deficient enzyme is expressed predominantly in muscles, the disease presents either as a pure myopathy or as a cardiomyopathy.

TABLE 30–5. **Glycogenoses**

Type	Disease Eponym	Enzyme Deficiency	Location	Gene	Inheritance
Ia	Von Gierke's	Glucose-6-phosphatase (G6P)	Liver	1p21	AR
Ib	Von Gierke's	G6P transporter 1	Liver	11	AR
II	Pompe's	Acid maltase	Liver, heart, muscle, brain		
III	Cori-Forbes's	Debranching enzyme	Muscle	1p21	AR
IV	Andersen's	Branching enzyme	Muscle, heart, liver, brain	3	AR
V	McArdle's	Myophosphorylase	Muscle	11	AR or AD
VI	Hers'	Phosphorylase	Liver	14	AR
VII	Tarui's	Phosphofructokinase	Muscle	1	AR
VIII	Hug's	Phosphorylase B kinase	Muscle	PHKA1: Xq12–q13	XR
			Liver	PHKA2: Xp22	XR
			Muscle	PHKB: 16q12–q13	AR
			Liver, muscle	PHKG1: 7p12–q12	AR
			Liver	PHKG2: 6p11–p12	AR
IX	Bresolin's	Phosphoglycerate kinase	Muscle	Xq13	XR
X	Tonin's	Phosphoglycerate mutase	Muscle	7p12–7p13	AR
XI	Tsujino's	Lactate dehydrogenase	Muscle	11	AR
XII	Kreuder's	Aldolase	Muscle	16q22–q24	AR

AD, Autosomal dominant; AR, autosomal recessive; XR, X-linked.

Epidemiology and Risk Factors. Most of the glycogenoses are inherited as autosomal recessive diseases. However, an X-linked inheritance has been demonstrated in the most frequent form of liver phosphorylase kinase deficiency (Hug's disease), in some patients with muscle phosphorylase kinase deficiency (Ohtani's disease), and in phosphoglycerate kinase deficiency (Bresolin's disease). An autosomal dominant transmission has been suggested in a few families with myophosphorylase deficiency (McArdle's disease). The genes responsible for most glycogenoses have been mapped (see Table 30–5). Several mutations have been identified for each disorder. The molecular heterogeneity of the glycogenoses frequently results in clinical heterogeneity. For instance, although in most patients with debranching enzyme deficiency (Cori-Forbes disease) the disease involves the liver and the muscle, some patients (about 15%) have only liver involvement without muscle disease. This rare clinical phenotype is associated specifically with exon 3 mutations. There are pockets of these diseases in certain populations. For instance, most patients with muscle phosphofructokinase deficiency (Tarui's disease) in the United States are related to Ashkenazi Jews. The most common mutations responsible for each disorder differ in various ethnic groups. For instance, the most common mutation in North American patients with McArdle's disease seems to be R49X. This mutation is only seen in a minority of Mediterranean patients and it has never been observed in Japan. Knowledge of the most common mutation in a specific ethnic group allows the use of molecular genetics analysis in the blood for diagnostic purposes, thus avoiding the need for a muscle biopsy. Autosomal recessive inheritance has been shown clearly in patients with Pompe's disease, in which the type 3 and 4 variants are possibly related to different alleles. The gene for human acid alpha-glucosidase is contained on chromosome 7q251–23.[53] Two types of mutant alleles were identified in one family in which both adults and infants had acid maltase deficiency.[54] One type resulted in reduced net production of active alpha-glucosidase with partial enzyme deficiency. An infant type of debrancher enzyme deficiency syndrome appears to be transmitted as an autosomal recessive trait, but the heterozygous state could not be diagnosed with certainty. Muscle glycogen concentrations appeared to be normal in another patient. Studies have confirmed that an autosomal recessive mode of inheritance occurred in the brancher enzyme disorder. The presence of enzymatic activity in cultured fibroblasts is lower in affected individuals than in normal controls, and the same is true (although less marked) in their parents, strongly suggesting that the trait is autosomal recessive. Tarui's disease is also transmitted in this way. Prenatal diagnosis and genetic research are indicated in further studies of these entities.

Clinical Features and Associated Disorders. In Von Gierke's disease (glycogenosis type I), hypoglycemia causes many of the clinical difficulties seen in patients during the first year of life. In this period seizures are frequent, and long-standing hemiplegia and mental retardation occur. Systemic features include failure to thrive and isolated hepatomegaly, whereas dermatological signs include xanthomas and excessive subcutaneous fat over the buttocks, breasts, and cheeks. Affected children usually have a protruding abdomen due to enlargement of the liver. Patients often have recurrent stomatitis and frequent infections and may have isolated chronic inflammatory bowel disease.

There are three phenotypes of acid maltase deficiency (glycogenosis type II).[55] The infantile form or Pompe's disease usually presents with hypotonia and associated weakness after a seemingly normal development during the first weeks or several months of life. A pseudohypertrophy of calf muscles is seen. Spontaneous movement declines, the cry becomes weak and struggling, and swallowing is poor. Respiratory difficulty results from the skeletal muscular weakness and inability to handle pooled nasopharyngeal secretions. Massive cardiomegaly develops, and a soft, systemic murmur is often heard at the left sternal border. Ultimately, hepatomegaly appears, and the tongue may be enlarged and protrude awkwardly. Palpation of the muscles reveals them to be firm, but muscle stretch reflexes are suppressed. Progressive debilitation occurs, and patients usually die by 1 to 2 years of age.

In the late infantile form of acid maltase deficiency or Smith's disease, symptoms and signs may simulate those of Duchenne's muscular dystrophy. In such patients, the gastrocnemius and deltoid muscles are firm and rubbery on palpation. There is accompanying hypertrophy of the gastrocnemius muscles, and Gowers' sign is often present. Toe walking develops with ankle contractures, and the gait is unsteady and wobbling owing to lumbar lordosis. Cardiomegaly is absent. In the adult form of acid maltase deficiency, or Engel's disease,[56] weakness of the muscles develops during the third through sixth decades of life. Weakness is more prominent proximally than distally, and the pelvic girdle is involved more than the shoulders. Intercostal and diaphragmatic muscles are involved in many patients. Adults do not show enlargement of the liver, heart, or tongue. Frequently, symptoms suggesting polymyositis or late-onset muscular dystrophy cause confusion in the initial clinical diagnosis.

Three types of debranching enzyme deficiency syndrome (glycogenosis type III) have been identified: infantile, childhood, and adult. In the infantile type, early symptoms are similar to, but less marked than, those typical of Von Gierke's disease, which is associated with hypoglycemia, failure to thrive, and hepatomegaly. Patients with the infantile type are hypotonic and weak with poor head control. Juvenile-onset debranching enzyme deficiency begins between the ages of 2 and 15 with exercise intolerance and associated heart failure. These patients are hypotonic and have a protuberant abdomen. Adult patients develop progressive chronic distal myopathy and neuropathy in middle age.

Clinical manifestations of the infantile branching enzyme deficiency (glycogenosis type IV), or Andersen's disease, are generally seen in the first 6 months of life and are related to weakness, feeding difficulties, muscle wasting, tachypnea, failure to thrive, and hepatosplenomegaly. Such patients have poor motor and mental development, muscular hypotonia, and hyporeflexia. More benign forms of this variant present later in life with only mild hepatomegaly and elevated liver enzymes The adult "polyglucosan body disease," characterized by diffuse peripheral and central involvement, is allelic to this disorder.[57]

Children affected with classic McArdle's disease (myophosphorylase deficiency) initially show decreased stamina and easy fatigability. Although onset usually occurs in childhood, neonatal presentations have been reported. Severe cramping pain, usually in the distal skeletal muscles, develops after exercise and is often associated with renal impairment. In adolescence and adulthood, patients may develop persistent weakness and moderate loss of muscle bulk. Patients with Hers' disease have no specific neurological or muscle findings but display varying degrees of growth retardation, hypoglycemia, ketosis, and hepatomegaly. In Tarui's disease,[58] motor development is normal during the first decade, but decreased muscle exercise tolerance, myoglobulinuria, and easy fatigability develop in childhood. An unusual infantile syndrome characterized by limb weakness, seizures, cortical blindness, and corneal opacifications occurs; microscopic studies reveal typical findings of neuron axonal dystrophy.[59]

Mild cases of liver phosphorylase kinase deficiency (Hug's disease)[60] have been associated with hepatomegaly, attacks of ketonuria with fasting, and intermittent diarrhea. Hypotonia in infancy can occur. Pure muscle disease with exercise intolerance, myalgia, cramps, and weakness is reported in some patients.

In patients with other glycogenosis defects, such as phosphoglycerate mutase, phosphoglycerate kinase, and lactate dehydrogenase deficiencies, exercise intolerance with myoglobinuria occurs. In patients with phosphoglycerate kinase deficiency, or Bresolin's disease,[61] the defect is sex-linked, and hemolytic anemia, seizures, mental retardation, and exercise intolerance with myoglobinuria are prominent features. In adults, phosphoglycerate mutase deficiency, or Tonin's disease,[62] has been associated with myalgia, cramps, and myoglobinuria following exercise. Lactate dehydrogenase deficiency, or Tsujino's disease,[63] has been reported in one patient who suffered from severe myoglobinuria with exercise.

Differential Diagnosis. Most of the glycogen storage disorders must be differentiated from various myopathies and muscular dystrophies. In the former, abnormalities are seldom limited to the muscle. Liver failure problems and other systemic symptoms are often obvious. Because of the liver problems present in most of these diseases, one must always consider other storage diseases such as the mucopolysaccharidoses, mucolipidoses, sphingomyelinoses, cerebrosidoses, and gangliosidoses in the differential diagnosis.

Evaluation. These diagnoses can usually be made by performing assays of enzymatic activity in the particular tissue most affected, such as the liver, peripheral white cells, muscle, and even brain. Since severe hypoglycemia is the best screening indicator of this class of diseases, postprandial and glucose tolerance tests are particularly useful. A variety of other biochemical tests, such as uric acid, cholesterol, fatty acids, triglycerides, lipid profiles, and liver function tests, should be performed, as well as bone studies in specific instances. Oligosaccharides are identified in urine of patients with Pompe's disease.[18]

Management, Prognosis, and Future Perspectives. Correction of Pompe's disease by enzyme replacement with a recombinant human acid maltase is presently under clinical trial, and initial results have been promising. Liver transplantation has been performed with apparent beneficial results in Von Gierke's disease, Forbes' disease, and Andersen's disease. Most therapies, however, remain supportive and address the particular syndrome involved. In Von Gierke's disease, for instance, small amounts of free glucose can be given to maintain normal glucose concentrations; dietary carbohydrates are also given, but because excessive glucose leads to glycogen storage in the liver and kidneys, small feedings of carbohydrates are the preferred method of treatment. Dietary substitution of medium-chain for long-chain triglycerides has been used, and diazoxide has been beneficial in some cases. Portal caval shunts bypass the liver and can be helpful in selected disorders. Preoperative intravenous hyperalimentation appears to eliminate some of the metabolic problems that occur following surgery.

In the debrancher syndromes, growth failure and hepatic dysfunction, including hypoglycemia, appear to improve with the administration of oral cornstarch. Similarly, symptoms can be controlled with frequent small carbohydrate meals in Hers' disease.

In patients with McArdle's disease and Tarui's disease, a ketogenic diet has shortened the muscle recovery period from an acute physical load. High-protein diet and aerobic exercise are also somewhat beneficial. Vitamin B_6 supplementation may be effective in McArdle's disease. Despite any of these interventions, the prognosis is guarded for patients with all of the glycogenoses.

Leukodystrophies

The leukodystrophies (Table 30–6) are genetic diseases that show morphological changes in the white matter of the CNS. Each of the leukodystrophies most likely represents an inborn error of metabolism due to a defective gene that produces an enzymatic abnormality and metabolic derangement affecting myelin. Myelin dysfunction is the basic feature of all these disorders, and demyelination or destruction of normally formed myelin can occur as well as loss of defective myelin, called dysmyelination. Simple demyelination is typical of many sudanophilic leukodystrophies. Dysmyelination is related to an underlying genetic or metabolic disturbance, and in this type of leukodystrophy, abnormal lipids incorporated into the defective myelin sheath tend to be metachromatic when stained. Leukodystrophies may be caused by enzymatic defects in peroxisomal or mitochondrial functions that induce demyelination or to enzymatic defects at specific points in the metabolic pathways of the sphingolipids.

PELIZAEUS-MERZBACHER SYNDROME

Pelizaeus-Merzbacher syndrome is a particular type of demyelinating sudanophilic leukodystrophy and has many subtypes.[64] In all, sudanophilia is produced when neutral fat stains such as Sudan black react with the neutral fat breakdown products of myelin. Since this breakdown of myelin is the result of a variety of metabolic or acquired insults, sudanophilia provides no useful information about the pathogenic origin of the insult. Most of the early reports were based on the pathological process rather than on the clinical picture, and the common denominator histologically is the presence in the CNS of patches of dysmyelination interspaced with perivascular islands of relatively intact myelin. This pattern produces a striped or tigroid appearance and is the origin of the term tigroid leukoencephalopathy, the pathological hallmark of all forms of Pelizaeus-Merzbacher syndrome.

TABLE 30–6. **Leukodystrophies**

Type	Name	Enzyme Defect	Storage Material	Genetics	Age of Onset	Special Comments
Pelizaeus-Merzbacher Syndrome						
1	Classical	Proteolipid protein	Sudanophilic material	X-linked	Infantile	Frequently confused with cerebral palsy (slow progression)
2	Connatal Seitelberger's disease	Not known	Sudanophilic material	Not known	Birth	More severe than type 1
3	Transitional Lowenberg-Hull disease	Not known	Sudanophilic material	Sporadic	Infantile	Death by age 5 to 10 years
4	Adult	Not known	Sudanophilic material	Autosomal dominant	Adult	No ocular abnormalities
5	Variant	Not known	Sudanophilic material	Not known	Variable	
Cockayne's Syndrome						
6	Classic	DNA repair	Sudanophilic material	Autosomal recessive	6 to 12 months	Dwarfism with CNS and PNS signs
Alexander's Disease						
7	Classic infantile	GFAP	GFAP	Sporadic	Infants	Psychomotor retardation, megalocephaly
8	Juvenile	GFAP	GFAP	Autosomal dominant or sporadic	Children 7 to 14 years	Prominent bulbar dysfunction with normal mentation
9	Adult	GFAP	GFAP	Autosomal dominant	Young adults	Presentation of multiple sclerosis
Canavan's Syndrome						
10	Classic infantile	Aspartoacylase	*N*-acetylaspartate in plasma	Autosomal recessive	Infants	Hypotonia, megalocephaly, blindness
11	Neonatal	Aspartoacylase	*N*-acetylaspartate in plasma	Sporadic	Newborns	Hypotonia, poor swallowing, death within first weeks of life
12	Juvenile	Aspartoacylase	*N*-acetylaspartate in plasma	Sporadic	Children 5 to teenage years	Ataxia, tremor, mental retardation with loss of vision, endocrine and cardiac disorders

Table continued on following page

TABLE 30–6. **Leukodystrophies** *Continued*

Type	Name	Enzyme Defect	Storage Material	Genetics	Age of Onset	Special Comments
Krabbe's Syndrome						
13	Classic, infantile	Galactocerebroside β-galactosidase	Galactocerebroside	Autosomal recessive	Infants	Irritability followed by hypertonicity, optic atrophy, and signs of neuropathy
14	Late onset	Galactocerebroside β-galactosidase	Galactocerebroside	Autosomal recessive	Usually childhood, but may be adults	Cortical blindness, optic atrophy, spasticity
Metachromatic Leukodystrophy						
15	Greenfield's, classical, or late infantile	Arylsulfatase or SAP-B	Sulfatide	Autosomal recessive	Late infantile 1 to 24 months	Ataxia, hypotonia, bulbar signs, intellectual decline, and peripheral neuropathy
16	Scholz's	Arylsulfatase A	Sulfatide	Autosomal recessive	Juvenile 4 to 10 years	Gait instability, tremor, ataxia, spasticity
17	Austin's	Arylsulfatase A	Sulfatide	Autosomal recessive	Adult	Mental instability, progressive dementia
Adrenoleukodystrophy						
18	Multiple peroxisomal enzyme deficiency, Zellweger's syndrome	Peroxins (1, 2, 5, 6, 12)	Excessive very long-chain fatty acids	Autosomal recessive	Neonatal	Dysmorphic features, hypotonia, seizures and feeding difficulties, with hepatosplenomegaly
19	Ulrich's disease Pseudoneonatal adrenoleukodystrophy (NALD)	Acyl-CoA oxidase	Excessive very long-chain fatty acids	Autosomal recessive	Neonatal	Coarse features, seizures, poor mental development, visual impairment
20	X-linked Siemerling-Creutzfeldt's	ABC protein	Excessive very long-chain fatty acids	X-linked recessive	Childhood onset is classic	Classic form: progressive psychomotor decline; variant can be adrenomyeloneuropathy with slowly developing spastic paraparesis of adulthood

CNS, Central nervous system; PNS, peripheral nervous system; GFAP, glial fibrillary acid protein; SAP-B, saponin B.

Classic Pelizaeus-Merzbacher disease (PMD) has a strong tendency to be more prominent in males, suggesting, but not proving, a sex-linked inheritance. This degenerative disorder is a primary genetic disorder of the oligodendrocytes, one of the major cell types in the CNS white matter. Each oligodendrocyte myelinates up to 50 axonal segments. The hallmark of the syndrome is the pathological finding of patchy losses of oligodendrocytes with little sudanophilic dysmyelination. Axonal degeneration accompanies dysmyelination and no axons are demonstrated where myelin sheaths are absent. Neurons are usually well preserved.[65] The X-linked PMD results from a defect in the oligodendrocytic synthesis of proteolipid protein (PLP), the major CNS myelin protein that makes up about 50 percent of the protein mass in myelin. In the peripheral nervous system, PLP is synthesized by Schwann cells and constitutes less than 1 percent myelin protein. PLP gene mutations on Xq22 cause PMD.[66] A prenatal diagnosis of the X-linked PMD has been made by DNA testing.[67] Contrary to the classic X-linked PMD, the transitional type of disorder (type 3) occurs sporadically. Lowenberg-Hill's disease (type 4) shows autosomal dominant transmission.

Classic PMD usually begins in the first few months of life, heralded by nystagmus and head tremor. Motor developmental delay occurs, and eventually ataxia, attention tremor, and choreoathetosis develop. Other signs include lower extremity spasticity, dysarthria, and optic atrophy. Motor and ocular impairments are severe compared with the mild degree of dementia. Deterioration assumes an even slower pace after 5 to 6 years of age. Clinical seizures (generalized or focal) usually appear during the later stages of the disease. Death is usually delayed until the second decade of life or early adulthood. Although not always present, a very characteristic early clinical finding may be a slow, rotary "cogwheel" nystagmus. As the patient becomes older, the nearly diagnostic ocular motility sign changes to a nonspecific movement disorder of the eyes. Jerk nystagmus is invariable.

Among the variants, in the connatal form, hypotonia is severe and accompanied by feeding difficulties. Laryngeal stridor is frequently noted. Optic atrophy can be identified early. The clinical deterioration rapidly leads to death within months to a few years of life. In transitional or type III disease (Seitelberger's disease), the clinical severity falls somewhere between that of the connatal and classic infantile forms. Invariably there is moderately severe mental retardation, and the average age of death is between 5 and 10 years. Lowenberg-Hill's disease, the adult form, has a very slow course. In contrast to all other forms, no ocular features are seen, and episodic psychotic events are characteristic. It is now well accepted that one of the X-linked forms of hereditary spastic paraplegia (SPG2) is allelic to PMD. Some patients present a pure form involving only the lower extremities while others have in addition nystagmus, dysarthria, and ataxia.[68]

Abnormalities of the brain stem auditory-evoked responses and sleep EEG are seen in some patients.[68] Cranial computed tomography (CT) scans in long-standing cases have demonstrated cerebellar atrophy and focal areas of demyelination. MRI demonstrates a decreased thickness of the corpus callosum, persistent myelin islands, and a reversal of the normal gray-white matter signal relationships consistent with dysmyelination.

All the leukoencephalopathies, genetic and nongenetic, should be included in the differential diagnosis. There is no specific curative therapy for PMD, and diligent supportive care is essential for both patients and families. While the search for treatment continues, specific clinical genetic characterization and research into the biochemical basis for the diseases continue.

COCKAYNE'S SYNDROME

Cockayne's syndrome (see Table 30–6) is sometimes classified as a variant of PMD because of the similar pattern of patchy demyelination among preserved islands of myelin.[64] However, in this disease there is pronounced involvement of multiple systems, suggesting a different pathogenic mechanism. The brain is small, and the white matter is atrophic. Calcifications are frequently present in the globus pallidus and cerebellum, along with mineralization of small arteries. The brain may contain a diffuse proliferation of astrocytes of bizarre appearance, predominantly in the cerebral cortex. Occasionally, Alzheimer-type neural fibrillary tangles are seen. The peripheral nervous system is also involved, with segmental demyelination with preservation of the axon cylinders. Patients with Cockayne's syndrome are hypersensitive to sunlight. Cultured cells are hypersensitive to UV radiation. The protein products deficient in the various forms of Cockayne's syndrome are involved in different aspects of the repair of damaged DNA. The common problem in patients with Cockayne's syndrome is a failure to repair oxidation-induced damage to DNA bases. Patients with Cockayne's syndrome suffer from defects in "transcription-coupled repair" (TRP).

Cockayne's syndrome can arise from mutations in one of five genes. Two genetic complementary groups have been isolated in classic Cockayne's syndrome. Cockayne's syndrome type A (CSA) is characterized by deficiencies in the WD repeat protein, a subunit of RNA polymerase II TFIIH. The CSA gene is encoded on chromosome 5. Cockayne's syndrome type B (CSB) is caused by deficiency in a helicase member of the SW12/SNF2 family of ATPases. Several mutations in the CSB gene have been described on chromosome 10q11. Another class of patients with Cockayne's syndrome shows concurrently clinical features of xeroderma pigmentosum (XP). Three mutated genes have been identified in this group of patients: XPB, XPD, and XPG.[69, 70] All forms of Cockayne's syndrome are inherited as an autosomal recessive trait. Both the central and the peripheral nervous system are involved.

Patients with this syndrome are often normal at birth, but in the first 6 months of life they develop a photosensitive dermatitis. In the second year, growth retardation, dwarfism, and kyphosis become apparent.[71] A facial rash and a facial-somatic dysplasia with a beaklike nose are part of the early picture. Microcephaly, mental retardation, retinitis pigmentosa, and optic atrophy soon develop. Following infancy, cerebellar dysfunction, sensorineural hearing loss, and upper motor neuron signs characterize the progressive neurological syndrome. Reflexes may be difficult to elicit, and other typical features are joint deformities, abnormally advanced bone age, dental caries, and renal disease. Ophthalmological findings include retinal involvement, poor pupillary response, lenticular cataracts, corneal opacities, and impaired lacrimation. Normal pressure hydrocephalus has been implicated as a possible mechanism for some of the neurological deterioration seen in these patients, although this has not been a consistent finding.[72]

Neuroimaging procedures reveal calcification of the basal ganglia and cerebellum, and neurophysiological testing shows nerve conduction velocity. It is probably easier to confuse this syndrome with a dysplastic cytogenetic disturbance than with the pediatric neurodegenerative disorders or other leukodystrophies because central demyelination is one of the least striking clinical manifestations. Case reports indicate that treatment of the normal pressure hydrocephalus, when it occurs, may be beneficial (see Chapter 28). No specific curative therapy is available, and only supportive treatment may be offered.

ALEXANDER'S DISEASE

This degenerative disorder is a primary genetic disorder of astrocytes, one of the major cell types in the CNS white matter (see Table 30–6). As a result, there is a global dysmyelination or demyelination of the CNS. The pathological hallmark of all forms of Alexander's disease is the presence in astrocytes of cytoplasmic eosinophilic hyaline bodies, called Rosenthal fibers. These inclusions are particularly numerous beneath the pial arachnoid membranes, beneath the ependyma, and around the cerebral blood vessels and are found throughout most of the brain. Rosenthal fibers contain the glial fibrillary acid protein (GFAP), an intermediate filament protein. Rosenthal fibers occur especially in the optic nerves, optic tracts, optic chiasm, cerebral peduncles, and spinal cord. Abnormal astrocytes are also observed in the basal ganglia, thalamus, and hypothalamus. Although the astrocytes become distended, there is no evidence of abnormal storage material within neurons. The white matter is soft and retracted and shows a variable loss of myelin, which appears more marked and diffuse in infantile cases. Axon cylinders are preserved. Rosenthal fibers in Alexander's disease result from molecular alterations and overproduction of GFAP. Alexander's disease has been shown to result from multiple mutations in the GFAP gene on chromosome 17.[73] In all patients, the GFAP mutations are dominant. The mutations usually arise de novo or from germinal mosaicism in cases with early onset. In adult forms, milder mutations are autosomal dominant.[74]

The rare neonatal form is characterized by early, often intractable, multifocal seizures. Hydrocephalus occurs and is due to three factors: aqueductal stenosis from the propagation of astrocytes containing excessive amounts of eosinophilic cytoplasmic material, lack of developmental maturation of the aqueductal area, and elevated protein content in the cerebrospinal fluid (CSF).[75]

The most common form of Alexander's disease is the infantile form, which has an average onset at 6 months of age. However, onset may occur at any time from shortly before birth to as late as 2 years of age. The average duration of disease is 2 to 3 years, but it can vary from a few months to several years. Psychomotor retardation predominates initially, but later progressive spasticity and seizures in the context of megalocephaly, with or without frank hydrocephalus, develop.

In the juvenile form, which is much less common than the infantile form, onset usually occurs between 7 and 14 years of age, and the duration is approximately 8 years. Bulbar and pseudobulbar dysfunction predominates, with dysphagia, dysarthria, nystagmus, ptosis, full facial palsy, and tongue atrophy.[76] Generalized spasticity and weakness may also occur, but unlike the severe mental retardation characteristic of the infantile form, mentation tends to remain intact. The adult form of Alexander's disease has an early stuttering course mimicking multiple sclerosis and characterized clinically by blurred vision, spasticity, nystagmus, dysarthria, and dysphagia. Other reported neurological manifestations include palatal and ocular myoclonus.[77]

CT changes include low attenuation in the deep cerebral white matter, most extensively in the frontal lobes and subependymal regions. The ventricles are variably enlarged. There is inconsistent abnormal enhancement of the caudate nuclei, anterior columns of the fornix, optic radiations, and periventricular areas.

Since the types of Alexander's disease are phenotypically distinct, the differential diagnosis varies by age. If one encounters an infant with chronically developing megalocephaly or macrocephaly with mild regression in psychomotor milestones in the absence of any other obvious cause, Alexander's disease is a highly probable diagnosis. Juvenile leukoencephalopathy must be considered in children and multiple sclerosis in adults.

No specific therapy is available for Alexander's disease. Much supportive care, however, is necessary, including good nutrition and generous use of antibiotics and antiepileptics. Despite these measures, the prognosis for infants and children with this disease at present is poor. Recent advances in positron-emission tomography scanning and single photon emission computed tomography indicate that there is an abnormal flow of spinal fluid through the blood-brain barrier. Clearer understanding of this disorder may aid in developing interventions.

CANAVAN'S SYNDROME

Canavan's syndrome (see Table 30–6) is a spongy degeneration of the CNS with abnormalities found particularly in the white matter. Vacuoles accumulate in a variety of brain cells, particularly astrocytes, and produce the spongy appearance. The vacuoles result from excessive fluid accumulation in astrocytes, apparently from metabolic disturbances that produce dysmyelination.[78] Chemical changes are limited to the white matter, notably myelin, and are nonspecific. There are increased water content and decreased total lipids in the white matter. Myelin breakdown products are not found. Dysmyelination is extensive, but axonal fibers and the oligodendroglia are not extensively affected. The precise cause of these abnormalities frequently remains uncertain.

The term Canavan's disease is used to describe an autosomal recessive spongy degeneration of the brain, occurring mainly among Ashkenazi Jewish individuals, and characterized by increased levels of *N*-acetylaspartic acid (NAA) in the urine and plasma and aspartoacylase deficiencies in cultured skin fibroblasts.[79] It is caused by a deficiency of aspartoacylase (ASPA), an enzyme playing a role in myelin synthesis. Elevated levels of NAA are found in urine, serum, and CSF. Canavan's disease results from mutations in the ASPA gene on chromosome 17p13.[80] DNA analysis is the method of choice for prenatal diagnosis.[81]

The three types of Canavan's disease are characterized by abnormal white matter signal on MRI and lack of involvement of peripheral nerves. Large amounts of NAA are found in urine (see Table 30–6). The infantile form, or classic Canavan's disease, begins within a few months of birth, and death generally occurs by 3 to 4 years of age. The infant initially is hypotonic and has poor head and neck control. Megalocephaly is common by 6 months of age, and arrested development is consistent. In the second 6 months, hypotonia is replaced by spasticity and often by decorticate and decerebrate posturing. Some hyper-reactivity is precipitated by auditory, visual, and tactile stimuli. Vision deteriorates as optic atrophy and nystagmus develop. Seizures of various types, including focal and myoclonic seizures, are usual, and choreoathetotic or dystonic movements can occur. Dysautonomia in the form of paroxysmal episodes of sweating, hyperthermia, vomiting, and hypotension are terminal manifestations.

The neonatal form of Canavan's disease is deadly within a few weeks and is characterized by lethargy, hypotonia, diminished spontaneous movement, and difficulty in swallowing. The rare juvenile form develops after 5 years of age and extends into adolescence. Ataxia, tremor, ptosis, and mental deterioration are characteristic. The course is characterized by progressive cerebellar symptoms, dysarthria, dementia, seizures, spasticity, and loss of vision. There is no correlation between the severity of the morphological white matter changes and the clinical presentation.[82] Gene therapy is under investigation. Symptomatic support includes nutritional therapy and generous use of antiepileptic drugs and antibiotics. Whereas currently the prognosis is poor, future research efforts utilizing cloistered populations with the disease, such as those found in Saudi Arabia, may lead to new discoveries.

KRABBE'S SYNDROME

In contrast to other leukodystrophies, Krabbe's syndrome appears to be purely neurological. In these patients, there is a deficiency of the lysosomal enzyme galactocerebroside-beta-galactosidase (GALC). The disease is inherited as an autosomal recessive trait. The various forms of the disease result from multiple mutations in the GALC gene on chromosome 14q24.3–q32.1.[83] Assays of amniotic fluid allow prenatal diagnosis, and enzymatic assays on white cells or serum may detect the carrier state. A saposin A deficiency is expected to be responsible for some cases of Krabbe's syndrome with near-normal GALC activity.

In the CNS, the white matter is decreased in mass and is gliotic, firm, and rubbery to palpation. In the areas of demyelination, oligodendroglial cells are severely reduced in number. Globoid cells, found deep in the white matter around and within vessels, are distinctive. Their abundant cytoplasm stains positively with periodic acid–Schiff (PAS) and only faintly with Sudan black. No metachromasia is present. The small globoid cells are round and mononuclear, while the large ones (varying from 20 to 50 microns) become irregular and multinucleated. Electron microscopy reveals within the cytoplasm of the cells cytoplasmic inclusions containing both electron-dense linear or curved tubular profiles, a distinctive sign in Krabbe's disease.[84] Neurons in the pons, thalamus, and dentate nuclei show varying degrees of degeneration, but the neuronal processes of the cerebral cortex are reasonably well preserved. Involvement of the peripheral nervous system varies, and segmental demyelination has been reported.[85] Globoid cells are not seen in peripheral nerves, but histiocytes with foamy cytoplasm and tubular inclusions have been demonstrated. Krabbe's disease is distributed worldwide and has no gender, racial, or ethnic proclivities.

There are two primary forms of Krabbe's disease, the early-onset or classic form and the late-onset form. The early-onset type usually appears clinically between the third and eighth months of life, although biochemical and pathological changes are present in the early gestational period. Initially, the patient is irritable and has intermittent fever for no discernible reason. Episodic limb or trunk rigidity may occur, and a heightened startle response to noise, light, or touch may be apparent. Feeding problems and seizures occur frequently. Myoclonic seizures may suggest infantile spasms. Macrocephaly is uncommon, and hepatosplenomegaly is absent. There are usually no cherry-red spots. Early in the course, EEG shows a severe slowing of the background activity and abundant paroxysmal discharges. By 6 months of age, the infant develops severe hypertonus with obvious opisthotonos and decorticate-decerebrate rigidity. Reflexes may be hyperactive or hypoactive if advanced peripheral neuropathy is present. Bilateral Babinski signs are usually present along with optic atrophy. By 9 months of age, the baby is usually blind and deaf. In light of these characteristic clinical features, there is very little confusion between the diagnosis of classic Krabbe's disease and other infantile-onset degenerative conditions.

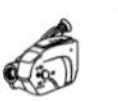

The late-onset type of Krabbe's disease is extremely uncommon. These patients first develop difficulties later in infancy, in childhood, or even in adult life.[86] The late infantile form is characterized by onset between 6 months and 3 years of developmental regression with ataxia and stiffness, feeding difficulties, irritability, and loss of vision. The juvenile or adult form is usually characterized by a progressive amaurosis starting in late childhood, followed years later by a progressive gait impairment with spasticity or dystonia, and finally dementia. Optic atrophy and peripheral neuropathy are consistent findings late in the course of the illness.

Periventricular hyperdensities demonstrated on CT scans have been reported, particularly in the terminal phases of the classic form. MRI scans demonstrate white matter involvement of the cerebrum and cerebellum,[87] and electrophysiological evidence of peripheral nerve demyelination is prominent. Treatment at this time is limited to allogenic hematopoietic stem cell transplantation that appears to slow the progression of the disease and improve MRI results. Studies using stem cells and viral vectors to transduce transplantable cells are under way.[88]

METACHROMATIC LEUKODYSTROPHIES

The metachromatic leukodystrophies (see Table 30–6), also known as sulfatide lipidoses, are a group of lysosomal storage disorders recognized by the accumulation of excessive amounts of lipid sulfatides. The term metachromatic, as a description of the diseases, derives from the staining properties of the stored lipid sulfatides, which develop a brown or gold hue with toluidine blue rather than the usual blue of myelin. In the CNS, the sulfatides are stored in lysosomes of microglia and neuronal cells. In the peripheral nervous system, the lysosomal storage of sulfatide within Schwann cells leads to a segmental demyelinating neuropathy. Outside of the nervous system, the sulfatide is stored in other organs and tissues such as the kidneys, pancreas, adrenal glands, liver, and gallbladder.[89]

In the classic form of metachromatic leukodystrophy, sulfatide content in the white matter is four to eight times that found in normal controls. Large amounts of sulfatides are found in the urine. The deficient enzyme in the classic metachromatic leukodystrophy is arylsulfatase A (ASA). A "sphingolipid activator protein" (SAP), saposin B, is a heat-stable nonenzymatic protein necessary for the normal catalytic function of ASA. The late infantile, juvenile, and adult forms of the syndrome are caused by mutations in the ASA gene located on chromosome 22q13.31.[90] Patients with metachromatic leukodystrophy due to saposin B deficiency (SAP-1 deficiency) have a near-normal ASA activity and, in addition to sulfatides, excrete globotriosylceramide and digalactosylceramide.[91] Saposin B deficiency is caused by specific mutations in the prosaposin gene on chromosome 10q21.[92] This condition is allelic to saposin C deficiency causing Gaucher's syndrome. All forms of metachromatic leukodystrophy are inherited as an autosomal recessive trait. Arylsulfatase A deficiency is not unique to metachromatic leukodystrophy and also occurs in the mucopolysaccharidosis multiple sulfatase deficiency, in which activity of the three isoenzymes of arylsulfatase (A, B, and C) is markedly reduced.

Epidemiology and Risk Factors. All forms of metachromatic leukodystrophy are inherited as autosomal recessive traits. This condition is globally distributed. The prevalence of all forms of metachromatic leukodystrophy is approximately 1 in 100,000 life births. The genes responsible for the various forms of metachromatic leukodystrophy have been mapped and several mutations have been identified for each disorder. The molecular heterogeneity of the metachromatic leukodystrophies frequently results in a clinical heterogeneity. For instance, two distinct types of arylsulfatase A mutations (type O and type R) can be distinguished. Type O mutations tend to eliminate completely any functional gene product. Patients homozygous or heterozygous for type O mutations invariably have the infantile form of metachromatic leukodystrophy. Type R mutations tend to be associated with a small amount of residual enzyme activity. Most patients homozygous for type R mutations present an adult form of metachromatic leukodystrophy. Mixed heterozygosity between type O and type R mutations most often results in a juvenile form. Only a single phenotype generally occurs in families with more than one affected member; the age of onset, clinical presentation, and progression of the illness are similar among members of a single family. Several ethnic groups have a higher frequency of this disease. The Habbanite Jewish community in Israel has a particularly high frequency of late infantile metachromatic leukodystrophy (1.3%).

Clinical Features and Associated Findings. According to the age of onset, three clinical forms of metachromatic leukodystrophy have been recognized. The late infantile form usually begins between the ages of 18 and 24 months, although onset may occasionally be delayed until as late as age 4 years.[93, 94] These children develop a gait disturbance that may appear as ataxia or weakness.[95] Hypotonia is very prominent during this time. A lazy eye may be the presenting complaint. Thereafter, a rather rapid decline continues over a period of 6 months or more causing serious gait and bulbar dysfunction. The hypotonia becomes much worse as the disease continues, and weakness dominates during these phases. Intellectual deterioration occurs reasonably rapidly over a 6- to 12-month period. By the terminal stage, hypotonia has reverted to hypertonia and frank spasticity. Involuntary movements may also occur. Another characteristic of the classic form that distinguishes it from other forms of metachromatic leukodystrophy is the presence of megalocephaly, although this finding is not as striking as it is in the gangliosidoses or in Alexander's and Canavan's syndromes.

A peripheral neuropathy may exist even in the early stages of this disease when absence of reflexes or hyporeflexia is evident. This is a result of peripheral segmental demyelination and the deposition of sulfatide within the nerve fibers. As the CNS sulfatide deposits increase with disease progression, one can account for the turnaround in muscle tone. The hypotonia is first accentuated because of suprasegmental shock influences. These in turn are altered when suprasegmental release occurs. This is the switching point of the change from clinical hypotonia to clinical hypertonia and its associated phenomena. Seizures are a late manifestation. Patients with the classic form often die by 8 to 10 years of age. Yet other patients reach a vegetative trough and live well into their teens. By this time, such patients are indistinguishable from those with the later-onset forms of the disease.

Onset in the juvenile form occurs between 4 and 10 years of age. The majority of patients show the first symptoms during their early years at school and these include bradykinesia and poor school performance. In the very early periods, daydreaming, confusion, and emotional lability are frequently reported. Where unsteadiness of gait due to pyramidal tract involvement may be noted, extrapyramidal dysfunction with postural abnormalities and tremor may also develop. Myotactic reflexes are usually increased even in the early stages, and there is little tendency for hypotonia to appear. The rate of deterioration is usually slow and is much more variable than that of the late infantile form of the syndrome. Patients often are not bedridden even 5 to 10 years after the initial symptoms appear. Dementia occurs but is slower to develop than in the late infantile form. Decerebrate posturing and generalized convulsions occur as a late manifestation. When the juvenile form is chronic, or even when the late infantile form is subacute, patients usually live for 20 years or longer.

Onset of the adult form occurs at any time after puberty. Initial symptoms frequently consist of personality and mental changes that signal the impending dementia. Other presenting symptoms include seizures and behavior changes. Patients may show a hypospontaneity and a blunted effect or inattention and hyperactivity. Such symptoms are often misdiagnosed as schizophrenia or manic-depressive illness. There are usually no clinical signs of peripheral neuropathy. Disorders of movement and posture appear later. Frank dementia becomes the central feature, occurring most frequently by the third or fourth decade of life. Often these mental symptoms in the adult are accompanied by progressive corticobulbar, corticospinal, and cerebellar changes. Visual and somatosensory evoked potentials are delayed. Even in this form, nerve conduction velocities are markedly lowered.

Differential Diagnosis. In any disorder showing progressive manifestations such as seizures, dementia, and motor failure, the diagnosis must be considered when signs of peripheral neuropathy are found. Many variants of metachromatic leukodystrophy as well as other conditions should be considered in the differential diagnosis. Multiple sulfatase deficiency that is not associated with striking leukodystrophy should not be confused with metachromatic leukodystrophy. Also, several subtypes in which there is no clear demonstration of a deficiency in the enzyme but in which there is a defect in the activator protein should be considered. Additionally, all leukodystrophies should be entered in the differential diagnosis. Consideration of other leukodystrophies depends on their phenotypic expression as well as a variety of peripheral neuropathies without prominent CNS symptoms.

Evaluation. Spinal fluid protein concentration is usually moderately elevated, with concentrations between 150 and 300 mg/100 mL. There are no qualitative abnormalities in the protein profile. Demonstration of a deficiency of ASA activity either in urine or in leukocytes confirms the diagnosis in the majority of cases. Decreased gallbladder function may be detected by a simple cholecystogram or ultrasonography examination and may be a useful adjunct in the workup. The presence of metachromatic granules in the urine is of some help and gross inspection of an office urine sample can be suggestive of the diagnosis. Brain stem auditory, visual, and somatosensory evoked responses show some abnormalities, but the results are variable. The most consistent finding is the characteristic decreased nerve conduction velocities found in almost all forms of metachromatic leukodystrophy.

Management. Bone marrow transplantation in patients with late infantile metachromatic leukodystrophy due to ASA deficiency or saposin B deficiency has had little impact on long-term outcome except perhaps in patients with juvenile or adult onset. The effectiveness and safety of this therapy need further evaluation.

PEROXISOMAL LEUKODYSTROPHIES: ADRENOLEUKODYSTROPHY

The peroxisomal leukodystrophies (see Table 30–6) represent a relatively new concept for neurologists. Peroxisomes are the subcellular organellae in the cell body that can be deranged by being absent, malformed, or dysfunctional. Resultant conditions include neonatal disorders such as Zellweger's disease and adrenoleukodystrophy as well as later-onset adult conditions such as Refsum's disease. The pioneering work of Moser, Schutgens, and associates on the peroxisomal entities has established the fact that peroxisomal dysfunction does not invariably produce the clinical or pathological features of leukodystrophy. The peroxisome is ubiquitous in its clinical and pathological expression. In an excellent short review of these disorders, Moser[96] gives a list of 14 major peroxisomal diseases to illustrate the two categories of peroxisomal defects. One of these categories is identified as a disorder of peroxisome biogenesis (PBG) or assembly. Another category encompasses disorders with a single peroxisomal enzyme defect, the prototypes being noninfantile Refsum's disease and sex-linked adrenoleukodystrophy (X-ALD).[97]

The pathological hallmark of the PBG disorders is the finding of ghost peroxisomes. As a result, there is a concomitant loss of activity in multiple peroxisomal enzymes. Multiple biochemical abnormalities are observed: plasma very long-chain fatty acids (VLCFAs), phytanic acid, and trihydroxy-cholestanoic acid (THCA) are increased and the plasmalogen synthesis is decreased. The overlapping phenotypes representative of this category are Zellweger's syndrome, Ulrich's disease or neonatal adrenoleukodystrophy, and infantile Refsum's disease. These autosomal recessive conditions have their onset early in life. Patients have severe neurological and hepatic dysfunction, craniofacial abnormalities, and hypotonia. Dysmorphic features are always present. Adrenal insufficiency is subclinical. Neuropathology shows a sudanophilic leukodystrophy with signs of brain (cerebral and/or cerebellar) dysgenesis. Mutations of either of five genes encoding peroxins (PEX1, PEX2, PEX5, PEX6, and PEX12) are responsible for most of these phenotypes.[98, 99]

Zellweger's disease is a severe, rapidly fatal disorder characterized by cerebrohepatorenal syndrome. Hepatomegaly, renal cysts, hypotonia, and seizures are accompanied by prominent dysmorphic features (giving these infants the premature appearance), eye findings (retinitis pigmentosa, glaucoma, cataract, and sometimes Brushfield's spots), deafness, aberrant calcific stippling of the patellae, and abnormal genitalia (hypoplasia of labia major or hypospadias). Neonatal adrenoleukodystrophy and infantile Refsum's disease differ from Zellweger's by their milder dysmorphic features and a very protracted course with failure to thrive and minimal psychomotor gains. Sensory hearing loss, retinal degeneration, and hepatomegaly may be present. Occasionally, the symptoms occur at a somewhat later period than expected.[97] Subdural hematoma may be the presenting symptom.[100] One patient presented at 23 months with frequent emesis and acute mental deterioration, followed very quickly by refractive seizures. A long history of developmental, mental, and motor delay had previously been observed in this child. There tends to be a staggering course, sometimes with developmental stagnation or regression preceded or followed by improvement in visual impairment, truncal hypotonia, and limb spasticity.

The pathological hallmark of all the peroxisomal disorders with single enzyme deficiency is the presence of peroxisomes and, in most cases, a normal plasmalogen synthesis. Only one peroxisomal enzyme is deficient, and therefore metabolic abnormalities are selective and generally involve only one metabolic pathway. However, when the deficient enzyme is necessary for the normal function of multiple metabolic pathways, the finding of multiple metabolic derangements may suggest a PBG disorder. Both bifunctional enzyme deficiency and oxoacyl-CoA thiolase deficiency are associated with VLCFA and THCA and present with the clinical phenotype of "pseudo-Zellweger's disease."

Acyl-CoA oxidase deficiency is responsible for a selective elevation of VLCFA and a phenotype called "pseudo-neonatal adrenoleukodystrophy." Patients have dysmorphic features, hypotonia, feeding difficulties, intractable neonatal seizures, and minimal psychomotor development during the first 2 years of life. Adrenal insufficiency is subclinical. Brain imaging may show contrast enhancement surrounding the demyelinated areas.[101]

In the X-ALD, the genetic abnormality has been mapped to the Xq28 region. The disease results from mutations in the ALDP gene, which encodes a peroxisomal membrane protein member of the ATP binding cassette family. It has been postulated that this protein transports acyl-CoA synthase to its site of action.[102] The saturated VLCFAs (C:25 and C:24) are increased. Adrenal insufficiency frequently leads to shin hyperpigmentation and/or addisonian crisis.

Among the variants of X-ALD, the childhood form is usually the more fulminating disorder. Patients are completely normal until 4 to 10 years of age, when behavioral problems such as failure in school develop. This first sign is the result of rapid regression of auditory discrimination, spatial orientation, speech, and fine motor skills. Seizures occur in less than a third of the patients reported by Naidu and Moser.[100] Typically, there is a rapid clinical deterioration to spastic paraparesis, swallowing difficulties, and visual loss, culminating in a vegetative state within 2 years of the appearance of symptoms. Neuroimaging typically demonstrates a symmetrical periventricular demyelination, more prominent initially over the occipital regions, with characteristic contrast enhancement at the rim of the lesion.

In the adolescent cerebral X-ALD syndrome, signs and symptoms of cerebral involvement are manifest, yet the onset of disease usually occurs between the ages of 10 and 21. The adult form usually presents with dementia, psychiatric disturbances, seizures, spinocerebellar degeneration, or spastic paraparesis with onset at some time after the age of 21. Such patients have presentations similar to those of other problems such as multiple sclerosis, schizophrenia, and brain tumor. They show a reasonably rapid regression. After many years, a demyelinating peripheral neuropathy may present the features of a hypertrophic neuropathy with oinon bulb formation.

Included in the differential diagnoses are most of the leukoencephalopathies and dystrophies as well as other processes, depending on the phenotypic expression of the disorder. All early-onset disorders in which there is degeneration and dysplastic status should be considered.

Very long-chain fatty acids in plasma and cultured fibroblasts are elevated in all forms of ALD and in Zellweger's syndrome. Probably the presence of VLCFAs and the other biochemical abnormalities noted previously are the major methods of making the diagnosis. However, all evaluations consistent with the severe dysmorphic and degenerative states of such patients are probably indicated.

The potential for therapy is limited for this group of diseases. In most cases, therapy is primarily directed toward supportive care. Treatment for liver dysfunction or the prothrombin deficiency with vitamin K is indicated in PBG disorders. Rehabilitative approaches are sometimes helpful. One should consider the probability of complications such as subdural hematoma and its treatment. Attempts to mediate some of the biochemical abnormalities with lipid therapy or dietary restriction of VLCFAs have been tried, but they do not normalize plasma levels of the VLCFAs, or red blood cell plasmalogen synthesis. Peroxisomal proliferators such as clofibrate do not induce formation of catalase-containing peroxisomes nor improve clinical status of PBG disorders.

Therapy for X-ALD is under active investigation at this time. Steroid replacement therapy is effective for adrenal insufficiency but does not alter the rate of progression of neurological disability. Dietary therapy with a 4:1 mixture of glyceryl trioleate and glyceryl trierucate (Lorenzo's oil) has normalized levels of VLCFAs and plasma within 4 weeks. The results in symptomatic patients, however, have been disappointing.[103] Therapeutic plasma exchanges are successful in reducing VLCFA but do not alter the clinical course. Various immunosuppressive therapies have been unsuccessful. Bone marrow transplantation is of benefit to patients with early neurological involvement.[104]

Other Lipidoses

FABRY'S DISEASE

This X-linked lipidosis is characterized biochemically by the intralysosomal accumulation of globotriaosylceramide, galabiosylceramide, and other glycosphingolipids. The enzymatic deficiency is alpha-galactosidase A. The molecular structure of the gene encoding the enzyme was first identified as the full-length cDNA clone and is localized to Xq21.33–q22.[105] Both point mutations and deletions have been described for this gene. The majority of the glycosphingolipids are synthesized in the liver or bone marrow and thereafter are transported to cells by lipoproteins. The major substrate burden in Fabry's disease appears to be on cellular membranes that depend on glycosphingolipids for their integrity and function. Organ storage occurs presumably because of permeable membranes that permit accumulation of high levels of circulating lipids.

In the majority of affected males, the clinical symptoms begin in late childhood or adolescence with the development of painful neuropathy, which is most pronounced in the extremities; syncopal episodes and hypohydrosis associated with heat intolerance and low-grade fever; corneal and lenticular opacities; and characteristic skin lesions, known as angiokeratoma. These dermatological features consist of ectatic blood vessels covered by thin skin and appear as discreet, slightly raised, blue or dark red spots that cluster in the groin, umbilical area, and thighs. The neurological signs are usually vascular in origin and include transient ischemic attacks, ischemic strokes, and cerebral hematomas. Renal failure and vasculopathy of the heart and brain lead to early death in adulthood. In the minority of affected males, the main manifestation is a hypertrophic cardiomyopathy. Most female carriers are asymptomatic. A minority presents with isolated acroparesthesia, cardiac symptoms, or corneal dystrophy. Pathologically, storage of glycolipids in the systemic vascular system leads to progressive cardiac, CNS, and renal involvements. The CNS shows lipid accumulation in the autonomic nervous system neurons and several other regions, including supraoptic, preoptic, and paraventricular nuclei. The nucleus basalis, anterior thalamus, and the hippocampus are also characteristically loaded with glycolipid, and when the cerebral cortex is involved, layers 5 and 6 demonstrate the neuronal lipid storage. In the peripheral nervous system, lipid accumulation can be observed in neurons of sensory and autonomic ganglia, in Schwann cells, and in endothelial cells and pericytes of endoneurial capillaries. Loss of small-caliber myelinated and unmyelinated fibers occurs.[106]

Because the disease is rare, carrier testing is not routinely performed. In affected pedigrees, however, alpha-galactosidase A analysis identifies affected males and often heterozygous females. Affected males cannot pass the disease to their sons, but all daughters are carriers.

The differential diagnosis includes conditions associated with angiokeratoma, including metabolic disorders such as neuraminidase deficiency, galactosialidosis, fucosidosis, and GM_1-gangliosidosis. Drugs that can cause corneal opacification include chloroquine and amiodarone. The treatment of Fabry's disease focuses primarily on abatement of the painful neuropathy, and carbamazepine and diphenylhydantoin, as well as neurotropin, have been used with success.[107] Renal transplantation has also been used in patients with severe renal failure. Recombinant alpha-galactosidase A replacement therapy clears microvascular endothelial deposits of globotriaosylceramide in affected tissues, reversing the chief clinical manifestations of the disease.[108]

NONINFANTILE REFSUM'S DISEASE

This autosomal recessive nonlysosomal lipidosis is characterized biochemically by an isolated peroxisomal phytanoyl-CoA alpha-hydroxylase (PAHX) deficiency resulting in a cytoplasmic accumulation of phytanic acid. The sequence of PAHX gene is known and localized on chromosome 10p. Both point mutations and deletions have been described in the PAHX associated with Refsum's disease.[109] Phytanic acid is a branched-chain fatty acid that is primarily derived from a diet rich in dairy products, some meat, and fish. The mechanism of phytanic acid toxicity is unclear.

Clinically, Refsum's disease is known as heredopathia atactica polyneuritiformis and is characterized by retinitis pigmentosa, peripheral neuropathy, cerebellar ataxia, and high protein levels in the CSF without pleocytosis. Cardiac involvement, anosmia, nystagmus, and nerve deafness occur in almost all patients as well. Ichthyosis and skeletal abnormalities, particularly pes cavus and the bilateral shortening or elongation of metatarsals and metacarpals, are inconsistent systemic features. The first clinical symptoms are usually night blindness and clumsiness. Most patients have a bilateral constriction of the visual fields by the time they present. Rapid weight loss, fever, and pregnancy have been associated with acute or subacute presentations mimicking Guillain-Barré syndrome and chronic inflammatory demyelinating neuropathy. Pupillary miosis makes the funduscopic exam difficult. Neuropathy develops slowly and is associated with proprioceptive sensory loss, absent myotactic reflexes, distal muscle wasting, and foot drop. Nerve conduction findings include slowed conduction velocities. Although neuropathy may contribute to some of the cerebellar findings, there appears to be true cerebellar ataxia in this condition. The age of neurological disability onset is highly variable from childhood to the sixth decade but usually occurs in adolescence and young adulthood. In association, cardiac involvement is of clinical significance, and tachycardia, systolic murmurs, and conduction disturbances occur. Fatal cardiac arrhythmias may be responsible for several cases of documented sudden deaths in untreated patients with Refsum's disease.

Markedly raised plasma levels of phytanic acid and occurrence of plasma phytanyl triglycerides are consistently present in noninfantile Refsum's disease. Phytanic acid accumulation is not unique to Refsum's disease, however, and is also seen in PBG defects (infantile Refsum's disease, neonatal adrenoleukodystrophy, Zellweger's syndrome, and rhizomelic chondrodysplasia punctata) and isolated peroxisomal branched-chain oxidation defects. In noninfantile Refsum's disease, pristanic acid is low/normal due to lack of production from phytanic acid, distinguishing this condition from PBG defects and from isolated peroxisomal branched-chain oxidation defects. Some patients with noninfantile Refsum's disease may have elevated pipecolic acid levels.[110] Pathologically, in noninfantile Refsum's disease, the peroxisomal structure is normal, distinguishing this condition from PBG defects characterized by an abnormal peroxisome. Nerve biopsy shows "onion bulb" formation and targetoid cytoplasmic inclusion in the Schwann cell. In the CNS, phytanic acid accumulates in neurons, glial cell of the globus pallidus and substania nigra, ependymal cell, choroid plexus, and leptomeninges.

The differential diagnosis of Refsum's disease includes other neurological syndromes with neuropathy and ataxia, such as some mitochondrial diseases (Friedreich's ataxia and neuropathy, ataxia, retinitis pigmentosa), abetalipoproteinemia, vitamin E deficiency, and Charcot-Marie-Tooth and their variants. Elevated plasma phytanic acid levels eliminate these diagnoses.

The diet should contain enough calories to prevent weight loss, and fish, beef, lamb, and dairy products should be avoided.[111] Improvement is slow, and plasmapheresis is used as an adjunct to hasten clinical recovery. Retinal damage and nerve deafness do not improve, but the other signs may substantially abate over a very prolonged period.

ABETALIPOPROTEINEMIA (BASSEN-KORNZWEIG SYNDROME)

This autosomal recessive lipid disorder is characterized biochemically by extremely low levels of serum cholesterol and triglycerides due to a defect in the intestinal microsomal triglyceride transfer protein (MTP), a protein necessary for the assembly of apolipoprotein B–containing lipoproteins (low-density lipoproteins and chylomicrons). Without MTP, the apolipoprotein B is not properly lipidated and undergoes presecretory degradation. The result is absence of plasma chylomicrons and very-low-density lipoproteins. Intestinal fat absorption is deficient. The MTP gene is sequenced and localized on chromosome 4q. Both point mutations and deletions in the MTP gene are responsible for abetalipoproteinemia.[112, 113]

Clinical manifestations develop in the first decade of life with steatorrhea, distal sensorimotor neuropathy, and retinitis pigmentosa. Ataxia is accompanied by dysarthria, areflexia, and proprioceptive sensory loss. The presence of extensor Babinski responses may suggest the diagnosis of Friedreich's ataxia. A generalized muscle weakness and wasting accompanied by ptosis and ophthalmoparesis may also develop.[114] Serum cholesterol and triglyceride levels are low, low-density lipoproteins are completely absent, and erythrocytes take on the appearance of acanthocytes. Because of the reduced chylomicrons, severe deficiencies of fat-soluble vitamins, namely A, K, and E, occur. Systemic signs can include cardiomyopathy and failure to thrive. Normal villi are seen in small bowel biopsies, but the mucosal cells are filled with lipid droplets.

The differential diagnosis includes disorders that have combined neuropathy and ataxia, and include Friedreich's disease and the hereditary sensorimotor neuropathies. Laboratory analysis and EMG studies suggesting axonal neuropathy are helpful in directing the clinician.[115] The differential diagnosis also includes those disorders with acanthocytes, namely neuroacanthocytosis, although typically the latter disorder has tics and dystonia rather than profound neuropathy and ataxia. Finally, the differential diagnosis includes all conditions associated with vitamin E deficiency because neurological abnormalities in Bassen-Kornzweig disease resemble vitamin E deficiency in other situations.

There is strong evidence, both clinically and in the laboratory, that the neurological findings relate directly to vitamin E deficiency. Vitamin E supplementation can arrest the progression of both retinal and neurological deficits.[116] Other dietary treatments are important to overall rehabilitation status and include restricted intake of long-chain fatty acids and supplementation of other fat-soluble vitamins.

AN-ALPHA-LIPOPROTEINEMIA (TANGIER'S DISEASE)

This autosomal recessive nonlysosomal lipid storage disorder is characterized biochemically by near or complete absence of circulating high-density lipoproteins and by the cytoplasmic accumulation of cholesteryl esters and phospholipids in histiocytes, Schwann cells, neurons (spinal ganglion and spinal cord), nevus cells, smooth muscle cells, and fibroblasts. The virtual absence of circulating plasma high-density lipoprotein is caused by molecular defects in the ATP binding cassette (ABC) transporter 1 (ABCA1), a permease belonging to one of the superfamilies of efflux pumps. The human ABCA1 gene maps on chromosome 9q31. Point mutations, insertions, and deletion in the ABCA1 gene cause Tangier's disease.[117]

Tangier's disease is associated with a nonspecific peripheral neuropathy that may be motor, sensory, or mixed in type. The neuropathy presents in childhood or adulthood, but the distinctive clinical feature of affected persons is their dramatically enlarged and orange-tinged tonsils. Atherosclerosis resulting in cardiovascular disease is a common systemic complication. Plasma HDL cholesterol is extremely low or absent.

Reviews and Selected Updates

Altarescu G, Sun M, Moore DF, et al: The neurogenetics of mucolipidosis type IV. Neurology 2002;59:306–313.

Amato AA: Acid maltese deficiency and related myopathies. Neurol Clin 2000;18:161–165.

Crochey AC, Farber S: Niemann-Pick disease: A review of 18 patients. Medicine 1958;37:1.

Dyken P: The neuronal ceroid-lipofuscinoses. J Child Neurol 1989;4:165–174.

Dyken P, Wisniewski K: Classification of the neuronal ceroid-lipofuscinoses: Expansion of the atypical forms. Am J Med Genet 1995;57:150–154.

Engel AG, Dale AJ: Glycogenosis of late onset with mitochondrial abnormalities. Proc Staff Mayo Clin 1968;43:233–279.

Moser HW: Pathogenetic mechanisms in peroxisomal disorders. Curr Opin Neurol 1996;9:473–476.

Swaiman K: Diseases associated with primary abnormalities in carbohydrate metabolism. *In* Swaiman K (ed): Pediatric Neurology: Principles and Practice, 2nd ed. Vol. 2. St. Louis, Mosby, 1994, p 1253.

Weibel TD, Brady RO: Systematic approach to the diagnosis of lysosomal storage disorders. Ment Retard Dev Disabil Res Rev 2001;7:190–199.

References

1. Zeman W, Dyken P: Neuronal ceroid-lipofuscinosis (Batten's disease). Relationship to amaurotic familial idiocy. Pediatrics 1969;44:170–183.
2. Bennett MJ, Hofman SL: The neuronal ceroid-lipofuscinoses (Batten disease): A new class of lysosomal storage diseases. J Inher Metab Dis 1999;22:535–544.
3. Palmer DN, Jolly RD, van Mil HC, Tyynelä J, Westlake VJ: Different pattern of hydrophobic protein storage in different forms of neuronal ceroid lipofuscinosis (NCL, Batten disease). Neuropediatrics 1997;28:45–48.
4. Boustany RN: Neurology of the neuronal ceroid-lipofuscinoses: Late infantile and juvenile types. Am J Med Genet 1992;42:533–535.
5. Wisniewski KE, Kida E, Golabek AA, al: Neuronal ceroid lipofuscinoses: Classification and diagnosis. Adv Genet 2001;45:1–34.
6. Dyken PR: Reconsideration of the classification of the neuronal ceroid-lipofuscinoses. Am J Med Genet Suppl 1988;5:69–84.
7. Berkovic SF, Carpenter S, Andermann F, et al: Kuf's disease: A critical reappraisal. Brain 1988;111:27–62.
8. Dyken PR, Bastian F, Nelson G, et al: Purkinje cell accumulation of lipopigments confirming a spinocerebellar degeneration due to neuronal ceroid-lipofuscinosis. Proc Child Neurol Soc 1989;18:236.
9. Hofmann SL, Das AK, Lu J-Y, Soyombo AA: Positional candidate gene cloning of CLN1. Adv Genet 2001;45:69–92.
10. Pshezhetsky AV, Ashmarina M: Lyzosomal multienzyme complex: Biochemistry, genetics, and molecular pathophysiology. Prog Nucl Acid Res Molec Biol 2001;69:81–114.
11. d'Azzo A, Andria G, Strisciuglio P, Galjaard H: Galactosialidosis. *In* Scriver CR, Beaudet AL, Sly WS, Valle D (eds): The Metabolic Basis of Inherited Disease, 7th ed. New York, McGraw-Hill, 1995, pp 2825–2837.
12. Gravel RA, Clarke JTR, Kaback MM, et al: The GM_2 gangliosidoses. *In* Scriver CR, Beaudet AL, Sly WS, Valle D (eds): The Metabolic Basis of Inherited Disease, 7th ed. New York, McGraw-Hill, 1995, pp 2839–2879.
13. Sakuraba H, Itoh K, Shimmoto M, et al: GM_2 gangliosidosis AB variant. Clinical and biochemical studies of a Japanese patient. Neurology 1999;52:372–376.
14. Dyken P, Maertens P, Gurbani S: Tay-Sachs disease in two Afro-American families in the Southern United States. J Child Neurol 1996;11:234.
15. Erwin RE, Al-Harbi H, Al-Harbi W, et al: Sandhoff variant GM_2 gangliosidosis in Saudi Arabia. Saud Med J 1989;10:526–527.
16. Norman RH, Ulrich H, Tingey AH, et al: Tay-Sachs disease with visceral involvement and its relationship to Niemann-Pick disease. J Pathol Bacteriol 1959;78:409–421.
17. Landing BH, Silverman IN, Craig JM: Familial neurovisceral lipidosis. Am J Dis Child 1964;108:503.
18. Klein A, Lebreton A, Lemoine J, et al: Identification of urine oligosaccharides by matrix-assisted laser desorption ionization time-of-flight mass spectrometry. Clin Chem 1998;44:2422–2428.
19. Suzuki K: Neuropathology of late onset gangliosidosis: A review. Rev Neurosci 1991;13:205–210.
20. Uyama E, Terasaki T, Watanabe S, et al: Type 3 GM_1 gangliosidosis: Characteristic MRI findings correlated with dystonia. Acta Neurol Scand 1992;86:609–615.
21. Swaiman K: Lysosomal diseases. *In* Swaiman K (ed): Pediatric Neurology: Principles and Practice, 2nd ed. Vol. 2. St. Louis, Mosby, 1994, pp 1275–1334.
22. Schulte FJ: Clinical course of GM_2 gangliosidosis: A correlative attempt. Neuropediatrics 1984;15:66–70.
23. Rapin I, Suzuki K, Valsamis M: Adult (chronic) GM.MDSD/2.MDNM/ gangliosidosis: Atypical spinocerebellar degeneration in a Jewish sibship. Arch Neurol 1976;33:120–130.
24. Oates CE, Bosch EP, Hart MN: Movement disorders associated with chronic GM_2 gangliosidosis: Case report and review of the literature. Eur Neurol 1986;25:154–159.
25. Karni A, Navon R, Sadeh M: Hexosaminidase A deficiency manifesting on spinal muscular atrophy of late onset. Ann Neurol 1988;24:451–453.
26. Hurowitz GI, Silver JM, Brin MF, et al: Neuropsychiatric reports of adult onset Tay-Sachs disease: Two case reports with several new findings. J Neuropsychiat Clin Neurol 1993;5:30–36.

27. Chow GCS, Clark JTR, Banwell BL: Late-onset GM_2 gangliosidosis presenting as burning dysesthesia. Pediatr Neurol 2001;25:59–61.
28. Blieden LC, Desnick RJ, Carter JB, et al: Cardiac involvement in Sandhoff's disease: Inborn error of glycosphingo-lipid metabolism. Am J Cardiol 1974;34:83–88.
29. Eiris J, Chabas A, Coll MJ, Castr-Gato M: Late infantile and juvenile form of GM_2-gangliosidosis variant B1. Revist Neurologica 1999;29:435–438.
30. Triggs-Raine BL, Mules EH, Kaback MM, et al: A pseudodeficiency allele common in non-Jewish Tay-Sachs carriers: Implications for carrier screening. Am J Hum Genet 1993;53:537–539.
31. Yamamoto L, Ninomiya H, Matsumoto M, et al: Genotype-phenotype relationship of Niemann-Pick disease type C: A possible correlation between clinical onset and levels of NPC1 protein in isolated skin fibroblasts. J Med Genet 2000;37:707–711.
32. Naureckiene S, Sleat D, Lackland H, et al: Identification of *HE1* as the second gene of Niemann-Pick C disease. Science 2000;290:2298–2301.
33. Greer WL, Riddell DC, Murty S, et al: Linkage disequilibrium mapping of the Nova Scotia Variant of Niemann-Pick disease. Clin Genet 1999;55:248–255.
34. Crochey AC, Farber S: Niemann-Pick disease: A review of 18 patients. Medicine 1958;37:1.
35. Kamoshita S, Aron AM, Suzuki K: Infantile Niemann-Pick disease: A chemical study with isolation and characterization of membranous cytoplasmic bodies and myelin. Am J Dis Child 1969;117:379–394.
36. Gaucher P: De l'épitheliome primitif de la rate. Thèse, Université de Paris, Paris, 1882.
37. Soffer D, Yamanaka T, Wenger DA, et al: Central nervous system involvement in adult-onset Gaucher's disease. Acta Neuropathol 1980;49:1–6.
38. Tayebi N, Callahan M, Madike V, et al: Gaucher disease and Parkinsonism: A phenotype and genotype characterization. Molec Genet Metab 2001;73:313–321.
39. Vellodi A, Bembi B, De Villemeur TB, al: Management of neuronopathic Gaucher disease: A European consensus. J Inherit Metab Dis 2001;24:319–327.
40. Matalon R, Kaul R, Michals K: Mucopolysaccharidoses and mucolipidoses. *In* Duchett S (ed): Pediatric Neuropathology. Baltimore, Williams & Wilkins, 1995, p 525.
41. Van de Kamp JJ, Neirmeijer MF, Von Figura K, Giesberts MA: Genetic heterogeneity and clinical variability in the Sanfilippo syndrome (Types A, B and C). Clin Genet 1981;20:152–160.
42. Lowry RB, Renwick DH: Relative frequency of Hurler and Hunter syndromes. N Engl J Med 1971;284:221–222.
43. Beesley CE, Young EP, Vellodi A, Winchester BG: Mutational analysis of Sanfilippo syndrome type A (MPSIIIA): Identification of 13 novel mutations. J Med Genet 2000;37:704–707.
44. Tessitore A, Villani GR, Di Domenico C, et al: Molecular defects in the alpha *N*-acetylglucosaminidase gene in Italian Sanfilippo type B patients. Hum Genet 2000;107:568–576.
45. Robertson DA, Callen DF, Baker EG, Morris CP, Hopwood JJ: Chromosomal localization of the gene for human glucosamine 6-sulphatase to 12q14. Hum Genet 1988;79:175–178.
46. Morquio L: Sur une forme de dystrophie osseuse familiale. Arch Med Eur 1929;32:129.
47. Nelson J, Thomas PS: Clinical findings in 12 patients with MPS IVA (Morquio's disease): Further evidence for heterogeneity. III. Odontoid dysplasia. Clin Genet 1988;33:126–130.
48. Rapin I, Goldfischer S, Katzman R, et al: The cherry-red spot—myoclonus syndrome. Ann Neurol 1978;3:234–242.
49. Mueller OT, Wasmuth JJ, Murray JC, et al: Chromosomal assignment of *N*-acetylglucosaminyl-phosphotransferase, the lysosomal hydrolase targeting enzyme deficient in mucolipidosis II and III (abstract). Cytogenet Cell Genet 1987;46:664.
50. Bach G: Mucolipidosis type IV. Molec Genet Metabol 2001; 73:197–203.
51. Tsujino S, Nonaka I, DiMauro S: Glycogen storage myopathies. Neurol Clin 2000;18:125–150.
52. Hirschhorn R, Reuser AJJ: Glycogen storage disease type II: Acid α-glucosidase (acid maltase) deficiency. *In* Scriver CR, Beaudet AL, Sly WS, et al (eds): The Metabolic and Molecular Bases of Inherited Disease, 8th ed. Vol. 3. New York, McGraw-Hill, 2001, pp 3389–3420.
53. Martiniuk F, Bodkin M, Tzall S, Hirschhorn R: Isolation and partial characterization of the structural gene for human acid α-glucosidasae. DNA Cell Biol 1991;10:283–292.
54. Hoefsloot LH, Vander Ploeg AT, Kroos MA, et al: Adult and infantile glycogenosis type II in one family, explained by allelic diversity. Am J Hum Genet 1990;46:45–52.
55. Smith J, Zellweger H, Afifi AK: Muscular form of glycogenosis type II (Pompe): Report of a case with unusual features. Neurology 1967;17:537–549.
56. Engel AG, Dale AJ: Autophagic glycogenosis of late onset with mitochondrial abnormalities: Light and electron microscopic observations. Proc Staff Mayo Clinic 1968;43:233–279.
57. Ziemssen F, Sindern E, Schroder JM, et al: Novel missense mutations in the glycogen-branching enzyme gene in adult polyglucosan body disease. Ann Neurol 2000;47:536–540.
58. Tarui S, Okuno G, Ikura Y: Phosphofructose deficiency in skeletal muscle: A new type of glycogenosis. Biochem Biophys Res Commun 1965;19:512.
59. Servidei S, Bonilla E, Diedrich RG, et al: Fatal infantile form of muscle phosphofructokinase deficiency. Neurology 1986;36:1465–1470.
60. Hug G, Schubert WK, Chuck G: Deficient activity of dephosphorylase kinase and accumulation of glycogen in liver. J Clin Invest 1969;48:704–715.
61. Bresolin N, Ro YI, Reyes M, et al: Muscle phosphoglycerate mutase (PGAM) deficiency: A second case. Neurology 1983;3:1049–1053.
62. Tonin P, Shanske S, Mirañda AF, et al: Phosphoglycerate kinase deficiency: Biochemical and molecular genetic studies in a new myopathic variant (PGK Alberta). Neurology 1993;43:387–391.
63. Tsujino S, Shanske S, Sakoda S, et al: The molecular genetic basis of muscle phosphoglycerate mutase (PGAM) deficiency. Am J Hum Genet 1993;52:472–477.
64. Seitelberger F, Urbanits S, Nave K-A: Pelizaeus-Merzbacher disease. *In* Vinken PJ, Bruyn GW (eds): Handbook of Clinical Neurology. New York, Elsevier, 1996, pp 559–579.
65. Merzbacher L: Eine eigenartige familiare Erknanbunsform (Aplosia extracorticalis congenita). Z Neurol Psychiatr 1910;3:1–138.
66. Garbern J, Cambi F, Shy M, Kamholz J: The molecular pathogenesis of Pelizaeus-Merzbacher disease. Arch Neurol 1999;56:1210–1214.
67. Regis S, Filocamo M, Mazzoti R, et al: Prenatal diagnosis of Pelizaeus-Merzbacher disease: Detection of proteolipid protein gene duplication by quantitative fluorescent multiplex PCR. Prenat Diagn 2001;21:668–671.
68. Garg BP, Markand ON, DeMeyer WE: Usefulness of BAER studies in the early diagnosis of Pelizaeus-Merzbacher disease. Neurology 1983;33:955–956.
69. Saugier-Veber P, Munnich A, Bonneau D, et al: X-linked spastic paraparesis and Pelizaeus-Merzbacher disease are allelic disorders at the proteolipid protein locus. Nat Genet 1994;6:257–262.
70. Hanawalt PC: DNA repair: The base for Cockayne syndrome. Nature 2000;405:415–416.
71. Dabbagh O, Swaiman K: Cockayne syndrome: MRI correlates of hypomyelination. Pediat Neurol 1988;4:113–116.
72. Brumback RA, Yoder FW, Andrews AD, et al: Normal pressure hydrocephalus (recognition and relationship to neurological abnormalities in Cockayne's syndrome). Arch Neurol 1978;35:337–345.
73. Brenner M, Johnson AB, Boespflug-Tanguy O, et al: Mutations in GFAP, encoding glial fibrillary acid protein, are associated with Alexander disease. Nat Genet 2001;27:117–120.
74. Rodriguez D, Gauthier F, Bertini E, et al: Infantile Alexander disease: Spectrum of GFAP mutations and genotype-phenotype correlation. Am J Hum Genet 2001;69:1134–1140.
75. Springer S, Erlewein R, Naegele T, et al: Alexander disease—classification revisited and isolation of a neonatal form. Neuropediatrics 2000;31:86–92.
76. Seil FJ, Schochet SS, Earle KM: Alexander's disease in an adult. Arch Neurol 1968;19:494–502.
77. Martidis A, Yee R, Azzarelli B, Biller J: Neuro-ophthalmic, radiologic, and pathologic manifestations of adult-onset Alexander disease. Arch Ophthalmol 1999;117:265–267.
78. Gascon GG, Ozand PT, Mahdi A, et al: Infantile CNS spongy degeneration—14 cases. Clinical update. Neurology 1990;40:1876–1882.
79. Matalon R, Michals K, Sebesta D, et al: Aspartoacylase deficiency and *N*-acetylaspartic aciduria in patients with Canavan disease. Am J Med Genet 1988;29:463–471.
80. Tahmaz FE, Sam S, Hoganson GE, Quan F: A partial deletion of aspartoacylase gene is the cause of Canavan disease in a family from Mexico. J Medic Genet 2001;38:E9.

81. Matalon R, Michals-Matalon K: Prenatal diagnosis of Canavan disease. Prenat Diagn 1999;19:669—670.
82. Brismar J, Brismar G, Gascon G, Ozand P: Canavan's disease: CT and MR imaging of the brain. Am J Neuroradiol 1990;11:805–810.
83. Wenger DA, Rafi MA, Luzi P, Datto J, Costantino-Ceccarini E: Krabbe disease: Genetic aspects and progress towards therapy. Molec Genet Metabol 2000;70:1–9.
84. Suzuki K: Ultrastructural study of experimental globoid cells. Lab Invest 1970;28:612–619.
85. Lake BD: Segmental demyelination of peripheral nerves in Krabbe's disease. Nature 1968;217:171–172.
86. Lyon G, Hagberg B, Evrard P, et al: Symptomatology of late onset Krabbe's leukodystrophy: The European experience. Rev Neurosci 1991;13:240–244.
87. Baram TZ, Goldman AM, Percy AK: Krabbe disease: Specific MRI and CT findings. Neurology 1986;36:111–115.
88. Krivit W, Aubourg P, Shapiro E, Peters C: Bone marrow transplantation for globoid cell leukodystrophy, adrenoleukodystrophy, metachromatic leukodystrophy, and Hurler syndrome. Curr Opin Hematol 1999;6:377–382.
89. Austin J: Metachromatic sulfatides in cerebral white matter and kidney. Proc Soc Exp Biol Med 1959;100:361.
90. Kolodny EH, Fluharty AL: Metachromatic leukodystrophy and multiple sulfatase deficiency: Sulfatide lipidosis. *In* Scriver CR, Beaudet AL, Sly WS, et al (eds): The Metabolic and Molecular Bases of Inherited Disease, 7th ed. Vol. 2. New York, McGraw-Hill, 1995, pp 2693–2739.
91. Schlote W, Harzer K, Christomanou H, et al: Sphingolipid activator protein 1 deficiency in metachromatic leukodystrophy with normal arylsulfatase activity. A clinical, morphological, biochemical and immunological study. Eur J Pediatr 1991;150:584–591.
92. Kao F-T, Law ML, Hartz J, et al: Regional localization of the gene coding for sphingomyelin activator protein SAP-1 on human chromosome 10. Somat Cell Mol Genet 1987;13:685–688.
93. Greenfield JG: A form of cerebral sclerosis in infants associated with primary degeneration of the interfascicular glia. J Neurol Psychopathol 1933;13:289–302.
94. Normam RM, Urich H, Tingley AH: Metachromatic leukodystrophy: A form of lipidosis. Brain 1960;83:369.
95. Hagberg B, Sourounder P, Svennerholm L, et al: Late infantile metachromatic leucodystrophy of the genetic type. Acta Paediatr 1960;49:135.
96. Moser HW: Peroxisomal disorders. *In* Dyken P (ed): Pediatric Neurodegenerative Diseases. American Academy of Neurology Program, 48th annual meeting, San Francisco, March 29, 1996.
97. Mobley WC, White CL, Tennelson G, et al: Neonatal adrenoleukodystrophy. Ann Neurol 1982;12:204.
98. Reuber BE, Germain-Lee E, Collins CS, et al: Mutations in PEX1 are the most common cause of peroxisomal biogenesis disorders. Nature Genet 1997;17:445–448.
99. Huhse B, Rehling P, Albertini M, et al: PEX 17p of *Saccharomyces cerevisiae* is a peroxin and component of peroxisomal protein translocation machinery. J Cell Biol 1998;140:49–60.
100. Naidu S, Moser H: Peroxisomal disorders. *In* Swaiman K (ed): Pediatric Neurology: Principles and Practice, 2nd ed. Vol. 2. St Louis, Mosby, 1994, pp 1357–1383.
101. Fournier B, Saudubray JM, Benichou B, et al: Large deletion of the peroxisomal acyl-CoA oxidase gene in pseudoneonatal adrenoleukodystrophy. J Clin Invest 1994; 94:526–531.
102. Moser HW, Smith KD, Watkins PA, Powers J, Moser AB: X-linked adrenoleukodystrophy. *In* Scriver CR, Beaudet AL, Sly WS, et al (eds): The Metabolic and Molecular Bases of Inherited Disease, 8th ed. Vol. 2. New York, McGraw-Hill, 2001, 3257–3301.
103. van Geel BM, Assies J, Haverkort EB, et al: Progression of abnormalities in adrenomyeloneuropathy and neurologically asymptomatic–linked adrenoleukodystrophy despite treatment with "Lorenzo's oil." J Neurol Neurosurg Psychiatry 199;67:290–299.
104. Shapiro E, Krivit W, Lockman L, et al: Long-term effect of bone-marrow transplantation in childhood-onset cerebral X-linked adrenoleukodystrophy. Lancet 2000;356:713–718.
105. Kornreich R, Desnick RJ, Bishop DF: Nucleotide sequence of human alpha-galactosidase A gene. Nucleic Acids Res 1989;17:3301–3302.
106. Cable WJL, Dvorak AM, Osage JE, Kolodny EH: Fabry disease: Significance of ultrastructural localization of lipid inclusions in dermal nerves. Neurology 1982a;32:347–353.
107. Inagaki M, Ohno K, Ohta S, et al: Relief of chronic burning pain in Fabry disease with neurotropin. Pediatr Neurol 1990;6:211–213.
108. Eng CM, Guffon N, Wilcox WR, et al: Safety and efficacy of recombinant human (alpha)-galactosidase A replacement therapy in Fabry's disease. N Engl J Med 2001;345:9–16.
109. Wills AJ, Manning NJ, Reilly MM: Refsum's disease. QJM 2001;94:403–406.
110. Baumgartner MR, Jansen GA, Vervoeren NM, et al: Atypical Refsum disease with increased pipecolic academia and abnormal catalase distribution. Ann Neurol 2000;47:109–113.
111. Hansen E, Refsum S: Heredopathia atactica polyneuritiformis. Phytanic acid storage disease (Refsum's disease). A biochemically well defined disease with a specific dietary treatment. *In* Huber A, Klein D (eds): Neurogenetics and Neuro-ophthalmology. Developments in Neurology, Vol. 5. New York, Elsevier, 1981, pp 333–339.
112. Ohashi K, Ishibashi S, Osuga J-i, et al: Novel mutations in the microsomal triglyceride transfer protein gene causing abetalipoproteinemia. J Lipid Res 2000;41:1199–1204.
113. Xiao Ping Y, Akihiro A, Kunimasa Y, Kouji K, Junji K, Hiroshi M: Abetalipoproteinemia caused by maternal isodisomy of chromosome 4q containing an intron 9 splice acceptor mutation in the microsomal triglyceride transfer protein gene. Arterioscl Thromb Vasc Biol 1999;19:1950–1955.
114. Guggenheim MA, Ringel SP, Silverman A, Grabert BE: Progressive neuromuscular disease in children with chronic cholestasis and vitamin E deficiency: Diagnosis and treatment with alpha tocopherol. J Pediatr 1982;100:51–58.
115. Brin MF, Pedley TA, Lovelace RE, et al: Electrophysiologic features of abetalipoproteinemia: Functional consequences of vitamin E deficiency. Neurology 1986;36:669–673.
116. Runge P, Muller DP, McAllister J, et al: Oral vitamin E supplements can prevent the retinopathy of abetalipoproteinemia. Br J Ophthalmol 1986;70:166–173.
117. Brousseau ME, Schaefer EJ, Dupuis J, et al: Novel mutations in the gene encoding ATP-binding cassette 1 in four Tangier disease kindreds. J Lipid Res 2000;41:433–441.

CHAPTER 31

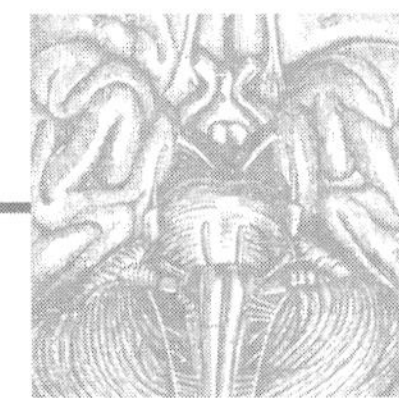

GENEROSO G. GASCON and PINAR T. OZAND

Aminoacidopathies and Organic Acidopathies, Mitochondrial Enzyme Defects, and Other Metabolic Errors

A large number of diseases, at least 70, involve the metabolism of organic and amino acids. Some diseases present as repeated episodes of acute metabolic decompensation, and the central nervous system (CNS) involvement is usually secondary to the accompanying acidosis, hypoglycemia, or hyperammonemia or to the elevated concentration of amino acids. Nevertheless, it is the secondary involvement of the CNS that is important and is the main problem requiring management. Another group of these disorders involves the CNS primarily, with the systemic disease being negligible. Such disorders are difficult to label at the time of initial encounter as either an organic or amino acid disorder because there are no episodes of acid-base disturbance or disturbance of glucose or ammonia metabolism. They can only be diagnosed by specialized biochemical tests. The recent advent of tandem mass spectrometry is changing the practice of neurometabolic diseases since it provides a rapid diagnosis.[1, 2] In many instances the child will become neurologically crippled before the diagnosis is suspected and ascertained. A third group of disorders impact both the CNS and peripheral tissues. Likewise, mitochondrial enzyme defects treated later in the chapter can be classified by age of presentation. Childhood disorders are classified in Table 31–1 according to their main presenting features and age.[1, 2] The porphyrias are primarily adult-onset disorders.

TABLE 31–1. **Different Clinical Presentations of Amino Acid and Organic Acid Disorders According to Age and Symptoms**

Neonatal Disorders with Devastating Metabolic Disease
Maple syrup urine disease (MSUD) (branched-chain aminoacidemia)
Urea cycle disorders
Nonketotic hyperglycinemia
Propionicacidemia, methylmalonicacidemia, and isovalericacidemia
Certain phenotypes of 3-hydroxy-3-methylglutaryl-CoA lyase deficiency
Holocarboxylase synthetase deficiency
Pyruvate dehydrogenase and pyruvate carboxylase deficiencies
Cytochrome-*c* oxidase deficiency
Carnitine/carnitine-acyl translocase deficiency
Long-chain acyl-CoA dehydrogenase (LCAD) deficiency
Medium-chain acyl-CoA dehydrogenase deficiency (MCAD) with early neonatal death
Multiple acyl-CoA dehydrogenase deficiency
Certain phenotypes of 3-methylglutaconicacidurias
Later Infancy Disorders with Recurrent Metabolic Decompensation
Intermittent, or intermediate MSUD
Late-onset urea cycle disorders
Arginase deficiency
Certain phenotypes of 3-hydroxy-3-methylglutaryl-CoA lyase deficiency
Certain phenotypes of propionicacidemia and methylmalonicacidemia
Ethylmalonicaciduria and malonicaciduria
Certain phenotypes of 3-methylglutaconicacidurias
β-Ketothiolase deficiency
Later Infancy and Childhood Disorders with Prominent Neurological Manifestations
Classic and biopterin-dependent hyperphenylalaninemia
Homocystinuria due to cystathionine β-synthase deficiency
Disorders of folate and vitamin B_{12} metabolism with homocystinuria
4-Hydroxybutyricaciduria
Glutaricaciduria type 1
Certain phenotypes of 3-methylglutaconicacidurias
Carnitine palmitoyl transferase (CPT) I and II deficiencies
Adenosine triphosphate synthetase deficiency
Certain phenotypes of MCAD and LCAD deficiencies
Biotinidase deficiency

Aminoacidopathies and Organic Acidopathies

NEONATAL DISORDERS

The Advent of Neonatal Screening Programs

It has been more than 35 years since a neonatal screening test program was established for phenylketonuria (PKU). These initial efforts were based on an inhibition assay developed by Dr. Robert Guthrie.[3] In the 1980s, several other diseases were added to such screening programs.[4] The major breakthrough came from the adoption and modification of a tandem mass spectroscopy system (MS/MS)[5, 6, 7] that now can fit the needs of mass screening programs.[8, 9, 10] The method is easy to use and yields rapid results. The analytic time is approximately 90 seconds and preparation time for a batch of 96 samples is approximately 2 hours. In one analytic panel, 30 or more organic and aminoacidemias can be screened (Table 31–2). The method is nearly always free of false-negative and false-positive results. Some abnormal values, either elevations or depressions, are very specific and pathognomic of inborn errors if other causes are excluded. For example, high octanoyl carnitine levels occur in medium-chain acyl-CoA dehydrogenase (MCAD) deficiency. Depressed methionine levels occur in methylenetetrahydrofolate reductase deficiency. Clinical interpretation is essential, however, because the biochemical results are extremely accurate but still do not always indicate a primary inborn error of metabolism. For example, elevation of octanoyl carnitine might also be observed under valproate treatment, and hypomethioninemia might also reflect general protein malnutrition. Therefore, these screening tests require clinical interpretation.

The impact of screening programs and early intervention are increasingly clear worldwide. Patients with glutaricaciduria identified in the early neonatal period are growing as normal children under treatment. A large number of children with organic and aminoacidemias detected by neonatal screening are today developing clinically as healthy children. Certain other disorders such as 3-hydroxy-3-methylglutaryl-CoA lyase deficiency, β-ketothiolase deficiency, methylenetetrahydrofolate reductase deficiency, isovalericacidemia, PKU of both types, methylmalonicacidemia, MCAD, citrullinemia, and argininosuccinicaciduria, when identified in the neonate, almost always can be treated with rewarding results. In spite of this progress, some identified disorders remain untreatable. Severe phenotypes of propionicacidemia and methylmalonicacidemia, severe phenotypes of other fatty acid oxidation disorders, and glutaricaciduria type 2 cases still experience severe morbidity or an early death despite management.

Maple Syrup Urine Disease

Pathogenesis and Pathophysiology. In 1962, Menkes and colleagues observed an unusual odor, like that of maple syrup, in the urine of four infants who died of progressive encephalopathy in the first few weeks of life (Fig. 31–1).[11] Maple syrup urine disease (MSUD) is a disorder of branched-chain amino acid (BCAA) metabolism, in which the

TABLE 31-2. **Disorders That Can Be Screened by Tandem Mass Spectroscopy (MS/MS)***

Organic Acidemias	Amino Acid and Other Disorders
Propionicacidemia	Hyperphenylalaninemia, classic
Methylmalonicacidemia	Hyperphenylalaninemia, biopterin dependent
Isovalericacidemia	Branched-chain amino acidemia (maple syrup urine disease); classic, intermittent, and intermediate variants
3-Hydroxy-3-methylglutaryl-CoA lyase deficiency	Citrullinemia
β-Ketothiolase deficiency	Argininemia
Multiple carboxylase deficiency	Argininosuccinicacidemia
Short-, medium-, and very long-chain acyl- CoA dehydrogenase deficiencies	Lysinuric protein intolerance
Carnitine/acylcarnitine translocase deficiency	Hyperlysinemia
Carnitine palmitoyl- CoA transferase deficiency types 1 and 2	Hyperprolinemia
Multiple acyl-CoA dehydrogenase deficiency	Nonketotic hyperglycinemia
Pyroglutamicaciduria	Homocystinuria
Pipecolicaciduria	Disorders due to cobalamin mutations
	Methylenetetrahydrofolate reductase deficiency

*Several of these disorders have been identified in the metabolic service of King Faisel Specialist Hospital and Research Center, Saudi Arabia, during the past 8 years through MS/MS.

concentrations of L-leucine, L-isoleucine, and L-valine, as well as their corresponding alpha-ketoacids, are elevated in body fluids. The branched-chain alpha-ketoacid dehydrogenase (BCKAD) is deficient, and the disorder is inherited as an autosomal recessive trait. It is a multienzyme complex that contains three major subunits: E1, a decarboxylase; E2, an acyltransferase; and E3, a lipoamide dehydrogenase (dihydrolipoic dehydrogenase). The activity of BCKAD is regulated either by inhibition of reaction products or substrate analogues by reversible phosphorylation/dephosphorylation of the E1 subunit or by the regulation of gene expression through such hormones as insulin and corticosteroids, or L-carnitine or by glucose. The chromosome location of the genes of the subunits and of complementary DNAs is

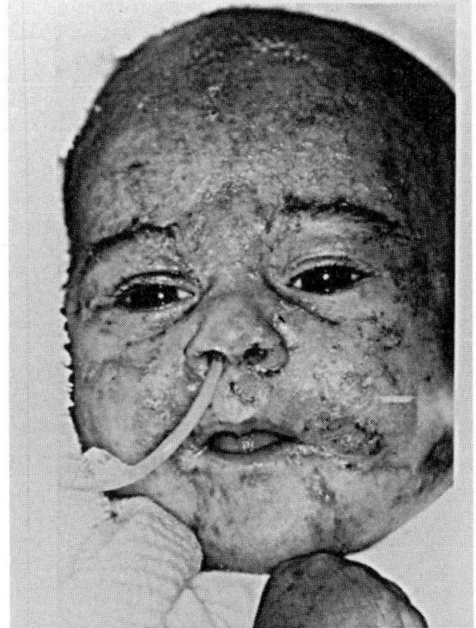

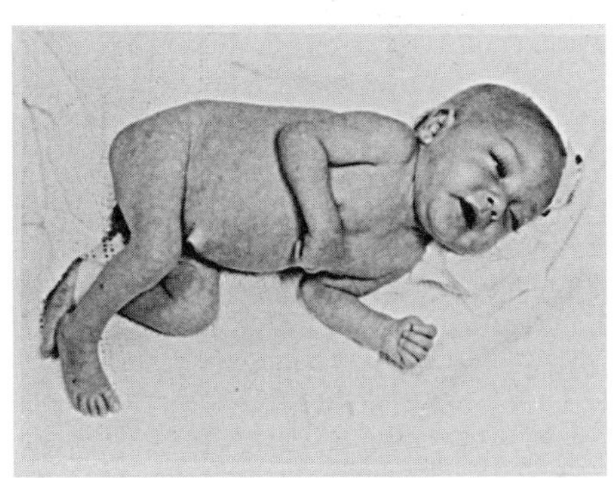

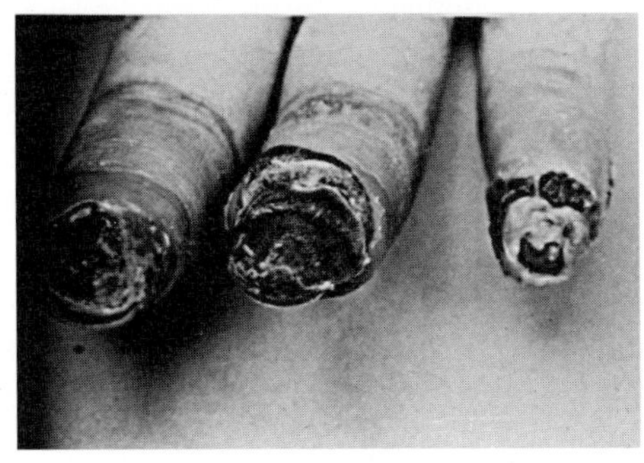

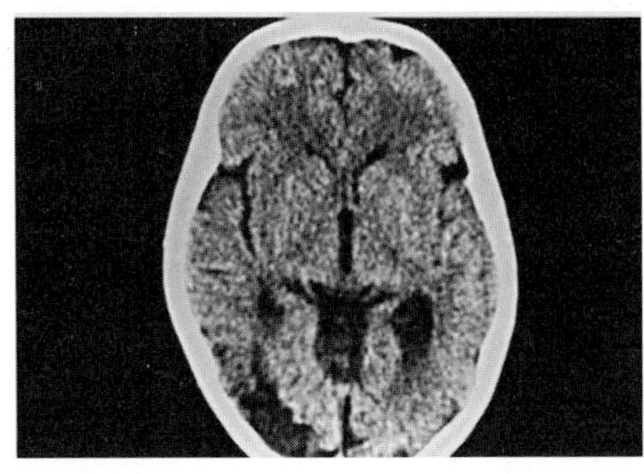

FIGURE 31–1. Maple syrup urine disease and homocystinuria. Clockwise, from left upper corner. The facial and generalized erythematous, scaly, weeping rash in acute, untreated maple syrup urine disease (MSUD). Spastic quadriparetic posture and increased fat pads in cheeks of an infant with poorly managed MSUD. CT of the brain showing left occipital infarct in patient with homocystinuria. Gangrenous fingertips in homocystinuria.

established (Table 31–3). Mutations of the subunits from different ethnic groups have been identified.

The severe CNS symptoms of the disease have been attributed to brain edema, caused by elevated BCAAs, particularly L-leucine. The neuropathological finding in patients who die is generalized spongy CNS degeneration, similar to other disorders such as nonketotic hyperglycinemia.

Epidemiology and Risk Factors. The worldwide frequency based on routine screening data from 26.8 million newborns is about 1 in 185,000.[12] The disease is common in consanguineous communities; for example, among the Mennonites of Pennsylvania, the incidence is 1 in 176. It is encountered frequently in the Middle East, particularly in the Arabian peninsula, where its frequency may be as high as 1 in 2000.

Clinical Features and Associated Disorders. The classical form of MSUD usually presents within the first 2 weeks of life and rarely beyond 1 month of age. The prodromal symptoms include refusal to feed, vomiting, increasing lethargy, and seizures, with eventual coma. Because the cerebral peduncles and the dorsal part of the brain stem are the earliest parts of the CNS involved, the patient develops opisthotonus and primitive reflexes are usually absent. The initial clinical diagnosis is commonly meningitis or sepsis; because such patients frequently have associated sepsis, the primary diagnosis may be missed for many days. Cerebral edema leads to tone disturbances, alternating between increased tone and hypotonia. Seizure activity is usually clonic or myoclonic with eyes rolling upward. Early optic atrophy is usual and recedes only if the therapeutic intervention is prompt. When the presence of disease is not recognized at this stage, or the neonate is not managed appropriately, the infant becomes blind and has severe spastic quadriplegia (see Fig. 31–1). Undiagnosed patients usually develop apnea and die. When treated appropriately, the symptoms will gradually disappear. In well-managed patients, mild to moderate hypotonia (particularly axial hypotonia) persists during the first year of life; eventually, mild to moderate cerebellar ataxia will remain as the only neurological sequela.

The symptoms of MSUD reappear as overwhelming illness and coma in patients with disorders that lead to protein catabolism, especially infections and diarrhea. When these conditions are not managed appropriately, they lead to further neurological deterioration or death. Clinical symptoms and the course of the disease are milder in infants who are diagnosed through neonatal screening and treated before the initial metabolic crisis. In contrast, a patient with late-diagnosed MSUD experiences frequent recurrent episodes, requires prolonged hospital care, and poses significant management problems without ever improving.

The odor of infants is that of burnt sugar, or maple syrup. It is easily recognized in the urine, hair, axillae, and perineum or in cerumen; it is best appreciated on frozen urine, because the smell is caused by compounds with oily characteristics accumulating on the frozen surface.

When the levels of BCAA are not monitored frequently during dietary management, abnormal ratios of leucine/isoleucine or of valine ensue. This situation manifests as severe dermatitis, described as scalded skin syndrome (see Fig. 31–1). The dermatitis will resolve when the ratios of amino acids are normalized. A number of MSUD variants have been described.[13]

Differential Diagnosis. Clinically, the most important differential diagnoses are other causes of neonatal coma, and many can be differentiated by clinical (Table 31–4) or by simple laboratory observations (Table 31–5). In the neonate, MSUD is almost always confused with sepsis or meningitis, and the disease is usually associated with either one. The diagnosis of MSUD is suspected only after the sepsis or meningitis workup reveals normal results. Precious therapeutic time will be lost, causing severe neurological crippling or death. MSUD must always be ruled out in any neonate with lethargy progressing to coma; with alternating tone changes; in the absence of changes in blood pH, glucose, and ammonia; and regardless of the presence of an infection. In variant forms of the disease, the diagnosis is usually reached when either blood amino acids or urine organic acids are studied in a child with periodic coma or in a child with pyramidal or cerebellar signs.

TABLE 31–3. **Chromosomal Locations of Diseases**

Disease and Enzyme(s)	Chromosome Location
Maple syrup urine disease: branched-chain alpha-ketoacid dehydrogenase (E1, E2, and E3 subunits)	$E_{1\alpha}$: 19q13/1–q13/2: $E_{1\beta}$: 6p21–p22; E2: 1p31; and E3: 7q31–q32
Propionicacidemia: propionyl-CoA carboxylase	α subunit: 13q32; β subunit 3q13–3q22
Methylmalonicacidemia: methylmalonyl-CoA mutase, hydroxycobalamin reductases, adenosyl transferase and cobalamin A–F groups	Mutase: 6p12–p21.2 Others are unknown
Urea cycle disorders: carbamoylphosphate synthetase (CPS), ornithine transcarbamylase (OTC), argininosuccinicacid (ASA) synthetase, ASA lyase	CPS: 2p OTC: Xp21.1 ASA synthetase: 9q34 ASA lyase: 7cen–p21
Classic PKU: phenylalanine hydroxylase	12q22–224.1
Biopterin-dependent PKU: GTP cyclohydrolase, 6-pyruvoyl-tetra-hydropterin synthase (6PTS), dihydropterin reductase (DHPR), and 4α-carbinolamine dehydratase (PCD) deficiencies	GTP cyclohydrolase: 14q22.1–q22.2 6PTS: cDNA available DHPR: 4p15.3 PCD: 10q22
Homocystinuria: cystathionine β-synthase	21q21–q22.1
Glutaricaciduria type 1: glutaryl-CoA dehydrogenase	19p13.2
Biotinidase deficiency: biotinidase	3p25

TABLE 31–4. **Differential Diagnoses of Coma in Neonate: Clinical Findings**

Disease	Tone	Seizures	Dysmorphia	Liver Disease	Infectious Complications
Maple syrup urine disease (MSUD)	Alternating tone	Myoclonic or clonic	Absent	Absent	Almost always present
MSUD (recurrent crisis)	Not specific	May be present	Absent	Absent	May be present
Urea cycle disorders	Severe hypertonia	Usually myoclonic	Absent	Absent	May be present
Various organic acidemias	Hypotonia (propionic-acidemia), hypertonia (methylmalonicacidemia and isovalericacidemia)	Myoclonic or clonic	Facial and CNS dysmorphia present in propionicacidemia and pyruvate dehydrogenase deficiency	Present in cytochrome-c oxidase deficiency or oxidative phosphorylation diseases	Almost always present
Fatty acid oxidation disorders	Myopathy or cardiomyopathy	As caused by hypoglycemia	Only type 2 glutaric aciduria	Only type 2 glutaric-aciduria	Usually absent
Nonketotic hyperglycinemia	Severe hypotonia, stridor, hiccups	Severe, usually myoclonic	CNS dysgenesis such as absent corpus callosum	Absent	Usually absent
Zellweger's syndrome	Severe hyopotonia	Severe, usually myoclonic	Facial, CNS dysgenesis, cysts in organs	Severe liver involvement	Usually absent
Nesidioblastosis	None	As caused by hypoglycemia	None	None	None

TABLE 31–5. **Differential Diagnoses of Coma in Neonate: Laboratory Findings**

Disease	Blood pH	Blood Glucose	Blood Ammonia	Blood Lactic Acid	Urine Ketones	Special Findings
Maple syrup urine disease (MSUD)	Normal	Normal	Normal	Normal	Trace or absent	Elevated branched-chain amino acids and branched-chain ketoacids in urine
MSUD (recurrent crisis)	Acidosis	Moderate/severe hypoglycemia	Normal	Normal	Moderate/severe ketonuria	As in neonatal period
Urea cycle disorders	Alkalotic or normal	Normal	Rapid elevation	High in argininosuccinic-aciduria and citrullinemia	Absent	Citrulline values differentiate various types; high oroticaciduria in certain types
Various organic acidemias	Overt/ compensated acidosis w/large-base excess	May be mild/ moderately low	Usually elevated	Usually elevated	Trace/strong (+) in various disorders	Urine organic acids, blood acylcarnitines
Fatty acid oxidation disorders	Usually normal	Usually moderately/ severely low	Variable, but usually normal	May be elevated	Absent	Urine organic acids, blood and urine acylcarnitines
Nonketotic hyperglycinemia	Normal	Normal	Normal	Normal	Normal	Elevated glycerine in blood and cerebrospinal fluid
Zellweger's syndrome	Normal	Normal	Normal	Normal	Normal	Elevated liver enzymes and very long-chain fatty acids in blood; pipecolic acid in urine
Nesidioblastosis	Normal	Low with inappropriately elevated insulin levels	Normal	Normal	Normal	Blood glucose and insulin determined at the same time

Evaluation. Test findings should be grouped into two age categories: one for neonatal and one for episodes after 6 months of age. In the neonatal period, the disease almost never causes significant hypoglycemia, nor acidosis, ketonuria, or hyperammonemia. Therefore, the presence of coma in a neonate who has nearly normal clinical biochemical findings should immediately suggest MSUD. Definite diagnosis is through determination of amino acids in plasma or in urine, which shows significant elevations of L-leucine, isoleucine, and valine. Leucine concentration in blood is always higher than that of the other BCAAs. BCAAs or BCKAD can be measured either by chromatographic techniques or more rapidly by MS/MS determinations. A quick spot test of the ketoacids in the urine is a strongly positive yellow flocculation when 2,3-dinitrophenylhydrazine is added. After 6 months of life, when recurrent acute metabolic decompensation occurs, it is accompanied by mild to moderate hypoglycemia, severe acidosis, and ketonuria.

The electroencephalogram (EEG) of the newborn with MSUD has a characteristic sharp wave pattern described as comblike rhythm.[14] After proper management, the EEG may be normal between attacks or there may be a generalized slowing of the background and paroxysmal discharges, indicative of the ongoing metabolic disease. In older patients, leucine loading may lead to EEG abnormalities. Even in well-controlled patients, seizure disorder may appear later during childhood, requiring anticonvulsive treatment.

Neuroimaging is a valuable tool, particularly when amino acid determination is not immediately available. In the neonate, it causes a characteristic appearance of white matter attenuation suggestive of brain edema that appears as early as 9 days of life despite dietary treatment. The MSUD edema initially involves the deep cerebellar matter, the dorsal part of the brain stem, the cerebral peduncles, and the dorsal limb of the internal capsule. Eventually, marked generalized diffuse edema appears in the central white matter and is particularly prominent in the frontal areas. The edema subsides after several months of treatment, with mild to severe atrophy of the brain remaining, as evidenced by enlarged ventricles and prominent sulci. The severity of these findings depends on the stage of the disease at which the treatment is initiated. In well-managed patients, the neuroradiological sequelae may be increased cerebellar foliation, cerebellar white matter disease, or cerebellar atrophy supporting the clinical presence of ataxia; this last finding may be the only neurological sequela in such children.

Management. Treatment consists of emergency reduction of increased BCAAs in blood. In patients diagnosed early, peritoneal dialysis or hemodialysis should be attempted. A secure central line must be placed, because intensive parenteral nutrition and antibiotics are used for several weeks to prevent catabolism and prompt anabolism. Specific amino acid solutions without BCAA for parenteral nutrition, in MSUD and other disorders of BCAAs, are available from PharmThera (Memphis, TN).[15] Insulin drip, using diluted insulin solutions, must be initiated to ensure anabolism. Blood levels of BCAAs must be measured initially once or twice daily to monitor the reduction of the level of BCAAs; this is best done by MS/MS. A simple clinical guideline to therapy is to follow weight gain in a nonedematous neonate. The treatment usually leads to daily weight increments for about 10 days, at which time the blood leucine level is reduced below 1000 μM. Oral intake of special mild formulas with restricted BCAAs must then be resumed, and parenteral nutrition must be discontinued gradually. A neonate with MSUD is usually difficult to feed, and either a nasogastric tube or temporary button gastrostomy may be used for this purpose.

Once the acute metabolic decompensation is controlled, the patient is placed on BCAA-restricted formulas such as Ketonex or other MSUD formulas. Chronic management is difficult because it requires provision of BCAAs in amounts that permit growth but that do not cause significant BCAA elevations. This requires frequent amino acid analysis and can be achieved only in tertiary care centers where easy access to high-performance liquid chromatography or MS/MS is available. Patients should receive thiamine supplementation and L-carnitine; when metabolic decompensation occurs, leucine should be restricted.

Prognosis, Prevention, and Prenatal Diagnosis. Prognosis depends on early detection and treatment. Patients whose disease is diagnosed before the initial metabolic attack will grow as nearly normal children, despite recurrent attacks in later infancy. Successfully managed patients will have a near-normal IQ and normal school performance.[16, 17] A neonatal screening should be mandatory in countries where the disease is prevalent. The safety window of classic MSUD is only a few days; therefore, newborns should be screened for this disease at 24 to 48 hours of life. This can be achieved either by a Guthrie test or, more easily, by MS/MS. The BCKAD activity can be measured in cultured amniotic cells.[18] If the mutation is known, this can be achieved by molecular genetic studies.

Urea Cycle Disorders

Pathogenesis and Pathophysiology. Recognized only during the past 40 years, the urea cycle disorders (UCDs) include argininosuccinicaciduria (ASA uria; ASA lyase deficiency),[19] citrullinemia (ASA synthetase deficiency),[20] ornithine transcarbamoylase (OTC) deficiencies,[21] and carbamoylphosphate synthetase (CPS) deficiency (Fig. 31–2).[22] Ammonia is detoxified through five synthetic enzymes and one enzyme that synthesizes an activator for the initial step. The initial three enzymes are in the mitochondria, and the latter three are in the cytosol. This cyclic process both generates and hydrolyzes L-arginine, which is an essential amino acid in infants and important for normal development of the brain. When only one of the activities on this pathway is deficient, hyperammonemia and CNS symptomatology ensue. This usually occurs during the first few days to weeks of life and is one of the major causes of devastating metabolic disease of the newborn.

The UCDs cause hyperammonemia, and the clinical picture is similar in all forms of neonatal UCD. The gene locations of urea cycle enzymes are shown in Table 31–3, and complementary DNA is available for most of them.

When any of the aforementioned enzymes is deficient, ammonia cannot be converted into urea, leading to hyperammonemia within the first week of life. Unlike hepatic coma, in which ammonia is only one of the many putative toxins, in neonatal UCD, ammonia is the only cause of encephalopathy. Blood ammonia concentrations exceeding 300 μM are highly

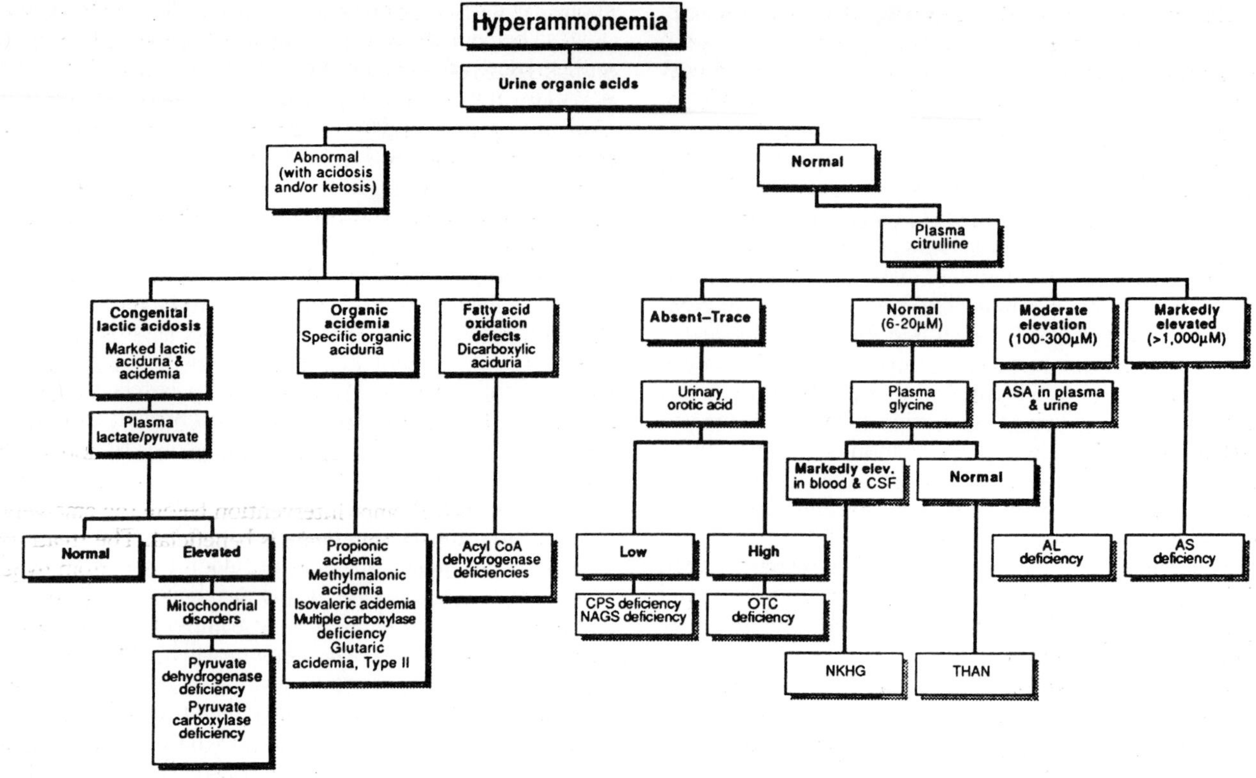

FIGURE 31–2. Algorithm for approach to neonatal-onset hyperammonemia. Abbreviations: NKHG, nonketotic hyperglycinemia; THAN, transient hyperammonemia of the newborn; CPS, carbamoylphosphate synthetase; OTC, ornithine transcarbamylase; AL, argininosuccinate lyase; AS, argininosuccinate synthetase; NAGS, *N*-acetylglutamate synthetase; ASA, arginosuccinic acid. (From Batshaw ML: Errors of Urea Synthesis. Ann Neurol 1994;35:133–141. Copyright © 1994 John Wiley & Sons. Reprinted by permission of John Wiley & Sons, Inc.)

neurotoxic, particularly when prolonged. Primate models with induced hyperammonemia closely mimic the clinical, neurophysiological, and neuropathological findings observed in human neonatal UCD. In late-onset forms of ASA synthetase and lyase deficiencies, levels of citrulline, ASA, and ASA anhydride are elevated between crises when the patient is asymptomatic. This suggests that the acute neonatal symptoms of these diseases are due to hyperammonemia and not to elevated levels of urea cycle amino acids. Support for this theory is the family reported by Issa and associates[23] in which one neonate with citrullinemia died with hyperammonemia while her twin brother remained asymptomatic with elevated levels of citrulline. This point is of paramount importance for the management and prognosis of UCDs.

The swelling of astrocytes in UCDs is due to hyperammonemia and might be caused by the concomitant elevation of glutamine. When glutamine synthetase is inhibited, cerebral edema caused by hyperammonemia can be prevented. In OTC deficiency, the hyperammonemia encephalopathy is shown to be related to brain glutamine accumulations, as demonstrated by magnetic spectroscopic studies.

Epidemiology and Risk Factors. Fortunately, the UCDs are rare disorders. All, except OTC deficiency, are inherited as autosomal recessive traits. The OTC gene is on chromosome X, and its severe form is encountered only in males. The heterozygote female is discussed among UCDs of late onset. The cumulative frequency of all types of neonatal UCDs in Japan is 1 in 46,000 births; and the frequency for OTC deficiency in Japan was reported to be 1 in 80,000. In the Massachusetts screening program, the incidence of ASA lyase deficiency was 1 in 70,000,[24] and in a Quebec screening program, it was 1 in 77,000.[25] Approximately 65 cases of ASA lyase deficiency have been reported. The incidence of ASA synthetase deficiency (citrullinemia) in the Quebec program was 1 in 250,000 births.[25] In the Middle East, the most common forms of neonatal UCD are ASA lyase and synthetase deficiencies and they might occur in 1 in 2000 to 3000 births.

Clinical Features and Associated Disorders. All forms of neonatal UCDs manifest nearly identical clinical symptoms. The infant is usually the product of normal pregnancy and delivery, with normal Apgar scores, and remains normal usually for 24 to 72 hours. Shortly thereafter, however, the infant becomes lethargic and refuses to feed; this quickly progresses to coma and is associated with hypothermia, hyperventilation, and respiratory alkalosis. Because cerebral edema appears early in the acute event, the bulging fontanelle erroneously leads to a diagnosis of meningitis with sepsis or pneumonia. If a coma workup is neglected, the neonate will die within a few days with a missed diagnosis. Brittle hair showing trichorrhexis nodosa in ASA lyase deficiency is encountered later during infancy and is not a prominent feature if the infant is given adequate amounts of L-arginine. Patients with ASA lyase deficiency might also have moderate to severe hepatomegaly. Phenotypical variability is the function of different mutations. Metabolic consequences also depend on the availability of compounds that might serve as an ammonia sink; for example, OTC deficiency is less severe than CPS deficiency and ASA synthesis that proceeds normally from citrulline might serve as a store for waste nitrogen.

Differential Diagnosis. The diagnosis is quickly reached by the uniform clinical presentation of the neonatal UCD. Differential diagnosis for neonatally important organic acidemias is by measurement of blood pH, lactic acid, ketone bodies, and glucose (see Tables 31–5 and 31–6). The hyperammonemia observed in organic acidemias is associated with overt or compensated metabolic acidosis, whereas in UCDs the blood pH is usually normal or alkalotic. Blood glycine and urine ketones are elevated in the major ketotic organic acidemias of the neonate, which is not the case in UCDs. It is important to differentiate various types of UCD from CPS and OTC deficiencies. This differential diagnosis is essentially reached by measurements of specific amino acids in plasma and of orotic acid in the urine. *N*-acetylglutamate (NAG) synthetase deficiency may be proven clinically by normalization of ammonia after administration of 250 to 500 mg/kg/day NAG in a suspect case. It is now possible to diagnose citrullinemia and ASA uria rapidly within a few hours in a suspected case by MS/MS. The simultaneous measurement of acylcarnitines with amino acids particularly eliminates any confusion rising from other diseases with co-existent lactic acidemia.

Evaluation. Any neonate with coma and devastating metabolic disease should receive a battery of clinical biochemical tests, including a determination of ammonia in addition to blood gases, pH, blood glucose, urea, and lactate (see Table 31–5). These data provide a provisional diagnosis of a UCD within hours, and a definite diagnosis can be made by the measurement of specific amino acids and orotic aciduria.

Management. Prompt intervention before the emergence of significant hyperammonemia is beneficial. The treatment consists of two phases: (1) rescue of the neonate from hyperammonemic coma and (2) maintenance of normal physical and intellectual growth between metabolic crises with recurrent hyperammonemia. The essential medications for both phases of treatment in UCD are phenylacetate or phenylbutyrate and L-arginine. These medications bind and remove ammonia through alternate pathways as hippurate (1 M ammonia per mole of benzoate) and phenylacetylglutamine (2 M of ammonia per mole of phenylacetate or phenylbutyrate). In ASA synthetase and lyase deficiencies, L-arginine is used because it is converted into citrulline and ASA, respectively, and thus provides an ammonia sink. To avoid cerebral edema, recurrent episodes of hyperammonemia should be treated vigorously at the earliest clinical sign of decline, such as lethargy, irritability, vomiting, or behavior change, or before the plasma ammonia level increases to three times its normal limit.[26]

Treatment between episodes of metabolic decompensation provides enough protein to ensure adequate growth but avoids hyperammonemia and elevated plasma glutamine levels. In CPS and OTC deficiencies, during the first 6 months of life, a diet that contains a 0.7-g/kg/day mixture of essential amino acids (using UCD formulas available from Mead Johnson, Princeton NJ, or Milupa, Hillington, Middlesex, UK) together with normal milk protein 0.7 to 2 g/kg/day is given and the plasma amino acid levels are monitored. More recently, orthoptic liver transplantation has been recommended for the definitive treatment of UCD; the rewarding results of this treatment in seven patients with UCD have been reviewed.[27]

Mortality relates directly or indirectly to the consequences of acute brain edema. Even if this complication is prevented, acute hyperammonemia either initially or intermittently can lead to intracerebral and subdural hemorrhage. No infant with a UCD should be given valproate because it may cause liver failure and death.[28]

Prognosis and Prevention. Neurological outcome and morbidity depend on early diagnosis and appropriate treatment. Long-term studies suggest that use of phenylbutyrate with diet therapy offers the best chance of survival. Hyperammonemia of acute decompensation in ASA lyase and synthetase deficiencies is easily controlled by intravenous or oral administration of L-arginine; with subsequent use of diet and phenylbutyrate, the survival rate is 90 percent.

TABLE 31–6. **Mitochondrial Enzyme Defects***

Infantile
Subacute necrotizing encephalopathy or Leigh's disease (I, II)
Progressive infantile poliodystrophy or Alpers' disease (IV)
Lethal infantile mitochondrial disease (I)
Others
Hypertrophic cardiomyopathy and myopathy (II)
Infantile bilateral striatal necrosis and Leber's hereditary optic neuropathy (II)
Mitochondrial myopathies (I)
Benign infantile mitochondrial myopathy and cardiomyopathy (I)
Lethal infantile cardiomyopathy, X-linked or Barth's syndrome (I)
Benign infantile mitochondrial myopathy (I)
Childhood
Myoclonic epilepsy and ragged red fiber disease (II)
Mitochondrial encephalomyopathy, lactic acidosis, and strokelike episodes (II)
Chronic progressive external ophthalmoplegia, autosomal dominant (I)
Kearns-Sayre syndrome, autosomal dominant (I)
Others
Mitochondrial myopathy (II, IV)
Idiopathic dystonia (IV)
Myoneurogastrointestinal disorder and encephalopathy (IV)
Luft's disease (nonthyroid hypermetabolism) with generalized myopathy (IV)
Adolescence
Leber's hereditary optic neuropathy (II)
Kearns-Sayre syndrome (III)
Chronic progressive external ophthalmoplegia (III)
Others
Leber's hereditary optic neuropathy plus multiple system degeneration (II)
Inherited exertional myoglobinuria (I)
Adulthood
Malignant migraine (III)
Neuropathy, ataxia, retinitis pigmentosa syndrome (II)
Others
Hypertrophic cardiomyopathy and myopathy (II)
Mitochondrial myopathy (II, IV)

*Diseases are listed by order of most likely age presentation. The molecular genetics class is given in parentheses.

The neurological outcome in CPS and OTC deficiencies, even when treated appropriately, is only fair, with an average IQ score of 53 ± 6.[29] Spastic gait is the eventual neurological sequela. The relatively poor prognosis in these two diseases is due to the unusual severity of hyperammonemia, its early onset, and its difficult management with frequent recurrent hyperammonemic episodes. On the other hand, both argininosuccinicaciduria and citrullinemia have a better neurological prognosis if they are identified before the initial acute metabolic decompensation and treated appropriately.

No large-scale study for the neonatal screening of UCD has been reported. The short safety window requires screening procedures that provide rapid results. The method should also have low false-negative results and be able to identify the milder forms of the disease. The newly described MS/MS procedure using dried blood spots has been able to identify both citrullinemia and argininosuccinicaciduria before the emergence of hyperammonemia and thus is useful for such mass screening of these two disorders. When the MS/MS-based orotic acid screen becomes possible, OTC deficiency should also be screenable. At present, there is no possibility of screening for the CPS deficiency. All subsequent newborns in a family with a previous newborn with UCD should be treated as such, until proven otherwise.

Propionicacidemia

Of the disorders that present as devastating neonatal metabolic disease listed in Table 31–1, propionicacidemia and methylmalonicacidemia are encountered more frequently than the others.

Pathogenesis and Pathophysiology. Propionicacidemia was first described by Nyhan and associates in an infant with episodic ketoacidosis, elevated plasma glycine (ketotic hyperglycinemia), and protein intolerance.[30] The disease is caused by the deficiency of propionyl-CoA carboxylase (PCC) and the inheritance is autosomal recessive. Propionyl-CoA is generated through the breakdown of L-isoleucine, valine, threonine, methionine, cholesterol, and odd chain–numbered fatty acids. The enzyme is a polymer composed of nonidentical subunits (alpha and beta), with the native enzyme being a hexamer. Its cofactor is biotin, which is bound to an epsilon-amino group of lysine in the alpha subunit. The chromosomal locations of subunits are known, and complementary DNA is available (see Table 31–3). The deficiency of either subunit causes propionicacidemia.

Deficiency of PCC results in the accumulation of propionyl-CoA, which passes into circulation as propionylcarnitine or propionylglycine. Alternate pathways generate methylcitric acid, 3-hydroxypropionic acid, and tiglic acid. The toxic effects in CNS, bone marrow, and other tissues may be due to the accumulation of excess propionyl-CoA, depletion of the intramitochondrial free CoA pool, or toxic effects of compounds formed secondarily. Hyperglycinemia may be nonspecific and be due to inhibition of glycine cleaving enzyme. Hyperammonemia might be due to the inhibition of CPS I by the accumulating propionyl-CoA. Hypoglycemia might be due to the inhibition of pyruvate carboxylase or malate shuttle by elevated intramitochondrial propionyl-CoA. Despite the association of severe ketoacidosis during metabolic crisis, the mechanism of excess ketone body generation is not clear.

Epidemiology and Risk Factors. The disease may be rare in the United States and Canada, affecting 1 in 250,000 to 500,000 births. However, in the Middle East, particularly in Saudi Arabia, it may be as high as 1 in 1000 births.

Clinical Features and Associated Disorders. The disease manifests from newborn to late infancy with acute decompensation as seen in other organic acidurias. A prodrome of vomiting and refusal to feed progresses to lethargy and coma within days. The infant becomes quickly dehydrated and may experience clonic, myoclonic, or grand mal seizures. Physical examination reveals severe central hypotonia, both during and in between crises. The oral mucosa, angles of the mouth, and perineal area usually show evidence of candidiasis. Facial appearance is usually typical, with depressed nasal bridge and long philtrum; there may be associated abnormalities of the nipple.[31] Vomiting may be so severe that the infant might be operated on for pyloric stenosis or intestinal obstruction. Approximately 30 percent of the infants might present with immune deficiency, seizure disorder, or acute extrapyramidal signs such as choreoathetosis and dystonia.[31]

Differential Diagnosis. Two organic acidemias, methylmalonicacidemia and isovalericacidemia, in the neonate cause severe ketoacidosis, but both show increased muscle tone, whereas the tone in propionicacidemia is severely decreased. Patients with isovalericacidemia in crisis usually have a "sweaty feet" smell known to be associated with the disease. Propionicacidemia associated with immune deficiency might be confused with other disorders with immune deficiency.[31] The urine and blood in infants with multiple carboxylase deficiency will show other intermediates, such as methylcrotonylglycine or isovalerylcarnitine.

All neonates with organic acidemia, all infants with symptoms suggestive of immune deficiency in association with thrombocytopenia or ketosis, and all infants with idiopathic seizure disorder or acute extrapyramidal tract signs should be tested for propionicacidemia, particularly where its prevalence is high.

Evaluation. In early neonatal form, hyperammonemia is severe, usually exceeding 1 mM; in repeated episodes, it is usually moderate, rarely exceeding 300 μM; there is severe acidosis with accumulation of massive amounts of ketone bodies. Lactic acidosis is mild, rarely exceeding 6 mM. Hypoglycemia is usually moderate, rarely decreasing below 2 mM. Propionicacidemia has serious deleterious effects on bone marrow cells; neutropenia and thrombocytopenia are common. The platelet count usually drops several days after the onset of coma, while ketonuria is waning.[31] If it is not appreciated, the patient will have bleeding, particularly intracranially. Propionicacidemia causes severe depletion of T lymphocytes, and the patient will experience frequent infections and sepsis due to unusual gram-negative organisms or *Candida*.

The diagnosis is made by detecting 3-hydroxypropionic acid, propionylglycine, and methylcitrate in the urine by gas chromatography/mass spectrometry or by estimating elevated glycine and propionylcarnitine and decreased free carnitine levels in blood through MS/MS. Propionylcarnitine will be elevated both in propionicacidemia and methylmalonicacidemia; if desired, PCC activity can be measured in leukocytes and cultured fibroblasts. Biochemical findings of propionicacidemia are also seen in multiple carboxylase deficiency owing to holocarboxylase synthetase or biotinidase deficiencies.

Management. Treatment of initial or acute crisis is by administration of high amounts of glucose and bicarbonate, together with insulin drip, intravenous L-carnitine (50 to 75/mg/kg every 6 hours), and optimum antibiotic coverage to treat sepsis, if present. When amino acid mixtures with restricted BCAAs are available, they can be added to the total parenteral nutrition. Vomiting during or between crises is controlled by intravenous or oral administration of ondansetron. Platelet count should be monitored daily during acute episodes; when it decreases below 50,000/μL, platelet transfusions should be given. It is advisable to place a gastrostomy with fundoplication during the first few years to manage chronic anorexia and vomiting. Once the patient's condition has stabilized, oral feeding with special propionicacidemia formula restricted in isoleucine and valine should be resumed, together with oral carnitine, 100 to 200 mg/kg/day, and Polycitra solution, 2 to 4 mL/kg/day. The patient should never be permitted to fast because excessive odd chain–numbered fatty acids stored in the adipose tissue of propionicacidemia patients will mobilize and prompt a crisis. Metronidazole at a dose of 7.5 mg/kg/day should be used to decrease intestinal sources of propionate. Human growth hormone has been used as an adjunctive treatment. Sepsis, intracranial bleeding, and pancreatitis are dreaded complications.

Prognosis and Prevention. The prognosis in propionicacidemia is usually poor, with 50 percent of the patients dying and at least 25 percent showing mental retardation. Chronic hypotonia causes delayed acquisition of motor milestones. A routine neonatal screening test is not uniformly available. Preliminary results of a tandem mass spectrometry–based procedure indicated its value in detecting the disease within 24 to 48 hours, before the initial crisis.

Methylmalonicacidemia

Pathogenesis and Pathophysiology. Methylmalonicacidemia was first described by Oberholzer and co-workers in 1967 in infants critically sick with profound ketoacidosis and accumulation of methylmalonic acid in blood and urine.[32] The disease is a family of disorders caused by defective activity of methylmalonyl-CoA mutase (mutase [0] or mutase [–] complementation groups) or by defective intramitochondrial processing of vitamin B_{12} (cblA and cblB complementation groups). Other disorders of vitamin B_{12} will cause methylmalonicaciduria but are not associated with the periodic acidotic crisis of methylmalonicacidemia. They are associated with homocystinuria and are presented in the section on neurological diseases associated with homocystinuria.[33]

Genetic heterogeneity of the disease is evidenced by some phenotypes being responsive to large doses of vitamin B_{12} whereas no response is observed in others. The defects in the mutase are either (0) with no, or (–) with little, residual activity. The cofactor of the enzyme is 5′-deoxyadenosylcobalamin, and complementation groups cblA and cblB represent its defective synthesis. The toxic effects of intracellular accumulating methylmalonyl-CoA are similar to those of propionyl-CoA. All variants of methylmalonicacidemia are determined by autosomal recessive genes. The chromosome location of the mutase is known, and its complementary DNA is available (see Table 31–3).

Epidemiology and Risk Factors. The incidence of methylmalonicacidemia in the Massachusetts screening program was 1 in 48,000.[24] The disorder is more common in the Middle East, probably occurring in 1 in 1000 or 2000 births.

Clinical Features and Associated Disorders. The usual presentation in the neonate is as a typical organic acidemia with overwhelming illness, similar to the presentation of propionicacidemia or isovalericacidemia. These episodes recur either as a consequence of excessive protein intake or from increased protein catabolism through vomiting or infections. The acidosis is usually so severe that the patient will be admitted in shock and might die. Mucocutaneous candidiasis is common, disappearing with appropriate management. The patient usually has increased muscle tone. Seizures, when present, are clonic or myoclonic. As in propionicacidemia, patients with methylmalonicacidemia are prone to a variety of infections and sepsis by unusual organisms. Facial dysmorphia includes high forehead, epicanthal folds, and a triangular mouth. Between episodes, the patient will appear normal, with only mild or no developmental delay.

Patients who are poorly managed, particularly those with vitamin B_{12}–unresponsive variants, might suffer infarcts (metabolic stroke) in the globus pallidus or internal capsule and may develop hemiplegia and acute dystonia. Failure to thrive and failure of linear growth are common. As in propionicacidemia, anorexia and chronic vomiting are usual. The patient may develop acute pancreatitis.[34] Poorly managed children with methylmalonicacidemia will develop nephropathy due to tubulointerstitial nephritis or less often to urate nephropathy.

Differential Diagnosis. Most considerations listed for propionicacidemia are also true for methylmalonicacidemia; both propionicacidemia and isovalericacidemia present with massive ketonuria during crisis, the differential diagnosis of which is given in the previous section on propionicacidemia. The same criteria that are listed under propionicacidemia should be used to evaluate any child for possible methylmalonicacidemia.

Evaluation. The acute episode is characterized by severe acidosis with massive ketone body accumulation. Initial episode in a newborn is always accompanied by significant hyperammonemia, whereas blood ammonia values are only mildly elevated in repeated episodes. Hypoglycemia is usually moderate and rarely below 3 mM. There may be mild elevation of plasma glycine levels. During acute episodes, neutropenia and thrombocytopenia are common. Poorly controlled patients show hyperuricemia. A definite diagnosis of the disease is made by detecting massive methylmalonicaciduria; a neonate may excrete up to 1 g/day (normal adult, <5 mg/day). Plasma concentrations of methylmalonic acid in crisis may be as high as 0.2 to 2.5 mM (normally not detectable). Levels of propionylcarnitine in blood are elevated both during and between crises. Other organic acids in urine are those seen in propionicacidemia. Mutase activity may be measured in a variety of ways in specialized laboratories. The cblA and cblB mutants are identified by complementation studies. Clinical follow-up is by determination of blood levels of methylmalonic acid.

Management. The treatment of acute metabolic crisis is similar to those measures described for propionicacidemia. Exceptions for methylmalonicacidemia are the use of overhydration with adequate calories and no requirement for insulin drips. A patient with methylmalonicacidemia in crisis should be given excessive amounts of intravenous fluids, to clear the circulation from methylmalonic acid. Acidosis in methylmalonicacidemia is usually more severe than in propionicacidemia, requiring very large amounts of bicarbonate, which might quickly lead to hypernatremia. In such instances, tromethamine (Tham) 40 mL/kg/day in six divided doses may be used for 2 to 3 days. The intravenous use of carnitine shortens the crisis significantly.

All patients with methylmalonicacidemia are restricted in their intake of isoleucine, valine, threonine, and methionine, using the same diet for patients with propionicacidemia. Every patient with methylmalonicacidemia should be tested for response to vitamin B_{12} by administering daily 1 mg hydroxocobalamin intramuscularly. Patients with cblA, methylmalonicacidemia with mutase (–), and half of the patients with cblB or mutase (0) will respond to vitamin B_{12}. The outcome in the responsive patient is favorable, requiring less stringent control of protein intake. Protein requirement of vitamin B_{12}–unresponsive patients must be individualized, providing a minimal amount of the restricted amino acids that will permit growth but that will not lead to frequent decompensation. Generous amounts of calories are supplied through lipids and carbohydrates. Management of unresponsive methylmalonicacidemia is not easy, requiring enormous effort from physician, dietitian, and parents. Other therapeutic measures include metronidazole, 7.5 mg/kg/day; oral carnitine, 100 to 200 mg/kg/day; Shohl's solution, 2 to 4 mL/kg/day; and intramuscular hydroxocobalamin, 1 mg every other day. Patients with methylmalonicacidemia tend to be short and obese; human growth hormone has been used to increase growth and lean body mass and to decrease adipose tissue.

There is no treatment for renal disease due to interstitial nephritis. Allopurinol may be used in patients with high uricacidemia. Patients with methylmalonicacidemia who have basal ganglia infarcts might have cblC or cblD mutations, and homocystinuria should always be investigated in any patient with methylmalonicacidemia. No therapeutic measures, other than standard supportive therapy, are available for pancreatitis.

Prognosis. The addition of L-carnitine and metronidazole to the management of this disorder has changed the prognosis. Van der Meer and colleagues[35] have pointed out that although most patients before 1985 died, those after 1985, when these drugs were introduced, survived with improved general health. The lifestyle of a well-managed patient with methylmalonicacidemia will be normal, without mental retardation, or developmental or motor delay.

DISORDERS OF LATER INFANCY WITH RECURRENT METABOLIC CRISES

Late-Onset Urea Cycle Disorders

Pathogenesis and Pathophysiology. Late-onset disease has been described in patients with CPS, OTC, ASA synthetase, AS lyase, and arginase deficiencies. They will appear from the first year of life to adulthood with abrupt episodes of acute hyperammonemia. Initial crisis will occur usually when the infant is weaned from breast milk or from low-protein formulas to cow's milk formulas. Decompensation can also occur when the patient ingests a high protein load or experiences increased catabolism (e.g., infection). These episodes readily abate with cessation of protein intake.

Epidemiology and Risk Factors. Patients with a late-onset UCD are rare. The heterozygote female for OTC deficiency is at risk of developing symptoms; when a male infant with OTC deficiency is born, the mother has to be instructed for possible late-onset disease. Terheggen and associates, in 1969,[36] described argininemia in two sisters with spastic paraplegia (arginase deficiency). Arginase deficiency is rare. The mechanism for the toxicity of excess arginine is not known. Whether this is due to impaired neurotransmitter metabolism or to excess nitric oxide production from elevated arginine is not clear. Two forms of arginase are known: A-I and A-II. The A-I isozyme contributes 98 percent of the liver activity and is deficient in patients with argininemia. It is inherited as autosomal recessive.

Clinical Features and Associated Disorders. The symptoms are remarkably similar among various types of late-onset UCD. Sudden hyperammonemia leads to such neurological signs as seizures and apnea. It may be preceded by vomiting and lethargy progressing to disorientation, ataxia, amblyopia, and eventually coma. The late-onset CPS deficiency is rare. On the other hand, OTC deficiency may be mild in a male and may first manifest as early as 6 weeks or as late as 6 years. Since infections trigger hyperammonemia, late-onset OTC deficiency may be confused with Reye's syndrome. In symptomatic heterozygotes or mild OTC deficiency, growth and mental retardation are seen in half of patients. The use of valproate in OTC carriers may also cause liver toxicity. Late-onset OTC deficiency causes high mortality.

ASA synthetase deficiency was first reported in a 9-month-old girl with mental retardation. In Japan, a variant form of this disease is found to occur as late as 48 years of age. The symptoms in such cases are nonspecific and include bizarre behavior, psychotic episodes, delusions, hallucinations, insomnia, and endocrine disturbances, such as delayed menarche. ASA lyase deficiency may also occur late in infancy or adults. These cases present as mental retardation or ataxia, or the patient might be totally asymptomatic. This heterogeneity might be explained by the studies of McInnes and colleagues, which indicated at least 12 allelic mutations leading to extensive genetic heterogeneity.[37] Immunoblot analysis shows a wide variation in size and amount of enzyme protein in patients. The presentation of arginase deficiency is heterogeneous. Early development is usually unremarkable, but developmental delay and psychomotor retardation will definitely appear by 3 years. Progressive spastic diplegia is by far the most common motor deficit, seen by 5 years.[38] Seizures are present in half of the patients and are often generalized tonic-clonic. These symptoms improve or regress on dietary restriction of arginine.

Differential Diagnosis. The clinical presentations of all of late-onset UCDs are alike, because only the laboratory findings will identify exact diseases. Oroticaciduria is a common feature except for partial CPS I deficiency. By definition, the mother of a patient with OTC deficiency is a carrier; the presence of the mutant gene in other females related to the mother must be ruled out by allopurinol testing, provided that other diseases that give a positive result are absent.[39] Although it is the most common presenting symptom of arginase deficiency, spastic diplegia has many other causes (e.g., periventricular hemorrhage in a premature infant or hypoxic brain injury). In these conditions, spasticity is either static or progresses slowly. When spastic diplegia is progressive, familial spastic paraplegia, worsening of an existing hydrocephalus, spinal cord cysts, or tumors should be ruled out.

Hyperammonemia is encountered in other disorders. Reye's syndrome can be differentiated by the elevated transaminase and high plasma lysine levels. Patients with liver failure usually have elevated plasma methionine and tyrosine levels, which are not observed in UCDs of various types. Patients with valproate toxicity have elevated valproylcarnitine levels and deficiency of free carnitine in studies with tandem mass spectrometry.

Any infant or child who develops sudden lethargy or coma after a high-protein meal, infection, and prodrome of vomiting should be immediately evaluated for changes in blood gases, ammonia, lactic acid, and ketones. Arginase deficiency should be ruled out in all children with spastic diplegia. The definite diagnosis of a UCD, or an organic acidemia, will be reached by using high-pressure liquid chromatography, gas chromatography/mass spectrometry, and MS/MS techniques in blood and urine samples. Any infant or child with psychomotor retardation or seizures with no clear cause, or with progressive encephalopathy, should be studied by measurement of plasma amino acids and in some cases by the study of urinary organic acids.

Evaluation. The laboratory findings are the same as those described for neonatal onset UCD, except the hyperammonemia and elevation of specific amino acid and orotic acid levels are only prominent during the acute metabolic crisis. Both ASA synthetase and ASA lyase deficiencies are readily diagnosed by the plasma amino acid profile during the acute episode. Plasma arginine is elevated 2 to 10 times normal in arginase deficiency, and arginase in red blood cells is deficient. Hyperammonemia is not a constant feature of arginase deficiency but is found during a catabolic event (e.g., an infection or consumption of high-protein diet). A urine sample may show oroticaciduria and increased excretion of arginine.

Management. The treatment is approximately the same as that for UCD in the neonatal period: protein restriction, sodium phenylbutyrate, and L-arginine in doses previously described. Such patients should receive low-protein diets. No specific treatment exists for arginase deficiency. Reduction of protein intake might lead to improvement of the continued disease progression and at times dramatic resolution of the symptoms. Cognitive dysfunction appears to be amenable to diet therapy, and improvement of spasticity has been observed in 30 percent of patients with arginase deficiency. Late-onset UCDs show the same complications as described for the acute neonatal form.

Prognosis and Prevention. Prognosis depends on rapid identification and adequate management. A survey of 12 patients with late-onset ASA lyase deficiency indicated no eventual impairment in intellectual and psychomotor development. Arginase deficiency may be managed with success and arrest of the disease. All subsequent newborns of a family with UCD should be investigated for the disease. The maternally related female members of the extended family with OTC deficiency must be investigated for the presence of the mutated gene either by molecular genetic studies or by allopurinol loading.

PROGRESSIVE DISEASES OF INFANCY AND CHILDHOOD

A large number of amino and organic acid disorders appear primarily with neurological symptoms. Only four disorders, phenylketonuria (classic form and biopterin-dependent variant), homocystinuria, glutaricaciduria type 1, and biotinidase deficiency are presented here.

Deficiency of Phenylalanine Hydroxylase

Pathogenesis and Pathophysiology. Although phenylalanine hydroxylase (PAH) is a liver enzyme, the clinical manifestations of classic PKU relate to the CNS. There are no abnormal metabolites formed in classic PKU but only excessive amounts of normal compounds. Therefore, it is logical to assume that elevated levels of blood phenylalanine are responsible for the toxicity. Both animal models and magnetic spectroscopic studies in human brain indicate that phenylalanine levels exceeding 1.3 mM affect the brain metabolism adversely and account for acute phenylalanine toxicity. The threshold for chronic toxicity may be much lower. Acute and chronic adverse effects of high blood phenylalanine on brain can be prevented by high doses of BCAAs. Because both phenylalanine and BCAA share the same transport system, it is conceivable that mutual competition of neutral amino acids at the L-transport system may account for some of these toxic effects. Some patients diagnosed to have mild hyperphenylalaninemia in the past might have had carbinolamine dehydratase deficiency. Fair features and hypopigmentation are caused by the inhibition of tyrosinase by hyperphenylalaninemia. Location of the PAH gene is given in Table 31–3, and its complementary DNA is available.

Epidemiology and Risk Factors. The disease occurs at varying frequency. The highest frequency is in Turkey with 1 in 2600 births; it is lower among Japanese at 1 in 140,000. Ashkenazic Jews and Finns each have an incidence of 1 in 200,000 births.

Clinical Features and Associated Disorders. PKU usually manifests after 1 year of age as mental retardation. The late emergence of physical findings is the rationale for screening tests in all newborns. The safety window is approximately 6 weeks; by 1 year of age, the untreated child might lose 50 percent on IQ measurements. The infant is usually born prematurely and has a fair complexion and eczematoid lesions. Myoclonic seizures might occur as early as 4 months of age, and developmental delay appears between 6 and 18 months of age. Some patients develop normally until 1 year but then lose the milestones. Despite severe CNS involvement, no pyramidal or extrapyramidal signs are usually detected.

Children with untreated or poorly managed PKU usually end up in institutions. A review of 51 never-treated patients followed for more than 20 years indicated 25 percent had seizure disorders, half were profoundly retarded, and about half were moderately impaired.[40] Approximately two thirds of untreated patients develop microcephaly. Autistic behavior may also emerge. Aggressive, hyperactive behavior is common in poorly managed patients, which becomes less noticeable on lowering the blood phenylalanine level. In well-controlled patients, ingestion of food with high phenylalanine content at any time during life will cause confusion and a clear-cut fall in school performance.

Differential Diagnosis. In neonates with severe liver disease, levels of most plasma amino acids, notably tyrosine and methionine, are elevated; at times, that of phenylalanine may also be moderately high. Occasionally, isolated elevation of the blood phenylalanine level (up to 250 μM) will occur transiently in a normal neonate. In such infants, a repeat study at 4 to 6 weeks usually indicates normal phenylalanine, and the infant will not develop any signs of PKU later in life. The reasons for this transient hyperphenylalaninemia remain obscure.

Other common causes of childhood mental retardation include hyperprolinemia, homocystinuria, and fragile-X syndrome. Clinically, hyperprolinemia cannot be distinguished from mild PKU except by the amino acid analysis. Patients with a missed diagnosis of homocystinuria will have its classic phenotype, which is not observed in classic PKU. Patients with fragile-X syndrome are mostly males with typical facial features of the disease, severe autism, or mental retardation; molecular genetic studies identify the disease.

Many developing countries do not have a neonatal PKU screening program. Therefore, any infant with seizures, developmental delay, or fair features in a community with dark complexion, and any child with mental retardation, hyperactivity, and aggressive behavior should be evaluated for classic PKU.

Evaluation. The blood phenylalanine level is elevated (>120 μM), usually more than 1 mM, and the blood phenylalanine/tyrosine ratio is higher than 2, as determined by high-protein liquid chromatography or tandem mass spectrometry techniques. The green color produced by acidic ferric chloride in the urine of PKU patients is caused by the presence of phenylpyruvic acid. This compound is labile, disappearing from urine stored cold or frozen in 1 to 2 days. This test must be done on freshly collected urine. Computed tomography (CT) or magnetic resonance imaging (MRI) reveals demyelination or dysmyelination in central white matter, disappearing on treatment and reappearing if treatment is discontinued.

Prognosis and Prevention. Well-controlled studies indicate that prognosis is extremely rewarding if treatment is started in the first month of life. The North American Collaborative Study of patients to 12 years of age indicates that the longest treated patients who had phenylalanine values less than 900 μM had the best IQ and psychological test scores.[41] Numerous studies indicated deterioration of IQ, deviant EEG findings, and emergence of demyelination on MRI if the treatment is discontinued at or about school age. It is prudent to continue the treatment as long as possible, well into adolescence. Parents should be warned that a well-treated patient will function normally in daily life but may show significant deficits in conceptual, visuospatial, and language-related tasks; in reading and arithmetic skills; in attention span; and in problem-solving abilities.

Classic PKU was one of the first inborn errors of metabolism for which neonatal screening was applied.[3] Hyperphenylalaninemia and disturbed ratio of phenylalanine/tyrosine in a neonate with classic PKU may be apparent as early as 24 hours but definitely by 3 to 7 days of life. Given the 6-week safety window, neonatal screening for PKU may be done during the first month. Any positive screening result should be rechecked within 1 month. The conventional procedure for PKU screening is the Guthrie test. The problem of false-positive results and the anxiety created in the family recalled for repeat testing led to the exploration of other techniques. More recently, MS/MS-based screening procedures have been described that have less problems with false-negative and false-positive results, because, in addition to phenylalanine estimation, they provide an accurate phenylalanine/tyrosine ratio.[1, 2]

The principle of treatment is to restrict dietary intake of phenylalanine. There are numerous formulas for this purpose that have been in use since the mid-1950s. Treatment should be monitored by monthly or bimonthly measurement of plasma amino acids, to ensure that phenylalanine and other essential amino acids are not lower than normal. Given the beneficial effects of BCAAs in preventing the adverse CNS manifestations of hyperphenylalaninemia, they may be used to supplement the diet. Patients with PKU should avoid consuming food or drinks that contain aspartame, an artificial sweetener (*N*-aspartylphenylalanine), because intestinal hydrolysis liberates phenylalanine.

Successful management of many females with PKU has resulted in normal lifestyle, marriages, and child bearing. Infants born to mothers with PKU, however, have numerous congenital defects, such as microcephaly, impaired somatic growth, and heart disease.[42] Because similar defects are not seen among offspring of fathers with PKU, it is apparent that high blood phenylalanine levels in the mother are the cause. Although no threshold is agreed on, fetal outcome is satisfactory if the maternal blood phenylalanine levels are maintained at less than 600 μM throughout the pregnancy.

Biopterin-Dependent Hyperphenylalaninemia

Pathogenesis and Pathophysiology. Defective synthesis of biopterin (BH_4) causes disruption in several biochemical functions. Deficiencies of the first two steps, that is, guanosine triphosphate cyclohydrolase (GTP-CH) and 6-pyruvoyl-tetra-hydropterin synthase (6PTS), are known as synthetic defects. The hydroxylase reacts with BH_4, converting it to its hydroxy form 4α-carbinolamine, which is then dehydrated by primapterin carbinolamine dehydratase (PCD) to quininoid dihydrobiopterin, which is labile and must be reduced back to BH_4 through a reaction that uses reduced nicotinamide adenine dinucleotide and is catalyzed by dihydropteridine reductase (DHPR). The deficiencies of the latter two enzymes are known as recycling defects. Because primapterin is excreted in PCD deficiency, the disease is also called primapterinuria. BH_4 is a cofactor for enzymes of the initial step in dopamine and serotonin synthesis; when it is not available, neurotransmitter and autonomic function, both in the CNS and periphery, are disturbed. In addition, BH_4 is a cofactor for the generation of nitric oxide in the CNS, which is a neurotransmitter/modulator. Deficiency of BH_4 causes severe autonomic irregularities and mental retardation and, ultimately, is not compatible with life. Severe cardiopulmonary dysrhythmia, fluctuating blood pressure, sleep irregularities, and early unexpected death may be explained by these considerations. Because 4α-carbinolamine can be spontaneously dehydrated, PCD deficiency does not cause severe disease. In BH_4-dependent PKU, neurological manifestations are severe in the presence of mild hyperphenylalaninemia, suggesting that trace BH_4 levels are sufficient to promote the phenylalanine hydroxylase reaction in liver but not high enough for adequate hydroxylation of tyrosine and tryptophan in the CNS. All four diseases are inherited as autosomal recessive. The location of their genes is shown in Table 31–3.

Epidemiology and Risk Factors. Hyperphenylalaninemia due to BH_4 deficiency is rare and accounts for 2 percent of all PKU cases. An international database in 1995 for abnormal BH_4 metabolism indicated the following[43]: 12 patients with GTP-CH deficiency, 182 with 6PTS deficiency, 87 with DHPR deficiency, and 12 with PCD deficiency. The overall frequency is estimated to be 1 in 10^6 births. In some parts of the world these defects occur more frequently (e.g., 10 percent in Italy, 15 percent in Turkey, 19 percent in Taiwan, and 68 percent in Saudi Arabia).

Clinical Features and Associated Disorders. The signs seen in this disorder are remarkably similar except for PCD deficiency.[44] The classic presentation is an infant, usually of low birth weight, who develops normally for 2 to 3 months. Then myoclonic seizures appear approximately at 3 months, probably due to serotonin depletion. Bradykinesia is apparent particularly when the infant is naked. The infant lies expressionless. Initially, there may be hypotonia, but soon after "lead pipe" or "cogwheel" rigidity appears (Fig. 31–3). These are parkinsonian features caused by deficient dopamine. In fact, extensor posturing of the extremities, opisthotonic arching of the back, and pronation of hands are common. Oculogyric crisis, involuntary dystonic movements, and tremors may be observed. Feeding is difficult owing to difficulties in swallowing, and the patient drools because of inability to manage secretions. Early failure to thrive and fair features of PKU are observed. Development arrests at 2 to 3 months, unless the disorder is treated. The patient suffers from severe bronchopneumonia from respiratory irregularities and is often admitted to an intensive care unit for cardiorespiratory difficulties, usually dying before 5 years of age. Those children who survive remain profoundly retarded. Episodes of hyperthermia without infection, fluctuating high blood pressure, and reversed diurnal rhythm of sleep have been described. Deficiency of DHPR, in general, shows a more severe progression of the disease, whereas GTP-CH deficiency might be milder and missed in some instances. The clinical picture of PCD deficiency is essentially that of a mild PKU, and it is not unusual for such a patient to be classified as having transient hyperphenylalaninemia.

Differential Diagnosis. All infants with parkinsonian signs, myoclonic seizures, unexpected fair features, unexplained failure to thrive, unexplained severe bronchopneumonia or cardiopulmonary arrest, unexplained hyperthermia, and fluctuating blood pressure should be studied for the presence of 6PTS and DHPR deficiencies. Blood amino acids, particularly phenylalanine, should be determined in all children with mental retardation. Even when mild hyperphenylalaninemia is found, BH_4 loading, DHPR activity in red blood cells, and pterin measurement in urine should be performed.

Evaluation. Hyperphenylalaninemia is usually not as severe as in classic PKU. The end products of catecholamine and serotonin metabolism in cerebrospinal fluid (CSF) and urine, such as 5-hydroxyindoleacetic, homovanillic, and vanillylmandelic acids, are considerably lower than normal. The characteristic findings are in the urinary pterin metabolites. In GTP-CH deficiency, both neopterin and biopterin are low in the urine. In 6PTS deficiency, the urine neopterin level is very high and that of biopterin is very low or

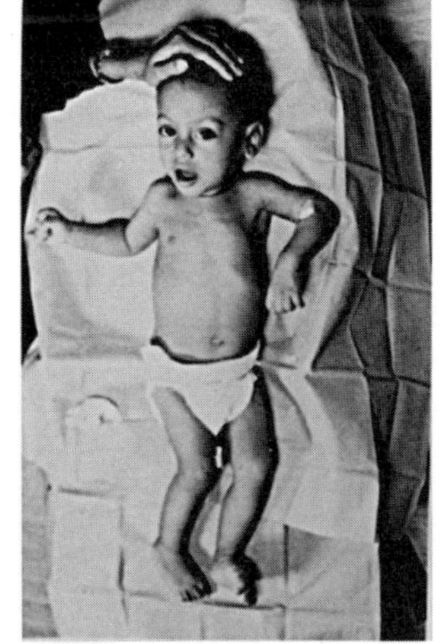

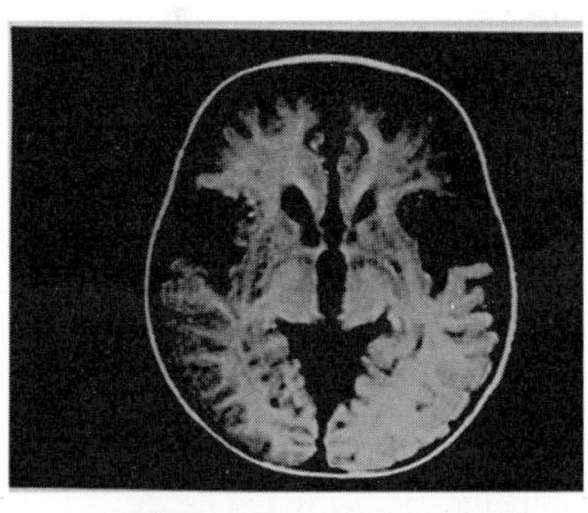

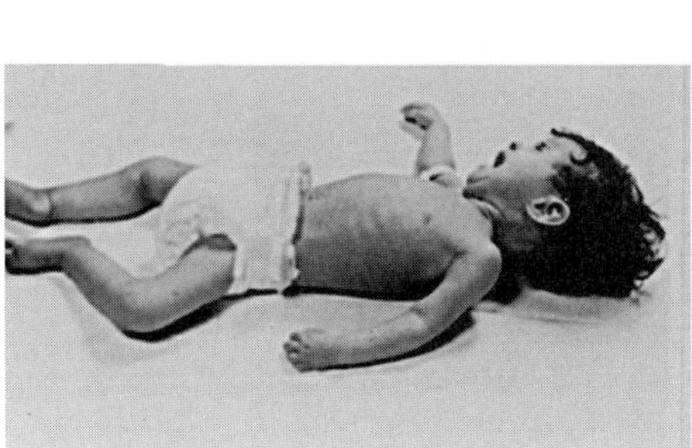

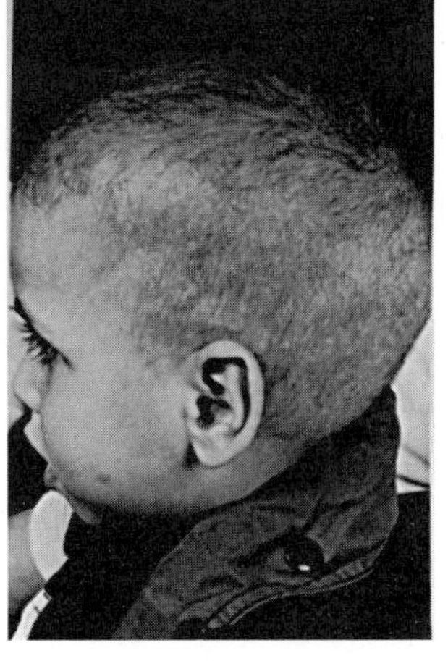

FIGURE 31–3. Glutaricaciduria, biotinidase deficiency, and biopterin-dependent phenylketonuria. Clockwise from left upper corner. Infant with glutaricaciduria type 1 (GAT1) showing dystonic posture and rigidity in flexion. MRI of the brain showing open operculum sign and frontotemporal atrophy in infant with GAT1. Alopecia in a biotinidase-deficient 9-month-old infant with frequent myoclonic seizures from age 3 months. Infant with biopterin-dependent phenylketonuria due to 6-pyruvoyl-tetra-hydropterin synthase (6PTS) deficiency showing dystonic grimacing and fisting of hands and hypotonic pithed frog posture of legs.

undetectable, leading to a greatly elevated neopterin/biopterin ratio. The urinary excretion of pterins may range from normal to massively elevated in DHPR deficiency. In PCD, an unusual pterin, primapterin, is detected in the urine. The pterin assay has been adapted to be used with dried urine spots on filter paper.[45]

Another option is to perform a BH_4 loading dose, given 2 mg/kg IV or 7.5 to 20 mg/kg orally in divided doses. This will lower plasma phenylalanine to within normal limits within 8 to 12 hours if a patient has BH_4-dependent PKU. In 6PTS deficiency, the excretion of neopterin will rapidly decrease on BH_4 loading. The BH_4 loading must be done while the patient is on a normal diet. An occasional patient with 6PTS deficiency with normal CSF finding but abnormal plasma and urine phenylalanine and pterin values has been described. This milder form of the disease is called the peripheral type. It is important to measure the red blood cell DHPR activity to rule out DHPR deficiency, because a BH_4 loading test might miss an occasional patient. Levels of prolactin are elevated in various forms of BH_4 deficiency and might provide a rapid clue to the presence of these diseases.

Management. The patients with BH_4 deficiency should be treated with BH_4, which is available from either Milupa, Hillington, Middlesex, UK, or Schirks Laboratories, Jona, Switzerland. The standard therapy is 20 mg/kg/day BH_4 given in three to four equal doses. All patients with proven diagnosis should be immediately placed on neurotransmitter precursors, which do not require hydroxylation. These are levodopa, 15 mg/kg/day and L5-hydroxytryptophan, 4 mg/kg/day, together with 2 to 4 mg/kg/day carbidopa. The best results are obtained when neurotransmitter therapy is combined with BH_4. Therapeutic results should be followed by plasma phenylalanine, prolactin and, when possible, urine pterins. Additional supplementation of folate is given in DHRP deficiency because it results in reduction of synthesis of tetrahydrofolate.

Prognosis and Prevention. Certainly the majority of the patients with 6PTS deficiency will respond well to the therapy and will grow as normal children. However, prognosis in all BH_4-dependent PKU is guarded, particularly in DHPR deficiency, because many patients have neurological impairment despite vigorous and early therapy. The hyperphenylalaninemia of various forms of BH_4 deficiency can be identified in routine screening tests; however, the diagnosis in a patient with GTP-CH deficiency was missed in the neonatal screening. Prenatal diagnosis has been achieved in DHPR and 6PTS deficiencies.

Homocystinuria: Cystathionine ß-Synthase Deficiency

Pathogenesis and Pathophysiology. Two important groups of diseases involving methionine metabolism are (1) homocystinuria due to the deficiency of cystathionine β-synthase (CBS) and (2) homocystinuric syndromes with abnormalities of folate or vitamin B_{12} metabolism with or without methylmalonicaciduria.[46] CBS deficiency, commonly known as homocystinuria, was reported in 1962.[47] The recognition of homocystinuric syndromes is more recent.[48]

The primary metabolic consequence of CBS deficiency is intracellular homocysteine accumulation. The cells then excrete the compound to plasma where the elevated levels exist either as free or as oxidized to homocystine, to mixed disulfides with cysteine, or with other sulfhydryl groups in proteins. When homocysteine is elevated in plasma, homocystine is excreted through the urine. Homocysteine is located at the crossroads of important biochemical reactions.

Homocysteine is an end product of biochemical reactions that utilize methylation. Biological methylations are achieved by activated methionine, S-adenosylmethionine. Once the methyl group is transferred, remaining S-adenosylhomocysteine is hydrolyzed into homocysteine and adenosine. Homocysteine must then either be reconverted into methionine or condensed with serine by CBS into cystathionine and excreted. These two paths are catalyzed by several different enzymes. The cystathionine synthesis is catalyzed by CBS, whereas the remethylation through the use of methyltetrahydrofolate is catalyzed by 5-methyltetrahydrofolate–homocysteine S-methyltransferase (methionine synthetase) or through other enzymes from betaine if the latter compound is used as a therapeutic agent. When CBS is deficient, homocysteine is elevated and thus hypermethioninemia and homocystinuria ensue; urine contains no cystathionine. Hypermethioninemia is due to increased methylation of homocysteine in liver by folate-dependent methylating enzymes. Numerous physiological disturbances account for the symptoms of CBS deficiency.

High homocysteine may cause undesirable disulfide crosslinkages, disrupting fibrillin. Among other vasoactive properties, homocysteine impairs the protein C–activating cofactor activity of thrombomodulin, and this feature may be involved in thrombotic events. In addition, both L-homocysteic acid and homocysteine-sulfinic acids derived from homocysteine are present in the urine of CBS-deficient patients. These two compounds are potent agonists for *N*-methyl-D-aspartate (NMDA) receptors and might cause neuronal damage as a result of excessive stimulation of NMDA receptors. Two primary groups of patients are identified, based on their response to pyridoxine. In pyridoxine-responsive patients, a small residual activity of CBS is present that is enhanced by large doses of pyridoxine. Although the control activity does not attain control levels, it becomes sufficient to maintain a low level of the homocysteine pool. The CBS gene is mapped (see Table 31–3).

In 1967, it was shown that the biochemical abnormalities in some patients with CBS deficiency could be corrected by administering large doses of pyridoxine.[49] Large international surveys indicate that approximately half of the patients are pyridoxine responsive. These patients are clinically heterogeneous, with some showing a clear-cut response and others a less dramatic response. Even the most responsive patient will have elevated plasma methionine and homocystinuria when loaded with methionine; therefore, they should be kept under continuous treatment.

Because of interactions between folate and vitamin B_{12} with homocysteine metabolism, homocystinuria occurs in acquired or inherited disorders of folate or vitamin B_{12}.

Epidemiology and Risk Factors. The cumulative frequency of CBS deficiency for countries with screening programs is 1 in 344,000. In parts of New South Wales in Australia this might be as high as 1 in 65,000 to 75,000. The disease is common in the Middle East, possibly occurring in 1 in 1000 to 2000 births. Approximately 75 patients with cblC and 30 with methylenetetrahydrofolate reductase deficiency are known.

Clinical Features and Associated Disorders. The phenotype of few diseases is as impressive as that of CBS deficiency, because numerous organs are involved. The main systems affected are the eye, the vascular system, the CNS, and the skeletal system.

EYE. Dislocation of the lens, ectopia lentis, is a constant feature but occurs usually after 2 years. The rate of lens dislocation is higher among patients who do not respond to pyridoxine. Marked myopia is associated with the loosened or subluxated lens. Cataracts, acute pupillary block glaucoma, and retinal degeneration may be additional complications.

VASCULAR SYSTEM. Thromboembolic phenomena are dreaded complications of the disease, accounting for morbidity and mortality (see Fig. 31–1). They can occur at any age and in any vessel. Thrombosis in CNS causes neurological signs, such as hemiplegia, dystonia, or seizures; in the eye, optic atrophy; and in the kidney, severe hypertension. The risk of thrombosis is less in pyridoxine-responsive patients.

CENTRAL NERVOUS SYSTEM. Mental retardation and neurological abnormalities are the main features. The developmental delay is usually apparent by the second year of life. Patients with pyridoxine-responsive disease are less affected. The degree of mental retardation varies between severe to normal, and it is not unusual to encounter an occasional pyridoxine-unresponsive child with normal or high IQ. Besides the neurological findings related to thrombotic events in the CNS, approximately 20 percent of the patients will suffer from seizures, mainly generalized convulsions. It is common for these individuals later in life to suffer from episodic depression, behavior disorders, and other personality disorders.

SKELETAL FINDINGS. Osteoporosis is a common late complication, and half of the patients will show some evidence of it by 20 years of age. It is more severe and appears earlier in pyridoxine-nonresponsive patients. Biconcave vertebrae are seen. The maturation of the skeleton is abnormal and leads to lengthening of the long bones (dolichostenomelia), which accounts for the marfanoid appearance of patients.

OTHER FEATURES. Females with CBS deficiency experience frequent fetal loss. The offspring of men with CBS deficiency are normal. The risk factors for early vascular disease among heterozygotes and those individuals with mild homocystinemia have been investigated in detail. Since the pioneering publication by Wilcken and Wilcken,[50] numerous reports and reviews support that preceding homocystinemia in normal subjects with mild homocystinemia may be responsible for vascular disease. However, most obligate heterozygotes do not have overt clinical atherosclerotic disease, and more studies are needed to conclude the risk factor for carriers.

Differential Diagnosis. Several symptoms of CBS are shared by other disorders. Lens abnormalities are encountered in a number of ophthalmological diseases. Another abnormality of sulfur metabolism, sulfite oxidase deficiency, also causes ectopia lentis. Thromboembolic phenomena and mental retardation are encountered in a large number of clinical conditions and are not detailed. The neurological symptoms of folate or vitamin B_{12} metabolic abnormalities are not specific. Their presence is first suspected either by macrocytic anemia or by a positive urine homocystine test.

All children with lens, vascular, and CNS signs of CBS deficiency should be evaluated for homocystinuria. Any child with macrocytic anemia or neurological symptoms associated with a positive urine homocystine test should be evaluated for a possible defect in folate or vitamin B_{12} metabolism.

Evaluation. The most consistent laboratory feature is homocystinuria. An easy test is urinary sodium nitroprusside reaction. If positive, homocystine should be identified by other procedures because most sulfur amino acids will yield a positive test. Some patients with pyridoxine-responsive disease will show marked responses to low doses of pyridoxine and the urine in such patients might give false-negative results. In most patients, blood methionine levels will be significantly elevated, which is a clue to CBS deficiency, unless a liver pathological process exists. Whereas in CBS deficiency homocystinuria is accompanied by elevated blood levels of methionine, other diseases associated with homocystinuria have accompanied hypomethioninemia and cystathioninuria. Some of these disorders show other laboratory findings, such as methylmalonicaciduria and megaloblastic anemia.

Management. The medical management of CBS deficiency requires correction of biochemical abnormalities, with the goal of preventing or halting the disease or improving the reversible clinical manifestations. This is best achieved in a newborn before any complication of the disease becomes apparent. Patients who are pyridoxine responsive require the administration of large amounts of pyridoxine. A patient should not be considered unresponsive until a dose of 500 to 1000 mg/day is given for several weeks. The dose of pyridoxine recommended varies from as little as 25 mg/day to as large as 1200 mg/day. The neuropathy and ataxia resulting from the toxic effect of pyridoxine is not encountered in doses of 500 mg/day for at least as long as 2 years. Although it is not uniformly agreed on, pyridoxine-responsive patients should be given a methionine-restricted, cystine-supplemented diet, since they have reduced tolerance for high doses of methionine. Folate repletion may be necessary for pyridoxine responsiveness, and folate, 5 to 10 mg/day, should be provided. The preventive use of anticoagulants such as aspirin is also controversial; if used they should be given in small quantities, such as 325 mg/day or less to an adolescent.

Patients who are not pyridoxine responsive and who are diagnosed later during childhood should be treated with large doses of betaine, 50 to 100 mg/kg/day. The compound increases the rate of homocysteine methylation by the action of a liver enzyme, betaine homocysteine methyltransferase. It reduces plasma homocystine and increases methionine. In conjunction with diet therapy, it usually improves the clinical condition and retards the progression of disease. The best results are obtained in newborns detected to have the disease by providing a diet restricted in methionine and supplemented with cystine. At least four such formulas are commercially available and, when used together with betaine, ensure normal growth and psychological development. Experience is limited for the outlook of pyridoxine-responsive infants identified neonatally.

Prognosis and Prevention. Untreated patients with CBS deficiency die as a result of thromboembolic phenomena; mortality is much less in pyridoxine-responsive patients. The outcome is excellent in early-diagnosed and treated pyridoxine-responsive children. The mental development is normal, and thromboembolic phenomena are minimal or absent. The best one can hope for in a pyridoxine-unresponsive patient diagnosed late is to arrest the progression of the disease by treatment. By strict adherence to the therapy outlined, it is possible to normalize mental development in neonatally diagnosed pyridoxine-unresponsive patients.

In other syndromes associated with homocystinuria, the prognosis depends on early detection, early treatment, and the degree of the responsiveness of the disease to treatment. The neurological prognosis for the cblG and methylenetetrahydrofolate reductase–deficient group is not as good as the others. Approximately 50 million newborns in the world, mainly in Japan and the United States, have been screened for CBS deficiency. The disease may be screened through blood methionine or urine homocystine tests. The drawback of methionine-based screening is that only a few patients with the pyridoxine-responsive variant have so far been identified, whereas these are the patients that will benefit most from early detection. Screening based on homocystine detection in urine has also been disappointing. The efficiency and false-positive and false-negative results of screening tests for CBS deficiency have not yet been settled.

Disorders of Lysine and Tryptophan Metabolism: Glutaricaciduria Type 1

Pathogenesis and Pathophysiology. Glutaricaciduria type 1 (GAT1) (see Fig. 31–3) was first described in 1975[51] and is caused by deficiency of glutaryl-CoA dehydrogenase (GCDH), which is on the catabolic pathways of L-lysine and L-tryptophan. The presence of glutaric, 3-hydroxyglutaric, and glutaconic acids in urine is pathognomonic for the disease. Excess glutaryl-CoA leads to the formation of glutarylcarnitine, which can be detected both in blood and urine. The concentration of acids in the blood is not high enough to disturb the acid-base balance; because there is no inhibition of ketone body and lactate utilization, or of urea formation, the disease does not usually cause acidosis or hyperammonemia. Its significant metabolic sequel is solely in the CNS. Chromosome location of GCDH is shown in Table 31–3.

The mechanism of toxicity of glutaric acid in the CNS, particularly to the striatal system, is not well understood. Neither the degree of GCDH deficiency nor the amount of glutaric aciduria correlates with the severity of the disease. Glutaric acid is toxic toward striatal cells in culture. Glutaric, glutaconic, and 3-hydroxyglutaric acids are competitive inhibitors of glutamate decarboxylase (GAD), the enzyme responsible for gamma-aminobutyric acid formation. Whether inhibition of GAD by itself accounts for neuronal death is uncertain. The block in GCDH might shift tryptophan metabolism to quinolinic acid, which is a potent neurotoxin.[52] Autopsy of brain in advanced cases shows severe neuronal loss and fibrous gliosis in basal ganglia, with some spongy degeneration of cortical white matter, indicating these as the target areas.

Epidemiology and Risk Factors. The disease is not rare but might be underdiagnosed. Over 100 patients have been described, 20 of whom are from the Middle East. It is estimated to affect 1 in 30,000 persons in Sweden. It is especially common in consanguineous communities, such as in Saudi Arabia, among the Saulteaux/Ojibway Indians in Canada, and in the United States among the Amish community in Pennsylvania.

Clinical Features and Associated Disorders. The infant is normal at birth, and the only detectable symptom might be macrocephaly. A typical history is rapid neurological deterioration and loss of developmental milestones after an infectious episode, which is usually mistaken for meningitis or encephalitis because a slight increased CSF protein level is usual. Seizures, dystonia (see Fig. 31–3), and choreoathetosis appear soon after and worsen, leading to a diagnosis of choreoathetoid cerebral palsy or postencephalitic cerebral palsy. Repeated viral infections each cause further deterioration, and the patient will eventually be severely crippled. Almost all patients show absolute or relative macrocephaly. In some patients, the clinical picture will be mild and no further deterioration will occur, particularly if no intercurrent viral infection takes place. An occasional infant identified through screening will show no or minimal neurological signs and will have macrocephaly and neuroradiological findings of GAT1, suggesting prenatal onset of the disease.

Evaluation. All infants with acute or chronic extrapyramidal signs should be investigated for GAT1. Results of routine blood cell counts, blood chemistries, and amino acid determinations are normal even in the most advanced patient; unless the neurologist suspects and orders special tests, the disease remains undiagnosed. The characteristic biochemical findings are the presence of glutaric, 3-hydroxyglutaric, and glutaconic acids in the urine and of glutarylcarnitine in blood and urine. Use of MS/MS to detect glutarylcarnitine in blood and urine has proved to be an unfailingly rewarding means of diagnosis.

The neuroradiological studies reveal a widened sylvian fissure or the "open opercular" sign (see Fig. 31–3), dense basal ganglia, total atrophy of the caudate heads in advanced disease, and evidence of mild white matter disease in the centrum ovale.[53] These occur before the emergence of neurological deterioration. Findings on MRI or CT of the brain are characteristic of GAT1, and an experienced neuroradiologist will report the presence of the disease before the results of biochemical tests become available.

Differential Diagnosis. Among infants and young children with striatal necrosis, some have other definable causes, such as 3-methylglutaconicaciduria, propionicacidemia, or oxidative phosphorylation disease. Their clinical and laboratory presentations are different, and macrocephaly and the wide opercular signs are absent. Other causes of macrocephaly in infancy include Canavan's disease, Alexander's disease, and L-2 hydroxyglutaricaciduria. These conditions are progressive pyramidal tract diseases and should not be confused with GAT1.

Management. Treatment may be rewarding if initiated before the clinical manifestations of the disease. The treatment of choice is reducing lysine and tryptophan intake. Such formulas are available. The medications used are L-carnitine orally, 100 to 200 mg/kg/day; riboflavin, 50 mg/kg/day; and baclofen, 5 to 10 mg three times daily. The exact mechanism of action of baclofen is not known, but it has been effective in some instances. In one patient, vigabatrin caused significant clinical improvement. All intercurrent infections, particularly those with viral etiology, demand immediate intervention by administering L-carnitine intravenously (50 to 100 mg/kg repeated every 6 hours) and providing adequate calories through glucose and insulin drip. These treatments will be of little value in patients who have already suffered significant damage to striatum.

Prognosis and Prevention. Prognosis is poor for patients who have been diagnosed late, although the treatment might slow the progression of the disease. Limited information is available for patients diagnosed early. Prenatal diagnosis of the disease is made through study of organic acids in amniotic fluid or by measuring GCDH in cultured amniotic cells. MS/MS-based neonatal screening identifies GAT1.

Biotinidase Deficiency

Biotinidase deficiency was first recognized in 1983, among patients with late-onset multiple carboxylase deficiency.[54] The worldwide frequency among 8 million newborns is 1 in 112,000.[55] Biotin is the cofactor for such carboxylases as propionyl-CoA, 3-methylcrotonyl-CoA, acetyl-CoA, and pyruvate carboxylase. The most important source of biotin is through biotinidase; hence, when biotinidase is absent, a state of biotin deficiency gradually emerges. Biotinidase activity in brain is very low,[56] and the brain totally depends on the transfer of biotin across the blood-brain barrier. When biotin is deficient, pyruvate carboxylase in the CNS might decrease, leading to localized lactic acidosis. Biotinidase-deficient patients suffer from central deafness before treatment, and hearing usually does not improve after treatment. The reason for selective targeting of the auditory center is unknown. Alopecia (see Fig. 31–3) and dermatitis in these patients are possible owing to depletion of fatty acids as a result of deficient acetyl-CoA carboxylase activity. Approximately 55 percent of patients develop clonic or myoclonic seizures, hypotonia, and developmental delay between 3 and 6 months of age. Hearing abnormality coincides with the emergence of seizures. Dermatitis, visual problems, and ataxia are the final events. The changes in acylcarnitines and organic acids appear only during acute decompensation, and the disease cannot be identified through these compounds. Individuals with partial deficiency might be at risk only for cutaneous symptoms. Immunological dysfunction manifests as candidal dermatitis as described for propionicacidemia and methylmalonicacidemia.

Colorimetric and fluorometric procedures are available for measurement in serum. Prenatal diagnosis has not yet been reported. During acute decompensation, the blood acylcarnitine and urine organic acid profiles are the same as seen in holocarboxylase synthetase (HCS) deficiency. Biotin-responsive mild forms of HCS deficiency and milder forms of propionicacidemia must be ruled out by clinical and laboratory observations. Alopecia and rash can be encountered in deficiency of zinc or essential fatty acids. Biotinidase deficiency might be confused with severe combined immune deficiency.

Deafness persists even in a well-treated patient, but alopecia and other symptoms disappear with treatment. As little as 5 to 30 mg of biotin will be curative.

Inherited Disorders Related to Vitamin Metabolism

Certain disorders result from inborn errors of metabolism involving vitamins. Some of these disorders lead to severe neurological crippling unless recognized early and treated. Three such disorders that are of neurological interest will be discussed.

BIOTIN-RESPONSIVE ENCEPHALOPATHY

Pathogenesis and Pathophysiology. This is a novel disease described recently.[57, 58] Recently, a gene locus on chromosome 4p has been shown. It is thought to be related to the biotin transporter in the brain (Gusella, personal communications).

Epidemiology and Risk Factors. The disease has been described among consanguineous communities of the Arabian peninsula and Middle East[57] (Saudi Arabia, Yemen, and Syria). Initially 10 patients were reported. More recently five more Saudi children with the disease were added to this list. The clinic files suggest that one or two new patients are diagnosed per year.

Clinical Features and Associated Disorders. This disorder usually presents with confusion, dysarthria, and signs of a subacute encephalopathy between ages 5 and 14 years. It evolves into rapid coma with seizures, pyramidal and extrapyramidal signs, such as facial paralysis, severe cogwheel rigidity, dystonic and oculogyric posturing, and choreoathetosis. The eye-grounds remain normal. In the Arab families in which the disease was described, 80 percent of the parents were products of first-cousin marriages, and the remaining of second-cousin marriages. When untreated the disease was lethal. In 80 percent of the families, additional childhood deaths could be attributed to this disease retrospectively, although the diagnosis was not specifically established. There were no significant co-morbid associations; in one family a brother had a tic disorder, in another the patient had a complex congenital heart disease, and in a third family there was a brother with mental retardation of unknown cause. This disease presents as an acute encephalopathic crisis that resolves within 1 or 2 days when the appropriate treatment is given. The acute neurological manifestations reappear within 1 month if treatment is discontinued. The longest follow-up is now 15 years. All of the patients except one remain neurologically healthy on treatment, and the older ones are either university students or are leading a successful professional life.

Differential Diagnosis. Several diseases of childhood should be considered, including DOPA-responsive dystonia,[59] idiopathic dystonia of childhood, and childhood parkinsonism resembling DOPA-responsive disease but without diurnal variation and only a mild response to DOPA.[60] Postinfectious benign acute basal ganglia destruction is preceded and precipitated by an infectious process. It is an extrapyramidal tract disease sharing many features of biotin-responsive encephalopathy, except chorea and seizures are absent. It usually disappears within 1 month. Finally, biotinidase deficiency[61] usually manifests with myoclonic seizures in early infancy with hair loss, rapid hearing loss, and dermatitis. In contrast to biotin-responsive encephalopathy, at presentation there are no extrapyramidal signs in biotinidase deficiency. The diagnosis is easily and rapidly diagnosed by the determination of biotinidase in serum.

Evaluation. The evaluation usually starts with the clinical assessment and a consideration of the differential diagnosis for other childhood extrapyramidal diseases. In this disorder, all chemistries, lactate, pyruvate, ammonia, amino acid profile, cholesterol, uric acid, very long-chain fatty acids, phytanic acid, biotinidase, MS/MS studies for blood, urine organic acids by gas chromatography/mass spectroscopy (GC/MS), EEG, brain stem auditory evoked potentials, visual evoked potentials, nerve conduction studies, electromyogram (EMG), and in fibroblasts, pyruvate carboxylase and propionyl-CoA carboxylase activities are unremarkable. The pathognomonic finding is the MRI of the brain that shows degeneration of the centers of the caudate heads and of putamina (Fig. 31–4). During an acute crisis, central white matter disease as well as these structures show edema. Upon treatment, the changes observed in the basal ganglia persist despite total resolution of the neurological manifestations. In the oldest patient, now 23 years of age, despite a normal neurological status, these changes are still present with no further deterioration.

Management The treatment is oral biotin 10 to 15 mg/kg/day. If detected early, even the most severe neurological signs will disappear within 24 to 48 hours with a return to normalcy. This response is not observed in any other basal ganglia disease of childhood. The symptoms will reappear within 1 month if the patient discontinues this treatment.

Prognosis and Prevention. The prognosis depends on provision of biotin. A missed diagnosis for more than 7 to 10 days after the first crisis or many repeated neurological crises due to noncompliance with biotin treatment results in permanent neurological crippling. As revealed by the family histories, a prolonged course of untreated disease leads to death. The pathognomonic MRI findings may be detected in totally asymptomatic siblings as early as 24 months. Such children must be placed on treatment by biotin to prevent a neurological crisis. At present there are three such cases, all siblings to an index case who are under treatment for 2 to 8 years without any abnormal neurological signs.

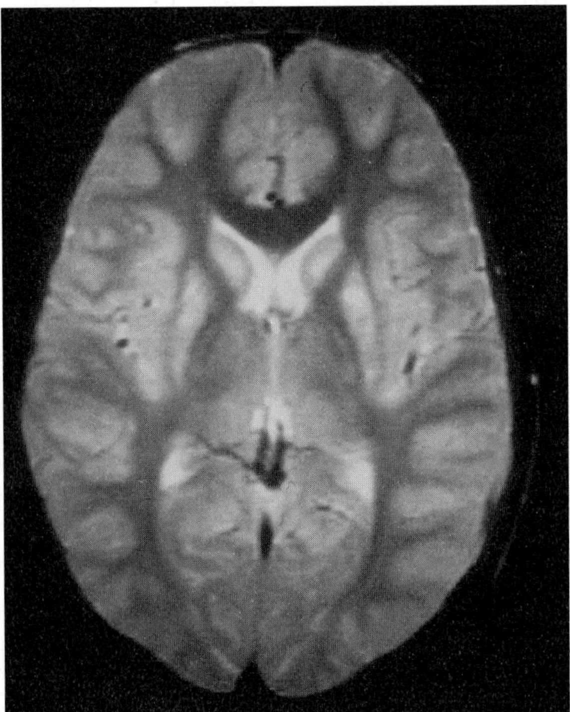

FIGURE 31–4. The brain MRI of a patient with biotin-responsive encephalopathy showing bilateral symmetrically increased T_2 signal intensity within the central parts of the caudate nuclei and in the putamen.

DISORDERS OF VITAMIN B_{12} METABOLISM

Pathogenesis and Pathophysiology. Vitamin B_{12} follows a complex metabolic route before its conversion into an active form that functions in the metabolism of methylmalonic acid and homocysteine. Intrinsic factor is necessary for gastrointestinal absorption. A specific receptor, cubilin, is required for its internalization and a specific globulin in plasma, transcobalamin II, is required for its transport to cells where it is stored in lysosomes as transcobalamin II–B_{12} complex. Defective cytoplasmic release leads to cobalamin (Cbl) F complementation with stored lysosomal B_{12}, causing a condition reminiscent of cystinosis. Vitamin B_{12} must be converted to a chemical form that can attach for further conversions (cobalamin C and D mutation groups) and then attach to a specific methyltransferase. Methyltransferase deficiency leads to absent methylcobalamin. Mitochondrial vitamin B_{12} participates in the formation of adenosylcobalamin, a cofactor for methylmalonyl-CoA mutase.

The defects in intrinsic factor, cubilin,[62] transcobalamin II, CblF, CblC, and CblD result in deficient methylation function as well as defective metabolism of methylmalonyl-CoA. Thus, such disorders are characterized by a combination of homocystinuria and methylmalonicaciduria. In contrast, defects in mitochondrial adenosyl-cobalamin formation (CblA and CblB) result only in methylmalonic-acidemia.

Among these disorders, cubilin defect (Imerslund-Graesbeck syndrome),[62] transcobalamin II deficiency,[63] and CblC deficiency[64] cause significant neurological morbidity.

Epidemiology and Risk Factors. The congenital deficiency of intrinsic factor has been described mainly in Mexican kindred. The prevalence of cubilin deficiency is high among Arabs[1] and Scandinavians; it is primarily a Finnish disease. The CblC deficiency accounts for most of the inborn errors of cobalamin metabolism. Because some of these disorders manifest in late childhood, a younger sibling might be asymptomatic and should be tested for the possible presence of the disorder.

Clinical Features and Associated Disorders. Phenotypic expression may be varied. In an early infantile form, the presentation includes failure to thrive, hypotonia, and lethargy with pancytopenia and hepatic dysfunction. Renal involvement includes thrombotic microangiopathy due to hyperhomocysteinemia. Diffuse hepatic steatosis, early pigmentary retinopathy, facial dysmorphia, congenital heart disease, microcephaly, hydrocephalus, and hip dislocation can be associated features.

In late-onset phenotype, the child develops normally in early life and may even start school in good health. In a typical case, school performance deteriorates and dysarthria, unsteady gait, pyramidal tract signs, and lethargy progress to dementia. Myelopathy develops with the pattern of subacute combined degeneration of the cord, leading to impaired vibration and position sense, and extensor Babinski responses.

Differential Diagnosis. The early infantile form can be confused with other infantile diseases that cause failure to thrive, especially mitochondriopathies, and peroxisomal diseases. The presence of dysmorphic features may suggest a chromosome abnormality but pancytopenia and abnormalities in urine homocystine screening tests will identify the CblC disease. Many disease features are also present in methylenetetrahydrofolate reductase deficiency (MTHFR). A GC/MS study, however, indicates methylmalonicaciduria and tandems/MS indicates elevated propionylcarnitine, which will be absent in MTHFR deficiency.

The later childhood phenotype in a boy will be confused mainly with X-linked adrenoleukodystrophy (X-ALD), X-linked adrenomyeloneuropathy, L-2-hydroxyglutaric-aciduria, childhood-onset metachromatic leukodystrophy, and amyotrophic lateral sclerosis. Megaloblastic anemia, thrombocytopenia, hypersegmented polymorphonuclear leukocytes, elevated lactate dehydrogenase, homocystinuria with elevated cystathioninemia and cystathioninuria, methylmalonicaciduria, elevated propionylcarnitine, and normal levels of C-26 fatty acids in blood and normal plasma corticotropin readily differentiate the CblC deficiency from these other diseases. The white matter changes on brain MRI of X-ALD cases are primarily localized around the posterior ventricular horns, whereas the leukodystrophy in CblC is generalized. Childhood-onset metachromatic leukodystrophy shows characteristic tigroid white matter on MRI; the leukodystrophy in CblC does not have a specific pattern. L-2-Hydroxyglutaricaciduria is associated with seizures and mental retardation but not with progressive mental deterioration. Pyramidal signs predominate the neurological examination. The brain MRI shows a centripetal leukodystrophy with loss of U-fibers.

Evaluation. Any infant with hypotonia or with a family history of prior infantile death should be studied for CblC disease. A simple urine homocystine determination and blood panel for pancytopenia will identify the general category of metabolic derangement; when these tests are positive, urine GC/MS for methylmalonicaciduria and blood MS/MS for propionylcarnitine and hypomethioninemia should be conducted. Because phenotypic manifestations overlap with other Cbl defects, fibroblast complementation studies should also be performed.[65]

Any child showing a late-onset encephalopathy should be evaluated for CblC disease. An MRI of the spinal cord is essential to document the subacute combined degeneration of the cord. Again, a positive test on the simple urine screen for homocystine justifies further workup.

Management. Treatment should include hydroxycobalamin injections, the active form of vitamin B_{12}, 1 mg daily. Carnitine 100 to 200 mg/kg/day should be provided to decrease the accumulation of propionylcarnitine. Homocystinemia should be managed by betaine 100 to 200 mg/kg/day. To stimulate methionine synthetase, folic or folinic acid must be given.

Prognosis. In a young infant, unless homocysteinemia can be managed, the disease will be lethal with hemolytic-uremic syndrome and kidney, liver, or respiratory failure. The prognosis in a late-onset disease varies.[65] When patients respond well to treatment, regression of neurological findings occurs rapidly. In other similarly treated subjects, no ameliorative response has been observed, presumably due to more complete metabolic derangements or involvement of pathways unaffected by available treatment agents.

METHYLENETETRAHYDROFOLATE REDUCTASE DEFICIENCY

Pathogenesis and Pathophysiology. MTHFR (EC 1.5.1.20) deficiency is an inborn error of metabolism of folic acid. MTHFR catalyzes the reduction of methylenetetrahydrofolate to methyltetrahydrofolate. The latter is one of the two cofactors for methionine synthetase (MeS), the enzyme that re-methylates homocysteine produced from the hydrolysis of S-adenosylmethionine (SAH). The SAH in turn is the end product of S-adenosylmethionine (SAM) used for several anabolic reactions of methylating nucleic acids and proteins. The remaining homocysteine residue must be methylated again and converted into methionine, which is used to synthesize SAM, and thus the cycle is completed. The MeS that catalyzes this reaction plays a pivotal role in the body, particularly in the brain, assuring a steady supply of methionine for protein synthesis and nucleic acid methylation. MeS requires two cofactors: methyltetrahydrofolate and methylcobalamin. Deficiency of methionine occurs either when the enzyme is deficient (very rare) or more commonly when there is a defect in the metabolism of folic acid or vitamin B_{12}. Among these latter possibilities, the absence of MTHFR causes a very severe neurological disease in an infant. A defect with similar consequences was discussed in the errors of vitamin B_{12} metabolism. The partial deficiency of MTHFR in an adolescent or young adult has been implicated in homocystinuria leading to strokes, miscarriages, and neural tube defects. While a low methionine arrests brain growth, hypermethioninemia can occur without any neurological symptoms.

Epidemiology and Risk Factors. Absence of MTHFR is panethnic and has been described in different populations. The partial deficiency is due to a thermolabile mutation in MTHFR and is observed frequently in many populations, especially Koreans. The disease process caused by such a mutation and its consequences in the young adult or adolescent populations are not included in this section. The severe infantile form is encountered frequently among Arabs in the Middle East.

Clinical Features and Associated Disorders. The phenotypic expression of this disorder varies from severe early infantile to late infantile forms. The severe early infantile presentation includes intractable hiccups, central hypotonia, myoclonic seizures associated with frequent apneic attacks, early onset microcephalus, microophthalmia, and retinitis.[66] This acute encephalopathy is rapidly progressive, leading to cessation of crying and swallowing. Because absent folic acid function also impairs leukocyte function, intercurrent fungal and bacterial infections are common. These complications as well as the severe encephalopathy lead to death by 3 to 4 months of age if the disease is untreated. The family history may include previous early infantile deaths with a similar presentation. The later-onset infantile form is more indolent and has such nonspecific symptoms as seizures, progressive pyramidal and cerebellar signs, and cognitive decline.[67, 68] No associated disorder was observed in four consanguineous families encountered in Saudi Arabia.

Differential Diagnosis. The early infantile form may be confused with nonketotic hyperglycinemia, 4-hydroxybutyricaciduria, multiple acyl-CoA dehydrogenase deficiency, molybdenum cofactor or sulfite oxidase deficiency, and peroxisomal and early-onset oxidative phosphorylation diseases. Rapid biochemical testing is available to identify MTHFR deficiency.

In MTHFR deficiency, there will be neutropenia and homocystinuria, both readily detectable in a clinical biochemistry laboratory. In contrast to classic homocystinuria due to a deficiency of cystathionine synthetase, in MTHFR deficiency, cystathioninuria and cystathioninemia occur. In nonketotic hyperglycinemia, which can be confused because of the constellation of hiccups, severe hypotonia, and early myoclonic seizures, the CSF glycine will be elevated. In 4-hydroxybutyricaciduria, the urine GC/MS assay for organic acids will identify the disease. Multiple acyl-CoA dehydrogenase deficiency usually presents as a devastating metabolic disease of the newborn with acidosis and hypoglycemia. In sulfite oxidase or molybdenum cofactor deficiency, the blood uric acid will be very low and the brain MRI reveals subcortical cysts. In early-onset mitochondrial diseases such as cytochrome-*c* oxidase deficiency, there will involvement of other systems such as heart and liver with prominent lactic acidosis. Finally, in neonatal forms of peroxisomal diseases, there will be hepatomegaly, patellar x-ray stippling, and brain ultrasound abnormalities showing corpus callosum hypogenesis and brain cysts.

Evaluation. A CBC for neutropenia and a homocystine screening test in the urine must immediately be secured in any newborn with evolving encephalopathy. If either of these tests is abnormal, an MS/MS or an amino acid profile should be obtained to detect hypomethioninemia. MS/MS is a unique procedure among all other screening tests because it can detect low levels of amino acids, including methionine.[66] Blood homocystine level must be determined because the renal threshold for homocystine is approximately 50 μM. Furthermore, blood MS/MS will indicate elevated propionylcarnitine in the case of a vitamin B_{12} metabolic defect; this elevation is not observed in MTHFR deficiency. If needed, urine GC/MS tests should be performed for methylmalonic and methylcitric acids to rule out a vitamin B_{12} defect. If other disorders are considered, additional studies should be performed as needed. If available, positron-emission tomography (PET) brain scans with ^{18}F-fluoro-2-deoxyglucose are advisable[66] and reveal absent cerebral and cerebellar glucose uptake. The metabolic pattern returns to normal gradually after appropriate treatment with methionine. The white matter changes on MRI are nonspecific.

Management. The two management goals are to provide enough methionine for adequate brain growth and to reduce homocystine levels in blood. These goals are achieved by providing 100 to 150 mg betaine/kg/day and 200 to 300 mg/kg/day methionine. The blood methionine level must be closely monitored biweekly to achieve a level of 200 to 400 μM.[66] Some physicians hesitate to use methionine for fear of producing high levels of homocysteine in the blood, but in the authors' experience, if enough betaine is used, hyperhomocysteinemia is not a major problem. On general principles, to stimulate a defective enzyme activity to an appreciable level, weekly injections of folinic acid 15 mg and vitamin B_{12} 1 mg may be added.

Prognosis and Prevention. The outcome depends on early detection and early, aggressive treatment. Unless an aggressive treatment is given, the infant will develop microcephaly. When the above protocol is not applied, the infant will likely suffer severe neurological crippling and will expire. With appropriate treatment, however, the child will develop normally or within near-normal limits. The authors are aware of three such normal children 1 to 5 years of age.

Mitochondrial Enzyme Defects

Mitochondrial DNA (mtDNA) was first discovered in 1963, and in the following 20 years the basic principles of mitochondrial genetics were established.[69] These are maternal inheritance, replicative segregation, threshold expression, high mtDNA mutation rate (compared with nuclear DNA genes), and accumulation of somatic mutations with aging.

The mtDNA of the mother is transmitted to all of her children through the egg cytoplasm, containing 200,000 to 300,000 mtDNAs. The number of mitochondria increases a hundredfold, whereas the mtDNA copy number per mitochondrion decreases from 2 to 10 to 1 to 2 mtDNAs during oogenesis. After fertilization, the early embryo goes through nuclear DNA replication and cell cleavage without significant increase in number of mitochondria or mtDNAs. The mtDNA copy number per mitochondrion varies according to cell type, with an inverse relationship between mitochondrial density and copy number. The highest mtDNA copy number is in brain mitochondria. Mutations in cellular mtDNAs result in mixed intracellular populations of mutant and normal genomes, a situation called heteroplasmy. When heteroplasmic cells divide, different mtDNAs partition randomly into daughter cells (replicative segregation), resulting in variation of cell genotypes.

What clinical phenotype a mitochondrial disease expresses depends on the severity of the mtDNA mutation, the percentage of mutant mtDNAs, and the differing energy requirements and reserve of tissues. Each tissue requires a different minimum level of mitochondrial adenosine triphosphate production (a threshold) to sustain normal cell function. In a family with heteroplasmic mtDNA mutations, different family members can inherit different percentages of mutant mtDNAs and therefore present with different clinical symptoms. The phenotypical effect of the mutations depends on the severity of the damage to the protein the gene encodes. Cells with the lowest potential to replicate, like neurons, appear to be the ones most susceptible to degenerative changes in proteins, lipids, nuclear DNA, and mtDNA. Which neurons accumulate mtDNA mutations is proportional to the metabolic rate. Thus, cerebral cortex, which in PET shows a high glucose utilization rate, and basal ganglia, which also have dopaminergic neurons that generate hydrogen peroxide and oxygen radicals, are the brain areas most susceptible to accumulation of mtDNA damage.

Among the many disorders of oxidative phosphorylation, clinical classifications that focus on the most severe organ system presentations are misleading.[69] Because the expression of mtDNA defects of oxidative phosphorylation depends on the quantitative principles stated earlier, complete phenotypes are rarely exhibited. Biochemical classifications have the same shortcomings because the type and severity of the enzyme defect varies with the percentage of mutant mtDNA in heteroplasmic families. A molecular genetic classification is therefore the most useful. It includes four categories: class I, nuclear DNA mutations; class II, mtDNA point mutations; class III, mtDNA deletions and duplications; and class IV, genetics not yet defined. In keeping with the previous section of aminoacidopathies and organic acidopathies, these diseases are listed in Table 31–6 by order of most likely age presentation. Only the major diseases are discussed here.

SUBACUTE NECROTIZING ENCEPHALOMYELOPATHY (LEIGH'S DISEASE)

Pathogenesis and Pathophysiology. At the molecular level, Leigh's disease can be caused by both mendelian (autosomal recessive nuclear coded DNA) and mtDNA defects.[70, 71] Areas affected are primarily the basal ganglia, brain stem, and cerebellum. The cerebral cortex and retinal pigment are less involved. Pathologically, there is spongy degeneration, demyelination, gliosis, necrosis, relative sparing of neurons, and capillary proliferation. Several enzyme complexes involved in mitochondrial respiratory metabolism show defects, singly or in combination. These are in cytochrome-c oxidase (COX; complex IV), NADH dehydrogenase (complex I), pyruvate dehydrogenase complex (PDHC), and pyruvate carboxylase. The most commonly reported defect is within the ATPase 6 gene at mtDNA position mt8993, a T to G or T to C mutation, resulting in severe defects of ATP production.[72] This is the same gene defect that causes the NARP syndrome (neuropathy, ataxia, and retinitis pigmentosa) in adults.

Epidemiology and Risk Factors. Leigh's disease is a relatively common neurometabolic disease. About one half of patients are diagnosed in the first year of life, usually before age 6 months; in a fourth, the onset is early in the second year of life. Males are predominantly affected. There is a juvenile and an adult form.

Clinical Features and Associated Disorders. The usual age at onset is before the age of 1 year, with death usually before 5 years. A previously healthy, normal infant exhibits a progressive encephalopathy, with an early characteristic central hypoventilation syndrome. Central hypotonia is prominent early and may later be followed by spasticity. Brain stem findings are shown as poor feeding, sucking, and swallowing and as nuclear or supranuclear ophthalmoplegia. There may be optic atrophy but also pigmentary degeneration of the retina. If the onset occurs after the infant has obtained some upright posture, ataxia becomes evident. Seizures occur in the early-onset form, particularly when due to PDHC deficiency or the NARP mt8993 mutation. Movement disorders may occur later in the course and consist often of multifocal myoclonus. Serial CSF lactate and pyruvate levels are elevated. The diagnosis can usually be made by the combination of a typical course, elevated CSF lactate and pyruvate, and typical lesions on MRI.

Differential Diagnosis. Included is any infantile-onset chronic or subacute progressive encephalopathy, but particularly the organic acidurias that present as progressive encephalopathy: glutaricaciduria type 1, biotinidase deficiency, and biopterin-dependent phenylketonuria. Other mitochondrial disorders—lethal infantile mitochondrial disease, atypical peroxisomal disorder, and infantile neuraxonal dystrophy—should be considered.

Evaluation (Fig. 31–5). In Leigh's disease, blood amino acid screening may show nonspecific aminoaciduria. Blood and, more definitively, CSF lactate and pyruvate levels are elevated, with lactate/pyruvate ratios not always at 25:1. Blood ammonia and glucose values are usually normal, as are those of urine organic acids. Other useful tests include serum biotinidase determination, blood sampling for very long chain fatty acids and red blood cell catalase, and pipecolic acid determination for excluding peroxisomal disorders. On T2-weighted sequences of brain MRI images, areas of increased intensity are seen in brain stem, cerebellum, and basal ganglia symmetrically. An EEG may show only background slowing consistent with a nonfocal encephalopathy. Nuclear MR spectrometry, if available, may show a decreased phosphocreatine-to-phosphate ratio in affected brain areas. Specific cause is investigated by enzyme analysis for COX and PDHC activity in cultured skin fibroblasts and/or muscle biopsy, and muscle biopsy is performed for mtDNA analysis (see Fig. 31–5).

Management. Supportive and symptomatic management includes nasogastric tube or gastrostomy for feeding problems to prevent aspiration, tracheostomy and ventilatory support for respiratory failure, prompt treatment of infections, frequent changes of position in bedridden patients to prevent skin ulceration, and the use of antiepileptic and antispastic drugs when appropriate. Metabolic treatment can be attempted, even while waiting for a definitive diagnosis, by starting with broad-spectrum cofactor supplementation therapy. This assumes that if the patient has a treatable mitochondrial disease, it will respond to factors that increase mitochondrial ATP production. Biotin (50 mg/day or more) and thiamine (300 mg/day or more) can be given in megadoses, in combination with the multivitamins. At least a 2-month trial should be given to determine therapeutic efficacy, although this approach is difficult to assess because of the phenotypical and genetic heterogeneity of these diseases. Dichloroacetate is available for lowering of lactic acid levels in research protocols, and it is hoped that it will soon be approved by the Food and Drug Administration. Doses of 15 to 200 mg/kg/day have been used in infants and children, with about a 20 percent fall in lactic acid levels. Coenzyme Q10, vitamin K, and vitamin C may also be tried.

Prognosis and Future Perspectives. The prognosis for Leigh's disease is grave: death is inevitable. The course at times may spontaneously remit, and therapies may seem to arrest the disease for periods of time. Death usually occurs by respiratory failure or complications such as sepsis.

PROGRESSIVE INFANTILE POLIODYSTROPHY (ALPERS' DISEASE)

Pathogenesis and Pathophysiology. CNS locations affected by Alpers' disease are the same as those of Leigh's disease, but in reverse order: most severe in cerebral cortex, then cerebellum, basal ganglia, and brain stem. Lesions show diffuse neuronal degeneration, characteristic spongiform or microcystic degeneration, and, in common with Leigh's disease, gliosis, necrosis, and capillary proliferation.[73] Biochemical abnormalities have not been specific and have included

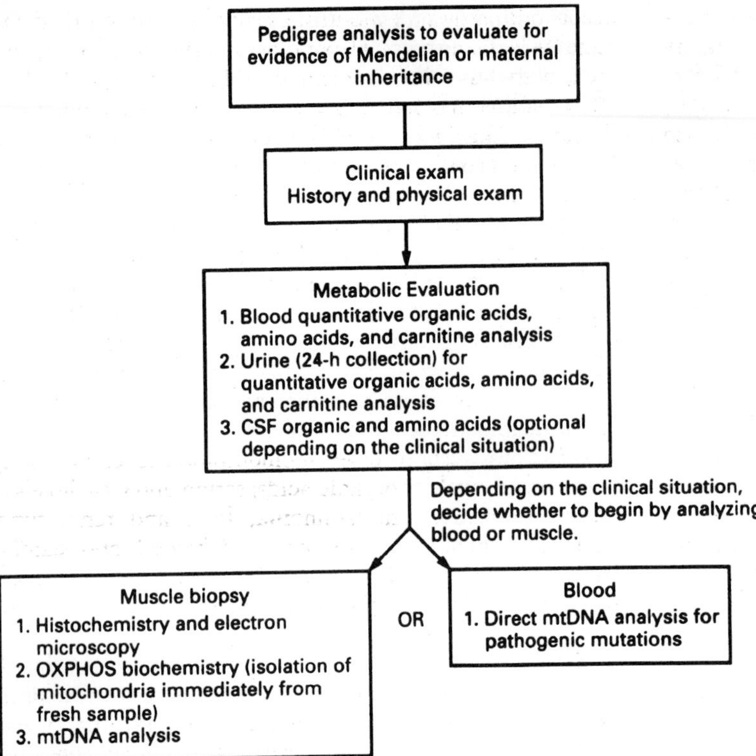

FIGURE 31–5. Algorithm for general approach to the investigation of diseases of oxidative phosphorylation. Reproduced with permission from The McGraw-Hill Companies, from Scriver C, ed: The Metabolic and Molecular Bases of Inherited Disease, 7th ed., New York, McGraw-Hill, 1995, p 1579.

decreased pyruvate dehydrogenase activity, decreased utilization of pyruvate and NADH, and citric acid cycle dysfunction. The genetic abnormality and mechanism of transmission is unknown. It is even disputed whether Alpers' disease is a mitochondrial disease at all. The cortical spongy degeneration appears similar to that of adult Creutzfeldt-Jakob disease, now recognized as a prion disease.

Epidemiology and Risk Factors. The epidemiology is unclear, because the recognition of the syndrome has been unclear, and there is no known gene defect despite the familial occurrence.

Clinical Features and Associated Disorders. Age at onset and duration are similar to those of Leigh's disease. However, there is usually psychomotor delay before the abrupt onset of seizures.[74] The seizures may be focal status epilepticus and epilepsia partialis continua, but they evolve into multifocal myoclonus. Areflexia and hypotonia are initially present, with some signs of spasticity later. Ataxia and nystagmus may worsen, with all other neurological signs and symptoms, during infections. Approximately 40 percent of patients have associated hepatic dysfunction. The course is rapidly progressive after onset of seizures. Blindness and optic atrophy occur late.

Differential Diagnosis. This includes any of the infantile or late infantile progressive encephalopathies with primary involvement of cortical gray matter and presentation with refractory epilepsy. Probably the most common of these diseases is neuronal ceroid lipofuscinosis (Jansky-Bielschowsky or Batten-Spielmeyer-Vogt presentations), which can be ruled out by looking for appropriate inclusion bodies in skin, conjunctival, or full-thickness rectal (ganglion cell) biopsy specimens with electron microscopy. Another mitochondrial disease with severe epilepsy is the myoclonic epilepsy and ragged red fibers (MERRF) syndrome (see subsequent section). Other storage diseases at this age, such as atypical GM_2-gangliosidosis (Tay-Sachs disease, Sandhoff's disease), infantile sialidosis, and galactosialidosis, could be diagnosed by testing for lysosomal enzyme activity, preferably on cultured skin fibroblasts, rather than blood. Other rare causes of a progressive encephalopathy with refractory seizures at this age, but important because they are treatable and reversible, are later-onset pyridoxine dependency and nonketotic hyperglycinemia (both usually neonatal-onset diseases), biotinidase deficiency, and disorders of biogenic amine metabolism, such as folate-responsive seizures. Sulfite oxidase deficiency and Menkes' disease usually present earlier in infancy. The former can be screened for by a commercially available sulfite oxidase urine dipstick test, the latter, by measuring serum copper and ceruloplasmin. Extremely rare at this age are slow virus (subacute sclerosing panencephalitis) diseases. Within the differential diagnosis are epileptic syndromes that appear to be progressive at the onset but that usually plateau into developmental arrest and retardation. These include the syndrome of severe myoclonic epilepsy and the Lennox-Gastaut syndrome.

Evaluation. Because there is no one pathognomonic clinical sign or laboratory study, Alpers' disease is a diagnosis of exclusion. Therefore, all rapidly progressive infantile encephalopathies need to be excluded by clinical story and/or laboratory tests. Measurement of amino acids, organic acids, lactate, and pyruvate should be done in CSF as well as in blood. Mitochondrial biochemical and DNA studies should be performed, looking specifically for the MERRF mutation, as well as functional neuroimaging studies (i.e., MR spectrometry, single photon emission computed tomography [SPECT], and PET if available), to garner evidence for defective energy metabolism and oxidative phosphorylation and to determine the biochemical geography. In Alpers' disease EEGs are markedly abnormal, showing a diffuse encephalopathy. A characteristic EEG pattern consists of high-voltage, very slow delta waves mixed with low-voltage polyspikes. Serial visual evoked potentials extinguish over time. Structural neuroimaging studies (CT, MRI) show progressive marked cortical atrophy. Results of liver function tests are abnormal at the onset of seizures, before clinical features of hepatic degeneration.

Management. There is no specific treatment. The broad-spectrum approach described earlier for Leigh's disease should be applied in order not to miss a treatable progressive encephalopathy. A trial of pyridoxine, 50 mg twice a day orally, can be done to rule out pyridoxine-dependent/deficient seizures. If the serum and CSF glycine levels are elevated, the glycine cleavage enzyme activity should be assessed by liver biopsy in a laboratory qualified to do this test; treatment should be started with dextromethorphan, leucovorin, and sodium benzoate for nonketotic hyperglycinemia. In symptomatic treatment of the seizures, valproic acid should be avoided, because the risk of accelerating the course and a resultant fatal toxic hepatitis is very high. Other treatments of refractory, nonsurgically treatable epilepsy at this age, such as corticotropin or prednisone, ketogenic diet, and intravenous IgG, are unproven and may be harmful.

Prognosis and Future Perspectives. This is a fatal disease. Future treatment approaches depend on elucidation of the underlying biochemical and molecular pathogenesis.

LETHAL INFANTILE MITOCHONDRIAL DISEASE OR CONGENITAL LACTIC ACIDOSIS

The oxidative phosphorylation defects associated with extreme neonatal lactic acidosis involve defects in multiple complexes (mostly complex I and IV but also III) and various cytochromes. There are probably several genetic mechanisms of lethal infantile mitochondrial disease (LIMD): tissue-specific depletions of mtDNA, mtDNA mutations, and abnormal expression of specific complex I or IV subunits. The genetics of the mtDNA depletion syndromes could be autosomal recessive or dominant with variable expressivity. Three hypotheses could explain these: (1) there is a defect in a nuclear gene that controls mtDNA replication and copy number; (2) there is abnormal timing of mtDNA replication (delayed) in embryogenesis; and (3) an mtDNA point mutation interacts with specific nuclear alleles and replication is impaired.

These are rare diseases, and the epidemiology is unknown. Because the respiratory chain is influenced by mitochondrial and nuclear genomes, inheritance is either mendelian or maternal.

Presentation is usually in or shortly after the neonatal period, with marked hypotonia and weakness, failure to thrive, respiratory difficulty, and severe lactic acidosis. The hypotonia/weakness is due to a myopathy with lipid and glycogen accumulation and abnormally shaped mitochondria without inclusions but only rare, ragged red fibers. Death occurs ordinarily by 5 months, usually because of the uncorrectable lactic acidosis. Hepatic dysfunction is highly associated, with lesser involvement of kidneys (proximal tubule abnormalities and generalized aminoaciduria) and a myocardiopathy. The brain itself is rarely involved, but when it is, bilateral basal ganglial abnormalities are shown on neuroimaging.

The differential diagnosis includes other infantile causes of lactic acidosis: primary defects of pyruvate metabolism, such as pyruvate dehydrogenase deficiency, or secondary disturbances, such as in various organic acidurias and fatty acid oxidation defects; Krebs' cycle defects; and defects of gluconeogenesis.[75] Before the serum lactic acid levels are known, the clinical picture resembles the hyperammonemia syndromes due to urea cycle defects.

Important tests to order include blood levels of amino acids; urine levels of organic acids; serum and CSF levels of lactate, pyruvate, and ammonia; liver and renal function tests; blood creatine kinase (skeletal and cardiac fractions); ultrasound evaluation of the heart; neuroimaging of the brain; and EEG to document a toxic/metabolic encephalopathy.

Supportive treatment of liver, renal, and cardiac failure is important, along with consultation with a center using experimental protocols. For respiratory chain defects, megadoses of vitamins K and C, coenzyme Q10, L-carnitine, and folic acid have all been tried with controversial benefit. If pyruvate dehydrogenase (PDH) deficiency is the cause, thiamine and lipoic acid may be therapeutic, because PDH requires these as cofactors. If biotinidase deficiency or multiple carboxylase deficiency is the cause, 50 mg of biotin daily can be given. Fructose-1,6-biphosphatase deficiency and glucose-6-phosphatase deficiency, both gluconeogenic defects, respond to frequent daily and continuous nocturnal feedings to prevent hypoglycemia. There is no effective treatment for pyruvate carboxylase (PC) deficiency or partial defects of the Krebs cycle. Correction of the metabolic acidosis and lowering of serum lactic acid is most effective with sodium dichloroacetate (DCA), 15 to 200 mg/kg/day administered intravenously or orally. DCA crosses the blood-brain barrier and inhibits the PDH-specific kinase, activating the PDHC and lowering brain and blood lactate levels.

LIMD is lethal. If definite nuclear gene mutations are identified in the future, prenatal diagnosis using chorionic villus sampling or amniocentesis should be feasible. The prognosis of the other congenital lactic acidoses depends on the underlying biochemical defects—best with biotinidase deficiency and the gluconeogenic defects, less with PDH, PC, and Krebs' cycle defects.

MYOCLONIC EPILEPSY AND RAGGED RED FIBERS SYNDROME

The majority of cases of MERRF syndrome have a heteroplasmic G to A point mutation at bp8344 in the $tRNA^{Lys}$ gene.[76] This results in protein synthesis defects involving primarily complexes I and IV, which have the greatest number of mtDNA-coded subunits. Any quantitative measure of energy metabolism—^{31}P-NMR, anerobic threshold determination, or biochemical analysis of skeletal muscle—shows decreased ATP-generating capacity. When mutant mtDNAs exceed 85 percent in a tissue, the patient becomes symptomatic.

Neuropathology shows degeneration of cerebellar cortex, substantia nigra, dentatorubral and pallidoluysian systems, locus ceruleus, inferior olivary nucleus, and pontine tegmentum.

The exact incidence is not known. Familial occurrence with maternal inheritance, usually before age 20, is the rule. Commonly, symptoms and signs overlap among MERRF, mitochondrial encephalopathy, lactic acidosis, and strokelike episodes (MELAS), and Kearns-Sayre syndrome (KSS).

The classic presentation is usually in late childhood, although it may begin in early adulthood, with progressive myoclonic epilepsy, ataxia, and action-induced polymyoclonus. Weakness and hypotonia due to a mitochondrial myopathy and a progressive dementia follow. Hearing loss may be associated. This presentation resembles the historical Ramsay Hunt syndrome of dysergia cerebellaris myoclonica.

MERRF is differentiated clinically from MELAS (see next section) by the lack of strokelike episodes in MERRF. Benign essential familial myoclonus is nonprogressive. The principal differential is with other causes of progressive myoclonic epilepsy in late childhood/early adolescence. These are storage diseases—neuronal ceroid lipofuscinosis (Kufs' type) and neuraminidase deficiency (sialidosis type 1); diseases of unknown etiology—Lafora's disease, Baltic myoclonus; and slow virus and prion diseases—subacute sclerosing panencephalitis and early-onset spongiform encephalopathy.

Tests to be ordered include serum and CSF lactate, pyruvate, and alanine levels; EEG and visual evoked potentials; MRI of the brain, which often shows areas of increased intensity in T2-weighted sequences; ^{31}P-NMR of muscle; muscle biopsy for biochemical tests of oxidative phosphorylation and for visualizing ragged red fibers, by light microscopy using the Gomori's trichrome stain, and by electron microscopy; and mtDNA analysis, looking for the MERRF and MELAS point mutations.

Seizures can be symptomatically treated with valproate (watching for carnitine deficiency) and clonazepam. There is a dearth of data as to whether measures for refractory myoclonic epilepsy—ketogenic diet, corticotropin or corticosteroids, or L-5-hydroxytryptophan plus carbidopa—have been effective. Corticosteroids have been used for the myopathy and improvement has been noted, but this is not generally recommended at present. Because coenzyme Q10 improves electron transfer from complex I and riboflavin serves as a cofactor for electron transport in complex I (and II), these agents are reasonable to try (see Fig. 31–5). Use of vitamin K (menadione and phytonadione) has less rationale.

The course is chronic and slowly progressive. Different family members may become symptomatic, with different phenotypes, at different ages, depending on the percentage of the mutant DNA in muscle and brain. It would be important for all maternal relatives to have blood analyses for the mutant DNA and, if negative on muscle, to determine the risk of becoming symptomatic with age. Prenatal diagnosis by amniocentesis or chorionic villus sampling for mtDNA point mutations is unreliable presently because the genotype of that tissue may not reflect that of the embryo's muscle and brain.

MITOCHONDRIAL ENCEPHALOPATHY, LACTIC ACIDOSIS, AND STROKELIKE EPISODES

About 80 percent of MELAS patients exhibit a heteroplasmic A to G point mutation in the dihydrouridine loop of the $tRNA^{Leu(UUR)}$ gene at mt3243.[77] Two other mutations in the same gene, at mt3250 and mt3271, have been identified in the remaining cases. The MELAS3243 mutation alters the dihydrouridine loop of the $tRNA^{Leu(UUR)}$ gene and changes a nucleotide at the binding site for a nuclear DNA-encoded transcription termination factor. It is hypothesized that the mutation reduces the binding affinity of the transcription termination factor. Another possibility is that this mutation impairs protein synthesis by interfering with polypeptide chain elongation. The cerebral infarcts are nonvascular, owing to transient dysfunction of oxidative phosphorylation within parenchyma. Areas of neuronal loss, demyelination, and astrocytic proliferation are found in the infarct-like brain areas. PET studies show reduced cerebral metabolic rates for oxygen but normal glucose utilization. Mitochondrial abnormalities of endothelial cells and smooth muscle cells produce a mitochondrial angiopathy. The vascular metabolic dysfunction may cause increased production of free radicals, which could damage vasodilators such as nitrous oxide, causing vasoconstriction.

The exact incidence is unknown. Most cases occur before age 20, and about a fourth of patients have a positive family history consistent with maternal inheritance.

Patients may present sporadically or in maternal pedigrees, in infancy, childhood, or adulthood. The overall course is of a progressive degenerative disease with strokelike episodes and a mitochondrial myopathy. Various symptoms appear singly or in combination and include hemiplegia, sudden cortical blindness, hemianopia, episodes of confusion and hallucination with fever, aphasia, migraine headaches in a maternal lineage preceding strokelike episodes, and maternally inherited diabetes mellitus type II and deafness. Multisystem complaints and signs include myalgia, fatigability, weakness, ophthalmoplegia, pigmentary retinal degeneration, cardiomyopathy, cardiac conduction defects and block, dementia, deafness, ataxia, myoclonus, seizures, lactic acidosis, and proximal renal tubule dysfunction.

Conditions to exclude include any other causes of stroke in childhood, infancy, or adulthood; other mitochondrial multisystem disorders, such as MERRF or KSS/chronic progressive external ophthalmoplegia (CPEO), or other uncharacterized disorders; and any neurological disease in adulthood with an overall progressive course but relapses that leave residuals, such as multiple sclerosis or other demyelinating diseases.

In the general diagnostic approach (see Fig. 31–5), the best diagnostic clues are found on CT and MRI, which show cortical infarcts that are not wedge shaped but cut across several vascular territories, usually located in the posterior quadrants initially. Basal ganglia calcifications, in particular, occur and are seen better by CT than MRI. Ventricular dilation and cortical atrophy are also seen. With a history of strokelike episodes, these neuroimaging findings, associated with lactic acidosis and a myopathy, should strongly suggest the diagnosis. Functional neuroimaging studies, such as SPECT using N-isopropyl-*p*-[^{123}I]-iodoamphetamine tracer can detect regional hypoperfusion when structural studies (CT, MRI) are unrevealing. SPECT is useful not only in delineating the lesion but also in following the course. Analysis of mtDNA for the known point mutations on blood and muscle confirms the diagnosis.

Coenzyme Q10 in doses up to 300 mg/day may be needed for optimal benefit, starting at 4.3 mg/kg/day.

Corticosteroids and a novel quinone not available in the United States, idebenone, have shown some benefit. MELAS is a progressive neurodegenerative disease with a guarded prognosis.

CHRONIC PROGRESSIVE EXTERNAL OPHTHALMOPLEGIA AND KEARNS-SAYRE SYNDROME

These conditions are discussed together because of a common overlap.[78] Most cases are spontaneous and have mtDNA deletions. Over 100 different deletions have been identified; 90 percent occur between the large arc between the two points of replication. Deleted mtDNAs localize to distinct regions along muscle fiber, whereas normal mtDNAs are evenly distributed, resulting in a periodic respiratory deficiency along the muscle fiber. The loss of tRNAs is rate limiting in these areas, causing deficits in protein synthesis and oxidative phosphorylation. Duplications may occur spontaneously or be maternally inherited and are detected in quiescent (muscle) and actively dividing tissue (lymphocytes). The mechanism of their generation is unclear. The exact incidence of these conditions is unknown. Most all cases are sporadic.

If ophthalmoplegia before the age of 20 years is accompanied by atypical retinitis pigmentosa, mitochondrial myopathy, along with cardiac conduction defects, a cerebellar syndrome, or elevated CSF protein (above 100 mg/dL), this constellation is termed KSS. Chronic progressive ophthalmoplegia with onset after age 20 is termed CPEO and, if coupled with a variety of other manifestations, CPEO-plus. These manifestations are many: lactic acidemia; eye and ear findings, including pigmentary retinopathy, optic atrophy, and hearing loss; cardiac conduction defects, arrhythmias, and dilated or hypertrophic cardiomyopathies; CNS dysfunction, including dementia, seizures, and ataxias; peripheral nervous system damage, including motor/sensory neuropathies; mitochondrial myopathy; and multisystemic organ involvement in the form of diabetes mellitus, hypoparathyroidism, glomerulosclerosis, proximal renal tubule dysfunction, gastrointestinal motility problems, and respiratory failure.

Conditions to exclude include other mitochondrial diseases, primarily MERRF and MELAS; any disease causing ophthalmoplegia when that is the sole presenting symptom, especially myasthenia gravis; other diseases that cause multisystem involvement, such as collagen vascular diseases, particularly systemic lupus erythematosus; and in the appropriate setting, Lyme disease (caused by infection with *Borrelia burgdorferi*) or Whipple's disease. The ultimate diagnosis is made by muscle biopsy and mtDNA analysis. There is no proven specific treatment, although coenzyme Q10 and carnitine have been used. Implanted cardiac pacemakers can be used for conduction defects. Associated endocrine abnormalities—growth hormone deficiency, diabetes mellitus, or hypoparathyroidism—can be treated medically. Although these conditions are considered chronic, complete heart block may result in sudden death.

LEBER'S HEREDITARY OPTIC NEUROPATHY

Leber's hereditary optic neuropathy (LHON) was the first human disease proven to be due to an mtDNA point mutation.[79] Pedigrees may be heteroplasmic or homoplasmic. Eleven different missense mutations have been identified. Approximately 80 percent are accounted for by mutations at bp11,778 and bp3460. There is much genetic heterogeneity, because the remaining cases reveal novel, complex mtDNA mutations that are primary or synergistic. Multifactorial etiopathogenesis probably exists.

The exact incidence of LHON is unknown. It is maternally inherited, has variable penetrance, and has male predominance. An X-chromosome locus has not been proven, with the sex differences being explained more by sex-related physiological differences.

LHON presents as loss of central visual acuity in adolescence or early adulthood, acutely or subacutely, although it rarely can occur in children. Funduscopic examination shows telangiectatic microangiopathy and swelling of the nerve fiber layer around the optic disc in acute presentations and optic atrophy in subacute to chronic presentations. Up to almost one fourth of patients regain vision. In addition to blindness, complex neurological features include signs suggestive of multiple sclerosis, multisystem atrophy, or MELAS. Extrapyramidal features like dystonia may develop with bilateral striatal necrosis.

The differential diagnosis includes other causes of optic neuritis, multiple sclerosis, MELAS, Leigh's disease, subacute combined degeneration due to vitamin B_{12} deficiency, Friedreich's-like ataxia, and other causes of multisystem degeneration. The general paradigm should be followed, but in leukocyte/platelet analysis, for major manifestations, MTNDI*LHON4160 and MTND4*LHON11778 should be assessed. For minor manifestations, MTND4*LHON11778 and MKTND1*LHON3460 and MTND6*LHON14484 are assessed. If any of these are positive, then haplotype analysis is indicated. Laboratory evaluations necessary to rule out disorders in the differential diagnosis should be done simultaneously. Recovery from blindness depends on the mutation involved—5 percent in the most common and 22 percent in the second most common mutation.

MALIGNANT MIGRAINE

Various oxidative phosphorylation defects occur in the brain, although how they relate to the production of migraine is speculative. Migraine affects as much as 25 percent of the population and is frequently seen in maternal relatives of patients with diseases of oxidative phosphorylation. Malignant migraine refers to three situations: migraine patients who turn out to have MELAS; migraine patients who are maternal relatives of patients with oxidative phosphorylation diseases and who are unresponsive to the usual prophylactic medications; and migraine patients who develop strokes. Blood should be tested for biochemical and mtDNA defects of oxidative phosphorylation. If the blood tests are negative, muscle biopsy should be done for routine pathology, histochemistry and electron microscopy, oxidative phosphorylation biochemistry, and mtDNA analysis to include Southern blot analysis for mtDNA rearrangements. Management is nonspecific. The prognosis is unknown and may depend on whether more specific mutations are found to be associated.

NEUROPATHY, ATAXIA, RETINITIS PIGMENTOSA SYNDROME

The neuropathy, ataxia, retinitis pigmentosa syndrome is due to a point mutation at bp8993 in the ATPase 6 gene (MTATP6*NARP8993), which changes a highly conserved leucine at position 156 to an arginine. The exact incidence is unknown, but this is a rare, functionally recessive, with variable systemic expression, adult-onset progressive disease. Presentation is with neuropathy or neurogenic weakness, ataxia, and pigmentary retinopathy. It can also be associated with dementia, generalized seizures, cerebellar and brain stem atrophy, and corticospinal degeneration. The first presentation is usually nyctalopia, followed by loss of peripheral vision. The differential diagnosis includes multisystem atrophy, familial ataxias in mid to late life; any other causes of retinitis pigmentosa, such as adult-onset neuronal ceroid lipofuscinosis; and peroxisomal disorders such as Refsum's disease. The evaluation includes specific analysis for MTATP6*NARP8993 and MTTL1*MELAS3243. Results of metabolic and muscle investigations are usually normal or slightly abnormal, with lactic acidemia only in the more severe cases.

MITOCHONDRIAL MYOPATHIES

Mitochondrial myopathies are a ubiquitous accompaniment of most diseases of oxidative phosphorylation in all classes (I to IV) but can occur as the sole symptom, owing to disorders of class I, II, and IV.[80] In class I there may be autosomal dominant or recessive presentations with tissue-specific presentations; in class II these may or may not have ragged red fibers; and in class IV the distribution of the myopathy is variable: fascioscapulohumeral, limb-girdle, generalized, with childhood, adolescent, and adult-onset forms. Class IV presents usually as singleton cases; familial cases suggest class I and II disorders. Darras and Friedman have prepared diagnostic algorithms to simplify the clinical and laboratory evaluation of mitochondrial myopathies.

REYE'S SYNDROME

Reye's syndrome is defined by the Centers for Disease Control and Prevention as an acute, noninflammatory encephalopathy with altered levels of consciousness and liver dysfunction.[81] The liver disease must include either fatty metamorphosis of the liver or at least a threefold increase in alanine aminotransferase, aspartate aminotransferase, or serum ammonia.

Pathogenesis and Pathophysiology. A growing body of evidence suggests that Reye's syndrome may be a multiorgan disease due to diffuse mitochondrial injury of unknown origin.[82, 83] Mitochondria in hepatocytes, brain capillary endothelial cells, neurons, cardiac and skeletal muscle fibers, and pancreatic cells show histological damage. Liver mitochondrial enzyme activity is low.[84] In one study, several depressed electron transport enzymes and lowered adenosine triphosphate/adenosine diphosphate ratios were documented.[81] Epidemiological studies strongly associate three virus infections (influenza B, influenza A, and varicella-zoster (see Chapter 41) with Reye's syndrome, although the mechanism of their involvement with the pathogenesis of the condition is unclear. There is no evidence of full viral replication in the two primary organs of damage: liver and brain. It has been suggested that viral proteins are toxic, that the infection causes release of toxins, or that the viral infection plus endogenous or exogenous cofactors, such as salicylates, aflatoxins, insecticides, or certain oils, combine to damage liver and brain.

Epidemiology and Risk Factors. Reye's syndrome occurs worldwide. In the United States, from 1982 to 1985, the incidence was approximately 0.3 in 100,000 persons, and the rate has been relatively stable since then.[81] There is no solid evidence to establish a genetic basis for Reye's syndrome, and only a few cases occur within families.[85] There may be two epidemiological patterns: (1) an epidemic form, not noted since the 1980s, that occurred mainly in winter and early spring, clustering in time and geographic region, and associated with outbreaks of influenza B and A, and (2) endemic Reye's syndrome with sporadic occurrence and associated with other viral infections, specifically varicella. Most Reye's syndrome cases associated with varicella occur in children between ages 5 and 9, whereas influenza type B–associated disease occurred in children aged 10 to 14. Salicylate usage has been associated with Reye's syndrome, and the reduction in cases seen in the past years has been specifically linked to reduced salicylate ingestion in children.[86]

Clinical Features and Associated Disorders. The clinical manifestations can be divided into a prodromal phase and the syndrome itself. During the prodrome, there is an upper respiratory tract infection in 60 to 80 percent of cases, and most documented cases have demonstrated influenza B, A, or varicella-zoster virus. During stage I of Reye's syndrome, vomiting is the primary feature. It is not known whether this effect is due to brain stem dysfunction or a systemic cause, but it is usually abrupt in onset and unremitting. The child becomes irritable and gradually lethargic. Most patients recover from this stage and never develop severe agitation and coma. With stage 2, restlessness and disorientation predominate, along with signs of dysautonomia, tachycardia, sweating, and dilated pupils. Seizures may develop, but status epilepticus is rare. With stage 3, coma ensues, with papilledema developing over 2 to 3 days but without lateralizing signs of focal neurological damage. Seizures develop in approximately half of these patients. In stage 4, there is cerebrate posturing and respiratory dysfunction. The coma of stage 5 is associated with flaccid tone and no response to painful stimuli. Brain stem reflexes, like cold caloric testing (see Chapter 1), are minimal or absent.

Evaluation and Differential Diagnosis. Laboratory studies during the prodromal phase are not diagnostic. Once vomiting develops, alanine aminotransferase and aspartate aminotransferase levels are often very high, often 20 to 30 times normal, but ammonia levels are in the normal range. As coma develops, ammonia levels increase threefold or more over the normal range. Other abnormalities of laboratory tests occur with increases in lactic acid and organic acids, suggesting a blend of respiratory alkalosis and metabolic acidosis, sometimes with hypoglycemia, especially in children younger than 3 years of age. Prolonged prothrombin times develop, but hemorrhaging is rare. The EEG is abnormal with diffuse slowing, and sometimes, burst suppression activity (see Chapter 24), but there is no specific pattern of diagnostic value. Liver biopsy shows highly characteristic fatty metamorphosis without inflammation. Neuroimaging with CT or MRI shows a normal brain or diffuse cerebral edema with ventricular compression. Diseases that should be excluded in the diagnosis are encephalitis and meningitis, UCDs, BCAA disorders, and other enzyme deficiency states, including propionicacidemia, glutaricaciduria, and disorders of ketogenesis. Finally, inadvertent intoxication with insecticides, salicylates, methyl bromide, margosa oil, and lead can give a combined picture of encephalopathy and hepatic damage in a young child.

Treatment and Prognosis. There is no specific therapy, and management is aimed at monitoring vital functions, correcting liver abnormalities, and controlling increased intracranial pressure until the disease runs its natural course. Hospitalization in an intensive care unit is recommended, because mental status and respiratory function can change abruptly. Salicylates must not be used, and serum glucose levels must be monitored. Vitamin K is often administered, and anticonvulsants are used to treat clinical seizures and sometimes subclinical epileptic activity that is evident on the EEG. Treatment of the hyperammonemia is particularly problematic because dialysis and exchange transfusions do not markedly reduce ammonia levels or improve outcome. Increased intracranial pressure is a major danger, and some centers use monitoring technology (see Chapter 26) to provide a constant assessment of shifts in pressure gradients. The goal is usually to keep intracranial pressure below 20 mm Hg with a mean cerebral perfusion pressure (mean blood pressure minus mean intracranial pressure) maintained at 60 to 90 mm Hg.

Overall, mortality currently is 30 to 35 percent. Predictors of poor outcome appear to be young age, especially infants younger than 2 years old; high clinical stage at the time of hospital admission; rapid progression from vomiting to coma; maximal clinical stage; high creatine kinase levels; and ammonia levels above 300 μg/dL at the time of hospital admission. In those surviving, hepatic recovery is full but nervous system residua are many. Behavioral problems include attention difficulties, retardation, and aggressive impulsivity. Neurological problems include hemiparesis and quadriparesis, dysarthria, cortical blindness, and seizures. Even among children believed to have full recovery, 34 percent had measurable deficits in school achievement, visuomotor integration, sequencing, and problem solving.[87]

Fatty Acid Oxidation Disorders

Besides the mitochondrial enzyme defects characterized by disordered oxidative phosphorylation, 12 disorders of fatty acid oxidation and ketogenesis are known (Table 31–7).[88] Medium-, long-, and short-chain acyl-CoA dehydrogenase deficiencies (MCAD, LCAD, SCAD) are caused by defects of the beta-oxidation spiral; the rest, except long-chain L-3 hydroxyacyl-CoA dehydrogenase (LCHAD) deficiency, are due to defects in the carnitine cycle. The mutations responsible for very long-chain acyl-CoA dehydrogenase (VLCAD) deficiency have recently been described.[89] In this class of disorders there are three main presentations: (1) acute toxic encephalopathy with episodes of nonketotic hypoglycemia in the first 2 years of life provoked by fasting (MCAD), (2) skeletal and/or cardiac myopathies with weakness and low plasma carnitine levels (carnitine palmitoyl transferase [CPT] I and II deficiencies, LCAD, LCHAD, and SCAD), and (3) the syndrome of nonketotic hypoglycemia plus very low plasma carnitine levels (<10 μM) and absent dicarboxylicaciduria (carnitine transport defect).

TABLE 31–7. **Fatty Acid Oxidation Disorders**

Infantile
Medium-chain acyl-CoA dehydrogenase deficiency (MCAD)* (newborn to 14 years)
Long-chain acyl-CoA dehydrogenase deficiency (LCAD, VLCAD)
Short-chain acyl-CoA dehydrogenase deficiency (SCAD)
CPT II deficiency (severe infantile form)
Childhood
Carnitine transport defect* (3 months to 7 years)
CPT I deficiency
Long-chain L-3 hydroxyacyl-CoA dehydrogenase (LCHAD, trifunctional enzyme)
Adulthood
CPT II deficiency (classical exercise-induced myoglobinuria)* (adult)

*Discussed in text.

As outlined by Treem, the clinical spectrum now also includes sudden infant death syndrome (SIDS), fulminant hepatic failure, and complications during pregnancy. Approximately 5 percent of 313 cases of SIDS were due to defects in fatty acid oxidation.[90] A careful protocol for postmortem diagnosis of fatty acid oxidation disorders has been published.[91] Because MCAD can be detected in asymptomatic siblings, all siblings of infants who die of SIDS should be tested for a fatty acid oxidation disorder.

Some patients with fatty acid oxidation defects can sustain severe liver injury with cirrhosis, necrosis, or liver failure, eventually leading to the need for liver transplantation.[92] Recent reports cite an association between fatty acid oxidation disorders and complications of pregnancy.[93, 94] All infants born of mothers with acute fatty liver of pregnancy or hemolysis, elevated liver enzymes, low platelet count (HELLP syndrome), often associated with severe pre-eclampsia, should be screened for fatty acid oxidation defects. A neonatal blood acylcarnitine profile analysis by MS/MS and genetic screening for the G1528C mutation in the alpha subunit of the trifunctional protein are available.

The diagnostic approach includes history; physical/neurological examination; routine laboratory studies, particularly including liver and urine function tests and determination of electrolytes, pH, lactate, pyruvate, ammonia, blood glucose, and urine ketones; blood free carnitine and acylcarnitines; and urine GS/MS for organic acids. These evaluations are followed by specialized techniques, including specific biochemical enzymatic analysis and molecular analysis. Because the enzymes in the beta-oxidation spiral exist in different forms with chain specificities that overlap and because oxidation of unsaturated fatty acids requires different enzymes, it is expected that other diseases of fatty acid oxidation involving enzymes in these steps will be described in the future.

MEDIUM-CHAIN ACYL-COA DEHYDROGENASE DEFICIENCY

The optimal chain length specificity of MCAD is 8 carbons. The ability to oxidize fatty acids beyond medium-chain length is impaired 20 percent or less of control rates in cultured fibroblasts. Light microscopy of liver in acute cases shows steatosis, which disappears on recovery. The hepatic mitochondria show increased matrix density and intracristal widening, giving a condensed appearance. There may be crystalloids in the matrix. These are in contrast to the findings of Reye's syndrome, in which electron microscopy shows matrix swelling and rarefaction. MCAD is the most common mitochondrial beta-oxidation disorder, with an estimated frequency being 1 in 10,000 to 20,000. Previous unexplained sibling deaths should raise MCAD as a possible diagnosis.

Most patients present between ages 3 and 15 months, rarely after 4 years. Phenotypical heterogeneity prevails, ranging from SIDS, to recurrent Reye's-like syndrome, to episodic nonketotic hypoglycemic coma. A common presentation is vomiting and lethargy, followed by fasting, associated with a prior viral respiratory or gastrointestinal infection. Presentation is usually to an emergency department as an acute toxic encephalopathy or coma, with hypoketotic hypoglycemia, hyperammonemia, and abnormal liver function tests. The serum carnitine value is low, and urine acylcarnitines are increased, with a specific profile. Enzyme assay for MCAD activity can be done on cultured skin fibroblasts, muscle, liver, or blood lymphocytes. The differential diagnosis includes other fatty acid oxidation disorders, exogenous toxic encephalopathies, and true Reye's syndrome. Specific management involves intravenous dextrose 10 percent, avoidance of fasting with frequent short feeds, L-carnitine 100 mg/kg/day in divided doses orally, and preventive management by neonatal screening of subsequent siblings and screening with acylcarnitine profiles of present siblings. The risk of death with the first episode (SIDS presentation) is about 20 percent. In delayed treatment, there is a risk for developmental retardation, speech and language delay, behavioral problems and attention deficit disorder, muscle weakness, seizures, and failure to thrive.

CARNITINE TRANSPORT DEFECT: PRIMARY GENERALIZED CARNITINE DEFICIENCY

Carnitine fails to be taken up in muscle, heart, and kidney but not liver, leading to insufficient carnitine to support fatty acid oxidation.[95] The kidney fails to conserve carnitine by reabsorption, resulting in very low plasma carnitine levels, which then causes decreased passive diffusion into liver, impairing ketogenesis. Accumulating acyl-CoA compounds become substrates for peroxisomal beta-oxidation, which produces medium-chain fatty acids and dicarboxylic acids, which do not require carnitine for mitochondrial entry. They are then completely oxidized in mitochondria, which is the reason for lack of dicarboxylicaciduria in disorders of the high-affinity carnitine transporter. Treatment with L-carnitine restores plasma levels to normal (40 to 60 μM) but not skeletal muscle. Muscle function can be restored, however, with less than 10 percent normal muscle carnitine levels. This is a rare disorder, and the exact incidence is unknown. There are two major types of presentation, an early one (3 months to 2 ½ years) with nonketotic hypoglycemia, and a later one (1 to 7 years) with cardiomyopathy. The nonketotic hypoglycemia in the early presentation is accompanied by hyperammonemia and elevated alanine and aspartate aminotransferase levels, which may present after a short fast, particularly if the patient is being fed a carnitine-free formula. The cardiomyopathy in the later presentation is progressive, with cardiac decompensation and respiratory distress, and is often accompanied by skeletal muscle weakness. Mild to moderate anemia, nonresponsive to iron, may be present. Very low plasma carnitine levels (<10 μM) and absent dicarboxylicaciduria are practically pathognomonic of a carnitine transporter defect. The differential diagnosis includes carnitine deficiencies secondary to other disorders of the carnitine cycle, in which medium- and long-chain acylcarnitines that accumulate from the metabolic block may induce a defect in tissue uptake of free carnitine. In this primary disorder the diagnosis is established by measuring carnitine uptake by fibroblasts and leukocytes (<10 percent of control rates). In the nonketotic hypoglycemia presentation, management involves the intravenous use of glucose and the long-term oral administration of L-carnitine at 100 to 120 mg/kg/day in two to three divided doses. Oral L-carnitine doses can be higher in the cardiomyopathy presentation, up to 175 mg/kg/day.

CARNITINE PALMITOYL TRANSFERASE II DEFICIENCY

In CPT II deficiency, long-chain acylcarnitines are transported across the inner mitochondrial membrane but cannot be converted to their corresponding long-chain acyl-CoAs. They accumulate in the mitochondrial matrix and are transported out into plasma. These elevated levels may produce cardiac arrhythmias. Dicarboxylicaciduria is absent, because of the same explanation given for carnitine transport defect. The exact incidence is unknown, but the adult form is more common than the infantile form. Risk factors are fasting and prolonged exercise.

There are two presentations: the adult muscular form, in which prolonged exercise induces weakness and myoglobinuria, and a severe infantile form, in which nonketotic hypoglycemic coma without dicarboxylicaciduria, seizures, hepatomegaly, cardiomegaly, and cardiac arrhythmia are accompanied by low plasma and tissue levels of carnitine with increase in long-chain acylcarnitines. The classic adult form is autosomal recessive and usually affects males between 15 and 30 years of age. The serum creatine kinase value is normal between episodes, carnitine levels are usually normal in plasma and tissues, and long-term muscle weakness is rare, although lipid storage may be seen on muscle biopsy. The differential diagnosis includes other carnitine cycle disorders. Management involves supportive treatment of the renal failure and measures to remove the myoglobin from kidney and avoidance of triggering factors—prolonged exercise, exposure to cold, infections, and fasting. Presentation in the neonatal period usually ends in death. In the adult form, about a fourth of patients develop renal failure secondary to the episodic myoglobinuria.

Other Metabolic Disorders

VARIOUS TRANSPORTER DEFECTS

Hartnup's Disease

Hartnup's disease is an autosomal recessive transport disorder of neutral amino acids, affecting the kidney and small intestine and leading to excessive neutral aminoaciduria 5 to 20 times normal.[96] These monoamino/monocarboxylic amino acids include alanine, glutamine, histidine, serine, phenylalanine, tyrosine, tryptophan, asparagine, leucine, isoleucine, and valine but not proline. Plasma levels are normal. These same amino acids, particularly tryptophan, are retained in the gut and broken down by bacteria; their breakdown products, indolic compounds, are excreted in the urine. Because tryptophan is excessively excreted in urine and not reabsorbed in the gut, it is not available for synthesis of niacin. Many subjects are discovered to have the aminoaciduria but have no clinical manifestations (Hartnup's disorder). When the disorder is symptomatic, it is called Hartnup's disease; the main clinical manifestations are probably due to niacin deficiency, although the excessive indolic compounds may contribute to a metabolicencephalopathy. The actual carrier in the transport system or the gene responsible has not been identified. The biochemical phenotype is common, occurring in 1 in 30,000 newborns screened. However, only 10 percent or less actually develop the classical clinical phenotype. To develop the disease, multiple factors are probably involved—environmental, such as poor nutrition or intestinal diarrhea, and polygenic, such as low plasma amino acid levels that interact with the primary monogenic defect. Males and females are equally affected. Consanguinity in parents and affected siblings occurs not uncommonly. The disorder is worldwide and not associated with other genetic disorders.

The earliest clinical findings are photosensitive skin, leading to the pellagra-like rash in late infancy or early childhood. Later, episodic neuropsychiatric symptoms appear—intermittent cerebellar ataxia and emotional lability to psychoses—together or separately and often triggered by poor nutrition and diarrhea, fever, or sun exposure. EEGs are nonspecific, and CSF studies are normal. Partial expressions, such as intestinal or renal tubular defects alone, may be seen. The differential diagnosis includes any cause of acute cerebellar ataxia in childhood: postinfectious cerebellitis, brain stem encephalitis, posterior fossa tumor, and vestibular neuronitis. When attacks are intermittent, particularly with the mental symptoms, episodic disturbances such as nonconvulsive status epilepticus, acute confusional migraine, other toxic-metabolic encephalopathies, or demyelinating disease should be considered. The rash with neurological signs should bring to mind other vitamin deficiency diseases, such as thiamine or biotinidase deficiency.

The evaluation involves simple urine amino acid chromatography, which will detect the neutral aminoaciduria, and oral loading tests with L-tryptophan, which will detect the indoluria. No consistent picture of abnormalities has arisen from brain CT, MRI, and PET studies. To treat symptomatic subjects, nicotinamide, rather than nicotinic acid, is given orally at 50 to 300 mg/day. Both the rash and ataxia respond. A high-protein diet may help prevent attacks in those with low plasma amino acid resting levels. Although mental retardation may occur, dementia does not. There may be learning difficulties, but most patients have normal mentation. Further specific therapy awaits elucidation of the specific membrane transport carrier system and whether the defect is of transport activation, regulation, or direct transporting, as well as mapping and cloning of the gene. As yet there are no animal models.

Menkes' Disease

Menkes' disease, an X-linked disorder in which insufficient intestinal absorption of copper leads to deficiency of copper-requiring enzymes, is now known to be due to a gene located at Xq13.3.[97] The gene product belongs to a highly conserved family of cation-transporting ATPases, which function in the transport of ions across cellular and intracellular membranes. The low serum copper levels, the high tissue levels (particularly intestinal mucosa, except liver), and studies from patients' cultured cells strongly suggest that the basic pathogenetic defect is the failure of a plasma membrane pump that usually extrudes copper from cells or the failure of a pump that ordinarily transports copper into an intracellular organelle-like endoplasmic reticulum. Deficient activity of copper-requiring enzymes explains the symptoms and signs. Deficiency of dopamine beta-hydroxylase, critical to the catecholamine synthesis pathway, may be related to autonomic abnormalities due to decreased sympathetic adrenergic function. Cytochrome-*c* oxidase deficiency probably can be related to hypotonia, weakness, and the lesions similar to those seen in Leigh's disease, without severe lactic acidosis associated with complex IV respiratory chain defects. Reduced lysyl oxidase activity relates to the arterial tortuosity and other connective tissue disorders. Reduced tyrosine hydroxylase leads to lack of pigmentation. Partial loss of copper-zinc superoxide dismutase (Cu-Zn SOD) could lead to oxidant stress and cytotoxicity because of lack of defense against oxygen free radicals. The incidence is estimated to be 1 in 100,000 to 250,000 live births, a rare condition. One third of the estimated 15 to 30 affected infants born annually in the United States are predicted to be nonfamilial new mutations.

Male infants usually present at 2 to 3 months with developmental arrest and regression, hypotonia, seizures, and failure to thrive. Seizures are an early presentation, are frequent, and are multifocal myoclonic jerks that are often stimulus-precipitated. Recurrent hypothermia and infections occur. The near-pathognomonic clinical sign is scarce, colorless, wiry, friable hair on scalp and eyebrows and, under the microscope, the characteristic appearance of pili torti (twisted hair shaft). Secondary microcephaly occurs later. A mild Menkes' disease variant occurs, with later onset and milder neurological findings. The occipital horn syndrome, another variant, has few mental or neurological signs but calcified occipital horns, changes in clavicles and long bones, and sometimes chronic diarrhea and arterial changes. The differential diagnosis includes any early infantile progressive encephalopathy presenting with seizures, such as storage disease (Tay-Sachs disease, Sandhoff's disease, infantile neuronal ceroid lipofuscinosis), aminoacidurias (nonketotic hyperglycinemia), disorders of biogenic amine metabolism (folinic acid–responsive seizures), mitochondrial diseases (Alpers' disease), sulfite oxidase deficiency, glucose transporter deficiency, or the nonprogressive infantile myoclonic epilepsies. To make the diagnosis, the clinical picture, along with typical radiological features (osteoporosis, scalloping of vertebral bodies, excessive wormian bone formation), microscopic examination of the hair, and very low levels of serum copper and ceruloplasmin after the neonatal period, is sufficient. Cultured skin fibroblasts show increased copper content. In families at risk, prenatal diagnosis and heterozygote carrier detection can be done by biochemical and mutational analysis of cultured amniocytes or chorionic villi. The therapeutic strategies must (1) bypass the block in intestinal copper absorption; (2) supply copper to intracellular enzymes that require it for a cofactor; and (3) identify and treat patients early, preferably presymptomatically. Intravenous copper histidine bypasses the intestinal block but produces no substantive neurological improvement nor increases life span. Therapy with vitamins C and E has been ineffective. Supportive care includes maximizing caloric intake, physical and occupational therapy, psychosocial support of families and, most importantly, genetic counseling. Children usually die by age 3. Future treatments might explore the principle that lipid-soluble complexes can increase copper transport through cellular membranes. Gene therapy would be difficult because of the widespread, multisystem involvement and awaits functional characterization of the transport protein and progress in developing gene delivery systems to the brain.

Glucose Transporter or GLUT1 Deficiency Syndrome (Devivo Disease)

The erythrocyte glucose transporter is homologous to that in the brain, with both facilitating the diffusion of glucose across lipophilic plasma membranes.[98] This condition is due to defective functioning of the type 1 glucose transporter (GLUT1) in brain microvessels at the blood-brain barrier, causing low CSF glucose (hypoglycorrhachia) and therefore decreased cerebral energy metabolism and brain function. GLUT1 is coded by a gene localized to chromosome 1 and is developmentally regulated, with the messenger RNA in brain increasing with increasing cerebral metabolic rate for glucose in infancy and childhood. Symptoms occur when this rate increases in early infancy, doubling or tripling that in the neonatal and fetal periods. This is a very rare condition, originally reported as sporadic, then associated with haploinsufficiency, but recently, behaving as an autosomal dominant disorder in cases of familial epilepsy.[99] Numerous mutations in the GLUT1(SLC2A1) gene, which encodes the major glucose transporter in mamallian blood-brain barrier, include deletions, missense mutations, insertions, splice site, and nonsense mutations.[100]

At about age 3 months, a perfectly normal infant develops seizures—myoclonic, atypical absence, or unclassifiable—that are refractory to antiepileptic drugs. Developmental delay occurs the longer seizures are uncontrolled and the diagnosis is undiscovered, which can culminate in mental retardation and secondary microcephaly. The differential diagnosis includes any disease or condition causing refractory seizures in early infancy (see section on Menkes' disease). In this disorder, CSF glucose is 30 mg/dL or lower, with a reduced CSF/blood glucose ratio (about 0.33). CSF lactate is also low (0.97 mM/L or less). EEGs and neuroimaging studies are normal. Treatment involves seizure control with a ketogenic diet, because the diet provides ketone bodies as an alternative source of fuel for brain metabolism. The prognosis for seizure control and normal development is excellent with early diagnosis and treatment. It is likely that the defect becomes less consequential with age as the cerebral metabolic rate for glucose slows down to adult levels.

LESCH-NYHAN DISEASE (HYPOXANTHINE-GUANINE PHOSPHORIBOSYLTRANSFERASE DEFICIENCY)

Lesch-Nyhan disease is an X-linked recessive disease involving abnormal purine metabolism. The disorder is due to complete deficiency of hypoxanthine-guanine phosphoribosyltransferase (HPRT), an enzyme necessary for the recycling of free purine bases and reconversion into their nucleotide forms, after nucleotides are metabolized during DNA or RNA synthesis or after serving as coenzymes.[101] Specifically, if HPRT is deficient, hypoxanthine, a free purine base, cannot be reconverted back to inosine 5′-monophosphate, from which adenosine 5′-monophosphate and guanosine 5′-monophosphate are synthesized by separate pathways. There is an acceleration of the de novo purine biosynthesis pathway, so hypoxanthine is converted by xanthine oxidase to uric acid, resulting in hyperuricemia. However, the hyperuricemia does not explain the neurological symptoms, the pathophysiology of which is essentially unknown. Based on animal models, speculation is that self-injurious behavior may be related to supersensitivity of the D_1 subclass of dopamine receptors. Autopsies have revealed no specific cerebral gross anatomical or histopathological findings.

Incidence is rare, perhaps 1 in 380,000 births. The disorder occurs in many racial groups equally and is not more frequent in consanguineous populations. Patients are normal at birth, but by 6 months, developmental delay is evident. Axial hypotonia but appendicular spasticity and choreoathetoid movements appear in late infancy, and "cerebral palsy" is usually diagnosed at this time. The diagnosis is usually suspected in the toddler and early childhood years, when various kinds of compulsive self-mutilation, usually biting of lips, cheeks, or fingers, occur. Dysarthria makes communication difficult, and excitation may stimulate opisthotonus or torsion dystonia. Compulsive aggression can be directed toward anyone near the patient, including family members, and includes hitting as well as abusive language. Associated disorders are various hematological disorders, growth retardation, renal stones, and gouty arthritis if patients survive to adulthood.

Before the self-mutilating symptoms, other causes of nonprogressive or progressive extrapyramidal "cerebral palsy" should be considered, such as kernicterus, glutaricaciduria type 1, biopterin-dependent phenylketonuria, or biotinidase deficiency. Although some severely mentally retarded children of any etiology have self-abusive behaviors, such as head-banging, the relentlessness and compulsiveness of the self-injurious behavior in Lesch-Nyhan disease is extreme and unique.

The main clinical sign is self-injurious behavior resulting in tissue loss. Enzyme activity of HPRT can be assayed by radiochemical methods from dried blood spots, cultured skin fibroblasts, and hair follicle cells in probands and suspected female carriers. Biochemical analysis must be confirmed by molecular genetic analysis, particularly for female carriers. The entire HPRT locus has been sequenced, and the mutations in Lesch-Nyhan disease are extremely heterogeneous. The majority are detected by polymerase chain reaction–based techniques, usually amplification of genomic DNA and direct sequencing. In a small percentage, Southern blot analysis using HPRT complementary DNA as a probe is necessary to detect translocations or duplications.

Allopurinol, a xanthine oxidase inhibitor, decreases blood uric acid effectively but has no effect on the neurological symptoms. The following have been ineffective: folate, glutamine, magnesium, chlorpromazine, L-tryptophan, and clomipramine. Treatment with L-5-hydroxytryptophan plus carbidopa has been temporarily beneficial, but self-injurious behaviors re-emerge after discontinuing treatment or tolerance develops. Behavior modification—extinction, reinforcement of alternative behavior, or aversion therapy—shows inconsistent results. Physical restraints to prevent tissue injury are the most effective and include upper extremity splints to keep the arms straight, tying legs to wheelchairs so they cannot be brought up to the mouth, and dental guards to avoid teeth extraction as an extreme preventive measure.

Most patients are mentally retarded and do not stand or walk. Death frequently occurs during childhood. A patient with Lesch-Nyhan disease should be an ideal candidate for gene replacement therapy. The problem is to transfect an appropriate vector that would target brain cells, because neurological signs would not likely be affected by simple transplantation of infected cultured bone marrow cells into receptive hosts. Prenatal diagnosis using mutation detection and linkage analysis can detect 100 percent of affected males and excludes women who are suspected carriers if that family's HPRT mutation is known.

CONGENITAL DISORDERS OF GLYCOSYLATION (CDG) (CARBOHYDRATE-DEFICIENT GLYCOPROTEIN SYNDROME)

Pathogenesis and Pathophysiology. These disorders are clinically and biochemically heterogenous. They result from impaired synthesis of N-linked oligosaccharides, complex multisugars attached to proteins that function in cell-to-cell recognition and glycoprotein turnover. Strokelike episodes may be due to coagulation factors and their inhibitors, many of which are N-linked glycoproteins. Decreased levels of antithrombin III and protein C and decreased activity of factor XI, protein S, and heparin cofactor II have been reported, particularly during catabolic challenges such as fever and infection. However, specific coagulopathies have not been associated with the actual strokelike episodes, and ischemia or vasculopathy have not been demonstrated by MRI/MRA. Type Ia is due to phosphomannomutase deficiency. At least 11 CDGs have been discovered.

Epidemiology and Risk Factors. These are rare disorders with undetermined incidence and prevalence, but they have probably been underrecognized.

Clinical Features and Associated Disorders. Affected infants develop severe CNS and other system deficits. Signs include not only developmental delay, hypotonia, failure to thrive, and mental retardation, but also oculomotor abnormalities, especially ocular bobbing, retinal pigmentary degeneration, cerebellar ataxia, and peripheral neuropathy. Systemic features are inverted nipples, female hypogonadism, abnormal fat distribution in perineal areas, and pericardial effusions without facial dysmorphia. Seizures and strokelike episodes occur in about one half of patients, often triggered by fever and infections. Recovery from stupor and coma is usually complete, but permanent residuals can occur.

Evaluation and Differential Diagnosis. Suggestive laboratory features are evidence of coagulopathy, elevated liver function tests, low albumin, and low thyroxine and thyroxine-binding globulin levels. The diagnosis is confirmed by a characteristic serum transferrin isoelectric focusing pattern measured on frozen serum. The initial differential diagnosis is wide and includes any causes of metabolic strokelike episodes and seizures. Mitochondrial oxidative phosphorylation disorders, such as MELAS and MERRF, can be exluded by normal lactate peaks on magnetic resonance spectroscopy (MRS). The decreased n-acetyl aspartic acid peak on MRS is nonspecific, and any of the epilepsy syndromes that present with febrile seizures or febrile status epilepticus are in the differential diagnosis: severe myoclonic epilepsy syndrome of Dravet, which itself is being conceptualized as part of the familial febrile seizures; generalized epilepsy syndrome; and subtle malformations of cortical development. Various neurometabolic diseases with stuttering or progressive courses should be considered, depending on symptom presentation. In case of coma, fatty acid oxidation disorders, some organic acidurias, and UCDs are possible. If ataxia and a small cerebellum are present, abetalipoproteinemia, ataxia-telangiectasia, or ataxia-oculomotor apraxia syndrome should be evaluated. When hypotonia and seizures occur, peroxisomal disorders such as neonatal adrenoleukodystrophy or infantile Refsum's disease are possible. Retinal pigmentary degeneration and refractory seizures may also suggest neuronal ceroid lipofuscinoses. Finally, in cases of recurrent hemiplegia, the syndromes of hemiplegic migraine or recurrent familial hemiplegia are within the differential diagnosis.

Treatment and Prognosis. There is no specific etiological treatment yet, except for oral D-mannose in CDG-Ib, so management is symptomatic and supportive. Such treatments include prompt defervescence of fever and treatment of infections; prevention of catabolic events; and intravenous lorazepam, fosphenytoin, and/or phenobarbital for status epilepticus or frequent repetitive convulsions. The course is usually that of a static encephalopathy from birth, punctuated by paroxysmal neurological events that may be followed by recovery or residual neurological deficit. However, normal early development with regression in infancy proceeding to severe motor and mental deficiency has been reported.[102–104]

PORPHYRIAS

Porphyrias are caused by enzymatic defects in the heme pathway. There are several forms, each with similar neurological findings, highlighted by abdominal pains and peripheral neuropathy. Those with autosomal dominant inheritance include acute intermittent porphyria (AIP), due to porphobilinogen deaminase deficiency, hereditary coproporphyria (HCP) due to coproporphyrinogen oxidase deficiency, and variegate porphyria (VP), due to protoporphyrinogen oxidase deficiency. An autosomal recessive condition characterized by deficiency in delta-aminolevulinic acid dehydratase has been described.

In AIP, although the enzymatic defect is constant throughout life, neuropathic crises are interspersed between long periods of near-normal function. Abdominal pain usually is the initial symptom of a neuropathic attack, followed by a subacute motor neuropathy that may ascend from the feet, resembling Guillain-Barré syndrome. Facial, bulbar, and extremity weakness develops in most cases. EMG studies help in distinguishing AIP from demyelinating neuropathy, since in the former, denervation and evidence of axonal neuropathy is more pronounced than slowed conduction velocities. In addition to these typical neuropathic signs, dysautonomia may be pronounced and lead to cardiac arrhythmias, blood pressure instability, and urinary retention. Neurobehavioral signs indicative of CNS involvement include psychotic behavior, delirium, and seizures, although the seizures are usually due to hyponatremia and inappropriate release of antidiuretic hormone.[105]

Although the crises of AIP may be spontaneous in onset, certain risk factors are identified, including infection, ingestion of alcohol, and use of a large variety of drugs, including anticonvulsant medications. The diagnosis of AIP depends on the clinical presentation of intermittent painful crises, behavioral alterations, and neuropathy with excessive urinary excretion rates of delta-aminolevulinic acid and porphobilinogen. Treatment involves special dietary changes at the earliest sign of an attack. Patients must immediately increase their carbohydrate intake; if this maneuver does not abort the crisis, intravenous dextrose and hematin should be given to prevent activation of hepatic delta-aminolevulinic acid synthetase. In light of the large number of drugs associated with exacerbation of AIP crises, the control of the painful abdominal cramps is problematic, although low-dose narcotics may be used in many patients, sometimes supplemented with very low doses of benzodiazepine derivatives.[106]

HCP is much rarer than AIP. The neuropathic and systemic clinical manifestations of the two conditions are the same, except that a distinctive cutaneous photosensitivity occurs in one third of the HCP patients. Like AIP, HCP is punctuated with crises of neurological dysfunction that are precipitated by drugs, infections, and alcohol. HCP has a characteristic metabolic profile with elevated urinary and fecal coproporphyrins. Similar to AIP, delta-aminolevulinic acid and porphobilinogen are found in the urine, but coproporphyrin, a product not found in AIP, is also present in urine. Enzyme assays for coproporphyrin oxidase will demonstrate the deficiency, but this test is not readily available.[107]

VP is particularly found in southern Africa. It mimics AIP and CHP clinically, and photosensitivity is common.[106] In addition, a variety of skin lesions, including hyperpigmentation, hypertrichosis, vesicles, and bullae, are seen in patients with VP. Excretion patterns are similar to those of HCP, except the excreted amount of porphobilinogen exceeds coproporphyrin in VP whereas they are approximately equal in HCP. Treatment is the same as for AIP and HCP.

Finally, delta-aminolevulinic acid dehydratase deficiency is unique in being an autosomal recessive disorder. Neurological findings, as well as systemic and dermatological signs, mimic those of the other porphyrias, and the differentiation is made exclusively on the biochemical findings of enzyme deficiency and the high urinary excretion of delta-aminolevulinic acid without porphobilinogen.[107]

Reviews and Selected Updates

Darras BT, Friedman NR: Metabolic myopathies: A clinical approach. Part I. Pediatr Neurol 2000;22:87–97, 171–181.

DiDonato S, Parini R, Uziel G: Metabolic Encephalopathies, Therapy and Prognosis. London, John Libbey & Co, 1995.

Elder GH, Hift RJ: Treatment of acute porphyria. Hosp Med 2001;62:422–425.

Gordon N: Carbohydrate-deficient glycoprotein syndromes. Postgrad Med J 2000;76:145–149.

Kazemi-Esfarjani P, Skomorowska E, Jensen TD, Haller RG, Vissing J: A nonischemic forearm exercise test for McArdle disease. Ann Neurol 2002; 52:153–159.

Korson MS: Advances in newborn screening for metabolic disorders: What the pediatrician needs to know. Pediatr Ann 2000;29:294–301.

Leonard JV, Morris AAM: Inborn errors of metabolism around time of birth. Lancet 2000;356:583–587.

Lindoz NM, Karnes PS: Initial assessment of infants and children with suspected inborn errors of metabolism. Mayo Clin Proc 1995;70:987–988.

Lyon G, Adams RD, Kolodny EH: Neurology of Hereditary Metabolic Diseases of Children, 2nd ed. New York, McGraw-Hill, 1996.

McKusick V: Mendelian Inheritance in Man, 11th ed. Baltimore, Johns Hopkins University Press, 1994.

Ozand PT, Gascon GG: Organic acidurias: A review: I and II. J Child Neurol 1991;6:96–219, 288–303.

Saudubray JM, Charpentier C: Clinical phenotypes: Diagnosis/algorithm. *In* Scriver CR, Beaudet AL, Sly WS, Valle D (eds): The Metabolic and Molecular Bases of Inherited Disease, 7th ed. New York, McGraw-Hill, 1995, pp 327–400.

Shoffner JM: Oxidative phosphorylation disease diagnosis. Ann NY Acad Sci 1999;893:42–60.

Treem WR: New developments in the pathophysiology, clinical spectrum, and diagnosis of disorders of fatty acid oxidation. Curr Opin Pediatr 2000;12:463–468.

References

1. Millington DS, Kodo N, Norwood DL, Roe CR: Tandem mass spectrometry: A new method for acylcarnitine profiling with potential for neonatal screening for inborn errors of metabolism. J Inherit Metab Dis 1990;13:321–324.
2. Rashed MS, Ozand PT, Bucknall MP, Little D: Diagnosis of inborn errors of metabolism from blood spots by acylcarnitines and amino acids profiling using automated electrospray tandem mass spectrometry. Pediatr Res 1995;38:324–331.
3. Guthrie R: Blood screening for phenylketonuria. JAMA 1961;178:863.
4. Guthrie R: Screening for "inborn errors of metabolism" in the newborn infant: A multiple test program. Birth Defects 1968;IV:92–98.
5. Hunt DF, Giordani ABB, Rhodes G, et al: Mixture analysis by rapid triple quadrupole mass spectrometry: Metabolic profiling of urinary carboxylic acids. Clin Chem 1982;28:2387–2392.
6. Millington DS, Norwood DL, Kodo N, et al: Biomedical applications of high performance liquid chromatography-mass spectrometry with continuous-flow fast atom bombardment. J Chromatogr 1991;562:175–190.
7. Rashed MS, Rahbeeni Z, Ozand PT: Application of electrospray tandem mass spectrometry to neonatal screening. Semin Perinatol 1999; 23:183–193.
8. Korson MS: Advances in newborn screening for metabolic disorders: What the pediatrician needs to know. Pediatr Ann 2000;29:294–301.
9. Chakrapani A, Cleary MA, Wraith JE: Detection of inborn errors of metabolism in the newborn. Arch Dis Child Fetal Neonatal 2001;84:F205–F210.
10. Chace DH, DiPerna JC, Naylor EW: Laboratory integration and utilization of tandem mass spectrometry in neonatal screening: A model for clinical mass spectrometry in the next millenium. Acta Paediatr Suppl 1999;88:45–47.
11. Menkes JH, Hurst PL, Craig HM: New syndrome: Progressive infantile cerebral dysfunction associated with unusual urinary substance. Pediatrics 1954;14:462–467.
12. Naylor EW: Newborn screening for maple syrup urine disease. *In* Therrell BL (ed): Laboratory Methods for Neonatal Screening. Washington, DC, American Public Health Association, 1993, pp 115–124.
13. Dancis J: Variants of maple syrup urine disease. *In* Nyhan WL (ed): Heritable Disorders of Amino Acid Metabolism. New York, John Wiley & Sons, 1974, pp 32–36.
14. Tharp BR: Unique EEG pattern (comb-like rhythm) in neonatal maple syrup urine disease. Pediatr Neurol 1992;8:65–68.
15. Berry GT, Heidenreich R, Kaplan P, et al: Branched-chain amino acid–free parenteral nutrition in the treatment of acute metabolic

decompensation in patients with maple syrup urine disease. N Engl J Med 1991;324:175–179.
16. Rabier D, Narcy C, Revillon HP, et al: Normalization of plasma branched-chain amino acids (BCAAs) after liver transplantation in maple syrup urine disease (MSUD). Abstracts of the 29th SSIEM Annual Symposium, London, September 10–13th, 1991, p 129.
17. Nord A, Van Doornick WJ, Greene C: Developmental profile of patients with maple syrup urine disease. J Inherit Metab Dis 1991;14:881–889.
18. Wendel U, Rudiger HW, Passarge E, Mikkelsen M: Maple syrup urine disease: Rapid prenatal diagnosis by enzyme assay. Humangenetik 1973;19:127–128.
19. Allan JD, Cusworth DC, Dent CE, Wilson VK: A disease, probably hereditary, characterized by severe mental deficiency and a constant gross abnormality of the amino acid metabolism. Lancet 1958;1:182–187.
20. McMurray WC, Mohyuddin F, Rossiter FJ, et al: Citrullinuria: A new aminoaciduria associated with mental retardation. Lancet 1962;1:138.
21. Russell A, Levin B, Oberholzer VG, Sinclair L: Hyperammonemia: A new instance of an inborn enzymatic defect of the biosynthesis of urea. Lancet 1962;2:699–700.
22. Freeman JM, Nicholson JF, Schimke RT, et al: Congenital hyperammonemia: Association with hyperglycinemia and decreased levels of carbamyl phosphate synthetase. Arch Neurol 1970;23:430–437.
23. Issa AR, Yadav G, Teebi AS: Intrafamilial phenotypic variability in citrullinemia: Report of a family. J Inherit Metab Dis 1988;11:306–307.
24. Levy HL, Coulombe JT, Shih VE: Newborn urine screening. *In* Bickel H, Guthrie R, Hammersen G (eds): Neonatal Screening for Inborn Errors of Metabolism. Berlin, Springer-Verlag, 1980, pp 89–103.
25. Lemieux B, Auray-Blais CH, Giguere R: Comparison between amino acids and orotic acid analysis in the detection of urea cycle disorders in the Quebec urinary screening program. Adv Exp Biol Med 1982;153:321–329.
26. Neu AM, Christenson MJ, Brusilow SW: Hemodialysis for inborn errors of metabolism. *In* Nissenson AR, Fine AR (eds): Dialysis Therapy, 2nd ed. Philadelphia, Hanley & Belfus, 1992, pp 371–372.
27. Todo S, Starzl TE, Tzakis A, et al: Orthoptic liver transplantation for urea cycle enzyme deficiency. Hepatology 1992;15:419–422.
28. Hjelm M, de Silva LVK, Seakins JWT, et al: Evidence of inherited urea cycle defect in a case of fatal valproate toxicity. BMJ 1986;292:23–24.
29. Msall M, Batshaw ML, Suss R, et al: Neurologic outcome in children with inborn errors of urea synthesis. N Engl J Med 1984;310:1500–1505.
30. Nyhan WL, Borden MA, Bard L, Cooke RE: Idiopathic hyperglycinemia, a new disorder of amino acid metabolism. Pediatrics 1961;27:530–550.
31. Ozand PT, Rashed M, Gascon GG, et al: Unusual presentations of propionic acidemia. Brain Dev 1994;16(Suppl):46–57.
32. Oberholzer VG, Levin B, Burgess EA, Young WF: Methylmalonic aciduria: An inborn error of metabolism leading to chronic acidosis. Arch Dis Child 1967;42:492–504.
33. Mudd SH, Levy HL, Abeles RH, Kennedy JP Jr: A derangement in B12 metabolism leading to homocystinemia, cystathioninemia and methylmalonic aciduria. Biochem Biopsy Res Commun 1969;35:121–126.
34. Kahler SG, Sherwood WG, Woolf D, et al: Pancreatitis in patients with organic acidemias. J Pediatr 1994;124:239–243.
35. Van der Meer SB, Poggi F, Spada M, et al: Clinical outcome of long-term management of patients with vitamin B12–unresponsive methylmalonic acidemia. J Pediatr 1994;125:903–908.
36. Terheggen HG, Schwenk A, Lowenthal A, et al: Argininemia with arginase deficiency. (Letter.) Lancet 1969;2:748–749.
37. McInnes RR, Shih V, Chilton S: Interallelic complementation in an inborn error of metabolism: Genetic heterogeneity in argininosuccinate lyase deficiency. Proc Natl Acad Sci USA 1984;81:4480–4484.
38. Terheggen HG, Lowenthal A, Colombo JP: Clinical and biochemical findings in argininemia. Adv Exp Med Biol 1982;153:111–119.
39. Hauser ER, Finkelstein JE, Valle D, Brusilow SW: Allopurinol-induced orotidinuria: A test for mutations at the ornithine transcarbamylase locus in women. N Engl J Med 1990;322:1641–1645.
40. Pitt DB, Danks DM: The natural history of untreated phenylketonuria. J Pediatr Child Health 1991;27:189–190.
41. Dobson JC, Kushida E, Williamson M, Friedman G: Intellectual performance of 36 phenylketonuria patients and their nonaffected siblings. Pediatrics 1976;58:53–58.
42. Lenke RR, Levy HL: Maternal phenylketonuria and hyperphenylalaninemia: An international survey of untreated and treated pregnancies. N Engl J Med 1980;303:1202–1208.
43. Blau N, Barnes I, Dhondt JL: International database of tetrahydrobiopterin deficiencies: An update. J SSIEM 1995;33:PO25.
44. Blau N, Barnes I, Dhondt JL: International database of tetrahydrobiopterin deficiencies. J Inherit Metab Dis 1996;19:8–13.
45. Blau N, Kierat L, Heizmann CW, et al: Screening for tetrahydrobiopterin deficiency in newborns using dried urine on filter paper. J Inherit Metab Dis 1992;15:402–404.
46. Ribes A, Vilaseca MA, Briones P, et al: Methylmalonic aciduria with homocystinuria. J Inherit Metab Dis 1984;7(Suppl):129–130.
47. Carson NAJ, Neill DW: Metabolic abnormalities detected in a survey of mentally backward individuals in Northern Ireland. Arch Dis Child 1962;37:505–513.
48. Qureshi AA, Rosenblatt DS, Cooper B: Inherited disorders of cobalamin metabolism. Crit Rev Onc Hematol 1994;17:133–151.
49. Barber GW, Spaeth GL: Pyridoxine therapy in homocystinuria. (Letter.) Lancet 1967;1:337.
50. Wilcken DEL, Wilcken B: The pathogenesis of coronary artery disease: A possible role for methionine metabolism. J Clin Invest 1976;57:1079–1082.
51. Goodman SI, Markey SP, Moe PG, et al: Glutaric aciduria: A "new" disorder of amino acid metabolism. Biochem Med 1975;12:12–21.
52. Heyes MP: Hypothesis: A role for quinolinic acid in the neuropathology of glutaric aciduria type 1. Can J Neurol Sci 1987;14:441–443.
53. Brismar J, Ozand PT: CT and MRI of the brain in glutaric acidemia type 1: A review of 59 published cases and a report of 5 new patients. AJNR 1995;16:675–683.
54. Wolf B, Grier RE, Allen RJ, Goodman SI, Kien CL: Biotinidase deficiency: The enzymatic deficit in late onset multiple carboxylase deficiency. Clin Chim Acta 1983;131:272–281.
55. Wolf B: Worldwide survey of neonatal screening for biotinidase deficiency. J Inherit Metab Dis 1991;14:923–927.
56. Suchy SF, Secor McVoy JR, Wolf B: Neurologic symptoms of biotinidase deficiency: Possible explanation. Neurology 1985;35:1510–1511.
57. Ozand PT, Gascon GG, Al-Essa M, et al: Biotin-responsive basal ganglia disease: A novel entity. Brain 1998;121:1267–1279.
58. Dabbagh O, Brismar, J, Gascon GG, et al: The clinical spectrum of biotin-treatable encephalopathies in Saudi Arabia. Brain Dev 1994;16(Suppl):72–80.
59. Nygaard TG, Marsden CD, Fahn S: Dope-responsive dystonia: Long-term treatment response and prognosis. Neurology 1991;41:174–181.
60. Narabayashi H, Yokochi M, Iizuka R, et al: Juvenile parkinsonism. *In* Vinken PJ, Bruyn GW, Klawans HL (eds): Handbook of Clinical Neurology. Vol. 49. Amsterdam, Elsevier Science, 1986, pp 153–165.
61. Wolf B: Disorders of biotin metabolism. *In* Scriver CR, Beaudet AL, Sly WS, Valle D (eds): The Metabolic and Molecular Bases of Inherited Disease, 7th ed. New York, McGraw Hill, 1995, pp 3151–3177.
62. Al-Essa M, Sakati A, Dabbagh O, et al: Inborn error of vitamin B_{12} metabolism: A treatable cause of childhood/dementia/paralysis. J Child Neurol 1998;13:239–242.
63. Kaikov Y, Wadsworth LD, Hall CA, Rogers PCJ: Transcobalamin II deficiency: Case report and review of literature. Eur J Pediatr 1991;150:841–843.
64. Enns GM, Barkovich AJ, Rosenblatt DS, et al: Progressive neurological deterioration and MRI changes in cblC: Methylmalonic acidaemia treated with hydroxycobalamin. J Inherit Metab Dis 1999;22:599–607.
65. Anderson HC, Marble M, Shapira E: Long-term outcome in treated combined methylmalonic acidemia and homocystinemia. Genet Med 1999;1:146–150.
66. Al-Essa M, Al-Amir A, Rashed M, et al: Clinical, fluorine-18 labeled 2-fluoro-2-deoxyglucose positron emission tomography of the brain, MR spectroscopy and therapeutic attempts in methylenetetrahydrofolate reductase deficiency. Brain Dev 1999;21:345–349.
67. Narisawa K, Wada Y, Saito T, et al: Infantile type of homocystinuria with N5,10-methylenetetrahydrofolate reductase defect. Tohoku J Exp Med 1977;121:185–294.
68. Shih VE, Salem MZ, Mud SH, et al: A new form of homocystinuria due to N(5,10)-methylenetetrahydrofolate reductase deficiency. Pediatr Res 1972;6:395.
69. Shoffner JM, Wallace DC: Oxidative phosphorylation diseases. *In* Scriver CR, Beaudet AL, Sly WE, Valle D (eds): The Metabolic and Molecular Bases of Inherited Disease, 7th ed. New York, McGraw-Hill, 1995, pp 1535–1610.
70. Shoffner JM, Wallace DC: Oxidative phosphorylation diseases. Disorders of two genomes. Adv Hum Genet 1990;19:267–330.
71. Leigh D: Subacute necrotizing encephalomyelopathy in an infant. J Neurol Neurosurg Psychiatry 1951;14:216–221.

72. Santorelli FM, Shanske S, Macaya A, et al: The mutation at nt8993 of mitochondrial DNA is a common cause of Leigh's syndrome. Ann Neurol 1993;34:827–834.
73. Alpers BJ: Diffuse progressive degeneration of the gray matter of the cerebrum. Arch Neurol Psychiatry 1931;25:469–505.
74. Harding BN: Progressive neuronal degeneration of childhood with liver disease (Alpers-Huttenlocher syndrome): A personal review. J Child Neurol 1990;5:273–287.
75. Alfonso I: Lactic acidemia in the newborn. Int Pediatr 1995;10(Suppl 1):40–43.
76. Shoffner JM, Lott MT, Lezza AMS, et al: Myoclonic epilepsy and ragged red fiber disease (MERRF) is associated with mitochondrial DNA $tRNA^{Lys}$ mutation. Cell 1990;61:931–937.
77. Hirano M, Pavlakis SG: Mitochondrial myopathy, encephalopathy, lactic acidosis and strokelike episodes (MELAS): Current concepts. J Child Neurol 1994;9:4–13.
78. Moraes CT, Di Mauro S, Zeviani M, et al. Mitochondrial DNA deletions in progressive external ophthalmoplegia and Kearns-Sayre syndrome. N Engl J Med 1989;320:1293–1299.
79. Wallace DG, Singh G, Lott MT, et al: Mitochondrial DNA mutation associated with Leber's hereditary optic neuropathy. Science 1988;1242:1427–1430.
80. Schon EA, Tritschler HJ, Moraes C, et al: Mitochondrial myopathies. Int Pediatr 1992;7:23–27.
81. Centers for Disease Control: Reye syndrome surveillance—United States, 1989. MMWR 1991;40:88–89.
82. Van Coster RN, DeVivo DC, Blake D, et al: Adult Reye's syndrome: A review with new evidence for a generalized defect in intramitochondrial enzyme processing. Neurology 1991;41:1815–1821.
83. DeVivo DC: Reye syndrome: A metabolic response to an acute mitochondrial insult? Neurology 1978;28:105–108.
84. Woodfin BM, Davis LE: Displacement of hepatic ornithine carbamoyltransferase from mitochondria to cytosol in Reye's syndrome. Biochem Med Metabol Biol 1991;46:255–262.
85. Wilson R, Miller J, Greene H, et al: Reye's syndrome in three siblings. Am J Dis Child 1980;134:1032–1034.
86. Forsyth BW, Horwitz RI, Acampora D, et al: New epidemiologic evidence confirming that bias does not explain the aspirin/Reye's syndrome association. JAMA 1989;261:2517–2524.
87. Kotagal S, Rolfe U, Schwartz KB, Escober W: "Locked-in" state following Reye's syndrome. Ann Neurol 1984;15:599–601.
88. Roe CR, Coates PM: Mitochondrial fatty acid oxidation disorders. *In* Scriver CR, Beaudet AL, Sly WS, Valle D (eds): The Metabolic and Molecular Bases of Inherited Disease, 7th ed. New York, McGraw-Hill, 1995, pp 1501–1525.
89. Mathur A, Sims HF, Gopalakrishnan D, et al: Molecular heterogeneity in very-long chain acyl-CoA dehydrogenase deficiency causing pediatric cardiomyopathy and sudden death. Circulation 1999;99:1337–1343.
90. Boles RG, Buck EA, Blitzer MG, et al: Retrospective biochemical screening of fatty acid oxidation disorders in postmortem livers of 418 cases of sudden death in the first year of life. J Pediatr 1998;132:924–933.
91. Rinaldo P, Hye-Ran Y, Yu C, et al: Sudden and unexpected neonatal death: A protocol for the postmortem diagnosis of fatty acid oxidation disorders. Semin Perinatol 1999;23:204–210.
92. Odaib AA, Shneider BL, Bennett MJ, et al: A defect in the transport of long-chain fatty acids associated with acute liver failure. N Eng J Med 1998;339:1752–1757.
93. Treem WR, Shoup ME, Hale DE, et al: Acute fatty liver of pregnancy, hemolysis, elevated liver enzymes, and low platelets syndrome, and long chain 3-hydroxyacyl-coenzyme A dehydrogenase deficiency. Am J Gastroenterol 1996;1:2293–2300.
94. Ibdah JA, Bennett, MJ, Rinaldo P, et al: A fetal fatty-acid oxidation disoder as a cause of liver disease in pregnant women. N Engl J Med 999;340:1723–1731.
95. DeVivo DG, Tein I: Primary and secondary disorders of carnitine metabolism. Int Pediatr 1990;5:134–141.
96. Levy HL: Hartnup disorder. *In* Scriver CR, Beaudet AL, Sly WE, Valle D (eds): The Metabolic and Molecular Bases of Inherited Disease, 7th ed. New York, McGraw-Hill, 1995, pp 3629–3639.
97. Kaler SG: Menkes disease. Adv Pediatr 1994;41:263–304.
98. DeVivo DC, Trifiletti RR, Jacobson RI, et al: Defective glucose transport across the blood-brain barrier as a cause of persistent hypoglycorrhachia, seizures and developmental delay. N Engl J Med 1991;325:703–709.
99. Brockman K, Wang D, Korenke CG, et al: Autosomal dominant Glut-1 deficiency syndrome and familial epilepsy. Ann Neurol 2001;50: 476–485.
100. Wang D, Kranz-Eble P, DeVivo DC: Mutational analysis of GLUT1 (SLC2A1) in Glut-1 deficiency syndrome. Hum Mutat 2000;16:224–231.
101. Rossiter BJF, Caskey TC: Hypoxanthine-guanine phosphoribosyl transferase deficiency: Lesch-Nyhan syndrome and gout. *In* Scriver CR, Beaudet AL, Sly WS, Valle D (eds): The Metabolic and Molecular Bases of Inherited Disease, 7th ed. New York, McGraw-Hill, 1995, pp 1679–1697.
102. Hagberg BA, Blennow G, Kristiansson B, Stibler H: Carbohydrate-deficient glycoprotein syndromes: Peculiar group of new disorders. Pediatr Neurol 1993;9:255–262.
103. Pearl P, Krasnewich D: Neurologic course of congenital disorders of glycosylation. J Child Neurol 2001;16:409–413.
104. Jaeken J: Congenital disorders of glycosylation. Annu Rev Genomics Hum Genet 2001;2:129–151.
105. Ridley A: The neuropathy of acute intermittent porphyria. Q J Med 1969;38:307–333.
106. Tefferi A, Solberg LA, Ellefson RD: Porphyrias: Clinical evaluation and interpretation of laboratory tests. Mayo Clin Proc 1994;69:289–290.
107. Elder GH, Smith SG, Smyth SJ: Laboratory investigation of the porphyrias. Ann Clin Biochem 1990;27:395–412.

CHAPTER 32

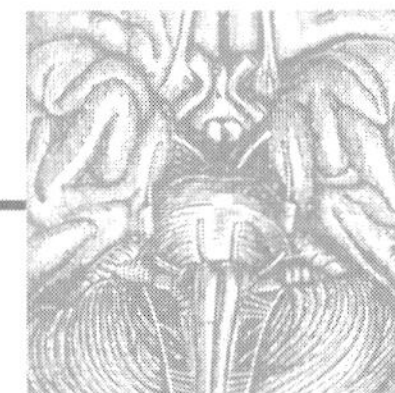

BRUCE O. BERG

Chromosomal Abnormalities and Neurocutaneous Disorders

History and Definitions

During the last several decades, information about chromosomal abnormalities has increased rapidly. Until recently, however, identified aberrations were limited to quantitative abnormalities of increased or decreased chromosomal material. Newer techniques have enabled us to identify numerous deletions and highly specific duplications, or translocations, which ultimately result in qualitative abnormalities of genes. Recombinant DNA techniques provide powerful tools for the definition of inherited neurological diseases and allow us to identify and define regulatory events that are the basis of cellular differentiation and embryogenesis.

Cognitive impairment is the primary neurological ramification of chromosomal abnormalities; however, most early reports of this finding were based on the study of individuals who were severely retarded. These individuals may have had multiple congenital anomalies with or without associated chromosomal disorders. Furthermore, various chromosomal anomalies may occur in seemingly normal adults with no obvious intellectual deficits.

This chapter focuses first on a number of clinical syndromes in which there are conspicuous neurological sequelae of chromosomal abnormalities and then on the most common neurocutaneous syndromes.

Chromosomal Anomalies

AUTOSOMAL ABNORMALITIES

Trisomy 21 (Down's Syndrome)

Pathogenesis and Pathophysiology. Several cytogenetic variants can produce Down's syndrome, and trisomy 21 is the most frequent. In this variant, Down's syndrome is due to an extra chromosome 21 or parts of it.[1] Trisomy of subbands 21q22.1 to 22.3 of the distal part of the long arm of chromosome 21 is the smallest component sufficient to cause Down's syndrome. In patients with trisomy 21, the genes on the extra segment of the chromosome are not found in a double dose as is normal but are tripled. In approximately 1 to 2 percent of cases, Down's syndrome occurs in the setting of mosaicism, in which there are two or more cell populations. Each cell population has a different karyotype, and one has a trisomy 21. The fusion of chromosome 21 with another acrocentric chromosome, most commonly chromosome 14, 21, or 22, may also result in a clinical syndrome that does not differ from that produced by the triplication of the subband 21q22. Finally, a rare familial form of Down's syndrome has been reported that may result from familial mosaicism, maternal trisomy 21, or other cytogenetic causes. The exact method by which these chromosomal anomalies cause the clinical sequelae of Down's syndrome has yet to be determined.

Epidemiology and Risk Factors. Down's syndrome is the most common autosomal chromosomal abnormality in human live births that results in structural malformations associated with developmental retardation. This disorder occurs in about 1 of 1000 neonates, and the frequency of trisomy 21 increases with maternal age. While familial forms of Down's syndrome are rare, the risk of a mother having a second affected infant is approximately 0.5 percent. In a child with a translocation, chromosomal karyotyping should be performed in both parents, since if one parent has the translocation, the risk of having a similarly affected child is much higher.

Clinical Characteristics and Associated Disorders. The physical characteristics of patients with Down's syndrome are commonly recognized in the first month of life, if not in the newborn nursery. Common features include brachycephaly with a round face, Brushfield's spots, a small mouth and a large protruding tongue, small ears, epicanthal folds with upslanting palpebral fissures, and a flattened or depressed nasal bridge. Although epicanthal folds and a transverse simian palmar crease are considered characteristic of Down's syndrome, they are found in only 50 percent of these patients. Brachydactyly and clinodactyly of the fifth finger are observed more commonly than the simian palmar crease. There is a widened space between the first and second toes.

In addition to the typical phenotypic features of the syndrome, associated congenital cardiac and gastrointestinal abnormalities may be present. A third to a half of patients with Down's syndrome have congenital cardiac defects, of which one third are endocardial cushion defects and the remainder are ventricular septal defects. Tetralogy of Fallot and atrial septal defects also occur, and there is an increased incidence of moyamoya disease. More than half of patients have bilateral hearing loss, of which many cases are attributable to anomalies of the inner and middle ear. Malformations of the gastrointestinal tract, including intestinal atresia and imperforate anus, occur in about 5 to 7 percent of patients, and there is a reported increased incidence of Hirschsprung's disease. Although abnormalities of T-lymphocyte function have been reported, no specific relationship of these to the infection rate has been established. Other associated abnormalities include gastroesophageal reflux, pulmonary hypertension, upper airway obstruction, obstructive sleep apnea, and an increased incidence of thyroid dysfunction, diabetes mellitus, cataracts, and leukemia.

The major neurological features of Down's syndrome are developmental delay and severe, diffuse muscular hypotonia, which affects most patients. Convulsive disorders are also more commonly present in these patients. The pathogenesis of the convulsive activity in this population is probably multifactorial and may result from a combination of medical risk factors and inherent neurological abnormalities. As individuals with Down's syndrome age, however, other neurological signs may appear. About 20 percent of patients complain of neck pain or discomfort, and they may demonstrate torticollis, gait impairment, or corticospinal tract dysfunction. These features are believed to be related to atlantoaxial subluxation and instability and result in compression of the medulla and spinal cord.

By about the fourth decade of life, additional deterioration of cognitive function may become apparent. This deterioration has been attributed to dementia, which results from a degenerative process that has neuropathological similarities to Alzheimer's disease.[2] Olfactory abnormalities may also appear, and these can pre-date the onset of dementia by 10 to 15 years.[3]

Differential Diagnosis. It is impossible to distinguish the clinical features of Down's syndrome resulting from the "typical" trisomy 21 from those resulting from translocation. Other chromosomal abnormalities should be considered, but the phenotypic features and neurological signs generally make the diagnosis clear.

Evaluation. The diagnosis of Down's syndrome is made by the presence of the typical physical abnormalities and can be confirmed by chromosomal karyotype. Radiological studies such as plain skull films may demonstrate a brachycephalic skull in which the anterior fontanelle and metopic suture close late. Computed tomography (CT) may show calcifications in the basal ganglia and a large opercula, while magnetic resonance imaging (MRI) reveals evidence of delayed myelination in some cases.[4] Other MRI studies have demonstrated smaller hippocampal and neocortical structures in patients with Down's syndrome compared to controls.[5] Additionally, these investigations suggest that patients with Down's syndrome develop signs associated with brain aging at an earlier age than normal; these signs include increased rates of ventricular dilatation, peripheral atrophy, and deep white matter lesions. The electroencephalogram (EEG) may be abnormal and can become progressively disorganized with the evolution of Alzheimer's type dementia. Reports of postmortem evaluations have noted the presence of a small, spherical brain and a cerebellum that is reduced in size. Microscopic abnormalities include reduced neuronal density in cortical regions, a loss of cortical interneurons, a reduction in the number of spines along pyramidal cells, and an accumulation of undifferentiated fetal cells in the cerebellum. Abnormalities in the basal nuclei of the brain include a reduced cell count that shows a continued steady decline with age. In nearly all subjects who die after reaching the age of 35, changes consistent with Alzheimer's disease are found.

Management and Prognosis. There is no specific treatment for Down's syndrome. Compared to the general population, these patients have increased morbidity and mortality, primarily from cardiac causes.

Trisomy 18 (Edwards' Syndrome)

Edwards' syndrome[6] is the second most common autosomal chromosomal abnormality associated with an extra autosome. The incidence of trisomy 18 is 0.3 per 1000 live births, and females are affected more often than males (3:1). In the majority of patients the entire chromosome 18 is trisomic, whereas other affected patients may have a mosaic state of partial trisomy. This anomaly is more frequent in the offspring of older mothers. A history of decreased in utero activity is typical, and there is an even distribution of premature, normal term, and postmature neonates with this disorder. Affected infants have a feeble cry, decreased adipose and subcutaneous tissue, and a paucity of muscle bulk. The face is generally small with a high nasal bridge, short palpebral fissures, ptosis, small mouth, narrow palate, and micrognathia.

The hands are clenched, with the second finger overriding the third and the fifth overriding the fourth. The nails are hypoplastic, especially those on the fifth fingers and toes. Other commonly associated findings include rocker-bottom feet, a short sternum, small pelvis, umbilical and inguinal hernias, and diastasis recti. The skin can be redundant, and hirsutism of the head and back is notable. Cardiac malformations include ventricular and atrial septal defects and patent ductus arteriosus.

No consistent central nervous system (CNS) abnormalities are found in this disorder, but agenesis of the corpus callosum is the most common anomaly and may be associated with cerebellar or cerebral white matter heterotopias. In those individuals who survive early infancy, severe mental retardation may occur. No specific therapy is available for patients with this syndrome. About half of patients expire before the age of 6 months, and only 10 percent survive 1 year.

Trisomy 13 (Patau's Syndrome)

The incidence of this trisomic syndrome, which occurs primarily in the offspring of older mothers, is approximately 1 in 7000, and it affects mainly females.[7] It should be noted that translocation can also result in this syndrome, but mothers of these children are usually younger. The clinical characteristics of this syndrome include multiple congenital anomalies with varying degrees of midfacial anomalies. Infants may have ophthalmic abnormalities including anophthalmia, cyclopia, microphthalmia, and colobomas. Facial defects, such as cleft palate and lip and micrognathia, can also occur. A variety of congenital cardiac abnormalities such as ventricular or atrial septal defects and patent ductus arteriosus may be present. Intestinal malrotation, Meckel's diverticulum, and a spectrum of urogenital structural abnormalities are commonly seen. Polydactyly, with the third and fifth fingers overlapping the fourth, occurs in most affected infants. Neurologically, patients have developmental retardation as well as an increased frequency of neural tube defects and microcephaly. Pathologically, the most common abnormalities include arrhinencephaly and holoprosencephaly, which can be associated with the absence of the interhemispheric fissure and the olfactory bulbs and tracts as well as with a single ventricle. Sample case reports have also noted the presence of corpus callosum lipomas and frontal cranial defects. As in infants with trisomy 18, heterotopias in the cerebellum and cerebral white matter may be observed. As is true of other trisomic conditions, no specific therapy is available. The average length of survival is about 9 months, and about 90 percent of affected patients die before the age of 12 months.

Prader-Willi Syndrome

The Prader-Willi syndrome is a sporadic disorder that occurs in about 1 in 20,000 live births and has a risk of recurrence in the same family of about 1 in 1000. The responsible abnormality on chromosome 15 can be documented by cytogenetic studies, and in about 50 percent of patients there is a deletion at 15q11–q13. The disorder that produces Angelman syndrome has the same gene locus. The use of cytogenetic techniques and DNA polymorphisms has made it possible to discern the origin of the parental deletion. Patients with Prader-Willi syndrome inherit the chromosomal disorder from their father, whereas patients with the Angelman syndrome inherit the chromosomal abnormality from their mother.[8]

Mothers of infants with the Prader-Willi syndrome note decreased in utero fetal activity, and often these neonates are born in breech presentation. The affected individuals are of short stature and have small hands and feet and a narrowed cranial bifrontal diameter.[9] Their eyes are almond-shaped, and they often have strabismus. The face is long, and nearly 50 percent of patients have hypopigmentation of the skin. Other common features include a small phallus, cryptorchidism, and hypogonadism with a small flat scrotum. Affected infants have a feeble suck and severe hypotonia, which commonly requires the use of a feeding tube. Near the end of the first year of life, however, the hypotonia may become less severe. The degree of mental retardation may seem more prominent in early life and may be correlated with the severity of the hypotonia. From 1 to 3 years of age, patients gain considerable weight and become obese because of hyperphagia. As the hypotonia becomes less severe, they also seem to be more mentally alert, yet the intelligence level usually ranges from an IQ of 40 to 60. Although the primary explanation for the short stature, hyperphagia, and hypogonadism has not been specifically defined, there is evidence that suggests the presence of primary hypothalamic dysfunction. Recent improvements in MRI scanning techniques have demonstrated anomalous cortical growth on the banks of the sylvian fissure in some children with Prader-Willi syndrome.[10] These "growths" are seen even more frequently in children with Angelman syndrome and are thought to represent misrouting of long projection axons. Electrophysiological studies and muscle biopsies have failed to reveal any clues to the cause of the severe hypotonia seen in these patients. At the present time, no direct therapy is available for the neurological aspects of this disorder.

SEX CHROMOSOMAL ABNORMALITIES

Klinefelter's Syndrome

This syndrome, characterized by a 47XXY chromosomal karyotype, is the most common human sex chromosomal aberration and is associated with the sex chromatin–positive form of seminiferous tubular dysgenesis. The frequency of the 47XXY karyotype is reported to be 0.9 in 1000; 0.15 in 1000 have a mosaic form. About half of patients with a 47XXY disorder die in utero.

Affected children have small, firm testes, and adult patients have azoospermia.[11] This disorder is a common cause of primary hypogonadism and male infertility. Although a male phenotype is typical, delayed or poorly developed secondary sex characteristics are present, and about half the patients have varying degrees of gynecomastia, androgen deficiency, and eunuchoid features. These patients tend to be tall and have long legs, and adults have an increased incidence of pulmonary disease, varicose veins, diabetes mellitus, and breast cancer.[12] Serum levels of follicle-stimulating hormone and luteinizing hormone are increased early in the second decade, whereas testosterone concentrations are normal to low. Plasma levels of estradiol are normal or high. Affected individuals have cognitive abnormalities, including impaired auditory sequential memory with delayed language development and associated learning disorders.[13] There is a slight lowering of the mean IQ and an increased incidence of behavioral and personality abnormalities. A higher than normal prevalence of postural tremor has been reported, but the findings have not been replicated.

If androgen deficiency is present, administration of testosterone may produce an improvement in the secondary sexual characteristics and increase the general well-being of the patient. Testosterone therapy may also lessen the degree of gynecomastia, but in those patients with notable breast enlargement, surgical reduction of the breast tissue may be important for cosmetic reasons.

XYY Syndrome

The incidence of this abnormal sex chromosomal karyotype is about 1 in 1000 live male births. These patients have a normal male phenotype, although cryptorchidism and hypogonadism have been known to occur. Tall stature and acneiform eruptions are common characteristics. Although earlier studies suggested that affected patients had inordinately aggressive, impulsive behavior, this finding has not been reliably substantiated. Most patients have normal behavior, and their intelligence tends to be low normal. Delayed acquisition of speech and language skills may also be present. Other minor neurological findings include postural tremor and motor incoordination.

Turner's Syndrome

Turner's syndrome, a form of gonadal dysgenesis resulting from a 45,X karyotype (X-chromosomal monosomy), is characterized by female phenotype, short stature, a shieldlike chest, a short and sometimes webbed neck, low-set ears, high-arched palate, small mandible, and sexual infantilism.[14] The frequency of 45,X in female live births is 0.1 to 0.6 per 1000. A variety of other malformations can be associated, including congenital lymphedema, particularly of the hands and feet, cardiac and renal defects, skeletal anomalies, and abnormalities of the nails. An increased number of pigmented nevi has also been reported. Other disorders have been associated with this disorder, including Hashimoto's thyroiditis, obesity, inflammatory bowel disease, and rheumatoid arthritis. Nerve deafness occurs in approximately half the patients, and olfactory as well as taste deficits have been described. Eighteen percent of patients studied in one series were mentally retarded, although this high prevalence may be due to selection bias. The absence of the X chromosome does not cause intellectual impairment per se, but the majority of these patients have right-left disorientation and defects in perceptual orientation.[15]

Psychological tests demonstrate that girls with Turner's syndrome perform poorly on visuospatial and intellectual measures and have difficulty with attention and social behaviors compared with age-matched controls.[16] Others have reported that Turner's syndrome patients have significantly lower scores on all the Wechsler adult intelligence scale tests except verbal comprehension and reading level.[17] The most significant difference is found in the visuospatial construction. Volumetric brain measures derived from MRI reveal no differences in overall cerebral or subcortical volume, yet the regional distribution of gray and white matter varies in the two groups. In general, girls with Turner's syndrome have a smaller proportion of tissue in the right and left parietal regions and a larger amount in the right inferior parietal-occipital region. Additional MRI studies have shown that measured volumes of the hippocampus; the caudate, lenticular, and thalamic nuclei; and the parieto-occipital brain matter bilaterally are smaller.[18]

Treatment of patients with Turner's syndrome is directed at facilitating growth by administering recombinant growth hormone,[19] correcting associated congenital anomalies, and carefully managing hormonal replacement therapy for sexual infantilism.

Fragile-X Syndrome

Second only to Down's syndrome, the fragile-X syndrome is the most common cause of mental retardation in males and has a frequency of about 1 in 1500 males. It is found in all ethnic groups and has been identified in patients with other chromosomal abnormalities. The higher incidence of mental retardation in males and reports of families in which only males are affected suggest a nonspecific X-linked inheritance, termed the Martin-Bell or Renpenning's syndrome.[20, 21] No cytogenetic abnormality had been found in this heterogeneous subgroup of the mentally retarded population until a fragile site in the terminal region of the long arm of the X chromosome (Xq27.3) was demonstrated when the cells were cultured without folic acid.

The hereditary transmission of the fragile-X syndrome has been described by Tarleton and Saul, and the fragile-X gene has been isolated, cloned, and characterized.[22] It contains a trinucleotide sequence (CGG) that repeats in the normal genome 6 to 45 times, whereas the repeat is expanded to several hundred copies in patients with fragile-X syndrome. Carriers of the fragile-X syndrome, who are asymptomatic, have about 50 to 230 copies of this sequence. The expansion of the CGG repeat sequence is associated with methylation-induced inactivation of a sequence (CpG island) that is contiguous but separate from the *FMR-1* gene.[23] This region is thought to initiate gene transcription. The degree of methylation correlates with the number of repeats, suggesting that the fragility of the site of the fragile-X (FRAXA) is related to the triplet repeats.

The characteristic physical features of affected males with fragile-X syndrome include a long face, prominent mandible, large ears, and macro-orchidism with no evidence of endocrine dysfunction. All signs may not be present in prepubertal males and are not always prominent in adults. Although affected children may be unusually tall, the adult male with fragile-X tends to be shorter than average. Other associated features include joint hyperextensibility, flat feet, scoliosis, mitral valve prolapse, and dilatation of the aortic root. Although no specific abnormality of connective tissue metabolism has been identified in patients with this syndrome, abnormal elastin fibrils have been observed in skin biopsies of some patients. Some heterozygote females may also have a long face, prominent ears, and joint hyperextensibility. These features are more commonly observed in mentally subnormal females than in those with normal intelligence.

The majority of adult males with fragile-X have mental abilities that are moderately retarded, but about 30 percent have severe mental impairment. A small number of males have low-normal or mildly retarded intelligence, albeit with a variety of specific learning disabilities. There may be a delay in acquisition of speech and language skills, and older patients often have a low-pitched, somewhat hoarse voice with features of perseveration, cluttering, and staccato speech. The degree of mental impairment in females is somewhat less than in males, with about a third of patients having mental abilities in the retarded range and about a half demonstrating specific learning disabilities. Attentional deficits, hyperactivity, and impulsive and aggressive behaviors are known to occur. Patients may additionally have macrocephaly, hypotonia, oculomotor dysfunction, and inordinate clumsiness with impairment of fine and gross motor movements.[24] An increased incidence of convulsive disorders may occur in nearly 25 percent of patients. These seizures are generally simple or partial complex seizures and tend to occur more frequently during the first 10 to 15 years of life. The seizures are usually well controlled by the administration of standard antiepileptic medications and appear to have no relationship to the degree of mental retardation. Tic disorders have also been reported in patients with fragile-X syndrome and their families.

There is no specific treatment for fragile-X syndrome other than providing special educational programs tailored to the specific disabilities of each patient. For patients with attentional deficit disorder and hyperactivity, these behaviors are sometimes improved by the administration of CNS stimulants.

Neurocutaneous Disorders

The neurocutaneous syndromes comprise a group of heterogeneous disorders characterized by dysplasia and a tendency to form tumors.[25, 26] The CNS and skin are primarily involved, but other organ systems can be affected. Since the skin and nervous tissue originate from the same germ layer, the ectoderm, these disorders have been variously called congenital ectodermoses and congenital neuroectodermal dysplasias. Van der Hoeve believed that the ocular findings of neurofibromatosis and tuberous sclerosis were similar and suggested that they be classified together under the inappropriate term phakomatosis (Greek *phakos*: lentil, mole, or birthmark).[27] He later added von Hippel-Lindau disease and Sturge-Weber syndrome to this category,[28, 29] and in 1941, Louis-Bar proposed that ataxia-telangiectasia should also be considered as one of the phakomatoses. During the last 50 years a wide variety of disorders, all of which are unusual and many of which lack dysplastic or neoplastic characteristics, have been considered to belong to this heterogeneous group of disorders. The major neurocutaneous syndromes are considered herein, and others are noted in Table 32–1.

AUTOSOMAL DOMINANT DISEASES

Neurofibromatosis (Von Recklinghausen's Disease)

Pathogenesis and Pathophysiology. Neurofibromatosis[30] is no longer considered a single clinical entity and has been divided into at least two distinct forms.[31] The common form, once known as peripheral neurofibromatosis (NF), is called NF-1, and the rare form, once termed central NF, is NF-2. Both are inherited as autosomal dominant traits, and the gene locus responsible for NF-1 is on chromosome 17 (17q11.2), whereas that for NF-2 is on chromosome 22 (22q11.1 to 22q13.1). These disorders are due to abnormalities in the development of neural crest cells that produce hyperplasia, neoplasia, and dysplasias of the neuroectodermal elements and their supporting structures. Recently, the gene for NF-1 was found to code for a large, ubiquitously expressed protein (neurofibromin).[32] This protein has structural and functional similarity to a family of proteins that has guanosine triphosphatase activation properties. This family of proteins is involved in the regulation of the proto-oncogene *ras*. It has been speculated that the functions of the NF-1 gene product may be related to its ability to regulate *ras*-mediated cell proliferation.

Epidemiology and Risk Factors. NF-1 occurs in approximately 1 in 4000 to 5000 individuals. About half the cases appear to be sporadic, and the mutation rate has been estimated at 1 in 10,000 gametes per generation, one of the highest mutation rates in humans. Approximately 50 percent of patients have affected relatives, and in nearly all instances the distribution of cases is consistent with an autosomal dominant mode of inheritance. NF-1 is observed in all regions of the world and affects men and women equally. The frequency of NF-2 is not known, and its natural history has been derived from studies of a large Pennsylvania family.

Clinical Features and Associated Disorders. NF-1 is characterized by cutaneous pigmentation, multiple tumors within the central and peripheral nervous systems, and lesions of the vascular and other organ systems[33, 34] (Table 32–2). Focal hyperpigmented areas and café au lait spots, ranging in size from a few millimeters to centimeters, are more commonly found on the trunk than on the limbs, and they are not found on the scalp, soles, or palms (Fig. 32–1). These spots are light brown and result from an aggregation of neural crest–derived pigmented melanoblasts in the basal layer of the epidermis. Café au lait spots are present at birth and become more apparent with time. The number of café au lait spots probably does not significantly increase after the first several years of life, although the degree of hyperpigmentation usually does. The presence of six or more café au lait spots larger than 15 mm in greatest diameter is required for a diagnosis of NF, a criterion that is most useful when applied to the postpubertal patient. It should be recognized, however, that about 10 percent of the general population have café au lait spots without other stigmata of the disease. Less frequent cutaneous changes in NF-1 include diffuse axillary or inguinal freckling and large areas of faintly increased pigmentation (melanoderma) (Fig. 32–2).

Fibroma molluscum, soft or firm papules found in or just below the dermis that vary in size from a few millimeters to one or more centimeters, may also occur (Fig. 32–3). They are violaceous in color and vary in configuration from flat or sessile forms to pedunculated or lobulated forms. When compressed, these skin lesions tend to invaginate into the subcutaneous tissue. Hypopigmented spots similar to those observed in patients with tuberous sclerosis, discrete areas of skin hypoplasia, and angiomas may also be present in NF-1. All dermatological abnormalities may appear well before any neurological signs or symptoms occur.

TABLE 32–1. **Selected Neurocutaneous Syndromes**

Disease	Clinical Features
Autosomal Dominant Inheritance	
Incontinentia pigmenti achromians (hypomelanosis of Ito)	Bilateral asymmetrical areas of hypopigmented whorls ("marbling"); central nervous system, eye, tooth, skin, nail, and bone anomalies
Rendu-Osler-Weber disease	Multiple angiomas of skin and mucous membranes that are dilations of capillaries and venules; bleeding from any site: nose, gastrointestinal, pulmonary, and urinary systems
Waardenburg's syndrome (I)	Frontal patch of white hair, heterochromia iridis, lateral displacement of inner canthus and, at times, cochlear deafness
Waardenburg's syndrome (II)	Clinical findings are similar to type I without the lateral displacement of inner canthus; deafness is more common
Autosomal Recessive Inheritance	
Ataxia-telangiectasia	Ataxia and telangiectasias of the bulbar conjunctivae, malar eminences, ear lobes, and upper neck; increased incidence of respiratory infections, lymphomas, Hodgkin's disease, acute leukemia, and a variety of cancers; thymus gland is hypoplastic or absent; there is decreased IgA and IgG; increased chromosomal breakage and increased sensitivity to ionizing radiation of fibroblasts and lymphocytes
Chédiak-Higashi syndrome	Rare, partial oculocutaneous albinism, photophobia, neuropathy, and recurring infection; giant cytoplasmic organelles are observed
Refsum's syndrome	Retinal pigmentary degeneration, polyneuropathy, and ataxia; sensorineural deafness, anosmia, and cardiomyopathy are usually present; abnormalities of the eyes, skin (icthyosis), and bone are often present
Rothmond-Thomson syndrome	Erythematous skin lesions in early life followed by telangiectasias, atrophy, hypo- and/or hyperpigmentation, ectodermal dysplasia; body hair is sparse or absent; cataracts, short stature, hypogonadism, and skeletal abnormalities are common; intelligence is normal
Rud's syndrome	Icthyosis and hypogonadism are major features; microcephaly, sensorineural deafness, polyneuropathy, and hypoplastic teeth and nails are less frequent
Sjögren-Larsson syndrome	Congenital icthyosis associated with mental subnormality and corticospinal tract dysfunction
Xeroderma pigmentosum	Defect in DNA repair results in premature aging of tissues exposed to sunlight; microcephaly, mental subnormality, ocular changes, corticospinal tract dysfunction, ataxia, and movement disorders may be present
X-Linked Inheritance	
Fabry-Anderson disease	A glycolipid lysosomal storage disease with a wide spectrum of clinical findings: angiokeratosis is a characteristic feature; lancinating limb pain is often the first symptom; joint pain may resemble that of juvenile rheumatoid arthritis; ocular, cardiac, and gastrointestinal symptoms may be present; cerebrovascular accidents can occur in young adults; neuropathy; renal disease manifests as inability to concentrate urine, urinary frequency, polyuria, and nocturia
Incontinentia pigmenti (Bloch-Sulzberger syndrome)	Seen almost entirely in females; characterized by skin lesions present during the first few weeks of life that are erythematous, macular, papular, vesicular, or bullous; second stage, skin lesions are variably verrucous, lichenoid, or keratotic; third stage, lesions are notable for hyperpigmentation; abnormalities of the eyes, central nervous system, hair, teeth, and bone are commonly associated

Lisch nodules are iridic melanocytic hamartomas that are age dependent and are found in 10 percent of patients less than 6 years of age, 50 percent of patients less than 30 years old, and in virtually all affected patients by the age of 50 years (Fig. 32–4). Optic gliomas, reported in 15 to 20 percent of patients, can present with decreased visual acuity or visual field defects.[35] These tumors can involve the optic chiasm and hypothalamus and rarely become manifest as the diencephalic syndrome of infancy. There is some controversy about the nature of the tumor, but optic gliomas of childhood are probably congenital, indolent, and slowly growing hamartomas. Congenital glaucoma may also be a complication of NF-1 and is sometimes associated with neurofibromas of the superior eyelid.

Neural tumors, or neurofibromas, can involve any nerve from the dorsal root ganglia to the terminal twigs of the peripheral nerves, and any organ can be involved (Fig. 32–5). Peripheral neurofibromas vary in size and occur more frequently on the trunk than on the limbs. Plexiform neuromas are composed of an overgrowth of neural elements of tumor and connective tissue that infiltrates normal tissue. These larger tumors can be superficial, affecting the skin and subcutaneous tissue, or deep, affecting visceral and adjacent tissues. Intracranial tumors occurring in NF-1 are primarily meningiomas and gliomas. There is an increased incidence of optic gliomas and neurofibromas in these patients, and schwannomas may also occur and may involve other cranial nerves. Intraspinal tumors can be present and are sometimes accom-

TABLE 32–2. **Diagnostic Criteria for Neurofibromatosis**

Diagnostic Criteria for Neurofibromatosis 1
Six or more café au lait macules over 5 mm in greatest diameter in prepubertal individuals and over 15 mm in greatest diameter in postpubertal individuals
Two or more neurofibromas of any type or one plexiform neuroma
Freckling in the axillary or inguinal region
Optic glioma
Two or more Lisch nodules (iris hamartomas)
Distinctive osseous lesion such as sphenoidal dysplasia or thinning of long bone cortex with or without pseudoarthrosis
First-degree relative (parent, sibling, or offspring) with neurofibromatosis 1 by these criteria

Diagnostic Criteria for Neurofibromatosis 2
Bilateral cranial nerve VIII masses seen with appropriate imaging techniques
First-degree relative with neurofibromatosis 2 and either unilateral cranial nerve VIII mass or two of the following: neurofibroma, meningioma, glioma, schwannoma, and juvenile posterior subcapsular lenticular opacity

panied by spinal cord anomalies. While most tumors in this disorder are benign, some neurofibromas may undergo malignant transformation.

The diagnostic criteria for NF-2 require one or more of the following: bilateral cranial nerve VIII masses; a parent, sibling, or child with NF-2; and either a unilateral cranial nerve VIII

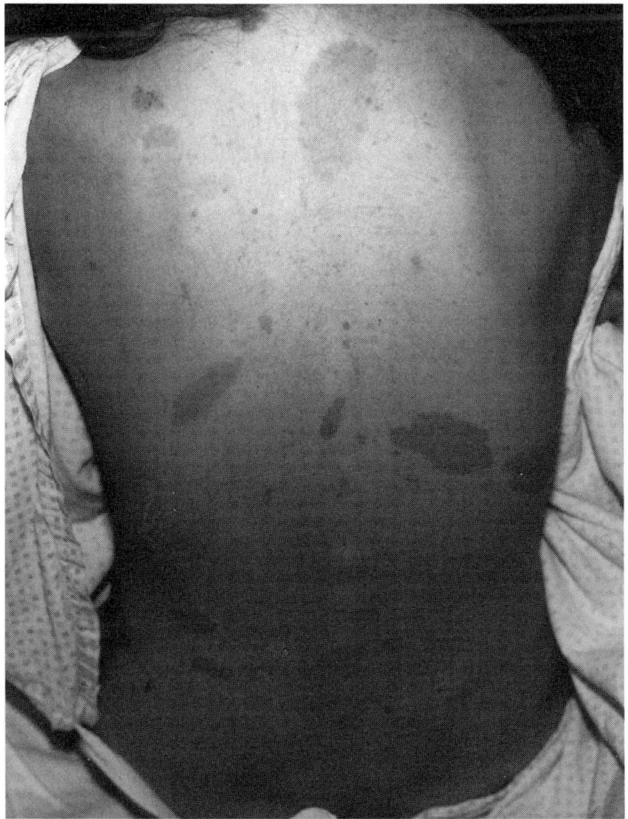

FIGURE 32–1. A 9-year-old patient with multiple café au lait spots of varying sizes, which are more common on the trunk than on the limbs.

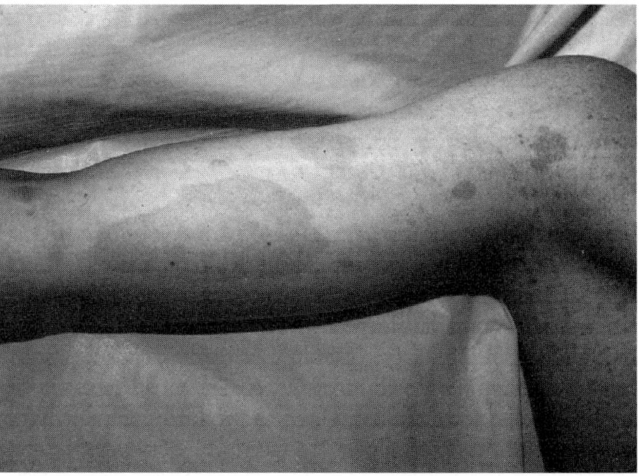

FIGURE 32–2. Axillary and inguinal region freckling, as observed in this patient, is common in patients with neurofibromatosis.

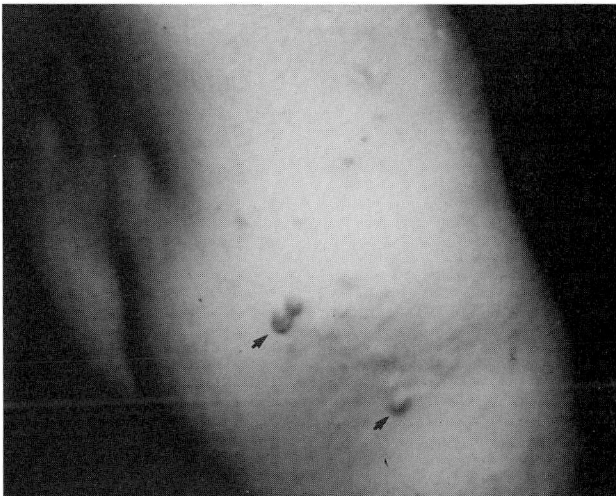

FIGURE 32–3. An example of fibroma molluscum, which is a soft or firm papular or polypoid lesion found in or just below the dermis and which ranges in size from a few millimeters to 1 cm or more. (Courtesy of Dr. Mary Williams, Department of Dermatology, University of California Medical Center, San Francisco.)

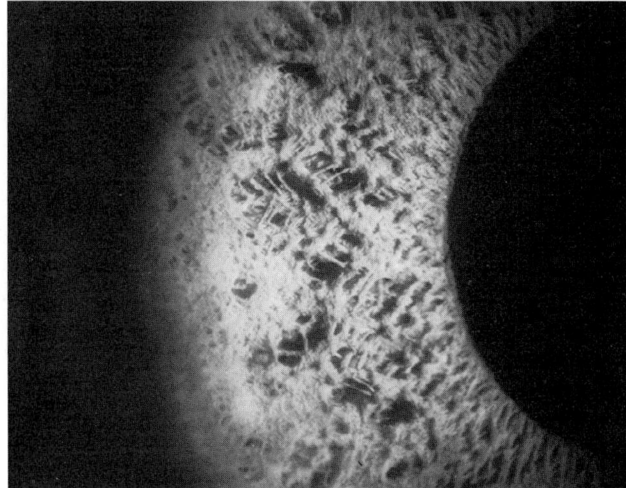

FIGURE 32–4. Lisch's nodules are age-dependent iridic melanocytic hamartomas that are commonly observed in patients with neurofibromatosis. (Courtesy of Dr. Creig Hoyt, Department of Ophthalmology, University of California Medical Center, San Francisco.)

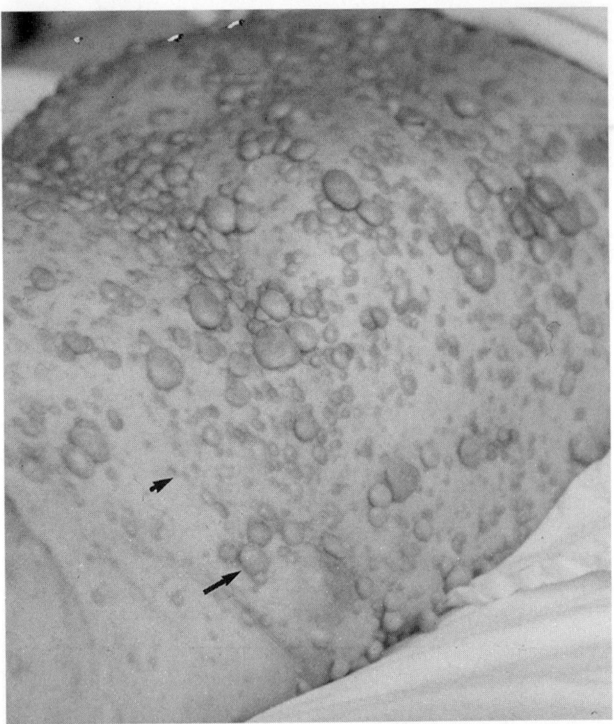

FIGURE 32–5. An older teenage patient with numerous neurofibromas *(short arrow)* as well as multiple lesions typical of fibroma molluscum *(long arrow)*.

mass or any two of the following: neurofibroma, meningioma, glioma, schwannoma, or juvenile posterior subcapsular lenticular opacity. Bilateral acoustic neuromas become manifest in over 95 percent of affected individuals. Symptoms of acoustic neuromas are usually referable to pressure on the vestibulocochlear and facial nerves, and patients may complain of tinnitus, buzzing, or background noise in the head. Alternatively, the initial symptom may be unilateral loss of hearing, which is noticed when the patient uses the telephone. Typically, symptoms begin in the second or third decade, but patients may become symptomatic in the first decade or as late as the ninth. Other features of NF-2 include café au lait spots and neurofibromas, although these are less commonly observed than in patients with NF-1. Presenile lens opacities or subcapsular cataracts have been found in nearly 50 percent of patients and may precede the symptoms of acoustic neuromas. Patients with NF-2 may have Schwann cell tumors of other cranial nerves or spinal roots, and meningiomas, astrocytomas, and ependymomas may present in the same patient. Optic gliomas, astrocytomas, and hamartomas are usually not found in this form of NF.

Associated features of NF include mental retardation or seizures, which occur in about 10 percent of NF patients, and about 40 percent have specific learning disabilities and hyperactivity. Occlusive cerebrovascular disease, although rare, can sometimes be demonstrated by angiography, which shows occlusive changes of the supraclinoid segment of the internal carotid artery associated with the telangiectasia characteristic of moyamoya disease.

Macrocephaly and short stature are reported in 10 to 40 percent of NF patients, and a variety of bony changes may also be present (including "ballooning" of the middle fossa, an enlarged or J-shaped sella, and dysplastic changes of the sphenoid). Patients with optic gliomas may have enlarged optic foramina, and bony defects of the orbit and other cranial bones are not uncommon. Scoliosis has been reported in 10 to 40 percent of patients and usually becomes manifest after the age of 6 years. Anterior meningocele, kyphosis, enlarged intervertebral foramina, bowing of the tibia and fibula, and bony overgrowth occur. Precocious puberty may occur in NF-1 patients with gliomas or hamartomas of the hypothalamus.

NF may be associated with a number of other neoplastic processes with a more than random frequency. These include leukemia, Wilms' tumor, neuroblastoma, multiple endocrine neoplasias, and pheochromocytoma. Of patients with pheochromocytomas, 4 to 23 percent are reported to have neurofibromatosis, whereas fewer than 1 percent of patients with neurofibromatosis have pheochromocytomas. Hypertension may also result from intimal proliferation and fibromuscular changes of the media of the small renal arteries, or from a pheochromocytoma.

Differential Diagnosis. The differential diagnosis of NF-1 is limited to the presence of a family history of the disease and the typical neurological and dermatological findings. NF-2 should be distinguished from sporadic, unilateral acoustic neuroma (SUAN). NF-2 usually presents prior to 40 years of age and is distinguished by the presence of brain and spinal tumors, café au lait spots, fibromas, and posterior capsular lens opacities. In contrast, SUAN presents after 40 years and has no associated findings.

Evaluation. The diagnostic tests used in patients with NF should be determined by the findings in the clinical examination because most studies will not be valuable in the asymptomatic NF patient. MRI can be useful in the evaluation of patients with possible intracranial, extracranial, and nerve root neoplasms. This neuroimaging study may also demonstrate incidental "bright areas" in patients with NF-1 that are consistent with "hamartomas" that may represent focal areas of heterotopic or dysplastic tissue. These focal areas of increased signal intensity on T2-weighted images are not associated with vasogenic edema and are primarily seen in the basal ganglia, internal capsule, midbrain, cerebellum, and subcortical white matter. They are not visualized on contrast-enhanced CT. MRI findings suggestive of gliomas include the presence of vasogenic edema, mass effect, cavitation, enhancement with gadolinium, and decreased signal intensity on T1-weighted images. When optic nerve gliomas are suspected, MRI with fat suppression techniques is a useful adjunctive study. The spine of a patient with NF-1 should also be imaged with MRI if there are symptoms or signs of intraspinal or nerve root compression. Isolated neurofibromas may involve the neural foramina and spinal canal, forming the so-called dumbbell tumor. Neoplasms involving the spinal canal and cord are best demonstrated with the use of gadolinium.

Patients who are at high risk for NF-2 should undergo MRI with gadolinium of the head, paying special attention to the cerebellopontine angle and internal acoustic meatus. Careful ophthalmic assessment should be performed to document the presence or absence of posterior capsular lenticular opacities and papilledema. Tests of vestibular and auditory function as well as brain stem auditory evoked potentials should be considered in the evaluation of these patients.

If symptoms suggest the presence of a pheochromocytoma, abdominal and mediastinal imaging should be performed, and neurotransmitter metabolites should be measured. Patients who are having problems with academic achievement should undergo neuropsychological studies to detect the presence and nature of any specific learning disabilities.

Management. Treatment of patients with NF is supportive and symptomatic. Patients with specific learning disabilities should receive the benefit of special education programs. Patients with seizures should be treated with standard antiepileptic agents. Peripheral neurofibromas are generally indolent and do not require surgical removal unless they are subjected to repeated trauma and abrasion or show rapid growth. Plexiform neuromas may be removed for strictly cosmetic reasons. Intracranial and intraspinal tumors should be treated with neurosurgical intervention, irradiation, or chemotherapy when appropriate. Most investigators suggest managing optic gliomas conservatively, with serial MRI scans and visual field and acuity examinations, rather than by immediate surgery or chemotherapy.[36, 37] The clinical course of patients with NF-2 may be relatively benign, and indications for acoustic neuroma surgery must be made on an individual basis. The presence of an acoustic neuroma does not inevitably lead to deafness and facial disfigurement; moreover, surgery in the region of the cerebellopontine angle is not without risk. Partial removal may be appropriate to preserve useful hearing in some cases. Counseling should address the issues of prognosis, genetics, and psychological and social adjustment.

Prognosis. Neurofibromatosis is a progressive disorder that requires continuous surveillance. The overall prognosis is determined by the location, number, and severity of the tumors that are present. It is important to note that most patients with the disease retain good function.

Tuberous Sclerosis

Pathogenesis and Pathophysiology. Tuberous sclerosis, or tuberous sclerosis complex (TSC), is inherited as an autosomal dominant trait. The TSC is the result of mutation of two genes, namely, TSC 1, which is cloned from human chromosome 9, and the TSC 2, which is cloned from chromosome 16. The TSC 1 and TSC 2 encoded proteins have been named *hamartin* and *tuberin*, respectively.[38] Other cases have been attributed to a gene mutation. Although the genetic basis of the disease has been established, the pathogenesis remains unknown. The lesions involve cells derived from the ectoderm and mesoderm, and the cellular elements demonstrate abnormalities in number and size.

Epidemiology and Risk Factors. Tuberous sclerosis has been identified in all races in all parts of the world. Both sexes are equally affected, and heredity is evident in 50 percent of cases. Prevalence is estimated at 1 in 50,000 to 1 in 300,000 people. This disorder accounts for nearly 1 percent of the institutionalized population in the United States and for 0.3 percent of patients with epilepsy.

Clinical Features and Associated Disorders. Though Bourneville[39, 40] is credited with the first description of the disease, probably von Recklinghausen described it initially. Bourneville believed that the cerebral "scleroses" and renal tumors were associated findings, but he failed to recognize the importance of the typical facial skin lesions. Vogt believed that a triad of clinical findings including seizures, mental retardation, and adenoma sebaceum were characteristic of the disease,[41] but the criteria for diagnosis have recently been revised (Table 32–3). TSC is characterized by a variety of clinical findings including seizures, varying degrees of mental subnormality, and dysplastic or neoplastic changes of the skin, nervous system, and other organ systems.

The clinical expression of the disease is dependent on which organs are affected and the extent of their involvement. Seizures, either partial or generalized, are the most common symptom of the disease, and infantile spasms are particularly frequent during the first several years of life. The

TABLE 32–3. **Diagnostic Criteria for Tuberous Sclerosis Complex (TSC)**

Primary Features
Facial angiofibromas
Multiple ungual fibromas
Cortical tuber (histologically confirmed)
Subependymal nodule or giant cell astrocytoma (histologically confirmed)
Multiple calcified subependymal nodules protruding into the ventricle (radiographical evidence)
Multiple retinal astrocytomas
Secondary Features
Affected first-degree relative
Cardiac rhabdomyoma (histologic or radiographic evidence)
Other retinal hamartomas or achromic patch
Cerebral tubers (radiographical confirmation)
Noncalcified subependymal nodules (radiographical confirmation)
Shagreen patch
Forehead plaque
Pulmonary lymphangiomyomatosis (histological confirmation)
Renal angiomyolipoma (radiographical or histological confirmation)
Renal cysts (histological confirmation)
Tertiary Features
Hypomelanotic macules
"Confetti" skin lesions
Renal cysts (radiographical evidence)
Randomly distributed enamel pits in deciduous or permanent teeth
Hamartomatous rectal polyps (histological confirmation)
Bone cysts (radiographical evidence)
Pulmonary lymphangiomyomatosis (radiographical evidence)
Cerebral white matter "migration tracts" or heterotopias (radiographical evidence)
Gingival fibromas
Hamartoma of other organs (histological confirmation)
Infantile spasms
Definite TSC
One primary feature, two secondary features, or one secondary plus two tertiary features
Probable TSC
Either one secondary plus one tertiary feature or three tertiary features
Suspect TSC
Either one secondary feature or two tertiary features

From Roach ES, Smith M, Hottenlocher P, et al: Report of the diagnostic criteria committee of the National Tuberous Sclerosis Association. J Child Neurol 1992;7:221.

early onset and severity of the seizure disorder are correlated with the degree of mental abnormality. Mental function is notably variable, however, and about a third of patients have normal intelligence. Some patients develop normally during their early years only to experience a deterioration in mental function in the latter part of the first decade.

The most common skin lesion is the hypopigmented macule, which is found in about 90 percent of patients[42] (Fig. 32–6). According to Fitzpatrick, the most frequent shape is the polygonal or "thumb-print" lesion, followed by the "ash leaf" spot, and finally by groups of multiple "confetti-like" hypopigmented macules.[43] Adenoma sebaceum, which is an angiofibromatous lesion, had been generally considered the most common skin change in tuberous sclerosis, but the lesions occur in only 50 percent of patients (Fig. 32–7). The lesions appear in patches or in a butterfly distribution about the nose, cheeks, and chin. They are rarely apparent at birth, are usually first observed between the ages of 1 and 4 years, and tend to enlarge over time. Other skin changes include the "shagreen" patch (a "leathery" plaque), which is usually found over the lumbosacral or gluteal region; café au lait spots; fibromas; and angiomas. Subungual or periungual fibromas (Koenen's tumors) are found in about 20 percent of patients and affect the toes more commonly than the fingers. These lesions are usually first noted during adolescence. Gingival fibromas also can occur as well as pitting of the dental enamel.

Retinal tumors, which seldom affect vision, can occur and are thought to be astrocytic hamartomas. They are nodular or mulberry-like in configuration and may be solitary or multiple; they tend to calcify. Other associated ocular findings include retinal gray-yellow glial patches, and iridic hypomelanotic spots, cataracts, and colobomas of the iris, lens, and choroid. Renal tumors occur in about half of patients with TSC and are primarily renal cysts or renal angiomyolipomas. These tumors can occur separately or in combination, and they are typically multiple, involving both kidneys. Although they can be symptomatic because of renal enlargement, they are usually indolent. Angiomyolipomas are also thought to be benign, yet they may result in hemorrhage and can cause serious morbidity or mortality. Early onset and severe hypertension can occur in patients with numerous renal cysts, and it has been suggested that patients with TSC have an increased risk of renal cell carcinoma. Cardiac rhabdomyomas are present in about half of patients and can be solitary, multiple, or infiltrative, diffusely affecting the myocardium. Newer techniques of echocardiography have facilitated early recognition of this tumor.

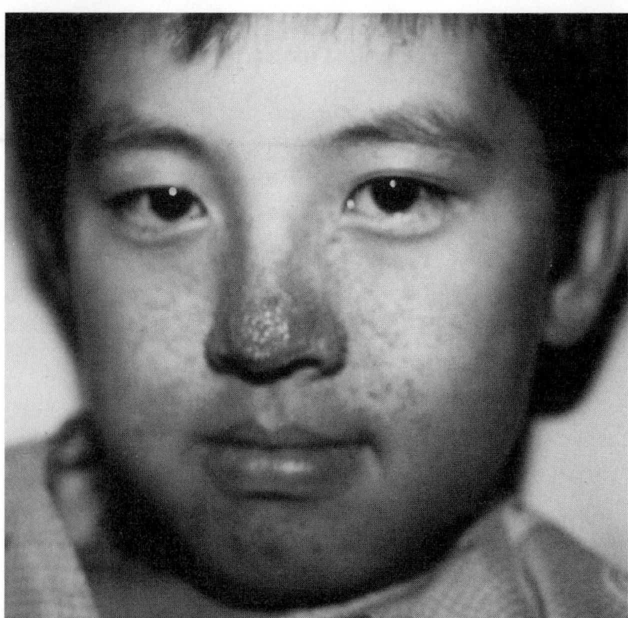

FIGURE 32–7. Adenoma sebaceum occurs as angiofibromatous lesions about the nose, the nasolabial folds, or chin; they are present in about 50 percent of patients with tuberous sclerosis.

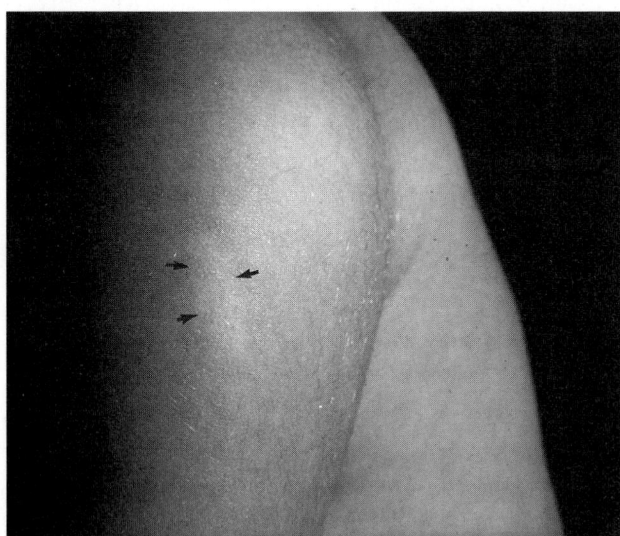

FIGURE 32–6. A typical ash leaf–shaped area of hypopigmentation (*arrows*) found in most patients with tuberous sclerosis.

The lungs can also be affected in patients with TSC; they demonstrate multicystic lesions that have been shown to be similar pathologically to lymphangiomyomatosis.[44] Pulmonary abnormalities occur almost entirely in females, presenting as dyspnea, spontaneous pneumothorax, and pulmonary hypertension. Endocrine abnormalities have also been reported.

Differential Diagnosis. The clinical features of TSC just described are characteristic, and although other neurocutaneous syndromes may have some similar features, it is rarely difficult to make the correct diagnosis. Infants who show developmental delay and intracranial calcifications and seizures should be evaluated for the possible presence of intrauterine infections such as toxoplasmosis and cytomegalovirus, among others.

Evaluation. Visualization of these hypomelanotic macules is enhanced by using a Wood light because melanin absorbs light of that frequency (360 nm), and areas deficient in melanin are visually accentuated. Imaging studies of affected patients can be effectively used to assist in diagnosis. Intracranial calcifications, commonly found in the region of the foramen of Monro or the periventricular region, are present in about 60 percent of skull radiographs in these patients. CT may demonstrate cerebral hamartomas, subependymal nodules, ventriculomegaly, and areas of demyelination. The calcified subependymal nodule (the tuber) is the most reliable finding on CT head scans, but periventricular calcifications can also be observed in patients with toxoplasmosis, cytomegalic inclusion disease, and Fahr's syndrome.[45] MRI demonstrates with greater specificity not only the uncalcified subependymal nodules but also the distortion of the normal cerebral cytoarchitecture.[46]

Other characteristic radiographic abnormalities include cystic changes of the phalanges and metacarpals, sclerotic areas in the long bones, and areas of increased or decreased bone density in the skull. Renal changes can be demonstrated by CT, MRI, or renal angiography, and the presence of a cardiac tumor is readily demonstrated by echocardiography. Patients with rare pulmonary involvement show a fine reticular infiltrate or multicystic changes on chest radiographs. EEG and examination of the cerebrospinal fluid are of little help in establishing the diagnosis.

The tubers can be located anywhere in the cerebral hemisphere but are commonly found in the cortical gyri. Smaller nodules can be located in the region of the sulcus terminalis or the basal ganglia, protruding into the ventricle. Those tubers situated in the region of the foramen of Monro or the aqueduct of Sylvius may become large enough to obstruct the normal flow of cerebrospinal fluid, resulting in hydrocephalus. The tuber is characterized pathologically by a decreased number of neurons with large, bizarre, and sometimes vacuolated "monster" neurons. A proliferation of fibrillary astrocytes, areas of demyelination, and abnormalities of cortical cytoarchitectonics are seen. Some vessel walls may show hyaline degeneration. The subependymal nodules are fibrocellular with round or oval cells and whorls of fibrillary glial tissue. Calcium and amyloid deposits may be present within the tuber or the subependymal nodule; cerebellar calcification rarely occurs.

Management. Convulsive disorders are treated by the administration of standard anticonvulsant medications; control, however, cannot be ensured. The individual TSC patient with recurrent partial seizures may experience some improvement with the excision of carefully identified epileptogenic foci. No specific treatment is available for the angiofibromatous lesions of adenoma sebaceum. They may be surgically removed if subject to repeated irritation or trauma, as is true, for example, of lesions obstructing the nares. Patients with TSC must not only receive careful medical management but should also be evaluated and followed by social workers and psychologists. Genetic counseling for the family is mandatory.

Von Hippel-Lindau Disease

Von Hippel-Lindau disease, which is inherited as an autosomal dominant trait, is characterized by hemangioblastomas of the retina and cerebellum. Von Hippel thought the retinal lesion was a hemangioblastoma, but he labeled it *angiomatosis retinae*.[47] Lindau first recognized the association between the retinal and cerebellar hemangioblastomas; moreover, he was aware that patients could have other lesions, including spinal cord angiomas and cystic tumors of the pancreas, liver, and epididymis.[48] Linkage analysis has localized the gene defect to chromosome 3p25–26.[49, 50] Additional findings include cysts of the pancreas, liver, and spleen as well as renal tumors. Compared with other neurocutaneous disorders, skin lesions are not associated with the disease.[51]

The retinal hemangioblastoma is one of the earliest manifestations of the disease, and although it is reported to occur in childhood, it is usually found during or after the third decade. Aneurysmal dilation of the peripheral retinal vessels appears to be the earliest characteristic feature of the lesion, but, later, tortuous vessels marked by an afferent arteriole and venule leading to a raised retinal lesion appear. Some retinal lesions are small and easily overlooked. The retinal abnormalities have been divided into three stages: first, a pinkish red vascular lesion found in the midperipheral retina with visible "feeder" vessels and variable exudate; second, a pale gray lesion in which the feeder vessels can be observed on fluorescein retinal angiography; and third, retinal vascular lesions that are similar to diabetic microaneurysms but have no retinal vascular connections. These peripheral retinal lesions may not result in any visual impairment; however, if the lesion involves the macula or optic disc, progressive visual loss can occur.

The diagnosis of a cerebellar hemangioblastoma is usually made during the third or fourth decade, but there are reports of its occurrence before puberty. The presenting signs and symptoms are those of cerebellar dysfunction and increased intracranial pressure. These tumors may also involve the medulla and spinal cord, and about 80 percent of patients have an associated syringomyelia. Supratentorial hemangioblastomas, while uncommon, have been reported in the region of the pituitary gland and the third ventricle as well as the cerebral hemispheres.

Associated renal lesions are found in von Hippel-Lindau disease and include benign cysts, angiomas, and hypernephromas, which are common and are a significant cause of morbidity and mortality in the disease. Benign cysts may also be found in the pancreas, adrenal gland, and epididymis; they are usually asymptomatic. There is an increased frequency of pheochromocytomas in patients with von Hippel-Lindau disease.[52] Retinal hemangioblastomas are recognized by careful ophthalmoscopy, and fluorescein angiography can show the vascular characteristics of the lesion. CT and MRI demonstrate the lesions of the cerebellum and spinal cord. The intra-abdominal lesions are shown by abdominal CT and ultrasonography.

Some retinal lesions are recognized because of visual impairment and retinal detachment.[53] Obliteration of these lesions has been accomplished with cryocoagulation or photocoagulation. Cerebellar hemangioblastomas are removed surgically in about 90 percent of patients, who have a risk of recurrence of about 15 percent. Small renal tumors should be judiciously removed because the presence of multiple tumors is a possibility. In patients with cystic renal disease, nephrectomy should be considered, followed by dialysis.

AUTOSOMAL RECESSIVE DISEASE

Ataxia-Telangiectasia

Syllaba and Henner[54] first reported three adolescent patients with progressive choreoathetosis and ocular telangiectasia in 1926, but it was not until 1964 that Martin recognized their clinical description as ataxia-telangiectasia (AT).[55] A second report in 1941 by Louis-Bar described a young boy with progressive cerebellar ataxia and extensive cutaneous telangiectasias; she identified the syndrome as one of the phakomatoses.[56] After the 1958 descriptions by Bean,[57] Boder and Sedgwick,[58, 59] and Centerwall and Miller,[60] AT became recognized as a distinct disease, and multiple reports appeared in the literature.

AT is an autosomal recessive disorder characterized by a constellation of signs and symptoms associated with progressive cerebellar dysfunction, conjunctival and cutaneous telangiectasias, severe immune deficiencies, premature aging, and a predisposition to cancer.[61] AT is inherited as a single mendelian locus on chromosome 11q22–23. Recent studies have identified the mutated gene in AT, and its identification provides answers to the link between the mutated gene product in AT and the signaling pathways that regulate the cell cycle.[62] In the normal cell cycle, surveillance checkpoints are used to arrest cells during the cell cycle, allowing either completion of certain events that are required at that point or repair of damage. During these delay periods, damaged DNA can be repaired so that subsequent cycles can occur normally.[63] Clinical and laboratory work has suggested that the AT gene product is involved in maintaining the integrity of chromosomal DNA and in signal transduction mechanisms that operate to regulate the cell cycle or DNA repair. The exact biochemical roles of the gene product in these processes, however, remain unknown.

AT occurs equally among the sexes and is reported in all races and in all parts of the world. The prevalence of this disorder ranges from 1 in 40,000 to 100,000 births. Although AT is a multisystem disorder, progressive neurological deterioration is the hallmark of the syndrome.[61] The early neurological features of AT are characterized by signs indicative of a progressive cerebellar degeneration, including ataxia and dysarthric speech. Ataxia is manifested by a swaying of the head and trunk and becomes apparent shortly after affected children begin to walk. It progresses and becomes severe enough to warrant the use of a wheelchair by 10 to 15 years of age. By this time, dyssynergia and intention tremor of the extremities interfere with normal activity. Speech is initiated slowly and slurred, and words are articulated poorly. Choreoathetosis can be present in older children and can even mask the ataxia. Myoclonic jerks, rigidity, dystonic posturing, muscular hypotonia, drooling, and arrest of cognitive development are also typical. These patients also have characteristic facies, described as relaxed, dull, sad, and inattentive when unstimulated. The examination also reveals oculomotor abnormalities, including slowly initiated voluntary horizontal movements of conjugate gaze with nystagmus-like jerks with fixation and refixation. The deep tendon reflexes are diminished, the plantar response is flexor, Romberg's sign is absent, and deep and superficial sensation is normal. Later neurological features may be dominated by spinal cord dysfunction, including abnormalities of position and vibratory sensation. Other patients demonstrate neuromuscular deficits with diffuse weakness, muscle atrophy, fasciculations, and absent tendon reflexes with intact sensory findings. Finally, in some patients there is a more mixed clinical picture including abnormalities of both sensory and motor function.

Non-neurological features vary and include vasculocutaneous, immunological, and neoplastic manifestations. The characteristic telangiectasias usually appear later than ataxia, typically at around 3 to 6 years of age in the region of the conjunctival angles of the eye. Once present, they steadily progress and spread in a symmetrical pattern across the exposed portion of the bulbar conjunctivae. These telangiectasias are bright red horizontal streaks that cause the eyes to look "bloodshot" and eventually involve the rest of the conjunctivae, eyelids, adjoining facial regions, external ears, neck, and antecubital and popliteal spaces. Rarely, the telangiectasias may be present on the dorsum of the hands and feet and on the mucosal surfaces of the palate. These abnormal vessels are not symptomatic and appear to be of venous origin, branching from subpapillary venous plexuses in the skin and dilated connecting venules in the conjunctivae.

Patients with AT also demonstrate progeric changes of the hair and skin, including early graying of the hair and atrophic, hidebound facial skin. Pigmentary changes are also frequent and consist of hyperpigmentation and hypopigmentation with cutaneous atrophy. A few patients may demonstrate partial albinism, vitiligo, and café au lait spots. Seborrheic dermatitis occurs in nearly all patients, and senile keratoses, atopic dermatitis, and eczema are also reported. Another prominent feature of AT is frequent sinopulmonary infections. These may range from infection of the ears, nose, and sinuses to chronic bronchitis and recurrent pneumonia. The latter two may result in bronchiectasis and pulmonary fibrosis. Chronic infections are typically due to common bacteria; however, they are sometimes poorly responsive to antibiotic therapy. The predisposition to infection is associated with the presence of an abnormal thymus and a marked deficiency of IgA, which is the predominant immunoglobulin in respiratory secretions. Neoplasms occur in an estimated 10 to 15 percent of patients with AT and are second only to pulmonary disorders as a cause of death. The most common neoplasms include Hodgkin's disease, malignant lymphomas, reticulum cell sarcoma, and histocytosarcomas. Various other tumors have been associated with AT, including medulloblastoma, basal cell carcinoma, acute lymphocytic leukemia, and gliomas, as well as others. These patients also have retarded somatic growth with dwarfing and various skeletal disorders. Endocrine abnormalities are also prominent, and female hypogonadism with sexual infantilism is found consistently. Male hypogonadism also occurs but is less prominent and is characterized by a delay in puberty, incomplete spermatogenesis, and decreased Leydig cells. Other studies report an unusual type of diabetes mellitus that appears in late adolescence as well as anterior lobe pituitary abnormalities.

The laboratory evaluation of patients with AT reveals normal results on routine studies of the urine, blood (except for lymphopenia), and spinal fluid. Although glucose studies may reveal evidence of an insulin-resistant diabetes mellitus, thyroid function studies are normal. Elevations in serum alpha-fetoprotein and plasma carcinoembryonic antigen are typically, but not invariably, present and are not required diagnostic criteria. Humoral or cellular immunological defects are also helpful in the diagnosis of AT, including low or absent levels of IgA, IgG2, and IgE, yet these are not invariable. Plain films of the skull may show decreased or absent nasopharyngeal adenoidal tissue, and CT and MRI studies of the head show cerebellar atrophy. Muscle and nerve biopsies may reveal evidence of denervation atrophy and axonal degeneration, respectively.

Treatment of patients with AT is supportive and includes treatment of infections and the use of sunscreens to retard the cutaneous progeric changes. Early institution of pulmonary physiotherapy and physical therapy is important. Prenatal diagnosis is possible through the measurement of alpha-fetoprotein levels in amniotic fluid and the documentation of increased spontaneous chromosomal breakage of amniotic cell DNA.

UNKNOWN INHERITANCE PATTERNS

Sturge-Weber Syndrome

Sturge is credited with the first report of this syndrome, which appeared in a 6-year-old girl who had a facial angioma, buphthalmos, and contralateral partial seizures.[64] Sturge surmised that she had an underlying cerebral angioma, but it was not until 18 years later that a cerebral angioma affecting the leptomeninges of these patients was first described. Weber reported the presence of intracranial calcifications in skull radiographs of these patients, Dimitri noted double serpentine calcifications, and Krabbe correctly pointed out that the calcifications were located primarily in the cerebral substance rather than in the vessel walls. Van der Hoeve believed that this syndrome was the "fourth phakomatosis."

Sturge-Weber syndrome (SWS) is characterized by a congenital facial angioma (nevus flammeus, port-wine stain) that is associated with signs and symptoms of an ipsilateral leptomeningeal angioma (Fig. 32–8). The facial angioma is usually unilateral, although it can be bilateral, and involves at least the upper face, superior eyelid, or periorbital region. Angiomas can also occur in other areas of the head including the nasopharynx, palate, lips, gingiva, and tongue, as well as the neck, trunk, and extremities. The facial angioma conforms to the sensory divisions of the trigeminal nerve, but its configuration may be determined by the embryological facial development. Leptomeningeal angiomas can also occur in the absence of any facial angioma. In this case, although the signs are similar to those of SWS, the patients should be considered to have a different disorder referred to as leptomeningeal angiomatosis. SWS has no known recognized pattern of inheritance, but there is one report of a father and son who had facial angiomas and glaucoma.

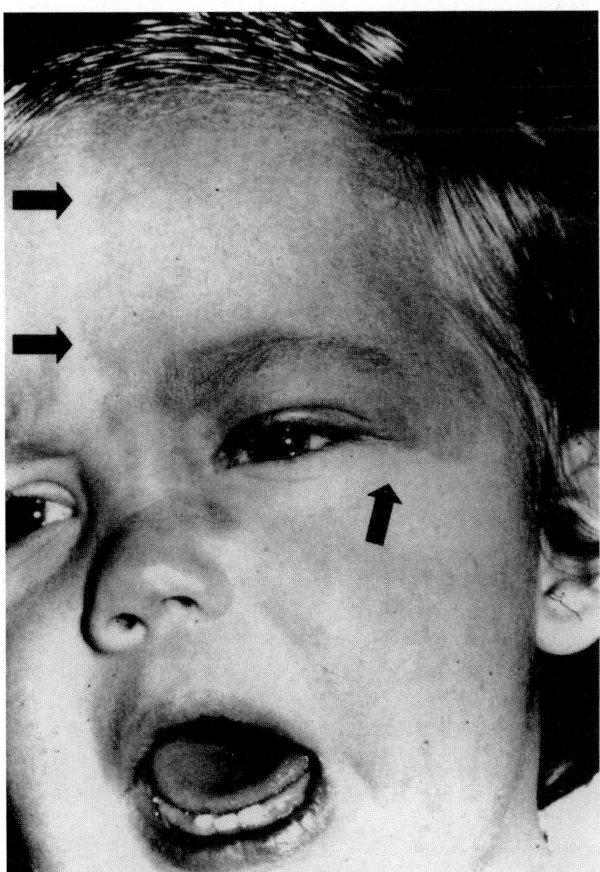

FIGURE 32–8. Fourteen-month-old male with "port-wine stain" angioma involving the upper face, primarily in the distribution of the ophthalmic division of the left cranial nerve V. In addition, he had glaucoma of the left eye and contralateral partial seizures.

Most patients with SWS have seizures, often beginning in infancy, that are primarily partial motor seizures, but some patients have secondary generalization. Other seizure types, such as myoclonic, tonic, and atonic seizures as well as infantile spasms, can occur less frequently. Earlier studies noted a seizure frequency of 70 to 90 percent. In a retrospective study of 102 patients, 88 patients had a leptomeningeal angioma affecting one cerebral hemisphere, and 14 patients had bilateral hemispheric involvement.[65] Seizures occurred in 75 percent of these patients. Among the patients with unilateral involvement, 63 had seizures, the mean age of seizure onset being 24 months. Thirteen of the 14 patients with bilateral involvement had seizures, the mean age of onset being 6 months.

At least half of patients with SWS are mentally subnormal, and behavioral problems are common. As seizures of early onset increase in frequency and severity, mental function and behavior often regress. In the retrospective study noted previously, 25 of 88 patients with unihemispheric leptomeningeal involvement who did not have seizures were of average intelligence; 1 of 14 patients with bilateral hemispheric involvement was unaffected by seizures, and that patient was of average intelligence. Others have documented that SWS patients with seizures have a notably higher incidence of developmental delay and emotional and behavioral problems, and these patients need special education. These observations are important considerations in patient management. Hemisensory deficits can occur but are sometimes difficult to document reliably in very young and mentally subnormal patients. Homonymous hemianopia has been noted in about one third of patients, and glaucoma secondary to choroidal angioma is found in one fourth. Other ocular abnormalities include iridic heterochromia in which the hyperpigmented iris is ipsilateral to the facial angioma, optic atrophy, and strabismus.

Electroencephalographic studies often show decreased amplitude and frequency of electrocerebral activity overlying the affected hemisphere. Other commonly noted abnormal EEG features include multiple and independent spike foci. Intracranial calcifications on skull radiographs are present in about 90 percent of patients, are usually found in the occipital or parieto-occipital region, and have a serpentine linear, parallel configuration ("tram sign"). They are rarely observed on plain skull radiographs during infancy but are present in most patients by the end of the second decade. CT of the head demonstrates intracerebral calcifications and cerebral atrophy more readily than do plain skull radiographs and has documented calcific deposits during the first few months of life. MRI, however, is the neuroimaging study of choice to show the extent of structural abnormalities of SWS.

Cerebral angiography demonstrates decreased cerebral venous drainage and dilation of the deep cerebral veins.[66, 67] A variety of vascular abnormalities, including thrombotic lesions, dural venous sinus abnormalities, and arteriovenous malformations, has been observed in about a third of patients. Positron-emission tomography (PET) can provide some measure of cerebral metabolic impairment, and serial PET scans can demonstrate the progression of the disease process.[68] Moreover, PET scans can provide important information that can be used to guide careful selection of patients for focal cortical resection or hemispherectomy.[69] Single photon emission computed tomography can also reveal useful information about cerebral perfusion.

Characteristic pathological features of SWS include thickened hypervascularized leptomeninges, which primarily affect the occipital, parietal, or temporo-occipital lobes. Meningeal vessels are small and tortuous, producing a dark, purplish blue color. These abnormal vessels rarely enter the underlying atrophic cerebral hemisphere. Calcific deposits are primarily located in the molecular and outer pyramidal cortical layers, but small calcific spicules can be found in some small cerebral vessels. The pathogenesis of calcium deposition in the brain substance is not well understood.

Management of patients with SWS requires careful attention not only to the patient's neurological deficits, but also to the associated behavioral and emotional problems.[70] Convulsive disorders are treated by administration of standard antiepileptic drugs, but seizures in some patients may be refractory to medical management. These patients should be considered for focal cerebral resection of the affected lobes or hemispherectomy.[71, 72] Management of the associated problems of mentally subnormal patients or those with behavioral or emotional disturbances requires the skills not only of the physician but of competent psychologists and social workers as well.

Reviews and Selected Updates

Berg BO: Principles of Child Neurology. New York, McGraw-Hill, 1996.

De Grouchy J, Turleau C: Clinical Atlas of Human Chromosomes, 2nd ed. New York, Wiley, 1984.

Rosenberg RN, Pettegrew JW: Genetic neurological diseases. *In* Rosenberg RN (ed): Comprehensive Neurology. New York, Raven Press, 1991.

Rosenberg RN, Prusiner SB, DiMauro S, et al: The Molecular and Genetic Basis of Neurological Disease, 2nd ed. Boston, Butterworth-Heinemann, 1997.

Schinzel A: Catalogue of Unbalanced Chromosome Aberrations in Man. Berlin, Walter de Gruyter, 1984.

References

1. LeJeune J, Gautier M, Turpin R: Etude des chromosomes somatiques de neuf enfants mongoliens. C R Acad Sci (Paris) 1959;248:1721.
2. Wisniewski KE, Dalton AJ, McLahlan C, et al: Alzheimer's disease in Down's syndrome: Clinicopathologic studies. Neurology 1985;35: 957–961.
3. McKeown DA, Doty RL, Perl DP, et al: Olfactory function in young adolescents with Down's syndrome. J Neurol Neurosurg Psychiatry 1996;61:412–414.
4. Muller F, Bussieres L: Magnetic resonance imaging evaluation of delayed myelination in Down syndrome: A case report and review of the literature. J Child Neurol 1992;7:417–421.
5. Emerson JF, Kesslak JP, Chen PC, Lott IT: Magnetic resonance imaging of the aging brain in Down's syndrome. Prog Clin Biol Res 1995;393:123–138.
6. Edwards J, Harnden D, Cameron A, et al: A new trisomic syndrome. Lancet 1960;1:787.
7. Patau K, Smith D, Therman E, et al: Multiple congenital anomaly caused by an extra autosome. Lancet 1960;1:790.
8. Fryburg JS, Breg WR, Lindgren V: Diagnosis of Angelman syndrome in infants. Am J Med Genet 1991;38:58–64.
9. Holm VA, Cassidy SB, Butler MG, et al: Prader-Willi syndrome: Consensus diagnostic criteria. Pediatrics 1993;91:398.
10. Leonard CM, Williams CA, Nicholls RD, et al: Angelman and Prader-Willi syndromes: Magnetic resonance imaging study of differences in cerebral structure. Am J Med Genet 1993;46:26–33.
11. Ratcliffe SG: Klinefelter's syndrome in adolescence. Arch Dis Child 1982;57:6–12.
12. Ratcliffe SG, Butler GE, Jones M: Edinburgh study of growth and development of children with sex chromosome abnormalities. IV. Birth Defects 1990;26:1–44.
13. Bender B, Fry E, Pennington B, et al: Speech and language development in 41 children with sex chromosome anomalies. Pediatrics 1983;71:262–267.
14. Turner HH: A syndrome of infantilism, congenital webbed neck and cubitus valgus. Endocrinology 1938;23:566–698.
15. Temple CM, Carney RA: Intellectual functioning of children with Turner syndrome: A comparison of behavioral phenotypes. Dev Med Child Neurol 1993;35:691.
16. Reiss AL, Freund L, Plotnick L, et al: The effects of X monosomy on brain development: Monozygotic twins discordant for Turner's syndrome. Ann Neurol 1993;34:95–107.
17. Murphy DG, DeCarli C, Daly E, et al: X-chromosome effects on female brain: A magnetic resonance imaging study of Turner's syndrome. Lancet 1993;342:1197–1200.
18. Reiss Al, Mazzocco MM, Greenlaw R, et al: Neurodevelopmental effects of X monosomy: A volumetric imaging study. Ann Neurol 1995;38:731–738.
19. Buchanan CR, Law CM, Milner RD: Growth hormone in short, slowly growing children and those with Turner's syndrome. Arch Dis Child 1987;62:912–916.
20. Martin JP, Bell J: Pedigree of mental defect showing sex-linkage. J Neurol Psychiatry 1943;6:154.
21. Renpenning H: Familial sex-linked mental retardation. Can Med Assoc J 1957;87:854.
22. Tarleton JC, Saul RA: Molecular genetic advances in fragile-X syndrome. J Pediatr 1993;122:169–185.
23. McConkie-Rosell A: Evidence that methylation of the FMR-1 locus is responsible for variable phenotypic expression of the fragile-X syndrome. Am J Hum Genet 1993;53:800–809.
24. Reiss AL, Aylward E, Freund LS, et al: Neuroanatomy of the fragile-X syndrome: The posterior fossa. Ann Neurol 1991;29:26–32.
25. Bielschowsky M: Über tuberose Sklerose und ihre Beziehungen nur Recklinghausen Krankheit. Z Gesamte Neurol Psychiatr 1914;26:133.
26. Bielschowsky M: Entwurf eines Systems der Heredodegenerationen des Zentralnervenssystems einschliesslich der zugehoren Striatumkrankungen. J Psychol Neurol 1919;14:48.
27. Van der Hoeve J: Eye diseases in tuberous sclerosis of the brain and in Recklinghausen disease. Trans Ophthalmol Soc UK 1923;43:534.
28. Van der Hoeve J: The Doyne Memorial Lecture: Eye symptoms in phakomatoses. Trans Ophthalmol Soc UK 1932;52:380.
29. Van der Hoeve J: Les phacomatoses de Bourneville, de Recklinghausen et de von Hippel-Lindau. J Belge Neurol Psychiatr 1933;33:752.
30. Von Recklinghausen F: Uber die multiplen Fibrome der Haut and ihre Beziehungen zu den multiplen Neuromen. Berlin, Hirschwald, 1882.
31. National Institutes of Health: Consensus Development Conference Statement 6: No. 12: Neurofibromatosis. Atlanta, National Institutes of Health, 1987, p 1.
32. Gutmann DH, Collins FS: Recent progress toward understanding the molecular biology of Von Recklinghausen neurofibromatosis. Ann Neurol 1992;31:555–561.
33. Crowe FW, Schull WJ, Neil JW: A Clinical, Pathological and Genetic Study of Multiple Neurofibromatosis. Springfield, IL, Charles C Thomas, 1956.
34. Riccardi VM, Eichner JE: Neurofibromatosis—Phenotype, Natural History and Pathogenesis. Baltimore, Johns Hopkins University Press, 1986.
35. Chutorian AM, Schwartz JF, Evans RA: Optic gliomas in children. Neurology 1964;14:83.
36. Hoyt WF, Baghdassarian SA: Optic glioma of childhood: Natural history and rationale for conservative management. Br J Ophthalmol 1969;53:793–798.
37. Imes RK, Hoyt WF: Childhood chiasmal gliomas: Update on the fate of patients in the 1969 San Francisco study. Br J Ophthalmol 1986;70: 179–182.
38. Cheadle JP, Reeve MP, Shannon JR, Kwiatkowski DJ: Molecular genetic advances in tuberous sclerosis. Hum Genet 2000;107:97–114.
39. Bourneville DM: Sclerose tubereuse des circonvolutions cerebrales: Idiotie et epilepsie hemiplegique. Arch Neurol (Paris) 1881;1:390.

40. Bourneville DM, Brissaud E: Idiotie et epilepsie symptomatiques de sclerose tubereuse ou hypertrophique. Arch Neurol (Paris) 1900;10:29.
41. Vogt H: Zur Diagnostik der tuberosen Sklerose. Z Erfrosch Behandl Jugendl Schwachsinns 1908;2:1.
42. Gold AP, Freeman JM: Depigmented nevi: The earliest sign of tuberous sclerosis. Pediatrics 1965;55:1003.
43. Fitzpatrick TB: History and significance of white macules, earliest visible sign of tuberous sclerosis. Ann NY Acad Sci 1991;615:26–35.
44. Torres VE, Bjornsson J, King BF, et al: Extrapulmonary lymphangioleiomatosis and lymphangiomatous cysts in tuberous sclerosis complex. Mayo Clin Proc 1995;70:641–648.
45. Maki Y, Enomoto T, Maruyama H, et al: Computed tomography in tuberous sclerosis: With special reference to relation between clinical manifestations and CT findings. Brain Dev 1979;1:38–48.
46. McMurdo SK Jr, Moore SG, Brant-Zawadski M, et al: Magnetic resonance imaging of intracranial tuberous sclerosis. AJR 1987;148:791–796.
47. Von Hippel E: Die anatomische Grundlage der von mir beschriebenen "sehr seltene Erkrankung der Netzhaut." Albrecht von Graefes Arch Ophthalmol 1911;79:350.
48. Lindau A: Studien uber Kleinhirncyten: Bau, Pathogenese und Beziehungen zur Angiomatosisretinae. Acta Pathol Microbiol Scand Suppl 1926;1:1.
49. Seizinger BR, Rouleau GA, Ozelius LJ, et al: Von Hippel-Lindau disease maps to the region of chromosome 3 associated with renal cell carcinoma. Nature 1988;332:268–269.
50. Seizinger BR, Smith DI, Filling-Katz MR, et al: Genetic flanking markers refine diagnostic criteria and provide insights into the genetics of von Hippel-Lindau disease. Proc Natl Acad Sci USA 1991;88:2864–2868.
51. Melmon KL, Rosen SW: Lindau's disease: A review of the literature and study of a large kindred. Am J Med 1964;36:595.
52. Atuk NO, Mcdonald T, Wood T, et al: Familial pheochromocytoma, hypercalcemia, and von Hippel-Lindau disease: A ten year study of a large family. Medicine (Baltimore) 1979;58:209–218.
53. Schirmer RS: Ein Fall von Telangiektasie. Albrecht von Graefes Arch Ophthalmol 1860;7:199.
54. Syllaba L, Henner K: Contribution à l'indépendance de l'athétose double idiopathique et congénitale. Atteinte familiale, syndrome dystrophique, signe du résau vasculaire conjonctival, intégrité psychique. Rev Neurol 1926;541:562.
55. Martin L: Aspect choréoathétosique du syndrome d'ataxie-télangiectasie. Acta Neurol Belg 1964;64:802–819.
56. Louis-Bar D: Sur un syndrome progressif comprenant des télangiectasies capillaires cutanées et conjonctivales symétriques, à disposition naevode et de troubles càràbelleux. Confin Neurol (Basel) 1941;4:32–42.
57. Bean WB: Vascular Spiders and Related Lesions of the Skin. Springfield, IL, Charles C Thomas, 1958, pp 160–162.
58. Boder E, Sedgwick RP: Ataxia-telangiectasia. A familial syndrome of progressive cerebellar ataxia, oculocutaneous telangiectasia and frequent pulmonary infection. Pediatrics 1958;21:526–554.
59. Boder E, Sedgwick RP: Ataxia-telangiectasia: Dermatological aspects. Trans Los Angeles Dermatol Soc Arch Dermatol 1958;78:402–405.
60. Centerwall WR, Miller MM: Ataxia, telangiectasia, and sinopulmonary infections. A syndrome of slowly progressive deterioration in childhood. Am J Dis Child 1958;95:385–396.
61. Sedgwick RP, Boder E: Ataxia-telangiectasia. *In* de Jong JMBV (ed): Hereditary Neuropathies and Spinocerebellar Atrophies. Handbook of Clinical Neurology, Vol. 60. Amsterdam, Elsevier Science, 1991, pp 347–423.
62. Savitsky K, Bar-Shira A, Gilad S, et al: A single ataxia telangiectasia gene with a product similar to Pl-3 kinase. Science 1995;268:1749–1753.
63. Shiloh Y: ATM and ATR: Networking cellular responses to DNA damage. Curr Opin Genet Dev 2001;11:71–77.
64. Sturge WA: A case of partial epilepsy, apparently due to a lesion of one of the vaso-motor centers of the brain. Trans Clin Soc (Lond) 1879; 12:162.
65. Bebin EM, Gomez MR: Prognosis in Sturge-Weber disease: Comparison of unihemispheric and bihemispheric involvement. J Child Neurol 1988;3:181–184.
66. Bentson JR, Wilson GH, Newton THE: Cerebral venous drainage pattern in Sturge-Weber syndrome. Radiology 1971;102:111–118.
67. Wagner EJ, Rao KC, Knipp HC: CT-angiographic correlations in Sturge-Weber syndrome. J Comput Assist Tomogr 1981;5:324–327.
68. Chugani HT, Mazziota JC, Phelps ME: Sturge-Weber syndrome: A study of cerebral glucose utilization with positron emission tomography. J Pediatr 1989;114:244–253.
69. Lee JS, Asano E, Muzik O, et al: Sturge-Weber syndrome: Correlation between clinical course and PET findings. Neurol 2001;57:189–195.
70. Rochkind S, Hoffman HJ, Hendricks ED: Sturge-Weber syndrome: Natural history and prognosis. J Epilep 1990;3:293.
71. Hoffman HJ, Hendricks EB, Dennis M, et al: Hemispherectomy for Sturge-Weber syndrome. Child's Brain 1979;5:233–248.
72. Arzimanoglou AA, Andermann F, Aicardi J, et al: Sturge-Weber syndrome: Indications and results of surgery in patients. Neurology 2000;55:1472–1479.

CHAPTER 33

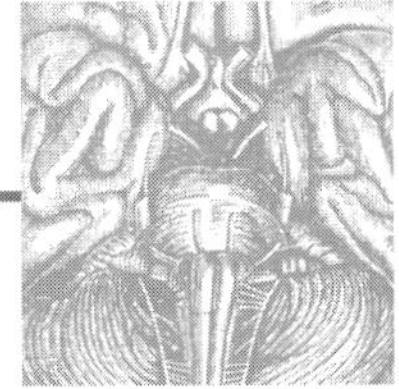

RICHARD J. CASELLI and BRADLEY F. BOEVE

The Degenerative Dementias

The term dementia has an intellectually constricting effect on differential diagnostic considerations and should be applied with care. A confused elderly person seen for the first time might be described as demented but may in fact be confused because of toxicity from a narcotic analgesic received postoperatively. A more generic term that is less diagnostically constricting is encephalopathy. Encephalopathy can be acute, subacute, or chronic, and there are reversible and irreversible etiologies. Dementia is a type (or types) of chronic encephalopathy that can have many causes, including irreversible degenerative and potentially reversible nondegenerative causes.

The most important diagnostic step in evaluating dementias is to determine whether a chronic encephalopathy results from a degenerative or other potentially reversible cause. Clues may exist at any level of the diagnostic ladder, although typically only a subset of clues is found in any one patient. Historical clues suggesting a reversible process include fluctuating severity, altered level of consciousness or hypersomnolence, and visual hallucinations (although fluctuating severity and visual hallucinations are also typical in dementia with Lewy bodies, which is a degenerative disease). Clues on mental status testing include finding the patient to be inattentive, disoriented, and somnolent but not particularly amnesic. Clues on physical examination include a variety of findings that may be common in elderly patients but are not part of the typical picture of Alzheimer's disease (AD) such as ataxia, hyper-reflexia, and tremulousness.

Laboratory evaluation should be directed toward common medical ailments, and a reasonably recent complete physical evaluation should be available or obtained in all patients suspected of having a significant brain-related disease. Practice parameters from the American Academy of Neurology for the diagnosis of dementia specify thyroid function studies and serum vitamin B_{12} levels be performed. Serological tests for syphilis should be considered in the appropriate medical setting, but are no longer routinely recommended. All patients being evaluated for dementia should undergo structural neuroimaging with computed tomography (CT) or magnetic resonance imaging (MRI) of the brain. When a nondegenerative-based chronic progressive encephalopathy is suspected, electroencephalography (EEG) may be helpful in demonstrating severe dysrhythmic slowing. Cerebrospinal fluid (CSF) examination may show an elevated IgG index and synthesis rate, and occasionally oligoclonal bands, suggesting an intrathecal inflammatory reaction. Autoimmune and paraneoplastic serologies may be helpful in such patients as well. Ultimately, if suspicion remains high based on noninvasive tests for a nondegenerative cause, cerebral angiography and meningeal and brain biopsy should be considered. In the absence of such invasive testing, an empirical therapeutic trial of prednisone could be considered in order to be certain that the steroid-responsive type of chronic inflammatory meningoencephalitis (CIME) does not exist.

If a degenerative disease is ultimately diagnosed, then it must be realized that an incurable, invariably progressive, and ultimately fatal condition has been diagnosed.

Chronic progressive encephalopathies can be divided into potentially reversible and irreversible diseases. More important than remembering a few specific diseases is to keep pathophysiological categories in mind. Some reversible causes of subacute and chronic widespread progressive encephalopathy include:

1. inflammatory: CIME, sarcoidosis, primary and secondary central nervous system (CNS) vasculitides, CNS complications of systemic lupus erythematosus, and paraneoplastic limbic encephalitis
2. infectious: chronic meningitis due to fungi, tuberculosis, *Listeria monocytogenes*, Lyme disease, syphilis, CNS Whipple's disease
3. nutritional: vitamin B_{12} deficiency
4. toxic: drugs (particularly prescription medications)
5. mass lesion: subdural hematoma, communicating (normal pressure) hydrocephalus, meningioma and other tumors
6. complex partial status epilepticus

Some irreversible causes of chronic widespread progressive encephalopathy include:

1. degenerative: AD, Pick's disease, asymmetrical cortical degeneration syndromes (ACDS), dementia with Lewy bodies (DLB), progressive supranuclear palsy (PSP), Huntington's disease (HD), Parkinson's disease (PD)
2. vascular: multi-infarct dementia, disseminated intravascular coagulation, Binswanger's disease, cerebral autosomal dominant arteriopathy with subcortical infarcts and leukoencephalopathy
3. metabolic: storage diseases, leukodystrophies
4. neoplastic: meningeal metastases, gliomatosis cerebri

With this perspective in mind, this chapter considers the subset of irreversible causes of chronic progressive encephalopathies referred to as neurodegenerative dementing diseases, which affect adults. They fall into three broad categories: cortical, subcortical, and mixed. Essentially all neurodegenerative dementias have both cortical and subcortical pathology, but those that primarily target the cerebral cortex are clinically distinguishable from those that primarily target subcortical structures, so the distinction has both heuristic and practical value. Finally, there are some diseases that have a more balanced cortical-subcortical mix pathologically and clinically.

Cortical Dementia

ALZHEIMER'S DISEASE AND ALZHEIMER'S DEMENTIA

The two terms are related but not synonymous. AD is the disease process that ultimately results in Alzheimer's dementia. Alzheimer's dementia has a characteristic cognitive pattern. Early in a patient's course, AD may cause memory loss of insufficient severity to warrant the designation of dementia. Other patients with AD may follow an atypical course with progressive aphasia or progressive apraxia rather than a typical Alzheimer's dementia. Most of the time, however, AD causes Alzheimer's dementia.

Pathogenesis and Pathophysiology. AD is characterized by generalized cerebral cortical atrophy (Fig. 33–1) with widespread cortical neuritic (or senile) plaques (NP) and neurofibrillary tangles (NFT) (Fig. 33–2). Other typical pathological findings include neuropil threads, granulovacuolar degeneration, lipochrome accumulation, and Hirano bodies. NPs are composed of an amyloid core surrounded by dystrophic neurites, whereas paired helical filaments are the major constituent in NFTs, neuropil threads, and dystrophic neurites. None of these histological findings individually are entirely specific for AD, because NPs can be seen in clinically nondemented patients,[1] and NFTs can occur in other neurodegenerative and prion disorders. The current neuropathological criteria for the diagnosis of AD is based on the frequency of NP and topography of NFT.[2]

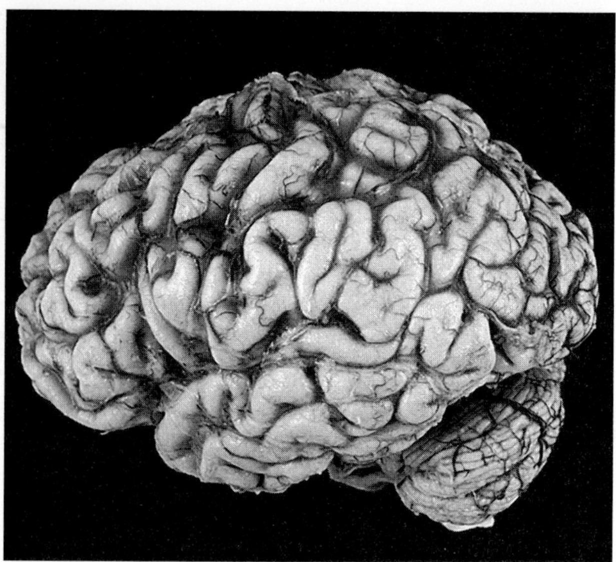

FIGURE 33–1. Alzheimer's disease. Note the generalized cerebral cortical atrophy. (Courtesy of JE Parisi, Mayo Clinic, Rochester, Minnesota.)

Synapse loss appears to be the most important correlate of dementia severity,[3] but the number of NPs and NFTs and the density of β-amyloid load have each been associated with dementia severity. Mesial temporal structures, particularly the hippocampal formation, are involved early in AD, and this accounts for the amnestic syndrome in these patients. AD produces a lamina-specific pattern of damage to the entorhinal cortex that disrupts cortical input to the hippocampal formation from association and limbic cortices and disrupts hippocampal outflow from the cornu Ammonis sectors and subiculum to the association cortices, diencephalon, basal forebrain, and amygdala. Hence, AD effectively disconnects the hippocampus from its major input and output pathways.[4]

The plaque core in AD in isolation or occurring with Down's syndrome is composed of insoluble β-amyloid,[5] and the gene for amyloid β precursor protein (βAPP) has been mapped to chromosome 21. The βAPP is normally expressed in multiple cells of neural and non-neural origin and has several putative cellular functions. The βAPP can be processed by nonamyloidogenic and amyloidogenic pathways. The fragment of βAPP formed by the latter pathway, termed β-amyloid or Aβ, is a soluble secretory product composed of 39 to 43 residues. This pathway may generate Aβ at the cell surface, in the lysosomes, or in the Golgi apparatus, and the precise mechanism of Aβ processing may be cell-type specific.[6] The form secreted in highest quantity is Aβ1-40, with lesser amounts being in the Aβ1-42 form. Each form is secreted in

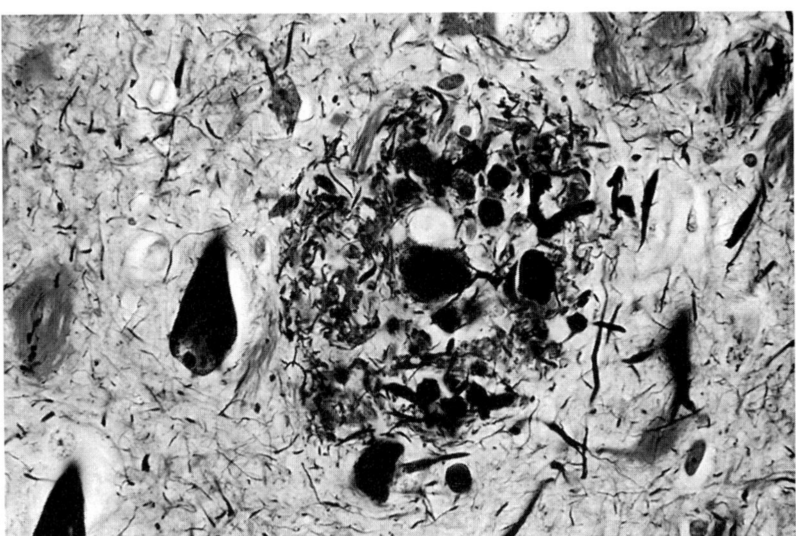

FIGURE 33–2. Photomicrograph of entorhinal cortex in Alzheimer's disease. The neuritic plaque is composed of an amyloid core surrounded by dystrophic neurites. The dark flame-shaped fibrillar structures are neurofibrillary tangles, which are chiefly made up of paired helical filaments. (Bielschowsky silver stain; 200×; courtesy of JE Parisi, Mayo Clinic, Rochester, Minnesota.)

varying amounts in cognitively normal and abnormal individuals, and levels of each can be measured in both plasma and CSF. The insoluble Aβ1-42 form is contained in plaques. Additional amyloid-associated proteins are believed to interact with Aβ, which can also promote amyloid fibril formation and deposition as plaques.

Plaques, in which amyloid deposition is diffuse and distended neurites are absent, have been termed diffuse nonneuritic plaques. These plaques are present in nondemented aged and Down's syndrome patients. With the appearance of distended neurites, the plaques are then classified as diffuse NPs. Insoluble amyloid fibrils surrounded by distended neurites constitute a dense-core NP, which is equivalent to the classic NP. A "burnt-out" plaque is a dense core of amyloid without the surrounding distended neurites. The accumulated evidence favors the amyloid cascade hypothesis in the pathogenesis of AD (Fig. 33–3). This hypothesis states that the initial abnormality in AD pathogenesis is amyloid deposition in the neuropil (forming plaques) and cerebral vessels (forming amyloid angiopathy).[6, 7] This deposition is neurotoxic, leading to cytoskeletal derangement with neurofibrillary tangle formation, leading, in turn, to neuronal degeneration. Studies from several laboratories suggest that Aβ1-42 is the crucial form of Aβ involved in this cascade. Aβ1-42 has been shown to form insoluble amyloid fibrils faster than Aβ1-40 in vitro. This form is deposited in the diffuse plaques of Down's syndrome patients far in advance of Aβ1-40, and this peptide is the primary form of Aβ deposition in the NPs of sporadic AD. Plasma Aβ1-42 is elevated in approximately 12 percent of patients, and CSF Aβ1-42 is reduced in patients with clinically diagnosed AD.[8] The reduction of Aβ1-42 presumably reflects diminished clearance and subsequent deposition. It is hoped that interfering with Aβ1-42 formation or deposition may impact AD pathogenesis.

The six human isoforms of the microtubule-associated protein tau are derived from a single gene on chromosome 17. Tau normally binds to microtubules when dephosphorylated or only partially phosphorylated. Hyperphosphorylated tau is the major component of paired helical filaments, which are the major constituents of NFTs, neuropil threads, and dystrophic neurites. Accumulated paired helical filaments or microtubule destabilization, or both, may disrupt axonal transport and lead to NFT formation and neuronal death. In AD, tau concentration is elevated in the CSF.[9]

The association between the type 4 allele of apolipoprotein E (ApoE ε-4) and late-onset familial[10, 11] and sporadic AD[11] was recognized in 1993. An increased risk of developing sporadic AD and a decreased age of onset has been associated with the ApoE ε-4 allele, whereas risk decreases and age of onset increases with the ApoE ε-2 allele.[12] However, ApoE ε-4 does not directly cause AD because it can occur in the absence of even one copy of the ApoE ε-4 allele, and two copies of this allele have been documented in cognitively and neuropathologically normal individuals. Disease progression does not appear to be associated with ApoE status.

ApoE is found in the NPs, vascular amyloid, and NFTs of AD. Amyloid deposition in NPs and blood vessels has correlated with ApoE ε-4 dosage (that is, whether there is one or two copies of the ApoE ε-4 allele), whereas the frequency of NFTs has not.[13] ApoE promotes amyloid filament formation in vitro.[14] ApoE ε-3, but not ApoE ε-4, binds to microtubule-associated protein tau, which may slow the rate of tau phosphorylation and self-assembly into parahelical filaments.

There are four types of ApoE receptors in the brain. One type, the low-density lipoprotein receptor–related protein, is found in hippocampal pyramidal cells and dentate granule cells. It is a highly conserved protein found also in nematodes, and it functions in membrane maintenance. LRP binds and internalizes not only ApoE but also several other ligands, all of which have been associated with NP. LRP internalization of its associated ligands may be impaired in AD, thus resulting in Aβ-ApoE complex aggregation and NP formation.[15] The specific interactions between the various ligands and ApoE isoforms remain to be determined, but the potential may exist for developing therapeutic interventions that manipulate these interactions.

Limited pathological, clinical, and epidemiological studies have supported a role for immunological activation as an intrinsic component of the neurodegenerative process.[16] The number of activated microglia is high in diffuse plaques and higher in diffuse NPs, but there are fewer microglia in more mature plaques with amyloid cores, suggesting that the inflammatory response may have a primary role in the early steps of plaque formation.

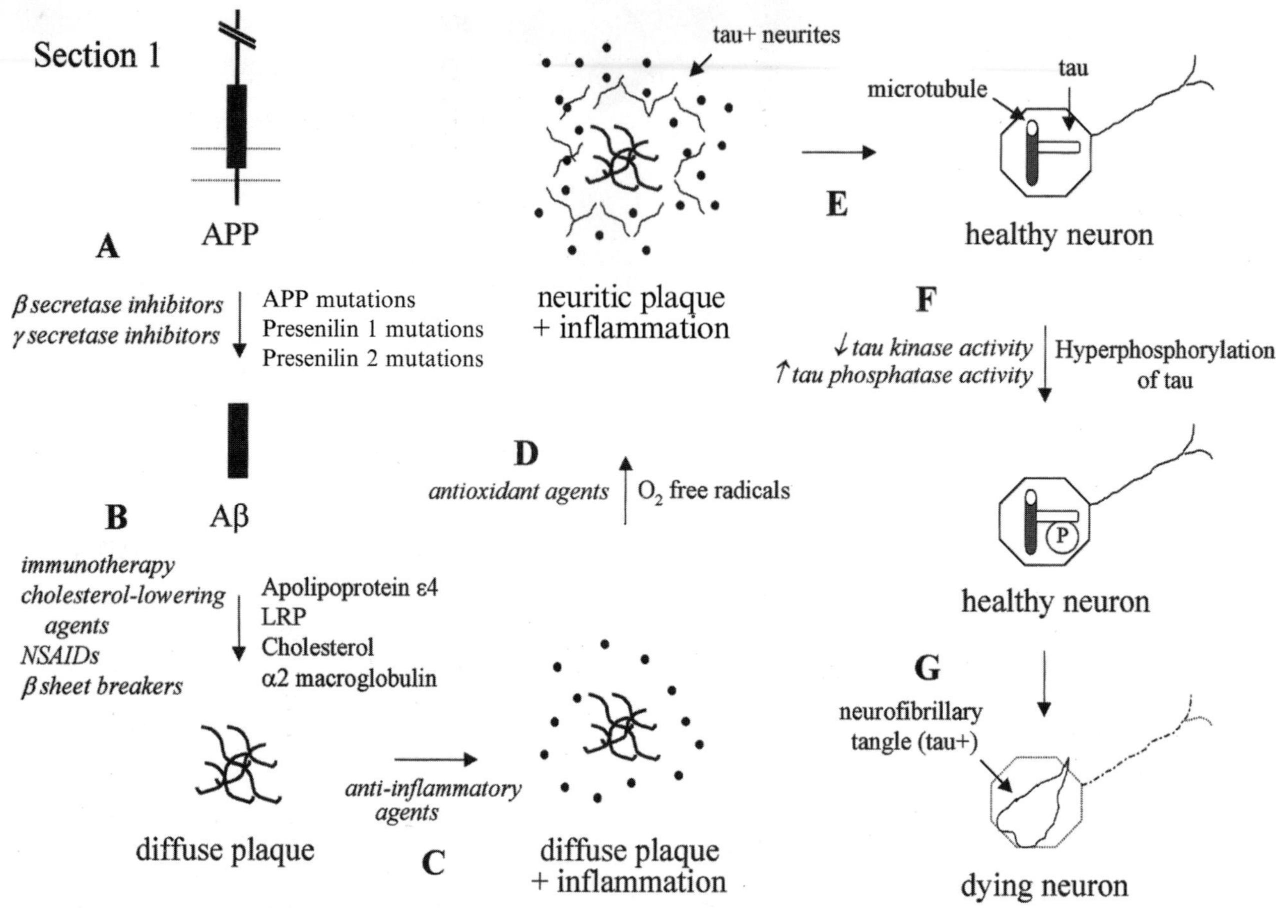

FIGURE 33–3. The amyloid cascade hypothesis of Alzheimer's disease (AD) pathogenesis and potential therapeutic targets. The amyloid precursor protein (APP) is a 770-amino acid protein whose normal physiologic function has not been defined. The APP can be cleaved by the enzymes α-, β-, and γ-secretase *(1A, 2A–2D)*. Presenilin likely requires nicastrin to allow γ-secretase activity to occur *(2D)*. The APP is cleaved into p3 by α-secretase; p3 is a soluble and nontoxic form of amyloid *(2A, 2B)*. β- and γ-secretase activity cleaves APP into β-amyloid (Aβ) which fibrillizes, aggregates, and deposits in the brain *(2C and 2D)*. The 42-amino acid fragment ($A\beta_{42}$) tends to deposit in the brain parenchyma and is the major constituent of amyloid plaques; the 40-amino acid fragment ($A\beta_{40}$) tends to deposit in blood vessels and cause amyloid angiopathy, thereby increasing friability and the tendency to hemorrhage. Mutations in APP, presenilin 1, and presenilin 2 all act to increase production of Aβ *(1A)*. Aβ interacts with apolipoprotein E ε-4, lipoprotein-related protein, cholesterol, α2 macroglobulin, and other compounds to increase aggregation and/or decrease clearance of amyloid or diffuse plaques *(1B)*. The plaques presumably lead to microglial activation and the associated inflammatory response and free radical formation *(1C, 1D)*. Tau-positive neurites then develop around the amyloid core resulting in neuritic plaques. The amyloid cascade hypothesis posits that the preceding series of events causes healthy neurons to degenerate *(1E)*; the mechanisms underlying this process have not yet been adequately characterized. The microtubule-associated protein tau becomes hyperphosphorylated *(1F)*, causing impaired intracellular processing and neurofibrillary tangle formation *(1G)*. The affected neurons degenerate, ultimately causing dementia.

Several steps in this cascade could potentially be manipulated to affect AD pathogenesis. β- and γ-secretase inhibitors may decrease Aβ production and potentially prevent the development, delay the onset, and delay the rate of progression of AD *(1A, 2C, 2D)*. Promotors of α-secretase activity *(2A)* could decrease the proportion of APP that is processed via steps 2C and 2D. Immunotherapy (i.e., amyloid vaccine), cholesterol-lowering agents, and β-pleated sheet breakers may decrease amyloid plaque development and/or increase amyloid clearance *(1B)*. Epidemiological studies have suggested that nonsteroidal anti-inflammatory drugs (NSAIDs) are protective against AD, which has been presumed to be due to their anti-inflammatory properties *(1C)*. Recent data indicate that certain NSAIDs actually decrease Aβ levels independent of their anti-inflammatory properties *(1B)*. There is continued hope that NSAIDs and other agents with anti-inflammatory properties may decrease the inflammatory response to amyloid plaques *(1C)*. Free radical scavengers such as α-tocopherol and selegiline have been shown to delay the rate of progression in patients with AD, presumably by affecting free radical formation *(1D)*. The complex interactions between amyloid and tau processing could be manipulated *(1E)*. Decreasing tau kinase activity and/or increasing tau phosphatase activity could decrease development of neurofibrillary tangles *(1F, 1G)*.

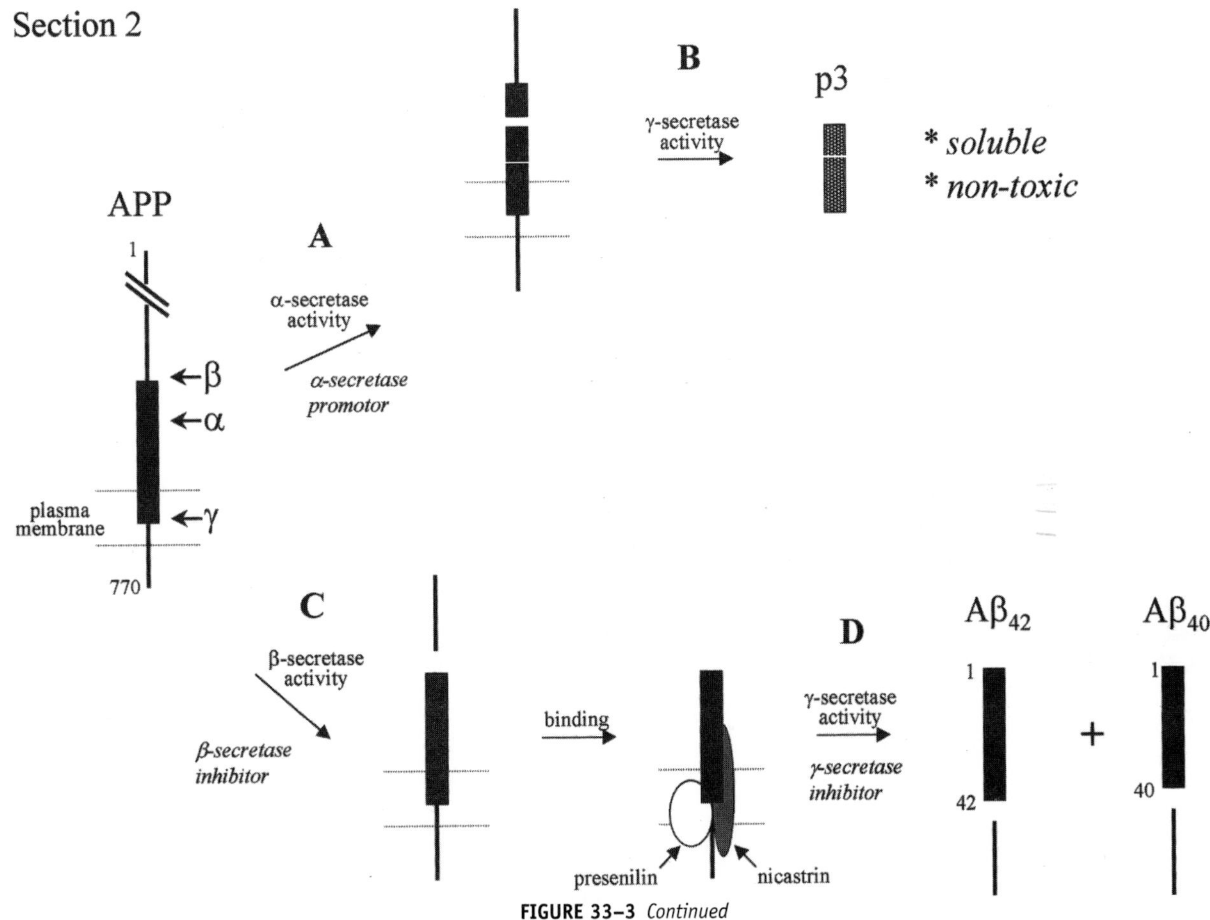

FIGURE 33–3 *Continued*

Chronic aluminum exposure was once thought to play a role in AD mainly due to encephalopathy occurring in dialysis patients who were exposed to toxic levels of aluminum. The possible mechanisms by which aluminum could lead to AD histopathology include promoting hyperphosphorylation of tau and subsequent formation of NFTs, altering processing of the βAPP, which would lead to the formation of NPs, and initiating the inflammatory response.[17] However, at present, aluminum exposure is not thought to be a major risk factor for AD.

The oxidative stress hypothesis of neurodegeneration holds that free radical generation from metabolism is neurotoxic, and there is some evidence that Aβ may promote free radical formation.[18] This has led some to propose the use of antioxidants clinically and in experimental trials in patients with clinically diagnosed AD.[16]

Levels of acetylcholine, noradrenaline, serotonin, gamma-aminobutyric acid (GABA), glutamate, somatostatin, neuropeptide Y, and substance P have all been documented to be reduced in the brains of AD patients. However, reductions in acetylcholine and choline acetyltransferase are the most profound, and therefore they have been thought to be the most important. Such reductions are due to neuronal loss in the basal forebrain, which is the major region from which cholinergic projections originate.[19] Only modest improvement in cognitive functions have been achieved with cholinergic agonists, presumably due to neuronal loss in the cortical targets that receive cholinergic input.

Pathological variants of AD include limbic AD, plaque-only AD (usually the Lewy body variant of AD[20]), and the Lewy body variant (LBV) of AD (though this has been lumped under the broader heading "dementia with Lewy bodies"). The pathophysiological relationship between LBV and AD and the appropriate nomenclature are still under debate (see Dementia with Lewy Bodies section).

There are four genetic variants of AD. AD1 results from a mutation in the APP gene on chromosome 21, resulting in increased amyloid formation and deposition in the brain, resulting, in turn, in familial late-onset AD, as well as cerebral vasculature with consequent amyloid angiopathy. AD2 is another genetic subtype of familial late-onset AD reflecting the type 4 allele of ApoE located on chromosome 19.[10] AD3 is a form of familial early-onset AD resulting from mutation of an integral membrane protein (presenilin-1) gene located on chromosome 14. Mutations in this gene may be responsible for more than 75 percent of cases of familial early-onset AD with a mean onset before age 50.[21] Finally, AD4 is another familial early-onset form of AD related to a mutation of another transmembrane protein (presenilin-2) located on chromosome 1 in seven related families of Volga German ancestry (and one Italian kindred) with autosomal dominant AD.[22] Recent evidence suggests that presenilin is the major component of γ-secretase. Additional loci on chromosome 10 and 12 have been associated with AD; the specific genes have not yet been identified.[23, 24] The genetic variants of AD1, AD3, and AD4 seem to exert their pathogenetic effect through increased production and deposition of insoluble β-amyloid.

Alzheimer's pathology has also been found in some patients with non–Alzheimer-type patterns of dementia,

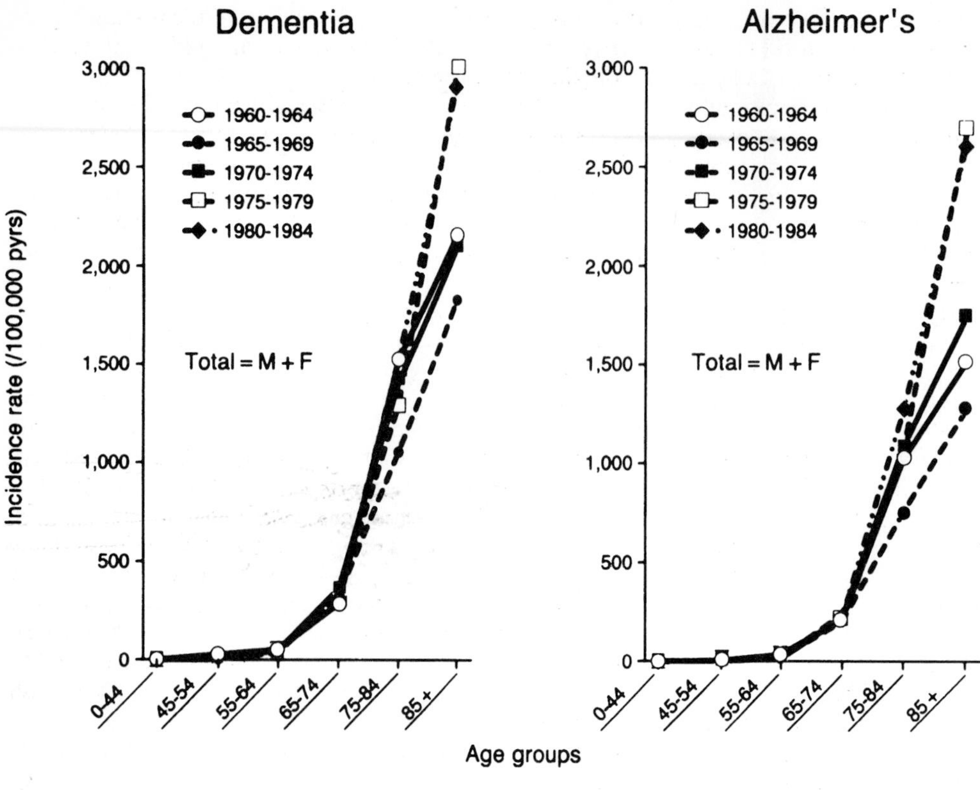

FIGURE 33–4. Incidence rates of dementia (all causes) and Alzheimer's disease in Olmsted County, Minnesota, by age for five quinquennial periods (1960 to 1984). pyrs = person years. (From Kokmen E, Beard CM, O'Brien PC, Kurland LT: Epidemiology of dementia in Rochester, Minnesota. Mayo Clin Proc 1996;71:275–282.)

including frontotemporal, aphasic, and perceptual-motor syndromes (see ACDS, later).

Epidemiology and Risk Factors. AD is the most common cause of dementia overall, accounting for more than half of all cases, and it increases in frequency with advancing age. Epidemiological age-specific estimates of incidence and prevalence vary by region and study due to differences in diagnostic criteria and population demographics. Figures 33–4 and 33–5 show the incidence and prevalence rates for dementia (all causes) and AD in particular in Olmsted

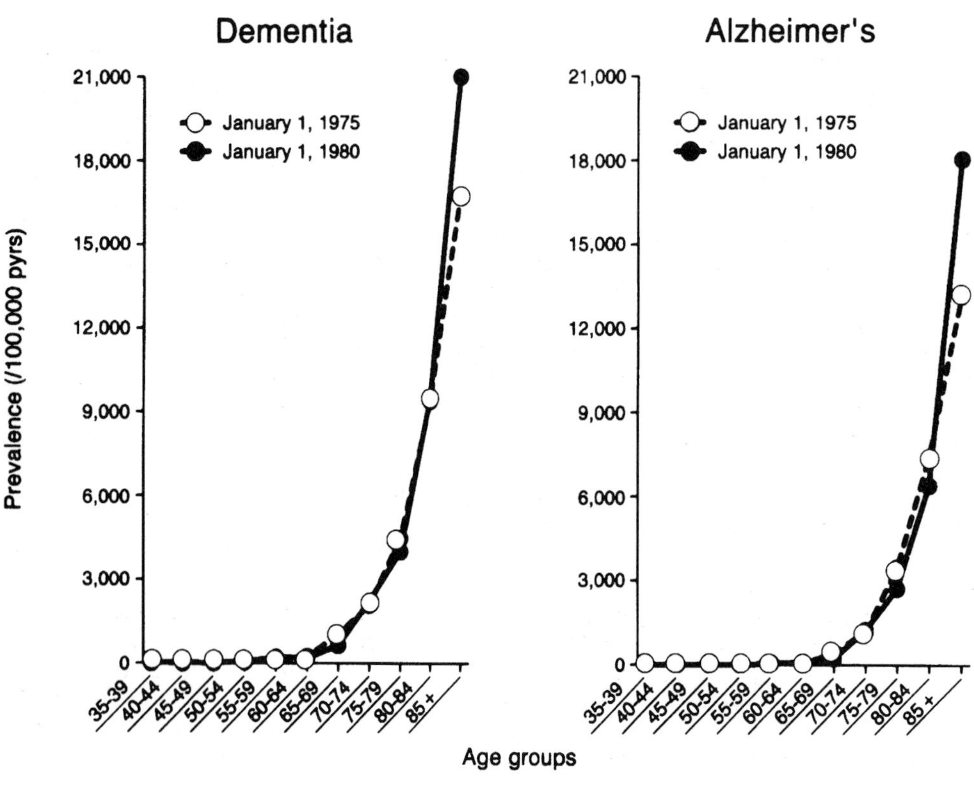

FIGURE 33–5. Prevalence rates of dementia (all causes) and Alzheimer's disease in Olmsted County, Minnesota, by age for two prevalence dates: January 1, 1975, and January 1, 1980. pyrs = person years. (From Kokmen E, Beard CM, O'Brien PC, Kurland LT: Epidemiology of dementia in Rochester, Minnesota. Mayo Clin Proc 1996;71:275–282.)

County, Minnesota.[25] There is an exponential increase in both with advancing age at least through the ninth decade. Whether this trend continues into the tenth decade is presently unknown. The prevalence of severe dementia over the age of 60 is estimated at 5 percent, and over the age of 85, between 20 and 50 percent. The lifetime risk of developing AD is estimated to be between 12 and 17 percent.[26, 27]

Following age, ApoE status is the second most important risk factor. In both familial late-onset[10] and sporadic[11] cases, the ApoE ε-4 allele increases risk and the ε-2 allele decreases risk.[12] The lifetime risk of AD in people without a family history increases from 9 percent without an ApoE ε-4 allele to 29 percent with one copy of the ApoE ε-4 allele.[27] ApoE ε-4 homozygotes make up roughly 2 percent of the population, but approximately 83 percent are estimated to develop AD in their lifetime,[28] similar to the 91 percent reported in familial late-onset cases.[10, 11] In limited populations, other genetic factors play a determining role, including Down's syndrome (trisomy 21),[29] familial early-onset Alzheimer's kindreds (chromosome 14),[21] and the Volga German kindreds of familial early-onset AD (chromosome 1).[22]

Other purported risk factors are weaker and some are more controversial in that not all well-controlled epidemiological studies have found them to be significant. These risk factors include limited education, depression, gender, estrogen replacement therapy, use of vitamin E, head trauma, use of anti-inflammatory drugs, and a history of thyroid disease.

Clinical Features and Associated Disorders. AD has been considered the paradigm of a cortical dementia syndrome. The hallmarks of cortical dementia include not only memory loss, which is common to many dementia syndromes, but also elements of aphasia, apraxia, and agnosia. Further, in general, there is an absence of subcortical features such as parkinsonism. Some patients with pathologically proven AD, however, also exhibit features of mild parkinsonism, emphasizing that diagnostic boundaries are relative, not absolute. Table 33–1 shows the National Institute of Neurological and Communicative Disorders and Stroke and the Alzheimer's Disease and Related Disorders Association (NINCDS-ADRDA) Work Group's diagnostic criteria for AD.[30] Definite AD is defined by tissue confirmation. Probable AD is defined by the clinical picture of dementia in the absence of certain atypical features such as focal neurological abnormalities and for which another cause cannot be found. Possible AD is defined by the clinical picture of dementia, but with either atypical features in the course of the illness or with a second potentially contributory disease not believed to be the primary cause. In the absence of histological confirmation, therefore, the clinical picture of dementia is the most important diagnostic feature.

Dementia is not a homogeneous clinical syndrome. It is defined as disabling impairment of multiple cognitive domains. Hence, memory loss alone does not equal dementia, even though it may be the heralding symptom of a dementing illness and is the most commonly impaired cognitive domain among all dementia syndromes (cortical and subcortical). Degenerative dementia further implies disease progression over time. The pattern and evolution of cognitive deficits defines the syndrome of Alzheimer's dementia, even though pathologically defined AD may rarely not present in this way. Nonetheless, the overall clinical-pathological correlation of Alzheimer's dementia with AD is now approximately 87 percent.[31]

Most clinical studies agree that the earliest clinical sign of AD is memory loss, which precedes the actual dementia. Abnormal cerebral metabolism, demonstrated by positron-emission tomography (PET), may precede even mild memory loss.[32] A few studies have correlated other relative cognitive inefficiencies occurring much earlier in life with the subsequent development of dementia, although interpretation of these findings has been a source of controversy.

Recent memory is easier to assess reliably than remote memory and is thought to be disproportionately severely involved. Nonetheless, remote memory is also abnormal, and there is a gradient effect regarding recall over a retrograde time interval: The oldest memories appear to be the best preserved, with proportionately greater forgetting as the retrograde interval shortens.[33] In contrast, procedural memory appears to be relatively spared. Alzheimer's patients are able to learn simple skills as easily as normal controls and better than patients with subcortical patterns of dementia or patients with various types of sensorimotor deficits.[34] Although apraxia is one of the defining features of cortical dementia, it is rarely severe in mild to moderate stages of AD and can be very difficult to distinguish from impaired comprehension in these patients. One very important skill that needs to be addressed clinically is driving. Despite the relative preservation of procedural memory, patients with mild Alzheimer's dementia have a higher rate of collisions and moving violations than age-matched controls,[35] although estimates of risk vary, especially during the first 2 years of the disease. Whether this actually results from impaired procedural memory, attentional factors, other cognitive aspects, or a combination is unclear, although visual tracking, memory, and Mini-Mental State score all correlate with a laboratory-based driving score.[35]

Memory loss is a cardinal feature of Alzheimer's dementia, but it is not the only abnormality in most patients. However, many patients present with a circumscribed, slowly progressive amnesic syndrome, which is sometimes referred to as "mild cognitive impairment" (MCI).[36] The criteria for the diagnosis of MCI are shown in Table 33–2. The memory loss in these patients should be distinguished from the milder memory problems of normal aging. MCI has the same profile of risk factors as AD, including advanced age and ApoE,[37] and patients who have come to autopsy often prove to have AD. Such patients also have radiologically demonstrable hippocampal atrophy. Over half of patients who present with MCI develop features of dementia over a 4- to 5-year period.[37] The practice parameter on MCI suggests that patients with forgetfulness should be evaluated and monitored.[38] Recognition of patients with MCI will become increasingly important as many agents will be tested to potentially delay the rate of progression of MCI to AD.

Aphasia, apraxia, and agnosia are the other categories of cognitive impairment that typically occur in cortical dementia syndromes and particularly in AD. In Alzheimer's dementia, these aspects do not dominate the clinical picture. A patient with a predominant aphasic syndrome (progressive aphasia) should not be assumed to have AD, though some do (see Asymmetrical Cortical Degeneration Syndromes). Rather, these aspects of cognitive pathology occur in discrete

TABLE 33–1. NINCDS-ADRDA Criteria for the Diagnosis of Alzheimer's Disease*

I. Clinical Diagnosis of Probable Alzheimer's Disease
  1. Dementia established by clinical examination and mental status testing and confirmed by neuropsychological testing
  2. Deficits in at least two cognitive domains
  3. Progressive cognitive decline, including memory
  4. Normal level of consciousness
  5. Onset between ages 40 and 90 (most common after 65) years
  6. No other possible medical or neurological explanation

II. Probable Alzheimer's Disease Diagnosis Supported by
  1. Progressive aphasia, apraxia, and agnosia
  2. Impaired activities of daily living
  3. Family history of similar disorder
  4. Brain atrophy on CT/MRI, especially if progressive
  5. Normal CSF, EEG (or nonspecifically abnormal)

III. Other Clinical Features Consistent with Probable Alzheimer's Disease
  1. Plateau in course
  2. Associated symptoms: depression; insomnia; incontinence; illusions; hallucinations; catastrophic verbal, emotional, or physical outbursts; sexual disorders; weight loss; during more advanced stages increased muscle tone, myoclonus, and abnormal gait
  3. Seizures in advanced disease
  4. CT normal for age

IV. Features That Make Alzheimer's Disease Uncertain or Unlikely
  1. Acute onset
  2. Focal sensorimotor signs
  3. Seizures or gait disorder early in course

V. Clinical Diagnosis of Possible Alzheimer's Disease
  1. Dementia with atypical onset or course in the absence of another medical/neuropsychiatric explanation
  2. Dementia with another disease not felt otherwise to be the cause of dementia
  3. For research purposes, a progressive focal cognitive deficit

VI. Definite Alzheimer's Disease
  1. Meets clinical criteria for probable Alzheimer's disease
  2. Tissue confirmation (autopsy or brain biopsy)

VII. Research Classification of Alzheimer's Disease Should Specify
  1. Familial?
  2. Early onset (before age 65)?
  3. Down's syndrome (trisomy 21)?
  4. Co-existent other neurodegenerative disease (e.g., Parkinson's disease)?

*National Institute of Neurological and Communicative Disorders and Stroke and the Alzheimer's Disease and Related Disorders Association Work Group's report summarizing the criteria for a diagnosis of Alzheimer's disease.
CSF, Cerebrospinal fluid; CT, computed tomography; EEG, electroencephalogram; MRI, magnetic resonance imaging study.
Reprinted from McKhann G, Drachman D, Folstein M, et al: Clinical diagnosis of Alzheimer's disease: Report of the NINCDS-ADRDA Work Group under the auspices of Department of Health and Human Services Task Force on Alzheimer's Disease. Neurology 1984;34:939–944. By permission of Little, Brown and Company (Inc.).

TABLE 33–2. Clinical Diagnosis of Mild Cognitive Impairment (MCI)[36]

Core Features
A memory complaint
Normal activities of daily living
Normal general cognitive functioning
Abnormal memory functioning for age
Patient is *not* demented by DSM-III-R criteria

apportionments that define the dementia syndrome as typical Alzheimer's dementia. In patients with such an apportionment, clinicopathological correlation rates are high.[31] In mild to moderate stages of dementia, anomia is prominent and readily detectable with neuropsychological testing using a variety of naming tests (see Chapter 27). Patients are, however, fluent and may have relatively good comprehension, so clinical detection is not always easy. As the disease progresses, the predominantly anomic aphasia gives way to a more fluent, or Wernicke's, type of aphasia with impaired comprehension. Nonfluent aphasia does not generally occur

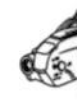

in AD, although preterminally patients become mute (see Chapter 6). This should not be the case in a patient who is still ambulatory, however.

Apraxia can be confused with impaired comprehension in mild to moderate stages of Alzheimer's dementia. Patients have difficulty performing tasks at which they were previously adept, such as repairing a household appliance or doing carpentry work. They also have difficulty learning new procedures such as operating a new car, new appliance, or remote control device. They have some difficulty pantomiming gestures in the office setting but also have constructional apraxia. In moderately advanced stages, patients have trouble dressing and performing other activities of daily living. Patients with clinically evident apraxia typically also have significant perceptual difficulties (see later) and definitely should not be driving a motor vehicle.

Anosognosia, the failure to recognize illness, is a cardinal feature of Alzheimer's dementia and is typically present, even in mild stages of the disease. It is a useful sign to distinguish progressive amnesic syndromes from Alzheimer's dementia. A typical patient with AD is brought or sent for evaluation rather than coming of his or her own accord. He or she may deny significant memory problems and will actively try to explain away the observations of concerned family members and friends, even to the point of becoming hostile and accusative. This is one of the most difficult aspects of the disease because such patients often should not be driving or managing their own finances but will do so anyway, sometimes to their detriment.

In moderate to advanced stages, patients exhibit other so-called agnosic types of disturbances. Arguably, the difficulty such patients have in recognizing familiar people reflects prosopagnosia, save that they are not reliably benefited by voice recognition either. Difficulty finding their way could be compared with topographagnosia, another visual agnosic syndrome, but again this is not occurring in the pure form given the wealth of other cognitive problems accompanying it. Rarely, patients with histologically documented AD present with a disabling, primarily visual syndrome termed simultanagnosia, in which there is an inability to view all parts of a complex visual scene in a single coherent time-space frame. Such patients fail to see a target object that is right in front of them, especially if it is surrounded by potentially distracting stray objects.[39] Strictly speaking, this is not an agnosic disorder, but another type of complex visual disturbance that resembles agnosia and can occur in this setting. It is rarely the presenting feature. More commonly, it is a mild accompanying feature.

Psychiatric symptoms include both affective and psychotic disturbances. Depression interferes with a person's functional status and an accurate cognitive assessment, erroneously leading to the diagnosis of dementia; such is the nature of pseudodementia, which has been estimated to account for 4 to 5 percent of dementia cases.[40] More commonly, depression may complicate the course of AD and other dementing illnesses. Antidepressant therapy should be strongly considered in such patients. Psychotic symptoms most commonly involve paranoid delusions and, less commonly, hallucinations. AD should be in the differential diagnosis of an elderly patient presenting de novo with an organic delusional syndrome or hallucinosis. Common paranoid themes involve infidelity and stealing. Hallucinations are generally complex, involving people (familiar or unfamiliar), animals, or both. The combination of anosognosia, paranoid delusions, and mild cognitive decline is potentially dangerous and very difficult to manage, especially if such individuals live alone, yet a significant minority of Alzheimer's patients have exactly that combination.

Two common vegetative groups of symptoms regard sleep disturbances and incontinence. Sleep-wake cycle disturbances are common and may be present even during relatively mild stages of the illness. They become more common and more severe during moderately severe stages. There are two aspects to the sleep-wake cycle disturbance. The first is the so-called sundowning effect, which means that the patient becomes more confused, agitated, and difficult to manage during the evening hours. The second regards either not sleeping at night, waking up during very early hours, or going to sleep very early in the evening. Sleep becomes fractionated into shorter segments throughout the 24-hour period. As the disease progresses to more advanced stages, patients may become generally less active, may sleep more, and, eventually, in terminal stages, are bedbound with little apparent conscious activity. Weight loss is common during the latter stages, as well. Incontinence (both urinary and fecal) is uncommon in mild stages but becomes increasingly frequent as the disease progresses and is universal in late stages. Early on, it may inadvertently result from voiding in the "wrong place" rather than actual sphincter control problems, but in later stages, sphincter control is lost.

Late and preterminal stage AD ensues after roughly a 5- to 10-year course but is highly variable and can be shorter or longer. In very advanced stages, patients are no longer ambulatory, become mute and incontinent, and are totally dependent on their caregiver or nursing attendant. Eventually dysphagia signals the terminal phase, and unless a feeding tube is placed, patients eventually die from inanition or aspiration, or both. Few patients live to these stages, with death resulting from intercurrent illnesses in most.

Down's syndrome has a strong association with AD. If a patient with Down's syndrome (trisomy 21) lives beyond the age of 40 years, it is a near certainty that there will be neuropathological evidence of AD at autopsy.[29] Clinical dementia increases with age and peaks at roughly 40 to 75 percent over the age of 60.[29] Analysis of the amyloid plaques has shown that trisomy 21 predisposes to larger plaques, presumably reflecting increased production of Aβ, in contrast to ApoE ε-4, which leads to greater numbers of plaques, presumably reflecting increased probability of senile plaque initiation.[41]

Not all neuropathologically defined cases of AD present with Alzheimer's dementia, as is elaborated in the discussion of ACDS. Patients with the syndromes of progressive aphasia, progressive apraxia (and other motor syndromes), and progressive simultanagnosia have all been reported, on occasion, to have Alzheimer-type pathology. Such cases raise questions regarding the nosology of degenerative cortical syndromes.

Differential Diagnosis. AD is one disease among many, both degenerative and nondegenerative, that can produce the categorical syndrome of a chronic progressive encephalopathy. All-encompassing, indiscriminant differential diagnostic inclusion of a hundred conditions encompassed by this broad category is inefficient and impractical.

So, too, is the reflex assumption that memory loss in an elderly individual equals dementia equals AD. Simply determining that a disease is degenerative already accomplishes the most important goal of excluding any possible or more effectively treated etiology.

Reversible forms of dementia are truly chronicencephalopathies and often cause one or several of the following: hypersomnolence, acute or subacute deterioration, fluctuating severity, severe EEG abnormalities, visual hallucinations, tremulousness, or unsteadiness, or it may be accompanied by non-neurological symptoms as well. Such symptoms may occur within the context of another disease process known to cause neurological problems sometimes, such as hypothyroidism, or may occur under specific circumstances such as immunosuppression. Irreversible forms of dementia are generally more slowly progressive (more than a year or two), fluctuate much less, do not occur within the context of another potentially causative disease, have recognizable clinical and cognitive profiles, and are not accompanied by many of the aforementioned clues of a reversible chronic encephalopathy. When analyzed in this way, a more realistic differential diagnosis of AD includes (1) other degenerative diseases, such as Pick's disease, nonspecific degeneration (dementia lacking distinctive histopathology), and dementia with Lewy bodies; and (2) vascular dementia resulting from small vessel disease due either to atherosclerotic small vessel disease or amyloid angiopathy. In mild to moderate stages, clinical cognitive patterns can be very helpful in distinguishing various dementing illnesses. In late stages, however, patients are more diffusely impaired both cognitively and somatically, making it difficult to tell one degenerative brain disease from another.

Evaluation. Because the recognition of distinctive clinical cognitive patterns can be difficult, a practical approach must take into account some of the chronic encephalopathic causes as well as degenerative and related causes. Neuroimaging is essential. MRI is preferred, if possible, but CT is generally adequate. Structural processes such as chronic (or subacute) subdural hematomas, tumors (frontal lobe meningiomas and temporal lobe gliomas in particular), cerebrovascular lesions, prior traumatic encephalomalacia, relevant focal atrophy (see ACDS section), and meningeal enhancement are among the many important diagnostic clues that mitigate against a diagnosis of AD. Bilateral medial temporal or more generalized atrophy may be discernible, but this is nonspecific, and in the absence of quantitation, it is difficult to use for diagnostic purposes. Physiological neuroimaging is not recommended for routine evaluation of patients suspected of having AD but may be helpful in ACDS (see later). Nonetheless, single photon emission computed tomography (SPECT) and PET have shown bilateral temporoparietal and posterior cingulate hypometabolism and hypoperfusion in AD.

Cognitive examination is essential, but whether formal neuropsychological assessment is required depends on the examining physician's skill in clinical cognitive assessment. In general, neuropsychological assessment is highly desirable in mild to moderate stages of dementia for both qualitative description of the dementia pattern (which has diagnostic significance) and quantitative estimation of cognitive disability. Although variable, a typical neuropsychological profile will show severe learning and memory impairment and anomia. Frequently, there is also evidence of impaired aural comprehension, a generally reliable indicator of significant cognitive disability. Psychomotor speed is generally preserved, although with longitudinal assessment, it also declines.

Basic laboratory and general health measures are also essential. Cognitive decline has very different implications in a smoker with active lung cancer, severe anemia, or disseminated intravascular coagulation, for example, than in a previously healthy octogenarian. Recent chest x-ray study, electrocardiogram, urinalysis, complete blood counts, and a chemistry profile (which should include electrolytes, calcium, fasting blood glucose, and renal and liver function tests) are not specifically neurological but can be very relevant if they disclose a severe abnormality. Thyroid function tests and vitamin B_{12} should be assessed. The actual frequency of vitamin B_{12} deficiency–related dementia is questionable, however. In patients with severe vitamin B_{12} deficiencies, anemia and combined systems disease with prominent myelopathic features seem to predominate. Cognitive decline in such a setting should certainly prompt consideration of B_{12} deficiency, but in cases of mild B_{12} deficiency without accompanying features, its significance is doubtful (see Chapter 40). CNS syphilis has become rare, but again should be screened with rapid plasma reagin or other syphilitic serological tests. The erythrocyte sedimentation rate is an arguably useful screening test for a variety of diseases that result in a systemic inflammatory response, and when the rate is highly elevated, it may be an important diagnostic clue.

The previously mentioned laboratory measures are the core tests to consider in essentially all patients. Additional tests that may not be necessary in every patient include EEG, spinal fluid examination, overnight oximetry, psychiatric evaluation, small bowel biopsy, Lyme disease serology, human immunodeficiency virus serology, various connective tissue disease serologies, and paraneoplastic serologies. Ultimately, invasive testing including cerebral angiography and meningeal or brain biopsy also have their place in the diagnostic armamentarium for chronic progressive encephalopathy but not when AD is the leading diagnostic consideration.

Degenerative diseases other than DLB (see DLB section) and depression are rarely accompanied by severe EEG disturbances. In contrast, EEG abnormalities are often severe (and usually nonspecific) in toxic, metabolic, inflammatory, infectious, and neoplastic encephalopathies. Complex partial status epilepticus and Creutzfeldt-Jakob disease may produce pathognomonic patterns. When in doubt, an EEG is a simple, noninvasive screening test for a wide variety of diseases, many of which are reversible. Patients suspected of having a chronic encephalopathy, perhaps reinforced by a severely abnormal EEG, should undergo spinal fluid examination, and tests should include immunological indices such as IgG index, IgG synthesis rate, and oligoclonal bands. Although these tests are nonspecific, they are markers of intrathecal inflammation, which does not generally occur in AD or any other degenerative neurological diseases. Other tests including cytology, cultures for fungi and mycobacteria, and routine tests such as total protein, glucose, cell count, and syphilis serology should also be obtained when a spinal tap is performed. Opening pressure should be recorded, especially in patients suspected of having communicating, normal pressure hydrocephalus.

Overnight oximetry is a useful screening test for obstructive sleep apnea, a common cause of hypersomnolence with secondary inattentiveness and mild memory impairment. Psychiatric evaluation should be considered if depression is suspected, and if psychotic symptoms complicate the clinical picture. Small bowel biopsy should be considered if CNS Whipple's disease is suspected. Various serological tests should be considered for specific infectious diseases (such as Lyme disease, particularly if a patient is from an endemic area), autoimmune diseases (including Sjögren's syndrome), and paraneoplastic conditions in patients with prior or known provocative malignancies (especially oat cell lung cancer and ovarian cancer).

Management. There is no known way to entirely protect against AD, but some beneficial trends have been noted among people who take vitamin E supplements (and possibly other antioxidants), take anti-inflammatory drugs, and have a highly educated background, although many college graduates and accomplished professionals who take anti-inflammatory drugs for arthritis and vitamin E to stay young still develop AD. Some studies have suggested that among postmenopausal women, there is a slight protective effect with estrogen replacement. On the other hand, more women than men have AD, and gender has itself been suggested as a risk factor.

There are few so-called memory tonics available to patients and physicians. At present, the only drugs with possible cognitive-enhancing effects in AD are centrally acting acetylcholinesterase inhibitors, which are thought to partially reverse the decline in cortically projected acetylcholine that results from degeneration of the cholinergic basal forebrain.[42] The first of this class to be released was tacrine, though its use has dropped off in favor of newer agents (donepezil, rivastigmine, and galantamine as of this writing), which have been less toxic and less complex to titrate despite similar efficacy. The symptomatic benefits of all of these drugs are modest, but rate of cognitive decline seems to slow somewhat for reasons that are not yet well understood, and so their use has been advocated even in the absence of overt symptomatic benefit. Nonetheless, they can result in functionally important gains in some patients and should be particularly considered in patients with mild to moderate stages of the disease. There is accumulating evidence that modest gains can occur in more advanced stages of disease, though their use in such patients remains controversial. Relatively common side effects include gastrointestinal upset such as nausea, anorexia, and diarrhea. More severe side effects are less common but generally reflect systemic cholinergic effects. They should either not be used or be used with great caution in patients with cardiac conduction defects, liver disease, or seizures. A sudden decline in cognitive status or other neurological function, such as ambulation, in a patient with AD generally implies a secondary disease process, often one that is non-neurological such as a urinary tract infection, pneumonia, and fluid and electrolyte disturbances. Medication side effects (particularly those associated with tricyclic antidepressants, benzodiazepines, and narcotic analgesics) or complications from improper medication administration should be sought, especially if the patient has continued to administer his or her own medications without adequate supervision. Common neurological causes include subdural hematoma, stroke, and complex partial seizures. The differential diagnosis is extensive and is that of an acute encephalopathy.

Although it is disabling and characteristic of AD, cognitive loss is not the greatest obstacle posed by patients to their caregivers. Paranoid delusions and other psychotic symptoms are disruptive, pose extraordinary obstacles to effective caregiving, and are probably the most common reasons patients are sent to nursing homes. Small doses of neuroleptic medications may produce sufficient relief as to permit caregivers to continue to keep the patient at home, and these medications should be part of the therapeutic armamentarium. Haloperidol at doses ranging from 0.5 mg to 2 mg a day is often sufficient, but sometimes higher doses are required. 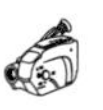 Extrapyramidal side effects, however, can become dose-limiting problems. Risperidone is a newer neuroleptic agent with additional effects on serotonergic systems and may be associated with fewer extrapyramidal side effects at equivalent doses of haloperidol. More recent atypical antipsychotic drugs include olanzepine and quetiapine, and the latter in particular may have a far lower rate of extrapyramidal side effects, making this class of antipsychotic preferable especially in patients with concurrent parkinsonism (for example, DLB).

Antidepressants with anticholinergic side effects, including all the tricyclic antidepressants, often exacerbate the confusion in these patients and are generally not recommended. Rather, selective serotonin reuptake inhibitors (SSRIs), such as fluoxetine, sertraline, and citalopram, can enhance energy levels (and possibly attentiveness as a result in some patients) and have antidepressant effects without the risk of anticholinergic side effects. They should not be used, however, in agitated patients or in patients with psychotic symptoms because SSRIs can exacerbate these behaviors. For anxiety, buspirone, although it is generally less effective than benzodiazepines, has much less risk of paradoxical agitation and should be tried first. Neuroleptic agents can also be considered for anxiety in some patients, especially if there are accompanying psychotic symptoms.

Sedative-hypnotic agents can be used in patients in whom sleep-wake disturbances are disrupting their home care. Agents that have few side effects or risks of exacerbating confusion and agitation include diphenhydramine, chloral hydrate, melatonin, trazodone, quetiapine, zolpidem, and zaleplon. Many patients fall asleep without difficulty but awaken at an early hour. In such instances, it is important that the sleeping aid be given when they waken. These medications help patients fall asleep, but they will not reliably keep them asleep for prolonged periods, which is in part why they are more advisable than longer-acting agents.

Treatment of the patient with AD ultimately means ensuring that their needs are met. Depending on what the patients cannot do for themselves, these things need to be done for them, or they need assistance with them. That includes dressing, cooking, bathing, eating, exercise (such as walking), and those problems listed earlier. The caregiver becomes an integral part of the patient's life and is vulnerable to depression, burnout, and associated problems. Support groups are important for caregivers, as is respite care to give the caregiver time away from the patient. Adult day care should be considered for patients at mild to moderate stages as a way to provide not only respite care for the caregiver but a supervised social outlet for the patient, too.

Prognosis and Future Perspectives. AD, like all degenerative neurological diseases, is relentlessly progressive. Because the patients are elderly and susceptible to a variety of other disease processes, AD itself is not the most common cause of death. However, if no other disease process supervenes, death usually ensues over roughly 6 to 10 years (there is great variability) after onset.

Increasing emphasis has been placed on early diagnosis in anticipation of preventive or retardant therapy. At the extreme of this approach is the fact that those individuals destined for AD have measurable differences throughout their lives,[43] and one such study correlated certain aspects of verbal skills at the mean age of 22 years with the subsequent development of AD 50 to 60 years later.[43] Other studies, however, still envision AD as a disease that begins in later life, but that various types of cognitive[44] and metabolic[32] derangements can be measured at least several years in advance of clinically evident cognitive decline. Possible strategies for preventive and retardant therapy include:

- interfering with a critical step in the amyloid/tau/ApoE pathway that results in plaque formation, or in the pathway that results in the hyperphosphorylation of tau leading to cytoskeletal disruption
- administration of ApoE ε-2 or analogue to promote whatever salutary effect it appears to have in preventing AD
- use of a large family of growth factor compounds that normally function during embryogenesis, some of which promote neuronal growth and retard neuronal death
- use of antioxidants to interfere with the generation of free radicals that cause cellular damage
- use of secretase inhibitors, particularly those affecting β-secretase, to decrease formation of β-amyloid and immunologic therapies such as vaccination against a key antigen such as β-amyloid

Strategies for symptomatic therapy include use of neurochemical cocktails that act on multiple neurochemical projection systems (e.g., an acetylcholinesterase inhibitor, an SSRI, and a noradrenergic agonist in combination).

Unless a very effective treatment or cure is found, the most important agenda item for the future lies not in the realm of science or medicine but in public policy. How to deal with the burgeoning elderly population and the growing number of Alzheimer's patients, many of whom require expensive chronic institutional care, will be issues of increasing societal and political focus.

ASYMMETRICAL CORTICAL DEGENERATION SYNDROMES

This is a heterogeneous group of disorders that produce distinctive cortical syndromes including aphasia, apraxia, and agnosia but that have a more focal appearance than

TABLE 33–3. **Asymmetrical Cortical Degeneration Syndromes Classification**

Syndrome	Major Topography	Main Pathology	Cognitive Signs	Other Early Neurological Signs
Progressive Aphasia				
Nonfluent	Dominant frontal operculum	Nonspecific	Nonfluent aphasia	Dysarthria, reflex asymmetry, memory loss
Fluent	Dominant temporal	Nonspecific	Fluent aphasia	Acalculia, apraxia, other parietal signs, memory loss
Anomic	Dominant anterior temporal	Pick's	Anomia	Abulia and other frontal lobe signs, memory loss
Mixed	Dominant perisylvian	Nonspecific	All aspects of speech disturbed	Memory loss, dysarthria, acalculia, apraxia
Perceptual-Motor Syndromes				
Visual	Asymmetrical bilateral P-T-O	Alzheimer's	Asimultanagnosia	Alexia, memory loss
Motor	Asymmetrical parietofrontal	CBD	Apraxia	Hemiakinetic-rigid syndrome, psychomotor slowing
Mixed	Asymmetrical P-F and P-O	CBD	Asimultanagnosia and apraxia	Memory loss, aphasia, and any of the above
Frontal Lobe Syndromes				
Neuropsychiatric	Asymmetrical bilateral prefrontal	Pick's, nonspecific	Abulia, disinhibition	Memory loss, anomia, anosognosia
Spasticity	Orbitofrontal	Nonspecific (PLS)	Psychomotor slowing	Spasticity, dysarthria
Mixed	Asymmetrical bilateral precentral gyrus Asymmetrical bilateral frontal	Unknown	Spastic-dementia syndrome	Dysarthria
Bitemporal Syndromes				
Amnesia	Bilateral mesial temporal	Alzheimer's	Memory loss	
Prosopagnosia	Right inferior temporal (bilateral?)	Unknown	Prosopagnosia	Memory loss, alexia
Neuropsychiatric	Bilateral anterior temporal	Unknown	Anomia, amnesia, abulia	Psychomotor slowing, anosognosia

CBD, Corticobasal degeneration; PLS, primary lateral sclerosis; P, parietal; T, temporal; F, frontal; O, occipital.
Adapted from Caselli RJ: Focal and asymmetric cortical degeneration syndromes. Neurologist 1995;1:1–19.

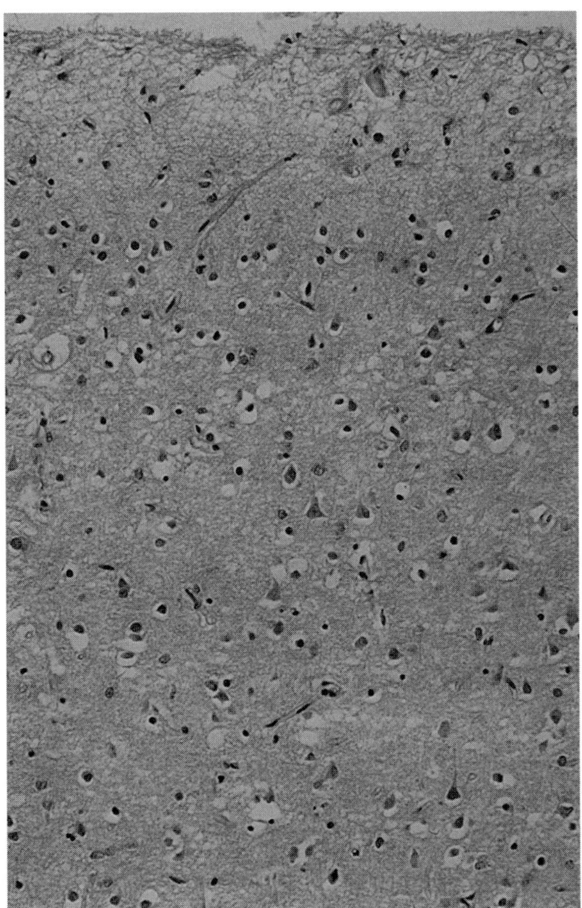

FIGURE 33–6. Photomicrograph of frontal cortex demonstrating nonspecific histology. Note the neuronal loss and gliosis, with spongiosis involving the superficial cortical layers. (Hematoxylin and eosin; 25×; courtesy of JE Parisi, Mayo Clinic, Rochester, Minnesota.)

Alzheimer's dementia. They can be roughly localized by the more focal features, though only a small subset are truly focal. There are four primary categories, each with several subtypes, including progressive aphasia, progressive frontal lobe/frontotemporal syndromes, progressive perceptual-motor syndromes, and progressive bitemporal syndromes (Table 33–3).

Pathogenesis and Pathophysiology. Despite the semiological and pathological diversity of the ACDS group, there is a common clinicopathological theme among all members: clinical presentation is dictated by the topographical distribution of degeneration. Nonspecific degenerative changes, consisting of neuronal loss, gliosis, and vacuolation of neuropil predominantly affecting superficial cortical laminae (Fig. 33–6), are common to all clinical subtypes and probably account for the overall majority of pathological findings in ACDS.

Progressive Aphasia

NONFLUENT APHASIA. The degenerative focus centers on anterior perisylvian language cortices (Broca's area). Neuropathology of progressive aphasia has included (1) nonspecific degenerative changes, including increased neuronal lipofuscin,[45] neuronal loss, astrocytosis, and perineuronal microvacuolation in superficial laminae with or without occasional amyloid plaques[46]; (2) tau-positive neuronal and/or glial pathology and nonspecific degenerative changes with focal accumulations of achromatic neurons[47]; and (3) unusual combinations of Pick/Alzheimer[48] and Alzheimer/Pick/Lewy body disease type pathology in one family (without Pick bodies).[48] The hippocampal formation is involved by the asymmetrical degeneration, but the nucleus basalis is spared.[46] Additionally, pigmented brain stem nuclei may be affected.[46]

FLUENT APHASIA. The degenerative focus is more posteriorly placed, including Wernicke's area, although usually the entire left temporal lobe appears atrophic. Neuropathology is similar to that of nonfluent aphasia, including nonspecific degenerative changes with moderate spongiosus of superficial cortical layers and involvement of the amygdala,[46] but some patients have been found to have AD.[49]

ANOMIC APHASIA. The responsible degenerative focus is in the left anterior temporal lobe. Neuropathologically, Pick's disease may cause generalized atrophy that is more severe in the left hemisphere, particularly the left anterior temporal lobe and insula, with sparing of the nucleus basalis of Meynert.[50]

MIXED APHASIA. Again, the degenerative focus appears to involve the left perisylvian cortices, particularly the left temporal lobe diffusely. Neuropathological findings include nonspecific degenerative changes with focal spongiosus of superficial cortical layers[51] and AD.[52]

Progressive Frontal Lobe Dementias (FLDs) and Frontotemporal Dementia (FTD) Syndromes (Pick's Disease). Arnold Pick originally introduced the concept of a lobar atrophy with relevant progressive focal symptoms in his description of a patient with progressive aphasic dementia, who at autopsy had, in addition to generalized cortical atrophy, focally accentuated atrophy of the left temporal lobe. The specific histological findings were later appreciated by Alzheimer in 1911, who observed distinctive intraneuronal inclusions, which were termed "Pick bodies." Swollen, ballooned, and poorly staining (chromatolytic) neurons were subsequently called "Pick cells."

Over the following decades, most investigators have included three pathological varieties of Pick's disease: lobar atrophy with swollen chromatolytic neurons (SCN) and Pick bodies (Pick's disease Type A), lobar atrophy with SCN but not Pick bodies (Pick's disease Type B), and lobar atrophy without SCN or Pick bodies (Pick's disease Type C, or nonspecific degeneration).[53] Whether the findings in Pick's disease Types B and C are indeed variants of Pick's disease or different disease processes is debated.

The cardinal pathological changes in Pick's disease Type A are lobar atrophy with corresponding neuronal loss that is most apparent in the first three cortical layers (Fig. 33–7). The maximally involved cortical gyri are very thin, and they are often described as walnut or knife-edge in appearance. When the temporal lobe atrophy is focally accentuated, the posterior one third of the superior temporal gyrus appears relatively preserved. Marked caudate and hippocampal atrophy are also typical findings. Variable degrees of co-existing subcortical gliosis and degeneration of other subcortical nuclei can occur as well, although the basal forebrain tends to be spared. Pick bodies are argentophilic, eosinophilic, rounded cytoplasmic masses that appear densely black on silver stains (Fig. 33–8). They are composed of 10- to 20-nm straight filaments that share antigenic properties with neurofilaments. Pick bodies tend to predominate in the most severely atrophic cortical regions and in the hippocampi. Pick cells

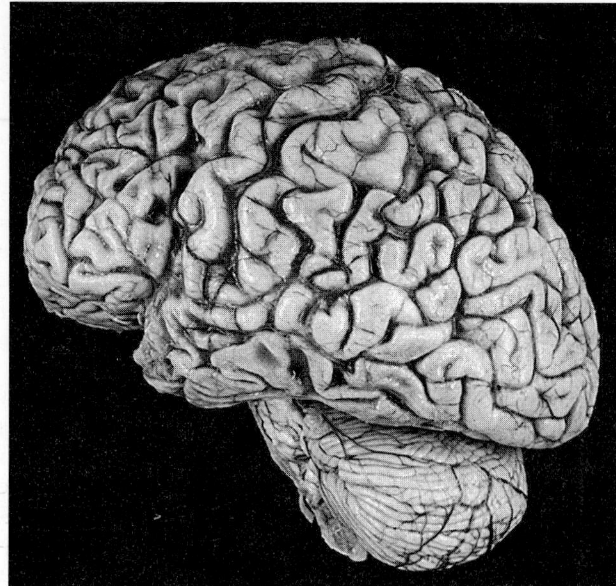

FIGURE 33–7. Pick's disease. Note the circumscribed frontotemporal cortical atrophy with relative sparing of the posterior one third of the superior temporal gyrus. The marked gyral thinning is often described as walnut or knife-edged in appearance. (Courtesy of JE Parisi, Mayo Clinic, Rochester, Minnesota.)

also immunostain positively to neurofilaments, but they are not regarded diagnostic of Pick's disease because similar-appearing cells have been observed in several other disorders. The nucleus basalis is spared or only mildly affected in both Pick's disease and in FLD.[54]

Pick's disease usually involves the frontal and anterior temporal lobes, but rare cases with preferential parietal lobe atrophy have also been described. Therefore, patients with Pick's pathology have exhibited the FLD and FTD syndromes, progressive aphasia syndrome,[50] and progressive perceptual-motor syndrome (corticobasal degeneration [CBD]).[55] There are a few kindreds with autosomal dominant Pick's disease with mutations in tau.[56]

Progressive Spasticity (Primary Lateral Sclerosis). Neuropathologically, there is highly circumscribed atrophy of the precentral gyrus with loss of Betz cells, decreased numbers of pyramidal neurons, and laminar gliosis in the external and internal pyramidal cell cortical layers.[57] No lower motor neuron abnormalities are typically found in hypoglossal or spinal gray nuclei, and the substantia nigra is generally unaffected.[57]

Progressive Perceptual-Motor Syndromes

VISUAL. To date, neuropathological studies of patients with dorsal visual syndromes have generally shown senile plaques and neurofibrillary tangles, which are typical of AD. The topographic distribution, however, differs from that seen in Alzheimer's dementia, with heaviest involvement of primary and association visual cortices in the occipital lobes and, to a slightly lesser degree, in the parietal lobes.[39] The nucleus basalis is involved in these cases.[39] Other pathologies include nonspecific degenerative changes (gliosis, neuronal loss, and vacuolation of superficial cortices),[58] and Creutzfeldt-Jakob disease (Heidenhain variant).[58] To date, there are no published pathological studies of patients with progressive ventral visual cortical disorders.

MOTOR. To date, most patients reported with this syndrome have had CBD with neuronal achromasia or nonspecific degenerative changes (see section on CBD). Other histological patterns have included Pick's disease,[55] AD with involvement of the nucleus basalis,[59] and PSP.[60] There is generalized but asymmetrical atrophy with the most severe focal degeneration generally occurring in superomedial frontoparietal regions, primary

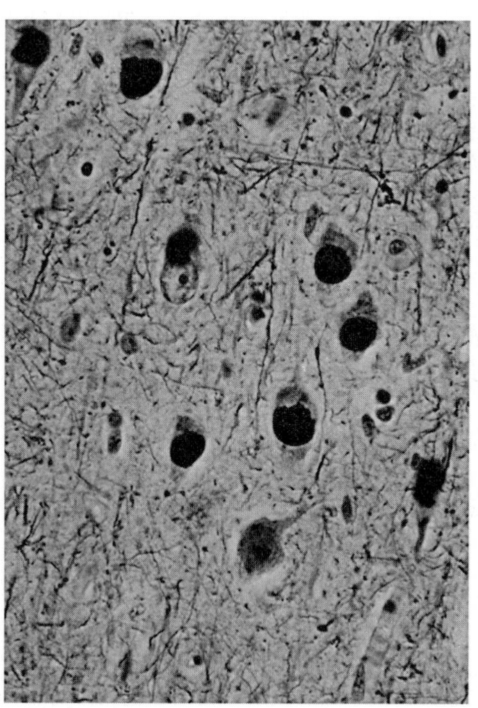

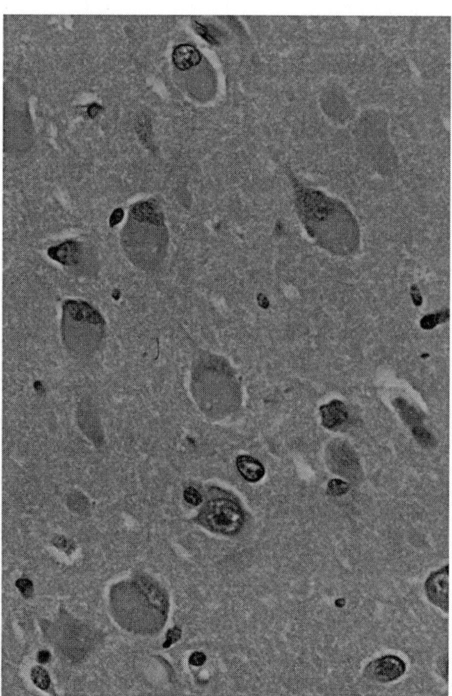

FIGURE 33–8. Photomicrograph of frontal cortex in classic Pick's disease (Pick's type A). The argentophilic, rounded cytoplasmic masses are Pick bodies, which are principally composed of 8- to 20-nm straight filaments. (Bielschowsky silver stain; 200×; courtesy of JE Parisi, Mayo Clinic, Rochester, Minnesota.)

motor cortex, and parietal convexity cortex, but other cortical regions, including Wernicke's area, sometimes can be severely involved as well. The substantia nigra is also involved, but the nucleus basalis is spared in the absence of AD.[61]

MIXED. Pathological findings include CBD and AD.

Progressive Bitemporal Syndromes

PROGRESSIVE AMNESIA. See discussion of Alzheimer's disease.

PROGRESSIVE PROSOPAGNOSIA. See discussion of progressive visual syndromes.

PROGRESSIVE BITEMPORAL NEUROPSYCHIATRIC SYNDROMES. On a clinical basis, patients with progressive bitemporal neuropsychiatric syndromes probably have either Pick's disease or AD, but neuropathological study is lacking.

Epidemiology and Risk Factors. There are no incidence and prevalence studies of this group of disorders, but clinical experience (at a tertiary care referral center) suggests that they are, as a group, perhaps a tenth as common as AD. Though many cases appear to be sporadic, studies of familial cases, some occurring in association with parkinsonism, have been associated with mutations of the tau gene on chromosome 17, and the term "tau-opathy" has since been coined. Kindreds can be quite complex and include diverse phenotypes.[62] Of the ACDSs, frontotemporal degeneration, progressive aphasia, and CBD (and PSP, which can mimic CBD) are all part of the tau-opathy spectrum.[63]

Clinical Features and Associated Disorders. There are four broad categories of ACDS, each of which can be further subdivided, and topographical and pathological correlations could be made for each (see Table 33–3). In most cases, there are three properties of the atrophy topography that are radiologically discernible: (1) there is a lateralized major atrophic focus; (2) there is a contralateral area of focal atrophy that is less severe than the primary focus, the homologous cortices; and (3) there is milder generalized atrophy. Metabolic abnormalities reflect this pattern as well.[64]

Several types of ACDS are associated with amyotrophic lateral sclerosis (ALS), including progressive aphasia,[65] frontal lobe syndromes including Pick's disease[66] and nonspecific frontal lobe degeneration,[67] and bitemporal syndromes.[68] In such cases, longevity is determined by the ALS component, and in the case of progressive aphasia with ALS, the disease course appears particularly rapid.[65] Occasional patients with apparent primary lateral sclerosis (PLS) may have mild lower motor neuron abnormalities, and they appear to have a slower course than typical ALS. Patients with a bitemporal or frontotemporal syndrome and ALS may have a more severe neuropsychiatric syndrome with features of Kluver-Bucy syndrome[68] compared with those without ALS. Finally, subtypes of ACDS may overlap in the same patient, such as progressive aphasia and a progressive perceptual-motor syndrome.

Progressive Aphasia. Although original credit should probably go to Arnold Pick for correlating lobar atrophy with aphasic dementia,[69] Mesulam's 1982 report of progressive aphasia[45] essentially refocused modern neurology on the relationship of focal cortical degeneration to a progressive cortical syndrome. Because most patients are left-hemisphere dominant for language, most patients have left-sided asymmetrical atrophy. However, occasional patients are found who are left handed and who have right-hemisphere asymmetrical atrophy accompanying progressive aphasia. Cognitive deficits other than those directly attributable to language may also occur, especially memory impairment and constructional apraxia.

Nonfluent progressive aphasia generally reflects anterior perisylvian cortical degeneration (Fig. 33–9). It should be readily distinguished from typical AD. Speech is effortful, halting, and sometimes dysarthric. Naming ability is marked by phonemic paraphasic errors (e.g., "calicopter" for helicopter), repetition is generally severely impaired, and although writing sometimes is easier than speaking, it is also usually abnormal. Aural and reading comprehension are less impaired in mild to moderate stages but deteriorate in most patients with disease progression. Some patients have orofacial apraxia but not gestural or limb apraxia. Verbal memory tests are difficult to administer, but verbal memory is typically

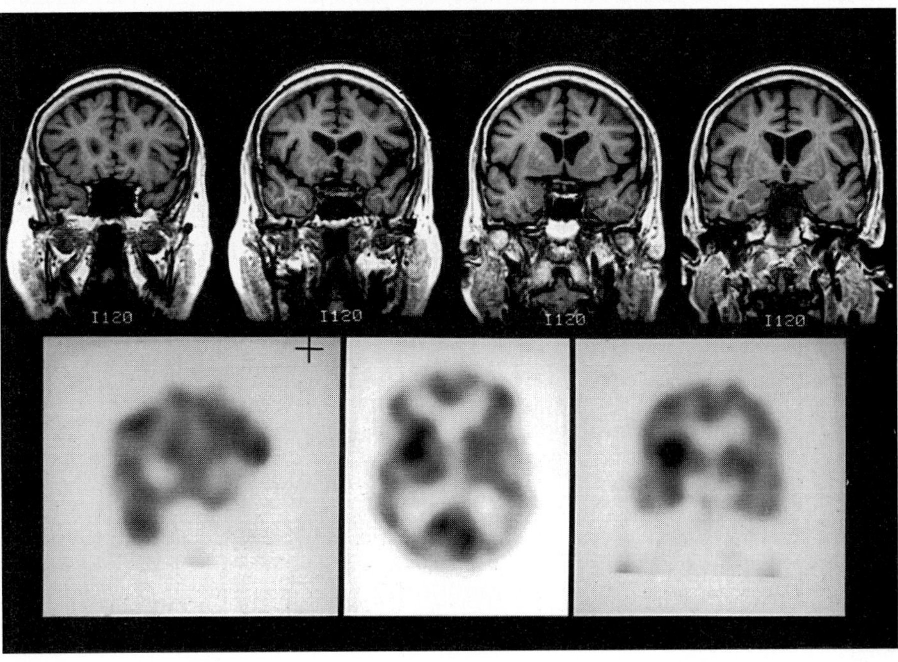

FIGURE 33–9. Progressive nonfluent aphasia. MRI *(top)* and SPECT *(bottom)* showing left frontal opercular atrophy. (Reprinted from Caselli RJ, Jack CR Jr: Asymmetric cortical degenerative syndromes: A proposed clinical classification. Arch Neurol 1992;49:770–780. By permission of Little, Brown and Company [Inc.].)

impaired. The criteria for the clinical diagnosis of progressive nonfluent aphasia are shown in Table 33–4.

Fluent aphasia involves degeneration of temporal and posterior perisylvian cortices. Contiguous involvement of neighboring cortices may complicate the clinical picture, making it difficult to distinguish a focal left temporoparietal syndrome (with aphasia, amnesia, apraxia, and acalculia) from a so-called diffuse cognitive disorder, or Alzheimer's dementia. The nonlanguage impairments, however, are much less disabling than the language impairment in progressive fluent aphasia. Fluency, articulation, and prosody are normal, but comprehension and naming are impaired. Sentence repetition appears to be impaired less consistently. The characteristic naming errors are semantic paraphasias, but phonemic paraphasias occur as well. Typically, a patient may recognize and describe the object or action he or she cannot name (e.g., "something that flies" for a helicopter), or give a generic descriptor. Spelling errors are frequent.

Anomic aphasia involves degeneration of anterior temporal cortices. Patients are fluent; comprehend well; and can repeat, read, and write with minimal difficulty, but, their speech lacks semantic precision. They substitute generic terms for specific words (e.g., "machine" for computer) and make semantic paraphasias (e.g., "staple" for paper clip). Anomia is a common feature of both AD and Pick's disease, but verbal memory is usually impaired even in the absence of dementia. Other investigators have applied the term "semantic dementia" to patients with prominent anomia associated with focal anterior temporal lobe atrophy; Table 33–5 shows the criteria for the diagnosis of sementic dementia.

Mixed progressive aphasia is a more nonspecific pattern involving degeneration of left temporal and perisylvian cortices. Patients with this condition have impairment of all aspects of language, making classification into a single taxonomic category impossible. They are nonfluent, with impaired comprehension, naming, repetition, writing, and reading.

Progressive Perceptual-Motor Syndromes. Although most patients have a mixed sensory-motor syndrome (including visual or somatosensory systems, or both), there are a few patients who have a pure sensory (typically visual) or pure motor syndrome (typically a hemiakinetic rigid syndrome). Progressive spasticity is considered under Asymmetrical Cortical Degeneration Syndromes.

Progressive visual syndromes involve degeneration of parieto-occipital or parietotemporal visual association cortices, or both. Visual association cortices can be broadly divided into dorsal (occipitoparietal) and ventral (occipitotemporal) pathways, and disorders of visual association cortices reflect this dichotomy. The occipitoparietal pathway is more concerned with localizing an object in space (where), and the occipitotemporal pathway is more concerned with object identification (what). Two broad types of complex visual disturbance have been described with ACDS. The more commonly reported is progressive simultanagnosia, reflecting dysfunction of the dorsal cortical visual pathway. Patients cannot integrate the numerous components of an ordinarily complex scene into a coherent whole. When viewing a street scene, for example, they might describe a car or a person or a lamppost but overlook the fact that it is an inner-city rush hour. Occasional associated problems that also reflect posterior parietal and temporal involvement include alexia, acalculia, right-left disorientation, and mild deficits of memory and language (fluent aphasia). Eventually, patients may be found to have inferior quadrantanopia, although typically visual field testing produces inconsistent responses.

The second type of complex visual disorder resulting from ACDS is visual agnosia, of which fewer examples are reported.[70, 71] Visual agnosia results from dysfunction of the ventral cortical visual pathway. Some patients have been described with progressive prosopagnosia, a failure to recognize familiar faces.[71] Rarely, patients may describe progressive topographagnosia, the inability to recognize familiar

TABLE 33–4. **Clinical Diagnosis of Progressive Nonfluent Aphasia**

Core Features
Insidious onset and gradual progression
Disorder of expressive language dominant feature initially and throughout the disease course
Nonfluent spontaneous speech with at least one of the following: agrammatism, phonemic paraphasias, anomia
Other aspects of cognition intact or relatively well preserved

Supportive Features
Speech and language:

- Stuttering or oral apraxia
- Impaired repetition
- Alexia, agraphia
- Early preservation of word meaning
- Late mutism

Behavior:

- Early preservation of social skills
- Late behavioral changes similar to frontotemporal dementia

Physical signs: late contralateral primitive reflexes, akinesia, rigidity, and tremor
Investigations:

- Neuropsychology: nonfluent aphasia in the absence of severe amnesia or perceptuospatial disorder
- Electroencephalography: normal or minor asymmetrical slowing
- Brain imaging (structural and/or functional): asymmetrical abnormality predominantly affecting dominant (usually left) hemisphere

Data from Neary et al, 1998.

TABLE 33–5. **Clinical Diagnosis of Semantic Dementia and Associative Agnosia**

Core Features
Insidious onset and gradual progression
Language disorder characterized by:

- Progressive, fluent, empty spontaneous speech
- Loss of word meaning, manifest by impaired naming and comprehension
- Semantic paraphasias

and/or

Perceptual disorder characterized by:

- Prosopagnosia: impaired recognition of identity of familiar faces
- Associative agnosia: impaired recognition of object identity

Preserved perceptual matching and drawing reproduction
Preserved single-word repetition
Preserved ability to read aloud and write to dictation orthographically regular words
Autobiographical memory intact or relatively well preserved

Supportive Features
Speech and language:

- Press of speech
- Idiosyncratic word usage
- Absence of phonemic paraphasias
- Surface dyslexia and dysgraphia
- Preserved calculation

Behavior:

- Loss of sympathy and empathy
- Narrowed preoccupations
- Parsimony

Physical signs:

- Absent or late primitive reflexes
- Akinesia, rigidity, and tremor

Investigations:

- Neuropsychology
- Profound semantic loss, manifest in failure of word comprehension and naming and/or face and object recognition
- Preserved phonology and syntax, and elementary perceptual processing, spatial skills, and day-to-day memorizing
- Electroencephalography: normal
- Brain imaging (structural and/or functional): predominant anterior temporal abnormality (symmetrical or asymmetrical)

Data from Neary et al, 1998.

places. In later stages, both ventral and dorsal visual pathways become involved, and a more globally encompassing visual agnosia results, as illustrated best by Oliver Sacks' Professor P.[70]

The term "posterior cortical atrophy" has also been applied to cases with dysfunction in the occipitoparietal pathway, and those with more occipitotemporal dysfunction have been termed "associative agnosia" (Table 33–6).

Progressive Motor Syndromes (see also CBD). Two major clinical characteristics, both slowly progressive in onset, make this disorder distinctive and easily recognized. The first are lateralized somatic deficits, including hemispasticity, hemiparesis, hemisensory impairment (usually in the form of astereognosis or tactile agnosia with less consistent impairment of more basic somatosensory modalities), and myoclonic jerks. Some patients may have a hemirigid or hemidystonic syndrome with tremor. The second is severe and disabling apraxia, including limb apraxia (inability to use the limb in a meaningful way, such as to use a comb), gestural apraxia (inability to pantomime or imitate symbolic movements), dressing apraxia, constructional apraxia, and apraxic agraphia. If the lateralized limb defects reflect dominant hemispheric dysfunction, then a mild fluent aphasia may be present that is milder than that seen in progressive fluent aphasia. When the lateralized limb defects reflect nondominant hemisphere dysfunction, it is uncommon (but possible) for a hemineglect syndrome to result.

Additional clinical abnormalities may include acalculia, psychomotor slowing, aphasia, and supranuclear oculomotor disturbances. Although patients with severe apraxia, psychomotor slowing, and mild aphasia may appear demented according to neuropsychological testing, they are usually rational, insightful, and upset by their condition. In late stages, patients can barely move or speak despite preserved consciousness.

Many patients have both a sensorimotor and a visuospatial disorder, combining features of both of the previously mentioned groups (Fig. 33–10).

Progressive Frontal Lobe and Frontotemporal Syndromes. The three main frontal lobe syndromes are a progressive neu-

TABLE 33–6. **Clinical Diagnosis of Frontotemporal Dementia (FTD)**

Core Features
Insidious onset and gradual progression
Early decline in social interpersonal conduct
Early impairment in regulation of personal conduct
Early emotional blunting
Early loss of insight
Instrumental functions of perception, spatial skills, praxis, and memory intact or relatively well preserved

Supportive Features
Behavioral disorder:

- Decline in personal hygiene and grooming
- Mental rigidity and inflexibility
- Distractibility and impersistence
- Hyperorality and dietary changes
- Perseverative and stereotyped behavior
- Utilization behavior

Speech and language:

- Altered speech output
- Aspontaneity and economy of speech
- Press of speech
- Stereotype of speech
- Echolalia
- Perseveration
- Mutism

Physical signs:

- Primitive reflexes
- Incontinence
- Akinesia, rigidity, and tremor
- Low and labile blood pressure

Investigations:

- Neuropsychology: significant impairment on frontal lobe tests in the absence of severe amnesia, aphasia, or perceptuospatial disorder
- Electroencephalography: normal on conventional EEG despite clinically evident dementia
- Brain imaging (structural and/or functional): predominant frontal and/or anterior temporal abnormality

Data from Neary et al, 1998.

ropsychiatric syndrome (frontal and frontotemporal dementia), a progressive spastic syndrome, and a mixture of these two.

The progressive neuropsychiatric syndrome is the best-known example of this group and has been referred to as frontal lobe or frontotemporal dementia (Fig. 33–11). Pick's disease is prominently represented in this group. More recently, Brun[72] and Gustafson[73] described a similar clinical syndrome in the absence of Pick bodies. The proposed criteria for the diagnosis of frontotemporal dementia are shown in Table 33–6. Although the clinical picture is characteristic, many clinicians have difficulty distinguishing these patients from those with Alzheimer-type dementia. Another common misdiagnosis is depression. The errors made by these patients tend to be omissions rather than commissions, and the term that describes this condition is abulia. They fail to change their clothes, to brush their teeth, to pursue their former interests, and to initiate many activities that constitute a normal day. Just as they fail to start something new, they may fail to stop what they are doing and perseveratively fixate, in a seemingly idiosyncratic fashion, on some particular activity, such as going to the bathroom, sorting through their wallet, or watching television. Some patients have greater disinhibition and emotional lability, crying at the least provocation, or laughing loud and long. They may complain that they are hungry yet be unmoved to fix themselves a snack. Some may perseveratively want to eat over and over. Memory and language (especially naming) are typically impaired. Despite their sometimes reduced temporal latency in responding to the examiner (they may start answering a question before the physician has finished asking it), their answers are brief and often consist of "I don't know." Patients with FLD may stick close to their caregiver and generally cause fewer disruptions than patients with AD, particularly in mild to moderate stages (although there are notable exceptions).

Associated clinical abnormalities reflect other frontal lobe dysfunctions, including spasticity and nonfluent aphasia. Because Pick's disease has a predilection for the temporal as well as the frontal lobe, some patients also develop signs referable to the temporal lobe, particularly anomia.

The syndrome of progressive spasticity has been termed PLS, and historically, the nosological focus has been on its relationship to ALS (see Chapter 36) rather than other frontal lobe degenerations. PLS reflects degeneration of the precentral gyrus and primary motor cortex.[57] Cognitive impairment is minimal but can include emotional lability, mild frontal lobe–related cognitive deficits, and mild memory impairment.[74]

Some patients present early in their course with a combination of both spasticity and FLD/FTD.[75] Conceivably, these patients have Pick's disease because Pick's disease produces spasticity late in the course of the illness, but patients with AD have also been reported to present (rarely) with progressive spasticity.

Progressive Bitemporal Syndromes. The three syndromes in this category are progressive amnesia, progressive prosopagnosia, and progressive neuropsychiatric syndrome. Progressive amnesia is discussed in the section on AD, and progressive prosopagnosia is discussed in the section on progressive visual syndromes because this entity overlaps both categories of ACDS. Patients with a progressive neuropsychiatric syndrome due to bitemporal degeneration (Fig. 33–12) have severe anomia and amnesia, relative indifference to their condition, and mild perseverative behaviors that are shared with patients in the frontal lobe group. Psychomotor speed is normal or only mildly impaired. Neuroimaging shows bilateral severe anterior temporal atrophy and hypoperfusion with relative sparing of the frontal lobes.

Differential Diagnosis. The two broad categories to consider are nondegenerative structural focal brain lesions, such as a slowly growing tumor and other degenerative conditions. Regarding the first, a slowly progressive neurological syndrome that can be reasonably localized could be neoplastic, whether malignant or benign. Rarely, high-grade arterial stenoses cause stuttering infarction mimicking a slowly progressive degenerative cortical syndrome, but this is very

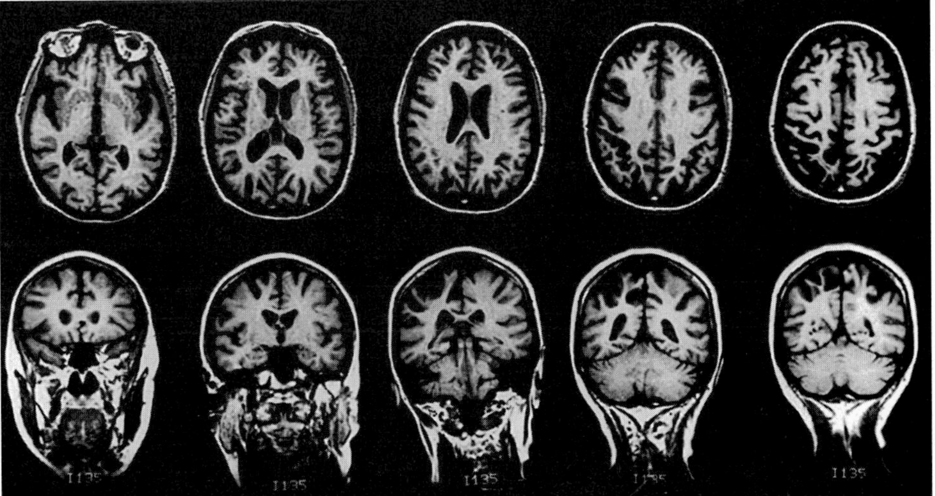

FIGURE 33–10. Progressive perceptual-motor syndrome. MRI *(top)* and SPECT *(bottom)* showing right greater than left parietal atrophy. (Reprinted from Caselli RJ, Jack CR Jr: Asymmetric cortical degenerative syndromes: A proposed clinical classification. Arch Neurol 1992;49:770–780. By permission of Little, Brown and Company [Inc.].)

uncommon. Other pathological processes that could occur focally, including infection or abscess and demyelinating or vasculitic conditions, should also be considered. Other degenerative illnesses include Creutzfeldt-Jakob disease in rapidly progressive cases and the wide variety of degenerative pathologies discussed earlier. For example, a patient suspected of CBD may have AD at autopsy. Among the frontal lobe, aphasic, and bitemporal varieties of ACDS, an association with ALS must also be considered.

Evaluation. The most important diagnostic test is adequate structural neuroimaging. MRI is preferable to CT, but either will generally suffice to evaluate the possibility of a tumor. In addition to excluding nondegenerative structural abnormalities, a magnetic resonance angiographic study could be included, if available, to search for a potentially relevant high-grade arterial stenosis. Patients with ACDS usually, but not invariably, have radiologically discernible focal atrophy in the symptomatic region. It is often subtle and of insufficient severity to permit blinded diagnosis of ACDS. However, in a patient with progressive anomic aphasia, for example, focal left anterior temporal atrophy should be considered important not only because of the absence of a tumor, but also because it shows the responsible lesion to be an atrophic one, presumably degenerative. Formal neuropsychological assessment can be helpful to assess quality and severity of cognitive impairment to a greater extent and usually demonstrates a pattern that is not typical for Alzheimer's dementia. It is also useful for monitoring disease progression. Other laboratory studies are less helpful because of the apparent focal nature of the ACDS. Metabolic encephalopathies do not usually cause the syndrome of slowly progressive aphasia, which is difficult to confuse with a diffuse encephalopathy. Nonetheless, it is still reasonable to make certain that basic laboratory data are normal, as was discussed for AD.

Management. Considerations similar to those discussed for AD are applicable here with minor additions. First,

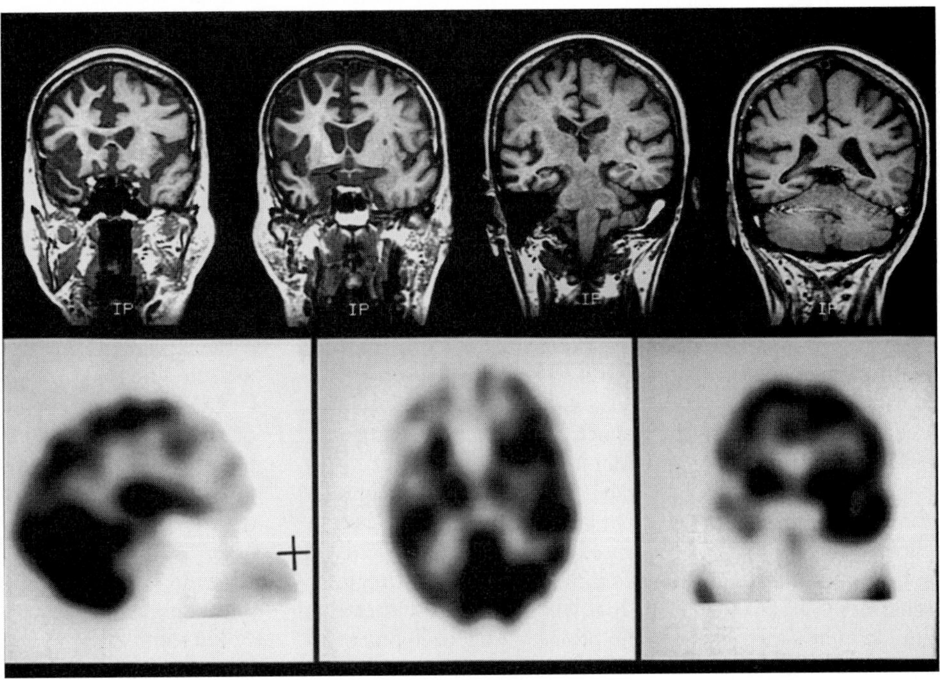

FIGURE 33–11. Progressive frontotemporal dementia. MRI *(top)* and SPECT *(bottom)* showing right greater than left frontal and anterior temporal atrophy in a patient with autopsy-documented Pick's disease. (Reprinted from Caselli RJ, Jack CR Jr: Asymmetric cortical degenerative syndromes: A proposed clinical classification. Arch Neurol 1992;49:770–780. By permission of Little, Brown and Company [Inc.].)

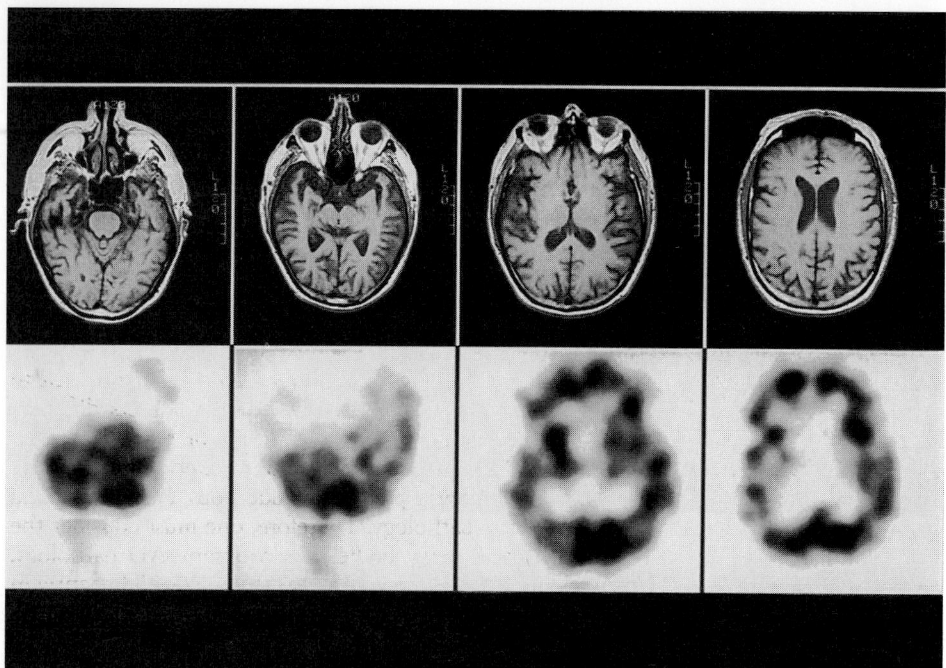

FIGURE 33–12. Progressive bitemporal neuropsychiatric syndrome: MRI *(top)* and SPECT *(bottom)* showing right greater than left anterior temporal atrophy. (From Caselli RJ: Focal andasymmetric cortical degeneration syndromes. Neurologist 1995;1:1–19.)

patients with ACDS are usually aware of their limitations and are not likely to get themselves in trouble unwittingly by wandering, refusing medications, and so forth. They require nursing home placement less often if a caregiver exists. Physical therapy is important for patients with CBD and PLS, especially because of the complications resulting from altered muscle tone and gait unsteadiness. Occupational therapy is particularly important for ACDS patients with apraxia and spatial disorders to assist with dressing, eating, and other activities of daily living. Speech therapy is appropriate to consider for progressive aphasia not only because of the aphasia but in later stages of nonfluent aphasia in particular, because of dysphagia as well. Late-stage complications are similar for AD but perhaps are most severe for CBD. In this condition, the combined impact of communication loss including speech and praxis, painful dystonic postures with contracture formation, and the relative preservation of insight, compounds suffering. Trials of carbidopa and levodopa (Sinemet) in CBD should be considered, even though it is usually of minimal efficacy at best. In patients with CBD with severe myoclonus, small doses of clonazepam can also be considered. Finally, in cases with severe dystonic posturing, especially hand closure, selective botulinum toxin injection can be considered to accomplish limited goals, such as allowing the hand to be opened for maintenance of skin hygiene and to retard contracture formation.

Prognosis and Future Perspectives. All of the ACDSs are progressive and follow a similar time course to AD. Most patients have a more generalized cortical degenerative process that becomes more significant in later stages, but occasionally, patients have a highly focal process with minimal evidence of generalized decline, even at the time of their death. Prognosis is better in the group with the highly focal process. Otherwise, ACDS of all types, like AD and other degenerative brain diseases, results in death after relentless progression.

ALS-DEMENTIA COMPLEX

Pathogenesis and Pathophysiology. The nosological distinction among frontotemporal lobe dementia (FTD), FTD with motor neuron disease (MND), and classic MND has been debated, with some arguing that FTD with MND is a distinct disorder and others suggesting each represents a phenotype along a continuum of the same disease.[76] The histological findings do not clarify nosology because in the majority of cases, they are nonspecific: neuronal loss, gliosis, and microvacuolation or spongiform changes predominantly affecting the superficial cortical layers and subcortical white matter. Degeneration is usually greatest in frontotemporal regions and, less commonly, in perisylvian language cortices. The nucleus basalis of Meynert appears normal, as do cortical levels of choline acetyltransferase and somatostatin.[77] Variable degrees of degeneration also occur in the amygdala, hippocampus, thalamus, caudate nucleus, and substantia nigra.

Epidemiology and Risk Factors. Dementia rarely occurs in patients with ALS, although known associations include the Parkinson-ALS-dementia complex of Guam, which occurs in the indigenous Chamorro population[78]; familial ALS[79]; and sporadic cases from both Eastern[80] and Western[65, 67, 68, 76] populations. Pathogenesis in most patients is uncertain, and histopathological features are generally nonspecific.

Clinical Features and Associated Disorders. Frontal lobe or frontotemporal dementia is the most common dementia pattern, followed by aphasic dementia. Clinical descriptions in the literature, however, have varied and include unqualified dementia,[80] dementia of the Alzheimer type, Pick's disease,[66] and dementia with Kluver-Bucy syndrome,[68] in addition to frontotemporal[67] and aphasic dementia.[65] Bulbar symptoms have been consistently prominent.

For some years, an association with Creutzfeldt-Jakob disease was suspected, but this is no longer thought to be the case.[81]

Differential Diagnosis. Certain types of the ALS-dementia complex may be rapidly progressive, with anarthria within 1 year and death within 2 years. Given the severity, rapid progression, and sometimes paucity of limb abnormalities, Creutzfeldt-Jakob disease should be considered. In rapidly progressive cases, carcinomatous meningitis can also cause encephalopathy and polyradiculopathy, which might be mistaken for ALS-dementia complex, so CSF evaluation can be useful. Head and neck tumors, particularly carcinoma of the posterior tongue with CNS metastases, can cause severe dysarthria and mental status changes, and they should not be overlooked particularly when dysarthria is the main finding. Finally, neuromuscular weakness due to ALS, myasthenia gravis, acid maltase deficiency, myotonic dystrophy, and any other disease of sufficient severity to compromise ventilatory capacity may lead to a hypoxic encephalopathy that, in the absence of a corroborating history, might be mistaken for ALS-dementia complex, so arterial blood gases should be considered in some cases.

Evaluation. Both the nature of the neuromuscular disorder and the cognitive disorder must be established. Electromyography is important for the neuromuscular disorder and an essential diagnostic step but may not be conclusive, especially in bulbar cases. Further evaluation of the ALS aspect of this disorder is considered in the section on ALS but may include acetylcholine receptor antibody and creatine kinase among other tests. Regarding the cognitive disturbance, formal mental status assessment is the first step, and if there is any doubt, formal neuropsychological assessment focusing particularly on frontal lobe and language function should be performed. Evaluation of the dementia should then proceed with similar considerations, as discussed for AD, with particular attention to neuroimaging. In this context, MRI is preferable to CT because imaging of lower brain stem structures in particular is better accomplished by MRI. In selected circumstances, as discussed earlier, additional consideration should be given to EEG, CSF examination, consultation with an otolaryngologist, and arterial blood gas evaluation.

Management. Treatment considerations overlap those for ALS (see the section on ALS). Caregiving for the demented patient is discussed under AD. This is a particularly difficult condition because of the combination of neuromuscular and cognitive problems that confront the patient.

Prognosis and Future Perspectives. As with other neurodegenerative diseases, progression is inevitable and generally more rapid than in AD, with death occurring within 3 to 5 years in typical cases. Unlike uncomplicated ALS, in which the mind is preserved, causing some individuals to opt for feeding tubes, external ventilatory support, and other life-sustaining measures, ALS-dementia complex also produces severe intellectual decline, making justification of such measures difficult.

Subcortical Dementia

PARKINSON'S DISEASE WITH DEMENTIA

There are several forms of primary degenerative parkinsonism, including idiopathic (or sporadic) PD, sporadic PD with superimposed pathological features of AD, familial PD (or parkinsonian syndromes), and Parkinson-ALS-dementia complex of Guam. Pathological substrates differ among these conditions, as do the frequency of cognitive disturbances. In patients with pathological evidence of AD, dementia is usually (but not invariably) present. In familial cases, genetic defects and pathological changes differ between kindreds, so it is difficult to generalize to sporadic PD. In each case of PD, however, when dementia is described, it is most consistent with a "subcortical pattern" to distinguish it from typical Alzheimer-type dementia.

Pathogenesis and Pathophysiology. Memory performance in nondemented and demented patients with PD is qualitatively different,[82, 83] suggesting that cognitive impairment in nondemented and demented PD patients reflects different anatomical or neurochemical systems,[82] or separate pathogenetic processes.[83] Histological components of the Parkinson's dementia picture include both Parkinson's and Alzheimer-type pathology. Therefore, one must consider the roles of cortical Lewy bodies, concomitant AD pathology, and cholinergic deficiency in the pathogenesis of dementia in PD (see the section on dementia with Lewy bodies). Recent studies using ubiquitin staining in previous pathologically diagnosed PD demonstrate that 76 percent of cases have neocortical Lewy bodies compared with only 32 percent of cases studied only with routine hematoxylin-eosin stains.[84] Concomitant AD changes meeting diagnostic criteria for AD diagnosis have been found in up to 50 percent of patients with PD dementia. Immunostaining with α-synuclein is more sensitive and specific than ubiquitin, and α-synuclein immunocytochemistry has rapidly become viewed as essential in the neuropathological characterization of demented individuals.

PD is characterized by nigral degeneration with Lewy bodies in the pigmented brain stem nuclei, but the contribution of medial substantia nigra neuronal loss, the most consistent pathological finding in PD, to dementia is unclear. The basal ganglia interface with the limbic system through a subset of structures collectively referred to as the ventral striatum and ventral pallidum. Cortical input to the ventral striatum is from the hippocampal formation through the precommissural fornix, and dopaminergic input comes from the ventral tegmental area (part of the mesocorticolimbic dopaminergic system). Analogous to the concept that the dorsal or neostriatum and its neocortical targets are part of a so-called motor loop, so, too, have the ventral striatum and its allocortical or paralimbic targets been termed a cognitive loop.[85] However, the role of the cognitive loop remains speculative, and it is unknown whether any cognitive alterations in PD or dementia reflect this loop.

Epidemiology and Risk Factors. Considering the heterogeneity of parkinsonian syndromes, potential co-occurrence of AD, and the cognitive side effects of antiparkinsonian treatment, estimates of dementia prevalence in PD vary considerably. Most range between 20 and 30 percent.[86] Based on autopsy studies, about half of demented parkinsonian patients have coincident AD pathology.[87]

Clinical Features and Associated Disorders. Although PSP was the original model for subcortical dementia, this model is applicable to PD, which is much more common than PSP. The concept was intended to distinguish subcortical dementia from the cortical dementia of AD. Subcortical dementia–related memory impairment is benefited more by cuing than is the memory disturbance of cortical dementia. Patients have equal or greater difficulty learning new material but have relatively less difficulty retrieving it, possibly due to disturbed frontal or frontostriatal function involved in attending to and organizing the memory task. Subcortical dementia is not usually accompanied by aphasia, apraxia, and agnosia. However, it is accompanied by psychomotor slowing, an early feature of Parkinson's dementia.[82, 83] Patients perform disproportionately poorly on timed tests whether the tests use motor responses (such as the digit symbol substitution subtest of the Wechsler Adult Intelligence Scale–Revised [WAIS-R]), or whether they are purely cognitive (such as the controlled oral word association test). PD results in disproportionately poor performances on visuospatial tasks, although this aspect does not seem to be a major source of clinical disability, and the cause is debated. Depression is more common in PD with or without dementia than in AD. Finally, the noncognitive (motor) parkinsonian features make distinction from AD and related cortical degenerative syndromes generally possible. The distinction has clinical value, despite overlap with cortical dementia on both clinical and pathological grounds that blur nosological boundaries. For example, a subset of patients with AD have mild extrapyramidal features,[82] and there is important subcortical pathology in the basal forebrain of AD. The coincidence of Alzheimer's pathology in patients with PD with so-called subcortical dementia has already been alluded to earlier. There are certain kindreds in which a parkinsonian syndrome is invariably accompanied by severe dementia. Nondegenerative quasiparkinsonian syndromes in which cognitive impairment is present can have many etiologies, including multi-infarct dementia, normal pressure hydrocephalus, and postencephalitic parkinsonism, and are discussed elsewhere.

Differential Diagnosis. The main question in patients presenting with parkinsonism and dementia is whether the entire picture is explained by PD and whether it will respond to levodopa therapy. The differential diagnosis of PD is extensive, and dementia can occur in many of the conditions discussed in the section on PD. Some of the differential diagnoses that are of particular note that are also degenerative include PSP, multiple system atrophy (MSA), DLB, and CBD. Occasionally, frontal lobe disorders may be mistaken for parkinsonian syndromes with dementia, including both degenerative etiologies, such as Pick's disease, and nondegenerative etiologies, such as frontal lobe meningiomas. Other progressive, nondegenerative diseases that have loosely fitting parkinsonian features include multi-infarct dementia and normal pressure hydrocephalus. Occasionally, parkinsonian features occur in patients with AD (see AD and DLB sections).

Evaluation. MRI is generally preferable to CT, in part because of the multifocal areas of increased T2 signal (often missed or poorly defined by CT) in periventricular, basal ganglia, and other locations that may signify a small vessel multi-infarct state. Evaluation is similar to that described for AD, save that response to therapy offers additional diagnostic information (see later).

Management. Dopaminergic therapy is discussed in the section on PD, but certain special considerations apply here. First, dopaminergic therapy is more likely to cause hallucinations and delusions in parkinsonian patients with dementia, as well as in patients with related parkinsonian syndromes, than in those with uncomplicated PD. Second, neuroleptic therapy is more likely to cause an exacerbation of parkinsonian symptoms. Third, so-called on-off motor fluctuations may be accompanied by mild fluctuations in cognitive status as well. There are no perfect solutions, and antipsychotic therapy with atypical agents such as quetiapine, which produce fewer parkinsonian side effects than standard agents, will need to be tried cautiously if absolutely required. Cholinesterase inhibitors could be considered, given the frequency of Alzheimer-type pathology, including cholinergic deficiency, although again there is at least the theoretical risk that increasing central cholinergic tone could mildly exacerbate the parkinsonian syndrome.

Prognosis and Future Perspectives. Prognostic considerations are similar to those discussed for AD except that the combination of parkinsonism and dementia is a more difficult management problem, and because dementia is usually a late complication of PD, it may signify a shorter life span than for patients with either uncomplicated PD or AD.

There is ongoing development of more highly selective neuroleptic agents with less toxicity than clozapine. One recent report suggested that selective serotonin receptor blockade may offer one such strategy. See the Movement Disorders section (Chapter 34).

MULTIPLE SYSTEM ATROPHY

This is an uncommon and heterogeneous group of disorders generally characterized by atypical, relative dopamine-unresponsive parkinsonism with variable degrees of cognitive impairment. MSA includes olivopontocerebellar atrophy (OPCA), striatonigral degeneration, and parkinsonism with orthostatic hypotension and dysautonomia (Shy-Drager syndrome).

Pathogenesis and Pathophysiology. Neuropsychological studies in both sporadic and familial cases of OPCA have demonstrated frontostriatal dysfunction.[88] A similar profile of frontostriatal impairment occurs in MSA with predominantly striatonigral degeneration features, which is qualitatively different from PD and PSP.[89] Therefore, it would appear the cognitive impairment in the various forms of MSA results, at least in part, from frontostriatal dysfunction. Cerebellar dysfunction may play an additional role in OPCA.

Epidemiology and Risk Factors. Of five clinical subtypes of OPCA that have been described on both genetic and sporadic bases, mild to moderate decline has been described in types III, IV, and V.[88] Approximately 60 percent of familial and 35 percent of sporadic cases have accompanying cognitive impairment[90] (also see Shy-Drager syndrome and striatonigral degeneration).

Clinical Features and Associated Disorders. Patients with dominantly inherited OPCA (type IV) have frontal lobe–related cognitive impairments,[88] but the apparent mild intellectual decline in most OPCA may be related more importantly to motor impairment and depression without actual dementia and without evidence of aphasia, agnosia, or apraxia.[91] MSA of the Shy-Drager variety has been less studied. Given the clinical similarities to other parkinsonian syndromes, as well as its clinical heterogeneity, mild "subcortical" patterns of cognitive impairment are possible, but it should not presently be regarded as a cause of severe dementia.

Management. Considerations are similar to those discussed for Parkinson's dementia, but successful treatment of psychotic symptoms in OPCA has been reported.

PROGRESSIVE SUPRANUCLEAR PALSY

Pathogenesis and Pathophysiology. Although the anatomical substrates underlying the parkinsonian and oculomotor disorder are relatively well understood (see Chapter 34), those underlying the cognitive symptoms are not. In addition to mesocorticolimbic dopaminergic alterations (see the section on Parkinson's disease dementia), there is evidence of more pronounced frontal lobe dysfunction than in other subcortical dementias on the basis of neuropsychological tests[92, 93] and PET.[94] These findings have been attributed to primary striatal damage, which disrupts normal processing in the frontostriatal "cognitive" circuit such that frontal deafferentation occurs.[92] Striatal damage could also explain disruption in the anterior cingulate attention and lateral-orbitofrontal social affect circuits.[92]

Rarely, patients with PSP have variable degrees of aphasia, anomia, alexia, apraxia, or hemineglect, and some have had a frank progressive perceptual-motor syndrome similar to CBD.[60] Anatomical distribution of degeneration is atypical in such cases and may be maximally present in the parietal cortex. All 10 cases in another report had neocortical tangles and neuropil threads; the density of tangles was highest in Brodmann area 4.[95] Pronounced transentorhinal and entorhinal cortical degeneration resulting in hippocampal-isocortex disconnection similar to that occurring in AD has rarely been observed in PSP with severe dementia.

In summary, the typical subcortical pattern of dementia probably reflects substrates that are similar to those found in Parkinson's dementia with greater physiological disruption of frontal lobe function, but atypical cases have presented as definite cortical patterns of dementia due to predominantly cortical patterns of pathology.

Epidemiology and Risk Factors. The incidence of PSP is roughly 3 new cases per million per year, and the prevalence is 1.5 cases per million, making it about 1 percent as common as PD.[96] Median survival after symptom onset is approximately 6 to 7 years.[96] Recent evidence suggests that PSP is a member of the tau-opathy family.

Clinical Features and Associated Disorders. In addition to the extrapyramidal and oculomotor abnormalities that characterize PSP (see Chapter 34), certain cognitive features that led to the characterization of subcortical dementia are discussed in the section on Parkinson's dementia. In addition, there are frontal lobe features that appear to be more prominent than in other types of subcortical dementia.[93]

Differential Diagnosis. PSP is part of the differential diagnosis of the patient with atypical parkinsonism with dementia (discussed in the PD dementia section) and is usually distinguished clinically on the basis of the oculomotor disturbance and levodopa unresponsiveness.

Evaluation. In addition to the evaluation outline for PD and AD, SPECT and PET may show frontal and basal ganglia hypometabolism.

Management. Severe dementia and psychosis is less common in PSP than in PD dementia, although treatment considerations are otherwise similar for Parkinson's dementia.

Prognosis and Future Perspectives. Disease progression is similar (relentless) to that of other neurodegenerative conditions. Median survival after symptom onset is 6 to 7 years, and patients are typically wheelchair bound at least a year before that.

HUNTINGTON'S DISEASE

Pathogenesis and Pathophysiology. The cognitive impairment in HD, like other subcortical dementias, primarily reflects frontostriatal dysfunction, and there is pathological evidence of both subcortical and cortical pathology. Grossly, the cortical gyri appear normal to slightly atrophic. Coronal sections reveal striking caudate greater than putamen and pallidum atrophy. Neuronal loss and gliosis follow the same regional distribution. The medium-sized spiny type I striatal neurons are preferentially affected, whereas the aspiny type I neurons that contain somatostatin and neuropeptide Y are unaffected. Several neurotransmitters are decreased in the striatum, most notably GABA and acetylcholine. Glutamic acid decarboxylase and choline acetyltransferase are also diminished.

Milder degenerative changes occur in the neocortex and thalamus. Cross-sectional areas within the frontal, temporal, and parietal lobes were decreased compared with controls, with atrophy in HD being greater than in PSP.[97] Quantitative analysis in HD patients compared with that of controls has revealed moderate to severe neuronal loss in the cortex and striatum, which was differentially distributed in the cortical laminae in primary sensory and association cortices.[98] Ubiquitin-reactive dystrophic neurites were identified in all cortical but no subcortical areas,[99] and these neurites have been hypothesized by some to correlate with dementia. Evidence exists for excitotoxic damage and mitochondrial DNA mutations and oxidative stress[100] in the pathogenesis of cortical pathology in HD.

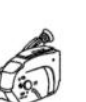

Clinical Features and Associated Disorders. Lieberman and associates found that 90 percent of patients were demented by a mean age of 48.3 years, and that dementia preceded the onset of chorea in 24 percent.[86] There are discrepant studies with regard to the existence of preclinical cognitive abnormalities, although preclinical metabolic abnormalities are detectable with PET.[101] Whether or not it is the critical determinant of cognitive decline, cognitive decline correlates pathologically and radiologically with degree of caudate atrophy[102] and hypometabolism.[103] Three areas of particular interest in the dementia of HD are frontal lobe–related or frontostriatal-related neuropsychiatric deficits, declarative memory impairment, and motor learning difficulties. Visuospatial disturbances have been demonstrated in some studies. With regard to frontostriatal neuropsychiatric deficits, patients may present initially with either primarily psychiatric or cognitive disturbances, although both may occur together. Regarding cognitive disturbances, prospective study of cognitive decline in early cases has shown that psychomotor slowing is a characteristic early feature,[104] and memory impairment, although present early on, does not deteriorate as rapidly, or correlate as well with caudate atrophy, as does psychomotor speed.[104] Patients with HD have greater perseveration and less initiation than AD patients, and they have greater problems with concentration and sustained attention. The overall pattern of frontal lobe–related deficits nonetheless appears qualitatively distinct from purely frontal cortical damage and has instead been attributed to frontostriatal dysfunction.

Regarding declarative memory impairment, much work has focused on the qualitative differences between HD and amnesic patients, including both AD and Korsakoff's patients. HD causes memory loss, but it appears to be less severe compared with that of AD at matched stages of dementia severity, although this factor has been more consistent at milder stages of dementia. Most studies have found that patients with HD have greater difficulty learning a task (such as a list of words), but they benefit more greatly by cued recall or recognition compared with free or unassisted recall. This has been thought to reflect greater impairment of retrieval than storage mechanisms, and it affects remote memory retrieval as well as more recently learned material.[33] There are many similarities in the memory disturbance between HD and PD, suggesting similarities between the subcortical dementia illnesses, but overlap is imperfect. For example, patients with HD have greater impairment of learning and free recall, better recognition memory, and more perseveration than PD patients.[105]

In contrast to the mild impairments of verbal learning, motor learning is severely impaired. There is a "double dissociation" between the performance of AD and HD patients on tests of these two memory systems: AD patients do poorly on verbal and well on motor learning, and HD patients do well on verbal and poor on motor learning.[34] Demented PD patients perform poorly on both,[34] which is interesting to consider in light of known overlap with AD pathology in a large subset of these patients. The most likely anatomical substrates, supported by the overlap with PD, are the basal ganglia, their frontal lobe connections, and related motor structures.

Differential Diagnosis. See Chapter 34. In the absence of chorea, the family history is critical in reaching a diagnosis. In the absence of both chorea and a family history, the differential diagnosis is that of other subcortical dementias and chronic progressive encephalopathies.

Evaluation. The clinical examination may provide compelling evidence for HD, which can be confirmed genetically. Ancillary tests include MRI or CT to ascertain caudate atrophy and (optionally) SPECT or PET to ascertain caudate hypometabolism. Neuropsychological assessment is useful to document the nature and severity of cognitive decline, particularly in mild to moderate stages of the illness. Other causes of chorea should be sought, as discussed in the Movement Disorders section (Chapter 34).

Management. See Chapter 34. Pharmacological management of dementia and chorea often involves dopaminergic antagonists including neuroleptic drugs but is far from adequate.

Prognosis and Future Perspectives. Death occurs within 10 to 20 years after onset, although suicide is more prevalent in at-risk and early-onset HD patients. Aspiration and inanition result from severe dysphagia, as well as from an apparent increased metabolic demand in patients with HD. See also the discussion of movement disorders in Chapter 34.

Mixed Cortical-Subcortical Dementias

CORTICOBASAL DEGENERATION

Pathogenesis and Pathophysiology. The characteristic pathological changes in CBD include asymmetrical frontoparietal cortical atrophy with corresponding neuronal loss and gliosis, substantia nigra degeneration, swollen achromatic neurons, and tau-positive neuronal and glial pathology.[106, 107] Variable degrees of degeneration in other subcortical nuclei also occur. The achromatic neurons immunostain positively to neurofilaments (Fig. 33–13). Some have regarded these neurons to be related to Pick cells, although immunohistochemical and ultrastructural analyses suggest that CBD can be differentiated from Pick's disease, PSP, and AD.[107] CBD is a diffuse cytoskeletal process characterized by the accumulation of pathologic tau proteins.[107] Impaired neurofilament phosphorylation, transportation, or degradation or distal axonal damage may be involved in the pathophysiology of neuronal achromasia. Neuronal achromasia may, therefore, represent the end result of one or more pathophysiological processes.

The profile of cognitive impairment reflects dysfunction predominantly of frontal and parietal cortices, including apraxia, psychomotor slowing, and visuoperceptual disturbances. Memory is also impaired. However, CBD pathology has also been observed in occasional patients with FTD and progressive aphasia.

Epidemiology and Risk Factors. CBD was originally described in 1967 by Rebeiz and colleagues.[108] There are few data regarding epidemiology or risk factors, although clinical experience suggests that the prevalence may be similar to that of PSP, or about 1 percent that of PD. There has been little evidence to date of a familial tendency.

Clinical Features and Associated Disorders. The vast majority of cases have exhibited a progressive perceptual-motor syndrome (see the section on ACDS, presented earlier), and the term progressive asymmetrical rigidity and apraxia syndrome has been proposed.[109] Less common presentations with a similar histology include frontotemporal dementia and progressive aphasia. Asymmetrical hyperreflexia, postural instability, frontal release signs, oculomotor impairment, and hypokinetic dysarthria commonly occur. Dysphagia begins insidiously in the latter stages of the disease, and eventually aspiration pneumonia and death ensue.

Characteristic CBD histological findings have been reported to co-exist with Pick's disease, PSP, and AD, and alternate presentations with the same histology have included FTD and progressive aphasia, as noted earlier.

Differential Diagnosis. See the section on ACDS. The most common misdiagnoses are stroke, PD, PSP, and perhaps AD. CBD falls within the spectrum of ACDS, and clinicopathological correlations are far from perfect, as previously discussed. Other degenerative histologies underlying a progressive apraxic or perceptual-motor syndrome include nonspecific degeneration, AD, Pick's disease, and PSP.

Evaluation. Neuroimaging is the single most important aspect in evaluating any focal-appearing cerebral syndrome, as discussed in the section on ACDS. A fairly consistent finding on CT and MRI is asymmetrical cortical atrophy, which

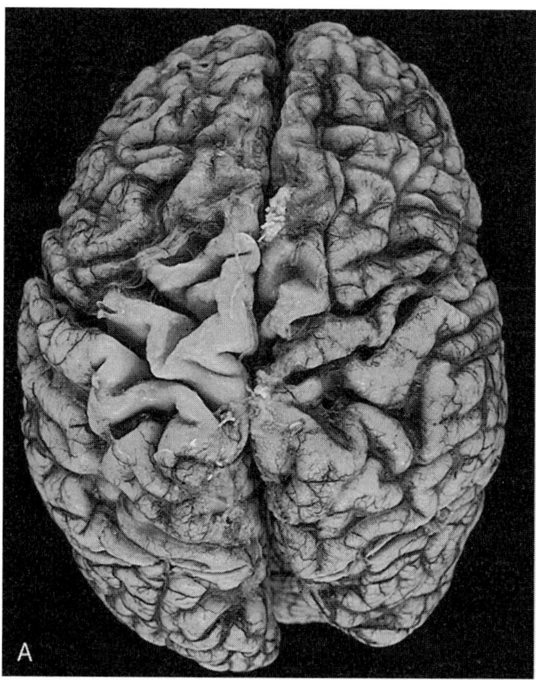

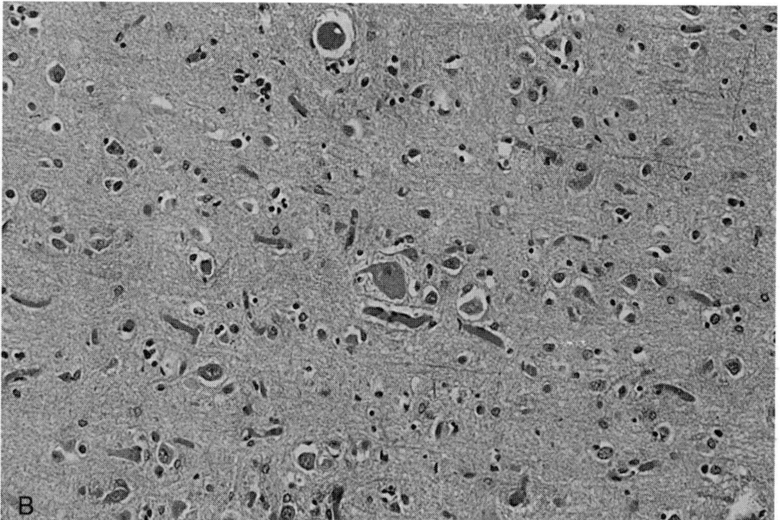

FIGURE 33–13. Corticobasal degeneration. *A,* Note the circumscribed perirolandic cortical atrophy. *B,* A ballooned achromatic neuron typical of corticobasal degeneration is shown in the center of the photomicrograph. (Hematoxylin and eosin; 50×; courtesy of JE Parisi, Mayo Clinic, Rochester, Minnesota.)

is predominantly parietal with variable involvement of contiguous regions in patients with a progressive perceptual-motor syndrome. The laterality of atrophy correlates with the laterality of clinical impairment.

Asymmetrical cortical (and subcortical) hypoperfusion on SPECT is usually more extensive than the MRI appearance of atrophy. Asymmetrical fluorodeoxyglucose cortical hypometabolism and asymmetrical striatal fluorodopa hypometabolism on PET are also found in this disorder, but these tests should be regarded as ancillary.

The neurological and neuropsychological pattern of deficits is distinctive and should not be mistaken for an Alzheimer- or Parkinson-type pattern of dementia.

Management. Pharmacotherapy generally provides minimal if any improvement in most symptoms,[110] but an empirical trial of levodopa is nonetheless reasonable and will occasionally result in modest symptomatic amelioration of rigidity. Clonazepam may yield modest improvement in myoclonus, but it may cause sedation with worsening of balance and cognitive function. Botulinum toxin injection can permit a clenched dystonic hand to be opened for hygiene maintenance. Pharmacotherapy should be supplemented with physical, occupational, and speech therapies. Passive range-of-motion exercises may retard the development of contractures. Ambulation becomes impaired in all individuals at some point, hence the need for gait assistance devices. Apraxia is often the most debilitating feature of the disorder. A home assessment by an occupational therapist can aid in determining which changes could be made to facilitate functional independence, although experience to date has been disappointing. Speech therapy and communication devices can optimize communication when dysarthria, apraxia of speech, or aphasia is present, although they are generally of minimal benefit. Therapists also counsel patients and families on swallowing maneuvers and food additives to minimize aspiration when dysphagia evolves. Decisions regarding placement of feeding gastrostomy tubes should be discussed before dysphagia becomes problematic.

Prognosis and Future Perspectives. Most patients succumb to the disease in 7 to 10 years. Death usually results from aspiration pneumonia or urosepsis.

The main focus of a recent symposium on CBD and other ACDS[109] regarded nosological status and terminology.

DEMENTIA WITH LEWY BODIES

Pathogenesis and Pathophysiology. Between 20 and 30 percent of brains of patients with a degenerative dementia have concomitant AD and PD changes, making Lewy body–related pathology the second most common histopathology behind AD. A much smaller percentage have diffuse Lewy bodies without AD changes. Therefore, the dementing disorders associated with Lewy bodies can be categorized into three groups: PD without cortical Lewy bodies or AD changes, PD with cortical Lewy bodies but not concomitant AD changes, and PD with cortical Lewy bodies and AD changes (previously termed the Lewy body variant of AD, LBV). The McKeith consensus criteria led to Dementia with Lewy Bodies as the preferred term for patients with cortical Lewy bodies and dementia with or without concurrent pathological evidence of AD.[111] Numerous data indicate that PD and AD have distinctly separate clinical, pathological, pathophysiological, and genetic correlates. However, there is a significant proportion of patients with combinations of the classic features of PD and AD, which suggests that there is a pathophysiological relationship between them.

Pathologically, the gross appearance of the brain is normal to slightly atrophic. The substantia nigra is pale. In the LBV of AD, there are sufficient numbers of NPs to apply the neuropathological diagnosis of AD. NFT counts are more variable. Lewy bodies, if present in the cortex, are almost invariably also present in the brain stem. The Lewy bodies in the brain stem are easily seen on sections stained with hematoxylin-eosin, where they tend to reside in the substantia nigra, locus caeruleus, and raphe nuclei. Cortical Lewy bodies often lack the surrounding halo that is typical of those in the brain stem and are more difficult to visualize unless immunostains for ubiquitin or α-synuclein are used (Fig. 33–14). The locations of maximal numbers of cortical Lewy bodies include the cingulate gyrus, insular cortex, and parahippocampal gyrus. Ubiquitin- and synuclein-positive neuritic changes are also present in the CA2/CA3 region of the hippocampus, whereas Lewy bodies are rarely found in the hippocampus. The degree of neuronal loss in the hippocampal CA subfields is variable in LBV and DLB. These findings suggest that the type of ubiquitin- and synuclein-positive changes may be site specific. The cholinergic neurons in the nucleus basalis are markedly depleted.

As noted earlier, a subgroup of AD cases with primarily plaque-only changes were found to have numerous extranigral Lewy bodies.[20] In those cases with more typical NPs and NFTs, the number of NFTs tends to be less in AD-plus-PD brains than in AD-only brains. All of these cases had sufficient numbers of NPs to apply the neuropathological diagnosis of AD. However, because frequent NPs have also been observed in cognitively normal individuals, debate has surrounded the issue of whether these cases represent a variant of AD (thus the name LBV of AD) or a distinct entity (thus the name DLB) with co-existing AD changes.

Katzman and colleagues[112] have provided several lines of evidence supporting the LBV of AD concept: (1) the clinical features of AD and LBV are similar, (2) the LBV has been observed in several familial AD1 cases, (3) the LBV has also been observed in rare Down's syndrome cases, and (4) the LBV is frequently observed in ApoE ε-4/ε-3 cases. Other investigators have observed an association between ApoE ε-4 dosage and PD-related changes, but interestingly, the severity of ubiquitin-positive neuritic changes in the hippocampus correlated with ApoE ε-4 dosage, whereas the frequency of cortical Lewy bodies did not.[113] It has been suggested that the LBV of AD may represent the result of a co-existent gene that promotes Lewy bodies rather than NFT in degenerating neocortical neurons.[112]

The cardinal features of DLB involve dementia and mild to moderate parkinsonism. The extrapyramidal symptoms reflect basal ganglia and nigral degeneration. The nature of cognitive impairment in DLB is likely multifactorial. The degree of neurofibrillary degeneration is less than in pure AD. Although supportive data are lacking, the presence and frequency of cortical Lewy bodies may be a contributor, and the effects of Lewy body and AD changes may be additive. Subcortical degenerative changes underlie the psychomotor slowing. Prominent hallucinations, delusions, illusions, and behavioral dyscontrol are also characteristic clinical features. It is unclear whether the neuropsychiatric features reflect unique qualities of cortical Lewy bodies themselves; the topographic distribution of Lewy body or cortical degeneration, or both; or neurochemical abnormalities.

The nucleus basalis atrophy and marked cholinergic deficiency in brains affected by LBV mirror that noted in brains affected by AD only, although findings in pure DLB without AD are less clear. Choline acetyltransferase activity has been found to be lower in patients with LBV than in those with AD only.[114] Reportedly, some patients with LBV with very low levels of this enzyme have improved while on tacrine therapy, but parkinsonism can worsen with tacrine. The brains of patients with AD- plus PD- changes have also been found to have reduced levels of dopamine and homovanillic acid compared with normal brains and those affected by AD only.

Epidemiology and Risk Factors. The relationship among DLB, AD, and PD is debated because there is evidence to support all points of view, that is, that DLB is related to AD and to PD and that it can be a distinct entity unrelated to either.

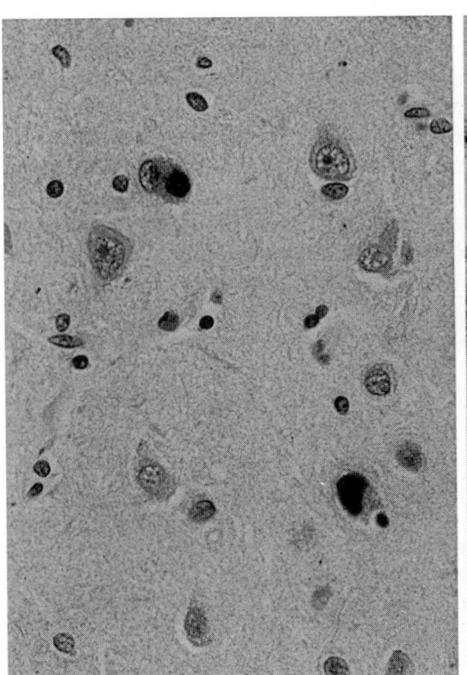

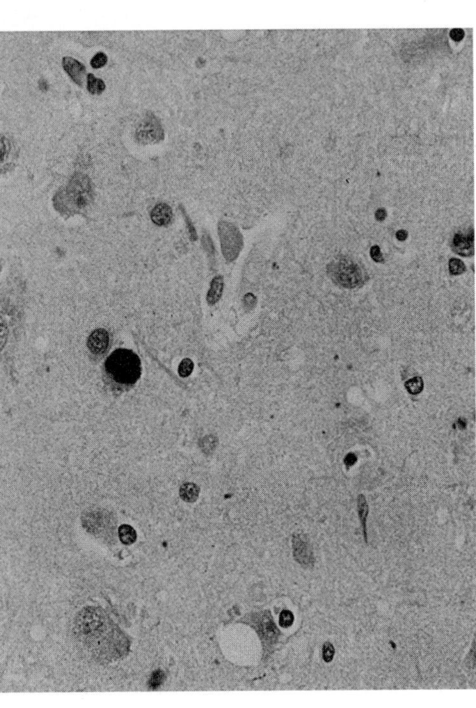

FIGURE 33–14. Photomicrograph of cortical Lewy bodies using an antiubiquitin immunostain. The core is composed of 7- to 8-nm filaments. (Hematoxylin and eosin; 400×; courtesy of JE Parisi, Mayo Clinic, Rochester, Minnesota.)

Hence, it is unclear whether epidemiological data that relate to AD and PD are relevant for DLB. There are no large epidemiological studies, but autopsy series suggest that the mean age of onset of DLB is 57 years, that it affects men more often than women (male-to-female ratio 1.7:1), and that death ensues after roughly 10 to 15 years.[115] In this series, there were 20 patients who died with PD and 8 who died with DLB, suggesting that the prevalence of DLB is, very roughly, 30 percent that of Parkinson's disease.[115] Extrapyramidal findings occur with increasing frequency as AD progresses (in close to 30 percent of patients[116]), but how often this reflects Lewy body–related pathology is uncertain. In an autopsy series of AD, 15 percent of patients had some type of Lewy body–related pathology.[117] The relationship of ApoE to DLB depends on how closely DLB is related to AD, and although ApoE genotype appears relevant, the relationship is weaker than for AD.[118]

Clinical Features and Associated Disorders. AD and PD are both part of the nosological spectrum of DLB, which seems to bridge the cortical and subcortical degenerative dementias. The literature is divided on whether parkinsonian or cognitive symptoms present first, but all investigators agree that both are important components.[115, 119] Although the published clinical criteria for the diagnosis of DLB continue to be debated, the proposed cardinal features of DLB include fluctuating cognition, visual hallucinations, and parkinsonism[111] (see Table 33–7). In general, the clinical picture of a mild parkinsonian syndrome with a more severe dementia and prominent visual hallucinations and paranoid delusions should prompt consideration of DLB. Although the parkinsonism can be levodopa responsive, levodopa may exacerbate the psychosis, and in the early to middle stages, the neuropsychiatric disturbance is generally the more disabling feature. As the disease progresses, however, both components worsen, and the patient may eventually develop severe parkinsonian symptoms and become wheelchair bound. Rest tremor is less frequent (about 29 percent of patients[115]) than in PD, but bradykinesia is a predictable feature. The quality of the dementia resembles the subcortical pattern with pronounced psychomotor slowing; absence of severe aphasia, agnosia, or apraxia; and concurrent parkinsonism. Atypical features, including impaired vertical gaze and progressive spasticity, have been described further, highlighting the clinicopathological overlap that occurs among many of the degenerative dementias.

Recent evidence suggests that rapid-eye-movement (REM) sleep behavior disorder is a frequently associated feature of DLB (as well as PD and MSA) but is rarely present in AD and the tau-opathies.[120, 121] REM sleep behavior disorder (RBD) is a parasomnia manifested by dream enactment behavior, in which the normal paralysis REM sleep is lost and patients appear to "act out their dreams."[122] Clinicians can usually elicit a history suggesting RBD by simply asking spouses whether their bed partners have repeatedly "acted out their dreams," even if such behavior was more frequent and severe years or decades earlier. The underlying neurologic substrates for RBD have not been adequately defined in humans.

Differential Diagnosis. The differential diagnosis of DLB is particularly broad because of its overlap with cortical and subcortical degenerative dementias, as well as the clinical similarities with nondegenerative dementing illnesses. Dementia and mild parkinsonism is perhaps the most common presenting symptom complex of small vessel–type multi-infarct dementia (another, and perhaps the most common, cause of subcortical dementia). Prominent visual hallucina-

TABLE 33–7. **Clinical Diagnosis of Dementia with Lewy Bodies (DLB)**

Core Features
Progressive cognitive decline that interferes with normal social and occupational functioning
Deficits on tests of attention/concentration, verbal fluency, psychomotor speed, and visuospatial functioning often prominent
Prominent or persistent memory impairment may not be present early in course of illness
Two of the following core features necessary for the diagnosis of *clinically probable* DLB, and one necessary for the diagnosis of *clinically possible* DLB:

- Fluctuating cognition or alertness
- Recurrent visual hallucinations
- Spontaneous features of parkinsonism

Supportive Features
Repeated falls
Syncope
Transient loss of consciousness
Neuroleptic sensitivity
Systematized delusions
Tactile or olfactory hallucinations
REM sleep behavior disorder
Depression

Features Suggesting Disorder Other Than DLB
Cerebrovascular disease evidenced by focal neurological signs and/or cerebral infarct(s) present on neuroimaging study
Findings on examination or on ancillary testing that another medical, neurological, or psychiatric disorder sufficiently accounts for clinical features

Data from McKeith IG, Galasko D, Kosaka K, et al: Consensus guidelines for the clinical and pathologic diagnosis of dementia with Lewy bodies (DLB): Report of the consortium on DLB international workshop. Neurology 1996;47:1113–1124; and McKeith et al, 1999.

tions can be an important clinical feature of certain reversible chronic progressive encephalopathies, including chronic inflammatory meningoencephalitis, chronic meningitides occurring on infectious or neoplastic bases, and many toxic-metabolic encephalopathies. Although they do occur in other degenerative dementias, including AD and PD, they are less frequent and should not be considered typical early features.

Evaluation. The neuropsychological pattern of impairment in DLB is quite different from that of AD, with significantly worse visual perceptual organization, sequencing, and letter fluency but significantly better confrontation naming and verbal memory.[123, 124] When diagnostic clarification for the diagnosis of RBD is necessary, particularly when the risk for injury is high, polysomnography (PSG) with simultaneous video-PSG monitoring is warranted. In addition to the usual tests for dementia evaluation (MRI, neuropsychological testing, and laboratory studies, as described in the section on AD), the EEG is particularly useful. Many reversible chronic progressive encephalopathies produce severe dysrhythmic slowing, whereas most degenerative diseases, at least in early stages, produce mild or no dysrhythmic slowing. Although a severely abnormal EEG can occur in DLB, it should prompt strong consideration of more exhaustive laboratory studies looking for unusual autoimmune causes and other systemic medical causes of encephalopathy, as well as a CSF examination. CSF tests should include microbiological, cytological, and immunological studies (including IgG index, IgG synthesis rate, and oligoclonal bands). These immunological studies may provide evidence of an intrathecal immunological response that, although nonspecific, may be more sensitive than fungal cultures or cytology and therefore may be the only sign of an autoimmune process. If the patient has a so-called psychotic delirium with minimal parkinsonian features, a severely dysrhythmic EEG, and a CSF profile that suggests an inflammatory mediated process, in the absence of another obvious cause, meningeal and brain biopsy should be considered, observing for CIME, CNS vasculitis, CNS infection, and meningeal carcinomatosis. Because CIME is very steroid responsive, an empirical trial of corticosteroid therapy could be considered, especially if there is reticence to perform a brain biopsy.

Management. As noted earlier, treatment of the parkinsonian syndrome may exacerbate the neuropsychiatric disorder, and treatment of the neuropsychiatric disorder may exacerbate the parkinsonian syndrome. A decision, therefore, must first be made regarding whether treatment is necessary at all, and if so, what symptoms warrant treatment. Generally, the neuropsychiatric syndrome is the most disabling aspect in mild to moderate stages, and selective neuroleptic therapy with quetiapine should be considered as a first choice. Treatment of the parkinsonian syndrome is similar to that of PD, generally beginning with Sinemet at a very low dose and gradually titrating the dose to symptoms and side effects. Other nonpharmacological aspects of caregiving are similar to those described for AD except that physical and occupational therapies are of greater importance at an earlier stage due to the extrapyramidal syndrome. Benefits, however, are generally modest.

Prognosis and Future Perspectives. As noted earlier, the mean age of onset of DLB is 57 years, and death ensues after roughly 10 to 15 years.[115] Treatment is difficult, often inadequate, and caregiving is especially difficult usually because of the psychosis.

DLB is an important nosological entity because it appears to occupy an intermediate position between AD and PD, two common degenerative diseases that are generally thought to have little in common. Therefore, understanding the genetics and disease mechanisms of DLB may provide important insights into its more frequent cousins as well. Also, this group of patients will be an important testing ground for newer antipsychotic agents with greater selectivity. Because RBD is often associated with DLB, and the onset of RBD often precedes (by decades in some cases) the onset of cognitive impairment or parkinsonism, isolated RBD may represent the earliest clinical manifestation of DLB (or PD or MSA). Thus, the presence of RBD may be particularly relevant early in the course of a neurodegenerative disease when intervention may be most critical; treatment of patients with isolated RBD could potentially delay or prevent the development of cognitive impairment or parkinsonism.

Reviews and Selected Updates

American Academy of Neurology Ethics and Humanities Subcommittee: Ethical issues in the management of the demented patient. Neurology 1996; 1180–1183

Caselli RJ: Focal and asymmetric cortical degeneration syndromes. Neurologist 1995;1:1–19.

Cummings J, Benson DF: Dementia: A Clinical Approach, 2nd ed. Stoneham, MA, Butterworth-Heinemann, 1992.

Doody RS, Stevens JC, Beck C, et al: Practice parameter: Management of dementia (an evidence-based review). Report of the Quality Standards Subcommittee of the American Academy of Neurology. Neurology 2001; 56:1154–1166.

Gomez-Isla T, Hollister R, West H, Mui S: Neuronal loss correlates with but exceeds neurofibrillary tangles in Alzheimer's disease. Ann Neurol 1997;41:17–24.

Katzman R: Diagnosis and management of dementia. *In* Katzman R, Rowe JW (eds): Principles of Geriatric Neurology. Philadelphia, F.A. Davis, 1992, pp 167–206.

Knopman DS, DeKosky ST, Cummings JL, et al: Practice parameter: Diagnosis of dementia (an evidence-based review). Report of the Quality Standards Subcommittee of the American Academy of Neurology. Neurology 2001;56:1143–1153.

Lang AE, Maraganore D, Marsden CD, Tanner C: Movement Disorder Society symposium on cortical-basal ganglionic degeneration (CBGD) and its relationship to other asymmetric cortical degeneration syndromes (ACDs). Mov Disord 1996;11:346–357.

Levy-Lahad E, Bird TD: Genetic factors in Alzheimer's disease: A review of recent advances. Ann Neurol 1996;40:829–840.

Lieberman A, Dziatolowski M, Neophytides A, et al: Dementias of Huntington's and Parkinson's disease. *In* Chase TN, Wexler NS, Barbeau A (eds): Advances in Neurology, Vol. 23, Huntington's Disease. New York, Raven Press, 1979, pp 273–280.

McKeith IG, Perry EK, Perry RH, et al: Report of the second dementia with Lewy bodies international workshop: Diagnosis and treatment. Neurology 1999;53:902–905.

Mendez MF, Cherrier M, Kent M: Frontotemporal dementia versus Alzheimer's disease. Neurology 1996;47:1189–1194.

Neary D, Snowden JS, Gustafson L, et al: Frontotemporal lobar degeneration: A consensus on clinical diagnostic criteria. Neurology 1998;51:1546–1554.

Terry R, Katzman R: Alzheimer's disease and cognitive loss. *In* Katzman R, Rowe JW (eds): Principles of Geriatric Neurology. Philadelphia, F.A. Davis, 1992, pp 207–265.

References

1. Crystal H, Dickson D, Fuld P, et al: Clinico-pathologic studies in dementia: Nondemented subjects with pathologically confirmed Alzheimer's disease. Neurology 1988;38:1682–1687.
2. The National Institute on Aging and Reagan Institute Working Group on Diagnostic Criteria for the Neuropathologic Assessment of

Alzheimer's Disease: Consensus recommendations for the postmortem diagnosis of Alzheimer's disease. Neurobiol Aging 1997;18(S4):S1–S2.

3. Terry R, Masliah E, Salmon D, et al: Physical basis of cognitive alterations in Alzheimer's disease: Synapse loss is the major correlate of cognitive impairment. Ann Neurol 1991;30:572–580.
4. Hyman BT, Van Hoesen GW, Damasio AR, Barnes CL: Alzheimer's disease: Cell-specific pathology isolates the hippocampal formation. Science 1984;225:1168–1170.
5. Masters C, Simms G, Weinman N, et al: Amyloid plaque core protein in Alzheimer's disease and Down syndrome. Proc Natl Acad Sci USA 1985;82:4245–4249.
6. Smith C, Anderton B: The molecular pathology of Alzheimer's disease: Are we any closer to understanding the neurodegenerative process. Neuropathol Appl Neurobiol 1994;20:322–338.
7. Hardy J, Higgins G: Alzheimer's disease—The amyloid cascade hypothesis. Science 1992;256:184–185.
8. Motter R, Vigo-Pelfrey C, Kholodenko D, et al: Reduction of β-amyloid peptide 42 in the cerebrospinal fluid of patients with Alzheimer's disease. Ann Neurol 1995;38:643–648.
9. Vigo-Pelfrey C, Seubert P, Barbour R, et al: Elevation of microtubule-associated protein tau in the cerebrospinal fluid of patients with Alzheimer's disease. Neurology 1995;45:788–793.
10. Corder EH, Saunders AM, Strittmatter WJ, et al: Gene dose of apolipoprotein E type 4 allele and the risk of Alzheimer's disease in late onset families. Science 1993;261:921–923.
11. Saunders AM, Strittmatter WJ, Schmechel D, et al: Association of apolipoprotein E allele ε4 with late onset familial and sporadic Alzheimer's disease. Neurology 1993;43:1467–1472.
12. Corder EH, Saunders AM, Risch NJ, et al: Protective effect of apolipoprotein E type 2 allele for late onset Alzheimer disease. Nat Genet 1994;7:180–184.
13. Schmechel D, Saunders A, Strittmatter W, et al: Increased amyloid B-peptide deposition in cerebral cortex as a consequence of apolipoprotein E genotype in late-onset Alzheimer disease. Proc Natl Acad Sci USA 1993;90:9649–9653.
14. Ma J, Yee A, Brewer H, et al: Amyloid-associated proteins alpha 1-antichymotrypsin and apolipoprotein E promote assembly of Alzheimer beta-protein into filaments. Nature 1994;6501:92–94.
15. Kounnas MZ, Moir RD, Rebeck GW, et al: LDL receptor–related protein, a multifunctional ApoE receptor, binds secreted B–amyloid precursor protein and mediates its degradation. Cell 1995;82:331–340.
16. McGeer PL, Rogers J: Anti-inflammatory agents as a therapeutic approach to Alzheimer's disease. Neurology 1992;42:447–449.
17. Armstrong R, Winsper S, Blair J: Aluminum and Alzheimer's disease: Review of possible pathogenic mechanisms. Dementia 1996;7:1–9.
18. Hensley K, Carney J, Mattson M, et al: A model for beta-amyloid aggregation and neurotoxicity based on free radical generation by the peptide: Relevance to Alzheimer disease. Proc Natl Acad Sci 1994;91:3270–3274.
19. Whitehouse P, Price D, Struble R, et al: Alzheimer disease and senile dementia: Loss of neurons in basal forebrain. Science 1982;215:1237–1239.
20. Hansen L, Masliah E, Galasko D, Terry R: Plaque-only Alzheimer disease is usually Lewy body variant, and vice versa. J Neuropathol Exp Neurol 1994;52:648–654.
21. Sherrington R, Rogaev EI, Liang Y, et al: Cloning of a gene bearing missense mutation in early-onset familial Alzheimer's disease. Nature 1995;375:754–760.
22. Levy-Lahad E, Wasco W, Poorkaj P, et al: Candidate gene for the chromosome 1 familial Alzheimer's disease locus. Science 1995;269:973–977.
23. Ertekin-Taner N, Graff-Radford N, Younkin LH, et al: Linkage of plasma Abeta42 to a quantitative locus on chromosome 10 in late-onset Alzheimer's disease pedigrees. Science 2000;290:2303–2304.
24. Wu WS, Holmans P, Wavrant-DeVrieze F, et al: Genetic studies on chromosome 12 in late-onset Alzheimer disease. JAMA 1998;280:619–622.
25. Kokmen E, Beard CM, O'Brien PC, Kurland LT: Epidemiology of dementia in Rochester, Minnesota. Mayo Clin Proc 1996;71:275–282.
26. Farrer LA, Cupples LA: Estimating the probability for major gene Alzheimer disease. Am J Hum Genet 1994;54:374–383.
27. Seshadri S, Drachman DA, Lippa CF: Apolipoprotein E ε4 allele and the lifetime risk of Alzheimer's disease. Arch Neurol 1995;52:1074–1079.
28. Poirer J, Davignon D, Bouthillier D, et al: Apolipoprotein E polymorphism and Alzheimer's disease. Lancet 1993;ii:697–699.
29. Wisniewski KE, Wisniewski HM, Wen GY: Occurrence of neuropathological changes and dementia of Alzheimer's disease in Down's syndrome. Ann Neurol 1985;17:278–282.
30. McKhann G, Drachman D, Folstein M, et al: Clinical diagnosis of Alzheimer's disease: Report of the NINCDS-ADRDA Work Group under the auspices of Department of Health and Human Services Task Force on Alzheimer's Disease. Neurology 1984;34:939–944.
31. Gearing M, Mirra SS, Hedreen JC, et al: The Consortium to Establish a Registry for Alzheimer's Disease (CERAD). Part X. Neuropathology confirmation of the clinical diagnosis of Alzheimer's disease. Neurology 1995;45:461–466.
32. Reiman EM, Caselli RJ, Yun LS, et al: Preclinical evidence of Alzheimer's disease in persons homozygous for the ε4 allele for apolipoprotein E. New Engl J Med 1996;334:752–758.
33. Beatty WW, Salmon DP, Butters N, et al: Retrograde amnesia in patients with Alzheimer's or Huntington's disease. Neurobiol Aging 1988;9:181–186.
34. Heindel WC, Salmon DP, Shults CW, et al: Neuropsychological evidence for multiple memory systems: A comparison of Alzheimer's, Huntington's, and Parkinson's disease patients. J Neurosci 1989;9:582–587.
35. Fitten LJ, Perryman KM, Wilkinson CJ, et al: Alzheimer and vascular dementias and driving: A prospective road and laboratory study. JAMA 1995;273:1360–1365.
36. Petersen RC, Smith GE, Waring SE, et al: Mild cognitive impairment: Clinical characterization and outcome. Arch Neurol 1999;56:303–308.
37. Petersen RC, Smith GE, Ivnik RJ, et al: Apolipoprotein E status as a predictor of the development of Alzheimer's disease in memory-impaired individuals. JAMA 1995;273:1274–1278.
38. Petersen RC, Stevens JC, Ganguli M, et al: Practice parameter: Early detection of dementia: Mild cognitive impairment (an evidence-based review). Neurology 2001;56:1133–1142.
39. Hof PR, Bouras C, Constantinidis J, Morrison JH: Balint's syndrome in Alzheimer's disease: Specific disruption of the occipito-parietal visual pathway. Brain Res 1989;493:368–375.
40. Clarfield AM: The reversible dementias: Do they reverse? Ann Intern Med 1988;109:476–486.
41. Hyman BT, West HL, Rebeck GW, et al: Quantitative analysis of senile plaques in Alzheimer disease: Observation of log-normal size distribution and molecular epidemiology of differences associated with apolipoprotein E genotype and trisomy 21 (Down syndrome). Proc Natl Acad Sci USA 1995;92:3586–3590.
42. Knapp MJ, Knopman DS, Solomon PR, et al for the Tacrine Study Group: A 30-week randomized controlled trial of high dose tacrine in patients with Alzheimer's disease. JAMA 1994;271:985–991.
43. Snowden DA, Kemper SJ, Mortimer JA, et al: Linguistic ability in early life and cognitive function and Alzheimer's disease in late life: Findings from the nun study. JAMA 1996;275:528–532.
44. Bondi MW, Salmon DP, Monsch AU, et al: Episodic memory changes are associated with the ApoE ε-4 allele in nondemented older adults. Neurology 1995;45:2203–2206.
45. Mesulam M: Primary progressive aphasia without generalized dementia. Ann Neurol 1982;11:592–598.
46. Snowden JS, Neary D, Mann DMA, et al: Progressive language disorder due to lobar atrophy. Ann Neurol 1992;31:174–183.
47. Lippa CF, Cohen R, Smith TW, Drachman DA: Primary progressive aphasia with focal neuronal achromasia. Neurology 1991;41:882–886.
48. Morris JC, Cole M, Banker BQ, Wright D: Hereditary dysphasic dementia and the Pick-Alzheimer spectrum. Ann Neurol 1984;16:455–466.
49. Popagar S, Williams R: Alzheimer's disease presenting as slowly progressive aphasia. Rhode Island Med J 1984;67:181–185.
50. Graff-Radford NR, Damasio AR, Hyman BT, et al: Progressive aphasia in a patient with Pick's disease: A neuropsychologic, radiologic, and anatomic study. Neurology 1990;40:620–626.
51. Kirshner HS, Tanridag O, Thurman L, Whetsell WO Jr: Progressive aphasia without dementia: Two cases with focal spongiform degeneration. Ann Neurol 1987;22:527–532.
52. Benson D, Zaias B: Progressive aphasia: A case with postmortem correlation. Neuropsych Neuropsychol Behav Neurol 1991;4:215–223.
53. Tissot R, Constantinidis J, Richard J: Pick's disease. *In* Vinken P, Bruyn G, Klawans H (eds): Handbook of Clinical Neurology, Vol. 46. Amsterdam, Elsevier, 1985, pp 233–246.
54. Mizukami K, Kosaka K: Neuropathological study on the nucleus basalis of Meynert in Pick's disease. Acta Neuropathol 1989;78:52–56.
55. Lang A, Bergeron C, Pollanen M, Ashby P: Parietal Pick's disease mimicking cortical-basal ganglionic degeneration. Neurology 1994;44:1436–1440.
56. Ghetti B, Murrell JR, Zolo P, Spillantini MG, Goedert M: Progress in hereditary tauopathies: A mutation in the Tau gene (G389R) causes a Pick disease-like syndrome. Ann NY Acad Sci 2000;920:52–62.

57. Pringle CE, Hudson AJ, Munoz DG, et al: Primary lateral sclerosis: Clinical features, neuropathology, and diagnostic criteria. Brain 1992;115:495–520.
58. Ross GW, Benson DF, Verity AM, Victoroff JI: Posterior cortical atrophy: Neuropathological correlations (abstract). Neurology 1990;40 (Suppl 1):200.
59. Jagust W, Davies P, Tiller-Borcich J, Reed B: Focal Alzheimer's disease. Neurology 1990;40:14–19.
60. Scully R, Mark E, McNeely W, McNeely B: Case records of the Massachusetts General Hospital (Case 46-1993). N Engl J Med 1993;329:1560–1567.
61. Riley DE, Lang AE, Lewis A, et al: Cortical-basal ganglionic degeneration. Neurology 1990;40:1203–1212.
62. Reed LA, Wszolek ZK, Hutton M: Phenotypic correlations in FTDP-17. Neurobiol Aging 2001;22(1):89–107.
63. Hutton M, Lendon CL, Rizzu P, et al: Association of missense and 5'-splice-site mutations in tau with the inherited dementia FTDP-17. Nature 1998;393:702–705.
64. Caselli RJ, Reiman EM, Timmann D, et al: Progressive apraxia in clinically discordant monozygotic twins. Arch Neurol 1995;52:1004–1010.
65. Caselli RJ, Windebank AJ, Petersen RC, et al: Rapidly progressive aphasic dementia and motor neuron disease. Ann Neurol 1993;33: 200–207.
66. Brion S, Psimaras A, Chevalier JF, et al: L'association maladie de Pick et sclerose laterale amyotrophique. L'Encephale 1980;6:259–286.
67. Neary D, Snowden J, Mann D, et al: Frontal lobe dementia and motor neuron disease. J Neurol Neurosurg Psychiatry 1990;53:23–32.
68. Dickson DW, Horoupian DS, Thal LJ, et al: Kluver-Bucy syndrome and amyotrophic lateral sclerosis: A case report with biochemistry, morphometrics, and Golgi study. Neurology 1986;36:1323–1329.
69. Pick A: On the relation between aphasia and senile atrophy of the brain. Translated by WC Schoene from Pick A: Über die Beziehungen der senilen Hirnatrophie zur Aphasie. Prager Medicinische Wochenschrift 17, 16 (1892), 165–167. *In* Rottenberg DA, Hochberg FH (eds): Neurological Classics in Modern Translation. New York, Hafner Press, 1977, pp 35–40.
70. Sacks O: The Man Who Mistook His Wife for a Hat, and Other Clinical Tales. New York, Harper Perennial, 1970.
71. Tyrrell PJ, Warrington EK, Frackowiak RSJ, Rossor MN: Progressive degeneration of the right temporal lobe studied with positron emission tomography. J Neurol Neurosurg Psychiatry 1990;53:1046–1050.
72. Brun A: Frontal lobe degeneration of non-Alzheimer type. 1. Neuropathology. Arch Gerontol Geriatr 1987;6:193–208.
73. Gustafson L: Frontal lobe degeneration of non-Alzheimer type. II. Clinical picture and differential diagnosis. Arch Gerontol Geriatr 1987;6:209–223.
74. Caselli RJ, Smith BE, Osborne D: Primary lateral sclerosis: A neuropsychological study. Neurology 1995;45:2005–2009.
75. Caselli RJ, Jack CR Jr: Asymmetric cortical degenerative syndromes: A proposed clinical classification. Arch Neurol 1992;49:770–780.
76. Hudson A: Amyotrophic lateral sclerosis and its association with dementia, parkinsonism and other neurologic disorders: A review. Brain 1981;104:217–247.
77. Horoupian D, Thal L, Katzman R, et al: Dementia and motor neuron disease: Morphometric, biochemical, and Golgi studies. Ann Neurol 1984;16:305–313.
78. Hirano A, Kurland LT, Krooth RS, Lessell S: Parkinsonism-dementia complex, an endemic disease on the island of Guam. I. Clinical features. Brain 1961;84:642–661.
79. Kurland LT, Mulder DW: Epidemiologic investigations of amyotrophic lateral sclerosis. 2. Familial aggregations indicative of dominant inheritance. Neurology 1955;5:182–196.
80. Morita K, Kaiya H, Ikeda T, Namba M: Presenile dementia combined with amyotrophy: A review of thirty-four Japanese cases. Arch Gerontol Geriatr 1987;6:263–277.
81. Salazar AM, Masters CL, Gajdusek DC, Gibbs CJ: Syndromes of amyotrophic lateral sclerosis and dementia: Relation to transmissible Creutzfeldt-Jakob disease. Ann Neurol 1983;14:17–26.
82. Stern Y, Richards M, Sano M, Mayeux R: Comparison of cognitive changes in patients with Alzheimer's disease and Parkinson's disease. Arch Neurol 1993;50:1040–1045.
83. McFadden L, Mohr E, Sampson M, et al: A profile analysis of demented and nondemented Parkinson's disease patients. *In* Battistin L, Scarlato G, Caraceni T, Ruggieri S (eds): Advances in Neurology, Vol. 69. Philadelphia: Lippincott-Raven, 1996, pp 339–341.
84. Sugiyama H, Hainfellner J, Yoshimura M, Budka H: Neocortical changes in Parkinson's disease, revisited. Clin Neuropathol 1994;13:55–59.
85. Nauta WJH: Circuitous connections linking cerebral cortex, limbic system, and corpus striatum. *In* Doane BK, Livingston KE (eds): The Limbic System: Functional Organization and Clinical Disorders. New York, Raven Press, 1986, pp 43–54.
86. Lieberman A, Dziatolowski M, Neophytides A, et al: Dementias of Huntington's and Parkinson's disease. *In* Chase TN, Wexler NS, Barbeau A (eds): Advances in Neurology, Vol. 23, Huntington's Disease. New York, Raven Press, 1979, pp 273–280.
87. Yoshimura M: Pathological basis for dementia in elderly patients with idiopathic Parkinson's disease. Eur Neurol 1988;28(Suppl 1):29–35.
88. Kish SJ, El-Awar M, Schut L, et al: Cognitive deficits in olivopontocerebellar atrophy: Implications for the cholinergic hypothesis of Alzheimer's dementia. Ann Neurol 1988;24:200–206.
89. Robbins T, James M, Owen A, et al: Cognitive deficits in progressive supranuclear palsy, Parkinson's disease, and multiple system atrophy in tests sensitive to frontal lobe dysfunction. J Neurol Neurosurg Psychiatry 1994;57:79–88.
90. Berciano J: Olivopontocerebellar atrophy: A review of 117 cases. J Neurol Sci 1982;53:253–272.
91. Berent S, Giordant B, Gilman S, et al: Neuropsychological changes in olivopontocerebellar atrophy. Arch Neurol 1990;47:997–1001.
92. Litvan I: Cognitive disturbances in progressive supranuclear palsy. J Neural Transm 1994;42(Suppl):69–78.
93. Pillon B, Dubois B, Ploska A, Agid Y: Severity and specificity of cognitive impairment in Alzheimer's, Huntington's, and Parkinson's diseases and progressive supranuclear palsy. Neurology 1991;41:634–643.
94. D'Antona R, Baron J, Samson Y, et al: Subcortical dementia: Frontal cortex hypometabolism detected by positron tomography in patients with progressive supranuclear palsy. Brain 1985;108:785–799.
95. Verny M, Duyckaerts C, Delaere P, et al: Cortical tangles in progressive supranuclear palsy. J Neural Transm 1994;42:179–188.
96. Golbe LI: The epidemiology of PSP. J Neural Transm 1994;42:263–273.
97. Mann D, Oliver R, Snowden J: The topographic distribution of brain atrophy in Huntington's disease and progressive supranuclear palsy. Acta Neuropathol 1993;85:553–559.
98. Heinsen H, Strik M, Bauer M, et al: Cortical and striatal neurone number in Huntington's disease. Acta Neuropathol 1994;88:320–333.
99. Jackson M, Gentleman S, Lennox G, et al: The cortical neuritic pathology of Huntington's disease. Neuropathol Appl Neurobiol 1995;21:18–26.
100. Storey E, Kowall N, Finn S, et al: The cortical lesion of Huntington's disease: Further neurochemical characterization, and reproduction of some of the histological and neurochemical features by *N*-methyl-D-aspartate lesion of rat cortex. Ann Neurol 1992;32:526–534.
101. Mazziotta JC, Phelps ME, Pahl JJ, et al: Reduced cerebral glucose metabolism in asymptomatic subjects at risk for Huntington's disease. New Engl J Med 1987;316:357–362.
102. Bamford KA, Caine ED, Kido DK, et al: Clinical-pathologic correlation in Huntington's disease: A neuropsychological and computed tomography study. Neurology 1989;39:796–801.
103. Berent S, Giordani B, Markel D, et al: Positron emission tomographic scan investigations of Huntington's disease: Cerebral metabolic correlates of cognitive function. Ann Neurol 1988;23:541–546.
104. Bamford KA, Caine ED, Kido DK, et al: A prospective evaluation of cognitive decline in early Huntington's disease: Functional and radiographic correlates. Neurology 1995;45:1867–1873.
105. Massman PJ, Delis DC, Butters N, et al: Are all subcortical dementias alike? Verbal learning and memory in Parkinson's and Huntington's disease patients. J Clin Exp Neuropsychol 1990;12:729–744.
106. Gibb W, Luthert P, Marsden CD: Corticobasal degeneration. Brain 1989;112:1171–1192.
107. Feany M, Dickson D: Widespread cytoskeletal pathology characterizes corticobasal degeneration. Am J Pathol 1995;146:1388–1396.
108. Rebeiz JJ, Kolodny EH, Richardson EP Jr: Corticodentatonigral degeneration with neuronal achromasia: A progressive disorder of late adult life. Trans Am Neurol Assoc 1967;92:23–26.
109. Lang AE, Maragonore D, Marsden CD, Tanner C: Movement Disorder Society Symposium on Cortical-Basal Ganglionic Degeneration (CBGD) and Its Relationship to Other Asymmetric Cortical Degeneration Syndromes (ACDs). Mov Disord 1996;11:346–357.
110. Kompoliti K, Goetz CG, Boeve BF, et al: Clinical presentation and pharmacologic therapy in corticobasal degeneration. Arch Neurol 1998;55:957–963.

111. McKeith IG, Galasko D, Kosaka K, et al: Consensus guidelines for the clinical and pathologic diagnosis of dementia with Lewy bodies (DLB): Report of the consortium on DLB international workshop. Neurology 1996;47:1113–1124.
112. Katzman R, Galasko D, Saitoh T, et al: Genetic evidence that the Lewy body variant is indeed a phenotypic variant of Alzheimer's disease. Brain Cogn 1995;28:259–265.
113. Gearing M, Schneider J, Rebeck G, et al: Alzheimer's disease with and without coexisting Parkinson's disease changes: Apolipoprotein E genotype and neuropathologic correlates. Neurology 1995;45:1985–1990.
114. Perry E, Haroutunian V, Davis K, et al: Neocortical cholinergic activities differentiate Lewy body dementia from classical Alzheimer's disease. Neuroreport 1994;5:747–749.
115. Louis ED, Goldman JE, Powers JM, Fahn S: Parkinsonian features of eight pathologically diagnosed cases of diffuse Lewy body disease. Mov Disord 1995;10:188–194.
116. Mayeux R, Stern Y, Spanton S: Heterogeneity in dementia of the Alzheimer type: Evidence of subgroups. Neurology 1985;35:453–461.
117. Joachim CL, Morris JH, Selkoe DJ: Clinically diagnosed Alzheimer's disease: Autopsy results in 150 cases. Ann Neurol 1988;24:50–56.
118. Lippa CF, Smith TW, Saunders AM, et al: Apolipoprotein E genotype and Lewy body disease. Neurology 1995;45:97–103.
119. Crystal HA, Dickson DW, Lizardi JE, et al: Antemortem diagnosis of diffuse Lewy body disease. Neurology 1990;40:1523–1528.
120. Boeve BF, Silber MH, Ferman TJ, et al: REM sleep behavior disorder and degenerative dementia: An association likely reflecting Lewy body disease. Neurology 1998;51:363–370.
121. Boeve BF, Silber MH, Ferman TJ, Lucas J, Parisi J: Association of REM sleep behavior disorder and neurodegenerative disease may reflect an underlying synucleinopathy. Mov Disord 2001;16:622–630.
122. Olson EJ, Silber MH, Boeve BF: REM sleep behavior disorder: Demographic, clinical, and laboratory findings in 92 cases. Brain 2000;123:331–339.
123. Salmon DP, Galasko D, Hansen LA, et al: Neuropsychological deficits associated with diffuse Lewy body disease. Brain Cogn 1996;31:148–165.
124. Ferman TJ, Boeve BG, Smith GE, et al: REM sleep behavior disorder and dementia: Cognitive differences when compared with AD. Neurology 1999;52:951–957.

CHAPTER 34

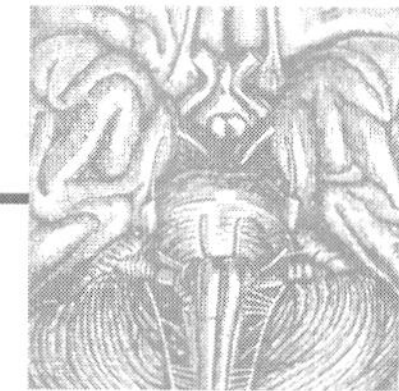

JOSEPH JANKOVIC

Movement Disorders

History

Because they attract visual attention, movement disorders have been described in both medical and nonmedical historical material for hundreds of years. Early etiological explanations reflected the knowledge and prejudices of their times, with various life forces and demonic possession being cited as common causes. The original clinical descriptions of these disorders, however, extend far beyond historical interest and are important documents rich in details of phenomenology and natural history. Gilles de la Tourette syndrome, although not named until the 19th century, was vividly described in the *Malleus Maleficarum* (1489), and Paracelsus described various forms of chorea in careful detail. Parkinson's disease, the prototypical movement disorder, was first reported by James Parkinson in 1817, and his succinct and vibrant description of the disease in the context of the pollution of London in the Industrial Revolution covered not only the major clinical features of the disease, but also suggested the possibility of a causative role of environmental toxins. Specifically, in the United States, the country practitioner George Huntington extensively described Huntington's chorea in the 1800s, basing his description on his and his father's experiences with a large New York kindred. Clear phenomenological descriptions occupied primary attention during the 19th century, largely steered by the supervision of Charcot and other European neurologists. In the first half of the 20th century, a clearer focus was placed on the basal ganglia due to early histological and biochemical studies. The molecular, biological, and physiological bases of both hypokinetic and hyperkinetic disorders have received primary attention during the past "decade of the brain."

Hypokinetic Movement Disorders

PARKINSON'S DISEASE

Pathogenesis and Pathophysiology. Pathological findings of Parkinson's disease (PD) include depigmentation and neuronal loss in the substantia nigra (SN) and the presence of Lewy bodies and pale bodies (Fig. 34–1). Because the degenerating cells in the SN normally synthesize the neurochemical dopamine, the pathophysiological hallmark of PD is dopaminergic underactivity at the site of these cells' axonal projection—that is, the striatum (caudate nucleus and putamen) (Fig. 34–2). Lewy bodies are eosinophilic inclusions composed of neurofilament, tubulin components, α-synuclein, and ubiquitin. Pale bodies are composed of neurofilament interspersed with vacuolar granules. Besides the substantia nigra, they are also present in the basal ganglia, cortex, brain stem, and spinal cord. Although characteristic of PD, Lewy bodies are also seen in Alzheimer's disease, Hallervorden-Spatz disease, ataxia-telangiectasia, and, rarely, in patients without clinical neurological disease.[1]

The mechanism of Lewy body formation and cell death in PD is not known, but the degenerative process is highly

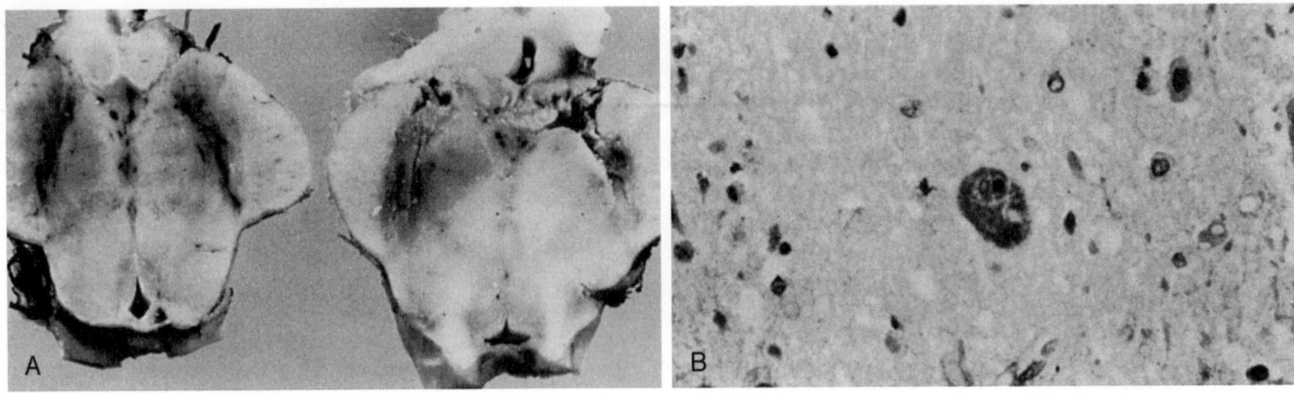

FIGURE 34–1. *A* and *B*, An isolated Lewy body, a distinctive eosinophilic cytoplasmic inclusion body found in the substantia nigra of Parkinson's disease.

localized at the beginning of the illness. Anatomical studies have found that the area first affected in the disorder is the pars compacta in the ventrolateral SN (SNpc) with its fibers projecting to the putamen. Neurochemical changes resulting from this selective neurodegeneration consist mainly of loss of dopamine (DA), and it is estimated that 60 to 85 percent of nigral neurons and striatal DA is lost prior to the development of PD symptoms.

The most actively studied hypothesis of the origin of PD has focused on the possibility that the natural proteasomal activity in the brains of patients with PD may be impaired, thus leading to abnormal protein aggregation. Postmortem studies of brains of patients with PD have provided evidence that proteasomal function is selectively impaired in the SN.[2] Aggresomes, centrosome-associated structures that sequester proteasomal components, normally localize in the perinuclear area presumably to guard the nucleus and protect other organelles from exposure to the potentially toxic proteins, but in PD the normal aggresome formation is impaired and therefore these cells do not benefit from the potentially cytoprotective response. This finding is one piece of growing evidence that inhibition of the ubiquitin-proteasome pathway leads to altered protein handling and Lewy body formation. Thus, as a result of an age-related or disease-related impaired proteasomal system, both normal and abnormal proteins accumulate and aggregate to form Lewy bodies, which in turn leads to neurodegeneration. The impaired proteasomal-ubiquitin process, coupled with selectively increased oxidative stress, leads to apoptosis and cell death. Metabolic pathways for DA generate numerous byproducts that include hydrogen peroxide, superoxide anions, and hydroxy-radicals. Interaction between these chemicals and membrane lipids leads to lipid peroxidation; membrane disruption; and, potentially, cell death. In support of this hypothesis, several observations are pertinent: (1) glutathione peroxidase, a tripeptide normally present in brain that is reduced with oxidative stress, is markedly reduced in the SN of patients with PD; (2) elemental iron, which can facilitate the formation of free radicals in the nervous system, is increased in the brains of PD patients; (3) the iron-chelating protein ferritin is decreased or of normal concentration in PD, so that compensatory increases to handle elemental iron do not occur; and (4) specific enzymatic activity defects in complex 1 of the mitochondrial respiratory chain appear to occur in the SN of the brains of patients with PD. Whereas all these events develop and probably reflect or provoke oxidative stress in the SN, the actual precipitant, whether genetic, environmental, dietary, or multifactorial, remains to be determined.

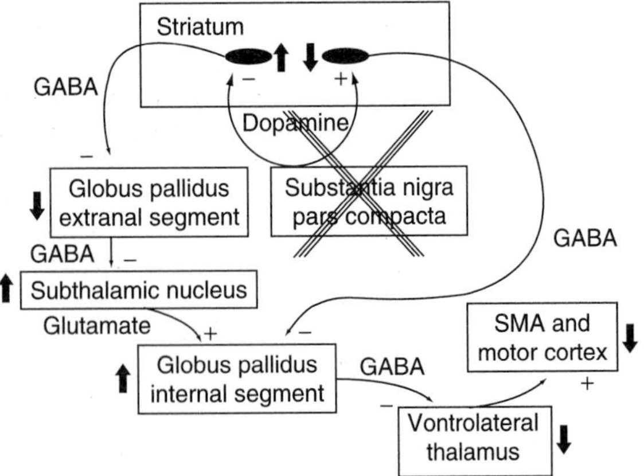

FIGURE 34–2. Basal ganglia circuitry relevant to pathogenesis of PD. GABA, Gamma-aminobutyric acid; SMA, supplementary motor area.

Although the primary lesion involves dopamine, other neurotransmitter systems are also affected. At the level of the striatum, muscarinic cholinergic function competes with dopaminergic activity, and hence in PD, there is a relative overactivity of acetylcholine. Also, other pigmented nuclei besides the SN degenerate, and changes in norepinephrine and serotonin result from changes in the locus caeruleus and dorsal raphe, respectively.

Epidemiology and Risk Factors. Population-based surveys in the United States, Portugal, and Italy have reported that the prevalence of PD ranges from 107 to 187 per 100,000 population.[3] A community study of the elderly in a suburb of Boston, however, found parkinsonian features in 159 of 467 (34 percent) individuals aged 65 years or older.[4] This study suggests that at least one third of the elderly exhibit some evidence of PD or other parkinsonian disorders.

Although both environmental and inherited factors have been implicated in the pathogenesis of PD, no specific cause has been found. Case-controlled studies have documented an increase in risk for PD associated with a family history of PD, insecticide exposure, herbicide exposure, rural residency at the time of diagnosis, well water exposure, and nut or seed eating 10 years prior to diagnosis.[5] Study of time trends over 15 years in the incidence of parkinsonism in Olmsted

County, Minnesota, found no evidence of major environmental risk factors for PD.[6] Exposure to hydrocarbon solvents has been associated with earlier onset of symptoms and more severe PD and other forms of parkinsonism.[7, 8] Welders with PD were found to have their onset of PD on the average 17 years earlier than a control population of PD patients, suggesting that welding, possibly by causing manganese toxicity, is a risk factor for PD.[9] Numerous reports suggest the possibility that the frequency of PD is decreased in patients with a history of cigarette smoking and caffeine consumption.[10–12] The best studied model of parkinsonism is that produced by 1-methyl-4-phenyl-1,2,3,6-tetrahydropyridine (MPTP), a meperidine analogue first developed during the production of an illicit drug. This compound, when injected intravenously, produces parkinsonism in humans and animals.[13]

Twin studies suggest that genetic predisposition may play a role in the development of PD,[14] and a number of parkinsonian pedigrees have been reported.[15–18] The gene locus in one autosomal dominant pedigree was isolated to chromosome 4q21.23 and was later found to involve Ala53thr substitution in the α-synuclein gene.[19] It has been hypothesized that this and other mutations cause the natively unfolded α-synuclein protein to alter its secondary structure, ubiquitinate, and self-aggregate.[20] In addition to mutations in the gene coding for α-synuclein, there is a growing number of parkinsonian disorders associated with specific genetic defects. For example, one of the most common causes of young-onset parkinsonism is an autosomal recessive form of PD (ARPD) due to mutations in the gene called Parkin (PARK2) on chromosome 6q25.2–27. This 500 kbase, 12-exon gene encodes a 465–amino acid protein containing an N-terminal ubiquitin-like motif and C-terminal RING finger motif. Multiple mutations have been identified in this gene among families with this levodopa-responsive form of PD.[21] Parkin, the protein product of the Parkin gene, is expressed in SN and other brain regions as well as in Lewy bodies of patients with PD.[22] Normal parkin is thus involved in ubiquitination and subsequent degradation of certain proteins, but mutated parkin protein loses this activity and thus may lead to an accumulation of proteins, yet to be identified. This process could cause a selective neural cell death without formation of Lewy bodies. In contrast to typical PD, patients with ARPD often present with a dystonic gait during early adulthood. The mean age at onset of this variant is 25, but the disease may not present until age 58. Parkin gene mutation phenotypes range from dopa-responsive dystonia to young-onset PD with early levodopa-induced dyskinesias, to otherwise typical PD. In one study, 36 of 73 (49 percent) families with PD onset at 45 or younger had a mutation in the Parkin gene: 10 of 13 (77 percent) patients with onset at 20 or before and 2 of 64 (3 percent) patients with onset at 30 or later.[23] Another gene locus for PD has been found on chromosome 2p13.[24] This locus (PARK3) was detected in a group of European families with a mean age at onset of 59 years. Although some members of the kindreds had prominent dementia, the autopsy in some cases confirmed the typical pathological features of PD, including Lewy bodies. An autosomal dominant, levodopa-responsive, Lewy body parkinsonism has been recently mapped to chromosome 4p15.7 (PARK4).[25] The haplotype also occurred in members of the family who did not have any clinical evidence of parkinsonism but rather exhibited postural tremor phenomenologically identical to essential tremor (ET). This finding and other data provide further evidence that PD and ET may be associated and genetically related.[26] The finding of a mutation in the deubiquinating enzyme ubiquitin carboxy-terminal hydrolase L1 (UCH-L1) gene on 4p14 in one German family with autosomal dominant PD (PARK5)[27] further supports the concept that an impairment of normal protein degradation is an important mechanism of neurodegeneration in PD. More recently, two loci on chromosome 1 have been found to be associated with autosomal recessive, early-onset parkinsonism: 1p35–36 (PARK6)[28] and 1p36 (PARK7).[29] In addition to these parkinsonism-related gene loci, there may be multiple genetic factors important in the pathogenesis of PD and other parkinsonian disorders. In a complete genomic screen of 174 families with multiple individuals diagnosed with PD involving a total of 870 family members (378 with PD), Scott and colleagues[30] found LOD scores ranging from 1.5 to 5.47 indicative of linkage to the following five chromosomal regions: 6 (in the Parkin gene), 17q (in the Tau gene), 8p, 5q, and 9q.

Clinical Findings and Associated Disorders. The cardinal features of PD include resting tremor, rigidity, bradykinesia, and postural instability. Many movement disorder specialists consider a good response to levodopa or dopamine agonists useful in clinically supporting the diagnosis. The rest tremor usually consists of an oscillatory movement of 4 to 7 Hz frequency that involves the limbs, jaw, face, and tongue but almost never involves the head itself. The tremor of the forearm is often pronating and supinating, while the hand tremor has been described as "pill-rolling." Early in the course of the disease, the tremors and other signs are usually asymmetrical but eventually become bilateral. In addition to the rest tremor that is so distinctive of PD, most patients also have a postural tremor, which is evident with the hands extended or in action. This postural tremor probably represents re-emergence of rest tremor or co-existent ET (see later discussion). Tremor in patients with ET, in contrast to PD, often involves not only the hands but also the head and voice, rarely affects the legs, and improves frequently with alcohol, propranolol, or primidone. Some PD patients or their relatives have an associated postural tremor that appears as ET and precedes the onset of PD symptoms by several years or decades, suggesting a possible link between the two conditions, at least in some families.

Bradykinesia (slowness of movement) or hypokinesia (poverty of movement) is manifested by slowing of activities of daily living such as dressing, feeding, brushing teeth, and bathing. Other features of bradykinesia or hypokinesia include masked facies (hypomimia), hypokinetic dysarthria, drooling, and slow and small handwriting (micrographia). On examination, rapid alternating movements are performed slowly and with decreasing amplitude. In more advanced stages, frequent arrests of movement, called "freezing" or "motor blocks," may be seen. These are manifested by an interruption in finger tapping or hand clasping, start hesitation such as an inability to initiate gait or other movements, and freezing when turning or walking through narrow passages.

Postural instability also often occurs in the more advanced stages of the disease. This gait and postural difficulty is frequently accompanied by small steps and festination, a tendency when standing or walking to propulse involuntarily or to retropulse and fall. In the distinctive "pull test" the

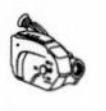

examiner stands behind the patient and tugs briskly on the shoulders; the PD subject takes several small steps backward, possibly falling into the examiner's arms.

Most of the other signs of PD represent variations of these cardinal characteristics: sialorrhea, dysphagia, difficulty in turning in bed, and ambulatory problems that become progressively worse. Sleep disruption is common in PD patients, who demonstrate fragmented sleep and frequent awakenings. Recent studies suggest that a distinctive sleep aberration, REM behavioral disorder (see Chapter 54), may be a frequent early element of PD. Additionally, akathisia, an uncomfortable feeling that drives the patient to move, can be a prominent and poorly appreciated aspect of untreated PD, and this behavior may be related to dopaminergic dysfunction. Besides motor symptoms, PD patients may also exhibit several behavioral changes, including depression in at least one third of patients, and dementia in an equal proportion. Frontal release, or "cortical disinhibition" signs, may be seen, but they are not specific for PD. Pain, burning, coldness, numbness, and other sensory symptoms, often wrongly attributed to bursitis or arthritis, are reported by about half of patients. Seborrhea, particularly that involving the face, is an example of systemic involvement in PD.

The mean age of clinical onset of PD is the mid-fifties, but the range is very wide, and some patients present in their twenties and thirties, while others show no signs until their eighties. Although there are many exceptions, young patients often present with tremor-predominant disease and elderly patients with gait dysfunction and akinesia. Juvenile PD is a childhood and adolescent disease, presenting with parkinsonism and dystonia, and has a different histological appearance than PD.

Differential Diagnosis. Besides PD, there are many other causes of parkinsonism (Table 34–1). The second most common group is the parkinsonism-plus syndromes (12 percent), a conglomerate term for a large number of degenerative disorders in which parkinsonism is one of several neurological features. Drug-induced parkinsonism (8 percent) and heredo-

TABLE 34–1. **Classification of Parkinsonism**

I. Primary Parkinsonism
   - Parkinson's disease
   - Juvenile parkinsonism

II. Multiple System Degenerations (Parkinsonism-Plus Syndromes)
   - Progressive supranuclear palsy (PSP)
   - Multiple system atrophy (MSA)
     - Striatonigral degeneration (SND)
     - Olivopontocerebellar atrophy (OPCA)
     - Shy-Drager syndrome (SDS)
   - Lytico-Bodig or parkinsonism-dementia-ALS complex of Guam (PDACG)
   - Cortical-basal ganglionic degeneration (CBGD)
   - Progressive pallidal atrophy

III. Hereditary Parkinsonism
   - Hereditary juvenile dystonia-parkinsonism
   - Autosomal dominant Lewy body disease
   - Huntington's disease (HD)
   - Wilson's disease (WD)
   - Hereditary ceruloplasmin deficiency
   - Hallervorden-Spatz disease (HSD), also known as neurodegeneration with brain iron accumulation Type I (NBIA-I)
   - Olivopontocerebellar and spinocerebellar degenerations (OPCA and SCA)
   - Familial amyotrophy-dementia-parkinsonism
   - Disinhibition-dementia-parkinsonism-amyotrophy complex
   - Gerstmann-Strausler-Scheinker disease
   - Familial progressive subcortical gliosis
   - Lubag (X-linked dystonia-parkinsonism)
   - Familial basal ganglia calcification
   - Mitochondrial cytopathies with striatal necrosis
   - Ceroid lipofuscinosis
   - Familial parkinsonism with peripheral neuropathy
   - Parkinsonian-pyramidal syndrome
   - Neuroacanthocytosis (NA)
   - Hereditary hemochromatosis

IV. Secondary (Acquired, Symptomatic) Parkinsonism
   - Infectious: postencephalitic, AIDS, SSPE, Creutzfeldt-Jakob disease, prior diseases
   - Drugs: dopamine receptor–blocking drugs (antipsychotic, antiemetic drugs), reserpine, tetrabenazine, alpha-methyldopa, lithium, flunarizine, cinnarizine
   - Toxins: MPTP, CO, Mn, Hg, CS_2, cyanide, methanol, ethanol
   - Vascular: multi-infarct, Binswanger's disease
   - Trauma: pugilistic encephalopathy
   - Other: parathyroid abnormalities, hypothyroidism, hepatocerebral degeneration, brain tumor, paraneoplastic diseases, normal pressure hydrocephalus, noncommunicating hydrocephalus, syringomesencephalia, hemiatrophy-hemiparkinsonism, peripherally induced tremor and parkinsonism, and psychogenic disorders

degenerative conditions, such as juvenile Huntington's disease, are less frequent. Cyanide intoxication and carbon monoxide poisoning associated with bilateral pallidal necrosis are examples of an acute cause of parkinsonism,[10] and other toxins such as carbon disulfide and manganese can also produce parkinsonism, the latter often preceded by psychiatric difficulties ("manganese madness"). Reversible parkinsonism is caused by drugs, especially neuroleptics and metoclopramide, and lesser known agents such as alpha-methyldopa, reserpine, amiodarone, and certain calcium channel blockers must also be considered in the differential diagnosis. Finally, patients in whom PD is suspected should be screened for potential illicit narcotic exposure, a travel history, or an underlying medical illness such as the acquired immunodeficiency syndrome that would predispose them to opportunistic infections including abscesses, and a family history of neurological disorders should be obtained as well. A past medical history of stroke or hypertension may suggest a subcortical vascular encephalopathy presenting with parkinsonian features, and old meningitis or head trauma could suggest normal pressure hydrocephalus presenting with freezing, festination, and a gait disorder sometimes confused with parkinsonism.

Evaluation. When all four cardinal characteristic signs are present, and the patient shows a brisk response to dopaminergic therapy, the diagnosis is straightforward. Part of the workup usually includes a magnetic resonance imaging (MRI) scan, looking for evidence of alternate diagnoses such as stroke, intoxications, or other degenerative disorders.[31] Although it is not yet firmly established, cerebrospinal fluid (CSF) homovanillic acid, the final metabolite of dopamine, especially when expressed as a ratio to CSF xanthine, may become a future marker of disease activity.

Management. The large array of drugs used in the treatment of PD is outlined in Table 34–2 with standard doses and side effects. Treatment of symptomatic PD is based primarily on restoring a deficiency of DA due to a loss of dopamine-producing cells in the SN.[31] This neurotransmitter is synthesized from the amino acid tyrosine. The conversion of tyrosine to levodopa is facilitated by the rate-limiting enzyme tyrosine hydroxylase; levodopa is in turn converted into dopamine by the nonspecific enzyme dopa-decarboxylase. These dopaminergic neurons synapse with cholinergic interneurons and gamma-aminobutyric acid (GABA)–ergic outflow neurons in the striatum.

Five subtypes of DA receptors have been identified; the D_1 and D_2 receptors are most prominent in the striatum, and the D_3, D_4, and D_5 receptors are present in the limbic system and other dopaminergic pathways. The D_1 receptor is linked to adenylate cyclase. In contrast, the D_2 receptor is activated by

TABLE 34–2. **Medications for Parkinson's Disease**

Medications	Dosage	Side Effects
Dopaminergic Drugs		
Precursor amino acid: levodopa		Nausea, hypotension, confusion, hallucinations, dyskinesia
Carbidopa/levodopa	10/100, 25/100, 25/250, 100–1000 mg/d	
Controlled release	25/100, 50/200, 200–1400 mg/d	
Dopamine agonists		Somnolence, confusion, hallucinations, hypotension
Bromocriptine	2.5–60 mg/d	
Pergolide	0.25–60 mg/d	
Pramipexole		
Ropinirole		
Monamine oxidase B inhibitor		Sleep disturbance, lightheadedness, hallucinations
Selegiline (deprenyl)	5–10 mg/d	
Indirect agonist		Hallucinations, dry mouth, livedo reticularis, ankle swelling, myoclonic encephalopathy in setting of renal failure
Amantadine	100–300 mg/d	
Catecholamine-O-Methyl Transferase inhibitor		Used in conjunction with levodopa: dyskinesia, lightheadedness
Tolcapone	300–600 mg/d	
Entacopone	200 mg, 2 to 8 times/day with each dose of carbidopa/levodopa	
Other Drug Classes		
Anticholinergics		Confusion, sleepiness, blurred vision, constipation
Trihexyphenidyl	2–15 mg/d	
Biperidine	1–8 mg/d	
Novel neuroleptics: used for psychosis and unusual tremor		
Clozapine	12.5–100 mg/d	Fatal neutropenia, somnolence
Quetiapine	12.5–100 mg/d	Somnolence, potential aggravated parkinsonism
Miscellaneous		
Amitriptyline: used for sleep fragmentation	10–50 mg/d at bedtime	Dry mouth, forgetfulness, blurred vision, constipation
Baclofen: used for dystonic cramps	10–80 mg/d	Sleepiness, dizziness

DA and DA agonists. The different roles of D_1 and D_2 receptors in regulation of striatal function have not been fully defined, but the D_2 receptor appears to be more important in mediating the parkinsonian symptoms. In the brain in PD, the D_1 receptors in the striatum appear to be reduced (downregulated), whereas the D_2 receptors are increased (upregulated).[15] As a result of nigrostriatal deficiency, activation of the indirect D_2-mediated, inhibitory (GABA) striatopallidal pathway is increased, resulting in disinhibition of the subthalamic nucleus and the globus pallidus internum (GP_i), the main output nucleus from the basal ganglia. The increased activation of the GP_i is further enhanced by disinhibition of the decreased activity of the direct D_1-mediated, inhibitory (GABA) striatopallidal pathway (see Fig. 34–2).

The most effective treatment for the symptoms of PD is levodopa, but the chronic use of levodopa is complicated by the development of two motor problems, namely, fluctuations and dyskinesias in about half the patients after 5 years of therapy. Fluctuations are irregular and clinically unpredictable responses to medications, and dyskinesias are involuntary, usually choreic, but sometimes dystonic movements that are drug induced. Levodopa is absorbed in the small intestine via a large neutral amino acid transporter system and is then converted to DA by the ubiquitous enzyme dopa-decarboxylase. Conversion to DA outside the blood-brain barrier activates the area postrema and is largely responsible for some of the early side effects of levodopa, particularly nausea and vomiting. The addition of dopa-decarboxylase inhibitors that do not cross the blood-brain barrier (e.g., carbidopa or benserazide) minimizes DA formation in the periphery and greatly improves patient tolerance to therapy. This is the concept behind the use of the carbidopa-levodopa combination (e.g., Sinemet), which is prescribed as a ratio of carbidopa to levodopa (25/100, 25/250, or 10/100) and more recently has become available in a controlled-release formulation (CR 50/200 or CR 25/100). Approximately 100 mg of carbidopa per day is needed for effective peripheral blockade. Although carbidopa is useful in preventing the "peripheral" side effects of levodopa, the motor side effects of fluctuations and dyskinesia as well as psychiatric reactions such as confusion, delusions, and visual hallucinations are not prevented or ameliorated by its addition to levodopa.

In the early stages of levodopa therapy, motor fluctuations correlate well with plasma levodopa levels. Initially, patients may report a "wearing-off" or end-of-dose deterioration in mobility, which is thought to result from a reduced duration of therapeutic plasma and brain levels of levodopa. A typical patient may also notice dyskinesias or involuntary movements related to peak plasma levodopa levels ("peak dose dyskinesia"). Most patients have this pattern of response characterized by improvement-dyskinesia-improvement (IDI). About 15 percent of patients who are treated chronically with levodopa experience initial dyskinesia within a few minutes after ingestion of levodopa; this is followed by an improvement in parkinsonian symptoms for 2 to 4 hours and then by subsequent recurrence of dyskinesia, usually in the form of dystonia. This diphasic dyskinesia pattern of dyskinesia-improvement-dyskinesia is referred to as the DID response. Treatment of these motor fluctuations is based on "smoothing out" the plasma concentration curves either by giving more frequent smaller doses of levodopa, converting to the controlled-release form of levodopa, or, in the patient with markedly advanced disease, titrating the medication by having the patient sip very small quantities of Sinemet dissolved in water or juice every 30 or 60 minutes throughout the waking day.[16] In patients with advancing disease who have had prolonged levodopa therapy, more complex and less predictable ("on-off") motor fluctuations occur. For instance, patients may change from relatively normal function to a frozen akinetic state in as little as 15 seconds (sudden on-off), or they may develop severe dyskinesia at both the peak effect of the levodopa dose and at the end of the dose (biphasic dyskinesia). The mechanism of these motor fluctuations and dyskinesias is not well understood, but there is a growing body of evidence supporting the notion that some of these problems arise from the combination of loss of presynaptic DA storage capacity and postsynaptic receptor alterations.[17]

In the 1980s, the monoamine oxidase-B (MAO-B) inhibitor deprenyl (selegiline) was reported to delay the clinical progression of PD. In a large multicenter trial, the Deprenyl and Tocopherol Antioxidative Trial of Parkinson's Disease (DATATOP), deprenyl but not tocopherol delayed the need for levodopa by approximately 9 months.[18] Whether this is due to deprenyl's beneficial effect on the parkinsonian symptoms or to a putative neuroprotective action is a subject of continued debate. Other MAO-B inhibitors, such as lazabemide, have been evaluated in PD as well, but long-term protocols aimed at defining neuroprotective mechanisms have not been carried out.

In the early stages of PD, anticholinergic (e.g., trihexyphenidyl) therapy may provide moderate improvement. This strategy is based on the neurochemical competition between DA and acetylcholine in the striatum. Amantadine, an antiviral agent, has mild dopaminergic activity and possibly anticholinergic action as well. Amantadine and anticholinergic agents may produce dry mouth, nausea, vomiting, blurring of vision, visual hallucinations, and other mental changes. Because of the anticholinergic side effects, patients with glaucoma, prostatic hypertrophy, and dementia may experience exacerbations of these conditions with these agents. Amantadine may also cause pitting edema and livedo reticularis, a purplish-reddish mottling of the skin, particularly the skin below the knees; it should be avoided in patients with impaired renal function.

Since the introduction of bromocriptine and pergolide, DA agonists, which are agents that stimulate dopamine receptors themselves, have played an increasingly important role in the treatment of PD. Because these medications have a relatively long half-life, they are used most frequently to prolong the effects of levodopa and thus smooth out motor fluctuations. While some movement disorder specialists advocate the use of DA agonists in the early phases of pharmacological therapy, others introduce DA agonists after the dose of levodopa has reached 300 to 600 mg/day or when levodopa-related fluctuations emerge. Side effects associated with DA agonists include nausea, drowsiness, confusion, hallucinations, orthostatic hypotension, exacerbation of dyskinesias, erythromelalgia and, rarely, pulmonary fibrosis. The latter two side effects have been attributed to the ergot structure of pergolide and bromocriptine, and they almost never occur with the non-ergoline DA agonists pramipexole and ropinirole.

As a result of new findings suggesting levodopa sparing and possibly neuroprotective effects of DA agonists, their role in the management of PD has shifted from being primarily used late in the disease in conjunction with levodopa (adjunctive therapy) to being also used as early symptomatic treatment. Several studies have now demonstrated that when introduced in early stages of PD, dopamine agonists provide adequate symptomatic benefit and delay the need for levodopa, thus minimizing the risk of levodopa-related dyskinesias and motor fluctuations.[32, 33]

Among DA agonists, apomorphine is the only short-acting compound. As an injectable DA agonist, it can be useful in "rescuing" some PD patients from sudden, unpredictable off periods. Because of the strong emetic response with this agent, however, coadministration of the peripheral DA receptor–blocking drug domperidone is usually necessary.

Another new class of drugs is the catechol-O-methyltransferase (COMT) inhibitors such as entacapone and tolcapone. By limiting DA metabolism, they increase levodopa bioavailability, prolong the "on" response to levodopa, reduce motor fluctuations effectively, and allow a reduction in daily levodopa dosage.[34]

Of particular interest in PD during the last several years has been the use of various surgical procedures, which have capitalized on a growing knowledge of basal ganglia anatomy and physiology (see Fig. 34–2).[35] The traditional ablative procedures are gradually giving way to newer strategies, particularly deep brain stimulation (DBS). Besides lower risks associated with surgery, DBS has the advantage of customizing the stimulating parameters to the needs of the individual patient. In a multicenter, prospective, double-blind, crossover study in 143 patients with advanced PD who received bilateral high-frequency stimulation of SN or GP_i, the Unified Parkinson's Disease Rating Scale (UPDRS) motor scores improved by 49 percent ($p < 0.001$) and 37 percent ($p < 0.001$), respectively, in comparison to the non-stimulated state.[36] Furthermore, 6 months following implantation as compared to baseline, the percent time "on" without dyskinesias increased from 27 to 74 ($p < 0.001$) and 28 to 64 ($p < 0.001$) with SN and GP_i DBS, respectively. Adverse events included intracranial hemorrhage in seven and lead displacement in two. While the levodopa dosage remained unchanged in the GP_i group, the daily levodopa dose equivalents were reduced by 37 percent in the SN DBS group ($p < 0.001$). Freed et al[37] reported the results of the first double-blind placebo-controlled trial of fetal graft transplantation for advanced PD. Forty patients, stratified by age into younger than and older than 60 years, with approximately a 7-year history of PD symptoms, were randomized to receive either four embryonic mesencephalons delivered via four needle passes to the left and right putamen or a sham operation (four drill holes to the forehead without dural penetration). After 1 year, the "sham-operated" patients were given the option to be implanted and were then followed in an open label manner; a total of 33 patients received an implant. Overall, there was no difference between the implanted versus sham patients with respect to the primary outcome variable, a global rating by the patients (from −3, PD markedly worse to +3, PD markedly improved). There was, however, a significant improvement in bradykinesia and rigidity, but only in the younger (<60 years old) patients. There was no improvement in freezing or motor fluctuations, and gait actually deteriorated. Although there were more adverse events in the implanted group, these were not considered directly related to the surgery. There was a marked placebo effect, sometimes lasting the whole year. Of 20 implanted patients, 17 had evidence of fiber outgrowth from the transplanted tissue as indicated by ^{18}F-fluorodopa positron-emission tomography (PET) scans, and in the younger patients, PET results and UPDRS improvements correlated. Most importantly, 5 of 33 patients who eventually received the implant experienced dyskinesias even during "off" periods. These dyskinesias are hypothesized to be the result of release of DA from the fetal implant. They have been successfully treated with GP_i DBS in three of the five patients.

Because of the remarkable array of options in the treatment of PD, it is reasonable to approach the treatment of each patient with a basic algorithm (Table 34–3). For all patients, education, exercise, and good nutrition are considered useful. If patients have no significant functional impairment in terms of independent living, consideration of a mild dopaminergic drug with a putatively neuroprotective strategy in the form of deprenyl can be considered. If additional symptomatic relief is needed, most movement disorder specialists add a DA agonist and later, when symptoms need urgent treatment to protect the patient's safety or job security, levodopa is introduced. If symptoms can be treated more slowly, the use of anticholinergic drugs in young patients with tremor-predominant PD is often helpful, and amantadine can be used as a mild dopaminergic drug to delay the need to start

TABLE 34–3. **An Algorithm for Managing Parkinson's Disease at Different Phases**

For All Patients: education, physical or exercise therapy, good nutrition

For Patients with No Clinically Significant Disability:
- Consider selegiline
- Consider referral to study centers for trials of new neuroprotective strategies

For Patients with Clinically Significant Disability:
- *Job security threatened or health endangered:*
  - Levodopa, usually controlled-release formulation
- *Job security NOT threatened and health NOT endangered:*
  - Young and tremor-predominant disease: Anticholinergic drugs, amantadine, selegeline
  - Older patients: amantadine, dopamine agonists
  - Elderly patients or cognitively impaired: levodopa

Above Patients with Progressive Disability:
- Add levodopa either as controlled-release or standard formulation
- Once on levodopa, if added prolongation of effect is needed, add selegiline if patient is not currently taking it or, in the future, catechol-O-methyl (COMT) transferase inhibitors may become available

Patients with Specific Complications:
- *Patients on levodopa who develop motor fluctuations:*
  - More frequent, small doses of levodopa or liquid Sinemet
  - Selegiline agonists (or COMT inhibitors)
  - Consider deep brain stimulation (DBS) of the subthalamic nucleus
- *Patients with unremitting tremor:*
  - Deep brain stimulation
- *Patients with hallucinations:*
  - Reduce medications. Stop all drugs except Sinemet
  - Consider Quetiapine, atypical neuroleptic

levodopa in other patients. In patients who are just starting levodopa/carbidopa, the controlled-release form is often selected to minimize the number of doses needed each day. As the disease progresses, combinations of drugs are usually needed, and most patients will require both an agonist and levodopa/carbidopa within the first 7 years of therapy. In elderly patients, especially those with hallucinations or dementia, however, levodopa/carbidopa alone, usually in the regular formulation, is often the most practical regimen because of its relative simplicity. In terms of referral to a movement disorder specialist, if patients develop complicated dyskinesias, a prominent behavioral problem, or additional neurological signs that suggest the presence of another parkinsonian disorder (parkinsonism-plus syndromes), they should be evaluated in a center that has expertise in these unusual problems with access to experimental drugs and surgical protocols.

One particularly difficult problem in managing PD patients is hallucinosis. Patients who are treated chronically with dopaminergic drugs develop visual hallucinations that can become frightening and severely disabling to the patient and caregiver. In this situation, the drug dosage should be reduced, and most patients are best managed on levodopa/carbidopa alone. In some instances, atypical neuroleptics with few extrapyramidal side effects can be used. Clozapine has been successful in abating hallucinations and psychotic behavior in PD patients, but it is an expensive drug and is associated with the potentially lethal side effect of agranulocytosis.[38] Other atypical antipsychotic drugs, particularly quetiapine, are often used to control drug-induced psychosis without aggravating underlying parkinsonism. Whenever a neuroleptic agent is introduced, however, careful monitoring is needed to ensure that parkinsonism is not exacerbated.

Prognosis and Future Perspectives. Survival of patients with PD has greatly improved since the development of levodopa. Prior to the advent of levodopa, mortality among PD patients was three times the normally expected rate. However, with the advent of levodopa and other medications, the life span of PD patients is almost the same as that of an age-matched control population without the disease.[39] Some studies have suggested that PD patients are more likely to die from infection than from cancer compared to an age-matched group of controls. Early, even presymptomatic, detection of disease is paramount to early intervention, and major efforts are currently aimed at identifying biological markers for both the presence of disease (trait marker) and disease activity (state marker).

PARKINSONISM-PLUS SYNDROMES

In addition to Parkinson's disease, parkinsonism is one of the major clinical features in several other primary neurodegenerative conditions. However, because they all have additional features not typical of Parkinson's disease and share an overall worse prognosis and poorer response to antiparkinsonian therapy, they are often grouped together under the conglomerate term parkinsonism-plus syndromes. Within this group, each condition has distinctive characteristics that must be recognized and distinguished from one another and from PD.

Progressive Supranuclear Palsy

Pathogenesis and Pathophysiology. Progressive supranuclear palsy (PSP) is the most common and best recognized entity among the parkinsonism-plus syndromes. PSP is an idiopathic condition with no known precipitant or strong genetic component. Postmortem analysis of the brains of PSP patients show neuronal loss, gliosis, and neurofibrillary tangles composed of straight and paired helical filaments.[40] The SN, subthalamic nucleus, globus pallidus, superior colliculus, pretectal area, and substantia innominata are the sites of maximum involvement. Dopaminergic, cholinergic, and adrenergic neurotransmitter systems are affected, provoking a far more diffuse degenerative process than that seen in Parkinson's disease.[13] There is a growing body of evidence that PSP is due to an alteration in the gene on chromosome 17 coding for the tau protein.[41]

Epidemiology and Risk Factors. A medically based survey in central New Jersey found that the age-adjusted prevalence of PSP was 1.38 per 100,000 population, and men appeared to be slightly more frequently affected than women.[42] Most patients experience the initial symptoms during their sixth and seventh decades. No clear geographic, occupational, or temporal clusters of PSP have been found. Although PSP is not considered a genetic disorder, rare familial clusters have been reported and Conrad and colleagues have identified an association with a particular tau genetic factor.

Clinical Features and Associated Disorders. PSP shares some clinical features with PD, such as bradykinesia, rigidity, dysarthria, dysphagia, and dementia. However, PSP patients rarely exhibit tremor and usually have much more profound postural instability. In addition, axial rigidity is more prominent than limb rigidity. Some patients with PSP also develop severe palilalia, emotional incontinence, and other evidence of bilateral frontal lobe dysfunction.[40]

The best known feature of PSP, vertical ocular gaze paresis, may be overcome by passive head movement, which activates the oculocephalic reflexes (hence the designation supranuclear). Riley and colleagues[43] reported five patients who presented with "pure akinesia" of gait, speech, and handwriting without rigidity, tremor, dementia, or eye movement abnormalities on clinical examination. None of the patients responded to levodopa, and four demonstrated subtle changes in vertical saccades on eyelid movement recordings.[43] The diagnostic criteria for PSP have been recently refined as a result of careful clinical-pathological correlative studies, and the greatest diagnostic confidence is placed in the combined clinical features of early frequent falls within the first year of clinical disease and vertical downward supranuclear paresis on examination.[44]

Differential Diagnosis. Whereas PSP is idiopathic, the same clinical syndrome has been associated with Alzheimer's disease, multiple strokes, multiple system atrophy (MSA), posthypoxic encephalopathy, and Whipple's disease. Parkinson's disease itself and the other parkinsonism-plus syndromes, including corticobasal ganglionic degeneration (CBD), Lewy body dementia, normal pressure hydrocephalus, and "multi-infarct parkinsonism" must also be considered. Rarely, other conditions such as dentatorubro-pallido-luysian atrophy, neuroacanthocytosis, progressive external ophthalmoplegia, and hydrocephalus may present with oculomotility disorders that are suggestive of PSP.

Evaluation. MRI should be performed in patients in whom PSP is suspected to rule out a multi-infarct state or hydrocephalus. Single photon emission computed tomography (SPECT) and PET demonstrate prefrontal hypoactivity and show evidence of severe involvement of the dopaminergic terminals as well as the postsynaptic DA receptors in the striatum.[45]

Management. Although PSP is associated with loss of multiple neurotransmitters, pharmacological therapies remain disappointing. Levodopa ameliorates the bradykinesia and rigidity in about a third of cases, but the benefit rarely persists beyond 1 or 2 years. DA agonists rarely provide additional benefit. If, however, the dopaminergic drugs improve the bradykinesia but have no impact on poor balance, the medicated patient may feel more agile and independent, only to fall more frequently, leading to consequently greater disability. Anticholinergic drugs and tricyclic antidepressants with anticholinergic effects (e.g., amitriptyline) may be helpful in treating emotional incontinence. Idazoxan, a noradrenergic drug, produced modest improvement in a small number of patients, but sympathomimetic and other side effects have limited further development of this drug.[46] Blepharospasm, occasionally associated with PSP, responds to botulinum toxin injection, and dry eyes may be treated with topical lubricants. Although physical, occupational, and speech therapy are of limited potential, these options may be beneficial in some patients and their families. Electroconvulsive therapy, adrenal implantation, and pallidotomy have been of no benefit.

Prognosis and Future Perspectives. The median interval from onset of the initial symptom, regardless of its nature, to onset of gait difficulty is estimated at 0.3 years; to the need for gait assistance, 3.1 years; to confinement to bed or wheelchair, 8.2 years; and to death, 9.7 years.[42] The problems that most frequently cause complications or death are falls and aspiration.

Multiple System Atrophy

Pathogenesis and Pathophysiology. The pathogenic mechanisms of MSA remain unknown, and in contrast to PD, there is no evidence that genetic factors play a role. Recent findings link MSA to PD and related neurodegenerative disorders as "α-synucleinopathies."[19] Whereas the initial neurodegenerative events are unclear, in well-established cases, the staining characteristics and distribution of oligodendroglial fibrillary cytoplasmic inclusions are distinctively different from the neurofibrillary tangles of Alzheimer's disease, PSP, postencephalitic parkinsonism, and others.[47] Highly variable neuronal loss and gliosis are seen in the substantia nigra, caudate, putamen, cerebellar cortex, pyramidal tract, Edinger-Westphal nucleus, locus caeruleus, inferior olives, dorsal motor nucleus of the vagus, Purkinje cells, intermediolateral cell column of the spinal cord, spinocerebellar tracts, and Onuf's nucleus. Reduced dopamine or norepinephrine levels occur in the nigra, nucleus accumbens, septum, hypothalamus, and locus caeruleus.[47]

Epidemiology and Risk Factors. In a review of autopsies of parkinsonism, Quinn reported frequencies ranging from 3.6 to 22 percent, with a mean of 8.2 percent (68/833 cases).[48] However, no study has been undertaken to determine the population prevalence of MSA. At one large referral center, 100 patients with MSA reported a median age at onset of 53 years (range, 33 to 76 years).[49]

Clinical Features and Associated Disorders. MSA encompasses three neurodegenerative syndromes, which in the past were considered clinically distinct: striatonigral degeneration (SND), olivopontocerebellar atrophy (OPCA), and Shy-Drager syndrome (SDS). All these conditions share similarities with one another and with PD. The hallmark features of MSA are parkinsonism that is poorly responsive to levodopa therapy and varying degrees of autonomic, cerebellar, and pyramidal dysfunction. SDS is diagnosed clinically when dysautonomia far outweighs the other signs, SND is designated when anterocollis and pyramidal dysfunction are prominent, and OPCA is used to characterize the patient with prominent cerebellar features of ataxia, limb dyssynergia, and kinetic tremor. For all MSA patients, autonomic insufficiencies include orthostatic hypotension, postprandial hypotension, anhidrosis with thermoregulatory disturbances, poor lacrimation and salivation, constipation, and impotence. Disturbances in bladder emptying and incontinence may also occur. In addition, emotional lability, pyramidal signs, supranuclear ophthalmoplegia, anterocollis, myoclonus, sleep apnea and other ventilatory dysrhythmias, respiratory stridor, polyneuropathy, amyotrophy, and dementia may be present in any of the forms.[44] The variety of clinical presentations is wide, and pure autonomic failure, sleep apnea syndromes, some forms of peripheral neuropathies, and conditions that clinically resemble amyotrophic lateral sclerosis all may represent forms of underlying MSA.

Differential Diagnosis. Parkinson's disease, particularly in patients with prominent postural instability and gait disturbance, may be difficult to distinguish from MSA.[50] PSP and other parkinsonism-plus syndromes can be particularly difficult to separate, especially in the first 5 years of clinical illness. Vascular encephalopathies with multiple subcortical strokes may produce a similar constellation of signs, and the condition of pure autonomic failure can be difficult to differentiate from MSA in the early course of illness.

Evaluation. MRI may be useful to rule out a multi-infarct state, normal pressure hydrocephalus, or other causes of parkinsonism. An MRI scan demonstrating marked hypointensity of the striatum and linear hyperintensity lateral to the putamen on T2-weighted images suggests iron deposition and supports the diagnosis of MSA.[48] PET scans of MSA are similar to those of PSP and usually confirm a decreased density of striatal D_2 receptors.[51] External urethral and rectal sphincter electromyography (EMG) is abnormal in almost all patients with MSA. Resting, supine, and standing norepinephrine levels are of questionable value, but supine and standing norepinephrine levels have been found to be slightly elevated in patients with MSA, whereas in those with pure autonomic failure they are usually decreased.[52]

Management. Levodopa may provide some relief, usually short term, for the rigidity, bradykinesia, and postural instability typical of MSA.[53] Patients with MSA usually require larger doses of levodopa than patients with PD, but side effects such as increased orthostatic hypotension and facial dystonia often limit the usefulness of levodopa. Patients rarely derive any meaningful benefit from DA agonists, anticholinergics, amantadine, or other antiparkinsonian drugs. Symptomatic orthostatic hypotension can be treated with sodium and volume repletion unless the patient is at risk of congestive heart failure or renal insufficiency. Ancillary measures such as wearing elastic stockings to increase central venous volume and elevating the head of the bed 6 inches may also be attempted but often prove uncomfortable. Fludrocortisone, a mineralocorticoid, often improves orthostatic symptoms by increasing vascular volume. Some patients benefit from the inhibition of vasodilator prostaglandin synthesis brought about by indomethacin and from the use of the alpha-adrenergic agonist clonidine and the peripheral vasoconstrictor ephedrine. Midodrine, an alpha-adrenergic agonist, has benefited some patients with moderate and severe orthostatic hypotension of various causes.[54] Urinary frequency or incontinence, if due to detrusor hyper-reflexia, may respond to peripherally acting anticholinergic agents such as oxybutynin or propantheline given at bedtime. Intranasal desmopressin at bedtime may offer relief from nocturnal urinary frequency. Impotence may respond to yohimbine, papaverine, or a penile implant. Constipation can be treated with cisapride, stool softeners, and bulk-forming agents. Hallucinations caused by dopaminergic therapeutic agents usually respond to a lower dose of dopaminergic medications or to clozapine at bedtime.[38] This latter therapy must be used cautiously, however, in patients with hypotension. All patients receiving this drug must be monitored for agranulocytosis with weekly white blood cell counts.

Prognosis and Future Perspectives. Based on autopsy-proven cases of MSA, the average survival time is expected to be less than a decade (mean survival 8.0 years,[48] median survival 9.5 years).[49] Future studies may focus on the role of iron and oxidative stress in this disorder and the pathological hallmark of glial cytoplasmic inclusion bodies.

Other Parkinsonism-Plus Syndromes

Corticobasal Degeneration. CBD is a distinctive parkinsonism-plus syndrome because specific cortical signs are associated with it and it has a particular pathological picture. Autopsy in patients with CBD reveals asymmetrical, focal frontoparietal atrophy, "ballooned" and enlarged cells in the cortex, depigmentation of the substantia nigra without Lewy bodies, and diffuse neuronal loss.[55] There is no familial predisposition, and no environmental factors increase the risk of disease. Clinically, patients usually develop symptoms after age 60, and neurological signs of CBD include focal or asymmetrical rigidity, bradykinesia, postural and action tremor, and marked dystonia, usually predominantly in one upper extremity. The most characteristic symptom, however, is limb apraxia, and the involved extremity can become so dysfunctional that it moves completely by itself and can be considered an "alien limb."[56] In most instances, the condition starts as an apparent case of PD, but the cortical sensory loss, dystonia, and apraxia are noticed quickly as distinctive. PSP and MSA can present with these signs and therefore must always be considered in the differential diagnosis. The parkinsonism can be treated with modest success in some cases by introducing levodopa or DA agonists, but the marked disability resulting from the limb dyspraxia is progressive, untreatable, and markedly disabling. Botulinum toxin can relieve elements of the dystonia. The condition usually progresses steadily, and death occurs within 10 years of diagnosis.[56]

Parkinsonism-Dementia Amyotrophic Lateral Sclerosis Complex (PDALS). This distinctive condition occurs on the island of Guam (locally known as Lytico-Bodig disease) and has been the focus of significant research because of the possibility that genetic and environmental causes may be contributive.[57] A study of over 2000 affected and nonaffected individuals in Guam showed that the incidence of this disorder peaked in the 1950s and has gradually declined since that time. The rapid decline in incidence of this disorder in Guam strongly supports the role of environmental factors in the pathogenesis of this disorder.[58] Early studies focusing on possible environmental dietary toxins were encouraging, but recent work has failed to identify any agent consistently, and the once-held hypothesis that native flour contains a causative neurotoxin is no longer considered tenable.[58] Pathologically, depigmentation, basophilic inclusion bodies, and cell loss in the substantia nigra are apparent in cases of PDALS. Neurofibrillary tangles without senile plaques are present in the substantia nigra, anterior horn cells, and pyramidal tracts.[58] Clinical findings in PDALS range from motor neuron disease in younger patients to parkinsonism with severe dementia in the older population. The amyotrophic lateral sclerosis (ALS) form is seen predominantly in the Chamorros, while the parkinsonism-dementia presentation may be seen in both Chamorro and Filipino residents. The ALS seen in Guam does not differ clinically from the motor neuron disease seen in the remainder of the world. Although no cause has been established, the co-existence of these neurodegenerative conditions in one population with overlapping signs supports the continuation of hypotheses based on a common cause. The differential diagnosis for PDALS includes Alzheimer's disease, diffuse Lewy body disease, postencephalitic parkinsonism, PD, the parkinsonism-plus syndromes, lower body parkinsonism and other causes of parkinsonism, as well as ALS and the various forms of motor neuron disease.[58] Regardless of its form of clinical presentation, the disorder is relentlessly progressive, and death usually occurs within 10 years of diagnosis.

Hemiatrophy/Hemiparkinsonism. Hemiatrophy/hemiparkinsonism (HA/HP) is an uncommon disorder that involves the onset of parkinsonism on one side of the body in association with a hemiatrophic face, arm, or leg in varying combinations. First described by Klawans,[59] the disease presents with unilateral parkinsonism; the hemiatrophy is completely unnoticed by the patient. In a hemiparkinsonian patient, therefore, comparative examination of the size of the hands and feet may be necessary to diagnose the condition. Compared to PD, the parkinsonism of HA/HP usually begins at a younger age and generally remains on the hemiatrophic side for several years before it sometimes becomes bilateral. Unilateral dystonic movements are a common early feature and may respond well to levodopa. The cause is unknown, but early birth injury from hypoxia or trauma has been suggested as a possibility, and there may be some relationship between this syndrome and a distinct form of dystonia termed dopa-responsive dystonia.[60] Hemiatrophy of the contralateral cortex may be seen on MRI in some patients.

STIFF-PERSON SYNDROME

Pathogenesis and Pathophysiology. Stiff-person syndrome (SPS) is believed to be an idiopathic disorder in some patients and an autoimmune disorder with functional impairment of spinal neurons due to antibodies directed against the enzyme glutamic acid decarboxylase (GAD) in others.[61] This enzyme is essential for the conversion of glutamic acid to GABA, an inhibitory neurotransmitter found throughout the central nervous system.[62] In a paraneoplastic form of SPS, amphiphysin, a protein associated with synaptic vesicles, has been implicated, and this product's gene has been mapped to 7p13–14.[63] Neurophysiological studies show continuous excessive firing of the motor unit, suggesting that the disorder is due to disinhibition of the descending pathways to the Renshaw cells or gamma motor system.[64] Autopsy information, albeit limited, has failed to demonstrate any abnormalities in the brain stem, spinal cord, peripheral nerve, or muscle.

Epidemiology and Risk Factors. The disorder is more common in women and is frequently associated with other autoimmune disorders (diabetes mellitus, thyroiditis, myasthenia gravis, pernicious anemia, and vitiligo).[64]

Clinical Features and Associated Disorders. Typically, SPS patients present with painful muscle cramps and severe lordosis secondary to chronic spasm of the paraspinal muscles. Although predominantly a disease of the axial muscles, cranial involvement has been reported in 25 percent of patients, and spread to the proximal limbs occurs. Examination reveals marked lumbar and thoracic muscle spasms. Stress or exertional activity may provoke painful spasms that may last for hours. Because of hypertonicity, the gait may resemble that of a "tin soldier."

Differential Diagnosis. Among the primary differential diagnoses are dystonia and orthostatic tremor. In both instances, patients may complain of tight cramping muscles and pain, especially when standing. Other rare conditions resembling SPS include tetanus, progressive encephalomyelitis with rigidity, and Isaac's syndrome. Tetanus secondary to infection with *Clostridium tetanii* is usually associated with a laceration injury and progresses from focal muscle spasm at the site of inoculation to bulbar and generalized spasms. Progressive encephalomyelitis usually begins with pain and sensory changes, and in these patients, a paraneoplastic disorder is possible. Isaac's syndrome is often familial and is associated with peripheral neuropathy, but most important, it usually causes more symptoms in the appendicular muscles than in the axial ones.

Evaluation. Electromyographic demonstration of continuous motor unit activity is essential to confirm the diagnosis of SPS. The presence of reduced motor activity after benzodiazepine administration is also important. Diagnostically, spinal fluid analysis may reveal increased immunoglobulin or oligoclonal bands, and the presence of GAD antibodies is helpful in confirming the autoimmune form of this diagnosis.

Management. Treatment is based on controlling rigidity; currently, diazepam (20 to 300 mg/day) is the most effective medication for this purpose. Baclofen, clonazepam, valproic acid, and clonidine have been reported to improve symptoms. The role of treatment for autoimmune conditions, such as plasmapheresis, corticosteroids, or azathioprine, has yet to be defined, but high-dose intravenous immunoglobulin has been found to be an effective, albeit costly, treatment.[65] Intrathecal baclofen and botulinum toxin may also be beneficial, but because of the rarity of this syndrome, controlled clinical trials of these drugs for this purpose have not been undertaken. Although these patients may be in pain, extreme caution must be used in mixing narcotic medications with benzodiazepine derivatives, especially if the patient's spasms induce respiratory acidosis because of the rigidity of the diaphragmatic muscles.

Prognosis and Future Perspectives. Without treatment, SPS progresses to total disability related to generalized rigidity and secondary musculoskeletal deformities. The pathogenetic autoimmune mechanisms remain to be elucidated.

Hyperkinetic Movement Disorders

HUNTINGTON'S DISEASE

This primary neurodegenerative disorder usually begins during adult life, often after the affected individuals have already borne their children. It is inherited in an autosomally dominant pattern, and the disorder has clinical manifestations that often vary among involved family members, and patients may have predominantly behavioral, cognitive, or movement disorder signs.

Pathogenesis and Pathophysiology. Huntington's disease (HD) is caused by a mutation on chromosome 4 consisting of an unstable expansion of CAG repeats. Normal individuals have between 11 and 34 repeats, whereas those with HD have between 37 and 86. The trinucleotide CAG codes for glutamine, and the increase in polyglutamine is thought to cause an overexpression of the gene whose protein is termed huntingtin. This product tightly binds with ubiquitin to form intranuclear inclusions and may subsequently interfere with normal mitochondrial bioenergetic mechanisms.[66] Huntingtin is associated with vesicle membranes and microtubules and as such probably has a role in endocytosis, intracellular trafficking, and membrane recycling. It is not yet clear whether HD results from a toxic property of the mutant protein (gain of function) or loss of neuroprotective activity of the normal huntingtin (loss of function).[67]

It is not known why the striatum is preferentially affected because the HD mRNA product has been found in all examined tissues.[68] Neuronal loss in the caudate and putamen has been correlated with a longer CAG trinucleotide repeat length, and the preproenkephalin medium spiny neuron seems to be particularly vulnerable.[69]

Pathological changes in the brain of patients with HD include generalized atrophy with neuronal degeneration in the cortex and severe loss of medium spiny projection neurons with preservation of cholinergic aspiny interneurons in the caudate and putamen. Marked caudate atrophy is the pathological hallmark of the disease, and this finding can be detected on MRI scans. MR spectroscopy demonstrates changes that reflect increased levels of lactic acid, suggesting a bioenergetic defect. Additional evidence, particularly in experimental models of HD, suggests that mitochondrial dysfunction may be a possible pathogenetic mechanism of neuronal cell death.[70]

Several important biochemical abnormalities have been noted in postmortem brain tissue, particularly in the striatum. These include decreases in choline acetyltransferase activity and acetylcholine, a reduction in the total number of cholinergic muscarinic receptors, and depletion of GAD, substance P, angiotensin-converting enzyme, cholecystokinin, enkephalin, and other peptides. In contrast, the concentrations of DA, norepinephrine, serotonin, neurotensin, somatostatin, and thyrotropin-releasing hormone are normal or increased.[70] The result of these changes suggests a functional overactivity of the cerebral glutaminergic and striatal dopaminergic systems and an underactivity of the GABAergic systems.

Epidemiology and Risk Factors. The estimated prevalence of HD is 5 to 10 per 100,000 people in the United States.[71] Because the CAG repeat length is unstable in sperm, affected fathers often transmit a very high repeat sequence, resulting in an early onset of disease in their offspring.

Clinical Features and Associated Disorders. Gradual onset of chorea, dementia, and behavioral abnormalities in a young or middle-aged adult should suggest the possibility of HD. Slowed saccadic eye movements are usually the first detectable clinical sign, and in 85 percent of patients chorea is the predominant movement disorder. Movements may start as fine, irregular body jerks that have no functional significance, but coordination, gait, and balance difficulties gradually supervene. In the juvenile form of HD, rigidity, bradykinesia, resting tremor, dystonic postures, ataxia, seizures, myoclonus, and mental retardation are more prominent, and this presentation is termed the Westphal variant of HD. Even in patients with adult-onset and prominent chorea, bradykinesia and postural reflex compromise can occur and may be sources of significant functional disability. In the terminal phases of HD, dysarthria, dysphagia, and respiratory difficulties become the most disabling and life-threatening problems.[70]

Cognitive impairment is a source of major disability in these patients. Memory difficulties, concentration problems, confusion, and forgetfulness can occur (see Chapter 33). In addition, depression and other emotional disturbances may be severe and can lead to erratic, impulsive behavior as well as suicidal ideation. Other psychiatric disturbances include delusional thoughts, paranoia, and hallucinations.[70] Eventually, patients become demented, and most require assistance and supervision in daily living activities.

Differential Diagnosis. Besides HD, other less common heredofamilial choreas include hereditary benign chorea and neuroacanthocytosis (see later discussion in this chapter). If a family history of choreic or psychiatric disorders is lacking, numerous other disorders should be considered, including tardive dyskinesia, CNS vasculitis, Wilson's disease, Sydenham's chorea, and toxin exposure. Drugs causing chorea include oral contraceptives, levodopa, CNS stimulants, neuroleptics, phenytoin, carbamazepine, and ethosuximide. If the diagnosis is approached from the perspective of genetic testing, other hereditary neurodegenerative conditions with expanded trinucleotide repeats of CAG include Kennedy's syndrome (X-linked spinal and bulbar muscular atrophy), myotonic dystrophy, spinocerebellar atrophy type 1, and DRPLA (Table 34–4).

Evaluation. In addition to taking a complete family history, blood should be drawn for DNA testing. Careful counseling about the implications of the diagnosis is essential when working with patients who are at risk for the disease. Issues of privacy are particularly important because giving subjects positive diagnostic information reveals information about the parents' genetic makeup. MRI scans can detect the presence of caudate and cerebral atrophy. When the family history is in doubt, an assiduous search of autopsy reports on relatives can sometimes unearth the diagnosis in the genealogy.

Management. DA receptor–blocking agents (e.g., haloperidol or fluphenazine) and dopamine-depleting agents (e.g., tetrabenazine, reserpine) reduce the choreic movements but may not improve other symptoms of Huntington's disease. Because of their potentially serious side effects, including tardive dyskinesia (neuroleptics), depression (dopamine-depleting drugs), and parkinsonism (both drug classes), the antidopaminergic drugs should be reserved for patients with disabling chorea or serious psychosis. The tricyclic antidepressants and selective serotonin reuptake inhibitors are often helpful in ameliorating the affective dis-

TABLE 34–4. **Etiological Classification of Chorea**

1. Developmental and aging choreas
   a. Physiological chorea of infancy
   b. Cerebral palsy—anoxic, kernicterus
   c. Minimal cerebral dysfunction
   d. Buccal-oral-lingual dyskinesia and edentulous orodyskinesia in elderly
   e. Senile chorea (probably several causes)
2. Hereditary choreas
   a. Huntington's disease
   b. Benign hereditary chorea
   c. Neuroacanthocytosis
   d. Other CNS "degenerations": Olivopontocerebellar atrophy, Azorean disease, ataxia-telangiectasia, tuberous sclerosis, Hallervorden-Spatz, dentato-rubral-pallido-lysian atrophy (DRPLA), familial calcification of basal ganglia, others
   e. Neurometabolic disorders: Wilson's disease, Lesch-Nyhan disease, lysosomal storage disorders, amino acid disorders, Leigh's disease, porphyria
3. Drug-induced choreas: neuroleptics (tardive dyskinesia), antiparkinsonian drugs, amphetamines, tricyclics, oral contraceptives, anticonvulsants, anticholinergics, others
4. Toxin-induced choreas: alcohol intoxication and withdrawal, anoxia, carbon monoxide, Mn, Hg, thallium, toluene
5. Metabolic causes
   a. Hyperthyroidism
   b. Hypoparathyroidism (various types)
   c. Pregnancy (chorea gravidarum)
   d. Hyper- and hyponatremia, hypomagnesemia, hypocalcemia
   e. Hypo- and hyperglycemia (latter may cause hemichorea, hemiballismus)
   f. Acquired hepatocerebral degeneration
   g. Nutritional—e.g., beriberi, pellagra, vitamin B_{12} deficiency in infants
6. Infectious causes
   a. Sydenham's chorea
   b. Encephalitis lethargica
   c. Various other infections and postinfectious encephalitides, including Creutzfeldt-Jakob disease

orders but may precipitate myoclonus. Antiglutaminergic drugs and facilitators of mitochondrial metabolism are currently being tested in clinical trials. Psychological support, genetic counseling, long-term planning, and access to social service agencies are important elements of patient management.

Prognosis and Future Perspectives. Despite recent advances in treatment, this disorder results in progressive functional decline and eventual death, usually within 12 to 15 years of onset. Neural transplantation with fetal striatal or other cell sources may become experimental options in the future.

OTHER FORMS OF CHOREA

Senile chorea (essential chorea) begins after age 60 and is unaccompanied by any particular neurobehavioral symptoms or a family history of chorea. Whereas some patients have caudate atrophy similar to that seen in HD, others have predominant putamenal degeneration. In occasional cases, genetic detection studies in these patients reveal that the correct diagnosis is actually HD. Treatment of the chorea is similar to that used for HD.

Paroxysmal dyskinesia is a chronic condition that becomes manifest by a sudden onset of transient choreoathetosis, dystonia, or both. The familial paroxysmal dyskinesias are subdivided into kinesigenic and nonkinesigenic disorders depending on whether or not they are induced by sudden voluntary movements.[72] In the familial (autosomal dominant or recessive) kinesigenic paroxysmal dyskinesia, the movements are brief, usually lasting less than 3 minutes, and occur many times daily, sometimes up to 100 times a day.[72] Nonkinesigenic and exertional paroxysmal dyskinesias may also be transmitted as autosomal dominant disorders, and the movements in these forms tend to be more dystonic than choreic in nature. The episodes of dyskinesia are usually more prolonged (lasting 2 minutes to 4 hours) and less frequent (occurring three to five times a day). Attacks are precipitated by alcohol, coffee, fatigue, stress, or excitement. Kinesigenic dyskinesias respond well to anticonvulsant medications such as phenytoin, carbamazepine, or phenobarbital. In contrast, the nonkinesigenic dyskinesias respond poorly to most medical therapy, although some patients improve with clonazepam.[72] Pathophysiologically, these conditions appear to be an interface between movement disorders and epilepsy, since in some conditions assiduous electrode placement over the frontal and frontocentral regions may reveal epileptic spikes and phase reversals.[73] Secondary paroxysmal dyskinesias may be associated with structural lesions of the premotor cortex or basal ganglia, and specific causes include multiple sclerosis and hypocalcemia.[72]

Neuroacanthocytosis is a rare disorder with autosomal dominant, recessive, or even X-linked inheritance and is manifested by chorea, tics, dystonia, parkinsonism, self-mutilatory behavior, amyotrophy, areflexia, elevated creatine kinase, and other symptoms.[74] One of the most distinguishing features of neuroacanthocytosis is an eating dysfunction that is due to orolingual dystonia and is manifested by expulsion of food from the mouth by a protruding tongue. Involuntary vocalizations and parkinsonism also occur. Although the mechanism of acanthocyte formation in neuroacanthocytosis is unknown, abnormal protein to fatty acid ratios and in some cases abnormal erythrocyte surface antigens have been found. It is possible that, as in the periodic ataxias, some of the paroxysmal dyskinesias represent abnormalities of the calcium channel or other channelopathies. Acanthocytes in most patients can be seen in fresh blood smears, but erythrocytes may require incubation in normal saline for 3 to 5 minutes prior to wet mount preparation. Computed tomography or MRI of the head may demonstrate cerebral or caudate atrophy. PET scans reveal 42 and 54 percent reductions in putamenal and caudate fluorodopa uptake, respectively, and a 65 and 53 percent reduction in the D_2 receptor density in these areas.[74] Treatment may involve the use of dopamine-blocking agents in the form of neuroleptics (haloperidol, fluphenazine) or dopamine-depleting drugs (reserpine, tetrabenazine). As the disease progresses, most care is supportive. Whereas the course of progression varies, death usually occurs within 15 years of diagnosis.

Sydenham's chorea (also known as St. Vitus' dance) develops following exposure to the bacteria *Streptococcus pneumoniae* and, in the age of antibiotic therapy, is rare.[68] Most typically, Sydenham's chorea is associated with infection and other sequelae of rheumatic fever. Autopsy studies of patients with Sydenham's chorea reveal edema, chromatolysis, and atrophy that affect primarily the striatum, but the cortex, thalamus, and other basal ganglial nuclei may be variably involved as well.[68] The clinical picture involves a child with diffuse chorea, motor impersistence, and variable degrees of weakness. Unlike arthritis and carditis, chorea may not develop for weeks or even months after acute infection has occurred. Children are often very distressed in the midst of the chorea, rest poorly, and can develop a number of behavioral abnormalities. In addition to high titers of antistreptolysin, approximately 50 percent of patients have IgG antibodies that react against neurons in the caudate and subthalamic nuclei. The condition is usually self-limited, but during the period of marked chorea, dopamine-blocking or -depleting agents (see earlier discussion) can be used. Because prolonged drug usage is usually not necessary, major concerns about the induction of tardive dyskinesia from neuroleptic drugs do not exist.

In the evaluation of these forms of primary choreic disorders, other secondary choreas must be considered. Chorea gravidarum and endocrine-metabolic choreas, such as birth control pill chorea, should be considered in appropriate women with hyperkinetic movements. Prior Sydenham's chorea may be a risk factor for these conditions. Estrogens may serve as a facilitator of dopamine pharmacology, either directly at the receptor sites or through second messengers. In pregnancy, DA receptor–blocking drugs (neuroleptics) should be avoided, particularly during the limb-genesis period of the first trimester. Benzodiazepines may be appropriate in the second and third trimesters, but fetal respiratory depression must be avoided. Hyperthyroidism, either primary or pituitary in origin, can be associated with various movement disorders, including chorea.

PRIMARY DYSTONIA

Pathogenesis and Pathophysiology. Dystonia consists of sustained, repetitive, patterned contractions of the muscles producing twisting (e.g., torticollis) or squeezing (e.g., blepharospasm) movements or abnormal postures that may be present at rest, when changing position, or when performing a specific motor activity.[75] The most frequently encountered form of generalized dystonia is primary dystonia, formerly referred to as dystonia musculorum deformans or idiopathic torsion dystonia. It is an autosomal dominant disorder in which the genetic defect consists of a three base pair deletion in a gene on chromosome 9q32–34 (DYT1), coding for an ATP-domain protein called TorsinA. The mutant protein forms multiple, large inclusions composed of endoplasmic reticulum–derived membrane whorls in cultured cells.[76] Rarer forms of pure dystonia unrelated to this defect or due to enzyme deficiencies have been described (Table 34–5) but are not well delineated.

Although autopsy studies have produced no reproducible histological or biochemical abnormalities in patients with primary dystonia, the disorder is thought to be due to altered

TABLE 34–5. **Etiological Classification of Dystonia**

- I. Idiopathic (primary) dystonia
  - A. Sporadic (idiopathic torsion dystonia, ITD)
  - B. Inherited (hereditary torsion dystonia)
    1. Classic autosomal dominant ITD (DYT1 gene, 9q34)
    2. Nonclassic autosomal dominant ITD (not DYT1 gene)
    3. Autosomal recessive tyrosine hydroxylase deficiency
- II. Secondary dystonia
  - A. Dystonia-plus syndromes
    1. Myoclonic dystonia (not DYT1 gene)
    2. Dopa-responsive dystonia (DRD, GTP cyclohydrolase I 14q22.1–q22.2 gene defect)
    3. Rapid-onset dystonia-parkinsonism (RDP)
    4. Early-onset parkinsonism with dystonia (EPD)
    5. Paroxysmal dystonia-choreoathetosis
  - B. Associated with neurodegenerative disorders
    1. Sporadic
       - Parkinson's disease
       - Progressive supranuclear palsy
       - Multiple system atrophy
       - Corticobasal ganglionic degeneration
       - Multiple sclerosis
       - Central pontine myelinolysis
    2. Inherited
       - Wilson's disease
       - Huntington's disease
       - Juvenile parkinsonism-dystonia
       - Progressive pallidal degeneration
       - Hallervorden-Spatz disease
       - Hypoprebetalipoproteinemia, acanthocytosis, retinitis pigmentosa, and pallidal degeneration (HARP syndrome)
       - Joseph's disease
       - Ataxia-telangiectasia
       - Neuroacanthocytosis
       - Rett's syndrome (?)
       - Intraneuronal inclusion disease
       - Infantile bilateral striatal necrosis
       - Familial basal ganglia calcifications
       - Spinocerebellar degeneration
       - Olivopontocerebellar atrophy
       - Hereditary spastic paraplegia with dystonia
       - X-linked dystonia-parkinsonism or Lubag (pericentromeric)
       - Deletion of 18q
  - C. Associated with metabolic disorders
    1. Amino acid disorders
       - Glutaricacidemia
       - Methylmalonicacidemia
       - Homocystinuria
       - Hartnup's disease
       - Tyrosinosis
    2. Lipid disorders
       - Metachromatic leukodystrophy
       - Ceroid lipofuscinosis
       - Dystonic lipidosis ("sea blue" histiocytosis)
       - Gangliosidoses GM_1, GM_2 variants
       - Hexosaminidase A and B deficiencies
    3. Miscellaneous metabolic disorders
       - Wilson's disease
       - Mitochondrial encephalopathies: Leigh's disease, Leber's disease
       - Lesch-Nyhan syndrome
       - Triosephosphate isomerase deficiency
       - Vitamin E deficiency
       - Biopterin deficiency
  - D. Due to a known specific cause
    - Perinatal cerebral injury and kernicterus: athetoid cerebral palsy, delayed onset dystonia
    - Infection: viral encephalitis, encephalitis lethargica, Reye's syndrome; subacute sclerosing panencephalitis; Creutzfeldt-Jakob disease; acquired immunodeficiency syndrome
    - Other: tuberculosis, syphilis, acute infectious torticollis
    - Paraneoplastic brain stem encephalitis
    - Cerebral vascular and ischemic injury
    - Brain tumor
    - Arteriovenous malformation
    - Head trauma and brain surgery
    - Peripheral trauma
    - Toxins: MN, CO < CS_2, methanol, disulfiram, wasp sting
    - Drugs: levodopa, bromocriptine, antipsychotics, metoclopramide, fenfluramine, flecainide, ergot, anticonvulsants, certain calcium channel blockers
- III. Other hyperkinetic syndromes associated with dystonia
  - A. Tic disorders with dystonic tics
  - B. Paroxysmal dyskinesias
    1. Paroxysmal kinesigenic choreoathetosis
    2. Paroxysmal dystonic choreoathetosis
    3. Intermediate paroxysmal dyskinesia
    4. Benign infantile paroxysmal dyskinesia
- IV. Psychogenic
- V. Pseudodystonia
  - Atlantoaxial subluxation
  - Syringomyelia
  - Arnold-Chiari malformation
  - Trochlear nerve palsy
  - Vestibular torticollis
  - Posterior fossa mass
  - Soft tissue neck mass
  - Congenital postural torticollis
  - Congenital Klippel-Feil syndrome
  - Isaac's syndrome
  - Sandiffer's syndrome
  - Satoyoshi syndrome
  - Stiff-person syndrome

physiological control of descending pathways from the basal ganglia and brain stem. Subtle changes on MRI have been reported in patients with primary dystonia, but in most patients no discernible abnormalities can be identified on imaging tests. PET studies have also failed to reveal consistent abnormalities. Studies using blink, acoustic, and vestibulo-ocular reflex testing, however, have revealed abnormalities suggesting that the brain stem reflexes have enhanced excitability.[77] Changes in norepinephrine, serotonin, and dopamine levels have been found in some patients.

Epidemiology and Risk Factors. Limited information is available about the epidemiology of primary dystonia, but data from Rochester, Minnesota, reveal a prevalence of 34 per million population; specific cultural groups are more likely to develop primary dystonia than others, however, and among Jews of eastern European ancestry the prevalence is at least double that seen in other groups.

Clinical Features and Associated Disorders. Primary dystonia may involve the entire body (generalized dystonia) or may be confined to one body part (focal dystonia), for example, the head (cranial dystonia) or neck (cervical dystonia); alternatively, it may involve contiguous body parts (segmental dystonia); for example, the neck, shoulder, and arm. The most common form of limb dystonia is dystonic writer's cramp.

Although primary dystonia is a highly variable condition, there are a number of important clinical patterns. First, primary dystonia, regardless of its eventual outcome (focal, segmental, or generalized), usually begins as a focal condition, and in children the legs and feet are the areas most commonly affected. Second, environmental conditions affect dystonia and, importantly, in the early stages of primary dystonia, dystonia is usually seen only during activity, for example, when walking or running (action dystonia). In addition, and related to exacerbation of disease with action, dystonic signs usually become prominent in the middle and later part of the day. This feature is most pronounced in a particular form of dystonia, termed dopa-responsive dystonia (see subsequent discussion), in which diurnal fluctuation in the gait disturbance may be so marked that the patient is almost normal in the early morning but becomes virtually crippled by late afternoon or evening. Third, the younger the age at onset, the more likely the dystonia is to become severe and spread to many body regions. Likewise, adult-onset primary dystonia is almost always focal or segmental and does not become generalized. Fourth, patients with primary dystonia often report that certain postures or sensory "tricks" or "gestes antagonistique" improve their dystonia. For example, gentle counterpressure by a hand against the chin in a patient with torticollis may enable the patient to maintain the primary or normal position of the head. Finally, one of the features in many patients with dystonia is an associated tremor in addition to the contorted posture. This tremor, termed dystonic tremor, involves the patient's attempt, conscious or not, to overcome the dystonia. It is most pronounced when the patient works maximally to resist the pull of the dystonic muscles and is least apparent when the patient permits the involved body part to drift with the dystonic spasm.

Differential Diagnosis. In addition to primary dystonia, the differential diagnosis of the dystonic patient (see Table 34–5) must include, first, dystonia-plus syndromes (see later discussion), a conglomerate term that includes other forms of primary dystonia associated with additional neurological deficits, and second, secondary forms of dystonia, in which the dystonia is related to underlying damage from a known pathological cause. In the latter category, causes of dystonia are numerous and include exposure to DA receptor–blocking drugs ("tardive dystonia"), hypoxic encephalopathy, head trauma, encephalitis, human immunodeficiency virus and other infections, peripheral or segmental nerve injury, inherited disorders (e.g., Wilson's disease), metabolic disorders and other inborn errors of metabolism, mitochondrial disorders, and chromosomal abnormalities.[74] Unilateral dystonia (hemidystonia) is usually not part of the clinical picture of primary dystonia but is associated with a structural lesion in the contralateral striatum, particularly the putamen.

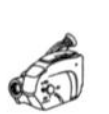

Evaluation. The diagnosis of primary dystonia should be considered in any patient with an abnormal posture and a family history of variable problems with cramps, spasms, tremors, and crippling conditions. In the initial evaluation the clinician should gather information about age at onset, initial and subsequent areas of involvement, course and progression of disease, tremor or other movement disorders, possible birth injury, developmental milestones, and exposure to neuroleptic medications, as well as a family history of dystonia, parkinsonism, or other movement disorders. Consanguinity or Jewish ancestry should be noted as well. Since the clinical expression of primary dystonia is highly variable even within families, the history and family tree may be extremely difficult to establish with confidence. Some family members may have severe problems and require extensive assistance with activities of daily living, while others may show only mild symptoms (e.g., writer's cramp).[75] Evidence of other conditions known to produce dystonia but associated with other neurological dysfunctions (e.g., cognitive, pyramidal, sensory, or cerebellar deficits) should be evaluated along with secondary causes of dystonia. The ceruloplasmin level should be obtained in all patients in whom onset of dystonia occurs before the age of 50, since Wilson's disease is highly treatable. Other blood tests, including genetic tests, depend on the clinical setting, and the various storage and metabolic disorders should be evaluated individually. An MRI scan is important in the evaluation of structural abnormalities, and skull, neck, and spine evaluations may be needed if there is evidence of a secondary myelopathy or scoliosis due to axial dystonia.

Management. In treating primary dystonia, high-dose anticholinergic therapy (e.g., trihexyphenidyl in doses of up to 70 mg/day) may be effective in ameliorating dystonia, particularly in younger patients. However, many patients are unable to tolerate such high doses because loss of memory, hallucinations, blurring of vision, and other anticholinergic side effects may occur. In addition, all patients with childhood-onset dystonia deserve a trial of levodopa, using Sinemet in doses of up to 100/1000 mg/day.[74] Other agents such as oral baclofen, carbamazepine, and tetrabenazine have been reported to be beneficial in some dystonic patients. Recent interest has focused on the use of intrathecal baclofen in patients with generalized and axial dystonia, but controlled trials of this usage have not been published.

Intramuscular injections of botulinum toxin type A or type B are the most effective treatment for focal dystonia and may be used in a limited form in patients with segmental or generalized dystonia.[78, 79] Because it acts at the presynaptic membrane, this botulinum toxin prevents release of acetylcholine at the nerve terminal, causing muscle weakness. Injection into dystonic muscles requires knowledge of the muscle anatomy and the site of muscle innervation, and some clinicians perform this procedure with the aid of EMG guidance. Treatment is necessary every 3 to 5 months in most patients, and this therapy has been used safely in some patients for more than 15 years. However, some patients develop resistance to the clinical response, and antibodies to the A toxin may develop. If the dose is limited to less than 300 units per procedure and the treatment is given no more frequently than every 3 months, the risk of immunoresistance is minimized.[80] Other types of botulinum toxins, namely B and F, are currently being investigated for the treatment of focal dystonia.

Thalamotomy and high-frequency thalamic or pallidal stimulation are occasionally performed in patients with otherwise medically intractable disease.[81] It is more effective for distal than for proximal dystonia.[82] Unfortunately, when these procedures are bilateral, patients may be left with severe dysarthria, dysphagia, and memory deficit. In this regard, pallidotomy may have some advantages. Cervical cord stimulation, peripheral nerve section, rhizotomy, and myotomy are occasionally effective.

Prognosis and Future Perspectives. Prognosis in primary dystonia is highly dependent on age of onset; the younger the age at onset, the higher the likelihood of spread and progression to generalized disabling dystonia. The biological markers and pathophysiological mechanisms of dystonia remain to be elucidated. It is likely that the gene or genes for primary dystonia will be identified, and the study of the gene product may provide clues to the pathogenesis of primary dystonia. Extensive information on subthalamic nucleus deep brain stimulation is not yet available.

OTHER FORMS OF PRIMARY DYSTONIA

Several other forms of primary inherited degenerative syndromes are associated with dystonia.[74] Like the parkinsonism-plus syndromes, the major hallmark in these dystonia-plus syndromes is dystonia, but this is accompanied by movement disorders. Dopa-responsive dystonia (DRD) is also an autosomal dominant disorder caused by a mutation in the GTP cyclohydrolase I gene on chromosome 14q, which causes a defect in dihydrobiopterin synthesis. These patients present with dystonia and parkinsonism that has a marked diurnal fluctuation. In the early morning they may be symptom-free or only mildly affected, but then a progressive gait disorder and cramping and rigidity develop during the day. These patients are markedly sensitive to low doses of levodopa, and often doses of Sinemet as low as 25/100 mg/day are effective in obliterating clinical signs. For this reason, it is particularly important to recognize DRD, and all children with dystonia and adults with leg or trunk dystonia deserve a trial of levodopa. Another syndrome, X-linked dystonia-parkinsonism, is much rarer and is confined largely to inhabitants of the Philippines.[75] These patients, mostly men, develop severe axial dystonia and a hunched parkinsonian posture. Falls, dysphagia, and voice compromise follow, and these signs usually are preludes to death. In contrast, myoclonic dystonia (see later section on essential myoclonus) is a benign autosomal dominant disorder marked by a combination of dystonia and jerking myoclonic movements, usually starting in the first or second decade of life without other neurological deficits. These patients show a dramatic response to alcohol[75] and are treated with this product combined with benzodiazepines with usually excellent results.[76]

HALLERVORDEN-SPATZ DISEASE

Pathogenesis and Pathophysiology. Hallervorden-Spatz disease (HSD) is a rare autosomal recessive disorder associated with excessive iron deposition in the globus pallidus (GP).[83] The most striking autopsy finding in HSD patients is the asymmetrical rust-brown pigmentation of the GP and zona reticulata of the SN. The iron pigmentation occurs both extracellularly and intracellularly but is predominantly found in astrocytes, microglia, and neurons. "Mulberry" concretions are also typically present in the extracellular space. Numerous and large spheroid bodies, identified by myelin staining and surrounded by pigment granules, are typically present throughout the medial GP, SN zona reticulata, cortex, and subthalamic nucleus.[84] The spheroid bodies apparently represent degenerating myelinated axons. Linkage analyses initially localized the HSD gene on 20p12.3–p13 and subsequently seven base pair deletion and various missense mutations were identified in the coding sequence of gene PANK2 with homology to pantothenate kinase.[85]

Clinical Features and Associated Disorders. HSD was initially described in a 1 family of 12 children, 3 of whom died at birth; 8 of the remaining 9 developed athetosis, tremor, and visual difficulties. Dystonia and rigidity are the major hallmarks of this childhood illness, but other associated features include gait and posture disturbances, chorea, athetosis, tremor, dysarthria, blindness with retinitis pigmentosa, intellectual decline, spasticity, and seizures. Myoclonus is rare and usually is a preterminal sign. Although the onset usually occurs in the first decade of life, rare patients with adult-onset HSD starting in the fourth to sixth decade and presenting as parkinsonism have been described.[84]

Differential Diagnosis. HSD has a wide spectrum of presentation and therefore a potentially large differential diagnosis. A disease of iron deposition in the basal ganglia, HSD shares some features with other disorders associated with deposition of metals, such as Wilson's disease and manganese toxicity. Other disorders with overlapping clinical features include juvenile Huntington's disease, neuroacanthocytosis, and neuronal ceroid lipofuscinosis.

Evaluation. CT scans reveal high signal intensity in the medial GP, and MRI demonstrates decreased signal intensity in the GP on T2- or proton density–weighted images; these abnormalities are produced by iron deposition bilaterally in the pallidum.[84] In some cases, the center is hyperintense, giving rise to the term "eye of the tiger" sign. Ophthalmological examination may be particularly helpful because it may show optic degeneration and retinitis pigmentosa.

Management. There is no specific treatment for HSD. Chelation therapy to remove excess iron accumulation in the basal ganglia has not been useful. Parkinsonism in some patients has responded to levodopa and bromocriptine therapies, but anticholinergic agents have failed to improve symptoms of tremor, dystonia, or bradykinesia. The choreoathetosis may benefit from benzodiazepines, but dopamine antagonists are generally not used because of the risk of worsening parkinsonism. Antiepileptic drugs are useful for the control of seizures. Supportive care and physical, occupational, and speech therapy should also be instituted when appropriate.[84]

Prognosis and Future Perspectives. The mean duration of the disease is 11 years, and 45 percent of patients die before reaching the age of 20 years.[83] Putative gene markers have been found recently, but further studies are needed before the gene mutation is characterized and the gene product is identified. Until then, the more appropriate term for this disorder is neurodegeneration with brain iron accumulation Type I (NBIA-I).

GILLES DE LA TOURETTE SYNDROME AND OTHER TIC DISORDERS

Pathogenesis and Pathophysiology. Tics are repetitive movements that usually involve the eyes, face, shoulders, neck, and vocal apparatus more than the rest of the body. When childhood-onset tics are multifocal, motor, and vocal, last longer than 1 year, and naturally wax and wane, the term Gilles de la Tourette syndrome (GTS) is applied.[86] Once considered a rare psychiatric condition, GTS is now recognized as a relatively common neurological disorder with both motor and behavioral manifestations. In approximately 60 percent of cases of GTS, a family history of similar disorders can be found, which suggests that it is an autosomal dominant disorder. No genetic marker, however, has yet been identified. Because tics respond to dopamine-depleting drugs and DA receptor antagonists (neuroleptics), striatal DA receptor supersensitivity and developmental striatal DA terminal hyperinnervation have been proposed as possible causes of GTS symptoms.[87] Some clinical data indicate that neurotransmitters other than DA may be involved in other aspects of GTS.[88] Obsessive-compulsive disorder (OCD), a condition thought to be related to serotonergic neurochemistry, is present in at least half of patients with GTS, and this observation suggests that the serotonergic pathways in GTS may be altered. There is also some support for the idea that the opiate or second-messenger system may be involved in this disorder.[87]

Epidemiology and Risk Factors. Because most children with GTS have mild and undiagnosed symptoms, past prevalence estimates may be low. One review of epidemiological prevalence data in children found that prevalence estimates ranged from 0.5 to 50 per 10,000 population.[89] Kurlan reported that the frequency of tics in children ranged from 4 to 24 percent and that 26 percent of children in special education classes had tics compared to 6 percent of children in regular classes.[90] These studies suggest that children requiring special education may represent a high-risk population for tics. Some worsening of tics during pregnancy has been observed. Although genetic factors are clearly the most important determinants, there is some evidence that perinatal complications increase the risk of GTS.

Recent studies have emphasized the familial nature of GTS, with approximately a third of probands having a positive family history of simple tics and another third having a positive family history of the full GTS.[87] Transmission is often bilenial, meaning that both parents are affected. Typically, the father has a history of tics that may or may not persist through adulthood, and the mother has features of OCD. This pattern suggests that GTS represents one part of a spectrum, of which the mildest manifestation is a simple or transient tic of childhood and the most severe manifestation is the full syndrome that includes motor as well as behavioral features. This clinical heterogeneity makes specific definition of GTS problematic for genetic studies.

Clinical Manifestations and Associated Disorders. Tics are defined as simple or complex repetitive movements that occur out of background of normal motor activity. They are usually fast (myoclonic) but can be slow (dystonic). They increase with fatigue and after stress and decrease with concentration.[91] GTS is characterized by chronic waxing and waning motor and vocal tics, usually beginning between the ages of 2 and 21 years. It affects boys more frequently than girls. About half the patients start with simple motor tics, such as frequent eye blinking, facial grimacing, head jerking, or shoulder shrugging, or with simple vocal tics such as throat clearing, sniffing, grunting, snorting, hissing, barking, or other noises. Complex motor tics include squatting, hopping, skipping, hand shaking, and ritualized movements such as compulsive touching of objects, people, or self. Complex vocal tics include semantically meaningful utterances, including shouting of obscenities and profanities (coprolalia). Although coprolalia and other disturbing or socially unacceptable phenomena (copropraxia, coprographia, and mental coprolalia) can occur, these features are not necessary to the diagnosis of GTS. Of great clinical importance, tics can be voluntarily suppressed for seconds to minutes, but this suppression may be followed by a rebound burst of exaggerated abnormal involuntary movements. For this reason, tics may not be seen in the doctor's office, even though they may be disabling at school or at home. Many patients also report a premonitory phenomenon prior to the onset of motor tic. This crescendo urge, tension, or abnormal sensation in the distribution of the tic is relieved with the performance of the involuntary movement. In addition to these motor and vocal tics, many patients develop behavioral disorders, especially OCD and attention deficit hyperactivity disorder (ADHD), impulsive and self-destructive behavior, sleep abnormalities, and alterations in mood and sexual behavior. Learning disability often overlaps with hyperactivity and ADHD.

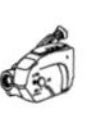

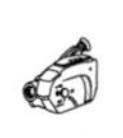

Differential Diagnosis. GTS is considered one end of a continuum of primary tic disorders[91] that includes transient tic disorder of childhood (tic or tics lasting less than 1 year) and chronic multiple tic disorder (motor or vocal tics, but not both). These semantic differences probably have no pathophysiological distinction, and therefore these primary tic disorders can be considered as clinical variants of one process. In contrast, several forms of secondary tics should be excluded, including hypoxic head injury, head trauma, encephalitis, carbon monoxide intoxication, Huntington's disease, neuroacanthocytosis, and startle disorders.[86] In these cases, tics are usually combined with other abnormal movements, often chorea, cognitive impairment, or other neurological deficits. Tics must also be differentiated from other hyperkinetic movement disorders, including myoclonus, blepharospasm, stereotypies, and hyperekplexia.[86] It may be difficult to differentiate complex motor tics and compulsions.

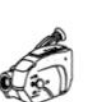

Evaluation. The diagnosis of GTS is usually made by the history and can be verified by neurological observation. However, given the voluntary supressibility of tics and the characteristic waxing and waning quality of the disease, it is possible that tics may be absent at the time of an examination. Asking the patient or the parents to bring a videotape of the movements taken during a period of relaxation and fatigue is often of greater diagnostic yield than several minutes of scrutiny in the doctor's office. Neuroimaging or other diagnostic studies are generally not required. A careful family history is critical, specifically as it relates to a history of tics, unusual habits or rituals, obsessive-compulsive symptoms, and other manifestations of GTS. Attention should be paid to the possibility of neonatal or perinatal injury and whether the child met developmental milestones appropriately. Blood tests in selected cases may include genetic testing for Huntington's disease and neuroacanthocytosis.

Management. Because most tic disorders are mild, the majority of patients require no pharmacological therapy. Education and identification of normal patterns of waxing and waning of symptoms are often the only interventions needed. Because of the fluctuating nature of GTS, however, at some point many patients require short-term drug therapy. In such cases, therapy should be targeted to the symptoms that are particularly troublesome for the patient, and distinctions should be made between tics, ADHD, and OCD. Tics most often respond to DA receptor blockers such as pimozide, fluphenazine, haloperidol, and risperidol. Many clinicians prefer pimozide (1 to 8 mg/day) and fluphenazine because they may be less sedating than other neuroleptic drugs. However, all neuroleptics carry a risk of tardive dyskinesia and require regular follow-up. Tetrabenazine, a monoamine depletor and DA receptor blocker, also improves tics, and, although it is not readily available in the United States, it does not carry a substantial risk of tardive dyskinesia. OCDs often respond to clomipramine, sertraline, fluoxetine, and paroxetine. Patients who have difficulty with OCD and also report problems in falling asleep or wetting the bed may be good candidates for the tricyclic antidepressant clomipramine. Clonidine, guanfacine, and methylphenidate are helpful for patients with ADHD, and lithium carbonate and carbamazepine are sometimes used for patients who have severe mood changes and impulse control problems.[92] Supportive individual or family counseling may help the patient and the family adapt to the many internal and external stresses associated with the GTS. In addition, neuropsychological testing to identify the patient's strengths and weaknesses usually allow the patient to reach his or her maximum academic potential. The local and national Tourette Syndrome Association can serve as an important resource for educational material and as a patient advocate in the school and work environment.

Prognosis and Future Perspectives. Most patients show a marked improvement after adolescence and have few or no clinically significant tics as adults. Ten to 30 percent continue to be symptomatic throughout early adulthood and middle age.[87] The pathogenic mechanism for GTS remains unknown, but current research focuses on the identification of genetic and biochemical mechanisms of this complex neurobehavioral disorder.

OTHER STEREOTYPIES

Stereotyped motor behavior can occur in normal children and in children with a variety of other primary neurodegenerative conditions. Repetitive head banging, an example of stereotypic activity, is seen in 15 percent of normal children.[93] In addition, thumb sucking, rocking, and other ritualistic behaviors are common during childhood. Most stereotypies, however, represent evidence of underlying brain dysfunction and hence require recognition. Stereotypic movements occur in at least a third of mentally retarded patients and are a characteristic feature of various autistic disorders such as infantile autism and Rett's, Angleman's, and Asperger's syndromes.[74] In all these conditions, stereotypies present as repetitive, coordinated, purposeless, involuntary movements such as chewing, lip smacking, body rocking, shoulder shrugging, marching in place, shifting of weight, and thrusting movements of the trunk and pelvis. Respiratory dyskinesia can produce grunting vocalizations, hyperventilation, and shortness of breath.

Rett's syndrome occurs only in girls and is believed to be linked to the X chromosome but is lethal in hemizygous males.[74] Some authors have suggested that Rett's syndrome is a result of disordered lipid metabolism, whereas others believe that these children have a derangement of the neuronal mitochondria. Typically, these children develop normally through the first 6 to 12 months of life, but then motor abnormalities (stereotypies, dystonia, chorea) emerge, accompanied by cognitive regression. The stereotypies observed most frequently in girls with Rett's syndrome include clapping, wringing, clenching, washing, patting, and rubbing behaviors. Other hyperkinetic disorders of movement include oromandibular dystonia, other dystonias, scoliosis, myoclonus, and choreoathetosis. All patients also have gait disturbances, and parkinsonian findings are manifest chiefly as hypomimia, rigidity, and bradykinesia.[74, 93]

Children with Angleman's syndrome have a jerky gait (puppet movements), a tendency to exhibit hand flapping stereotypies, and laughter with minimal stimulus. Patients with Angleman's syndrome and Prader-Willi syndrome both have a similar 15q11–13 chromosomal deletion, and parental origin of the chromosomal abnormality has been postulated to play a role. The children have psychomotor and cognitive delay and ataxia; speech is almost completely absent.[94] Seizures are present in nearly all patients, and 72 percent have early feeding problems. Eventually, 70 percent of these children learn to walk, and many are able to help with household chores. The most characteristic movement in this disorder is hand flapping with elbow and wrist flexion, but athetosis and tremulousness may also be present.

Asperger's syndrome is an autistic disorder manifested by poor reciprocal interaction, inappropriate emotional expression, impaired nonverbal communication, circumscribed interests, and repetitive activities. These children generally function at a higher intellectual level than most patients with pervasive developmental disorders. Like other autistic patients, they have stereotyped motor behavior, clumsiness, and tics.[74] Abnormalities in patients with Asperger's syndrome include cortical atrophy with widened Sylvian fissure anomalies (the opercular sign). Increased lipofuscin is present in the brain, conjunctiva, and muscle, and the substantia nigra has reduced pigmentation.

Because many children in the preceding categories receive treatment with chronic neuroleptic agents, their primary stereotypies must be distinguished from drug-induced tardive dyskinesia. Prominent lingual-facial buccal movements are typical of the latter condition and are less characteristic of the primary stereotypies.

In all these disorders routine laboratory data, spinal fluid analysis, and chromosomal studies are usually normal. No consistent neurochemical abnormalities have been found. Postmortem studies in patients with Rett's and Angleman's syndromes reveal microcephaly and mild neuronal loss with diffuse gliosis.[74] Evaluation for Asperger's syndrome by MRI may reveal abnormalities.[94] In all instances, therapy for patients with stereotypies is empirical and involves primarily the use of neuroleptic agents or dopamine-depleting drugs such as reserpine and tetrabenazine.

RESTLESS LEGS SYNDROME

Restless legs syndrome (RLS) is one of the most common movement disorders, affecting about 5 to 10 percent of the general population.[95, 96] Clinical criteria established by the International Restless Legs Syndrome Study Group include a set of four symptoms that establish the diagnosis of RLS: (1) a desire to move the limbs, often associated with unpleasant sensations; (2) restlessness: (3) worsening of symptoms at rest and at least temporary relief with movement; and (4) worsening of symptoms in the evening or night.

The sensations that people feel are always unpleasant but not necessarily painful. The most common descriptions used include such words as "need to move," "crawling," "tingling," "restless," "cramping," "creeping," "pulling," "painful," "electric," "tension," "discomfort," and "itching." Despite the name, these sensations can also be felt in the arms, although the legs are almost always more severely affected. Another feature that many patients with RLS have is called periodic limb movements while asleep. These are kicking movements of the legs while patients are asleep; these movements may be irregular and simple or rhythmic and more complex, resembling bicycling movements. Several surveys have now shown how prevalent RLS symptoms are, and the disorder increases with age. RLS patients often do not see a physician until mid- to later life but report subtle symptoms dating from much earlier in their life. These symptoms typically worsen over time.

The exact cause of RLS is not known, but in most cases it appears to be inherited in an autosomal dominant pattern. Secondary RLS may be associated with neuropathy, kidney failure, iron deficiency, and pregnancy. The most consistently effective treatments for RLS are dopaminergic medications, such as levodopa or DA agonists, including pramipexole, ropinirole, pergolide, bromocriptine, and cabergoline. Opioids may also help RLS symptoms.

PAINFUL LEGS–MOVING TOES SYNDROME

Painful legs–moving toes syndrome (PLMTS) is a movement disorder associated with significant sensory symptoms. The condition is idiopathic in origin but usually develops in association with back pain and often in the context of prior back injury or surgery. No specific pathophysiological mechanisms have been elucidated, and although a spinal cord or peripheral nervous system origin has been proposed, electrophysiological studies are often normal.[97] Because the condition sometimes follows herpes zoster infection, primary involvement of the posterior roots and ganglia has been suggested to explain the syndrome. The movements are not a response to the pain because even after local anesthesia or sympathetic blockade, the movements persist. Clinically, the condition involves continuous writhing movements of the toes and pain in the legs. The pain may range from mildly irritating to excruciatingly severe.[98] In most cases, it has a constant, boring quality, but it can be burning or crushing. It does not, however, have a shooting or electric quality like a radicular irritation. The toe movements are sinuous and crawling, usually continuous throughout the waking hours and incessantly repetitive. Unlike akathisia, the patient feels no relief in moving and instead tires from fruitless attempts to stop the movement. There is no effective treatment for PLMTS, but sympathetic blockade and anticonvulsants have been used.[98]

ACTION OR NONREST TREMORS (Table 34–6)

Essential tremor (ET) is the most frequent hyperkinetic movement disorder. Its age-adjusted prevalence is 2 to 5 percent,[26] and, as a lifelong illness, ET may affect any age group. It has a bimodal distribution of age at onset, with two peaks, adolescence and the fourth to fifth decade of life. In many families, ET is inherited in an autosomally dominant pattern, and in these patients, the term *familial tremor* can be used interchangeably with ET. Although central mechanisms are thought to be causative, no specific structural abnormality has been noted in the brains of patients with ET. Because ET can be exacerbated by hyperthyroidism and by caffeine and noradrenergic drugs, alterations in the central norepinephrine chemistry have been suggested.

In contrast to the resting tremor characteristic of PD, ET is a *postural* tremor, which is characteristically present during maintenance of a position. This tremor is typically an alternating flexion-extension movement, whereas supination-pronation oscillation is more characteristic of Parkinson's tremor. ET is also faster (7 to 10 Hz) than the PD tremor (4 to 7 Hz), and when fully developed, it usually involves the head, neck, and voice. Tremor often interferes with handwriting, drawing, holding a spoon, using a drinking cup, and manipulating tools.[26] The vocal cords may be affected, resulting in a wavering voice. Although ET usually occurs in isolation, it can be associated with various other neurological conditions including dystonia, parkinsonism, and certain inherited peripheral neuropathies (e.g., Charcot-Marie-Tooth disease). The differential diagnosis includes normal physiological tremor and the tremors associated with anxiety, thyrotoxicosis, and alcohol withdrawal as well as druginduced tremors resulting from bronchodilator use, corticosteroids, various CNS stimulants, lithium, and sodium valproate. ET diminishes with rest, ethanol, beta-noradrenergic blockers (usual dose, propranolol 80 to 240 mg/day), primidone (25 to 750 mg/day), and benzodiazepines. In addition, some patients may benefit from gabapentin and injections of botulinum toxin directly into the contracting muscles.[78] Thalamotomy or high-frequency thalamic stimulation may be an option in patients with severe tremors that are refractory to other treatment.[99]

Orthostatic tremor and primary writer's tremor are two particular forms of tremor that are highly dependent on posture. In the former, patients can usually walk with only mild discomfort, but when asked to stand in place for several seconds, they develop hard and cramping calves and thighs that shake uncontrollably. Although considered by some to be a variant of ET, this tremor does not respond to the usual

TABLE 34-6. Classification and Differential Diagnosis of Tremors

1. Rest tremors
   a. Parkinson's disease
   b. Other parkinsonian syndromes (less commonly)
   c. Midbrain ("rubral") tremor: rest < postural < kinetic
   d. Wilson's disease (also acquired hepatocerebral degeneration)
   e. Essential tremor—only if severe: rest < < postural and action
2. Postural and action ("terminal") tremors
   a. Physiological tremor
   b. Exaggerated physiological tremor (these factors can also aggravate other forms of tremor)
      i. Stress, fatigue, anxiety, emotion
      ii. Endocrine: hypoglycemia, thyrotoxicosis, pheochromocytoma, adrenocorticosteroids
      iii. Drugs and toxins: beta agonists, dopamine agonists, amphetamines, lithium, tricyclic antidepressants, neuroleptics, theophylline, caffeine, valproic acid, alcohol withdrawal, mercury ("Hatter's shakes"), lead, arsenic, others
   c. Essential tremor (familial or sporadic) ?subtypes
   d. Primary writing tremor
   e. With other CNS disorders
      i. Parkinson's disease
      ii. Other akinetic-rigid syndromes
      iii. Idiopathic dystonia, including focal dystonias
   f. With peripheral neuropathy
      i. Charcot-Marie-Tooth syndrome (controversial whether to call this the Roussy-Levy syndrome)
      ii. Variety of other peripheral neuropathies (especially dysgammaglobulinemia)
   g. Cerebellar tremor
3. Kinetic (intention) tremor
   Disease of cerebellar "outflow" (dentate nucleus and superior cerebellar peduncle): multiple sclerosis, trauma, tumor, vascular disease, Wilson's acquired hepatocerebral degeneration, drugs, toxins (e.g., mercury), others
4. Miscellaneous rhythmical movement disorders
   a. Psychogenic tremor
   b. Orthostatic tremor
   c. Rhythmical movements in dystonia (dystonic tremor)
   d. Rhythmical myoclonus (segmental myoclonus—e.g., palatal or branchial myoclonus, spinal myoclonus, limb myorhythmia)
   e. Oscillatory myoclonus
   f. Asterixis
   g. Clonus
   h. Epilepsia partialis continua
   i. Hereditary chin quivering
   j. Spasmus nutans
   k. Head bobbing with third ventricular cysts
   l. Nystagmus

Modified from Weiner WJ, Lang AE: Movement Disorders: A comprehensive survey. New York, Futura, 1989.

drugs described previously, and clonazepam (1 to 10 mg/day) is usually far more effective. Baclofen can also be used. The differential diagnosis includes dystonia and stiff-person syndrome. Similarly, primary writer's tremor does not occur outside the very specific activity of writing. It is thought that the complicated posture and muscle activation of writing induces the contractions in the agonist and antagonist hand muscles that induce the tremor. Sometimes the hand cramps at the same time, suggesting the presence of an underlying dystonia. The handwriting becomes sloppy, shaky, and large. Patients may respond to the medications used for ET, but often they improve more with anticholinergic medicines, again suggesting that dystonia may underlie these tremulous movements. Importantly, changing to a large, fat pen that requires different muscles for holding and writing with it or switching to typing is often the most helpful of all therapies.

Cerebellar kinetic tremor, sometimes referred to as an intention tremor, is most apparent during a goal-directed limb movement such as that used in the finger-to-nose or heel-to-shin test. In contrast to postural tremor, the patient's greatest disability occurs at the "endpoint," when a sudden destabilization occurs with severe shaking. This tremor is usually caused by a lesion in the cerebellar outflow (dentatorubral) tracts,[26] and therefore it is seen most typically in patients with multiple sclerosis, cerebrovascular accidents, or primary cerebellar disorders. Likewise, rubral tremor, a tremor that mixes rest, postural, and kinetic tremors, is generally not an idiopathic tremor and is induced by structural disease in the midbrain or fiber pathways connecting this region with the cerebellar and thalamic nuclei. Treatment of these tremors is frustrating, and no reliable pharmacological success has been reported. Because these patients are generally not weak and overshoot their targets as they move, stabilization of the involved limbs with wrist weights can reduce the amplitude and disability of the tremor.

Dystonic tremor is a prominent form of shaking that occurs as a compensation for dystonic spasms and must be recognized so that the underlying dystonia can be treated (see earlier discussion). Finally, palatal tremor, also termed *palatal myoclonus*, is characterized by continuous and synchronous contractions of the soft palate that occur at frequencies of 100 to 150 per minute (range, 20 to 600 per minute). Patients may not notice the jerking movements unless they are accompanied by persistent ear clicks caused by the repetitive opening and closing of the eustachian tubes. Concomitant contractions of other muscles, including the larynx, extraocular muscles, neck, diaphragm, tongue, and face, may be observed. These patients may have additional symptoms including postural tremor, oscillopsia, dysphagia, and dysarthria. The movements, which generally persist throughout life with infrequent remissions, may be idiopathic or due to brain stem or cerebellar disease. The anatomical and physiological bases underlying palatal tremor involve the hypertrophic degeneration of the olivary nucleus located within the medulla oblongata. The alteration of the inferior olive develops secondary to a lesion within the Guillain-Mollaret triangle, a pathway extending from the contralateral dentate nucleus via the superior cerebellar peduncle and ipsilateral central tegmental tract. Palatal tremor is usually resistant to therapy, which is unnecessary in most patients. 5-Hydroxytryptophan, the serotonin precursor, and carbamazepine are variably effective. Others have reported success with clonazepam, tetrabenazine, and trihexyphenidyl. Surgical intervention, including perforation of the tympanic membrane and tamponade of the eustachian tubes, is unsuccessful.

WILSON'S DISEASE

Pathogenesis and Pathophysiology. Wilson's disease (WD), or hepatolenticular degeneration, is an autosomal recessive disorder of copper metabolism. The specific genetic biochemical defect appears to be an abnormality of a copper-binding, membrane-associated adenosine triphosphatase–associated protein, and the allele for this protein has been localized to the long arm of chromosome 13.[100] It is postulated that most of the symptoms result from excess deposition of copper in tissues, particularly in the brain and liver.

Epidemiology and Risk Factors. This rare neurodegenerative movement disorder occurs in approximately 1 in 40,000 people. Although the disorder may not become clinically evident until the fourth or fifth decade of life, the initial presentation most often appears in the early twenties.[100]

Clinical Features and Associated Disorders. Clinical features are age-dependent. Children with WD exhibit a typical facies (so-called sardonic smile), behavioral abnormalities, and various motor disorders.[101] These include tremor (particularly in a wing-beating position), dystonia, rigidity, postural instability, dysarthria, and ataxia.[102] Some patients also exhibit mental and behavioral changes and seizures. Almost all patients show evidence of hepatic dysfunction. The adult patient usually presents with parkinsonian features, dystonia, athetosis, and slow (myorhythmic) or coarse postural (so-called wing-beating) tremor. In adults, the neurological symptoms predominate over the hepatic dysfunction, and the disorder appears to be less rapidly progressive. Approximately a third of patients present with psychiatric symptoms. These range from irritability and loss of impulse control to mania and depression, sometimes with catatonic symptoms.

The clinical hallmark of the disorder is the presence of a brownish-golden ring at the corneal rim (Kayser-Fleischer ring), which is due to the deposition of copper in the cornea. This sign is seen in almost all patients with neurological or psychiatric manifestations of WD, although slit-lamp examination is sometimes necessary to detect the copper deposition.[101] Other ocular abnormalities seen in Wilson's disease include "sunflower" subcapsular cataracts, retinitis pigmentosa, optic nerve atrophy, and loss of smooth pursuit.

Differential Diagnosis. The differential diagnosis of WD depends on the phenotypical presentation. In children, evaluation usually centers around hepatic disorders, whereas in adults, diagnostic considerations center around the type of movement disorder seen (tremor, chorea, dystonia, or parkinsonism). Although Kayser-Fleischer rings are extremely helpful in confirming this diagnosis clinically, they are also seen in patients with silver intoxication, primary biliary cirrhosis, Addison's disease, carotinemia, and chalcosis as a result of unilateral trauma to the eye with copper-containing foreign bodies.[101]

Evaluation. All patients should be evaluated by an ophthalmologist for the presence of the Kayser-Fleischer ring. Decreased serum ceruloplasmin (<20 mg/dL) in 90 percent of patients, increased urinary copper excretion (>100 μg/mL), impaired hepatic and renal function, hemolytic anemia, and aminoaciduria may also be present. In most cases a 24-hour urinary copper screen will detect elevated urinary copper levels (>100 μg/24 hours). If these tests are not diagnostic, liver biopsy should be performed with copper measurements (copper greater than 200 μg/g dry weight).[26] T2-weighted MRI scans may show the "face of the panda" sign in the midbrain due to hypodensity of the superior colliculi and hyperdensity in the medial substantia nigra and tegmentum. Fluorodopa PET scans are abnormal in symptomatic patients, demonstrating evidence of nigrostriatal damage.

Management. Because good recovery of hepatic and neurological function is possible in most patients, treatment must be instituted quickly. The goal of therapy is to reduce copper intake by means of a low-copper diet and increase copper excretion. D-Penicillamine is the chelating agent most often used; its side effects are potentially serious but preventable. These include nephrotic syndrome, fever, thrombocytopenia, dermatitis, vitamin B_6 deficiency, seizures, and zinc deficiency, which causes impairment of taste and smell. Pyridoxine should be administered along with penicillamine. Some investigators suggest using tetrathiomolybdate, a drug that both blocks copper absorption and binds to blood-borne copper, as an initial therapy. In addition, zinc acetate may be used as a maintenance therapy because of its low potential for serious side effects other than gastrointestinal effects. Dietary education about foods containing high levels of copper should be undertaken, and specific restrictions should be placed on liver and shellfish.[101] In patients who have sustained severe liver damage at the time of treatment, liver transplantation may be considered but remains controversial.

Since the disorder is inherited as an autosomal recessive trait, it is important to screen other members of the family with a neurological examination, serum ceruloplasmin level, and slit-lamp examination of the cornea. The clinical manifestations of the disorder and progression of disease may be prevented by early institution of copper chelation therapy.

Prognosis and Future Perspectives. If WD is recognized early in the course of the illness and is treated aggressively with initial and maintenance chelation therapy, it is potentially a curable disorder. Without treatment, patients progress to disability and death. The gene for WD has been identified on chromosome 13, but several mutations within the gene have been found, and therefore, DNA testing is not yet practical.[101]

HEMIFACIAL SPASM

Hemifacial spasm (HFS) is characterized by intermittent twitching of the muscles supplied by one facial nerve. It is thought to result from compression of the facial nerve at its junction with the brain stem by an aberrant or ectopic posterior fossa artery. Whereas many cases are idiopathic in origin, compression by vascular structures was responsible in over 90 percent of cases; other rare causes include tumors and bony or other abnormalities.[103] The average age-adjusted annual incidence for patients of all ages is 0.78 per 100,000, and the prevalence has been estimated at 14.5 per 100,000 in women and 7.4 per 100,000 in men.[104] Onset generally occurs between the second and eighth decades of life, the average age at onset being 45 to 51. Onset during infancy is atypical and usually indicates an underlying tumor, anomaly, or other pathology. Women are more commonly affected than men, and Asians have a particularly high risk compared with other populations. Although familial cases have been reported, most are sporadic. Trigeminal neuralgia can be associated with the development of HFS, suggesting that ephaptic transmission may underlie the pathophysiology of these two syndromes.

Clinically, symptoms begin in the periorbital region and spread to the ipsilateral facial muscles during the next few months. Spasm occurs spontaneously, is almost always unilateral, and is exacerbated by voluntary facial movements such as lip pursing, stress, fatigue, anxiety, or a change in head position. The movements often persist during sleep. Stapedius muscle contraction frequently accompanies contraction of the muscles of facial expression and may produce ipsilateral tinnitus.[103]

HFS must be differentiated from other conditions that cause involuntary facial movements. Blepharospasm and other forms of facial dystonia are almost always bilateral. Postparalytic facial spasms generally reflect either fixed contraction of the facial muscles or synkinesis or both. There is always a history of preceding facial weakness (e.g., Bell's palsy), and spontaneous spasms are generally absent. Spastic paretic facial contracture may be confused with HFS. The involved side is weak and contracted, unlike the situation in HFS, in which the facial muscles are relaxed between twitches. Facial myokymia is characterized clinically by undulating movements of the facial muscles. Facial tics are rapid, stereotyped, and relatively well coordinated movements that may also occur in regions distant from the face. Hemimasticatory spasm involves muscles innervated by both the facial and trigeminal nerves.

In the patient with normal results on neurological examination, including careful attention to brain stem testing (e.g., blink reflex and extraocular motility), further workup is usually not needed. If, however, neurological abnormalities, such as facial sensory deficits or an abnormal corneal blink reflex, are present, MRI and possibly MR angiography are suggested. Specific attention to the cerebellopontine angle and brain stem is required to detect possible tumors or arteriovenous malformations.

Although some clinicians treat HFS first with clonazepam, botulinum toxin injection to the involved muscles is now the treatment of choice.[103] The role of surgical decompression has diminished with the advent of this therapy, but surgery is still performed in some clinical settings. Endoscopic surgical correction may offer a permanent treatment with less morbidity than posterior fossa exploration. Myectomies, nerve sectioning, and phenol injections have essentially been replaced by botulinum toxin injections.

ESSENTIAL MYOCLONUS

As with other movement disorders, myoclonus may be classified in several ways, including phenomenologically, anatomico-physiologically (see Chapter 16), and etiologically. The etiological divisions are physiological, essential, epileptic, and symptomatic myoclonus. Physiological forms include benign hiccups and hypnic jerks, which are sudden movements experienced by many normal individuals when falling asleep. These two phenomena rarely require evaluation or treatment.[105] Because epileptic myoclonus and the vast array of symptomatic causes of myoclonus are described in the appropriate etiological chapters in this book, this section reviews only the hereditodegenerative (essential) forms of myoclonus.

Pathogenesis and Pathophysiology. Using the term paramyoclonus multiplex, Friedreich presumably was first to describe a patient with essential myoclonus. Although myoclonus has been clinically well defined, there has been no biochemical investigation that has explained the pathophysiological mechanism underlying essential myoclonus. Cerebral blood flow studies utilizing SPECT and xenon-133 or [technetium-99m]-d,l-hexamethylpropyleneamineoxime have revealed focal asymmetries in cerebral blood flow patterns consisting of relative hypoperfusion of the left cerebral hemisphere combined with an associated crossed cerebellar diaschisis.[106] This pattern could result from small lesions in the brain stem or basal ganglia, with secondary deafferentation of the ipsilateral frontal lobe and contralateral cerebellum, suggesting that essential myoclonus has a subcortical origin. Electrophysiological studies also suggest a subcortical origin for this form of myoclonus.

Epidemiology and Risk Factors. Essential myoclonus is a rare disorder; however, the overall prevalence in the population is unknown.

Clinical Features and Associated Disorders. Since its initial description, the diagnostic criteria for this form of myoclonus have evolved to the present state (Table 34–7). The jerks in essential myoclonus are brief (50 to 200 msec) and may be generalized, multifocal, segmental, or unilateral. Myoclonic jerks mainly involve the muscles of the neck or upper body and are exacerbated by action, particularly writing or outstretching of the arms. The jerks abate during sleep and are ameliorated by alcohol. The beneficial effects of the latter are at times dramatic and nearly diagnostic; however, following withdrawal of alcohol, the condition frequently becomes worse on the rebound.[107]

Some individuals with essential myoclonus have associated dystonic movements, including spasmodic torticollis and blepharospasm. The presence of dystonia is an exception to the diagnostic criteria, as noted previously. Further complicating these diagnostic criteria is the occurrence of myoclonus in patients with hereditary dystonia, so-called myoclonic dystonia or dystonia with alcohol-responsive lightening-like jerks. Whether these entities represent different disorders remains to be elucidated by future genetic studies.[108]

In contrast to the hereditary form, the characteristics of sporadic essential myoclonus are more heterogeneous. Patients with this disorder range in age from 2 to 64 years at onset, have normal neurological findings on examination, and have normal EEG results. The myoclonic jerks may be oscillatory, rhythmical segmental, nonrhythmical segmental, or nonrhythmical multifocal; the trunk and proximal limb muscles, followed by the muscles of the neck and face, are

TABLE 34–7. **Diagnostic Criteria for Essential Myoclonus**

1. Onset of myoclonus in first or second decade
2. Males and females equally affected
3. Benign course
4. Dominant mode of inheritance with variable severity
5. Absence of seizures, dementia, gross ataxia, or other deficit
6. Normal EEG
7. Normal somatosensory evoked potentials

TABLE 34–8. **Symptomatic Myoclonus**

I. Metabolic—endogenous
 Hypoxia, uremia, chronic hemodialysis, hepatic failure, hypercarbia, hypoglycemia, hyponatremia, nonketotic hyperglycemia
II. Metabolic—exogenous
 Bismuth, cocaine, organic mercury, methylbromide, strychnine, tetraethyl lead, tetanus
III. Degenerative
 Dementias—Alzheimer's disease
 Movement disorders—corticobasal degeneration, multiple system atrophy, progressive supranuclear palsy, Hallervorden-Spatz disease, Huntington's disease
IV. Neurovascular
 Ischemia
 Hemorrhagic
V. Infectious
 Transmissible spongiform encephalopathies—Creutzfeldt-Jakob disease, kuru, viral—measles, Epstein-Barr virus, etc.
VI. Neoplastic
 Neuroblastoma
 Paraneoplastic disorders—ovarian, lung, breast
VII. Autoimmune—multiple sclerosis
VIII. Traumatic
 Penetrating trauma—brain, spinal cord
 Heat stroke
 Electric shock
 Decompression illness
IX. Iatrogenic
 Medications (amantadine, etomidate, penicillin, buspirone, diclofenac, lithium, metoclopramide, tricyclic antidepressants, levodopa, dopamine agonists)
 Procedures (water-soluble contrast media, post-thalamotomy)

most affected. Generally, patients do not demonstrate marked progression of symptoms or disability.

Differential Diagnosis. Because essential myoclonus has no known cause, its diagnosis is one of exclusion, and other causes must be evaluated. The co-existence of myoclonus and epilepsy suggests the presence of a form of epileptic myoclonus, which may present with either focal or generalized myoclonus. In these patients epilepsy is the dominant feature, the syndrome is generally age-related, and in most cases EEG abnormalities are associated (see Chapter 52). Myoclonic syndromes associated with underlying diseases that cause a predominant encephalopathy, ataxia, dementia, or pyramidal or extrapyramidal signs as major features of the illness are termed symptomatic myoclonias. Syndromes comprising symptomatic myoclonus with seizures are termed progressive myoclonic epilepsies (PME) (see Chapter 52), although the seizures are generally minor or late developments. Symptomatic causes of myoclonus include a variety of disorders (Table 34–8).

Evaluation. The evaluation of essential myoclonus relies on a detailed history and a thorough neurological examination. Neuroimaging studies (head MRI and CT) in patients with essential myoclonus are normal, but these studies are helpful in patients with alternative diagnoses such as stroke, degenerative disorders, and trauma. Electrophysiological tools, including EMG, EEG, and somatosensory evoked potentials (SEPs), can be particularly valuable in distinguishing the levels of neural dysfunction in patients with myoclonic syndromes. In essential myoclonus, these studies are normal; however, EEG results are generally abnormal in patients with epileptic myoclonus and the PMEs, showing epileptiform discharges. Patients with metabolic or toxic causes of myoclonus may also show diffuse slowing on EEG. SEPs are also normal in patients with essential myoclonus, as well as subcortical and spinal forms of myoclonus, but are abnormal in those syndromes originating in the cortex, including most PMEs. Blood, cerebrospinal fluid, and tissue biopsies, although normal in patients with essential myoclonus, should be used in the appropriate clinical settings.

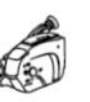

Treatment. Despite its nonprogressive, benign nature, essential myoclonus can significantly impair the performance of routine daily activities, and symptomatic treatment of the myoclonic jerks can result in substantial improvement in the patient's quality of life. Although alcohol has been shown to alleviate the movements in a number of patients with essential myoclonus, the limitations of this pharmacological therapy are obvious. Manipulation of brain serotonin levels, although beneficial in some forms of myoclonus, has generally been unsuccessful in the treatment of essential myoclonus. A variety of medications may be used in this and other myoclonic disorders (Table 34–9). The benzodiazepines, particularly clonazepam, are the most consistently effective medications used for the treatment of essential myoclonus. In addition, favorable treatment results have been observed with certain anticholinergic medications

TABLE 34–9. **Medications for the Treatment of Myoclonus**

Medication	Common Initial Dose	Usual Maximum Dose	Clinical Uses
Chlorpromazine	25–50 mg intravenously	50 mg by mouth t.i.d.	Hiccups
Clonazepam	0.5–1.5 mg/d	20 mg/d by mouth	Most forms of myoclonus
L-5-Hydoxytryptophan	25 mg by mouth q.i.d.	500 mg by mouth q.i.d.	Posthypoxic myoclonus
with carbidopa	25 mg by mouth q.i.d.	50 mg by mouth q.i.d.	
Levetiracetam	500 mg b.i.d.	1500 mg b.i.d.	Cervical myoclonus
Metoclopramide	10 mg intravenously	10 mg by mouth t.i.d.	Hiccups
Piracetam	7.2 g/d by mouth	16 g/d by mouth	Cortical myoclonus
Tetrabenazine	25–50 mg/d by mouth	200 mg/d by mouth	Segmental myoclonus
Valproic acid	15 mg/kg/day by mouth	2000 mg/d	Most forms of myoclonus

including benztropine and trihexyphenidyl. Piracetam and the structurally related drug levetiracetam have been also reported to be effective in the treatment of cortical myoclonus.[109]

STARTLE SYNDROMES

The startle syndromes are characterized by an exaggerated motor response to unexpected auditory, and at times somesthetic or visual, stimuli. Confusion has overtaken the classification of these syndromes as various terms have been introduced. Hyper*ek*plexia has often been used synonymously with any startle disorder; however, the word hyperexplexia (to jump excessively) was used to describe the autosomal dominantly inherited exaggerated startle reflexes in a large Dutch kindred. Matsamuto and Hallett have advocated the use of the proper Greek term hyperexplexia to denote any movement disorder in which there is a physiological demonstration of exaggerated startle reflexes and have incorporated this terminology in dividing the startle syndromes into five main types (Table 34–10).[110]

The pathophysiology of hyperexplexia has been recently elucidated, and now there is general agreement that the motor response in patients with hereditary and symptomatic hyperexplexia is a pathological exaggeration of the normal startle reflex.[111] To elicit a startle response in normal humans, an acoustic stimulus must have a volume of approximately 100 dB and a rise time of less than 5 msec. The response to such an unexpected stimulus varies in normals, and eye blinking may be the only visible reaction. Typically, however, facial grimacing, head flexion with shoulder abduction, elbow flexion, pronation of the forearms, and fist clenching occur. In normals, habituation (a decrease in magnitude of response with repetition of the stimulus) occurs with four to five repeated stimuli. Electrophysiologically, surface EMG recordings demonstrate a bilaterally symmetrical response composed of a blink response and activation of other craniocervical muscles with variable limb muscle recruitment. The overall pattern of muscle recruitment suggests that the normal human auditory startle reflex originates in the caudal brain stem. The audiogenic jumps seen in hyperexplexias are believed to be generated by the normal startle circuit underheightened excitability, perhaps of cerebral origin. Hereditary hyperexplexia is inherited as an autosomal dominant trait caused by mutations in the alpha-1 subunit of the inhibitory glycine receptor, which is localized to chromosome 5q.[112]

The hallmark of hyperexplexia is an exaggerated startle response to a sudden, unexpected stimulus. Children with hyperexplexia are born with continuous stiffness and demonstrate a flexor posture, both of which disappear with sleep. Severely affected children startle excessively to sudden stimuli, and infants characteristically flex rather than extend their arms as seen with the normal Moro response. Apnea and cardiorespiratory arrest can occur, perhaps due to stiffness of the chest wall. The increased tone gradually disappears during the first several months of life, yet the startle response can interfere with walking and may result in trauma from falls. Severely affected patients have startle attacks throughout life; they often become worse during adolescence, and variable improvement occurs later in life. Other affected individuals may have infrequent attacks that may become worse with stress or illness. Violent bilateral flexion of the legs can occur during descent into slow-wave sleep or rarely during the daytime. Abdominal muscle involvement has been postulated to result at times in inguinal and abdominal hernias.

Other cerebral (perinatal anoxia), diencephalic (stroke), and brain stem (inflammatory, hemorrhage) lesions have also been associated with hyperexplexia, but most reports lack the physiological investigations necessary to prove that the startle reflex was involved. Certain psychiatric diseases including post-traumatic stress disorder may be associated with evidence of hyperarousal and an exaggerated startle reflex. Others have observed increased startle reactions in catatonic schizophrenics, patients with GTS, and newborns following in utero exposure to cocaine. The majority of acquired cases of exaggerated startle, however, are idiopathic and have no identifiable cause. An additional differential diagnostic consideration in the presence of exaggerated startle is startle epilepsy. Characterized by epileptic seizures triggered by sudden unexpected stimuli preceded by a startle, this disorder has been described in patients with severe brain damage, most commonly perinatal anoxic encephalopathy, but also in those with Down's syndrome, Sturge-Weber syndrome, and Tay-Sachs disease. Finally, a group of behaviors including "jumping," latah, and myriachit have been considered to represent startle phenomena, but others suggest that these entities are merely culturally based, conditioned behaviors. As a group, individuals with these behaviors demonstrate an initial violent start in response to a sudden stimulus that is variably followed by automatic speech (echolalia, echopraxia, or coprolalia) and the exhibition of aggressive gestures or defensive postures.

Clonazepam and other benzodiazepines are considered the drugs of choice for the treatment of hyperexplexia; when effective, they reduce the severity and frequency of the startle reactions. Valproic acid, 5-hydroxytryptophan, and piracetam have also been successful in certain patients.

TABLE 34–10. **Startle Syndromes**

I. Hereditary hyperekplexia
II. Symptomatic hyperekplexia
III. Startle epilepsy
IV. Jumping, latah, myriachit
V. Psychogenic startle

Reviews and Selected Updates

American Academy of Neurology Quality Standards Subcommittee: Practice parameters: Initial therapy of Parkinson's disease. Neurology 1993;43:1296–1297.

Cardoso F, Eduardo C, Silva AP, Mota CC: Chorea in 50 consecutive patients with rheumatic fever. Mov Disord 1997;12:701–703.

Conrad C, Andreadis A, Trojanowski JQ, et al: Genetic evidence for the involvement of tau in progressive supranuclear palsy. Ann Neurol 1997;41:277–281.

Jankovic J: Therapeutic strategies in Parkinson's disease. *In* Jankovic J, Tolosa E (eds): Parkinson's Disease and Movement Disorders, 4th ed. Philadelphia, Lippincott, Williams & Wilkins, 2002, pp 116–151.

Jankovic J: Tourette's syndrome. N Engl J Med 2001;345:1184–1192.

Jankovic J, Beach J: Long-term effects of tetrabenazine in hyperkinetic movement disorders. Neurology 1997;48:358–362.

Jankovic J, Fahn S: Dystonic disorders. *In* Jankovic J, Tolosa E (eds): Parkinson's Disease and Movement Disorders, 4th ed. Philadelphia, Lippincott, Williams & Wilkins, 2002, pp 331–357.

Litvan I, Agid Y, Goetz C, et al: Accuracy of the clinical diagnosis of corticobasal degeneration: A clinicopathologic study. Neurology 1997;48:119–125.

Olanow CW, Watts RL, Koller WC: An algorithim (decision tree) for the management of Parkinson's disease (2001): Treatment guidelines. Neurology 2001;56 (Suppl 5):S1–S88.

Ozelius LJ, Hewett JW, Page CE, et al: The early onset torsion dystonia gene [DYT1] encodes an ATP-binding protein. Nature Genet 1997;17:40–48.

Therapeutics and Technology Assessment Subcommittee: Assessment: Training guidelines for the use of botulinum toxin for the treatment of neurologic disorders. Neurology 1994;44:2401–2403.

References

1. Gibb WRG, Lees AJ: Pathological clues to the cause of Parkinson's disease. *In* Marsden CD, Fahn S (eds): Movement Disorders, 3rd ed. Oxford, Butterworth, 1994, pp 147–166.
2. McNaught KSP, Jenner P: Proteasomal function is impaired in substantia nigra in Parkinson's disease. Neurosci Lett 2001;297:191–194.
3. Mayeux T, Marder K, Cote LJ, et al: The frequency of idiopathic Parkinson's disease by age, ethnic group, and sex in northern Manhattan, 1988–1993. Am J Epidemiol 1995;142:820–827.
4. Bennet DA, Beckett CA, Murray AM, et al: Prevalence of parkinsonian signs and associated mortality in a community population of older people. N Engl J Med 1996;334:71–76.
5. Koller W, Vetere-Overfield B, Gray C: Environmental risk factors in Parkinson's disease. Neurology 1990;40:1218–1221.
6. Rocca WA, Bower JH, McDonnell SK, et al: Time trends in the incidence of parkinsonism in Olmsted County, Minnesota. Neurology 2001;57:462–467.
7. Pezzoli G, Canesi M, Antonini A, et al: Hydrocarbon exposure and Parkinson's disease. Neurology 2000;55:667–673.
8. Hanna P, Jankovic J, Kilkpatrick J: Multiple system atrophy: The putative causative role of environmental toxins. Arch Neurol 1999;56:90–94.
9. Racette BA, McGee-Minnich L, Moerlein SM, et al: Welding-related parkinsonism: Clinical features, treatment, and pathophysiology. Neurology 2001;56:8–13.
10. Rosenow F, Herholz K, Lanfermann H, et al: Neurological sequelae of cyanide intoxication—the patterns of clinical, magnetic resonance imaging and positron emission tomography findings. Ann Neurol 1995;38:825–827.
11. Hernán MA, Takkouche B, Caamano-Isorna F, et al: A meta-analysis of coffee drinking, cigarette smoking, and the risk of Parkinson's disease. Ann Neurol 2002;52:276–284.
12. Ascherio A, Zhang S, Hernán MA, et al: Prospective study of caffeine consumption and risk of Parkinson's disease in men and women. Ann Neurol 2001;50:56–63.
13. Jankovic J: Classification and epidemiology of movement disorders. *In* Krauss JK, Jankovic J, Grossman RG (eds): Surgery for Parkinson's Disease and Movement Disorders. Philadelphia, Lippincott, Williams & Wilkins, 2001, pp 3–23.
14. Johnson WG, Hodge S, Duvoisin RC: Twin studies and the genetics of Parkinson's disease: A reappraisal. Mov Disord 1990;5:187–194.
15. Seeman P, Van Tol HHM: Dopamine receptor pharmacology. Trends Pharmacol Sci 1994;15:264–270.
16. Pappert EJ, Goetz CG, Niederman FG, et al: Liquid levodopa/carbidopa produces significant improvements in motor function without dyskinesia exacerbation. Neurology 1996;47:1493–1495.
17. Nutt JG, Holford NHG: The response to levodopa in Parkinson's disease: Imposing pharmacological law and order. Ann Neurol 1996;39:561–573.
18. The Parkinson Study Group: Effects of tocopherol deprenyl on the progression of disability in early Parkinson's disease. N Engl J Med 1993; 328:176–183.
19. Galvin JE, Lee VMY, Trojanowski JQ: Synucleinopathies: Clinical and pathological implications. Arch Neurol 2001;58:186–190.
20. Chung KKK, Dawson VL, Dawson TM: The role of the ubiquitin-protasomal pathway in Parkinson's disease and other neurodegenerative disorders. TINS 2001;24(Suppl):S7–S14.
21. Terreni L, Calabrese E, Calella AM, et al: New mutation (R42P) of the parkin gene in the ubiquitinlike domain associated with parkinsonism. Neurology 2001;56:463–466.
22. Shimura H, Hattoi N, Kubo S-I, et al: Familial Parkinson disease gene product, parkin, is a ubiquitin-protein ligase. Nat Genet 2000; 25:302–305.
23. Lücking CB, Dürr A, Bonifati V, et al: Association beween early-onset Parkinson's disease and mutations in the parkin gene. N Engl J Med 2000;342:1560–1567.
24. Gasser T, Müller-Myhsok B, Wszolek ZK, et al: A susceptibility locus for Parkinson's disease maps to chromosome 2p13. Nat Genet 1998;18: 262–265.
25. Farrer M, Gwinn K, Muenter M, et al: A chromosome 4p haplotype segregating with Parkinson's disease and postural tremor. Hum Mol Genet 1999;8:81–85.
26. Jankovic J: Essential tremor: Aeterogeneous disorder. Mov Disord 2002; 17:638–644.
27. Leroy E, Boyer R, Auberger G, et al: The ubiquitin pathway in Parkinson's disease. Nature 1998;395:451–452.
28. Valente EM, Brancati F, Ferraris A, et al: PARK6-linked parkinsonism occurs in several European families. Ann Neurol 2002;51:14–18.
29. Van Duijn CM, Dekker CJ, Bonifati V, et al: PARK7, a novel locus for autosomal recessive early-onset parkinsonism, on chromosome 1p36. Am J Hum Genet 2001;69:629–634.
30. Scott WK, Nance MA, Watts RL, et al: Complete genomic screen in Parkinson disease: Evidence for multiple genes. JAMA 2001;286: 2239–2244.
31. Stacy M, Brownlee J: Treatment options for early Parkinson's disease. Am Fam Phys 1996;53:1281–1287.
32. Rascol O, Brooks DJ, Korczyn AD, et al: A five-year study of the incidence of dyskinesia in patients with early Parkinson's disease who were treated with ropinirole or levodopa. 056 Study Group. N Engl J Med 2000;18:1484–1491.
33. The Parkinson Study Group: Pramipexole vs levodopa as initial treatment for Parkinson's disease. A randomized controlled trial. JAMA 2000;284:1931–1938.
34. Nutt JG, Woodward WR, Beckner RM, et al: Effect of peripheral catechol-O-methyl transferase inhibition on the pharmacokinetics and pharmacodynamics of levodopa in parkinsonian patients. Neurology 1994;44:913–919.
35. Jankovic J: Surgery for Parkinson's disease and other movement disorders: Benefits and limitations of ablation, stimulation, restoration, and radiation. Arch Neurol 2001;58:1970–1972.
36. The Deep-Brain Stimulation for Parkinson's Disease Study Group: Deep-brain stimulation of the subthalamic nucleus or the pars interna of the globus pallidus in Parkinson's disease. N Engl J Med 2001;345:956–963.
37. Freed CR, Greene PE, Breeze RE, et al: Transplantation of embryonic dopamine neurons for severe Parkinson's disease. N Engl J Med 2001;344:710–719.
38. Factor SA, Brown D, Mohlo EX, et al: Clozapine: A 2-year open trial in Parkinson's disease with psychosis. Neurology 1994;44:544–546.
39. Uitti RJ, Ahlskog JE, Maraganore DM, et al: Levodopa therapy and survival in idiopathic Parkinson's disease: Olmsted County project. Neurology 1993;43:1918–1926.
40. Hauw J-J, Daniel SE, Dickson D, et al: Preliminary NINDS neuropathologic criteria for Steele-Richardson-Olszewski syndrome (progressive supranuclear palsy). Neurology 1994;44:2015–2019.
41. Albers DS, Augood SJ: New insights into progressive supranuclear palsy. Trends Neurosci 2001;24:347–353.
42. Golbe LI, Davis PH, Schoenberg BS, et al: Prevalence and natural history of progressive supranuclear palsy. Neurology 1988;38:1031–1034.
43. Riley DE, Fogt N, Leigh RJ: The syndrome of "pure akinesia" and its relationship to progressive supranuclear palsy. Neurology 1994;44:1025–1029.
44. Litvan I, Agid Y, Jankovic J, et al: Accuracy of clinical criteria for the diagnosis of progressive supranuclear palsy (Steele-Richardson-Olszewski syndrome). Neurology 1996;47:1–9.
45. Burn DJ, Sawle GV, Brooks DJ: Differential diagnosis of Parkinson's disease, multiple system atrophy, and Steele-Richardson-Olszewski syndrome: Discriminant analysis of striatal 18F-dopa PET data. J Neurol Neurosurg Psychiatry 1994;57:278–284.
46. Ghika J, Tennis M, Hoffman E, et al: Idazoxan treatment in progressive supranuclear palsy. Neurology 1991;41:986–991.
47. Papp ML, Lantos PL: The distribution of oligodendroglial inclusions in multiple system atrophy and its relevance to clinical symptomatology. Brain 1994;117:235–243.
48. Gilman S: Multiple system atrophy. *In* Jankovic J, Tolosa E (eds): Parkinson's Disease and Movement Disorders, 4th ed. Philadelphia, Lippincott, Williams & Wilkins, 2002.
49. Wenning GK, Ben Shlomo Y, Magalhaes M, et al: Clinical features and natural history of multiple system atrophy: An analysis of 100 cases. Brain 1994;117:835–845.

50. Jankovic J, McDermott M, Carter J, et al: Variable expression of Parkinson's disease: A baseline analysis of the DATATOP cohort. Neurology 1991;41:1529–1534.
51. Brooks DJ, Ibanez V, Sawle GV, et al: Striatal D2 receptor status in patient with Parkinson's disease, striatonigral degeneration, and progressive supranuclear palsy, measured with 11C-raclopride and positron emission tomography. Ann Neurol 1992;31:184–192.
52. Polinsky RJ: Shy-Drager syndrome. *In* Jankovic J, Tolosa E (eds): Parkinson's Disease and Movement Disorders. Baltimore, Williams & Wilkins, 1993, pp 191–204.
53. Hughes AJ, Colosimo C, Kleedorfer B, et al: The dopaminergic response in multiple system atrophy. J Neurol Neurosurg Psychiatry 1992;55:1009–1013.
54. Jankovic J, Gilden JL, Hiner BC, et al: Neurogenic orthostatic hypotension: A double-blind placebo-controlled study with midodrine. Am J Med 1993;93:38–48.
55. Rinne JO, Lee MS, Thompson PD, Marsden CD: Corticobasal degeneration: A clinical study of 36 cases. Brain 1994;117:1183–1196.
56. Doody RS, Jankovic J: The alien hand and related signs. J Neurol Neurosurg Psychiatry 1992;55:806–810.
57. Lilienfield DE, Perl DP, Olanow CW: Guam neurodegeneration. *In* Calne DB (ed): Neurodegenerative Diseases. Philadelphia, WB Saunders, 1994, pp 895–908.
58. Galasko D, Salmon DP, Craig UK, et al: Clinical features and changing patterns of neurodegenerative disorders on Guam, 1997–2000. Neurology 2002;58:90–97.
59. Klawans HL: Hemiparkinsonism as a late complication of hemiatrophy: A new syndrome. Neurology 1981;31:625–628.
60. Lang AE: Hemiatrophy, juvenile-onset exertional alternating leg paresis, hypotonia and hemidystonia and adult-onset hemiparkinsonism: The spectrum of hemiparkinsonism-hemiatrophy syndrome. Mov Disord 1995;10:489–495.
61. Brashear HR, Phillips LH: Autoantibodies to GABAergic neurons and response to plasmapheresis in stiff-man syndrome. Neurology 1991;41:1588–1592.
62. Darnell RB, Victor J, Rubin M, et al: A novel antineuronal antibody in stiff-man syndrome. Neurology 1993;43:114–120.
63. Yamamoto R, Xi L, Francke U, et al: Primary structure of human amphiphisin, the dominant autoantigen of paraneoplastic stiff-man syndrome, and mapping of its gene (AMPH) to chromosome 7p13–p14. Hum Mol Genet 1995;4:265–268.
64. Thompson PD: Stiff people. *In* Marsden CD, Fahn S (eds): Movement Disorders, 3rd ed. Oxford, Butterworth, 1994, pp 373–405.
65. Dalakas MC, Fujii M, Li M, et al: High-dose intravenous immune globulin for stiff-person syndrome. N Engl J Med 2001;345:1870–1876.
66. DiFiglia M, Sapp E, Chase KO, et al: Aggregation of huntingtin in neuronal intranuclear inclusions and dystrophic neurites in brain. Science 1997;277:1990–1993.
67. Cattaneo E, Rigamonti D, Coffredo D, et al: Loss of normal huntingtin function: New developments in Huntington's disease research. Trends Neurosci 2001;24:182–188.
68. Nance MA: Huntington's disease another chapter rewritten. Am J Hum Genet 1996;59:1–6.
69. Ritchfield EK, Maguire-Zeiss KA, Vonkeman HE, et al: Preferential loss of preproenkephalin neurons from the striatum of Huntington's disease patients. Ann Neurol 1995;38:852–861.
70. Penney JB, Young AB: Huntington's disease. *In* Jankovic J, Tolosa E (eds): Parkinson's Disease and Other Movement Disorders, 3rd ed. Baltimore, Williams & Wilkins, 1998.
71. Huntington's Disease Collaboration Research Group: A novel gene containing a trinucleotide repeat that is expanded and unstable on Huntington's disease chromosomes. Cell 1993;72:971–983.
72. Jankovic J, Demirkiran M: Classification of paroxysmal dyskinesias and ataxias. *In* Frucht S, Fahn S (eds): Myoclonus and Paroxysmal Dyskinesias, Advances in Neurology. Philadelphia, Lippincott, Williams & Wilkins, 2002; pp387–400.
73. Bennett DA, Goetz CG: Acquired paroxysmal dyskinesia. *In* Joseph AB, Young RR (eds): Movement Disorders in Neurology and Neuropsychiatry. Oxford, Blackwell Scientific Publications, 1992, pp 548–556.
74. Stacy M, Jankovic J: Rare movement disorders associated with metabolic and neurodegenerative diseases. *In* Robertson MM, Eapen V (eds): Movement and Allied Disorders of Childhood. Chichester, John Wiley & Sons, 1995, pp 177–198.
75. Stacy M, Jankovic J: Differential diagnosis and treatment of childhood dystonia. Pediatr Ann 1993;22:353–358.
76. Breakfield XO, Kamm C, Hanson PI: TorsinA: Movement at many levels. Neuron 2001;31:9–12.
77. Lew H, Jordan C, Jerger J, Jankovic J: Acoustic reflex abnormalities in cranial-cervical dystonia. Neurology 1992;42:594–597.
78. Jankovic J, Brin MF: Therapeutic uses of botulinum toxin. N Engl J Med 1991;324:1186–1194.
79. Tintner R, Jankovic J: Botulinum toxin for the treatment of cervical dystonia. Exp Opin Pharmacother 2001;2:1985–1994.
80. Jankovic J: Botulinum toxin: Clinical implications of antigenicity and immunoresistance. *In* Brin MF, Hallett M, Jankovic J (eds): Scientific and Therapeutic Aspects of Botulinum Toxin. Philadelphia, Lippincott, Williams & Wilkins, 2002, pp 409–416.
81. Vercueil L, Pollak P, Fraix V, et al: Deep brain stimulation in the treatment of severe dystonia. J Neurol 2001;248:695–700.
82. Cardoso F, Jankovic J, Grossman RG, Hamilton WJ: Outcome after stereotactic thalamotomy for dystonia and hemiballismus. Neurosurgery 1995;36:501–508.
83. Swaiman KF: Hallervorden-Spatz and brain iron metabolism. Arch Neurol 1991;48:1285–1293.
84. Olanow CW: Hallervorden-Spatz syndrome: An iron storage disease. *In* Calne DB (ed): Neurodegenerative Diseases. Philadelphia, WB Saunders, 1994, pp 807–823.
85. Zhou B, Westaway SK, Levinson B, et al: A novel pantothenate kinase gene (PANK2) is defective in Hallervorden-Spatz syndrome. Nature Genet 2001;28:345–349.
86. Jankovic J: Tourette's syndrome. N Engl J Med 2001;345:1184–1192.
87. Singer HS: Neurobiology of Tourette syndrome. *In* Jankovic J (ed): Tourette Syndrome. Neurol Clin North Am 1997;15:357–380.
88. Leckman JF, Peterson BS, Anderson GM, et al: Pathogenesis of Tourette's syndrome. J Child Psychol Psychiatry 1997;38:119–142.
89. Tanner CM, Goldman SM: Epidemiology of Tourette syndrome. *In* Jankovic J (ed): Tourette Syndrome. Neurol Clin North Am 1997;15:357–380.
90. Kurlan R: Tourette's syndrome in a special education population: Hypothesis. Adv Neurol 1992;58:75–81.
91. Tourette Syndrome Classification Study Group: Definitions and classification of tic disorders. Arch Neurol 1993;50:1013–1016.
92. Kurlan R: Tourette's syndrome. *In* Jankovic J (ed): Neurobase. San Diego, Arbor Publishing, 1996.
93. Jankovic J: Stereotypies. *In* Marsden CD, Fahn S (eds): Movement Disorders, 3rd ed. Oxford, Butterworth, 1994, pp 503–517.
94. Clayton-Smith J: Clinical research on Angelman syndrome in the United Kingdom: Observations on 82 affected individuals. Am J Med Genet 1993;46:12–15.
95. Chokroverty S, Jankovic J: Restless legs syndrome: A disease in search of identity. Neurology 1999;52:907–910.
96. Ondo WG, Vuong DK, Jankovic J: Exploring the relationship between Parkinson's disease and restless legs syndrome. Arch Neurol 2002;59:421–424.
97. Dressler D, Thompson PD, Gledhill RF, Marsden CD: The syndrome of painful legs and moving toes. Mov Disord 1994;9:13–21.
98. Goetz CG, Buchman AS: Painful legs/moving toes syndrome. *In* Joseph AB, Young RR (eds): Movement Disorders in Neurology and Neuropsychiatry. Oxford, Blackwell Scientific Publications, 1992, pp 557–564.
99. Benabid AL, Pollack P, Gao D, et al: Chronic electrical stimulation of the ventralis intermedius nucleus of the thalamus as a treatment of movement disorders. J Neurosurg 1996;84:203–214.
100. Tanzi RE, Petrukin K, Chernov I: The Wilson's disease gene is a copper transporting ATPase with homology to the Menke's disease gene. Nat Genet 1993;5:344–350.
101. Demirkiran M, Jankovic J, Lewis RA, Cox DW: Neurologic presentation of Wilson's disease without Kayser-Fleisher ring. Neurology 1996;46:1040–1043.
102. Svetel M, Kozic D, Stefanoval E, et al: Dystonia in Wilson's disease. Mov Disord 2001;16:719–723.
103. Wang A, Jankovic J. Hemifacial spasm: Clinical correlates and treatments. Muscle Nerve 1998;21:1740–1747.
104. Auger RG, Whisnant JP: Hemifacial spasm in Rochester and Olmsted County, Minnesota, 1960 to 1984. Arch Neurol 1990;47:1233–1234.
105. Pappert EJ, Goetz CG: Treatment of myoclonus. *In* Kurlan R (ed): Treatment of Movement Disorders. Philadelphia, JB Lippincott, 1995, pp 247–336.
106. Delecluse F, Waldmar G, Vestermark S, et al: Cerebral blood flow deficits in hereditary essential myoclonus. Arch Neurol 1992;49:179–182.

107. Fahn S, Sjaastad O: Hereditary essential myoclonus in a large Norwegian family. Mov Disord 1991;3:237–247.
108. Quinn NP: Essential myoclonus and myoclonic dystonia. Mov Disord 1996;11:119–124.
109. Frucht SJ, Louis ED, Chuang C, Fahn S: A pilot tolerability and efficacy study of levetiracetam in patients with chronic myoclonus. Neurology 2001;57:1112–1114.
110. Matsumoto J, Hallett M: Startle syndromes. *In* Marsden CD, Fahn S (eds): Movement Disorders, 3rd ed. Oxford, Butterworth, 1994, pp 418–433.
111. Matsumoto J, Fuhr P, Nigro M, Hallett M: Physiological abnormalities in hereditary hyperexplexia. Ann Neurol 1992;32:41–50.
112. Shiang R, Ryan SG, Zhu Y, et al: Mutations in the alpha$_1$ subunit of the inhibitory glycine receptor cause the dominant neurological disorder hyperexplexia. Nat Genet 1993;5:351–357.

CHAPTER 35

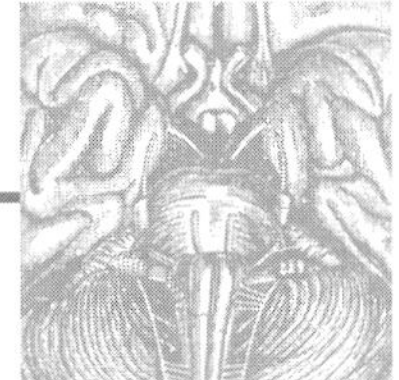

THOMAS KLOCKGETHER

Ataxias

History and Definitions

The degenerative and congenital ataxias comprise a wide spectrum of disorders with ataxia as the prominent symptom. The neuropathological hallmark of these diseases is degeneration or malformation of the cerebellar cortex and of the spinal pathways. In many cases, there is additional involvement of the brain stem and the basal ganglia.

Traditionally, classifications of ataxia were based on neuropathological criteria. Thus, Holmes distinguished between spinocerebellar degeneration, degeneration of the cerebellar cortex, and olivopontocerebellar atrophy.[1] More recently, a clinical classification introduced by Harding gained wide acceptance.[2] This classification distinguishes between congenital, hereditary, and nonhereditary ataxias. Hereditary ataxias are further subdivided into ataxias with autosomal recessive inheritance such as Friedreich's ataxia (FRDA), and ataxias with autosomal dominant inheritance, which are now usually named spinocerebellar ataxias (SCA). In recent years, the causative mutations of most hereditary ataxias have been identified, allowing a rational classification of hereditary ataxias. The nonhereditary ataxias comprise diseases with unknown etiology and symptomatic ataxias with a known cause. The symptomatic ataxias, many of which are due to alcoholism or malignant disease, are covered in other chapters (Table 35–1).

Congenital Ataxias

Pathogenesis and Pathophysiology. Cerebellar malformations are often part of complex malformation syndromes affecting diverse structures of the central nervous system (CNS). In addition, there are cerebellar malformations that are more or less limited to the cerebellum. In these latter forms, congenital ataxia is often a prominent clinical feature although ataxia may be associated with other symptoms such as mental retardation, spasticity, and seizures. In some cases of severe cerebellar malformation ataxia is surprisingly mild (see Chapter 28).

The etiology of congenital ataxia is poorly understood. Occasional appearance of congenital ataxia in siblings suggests that it may be autosomal recessively inherited. The molecular genetic basis of congenital ataxia, however, is incompletely explored. Sporadic cases of congenital ataxia outnumber familial cases by far. Whether sporadic cases are also due to recessive mutations or whether they have other causes is unknown. Animal experimental studies show that a variety of exogenous factors such as toxins, viral infection, hypoxia, and irradiation may lead to cerebellar malformation.[3]

Epidemiology and Risk Factors. Congenital ataxia due to cerebellar malformation is a rare condition. Precise information on the epidemiology of congenital ataxia is not available.

Clinical Features and Associated Disorders. *Cerebellar aplasia* seldom occurs alone. It is characterized by complete or near complete absence of the cerebellum. The clinical picture of cerebellar aplasia is variable. Life expectancy of patients with cerebellar aplasia ranges from a few weeks to a normal life span. In general, patients with cerebellar agenesis have profoundly impaired motor development and persistent motor deficits. But there are reports on patients with subtotal cerebellar aplasia who learned to stand, walk, and run. Compensation appears to be best if intelligence is normal.[4]

Vermian aplasia is often associated with reduction in the size of the cerebellar hemispheres and anomalies of the cerebellar and olivary nuclei. As in cerebellar aplasia, survival ranges from a few weeks to a normal life span. The clinical picture of vermal aplasia is not uniform. It may be associated with a nonprogressive cerebellar syndrome, or it may be completely asymptomatic. If vermal aplasia is associated with other malformations, a neurological syndrome without features of cerebellar dysfunction may be present.

Joubert's syndrome is an autosomal recessive disorder with a distinctive clinical picture. It is genetically heterogeneous

TABLE 35-1. **Classification of Ataxia**

Congenital Ataxias

Hereditary Ataxias

Autosomal Recessive Ataxias
- Friedreich's ataxia (FRDA)
- Ataxia-telangiectasia (AT)
- Autosomal recessive spastic ataxia of Charlevoix-Saguenay (ARSACS)
- Abetalipoproteinemia
- Ataxia with isolated vitamin E deficiency (AVED)
- Refsum's disease
- Cerebrotendinous xanthomatosis
- Autosomal recessive ataxia with oculomotor apraxia (AOA)
- Autosomal recessive ataxia linked to chromosome 9q
- Autosomal recessive ataxia with hearing impairment and optic atrophy
- Infantile onset spinocerebellar ataxia (IOSCA)
- Early onset cerebellar ataxia (EOCA)

Autosomal Dominant Ataxias
- Spinocerebellar ataxias (SCA)
- Dentatorubral-pallidoluysian atrophy (DRPLA)
- Episodic ataxias (EA)

Nonhereditary Degenerative Ataxias
- Multiple system atrophy, cerebellar type (MSA-C)
- Sporadic adult-onset ataxia of unknown etiology

Symptomatic Ataxias
- Alcoholic cerebellar degeneration
- Ataxia due to other toxic reasons (antiepileptics, lithium, solvents)
- Paraneoplastic cerebellar degeneration
- Other immune-mediated ataxias (gluten ataxia, ataxia associated with anti-GAD antibodies)
- Acquired vitamin E deficiency
- Hypothyroidism
- Ataxia due to physical causes (heat stroke, hyperthermia)

with one locus on chromosome 9q.[5] Joubert's syndrome comprises episodes of hyperpnea alternating with apnea, abnormal eye movements, ataxia, and mental retardation. Most patients die before the age of 3 years. Neuropathologically, complete or partial vermal aplasia is found along with changes in the cerebellar cortex and dentate nucleus.[6]

Cerebellar hypoplasia is characterized by reduced size of the entire cerebellum or parts of it. Cerebellar hypoplasia may be detected by chance in neurologically healthy individuals. Often, however, cerebellar hypoplasia is associated with congenital ataxia. In affected children, motor milestones are delayed. When the child begins to walk, the gait is ataxic with frequent falls. Limb movements and speech may be also affected.[7]

The *Dandy-Walker malformation* is a complex malformation of the CNS characterized by partial or complete aplasia of the cerebellar vermis associated with a large posterior fossa cyst. Other abnormalities include enlargement of the posterior fossa, abnormally high placement of the tentorium, and elevation of the transverse sinuses. The Dandy-Walker malformation is almost always associated with hydrocephalus. The clinical syndrome of the Dandy-Walker malformation is related to the extent of the hydrocephalus. Despite the presence of vermal aplasia congenital ataxia is not a typical feature of the Dandy-Walker malformation.

Chiari malformations consist of caudal herniation of parts of the cerebellum and brain stem into the upper cervical canal. Although these malformations affect the cerebellum, they do not lead to congenital ataxia.

Differential Diagnosis and Evaluation. Congenital ataxia can be distinguished from other types of early-onset ataxias by the nonprogressive nature of the disorder. A clinical distinction among the various cerebellar malformations that underlie congenital ataxia is impossible.

Magnetic resonance imaging (MRI) is the method of choice for evaluation of patients with congenital ataxia. MRI clearly shows the size of the cerebellum and the presence of any associated anomalies such as cysts and hydrocephalus.[8] Electrophysiological investigations do not reveal consistent abnormalities.

Management, Prognosis, and Future Perspectives. There is no specific treatment for congenital ataxia. If cerebellar malformations occur in combination with hydrocephalus, surgical shunting is required.

Congenital ataxia itself is a nonprogressive and benign condition. Children with normal intelligence will compensate cerebellar defects particularly well. However, the cerebellar malformations that underlie congenital ataxia are often associated with other malformations of the CNS. These may lead to mental retardation, epilepsy, disorders of breathing, and noncerebellar motor symptoms. Prognosis in children affected by complex malformation syndromes is poor, and many of them die in the first weeks of life.

Hereditary Ataxias

AUTOSOMAL RECESSIVE DISORDERS

Friedreich's Ataxia (FRDA)

Pathogenesis and Pathophysiology. FRDA is an autosomal recessive disease. In most cases of FRDA, the causative mutation is a homozygous, intronic GAA repeat expansion in a gene coding for a mitochondrial protein named frataxin. Less than 4 percent of FRDA patients are compound heterozygotes with one allele carrying the GAA repeat expansion and the other a point mutation.[9, 10] FRDA patients have low frataxin mRNA levels suggesting that reduced frataxin levels are the primary cause of neurodegeneration and cardiomyopathy in FRDA. Loss of frataxin has been shown to lead to mitochondrial iron overload, increased production of free radicals, and impaired utilization of iron for synthesis of iron-sulphur clusters resulting in decline of mitochondrial respiratory activity.[11]

The first pathological changes in FRDA are thought to occur in the dorsal root ganglia with loss of large sensory neurons. In advanced cases, the neuropathological abnormalities include axonal sensory and motor neuropathy, degeneration of spinal tracts (spinocerebellar tracts, posterior columns, pyramidal tract), and hypertrophic cardiomyopathy. There is only occasional involvement of the cerebellum with loss of Purkinje cells and moderate cerebellar atrophy.

Epidemiology and Risk Factors. Prevalence rates of FRDA range from 0.4 to 4.7 per 100,000. As in other recessive disorders, birth from a consanguineous marriage is a major risk factor for FRDA. In families with one affected child, each of the remaining children carries a risk of 25 percent to develop FRDA. Children descending from an unaffected sibling of an FRDA patient and a nonconsanguineous spouse have an estimated risk of about 1:1000 to develop FRDA.

Clinical Features and Associated Disorders. FRDA usually starts before the age of 25 years, most often between ages 10 and 15 years. In most patients, ataxia of gait and stance is the first manifestation of the disease. In others, skeletal deformities, in particular scoliosis, are present prior to the onset of ataxia. There are a number of clinical symptoms that are present from the beginning of the disease in virtually all patients. These include progressive ataxia and impaired vibration or position sense. Most patients have areflexia of lower extremities, about two thirds extensor plantar responses. There is progressive weakness of the extremities, which is due to pyramidal tract dysfunction and to distal muscle atrophy. Despite pyramidal involvement muscle tone is usually normal or decreased. However, some patients may suffer from spontaneous flexor spasms. Less than 10 percent of FRDA patients experience reduced appreciation of pain and light touch. Oculomotor disturbances are a frequent finding in FRDA. Typically, they include fixation instability with square wave jerks and reduced gain of vestibulo-ocular reflex. In contrast to cerebellar disease, gaze-evoked nystagmus is an unusual finding. In the course of the disease, all FRDA patients develop dysarthria characterized by slow, hesitating, and scanning speech. In later stages of the disease, optic atrophy with reduced visual acuity and progressive sensorineural hearing loss can occur. Bladder function is usually unimpaired, although some patients complain of frequency and urgency in late stages of the disease. There is no evidence that FRDA is associated with cognitive impairment. FRDA is associated with a number of non-neurological symptoms that include skeletal deformities, such as scoliosis and pes cavus, and hypertrophic obstructive cardiomyopathy. Ten percent of the patients have diabetes mellitus.[12–14] The advent of molecular diagnostic tests for FRDA has allowed identification of atypical variants of FRDA. These include late-onset cases with disease onset beyond the age of 25 years and cases where tendon reflexes are retained or exaggerated.[14, 15]

Differential Diagnosis. A number of early-onset recessive ataxias, including ataxia-telangiectasia, abetalipoproteinemia, ataxia with isolated vitamin E deficiency, and Refsum's disease, may cause confusion with FRDA. To exclude these diseases, serum levels of α-fetoprotein, phytanic acid, and vitamin E should be measured, and a lipid electrophoresis performed. In most instances, however, FRDA can be clearly distinguished from other disorders by its highly characteristic clinical phenotype. To aid diagnosis, a number of typical diagnostic criteria have been proposed. These include (1) progressive ataxia with an onset before the age of 25 years, (2) lower limb areflexia, (3) decrease of position or vibration sense in lower limbs, and (4) dysarthria within 5 years after onset of ataxia.[12, 13] In atypical cases of FRDA with retained tendon reflexes or late disease onset, a definite diagnosis of FRDA can be made only by genetic testing.

Hereditary motor-sensory neuropathies (HMSN) may mimick the phenotype of FRDA although these patients do not develop oculomotor abnormalities, dysarthria, or cardiomyopathy. HMSN has been subdivided on the basis of motor nerve conduction velocity (MNCV) in type I (MNCV < 37 m/s; demyelinating form) and type II (MNCV > 37 m/s; axonal form). Since motor nerve conduction velocity is usually normal in FRDA, nerve conduction tests can be used to distinguish between HMSN type I and FRDA. However, nerve conduction findings in HMSN type II are essentially the same as in FRDA. This may lead to considerable diagnostic confusion that requires genetic testing to resolve.

Evaluation. Nerve conduction studies in FRDA show signs of sensory axonal neuropathy. Sensory nerve action potentials (SNAPs) are absent in more than 90 percent of FRDA patients. In the remaining, SNAPs are reduced in amplitude. MNCVs are either normal or moderately reduced.[16] Motor evoked potentials (MEPs) to transcranial magnetic stimulation are abnormal in almost all FRDA patients with loss of responses or increased central motor conduction time (CMCT) indicating pyramidal tract involvement. Somatosensory evoked potentials (SEPs) are always abnormal in FRDA. Cortical N20 responses after median nerve stimulation are absent or delayed. P40 responses after tibial nerve stimulation are usually missing, whereas positive waves with latencies of 60 to 80 ms may be recorded in some patients. Brain stem auditory evoked potentials (BAEPs) are often abnormal in FRDA. Abnormalities consist of absence or delay of wave III and V, whereas wave I is usually preserved suggesting pathological conduction along the central auditory pathways.[17] Visual evoked potentials (VEPs) are abnormal in about two thirds of FRDA patients with absence or increased latency of P100 responses.[18] MRI is the method of choice to study the atrophy changes underlying FRDA. Typically, MRIs show severe atrophy of the cervical spinal cord, while there is little evidence of cerebellar atrophy (Fig. 35–1).[19]

Electrocardiography and echocardiography are useful to study cardiac involvement in FRDA. The most common electrocardiographic abnormality in FRDA is presence of T-wave inversion. Echocardiography may reveal interventricular septal hypertrophy, left ventricular wall hypertrophy, and reduction of left ventricular dimension. A molecular diagnosis of FRDA can be made by demonstration of homozygosity for the GAA repeat expansion by polymerase chain reaction.

Management. Since frataxin deficiency leads to increased production of free radicals, free radical scavengers are currently investigated in FRDA. Rustin and colleagues recently reported that idebenone (5 mg/kg per day), a short-chain quinone analogue acting as a free radical scavenger, given over 4 to 9 months decreased the left ventricular mass index in three FRDA patients.[20] Randomized, controlled trials with this compound have not yet been completed. Antiataxic drugs such as 5-hydroxytryptophan, buspirone, and amantadine are ineffective or only marginally effective in FRDA. Physiotherapy and speech therapy are generally recommended. Patients with clinically relevant cardiomyopathy and diabetes mellitus should receive standard medical treatment.

Prognosis and Future Perspectives. FRDA is a progressive disorder. On average, FRDA patients become wheelchair-bound 10 to 12 years after disease onset. Median survival after disease onset is approximately 35 years.[21]

Early-Onset Cerebellar Ataxia with Retained Tendon Reflexes

Pathogenesis and Pathophysiology. Early-onset cerebellar ataxia with retained tendon reflexes (EOCA) denotes a type

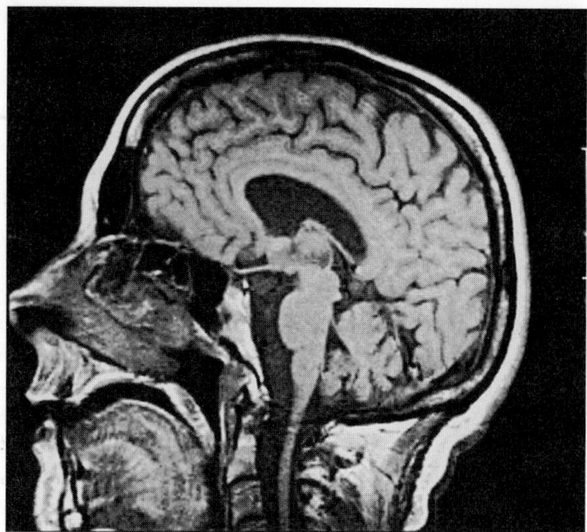

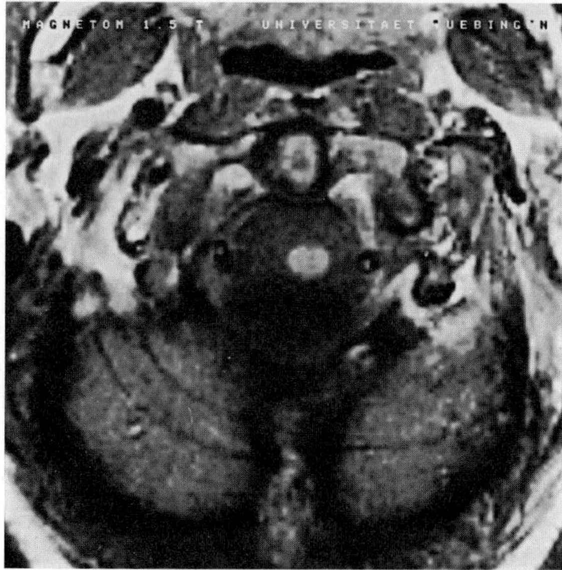

FIGURE 35–1. T1-weighted MRIs of infratentorial brain structures and cervical spinal cord in FRDA. The images show the posterior fossa in the midsagittal plane *(upper panel)* and an axial slice at the level of the dens axis *(lower panel)*. There is severe shrinkage of the cervical spinal cord. In contrast, the cerebellum and brain stem have normal size.

of degenerative ataxia with disease onset before age 25 that is distinguished from FRDA in that patients with EOCA retain tendon reflexes.[22] The occurrence of EOCA in siblings suggests an autosomal recessive disorder. Segregation analysis performed in EOCA patients, however, yielded segregation ratios that were lower than the expected value of 0.25 for autosomal recessive inheritance, suggesting that genetic heterogeneity exists among EOCA patients.[17] Other cases appear to be nonhereditary and idiopathic. The high proportion of male patients in most series of EOCA patients suggests the possibility that inheritance is based on the X chromosome in some cases. The molecular genetic basis of EOCA is unknown. The major neuropathological abnormality in EOCA is diffuse cerebellar atrophy. Occasionally, additional degeneration of brain stem nuclei and medial cerebellar peduncles occurs, suggesting the presence of OPCA.

Epidemiology and Risk Factors. The prevalence of EOCA has been reported to be 0.5 to 2.3 per 100,000.[23] As in other recessive hereditary disorders, birth from a consanguineous marriage is a risk factor for EOCA. In families in which one child is affected by EOCA, the remaining children have an increased risk of developing the disorder. However, this risk appears to be smaller than the estimated risk of 25 percent for an autosomal recessive disorder.

Clinical Features and Associated Disorders. By definition, EOCA starts before the age of 25 years. On average, disease onset occurs at the age of 17 years. All EOCA patients suffer from a progressive cerebellar syndrome marked by ataxia of gait and stance, ataxia of limb movements, dysarthria, and cerebellar oculomotor abnormalities (gaze-evoked nystagmus, saccade hypermetria, broken smooth pursuit, reduced optokinetic nystagmus, and impaired suppression of vestibulo-ocular reflexes by fixation). About half of the patients have an impaired vibration or position sense. Other noncerebellar symptoms, such as pyramidal tract signs, skeletal muscle atrophy, pale optic discs, cardiomyopathy, diabetes mellitus, and skeletal deformities, are rare or absent.[17, 22]

Differential Diagnosis. There are a number of rare types of early-onset cerebellar ataxia of unknown etiology that resemble EOCA in many respects but have characteristic additional features. These disorders include *early-onset cerebellar ataxia with hypogonadism* (Holmes' syndrome), *with optic atrophy and spasticity* (Behr's syndrome), *with cataract and mental retardation* (Marinesco-Sjögren's syndrome), *with retinal degeneration and deafness* (Hallgren's syndrome), and *with myoclonus* in the absence of severe epilepsy and dementia (Ramsay Hunt syndrome).

Evaluation. EOCA can be distinguished clinically from FRDA by the presence of tendon reflexes. In addition, the oculomotor abnormalities in FRDA and EOCA patients are different, and EOCA patients usually do not have cardiomyopathy. On MRI, EOCA patients are found to have cerebellar atrophy, whereas FRDA patients have isolated cervical spinal cord atrophy. Nevertheless, the differentiation of FRDA and EOCA may be difficult in exceptional cases of FRDA with retained tendon reflexes. In these cases, a molecular genetic test for FRDA must be performed.

EOCA may be confused with other early-onset disorders associated with ataxia, such as ataxia telangiectasia, abetalipoproteinemia, Refsum's disease, ataxia with isolated vitamin E deficiency, juvenile and adult forms of GM_2-gangliosidosis, adrenoleukodystrophy, and mitochondrial encephalomyopathies. To exclude these disorders, the workup of an EOCA patient should include determination of the serum levels of α-fetoprotein, serum lipids, phytanic acid, vitamin E, hexosaminidase A, and very long-chain fatty acids. In addition, cerebrospinal fluid lactate levels should be measured. In some cases, a muscle and skin biopsy may be helpful to exclude mitochondrial encephalomyopathies and lipid storage diseases.

Nerve conduction studies show evidence of axonal neuropathy in the majority of EOCA patients. Nerve conduction velocity (NCV) is usually normal or mildly reduced. However, there are exceptional cases in which the NCV is as low as 20 m/sec. Cortical potentials of SEPs are absent or moderately delayed. Abnormal BAEPs are found in more than half of EOCA patients. The abnormalities include loss of waves I, III, and V and delay of waves III and V, suggesting pathology of the auditory nerve and the central auditory pathways. MRI usually shows cerebellar atrophy. In some cases, the brain stem is also atrophic, suggesting the presence of OPCA. Spinal cord atrophy is not a typical feature of EOCA.[17]

Management, Prognosis, and Future Perspectives. At present, there is no specific treatment for EOCA. As in FRDA, 5-hydroxytryptophan, amantadine, or buspirone may be tried, although there are no controlled trials that clearly demonstrate the efficacy of these drugs in relieving ataxia. Physical therapy is recommended. Many EOCA patients become dependent on canes or wheelchairs within years after the onset of disease. EOCA is a progressive disorder; however, it progresses more slowly than FRDA. On average, EOCA patients become wheelchair-bound about 20 years after disease onset. Reliable data concerning survival in EOCA are not available.

Ataxia-Telangiectasia

Ataxia-telangiectasia (AT) is the second most common recessive ataxia. It is a multisystemic disorder characterized by a progressive ataxia starting in early childhood, occurrence of oculocutaneous telangiectasia, a high incidence of neoplasia, radiosensitivity, and recurrent infections. The gene affected in AT, ATM (ataxia-telangiectasia mutated), encodes a member of the phosphoinositol-3 kinase family involved in cell cycle checkpoint control and DNA repair.[24] AT is covered in more detail in Chapter 32.

Autosomal Recessive Spastic Ataxia of Charlevoix-Saguenay

Autosomal recessive spastic ataxia of Charlevoix-Saguenay (ARSACS) is an autosomal recessive ataxia with a distinctive phenotype that is prevalent in a restricted area in Quebec in Canada. ARSACS is due to mutations in a large, single exon gene encoding a novel protein named sacsin. The most frequent mutation accounting for more than 90 percent of all mutations is a deletion leading to protein truncation. Sacsin contains a heat-shock domain suggesting that it subserves chaperone function.[25] Autopsies of ARSACS patients showed cortical atrophy, pyramidal degeneration, atrophy of the upper cerebellar vermis, and loss of motoneurons. Immunocytochemical studies revealed abnormal accumulations of neurofilaments (Y. Robitaille, personal communication). The CNS abnormalities are accompanied by a mixed sensorimotor neuropathy.

ARSACS is characterized by the combination of progressive cerebellar ataxia and spasticity. Muscle reflexes are exaggerated and plantar responses are extensor. With progression of the disease, the ankle jerks disappear, and distal wasting of foot muscles develops. A highly characteristic ocular sign is the presence of prominent myelinated fibres radiating from the optic disc at fundoscopy.

A genetic test for ARSACS has been established at the Genetic Service of the St. Justine Hospital in Montreal (A. Richter, personal communication). ARSACS typically starts at the age of 1 to 2 years. On average, patients become wheelchair-bound around the age of 40 years. There is no effective therapy for ARSACS. A minority of patients with pronounced spasticity may benefit from antispastic drugs.

Abetalipoproteinemia

Abetalipoproteinemia is a rare, autosomal recessive disorder characterized by onset of diarrhea soon after birth and slow development of a neurological syndrome thereafter. The neurological syndrome consists of ataxia, weakness of the limbs with loss of tendon reflexes, disturbed sensation, and retinal degeneration. Abetalipoproteinemia is caused by mutations in the gene encoding a subunit of a microsomal triglyceride transfer protein.[26] As a consequence, circulating apoprotein B–containing lipoproteins are almost completely missing, and the patients are unable to absorb and transport fat and fat-soluble vitamins. The neurological symptoms are due to vitamin E deficiency. Management of abetalipoproteinemia consists of a diet with reduced fat intake and oral vitamin E supplementation (50 to 100 mg/kg per day) (see Chapter 30).

Ataxia with Isolated Vitamin E Deficiency

Ataxia with isolated vitamin E deficiency (AVED) is a rare, autosomal recessive disorder with a phenotype resembling FRDA. AVED patients carry homozygous mutations of the gene encoding the α-tocopherol transport protein, a liver-specific protein that incorporates vitamin E into very low-density lipoproteins.[27] As a consequence, vitamin E is rapidly eliminated. AVED is a frequent cause of recessive ataxia in North African countries but is rarely encountered in other parts of the world. Because there is no absorption deficit, oral supplementation of vitamin E at a dose of 800 to 2000 mg/day is recommended.

Refsum's Disease

Refsum's disease is a rare, autosomal recessive disorder due to mutations in the gene encoding phytanoyl-CoA hydroxylase that is involved in the α-oxidation of phytanic acid.[28] The clinical phenotype of Refsum's disease is caused by accumulation of phytanic acid in body tissues. Clinically, Refsum's disease is characterized by ataxia, demyelinating sensorimotor neuropathy, pigmentary retinal degeneration, deafness, cardiac arrhythmias, and ichthyosis-like skin changes. Whereas ocular and hearing problems are usually slowly progressive, there may be acute exacerbations of ataxia which are precipitated by low caloric intake and mobilization of phytanic acid from adipose tissue.

Refsum's disease is treated by dietary restriction of phytanic acid from the 50 to 100 mg contained in a normal Western diet to less than 10 mg per day. With good dietary supervision, ataxia and neuropathy may improve. In contrast, the progressive loss of vision and hearing cannot be prevented. In acute exacerbations, plasma exchange is effective in lowering phytanic acid levels and improving neurological and cardiac function (see Chapter 30).

Cerebrotendinous Xanthomatosis

Cerebrotendinous xanthomatosis is a rare, autosomal recessive lipid storage disorder with accumulation of cholestanol and cholesterin in various tissues. The disorder is due to mutations of the gene encoding sterol 27-hydroxylase.[29] The clinical syndrome includes xanthomatous swelling of the tendons, cataracts, and slowly progressive neurological symptoms, including ataxia, pyramidal signs, and cognitive decline. Cerebrotendinous xanthomatosis is treated by oral administration of chenodeoxycholate (750 mg/day). Treatment can be further improved by addition of HMG-CoA reductase inhibitors such as simvastatin or lovastatin.

Autosomal Recessive Ataxia with Oculomotor Apraxia

Autosomal recessive ataxia with oculomotor apraxia (AOA) is a rare, autosomal recessive ataxia caused by mutations in a gene coding for a novel protein named aprataxin.[30,31] The neurological presentation of AOA is variable. The gene has been simultaneously found by two research groups, one studying Portuguese families with an AT-like phenotype including progressive ataxia, oculomotor apraxia, and peripheral neuropathy, and another studying Japanese families with ataxia and hypalbuminemia. In contrast to AT, telangiectasias, neoplasias, and immunodeficiency are always absent. Disease onset ranges from early childhood to adolescence. Patients survive into middle or late adulthood albeit in a severely disabled state.[32]

Autosomal Recessive Ataxia Linked to Chromosome 9q

Recently, linkage to chromosome 9q was demonstrated in a consanguineous Japanese family with ataxia associated with elevated levels of serum creatine kinase, γ-globulin, and α-fetoprotein.[33] Another family with the clinical phenotype of ataxia with oculomotor apraxia was mapped to the same chromosomal region.[34]

Autosomal Recessive Ataxia with Hearing Impairment and Optic Atrophy

Linkage to chromosome 6p was demonstrated in an Israeli family with early-onset recessive ataxia. Patients subsequently developed hearing impairment as well as optic atrophy.[33]

Infantile Onset Spinocerebellar Ataxia

Infantile onset spinocerebellar ataxia (IOSCA) is an early-onset recessive ataxia linked to a locus on chromosome 10q that has been described in Finnish families. The disease manifests around the age of 1 year as acute or subacute clumsiness, athetoid movements in hands and face, hypotonia, and loss of deep tendon reflexes in the legs. Ophthalmoplegia and a sensorineural hearing deficit are found by school age, sensory neuropathy and optic atrophy by the age of 10 to 15 years, and female hypogonadism and epilepsy by the age of 15 to 20 years. Most patients are wheelchair-bound by the age of 20 years.[35]

AUTOSOMAL DOMINANT DISORDERS

Spinocerebellar Ataxias (SCA)

The SCA are a genetically heterogeneous group of autosomal dominan progressive ataxia disorders. Up to now, 15 different gene loci (SCA1-8,10-14,16,17) have been found in association with SCA. SCA9 and 15 have been reserved for new loci that have not been published yet (Table 35–2).

All mutations that have been identified so far (SCA1-3,6,8,10,12,17) are expanded repeats. In six of them (SCA1-3,6,7,17), the mutation is a translated CAG repeat expansion coding for an elongated polyglutamine tract within the respective proteins (Fig. 35–2A). These disorders belong to a larger group of polyglutamine disorders that also includes Huntington's disease, DRPLA, and spinobulbar muscular atrophy. In all polyglutamine disorders, there is an inverse correlation between age of onset and CAG repeat length (Fig. 35–2B). It is assumed that the polyglutamine disorders share important pathogenetic features. In other SCAs, the repeat expansion is found in the 5′ untranslated region (SCA12), in an intron (SCA10), and in the 3′ untranslated region (SCA8) (see Table 35–2).

SCA1, SCA2, SCA3, and SCA6 are the most frequent mutations, accounting for 50 to 70 percent of all families with dominant ataxia. SCA1, SCA2, and SCA3 are multisystemic disorders with a clinical syndrome suggesting widespread involvement of the central and peripheral nervous system going far beyond the cerebellum and spinal cord. Clinically, they usually present with progressive ataxia accompanied by a variety of additional symptoms. Correspondingly, neuropathological studies show neurodegeneration not only in the spinocerebellar system, but also in the cortex, basal ganglia, and brain stem. In Harding's classification, this group of disorders was named autosomal dominant cerebellar ataxia type I (ADCA-I).[2] SCA6 is the prototype of an (almost) purely cerebellar disorder with a later disease onset and a more favorable prognosis, corresponding to ADCA-III of Harding's classification. SCA7, formerly ADCA-II, is distinct in having the additional feature of progressive visual loss due to retinal degeneration. All other SCA mutations are extremely rare and have been observed only in a small number of or even in single families.

Spinocerebellar Ataxia Type 1

PATHOGENESIS AND PATHOPHYSIOLOGY. SCA1 is an autosomal dominant disorder with a disease locus on chromosome 6p in both Japanese and American families. In 1993, Orr and colleagues isolated the SCA1 gene and showed that the mutation is an unstable CAG trinucleotide repeat expansion within a translated region of the gene.[36] The repeat length in normals varies between 6 and 39 trinucleotides, whereas SCA1 patients have one allele within a range of 40 to 81 repeat units. The mutated SCA1 genes contain uninterrupted CAG stretches. In contrast, normal alleles have a midstream CAT interruption.[37] Repeat length and the presence or absence of the interruption appear to be critical for the stability of trinucleotide repeats. Repeats in the normal size range containing a CAT interruption are stable in parent-to-offspring transmission. Expanded uninterrupted repeats occurring in SCA1 patients are unstable with a tendency to further expansion during meiosis, in particular

TABLE 35–2. **Mutations and Clinical Phenotypes of Spinocerebellar Ataxias (SCA)**

Disorder	Mutation	Gene Product	Clinical Phenotype
SCA1	Translated CAG repeat expansion	Ataxin-1	Ataxia, pyramidal signs, neuropathy, dysphagia, restless legs syndrome
SCA2	Translated CAG repeat expansion	Ataxin-2	Ataxia, slow saccades, neuropathy, restless legs syndrome
SCA3 (Machado-Joseph disease)	Translated CAG repeat expansion	Ataxin-3	Ataxia, pyramidal signs, ophthalmoplegia, neuropathy, dystonia, restless legs syndrome
SCA4	Unknown	Unknown	Ataxia, neuropathy
SCA5	Unknown	Unknown	Almost pure cerebellar ataxia
SCA6	Translated CAG repeat expansion	Calcium channel subunit (CACNA1A)	Almost pure cerebellar ataxia
SCA7	Translated CAG repeat expansion	Ataxin-7	Ataxia, ophthalmoplegia, visual loss
SCA8	Untranslated CTG repeat expansion	Unknown	Almost pure cerebellar ataxia
SCA10	Intronic ATTCT repeat expansion	Unknown	Ataxia, epilepsy
SCA11	Unknown	Unknown	Almost pure cerebellar ataxia
SCA12	Untranslated CAG repeat expansion	Phosphatase subunit (PP2A-PR55ß)	Ataxia, tremor
SCA13	Unknown	Unknown	Ataxia, mental retardation
SCA14	Unknown	Unknown	Ataxia, myoclonus
SCA16	Unknown	Unknown	Almost pure cerebellar ataxia
SCA17	Translated CAG repeat expansion	TATA binding protein	Ataxia, dystonia

during spermatogenesis. This mechanism leads to larger expansion in offspring of affected males.

In SCA1, there is an inverse correlation between the length of the CAG repeat and the age of onset, with the largest alleles occurring in patients with juvenile disease onset. As a consequence of the instability of expanded repeats during gametogenesis, age of onset is variable with features of anticipation. Anticipation is most pronounced in offspring of affected males.

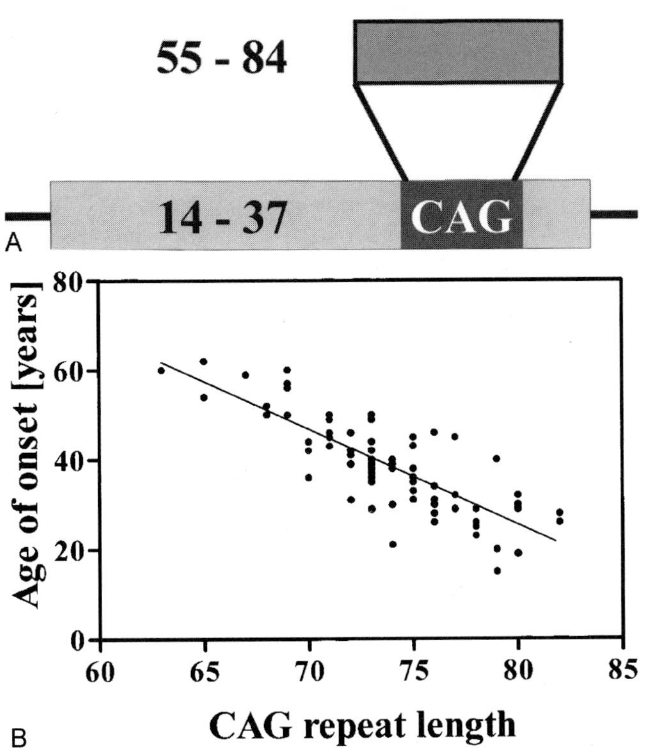

FIGURE 35–2. *A,* Diagrammatic representation of the SCA3 gene mutation. Normals have a CAG trinculeotide repeat within one of the exons ranging from 14 to 37 trinculeotides. In patients, the repeat is expanded to 55 to 84 units. *B,* Relationship between age of onset and CAG repeat length in SCA3.

Ataxin-1 is expressed ubiquitiously within the central nervous system. Its physiological function is poorly understood. SCA1 knock-out mice have mild learning disturbances, but are otherwise normal. This observation makes it highly improbable that SCA1 is caused by a loss of ataxin-1 function. Rather, it is assumed that the pathogenesis of SCA1 is due to a novel deleterious function of the elongated ataxin-1 protein. To study the pathogenesis of SCA1, transgenic mouse models have been created. Mice carrying an expanded ataxin-1 allele whose expression is directed specifically to Purkinje cells develop Purkinje cell pathology and an associated ataxia.[38] A highly characteristic feature of SCA1 transgenic mice is the occurrence of neuronal intranuclear inclusions in Purkinje cells containing aggregated ataxin-1. However, these inclusions do not appear to be a prerequisite for neurodegeneration.[39]

Numerous observations suggest that abnormal folding and aggregation of mutated ataxin-1 are essential for the pathogenesis of SCA1. The most persuasive evidence comes from experiments showing that overexpression of chaperones, intracellular proteins that serve to refold proteins and prevent aggregation, prevents the development of neuropathology in SCA1 transgenic mice. The abnormally folded ataxin-1 is thought to interact with a variety of proteins, among them transcription factors resulting in transcriptional dysregulation.

Neuropathological findings in SCA1 are variable. In most cases, there is olivopontocerebellar atrophy and degeneration of ascending spinal pathways with minor degeneration of the pyramidal tract. In the cerebellar cortex, Purkinje cells are primarily affected. Often, there is additional cell loss in the caudal cranial nerve nuclei.[40] In surviving neurons of the nucleus centralis pontis, the presence of ubiquitin-positive nuclear inclusions containing ataxin-1 has been demonstrated.

EPIDEMIOLOGY AND RISK FACTORS. The prevalence of dominant ataxias has been reported to be 1.2:100,000 with large regional variation due to founder effects.[41] A recent nationwide study reported a frequency of 3 percent of SCA1 among 149 families.[42] SCA1 is a genetically determined disorder without any known environmental risk or precipitation factors. Children from an SCA1 patient carry a 50 percent risk to develop the disease.

CLINICAL FEATURES AND ASSOCIATED DISORDERS. Disease onset in SCA1 varies and can occur between adolescence and late adulthood with features of anticipation. On average, the disease starts around age 35 years. All SCA1 patients suffer from a progressive cerebellar syndrome with ataxia of gait and stance, ataxia of limb movements, dysarthria, and cerebellar oculomotor abnormalities (gaze-evoked nystagmus, saccade hypermetria, broken up smooth pursuit, reduced optokinetic nystagmus, impaired suppression of vestibulo-ocular reflex by fixation). In the majority of patients, there are additional noncerebellar symptoms. Pyramidal tract signs, skeletal muscle atrophy, and pale discs are found in more than 50 percent of SCA1 patients. Gaze palsy, slow saccades, decreased vibration sense, and bladder dysfunction occur less frequently, while basal ganglia symptoms and dementia are rare symptoms in SCA1. Dysphagia is a typical feature of late disease stages.[43, 44]

DIFFERENTIAL DIAGNOSIS AND EVALUATION. Diagnosis of SCA1 is made by demonstration of CAG repeat expansion at the SCA1 locus. Clinically, SCA1 cannot be distinguished with certainty from other SCAs. However, the presence of pyramidal tract signs, pale discs, and dysphagia is suggestive for SCA1 because these symptoms are found less frequently in other SCA mutations.

NCVs are in the normal range or moderately reduced. SNAPs are reduced in almost all patients, suggesting sensory axonal neuropathy. Patients having widespread atrophy of skeletal muscles demonstrate chronic neurogenic electromyographic (EMG) features. MEPs to transcranial magnetic stimulation are abnormal in almost all SCA1 patients with loss of responses or increased CMCT indicating pyramidal tract involvement. SEPs due to tibial nerve stimulation are usually delayed or absent. Similarly, VEPs are abnormal in almost all SCA1 patients with loss or delay of P100. Abnormalities of BAEPs with delay of peaks I, III, and V and increased interpeak latencies are found in about half of SCA1 patients.[45] MRI shows diffuse cerebellar atrophy, brain stem atrophy, and shrinkage of the cervical spinal cord.[46]

MANAGEMENT. At present, there is no specific treatment for SCA1. As in other types of ataxias, a trial with 5-hydroxytryptophan, amantadine, or buspirone may be done, although the efficacy of these compounds in relieving ataxia has not been convincingly proven. Physical therapy is recommended. Many SCA1 patient are dependent on canes or wheelchairs within years after disease onset. Patients with severe dysphagia should be fed via gastric tubing to avoid undernourishment and aspiration.

PROGNOSIS AND FUTURE PERSPECTIVES. SCA1 is a progressive disorder. On average, SCA1 patients become wheelchair-bound about 13 years after disease onset. Median survival after disease onset is 18 to 20 years.

Spinocerebellar Ataxia Type 2

PATHOGENESIS AND PATHOPHYSIOLOGY. The mutation causing SCA2 is a translated CAG repeat expansion in a gene coding for ataxin-2. The repeat length in normals varies between 6 and 31 trinucleotides with more than 90 percent of control alleles having 22 or 23 repeats. SCA2 patients have one allele within a range of 36 to 63 repeat units. Alleles with a length of 30 to 34 repeats represent an intermediate range that may give rise to expansion in the offspring. Normal alleles have CAA interruptions. Expanded alleles are unstable with a tendency to further expansion, particularly in father-to-child transmission.[47]

Recently, transgenic mice overexpressing an expanded SCA2 allele in cerebellar Purkinje cells have been generated. These mice show progressive incoordination and morphological alterations of Purkinje cells. In contrast to SCA1, nuclear localization of the abnormal protein is not necessary for the development of the disease.[48]

Autopsy studies of SCA2 patients consistently show olivopontocerebellar atrophy with marked reduction of Purkinje cells, degeneration of the inferior olives, pontine nuclei, and pontocerebellar fibers. In most cases, there is additional degeneration of posterior columns and spinocerebellar pathways, and cell loss in the substantia nigra. Ubiquitinated nuclear inclusions have not been observed in SCA2.

EPIDEMIOLOGY AND RISK FACTORS. The incidence and prevalence of SCA2 are unknown. There are large regional variations due to founder effects. Large SCA2 families have been found in Cuba, Tunisia, Martinique, Austria, Germany and Italy. SCA2 is a genetically determined disorder without any known environmental risk or precipitation factors. Children from SCA2 patients carry a 50 percent risk to develop the disease.

CLINICAL FEATURES AND ASSOCIATED DISORDERS. Disease onset in SCA2 varies, occurring between early childhood and late adulthood with features of anticipation. On average, the disease starts around the age of 35 years. All SCA2 patients suffer from a progressive cerebellar syndrome with ataxia of gait and stance, ataxia of limb movements, and dysarthria. Saccade slowing is a highly characteristic feature that is observed in the majority of SCA2 patients. About half of the patients have vertical or horizontal gaze palsy. Cerebellar oculomotor abnormalities are rarely found in SCA2. Typically, tendon reflexes are absent or decreased. Pyramidal tract signs are present in less than 20 percent of the patients. Vibration sense is decreased in most patients, but sensation is otherwise normal. Dementia, basal ganglia symptoms, pale discs, and bladder dysfunction are usually absent.[42, 49, 50]

DIFFERENTIAL DIAGNOSIS AND EVALUATION. Diagnosis of SCA2 is made by demonstration of CAG repeat expansion at the SCA2 locus. Clinically, SCA2 cannot be distinguished with certainty from other SCAs. However, the presence of slow saccades, axonal neuropathy, and severe pontine atrophy in MRI is suggestive for SCA2. Nerve conduction findings are similar to SCA1 with low amplitudes of SNAPs and normal or slightly reduced NCVs. In contrast to SCA1, MEPs to transcranial magnetic stimulation and VEPs are usually normal in SCA2. BAEPs reveal abnormalities in less than half of SCA2 patients. SEPs after tibial nerve stimulation are usually abnormal. MRIs show diffuse cerebellar atrophy with marked brain stem atrophy suggesting the presence of olivopontocerebellar atrophy. In addition, the cervical spinal cord is atrophic in most patients (Fig. 35–3).[46]

MANAGEMENT. At present, there is no specific treatment for SCA2. Principles of symptomatic and palliative therapy are identical to those in SCA1.

PROGNOSIS AND FUTURE PERSPECTIVES. SCA2 is a progressive disorder. On average, SCA2 patients become

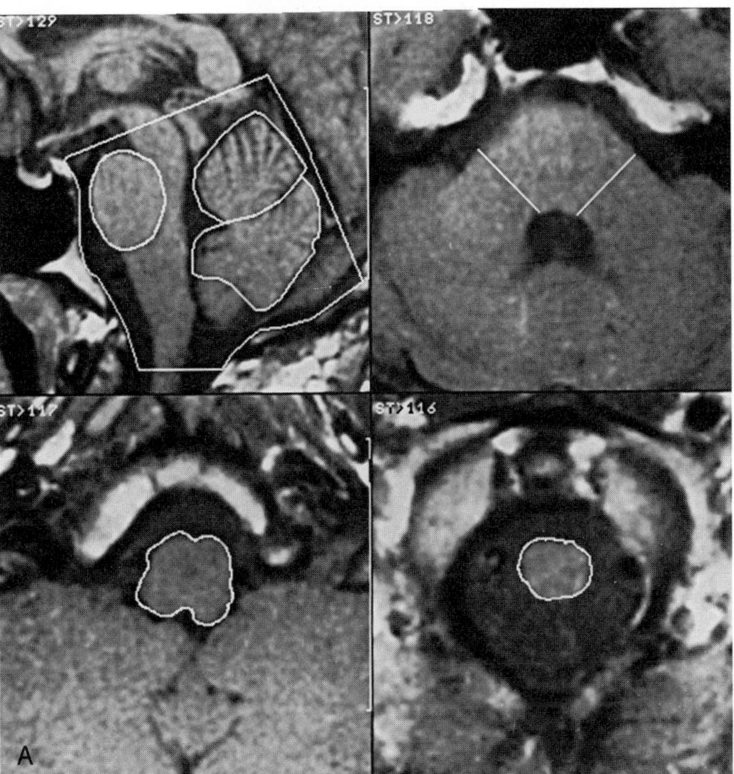

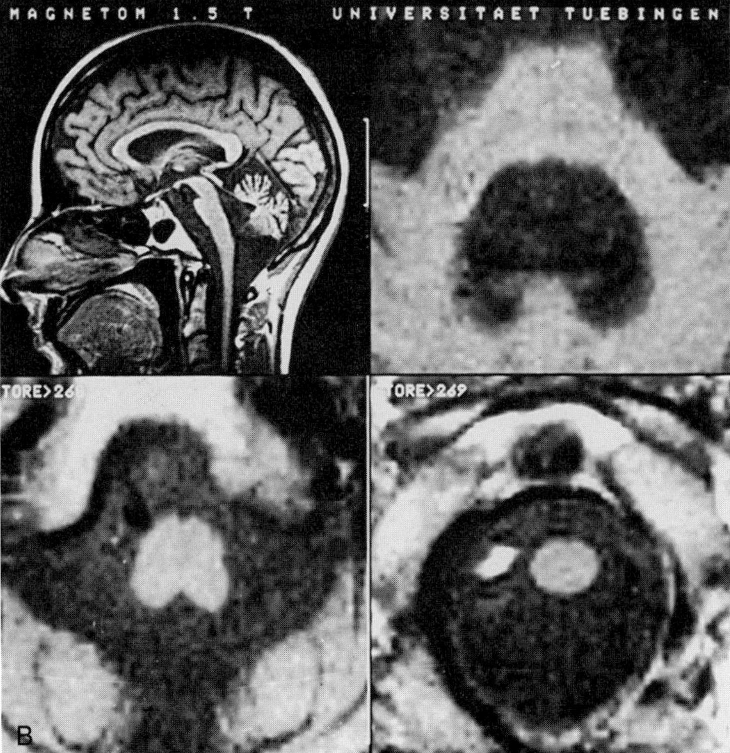

FIGURE 35–3. T1-weighted MRIs of infratentorial brain structures and cervical spinal cord in different types of degenerative ataxia. The images show the posterior fossa in the midsagittal plane *(upper left)* and axial slices at the level of the middle cerebellar peduncles *(upper right)*, inferior olive complex *(lower left)*, and dens axis *(lower right)*. *A,* Normal. *B,* SCA2. There is severe cerebellar and brain stem shrinkage, suggesting the presence of OPCA. In addition, the cervical spinal cord is atrophic.

Figure continued on following page

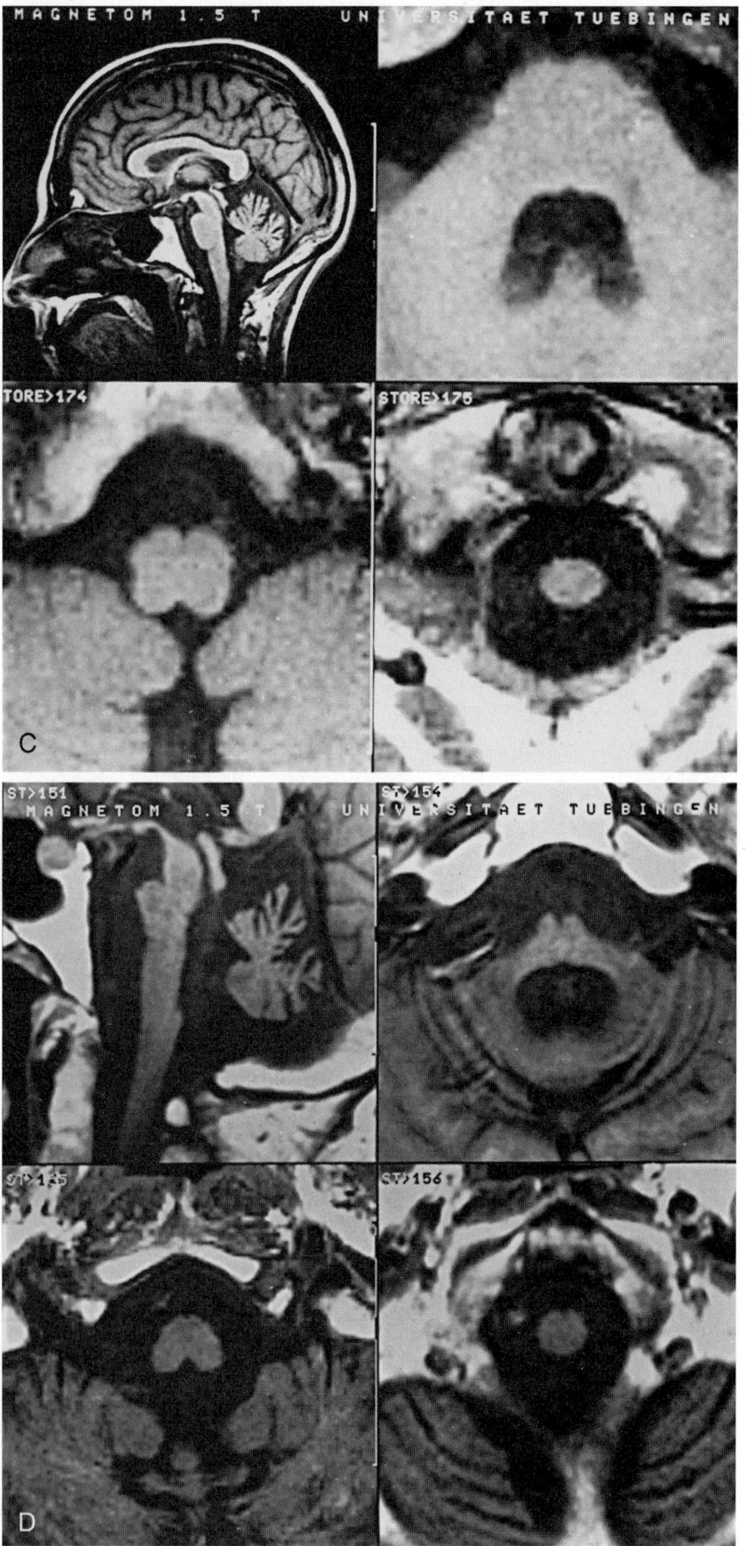

FIGURE 35–3 *Continued. C,* SCA3. There is only mild cerebellar vermal atrophy with additional involvement of the spinal cord. *D,* MSA-C. There is severe cerebellar and brain stem shrinkage, suggesting the presence of OPCA. The cervical spinal cord has normal size.

wheelchair-bound about 15 years after disease onset. Median survival after disease onset is approximately 25 years. Patients with disease onset in childhood appear to have a worse prognosis.

Spinocerebellar Ataxia Type 3

PATHOGENESIS AND PATHOPHYSIOLOGY. The mutation causing SCA3 is a translated CAG repeat expansion in a gene coding for ataxin-3.[51] The SCA3 mutation was initially found in families with the Machado-Joseph disease phenotype. Machado-Joseph disease is an historical term used to denote a dominantly inherited ataxic disorder with large phenotypical variation that was first described in patients of Azorean descent.[52] After discovery of the gene mutation it was found that this mutation is frequently found in ataxia families of non-Azorean origin.

While the repeat length of the SCA3 gene in normals varies between 14 and 37 trinucleotides, SCA3 patients have one allele within a range of 55 to 84 repeat units (see Fig. 35–2A). Both the normal and mutated SCA3 genes contain uninterrupted CAG stretches. Expanded SCA3 alleles display intergenerational instability with a tendency to further expansion. As shown by a worldwide haplotype analysis, the majority of abnormal alleles are derived from two founder mutations that originated in Portuguese families settling on the Azores.[53]

As in SCA1, abnormal folding and aggregation of the expanded disease protein appear to be of importance for pathogenesis. Overexpression of a chaperone in Drosophila model of SCA3 prevents neurodegeneration.[54] Expanded ataxin-3 has been shown to interact with a variety of transcription factors resulting in transcriptional dysregulation.[55]

SCA3 is a multisystemic disorder characterized by degeneration of spinocerebellar tracts, dentate nucleus, pontine and other brain stem nuclei, substantia nigra, and pallidum. In contrast to most other SCA, the cerebellar cortex and the inferior olives are widely spared. Nuclear inclusions containing expanded ataxin-3 have been found in neurons of affected brain regions.

EPIDEMIOLOGY AND RISK FACTORS. The prevalence of all dominant ataxias has been reported to be 1.2:100,000 with large regional variation due to founder effects. A recent nationwide study reported a frequency of SCA3 of 21 percent among 149 families.[42] SCA3 is a genetically determined disorder without any known environmental risk or precipitation factors. Children from SCA3 patients carry a 50 percent risk to develop the disease.

CLINICAL FEATURES AND ASSOCIATED DISORDERS. Disease onset in SCA3 varies, occurring between early childhood and late adulthood with features of anticipation. On average, the disease starts around the age of 40 years. Age at disease onset is inversely correlated with CAG repeat length (see Fig. 35–2B). The clinical picture of SCA3 is characterized by a wide range of clinical manifestations, the precise nature of which partly depends on repeat length. All SCA3 patients suffer from a progressive syndrome with ataxia of gait and stance, ataxia of limb movements, and dysarthria. Vertical or horizontal gaze palsy are frequent additional findings, which occur independently of age of onset. Saccade velocity is usually normal. Dementia, basal ganglia symptoms, pale discs, and bladder dysfunction are absent in most cases. Patients with a repeat length of more than 74 have an early disease onset, usually before 30 years, and clinical features of pyramidal tract and basal ganglia involvement. Most of these patients have increased tendon reflexes, extensor plantar responses, spasticity, and dystonia. Patients with an intermediate repeat length of 71 to 74 units have a disease onset in middle age and show mainly ataxia and gaze palsy. Patients with a repeat length of less than 71 have a later disease onset and show signs of peripheral neuropathy with loss of tendon reflexes, amyotrophy, and decreased vibration sense. However, the boundaries between these clinical syndromes are vague, and the clinical phenotype of an individual may change with progression of the disease. Therefore, we do not advocate dividing SCA3/MJD patients into clinical subtypes.[43, 56–58]

DIFFERENTIAL DIAGNOSIS AND EVALUATION. Diagnosis of SCA3 is made by demonstration of CAG repeat expansion at the SCA3 locus. Clinically, SCA3 cannot be distinguished with certainty from other SCAs.

The results of electrophysiological investigations resemble those in SCA2 with evidence for peripheral axonal neuropathy and posterior column involvement, while MEPs to transcranial magnetic stimulation and VEPs are normal in most patients. On MRI, the cerebellum and brain stem appear normal or only moderately shrunken. As in SCA1 and SCA2, the cervical spinal cord is atrophic in most patients (Fig. 35–3).

MANAGEMENT. At present, there is no specific treatment for SCA3. Principles of symptomatic and palliative therapy are identical to those in SCA1.

PROGNOSIS AND FUTURE PERSPECTIVES. SCA3 is a progressive disorder. On average, SCA3 patients become wheelchair-bound about 15 years after disease onset. Median survival is 25 to 30 years. Progression is faster in patients with long repeats and early disease onset.

Spinocerebellar Ataxia Type 6

PATHOGENESIS AND PATHOPHYSIOLOGY. The mutation causing SCA6 is a CAG repeat expansion in the 3′ translated region of the CACNA1A gene coding for the α_{1A} voltage-dependent calcium channel subunit.[59] Calcium channels containing the α_{1A} subunit mediate P- and Q-type currents. The α_{1A} subunit is expressed throughout the brain with highest expression levels in cerebellar Purkinje cells. In contrast to other CAG repeat mutations, the expansions causing SCA6 are relatively short ranging between 21 and 27 and do not undergo intergenerational length changes.[60]

The pathogenesis of SCA6 is not completely understood. One hypothesis says that SCA6 is due to a gain of function mechanism resembling that of other polyglutamine disorders. On the other hand, there is evidence for altered calcium channel function in SCA6 resulting in excessive entry of calcium ions into cerebellar Purkinje cells.[61] The view that altered calcium channel function may be sufficient to cause progressive ataxia is supported by the observation that a missense mutation in the CACNA1A gene may cause progressive ataxia without episodic features.[62] Both pathogenetic mechanisms, polglutamine-induced gain of function and altered calcium channel function do not appear to be mutually exclusive.

Autopsy studies of SCA6 patients consistently show a pure cerebellar degeneration with prominent loss of cerebellar Purkinje neurons. In contrast to other polyglutamine disease, neurons do not contain ubiquitinated nuclear inclusions, but rather cytoplasmic inclusion containing channel protein.[63]

EPIDEMIOLOGY AND RISK FACTORS. The prevalence of all dominant ataxias has been reported to be 1.2:100,000 with large regional variation due to founder effects. The proportion of SCA6 among all dominant ataxias varies from 1 to 30 percent in different populations. SCA6 is the most frequent cause of dominant ataxias with a pure cerebellar presentation. SCA6 is a genetically determined disorder without any known environmental risk or precipitation factors. Children from SCA6 patients carry a 50 percent risk to develop the disease.

CLINICAL FEATURES AND ASSOCIATED DISORDERS. Disease onset in SCA6 is later than in other SCAs and varies, occurring between ages 30 and 75 years. Most patients become ataxic in their fifties. SCA6 patients suffer from a progressive cerebellar syndrome with ataxia of gait and stance, ataxia of limb movements, and dysarthria. Horizontal gaze-evoked nystagmus is almost universally present, and downbeat nystagmus is found in more than half of SCA6 patients. Other cerebellar oculomotor findings are also common such as impaired smooth pursuit and dysmetric saccades. With disease progression, some SCA6 patients have clinical evidence of noncerebellar involvement, including pyramidal signs and mild sensory disturbances.[64]

DIFFERENTIAL DIAGNOSIS AND EVALUATION. Diagnosis of SCA6 is made by demonstration of CAG repeat expansion of the CACNA1A gene. Clinically, SCA6 cannot be distinguished with certainty from other SCAs. Pure cerebellar presentation and late disease onset are suggestive of SCA6.

MANAGEMENT. At present, there is no specific treatment for SCA6. Principles of symptomatic and palliative therapy are identical to those in SCA1.

PROGNOSIS AND FUTURE PERSPECTIVES. SCA6 is a progressive disorder leading to physical disability. Compared to the other common SCAs, however, prognosis is better, and life expectancy is not shortened.

Spinocerebellar Ataxia Type 7

PATHOGENESIS AND PATHOPHYSIOLOGY. SCA7 is a rare, autosomal dominant ataxia that is distinct from all other SCAs in having the constant additional feature of retinal degeneration. The causative gene mutation is a translated CAG repeat expansion in a gene coding for ataxin-7. The normal range is 7 to 19 repeats, and the pathogenic alleles range from 37 to more than 300 repeats.[65] Expanded alleles are unstable with a strong tendency to further expansion, particularly in father to child transmission. SCA7 patients with childhood onset have almost always inherited the disease from their father. Ataxin-7 is widely expressed through the brain and localized in the cytoplasm of neurons. In patients, ataxin-7 is redistributed to the nucleus to form ubiquitinated intranuclear inclusions. A transgenic mouse model of SCA7 has been created that replicates important features of the disease.[66]

Neuropathological examinations of SCA7 patients consistently revealed olivopontocerebellar atrophy. All patients have primarily macular degeneration which then spreads to involve the retina. There is often secondary atrophy of the optic nerve.

EPIDEMIOLOGY AND RISK FACTORS. SCA7 is a rare disease occurring only in a small number of families. Information on the incidence and prevalence of SCA7 is not available. SCA7 is a genetically determined disorder without any known environmental risk or precipitation factors. Children from SCA7 patients carry a 50 percent risk to develop the disease.

CLINICAL FEATURES AND ASSOCIATED DISORDERS. Disease onset in SCA7 varies between childhood and late adulthood with features of anticipation. Anticipation is greater when the disease is transmitted by males. On average, SCA7 starts around the age of 25 years. The clinical picture and the course of the disease depend on the age of onset. In patients with late disease onset after the age of 40 years, cerebellar ataxia is the first symptom. There are some exceptional cases who never develop visual problems. In most patients, however, ataxia is followed by progressive loss of vision. In about half of the patients with late disease onset, there is no evidence of retinal degeneration or optic atrophy, suggesting that retinopathy only affects the macula. All patients with earlier disease onset before the age of 40 years have visual problems, starting either prior to or at the same time as cerebellar ataxia. The majority of these patients have retinal degeneration, some of them also optic atrophy. Tendon reflexes are usually absent. There are a number of additional symptoms that occur in less than half of the patients, and that tend be more frequent in patients with long disease duration. These symptoms include gaze palsy, dysphagia, hearing loss, and muscle weakness. Dementia and basal ganglia symptoms are not typical features of SCA7.[67]

DIFFERENTIAL DIAGNOSIS AND EVALUATION. Diagnosis of SCA7 is made by demonstration of CAG repeat expansion of the SCA7 gene. SCA7 is highly probable in patients with ataxia in combination with progressive visual loss and a positive family history suggesting autosomal dominant inheritance.

MRIs show cerebellar and brain stem atrophy suggesting the presence of olivopontocerebellar atrophy. Electroretinography may be used for early detection of retinal degeneration.

MANAGEMENT. There is no specific treatment for SCA7.

PROGNOSIS AND FUTURE PERSPECTIVES. SCA7 is a progressive disorder. Disease progression is more rapid in patients with early disease onset. On average, patients with juvenile disease onset die 5 years after disease onset, while patients with adult onset survive for about 15 years.

Dentatorubral Pallidoluysian Atrophy (DRPLA)

Pathogenesis and Pathophysiology. DRPLA is an autosomal dominant disease occurring mainly in Japan. The DRPLA gene is localized on chromosome 12p. DRPLA patients show an unstable expanded CAG repeat within a coding region of the gene. While the repeat length in normals varies between 7 and 23 trinucleotides, DRPLA patients have one allele within a range of 49 to 79 repeat units. As in other trinucleotide repeat disorders, DRPLA alleles display intergenerational instability with a tendency to further expansion. Larger expansions frequently occur with paternal transmission. There is an inverse correlation between the length of the CAG repeat and the age of onset with the largest alleles occurring in patients with juvenile disease onset. As a consequence of the intergenerational instability of expanded repeats, age of onset is variable with features of anticipation.[68]

The degenerative pathological changes seen in DRPLA mainly affect the dentate nucleus, with its projection to the red nucleus, and the external pallidum, with its projection to the subthalamic nucleus. Usually, the dentatorubral system is more severely affected. Atrophy may be also present in other basal ganglia nuclei, the thalamus, and the inferior olives. In several cases, degeneration of posterior columns and spinocerebellar tracts has been described. Involvement of the pontine tegmentum has been also found, and this appears to correlate with oculomotor abnormalities.

Epidemiology and Risk Factors. DRPLA has been predominantly reported in Japan, but diseases with similar features have been occasionally observed in non-Japanese families. The Haw River syndrome, a hereditary disease occurring in an African-American family, is genetically identical with DRPLA.[69] In Japan, the prevalence rate of DRPLA has been estimated to be 0.1 per 100,000.[70]

Clinical Features and Associated Disorders. Disease onset in DRPLA varies between infancy and late adulthood with features of anticipation. On average, the onset of clinical features begins around the age of 30 years. The clinical picture of DRPLA is characterized by a wide range of clinical manifestations, the precise nature of which depend on age of onset and repeat length. The most constant clinical findings in DRPLA are cerebellar ataxia, dysarthria, and progressive dementia. These features are present in almost all patients irrespective of age of onset and repeat length. Patients with disease onset before the age of 21 years and large expansions show the clinical syndrome of progressive myoclonus epilepsy. Some of them have opsoclonus. In patients with later disease onset and shorter expansions, myoclonus and seizures are less prominent. Instead, many of these patients have involuntary choreic or dystonic movements and psychiatric abnormalities, including personality changes, hallucinations, and delusional ideas. Various oculomotor disturbances have been described, including gaze-evoked nystagmus, broken up smooth pursuit, square wave jerks, and vertical gaze palsy.[71]

Differential Diagnosis and Evaluation. The diagnosis of DRPLA is made by demonstration of an expanded CAG repeat at the DRPLA locus. The differential diagnosis of juvenile-onset cases presenting with progressive myoclonus epilepsy includes Unverricht-Lundborg disease, mitochondrial encephalomyopathy with ragged red fibers, neuronal ceroid-lipofuscinosis, Lafora body disease, and sialidosis. Adult-onset cases of DRPLA may be confused with Huntington's disease. Clinically, the presence of ataxia and seizures makes Huntington's disease unlikely and points to a diagnosis of DRPLA. DRPLA is distinct from SCAs in having the clinical feature of dementia. A syndrome of ataxia, myoclonus, and rapid cognitive decline similar to that in DRPLA may occur in Creutzfeldt-Jakob disease. Compared to DRPLA, however, progression is usually faster in Creutzfeldt-Jakob disease. In exceptional cases, DRPLA may be mistaken for schizophrenia.

Molecular studies have shown that DRPLA and the Haw River syndrome are identical.

The electroencephalographic (EEG) background activity is slowed in almost 80 percent of DRPLA patients. More than half have epileptiform EEG patterns, and in about one third EEG reveals photosensitivity.[72] MRIs of DRPLA patients show atrophy of the superior cerebellar peduncles. In addition, T2-weighted images show high-intensity signals in the pallidum.[73]

Management. At present, there is no specific treatment for DRPLA. DRPLA patients with epilepsy require standard antiepileptic treatment. Phenytoin should be avoided because it may worsen ataxia.

Prognosis and Future Perspectives. DRPLA is a progressive disorder. Quantitative data concerning rate of progression in DRPLA are not available.

Episodic Ataxia (EA)

Episodic Ataxia-type 1 (EA-1)

PATHOGENESIS AND PATHOPHYSIOLOGY. EA-1 is an autosomal dominant disorder. EA-1 is due to a missense mutation in the potassium channel gene, KCNA1, on chromosome 12p leading to inefficient repolarization of the nerve cell membrane subsequent to an action potential.[74]

EPIDEMIOLOGY AND RISK FACTORS. EA-1 is a rare familial disorder. Information concerning the epidemiology of this disorder is not available.

CLINICAL FEATURES AND ASSOCIATED DISORDERS. Disease onset of EA-1 occurs in early childhood. Clinically, EA-1 is characterized by brief attacks of ataxia and dysarthria. The attacks last for seconds to minutes and may occur several times per day. They are often provoked by movements and startle. Apart from ataxia, the attacks may have dystonic or choreic features. EA-1 is associated with interictal myokymia (i.e., twitching of small muscles around the eyes or in the hands). Ataxia or gaze-evoked nystagmus are absent between attacks.[75]

DIFFERENTIAL DIAGNOSIS AND EVALUATION. A routine molecular genetic test for EA-1 is not available because different point mutations within the KCNA1 gene may lead to the disorder. Clinically, EA-1 can be differentiated from EA-2 (see later discussion) by the shorter duration of the attacks, the presence of myokymia, and the absence of interictal ataxia and nystagmus. A number of rare metabolic defects of autosomal recessive inheritance may give rise to intermittent ataxia. These disorders include metabolic syndromes with hyperammonemia, aminoacidurias without hyperammonemia, and disorders of pyruvate and lactate metabolism.

Interictal EMG of muscles displaying myokymia shows spontaneous repetitive discharges which subside after nerve blockade. These abnormalities have been also termed neuromyotonia.[75] Nerve conduction and evoked potential studies do not reveal additional abnormalities. MRIs of the head are normal.

MANAGEMENT. Acetazolamide (2 × 250 mg/day) is of benefit in reducing attacks in some but not all kindreds. Anticonvulsants are used to reduce myokymia.

PROGNOSIS AND FUTURE PERSPECTIVES. EA-1 has a favourable prognosis in that attacks tend to abate after early childhood.

Episodic Ataxia-type 2 (EA-2)

PATHOGENESIS AND PATHOPHYSIOLOGY. EA-2 is a rare disorder caused by nonsense mutations causing truncation of the CACNA1A gene coding for the α_{1A} voltage-dependent calcium channel subunit.[76] Missense mutations of the same gene are associated with familial hemiplegic migraine, while a CAG repeat expansion in the 3′ end of the gene causes SCA6.[59, 76]

EPIDEMIOLOGY AND RISK FACTORS. EA-2 is a rare familial disorder. Information concerning the epidemiology of this disorder is not available.

CLINICAL FEATURES AND ASSOCIATED DISORDERS. Clinical onset of EA-2 is usually during childhood, varying from 6 weeks to 30 years. EA-2 is clinically characterized by recurrence of acute attacks of ataxia of gait and stance, limb ataxia, and dysarthria. The attacks last from several hours to a day or more. Emotional stress, exercise, and fatigue but not movements or startle may precipitate the attacks. The frequency of attacks varies widely from several times per day to less than once per month. Neurological examination between attacks discloses mild gait ataxia and gaze-evoked nystagmus. Some patients develop progressive ataxia and dysarthria.[77]

DIFFERENTIAL DIAGNOSIS AND EVALUATION. Because a genetic test for EA-2 is not routinely available, the diagnosis is based on a carefully taken history and clinical examination. Compared to EA-1, attacks in EA-2 last longer and are not provoked by movements or startle. In addition, EA-2 patients may have mild interictal ataxia. The differential diagnosis of EA-2 corresponds to that in EA-1.

EA-2 is often associated with MRI abnormalities. In particular, patients with progressive interictal ataxia show atrophy of the cerebellar vermis.[78] In addition, MR spectroscopy shows an elevated cerebellar pH in these patients.[79] Electrophysiological investigations do not show consistent abnormalities.

MANAGEMENT. Continued acetazolamide (2 × 250 mg/day) therapy completely abolishes episodes of ataxia in EA-2. Cessation of acetazolamide usually prompts rapid recurrence of the attacks.[80]

PROGNOSIS AND FUTURE PERSPECTIVES. Experience with EA-2 families treated with acetazolamide suggests that acetazolamide remains effective in reducing attacks for up to 20 years. It is not clear whether acetazolamide is also effective in slowing the progressive ataxia occurring in some of the family members.

Nonhereditary, Idiopathic Cerebellar Ataxia

MULTIPLE SYSTEM ATROPHY (MSA)

Pathogenesis and Pathophysiology. Multiple system atrophy (MSA) is a sporadic, adult-onset disease characterized by neurodegeneration in the basal ganglia, brain stem, cerebellum, and intermediolateral cell columns of the spinal cord. MSA encompasses the former disease categories striatonigral degeneration, sporadic olivopontocerebellar atrophy, and Shy-Drager syndrome. The ultrastructural hallmark of MSA is the presence of oligodendroglial cytoplasmic inclusions. MSA patients present with various combinations of parkinsonism, cerebellar ataxia, and autonomic failure (orthostatic hypotension, urinary incontinence).[81] Cerebellar ataxia is present in more than half of MSA patients.[82] According to the prominent clinical presentation, MSA has been subdivided into a parkinsonian type (MSA-P) and a cerebellar type (MSA-C). The etiology of MSA is unknown.

Epidemiology and Risk Factors. The age-adjusted prevalence of MSA is 4.4 per 100,000.[83] There are no known genetic or environmental risk factors for MSA.

Clinical Features and Associated Disorders. On average, MSA starts around the age of 55 years. MSA-C is clinically characterized by a progressive cerebellar syndrome with ataxia of gait and stance, ataxia of limb movements, dysarthria, and cerebellar oculomotor abnormalities (gaze-evoked nystagmus, saccade hypermetria, broken up smooth pursuit, reduced optokinetic nystagmus, impaired suppression of vestibulo-ocular reflex by fixation). In addition, MSA-C patients have autonomic failure, including orthostatic hypotension, bladder dysfunction, and erectile dysfunction in male. Neurological noncerebellar symptoms include akinetic-rigid parkinsonism, pyramidal tract signs, and myoclonus. Autonomic symptoms may be present years before manifestation of ataxia, may occur simultaneously with ataxia, or may develop later.[84, 85]

Differential Diagnosis and Evaluation. The clinical phenotype of advanced MSA-C consisting of ataxia, parkinsonism, and autonomic failure is highly characteristic and will rarely give rise to confusion with other disorders. In contrast, incomplete or beginning forms of MSA-C must be carefully distinguished from sporadic ataxia of unknown etiology and symptomatic cerebellar ataxia. Degeneration of the cerebellar cortex with chronic cerebellar ataxia may be due to alcoholism, various toxic causes (antiepileptic drugs, cytostatic drugs, lithium, solvents, heavy metals), remote effects of malignancy (paraneoplastic cerebellar degeneration), malabsorption with vitamin E deficiency, increased body temperature (heat shock, neuroleptic malignant syndrome, sepsis), and hypothyrosis.

On MRI, MSA patients have olivopontocerebellar atrophy with diffuse cerebellar atrophy and additional shrinkage of the base of the pons and the middle cerebellar peduncles (Fig. 35–4A). T2-weighted images in MSA often show hypointense signal in the putamen suggesting basal ganglia involvement. In addition, there are hyperintensities in the pons and middle cerebellar peduncles reflecting degeneration and gliosis of pontocerebellar fibers (Fig. 35–4B). However, these are not early signs, and their absence does not exclude a diagnosis of MSA.[86, 87]

Management. There is no curative or preventive treatment for MSA. Among the cardinal symptoms of MSA–cerebellar ataxia, parkinsonism, and autonomic failure—ataxia is the most difficult to treat. As in other types of ataxias, a trial with 5-hydroxytryptophan, amantadine, or buspirone may be done, although there are no controlled trials that clearly demonstrate the efficacy of these drugs in relieving ataxia. Physical therapy is recommended. Parkinsonism and autonomic failure in MSA require adequate symptomatic treatment. Parkinsonian symptoms in MSA respond to dopaminergic medication, although the response is less robust than in idiopathic Parkinson's disease. Many patients develop urinary retention and have to be supplied with suprapubic catheters. For management of orthostatic hypotension, elastic stockings and oral treatment with mineralocorticoids are recommended.

Prognosis and Future Perspectives. MSA has a poor prognosis. Patients become wheelchair-bound approximately

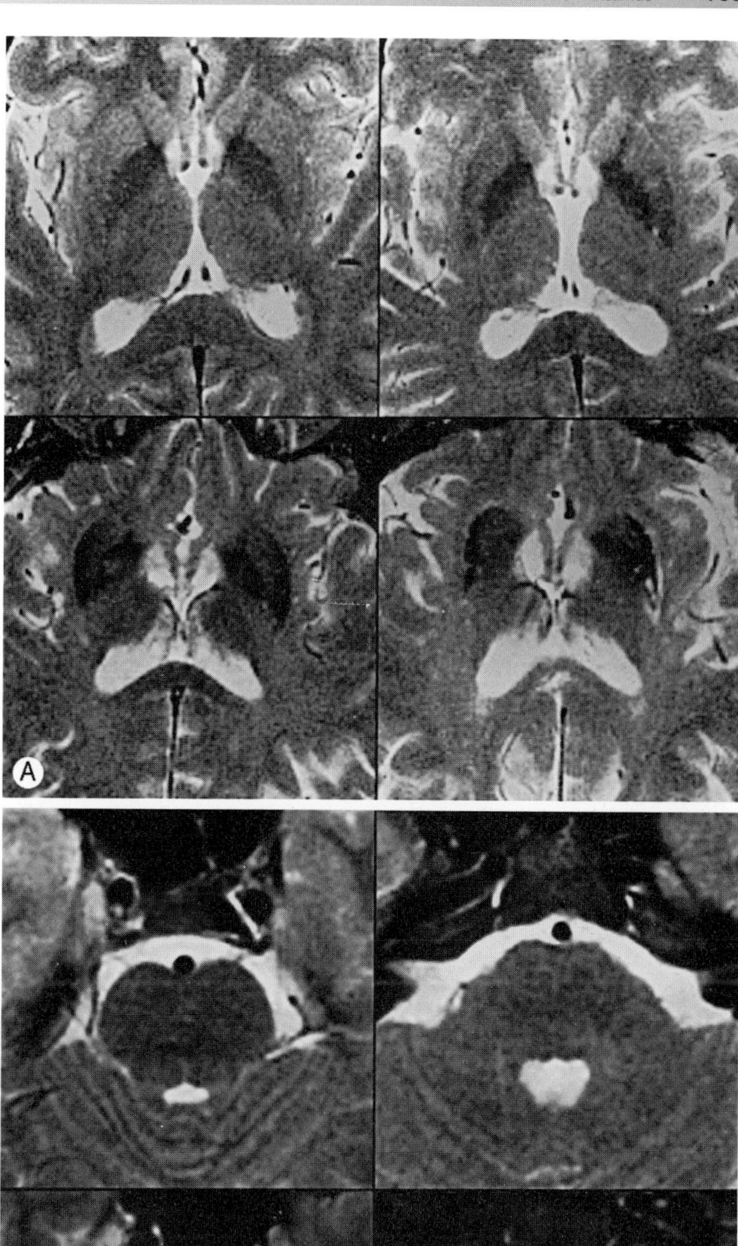

FIGURE 35–4. T2-weighted MRIs of the basal ganglia, pons, and middle cerebellar peduncles in MSA-C. *A,* Hypointensities of basal ganglia. Upper left part: Normal. Upper right part: Hypointensity at the dorsolateral margin of the putamen in beginning MSA-C. Lower left part: Strong hypointensity extending through part of the body of putamen in MSA-C. Lower right part: Hypointensity extending throughout the putamen, with intensity exceeding that in globus pallidus in late-stage MSA-C. Note the hyperintensity at the lateral putaminal border. *B,* Hyperintensities in the upper pons *(left side)* and middle cerebellar peduncles *(right side)*. Upper panel: Normal. Lower panel: Hyperintensities of the transverse pontine fibers between tegmentum and the base of pons *(left)* and in the middle cerebellar peduncles *(right)* in MSA-C.

5 years after disease onset. Median survival after disease onset is 8 to 10 years.[21]

SPORADIC ADULT-ONSET ATAXIA OF UNKNOWN ETIOLOGY

In many patients with sporadic adult-onset progressive ataxia, the underlying cause remains unknown. According to a recent study, this disorder is twice as frequent as MSA-C.[88] Cerebellar ataxia is the prominent symptom of sporadic ataxia, but more than one half have clinical features suggesting additional involvement of pyramidal tracts, posterior columns, and peripheral nervous system. Age of onset is around 55 years, and life expectancy is almost normal.[89]

The diagnosis of sporadic ataxia of unknown etiology is made by exclusion. As in MSA, symptomatic causes of cerebellar ataxia have to be carefully excluded. Sporadic ataxia of unknown etiology is distinguished from MSA by the absence of autonomic failure and parkinsonism. In early disease stages, a distinction between MSA-C and sporadic ataxia of unknown etiology is often impossible. Most of the patients have isolated cerebellar atrophy with little or no involvement of the brain stem. There are no specific treatment approaches for sporadic adult-onset ataxia.

Reviews and Selected Updates

Klockgether T: Handbook of Ataxia Disorders. New York, Marcel Dekker, 2000.

Pandolfo M: Molecular basis of Friedreich ataxia. Mov Disord 2001;16:815–821.

Surtees R: Inherited ion channel disorders. Eur J Pediatr 2000;159 Suppl 3:S199–S203.

Wenning GK, Seppi K, Scherfler C, Stefanova N, Puschban Z: Multiple system atrophy. Semin Neurol 2001;21:33–40.

Zoghbi HY, Orr HT: Glutamine repeats and neurodegeneration. Annu Rev Neurosci 2000;23:217–247.

References

1. Holmes G: An attempt to classify cerebellar disease, with a note on Marie's hereditary cerebellar ataxia. Brain 1907;30:545–567.
2. Harding AE: Classification of the hereditary ataxias and paraplegias. Lancet 1983;1:1151–1155.
3. Macchi G, Bentivoglio M: Agenesis or hypoplasia of cerebellar structures. *In* Vinken PJ, Klawans HL (eds): Handbook of Clinical Neurology, Vol 50. Amsterdam, Elsevier Science, 1987, pp 175–96.
4. Glickstein M: Cerebellar agenesis. Brain 1994;117:1209–1212.
5. Saar K, Al Gazali L, Sztriha L, et al: Homozygosity mapping in families with Joubert syndrome identifies a locus on chromosome 9q34.3 and evidence for genetic heterogeneity. Am J Human Genet 1999;65:1666–1671.
6. Joubert M, Eisenring JJ, Robb JP, Andermann F: Familial agenesis of the cerebellar vermis. A syndrome of episodic hyperpnea, abnormal eye movements, ataxia, and retardation. Neurology 1969;19:813–825.
7. Sarnat HB, Alcala H: Human cerebellar hypoplasia: A syndrome of diverse causes. Arch Neurol 1980;37:300–305.
8. deSouza N, Chaudhuri R, Bingham J, Cox T: MRI in cerebellar hypoplasia. Neuroradiology. 1994;36:148–151.
9. Campuzano V, Montermini L, Moltò MD, et al: Friedreich's ataxia: Autosomal recessive disease caused by an intronic GAA triplet repeat expansion. Science 1996;271:1423–1427.
10. Cossee M, Dürr A, Schmitt M, et al: Friedreich's ataxia: Point mutations and clinical presentation of compound heterozygotes. Ann Neurol 1999;45:200–206.
11. Puccio H, Simon D, Cossee M, et al: Mouse models for Friedreich ataxia exhibit cardiomyopathy, sensory nerve defect and Fe-S enzyme deficiency followed by intramitochondrial iron deposits. Nat Genet 2001;27:181–186.
12. Harding AE: Friedreich's ataxia: A clinical and genetic study of 90 families with an analysis of early diagnostic criteria and intrafamilial clustering of clinical features. Brain 1981;104:589–620.
13. Geoffroy G, Barbeau A, Breton G, et al: Clinical description and roentgenologic evaluation of patients with Friedreich's ataxia. Can J Neurol Sci 1976;3:279–286.
14. Dürr A, Cossee M, Agid Y, et al: Clinical and genetic abnormalities in patients with Friedreich's ataxia. N Engl J Med 1996;335:1169–1175.
15. Klockgether T, Chamberlain S, Wüllner U, et al: Late-onset Friedreich's ataxia: Molecular genetics, clinical neurophysiology, and magnetic resonance imaging. Arch Neurol 1993;50:803–806.
16. McLeod JG: An electrophysiological and pathological study of peripheral nerves in Friedreich's ataxia. J Neurol Sci 1971;12:333–349.
17. Klockgether T, Petersen D, Grodd W, Dichgans J: Early onset cerebellar ataxia with retained tendon reflexes. Clinical, electrophysiological and MRI observations in comparison with Friedreich's ataxia. Brain 1991; 114:1559–1573.
18. Carroll WM, Kriss A, Baraitser M, Barrett G, Halliday AM: The incidence and nature of visual pathway involvement in Friedreich's ataxia. A clinical and visual evoked potential study of 22 patients. Brain 1980;103:413–434.
19. Wüllner U, Klockgether T, Petersen D, Naegele T, Dichgans J: Magnetic resonance imaging in hereditary and idiopathic ataxia. Neurology 1993;43:318–325.
20. Rustin P, von Kleist Retzow JC, Chantrel Groussard K, et al: Effect of idebenone on cardiomyopathy in Friedreich's ataxia: A preliminary study. Lancet 1999;354:477–479.
21. Klockgether T, Lüdtke R, Kramer B, et al: The natural history of degenerative ataxia: A retrospective study in 466 patients. Brain 1998;121:589–600.
22. Harding AE: Early onset cerebellar ataxia with retained tendon reflexes: A clinical and genetic study of a disorder distinct from Friedreich's ataxia. J Neurol Neurosurg Psychiatry 1981;44:503–508.
23. Filla A, DeMichele G, Santorelli, et al: Epidemiological survey of hereditary ataxias and spastic paraplegias in Molise, Italy. *In* Lechtenberg R (ed): Handbook of Cerebellar Diseases. New York, Marcel Dekker, 1993, pp 407–414.
24. Savitsky K, Bar-Shira A, Gilad S, et al: A single ataxia telangiectasia gene with a product similar to PI-3 kinase. Science 1995;268:1749–1753.
25. Engert JC, Berube P, Mercier J, et al: ARSACS, a spastic ataxia common in northeastern Quebec, is caused by mutations in a new gene encoding an 11.5-kb ORF. Nat Genet 2000;24:120–125.
26. Sharp D, Blinderman L, Combs KA, et al: Cloning and gene defects in microsomal triglyceride transfer protein associated with abetalipoproteinaemia. Nature 1993;365:65–69.
27. Ouahchi K, Arita M, Kayden H, et al: Ataxia with isolated vitamin E deficiency is caused by mutations in the α-tocopherol transfer protein. Nat Genet 1995;9:141–145.
28. Jansen GA, Ofman R, Ferdinandusse S, et al: Refsum disease is caused by mutations in the phytanoyl-CoA hydroxylase gene. Nat Genet 1997;17:190–193.
29. Leitersdorf E, Reshef A, Meiner V, et al: Frameshift and splice-junction mutations in the sterol 27-hydroxylase gene cause cerebrotendinous xanthomatosis in Jews or Moroccan origin. J Clin Invest 1993;91:2488–2496.
30. Moreira MC, Barbot C, Tachi N, et al: The gene mutated in ataxia-ocular apraxia 1 encodes the new HIT/Zn-finger protein aprataxin. Nat Genet 2001;29:189–193.
31. Date H, Onodera O, Tanaka H, et al: Early-onset ataxia with ocular motor apraxia and hypoalbuminemia is caused by mutations in a new HIT superfamily gene. Nat Genet 2001; 29:184–188.
32. Barbot C, Coutinho P, Chorao R, et al: Recessive ataxia with ocular apraxia: Review of 22 Portuguese patients. Arch Neurol 2001; 58:201–205.
33. Bomont P, Watanabe M, GershoniBarush R, et al: Homozygosity mapping of spinocerebellar ataxia with cerebellar atrophy and peripheral neuropathy to 9q33-34, and with hearing impairment and optic atrophy to 6p21-23. Eur J Human Genet 2000;8:986–990.
34. Nemeth AH, Bochukova E, Dunne E, et al: Autosomal recessive cerebellar ataxia with oculomotor apraxia (Ataxia-telangiectasia-like syndrome) is linked to chromosome 9q34. Am J Human Genet 2000; 67:1320–1326.
35. Lonnqvist T, Paetau A, Nikali K, von Boguslawski K, Pihko H: Infantile onset spinocerebellar ataxia with sensory neuropathy (IOSCA): Neuropathological features. J Neurol Sci 1998;161:57–65.
36. Orr HT, Chung MY, Banfi S, et al: Expansion of an unstable trinucleotide CAG repeat in spinocerebellar ataxia type 1. Nat Genet 1993;4:221–226.
37. Chung MY, Ranum LP, Duvick LA, Servadio A, Zoghbi HY, Orr HT: Evidence for a mechanism predisposing to intergenerational CAG repeat instability in spinocerebellar ataxia type I. Nat Genet 1993;5:254–258.
38. Burright EN, Clark HB, Servadio Aet al: SCA1 transgenic mice: A model for neurodegeneration caused by an expanded CAG trinucleotide repeat. Cell 1995;82:937–948.
39. Klement IA, Skinner PJ, Kaytor MD, et al: Ataxin-1 nuclear localization and aggregation: Role in polyglutamine-induced disease in SCA1 transgenic mice. Cell 1998;95:41–53.
40. Genis D, Matilla T, Volpini V, et al: Clinical, neuropathologic, and genetic studies of a large spinocerebellar ataxia type 1 (SCA1) kindred: $(CAG)_n$ expansion and early premonitory signs and symptoms. Neurology 1995;45:24–30.
41. Polo JM, Calleja J, Combarros O, Berciano J: Hereditary ataxias and paraplegias in Cantabria, Spain. An epidemiological and clinical study. Brain 1991;114:855–866.
42. Moseley ML, Benzow KA, Schut LJ, et al: Incidence of dominant spinocerebellar and Friedreich triplet repeats among 361 ataxia families. Neurology 1998;51:1666–1671.

43. Bürk K, Abele M, Fetter M, et al: Autosomal dominant cerebellar ataxia type I: Clinical features and MRI in families with SCA1, SCA2 and SCA3. Brain 1996;119:1497–1505.
44. Dubourg O, Dürr A, Cancel G, et al: Analysis of the SCA1 CAG repeat in a large number of families with dominant ataxia: Clinical and molecular correlations. Ann Neurol 1995;37:176–180.
45. Abele M, Bürk K, Andres F, et al: Autosomal dominant cerebellar ataxia type I. Nerve conduction and evoked potential studies in families with SCA1, SCA2 and SCA3. Brain 1997;120:2141–2148.
46. Klockgether T, Skalej M, Wedekind D, et al: Autosomal dominant cerebellar ataxia type I: MRI-based volumetry of posterior fossa structures and basal ganglia in spinocerebellar ataxia types 1, 2 and 3. Brain 1998;121:1687–1693.
47. Pulst SM, Nechiporuk A, Nechiporuk T, et al: Moderate expansion of a normally biallelic trinucleotide repeat in spinocerebellar ataxia type 2. Nat Genet 1996;14:269–276.
48. Huynh DP, Figueroa K, Hoang N, Pulst SM: Nuclear localization or inclusion body formation of ataxin-2 are not necessary for SCA2 pathogenesis in mouse or human. Nat Genet 2000;26:44–50.
49. Orozco-Diaz G, Nodarse-Fleites A, Cordoves-Sagaz R, Auburger G: Autosomal dominant cerebellar ataxia: clinical analysis of 263 patients from a homogeneous population in Holguin, Cuba. Neurology 1990; 40:1369–1375.
50. Riess O, Laccone FA, Gispert S, et al: SCA2 trinucleotide expansion in German SCA patients. Neurogenetics 1997;1:59–64.
51. Kawaguchi Y, Okamoto T, Taniwaki M, et al: CAG expansions in a novel gene for Machado-Joseph disease at chromosome 14q32.1. Nat Genet 1994;8:221–228.
52. Rosenberg RN: Machado-Joseph disease: An autosomal dominant motor system degeneration. Mov Disord 1992;7:193–203.
53. Gaspar C, Lopes Cendes I, Hayes S, et al: Ancestral origins of the Machado-Joseph disease mutation: A worldwide haplotype study. Am J Hum Genet 2001;68:523–528.
54. Warrick JM, Chan HY, GrayBoard GL, Chai YH, Paulson HL, Bonini NM: Suppression of polyglutamine-mediated neurodegeneration in Drosophila by the molecular chaperone HSP70. Nat Genet 1999; 23:425–428.
55. Evert BO, Vogt IR, Kindermann C, et al: Inflammatory genes are upregulated in expanded ataxin-3-expressing cell lines and spinocerebellar ataxia type 3 brains. J Neurosci 2001;21:5389–5396.
56. Maciel P, Gaspar C, DeStefano AL, et al: Correlation between CAG repeat length and clinical features in Machado-Joseph disease. Am J Hum Genet 1995;57:54–61.
57. Matilla T, McCall A, Subramony SH, Zoghbi HY: Molecular and clinical correlations in spinocerebellar ataxia type 3 and Machado-Joseph disease. Ann Neurol 1995;38:68–72.
58. Dürr A, Stevanin G, Cancel G, et al: Spinocerebellar ataxia 3 and Machado-Joseph disease: Clinical, molecular, and neuropathological features. Ann Neurol 1996;39:490–499.
59. Zhuchenko O, Bailey J, Bonnen P, et al: Autosomal dominant cerebellar ataxia (SCA6) associated with small polyglutamine expansions in the α_{1A}-voltage-dependent calcium channel. Nat Genet 1997;15:62–69.
60. Matsuyama Z, Kawakami H, Maruyama H, et al: Molecular features of the CAG repeats of spinocerebellar ataxia 6 (SCA6). Hum Mol Genet 1997;6:1283–1287.
61. Restituito S, Thompson RM, Eliet J, et al: The polyglutamine expansion in spinocerebellar ataxia type 6 causes a beta subunit-specific enhanced activation of P/Q-type calcium channels in Xenopus oocytes. J Neurosci 2000;20:6394–6403.
62. Yue Q, Jen JC, Nelson SF, Baloh RW: Progressive ataxia due to a missense mutation in a calcium-channel gene. Am J Human Genet 1997;61:1078–1087.
63. Ishikawa K, Fujigasaki H, Saegusa H, et al: Abundant expression and cytoplasmic aggregations of α_{1A} voltage-dependent calcium channel protein associated with neurodegeneration in spinocerebellar ataxia type 6. Hum Mol Genet 1999;8:1185–1193.
64. Geschwind DH, Perlman S, Figueroa KP, Karrim J, Baloh RW, Pulst SM: Spinocerebellar ataxia type 6: Frequency of the mutation and genotype-phenotype correlations. Neurology 1997;49:1247–1251.
65. David G, Abbas N, Stevanin G, et al: Cloning of the SCA7 gene reveals a highly unstable CAG repeat expansion. Nat Genet 1997;17:65–70.
66. Yvert G, Lindenberg KS, Picaud S, Landwehrmeyer GB, Sahel JA, Mandel JL: Expanded polyglutamines induce neurodegeneration and trans-neuronal alterations in cerebellum and retina of SCA7 transgenic mice. Hum Mol Genet 2000;9:2491–2506.
67. Enevoldson TP, Sanders MD, Harding AE: Autosomal dominant cerebellar ataxia with pigmentary macular dystrophy. A clinical and genetic study of eight families. Brain 1994;117:445–460.
68. Koide R, Ikeuchi T, Onodera O, et al: Unstable expansion of CAG repeat in hereditary dentatorubral-pallidoluysian atrophy (DRPLA). Nat Genet 1994;6:9–13.
69. Burke JR, Wingfield MS, Lewis KE, et al: The Haw River Syndrome: Dentatorubropallidoluysian atrophy (DRPLA) in an African-American family. Nat Genet 1994;7:521–524.
70. Kita K: Spinocerebellar degeneration in Japan—the feature from an epidemiological study. Rinsho Shinkeigaku 1993;33:1279–1284.
71. Ikeuchi T, Koide R, Tanaka H, et al: Dentatorubral-pallidoluysian atrophy: Clinical features are closely related to unstable expansions of trinucleotide (CAG) repeat. Ann Neurol 1995; 37:769–775.
72. Inazuki G, Baba K, Naito H: Electroencephalographic findings of hereditary dentatorubral-pallidoluysian atrophy (DRPLA). Jpn J Psychiatry Neurol 1989;43:213–220.
73. Imamura A, Ito R, Tanaka S, et al: High-intensity proton and T2-weighted MRI signals in the globus pallidus in juvenile-type of dentatorubral and pallidoluysian atrophy. Neuropediatrics 1994;25:234–237.
74. Browne DL, Gancher ST, Nutt JG, et al: Episodic ataxia/myokymia syndrome is associated with point mutations in the human potassium channel gene, *KCNA1*. Nat Genet 1994;8:136–140.
75. Brunt ER, van-Weerden TW: Familial paroxysmal kinesigenic ataxia and continuous myokymia. Brain 1990;113:1361–1382.
76. Ophoff RA, Terwindt GM, Vergouwe MN, et al: Familial hemiplegic migraine and episodic ataxia type-2 are caused by mutations in the Ca^{2+} channel gene CACNL1A4. Cell 1996;87:543–552.
77. Baloh RW, Yue Q, Furman JM, Nelson SF: Familial episodic ataxia: Clinical heterogeneity in four families linked to chromosome 19p. Ann Neurol 1997;41:8–16.
78. Vighetto A, Froment JC, Trillet M, Aimard G: Magnetic resonance imaging in familial paroxysmal ataxia. Arch Neurol 1988;45:547–549.
79. Sappey Marinier D, Vighetto A, Peyron R, Broussolle E, Bonmartin A: Phosphorus and proton magnetic resonance spectroscopy in episodic ataxia type 2. Ann Neurol 1999;46:256–259.
80. Griggs RC, Moxley RT, Lafrance RA, McQuillen J: Hereditary paroxysmal ataxia: Response to acetazolamide. Neurology 1978;28:1259–1264.
81. Gilman S, Low PA, Quinn N, et al: Consensus statement on the diagnosis of multiple system atrophy. J Neurol Sci 1999;163:94–98.
82. Wenning GK, Tison F, Ben Shlomo Y, Daniel SE, Quinn NP: Multiple system atrophy: A review of 203 pathologically proven cases. Mov Disord 1997;12:133–147.
83. Schrag A, Ben Shlomo Y, Quinn NP: Prevalence of progressive supranuclear palsy and multiple system atrophy: A cross-sectional study. Lancet 1999;354:1771–1775.
84. Schulz JB, Klockgether T, Petersen D, et al: Multiple system atrophy: Natural history, MRI morphology, and dopamine receptor imaging with 123IBZM-SPECT. J Neurol Neurosurg Psychiatry 1994;57:1047–1056.
85. Wenning GK, Ben Shlomo Y, Magalhaes M, Daniel SE, Quinn NP: Clinical features and natural history of multiple system atrophy. An analysis of 100 cases. Brain 1994;117:835–845.
86. Schulz JB, Skalej M, Wedekind D, et al: Magnetic resonance imaging-based volumetry differentiates idiopathic Parkinson's syndrome from multiple system atrophy and progressive supranuclear palsy. Ann Neurol 1999;45:65–74.
87. Schrag A, Good CD, Miszkiel Ket al: Differentiation of atypical parkinsonian syndromes with routine MRI. Neurology 2000;54:697–702.
88. Gilman S, Little R, Johanns J, et al: Evolution of sporadic olivopontocerebellar atrophy into multiple system atrophy. Neurology 2000;55:527–532.
89. Abele M, Bürk K, Schöls L, et al: The aetiology of sporadic adult-onset ataxia. Brain 2002 125:961–968.

CHAPTER 36

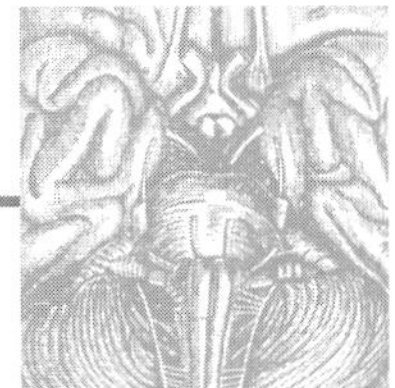

NAILAH SIDDIQUE, ROBERT SUFIT, and TEEPU SIDDIQUE

Degenerative Motor, Sensory, and Autonomic Disorders

History and Definitions

The disorders discussed in this chapter have been characterized by several generations of clinicians and scientists according to clinical presentation, muscle and nerve histochemistry, and electrophysiology. With the application of molecular biology techniques starting in the mid-1980s, the door has opened to understanding these diseases at the molecular level. Several of them are clearly monogenic in origin, such as Duchenne and Becker muscular dystrophy, whereas others, like sporadic amyotrophic lateral sclerosis, most likely result from the interaction of several genes with environmental factors. Work is rapidly progressing in identifying genes and gene products and function that will eventually lead to prophylactic as well as therapeutic intervention for these disorders.

Upper and Lower Motor Neuron Degenerative Disorders

AMYOTROPHIC LATERAL SCLEROSIS

Amyotrophic lateral sclerosis (ALS), which is also called motor neuron disease, Charcot's disease, or Lou Gehrig's disease, is an age-dependent and generally fatal paralytic disorder caused by the degeneration of motor neurons in the motor cortex, brain stem, and spinal cord. About 10 percent of cases are familial (FALS) and the rest are sporadic (SALS).

Pathogenesis and Pathophysiology. ALS is a primary disorder of motor cells and their axons. The hallmark of ALS is atrophy, degeneration, and loss of motor neurons in the lower brain stem and anterior horn of the spinal cord, followed by glial replacement. There is loss of pyramidal cells from the motor cortex of the prefrontal gyrus and large myelinated fibers of the anterior and lateral columns of the spinal cord, the brain stem, and the cerebrum. The posterior columns are usually spared in SALS. Lower brain stem nuclei are more often and more extensively involved than upper nuclei (Fig. 36–1). Therefore, oculomotor nuclei loss is modest and rarely demonstrable clinically, whereas the hypoglossal nuclei are prominently degenerated. Previously, it was thought that Clarke's nucleus was unaffected, but it is now recognized that those neurons may also degenerate. In patients who have an extended disease course due to parenteral nutrition and

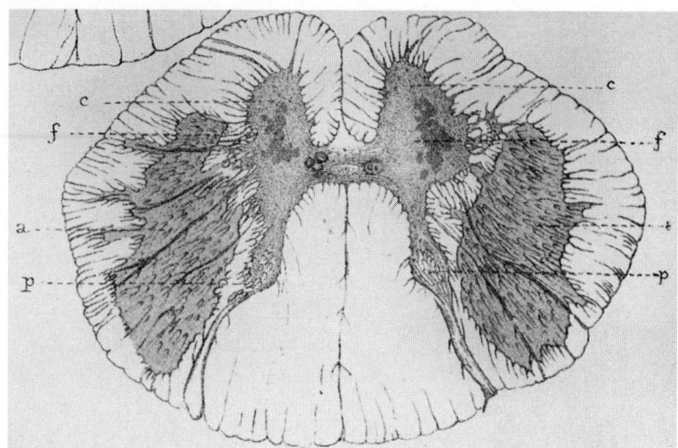

FIGURE 36–1. Spinal cord section from J-M Charcot's original presentations on amyotrophic lateral sclerosis, showing the combined anterior horn cell degeneration (*f*) and the sclerosis of the lateral columns (*a*). Anterior (*c*) and posterior (*p*) horn regions as normal anatomical landmarks inserted as reference points by Charcot. (From Charcot J-M: Oeuvres Complètes. Paris, Bureau du Progrès Meádical, 1873.)

artificial ventilation, there may be late involvement of oculomotor and sacral nuclei.

Several cytoplasmic and ultrastructural abnormalities are associated with ALS. Spheroids with a strongly argentophilic fibrillary pattern develop in conjunction with cell soma atrophy, suggesting they may be complementary processes. Ultrastructurally, the spheroids are neurofilament bundles that may contain other cytoplasmic structures, such as mitochondria. Some investigators hypothesize that the reported increase in phosphorylated neurofilaments identified using monoclonal antibodies reflects premature or excessive neurofilament phosphorylation that may be associated with impaired neurofilament transport. Other identified structures include Bunina bodies, tiny round eosinophilic structures that may be found in neuronal cytoplasm, and Lewy body–like eosinophilic inclusions found in both SALS and FALS. The latter are immunoreactive to neurofilaments, ubiquitin, and Cu/Zn superoxide dismutase (*SOD1*).[1]

Genetic linkage has identified *SOD1* at 21q22.1 as the cause in 20 percent of autosomal dominant familial cases (genetic nomenclature, *ALS1*). This finding has provided the first opportunity to study a type of ALS with a proven etiology. Because SALS is not associated with mutations in *SOD1* but is clinically indistinguishable from ALS1 and pathologically very similar, authorities assume there may be a common pathway involved in the two diseases. Therefore, the ALS phenotype may result from a variety of disruptions in the events required for motor neuron maintenance. Consequently, much research on the pathogenesis of motor neuron disease has focused on SOD1, an endogenous free radical scavenger enzyme. It functions as a dismutase, converting superoxide to oxygen and hydrogen peroxide, and is thought to have peroxidase and Cu sequestration properties. Superoxide is an unstable and highly active molecule that causes oxidation of cell constituents either directly or through toxic and stable derivatives. There is a 35 to 75 percent reduction in activity of mutant *SOD1* in ALS1, but there is no reduction in *SOD1* activity in non–chromosome 21 FALS. In most instances, loss of SOD1 enzyme activity appears to be due to structural instability, resulting in a shortened half-life of the mutant SOD1 protein.

Exploration of mechanisms by which mutant *SOD1* causes motor neuron degeneration has focused on exaggerated or disturbed functions of *SOD1*. Experiments with transgenic mice expressing different mutations suggest that it is unlikely that the disease phenotype is caused by a position effect of the mutations in the *SOD1* gene. Rather, it is more likely that gain of a toxic function of mutant *SOD1* leads to motor neuron death. Such a toxic mechanism may also underlie FALS in humans.[2]

Although *SOD1* activity serves as an antioxidant defense, the effects of conversion of O_2^- to H_2O_2 on the viability of cells may be double-edged. Hydrogen peroxide and its derivatives are directly toxic to cells and may signal apoptosis. Because *SOD1* activity is reduced in ALS1, it is conceivable that increased superoxide free radical could contribute to the disease. Although this hypothesis is supported by a number of in vitro studies, it is not fully defensible. First, not all mutations of the *SOD1* gene cause a decrease in the steady state of cytosolic *SOD1* activity. Second, transgenic mice overexpressing FALS-linked mutations in the *SOD1* gene on normal mouse background develop disease similar to ALS in humans, whereas those overexpressing normal *SOD1* remained phenotypically unaffected. Observations from overexpression transgenic mouse models and those from *SOD1* "knockout" mice strongly refute a loss of function hypothesis while supporting a gain of toxic function hypothesis. Firm conclusions are not yet possible, but increased peroxidase activity of mutant *SOD1* may play some role in the pathogenesis of ALS1.[2]

Preliminary studies on protein structure using antibodies against *SOD1* suggest that a common conformational change occurs in the mutants *A4V*, *G37R*, and *H46R* coded by exon 3 that may affect the lower rim of its electrostatic guidance channel. Structural mapping predicts that ALS1 mutations lead to structural changes in SOD1 that may distort the lower rim of this channel, allowing the catalytic site to become shallower and more exposed. As a result, molecules normally excluded may gain access to the catalytic reactive site.[2] Beckman and colleagues have proposed that cell injury occurs when the mutant *SOD1* reacts with peroxynitrite ($ONOO^-$) formed from superoxide and nitric oxide with resultant nitration of tyrosine residues of critical cytosolic proteins.[3] The access of peroxynitrite would be in keeping with the model of promiscuous accessibility to the copper site.

It has been proposed that mutant *SOD1* may exhibit metal-mediated cytotoxicities by disrupting the intracellular homeostasis of copper and zinc. It is well known that copper and zinc are potential neurotoxins, and sudden en masse release of zinc from *SOD1* aggregates in motor neurons may lead to cell death.[2] However, recent studies with mice lacking the gene for copper chaperone of *SOD1* suggest that copper does not play an important role in the pathogenesis of ALS.[4]

Different *SOD1* mutations of ALS1 do not seem to influence age of onset, but they do influence the progression of the disease, with the *A4V* mutation duration averaging 1.2 years, the *E100G* mutation 4.7 years, and the *H46R* and *G37R* mutations averaging 18 to 20 years.[2]

In genetic research, the risk to relatives of an affected person as compared to the general population can be calculated, with greater estimates corresponding to larger genetic control of trait variation. The estimated risk to siblings of ALS patients suggests that there is a significant genetic contribution. ALS1 represents a large genetic effect in a small ALS population (2.5% of ALS cases). Conversely, SALS may result from a genetic predisposition due to multiple small effects in larger ALS populations. Thus, newer techniques of identifying these effects, such as the transmission disequilibrium test, are being applied to SALS. Genes for glutamate transporters calcium homeostasis, apoptosis, mitochondrial dysfunction, or intracellular protein cargo transport are reasonable candidates for evaluation.[2, 5]

Rare recessive familial ALS (RFALS), which produces three different phenotypes classified according to type and timing of motor neuron involvement, has been identified in highly consanguineous families. The gene for RFALS type 3 (genetic nomenclature, *ALS2*) has recently been identified on chromosome 2. It codes for the protein alsin, which is expressed in various tissues in the body, including the brain, liver, and spinal cord. It is postulated there is a loss of normal function with an ALS phenotype occurring from mutations that affect both long and short transcripts of alsin and a milder primary lateral sclerosis (PLS) phenotype occurring from more distal mutations resulting in an intact short protein that may allow the preservation of some function.[6] RFALS type 1 (genetic nomenclature, *ALS5*) has been linked to chromosome 15,[7] and several other families remain unlinked. A slowly progressive autosomal dominant form of ALS that does not include bulbar involvement (genetic nomenclature, *ALS4*) has been mapped to 9q34.[8] Recent work suggests that deletions of the heavy neurofilament subunit tail may be a primary, although extremely rare, occurrence in both SALS and FALS.[9] The relationship between such deletions and ALS is still unclear.

FALS with dementia, a disinhibition dementia-parkinsonism-amyotrophy complex, has been linked to a region on chromosome 17q21–22[10] (see Chapter 33), and FALS associated with frontotemporal dementia has been linked to chromosome 9.[11]

A number of abnormalities in metabolism of the excitatory neurotransmitter glutamate have been identified in ALS, including alterations in tissue glutamate levels, transporter proteins, postsynaptic receptors, and indications of possible toxic agonists. Whether these are primary or secondary events and how they relate to the genesis of ALS is unclear but is under intense investigation.[12]

Epidemiology and Risk Factors. Broadly, there are three types of ALS usually considered in epidemiological studies: SALS, FALS, and a variant of ALS, sometimes called Guamanian ALS, found in the Western Pacific and characterized by the occurrence of parkinsonism, dementia, or both. SALS has a worldwide incidence of 1 to 2 in 100,000 persons, with fairly uniform distribution worldwide and equal representation among racial groups. The occurrence of ALS before the age of 40 years is uncommon. The incidence is greatest between the ages of 50 and 70 years, and it seems to decline thereafter. The male-to-female ratio is about 1.3:1. Clusters of the disease have been identified, particularly in the Kii peninsula of Japan and the Mariana Islands. The only indisputable risk factor other than age and gender is genetic susceptibility, with familial cases occurring in about 10 percent of most case series. Many isolated potential etiologies have been proposed for SALS, with the only consistent associations thus far being long-term exposure to heavy metals, particularly lead, and a family history of parkinsonism and dementia. There is recent evidence of association between increased dietary fat and cigarette smoking.[13–15] Curiously, cigarette smoking is negatively associated with the development of Parkinson's disease. Electrical injury has also been reported to increase the risk of ALS.[16]

Clinical and Associated Disorders. ALS is a syndrome of upper and lower motor neuron dysfunction at several levels of the neuraxis without involvement of other neurological systems. There is no definitive test that can diagnose ALS. In 1994, the El Escorial criteria were developed to standardize its diagnosis (Table 36–1).[17] Although the disease may present in many different ways and in different parts of the body, generally the patient seeks attention because of symptomatic weakness. Alternatively, there may be a history of fasciculations, muscle cramping, and atrophy before weakness is apparent. A frequent diagnostic feature is the presence of hyper-reflexia in segmental regions where muscles are starting to atrophy and an absence of sensory disturbance in the same distribution. Limb involvement occurs more often than bulbar involvement, and upper limbs are more often affected than lower limbs in SALS; this pattern is reversed in FALS. However, the pattern of involvement is frequently asymmetrical or focal. If more upper motor neurons are affected, the symptoms will be primarily clumsiness, stiffness, and fatigue, whereas lower motor neuron degeneration will present as weakness or atrophy and occasionally fasciculations. Bulbar symptoms include hoarseness, slurring of speech, choking on liquids, and difficulty initiating swallowing. Paresthesias and sensory symptoms affect up to 25 percent of patients, but if present, these complaints are mild. There is wide variation in disease progression and duration, neither of which can be

TABLE 36–1. **Summary of El Escorial Criteria for the Diagnosis of Amyotrophic Lateral Sclerosis**

The diagnosis of ALS requires the *presence* of signs of lower motor neuron (LMN) degeneration by clinical, electrophysiological, or neuropathological examination and signs of upper motor neuron (UMN) degeneration by clinical examination, and the progressive spread of these signs within a region or to other regions, together with the *absence* of electrophysiological or neuroimaging evidence of other disease processes that might explain these signs.

Suspected ALS
LMN signs only in at least two regions

Possible ALS
UMN and LMN signs in only one region, or UMN signs only in at least two regions, or LMN signs rostral to UMN signs
Special cases: monomelic ALS, progressive bulbar palsy without spinal UMN and/or LMN signs, primary lateral sclerosis without spinal LMN signs

Probable ALS
UMN signs in at least two regions, with some UMN signs above LMN signs

Definite ALS
UMN signs and LMN signs in bulbar region and at least two spinal regions, or UMN and LMN signs in three spinal regions

accurately predicted from age or site of onset, although generally elderly patients have a shorter survival. Bowel, bladder, and sexual functioning are usually spared, with about 4 percent of patients experiencing loss of sphincter control. ALS patients have diminished skin elasticity and rarely develop bedsores, seemingly because of the accumulation of a basic protein there.[1, 18] Although fasciculations, especially of the tongue, are considered by some to be specifically associated with ALS, they may actually be seen in any disorder affecting the motor neuron or their axons. Remote effect of radiation damage to the hypoglossal nerve is a case in point.

There has been controversy over the years whether syndromes that are confined to one type of motor neuron are distinct from ALS or are a variant of ALS. Primary lateral sclerosis and progressive pseudobulbar palsy are both syndromes confined to the upper motor neuron, whereas progressive muscular atrophy and progressive bulbar palsy affect only the lower motor neuron. Because all of these phenotypes are sometimes produced by the same mutation in the *SOD1* gene, and mutations in the gene for alsin can produce either ALS or PLS, it is generally now accepted that these phenotypes can be different manifestations of a similar process.

FALS with dementia (see Chapter 33), characterized by the association of frontal lobe dementia with parkinsonism and amyotrophy, has a marked variability of clinical symptoms among patients as a prominent feature. Whereas disinhibition and frontal lobe dementia are common features, the amyotrophy may be the most prominent feature in some patients and absent in others.[10]

Guamanian ALS first came to the attention of the medical community in the early 1950s when it was detected in a several-fold higher incidence in Guam than elsewhere (see Chapter 34). It is associated with parkinsonism and dementia in some patients. The incidence has been declining in the intervening years, but there has been an increase in the number of recognized persons with parkinsonism and dementia. This syndrome may include supranuclear gaze paresis. Its etiology is unclear. There has been interest in cycad flour as the source of an excitatory amino acid that causes a motor neuron disease in cynomolgus monkeys, but the amounts eaten by Guamanians in their flour appear insufficient to cause the disease. It has also been proposed that low levels of calcium and magnesium in the local environment may lead to chronic mild hyperparathyroidism with intraneuronal depositions of calcium hydroxyapatite and aluminum.[13] Only recently has examination into the possible genetic origins of the syndrome begun (see Chapters 33 and 34).

Differential Diagnosis and Evaluation. Within disorders of the motor neuron, the most difficult distinctions are among progressive muscular atrophy (PMA), proximal spinal muscular atrophy (SMA), spinobulbar muscular atrophy (SBMA or Kennedy disease), PLS, and hereditary spastic paraplegia (HSP) when there is no clear family history. Generally, progressive muscular atrophy is a progressive, asymmetrical lower motor neuron degeneration that has a later onset and can affect distal and proximal muscle, resulting in severe disability. The *A4V* mutation in *SOD1* leads to PMA and death within 12 months. SMA usually occurs in younger people and is symmetrical (see later discussion in this chapter). SBMA may have gynecomastia. HSP may be distinguished from primary lateral sclerosis by spasticity restricted to the lower extremities, normal upper extremity function, hyper-reflexia and the presence of flexor plantar response, and brisk superficial abdominal reflexes. Generally PLS is a disease of later onset that affects all extremities and bulbar function.

Electromyographic (EMG) features commonly seen include fibrillation, positive sharp waves, and complex repetitive discharges that indicate denervation. Simultaneously, reduced numbers and increased amplitude and duration of motor unit potentials indicate reinnervation. Multifocal fasciculations are also characteristic of the disease. Increased jitter on single-fiber EMG reflects immature endplates and inefficient reinnervation. Cerebrospinal fluid examination either is normal or shows mildly elevated protein (<100 mg/dL). There may be a moderate increase in creatine kinase (CK) of the muscle enzyme type.

Muscle biopsy demonstrates pyknotic nuclear clumps and small angulated fibers, small or large groups of atrophic fibers, and evidence of type grouping on ATPase staining and target fibers of NADH-TR.[1]

Management and Future Perspectives. Thus far, only the benzothiazole riluzole has been shown to extend life span, although in double-blind studies, the extension averages only 3 months and mortality rates are unaffected. In larger follow-up studies, the increase in life may be as long as 12 months.[19] Riluzole acts to block voltage-activated sodium channels and to protect against glutamate toxicity.[19] The life span of transgenic mice expressing mutant human SOD1 was prolonged by 22 percent with intrathecal administration of a caspase inhibitor,[20] and human clinical trials are planned. Although there is no truly effective pharmacological treatment yet available for ALS, a supportive multidisciplinary team can provide care and symptom management that significantly improves the patient's quality of life. Drugs such as baclofen, quinine, and phenytoin can be used to reduce cramping; anticholinergic agents can be used to control sialorrhea. Amitriptyline or selective serotonin reuptake inhibitors may help control pseudobulbar symptoms in some patients. Occupational therapy can provide techniques and orthotics that can extend the patient's ability to function independently. A speech pathologist can provide instruction to prolong the patient's ability to communicate and swallow. Augmentative communication devices are now covered by Medicare but require formal evaluation. Durable medical equipment (e.g., power-driven wheelchairs, hospital beds) allow most patients to remain at home. Open, sympathetic discussion of feeding and ventilatory support options is required with the patient and family. Bilevel positive airway pressure may provide at least short-term symptomatic relief of respiratory fatigue and sleep apnea. Algorithms for nutritional and respiratory management are available at the Web site of the American Academy of Neurology (*www.aan.com*). ALS remains a fatal disease, with a mean survival of 3 years after the onset of symptoms.[1]

SPINAL MUSCULAR ATROPHIES

The SMAs are diseases of the motor neurons of the medulla and spinal cord that most often present with muscle weakness in infancy and childhood. They may present with either proximal or distal weakness from the antenatal period onward. The inheritance pattern is most commonly autosomal recessive, but there are forms that are dominant and X linked (Table 36–2).

TABLE 36–2. **Types of Spinal Muscular Atrophy**

Type	Inheritance Pattern	Age of Onset	Presenting Symptoms	Hallmark	Prognosis
SMA type I (severe infantile SMA, acute or fatal SMA, Werdnig-Hoffman, Oppenheim disease, amyotonia congenita)	AR	In utero to 6 months	Hypotonia and weakness; problems with sucking, swallowing, and breathing	Never able to sit	Average life months, expectancy is 8 months, 95 percent dead before age 1
SMA type II (intermediate)	AR	Generally between 3 and 15 months	Proximal leg weakness, fasciculations, fine hand tremor	Never able to stand; facial muscles spared	Dependent on extent of timing of respiratory complications
SMA type III (chronic SMA, Kugelberg-Welander)	AR, AD	15 months to teen years	Proximal leg weakness, delayed motor milestones		Dependent on extent and timing of respiratory complications
SMA type IV (adult-onset SMA)	AD, AR, or very rarely X-linked recessive	Median age of onset, 37 years	Proximal weakness; variable within families; more severe in AD form		Life expectancy not markedly reduced
Distal SMA (progressive SMA, Charcot-Marie-Tooth–type SMA)	AR, AD	AR: birth or infancy; AD: adulthood	Distal weakness		Very slow clinical progression; does not alter life span

AD, Autosomal dominant; AR, autosomal recessive.

Pathogenesis and Pathophysiology. Information about the molecular basis for these disorders has exploded in the past 5 years. Both the severe and milder forms of autosomal recessive SMA have been linked to chromosome 5q11.3–13.1, a region that contains multiple copies of genes and pseudogenes and is characterized by instability. Deletions, truncations, or point mutations in what is now called the gene for survival of motor neurons (*SMN*) have been identified in SMA types I, II, and III.[21] Its protein product has no known homolog and its function is not yet fully known. It appears to be associated with RNA processing/translocation in the nucleus. Although there is no correlation between genotype and phenotype, most affected siblings exhibit the same phenotype, suggesting that there may be additional modifying factors, one of which could be another gene tightly linked to the pathogenic gene. Though several genes in the SMA locus have been implicated in the pathogenesis of SMA, it has become clear that *SMN* is the gene primarily responsible for the disease. It exists in two or more copies, the centromeric copy, ^{c}*SMN*, and the telomeric copy, ^{t}*SMN*. The ^{c}*SMN* does not produce a full-length transcript most of the time. Human study and conditional knockout models of SMA show that the SMA phenotype is dependent on the dosage of *SMN* product: the higher the level of *SMN*, the milder the phenotype.[22] Conditional knockout models affecting only the expression of *SMN* in muscle show dystrophic change correlating with increased CK and calf hypertrophy in juvenile SMA.[23]

Epidemiology and Risk Factors. The autosomal recessive SMAs are the most common heritable cause of death in infancy, with incidence estimates of 1 in 10,000 to 25,000 for type I in the Western world. Similar numbers are affected with the milder forms and forms with a later onset. Distal SMA of recessive inheritance is more common with consanguineous parents, whereas the dominant form is rare. X-linked adult SMA is also rare[24] and can be confused with Kennedy disease.

Clinical Features and Associated Disorders. The three clinical hallmarks of this disorder are hypotonia, weakness, and cranial nerve palsies (Fig. 36–2), though the facial muscles

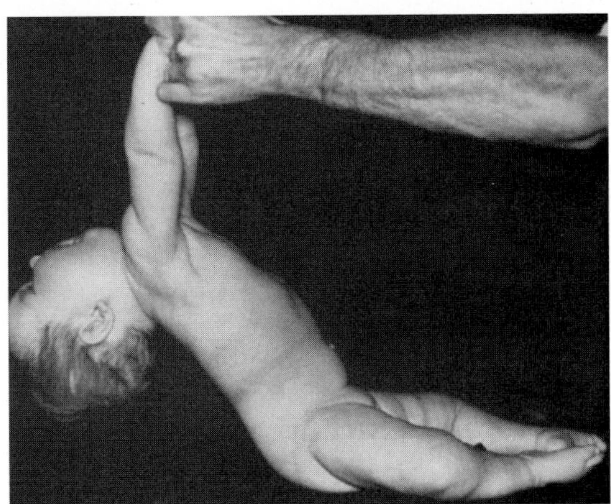

FIGURE 36–2. A baby with spinal muscular atrophy, showing the flaccid head lag in the supine position. (From Dubowitz V: Muscle Disorders in Childhood. Philadelphia, WB Saunders, 1995.)

are usually spared. Generally, SMA has an insidious onset of symmetrical weakness. Proximal muscles are weakened more than distal ones, and the legs become markedly weak before the arms are severely involved. Patients with the later-onset forms decline less rapidly than those with earlier onset. An interesting difference between the SMAs and other neurodegenerative disorders is that in the SMAs the greatest decline in muscular power occurs at onset and then slows, implying great loss of motor neurons initially, followed by a stabilization in any remaining neurons. This phenomenon results in a large number of complications owing to greater demands on remaining strength, such as scoliosis, contractures, and disuse atrophy, as well as respiratory, nutritional, and sleep problems. Arthrogryposis multiplex congenita, a disorder characterized by congenital limitation of motion in all joints except the temporomandibular and vertebral joints, is sometimes secondary to loss of anterior horn cells. A deletion of *SMN* has been found in half of such cases examined thus far.[25]

Progressive bulbar palsy of childhood, or Fazio-Londe disease, involves brain stem motor neuron degeneration that presents most often with stridor followed by ptosis, dysarthria, facial palsy, and dysphagia. Death generally occurs in early childhood.

An autosomal dominant scapuloperoneal SMA has been reported with fasciculations, weakness, and atrophy in that distribution. Autopsy findings included degeneration of anterior horn cells and motor neurons of cranial nerves VII, IX, and X. A few families with adult-onset, autosomal dominant facioscapulohumeral and scapulohumeral distribution SMA have been reported.[26]

Kennedy disease is a spinobulbar neuropathy with midlife onset, normal life span, and associated gynecomastia. It occurs in men only and is caused by the expansion of trinucleotide repeats in the androgen receptor (AR) gene located on the X chromosome.[27] This was a particularly important discovery because it paved the way for identification of trinucleotide repeats as the cause of several other neurological diseases. Trapping of important acetylation enzymes in aggregates of the AR may be the major cause of degeneration in the CAG repeat diseases.[28]

Differential Diagnosis and Evaluation. Because many disorders can mimic the clinical picture of the SMAs, it is essential to verify a neurogenic process with EMG and muscle biopsy. In children, the differential diagnosis is particularly wide (Table 36–3).

Homozygous deletion of SMN is a sensitive test for confirming the clinical diagnosis in almost all cases, including isolated cases and those with unusual features. A method for preimplantation diagnosis for couples at risk has recently been reported.[29] After genetic testing, the most revealing studies are EMG and muscle histochemistry, both of which will confirm a neurogenic process involving muscle. Fibrillation and normal-sized residual motor units are commonly seen in the acutely denervated muscle fibers of SMA I. Additionally, there is an abnormal rhythmical motor unit discharge during sleep. SMA II and III produce very large motor units and absence of spontaneous activity. Serum CK can be elevated, and it correlates positively with duration of illness.

Management and Future Perspectives. There is no specific treatment for any of the SMAs. Recent work suggests

TABLE 36–3. **Selected Differential Diagnosis of Motor Neuron Diseases of Children According to Some Presenting Symptoms**

Hypotonia
Hereditary motor and sensory neuropathies
Neuromuscular transmission defects
- Transient neonatal myasthenia
- Congenital myasthenic syndromes
- Infantile botulism

Congenital myopathies with distinguishing structural abnormalities
- Central core disease
- Nemaline myopathy
- Centronuclear myopathy

Muscular dystrophies
Metabolic myopathies
- Glycogen storage diseases
- Lipid storage myopathies
- Mitochondrial myopathies

Inflammatory myopathies
- Dermatomyositis/polymyositis

Connective tissue disorders
- Osteogenesis imperfecta
- Marfan disease
- Ehlers-Danlos syndrome

Metabolic diseases
- Aminoacidopathies
- Organicacidurias
- Renal reabsorption defects
- Endocrinopathies
- Prader-Willi syndrome
- Nutritional disorders

Progressive Muscle Weakness
Peripheral neuropathies
Subacute inflammatory polyradiculoneuropathy
- Hereditary motor neuropathies

Muscular dystrophies
Metabolic myopathies
- Glycogen storage diseases
- Lipid storage myopathies

Inflammatory myopathies
- Dermatomyositis/polymyositis

Progressive Cranial Nerve Paralysis
Neoplasms
- Brain stem glioma
- Extrinsic posterior fossa tumor
- Nasopharyngeal neoplasm

Neuromuscular transmission defect
- Botulism
- Myasthenia gravis
- Congenital myasthenic syndromes

Myopathies
- Ocular myopathies
- Ophthalmoplegia plus syndromes

Intracranial infections
- Tuberculosis

sodium butyrate may be helpful. In lymphoid cell lines from SMA patients, it increased the amount of SMN protein to normal. Administration to homozygous knockout transgenic SMA-like mice decreased the birth rate of the more severe type of SMA and ameliorated some symptoms.[30] Perhaps most important is recent work demonstrating in mice that deletion of murine SMN exon 7 directed to skeletal muscle results in ongoing muscle necrosis with a dystrophic phenotype that progresses to muscle paralysis and death, suggesting that primary involvement of skeletal muscle in SMA may contribute to motor deficits. This provides a new avenue to explore for intervention.[31]

A multidisciplinary approach aimed at preventing contractures, skeletal deformities, respiratory complications, and social isolation is imperative. Genetic counseling of parents of young SMA patients or SMA patients approaching childbearing age is appropriate. Thus far, prenatal testing for *SMN* deletion is available only on a research basis. The prognosis varies according to type, ranging from the early fatality of SMA I to the basically unaltered life span of SMA III.

HEREDITARY SPASTIC PARAPLEGIAS

The HSPs, also known as Strümpell-Lorrain syndrome and the familial spastic paraplegias, are a broad group of genetically and clinically diverse disorders characterized by lower extremity spasticity and weakness. Generally, they are classified according to mode of inheritance and symptoms. The more common uncomplicated or so-called pure HSP indicates progressive spasticity of the lower extremities that may be accompanied by a mild decrease in proprioception and urinary sphincter dysfunction, whereas complicated HSP denotes the presence of other neurological problems.

Pathogenesis and Pathophysiology. Information about the genetic basis for these disorders is mushrooming. It has been well established that uncomplicated autosomal dominant, autosomal recessive, and X-linked HSPs are heterogeneous disorders. Because families with strong similarities in phenotype are linked to different genetic loci, there may be various points of disturbance in a common biochemical pathway that leads to degeneration of the most distal portions of the longest ascending and descending central nervous system (CNS) axons, particularly the corticospinal tracts from the motor cortex to the legs, the fasciculus gracilis fibers, and the spinocerebellar fibers (Table 36–4).[32–48] Genetic penetrance is age dependent and nearly complete.[49]

Clinical Features and Associated Disorders. The patient generally presents with leg stiffness, weakness in the hip flexors, and impaired foot dorsiflexion in the second through fourth decades, although symptoms may be apparent in infancy or not until late adulthood. The gait disturbance progresses insidiously and continuously. Patients may also have paresthesia and mildly decreased vibratory sense below the knees and urinary urgency and incontinence late in the disease. On neurological examination, generally there are no abnormalities of the corticobulbar tracts or upper extremities, except possibly brisk deep tendon reflexes. In the lower extremities, deep tendon reflexes are pathologically increased and there is decreased hip flexion and ankle dorsiflexion. Crossed adductor reflexes, ankle clonus, and extensor plantar responses are present. Hoffman's and Tromner's signs, as well as pes cavus, may be present. Occasionally, slight dysmetria may be seen on finger-to-nose testing in patients with long-standing disease.

TABLE 36-4. **Hereditary Spastic Paraplegia (SPG), Gene Locus, and Protein Product**

Genetic Nomenclature	Inheritance	Gene Locus	Product
SPG1	X-linked	Xq28	L1CAM[32]
SPG2	X-linked	Xq28	Proteolipoprotein[33, 34]
SPG3	AD	14q12–q21	Atlastin[35]
SPG4	AD	2p24–21	Spastin[36]
SPG5A	AR	8p11–q13[37]	?
SPG5B	AR	?	?
SPG6	AD	15q11–1[38]	?
SPG7	AR	16q24.3	Paraplegin[39]
SPG8	AD	8q23–q24[40]	?
SPG9	AD	10q23–q24[41]	?
SPG10	AD	12q13[42]	?
SPG11	AR	15q13–q15[43]	?
SPG12	AD	19q13[44]	?
SPG13	AD	2q24–q34[45]	?
SPG14	AR	3q27–28[46]	?
SPG16	X-linked	Xq11.2[47]	?
SPG17	AD	11q12–q14[48]	?

AR, Autosomal recessive; AD, autosomal dominant; L1CAM, L1 cell adhesion molecule.

The designation *complicated HSP* indicates spasticity with additional neurological impairment, such as optic neuropathy, retinopathy, extrapyramidal disturbance, dementia, ataxia, ichthyosis, mental retardation, and deafness.[49]

Differential Diagnosis and Evaluation. The HSPs are diagnoses of exclusion. Particular care is necessary if the family history is not revealing or if there are numerous complications or atypical features. Because HSP can mimic treatable disorders, such as vitamin B_{12} deficiency, dopa-responsive dystonia, cervical spondylosis, early PLS, or multiple sclerosis, exhaustive evaluation is justified.[49]

Molecular diagnosis is available clinically only for proteolipoprotein (genetic nomenclature, *SPG2*), while testing for L1 cell adhesion molecule *(SPG1)*, atlastin *(SPG3)*, spastin *(SPG4)*, and paraplegin *(SPG7)* is available at some research facilities. Additional testing is available only to family members within kindreds linked to an identified locus. Electrophysiological studies are the most revealing. Somatosensory evoked potentials of the lower extremities show conduction delay in the dorsal column fibers, whereas cortical evoked potentials show reduced conduction velocity and amplitude in lumbar spinal segment muscles. Cortical evoked potentials of the arms are either normal or mildly slow. Nerve conduction studies are most often normal, although there may be subclinical sensory impairment of peripheral nerves and spinal pathways.

Magnetic resonance imaging of the brain and spinal cord as well as plasma very long-chain fatty acid analysis should be performed.[49]

Management and Prognosis. There is no treatment available to address the underlying process in HSP. Treatments to combat the problems associated with chronic paraplegia can be helpful, particularly oral or intrathecal baclofen or less commonly oral dantrolene for the lower extremity spasticity, and oxybutynin or tolterodine for bladder spasticity. Caution should be exhibited in counseling regarding the course of the disease because there is variation in severity of phenotype reported.

At this time, although the phenotypes of the various autosomal dominant HSPs are very similar, it does seem to be more severe in the families linked to chromosome 15q, in which more patients require wheelchairs by the fourth decade. Families with mutations in spastin show more variation, including a less common childhood onset and a relatively nonprogressive course.[36]

Degenerative Muscular Disorders

The muscular dystrophies are degenerative hereditary disorders, with the most common being the dystrophinopathies and disorders of dystrophin-associated proteins. In 1987, with the identification of a defect in the dystrophin gene as the cause of Duchenne muscular dystrophy (DMD), Monaco and Kunkel opened the door for research into the role of dystrophin and functionally related proteins in muscle function and maintenance.[50]

Dystrophin is controlled by a very large gene, at least 2300 kb and 79 exons, that encodes a 3685 amino acid protein product with four distinct domains. It has an I-beam shape with globular domains at each end and a rodlike segment in the middle (Fig. 36–3). At the amino-terminal end, it binds to cytoplasmic actin filaments; at the other end, it binds to a complex of proteins and glycoproteins called dystrophin-associated proteins and dystrophin-associated glycoproteins. Transcripts, each with its own promotor, suggest that dystrophin influences a number of distinct functions. Muscle dystrophin is found on the plasma membrane surface in skeletal muscle fibers, on the surfaces of plasma membrane and transverse tubules of cardiac muscle fibers, and on smooth muscle membranes. Cortical dystrophin is found in the hippocampus, amygdala, thalamus, hypothalamus, and neocortex, and a Purkinje cell isoform is found in the cerebellum.[51–53] A second protein product of the DMD gene, which is structurally different from dystrophin, has not been found in muscle, but its level in other tissues is comparable to that of dystrophin in muscle.[54]

It is now known that there are at least three subcomplexes that form the glycoprotein complex involved with dystrophin in muscle support. Several components of these subcomplexes have now been identified and some of their relationships determined. The dystroglycan subcomplex consisting of

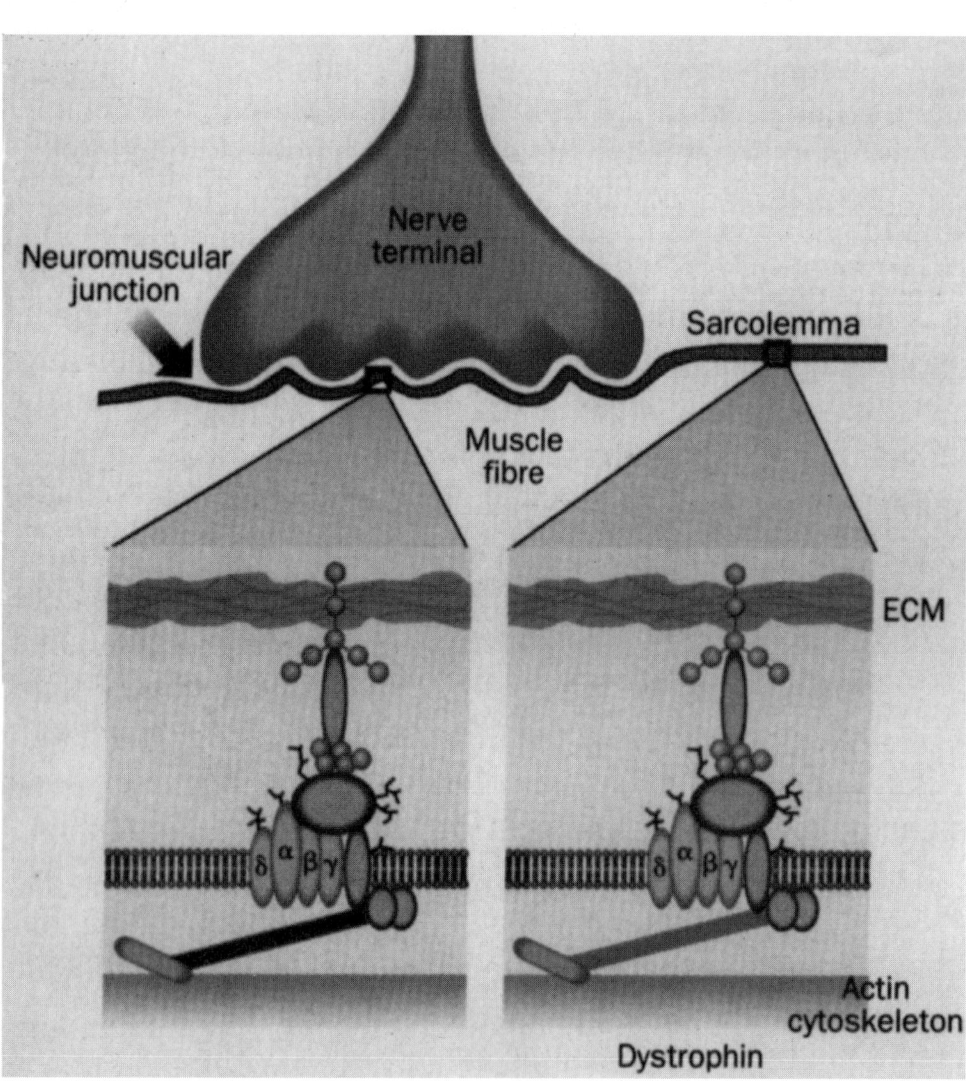

FIGURE 36–3. Localization of dystrophin and utrophin in the muscle cell. Dystrophin is found throughout the sarcolemma, whereas utrophin is confined to the neuromuscular junction. Both proteins are associated with a glycoprotein complex that binds to the extracellular matrix. (Reprinted with permission from Campbell KP, Crosbie RH: The structure of dystrophin. Nature 1996;384:308. Copyright 1996 MacMillan Magazines Limited.)

α-dystroglycan and β-dystroglycan functions as a connecting axis, called the dystrophin-axis, between the extracellular matrix and the subsarcolemma cytoskeleton. These dystroglycans are ubiquitously expressed in various tissues. The basal lamina is a network of several components, including laminin, that surrounds each muscle fiber in fixed contact with the sarcolemma and provides protection from mechanical damage. α-Dystroglycan is an extracellular protein that binds to the laminin subunit merosin in the basement membrane, as well as to β-dystroglycan, a transmembrane protein, which, in turn, binds to the cysteine-rich and carboxyl-terminus domains of dystrophin within the cell. Then the *N*-terminus domain of dystrophin binds to actin filaments, which forms the cytoskeleton of the subsarcolemma.[53] Utrophin, a dystrophin homolog, binds to actin and most likely the dystroglycan complex.[55] It is possible that utrophin and these proteins form a utrophin axis similar to the dystrophin axis.

Four other transmembrane glycoproteins, called the sarcoglycans, have been identified: α-sarcoglycan (in some sources called 50DAG, A2, and adhalin), β-sarcoglycan (43DAG, A3b), γ-sarcoglycan (35DAG, A4), and δ-sarcoglycan. It has been proposed that the sarcoglycan complex is fixed to the dystrophin axis by lateral association, although the binding site is not yet known. The sarcoglycan complex is expressed specifically in skeletal and cardiac muscle.[52]

Finally, the cytoplasmic complex consists of two families of proteins, the syntrophins that bind to the distal part of the carboxy-terminal domain of dystrophin[52] and dystrobrevin that co-localizes with dystrophin and DAPs.[56] The syntrophins are composed of at least three subclasses—α-syntrophin, specifically localized in muscle; β1-syntrophin, with a ubiquitous distribution; and β2-syntrophin, localized to the neuromuscular junction.

In the past few years, disruptions in these proteins and glycoproteins have been implicated in several types of muscular dystrophy (Table 36–5).

DYSTROPHINOPATHIES

Different mutations in the dystrophin gene produce different allelic disorders, most commonly either the lethal DMD or Becker muscular dystrophy (BMD), a milder myopathy. Very rarely, patients with cardiomyopathy with mild weakness, dilated cardiomyopathy without weakness, exercise intolerance associated with myalgias, muscle cramps, or myoglobinuria and asymptomatic elevation of serum CK have also been identified.[57]

Pathogenesis and Pathophysiology. Large mutations in the dystrophin gene are identified in about 75 percent of patients with DMD and 87 percent of patients with BMD. Most large mutations are deletions, and they tend to occur in regions where the introns are longer. The deletion breakpoints seem to be at sites where recombination events occur in healthy individuals. Large deletions are also common in BMD, whereas large duplications are rare. Small mutations account for about 30 percent of DMD cases and 15 percent of BMD cases. Mutations that shift the mRNA transitional reading frame usually produce a truncated dystrophin molecule missing the carboxy terminus, which in turn does not bind adequately to dystrophin-associated proteins at the cell membrane, resulting in severe dystrophin deficiency in the Duchenne phenotype. Either no dystrophin is made or the aborted molecule is degraded rapidly. Nonframeshifting mutations produce a dystrophin molecule with a preserved carboxy terminus in which more dystrophin remains and the phenotype is the milder form of BMD.[58] In-frame deletions alter the clinical presentation depending on where they occur. Deletions that involve the cysteine-rich and carboxy-terminus domains required for attachment to the dystrophin-associated proteins confer the Duchenne phenotype, whereas deletions in the proximal portion of the rod domain produce a very mild phenotype.[59] Deletions in the distal region present the BMD phenotype and produce 40 to 70 percent of the normal amount of dystrophin.[60] There are rare cases to

TABLE 36–5. **Limb Girdle Muscular Dystrophy**

Type	Inheritance	Gene Locus	Gene Product	Unusual Features	Disease Name
1A	AD	5q31–33	Myotilin[82]	Palatal weakness	
1B	AD	?	Lamin A/C[83]	Cardiac involvement, sudden death	Also called AD Emery-Dreifuss
1C	AD	3p25	Caveolin[84]		Caveolinopathy
1D	AD	6q23[85]	?	Dilated cardiomyopathy	
1E	AD	7q[86]	?	Dysphagia, Pelger-Hunt anomaly	
2A	AR	15q	Calpain-III[87]		Calpainopathy
2B	AR	2p13	Dysferlin[88]	Distal extremity weakness and wasting	Dysferlinopathy or Miyoshi neuropathy
2C	AR	13q12	γ-Sarcoglycan[89]	Cardiac involvement, abdominal, neck flexor and intercostal muscles affected, malignant course	γ-Sarcoglycanopathy (formerly SCARMD)
2D	AR	17q.33	α-Sarcoglycan (Adhalin)[90]		α-Sarcoglycanopathy
2E	AR	4q12	β-Sarcoglycan[91]		β-Sarcoglycanopathy
2F	AR	5q33	δ-Sarcoglycan[92]		δ-Sarcoglycanopathy
2G	AR	17q	Telethonin[93]	Early involvement of distal muscles	Telethonopathy
2H	AD	9q[94]	?		
2I	AR	19q13.3[95]	?		

AD, Autosomal dominant; AR, autosomal recessive.

which these generalizations do not apply: out-of-frame deletions that can result in DMD, BMD, or an intermediate phenotype and situations in which there is no correlation between the degree of dystrophin deficiency and the severity of phenotype.[57, 58]

Epidemiology and Risk Factors. DMD is the most common neuromuscular disease of childhood, with an estimated overall prevalence of 63 cases per million, whereas BMD has an overall prevalence of 24 cases per million.[61] Because dystrophin is at Xp21.1, nearly all patients are male. As many as 20 percent of new DMD cases and an unknown number of BMD cases are caused by gonadal mosaicism.[57]

Clinical Features and Associated Disorders. The hallmarks of DMD are progressive proximal muscle weakness with pseudohypertrophy of the calves. The myocardium is involved, whereas bulbar muscles are spared. There may be mild mental retardation. DMD is universally fatal, usually either from respiratory or cardiac complications.

As early as 1868, Duchenne had established criteria for the diagnosis of what would later be called DMD. These features still serve as an accurate description of the clinical picture: (1) weakness, appearing first in the lower extremities; (2) wide-based gait and stance, with lordosis; (3) subsequent hypertrophy of weakened muscles; (4) loss of muscle contractility with electrical stimulation; and (5) intact sensation and bowel and bladder function, with a (6) progressive, deteriorating course.

Usually, the child is asymptomatic in the neonatal period, with the earliest problems perceived by caregivers being developmental delays, particularly in walking and climbing, and the appearance of enlarged calf muscles. Between the ages of 3 and 6, the gait becomes waddling and lordotic. Gowers' sign appears, in which the child stands from a prone position by a process of climbing up the legs, using the hands first on the knees and then on the thighs to support her- or himself (Fig. 36–4). Usually by the age of 6 years, there is enlargement of calf, gluteal, lateral vastus, deltoid, and infraspinatus muscles, and weakness is readily apparent, with the proximal extremities more severely affected than the distal extremities, and lower extremities and torso more severely affected than the upper extremities (Fig. 36–5). Weakness of the arms may be present but is not obvious without careful examination. The strength of limb and torso muscles continues to decline steadily from ages 6 though 11 years. Proximal muscles continue to be more severely affected than distal muscles, with neck flexors becoming more involved than extensors, wrist extensors more than flexors, biceps and triceps more than deltoid, quadriceps more than hamstrings, and the tibialis posterior and peroni more than the gastrocnemius, soleus, and tibialis anterior. Tendon reflexes decrease and disappear as muscle weakness progresses. By the age of 10 years, 50 percent of patients have lost biceps, triceps, and knee reflexes, in contrast with the ankle reflex, which remains in one third of patients even in end-stage disease. Significant contractures of the iliotibial bands, hip flexors, and heel cords are present in 70 percent of the children by the age of 10 years. The children tend to have relatively mild functional impairment until they are about 8 years old, when they then decline more rapidly over the next 2 to 3 years. The second decade brings progressive kyphoscoliosis from weakened paraspinal muscles and decreased vital and total lung capacities and maximal inspiratory and expiratory pressures from weakened respiratory muscles. These problems first appear

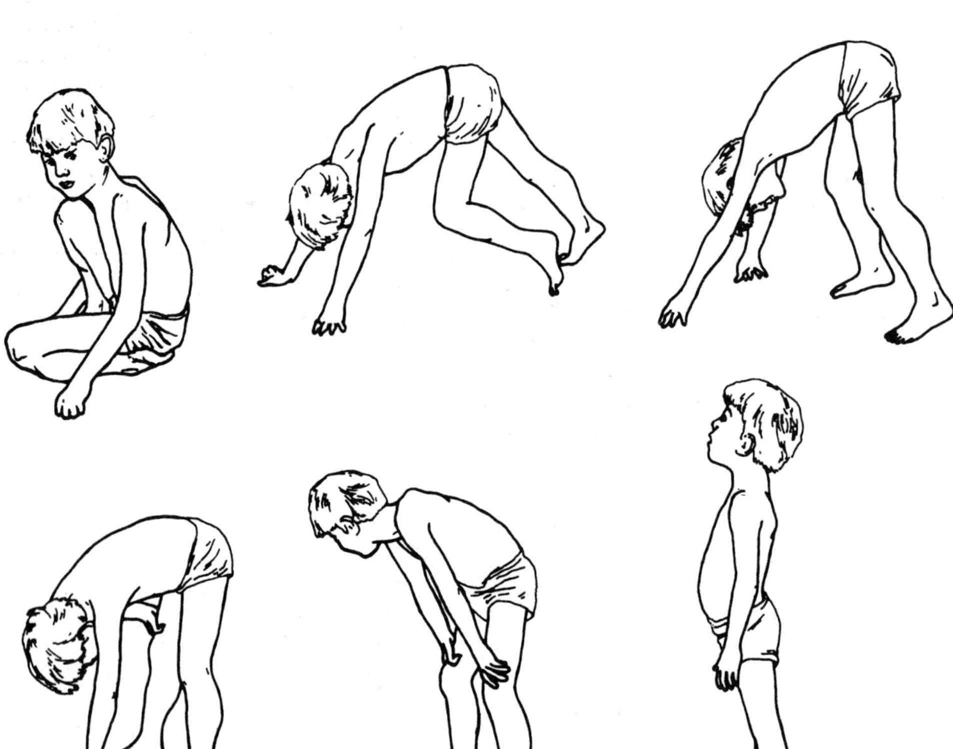

FIGURE 36–4. Gower's sign. (From Siegel IM: Muscle and Its Diseases: An Outline Primer of Basic Science and Clinical Method. Chicago, Yearbook Medical Publishers, 1986.)

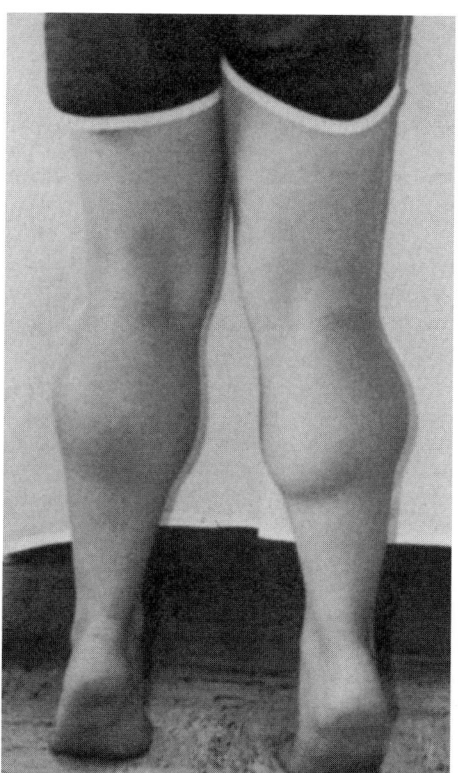

FIGURE 36–5. Enlarged calf muscles in a patient with Duchenne muscular dystrophy. (From Fenichel GM: Clinical Pediatric Neurology. Philadelphia, WB Saunders, 1997.)

between the ages of 8 and 9 years and progress as functional status deteriorates.

The mean age of death in a survey of 176 patients who died between 1970 and 1984 was 18.3 +/– 3 years. It was slightly increased to 20 +/– 3.9 years in the subset of 48 patients who died between 1980 and 1984. About 40 percent died of respiratory failure, and 10 to 40 percent died of cardiac complications. Although cardiac rate, rhythm, and conduction defects occur in up to 90 percent of DMD patients, they tend to be stable or slowly progressive problems.[57]

In BMD, disease is later in onset and slower in progression. As early as the mid-1950s, Becker proposed that these cases represented a variation of DMD. Now that it is known that DMD and BMD are allelic disorders, it is apparent that BMD phenotypes range from myalgias and muscle cramps to symptoms clinically indistinguishable from DMD.

Age of onset ranges from 1 to 70 years of age, with a mean of 12 years. Ninety percent of patients are affected by age 20. Lower extremity weakness appears on average by age 11, with upper extremity weakness by age 20. Loss of ambulation generally occurs around 40 but can occur as early as age 12. Age at death ranges from 23 to 89 years of age, with the average being 42.

Cardiac problems similar to those associated with DMD are present in about half of the patients with BMD. The extent of cardiac involvement does not correlate with degree of myopathy. Myocardial pathology includes degeneration of cardiac muscle and fibrous replacement of myocardiocytes, particularly in the posterobasal region and the adjacent lateral wall of the left ventricle.

In comparison with their unaffected brothers, 10 to 79 percent of these patients have fertility problems, and the severity of infertility correlates positively with severity of phenotype. Fatty infiltration of smooth muscle may result in delayed gastric emptying with emesis, abdominal pain, and distention. Adverse reactions to succinylcholine and halothane have been reported, which ranged from marked elevation of CK in the postoperative period to cardiac arrest.[57]

Differential Diagnosis and Evaluation. The diagnosis of DMD and BMD has become considerably more reliable with the advent of molecular genetics. When the clinical presentation, elevation of CK, muscle biopsy, EMG findings, and inheritance pattern are consistent with a dystrophinopathy, the patient's white blood cells or muscle should be examined for deletions or duplications in the dystrophin gene. Multiplex polymerase chain reaction (PCR) amplification of commonly deleted exons detects 98 percent of the deletions that cause more than 65 percent of the dystrophinopathies. Quantitative Southern blot analysis may be needed to detect partial gene duplication because it is more sensitive.[62, 63] Immunoblot analysis of muscle homogenates with dystrophin antibodies confirms abnormalities in at least 95 percent of DMD patients and differentiates DMD from BMD. Analysis of restriction length polymorphisms and a nonradioactive direct test based on PCR amplification provides rapid, precise carrier diagnosis in women whose relatives have a known deletion. Sisters and daughters of mothers who have given birth to boys with isolated cases of DMD or BMD should also be tested and counseled. Such mothers should also consider prenatal diagnosis because the risk for recurrence in additional sons is estimated at 7 percent. Prenatal diagnosis can be performed as early as 8 weeks' gestation.[64]

The EMG changes seen are those common to all myopathic disorders. Motor units fire at a relatively high rate for the degree of effort, with a higher number activated than would be in a muscle of comparable strength in a neurogenic problem. As the disease progresses, fewer and fewer motor units can be activated. An increased number of motor unit potentials are polyphasic with one or more late components, as well as components reduced in duration. Fibrillation potentials are often observed. Nerve conduction velocities are normal.

Similar pathological changes are present in BMD and DMD, particularly necrotic and regenerating fibers, branching fibers, abnormal fiber size, and endomysial fibrosis. Generally there are more necrotic, hypercontracted, and regenerating fibers with a more severe phenotype. Additionally, inflammatory cells are evident at perivascular, endomysial, and perimysial sites in DMD. Plasma membrane defects that lead to segmental fiber necrosis and eventual regeneration are observed with electron microscopy. Extensive discussion of morphological and electron microscopy studies is available in Engel.[57]

Serum CK is the most useful of the serum enzyme tests, with CK increased up to two orders of magnitude during the first 3 years when it peaks and then declines exponentially by about 20 percent annually. Myoglobinemia is roughly correlated with elevations in CK. Ambulatory DMD patients have diurnal fluctuations in myoglobin and CK, with increases corresponding to physical activity.[65] In the CSF, protein fractions are increased in most dystrophies and γ-globulin is decreased. Because excretion of total creatinine declines with decreasing functional muscle mass, urinary creatinine is 40 to

90 percent below normal.[66] Urinary creatinine excretion is about twice normal between ages 6 and 11, and it increases with age.

It is essential to evaluate the heart. Ninety percent of patients with DMD have myocardial fibrosis, revealed by elevated right precordial R waves and deep Q waves in left precordial and limb leads on electrocardiography (ECG).[67] Persistent or labile sinus tachycardia, sinus arrhythmias, and interatrial conduction defects are also common abnormalities. Echocardiography demonstrates small internal ventricles, hypokinesis of the posterobasal ventricular wall, and slowed ventricular relaxation.

Examination of dystrophin can prevent misdiagnosis in patients with disorders that mimic the clinical presentation of DMD and BMD, particularly the SMAs, congenital muscular dystrophy, acid maltase deficiency, and Emery-Dreifuss muscular dystrophy (ED MD). Dystrophin should also be evaluated in males with dilated cardiomyopathy, even in the absence of muscle weakness, and in girls with symptoms of DMD.

Management and Prognosis. Thus far, the only medication to improve functioning of boys with DMD when evaluated in carefully controlled trials is a regimen of alternate-day prednisone with a dosage range of 0.75 to 1.5 mg/kg/d. Improvement began about 1 month after beginning treatment and peaked by 3 months, with significant and sustained benefits still evident at 3 years. With treatment, the progressive decrease in muscle strength and increase in muscle mass were slower than expected, and the extent of disability was less. Side effects included those common to all steroids: altered behavior, cushingoid appearance, gastrointestinal disturbance, rashes, and hirsutism.[68]

Effective gene therapy remains elusive. A carefully controlled study determined that injecting normal myoblasts into affected muscle did not increase muscle force generation or the amount of dystrophin in muscle.[69]

Much of the management of the dystrophinopathies remains supportive, and there is controversy regarding appropriate active exercise regimens in the dystrophinopathies. The review by Spenser and Vignos provides a balanced discussion of the role of active exercise in DMD.[70] In one short-term controlled study, resistance exercises neither hastened physical deterioration, as has been proposed, nor maintained strength any better than free exercises. More clearly, passive exercises and joint stretching are important in delaying the onset of contractures. Maintaining ambulation as long as possible is crucial because its loss is associated with contractures and scoliosis, which, in turn, is associated with restrictive respiratory syndrome. Release of hip and ankle contractures by subcutaneous tenotomy while the patient is still ambulatory has been shown to preserve ambulation for about 2 additional years.[71]

Inspiratory resistive exercises have been shown to increase endurance of respiratory muscles but not vital capacity.[72] When indicated, intermittent ventilatory assistance ameliorates symptoms of hypoventilation but does not slow the deterioration of respiratory function. If assisted ventilation is employed when vital capacity falls below 10 percent of normal, it can prolong survival by 3 to 4 years.[57]

Bregman has outlined strategies that families can employ in managing childhood neuromuscular disorders: (1) maintaining a regular schedule of activities for both the affected child and other family members, (2) providing interesting activities appropriate to the degree of disability that enhance the affected child's experiences, (3) assisting the affected child in setting realistic goals, (4) encouraging as much independence as possible in the affected child, (5) employing stress reduction strategies, (6) including all family members in decision making, and (7) maintaining active relationships with the primary physician and support groups in the community.[73]

Data indicate that DMD patients are living somewhat longer than they used to, probably because of more aggressive respiratory and cardiac care, but as yet, nothing reverses the basically relentless course of either the Duchenne or Becker phenotype.

Future Perspectives. Recent work suggests that a disruption of basement membrane organization occurring in rare homozygotes for a null allele of dystroglycan may be the common feature of muscular dystrophies associated with the dystroglycan complex.[74] Effective treatment may involve either replacement of dystrophin or upregulation of a related protein, such as utrophin. Two recent papers report the development of adenoviral vectors from which protein-producing genes have been removed, allowing transport of more DNA and eliminating proteins that trigger the host response.[75, 76] Although upregulation of utrophin theoretically could occur pharmacologically, recent work with the utrophin transgene is very exciting. High expression of the utrophin transgene in skeletal and diaphragmatic muscle of the dystrophin-deficient *mdx* mouse markedly reduced dystrophic pathology.[77] It has been demonstrated that transgenic mice with premature stop codons in syntrophin produced normal dystrophin in muscle and had less muscle degeneration when treated with aminoglycosides than untreated mice with the same mutation, which may open an avenue for treatment.[78] It has been proposed that introduction of particular antisense oligoribonucleotides to modify the processing of dystrophin pre-mRNA may reduce the severity of symptoms. It was recently demonstrated in transgenic mice that upregulation of the protein alpha 7 integrin may compensate for dystrophin and utrophin deficiency.[79] Bone marrow transplantation in the *mdx* mouse demonstrated that bone marrow or muscle stem cells appear to provide a means for systemic repair of muscle.[80] Chaubourt and colleaques propose the use of nitric oxide donors as a palliative treatment in combination with gene and molecular therapy.[81]

LIMB GIRDLE MUSCULAR DYSTROPHIES

The limb girdle muscular dystrophies (LGMDs) are being reclassified on a genetic basis as their underlying pathologies are unraveled. The genes and their products or actions identified thus far again point to disturbances in the structural support system of muscle, particularly of the sarcoglycan complex. It may be that a disturbance in the sarcolemma–extracellular matrix interaction is the molecular basis for muscle fiber necrosis (see Table 36–5).[82–95] Emery estimates LGMD prevalence to be 1 in 100,000. As early as 1960, Morton proposed that homozygosity at either of two loci could produce LGMD and that about 1.6 percent of the normal population is heterozygous for an LGMD gene.[96]

With the exception of gamma-sarcoglycanopathy, previously known as severe childhood autosomal recessive muscular dystrophy (SCARMD) found primarily in North Africa, the LGMDs all fall within a clinical spectrum that includes weakness of proximal lower extremities, which is usually symmetrical, appearing any time from the first decade until middle age, generally followed by weakness in the shoulder girdle region. Occasionally, shoulder girdle weakness may precede the pelvic girdle weakness. Facial muscles are uninvolved. The progression is generally slow, with loss of ambulation occurring 10 to 30 years after onset. Cardiac involvement is not reported, except in the newly recognized autosomal dominant form reported from the Netherlands, known as LGMD-1B.

The features of gamma-sarocoglycanopathy have been well described by Ben Hamida and associates.[97] Pelvic girdle weakness precedes pectoral girdle weakness, with onset occurring between ages 3 and 12. Abdominal, neck flexor, and intercostal muscles are often affected, whereas external ocular, facial, lingual, and pharyngeal muscles are spared. Seventy-five percent of patients are unable to walk by their thirties. Contractures form and reflexes are lost as the disease progresses. Cardiomegaly and ECG abnormalities are common by the intermediate stages of the illness. There is no cognitive impairment.

If sufficient informative family members are available, linkage analysis can provide a genetic diagnosis if the patient has one of the previously linked types of LGMD. SCARMD can be diagnosed by a negative sarcolemmal immunostain for adhalin.[98]

There are several nonspecific findings associated with the LGMDs. Serum CK is mildly to moderately elevated, except in SCARMD, in which the levels may rival those of DMD.[98] Creatinuria and hypocreatinuria are nonspecific indicators of muscle destruction that may be present. The EMG shows nonspecific myopathic changes, including short duration, low-amplitude motor unit potentials, increased proportion of polyphasic potentials, and rapid recruitment. Fibrillation and positive sharp waves may occur with denervation caused by muscle fiber necrosis. Muscle biopsy pathology also is nonspecific, with morphology like that of other myopathies.[96]

The LGMDs have relatively common and nonspecific clinical and laboratory findings that may be seen in other neuromuscular disorders. Therefore, care must be taken in evaluation. As an example, in a Japanese series, 17 percent of patients with clinically diagnosed LGMD actually had a dystrophinopathy when muscle dystrophin content was analyzed, which emphasizes the need for examination of dystrophin protein and gene studies for accurate diagnosis (Table 36–6).[99] Protein testing by immunostaining of muscle tissue can establish the diagnosis of sarcoglycanopathy, calpainopathy, dysferlinopathy, and telethoninopathy. Mutation studies of the corresponding genes are so far available only on a research basis.

There are no specific treatments for any of the LGMDs. The physician's goal is to preserve as much function for as long as possible through the use of physical and occupational therapy and psychological support.

Research into the pathogenesis of these disorders is proceeding rapidly. A missense mutation in myotilin, a sarcomeric protein that binds to α-actin associated with the Z line does not disrupt α-actin binding, but does result in Z line streaming.[82] Missense mutations in the caveolin gene lead to an accumulation of caveolin in the Golgi apparatus, an example of a dominant-negative effect.[100] The sarcogylcanopathies involve four different genes that encode proteins which form a tetrameric complex at the muscle cell plasma membrane. Its function is to stabilize the association of dystrophin with the dystroglycans and stabilize the plasma membrane cytoskeleton. Mutations in each sarcoglycan gene are consistent with complete or partial loss of the complex.[101] Congenital muscular dystrophy has the pathological appearance of far-advanced dsytrophinopathies. In half of those cases the laminin merosin is absent, which makes some sense in that merosin forms a connection between the DAG and the basal lamina.[102] As the relationships and workings of the genes and complexes are better understood, it may be possible to offer a rational treatment for these disorders.

TABLE 36-6. **Differential Diagnoses in Limb Girdle Muscular Dystrophy**

Acid maltase deficiency
Becker muscular dystrophy
Carnitine deficiency
Central core disease
Centronuclear myopathy
Congenital fiber-type disproportion
Debrancher enzyme deficiency
Duchenne muscular dystrophy
Duchenne manifesting carrier
Emery-Dreifuss muscular dystrophy
Facioscapulohumeral dystrophy
Fingerprint myopathy
Inclusion body myositis
McArdle's disease
Mitochondrial myopathy
Multicore disease
Myopathy with tubular aggregates
Myopathy with cytoplasmic bodies
Nemaline rod disease
Reducing body myopathy
Sarcotubular myopathy
Scapuloperoneal dystrophy
Spinal muscular atrophy

FACIOSCAPULOHUMERAL MUSCULAR DYSTROPHY

Facioscapulohumeral muscular dystrophy (FSH MD), or Landouzy-Dejerine muscular dystrophy, is slowly progressive degenerative myopathy that affects particular facial, torso, and extremity muscles. Deletions in polymorphic fragments of the *FRG1* gene at 4q35 cause FSH MD in the majority of families, with fragments of less than 35 kb clearly associated with disease. Fragments between 48 kb and 300 kb are found in healthy individuals.[103, 104] About 15 percent of other clinically indistinguishable families remain unlinked.[105] Although isolated cases have been identified, generally with careful evaluation of the family there is a clear autosomal dominant inheritance pattern with a penetrance of 95 percent by the time the individuals reach their twenties. Prevalence is about 1 in 20,000.[106]

Onset has been reported from infancy until middle age. There is significant variability in the severity of symptoms within families, with some individuals having symptoms that are so mild that they are unaware they have the disease until other family members are diagnosed. Generally, the patient first notices asymmetrical weakness in an upper extremity, although facial weakness may have been present for some time. The facial weakness appears insidiously in the orbicularis oculi, zygomaticus, and orbicularis orbis muscles. The weakness generally progresses slowly and in a descending pattern from facial muscles to shoulder girdle to upper arms and then pelvic girdle muscles (Fig. 36–6). A recent report suggests mental retardation and epilepsy may occur in patients with very early onset.[107] There may be plateaus and even occasional arrest of the disorder.

Emery recommends that four criteria be present for the diagnosis of FSH MD: (1) onset in facial and shoulder muscles, with sparing of extraocular, pharyngeal, lingual, and cardiac muscles; (2) autosomal dominant inheritance pattern; (3) facial weakness in half or more of affected family members; and (4) myopathic changes, including polyphasic motor units of low amplitude and short duration on EMG and variation in fiber diameter, centrally located nuclei, and motheaten fibers on muscle biopsy. The unevenness of the disease process may extend to individual muscles.[108]

Several other problems have been identified in FSH MD, particularly in patients with early onset and relatively rapid progression. Hearing loss in the 4000- to 6000- Hz range and retinal capillary abnormalities (Coat's disease) have been reported. Although it is not usually clinically apparent, abnormal atrioventricular node or intranodal conduction also occur.[109]

There is no definitive treatment for FSH MD. Steroids may provide transient benefit if there are inflammatory changes on the muscle biopsy. Physical and occupational therapy are useful for maintaining optimal functioning. Orthotics and bracing may be helpful, as may surgical stabilization of the scapulae. Early photocoagulation of retinal abnormalities is recommended.[108] Large families who have been linked to the chromosome 4 locus may have their diagnosis verified by genetic testing. The course is relatively benign; most patients remain ambulatory, and life span is not significantly decreased.[109]

SCAPULOPERONEAL SYNDROMES

The scapuloperoneal syndromes (SPSs) are heterogeneous disorders characterized by weakness of both shoulder girdle and peroneal muscles. Both a neurogenic form (scapuloperoneal spinal muscular atrophy [SPSMA]) and a myopathic form (scapuloperoneal muscular dystrophy [SP MD]) have been identified. The neurogenic SPSMA was linked to chromosome 12q24.1–q24.31, which is a region about 20 cM telomeric to the location of the gene for the myopathic SP MD.[110]

These are uncommon disorders, with heated debate as to whether the SPSs are all distinct entities. Autosomal dominant, autosomal recessive, and sex-linked recessive patterns of inheritance have been reported, as well as sporadic cases. Genetic studies will undoubtedly eventually clarify the situation.

The clinical features of both the myopathic and neurogenic types are similar. Age of onset reported ranges from infancy to adulthood, most commonly late childhood or young adulthood. The usual presentation is weakness in shoulder girdle muscles, progressing to weakness in the anterior tibial muscles, followed by weakness in pelvic girdle mus-

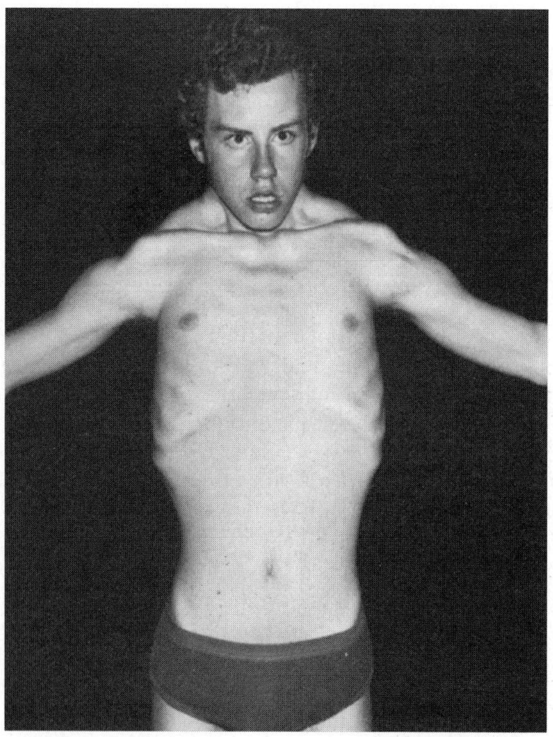

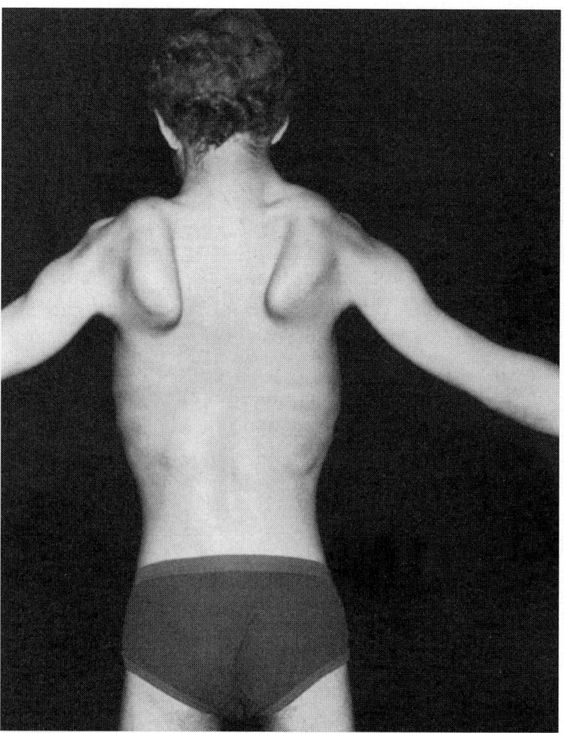

FIGURE 36–6. Facioscapulohumeral dystrophy in a 15-year-old boy. There is marked facial weakness on frontal view and dramatic scapular winging with arm abduction on the posterior view. (From Dubowitz V: Muscle Disorders in Childhood. London, WB Saunders, 1995.)

cles. When facial involvement occurs, it is mild and late in onset.

Although there are a few neuromuscular disorders that may present with weakness in the scapuloperoneal distribution, particularly Charcot-Marie-Tooth disease and FSH MD, a comprehensive neuromuscular workup based primarily on EMG and muscle and nerve biopsies screens out most of them.

Davidenkow's syndrome, which includes scapuloperoneal weakness, may be confused with the SPSs. However, it also has pes cavus deformities and progressive distal sensory loss with early depression of reflexes, as well as impaired sensory and motor nerve conduction velocities.[111]

ED MD may also produce weakness in the scapulohumeral distribution, but it has characteristic contractures and cardiac conduction abnormalities not present in the SPSs. The weakness tends to progress very slowly, and patients become only mildly disabled. It generally does not affect the life span.[112]

MYOTONIC DYSTROPHY

Myotonic dystrophy (DM), or Steinert's disease, is an autosomal dominant multisystem degenerative disease characterized by myotonia, progressive muscular weakness, gonadal atrophy, cataracts, and cardiac arrhythmias.

Pathogenesis and Pathophysiology. The molecular basis of DM is an unstable trinucleotide repeat sequence—cytosine, thymine, and guanidine (CTG)—in the protein kinase–encoding gene *(DMK)* located at 19q13.3. The repeat is present 50 to several thousands of times in patients with DM, compared to 5 to 30 times in the normal population. The size of the repeat is correlated roughly with severity of symptoms, with more affected patients having greater numbers of repeats.[113] The repeat expansion also may account for the anticipation seen in families with DM, in which the severity of symptoms increases and the age of onset decreases with subsequent generations.[114] It was demonstrated that the DMK protein is localized to the postsynaptic side of the neuromuscular junction in skeletal muscle and the intercalated discs in cardiac muscle in humans. Additionally, DMK protein is present in specific structures in rat brain, supporting the hypothesis that it may have selective actions in the CNS.[115] There have been widely conflicting results in the effort to unravel the precise effect of the expanded repeats; some data support the theory that there is a loss of function of the mutant allele, whereas other data favor increased expression of the allele. Recent work supports a new interpretation of the data. Both normal and expanded *DMK* genes are transcribed in patient muscle, but the expanded RNA has a dominant effect on RNA metabolism by preventing transport of poly(A)+ RNA out of the nucleus.[116]

Epidemiology and Risk Factors. There is an estimated prevalence of 3 to 5 per 100,000 population and an incidence of 1 in 8000 live births, making it the most common adult muscular dystrophy. Although a few isolated populations have an exceptionally high prevalence, DM has been found in all racial groups.[117]

Clinical Features and Associated Findings. The phenotype is correlated with the length of the CTG repeat and thus is widely variable, ranging from the single manifestation of cataracts that present in the middle years to severe neonatal hypotonia that can lead to death if respiratory support is not provided. Traditionally, these different types of symptoms have resulted in the designation of either congenital or noncongenital DM.

The classic presentation of noncongenital DM, which is well described by Harper, includes marked weakness in the face, jaw, and neck muscles and milder distal extremity weakness (Fig. 36–7).[117] Weakness of the extremities is often the first problem perceived by the patient, even when a careful evaluation may reveal a clear history of myotonia (sometimes termed muscle stiffness or cramping by patients), facial weakness, and nasal speech. Patients frequently seem unaware of their illness and symptoms, both in themselves and in family members. Using a percussion hammer, myotonia can be elicited in patients with DM with a brisk tap on the thenar muscle, causing flexion-opposition of the thumb with slow relaxation.

The person with advanced DM has a characteristic appearance: a long, thin face with sunken cheeks due to temporal and masseter wasting, a so-called "swan neck" because of sternocleidomastoid wasting, and ptosis, with relatively strong muscles in the posterior neck and shoulder girdle.

Congenital DM presents a distinctive picture that is different from other disorders. Facial diplegia and jaw weakness without concomitant extremity weakness are hallmarks. Weakness of the respiratory muscles with respiratory distress is present in at least 50 percent of patients and is the most common cause of death in these infants. Hypotonia is present in severely affected neonates, but it may disappear within weeks. Clinical myotonia is generally absent and is usually detectable only by EMG.[117]

A recent prospective study followed patients of both types for 10 years, with the conclusion that muscle weakness was relatively mild in both types, although it was progressive in the noncongenital form. Weakness was generalized in both types, with no significant differences found in distribution. Additionally, 75 percent of the noncongenital patients and 81 percent of the congenital patients had cardiac abnormalities, primarily conduction defects, demonstrated on ECG. Intellectual function was frequently and severely impaired

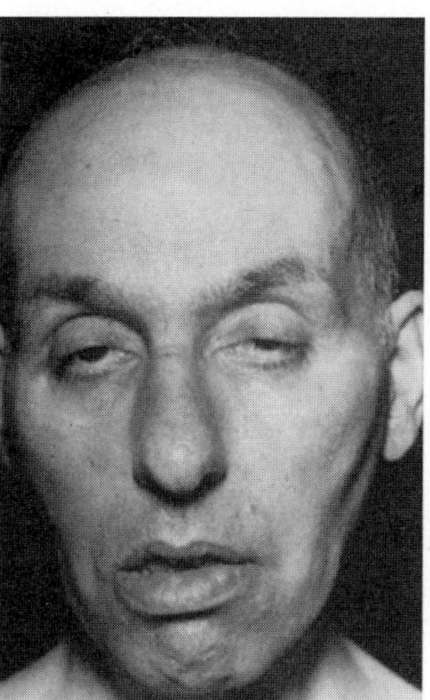
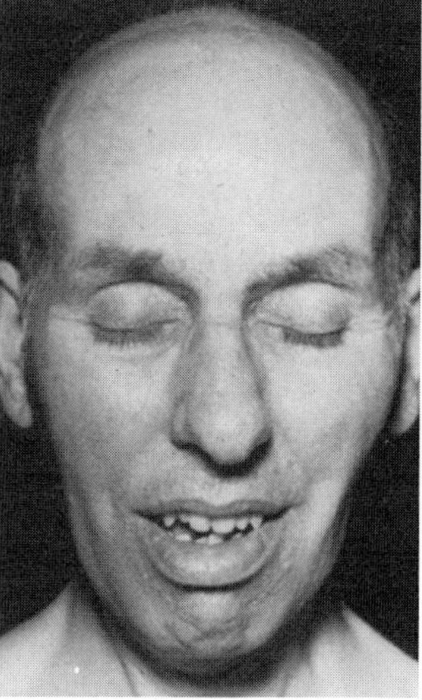

FIGURE 36–7. Myotonic dystrophy with typical myopathic facies, frontal balding, and sunken cheeks. (From Dubowitz V: Muscle Disorders in Childhood. Philadelphia, WB Saunders, 1995.)

in the congenital type, whereas only about a third of the noncongenital patients were mildly impaired.[118]

It cannot be overemphasized that DM is a multisystem disorder. The heart is prominently involved, and the severity of cardiac symptoms does not correlate with severity of other symptoms in this disorder. All patients with DM need to undergo ECG evaluation, because sudden death is well documented, and as many as 90 percent of patients have conduction defects, particularly first-degree heart block and atrial arrhythmias. Both the diaphragm and intercostal muscles may be myotonic and weak, which leads to alveolar hypoventilation. In addition, there are smooth muscle abnormalities throughout the gastrointestinal system. Particularly important are the delayed relaxation of the pharynx and reduced motility in the esophagus that may lead to aspiration, constipation, and anal sphincter abnormalities in children.

Central nervous system involvement includes generalized atrophy and ventricular dilatation, but structural changes in the brain do not seem to be common, even in patients with congenital disorders. However, there are well-known behaviors associated with DM that range from apathy and inertia, with concomitant lower socioeconomic status, to hypersomnolence that is often present without detectable respiratory problems. In addition, numerous endocrinological abnormalities have been reported, several with clinical importance. Hyperinsulinism and reduced numbers of insulin receptors are common, but diabetes is not. Elevations of pituitary follicle–stimulating hormone and luteinizing hormone occur frequently.

In males, testicular atrophy, Leydig cell hyperplasia, and slightly reduced serum testosterone are common. In females, no consistent ovarian problems have been documented, but the spontaneous abortion rate is high. Fertility in both sexes seems to be reduced to about 75 percent of normal. Finally, in the ocular system, cataracts with characteristic multicolored crystalline subcapsular opacities have been documented since the recognition of DM as an entity. Retinal degeneration, low intraocular pressure, and saccadic eye movement defects have been reported.[117]

Evaluation and Differential Diagnosis. The condition most clinically similar to DM is proximal myotonic myopathy, a multisystem disorder with predominantly proximal weakness, myotonia, and cataracts with autosomal dominant inheritance and a normal number of CTG repeats in the *DMK* gene.[119] Facioscapulohumeral dystrophy may have the same distribution of weakness, but there is no myotonia. More rarely, some of the LGMDs may have a similar distribution of weakness, again without myotonia. Molecular analysis can distinguish DM from these disorders, as well as those with marked myotonia, such as myotonia congenita and paramyotonia.

Sometimes the clinical presentation of DM is so distinctive that the experienced clinician uses tools only to confirm a diagnosis already made. EMG should be employed in suspected DM when myotonia is clinically equivocal or absent. The typical pattern is of long-lasting runs with declining frequency and amplitude, with the distal muscles of the upper extremities and the orbicularis orbis most often being involved. A careful slit-lamp evaluation will ascertain characteristic posterior lenticular opacities and should be performed on any patient suspected of having this condition. Muscle biopsy may show a constellation of abnormalities, including increased central nuclei, nuclear chains, ringed fibers, sarcoplasmic masses, atrophy of type I fibers, increased numbers of fibers in spindles, and increased arborization at the terminal.[117] Nerve biopsy shows increased arborization. Other conditions associated with myotonia, such as myotonia congenita (see Chapter 37) and drug-induced myotonia (see Chapter 55), need to be considered.

Management and Prognosis. Because there is no cure for DM, current management focuses on treatment of the myotonia and associated systemic problems, monitoring of pregnancy, and genetic counseling. Because patients frequently do not perceive their myotonia as being problematic, they may not follow a treatment plan. However, 100 mg of phenytoin taken three times daily is effective in reducing myotonia and does not produce the cardiosuppressive complications of either quinine or procainamide. Anesthesia should be used for these patients only when it cannot be avoided. Myotonia may be increased by the depolarizing relaxants used for inducing anesthesia or the anticholinesterases used to terminate relaxation, although the barbiturates, benzodiazepines, and opiates may produce apnea. Cases have been reported in which the diagnosis of DM has been made only after the patient experienced postoperative apnea. Harper provides a comprehensive discussion of anesthetic management in DM.[117] A bracelet that identifies the patient as having DM may be helpful.

Because cardiac complications may be life threatening, careful evaluation, including a His bundle electrogram, must be performed to ascertain conduction defects that need pacemakers. Some respiratory problems may be avoided by upright positioning during meals and by spacing meals well ahead of bedtime.

There is increased risk of spontaneous abortion in myotonic mothers, as well as complications during labor and delivery. There may be incoordination of contractions during labor that prolong the first stage, a retained placenta, and postpartum hemorrhage, as well as the previously cited anesthetic sensitivity.

Presymptomatic and prenatal genetic counseling, including a discussion of the increased risks of pregnancy to an affected or carrier mother as well as to the fetus, the phenomenon of anticipation, and congenital DM, should be provided to families with a history of DM. It should be remembered that although a significant number of persons with DM are mentally impaired, some who are not may be perceived as such because of facial weakness.

OCULOPHARYNGEAL MUSCULAR DYSTROPHY

Oculopharyngeal muscular dystrophy is a disorder of late adult onset characterized by progressive ptosis and dysphagia. It is caused by short GCG expansions in the the poly(A)-binding protein gene on chromosome 14. Most often the disease is dominant, with a more severe phenotype observed in compound heterozygotes for the GCG 9 mutation and the GCG 7 allele. Homozygosity for that same allele may produce recessive disease.[120] The highest prevalence of oculopharyngeal muscular dystrophy continues to be in Quebec, but families have now been identified in more than 20 countries.

Asymmetrical weakness of the levator palpebrae and pharyngeal muscles is the initial presentation, generally after the age of 50. Eventually all extraocular muscles may become involved. There is no cardiac involvement. The EMG shows myopathic changes. Muscle biopsy reveals changes found in other muscular dystrophies: loss of muscle fibers, variation in fiber size, increased numbers of nuclei and internal nuclei, and increased fibrous and fatty connective tissue. On histochemistry, there are small angulated fibers that react strongly for oxidative enzymes and "rimmed" vacuoles, particularly in type I fibers from extremity muscles rather than extraocular muscles. On electron microscopy, there are unique intranuclear tubular filaments.[121]

Oculopharyngeal muscular dystrophy can be distinguished from inclusion body myositis, which presents as dysphagia. It also has rimmed vacuoles, but the filaments seen are larger and are present in the cytoplasm as well as the nucleus; there are no ocular palsies. Ocular myasthenia gravis without waxing and waning of symptoms may produce weakness in the same distribution as oculopharyngeal muscular dystrophy, but it generates demonstrable neuromuscular junction transmission defects on EMG and neuromuscular junction abnormalities on morphological studies. Although late onset of the mitochondrial myopathy, Kearns-Sayre syndrome, or oculocraniosomatic disease may present with ptosis, histochemical and ultrastructural studies of muscle show biochemical defects in the respiratory chain and mitochondrial DNA deletions.

Interventions, such as eyelid crutches to alleviate the ptosis and a feeding tube to provide adequate nutrition, are palliative. If the patient does not receive a feeding tube, the dysphagia will lead to early death by malnutrition and starvation.

EMERY-DREIFUSS MUSCULAR DYSTROPHY

ED MD, which is characterized by early contractures and cardiomyopathy, was first identified as a distinct form of muscular dystrophy in a large Virginia family in 1966.[122] Generally it is X-linked recessive, although there are very rare autosomal dominant and recessive forms.[123] The incidence of the X-linked type is estimated to be about 1 in 100,000. One of 10 new X-linked cases may be a new mutation.[124]

In 1994 the gene for the X-linked ED MD was identified as STA at Xq28.[123] It codes for emerin, a serine-rich protein of 254 amino acids, which resembles membrane proteins of the secretory pathway involved in vesicular transport.[125] Several different mutations have been reported that result in lack of emerin in skeletal and cardiac muscle.[126, 127] Although the lack of emerin seems to cause the disease, the pathway remains to be established. In 1999 mutations in the lamin A/C gene on chromosome 8, which encodes for two proteins of the nuclear lamina, were identified in dominantly inherited ED MD.[128] This was the first time mutations in a component of nuclear lamina had been implicated in an inherited muscle disorder. There is a recent report of an individual with ED MD with a homozygous mutation in this same gene. His heterozygous parents are totally asymptomatic, which demonstrates that heterozygous mutations produce a broad range of phenotypes.[129]

The classic symptoms of ED MD include (1) contractures of elbows, Achilles' tendon, and postcervical muscles before weakness is present; (2) slowly progressive weakness and muscle wasting, generally starting in the humeroperoneal muscles; and (3) a cardiomyopathy that frequently presents as heart block. A similar disorder, X-linked scapuloperoneal syndrome that includes color blindness has been linked to Xq28 and may be allelic to ED MD.[121] It has been demonstrated that LGMD1B is allelic to the dominant form of ED MD.[130]

The early contractures and heart conduction block are features that are helpful in distinguishing this from other muscular dystrophies that may have weakness in the same distribution and the same pattern of inheritance. The main features of the cardiac involvement are impairment of impulse-generating cells, variable sinoatrial and atrioventricular conduction defects, increased atrial and ventricular heterotopia, and functional impairment of the myocardium. Rigid spine syndrome can be confused with ED MD but occurs sporadically, has contractures that are limited to the spinal musculature, and usually does not involve cardiac problems.[131]

In ED MD, the muscle biopsy has nonspecific myopathic or dystrophic changes, including variation in fiber size and fiber necrosis, and endomysial and perimysial fibrosis. Unlike DMD and BMD, there is no alteration in dystrophin.[132]

The care provided to the patient is similar to that for the other muscular dystrophies, with the notable exception of cardiac intervention. Merlini documented that up to 40 percent of patients with ED MD die suddenly, many of them without any preceding cardiac symptoms. Therefore, a thorough cardiac evaluation and insertion of a pacemaker when indicated is essential. Asymptomatic female carriers should be evaluated because they may also have cardiac abnormalities.[133]

The function of emerin needs to be determined. A recent paper suggests the small size of the STA gene and its housekeeping pattern of expression may make gene therapy possible in ED MD.[134]

DISTAL MYOPATHIES

The distal myopathies are a rare heterogeneous group of disorders characterized by progressive muscular weakness and atrophy beginning in the hands or feet (Table 36–7).[135–140] Several types of distal myopathies have been differentiated clinically, distinguished either by site of onset or mode of inheritance or by differences seen on muscle biopsy, but as their genetics emerge, reclassification is taking place on that basis.

The late adult–onset distal autosomal dominant myopathy that first appears in the hands, also called Welander distal myopathy or Swedish-type distal myopathy, has been linked to chromosome 2p.[135] It has a mean onset of 47 years (range, 20 to 77 years), with weakness in the hands that generally presents as clumsiness in the thumb and forefinger that spreads to other fingers. Eventually, patients develop distal leg weakness, more often in the extensors. Fewer than 20 percent of patients develop proximal extremity weakness, while more than 90 percent complain of vasomotor disturbances, primarily a sensation of cold, in the hands and feet. Another late adult–onset autosomal dominant disease found in Finland first involves weakness in the anterior tibial muscles, followed by weakness of the long toe extensor muscles and proximal leg weakness in about half the patients. There is no

TABLE 36–7. **Distal Myopathies: Distinctions in Different Types**

Age of Onset	Type	Site of Onset	Gene Locus	Inheritance
Late adulthood	Welander	Hands	2p13[135]	AD
	Finnish	Legs	2q31–32[136]	AD
	Markesberry-Griggs	Legs	?	AD
Early adulthood	Type I: Nonaka	Anterior compartment of legs	9p1–q1[137]	AR
	Type II: Miyoshi	Posterior compartment of legs	2p13.3–p13.1[138]	AR
	Type III: Laing	Anterior compartment of legs, distal weakness with sternocleidomastoid weakness	14q[139]	AD
	Desmin storage	Distal weakness with respiratory and bulbar involvement	2q35[140]	AD
Childhood (ages 5 to 15)	Juvenile	Feet, then hands		AD
Infancy (<2 years)	Infantile	Hands and feet		AD

AD, Autosomal dominant; AR, autosomal recessive.

weakness in the hands. Yet another late-onset autosomal dominant distal myopathy, known as Markesberry-Griggs myopathy, has been described in which proximal weakness is also common and the intrinsic foot muscles are affected. Cardiomyopathy in non-Scandinavian middle-aged adults can also occur.

The early adult–onset autosomal recessive myopathies begin with leg weakness. Type I starts in the anterior compartment, usually presenting with footdrop, whereas type II starts in the gastrocnemius muscles. These types are assumed to be different entities owing to differences seen on muscle biopsy as well as their different loci. There are two other early adult–onset forms that are autosomal dominant. Laing myopathy, linked to chromosome 14, includes facial and shoulder weakness in addition to distal weakness.[139] Desmin storage myopathy has respiratory, cardiac, and bulbar musculature involvement as well as prominent hand and foot involvement. The gene that codes for desmin, a muscle-specific subunit of the cytoskeletal elements of the intermediate filaments, has been identified on chromosome 2.[140]

Two early-onset forms have also been described in Dutch and British families. The infantile-onset form spreads from the feet to the hands but does not progress after age 18. The juvenile-onset form starts simultaneously in the hands and feet and slowly progresses until about age 50 years.[141]

The differential diagnosis includes myopathies and neuropathies. Whereas most myopathies predominantly affect proximal muscles, a few that can present distally include various metabolic myopathies and inclusion body myositis. Laing myopathy can resemble FSH MD. Although distal weakness may suggest neuropathic disorders, EMG and muscle studies establish the myopathic changes. Serum CK activity is markedly increased, often 50 times the normal value. Electrical studies demonstrate signs of myopathy in the involved areas of weakness, where nerve conductions are normal. Muscle biopsy shows dystrophic changes of variable severity. Rimmed vacuoles are frequently observed, suggesting a link between distal myopathies and inclusion body myositis. Patients with Welander's disease also show angulated fibers, whereas desmin storage is typical of the early adult–onset form with respiratory muscle involvement. DM can present without clinically apparent myotonia, and the neuronal late-onset type of Charcot-Marie-Tooth disease (CMT) may look similar.[141]

Thus far, no medical interventions have improved these conditions. Appropriate orthotics and physical and occupational therapy provide the most assistance. By and large, these are slowly progressive disorders that sometimes plateau, and they are not life threatening.

Degenerative Neuropathies

HEREDITARY SENSORY AND MOTOR NEUROPATHIES

In general, the hereditary sensory and motor neuropathies are peripheral neuropathies that affect autonomic nerves, sensory nerves, motor fibers, or a combination thereof. The molecular genetics of these disorders is being ardently pursued, and the mechanisms underlying them are rapidly being unraveled. However, to date there is overlapping terminology used when they are described (Table 36–8). This discussion is organized according to the classification that is emerging based on genetics (Table 36–9).[142–156] CMT is the most common hereditary sensory and motor neuropathy, and CMT

TABLE 36–8. **Types of Hereditary Sensory and Motor Neuropathy**

Type	Other Names	Particular Characteristics
HSMN I	CMT 1	Hypertrophic demyelinating neuropathy
HSMN II	CMT 2	Axonal neuropathy with normal or near-normal nerve conduction velocities
HSMN III	CMT 3, Dejerine-Sottas	Severe hypertrophic demyelinating neuropathy with onset in infancy

CMT, Charcot-Marie-Tooth.

TABLE 36–9. Genes and Gene Products in the Hereditary Sensory and Motor Neuropathies

Disorder	Inheritance	Gene Locus	Gene Product
CMT 1A	AD	Duplication (or rarely, point mutation) at 17p11.2–12	PMP-22[142]
HNPP	AD	Deletion at 17p11.2	PMP-22[143]
CMT 1B	AD	1q22.3	P0[144]
CMT 1C	AD	?	
CMT 2A	AD	1p36–P35	KIFIBβ[145]
CMT 2B	AD	3q[146]	?
CMT 2C	AD	2q14[147]	?
CMT 2D	AD	7p14[148]	?
CMT 2E	AD	8p21	NF-L[149]
CMT X	X-linked	Xq13.1	Connexin 32[150]
CMT 4A	AR	8q13[151]	?
CMT 4B	AR	11q23	MTRP2[152]
CMT 4C	AR	5q23–33[153]	?
CMT 4D	AR	8q24	NDRG1[154]
CMT 4E	AR, AD	10q21–q22	EGR2[155]
CMT 4F	AR	19q13	Periaxin[156]

AD, Autosomal dominant; AR, autosomal recessive; CMT, Charcot-Marie-Tooth disease; HNPP, hereditary neuropathy with liability to pressure palsies; P0, myelin protein zero; PMP, peripheral myelin protein; KIF1Bβ, kinesin superfamily motor protein β; NF-L, neurofilament protein-light polypeptide; MTRP2, myotubularin-related protein 2; NDRG-1, N-myc downstream-regulated gene; EGR2, early growth response 2 transcription factor.

type 1A is the most common form of CMT, accounting for more than 50 percent of all CMT cases.

Pathogenesis and Pathophysiology. Pathological changes seen in CMT include loss of myelinated fibers and sclerosis in the posterior column of the spinal cord, particularly in the fasciculus gracilis in its upper regions. Peripheral nerves show fewer myelin sheaths, with the extent of the decrease correlating with the severity of clinical disease. There is also loss of large axons and an increase in transverse fascicular area, especially in the auricular and sural nerves. Onion bulbs, made up of circumferentially directed Schwann cells and their processes, can be seen at myelinated internodes, demyelinated internodes, or former sites of myelinated fibers.

There has been considerable controversy over the years whether the primary defect in CMT originates in the neuron and its axon or in the Schwann cell. The primary histopathological changes involve demyelination, whereas the clinical picture of muscle weakness and atrophy is evidence of muscle denervation and axonal loss and of axons with calibers reduced out of proportion to the extant of myelin loss.[157]

The gene defects and their products associated with the CMTs are beginning to resolve this question. Peripheral myelin protein 22, which has been implicated in several of the CMTs (see Table 36–9), is present as a protein in all myelinated fibers of the peripheral nervous system and is localized to compact myelin. Studies in the trembler mouse, an animal model that also has a gene defect in peripheral myelin protein 22, indicate that Schwann cells can modulate axon caliber, neurofilament phosphorylation, and neurofilament density within the axoplasm. Therefore, abnormal expression of peripheral myelin protein 22 could account for both the neuronal and Schwann cell alterations seen in CMT.[158]

Myelin protein zero is the major component of peripheral nervous system myelin. It is an integral membrane glycoprotein, and its expression is confined to myelinated Schwann cells. A major role of the protein zero extracellular domain is compaction of peripheral myelin, while the cytoplasmic domain is thought to interact with a component of the opposing membrane of the compact myelin, holding these membranes together.[159]

Connexin 32 is a gap junction protein. Before its identification as a gene for X-linked CMT (CMT X), it was not known there were gap junctions in human peripheral nerve. It has now been detected at the nodes of Ranvier and the Schmidt-Lanterman incisures, which may mean it forms intracellular gap junctions between the folds in Schwann cell cytoplasm.[160]

Epidemiology and Risk Factors. The hereditary sensory and motor neuropathies occur worldwide, with an estimated prevalence ranging from 4.7 to 36 per 100,000, and an approximate incidence of 1 in 25,000 persons. Autosomal dominant, autosomal recessive, and X-linked dominant and recessive inheritance patterns have been reported (see Table 36–9).

Clinical Features and Associated Disorders. Although there is wide intrafamilial variability in phenotype, it is generally accepted that clinical presentations of CMT 1A and 1B are similar, although they are distinguishable, and CMT 1A may have a milder clinical course than 1B. Age of onset ranges from childhood to early adulthood, with symmetrical insidious weakness and atrophy of the intrinsic foot and peroneal muscles occurring first, associated with varus deformity of the feet and a steppage gait. Calf, intrinsic hand, and thigh muscles may be involved later (Fig. 36–8). Atrophy tends to occur at the distal ends of the gastrocnemius, soleus, and quadriceps muscles. Cramps and fasciculations are often reported after exercise. Stretch reflexes disappear first in the gastrocnemius and soleus, then the quadriceps, and finally the arms.

Although patients generally do not report sensory disturbances, a careful examination reveals abnormalities in all modalities. Pes cavus and hammertoes are present in up to two thirds of patients. Decreased skin temperature over the distal leg is common, and decreased sweating has been reported. Enlargement and hardening of nerves, particularly those between the shoulder and elbow, have been observed in up to one fourth of patients. Pain, primarily in the feet, is reported by 20 to 30 percent of CMT 1 patients.[161]

Hereditary neuropathy with liability to pressure palsies, also called "tomaculous neuropathy," is a syndrome characterized by a tendency toward the development of recurring sensory and motor nerve palsies brought on by mild pressure or trauma to a particular peripheral nerve bundle. Some of these patients have a deletion of PMP-22.[143] An insult from which a normal person would quickly recover results in residual nerve damage that may take days or even months to resolve. Some of these patients go on to develop CMT, whereas other family members may have only the HNPP phenotype.

Dejerine-Sottas syndrome, sometimes called progressive hypertrophic neuropathy, is a more severe form of peroneal muscular atrophy with presentation in infancy of progressive

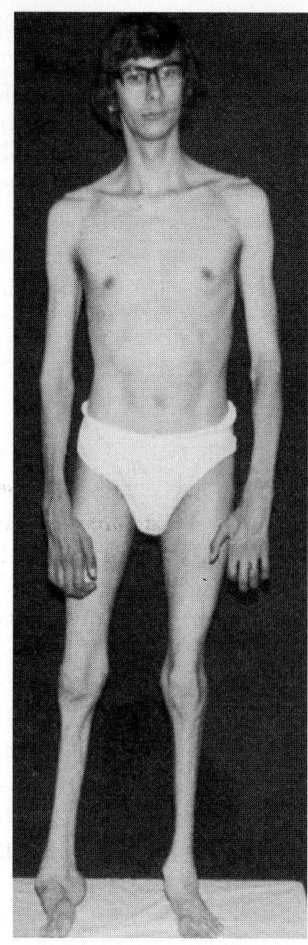

FIGURE 36–8. Patient with Charcot-Marie-Tooth disease showing marked wasting of calf muscles and intrinsic foot muscles. (From Dubowitz V: Muscle Disorders in Childhood. Philadelphia, WB Saunders, 1995.)

generalized muscle weakness, severe sensory loss, limb ataxia, and marked hypertrophy of peripheral nerves. Both dominant and recessive inheritance patterns have been reported. Molecular genetic studies indicate that Dejerine-Sottas syndrome is a variation of CMT with a generally more malignant phenotype.

About 10 percent of cases of CMT are X-linked, in which primarily male family members are affected through maternal transmission. Again there is intrafamilial variation in severity, but generally onset occurs in childhood, with slowly progressive distal weakness and sensory disturbance that tends to be more severe than that seen in CMT 1. Carrier females may have mild, variable clinical disease.

In Roussy-Levy syndrome, peroneal muscular atrophy is associated with essential tremor. Although originally described as a separate disorder, it has recently been shown to be a phenotypic variant of CMT 1A.[162]

Differential Diagnosis and Evaluation. Other mixed polyneuropathies of nutritional, infectious, toxic, autoimmune, and vasculitic origin should be considered. Both axonal and demyelinating neuropathies need to be included in the differential diagnosis. At present, genetic confirmation of this disorder is available only for CMT 1A and 1B, CMT 2E, CMT X, and hereditary neuropathy with liability to pressure palsies. CK is normal. On EMG, nerve conduction velocities are slowed in peripheral nerves. The extent of velocity reduction is no longer an accepted criterion for diagnosing the type of CMT. On nerve biopsy, there is a moderate increase in epineurium and perineurium and a variable decrease in the number of myelinated fibers that correlates with the severity of disease. Onion bulb formation is visible around myelinated and demyelinated internodes.[157]

Management. There is no cure or effective treatment for these disorders. Physical therapy, occupational therapy, and orthotic devices can help maintain optimal function. Genetic counseling is an obvious and important component of care for these patients.

Prognosis and Future Perspectives. Although large studies are not available, several series conclude that life expectancy is not reduced in CMT 1 and that generally those with CMT 1A remain ambulatory throughout their lives. A 20-year follow-up study of a family with CMT 1B demonstrated that patients remained ambulatory with a normal life span. Autopsy studies included a 92-year-old family member.[163]

HEREDITARY SENSORY AND AUTONOMIC NEUROPATHIES

The hereditary sensory and autonomic neuropathies (HSANs) are conditions in which primary sensory and autonomic neurons either fail to develop or undergo system atrophy and degeneration. Dyck proposes the comprehensive subdivision seen in Table 36–10. These disorders have been called by a large variety of names because their symptoms

TABLE 36–10. **Hereditary Sensory and Autonomic Neuropathies**

Type	Hallmark	Inheritance Pattern
HSAN I (hereditary sensory radicular neuropathy)	Insensitivity to pain in feet and ensuing tissue complications	Primarily autosomal dominant
HSAN II (congenital sensory neuropathy)	Early onset of loss of sensation in all modalities	Autosomal recessive
HSAN III (familial dysautonomia, Riley-Day)	Early onset, predominantly autonomic symptoms, absence of fungiform papillae on the tongue	Autosomal recessive, predominantly Jewish (gene on D9S58)
HSAN IV (familial sensory neuropathy with anhidrosis, congenital insensitivity to pain)	Mild mental retardation, episodes of fever related to environment rather than infection	Rare
HSAN V (congenital sensory neuropathy with selective loss of small myelinated fibers)	Congenital insensitivity to pain in extremities, normal strength and tendon reflexes, abnormality of nociception	Fewer than 10 cases reported

were described by various investigators. Types I, II, and III are discussed here. Within this classification there are two large divisions: HSAN I is a progressive disorder with symptom onset usually occurring in the second decade or later with primarily lower extremities affected. HSANs II to V are static congenital disorders that are more generalized. A common thread among all the types is insensitivity to pain.[164]

Hereditary Sensory and Autonomic Neuropathy Type I

HSAN I is a disorder in which sensory disturbances and associated tissue complications outweigh its motor and autonomic manifestations. HSAN I is a rare disorder that is usually autosomal dominantly inherited, although recessive and X-linked pedigrees have been identified.[163] There is chronic axonal atrophy, myelin remodeling, and axonal degeneration with sparing of the CNS and non-neural tissues. HSAN I is caused by missense mutations in the *SPTLC1* gene at 9q22. These mutations increase de novo glucosylceramide synthesis in lymphoblast cell lines, which triggers apoptosis, causing massive cell death during neural tube closure, which may be the mechanism of neural degeneration seen in HSAN I.[165]

Although there are different phenotypes, typically the disorder presents in one of the following ways: (1) foot complications, such as plantar ulcers, recurring paronychia of toes, stress fractures of foot bones, recurrent cellulitis, and resorption of foot bones; (2) spontaneous pain, either burning or aching of the feet that is worsened with weight bearing and decreased at night, or disabling lancinating pain in deep tissues of the feet, legs, or shoulder; or (3) symptoms of sensory and autonomic neuropathy.

The complications of HSAN I may be of sudden, overwhelming onset, with ulcers first developing over pressure points on the foot. When these ulcers are neglected, they do not heal and are associated with the complications previously described. Phenotypes have been reported in which HSAN is associated with deafness, leg weakness and atrophy, burning feet, restless legs, and neuropathic atrophy. HSAN is a slowly progressive disorder that does not seem to decrease the life span. It cannot be emphasized enough that proper foot care can prevent complications that can lead to foot amputation and sepsis.

HSAN I may be distinguished from other varieties of HSAN because it starts later, usually in the second or third decade; is slowly progressive; and preferentially affects lower limbs. It is closest in presentation to HSAN II, although in that condition, the motor and autonomic symptoms outweigh the sensory symptoms and deficits of type I. Spinocerebellar degeneration can be distinguished from HSAN I because of its kinesthetic and mechanoreceptor loss, cerebellar ataxia, and relatively less small-fiber sensory and autonomic dysfunction. Familial amyloidosis may include sexual and sphincter dysfunction, which are not found in HSAN I, and porphyria with neuropathy has a more acute onset associated with changes in mental status.

Typically, touch-pressure threshold, thermal discrimination, and nociception are abnormally elevated in the foot and leg, although they may be altered in the arm and hand as well. Paresthesias are not present. Loss of sweating in the distal leg is common. Sural nerve amplitudes are reduced, with small myelinated fibers being primarily affected. A decrease in the Achilles tendon reflex is common, followed most often by a decrease in the quadriceps reflex.[164]

There is no effective treatment. The main goal is the prevention of foot ulcers. The feet should be inspected regularly for signs of pressure points, soaked daily, and treated with petrolatum lotion applied to seal in moisture. Shoes should be chosen carefully to avoid pressure points. Any ulcers should be treated promptly with cleaning and debridement, if necessary. The appropriate antibiotic should be used for cellulitis or septicemia. Genetic counseling should include information about phenotypic variation and degree of risk.

Hereditary Sensory and Autonomic Neuropathy Type II

HSAN II is characterized by an early onset of loss of sensation in all modalities. This is a rare disorder, in which cases reported are either sporadic or within a sibship, suggesting an autosomal recessive pattern of inheritance. There is profound loss of myelinated fibers in cutaneous nerves, especially the sural nerve. Dyck proposes that the degenerative process begins in utero or in infancy.[164] There are fewer nerve fibers at the ankle than the midcalf, marked denervation of the extensor digitorum brevis, evidence of segmental demyelination and remyelination, and electron microscopic abnormalities within axis cylinders.[164] As yet, no gene locus has been identified.

Symptoms first appear in infancy or early childhood and may be widespread. Paronychia, whitlows, ulcers of the fingers and feet, and previously undetected fractures of the foot and hand are common and result directly from underlying sensory disturbance (Fig. 36–9). There have been pedigrees reported with HSAN II and other dysautonomic features, as well as retinitis pigmentosa or tonic pupils. There is sensory loss affecting all modalities in the lower and upper limbs and

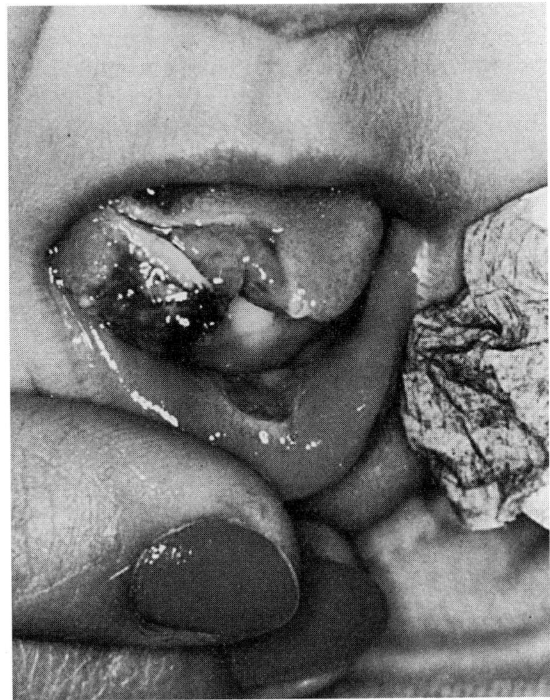

FIGURE 36–9. Child with hereditary sensory neuropathy type II showing destruction of tongue tissue due to insensitivity to pain. (Courtesy of Dr. J. Sarlangue, Hôpital Pelligrin Enfants, Bordeaux, France.)

sometimes in the trunk. Tendon reflexes are generally absent or diminished in all limbs. There is loss of sweating over acral parts. However, there is no prominent muscle weakness, postural hypotension, or sphincter disturbance.

Generally, there are no sensory nerve action potentials elicitable in the ulnar, median, or sural nerves, while the conduction velocities of motor fibers of the same nerves are at or just below the lower end of normal. Minimal fibrillation may be found in the extensor digitorum brevis, which has a decreased number of motor unit potentials, a large number of which are polyphasic.[164]

Complications are much more difficult to prevent in HSAN II owing to its early onset at an age when patients cannot understand the problem or cooperate with preventive regimens. In addition, complications are frequent because the hands are so seriously affected. Preventive care, which is similar to that of HSAN I, needs to be as aggressive as possible because complications may be life threatening. Special attention should be given so that these children have adequate educational opportunities to develop their intellectual potential in spite of severe physical handicaps. Genetic counseling should be provided.

Hereditary Sensory and Autonomic Neuropathy Type III (Riley-Day Syndrome, Familial Dysautonomia)

HSAN III is present almost exclusively in Ashkenazi Jews. Some investigators argue that those who are not Jewish in fact have a different type of neuropathy. The gene frequency has been estimated at 0.01 per 100,000 Jews in the United States.[166] Mutations in the gene that codes for IKAP, a scaffold protein and regulator for three different kinases involved in proinflammatory signaling, have recently been identified.[167] Postmortem studies have varied widely; some have shown no nervous system lesions at all, whereas others show extensive damage, particularly in the brain stem reticular formation, the cortex, and the long tracts of the cord. There is a marked decrease in the number of unmyelinated fibers of the cutaneous nerves.[164]

Usually, HSAN III presents at birth. Axelrod proposes that it should be suspected in a child of Eastern European Jewish extraction with breech delivery, meconium staining, poor suck, hypotonia, or hypothermia. There is difficulty feeding and a failure to thrive, along with unexplained fevers, lack of tearing, paroxysmal hypertension, increased sweating, cold hands and feet, erythematous blotching of the skin, and drooling. There is also a lack of fungiform papillae on the tongue, a feature that is highly distinctive of this disorder. Although there is overlap between symptoms and signs of this and other types of HSAN, examination of the tongue leads to the exclusion or inclusion of this diagnosis. If the disorder presents later, it may be observed as delayed development or stunted growth with decreased pain sensation and ataxia. Abnormalities in cutaneous temperature discrimination and nociception are present in most patients, whereas fewer have abnormalities in joint position and vibratory sensation.

Recurrent vomiting is common in the early years. Several gastrointestinal abnormalities have been identified: megaesophagus, pylorospasm, gastric ulcer, jejunal distention, and megacolon. Corneal abrasions may occur secondary to corneal insensitivity, whereas neuropathic or Charcot's joints may occur secondary to pain insensitivity. About half of the patients develop kyphosis, scoliosis, or both. Pulmonary complications, profound hypotension, and prolonged respiratory depression from the administration of anesthesia have been reported.[164]

Clinical and laboratory diagnosis may be based on the presence of five signs: (1) lack of the normal flare after intradermal injection of histamine, (2) absence of fungiform papillae on the tongue, (3) miosis of the pupil after conjunctival instillation of 2.5 percent methacholine chloride, (4) absent deep tendon reflexes, and (5) diminished tear flow. Sural nerve biopsy shows markedly decreased unmyelinated fibers, no active fiber degeneration, and fewer Schwann cell cytoplasmic clusters than other types of neuropathy. Nerve conduction velocity studies have mixed nerve velocities within the normal range.[168]

Treatment remains supportive and is best provided by an interdisciplinary team that includes a genetic counselor. Prenatal diagnosis is available for informative families.[169] Most patients do not survive to adulthood, succumbing to either recurrent infections or hyperpyrexia. The oldest surviving patient in one series was 38 years old, with one third of the patients in that series being 20 years or older.[170]

Hereditary Sensory and Autonomic Neuropathy Type IV

This rare condition, in which there is a sensory neuropathy accompanied by unexplained fevers, congenital insensitivity to pain, anhidrosis, and mental retardation, generally causes death from hyperpyrexia by age 3.[171] Mutations in the *NTRK1* gene, which codes for the tyrosine kinase nerve growth factor receptor, have recently been identified as the cause,[172] which suggests this factor plays a crucial role in the development and function of the nociceptive reception system as well as thermal regulation.

AUTONOMIC NEUROPATHY OF MULTIPLE SYSTEM ATROPHY (SHY-DRAGER SYNDROME)

In 1960, Shy and Drager first described the combination of progressive autonomic failure and multiple system atrophy that manifested as orthostatic hypotension, akinesia, and rigidity that led to incapacity in a few years (see Chapter 34). In the ensuing years, conditions including striatonigral degeneration and forms of olivopontocerebellar atrophy have been combined with Shy-Drager syndrome under the larger category of degenerative processes called multiple system atrophy. This discussion focuses on the phenotype with prominent dysautonomia that was described by Shy and Drager.

Shy-Drager syndrome affects men more often than women, most often in middle age or later. A Japanese series calculated the prevalence to be 0.3 per 100,000.[173] There have been reports of families with autosomal dominant inheritance. A genetic basis was postulated in 1983 when an association was found between HLA antigen Aw32 and autonomic failure.[174] Thus far, no gene has been identified. Recent work with alpha1-B-adrenergic receptors (alpha1-BARs) in transgenic mice that overexpress either wild-type or constitutively active alpha1-BARs produced granulovacuolar degeneration similar to that seen in Shy-Drager syndrome.[175, 176] There is degeneration of both pigmented catecholamine-containing cells in the brain stem and cholinergic cells in the intermediolateral columns, along with distal ganglionic and postganglionic degeneration. The abnormality in sympathetic function leads to depressed circulating norepinephrine responses to standing and exertion. There is enhanced blood pressure response to norepinephrine administration, along with evidence of increased α and β receptor concentrations, which correlates to supersensitivity to norepinephrine. Basal norepinephrine levels are normal. Generally, catecholamine is depleted in sympathetic nerve endings around blood vessels.[177]

Often in the male, the first symptom is impotence and loss of libido, with disturbance in micturition being common in both sexes. The characteristic orthostatic hypotension may be seen either as so-called drop attacks or as a gradual loss of consciousness over about a minute that is often associated with a neckache that radiates to the occiput and shoulders. Generally, there is at least partial loss of thermoregulatory sweating. Respiratory disturbance occurs as involuntary gasping, cluster breathing, and laryngeal stridor that may lead to obstructive sleep apnea and even death, or to central sleep apnea.

On neurological examination, abnormalities of the pupil, including Horner's syndrome, alternating anisocoria, and abnormal responses to drugs, may be seen. Mild parkinsonian features or cerebellar ataxia may accompany the condition, but dysautonomia is the predominant dysfunction. In the striatonigral degeneration variant, or multiple system atrophy, rigidity with little tremor, progressive loss of facial expression, limb akinesias, anterocollis, and gait instability predominate (see Chapter 34).There is difficulty walking, standing, turning, and feeding oneself, and the speech is faint and slurred. With pyramidal lesions, there may be an increase in tone, along with impaired rapid hand and foot movements and exaggerated deep tendon reflexes and bilateral extensor responses. Primitive reflexes may be present, and amyotrophy is common. Dementia is not seen more often than would be expected by chance owing to the age of this population. When the olivopontocerebellar variant is present, ataxia and limb tremor develops.[178]

Differential Diagnosis. Pure autonomic failure (Bradbury-Eggleston syndrome) may present with the same autonomic disturbance as Shy-Drager syndrome, but it does not have any other neurological symptoms. Amyloidosis may also look similar but generally is associated with a greater degree of bowel involvement and pain (see Chapter 37). Familial dysautonomia (Riley-Day syndrome, or HSAN III) presents in children and therefore is distinguishable from Shy-Drager syndrome.

Management. Several general actions may help the patient avoid aggravation of orthostatic hypotension: maintenance of adequate blood volume with fluid intake of 2 to 2.5 L/day, sleeping in a semirecumbent position, and rising slowly to standing. In addition, patients should avoid excessive warmth (in bathing and climate); do moderate rather than vigorous exercise; eat small, frequent meals; and avoid vasodilators, such as alcohol and nitroglycerin. Mechanical support may be provided by Jobst's stockings in combination with abdominal binding. Severe orthostatic hypotension has been successfully managed with an air force anti-gravity suit.[177] The most common pharmacological agent used is fludrocortisone, which increases blood volume and maintains venous return to the heart. Second-line drugs are the vasoconstrictors, such as phenylephrine and ephedrine, with the prostaglandin inhibitors being the next choice, followed by β-1 agonists. There is a recent report of a single patient responding favorably to octreotide, a splanchnic venoconstrictor.[179] Early tracheostomy for laryngeal stridor may prevent premature death. A recent Japanese study concluded that 90 percent of patients are alive 3 years after their first symptoms and 54 percent are alive after 6 years. Earlier onset of more extensive autonomic disturbance was associated with a poorer prognosis.[180]

Reviews and Selected Updates

Bird TD, Kraft GH, Lipe HP, et al: Clinical and pathological phenotype of the original family with Charcot-Marie-Tooth Type 1B: A 20-year study. Ann Neurol 1997;41:463–469.

Biros I, Forrest S: Spinal muscular dystrophy: Untangling the knot? J Med Genet 1999;36:1–8.

Burke B, Mounkes LC, Stewart CL: The nuclear envelope in muscular dystrophy and cardiovascular diseases. Traffic 2001;2:675–683.

Bushby K: The limb-girdle muscular dystrophies—multiple genes, multiple mechanisms. Hum Mol Genet 1999;8:1875–1882.

Carter GT, Galer BS: Advances in the management of neuropathic pain. Phys Med Rehabil Clin N Am 2001;12:447–459.

Emery AE: Emery-Dreifuss muscular dystrophy—a 40-year retrospective. Neuromuscul Disord 2000;10:228–232.

England JD, Garcia CA: Electrophysiological studies in the different genotypes of Charcot-Marie-Tooth disease. Curr Opin Neurol 1996;9:338–342.

Ganzini L, Johnston WS, Silveira MJ: The final month of life in patients with ALS. Neurology 2002;59:428–431

Gutmann L, Mitsumoto MD: Advances in amyotrophic lateral sclerosis. Neurology 1996;47:S17–S135.

Kakulas BA: The differential diagnosis of the human dystrophinopathies and related disorders. Curr Opin Neurol 1996;9:380–388.

Miller RG, Rosenberg JA, Gelinas DF, et al: Practice parameter: The care of the patient with amyotrophic lateral sclerosis (an evidence-based review). Report of the Quality Standards Subcommittee of the American Academy of Neurology. Neurology 1999;52:1311–1323.

Quality Standards Subcommittee of the American Academy of Neurology: Practice advisory on the treatment of amyotrophic lateral sclerosis with riluzole. Neurology 1997;49:657–659.

Siddique T: Motor neuron disease. Clin Neurosci 1995/1996;3:6.

Siddique T, Nijhawan D, Hentati A: Molecular genetic basis of familial ALS. Neurology 1996;47:S27–S34.

Straub V, Campbell KP: Muscular dystrophies and the dystrophin-glycoprotein complex. Curr Opin Neurol 1997;10:168–175.

References

1. Williams DB, Windebank AJ: Motor neuron disease. *In* Dick PJ, Thomas PK, Griffen JW, et al (eds): Peripheral Neuropathy, 3rd ed. Vol. 2. Philadelphia, WB Saunders, 1993, pp 1028–1050.
2. Siddique T: ALS: Molecular clues to the jigsaw puzzle of neuronal degeneration. Cold Spring Harbor Symposia on Quantitative Biology, Vol. LXL. Cold Spring Harbor Laboratory Press, 1996, pp 105–115.
3. Beckman JS, Chen J, Crow JP, Ye YZ: Reactions of nitric oxide, superoxide and peroxynitrite with superoxide dismutase in neurodegeneration. Prog Brain Res 1994;103:371–380.
4. Subramaniam JR, Lyons WE, Liu J, et al: Mutant SOD1 causes motor neuron disease independent of copper chaperone-mediated copper loading. Nat Neurosci 2002;5:301–307.
5. Beal MF: Mitochondria and the pathogenesis of ALS. Brain 2000;123: 1291–1292.
6. Yang Y, Hentati A, Deng H-X, et al: The gene encoding alsin, a protein with three guanine-nucleotide exchange factor domains, is mutated in a form of recessive amyotrophic lateral sclerosis. Nat Genet 2001;29:160–165. [Erratum: Nat Genet 2001;29:352.]
7. Hentati A, Ouahchi, K, Pericak-Vance MA, et al: Linkage of a commoner form of recessive amyotrophic lateral sclerosis to chromosome 15q15-q22 markers. Neurogenet 1998;2:55–60.
8. Chance PF, Rabin BA, Ryan SG, et al: Linkage of the gene for an autosomal dominant form of juvenile amyotrophic lateral sclerosis to chromosome 9q34. Am J Hum Genet 1998;62:633–640.

9. Al-Chalabi A, Andersen PM, Nilsson P, et al: Deletions of the heavy neurofilament subunit tail in amyotrophic lateral sclerosis. Hum Molec Genet 1999;8:157–164.
10. Wilhelmson KC, Lynch T, Pavlou E, et al: Localization of disinhibition-dementia-parkinsonism-amyotrophy complex to 17q21–22. Am J Hum Genet 1994;55:1159–1165.
11. Hosler BA, Siddique T, Sapp PC, et al: Linkage of familial amyotrophic lateral sclerosis with frontotemporal dementia to chromosome 9q21-q22. JAMA 2000;284:1664–1669.
12. Rothstein JD: Excitotoxicity and neurodegeneration in amyotrophic lateral sclerosis. Clin Neurosci 1996;3:348–359.
13. Nelson LM: Epidemiology of ALS. Clin Neurosci 1996;3:327–331.
14. Nelson LM, Matkin C, Longstreth WT Jr, McGuire V: Population-based case-control study of amyotrophic lateral sclerosis in western Washington State. II. Diet. Am J Epidemiol 2000;151:164–173.
15. Nelson LM, McGuire V, Longstreth WT Jr, Matkin C: Population-based case-control study of amyotrophic lateral sclerosis in western Washington State. I. Cigarette smoking and alcohol consumption. Am J Epidemiol 2000;151:156–163.
16. Sirdofsky MD, Hawley RJ, Manz H: Progressive motor neuron disease associated with electrical injury. Muscle Nerve 1991;14:977–980.
17. El Escorial: World Federation of Neurology. Criteria for the diagnosis of amyotrophic lateral sclerosis. J Neurol Sci 1994;124(Suppl):96–107.
18. Bradley WG: Overview of motor neuron disease: Classification and nomenclature. Clin Neurosci 1996;3:323–326.
19. Brooks BR: Emerging directions in ALS therapeutics: Palliative therapies at the advent of the twenty-first century. Clin Neurosci 1996;3:368–392.
20. Li M, Ona VO, Chen M, et al: Functional role and therapeutic implications of neuronal caspase-1 and -3 in a mouse model of traumatic spinal cord injury. Neurosci 2000;99:333–342.
21. Lefebvre S, Burglen L, Reboullet S, et al: Identification and characterization of a spinal muscular atrophy–determining gene. Cell 1995;80:155–165.
22. Campbell L, Potter A, Ignatius J, et al: Genomic variation and gene conversion in spinal muscular atrophy: Implications for disease process and clinical phenotype. Am J Hum Genet 1997;61:40–50.
23. Hsieh-Li HM, Chang J-G, Jong Y-J, et al: A mouse model for spinal muscular atrophy. Nature Genet 2000;24:66–70.
24. Pearn J: Incidence, prevalence, and gene frequency studies of chronic childhood spinal muscular atrophy. J Med Genet 1978;15:409–413.
25. Burglen L, Amiel J, Viollet L, et al: Survival motor neuron gene deletion in the arthrogryposis multiplex congenita–spinal muscular atrophy association. J Clin Invest 1996;98:1130–1132.
26. Gomez MR: Motor neuron disease in children. *In* Engel AG, Franzini-Armstrong C (eds): Myology, 2nd ed. Vol. 2. New York, McGraw-Hill, 1994, pp 1836–1853.
27. La Spada AR, Roling DB, Harding AE, et al: Meiotic stability and genotype-phenotype correlation of the trinucleotide repeat in X-linked spinal and bulbar muscular atrophy. Nat Genet 1992;2:301–304.
28. McCampbell A, Taye AA, Whitty L, et al: Histone deacetylase inhibitors reduce polyglutamine toxicity. Proc Natl Acad Sci USA 2001;98:15179–15184.
29. Georgiou I, Sermon K, Lissens W, et al: Preimplantation genetic diagnosis for spinal and bulbar muscular atrophy (SBMA). Hum Genet 2001;108:494–498.
30. Chang J-G, Hsieh-Li H-M, Jong Y-J, et al: Treatment of spinal muscular atrophy by sodium butyrate. Proc Natl Acad Sci USA 2001;98:9808–9813.
31. Cifuentes-Diaz C, Frugier T, Tiziano F, et al: Deletion of murine SMN exon 7 directed to skeletal muscle leads to severe muscular dystrophy. J Cell Biol 2001;152:1107–1114.
32. Jouet M, Rosenthal A, Armstrong G, et al: X-linked spastic paraplegia (SPG1), MASA syndrome and X-linked hydrocephalus result from mutations in the L1 gene. Nat Genet 1994;7:402–407.
33. Fryns JP, Spaepen A, Cassiman JJ, van den Berghe N: X-linked complicated spastic paraplegia, MASA syndrome, and X-linked hydrocephaly due to congenital stenosis of the Aqueduct of Sylvius: A variable expression of the same mutation at Xq28. J Med Genet 1991;28:429–431.
34. Willard HF, Riordan JR: Assignment of the gene for myelin proteolipid protein to the X chromosome: Implications for X-linked myelin disorders. Science 1985;230:940–942.
35. Zhao X, Alvarado D, Rainier S, et al: Mutations in a newly identified GTPase gene cause autosomal dominant hereditary spastic paraplegia. Nat Genet 2001;29:326–331.
36. Hazan J, Fonknechten N, Mavel D, et al: Spastin, a new AAA protein, is altered in the most frequent form of autosomal dominant spastic paraplegia. Nat Genet 1999;23:296–303.
37. Hentati A, Pericak-Vance MA, Hung WY, et al: Linkage of "pure" autosomal recessive familial spastic paraplegia to chromosome 8 markers and evidence of genetic locus heterogeneity. Hum Mol Genet 1994;3:1263–1267.
38. Fink JK, Wu C, Jones SM, et al: Autosomal dominant familial spastic paraplegia: Tight linkage to chromosome 15q. Am J Hum Genet 1995;56:188–192.
39. Casari G, Fusco M, Ciarmatori S, et al: Spastic paraplegia and OXPHOS impairment caused by mutations in paraplegin, a nuclear-encoded mitochondrial metalloprotease. Cell 1998;93:973–983.
40. Hedera P, Rainier S, Alvarado D, et al: Novel locus for autosomal dominant hereditary spastic paraplegia on chromosome 8q. Am J Hum Genet 1999;64:563–569.
41. Seri M, Cusano R, Forabosco P, et al: Genetic mapping to 10q23.3–q24.2, in a large Italian pedigree, of a new syndrome showing bilateral cataracts, gastroesophageal reflux, and spastic paraparesis with amyotrophy. Am J Hum Genet 1999;64:586–593.
42. Reid E, Dearlove AM, Rhodes M, Rubinsztein DC: A new locus for autosomal dominant "pure" hereditary spastic paraplegia mapping to chromosome 12q13 and evidence for further genetic heterogeneity. Am J Hum Genet 1999;65:757–763.
43. Martinez-Murillo F, Kobayashi H, Pegoraro E: Genetic localization of a new locus for recessive spastic paraplegia to 15q13–15. Am J Hum Genet 1999;63:A300.
44. Reid E, Dearlove AM, Osborn M, et al: A locus for autosomal dominant "pure" hereditary spastic paraplegia maps to chromosome 19q13. Am J Hum Genet 2000;66:728–732.
45. Fontaine B, Davoine CS, Durr A, et al: A new locus for autosomal dominant pure spastic paraplegia, on chromosome 2q24–q34. Am J Hum Genet 2000;66:702–707.
46. Vazza G, Zortea M, Boaretto F, et al: A new locus for autosomal recessive spastic paraplegia associated with mental retardation and distal motor neuropathy, SPG14, maps to chromosome 3q27–q28. Am J Hum Genet 2000;67:504–509.
47. Tamagaka A, Shima M, Tomita R, et al: Segregation of a pure form of spastic paraplegia and NOR insertion into Xq11.2. Am J Med Genet 2000;94:5–8.
48. Patel H, Hart PE, Warner TT, et al: The Silver syndrome variant of hereditary spastic paraplegia maps to chromosome 11q12–q14, with evidence for genetic heterogeneity within this subtype. Am J Hum Genet 2001; 69:209–215.
49. Fink JK, Hieman-Patterson T, for the Hereditary Spastic Paraplegia Working Group: Hereditary spastic paraplegia: Advances in genetic research. Neurol 1996;46:1507–1514.
50. Monaco AP, Kunkel LM: Cloning of the Duchenne/Becker muscular dystrophy locus. Adv Hum Genet 1988;17:61–98.
51. Ahn AH, Kunkel LM: The structural and functional diversity of dystrophin. Nat Genet 1993;3:283–291.
52. Ozawa E, Yoshida M, Suzuki A, et al: Dystrophin-associated proteins in muscular dystrophy. Hum Molec Genet 1995;4:1711–1716.
53. Worton R: Muscular dystrophies: Diseases of the dystrophin-glycoprotein complex. Science 1995;270:755–756.
54. Lederfein D, Yaffe D, Nudel U: A housekeeping type promoter, located in the 3-prime region of the Duchenne muscular dystrophy gene, controls the expression of Dp71, a major product of the gene. Hum Molec Genet 1993;2:1883–1888.
55. Matsumura K, Tome FM, Collin H, et al: Deficiency of the 50K dystrophin-associated glycoprotein in severe childhood autosomal recessive muscular dystrophy. Nature 1992;359:320–322.
56. Metzinger L, Blake DJ, Squier MV, et al: Dystrobrevin deficiency at the sarcolemma of patients with muscular dystrophy. Hum Molec Genet 1997;6:1185–1191.
57. Engel AH, Yamamoto M, Fischbeck KH: Muscular dystrophies. *In* Engel AH, Franzini-Armstrong C (eds): Myology, 2nd ed. New York, McGraw-Hill, 1994, pp 1130–1187.
58. Monaco AP, Bertelson CJ, Liechti-Gallati S, et al: An explanation for the phenotypic differences between patients bearing partial deletions of the DMD locus. Genomics 1988;2:90–95.
59. Matsumura K, Tome FM, Ionaescu V, et al: Deficiency of dystrophin-associated proteins in Duchenne muscular dystrophy patients lacking the COOH-terminal domains of dystrophin. J Clin Invest 1993;92:866–871.
60. Beggs AH, Hoffman EP, Snyder JR, et al: Exploring the molecular basis for variability among patients with Becker muscular dystrophy: Dystrophin gene and protein studies. Am J Hum Genet 1991;49:54–67.
61. Emery AEH: Population frequencies of inherited neuromuscular diseases—a world survey. Neuromuscul Disord 1991;1:19–29.

62. Hu XY, Ray PN, Worton RG: Mechanisms of tandem duplication in the Duchenne muscular dystrophy gene include both homologous and nonhomologous intrachromosomal recombination. EMBO J 1991;10:2471–2477.
63. Laing NG, Siddique T, Bartlett R, et al: Duchenne muscular dystrophy: Detection of deletion carriers by spectrophotometric densitometry. Clin Genet 1989;35:393–398.
64. Florence JM, Fox PT, Planer GJ, Brooke MH: Activity, creatine kinase, and myoglobin in Duchenne muscular dystrophy: A clue to etiology? Neurology 1985;35:758–761.
65. Griggs RC, Forbes G, Moxley RT, Herr BE: The assessment of muscle mass in progressive neuromuscular disease. Neurology 1983;33:158–165.
66. Perloff JK, Roberts WC, deLeon AC Jr, O'Doherty D: The distinctive electrocardiogram of Duchenne's progressive muscular dystrophy: An electrocardiographic-pathologic correlative study. Am J Med 1967;42:179–188.
67. Mendell JR, Moxley RT, Griggs RC, et al: Randomized, double-blind six-month trial of prednisone in Duchenne's muscular dystrophy. N Engl J Med 1989;320:1592–1597.
68. Karpati G, Ajdukovic D, Arnold D, et al: Myoblast transfer in Duchenne muscular dystrophy. Ann Neurol 1993;34:8–17.
69. Vignos PJ Jr : Physical models of rehabilitation in neuromuscular disease. Muscle Nerve 1983;6:323–328.
70. Spencer GE, Vignos PJ: Bracing for ambulation in childhood progressive muscular dystrophy. J Bone Joint Surg Am 1962;44:234–242.
71. DiMarco AF, Kelling JS, DiMarco MS, et al: The effects of inspiratory resistive training on respiratory muscle function in patients with muscular dystrophy. Muscle Nerve 1985;8:284–290.
72. Fukunaga H, Okubo R, Moritoyo T, et al: Long-term follow-up of patients with Duchenne muscular dystrophy receiving ventilatory support. Muscle Nerve 1993;16:554–558.
73. Bregman AM: Living with progressive childhood illness: Parental management of neuromuscular disease. Soc Work Health Care 1980;5:387.
74. Williamson RA, Henry MD, Daniels KJ, et al: Dystroglycan is essential for early embryonic development: Disruption of Reichert's membrane in Dag1-null mice. Hum Molec Genet 1997;6:831–841.
75. Kumar-Singh R, Chamberlain JS: Encapsidated adenovirus minichromosomes allow delivery and expression of a 14 kb dystrophin cDNA to muscle cells. Hum Molec Genet 1996;5:913–921.
76. Kochanek S, Clemens PR, Mitani K, et al: A new adenoviral vector: Replacement of all viral coding sequences with 28 kb of DNA independently expressing both full-length dystrophin and β-galactosidase. Proc Natl Acad Sci USA 1996;93:5731–5736.
77. Tinsley JM, Potter AC, Phelps SR, et al: Amelioration of the dystrophic phenotype of *mdx* mice using a truncated utrophin transgene. Nature 1996;384:349–353.
78. Barton-Davis ER, Cordier L, Shoturma DI, et al: Aminoglycoside antibiotics restore dystrophin function to skeletal muscles of *mdx* mice. J Clin Invest 1999;104:375–381.
79. Burking DJ, Wallace GQ, Nicol KJ, et al: Enhanced expression of the alpha 7 beta 1 integrin reduces muscular dystrophy and restores viability in dystrophic mice. J Cell Biol 2001;152:1207–1218.
80. Gussoni E, Soneoka Y, Strickland CD, et al: Dystrophin expression in the *mdx* mouse restored by stem cell transplantation. Nature 1999;401:390–394.
81. Chaubourt E, Voisin V, Fossier P, et al: Muscular nitric oxide synthase (muNOS) and utrophin. J Physiol Paris 2002;96:43–52.
82. Hauser MA, Horrigan SK, Salmikangas P, et al: Myotilin is mutated in limb girdle muscular dystrophy 1A. Hum Mol Genet 2000;9:2141–2147.
83. van der Kooi AJ, Ledderhof TM, de Voogt WG, et al: A newly recognized autosomal dominant limb girdle muscular dystrophy with cardiac involvement. Ann Neurol 1996;39:636–642.
84. Minetti C, Sotgia F, Bruno C, et al: Mutations in the caveolin-3 gene cause autosomal dominant limb-girdle muscular dystrophy. Nat Genet 1998;18:365–368.
85. Messina DN, Speer MC, Pericak-Vance MA, McNally EM: Linkage of familial dilated cardiomyopathy with conduction defect and muscular dystrophy to chromosome 6q23. Am J Hum Genet 1997;61:909–917.
86. Speer MC, Vance JM, Grubber JM, et al: Identification of a new autosomal dominant limb-girdle muscular dystrophy locus on chromosome 7. Am J Hum Genet 1999;64:556–562.
87. Richard I, Broux O, Allamand V, et al: Mutations in the proteolytic enzyme calpain 3 cause limb-girdle muscular dystrophy type 2A. Cell 1995;81:27–40.
88. Liu J, Aoki M, Illa I, et al: Dysferlin, a novel skeletal muscle gene, is mutated in Miyoshi myopathy and limb girdle muscular dystrophy. Nature Genet 1998;20:31–36.
89. McNally EM, Duggan D, Gorospe JR, et al: Mutations that disrupt the carboxyl-terminus of gamma-sarcoglycan cause muscular dystrophy. Hum Molec Genet 1996;5:1841–1847.
90. Duggan DJ, Gorospe JRM, Fanin M, Hoffman EP, Angelini C: Mutations in the sarcoglycan genes in myopathy patients. N Engl J Med 1997;336:618–624.
91. Bonnemann CG, Passos-Bueno MR, McNally EM, et al: Genomic screening for beta-sarcoglycan gene mutations: Missense mutations may cause severe limb-girdle muscular dystrophy type 2E (LGMD 2E). Hum Molec Genet 1996;5:1953–1961.
92. Nigro V, de Sa Moreira E, Piluso G, et al: Autosomal recessive limb-girdle muscular dystrophy, LGMD2F, is caused by a mutation in the delta-sarcoglycan gene. Nat Genet 1996;14:195–198.
93. Moreira ES, Wiltshire TJ, Faulkner G, et al: Limb-girdle muscular dystrophy type 2G is caused by mutations in the gene encoding the sarcomeric protein telethonin. Nat Genet 2000;24:163–166.
94. Weiler T, Greenberg CR, Zelinski T, et al: A gene for autosomal recessive limb-girdle muscular dystrophy in Manitoba Hutterites maps to chromosome region 9q31-q33: Evidence for another limb-girdle muscular dystrophy locus. Am J Hum Genet 1998;63:140–147.
95. Driss A, Amouri R, Ben Hamida C, et al: A new locus for autosomal recessive limb-girdle muscular dystrophy in a large consanguineous Tunisian family maps to chromosome 19q13.3. Neuromuscul Disord 2000;10:240–246.
96. Shields RW Jr: Limb girdle syndromes. *In* Engel AG, Franzini-Armstrong C (eds): Myology, 2nd ed. New York, McGraw-Hill, 1994, pp 1258–1274.
97. Ben Hamida M, Fardeau M, Attia NL: Severe childhood muscular dystrophy affecting both sexes and frequent in Tunisia. Muscle Nerve 1983;6:469–480.
98. Matsumura K, Tome FM, Collin H, et al: Deficiency of the 50K dystrophin-associated glycoprotein in severe childhood autosomal recessive muscular dystrophy. Nature 1992;359:320–322.
99. Arikawa E, Hoffman EP, Kaido M, et al: The frequency of patients with dystrophin abnormalities in a limb-girdle patient population. Neurology 1991;41:1491–1496.
100. Galbiati F, Volont D, Minetti C, et al: Phenotypic behavior of caveolin-3 mutations that cause autosomal dominant limb girdle muscular dystrophy (LGMD-1C): Retention of LGMD-1C caveolin-3 mutants within the golgi complex. J Biol Chem 1999;274:26732–26741.
101. Nigro V, Piluso G, Belsito A, et al: Identification of a novel sarcoglycan gene at 5q33 encoding a sarcolemmal 35 kDa glycoprotein. Hum Molec Genet 1996;5:1179–1186.
102. Tome FMS, Evangelista T, Leclerc A, et al. Congenital muscular dystrophy with merosin deficiency. Comp Rend Acad Sci (Paris) 1994;317:351–357.
103. van Deutekom JCT, Lemmers RJLF, Grewal PK, et al: Identification of the first gene (FRG1) from the FSHD region on human chromosome 4q35. Hum Molec Genet 1996;5:581–590.
104. Vitelli F, Villanova M, Malandrini A, et al: Inheritance of a 38-kb fragment in apparently sporadic facioscapulohumeral muscular dystrophy. Muscle Nerve 1999;22:1437–1441.
105. Gilbert JR, Stajich JM, Wall S, et al: Evidence for heterogeneity in facioscapulohumeral muscular dystrophy. Am J Hum Genet 1993;53:401–408.
106. Lunt PW, Compston DA, Harper PS: Estimation of age dependent penetrance in facioscapulohumeral muscular dystrophy by minimizing ascertainment bias. J Med Genet 1989;26:755–760.
107. Miura K, Kumagai T, Matsumoto A, et al: Two cases of chromosome 4q35-linked early onset facioscapulohumeral muscular dystrophy with mental retardation and epilepsy. Neuroped 1998;29:239–241.
108. Munsat TL: Facioscapulohumeral disease and the scapuloperoneal syndrome. *In* Engel AG, Franzini-Armstrong C (eds): Myology, 2nd ed. New York, McGraw-Hill, 1994, pp 1220–1232.
109. Padberg GW: Facioscapulohumeral muscular dystrophy. Doctoral thesis. University of Leiden, Intercontinental Graphics, 1982.
110. Isozumi K, DeLong R, Kaplan J, et al: Linkage of scapuloperoneal spinal muscular atrophy to chromosome 12q24.1–q24.31. Hum Molec Genet 1996;9:1377–1382.
111. Schwartz MS, Swash M: Scapuloperoneal atrophy with sensory involvement: Davidenkow's syndrome. J Neurol Neurosurg Psychiatry 1975;38:1063–1067.
112. Feigenbaum JA, Munsat TL: A neuromuscular syndrome of scapuloperoneal distribution. Bull Los Angeles Neurol Soc 1970;35:47–57.
113. Lavedan C, Hoffman-Radvanyi H, Shelbourne P, et al: Myotonic dystrophy: Size and sex dependent dynamics of CTG meiotic instability and somatic mosaicism. Am J Hum Genet 1993;52:875–883.

114. Redman JB, Fenwick RG, Fu YH, et al: Relationship between parental trinucleotide CGT repeat length and severity of myotonic dystrophy in offspring. J Am Med Assoc 1993;269:1960–1965.
115. Whiting EJ, Waring JD, Tamai K, et al: Characterization of myotonic dystrophy kinase (DMK) protein in human and rodent muscle and central nervous tissue. Hum Molec Genet 1995;4:1063–1072.
116. Wang J, Pegoraro E, Menegazzo E, et al: Myotonic dystrophy: Evidence for a possible dominant-negative RNA mutation. Hum Molec Genet 1995;4:599–606.
117. Harper PS, Rudel R: Myotonic dystrophy. *In* Engel AG, Franzini-Armstrong C (eds): Myology, 2nd ed. New York, McGraw-Hill, 1994, pp 1192–1219.
118. Johnson ER, Abresch RT, Gregory GT, et al: Profiles of neuromuscular diseases. Myotonic dystrophy. Am J Phys Med Rehabil 1995; 74:S104–S116.
119. Meola G, Sansone V, Rotondo G, et al: PROMM in Italy: Clinical and biomolecular findings. Acta Myo 1998;2:21–26.
120. Brais B, BouchardJ-P, Xie Y-G, et al: Short GCG expansions in the PABP2 gene cause oculopharyngeal muscular dystrophy. Nature Genet 1998;18:164–167.
121. Tome FMS, Fardeau M: Oculopharyngeal muscular dystrophy. *In* Engel AG, Franzini-Armstrong C (eds): Myology, 2nd ed. New York, McGraw-Hill, 1994, pp 1233–1245.
122. Emery AE, Dreifuss FE: Unusual type of benign X-linked muscular dystrophy. J Neurol Neurosurg Psychiatry 1966;29:338–342.
123. Becker PE: Dominant autosomal muscular dystrophy with early contractures and cardiomyopathy (Hauptman-Tannhauser). Hum Genet 1986;74:184.
124. Grimm T, Janka M: Emery-Dreifuss muscular dystrophy. *In* Engel AK, Franzini-Armstrong C (eds): Myology, 2nd ed. New York: McGraw-Hill, 1994, pp 1188–1191.
125. Kutay U, Hartmann E, Rapoport TA: A class of membrane proteins with a C-terminal anchor. Trends Cell Biol 1993;3:72–75.
126. Kress W, Muller E, Kausch K, et al: Multipoint linkage mapping of the Emery-Dreifuss muscular dystrophy gene. Neuromuscul Disord 1992;2:111–115.
127. Voit T, Krogmann O, Leonard HG, et al: Emery-Dreifuss muscular dystrophy: Disease spectrum and differential diagnosis. Neuropediatrics 1988;19:62–71.
128. Bonne G, Di Barletta MR, Varnous S, et al: Mutations in the gene encoding lamin A/C cause autosomal dominant Emery-Dreifuss muscular dystrophy. Nature Genet 1999;21:285–288.
129. Raffaele-Di Barletta M, Ricci E, Galluzzi G, et al: Different mutations in the LMNA gene cause autosomal dominant and autosomal recessive Emery-Dreifuss muscular dystrophy. Am J Hum Genet 2000; 66:1407–1412.
130. Muchir A, Bonne G, van der Kooi AJ, et al: Identification of mutations in the gene encoding lamins A/C in autosomal dominant limb girdle muscular dystrophy with atrioventricular conduction disturbances (LGMD1B). Hum Molec Genet 2000;9:1453–1459.
131. Goto I, Nagasaka S, Nagara H, Kuroiwa Y: Spine syndrome. J Neurol Neurosurg Psychiatry 1979;42:276–279.
132. Patel K, Voit T, Dunn MJ, et al: Dystrophin and nebulin in the muscular dystrophies. J Neurol Sci 1988;87:315–326.
133. Emery AE: Emery-Dreifuss syndrome. J Med Genet 1989;26:637–641.
134. Bione S, Maestrini E, Rivella S, et al: Identification of a novel X-linked gene responsible for Emery-Dreifuss muscular dystrophy. Nat Genet 1994;8:323–327.
135. Ahlberg G, von Tell D, Borg K, et al: Genetic linkage of Welander distal myopathy to chromosome 2p13. Ann Neurol 1999; 46:399–404.
136. Haravuori H, Makela-Bengs P, Udd B, et al: Assignment of the tibial muscular dystrophy locus to chromosome 2q31. Am J Hum Gene 1998;62:620–626.
137. Ikeuchi T, Asaka T, Saito M, et al: Gene locus for autosomal recessive distal myopathy with rimmed vacuoles maps to chromosome 9. Ann Neurol 1997;41:432–437.
138. Bejaoui K, Liu J, McKenna-Yasek D, et al: Genetic fine mapping of the Miyoshi myopathy locus and exclusion of eight candidate genes. Neurogenet 1998;1:189–196.
139. Laing NG, Laing BA, Meredith C, et al: Autosomal dominant distal myopathy: Linkage to chromosome 14. Am J Hum Genet 1995;56: 422–427.
140. Goldfarb LG, Park K-Y, Cervenakova L, et al: Missense mutations in desmin associated with familial cardiac and skeletal myopathy. Nature Genet 1998;19:402–403.
141. Griggs RC, Markesberry WR: Distal myopathies. *In* Engel AG, Franzini-Armstrong C (eds): Myology, 2nd ed. New York, McGraw-Hill, 1994, pp 1233–1245.
142. Lupski JR, Wise CA, Kuwano A, et al: Gene dosage is a mechanism for Charcot-Marie-Tooth disease type 1A. Nature Gene 1992;1:29–33.
143. Chance PF, Alderson MK, Leppig KA, et al: DNA deletion associated with hereditary neuropathy with liability to pressure palsies. Cell 1993;72:143–151.
144. Hayasaka K, Himoro M, Sato W, et al: Charcot-Marie-Tooth neuropathy type 1B is associated with mutations of the myelin P(0) gene. Nature Genet 1993;5:31–34.
145. Zhao C, Takita J, Tanaka Y, et al: Charcot-Marie-Tooth disease type 2A caused by mutation in a microtubule motor KIF1B-beta. Cell 2001;105:587–597.
146. Pericak-Vance MA, Speer MC, Lennon F, et al: Confirmation of a second locus for CMT2 and evidence for additional genetic heterogeneity. Neurogenet 1997;1:89–93.
147. McEntagart M, Norton N, Williams H, et al: Localization of the gene for distal hereditary motor neuronopathy VII (dHMN-VII) to chromosome 2q14. Am J Hum Genet 2001;68:1270–1276.
148. Ionasescu V, Searby C, Sheffield VC: Autosomal dominant Charcot-Marie-Tooth axonal neuropathy mapped on chromosome 7p (CMT2D). Hum Molec Genet 1996;5:1373–1375.
149. Mersiyanova IV, Perepelov AV, Polyakov AV: A new variant of Charcot-Marie-Tooth disease type 2 is probably the result of a mutation in the neurofilament-light gene. Am J Hum Genet 2000;67:37–46.
150. Bergoffen J, Scherer SS, Wang S, et al: Connexin mutations in X-linked Charcot-Marie-Tooth disease. Science 1993;262:2039–2042.
151. Ben Othmane K, Hentati F, Lennon F, et al: Linkage of a locus (CMT4A) for autosomal recessive Charcot-Marie-Tooth disease to chromosome 8q. Hum Molec Genet 1993;2:1625–1628.
152. Bolino A, Muglia M, Conforti FL: Charcot-Marie-Tooth type 4B is caused by mutations in the gene encoding myotubularin-related protein-2. Nature Genet 2000;25:17–19.
153. LeGuern E, Guilbot A, Kessali M, et al: Homozygosity mapping of an autosomal recessive form of demyelinating Charcot-Marie-Tooth disease to chromosome 5q23-q33. Hum Molec Genet 1996;5:1685–1688.
154. Kalaydjieva L, Gresham D, Gooding R, et al: N-myc downstream-regulated gene 1 is mutated in hereditary motor and sensory neuropathy-Lom. Am J Hum Genet 2000;67:47–58.
155. Warner LE, Mancias P, Butler IJ, et al: Mutations in the early growth response 2 (EGR2) gene are associated with hereditary myelinopathies. Nature Genet 1998;18:382–384.
156. Boerkoel CF, Takashima H, Stankiewicz P, et al: Periaxin mutations cause recessive Dejerine-Sottas neuropathy. Am J Hum Genet 2001;68:325–333. [Erratum: Am J Hum Genet 2001;68:557.]
157. Dyck PJ, Chance P, Lebo R, Carney JA: Hereditary motor and sensory neuropathies. *In* Dyck PJ, Thomas PK, Griffen JW, et al (eds): Peripheral Neuropathy, 3rd ed. Vol. 2. Philadelphia, WB Saunders, 1993, pp 1094–1136.
158. Suter U, Snipes GJ: Peripheral myelin protein 22: Facts and hypotheses. J Neurosci Res 1995;40:145–151.
159. Meijerink PH, Hoogendijk JE, Gabreels-Festen AA, et al: Clinically distinct codon 69 mutations in major myelin protein zero in demyelinating neuropathies. Ann Neurol 1996;40:672–675.
160. Harding AE: From the syndrome of Charcot, Marie and Tooth to disorders of peripheral myelin proteins. Brain 1995;118:809–818.
161. Carter GT, Jensen MP, Galer BS, et al: Neuropathic pain in Charcot-Marie-Tooth disease. Arch Phys Med Rehabil 1998;79:1560–1564.
162. Auer-Grumbach M, Strasser-Fuchs S, Wagner K, et al: Roussy-Levy syndrome is a phenotypic variant of Charcot-Marie-Tooth syndrome IA associated with a duplication on chromosome 17p11.2. J Neurol Sci 1998;154:72–75.
163. Bird TD, Kraft GH, Lipe HP, et al: Clinical and pathological phenotype of the original family with Charcot-Marie-Tooth type 1B: One 20-year study. Ann Neurol 1997;41:463–469.
164. Dyck PJ: Neuronal atrophy and degeneration predominantly affecting peripheral sensory and autonomic neurons. *In* Dyck PJ, Thomas PK, Griffen JW, et al (eds): Peripheral Neuropathy, 3rd ed. Vol. 2. Philadelphia, WB Saunders, 1993, pp 1065–1093.
165. Dawkins JL, Hulme DJ, Brahmbhatt SB, et al: Mutations in SPTLC1, encoding serine palmitoyltransferase, long chain base subunit-1, cause hereditary sensory neuropathy type I. Nature Genet 2001; 27:309–312.
166. Brunt PW, McKusich VA: Familial dysautonomia: A report of genetic and clinical studies, with a review of the literature. Medicine (Baltimore) 1970;49:343–374.

167. Anderson SL, Coli R, Daly IW, et al: Familial dysautonomia is caused by mutations of the IKAP gene. Am J Hum Genet 2001;68:753–758.
168. Axelrod FB, Pearson J, Tepperberg J, Ackerman BD: Congenital sensory neuropathy with skeletal dysplasia. J Pediatr 1983;102:727–730.
169. Oddoux C, Riech E, Axelrod F, et al: Prenatal diagnostic testing for familial dysautonomia using linked genetic markers. Prenat Diagn 1995;15:817–826.
170. Axelrod FB, Abularrage JJ: Familial dysautonomia. J Pediatr 1982;101: 234–236.
171. Rosemberg S, Nagahashi Marie SK, Kliemann S: Congenital insensitivity to pain with anhidrosis (hereditary sensory and autonomic neuropathy type IV). Pediat Neurol 1994;11:50–56.
172. Shatzky S, Moses S, Levy J: Congenital insensitivity to pain with anhidrosis (CIPA) in Israeli-Bedouins: Genetic heterogeneity, novel mutations in the TRKA/NGF receptor gene, clinical findings, and results of nerve conduction studies. Am J Med Genet 2000;92:353–360.
173. Hirayama K, Takayanagi T, Nakamura R, et al: Spinocerebellar degeneration in Japan: A nationwide epidemiological and clinical study. Acta Neurol Scand 1994;89:1–22.
174. Bannister R, Mowbray J, Sidgwick A: Genetic control of progressive autonomic failure: Evidence for association with an HLA antigen. Lancet 1983;1:1017.
175. Zuscik MJ, Sands S, Ross SA, et al: Overexpression of the alpha1B-adrenergic receptor causes apoptotic neurodegeneration: Multiple system atrophy. Nat Med 2001;7:132.
176. Johnson RH, Lambie DG, Spalding JMK: The autonomic nervous system. *In* Joynt RJ, Griggs RC (eds): Clinical Neurology, Vol. 4. Philadelphia, Lippincott-Raven, 1986, pp 1–94.
177. Brook WH: Postural hypotension and the anti-gravity suit. Aust Fam Physician 1994;10:1948–1949.
178. Bannister R: Clinical features in autonomic failure. *In* Bannister R (ed): Autonomic Failure: A Textbook of Clinical Disorders of the Autonomic Nervous System, 2nd ed. Oxford, Oxford University Press, 1988, pp 267–288.
179. Lamarre-Cliche M, Cusson J: Octreotide for orthostatic hypotension. Can J Clin Pharmacol 1999;6:213–215.
180. Saito Y, Matsucka Y, Takahashi A, Ohno Y: Survival of patients with multiple system atrophy. Intern Med 1994;33:321–325.

CHAPTER 37

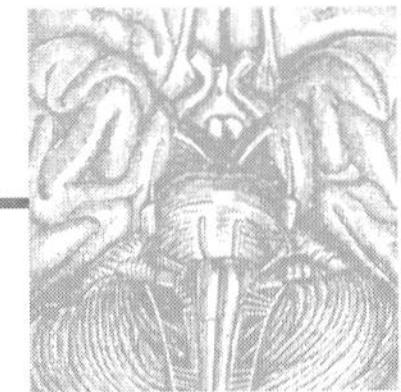

MICHAEL ROSE and ROBERT C. GRIGGS

Hereditary Nondegenerative Neuromuscular Disease

Muscle Channelopathies (Myotonias and Periodic Paralysis)

The neurological channelopathies are disorders of ion channels that result in abnormal excitability of cellular membranes in either the central or peripheral nervous system. A disturbance of ion channel function may result in either muscle membrane hyperexcitability leading to myotonia as the dominant feature, or alternatively in muscle membrane hypoexcitability leading to the episodic weakness seen in periodic paralysis. The muscle channelopathies can be grouped into sodium, chloride, calcium, and potassium channel disorders. Additional diseases are likely to be channelopathies but have not been firmly established to belong to this class (Table 37–1). Although the focus of this chapter is on the inherited channelopathies, acquired, usually autoimmune, channelopathies also result in nerve and muscle disease.

Traditionally the myotonias have been divided into dystrophic and nondystrophic disorders. The dystrophic myotonias have myotonia as one of several muscle symptoms, and muscle atrophy and weakness are prominent. These include dystrophia myotonica and proximal myotonic myopathy.[1, 2] By contrast, nondystrophic myotonias have myotonia as their most prominent symptom with little or no atrophy and weakness. These nondystrophic disorders result from a gene lesion in a muscle channel protein.

In the past, the periodic paralyses were divided on the basis of phenotype into those associated with a high or normal serum potassium (i.e., hyperkalemic periodic paralysis) and those associated with a low serum potassium concentration (hypokalemic periodic paralysis). In fact, serum potassium concentration is clearly the consequence rather than the cause of the periodic paralysis. Nevertheless, early genetic studies supported the traditional nosological separation,

TABLE 37–1. **Skeletal Muscle Channelopathies**

Channel/Disease	Chromosome
Skeletal Muscle Sodium α-Subunit	
Hyperkalemic periodic paralysis	17q23–25
With myotonia	
Without myotonia	
With paramyotonia congenita	
Hypokalemic periodic paralysis	17q23–25
Paramyotonia congenita	17q23–25
Sodium channel myotonia	17q23–25
Myotonia fluctuans	
Myotonia permanans	
Acetazolamide-responsive myotonia	
Skeletal Muscle Calcium Channel α1-Subunit (DHP sensitive)	1q31–32
Hypokalemic periodic paralysis	
Skeletal Muscle Chloride Channel	7q32
AD myotonia congenita (Thomsen's disease)	
AR myotonia congenita (Becker's disease)	
Potassium Channel	
Andersen's syndrome	17q23
Periodic paralysis	11q
Potential Channelopathy	
Schwartz-Jampel syndrome	

because hypokalemic periodic paralysis is a calcium channel disorder and hyperkalemic periodic paralysis is a sodium channel disorder. Of late, this tidy correlation of phenotype with genotype has been challenged by the recognition that some cases of hypokalemic periodic paralysis are due to sodium channel disorders and even rarer cases may be associated with a potassium channel mutation. Potassium channel mutations also account for Andersen's syndrome, a condition that includes periodic paralysis.

The two clinical hallmarks of channelopathies are myotonia and periodic paralysis. Disorders of sodium, chloride, calcium, and potassium are described in this section with attention not only to clinical descriptions, but also to disease-specific genetic and pathophysiological mechanisms. After the various individual channelopathies are described, later sections will deal with them again collectively, discussing differential diagnosis, evaluation, and management of the two clinical hallmarks, myotonia and paralysis.

It is difficult to get precise incidence figures for these conditions. They are undoubtedly underdiagnosed, because patients with mild symptoms may be misdiagnosed or may not seek medical attention. Finnish and Danish studies of hypokalemic periodic paralysis give an incidence of between 0.4 and 1.25 per 100,000.[3] For autosomal dominant myotonia congenita (Thomsen's disease), an incidence of between 0.25 and 4.0 per 100,000 has been quoted.[4]

SODIUM CHANNELOPATHIES

Disorders of the α-subunit of the muscle sodium channel result in four major distinct disorders: hyperkalemic periodic paralysis, hypokalemic periodic paralysis, paramyotonia congenita, and sodium channel myotonias. There is some phenotypic overlap of the sodium channelopathies, suggesting that they may be a continuum of disorder rather than rigidly demarcated clinical entities. Previous literature also includes normokalemic and myotonic periodic paralyses in this category, but since most, if not all, of these are potassium sensitive in exactly the same way as hyperkalemic periodic paralysis, it is likely that they represent sodium channel disorders.

Most, if not all, of the preceding disorders result from allelic point mutations in the same sodium channel gene that is situated on the long arm of chromosome 17. More than 25 different point mutations have been found that result in amino acid substitutions in conserved portions of the gene. Strict phenotypic-genotypic correlations for these point mutations are not yet defined because many have variable phenotypic expression. Physiologically these mutations result in reduced inactivation of the sodium channel, resulting in either increased muscle excitability with myotonia or increased muscle inexcitability with hyperkalemic periodic paralysis. In cases of hyperkalemic periodic paralysis, this physiological abnormality is accentuated by increasing the extracellular potassium concentration; in paramyotonia congenita, it is sensitive to cooling, thus accounting for the worsening of symptoms with these factors. It remains unclear how the sodium channel mutations may result in hypokalemic periodic paralysis.[5]

Paramyotonia Congenita

This disease is autosomal dominant, inherited with complete penetrance. The predominant symptom is paradoxical myotonia, usually present from birth and persisting throughout life. The myotonia is paradoxical because unlike classical myotonia, it increases with repetitive movements. Cold temperature exacerbates myotonia and can cause weakness. The myotonia particularly affects the face, neck, and forearm. Typically on relief of the myotonia, either spontaneously or on warming, there is a variable degree of weakness that persists for several hours. In a warm environment patients may have no symptoms at all. In some families with this disorder, there is a tendency for attacks of paralysis to occur independently of the myotonia. In many patients, these attacks are precipitated by potassium ingestion, in much the same way as hyperkalemic periodic paralysis. Occasional patients, usually adolescents, are weakened by hypokalemia.

Hyperkalemic Periodic Paralysis

As with paramyotonia congenita, hyperkalemic periodic paralysis normally appears in infancy or early childhood with frequent episodes of paralysis that are generally brief and mild, lasting between 15 minutes and 4 hours. Attacks are often precipitated by rest following exercise, by ingestion of potassium-rich foods, or by administration of potassium compounds. They commonly start in the morning before breakfast. Stress tends to make the attacks more easily provoked. Weakness is mainly proximal, but distal muscles can be involved. There is usually no ocular or respiratory muscle weakness. Examination of a patient during a severe attack reveals a flaccid tetraparesis with absent reflexes and normal sensory examination. The potassium may rise during the attack but not necessarily above the upper limit of normal range and rarely to levels that cause cardiac arrhythmia.

Generally between attacks, patients maintain normal strength, but in a few cases there is persistent mild weakness. The frequency of attacks may decline as the patient gets older. In some families with hyperkalemic periodic paralysis, there is co-existent mild myotonia. In these patients, cooling may provoke weakness as seen in paramyotonia congenita, but it does not worsen myotonia.

Hypokalemic Periodic Paralysis

Clinically, cases of hypokalemic periodic paralysis associated with sodium channel mutations have identical signs to those with the more common calcium channel–related hypokalemic periodic paralysis.[5] The clinical features are therefore given later under calcium channelopathies.

Sodium Channel Myotonias

This group of recently classified myotonias are related to sodium channel gene mutations but do not have the features of paramyotonia congenita nor episodes of periodic paralysis. In some cases, the myotonia is worsened by the cold but without associated weakness and the myotonia is responsive to acetazolamide.[6] In other families myotonia fluctuates on a daily basis and is provoked by exercise, termed "myotonia fluctuans."[7] Another sodium channel myotonia causes permanent and very severe myotonia, termed "myotonia permanans."[8]

CHLORIDE CHANNELOPATHIES

Two similar forms of myotonia congenita are now known to be due to disorders of the chloride channel. One is inherited as an autosomal dominant disease (Thomsen's disease) and the other as an autosomal recessive disease (Becker's disease).

In both forms of myotonia congenita, the characteristic feature is that of a reduced muscle membrane chloride conductance, which results in muscle membrane hyperexcitability with after-depolarization and repetitive firing leading to the myotonia. This abnormal physiology can be reproduced by chloride channel blockers or the substitution of impermeable ions for chloride. These diseases are linked to chromosome 7q32 in a region that encodes a chloride channel gene (*CLC9I*). Thomsen's and Becker's diseases are allelic disorders with nearly 50 mutations having been described so far. However, these mutations only account for 30 to 40 percent of cases, and undoubtedly other chloride channel mutations will emerge.[9]

Autosomal Dominant Myotonia Congenita (Thomsen's Disease)

The main symptom of this channelopathy is painless generalized myotonia, perceived as muscle stiffness, that usually appears in the first and second decades of life. It is provoked by exertion following rest and thus can be demonstrated by asking the patient to rise from a seated position after a period of repose. The myotonia improves with exercise. Patients have well-developed muscles with particular hypertrophy of the lower limbs, with a resultant athletic appearance. Muscle strength can be normal, possibly even stronger than normal, giving subjects advantage in power sports where speed is not a requisite. They have normal reflexes. Eyelid, grip, and percussion myotonia can usually be demonstrated.

Autosomal Recessive Myotonia Congenita (Becker's Disease)

This disorder is very similar to Thomsen's disease. The myotonia comes on later in the first decade but can be more severe than in Thomsen's disease. In addition to severe myotonic stiffness, patients can also have disabling transient weakness that is not seen in Thomsen's disease. After rest, their muscles are initially weak, and it takes a period of activity before full strength returns. At times, this weakness is so severe that patients require assistance to start ambulation; persistent weakness may occur. As in Thomsen's disease, there may be muscle hypertrophy, particularly of the legs and buttocks, with some hyperlordosis of the spine.

CALCIUM CHANNELOPATHIES

Mutations of the skeletal muscle dihydropyridine receptor (part of the calcium channel) cause primary hypokalemic periodic paralysis. An identical hypokalemic periodic paralysis, however, results from a sodium channel mutation or in rarer instances from a potassium channel mutation (see relevant sections). Secondary causes for hypokalemic periodic paralysis are more common than the hereditary form (see Differential Diagnosis).

In hypokalemic periodic paralysis, the weakness results from an abnormality of muscle membrane excitability. An influx of potassium into the muscle fiber occurs, with an accompanying influx of extracellular water. There is increased sensitivity to the effect of insulin on the movement of potassium into cells independently of the glucopenic action of insulin. This influx of potassium may account for the precipitation of hypokalemic periodic paralysis with large carbohydrate meals. In contrast to normal muscle fibers, the influx of potassium in hypokalemic periodic paralysis causes the muscle fibers to become depolarized and inexcitable. Calcium channel–related hypokalemic periodic paralysis is due to mutations of a gene on chromosome 1q coding for a skeletal muscle dihydropyridine receptor $\alpha 1$ subunit, which functions as a calcium channel (*CACNL1A3*). Three *CACNL1A3* mutations account for over 50 percent of cases of hypokalemic periodic paralysis, and these mutations are all in a highly conserved region of the gene that codes for the voltage sensor region of the channel.[10] The dihydropyridine receptor has a primary role in electrocontraction coupling with opening of the calcium channels of the sarcoplasmic reticulum allowing an influx of calcium into the muscle sarcoplasm and the triggering of muscle contraction. Although the mutations described in calcium channel–related hypokalemic periodic paralysis lead to loss of function of the dihydropyridine receptor, the precise relationship between receptor function failure and the abnormal response of muscle fibers to insulin, consequent hypokalemia and weakness, remain unclear.

Primary hypokalemic periodic paralysis due to calcium channelopathy is an autosomal dominant disorder but is more common in males and has variable penetrance in females. Attacks of episodic weakness usually start by adolescence and invariably before the age of 30 years. They often occur at night, so that patients awake with weakness. Attacks may be precipitated by carbohydrate or alcohol intake, rest after exercise, or emotional stress. The frequency of attacks is generally less than that seen in hyperkalemic periodic paralysis and can vary from daily or only one or two in a lifetime. Typically, attacks last between 1 and 4 hours, but occasionally they can persist for up to 3 days. Prodromal symptoms of muscle stiffness, heavy limbs, or sweating may occur followed by proximal lower limb weakness that spreads to tetraparesis. There is rarely ocular or bulbar involvement. Fatalities are rare and usually result from injudicious treatment, especially in the case of hypokalemia-induced cardiac arrhythmias. Oliguria is typical during attacks and results from the sequestration of water intracellularly.

In younger subjects the only detectable interictal abnormality is eyelid myotonia, seen in approximately 50 percent of patients. In older subjects, attacks frequently decrease, but patients may have persistent weakness. During severe attacks, patients are flaccid, paralyzed, and areflexic.

POTASSIUM CHANNELOPATHIES

One publication has described mutations in a potassium gene *KCNE3* on chromosome 11q, coding for a auxiliary subunit of the Kv3.4 potassium channel, occurring in two families with periodic paralysis. The periodic paralysis appeared to be hypokalemic in one of the families and hyperkalemic in the other.[11] In addition, Andersen's syndrome with a triad of periodic paralysis, cardiac arrhythmias, and dysmorphic features is a potassium channelopathy. Not only is periodic paralysis known to result from a channelopathy, but so are ventricular arrhythmias, as evidenced by the proven channel mutations seen in long QT syndromes. Thus it was suspected that Andersen's syndrome is also a channelopathy, but no linkage to the genes responsible for hypokalemic or hyperkalemic periodic paralysis or to the long QT syndromes has been found. Now the mutation has been described in a potassium channel gene. Thirteen out of 16 families with Andersen's syndrome have been shown to have mutations of the *KCNJ2* gene on 17q coding for the Kir 2.1 potassium channel with expression studies confirming the pathophysiological effects of these mutations.[12] Of interest is the recognition that fixed skeletal defects such as seen in Andersen's syndrome may result from channel gene mutations. Heretofore, the main effects of channelopathies appeared to be restricted to excitable tissues (e.g., muscle and nerve).

Potassium channelopathies can present as episodic weakness in association with hypokalemia, hyperkalemia, or Andersen's syndrome. The periodic paralysis of Andersen's syndrome does not neatly fit into the hypo- or hyperkalemic classification. During attacks of periodic paralysis, the potassium may rise, fall, or remain normal in these patients. The attacks may be provoked by either hyperkalemic or hypokalemic challenges or by neither. In some, the attacks have been unrecognized with the cardiac features being more prominent. Many cases show mild proximal weakness even between attacks. Cardiac involvement can be severe and result in episodes of syncope or cardiac arrest. A variety of ventricular arrhythmias may occur including a long QTc interval and bidirectional ventricular tachycardia, but at times the electrocardiogram (ECG) is normal. Asymptomatic family members, however, may harbor a long QTc interval and be at risk of cardiac arrhythmia. The dysmorphic features of Andersen's syndrome are subtle and often need an index of suspicion for recognition. They may include facial features of broad forehead and nose low-set ears, small mouth and jaw, a broad neck, and hand features such as clinodactyly or syndactyly.[13]

POSSIBLE MUSCLE CHANNELOPATHY: SCHWARTZ-JAMPEL SYNDROME

Schwartz-Jampel syndrome (SJS) is a rare autosomal recessive myotonic disorder with an unknown etiology. Previously described autosomal dominant cases of SJS probably have a sodium channel mutation and represent cases of myotonia permanans.[8] Autosomal recessive SJS is genetically heterogenous, with some cases having mutations in the *HSPG2* gene on chromosome 1p35–36.1.[14, 15] This gene encodes for perlecan, a ubiquitous protein that constitutes 50 percent of the extracellular matrix of all tissues. It is speculated that loss of function mutations in perlecan result in abnormal development of cartilage and also affect muscle excitability perhaps because there is faulty distribution of acetylcholinesterase.[14]

Symptom onset is before age 3, with severe continuous motor activity and muscle stiffness particularly in the face and in the thighs. Patients have an unusual masklike face with blepharospasm and continuous motor activity of the chin and lips. Hypertrophy of the thigh muscles occurs. They have radiological evidence of osteochondrodysplasia, often resulting in reduced stature, kyphoscoliosis, bowing of the diaphyses, and irregular epiphyses.[16] When all the preceding features are present, then mutations in the perlecan gene are more likely to be found. This is not the case with neonatal onset or when osteochondrodysplasia is absent.[14]

Differential Diagnosis

MYOTONIA. The principle symptom of myotonia is that of muscle stiffness and an inability to relax contracted muscle. In most cases, myotonia is painless, although occasionally sodium channel–related myotonia causes discomfort. Stiffness can be confused with spasticity or rigidity. Muscle cramps are often a feature of a peripheral nerve disorder and are readily differentiated on electromyography (EMG). Dystonia results in abnormal posture and is the result of abnormal discharge of whole motor units rather than individual muscle fibers. Painless, electrically silent contractures may be a feature of metabolic myopathy such as McArdles' disease. Pseudomyotonia or impaired muscle relaxation without electrical evidence of myotonia occurs in acid maltase deficiency and Brody's disease. True myotonia may be part of a generalized disorder as in dystrophia myotonia, but in such disorders myotonia is not usually the presenting symptom. The different nondystrophic myotonias are usually distinguished clinically, but sometimes gene analysis is needed to come to a final diagnosis.

PERIODIC PARALYSIS. The differential diagnosis of periodic paralysis must include other causes of a flaccid areflexic tetraparesis without sensory signs. Metabolic causes such as hypercalcemia, hypocalcemia, hypophosphatemia, hypomagnesemia, and rhabdomyolysis need to be excluded. Diseases such as Guillain-Barré syndrome, myasthenic syndromes, and acute poliomyelitis can also produce a similar clinical picture. In many cases, the history and associated features will point to the correct diagnosis. Secondary hypokalemic periodic paralysis usually results from intracellular potassium depletion from either renal, endocrine, gastrointestinal, or drug-induced mechanisms (Table 37–2). Usually these underlying conditions are obvious, but in less clear cases the recurrent episodes of transient weakness can be difficult to distinguish from primary hypokalemic periodic paralysis. Late-onset hypokalemic periodic paralysis raises strong suspicions of secondary rather than primary periodic paralysis. Thyrotoxic periodic paralysis results from alteration of muscle membrane permeability and is much more prevalent in Japanese, Chinese, and other Asian populations, though it occurs in Caucasians. The clinical presentation is often indistinguishable from hypokalemic periodic paralysis but with the additional, sometimes subtle, evidence of hyperthyroidism.[17] Paralytic episodes may precede the occurrence of any other clinical feature of hyperthyroidism.

Evaluation of Channelopathies

MYOTONIA. Creatine kinase (CK) is usually normal, but there may be two- to fivefold elevations in Thomsen's and Becker's diseases, perhaps reflecting the degree of muscle hypertrophy. EMG shows spontaneous myotonic discharges, but in paramyotonia congenita, provocation by cooling of the examined limb may be required to demonstrate this phenomenon. There is also decrement in the compound motor action potential (CMAP) with exercise or with high-frequency 30-Hz stimulation, particularly in cases of myotonia congenita.[18, 19] The decrement in the CMAP is particularly marked in Becker's disease, and this is presumably the cause of the transient weakness seen in that condition.[19] In Schwartz-Jampel syndrome the EMG shows continuous spontaneous motor activity with little of the fluctuation of the frequency and amplitude that is seen with other myotonias and may be myogenic or neurogenic in origin. In phenotypically similar cases where the electrical activity does more closely resemble myotonia, the diagnosis may be that of myotonia permanans.[8] Muscle biopsy may show little abnormality. Variation in fiber size with fiber hypertrophy and increased central nuclei may be found. In paramyotonia congenita with hyperkalemic periodic paralysis, vacuolated fibers and necrotic fibers may be seen. In myotonia congenita there may be a lack of 2B fibers. Study of family members may be valuable since there may be clinical or EMG evidence of disease in apparently asymptomatic individuals, which clarifies the mode of inheritance.

PERIODIC PARALYSIS. During an episode of weakness, serial blood tests should be taken for potassium, calcium, magnesium, phosphate, and CK to exclude the other previously mentioned causes of weakness. Since the potassium level may be normal during hyperkalemic periodic paralysis and occasionally in hypokalemic periodic paralysis, the potassium level needs to be checked sequentially every 15 to 30 minutes in order to determine the direction of change at a time when muscle strength is either worsening or improving. An ECG may show changes consistent with hypo- or hyperkalemia and may also forewarn of cardiac complications. EMG shows reduced CMAP proportionate to the degree of weakness. Nerve conduction studies are normal. The neurophysiology also serves to exclude other causes of paralysis such as the Guillain-Barré syndrome or myasthenia gravis.

Patients who are seen between attacks need investigation to exclude causes of secondary hypokalemia. EMG may be helpful in showing evidence of myotonia, which would favor hyperkalemic periodic paralysis. In those patients in whom fixed weakness has developed, the EMG may be myopathic. Even in those with an initially normal EMG, there may be a exaggerated increment followed by decline of the CMAP with high-frequency 30-Hz stimulation or following repetitive muscle contraction.[20] Muscle biopsy is often abnormal between attacks of hypokalemic periodic paralysis with pathognomonic changes of large central vacuoles and occasional necrotic fibers. In hyperkalemic periodic paralysis, smaller vacuoles may be present and tubular aggregates may be seen. Provocative testing may be required to confirm the diagnosis. This must be performed with careful supervision, including monitoring of the potassium and the ECG. Hypokalemic challenge can be performed by giving intravenous glucose with or without insulin.[21] Hyperkalemic challenge can be performed by giving repeated doses of oral potassium.[21] Where available, genetic testing may be the preferred investigation, but its effectiveness depends on the screening strategy employed.

Management of Channelopathies

MYOTONIA. Myotonia can be exacerbated by some muscle relaxant drugs and by anticholinesterase drugs, and anesthesia for these patients needs to be planned accordingly. Potassium administration can exacerbate myotonia, and thus potassium supplementation should only be given where necessary and with caution. The treatment of myotonia congenita relies on membrane-stabilizing drugs such as procainamide and quinine; these can be used intermittently on an as-needed basis. Phenytoin is more useful for chronic

TABLE 37–2. Secondary Causes of Hypokalemic Periodic Paralysis

Endocrine
Primary hyperaldosteronism (Conn's syndrome)
Thyrotoxic periodic paralysis

Renal
Juxtaglomerular apparatus hyperplasia (Bartter's syndrome)
Renal tubular acidosis
Fanconi's syndrome

Gastrointestinal
Laxative abuse
Villous adenoma
Gastrointestinal fistula

Drug-Induced
Amphotericin B
Licorice
Corticosteroids
p-Aminosalicylic acid
Carbenoxalone
Potassium-depleting diuretics

administration and is less likely to have cardiac side effects. Occasional cases of myotonia are responsive to acetazolamide, and mexiletine is useful for both the myotonia and the weakness associated with paramyotonia congenita.

PERIODIC PARALYSIS. Attacks of hypokalemic periodic paralysis may be partially prevented by a low-carbohydrate and low-sodium diet. Where hypokalemic periodic paralysis is secondary to thyrotoxicosis, this needs to be treated. In the interim the paralytic attacks and persistent weakness can be very effectively treated with β-adrenergic blocking agents. During acute attacks, emergency treatment may be required, but the preference is very much in favor of oral potassium since potassium concentration usually declines with parenteral potassium because of the diluents employed. The ECG should be carefully monitored during attacks for cardiac arrhythmias.

In hyperkalemic periodic paralysis, attacks are usually mild but are still worth treating to prevent the onset of permanent weakness. Thiazide diuretics are effective treatment. During acute attacks, treatment is seldom needed, but carbohydrate-containing food and fluid may aggravate the weakness and potassium-containing foods should be avoided. Inhaled β-adrenergic agonists such as salbutamol are effective treatments but may be contraindicated if there is a co-existing cardiac arrhythmia.

Both acetazolamide and dichlorphenamide can prevent paralytic attacks and may improve residual weakness between attacks.[22]

Congenital Myopathies

Pathogenesis and Pathophysiology. The initial definition of the congenital myopathies implied the onset at birth of a nonprogressive primary myopathy that could not be explained on the basis of a dystrophic or metabolic abnormality. However, in some morphologically and genetically identical cases, symptoms are not present at birth and are of later onset. Furthermore, some cases of congenital myopathies such as nemaline myopathy and centronuclear myopathy show progressive weakness with a fatal outcome. The assumption that all of these congenital myopathies have no metabolic basis reflected ignorance as to their etiology. The various congenital myopathies continued to be diagnosed in most instances on the basis of their morphological characteristics as seen in muscle biopsy. In some of these, there is a large body of literature that defines a clear phenotype, but in others only one or two case reports have been described, and the lack of morphological specificity casts doubt on their validity as separate disease entities. The recent descriptions of the gene lesion for most of the disorders are rapidly changing their classification.

Epidemiology. All of the congenital myopathies are rare with an incidence of less than 1 per 100,000.

Clinical Features. The diagnostic label itself implies that there is muscle weakness present at birth, but some of them are of late childhood or adult onset, as specified in the following sections. Presentation may be in utero with reduced fetal movements. There may be delayed second stage of labor and a higher incidence of assisted delivery with its consequent complications resulting from fetal hypotonia. The most common presentation is that of a floppy baby who has delayed motor milestones. In school these individuals usually have difficulty in keeping up with their peers, either in sporting activities or simply in running or walking. Early weakness may manifest as difficulty rising from a chair or the floor and in managing stairs. In some congenital myopathies, as specified in the following sections, there is facial weakness and ophthalmoplegia. The muscle weakness can give rise to skeletal defects causing dysmorphic features, kyphoscoliosis, and pes cavus. Diaphragmatic or chest wall involvement can give rise to respiratory weakness with carbon dioxide retention, particularly at night, causing morning headaches or daytime somnolescence. Such respiratory weakness is usually a late feature in the congenital myopathies, but nemaline myopathy is a notable exception for its early onset. As a rule the congenital myopathies are stable or only slowly progressive, and many patients are remarkably active despite their weakness. Specific clinical features of the individual congenital myopathies will be highlighted, and differential diagnosis, evaluation, and management will be considered collectively afterward.

NEMALINE MYOPATHY

This particular congenital myopathy is defined on the basis of the presence of rods in the muscle biopsy. These are seen as red-staining structures using the Gomori trichrome stain, and it is their threadlike appearance that gives this condition its name, *nema* being Greek for thread.

The usual picture is one of mild and progressive myopathy present from birth. However, there are some more severely affected individuals, with early fatalities. In addition some adult-onset cases appear to have profuse rods on muscle biopsy but without the usual clinical phenotype. Typical cases usually have generalized reduction of muscle bulk, generalized limb weakness, mild facial weakness but no ocular involvement. Cardiac involvement is unusual. The facial appearance is characteristic with high arched palate and a long thin face. Respiratory failure due to involvement of the diaphragm is an early feature that can have a major impact on the prognosis.

Electron microscopy shows that the rods represent an abnormal deposition of Z band material. The etiology of this and its relevance to the subsequent development of nemaline myopathy is unknown. Rods are not exclusive to nemaline myopathy and can be seen as an occasional feature in other muscle disorders, including polymyositis, HIV-related myopathy, and in muscle injured by tenotomy. There are many sporadic cases, but autosomal dominant cases have shown mutations of the a tropomyosin (*TPM3*) on chromosome lq21,[23] and autosomal recessive cases and some sporadic cases have shown mutations of three further genes, including the nebulin gene on chromosome 2q21–22,[24] the skeletal muscle alpha-actin gene (*ACTA 1*) on chromosome 19q42,[25] and the slow skeletal muscle troponin T gene (*TNNT1*) on chromosome 19q13.4.[26] The last of these mutations was found in a form of nemaline myopathy common in the Amish population. Other genes will undoubtedly be found as cases of nemaline myopathy exist that show no linkage to any of these chromosome loci.

MYOTUBULAR/CENTRONUCLEAR MYOPATHY

The key morphological abnormality is the presence of central nuclei that occupy between 25 to 80 percent of the muscle fibers, more often in the type 1 fibers, which usually predominate. There is often a halo around the central nuclei, which shows increased oxidative enzyme activity and glycogen staining with reduced amounts of ATPase staining. The original term, *myotubular myopathy*, was based on the resemblance of these morphological abnormalities to that of myotubules. The later and preferred term of *centronuclear myopathy* is more descriptive and avoids assumptions about the etiology of the abnormality.

Prominent ptosis and ophthalmoplegia distinguish this disease from the other congenital myopathies. Cardiac involvement is not common. A variety of skeletal malformations occur, resulting in a Marfanoid habitus with a long narrow face and high arched palate. A more severe X-linked variety is recognized with in utero and neonatal presentation and severe generalized weakness with bulbar and respiratory involvement but less ptosis and ophthalmoparesis.[27] With intensive initial support some improvement may occur, but patients remain severely disabled and prone to sudden death due to aspiration. A late childhood- or adult-onset variant is seen, which presents with mild limb weakness without ptosis, ophthalmoparesis, or dysmorphic features.

Because of the resemblance to myotubules, these diseases are felt to represent a maturational arrest with failure of the normal peripheral migration of nuclei during differentiation. However, the morphological similarities with myotubules are only superficial, and central nuclei can appear after infancy. Many of these cases are hereditary, and autosomal recessive, autosomal dominant, and X-linked varieties have been described. The X-linked variety has been shown to be due to mutations in the myotubularin gene (*MTM1*) with the number of known mutations into triple figures, although three mutations occur in 17 percent of X-linked cases.[28]

CENTRAL CORE DISEASE

In this disorder, the key morphological abnormality is the presence of central or eccentric cores that do not stain for glycogen or oxidative enzymes but sometimes for ATPase. The cores have a predilection for type 1 fibers that are the predominant fiber type on biopsy.

Distinguishing clinical features of central core disease are the lack of cranial involvement, apart from occasional mild facial weakness, the frequency of congenital dislocation of the hip, and the occasional co-existence of malignant hyperthermia. Anesthetic precautions are required to avoid the risk of hyperthermic crises in this disease.

The etiology is unknown. The resemblance of cores to target fibers suggests that central core disease may be a disorder of innervation. Cases are autosomal dominant or occasionally sporadic. This disease may be allelic, with malignant hyperthermia also having point mutations of the ryanodine receptor on chromosome 19q13.1.[29]

OTHER CONGENITAL MYOPATHIES

There are a variety of other morphological abnormalities that have been described in cases with a presentation typical of congenital myopathy with names to match: minicore, multicore, finger print body, zebra body, sarcotubular, and hyaline body myopathies. There are too few case reports of these myopathies to discern a distinctive or diagnostic phenotype for each and to be sure that each necessarily represents distinct myopathy.

CONGENITAL FIBER-TYPE DISPROPORTION

This description arose from a survey of congenital myopathies by Brooke who found several subjects in whom the type 1 fibers were at least 12 percent smaller than the type 2 fibers.[30] This finding was isolated in some cases; in others it co-existed with other more striking pathological abnormalities. Later workers have suggested a tightening of the pathological criteria to include normal or increased size of type 2 fibers so that this diagnosis can be separated from mild spinal muscular atrophy.[31] Even with these requirements, there remains considerable doubt as to whether this entity represents a distinct form of congenital myopathy.

There are no specific clinical features to define the condition, and the severity can be quite variable. Initially it was suggested that these pathological appearances had some prognostic value in that all the cases in Brooke's original series showed no progression of their weakness beyond 2 years of age, and some even improved. This pattern, however, has not been borne out by subsequent studies. No specific pathophysiological explanation has been advanced for the pathological picture, and there is no genetic marker for it.

Differential Diagnosis of Congenital Myopathies. The differential diagnosis of congenital myopathy includes all causes of a floppy infant including central, neurogenic, and myopathic. The neurogenic causes are usually central, although hereditary neuropathies causing dysmyelination or hypomyelination and anterior horn disease also present similarly. CNS disorders may show upper motor neuron features, seizures, or intellectual impairment, but recognition of some of these features may be difficult. Of the myopathic causes, a distinction needs to be made between the congenital muscular dystrophies, congenital myotonic dystrophy, congenital myasthenia (see later discussion), and the metabolic myopathies.

Evaluation of Congenital Myopathies. CK level is normal or only mildly elevated, in distinct contrast to many early-onset muscular dystrophies. Neurophysiology tests allow exclusion of the neuropathies and myasthenias. Nerve conduction studies are normal, and the EMG may show mild nonspecific myopathic features. The definitive diagnosis of a congenital myopathy rests on the morphological characteristics seen at muscle biopsy. These morphological abnormalities need to be present in reasonable number in order to make the diagnosis, as any of them may be nonspecific findings in other neuromuscular disorders. In some cases of congenital myopathy, the muscle biopsy may show only minor nonspecific myopathic features. This pattern may reflect a selectivity of muscle involvement, and when other causes have been excluded, a label of "nonspecific congenital myopathy" may be applied.

Management. There is no specific treatment for any of the congenital myopathies. The association of central core disease with malignant hyperthermia make it prudent to avoid precipitating factors (see later discussion). Otherwise the management of the congenital myopathies is supportive, with particular regard to the prevention of secondary complications such as contractures and progressive kyphoscoliosis. Bracing may be an effective means of maintaining ambulation but is usually unsatisfactory. Respiratory and cardiac function needs to be regularly assessed and appropriate support given.

Congenital Myasthenias

The onset of myasthenic symptoms at birth, especially in the presence of a family history, makes congenital forms of myasthenia a diagnostic possibility. With the advent of the acetylcholine receptor (AChR) and calcium channel antibody tests as markers for myasthenia gravis and Lambert-Eaton myasthenia, it has become apparent that congenital myasthenia, like the congenital myopathies, may also present later in life, and at times without a family history.

Pathogenesis and Pathophysiology. Congenital defects of the neuromuscular junction can be divided into presynaptic, synaptic, and postsynaptic defects (Table 37–3). Presynaptic defects include defects in the synthesis of acetylcholine or in the packaging of acetylcholine into the presynaptic vesicles, thereby reducing the amount of acetylcholine available for release. Synaptic defects include deficiency of acetylcholinesterase. Postsynaptic defects consist of abnormal function or altered numbers of acetylcholine receptors. Not all of the congenital myasthenic syndromes have a well-defined cause. Some appear to be sporadic, but, of the inherited cases, autosomal recessive inheritance is most common. The slow channel syndrome is inherited as an autosomal dominant.

TABLE 37–3. **Classification of the Congenital Myasthenias**

Preynaptic Defects
Defect of ACh resynthesis or packaging
Paucity of synaptic vesicles and reduced quantal release

Pre- and Postsynaptic Defects
Endplate AChE deficiency

Postsynaptic Defects
Kinetic abnormalities of AChR with AChR deficiency
- Classic slow channel syndrome
- Epsilon subunit mutations
- AChR deficiency and short channel open time

Kinetic abnormalities of AChR without AChR deficiency
- High-conductance fast channel syndrome
- Syndrome attributed to abnormal interaction of ACh with AChR

Partially Characterized Syndromes
Other AChR deficiencies
Congenital myasthenic syndrome resembling LEMS
Congenital myasthenic syndrome with facial malformations
Familial limb girdle myasthenia

ACh, Acetylcholine; AChE, acetylcholinesterase; AChR, acetylcholine receptor; LEMS, Lambert-Eaton myasthenic syndrome.

Epidemiology and Risk Factors. Precise incidence figures are not available, but the congenital myasthenias represent a minority of patients with myasthenia, making them rare diseases. There are undoubtedly cases of myasthenia that mistakenly remain undiagnosed as congenital when presumed to be serologically negative cases of autoimmune myasthenia, particularly when they respond well to anticholinesterase treatment.

Clinical Features. Only the broad clinical features of the congenital myasthenias will be described here. The individual syndromes are listed in Table 37–3, and further detail can be found in several reviews.[32–34] The presentation of congenital myasthenias can be similar to that of congenital myopathies, with a floppy baby, showing difficulties with feeding, delayed motor milestones, and persistent or sometimes progressive limb weakness. Skeletal abnormalities can result from this weakness. Ocular, bulbar, and respiratory weakness may occur, but some of the syndromes are notable for lack of ocular involvement. Other syndromes characteristically have a later onset, typically in the second or third decade. The distinguishing feature of the weakness is its fluctuating nature, usually worsening with activity such as feeding, crying, or moving. With some of the myasthenic syndromes, episodic exacerbations occur with fever, with emotional upset, or for no obvious reason. The autosomal recessive inheritance of most of these syndromes means that there may not be a family history. Examination is characterized by fatigable weakness. Fixed weakness is usually generalized, but very selective weakness is described. Delayed pupillary responses occur in some cases. Reflexes are generally but not invariably preserved.

Differential Diagnosis. The differential diagnosis is the same as that for congenital myopathies. Clinical distinction from mitochondrial myopathy may be difficult as the latter can also present with fatigable weakness. Neonatal botulism needs to be excluded. Once the diagnosis of a myasthenic syndrome has been made, differentiating congenital from acquired autoimmune myasthenia may be required, particularly in late-onset cases lacking a family history. Neonatal myasthenia from passive placental transfer of AChR antibodies usually occurs in the offspring of obviously affected AChR antibody-positive mothers.

Evaluation. A positive AChR antibody test excludes congenital myasthenia, but because there are cases of AChR antibody-negative myasthenia gravis, a negative test is not specifically diagnostic. A positive edrophonium test confirms a myasthenic syndrome but does not differentiate congenital myasthenia from myasthenia gravis. A negative test occurs in some cases of congenital myasthenia when there is a deficiency of acetylcholinesterase. EMG studies may show a decrement in the compound muscle action potential to repetitive stimulation but at 10 Hz rather than the usual 3 Hz. Single-fiber EMG may show excess jitter and blocking. Morphological, immunostaining, and immunochemical techniques and in vitro neurophysiological analysis on intercostal muscle containing motor endplates are research methods for confirming and characterizing the nature of a congenital myasthenia.[32, 34] Genetic analysis may show mutations of genes encoding for subunits of AChR.[32]

Management. Respiratory and bulbar complications require appropriate supportive measures. Depending on the precise nature of the congenital myasthenia, some cases may respond to chronic anticholinesterase treatment. Those who do not respond to anticholinesterase therapy may gain benefit from treatment with 3,4, diaminopyridine.[35]

Malignant Hyperthermia

Malignant hyperthermias are hereditary skeletal muscle diseases, characterized by a hypercatabolic reaction of muscle to anesthetic agents or to physical or emotional stress.

Pathogenesis and Pathophysiology. The central event appears to be an increase in the calcium concentration that results in continuous activation of the actin-myosin contraction apparatus and sustained muscle contraction. This increase in calcium level is due to an increased release of calcium from the sarcoplasmic reticulum of the muscle together with a reduction in calcium reuptake. The continuous muscle activity results in muscle rigidity, muscle necrosis, hyperpyrexia, and hypermetabolism. Linkage has been found to chromosome 19q13.1. A ryanodine receptor gene in this region has been shown to have mutations in 50 percent of cases.[29] The ryanodine receptor is a calcium-release channel involved in calcium homeostasis. Linkage has also been found to chromosomes 7q and 3q and to chromosome 17q1.2–24, which codes for the α-subunit of the sodium channel.[36, 37]

Epidemiology. Malignant hyperthermia has a worldwide distribution with an incidence in 1 in 12,000 anesthetic incidents in children and 1 in 50,000 anesthetic events in adults.[38] However, many mild cases likely go unrecognized and are mistaken as other anesthetic complications. Males are more affected than females and there is a peak incidence at age 30 years. Thereafter, the incidence declines such that cases are virtually unheard of beyond the age of 75 years.[38]

Clinical Features. The most common precipitating event is that of halothane general anesthesia. The muscle relaxant succinylcholine is a milder trigger of attacks when used alone, but a more potent one when combined with halothane. The likelihood of triggering an attack with these agents is increased if the patient has been exercising vigorously beforehand or is under stress at the time of anesthetic induction.

In between attacks of malignant hyperthermia, patients rarely have any muscle symptoms, though some muscle diseases are associated with attacks of malignant hyperthermia (see later discussion). In 50 percent of cases, patients may have had previous anesthesia without any complications.[38] Attacks start often with jaw spasm followed by generalized muscle spasm and rigidity. Associated findings include hyperventilation, tachycardia, and an unstable blood pressure. A mottled, flushed, and cyanotic skin rash may appear, and after an interval of 15 to 16 minutes, the body temperature may start to rise precipitously. Metabolic and respiratory acidosis, hypoxemia, generalized vasoconstriction, and an increased cardiac output occur. The serum potassium may rise and the CK may increase a hundredfold. Consequent complications of myoglobinuria and disseminated intravascular coagulation may occur, leading to renal failure. During recovery, patients may have a further relapse.

Differential Diagnosis. The condition most closely resembling malignant hyperthermia is the neuroleptic malignant syndrome, an abnormal response to dopamine blocking agents. Patients develop rigidity with hyperthermia and share many of the biochemical features seen in malignant hyperthermia. Neuroleptic malignant syndrome usually occurs in the setting of psychiatric disease with the use of neuroleptic drug treatment. Acute dystonic reactions to drugs such as neuroleptics or antiemetics can produce a similar picture of rigidity. Patients with myotonia may develop rigidity with depolarizing agents during anesthetic induction.

Evaluation. During the acute illness, the main emphasis of the evaluation is monitoring possible hyperkalemia and cardiac, respiratory, and renal complications so that appropriate measures can be taken. Evaluation of well patients thought to be at risk of developing malignant hyperthermia can be difficult. Only a few have a raised CK. The genetic heterogeneity and the fact that even the recognized point mutations only cover a small percentage of the patients at risk limit the value of genetic testing. A variety of in vivo tests have been purported to highlight at-risk individuals, but these are not particularly reliable. The recognized screening test is the in vitro caffeine and halothane contracture test, which detects an exaggerated response to caffeine or halothane in freshly isolated muscle. This test is performed only in specialized centers, and even this test shows overlap between normal and affected individuals, causing false-positive readings.[39]

Management. Preventive measures include the avoidance of precipitating agents, namely halothane and succinylcholine, but many other agents have some risk in susceptible subjects. Patients with known malignant hyperthermia should be advised to wear medical alert bracelets to warn of their susceptibility. Narcotics, barbiturates, benzodiazepines, nitrous oxide, and nondepolarizing muscle relaxants are generally safe to use. Acute management consists of the removal of the triggering agents and supportive measures as required. Body cooling may be required in response to the hyperthermia that aggravates the metabolic derangement. Dantrolene is the mainstay of treatment and, when given intravenously, results in reversal of the abnormalities. Mortality has dropped since its regular use.

Prognosis. The improved recognition of this complication, better supportive measures, and widespead availability of dantrolene have resulted in a dramatic drop in mortality from 65 percent to 2 percent.

Brody's Disease

This disorder, first described by Brody in 1969,[40] clinically resembles myotonia, but the EMG of affected muscle does not show any myotonic discharges.

Pathogenesis and Pathophysiology. The pseudomyotonia is thought to be the result of abnormalities in sarcoplasmic reticulum Ca^{2+} ATPase, a transmembrane protein responsible for extruding calcium out of the cytoplasm and into the sarcoplasmic reticulum. This 100-kD protein is coded on chromosome 16 and is deficient in amount or activity, particularly in the type 2 muscle fibers.[41] Genetic heterogeneity was suggested by reports of variable patterns of inheritance, including autosomal dominant, recessive, and X-linked. This heterogeneity has been confirmed by the fact that some cases with recessive inheritance have mutations in the *ATP2A1* gene encoding SERCA1, the fast-twitch skeletal muscle sarcoplasmic reticulum Ca^{2+} ATPase, whereas others do not.[42–45]

Epidemiology. This is a rare disorder and only about 20 cases have been recorded in the literature.[41]

Clinical Features. The disease usually begins in childhood. Patients often have difficulty in keeping up with their peers in physical activities. They develop poor relaxation of muscles, initially in the limbs, but then in the face and the trunk. This pseudomyotonia is worsened by exercise and cold weather. In some myoglobinuria occurs. On examination they have eyelid and grip, but not percussion, myotonia. There may be mild muscle atrophy and weakness in the final stages of the disease.

Differential Diagnosis. The differential diagnosis of Brody's disease is that of myotonia and pseudomyotonia as detailed for the preceding myotonias.

Evaluation. CK may be normal or slightly elevated, particularly in patients with associated myoglobinuria. Muscle biopsy shows type 2 A and B atrophy with angulated fibers. EMG shows electrical silence during the time of apparent myotonia. Biochemical and immunological assays of sarcoplasmic reticulum Ca^{2+} ATPase may be employed to make the diagnosis.

Management. Empirical treatment with dantrolene and calcium channel blockers has been used with varying success.

Prognosis. The disease is slowly progressive or stationary over years, but in some individuals exercise-induced pseudomyotonia worsens as they get older.

Familial Amyloid Polyneuropathy

In amyloidosis, extracellular deposition of amyloid occurs in a variety of organs such as the heart, intestinal tract, liver, and kidneys. In amyloid neuropathy, the peripheral nerve deposition predominates. Amyloid neuropathy may be due to acquired, usually immunoglobin-derived, amyloid, or it may be hereditary, as in familial amyloid polyneuropathy. Amyloid is a class of glycoproteins that have a fibrillar β sheet structure likely derived from a variety of precursor proteins. In familial amyloid polyneuropathy (FAP) the dominant form of amyloid is derived from transthyretin (TTR), but amyloid formed from apolipoprotein A1 and gelosin is also seen. Initially, FAP was described on a clinical basis with four types recognized. Despite overlap with the increasing discoveries of specific mutations, this original classification is still useful (Table 37–4).

Pathogenesis and Pathophysiology. All of these amyloid neuropathies result from the deposition of amyloid, derived from various precurser proteins, within the substance of the nerve. To date, 80 mutations of the TTR gene have been described as well as mutations of the apolipoprotein A1 and gelosin protein genes. All are autosomal dominant conditions with reduced penetrance. Most individuals are heterozygous for the given mutation. Some homozygous individuals for the *Met 30* TTR mutation have been described but without any difference in the clinical phenotype from the heterozygous individuals. The *Met 30* mutation has arisen spontaneously in different parts of the world.[46] By contrast the *Ala 60* TTR mutation, which was first described in a family in the Appalachian region, has been found to be due to a founder effect with its origin in Ireland.[47]

The deposition of amyloid may occur within the nerve without being derived from circulating amyloid. In the TTR-associated FAP with the *Met 30* mutation, axonal loss occurs first in the small and later in the large unmyelinated fibers. Although axonal degeneration is the predominant pathological finding, there is also evidence of segmental demyelination. The amyloid may be either diffusely or patchily distributed, making a standard distal nerve biopsy of little diagnostic value in cases with involvement restricted to proximal nerves. Amyloid deposition can occur in the connective tissue of the peripheral nerves, in the endoneurial tissue, and in the vasa nervorum.

The mechanism by which amyloid deposition leads to neuropathy is unclear. Some have argued that the neuropathy results from a generalized metabolic disorder and that amyloid deposition is a secondary event. Deposition within the endoneurial vessels might result in ischemic nerves but would not fully explain the selectivity of small fiber involvement. The endoneurial blood vessel deposition of amyloid might alter vascular permeability with consequent endoneurial edema, contributing to the compressive damage on the nerves. Compressive damage may also result from the deposition of amyloid in the connective tissue surrounding the peripheral nerve. Although the presence of segmental demyelination favors a compressive etiology, this finding is not the dominant feature of the disorder and so likely is not a primary mechanism of neuropathic change.

Epidemiology. The most common FAP is the TTR-associated form with a *Met 30* mutation described in 500 Portuguese families.[48] The gelosin-derived FAP has been described in 200 Finnish families.[48] By contrast, some FAP mutations have been confined to a single family.

TABLE 37–4. **Classification of Familial Amyloid Polyneuropathies (FAP)**

FAP Type	Clinical Phenotype	Amyloid Precursor	Common Mutation
Type 1 (Portuguese)	Lower limb neuropathy	Transthyretin	Met 30 (plus others)
(Irish/Appalachian)		Transthyretin	Ala 60
Type 2 (Indiana)	Upper limb neuropathy	Transthyretin	Ser 84, His 58 plus others
Type 3 (Iowa)	Lower limb neuropathy Nephropathy Gastric ulcers	Apolipoprotein A1	Arg 26
Type 4 (Finnish)	Cranial neuropathy Corneal dystrophy	Gelosin	Asp 187, Tyr 187

FAP TYPE 1 (PORTUGUESE)

TTR-derived FAP was originally described in Portugal but has now been found in a wide variety of countries, including Scandinavian and Mediterranean regions as well as North and South America and Japan. The age of onset varies with the ethnic origin; the Portuguese develop symptoms in their twenties and thirties, whereas the Swedes and the French generally develop symptoms in their late fifties. The initial symptom is painful dysesthesia with attacks of stabbing pain in the lower limbs. Early small fiber involvement causes loss of pain and temperature sensation, making patients prone to foot ulcers, osteomyelitis, Charcot joints, and trophic skin changes. The neuropathy slowly progresses with the eventual involvement of all nerve fiber types and all sensory modalities. Subsequent motor involvement results in muscle wasting and weakness with loss of reflexes. Months or years after lower limb involvement, the upper limbs can become impaired. Carpal tunnel syndrome may occur but is rarely a presenting feature. Autonomic neuropathy is frequent and can be severe with postural hypotension, impotence, gastrointestinal upset, urinary difficulties, and dry skin. Cardiac amyloid deposition may be asymptomatic but can result in arrrhythmias and either a restrictive or hypertrophic cardiomyopathy. Occasionally, renal involvement is severe.

The majority of cases with this clinical picture have the common TTR *Met 30* mutation, but there are a large number of other point mutations in the TTR gene that give rise to a similar clinical picture. The *Ala 60 Thr* TTR point mutation gives rise to an Irish/Appalachian variant of FAP with the distinguishing features of later onset (the sixth and seventh decade), prominent motor and large fiber sensory involvement, and more severe and symptomatic cardiac involvement.

FAP TYPE 2 (INDIANA)

This was originally described in families of Swiss origin in Indiana and families of German origin in Maryland. Patients present in middle life, commonly with bilateral carpal tunnel syndrome and vitreous opacities. Some patients, particularly men, may develop a mild and generalized neuropathy with motor features appearing first in the upper limbs then spreading to the lower limbs. Autonomic neuropathy can also occur. Regardless of its form, neuropathy is rarely disabling. Hepatosplenomegaly may occur. The vitreous abnormalities can cause severe visual impairment. The original cases had a *Ser 84* or *His 58* TTR point mutation, but a variety of other mutations have been described.[49, 50]

FAP TYPE 3 (IOWA)

This form of amyloidosis has many features in common with FAP type 1. Upper and lower extremities are affected, but usually carpal tunnel syndrome does not occur. The peripheral neuropathy can be severe, but the autonomic neuropathy is less prominent. Systemic signs include peptic ulceration and renal involvement that often results in hypertension and uremia. Amyloid deposition also occurs in the liver, adrenal glands, and testes. This type of FAP is associated with apolipoprotein Al–derived amyloid, and a substitution of arginine for glycine has been found in nucleotide 26 of the gene.

FAP TYPE 4 (FINNISH)

This form was first described in a Finnish family but has since been identified in Dutch, Japanese, and Irish-American families. Corneal dystrophy may begin in the fourth decade but is usually asymptomatic. A progressive cranial neuropathy then usually occurs with the facial nerve most frequently affected, although the trigeminal, hyperglossal, and vestibular nerves can also be involved. The facial skin becomes initially thickened and then atrophic. A mild generalized sensory and autonomic neuropathy ensues. Although cardiac deposition of amyloid occurs, patients only rarely have symptoms of cardiac disease. In this disorder, the amyloid precursor protein is gelosin, and two mutations have been described in this gene thus far.[51, 52]

Differential Diagnosis of FAP. Differential diagnosis of FAP varies with the presentation and is wider when there is no family history. Presentation with a painful distal mainly sensory neuropathy of small fiber type poses considerations of leprosy, diabetes, vasculitis, or paraneoplastic-associated neuropathies. Familial small fiber neuropathies include type 1 hereditary sensory neuropathy and the neuropathy associated with Tangier's disease. Presentation with carpal tunnel syndrome raises the diagnostic possibilities of hypothyroidism, diabetes, osteoarthritis, and acromegaly. Carpal tunnel syndrome may also occur in patients undergoing hemodialysis with deposition of β-microglobulin-derived amyloid. Presentation with prominent autonomic symptoms may require differentiation from other hereditary diseases such as familial dysautonomia (Riley-Day syndrome), dopamine β-hydroxylase deficiency, and Fabry's disease.

Evaluation of FAP. Hematological and biochemical tests may reflect hepatic, renal, or gastrointestinal infiltration with amyloid. In isolated cases of amyloid neuropathy, a careful search for monoclonal antibodies is required to exclude acquired amyloidosis. Urine and serum should be screened with special attention to γ-chains, the predominant monoclonal species.[48] ECG may show evidence of cardiac involvement, including heart block, other conduction defects, and widespread Q-wave and T-wave repolarization changes. Echocardiography may show either a restrictive or hypertrophic cardiomyopathy. Autonomic function tests may reveal abnormal responses of blood pressure and heart rate to postural change and other provocative measures. Neurophysiology studies show evidence of an axonal neuropathy, but in the early stages when only small diameter fibers are involved, sensory nerve actual potentials may be preserved. Sensory and motor conduction velocities are usually normal or only slightly reduced. EMG shows evidence of chronic partial denervation in long-standing cases. In FAP type 4, EMG shows evidence of both axonal degeneration and demyelination with slow nerve conduction velocities and prolonged distal motor latencies. The diagnosis of amyloid requires pathological demonstration of amyloid deposition detected by staining with Congo red and demonstrating the characteristic green birefringence with polarizing filters. Electromicroscopy can also demonstrate the characteristic fibrillar appearance of the protein. For biopsy, rectal tissue is the most accessible tissue to sample. Immunohistochemistry can usually characterize the nature of the amyloid, although there may be technical difficulties when only small amounts of amyloid are present. TTR antibody immunohistochemistry will be negative in some cases if TTR is not the precursor for the amyloid. It is also possible to detect variant TTR in the blood using autoimmune assay and enzyme-linked immunosorbent assay techniques. Screening for the common TTR mutations is available; if these tests are negative, but a high index of suspicion remains, sequencing the entire TTR gene may be justified.

Management. Treatment is supportive in terms of autonomic, renal, gastrointestinal, and vitreous complications. Plasma exchange intending to remove the circulating amyloid protein has not been successful. Because over 90 percent, of TTR is synthesized in the liver, some patients have undergone liver transplantation. This treatment is associated with a significant decline in the circulating TTR levels with some stabilization of symptoms, including those linked to neuropathy.[53] However, neurological benefit may not be accompanied by an arrest or slowing in the progression of the cardiomyopathy.[54] Liver transplantation remains a hazardous procedure particularly in those with autonomic involvement.[55,56] Mortality may reach 20 percent, usually in the first 6 months from infection and rejection. The risk/benefit ratio may be acceptable if performed early in the course of the disease.

Prognosis. The different forms of FAP vary in their prognosis. In FAP type 1, death from sepsis and systemic disease occurs about 15 years after onset; in late-onset cases, the disease progression may be slower. In FAP type 2, the peripheral neuropathy and the autonomic involvement are not severe, and individuals may survive as long as 35 years with only modest disability. However, the vitreous disposition may lead to severe visual loss. In FAP type 3, peripheral neuropathy becomes disabling over the course of 10 years, and death is the result of renal failure.

Future Perspectives. Further experience with liver transplantation will define the success rates and phenotypic features most predictive of good surgical outcome.

Giant Axonal Neuropathy

Most cases with this rare condition occur spontaneously, but occasional autosomal recessive inheritance has been documented.[57] Symptoms begin in childhood with a slowly progressive peripheral motor and sensory neuropathy. Patients often have very tight, curly black hair. There may be associated CNS involvement with intellectual impairment, optic atrophy, cerebellar ataxia, nystagmus, and corticospinal disturbance. Death usually occurs in adolescence. Investigations may show mildy reduced motor conduction velocities and sensory nerve action potentials. Diagnosis is made by nerve biopsy, where there is evidence of axonal loss with focal swellings along the nerve seen on electron microscopy to contain neurofilament accumulations.

Intermediate filaments in a variety of cell types suggest that the abnormality is not confined to axons and hair.[58] Decreases in disulfides and increases in thiol groups have been noted in hair samples from patients.[59] In some cases, mutations have been described in the giant axonal neuropathy gene (GAN) on chromosome 16q24.1 encoding for a novel, ubiquitously expressed cytoskeletal protein called gigaxonin.[60,61]

The differential diagnosis is that of an axonal neuropathy not necessarily having a family history but with the abnormal kinky hair being the distinguishing feature.

The management is supportive, there being no specific treatment.

Isaac's Disease

The hallmark of this disorder is neuromyotonia or hyperexcitability of peripheral nerves that result in spontaneous and continuous muscle electrical activity. Though some cases are inherited, the majority are acquired. The syndrome is rare, and assessment of its frequency and of its definitive clinical features is hampered by variable names given to it in the past.

Typical patients have muscle stiffness, cramps, and myokymia with some having generalized weakness and sweating. Onset can be any time during life, and the condition tends to be chronic. Motor features are most prominent in the limbs and trunk. Respiratory muscle involvement can cause breathing difficulties, and laryngeal involvement can cause stridor. Examination may reveal mild weakness with reduced or absent tendon reflexes and evidence of myokymia with occasional muscle hypertrophy as a result.

The continuous discharges may originate anywhere along the length of the peripheral nerve. The acquired autoimmune disease may be associated with antibodies against potassium channels.[62] In hereditary cases, there is a likely genetic defect in the potassium channel, an assumption clinically strengthened by the co-existence of myokymia in another condition with a well-established potassium channel defect, autosomal dominant episodic ataxia type I.[63]

Myokymia can arise from peripheral nerve damage. It is also a feature of autosomal dominant episodic ataxia type I. The features of cramps and stiffness raise the differential of Brody's disease, stiff person syndrome, and the myotonias.

EMG gives confirmation of the diagnosis in showing doublet, triplet, or multiple spontaneous motor unit discharges that may be present even in the absence of visible myokymia. Nerve and muscle biopsies show nonspecific features. In a few cases, oligoclonal IgG has been found in the CSF.[64]

Management. Anticonvulsant medications such as phenytoin and carbamazepine have been the primary treatment. Plasma exchange may be appropriate when an autoimmune etiology is considered probable. In some of these latter cases, immune suppression with corticosteroids and azathioprine has been tried.[64]

Reviews and Selected Updates

Chinnery PF, Walls TJ, Hanna MG, et al: Normokalemic periodic paralysis revisited: Does it exist? Ann Neurol 2002;52:251–252.

Dubowitz V: Muscle Disorders in Childhood, 2nd ed. London, WB Saunders, 1995.

Dyck PJ, Thomas PK: Peripheral Neuropathy. Philadelphia, WB Saunders, 1993.

Engel AG, Franzini-Armstrong C: Myology, 2nd ed. New York, McGraw-Hill, 1994.

Griggs RC, Mendell JR, Miller RG: Evaluation and Treatment of Myopathies. Philadelphia, F.A. Davis, 1995.

Karpati G, Hilton-Jones D, Griggs RC: Disorders of Voluntary Muscle, 7th ed. Cambridge, Cambridge University Press, 2001.

Mendell JR, Kissel JT, Cornblath DR: Diagnosis and Management of Peripheral Nerve Disorders. Oxford, Oxford University Press, 2001.

Rose MR, Griggs RC: Channelopathies of the Nervous System. Oxford, Butterworth Heinemann, 2001.

References

1. Ricker K, Koch MC, Lehmann-Horn F, et al: Proximal myotonic myopathy. Clinical features of a multisystem disorder similar to myotonic dystrophy. Arch Neurol 1995;52:25–31.
2. Ricker K, Koch MC, Lehmann-Horn F, et al: Proximal myotonic myopathy: A new dominant disorder with myotonia, muscle weakness, and cataracts. Neurology 1994;44:1448–1452.
3. Johnsen T: Familial periodic paralysis with hypokalaemia. Experimental and clinical investigations. Dan Med Bull 1981;28:1–27.
4. Becker PE: Myotonia Congenita and Syndromes Associated with Myotonia. Stuttgart, Thieme, 1977.
5. Jurkat-Rott K, Mitrovic N, Hang C, et al: Voltage-sensor sodium channel mutations cause hypokalemic periodic paralysis type 2 by enhanced inactivation and reduced current. Proc Natl Acad Sci USA 2000;97:9549–9554.
6. Ptacek LJ, Tawil R, Griggs RC, et al: Sodium channel mutations in acetazolamide-responsive myotonia congenita, paramyotonia congenita, and hyperkalemic periodic paralysis. Neurology 1994;44:1500–1503.
7. Ricker K, Moxley RT, Heine R, Lehmann-Horn F: Myotonia fluctuans. A third type of muscle sodium channel disease. Arch Neurol 1994;51:1095–1102.
8. Lerche H, Heine R, Pika U, et al: Human sodium channel myotonia: Slowed channel inactivation due to substitutions for a glycine within the III–IV linker. J Physiol 1993;470:13–22.
9. Zhang J, George AL, Griggs RC, et al: Mutations in the human skeletal muscle chloride channel gene (CLCN1) associated with dominant and recessive myotonia congenita. Neurology 1996;47:993–998.
10. Fouad G, Dalakas M, Servidei S, et al: Analysis of the DHP receptor α-1 subunit gene for mutations causing hypokalemic periodic paralysis. Neuromuscul Disord 1997;7:33–38.
11. Abbott GW, Sesti F, Splawski I, et al: MiRP2 forms potassium channels in skeletal muscle with Kv3.4 and is associated with periodic paralysis. Cell 2001;104:217–231.
12. Plaster NM, Tawil R, Tristani-Firouzi M, et al: Mutations in Kir2.1 cause the developmental and episodic electrical phenotypes of Andersen's syndrome. Cell 2001;105:511–519.
13. Sansone V, Griggs RC, Meola G, et al: Andersen's syndrome: A distinct periodic paralysis. Ann Neurol 1997;42:305–312.
14. Nicole S, Davoine CS, Topaloglu H, et al: Perlecan, the major proteoglycan of basement membranes, is altered in patients with Schwartz-Jampel syndrome (chondrodystrophic myotonia). Nat Genet 2000;26:480–483.
15. Fontaine B, Nicole S, Topaloglu H, et al: Recessive Schwartz-Jampel syndrome (SJS): Confirmation of linkage to chromosome 1p, evidence of genetic homogeneity and reduction of the SJS locus to a 3-cM interval. Hum Genet 1996;98:380–385.
16. Spaans F, Theunissen P, Reekers AD, Smit L, Veldman H: Schwartz-Jampel syndrome: I. Clinical, electromyographic, and histologic studies. Muscle Nerve 1990;13:516–527.
17. Griggs RC, Bender AN, Tawil R: A puzzling case of periodic paralysis. Muscle Nerve 1996;19:362–364.
18. Streib EW: AAEE minimonograph #27: Differential diagnosis of myotonic syndromes. Muscle Nerve 1987;10:603–615.
19. Aminoff MJ, Layzer RB, Satya-Murti S, Faden AI: The declining electrical response to muscle to repetitive nerve stimulation in myotonia. Neurology 1977;27:812–816.
20. McManis PG, Lambert EH, Daube JR: The exercise test in periodic paralysis. Muscle Nerve 1986;9:704–710.
21. Griggs RC, Mendell JR, Miller RG (eds): Evaluation and Treatment of Myopathies. Philadelphia, F.A. Davis, 1995.
22. Tawil R, McDermott MP, Brown R, et al: Randomized trials of dichlorphenamide in the periodic paralyses. Working Group on Periodic Paralysis. Ann Neurol 2000;47:46–53.
23. Laing NG, Wilton SD, Akkari PA, et al: A mutation in the alpha tropomyosin gene TPM3 associated with autosomal dominant nemaline myopathy. Nat Genet 1995;9:75–79.
24. Pelin K, Hilpela P, Donner K, et al: Mutations in the nebulin gene associated with autosomal recessive nemaline myopathy. Proc Natl Acad Sci 1999;96:2305–2310.
25. Nowak KJ, Wattanasirichaigoon D, Goebel HH, et al: Mutations in the skeletal muscle alpha-actin gene in patients with actin myopathy and nemaline myopathy. Nat Genet 1999;23:208–212.
26. Johnston JJ, Kelley RI, Crawford TO, et al: A novel nemaline myopathy in the Amish caused by a mutation in troponin T1. Am J Hum Genet 2000;67:814–821.
27. Barth PG, Van Wijngaarden GK, Bethlem J: X-linked myotubular myopathy with fatal neonatal asphyxia. Neurology 1975;25: 531–536.
28. Laporte J, Biancalana V, Tanner SM, et al: MTM1 mutations in X-linked myotubular myopathy. Hum Mutat 2000;15:393–409.
29. McCarthy TV, Quane KA, Lynch PJ: Ryanodine receptor mutations in malignant hyperthermia and central core disease. Hum Mutat 2000;15:410–417.
30. Brooke MH: Clinical studies in myology. *In* Kakulas BA (ed): Proceedings of the Second International Congress on Muscle Diseases. Perth, Australia. Amsterdam, Excerpta Medica, 1973.
31. Dubowitz V: Muscle Disorders in Childhood. London, WB Saunders, 1995.
32. Vincent A, Newland C, Croxen R, Beeson D: Genes at the junction—candidates for congenital myasthenic syndromes. Trends Neurosci 1997;20:15–22.
33. Middleton LT: Congenital myasthenic syndromes. Neuromusc Disord 1996;6:133–136.
34. Engel AC: Congenital myasthenic syndromes. *In* Engel AC, Franzini-Armstrong C (eds): Myology, New York, McGraw Hill, 1994, pp 1806–1835.
35. Palace J, Wiles CM, Newsom-Davis J: 3,4-Diaminopyridine in the treatment of congenital (hereditary) myasthenia. J Neurol Neurosurg Psychiatry 1991;54:1069–1072.
36. Iles DE, Lehmann-Horn F, Scherer SW, et al: Localization of the gene encoding the alpha 2/delta-subunits of the L-type voltage dependent calcium channel to chromosome 7q and the analysis of the segregation of flanking markers in malignant hyperthermia susceptible families. Hum Mol Genet 1994;3:969–975.
37. Sudbrak R, Procaccio V, Klausnitzer M, et al: Mapping of a further malignant hyperthermia susceptibility locus to chromosome 3q13.1. Am J Hum Genet 1995;56:684–691.
38. Britt BA: Malignant hypethermia. *In* Lane RJM (ed): Handbook of Muscle Disease. New York, Marcel Dekker, 1996, pp 451–471.
39. Hopkins PM, Halsall PJ, Ellis FR: Diagnosing malignant hyperthermia susceptability. Anaesthesia 1994;49:373–375.
40. Brody I: Muscle contracture induced by exercise: A syndrome attributable to decreasing relaxing factor. New Engl J Med 1969;281: 187–192.
41. Hiel JAP, Jongen PJH, Poels PJE, et al: Sarcoplasmic reticulum Ca^{2+} adenosine triphosphatase deficiency (Brody's disease). *In* Lane RJM (ed): Handbook of Muscle Disease. New York, Marcel Dekker, 1996, pp 473–478.
42. Odermatt A, Taschner PE, Scherer SW, et al: Characterization of the gene encoding human sarcolipin (SLN), a proteolipid associated with SERCA1: Absence of structural mutations in five patients with Brody disease. Genomics 1997;45:541–553.
43. Odermatt A, Taschner PE, Khanna VK, et al: Mutations in the gene-encoding SERCA1, the fast-twitch skeletal muscle sarcoplasmic reticulum Ca^{2+} ATPase, are associated with Brody disease. Nat Genet 1996;14:191–194.
44. Odermatt A, Barton K, Khanna VK, et al: The mutation of Pro789 to Leu reduces the activity of the fast-twitch skeletal muscle sarco(endo)plasmic reticulum Ca^{2+} ATPase (SERCA1) and is associated with Brody disease. Hum Genet 2000;106:482–491.
45. Zhang Y, Fujii J, Phillips MS, et al: Characterization of cDNA and genomic DNA encoding SERCA1, the Ca(2+)-ATPase of human fast-twitch skeletal muscle sarcoplasmic reticulum, and its elimination as a candidate gene for Brody disease. Genomics 1995;30:415–424.
46. Ii S, Sommer SS: The high frequency of TTR M30 in familial amyloidotic polyneuropathy is not due to a founder effect. Hum Molec Genet 1993;2:1303–1305.
47. Reilly MM, Staunton H, Harding AE: Familial amyloid polyneuropathy (TTR ala 60) in northwest Ireland: A clinical, genetic, and epidemiological study. J Neurol Neurosurg Psychiatry 1995;59:45–49.
48. Demirkiran M, Jankovic J: Paroxysmal dyskinesias: Clinical features and classification. Ann Neurol 1995;38:571–579.
49. Dwulet FE, Benson MD: Characterization of a transthyretin (prealbumin) variant associated with familial amyloidotic polyneuropathy type II (Indiana/Swiss). J Clin Invest 1986;78:880–886.

50. Nichols WC, Liepnieks JJ, McKusick VA, Benson MD: Direct sequencing of the gene for Maryland/German familial amyloidotic polyneuropathy type II and genotyping by allele-specific enzymatic amplification. Genomics 1989;5:535–540.
51. de la Chapelle A, Tolvanen R, Boysen G, et al: Gelsolin-derived familial amyloidosis caused by asparagine or tyrosine substitution for aspartic acid at residue 187. Nature Genetics 1992;2:157–160.
52. Levy E, Haltia M, Fernandez-Madrid I, et al: Mutation in gelsolin gene in Finnish hereditary amyloidosis. J Exp Med 1990;172:1865–1867.
53. Adams D, Samuel D, Goulon-Goeau C, et al: The course and prognostic factors of familial amyloid polyneuropathy after liver transplantation. Brain 2000;123:1495–1504.
54. Dubrey SW, Davidoff R, Skinner M, Bergethon P, Lewis D, Falk RH: Progression of ventricular wall thickening after liver transplantation for familial amyloidosis. Transplantation 1997;64:74–80.
55. Skinner M, Lewis WD, Jones LA, et al: Liver transplantation as a treatment for familial amyloidotic polyneuropathy. Ann Intern Med 1994;120:133–134.
56. Holmgren G, Ericzon BG, Groth CG, et al: Clinical improvement and amyloid regression after liver transplantation in hereditary transthyretin amyloidosis. Lancet 1993;341:1113–1116.
57. Dyck PJ, Chance P, Lebo R, Carney JA: Hereditary motor and sensory neuropathies. *In* Dyck PJ, Thomas PK (eds): Peripheral Neuropathy. Philadelphia, WB Saunders, 1993, pp 1094–1136.
58. Beressi A, Sunheimer RL, Huish S, Finck C, Pincus MR: Acute severe rhabdomyolysis in an human immunodeficiency virus-seropositive patient associated with rising anti-coxsackie B viral titers. Ann Clin Lab Sci 1994;24:278–281.
59. Carpenter S, Karpati G, Andermann F, Gold R: Giant axonal neuropathy. A clinically and morphologically distinct neurological disease. Arch Neurol 1974;31:312–316.
60. Cavalier L, Ben Hamida C, Amouri R, et al: Giant axonal neuropathy locus refinement to a <590 kb critical interval. Eur J Hum Genet 2000;8:527–534.
61. Bomont P, Cavalier L, Blondeau F, et al: The gene encoding gigaxonin, a new member of the cytoskeletal BTB/kelch repeat family, is mutated in giant axonal neuropathy. Nat Genet 2000;26:370–374.
62. Hart IK, Waters C, Vincent A: Autoantibodies detected to expressed K+ channels are implicated in neuromyotonia. Ann Neurol 1997; 41:238–246.
63. Browne DL, Brunt ER, Griggs RC, et al: Identification of two new KCNA1 mutations in episodic ataxia/myokymia families. Hum Mol Genet 1995;4:1671–1672.
64. Hart IK, Newsom-Davis J: Neuromyotonia (Isaac's syndrome). *In* Lane RJM (ed): Handbook of Muscle Disease. New York, Marcel Dekker, 1996, pp 355–363.

CHAPTER 38

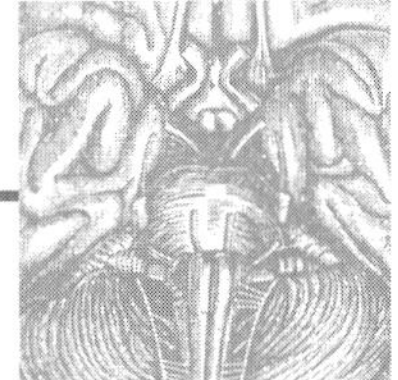

MARK A. FERRANTE

Endogenous Metabolic Disorders

Electrolyte Abnormalities

SODIUM DISORDERS

Although dietary intake varies, body fluid composition and volume remain fairly constant, a reflection of multiple compensatory mechanisms. Although it is frequently cited that total body water (TBW) constitutes approximately 60 percent of body weight, the percentage varies with age, gender, and body habitus from 42 percent (obese, elderly female) to 75 percent (infant).[1] The cell membrane serves as an interface between the intracellular fluid and extracellular fluid (ECF) compartments; their ratio is roughly 2 to 1. About three fourths of ECF is interstitial, while the remaining one fourth is intravascular (blood volume). The blood volume consists of plasma and formed elements, with plasma volume being approximately 95 percent water and 5 percent macromolecules (e.g., albumin). The interface between the interstitial and intravascular compartments is the capillary, which does not permit crossing of macromolecules. For that reason, the interstitial fluid is an ultrafiltrate of the plasma, and therefore their electrolyte concentrations are similar.

Starling forces determine the direction of water flow between compartments. Because the cell membrane is water permeable, whenever an intercompartmental osmolal gradient develops, water passively moves down its concentration gradient, from an area of lower osmolality to one of higher osmolality, thereby maintaining osmolal equilibrium. Solutes that are freely permeable across the membrane (e.g., urea, ethanol) are referred to as ineffective osmoles, because they do not form significant osmolal gradients across the membrane. Conversely, membrane impermeable solutes (e.g., glucose, sodium [Na], mannitol, glycerol) are referred to as effective osmoles because they do create osmolal gradients across the membrane.[1] Translocational hyponatremia is most commonly caused by hyperglycemia.[2] Because the different fluid compartments are in osmolal equilibrium, the serum osmolality is a good reflection of the intracellular osmolality and can be approximated using the following formula[3]:

$$\text{Serum osmolality} = 1.86\ \text{Na} + \text{BUN}/2.8 + \text{Glucose}/18 + 9,$$

where Na concentration is expressed in milliequivalents per liter (mEq/L) and blood urea nitrogen (BUN) and glucose concentrations are expressed in milligrams per deciliter (mg/dL). A discrepancy between *calculated* and *measured* osmolality indicates the presence of other serum osmoles. When sufficient amounts of ineffective osmoles are present, hypo-osmolal hyponatremia can be associated with normal or even high serum osmolality. In this setting, the risks of hypo-osmolality are the same because the solutes are ineffective osmoles.[2] By monitoring the osmolality and volume of the ECF, the body maintains its fluid composition and volume fairly constant.[4,5]

Hyponatremia

Pathogenesis and Pathophysiology. Hyponatremia reflects an excess of water, relative to Na. Because Na is an effective osmole, intercompartmental Na imbalances must be corrected by water movement. This can produce brain edema, which, in turn, may produce pulmonary edema, central diabetes insipidus (DI), cerebral infarction, cortical blindness, persistent vegetative state, respiratory arrest, and coma.[1] Hyponatremic patients can be subdivided into hyperosmolal, normo-osmolal, and hypo-osmolal types. The hypo-osmolal type is the most frequent category and is usually further subdivided, based on ECF volume, into hypervolemic, normovolemic, and hypovolemic (Table 38–1).

The neurological symptoms associated with hyponatremia primarily reflect central nervous system (CNS) involvement (e.g., encephalopathy, seizures) and are related to the rapidity of the onset of the lowered Na level. Brain cell compensatory mechanisms exist to counter hyponatremia (see Clinical Features and Associated Disorders) but require time to occur. When hyponatremia occurs acutely, water passively flows down its concentration gradient, resulting in its entry into the brain cells, thereby producing cerebral edema. The causes of peripheral neurological symptoms and signs (cramping, muscle twitching, and fasciculations) are most likely related to altered ion conductances and abnormal discharges of the peripheral nerves.

Epidemiology and Risk Factors. Among hospitalized patients, the incidence of hyponatremia is about 1 percent and its prevalence is about 2.5 percent.[6,7] Postoperative patients account for roughly 25 percent of all hyponatremic episodes.[8] It is important to note that although the incidence of hyponatremia is similar between the sexes, premenopausal women have a significantly greater incidence of brain damage than do men or postmenopausal women.[1] This is a reflection of Na/K-ATPase pump inhibition (which blocks the first line of defense against hyponatremia) and antidiuretic hormone (ADH) release stimulation (which contributes to water retention) by the sex hormones.[1]Another significant risk factor for hyponatremia-induced brain damage is hypoxia, a reflection of its inhibitory effect on Na/K-ATPase transport activity, which, therefore, compromises the brain's ability to compensate for the hyponatremia.[1] Other high-risk populations are patients with acquired immunodeficiency syndrome, syndrome of inappropriate antidiuretic hormone (SIADH; pulmonary disease, intracranial disease, drug-induced), adrenal insufficiency, and isotonic fluid loss (emesis, diarrhea).[8] Among pregnant patients, the misuse of oxytocin is the most common cause of hyponatremia.[9] Severe, symptomatic hyponatremia can result when procedures requiring large quantities of irrigant solutions (e.g., transurethral prostatectomy) are performed using irrigant solutions that do not contain sodium.[2]

TABLE 38–1. Major Causes of Hyponatremia

Iatrogenic
Factitious (blood drawn proximal to hypotonic infusion)
Hyperosmolal (glucose, mannitol, radiocontrast)
Normo-osmolal (hyperlipidemia, hyperproteinemia)
Hypo-osmolal
- *Hypervolemic* (decreased cardiac output, increased vascular compliance, water shift)
- *Normovolemic* (SIADH, drugs, hypothyroidism)
- *Hypovolemic* (renal, extrarenal [e.g., gastrointestinal, cutaneous, hemorrhage])

Data from Votey SR, Peters AL, Hoffman JR: Disorders of water metabolism: Hyponatremia and hypernatremia. Emerg Med Clin North Am 1989;7:749–769; and Riggs JE: Neurological manifestations of electrolyte disorders. *In* Aminoff MJ (ed): Neurology and General Medicine, 2nd ed. New York, Churchill Livingstone, 1995, pp 321–331.

Clinical Features and Associated Disorders. The most common clinical features of hyponatremia are gastrointestinal (GI) (e.g., nausea, vomiting, anorexia) and neurological, with CNS abnormalities predominating. The CNS symptoms reflect cerebral edema due to the passive movement of water from the hypo-osmolal ECF into the brain cells. Initial water entry into the cell stimulates solute extrusion, initially by the Na/K-ATPase pump, which limits the amount of water entry required to restore osmotic equilibrium and may render the patient asymptomatic.[1] The most common CNS manifestation is encephalopathy, ranging from mild confusion to coma, depending on the degree of cerebral edema, its rapidity of onset, and its absolute magnitude. Sodium levels above 125 mEq/L are usually associated with GI symptoms, whereas seizures, coma, and permanent neurological sequelae are typically only observed with levels below 115 mEq/L. Neurological features due to hyponatremia of slow onset may be much less apparent, although impaired cognition is typical with Na levels below 120 mEq/L.[3] Asterixis, ataxia, and multifocal myoclonus may also be observed in acute hyponatremic encephalopathy but are less frequent than in uremic encephalopathy (UE).[3] Focal neurological features may also be seen and usually remit with correction of the hyponatremia. These findings may represent underlying focal pathologies with a resultant lower threshold for clinical expression. Other reported neurological features of hyponatremia include headache, respiratory depression, bizarre behavior, nystagmus, increased tone, and hallucinations. Opisthotonic posturing, respiratory arrest, and fixed and dilated pupils suggest cerebral herniation.[8] Muscle cramping may occur, but fasciculations, tremor, and twitching are uncommon.[10] An associated disorder related to hyponatremia, or rather its treatment, is central pontine myelinolysis (discussed later).

Differential Diagnosis. The principal causes of hyponatremia include primary dilutional hyponatremia, SIADH, diuretic usage, and water intoxication. Dilutional hyponatremia can be seen in edematous states, such as cirrhosis, nephrosis, and congestive heart failure, as well as with excessive water intake in the presence of renal failure (RF), Addison's disease, myxedema, and nonosmotic ADH secretion. The possibility of adrenal insufficiency must always be excluded in the presence of hyperkalemia. Among hospitalized patients, the most common cause of acute hyponatremia is iatrogenic overhydration (e.g., excessive intravenous [IV] fluid administration) in the presence of impaired water elimination.[6] SIADH occurs with oat cell carcinoma of the lung, a variety of CNS and pulmonary disorders, the Guillain-Barré syndrome, and acute intermittent porphyria and may also be idiopathic. The differential diagnosis also should include drug intoxications, infections, endocrinopathies, and other electrolyte disorders.

Evaluation. When hyponatremia is identified, the possibility of an error, either by the laboratory or by the phlebotomist (e.g., sampling proximal to a hypotonic fluid infusion), should be considered. If hyponatremia is verified, the patient's past medical history and medication profile should be reviewed, because they may suggest the cause. A careful physical examination should be performed and, if possible, the ECF volume status should be ascertained, along with serum electrolytes, BUN, creatinine (Cr), and osmolality. Uric acid is inversely proportional to the volume status and, therefore, may be helpful in determining hypervolemic and hypovolemic states. The serum osmolality should be calculated and compared with the measured osmolality and, if a discrepancy exists, the presence of an unidentified serum osmole (e.g., mannitol) is suggested. Other studies to consider include thyroid functions, adrenal studies, and the evaluation of urine Na, fractional excretion of Na, osmolality, and pH.

Management. In all cases of hyponatremia, the underlying cause must be identified and treated, and iatrogenic hyponatremia prevented (e.g., avoidance of free water and hypotonic solutions [D_5W, ½ normal saline (NS)] in postoperative patients). Initial management is based on the type of symptoms, their rapidity of onset, and the underlying etiology. Acute-onset hyponatremia is usually associated with a marked increase in brain water and a risk of cerebral herniation; for that reason, the condition requires rapid treatment. This is especially true if seizures or a decreased level of alertness is present. If the condition is left untreated, acute hyponatremia is nearly always fatal. Unfortunately, a lack of consensus regarding the optimal treatment of symptomatic hyponatremia remains.[2] Water restriction in acute hyponatremia is never indicated, and hypertonic saline is given in an intensive care setting. In patients with chronic hyponatremia, however, hypertonic saline is not always indicated and may even be dangerous. Its management should be based on the presence of symptoms. Asymptomatic patients with volume depletion require repletion (with NS), and those with hormone deficiency (e.g., hypothyroidism, adrenal insufficiency) require hormone replacement. Patients with drug-induced hyponatremia require the discontinuation of the offending agent. Water restriction may be appropriate for some patients with asymptomatic hyponatremia. Demeclocycline, a tetracycline antibiotic that produces nephrogenic DI, can be used for the long-term management of patients with stable asymptomatic hyponatremia (e.g., SIADH).[11]

Hyponatremic-induced seizures can be treated with IV 3 percent hypertonic saline at a dose of 4 to 6 mL/kg body weight.[12] This dosage rapidly raises the serum Na level by about 3 to 5 mEq/L and avoids the risk of respiratory embarrassment associated with benzodiazepines and phenobarbital. Hyponatremic-induced seizures are more commonly associated with acute hyponatremia, in which case rapid normalization to a level of 120 to 125 mEq/L can be accomplished without risk of neurological complications. The serum Na concentration need not be corrected to normal to obtain seizure control, and overcorrection can be harmful. Therapy with hypertonic saline should be discontinued when the patient becomes asymptomatic or the plasma Na concentration increases by 20 mEq/L or reaches a value in the range of 120 to 125 mEq/L.[1] To avoid potential complications, the plasma Na should never be acutely elevated to normonatremic levels and should not be increased by more than 25 mEq/L during the first 48 hours of therapy.[13] One of the most recent recommendations is that the elevation be limited to 8 mEq/L on any day of treatment (e.g., 1 to 2 mEq/L per hour × 4 hours with severe symptoms) and be cautiously exceeded only when severe symptoms do not respond since, at that point, the risk of hypotonicity would outweigh the potential risk of osmotic myelinolysis.[2] In the setting of chronic hyponatremia, seizures are less common. Loop diuretics (e.g., furosemide) result in solvent loss greater than solute loss (i.e., net water loss) and can be used, in addition to the hypertonic saline, to raise the serum Na concentration.

Central pontine myelinolysis refers to the demyelinating lesions noted in the pons of patients with hyponatremia, which were previously believed to occur when the serum Na concentration was corrected too rapidly (discussed later; Fig. 38–1). Because myelinolysis also occurs outside of the pons, the term *osmotic myelinolysis* is also used by some physicians.[14] Central pontine myelinosis was first described in 1959[15] in malnourished alcoholics and was later noted in hospitalized patients undergoing hydration.[16] In 1980, Leslie and colleagues[17] suggested that central pontine myelinosis was due to rapid correction of hyponatremia. This led some physicians to suggest that the rate of hyponatremia correction should not exceed 12 mEq/L per day.[18] Others have suggested that the magnitude of correction determines whether or not neurological complications occur.[13] Based on several prospective studies, Griggs proposed that cerebral demyelination is not a manifestation of the rapid correction of *acute* hyponatremia,[8] and studies have not confirmed that the demyelination associated with hyponatremia is related to rapid correction.[19] In fact, the majority of brain lesions observed among patients with symptomatic hyponatremia result from a delay in the initiation of therapy, which, in turn, results in respiratory insufficiency.[20] Cerebral demyelinating lesions also occur with improper therapy, but they are unrelated to its *rate* of correction.[13] It has been reported that cerebral demyelination occurs only when patients with hyponatremia are overcorrected (i.e., patients are made hypernatremic), have an *absolute* increase in plasma Na concentration exceeding 25 mEq/L during the first 24 to 48 hours of therapy, suffer a hypoxic event, or have underlying severe liver disease.[1] A review on myelinolysis suggested that chronic hyponatremia should be corrected at a rate below 10 mEq/L during any 24-hour period.[21]

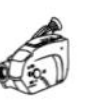

Prognosis and Future Perspectives. The prognosis is much better for patients with chronic hyponatremia than for those with acute hyponatremia. Acute hyponatremia is associated with substantial morbidity and mortality, with a mortality rate of 50 percent in one series.[3] In addition to a higher mortality, patients with hyponatremia-induced seizures frequently show persistent neurological deficits.[3] Diuretic-induced hyponatremia, hypoxia, alcoholism, malnutrition, liver disease, and female gender are risk factors for a poor neurological outcome.[4] Because volume-induced ADH release occurs with significant blood volume reductions, treatment of hypervolemic hypo-osmolal hyponatremia carries an ominous prognosis.[4] In the future, the treatment of central pontine myelinolysis—a disorder currently not cor-

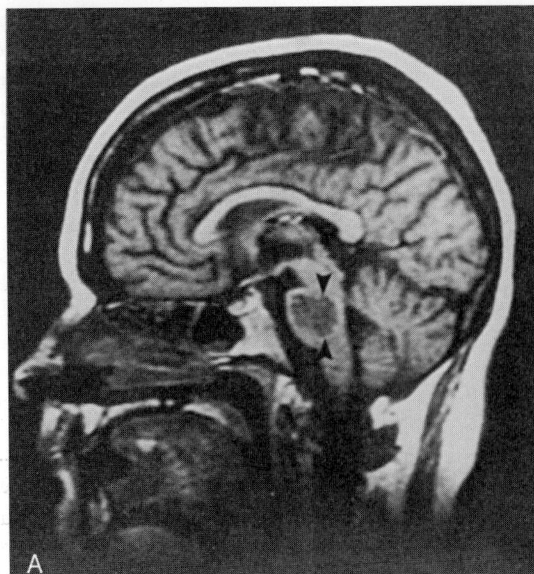

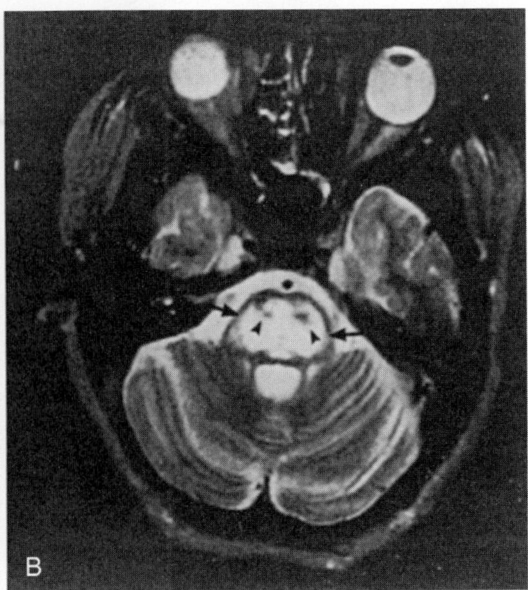

FIGURE 38–1. A 30-year-old woman with a history of alcoholism presented with confusion and disorientation following a seizure. The patient's serum sodium was 99 mmol/L, and she was treated with an infusion of normal saline. This resulted in a sodium value of 125 mmol/L 24 hours later. The patient initially had dysarthria and slow response on finger-to-nose testing and was interactive on examination. On day 7 of admission, the patient became unresponsive and had new Babinski's signs. Brain magnetic resonance imaging demonstrated central pontine myelinolysis with a region of low signal intensity on a sagittal T1-weighted image *(A)* and high signal intensity on an axial T2-weighted image, which is marked by the arrows *(B)*. The arrowheads in *B* show the relative preservation of the corticospinal tracts. (From Hart BL, Eaton RP: Images in clinical medicine–Osmotic myelinolysis. N Engl J Med 1995;333:1259.)

rectable—may include reinduction of the hyponatremic state.[22]

Hypernatremia

Hypernatremia is defined as a serum Na concentration above the normal range (135 to 145 mEq/L) and represents a relative increase in total body Na relative to TBW. This may be caused by either water loss or Na gain and is usually encountered when water losses exceed Na losses (i.e., hypo-osmolal fluid loss) along with decreased water intake (e.g., limited access to water, loss of thirst).

Pathogenesis and Pathophysiology. The primary cause of hypernatremia is water loss, either renal, extrarenal, or both, along with limited water intake (e.g., decreased thirst, or a comatose or debilitated condition). Disorders causing renal water loss include DI, osmotic diuresis, hypokalemia and hypercalcemia (which may impair the concentrating capacity of the kidney), and renal parenchymal disease (e.g., sickle cell anemia). Those disorders causing nonrenal water losses include excessive sweating and other insensible losses, diarrhea, and disordered thirst. Central DI (i.e., pituitary deficiency of ADH) most commonly results from pituitary region tumors, their surgical treatment, and cranial trauma,[23] and less frequently from infiltrative disorders (e.g., sarcoidosis). Impaired ADH synthesis is the underlying problem in some patients, whereas others have impaired ADH release in response to osmotic stimuli. Nephrogenic DI (renal ADH unresponsiveness) is usually acquired (e.g., drugs, such as amphotericin B, lithium, and fluorocarbon anesthetics), and a transient form of DI can be seen in late pregnancy and tends to remit postpartum. Less common etiologies include excessive Na intake with limited water access (seen with water loss due to peritoneal dialysis), high dietary Na, seawater consumption, and iatrogenic errors in IV fluid delivery or total parenteral nutrition formulation. Essential hypernatremia has also been attributed to an impaired osmoreceptor set point.

Although the pathophysiology of hypernatremia is similar to that of hyponatremia (the movement of water along its concentration gradient to restore osmolal equilibrium), the pathology is different (cerebral dehydration occurs rather than cerebral edema). When the hypernatremia develops slowly, brain cells may be able to compensate by increasing the influx of electrolytes across the cell membrane, decreasing the intracellular electrolyte binding, and increasing the intracellular amino acid concentration.[23–25] In doing so, the brain increases its intracellular osmolality to avoid water loss (dehydration).

Epidemiology and Risk Factors. The incidence of hypernatremia among hospitalized adults ranges from 0.7 to 2.3 percent and is even greater among children.[8] It is usually seen among patients at the extremes of age, in whom it is most frequently caused by gastroenteritis (infants) and limited water intake due to debilitation.[10] Common causes of hypernatremia among the elderly include surgery (21 percent), febrile illness (20 percent), infirmity (11 percent), and diabetes mellitus (11 percent).[8] The elderly are at further risk because they have a diminished capacity for urine concentration and a depressed thirst response.[8, 26]

Closed head injury is also a risk factor for the development of DI and hypernatremia, with an incidence of 2 percent after severe closed head injury; the incidence is greater if the sella turcica region is involved.[23] Also, hypernatremia is often induced by IV mannitol, which is used to decrease intracranial pressure (ICP); when mannitol therapy is discontinued, fluid therapy quickly restores the Na concentration.[27]

Clinical Features and Associated Disorders. The most common neurological manifestations reflect CNS involvement and range from mild confusion to coma, the severity typically correlating with the degree of hypernatremia and the rapidity of its onset. A history of a strong sense of thirst and signs of dehydration should be sought.[8]

When the onset of hypernatremia is acute, early symptoms typically occur at an osmolality of 320 to 330 mOsm/kg body water, whereas coma and respiratory arrest more commonly occur at values exceeding 360 mOsm/kg body water.[4] As with hyponatremia, seizures are usually seen with acute-onset hypernatremia and tend to be generalized. Focal neurological features likely reflect focal dysfunction. In the setting of rapid brain dehydration, tearing of the bridging veins may result in subdural hemorrhages. Subarachnoid hemorrhage and intraparenchymal hemorrhages may also occur. Similar to other metabolic encephalopathies, myoclonus, asterixis, and tremor occur and muscle cramping is frequently reported. Seizures are infrequent in chronic hypernatremia, except when it is too rapidly corrected.

Differential Diagnosis and Evaluation. With the clinical syndrome of confusion or coma, other disorders in addition to hypernatremia should be considered in the differential diagnosis, including other electrolyte abnormalities, endocrinopathies, drug or toxin exposure, stroke, cerebral masses, trauma, and infection. The underlying cause of the hypernatremia should be identified and treated. In the case of nonrenal water losses, the etiology should be obvious, and the urine should be concentrated and of low volume. A history, thorough physical examination, and the same laboratory tests used in the evaluation of hyponatremia should be obtained. The presence of a hypotonic urine in the face of dehydration and hypernatremia is diagnostic of DI, either central or nephrogenic. In nonketotic hyperosmolar hyperglycemia (NKHH), the serum osmolality and glucose are markedly elevated, ketone bodies are absent, and the patient is dehydrated (see Hyperglycemia). Because focal neurological findings may be produced by intraparenchymal, subdural, or subarachnoid hemorrhages, brain neuroimaging with computed tomography (CT) should be considered. In this setting, other etiologies associated with focal neurological signs should be contemplated, including stroke, arteriovenous malformation, and post-traumatic sequelae.

Management. Management necessitates identification of the underlying cause and correction of the hypertonic state. After the patient is stabilized, water replacement is usually the initial management. Importantly, free water cannot be given IV, because the rapid lowering of plasma osmolality at the injection site causes massive hemolysis. D_5W is roughly isotonic with plasma, but isotonic saline solutions offer several advantages, including quicker correction of hypovolemia and a less rapid correction of serum Na concentration. A patient with a fixed urinary concentrating defect due to central or nephrogenic DI will develop the excretion of free water and worsening of hypernatremia when isotonic saline is administered. The amount of water deficit can be estimated by the following formula:

$$\text{Water Deficit} = \text{TBW}\ (1 - 140\ \text{mEq/L} / \text{actual Na}),$$

where TBW is in liters, and Na concentration is in mEq/L. However, Adrogue and Madias have recently recommended that this approach be abandoned because, although it adequately estimates the water deficit in patients with hypernatremia secondary to pure water loss, it underestimates the deficit in patients with hypotonic fluid loss and, in addition, it is not useful when both Na and K must be administered. In their recent review, they provide formulas to estimate the effect of 1 liter of infusate on serum Na based on the Na concentration of the particular infusate. In acute hypernatremia, the risk of tissue dehydration (e.g., brain) is significant and fluid replacement should begin immediately. The risk of cerebral edema is not a concern because the brain rapidly extrudes any accumulated electrolytes and, consequently, a rate of reduction of 1 mEq/L/hour is acceptable. Importantly, among patients with chronic hypernatremia, correction should occur over a 48-hour period and not exceed a rate of 0.5 mEq/L per hour, otherwise seizures or cerebral edema might be precipitated.[4] This reflects the increased hyperosmolality of brain cells brought about via compensatory mechanisms to avoid dehydration. When hypernatremia is aggressively treated with hypotonic fluids, cerebral edema occurs; subsequent seizures, coma, or death may result.

Prognosis and Future Perspectives. Hypernatremia, either acute or chronic in onset, is associated with a high rate of mortality and severe morbidity.[4] Among children with severe hypernatremia, an initial mortality rate of 20 percent, as well as an incidence of permanent brain damage exceeding 33 percent, has been reported.[10, 28] The mortality rate from hypernatremia in hospitalized adults is about 50 percent,[8] although the existence of severe concomitant disease makes it difficult to determine the exact cause of the mortality.

POTASSIUM DISORDERS

The total body content of potassium (K) is about 3500 mEq,[29] and roughly 98 percent is intracellular, two thirds of which is intramuscular.[10] Because cell membranes are more permeable to K than to Na and Cl, K is primarily responsible for the resting transmembrane potential and is therefore critical to the function of excitable tissue.

Hypokalemia

Hypokalemia, the most frequent electrolyte disorder encountered by the clinician, is defined as a plasma K concentration below the normal range (3.5 to 5.5 mEq/L).

Pathogenesis and Pathophysiology. Whenever K losses exceed intake, total body K decreases and hypokalemia results. Each 1-mEq/L decrement in the plasma K level roughly correlates to a total body K decrease of 100 to 300 mEq (Table 38–2). K influx increases intracellular positivity,

TABLE 38–2. Major Causes of Hypokalemia

Inadequate intake
Transcellular shifts (systemic alkalosis, thyrotoxic and hypokalemic periodic paralysis)
Renal loss
Gastrointestinal losses
Other (drugs, head trauma, burns, hypomagnesemia, hypocalcemia)

Modified from Zull DN: Disorders of potassium metabolism. Emerg Med Clin North Am 1989;7:771–794.

thereby producing a mild depolarization. This lessened state of electrical excitability underlies the muscle weakness and hyporeflexia that can be seen clinically.

Epidemiology and Risk Factors. Approximately 2 percent of normal adults, 21 percent of hospitalized patients, 25 percent of patients taking 50 mg of hydrochlorothiazide daily, and nearly 100 percent of patients taking more than one class of diuretic have hypokalemia.[29] Although acute hypokalemia is an uncommon cause of weakness, certain scenarios increase its risk of development, including rapid correction of systemic acidosis (e.g., hyperventilation, bicarbonate administration), postoperative patients unable to take food by mouth (because K excretion cannot be stopped), and the chronic use of beta-2 agonists (e.g., asthmatics).

Clinical Features and Associated Disorders. The clinical features of hypokalemia are predominantly muscular and occur more frequently when the extracellular K level changes rapidly. The magnitude is also influential.[10] K levels of 3 to 3.5 mEq/L are associated with weakness, myalgias, and easy fatigability; those of 2.5 to 3.0 mEq/L are associated with more pronounced weakness; and those below 2.5 mEq/L (and especially if below 2.0 mEq/L) are associated with structural muscle damage (rhabdomyolysis and myoglobinuria). Areflexic quadriplegia and respiratory insufficiency may also occur at these lowest levels. The cranial musculature is rarely involved. Tetany may be observed in some hypokalemic patients, especially those with concomitant systemic alkalosis. Because hypokalemia can mask the tetany of hypocalcemia, tetany may appear as the hypokalemia is corrected.[10] Sensory disturbances and encephalopathic features are not expected in hypokalemia and, when present, should prompt a search for an underlying cause. Because hypokalemia can increase renal ammonia production, it can aggravate a pre-existing hepatic encephalopathy (HE).[30]

Differential Diagnosis and Evaluation. Frequently, the cause of hypokalemia is apparent by history, and a full general and neurological examination, with particular emphasis on muscle strength and deep tendon reflexes, is necessary. The possibility of Cushing's syndrome or hyperaldosteronism is suggested by hypertension, and the presence of thyrotoxic periodic paralysis (TPP) is indicated by evidence of hyperthyroidism. Laboratory evaluation should include Na, K, Cl, bicarbonate, BUN, Cr, glucose, calcium (Ca), and magnesium (Mg), as well as an arterial blood gas (ABG) and an electrocardiogram (ECG). Thyroid function tests (TFTs) identify the rare TPP, and muscle biopsy may demonstrate vacuolar change but generally is not indicated.

Management. Therapy includes correction of the underlying cause and replacement therapy. Replacement therapy is usually recommended once the K level is below 3.5 mEq/L. Oral supplementation is preferred, but IV supplementation may be required when GI dysfunction exists or when the K deficiency is severe (with arrhythmias and neuromuscular manifestations).

Prognosis and Future Perspectives. Although respiratory failure and death can occur when hypokalemia goes unrecognized, complete recovery is expected when K replacement can be provided and the underlying disorder corrected. For disorders that cannot be corrected (e.g., aldosterone-secreting tumors), the prognosis is related to the underlying disorder.

Hyperkalemia

Pathogenesis and Pathophysiology. Hyperkalemia may result in three ways: (1) increased entry of K into the ECF, (2) intracellular K efflux, or (3) decreased K output. Of these three processes, intracellular K efflux and decreased K output predominate. Because the renal capacity for kaliuresis adapts to increasing K intake, hyperkalemia usually is not seen unless a massive amount of K is ingested, parenteral replacement is provided too rapidly, or co-existent adrenal or renal dysfunction exists. Even in the setting of complete RF, the rise in serum K is slow, ranging from 1 mEq/L per week to 0.5 mEq/L per day.[31] In the setting of hyperkalemia, the intercellular gradient for K efflux is lessened and, therefore, intracellular positivity increases. This results in a minimal depolarization which, in turn, makes the tissue less excitable by causing a reduction in Na influx.

Epidemiology and Risk Factors. Among hospitalized patients, the incidence of hyperkalemia approaches 10 percent, one fifth of which is above 6.0 mEq/L.[29] Risk factors for the development of hyperkalemia include (1) renal or adrenal insufficiency, (2) K supplementation at rates and quantities above the suggested values, (3) situations resulting in tissue destruction (e.g., induction of chemotherapy), and (4) the use of beta-2 antagonists (e.g., propranolol) or other medications known to cause hyperkalemia (e.g., heparin, K-sparing diuretics).

Clinical Features and Associated Disorders. The usual manifesting feature of hyperkalemia is cardiac toxicity.[10] ECG features include peaked T waves, increased PR (atrioventricular block) and QRS (interventricular block) intervals, and arrhythmias. Cardiac arrest represents the major problem and may be the initial symptom.[29] Like hypokalemia, the major neurological manifestations of hyperkalemia are peripheral. Hyperkalemia may cause loss of strength and deep tendon reflexes, although this is observed less commonly than with hypokalemia. Muscle cramping is not uncommon, and both paresthesias[29] and focal neurological signs[32] have been reported.

Differential Diagnosis and Evaluation. Systemic acidosis and adrenal or renal insufficiency are the more frequently encountered etiologies of hyperkalemia. Once hyperkalemia is noted, an ECG must be obtained, followed by continuous cardiac monitoring until causes of pseudohyperkalemia are excluded. This requires a complete blood count (CBC) with smear for the presence of red blood cell hemolysis, thrombocytosis (> 500,000/μL), or leukocytosis (> 50,000/μL). Tourniquet-induced stasis and forearm exercise may also produce hyperkalemia.[3]

Management. The treatment of hyperkalemia includes addressing its cardiac manifestations, reversing the underlying disorder, decreasing the K input, increasing the intracellular influx of K, and increasing K excretion.

CALCIUM DISORDERS

Ninety-nine percent of total body Ca is contained in bone, making the skeleton a Ca reservoir; the remaining 1 percent is distributed in the intracellular and ECF compartments. Because 1 percent of skeletal Ca is freely exchangeable with the ECF, it can help buffer acute changes in the serum Ca, whereas the kidney regulates calciuresis.[33] Among normal adults with average calcium intake, urinary calcium excretion ranges between 100 and 400 mg/day.[34] Total serum Ca reflects dietary intake, GI absorption, calciuresis, and transfer from the bone to the ECF. Parathyroid hormone (PTH), 1,25-dihydroxycholecalciferol (DHCC), and calcitonin regulate both Ca absorption from the gut and calciuresis. PTH causes tubular cells to reabsorb calcium and stimulates renal parenchymal cells to hydroxylate vitamin D into its active form (DHCC).[34] PTH is released whenever the serum ionized Ca level falls; conversely, hypercalcemia suppresses the release of PTH. In addition to the nearly instantaneous changes in PTH secretion brought about by shift in serum Ca concentration, Marx emphasized that changes in PTH mRNA (over a period of hours) and changes in the size of the parathyroid glands (days to months) also contribute to the regulation of the serum Ca level. Because PTH promotes the synthesis of 1,25-DHCC, it indirectly influences GI absorption.

Hypocalcemia

Although ionized Ca is the physiologically active form, total serum Ca is the laboratory parameter usually measured. This value reflects the ionized (unbound, 50 percent), the bound (mostly to albumin, 40 percent), and the chelated (10 percent) fractions. In the presence of normal serum protein levels, hypocalcemia exists when the total serum Ca value is below the normal range of 8.8 to 10.4 mg/dL. However, in the setting of hypoalbuminemia, although the measured total serum Ca is low, the patient is asymptomatic because the physiologically active, ionized fraction is normal.[35] Although the total serum Ca value may be corrected for hypoalbuminemia (e.g., by adding 0.8 mg/dL to the measured Ca value for every 1.0-g/dL decrement in the serum albumin value), this correction formula may be inaccurate in critically ill patients.[36] For that reason, it is best to measure the ionized Ca value in this patient population.

Pathogenesis and Pathophysiology. Hypocalcemia may be caused by PTH or 1,25-DHCC deficiency, as well as by end-organ resistance to their actions and other conditions (Table 38–3). In the setting of chronic renal failure, decreased renal synthesis of 1,25-DHCC and hyperphosphatemia cause hypocalcemia with resultant secondary hyperparathyroidism. Ionized Ca is important for presynaptic neurotransmitter release and stabilization of nerve and muscle membranes (divalent cations stabilize the cell membranes of nerve and muscle).[33] Thus, it is not surprising that disturbances of ionized Ca result in neuromuscular manifestations.

TABLE 38–3. Major Causes of Hypocalcemia

Hypoparathyroidism
Normal or increased parathyroid function (renal failure, vitamin D deficiency)
Protein binding and anion chelation of ionized calcium
Medications (anticalcemic and antineoplastic agents)
Multifactorial (gram-negative sepsis)

Modified from Spiegel AM: The parathyroid glands, hypercalcemia, and hypocalcemia. *In* Bennett JC, Plum F (eds): Cecil Textbook of Medicine, 20th ed. Philadelphia, WB Saunders, 1995, pp 1364–1373.

Neurologically, both the peripheral nervous system (PNS) and CNS may be involved. Tetany, a PNS manifestation, is thought to be caused by repetitively generated nerve fiber action potentials, possibly related to the spontaneous depolarization of the nerve cell membrane in the setting of hypocalcemia. When the rate of sequential muscle fiber depolarization does not permit Ca reuptake by the sarcoplasmic reticulum, tetany occurs. The instability of the neuromuscular membranes may explain why the clinical features of hypocalcemia are positive in nature (e.g., perioral and acral paresthesias, and muscle spasms).

Epidemiology and Risk Factors. Except in neonates and patients with RF, hypocalcemia is relatively rare. The most likely cause of hypocalcemia among patients presenting to an emergency room is hypomagnesemia.[33] Risk factors include past thyroidectomy, neck trauma, a family history of hypocalcemia, malabsorption syndromes, antiepileptic drug usage, severe liver or kidney disease (decreased 1-alpha-hydroxylation of vitamin D), and pancreatitis. The incidence of postsurgical hypoparathyroidism (usually thyroidectomy) varies with the expertise of the surgeon.[37] The decrease in total serum Ca during pregnancy reflects dilutional hypoalbuminemia and, for that reason, the ionized Ca concentration is unchanged.[38]

Clinical Features and Associated Disorders. The clinical features of hypocalcemia are primarily neuromuscular, regardless of the underlying disorder, and are dependent on its rapidity of onset and magnitude. The earliest PNS symptoms include perioral and acral paresthesias, as well as tetany (tonic muscle spasms), the most characteristic and frequently recognized sign of hypocalcemia.[10] Tetany can be overt or latent, and provocative tests may be necessary to elicit latent tetany. Provocative tests include Chvostek's sign, the contraction of ipsilateral facial muscles in response to light percussion over the facial nerve (just anterior to the ear), and Trousseau's sign, carpal spasm in response to ischemia (e.g., 3-minute application of blood pressure cuff maintained just above systolic pressure). The carpal spasm produced is first preceded by acral paresthesias, followed by sensations of spasm, and then carpal spasm, paralleling the sequence of development of tetany.[39] Latent tetany may also become overt in the setting of alkalosis (e.g., hyperventilation or Na bicarbonate administration), a reflection of increased binding between ionized Ca and albumin. When tetany is severe, lower extremity and pedal spasms, as well as laryngeal stridor, may be observed. Opisthotonos may occur if spasms involve the trunk. A history of preceding muscle cramps, or generalized muscle aching, is frequently obtained.

CNS manifestations include irritability, delirium, delusions, hallucinations, depression, and dementia. When the onset of hypocalcemia is slow and insidious, dementia may be the initial manifestation. Seizures may occur and can be the presenting sign when hypocalcemia is severe. They are usually generalized but may be focal.[39] Intracerebral calcifications, seen most frequently with idiopathic hypoparathyroidism and pseudohypoparathyroidism, are usually asymptomatic. Although the basal ganglia are frequently affected, parkinsonism, athetosis, and chorea have been reported only rarely.[40] When the condition is persistent, cataract formation may occur. CHF and papilledema with increased ICP (idiopathic intracranial hypertension) are rarely observed.[37]

Differential Diagnosis. The etiologies of hypocalcemia are listed in Table 38–3. The most common cause of hypoparathyroidism is surgical (e.g., thyroidectomy) and is usually transient, becoming permanent in less than 3 percent of patients. Severe hypomagnesemia may cause hypocalcemia by inducing deficient PTH secretion and causing end-organ resistance to PTH. This explains why hypomagnesemia causes many of the same clinical manifestations as hypocalcemia.

Evaluation. Serum electrolyte, BUN, Cr, Ca (total and ionized), Mg, phosphorus, alkaline phosphatase, and albumin levels should be determined. An ABG identifies whether a hyperventilation syndrome is present. An ECG and continuous cardiac monitoring may be required. More specific tests for intestinal malabsorption may also be necessary. In osteomalacia or rickets, the serum alkaline phosphatase is elevated. CT imaging of the head may reveal intracranial calcifications, especially in the basal ganglia region. When hypocalcemia and hyperphosphatemia co-exist in the presence of normal renal function, the diagnosis of hypoparathyroidism is strongly suggested and the appropriate laboratory evaluation is required. Hypocalcemia coupled with a normal or low serum P level suggests vitamin D deficiency, malabsorption, or another cause of secondary hypoparathyroidism. Steatorrhea is frequently associated with hypomagnesemia and may serve as a clue to its presence.

Management. Acute, symptomatic hypocalcemia requires emergency treatment with IV Ca until symptoms resolve. Hypertension, bradycardia, cardiac conduction block, and digitalis toxicity may be precipitated if the infusion is provided too rapidly, and so monitoring is required.[23] Because this form of treatment lasts only a few hours, it must be repeated, or the patient must be provided with a continuous infusion. In less urgent settings (e.g., postsurgical hypocalcemia), elemental Ca may be given as a continuous infusion over 4 to 10 hours and Ca monitored. In the setting of mild hypocalcemia, treatment with oral Ca replacement alone may suffice. Ca carbonate, up to 1200 mg orally three times daily, may safely be given.[23] Definitive resolution of hypocalcemia, however, requires identification and treatment of the underlying disease. For patients requiring long-term Ca supplementation, monitoring for evidence of toxicity is required (e.g., hypercalcemia, hypercalciuria).

Hypercalcemia

Pathogenesis and Pathophysiology. Hypercalcemia occurs when serum Ca entry (from bone resorption and GI absorption) exceeds calciuresis. In the presence of normal serum proteins, hypercalcemia exists when the serum Ca concentration is above the normal range. However, physiological hypercalcemia is present only when the ionized Ca is above its normal range. The ionized Ca value can be calculated, based on the serum albumin level, or directly measured in most laboratories. In the setting of hypoalbuminemia, although the total serum Ca value may be normal, ionized Ca may be significantly elevated and require emergent treatment. In addition to serum protein binding, consideration of chelation (anions) and acid-base status is also important.

Epidemiology and Risk Factors. Approximately 40 percent of hypercalcemic patients develop neurological manifestations.[10, 41] Nearly all patients with hypercalcemia have a malignancy or hyperparathyroidism, or are using thiazide diuretics (Table 38–4). Malignancies are most common among hospitalized patients, and hyperparathyroidism is common among ambulatory patients.[42] The incidence of primary hyperparathyroidism in the United States is approximately 25 cases per 100,000 people and increases significantly when only the elderly population is considered; about 50,000 new cases present annually.[34] Malignancy-induced hypercalcemia occurs predominately in patients with bone metastases, such as lung (especially squamous cell), breast, ovarian, renal, hematological, head and neck, and GI cancers.[33, 43] Through increased calciuresis, the majority of these patients do not develop hypercalcemia. However, in the setting of renal dysfunction, hypercalcemia is readily provoked. Disorders that result in prolonged immobilization (paralysis, coma, or trauma) can cause hypercalcemia, especially in patients undergoing bone remodeling (normal growth in a young patient, osteoporosis in the elderly, Paget's disease). Infrequently, humoral hypercalcemia of malignancy (i.e., PTH-related peptide excretion by the tumor) is observed. This topic recently has been reviewed by Epstein.

Clinical Features and Associated Disorders. The presentations of hypercalcemia vary with the patient's age, underlying disorder, magnitude of hypercalcemia, albumin level, and rapidity of onset. Individuals with mild hypercalcemia are frequently asymptomatic (identified by routine blood testing), whereas those with severe hypercalcemia may present in coma and rapidly progress to death. General features may reflect the underlying disorder, such as weight loss and cachexia with malignancy, or abdominal pain with acute pancreatitis. Less specific features include dehydration, polyuria, polydipsia, nocturia, hypercalciuria, urolithiasis, nephrolithiasis, nephrocalcinosis, renal impairment, GI disorders (anorexia, constipation, ileus, nausea, vomiting), pruritus, hypertension, and soft tissue deposition.

Neurologically, CNS symptoms predominate and can include headache, fatigue, apathy, depression, agitation, insomnia, hallucinations, psychosis, confusion, lethargy, obtundation, coma, and, rarely, seizures. The mental status changes are directly related to the degree of hypercalcemia and are more frequent at Ca levels exceeding 14 mg/dL. All CNS signs are reversible with treatment. PNS manifestations

TABLE 38–4. **Major Causes of Hypercalcemia**

Common Causes
Malignancy, hyperparathyroidism, thiazide diuretics
Less Common Causes
Familial hypocalciuric hypercalcemia
Vitamin D mediated
Calcium carbonate ingestion
Thyrotoxicosis and hypoadrenalism
Immobilization
Drugs (hypercalcemic agents, lithium, tamoxifen)
Artifactual (elevated serum proteins)

Data from Olinger ML: Disorders of calcium and magnesium metabolism. Emerg Med Clin North Am 1989;7:795–822; Spiegel AM: The parathyroid glands, hypercalcemia, and hypocalcemia. *In* Bennett JC, Plum F (eds): Cecil Textbook of Medicine, 20th ed. Philadelphia, WB Saunders, 1995, pp 1364–1373; and Lipsky MS: Hypercalcemia. *In* Rakel RE (ed): Saunders Manual of Medical Practice, Philadelphia, WB Saunders, 1996, pp 663–664.

reflect decreased neuromuscular excitability, and although they are common, these manifestations are nonspecific. Weakness is generally subjective with few objective signs.[42]

Differential Diagnosis and Evaluation. Before the realization that the observed clinical features reflect hypocalcemia, other etiologies must be considered. The particular cerebral manifestations, such as seizures and encephalopathic features, also dictate specific evaluation. The differential diagnoses of these central manifestations are lengthy and not addressed here (see Chapter 52). In the clinical setting of tetany, consideration should be given to disorders associated with cramping such as congenital myopathies and dystrophies (e.g., Duchenne's muscular dystrophy), cramp-myalgia syndrome (a dystrophinopathy), benign cramp syndrome (pseudotetanus), disorders producing contractures (e.g., McCardle's disease), and disorders producing continuous muscle activity (neuromyotonia).

The differential diagnosis of hypercalcemia is extensive. Frequently, the history, physical examination, initial laboratories, and routine radiographs identify the cause of hypercalcemia. A thorough examination may disclose features indicating the underlying disorder (e.g., breast mass, lymphadenopathy). Important laboratory evaluations include serum PTH level, urine Ca, CBC, chemistries (total and ionized serum Ca, Mg, P, alkaline phosphatase), urinalysis, stool for occult blood, ECG, and chest x-ray study. Other considerations include tests of adrenal and thyroid function, serum and urinary immunoelectrophoresis (for myeloma), vitamin D metabolite levels, and immunoassay for PTH-related peptide. A bone scan may be required in some patients, including those with suspected multiple myeloma (e.g., abnormal serum protein electrophoresis, anemia, increased plasma cells on blood smear). Also, 24-hour urinary excretion of calcium can be measured when familial hypocalciuric hypercalcemia (rare) is suspected.[34]

Management. Prevention of hypercalcemia in immobilized patients includes early mobilization and hydration, which increases calciuresis and dilutes the urine. High Ca–containing dietary products should be avoided. Although the underlying cause is the most important consideration for definitive treatment, the initial management of hypercalcemia depends on its magnitude and symptoms and may need to be initiated without a specific diagnosis. The major treatment modalities act by decreasing bone resorption, decreasing GI absorption, and increasing calciuresis. Mild hypercalcemia (<11.5 mg/dL) may require only recognition of the underlying disorder, recommendations to increase fluid intake, and careful follow-up. Conversely, in the setting of severe hypercalcemia (>15 mg/dL or severe clinical signs), urgent treatment is usually required and, in the setting of normal renal function, typically consists of volume replacement using IV normal saline, furosemide, and careful monitoring of therapy.

Prognosis and Future Perspectives. The prognosis for patients with hypercalcemia is related to the underlying disorder resulting in the hypercalcemia. Although cancer patients with hypercalcemia have a poor prognosis and usually die within a few months, hypercalcemic treatment usually improves their quality of life.

MAGNESIUM DISORDERS

Although magnesium (Mg) is the fourth most common cation in the body, less than 0.5 percent is present in the serum,[44] of which about 30 percent is protein bound, 15 percent is chelated to serum anions, and 55 percent exists in the ionized (physiologically active) form.[33] The amount of protein-bound Mg is directly proportional to the serum albumin concentration and the pH and is inversely proportional to the serum anion concentration. In addition, transcellular shifting between the intracellular and extracellular compartments can occur. Although the Mg contained in bone is not readily exchangeable with that present in the serum, a shift of Mg from the ECF to the intracellular fluid occurs with insulin administration[45] and the correction of acidosis.[33] Intracellular Mg functions as an essential co-factor in hundreds of important enzymatic reactions. Mg balance is regulated by the GI tract and the kidney, which maintains the serum Mg concentration between 1.6 and 2.1 mEq/L. An interrelationship exists between Mg and Ca, as evidenced by the development of hypocalcemia in response to Mg depletion.[46] In fact, Mg depletion is the most common cause of hypocalcemia in a general hospital population.[47] An interrelationship also exists between Mg and K, and although the mechanism is unknown, it may be related to the Mg requirement of the Na/K-ATPase enzyme system.[48]

Hypomagnesemia

Because the serum Mg concentration contributes less than 0.5 percent of total body Mg, the terms hypomagnesemia and Mg deficiency are defined separately. Hypomagnesemia refers to a serum Mg concentration below the normal range, whereas Mg deficiency refers to a decrease in the total body or intracellular Mg contents. In the clinical setting of severe tissue Mg deficiency, the serum Mg may be normal or even elevated. Conversely, in the setting of normal tissue stores, hypomagnesemia may be present.

Pathogenesis and Pathophysiology. Mg affects both the PNS and CNS. Peripherally, Mg has a curare-like action at the neuromuscular junction, an action counteracted by acetylcholinesterase inhibitors and Ca.[39] Mg is both a Ca channel antagonist (opposes Ca) and a membrane stabilizer (acts synergistically with Ca).[33] Centrally, Mg has a depressant effect (interestingly, hibernating animals are hypermagnesemic), which is opposed by pentylenetetrazol (Metrazol).[39]

Epidemiology and Risk Factors. Among hospitalized patients, the prevalence of hypomagnesemia is about 10 percent; it is approximately 20 percent when only intensive care unit patients are considered.[47] Because Mg deficiency is more common than hypomagnesemia,[33] the true incidence of Mg deficiency must exceed 10 percent. Risk factors for the development of hypomagnesemia include chronic diarrheal disorders, ketoacidosis, loop diuretic or digitalis usage, and alcoholism (Table 38–5).[33] Among patients with steatorrheic states, the prevalence of Mg depletion is about one third; the correlation between fecal Mg and fat content suggests that Mg depletion may be due to formation of a complex between Mg and fat. The recommended daily allowance of Mg (1200 mg) for pregnant and lactating women is 50 percent greater than that for nonpregnant women.[49]

Clinical Features and Associated Disorders. Hypomagnesemia may be asymptomatic, yet when it is symptomatic, the neurological manifestations include agitation, tremor, myoclonus, seizures (rarely), confusion, coma, paresthesias, muscle fasciculations, weakness, presence of Chvostek's and

TABLE 38–5. **Major Causes of Hypomagnesemia**

Hypoalbuminemia
Redistribution (correction of acidotic state)
Nutritional deficiencies
Gastrointestinal tract losses (chronic diarrhea)
Renal excretion (osmotic diuresis)
Drug induced:
  Acetazolamide, alcohol, aminoglycosides, amphotericin-B, cisplatin, digoxin, ethacrynic acid, furosemide, mannitol, methotrexate, pentamidine, theophylline, thiazides
Endocrine disorders (hyperthyroidism, hyperparathyroidism and hypoparathyroidism, ketoacidosis)
Multifactorial (chronic alcoholism, diabetic ketoacidosis)

Data from Olinger ML: Disorders of calcium and magnesium metabolism. Emerg Med Clin North Am 1989;7:795–822; Tosiello L: Hypomagnesemia and diabetes mellitus. Arch Intern Med 1996;156:1143–1148; and Alfrey AC: Disorders of magnesium metabolism. *In* Bennett JC, Plum F (eds): Cecil Textbook of Medicine, 20th ed. Philadelphia, WB Saunders, 1995, pp 1137–1138.

Trousseau's signs, tetany, and hyper-reflexia.[23, 47, 50, 51] In addition, a cardioskeletal mitochondrial myopathy has been described in association with chronic hypomagnesemia.[52] Athetoid and choreiform movements have also been reported during hypomagnesemia, although these signs may have reflected co-existent liver disease.[39] Unfortunately, the association of hypomagnesemia with hypokalemia, hypocalcemia, and other metabolic disorders makes it difficult to state with certainty which manifestations truly reflect hypomagnesemia. Importantly, the efficacy of Mg repletion in relieving manifestations of neuromuscular irritability may reflect its curare-like action (i.e., a therapeutic effect rather than reversal of deficiency symptoms). When the clinical manifestations of Mg deficiency are determined by induction of deficiency in human volunteers, GI features (anorexia, nausea, and vomiting), CNS features (lethargy, weakness, and personality change), PNS features (positive Trousseau's and Chvostek's signs, carpopedal spasm), tremor, and muscle fasciculations may be observed. Unfortunately, these features correlate with the development of hypocalcemia and hypokalemia.

Differential Diagnosis and Evaluation. Although the differential diagnosis of hypomagnesemia is long, it most commonly reflects an inadequate intake superimposed on impaired renal reabsorption or GI absorption. The two major problems in diagnosing Mg deficiency are that the serum Mg content represents only 0.5 percent of the total body content, and that the relationship between the serum level and the intracellular and total body content is poor. Thus, it is not uncommon to suspect hypomagnesemia and be faced with a normal serum Mg level. In this situation, a Mg loading test has been suggested.[45] The presence of either hypokalemia or hypocalcemia, especially when it is resistant to treatment, makes the likelihood of symptomatic hypomagnesemia even greater, and for that reason, the concentrations of these two electrolytes should be determined. A urine Mg level helps differentiate renal from nonrenal etiologies.

Mg, like Ca, affects both the CNS and the PNS. Because Mg functions as a membrane stabilizer (synergistic with Ca), hypomagnesemia (like hypocalcemia) produces membrane instability. For that reason, it should always be considered in the neurological differential diagnosis of hypocalcemia, especially when hypocalcemia is unresponsive to treatment. Diagnostic considerations to entertain vary with the clinical manifestations; they parallel those of hypocalcemia.

Management. The treatment of Mg deficiency depends on the underlying disorder, the clinical status of the patient, and the degree of deficit. In an emergency setting (e.g., seizure), Mg sulfate heptahydrate solution may be infused.[47] In the nonemergent setting, when hypomagnesemia is severely decreased, treatment may be IV or intramuscular. The intramuscular route is safer and preferred, when possible. Because serum Mg equilibrates with intracellular Mg slowly, rapid replacement may cause transient hypermagnesemia. Consequently, total body Mg repletion may require several days of treatment. Finally, in nonemergent settings when the degree of hypomagnesemia is not severe, oral replacement therapy can be undertaken using Mg oxide. In mild, asymptomatic cases, dietary modification to include high Mg–containing foods (e.g., dried fruits, grains, legumes, green leafy vegetables, and unprocessed cereals) may suffice. During Mg replacement therapy, the serum Mg level should be monitored frequently and treatment continued until a normal serum Mg level is achieved. Because Mg is a neuromuscular depressant, tendon reflexes should be monitored for evidence of overtreatment (diminished reflexes); the infusion should be discontinued if either hypermagnesemia or hyporeflexia is observed.[39] When Mg is replaced intravenously, Ca gluconate should be on hand to counteract transient hypermagnesemic-induced problems, such as apnea caused by respiratory muscle paralysis.[10]

Hypermagnesemia

Because the kidney is the major regulator of serum Mg levels, hypermagnesemia is frequently observed in patients with renal impairment, especially when the condition is combined with increased Mg intake. By blocking the presynaptic Ca channels, Mg acts to limit depolarization-induced Ca influx. Because exocytosis of acetylcholine-containing vesicles is Ca dependent, neuromuscular depression occurs. Symptomatic hypermagnesemia is infrequently encountered.

In contrast to the neuromuscular irritability observed with hypomagnesemia, the neurological manifestations of hypermagnesemia are characterized by nervous system depression. The predominant neuromuscular manifestation is muscle weakness (or paralysis) due to neuromuscular junction transmission blockade.[53] The manifestations of hypermagnesemia, both neurological and non-neurological, have been studied in experimental animals and human patients and reflect the degree of elevation of the serum Mg level. In general, patients are asymptomatic until the serum Mg level exceeds 4 mEq/L.[47] Blood pressure depression begins at levels between 3 and 5 mEq/L,[54] at which time the reflexes may be slightly depressed[47] and responsiveness may be slightly impaired.[39] As the serum Mg level increases further, hypotension becomes more pronounced. At levels between 7 and 10 mEq/L, the reflexes diminish and weakness and ataxia appear.[39] At this level, lethargy and confusion have been reported,[10] although this is controversial. In one study, levels as high as 12.4 mEq/L resulted in profound paralysis without significant changes in level of consciousness.[55] Possible explanations for the mental decline observed in patients with hypermagnesemia include chronicity, which permits the

CNS Mg level to rise; hypermagnesemia-induced hypoxic-ischemic encephalopathy; or neuromuscular junction blockade mistaken for mental status decline.[33] At 10 mEq/L, respiratory impairment appears with resultant hypoxia and hypercapnia.[39] At levels of 10 to 15 mEq/L, reflexes disappear and a flaccid quadriplegia may develop,[47] and as respiratory embarrassment worsens, CNS narcosis results in coma and death. Other symptoms associated with hypermagnesemia include nausea, lethargy, dilated pupils, bradycardia, and, rarely, complete heart block and cardiac arrest.[47]

The underlying cause of the hypermagnesemia, as well as its neurological and cardiovascular manifestations, should be identified. Respiratory, cardiac, and renal status should be determined. In the setting of hypermagnesemia, sources of Mg should be identified and discontinued. In asymptomatic patients with normal or mildly impaired renal function, this action alone may suffice. Because natriuresis enhances urinary Mg excretion, furosemide may be administered and the urine volume replaced.[47] Of course, this may induce hypocalcemia. In life-threatening situations, Ca salts can be administered to counteract the neuromuscular blockade and cardiotoxicity. Hemodialysis, using an Mg-free dialysate, is the most effective way of reducing serum Mg levels.[47]

Oxygen and Carbon Dioxide Abnormalities

Conditions causing hypoxemia include a low inspired oxygen (O_2) concentration, ventilation-perfusion mismatch, right-to-left shunting, impaired diffusion, and hypoventilation; those causing hypercapnia include the breathing of a carbon dioxide (CO_2)–containing gas, ventilation-perfusion mismatch, and hypoventilation. Because neuromuscular dysfunction produces hypoventilation, which, in turn, produces both hypoxemia and hypercapnia, distinguishing which neurological features are related to which condition is difficult. Although isolated hypoxic encephalopathy is seldom seen in humans[56] (e.g., mountain sickness), an understanding of its pathophysiological basis is important. Thus, this section is divided into three parts: hypoventilation, hypoxia, and hypocapnia.

HYPOVENTILATION

The respiratory system consists of the lungs and chest wall and has two functions: ventilation and gas exchange. Ventilation refers to the movement of air into and out of the lungs and is required for effective gas exchange. Ventilation requires the synchronized activities of both nervous and muscle tissue. The muscles of respiration (and their innervation) are typically divided into the inspiratory group (diaphragm [C3–C5], external intercostals [T1–T12], and scalenes [C4–C8]) and the expiratory group (abdominals [T7–L1] and internal intercostals [T1–T12]). During quiet breathing, the inspiratory muscles are active, with the diaphragm generating most of the tidal volume, and expiration is predominantly passive. When quiet breathing is unable to keep pace with the metabolic demands of the body (e.g., during exercise or respiratory muscle failure), the accessory muscles of inspiration (trapezii, sternocleidomastoids, serrati, pectorals, levator scapulae, and the costal levators) are recruited and expiration becomes active; thus, ventilation increases.

All levels of the neuraxis are involved in respiration, and for the most part, it occurs without voluntary effort (i.e., it is automatic). Automatic respiration occurs via two neuronal groups located within the brain stem: one is situated near the floor of the fourth ventricle (the medullary center), and the other is located within the pons (the pontine pneumotaxic center). The medullary neurons have inherent automaticity, and the pontine neurons help coordinate the cyclical respirations. Through synapses with motor neurons innervating respiratory muscles, these neurons are responsible for spontaneous respiration. Voluntary respiration, which involves corticospinal tract innervation of the same respiratory motor neurons, can override automatic breathing. Under normal circumstances, respiratory regulation reflects the $PaCO_2$ and pH and, to a lesser extent, the PaO_2. Chemoreceptors within the carotid and aortic bodies transmit this information to the respiratory centers in the brain stem (via cranial nerves IX and X, respectively), and respiration is adjusted accordingly.

The term *hypoxic encephalopathy* refers to the neurological findings resulting from impaired gas exchange or ventilation (e.g., anoxic anoxia, anemic anoxia, and histotoxic anoxia) and differs from the term *hypoxic-ischemic encephalopathy*, which refers to neurological dysfunction related to cerebral hypoperfusion (i.e., ischemic anoxia). With hypoxic-ischemic encephalopathy, in addition to hypoxia, there is loss of substrate (e.g., glucose) and impaired waste removal. Anoxic anoxia refers to reduced PaO_2 (e.g., at high altitudes), whereas anemic anoxia relates to reduced hemoglobin availability for O_2 transport (e.g., in anemia and carbon monoxide intoxication). Histotoxic anoxia occurs when, in the setting of adequate O_2 availability, the tissue's ability to use O_2 is impaired (e.g., cyanide toxicity).

Pathogenesis and Pathophysiology. Ventilatory failure results in hypercapnia as well as hypoxemia, a combination that causes cerebral vasodilation, increased cerebral blood flow (CBF), and, occasionally, increased ICP. Although hypoxemia probably contributes to the observed neurological features, the degree of CO_2 retention is more closely correlated.[56] Acute, moderate hypercapnia (5 to 10 percent CO_2 in the inspired air) increases arousal and excitability. At higher levels of CO_2, an anesthetic effect occurs, followed by a convulsant effect at the highest levels.[56, 57] Because CO_2 freely crosses the blood-brain barrier (BBB), thereby producing a cerebrospinal fluid (CSF) acidosis, respiratory acidosis is more neurologically disabling than is metabolic acidosis. Fortunately, several compensatory mechanisms exist to enhance the nervous system's tolerability of respiratory insufficiency. The CNS compensates by increasing O_2 extraction, CO_2 release, and CBF. These processes arise in conjunction with systemic alterations at the level of the kidney and with polycythemia.[58] Should compensatory mechanisms fail, hypoxia, hypercapnia, and acidosis develop and produce neurological sequelae. Sustained hypoxia produces brain edema and cell death, abnormalities that can precipitate cardiac arrhythmias and hypotension. Again, isolated hypoxic encephalopathy is seldom seen in humans.[56]

Clinical Features and Associated Disorders. Pulmonary disease causes both hypoxemia and hypercapnia, and distinguishing which neurological features are related to which state is difficult. The clinical features observed reflect the body's ability to compensate and the acuteness of the situation. The neurological manifestations are most closely related to the rapidity of onset and degree of hypercapnia, although hypoxia and cerebral edema may also contribute.[59] Compensatory mechanisms may render individuals asymptomatic, even in the setting of significant degrees of hypoxia and hypercapnia. When these mechanisms cannot keep pace, clinical features of respiratory insufficiency manifest. Initially, patients with respiratory insufficiency may complain of sleep disturbances, daytime somnolence, and early morning headache, a reflection of nocturnal hypoventilation with resultant CO_2 retention and vasodilation; however, these symptoms are nonspecific and can occur with CHF or respiratory muscle weakness.[60] Mental status changes are common early and include drowsiness, forgetfulness, and inattentiveness. Later, lethargy, obtundation, and coma may appear.[58] Tremor and asterixis are frequently seen, whereas myoclonus and seizures are uncommon and are observed only with severe and prolonged respiratory insufficiency.[59] Tendon reflexes may be brisk or depressed, upper motor neuron features may be present, and papilledema occurs in up to 10 percent of patients.[58]

Differential Diagnosis and Evaluation. Respiratory impairment may be caused by dysfunction of gas exchange or ventilation (Table 38–6). Differentiation between these two categories is important and is usually afforded by a thorough history, physical examination, and laboratory evaluation.

TABLE 38–6. **Major Causes of Respiratory Insufficiency**

Extrapulmonary Causes
Central nervous system (parenchymal disorders, increased intracranial pressure, sleep apnea)
Neuromuscular disorders
Spinal cord: tetanus, trauma
Anterior horn cell: amyotrophic lateral sclerosis, poliomyelitis, rabies
Nerve: Guillain-Barré syndrome, diphtheria, porphyria, ciguatoxin, saxitoxin, tetrodotoxin, thallium intoxication, acute hyperkalemic paralysis, buckthorn polyneuropathy
Neuromuscular junction: myasthenia gravis, congenital myasthenic syndromes, botulism, hypermagnesemia, organophosphate poisoning, tick paralysis, snake bite
Muscle: polymyositis, inclusion body myositis, myotonic dystrophy, limb girdle muscular dystrophies, hypophosphatemia, stonefish myotoxin, nemaline myopathy, centronuclear myopathy, rhabdomyolysis
Other: kyphoscoliosis, ankylosing spondylitis, chest trauma, extreme obesity, pleural diseases

Pulmonary Causes
Chest bellows (non-neurological)
Primary muscle fatigue
Secondary muscle dysfunction: electrolyte disturbances, malnutrition, reduced respiratory drive: metabolic alkalosis, sedation
Other (e.g., pulmonary parenchymal or airway disorders, cardiac failure)

Modified from Jozefowicz RF: Neurologic manifestations of pulmonary disease. Neurol Clin 1989;7:605–616; and Bennett DA, Bleck TP: Diagnosis and treatment of neuromuscular causes of acute respiratory failure. Clin Neuropharmacol 1988;11:303–347.

Unlike motor unit disorders that produce hypoventilation, CNS disorders produce abnormal respiratory patterns, such as Cheyne-Stokes (forebrain and diencephalic damage), central neurogenic hyperventilation (hypothalamic and midbrain damage), apneustic (inspiratory breath holding related to pontine tegmental damage), cluster (irregular bursts of rapid breathing alternating with apneic periods), and ataxic (irregular breathing related to medullary damage) breathing patterns. The respiratory impairment associated with spinal cord disorders is predominantly a reflection of its location. Lesions at C3 affect diaphragmatic and intercostal function and spare only the accessory muscles of inspiration innervated by cranial nerve XI. Lesions at C4 or C5 produce lesser degrees of diaphragmatic impairment. Low cervical and high thoracic lesions spare the diaphragm but affect the intercostal and abdominal muscles, thereby limiting full inspiration and active expiration. Midthoracic lesions affect only the abdominal muscles and therefore interfere only with active expiration. Respiratory impairment due to diaphragmatic weakness is worse in the supine position and improved in the erect position, a reflection of the effect of gravity on the abdominal contents. These features should be sought on physical examination. The electroencephalographic (EEG) changes associated with pulmonary encephalopathy are nonspecific and similar to those observed in patients with other forms of metabolic encephalopathy (i.e., diffuse slowing and slowing of the posterior dominant rhythm).

It is important to determine whether or not respiratory impairment reflects neurological dysfunction. Helpful studies for this discrimination include an ABG, pulmonary function tests, and electromyographic examination. Neuromuscular system dysfunction impairs ventilation and is associated with both hypercapnia and hypoxemia. Non-neurological mechanisms of respiratory insufficiency (e.g., impaired gas exchange) initially produce hypoxemia without hypercapnia. This reflects the nonlinear hemoglobin dissociation curve of O_2 versus the essentially linear loading curve of CO_2. Thus, high-ventilation areas of the lung are able to compensate for low-ventilation areas until pulmonary disease is severe. In summary, hypoxemia in the presence of a normal or decreased $PaCO_2$ is indicative of a parenchymal process. Neurological versus non-neurological respiratory impairment may also be differentiated by determining the A-a gradient (i.e., the gradient between alveolar [A] and arterial [a] O_2 tensions), a value that is easily determined. The PaO_2 and $PaCO_2$ are obtained from the ABG, and the PAO_2 is obtained from the following equation:

$$PAO_2 = [(PB - 48) \times FIO_2] - PaCO_2/R,$$

where PB is the barometric pressure (760 mm Hg at sea level), FIO_2 is the fraction of O_2 in the inspired air (0.21 in room air), and R is the respiratory quotient (0.8). On room air, an A-a gradient above 20 to 30 mm Hg always indicates intrapulmonary pathology, whereas an A-a gradient below 10 mm Hg suggests extrapulmonary causes of hypoxemia (e.g., hypoventilation). Pulmonary function test parameters indicative of respiratory muscle weakness include reduced vital capacity, reduced maximum voluntary ventilation, and increased residual volume. Of these parameters, only the vital capacity can be measured outside of the pulmonary function test laboratory. Maximum expiratory and inspiratory pressures are better parameters for identifying respiratory muscle weakness[61]; maximum expiratory pressure is the most sensitive indicator for patients with neuromuscular disease. Although it is less useful for identifying respiratory muscle weakness, forced vital capacity is useful for the serial assessment of patients with known neuromuscular disorders. When the vital capacity drops below 25 mL/kg body weight, the ability to cough is impaired and oropharyngeal secretion accumulation occurs. Thus, the risk of aspiration pneumonia is significantly increased. Routine nerve conduction studies (NCS) (including phrenic NCS), repetitive nerve stimulation, and needle electrode examination (including the diaphragm) can be of great assistance in identifying both the nature (e.g., demyelinating neuropathy) and the site (e.g., nerve, neuromuscular junction, or muscle) of the underlying disorder.

Management. If the condition is left untreated, encephalopathy related to pulmonary dysfunction may lead to coma and death. The mainstays of treatment are to improve gas exchange and ventilation. In patients with chronic hypercapnia, in whom hypoxia-stimulated respiratory drive exists, high-concentration O_2 administration may produce clinical deterioration due to CO_2 retention. The O_2 affinity of hemoglobin and cytochrome is not as great as the affinity for carbon monoxide (CO) and cyanide, respectively. For that reason, CO and cyanide toxicity may require hyperbaric O_2 therapy.[62–64]

Prognosis and Future Perspectives. Because cerebral O_2 delivery depends on the mean arterial blood pressure and autoregulation, and because compensatory mechanisms exist, it is difficult to determine the severity of hypoxia a patient has experienced. When there is no loss of consciousness, there is rarely if ever any permanent nervous system damage.[62] When hypoxia induces hypoperfusion (e.g., cardiac arrest) and hence ischemic anoxia, the prognosis worsens.

HYPOXIA

Hypoxia increases CBF, glucose use, and brain lactate concentration, whereas energy metabolite (e.g., adenosine triphosphate [ATP], adenosine diphosphate [ADP], and adenosine monophosphate [AMP]) levels remain close to normal, even during severe hypoxia.[65] Breathing 10 percent O_2 for 15 to 30 minutes increases the CBF by 35 percent, whereas breathing 7 percent O_2 (PaO_2 35 mm Hg) for 15 minutes increases CBF by 75 percent.[65] Once the PaO_2 drops below 25 mm Hg, ATP decreases, AMP and ADP increase, and the EEG is markedly slowed or nearly isoelectric.[65] In addition, changes in ion homeostasis are induced by hypoxia. Unlike ischemic anoxia, in which Ca uptake is increased, hypoxia diminishes Ca uptake, thereby decreasing Ca-dependent acetylcholine release; this can be overcome by agents that enhance Ca uptake at the nerve terminals.[66] Finally, neurotransmitter metabolism is also affected by hypoxia. Acetylcholine synthesis is O_2 dependent, and brain acetylcholine levels are decreased in the setting of hypoxia. However, because acetylcholine release in some brain regions is Ca dependent, the lowered brain acetylcholine levels may reflect the effect of hypoxia on Ca metabolism. Changes in amino acid, catecholamine, and serotonin neurotransmitter levels, as well as adenosine, cyclical nucleotides, and fatty acids, have also been reviewed.[65]

Compensatory physiological mechanisms (e.g., increased erythropoiesis and O_2 dissociation curve shifts) permit adaptation to hypoxia, thereby making the effects of hypoxia time dependent and necessitating separate discussions for acute and chronic hypoxic states. Healthy human volunteers subjected to rapid decompression hypoxia (analogous to acute hypoxia, clinically) demonstrate an association between the PaO_2 level and the neurological features observed.[56] New skill learning and the processing of complex information are the most vulnerable to hypoxia.[65] At a PaO_2 of 80 mm Hg, impaired dark adaptation is noted; at 55 to 45 mm Hg, impaired learning and short-term memory occurs, whereas measures of selective attention are normal; at 40 to 30 mm Hg, loss of judgment, euphoria, delirium, and muscular incoordination occurs; additionally, twice as much light is required for visual perception; below 25 to 20 mm Hg, consciousness is rapidly lost.[56, 65] High altitude sickness begins shortly after ascending above 10,000 feet and is characterized by headache, decreased concentration, sleep disturbances, anorexia, nausea, and lassitude (see Chapter 51).

The clinical features of acute CO toxicity include prominent headache, nausea, vomiting, and encephalopathic features. The cherry-red lip appearance often described with this disorder is only present at high CO levels in comatose patients (see Chapter 39).

Several posthypoxic neurological syndromes have been described, including myoclonus, delayed anoxic encephalopathy, parkinsonism, and cerebral palsy. Global cerebral hypoxia of any etiology can result in myoclonus, as well as other neurological deficits. Posthypoxic myoclonus presents in two different clinical forms. Immediately following the hypoxic event, while the patient remains comatose, myoclonic jerks can appear. This acute form is transient and characterized by spontaneous jerks that involve the face predominately, yet may be generalized. Little is known about the electrophysiological properties of this acute posthypoxic myoclonus, but the prognosis associated with this sign is poor. In those patients who survive the hypoxic event and regain consciousness, a second type of delayed posthypoxic myoclonus may develop. Lance and Adams described this delayed form in patients demonstrating stimulus-sensitive intention or action myoclonus (posthypoxic action myoclonus [PHAM]) following cardiac or respiratory arrest.[67] The characteristic feature of PHAM is the occurrence of myoclonus, both positive and negative, with voluntary movement, especially walking and movements requiring precision. Patients may be unable to walk when negative myoclonus occurs during ambulation. Fahn summarized the clinical findings of 88 patients (permanent in 87) with PHAM.[68] All were acutely comatose with a median duration of unconsciousness of 4 days (range, 1 to 120 days). The duration of coma did not correlate with the subsequent severity of the action myoclonus. Anesthesia-related mishaps were the single most common cause of cerebral hypoxia, with other etiologies including myocardial damage, drug overdose, and airway obstruction. Other neurological abnormalities, including cerebellar dysfunction, spasticity, dementia, and cortical blindness, were observed in these patients following the resolution of coma. EEG recordings may reveal generalized symmetrical or asymmetrical sharp waves, or spikes with slow waves may be detected.

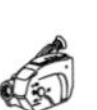

Alternatively, moderate- to high-voltage fast activity, occurring centrally, can be observed. Other patients have slowing of the background or even normal EEGs. Somatosensory evoked potentials in patients with PHAM may initially be enlarged, yet decrease in size following initiation of therapy. The pathophysiological basis of PHAM is a matter of conjecture. Only a few pathological investigations exist and are not significantly helpful in the understanding of the pathophysiology of PHAM. 5-Hydroxytryptophan (5-HTP), the serotonin precursor, has been shown to be beneficial in PHAM and has generated considerable interest in the possible role of brain serotonin in this form of myoclonus. 5-HTP alone and with carbidopa has been effective in reducing the amplitude of the myoclonic jerks. 5-HTP is started at 100 mg/day in four divided doses and is increased by 100 mg every 3 to 5 days, slower if side effects occur. Maximum daily dosage ranges from 1000 to 2000 mg. Carbidopa is given at 25 to 50 mg four times daily and should not be stopped before the discontinuation of 5-HTP. Lower doses of 5-HTP (400 to 500 mg) may suffice when administered with either fluoxetine or paroxetine, serotonin uptake inhibitors, and carbidopa. Despite the use of carbidopa, systemic side effects are nearly universal and frequently necessitate 5-HTP dose reduction or discontinuation. Common side effects include diarrhea, nausea, vomiting, abdominal pain, euphoria, insomnia, and blurred vision. Other medications with some utility in the treatment of PHAM, either alone or in combination, include valproate, piracetam, and clonazepam. The other benzodiazepines, phenobarbital, and phenytoin are usually of no benefit.

Postanoxic encephalopathy is an unexplained phenomenon that is observed during recovery (1 to 4 weeks) from an anoxic insult. It is characterized by irritability, confusion, apathy, and occasionally agitation or mania.[69] Although most patients with this disorder survive for a period, serious mental and motor disturbances are reported, and many patients develop diffuse rigidity, spasticity, weakness, a shuffling gait, incontinence, coma, and death after 1 to 2 weeks.[69] At autopsy, the major pathological finding is widespread cerebral demyelination.[62] Uncommonly, rigidity, muteness, and helplessness develop over a period of weeks to months, and, in these cases, autopsy reveals the basal ganglia to be more affected than the cerebral white matter and cortex.[62, 70]

Parkinsonism following cerebral anoxia is usually accompanied by a large number of other neurological sequelae, a reflection of the cerebral structures most susceptible to anoxic insult (i.e., Sommer's sector of Ammon's horn, Purkinje's cells, the cerebral cortex [especially layer 3], the striatum, and the globus pallidus). For that reason, a "pure" parkinsonian syndrome is unexpected. It has been reported in CO intoxication, in both the acute and chronic settings.[71]

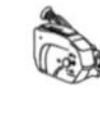

Cerebral palsy refers to a syndrome of acquired, nonprogressive perinatal encephalopathy due to a variety of insults, including anoxia, hypoperfusion, trauma, vascular events, congenital abnormalities, and kernicterus (less common today). Asphyxia accounts for only a minority of cases, the most common cause reflecting prenatal factors that are difficult to identify with certainty.[72] Cerebral palsy may be classified based on the type of motor impairment, and its distribution is segregated into spastic types and hypotonic types. Spastic types include spastic diplegia (legs more involved than arms), which is more common in premature infants; spastic hemiplegia, which is the most common form acquired after birth; and spastic quadriplegia (usually asymmetrical with arms more involved than legs), which is sometimes termed *double hemiplegia*. The hypotonic types include athetoid (predominant basal ganglia development) and ataxic (predominant cerebellar involvement). The spectrum of intellectual and motor deficit ranges from normal intelligence with mild motor deficits to severe retardation without the ability to walk.

HYPOCAPNIA

Hyperventilation is defined as breathing in excess of metabolic demands and, therefore, is purely a respiratory disturbance. It produces hypocapnia, respiratory alkalosis, cerebral vasoconstriction (which, in turn, reduces the CBF), a reduction in the availability of O_2 peripherally (through shifts of the O_2 dissociation curve), a reduction in the level of ionized serum Ca, and, when sustained, significant hypophosphatemia.[58] Thus, neurological features are frequent, and patients with hyperventilation disorders are frequently referred to neurologists. Symptoms associated with hyperventilation vary widely and include lightheadedness, acral and perioral paresthesias (which may be painful), syncope and, less commonly, carpopedal spasms, muscle cramps, blurred vision, headache, dyspnea, and chest pain.[57, 58] Other reported symptoms include sweating of the hands, cold extremities, giddiness, ataxia, tremor, tinnitus, hallucinations, epigastric pain, a bloated feeling, vomiting, and unilateral somatic symptoms, which may result in the misdiagnosis of cerebral ischemia, seizure, or complicated migraine.[73] Once it is induced, hypocapnia can be maintained with only an occasional sigh, thereby making its visual recognition difficult.[74] These symptoms probably arise from a reduction in CBF and are associated with significant cerebral hypoxia.[73] For every 1 mm Hg drop in $PaCO_2$, the CBF drops by 2 percent.

Disorders associated with hyperventilation can be subdivided into psychogenic (e.g., anxiety, panic, sighing, air hunger, or factitious disorders), organic (usually multifactorial including respiratory disease, CNS disorders, pain, aspirin overdose), and physiological (progesterone ingestion, prolonged conversation, hypoxic stimulation of chemoreceptors at high altitude, pyrexia).[73] Hyperventilation is frequently reported in anxious individuals without any identifiable systemic disease.[58] However, because isolated anxiety (i.e., in the absence of hyperventilation) has no effect on CBF, it should not produce these symptoms.[75] Patients with organic disorders (e.g., asthma) can present with hyperventilation. Additionally, disorders producing anxiety (e.g., angina) can cause hyperventilation. Thus, the identification of hyperventilation should never be considered synonymous with anxiety, nor should these patients be taken less seriously. For that reason, whenever hyperventilation is recognized, organic etiologies should be excluded and treatment initiated.

Endocrine Abnormalities

An interdependence exists between the endocrine and nervous systems, as demonstrated by the influence of hormones on the nervous system and the requirement of an intact nervous system for endocrine activity. Endocrine disorders may initially present with signs and symptoms of neurologic disease, whereas pre-existing neurologic disorders may worsen in the setting of endocrine dysfunction. In the past, when early screening was not commonplace and treatment was not an option, the neurological features ascribed to endocrine dysfunction were much more pronounced. However, because these disorders are now diagnosed earlier, the clinical features are often much more subtle. The early recognition of endocrine-related neurological dysfunction is important because the condition is frequently reversible.

THYROID DISORDERS

The thyroid gland synthesizes and secretes tetraiodothyronine (T_4) and, in much smaller quantities, triiodothyronine (T_3), which is at least two to four times more potent than T_4. Both of these hormones regulate tissue metabolism. Iodine is bound to tyrosine residues of thyroglobulin in the thyroid gland (organification), and these iodinated residues are then coupled to form T_4 and T_3. Both protein-bound (inactive) and unbound (active) thyroid hormone fractions exist in serum. In the periphery, T_4 is deiodinated to T_3, accounting for about 80 percent of T_3 production[76]; otherwise it is converted into reverse T_3 (rT_3), a metabolically inactive product.

Hypothyroidism

Pathogenesis and Pathophysiology. Hypothyroidism can be related to thyroid gland dysfunction (i.e., primary hypothyroidism), to a disturbance outside of the thyroid gland (i.e., central hypothyroidism), or to peripheral resistance to thyroid hormone.[77] Hypothyroidism is the most common disorder of thyroid function and is most often caused by primary hypothyroidism rather than by secondary hypothyroidism. Mechanisms of thyroid gland dysfunction include parenchymal destruction (viral or autoimmune), chronic inflammation with lymphocytic infiltration (Hashimoto's thyroiditis), cell death (radiation damage), or defective hormonogenesis. Defective hormonogenesis may occur due to inadequate iodine intake (i.e., endemic goiter), excessive ingestion of goitrogens (e.g., turnips), intrinsic defects in thyroid hormone production (e.g., rare enzymopathies), as well as medication-induced thyroid hormone synthesis disturbance (e.g., lithium, thionamides, amiodarone). In some patients, iodine loading may cause significant hypothyroidism (Wolff-Chaikoff effect). In addition, the hypothalamic-pituitary-thyroid axis can be disturbed following head injury[78] or pituitary apoplexy.[79]

Although the pathogenesis and pathophysiology of many of the peripheral neurological manifestations of the hypothyroid state are known, most of the CNS manifestations are unexplained. Although hypothyroid-induced seizures may be related to hyponatremia, coma likely represents a multifactorial process.[80] Direct metabolic effects or entrapment by adjacent tissue (e.g., myxedematous infiltration) may cause peripheral and cranial mononeuropathies.[76, 77] Persistent percussion-induced local muscle contraction is referred to as myoedema and is caused by delayed Ca reuptake by the sarcoplasmic reticulum, thereby prolonging the contraction.[81] A reduction in myosin ATPase activity contributes to slowed contraction, and delayed reuptake of Ca by the sarcoplasmic reticulum contributes to delayed relaxation.[82] Also, a shift in muscle fiber type distribution from fast twitch to slow twitch may contribute to slowed muscle contraction and relaxation.[83] In addition, a reduction in muscle mitochondrial oxidative capacity and beta-adrenergic receptors, as well as the induction of an insulin-resistant state, may contribute to weakness, fatigue, and exertional pain.[83] The pathophysiology of the muscle enlargement, a feature more commonly observed in children (Kocher-Debré-Sémélaigne syndrome), is uncertain, although work hypertrophy related to prolonged contraction is suspected.[82]

Epidemiology and Risk Factors. The incidence of primary hypothyroidism is much greater in women than in men,[76, 84] especially among women between the ages of 40 and 60 years. Central hypothyroidism (e.g., hypothalamic- and pituitary-related), on the other hand, is more commonly observed among the neurosurgical population.[27] Primary hypothyroidism is much more common than secondary hypothyroidism and is usually caused by autoimmune destruction (e.g., Hashimoto's thyroiditis), irradiation, or surgically treated hyperthyroidism. Pituitary and hypothalamic disease contribute less than 10 percent of cases of hypothyroidism.[80] Myxedema coma is extremely rare, and its incidence is higher in elderly women, especially those over 60 years.[77] Risk factors for myxedema coma include noncompliance with levothyroxine therapy, infection, surgery, drugs, hyponatremia, and the winter months.[77, 80] Although complex changes in thyroid function occur during pregnancy, the normal pregnant woman is euthyroid,[85] and the incidence of hypothyroidism is not influenced by pregnancy.[38]

Clinical Features and Associated Disorders. Clinically, the onset of hypothyroidism may range from subtle and insidious findings to florid psychosis. The general examination features of hypothyroidism are numerous (Table 38–7). CNS features include forgetfulness, inattention, apathy, and slowing of speech, movement, and mentation. These features may

TABLE 38–7. **General Features of Hypothyroidism**

Subjective	Objective
Fatigue, somnolence, cold intolerance, syncope, exertional dyspnea, weight gain, arthralgias, nausea, anorexia, indigestion, constipation, menstrual abnormalities	Bradycardia, hair changes (sparse, coarse, dry, brittle), puffy face, loss of lateral aspects of the eyebrows, periorbital edema, macroglossia, voice deepening and hoarsening, skin changes (scaly, thick, doughy, coarse, dry, carotenemia), brittle nails, nonpitting edema, galactorrhea, effusions

Data from Mitchell JM: Thyroid disease in the emergency department: Thyroid function tests and hypothyroidism and myxedema coma. Emerg Med Clin North Am 1989;7:885–902; Mazzaferri EL: Adult hypothyroidism: I. Manifestations and clinical presentation. Postgrad Med 1986;79:64–72; Myers L, Hays J: Myxedema coma. Crit Care Clin 1991;7:43–56; and Kaminski HJ, Ruff RL: Neurologic complications of endocrine diseases. Neurol Clin 7:489–508.

mimic depression. Seizures, personality changes, psychotic states, coma, and dementia may also be clinically apparent. Cerebellar ataxia is seen in 5 to 10 percent of patients[86] and may be the presenting sign (so-called myxedema staggers); its pathophysiology remains unknown. A psychotic presentation (myxedema madness) characterized by agitation, disorientation, delusions, hallucinations, paranoia, and restlessness is observed in approximately 3 to 5 percent of patients.[76] Myxedema coma is extremely rare, and its characteristic features include extreme hypothermia, seizures (the presenting manifestation in nearly 20 percent of patients[80]), respiratory depression, and areflexia. Death can occur when early recognition and prompt treatment are lacking. Dementia may develop when hypothyroidism is severe. Except for the marked increase in the number of hours these patients remain asleep or resting, the clinical features of the dementia are similar to those secondary to other causes.[87] The pathophysiology of Hashimoto's encephalopathy is unknown but may reflect an inflammatory vasculitis of the CNS. As emphasized by Doherty, its clinical features include rapidly progressive dementia, seizures, extrapyramidal rigidity, myoclonus, and, on occasion, focal CNS features. It and the EEG features associated with it may mimic a prion disease. Often, the patient is biochemically euthyroid with elevated thyroid peroxidase antibodies as the only marker.[88, 89]

Peripheral neuromuscular features include cranial and peripheral neuropathies, prolonged reflex relaxation time (up to 85 percent of hypothyroid patients),[76, 77] and myopathy. Visual field defects can occur when pituitary enlargement causes hypothyroidism with concomitant chiasmal compression. A facial mononeuropathy, due to nerve entrapment in the fallopian canal of the temporal bone, may rarely occur.[90] Although sensorineural hearing loss has been reported to correlate with the degree of hypothyroidism and has a high incidence among patients with congenital hypothyroidism,[87] its reported incidence among adult hypothyroid patients varies.[91] Minor evidence of polyneuropathy, such as distal lower extremity sensory dysfunction and absent ankle jerks, is observed in approximately 10 percent of patients,[82] and, rarely, a moderately severe sensorimotor polyneuropathy has been described. Carpal tunnel syndrome (i.e., median mononeuropathy at the wrist) occurs in 15 to 30 percent of hypothyroid patients, is usually bilateral, and is the most common mononeuropathy encountered.

Myopathy can be a feature of hypothyroidism and manifests with proximal muscle weakness. Regardless of the cause of the hypothyroidism, weakness is observed in about one third of these patients.[81] Increased muscle size and firmness, which is most obvious in the limb musculature, as well as slowed muscle contraction are important features to identify. Exertional pain, stiffness, and cramps may be noted, and myoedema may be observed. Hoffman syndrome is a myopathic syndrome characterized by firm, large, well-developed muscles and prominent myotonia that can be seen in adults with hypothyroidism. Myoedema, a mounding of the muscle in response to direct percussion, is painless and electrically silent and occurs in one third of hypothyroid patients.[81] Difficulty relaxing the hand grip and exacerbation by cold weather may suggest myotonia. However, unlike myotonia, hypothyroid myopathy involves a slowness of muscle relaxation and contraction and resolves with correction of the hypothyroid state.[87] In patients with newly detected hypothyroidism, skeletal muscle is less frequently affected, despite the fact that 25 percent of patients with hypothyroidism have muscle symptoms. Although sleep apnea is usually of the obstructive type, other possibilities include a central abnormality, chest muscle weakness, and blunted responses to hypoxia and hypercapnia.[76] Reports have associated hypothyroidism with SIADH,[27] idiopathic intracranial hypertension,[92] and myasthenia gravis.

Differential Diagnosis. The differential diagnosis of hypothyroidism includes nonthyroidal illness (i.e., decreased T_3 or T_4, or both, without clinical hypothyroidism), euthyroid hypothyroxinemia (decreased T_4 caused by decreased thyroid-binding globulin), and drugs that inhibit T_4 binding (salicylates, phenytoin, and phenobarbital). Once hypothyroidism has been diagnosed, the most important clinical distinction is between primary and secondary hypothyroidism. The clinical and laboratory similarities between myxedema coma and other life-threatening causes of the comatose state may make its diagnosis extremely difficult. Regarding hypothyroid myopathy, the muscular appearance, stiffness, and exacerbation by cold may suggest a mild form of myotonia congenita, which can present in adulthood. Although the stiffness noted in patients with pyramidal and extrapyramidal diseases may appear similar to that of hypothyroid myopathy, the characteristic history, appearance, and laboratory studies usually permit the diagnosis of hypothyroidism.

Evaluation. The combination of a low T_4 level and an elevated thyroid-stimulating hormone (TSH) level is virtually diagnostic of primary hypothyroidism, because TSH elevation does not occur in central hypothyroidism. Further delineation between primary and secondary hypothyroidism is dependent on history, examination, and other laboratory studies. In addition to TFTs, other laboratory abnormalities have been described, including anemia (normocytic-normochromic, microcytic-hypochromic, or macrocytic) and hyponatremia (factitious due to hyperlipidemia or secondary to impaired free water excretion), as well as elevated serum creatine kinase (CK), myoglobin,[83] and prolactin. Although elevated CK levels are frequently observed in patients with hypothyroidism, when patients with predominantly subclinical and mild hypothyroidism are studied, elevated CK levels are much less frequent (about 3 percent). Because of the possibility of concomitant adrenal insufficiency, a serum cortisol level should also be obtained. The EEG may show slowing of the posterior dominant rhythm and a generalized voltage decrease, as well as triphasic waves that disappear with replacement therapy.[93] CSF analysis may reveal an elevated protein content which may exceed 100 mg/dL.

Management. The treatment of hypothyroidism, regardless of cause, consists of thyroid hormone replacement. Thyroxine dosages may need to be increased when females with hypothyroidism are placed on estrogen therapy.[89] Even in the setting of hypothyroid-induced seizures, achievement of the euthyroid state facilitates control.[86] Precipitants of myxedema coma (e.g., infection, cold exposure, certain drugs [phenothiazines, narcotics, and sedative-hypnotics, phenytoin, rifampin], and other stressors [surgery, trauma]) require correction.[76]

Prognosis and Future Perspectives. With early recognition and treatment, as well as improved intensive supportive care, the mortality rate of myxedema coma has decreased from roughly 50 to 70 percent to around 15 to 20 percent.[94]

Without early recognition and prompt institution of replacement therapy, the prognosis is grave.[95]

Hyperthyroidism

Pathogenesis and Pathophysiology. Thyroid hormones affect mitochondrial oxidative capacity, protein synthesis and degradation, tissue sensitivity to catecholamines, muscle fiber differentiation, and capillary growth.[96] Excess thyroid hormone produces accelerated muscle protein catabolism and enhanced lysosomal protease activity and interferes with the anabolic effects of insulin on muscle.[81] Despite this understanding, the exact pathophysiology of thyrotoxic myopathy remains unknown. CNS observations include elevated rates of cerebral circulation, faster posterior dominant rhythms, alterations in the sensitivity of some brain enzymes and neurotransmitter systems, and altered metabolic responses.[96] At present, the specific pathophysiological processes causing these manifestations remain unknown. It has been proposed that alterations in central and peripheral beta-adrenergic tone may be responsible for hyperthyroid-related tremor and chorea and that brisk tendon reflexes may reflect faster muscle contraction and relaxation times. As outlined by Weetman, Graves' disease is caused by thyroid-stimulating antibodies that activate the thyrotropin receptor on thyroid cells, causing thyroid hypersecretion, hypertrophy and hyperplasia of thyroid follicles, and the characteristic diffuse goiter.

Epidemiology and Risk Factors. Hyperthyroidism is more common in women than in men (10:1 ratio) and often shows a strong familial predisposition. During pregnancy, hyperthyroidism occurs more commonly than hypothyroidism, with an incidence ranging from 0.05 to 0.2 percent, most commonly related to Graves' disease, acute (i.e., subacute) thyroiditis, toxic nodular goiter, and toxic adenoma.[38, 85] The incidence of low-birth-weight infants is significantly increased, and neonatal mortality is slightly increased.[85]

Clinical Features and Associated Disorders. The general clinical features of thyrotoxicosis are numerous (Table 38–8). Neuropsychiatric signs include impaired attention, concentration, and memory, as well as emotional lability, nervousness, hypervigilance, lethargy, depression (i.e., apathetic hyperthyroidism), mania, psychosis, insomnia, and agitated delirium.[86] Apathetic hyperthyroidism most frequently occurs in the elderly, lacks the usual hyperadrenergic features, and may easily be confused with depression or dementia.

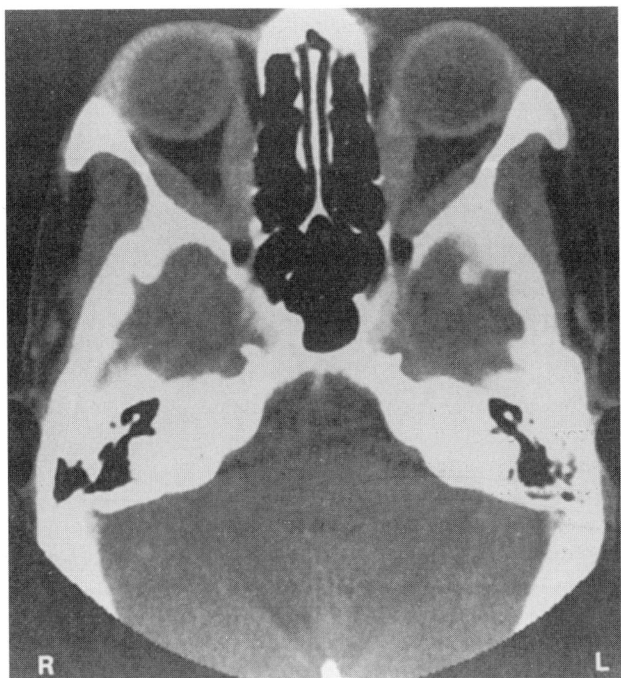

FIGURE 38–2. A 40-year-old woman who presented with complaints of double vision. This brain computed tomography of the orbits demonstrates enlarged extraocular muscles bilaterally associated with Graves' ophthalmopathy. (From Kennell T, Levy JM, Stegman CJ: Radiologic case. West J Med 146:241, 1987. Reprinted by permission of The Western Journal of Medicine.)

Although new-onset adulthood seizures are rarely related to hyperthyroidism, the seizure incidence among thyrotoxic patients ranges from 1 to 9 percent.[83] Movement disorders, such as tremor (usually enhanced physiological tremor) and choreoathetosis, as well as upper motor neuron signs, including spasticity, hyper-reflexia, clonus, and Babinski's signs, may also be observed.[71, 97] 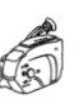

Peripheral neurological features include cranial and peripheral neuropathies, as well as neuromuscular junction and muscle disturbances (Fig. 38–2). Ocular features include lid lag, stare, widened palpebral fissures, extraocular muscle dysfunction with diplopia, and optic nerve compression with visual impairment. Eyelid retraction manifests in several

TABLE 38–8. General Features of Thyrotoxicosis

Subjective	Objective
Impaired concentration and memory, emotional lability, nervousness, irritability, palpitations, heat intolerance, increased sweating and appetite, weight loss, frequent defecation, menstrual abnormalities, insomnia, headaches	Impaired attention span and memory, hypervigilance, systolic flow murmurs, skin changes (warm, moist, smooth), ECG changes (sinus tachycardia, atrial fibrillation), psychiatric problems (depression, mania, bipolar disorder, manic psychosis), chorea, thyrotoxic periodic paralysis, thyroid storm, ocular features

Data from Weiner WJ, Lang AE (eds): Movement Disorders: A Comprehensive Survey. New York, Futura, 1989; Kaminski HJ, Ruff RL: Neurologic complications of endocrine diseases. Neurol Clin North Am 1989;7:489–508; Abend WK, Tyler HR: Thyroid disease and the nervous system. *In* Aminoff MJ (ed): Neurology and General Medicine, 2nd ed. New York, Churchill Livingstone, 1995, 333–347; and Shahar E, Shapiro MS, Shenkman L: Hyperthyroid-induced chorea: Case report and review of the literature. Isr J Med Sci 1988;24:264–266.

ways: (1) Stellwag's sign, a staring expression with infrequent blinking; (2) Dalrymple's sign, a widened palpebral fissure due to retraction of both the upper and lower lids; (3) von Graefe's sign, a larger than normal portion of visible sclera with downward eye movement; (4) Joffroy's sign, a lack of frontalis muscle contraction with upgaze; and (5) Möbius' sign, sympathetic overactivity-induced exophthalmos with resultant limited convergence.[86] Although reports of a distal sensorimotor polyneuropathy in thyrotoxic patients are rare, improvement of the neuropathic features with attainment of the euthyroid state indicates that these features are manifestations of hyperthyroidism.[98] Myasthenia gravis (MG) can be associated with hyperthyroidism, although some of the reported cases may have been secondary to coincident MG.[83] Also, when bulbar weakness responds to treatment of the hyperthyroid state, it is more likely related to hyperthyroidism.[99] When MG co-exists with thyrotoxic myopathy, the clinical findings do not differ from those in euthyroid patients, although the patients may be weaker due to the co-existence of two motor disorders. Thyrotoxic myopathy is characterized by the gradual onset of proximal limb weakness, which may be accompanied by myalgias, easy fatigability, and prominent atrophy. Although the muscular atrophy may be severe, most patients remain ambulatory. Shoulder girdle muscles can be more severely affected than the hip girdle muscles, with prominent atrophy and scapular winging.[81, 82] Distal limb muscles are also affected, the facial muscles may be affected, and, rarely, bulbar and ocular muscles are involved.[82, 96] Thyroid-associated ophthalmopathy refers to the exophthalmos and ocular muscle dysfunction associated with thyroid disease. It is seen in most patients with Graves' disease but is also seen in 5 percent of patients with Hashimoto's thyroiditis. It is not correlated with the onset of Graves' disease,[100] having been reported to precede (rarely), occur concomitantly with, or develop after its treatment. It also does not correlate with the level of circulating thyroid hormone and may occur in euthyroid patients or in patients with hypothyroid Graves' disease.[86] When it is prominent, thyroid-associated ophthalmopathy may cause exposure keratopathy (due to marked proptosis), as well as optic nerve compression. Thyrotoxic periodic paralysis refers to recurrent attacks of flaccid paralysis of the limbs and trunk (the oculobulbar muscles are usually spared or involved to a lesser degree) due to secondary hypokalemia.

Differential Diagnosis. The differential diagnosis of thyrotoxicosis includes other hypermetabolic disorders, euthyroid hyperthyroxinemia, and nonthyroidal causes. Occasionally, recognition that myopathic features are due to thyrotoxicosis can be difficult, especially if the myopathy is the presenting feature (rare), when exophthalmos is minimal, or when an apathetic state is present.[101] When it is present, the observation of hyper-reflexia is helpful, because this feature is not observed in other metabolic myopathies. Thyrotoxic myopathy with pronounced muscular atrophy should be differentiated from progressive muscular atrophy by the presence of fasciculations and more profound weakness in the latter. When thyrotoxic myopathy involves the ocular and bulbar musculature, it must be differentiated from MG. In thyrotoxic myopathy, rapid muscle fatigue and recovery with rest is not appreciated, a response to anticholinesterases is not observed, and decrement is not apparent on EMG; in MG, ocular and bulbar muscle involvement is more pronounced and atrophy is not present.[96] Also, myasthenia gravis is painless, without orbital congestion, lid lag, lid retraction, or exophthalmos. The ophthalmoplegia is paretic, rather than restrictive, and usually there is lid ptosis, diurnal variation, and Cogan's lid twitch, as well as normal orbital imaging studies.[102] Conversely, with thyroid ophthalmopathy, mild orbital discomfort, orbital congestion, lid lag, lid retraction, exophthalmos, restrictive ophthalmoplegia (often late), and absence of ptosis, diurnal variation, and Cogan's lid twitch are observed. Also, a positive forced duction test and enlarged extraocular muscles on imaging studies of the orbits are characteristic.[102] These two conditions may co-exist. Polymyositis should also be considered and is differentiated by EMG and muscle biopsy. In the setting of episodic weakness, thyrotoxic periodic paralysis should be considered. The latter is a sporadic disorder that is much more frequent among the Asian population, is much more frequent in males, typically begins in the second decade of life, affects the lower extremities more frequently than the upper extremities, and spares the oculobulbar muscles.[102] Vigorous exercise and high-carbohydrate meals may precipitate acute attacks.

Evaluation. TFTs can confirm thyrotoxicosis, typically demonstrating an elevated free T_4, total T_4, T_3RU, free thyroxine index, free T_3, total T_3, and a suppressed (usually undetectable) TSH. A normal or elevated TSH in the face of unequivocal clinical thyrotoxicosis should raise suspicion for a TSH-secreting pituitary adenoma. Other laboratory features may include anemia, hypokalemia, hypercalcemia, and an elevated erythrocyte sedimentation rate. Roughly half of hyperthyroid patients demonstrate EEG changes, most commonly generalized slowing or excessive fast activity, both of which resolve with attainment of the euthyroid state.[83] Magnetic resonance imaging (MRI) with gadolinium may demonstrate the characteristic features of thyroid ophthalmopathy including multiple extraocular muscle involvement, smooth margins gradually tapering into the tendon insertions, and uniform enhancement when contrast is administered. These features are readily displayed with fat saturation techniques that de-emphasize intraocular fat. Optic nerve impingement may also be visualized with a similar approach. MRI may also be useful in ruling out orbital pseudotumor, Tolosa-Hunt syndrome, orbital lymphoma, Wegener's granulomatosis, and orbital aspergillosis.[103]

When co-existent MG is considered, acetylcholine receptor antibodies in response to edrophonium (Tensilon) may be helpful in its evaluation. Although the Tensilon test may be normal in MG (false-negative result) and may lead to improvement of dysthyroid orbitopathy (false-positive result),[86] patients with thyrotoxic bulbar features typically do not have immunological, electrophysiological, or pharmacological evidence of MG.[82]

Management. Almost all of the clinical features of thyroid dysfunction, with the exception of thyroid-associated ophthalmopathy, resolve once the euthyroid state is achieved.[96, 104] Medical treatment of thyrotoxicosis includes the use of beta-blockers; antithyroid, anti-inflammatory, and immunosuppressive drugs; radioactive iodine-131; and iodine-containing compounds. Beta-blockers, in addition to decreasing the beta adrenergic–mediated features of thyrotoxicosis, may decrease the peripheral conversion of T_4 to T_3. Beta-blockers are also useful in the prophylactic treatment of TPP while attainment of the euthyroid state is awaited. A typical dosage regimen is propranolol, 40 mg four times daily.[82] Prophylaxis against further attacks includes avoidance of identified precipitants and acetazolamide until restoration of the euthyroid state is achieved. In hyperthyroid patients with co-existent MG, beta-blockers should be used cautiously because of their neuromuscular blocking properties.[82] Higher-grade orbital features typically require either systemic corticosteroids (with or without cyclosporine), irradiation, or orbital decompression,[105] yet some believe surgery is rarely indicated because the dysthyroid orbitopathy usually spontaneously arrests before a serious degree of ophthalmopathy has been reached.[106] One of the most frequent complications of thyroid surgery is recurrent laryngeal nerve paralysis.[107] A more limited surgery involving partial lid suturing may be required to protect the cornea. When an undetectable serum thyrotropin concentration is identified in the presence of normal serum T_3 and T_4 concentrations, the term *subclinical hyperthyroidism* is applied. Toft provided recommendations on its management. Significant depression can be associated with subclinical hyperthyroidism.

PARATHYROID DISORDERS

See the sections on hypocalcemia and hypercalcemia.

ADRENAL DISORDERS

Hypoadrenalism

Pathogenesis and Pathophysiology. The adrenal gland is the effector organ of the hypothalamic-pituitary-adrenal (HPA) axis and secretes cortisol in response to stimulation by pituitary-derived corticotropin (adrenocorticotropic hormone [ACTH]). Pituitary function, in turn, is under the control of corticotropin-releasing hormone from the hypothalamus. Dysfunction anywhere in the HPA axis may result in adrenal insufficiency. Primary adrenal insufficiency (PAI) is due to bilateral adrenal gland destruction, and secondary adrenal insufficiency (SAI) results from hypothalamic or pituitary dysfunction. Although brain injury affects the HPA axis, the most frequent cause of adrenal insufficiency is iatrogenic SAI following the withdrawal of exogenously administered steroids.[78] The fatigue and weakness associated with hypoadrenalism reflect the associated hypotension as well as the water and electrolyte disturbances. The role of glucocorticoids in catabolic energy mobilization likely also contributes.

Epidemiology and Risk Factors. PAI is relatively rare, may occur at any age, and affects both sexes equally.[108] Acquired immunodeficiency syndrome and active tuberculosis are significant risk factors for PAI. Major risk factors for SAI include prior administration of exogenous corticosteroids, especially prolonged, high-dose courses, and any destructive lesion of the pituitary or hypothalamus.

Clinical Features and Associated Disorders. The clinical features of adrenal insufficiency are influenced by the site of dysfunction, because PAI affects all of the adrenocortical hormones, whereas SAI only affects glucocorticoids. Thus, hyperpigmentation, salt craving, and hyperkalemia are unique to patients with PAI. Patients with adrenal insufficiency may present acutely or as a chronic condition. Acute adrenal insufficiency is a medical emergency (so-called addisonian crisis) characterized by mental status changes, fever, hypotension, volume depletion, arthralgias, myalgias, and abdominal pain that may mimic an acute abdomen.[109] Chronic adrenal insufficiency may present more insidiously with fatigue, weakness, GI symptoms, amenorrhea, decreased libido, salt craving, arthralgias, and hypoglycemic symptoms. Neurological manifestations can include confusion, apathy, depression, psychosis, paranoia, and myalgias, as well as hypoglycemic symptoms.[110] In addition, a past medical history of cancer, recent tuberculosis exposure or steroid usage, immunosuppression, a history of treated Cushing's syndrome, features of hypothalamic/pituitary disease, or other endocrine deficiencies, as well as a family history of a sex-linked recessive disorder, should be sought.

Differential Diagnosis. In the industrialized world, approximately 70 percent of cases of PAI are autoimmune in etiology (due to the polyendocrine deficiency syndrome), 20 percent are related to tuberculosis (most common cause worldwide), and the remaining 10 percent are due to other causes (Table 38–9).[109] SAI commonly follows exogenous steroid withdrawal and the surgical treatment of Cushing's syndrome; it is uncommonly related to hypothalamic or pituitary lesions.[109] The neurological differential diagnosis relates to the rapidity of onset of the hypoadrenalism. In the setting of acute adrenal insufficiency (i.e., addisonian crisis), the differential diagnosis of acute-onset encephalopathy must be entertained in addition to those disorders that produce septic shock. With a more chronic presentation, the differential diagnosis varies with the clinical manifestations and includes those disorders associated with encephalopathy, fatigue, weakness, or myalgias.

Evaluation. The evaluation of patients with suspected adrenal insufficiency serves to determine the adequacy of cortisol production and to localize the process within the HPA axis (i.e., PAI versus SAI). Tests to assess cortisol production include the serum cortisol level, ACTH (Cortrosyn) stimulation test, insulin tolerance test, and the metyrapone test. The plasma ACTH level is the principal localizing test,[111] and in severely stressed patients with normal adrenal function, serum cortisol levels range from 20 to 120 μg/dL.[109] In unstressed patients, the normal cortisol level overlaps with that observed in patients with adrenal insufficiency, making random cortisol testing less useful in this group.

TABLE 38–9. **Major Causes of Adrenal Insufficiency**

Primary adrenal insufficiency
Autoimmune
Infections
Hemorrhage
Metastatic disease
Drugs
Infiltrative
Bilateral adrenalectomy
Adrenoleukodystrophy; adrenomyeloneuropathy; congenital adrenal hypoplasia
Secondary adrenal insufficiency
Suppression of the hypothalamic-pituitary-adrenal axis
Lesions of the pituitary or hypothalamus

Modified from Loriaux DL: Adrenocortical insufficiency. *In* Becker KL, Bilezikian JP, Brenner WJ, et al (eds): Principles and Practice of Endocrinology and Metabolism, 2nd ed. Philadelphia, JB Lippincott, 1995, pp 682–686; and Rone JK: Adrenal insufficiency. *In* Rakel RE (ed): Saunders Manual of Medical Practice, Philadelphia, WB Saunders, 1996, pp 653–656.

Management. In patients receiving exogenous glucocorticoids, the prevention of HPA axis suppression is aided by using the lowest possible dosage, shortest duration, and an every-other-day dosing schedule, when possible. The treatment of adrenal insufficiency is hormone replacement. In general, in acute adrenal insufficiency, IV hydrocortisone is administered and fluid, Na, and glucose are replaced. In chronic adrenal insufficiency, the preferred replacement glucocorticoid is also hydrocortisone, because it has a short half-life and is therefore less likely to produce Cushing's syndrome or osteoporosis.[110] A typical regimen is hydrocortisone, 20 mg in the morning and 10 mg in the evening. Mineralocorticoid replacement may be required in PAI and is usually provided by fludrocortisone (Florinef), 0.05 to 0.1 mg/day, along with the recommendation for a high-Na diet. The management of an uncommon endocrine emergency, pituitary apoplexy, recently has been reviewed.[79]

Hyperadrenalism

Hyperadrenalism refers to hypersecretory disorders of the adrenal medulla (e.g., pheochromocytoma) and cortex (e.g., aldosteronism and Cushing's syndrome). *Pheochromocytomas* are catecholamine-secreting tumors of neural crest (neuroectoderm) origin that may be sporadic or familial. In adults, approximately 10 percent of these tumors are malignant, 10 percent are extra-adrenal (i.e., 90 percent occur within the adrenal glands), and 10 percent are bilateral.[112]

The major clinical features of pheochromocytoma are headaches, palpitations, diaphoresis, hypertension, hypotension, pallor, weight loss, chest pain, and abdominal pain.[112] Other features include dizziness, anxiety, nausea, vomiting, diarrhea, mydriasis, tachycardia, pulmonary edema, and CHF.[106] A more serious neurological feature is intracranial hemorrhage. *Pheochromocytoma multisystem crisis* is a serious and rare presentation that is characterized by encephalopathic features, multiple organ failure, fever, and labile blood pressure.[113] Pheochromocytoma can be associated with multiple endocrine neoplasia type II, neurofibromatosis, and von Hippel–Lindau disease.[106]

The differential diagnosis of hypertension associated with hyperadrenergic symptoms is extensive and includes thyrotoxicosis, anxiety and panic disorders, hypoglycemia, diencephalic epilepsy, acute myocardial infarction, abrupt clonidine withdrawal, and drug usage (e.g., monoamine oxidase inhibitors, cocaine, decongestants). Although pheochromocytoma is rare, its life-threatening status requires consideration and exclusion whenever hypertension is associated with suggestive symptoms, especially the triad of headache, palpitations, and diaphoresis.

A total plasma catecholamine (epinephrine plus norepinephrine) level, drawn 30 minutes after supine rest, can be diagnostic. Values above 2000 pg/mL are pathognomonic for pheochromocytoma, whereas those below 1000 pg/mL exclude pheochromocytoma. Twenty-four–hour urine studies (metanephrines, normetanephrines, and vanillylmandelic acid) and clonidine suppression testing are required when values between these levels are obtained.[112] Twenty-four–hour urine studies are diagnostic in up to 90 percent of patients with pheochromocytoma.[106] Once the diagnosis of pheochromocytoma is confirmed, tumor localization becomes the priority and is best evaluated by abdominal CT.

For neurologists, it is important to consider pheochromocytomas in patients with headaches and other suggestive symptoms. Serious morbidity and mortality may occur when these patients present with headache and beta-blocker therapy is begun, which allows unopposed alpha-adrenergic stimulation. This may result in CHF, myocardial or cerebral infarction, malignant hypertension, or death. When pheochromocytoma is considered to be a diagnostic possibility, referral to an endocrinologist for further evaluation and treatment is appropriate. With the widespread availability of imaging (CT, MRI) and biochemical assays, the incidence of undiagnosed pheochromocytoma has dropped significantly.[112] With surgery, most pheochromocytomas are cured. However, 10 percent are malignant and current treatments for widespread metastases are unsatisfactory.

Aldosteronism results from the overproduction of aldosterone by the adrenal cortex and can be primary or secondary. Primary aldosteronism refers to aldosteronism related to adrenal gland disorders such as aldosterone-secreting adrenal adenomas (Conn's syndrome) and functional overactivity of both adrenal glands (idiopathic hyperaldosteronism). Secondary aldosteronism refers to stimulation of aldosterone production by extra-adrenal influences, such as occurs in CHF, cirrhosis, volume depletion (or other conditions of decreased effective renal perfusion), and Barrter's syndrome, a rare disorder characterized by hyper-reninemia, hypokalemia, and normal blood pressure. Aldosteronism, both primary and secondary, results in hypokalemia and metabolic alkalosis, which, in turn, may cause neurological symptoms. Primary aldosteronism is approximately twice as common in women, occurs between the ages of 30 and 50 years, and is found in approximately 1 percent of hypertensive patients.[108] It is the most common endocrine cause of secondary hypertension.

Aldosteronism-induced hypokalemia may trigger episodic attacks of severe muscular weakness (similar to periodic paralysis), tetany, paresthesias, polyuria, and hypertension.[114] The episodic attacks of weakness are similar to both the familial and thyrotoxic forms of periodic paralysis, although respiratory paralysis is more common.[82] Unlike the familial form, hypokalemia and alkalosis may be present between attacks.[82] In addition to episodic weakness, a subacute or chronic myopathy may develop. In this setting, serum creatinine kinase may be moderately elevated and EMG examination discloses myopathic features that are often accompanied by fibrillation potentials.[82] Rarely, rhabdomyolysis and myoglobinuria occur. Laboratory features include an inability to concentrate the urine, hypernatremia, hypokalemia, metabolic alkalosis, and hypokalemic-induced ECG changes. The plasma renin activity should be measured, because this factor allows the differentiation between primary (suppressed) and secondary (elevated) aldosteronism.

The etiology dictates the treatment. In idiopathic hyperaldosteronism, medical therapy is primary, whereas hyperaldosteronism due to an adenoma is typically treated by surgical excision, although medical treatment with spironolactone (an aldosterone antagonist) and dietary Na restriction may be effective (antihypertensives may also be required).

Cushing's syndrome is the clinical expression of chronic excess adrenal corticosteroids (i.e., hypercortisolism) and can be classified into ACTH-dependent and ACTH-independent etiologies.[115] Disorders belonging to the ACTH-dependent category overproduce cortisol in response to excessive ACTH release, whereas those in the ACTH-independent category produce cortisol without ACTH stimulation. ACTH-dependent causes account for 80 percent of the cases of endogenous Cushing's syndrome and include ACTH-producing pituitary tumors (Cushing's disease; 65 percent), as well as both ACTH-producing (15 percent) and corticotropin-releasing hormone–producing (rare) ectopic tissue.[116] ACTH-independent etiologies account for 20 percent of the cases of Cushing's syndrome and include adenoma and carcinoma of the adrenal gland, nodular hyperplasia, and cortisol-secreting tumors.[116] In addition to these endogenous etiologies, prolonged administration of exogenous glucocorticoids can cause a nearly identical syndrome.

The clinical features of Cushing's syndrome vary with the underlying etiology and are dependent on the amount of ACTH, cortisol, and other adrenocortical steroids secreted (Table 38–10). Neuropsychiatric manifestations can include irritability, emotional lability, depression, and psychotic episodes.[83, 106] Approximately 50 percent of the patients with Cushing's disease have muscle weakness.[82] Other possible neurological signs are mental status changes and visual field defects as well as optic neuropathy when pituitary adenomas extend beyond the confines of the sella turcica. Rarely, the accumulation of fat epidurally can result in the development of a myelopathy. An association with idiopathic intracranial hypertension has also been reported (see Chapter 53).

Cushing's syndrome must be differentiated from disorders producing secondary hypercortisolism (e.g., obesity, major depression, alcoholism). Initial evaluation usually includes an overnight dexamethasone suppression test and a 24-hour urine collection for free cortisol. Free cortisol typically exceeds 90 μg/day in Cushing's syndrome. The overnight dexamethasone suppression test assesses the patient's ability to suppress cortisol production in response to a low dose of dexamethasone. Typically, 1 mg of dexamethasone is administered at 11 PM, and a blood sample for serum cortisol is drawn at 8 AM. Serum cortisol is suppressed to below 5 μg/dL in normal individuals, whereas it is above 10 μg/dL in patients with Cushing's syndrome. False-positive results may be noted with physiological stress, estrogen or antiepileptic drug use, RF, and endogenous depression.[116]

Basic laboratory studies may identify glucose intolerance, leukocytosis with lymphopenia, polycythemia, and hypokalemia. Hypokalemia is unusual in Cushing's disease (10 percent) but is much more common in the ectopic ACTH syndrome (60 percent).[116] An MRI scan of the pituitary is the procedure of choice for the identification of pituitary adenomas. Abdominal CT scanning for the presence of an adrenal tumor is indicated in ACTH-independent syndromes. The treatment of endogenous Cushing's syndrome depends on the underlying etiology.

TABLE 38–10. The Clinical Features of Cushing's Syndrome and Disease

Cushing's Syndrome	Cushing's Disease
Hypertension, diabetes, hyperphagia, central obesity, moon facies, dorsocervical fat deposition (buffalo hump; may cause myelopathy), hirsutism, acne, menstrual disorders, evidence of protein catabolism (e.g., easy bruising, myopathy, osteopenia), cutaneous lesions (hyperpigmentation; wide, purple striae), psychiatric manifestations	Mental status changes, idiopathic intracranial hypertension, visual field defects, optic neuropathy

Data from Layzer RB: Neuromuscular manifestations of endocrine disease. *In* Becker KL, Bilezikian JP, Bremner WJ, et al (eds): Principles and Practice of Endocrinology and Metabolism, 2nd ed. Philadelphia, JB Lippincott, 1995, pp 1762–1770; and Schteingart DE: Cushing syndrome. *In* Becker KL, Bilezikian JP, Bremner WJ, et al (eds): Principles and Practice of Endocrinology and Metabolism, 2nd ed. Philadelphia, JB Lippincott, 1995, pp 667–682.

GROWTH HORMONE DISORDERS

Growth hormone (GH; somatotropin) is secreted by the anterior pituitary in response to hypothalamic GH-releasing hormone (GHRH). GH promotes linear growth and has both anabolic and catabolic effects. Hypersecretion of GH causes gigantism when it occurs before epiphyseal closure and acromegaly when it begins afterward. Hyposecretion causes short stature in childhood and possibly a chronic fatigue-like syndrome in adults. GH acts indirectly through insulin-like growth factors (IGFs, somatomedins), with IGF-1 (formerly somatomedin C) being the most important for growth. Prolonged exposure to elevated levels of GH and IGF-1 results in the insidious onset of skeletal and soft tissue overgrowth, the latter of which is most pronounced in tissues containing large amounts of cartilage proteoglycans.[117] Cortical bone density is increased and trabecular bone (e.g., vertebral) density is decreased, probably because of co-existent hypogonadism.[117] Soft tissue hypertrophy may result in compression neuropathies, radiculopathies, and, rarely, myelopathy.[81]

More than 98 percent of cases of acromegaly are due to GH hypersecretion by a pituitary adenoma.[118] Rare etiologies include increased hypothalamic production of GHRH, ectopic pharyngeal pituitary tissue, and ectopic hormone (GH, GHRH)–secreting tumors (e.g., hypothalamic gangliocytoma; breast, stomach, and lung tumors).[117] GH-secreting pituitary adenomas are relatively rare, with an incidence of 3 to 4 per million and a prevalence of 50 to 70 per million.[118] There is no sexual predilection, and the majority of patients are diagnosed in their fourth or fifth decade, after a mean delay of 8.7 years.[119]

If it is present, an enlarging pituitary adenoma may produce headaches, visual changes (e.g., bitemporal hemianopia due to optic chiasm compression), and hypopituitarism (e.g., decreased ACTH or TSH levels due to anterior pituitary destruction), as well as DI (posterior pituitary involvement) and diplopia (due to cavernous sinus invasion). The lack of correlation between headache and tumor size reported in some series[119] suggests that headache may also be a feature of GH hypersecretion.

The hypersecretion of GH produces various forms of disfigurement and other physical changes (Table 38–11). Central sleep apnea has been reported in one third of acromegalic patients with sleep apnea.[120] Importantly, the presence of sleep apnea increases the risk for hypertension, myocardial infarction, and stroke, as well as accident susceptibility due to daytime sleepiness.[118] Mononeuropathies,

TABLE 38–11. **General Features of Growth Hormone Hypersecretion**

Growth Hormone Hypersecretion
Musculoskeletal: Increasing hat, glove, or shoe sizes; prognathism; prominent supraorbital ridges; coarsening of facial features (e.g, large bulbous nose, thick lips, separated teeth)
Endocrine: Hyperhidrosis, fatigue, exercise intolerance, hoarseness, sleep apnea (peripheral and central)
Cardiopulmonary: Hypertension, hyperlipidemia, cholelithiasis, carbohydrate intolerance, overt diabetes, heart disease (e.g., arrhythmias, congestive heart failure, coronary artery disease)
Other: Arthralgias, slight kyphosis, visceromegaly, reproductive problems (women: amenorrhea, galactorrhea, anovulatory problems; men: decreased libido, hypogonadism), hyperprolactinemia, adenomatous polyps and colon cancer, esophageal and gastric cancer, parathyroid and pancreatic islet cell adenomas (MEN-I syndrome)

Pituitary Gland Enlargement
Headaches, visual changes (e.g., bitemporal hemianopsia due to optic chiasm involvement), hypopituitarism, diabetes insipidus, diplopia

MEN-I, Multiple endocrine neoplasia, type I.
Data from Kissel JT: Endocrine myopathies, *In* Update on Neuromuscular Disease. Course 423 of the AAN Annual Meeting, Washington, DC, May, 1994, pp 34–35; Maugans TA, Coates ML: Diagnosis and treatment of acromegaly. Am Fam Phys 1995;52:207–213; Molitch ME: Clinical manifestations of acromegaly. Endocrinol Metab Clin North Am 1992;21:597–614; and Grunstein RR, Ho KY, Sullivan CE: Sleep apnea in acromegaly. Ann Intern Med 1991;115:527–532.

especially compression neuropathies such as carpal tunnel syndrome (CTS), may be noted. CTS occurs in 50 percent of patients and is noted in 75 percent when EMG testing is performed.[82] Objective weakness, in a myopathic pattern, is observed in about 40 percent of acromegalic patients.[82] The weakness typically has an insidious onset and is a late manifestation, correlating best with the duration of acromegaly.[81] Polyneuropathies, nerve root and spinal cord compression, headaches, and visual changes have also been described.[81]

The most sensitive and specific screening test for acromegaly is the IGF-1 level. The pulsatile nature of GH secretion may result in a randomly high GH level being obtained in a normal person, as may physical stressors, making this a less useful test. All patients with elevated IGF-1 levels should have an oral glucose tolerance test, the gold standard for acromegaly. MRI can confirm the suspicion of a pituitary adenoma. When MRI is negative in an acromegalic patient, consideration should be given to the rarer etiologies of acromegaly.

The prevention of many of the sequelae of disorders associated with acromegaly (e.g., hypertension, cardiovascular disease, stroke, sleep apnea, diabetes, arthropathy) requires early identification and treatment. The management of acromegaly includes the identification of the source of the excess GH secretion and its excision, irradiation, or medical suppression. The somatostatin analog octreotide is a highly effective pharmacological means of controlling GH secretion[106] but has the disadvantage of high cost and the need for multiple daily injections.

GLUCOSE METABOLISM DISORDERS

Hypoglycemia

Pathogenesis and Pathophysiology. Unlike other body tissues, the CNS relies almost exclusively on glucose as an energy substrate. CNS features that promote its vulnerability to hypoglycemia include its low glucose level (about 25 percent of the serum glucose value), its inability to store significant glucose as glycogen, and the high cerebral metabolic rate (5 mg/100 g brain tissue/min) for glucose.[121] Thus, for a 1400-g brain, the glucose requirement is 70 mg/min. The brain's dependence on glucose, coupled with its limited glycogen stores, results in rapid CNS dysfunction when hypoglycemia occurs and permanent neurological sequelae if it is prolonged. The glucose level at which CNS dysfunction occurs depends on its rapidity of onset, the current level of CNS activity, the quantity of CNS glycogen, and the availability of alternative fuels. The immediate cause of CNS dysfunction is unknown. Although it was initially believed to be due to tissue energy depletion, high-energy organic phosphates are normal during the early stages of symptomatic hypoglycemia.[56] Alternative explanations include accumulation of metabolic byproducts of nonglucose metabolism, impaired acetylcholine synthesis, and changes in neurotransmitter levels, such as those of glutamate, aspartate, and gamma-aminobutyric acid.[56] When glucose slowly decreases, the CNS can use nonglucose substrates, especially ketoacids and glucose metabolism intermediaries,[62] as well as several amino acids.[56]

Epidemiology and Risk Factors. Hypoglycemia is a common problem without predilection for any age, gender, or ethnic group. Although excessive insulin administration is the most common cause of hypoglycemia,[57] excessive use of oral hypoglycemic agents is another common cause. The major risk factor for the development of reactive hypoglycemia (infrequent) is GI surgery (e.g., vagotomy and pyloroplasty, gastrectomy, or gastrojejunostomy).

Clinical Features and Associated Disorders. Symptoms of hypoglycemia can be divided into adrenergic and neuroglycopenic (low CNS glucose). The adrenergic symptoms (e.g., diaphoresis, tachycardia, enhanced physiological tremor) are inversely correlated to the rate of development of hypoglycemia, being most pronounced with acute onsets. Hunger, visual disturbances, and altered temperature perceptions are other possible adrenergic features. The neuroglycopenic features include headache, malaise, impaired concentration, confusion, disorientation, irritability, lethargy, stupor, coma, generalized seizures, myoclonus, and psychiatric disturbance. Focal CNS dysfunction, including focal seizures, hemiplegia, paroxysmal choreoathetosis, and patchy brain stem and cerebellar involvement mimicking basilar artery thrombosis, have also been reported.[122] With subacute onsets, drowsiness, lethargy, decreased psychomotor activity, and confusion may be observed,[62] and when chronic, the insidious onset of memory, personality, and behavioral disturbances may suggest dementia.[123] The medullary phase of hypoglycemia, characterized by deep coma, pupillary dilatation, shallow breathing, bradycardia, and hypotonicity, occurs at a blood glucose level of around 10 mg/dL.[62]

Adrenergic features, when present, precede neurobehavioral features, thereby functioning as an early warning system. However, when sympathetic dysfunction (e.g., diabetic autonomic neuropathy) exists or when adrenergic blockers are being used, these features may be inapparent.

Differential Diagnosis and Evaluation. Hypoglycemia may be divided into fasting (the overwhelming majority), reactive (uncommon), and artifactual (Table 38–12). Fasting hypoglycemia is usually the result of exogenous insulin or oral hypoglycemic administration by diabetic patients. Drug-induced hypoglycemia can be caused by pentamidine, nonsteroidal anti-inflammatory drugs, salicylates, sulfonamides, clofibrate, phenytoin, rifampin, thyroid hormone, anabolic steroids, and probenecid. Enzyme defects causing hypoglycemia are rare and typically begin in childhood. By prolonging the half-life of insulin and oral agents, RF may result in hypoglycemia. Liver disease may also cause hypoglycemia in this way while also impairing glucose production and glycogen storage. Disorders of fatty acid utilization increase the need for glucose and may rapidly result in hypoglycemia. Reactive hypoglycemia is most commonly caused by surgical procedures (iatrogenic) that result in rapid gastric emptying, which, in turn, stimulates excessive insulin release, thereby causing hypoglycemia.[124]

The neurological symptoms associated with hypoglycemia primarily reflect CNS involvement (e.g., encephalopathy and seizures) and are related to the rapidity of onset. Diagnostic considerations of patients with hypoglycemia depend on the presenting manifestations (e.g., disorders known to produce seizures, when hypoglycemia is associated with such, or disorders known to produce encephalopathy, when hypoglycemia is associated with confusion).

Evaluation. Whipple's triad (hypoglycemic features, laboratory confirmation of a low serum glucose, and resolution of symptoms with glucose replacement) is diagnostic of hypoglycemia. To identify the underlying cause of hypoglycemia, other studies, including serum studies for C-peptide, proinsulin and insulin levels, antibodies to insulin or its receptor, and sulfonylurea levels, may be required in addition to routine laboratories. Abdominal imaging (CT or MRI) and arteriography, for tumor localization, may be useful. In the evaluation of related neurological symptoms, the EEG reveals generalized slowing, unless the degree of hypoglycemia is mild. In this setting, hyperventilation-induced slowing may persist after hyperventilation is discontinued. In the setting of symptomatic hypoglycemia, the confusional state correlates with EEG slowing. Additionally, seizure activity may be observed. As the glucose level drops further, the comatose state supervenes and burst-suppression activity is demonstrated on the EEG. Intravenous administration of glucose can reverse hypoglycemic seizure activity and coma.

TABLE 38–12. Major Causes of Hypoglycemia

Fasting
Inadequate glucose supply, excessive glucose demand
Reactive
Iatrogenic (abrupt discontinuation of total parenteral nutrition)
Fructose and leucine intolerance and galactosemia
Idiopathic
Artifactual (lymphoproliferative disorders)

Data from Bleck TP: Metabolic encephalopathies. *In* Weiner WJ (ed): Emergent and Urgent Neurology. Philadelphia, JB Lippincott, 1992, pp 27–57; Lockwood AH: Toxic and metabolic encephalopathies. *In* Bradley WG, Daroff RB, et al (eds): Neurology in Clinical Practice, 2nd ed. Boston, Butterworth-Heinemann, 1996, pp 1355–1372; and Yealy DM, Wolfson AB: Hypoglycemia. Emerg Med Clin North Am 1989;7:837–848.

Regarding symptom resolution with glucose replacement, although catecholamine-mediated features usually respond within minutes, the CNS-related features may require longer for resolution.[124] If the CNS features do not resolve within an hour, permanent CNS damage may have occurred. In addition, the possibility that the hypoglycemia is related to another disorder should be considered.

Management. Prevention of serious morbidity and mortality requires early recognition of hypoglycemia and prompt glucose replacement, regardless of etiology. To avoid masking of the autonomic (warning) features of hypoglycemia, beta-blockers should be avoided in patients taking hypoglycemic agents. To prevent the development of Wernicke-Korsakoff syndrome in alcoholic and malnourished patients, thiamine supplementation (1 mg/kg) should also be administered before giving glucose. Malnourished patients should also receive niacin to prevent pellagra. Depending on the etiology, more specific therapies may be indicated (e.g., corticosteroid replacement for adrenal insufficiency).

Prognosis and Future Perspectives. Hypoglycemia is associated with a substantial morbidity, primarily related to accidents (e.g., vehicular) and seizures with resultant injuries.[121] In the setting of hypoxic encephalopathy, premature prognostication should be avoided, given that slow improvement may continue for 1 to 2 years.[62] When glucose is replaced before the medullary phase is reached, the features may be reversible. After this point, especially if treatment was delayed, recovery may be protracted or incomplete.[62] The potential risk of glucose administration to euglycemic and hyperglycemic patients is small compared with the potentially substantial benefit. However, the possibility of cerebral ischemia must be considered, because hyperglycemia at the onset of brain ischemia worsens the postischemic outcome, whereas hyperglycemia occurring *after* experimental cerebral infarction does not.[57, 125]

Hyperglycemia

Diabetic ketoacidosis (DKA) and NKHH, two hyperglycemic syndromes occurring among patients with diabetes, can both present with encephalopathy. In addition, patients with NKHH frequently present in coma or with new-onset seizures. Thus, because neurologists are often summoned early, they must be familiar with these disorders.

Pathogenesis and Pathophysiology. Although the brain tolerates hyperglycemia better than hypoglycemia, encephalopathic features still develop, usually as a reflection of cerebral dehydration (e.g., intravascular hyperosmolality) or cerebral edema (e.g., too-rapid correction of the hyperglycemia). A correlation between the degree of encephalopathy and the serum osmolality exists, the pathophysiology of which has been discussed (see Hyponatremia). In addition to osmotic effects, intravascular coagulation related to hyperviscosity may occur.[59]

The primary problem in DKA is insulin deficiency. This results in an increased ratio of glucagon to insulin, accelerated gluconeogenesis, enhanced glycogenolysis, and reduced glucose clearance, thereby producing hyperglycemia.[126] In addition, insulin deficiency leads to increased fatty acid mobilization and the increased glucagon-to-insulin ratio induces fatty acid oxidation.[126] Therefore, lipolysis and ketone body formation occur. Once the renal threshold is exceeded, glucosuria occurs,[121] which promotes polyuria, due to osmotic diuresis, and polydipsia. In the setting of NKHH, insulin production is usually sufficient to inhibit lipolysis (i.e., nonketotic) but insufficient to prevent hyperglycemia. As the serum osmolality slowly rises, cerebral idiogenic osmole formation occurs (to prevent dehydration), thereby making the patient susceptible to cerebral edema during rehydration.

Epidemiology and Risk Factors. The major risk factor for the development of hyperglycemia is diabetes mellitus, with a prevalence of about 1 percent in the United States. NKHH accounts for 10 to 20 percent of all cases of severe hyperglycemia,[127] a value that is decreasing due to earlier detection of uncontrolled hyperglycemia.[128] Because of the high glucose content of total parenteral nutrition, patients receiving this type of therapy are also at risk of developing hyperglycemia. The incidence of gestational diabetes (carbohydrate intolerance that is present only during pregnancy) ranges from 1 percent in predominantly rural areas to 12 percent in racially mixed urban areas.[129]

Clinical Features and Associated Disorders. The general medical features of hyperglycemia include polyuria, polydipsia, and anorexia. Patients with DKA tend to be younger, type I diabetics, with a symptom onset measured in days. At onset, the mental status varies from normal (20 percent) to comatose (10 percent) and correlates most to the level of hyperosmolality.[126] DKA is frequently precipitated by infection or noncompliance with insulin therapy. Patients with NKHH tend to be older, type II diabetics with more pronounced dehydration. Unlike patients with DKA, focal neurological abnormalities, seizures (both focal and generalized), and coma are commonly observed. The most common precipitants of NKHH are infection, chronic renal insufficiency, GI bleeding, pancreatitis, stroke, burns, and certain medications.[128]

Differential Diagnosis. Although patients who present with encephalopathy may easily be diagnosed with hyperglycemia as the cause, diagnostic difficulty arises when encephalopathic patients present without a history of diabetes. Blood glucose determinations must be performed on all encephalopathic patients, and when they are shown to be hyperglycemic, DKA and NKHH, in addition to uremia, hepatic failure, toxin ingestion, starvation ketosis, alcoholic ketoacidosis, lactic acidosis, and other causes of encephalopathy, must be excluded. A history of ethanol abuse and, typically, a lack of hyperglycemia helps differentiate alcoholic ketoacidosis. Evidence of renal dysfunction and the absence of ketones helps differentiate uremia, and starvation ketosis is not associated with hyperglycemia.

Evaluation. In evaluating patients with hyperglycemic-induced encephalopathy, precipitating factors and secondary disturbances should be sought, including electrolyte disturbances (hypokalemia, hypophosphatemia, hypomagnesemia), infection (leukocytosis, urinalysis, chest x-ray study, blood and urine cultures), and hypokalemic-induced ECG changes. In addition, ABGs and serum osmolality, as well as renal and hepatic function, should be assessed. Hyperamylasemia, seen in nearly 80 percent of patients with DKA, may result in an incorrect diagnosis of pancreatitis.[126] Typical laboratory features in patients with DKA include blood glucose above 400 mg/dL, arterial blood pH below 7.2, bicarbonate below 10 mEq/L, and an elevated serum osmolality (usually below 350 mOsm/L). Ketone bodies and beta-hydroxybutyrate are elevated in the blood and urine, and there is a marked glycosuria.[121] In patients with NKHH, the blood glucose level is usually above 800 mg/dL and the osmolality above 350 mOsm/L.[59]

Management. If encephalopathic features are noted in a known diabetic, 25 g of dextrose should be administered intravenously because hypoglycemia is the most common cause of mental status changes and this dosage will not cause harm in the setting of DKA.[130] The primary treatment of DKA is insulin replacement, which facilitates glucose uptake and glycogen formation and reduces the rate of ketone body formation. Volume repletion initially requires NS, because most patients have TBW deficits of roughly 5 L.[126] This also lessens the degree of cerebral edema. Half-normal saline can be substituted once the orthostasis resolves, and 5 percent dextrose can be added after the glucose drops to 250 mg/dL or below. Although cerebral edema is a concomitant of treatment, a malignant increase in cerebral edema may occur, with resultant increased ICP, rapid deterioration, and death.[121] In this setting, aggressive treatment of cerebral edema must be undertaken, typically with hyperventilation, mannitol administration, and ICP monitoring. Because the major problem in patients with NKHH is dehydration, the primary treatment is rehydration, followed by insulin therapy and correction of underlying illnesses. Normal saline is the fluid of choice, and once blood glucose levels reach 250 mg/dL, 5 percent dextrose is provided to avoid hypoglycemia.

Seizure control requires normalization of serum osmolality and glucose. Standard antiepileptic drugs are ineffective; furthermore, some antiepileptic drugs, such as phenytoin, can inhibit the release of endogenous insulin.[127] In DKA, the rate of patient mortality remains significant (6 to 9 percent), with most deaths related to cardiovascular or cerebral complications, or the precipitating factor.[121] Mortality rates as high as 40 to 70 percent are reported for NKHH.

DIABETES

The neurological complications of diabetes were first recognized in 1798, and until 1864, diabetes was considered an effect of neuropathy.[131] For discussion purposes, the neurological complications of diabetes can be divided into CNS, cranial nerve, and PNS disturbances, of which PNS disturbances predominate. These disorders involve different parts of the nervous system and therefore produce different clinical manifestations.

Central Nervous System Complications of Diabetes

The brain, although not frequently discussed as a target of the complications of chronic diabetes, is nonetheless affected by this disorder. In addition to the neurological complications of glycemic extremes previously discussed (see Hypoglycemia and Hyperglycemia), patients with diabetes have an increased stroke incidence, increased stroke severity and, possibly, a chronic encephalopathy.[132] Regarding stroke, diabetes increases the risk of large, medium, and small vessel atheroma, as well as arteriolar and capillary microangiopathy, even after other concomitant risk factors (e.g., hypertension) are excluded.[133] In addition, studies have shown that the presence of hyperglycemia at the time of stroke results in more severe brain injury and, hence, a poorer stroke outcome (see Hyperglycemia). CNS abnormalities reported in patients with diabetes include increased P-300 latency, abnormal psychometric tests, and, among children with diabetes, lower school achievement test scores.[133] Potential causes for encephalopathy in patients with diabetes include vascular (e.g., stroke, altered BBB function, and cerebrovascular reactivity), metabolic (e.g., altered glycemia, ketosis, hypoxia, electrolyte changes, and neurotransmitter changes), and the co-existence of other disorders (e.g., hypertension, RF).[132]

Spinal cord abnormalities include infarction and pseudotabes diabetica. Pseudotabes diabetica reflects dorsal root ganglia disease, which, in turn, causes posterior column degeneration. Thus, this actually represents a disorder with a PNS onset resulting in secondary distal axon degeneration (i.e., the dying back phenomenon) causing posterior column degeneration.

Cranial Nerve Complications of Diabetes

The cranial mononeuropathies complicating diabetes primarily involve the oculomotor nerves (i.e., oculomotor [cranial nerve (CN) III], trochlear [CN IV], and abducens [CN VI]). Facial neuropathy and anterior ischemic optic neuropathy are briefly discussed, because these items are reviewed elsewhere in this text. Although peripheral nerve infarction has been the presumed mechanism of cranial mononeuropathies among diabetic patients, microinfarction-induced fascicular disruption within the brain stem parenchyma has been identified in many of these patients.[134] Diabetic oculomotor cranial mononeuropathies primarily involve CN III, followed by CN VI; CN IV is uncommonly affected alone. Clinically, patients notice the onset of eye pain or headache, followed by diplopia. The ophthalmoplegia reflects muscle weakness in the distribution of a single oculomotor nerve. Typically, in the setting of CN III involvement, pupillary sparing is noted. This likely reflects the peripheral location of the pupillomotor fibers, which are therefore supplied by external larger vessels, rather than internal small vessels. However, this is not always the case. Pupillary involvement is found in 10 to 20 percent of patients with vasculopathic (e.g., diabetes) cranial mononeuropathies, and pupillary sparing is found in 8 to 15 percent of patients with aneurysms.[135, 136] Concerning the latter, pupillary involvement usually appears within 3 to 5 days.[136] Even patients with complete paralysis tend to recover without residual weakness, usually within 3 months.[131] Among patients with diabetes, facial mononeuropathies occur with increased frequency and a poor outcome may be observed.[131] Thus, the facial mononeuropathy associated with diabetes may be secondary rather than idiopathic. Differences noted in diabetic patients with facial mononeuropathies support this statement and include (1) normal taste (argues for a different lesion site), (2) more frequent recurrent or bilateral facial nerve involvement, and (3) more frequent axon loss as the underlying pathophysiology rather than demyelinating conduction block,[137] which explains the poorer outcome. Clinically, patients with CN II involvement and an anterior ischemic optic neuropathy suffer acute visual loss, visual field defects (usually inferior altitudinal), or both. Ophthalmologically, a pale and swollen optic disc (usually superiorly), accompanied by flame-shaped hemorrhages within the optic disc or the peripapillary retina, is observed. In addition, most of these patients have a small optic disc, no central cup, and anomalous branching patterns of the optic disc vessels, a triad referred to as the *disc at risk*.[135] Importantly, there is a 40 percent chance of a similar episode in the contralateral eye and a 2 to 4 percent chance of a recurrent episode in the same eye.[135] Among this patient population, the occurrence of diabetes mellitus is increased (20 percent).[135] However, this may reflect the increased prevalence of hypertension among the diabetic population.

Peripheral Nervous System Complications of Diabetes

A great variety of PNS disorders are observed among patients with diabetes, and these disorders can be divided into focal, segmental, and generalized.

Focal Peripheral Nervous System Disorders. The focal PNS disorders include focal myopathies and mononeuropathies. The etiologies of focal myopathies include traumatic (associated with insulin injection injury) and vascular (related to thigh muscle infarction). Mononeuropathies may be divided into those affecting the cranial nerves (discussed earlier) and those affecting the somatic nerves. Somatic mononeuropathies result from entrapment or compression and nerve infarction. Entrapment and compression tend to occur in the same nerves and at the same sites as among the nondiabetic population—median mononeuropathies at the wrist (i.e., CTS), ulnar mononeuropathies at the elbow, and common peroneal mononeuropathies at the fibular head. The prevalence of CTS among diabetics, as among the nondiabetic population, increases in the presence of polyneuropathy.[138] An increased incidence of ulnar neuropathy also exists, whereas the occurrence of a common peroneal mononeuropathy at the fibular head is likely coincidental.[138] Concerning the lower extremity, although femoral mononeuropathies are the most frequently reported lower extremity mononeuropathies among diabetic patients, they are extremely rare. The initial publications on diabetic femoral neuropathies likely represent mislabeled diabetic amyotrophy (discussed later), and in subsequent publications, these authors noted that the lesions were located more proximally.[137] Thus, common peroneal mononeuropathies are the most common lower extremity mononeuropathy. These lesions occur unilaterally or bilaterally and can be caused by either compression or nerve infarction.[137] In patients with nerve infarction, the onset is acute and painful, the pathophysiology reflects axon loss, and recovery is often slow and suboptimal. The poor outcome reflects several features, including (1) the lesions tend to be complete, and robust collateral sprouting cannot occur; (2) the lesions tend to involve the nerve trunks proximally or in their midportion, and the distance required for proximodistal regeneration is greater; and (3) the lesions tend to occur in elderly patients.[137] Unlike nerve infarction, which produces solely axon loss, compressive lesions may produce demyelinating conduction block, axon loss, or a combination of the two, and, therefore, it is not unexpected that, in general, patients with compressive lesions tend to have a better outcome. Except for an attempt to control the serum glucose concentration better, the mononeuropathies occurring among diabetic patients are treated in the same manner as those occurring among nondiabetic patients.

Segmental Peripheral Nervous System Disorders. The diabetic polyradiculopathy syndromes belong to this category. The term *diabetic myelopathy* was introduced by Bruns in 1890 and was displaced by Garland in 1955 when it became clinically and pathologically apparent that the disease process was not a myelopathy.[131] Garland suggested the intentionally nonlocalizing term *diabetic amyotrophy*. Several years later, Sullivan suggested the term *asymmetrical* (motor) *proximal neuropathy*, variations of which appear in most current discussions.[139] Historically, at least 20 synonyms for this entity have been used, which is a reflection of its varied presentations.[137] The term diabetic *thoracoabdominal neuropathy* (discussed later) has at least 10 synonyms.[137] In 1981, Bastron and Thomas proposed the more general term *diabetic polyradiculopathy* for all of the diabetic neuropathies other than distal symmetrical polyneuropathy,[140] thereby incorporating several of the various diabetic polyradiculopathy syndromes into a single entity (e.g., diabetic amyotrophy and diabetic thoracoabdominal neuropathy). In addition, they coined the term *territorial extension* to describe the cephalad, caudal, or contralateral progression of this process from one root region to another. Based on this framework, Wilbourn drew several important conclusions, including (1) the root level is primarily attacked; (2) single or contiguous roots are attacked most severely; (3) territorial extension occurs in approximately two thirds of patients; (4) some root regions are more likely to be affected than others; (5) when uncommon root regions are involved, they generally follow involvement of the more typical root region; (6) the predominant pathophysiology is axon loss; and (7) the majority of patients have co-existing diabetic distal symmetrical polyneuropathy (DDSPN).[137] Thus, the commonly observed diabetic amyotrophy reflects isolated root involvement of the L2–L4 root levels, whereas diabetic thoracoabdominal neuropathy reflects isolated root involvement of the mid- to lower thoracic root levels. Also, when patients with diabetic amyotrophy develop foot drop, it most likely reflects territorial extension into the L5 level, and should it progress more caudally, global leg muscle involvement will develop. Bilateral shoulder girdle weakness is occasionally observed.[137]

Generalized Peripheral Nervous System Disorders. Disorders included in this category are DDSPN and diabetic autonomic neuropathy. DDSPN is the most common form of diabetic neuropathy and resembles the polyneuropathies caused by numerous other disorders. Different diagnostic criteria and methods of detection, applied to patients with diabetes of varying duration (i.e., patient selection bias), have led to a wide variation in its reported incidence and prevalence. Typically, paresthesias and numbness begin in the toes and ascend proximally in a stocking-like distribution. When the ascent reaches the upper tibia, the hands begin to become involved. Once involved, the upper extremity disturbance also progresses proximally in a glovelike distribution. This distribution pattern, in which the longest nerves are first affected, is often referred to as a dying-back neuropathy. At this time, diminished or absent ankle reflexes and foot intrinsic muscle weakness are evident. Even anhidrosis follows this pattern, which typically begins in the foot and predisposes patients to foot ulcers. The electrodiagnostic abnormalities

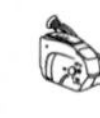

also show a distal to proximal gradient. The most sensitive NCS are the plantar mixed NCS, followed by the superficial peroneal and sural sensory NCS, followed by the upper extremity sensory NCS. The motor NCS abnormalities and needle electrode examination abnormalities follow this same pattern. When one considers that a nerve is made of sensory, motor, and autonomic axons ranging in size from small to large, it is easy to envision the range of clinical symptoms this disorder produces. Small fiber sensory disruption causes loss of pain and temperature perception, as well as more prevalent features of dysautonomia. Large fiber sensory involvement impairs proprioception, vibratory perception, gait (sensory ataxia), and reflexes. Motor axon dysfunction produces weakness, and autonomic axon involvement produces various dysautonomic features. Occasionally, patients present with disproportionate small fiber or large fiber sensory involvement or autonomic involvement. As pointed out by Dyck and colleagues, a continuum of fiber involvement is most common, with the disproportionate cases representing the extremes of a normal distribution.[131, 138] Thus, diabetic autonomic neuropathy can present in isolation, although uncommonly, and the symptoms reflect the wide distribution of autonomic fibers: pupillary (miotic pupils with sluggish light reflex), cardiovascular (resting tachycardia, orthostatic hypotension), GI (constipation), genitourinary (impotence, reduced vaginal lubrication), and sudomotor (distal anhidrosis) systems.[133] The symptoms, evaluation, and management of diabetic autonomic neuropathy have been reviewed.[141] Hyperglycemic polyneuropathy refers to transient, distal paresthesias or dysesthesias occurring just before the diagnosis of diabetes or following ketoacidotic coma. The treatment of painful diabetic neuropathy is often the major management problem and can be challenging. For mild cases, simple analgesics may suffice, as may cold water soaks and the use of support stockings for evening pain. The potential for nephrotoxicity limits the usefulness of chronic nonsteroidal anti-inflammatory drugs, and the potential for addiction (as well as the occurrence of tolerance) limits the utility of narcotics. Tricyclic antidepressants, such as amitriptyline and nortriptyline, desipramine, carbamazepine (perhaps the drug of choice if the pain is lancinating or paroxysmal), gabapentin, and mexiletine have been shown to be of value. The anticholinergic side effects associated with the tricyclic antidepressants limit their utility for patients with accompanying autonomic dysfunction. These agents, as well as others, have been reviewed.[133]

Organ Failure

HEPATIC FAILURE

Because of the complexity of liver metabolism, patients with liver disease may develop many complications, including neurological dysfunction. This problem can be expected, considering the important role the liver plays in both nutrient metabolism (glycolysis, nutrient biosynthesis) and detoxification. The term *hepatic encephalopathy* (HE) refers to diffuse cerebral dysfunction occurring secondary to liver disease. When HE develops acutely in patients with liver disease of less than 8 weeks' duration, the term *fulminant hepatic failure* (FHF) is used, whereas the term *portal-systemic encephalopathy* (PSE) is used when HE develops in patients with chronic liver disease. This differentiation has therapeutic implications because a number of treatments exist for patients with PSE, whereas no specific form of treatment has been proven beneficial in FHF, except urgent liver transplantation.

Pathogenesis and Pathophysiology. Although neither the responsible toxin nor the pathogenesis of HE is known, it is believed to result from impaired hepatic degradation of neurotoxic substances arising from the GI metabolism of nitrogenous compounds. Normally, these GI products are delivered to the liver by the portal vein. There are two mechanisms by which hepatic impairment may result in the systemic accumulation of these gut-derived substances: (1) direct entry of portal vein–derived blood into the systemic circulation (shunting) secondary to the formation of portal-systemic collaterals (e.g., PSE) and (2) impaired detoxification secondary to hepatocyte dysfunction (e.g., FHF). HE results in increased BBB permeability, which, in turn, enhances the entry of these substances into the CNS, facilitating the development of HE. This may explain the reason patients with liver disease can become symptomatic with only minimal hyperammonemia and their sensitivity to precipitation by ammonia-producing processes.[142] Normally, the brain removes ammonia by converting it to glutamine. If glutamine accumulates rapidly, the increased intracellular osmolality of the brain can cause cerebral edema.[143]

A variety of substances have been implicated in the pathogenesis of HE, including ammonia, endogenous benzodiazepines, Na/K-ATPase inhibitors (e.g., glutamine, short-chain fatty acids, aromatic amino acids, and mercaptans), false neurotransmitters (e.g., octopamine), and gamma-aminobutyric acid.[144] The leading hypothesis relates to the effects of ammonia and states that HE results from its systemic accumulation. Findings supporting this hypothesis include (1) patients with HE usually have elevated arterial ammonia levels, (2) the degree of hyperammonemia correlates with the depth of coma, (3) ammonia metabolites (alpha-ketoglutarate and glutamine) are elevated in the brains and CSF of patients with HE, (4) the BBB permeability increases for ammonia, (5) the cerebral metabolic rate increases for ammonia, (6) experimental administration of ammonium salts results in reversible HE, (7) ammonia-forming compounds in the GI tract (e.g., protein meals, blood) reproducibly precipitate coma, (8) all proven treatments reduce blood ammonia levels, and (9) patients with urea cycle enzyme defects develop hyperammonemia and encephalopathy in the setting of normal liver function.[142, 143, 145] A second hypothesis is the false neurotransmitter theory. This theory suggests that the increased ratio of aromatic to branched-chain amino acids occurring in liver failure causes an increased entry of aromatic amino acids into the brain (i.e., less competition). The enhanced entry of aromatic amino acids, in turn, increases the synthesis of serotonin and false neurotransmitters (e.g., octopamine). The increased quantities of false neurotransmitters could theoretically competitively inhibit the normal function of true neurotransmitters. However, although false neurotransmitters do accumulate in PSE, there is no evidence that they are responsible for the encephalopathy. Because the pathogenesis of HE is probably not due to the accumulation of any single cerebral toxin, a multifactorial process is more likely, with the accumulation of multiple substances synergistically contributing to its development.

Epidemiology and Risk Factors. FHF is rare, with an incidence of approximately 2000 cases per year in the United States.[146] Viral hepatitis, usually hepatitis B or hepatitis C, is the most common cause of FHF in the United States and accounts for approximately 75 percent of cases.[146] Among patients with hepatitis B, approximately 1 percent develop FHF. Drug-induced liver dysfunction is second in frequency.[143] Abnormalities associated with liver disease, such as hypoxia, acid-base disturbances, and electrolyte abnormalities, predispose patients to the development of encephalopathy. Retrospective epidemiological studies have shown a correlation between intracranial hemorrhage and hepatic disease, with the relative risk for intracranial hemorrhage increased roughly fivefold among patients with liver disease.

Clinical Features and Associated Disorders. The neurological manifestations of HE range from subtle psychomotor abnormalities to coma and death. The exact clinical picture depends on the rapidity of onset, the degree of liver dysfunction, and the degree of portal-systemic shunting. PSE, the much more commonly encountered form, is mostly observed among patients with chronic liver disorders (e.g., cirrhosis). In addition to the neurological features, these patients may have numerous other clinical findings (Table 38–13). PSE is typically precipitated by ammonia-producing processes, such as GI bleeding, increased dietary protein, constipation, and azotemia. Other known precipitants include infection, hypokalemia, hypoglycemia, hypoxia, and medications (e.g., sedative-hypnotics, analgesics).[145] Usually, the onset of encephalopathy is slow and insidious, often beginning with anxiety, altered sleep patterns and mood, agitated delirium, or a decreased attention span. Eventually, lethargy progresses to stupor and coma.[145] Asterixis is almost always present, and as the encephalopathy progresses, increased muscle tone, hyper-reflexia, and extensor plantar responses are commonly noted. As part of the coma, decorticate and decerebrate posturing may also be observed. Unless a superimposed acute event occurs, cerebral edema is uncommon in these patients.[144] Unlike Uremic encephalopathy, seizures are infrequent and suggest the presence of a co-existent disorder.

The onset of FHF is much more rapid and is typically associated with severe liver disease. Mental status changes, such as agitation, inappropriate behavior, and impaired judgment, appear early and may quickly progress to stupor and coma. Unlike PSE, cerebral edema with increased ICP is common and may result in cerebral herniation and death. Seizures and

TABLE 38–13. **Clinical Features of Chronic Liver Disease**

Subjective	Objective
Anorexia, fatigue	Jaundice, scleral icterus, Kayser-Fleischer rings (Wilson's disease, primary biliary cirrhosis), fetor hepaticus (musty, sweet breath odor), spider nevi, gynecomastia, caput medusa (dilation of the umbilical vessels), splenomegaly, ascites, xanthomas, palmar erythema, Dupuytren's contractures of the hands and feet

focal neurological signs are uncommon and suggest a coexistent process (e.g., subdural hematoma [SDH]).

In addition to developing encephalopathy, some patients with chronic liver disease develop hepatocerebral degeneration, a slowly progressive and irreversible neurodegenerative syndrome associated with extensive portal-systemic shunting. It is characterized by tremor, rigidity, bradykinesia, ataxia, dysarthria, choreoathetosis, and dementia. Studies have shown a selective loss of dopaminergic D_2 (postsynaptic) receptors in the globus pallidus of patients with PSE, suggesting that these extrapyramidal signs may reflect dopaminergic neuronal dysfunction.[145] Rarely, spinal cord degeneration (hepatic myelopathy), characterized by spastic paraparesis, hyper-reflexia, and extensor plantar responses, is observed.[147] The presence of polyneuropathy has been variably reported. When they are present, these signs are typically mild or asymptomatic. It is not known whether these neuropathic changes are directly related to hepatic dysfunction (e.g., from toxin accumulation) or to the disease process causing the liver impairment (e.g., alcohol abuse, hemochromatosis).

Differential Diagnosis and Evaluation. Any disorder resulting in liver failure may cause HE. Viral hepatitis is the most common cause of FHF in the United States, followed by drug-induced liver dysfunction (e.g., acetaminophen, isoniazid, rifampin, methyldopa [Aldomet], halothane), fatty infiltration, Reye's syndrome, infiltrative diseases, and less common causes.[139, 146]

The diagnosis of HE is clinical and depends on the identification of precipitating factors and the observation of a good response to empirical treatment.[148] Unfortunately, there are no pathognomonic features of HE, and all of its typical features may be noted with encephalopathies of other etiologies. Patients suspected of having HE require a thorough neurological examination. Laboratory studies help exclude alternative etiologies of encephalopathy and identify other complications related to hepatic disease. Potentially helpful laboratory studies include a CBC, electrolytes, BUN, Cr, glucose, Ca, drug screen, vitamin B_{12} level, ABGs, and liver function tests. There is no correlation between the degree of HE and the degree of liver function test abnormality. In fact, liver function tests may be normal in the setting of severe, chronic liver disease. An arterial blood ammonia level should be drawn, placed on ice, and immediately assayed. Venous samples are unacceptable because tourniquet-induced muscle ischemia can result in the release of ammonia from muscle (possible false-positive result), and muscle itself can take up variable amounts of ammonia, producing false-negative results.[142] Although it is infrequent, a normal value does not exclude HE, especially in the fasting state.[144, 148] Although its absolute value does not correlate with the degree of HE, the ammonia level is useful in following the individual patient's course and response to therapy.

The EEG typically reveals generalized slowing, and triphasic waves may also be seen. Triphasic waves, although characteristic of HE, are not specific for this disorder and can be observed in a wide variety of encephalopathic states and structural processes (Fig. 38–3). Because the degree of slowing is proportional to the severity of encephalopathy, serial EEGs allow for the assessment of the subsequent clinical course and response to treatment. If the patient is febrile or if meningismus is observed, CSF analysis should be cautiously performed, because increased ICP or a coagulopathy may also be present in this patient population. The opening pressure should be recorded and routine CSF studies obtained. In HE, the CSF protein may be mildly elevated, and glutamine levels are usually elevated. The glutamine level has been cited as the biochemical parameter most closely correlated to the degree of HE.[143, 149]

Once HE is diagnosed, the degree of impairment should be clinically graded and used as a baseline for future compar-

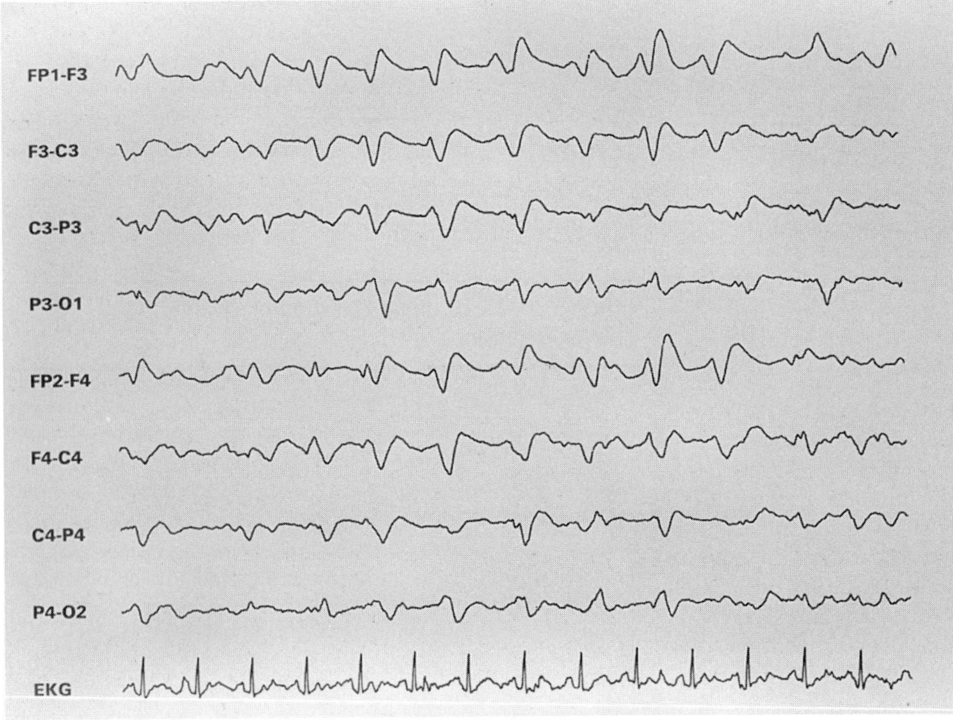

FIGURE 38–3. A 58-year-old patient with hepatic encephalopathy. The patient's EEG demonstrates classic triphasic waves that are more prominent anteriorly. (From Lüders HO, Koechter S: Atlas und Klassifikation der Elektroenzephalopgraphie, Verlag, CIBA-Geigy 1994, p 118.)

isons. Daily handwriting samples, number connection tests (e.g., trail making), and mental status examinations are helpful in the daily assessment of patients with HE.[144] The most widely used grading system categorizes patients into one of four stages, based primarily on alterations in mentation and the EEG.[143] Stage I is characterized by subtle changes in thought processes and personality, such as dyscalculia, poor handwriting, impaired construction of simple figures, difficulty connecting a series of numbers, and sloppiness. At this stage, any abnormalities on the EEG are subtle. In stage II, more obvious changes in thought processes, such as confusion, inappropriate behavior, decreased attention, drowsiness, and abnormal sleep patterns, are noted. Asterixis and hyper-reflexia are usually present, and clonus as well as extensor plantar responses may also be observed. The EEG shows generalized slowing. In stage III, further worsening of thought processes occurs, with confusion and an even shorter attention span. The patient is unable to perform fine motor movements and remains asleep most of the time. Asterixis is present, and the EEG shows more pronounced slowing; in addition, triphasic waves may be observed. In stage IV, the patient is comatose. Brain stem reflexes persist until the deepest stages of coma are reached. The EEG shows generalized delta frequency slowing. ICP monitoring can be helpful in the management of patients in stages III and IV by guiding therapy, facilitating the early detection of rising ICP, and identifying patients with sustained ICP elevations, so that they may be excluded from emergency liver transplantation procedures.[143] When ICP monitoring cannot be performed, the patient must be followed closely for evidence of cerebral herniation so that treatment can be provided at a time when the process may be reversible.

In HE, focal neurological features are unexpected and suggest a co-existent structural abnormality (e.g., SDH) or focal metabolic abnormality (e.g., postictal state). In these cases, CT or MRI studies of the head are warranted. In patients with hepatocerebral degeneration, reversible MRI abnormalities, which are most pronounced in the globus pallidus, may be seen. Proton magnetic resonance spectroscopy can be used to detect specific metabolic abnormalities in this region of the brain, thereby constituting an early marker of metabolic alteration.[150]

Management. Prevention is an important aspect of treatment among patients with chronic liver disease. Known precipitants of HE should be avoided and, if they are identified, reversed. Because the onset of PSE is slow, insidious, and often subclinical, patients with chronic liver disease should undergo periodic psychometric testing.[151] As many as 70 percent of patients with cirrhosis and without evidence of an overt encephalopathy have significant impairment when tested.[142] Because the visuospatial sphere is the most frequently affected, the Reitan Trials A and B, Block Design, and Symbol-Digit subtests of the Wechsler Adult Intelligence Scale-Revised (WAIS-R), as well as the Purd Pegboard test, are frequently employed and commonly found to yield abnormal results.[142]

In the patient with HE, empirical therapy should be initiated while causes of encephalopathy are being excluded and precipitating factors are being sought. Thiamine hydrochloride, 100 mg IV, is administered and should be followed by a daily dosage of 50 mg PO to prevent Wernicke-Korsakoff syndrome.

General measures in the treatment of HE include maintaining adequate nutrition, good renal function, and acid-base status, as well as reducing colonic ammonia production. Because normal brain pH is 6.95 and blood pH is 7.4, there is a tendency for ammonia to enter the brain. By minimizing the interaction between enteric bacterial flora and nitrogenous substances, colonic ammonia production is reduced. Dietary protein restriction, avoidance of constipation, and GI tract evacuation are helpful in this respect. The GI tract is evacuated through the use of cathartics (e.g., lactulose) and enemas. Lactulose is a synthetic disaccharide capable of reducing arterial ammonia levels. In the colon, it is converted into acidic metabolites, which create a pH gradient across the intestinal wall. Colon acidification was thought to select for bacteria that did not contain urease. Instead, colon acidification decreases blood ammonia by trapping it in the acidified feces, thereby making it unavailable for absorption.[152] In addition, the pH gradient causes movement of ammonia into the colon. The dosage is usually titrated to yield 2 to 3 soft bowel movements per day, typically requiring 30 to 40 g four times daily. If the patient is comatose, hourly doses of 20 to 30 g are provided until a catharsis is produced, after which the dosage can be reduced.[142] Some patients do not tolerate lactulose, presumably because of the associated contaminants, such as lactose, galactose, and other carbohydrates. Lactitol, another synthetic disaccharide, is better tolerated. It is purer than commercial lactulose and, therefore, has fewer adverse effects such as nausea, diarrhea, and intestinal cramping. Unfortunately, it is more expensive and is not available in the United States. Neomycin, a nonabsorbable antibiotic, kills colonic bacteria and thereby decreases both the bacterial nitrogen content and the synthesis of urea. Compared with lactulose, it has more side effects without increased efficacy. In addition, there is some evidence that aminoglycosides contribute to the development of hepatorenal syndrome, and for that reason, they are rarely used today. In the setting of neomycin resistance, metronidazole is an alternative. Dietary protein restriction (less than 1 g/kg dry weight of high biological value protein) and the administration of multivitamins, folate and thiamine supplements, vitamin K, and at least 2000 calories per day should be provided.[146, 151] Therapies considered to be nonbeneficial include branched-chain amino acid solutions, serotonin reuptake inhibitors, L-dopa, and bromocriptine.[145] Sodium benzoate was also shown to reduce blood ammonia levels in a double-blinded and randomized trial of 38 patients with PSE.[153] Improvement within 1 to 3 days of starting empirical therapy is expected. Failure to respond suggests the wrong diagnosis, a missed precipitant, multiple causes of the encephalopathy, or, the most common cause, a missed nosocomial infection.[148] In addition to the general measures listed earlier, more specific treatments may be required. Orthotopic liver transplantation (OLT) represents an alternative for patients with little chance of recovery. A review of the patients undergoing OLT reported a number of neurological sequelae, including severe quadriplegia, perioperative mononeuropathies, and herpes zoster–related radiculopathies.[154] A recent review of the causes and outcome of seizures in the post-OLT patient population revealed that the majority of new-onset seizures after OLT were related to immunosuppressive treatment, did not require antiepileptic drug (AED) therapy for favorable long-term outcome, and were not as ominous as previously thought.[155]

Prognosis and Future Perspectives. The mortality rate for patients with FHF, despite aggressive therapy, is approximately 85 percent.[142] Age, etiology, and degree of encephalopathy influence survival in FHF. Younger patients have a more favorable outcome, with the discriminatory age lying between 30 and 50 years.[156] Recovery from FHF is expected when the condition is due to hepatitis A and acetaminophen hepatotoxicity, yet the rate is only 40 percent when it is associated with hepatitis B and 20 percent when it is associated with hepatitis C or drug-induced hepatitis. When FHF is associated with Wilson's disease, recovery almost never occurs.[143, 157] The recovery rate approaches 75 percent for patients who do not progress beyond stage II, whereas less than 20 percent of those patients reaching stage IV survive.[143] In patients with FHF, death is commonly caused by complications involving other organ systems, two thirds of which are neurological.[146] OLT has increased the survival rate significantly (50 to 90 percent) and, in the case of patients with cirrhosis, can normalize their neuropsychiatric status. Ultimately, the prognosis is related to the ability of the liver to regenerate or the availability of livers for transplantation.

Typically, patients with PSE have a good prognosis for full recovery, especially if a precipitating factor can be identified and reversed. When the cause cannot be reversed, continuous therapy is required (e.g., surgical portacaval shunts). Still, the underlying etiology, the occurrence of secondary complications, and the degree of encephalopathy affect survival. Favorable prognosticators include an identifiable and treatable precipitant, mild encephalopathy, and lack of secondary complications.[142]

RENAL FAILURE

The kidney is one of the principle homeostatic organs of the body and is involved in the regulation of water, electrolyte, and acid-base balance; the excretion of metabolic waste products; and the synthesis of erythropoietin, renin, and 1,25-DHCC. This section focuses on the neurological manifestations of renal failure, both acute (ARF) and chronic (CRF), and the neurological complications of its treatment.

Pathogenesis and Pathophysiology. Uremic encephalopathy (UE) regularly occurs when the glomerular filtration rate falls below 10 percent of normal, regardless of whether it occurs with ARF or CRF.[158] The fact that dialysis can rapidly clear UE suggests that the responsible molecules causing UE are water soluble and small to moderate in size. However, because renal insufficiency causes a spectrum of biochemical abnormalities, the individual significance of any single abnormality is indeterminable.

Although water, osmolality, acid-base, and electrolyte abnormalities are commonly observed in patients with RF, they do not appear to contribute substantially to the development of UE. The brain water content in uremic patients is normal,[159–161] and an absence of brain edema in animals with acute uremia[160] further argues against water toxicity as the cause of UE. Although the increase in brain osmolality (from 310 to 350 mOsm/kg water) noted in ARF patients is due to urea, this compound is nontoxic, even at high concentrations.[56] Among CRF patients, urea constitutes only half of the osmotically active particles, with the unidentified remainder referred to as idiogenic osmoles.[162] The lack of a significant gradient between the blood, CSF, and brain urea concentrations[163] also argues against osmolality variability as the primary cause of UE.

The accumulation of toxic organic acids in the CNS has been proposed as a possible mechanism of UE.[63] However, studies of CSF acidity in uremic patients[164] and of acid-base balance in the CSF, blood, brain, and skeletal muscle of uremic dogs[165] have been normal. Although the permeability of the BBB is increased toward insulin and sucrose, its permeability toward weak acids is decreased.[56]

Cooper and associates[161] studied the brains of 10 patients who had died of uremia and noted the brain content to be normal for K, Cl, and Mg; slightly decreased for Na; and approximately doubled for Ca. In experimental uremia, increased brain Ca levels have been associated with an increase in the PTH level.[161] In addition, the increase coincided with the onset of EEG abnormalities, with both appearing about 2 days after onset of the RF. In a study of 20 dialysis patients with EEG slowing, a direct correlation was noted between the plasma concentration of the *N*-terminal fragment of PTH and the degree of EEG slowing.[166, 167] Administration of PTH to normal dogs produces EEG changes similar to those seen in uremic animals. The EEG abnormalities, as well as the increased brain Ca, can be prevented by performing a parathyroidectomy before the induction of RF.[56] PTH accumulation probably affects the Ca pump,[168] suggesting that this hormone is a uremic toxin.[169] Although more recent studies have corroborated the relationship between PTH and brain Ca content abnormalities,[170] the fact that this hormone is not dialyzable argues against it as the uremic toxin responsible for UE. Ca content may be affected by other system abnormalities.

Uremic neuropathy (UN) is the most common neurological manifestation observed among CRF patients. It is pathologically characterized by axon loss. Its pathogenesis is unknown but, like UE, improvement occurs following dialysis, suggesting that the responsible substances are dialyzable. Because some patients experience neuropathic improvement only when their dialysis time is increased, it is postulated that the responsible substances are larger than urea (because larger molecules require more time to cross dialysis membranes). Hypotheses concerning the role of PTH and Ca metabolism in UN have been advanced and are supported by the following features: (1) PTH increases the Ca content of nerve; (2) increased nerve Ca content slows its conduction velocity; (3) the observed slowing is prevented by performing parathyroidectomy before the administration of PTH; and (4) the PTH level is inversely related to the nerve conduction velocity in uremic patients. Like UE, the strongest argument against PTH as the mediator of UN is its nondialyzability. Also, hyperparathyroidism is not typically associated with a neuropathy.

Epidemiology and Risk Factors. In the United States, although the frequency of ARF is low (roughly 30 patients/million/year),[171] the prevalence of end-stage renal disease increased from 45,000 in 1977 to greater than 165,000 in 1990.[172] In the United States, hypertension and diabetes are the leading causes of CRF.[172] The most important risk factors for the development of UN are the duration and severity of the RF.[166] In recent years, the appearance of neuropathy in chronic hemodialysis patients has become rare,[173] which is the result of earlier treatment, more intensive dialysis, and technical improvements in dialysis membranes (thinner, with greater clearance properties).[174]

Clinical Features and Associated Disorders. The clinical features of UE are similar to those of other metabolic encephalopathies. The typical progression of clinical features begins with inattentiveness, impaired concentration, fatigue, apathy, and irritability, which is usually accompanied by motor manifestations (e.g., tremor, asterixis, and myoclonus). Tetany, seizures (focal and generalized), focal neurological signs, and meningeal features are also common.[121, 175] One or more of these features may predominate, and symptom fluctuation is typical. Without treatment, coma develops and Kussmaul breathing may be followed by Cheyne-Stokes breathing. Simultaneous evidence of CNS depression (lethargy, obtundation, coma) and excitation (agitation, myoclonus, seizures) are important features of UE.[166] In CRF patients, personality changes and features of polyneuropathy may be the earliest features, because the encephalopathic manifestations may not appear until the process is advanced.[57, 176]

Asterixis, first described by Adams and Foley[177] in patients with PSE and later noted by Tyler in uremic patients,[178] is a nonspecific feature of metabolic encephalopathies typically present once higher cortical function is affected.[175, 179] In patients incapable of voluntarily maintaining a posture (e.g., comatose patients), the examiner can position the ankles of a supine patient near the buttocks and observe for abduction-adduction movements at the hip joints.[180] Myoclonus is often multifocal and is more common in the deeper stages of encephalopathy.[174, 175] Uremic twitching (severe asterixis with myoclonus) can be continuous and evident during both wakefulness and sleep[62] and may simulate a multifocal seizure disorder,[175] chorea, or ballismus.[181] Other motor system abnormalities include muscle cramping and tetany, which may be overt or latent.[166, 175]

Seizures, which are relatively uncommon in other metabolic encephalopathies,[174] occur in approximately 25 percent of patients with UE. The seizures are usually generalized,[174] although focal motor seizures may also be seen.[166, 181] Seizures occur earlier and more frequently (40 percent) among ARF patients than among CRF patients (10 percent).[174] In addition, seizures may occur due to dialysis disequilibrium syndrome (see later), hypertensive encephalopathy, water intoxication, or other metabolic encephalopathies.

Unlike the flaccidity characterizing some metabolic encephalopathies, limb tone is usually increased in UE and may even be asymmetrical.[174, 175] As the disorder progresses, opisthotonic or decorticate posturing may be observed.[182] Cranial nerve reflexes (e.g., corneal, oculocephalic, and pupillary) are normal, unless the patient is deeply comatose.[166] Sensory examination abnormalities in a stocking-glove distribution and hyporeflexia suggest the presence of UN. Wernicke's encephalopathy has been reported in hemodialysis patients, which is a reflection of the water-soluble, and hence dialyzable, nature of thiamine.

UN is a symmetrical, sensorimotor, axon loss, dying-back (i.e., it has a distal-proximal gradient) polyneuropathy that is clinically indistinguishable from other polyneuropathies that have a stocking-glove distribution. Although lower extremity vibratory sensation impairment[183] and loss of deep tendon reflexes[178] have been reported as early features, suggesting early large fiber involvement, a wide spectrum of clinical patterns has been observed. The sensory aspects of UN were recently studied, and paradoxical heat sensation (i.e., the perception of heat in response to low temperature stimulation) was identified in 15 of 36 (42 percent) patients,[184] more than fourfold greater than the normal population.[185] Although burning dysesthesias have been frequently cited as a characteristic feature of UN, Asbury has reported them to be rare, a likely reflection of routine supplementation with thiamine and other water-soluble vitamins. Autonomic symptoms, such as orthostasis, impotence, diarrhea, and hyperhidrosis, are commonly reported.[186] An acute, flaccid quadriplegia has also been reported.[187] The restless legs syndrome (see Chapter 54) occurs in over 40 percent of uremic patients[188–190] and may be a harbinger of polyneuropathy. Although distal lower extremity cramping has also been suggested to herald polyneuropathy, cramps occur in patients without neuropathic features and are more frequent among patients with ARF.[174] Other features reported in uremic patients include myopathy,[63, 191] optic neuropathy, isolated mononeuropathies, flaccid quadriparesis (due to hyperkalemia), and vestibulocochlear and neuromuscular junction disturbances (due to aminoglycoside antibiotics). CTS is another manifestation of uremia that may result from the deposition of amyloid fibrils. The amyloid fibrils are composed of beta-2 microglobulin, a substance that is poorly dialyzed and builds up over time in chronically hemodialyzed patients (healthy kidneys are capable of catabolizing beta-2 microglobulin). The shoulder joints and carpal bones are frequently involved and abnormalities may be seen on plain films of these areas.

Differential Diagnosis and Evaluation. When patients with known RF present with encephalopathic features, concomitant medical problems, such as DKA, hypertensive encephalopathy, hypertensive intracranial hemorrhage, intracranial abscess, infectious meningitis, primary CNS lymphoma, and hepatic or pulmonary insufficiency, should be sought. Current medications should be reviewed for drugs that are metabolized or excreted by the kidney, especially those known to have neurological manifestations. For patients receiving dialysis treatments, determine (1) the temporal relationship between the last dialysis session and the onset of encephalopathic features, (2) the current dialysis regimen, (3) occurrence of neurological symptoms with previous dialysis sessions, and (4) the length of time the patient has been undergoing maintenance dialysis. Initial laboratory studies should include CBC with differential, prothrombin time, partial thromboplastin time, electrolytes, BUN and Cr, glucose, liver function tests, Ca, Mg, Phosphorus and urinalysis. Finally, if infection is suspected and a source is not immediately apparent, lumbar puncture for CSF analysis should be performed.

Patients with RF who have focal neurological findings or seizures require additional evaluation with head CT or MRI to evaluate for SDH, intracerebral hemorrhage, infarction, abscess, neoplasm, or other focal processes. An EEG is also helpful and typically shows diffuse slowing (indicative of an encephalopathy), may show triphasic waves (consistent with a metabolic process), and sometimes shows paroxysmal activity that includes spikes or sharp waves.[59] Electrodiagnostic testing helps characterize an identified polyneuropathy and may be used to monitor the course of disease after dialysis has been initiated. Secondary hyperparathyroidism should be considered in those patients noted to have proximal extremity muscle weakness and the appropriate laboratories ordered.[174]

Management. Because drugs requiring renal metabolism or excretion can accumulate to toxic levels in patients with RF, medication selection is important for the prevention of neurological side effects. In this population, aminoglycoside antibiotics are commonly used but may cause cochlear, vestibular, or neuromuscular junction disturbances. The use of B vitamin supplementation in those patients undergoing maintenance dialysis can help prevent UN.

UE requires definitive treatment and is directed toward correcting its cause (e.g., urinary tract obstruction), when possible. Otherwise, dialysis is required to manage fluid, electrolyte, and acid-base imbalances commonly seen in this setting. A nutritionist, to recommend dietary guidelines (e.g., salt, protein), can be very helpful. Because tremulousness, asterixis, and myoclonus tend to resolve as the UE improves, they usually do not require specific treatment. When they are severe, asterixis and myoclonus may respond to clonazepam or valproic acid.

The management of seizures in this patient population warrants separate discussion because changes in plasma protein binding and AED metabolism complicate its management. For highly protein-bound AEDs, such as phenytoin, decreased plasma protein binding increases the percentage of unbound (free, active) drug. Normally, phenytoin is about 90 percent protein bound and 10 percent unbound, yet in uremic patients, the percentage of unbound phenytoin may approach 25 to 75 percent.[121, 192] Because the rate of AED diffusion into the brain is proportional to the unbound fraction,[193] the CNS concentration increases[194] and adjustments may be required. Because the therapeutic range of total phenytoin is 10 to 20 μg/mL and nonuremic patients have 10 percent in the unbound state, the therapeutic range of free phenytoin is 1 to 2 μg/mL. Therefore, when uremic patients require phenytoin, the required dosage is best determined by following the free phenytoin level. Because phenytoin is not dialyzable, supratherapeutic levels should be used only when necessary for seizure control. A potential for cross-reactivity between phenytoin and its metabolites exists whenever immunological methods are used to determine free phenytoin levels and can result in falsely elevated levels.[195] For any given phenytoin dose, the drug level is lower in patients with RF,[196] a reflection of the increased volume of distribution[197] and rate of metabolism.[198, 199] The rate of metabolism reduces the half-life of phenytoin to 8.1 hours in uremics.[198] The increased proportion of free phenytoin balances the greater volume of distribution and shorter half-life; thus, the same loading and maintenance doses used in nonuremic patients are used in this clinical situation. However, because the half-life is decreased, a dosage regimen of three times a day is favored over a twice-daily regimen.

Although phenobarbital is renally excreted, it is a useful AED for the treatment of epilepsy in this patient population, provided that sedation can be avoided. Because phenobarbital is only 40 to 60 percent protein bound, its level can be decreased by dialysis. When phenobarbital is used, a postdialysis serum phenobarbital level should be obtained and a supplemental dosage provided. Valproic acid is useful for myoclonus and generalized seizures. Seizures occurring during or up to 8 hours after a dialysis run can be a manifestation of the dialysis disequilibrium syndrome. In these patients, prophylactic AEDs are recommended until uremia is controlled.[179] Also, decreasing the blood flow rate and duration of dialysis, increasing dialysis frequency, and administering hypertonic mannitol during dialysis can help with seizure control.

Treatment of the RF improves the UN, and patients with mild UN typically recover completely with maintenance dialysis. Conversely, patients with severe UN rarely recover, even after several years of treatment, and the slowed nerve conduction velocities are only mildly improved by dialysis.[174] Renal transplantation is much more effective at relieving neuropathic symptoms than is maintenance dialysis.[200, 201] NCS show improvement within days of transplantation,[202] and the improvement continues with complete recovery at times.[200, 201] Neuropathic pain associated with RF can be treated as well with tricyclic antidepressants or antiepileptic drugs (e.g., gabapentin, carbamazepine; see Chapter 20). Uremic optic neuropathy causes rapidly progressive visual loss that responds to hemodialysis and corticosteroid treatment.[63]

Neurological Complications of Dialysis

Complications associated with dialysis include dialysis disequilibrium syndrome (DDS), dialysis dementia, SDH, dialysis headaches, exacerbation of migraine headaches, muscle cramping, neurological vitamin deficiency syndromes, ischemic neuropathy due to the presence of an arteriovenous fistula, and CTS (Table 38–14).

DDS refers to a transient form of encephalopathy related to dialysis. Although its pathogenesis is unknown, it most likely results from a shift of water into the brain (i.e., cerebral edema) in response to the rapid reduction of serum osmolality occurring with dialysis. The duration of symptoms reflects the time required for the brain to decrease its own osmolality. In the predialysis state, idiogenic osmoles allowed the brain to protect itself against dehydration (i.e., it countered the increased serum osmolality). Conversely, in the postdialysis state, this previously protective feature becomes detrimental. Arieff and colleagues[163] compared different rates of hemodialysis in uremic dogs and showed that the amount of cerebral edema was greater in the more rapidly hemodialyzed group. This hypothesis is further supported by the appearance of DDS during the early phases of a hemodialysis program rather than after routine maintenance dialysis has begun. This likely reflects the greater net difference between the predialysis and postdialysis serum concentrations of dialyzable mol-

TABLE 38–14. **The Neurological Complications of Dialysis**
Dialysis disequilibrium syndrome
Dialysis dementia
Subdural hemorrhage
Dialysis headaches
Exacerbation of pre-existing migraine headaches
Muscle cramping
Vitamin deficiency
Ischemic monomelic neuropathy
Carpal tunnel syndrome

ecules occurring with the earlier dialysis treatments. The onset of DDS is usually around the third or fourth hour of a dialysis run (sometimes up to 24 hours after) and typically lasts several hours. Although DDS is seen in all age groups, it is more common at the extremes of age. Delirium, although infrequently precipitated, often lasts several days.[203] Symptoms of DDS are usually self-limited and include headache, anorexia, nausea, emesis, hypertension, disorientation, tremors, twitching, blurred vision, fatigue, muscle cramps, restlessness, and dizziness.[204] More serious neurological sequelae, such as seizures, coma, and death, were not uncommon before 1970, when aggressive dialysis was used. Uncommon features, including exophthalmos, increased intraocular pressure,[205] papilledema,[63] and increased ICP, have been reported.[166] If muscle cramping occurs, it may respond to quinine sulfate, 320 mg PO, at the beginning of each dialysis.

The differential diagnosis of DDS includes malignant hypertension, Wernicke's encephalopathy, UE, dialysis dementia, SDH, hyponatremia, hypercalcemia, hypoglycemia, NKHH, hypoxic-ischemic processes, copper and nickel intoxication, and excessive ultrafiltration.[158] DDS may respond to an extension of the dialysis period from 4 to 6 hours, or switching to peritoneal dialysis.

Dialysis dementia, also called dialysis encephalopathy, is a rare, subacutely progressive, irreversible, and fatal encephalopathy that was initially described in 1972 in chronic hemodialysis patients.[206] The disorder usually begins with memory problems and dysarthric, stuttering, hesitant speech, progressing to mutism, asterixis, myoclonus, dementia, coma, and death.[57] The speech disorder is initially intermittent, appearing during and just after dialysis but eventually becomes permanent.[62, 175] Other features include personality and behavioral changes and occasionally apraxia of speech.[62] Delusions, hallucinations, gait disturbances,[63] and focal neurological abnormalities[175] may also be seen. Seizures are common and usually multifocal.[207]

It is now strongly suspected that dialysis dementia is caused by high brain aluminum content. In 1976, Alfrey and co-workers[208] reported that the brain aluminum content was greater in patients with dialysis dementia than it was in normal controls. Although oral P-binding drugs were initially considered to be the source of exogenous aluminum, this did not explain the geographic variation in the incidence of the disorder. Researchers discovered a difference in dialysate aluminum content among various dialysis centers,[209] and epidemiological studies linked dialysis dementia to municipal water supplies with high aluminum levels.[210] Unexplained sporadic cases in centers with low aluminum dialysate content, however, have been reported.[210] The high blood aluminum levels in these sporadic cases suggest that the GI absorption of aluminum (oral P-binding drugs) may occasionally cause this syndrome.

In evaluating these patients, it is important to remember that dialysis dementia is rare and should always be a diagnosis of exclusion. The differential diagnosis includes DDS, hypertensive encephalopathy, structural lesions (e.g., SDH, stroke), and metabolic encephalopathies such as drug intoxications. Trace element intoxications, decreased glucose, electrolyte disorders (increased Ca, decreased Na or phosphorus), hyperosmolal states, hyperparathyroidism, and UE should also be considered.[158] Changes in dialysis schedule, a change in baseline metabolic status, infection (e.g., dialysis shunt, brain abscess, hepatitis), and treatable encephalopathies (vitamin B_{12}, folate, TFTs) can present similarly.[209] Routine laboratory studies, urinalysis, chest x-ray study, and neuroimaging, when focal neurological abnormalities are identified, are also required. If an infectious cause is suspected, CSF examination may be required. The EEG is invariably abnormal, showing characteristic bursts of frontal slowing and epileptiform spikes.

Dialysis dementia does not respond to an increase in weekly dialysis time or renal transplantation. Because deferoxamine crosses the BBB, binds aluminum with greater affinity than do plasma proteins, and results in a dialyzable complex, it can be used to treat this disorder.[211] The CSF aluminum content increases with deferoxamine treatment, a finding that correlates with deterioration,[209] and it has been associated with visual and auditory disturbances.[63] Several dosing protocols have been reported, and treatment duration has not yet been determined.[209, 212, 213] Seizures are treated similarly to those in other patients with RF.

On average, dialysis dementia begins 37 months (range, 9 to 84 months) after hemodialysis is initiated and has an average survival of 6 months (range, 1 to 15 months).[214] However, waxing and waning courses, several-year survivals, and transient symptoms have also been reported.[215, 216] Reports from Europe and the United States have suggested that dialysis dementia might be part of a larger syndrome, including anemia, bone disease, and a proximal myopathy.[217]

Acknowledgments

The author wishes to thank Dr. James K. Rone, Endocrinology; Dr. Kristin Joyner, Nephrology; and Dr. Brian Robinson (deceased), Gastroenterology, for the helpful criticisms and useful suggestions they provided in the first edition of this textbook.

Reviews and Selected Updates

Adrogue HJ, Madias NE: Hypernatremia. New Engl J Med 2000;342: 1493–1499.

Epstein FH: The physiology of parathyroid hormone-related protein. New Engl J Med 2000;342:177–185.

Hartl E, Finsterer J, Grossegger C, et al: Relationship between thyroid function and skeletal muscle involvement in subclinical and overt hypothyroidism. Endocrinologist 2001;11:217–221.

Marx SJ: Hyperparathyroid and hypoparathyroid disorders. New Engl J Med 2000;343:1863–1875.

Toft AD: Subclinical hyperthyroidism. New Engl J Med 2001;345:512–516.

Weetman AP: Graves' disease. New Engl J Med 2000;343:1236–1248.

References

1. Fraser CL, Arieff AI: Epidemiology, pathophysiology, and management of hyponatremic encephalopathy. Am J Med 1997;102:67–77.
2. Adrogue HJ, Madias NE: Hyponatremia. New Engl J Med 2000;342: 1581–1589.
3. Griggs RC: Treatment and Prevention of Electrolyte and Acid Base Disorders. Course 145, Internal Medicine for the Neurologist. 46th Annual Meeting of the American Academy of Neurology, Washington, DC, 1994, pp 31–48.
4. Votey SR, Peters AL, Hoffman JR: Disorders of water metabolism: Hyponatremia and hypernatremia. Emerg Med Clin 1989;7:749–769.
5. Robertson GL, Aycinena P, Zerbe R: Neurogenic disorders of osmoregulation. Am J Med 1982;72:339–353.

6. Anderson RJ: Hospital-associated hyponatremia. Kidney Int 1986;29:1237–1247.
7. Anderson RJ, Chung HM, Kluge R, Schrier RW: Hyponatremia: A prospective analysis of its epidemiology and the pathogenetic role of vasopressin. Ann Intern Med 1985;102:164–168.
8. Arieff A: Treatment of acid-base and electrolyte disorders. Internal Medicine for the Neurologist. 44th Annual Meeting of the American Academy of Neurology, San Diego, CA, 1992.
9. Donaldson JO: Neurology of Pregnancy, 2nd ed. Philadelphia, WB Saunders, 1989.
10. Riggs JE: Neurological manifestations of electrolyte disorders. *In* Aminoff MJ (ed): Neurology and General Medicine, 3rd ed. New York, Churchill Livingstone, 2001, pp 307–316.
11. DeFronzo RA, Arieff AI: Hyponatremia: Pathophysiology and treatment. *In* Arieff AI, DeFronzo RA (eds): Fluid, Electrolyte, and Acid-base Disorders, 2nd ed. New York, Churchill Livingstone, 1995, pp 255–303.
12. Sarnaik AP, Meert K, Hackbarth R, Fleischmann L: Management of hyponatremic seizures in children with hypertonic saline: A safe and effective strategy. Crit Care Med 1991;19:758–762.
13. Ayus JC, Krothapalli RK, Arieff AI: Treatment of symptomatic hyponatremia and its relation to brain damage: A prospective study. N Engl J Med 1987;317:1190–1195.
14. Riggs JE, Schochet SS Jr: Osmotic stress, osmotic myelinolysis, and oligodendrocyte topography. Arch Pathol Lab Med 1989;113: 1386–1388.
15. Adams RD, Victor M, Mancall EL: Central pontine myelinolysis: A hitherto undescribed disease occurring in alcoholic and malnourished patients. Arch Neurol Psychiatry 1959;81:154–172.
16. Paguirigan A, Lefken EB: Central pontine myelinolysis. Neurology 1969;19:1007–1011.
17. Leslie KO, Robertson AS, Norenberg MD: Central pontine myelinolysis: An osmotic gradient pathogenesis. J Neuropathol Exp Neurol 1980;39:370.
18. Sterns RH, Riggs JE, Schochet SS Jr: Osmotic demyelination syndrome following correction of hyponatremia. N Engl J Med 1986;314:1535–1542.
19. Tien R, Arieff AI, Kucharczyk W, et al: Hyponatremic encephalopathy: Is central pontine myelinolysis a component? Am J Med 1992;92:513–522.
20. Ayus JC, Arieff AI: Pulmonary complications of hyponatremic encephalopathy: Noncardiogenic pulmonary edema and hypercapnic respiratory failure. Chest 1995;107:517–521.
21. Laureno R, Karp BI: Myelinolysis after correction of hyponatremia. Ann Intern Med 1997;126:57–62.
22. Oya S, Tsutsumi K, Ueki K, Kirino T: Reinduction of hyponatremia to treat central pontine myelinolysis. Neurology 2001;57:1931–1932.
23. Andrews BT: Fluid and electrolyte disorders in neurosurgical intensive care. Neurosurg Clin 1994;5:707–723.
24. Darby JM, Nelson PB: Fluid, electrolyte, and acid-base balance in neurosurgical intensive care. *In* Andrews BT (ed): Neurosurgical Intensive Care. New York, McGraw-Hill, 1993, pp 133–162.
25. Cserr HF, dePasquale M, Patlak CS: Volume regulatory influx of electrolytes from plasma to brain during acute hyperosmolality. Am J Physiol 1987;253:530–537.
26. Phillips PA, Rolls BJ, Ledingham JG, et al: Reduced thirst after water deprivation in healthy elderly men. N Engl J Med 1984;311:753–759.
27. Kliman B: Metabolic derangements. *In* Ropper AH (ed): Neurological and Neurosurgical Intensive Care, 3rd ed. Rockville, MD, Aspen, 1993, pp 119–128.
28. Morris-Jones PH, Houston IB, Evans RC: Prognosis of the neurological complications of acute hypernatremia. Lancet 1967;2:1385–1389.
29. Zull DN: Disorders of potassium metabolism. Emerg Med Clin 1989;7:771–794.
30. Gabow PA, Peterson LN: Disorders of potassium metabolism. *In* Schrier RW (ed): Renal and Electrolyte Disorders, 3rd ed. Boston, Little, Brown, and Company, 1986, pp 207–249.
31. Pestana C: Fluids and Electrolytes in the Surgical Patient, 5th ed. Philadelphia, Lippincott, Williams & Wilkins, 2000.
32. Lee KS, Powell BL, Adams PL: Focal neurological signs associated with hyperkalemia. South Med J 1984;77:792–793.
33. Olinger ML: Disorders of calcium and magnesium metabolism. Emerg Med Clin 1989;7:795–822.
34. Singhal S, Johnson CA, Udelsman R: Primary hyperparathyroidism: What every orthopedic surgeon should know. Orthopedics 2001; 24:1003–1009.
35. Zaloga GP, Chernow B, Cook D, et al: The importance of measured serum ionized calcium levels in critically ill patients. Crit Care Med 1984;12:236.
36. Zaloga GP, Wilkens R, Tourville J, et al: A simple method for determining physiologically active calcium and magnesium concentrations in critically ill patients. Crit Care Med 1987;15:813–816.
37. Spiegel AM: The parathyroid glands, hypercalcemia, and hypocalcemia. *In* Bennett JC, Plum F (eds): Cecil Textbook of Medicine, 20th ed. Philadelphia, WB Saunders, 1995, pp 1364–1373.
38. Hess LW, Morrison JC, Hess DB: General medical disorders during pregnancy. *In* DeCherney AH, Pernoll ML (eds): Current Obstetrics and Gynecologic Diagnosis and Treatment, 8th ed. Norwalk, CT, Appleton & Lange, 1994, pp 468–492.
39. Fishman RA: Neurologic manifestations of magnesium metabolism. Course 211, Neurologic Manifestations of Electrolyte Disorders. 45th Annual Meeting of the American Academy of Neurology, New York, 1993, pp 1–5.
40. Agus ZS, Wasserstein A, Goldfarb S: Disorders of calcium and magnesium homeostasis. Am J Med 1982;72:473–488.
41. Koeze TH, Klingon GH: Acquired toxoplasmosis: Case with focal neurologic manifestations. Arch Neurol 1964;11:191–197.
42. Lipsky MS: Hypercalcemia. *In* Rakel RE (ed): Saunders Manual of Medical Practice. Philadelphia, WB Saunders, 1996, pp 663–664.
43. Dent DM, Miller JL, Klaff L, et al: The incidence and causes of hypercalcemia. Postgrad Med J 1987;63:745–750.
44. Elin RJ: Assessment of magnesium status. Clin Chem 1987;33:1965–1970.
45. Tosiello L: Hypomagnesemia and diabetes mellitus. Arch Intern Med 1996;156:1143–1148.
46. Shils ME: Experimental human magnesium depletion. Medicine (Baltimore) 1969;48:61–85.
47. Alfrey AC: Disorders of magnesium metabolism. *In* Bennett JC, Plum F (eds): Cecil Textbook of Medicine, 20th ed. Philadelphia, WB Saunders, 1995, pp 1137–1138.
48. McLean RM: Magnesium and its therapeutic uses: A review. Am J Med 1994;96:63–76.
49. Pernoll ML, Taylor CM: Normal pregnancy and prenatal care. *In* DeChaney AH, Pernoll ML (eds): Current Obstetrics and Gynecologic Diagnosis and Treatment, 8th ed. Norwalk, Appleton & Lange, 1994, pp 183–201.
50. Chernow B, Smith J, Rainey TG, et al: Hypomagnesemia: Implications for the critical care specialist. Crit Care Med 1982;10:193.
51. Fishman RA: Neurological aspects of magnesium metabolism. Arch Neurol 1965;12:562–569.
52. Riggs JE: Cardioskeletal mitochondrial myopathy associated with chronic magnesium deficiency. Neurology 1992;42:128–130.
53. Swift TR: Weakness from magnesium-containing cathartics: Electrophysiologic studies. Muscle Nerve 1979;2:295–298.
54. Reinhart RA: Magnesium metabolism: A review with special reference to the relationship between intracellular content and serum levels. Arch Intern Med 1988;148:2415–2420.
55. Somjen G, Hilmy M, Stephen CR: Failure to anesthetize human subjects by intravenous administration of magnesium sulfate. J Pharmacol Exp Ther 1968;154:652–659.
56. Pulsinelli WA, Cooper AJL: Metabolic encephalopathies and coma. *In* Siegel G, Agranoff B, Albers RW, Molinoff P (eds): Basic Neurochemistry, 4th ed. New York, Raven Press, 1989, pp 765–781.
57. Bleck TP: Metabolic encephalopathies. *In* Weiner WJ (ed): Emergent and Urgent Neurology. Philadelphia, JB Lippincott, 1992, pp 27–57.
58. Jozefowicz RF: Neurolgic manifestations of pulmonary disease. Neurol Clin 1989;7:605–616.
59. Simon RP, Aminoff MJ, Greenberg DA: Disorders of cognitive function: Approach to diagnosis and acute confusional states. *In* Simon RP, Aminoff MJ, Greenberg DA (eds): Clinical Neurology. Norwalk, CT, Appleton & Lange, 1989, pp 1–40.
60. Bennett DA, Bleck TP: Diagnosis and treatment of neuromuscular causes of acute respiratory failure. Clin Neuropharmacol 1988;11:303–347.
61. Bates DV: The respiratory muscles and their disorders. *In* Bates DV (ed): Respiratory Function in Disease, 3rd ed. Philadelphia, WB Saunders, 1989, pp 369–381.
62. Adams RD, Victor M: The acquired metabolic disorders of the nervous system. *In* Adams RD, Victor M (eds): Principles of Neurology, 5th ed. New York, McGraw-Hill, 1993, pp 877–902.
63. Aminoff MJ: Neurological complications of systemic disease in adults. *In* Bradley WG, Daroff RB, et al (eds): Neurology in Clinical Practice, 2nd ed. Boston, Butterworth-Heinemann, 1996, pp 905–930.

64. Myers RAM, Snyder SK, Emhoff TA: Subacute sequelae of carbon monoxide poisoning. Ann Emerg Med 1985;14:1163–1167.
65. Gibson GE: Hypoxia. *In* McCandless DW (ed): Cerebral Energy Metabolism and Metabolic Encephalopathy. New York, Plenum, 1985, pp 43–78.
66. Gibson GE, Peterson C: Decreases in the release of acetylcholine in vitro with low oxygen. Biochem Pharmacol 1982;31:111–115.
67. Lance JW, Adams RD: The syndrome of intention or action myoclonus as a sequela to hypoxic encephalopathy. Brain 1963;86:111–136.
68. Fahn S: Posthypoxic action myoclonus: Literature review update. Adv Neurol 1986;43:157–169.
69. Choi IS: Delayed neurologic sequelae in carbon monoxide intoxication. Arch Neurol 1983;40:433–435.
70. Dooling EC, Richardson EP Jr: Delayed encephalopathy after strangling. Arch Neurol 1976;33:196–199.
71. Weiner WJ, Lang AE (eds): Movement disorders: A comprehensive survey. New York, Futura, 1989.
72. Fenichel GM: Paraplegia and quadriplegia. *In* Fenichel GM (ed): Clinical Pediatric Neurology: A Signs and Symptoms Approach. Philadelphia, WB Saunders, 1988, pp 263–278.
73. Gardner WN: The pathophysiology of hyperventilation disorders. Chest 1996;109:516–534.
74. Saltzman HA, Heyman A, Sieker HO: Correlation of clinical and physiologic manifestations of sustained hyperventilation. N Engl J Med 1963;268:1431–1436.
75. Mountz JM, Modell JG, Wilson MW, et al: Positron emission tomographic evaluation of cerebral blood flow during state anxiety in simple phobia. Arch Gen Psychiatry 1989;46:501–504.
76. Mitchell JM: Thyroid disease in the emergency department: Thyroid function tests and hypothyroidism and myxedema coma. Emerg Med Clin 1989;7:885–902.
77. Mazzaferri EL: Adult hypothyroidism: I. Manifestations and clinical presentation. Postgrad Med 1986;79:64–72.
78. Eledrisi MS, Urban RJ, Lieberman SA: Brain injury and neuroendocrine function. Endocrinologist 2001;11:275–281.
79. Vella A, Young WF Jr: Pituitary apoplexy. Endocrinologist 2001;11: 282–288.
80. Myers L, Hays J: Myxedema coma. Crit Care Clin 1991;7:43–56.
81. Kissel JT: Endocrine Myopathies. Update on Neuromuscular Disease. Course 423 of the AAN Annual Meeting, Washington, DC, 1994, pp 34–55.
82. Layzer RB: Neuromuscular manifestations of endocrine disease. *In* Becker KL, Bilezikian JP, Bremner WJ, et al (eds): Principles and Practice of Endocrinology and Metabolism, 2nd ed. Philadelphia, JB Lippincott, 1995, pp 1762–1770.
83. Kaminski HJ, Ruff RL: Neurologic complications of endocrine diseases. Neurol Clin 1989;7:489–508.
84. Bagchi N, Brown TR, Parish RF: Thyroid function in adults over age 55 years: A study in an urban US community. Arch Intern Med 1990;150:785–787.
85. Burrow GN: The thyroid gland and reproduction. *In* Yen SSC, Jaffe RB (eds): Reproductive Endocrinology, 2nd ed. Philadelphia, WB Saunders, 1986, pp 424–440.
86. Abend WK, Tyler HR: Thyroid disease and the nervous system. *In* Aminoff MJ (ed): Neurology and General Medicine, 2nd ed. New York, Churchill Livingstone, 1995, pp 333–347.
87. DeLong GR, Adams RD: The neuromuscular system and brain in hypothyroidism. *In* Braverman LE, Litiger RD (eds): Werner and Ingbar's The Thyroid: A Fundamental and Clinical Text, 6th ed. New York, JB Lippincott, 1991, pp 1027–1039.
88. Doherty C: Neurologic manifestations of thyroid disease. Neurologist 2001;7:147–157.
89. Arafah BM: Increased need for thyroxine in women with hypothyroidism during estrogen therapy. New Engl J Med 2001:344:1743–1749.
90. Earll JM, Kolb FO: Facial paralysis occurring with hypothyroidism: A report of two cases. Calif Med 1967;106:56–58.
91. Van't Hoff W, Stuart DW: Deafness in myxedema. Q J Med 1979;48:361–367.
92. Kurupath R, Ahlskog E, Garrity JA, Kurland LT: Idiopathic intracranial hypertension. Mayo Clin Proc 1994;69:169–180.
93. River Y, Zelig O: Triphasic waves in myxedema coma. Clin Electroencephalogr 1993;24:146–150.
94. Arlot S, Debussche X, Lalaw JD, et al: Myxedema coma: Responses of thyroid hormone with oral and intravenous high-dose l-thyroxine treatment. Intens Care Med 1991;19:16–18.
95. Tsitouras PD: Myxedema coma. Clin Geriat Med 1995;11:251–258.
96. DeLong GR, Adams RD: The neuromuscular system and brain in thyrotoxicosis. *In* Braverman LE, Litiger RD (eds): Werner and Ingbar's The Thyroid: A Fundamental and Clinical Text, 6th ed. New York, JB Lippincott, 1991, pp 793–802.
97. Shahar E, Shapiro MS, Shenkman L: Hyperthyroid-induced chorea: Case report and review of the literature. Isr J Med Sci 1988;24: 264–266.
98. Feibel JH, Campa JF: Thyrotoxic neuropathy (Basedow's paraplegia). J Neurol Neurosurg Psychiatry 1976;39:491–497.
99. Kammer GM, Hamilton CR: Acute bulbar muscle dysfunction and hyperthyroidism: A study of four cases and review of the literature. Am J Med 1974;56:464–470.
100. Gorman CA: Temporal relationship between onset of Graves' ophthalmopathy and diagnosis of thyrotoxicosis. Mayo Clin Proc 1983;58:515–519.
101. Feinberg WD, Underdahl LO, Eaton LM: Myasthenia gravis and myxedema. Mayo Clin Proc 1957;32:299–305.
102. Selim MH: Neurologic aspects of thyroid disease. Neurologist 2001;7:135–146.
103. Gittinger JW Jr: Eye diseases. *In* Wyngaarden JB, Smith LH Jr (eds): Cecil Textbook of Medicine, 18th ed. Philadelphia, WB Saunders, 1988, pp 2289–2299.
104. Bahn RS, Garrity JA, Gorman CA: Diagnosis and management of Graves' ophthalmopathy. J Clin Endocrinol Metab 1990;71:559–563.
105. Trobe JD, Glaser JS, Laflamme P: Dysthyroid optic neuropathy. Arch Ophthalmol 1978;96:1199–1209.
106. Zimmerman EA: Endocrine diseases. *In* Rowland LP (ed): Merritt's Textbook of Neurology, 8th ed. Philadelphia, Lea & Febiger, 1989, pp 823–844.
107. Jatzko GR, Lisborg PH, Muller MG, et al: Recurrent nerve palsy after thyroid operations: Principal nerve identification and a literature review. Surgery 1994;115:139–144.
108. Williams GH, Dluhy RG: Diseases of the adrenal cortex. *In* Braunwald E, Isselbacher KJ, Petersdorf RG, et al (eds): Harrison's Principles of Internal Medicine, 11th ed. New York, McGraw-Hill, 1987, pp 1753–1774.
109. Loriaux DL: Adrenocortical insufficiency. *In* Becker KL, Bilezikian JP, Brenner WJ, et al (eds): Principles and Practice of Endocrinology and Metabolism, 2nd ed. Philadelphia, JB Lippincott, 1995, pp 682–686.
110. Rone JK: Adrenal insufficiency. *In* Rakel RE (ed): Saunders Manual of Medical Practice. Philadelphia, WB Saunders, 1996, pp 653–656.
111. Grinspoon SK, Biller BMK: Laboratory assessment of adrenal insufficiency. J Clin Endocrinol Metab 1994;79:923–931.
112. Rusnak RA: Adrenal and pituitary emergencies. Emerg Med Clin 1989;7:903–925.
113. Newell KA, Prinz RA, Pickleman J, et al: Pheochromocytoma multisystem crisis: A surgical emergency. Arch Surg 1988;123:956–959.
114. Schipper HM, Abrams GM: Other endocrinopathies and the nervous system. *In* Aminoff MJ (ed): Neurology and General Medicine, 2nd ed. New York, Churchill Livingstone, 1995, pp 383–400.
115. Schteingart DE: Cushing syndrome. *In* Becker KL, Bilezikian JP, Bremner WJ, et al (eds): Principles and Practice of Endocrinology and Metabolism, 2nd ed. Philadelphia, JB Lippincott, 1995, pp 667–682.
116. Norton AJ: Cushing's syndrome/disease. *In* Rakel RE (ed): Saunders Manual of Medical Practice. Philadelphia, WB Saunders, 1996, pp 651–652.
117. Maugans TA, Coates ML: Diagnosis and treatment of acromegaly. Am Fam Phys 1995;52:207–213.
118. Melmed S, Ho K, Klibanski A, et al: Recent advances in pathogenesis, diagnosis, and management of acromegaly. J Clin Endocrinol Metab 1995;80:3395–3402.
119. Molitch ME: Clinical manifestations of acromegaly. Endocrinol Metab Clin 1992;21:597–614.
120. Grunstein RR, Ho KY, Sullivan CE: Sleep apnea in acromegaly. Ann Intern Med 1991;115:527–532.
121. Lockwood AH: Toxic and metabolic encephalopathies. *In* Bradley WG, Daroff RB, Fenichel GM, et al (eds): Neurology in Clinical Practice, 2nd ed. Boston, Butterworth-Heinemann, 1996, pp 1355–1372.
122. Rother J, Schreiner A, Wentz KU, Hennerici M: Hypoglycemia presenting as basilar artery thrombosis. Stroke 1992;23:112–113.
123. Lockwood AH: Hypoglycemia. *In* Feldmann E (ed): Current Diagnosis in Neurology. St. Louis, Mosby, 1994, pp 214–216.
124. Yealy DM, Wolfson AB: Hypoglycemia. Emerg Med Clin North Am 1989;7:837–848.

125. Wass CT, Lanier WL: Glucose modulation of ischemic brain injury: Review and clinical recommendations. Mayo Clin Proc 1996;71: 801–812.
126. Israel RS: Diabetic ketoacidosis. Emerg Med Clin North Am 1989;7:859–871.
127. Podolsky S: Hyperosmolar nonketotic coma in the elderly diabetic. Med Clin North Am 1978;4:815–828.
128. Pope DW, Dansky D: Hyperosmolar hyperglycemic nonketotic coma. Endo Metab Emerg 1989;7:849–857.
129. Palmer SM: Diabetes mellitus. *In* DeChaney AH, Pernoll ML (eds): Current Obstetrics and Gynecologic Diagnosis and Treatment, 8th ed. Norwalk, CT, Appleton & Lange, 1994, pp 368–379.
130. Hare JW, Rossini AA: Diabetic comas: The overlap concept. Hosp Pract 1979; May: 95–108.
131. Tarsy D, Freeman R: The nervous system and diabetes. *In* Kahn CR, Weir GC (eds): Joslin's Diabetes Mellitus, 13th ed. Philadelphia, Lea & Febiger, 1994, pp 794–816.
132. McCall AL: The impact of diabetes on the CNS. Diabetes 1992;41:557–570.
133. Harati Y: Diabetes and the nervous system. Endocrinol Metab Clin North Am 1996;25:325–359.
134. Hopf HC, Gutmann L: Diabetic 3rd nerve palsy: Evidence for a mesencephalic lesion. Neurology 1990;40:1041–1045.
135. Burde RM: Neuro-ophthalmic associations and complications of diabetes mellitus. Am J Ophthalmol 1992;114:498–501.
136. Kissel JT, Burde RM, Klingele TG, Zeiger HE: Pupil-sparing oculomotor palsies with internal carotid-posterior communicating artery aneurysms. Ann Neurol 1983;13:149–154.
137. Wilbourn AJ: Diabetic neuropathies. *In* Brown WF, Bolton CF (eds): Clinical Electromyography, 2nd ed. Boston, Butterworth-Heinemann, 1993, pp 477–515.
138. Dyck PJ, Lais A, Karnes JL, et al: Fiber loss is primary and multifocal in sural nerves in diabetic polyneuropathy. Ann Neurol 1986;19:425–429.
139. Sullivan JF: The neuropathies of diabetes. Neurology 1958;8:243–249.
140. Bastron JA, Thomas JE: Diabetic polyradiculopathy. Mayo Clin Proc 1981;56:725–732.
141. Low PA: Diabetic autonomic neuropathy. Semin Neurol 1996;16:143–151.
142. Lockwood AH: Hepatic encephalopathy. *In* Aminoff MJ (ed): Neurology and General Medicine, 3rd ed. New York, Churchill Livingstone, 2001, pp 233–246.
143. McDonald M, Ralph DD, Carithers RL Jr: Severe liver disease. *In* Shoemaker WC, Ayres SM, Grenvik A, et al (eds): Textbook of Critical Care, 3rd ed. Philadelphia, WB Saunders, 1995, pp 991–1003.
144. Wolke A, Van Ness MM: Hepatic encephalopathy. *In* Chobanian SJ, Van Ness MM (eds): Manual of Clinical Problems in Gastroenterology. Boston, Little, Brown, and Company, 1988.
145. Butterworth RF: Hepatic encephalopathy. Neurologist 1995;1:95–104.
146. Eastwood GL, Avunduk C: Fulminant hepatic failure and encephalopathy. *In* Eastwood GL, Avunduk C (eds): Manual of Gastroenterology: Diagnosis and Therapy. Boston, Little, Brown, and Company, 1988, pp 87–93.
147. Zieve L, Mendelson DF, Goepfert M: Shunt encephalomyelopathy. II. Occurrence of permanent myelopathy. Ann Intern Med 1960;53:53–63.
148. Mullen KD, Cole M: Hepatic encephalopathy. *In* Feldmann E (ed): Current Diagnosis in Neurology. St. Louis, Mosby, 1994, pp 221–226.
149. Lavoie J, Gigre JF, Pomier LG, et al: Amino acid changes in autopsied brain tissue from cirrhotic patients with hepatic encephalopathy. J Neurochem 1987;49:692–697.
150. Pujol J, Kulisevsky J, Moreno A, et al: Neurospectroscopic alterations and globus pallidus hyperintensity as related magnetic resonance markers of reversible hepatic encephalopathy. Neurology 1996;47:1526–1530.
151. Cole M, Mullen KD: Hepatic coma and portal-systemic encephalopathy. *In* Johnson RT, Griffin JW (eds): Current Therapy in Neurologic Disease, 4th ed. St. Louis, Mosby, 1993, pp 326–329.
152. Castell DO, Moore EW: Ammonia absorption from the human colon: The role of non-ionic diffusion. Gastroenterology 1971;60:33–42.
153. Sushma S, Dasarathy S, Tandon RK, et al: Sodium benzoate in the treatment of acute hepatic encephalopathy: A double-blind randomized trial. Hepatology 1992;16:138–144.
154. Wijdicks EFM, Litchy WJ, Wiesner RH, Krom RAF: Neuromuscular complications associated with liver transplantation. Muscle Nerve 1996;19:696–700.
155. Wijdicks EFM, Plevak DJ, Wiesner RH, Steers JL: Causes and outcome of seizures in liver transplant recipients. Neurology 1996;47:1523–1525.
156. Tygstrup N, Ranek L: Assessment of prognosis in fulminant hepatic failure. Semin Liver Dis 1986;6:129–137.
157. O'Grady JG, Gimson AES, O'Brien CJ, et al: Controlled trials of charcoal hemoperfusion and prognostic factors in fulminant hepatic failure. Gastroenterology 1988;94:1186–1192.
158. Fraser CL, Arieff AI: Nervous system manifestations of renal failure. *In* Schrier RW, Gottschalk CW (eds): Diseases of the Kidney, 5th ed. Boston, Little, Brown, and Company, 1992, pp 2789–2816.
159. Olsen S: The brain in uremia. Acta Psychiatr Neurol Scand Suppl 1961;156:1–128.
160. Fishman RA, Raskin NH: Experimental uremic encephalopathy: Permeability and electrolyte metabolism of brain and other tissues. Arch Neurol 1967;17:10–21.
161. Cooper JD, Lazarowitz VC, Arieff AI: Neurodiagnostic abnormalities in patients with acute renal failure: Evidence for neurotoxicity of parathyroid hormone. J Clin Invest 1978;61:1448–1455.
162. Mahoney CA, Arieff AI: Central and peripheral nervous system effects of chronic renal failure. Kidney Int 1983;24:170–177.
163. Arieff AI, Masry SG, Barrientos A, et al: Brain water and electrolyte metabolism in uremia: Effects of slow and rapid hemodialysis. Kidney Int 1973;4:177–187.
164. Posner JB, Swanson AG, Plum F: Acid-base balance in cerebrospinal fluid. Arch Neurol 1965;12:479–496.
165. Arieff AI, Guisado R, Massry SG, Lazarowitz VC: Central nervous system pH in uremia and the effects of hemodialysis. J Clin Invest 1976;58:306–311.
166. Lockwood AH: Neurologic complications of renal disease. Neurol Clin 1989;7:617–627.
167. Goldstein DA, Feinstein EI, Chui LA, et al: The relationship between the abnormalities in electroencephalogram and blood levels of parathyroid hormone in dialysis patients. J Clin Endocrinol Metab 1980;51:130–134.
168. Arieff AI, Massry SG: Calcium metabolism of brain in acute renal failure. J Clin Invest 1974;53:387–392.
169. Massry SG: Current status of the role of parathyroid hormone in uremic toxicity. Contrib Nephrol 1985;49:1–11.
170. Fraser CL, Sarnacki P: Parathyroid hormone mediates changes in calcium transport in uremic rat brain synaptosomes. Am J Physiol 1988;254:837–844.
171. Kjellstrand CM, Solez K: Treatment of acute renal failure. *In* Schrier RW, Gottschalk CW (eds): Diseases of the Kidney, 5th ed. Boston, Little, Brown, and Company, 1992, pp 1371–1404.
172. Warnock DG: Chronic renal failure. *In* Bennett JC, Plum F (eds): Cecil Textbook of Medicine, 20th ed. Philadelphia, WB Saunders, 1996, pp 556–563.
173. Manis T, Friedman EA: Dialytic therapy for irreversible uremia. N Engl J Med 1979;301:1321–1328.
174. Raskin NH: Neurological complications of renal failure. *In* Aminoff MJ (ed): Neurology and General Medicine, 2nd ed. New York, Churchill Livingstone, 1995, pp 303–319.
175. Raskin NH: Renal disease. *In* Rowland LP (ed): Merritt's Textbook of Neurology, 8th ed. Philadelphia, Lea & Febiger, 1989, pp 867–871.
176. Biasioli S, D'Andrea G, Feriani M, et al: Uremic encephalopathy: An updating. Clin Nephrol 1986;25:57–63.
177. Adams RD, Foley JM: The neurologic changes in the more common types of severe liver disease. Trans Am Neurol Assoc 1949;74:217–219.
178. Tyler HR: Neurologic disorders in renal failure. Am J Med 1968; 44:734–748.
179. Sagar SM: Toxic and metabolic disorders. *In* Samuels MA (ed): Manual of Neurologic Therapeutics, 5th ed. Boston, Little, Brown, and Company, 1995, pp 288–326.
180. Noda S, Ito H, Umezaki H, Minato S: Hip flexion-abduction to elicit asterixis in unresponsive patients. Ann Neurol 1985;18:96–97.
181. Raskin NH, Fishman RA: Neurologic disorders in renal failure. N Engl J Med 1976;294:143–148, 204–210.
182. Tyler HR: Neurological disorders seen in renal failure. *In* Vinken PJ, Bruyn BW (eds): Handbook of Clinical Neurology, Vol 27: Metabolic and Deficiency Diseases of the Nervous System. Amsterdam, North-Holland, 1976, pp 321–348.
183. Nielsen VK: The peripheral nerve function in chronic renal failure: IV. An analysis of the vibratory perception threshold. Acta Med Scand 1972;191:287–296.

184. Yosipovitch G, Yarnitsky D, Mermelstein V, et al: Paradoxical heat sensation in uremic polyneuropathy. Muscle Nerve 1995;18:768–771.
185. Hamalainen H, Vartiainen M, Karavanan L, Jarivilehto T: Paradoxical heat sensation during moderate cooling of the skin. Brain Res 1982;251:77–81.
186. Zucchelli P, Sturani A, Zuccala A, et al: Dysfunction of the autonomic nervous system in patients with endstage renal failure. Contrib Nephrol 1985;45:69–81.
187. Ropper AH: Accelerated neuropathy of renal failure. Arch Neurol 1993;50:536–539.
188. Nielsen VK: The peripheral nerve function in chronic renal failure: II. Intercorrelation of clinical symptoms and signs and clinical grading of neuropathy. Acta Med Scand 1971;190:113–117.
189. Guilleminault C, Cetel M, Philip P: Dopaminergic treatment of restless legs and rebound phenomenon. Neurology 1993;43:445.
190. Hening W: Motor disturbances of sleep. Update on the Neurology of Sleep. Course 443 of the 46th Annual Meeting of the American Academy of Neurology, Washington, DC, 1994, pp 89–124.
191. Lazaro RP, Kirshner HS: Proximal muscle weakness in uremia. Arch Neurol 1980;37:555–558.
192. Gilmore RL: Seizures associated with nonneurologic medical conditions. *In* Wyllie E (ed): The Treatment of Epilepsy: Principles and Practice. Philadelphia, Lea & Febiger, 1993, pp 667–677.
193. Martin BK: Potential effect of the plasma proteins on drug distribution. Nature 1965;207:274–276.
194. Campion DS: Decreased drug binding by serum albumin during renal failure. Toxicol Appl Pharmacol 1973;25:391–397.
195. Nandedkar AKN, Williamson R, Kutt H, et al: A comparison of plasma phenytoin level determination by EMIT and gas-liquid chromatography in patients with renal insufficiency. Ther Drug Monit 1980;2:427–430.
196. Odar-Cederlof I, Borga O: Kinetics of diphenylhydantoin in uremic patients: Consequences of decreased plasma protein binding. Eur J Clin Pharmacol 1974;7:31–37.
197. Burgess ED, Friel PN, Blair AD, Raisys VA: Serum phenytoin concentrations in uremia. Ann Intern Med 1981;94:59–60.
198. Letteri JM, Mellk H, Louis S, et al: Diphenylhydantoin metabolism in uremia. N Engl J Med 1971;285:648–652.
199. Borga O, Hoppel C, Odar-Cederlof I, Garle M: Plasma levels and renal excretion of phenytoin and its metabolites in patients with renal failure. Clin Pharmacol Ther 1979;26:306–314.
200. Bolton CF, Baltzan MA, Baltzan RB: Effects of renal transplantation on uremic neuropathy. N Engl J Med 1971;284:1170–1175.
201. Nielsen VK: The peripheral nerve function in chronic renal failure: VIII. Recovery after renal transplantation: Clinical aspects. Acta Med Scand 1974;195:163–170.
202. Oh SJ, Clements RS Jr, Lee YW, Diethelm AG: Rapid improvement in nerve conduction velocity following renal transplantation. Ann Neurol 1978;4:369–373.
203. Tyler HR: Neurological complications of dialysis, transplantation, and other forms of treatment in chronic uremia. Neurology 1965;15:1081–1088.
204. Teschan PE, Arieff AI: Uremic and dialysis encephalopathies. *In* McCandless DW (ed): Cerebral Energy Metabolism and Metabolic Encephalopathy. New York, Plenum, 1985, pp 263–285.
205. Sitprija V, Holmes JH: Preliminary observations on the changes in intracranial pressure and intraocular pressure during hemodialysis. Trans Am Soc Artif Intern Organs 1962;8:300–308.
206. Alfrey AC, Mishell JM, Burks J, et al: Syndrome of dyspraxia and multifocal seizures associated with chronic hemodialysis. Trans ASAIO 1972;18:257–265.
207. Mahurkar SD, Dhar SK, Salta R, et al: Dialysis dementia. Lancet 1973;1:1412–1415.
208. Alfrey AC, Le Gendre GR, Kaehny WD: The dialysis encephalopathy syndrome: Possible aluminum intoxication. N Engl J Med 1976; 294:184–188.
209. Hainline B: Dialysis encephalopathy. *In* Feldmann E (ed): Current Diagnosis in Neurology. St. Louis, Mosby, 1994, pp 209–214.
210. Alfrey AC: The toxicity of the aluminum burden. Semin Nephrol 1983;3:329–334.
211. Swartz RD: Deferoxamine and aluminum removal. Am J Kidney Dis 1985;6:358–364.
212. Van de Vyver FL, Silva FJE, D'Haese PC, et al: Aluminum toxicity in dialysis patients. Contrib Nephrol 1987;55:198–220.
213. Ackrill P, Ralston AJ, Day JP, et al: Successful removal of aluminum from patients with dialytic encephalopathy. Lancet 1980;2:692–693.
214. Chui HC, Damasio AR: Progressive dialysis encephalopathy ("dialysis dementia"). J Neurol 1980;222:145–157.
215. Lederman RJ, Henry CE: Progressive dialysis encephalopathy. Ann Neurol 1978;4:199–204.
216. Nadel AM, Wilson WP: Dialysis encephalopathy: A possible seizure disorder. Neurology 1976;26:1130–1134.
217. Arieff AI: Metabolic encephalopathy: Uremia and dysmolar states. Course 231, Internal Medicine for the Neurologist II. 48th Annual Meeting of the American Academy of Neurology, San Francisco, 1996.

CHAPTER 39

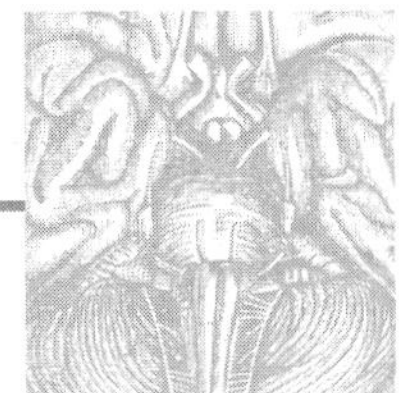

KAREN I. BOLLA and JEAN LUD CADET

Exogenous Acquired Metabolic Disorders of the Nervous System: Toxins and Illicit Drugs

History and Overview

Individual cases of lead poisoning were reported as early as 200 BC. However, it was not until the 20th century that industrialization and modernization resulted in a need for medical evaluation and treatment of health effects caused by exposure to harmful chemicals. To meet this need, a new medical specialty was developed called occupational and environmental medicine. Unfortunately, the number of physicians in this specialty is too few to treat the number of patients requiring evaluation and treatment. Even in academic and workplace settings that offer this expertise, neurological input is paramount because many of the health effects due to chemical exposure are related to the central and peripheral nervous systems. Whereas some health effects such as pulmonary distress and gastrointestinal symptoms are noticed easily by the affected individual, some nervous system effects may be unrecognized. Acute, high-level exposure to a toxicant often results in clearly identifiable signs (e.g., delirium, seizures, or unconsciousness), but the residual effects, involving cognition, mood, and personality, are usually quite subtle. The most common clinical presentation is one of poor concentration, short-term memory loss, depressed mood, anxiety, restlessness, loss of interest in work and hobbies, decreased libido, irritability, headaches, weakness, and sleep disturbances ranging from insomnia to somnambulism.[1, 2] Patients may also report symptoms consistent with peripheral neuropathy.

The diagnosis of neurotoxicant-related damage is one of exclusion. Therefore, other causes of central and peripheral nervous system dysfunction must be ruled out, and a history of significant exposure must be substantiated. The neurological examination, electroencephalogram (EEG), computed tomography (CT) scan, and magnetic resonance imaging (MRI) scan are generally not helpful in making a specific diagnosis of toxic encephalopathy but are helpful in ruling out other causes of the patient's symptoms. In contrast, nerve conduction studies are useful in detecting peripheral neuropathies that are often associated with exposure to specific chemicals. Central nervous system (CNS) effects are best discovered with neuropsychological assessment. However, interpretation of decrements in performance on these tests is often erroneous if made by individuals who lack specific expertise in neurobehavioral toxicology. The reader is referred to Bolla[3] for an in-depth discussion of the use and limitations of neuropsychological methods for the detection of alterations in the CNS following chemical exposure.

Once health effects have been detected, it can be problematic to relate these in a causal fashion to a specific chemical exposure. Because biomarkers for many chemicals are either difficult to obtain or do not exist, it is difficult to determine the intensity of current and past exposure, or even if an individual has been exposed to a toxic chemical. In instances of mass poisonings, this association can be made more readily. Also, for the evaluating clinician, a knowledge of the patient's baseline neurological function prior to exposure is important to ascertain whether there has been a change in neurological status, but it is rarely available.

Evaluation of the direct toxic effects on the CNS must also be considered in the context of the emotional state and personality characteristics of the patient. Psychological disturbance may be a primary or secondary sequela of chemical exposure. Emotional reactions to exposure may be as important as the direct physiological effects of the chemicals, especially when one is considering the cause and persistence of symptoms. In addition, specific inherent personality characteristics may predispose an individual to the development of physical, cognitive, and psychological symptoms even in the absence of any direct toxic effects on the nervous system. Certain individuals' expectations about the adverse health effects of suspected chemical exposure may result in an enhanced awareness of normal bodily sensations. The degree to which an individual is hypersensitive to endogenous stimuli (normal bodily sensations) may determine the duration and intensity of the symptoms.

This chapter focuses on the clinical manifestations subsequent to exposure to specific chemicals. The reader should be aware that the clinical symptoms reported in this chapter have been described in some studies, whereas other studies have failed to find significant symptoms associated with specific chemicals. In addition, not all symptoms listed for a given chemical are observed in one individual. Therefore, the association between symptoms and exposure to a given chemical is still controversial. In this chapter, the chemicals are organized by class (e.g., metals, organic solvents). Table 39–1 lists the occupations and job-related sources associated with a number of different chemicals. As with any diagnostic process, the ability to make a differential diagnosis between neurotoxicant exposure, neurological disease, psychiatric disturbance, or malingering is based on the combined evidence taken from the occupational, medical, social, and academic histories; the physical and neurological examinations; biological monitoring; nerve conduction studies, EEG, CT/MRI; and the neuropsychological evaluation.

Metal Intoxication

ARSENIC

Pathogenesis and Pathophysiology. Although arsenic is rapidly absorbed through the mucous membranes and the skin, the most common route is ingestion. Arsenic rapidly leaves the bloodstream for storage in the liver, kidneys, intestines, spleen, lymph nodes, and bones, and within 2 weeks it is deposited in the hair, remaining there for years. It also remains in the bones for extended periods of time. Excretion through the kidneys and feces is slow. A single dose may require up to 10 days to be excreted. Pathways involved in oxidative metabolism are sensitive to arsenic toxicity. Arsenic also prevents the transformation of thiamine into acetyl-CoA, causing patients to become clinically thiamine deficient. Organic arsenicals release the poison slowly and are therefore less likely to produce acute symptoms than the elemental form. Neuropathological findings in patients with fatal arsenic encephalopathy include cerebral congestion, multiple hemorrhagic lesions throughout the white matter, and areas of necrosis. Decreased numbers of myelinated fibers are seen in the peripheral nerves, and degenerative changes, consisting of swelling, granularity, and a reduction in the number of axons, are present.

Epidemiology and Risk Factors. Occupational and job-related sources of arsenic are listed in Table 39–1. The National Institute for Occupational Safety and Health (NIOSH) estimates that about 900,000 workers have potential daily exposure to arsenic.

Clinical Features and Associated Findings. Acute toxicity is associated with a sudden rise in temperature accompanied by headache, vertigo, nausea and vomiting, nervousness, and apprehension. Convulsions are common. Tendon reflex changes are variable and are frequently exaggerated.

TABLE 39–1. **Occupations and Job-Related Sources of Chemical Exposure**

	Alu-minum	Arse-nic	Lead	Manga-nese	Mer-cury	Thal-lium	Ace-tone	Ben-zene	Carbon Tetra-chloride	Eth-ylene Glycol	For-malde-hyde	Gas-oline	Iso-propyl Alcohol	MBK	Methyl Alco-hol	*N*-Hex-ane	TCE	Tetra-chlor-ethane	Tolu-ene	Turpen-tine
Airplane hangars								X	X			X								
Aircraft manufacture and maintenance	X																			
Alcohol distillation (brewing)					X			X			X				X					
Antifreeze										X					X					
Artificial flowers		X	X		X										X					
Artificial leathers		X					X	X							X					
Artificial pearls			X				X								X					
Automobile painting								X							X					
Automobile manufacture and repair			X					X				X			X					
Bookbinding		X	X												X					
Brass and bronze		X	X	X				X							X					
Brickmaking			X	X																
Cement-plastic mixing			X				X	X				X								
Can sealing								X												

Table continued on following page

TABLE 39–1. **Occupations and Job-Related Sources of Chemical Exposure** *Continued*

	Alu-minum	Arse-nic	Lead	Manga-nese	Mer-cury	Thal-lium	Ace-tone	Ben-zene	Carbon Tetra-chloride	Eth-ylene Glycol	For-malde-hyde	Gas-oline	Iso-propyl Alcohol	MBK	Methyl Alco-hol	*N*-Hex-ane	TCE	Tetra-chlor-ethane	Tolu-ene	Turpen-tine
Cosmetics	X	X			X								X							
Deodorants	X																			
Degreasing and scouring							X	X	X			X					X	X	X	
Dentistry			X		X															
Dry cleaning								X	X						X		X	X		X
Disinfectants		X			X						X									
Dyes		X	X		X		X	X	X		X			X	X	X	X			X
Enamels		X	X					X										X		X
Etching		X	X		X			X							X		X			X
Explosives	X		X				X	X		X	X				X					
Feathers		X						X							X					X
Fertilizers		X		X				X												
Fire extin-guishers									X									X		
Furniture polish								X	X					X	X	X		X	X	X
Fuel (airplane, auto)			X					X				X							X	X
Gardening		X	X																	
Glass			X	X											X			X		X
Glue							X	X						X		X	X		X	X
Insecticides		X	X						X											
Insulators		X						X	X											
Lacquer		X					X	X	X	X	X		X		X		X	X		X
Leather-tannery goods			X		X			X	X		X				X		X	X		
Linoleum		X	X	X				X	X						X					X
Millinery (hats)					X			X			X				X			X		X
Mining				X																

Metal cleaners, polishers							X	X			X			X		X			X
Paints	X	X	X	X	X	X	X	X					X	X	X	X	X		X
Paper workers			X		X					X									
Perfumes						X	X	X				X		X		X			
Pharma-ceuticals		X	X	X	X	X	X	X								X	X		X
Painting and lithog-raphy		X	X		X		X	X						X			X		X
Plastics			X			X	X	X						X			X		
Plumbing			X																
Pottery/ ceramics			X	X	X														
Rayon						X	X			X				X			X		
Refineries (petro-leum)			X			X	X									X	X	X	X
Rubber		X	X			X	X			X				X		X	X		
Shoe manu-facture and repair			X			X	X	X					X	X	X	X	X	X	X
Soaps, deter-gents		X		X			X	X		X				X		X	X		
Storage batteries		X	X		X														
Taxidermy		X			X														
Tobacco							X		X							X			
Vegetable oil extrac-tion													X		X	X			
Water-proofing							X	X		X									
Wax		X					X									X	X		X
Welding	X		X	X		X													

Nystagmus, paralysis, or incontinence may also be observed. Kernig's sign is often positive with neck stiffness. Mee's lines (white lines in the nails) usually appear 2 to 3 weeks after acute exposure to arsenic (Fig. 39–1). Encephalopathy with marked excitement followed by lethargy and coma occur, and signs of acute peripheral neuropathy can develop within hours. In patients with fatal acute poisoning, death ensues within a few days. With subacute and chronic arsenic encephalitis, continuous progressive headaches, physical and mental fatigue, vertigo, restlessness, mild somnolence, and focal paresis develop. Spinal cord involvement leads to weakness, sphincter disturbances, motor and sensory impairment, and trophic changes. Optic neuritis manifested by cloudy vision and visual field defects may also be observed subacutely but can be delayed for as long as 2 years. Generally, a mixed sensory and motor neuropathy develops within 7 to 10 days after ingestion of toxic amounts of arsenic, and patients often complain of severe burning in the soles of the feet (Fig. 39–2). Long-standing cognitive changes have been reported.[4]

Differential Diagnosis and Evaluation. Arsenic intoxication is suggested when a patient presents with severe abdominal pain, dermatitis, painful peripheral neuropathy, and seizures. A history of arsenic exposure and toxic levels in the hair, urine, or nails confirm the diagnosis. Arsenic is poorly tolerated in the presence of alcohol. Therefore, patients with alcohol-related disease may be at greater risk for developing associated arsenic neuropathy. Although hair and nails may be useful, urinary arsenic is the major biomarker; Table 39–2 shows the threshold levels. A level of arsenic in urine (24 hr) greater than 50 μg/g creatinine is considered to be elevated. However, a high urinary level may be seen after ingestion of seafood and thus a dietary history should be obtained. If urinary arsenic comes back elevated and is not fractionated, wait 3 days without seafood intake and repeat. A better measurement can be obtained from the inorganic arsenic metabolites, monomethylarsonic acid and dimethylarsinic acid in the urine. Although these screening guidelines are clinically useful, arsenic toxicity may occur even when blood and urine concentrations are normal.

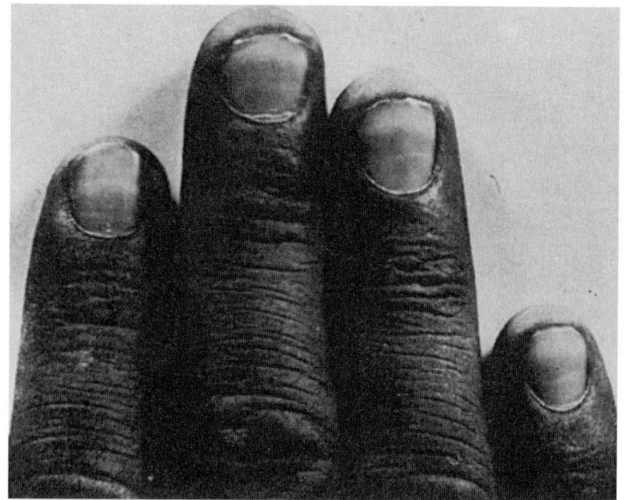

FIGURE 39–1. Double set of Mee's lines in a patient with arsenic intoxication. (Reprinted from Chhuttani PN, Chopra JS. Arsenic poisoning. *In* Vinken PJ, Bruyn GW, Cohen MM, Klawans HL [eds]: Intoxications of the Nervous System. Handbook of Clinical Neurology, Vol 36. Amsterdam, Elsevier, 1979, p. 202, with kind permission from Elsevier Science–NL, Sara Burgerhartstraat 25, 1055 KV Amsterdam, The Netherlands.)

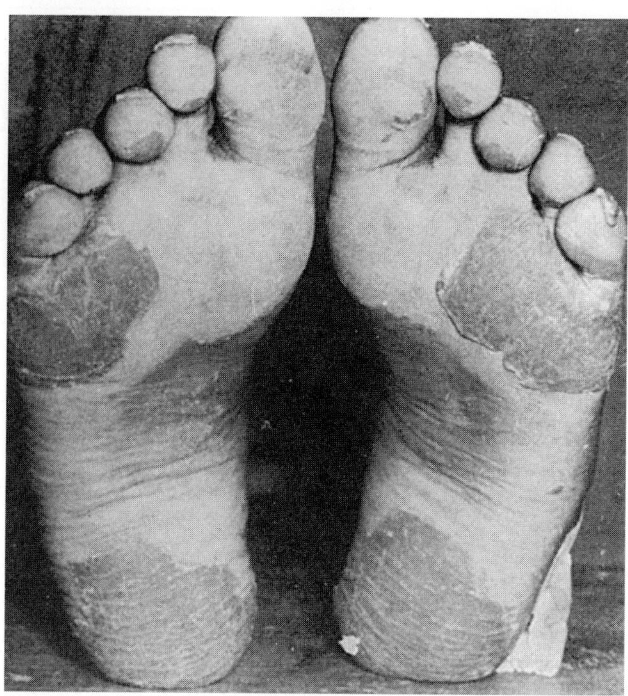

FIGURE 39–2. Hyperkeratosis of the skin of soles with exfoliation in a patient with peripheral neuropathy and arsenic intoxication. (Reprinted from Chhuttani PN, Chopra JS: Arsenic poisoning. *In* Vinken PJ, Bruyn GW, Cohen MM, Klawans HL [eds]: Intoxications of the Nervous System. Handbook of Clinical Neurology, Vol 36. Amsterdam. Elsevier, 1979, p. 202, with kind permission from Elsevier Science–NL, Sara Burgerhartstraat 25, 1055 KV Amsterdam, The Netherlands.)

Management. In patients with acute oral ingestion of arsenic, gastric lavage with electrolyte replacement is recommended. Also, excretion of absorbed arsenic can be enhanced by chelation using dimercaprol (British antilewisite [BAL]), D-penicillamine, or dimercaptosuccinic acid. Chelators essentially reverse or prevent the attachment of heavy metals to various essential body chemicals. While chelation may alleviate the acute symptoms, there is no evidence indicating that it improves chronic symptoms such as peripheral neuropathy or encephalopathy. In fact, once neuropathy occurs, BAL treatment is not considered effective. Intravenous fluids for dehydration and morphine for abdominal pain should also be given. In alcoholics who develop arsenic encephalopathy, vitamins should be administered to replace nutritional deficits.

Prognosis and Future Perspectives. Prognosis with severe arsenic poisoning is poor, with a mortality rate of 50 to 75 percent, usually within 48 hours. Intoxication during pregnancy carries a particularly poor prognosis. Follow-up studies after acute intoxication are few. A cohort of eight patients with arsenic ingestion at a local festival in Wakayama, Japan, were followed for a 1-year period. Sixty-seven patients in total were exposed to the arsenic. Arsenic intake was calculated from urinary amounts. Each patient underwent peripheral nerve testing at 1, 3, and 12 months. Six patients developed numbness and tingling of the extremities within 2 to 4 weeks. In three patients, symptoms were persistent at 1 year. Electrodiagnostic testing revealed a sensory neuropathy and delayed or absent F-wave responses. Motor nerve conduction velocities and compound muscle

TABLE 39–2. **Symptoms Associated with Heavy Metal Exposure**

Metal	Proposed Toxic Mechanism	Tissue Assessed and Toxic Levels*	Associated Symptoms	Clinical Findings†	Specific Treatments	Pathology
Aluminum	Decrease in glucose utilization; reduction of acetylcholine	Blood 6 μg/L† (*NC*) Urine (24 hr) 20 μg/L (*NC*)	Respiratory dysfunction	Cognitive decline; halting speech; ataxia	Deferoxamine (DFO)	
Arsenic Acute	Prevents thiamine transformation into acetylcholine; affects pathways involved in oxidative metabolism	Blood, unreliable Urine (24 hr) 50 μg/g creatine (*B, D, NC*)	GI distress; respiratory distress; cardiac distress; elevated temperature; Mee's lines	Headache; nervousness; vertigo; paralysis, seizures; myelopathy; hyperreflexia; neuropathy	Chelation; gastric lavage with electrolyte replacement; morphine for abdominal pain; IV fluids for dehydration	Cerebral congestion; white matter hemorrhagic lesions; demyelinization of peripheral nerves; reduction in number of axons
Chronic	Prevents thiamine transformation into acetylcholine; effects pathways involved in oxidative metabolism	Blood, unreliable Urine (24 hr) 50 μg/g creatine (*B, D, NC*)	Abdominal pain; dermatitis; increased risk of cancer	Headaches; fatigue; restlessness; vertigo; cognitive decline; visual changes or optic neuropathy; seizures; painful sensorimotor peripheral neuropathy		Cerebral congestion; white matter hemorrhagic lesions; demyelinization of peripheral nerves; reduction in number of axons
Lead Acute Children	Changes in neurotransmitters; inhibits NMDA receptor complex	Blood 10 μg/dL‡ (*B, CW*)	Respiratory distress	Lethargy; cognitive decline; gait disorder; ataxia; seizures	Removal from exposure; chelation with IV calcium disodium-EDTA, succimer (DMSA), or oral penicillamine	Unclear
Adults	Changes in neurotransmitters; inhibits NMDA receptor complex	Blood 30 μg/dl‡ Urine (24 hr) 150 μg/g creatine (*B, CW*); Zinc protoporphyrin in blood: 250 μg/dL erythrocytes or 100 μg/dL blood	GI distress; miscarriages; joint pain	Fatigue; delirium; seizures	Removal from exposure; chelation with IV calcium disodium-EDTA, succimer (DMSA), or oral penicillamine	Unclear

Table continued on following page

TABLE 39–2. **Symptoms Associated with Heavy Metal Exposure** *Continued*

Metal	Proposed Toxic Mechanism	Tissue Assessed and Toxic Levels*	Associated Symptoms	Clinical Findings[†]	Specific Treatments	Pathology
Chronic Children	Changes in neurotransmitters; inhibits NMDA receptor complex	Blood 10 μg/dL[‡] (*B, CW*)	Changes in auditory threshold; behavioral problems; cognitive decline; learning disabilities; attention deficit hyperactivity disorder	Learning disorders	Removal from exposure; chelation	Unclear
Adults	Changes in neurotransmitters; inhibits NMDA receptor complex	Blood 30 μg/dL[‡] Urine (24 hr) 150 μg/g creatine (*B, CW*); Zinc protoporphyrin in blood 250 μg/dL erythrocytes or 100 μg/dL blood	Miscarriage/stillbirth; arthralgia; anemia; hypertension; gout; renal effects; decreased sperm count	Scotopic visual effects; depression; irritability; sleep disturbance; decline in libido; decreased cognition (learning and memory); fasciculations; paresthesias; sensorimotor polyneuropathy; changes in auditory threshold	Removal from exposure; chelation	Punctate hemorrhages; dilation of vessels and ventricles; involvement of ganglion cells; histological changes in hippocampus and cerebellum; demyelinization of peripheral nerves
Manganese	Promotes formation of cytotoxic free radicals; oxidative stress; mitochondrial toxin	24 hour urine 3 μg/L (*NC*); Blood 2 μg/dL (*NC*)	Anorexia; manganese pneumonia	Headaches; apathy; fatigue; depression; hyperexcitability; dysarthria; psychotic behavior; tremor; gait disorders; micrographia; parkinsonism	Removal from exposure; for chronic movement disorders; levodopa, 5-hydroxytryptophan	Histological changes of ganglion cells; damage to substantia nigra and globus pallidus; nerve cell changes in basal nuclei, frontal and parietal cortex, cerebellum, hypothalamus
Mercury *Inorganic* Acute	Alters cell membranes; causes combination of: metabolic disturbance, disturbance of Ca^+ homeostasis, oxidative injury, aberrant protein phosphorylation	Blood 15 μg/L[†] Urine 35 μg/g creatine (*B, NC*)	Bronchial irritation; chills; gingivitis; GI distress; bloody diarrhea; brownish mouth lesions; metallic breath; respiratory distress; renal failure	Weakness; irritability; delirium; psychosis	Removal from exposure	Lesions in cerebral gray matter, cerebellum, brain stem nuclei

Chronic	Alters cell membranes; causes combination of metabolic disturbance, disturbance of Ca^{+} homeostasis, oxidative injury, aberrant protein phosphorylation	Blood 15 μg/L[†] Urine 35 μg/g creatine (*B*, *NC*)	Salivary gland swelling; excessive salivation; gingivitis; renal dysfunction	Shyness; fatigue; weakness; personality changes; hyperirritability; insomnia; depression; cognitive decline; visual disturbances; intentional tremor; parkinsonism; seizures; painful paresthesias; peripheral polyneuropathy (sensorimotor axonopathy)	Removal from exposure; chelation	Neuronal loss and gliosis of the calcarine cortex; atrophy of cerebellum, especially inferior vermis
Organic	Alters cell membranes; causes combination of metabolic disturbance, disturbance of Ca^{+} homeostasis, oxidative injury, aberrant protein phosphorylation	Blood 15 μg/L[†] (*D*, *NC*) Urine (24 hr) unreliable Hair 50 μg/g	Primarily affects the nervous system	Cognitive decline; neurasthenia; paresthesias; ataxia; restricted visual fields; cortical blindness; peripheral polyneuropathy; intention tremor, motor neuron disease (ALS-like)	Chelation with D-penicillamine, BAL, or DMSA; selenium; vitamin E	Damages primary visual cortex, cerebellar cortex, pre- and postcentral gyri, transverse gyrus, and putamen
Thallium	Affects Na^{+}/K^{+}-ATPase, porphyrin metabolism and SH groups	Urine (24 hr) 1 μg/g creatine (*NC*)	GI distress; alopecia	Irritability; fatigue; depression; confusion; movement disorder; optic abnormalities; sensory neuropathy; ascending weakness (Guillain-Barré, poliolike)	BAL; Prussian blue (potassium fermihexacycinoferrate); combined hemoperfusion and hemodialysis	Ganglion cell changes in cortex; demyelinization; axonal degeneration; segmental myelin degeneration in peripheral nerves

*Biological exposure indices (BEIs). American Conference of Governmental Industrial Hygienists (ACGIH) values from ACGIH: Threshold Limit Values and Biological Exposure Indices for 1994–1995. Cincinnati, ACGIH, 1994.

†Serum.

‡Whole blood.

NC, Level correlates poorly with clinical symptoms; *D*, diet significantly influences the measurement; *B*, present in significant amounts in individuals not occupationally exposed; *CW*, correlates well with clinical symptoms. GI distress: nausea, vomiting, stomach cramps; BAL, British antilewisite; DMSA, dimercaptosuccinic acid.

action potentials were normal. The amount of nervous system involvement was directly correlated with the amount of arsenic ingestion.[5]

INORGANIC LEAD

Pathogenesis and Pathophysiology. In the human body, inorganic lead is not metabolized but is absorbed, distributed, and excreted unchanged. The rate of absorption is influenced by nutritional status and age. The amount of lead absorbed increases significantly with iron or calcium deficiency and under fasting conditions. Once absorbed, lead travels bound by erythrocytes. It is then distributed primarily into blood, soft tissues (kidney, bone marrow, liver, and brain), and mineralized tissues (bones and teeth). In adults, approximately 95 percent of the total body burden of lead is contained in bones and teeth. In conditions of physiological stress, such as pregnancy, lactation, menopause, or chronic disease, lead can be mobilized from the bones, thus increasing the level of lead in the blood. The turnover rate of lead in cortical and trabecular bone is slow; although quantitative estimates of its half-life vary, there is a consensus that it is on the order of years or even decades.[6] Measures of the bone content of lead thus reflect the integrated or chronic lifetime lead exposure.[7] Unbound lead is excreted by the kidneys or through the biliary system into the gastrointestinal tract. In single exposed studies in adults, lead has a half-life of approximately 25 days in blood, about 40 days in soft tissue, and more than 25 years in bone. Therefore, while a person's blood level may begin to return to normal after a single exposure, the total body burden of lead may still be elevated. For lead poisoning to occur, significant acute exposures are not necessary. Since the body accumulates lead over time and releases it slowly, even small amounts can cause lead poisoning.

The nervous system is the most sensitive target of lead poisoning. Lead encephalopathy has been associated with softening and flattening of convolutions in the brain. At times punctate hemorrhages, dilation of the vessels, and dilation of the ventricular system, are seen, especially in the frontal portions of the brain. Histologically, extensive involvement of the ganglion cells is seen. The developing brain appears to be especially sensitive to levels of lead that were once thought to cause no harmful effects.

Epidemiology and Risk Factors. Lead poisoning has a very long clinical history.[8] Although lead as an etiological factor was identified as early as 200 BC, it remains a common entity even today. More than 1 million workers in over 100 different occupations have been exposed to lead (see Table 39–1). In lead-related industries, workers not only inhale lead dust and lead oxide fumes but may eat, drink, and smoke in or near contaminated areas, increasing the probability of lead ingestion. If the worker does not properly "clean up" before leaving work, he can bring lead dust home on his skin, shoes, and clothing, thus exposing family members. Sources of lead exposure for nonoccupational populations include air, food, water, certain consumer products, surface dust, and oils. Automobile emissions had been an important source of lead exposure, especially for urban residents. However, the deleading of gasoline has significantly altered environmental levels of lead. Periodic assessment of national blood lead levels support this inference. From 1976 to 1978, median blood levels for adults in the United States were approximately 13 μg/dL[9]; in 1991 lead levels were estimated at 6 μg/dL (Environmental Protection Agency, National Advisory Council for Environmental Policy and Technology [NACEPT] committee, 1993). The current major sources of lead in the environment appear to be lead paint in homes built prior to 1950 and lead used in plumbing (which was not restricted until 1986).

Children are especially vulnerable to the effects of lead, especially before the age of 5. Elevated lead levels in children are due to pica (compulsive eating of nonfood items) or to the mouthing of items contaminated with lead from paint dust. In addition, children absorb and retain more lead in proportion to their weight than adults. Young children also have a greater prevalence of iron deficiency, a condition that can increase gastrointestinal absorption of lead. Lead absorption from the gastrointestinal tract appears to differ with age. For example, in adults, approximately 10 percent of ingested lead is absorbed. However, in children, it is estimated that 40 to 50 percent of ingested lead is absorbed. Fetuses are at risk, because lead readily crosses the placenta. Exposure in utero can cause adverse neurological effects in the developing child.

Clinical Features and Associated Findings. Acute signs of lead toxicity in children include listlessness, drowsiness with clumsiness, and possibly ataxia. With very high levels of lead, convulsions, coma, and respiratory arrest may occur. Therefore, a diagnosis of lead toxicity in a child should be considered when a child presents with a change in mental status, gait disorder, or a history of seizures. Chronic low-level lead exposure in children may result in behavioral disturbances, learning disabilities, attention deficit hyperactivity disorder, or cognitive decline.

Currently, acute lead encephalopathy due to industrial lead exposure is rare. Symptoms generally include delirium, combative irrational behavior, and seizures. Early signs of lead exposure include sleep disturbances, decreased libido, increased distractibility, increased irritability, and mental status changes marked by psychomotor slowing and memory dysfunction.

Both sensory and motor peripheral nerve involvement is seen in adults with chronic lead intoxication. Sensory complaints include paresthesias and spontaneous pain. Motor signs include local weakness, atrophy, and fasciculations. In severe cases of lead toxicity, wrist drop and foot drop have been well documented. Extensive bilateral neuropathy involving the hands, fingers, deltoids, biceps, and triceps may also occur. In individuals with predominantly motor findings, nerve conduction velocity may not be altered even after significant occupational exposure. However, in other cases mild slowing in nerve conduction velocity has been reported even in asymptomatic lead workers.

Anemia may be seen in patients with chronically elevated lead levels. Long-term lead exposure may have a direct effect on kidney function and may be associated with hypertension and gout. Increased frequencies of miscarriage and stillborn births have been documented in women working in the lead trades. Low prenatal lead exposure may produce low birth weight and premature birth. Lead affects the male reproductive system by reducing sperm counts and sperm motility.

In one series of studies an association was found between the body burden of lead, corresponding to blood lead levels of 25 to 55 μg/dL, and a drop in mean verbal IQ score of 4.5 points in exposed children.[10,11] In another study of total body burden, primary school children with high lead levels in teeth but no known history of lead poisoning had larger deficits in psychometric intelligence scores, speech and language processing, attention, and classroom performance than children with lower levels of lead. In a 1990 follow-up report of children who 11 years previously had been found to have elevated lead levels in their teeth, a sevenfold increase was noted in the odds of failure to graduate from high school, lower class standing, greater absenteeism, reading disabilities, and deficits in vocabulary, fine motor skills, reaction time, and eye-hand coordination. In studies with adults, patients with occupational exposure to lead underwent cognitive testing to determine if exposure had effects on cognitive function. 535 patients with known lead exposure were compared to 188 control patients. Tibia lead levels as measured by x-ray fluorescence were directly correlated with diminished performance on tests of visuoconstructive ability, verbal memory, and learning. This study suggests that cognitive function can be affected from early exposure to neurotoxins.[12]

Differential Diagnosis and Evaluation. The laboratory pattern typical of patients with lead intoxication includes elevations in whole blood lead levels, free erythrocyte protoporphyrins (FEP), and urinary coproporphyrins. The blood lead level reflects more recent exposure to lead, while the FEP level tends to reflect more chronic levels of exposure. Blood lead levels greater than 10 μg/dL in children and 30 μg/dL in adults are considered elevated. FEP levels begin to rise in adults once blood lead levels reach 30 to 40 μg/dL. Once elevated, the FEP remains so for several months even after exposure has ceased and the blood lead level has fallen. The threshold blood zinc protoporphyrin level is 100 μg/dL. Both blood lead level and zinc protoporphyria should be obtained to determine the presence of significant lead exposure. The most widely available method for measuring body burden of lead is diagnostic chelation. Urinary lead excretion is measured after infusion of 1 g calcium ethylenediamine-tetra-acetic acid (EDTA). Urinary excretion of more than 600 g of lead over a period of 72 hours is considered elevated. A new noninvasive method of measuring the body burden of lead in bone is x-ray fluorescence (XRF).[13] XRF promises in the future to become the noninvasive gold standard for estimating the total body burden of lead. Except for patients with acute high exposure, an EEG is not generally useful. In addition, neither CT nor MRI reveal any abnormalities. The neuropsychological evaluation may prove useful in assessing specific cognitive deficits in individuals exposed to lead. In some studies, workers with lead blood levels below 30 μg/dL have demonstrated decreased muscle strain and affective complaints as well as decrements in visuomotor integration and psychomotor speed, short-term visual and verbal memory, attention or concentration, and problem-solving skills.[14–16] Nevertheless, it should be noted that a recent comprehensive review of the published literature on the neurobehavioral performance of individuals exposed to inorganic lead failed to find enough evidence to draw definitive conclusions on the negative influence of lead on human performance on neurobehavioral tests.[17]

Management. In both children and adults with substantial lead levels, immediate removal from the sources of exposure to lead and administration of chelating agents presently comprise the treatment of choice. Specific chelating agents for lead include intravenous calcium disodium-EDTA and a new oral agent called succimer (dimercaptosuccinic acid, DMSA). Chelation with oral penicillamine may be used (up to 2 g/day). Multiple chelation cycles may be necessary, and at least 24 hours of rest between cycles is suggested. Adequate hydration should be maintained because chelating agents have been associated with renal toxicity and may dramatically increase circulating levels of lead owing to their ability to unbind lead from the bones. DMSA is a relatively new oral chelating agent that is reported to be safer than EDTA and penicillamine. Common side effects are renal sequelae and hypertension. The latest guidelines for treating children suggest starting chelation therapy for children with blood lead levels above 45 μg/dL. While chelation therapy may reduce symptoms of acute lead poisoning, amelioration of the neurological and renal sequelae of both acute and chronic lead intoxication is less likely. Prevention of lead toxicity in children includes removal of young children from contaminated environments, such as houses with peeling paints. Individuals who work in occupations where they might be exposed to lead should use mandatory personal protective equipment. Routine monitoring for lead levels is also advised.

Prognosis and Future Perspectives. As the work of Needleman and colleagues suggests,[11] complete recovery of higher cognitive functions may not occur in children with early childhood exposure to lead. Likewise, it is unclear how much CNS function is recovered in adults, because research in this area is limited.

ORGANIC LEAD

Organic lead (tetraethyl lead, TEL) is used as an antiknock agent in gasoline and jet fuels. TEL is absorbed rapidly from the skin as well as the lungs and gastrointestinal tract and is converted to triethyl lead in the body. This form of lead may be responsible for its toxic effects. Due to its highly lipophilic nature, TEL passes the blood-brain barrier readily. It is soluble in CNS structures, especially the limbic forebrain, frontal cortex, and hippocampus. Symptoms of acute high-level exposure include delirium, nightmares, irritability, and hallucinations. Chronic effects of TEL, as measured by peak tibia lead in organolead workers, was associated with poorer neurobehavioral test scores in the domains of manual dexterity, executive ability, and verbal memory.[18] Treatment is mainly supportive, but chelation may be helpful.

MANGANESE

Pathogenesis and Pathophysiology. Inhalation is the primary source of exposure. Neuropathologically, ganglion cells, including cells of the pallidum, show histological changes. Damage to the substantia nigra has also been seen, as have nerve cell alterations in the basal nuclei, frontal and parietal cortex, cerebellum, and hypothalamus.

Epidemiology and Risk Factors. The neurological syndrome manganism was first described in 1837. Since that time, hundreds of cases have been reported in the medical literature. Mining dust and industry are the primary sources of manganese (see Table 39–1). Like organic lead, manganese is also an antiknock additive in gasoline.

Outside the occupational setting, hospitalized patients receiving total parenteral nutrition (TPN) therapy that includes manganese can develop distinctive T1-weighted hyperintense patterns in the region of the globus pallidum. These apparent lesions disappear after cessation of TPN, but in some patients their presence correlates with clinical signs of parkinsonism and high blood levels of manganese.

Clinical Features and Associated Findings. The onset of symptoms is extremely variable from individual to individual and depends on the intensity of exposure, individual susceptibility, and possibly the type of ore involved. Symptoms may appear after only 1 or 2 months or after 20 years of exposure. The earliest signs of manganism include anorexia, asthenia, apathy, somnolence, headaches, and social withdrawal. Personality changes are common and consist of irritability, emotional lability, and periods of hyperexcitability (manganese psychosis). With continued exposure, moderate to high-level exposure symptoms characteristic of parkinsonism develop, including "masked facies" and bradykinesia). Speech is affected, becoming faint, monotonous, disjointed, occasionally unintelligible, and even mute. Other symptoms include weakness and fatigue, which increase until the worker is unable to go to work. Symptoms are generally confined to the extrapyramidal system, and gait difficulties are observed as retropulsion on rising and propulsion on walking, awkwardness and fine or coarse tremor of the hands, and gross rhythmical movements of the trunk and head. Micrographia in writing samples may also be evident. Whereas individuals with classic cases of severe manganism have more diffuse signs than those typical of Parkinson's disease, there are some concerns that chronic low or moderate exposure during occupations like welding could be a risk factor for typical Parkinson's disease.[19]

Differential Diagnosis and Evaluation. Diagnosis requires a history of exposure to manganese in combination with physical findings. About 43 percent of the body burden of manganese is in the bone. Excretion is biphasic, consisting of a rapid phase with a half-life of 4 days and a second slower phase that has a half-life of 39 days. Methods of biological monitoring are poor, and individual manganese levels in blood and urine do not correlate with either present or past exposure. Diagnostic chelation with EDTA is not useful.

Management. Management involves removal of the patient from exposure. The chronic movement disorder may respond to the use of levodopa and 5-hydroxytryptophan. Patients studied by Mena and colleagues[20] responded well to levodopa doses of more than 3 g/day, showing a marked reduction in rigidity and all other symptoms except speech disorders. Traditional chelation therapy has not proved helpful.

Prognosis and Future Perspectives. Manganism is usually progressive once the syndrome develops. In the very early stages, symptoms may improve over a period of many months after the patient has been removed from exposure. This improvement is not thought to be correlated with a reduction in the concentration of manganese.[21]

INORGANIC MERCURY

Pathogenesis and Pathophysiology. Elemental mercury is transported in blood plasma, proteins, and hemoglobin. In the appropriate conditions, mercury may be incorporated rapidly into the brain. Once incorporated into the body, mercury can be found in the urine as long as 6 years after exposure has ceased. Inorganic mercury has the greatest affinity for the kidney. Although concentrations are lower in the CNS, they may still be significant. In the brain, animal studies have shown that the highest concentrations of mercury occur in the brain stem, followed by the cerebellum, cerebral cortex, and hippocampus.

Inorganic mercury exerts its neurotoxic effects by altering membranes. A paucity of information is available on the pathological events resulting from inorganic mercury intoxication. Very few postmortem studies have been published, and results vary from normal to slight neuronal damage with evidence of intracellular mercury.

Epidemiology and Risk Factors. Historically, inorganic mercury compounds have been used as antiseptics, disinfectants, purgatives, and components in the industrial manufacture of felt. Mercury was also used formerly in the form of cinnabar, a red pigment used for painting and coloring. Works of art containing cinnabar can be found in ancient Egyptian and Pakistanian ruins.

By current NIOSH estimates, 65,000 workers are potentially exposed to mercury. The occupations significantly at risk for mercury intoxication are listed in Table 39–1. Mercury is also one of the most serious environmental pollutants in air and water. Between 1953 and 1956, an epidemic of methyl mercury poisoning occurred in Japan when a large number of villagers developed chronic mercurialism (Minamata disease) from ingesting fish contaminated with methyl mercury from industrial waste. There appears to be a wide range of individual susceptibility to the toxic effects of mercury; these may depend on the form of mercury involved, hygiene, diet (including vitamin deficiency), and some intrinsic differences in mercury metabolism. Metallic mercury becomes volatile at room temperature and thus generally enters the body through the inhalation of mercury vapors.

Clinical Features and Associated Findings. Acute mercury poisoning usually results from accidental ingestion of an antiseptic in the medicine cabinet. Symptoms of acute inorganic mercury poisoning consist of massive gastrointestinal vomiting and colitis with renal failure. The breath has a metallic odor. A brownish mercurial linear streak may be visible along the margin of the teeth. Symptoms of irritability, rapid onset of weakness in the lower limbs, psychotic episodes with delirium, hallucinations, and motor hyperactivity have been reported. The major threat to these patients is gastrointestinal hemorrhage, but after 24 hours renal failure becomes the predominant cause of morbidity.

Chronic mercury toxicity can result in tremor and weakness of the limbs or progressive personality changes. Mercury-induced tremors, also known as "hatter's shakes" or "Danbury shakes," consist of fine and regular tremors interrupted by much coarser myoclonic jerks. These tremors can be seen at rest and often diminish with activity. In the later stages of intoxication, gait and balance may be altered because of the continuous trembling. In addition, dyskinetic movements, paresis, and convulsions have been reported. At times, these patients present a typical picture of parkinsonism. Mercury can also cause peripheral polyneuropathy (sensorimotor axonopathy), which affects the lower extremities more than the upper ones. Paresthesias with extreme pain or peripheral neuropathy with muscle atrophy may also occur. Cognitive decline, vertigo, nystagmus, blurred vision, narrowing of the visual fields, optic neuritis, optic atrophy, sensory ataxia with a positive Romberg's sign, seizures, and vegetative disturbances have also been observed.

Personality changes can develop before neurological signs appear. So-called "mercurial neurasthenia" may develop for weeks or months before the patient seeks treatment. This syndrome consists of extreme fatigue, hyperirritability, insomnia, pathological shyness, and depression. The hyperirritability may become so severe that extremely violent behavior develops, possibly including homicidal acts.

Acrodynia, chronic mercury toxicity in children, is a syndrome consisting of painful neuropathy that involves significant autonomic changes. This syndrome includes redness and coldness in the hands and feet, pain in the limbs, profuse sweating of the trunk, severe constipation, and weakness. Tremors similar to those found in adults and personality changes may also occur. Case reports of children with acrodynia and a syndrome mimicking signs of a pheochromocytoma have been described in association with inorganic mercury intoxication. The mercury may interfere with the normal catabolic processing of catecholamines via the cytosolic enzyme catecholamine-O-methyltransferase. Catecholamine-O-methyltransferase requires the use of the methyl group provided by coenzyme S-adenosylmethionine (SAM). Mercury inactivates SAM and leads to elevated levels of norepinephrine, dopamine, and epinephrine. The elevation of catecholamines leads to the pheochromocytoma-like syndrome.[22]

Differential Diagnosis and Evaluation. Serum concentrations of mercury are unreliable indicators of inorganic and organic mercury toxicity because blood levels vary greatly between individuals and in the same individual. The threshold biological exposure index (BEI) for blood is 15 μg/L, and for urine it is 35 μg/g creatine. However, urinary excretion is not a good measure of toxicity, since there seems to be little correlation between symptomatology and the amount of mercury excreted in the urine. Although the early differential diagnosis might include Parkinson's disease, the tremor seen with mercurial intoxication is not solely a resting tremor and is usually coarser than that found in patients with Parkinson's disease. Because the signs of mercury intoxication may mimic those of some common neurological syndromes, the correct diagnosis is dependent on a good occupational history, clinical symptomatology, and documentation of mercury in the patient's blood, urine, or hair.

Management and Prognosis. Removal of the patient from the sources of exposure and chelation with *N*-acetyl-D-penicillamine is recommended.

Prognosis and Future Perspectives. Follow-up of the survivors with Minamata disease years after poisoning occurred revealed decreased bilateral attenuation on CT scans in the visual cortex and diffuse atrophy of the cerebellum, especially the vermis.

ORGANIC MERCURY

Pathogenesis and Pathophysiology. Organic mercury readily crosses the blood-brain barrier, and its turnover in the brain is slow. In cases of chronic exposure, approximately 10 percent of the body burden localizes in the brain. Less than 3 percent is degraded into inorganic mercury. In a single case study, histological changes and high mercurial content were noted in the corpus callosum. Excretion occurs primarily through the gastrointestinal tract, mostly through biliary secretion, and the mercury then undergoes almost immediate gastrointestinal reabsorption into the bloodstream. Neuropathological changes noted in 10 cases included damage to peripheral neurons in the myelin sheath accompanied by glial proliferation and mobilization of phagocytes.[23] Anatomically, the most severe damage was found in the primary visual cortex, followed by the cerebellar cortex, the pre- and postcentral gyri, the transverse gyrus, and the putamen.

Epidemiology and Risk Factors. Sources of organic mercury include contaminated seafood or exposure to alkyl mercury (used in antifungal treatment of seed grains). There have been reports of massive intoxications resulting from ingestion of fish containing methyl mercury or from eating homemade bread prepared from seed treated with methyl mercury fungicide. Ingestion of livestock that have been fed grain treated with mercury-containing fungicides is an additional source.

Routes of absorption of organic mercury are primarily dermal and gastrointestinal. Organic mercury is slowly excreted through the kidneys, and its half-life varies from 40 to 105 days. Organic mercury readily crosses the placenta, resulting in blood concentrations in the fetus that are equal to or greater than those in the maternal blood. There have been several reports of fetal methyl mercury poisoning in asymptomatic mothers. Methyl mercury is also secreted in breast milk.

Clinical Features and Associated Findings. The clinical triad of organic mercury toxicity consists of peripheral neuropathy, ataxia, and cortical blindness. There may be a delay of 2 weeks to several months before symptoms appear after mercury exposure. The earliest symptoms may be paresthesias of the extremities, beginning distally and extending in a glove-stocking distribution. Touch and pain sensations are most impaired. Constriction of the visual fields is generally seen.[24]

In infants born of intoxicated mothers, severe brain damage may develop including retardation and cerebral palsy. Motor neuron disease resembling amyotrophic lateral sclerosis is another notable and prominent clinical pattern. In these patients, gradual weakness develops with features of both upper motor neuron disease (increased reflexes and prominent jaw jerk) and lower motor neuron disease (fasciculations and atrophy).

Differential Diagnosis and Evaluation. It is difficult to diagnose mercury toxicity from laboratory data because the blood and urine measurements vary widely. While measurements in blood and hair are less variable than those in urine, these do not necessarily reflect the degree of mercury toxicity. Hair samples must be collected according to specific protocols. For example, samples must be taken close to the scalp and then washed to remove contaminants such as hair dyes or hair treatments. The advantage of hair samples is that they provide exposure information for the past year. Hair sample levels are usually 300 to 500 times those seen in blood.

Management. Management of mercury toxicity depends first on eliminating the exposure. Other remedies include the use of mercury-binding chelators such as D-penicillamine, BAL, or DMSA, which may accelerate the excretion of mercury. However, because chelation mobilizes mercury from bones, it may cause the clinical symptoms to become worse and allow further deposits of mercury into the brain (especially BAL). Penicillamine may be more effective in improving the CNS effects of mercury. However, the side effects of penicillamine treatment may include hematopoietic suppression, alterations in cognitive and renal function, symptoms of myasthenia gravis, occasional hepatitis, and allergic reactions such as pruritus and swelling. With chelation, blood concentrations usually begin to decline after approximately 3 days. In asymptomatic individuals with increased blood concentrations of mercury, administration of selenium and vitamin E may prevent the development of symptoms. In patients with mild contractures, physical therapy can be helpful.

Prognosis and Future Perspectives. Most patients with severe mercury poisoning die within a few weeks of symptom onset. Some may survive with major neurological disability. In those with mild or moderate neurological symptoms, improvement may occur within the first 6 months, mostly in children and young adults. Isolated cases have been reported in which bedridden individuals regained the ability to walk, and some children who were totally blind regained vision.

Follow-up of the survivors with Minamata disease years after poisoning revealed decreased bilateral attenuation on CT scans in the visual cortex and diffuse atrophy of the cerebellum, especially the vermis.

ALUMINUM, THALLIUM, AND OTHER METALS

See Tables 39–1 and 39–2.

Organic Solvents (Table 39–3)

MIXED SOLVENTS

Pathogenesis and Pathophysiology. Organic solvents are lipophilic and very volatile. Lipophilicity influences the anatomical distribution of the solvents to organs rich in lipids (brain and adrenals). Lipophilic compounds are eliminated through the kidneys after several osmotic conversions have occurred to make them more water soluble. The resulting metabolites can be more toxic than the original compounds. Reports of synergistic effects between organic solvents and alcohol are found in the literature. Paint "huffers" show signs of acute denervation in the peripheral nervous system and show evidence of frontal lobe atrophy on MRI.[25] At high dose levels, depending on the specific chemical, solvents may act as anesthetics (e.g., trichloroethylene [TCE]), convulsants (e.g., fluorothyl), anticonvulsants (e.g., toluene), anxiolytics (e.g., toluene), antidepressants (e.g., benzyl chloride), and narcotics (e.g., TCE). However, the mechanisms involved in solvent neurotoxicity are generally unknown. For many solvents it is not known which are neurotoxins, whether or not they require bioactivation to become toxic to the nervous system, and what targets within the nervous system are critical. It is also unknown how the toxic metabolites produce cellular changes that result in human health effects. A wide variety of mechanisms related to the effects of organic solvents have been proposed. Neurotoxicity may result from effects on neurotransmitters such as dopamine and gamma-aminobutyric acid (GABA), although it is not known whether this occurs at specific receptor sites, at the bilipid layer surrounding the receptors, or at ion channels.

Epidemiology and Risk Factors. Due to the proliferation of the plastic and chemical industries, large segments of the population have been exposed to organic solvents. NIOSH estimates that in 1970, 9.8 million workers were exposed to solvents in the United States. Since solvents are highly volatile, and volatility corresponds to the amount of solvent that becomes airborne, the respiratory system is the primary mode of solvent absorption. The amount of uptake is modified by work load, respiratory rate, use of respirators, and adequacy of workplace ventilation. Because most solvents that cause health problems are mixtures of solvents, we will first discuss the neurological sequelae of exposure to organic solvents in general. Then we will describe briefly some of the more highly toxic individual organic solvents. Occupational settings of potential exposure to organic solvents are numerous and are shown in Table 39–1. At present, it appears that the number of workers suffering adverse effects from exposure to organic solvents has decreased. This is due to closer adherence by industry to appropriate levels of safe airborne concentrations as well as to the mandatory use of personal protective equipment by workers. Unfortunately, the abuse of solvents in the form of "huffing" remains a public health concern. In these cases, substances such as paint, airplane glue, and gasoline are placed in plastic bags, which are then placed over the face and inhaled to produce a "high."

Clinical Features and Associated Findings. The digestive, hepatic, renal, and nervous systems are all affected by organic solvents. All solvents have nasal mucosal irritant effects. Symptoms of acute high-level exposure include headache, dysphoria, dizziness, euphoria, excitation, and exhilaration. However, with discontinuation of exposure, symptoms of acute exposure abate within hours. With extremely high levels of exposure such as those obtained during paint huffing, the later stages of intoxication include somnolence and coma followed by death.

Chronic low-level exposure is generally seen in industrial settings. In these cases, development of symptoms is insidious. Headaches are the most commonly reported symptom. Characteristically, these begin shortly after arriving at work and disappear at night, on weekends, and during vacations when patients are not in the vicinity of the organic solvents. Other complaints include irritability, personality changes, depression, memory loss, poor attention or concentration, sleep difficulties, decreased libido, and pain and numbness starting in the feet and then progressing to the hands (peripheral neuropathy). Neurobehavioral findings are most notable in activities demanding manual dexterity, executive or motor functioning, and olfaction.[26]

Differential Diagnosis. Diagnosis of solvent encephalopathy is generally confirmed by the presence of a positive exposure history, objective findings on neurobehavioral tests, and negative findings on neurological examination with the exception of the possible presence of a polyneuropathy. There are few reliable or easily attainable biomarkers of solvent exposure. Therefore, this diagnosis is often one of exclusion. The differential diagnosis includes other neuropathological conditions (e.g., cerebrovascular disease, tumor), heavy alcohol use, and neuropsychiatric disorders (e.g., affective disorders, anxiety, somatoform disorders). Often, individuals who have been exposed to chemicals with strong odors misinterpret normal body sensations as pathological symptoms. Subsequently, these symptoms are misattributed to chemical exposure because of reports by the news media exaggerating the dangers of commonly encountered environmental chemicals.

TABLE 39–3. **Symptoms Associated with Organic Solvent Exposure**

Organic Solvents	Proposed Toxic Mechanism	Tissue Assessed and Toxic Levels*	Associated Symptoms	Clinical Findings	Specific Treatments	Pathology
Mixtures	Generally unknown, acts on neurotransmission	Not available	Irritant effects; contact dermatitis	Headaches; fatigue; irritability; depression; sleep difficulties; cognitive decline; decreased olfaction; peripheral neuropathy; myopathy	Removal from exposure	Atrophy (paint huffers)
Acetone	Unclear	Urine 50 mg/L	GI distress; irritant effects	Nausea; vomiting; headache; dysphoria; bad dreams; vertigo	Removal from exposure	Unclear
Benzene	Increases levels of GABA in cerebellum and pons; increases levels of glutamic acid decarboxylase (GAD); affects porphyrin metabolism	Urine 50 μg/g creatine; Exhaled air mixed: 0.08 ppm; S-phenylmecapturic acid in urine 20 μg/g creatinine; +, + muccnic acid in urine 500 μg/g creatinine	Increased risk of cancer; pancytopenia	Ataxia; inebriation; muscular twitching; paralysis; seizures; unconsciousness; peripheral neuropathy in cases with associated toluene exposure	Removal from exposure; lecithin, vitamin C, pentanucleotide, folic acid, pyridoxine	Denervation and clinical atrophy
Carbon Disulfide	Alkylation of proteins	Urine 5 mg/g creatine	Pulmonary and dermal irritant; cardiac effects; toxic threshold lowered in alcoholism, diabetes mellitus, renal/hepatic disease	Headache; irritability; cognitive decline; psychosis; delirium; hearing loss; loss of corneal reflex; parkinsonism; peripheral polyneuropathy	Removal from exposure	Chromatolysis and vacuolation in frontal lobe, globus pallidum, and putamen; peripheral nerve myelin swelling and fragmentation
Carbon Tetrachloride	Unclear	Not available	GI distress; hiccups; liver and kidney damage; toxic threshold lowered in alcoholism, obesity, diabetes, liver and kidney disease	Intoxication; headaches; vertigo; delirium; seizures; parkinsonism; optic atrophy; visual difficulties	Calcium gluconate and hemodialysis	Purkinje cell damage; cerebellar venous thrombosis and hemorrhagic infarcts; brain edema; neuronal loss; astrocytosis
Ethylene Glycol	Metabolized to aldehydes and oxalate	100 mL	Renal effects; cardiopulmonary effects	Restlessness; agitation; seizures; absent corneal reflexes; coma	Early dialysis to correct acidosis	Cerebral edema; vascular engorgement; hemorrhage

Table continued on following page

TABLE 39–3. **Symptoms Associated with Organic Solvent Exposure** *Continued*

Organic Solvents	Proposed Toxic Mechanism	Tissue Assessed and Toxic Levels*	Associated Symptoms	Clinical Findings	Specific Treatments	Pathology
Methyl Alcohol (Methanol)	Oxidation to formaldehyde and formic acid	Urine 15 mg/L (*B*, *NS*); Formic acid in urine 80 μg/g creatine (*B*, *NS*)	GI distress	Headache; weakness; incoordination; delirium; hallucinations; visual loss; stupor; seizures; parkinsonism; death	Administration of ethyl alcohol, folic acid, or bicarbonate; frequent measures of blood methanol, CO_2, bicarbonate, and PH; monitor serum potassium; peritoneal/hemodialysis	Shrinkage and degeneration of neurons, primarily in parietal cortex
Methyl-N-Butyl Ketone (MBK)	Metabolized to 2,5 hexanedine	No specific findings	Euphoria	Weight loss; sensorimotor polyneuropathy	Removal from exposure	Multifocal axonal degeneration; myelin thinning
N-Hexane	Metabolized to 2,5 hexanedine; inhibits glycolytic enzymes	Urine 5 μg/g creatinine (*NS*)	Euphoria	Headaches; poor appetite; mild euphoria; mostly peripheral polyneuropathy	Removal from exposure	Degeneration of peripheral nerve axons
Toluene (Methyl Benzene)	Toxic effects similar to benzene	Hippuric acid in urine 1.6 g/g creatine (*B*, *NS*); Venous blood 0.05 mg/L O-cresol in urine 0.5 mg/L	Pulmonary effects; cardiac effects	Euphoria; fatigue; ataxia; dizziness; tremor; cognitive decline; seizures; delirium; decreased olfaction; optic atrophy; hearing loss; peripheral neuropathy (in cases w/associated *N*-hexane exposure); alcohol intolerance	Removal from exposure	Cortical and cerebral atrophy
Trichlor-ethylene (TCE)	Unknown. Toxic effects potentiated by alcohol	Trichloroacetic acid in urine 100 mg/g creatine (*NS*); Trichloracetic acid and trichloroethanol in urine 300 mg/g creatine (*NS*) Blood free trichloroethanol in blood 4 mg/L (*NS*)	Cardiopulmonary effects; toxic threshold reduced with alcohol	Headaches; insomnia; fatigue; anxiety; trigeminal nerve damage; neuro-ophthalmological findings; alcohol intolerance; cognitive decline; hearing loss; peripheral neuropathy	Removal from exposure	Myelin and axonal degeneration

*Biological exposure indices (BEIs). American Conference of Governmental Industrial Hygienists (ACGIH) values from ACGIH: Threshold Limit Values and Biological Exposure Indices 2001. Cincinnati, ACGIH, 2001.

B, Present in significant amounts in individuals not occupationally exposed; *NS*, Nonspecific; may be observed after exposure to some other chemicals; GABA, gamma-aminobutyric acid.

Evaluation. In 1985 an attempt was made to develop a rating classification system for individuals who were exposed to organic solvents. The following categories were proposed: Type I—Subjective nonspecific symptoms only. Patients complain of fatigue, memory and concentration difficulties, and changes in mood and sleep patterns. However, there is no objective evidence of neurobehavioral dysfunction. After discontinuation of exposure, symptoms completely disappear within 6 months to 1 year. Type IIa—Sustained personality and mood change. Affective changes are noted. These include depression, aggressiveness, fatigue, poor impulse control, and anhedonia. Neurobehavioral findings are negative. It is unclear if these symptoms are reversible. Type IIb—Impairment of intellectual function documented by objective neurobehavioral test results with possible mild neurological signs. Difficulty in concentration, memory loss, and a decline in learning capacity may be objectively detectable. After removal from exposure, these symptoms may remain stable or improve but should not become worse. Type III—Dementia, with neurological signs and/or neuroradiological findings. Neurobehavioral test results are significantly affected. Type III is related to repeated severe exposure (e.g., paint huffers). It is poorly reversible but generally does not progress once exposure is stopped.[27]

Nerve conduction studies can be extremely useful because many organic solvents affect the peripheral nervous system (PNS) before the CNS. Sensory polyneuropathy, more pronounced in the feet than in the hands, is characteristic of exposure to chronic organic solvents.

Management. Management consists of removal from the source of exposure. In addition, the anxiety and depression typically seen in these individuals can be treated with psychotropic medications and supportive psychotherapy.

Prognosis and Future Perspectives. Once removed from the source of exposure, symptoms should remain stable or improve over time. However, deterioration in function is often seen and can be attributed to psychological disorders that develop secondary to the organic solvent exposure.

METHYL ALCOHOL

Methyl alcohol (methanol, wood alcohol) is used as a solvent, a component of antifreeze, and an adulterant of alcoholic beverages. While this chemical is only mildly toxic, it is oxidized to formaldehyde and formic acid, which produce severe acidosis and are responsible for the symptoms of methanol abuse. Neuropathological changes in the form of shrinkages and degeneration of neurons, primarily in the parietal cortex, have been reported.[28] The oxidation and excretion of methyl alcohol is so slow that toxic symptoms do not develop for 12 to 48 hours, although they may last for several days. Once apparent, toxic symptoms involve the visual apparatus, CNS, and the gastrointestinal and respiratory tracts. Early symptoms include nausea, vomiting, weakness, abdominal pain, vertigo, and headache. Additional symptoms may include restlessness, uncoordination and, in severe cases, delirium and hallucinations. Confusion and memory deficits are also reported. In severe cases, stupor, coma, tonic muscle contractions, hyperactive reflexes, visual loss, Parkinson-like extrapyramidal syndrome, and convulsions may also be seen. In the most severe cases, death occurs from respiratory failure.

Treatment involves frequent measurements of blood methanol, carbon dioxide, bicarbonate, and pH. Ethyl alcohol may be administered to retard the conversion of methanol into toxic formaldehyde and formic acid. Bicarbonate can be given to correct severe acidosis. Serum potassium levels should be monitored because bicarbonate tends to decrease potassium. Administration of folic acid may accelerate the metabolism of formic acid to carbon dioxide. Either peritoneal dialysis or hemodialysis can be used in patients with methanol blood concentrations of over 50 mg.

ETHYLENE GLYCOL

Antifreeze is the most common source of ethylene glycol. Due to its inebriant properties, ingestion of ethylene glycol can be fatal and accounts for about 40 to 60 deaths per year. While ethylene glycol itself is not toxic, it metabolizes to aldehydes and oxalate. The toxic dose is approximately 100 mL, and death is due to renal or cardiopulmonary mechanisms. After ingestion, symptoms may appear rapidly or may take hours to develop. Initial symptoms include restlessness and agitation, followed by somnolence, stupor, coma, and convulsions. The patient becomes cyanotic, pupils are nonreactive, and corneal reflexes are absent. In milder cases, fatigue, personality change, and depression are present. Ethylene glycol poisoning should be suspected when an apparently inebriated patient has no alcohol on the breath. Neuropathological changes have been reported and include cerebral edema, vascular engorgement, and hemorrhage. Treatment consists of correcting the acidosis and using early dialysis to remove the ethylene glycol, oxalate, and aldehyde and also treat the associated uremia. Patients with ethylene glycol intoxication who present with normal creatine levels and an absence of metabolic acidosis may benefit from administration of fomepizole without hemodialysis.[29]

N-HEXANE AND METHYL-*N*-BUTYL KETONE

N-hexane is a component of a number of glues. Therefore, exposure is likely to come from inhalant abuse. With acute exposure, *N*-hexane causes euphoric effects. Pronounced peripheral polyneuropathy may occur after chronic intoxication. Hexane is metabolized to 2,5-hexanedione (2,5-HD), which is responsible for much of the neurotoxicity related to this compound.

Unlike toluene, hexane does not produce significant central neurological symptoms. Lightheadedness, headache, decreased appetite, and mild euphoria as well as occasional hallucinations may occur acutely, but seizures and delirium are not associated with *N*-hexane exposure. The predominant neurological feature of *N*-hexane exposure appears to be peripheral neuropathy. Symmetrical sensory dysfunction in the hands and feet is the usual presenting complaint. Decreased response to pin, vibration, and thermal stimulation is found on examination. Glue huffers may develop proximal weakness. The most prominent electrophysiological feature is slowing of motor and nerve conduction velocities, which occurs in proportion to the intensity of clinical disease.[30]

More recent concerns regarding *N*-hexane and petroleum derivatives have focused on parkinsonism. Cases of well-described intoxication have been associated with rigidity, bradykinesia, tremor, and postural reflex compromise. A large cohort of patients with clinically diagnosed Parkinson's disease were screened for hydrocarbon exposure. Of the 990 interviewed, 188 patients reported hydrocarbon exposure and these patients were age and gender matched to patients with no reported exposure. The patients with exposure as determined by an industrial hygienist had an earlier onset age and more motoric impairment than the control patients.[31] Furthermore, animal experiments demonstrate that *N*-hexane exposure lowers brain dopamine and homovanillic acid, the central metabolite of dopamine.[32] Because *N*-hexane is a common environmental contaminate and hydrocarbons can be byproducts of endogenous metabolic pathways, these compounds are a focus of pathogenic research efforts in movement disorders. Although chemically dissimilar from carbon disulfide, *N*-hexane is metabolized to the gamma-diketone 2,5-hexanedione, which induces histologic neurofilament-filled swelling in distal axons of the CNS and PNS similarly to carbon disulfide. This observation suggests that these two neurotoxins may share some pathogenic features and serve as a unifying model for the study of chemicals that adversely affect both PNS and CNS axons.

Methyl-*N*-butyl ketone (MBK) is used as a paint thinner, cleaning agent, and solvent for dye printing. Exposure to MBK is associated with sensorimotor polyneuropathy, which may begin several months after continued chronic exposure. In the later stages, axonal degeneration occurs distally.

There is no specific treatment for *N*-hexane and MBK neuropathy other than removal from the source of exposure. After removal, recovery (regeneration of peripheral nerve axons) may occur over a period of weeks.

TOLUENE (METHYL BENZENE)

Toluene is a widely used solvent and is employed as a paint and lacquer thinner and as a cleaning and dying agent. It is also a constituent of motor and aviation fuels. Toluene is a major constituent of the glue used by paint huffers and has thus been implicated as the chemical responsible for the neurotoxic syndrome seen in this group of solvent abusers. Toluene's toxic effects are similar to those of benzene, although more mental status changes are seen.

With acute exposure, clinical signs include early exhilaration followed by fatigue, mild confusion, ataxia, and dizziness. With chronic use, exhilaration, euphoria, disinhibition, and tremor are common. Neurobehavioral effects include declines in performance IQ, decreased memory, poor motor control, decreased visuospatial functioning, and dementia.[33] Toluene appears to affect the CNS more readily than the PNS. Treatment primarily involves removal from exposure.

TRICHLORETHYLENE

Trichlorethylene (TCE) is used extensively in dry cleaning and for degreasing metal parts and extracting oils and fats from vegetable products. It is also used as an adhesive in the leather industry and occasionally in medicine as an anesthetic. A number of workers have become addicted to the fumes, since deliberate inhalation produces rapid euphoria. Fatalities resulting from bronchial constriction, pulmonary edema, and myocardial irritation have been reported.

TCE toxicity is associated with cranial and peripheral neuropathies. Mixed sensory and motor involvement of the trigeminal and facial nerves is characteristic of high-level TCE exposure. Neuro-ophthalmological findings include retrobulbar neuropathy, optic atrophy, and oculomotor disturbances. Peripheral neuropathy is common, usually mixed and predominantly distal. Neuropathological examination has revealed extensive myelin and axonal degeneration. TCE may act as a demyelinating agent because of its lipid solvent qualities. The effects of TCE appear to be potentiated by alcohol.

Clinically, a history of possible TCE exposure should be investigated in any patient with trigeminal neuralgia or trigeminal dysfunction. Long-term exposure or acute high-level exposure also produces disturbances in memory. When a human volunteer was exposed to 2, 3, and 500 ppm for more than 2 hours, his major complaint was drowsiness.[34] At 500 ppm, however, a pronounced decrease in neuropsychological functioning was observed. General CNS symptoms include headaches, dizziness, fatigue, alcohol intolerance, neurasthenia, anxiety, and insomnia. Neurobehavioral effects include poor concentration and memory, decreased manual dexterity and visuospatial accuracy, and a slowed reaction time. As with the other organic solvents, treatment primarily involves removal from exposure.

ACETONE, BENZENE, CARBON DISULFIDE, CARBON TETRACHLORIDE

See Table 39–3.

Gases (Table 39–4)

CARBON MONOXIDE

Pathogenesis and Pathophysiology. Carbon monoxide enters the bloodstream through pulmonary absorption and binds reversibly to hemoglobin. The affinity of hemoglobin for carbon monoxide is about 225 times greater than that for oxygen. Thus, exposure to carbon monoxide resulting in increased carboxyhemoglobin decreases the amount of oxygen carried by the red blood cell. This results in pronounced tissue oxygen deprivation. Pathoclinical correlates generally show globus pallidus lucency and atrophy on CT scan (Fig. 39–3).[35]

Epidemiology and Risk Factors. Carbon monoxide is an odorless, nonirritating gas, acute exposure to which accounts for over 3000 accidental or suicidal deaths each year and 10,000 episodes of illness. Industrial sources include portable kerosene heaters, hot water heaters, and furnaces. At home, inadequately vented fireplaces are a common source. However, the major source of carbon monoxide is automobile exhaust fumes, which have concentrations of approximately 50,000 ppm. While cigarette smoke may be a major source of carbon monoxide, it is diluted with air, making it significantly less toxic. The threshold limit value of carbon monoxide is 50 ppm, which causes a carboxyhemoglobin saturation of 8 to 10 percent after an 8-hour exposure. Carboxyhemoglobin levels of more than 50 percent are considered threatening, and levels of 70 to 75 percent are usually

TABLE 39-4. **Symptoms Associated with Exposure to Gases**

Gas	Proposed Toxic Mechanism	Tissue Assessed and Toxic Levels*	Associated Symptoms	Clinical Findings	Specific Treatments	Pathology
Carbon Monoxide	Binds to hemoglobin, creating tissue oxygen deprivation; mitochondrial toxin	Blood 3.5% of hemoglobin Exhaled air 20 ppm	None	Headaches; irritability; dizziness; cognitive decline; impaired vision; blindness; deafness; seizures; parkinsonism; coma	Removal from exposure; 100% oxygen; hyperbaric oxygen	Cerebral atrophy; globus pallidus lucency
Cyanide	Mitochondrial toxin	Blood 0.2 μg/L Urine thiocyanate level	Bitter almond taste; mucosal irritation; GI distress; cardiopulmonary distress	Agitation; panic attacks; headaches; dizziness; decreased consciousness	Administration of antidote; supportive ventilation	Demyelination and cellular damage in stratum cortex and cerebellum
Ethylene Oxide	Not known	Not established	Skin lesions; mucosal irritation; pulmonary edema; GI distress	Headaches; nausea; vomiting; decreased level of consciousness; peripheral neuropathy; axonal degeneration	Removal from exposure	Axonal neuropathy
Nitrous Oxide	Interferes with cobalamin-dependent enzymatic reactions	Not established	Vitamin B_{12} deficiency	Decline in manual dexterity; cognitive decline; polyneuropathy; axonal degeneration; gradual progressive numbness in extremities followed by weakness, gait disturbance, and loss of sphincter control	Removal from exposure; good nutrition; vitamin B_{12} treatment	Axonal degeneration

*Biological exposure indices (BEIs). American Conference of Governmental Industrial Hygienists (ACGIH) values from ACGIH: Threshold Limit Values and Biological Exposure Indices for 1994–1995. Cincinnati, ACGIH, 1994.

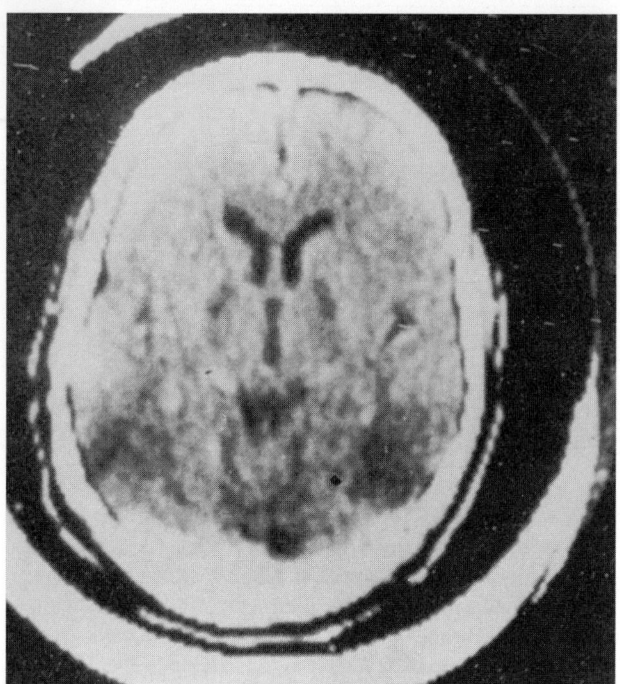

FIGURE 39–3. CT scan from a patient with carbon monoxide intoxication showing cystic lucencies in both globus palladi. (From Klawans HL, Stein RW, Tanner CM, Goetz CG: Pure parkinsonian syndrome following acute carbon monoxide intoxication. Arch Neurol 1982;39:302.)

fatal. Saturation may be obtained by either very high acute exposure or prolonged exposure to lower concentrations.

Clinical Features. Neurological signs of mild carbon monoxide poisoning include dizziness, headache, and impaired vision. As poisoning becomes more severe, symptoms develop into severe throbbing headaches, convulsions, and coma. Persistent chronic exposure, as occurs, for example, with inadequately vented heaters in the home, leads to blindness, deafness, pyramidal signs, extrapyramidal signs, and convulsive disorders.

Mild neurological effects may be transient to persistent and may appear immediately or days to weeks following exposure.[35] Behavioral and psychiatric changes include irritability, violent behavior, personality disturbances, euphoria, confusion, and impaired judgment. Neurobehavioral sequelae include difficulties with visual and verbal memory, spatial deficits, and declines in cognitive efficiency and flexibility.[36]

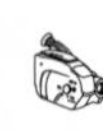

Parkinsonism has also been reported after acute and chronic exposure.

Differential Diagnosis and Evaluation. Both clinical symptoms and a history of exposure to carbon monoxide are necessary for a diagnosis. In suspected cases of carbon monoxide exposure, blood levels of carboxyhemoglobin can be determined. However, the current level of carbon monoxide in the blood is not indicative of the severity of poisoning because carboxyhemoglobin may rapidly decline after exposure ceases. If a patient dies of carbon monoxide poisoning, however, the level of carboxyhemoglobin determined at postmortem represents the actual level of carbon monoxide at the moment of death, since carbon monoxide cannot be excreted without active respiration.

Management. Treatment involves removal of the patient from the contaminated environment as well as administration of 100 percent oxygen. Hyperbaric oxygen reduces the half-life of carboxyhemoglobin to less than 25 minutes and is considered the treatment of choice for all patients with severe carbon monoxide intoxication. However, CNS oxygen toxicity is a potential risk of hyperbaric oxygen therapy. Additionally, hypothermia has been advocated to decrease the tissue demands of oxygen. Patients may be covered in ice for 8 to 12 hours at a temperature of 30 to 32° C.

Prognosis and Future Perspectives. The prognosis for patients with significant carbon monoxide poisoning varies. However, follow-up has shown the presence of neurological sequelae, consisting of cortical blindness, seizures, cognitive impairment with amnesia, polyneuropathy, and a parkinsonian syndrome. In a follow-up study performed 3 years after carbon monoxide poisoning, 43 percent of patients had impaired memory, 33 percent showed a deterioration of personality, and 13 percent showed neuropsychiatric damage.

CYANIDE, ETHYLENE OXIDE, NITROUS OXIDE

See Table 39–4.

Pesticides (Table 39–5)

ORGANOPHOSPHATE INSECTICIDES

Pathogenesis and Pathophysiology. Organophosphates inhibit acetylcholinesterase and pseudocholinesterase. Insecticides that are cholinesterase inhibitors include chlorpyrifos (Dursban), diazinon, malathion, ethyl and methyl parathion, and trichlorofon.[37] The neurotoxicity of these compounds is related to their ability to inhibit acetylcholinesterase, which occurs in the brain, spinal cord, myoneural junctions, pre- and postganglionic parasympathetic synapses, and preganglionic and some postganglionic sympathetic nerve endings. The resulting increase in acetylcholine overstimulates the postsynaptic receptors in the cholinergic system, thus differentially stimulating nicotinic receptors (skeletal muscle and autonomic ganglia) and muscarinic receptors (secretory glands and postganglionic fibers in the parasympathetic nervous system).

Epidemiology and Risk Factors. Organophosphate insecticides are highly toxic to insects but are relatively less so to man and domestic animals. Although specific organophosphates such as triorthocresyl phosphate, nipafox, and trichlorofon compounds are obviously neurotoxic, the situation is less clear for other organophosphate pesticides. At risk are factory workers involved in the production of these compounds and agricultural workers who use them to spray crops. The occurrence of organophosphate poisoning in the United States is low, although epidemics have been reported in some Third World countries. It should be noted, however, that 1754 pesticide related cases were reported in California in 1987. California accounts for about one third of the agricultural workforce in the United States. Organophosphates are absorbed through the skin and respiratory tracts. In addition, small amounts may be ingested by eating foods that have been sprayed with organophosphates.

Clinical Features and Associated Findings. Clinically, patients with acute mild symptoms complain of vague fatigue,

TABLE 39–5. **Symptoms Associated with Pesticide Exposure**

Pesticide	Proposed Toxic Mechanism	Tissue Assessed and Toxic Levels*	Associated Symptoms	Clinical Findings	Specific Treatments	Pathology
Methyl Bromide		Blood 2.8 μg/dL	Pulmonary and dermal irritant; renal effects; pulmonary effects; cardiac effects; GI distress; garlic or rotten fish odor	Mania; hallucinations; delirium; headache; vertigo; cognitive decline; amnesia; aphasia; incoordination; myoclonus; tremors	Removal from exposure	Affects cortical, cerebellar, and basal ganglia structures
Organochlorines (DDT)	Excessive and spontaneous release of acetylcholine		Metallic taste; thirst; burning eyes	Resembles Reye's syndrome in children; drowsiness; optic neuropathy; night blindness; tremors; seizures; mononeuropathy; polyneuropathy	Anticonvulsants for patients with seizures	With chlordecone, electron-dense particle accumulation in Schwann cells
Organophosphates	Inhibits acetylcholinesterase and pseudocholinesterase	Blood low cholinesterase activity (70% of baseline)	GI distress; excessive sweating and salivation; hypothermia; liver dysfunction	Headache; fatigue; dizziness; decreased consciousness; sleep disturbance; cognitive decline; blurred vision; absent pupillary response; muscular fasciculations; tremor; delayed polyneuropathy (OPIDP)	Administer atropine sulfate and pralidoxime	Axonal neuropathy and nonspecific CNS changes
Strychnine	Central analeptic agent; GABA antagonist; postsynaptic inhibitor		GI distress; respiratory failure	Irritability; excitement; decreased consciousness; paresthesias; muscular stiffness; fasciculations; seizures; rigidity	Respiratory support; seizure prevention; administer diazepam; morphine and apomorphine are contraindicated	Small subarachnoid hemorrhages; capillary proliferation; demyelinization

*Biological exposure indices (BEIs). American Conference of Governmental Industrial Hygienists (ACGIH) values from ACGIH: Threshold Limit Values and Biological Exposure Indices for 1994–1995. Cincinnati, ACGIH, 1994.

CNS, Central nervous system; GABA, gamma-aminobutyric acid; GI, gastrointestinal.

headache, dizziness, increased salivation, nausea and vomiting, diaphoresis, and abdominal cramps. Symptoms always develop within 24 hours after exposure. Difficulty with speaking or swallowing, shortness of breath, and muscular fasciculations have been reported in patients with more moderate poisoning. With increased severity of poisoning, more intense signs and symptoms can appear. These may include depressed levels of consciousness and marked myosis with no pupillary response. After initial recovery from acute severe intoxication, an organophosphate-induced delayed polyneuropathy (OPIDP) may develop. OPIDP is a distal dying back axonopathy characterized by cramping muscle pain in the legs, paresthesias, and motor weakness beginning 10 days to 3 weeks after the initial exposure. OPIDP-associated signs include foot drop, weakness of the intrinsic hand muscles, absent ankle jerk, and weakness of the hip and knee flexors.[38] Chronic low-level exposure has been associated with weakness, malaise, headache, and lightheadedness. Anxiety, irritability, altered sleep, tremor, numbness and tingling of the extremities, and small pupils may also be observed.[39] Neurobehavioral findings include decreased capacity for information processing, decreased memory and learning abilities, and poor visuoconstructional skills.

A cohort of 90 patients with chronic low-level exposure to organophosphates were clinically examined and found to have decreased vibratory sense as compared to a matched sample group. Nine of these patients underwent electrophysiological testing, and five of them were found to have abnormalities consistent with a peripheral neuropathic condition. This study suggests that low-level organophosphate exposure may be particularly toxic to the PNS.[40] Five cases of acute parkinsonism following acute exposure to organophosphates have been described. Each of these patients resembled the clinical picture of Parkinson's disease but did not respond to levodopa. After the offending agent was removed, four of the patients recovered without sequelae. Upon reexposure to the organophosphate, one patient had reoccurrence of parkinsonian symptoms. These case reports suggest a causal link between organophosphate exposure and parkinsonism.[41]

Differential Diagnosis and Evaluation. Diagnosis depends on exposure history, clinical symptoms, and abnormally low cholinesterase activity in the blood (BEI, 70 percent of baseline level). Serial cholinesterase levels that show a rise after removal from exposure are diagnostic of exposure. Fasciculations with miosis, although not always present, are also diagnostic of organophosphate poisoning. Also, improvement of acute symptoms can be expected after administration of atropine sulfate.

Management. At the time of ingestion, vomiting should be induced. The primary treatment for mild to moderate organophosphate poisoning is the administration of atropine sulfate (1 mg intravenously or intramuscularly) and pralidoxime (Protopam, 2-PAM, 1 g intravenously). However, potential complications of atropine toxicity include flushed, hot, and dry skin, fever, and delirium. Also, 2-PAM may cause dangerous increases in blood pressure.[37] In patients with very severe organophosphate poisoning, intravenous administration of pralidoxime will restore consciousness within 40 minutes.

Prognosis and Future Perspectives. Prolonged high exposure and the appearance of CNS and PNS symptoms may be associated with an incomplete recovery. However, recovery is complete within weeks to months after lower levels of exposure.

ORGANOCHLORINE INSECTICIDES

Pathogenesis and Pathophysiology. The neurotoxic mechanisms for dichlorodiphenyltrichloroethane (DDT) and other organochlorine insecticides is not well defined but may involve the excessive and spontaneous release of acetylcholine. This is in contrast to the acute actions of organophosphates, which block the metabolism of acetylcholine extracellularly. Interestingly, because exposure to both organochlorines and organophosphates produces cholinergic overactivation, these chemicals can cause similar symptomatology.

Epidemiology and Risk Factors. Chlorinated hydrocarbon insecticides are highly soluble in fats and oils. In addition, they last an extremely long time in the environment, thus contributing to chronic toxicity. Commonly used organochlorine insecticides include aldrin, chlordane, DDT, endrin, heptachlor, chlordecone (kepone), and lindane. Most of these insecticides have been banned or restricted in the United States because of their persistence in the food chain, which leads to deleterious effects on wildlife. DDT was banned in the United States in 1973 but is still used in the Third World. Absorption may occur through respiration or through the oral or skin route.

Clinical Features and Associated Findings. Clinical manifestations of organochlorine neurotoxicity have been associated with an oral dose of 10 mg/kg. With acute DDT toxicity, patients report a metallic taste in the mouth. Within 1 hour they complain of dryness of the mouth and extreme thirst. Drowsiness or extreme insomnia, burning eyes, and a gritty sensation in the eyelid are also reported. Other symptoms may include aching of the limbs, muscular spasms, tremors, stiffness and pain in the jaw, difficulty with concentration, and night blindness. Chronic exposure to these compounds can cause tremor and convulsions. Upper extremity weakness, which progresses to wrist drop, may also occur. Mononeuropathy, optic neuropathy, and polyneuropathy have all been described in patients with chronic exposure. In workers in industrial settings that produce DDT and other chlorinated hydrocarbon insecticides, abnormal EEGs marked by bitemporal, sharp wave activity and shifting lateralization have been reported.[42] A cohort of 59 males with chronic exposure to DDT were compared to matched controls using neurobehavioral testing. The group with chronic exposure to DDT scored consistently lower on cognitive testing and was directly related to years of exposure. The exposure group also had more neuropsychological and psychiatric symptoms than the matched controls.[43]

Differential Diagnosis and Evaluation. The diagnosis is made by the history. Although organochlorines and their metabolites can be found in the blood, this test is generally unavailable.

Management. Treatment is supportive. For patients with intractable seizures, diazepam and pentobarbital may be useful. Pentobarbital may also accelerate the metabolism of organochlorines. Atropine and adrenergic amines are contraindicated because they may potentiate myocardial irritability.

Prognosis. With the exception of anticonvulsants in patients in whom seizures are prominent features, there are no specific antidotes for DDT.

OTHER PESTICIDES: METHYL BROMIDE, PICROTOXIN, AND STRYCHNINE

See Table 39–5.

Animal Toxins

SNAKE, SCORPION, AND SPIDER VENOMS

Pathogenesis and Pathophysiology. Most animal neurotoxins affect the cholinergic system through either enhancement or blockade. Snake venoms are extremely toxic to cardiac muscle, coagulant pathways, and the nervous system.[44] Snake venom acts either presynaptically as a toxin that inhibits the release of acetylcholine from presynaptic cells in the neuromuscular junction or postsynaptically as an agent that produces a nondepolarizing neuromuscular block. The resulting effect is a depression of cholinergic function at the neuromuscular junction. There is little evidence that snake bites act directly on the nervous system. Spider venom causes a release of acetylcholine, producing tetanic spasms followed by paralysis.

Epidemiology and Risk Factors. Poisonous snakes include vipers, rattlesnakes, cobras, kraits, mambas, and the American coral snake. Pit vipers are the snakes of most concern in North America. The rattlesnakes, moccasins, cottonmouths, and copperheads comprise 95 percent of the annual snakebites in the United States.[45] Spiders such as the black widow probably account for most of the neurotoxic syndromes that occur after spider bites. Fatalities associated with spider bites occur in approximately 2.5 to 6 percent of cases.[46] Tarantula bites are probably similar to those of the black widow spider.

Clinical Features and Associated Findings. The clinical presentation of persons with a snake bite include localized pain and swelling, headache, vomiting, loss of consciousness, paresthesias, ptosis, loss of vision secondary to coagulation disturbances, and hemorrhage into the retina. Symptoms after snake bite may develop in from 1 to 10 hours. Beginning signs of paralysis include difficulty with swallowing and opening the mouth. Depending on the species, scorpion stings may include both local and systemic complications. Early symptoms include pain, swelling, excessive salivation, sweating, and abdominal pain. Death may result from hypertension, peripheral circulatory collapse, and cardiac failure. Neurological sequelae are more common in children than in adults and include overexcitement, muscle rigidity, convulsions, and alteration of mental status, which is probably secondary to hypoxia. In those with spider bites, neurological sequelae include paresthesias, fasciculations, tremor, and hyper-reflexia during the excitatory phase.

Differential Diagnosis and Evaluation. In patients with snake bites it is especially important to attempt to identify the specific snake involved, since a number of antivenins have been developed against specific poisons.

Management. Treatment of snake bites involves administration of anticholinesterases and specific antivenin as early as possible after the bite. Antivenom use carries the risk of adverse effects, including fatal anaphylaxis. To avoid this problem, pretreatment with diphenhydramine, steroids, and adrenaline has been advocated. In a prospective, placebo-controlled, randomized study of the use of 0.25 mL of adrenaline in 105 snakebite victims about to receive antivenom treatment, those patients receiving the adrenaline showed a significant reduction in adverse effects, including intracerebral hemorrhage.[47] If these are administered prior to the development of major weakness, both pre- and postsynaptic toxic effects can be aborted. Mechanical respiration may also be warranted. During the acute stages after a spider bite, atropine can be administered to control the cardiac muscle effort; gradual recovery will occur over approximately 2 days. Treatment for scorpion bites focuses primarily on supportive respiratory and cardiac measures and attention to coagulation.[48]

Prognosis and Future Perspectives. Survival depends heavily on the control of cardiac and coagulation defects.[49] The development of effective antitoxins and more rapid access to supportive care centers may improve the prognosis.

TICK PARALYSIS

Tick paralysis is a flaccid ascending paralysis caused by the bite of certain female ticks, specifically in North America, *Dermacentor andersoni*, *D. variabilis*, *D. occidentalis*, *Amblyomma americanum*, and *A. maculatum*, which are found commonly in areas west of the Rocky Mountains. The toxin producing the disease is presumably excreted in the saliva of the mature female tick during engorgement. Although persons of any age may be affected, small children are particularly likely to become paralyzed.[50] The head and neck are the most common sites of tick attachment, although any part of the body may be involved. There is some indication of an association between the proximity to the brain of the site of attachment and the severity of the disease. The toxin acts either by causing a failure to liberate acetylcholine at the neuromuscular junction or by causing a generalized depression of all excitable tissues, including the neurons of the spinal cord and brain stem. The course of tick paralysis depends on how soon the tick is found and removed. If it is removed before bulbar symptoms begin, improvement occurs within hours and is complete by 1 week. If bulbar symptoms have begun, death often occurs despite intensive therapy.[51] A polyclonal dog antiserum is available, but is expensive and effective only in the very early stages of paralysis. Recombinant veterinary vaccines based on the tick neurotoxin peptide sequences are currently being investigated.[52]

Plant Toxins (Table 39–6)

CHICKPEA (LATHYRISM)

Lathyrism is related to a neurotoxin acting through the glutaminergic system. Spastic paraplegia has been observed in Europe and India following consumption of different varieties of chickpea.[53] Development of human lathyrism is associated with two potent neurotoxins found in the peas:

TABLE 39–6. **Botanical Toxins**

Plant	Chemical	Mechanism of Toxicity	Physiological Changes
Amanita muscaria mushroom (fly agaric)	Ibotenic acid	Activates NMDA receptors	Marked depolarization with excitation and excitotoxicity
Clitobyte acromelalga mushroom	Acromelic acid Muscarine	Activates kainic acid receptors Activates cholinergic parasympathetic endings	Spasms, excitation, seizures Severe sweating, salivation, and hypertension
Cycad	Beta-*N*-Methyl-amino-*l*-alanine (BMAA)	Activates NMDA receptors	Associated with ALS-Guamanian-PD-dementia complex
Chickpea: Lathyrus	Beta-*N*-Oxalyl-amino-*l*-alanine (BOAA)	Acts as an agonist of AMPA receptors in spinal neurons	Induces spastic paralysis of lower limbs termed neurolathyrism
Betel nut	Arecoline	Stimulates parasympathetic receptors and causes CNS arousal	Excitation, salivation, slowed heart rate
Henbane	Scopolamine	Antagonizes muscarinic cholinergic receptors	Rapid heart rate, sedation and confusion, dilated pupils
Deadly nightshade, Jimson weed	Atropine	Antagonizes muscarinic cholinergic receptors	Rapid heart rate, sedation and confusion, dilated pupils

NMDA, *N*-methyl D-aspartate; ALS, amyotrophic lateral sclerosis; PD, Parkinson's disease; AMPA, alpha-amino-3 hydroxy-5-methyl–4-isoxazoleproprionic acid.

alpha-amino beta oxalylaminopropionic acid and alpha-amino gamma oxalylaminobutyric acid.[54]

Toxic neurological signs are seen when 30 percent or more of the diet consists of chickpeas. Men tend to be affected more than women. The onset is subtle, with pain in the lumbar region and stiffness and weakness of the lower extremities on awakening in the morning. A slight fever may be present. Paresthesias and weakness may develop during the next several days. The legs become spastic and exhibit clonic tremor. The upper extremities may also be involved in patients with severe disease. Within 1 to 2 weeks the pain and paresthesias usually disappear, although relapses sometimes occur. In addition to the more common spastic paraplegia, polyneuropathy and peripheral mononeuropathy may be present.[55]

MUSHROOMS

Amanita mushrooms have strong anticholinergic effects due to their concentration of ibotenic acid, muscazone, and muscimol. Clinically, intoxication takes the form of agitation, muscle spasms, ataxia, mydriasis, and even convulsions. Additional indole compounds may account for the hallucinosis that is often seen with intoxication. The genera *Inocybe* and *Clitocybe* contain muscarine and cause cholinergic excitation at all parasympathetic nerve endings except those of the neuromuscular junctions and nicotinic sites. *Coprius atramentarius*, or Inky Cap, is a common mushroom that is generally considered edible. Its consumption in combination with alcohol, however, results in a severe toxic reaction similar to that seen with disulfiram. The syndrome includes facial flushing, paresthesias, and severe nausea and vomiting. The responsible toxin is coprine, which acts to increase acetaldehyde blood levels. *Amanita* mushrooms are responsible for about 95 percent of fatalities associated with mushroom ingestion, reaching several hundred per year globally. Although most cases are sporadic, clusters of intoxicated victims are intermittently identified. The clinical course begins 6 to 8 hours after ingestion. Symptoms include massive emesis and bloody cholera-like diarrhea. Patients often die during this phase from electrolyte imbalance, but the most dangerous phase of hepatorenal failure does not occur until after 3 to 5 days. Secondary neurologic manifestations include a gradual decline of mental status with confusion, asterixis, and eventually hepatic coma and death. Treatment is mainly supportive and includes careful regulation of fluid status and electrolyte balance, correction of hypoglycemia, and monitoring of coagulation, renal, and liver function. Additionally, hemodialysis, often with exchange transfusion or plasma phoresis can be used, although mortality rates are 30 to 40 percent; when acute liver failure appears, 70 percent or more patients fail to survive.[56, 57]

Bacterial Toxins

DIPHTHERIA

Pathogenesis and Pathophysiology. Diphtheria is an acute infectious disease caused by the bacteria *Corynebacterium diphtheria*. Diphtheria is transmitted by respiratory droplets from infected persons or asymptomatic carriers. There are two forms, oropharyngeal and cutaneous, and the incubation period is from 1 to 4 days. The bacteria affects the respiratory tract and often the heart, kidneys, and nervous system as well. In the immediate area of the infection, usually the nose and throat, the bacteria produce a toxin that causes tissue damage and can spread via the bloodstream to other organs. Muscle and myelin are preferentially affected by this powerful exotoxin. Neurological symptoms result from either direct damage to muscle and peripheral nerve or from indirect damage caused by hypoxia and airway obstruction. Fortunately, the exotoxin does not penetrate the blood-brain barrier, and therefore the CNS is not directly affected.[58] Pathological signs include demyelinization of the ganglia of the peripheral nerves, especially the node of Ranvier, and the cranial and somatic nerves.

Epidemiology and Risk Factors. Diphtheria is now rare in many parts of the world owing to immunization. Potential risk factors for this disease are lack of immunization, crowding, and poor hygiene. In the United States, only five cases of diphtheria were reported in 1991. However, because of a drop in routine child immunizations in the U.S.S.R., a diphtheria epidemic that included more than 50,000 cases was reported in 1993 and 1994.

Clinical Features and Associated Findings. The clinical course follows a predictable pattern. Between the fifth and twelfth days of the illness the initial symptoms are sore throat, fever, a gray to black throat membrane, nasal voice, regurgitation, and dysphagia. At about this time the trigeminal, facial, vagus, and hypoglossal cranial nerves may be affected. In approximately half the patients who have postdiphtheria neurological dysfunction, ocular involvement and paralysis of accommodation were noted in the second or third week. Mononeuropathies can also occur within 2 weeks of onset, and further peripheral neuropathy, predominantly sensory polyneuropathy, or proximal motor neuropathy extending distally is characteristic in the sixth and seventh weeks of the illness. Sometimes toxic encephalopathy, consisting of a change in mental status, drowsiness, and possibly convulsions, is seen.

Differential Diagnosis and Evaluation. The diagnosis must be based on the clinical history and clinical presentation. Physical examination may show a characteristic gray membrane in the throat, enlarged lymph glands, and swelling of the neck and larynx. In patients with a clinical picture of Guillain-Barré syndrome with visual blurring and palatal involvement, a diagnosis of diphtheria should be questioned. Diphtheric polyneuropathy can be distinguished from all other polyneuropathies by the early bulbar symptoms, unique ciliary paralysis, and subacute evolution of a delayed symmetrical sensorimotor peripheral polyneuropathy. Diagnostic testing should include Gram stain of the infected membrane, a throat culture, and an electrocardiogram, which will show evidence of myocarditis.

Management. There is no specific treatment for the neurological symptoms of diphtheria. Treatment generally involves administration of antitoxin within 48 hours of the earliest signs of infection, rest, and maintenance of proper airway and cardiac function. All contacts of the infected person should be immunized, since protective immunity is not present longer than 10 years after the last vaccination. Diphtheria is preventable through immunization at the age of 3 months. Booster doses at 1 year and before the child enters school are suggested.

Prognosis. The death rate is 10 percent. If the patient does not expire because of respiratory distress or cardiac failure, he or she stabilizes and slowly recovers completely. Therefore, activities should be slowly resumed.

TETANUS

Pathogenesis and Pathophysiology. Tetanus is caused by a powerful exotoxin, *Clostridium tetani*, which produces spores. The spores can remain dormant in the soil or in animal excrement for many years until they enter the body and produce a toxin. In patients with tetanus toxicity, both the CNS and the PNS as well as the musculature are involved.[59] The major CNS effect occurs through disinhibition on gray matter gangliosides and through presynaptic antagonism of GABA. At high concentrations, tetanus toxin acts like botulism toxin in that it inhibits the release of acetylcholine at cholinergic synapses. The nervous system is infected by tetanus through retrograde axonal transport from the site of infection. The incubation period may range from 5 to 25 days but can be only a few hours. Early in the illness, pathological changes include changes in the nerve cells of the cortex and brain stem. If the illness lasts for more than 5 days, demyelination and gliosis may occur, and in the most severe cases, hemorrhages can occur.

Epidemiology and Risk Factors. In Third World countries, tetanus is still an important cause of morbidity and mortality. The bacteria can be transmitted in the anaerobic conditions of wounds, through soil-contaminated injuries, and, less commonly, by unclean needles used by drug abusers. In adults, tetanus is seen only in those who have not been immunized. About 50 to 100 cases are reported in the United States each year, and 60 percent of those cases occur in adults over the age of 60. Although neonatal tetanus due to infection of the stump of the umbilical cord is thought to be of only historical interest, worldwide it remains the second leading cause of vaccine-preventable death among children.[60]

Clinical Features and Associated Findings. The clinical course consists of early symptoms of chills, headache, restlessness, and pain at the site of injury. Tightness in the jaw and mild stiffness and soreness in the neck are usually noticed within a few hours. As symptoms develop, the jaw becomes stiff and tight (lockjaw). Muscular involvement then progresses to the throat and facial muscles. Muscular rigidity may then become generalized and may include the trunk and extremities. Rigidity in the abdominal muscles can result in a forward arching at the back. The tetanic contractions occur periodically and can cause severe pain. In the most severe cases, convulsions and marked dyspnea with cyanosis can occur, terminating in asphyxia and sudden death. Mental status remains intact. However, the patient suffers from anxiety and mental and physical agony.

Differential Diagnosis and Evaluation. A diagnosis of tetanus can be made by a positive history of a prior wound, a high titer of serum antibody to tetanus, a history of partial immunization, and clinical symptoms as just outlined. Tetanus must be differentiated from the stiff-person syndrome and the Moersch-Woltman syndrome. Trismus is not typical of stiff-person syndrome.

Management. Patients should be hospitalized and external stimuli kept to a minimum. The infected wound should be debrided. Muscle relaxation can be initiated by the use of barbiturates or diazepam. Although antiserum does not neutralize the toxins fixed in the nervous system, human tetanus immunoglobulin should be given. One dose of 3000 to 6000 units given intramuscularly into three sites simultaneously is recommended. If human antitoxin is unavailable, equine antiserum can be given. Tetanus is prevented by immunization. Children should be immunized at 2 months to 6 years of age. In adults, tetanus boosters last approximately 10 years.

Prognosis and Future Perspectives. The prognosis is poor. The fatality rate is approximately 65 percent. Death generally occurs rapidly between the third and fifth day of illness and is due to exhaustion, medullary failure, asphyxia resulting from spasm, or circulatory failure resulting from exertion on the heart. Occasionally, tetanus antitoxin produces an adverse reaction involving primarily the PNS. After 6 months, recovery is usually complete.

BOTULISM

Pathogenesis and Pathophysiology. Botulism is the most potent poison known to man. It is produced by the spores of *Clostridium botulinum*. Three distinct varieties of the disease exist. Foodborne botulism results primarily from the ingestion of contaminated home-canned fruits and vegetables. Since this type of botulinum toxin is produced by spores that are already formed and ingested, toxic signs appear rapidly, usually between 8 and 36 hours after ingestion, and an incubation period is not required. After ingestion of the botulinum toxin, neurological signs appear within hours or at most 1 week. Wound botulism is both an infection and an intoxication. The organism enters through the wound site, and the spores may germinate locally in the tissues, producing a potent exotoxin. The third form of botulism is infantile botulism, which occurs in the first 6 months of life. In this situation, spores germinate in the infant's intestine and produce the toxin in vivo. The basic pathophysiological mechanism of botulism neurotoxicity is inhibition of acetylcholine release.

Epidemiology and Risk Factors. Each year, approximately 20 cases of foodborne botulism in adults and 250 cases of infantile botulism are reported. Infantile botulism produces a very different clinical syndrome from that outlined following. This disease has been reported only within the last decade. Interestingly, botulinum toxicity has been offered as a possible explanation for the sudden infant death syndrome (SIDS). The age distribution is the same, and 10 infants with SIDS in California in 1977 also had evidence of intestinal infection with *C. botulinum*. Botulism may cause sudden infant death by producing flaccidity of the upper airway or tongue muscles, leading to airway obstruction during sleep.[61] The introduction of botulinum toxin for the treatment of dystonia, hemifacial spasm, and spasticity raises the possibility of iatrogenic treatment as a risk factor for botulism. A botulism-like syndrome of generalized weakness has been reported after injections of botulinum toxin likely due to systemic spread of toxin.[62, 63]

Clinical Features and Associated Findings. Early signs of toxicity include nausea and vomiting with abdominal pain, and diarrhea. Other symptoms include ptosis, extraocular paresis, and progressive weakness suggestive of myasthenia gravis. Cranial nerve symptoms most commonly involve the eyes. Additional symptoms include dryness of the mucous membranes, vertigo, deafness, dysphasia, swallowing difficulties, breathing difficulty that may lead to respiratory failure, speech impairment, absent or decreased gag reflex, and absent or decreased deep tendon reflexes. By the second to fourth day of the illness, muscular weakness develops. Often muscular involvement is limited to the neck muscles, resulting in an inability of the patient to raise the head.[64]

In infants symptoms consist of constipation, weakness with loss of muscle tone, and an alert but weak appearance.[65]

Differential Diagnosis. Weakness can usually be differentiated from Guillain-Barré syndrome because the weakness associated with botulism toxicity is descending, so the proximal muscles are affected before the distal extremities. The progressive weakness is suggestive of myasthenia gravis; however, the pupillary dilation seen in botulism is not characteristic of myasthenia. Stimulation single fiber EMG may be particularly useful in establishing the diagnosis and monitoring clinical progression.[66] Botulism should be considered in cases of SIDS, when asphyxia is thought to be due to upper airway or tongue flaccidity.

Evaluation. Confirmation of the diagnosis depends on detection of the toxin either in the patient (blood) or in the implicated food. A stool culture is often useful.

Management. Once the patient has been admitted to the hospital, respiration should be monitored. Trivalent ABE antitoxin is recommended.

Prognosis and Future Perspectives. In severe cases, a downward course is rapid and terminates in death. Death occurs in 70 percent of untreated cases. If the patient survives, recovery begins within a few weeks.

Illicit Drugs (Table 39–7)

COCAINE

Pathogenesis and Pathophysiology. Blockade of the uptake of monoamines into the presynaptic terminals is probably responsible for the acute effects produced by cocaine. Depending on the affected system, this blockade leads to increased levels of dopamine (DA), norepinephrine, or serotonin in the synaptic cleft. The increase in neurotransmitters is associated with overstimulation of postsynaptic receptors, activation of transcription factors, and increased or decreased expression of specific target genes.

TABLE 39–7. **Summary of Neurologic Signs and Symptoms of Drug Abuse**

Signs or Symptoms	Drugs
Cranial Nerves	
Pupils	
Pinpoint	Opiates
Dilated	Stimulants
Sluggish	Hallucinogens
Reactive	Opiate withdrawal
Extraocular Muscles	
Nystagmus	Depressants, phencyclidine (PCP)
Speech	
Slow	Opiates
Slurred	Depressants, opiates
Rapid	Stimulants
Motor	
Tremor (fine)	Hallucinogens, stimulants
Tremor (coarse)	Depressants
Reflexes	
Increased	Stimulants
Decreased	Depressants
Seizures	Opiates, stimulants, over-the-counter drugs

Cocaine can cause strokes when taken either intranasally, intravenously, or intramuscularly.[67, 68] The effects of cocaine on the cerebral circulation are due primarily to direct vasoconstriction, probably related to stimulation of noradrenergic receptors by increased levels of norepinephrine. This is exemplified by the markedly increased blood flow and vascular resistance that follows acute administration of cocaine. In addition, cocaine can enhance platelet response to arachidonic acid, thus promoting aggregation.

Cocaine-induced strokes may be ischemic or hemorrhagic. Cocaine-associated ischemic strokes can present as transient ischemic attacks. Infarctions in the distribution of all major arteries have been described. Cocaine-induced strokes in young patients have increased remarkably.[69] Although cerebral infarction has often been attributed to vasculitis and vasospasm, there are actually few documented examples of vasculitis in autopsied cases.[70, 71]

Intracerebral or subarachnoid hemorrhages may also be associated with cocaine use. The majority of these cases occur in the presence of saccular aneurysms or vascular malformations. Infarctions and hemorrhages have been reported in newborns whose mothers had used cocaine prior to delivery.

The mechanisms of cocaine-related stroke are unclear. However, it has been reported that cocaine hydrochloride is more often associated with hemorrhagic stroke than with occlusive stroke, whereas hemorrhagic and occlusive strokes occur with roughly equal frequency in patients who use cocaine alkaloid ("crack"). Acute hypertension can lead to intracranial hemorrhage, especially in subjects with underlying aneurysms or vascular malformations. Myocardial infarction, cardiac arrhythmia, and cardiomyopathy carry a very high risk of embolic stroke.

Acute cocaine exposure provokes cerebral vasoconstriction that may be a cause of occlusive stroke.[72] Cocaine metabolites also cause cerebral vasospasm, and these metabolites may be detectable in the chronic user's urine for weeks. Chronic cocaine abusers show increased distal arteriolar resistance that persists after a month of drug abstinence.[72] These findings demonstrate that chronic cocaine abuse increases the risk of thromboembolic strokes independent of acute use of the drug.[72]

The neuropsychological effects of chronic cocaine exposure are thought to be due to decreased DA levels in the brain. This hypothesized dopamine decrease may be secondary to long-term depletion of DA, which occurs with repeated drug administration. However, there is very little direct evidence to support this view and other data suggest that chronic cocaine exposure may induce structural changes in neuroanatomy. A CT study has shown that habitual cocaine users (those who use the drug at least twice weekly for 2 years or more) have significant degrees of cerebral atrophy with enlargement of the lateral ventricles and widening of the sylvian fissures compared with first-time users and nonusers. Studies examining the consequences of chronic cocaine abuse in abstinent cocaine abusers have shown that cerebral metabolism in the medial orbitofrontal cortex and basal ganglia during the first week of abstinence from cocaine is higher than that in normal subjects but then falls below normal levels and remains so for at least 3 months.[73] In another positron-emission tomography (PET) study, glucose metabolism in the entire cerebral cortex, thalamus, and midbrain was reduced following acute administration of cocaine.[74] In an O^{15} PET activation study conducted after 4 weeks of abstinence, cocaine users showed less activation in the left anterior cingulated cortex (ACC) and lateral prefrontal cortex bilaterally compared to controls during performance on a task aimed to activate these brain regions selectively[75] (Fig. 39–4). Because these brain regions play a role in performance monitoring[76] and the suppression of inappropriate responses of incorrect actions,[77] circuitry disruption could

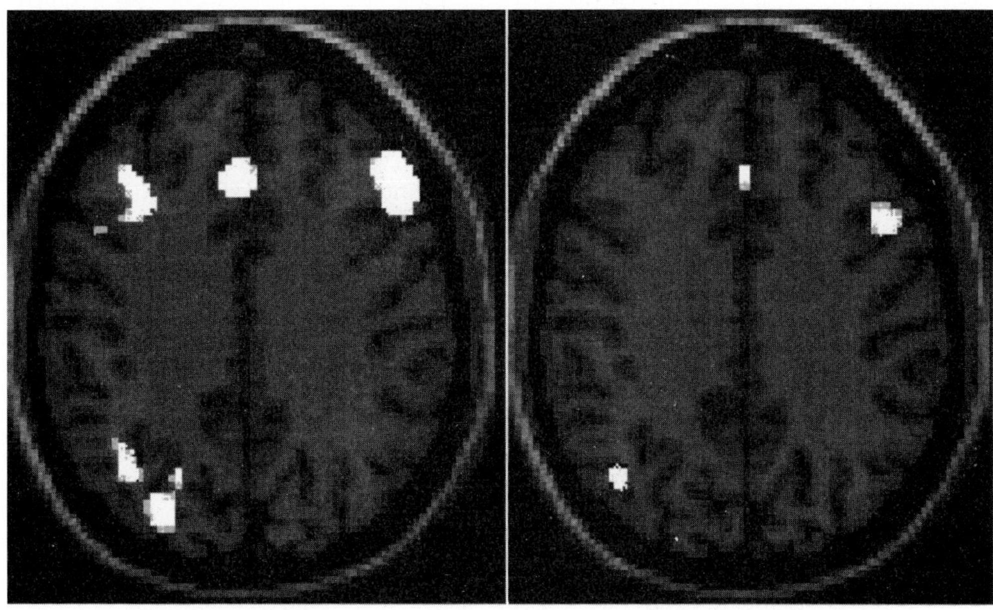

FIGURE 39–4. Oxygen^{15} positron-emission tomography (PET) scans, comparing non-drug-using individuals with cocaine abusers. While performing the Stroop task, non–drug users show greater activation in the left anterior cingulate cortex and lateral frontal cortex bilaterally than the cocaine abusers (Bolla et al, Society for Neuroscience Abstract. New Orleans LA, November, 2000).

impair a drug abuser's ability to discontinue drug-seeking behavior.

Epidemiology and Risk Factors. Cocaine was first used by South American Indians between 2000 and 1500 BC. From the 1920s to the 1960s, recreational use of cocaine in the United States was limited to jazz musicians and the "cultural avant garde." In the mid-1980s, the development of crack cocaine caused a marked increase in the number of new cocaine users to an estimated 5000 new users a day, 6 million regular users, and 1 million compulsive users. Recently, however, the use of cocaine has declined dramatically from an estimated 5.7 million current users in 1985 to an estimated 1.2 million current users in 2000.[78] Nevertheless, the epidemic of cocaine use with its associated medical and neurological sequelae makes cocaine use a major public health concern.

Clinical Features and Associated Findings. Cocaine produces a brief rush, which peaks at 1.5 to 2 minutes. This rush is followed by euphoria, excitability, and hypervigilance. The acute administration of cocaine causes both psychiatric and neurological symptoms. Acute psychiatric symptoms include anxiety, insomnia, paranoia, agitation, and psychosis. Neurological symptoms include stereotypy, bruxism, chorea, dystonia, myoclonus, seizures, lethargy, strokes, and coma. In addition, high doses of cocaine cause tachycardia, tachypnea, and hypertension. Parenteral cocaine users are also at risk for stroke related to infection, such as endocarditis and the acquired immunodeficiency syndrome (AIDS).

Differential Diagnosis and Evaluation. The clinical presentation of a cocaine-induced neurological disorder can mimic a number of other neurological abnormalities. However, a cocaine-related stroke or other neurological disorder can be diagnosed if a urine toxicology screen is positive for cocaine. It is important to perform the toxicology screen within the first 24 hours of presentation because of the short half-life of cocaine in the urine. However, urinary cocaine metabolites such as norcocaine and benzoyl ecgonine may remain positive for several days. Urine toxicology screening is indicated in all patients who present to the emergency room with an acute neurological syndrome because a very high prevalence of cocaine use exists in many communities, including suburban areas.

Management. Treatment of cocaine-induced neurological abnormalities depends on the clinical presentation. In patients with acute paranoia or psychosis, neuroleptics are indicated. However, it is important to note that cocaine abusers may be at increased risk for acute dystonic reaction secondary to antipsychotic drugs. In these cases, anxiolytics can be very helpful. Other complications, including strokes, are treated according to the clinical presentation.

AMPHETAMINE ANALOGS

Pathogenesis and Pathophysiology. The pathophysiological basis for the complications associated with amphetamine use are not well understood. Amphetamine-induced cerebral vasculitides cause occlusive as well as hemorrhagic strokes. Methamphetamine use can cause necrotizing angiitis. Also, cerebral arteritis with multiple occlusions of arterioles was reported in young abusers of intravenous methamphetamine who were hospitalized because of coma or stroke.[79] Angiographic studies in such patients have shown occlusions or beading of vessels in the internal carotid, distal middle cerebral, and lenticulostriate arteries.[80]

To test the role of methamphetamine in the etiology of vasculitis, monkeys were given methamphetamine intravenously and then underwent serial angiograms.[81] Some of the animals showed beading of small and large vessels that persisted or progressed over a 2-week period. Hypertension and behavioral changes were also seen. At autopsy, subarachnoid hemorrhages were found in some animals as well as brain petechiae, infarcts, microaneurysms, and perivascular white cell cuffing. More severe vasculitides were reported in another study of monkeys that received intravenous methamphetamine three times weekly for up to a year.[82] Angiographic and histological changes have also been reported in monkeys given intravenous methylphenidate.[82] Sural nerve biopsy showed hypersensitivity angiitis of medium and small arteries and veins in an adolescent amphetamine abuser who presented with mononeuritis multiplex.[83]

Epidemiology and Risk Factors. Amphetamines have been used for many decades to promote weight loss. They are also used in the treatment of attention deficit disorder and narcolepsy and as an adjunctive treatment in patients with treatment-resistant depression. During the 1960s and early 1970s, amphetamines were widely abused by people involved in the so-called counterculture movement. During the 1980s and 1990s, most of these drugs were replaced by cocaine. Nevertheless, prescribed amphetamines remained a significant source of abusable drugs. More recently, drugs such as methamphetamine ("meth," Ice) and methylenedioxymethamphetamine (MDMA, Ecstasy) have undergone a major resurgence among adolescents and young people in their early twenties. MDMA is used frequently at "raves" and has become a major public health issue in some communities. "Meth" is also widely used in California and in some midwestern states, where it is synthesized in basement laboratories. In Japan, "meth" abuse has been rampant since the end of World War II.

Clinical Features and Associated Findings. The amphetamine analogues tend to produce very similar signs and symptoms. These include hyperalertness, euphoria, hyperactivity, and greater physical endurance. Higher doses of these drugs can cause dysphoria, headaches, and confusion.[84] Unlike cocaine, these drugs can produce a prolonged rush when taken intravenously, and inhalation of "meth" can sometimes cause a more rapid rush. These responses are due to their longer half-lives; also, the psychological response to amphetamine analogs usually lasts longer than that of cocaine. In fact, "meth" can induce psychotic symptomatology that is often indistinguishable from that of an acute schizophrenic break. "Meth"-induced psychosis is quite common in Japan.

Gilles de la Tourette syndrome can be exacerbated and precipitated by amphetamine, methylphenidate, and pemoline; it sometimes clears with discontinuation of the drug but occasionally persists.[85, 86] The bruxism and choreiform movements that develop with chronic amphetamine use may also persist after the drug has been discontinued.

Strokes are also frequent complications of amphetamine abuse. Intracerebral hemorrhages have been reported after either nasal or intravenous use of these drugs. Often, strokes are preceded by complaints of severe headaches. Blood pressure is elevated in more than half the subjects who come to medical attention; diastolic pressure has been reported to be as high as 120 mm Hg. CT scans have shown intracerebral, intraventricular, or subarachnoid hemorrhage. Cerebral angiography shows irregular narrowing of the distal cerebral vessels; this is consistent with the presence of vasculitis.

Management. In patients who present with acute psychotic symptomatology, antipsychotic drugs may be indicated. It is very important to pay close attention to the patient's vital signs because amphetamines can cause a marked increase in body temperature. These patients may be more prone to develop the neuroleptic malignant syndrome. In such cases, it might be more beneficial to use a quiet, cool room for treatment rather than pharmacological agents. If this is not possible, anxiolytic agents are recommended. The clinical presentation of the patient should determine the exact method of management.

Prognosis and Future Perspectives. Whether the amphetamines can cause permanent psychiatric or cognitive disturbances is uncertain. Ten users of amphetamines reported decreased memory or poor concentration ability after they achieved abstinence. There are also reports of lasting psychosis or dementia. Formal studies of cognitive performance in chronic abusers of amphetamine analogs are presently under way in our clinical laboratory.

METHYLENEDIOXYMETHAMPHETAMINE

MDMA is a derivative of methamphetamine. The use of MDMA in the United States has reached epidemic proportions. In 1998, 3.4 million Americans had tried Ecstasy at least once, by 2000 this number had almost doubled to 6.5 million.[78] While not thought to be physically addicting, MDMA is reported to cause severe damage to the serotonergic neurons in nonhuman primates and decreases in the serotonin metabolite 5-hydroxyindoleacetic acid in the cerebrospinal fluid of humans who have abused the drug.[87] MDMA has properties similar to both stimulants and to hallucinogens. It is abused by individuals who wish to intensify their emotional and sensory experiences. MDMA and a close congener, methylenedioxyamphetamine (MDA), are reported to cause individuals to become more empathic. Before MDMA and MDA were made illegal in 1985, psychiatrists experimented with these drugs to facilitate psychotherapy, especially in patients who had difficulty in expressing their emotions. Just recently, the Food and Drug Administration has approved a protocol to study MDMA-assisted psychotherapy for the treatment of patients suffering from post-traumatic stress disorder.

MDMA and MDA can cause increases in blood pressure and heart rate, anxiety, and locomotor hyperactivity. Mild neurological side effects include pupillary dilatation and tremors, but more serious consequences include seizures, strokes, and coma. A number of studies have shown dose-related neurobehavioral deficits in memory with heavy MDMA use.[88–90] Public education efforts have focused especially on young adults to communicate the medical and neurotoxic concerns related to memory deficits and their potential irreversibility.

OPIOID AGONISTS

Pathogenesis and Pathophysiology. Opioid drugs can cause respiratory suppression because of the high density of opioid receptors in the brain stem nuclei. These receptors subserve respiration. CT studies have revealed cerebral and cerebellar white matter lucencies in patients who present with pseudobulbar palsy and quadriparesis. Postmortem studies have also shown edema and spongiform-type changes in the white matter of heroin abusers.[91] It is possible that these pathological changes may be secondary to the adulterants used with these drugs, such as chloroquine. This adulterant is often used in conjunction with heroin.

A large number of heroin abusers develop AIDS. At autopsy, neuropathological abnormalities consistent with AIDS are found. Almost all had neurological symptoms and signs prior to death. Retrospective surveys of AIDS cases suggest that parenteral drug abusers are more likely than other high-risk groups to have cryptococcal meningitis and CNS toxoplasmosis. No differences were found between parenteral drug abusers and nondrug-abusing homosexuals in the prevalence of these infections or of neurological symptoms, including dementia, seizures, or peripheral neuropathy. On the other hand, Kaposi's sarcoma is rare in drug abusers. Neuropsychological studies of asymptomatic HIV-seropositive parenteral drug abusers found no evidence of significant cognitive impairment, a finding that needs to be evaluated further.

Epidemiology and Risk Factors. The poppy has been used for its opioid content for more than a few thousand years. Opium has been available in Europe since the middle of the 16th century. By the 19th century, opium was popular in many countries as a euphoriant. After the Civil War, opioid use became widespread in the United States, and opium was present in a number of over-the-counter remedies, including Dover's powder, Godfrey's cordial, and Darby's carminative. The number of Americans reportedly addicted to opioids at the beginning of the 20th century ranges from 200,000 to more than 1 million. Most were white middle-aged women who took opium in medicines. More recently, opioid agonists have been used for their acute euphoric effects. Three milligrams of heroin are equivalent to about 10 mg of morphine. Until the advent of crack cocaine, heroin was probably the most common illicit drug used in many metropolitan areas. In the late 1960s, heroin-related fatalities were a very common cause of death in New York City men aged 15 to 35. In 1985, there was a striking rise in the number of fatal heroin overdoses in New Mexico; this was attributed to the availability of Mexican "black tar" heroin. Heroin (diacetylmorphine) is metabolized to 6-acetylmorphine and morphine.

Clinical Features and Associated Findings. The acute effects of opiates include euphoria and drowsiness.[92] Parenteral heroin produces a "hit" that lasts for about a minute. It is often compared to orgasm. The user then experiences a dreamlike and pleasant drowsiness. Visual hallucinations have been reported after morphine or heroin administration. Nausea and vomiting can also occur. Drug abusers often experience dryness of the mouth, pruritus, suppression of the cough reflex, respiratory depression, hypothermia, postural hypotension, and constipation.

Pentazocine (Talwin) and tripelennamine (Pyribenzamine) were widely abused in some American cities in the 1970s.[93] Cerebral hemorrhages resulted from the injection of crushed oral tablets that were suspended in water and passed through a cigarette filter. Pulverized meperidine tablets have caused seizures and fundal hemorrhages. Cerebral vasculitides have also been reported in users of these drugs.

The chronic use of heroin can result in myelopathy, which is probably of vascular origin.[94] Acute paraparesis, sensory loss, and urinary retention usually occur shortly after administration of the drug. Possible causes of spinal lesions include hypotension, embolism of foreign objects, and direct toxic effects of the drugs. Vasculitis affecting mainly the small arteries and arterioles has been reported. Also noted is an anterior spinal artery syndrome with quadriplegia that follows supraclavicular heroin injection.

A number of other neurological complications affect heroin users. Peripheral neuropathy can present as a Guillain-Barré syndrome.[95] The peripheral nerves may also be damaged secondary to direct injection or to pressure palsies. Ulnar and femoral neuropathies have also been observed. Painful brachial and lumbosacral plexopathies are also common; these can result from a septic aneurysm affecting the subclavian or axillary arteries. Vocal cord paralysis can follow repeated jugular vein injections.

Adulteration of heroin with chloroquine can cause headache, confusion, and visual disturbances. Spongiform encephalopathy has also been reported. In these patients, there were symptoms of apathy, bradyphrenia, dysarthria, and ataxia. There are also signs of spastic hemiparesis or quadriparesis, tremor, chorea, myoclonus, pseudobulbar palsy, fever, and blindness. Heroin use is also a risk factor for new-onset seizures independent of head injury, infection, stroke, or alcohol. Infections are a common cause of morbidity in heroin users. Osteomyelitis is associated with back or neck pain, radiculopathy, and sometimes even cord compression. Cervical infection is especially common among addicts who inject into the jugular vein. Symptoms frequently precede diagnosis by several weeks. *Staphylococcus aureus* and *Pseudomonas* are common etiological factors in these infections. Bacterial endocarditis can lead to intraparenchymal or extraparenchymal abscess of the brain or spinal cord, meningitis, cerebral infarction, diffuse vasculitis, and subarachnoid hemorrhage from rupture of septic mycotic aneurysms. Progressive neurological symptoms, including headache, fever, syncope, hemiparesis, and aphasia, are a common presentation of mycotic aneurysms.

Tetanus has been reported in skin poppers who suffer from multiple skin abscesses.[96] Among drug users, curarization is frequently necessary to control symptoms. Botulism with dysphagia, blurred vision, dysphonia, and descending paralysis has also occurred in parenteral heroin abusers.

Coma is a common presentation of opioid overdose. In some comatose patients, pulmonary edema is frequently present. These patients do not respond to naloxone. In milder cases, overdose of heroin can be associated with spastic quadriparesis, deafness, seizures, and dystonia. Postanoxic encephalopathy has also been reported. Death can follow very small amounts of heroin or methadone. Some of these complications may be due to adulterants. For example, quinine causes cardiac conduction abnormalities and ventricular fibrillation. The combination of heroin, ethanol, and quinine might synergize to cause sudden death.

Management. The treatment of opioid-related complications is based on the clinical presentation. Naloxone (2 mg) is initially administered for patients with respiratory depression. Increments of 2 to 4 mg can be repeated up to a total dose of 20 mg, depending on the clinical status of the patient. Higher doses are often used for those with propoxyphene, pentazocine, diphenoxylate, nalbuphine, or butorphanol toxicity. It is often necessary to administer naloxone intramuscularly or subcutaneously because of the bad veins of these patients. The clinician must be aware of the potential for precipitating withdrawal symptoms with overdosage of an antagonist. Based on the clinical status of the subject, it may be necessary to titrate a naloxone infusion because methadone and propoxyphene have long half-lives.

If heroin is taken in combination with cocaine or amphetamine, paranoid psychosis can be unmasked through the use of naloxone. Opioids taken in combination with barbiturates or ethanol can produce a coma that does not respond to naloxone.

HALLUCINOGENS

Hallucinogens (psychedelics) have been used and abused since time immemorial. Many of these compounds, including mescaline (peyote cactus) and psilocybin (mushrooms), are used in religious ceremonies by Native Americans. These drugs were used actively during the 1960s and early 1970s. In the 1980s they were displaced by cocaine, but there has been a resurgence in their use, especially among teenagers.

The most commonly abused hallucinogen in the United States is lysergic acid diethylamide (LSD). LSD is made from lysergic acid found in the fungus, ergot, which can grow on grains. Many of the hallucinogens are structurally similar to serotonin, which suggests that this class of drugs exerts its effects by altering this neurotransmitter. LSD also alters adrenergic mechanisms in the periphery and acts as a partial dopaminergic agonist. It is the most powerful hallucinogen and produces symptoms at doses varying from 25 to 50 μg. LSD is sold in a variety of forms, including small sticky pieces of paper that contain as much as 300 μg of the drug. LSD is readily absorbable after oral administration. Its effects peak after 2 to 4 hours and may last for several hours.

Symptoms consist of euphoria, intensive arousal, panic, or even depression. Perceptual distortions are very common, as are hallucinations. Neurological abnormalities include papillary dilatation, lacrimation, and hyperreflexia. Patients report visual changes consisting of increased intensity of colors and alterations in shapes. No toxic fatalities have been reported with LSD use. A number of LSD users have recurring episodic visual disturbances, which include flashes of color, geometric pseudohallucinations, and fleeting perceptions in the peripheral visual fields. Formerly known as "flashbacks," these have been renamed the hallucinogen persisting perception disorder. Some chronic heavy users of LSD have been reported to suffer from impaired memory, poor attention span, and confusion.

Users of LSD may require treatment because they experience severe anxiety, intense depression, or suicidal ideation. Therapy consists of "talking the patient down," which is a highly effective approach. If medication is required, diazepam given orally is the drug of choice.

METHYL-PHENYL-TETRAHYDROPYRIDINE

The first case of methyl-phenyl-tetrahydropyridine (MPTP)–induced parkinsonism was reported in 1979.[97] The subject later died of a drug overdose. At autopsy, destruction of the substantia nigra zona compacta was evident; other areas usually involved in Parkinson's disease such as the locus ceruleus were not affected. This article lay dormant until parkinsonism began appearing in the San Francisco Bay area among users of MPTP, sold as "synthetic heroin." The responsible chemical was identified as a byproduct of meperidine synthesis, 1-methyl-4-phenyl-1,2,3,6-tetrahydropyridine.[98]

The cerebrospinal fluid of affected patients contains decreased homovanillic acid levels similar to those observed in patients with Parkinson's disease.[99] PET using 18F-dopa of asymptomatic drug users exposed to MPTP showed decreased dopa uptake, which suggests that the numbers of DA terminals and, by extension, the nigral cell bodies were decreased. The MPTP model of dopamine depletion has been helpful in mechanistic studies of the degenerative and regenerative potential of the nigrostriatal DA system. MPTP is metabolized to 1-methyl-4-phenylpyridinium (MPP+) by monoamine oxidase B. MPP+ is then taken up into DA terminals, where it blocks complex I of the mitochondrial respiratory chain. This blockage may lead to adenosine triphosphate depletion with secondary cellular demise due to energy crisis. The possibility that abnormalities in the respiratory chain could also lead to cytotoxic oxygen-based free radicals has also been put forward.[100]

MPTP has also caused parkinsonism in laboratory workers who were accidentally contaminated through inhalation or skin contact. Bradykinesia and rigidity can be very severe, with muteness and inability to swallow. As in idiopathic Parkinson's disease, levodopa/carbidopa and bromocriptine can provide dramatic relief in these patients. Patients develop typical side effects of these drugs, including dyskinesia, on-off phenomenon, and psychiatric symptoms.

PHENCYCLIDINE

Phencyclidine (PCP) was developed initially as an anesthetic. However, a large number of patients developed postoperative psychosis after its administration. These occurrences stopped its use for this purpose in humans. Significantly, PCP affects all neurotransmitter systems. During the 1970s PCP was sold as "angel dust," and its use was rampant. At present, PCP is mainly used by lower middle class white men in a very few localities. It can be injected, snorted, smoked, or eaten, and has been found in samples of LSD, amphetamines, and marijuana. PCP has been sold as mescaline or as one of the hallucinogens.

PCP can cause a mixed euphoric-dysphoric syndrome with increasing doses of the drug. Users have reported sensations of time slowing, relaxation, and numbness. High doses of PCP can cause a psychotic picture similar to that of schizophrenia, with increasing agitation, hallucinations, and bizarre and violent behaviors. Catatonia has also been reported. Patients with PCP-induced psychosis may show increased body temperature, hypertension, and increased sweating. Neurological abnormalities include miosis, horizontal and vertical nystagmus, and ataxia. Increased muscle tone, hyper-reflexia, and tremors have also been reported. Very high doses of the drug have been reported to cause seizures and even coma. Delirium lasting for several days is common in patients recovering from PCP-induced coma.

Treatment of an intoxicated PCP user involves putting the subject in a very calm environment. Neuroleptic drugs are relatively contraindicated because they have the potential to cause development of the neuroleptic malignant syndrome or to precipitate seizures. Benzodiazepines are the drugs of choice in treatment of PCP-induced intoxication. Enhancement of PCP clearance by acidification of the urine is recommended in comatose patients.

CANNABINOL (MARIJUANA)

Marijuana is one of the most commonly abused drugs. It was used as early as 3000 BC in cultures as diverse as those found in the Middle East and Asia. The drug is known by a number of names, including hashish, ganja, and bhang. Low to moderate doses of the drug cause very few psychological and physiological symptoms. The pharmacological actions and the long-term effects of chronic use are still unclear.

Delta-tetrahydrocannabinol (THC) is derived from the marijuana plant, *Cannabis sativa*. The drug can be smoked, eaten, or taken intravenously. Its potency varies greatly. When smoked, the peak plasma level of the drug is reached within 10 minutes, although psychological effects do not develop until 20 to 30 minutes. The effects can last up to 3 hours. However, THC is absorbed and accumulates in tissues such as the testes and the brain. In very heavy users of marijuana, urinary clearance can take as long as 30 days.

THC causes euphoria, feelings of relaxation, and heightened sexual arousal. Some individuals experience increased hunger; others report increased suspiciousness, paranoia, and aggressiveness, and still others become quite withdrawn socially.

Neurological signs and symptoms include confusion, disorientation, and an organic delusional syndrome. Some recurrent users develop short-term memory deficits that persist for at least 1 month even in the context of abstinence. Transcranial Doppler sonography shows that cerebrovascular resistance and systolic velocity increase in marijuana abusers compared to controls. In fact, cerebral perfusion in 18- to 30-year-old marijuana abusers is comparable to that of normal 60-year-olds. This finding suggests that that marijuana abusers may be at increased risk for stroke.[101] Nystagmus, ataxia, and tremors have also been reported. The drug can precipitate seizures in patients with known seizure disorders. Life-threatening neurological abnormalities are very rare.

Treatment of patients with acute toxic reactions involves reassurance that the problems will clear up within a few hours. Because of the possible high concentration of the drug in various tissues, the neurological effects of the drug may take up to 8 hours to clear. No specific drug is necessary, although a benzodiazapine may be useful. In patients in acute psychotic states, haloperidol 5 to 20 mg/day in divided doses is recommended.

Acknowledgment

The authors would like to thank Regina Hess for her assistance in the preparation of this chapter.

Reviews and Selected Updates

ACGIH: Threshold Limit Values and Biological Exposure Indices for 2001. Cincinnati, American Conference of Governmental Industrial Hygienists, 2001.

Baker SR, Williamson CF: The Effects of Pesticides on Human Health. Advances in Modern Environmental Toxicology. Princeton, NJ, Princeton Scientific Co, 1990.

Chang LW, Dyer RS (eds): Handbook of Neurotoxicology. New York, Marcel Dekker, 1995.

Goetz CG: Neurotoxins in Clinical Practice. New York, Spectrum Publications, 1985.

Goetz CG, Meisel E: Biological neurotoxins. Neurol Clin 2000;18:719–740.

Hartman DE: Neuropsychological Toxicology: Identification and Assessment of Human Neurotoxic Syndromes. New York, Pergamon Press, 1988.

National Advisory Council for Environmental Policy and Technology Report of Environmental Protection Agency. Washington, DC, US Government Printing Office, 1993.

Rosenstock L, Cullen MR (eds): Textbook of Clinical Occupational and Environmental Medicine. Philadelphia, WB Saunders, 1994, pp 847–865.

References

1. Goetz CG: Neurotoxins in Clinical Practice. New York, Spectrum Publications, 1985.
2. Hartman D: Neuropsychological Toxicology: Identification and Assessment of Human Neurotoxic Syndromes. New York, Pergamon Press, 1988.
3. Bolla KI: Neuropsychological evaluation for detecting alterations in the central nervous system after chemical exposure. Regul Toxicol Pharmacol 1996;24:548–551.
4. Bolla-Wilson K, Bleecker ML: Neuropsychological impairment following inorganic arsenic exposure. J Occup Med 1987;29:500–503.
5. Kishi Y, Sasaki H, Yamasaki H, et al: An epidemic of arsenic neuropathy from a spiked curry. Neurology 2001;56:1417–1418.
6. Wittmers Jr LE, Wallgren J, Alich A, et al: Lead in bone. IV. Distribution of lead in the human skeleton. Arch Environ Health 1988;43:381–391.
7. Somervaille LJ, Chettle DR, Scott MC, et al: In vivo tibia lead measurements as an index of cumulative exposure in occupationally exposed subjects. Br J Ind Med 1988;45:174–181.
8. Davis JM, Elias RW, Grant LD: Current issues in human lead exposure and future development in the regulation of lead. Neurotoxicology 1993;14:15–28.
9. Annest JL, Pirkle JL, Makuc D, et al: Chronological trend in blood levels between 1976 and 1980. N Engl J Med 1983;308:1373–1377.
10. Bellinger D, Levinton A, Waternaux C, et al: Longitudinal analyses of prenatal and postnatal lead exposure and early cognitive development. N Engl J Med 1987;316:1037–1043.
11. Needleman HL, Schell A, Bellinger D, et al: The long-term effects of exposure to low doses of lead in childhood: An 11 year follow-up report. N Engl J Med 1990;322:83–88.
12. Schwartz BS, Stewart WF, Bolla KI, et al: Past adult lead exposure is associated with longitudinal decline in cognitive function. Neurology, 2000;55:1144–1150.
13. Todd AC, McNeill FE, Palethorpe JE, et al: In vivo x-ray fluorescence of lead in bone using K x-ray excitation with ^{109}Cd sources: Radiation and dosimetry studies. Environ Res 1992;57:117–132.
14. Hanninen H, Hernberg S, Mantere P, et al: Psychological performance of subjects with low exposure to lead. J Occup Med 1978;20:683.
15. Baker EL, Feldman RG, White RF, et al: The role of occupational lead exposure in the genesis of psychiatric and behavioral disturbances. Acta Psychiatr Scand 1983;303:38–48.
16. Ryan CM, Morrow L, Parkinson D, et al: Low level lead exposure and neuropsychological functioning in blue collar males. Int J Neurosci 1987;36:29–39.
17. Balbus-Kornfeld J, Stewart W, Bolla KI, et al: The effect of cumulative lead exposure on neurobehavioral test performance in adults. J Occup Environ Med 1995;52:2–12.
18. Stewart W, Schwartz BS, Simon D, Bolla KI, Todd AC, Links J: Neurobehavioral function and tibial and chelatable lead levels in 543 former organolead workers. Neurology 1999;52:1610–1617.
19. Racette BA, McGee-Minnich L, Moerlien SM, et al: Welding-related parkinsonism: Clinical features, treatment, and pathophysiology. Neurology 2001;56:8–13.
20. Mena I, Court J, Fuenzalida S, et al: Modification of chronic manganese poisoning treatment with L-dopa or 5-OH tryptophane. N Engl J Med 1970;282:5–10.
21. Cotzias GC, Horiuchi K, Fuenzalida S, et al: Chronic manganese poisoning: Clearance of tissue manganese concentrations with persistence of the neurological picture. Neurology 1968;18:376–382.
22. Torres AD, Ashok NR, Hardiek ML: Mercury intoxication and arterial hypertension: Report of two patients and review of the literature. Pediatrics 2000;105:E34.
23. Shiraki H: Neuropathological aspects of organic mercury intoxication. *In* Vinken PJ, Bruyn GW (eds): Handbook of Clinical Neurology. Amsterdam, North-Holland, 1979, pp 83–146.
24. Chang LW, Dyer RS (eds): Handbook of Neurotoxicology. New York, Marcel Dekker, 1995.
25. Hormes J, Filley C, Rosenberg N: Neurologic sequelae of chronic solvent vapor abuse. Neurology 1986;36:698–702.
26. Bolla KI, Schwartz BS, Stewart W, et al: A comparison of neurobehavioral function in workers exposed to a mixture of organic and inorganic lead and in workers exposed to solvents. Am J Ind Med 1995; 27:231–246.
27. Cranmer JM, Goldberg L: Human aspects of solvent neurobehavioral effects. Report of the workshop session on clinical and epidemiological topics. Proceedings of the Workshop on Neurobehavioral Effects of Solvents. Neurotoxicology 1986;7:45–56.
28. Mittal BV, Desai AP, Khade KR: Methyl alcohol poisoning: An autopsy study of 28 cases. J Postgrad Med 1991;37:9–13.
29. Sivilotti ML, Burns M, McMartin K, Brent J, for the Methylpyrazole for Toxic Alcohols Study Group: Toxicokinetics of ethylene glycol during fomepizole therapy: Implications for management. Ann Emerg Med 2000; 36:114–125.
30. Spencer PS, Couri D, Schaumburg HH: *N*-Hexane and methyl *n*-butyl ketone. *In* Spencer PS, Schaumberg HH (eds): Experimental and Clinical Neurotoxicology. Baltimore, Williams & Wilkins, 1980, pp 456–475.
31. Pezzoli G, Canesi M, Antonini A, et al: Hydrocarbon exposure and Parkinson's disease. Neurology 2000;55:667–673.
32. Pezzoli G, Strada O, Silani V, et al: Clinical and pathological features in hydrocarbon-induced parkinsonism. Ann Neurol 1996;40: 922–925.
33. Benignus VA: Neurobehavioral effects of toluene: A review. Neurobehav Toxicol Teratol 1981;3:408–415.
34. Feldman RG: Trichlorethylene. *In* Vinken PJ, Bruyn GW (eds): Handbook of Clinical Neurology. Amsterdam, North-Holland, 1979, pp 457–464.
35. Min SK: A brain syndrome associated with delayed neuropsychiatric sequelae following acute carbon monoxide intoxication. Acta Psychiatr Scand 1986;73:80–86.
36. Gordon MF, Mercandetti M: Carbon monoxide poisoning producing purely cognitive and behavioral sequelae. Neuropsychiatr Neuropsychol Behav Neurol 1989;2:145–152.
37. McConnell R: Pesticides and related compounds. *In* Rosenstock L, Cullen MR (eds): Textbook of Clinical Occupational and Environmental Medicine. Philadelphia, WB Saunders, 1994, pp 847–865.
38. Senanayake N, et al: Acute polyneuropathy after poisoning by a new organophosphate insectide. N Engl J Med 1982;306:155–157.
39. Baker SR, Williamson CF: The Effects of Pesticides on Human Health. Advances in Modern Environmental Toxicology. Princeton, NJ, Princeton Scientific Co, 1990.
40. Horowitz SH, Stark A, Marshall E, et al: A multi-modality assessment of peripheral nerve function in organophosphate-pesticide applicators. J Occup Environ Med 1999;41:405–408.
41. Bhatt MH, Elias MA, Mankodi AK: Acute and reversible parkinsonism due to organophosphate pesticide intoxication: Five cases. Neurology 1999;52:1467–1471.
42. Mayersdorf A, Israeli R: Toxic effects of chlorinated hydrocarbon insecticides on the human electroencephalogram. Arch Environ Health 1974;28:159–163.
43. Van Wendel de Joode B, Wesseling C, Kromhout H, et al: Chronic nervous-system effects of long-term occupational exposure to DDT. Lancet 2001;357:1014–1016.
44. Russell FE: Snake venom poisoning. Vet Human Toxicol 1991;33: 584–586.
45. Bond GR: Snake, spider and scorpion envenomation in North America. Ped Rev 1999;20:147–150.
46. Rodichok LD, Barron KD: Neurologic complications of bee sting, tick bite, spider bite, and scorpion sting. *In* Vinken PJ, Bruyn GW (eds): Handbook of Clinical Neurology. Amsterdam, North-Holland, 1979, pp 107–114.

47. Premawardhena AP, de Silva CE, Fonseka MM, et al: Low dose subcutaneous adrenaline to prevent acute adverse reactions to antivenom serum in people bitten by snakes: Randomized, placebo controlled trial. BMJ 1999;318:1041–1043.
48. Gueron M, Ilia R, Sofer S: The cardiovascular system after scorpion envenomation. J Toxicol Clin Toxicol 1992;30:245–258.
49. Gueron M, Ilia R, Margulis G: Arthropod poisons and the cardiovascular system. Am J Emerg Med 2000;18:708–714.
50. Schaumburg HH, Herskovitz S: The weak child—a cautionary tale. N Engl J Med 2000;342:127–129.
51. Hovell WH: Tick paralysis: A review. Mayo Clin Proc 1943;18:39–49 (Abstract).
52. Masina S, Broady KW: Tick paralysis: Development of a vaccine. Int J Parasitol 1999;29:535–541.
53. Misra UK, Sharma VP: Peripheral and central conduction studies in neurolathyrism. J Neurol Neurosurg Psychiatry 1994;57:572–577.
54. Weaver AL: Lathyrism: A review. Arthritis Rheum 1967;10:470–474.
55. Getahun H, Mekonnen A, Tekle-Haimanot R, et al: Epidemic of neurolathyrism in Ethiopia. Lancet 1999;354:306–307.
56. Gussow L: The optimal management of mushroom poisoning remains undetermined. West J Med 2000;173:317–318.
57. Jander S, Bischoff J, Woodcock BG: Plasmapheresis in the treatment of *Amanita phalloides* poisoning. II. A review and recommendations. Ther Apher 2000;4:308–312.
58. Waksman BH: Experimental study of diphtheric polyneuritis. J Neuropathol Exp Neurol 1961;20:35–45.
59. Weinstein L: Tetanus. N Engl J Med 1973;289:1293.
60. World Health Organization: Progress towards the global elimination of neonatal tetanus, 1990–1998. Wkly Epidemiol Rec 1999;74:73–80.
61. Arnon SS, Midura TF, Damus K, et al: Honey and other environmental risk factors for infant botulism. J Pediatr 1979;94:331–336.
62. Cobb DB, Watson WA, Fernandez MC: Botulism-like syndrome after injections of botulinum toxin. Vet Human Toxicol 2000;42:163.
63. Bhatia KP, Munchau A, Thompson PD, et al: Generalized muscular weakness after botulinum toxin injections for dystonia: a report of three cases. J Neurol Neurosurg Psychiatry 1999;67:90–93.
64. Barrett DH: Endemic food-borne botulism: Clinical experience 1973–1986 at Alaska Native Medical Center. Alaska Med 1991;33:101–108.
65. Urdaneta-Carruyo E, Suranyi A, Milano M: Infantile botulism: Clinical and laboratory observations of a rare neuroparalytic disease. J Paediatr Child Health 2000;36:193–195.
66. Chaudhry V, Crawford TO: Stimulation single-fiber EMG in infant botulism. Muscle Nerve 1999;22:1698–1703.
67. Levine SR, Brust JCM, Futrell N, et al: Cerebrovascular complications of the "crack" form of alkaloidal cocaine. N Engl J Med 1990;323:699.
68. Kaku DA, Lowestein DH: Emergence of recreational drug abuse as a major risk factor for stroke in young adults. Ann Intern Med 1990;113:821.
69. Sloan MA, Kittner SJ, Rigamonti D, et al: Occurrence of stroke associated with use/abuse of drugs. Neurology 1991;41:1358.
70. Krendel DA, Ditter SM, Frankel MR, et al: Biopsy-proven cerebral vasculitis associated with cocaine abuse. Neurology 1991;40:1092.
71. Fredericks RK, Lefkowitz DS, Challa VER, et al: Cerebral vasculitis associated with cocaine abuse. Stroke 1991;22:1437.
72. Herning RI, King DE, Better WE, Cadet J-L: Neurovascular deficits in cocaine abusers. Neuropsychopharmacology 1999;21:110–118.
73. Volkow ND, Fowler JS, Wolf AP, et al: Metabolic studies of drugs of abuse. *In* Harris L (ed): Problems of Drug Dependence 1990. NIDA Research Monograph 105. Washington, DC, Department of Health and Human Services, 1991, p 47.
74. London ED, Cascella NG, Wong DF, et al: Cocaine-induced reduction of glucose utilization in human brain. Arch Gen Psychiatry 1990;47:567–574.
75. Bolla KI, Ernst M, Mouratidis M, et al: Reduced brain activation in chronic cocaine abusers during performance on the Stroop Color-Word Interference Task. Society for Neuroscience Abstract. New Orleans LA, November, 2000.
76. MacDonald AW, Cohen JD, Stenger VA, Carter CS: Dissociating the role of the dorsolateral prefrontal and anterior cingulate cortex in cognitive control. Science 2000;288:1835–1838.
77. Bush G, Frazier JA, Rauch SL, et al: Anterior cingulate cortex dysfunction in attention-deficit/hyperactivity disorder revealed by fMRI and the counting stroop. Biol Psych 1999;45:1542–1552.
78. U.S. Department of Health and Human Services: National Household Survey on Drug Abuse, 2000 [on-line]. Available: www.samhsa.gov. Rockville, MD.
79. Rumbaugh CL, Bergeron T, Gang HCH, et al: Cerebral angiographic changes in the drug abuse patient. Radiology 1971;101:335.
80. Rothrock JF, Rubenstein R, Lyden PD: Ischemic stroke associated with methamphetamine inhalations. Neurology 1988;38:589–592.
81. Rumbaugh CL, Bergeron T, Scanlon RL, et al: Cerebral vascular changes secondary to amphetamine abuse in the experimental animal. Radiology 1971;101:345.
82. Rumbaugh CL, Fang HCH, Higgins RE, et al: Cerebral microvascular injury in experimental drug abuse. Invest Radiol 1976;11:382–394.
83. Stafford CR, Bodganoff BM, Green L, et al: Mononeuropathy multiplex as complication of amphetamine angiitis. Neurology 1975;25:570–572.
84. Martin WR, Sloan JW, Sapira JD, et al: Physiologic, subjective, and behavioral effects of amphetamine, methamphetamine, ephedrine, phenmetrazine, and methylphenidate in man. Clin Pharmacol Ther 1971;12:245.
85. Pollack MA, Cohen NL, Friedhoff AG: Gilles de la Tourette's syndrome: Familial occurrence and precipitation by methylphenidate therapy. Arch Neurol 1977;34:630–632.
86. Bonthala CM, West A: Pemoline induced chorea and Gilles de la Tourette's syndrome. Br J Psychiatry 1983;143:300–302.
87. McCann UD, Ridenour A, Shaham Y, Ricaurte G: Serotonin neurotoxicity after (±) 3,4-methylenedioxymethamphetamine (MDMA, Ecstasy): A controlled study in humans. Neuropsychopharmacology 1994;10:129–138.
88. Bolla KI, Ricaurte G: Memory impairment in abstinent MDMA ("Ecstasy" users). Neurology 1998;51:1532–1537.
89. Gouzoulis-Mayfrank E, Daumann J, Tuchtenhagen F, et al: Impaired cognitive performance in drug-free recreational ecstasy (MDMA) users. J Neurol Neurosurg Psychiatry 2000;68:719–725.
90. Parrott AC: Human research on MDMA (3,4-methylenedioxymethamphetamine) neurotoxicity: Cognitive and behavioural indices of change. Neuropsychobiology 2000;42:17–24.
91. Shiffer D, Brignolio F, Giordena MT, et al: Spongiform encephalopathy in addicts inhaling preheated heroin. Clin Neuropathol 1985;4:174.
92. Martin WR, Frazer HF: A comparative study of physiological and subjective effects of heroin and morphine administered intravenously in post addicts. J Pharmacol Exp Ther 1961;133:388.
93. Lahmeyer HW, Steingold RG: Pentazocine and tripelennamine: A drug abuse epidemic? Int J Addict 1980;15:1219–1232.
94. Goodhart LC, Loizou LA, Anderson M: Heroin myelopathy. J Neurol Neurosurg Psychiatry 1982;45:562–563.
95. Loizou LA, Boddie HG: Polyradiculoneuropathy associated with heroin abuse. J Neurol Neurosurg Psychiatry 1978;41:855–587.
96. Brust JCM, Richter RW: Tetanus in the inner city. NY State J Med 1974;74:1735.
97. Davis GC, Williams AC, Markey SP, et al: Chronic Parkinsonism secondary to intravenous injection of meperidine analogs. Psychiatry Res 1979;1:249.
98. Langston JW, Ballard P, Teturd JW, et al: Chronic Parkinsonism due to a product of meperidine analog synthesis. Science 1983;219:979–980.
99. McCrodden JM, Tipton KF, Sullivan JP: The neurotoxicity of MPTP and the relevance to Parkinson's disease. Pharmacol Toxicol 1990; 67:8–13.
100. Cadet JL, Brannock C: Free radicals and the pathobiology of brain dopamine systems. Neurochem Int 1998;32:117–131.
101. Herning RI, Better WE, Tate K, Cadet J-L: Marijuana abusers are at increased risk for stroke. Ann NY Acad Sci 2001;939:413–415.

CHAPTER 40

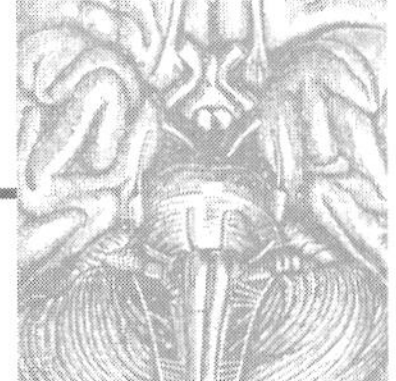

LAURENCE J. KINSELLA and DAVID E. RILEY

Nutritional Deficiencies and Syndromes Associated with Alcoholism

History and Definitions

The study of nutritional disorders of the nervous system is complex for several reasons. First, multiple deficiencies may coexist in the same patient in certain settings, such as malnutrition and malabsorption states. Second, nutritional disorders can occur with the ingestion of potentially toxic agents as in alcohol, making it difficult to separate the neurotoxic effects from a specific dietary deficiency. Third, in several disorders a single so-called biochemical lesion has not been identified, such as in Marchiafava-Bignami disease, central pontine myelinolysis, Strachan's syndrome, and deficiency amblyopia. Fourth, the rapidity of onset of some syndromes may not be interpreted as nutritional. Instead of evolving in a slowly progressive fashion, some deficiency states may become acutely symptomatic when triggered by an environmental stressor or sudden increase in metabolic demands for the deficient nutrient. The administration of intravenous glucose to a thiamin-depleted alcoholic patient may precipitate acute Wernicke-Korsakoff syndrome (WKS) owing to the sudden increase in thiamin-dependent carbohydrate catabolism. Intractable vomiting due to hyperemesis gravidarum may also cause WKS. Similarly, nitrous oxide administration to patients with asymptomatic cobalamin deficiency may cause an acute myeloneuropathy. Additionally, sudden changes in tissue osmolarity, such as the rapid correction of hyponatremia, may lead to central pontine myelinolysis (Table 40–1).

Fifth, at times, the same deficient nutrient may not affect patients uniformly. Thiamin deficiency leads to capillary proliferation, petechiae, and microglial degeneration of midline central nervous system (CNS) nuclei in some patients; in others, it leads to peripheral nerve axonal degeneration.

TABLE 40–1. **Acute and Subacute Presentation of Nutritional Deficiency Syndromes**

Syndrome	Clinical Setting
Wernicke-Korsakoff syndrome	Administration of intravenous glucose to a thiamine-deficient alcoholic patient
Wernicke-Korsakoff syndrome	Intractable vomiting due to hyperemesis gravidarum or gastroplasty
Postgastroplasty neuropathy	Intractable vomiting and severe weight loss in patients following weight reduction surgical procedures
Vitamin B_{12} myeloneuropathy	Nitrous oxide administration in cobalamin-deficient patients
Central pontine myelinolysis	Sudden change in tissue osmolarity in critically ill patients or alcoholics

Neurological symptoms and signs of individual deficiency states often overlap, making clinical distinction difficult. For example, encephalopathy may be seen in deficiencies of thiamin, cobalamin, and niacin; myeloneuropathy may be present in deficiencies of cobalamin and vitamin E; neuropathy can result from deficiency of B complex vitamins (thiamin, pyridoxine, and cobalamin) and pyridoxine excess; and optic neuropathy may be seen in cobalamin deficiency, vitamin A excess, or a combined deficiency of B complex vitamins, such as in deficiency amblyopia.

Sixth, the under-recognition of nutritional disorders in industrialized countries has led to difficulties in diagnosis, and these deficiencies may be more common than has been clinically appreciated. Although the incidence of WKS has traditionally ranged from 1 to 3 percent, autopsy data suggest a higher incidence,[1,2] and others report thiamin deficiency in up to 17 percent of elderly patients hospitalized for non-neurological reasons.[3] One study of thiamin-deficient alcoholics showed that over 50 percent of patients were also riboflavin deficient, and 2 percent had a concomitant deficiency of pyridoxine.[4] Cobalamin deficiency occurs in 5 to 14 percent of ambulatory elderly,[5,6] and up to 27 percent of hospitalized elderly develop protein-energy malnutrition (PEM) during their hospital stay.[7]

Finally, several inherited enzyme deficiency disorders, although not accompanied by a vitamin deficiency, may nonetheless be vitamin responsive (Table 40–2). Homocysteinemia responds to pharmacological doses of folate, cobalamin, and pyridoxine, whereas methylmalonicacidemia responds to cobalamin. Maple syrup urine disease, a branched-chain aminoaciduria, may be responsive to high-dose thiamin by inducing the enzyme alpha-ketoacid decarboxylase, promoting metabolism of branched-chain amino acids. Beta-methylcrotonylglycinuria and propionicacidemia may be responsive to biotin replacement; Hartnup's disease, a disorder of tryptophan metabolism, is also responsive to niacin.

Vitamin Deficiencies

THIAMIN

The discovery and isolation of vitamins began with the study of beriberi in the 19th century. Although beriberi has been recognized for centuries, it was not until the Industrial Revolution that the disease reached epidemic proportions. Grain mills began producing polished rice, which was mechanically stripped of the nutrient-rich husk. Epidemics of painful polyneuropathy and heart failure rapidly developed in regions where rice was the major source of carbohydrate, particularly in Asia. In 1897, Eijkman demonstrated the disease in pigeons after feeding the birds polished rice; he then cured the disease by feeding the same birds crude, unpolished rice. A search then began for the antineuritic factor within the rice husks. Funk thought he had identified the antiberiberi factor in 1911 as an amine within rice bran extracts and coined the term vitamine. Elvehjem later identified Funk's substance as the antipellagra factor nicotinic acid amide (niacin). The antiberiberi factor was synthesized in 1936, and the name was changed to thiamin to reflect the molecule's sulfur content.[8]

TABLE 40–2. **Characteristics of Disorders Responding to Large Doses of Vitamins and Cofactors**

Vitamin	Disorder	Affected Enzyme	Therapeutic Dose
Thiamine (vitamin B_1)	Branched-chain ketoaciduria (maple syrup urine disease)	Branched-chain ketoacid decarboxylase	5 to 20 mg
	Lactic acidosis	Pyruvate carboxylase	5 to 20 mg
	Pyruvicacidemia	Pyruvate dehydrogenase	5 to 20 mg
Cobalamin (vitamin B_{12})	Methylmalonicaciduria	Methylmalonyl-CoA mutase apoenzyme	2000 μg
	Homocystinuria	Defects in adenosyl-cobalamin and methyl-cobalamin synthesis	500 to 1000 μg
Pyridoxine (B_6)	Homocystinuria	Cystathionine synthase	200 to 1200 μg
	Pyridoxine-responsive infantile seizures	Glutamic acid decarboxylase	10 to 50 mg
Niacin	Hartnup's disease	Intestinal malabsorption of tryptophan	>400 mg
Folic acid	Homocystinuria	Methylenetetrahydrofolate reductase	>10 mg
Biotin	Beta-methylcrotonylglycinuria	Beta-methylcrotonyl-CoA carboxylase	5 to 10 mg
	Propionicacidemia	Propionyl-CoA carboxylase	5 to 10 mg

Adapted from Moser H: Genetic and metabolic diseases. *In* Asbury AK, McKhann GM, McDonald WI (eds): Diseases of the Nervous System: Clinical Neurobiology, 2nd ed. Philadelphia, WB Saunders, 1992, p 676.

Pathogenesis and Pathophysiology. The metabolically active form of thiamin, called thiamin pyrophosphate (TPP), is critical in the intermediary metabolism of carbohydrate. TPP is involved in three enzyme systems: (1) pyruvate dehydrogenase, which converts pyruvate to acetyl coenzyme A; (2) α-ketoglutarate dehydrogenase, which catalyzes the conversion of α-ketoglutarate to succinate in the Krebs cycle; and (3) transketolase, which catalyzes the pentose monophosphate shunt (Fig. 40–1). A deficiency of TPP leads to elevated levels of serum pyruvate and occasionally lactate, reduced red blood cell (RBC) transketolase activity, and a corresponding increase in transketolase activity in response to added TPP (TPP effect). It is not understood how TPP deficiency leads to the hallmark pathology.

Pathologically, patients with WKS show capillary proliferation and petechiae; spongy degeneration of astrocytes with neuronal preservation occurs in midline structures of the brain, such as the medial thalamic nuclei, mammillary bodies, periaqueductal gray area of the mesencephalon, and pontine tegmentum (Fig. 40–2). Degeneration of the superior cerebellar vermis is usually present. The lesions in the thalami and mammillary bodies probably account for the confusion, memory loss, and confabulation. The pontine tegmental lesions may cause the oculomotor palsies, and the truncal ataxia may result from the midline cerebellar degeneration. Cellular injury in these regions may be due to the inhibition of adenosine triphosphate (ATP) synthesis and the induction of abnormal carbohydrate metabolism. With thiamin deficiency polyneuropathy, the nerve shows axonal degeneration with secondary demyelination. Because of the frequency of this neuropathy in alcoholics, there is debate as to whether the cause is alcohol toxicity or thiamin deficiency. It has been theorized that the neuropathy of dry beriberi may be related to TPP deficiency–induced impairment of nerve excitability and conduction.[9]

Epidemiology and Risk Factors. Thiamin is most abundant in yeast, pork, legumes, cereal grains, and rice, and the recommended daily allowance (RDA) of this vitamin is 0.5 mg/1000 kcal.[10] The total body store is 30 to 100 mg, and it is present in heart, skeletal muscle, liver, kidneys, and brain. Because there is a limited quantity stored, the supply must be constantly replenished. The half-life of thiamin is approximately 2 weeks, and patients may suffer severe neurological complications and even death after 6 weeks of total thiamin depletion. Patients at high risk for deficiency include adults who derive most of their carbohydrate from milled rice, alcoholics, and infants breast fed by malnourished mothers. Other potentially thiamin-deficient states include prolonged total parenteral nutrition,[11] hyperemesis gravidarum,[12] anorexia nervosa, gastric or jejunoileal bypass,[13] intractable vomiting following gastric stapling for morbid obesity,[14] and severe malabsorption. Thiamin deficiency is also found in

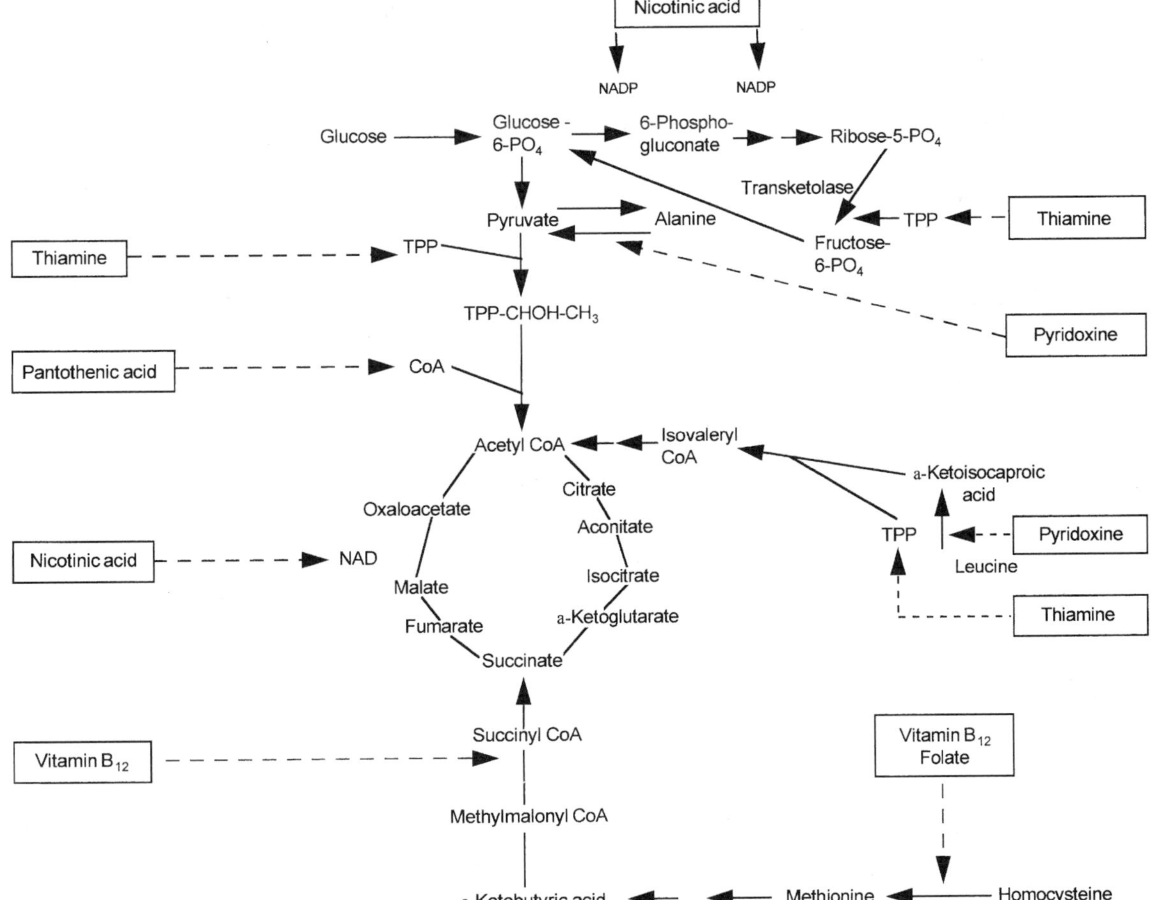

FIGURE 40–1. Major metabolic pathways involving coenzymes formed from water-soluble vitamins. (Modified from Marcus R, Coulston AM: Water soluble vitamins. *In* Goodman LS, Gilman A, Gilman AG [eds]: The Pharmacologic Basis of Therapeutics, 7th ed. New York, McGraw-Hill, 1985, p 1556.)

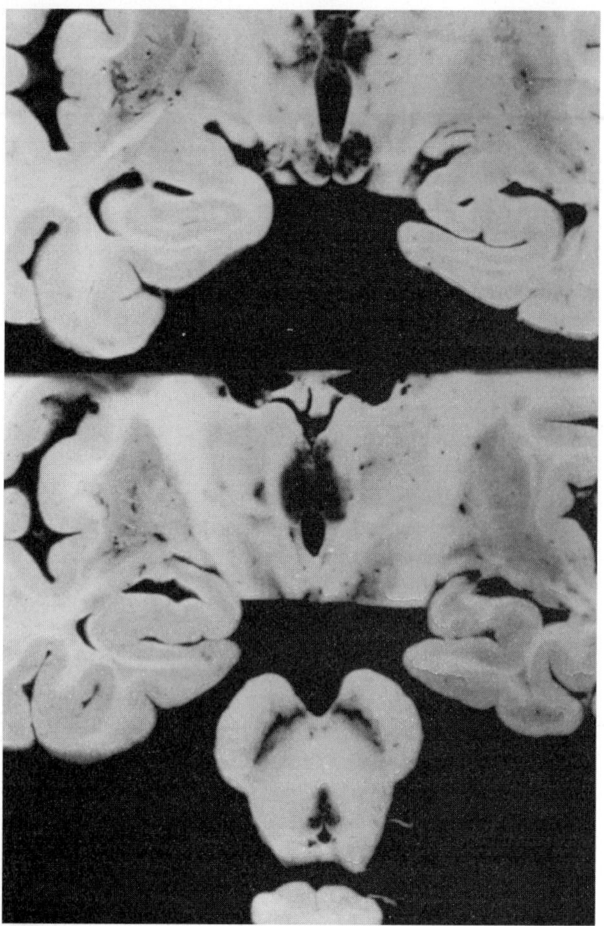

FIGURE 40–2. Wernicke's encephalopathy. Gross appearance characterized by petechial hemorrhages in the typical locations. (Reprinted with permission from Okazaki H: Fundamentals of Neuropathology, 2nd ed. New York, Igaku Shoin, 1989, p 192.)

those who are prisoners of war[12] or those who engage in a hunger strike. Thiamin deficiency has also been reported after long-standing peritoneal dialysis and hemodialysis.[15, 16]

Clinical Features and Associated Disorders. WKS and polyneuropathy (dry beriberi) are the two neurological disorders resulting from thiamin deficiency. Wernicke's disease and Korsakoff's psychosis often overlap, with Wernicke's disease having acute features of confusion, ataxia, and oculomotor palsies and nystagmus and Korsakoff's psychosis having delayed and often irreversible anterograde and retrograde memory impairment. Korsakoff's dementia may follow one or more episodes of Wernicke's encephalopathy. Although prospective clinical studies, including those of Victor,[8] suggest a high incidence of the classic triad in WKS, other autopsy series have found pathological evidence for the disorder in many patients with only one or two symptoms during life.[2]

The frequency of WKS from autopsy series ranges from 0.8 to 2.8 percent. The disorder is probably underdiagnosed during life. WKS is most common in alcoholics because patients are particularly susceptible to thiamin deficiency due to a combination of poor diet, inadequate intake and impaired absorption of vitamins, and overdependence on alcohol as a source of calories. Certain individuals may also have a genetic predisposition toward the development of WKS owing to an abnormality of thiamin-dependent enzymes.[17, 18]

Patients with thiamin deficiency may become acutely symptomatic when challenged with large doses of carbohydrate. An example is the alcoholic patient receiving intravenous glucose who then becomes agitated, confused, and ataxic. Acute attacks may also be produced by excessive vomiting, such as that associated with hyperemesis gravidarum, presumably due to markedly increased metabolic demands in the setting of decreased consumption.[8]

Mental status changes may include a global confusional state, memory loss, and agitation. Rarely, patients develop stupor and coma. Ocular abnormalities include nystagmus, lateral rectus palsies, conjugate gaze palsy, ptosis, retinal hemorrhages, pupillary abnormalities, and scotomas. Ataxia may be severe, preventing an affected patient from standing without assistance. Finger-to-nose and heel-to-shin tests are often normal when the patient is tested in the bed. Truncal ataxia often becomes obvious only on standing or sitting, reflecting the midline degeneration of the superior division of the vermis.

Polyneuropathy is present in over 80 percent of patients with WKS. It presents with slowly progressive muscular weakness and sensory and reflex loss, accompanied by burning feet and lancinating pains. Calf tenderness is a prominent feature. Bilateral footdrop and even wristdrop may be present (Fig. 40–3). Patients may also develop an autonomic neuropathy with orthostatic hypotension.

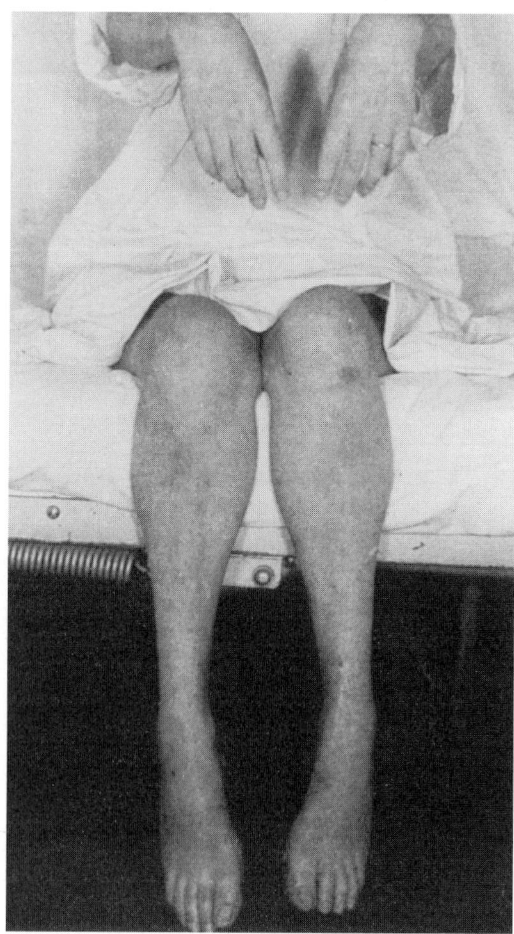

FIGURE 40–3. Bilateral wristdrop and footdrop in a 40-year-old woman with Wernicke-Korsakoff syndrome and polyneuropathy. (From Victor M, Adams RD, Collins GH: The Wernicke-Korsakoff Syndrome. Philadelphia, F.A. Davis, 1971.)

Differential Diagnosis. The presence of mild peripheral edema with a peripheral neuropathy may be a helpful physical sign to suggest thiamin deficiency with co-existing cardiac failure (wet beriberi). Thiamin deficiency should be considered in the differential diagnosis of an axonal polyneuropathy and be distinguished from diabetes, uremia, autoimmune and inflammatory conditions, and hereditary neuropathies. Other considerations in patients presenting with confusion, ataxia, and oculomotor disturbances should include hypoxic-ischemic encephalopathy, Leigh's encephalomyelopathy, adrenoleukodystrophy, metachromatic leukodystrophy, brain stem encephalitis, and certain infectious disorders (syphilis and human immunodeficiency virus [HIV]). Other nutrients deficient among alcoholics may include folic acid, pyridoxine, and niacin.[19]

Evaluation. The evaluation of patients with thiamin deficiency begins with a high index of suspicion, and the clinician must recognize that the disorder is not restricted to alcoholics. Several tests, including RBC transketolase activity assay, TPP stimulation of RBC transketolase (the TPP effect), and 24-hour urinary excretion of thiamin are used to assess thiamin status. Serum thiamin levels lack sufficient sensitivity and specificity to be used alone. RBC transketolase activity, with or without TPP challenge, is the most accurate assessment tool.[20] This test, however, is increasingly difficult to find commercially. Magnetic resonance imaging (MRI) may show abnormal signal in the midline nuclei corresponding to the pathological lesions described (Fig. 40–4).[11, 21]

Management. Treatment of suspected WKS begins with the immediate administration of at least 100 mg intravenous thiamin, followed by 100 mg IM daily for 3 to 5 days. Patients should then be maintained on 50 mg oral thiamin and daily multivitamins.

Prognosis and Future Perspectives. Whereas early recognition and treatment may reverse all symptoms, in practice, WKS often goes unrecognized until late in the disease, and therapy rarely reverses all of its manifestations. The oculomotor disturbances respond best to treatment and may show improvement within hours. Confusion and ataxia are more resistant. The peripheral neuropathy is often resistant to therapy unless it is treated early. Despite treatment, the mental changes of WKS may progress to permanent and disabling dementia.[22] Recent work by Gold and colleagues has found abnormalities of thiamin metabolism in patients with Alzheimer's disease.[23] Molecular genetics may help identify patients and families with a hereditary predisposition toward the development of WKS. Further characterization of the role of thiamin in the sodium-potassium ATPase pump may further our understanding of its role in nerve excitability and conduction, increasing our understanding of the pathogenesis of the neuropathy.[9] Some countries have experimented with fortification of food substances with thiamin to reduce the incidence of WKS, and fortification of alcoholic beverages has been advocated.

NIACIN AND NICOTINIC ACID

Nicotinic acid deficiency was found to be the causative agent of pellagra in 1937, yet the name was changed to niacin in order to prevent confusion with the tobacco derivative, nicotine. Niacin includes both nicotinic acid and nicotinamide, which form the metabolically active nicotinamide adenine dinucleotide (NAD) and NAD phosphate (NADP), an end product of tryptophan metabolism. More than 200 enzymes are dependent on NAD and NADP to carry out oxidation and reduction reactions, and these enzymes are involved in the synthesis and breakdown of all carbohydrates, lipids, and amino acids. Although niacin is endogenously produced in humans, exogenous intake is required in order to prevent deficiency. Niacin is found in meats, liver, fish, legumes, peanuts, enriched bread, coffee, and tea.

Pellagra continues to occur in portions of Africa and Asia, especially in populations dependent on corn as the principle source of carbohydrate. When corn is first soaked in lime

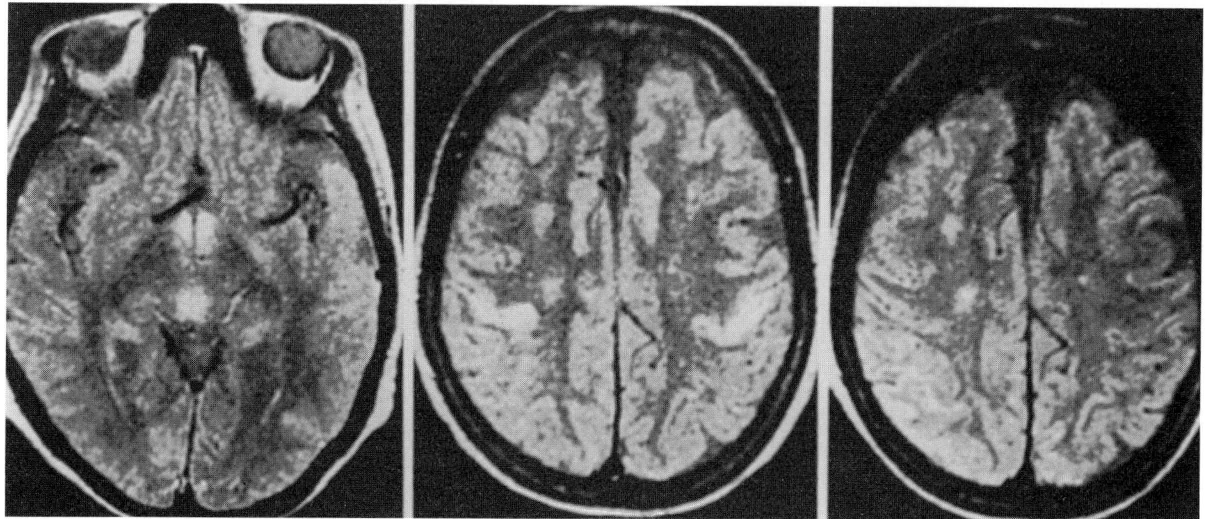

FIGURE 40–4. T2-Weighted magnetic resonance imaging of a patient with Wernicke-Korsakoff syndrome, demonstrating symmetrically increased signal intensity in the periaqueductal gray and midline structures. (From Yamashita M, Yamamoto T: Wernicke encephalopathy with symmetric pericentral involvement: MR findings. J Comput Assist Tomogr 1995;19:307.)

water, as is done in Mexico when tortillas are prepared, niacin is liberated and deficiency occurs less commonly. In the United States, niacin deficiency is seen in alcoholics and in those taking isoniazid. There is a single case report of a patient developing nicotinic acid deficiency after valproic acid therapy.[24] Pregnant women are protected from niacin deficiency owing to their enhanced ability to convert tryptophan to niacin endogenously, particularly in the third trimester.

Pellagra, or rough skin, affects the skin, the gastrointestinal system, and the CNS. Hence, the classic triad of the "three Ds"—dermatitis, diarrhea, and dementia. In industrialized countries, particularly among alcoholics, niacin deficiency may present only with encephalopathy.[25–27] Patients may have altered sensorium, diffuse rigidity of the limbs, and grasping and sucking reflexes. Dementia and confusion are the most constant findings, followed by diarrhea (50 percent) and dermatitis (30 percent).[27] Spinal cord and peripheral nerve defects have also been reported, particularly in prisoners of war.[12] Co-existing deficiencies of thiamin and pyridoxine are common, especially in alcoholics. Hartnup's disease, an autosomal recessive defect in tryptophan absorption by the gut and kidney, can give a clinical picture identical to pellagra that is responsive to niacin administration. Carcinoid syndrome can also produce niacin deficiency. Because all tryptophan is diverted to the production of serotonin in this disorder, none is available for the production of nicotinic acid, thereby predisposing to deficiency in the absence of supplementation.

Superphysiological doses of niacin (1.5 to 3 g daily) have been used successfully in the treatment of hypercholesterolemia, and this practice diminishes mortality by reducing a coronary artery disease risk factor. Side effects of high-dose niacin include flushing, hyperuricemia, hyperglycemia, and elevations in liver enzymes.

In the evaluation of potential niacin deficiency, nicotinic acid metabolites can be detected in the urine; however, clinical suspicion and ease of treatment make this measurement impractical and unnecessary. The administration of 40 to 250 mg of niacin daily is adequate to reverse most of the signs and symptoms of niacin deficiency. With proper therapy, the prognosis for the resolution of neurological symptoms is good.

COBALAMIN (VITAMIN B_{12})

Pathogenesis and Pathophysiology. Vitamin B_{12} deficiency produces neurological and hematological effects by impairing the function of two enzyme systems (Fig. 40–5).[6, 28] Methylcobalamin is a cofactor of methionine synthase, a cytosolic enzyme that catalyzes the conversion of homocysteine and methyltetrahydrofolate to produce methionine and tetrahydrofolate. Methionine is further metabolized to S-adenosylmethionine, which is necessary for methylation of myelin sheath phospholipids and proteins. Tetrahydrofolate is the required precursor for purine and pyrimidine synthesis. In the mitochondria, adenosylcobalamin catalyzes the conversion of L-methylmalonyl-CoA to succinyl-CoA.

In deficiency states, serum levels of homocysteine and methylmalonic acid rise. Although the mechanism of megaloblastic changes in both folate and cobalamin deficiency is reasonably well understood, the biochemical basis of the neurological damage that occurs in cobalamin deficiency remains uncertain. Of the two reactions that require cobalamin, the methionine synthase reaction is considered more likely to play a critical role in nervous system function. Rarely, neurological complications have also been reported in folate deficiency, because methionine synthase also requires this cosubstrate.[29] It has been proposed that the accumulation of methylmalonate and propionate provide abnormal substrates for fatty acid synthesis, resulting in abnormal odd-carbon and branched-chain fatty acids, so-called "funny fatty acids," which may be incorporated into the myelin sheath and interfere with impulse conduction.

Vitamin B_{12} deficiency results in demyelination of the posterior columns, corticospinal tracts, and white matter of the cerebral hemispheres (Fig. 40–6).[30] Less commonly, a sensorimotor and autonomic neuropathy that is axonal and demyelinating in nature may also be present.[31] These lesions lead to a constellation of symptoms, including cognitive and affective disorders, ataxia, spasticity, and paresthesias.

Epidemiology and Risk Factors. The total body store of cobalamin is 2000 to 5000 μg, half of which is stored in the liver. The recommended daily allowance is 6 μg/day, and the average diet provides 20 μg/day. Because the vitamin is tightly conserved through enterohepatic circulation, 2 to 5

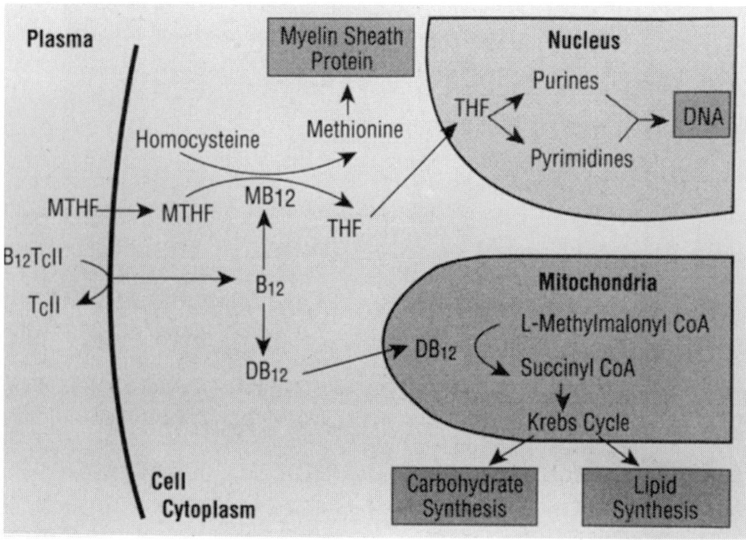

FIGURE 40–5. Intracellular vitamin B_{12} interactions. See the text for description. B_{12} indicates vitamin B_{12} (cyanocobalamin); MB_{12}, methylcobalamin; DB_{12}, deoxyadenosylcobalamin; TcII, transcobalamin II; B_{12}TcII, transcobalamin II-bound cobalamin; MTHF, methyltetrahydrofolate; THF, tetrahydrofolate; and CoA, coenzyme A. (From Flippo TS, Holder WD Jr: Neurologic degeneration associated with nitrous oxide anesthesia in patients with vitamin B_{12} deficiency. Arch Surg 1993;128:1391–1395.)

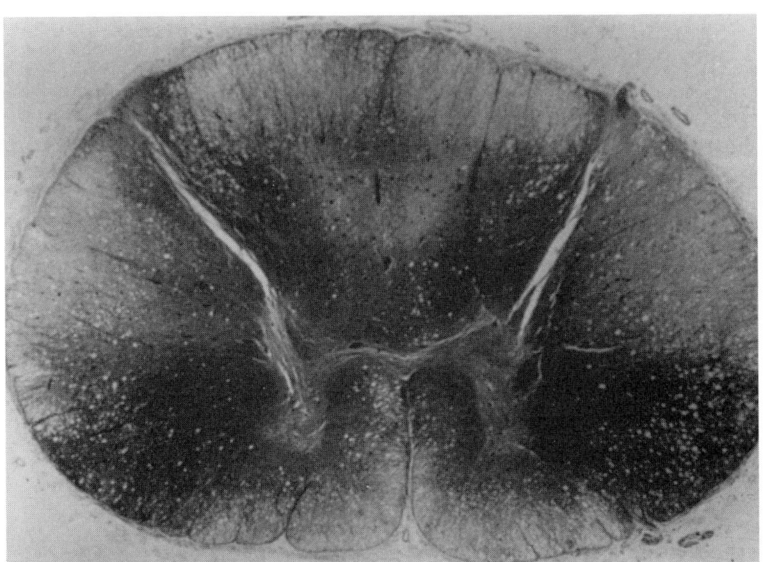

FIGURE 40–6. Subacute combined degeneration of the spinal cord. A thoracic cord segment showing spongy degeneration of the white matter in a typical distribution (Weil's stain). (From Okazaki H: Fundamentals of Neuropathology, 2nd ed. New York, Igaku Shoin, 1989, p 195.)

years elapse before a subject develops cobalamin deficiency from malabsorption, and as long as 10 to 20 years are needed to induce a dietary deficiency from a strict vegetarian diet.

The most common cause of vitamin B_{12} deficiency is pernicious anemia or autoimmune parietal cell dysfunction (Table 40–3).[32] The mean age of diagnosis is 60 years, and the female-to-male ratio is approximately 1.5:1. In white populations, the incidence of the disease increases with increasing age, peaking after age 65. In Hispanic and African populations, there is an overall younger age distribution, especially among women. When using radioassay-derived serum cobalamin levels below 200 pg/mL or elevated levels of homocysteine and methylmalonic acid as diagnostic criteria, the prevalence of vitamin B_{12} deficiency from all causes ranges from 7 to 16 percent.[5]

The majority of patients, roughly 50 to 78 percent, have autoimmune parietal cell dysfunction (pernicious anemia).[32]

TABLE 40–3. **Causes of Cobalamin Deficiency**

Etiology	Percent
Pernicious anemia	
Proven*	66
Probable†	12
Tropical sprue	6
Gastric resection	4
Ileal resection	3
Jejunal diverticula	2
Dietary cobalamin malabsorption	
Probable‡	2
Multiple etiologies	3
Unknown	2

*Intrinsic factor antibodies present, or, correction of abnormal Part I Schilling test with intrinsic factor.

†Evidence of achlorhydria (elevated serum gastrin) with abnormal Part I Schilling test in some, but evaluation incomplete.

‡Evidence of achlorhydria (elevated serum gastrin) with a normal Part I Schilling test.

Reprinted with permission from Healton EV, Savage DG, Brust JCN, et al: Neurologic aspects of cobalamin deficiency. Medicine (Baltimore) 1991;70:229–244.

Another 10 to 40 percent have food-bound cobalamin malabsorption due to achlorhydria.[33] The rest have a variety of etiologies, mainly due to malabsorption from medical, surgical, or pharmacological interruptions of gastric acid secretion or intrinsic factor secretion. These include patients following gastric surgery,[34] bypass procedures for weight reduction,[35] as well as those on long-term histamine-2 (H_2) blocker therapy, due to inhibition of acid secretion.[36] Nitrous oxide administration may precipitate acute vitamin B_{12} deficiency in patients with asymptomatic low cobalamin levels.[37] Other causes of vitamin B_{12} deficiency include ileal resection, parasitic infestations from *Diphyllobothrium latum*, Crohn's disease and other malabsorption states, short gut syndrome, veganism, chronic alcoholism with poor diet, and rare congenital enzyme deficiencies.

Clinical Features and Associated Disorders. Subacute combined degeneration of the spinal cord, peripheral nerve dysfunction, and cerebral dysfunction are classic features of the disorder. Many patients present without accompanying anemia or macrocytosis. Healton and associates reviewed 143 patients who had 153 episodes of cobalamin deficiency.[38] Seventy-four percent of the episodes presented with neurological symptoms, including paresthesias, numbness, gait ataxia, fecal incontinence, leg weakness, impaired manual dexterity, impaired memory, and impotence. Rarely, patients had orthostatic lightheadedness, anosmia, diminished taste, paranoid psychosis, and diminished visual acuity. The remaining 26 percent presented with non-neurological symptoms classically associated with pernicious anemia, including tiredness, syncope, palpitations, sore tongue, diarrhea, and other bowel disturbances.

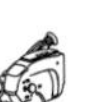

On examination, patients demonstrate a neuropathy in 25 percent, isolated myelopathy in 12 percent, and a combined neuropathy and myelopathy in 41 percent. Peripheral neuropathic symptoms and signs were combined with other manifestations such as myelopathy, cortical dysfunction, and autonomic dysfunction in 65 percent. Only 3 percent have a neuropathy as the only abnormality. Memory dysfunction and affective and behavioral changes were seen in 8 percent. Cognitive deficits included psychosis, affective disturbances, and memory disturbances, as well as changes in personality.

Orthostatic hypotension has been reported and is thought to be due to a disordered release of norepinephrine.[39, 40] Fourteen percent had normal examinations.

There have been several reports of patients developing a myeloneuropathy after exposure to nitrous oxide.[28, 37, 41] This occurs in two populations: those with normal cobalamin levels, but who chronically abuse the anesthetic gas for recreational purposes, and those with a subclinical vitamin B_{12} deficiency who, after a short exposure to nitrous oxide for a dental or surgical procedure, develop paresthesias, burning feet, and ataxia. Nitrous oxide is a potent oxidizing agent, which irreversibly oxidizes the cobalt core of cobalamin from a 1+ valence state to 3+ valence state, rendering methylcobalamin inactive. This effectively inhibits the conversion of homocysteine to methionine, thus interdicting the supply of S-adenosylmethionine.

Low cobalamin levels have also been found in occasional patients with multiple sclerosis[42] and HIV infection[43]; however, no pathogenic relationship or treatment response has been established in either disorder.

Differential Diagnosis. The diagnostic criteria for vitamin B_{12} deficiency include a consistent clinical syndrome of ataxia, paresthesias, cognitive dysfunction, and evidence of neuropathic or myelopathic dysfunction. A megaloblastic anemia is often missing in patients with neurologic symptoms.[32] In fact, a quarter have no anemia or macrocystosis.[38] The most characteristic presentation is gait dysfunction and paresthesias in an elderly individual. The hallmark finding of a myeloneuropathy, absent ankle reflexes and extensor plantar responses, is present in only 41 percent.[38] Vitamin B_{12} deficiency must be differentiated from other causes of myelopathy and neuropathy. Myelopathy and mental decline may also be seen in multiple sclerosis, but the other neuropathic signs of vitamin B_{12} deficiency should clarify the likely diagnosis. Other disorders that may have both central and peripheral manifestations include syphilis, amyotrophic lateral sclerosis, Friedreich's ataxia, vitamin E deficiency, metachromatic leukodystrophy, adrenomyeloneuropathy, mitochondrial cytopathy, and ceroid lipofuscinosis. These diagnoses should be considered in patients with the paradoxical findings of absent ankle reflexes and extensor plantar responses. Cervical spondylitic myelopathy with lumbar osteoarthropathy and cauda equina compression may also give a similar clinical pattern.

Evaluation. An algorithm for the diagnosis and treatment of cobalamin deficiency has been established (Fig. 40–7). It is based on two assumptions: (1) a normal cobalamin assay does not fully exclude cobalamin deficiency; and (2) the normal range may vary depending on the assay type. Many laboratories are switching from radioassay to chemiluminescence assay, which may have a higher normal reference range (250 to 1100 pg/mL).

In a patient with signs and symptoms of cobalamin deficiency, a cobalamin assay should be ordered initially. If the assay result is less than the lower limit of normal, intrinsic factor antibodies should be measured. In pernicious anemia, additional laboratory evidence of an autoimmune process is often found. Serum antibodies are present against parietal cells in 90 percent and against intrinsic factor in 60 percent of patients with pernicious anemia. Unfortunately, false-positive results for the gastric parietal cell test are common (found in 10 percent of people older than 70 years of age), and although the test for intrinsic factor antibodies lacks sensitivity, it is much more specific. If this test is positive, confirmation of the diagnosis of pernicious anemia with a Schilling test (see later) is not necessary.

In patients with serum cobalamin levels in the lower normal range, but in whom one still suspects cobalamin deficiency, the measurement of metabolite levels is appropriate. If either is elevated, then serum intrinsic factor antibodies should be measured. If the test for intrinsic factor antibodies is negative, then measurement of the serum gastrin level may be useful for establishing the presence of achlorhydria, which is almost invariably associated with pernicious anemia. The presence of hypersegmentation may be a sensitive marker for cobalamin deficiency, even in the absence of anemia or macrocytosis.

If metabolites or the serum gastrin levels are elevated, a Schilling test should be performed to evaluate for the presence of cobalamin malabsorption. Technically, patients with classic pernicious anemia have an abnormal test result when radioactive cobalamin alone is given by mouth (Part I of the Schilling test). This abnormality is corrected when the test is repeated with intrinsic factor (Part II of the Schilling test). Abnormally low secretion of cobalamin in Part II of the Schilling test indicates an intestinal cause for the cobalamin malabsorption, such as inflammatory bowel disease. Part II of the Schilling test may be repeated, after giving antibiotics or vermicides to exclude bacterial overgrowth (so-called blind loop syndrome) or fish tapeworm infestation due to *Diphyllobothrium latum*. Normal results on Part I of the test in a patient with cobalamin deficiency may be observed in total vegetarians. It may also occur in patients with food-cobalamin malabsorption who show normal absorption of crystalline cobalamin but are unable to digest and absorb cobalamin present in food due to achlorhydria. This defect can be identified using a modified Schilling test in which radioactive cobalamin is administered with food.

Management. Treatment may begin with intramuscular (IM) injections of 1000 μg of cobalamin per day for 5 days, then 500 to 1000 μg IM every month. Oral replacement is an alternative for patients who cannot tolerate intramuscular injections or for whom they are impractical. Recently, Kusiminski has demonstrated that 2000 μg vitamin B_{12} is as effective or more effective than intramuscular injections given monthly for maintaining normal serum vitamin B_{12} levels and correcting elevation in serum methylmalonic acid, with a comparable onset of action.[44] This effect occurred regardless of etiology and included patients with pernicious anemia, food-cobalamin malabsorption, and a history of gastric surgery. A loading dose was not necessary for oral replacement as serum metabolite elevations normalized as rapidly as did those patients receiving intramuscular loading doses.

Because 1 percent of all ingested cobalamin may be absorbed by passive diffusion, cobalamin requirements can be satisfied with oral therapy, even in patients with pernicious anemia, as long as the dose is sufficient. A dose of 1000 μg/day will yield 10 μg of absorbed cobalamin, which exceeds the recommended daily allowance. It may be practical to replenish cobalamin stores first using injections of cyanocobalamin for 1 week and then to maintain patients using a 1000 μg daily oral supplement.

Prognosis and Future Perspectives. The earlier intervention begins, the more likely the patient is to have a complete

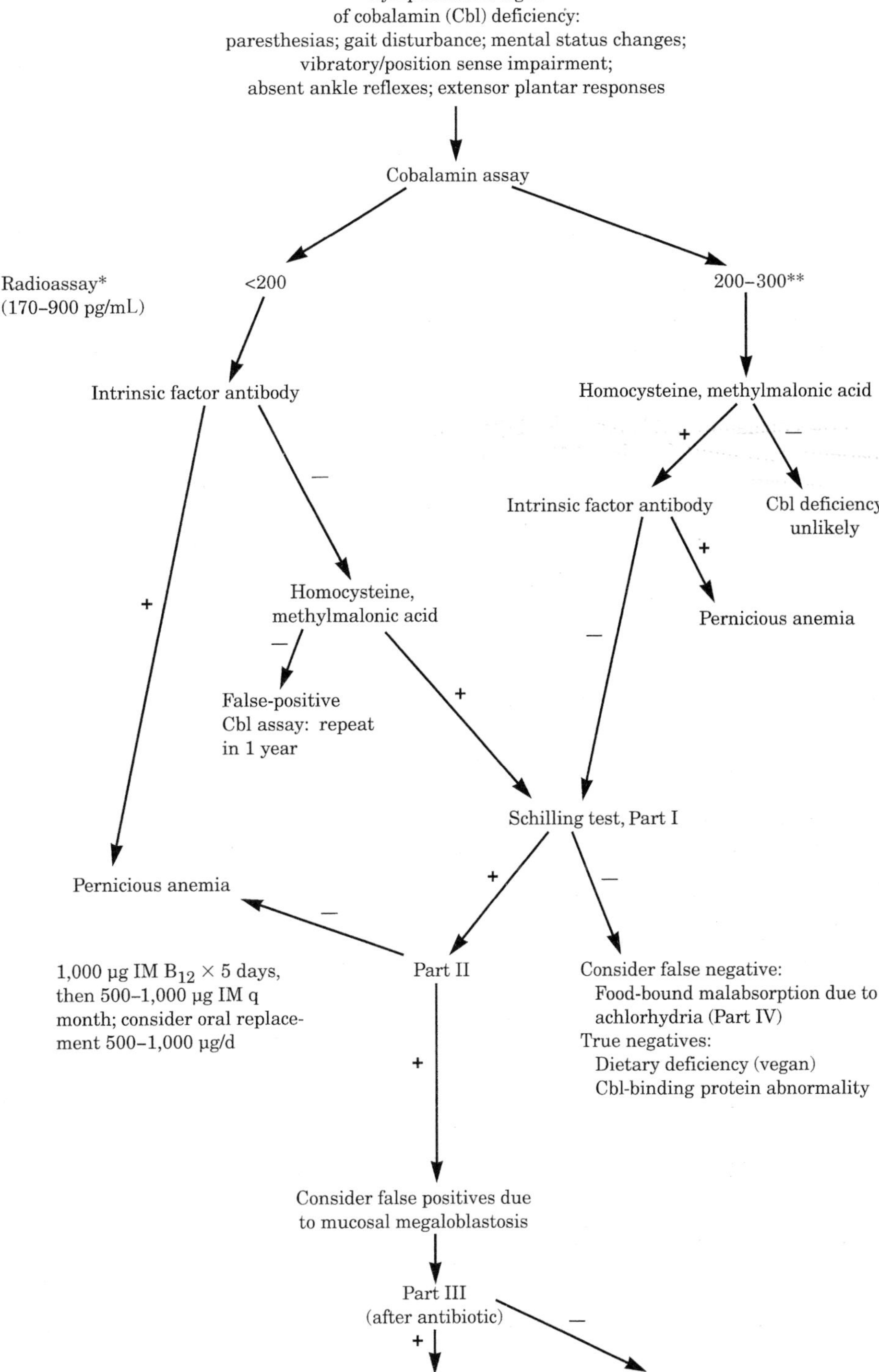

FIGURE 40–7. Algorithm for cobalamin deficiency diagnosis and treatment. A higher normal reference range should be applied if chemiluminescence or other non-radioisotopic ligand-binding assays are used. If the clinical picture is suggestive of possible cobalamin deficiency, patients with serum B_{12} greater than 300 pg/mL should be investigated similarly. IM, intramuscular. (From Green R, Kinsella LJ: Current concepts in the diagnosis of cobalamin deficiency. Neurology 1995;45:1435–1440.)

recovery.[38, 45] Paresthesias often improve within several weeks, whereas spinal cord dysfunction may require several months. About 2 percent of patients experience an acute worsening of paresthesias immediately following vitamin B_{12} supplementation, but this addition does not impair the long-term response to therapy. Folate supplementation may reverse the hematological abnormalities but will not prevent neurological deterioration. With early recognition, patients may resume a normal lifestyle with limited impairment of gait or cognition. Spasticity due to spinal cord dysfunction, when it is established, is often difficult to reverse but may continue to improve over many months to years. There are a variety of reports of neuroimaging in vitamin B_{12} deficiency, showing classic white matter changes in the posterior and lateral columns of the spinal cord. Resolution of the abnormalities on MRI may occur following replacement therapy.[46, 47]

Ten to twenty percent of patients may relapse owing to noncompliance with long-term supplementation. These patients often develop identical symptoms that respond equally well to repeat treatment.[45]

Hyperhomocysteinemia has been directly linked to an increasing incidence of coronary and cerebrovascular disease. It is present in cobalamin, pyridoxine, and folate deficiencies; renal failure; and heterozygous homocysteinemia. Therefore, vitamin B_{12} deficiency, as well as folate and pyridoxine deficiencies, may be independent risk factors for the development of carotid and coronary disease. This association awaits further study. Approximately 40 percent of patients with biochemical cobalamin deficiency may be asymptomatic. A high index of suspicion for vitamin B_{12} deficiency is warranted in view of its high prevalence in the elderly.

PYRIDOXINE (VITAMIN B_6)

Pyridoxal phosphate is the active biochemical form of pyridoxine. It is a coenzyme of amino acid metabolism, particularly tryptophan and methionine. By inhibiting methionine metabolism, excessive S-adenosylmethionine accumulates, which inhibits nerve lipid and myelin synthesis.[10] Because tryptophan is required in the production of niacin, pyridoxine deficiency can produce a secondary niacin deficiency indistinguishable from primary pellagra. Pyridoxine is also involved in lipid and neurotransmitter synthesis. Dopamine, serotonin, epinephrine, norepinephrine, and gamma-aminobutyric acid (GABA) all require pyridoxine for their production. Lott and associates have documented reduced pyridoxal phosphate and GABA concentrations in the brain of a child dying with pyridoxine-responsive seizures.[48]

The RDA of pyridoxine is 2 mg. It is found most abundantly in enriched breads, cereals and grains, chicken, orange and tomato juice, bananas, and avocados. Patients at risk for pyridoxine deficiency include those with general malnutrition, prisoners of war, refugees, alcoholics, infants of vitamin B_6–deficient mothers, and patients using isoniazid and hydralazine. Surveys of hospitalized elderly patients have shown that up to 5 percent may have a vitamin B_6 deficiency.[4] A rare autosomal recessive disorder of pyridoxine-responsive or pyridoxine-dependent neonatal seizures also exists.

Pyridoxine is unique in that both the deficiency and toxic states result in a peripheral neuropathy. Deficiency affects the blood, skin, and nervous system. The skin changes are indistinguishable from pellagra, probably due to the close interaction of niacin and pyridoxine. Pyridoxine improves the microcytic anemia of alcoholics as well as the anemia associated with pyridoxine-responsive seizures in infants. Pyridoxine-deficient peripheral neuropathy is seen primarily in patients on isoniazid or hydralazine, and it is characterized by sensory loss in distal limbs, weakness, and reflex changes. Patients describe burning feet and painful paresthesias. CNS manifestations include depression, irritability, and confusion.[49] Infants born to pyridoxine-deficient mothers may develop neonatal seizures[50] as part of their vitamin deficiency state, a condition distinct from hereditary pyridoxine-responsive seizures. Up to 10 percent of patients who are on isoniazid and have tuberculosis may develop a peripheral sensory neuropathy. Isoniazid promotes increased pyridoxine excretion in the urine, resulting in a deficiency state. Similar changes are seen in patients on hydralazine.

Excess pyridoxine also results in a peripheral neuropathy. Megadoses of pyridoxine produce a sensory neuropathy, generally in excess of 2 g/day but has been reported with long-standing use of as little as 200 mg/day.[51, 52] Symptoms of paresthesias, ataxia, and burning feet occur 1 month to 3 years after starting pyridoxine. Sural nerve biopsies show reduced myelin fiber density and myelin debris, suggesting axonal degeneration. After stopping pyridoxine, all patients improve, but the condition resolves entirely in only a few. Contrary to claims in the lay press, such cases demonstrate that not all B vitamins, even though they are water soluble and are excreted in the urine, are benign when taken in megadoses.

Urinary assays for xanthurenic acid and other pyridoxine metabolites may be performed following tryptophan loading in patients suspected of having pyridoxine deficiency. In the serum, cystathionine levels may also be elevated in this condition.

Daily intake of vitamin B_6 (150 to 450 mg) prevents the neuropathy of isoniazid and should be used by patients on this drug. Once it is established, the neuropathy does not entirely resolve but may improve with replacement vitamin B_6.

VITAMIN E

Alpha-tocopherol is the most active form of vitamin E present in humans. Tocopherol is absorbed and incorporated into chylomicrons in the small intestine. It is carried in portal blood to the liver and alpha-tocopherol transfer protein (α-TTP) binds and recycles vitamin E in the liver for incorporation into low-density lipoproteins and very low-density lipoproteins.[53] Once it is delivered to the cells, alpha-tocopherol serves as an antioxidant, preventing free radical peroxidation and injury to cell membranes. It is stored in adipose tissue, liver, and muscle. Deficiency can occur at any stage of tocopherol metabolism: reduced intake, fat malabsorption, inhibition of enterohepatic circulation, mutation of α-TPP, and abetalipoproteinemia. Vitamin E deficiency leads to axonal membrane injury, with resultant axonal degeneration of peripheral nerve, dorsal root ganglia, and posterior columns (Figs. 40–8 and 40–9).[54] Superficially, the spinal cord abnormalities bear a striking resemblance to those found with subacute combined degeneration of vitamin B_{12} deficiency. However, the lesions of vitamin B_{12} deficiency are due to spongy demyelination of the posterior columns and lateral tracts, whereas those of vitamin E deficiency are the result of swollen and dystrophic axons, or spheroids, and astrocytosis in the posterior columns, dorsal root ganglia, and Clarke's column.

Vitamin E is fat soluble and found in abundance in vegetable oils and wheat germ. The RDA is 10 mg (10 IU) for men and 8 mg (10 IU) for women. Patients at risk for the development of vitamin E deficiency include those who have the following clinical conditions: hypobetalipoproteinemia or abetalipoproteinemia (Bassen-Kornzweig syndrome); other disorders of the pancreas and liver, such as cystic fibrosis and primary biliary atresia; PEM; familial vitamin E deficiency due to a defect in α-TTP; and other malabsorptive states that result in cholestasis (Crohn's disease, ulcerative

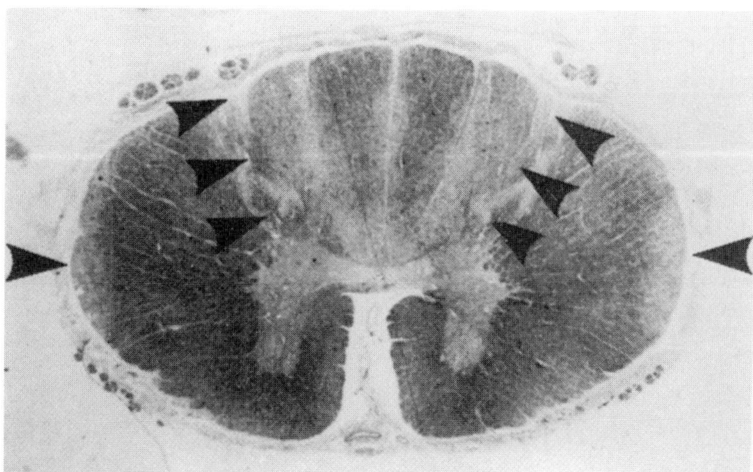

FIGURE 40–8. Vitamin E deficiency myelopathy. Cross section of cervical spinal cord. The triple arrowheads denote light-staining symmetrical areas of degeneration involving the posterior columns. The two single arrowheads indicate involvement of the dorsal and ventral spinocerebellar tracts. In the posterior columns, the fasciculus cuneatus is affected to a greater extent than the gracilis. Microscopically, numerous swollen and dystrophic axons (spheroids) and astrocytosis are present in the posterior columns, and nerve cell loss is seen in the dorsal root ganglia (luxol-fast blue–periodic acid–Schiff). (From Rosenblum JL, Keating JP, Prensky AL, Nelson JS: A progressive neurologic syndrome in children with chronic liver disease. N Engl J Med 1981;304:506.)

colitis, and celiac disease) (Table 40–4). Pregnancy increases vitamin E serum concentrations, but premature infants often have low levels of vitamin E due to a lack of adipose tissue as well as difficulty in transplacental migration of the vitamin. The majority of patients who have vitamin E deficiency are those with severe malabsorptive states present since birth or rare familial vitamin E deficiency due to transfer protein abnormalities.

Patients develop areflexia, cerebellar ataxia, cutaneous sensory impairment, position and vibratory sense abnormalities, and, less commonly, ophthalmoplegia, muscle weakness, nystagmus, extensor plantar responses, ptosis, and dysarthria (Table 40–5).[55] Acanthocytosis and pigmentary retinopathy is seen primarily in patients with abetalipoproteinemia. Patients with abetalipoproteinemia and congenital malabsorption develop symptoms in childhood and adolescence. Occasionally, adults with acquired malabsorption present with progressive ataxia. The familial vitamin E deficiency phenotype is indistinguishable from Friedreich's ataxia (Fig. 40–10). Autosomal recessive familial vitamin E deficiency has been studied extensively and found to be due to a frame shift mutation within the α-TTP gene on chromosome 8. Defective α-TTP prevents incorporation of vitamin E into very low-density lipoproteins.[56, 57]

Friedreich's ataxia, Machado-Joseph disease, and other familial spinocerebellar ataxias[58] should be considered in the differential diagnosis of patients presenting with this constellation of signs and symptoms.

Serum alpha-tocopherol is a reliable indicator of body vitamin E content. Tocopherol isomers can also be assessed using thin layer chromatography. Approximately 90 percent or more of vitamin E is alpha-tocopherol, which can be directly measured in the serum. Occasional patients with hyperlipidemia may have a falsely low alpha-tocopherol level. Vitamin E deficiency may result in electrophysiological abnormalities, including low-amplitude sensory nerve action potentials, slowed conductions, and abnormal somatosensory evoked potentials.[59]

Administration of alpha-tocopherol (400 mg bid) may reverse or prevent the progression of the effects of a deficiency state. Doses of up to 100 mg/kg/day may be required in those with abetalipoproteinemia and the familial vitamin E deficiency syndrome. Whereas oral doses of alpha-tocopherol correlate well with plasma levels, comparable increases in the

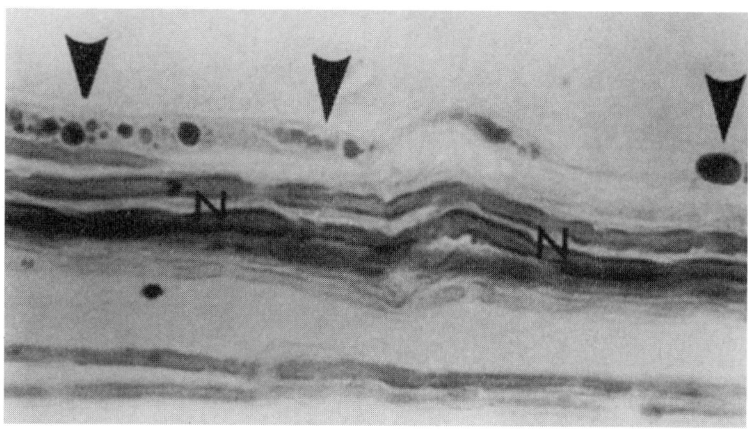

FIGURE 40–9. Teased nerve preparation in a patient with vitamin E deficiency, demonstrating axonal degeneration (sural nerve, osmium impregnation). (From Rosenblum JL, Keating JP, Prensky AL, Nelson JS: A progressive neurologic syndrome in children with chronic liver disease. N Engl J Med 1981;304:507.)

TABLE 40–4. **Vitamin E Deficiency–Associated Disorders**

Abetalipoproteinemia (Bassen-Kornzweig disease)
Celiac disease
Chronic pancreatitis
Chronic cholestatic liver disease
Cystic fibrosis
Familial vitamin E deficiency (alpha-tocopherol transfer protein mutation)
Homozygous hypobetalipoproteinemia
Inflammatory bowel disease
Intestinal lymphangiectasia
Malnutrition
Postgastrectomy
Short bowel syndromes
Total parenteral nutrition
Tropical sprue
Whipple's disease

Adapted with permission from Jackson CE, Amatao AA, Barohn RJ: Isolated vitamin E deficiency. Muscle Nerve 1996;19:1162. Reprinted by John Wiley & Sons, Inc.

ventricular cerebrospinal fluid do not occur, suggesting that CNS penetration may be exceedingly low.[60] An injectable vitamin E preparation is available for those who cannot absorb oral medication. The prognosis for recovery depends on the duration of symptoms before the initiation of treatment.

PANTOTHENIC ACID, VITAMIN A, AND VITAMIN D

Pantothenic acid is part of coenzyme A, an essential element of carbohydrate and fatty acid synthesis and degradation. Because of its ubiquity, no single neurological syndrome is known to be caused by pantothenate deficiency, with the exception of generalized malaise.[61]

Vitamin A, derived from β-carotene, is necessary for normal vision and reproduction. Deficiency leads to night blindness and corneal ulceration.[62] Hypervitaminosis of 25,000 IU daily for 1 to 2 years may cause symptoms of pseudotumor cerebri, including raised intracranial pressure and visual disturbances.[63, 64] Hypervitaminosis in pregnant mothers may lead to birth defects and learning disabilities.

Vitamin D is necessary for calcium absorption in the gut. Deficiency leads to osteomalacia, hypocalcemia, and hypophosphatemia.[65] The reason why muscle weakness occurs in such patients is unclear, and the phenomenon is explained only in part by low serum calcium.[66, 67]

TABLE 40–5. **Neurological Findings in Vitamin E Deficiency**

Truncal and appendicular ataxia
Areflexia
Abnormal vibration sense and proprioception
Ophthalmoplegia
Retinitis pigmentosa and acanthocytosis (in patients with abetalipoproteinemia)
Dysarthria
Generalized weakness
Extensor plantar responses

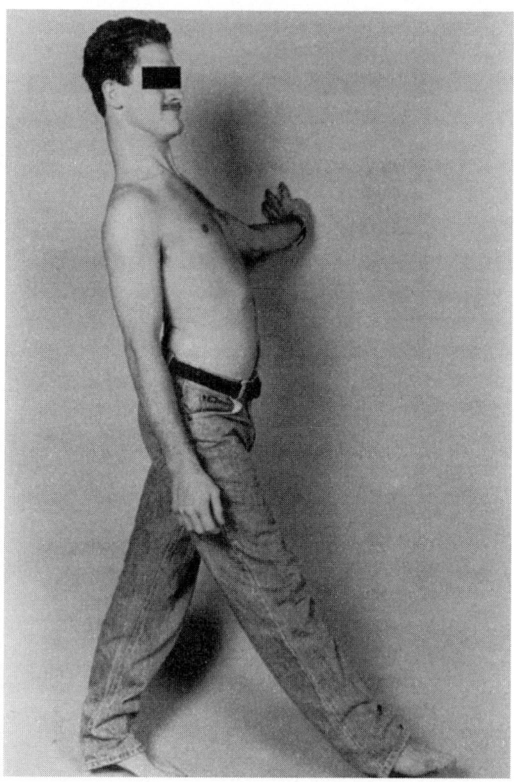

FIGURE 40–10. Patient with isolated vitamin E deficiency demonstrating gait characterized by pseudodystonic extension of the knees, as well as prominent lordosis, and genu recurvatum. (From Jackson CE, Amato AA, Barohn RJ: Isolated vitamin E deficiency. Muscle Nerve 1996;19:1163. Reprinted by John Wiley & Sons, Inc.)

Protein-Energy Malnutrition

In acute starvation, the nervous system sustains itself first on glucose derived from alanine, then on ketone bodies from the breakdown of fats. This process continues until fat is depleted, and then catabolism returns to visceral proteins. Death results from cardiac muscle resorption and eventual cardiac failure. In chronic PEM, the nervous system adapts poorly, and a retarded rate of brain growth, hypomyelination, and slowed conduction velocities of peripheral nerves results.

Chronic PEM has traditionally been a disease of the Third World, particularly Africa and Asia. In industrialized countries, it is seen in young children in poverty, the elderly, alcoholics, or children born to malnourished mothers. By a strict definition of acute loss of 10 percent body weight, PEM also occurs in hospitalized elderly, particularly those suffering from sepsis, burns, or other serious illnesses that preclude a normal diet. Up to 27 percent of hospitalized elderly develop PEM during their hospital stay, with an associated increased risk of mental status changes, depression, and prolonged length of stay.[7] In patients with third-degree burns, up to 500 g of muscle may be lost in a day, and death from malnutrition may occur in 2 to 3 weeks.

Traditionally, PEM has been viewed as either a primary protein deficiency (kwashiorkor) or an energy deficiency (marasmus). Kwashiorkor occurs in children older than 18 months and is often associated with diarrheal illnesses or other infectious diseases. Owing to the severe protein deficiency, circulating serum proteins are inadequate to maintain normal oncotic pressure, leading to marked peripheral edema. Marasmus occurs in children younger than 1 year of age and is not accompanied by edema. PEM may cause mental changes, including apathy and irritability, muscle wasting, generalized weakness, hypotonia, hyporeflexia, and gait impairment. Following a return to a normal diet, an acute encephalopathy has been described in some patients with PEM marked by rigidity, tremors, asterixis, and mental confusion.[68, 69] Infectious diseases may precipitate kwashiorkor in a patient with borderline malnutrition. PEM needs to be distinguished from other wasting conditions and edematous states such as thiamin deficiency, HIV infection, and the cachexia of malignancy.

The patient's nutritional status should be assessed by a careful dietary history. Energy malnutrition is defined as a 10 percent loss of ideal body weight.[7] Protein malnutrition requires assessment of serum proteins, including albumin, prealbumin, and total lymphocyte count. Because asterixis may be seen in some patients recovering from kwashiorkor and may be mistaken for hepatic encephalopathy, measurement of serum ammonia is often helpful to exclude this diagnosis.

Nutritious food and vitamin supplements generally lead to a complete recovery. Whether PEM results in long-term growth retardation and delayed intellectual development is controversial.[70] This condition is best prevented by education of affected family members on proper nutrition. In the United States, hospitalized elderly are perhaps at the greatest risk for PEM, and nutritional assessments of all patients at risk should be undertaken at admission to prevent serious malnutrition and to reduce the incidence of morbidity and mortality.

Other Nutritional Deficiencies

STRACHAN'S SYNDROME

In 1888, Henry Strachan, a British medical officer stationed in Jamaica, described a syndrome of painful peripheral neuropathy, ataxia, optic neuropathy, and stomatitis among sugar cane workers.[71] Denny-Brown and others found similar ailments among Allied troops liberated from prisoner-of-war camps after World War II.[12] In these patients, other symptoms included sensorineural deafness, dizziness, confusion, spastic leg weakness, foot drop, Wernicke's encephalopathy, and rare cases of neck extensor weakness and myasthenic bulbar weakness. Poor nutrition, hard physical labor, and concurrent infection were thought to be exacerbating factors. In Fisher's autopsy series of Canadian prisoners of war, the most prominent pathological finding was demyelination of the posterior columns of the thoracic and cervical spinal cord.[72] This demyelination accounted for the loss of vibratory and position sense and sensory ataxia. Pathologically, the optic and auditory nerves showed moderate to severe demyelination.

More recently, an outbreak of optic and peripheral neuropathy closely resembling Strachan's syndrome occurred in Cuba in 1992 to 1993, following the loss of food and fuel exports.[73] Fifty thousand people developed isolated or combinations of optic neuropathy, painful sensory neuropathy, dorsolateral myelopathy, sensorineural deafness, spastic paraparesis, dysphonia, and dysautonomia. Almost half (45 percent) developed centrocecal scotoma and optic neuropathy only, often following a period of weight loss. Optic neuropathy and myeloneuropathy were seen in 24 percent, optic neuropathy and sensorineural hearing loss in 14 percent, and peripheral and optic neuropathies with hearing loss in 7 percent.[73] Proposed mechanisms included vitamin B complex and thiamin deficiency, cyanide intoxication, viral infection, and mitochondrial deletion. Infections appeared to precipitate or exacerbate symptoms. Almost all patients responded to early supplementation with B complex vitamins. Evidence for peripheral nerve involvement has been mixed. Clinical evidence of neuropathy is often lacking despite severe symptoms. Fisher examined the peripheral nerves in 2 of 11 patients at postmortem and found no abnormalities; however, nerve teasing and modern histopathological techniques were not used. Osuntokun documented peroneal nerve conduction slowing and normal conductions of the median and ulnar nerves,[74] whereas Borrajero found abnormal sural nerve action potentials only in the most severely affected individuals.[75] Sural nerve biopsies showed axonal degeneration of large myelinated fibers.

Extensive study of the epidemiology of the Cuban outbreak revealed smoking, weight loss, sugar consumption, and excessive alcohol intake as risk factors. Urban men 25 to 64 years of age were most affected. Pregnant women, children, and the elderly were minimally affected; however, these groups were targeted for supplementation before the outbreak. Women were more likely to develop paresthesias in the feet, whereas men were more likely to develop optic neuropathy.[76] In Africa, pregnant women are most vulnerable,[74] and smoking and weight loss were the strongest risk factors for the optic neuropathy variant.

This clinical syndrome should be distinguished from beriberi, vitamin B_{12} deficiency, pellagra, tropical spastic paraparesis (human T-cell lymphotropic virus-1 [HTLV-1]), tropical ataxic neuropathy of Africa, subacute myelo-optic neuropathy, clioquinol ingestion in Japan, Leber's optic neuropathy, and nutritional amblyopia. In order to do so, dietary and family histories; vitamin B_{12}, folate, and transketolase levels; medication history; and an HTLV-1 assay should be obtained.

Treatment consists of re-establishing a balanced diet with B complex vitamin and vitamin A supplementation. In the Cuban experience, long-term sequelae were rare, because most had early treatment with nutritional supplements, including B complex and vitamin A. In prisoners of war with long-standing symptoms, persistent ataxia, burning feet, and visual defects often persisted despite adequate supplementation.

POSTGASTROPLASTY POLYNEUROPATHY

Some patients undergoing bariatric, or weight reduction, surgery develop a syndrome of acute or subacute sensory loss, weakness, and areflexia in the limbs, usually following a period of dramatic weight loss and repeated bouts of protracted vomiting.[77] A few patients have also developed a type of encephalopathy that is clinically and pathologically identical to WKS, with or without an associated polyneuropathy.[14] Indeed, Wernicke and Korsakoff each described young women with intractable vomiting in their original reports: One woman had attempted suicide by drinking sulfuric acid, whereas the other had hyperemesis gravidarum.[8]

Of 37 cases of postgastroplasty polyneuropathy reviewed, 26 developed neuropathy alone, 2 had encephalopathy, and 9 had features of both.[13, 14, 77–81] One patient developed blindness and optic neuropathy. Intractable vomiting is a constant feature. The syndrome may present suddenly several months after surgical procedures that include gastrojejunostomy, gastric stapling, vertical banding gastroplasty, and gastrectomy with Roux-en-Y anastomosis.[13] Following a period of recurrent vomiting and precipitous weight loss, patients develop numbness and tingling in the soles of the feet, calves, and thighs. Distal or proximal weakness may develop, and the patient may have difficulty arising from a chair or climbing stairs. Pain is not a dominant feature, unlike nutritional neuropathy, in which the calves are often exquisitely tender. Examination shows symmetrical sensory loss in the legs more than the arms, muscle weakness, and areflexia. Patients may develop quadriparesis and prolonged or permanent disability. When the condition is accompanied by encephalopathy, patients may demonstrate confusion, memory loss, and affective disturbances. Many patients have been mistakenly diagnosed early in their course as having a conversion disorder.

In this setting, Guillain-Barré syndrome, cobalamin myeloneuropathy, critical illness polyneuropathy, compressive radiculopathy, WKS, beriberi, Strachan's syndrome, hypocalcemia, and hypomagnesemia should be considered in the differential diagnosis.

Nerve conduction studies show severe reduction of sensory and motor action potentials, variable slowing, and absent or prolonged late responses in this disorder. Needle examination shows diffuse denervation with fibrillations, consistent with an axonal and demyelinating sensorimotor polyneuropathy. The polyneuropathy is axonal and demyelinating in type, acute in onset, and slow to resolve. Pathological studies have shown lipid-laden neurons and Schwann cells surrounding demyelinating and degenerating axons.[77]

Although thiamin deficiency has been suggested as the cause, reports documenting low thiamin activity are lacking. Furthermore, the pathology of the peripheral nerve is unlike any known nutritional neuropathy, and some patients have developed the neuropathy despite adequate nutritional supplementation.[81] The pathophysiology of this disorder is unknown, but may be related to the rapid mobilization of lipid in the surgically starved. Controversy exists whether vitamin and nutritional supplementation alone or reversal of the surgical procedure is most helpful in resolving the neuropathy. All patients following bariatric surgery should adhere to a strict dietary regimen with additional vitamins. If vomiting develops, patients should receive parenteral nutrition, vitamins, and thiamin. Most patients recover fully, but some have residual weakness and sensory loss. The degree of disability appears to depend on the duration and severity of symptoms before diagnosis and treatment.

Alcohol and the Nervous System

OVERVIEW AND PHARMACOLOGY

Alcohol is one of the most widely used psychoactive drugs, and alcoholism is characterized by the chronic, repetitive, excessive use of alcohol such that it interferes with the health, personal relationships, and livelihood of the drinker. In pharmacological terms, alcoholism is the addiction to alcohol. Although the cause of alcoholism is unknown, there clearly are genetic, environmental, and cultural factors involved. In the United States, the incidence of alcoholism cannot be determined specifically, but it is estimated that 10 percent of adult Americans are affected by alcohol abuse and dependence.

The active ingredient in most common alcoholic beverages is ethanol or ethyl alcohol, yet other impurities, including enanthic ethers, amyl alcohol, and acetaldehyde, may be contained in some liquors. Alcohol is absorbed from the stomach as well as the duodenum and jejunum and can be detected in the blood within 5 minutes of ingestion. Absorption rates are faster in patients with gastrectomies and in those individuals who are habituated to alcohol. Once it is in the bloodstream, alcohol enters other organs and can be detected in the cerebrospinal fluid, urine, and alveolar air. Alcohol is metabolized mainly in the liver, where it is oxidized to acetaldehyde via multiple enzymes but most importantly through the actions of alcohol dehydrogenase. Oxidation may also occur through peroxisomal and mitochondrial catalases, as well as by the microsomal ethanol-oxidizing system. Acetaldehyde itself may have effects independent from those of alcohol in the development of intoxication and addiction, although this remains speculative. As an end product, acetaldehyde is probably converted to acetate through the action of aldehyde dehydrogenase, but the exact degradation product of acetaldehyde is unknown. Once alcohol absorption ceases and equilibration within tissue has occurred, alcohol is metabolized at a constant rate without correlation to its blood concentration. This contrasts with acetaldehyde metabolism, which does depend on the tissue concentration of this metabolite. The rate of metabolism of alcohol can be enhanced by the administration of insulin, amino acids, and fructose, whereas starvation has the opposite effect.

The mechanism of action of alcohol on the nervous system has been debated for decades, and since the turn of the century, some investigators have speculated that alcohol acts as a nonspecific drug, producing its actions via perturbation of neuronal membrane lipids. More recently, it has been suggested that ethanol acts at the interface between membrane lipids and integral membrane proteins.[82] Neurotransmitter-gated ion channels have also been the focus of attention regarding the potential sites of alcohol action, including nicotinic acetylcholine, $GABA_A$, and *N*-methyl-D-aspartate (NMDA) receptor-ion channels. Alcohol affects the function of these receptor-ion channels mostly via direct interactions, yet the molecular structure of the alcohol-binding site has yet to be determined.

Tolerance to alcohol is defined as an acquired resistance to the effects of the drug, which can be related to pharmacokinetic, pharmacodynamic, environmental, and behavioral factors. It has been hypothesized that tolerance represents an adaptive change in the CNS with mechanistic similarities to learning or memory function. Recently, Szabo and Hoffman demonstrated that daily intracerebral injections of human recombinant brain-derived neurotrophic factor, neurotrophin-3, and neurotrophin-4/5, following ethanol withdrawal, maintained ethanol tolerance as compared with controls.[83] The authors suggest that some neurotrophins may modulate neuroadaptation to ethanol through their actions as either growth factors or the modulation of the function of postmitotic neurons. These actions could ultimately result in alterations in gene expression, producing the observed behavioral consequences. Tolerance to alcohol may also involve adaptive changes in neuronal membrane lipids, neurotransmitter receptors, ion channels, or intracellular secondary messengers that serve to counteract the short-term effects of alcohol.

ACUTE INTOXICATION

In the nervous system, alcohol acts as a depressant, and small doses may lead to disinhibition or a slight euphoria. The toxic effects of alcohol become more prominent with rising blood levels, yet through repeated consumption, humans can become habituated rapidly. Although blood levels of 100 mg/dL typically cause drunkenness in occasional imbibers, chronic alcohol abusers can tolerate levels up to 500 mg/dL without any apparent effects. The toxic effects of alcohol can be produced in any individual who ingests sufficient quantities of the substance. The state of drunkenness or acute intoxication is recognized by slurred speech, an erratic gait, and disinhibited verbosity and behavior. The phenomenon of acute intoxication depends on the blood alcohol concentration, the rate at which it has been attained, and the time during which it has been maintained.[84] Pathological intoxication refers to an episode of uncharacteristic behavior during a drinking bout. This behavior may include violence and is mainly attributable to the disinhibiting effect of a heavy consumption of alcohol. This behavior typically abates as the blood alcohol level falls, but at times, the use of restraints and sedation may be necessary. Parenteral sedatives, including phenobarbital and benzodiazepines, may be used.

An alcoholic blackout refers to a period of time during acute alcoholic intoxication that a person subsequently does not recall. It is a blank space in the continuum of a person's memory and objectivity, and there are no outward signs other than those of typical drunkenness. The blackouts may be complete or partial. These blackout periods correlate poorly with withdrawal symptoms and are not associated with chronic memory disturbances or the alcoholic dementia seen in some individuals. Blackout periods are associated with a high blood alcohol level and may occur in both the social and dependent drinker. Management includes supportive therapy and education.

The syndrome of drunkenness is so well recognized, even among lay people, that the main challenge for physicians is not to overlook concomitant intoxication with other drugs or other causes for ataxic gait, stupor, and coma. A blood alcohol level is the most important laboratory test to support a diagnosis of alcohol intoxication. However, because habituated alcoholics can tolerate several times the levels of nonhabituated individuals, the test result must be interpreted in light of the person's status in this regard.

The most important therapeutic problem in the setting of acute intoxication is respiratory depression. With higher blood alcohol levels, stupor and coma can occur, yet there are no distinctive clinical characteristics of alcoholic coma. The diagnosis should be suggested by the clinical setting. Respiratory depression is an early feature, so the diagnosis must be made promptly and should be treated in an intensive care unit. Mechanical ventilatory support should be instituted when necessary, and hypovolemia, acid-base balance, electrolyte, and temperature abnormalities must be corrected. Glucose (50 mL of 5% solution) with 100 mg intravenous and 100 mg intramuscular thiamin should be given if hypoglycemia is suspected. Because alcohol is absorbed rapidly, gastric lavage with activated charcoal is not likely to be of value in preventing a deeper intoxication. Death has occurred with blood alcohol levels of 4000 mg/L, and a level of 5000 mg/L is lethal in 50 percent of patients.[85] Recovery from alcohol-induced coma with high blood alcohol levels can be hastened with hemodialysis, but this measure is rarely indicated.[86] Unless the patient develops fatal coma or suffers trauma as a result of incoordination, virtually all episodes of acute alcohol intoxication resolve without sequelae.

WITHDRAWAL SYNDROMES

The manifestations of alcohol withdrawal occur when a person decreases or stops a high level of alcohol intake, either after a binge lasting a matter of days or after the regular ingestion of alcohol sustained over many months. Although the exact mechanisms are not known, most symptoms appear related to overactivity of various portions of the nervous system resembling a "rebound" phenomenon after profound suppression, and its basis may relate to alterations in the function of GABA or NMDA receptor systems. The earliest findings of alcohol withdrawal typically occur within 6 to 8 hours of alcohol cessation.[87] Tremulousness is the earliest and most common complaint, and many alcoholics view their so-called shakes as an indication that it is time to resume drinking in order to avoid more severe complications of withdrawal. Tremor appears within hours of cessation of alcohol ingestion and gradually increases to a peak within 1 or 2 days.[88] The tremor is postural and appears to be irregular due to its variable but large amplitude. The amplitude may increase at the end points of an action, and the typical frequency varies from 6 to 11 Hz.[89] This movement abnormality mainly involves the hands yet can cause titubation. The tremor remits during relaxation and sleep but often persists for weeks after discontinuation of alcohol consumption. The pathophysiological mechanisms of the tremor are not known, but it probably represents an exaggerated physiological tremor.[90] The tremulousness is associated with hyperacuity of all sensory modalities, hyper-reflexia, hypervigilance, anxiety, tachycardia, hypertension, and insomnia. The severity of these signs and symptoms vary with the intensity and duration of the previous alcohol exposure. In mild forms of withdrawal, the signs and symptoms usually resolve after 48 hours.

In severe reactions, patients may experience additional symptoms including auditory hallucinations, which usually take the form of identifiable voices saying critical or threatening things to the patient. When they occur, hallucinations generally appear within 24 hours of withdrawal. At first, patients tend to accept the voices as real and react accordingly, but as the intensity of the hallucinations wanes, they recognize their true origin. The hallucinosis may be accompanied by global confusion, and the autonomic hyperactivity continues and may become more pronounced.

Between 6 and 48 hours following alcohol discontinuation, seizures occur in approximately 3 to 4 percent of untreated patients.[91, 92] Although the seizures are almost always multiple with short interictal intervals over a few hours, there may be only a single seizure.[91] The seizures are generalized tonic-clonic, and focal seizures should suggest the presence of a focal lesion in addition to the effects of the alcohol. Alcoholics may also develop seizure disorders as a result of acute head trauma, the presence of a subdural hematoma, or other causes seen in nonalcoholics. Alcohol withdrawal itself may also potentially aggravate any pre-existing seizure disorder unrelated to the alcohol abuse. Thirty to forty percent of patients with seizures progress to delirium tremens if they are left untreated.[87, 93] One quarter of these individuals do so without an interceding lucid period. The remaining individuals have a period of improvement ranging between 12 hours and 5 days.[87, 93, 94]

Delirium tremens comprises a combination of psychic and autonomic hyperactivity, occurring usually after 3 to 5 days of alcohol abstinence but may be seen as late as 14 days. Only 5 to 6 percent of untreated patients withdrawing from alcohol develop this syndrome.[94] Patients with delirium tremens are agitated, hallucinating, and confused. The hallucinations are frequently of a visual nature, but other types occur. In addition, fever, tachycardia, diaphoresis, hypertension, and confusion are typical. Seizures are uncommon during this phase of withdrawal. Once it is present, the delirium typically lasts for 3 days.

Often by the time patients reach the hospital, alcohol is no longer detectable in the blood. Therefore, the diagnosis depends on the history and documentation of other clinical signs that are suggestive of chronic alcoholism (e.g., liver disease). Those patients with seizures or delirium tremens require laboratory screening for superimposed metabolic disorders that may contribute to the clinical picture. Additionally, individuals with clinically uncharacteristic seizures should undergo computed tomography scan of the brain to rule out focal trauma, stroke, or hemorrhage. The electroencephalogram (EEG) may also be helpful in this setting because it may demonstrate focal slowing or epileptiform activity. Generally, the EEG shows a sequence of changes induced by alcohol beginning with a decrease in the frequency during chronic intoxication, followed by a return to normal with alcohol cessation. During the awake EEG, withdrawal seizures may be precipitated by photic stimulation.

Febrile, delirious patients should have close monitoring of their vital signs, preferably in an intensive care unit, while a search is conducted for possible sources of infection that may cause or contribute to the clinical presentation. Volume repletion is often necessary due to excessive perspiration. Owing to possible nutritional deficiencies, 100 mg IV and 100 mg of intramuscular thiamin should be provided before the administration of glucose in order to prevent the acute precipitation of WKS. Intravenous fluids should also be supplemented by daily B complex vitamins. Benzodiazepines are helpful in reducing anxiety and tremulousness and may be useful in the prevention of seizure activity during withdrawal.[95] Chlordiazepoxide and diazepam are long-acting drugs with pharmacologically active metabolites, and repeated daily dosages can result in accumulation of these agents. Oxazepam, in contrast, is rapidly converted to an inactive compound and does not accumulate and contribute to excessive CNS depression.

Beta-blockers or clonidine can be used to treat the associated tachycardia and hypertension.[96, 97] Because withdrawal seizures are typically self-limited, treatment is generally not required. Furthermore, the value of phenytoin in uncomplicated withdrawal seizures has not been demonstrated, and the long-term administration of anticonvulsants is usually ineffective in preventing recurrences. Some studies have reported better control of seizures in patients with a previous history of seizures when phenytoin is added to benzodiazepine administration. Evidence from other reports has conflicted with this finding. Status epilepticus is rare in alcohol withdrawal but should be treated in a manner similar to the one used when it is found in other clinical settings.

As a group, the alcohol withdrawal syndromes represent self-limited episodes that resolve with no residual effects. However, delirium tremens carries a measurable mortality rate (perhaps 10 to 20%) due to autonomic dysfunction. The obvious means of preventing these disorders is drinking alcohol only in moderation. For those who are abusing alcohol already, the only sure way to prevent withdrawal syndromes is to continue the alcohol, which is rarely practical in a hospital setting.

ALCOHOLIC DEMENTIA AND CEREBRAL ATROPHY

Some authorities have contended that chronic excess ingestion of alcohol leads to cerebral atrophy and alcoholic dementia. However, the notion that alcohol has a direct toxic effect on cerebral tissue is greatly disputed. Most cases of dementia in alcoholics can be explained on the basis of Korsakoff's disease, other nutritional deficiencies, or medical causes. This syndrome has been described only in long-standing alcohol abusers, and the essential clinical features of this putative syndrome are the combination of cognitive and behavioral deficits including impaired memory and judgment, loss of social refinements, and paranoid ideation. Symptoms and signs develop gradually and continue to progress as long as alcohol abuse continues. Patients often show other stigmata of long-standing alcohol abuse. The major diagnostic distinction is with a slowly evolving form of Korsakoff's psychosis. Other considerations when encountering an impaired intellect in alcoholics include hepatic encephalopathy, subdural hematoma, hydrocephalus (from prior trauma or meningitis), or anoxic encephalopathy. Other dementing illnesses unrelated to alcoholism, such as Alzheimer's disease, should be considered. Brain imaging may reveal shrinkage of cerebral volume, especially in the frontal lobes. This finding is potentially reversible if patients can cease alcohol intake. To the extent that some cases represent a slowly evolving form of Korsakoff's disease, regular ingestion of thiamin supplements should help prevent the development of dementia. Once it is established, the dementia tends to remain static if alcohol consumption decreases, whereas it may progress if there is no change in lifestyle.

DEFICIENCY AMBLYOPIA

This disorder is most likely related to the depletion of one or more B vitamins, although none has been specifically implicated. Deficiency amblyopia occurs only after severe and prolonged nutritional deprivation. The strict dietary deficiencies required to produce amblyopia are known to occur mainly in mistreated prisoners of war and alcoholics. Smoking tobacco was once considered another risk factor (hence, the alias tobacco-alcohol amblyopia), but this is no longer believed to be true.

Patients with this disorder experience the subacute onset (over days to weeks) of symmetrical loss of visual acuity, and colors perceived appear to be washed out. On examination, the central portion of vision is especially impaired, and occasionally patients exhibit pallor of the optic discs. Patients often have evidence of other syndromes of nutritional deficiency, including a predominantly sensory polyneuropathy. The possible causes of optic neuropathy are legion, and most are much more common than deficiency amblyopia. The diagnosis should be suggested by the clinical setting.

The most valuable test in the evaluation of these patients is perimetry, which allows for the confirmation of the central or centrocecal distribution of the visual field defect. The diagnosis can be solidified, retrospectively, by a positive response to treatment. Because this disorder results from extreme nutritional deprivation, prevention is relatively easy. Any reasonably balanced diet should provide sufficient vitamin intake for this purpose. Substantial recovery is possible in most cases by eating a nutritious diet supplemented by multivitamins. The majority of patients recover if proper treatment is instituted and the degree of recovery is inversely proportional to the duration of nutritional deprivation.

CEREBELLAR DEGENERATION

Although a definite association between cerebellar degeneration and nutritional deficiency is not established in alcoholism, thiamin deficiency is suggested by the clinical and pathological resemblance to the cerebellar involvement in Wernicke's disease. Alcoholism is the chief risk factor for the development of this disorder, and males are affected more often than females. The main clinical manifestation is a disorder of gait characterized by instability and a widened base. Patients are unable to walk with one foot placed in front of the other and occasionally there is frank ataxia of the lower extremities, which is best appreciated on a heel-to-shin test. The gait disorder develops gradually, or occasionally in a stepwise fashion. The upper limbs are only rarely involved.

Because this disorder is associated with alcoholism, many patients have evidence of other complications of nutritional deficiency, particularly a polyneuropathy. In alcoholics, alternative causes of gait ataxia include Wernicke's disease, acquired hepatocerebral degeneration, and the effects of head trauma. Cerebellar syndromes featuring prominent speech or oculomotor deficits should suggest another cause for the ataxia, even in alcoholics.

MRI may demonstrate atrophy of the anterosuperior vermis, which is best seen on a midline sagittal image. With the uncertain pathogenesis, the only known effective preventive measure is the treatment of alcoholism. However, it is likely that avoiding nutritional deficiency would eliminate the risk of alcoholic cerebellar degeneration. The utility of vitamin supplementation after the cerebellar degeneration has occurred is unproven. In most cases, the gait disorder progresses over weeks to months, and then persists indefinitely. A small number of patients show only brief manifestations with spontaneous resolution.

MARCHIAFAVA-BIGNAMI DISEASE

The majority of the pathological changes in this disease occur in the middle lamina of the corpus callosum. The mechanism responsible for the white matter damage and the reason for the particular vulnerability of the corpus callosum are unknown. Long-standing alcohol abuse is clearly a risk factor, but Marchiafava-Bignami disease has also been described in nonalcoholics. The rarity of this disorder when measured against the prevalence of alcoholism also suggests that other factors are involved. Originally thought to selectively affect Italians, Marchiafava-Bignami has been found in other populations as well.

There is no consistent or typical clinical presentation, but manifestations usually encompass both cognitive and behavioral aspects. Many patients appear to become progressively demented, disinhibited, or aggressive. Transient neurological deficits, often focal in nature, may form part of the clinical picture. Seizures and impaired consciousness may be terminal events. Because chronic alcoholism is present in most cases, other typical findings in this population include polyneuropathy or ataxia. Hospital admissions, however, are usually precipitated by complications of alcohol withdrawal. Korsakoff's psychosis, alcoholic dementia, hepatic encephalopathy, and subdural hematoma form a partial list of conditions causing dementia or behavioral disorders in alcoholics and should be considered in the differential diagnosis. Brain MRI scans may show lesions in the corpus callosum. In most cases, the disorder progresses slowly, sometimes taking years to lead to stupor, coma, and death.

ALCOHOLIC MYOPATHY

There are two forms of alcoholic muscle disease: (1) an acute, painful myopathy associated with weakness, cramps, swollen and tender muscles, high creatine kinase (CK), and rhabdomyolysis with or without myoglobinuria; and (2) a chronic myopathy that is painless and often unnoticed by the patient, causing proximal weakness and type II fiber atrophy on nerve biopsy. In addition to skeletal muscle involvement, patients may have an associated cardiomyopathy.[98]

Proposed mechanisms of alcoholic injury have included mitochondrial dysfunction, phosphorus and potassium depletion, and rhabdomyolysis induced by either alcohol-related seizures or limb compression from alcoholic stupor. Alcohol may also act synergistically with nutritional deficiencies to disrupt energy metabolism, although a mitochondrial defect has not been demonstrated.[99] The acute myopathy may require an additional insult, such as hypokalemia, fasting, seizures, delirium tremens, or prolonged limb compression. In chronic myopathy, type IIb fiber atrophy and fiber size variability are present.[100] In acute myopathy, necrosis with or without inflammation, regenerating fibers, and type I atrophy are seen pathologically. Women are more susceptible than men to develop this complication due to a 40 percent lower dose of alcohol required to produce cardiac and skeletal myopathy.[98] Women may metabolize alcohol more slowly, leading to higher blood levels, possibly due to decreased gastric alcohol dehydrogenase and liver metabolism.

Acute necrotizing myopathy and rhabdomyolysis cause severe painful swelling of one or more muscles with induration of the skin and soft tissues. CK levels may be elevated, and myoglobinuria may result in acute renal failure. Acute attacks resolve in days to weeks after abstaining, and long-term disability is uncommon unless the patient has repeated attacks.[101] Chronic myopathy is painless weakness of proximal muscles. Cardiomyopathy, peripheral and autonomic neuropathies, and other complications of alcohol abuse may be concomitantly present in these patients. Other myopathic processes, including inflammatory (polymyositis/dermatomyositis), endocrine (thyroid, cortisol), electrolyte disorders (low potassium, phosphorus, calcium, and magnesium), toxins (colchicine), and infectious agents (legionella, mycoplasma, viral), should be considered in this clinical setting.

Martin and colleagues performed muscle biopsies in 151 consecutive inpatient alcoholics. Only half had weakness, and 15 percent had an elevated CK level. Chronic myopathy was observed in 60 percent, and 5 percent had necrosis, suggesting an acute myopathy on muscle biopsy. Clinical evidence of peripheral neuropathy was suggested in 65 percent, yet half were asymptomatic.[100]

In the evaluation of these patients, laboratory studies should include CK, aldolase, electrocardiograph, and echocardiogram. In one series of patients, the aldolase level was more commonly elevated than CK and may be more helpful in the diagnosis.[99] Rarely, when the diagnosis is in question, a muscle biopsy is warranted. Management includes strict abstinence from alcohol, intravenous saline diuresis to prevent renal failure from myoglobinuria, and thiamin and multivitamin supplementation.

ALCOHOLIC NEUROPATHY

Alcoholic neuropathy is difficult to separate from nutritional, specifically thiamin-deficient, neuropathy.[102] The clinical pattern and pathology of axonal degeneration is virtually identical to beriberi. The incidence ranges from 9 to 30 percent among hospitalized alcoholics,[103, 104] and up to 93 percent of ambulatory alcoholics may have electrophysiological evidence of neuropathy.[105] Victor and associates found signs of polyneuropathy in 82 percent of 230 patients with WKS,[8] and 84 percent of patients, who were able to give a dietary history, reported at least a 20-pound weight loss in the previous year. Alcoholic neuropathy occurs in those patients consuming at least 100 g of alcohol daily for several years. It is potentiated by nutritional deficiency. Men outnumber women, but women may be more susceptible at lower doses than men.[106] Although it is not known how alcohol injures peripheral nerves, theories include altered membrane lipid permeability[107] and oxidation injury from free radical formation.[108] How nutritional deficiency may potentiate the toxicity of alcohol awaits further study.

Attempts to control for the influences of alcohol and nutrition have yielded conflicting results. Alcoholics with neuropathy were allowed to continue drinking while receiving a nutritious diet with vitamin supplementation, and all noted improvement in symptoms.[109] Hallet and co-workers were unable to produce neuropathy in monkeys after 3 to 5 years of a high-alcohol diet.[110] However, Behse and Buchthal reported 37 cases of alcoholic neuropathy in patients drinking about 3 L of thiamin- and pyridoxine-fortified beer daily, the equivalent of 100 mL of ethanol.[106] Fourteen of 37 (37%) had marked weight loss. All patients had normal serum vitamin levels, except for one with thiamin deficiency and three with folate deficiency. The pattern and severity of the neuropathy did not differ between those with and without adequate nutrition. Similarly, Monforte and colleagues found no relationship between the nutritional status and the incidence of autonomic and peripheral neuropathies in alcoholics.[111] Pathologically, the peripheral nerve undergoes axonal degeneration with loss of large and small myelinated fibers in autonomic,[112] sensory, and motor nerves.[106]

The neuropathy is often asymptomatic until it is pointed out to the patient. The symptoms begin with paresthesias and burning feet, and later, painful calves, numbness, cramps, weakness, and sensory ataxia may develop. On examination, patients may have sensory loss (vibratory and deep sensation) in the distal legs, motor weakness, areflexia, calf tenderness, and orthostatic hypotension.[112] The skin of the legs becomes shiny, swollen, and subject to trauma and ulceration. Neuropathic joint degeneration may occur with bony resorption and deep tissue infection.[103] Other neurological processes including beriberi, inflammation, or metabolic disturbances should be ruled out. Blood studies and neurophysiological studies are useful in evaluating these patients and establishing the diagnosis.

These individuals are best managed by recommending abstinence from alcohol intake and enhancing their diet with vitamin supplements. Supplemental thiamin and pain control may be warranted in selected individuals. The prognosis depends on the severity and duration of symptoms. Behse and Buchthal found no evidence of clinical improvement or regeneration on nerve biopsy in 17 patients studied 2 years later.[106] The earlier patients abstain and establish regular diets, the more likely they are to recover from the neuropathy. Alcoholics with autonomic neuropathy have a reduced life expectancy.[113]

ALCOHOLISM AND MOVEMENT DISORDERS

In addition to the classic postural tremor associated with alcohol withdrawal, other movement disorders can occur in the setting of alcohol abuse and withdrawal.[114] A rare, slow tremor of the lower extremities can also occur in alcoholics and is produced by the synchronous flexion-extension of the muscles of the hip girdle.[115] This 3-Hz tremor is associated with alcoholic cerebellar degeneration affecting the anterior superior vermis and cerebellar hemispheres.[116] When they are supine, patients with this form of tremor may reveal a kicking movement when the legs are elevated and the knee and hip joints are flexed 90 degrees. It can be best observed when the patient stands with the feet together and the knees partially bent. This results in a slow up and down movement of the body.

Transient parkinsonism may rarely appear in the setting of alcohol abuse or withdrawal in patients with no liver dysfunction.[117, 118] This typically occurs a few days after alcohol cessation and is characterized by bradykinesia, stooped posture, and a coarse resting tremor in the hands. Cogwheel rigidity of the limbs can also be appreciated. These episodes may occur during alcohol withdrawal. These signs may last for a few weeks or months, yet they do not persist. Transient dyskinesias with lingual-oral, neck, or limb movements have been reported in some alcoholics.[119, 120]

With chronic abuse of alcohol, hepatic inflammation and fibrosis can occur and may be associated with encephalopathy. In this setting, patients have an altered level of consciousness with diffuse slowing and at times triphasic waves on an EEG. Asterixis, or so-called negative myoclonus, is a classic finding in these patients and is characterized by clusters of brief irregular lapses of sustained posture.[121, 122] On examination, this may be best demonstrated by asking the patient to hold out his or her upper extremities and extend the hands at the wrist. The involuntary lapses in posture are associated with 50- to 200-msec periods of electrical silence in muscles that are tonically active. The mechanisms of this movement are unknown. Chronic or persistent choreiform movements may also occur with alcoholic liver disease.[45]

FETAL ALCOHOL SYNDROME

The mechanism by which the abnormalities of the fetal alcohol syndrome are produced is unknown, but it is thought to be due to a direct teratogenic effect. There is no general agreement regarding the limits of vulnerability of the fetus in terms of gestational age. To date, this syndrome has been described only in children of mothers who drank alcohol frequently during their pregnancy. Fetal alcohol syndrome results in low birth weight and small head circumference. Cranial and joint deformities are common, and the children feed poorly and are "colicky" and tremulous. The infant mortality rate associated with this condition is high, and survivors suffer an increased risk of mental retardation. Many, but not all, of the mothers of affected babies suffered from withdrawal seizures, delirium tremens, or hepatic encephalopathy during the pregnancy. Infants with fetal alcohol syndrome have a higher incidence of various congenital brain malformations.

Because addicts often abuse several drugs, it is important to consider that an irritable, tremulous, small baby may also result from use of crack cocaine or other agents during pregnancy . There are no laboratory tests of value to support or refute the diagnosis of fetal alcohol syndrome. Maternal education regarding the toxic effects of alcohol is of paramount importance in preventing the fetal alcohol syndrome. There is no safe minimum amount of alcohol consumption that can be guaranteed not to be toxic to a fetus, so mothers-to-be are urged to abstain entirely from alcohol throughout their pregnancy. There is no direct treatment for the effects of the fetal alcohol syndrome, although proper postnatal nutrition and care will help affected babies as they do unaffected ones. Approximately one in six babies born with this syndrome die. Of the remainder, about half suffer permanent physical or mental handicaps.

Acknowledgment

We thank Monroe Cole, MD, for his thoughtful review of the manuscript.

Reviews and Selected Updates

Bartolomei F, Suchet L, Barrie M, Gastaut JL: Alcoholic epilepsy: A unified and dynamic classification. Eur Neurol 1997;37:13–17.

Brailowsky S, Garcia O: Ethanol, GABA, and epilepsy. Arch Med Res 1999;30:3–9.

Langlais PJ, Zhang SX: Cortical and subcortical white matter damage without Wernicke's encephalopathy after recovery from thiamin deficiency in the rat. Alcohol Clin Res 1997;21:434–443.

Manzo L, Locatelli C, Candura SM, Costa LG: Nutrition and alcohol neurotoxicity. Neurotoxicology 1994;15:555–565.

Nicolas JM, Estruch R, Salamero M, Orteu N: Brain impairment in well-nourished chronic alcoholism is related to ethanol intake. Ann Neurol 1997;41:590–598.

Rosenberg NR, Portegies P, de Visser M, Vermeulen M: Diagnostic investigation of patients with chronic polyneuropathy: Evaluation of a clinical guideline. J Neurol Neurosurg Psychiatry 2001;71:205–209.

Yamashita K, Kobayashi S, Yamaguchi S, Koide H, Nishi K: Reversible corpus callosum lesions in a patient with Marchiafava-Bignami disease: Serial changes on MRI. Eur Neurol 1997;37:192–193.

References

1. Harper C: The incidence of Wernicke's encephalopathy in Australia—a neuropathological study of 131 cases. J Neurol Neurosurg Psychiatry 1983;46:593–598.
2. Harper C, Giles M, Finlay-Jones R: Clinical signs of the Wernicke-Korsakoff complex: A retrospective analysis of 131 cases diagnosed at necropsy. J Neurol Neurosurg Psychiatry 1986;49:341–345.
3. O'Keefe ST, Tormey WP, Glasgow R, Lavan GN: Thiamin deficiency in hospitalized elderly patients. Gerontology 1994;40:18–24.
4. Langohr HD, Petruch F, Schroth J: Vitamin B_1, B_2, and B_6 deficiency and neurological disorders. J Neurol 1981;225:95–108.
5. Green R, Kinsella LJ: Current concepts in the diagnosis of cobalamin deficiency. Neurology 1995;45:1435–1440.
6. Joosten E, Van Den Berg A, Riezler R, et al: Metabolic evidence of deficiencies of vitamin B_{12}, folate, and vitamin B_6 occur commonly in elderly people. Am J Nutr 1993;58:468–476.
7. Incalzi RA, Gemma A, Capparella O, et al: Energy intake and in-hospital starvation, a clinically relevant relationship. Arch Intern Med 1996;156:425–429.
8. Victor M, Adams RD, Collins GH: The Wernicke-Korsakoff Syndrome. Philadelphia, F.A. Davis, 1971.
9. Haas RH: Thiamin and the brain. Ann Rev Nutr 1988;8:483–515.
10. Marcus R, Coulston AM: Water soluble vitamin, the vitamin B-complex and ascorbic acid. *In* Shils ME, Olson JA, Shike M (eds): Modern Nutrition in Health and Disease, 8th ed. Philadelphia, Lea & Febiger, 1994, pp 1547–1590.
11. Vortmeyer AO, Hagel C, Laas R: Hemorrhagic thiamin deficient encephalopathy following prolonged parenteral nutrition. J Neurol Neurosurg Psychiatry 1992;55:826–829.
12. Denny-Brown D: Neurological conditions resulting from prolonged and severe dietary restriction. Case reports in prisoners of war, and general review. Medicine (Baltimore)1947;26:41–113.
13. Peltier G, Hermreck AS, Moffat RE, et al: Complications following gastric bypass procedure for morbid obesity. Surgery 1979;86:648–654.
14. Paulson GW, Martin EW, Mojzisik C, Carey LC: Neurologic complications of gastric partitioning. Arch Neurol 1985;42:675–677.
15. Jagadha V, Deck JHN, Halliday WC, Smyth HS: Wernicke's encephalopathy in patients on peritoneal dialysis or hemodialysis. Ann Neurol 1987;21:78–84.
16. Descombes E, Dessibourg CA, Felly G: Acute encephalopathy due to thiamin deficiency (Wernicke's encephalopathy) in a chronic hemodialyzed patient: A case report. Clin Nephrol 1991;35:171–175.
17. Martin PR, McCool BA, Singleton CK: Molecular genetics of transketolase in the pathogenesis of the Wernicke-Korsakoff syndrome. Metab Brain Dis 1995;10:45–55.
18. Nixon PF: Is there a genetic component to the pathogenesis of the Wernicke-Korsakoff syndrome? Alcohol Alcohol 1984;19:219–221.
19. Hoyumpa AN: Mechanisms of vitamin deficiencies in alcoholism. Alcohol Clin Exp Res 1986;10:573–581.
20. Leigh D, McBurney A, McIlwain H: Erythrocyte transketolase activity in the Wernicke-Korsakoff syndrome. Br J Psychol 1981;138:153.
21. Yamashita M, Yamamoto T: Wernicke's encephalopathy with symmetric pericentral involvement: MR findings. J Comp Assist Tomogr 1995;19:306–308.
22. Rueler JB, Girard DE, Cooney TG: Wernicke's encephalopathy. N Engl J Med 1985;312:1035–1039.
23. Gold M, Chen MF, Johnson K: Plasma and red blood cell thiamin deficiency in patients with dementia of the Alzheimer's type. Arch Neurol 1995;52:1081–1086.
24. Skelton WP, Skelton, NR: Nutritional depletion polyneuropathy and valproic acid. Arch Intern Med 1993;153:902–905.

25. Teare JP, Hyamas G, Pollock S: Acute encephalopathy due to coexistent nicotinic acid and thiamin deficiency. Br J Clin Pract 1993;47:343–344.
26. Jollife N, Bowman KN, Rosenblum LA, Fein HD: Nicotinic acid deficiency encephalopathy. JAMA 1940;114:307–312.
27. Ishii N, Nishihara Y: Pellagra among chronic alcoholics: Clinical and pathologic study of 20 necropsy cases. J Neurol Neurosurg Psychiatry 1981;44:209–215.
28. Flippo TS, Holder WD Jr: Neurologic degeneration associated with nitrous oxide anesthesia in patients with vitamin B_{12} deficiency. Arch Surg 1993;128:1391–1395.
29. Lever EG, Elwes RDC, Williams A, Reynolds EH: Subacute combined degeneration of the cord due to folate deficiency: Response to methyl folate treatment. J Neurol Neurosurg Psychiatry 1986;49:1203–1207.
30. Pant SS, Ashbury AK, Richardson EP: The myelopathy of pernicious anemia: A neuropathological reappraisal. Acta Neurol Scand 1968;44(Suppl 35):1–36.
31. McCombe PA, McLeod JC: The peripheral neuropathy of vitamin B_{12} deficiency. J Neurol Sci 1984;66:117–126.
32. Lindenbaum J, Healton ES, Savage DG, et al: Neuropsychiatric disorders caused by cobalamin deficiency in the absence of anemia or macrocytosis. N Engl J Med 1988;318:1720–1728.
33. Carmel R: Cobalamin, the stomach, and aging. Am J Clin Nutr 1997;66:750–759.
34. Sumner AE, Chin MM, Abrahm JL, et al: Elevated methylmalonic acid and total homocysteine levels show high prevalence of vitamin B_{12} deficiency after gastric surgery. Ann Intern Med 1996;124:469–476.
35. Halverson JD: Micronutrient deficiencies after gastric bypass for morbid obesity. Am Surgeon 1986;52:594–598.
36. Marcuard SP, Albernaz L, Khazanie PG: Omeprazole therapy causes malabsorption of cyanocobalamin (vitamin B_{12}). Ann Intern Med 1994;120:211–215.
37. Kinsella LJ, Green R: Anesthesia paresthetica: Nitrous oxide-induced cobalamin deficiency. Neurology 1995;45:1608–1610.
38. Healton EV, Savage DG, Brust JCN, et al: Neurologic aspects of cobalamin deficiency. Medicine (Baltimore) 1991;70:229–244.
39. White WB, Reik L Jr, Cutlip DE: Pernicious anemia seen initially as orthostatic hypotension. Arch Intern Med 1991;141:1543–1544.
40. Eisenhofer G, Lambie DG, Johnson RH, Tan ETH, Whiteside EA: Deficient catecholamine release as the basis of orthostatic hypotension in pernicious anemia. JNNP 1982;45:1053–1155.
41. Layzer RB: Myeloneuropathy after prolonged exposure to nitrous oxide. Lancet 1988;2:1227–1230.
42. Reynolds EH, Bottiglieri T, Laundy M, et al: Vitamin B_{12} metabolism in multiple sclerosis. Arch Neurol 1992;49:649.
43. Herbert V: Vitamin B_{12} deficiency neuropsychiatric damage in acquired immunodeficiency syndrome. Arch Neurol 1993;50:569.
44. Kuzminski AM, Del Giacco EJ, Allen RH, Stabler SP, Lindenbaum J: Effective treatment of cobalamin deficiency with oral cobalamin. Blood 1998;92:1191–1198.
45. Savage DG, Lindenbaum J: Neurological complications of acquired cobalamin deficiency: Clinical aspects. Ballieres Clin Haematol 1995;8:657–678.
46. Hemmer B, Glocker FX, Schumacher M, et al: Subacute combined degeneration: Clinical, electrophysiological, and magnetic resonance imaging findings. JNNP 1998;65:822–827.
47. Timms SR, Cure JK, Kurent JE: Subacute combined degeneration of the spinal cord: MR findings. Am J Neuroradiol 1993;14:1224–1227.
48. Lott IT, Coulombe T, DiPaolo RV, et al: Vitamin B_6–dependent seizures: Pathology and chemical findings in brain. Neurology 1978;28:47–54.
49. Brent J: Reversal of prolonged isoniazid-induced coma by pyridoxine. Arch Intern Med 1990;150:1751–1753.
50. Molony CJ, Parmelee AH: Convulsions in young infants as a result of pyridoxine deficiency. JAMA 1954;154:405–408.
51. Dalton K, Dalton MJT: Characteristics of pyridoxine overdose neuropathy syndrome. Acta Neurol Scand 1987;76:8–11.
52. Parry GJ, Bredesen DE: Sensory neuropathy with low dose pyridoxine. Neurology 1985;35:1466–1468.
53. Bier JG, Corash L, Hubbard VS: Medical uses of vitamin E. N Engl J Med 1983;308:1063–1071.
54. Rosenblum JL, Keating JP, Prensky AL, Nelson JS: A progressive neurologic syndrome in children with chronic liver disease. N Engl J Med 1981;304:503–508.
55. Muller DPR, Lloyd JK, Wolff OH: Vitamin E and neurological function. Lancet 1983;i:225–227.
56. Gotoda T, Arita M, Arai H, et al: Adult onset spinocerebellar dysfunction caused by a mutation in the gene for the alpha-tocopherol transfer protein. N Engl J Med 1995;333:1313–1318.
57. Harding AE, Matthews S, Jones S, et al: Spinocerebellar degeneration associated with a selective defect of vitamin E absorption. N Engl J Med 1985;313:32–35.
58. Rosenberg RN: Spinocerebellar ataxias and ataxins. N Engl J Med 1995;333:1351–1352.
59. Brin MF, Pedley TA, Lovelace RE, et al: Electrophysiologic features of abetalipoproteinemia: Functional consequences of vitamin E deficiency. Neurology 1986;36:669–673.
60. Pappert EJ, Tangney CC, Goetz CG, et al: Alpha-tocopherol fails to increase ventricular CSF alpha-tocopherol levels in Parkinson's disease patients. Neurology 1996;47:1037–1042.
61. Tahiliani AG, Beinlich CJ: Pantothenic acid in health and disease. Vitam Horm 1991;46:165–228.
62. Goodman DS: Vitamin A and retinoids in health and disease. N Engl J Med 1984;310:1023.
63. Farris WA, Erdman JW: Protracted hypervitaminosis A following long-term, low level intake. JAMA 1982;247:317–318.
64. Herbert V: Toxicity of 25,000 international units of vitamin A supplements in health food users. Am J Clin Nutr 1982;36:185–186.
65. Schott DG, Wills MR: Myopathy and hypophosphatemic osteomalacia presenting in adult life. J Neurol Neurosurg Psychiatry 1975;38:297–304.
66. Skaria J, Katiyar BC, Srivastava TP, Dube B: Myopathy and neuropathy associated with osteomalacia. Acta Neurol Scand 1975;51:37–58.
67. Weber GA, Sloan P, Davies D: Nutritionally induced peripheral neuropathies. Clin Pediatr Med Surg N Am 1990;7:107–128.
68. Kahn E, Falcke AC: A syndrome simulating encephalitis affecting children recovering from malnutrition (kwashiorkor). J Pediatr 1956;49:37–45.
69. Balmer S, Howells G, Wharton B: The acute encephalopathy of kwashiorkor. Dev Med Child Neurol 1968;10:766–771.
70. Scoch MB, Smythe PN: 15-Year developmental study on effects of severe undernutrition during infancy on subsequent physical growth and intellectual functioning. Arch Dis Child 1976;51:327–336.
71. Strachan H: On a form of multiple neuritis prevalent in the West Indies. Practitioner 1897;59:477–484.
72. Fisher M: Residual neuropathological changes in Canadians held prisoner of war by the Japanese (Strachan's disease). Can Serv Med J 1955;11:157–199.
73. Roman GC: An epidemic in Cuba of optic neuropathy, sensorineural deafness, peripheral sensory neuropathy and dorsal lateral myeloneuropathy. J Neurol Sci 1994;127:11–28.
74. Osuntokun BO: An ataxic neuropathy in Nigeria: A clinical biochemical and electrophysiological study. Brain 1968;91:215–248.
75. Borrajero I, Perez JL, Dominguez C, et al: Epidemic neuropathy in Cuba: Morphological characterization of peripheral nerve lesions in sural nerve biopsies. J Neurol Sci 1994;127:68–76.
76. Thomas PK, Plant GT, Baxter P, et al: An epidemic of optic neuropathy and painful sensory neuropathy in Cuba: Clinical aspects. J Neurol 1995;242:629–638.
77. Feit H, Glasberg MR, Ireton C, et al: Peripheral neuropathy and starvation after gastric partitioning for morbid obesity. Ann Intern Med 1982;96:453–455.
78. Sassaris M, Meka R, Miletello G, et al: Neuropsychiatric syndromes after gastric partition. Am J Gastroenterol 1983;78:321–323.
79. Somer H, Bergstrom L, Muscajoki P, Rovamo L: Morbid obesity, gastric plication and a severe neurological deficit. Acta Med Scand 1985;217:575–576.
80. Harwood SC, Chodoroff G, Ellenberg MR: Gastric partitioning complicated by peripheral neuropathy with lumbosacral plexopathy. Arch Phys Med Rehabil 1987;68:310–312.
81. May WE: Nutritional sensory neuronopathy: An emerging new syndrome. Arch Neurol 1984;41:559–560.
82. Peoples RW, Li C, Weight FF: Lipid vs protein theories of alcohol action in the nervous system. Annu Rev Pharmacol Toxicol 1996;36:185–201.
83. Szabo G, Hoffman PL: Brain-derived neurotrophic factor, neurotrophin-3 and neurotrophin-4/5 maintain functional tolerance to ethanol. Eur J Pharm 1995;287:35–41.
84. Perrin RG, Hockman CH, Kalant H, et al: Acute effects of ethanol on spontaneous and auditory evoked electrical activity in cat brain. Electroencephalogr Clin Neurophysiol 1974;36:19–31.
85. Maling HM: Toxicology of single doses of ethyl alcohol. *In* J Tremolieres (ed): International Encyclopedia of Pharmacology and Therapeutics, Vol II, Alcohols and Derivatives. Oxford, Pergamon Press, 1970, pp 277–299.

86. Marc-Aurele J, Schreiner GE: The dialysance of ethanol and methanol: A proposed method for the treatment of massive intoxication by ethyl or methyl alcohol. J Clin Invest 1960;39: 802–807.
87. Victor M, Adams RD: The effect of alcohol on the nervous system. Res Publ Assoc Res Nerv Ment Dis 1953;32:526–573.
88. Friedlander WJ: Characteristics of postural tremor in normal and in various abnormal states. Neurology 1956;6:716–724.
89. Koller W, O'Hara R, Dorus W, Bauer J: Tremor in chronic alcoholism. Neurology 1985;35:1660–1662.
90. Marsden CD: The mechanisms of physiological tremor and their significance for pathological tremors. Prog Clin Neurophysiol 1978;5:1–16.
91. Victor M, Brausch C: The role of abstinence in the genesis of alcoholic epilepsy. Epilepsia 1967;8:1–20.
92. Isbell H, Graser HF, Wikler A, et al: An experimental study of the etiology of "rum fits" and delirium tremens. Q J Stud Alcohol 1955;16:1–33.
93. Victor M: The alcohol withdrawal syndrome. Postgrad Med 1970;47:68–72.
94. Thompson WL: Management of alcohol withdrawal syndromes. Arch Intern Med 1978;138:278–283.
95. Solomon J, Rouck LA, Koepke HH: Double-blind comparison of lorazepam and chlordiazepoxide in the treatment of the acute alcohol abstinence syndrome. Clin Ther 1983;6:52–58.
96. Kraus ML, Gottlieb LD, Horwitz RI, Anscher M: Randomized clinical trial of atenolol in patients with alcohol withdrawal. N Engl J Med 1985;313:905–909.
97. Baumgartner GR, Rowen RC: Clonidine vs chlordiazepoxide in the management of acute alcohol withdrawal syndrome. Arch Intern Med 1987;147:1223–1226.
98. Urbano-Marquez A, Estruch R, Fernandez-Sola J, et al: The greater risk of alcoholic cardiomyopathy and myopathy in women compared to men. JAMA 1995;274:149–154.
99. Cardellach F, Grau JM, Casademont J, et al: Oxidative metabolism in muscle mitochondria from patients with chronic alcoholism. Ann Neurol 1992;31:515–518.
100. Martin F, Ward K, Slavin G, et al: Alcoholic skeletal myopathy, a clinical and pathological study. Q J Med 1985;218:233–251.
101. Charness ME, Simon RP, Greenberg DA: Ethanol and the nervous system. N Engl J Med 1989;321:442–454.
102. D'Amour ML, Butterworth RF: Pathogenesis of alcoholic peripheral neuropathy: Direct effect of ethanol or nutritional deficit? Metab Brain Dis 1994;9:133–141.
103. Thornhill HL, Richter RW, Shelton ML, Johnson CA: Neuropathic arthropathy (Charcot forefeet) in alcoholics. Ortho Clin North Am 1973;4:7–20.
104. Victor M: Polyneuropathy due to nutritional deficiency and alcoholism. *In* Dyck PJ, Thomas PK, Lambert EH, Bunge RP (eds): Peripheral Neuropathy. Philadelphia, WB Saunders, 1984, p 1899.
105. Lefebvre D'Amour M, Shahani BT, Young RR, Bird KT: The importance of studying sural nerve conduction and late responses in the evaluation of alcoholic patients. Neurology 1979;29:1600–1604.
106. Behse F, Buchtal F: Alcoholic neuropathy: Clinical, electrophysiological, and biopsy findings. Ann Neurol 1977;2:95–110.
107. Stubbs CD, Williams BW, Pryor CL, Rubin E: Ethanol-induced modifications to membrane lipid structure: Effect on phospholipase A_2–membrane interactions. Arch Biochem Biophys 1988;262: 560–573.
108. Rooprai HK, Pratt OE, Shaw GK, Thomson AD: Superoxide dismutase in the erythrocytes of acute alcoholics during detoxification. Alcohol 1989;24:503–507.
109. Strauss MB: Etiology of "alcoholic" polyneuritis. Am J Med Sci 1935;189:378–382.
110. Hallet M, Fox JG, Rogers AE, et al: Controlled studies on the effects of alcohol ingestion on peripheral nerves of macaque monkeys. J Neurol Sci 1987;80:65.
111. Monforte R, Estruch R, Valls-Sole J, et al: Autonomic and peripheral neuropathies in patients with chronic alcoholism. Arch Neurol 1995;52:45–51.
112. Bischoff A: Dtsch Med Wochenschr 1971;96:317–322, as quoted in Layzer RB: Neuromuscular Manifestations of Systemic Disease. Philadelphia, F.A. Davis, 1985, p 345.
113. Johnson RH, Robinson BJ: Mortality in alcoholics with autonomic neuropathy. J Neurol Neurosurg Psychiatry 1988;51:476–480.
114. Neiman J, Lang AE, Fornazzari L, Carlen PL: Movement disorders in alcoholism: A review. Neurology 1990;40:741–746.
115. Silverskiold BP: A 3/sec leg tremor in a cerebellar syndrome. Acta Neurol Scand 1977;55:385–393.
116. Silverskiold BP: Cortical cerebellar degeneration associated with a specific disorder of standing and locomotion. Acta Neurol Scand 1977;55:257–272.
117. Carlen PL, Lee MA, Jacob MA, Livishits O: Parkinsonism provoked by alcoholism. Ann Neurol 1981;9:84–86.
118. Lang AE, Marsden CD, Obeso JA, Parkes JD: Alcohol and Parkinson disease. Ann Neurol 1982;12:254–256.
119. Mullin PJ, Kershaw PW, Bolt JMW: Choreoathetotic movement disorder in alcoholism. BMJ 1970;4:278–281.
120. Fornazzari L, Carlen PL: Transient choreiform dyskinesias during alcohol withdrawal. Can J Neurol Sci 1982;9:89–90.
121. Leavitt S, Tyler HR: Studies in asterixis. Arch Neurol 1964;10:360–368.
122. Young RR, Shahani BT: Asterixis: One type of negative myoclonus. Adv Neurol 1986;43:137–157.

CHAPTER 41

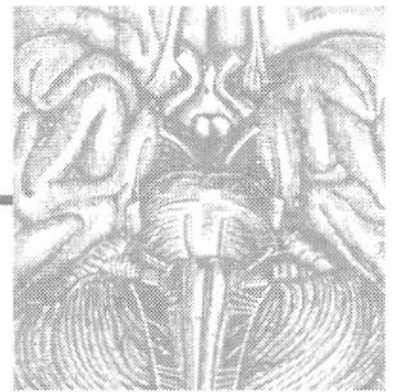

KAREN L. ROOS

Viral Infections

The diagnosis and therapy of central nervous system (CNS) viral infections is one of the most rapidly evolving and exciting areas in neurology. Viruses gain access to the CNS either through the bloodstream or through an intraneuronal route from the peripheral nerves. Viruses may cause acute CNS disease such as meningitis or encephalitis, a delayed complication of an acute infection such as postinfectious polyneuritis or autoimmune encephalomyelitis, latent infections with recurrence of disease from time to time, or slowly progressive neurological disorders. The important human nervous system viruses are listed in Table 41–1. The most common acute CNS viral infections are meningitis and encephalitis. The classic clinical presentation of viral meningitis includes fever, headache, photophobia, myalgias, and nausea and vomiting. There is no alteration in the level of consciousness. The viral etiological agents of meningitis are listed in Table 41–2, and Table 41–3 lists a differential diagnosis of aseptic meningitis. Viral encephalitis is characterized by fever, an altered level of consciousness, headache, and seizure activity. The etiological agents of viral encephalitis are listed in Table 41–4. In addition, viral encephalitis may present as a focal encephalitis with focal neurological deficits and focal seizure activity. The etiological agents of focal encephalitis are listed in Table 41–4.

In addition to meningitis and encephalitis, CNS enteroviral infections may present as an acute transverse myelitis (characterized by abrupt onset of weakness of the limbs progressing to flaccid paralysis in association with a sensory level), single or multiple limb paralysis, cerebellar ataxia (a common presentation of enteroviral CNS infection in children), a chronic meningoencephalitis (Table 41–5), or a postinfectious polyneuritis. Measles and rubella viruses can cause a slowly progressive neurological disease that presents several years after the acute viral illness has occurred. Other viruses, such as the human T-cell lymphotropic virus type 1 (HTLV-1), can cause a slowly progressive neuromyelopathy in adulthood with no prior history of apparent infection. Human herpesviruses, herpes simplex virus and varicella-zoster virus, are the prototypical viruses that establish lifelong latent infections in human peripheral and CNS sensory ganglia that may episodically reactivate, resulting in acute infection. This chapter reviews the epidemiology, pathogenesis, clinical features, diagnosis, and management of the human nervous system viruses listed in Table 41–1.

RNA Viruses

ENTEROVIRUSES (ECHOVIRUSES AND COXSACKIEVIRUSES)

Epidemiology and Risk Factors. Enteroviral infections occur primarily in the summer and autumn months in temperate climates; infants, young children, and immunocompromised patients are at greatest risk of infection. The enteroviruses comprise a total of 68 distinct serotypes of human pathogens, but the most common enteroviruses that cause aseptic meningitis are the coxsackieviruses B5, B3, B4, and A9; the echoviruses 30, 11, 7, 9, 6, 4, and 18; and

TABLE 41–1. Classification of Human Nervous System Viruses

RNA Viruses
Picornaviridae
  Coxsackieviruses
  Echoviruses
  Enterovirus 70 and 71
  Polioviruses
Paramyxoviridae
  Mumps virus
  Measles virus
Togaviridae: alphaviruses
  Western equine encephalitis virus
  Eastern equine encephalitis virus
  Venezuelan equine encephalitis virus
  Nonarthropod-borne togavirus: rubella virus
Flaviviridae
  Mosquito-borne
    St. Louis encephalitis virus
    Japanese encephalitis virus
    West Nile virus
    Dengue viruses
  Tick-borne
    Powassan virus
Bunyaviridae
  California encephalitis virus
Reoviridae
  Colorado tick fever
Retroviridae
  HIV-1
  HTLV-1
Arenoviridae
  Lymphocytic choriomeningitis virus
Orthomyxoviridae
  Influenza viruses

DNA Viruses
Herpesviridae
  Herpes simplex virus types 1 and 2
  Varicella-zoster virus
  Human herpesvirus-6
  Cytomegalovirus
  Epstein-Barr virus
Papovaviridae
  JC virus

Adapted from Bale JF: Viral encephalitis. Med Clin North Am 1993;77:25–42.

enteroviruses 70 and 71.[1, 2] The clinical signs and symptoms observed during enterovirus CNS infection depend to some extent not only on the patient's age, but also on the state of the individual's immune system. Neonates are at greatest risk for severe infection, either meningitis or meningoencephalitis. Enteroviral infection in agammaglobulinemic individuals may cause a chronic meningitis or meningoencephalitis. Enteroviral CNS infection in infants older than 2 weeks of age and in children and adults is rarely associated with severe disease and is most often an aseptic meningitis.

Pathogenesis and Pathophysiology. Enteroviruses may enter the host through the mucosal surfaces of the gastrointestinal or respiratory tract. Enteroviruses are acquired most commonly by fecal-oral contamination and, less commonly, via aerosolized respiratory droplets. Enteroviruses may also enter through the conjunctiva of the eye, initially producing a conjunctivitis before they spread to the CNS. When enteroviruses enter the host through the nasopharynx, the initial spread and replication of virus may take place in the upper respiratory tract lymphatics, but more often the viral inoculum is swallowed.[2] Once in the alimentary tract, the virus may infect the intestinal lining cells and remain limited to the gastrointestinal tract, causing symptoms of gastroenteritis and diarrhea, or it may traverse the intestinal lining cells, replicate in Peyer's patches in the mucosa of the lamina propria, and then disseminate to other organs, including the CNS.[2, 3] Most enteroviruses spread to the CNS via the bloodstream, but a small percentage may reach the CNS by direct neural spread from nerves terminating in the intestinal tissue. Virus traverses the blood-brain barrier either at the choroid plexus, where it may infect endothelial cells and spread into the cerebrospinal fluid (CSF), causing a meningitis, or at the endothelium of the cerebral capillary cells in the brain parenchyma, causing an encephalitis.[2]

Although viremia typically occurs 2 to 3 days after the enterovirus has infected the alimentary tract, signs and symptoms of CNS disease typically develop 5 to 16 days after the initial infection and may be biphasic, with minor illness preceding the onset of neurological disease.[3] Unlike most viral infections, in which cell-mediated immunity is the primary host defense against infection, clearance of enteroviral infection by the host is antibody mediated. For this reason, infants and young children and individuals with antibody deficiencies, particularly patients with X-linked agammaglobulinemia, are prone to severe or chronic enteroviral meningitis or meningoencephalitis.[4]

Clinical Features and Associated Findings. Enteroviral CNS infection may be an aseptic meningitis, an encephalitis, a focal encephalitis (group A coxsackieviruses), an acute transverse myelitis, single or multiple limb paralysis (poliomyelitis syndrome), Guillain-Barré syndrome, cerebellar ataxia, or a chronic meningoencephalitis.[2, 4–7]

ASEPTIC MENINGITIS. Enteroviruses are presently the most common cause of aseptic meningitis, accounting for 80 to 92 percent of all cases of aseptic meningitis for which an etiologic agent is identified.[2] Certain serotypes (group B coxsackieviruses and the echoviruses) are associated with a greater frequency of meningitis than other serotypes.[8, 9] In a review of aseptic meningitis in 274 children less than 2 years

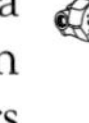

TABLE 41–2. Etiological Agents of Viral Menengitis

Herpes simplex virus types 1 and 2
Enteroviruses
Mumps
HIV
St. Louis encephalitis virus
West Nile virus
California encephalitis virus
Western equine encephalitis virus
Venezuelan equine encephalitis virus
Colorado tick fever
Lymphocytic choriomeningitis virus
Epstein-Barr virus
Influenza virus types A and B

TABLE 41–3. **Differential Diagnosis of Aseptic Meningitis**

Viral Infection
Enteroviruses (poliovirus, coxsackievirus types A and B, echovirus, human enterovirus 68 to 72)
Mumps
Herpes simplex virus types 1 and 2
Varicella-zoster virus
Human immunodeficiency virus
Arboviruses
Epstein-Barr virus
Lymphocytic choriomeningitis virus
Colorado tick fever

Bacterial Infection
Partially treated bacterial meningitis
Bacterial meningitis in cancer patient
Parameningeal infection
Listeria monocytogenes
Mycoplasma pneumoniae
Mycobacterium tuberculosis
Human monocytic ehrlichiosis
Human granulocytic ehrlichiosis

Spirochetes
Borrelia burgdorferi
Treponema pallidum

Fungal Infection
Cryptococcus neoformans
Histoplasma capsulatum
Coccidioides immitis
Blastomyces dermatitidis

Systemic Disease
Sarcoidosis
Leukemia, lymphoma
Adenocarcinoma, malignant melanoma, small cell lung cancer
Systemic lupus erythematosus
Behçet's disease
Endocarditis

Drugs
Nonsteroidal anti-inflammatory agents
OKT3
Azathioprine (Imuran)
Trimethoprim-sulfamethoxazole
Isoniazid
Intravenous immune globulin

Other
Migraine
Measles-mumps-rubella vaccine
Vasculitis
Parainfectious syndrome (acute disseminated encephalomyelitis)

of age, the group B coxsackieviruses and the echoviruses were the etiologic agents in 156 (92%) of the 169 laboratory-diagnosed cases.[10] The clinical presentation of aseptic meningitis includes fever (100° to 104° F [38° to 40° C]), severe headache, nausea and vomiting, photophobia, and nuchal rigidity. Neurological abnormalities are rare, and enteroviral meningitis in otherwise healthy children and adults is rarely associated with severe disease or poor outcome.[2]

ENCEPHALITIS. Enteroviral CNS infection may be severe, fatal, or protracted in infants and in individuals with agammaglobulinemia. In neonates, the illness begins with fever and nonspecific signs such as vomiting, anorexia, rash, or upper respiratory findings. Signs of meningeal inflammation may or may not be present at this stage. As the disease progresses, hepatic necrosis, myocarditis, necrotizing enterocolitis, disseminated intravascular coagulation, and other signs of

TABLE 41–4. **Etiological Agents of Viral Encephalitis**

Herpes Simplex Viruses
Herpes simplex virus type 1
Herpes simplex virus type 2 (neonates)

Arthropod-Borne
Mosquito-borne
- California encephalitis virus
- St. Louis encephalitis virus
- West Nile virus
- Japanese B encephalitis virus
- Eastern equine encephalitis virus
- Western equine encephalitis virus
- Dengue viruses

Tick-borne
- Powassan virus
- Colorado tick fever

Enteroviruses (Neonates, Young Adults, Agammaglobulinemic Patients)
Coxsackieviruses
Echoviruses
Enteroviruses 70 and 71

Immunocompromised
Varicella-zoster virus
Epstein-Barr virus
Cytomegalovirus
Human herpesvirus type 6
Measles virus (postmeasles encephalomyelitis, subacute sclerosing panencephalitis)
Rubella virus
Lymphocytic choriomeningitis virus

Focal Encephalitis
Herpes simplex virus
Enterovirus
California encephalitis virus
Powassan virus
Measles (subacute measles encephalitis)
Human herpesvirus type 6
Varicella-zoster virus

TABLE 41-5. **Causes of Chronic/Relapsing Meningoencephalitis**

Enteroviruses (agammaglobulinemic patients)
Measles (SSPE)
Rubella virus (progressive rubella panencephalitis)

"sepsis" may develop. The onset of encephalitis is characterized by an altered level of consciousness, seizures, and focal neurological deficits.[2] Unlike enteroviral aseptic meningitis, neonatal enteroviral meningoencephalitis may be fatal or associated with long-term sequelae. The infected neonate appears to be at greatest risk for severe morbidity and death when signs and symptoms develop in the first days of life, an onset suggestive of intrauterine or parturient exposure caused by maternal infection.[2] Chronic enteroviral meningoencephalitis has been reported in patients with agammaglobulinemia. The disease is most frequently caused by echoviruses, and the typical clinical presentation is that of a slowly progressive neurological disease with ataxia, headache, seizures, paresthesias, and loss of cognitive skills. This change in cognitive skills may be marked by loss of developmental milestones, episodic confusional states, and personality changes. Some patients also have non-neurological manifestations of chronic enteroviral infection, including fever, dermatomyositis-like syndrome, rashes, and hepatitis.[4] An enterovirus may also cause a focal encephalitis, but unlike patients with herpes simplex virus encephalitis, patients with enteroviral focal encephalitis typically improve spontaneously within 1 or 2 days of admission. The association of a macular or maculopapular rash with the clinical signs and symptoms as described earlier warrants the inclusion of enterovirus in the differential diagnosis of a focal encephalitis.

PARALYSIS. Coxsackieviruses and echoviruses have been implicated as the etiological agents of acute transverse myelitis, which is characterized by the abrupt onset of weakness of the limbs that progresses to flaccid paralysis, and diminished and then absent deep tendon reflexes, in association with a sensory level.[6, 11] Nonpolio enteroviruses may also cause paralysis of a single limb or multiple limbs that may resemble poliomyelitis.[7] The clinical disease and pathology associated with coxsackievirus and echovirus paralytic disease are generally much less severe than those seen with poliovirus. Echovirus type 70, the cause of epidemics of acute hemorrhagic conjunctivitis, has been associated with acute paralytic disease in Asia, Africa, and Latin America. Echovirus type 71, the usual etiological agent of hand-foot-mouth disease, has been responsible for epidemics of paralytic disease in Bulgaria, Hungary, and the United States.[12, 13] Infection of the anterior horn cells by a nonpolio enterovirus may contribute to disease in patients with postpolio syndrome, causing slowly progressive motor neuron damage.[12]

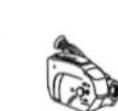

Differential Diagnosis. The diagnosis of enteroviral aseptic meningitis is based on examination of the CSF. The opening pressure should be normal or slightly increased, and there is a mild lymphocytic pleocytosis, a normal or slightly increased protein concentration, and a normal glucose concentration. The white blood cell (WBC) count typically is less than 1000 cells/mm^3.

Because enteroviral meningitis is quite common in neonates, it is important to emphasize the normal values for the CSF total WBC count and protein concentration in neonates (0 to 4 weeks), older neonates (4 to 8 weeks), and children and adults. The upper limit of normal for the CSF total WBC count is 22/mm^3 in infants 0 to 4 weeks old, 15/mm^3 in infants 4 to 8 weeks old, and 5/mm^3 in those older than 8 weeks of age.[15, 16] In normal uninfected CSF in newborns, about 60 percent of the cells are polymorphonuclear leukocytes and 40 percent are mononucleated cells.[16] In uninfected CSF in children and adults, the normal WBC count ranges from 0 to 5 mononuclear cells (lymphocytes and monocytes) per microliter. In normal uninfected CSF in children and adults, there should be no polymorphonuclear leukocytes; however, with use of the cytocentrifuge, an occasional polymorphonuclear leukocyte may be seen. If the total WBC count is less than 5/mm^3, the presence of a single polymorphonuclear leukocyte may be considered normal.[16] The normal protein concentration in neonates and older neonates is greater than that in children and adults. A CSF protein concentration as high as 150 mg/dL is considered normal in the neonate. By 1 year of age, the normal value for the lumbar CSF protein concentration is 45 mg/dL.[16] The upper range of normal for the lumbar CSF protein concentration in the adult is 50 mg/dL. The CSF WBC count is often higher in those with coxsackievirus aseptic meningitis than in patients with echovirus aseptic meningitis, and counts as high as 2000/mm^3 have been reported. A predominance of polymorphonuclear leukocytes may be seen early in the disease course with a transition to a lymphocytic pleocytosis as the disease progresses. In addition, hypoglycorrhachia has been reported in some patients with enteroviral aseptic meningitis.[17]

At the present time, isolation of an enterovirus by CSF viral culture is the gold standard for diagnosis of an enteroviral CNS infection. When an enterovirus is isolated from a non-CSF site (throat, stool, serum, urine) in conjunction with a CSF pleocytosis and an absence of bacteria by Gram's stain or the latex agglutination technique, enteroviral meningitis is the presumptive diagnosis. An enterovirus isolated from a non-CSF site may, however, be unrelated to the CNS infection.[18] CSF can be examined by the reverse transcriptase polymerase chain reaction (RT-PCR) for enteroviral RNA. As a general rule, CSF viral culture is negative in approximately 25 to 33 percent of CSF specimens from patients with enteroviral meningitis. In these patients, approximately two thirds of CSF specimens are found to be positive for enterovirus by RT-PCR.[1, 2]

An enterovirus is the likely etiological agent in the patient with a clinical presentation of aseptic meningitis, CSF findings of a lymphocytic pleocytosis with a normal glucose concentration, and a fourfold or greater increase in antiviral IgG antibody between acute and convalescent sera or the first-time appearance of virus-specific IgM antibodies.

Management. Because the majority of enteroviral infections are spread by the fecal-oral route, enteroviral infections are best prevented by proper handwashing techniques. Infants and children are at particular risk for these infections, and good hygiene, including parental handwashing after urine and stool diaper changes and washing the hands of the infant or child before eating, can reduce the transmission of these infections. Children and adolescents should be discouraged from sharing water bottles and drinking cups during athletic events.

Pleconaril is a new antipicornavirus agent that inhibits viral replication by blocking the viral uncoating process and viral attachment to host cell receptors. In a double-blind placebo-controlled trial, 130 patients with enteroviral meningitis between the ages of 14 and 65 years were treated with either 200 mg of Pleconaril three times per day or a placebo. Those receiving Pleconaril had a shorter duration of headache and returned to work and school earlier than untreated patients.[19] Intravenous immune globulin has been used to treat enterovirus infections in newborns and in patients with agammaglobulinemia and other immunodeficiency states with good success, but it is not recommended in children and adults with uncomplicated enteroviral aseptic meningitis.[4, 20, 21]

Prognosis and Future Perspectives. With the exception of neonates and patients with agammaglobulinemia, the majority of patients with enteroviral aseptic meningitis have a benign self-limited course of disease. As discussed previously, neonates and patients with agammaglobulinemia may have a severe, fatal, or protracted course of enteroviral meningoencephalitis. The prognosis of patients with acute transverse myelitis due to an enteroviral infection is generally good.[6, 12] The prognosis of limb paralysis due to a coxsackievirus or echovirus infection is generally much better than that due to poliovirus.[7]

POLIOVIRUS

Epidemiology and Risk Factors. Poliomyelitis was the most frightening infectious disease during the first half of the 20th century. Large epidemics led to extensive research in the epidemiology and pathogenesis of the disease. The poliovirus was first isolated in 1908 by inoculation of monkeys with a cell-free extract made from the spinal cord of a patient with fatal poliomyelitis.[22, 23] It was not until 1937, however, that the virus was isolated from intestinal washings, and by 1941 it was clear that the gastrointestinal tract played a major role in the pathogenesis of this infection.[24] Shortly thereafter it was recognized that the majority of poliovirus infections are a form of acute gastroenteritis. Paralysis develops in less than 1 in 100 individuals infected with the poliovirus.[25] In 1949 Enders, Weller, and Robbins made the major discovery that the poliovirus could be grown in tissue cultures of human embryonic skin, muscle cells, and intestinal tissue. Prior to that the only source of the poliovirus was nervous tissue from infected monkeys, an unacceptable inoculum in humans.[22] The work of Enders and his colleagues, combined with the efforts of the National Foundation for Infantile Paralysis, led to the recognition that there were only three serotypes of poliovirus and laid the groundwork for the development of the killed virus vaccine by Jonas Salk in 1955 and the oral live attenuated virus vaccine by Albert Sabin in 1961.[22–26] Poliomyelitis has been nearly eradicated from North America and Europe, but outbreaks of the disease continue to occur in the Indian subcontinent, the Eastern Mediterranean, and Africa.[27]

Pathogenesis and Pathophysiology. Poliovirus is a member of the Picornaviridae. There are three immunologically defined serotypes of poliovirus, all of which are capable of causing paralytic disease. The poliovirus is a single-stranded RNA enterovirus.[23] Natural polio infection occurs through ingestion of the virus, which initially multiplies in the oropharyngeal and intestinal mucosa. Poliovirus either enters the CNS via the bloodstream or, alternatively, may be transmitted to the CNS through vagal autonomic nerve fibers in the intestinal lumen.[23] A temporal association corresponding to the incubation period of the disease was observed between tonsillectomy and the development of bulbar poliomyelitis, suggesting that the exposure of nerve endings via tonsillectomy could transmit poliovirus to the CNS.[28] A third hypothesis is that ingested poliovirus initially replicates in the gastrointestinal tract; then a viremia ensues, and disseminated virus replicates at an extraneural site (i.e., skeletal muscle cells). Virus is then transported from the muscle cells via the peripheral nerves to the CNS. The hypothesis that poliovirus replicates in muscle cells and then enters the CNS through the peripheral nerves has been supported by the clinical observations that vigorous exertion or injury of a limb was temporally associated with limb paralysis.[23] In the Cutter incident, children inoculated intramuscularly with incompletely inactivated polio vaccine developed focal limb paralysis.[29, 30] Poliovirus replicates in the muscles of monkeys after intramuscular injection and causes limb paralysis of the injected limb.[29] The poliovirus receptor (PVR), a member of the immunoglobulin superfamily of proteins, is present at the motor endplate. During acute infection, the poliovirus may bind to the PVR-expressing motor endplate and travel by way of endocytosis and retrograde transport to the anterior horn cells in the spinal cord and brain stem.[29] Acute paralytic poliomyelitis is then characterized pathologically by severe anterior horn inflammation with loss of spinal and bulbar motor neurons.[31]

In his classic work on acute polio infection, Bodian noted evidence of a marked scarcity of normal-appearing neurons, even in cases of very mild paralysis, suggesting that acute paralytic polio was a generalized neuronal disease. The earliest cellular change in the motor neurons was dissolution of the cytoplasmic Nissl substance (chromatolysis). Infected neurons that exhibited only a mild degree of diffuse chromatolysis survived and continued to support motor units; in contrast, neurons that had severe chromatolysis followed by nuclear invagination and perinuclear chromatin aggregation could not support motor units, and subsequently permanent loss of function occurred in these muscle groups.[31, 32]

Postpolio syndrome, defined as "the development of new muscle weakness and fatigue in skeletal or bulbar muscles, unrelated to any known cause, that begins 25 to 30 years after an acute attack of paralytic poliomyelitis," is most likely explained by the status of the motor neurons that survived the initial infection. The surviving motor neurons, in an attempt to reinnervate the muscle fibers orphaned by the death of their parent motor neurons, adopt in their motor unit territory additional muscle fibers, so that the number of muscle fibers innervated by a single motor neuron may be four to five times the normal number. This puts metabolic stress on the neuronal cell bodies that, after a number of years, leads to a slow deterioration of nerve terminals. As each terminal dies, muscle fibers drop out, and weakness slowly progresses.[32]

Clinical Features and Associated Findings

NONPARALYTIC OR PREPARALYTIC. As stated previously, the majority of poliovirus infections were asymptomatic or characterized by a nonspecific viral syndrome of malaise, myalgias, and low-grade fever.

PARALYTIC. Patients who developed paralytic poliomyelitis may initially have had clinical symptoms of fever, malaise, headache, and gastrointestinal or upper respiratory tract symptoms. These symptoms subsided, only to recur after several days in association with increasing signs of meningeal irritation, headache, and stiff neck. When the illness progressed to the paralytic form, muscle soreness was prominent, particularly in the back and neck. Patients who developed paralysis usually did so on the second to fifth day after meningeal signs and fever became evident. Once weakness began, it typically progressed for only the first few days after its onset. The fever persisted for several days but often subsided before the paralysis was complete. Patients complained of severe muscle pain and spasms with asymmetrical flaccid muscle weakness that usually affected a lower extremity. Severe bulbar weakness occurred in 10 to 15 percent of patients with paralysis. The disease was most common in infants and children between the ages of 6 months and 10 years, and was more common in the late summer and autumn months. Acute mortality usually resulted from respiratory or bulbar involvement.[25]

POSTPOLIO SYNDROME. The following criteria are necessary for a diagnosis of postpolio syndrome as the cause of progressive weakness: (1) a history of documented acute paralytic poliomyelitis in childhood or adolescence as evidenced by a well-documented acute febrile paralytic attack during a polio epidemic that resulted in residual lower motor neuron weakness; (2) partial recovery of motor function and functional stability or recovery for at least 15 years; (3) residual asymmetrical muscle atrophy with weakness, areflexia, and normal sensation in at least one limb; and (4) normal sphincteric function.[33]

Differential Diagnosis. Although the poliovirus now can be recovered from stool, throat washings, CSF, and blood, during the polio epidemic in this century, virological confirmation was not available. The diagnosis was based on the clinical syndrome of fever with paralysis and residual lower motor neuron weakness. Examination of the CSF in the preparalytic stage showed an increase in the opening pressure and an increase in the WBC count that initially might be a predominance of polymorphonuclear leukocytes, but within a few days' time was characterized by a predominance of lymphocytes. WBC counts of 10 to 1000/mm^3 were typically seen. The protein concentration in the CSF at the onset of illness might be normal or slightly increased. Patients who developed paralysis had a higher number of WBCs in the CSF and a higher protein concentration than patients who did not develop paralysis.[25]

Needle examination shows a reduced number of voluntary motor unit potentials in the initial phase of paralysis, but in subsequent months, as the patient improves, the motor units become markedly enlarged, reflecting the reinnervation of the denervated muscle fibers.

Management. The management of patients with poliomyelitis and the postpolio syndrome is largely supportive. The treatment of bulbar poliomyelitis was significantly improved by the development of the "iron lung" in the 1930s. Patients with lower extremity weakness were initially treated with splints and plaster casts. Prolonged casting, often for months at a time, was typically employed. Eventually, the use of splinting and casting was replaced by physical therapy, braces, and other assistive ambulatory devices.[25] Anticholinesterase therapy has been beneficial in the treatment of symptoms of weakness and fatigue in patients with postpolio syndrome.[34]

In 1995, the Advisory Committee on Immunization Practices (ACIP) of the United States Public Health Service recommended that the United States adopt a sequential poliomyelitis immunization schedule—two doses of inactivated polio vaccine (IPV) followed by two doses of live oral polio vaccine (OPV) in order to reduce the occurrence of vaccine-associated polio from the live oral poliovirus vaccine.[35, 36] Although OPV is among the safest of vaccines, one case of vaccine-associated polio occurs for every 2.5 million doses of OPV administered. The proposed sequential schedule recommended by the ACIP was a compromise that sought to retain the advantages of OPV while preventing half of the 8 to 10 vaccine-related cases that occurred every year in the United States.[36] In order to totally eliminate the risk of vaccine associated poliomyelitis, in July 1999, the ACIP recommended that IPV be used exclusively in the United States beginning in 2000. An all-IPV schedule is presently the recommended schedule for polio vaccination of infants and children in the United States. The OPV continues to be used for routine immunization and to achieve polio eradication in countries throughout the world.[37]

MUMPS

Epidemiology and Risk Factors. Mumps is a member of the Paramyxoviridae group and is an enveloped virus containing a single-stranded RNA genome.[38] Prior to the widespread use of the trivalent measles-mumps-rubella (MMR) vaccine, mumps was an epidemic disease that occurred in the winter and spring months. Mumps was the most common cause of viral meningitis and encephalitis in many countries, the frequency of aseptic meningitis being estimated at 1 per 1000 cases of clinical mumps with much higher figures observed during epidemics.[39] In some countries, mumps was the most common cause of meningoencephalitis in children under 15 years of age.[40]

The live mumps vaccine has a 95 percent protection rate, and the MMR vaccine containing the Jeryl Lynn strain of mumps virus has nearly eliminated meningitis and meningoencephalitis due to mumps. In 1989, the ACIP in the United States estimated that the incidence of postvaccination encephalitis within 30 days of vaccination was 0.4 cases per 1 million doses administered.[41, 42]

The use of the Urabe Am 9 mumps vaccine was associated with a number of cases of aseptic meningitis in Canada and Japan, with an estimated rate of one case per several thousand vaccinations. The vaccine-associated cases of aseptic meningitis were mild and were rarely associated with sequelae, but the occurrence of aseptic meningitis with the vaccine containing the Urabe strain led to replacement of this strain of mumps virus with the Jeryl Lynn strain in many mass vaccination programs.[38]

Pathogenesis and Pathophysiology. Mumps virus spreads by respiratory droplets. After local replication occurs in the respiratory mucosa, viremia ensues. Parotitis occurs because the virus has an affinity for parotid ductal epithelial cells.[43] The mumps virus is neurotropic and meningotropic, and the

CNS is infected in the course of the viremia.[42] Virus infects the endothelial cells of the choroid plexus.

Clinical Features and Associated Findings. The mean incubation period for mumps is 16 to 18 days, and symptoms develop in 60 to 70 percent of those infected. Thirty to 40 percent of natural mumps infections are asymptomatic.[42] When symptomatic, an initial febrile illness with parotitis occurs in 95 percent of patients, and orchitis occurs in 25 percent of males.[43] Although many children with wild mumps meningitis have parotitis, clinical evidence of parotitis is not absolute.[44] CNS infection occurs in the absence of parotitis in 36 to 50 percent of cases.[43]

Mumps meningitis is characterized by fever, headache, vomiting, and signs of meningeal irritation. The clinical presentation of mumps encephalitis includes seizures, altered consciousness, behavioral abnormalities, sensory abnormalities, and difficulty with balance.[43] Mumps is a well-recognized cause of acquired deafness due to sensorineural hearing loss, which is typically unilateral and has been attributed to a cochlear neuritis with or without labyrinthine inflammation.[45] Mumps can cause an epididymo-orchitis, with subsequent infertility, pancreatitis, juvenile diabetes mellitus, fatal myocarditis, and abortions.[39]

Differential Diagnosis. The diagnosis of mumps aseptic meningitis is suggested by the clinical appearance of parotitis and meningitis and is established by examination of the CSF. The classic CSF abnormalities are a lymphocytic pleocytosis (300 to 600 cells/mm^3) and either a normal or decreased glucose concentration.[46] A positive CSF viral culture establishes the diagnosis. A fourfold rise in mumps antiviral antibody in convalescent sera compared to acute sera is also diagnostic, except in patients who have recently been immunized, in which case a fourfold rise in mumps-specific IgG may simply represent successful immunization. The diagnosis of mumps meningoencephalitis is made similarly by isolating the virus from the CSF and/or by noting a fourfold rise in mumps antiviral antibody between the acute and convalescent sera. The electroencephalogram (EEG) is reported to be abnormal in 100 percent of patients with mumps meningoencephalitis.[43, 47]

Management. No antiviral therapy is available for mumps meningitis or meningoencephalitis. Fortunately, these neurological complications have largely been eradicated through the widespread use of the MMR vaccine. As described earlier, there have been no cases of postvaccine meningitis with use of the Jeryl Lynn strain of mumps virus vaccine. The propensity of the vaccine to cause meningitis appears to have been associated with the Urabe strain, and a reported reduction in vaccine-associated aseptic meningitis in Canada following the change from the Urabe to the Jeryl Lynn mumps virus-containing MMR vaccine supports this observation.[44]

ARTHROPOD-BORNE VIRUSES

Epidemiology and Risk Factors. The arthropod-borne viruses (arboviruses) are transmitted to humans by the bite of a mosquito or tick. The epidemiology of arthropod-borne viral encephalitis is influenced by the season; the geographic location; the regional climatic conditions, such as the amount of spring rainfall; and the patient's age. LaCrosse virus is the most important arboviral cause of pediatric encephalitis in the United States.[48] The midwestern states of the United States report the highest incidence of LaCrosse virus infections. The LaCrosse virus belongs to the California group of encephalitis viruses. It is responsible for nearly all infections due to California group viruses in the United States. Most cases occur in late summer to early fall. The vector, *Aedes triseriatus*, is a forest-dwelling mosquito, and the risk of infection is associated with outdoor activities in woodland areas.[49] St. Louis encephalitis (SLE) occurs as periodic focal outbreaks of encephalitis in the midwestern, western, and southeastern United States, followed by years of sporadic cases. St. Louis encephalitis virus has caused large urban epidemics of encephalitis.[49, 50] Western equine encephalitis virus is an alphavirus that infects horses and humans in western North America, with most cases occurring between April and September. Eastern equine encephalitis (EEE) virus is also an alphavirus that infects horses and humans, primarily along the eastern seaboard and the gulf coast; its peak activity occurs in August and September. Eastern equine encephalitis virus has been isolated from species other than horses, including pheasants, piglets, and litters of puppies.[50] It causes a much more severe encephalitis than western equine encephalitis virus. Venezuelan equine encephalitis virus is endemic in South America and has caused rare cases of encephalitis in Central America and the southwestern United States, particularly in Texas.

Japanese encephalitis virus is a member of the St. Louis complex of flaviviruses and is the most common cause of arthropod-borne human encephalitis worldwide. Epidemic disease occurs in China and the northern parts of Southeast Asia, as well as in areas of India and Sri Lanka.[51] The principal vector is a rice-field-breeding culicine mosquito. There is no seasonal pattern to Japanese encephalitis except in some instances when outbreaks are associated with rainfall, irrigation, or floods.[52] Like St. Louis encephalitis virus and Japanese encephalitis virus, West Nile virus is a member of the Flaviviridae and is transmitted to humans by mosquito bites. Human cases of West Nile virus meningitis or encephalitis have been reported in Africa, Europe, the Middle East, West and Central Asia. As of autumn 2002, human, avian, animal or mosquito cases of West Nile virus infection have been reported in every state in the United States with the exception of Idaho, Washington, Oregon, Nevada, Utah, and Arizona. Dengue, a mosquito-borne flavivirus infection that is hyperendemic in Thailand, is a leading cause of hospitalization of children in Southeast Asia.[53] The principal vector is the mosquito *Aedes aegypti*, which breeds indoors in clean water, mainly in artificial water containers.[52]

The most important tick-borne causes of viral encephalitis in North America are Powassan (POW) virus and Colorado tick fever (CTF) virus. Powassan virus is a flavivirus most closely related to Russian spring-summer and Central European encephalitis viruses. The POW virus is widely distributed in the United States, but human infections with POW virus occur infrequently. In the years 1958 to 1994, a total of 24 confirmed POW cases among humans was reported in North America. The risk of infection is highest in wooded areas, where the potential for contact with infected ticks is highest.[50] Colorado tick fever virus is a member of the family Reoviridae. This virus has caused human infections in Colorado, Utah, Montana, California, Wyoming, Idaho, Oregon, South Dakota, Washington, New Mexico, Nevada, and southern Alberta and British Columbia, Canada. The primary risk of acquiring CTF is through exposure to infected *Dermacentor andersoni* ticks during outdoor recreational activities in mountain areas where the CTF virus is endemic in the months of April through June.[48]

Pathogenesis and Pathophysiology. Arboviral infections are transmitted to humans by a mosquito or tick bite. After local replication of the organism at a skin site, a viremia occurs with seeding of the reticuloendothelial system, including the liver, spleen, and lymph nodes. With continued viral replication at these sites, a secondary viremia occurs, seeding the CNS.[54] The probability of CNS infection depends on the efficiency of viral replication at the extraneural sites and the degree of the ensuing viremia. The arboviruses can invade the CNS through the cerebral capillary endothelial cells of the cerebral blood vessels or through the choroid plexus.[49]

Clinical Features and Associated Findings

CALIFORNIA GROUP VIRUS ENCEPHALITIS. Virtually all cases of California group virus encephalitis in the United States are caused by the LaCrosse strain. This virus typically produces clinically recognizable disease only in children and adolescents (aged 4 to 11 years). The LaCrosse virus may produce aseptic meningitis or a mild encephalitic illness. A distinct prodromal phase characterized by fever, chills, headache, nausea, vomiting, and abdominal pain lasting 1 to 4 days commonly precedes the onset of symptoms of encephalitis.[55] Encephalitis is characterized by fever, somnolence, and obtundation; seizures occur in approximately 50 percent of children and focal neurological signs in 20 percent, raising consideration of encephalitis due to herpes simplex virus type 1.[49] In adults, infection either is asymptomatic or causes a benign febrile illness or aseptic meningitis.[56]

ST. LOUIS ENCEPHALITIS. St. Louis encephalitis virus may cause a mild febrile illness with headache, an aseptic meningitis, or an encephalitis. The onset of encephalitis may be abrupt or preceded by an influenza-like prodrome of malaise, myalgias, and fever. The onset of encephalitis is characterized by symptoms of headache, nausea, vomiting, confusion, disorientation, irritability, stupor, tremors, and, occasionally, convulsions. The severity of illness increases with increasing age, and almost 90 percent of elderly individuals develop encephalitis.[49] A unique clinical feature of this form of encephalitis is the syndrome of inappropriate antidiuretic hormone secretion with hyponatremia, which can complicate this infection.[56]

WEST NILE VIRUS. West Nile virus infection begins as a febrile, influenza-like illness with headache, sore throat, malaise, myalgias, fatigue, and conjunctivitis. There may be a maculopapular or roseolar rash. This is followed by nausea, abdominal pain and diarrhea, and symptoms of encephalitis. There may also be a mild carditis, hepatitis, or pancreatitis. Some cases of encephalitis are associated with an axonal neuropathy. The association of encephalitis and an axonal neuropathy is a unique and distinguishing feature of West Nile virus infection. The only other neurological disease that causes encephalitis and an axonal neuropathy is a paraneoplastic syndrome.

WESTERN EQUINE ENCEPHALITIS. Western equine encephalitis tends to occur in children younger than age 1 year and in adults over age 50.[54] Inapparent infections with western equine encephalitis virus are more common than symptomatic cases. Like the other arthropod-borne encephalitides, western equine encephalitis begins with an influenza-like syndrome of fever, malaise, myalgias, pharyngitis, and vomiting. As the disease progresses, irritability, convulsions, or coma develops.[49]

EASTERN EQUINE ENCEPHALITIS. Eastern equine encephalitis virus causes a much more severe form of encephalitis than western equine encephalitis virus. Encephalitis is more common in infants and children. There may be an influenza-like prodrome with fever, headache, vomiting, malaise, and lethargy, but more typically patients with eastern equine encephalitis have an abrupt onset of high fever and convulsions and a rapid progression from stupor to coma.[49, 57] Eastern equine encephalitis may present with focal signs or focal seizure activity, thus mimicking herpes simplex virus encephalitis.[49]

In the series by Deresiewicz and colleagues, the mortality rate was 36 percent, and 35 percent of survivors had moderate or severe residual disability. Distinctive radiographic features by computed tomography (CT) or magnetic resonance imaging (MRI) of early basal ganglion and thalamic involvement help distinguish this type of encephalitis from herpes simplex encephalitis.

VENEZUELAN ENCEPHALITIS. Infection with Venezuelan encephalitis virus is typically mild, and encephalitis occurs only rarely. Children and the elderly are at greatest risk for encephalitis. Pharyngitis is a unique clinical feature of this form of arthropod-borne encephalitis.[54]

JAPANESE ENCEPHALITIS. The incubation period of Japanese encephalitis after a mosquito bite varies from 5 to 15 days. The onset of disease is characterized by a high fever with malaise, headache, nausea, and vomiting. These symptoms last from 1 to 6 days and may resolve or progress to a severe fulminant encephalitis with fever, vomiting, convulsions, and coma. Children most frequently have an encephalitis syndrome.[52]

DENGUE ENCEPHALITIS. The neurological features of encephalitis due to the dengue viruses include headache, seizures, nuchal rigidity, altered level of consciousness, behavioral disorders, delirium, paralysis, and cranial nerve palsies. The neurological manifestations of CNS dengue virus infection were previously thought to be secondary to vasculitis with cerebral edema, hypoperfusion, hyponatremia, and multiorgan failure, but recently this theory has been challenged by evaluation of a number of cases in which encephalitis occurred early in the illness coinciding with the viremic phase, suggesting that encephalitis is due to direct involvement of the brain by the virus itself.[58]

TICK-BORNE ENCEPHALITIS. The onset of encephalitis due to the POW virus is abrupt, with headache and fever to 104° F (40° C) and convulsions. There may be a prodromal phase of sore throat, lethargy, and headache. The encephalitis may be associated with focal neurological signs and may thus mimic herpes simplex virus encephalitis.[48] Infection with the Colorado tick fever virus is typically a biphasic illness. The onset of illness is characterized by fever, chills, arthralgias, myalgias, severe headache, ocular pain, conjunctival injection, nausea, and occasionally vomiting. A petechial or maculopapular rash may be seen. Defervescence may then occur, only to be followed by the recurrence of fever in 2 to 3 days. Aseptic meningitis and encephalitis occur primarily in children and may be associated with a petechial or maculopapular rash or a more severe rash with purpura and petechiae.

Disseminated intravascular coagulation and gastrointestinal bleeding may complicate the course of the illness.[48]

Differential Diagnosis. Based on criteria established by the Centers for Disease Control and Prevention (CDC), a confirmed case of arboviral disease is defined as a febrile illness with mild neurological symptoms, aseptic meningitis, or encephalitis with onset during a period when arbovirus transmission is likely to occur, plus at least one of the following: (1) fourfold or greater rise in viral antibody titer between acute and convalescent sera; (2) viral isolation from tissue, blood, or CSF; or (3) specific immunoglobulin M (IgM) antibody in CSF. A presumptive case is defined as a compatible illness plus either a stable elevated antibody titer to an arbovirus (≥320 by hemagglutination inhibition, ≥128 by complement fixation, ≥256 by immunofluorescent assay, or ≥160 by plaque-reduction neutralization test) or specific IgM antibody in serum by enzyme immunoassay.[50] The differential diagnosis of arboviral encephalitis includes herpes simplex virus encephalitis; bacterial, tuberculous, and fungal meningoencephalitis; brain abscess; rickettsial infections; infective endocarditis; CNS vasculitis; and carcinomatous meningitis.

The characteristic abnormalities found on examination of the CSF in patients with arboviral meningitis or encephalitis are: (1) a normal or mildly elevated opening pressure; (2) an initial polymorphonuclear leukocytic pleocytosis early in infection with a shift to a lymphocytic or mononuclear pleocytosis later in the illness; (3) a normal glucose concentration; and (4) a normal or mildly elevated protein concentration. LaCrosse virus has not been isolated from CSF. St. Louis encephalitis virus, EEE virus, and western equine encephalitis virus are rarely isolated from CSF.[48] A few distinguishing features of the laboratory diagnosis of arboviral meningitis or encephalitis deserve comment. Eastern equine virus encephalitis is the arboviral infection with the highest CSF WBC count. The CSF in patients with eastern equine virus encephalitis has 200 to 2000 cells/mm^3, 60 to 90 percent of which are polymorphonuclear leukocytes. The typical cell count in the CSF of SLE infection is fewer than 200 cells/mm^3; however, infection with this virus may be suggested by laboratory evidence of hyponatremia due to the inappropriate secretion of antidiuretic hormone.

Although the CDC criteria for arboviral infection are described above, for general clinical purposes the diagnosis is made by detecting a fourfold or greater increase in virus-specific IgG between the acute and convalescent sera and/or by identifying virus-specific IgM in the serum or CSF.[49] West Nile virus can be identified in CSF by culture or by PCR. The CSF in Japanese encephalitis usually has a pleocytosis with WBC counts of 10 to 1000/mm^3, and viral-specific IgM antibodies can be demonstrated in CSF in 80 percent of patients at the time of admission.[52] Dengue viruses can be isolated from the CSF and detected by PCR.[58] Neutralizing antibody is usually detectable at the time of onset of illness with POW virus. Virus has been isolated from the basal ganglia, cortex, and cerebellum of brain tissue in fatal cases. Colorado tick fever is characterized by leukopenia and in some instances thrombocytopenia. Early in the disease, Colorado tick fever virus can be isolated from serum, but later on it is more easily isolated from blood clots and from erythrocytes. Viremia may last for several months.[48]

Management and Prognosis. There is no antiviral therapy for the arboviral encephalitides, with the exception of La Crosse virus encephalitis. Ribavirin inhibits the replication of LaCrosse virus by inhibiting viral polymerase activity and has been reported to be efficacious in isolated cases of pediatric LaCrosse virus encephalitis.[59] There are ongoing clinical trials. The treatment of the other arboviral encephalitides consists primarily of supportive care with management of the neurological complications of seizures and increased intracranial pressure.

The majority of patients with California encephalitis recover completely, but 15 percent experience sequelae of behavioral abnormalities or recurrent seizures.[56] Mortality is low, less than 1 percent.[54] Sequelae occur in 20 percent of survivors of St. Louis encephalitis, consisting of irritability, memory loss, and occasionally seizures or motor deficits.[49, 54] The mortality rate is 2 to 20 percent, with the higher figure occurring in the elderly.[56] Western equine encephalitis has a mortality rate of 5 to 15 percent. Neurological sequelae are rare except in children who develop the disease when they are younger than 6 months of age. In young children, long-term sequelae consist of seizure disorders, paralysis, and developmental delay. Postencephalitic parkinsonism has been reported in some adult survivors of western equine encephalitis.[49, 54, 56] The mortality rate from eastern equine encephalitis is 60 to 75 percent, and neurological sequelae, consisting of mental retardation, seizures, spastic paralysis, and behavioral abnormalities, are common in those that survive.[54, 57] Mortality is less than 1 percent from Venezuelan equine encephalitis, and neurological sequelae are rare.[54] Vaccines for pre-exposure prophylaxis are available for western equine encephalitis, EEE, and Venezuelan equine encephalitis viruses, but not for SLE or LaCrosse virus.[48]

High-dose dexamethasone therapy has been utilized in the treatment of acute encephalitis due to Japanese encephalitis virus, but it appears to have little effect on outcome. A clinical trial of interferon-alpha in Japanese encephalitis patients in Thailand has produced promising results.[52] The intrathecal synthesis of IgM antibody appears to be an important determinant of survival. The majority of patients who have antibodies in their spinal fluid on the day of admission survive; a large proportion of those who do not, die.[51] Japanese encephalitis is preventable through vaccination. For primary immunization, two doses of inactivated Japanese encephalitis virus vaccine are administered at intervals of 7 and 14 days. A third injection is given a few months after primary vaccination to ensure full protection. This vaccination protocol may be all that is necessary for people who live in endemic areas; however, those in nonendemic areas may need further periodic booster injections.[52]

The management of dengue encephalitis is nearly always complicated by the systemic effects of this virus, including vasculopathy, thrombocytopenia, and coagulopathy. The majority of patients require transfusion of whole blood, fresh frozen plasma, and platelets. When disseminated intravascular coagulopathy complicates this infection, the mortality rate is high. Full recovery is possible.[52, 58] Of the 24 total cases of POW virus encephalitis that occurred in North America from 1958 to 1994, 4 of the acute infections were fatal, and 2 patients died 1 and 3 years after onset because of sequelae that were reported to be directly related to the disease.[50] Sequelae are common in patients who survive this infection, the most common of which is hemiplegia. Paralysis and atrophy of the shoulder muscles has also been reported.[48] Few fatalities and minimal sequelae have been reported in cases of Colorado tick fever encephalitis.[48]

INFLUENZA VIRUS

Epidemiology and Risk Factors. The term *influenza* derives from a flu epidemic in the 15th century that was attributed to an influence of the stars. Influenza viruses are single-stranded RNA viruses that are members of the orthomyxovirus family.[60] Influenza A virus is a major cause of respiratory disease in children and adults.[61] Influenza B and varicella-zoster virus are the most common antecedent infections in patients with Reye's syndrome. Influenza-type illnesses have been reported to precede the development of acute ascending paralysis, the Guillain-Barré syndrome. In utero exposure to the influenza virus has been suggested as a contributing factor to the development of schizophrenia.[62–64] The occurrence of influenza in mothers in the first trimester of pregnancy has been associated with an increased risk of neural tube defects.[65] A reversible paralytic syndrome and the Guillain-Barré syndrome have been associated with influenza immunizations.[66, 67]

Pathogenesis and Pathophysiology. The influenza virus is transmitted from person to person by aerosolized or respiratory droplets. The virus attaches to and replicates in ciliated columnar epithelium of the upper and lower respiratory tracts, following which a viremia ensues.[60] The major neurological complications of influenza are Reye's syndrome, postinfectious polyneuritis, and acute viral myositis.

Clinical Features and Associated Findings

INFLUENZA. The symptoms of influenza begin rapidly with fever, usually 101° to 102° F (38° to 39° C), associated with myalgias, headache, lethargy, and respiratory tract symptoms of dry cough, rhinorrhea, and sore throat. Eye pain and photophobia may occur. Influenza rarely causes gastrointestinal symptoms in adults; however, up to 50 percent of children have nausea, vomiting, and abdominal pain. Systemic symptoms and fever usually last 2 to 3 days and rarely more than 5 days.[60]

REYE'S SYNDROME. Reye's syndrome occurs primarily in children, most often in association with influenza B and varicella-zoster infections. Reye's syndrome is an acute, noninflammatory encephalopathy associated with hepatic dysfunction due to microvesicular fatty infiltration of the liver.[68] Reye's syndrome usually begins with severe vomiting, and this is one of the cardinal features of this syndrome. Vomiting is followed by or associated with lethargy progressing to stupor and coma.[60] The CDC's criteria for Reye's syndrome include (1) an alteration in the level of consciousness with the CSF containing less than 8 cells/mm^3; or (2) an alteration in the level of consciousness and cerebral edema without perivascular or meningeal irritation; and (3) either microvesicular fatty infiltration of the liver or a greater than threefold rise in serum aspartate aminotransferase level or ammonia.[69]

POSTINFECTIOUS POLYNEURITIS. The clinical picture of Guillain-Barré syndrome following an influenza virus infection is indistinguishable from Guillain-Barré syndrome of other causes.

ACUTE VIRAL MYOSITIS. Influenza A and B have been associated with myositis. Benign acute myositis is characterized by transient severe pain and weakness affecting the calves; it primarily affects children and occurs during epidemics of influenza.[70]

Differential Diagnosis. The influenza virus can be cultured from throat and nasopharyngeal swabs obtained within 3 days of onset of illness. Acute and convalescent sera should be sent to the laboratory to detect seroconversion or a fourfold or greater increase in virus-specific IgG between the serum samples. A fourfold rise in antibody titer indicates that the patient was recently infected with the influenza virus but is not definitive proof that the influenza virus is the etiological agent of the neurological syndrome.

Management and Prognosis. The majority of acute influenza infections are self-limited. The use of salicylates (e.g., aspirin) should be avoided in children with flulike symptoms to decrease the risk of Reye's syndrome.

Inactivated and live attenuated influenza vaccines are available. Vaccination is presently recommended for individuals who are at risk for influenza-related complications (e.g., pneumonia, myocarditis, exacerbation of chronic medical conditions); these include individuals older than age 65, persons with chronic cardiopulmonary disease including children with asthma, and residents of chronic care facilities. In addition, persons with chronic illnesses such as diabetes or renal disease and those compromised by immunosuppression should be vaccinated. Individuals who can transmit influenza to high-risk persons such as health care workers, nursing home and chronic care facility employees, and household members of high-risk persons should also be vaccinated.[60]

MEASLES

Epidemiology and Risk Factors. Measles is one of the three major infectious diseases worldwide and causes about 1.5 million childhood deaths per year.[71] In the 1960s, prior to routine childhood immunization, more than 400,000 cases of measles were reported annually; in comparison, less than 4000 cases were reported annually in the early 1980s. From 1988 to 1990, the incidence of measles increased eightfold.[72] Between 1987 and 1990, 52,846 cases of measles were reported to the CDC.[73] This marked increase in the number of cases of measles was attributed to outbreaks among unvaccinated preschool-age children and to outbreaks among vaccinated school-age children who had received only a single dose of measles vaccine.[73]

Encephalitis is a rare complication of measles infection. It occurs in one of three distinct types: (1) postinfectious or autoimmune encephalomyelitis, which presents as a sudden recurrence of fever with an altered level of consciousness, seizure activity, and multifocal neurological signs during convalescence from measles; (2) subacute sclerosing panencephalitis (SSPE), which presents after a latent period of 6 years or more from an acute measles infection and has an insidious onset of neurological dysfunction associated with myoclonus and seizure activity, and it progresses to coma and death within 1 to 2 years; and (3) subacute measles encephalitis (subacute inclusion body encephalopathy, progressive infectious measles encephalitis), which most commonly occurs in immunosuppressed individuals after a latent period of 1 to 10 months between the measles-like illness and the encephalitis.[74–76] Encephalomyelitis occurs in 1 per 1000 individuals who develop measles (mostly in older persons), and between 5 and 10 children per million who contract measles develop SSPE.[77]

Pathogenesis and Pathophysiology. Measles virus is spread by respiratory droplets, and only a small amount of virus is required to produce the infection. Virus replicates in the respiratory tract and then spreads to the local lymphatic tissues. Amplification of virus in the lymph nodes produces a primary viremia that results in the spread of virus to multiple lymphoid tissues and the skin, kidney, gastrointestinal tract, and liver. In these organs, the virus replicates in endothelial cells, epithelial cells, and monocytes and macrophages. Measles virus can be detected in peripheral blood leukocytes at the time of onset of prodromal symptoms and for several days after the onset of the rash. The fusion of the measles virus–infected cells leads to the formation of multinucleated giant cells, a pathological hallmark of this infection.[76]

Postmeasles encephalomyelitis (postinfectious encephalomyelitis, autoimmune encephalomyelitis) is a perivenular demyelinating disease rather than an inclusion body encephalitis. Histologically, the lesions resemble those induced experimentally by injection of animals with myelin proteins with adjuvant, that is, experimental, autoimmune encephalomyelitis.[71] There is little evidence of virus in the brain, as assessed either by virus isolation and antigen and RNA detection or by the appearance of measles virus–specific antibody in the CSF.[76]

The pathogenesis of SSPE and of subacute measles encephalitis has, however, been attributed to measles virus persistence in the CNS.[75, 78] The histological features of SSPE include inflammatory infiltrates, glial nodules, degeneration of neurons, hyperplasia of astrocytes and microglia, and intranuclear inclusion bodies of Cowdry type A with abundant measles virus antigen.[74] The histological diagnostic features of subacute measles encephalitis include intranuclear eosinophilic, and sometimes intracytoplasmic, inclusion bodies in neurons and oligodendrocytes with abundant paramyxovirus nucleocapsids and measles virus antigen.[74, 75]

Clinical Features and Associated Findings

MEASLES. The onset of measles is characterized by fever, cough, coryza, and conjunctivitis associated with Koplik's spots, which are small, white punctate lesions on the buccal mucosa. A maculopapular rash appears 2 to 3 days later, first on the face and behind the ears and then spreading in a centrifugal fashion to the trunk and extremities.[76] The cephalocaudal spread of the maculopapular rash is quite characteristic of measles.

POSTINFECTIOUS ENCEPHALOMYELITIS. Postmeasles encephalomyelitis usually occurs within 2 weeks after the onset of the rash. There is a sudden recurrence of fever associated with a decrease in consciousness, seizures, and multifocal neurological abnormalities. Mortality is approximately 20 percent, and sequelae are common in survivors.[71, 76]

SUBACUTE SCLEROSING PANENCEPHALITIS. SSPE is a progressive CNS disorder that begins several years after measles infection in early childhood and is characterized by behavioral abnormalities, intellectual deterioration, motor rigidity, and myoclonic jerks that progress to coma and death.

SUBACUTE MEASLES ENCEPHALITIS. Neurological signs resulting from subacute measles encephalitis typically develop 1 to 9 months after exposure to measles or from the time of onset of clinical measles. The disease is characterized by seizure activity, an alteration in the level of consciousness, and focal neurological deficits including hemiparesis, ataxia, and disturbances of language and vision. Seizure activity may be focal or generalized, and epilepsia partialis continua is a prominent feature.[75, 77] The majority of patients who develop subacute measles encephalitis are immunosuppressed.

Differential Diagnosis. The differential diagnosis of measles includes illnesses associated with fever and an erythematous maculopapular rash, such as scarlet fever, rubella, meningococcemia, Kawasaki's disease, toxic shock syndrome, and erythema multiforme due to a hypersensitivity to medications.[79, 80]

During the viremia of measles infection, measles virus can be isolated from peripheral blood mononuclear cells.[81] The clinical diagnosis, however, is more typically based on the presence or a history of the characteristic findings of fever, an erythematous maculopapular rash demonstrating a cephalocaudal spread, coryza, cough, conjunctivitis, and Koplik's spots. Laboratory results that support a diagnosis of measles are the detection of measles IgM and a fourfold increase in measles IgG between acute and convalescent sera.[79] The diagnosis of postmeasles encephalomyelitis is based on the occurrence of encephalitis within 2 weeks of the rash of measles associated with a recurrence of fever.

The diagnosis of SSPE is typically based on the characteristic clinical appearance as described earlier and the appearance of periodic complexes on the EEG; clinical myoclonic jerks have a one-to-one relationship with the periodic EEG complexes.[82] Measles antibody titers in CSF are typically elevated in patients with SSPE.

The diagnosis of subacute measles encephalitis can be confirmed only by brain biopsy but is suggested by the following: (1) a history of measles or exposure to measles within 1 to 10 months of presentation; (2) an immunocompromised state; (3) refractory focal seizures (epilepsia partialis continua) as part of the neurological symptomatology; and (4) absence of fever.[75] Examination of the CSF reveals a mild mononuclear pleocytosis and a mild elevation in the protein concentration, but in about a third of the patients the CSF is entirely normal. The EEG is slow with nonspecific abnormalities. Detection of measles virus RNA by PCR technology may make the diagnosis of subacute measles encephalitis considerably easier.

Management and Prognosis. The dramatic increase in measles from 1987 to 1990 led to two principal changes in the recommendations for measles vaccination made by both the ACIP and the American Academy of Pediatrics Committee on Infectious Diseases of the CDC: (1) the age for the initial measles vaccination was changed from 15 months to 12 months, and (2) a second dose of measles vaccine was recommended at either 4 to 6 years or at the time of entry to middle or junior high school.[73] The vaccine in use today is a live attenuated measles virus that was developed from the original Edmonston strain of measles virus isolated by Enders in 1954.[76]

Measles during pregnancy has a more severe clinical course and is associated with an increased risk of premature labor or spontaneous abortion.[72, 83] Pregnancy is a significant risk factor for mortality during measles.[72] Measles infection in pregnancy does not, however, appear to be associated with an increased risk of congenital anomalies, leading to the suggestion that although infection with measles increases the risk of premature termination of pregnancy within the first 2 weeks of onset of the rash, if pregnancy continues, the likelihood of a favorable outcome is high.[83] It is recommended that susceptible pregnant women exposed to a person with active measles receive serum immune globulin (gamma globulin 16.5 percent) within 6 days of exposure to prevent or modify subsequent disease. All infants born to mothers with active measles in the 6 days before delivery should also receive intravenous immunoglobulin prophylaxis (500 mg/kg) immediately after birth and again 1 week later.[72, 83, 84] Ribavirin has been shown to be effective against measles virus in vitro. It has been suggested that ribavirin might be useful as therapy for immunocompromised patients with measles, although anecdotal case reports in which intravenous ribavirin was used have not demonstrated a therapeutic effect. Ribavirin does cross the placenta and is present in amniotic fluid in potentially therapeutic levels. Teratogenic effects have been reported in rats (but not primates) given high doses of ribavirin during pregnancy; therefore, there is some concern about the possible teratogenicity of this drug.[72]

Treatment of the encephalitis syndrome described earlier that may complicate measles infection is primarily supportive. There are a few favorable case reports of the use of ribavirin in patients with subacute measles encephalitis; however, firm recommendations cannot be made at this time.[75, 85] There are reports of clinical improvement in patients with SSPE who were treated with inosiplex and intrathecal interferon-alpha, as well as reports of patients who showed no improvement with this therapy. No firm recommendations can be made at this time.

ARENAVIRUS (LYMPHOCYTIC CHORIOMENINGITIS VIRUS)

Epidemiology and Risk Factors. The natural reservoir for the lymphocytic choriomeningitis virus (LCMV) is the common house mouse. Hamsters and laboratory animals can also be infected with this virus. Most human infections result from contact with house mice.[86, 87] Four clinical syndromes due to infection with LCMV have been described: (1) subclinical asymptomatic infection, (2) nonmeningeal influenza-like illness, (3) aseptic meningitis, and (4) meningoencephalomyelitis. The LCMV was the first specific etiological agent of the aseptic meningitis syndrome to be identified.[87]

Pathogenesis and Pathophysiology. The LCMV is a member of the arenavirus family and is maintained in nature primarily by vertical intrauterine infection in mice, hamsters, and rodents, producing a chronic asymptomatic infection in the offspring. These animals shed the virus in saliva, nasal secretions, semen, milk, urine, and feces.[87] The route of transmission to humans remains unknown but is presumed to occur through contamination of open cuts or aerosolized spread of virus. There is no evidence of person-to-person transmission of LCMV infection.[86] Local replication of LCMV is followed by dissemination to the reticuloendothelial system with a subsequent viremia. The CNS is infected during the course of the viremia.

Clinical Features and Associated Findings. Clinical manifestations of acute LCMV infection in children and adults range from asymptomatic seroconversion to an influenza-like illness to an aseptic meningitis, and rarely to a meningoencephalomyelitis. In patients with aseptic meningitis, there is often a history of a biphasic illness. The first stage resembles an influenza-like illness. This is then followed by a symptom-free period of time varying from a few days to 3 weeks, which is followed in turn by the acute onset of high fever, headache, vomiting, and signs of meningeal irritation.[86] Although the clinical presentation of CNS infection with LCMV is most frequently an aseptic meningitis, it may also be a meningoencephalitis. Congenital LCMV infection can result in intrauterine or early neonatal death, hydrocephalus, chorioretinitis, and psychomotor retardation.[88]

Differential Diagnosis. The diagnosis of LCMV infection can be made by the appearance of IgM antibodies in a serum sample or by a fourfold or greater rise in antibody titer between the acute and convalescent serum samples. The classic CSF abnormalities include the following: (1) a lymphocytic pleocytosis of 300 to 3000 cells/mm^3, and (2) hypoglycorrhachia.[86] LCMV is one of the few etiological agents of an aseptic meningitis with hypoglycorrhachia. LCMV can be isolated from the CSF. The diagnosis of congenital LCMV infection is based on the clinical presentation and laboratory evidence of persistently high IgG immunofluorescent antibody (IFA) titers.[89]

Management. Prevention of LCMV infection is the priority. Laboratory animals acquired from areas where arenaviruses are indigenous should be tested for LCMV infection. Pregnant women should avoid contact with laboratory and household mice and hamsters. LCMV aseptic meningitis in children and adults is self-limited, and complete recovery is the rule.

RUBELLA

Epidemiology and Risk Factors. Since the rubella vaccine became available in 1969, rubella and the neurological complications of rubella have been due primarily to periodic outbreaks of the disease. The neurological syndromes associated with rubella virus infection include (1) the congenital rubella syndrome, (2) acute encephalitis complicating rubella, (3) postrubella polyradiculoneuritis, and (4) progressive rubella panencephalitis.[90, 91] Acute encephalitis is a rare complication of rubella infection, with a reported incidence of 1 in 5000 to 1 in 24,000 cases.[91] Postrubella polyradiculoneuritis complicates rubella in an estimated 4 percent of patients. Only five cases of acute postrubella polyradiculoneuritis have been reported in the past 30 years.[91] The most common neurological complication of rubella infection is the congenital rubella syndrome. The gestational age at the time of infection determines the risk of fetal anomaly.[92] The risk of congenital rubella syndrome is greatest when infection occurs during the first trimester. Progressive rubella panencephalitis is a slow virus disease of the CNS that has many clinical similarities to SSPE caused by measles virus and is an uncommon late-onset manifestation of congenital rubella.[93]

Pathogenesis and Pathophysiology. The rubella virus is a single-stranded RNA virus. Infection is acquired by droplet inhalation; viral replication occurs in the nasopharynx with a subsequent viremia. The CNS is infected in the course of the viremia. Maternal viremia during the first trimester of pregnancy can infect the placenta and spread to the fetus.[94] Disease in the fetus exposed to this virus during the first trimester is severe.[95]

Clinical Features and Associated Findings

RUBELLA. Rubella is a generalized maculopapular exanthem associated with fever. Arthralgias, lymphadenopathy, and conjunctivitis may also be associated with the acute illness.

ACUTE ENCEPHALITIS. Acute encephalitis is a rare complication of rubella infection. Symptoms usually appear within 1 to 6 days after the typical maculopapular rash develops and are characterized by headache, dizziness, lethargy, behavioral abnormalities, coma, and generalized or focal seizures in as many as 50 percent of cases. The case fatality rate of acute rubella encephalitis is low, and most nonfatal cases recover rapidly with minimal or no sequelae.[90]

POSTRUBELLA POLYRADICULONEURITIS. Postrubella polyradiculoneuritis develops abruptly as the exanthem of rubella fades and has the clinical features of the Guillain-Barré syndrome. The duration of the illness is usually brief.[91]

CONGENITAL RUBELLA SYNDROME. Features of the congenital rubella syndrome include intrauterine growth retardation, sensorineural deafness, cataracts, congenital glaucoma, patent ductus arteriosus, pulmonic stenosis, microcephaly, mental retardation, meningoencephalitis, purpuric rash, hepatosplenomegaly, and radiolucent bone densities.[96] In addition to these clinical signs, which are present at birth, children with congenital rubella syndrome may develop delayed-onset progressive rubella panencephalitis, a slow virus disease of the CNS that has many clinical similarities to SSPE caused by measles virus.[93] This syndrome may also follow childhood rubella in rare instances.[97] Symptoms typically begin between ages 8 and 19 years with deterioration in school performance and behavior sometimes associated with seizures. The neurological deterioration progresses to a global dementia with ataxia, spasticity of gait, dysarthria, and dysphagia. Progressive pallor of the optic discs and a maculopathy occur.[97]

Differential Diagnosis. Examination of the CSF in patients with rubella encephalitis may be normal or may demonstrate a mild to moderate mononuclear cell pleocytosis and an elevated protein concentration. Virus is rarely isolated from the CSF in patients with rubella encephalitis. Electroencephalography may demonstrate diffuse or focal abnormalities. Diagnosis is made by detection of rubella-specific IgM antibodies in serum or by demonstration of a fourfold rise in rubella-specific IgG in the convalescent sera compared to the acute sera.[90] Similarly, the diagnosis of postrubella polyradiculoneuritis is based on the findings of a demyelinating peripheral neuropathy following an exanthematous illness. One of the characteristics of the rash of rubella is that the maculopapular rash almost invariably begins on the face before it becomes generalized, and it is often associated with posterior cervical adenopathy.[97] A description of this type of rash preceding the clinical syndrome of polyradiculoneuritis is suggestive of rubella. By the time the polyradiculoneuritis develops, serum for IgM antibodies to rubella virus may be negative. A single elevated rubella IgG titer is suggestive but not diagnostic of a recent rubella infection, but when associated with a history of the rubella rash as described previously, it is quite compatible with the diagnosis.

In infants who have clinical evidence of the congenital rubella syndrome at birth, serum IgM antibody to rubella virus and viral cultures should be obtained. Other laboratory abnormalities supporting the diagnosis of congenital rubella syndrome include hyperbilirubinemia, thrombocytopenia, elevated serum transaminase levels, and long-bone radiographs demonstrating metaphyseal lucencies. Neuroimaging studies reveal intracranial calcifications, delayed myelination, or ventriculitis.[98] Several different methods have been used to make an intrauterine diagnosis of rubella infection, including isolation of the rubella virus in the amniotic fluid obtained by amniocentesis, cordocentesis, use of the PCR method on extracts from chorionic villi and placenta, and ultrastructural examination of amniotic fluid cells using transmission and scanning electron microscopy.[99] Examination of the CSF in progressive rubella panencephalitis demonstrates a mild lymphocytic pleocytosis (0 to 37 cells/mm^3), a moderate increase in the protein concentration (60 to 142 mg/mL), and intrathecal immunoglobulin synthesis.[97]

Management and Prognosis. The key to management of the neurological complications of rubella is prevention. The rubella vaccine licensed for use in the United States is a live attenuated RA 27/3 rubella virus.[94] The immunogenicity of the vaccine is reduced by whole blood transfusion; therefore, it is recommended that rubella vaccine not be given for 3 months after immunoglobulin or whole blood transfusion.[92] The incidence of arthritis after vaccination is low when the RA 27/3 strain of rubella vaccine is used. Breast feeding is not a contraindication to postpartum immunization. Infants infected with the rubella virus through breast milk may experience a mild rash, but the majority remain asymptomatic, and no serious adverse effects have been reported.[96] Currently, the first dose of rubella vaccine is given to children as part of the MMR vaccine at 12 to 15 months of age. A second dose of the MMR vaccine is recommended when the child first enters school or later when he or she enters middle school.[94]

HUMAN T-CELL LYMPHOTROPIC VIRUS TYPE 1

Epidemiology and Risk Factors. The human T-cell lymphotropic virus type 1 (HTLV-1) causes a rapidly progressive adult T-cell leukemia or lymphoma and a slowly progressive neuromyelopathy known as HTLV-1–associated myelopathy-tropical spastic paraparesis (HAM-TSP).[100, 101] The distribution of HTLV-1 infection is worldwide with major foci of endemic infection in southwestern Japan, the Caribbean, Central and South America, sub-Saharan Africa, the Middle East, and Melanesia. It is estimated that between 10 and 20 million people are infected with HTLV-1. In the United States and Europe, HTLV-1 is found primarily in intravenous drug abusers.[100] Transmission of HTLV-1 can occur from mother to child primarily by breast milk, between intravenous drug addicts through the sharing of contaminated needles and syringes, by sexual contact, and by the transfusion of contaminated blood products. Vertical transmission of HTLV-1 from mother to child has been reported to occur in 15 to 20 percent of children born to HTLV-1 positive mothers. Breast milk appears to be the principal route because seroconversion rates are 14 to 20 percent for breast-fed infants compared to 3 to 5 percent for bottle-fed infants.[102] Sexual transmission of HTLV-1 is fairly inefficient compared to transmission of the human immunodeficiency virus

(HIV). Blood transfusion is, however, a very efficient means of transmission of HTLV-1, and the greatest risk is incurred by recipients who receive seropositive blood stored for less than 1 week, who require multiple transfusions, or who receive immunosuppressive therapy at the time of the transfusion.[103]

Pathogenesis and Pathophysiology. There are presently two major theories of the pathogenesis of HAM-TSP, an autoimmune model and a cytotoxic model. In the autoimmune model, HTLV-1 activates autoreactive T cells, which then migrate to the CNS, penetrate the blood-brain barrier, and stimulate the production of inflammatory cytokines, leading to subsequent tissue destruction.[101, 104] In the cytotoxic model, tissue destruction is caused by a CD8-mediated cytolytic attack against HTLV-1–infected CNS cells or infected CD4 T cells in the CNS. An early event in HAM-TSP appears to be a breakdown of the blood-brain barrier, leading to perivascular influx of mononuclear cells. CD4 T cells are the predominant cell type early in disease, but CD8 T cells are found almost exclusively in the later stages of disease. As the duration of HAM-TSP progresses, an increasing number of CD8 cells infiltrate the CNS. This infiltration is associated with an upregulation of HLA class 1 and class 2 molecules and an increased expression of cytokines. The end result is demyelination with axonal involvement that is widespread in the spinal cord, and the corticospinal tracts tend to be more affected than the more heavily myelinated posterior columns. The thoracic spinal cord is the area of maximum involvement.[101, 105]

Clinical Features and Associated Findings. HTLV-1–associated myelopathy-tropical spastic paraparesis is a slowly progressive spastic paraparesis marked by hyperreflexia, bladder dysfunction, constipation, and impotence in males. Sensory abnormalities due to demyelination of the posterior columns occur less frequently than motor abnormalities and present primarily as paresthesias of the lower extremities.[103]

Differential Diagnosis. The differential diagnosis includes myelopathy due to a compressive lesion of the cord from a disc, tumor, or infection; subacute combined degeneration resulting from vitamin B_{12} deficiency; HIV-1 myelopathy; multiple sclerosis; and syphilis.

Serological testing should be performed to detect HTLV-1 antibodies in serum. MRI of the brain may demonstrate hyperintense lesions in the subcortical white matter on T2-weighted scans, resembling the lesions of multiple sclerosis.[106] MRI of the spinal cord may show hyperintense lesions in the thoracic spinal cord. Elevated antibody titers to HTLV-1 can be detected in blood and CSF of patients with HAM-TSP.

Management and Prognosis. The presence of inflammatory cells, including macrophages and T cells, in HAM-TSP spinal cord material, in addition to the upregulation of HLA and cytokine molecules, suggests that an increase in immunological activity in the CNS is the basis of the pathogenesis of HAM-TSP.[105] Immunosuppressive therapy is the only modality presently available to treat HAM-TSP. There is no specific antiviral therapy. The best means of treatment may be prevention through an HTLV-1 vaccine, and it has been suggested that the development of vaccination against the HTLV-1 retrovirus would serve as a pathfinder for the development of a vaccine against HIV.[100]

DNA Viruses

HERPES SIMPLEX

Epidemiology and Risk Factors. Herpes simplex virus (HSV) infections of the CNS are of several types: (1) an acute encephalitis, (2) a benign recurrent lymphocytic meningitis, (3) an acute facial nerve paralysis, (4) recurrent ascending myelitis, and (5) a neuritis localized to a single sensory nerve. Neonatal HSV infections occur at a rate of approximately 1 in 3500 to 5000 deliveries per year in North America. Three forms of infection of the newborn are recognized: infection localized to the skin, eye, and mouth; encephalitis; and disseminated disease with involvement of the CNS. Neonatal HSV infections are usually caused by HSV type 2 (HSV-2).[107]

In children age 6 months or older and in adults, HSV type 1 (HSV-1) is the most common cause of sporadic fatal encephalitis. Herpes simplex encephalitis is estimated to occur in 1 in 250,000 to 500,000 persons per year.[108] HSV-2 is increasingly recognized as the etiological agent of benign recurrent lymphocytic meningitis, and HSV-1 as the etiological agent of acute facial nerve paralysis, Bell's palsy.

Pathogenesis and Pathophysiology. The human herpesviruses are neurotropic viruses that are able to establish active and latent infections in the CNS and can cause tissue damage through viral replication in nervous tissue and reactivation from the latent state.[109] The pathogenesis of neonatal HSV disease is different from that of HSV disease in older infants, children, and adults. Neonatal HSV infection is acquired most commonly when the fetus comes in contact with infected maternal genital secretions. The type of maternal infection, whether primary or recurrent, has a significant influence on the risk of infection to the fetus. Maternal primary infection at the time of delivery is associated with a fetal risk of infection of approximately 35 percent. Maternal recurrent infection at the time of delivery is associated with a significantly lower risk to the fetus of approximately 3 percent.[107]

There are two forms of HSV encephalitis during the neonatal period. In babies with encephalitis alone, the illness begins, on average, within 2 weeks of birth. Infection of the CNS by HSV in these neonates is thought to occur by intraneuronal routes. The majority of these babies do not develop skin lesions, and brain disease is often localized to one or both temporal lobes, but it can progress to involve other areas of the brain. In contrast, in newborns with encephalitis resulting from disseminated disease, symptoms of brain involvement begin at the age of 7 to 9 days or earlier. The CNS becomes infected through blood-borne spread of the virus, and neuroimaging procedures reveal multiple areas of hemorrhagic necrosis throughout the cerebral cortex.[107, 108]

In children and adults, HSV-1 encephalitis occurs as either an acute infection or as reactivation of latent infection in the trigeminal ganglion. Infection most commonly involves the temporal cortex, the orbital-frontal cortex, and the limbic structures. In most cases the initial infection begins in the oral cavity, and the virus spreads transneuronally along a division of the trigeminal nerve to the trigeminal ganglion.[109] In experimental animal models of HSV-1 encephalitis, intranasal inoculation leads to viral entry via the olfactory nerve with subsequent infection of the olfactory bulb. Infection then develops in the temporal cortex analogous to human disease; however, the olfactory bulb is rarely affected in humans, and therefore the olfactory nerve is less likely to be the site of viral entry in humans.[110] The extent and severity of CNS disease is related to the neurovirulence of the virus, the degree of viral inoculum, the immunocompetence of the individual, and possibly genetic determinants of susceptibility to HSV infection.[111]

The human herpesviruses have the ability to establish lifelong latent infection in the peripheral sensory ganglia (PSG), in the trigeminal ganglion, and in the motor neurons of the hypoglossal nucleus. During acute infection, cells that are infected with HSV-1 ultimately die. The pathogenesis of virus that establishes latency is fundamentally different. Following peripheral inoculation, HSV-1 DNA viral particles are carried by retrograde axonal flow to the PSG. Since HSV is a lytic virus and replication within a cell results in cell death, latency cannot be established in cells in which the virus has completed a full replication cycle. During attachment of HSV-1 to the axonal membrane of the peripheral nerve, the virus loses its envelope, and the contents of the tegument as well as the capsid are transported to the neuronal nucleus. Vmw65, an HSV-1 transactivating protein that is a component of the viral tegument, has a role in this process. The amount of Vmw65 that is carried with the virus to the cell nucleus eventually determines the fate of the infection. If sufficient amounts reach the neuronal cell body, a replication cycle ensues, and the cell dies; if, however, the amount of Vmw65 is insufficient, no replication cycle begins, and latent infection is established.[109] No infectious viral particles are present during latent infection. During latent HSV-1 infection the linear DNA is present as a circular molecule that is not integrated into the host cell DNA.[112] External stimuli triggering reactivation of HSV include injury to tissues innervated by the neurons harboring latent infection and the systemic conditions of exposure to sun, fever, malignancy, and immunosuppression. Even after numerous repeated bouts of reactivation, most patients do not have permanent sensory loss or any other neurological deficit in the affected dermatome, presumably because reactivation is not associated with significant destruction of latently infected neurons.[109–112]

The nature of the latent state of the HSV infection in the trigeminal ganglion is not as well understood as HSV infection in the peripheral nervous system. CNS disease as a result of HSV-1 infection—herpes encephalitis—in immunocompetent individuals is a very rare single event, whereas HSV infection in the peripheral nervous system may recur many times during an individual's lifetime. It is estimated that in approximately a third of patients, HSV-1 encephalitis occurs during the primary viral infection, and that in the other 70 percent, HSV-1 encephalitis is due to reactivation of latent infection in the trigeminal ganglion.[109] The pathogenesis of herpes simplex virus infection as a cause of benign recurrent lymphocytic meningitis is postulated to be due to HSV-2 primary infection or to reactivation in a sacral dorsal root ganglion that seeds the CSF subarachnoid space and produces meningitis.[113] The pathogenesis of herpes simplex viral infection in acute facial nerve paralysis is presumed to be reactivation of latent infection in the geniculate ganglion.[114]

Clinical Features and Associated Findings

ACUTE ENCEPHALITIS. As discussed in the preceding section on pathogenesis, HSV encephalitis typically involves the temporal lobe or lobes, the orbital-frontal cortex, and the limbic structures. The clinical presentation is that of a focal encephalitis characterized by focal neurological deficits (hemiparesis in approximately a third of patients), focal seizure activity often involving the temporal lobe, headache, altered behavior, personality changes, fever, and altered levels of consciousness. The classic paper on diseases that mimic herpes simplex encephalitis appeared in *JAMA* in 1989.[115] This study, which included a total of 432 patients who underwent brain biopsy for presumptive herpes simplex encephalitis, predated the routine use of MRI and the availability of CSF PCR. Today the differential diagnosis of acute focal encephalitis with fever, after neuroimaging and CSF analysis, is that of a focal viral encephalitic process. The causes of a focal viral encephalitic process are listed in Table 41–4.

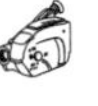

RECURRENT LYMPHOCYTIC MENINGITIS. HSV-2 is an etiological agent of benign recurrent lymphocytic meningitis (Mollaret's meningitis).[113] This meningitis is characterized by recurrent attacks of fever, headache, and meningeal irritation that last from 2 to 5 days. There may also be symptoms of a sacral radiculitis.

BELL'S PALSY. HSV is an etiological agent of acute facial nerve paralysis.[114]

Differential Diagnosis. MRI is preferred over the CT scan for demonstration of the early lesions of herpes simplex virus encephalitis. On T2-weighted and fluid-attenuated inversion recovery images, high signal intensity lesions are seen in the medial and inferior temporal lobes, which may extend up into the insula. The CSF is under increased pressure, the protein concentration is mildly to moderately elevated, and a lymphocytic pleocytosis is present, as are red blood cells and/or xanthachromia, which reflect the hemorrhagic necrotic nature of the encephalitis; the glucose concentration is normal or mildly decreased. CSF viral cultures for HSV-1 are almost always negative.

The PCR technique, a highly sensitive and specific test for herpes simplex virus encephalitis, may be negative initially in the first 24 to 48 hours of infection but then becomes positive and remains positive for at least 2 weeks. HSV DNA was detected by PCR in the CSF of 53 (98%) of 54 patients with biopsy-proven HSV encephalitis. Positive results were found in 3 (6%) of 47 patients whose brain tissue was culture negative.[116] False-positive PCR analysis for HSV DNA has been reported, and a laboratory with expertise in the PCR technique should be used.[117] PCR should not be performed on bloody CSF. Porphyrin compounds derived from the degradation of heme in erythrocytes may inhibit the PCR reaction, giving a false-negative result. CSF and serum should also be sent for HSV antibody assay. The intrathecal synthesis of HSV-specific antibody can be detected, usually within 3 to 10 days or more after the onset of symptoms, and antibodies can be detected for as long as 3 months after the onset of symptoms. A serum-to-CSF ratio of less than 20:1 suggests intrathecal production of antibodies to HSV-1. The EEG may also contribute to the diagnosis by showing periodic focal or unilateral high-amplitude complexes consisting of a single wave or a group of waves that repeat at fairly regular intervals and are expressed maximally over the involved temporal lobe. For the diagnosis of benign recurrent lymphocytic meningitis, CSF should be analyzed by the PCR method for HSV-2 and/or HSV-1.[113]

Establishing the etiological agent of a facial nerve paralysis is typically difficult except when the characteristic lesions of the Ramsay Hunt syndrome are present. The PCR technique has been used to detect HSV DNA in facial nerve endoneurial fluid and in patients with Bell's palsy, thus identifying HSV-1 as an etiological agent.[118]

Management. Acyclovir is the drug of choice for neonates with HSV infections of the CNS and for patients with herpes simplex virus encephalitis. While the standard of care has been a dose of 10 mg/kg three times daily (for a total of 30 mg/kg/day) for a minimum of 14 days, higher dosages and longer courses (3 weeks followed by an oral antiviral agent) are being investigated. Approximately 5 to 10 percent of patients with herpes simplex encephalitis show a relapse clinically.[108] It is recommended that the use of brain biopsy be reserved for patients in whom the diagnosis remains unclear despite the previously described diagnostic studies and for those in whom progressive neurological deterioration occurs despite acyclovir therapy.[108] Patients with HSV-related Mollaret's meningitis may benefit from prophylactic acyclovir because this treatment has been demonstrated to be effective in preventing recurrent genital herpes.[119] A combination of oral acyclovir and prednisone has also been recommended for the treatment of acute idiopathic facial nerve palsy, but firm recommendations cannot be made at this time.

VARICELLA-ZOSTER VIRUS

Epidemiology and Risk Factors. Varicella-zoster virus (VZV) is the etiological agent of chickenpox. Von Bokay was the first to observe that susceptible children might develop varicella after exposure to the herpes zoster virus. Joseph Garland, a long-term editor of the *New England Journal of Medicine*, was the first to suggest that zoster reflected activation of a latent varicella virus.[120] In 1954, Thomas Weller confirmed von Bokay's observation that children develop varicella following exposure to patients with herpes zoster by demonstrating, with tissue culture and antibody studies, that the two diseases were caused by the same virus.[121] The likelihood of developing zoster increases with advancing age, a phenomenon attributed to immune senescence and a decline in the VZV-specific T-lymphocyte population.[122] Varicella, or chickenpox, results from the initial exposure to VZV, and approximately 1 in 1000 to 4000 patients with varicella develop neurological complications of encephalitis (which most often presents as an acute cerebellar ataxia), aseptic meningitis, polyneuritis, multiple cranial neuropathies, or Reye's syndrome.[121] Post-herpetic neuralgia is the most common neurological complication of zoster. VZV is also the etiological agent of the Ramsay Hunt syndrome. J. Ramsay Hunt introduced the term herpes zoster oticus in 1907 to refer to a herpetic inflammation of the geniculate ganglion.[123] Varicella-zoster virus encephalitis is increasingly recognized in immunosuppressed individuals, particularly those with the acquired immunodeficiency syndrome (AIDS), and is characterized by multifocal ischemic and hemorrhagic infarctions associated with demyelination.[124]

Pathogenesis and Pathophysiology. VZV is a double-stranded DNA virus. Initial infection occurs in the mucosa of the upper respiratory tract and/or in the conjunctivae. The initial site of replication of the virus is unknown but most likely includes adenoid-tonsillar tissues of the head and neck. A primary viremia occurs 4 to 6 days later. The virus then undergoes a second cycle of replication at multiple sites within the host. Thereafter, a second viremia occurs with infection of the capillaries of the skin and the appearance of the characteristic vesicular lesions of chickenpox.[125]

The mechanism by which VZV establishes latency in the sensory ganglia is not as well understood as the mechanism by which HSV establishes latency. However, by analogy to HSV, it is presumed that viral multiplication in epithelial cells extends locally to involve the distal ramifications of sensory nerves. The virus then travels by axonal transport along the sensory nerves to the neuronal cell body in the sensory ganglia. VZV may also arrive at the sensory ganglia via a hematogenous route during the viremic stage of chickenpox. Once in the ganglia, VZV establishes a lifelong latent infection. Non-neuronal cells are also involved in the pathogenesis of VZV latency. In contrast, in primary HSV infection few non-neuronal cells are infected. Zoster exhibits a predilection for the mid to lower thoracic (T3–T12), upper lumbar (L1–L2), and ophthalmic (V1) dermatomes. The propensity for zoster to occur in these dermatomes is attributed to the fact that chickenpox lesions are concentrated in these regions; thus, there is a greater proportion of cells in the corresponding sensory ganglia that become latently infected via neural transport.[122] In an autopsy series of 14 adults in which the PCR technique was used to detect VZV DNA in the sensory ganglia, VZV DNA was detected in the trigeminal ganglia in 10 of 11 (91%) adults and in the thoracic ganglia in 12 of 14 (86%) adults.[126] Reactivation of VZV from the sensory ganglia leads to centrifugal migration of the virus through the nerve to the epithelial surface of the corresponding dermatome, yielding the classic vesicular eruption.[122] Pathological studies of sensory ganglia during herpes zoster show extensive necrosis and neuronal destruction, and it has been suggested that zoster-associated neuralgia may be a consequence of this extensive cytopathology.[112, 122]

Clinical Features and Associated Findings. As described earlier, the neurological complications of varicella include encephalitis, aseptic meningitis, polyneuritis, multiple cranial neuropathies, and Reye's syndrome.

ENCEPHALITIS. Approximately 1 in 4000 children with varicella under the age of 15 develop acute cerebellar ataxia days to a week after the appearance of the varicella rash. There is a 5 percent mortality rate and a 17 percent morbidity rate, including mental retardation, seizures, and ataxia.[121]

Varicella-zoster virus encephalitis in immunosuppressed patients occurs days to months following zoster or may develop without any history of a vesicular rash. The symptoms of encephalitis include fever, seizures, focal neurological deficits, and an alteration in consciousness. There is radiological evidence of multifocal ischemic and hemorrhagic infarctions that involve white matter more than gray matter and are often concentrated at the gray-white matter junction. Small demyelinative lesions with preservation of axons are also seen and are attributed to small vessel vasculopathy.[124]

FACIAL NERVE PARALYSIS. Both HSV and VZV are etiological agents of Bell's palsy. VZV is more likely than HSV to cause a complete cranial nerve VII paralysis with concomi-

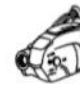

tant severe pain and sensorineural hearing loss. Complete recovery of facial function may not occur.[123]

REYE'S SYNDROME. Reye's syndrome is discussed in the earlier section on influenza virus in this chapter.

NEURALGIA. Pain is the most common symptom of zoster and may precede the eruption by days to weeks. It may occasionally be the only manifestation—the so-called zoster sine herpete.[127] The pain of zoster tends to resolve with time, or it may be associated with or followed by post-herpetic neuralgia. The latter is defined as the presence of pain for more than a month after the onset of the zoster eruption.[127] Post-herpetic neuralgia is the most common neurological complication of VZV.

THROMBOTIC CEREBROVASCULOPATHY. The neurological syndrome of thrombotic cerebrovasculopathy associated with herpes zoster infection presents as a herpes ophthalmicus eruption followed by headache and the apoplectic onset of hemiplegia. On neuroimaging there is evidence of infarction in the distribution of the anterior or middle cerebral arteries, which on angiography is seen to be due to multifocal thrombosis. The pathogenesis of this syndrome appears to be direct viral invasion of the arterial walls via viral spread along the intracranial branches of the trigeminal cranial nerve. This syndrome is extremely rare.[121]

Differential Diagnosis. The diagnosis of VZV encephalitis is suggested by the clinical presentation, supported by the preceding neuroimaging abnormalities, and associated with a CSF lymphocytic pleocytosis. Varicella-zoster antibody measured by indirect immunofluorescence is present in a titer of 1:2 or more in the CSF in 94 percent of patients.[121] Detection of VZV DNA in CSF by PCR can confirm the diagnosis.[124] The diagnosis of Bell's palsy due to VZV is suggested by the classic vesicular eruption on the pinna, or the ear may be reddish and have a hyperemic concha or helix.[123] The diagnosis of post-herpetic neuralgia is made on clinical grounds.

Management and Prognosis. VZV encephalitis is treated with intravenous acyclovir (Table 41–6). Early treatment with prednisone and acyclovir appears to improve the outcome in patients with Bell's palsy due to VZV.[123] Prednisone also appears to be beneficial in the treatment of neuritis due to zoster but does not appear to have any effect on the development of post-herpetic neuralgia. Similarly, oral acyclovir (800 mg five times daily) appears to reduce the pain associated with a zoster rash but does not have an effect on the development of post-herpetic neuralgia.[127] Valaciclovir (1.0 g orally three times per day) and acyclovir (800 mg orally five times per day) were approximately equal in their ability to decrease virus shedding and accelerate the time to cutaneous healing of zoster.[128] Valaciclovir is a prodrug of acyclovir and achieves by oral administration plasma acyclovir concentrations similar to those achieved only with intravenous acyclovir.[127] Famciclovir is a prodrug of penciclovir, an acyclic guanine derivative that is similar to acyclovir in terms of structure, spectrum of activity, and mechanism of action.[128] A trial comparing famciclovir (at doses of 250 mg, 500 mg, or 750 mg three times daily) with acyclovir (800 mg five times per day) in 544 immunocompetent adults with herpes zoster demonstrated that famciclovir was equivalent to acyclovir in terms of acceleration of cutaneous healing, loss of acute pain, safety, and tolerance.[128] If begun within 72 hours after the appearance of the rash, famciclovir, valaciclovir, or acyclovir reduces the acute pain in patients with zoster. At this time, no single drug can be recommended over another except to say that famciclovir and valaciclovir can be given less often than acyclovir. Corticosteroids appear to improve the quality of life after zoster even though they do not alter the course of post-herpetic neuralgia; therefore, their administration in combination with an antiviral agent is recommended in individuals in whom they are not contraindicated.[127] Post-herpetic neuralgia can be treated with topical lidocaine-prilocaine cream or 5 percent lidocaine gel. Topical capsaicin cream is not recommended because of the burning that occurs with its application. A tricyclic antidepressive agent such as amitriptyline or desipramine can be started at a low dose (12.5 to 25 mg) at bedtime. Patients should be advised that it takes several weeks to achieve maximum benefit from an antidepressant drug. Anticonvulsant drugs, specifically carbamazepine, can reduce the lancinating component of the neuropathic pain.[127]

CYTOMEGALOVIRUS

Epidemiology and Risk Factors. Cytomegalovirus (CMV) is the most common life- and sight-threatening opportunistic viral infection in patients with AIDS.[129] Central nervous system infection by CMV in patients with AIDS may take the form of one or more of five distinct neurological syndromes: retinitis, polyradiculomyelitis, encephalitis with dementia,

TABLE 41–6. **Antiviral Agents**

Antiviral Agent	Dosage	Indications	Adverse Effects
Acyclovir	1. 10 mg/kg intravenously every 8 hours 2. 800 mg orally 5 times/day	1. Herpes simplex virus encephalitis 2. Zoster	Renal toxicity, nausea, confusion Headache, nausea, diarrhea
Valaciclovir	1.0 g orally tid	Zoster	
Famciclovir	750 mg orally tid	Zoster	
Ganciclovir	Induction therapy: 5 mg/kg bid intravenously Maintenance therapy: 6 mg/kg once daily intravenously	CMV	Neutropenia, thrombocytopenia, confusion, convulsions, dizziness, headaches, nausea
Foscarnet	Induction therapy: 60 mg/kg intravenously every 8 hours Maintenance therapy: 100–120 mg/kg intravenously daily	CMV	Renal toxicity, anemia, hypocalcemia, hypophosphatemia, seizures

ventriculoencephalitis, and mononeuritis multiplex.[130] Organ transplant recipients are also at risk for encephalitis due to CMV. Newborns with congenital CMV infection may have seizures, spasticity, microcephaly, chorioretinitis or optic atrophy, and neuroradiographical evidence of intracerebral calcifications and cerebral atrophy.[131]

Cytomegalovirus is a DNA virus and a member of the herpesvirus group, which includes VZV, HSV types 1 and 2, and Epstein-Barr virus. All of these viruses have a propensity to assume a latent state in humans and to undergo reactivation.[131] Primary infection with CMV is usually benign; approximately 80 percent of adults in the United States have complement fixation antibodies to CMV by the age of 40, but under conditions of immune suppression, latent virus may be reactivated, producing a variety of systemic and neurological syndromes.

Pathogenesis and Pathophysiology. CMV is acquired by close personal contact through saliva, cervical secretions, and semen, and through blood transfusion. In congenital CMV infections, the fetus acquires the infection transplacentally. Symptomatic congenital CMV infection is a complication only of primary maternal infection; infants born to immune mothers may be infected but appear to be asymptomatic in the newborn period. Perinatal infection in infants occurs either through contact with CMV-infected uterine cervical secretions or through transmission of CMV in breast milk. Infection of the CNS results from viremia, and CMV has a predilection to infect the ependymal cells lining the ventricles and the gray matter in the cortex, basal ganglia, brain stem, and cerebellum.[130, 131] The CNS symptoms and neuropathological abnormalities observed in CMV-infected fetuses have been attributed to chronic intrauterine CMV encephalitis.[131]

Clinical Features and Associated Findings. As stated earlier, CMV may cause congenital disease, retinitis, lumbosacral polyradiculopathy and myelitis, encephalitis with dementia, ventriculoencephalitis, mononeuritis multiplex, and infectious polyneuritis—the Guillain-Barré syndrome.

CONGENITAL CMV INFECTION. The clinical spectrum of congenital CMV infection varies from an asymptomatic infant to one who has the signs and symptoms of disseminated disease. In the most severe form of congenital CMV infection, the virus affects multiple organs, and the infant has hepatitis, splenomegaly, pneumonitis, jaundice, thrombocytopenia, chorioretinitis, hemolytic anemia, petechial or purpuric rash, seizures, spasticity, microcephaly, optic atrophy, and neuroimaging evidence of intracerebral calcifications and cerebral atrophy.[131]

RETINITIS. The presenting complaint of CMV retinitis is usually unilateral "floaters" or decreased visual acuity. Ophthalmological examination demonstrates large white-colored areas with perivascular exudates and hemorrhages. Initially these abnormalities are found at the periphery of the fundus, but if left untreated, lesions progress to involve the macula and the optic disc.[132]

LUMBOSACRAL POLYRADICULOPATHY AND MYELITIS. The presentation of this syndrome is characterized by a subacute onset of weakness, areflexia, and sensory loss in the legs in association with bladder- or anal-sphincter dysfunction. The disease evolves as an ascending paraparesis.[130] Clinical evidence of lower extremity weakness, areflexia, and bilateral Babinski's signs (if the spinal cord is involved) suggests this syndrome.

ENCEPHALITIS. Patients with AIDS and encephalitis due to CMV present with forgetfulness, memory impairment, apathy, and withdrawal like patients with HIV encephalitis, except that patients with CMV encephalitis have had AIDS longer and have lower mean CD4 lymphocyte counts at presentation. Patients with CMV encephalitis also have rapidly progressive cognitive impairment, and their survival is markedly shorter than that of patients with HIV dementia. CMV encephalitis is characterized by multifocal, diffusely scattered, small microglial nodules and inclusion-bearing cytomegalic cells that are concentrated in the gray matter in the cortex, basal ganglia, brain stem, and cerebellum. There is a strikingly high incidence of hyponatremia, hyperkalemia consistent with an addisonian state, dilutional hyponatremia with hypo-osmolality, or hypernatremia due to dehydration in patients with CMV encephalitis.[130]

VENTRICULOENCEPHALITIS. A distinction is made between CMV encephalitis, described earlier, and CMV ventriculoencephalitis, which is characterized by necrosis of the cranial nerves and of the periventricular parenchyma.[130] This syndrome presents as a rapidly fatal delirium with oculomotor palsies and nystagmus, and a linear homogeneous increased signal on T2-weighted MRI scans around the ventricles with ventriculomegaly.

MONONEURITIS MULTIPLEX. CMV mononeuritis results from focal necrotizing vasculitis of the epineural arteries and presents as a multifocal or asymmetrical sensory or motor deficit in the distribution of a peripheral or cranial nerve.[130]

Differential Diagnosis. The diagnosis of congenital CMV infection is made by recovery of infectious virus from urine, saliva, buffy coat leukocytes, or CSF. Demonstration of seroconversion or a fourfold increase in CMV antibody titers between the acute and convalescent sera strongly supports recent CMV infection. CT scan demonstrates intracerebral calcifications and cerebral atrophy in newborns with CNS symptoms.[131] The diagnosis of CMV retinitis is made clinically because it is impractical to obtain fluid or tissue from the eye for culture or microscopic examination. Blood, urine, or semen can be cultured to document active CMV infection in the patient, but the relevance of these cultures is questionable because patients without retinitis have positive cultures.[132] In patients with CMV lumbosacral polyradiculopathy, the CSF often demonstrates a pleocytosis with a neutrophilic predominance, the protein concentration is elevated, and the glucose concentration may be low or normal. Culture of CSF for CMV is the gold standard, but this test is insensitive (positive in 60% of patients), and CSF should also be analyzed by the PCR technique.[133, 134] MRI may reveal enlargement of the conus medullaris, clumping of lumbosacral rootlets, or enhancement (with gadolinium) of the leptomeninges of the lower spinal cord.[130] In patients with CMV encephalitis there may be a mild mononuclear pleocytosis and an elevated protein concentration. CSF should be analyzed for CMV DNA by PCR. In patients with CMV ventriculoencephalitis, MRI (as described previously) may demonstrate increased periventricular signal intensity on T2-weighted images. In all patients in whom a CMV neurological syndrome is suspected, culture of the CSF and analysis of CSF by PCR to detect CMV DNA should be performed.

Management. Ganciclovir and foscarnet are the two antiviral agents that have been proved effective in the treatment of CMV retinitis. CMV polyradiculopathy, encephalitis, and ventriculoencephalitis have been treated with dosing regimens that are identical to those used for CMV retinitis, although their clinical efficacy has not been established (see Table 41–6). Ganciclovir 5 mg/kg intravenously is given twice daily during "induction" therapy for a minimum of 2 to 3 weeks. This is followed by maintenance therapy at a dose of 6 mg/kg intravenously qd. Foscarnet is given in a dose of 60 mg/kg administered intravenously every 8 hours for induction therapy for a minimum of 2 to 3 weeks, followed by maintenance therapy of 100 to 120 mg/kg given intravenously qd. The doses of ganciclovir and foscarnet must be reduced when renal function is impaired or renal toxicity develops. A reversible leukopenia is an adverse effect of ganciclovir, as is a thrombocytopenia. Adverse effects of foscarnet include renal toxicity, anemia, hypocalcemia, hypophosphatemia, and seizures.[132] Both CMV encephalitis and ventriculoencephalitis have been reported in patients receiving maintenance therapy for CMV retinitis even when the retinitis remains under control.[129, 130]

HUMAN HERPESVIRUS-6

Epidemiology and Risk Factors. Human herpesvirus-6 (HHV-6) is the causative agent of the common childhood infection roseola infantum (exanthem subitum).[135] The virus was first isolated in 1986 from the peripheral blood lymphocytes of patients with AIDS and those with lymphoproliferative disorders. It is a member of the human herpesvirus family and shares some DNA sequence homology with CMV.[136] Saliva may be the major mode of transmission of HHV-6. Primary infection may be symptomatic or asymptomatic; the virus is then able to become latent in the host and reactivates in the presence of immunosuppression. The majority of the population is exposed to HHV-6 in infancy; by age 2 years, most children are seropositive.[136]

Pathogenesis and Pathophysiology. HHV-6 DNA has been detected by PCR in 6 of 9 (66%) normal brain tissue specimens in one study and in the CSF of 9 of 10 patients with exanthem subitum and neurological symptoms.[137, 138] Human T-lymphocytes are the primary cell type infected by HHV-6, but HHV-6 has also been shown to infect cells of neuronal and glial origin in vitro.[137] The detection of HHV-6 DNA by PCR in children with exanthem subitum and neurological symptoms suggests that HHV-6 invades the brain during acute infection.[138] The presence of HHV-6 DNA in normal brain tissue specimens is evidence of the persistence or latency of HHV-6 in the CNS.[137] Reactivation of latent HHV-6 infection has been demonstrated in children and in immunocompromised adults.[139, 140]

Clinical Features and Associated Findings. As previously stated, HHV-6 is the etiological agent of childhood exanthem subitum. The most common CNS complications of primary HHV-6 infection are seizures, meningoencephalitis, and encephalopathy.[139] HHV-6 has been reported as the etiological agent of focal encephalitis in bone marrow transplant recipients and in immunocompetent adults with focal encephalitis in whom the clinical presentation suggested herpes simplex virus encephalitis.[136, 140] CNS infection with HHV-6 has also been associated with diffuse or multifocal demyelination and a clinical picture of fulminant multiple sclerosis.[141] Disseminated HHV-6 infection has been reported in children and adults with AIDS.[142, 143]

EXANTHEM SUBITUM. Roseola infantum or exanthem subitum is a common disease of infancy characterized by high fever for a few days followed by the appearance of a generalized maculopapular rash when the fever subsides. Febrile convulsions in this disease have a reported incidence of 13 to 30 percent, children 12 to 15 months of age being at highest risk.[135, 138]

ENCEPHALITIS AND FOCAL ENCEPHALITIS. HHV-6 DNA has been recovered from the brain of a patient at autopsy who died of encephalitis 5 months after undergoing allogeneic bone marrow transplantation.[140] Three of 37 patients with a clinical presentation suggestive of herpes simplex encephalitis and 6 of 101 patients with clinical and laboratory evidence of herpes simplex encephalitis were found to have HHV-6 DNA in their CSF when samples of CSF were sent to the University of Alabama for the purpose of undergoing diagnostic PCR analysis for possible herpes simplex encephalitis. The spectrum of disease ranged from mild encephalitis with complete resolution to severe neurological dysfunction and death.[136] A dense and disseminated active HHV-6 infection was found in the brain tissue of a young woman with a fulminant demyelinative disease that was clinically and histopathologically diagnosed as acute multiple sclerosis.[141]

Differential Diagnosis. Primary HHV-6 infection is diagnosed by culture of peripheral blood mononuclear cells and a concomitant fourfold or greater rise in IgG titer between the acute and convalescent sera. CSF can be analyzed by PCR to detect HHV-6 DNA. IgM antibody may be present during reactivation, and therefore its presence does not differentiate a primary infection from reactivation.[139]

Management. Limited information is available on the susceptibility of HHV-6 to antiviral agents. The pattern of antiviral inhibition of HHV-6, however, resembles that of the human cytomegalovirus, suggesting that ganciclovir and foscarnet may be effective for the treatment of HHV-6 infections.[144]

EPSTEIN-BARR VIRUS

Epidemiology and Risk Factors. Epstein-Barr virus (EBV) is a human B-lymphotropic virus, the causative agent of infectious mononucleosis. The major route of transmission of EBV is through saliva, and EBV infects the epithelial cells of the oropharynx and adjacent structures as well as those of the uterine cervix. Epithelial cells may play a major role in the persistence of EBV by allowing chronic viral replication and release of infectious particles throughout the lifetime of a virus-infected host. Eighty to 90 percent of children in developing countries are seropositive for EBV between 2 and 3 years of age. By the third decade, nearly 100 percent of adults have EBV serum antibodies.[145]

Pathogenesis and Pathophysiology. EBV is a lymphotropic virus that selectively infects B-lymphocytes. B-lymphocytes are infected by EBV during their passage through the chronically EBV-infected oropharyngeal epithelium. EBV has the unique biological property of being able to induce dysregulated activation and growth of a subpopulation of the infected B cells that then grow continuously as lymphoblastoid cell lines that secrete immunoglobulins.[145, 146] CNS invasion by infected B-lymphocytes appears to be important in the pathogenesis of CNS disease.[147]

Clinical Features and Associated Findings. Infectious mononucleosis is the only known disease caused by acute EBV infection. The neurological complications of infectious mononucleosis include meningoencephalitis, Guillain-Barré syndrome, cerebellitis, transverse myelitis, cranial nerve palsies (of which the most common is cranial nerve VII palsy), and a variety of optic nerve abnormalities (papilledema, optic neuritis, retrobulbar neuritis).[148] EBV infection is almost universally associated with primary CNS lymphomas in patients with AIDS.[149] Persistent viral activity or reactivation of EBV has been studied in the etiology of chronic fatigue syndrome.

INFECTIOUS MONONUCLEOSIS. The term *infectious mononucleosis* was first used in 1920 to describe the clinical findings of medical students attending Johns Hopkins University who had the typical clinical picture of this disease associated with atypical mononuclear cells.[148] The clinical course of infectious mononucleosis is characterized by a 7-day prodromal illness followed by a 4-day to 3-week acute illness characterized by fever, headache, malaise, pharyngitis, cervical lymphadenopathy, and mononuclear leukocytosis with atypical lymphocytes. Splenic and hepatomegaly may be present with transient hepatic dysfunction.[145, 148] The neurological complications of infectious mononucleosis include the Guillain-Barré syndrome, an aseptic meningitis or encephalitis of which nonfebrile seizures are a common presenting manifestation, and cranial nerve palsies, the most common of which is an isolated or bilateral facial nerve palsy.[148] Overall, meningoencephalitis is the most common neurological complication, whereas transverse myelitis is the least common.

CNS LYMPHOMA. EBV is detectable from a majority of primary CNS lymphomas in AIDS patients and to a lesser degree from primary CNS lymphomas in immunocompetent individuals.[149] The clinical presentation is that of progressive personality changes, seizures, and signs of increased intracranial pressure.[150]

CHRONIC FATIGUE SYNDROME. Chronic fatigue syndrome is characterized by debilitating fatigue accompanied by a variety of symptoms, including cognitive difficulty, myalgias, and arthralgias.[151]

Differential Diagnosis. The diagnosis of infectious mononucleosis is based on a positive heterophil antibody test, the appearance of atypical lymphocytes in the blood at 1 to 4 weeks after onset of disease, and/or by changes in EBV-specific antibodies. An acute infection is documented by detection of antiviral capsid antigen (VCA) titers of 1:320 or higher, the presence of anti-D (i.e., diffuse component of EBV-induced early antigen complex), or EBV VCA IgM antibodies and the absence of antibodies to virus-associated nuclear antigen (anti-EBNA IgG). In acute and convalescent paired sera, fourfold or greater increments in anti-VCA or anti-D titers, or a late decrease in anti-VCA titers or loss of anti-D titers, and the appearance of anti-EBNA IgG denote a recent infection. Anti-VCA titers peak early and then decline to persistent lower levels. Anti-D responses and virus-specific IgM antibodies are present for only a few weeks. Anti-EBNA antibodies appear late in convalescence and persist for life.[148] In patients in whom neurological complications of infectious mononucleosis are suspected, the combination of serological tests and PCR performed on CSF for the EBV DNA genome is recommended. If PCR for EBV DNA on CSF is negative, an acute EBV infection can be documented by evidence of positive IgM antibody titers to the viral capsid antigen early in the disease course, with a fourfold decrease in IgG antibody titers to the viral capsid antigen corresponding to a fourfold or greater increase in antibody to Epstein-Barr nuclear antigen between the acute and convalescent sera. A distinction between latent and symptomatic EBV infection cannot be made based strictly on positive results of PCR on CSF for EBV DNA.[152]

The diagnosis of primary CNS lymphoma is based on CT or MRI evidence of a focal enhancing mass lesion or lesions, and typically an unsuccessful response to antitoxoplasma therapy, because the neuroimaging appearance of *Toxoplasma gondii* encephalitis and primary CNS lymphoma is similar. The gold standard for the diagnosis has been brain biopsy; however, the PCR technique is both sensitive and specific in making the diagnosis. EBV DNA was detected by PCR in the CSF from 7 of 8 patients with primary CNS lymphoma diagnosed by brain biopsy (87.5% sensitivity) but in none of the 11 controls with brain mass lesions (100% specificity).[149]

Although there are reports of patients with chronic fatigue syndrome and high antibody titers to viral capsid antigen and early antigen of EBV, to date there is no scientific evidence that the reactivation of EBV is involved in the chronic fatigue syndrome.[153]

Management. Although there are no EBV antiviral agents, ganciclovir is known to inhibit EBV replication in vitro, and there are a few reports of successful treatment of EBV meningoencephalitis with ganciclovir in transplant recipients.[154] Primary CNS lymphoma is treated with radiation therapy.

VARIOLA VIRUS (SMALLPOX)

Epidemiology and Risk Factors. No infectious disease in history has been more lethal than smallpox. In the 20th century, smallpox killed 300 million people worldwide. Through an effective immunization program, the World Health Organization was able to eliminate smallpox. One of the last outbreaks occurred in Iran, then spread to northern Iraq and to Syria in the mid-1970s. In 1980, the World Health Assembly recommended that all countries cease vaccination. Several vials of virus were to be retained in two designated laboratories, the Institute of Virus Preparations in Moscow, Russia, and the CDC in Atlanta, Georgia. The Fifty-second World Health Assembly established a deadline of December 31, 2002, to destroy all remaining stocks of variola virus.[155, 156] Terrorist groups are believed to have obtained smallpox. Specimens were taken from patients in Iran, Iraq, and Syria, and smallpox was isolated. The whereabouts of these specimens of smallpox are not known.

Pathogenesis and Pathophysiology. Smallpox spreads from person to person by droplet nuclei from oropharyngeal secretions and can be spread by contaminated clothing and beds.[157] The infectious dose is very small; for this reason, disease can spread quickly.

Clinical Features and Associated Findings

SMALLPOX. The incubation period is 7 to 17 days between the time the virus attaches to the oropharyngeal or respiratory mucosa and the onset of high fever, sore throat, headache, and backache. A maculopapular rash appears on the mucosa of the mouth and oropharynx, face, and forearms and spreads to the trunk and legs. The lesions become vesicular then pustular (small boils). The lesions are more dense on the face and extremities than on the trunk. The lesions are all in the same stage at the same time, and thus appear similar to each other. Patients are most infective when they have lesions in their mouth because virus titers in saliva are highly infectious at this time.[157] Smallpox can be complicated by encephalitis and postinfectious encephalomyelitis.

HEMORRHAGIC SMALLPOX. This form of smallpox presents with high fever, headache, backache, and abdominal pain, followed by petechial and hemorrhagic lesions in the skin and mucous membranes. The skin rash initially has the appearance of meningococcemia. Pregnant women are particularly susceptible, and this is uniformly fatal.[157]

POSTVACCINIAL ENCEPHALOMYELITIS. Postvaccinial encephalomyelitis, also called postinfectious encephalomyelitis, acute disseminated encephalomyelitis, and acute demyelinating encephalomyelitis, is an acute inflammatory, demyelinating disease of the brain, optic nerves, and spinal cord that historically was a major complication of smallpox vaccination. The illness is characterized by the abrupt onset of fever, altered level of consciousness, and multifocal neurological deficits.

Diagnosis. Smallpox is a DNA virus that is a member of the orthopoxviruses. Smallpox infection can be rapidly diagnosed in the laboratory by the electron microscopic appearance of brick-shaped virions from vesicular or pustular fluid that is collected from an open lesion or by an examination of a specimen from scabs. The characteristic abnormalities on MR scan in postvaccinial encephalomyelitis are multifocal areas of hyperintensity on T2-weighted images consistent with a multifocal demyelinating disease.

Management. The care of patients with smallpox is primarily supportive. Patients should be isolated; those caring for them should wear gowns, gloves, and masks; and bed linens should be autoclaved. All close contacts of any person with smallpox should be promptly vaccinated. Vaccination that is administered within 4 days of exposure has been shown to offer some protection against acquiring infection.[157]

JC VIRUS

Epidemiology and Risk Factors. The JC virus is ubiquitous; antibodies to the virus are present in up to 85 percent of individuals by the age of 9 years.[158] The JC virus is the etiological agent of progressive multifocal leukoencephalopathy (PML).

Pathogenesis and Pathophysiology. The kidneys are thought to be the site of latent JC viral persistence. Reactivation of the virus associated with immunosuppression results in hematogenous dissemination of the virus to the brain. Foci of PML are frequently located in proximity to blood vessels.[159] Progressive multifocal leukoencephalopathy occurs in patients with impaired cell-mediated immunity such as those with AIDS, chronic lymphocytic leukemia, Hodgkin's disease, other lymphomas, systemic lupus erythematosus, organ transplantation, and sarcoidosis.[158, 159] The virus preferentially infects the myelin-producing oligodendrocytes, resulting in cell lysis and demyelination.[159]

Clinical Features and Associated Findings. Focal neurological deficits (hemiparesis, dysarthria, and cerebellar limb and gait ataxia), seizure activity, and cognitive impairment characterized by memory impairment, psychomotor retardation, and inattentiveness characterize the clinical presentation of PML.[159]

Differential Diagnosis. On CT scan, PML appears as single or multiple nonenhancing, hypodense lesions in the white matter, most commonly in the parietal-occipital regions. On T2-weighted MRI scans, the lesions have increased signal intensity and do not enhance after contrast administration. Examination of the CSF is usually normal.[159] The PCR technique can detect JC virus DNA in CSF with a reported sensitivity of 75 percent and a specificity of 96 percent.[160] Serum and CSF antibody titers for JC virus are not useful in establishing the diagnosis of PML because 80 percent of the population show antibodies to JC virus by adulthood.[159] Brain biopsy should be used for diagnosis in patients who have suspicious white matter lesions on MRI and in whom JC virus is not detected by PCR on CSF.[160]

Management. There is no proven therapy for PML, but clinical trials are ongoing. There is a correlation between the CD4 T-cell count and survival, in that patients with higher CD4 T-cell counts survive longer. Notable improvement in PML has been observed in AIDS patients treated with high-dose 3-azido-3-deoxythymidine (AZT), and it is hypothesized that the AZT-induced elevation of CD4 T-cell counts improves cell-mediated immunity sufficiently to resist the JC virus infection.[159] The average length of survival from the onset of symptoms to death is 1 to 4 months, but a small percentage of patients reportedly have improved spontaneously and survived for several years.[159]

Acknowledgment

The assistance of Mrs. Linda Hagan in the preparation of this manuscript is greatly appreciated.

Reviews and Selected Updates

Bale JF: Perinatal viral infections. *In* Roos KL (ed): Central Nervous System Infectious Diseases and Therapy. New York, Marcel Dekker, 1997, pp 1–24.

Deresiewicz RL, Thaler SJ, Hsu L, Zamani AA: Clinical and neuroradiographic manifestations of eastern equine encephalitis. N Engl J Med 1997;336:1867–1874.

Jackson AC: Update on rabbies. Curr Opin Neurol 2002;13:327–331.

Lakeman FD, Whitley RJ: NIAID-Collaborative Antiviral Study Group: Diagnosis of herpes simplex encephalitis: Application of polymerase chain reaction to cerebrospinal fluid from brain-biopsied patients and correlation with disease. J Infect Dis 1995;171:857–863.

Roos KL: Encephalitis. Neurol Clin 1999;17:813–834.

Rotbart HA: Viral meningitis. Semin Neurol 2000;3:277–292.

References

1. Rotbart HA, Sawyer MH, Fast S, Lewinski C: Diagnosis of enteroviral meningitis by using PCR with a colorimetric microwell detection assay. J Clin Micro 1994;32:2590–2592.
2. Rotbart HA: Enteroviral infections of the central nervous system. Clin Infect Dis 1995;20:971–981.
3. Morrison LA, Fields BN: Parallel mechanisms in neuropathogenesis of enteric virus infections. J Virol 1991;65:2767–2772.
4. McKinney RE, Katz SL, Wilfert CM: Chronic enteroviral meningoencephalitis in agammaglobulinemic patients. Rev Infect Dis 1987;9:334–356.

5. Modlin JF, Dagan R, Berlin LE, et al: Focal encephalitis with enterovirus infections. Pediatrics 1991;88:841–845.
6. Jadoul C, Goethem JV, Martin JJ: Myelitis due to coxsackievirus B infection. Neurology 1995;45:1626–1627.
7. Yui LA, Gledhill RF: Limb paralysis as a manifestation of coxsackie B virus infection. Dev Med Child Neurol 1991;33:427–438.
8. Leonardi GP, Greenberg AJ, Costello P, Szabo K: Echovirus type 30 infection associated with aseptic meningitis in Nassau County, New York, USA. Intervirology 1993;36:53–56.
9. Yamashita K, Miyamura K, Yamadera S, et al: Epidemics of aseptic meningitis due to echovirus 30 in Japan. Jpn J Med Sci Biol 1994;47:221–239.
10. Berlin LE, Rorabaugh ML, Heldrich F, Roberts K: Aseptic meningitis in infants 2 years of age: Diagnosis and etiology. J Infect Dis 1993;168:888–892.
11. Takahashi S, Miyamoto A, Oki J, et al: Acute transverse myelitis caused by echo virus type 18 infection. Eur J Pediatr 1995;154:378–380.
12. Bartfeld H, Donnenfeld H, Kascsak R: Relevance of the post-polio syndrome to other motor neuron diseases: Relevance to viral (enteroviral) infections. Ann NY Acad Sci 1995;753:237–244.
13. Alexander JP, Baden L, Pallansch MA, Anderson LJ: Enterovirus 71 infections and neurologic disease—United States, 1977–1991. J Infect Dis 1994;169:905–908.
14. Connolly KJ, Hammer SM: The acute aseptic meningitis syndrome. Infect Dis Clin North Am 1990;4:599–622.
15. Bonadio WA, Stanco L, Bruce R, et al: Reference values of normal cerebrospinal fluid composition in infants ages 0 to 8 weeks. Pediatr Infect Dis J 1992;11:589–591.
16. Roos KL: Cerebrospinal fluid. *In* Roos KL: Meningitis: 100 Maxims in Neurology. London, Arnold, 1996, pp 36–52.
17. Severien C, Jacobs KH, Schoenemann W: Marked pleocytosis and hypoglycorrhachia in coxsackie meningitis. Pediatr Infect Dis J 1994;13:322–323.
18. Johnson GM, McAbee GA, Seaton ED, Lipson SM: Suspect value of non-CSF viral cultures in the diagnosis of enteroviral CNS infections in young infants. Dev Med Child Neurol 1992;34:876–884.
19. Shafran SD, Halota W, Gilbert D, et al: Pleconaril is effective for enteroviral meningitis in adolescents and adults: A randomized placebo-controlled multicenter trial [abstract 1904]. Abstracts of the 39th Interscience Conference on Antimicrobial Agents and Chemotherapy, 1999, San Francisco, CA. American Society for Microbiology, 1999:436.
20. Abzug MJ, Keyserling HL, Lee ML, Levin MJ: Neonatal enterovirus infection: Virology, serology, and effects of intravenous immune globulin. Clin Infect Dis 1995;20:1201–1206.
21. Geller TJ, Condie D: A case of protracted coxsackie virus meningoencephalitis in a marginally immunodeficient child treated successfully with intravenous immunoglobulin. J Neurol Sci 1995;129:131–133.
22. Horstmann DM: Three landmark articles about poliomyelitis. Medicine (Baltimore) 1992;71:320–325.
23. Racaniello VR, Ren R: Poliovirus biology and pathogenesis. Curr Top Microbiol Immunol 1996;206:305–325.
24. Paul JR: The clinical epidemiology of poliomyelitis. Medicine (Baltimore) 1941;20:495–520.
25. Mulder DW: Clinical observations on acute poliomyelitis. Ann NY Acad Sci 1995;753:1–10.
26. Enders JF, Weller TH, Robbins FC: Cultivation of the Lansing strain of poliomyelitis virus in cultures of various human embryonic tissues. Science 1949;109:85–87.
27. Sabin AB: My last will and testament on rapid elimination and ultimate global eradication of poliomyelitis and measles. Pediatrics 1992;90:S162–S169.
28. Aycock WL: Tonsillectomy and poliomyelitis. Medicine (Baltimore) 1942;21:65–94.
29. Illa I, Leon-Monzon M, Agboatwalla M, et al: Role of the muscle in acute poliomyelitis infection. Ann NY Acad Sci 1995;753:58–67.
30. Nathanson N, Langmuir AD: The Cutter incident: Comparison of the clinical character of vaccination and contact cases occurring after use of high rate lots of Cutter vaccine. Am J Hyg 1963;78:61–69.
31. Bodian D: Poliomyelitis: Pathologic anatomy. *In* Poliomyelitis: Papers and Discussions. Proceedings of the First International Poliomyelitis Conference. Philadelphia, JB Lippincott, 1962, pp 62–84.
32. Dalakas MC: Pathogenetic mechanisms of post-polio syndrome: Morphological, electrophysiological, virological, and immunological correlations. Ann NY Acad Sci 1995;753:167–185.
33. Dalakas MC: The post-polio syndrome as an evolved clinical entity: Definition and clinical description. Ann NY Acad Sci 1995;753:68–80.
34. Trojan DA, Cashman NR: Anticholinesterases in post-poliomyelitis syndrome. Ann NY Acad Sci 1995;753:285–295.
35. Frankel D: US group urges immunization change. Lancet 1995;346:1151.
36. Hull HF, Lee JW: Sabin, Salk or sequential? Lancet 1996;347:630.
37. Hull HF, Ward NA, Hull BP, et al: Paralytic poliomyelitis: Seasoned strategies, disappearing disease. Lancet 1994;343:1331–1337.
38. Forsey T: Mumps vaccines—current status. J Med Microbiol 1994;41(1):1–2.
39. Peltola H: Mumps vaccination and meningitis. Lancet 1993;341:994–995.
40. Noah ND, Urquhart AM: Virus meningitis and encephalitis in 1979. J Infect Dis 1980;2:379–383.
41. Mumps prevention. Recommendations of the Immunization Practices Advisory Committee (ACIP). MMWR 1989;38:388–400.
42. Mumps meningitis and MMR vaccination. Lancet 1989;2(8670):1015–1016.
43. Swoveland PT, Johnson KP: Subacute sclerosing panencephalitis and other paramyxovirus infections. *In* McKendall RR (ed): Handbook of Clinical Neurology, Vol. 12(56): Viral Disease. Amsterdam, Elsevier Science, 1989, pp 417–438.
44. Miller E, Goldacre M, Pugh S, et al: Risk of aseptic meningitis after measles, mumps, and rubella vaccine in UK children. Lancet 1993;341:979–982.
45. Yamamoto M, Watanabe Y, Mizukoshi K: Neurotological findings in patients with acute mumps deafness. Acta Otolaryngol (Stockh) 1993;(Suppl 504):94–97.
46. Johnstone JA, Ross CAC, Dunn M: Meningitis and encephalitis associated with mumps infection. Arch Dis Child 1972;47:647–651.
47. Koskiniemi M, Donner M, Pettay O: Clinical appearance and outcome in mumps encephalitis in children. Acta Paediatr Scand 1983;72:603–609.
48. Calisher CH: Medically important arboviruses of the United States and Canada. Clin Microbiol Rev 1994;7:89–116.
49. Bale JF: Viral encephalitis. Med Clin North Am 1993;77:25–42.
50. Arboviral disease—United States, 1994. MMWR 1995;44:641–644.
51. Johnson RT: The pathogenesis of acute viral encephalitis and post-infectious encephalomyelitis. J Infect Dis 1987;155:359–364.
52. Thisyakorn U, Thisyakorn C: Diseases caused by arboviruses—dengue haemorrhagic fever and Japanese B encephalitis. Med J Aust 1994;160:22–26.
53. Thaithumyanon P, Thisyakorn U, Deerojnawong J, Innis BL: Dengue infection complicated by severe hemorrhage and vertical transmission in a parturient woman. Clin Infect Dis 1994;18:248–249.
54. Whitley RJ: Viral encephalitis. N Engl J Med 1990;323:242–250.
55. Johnson KP, Lepow ML, Johnson RT: California encephalitis: Clinical and epidemiological studies. Neurology 1968;18:250–254.
56. Hanley DF, Ray CG: Viral encephalitis: When it's likely. Patient Care 1992;June 15:293–311.
57. Feemster RF: Equine encephalitis in Massachusetts. N Engl J Med 1957;257:701–704.
58. Lum LCS, Lam SK, Choy YS, et al: Dengue encephalitis: A true entity? Am J Trop Med Hyg 1996;54(3):256–259.
59. McJunkin JE, Khan R, de los Reyes EC, et al: Treatment of severe LaCrosse encephalitis with intravenous ribavirin following diagnosis by brain biopsy. Pediatrics 1997;99:261–267.
60. LaForce FM, Nichol KL, Cox NJ: Influenza: Virology, epidemiology, disease, and prevention. Am J Prev Med 1994;(Suppl 10):31–44.
61. Gruber WC, Belshe RB, King JC, et al: Evaluation of live attenuated influenza vaccines in children 6–18 months of age: Safety, immunogenicity, and efficacy. J Infect Dis 1996;173:1313–1319.
62. Wright P, Murray RM: Schizophrenia: Prenatal influenza and autoimmunity. Ann Med 1993;25:497–502.
63. Wright P, Gill M, Murray RM: Schizophrenia: Genetics and the maternal immune response to viral infection. Am J Med Genet 1993;48:40–46.
64. Takei N, Murray RM, Sham P, O'Callaghan E: Schizophrenia risk for women from in utero exposure to influenza. Am J Psych 1995;152(1):150–151.
65. Lynberg MC, Khoury MJ, Lu X, Cocian T: Maternal flu, fever, and the risk of neural tube defects: A population-based case-control study. Am J Epidemiol 1994;140:244–255.
66. Aggarwal A, Lacomis D, Giuliani MJ: A reversible paralytic syndrome with anti-GD_{1b} antibodies following influenza immunization. Muscle Nerve 1995;18:1199–1201.
67. Roscelli JD, Bass JW, Pang L: Guillain-Barré syndrome and influenza vaccination in the US Army, 1980–1988. Am J Epidemiol 1991;133:952–955.

68. Hukin J, Junker AK, Thomas EE, Farrell K: Reye syndrome associated with subclinical varicella zoster virus and influenza A infection. Pediatr Neurol 1993;9:134–136.
69. Gilden DH, Vafai A: Varicella-zoster. *In* McKendall RR (ed): Handbook of Clinical Neurology, Vol. 12(56): Viral Disease. Amsterdam, Elsevier Science, 1989, pp 229–247.
70. Ruff RL: Acute viral myositis, virus-induced immune complex myositis and myoglobinuria. *In* McKendall RR (ed): Handbook of Clinical Neurology, Vol. 12(56): Viral Disease. Amsterdam, Elsevier Science, 1989, pp 193–206.
71. Johnson RT: The virology of demyelinating diseases. Ann Neurol 1994;36:S54–S60.
72. Atmar RL, Englund JA, Hammill H: Complications of measles during pregnancy. Clin Infect Dis 1992;14:217–226.
73. Hutchins S, Markowitz L, Atkinson W, et al: Measles outbreaks in the United States, 1987 through 1990. Pediatr Infect Dis J 1996;15:31–38.
74. Budka H, Urbanits S, Liberski PP, et al: Subacute measles virus encephalitis: A new and fatal opportunistic infection in a patient with AIDS. Neurology 1996;46(2):586–587.
75. Mustafa MM, Weitman SD, Winick NJ, et al: Subacute measles encephalitis in the young immunocompromised host: Report of two cases diagnosed by polymerase chain reaction and treated with ribavirin and review of the literature. Clin Infect Dis 1993;16: 654–660.
76. Griffin DE, Ward BJ, Esolen LM: Pathogenesis of measles virus infection: A hypothesis for altered immune responses. J Infect Dis 1994;170(Suppl 1):S24–S31.
77. Hughes I, Jenney ME, Newton RW, et al: Measles encephalitis during immuno-suppressive treatment for acute lymphoblastic leukemia. Arch Dis Child 1993;68(6):775–778.
78. Billeter MA, Cattaneo R, Spielhofer P, et al: Generation and properties of measles virus mutations typically associated with subacute sclerosing panencephalitis. Ann NY Acad Sci 1994;724:367–377.
79. Makhene MK, Diaz PS: Clinical presentations and complications of suspected measles in hospitalized children. Pediatr Infect Dis J 1993;12: 836–840.
80. McNutt NS, Kindel S, Lugo J: Cutaneous manifestations of measles in AIDS. J Cutan Pathol 1992;19:315–324.
81. Forthal DN, Aarnaes S, Blanding J, et al: Degree and length of viremia in adults with measles. J Infect Dis 1992;166:421–424.
82. Markand ON, Panszi JG: The electroencephalogram in subacute sclerosing panencephalitis. Arch Neurol 1975;32:719–726.
83. Eberhart-Phillips JE, Frederick PD, Baron RC, Mascola L: Measles in pregnancy: A descriptive study of 58 cases. Obstet Gynecol 1993;82:797–801.
84. Kamaci M, Zorlu CG, Belhan A: Measles in pregnancy. Acta Obstet Gynecol Scand 1996;75:307–309.
85. Ross LA, Kim KS, Mason WH Jr, Gomperts E: Successful treatment of disseminated measles in a patient with acquired immunodeficiency syndrome: Consideration of antiviral and passive immuno-therapy. Am J Med 1990;88:313–314.
86. Roebroek RMJA, Postma BH, Dijkstra UJ: Aseptic meningitis caused by the lymphocytic chorio-meningitis virus. Clin Neuro Neurosurg 1994;96:178–180.
87. Jahrling PB, Peters CJ: Lymphocytic choriomeningitis virus: A neglected pathogen of man. Arch Pathol Lab Med 1992;116:486–488.
88. Larsen PD, Chartrand SA, Tomashek KM, et al: Hydrocephalus complicating lymphocytic choriomeningitis virus infection. Pediatr Infect Dis J 1993;12:528–531.
89. Barton LL, Budd SC, Morfitt WS, et al: Congenital lymphocytic choriomeningitis virus infection in twins. Pediatr Infect Dis J 1993;12: 942–946.
90. Dwyer DE, Hueston L, Field PR, et al: Acute encephalitis complicating rubella virus infection. Pediatr Infect Dis J 1992;11:238–240.
91. Aguado JM, Posada I, Gonzalez M, Lizasoain M: Meningoencephalitis and polyradiculoneuritis in adults: Don't forget rubella. Clin Infect Dis 1993;17:785–786.
92. Robinson J, Lemay M, Vaudry WL: Congenital rubella after anticipated maternal immunity: Two cases and a review of the literature. Pediatr Infect Dis J 1994;13:812–815.
93. Chantler JK, Smyrnis L, Tai G: Selective infection of astrocytes in human glial cell cultures by rubella virus. Lab Invest 1995;72:334–340.
94. Edwards KM: Pediatric immunizations. Curr Prob Pediatr 1993;23(5): 186–209.
95. Congenital rubella syndrome among the Amish—Pennsylvania, 1991–1992. JAMA 1992;268:859–860.
96. Lee SH, Ewert DP, Frederick PD, Mascola L: Resurgence of congenital rubella syndrome in the 1990s: Report on missed opportunities and failed prevention policies among women of childbearing age. JAMA 1992;267:2616–2620.
97. Wolinsky JS: Progressive rubella panencephalitis. *In* McKendall RR (ed): Handbook of Clinical Neurology, Vol. 12(56): Viral Disease. Amsterdam, Elsevier Science, 1989, pp 405–416.
98. Bale JF, Murph JR: Congenital infections and the nervous system. Pediatr Clin North Am 1992;39:669–690.
99. Straussberg R, Amir J, Harel L, Djaldetti M: Ultrastructural alterations of the amniocytes in 2 patients with rubella during the first trimester of pregnancy. Fetal Diagn Ther 1995;10:60–65.
100. De The G, Bomford R: An HTLV-1 vaccine: Why, how, for whom? AIDS Res Hum Retroviruses 1993;9:381–386.
101. Hollsberg P, Hafler DA: What is the pathogenesis of human T-cell lymphotropic virus type 1-associated myelopathy/tropical spastic paraparesis? Ann Neurol 1995;37:143–145.
102. De Mistro A, Chotard J, Hall AJ, et al: HTLV-I/II seroprevalence in the Gambia: A study of mother-child pairs. AIDS Res Hum Retroviruses 1994;10:617–620.
103. Bentrem DJ, McGovern EE, Hammarskjold ML, Edlich RF: Human T-cell lymphotropic virus type-1 (HTLV-1) retrovirus and human disease. J Emerg Med 1994;12:825–832.
104. Puccioni-Sohler M, Rieckmann P, Kitze B, Lange P: A soluble form of tumor necrosis factor receptor in cerebrospinal fluid and serum of HTLV-1-associated myelopathy and other neurological diseases. J Neurol 1995;242:239–242.
105. Lehky TJ, Fox CH, Koenig S, et al: Detection of human T-lymphotropic virus type 1 (HTLV-1) tax RNA in the central nervous system of HTLV-1-associated myelopathy/tropical spastic paraparesis patients by in situ hybridization. Ann Neurol 1995;37:167–175.
106. Godoy AJ, Kira J, Hasuo K, Goto I: Characterization of cerebral white matter lesions of HTLV-I-associated myelopathy/tropical spastic paraparesis in comparison with multiple sclerosis and collagen-vasculitis: A semiquantitative MRI study. J Neurol Sci 1995;133:102–111.
107. Whitley RJ: Neonatal herpes simplex virus infections: Pathogenesis and therapy. Pathobiology 1992;40:729–734.
108. Whitley RJ, Lakeman F: Herpes simplex virus infections of the central nervous system: Therapeutic and diagnostic considerations. Clin Infect Dis 1995;20:414–420.
109. Steiner I, Kennedy PGE: Molecular biology of herpes simplex virus type 1 latency in the nervous system. Mol Neurobiol 1993;7:137–159.
110. Barnett EM, Jacobsen G, Evans G, et al: Herpes simplex encephalitis in the temporal cortex and limbic system after trigeminal nerve inoculation. J Infect Dis 1994;169:782–786.
111. Bravo FJ, Myers MG, Stanberry LR: Neonatal herpes simplex infection: Pathogenesis and treatment in the guinea pig. J Infect Dis 1994;169:947–955.
112. Kennedy PGE, Steinert I: A molecular and cellular model to explain the differences in reactivation from latency by herpes simplex and varicella-zoster viruses. Neuropathol Appl Neurobiol 1994;20:368–374.
113. Tedder DG, Ashley R, Tyler KL, Levin MJ: Herpes simplex virus infection as a cause of benign recurrent lymphocytic meningitis. Ann Intern Med 1994;121:334–338.
114. Barringer JR: Herpes simplex virus and Bell palsy. Ann Intern Med 1996;124:63–65.
115. Whitley RJ, Cobbs GC, Alford CA, et al: Diseases that mimic herpes simplex encephalitis: Diagnosis, presentation, and outcome. JAMA 1989;262:234–239.
116. Lakeman FD, Whitley RJ, et al: Diagnosis of herpes simplex encephalitis: Application of polymerase chain reaction to cerebrospinal fluid from brain-biopsied patients and correlation with disease. J Infect Dis 1995;171:857–863.
117. Landry ML: To the editor: False-positive polymerase chain reaction results in the diagnosis of herpes simplex encephalitis. J Infect Dis 1995;172:1641–1643.
118. Murakami S, Mizobuchi M, Nakashiro Y, Doi T: Bell palsy and herpes simplex virus: Identification of viral DNA in endoneurial fluid and muscle. Ann Intern Med 1996;124:27–30.
119. Picard FJ, Dekaban GA, Silva J, Rice GPA: Mollaret's meningitis associated with herpes simplex type 2 infection. Neurology 1993; 43:1722–1727.
120. Weller TH: Varicella and herpes zoster: A perspective and overview. J Infect Dis 1992;166(Suppl 1):S51–S56.
121. Elliott KJ: Other neurological complications of herpes zoster and their management. Ann Neurol 1994;35:S57–S61.

122. Meier JL, Straus SE: Comparative biology of latent varicella-zoster virus and herpes simplex virus infections. J Infect Dis 1992;166(Suppl 1):S13–S23.
123. Adour KK: Otological complications of herpes zoster. Ann Neurol 1994;35:S62–S64.
124. Amlie-Lefond C, Kleinschmidt-DeMasters BK, et al: The vasculopathy of varicella-zoster virus encephalitis. Ann Neurol 1995;37:784–790.
125. Grose C, Ng TI: Intracellular synthesis of varicella-zoster virus. J Infect Dis 1992;166(Suppl 1):S7–S12.
126. Mahalingam R, Wellish MC, Dueland AN, et al: Localization of herpes simplex virus and varicella zoster virus DNA in human ganglia. Ann Neurol 1992;31:444–448.
127. Kost RG, Straus SE: Postherpetic neuralgia—pathogenesis, treatment, and prevention. N Engl J Med 1996;335:32–42.
128. Gnann JW: New antivirals with activity against varicella-zoster virus. Ann Neurol 1994;34:S69–S72.
129. Berman SM, Kim RC: The development of cytomegalovirus encephalitis in AIDS patients receiving ganciclovir. Am J Med 1994;96:415–419.
130. McCutchan JA: Cytomegalovirus infections of the nervous system in patients with AIDS. Clin Infect Dis 1995;20:747–754.
131. Bale JF: Human cytomegalovirus infection and disorders of the nervous system. Arch Neurol 1984;41:310–320.
132. Drew WL: Cytomegalovirus infection in patients with AIDS. Clin Infect Dis 1992;14:608–615.
133. Kalayjian RC, Cohen ML, Bonomo RA, Flanigan TP: Cytomegalovirus ventriculoencephalitis in AIDS: A syndrome with distinct clinical and pathologic features. Medicine (Baltimore) 1993;72:67–77.
134. Holland NR, Power C, Mathews VP, et al: Cytomegalovirus encephalitis in acquired immunodeficiency syndrome (AIDS). Neurology 1994;44:507–514.
135. Caserta MT, Hall CB, Schnabel K, et al: Neuroinvasion and persistence of human herpesvirus 6 in children. J Infect Dis 1994;170:1586–1589.
136. McCullers JA, Lakeman FD, Whitley RJ: Human herpesvirus 6 is associated with focal encephalitis. Clin Infect Dis 1995;21:571–576.
137. Luppi M, Barozzi P, Maiorana A, et al: Human herpesvirus-6: A survey of presence and distribution of genomic sequences in normal brain and neuroglial tumors. J Med Virol 1995;47:105–111.
138. Kondo K, Nagafuji H, Hata A, et al: Association of human herpesvirus 6 infection of the central nervous system with recurrence of febrile convulsions. J Infect Dis 1993;167:1197–2000.
139. Hall CB, Long CE, Schnabel KC, et al: Human herpesvirus-6 infection in children: A prospective study of complications and reactivation. N Engl J Med 1994;331:432–438.
140. Drobyski WR, Knox KK, Majewski D, Carrigan DR: Brief report: Fatal encephalitis due to variant B human herpesvirus-6 infection in a bone marrow-transplant recipient. N Engl J Med 1994;330:1356–1360.
141. Carrigan DR, Harrington D, Knox KK: Subacute leukoencephalitis caused by CNS infection with human herpesvirus-6 manifesting as acute multiple sclerosis. Neurology 1996;47:145–148.
142. Knox KK, Carrigan DR: Active human herpesvirus six (HHV-6) infection of the central nervous system in patients with AIDS. J Acquir Immune Defic Syndr Hum Retrovirol 1995;9:69–73.
143. Saito Y, Sharer LR, Dewhurst S, et al: Cellular localization of human herpesvirus 6 in the brains of children with AIDS encephalopathy. J Neurovirol 1995;1:30–39.
144. Caserta MT, Hall CB: Human herpesvirus-6. *In* Scheld WM, Whitley RJ, Durack DT (eds): Infections of the Central Nervous System, 2nd ed. Philadelphia, Lippincott-Raven, 1997, pp 129–138.
145. Schuster V, Kreth HW: Epstein-Barr virus infection and associated diseases in children: Pathogenesis, epidemiology and clinical aspects. Eur J Pediatr 1992;151:718–725.
146. Case 7–1995: Case records of the Massachusetts General Hospital. N Engl J Med 1995;332:663–671.
147. Cotton MF, Reiley T, Robinson CC, et al: Acute aqueductal stenosis in a patient with Epstein-Barr virus infectious mononucleosis. Pediatr Infect Dis J 1994;13:224–227.
148. Connelly KP, DeWitt LD: Neurologic complications of infectious mononucleosis. Pediatr Neurol 1994;10:181–184.
149. De Luca A, Antinori A, Cingolani A, et al: Evaluation of cerebrospinal fluid EBV-DNA and IL-10 as markers for in vivo diagnosis of AIDS-related primary central nervous system lymphoma. Br J Haematol 1995;90:844–849.
150. Bashir RM, Hochberg FH, Wei MX: Epstein-Barr virus and brain lymphomas. J Neurooncol 1995;24:195–206.
151. Mawle AC, Nisenbaum R, Dobbins JG, et al: Immune responses associated with chronic fatigue syndrome: A case-control study. J Infect Dis 1997;175:136–141.
152. Landgren M, Kyllerman M, Bergstrom T, Dotevall L: Diagnosis of Epstein-Barr virus-induced central nervous system infections by DNA amplification from cerebrospinal fluid. Ann Neurol 1994;35:631–635.
153. Swanink CMA, van der Meer JWM, Vercoulen JHMM, et al: Epstein-Barr virus (EBV) and the chronic fatigue syndrome: Normal virus load in blood and normal immunologic reactivity in the EBV regression assay. Clin Infect Dis 1995;20:1390–1392.
154. Dellemijn PLI, Brandenburg A, Niesters HGM, et al: Successful treatment with ganciclovir of presumed Epstein-Barr meningoencephalitis following bone marrow transplant. Bone Marrow Transplant 1995;16:311–312.
155. Henderson DA, Fenner F: Recent events and observations pertaining to smallpox virus destruction in 2002. CID 2001;33:1057–1059.
156. Fifty-Second World Health Assembly: Smallpox eradication: Destruction of variola virus stocks. 1999; Resolution 52.10.
157. Henderson DA, Inglesby TV, Bartlett JG, et al: Smallpox as a biological weapon: Medical and public health management. JAMA 1999;281:2127–2137.
158. Case 20–1995: Case records of the Massachusetts General Hospital. N Engl J Med 1995;332:1773–1780.
159. von Einsiedel RW, Fife TD, Aksamit AJ, Cornford ME: Progressive multifocal leukoencephalopathy in AIDS: A clinicopathologic study and review of the literature. J Neurol 1993;240:391–406.
160. Fong IW, Britton CB, Luinstra KE, et al: Diagnostic value of detecting JC virus DNA in cerebrospinal fluid of patients with progressive multifocal leukoencephalopathy. J Clin Microbiol 1995;33:484–486.

CHAPTER 42

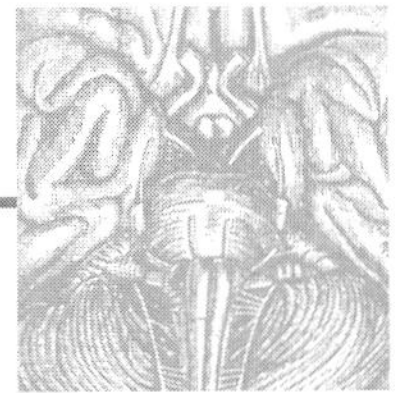

KAREN L. ROOS

Nonviral Infections

Bacterial Infections

ACUTE BACTERIAL MENINGITIS

Epidemiology and Risk Factors. There are approximately 25,000 cases of bacterial meningitis in the United States each year, but this disease is much more prevalent in developing countries. Group B streptococci and gram-negative enteric bacilli are the etiological organisms of the majority of cases of bacterial meningitis during the neonatal period in developed countries. In underdeveloped countries, gram-negative bacilli, predominantly *Escherichia coli*, are the most common pathogens.[1] Risk factors that predispose the newborn to bacterial meningitis include maternal infections, particularly of the urinary tract and uterus; obstetrical risk factors, including prolonged rupture of membranes and birth trauma; prematurity; low birth weight (< 2500 g); congenital anomalies; perinatal hypoxia/asphyxia; cardiopulmonary resuscitation and monitoring; prolonged ventilatory support; and intravenous lines.[1] After the neonatal period, *Streptococcus pneumoniae* and *Neisseria meningitidis* are the most common etiological agents of bacterial meningitis. *Haemophilus influenzae* type b (Hib) was the leading cause of bacterial meningitis in young children before the widespread use of the Hib conjugate vaccine. The latter has resulted in a marked reduction in the incidence of invasive infections caused by Hib in the United States. *N. meningitidis* causes meningitis primarily in children and young adults, with the majority of cases occurring in individuals under age 30. Major epidemics are heralded by disease occurring in older age groups. The "meningitis belt" of sub-Saharan Africa refers to areas of Africa where there are repeated epidemics of serogroup A meningococcal meningitis.[2] Annual outbreaks of meningitis occur in the meningitis belt in late April and early May when the dry desert winds have ceased and temperatures are high throughout the day. The epidemic tends to end with the onset of the rainy season. Transmission of meningococci is facilitated by airborne droplets, and the nasopharynx is the natural reservoir for this organism. During periods of low humidity, an alteration in the nasopharyngeal mucosal barrier predisposes the individual to infection. In addition, crowding, the presence of other respiratory pathogens, poor hygiene, and other poorly defined environmental factors contribute to the development of an epidemic of meningococcal meningitis.[2] Colonization of the nasopharynx in an individual may result in an asymptomatic carrier state or invasive infection.

S. pneumoniae is the most common causative organism of community-acquired bacterial meningitis in the adult. Pneumonia and acute and chronic otitis media are important antecedent events. Chronic disease, specifically alcoholism, sickle cell anemia, diabetes, renal failure, cirrhosis, splenectomy, hypogammaglobulinemia, and organ transplantation are predisposing conditions for pneumococcal bacteremia and meningitis. The pneumococci are a common cause of recurrent meningitis in patients with head trauma and cerebrospinal fluid (CSF) rhinorrhea. In the older adult (age 50 years and older), *S. pneumoniae* is likely to cause meningitis in association with pneumonia or otitis media, and gram-negative bacilli are the likely organisms to cause meningitis in association with chronic lung disease, sinusitis, a neurosurgical procedure, or a chronic urinary tract infection.[3, 4] The most common gram-negative bacilli causing meningitis in the older adult are *E. coli*, *Klebsiella pneumoniae*, *H. influenzae*, *Pseudomonas* organisms, *Enterobacter* species, and *Serratia* species.[3, 5, 6] *Listeria monocytogenes* is an important causative organism of neonatal meningitis and of meningitis in patients that are diabetic, alcoholic, elderly, or immunosuppressed, especially transplant recipients.[2] Infection with *L. monocytogenes* may be acquired through the consumption of soft cheeses, raw vegetables, seafood, cole slaw, and undercooked chicken and delicatessen meats. The staphylococci are the etiological organisms of meningitis primarily in the neurosurgical patient. *S. aureus* and coagulase-negative staphylococci are the predominant organisms causing infections in patients with CSF shunts or subcutaneous Ommaya reservoirs.

Pathogenesis and Pathophysiology. The most common bacteria that cause meningitis, *N. meningitidis* and *S. pneumoniae*, initially colonize the nasopharynx by attaching to the nasopharyngeal epithelial cells. The organisms are able to attach to the nasopharyngeal epithelial cells via an interaction between bacterial surface structures, such as the fimbriae of *N. meningitidis* and host cell surface receptors. The bacteria are then either carried across the cell in membrane-bound vacuoles to the intravascular space or invade the intravascular space by creating separations in the apical tight junctions of columnar epithelial cells.[7, 8] *S. pneumoniae* and *N. meningitidis* are both encapsulated bacteria, and once they gain access to the bloodstream, they are successful in avoiding phagocytosis by neutrophils and classic complement-mediated bactericidal activity because of the presence of the polysaccharide capsule. Bacteria that are able to survive in the circulation enter the CSF from the bloodstream through the choroid plexus of the lateral ventricles and other areas of altered blood-brain barrier permeability. The CSF is an area of impaired host defense because of a lack of sufficient numbers of complement components and immunoglobulins for the opsonization of bacteria.[7] Normal uninfected CSF contains no phagocytic cells, has a low protein concentration, contains no IgM, and has low concentrations of C_3 and C_4.[9] In addition, the fluid medium of the CSF impairs the phagocytosis of bacteria by neutrophils.[9, 10] Bacteria multiply rapidly in the subarachnoid space. Both the multiplication of bacteria and the lysis of bacteria by bactericidal antibiotics result in the release of bacterial cell wall components. These induce the formation of the inflammatory cytokines, interleukin-1 (IL-1) and tumor necrosis factor (TNF), by monocytes, macrophages, brain astrocytes, and microglial cells, which leads to altered blood-brain barrier permeability and the recruitment of polymorphonuclear leukocytes. This process results in the formation of a purulent exudate in the subarachnoid space, which is the basis for the neurological complications of bacterial meningitis. The inflammatory cytokines, IL-1 and TNF, which are produced in response to the release of bacterial cell wall components induce the formation of leukocyte adhesion molecules on vascular endothelial cells. The adherence of neutrophils to vascular endothelial cells is a necessary prerequisite for neutrophils to traverse the blood-brain barrier. It is not clear what role, if any, neutrophils play in eradicating the infection in the subarachnoid space. Large numbers of leukocytes in the subarachnoid space contribute to the purulent exudate and obstruct the flow of CSF. Adherence of leukocytes to the cerebral capillary endothelial cells increases the permeability of blood vessels, allowing for the leakage of plasma proteins through open intercellular junctions that lead to vasogenic brain edema. The leukocytes that successfully migrate into the CSF can subsequently be stimulated by the inflammatory cytokines to degranulate and release toxic oxygen metabolites, producing cytotoxic cerebral edema. IL-1 is a chemoattractant for neutrophils.[7, 11] IL-1 may also have a role in the altered level of consciousness and the production of fever in bacterial meningitis. It has been demonstrated that IL-1 facilitates slow-wave sleep and produces fever by its effect on the hypothalamus.[12, 13] Other inflammatory cytokines, including interleukin-6 and interleukin-8, also have a role in the induction of meningeal inflammation, but the role of these cytokines has not been studied as extensively as that of IL-1 and TNF. Platelet activating factor also has a prominent role in increasing blood-brain barrier permeability.[14]

The alteration in blood-brain barrier permeability during bacterial meningitis results in vasogenic cerebral edema, which contributes to increased intracranial pressure. It also allows for the leakage of plasma proteins into the CSF that contribute to the inflammatory exudate in the subarachnoid space.[8] The purulent exudate in the subarachnoid space interferes with the resorptive function of the arachnoid granulations. As resorption is obstructed, CSF dynamics are altered, and there is transependymal movement of fluid from the ventricular system into the brain parenchyma, which contributes to interstitial edema. The purulent exudate in the basal cisterns obstructs CSF outflow through the ventricles, also contributing to interstitial edema.

An increase in intracranial pressure (ICP) affects cerebral perfusion pressure (CPP), which is defined as the difference between the mean arterial pressure (MAP) and the ICP (CPP = MAP–ICP). Cerebral perfusion pressure is also adversely affected by a loss of cerebral autoregulation. Cerebral blood flow is initially increased in bacterial meningitis; however, shortly thereafter cerebral blood flow begins to decrease. Cerebral blood flow is normally protected through cerebrovascular autoregulation. There is dilatation or constriction of cerebral resistance vessels in response to alterations in CPP, as a result of either changes in the MAP or changes in ICP.[15] The loss of cerebral autoregulation means that cerebral blood flow decreases when systemic blood pressure decreases and increases when systemic blood pressure increases. Because patients with bacteremia and bacterial meningitis are at risk for hypotension, the loss of cerebral autoregulation also puts them at risk for decreased cerebral blood flow. Cerebral blood flow is also affected by narrowing of large arteries at the base of the brain due to encroachment by the purulent exudate in the subarachnoid space. Furthermore, infiltration of the arterial walls by inflammatory cells with secondary intimal thickening, and thrombosis of the major sinuses and thrombophlebitis of the cerebral cortical veins contribute to diminished cerebral blood flow.

Clinical Features and Differential Diagnosis. The classic presentation of bacterial meningitis is headache, fever, stiff neck, and an altered level of consciousness, but the clinical symptoms and signs may vary depending on the age of the patient and the duration of illness before presentation. The symptoms and signs of bacterial meningitis in the neonate are often subtle and typically nonspecific, and include fever or hypothermia, lethargy, seizures, irritability, bulging fontanel, poor feeding, vomiting, and respiratory distress. Meningitis should always be considered when sepsis is suspected in the neonate.[1, 16] In children and adults, the symptoms and signs of bacterial meningitis are fever, headache, vomiting, photophobia, nuchal rigidity, lethargy, confusion, or coma. Meningitis in children typically presents as either a subacute infection that gets progressively worse over several days, following an upper respiratory tract or ear infection, or as an acute fulminant illness that develops rapidly in a few hours. The typical rash of meningococcemia is a petechial-purpuric rash that develops on the trunk, lower extremities, mucous membranes, conjunctiva, and occasionally on the palms and soles. A petechial, purpuric, or erythematous maculopapular rash is also seen in enteroviral meningitis, *N. gonorrhoeae* sepsis, *H. influenzae* type b and pneumococcal meningitis, Rocky Mountain spotted fever, and *S. aureus* endocarditis. Children with bacterial meningitis may also be ataxic as a result of labyrinthine dysfunction or vestibular neuronitis. In adults, an upper respiratory tract infection frequently precedes the development of meningeal symptoms, and its presence should be sought in the history.[7, 16] Adults typically complain of headache, photophobia, and stiff neck, and they may have a rapid progression from lethargy to stupor and coma. The clinical presentation of meningitis in an older adult consists of fever and confusion, stupor, or coma.

Cranial nerve palsies, and most notably sensorineural hearing loss, are a common complication of bacterial meningitis and may be present early in the course of the illness. A stiff neck is the pathognomonic sign of meningeal irritation, resulting from a purulent exudate or hemorrhage in the subarachnoid space. Nuchal rigidity or meningismus is present when the neck resists passive flexion. Kernig's sign is also a classic sign of meningeal irritation, and as originally described by Kernig, it requires the patient to be in the seated position. Kernig noted that attempts to passively extend the knee while the patient was seated were met with resistance in the presence of meningitis so that a contraction of the extremities was maintained.[17, 18] Jozef Brudzinski described at least five different meningeal signs. His best known sign, the nape of the neck sign, is elicited with the patient in the supine position and is positive when passive flexion of the neck results in spontaneous flexion of the hips and knees.[18, 19]

Seizures occur in 40 percent of patients with bacterial meningitis, typically during the first week of illness. The etiology of seizure activity can be attributed to either one or a combination of the following: (1) fever; (2) cerebrovascular disease consisting of either focal arterial ischemia, infarction, or cortical venous thrombosis with hemorrhage; (3) hyponatremia; (4) subdural effusion or empyema producing a mass effect; and (5) antimicrobial agents (e.g., imipenem, penicillin).[16] Raised ICP is an expected complication of bacterial meningitis and presents as one or a combination of the following clinical signs: (1) an altered level of consciousness; (2) the Cushing reflex—bradycardia, hypertension, and irregular respirations;[20] (3) dilated, nonreactive pupil or pupils; (4) unilateral or bilateral cranial nerve VI palsies; (5) papilledema; (6) neck stiffness; (7) hiccups; (8) projectile vomiting; and (9) decerebrate posturing.[16] Acute ischemic stroke may occur in the course of bacterial meningitis as a result of narrowing of the large arteries at the base of the brain. This may occur from encroachment by a purulent exudate in the subarachnoid space or infiltration of the arterial wall by inflammatory cells (vasculitis). Vasospasm, thrombotic or stenotic occlusion of branches of the middle cerebral artery, and septic venous sinus thrombosis with thrombophlebitis of cortical veins may also occur.[7]

The differential diagnosis of this clinical presentation includes viral meningoencephalitis, fungal meningitis, tuberculous meningitis, focal intracranial mass lesions, subarachnoid hemorrhage, Rocky Mountain spotted fever, and neuroleptic malignant syndrome.

Evaluation. The gold standard for the diagnosis of bacterial meningitis is the examination of the CSF. The classic CSF abnormalities in bacterial meningitis are (1) an increased opening pressure; (2) a polymorphonuclear leukocytic pleocytosis; (3) a decreased glucose concentration; and (4) an increased protein concentration. Raised ICP is an expected complication of bacterial meningitis and can theoretically contribute to brain herniation following lumbar puncture. When there are clinical signs of raised ICP and urgent lumbar puncture is indicated, a bolus of mannitol 1 g/kg of body weight can be given intravenously and the lumbar puncture can be performed 20 minutes later. In addition, the patient can be intubated and hyperventilated. Alternatively, lumbar puncture can be deferred and blood cultures obtained until the raised ICP can be treated. Regardless, the lumbar puncture should be performed with a 22-gauge needle.[21] When obtaining CSF for analysis it is important to remember that adults have approximately 150 mL of CSF, but infants and children have smaller amounts, in the range of 30 to 60 mL in the neonate and 100 mL in the adolescent.[22] The volume of CSF in a child 4 to 13 years of age is in the range of 65 to 140 mL, with an average volume of 90 mL.[23] Approximately 10 to 12 mL of CSF should be withdrawn from an adult, and the withdrawal of 3 to 5 mL is recommended in the neonate and child.[22] The CSF glucose concentration is low when the value is less than 40 mg/dl or when the CSF/blood glucose ratio is less than 0.6. When an ampule of 50 ml of 50 percent glucose (D50) has been given en route to the emergency room, 30 minutes is required for the ampule of D50 to influence the CSF glucose concentration. The CSF white blood cell (WBC) count is usually more than 100 cells/mm^3 and is often more than 1000 WBCs/mm^3 in bacterial meningitis. Although there is typically a predominance of polymorphonuclear leukocytes in the CSF in bacterial meningitis, a predominance of lymphocytes has been reported in cases of acute bacterial meningitis when the CSF WBC concentration was less than 1000/mm^3 and in bacterial meningitis due to *L. monocytogenes*.[24, 25] The initial CSF examination in neonatal bacterial meningitis may have an absence of pleocytosis and normal glucose and protein concentrations. A Gram's stain of the CSF should be examined carefully, and a high index of suspicion for meningitis should be maintained in the neonate with fever, seizure activity, irritability, lethargy, and/or respiratory distress.[26, 27] Oral antimicrobial therapy administered before lumbar puncture will not significantly alter the CSF WBC count or glucose concentration but will decrease the likelihood of identifying the organism on Gram's stain or isolating it in culture.[21] The latex particle agglutination test for the detection of bacterial antigens of *H. influenzae* type b, *S. pneumoniae*, *N. meningitidis*, group B streptococcus, and *E. coli* K1 strains in the CSF is very useful in making a rapid diagnosis of bacterial meningitis. It is also helpful in making the diagnosis of bacterial meningitis in patients who were pretreated with antibiotics and in the patient whose Gram's stain and CSF culture are negative. The Limulus amebocyte lysate test is very sensitive in detecting gram-negative bacterial meningitis. It has a 77 to 99 percent sensitivity for the detection of gram-negative endotoxin in the CSF.[21] A good rule is that the Gram's stain and bacterial culture should be negative in the CSF obtained 24 hours after the initiation of intravenous antimicrobial therapy, if the organism is sensitive to that antibiotic.

Management. Empirical therapy of bacterial meningitis in the neonate should include the combination of ampicillin (50 mg/kg q 6 to 8 hr) and either cefotaxime (50 mg/kg q 8 to 12 hr) or an aminoglycoside, such as gentamicin (2.5 mg/kg q 8 to 12 hr) or amikacin (10 mg/kg q 8 to 12 hr).[1] Empirical therapy of bacterial meningitis in infants 4 to 12 weeks of age requires antimicrobial agents that are active against the likely pathogens of the neonatal age group as well as those that cause infection in infants and children. An appropriate regimen in this age group is ampicillin and either cefotaxime or ceftriaxone (100 mg/kg/d intravenously in divided doses q 12 hr). A third-generation cephalosporin, either cefotaxime (225 mg/kg/d intravenously in divided doses q 6 hr) or ceftriaxone (100 mg/kg/d intravenously in divided doses q 12 hr) plus vancomycin (40 mg/kg/d intravenously in divided doses q 6 hr) is recommended for empirical therapy of bacterial meningitis in the older infant and child. Empirical therapy of bacterial meningitis in adults should include a combination of ceftriaxone (2 g intravenously bid) or cefotaxime (8 to 12 g/d intravenously in divided doses q 4 hr) or cefepime (2 g intravenously bid) plus vancomycin (500 mg intravenously q 6 hr). In the older adult and in the immunocompromised adult in whom *L. monocytogenes* may be the etiological organism, ampicillin (12 g/d in divided doses q 4 hr) should be added to this regimen. In patients who have recently undergone a neurosurgical procedure or who are immunocompromised, *Pseudomonas aeruginosa* may be the etiological agent, and ceftazidime (6 g/d intravenously in divided doses q 8 hr) should be substituted for cefotaxime or ceftriaxone. Once the causative organism has been identified, antimicrobial therapy can be modified based on the recommendations for that specific organism. Recommendations for antimicrobial therapy based on the infecting organism are listed in Table 42–1.

TABLE 42–1. **Antimicrobial Therapy Based on Etiological Organism**

	Antibiotic and Dose (Intravenous Unless Indicated)		
Organism	**Infants (>2000 g)**	**Children**	**Adults**
Group B streptococcus	Ampicillin 50 mg/kg q 6 hr plus amikacin 10 mg/kg q 8 hr or gentamicin 2.5 mg/kg q 8 hr		
Neisseria meningitidis		Penicillin G 250,000 to 400,000 U/kg/d (divided q 4 hr) plus (at end of therapy) oral rifampin, older than 1 yr: 10 mg/kg q 12 hr for 2 d. Younger than 1 yr: 5 mg/kg q 12 hr for 2 d	Penicillin G 20 to 24 million U/d (divided q 4 hr) plus (at end of therapy) oral rifampin 600 mg q 12 hr for 2 d
Streptococcus pneumoniae		Cefotaxime 225 mg/kg/d (divided q 6 hr) or ceftriaxone 100 mg/kg/d (in a once or twice daily dosing interval) *plus* vancomycin 40 mg/kg/d (q 6 hr dosing interval)	Cefotaxime 8 to 12 g/d (divided q 4 hr) or ceftriaxone 4 g/d (2 q 12 hr) *plus* vancomycin 2 g/d (in a 6- or 12-hr dosing interval)
Enteric gram-negative bacilli (except *Pseudomonas aeruginosa*)	Cefotaxime 50 mg/kg q 8 hr plus amikacin or gentamicin	Cefotaxime or ceftriaxone (as above)	Cefotaxime or ceftriaxone (as above)
Pseudomonas aeruginosa	Ceftazidime 50 mg/kg q 8 hr	Ceftazidime 150 mg/kg/d (q 8-hr dosing interval)	Ceftazidime 6 g/d (q 8-hr dosing interval)
Listeria monocytogenes	Ampicillin 50 mg/kg q 6 hr plus amikacin or gentamicin for 3 to 5 d	Ampicillin 150 to 200 mg/kg/d (q 4-hr dosing interval)	Ampicillin 12 g/d (divided q 4 hr) +/– gentamycin 6 mg/kg/d divided q 8 hrs in critically ill patients
Haemophilus influenzae type b	Cefotaxime	Cefotaxime or ceftriaxone	Cefotaxime or ceftriaxone
Staphylococcus aureus Methicillin-sensitive	Methicillin 50 mg/kg q 6 hr	Oxacillin 200 to 300 mg/kg/d (divided q 4 hr)	Oxacillin 12 g/d (divided q 4 hr)
Staphylococcus aureus Methicillin-resistant	Vancomycin 15 mg/kg q 8 hr	Vancomycin 40 mg/kg/d (divided q 6 hr)	Vancomycin 2 g/d (divided q 6 hr)

The American Academy of Pediatrics recommends the consideration of dexamethasone for bacterial meningitis in infants and children 2 months of age and older. The recommended dose is 0.6 mg/kg/d in four divided doses (0.15 mg/kg/dose) given intravenously for the first 4 days of antimicrobial therapy.[28] The first dose of dexamethasone should be administered several minutes before the first dose of antimicrobial therapy. Dexamethasone is beneficial in preventing the neurological complications of bacterial meningitis by decreasing meningeal inflammation. Dexamethasone inhibits the synthesis of the inflammatory cytokines IL-1 and TNF, that are produced by brain astrocytes and microglial cells in response to bacterial cell wall components in the subarachnoid space. As discussed earlier, the inflammatory cytokines increase the permeability of the blood-brain barrier and recruit polymorphonuclear leukocytes from the bloodstream to the CSF. The result is the production of a purulent exudate in the subarachnoid space. Although the majority of patients in the clinical trials evaluating the efficacy of dexamethasone in bacterial meningitis have been infants and children, the available experimental and clinical data on dexamethasone in pneumococcal meningitis justifies the recommendation for the use of dexamethasone in adults with pneumococcal meningitis. The recommended dose is 8 to 10 mg intravenously every 8 hours for 4 days. In a clinical trial that evaluated the efficacy of dexamethasone in pneumococcal meningitis in adults, patient mortality was reduced despite the use of an ampicillin dose that is now considered subtherapeutic.[29] Dexamethasone appears to be reasonably safe. The third-generation cephalosporins penetrate the CSF extremely well even in the presence of dexamethasone.[30, 31] The penetration of vancomycin, however, may be adversely affected by dexamethasone therapy because meningeal inflammation improves the penetration of vancomycin into the CSF. The clinical significance of this is unclear. Consideration should therefore be given to the use of higher doses of vancomycin (60 mg/kg/d in divided doses q 6 hr) or intrathecal vancomycin in cases of highly penicillin-resistant and cephalosporin-resistant pneumococcal meningitis when dexamethasone is used concomitantly with antimicrobial therapy. The use of a histamine-2 antagonist with dexamethasone is recommended to avoid gastrointestinal bleeding.

The majority of children with bacterial meningitis are hyponatremic with serum sodium concentrations less than 135 mEq/L at the time of admission owing to the syndrome of inappropriate antidiuretic hormone secretion (SIADH). The time-honored treatment of SIADH was fluid restriction. This practice, however, has received renewed attention because of the knowledge that autoregulation of cerebral blood flow is lost in the course of bacterial meningitis. A decrease in the mean systemic arterial pressure is therefore associated with a decrease in the cerebral blood flow. In experimental pneumococcal meningitis, fluid-restricted rabbits had a greater decrease in MAP and cerebral blood flow than did euvolemic rabbits.[32] The present recommendations are to limit the initial rate of intravenous fluid administration to approximately three quarters of the normal maintenance requirements (or 1000 to 1200 mL/m^2/24 hr). The intravenous fluid should be a multielectrolyte solution containing between one quarter and one half normal saline and potassium at 20 to 40 mEq/L in 5 percent dextrose. Once the serum sodium concentration increases above 135 mEq/L, the volume of the fluids administered can be gradually increased.[33, 34]

The development of seizure activity should be anticipated in the patient with bacterial meningitis. Seizure activity occurs in approximately 30 to 40 percent of children with acute bacterial meningitis and in more than 30 percent of adults with pneumococcal meningitis, typically occurring in the first few days of the illness. There is an increased risk of epilepsy following bacterial meningitis especially in those individuals who have seizures in the first few days of infection.[35] Raised ICP is an expected complication of bacterial meningitis and should be anticipated at the time of the initial lumbar puncture. The ICP should be measured by an ICP monitoring device. The treatment of raised ICP in bacterial meningitis includes one or more of the following: (1) elevation of the head of the bed 30 degrees; (2) hyperventilation to maintain the $PaCO_2$ between 25 and 33 mm Hg; (3) mannitol 1.0 g/kg bolus intravenous injection, then 0.25 to 0.5 g/kg intravenous every 3 to 5 hours to achieve a serum osmolarity of 295 to 320 mOsm/L; (4) dexamethasone 0.15 mg/kg q 6 hr; and (5) pentobarbital coma with a loading dose 5 to 10 mg/kg administered intravenously at a rate of 1 mg/kg/min and a maintenance dose of 1 to 3 mg/kg/hr.[36, 37] Subdural effusions commonly develop in the course of bacterial meningitis in children when the infection in the adjacent subarachnoid space leads to an increase in the permeability of the thin-walled capillaries and veins in the inner layer of the dura. The result is leakage of albumin-rich fluid into the subdural space. This is usually a self-limited process, and as the inflammatory process subsides, fluid formation ceases and the fluid in the subdural space is reabsorbed.[34, 38, 39] The indications for aspiration of a subdural fluid collection include the clinical suspicion of infected fluid (prolonged fever), a rapidly enlarging head circumference in a child without hydrocephalus, focal neurological findings, or clinical signs of increased ICP.[34]

BRAIN ABSCESS

Epidemiology and Risk Factors. Brain abscess is a rare disease in immunocompetent individuals. In adults, otitis media and paranasal sinusitis (frontal, ethmoidal, or sphenoidal sinuses) are the most common predisposing conditions for brain abscess formation. In children, otitis media and cyanotic congenital heart disease are the most common predisposing conditions for brain abscess formation. Individuals with the acquired immunodeficiency syndrome (AIDS) are at increased risk for focal intracranial infections caused by *Toxoplasma gondii* (see Chapter 44). Organ transplant recipients are at risk for brain abscesses caused by *Aspergillus fumigatus*. Patients receiving chronic corticosteroid therapy and those who are immunosuppressed from bone marrow transplantation are at a particular risk for central nervous system (CNS) candidiasis manifested as multiple intraparenchymal microabscesses, mainly in the territory of the middle cerebral artery. Brain abscesses may develop as a result of cranial trauma, either penetrating brain injuries or neurosurgical procedures, of which the most common is craniotomy. The reported incidence of brain abscess following clean neurosurgical procedures is 6 to 7 per 10,000 cases.[40] A brain abscess may develop as the result of hematogenous spread of infection from a remote site such as chronic pyogenic lung diseases, wound and skin infections, osteomyelitis, intra-abdominal and pelvic infections, and endocarditis. Finally, pulmonary arteriovenous malformation is a predisposing condition for brain abscess formation.

Pathogenesis and Pathophysiology. A brain abscess may develop in association with any of the following: (1) direct spread from a contiguous cranial site of infection such as otitis media, odontogenic infections, sinusitis or mastoiditis, or retrograde septic thrombophlebitis from these sites as well as facial and scalp infections; (2) following cranial trauma; (3) hematogenous spread from a remote infection site; and (4) immunosuppression either from neutropenia, organ or bone marrow transplantation, lymphoma, leukemia, or AIDS. Approximately 20 percent of brain abscesses are said to be cryptogenic, with no predisposing factor. The results of animal experiments suggest that in order for brain abscesses to form, there must be a pre-existing area of ischemia, necrosis, or hypoxia in brain tissue.[41] Intact brain parenchyma is relatively resistant to infection.[42] Once bacteria have established an infection, brain abscess formation evolves through four stages regardless of the infecting organism. These stages were described in animal models of brain abscesses, and have been shown to correlate with human brain abscess evolution observed by computed tomography (CT) imaging. These stages are early cerebritis, late cerebritis, early capsule formation, and late capsule formation. The early cerebritis stage (days 1 to 3 following intracerebral inoculation with alpha-hemolytic streptococci in dogs) is characterized by perivascular infiltration of inflammatory cells composed of polymorphonuclear leukocytes, plasma cells, and mononuclear cells that surround a central core of coagulative necrosis. Marked cerebral edema surrounds the lesion at this stage.[43, 44] The CT scan reveals a low-density lesion with faint contrast enhancement at its edge. The late cerebritis stage (days 4 to 9) is characterized by a lesion with a necrotic center surrounded by an inflammatory infiltrate of macrophages and fibroblasts. Rapid new vessel formation occurs around the developing abscess. A thin capsule of fibroblasts and reticular fibers gradually develops, and the area is surrounded by cerebral edema. The CT scan image demonstrates a low-density lesion surrounded by a prominent ring of enhancement following contrast administration. In the stage of early capsule formation (days 10 to 13), the necrotic center decreases in size, and the inflammatory infiltrate changes in character and contains an increasing number of fibroblasts and macrophages. Mature collagen evolves from reticulin precursors, forming a capsule that is better developed on the cortical than the ventricular side of the lesion. The CT scan image shows an area of low density, and the diameter of ring-contrast enhancement has decreased in size. The stage of late capsule formation (day 14 and later) is characterized by a well-formed necrotic center surrounded by a dense collagenous capsule. On the CT scan image, the low-density lesion is surrounded by a sharply demarcated, dense ring of contrast enhancement. The preceding description of brain abscess formation may be modified slightly by different microorganisms and altered in the immunocompromised host. Depending on the etiological organism and the predisposing condition leading to infection, there may be delayed or incomplete encapsulation of the abscess cavity or the abscess may enlarge more quickly than described earlier.[40]

Clinical Features and Differential Diagnosis. A brain abscess presents as an expanding focal infectious mass lesion. The most common clinical presentation is headache, either hemicranial or generalized; fever; vomiting; a focal neurological deficit; or focal or generalized seizure activity. The findings on neurological examination are related both to the site of the abscess and to the degree of raised ICP. Patients with increased ICP will have alterations in consciousness ranging from lethargy to irritability, confusion, or coma. There may be papilledema and deficits of cranial nerves III or VI, or both. If the abscess has ruptured into the ventricular system or if there has been spread of infection to the subarachnoid space, there may be signs of meningitis. The differential diagnosis of this clinical presentation includes herpes simplex virus encephalitis, subdural empyema, cranial epidural abscess, a focal cerebral infarction with edema, a cerebral hemorrhage, a primary neurological tumor, or a metastatic tumor.

Evaluation. The diagnosis of a brain abscess is made through neuroimaging using either a cranial CT or magnetic resonance imaging (MRI) scan that demonstrates a ring-enhancing lesion. Typically, the cranial CT scan demonstrates the abscess as a low-density lesion with a sharply demarcated, dense ring of contrast enhancement surrounded by a variable hypodense region of edema. In the early and late stages of cerebritis, there is often diffusion of contrast medium into the low-density center of the abscess on delayed scans obtained 30 minutes after the administration of intravenous contrast. As the abscess matures, its margin becomes more defined and the enhancement around the abscess becomes more homogeneous. In the early and late stages of capsule formation, there is no significant inward diffusion of contrast on delayed scans. Cranial MRI scanning is superior to cranial CT scanning in detecting a lesion in the early cerebritis stage. On this type of image, the abscess appears as an area of hypointensity on T1-weighted images and hyperintensity on T2-weighted images with indistinct margins. When the abscess becomes encapsulated, it appears as a lesion of low intensity surrounded by an area of isointensity or hyperintensity on T1-weighted images. The T2-weighted MRI images reveal a hyperintense lesion surrounded by a rim of hypointensity with surrounding area of hyperintensity that represents edema. The T1-weighted MRI images obtained after intravenous gadolinium administration demonstrate ring enhancement of the abscess capsule.[40] Patients with a brain abscess may have a peripheral leukocytosis or an elevated erythrocyte sedimentation rate; however, in a significant number of patients, the laboratory criteria for infection will be lacking. The serum C-reactive protein (CRP) concentration has been reported to be useful in distinguishing brain abscess from brain tumor. Patients with brain abscesses have an elevated CRP level, whereas those with a brain tumor will have low levels.[40, 45] Indium-111-labeled leukocyte scintigraphy may also be useful in distinguishing between a brain abscess and tumor. This scan uses radiolabeled leukocytes to detect areas of active inflammation. False-positive results may occur when there has been leukocytic infiltration into a brain tumor, especially those with severe necrosis. A lumbar puncture is contraindicated in a patient with a brain abscess because of the risk of herniation. The etiological organism is rarely identified from CSF cultures obtained by lumbar puncture, but it can be identified by

CT- or MRI-guided stereotactic aspiration of the abscess. This approach is the procedure of choice for the identification of the infectious organism. All patients should also have a chest x-ray. Additionally, a CT scan of the head with bony windows for the evaluation of the paranasal sinuses, middle ear, and mastoids should be done when a contiguous site of infection is suspected as the source of the brain abscess. Blood cultures should be obtained when hematogenous dissemination from a remote site of infection is the likely etiology.

Management. The management of a brain abscess is directed at decreasing the mass effect associated with the abscess, draining the pus, and using antimicrobial therapy to treat the abscess and the primary source of infection.[40] Surgical management of a brain abscess involves either complete extirpation of the abscess or aspiration of the abscess cavity through a burr hole with or without placement of a drainage catheter into the abscess cavity. The purulent material obtained at the time of aspiration allows for the identification of the infecting organism. Aspiration of the contents of an abscess cavity has a lower morbidity and a lower risk of seizures compared with complete excision. Complete excision removes the lesion from the parenchyma of the brain and allows for a rapid decompression but may cause damage to brain parenchyma. Complete excision is recommended when gas is present within the abscess cavity and for an abscess due to *Nocardia* species.

In the majority of patients with a brain abscess, stereotactic aspiration of the abscess should be performed for Gram's stain and bacterial culture, as well as fungal smear and culture. In patients with AIDS, however, the majority of focal infectious CNS lesions are caused by *T. gondii*, and in such cases, serum should be sent for antitoxoplasma IgG. The lesions of *T. gondii* are typically located at the gray-white junction in the cerebral hemispheres, in the deep white matter, and in the thalamus and basal ganglia. With contrast administration, the majority of lesions enhance in a ringed, nodular, or homogeneous pattern and are surrounded by edema. Cranial MRI scanning is superior to CT scanning in detecting the multiple lesions of toxoplasma abscesses. Thallium single-photon emission computed tomography (SPECT) imaging may be helpful in distinguishing cerebral toxoplasmosis from primary CNS lymphoma. Focal areas of increased uptake are seen in patients with lymphoma. In patients with a detectable toxoplasma serology and more than one enhancing lesion on neuroimaging, a presumptive diagnosis of toxoplasma encephalitis can be made and a treatment trial with pyrimethamine and sulfadiazine or pyrimethamine and clindamycin can be initiated. The other group of patients that provide an exceptional diagnostic and therapeutic challenge are those not infected with human immunodeficiency virus (HIV) but who have multiple brain abscesses. In these patients, stereotactic aspiration of the largest lesion for purulent material for culture is recommended.

The etiological organism of a brain abscess can be predicted to some degree based on the location of the abscess and the predisposing condition. Streptococci, specifically *S. milleri*, are the most frequent organisms isolated from frontal lobe abscesses associated with chronic sinusitis. Temporal lobe abscesses are most frequently secondary to chronic infections of the ear, and streptococci (anaerobic or aerobic), Enterobacteriaceae, and Bacteroides species are the most commonly isolated bacteria. A brain abscess owing to chronic otitis media frequently yields multiple organisms in culture. The majority of brain abscesses secondary to trauma or craniotomy are caused by *S. aureus*.[40] Viridans, anaerobic, and microaerophilic streptococci are the usual organisms isolated from brain abscesses caused by cyanotic congenital heart disease. A brain abscess in an immunocompromised individual may be from *Candida* species, *Nocardia asteroides*, *Aspergillus*, Zygomycetes, Enterobacteriaceae or *P. aeruginosa*.

A combination of vancomycin (2 g/d intravenously in an adult, 40 to 60 mg/kg/d in a child), a third-generation cephalosporin (cefotaxime, ceftriaxone, or ceftazidime), and metronidazole (500 mg q 6 hr intravenously for an adult and 7.5 mg/kg q 8 hr for a child) is the recommended empirical therapy for immunocompetent patients with brain abscesses. The final culture results and organism sensitivities are used to make the antibiotic coverage more specific. Aspergillosis should be considered in immunosuppressed patients with unremitting fever and multiple brain abscesses. A chest x-ray study may demonstrate pulmonary infiltrates and bronchoscopy may identify the infecting organism in some cases. Fungal brain abscesses are treated with amphotericin B; liposomal amphotericin B should be used for brain abscesses due to *Aspergillus* species. Corticosteroid therapy is recommended for the treatment of vasogenic cerebral edema that surrounds a brain abscess and to treat any mass effect. Because steroid therapy may decrease the penetration of antibiotics into brain tissue, it should be discontinued when the edema and mass effect improve or resolve. Abscesses that enlarge or do not become smaller during antimicrobial therapy may need repeat aspiration or excision.

CRANIAL AND SPINAL SUBDURAL EMPYEMA

Epidemiology and Risk Factors. Subdural empyema is a pyogenic infection in the space between the dura mater and the arachnoid and represents 13 to 20 percent of localized intracranial infections. The arachnoid is not a very strong barrier, and subdural empyema may breach the arachnoid and cause subpial infection.[46] The most common predisposing condition that leads to the development of a subdural empyema is paranasal sinusitis, especially frontal sinusitis. Paranasal sinusitis is the primary cause of a subdural empyema in 50 to 80 percent of patients, and otitis media is the primary cause in 10 to 20 percent.[47, 48] Superficial infections of the scalp and skull, craniotomy, or septic thrombophlebitis from sinusitis, otitis, or mastoiditis may extend to the subdural space, causing empyema.[46] Subdural empyema in infants usually represents an infected subdural effusion complicating a bacterial meningitis.[49, 50] An empyema may rarely develop in the subdural area of the spinal cord.

Pathogenesis and Pathophysiology. The most important pathophysiological antecedent of a subdural empyema is septic thrombophlebitis of the mucosal veins of the sinuses that results in retrograde extension of infection with drainage of bacteria into the regional dural veins, and then into the superior sagittal sinus.[48, 51] Subdural empyema may also result from the direct infection of the subdural space during a neurosurgical procedure. Once the infection is established in the subdural space, evolution of an empyema tends to be remarkably rapid because the subdural space has no barriers. The infection can spread medially over the tentorium toward the falx and posteriorly to the infratentorial area.[46, 51] Septic thrombophlebitis extends in a retrograde fashion from the dural sinuses to the cortical veins. Cortical venous infarction may follow and is largely responsible for the severe symptoms, particularly the focal signs, that develop during the course of the illness.[51, 52] Cortical venous thrombosis and infarction cause hemorrhagic and ischemic necrosis of brain parenchyma that subsequently permits brain abscess formation. A co-existent cerebral abscess has been reported in up to 24 percent of cases of subdural empyema.[48, 53] Spinal subdural empyema may be the result of hematogenous spread of infection from a distant site, trauma, spine surgery, or a dermal sinus tract that connects the skin and the dura.

Clinical Features. A patient with a cranial subdural empyema appears acutely ill with headache that is often localized initially to the side of infection and has fever, chills, and nuchal rigidity. In children and adults, the triad of sinusitis, fever, and an acute neurological deficit should be treated with a high index of suspicion for a subdural empyema.[46] A progressive disturbance of consciousness occurs as the subdural empyema produces a mass effect that results in increased ICP. Focal neurological deficits are present in 80 to 90 percent of patients and are caused by mass effect from the subdural collection of fluid and cortical vein thrombophlebitis. Periorbital edema and erythema may be present in patients with a subdural empyema originating from the frontal sinus.[48, 52] Seizures, which are typically focal, occur in 30 to 60 percent of patients.[46] Infants with subdural empyemas usually have an increase in their head size, a bulging fontanel, irritability, poor feeding followed by hemiparesis, convulsions, stupor, and coma.[47] A spinal subdural empyema presents as fever with signs of rapidly progressive spinal cord compression. Backache may be present, but it is not as characteristic of the presentation of a spinal subdural empyema as it is of the presentation of spinal epidural abscess.

Differential Diagnosis and Evaluation. The differential diagnosis of the signs and symptoms of a cranial subdural empyema includes bacterial meningitis, superior sagittal sinus thrombosis, epidural abscess, and cerebral abscess.[51] A lumbar puncture should not be performed in patients with the clinical signs of raised ICP or focal neurological deficits. In most series, bacteria are not demonstrated by microscopic examination or culture of CSF obtained by lumbar puncture in patients with a subdural empyema.[51–53] Cranial MRI is the diagnostic procedure of choice to demonstrate the presence of a subdural empyema. The subdural empyema will have a mildly increased signal intensity on MRI T1-weighted images and a markedly increased signal intensity on T2-weighted images when compared with ventricular CSF.[46] A benign subdural effusion can also be differentiated from an infected subdural empyema using a cranial MRI scan. A subdural effusion is isointense compared with CSF on MRI T1- and T2-weighted images, and a subdural empyema is hyperintense when compared with CSF on T2-weighted images.[46] On a CT scan, a subdural empyema has the appearance of a crescent or lentiform-shaped area of low density adjacent to the inner border of the skull.[54] The empyema consists of an inflammatory exudate and appears denser than CSF. MRI is the best neuroimaging procedure to demonstrate the presence of a spinal subdural empyema.

Management. The treatment of subdural empyema consists of intravenous antibiotic therapy, surgical drainage of the empyema and infected sinuses, and management of increased ICP when present. The majority of cranial subdural empyemas are caused by those organisms typically isolated from patients with chronic sinusitis or otitis. Aerobic streptococci are the causative organisms in 30 to 50 percent of patients with subdural empyema. Anaerobic organisms, particularly anaerobic and microaerophilic streptococci, are isolated from 15 to 25 percent of cases; staphylococci are isolated from 15 to 25 percent of cases; and aerobic gram-negative bacilli are isolated from 5 to 10 percent of cases.[47, 48] Empirical therapy must cover aerobic and anaerobic streptococci, staphylococci, and gram-negative bacilli. A combination of penicillin G (20 to 24 miU/d adults, 400,000 U/kg/d for children and infants) or a third-generation cephalosporin (ceftriaxone or cefotaxime), metronidazole (600 mg/d adults, 22.5 mg/kg/d infants and children), and nafcillin (9 to 12 g/d adults, 200 mg/kg/d infants and children) or vancomycin is recommended (Table 42–2). Surgical drainage can be accomplished by either craniotomy or multiple burr holes.[46]

TABLE 42–2. **Antimicrobial Therapy for Subdural Empyema**

Organism	Adult	Dosing Interval	Child	Dosing Interval
Staphylococcus aureus Methicillin-sensitive	Nafcillin 9 to 12 g/d	Every 4 hr	Nafcillin 200 mg/kg/d	Every 4 hr
Staphylococcus aureus Methicillin-resistant	Vancomycin 2 g/d	Every 12 hr	Vancomycin 40 to 60 mg/kg/d	Every 12 hr
Streptococci	Penicillin G 20 to 24 MU/d	Every 4 hr	Penicillin G 250,000 to 400,000 U/kg/d	Every 4 to 6 hr
Gram-negative bacilli	Ceftriaxone 4 to 6 g/d	Every 12 hr	Ceftriaxone 80 to 100 mg/kg/d	Every 12 hr
	or		*or*	
	Cefotaxime 8 to 12 g/d	Every 4 hr	Cefotaxime 200 mg/kg/d	Every 6 hr
	or		*or*	
	Ceftazidime 6 g/d	Every 8 hr	Ceftazidime 125 to 150 mg/kg/d	Every 8 hr
Anaerobes	Metronidazole 600 mg/d	Every 8 hr	Metronidazole 22.5 mg/kg/d	Every 8 hr
	or		*or*	
	Chloramphenicol 4 g/d	Every 6 hr	Chloramphenicol 100 mg/kg/d	Every 6 hr

Reproduced with permission from Shapiro S: Cranial epidural abscess and cranial subdural empyema. *In* Roos KL (ed): Central Nervous System Infectious Diseases and Therapy. New York, Marcel Dekker, 1997, pp 499–506.

Intravenous antibiotics should be continued for at least 3 weeks after surgical drainage, and then oral antibiotic therapy can be substituted to complete a 6-week course of therapy. Reoperation for further irrigation and drainage of loculated pockets of pus is typically necessary. It is therefore recommended that the patient undergo frequent CT or MRI scans to evaluate whether resolution of the infection has occurred.[46]

S. aureus is the causative organism in the majority of cases of spinal subdural empyema and such cases should undergo a laminectomy and dural incision with drainage. Extensive irrigation of the subdural space with bacitracin and either vancomycin or gentamicin is recommended. Intravenous antimicrobial therapy for 4 to 8 weeks, and often longer, is also recommended.[55]

CRANIAL AND SPINAL EPIDURAL ABSCESS

Epidemiology and Risk Factors. Cranial epidural abscesses develop in the space between the dura and inner table of the skull and are usually caused by the spread of infection from the frontal sinuses, middle ear, mastoid, or orbit.[48] Epidural abscesses may also develop as a complication of a craniotomy or compound skull fracture. At present, the most common cause of a cranial epidural abscess is craniotomy that has been complicated by an infection of the wound, bone flap, or epidural space.[46] Epidural abscesses may result from or be associated with an area of osteomyelitis.

A spinal epidural abscess develops in the space outside the dura mater but within the spinal canal. The spinal epidural space is only a true space posterior to the spinal cord and the spinal nerve roots. The anteroposterior width of the epidural space is greatest in the area where the spinal cord is smallest; i.e., from approximately T4 to T8 and from L3 to S2.[56, 57] The most common location for an epidural abscess is the posterior midthoracic region between the fourth and eighth thoracic vertebrae.[58] The anterior epidural space is only a potential space because the dura is virtually adherent to the posterior surface of the vertebral bodies along the ventral aspect of the spinal canal from the first cervical to the second sacral vertebrae. Anterior abscesses usually occur at cervical levels.[59] The most common etiology of a spinal epidural abscess is hematogenous spread of bacteria from a remote site of infection to the epidural space. This includes such sites as the skin, urinary tract, lungs, pelvis, cardiac valves, and pharynx. An epidural abscess may also develop by direct extension from a contiguous infection such as vertebral osteomyelitis. The latter disorder is a particularly common etiology for spinal epidural abscess formation in intravenous drug abusers. Immunosuppression from any cause, but most commonly from AIDS or diabetes mellitus, is a predisposing condition in approximately 50 percent of cases of spinal epidural abscesses.[55] The formation of a small hematoma owing to mild blunt trauma may also provide a *locus minoris resistentiae* that may allow for hematogenous seeding of infection resulting in the formation of a spinal epidural abscess.

Pathogenesis and Pathophysiology. Infection in the frontal sinuses, middle ear, mastoid, or orbit is able to reach the epidural space through the retrograde spread of thrombophlebitis in the emissary veins that drain these areas, by way of direct spread of the infection through bone (osteomyelitis), or through direct infection of the epidural space during craniotomy.[60] As stated earlier, hematogenous spread to the epidural space from a remote site of infection is an extremely rare cause of cranial epidural abscess but an extremely common cause of spinal epidural abscess.

A spinal epidural abscess may develop as a result of the hematogenous spread of infection from a distant focus of infection to the epidural space. There may also be hematogenous spread of infection to a vertebral body or disc that results in discitis and/or osteomyelitis that subsequently extends into the spinal epidural space. Infection of the epidural space may also occur from direct extension of infection from decubitus ulcers, infected abdominal wounds, or psoas abscesses.[55] The pathophysiology of spinal cord dysfunction from spinal epidural abscess has been investigated in a rabbit model.[61, 62] The gross appearance of the spinal cord at the level of the epidural abscess is usually normal. Microscopically, scattered areas of softening, vacuolization of the cord, areas of necrosis with the disappearance of cells, loss of myelin, and axonal swelling are frequently seen. Myelomalacia occurring in the spinal cord beneath an epidural abscess results from the direct compression of neural tissue and inflammatory thrombosis in the intraspinal vessels with subsequent infarction.

Clinical Features. The clinical presentation of an intracranial epidural abscess is an unrelenting hemicranial headache or persistent fever that develops during or after treatment for frontal sinusitis, mastoiditis, or otitis media. Focal neurological deficits, seizures, and signs of increased ICP do not develop until the infection extends into the subdural space.[51] Approximately 10 percent of epidural abscesses are associated with a subdural empyema.[46] An epidural abscess that develops near the petrous bone and involves cranial nerves V and VI presents with ipsilateral facial pain and lateral rectus weakness (Gradenigo's syndrome). A spinal epidural abscess presents as fever and pain at the affected spinal level. Heusner[63] described a characteristic clinical pattern of symptom progression. Back pain is the initial symptom, which is followed by radicular pain in the extremities or pain in an intercostal thoracic dermatomal pattern within 2 to 3 days. As the disease progresses, paresis of appendicular muscles is associated with loss of sensation below the level of the lesion and the loss of bowel and bladder control. Finally, there is complete paralysis of appendicular muscles and a loss of all sensory modalities below the level of the lesion.

Evaluation. The MRI is the diagnostic procedure of choice to demonstrate a cranial epidural abscess because it is free from bony artifacts adjacent to the inner table of the skull and is easily able to demonstrate extracerebral fluid collections. The epidural fluid will be of higher signal intensity on both MRI T1- and T2-weighted images than the ventricular CSF. Following the administration of gadolinium, a significant enhancement of the dura on MRI T1-weighted images is seen.[46] On the noncontrasted CT scan, an epidural abscess has the appearance of a poorly defined lentiform area of low density adjacent to the inner table of the skull. After the administration of contrast, the convex inner side of the low-density lesion enhances. This represents the inflamed dural membrane.[51]

MRI is also the procedure of choice to demonstrate a spinal epidural abscess. A spinal epidural abscess extends three spinal segments on average and may extend for as long as 13 segments.[55] MRI is able to visualize the entire extent of the epidural abscess in all directions and the degree of spinal cord compression. An epidural abscess is isointense to CSF on MRI T1-weighted images and hyperintense as compared with CSF on MRI T2-weighted images. Following the administration of gadolinium, enhancement of the lesion occurs. Because spinal epidural abscess is usually a result of the hematogenous seeding of the epidural space, there may be evidence of systemic illness with a peripheral leukocytosis or an elevation in the erythrocyte sedimentation rate. The examination of the CSF may be useful to determine the infecting organism. A lumbar puncture should not be performed when the possibility of a lumbar abscess exists, however, because of the risk for spread of the infection from the epidural space to the subarachnoid space.

Management. The primary treatment of a cranial epidural abscess is surgical debridement, Gram's stain and culture of the purulent material, and intravenous antibiotic therapy. Recommendations for the choice of empirical antibiotic therapy are the same as those described for empirical therapy of subdural empyema and should cover aerobic and anaerobic streptococci, staphylococci, gram-negative bacilli, and anaerobes.

An acute spinal epidural abscess must be managed with an immediate laminectomy and decompression and drainage of the epidural space, followed by 4 to 6 weeks of intravenous antibiotic therapy and then 2 to 3 months of oral antibiotic therapy.[55] Empirical antibiotic therapy should include coverage for *S. aureus* because this organism is the etiological agent in the majority of spinal epidural abscesses. There is an increasing incidence, however, of spinal epidural abscess due to gram-negative aerobic bacilli, aerobic streptococci, anaerobes, and *Mycobacterium tuberculosis*. Empirical therapy should also include antituberculous chemotherapy, including isoniazid, rifampin, ethambutol, pyrazinamide, and either streptomycin, rifabutin, or clofazime. A tuberculous spinal epidural abscess is usually associated with vertebral osteomyelitis.

CAT-SCRATCH DISEASE

Cat-scratch disease is caused by the bacterium *Bartonella henselae* and begins with a cutaneous papule or pustule at the site of inoculation, usually a kitten scratch or bite, within a week of the injury. A regional adenopathy involving the head, neck, and upper extremity follows in 1 to 7 weeks. Fever and malaise occurs in approximately one third of patients. The diagnosis is made by demonstrating pleomorphic bacilli by Warthin-Starry silver stain of a lymph node biopsy or by polymerase chain reaction (PCR) amplification techniques on lymph node tissue. The neurological and ophthalmological manifestations associated with cat-scratch disease include (1) encephalopathy (in 2 to 4 percent of patients with cat-scratch disease) characterized by headache, restlessness, irritability, focal or generalized seizure activity, confusion, disorientation, and coma; possible focal neurological deficits, including disturbances of language, cranial nerve palsies, hemiplegia, and ataxia; and (2) neuroretinitis, characterized by a painless, unilateral, sudden loss of visual acuity. On examination, papilledema is associated with macular exudates in a star formation. There is mounting evidence implicating *B. henselae* in HIV dementia and HIV-associated focal brain lesions, aseptic meningitis, and neuropsychiatric disease. The serological test for anti-*Bartonella* antibodies cannot discriminate between anti-*Bartonella henselae* and anti-*Bartonella quintana* (the etiological agent of trench fever) antibodies. Examination of the CSF in cases of cat-scratch disease encephalopathy demonstrates an elevated protein concentration, a lymphocytic and rarely a leukocytic pleocytosis, and a normal glucose concentration. CSF cultures for *B. henselae* are negative. In patients with lymphadenopathy, biopsy of a lymph node may reveal the typical features of cat-scratch disease. Skin tests with the Hanger-Rose cat-scratch disease antigen are positive in the majority of patients. In a few patients with neuroretinitis associated with cat-scratch disease, *B. henselae* has been isolated from blood. Gram's stain reveals small, gram-negative, slightly curved rods. The physician should question the patient about the history of a scratch by a kitten or a cat and the appearance of any skin lesion. No clear guidelines exist for which patients should be treated and what antibiotic should be used. The majority of patients with cat-scratch disease without an associated neurological manifestation have a self-limited illness. The demonstration of *B. henselae* bacteremia associated with neuroretinitis has led to the recommendation that antimicrobial therapy with either erythromycin, doxycycline, azithromycin, clarithromycin, or ofloxacin be considered in these patients. As stated earlier, an increasing amount of evidence exists for *B. henselae* as an etiological agent in a small proportion of cases of HIV-associated dementia, neuropsychiatric illness, focal brain lesions, and aseptic meningitis. Antimicrobial therapy may benefit these patients, but firm recommendations cannot be made at this time.[64]

WHIPPLE'S DISEASE

Whipple's disease is caused by the rod-shaped bacillus *Tropheryma whippelii* and presents with arthralgias, abdominal pain, fever, diarrhea, malabsorption, and weight loss.[65, 66] Whipple's disease occurs predominantly in middle-aged men and most often in farmers. Approximately 6 to 7 percent of patients with Whipple's disease have neurological manifestations, but many cases of CNS involvement in Whipple's disease go unrecognized.[66] The characteristic triad of Whipple's disease is dementia, ophthalmoplegia, and myoclonus.[66] Nearly all cases of ophthalmoplegia involve a conjugate vertical gaze palsy. A peculiar mixture of smooth convergent-divergent pendular oscillations of the eyes with synchronous rhythmical contractions of the jaw, oculomasticatory myorhythmia, is thought to be unique to Whipple's disease. The diagnosis of CNS Whipple's disease is difficult. Examination of the CSF may be normal or may demonstrate a mild pleocytosis. Para-aminosalicylic acid–positive cells are rarely identified in CSF, but if they are, CNS Whipple's disease is a strong possibility. Para-aminosalicylic acid staining of a CSF cytocentrifuged pellet should therefore be performed in all patients in whom CNS Whipple's disease is suspected.[66] The para-aminosalicylic acid reagents will also stain *Mycobacterium avium* complex, *Histoplasma capsulatum*, and nonmicrobial glycoprotein. The PCR technique has allowed for the identification of *T. whippelii* from small intestinal biopsy tissue, lymph node tissue, and CSF.[67] Brain biopsy is not routinely recommended for CNS Whipple's disease. *T. whippelii* infection of the duodenal mucosa can be detected by

PCR in patients in whom an isolated extraintestinal disease exists and in patients with isolated CNS disease. It has been suggested, therefore, that a patient with suspected CNS Whipple's disease should undergo a duodenal tissue biopsy by endoscopy, and the material obtained should be examined by PCR for *T. whippelii*. PCR-based Whipple's disease diagnostic tests, however, are not yet standardized.[66] Trimethoprim-sulfamethoxazole appears to be the most effective therapy for the treatment and prevention of CNS Whipple's disease. Treatment should be initiated with trimethoprim-sulfamethoxazole 160 mg/800 mg by mouth two to three times daily, procaine penicillin G 1.2 million units intramuscular injection daily, and streptomycin 1 g by intramuscular injection daily. Penicillin and streptomycin are continued for a total of 14 days. Trimethoprim-sulfamethoxazole should be continued for at least 1 year. Some clinicians continue antibiotic therapy for CNS Whipple's disease for at least 2 years, and some indefinitely.[66]

Mycobacterial Infections

MYCOBACTERIUM TUBERCULOSIS

Epidemiology and Risk Factors. Chopin, Keats, Thoreau, Paginini, Modigliani, Elizabeth Browning, and Thomas Wolfe died of tuberculosis.[68–70] In the beginning of the 20th century, tuberculous meningitis was common; then after World War II a dramatic decrease in the incidence of tuberculosis occurred in the United States and Europe, although tuberculosis and CNS tuberculosis continued to be prevalent in developing countries. Beginning in 1985, however, the incidence rates of tuberculosis began to increase in the United States. This resurgence of disease was concentrated among males, 25 to 44 years of age, and particularly among immigrants from areas with a high prevalence of tuberculosis infection. A marked increase in the incidence of tuberculosis in long-term residents of American nursing homes was also noted. CNS tuberculosis is considerably more frequent in individuals with AIDS and tuberculosis involving other organ systems than in immunocompetent persons with tuberculosis. In some parts of the world, the most common AIDS-associated CNS infection is tuberculous meningitis.[71]

Pathogenesis and Pathophysiology. Tuberculous meningitis does not develop acutely from the hematogenous spread of tubercle bacilli to the meninges from a pulmonary source of acute infection. Isolated miliary tubercles form in the parenchyma of the brain or the meninges during the hematogenous dissemination of tubercle bacilli during the course of the primary infection or episodically from the endogenous reactivation of latent tuberculosis elsewhere in the body. The tubercles tend to enlarge and are usually caseating.[72] The fate of these tubercles and the subsequent course of infection are at least, in part, a function of the immunological capacity of the host. Minute caseous foci may be completely eliminated by macrophages, leaving no residua of infection. Larger caseous foci may shelter viable mycobacteria that cause reactivated disease only in the presence of impaired host immunity.[71] The propensity for a caseous lesion to produce meningitis is determined by its proximity to the subarachnoid space, the rate at which fibrous encapsulation develops, and the rate at which the lesions enlarge. Organisms proliferate in the caseous centers, eventually leading to the rupture of the tubercle. Subependymal caseous foci may remain quiescent for months or years but then cause meningitis through the discharge of bacilli and tuberculous antigens into the subarachnoid space.[72, 73] The neurological complications of tuberculous meningitis are initiated by a hypersensitivity reaction that occurs in the subarachnoid space when tuberculoproteins are released by the rupture of a caseous lesion. The exudate is located predominantly in the basilar cisterns and surrounds the cranial nerves and major blood vessels at the base of the brain. As the basilar cisterns are filled with a purulent exudate, the flow of CSF is blocked and an obstructive hydrocephalus may develop. The inflammatory exudate also obstructs the resorption of CSF by the arachnoid granulations, the result of which is a communicating hydrocephalus. Cerebral ischemia and infarction occur either as the result of vasculitis caused by direct invasion of the arterial walls by mycobacteria and inflammatory cells or by the compression of the blood vessels at the base of the brain from the inflammatory exudate.[72, 74] Cranial nerve abnormalities resulting from tuberculous meningitis may result from either mechanical compression of the nerve by the purulent exudate or as a result of vasculitic infarction of the nerve.[68] Border-zone encephalitis describes an inflammatory reaction in the brain tissue underlying areas of thick, adherent exudate.[68–71] Tuberculous encephalopathy refers to the development of cerebral edema, occasionally with perivascular demyelination or hemorrhagic leukoencephalopathy deep in the white matter of the brain at a distance from vascular abnormalities and purulent exudate. It is hypothesized that this is a purely allergic phenomenon mediated by tissue hypersensitivity, either to the bacilli or their antigens or possibly to a myelin-related antigen of brain tissue itself.[71]

Clinical Features. The clinical presentation of tuberculous meningitis is either an acute meningoencephalitis characterized by coma, raised ICP, seizures, and focal neurological deficits or a slowly progressive illness with persistent and intractable headache followed by confusion, lethargy, and cranial nerve deficits. Fever may or may not be present in the course of this infection. 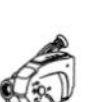 Cranial nerve VI is the most frequently affected by tuberculous meningitis followed by cranial nerves III, IV, VII, and less commonly cranial nerves II, VIII, X, XI, and XII.[71] Hemiparesis may develop as a result of ischemic infarction in the medial striate and thalamoperforating arteries. The most commonly reported symptoms in children include nausea, vomiting, and behavioral changes. Seizures are an infrequent presenting sign, although more than 50 percent develop seizures during the initial hospitalization.[71] In patients with an acute meningoencephalitis syndrome, coma may evolve rapidly because of increased ICP from both cerebral edema and communicating and obstructive hydrocephalus. The clinical syndrome of tuberculous encephalopathy is characterized by convulsions, stupor, coma, involuntary movements, paralysis, and decerebrate spasms or rigidity with or without clinical signs of meningitis or CSF abnormalities of tuberculous meningitis.[75] The clinical presentation of tuberculous meningitis in HIV-infected individuals is similar to the clinical presentation in immunocompetent patients; however, HIV-infected patients are more likely to have an acellular spinal fluid at presentation and have a higher incidence of intracerebral mass lesions.[71]

Evaluation. The combination of an unrelenting headache (with or without low grade fever) with malaise and anorexia and a CSF lymphocytic pleocytosis with a mild decrease in the glucose concentration is suggestive of tuberculous meningitis. The initiation of therapy should not await bacteriological proof of tubercle bacilli by smear or culture. The development of hydrocephalus and the clinical scenario just described is additional strong evidence for tuberculous meningitis. The absence of radiographical evidence of pulmonary tuberculosis and/or a negative tuberculin skin test does not exclude the possibility of tuberculous meningitis. The classic "Ghon complex" refers to Anton Ghon's observation from autopsy specimens that the primary lesion of tuberculosis is in the lung with secondary infection in the tracheobronchial lymph nodes.[76] In addition to the primary complex, chest radiographic abnormalities suggestive of pulmonary tuberculosis are hilar adenopathy, a miliary pattern, upper lobe infiltrate, cavitations, and lobar consolidation. CNS disease may develop from caseous foci in organs other than the lung with subsequent hematogenous dissemination of virulent tubercle bacilli to the CNS. The adrenal gland, bone, genitourinary tract, and the mediastinal and abdominal lymph nodes are all potential sources of caseous foci, which may serve as "seed beds" for the later development of hematogenous dissemination of tubercle bacilli.[77] The intradermal tuberculin skin test is negative in 50 to 70 percent of patients with tuberculous meningitis and often becomes positive during the course of therapy.[73, 78] The classic CSF abnormalities in tuberculous meningitis are as follows: (1) an elevated opening lumbar pressure; (2) increased WBC count between 10 and 500 cells/mm^3 with a predominance of lymphocytes; (3) an elevated protein concentration in the range of 100 to 500 mg/dL; (4) a decreased glucose concentration (the median glucose concentration is approximately 40 mg/dL); and (5) a positive culture in 75 percent of patients requiring 3 to 6 weeks for growth. A cobweb-like "skin" may form at the top of the CSF specimen and is the classic pellicle of tuberculous meningitis. Tubercle bacilli may become entangled in the skin of the pellicle and are more easily located by smear or culture of the pellicle than elsewhere in the CSF.[71] The last tube of CSF collected should be sent for acid-fast bacilli smear. Positive smears are typically reported in only 10 to 40 percent of patients with tuberculous meningitis. The CSF chloride concentration and the bromide partition test have been disappointing in their ability to differentiate tuberculous meningitis from other etiologies of lymphocytic meningitis. The CSF chloride concentration typically decreases as the CSF protein concentration increases; therefore, this is a rather nonspecific test. The bromide partition test measures the ratio of serum to CSF bromide 24 hours after the oral administration of sodium bromide or the intravenous injection of radioactive bromide.[79] A low bromide partition ratio is seen in any infectious or inflammatory CNS disease that increases the permeability of the blood-CSF barrier. The concentration of tuberculostearic acid in CSF has been reported to be a sensitive marker for CNS tuberculosis and enjoyed a brief period of popularity, even though it was extremely difficult to find a laboratory that was able to run this assay. The PCR technique and other molecular diagnostic techniques for the detection of M. *tuberculosis* DNA in the CSF hold the greatest promise.[67] The sensitivity of the PCR technique for the detection of M. *tuberculosis* DNA in CSF is approximately 54 percent; however, false-positive results occur with rates of 3 to 20 percent.[71]

Management. The American Academy of Pediatrics recommends a combination of isoniazid (INH), rifampin, pyrazinamide, and streptomycin as the initial therapy of tuberculous meningitis in children.[80] The doses are listed in Table 42–3. When antimicrobial sensitivities are known, the treatment regimen may be altered. Standard therapy uses four drugs for 2 months followed by INH and rifampin alone for 6 to 9 months. Most drug regimens include INH, rifampin, and pyrazinamide and either ethambutol or streptomycin (in children too young to be monitored for visual acuity).[81] When the results of drug susceptibility studies are available, and if the organism is sensitive to INH and rifampin, ethambutol and pyrazinamide are continued for only 2 months, and then INH and rifampin are continued for a total of 9 to 12 months. Empirical therapy for tuberculous meningitis in HIV-infected individuals should include a combination of INH, pyridoxine, and rifampin plus ethambutol or pyrazinamide and either streptomycin or rifabutin or clofazimine (Table 42–4). Corticosteroid therapy decreases meningeal inflammation. Isoniazid and pyrazinamide penetrate the CSF with or without meningeal inflammation, but the penetration of rifampin, streptomycin, and ethambutol is considerably better in the presence of meningeal inflammation. Dexamethasone therapy is recommended for patients with altered consciousness, papilledema, focal neurological signs, impending herniation, spinal block, and hydrocephalus. In addition, as patients are treated for tuberculous meningitis, the slow resolution of the inflammatory exudate in the basilar cisterns may obstruct the flow and resorption of CSF with the subsequent development of hydrocephalus. These patients may benefit from a short course of oral prednisone. A basic principle of management for patients with organisms that are resistant to one or more drugs is the administration of at least two agents to which a demonstrated susceptibility exists. For example, for patients with isolated INH resistance, INH should be discontinued and pyrazinamide and rifampin continued for the entire course of therapy.[81]

TABLE 42–3. **Empirical Therapy for Tuberculous Meningitis**

	Dosage	
Drug	**Children**	**Adults**
Isoniazid (INH)	10 mg/kg/d once daily	300 mg/d
Pyridoxine		50 mg/d
Rifampin	10 mg/kg/d	600 mg/d
Pyrazinamide	30 mg/kg/d	30 mg/kg/d
Ethambutol*	15 to 25 mg/kg/d	15 to 25 mg/kg/d
Streptomycin†	20 to 40 mg/kg/d	
Corticosteroids		
Dexamethasone‡	0.15 mg/kg q 6 hr	0.15 mg/kg q 6 hr
Prednisone§	1 mg/kg/d	1 mg/kg/d

*When antimicrobial resistance is suspected.
†The American Academy of Pediatrics recommends a combination of INH, rifampin, pyrazinamide, and streptomycin for tuberculous meningitis in children.
‡For altered consciousness, papilledema, focal neurological signs, impending herniation, spinal block, hydrocephalus.
§For intractable headache, papilledema with otherwise normal neurological examination.

TABLE 42-4. **Antituberculous Chemotherapy in HIV-Infected Individuals**

Isoniazid	10 to 15 mg/kg/d
Rifampin	10 to 15 mg/kg/d
Pyridoxine	50 mg/d
plus	
Ethambutol	25 mg/kg/d
or	
Pyrazinamide	20 to 30 mg/kg/d
plus	
Streptomycin	20 to 40 mg/kg/d
or	
Rifabutin	300 mg/d
or	
Clofazimine	300 mg/d

MYCOBACTERIUM AVIUM

CNS disease from M. *avium* is a result of the hematogenous dissemination of this organism from a respiratory or gastrointestinal source of infection. M. *avium* and M. *intracellulare* are separate species, but their separation has no clinical value; therefore, they are considered together in this section. Infection with these species of mycobacteria occurs primarily in patients with advanced HIV disease, generally in patients with fewer than 50 $CD4^+$ cells/mm^3. Infection of the CNS can present as meningitis, meningoencephalitis, rhombencephalitis, brain abscess, or cranial neuropathies. Neuroimaging may demonstrate meningeal enhancement, hydrocephalus, or single or multiple enhancing lesions. Diagnosis is made by acid-fast smear and culture of the CSF or brain abscess aspirate. There have been few randomized, comparative controlled treatment trials for M. *avium* and M. *intracellulare* CNS infections. Clarithromycin and azithromycin have excellent activity in the therapy of disseminated M. *avium* disease in HIV-infected individuals, but their therapy in M. *avium* CNS infections has not been studied. Rifabutin is efficacious for the prophylaxis of disseminated M. *avium* infection in HIV patients and has been shown to increase survival in HIV-infected individuals with disseminated disease when used at higher doses (450 to 600 mg). The treatment of a CNS complication of disseminated disease should include at least a four-drug regimen, which at present is clarithromycin (500 mg bid), rifampin (600 mg daily), ethambutol (25 mg/kg/d for 2 months then 15 mg/kg/d), and streptomycin (0.75 to 1.0 g at least three times per week). A combination of azithromycin (250 mg/d), rifabutin (300 mg daily), and ethambutol and streptomycin has been recommended as an alternative treatment regimen. Treatment is continued until cultures are negative for at least 12 months and will likely need to be continued for the life of the patient.[82]

Spirochete Infections

NEUROSYPHILIS

The origin of the name *syphilis* is from a poem titled "Syphilis sive morbus Gallicus" by an Italian physician, Girolamo Fracastoro. The poem is about a shepherd boy named Syphilus who lives in the time of King Alcithous of Haiti. When Syphilus loses his sheep because of a drought, he blames the Sun God and convinces the natives of Haiti to offer sacrifices to King Alcithous, rather than to the Sun God. The angered Sun God revenges himself by sending a plague to the island natives. The shepherd boy Syphilus is, of course, the very first victim.[83] One of the Pinzon brothers who sailed with Christopher Columbus as captains of the Niña and the Pinta is historically blamed for bringing syphilis to Spain. The first documented case of syphilis in the colonized New World occurred in Connecticut in 1646.[83] The term *neurosyphilis* describes any of six neurosyphilitic syndromes, including asymptomatic neurosyphilis, acute symptomatic syphilitic meningitis, meningovasculitis, parenchymatous neurosyphilis (dementia paralytica or tabes dorsalis), CNS gummata, and congenital neurosyphilis.[84]

Epidemiology and Risk Factors. In the preantibiotic era, tabes dorsalis was the most common form of neurosyphilis. Over the past decade, an increasing number of patients with asymptomatic or symptomatic syphilitic meningitis, meningovasculitis, and syphilitic eye disease have been reported. The increasing number of cases of early neurosyphilis is occurring in individuals infected with HIV.[85–88]

Pathogenesis and Pathophysiology. Primary syphilis is defined by the appearance of a painless chancre at the site of inoculation. If untreated, the chancre will heal within 3 to 6 weeks, after which most patients progress to the secondary stage of disease in which systemic spirochetemia becomes manifest by skin rash and flulike symptoms with lethargy, fever, headache, and sore throat. The skin rash is typically nonpruritic and widespread but is most marked on the palms and soles. There may be generalized lymphadenopathy. Untreated, secondary syphilis also resolves over a period of weeks to months. A period of latency during which there are no clinical manifestations of syphilis occurs, but there is historical and serological evidence of syphilis. About one third of patients with untreated latent syphilis develop tertiary manifestations of the disease after a variable period ranging from months to years. Tertiary syphilis may present as either cardiovascular syphilis, gummatous syphilis, or neurosyphilis.[89, 90] Invasion of the CNS by *T. pallidum* occurs early in the course of infection. Clinical neurosyphilis may present at any point in the natural history of infection beyond the primary stage.[90] During the early stages of *T. pallidum* CNS infection, pathological changes are limited to perivascular infiltration of the meninges with lymphocytes and plasma cells. Focal meningeal inflammation may lead to the formation of hypertrophic meninges or gummata. Inflammatory cells invade blood vessel walls causing arteritis and eventually luminal occlusion by thrombosis, ischemia, and infarction.[90, 91] Parenchymal involvement occurs in late neurosyphilis and is characterized by neuronal degeneration and loss, and gliosis. The brain becomes atrophic, and the meninges are thickened and cloudy.[91] In tabes dorsalis the preganglionic portion of the dorsal roots are infiltrated with lymphocytes and plasma cells, and the posterior columns of the spinal cord become atrophic.[91]

Clinical Features and Evaluation. Asymptomatic neurosyphilis is defined by an abnormal CSF evaluation including a mild lymphocytic or mononuclear pleocytosis, an elevated protein concentration, and a reactive CSF Venereal Disease Research Laboratory (VDRL) test in a patient without neurological signs or symptoms.[85, 91]

Acute symptomatic syphilitic meningitis was first described by H. Houston Merritt in 1935.[92] The most common symptoms of syphilitic meningitis are headache, nausea and vomiting, and stiff neck. In Merritt's review, papilledema was frequently present resulting from acute hydrocephalus associated with meningeal inflammation with increased ICP. Papilledema is not a common finding today. Abnormalities of cranial nerves II, VI, VII, and VIII are common. The meningeal symptoms typically develop within 1 to 2 years of the initial infection.[85] Examination of the CSF in cases of syphilitic meningitis reveals an increased opening pressure, a lymphocytic pleocytosis, a normal or slightly decreased glucose concentration, an elevated protein concentration, and a positive VDRL test. A nonreactive CSF-VDRL test does not rule out neurosyphilis. A reactive CSF-VDRL test virtually confirms the diagnosis of neurosyphilis except when the CSF is blood tinged. Blood in the CSF may give a false-positive CSF-VDRL test.[84, 85, 88, 92]

Meningovascular syphilis is defined by the appearance of focal neurological signs from an inflammatory, obliterative endarteritis involving small and medium-sized arteries associated with signs of meningeal inflammation. The middle cerebral artery is commonly involved and its involvement is clinically manifest by the so-called luetic hemiplegia. Examination of the CSF may reveal an isolated elevation of protein concentration or a mild pleocytosis and a reactive VDRL. Cerebral angiography may demonstrate a nonspecific pattern of diffuse narrowing of intracerebral arteries and arterioles. Neuroimaging may demonstrate multiple areas of infarction. The peak incidence for the development of meningovascular syphilis is 5 to 7 years after the primary infection.[89] Syphilitic arteritis can also develop in any intraspinal artery, resulting in acute transverse myelitis with paraplegia, sensory level, and loss of sphincter control.[91]

Dementia paralytica is manifest as a slow deterioration in cognitive functioning with impaired memory, loss of insight and judgment, language abnormalities, loss of appendicular strength, tremor of the tongue and hands, pupillary abnormalities, and loss of bowel and bladder control. The syndrome of dementia paralytica typically occurs 10 to 20 years after primary infection. Examination of the CSF at this stage demonstrates one or a combination of the following: (1) a positive VDRL test, (2) lymphocytic pleocytosis, or (3) an elevated protein concentration.[85]

Tabes dorsalis is characterized by paresthesias or dysesthesias in a radicular distribution.[91] As the disease progresses, proprioceptive and vibratory sense is lost due to neuronal degeneration and infiltration of inflammatory cells into the dorsal columns and posterior spinal nerve roots of the spinal cord. Loss of the pupillary reaction to light with preservation of pupillary constriction to accommodation—the Argyll-Robertson pupillary abnormality—may be present. The patient has a broad-based, foot-slapping gait. The peak incidence for tabes dorsalis is 15 to 20 years after the primary infection.[89] It has been suggested that the lancinating pains typically attributed to tabes dorsalis in the past were due to the heavy metal therapy used to treat neurosyphilis in the preantibiotic era and not the primary infection.[91]

Gummatous neurosyphilis is characterized by gummata located in the basal cisterns, leptomeninges, or within the parenchyma. They produce focal neurological deficits and cranial nerve palsies by exerting pressure on adjacent structures.[91]

Diagnosis. The serological tests for syphilis can be grouped into two categories: treponemal tests that detect specific antibodies against *T. pallidum* and which include the fluorescent treponemal antibody absorption test (FTA-ABS) and the microhemagglutination–*Treponema pallidum* test (MHA-TP), and nontreponemal tests, which detect antibodies to lipids found on the membranes of *T. pallidum* using cardiolipin-lecithin-cholesterol antigens. The nontreponemal tests in routine use today include the VDRL and the rapid plasma reagin test. The FTA-ABS test is the first serological test to become positive after inoculation. The FTA-ABS and the MHA-TP tests are nonquantitative; they are either positive or negative. The VDRL test may be quantitated by serial dilutions of serum, and the titer is reported as the greatest serum dilution that produces a positive result. The VDRL titer reaches low levels in late syphilis and may eventually become nonreactive.[85] The causes of biological false-positive VDRL and FTA-ABS tests are listed in Table 42–5. Most false-positive VDRL tests have a low titer of 1:8 or less.[85] In a patient with presumed neurosyphilis, a serological test for syphilis, either the FTA-ABS test or the MHA-TP test, is performed initially. Because the VDRL test may become nonreactive in later stages of syphilis, only about 70 percent of patients with neurosyphilis have a positive VDRL test. A CSF examination should be performed in patients with a reactive MHA-TP or FTA-ABS. The diagnosis of neu-

TABLE 42–5. **Causes of False-Positive Serological Tests for Syphilis**

False-Positive Fluorescent Treponemal Antibody Absorption (FTA-ABS) Test
Technical error
Lyme borreliosis
Genital herpes simplex
Lupus erythematosus
Scleroderma
Mixed connective tissue disease
Cirrhosis
Nonvenereal treponematoses
Transient (< 6 Months) False-Positive Venereal Disease Research Laboratory (VDRL) Test
Mycoplasma pneumoniae
Enterovirus infection
Infectious mononucleosis
Tuberculosis
Viral pneumonia
Leptospirosis
Measles
Mumps
Chronic False-Positive VDRL Test (Lasting Longer Than 6 Months)
Systemic lupus erythematosus and other connective tissue disorders
Intravenous drug use
Rheumatoid arthritis
Reticuloendothelial malignancy
Age (elderly person)
Hashimoto's thyroiditis

From Roos KL: Syphilitic meningitis. *In* Meningitis: 100 Maxims in Neurology. London, Arnold, 1997, pp 171–181. Reproduced by permission.

rosyphilis is made in the presence of a reactive serological test with either neurological manifestations consistent with neurosyphilis or CSF evidence of a lymphocytic pleocytosis and an elevated protein concentration, and/or a positive CSF-VDRL test. Most clinicians treat patients for neurosyphilis when they have a positive serological test and a CSF lymphocytic pleocytosis with an elevated protein concentration whether the CSF-VDRL is reactive or not. A reactive CSF-VDRL establishes the diagnosis but a nonreactive test does not exclude the diagnosis.

Screening for the presence of syphilis in HIV-1-infected individuals should be performed by the serum FTA-ABS test as the nontreponemal tests for syphilis may be falsely negative in HIV-infected individuals. A loss of reactivity to the treponemal tests occurs in individuals infected with HIV-1 with advanced immunosuppression.[88] In HIV-infected individuals with neurosyphilis, the CSF should demonstrate a lymphocytic pleocytosis and an elevated protein concentration. When the CSF-VDRL is negative, a CSF FTA-ABS or CSF MHA-TP should be obtained. The lack of CSF FTA-ABS or CSF MHA-TP reactivity excludes a diagnosis of neurosyphilis. The CSF FTA-ABS and CSF MHA-TP are not routinely recommended for the screening of neurosyphilis in non-HIV-infected individuals because reactivity of these tests on CSF does not establish the diagnosis of neurosyphilis.[91]

Management. Primary, secondary, and latent syphilis are treated with benzathine penicillin; neurosyphilis is treated with intravenous aqueous crystalline penicillin G 3 to 4 million units every 4 hours for 10 to 14 days. An alternative regimen is procaine penicillin, 2.4 million units intramuscularly daily with probenecid, 500 mg orally four times a day, both for 10 to 14 days. Patients with a history of penicillin allergies should be skin tested and desensitized if necessary.[85, 91] The frequency with which intravenous antibiotics are unsuccessful in the therapy of neurosyphilis is extremely low. In those instances in which a progression of clinical disease or persistence of a CSF lymphocytic pleocytosis or a reactive CSF-VDRL is present, retreatment of the patient with an additional 24 million units/d for 10 days is reasonable. The initial CSF pleocytosis will resolve 6 months after penicillin therapy in 80 percent of patients. Serial CSF-VDRL titers should decrease with treatment. Re-examination of the CSF should occur in HIV-infected patients with neurosyphilis.

LYME DISEASE

Epidemiology and Risk Factors. The Swedish dermatologist, Afzelius, first described an expanding ringlike skin lesion following a tick bite in 1910. He called this lesion erythema chronicum migrans.[93, 94] The first case report of erythema migrans in the United States involved a physician in Wisconsin who was bitten by a tick while hunting. This was reported in 1970.[95] In the mid-1970s a number of children and adults from Lyme, Old Lyme, and Haddam, Connecticut, presented with recurrent attacks of asymmetrical large joint pain and swelling that was often preceded by an erythematous expanding plaque-like skin lesion with central clearing.[96] This disease was termed Lyme arthritis. Lyme arthritis was later renamed Lyme disease. In 1979, Andrew Spielman, while searching for the tick vector of human babesiosis, named one tick suspect, *Ixodes dammini*, in honor of the distinguished Harvard pathologist Gustave Dammin.[96, 97] This tick would later be identified as the vector of Lyme disease.[96] In 1981, Willi Burgdorfer isolated the Lyme spirochete from ticks collected on Shelter Island.[98] By 1983, two separate groups headed by Steere[99] and Benach[100] cultured *Borrelia burgdorferi* from patients with Lyme disease, conclusively establishing this organism as the infectious agent.[94, 96]

In Canada, Lyme disease occurs in Ontario and Manitoba; in the United States the highest incidence of Lyme disease has been reported in Connecticut, Delaware, Maryland, New Jersey, New York, Pennsylvania, Rhode Island, and Wisconsin. The tick vector in the Northeast and Midwest is the black-legged tick, *I. scapularis*, which has a northern (*I. dammini*) and southern form.[94] The usual vector of Lyme disease on the West Coast is *I. pacificus*; the frequency of Lyme disease is much lower on the West Coast than in the Northeast.

Pathogenesis and Pathophysiology. Lyme disease is caused by invasion of the CNS by the spirochete *B. burgdorferi*. The pathophysiology of Lyme disease bears several similarities to the pathophysiology of syphilis. The organism initially invades the body through intradermal inoculation. This occurs through a painless tick bite. *B. burgdorferi* is transmitted through the mouth parts of the tick, and transmission of infection occurs only after prolonged attachment and feeding over 24 hours. Humans are most likely to be bitten in the late spring and early summer.[94] Similar to syphilis, inoculation is followed by a spirochetemia with wide dissemination, and like syphilis, invasion of the CNS initially presents as a meningitis. The various neurological syndromes are felt to result not only from infection of the CNS by *B. burgdorferi*, but also from the reaction of the immune system to the spirochete and the associated inflammatory response. The spirochetes activate T-cell subsets and induce cytokine production (including interleukins 1 and 6, and tumor necrosis factor alpha). In addition, they cause production of autoantibodies to axonal proteins, gangliosides, neurons, myelin components, and cardiolipin.[94]

Clinical Features. The neurological manifestations of Lyme disease are classically divided into early syndromes and late syndromes. The early syndromes include meningitis, facial nerve and other cranial nerve palsies, and radiculoneuritis. Delayed syndromes include sensorimotor polyradiculoneuropathy, encephalopathy, and encephalomyelitis.[94, 101, 102]

MENINGITIS. Signs and symptoms of meningitis may develop while the characteristic skin lesion, erythema migrans, is still present and typically occur within 12 weeks of infection. Most patients complain of headache and fatigue; some may have severe pain between the scapulae, severe fatigue, myalgias, and arthralgias. The diagnosis of Lyme disease is made by examination of the CSF that demonstrates a lymphocytic pleocytosis with a normal glucose concentration and a mildly to moderately elevated protein concentration. Paired samples of serum and CSF should be sent to detect the intrathecal production of *B. burgdorferi* antibody (usually IgG or IgA). Intrathecal anti–*Borrelia burgdorferi* antibody production can be detected in 50 to 90 percent of cases. CSF PCR can be used to amplify *B. burgdorferi* DNA and is positive in 30 to 40 percent of patients with Lyme meningitis.[94, 101] Culture of the organism from CSF is rarely positive.

FACIAL NERVE AND OTHER CRANIAL NERVE PALSIES. The most frequent neurological abnormality in patients with

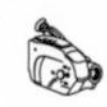

Lyme disease is facial nerve palsy that is unilateral or bilateral and most often occurs within 4 weeks of the appearance of erythema migrans. Patients may also complain of headache and fatigue. Other cranial nerves may also be involved in Lyme disease, including cranial nerves II, III, IV, V, VI, VIII, and IX to XII, although such involvement is rare.[94] The most useful diagnostic tests for patients with a facial nerve palsy are a serum Lyme enzyme-linked immunosorbent assay (ELISA), Western blot, and a CSF examination. The CSF may demonstrate a lymphocytic pleocytosis and intrathecal antibody production of anti–*Borrelia burgdorferi* antibodies. In patients with a facial nerve palsy and a normal CSF examination, oral doxycycline (100 mg bid for 2 weeks) can be used; however, patients with facial nerve palsy and CSF pleocytosis should be treated with intravenous ceftriaxone.[101]

RADICULONEURITIS. Early in the course of spirochetemia, patients may complain of severe sharp, jabbing, or deep and boring pain in a radicular nerve distribution. Often, the limb that was the site of the tick bite is the site of the pain.[102] Within days to weeks there may be sensory loss, weakness, or hyporeflexia in the limb. There may be clinical signs of an associated myelitis characterized by sphincter dysfunction or Babinski's sign. Patients may also have a facial nerve palsy. The diagnosis is made by the examination of CSF and through electromyography (EMG). The majority of patients have a CSF lymphocytic pleocytosis, an increased CSF protein concentration, and evidence of intrathecal production of anti–*Borrelia burgdorferi* antibody.[102] The majority of patients also have a positive Lyme serology and Western blot.[101] The abnormalities on EMG are consistent with a polyradiculopathy with a predominantly axonal process.[94] Some patients may have a clinical presentation suggestive of the Guillain-Barré syndrome with areflexia and a predominantly motor involvement. EMG findings of a primarily axonal process and CSF evidence of a lymphocytic pleocytosis, however, are not consistent with a diagnosis of Guillain-Barré. Guillain-Barré syndrome may occur as a postinfectious complication of Lyme disease. In these patients, the EMG does show changes typical of a demyelinating process, and examination of the CSF demonstrates the characteristic cytoalbuminological dissociation.[94]

ENCEPHALOPATHY. Encephalopathy was initially described in patients with systemic manifestations of Lyme disease and in particular, arthritis. The patients have a mild confusional state characterized by difficulty with memory and cognitive slowing often accompanied by fatigue and malaise. Neuropsychological testing is abnormal, but CSF abnormalities may or may not be present. Pleocytosis is reported in 5 percent of patients, and intrathecal anti–*Borrelia burgdorferi* antibody production is present in less than 50 percent of patients.[94, 102] Active neurological involvement that is suggested by CSF abnormalities, the psychological consequences of chronic illness, and possibly residual neurological deficits of a past infection with Lyme disease may affect a patient's perception of cognitive dysfunction. In addition, evidence from quantitative analysis of SPECT scans suggests that Lyme encephalopathy patients with measurable memory deficits have reduced perfusion affecting primarily subcortical frontotemporal white matter and basal ganglia.[103]

SENSORIMOTOR POLYRADICULONEUROPATHY. Patients with chronic Lyme radiculoneuropathy present with sensory symptoms, particularly distal paresthesias in a stocking and glove or a stocking distribution. A less common presentation is pain in the distribution of the cervical, thoracic, or lumbosacral dermatomes. This syndrome is distinct from the painful symptoms of radiculoneuritis that occurs within a few weeks of infection with *B. burgdorferi*. Although patients with a chronic radiculopathy complain of pain, it is much less severe than in the acute radiculoneuritis form. Electrophysiological studies demonstrate a mild sensorimotor radiculoneuropathy with axonal loss, minor decreases in the distal compound action potential amplitudes (sensory greater than motor), little or no slowing of nerve conduction velocities, and mild to moderate distal and paraspinal muscle denervation.[101] In patients who complain of paresthesias, mildly prolonged distal motor or sensory latencies and mild slowing of distal motor conduction velocities is present.[94] These patients do not typically have a facial nerve palsy, and examination of the CSF is usually normal.[94]

ENCEPHALOMYELITIS. A very rare, late neurological syndrome in North American Lyme disease affects both the brain and spinal cord white matter. Examination of the CSF demonstrates a lymphocytic pleocytosis, a mildly elevated protein concentration and the intrathecal production of anti–*Borrelia burgdorferi* antibodies.[102]

Evaluation. The diagnosis of CNS Lyme disease begins with asking the patient about a history of a tick bite, whether there was travel to an endemic area, and if the skin lesion was characteristic of erythema migrans. This lesion begins as a painless macule, which continues to expand until it becomes an annular erythematous plaque. It occurs at the site of a tick bite an average of 8 to 9 days after infection. As the lesion expands, the center may become clear, vesicular, or edematous forming a bull's-eye lesion.[94] Serum should be sent for ELISA and Western blot testing. A positive serology is indicative of exposure to the organism and should not be considered proof of active infection.[102] Interpretation of the serological test is further confounded by the evidence that seronegative Lyme cases exist. CNS infection is most readily confirmed if the paired serum and CSF anti–*Borrelia burgdorferi* antibody titer demonstrates the intrathecal production of these antibodies. This occurs when the antibody titer in the CSF is greater than the antibody titer in serum. Other CSF abnormalities suggestive of Lyme disease are a mononuclear or lymphocytic pleocytosis, an elevated protein concentration, and a normal glucose concentration. As described in the specific clinical features of each neurological syndrome, the CSF is almost always abnormal in Lyme meningitis and early radiculoneuritis. The CSF is at times abnormal with an isolated facial nerve palsy or with encephalomyelitis and can be normal or abnormal when encephalopathy is present. The CSF is typically normal in chronic Lyme disease sensorimotor polyradiculoneuropathy.[94]

Management. Facial nerve palsy without CSF abnormalities may be treated with oral doxycycline 100 mg twice a day for 2 weeks. Intravenous ceftriaxone is the drug of choice for all other neurological syndromes of Lyme disease. The adult dose is 2 g/d, and the pediatric dose is 75 to 100 mg/kg/d. Treatment with ceftriaxone should be continued for at least 2 weeks, and many physicians prefer 4 weeks of therapy.[101] A vaccine made of a lipidated outer surface protein of *B. burgdorferi* is now available.

Other Tickborne Infections

EHRLICHIOSIS

Ehrlichia are small gram-negative pleomorphic coccobacilli that primarily infect circulating leukocytes and other cells derived from the hematopoietic system.[104] There are two species of ehrlichia that cause human disease. *Ehrlichia chaffeensis* is the causative organism of human monocytic ehrlichiosis, and an organism that is closely related to or nearly identical to *E. equi* and *E. phagocytophila* is the causative agent of granulocytic ehrlichiosis.[104–106] *E. chaffeensis* infects mononuclear phagocytes in the blood and tissues, and the granulocytic *Ehrlichia* species infects granulocytic phagocytes in blood and tissues.[104] The infectious agents of human ehrlichiosis and Lyme disease are both transmitted by tick bites. Most cases of human granulocytic ehrlichiosis have been identified in Wisconsin, Minnesota, New York, Connecticut, and Massachusetts, and most cases of human monocytic ehrlichiosis have been identified in the southeastern and south-central United States.[106]

The pathogenesis of the diseases caused by ehrlichiae are not well understood at this time. It is clear, however, that the ehrlichiae damage and lyse host phagocytic cells once they have attached to these cells, resulting in leukopenia and thrombocytopenia.[106]

Patients with human granulocytic ehrlichiosis present with a febrile illness associated with myalgia, headache, malaise and occasionally nausea, vomiting, or a cough. The clinical presentation may be helpful in distinguishing Lyme disease from human granulocytic ehrlichiosis. Nausea, vomiting, and cough are very infrequent in Lyme disease. Fatigue is more often a complaint with Lyme disease than with human granulocytic ehrlichiosis.[106] The incubation period is approximately 7 days following a tick bite, and approximately 20 percent of patients with ehrlichiosis have a rash that consists of a maculopapular eruption or petechiae.[107] Despite the different causative agents of monocytic and granulocytic ehrlichioses, the clinical and laboratory manifestations of the infections are similar. Neurological manifestations of both include severe headache, lethargy, confusion, coma, and seizure activity. The most common CSF abnormalities are lymphocytic pleocytosis with an elevated protein concentration and a borderline low CSF glucose concentration.[108] Laboratory evidence of leukopenia, thrombocytopenia, and anemia, and mild to moderate elevations in levels of aspartate and alanine aminotransferases, alkaline phosphatase, and lactate dehydrogenase are present.[104]

Monocytic and granulocytic ehrlichiosis are separate diseases caused by different etiological agents; therefore, laboratory diagnosis requires different tests for each. The current CDC recommendation for the serological diagnosis of monocytic ehrlichiosis is a fourfold increase in *E. chaffeensis* antibody titer (a minimum titer of 64) or a single high-serum antibody titer (greater than or equal to 128) in patients with a clinically compatible history. The current CDC recommendation for serological confirmation of human granulocytic ehrlichiosis requires a serological reaction or a four-fold increase in titer to *E. equi* antigen. A minimum titer of 80 is required.[104] Diagnosis during the acute phase of the illness can also be made by PCR amplification of the agent of human granulocytic ehrlichiosis DNA from blood.[106] Wright's or Giemsa staining of a blood smear may also demonstrate morulae in lekocytes. Co-infections with *B. burgdorferi* and the agent of human granulocytic ehrlichiosis can occur.

Ehrlichioses are treated with doxycycline. *E. chaffeensis* is susceptible to doxycycline and rifampin. Doxycycline is the recommended agent for human granulocytic ehrlichiosis. The recommended dose in children and adults is 100 mg twice daily for adults or 3 mg/kg/d in two divided doses for children. Doxycycline can be given by either the oral or intravenous route.[104]

ROCKY MOUNTAIN SPOTTED FEVER

Rocky Mountain spotted fever is a rickettsial disease caused by *Rickettsia rickettsii*, a small intracellular parasite. Infection is acquired by a tick bite. The majority of infections are acquired in the south Atlantic coastal and the western and southern central states with the highest incidence in Virginia, North Carolina, South Carolina, Oklahoma, and Tennessee. The disease typically occurs during spring and summer. Fever, rash, and a history of exposure to ticks is the classic triad of Rocky Mountain spotted fever. The illness usually begins 5 to 7 days after the tick bite. The majority of patients have fever, severe frontal headache, malaise, myalgia, and vomiting. An altered level of consciousness and meningismus may develop during the course of the illness in addition to abdominal pain, hepatosplenomegaly, respiratory failure, renal dysfunction, and myocarditis.

The classic rash of Rocky Mountain spotted fever first appears as macules on the wrists and ankles and subsequently spreads to involve the trunk, face, palms, and soles. The rash appears 1 to 15 days after the onset of the illness.[107] The rash is initially a diffuse erythematous maculopapular rash that blanches with pressure. It progresses to a petechial rash, then to a purpuric rash and, if untreated, to skin necrosis or gangrene. The rash begins on the wrists and ankles and then spreads distally and proximally within a few hours. Ten percent of patients do not have a rash (spotless Rocky Mountain spotted fever). Neurological manifestations of Rocky Mountain spotted fever include severe bifrontal headache that is unresponsive to common analgesics, delirium, confusion, seizures, coma, hyper-reflexia, spastic paraparesis or quadraparesis, facial diplegia, nystagmus, and/or ataxia. Stupor and coma occur in approximately 25 percent of patients and are associated with a poorer prognosis than those cases without signs of encephalitis. Laboratory abnormalities in patients with Rocky Mountain spotted fever include thrombocytopenia, hyponatremia, and elevated liver enzyme abnormalities. CSF abnormalities include a mild (rarely more than 100 cells/mm^3) lymphocytic pleocytosis and an elevated protein concentration. In the acute stage, the diagnosis of Rocky Mountain spotted fever can be made by skin biopsy with the demonstration of rickettsiae in the endothelial cells of blood vessels by immunofluorescence. Serological tests are useful for the confirmation of the diagnosis and include an indirect immunofluorescent antibody assay (IFA), an indirect hemagglutination assay (IHA), latex agglutination (LA), and complement fixation (CF). According to the Centers for Disease Control and Prevention, diagnostic titers for Rocky Mountain spotted

TABLE 42–6. **Recommended Antimicrobial Therapy of Rocky Mountain Spotted Fever**

Antibiotic	Dosage	Duration of Therapy
Tetracycline–Child*	25 to 50 mg/kg/d (oral dose) in 4 divided doses	7 to 10 days
Tetracycline–Adult	500 mg (oral dose) qid	7 to 10 days
Doxycycline–Adult	100 mg (oral dose) bid	7 to 10 days
Chloramphenicol (for children under 8 years of age)	50 mg/kg/d IV in 4 divided doses	7 to 10 days

*Not recommended for children under age 8 years to avoid staining of the teeth.

Reproduced with permission from Pourmand, Roos KL: Seasonal (spring-summer) encephalitides. *In* Roos KL (ed): Central Nervous System Infectious Diseases and Therapy. New York, Marcel Dekker, 1997, pp 193–211.

fever include a titer of 1:64 for IFA, 1:16 for CF, and a fourfold increase between acute and convalescent sera for LA and IHA. The PCR is also under development for the diagnosis of this disease. The treatment of Rocky Mountain spotted fever is outlined in Table 42–6.[109]

BABESIOSIS

Babesiosis is a malaria-like illness caused by a protozoan parasite and transmitted by a tick bite. Most human cases of babesiosis have occurred during the summer months in the northeastern United States, Maryland, Virginia, Georgia, Wisconsin, Minnesota, California, and Washington. Symptoms of babesiosis typically begin approximately 1 week after a tick bite and include malaise, anorexia, and fatigue followed several days later by fever, drenching sweats, myalgia, and headache. The clinical spectrum ranges from a mild self-limited illness to a serious disease with hemolytic anemia, renal failure, and hypotension, primarily in patients of advanced age or in those with underlying chronic disease. Babesiosis can be diagnosed by examining Wright-stained or Giemsa-stained peripheral blood smears. The parasites invade erythrocytes and appear as small intraerythrocytic ring forms resembling the causative organism of malaria, *Plasmodium falciparum*. An indirect immunofluorescence test titer of greater than or equal to 1:64 is considered positive for babesiosis, although most patients with acute illness have titers of greater than or equal to 1:1024. The recommended treatment for this illness consists of a 7-day course of oral quinine plus clindamycin (by the intravenous or oral route).[107]

Fungal Infections

As a general rule, fungal infections occur in individuals who are immunosuppressed as a result of (1) AIDS; (2) organ transplantation; (3) immunosuppressive chemotherapy or chronic corticosteroid therapy; or (4) chronic disease. The single exception to this generalization is cryptococcal meningitis, which may occur in healthy individuals. The fungus-causing infection can be predicted to some degree based on the predisposing condition. For example, individuals with AIDS are at risk for meningitis due to *Cryptococcus neoformans* and *Histoplasma capsulatum*. Cryptococcal meningitis is the most common life-threatening opportunistic fungal infection in patients with AIDS and occurs in 5 to 10 percent of patients, typically when their circulating CD4+ T lymphocyte count is less than 100 cells/mm^3.[110] Two fungi are responsible for the majority of CNS fungal infections in patients who have undergone organ transplantation. Fungal meningitis in these patients is typically due to *C. neoformans*, and fungal brain abscesses are often due to *Aspergillus fumigatus*. Patients receiving chronic corticosteroid therapy and patients who have received bone marrow transplantation are at risk for cryptococcal meningitis and CNS candidiasis. *Candida* tend to cause intraparenchymal microabscesses, mainly in the territory of the middle cerebral artery. Individuals with granulocytopenia for any reason are at risk for infections due to *Candida*, *Aspergillus fumigatus*, and the Zygomycetes organisms (mucormycosis).[111] Intravenous drug abusers are at a particular risk for fungal brain abscesses due to Zygomycetes and *Candida*. *Coccidioides immitis* is a dimorphic fungus that is endemic to the desert areas of the Southwest, specifically California, Arizona, New Mexico, and Texas. The disease is acquired by inhaling the infectious particles, but less than 1 percent of individuals who develop a primary infection develop disseminated disease. Coccidioidomycosis should be considered in the differential diagnosis of any febrile illness in a transplant recipient in an endemic area for this fungus.[112] The fungus *Blastomyces dermatitidis* is found principally in North America in the Mississippi, Ohio, and St. Lawrence river basins; the Great Lakes area; and the southeastern United States. Infection is most likely to be acquired as a result of occupational exposure to contaminated soil.[113] CNS involvement by this fungus is nearly always the result of hematogenous spread from a pulmonary source or occurs as result of infection in contiguous structures or with osteomyelitis.[114]

CRYPTOCOCCUS NEOFORMANS

Cryptococcus neoformans is an encapsulated yeastlike fungus. Infection is acquired through direct exposure to bird droppings. The infection is initially characterized by a localized pneumonitis, but when dissemination occurs the CNS is a preferential site for disease, presumably because the CSF is a good culture media for cryptococci.[115] The most common symptoms of cryptococcal meningitis are headache, fever, and malaise, but cryptococcal meningitis may also present with nausea and vomiting, meningeal signs, altered mental status, and cranial nerve palsies. Cryptococcal skin lesions may precede the development of meningitis; when present, they are an indication for lumbar puncture, even in the absence of signs and symptoms of meningitis.[116] Diagnosis is made by examination of the CSF, and the following are typical abnormalities: (1) normal or slightly elevated opening pressure; (2) lymphocytic pleocytosis; (3) elevated protein concentration; (4) decreased glucose concentration; and (5) positive cryptococcal antigen. The cryptococcal antigen is a highly sensitive and specific test and should be performed on all CSF specimens. A reactive CSF cryptococcal antigen test establishes the diagnosis. *C. neoformans* can also be grown in culture of CSF.

The treatment of cryptococcal meningitis in immunocompetent patients includes either a combination of intravenous amphotericin B (0.5 to 0.7 mg/kg/d) plus oral flucytosine (25 mg/kg qid) or Ambisome 5 mg/kg/day. A combination of amphotericin B plus flucytosine or Ambisome monotherapy is used for 2 weeks or until the CSF culture is sterile. This induction therapy is followed by fluconazole 400 to 800 mg/day, which is continued for 8 to 10 weeks. The therapy of cryptococcal meningitis in patients with AIDS includes a combination of intravenous amphotericin B (0.7 to 1.0 mg/kg/d) with flucytosine (100 mg/kg/d in four divided doses) for at least 2 weeks or until the CSF culture is sterile followed by fluconazole (400 mg/d) for 10 to 12 weeks, at which point the CSF should be recultured. When the CSF culture is sterile, the patient is switched to maintenance fluconazole (200 mg/d) therapy for life.

The management of increased ICP is critical to successful outcome from cryptococcal meningitis. ICP should be measured at the initial lumbar puncture, at the completion of induction therapy, and anytime during the course of the illness when the patient has a change in mental status or a change in the neurological examination (gait abnormalities, pathologically brisk reflexes, cranial nerve abnormalities, visual changes). The increased ICP is due to altered CSF hemodynamics and should be managed with either daily lumbar punctures (to decrease CSF pressure by 50 percent and maintain CSF pressure at less than 300 mm H_2O), a ventriculostomy, or a ventriculoperitoneal shunt. Corticosteroid therapy should not be used in cryptococcal meningitis.

The most common adverse reaction to amphotericin B is fever, chills, and hypotension 1 to 3 hours after initiation of the IV infusion. Renal insufficiency and anemia are common adverse reactions during the course of therapy, and renal insufficiency may necessitate interruption of therapy or reduction of dose. The most common adverse reaction to flucytosine is leukopenia. The most common adverse reactions to fluconazole are nausea, vomiting, and elevated serum transaminases.

HISTOPLASMA CAPSULATUM

Histoplasma capsulatum is a dimorphic fungus that is endemic to the Ohio and Mississippi River valleys of the central United States. The fungus is acquired by inhalation. Dissemination is rare and occurs primarily in patients with defective cellular immunity, such as patients with AIDS, patients with lymphoreticular malignancies, and organ transplant recipients.[115] The most common presentation of CNS histoplasmosis is meningitis. The typical presentation includes fever, sweats, weight loss, headache, mental status abnormalities (including decreased level of consciousness, confusion, personality changes, and/or memory impairment), cranial nerve palsies, stroke, or seizures.[115] CNS histoplasmosis may also be a solitary abscess or multiple lesions, but meningitis is the much more common presentation. The majority of patients with CNS histoplasmosis have an abnormal neuroimaging study with meningeal enhancement, hydrocephalus, solitary or disseminated contrast-enhancing lesions, or various combinations of these entities. Chest radiographs should be obtained. The most common x-ray abnormalities in histoplasmosis are diffuse or focal pulmonary infiltrates. *Histoplasma* polysaccharide antigen (HPA) in urine, blood, and CSF may allow for a rapid diagnosis. The presence of the HPA in CSF is a reliable indicator of CNS involvement; however, cross reactions with *C. immitis*, *C. neoformans*, and *Candida* have been reported.[115] Serological tests for anti-*Histoplasma capsulatum* antibodies may be helpful. They may also be misleading and can be negative in 10 to 25 percent of patients with disseminated histoplasmosis or falsely positive in patients with other fungal diseases or tuberculosis. Antibodies remain elevated for several years despite resolution of histoplasmosis and may lead to a misdiagnosis of patients with neurological illnesses caused by other diseases.[117] Examination of the CSF typically reveals a lymphocytic pleocytosis ($\leq$ 100 cells/mm^3), although a predominance of polymorphonuclear leukocytes may also occur. The CSF protein concentration is increased, and the CSF glucose concentration is usually decreased. It is rare to identify the fungus on CSF India ink stain. The CSF culture, however, is frequently positive, as are blood, bone marrow, and urine cultures. In general, when fungal meningitis is suspected, multiple cultures of lumbar fluid should be obtained to identify the organism. Consideration should also be given to obtaining CSF by a cisternal puncture. In cases of *H. capsulatum* meningitis, one CSF culture out of several is typically positive, stressing the need for repeated attempts to isolate the fungus using large volumes of centrifuged CSF.[115] Intravenous amphotericin B (0.75 to 1.0 mg/kg/d) remains the mainstay of treatment of CNS histoplasmosis. A total dose of 30 mg/kg is recommended. A course of amphotericin B is followed by oral itraconazole 200 mg twice daily for 6 months to 1 year. Itraconazole is the antifungal agent of choice for chronic suppressive therapy in patients with AIDS.[115]

COCCIDIOIDES IMMITIS

Coccidioides immitis is a dimorphic fungus that is endemic to the desert areas of the Southwest, specifically California, Arizona, New Mexico, and Texas. *C. immitis* grows as a mycelia that releases air-borne arthroconidia, which when inhaled and in the alveoli transform into spherules containing endospores. Infection is most often either asymptomatic or a limited pneumonitis with fever and cough. Dissemination occurs in less than 1 percent of patients, and CNS disease is primarily a meningitis. A predisposition to disseminated disease has been associated with the following: (1) pregnancy—infection that is acquired during the third trimester is associated with an increased risk of severe disease; (2) hemodialysis; (3) immunosuppressive therapy; (4) extremes of age; (5) race—patients of African-American, Hispanic, and Filipino descent have a higher risk of dissemination; (6) AIDS; and (7) organ transplantation.[115] Meningitis is a common initial presentation of coccidioidomycosis in AIDS patients. The most common symptoms and signs of *C. immitis* meningitis are headache, change in mental status (particularly lethargy and confusion), low-grade fever, and weight loss.[112] There may be evidence of skin lesions, and biopsy of these with visualization of typical *C. immitis* spherules makes the diagnosis. The coccidioidal skin test has no role in the diagnostic evaluation of a CNS infection because false-negative results are common, and positive results only indicate prior exposure to the fungus.[115] The diagnosis of *C. immitis* meningitis is made by examination of the CSF. The complement fixation antibody test on CSF is reported to have a specificity of 100 percent and a sensitivity of 75 percent in the setting of active disease.[113] Coccidioidal meningitis can present as an eosinophilic meningitis.[115] Positive cultures may be obtained in up to one third of patients. *C. immitis* meningitis is treated with a combination of intravenous amphotericin B (0.5 to 0.75 mg/kg/d) plus intrathecal amphotericin B (0.25 to 0.75 mg/d three times weekly). Intravenous amphotericin B is continued for at least a year after obtaining a normal CSF. Intrathecal amphotericin B is continued for 3 months, followed by a tapering course. The CSF glucose and protein concentrations can remain abnormal for years, and the CSF cell count is unreliable because it may decrease spontaneously in untreated CNS coccidioidomycosis. A sudden rise in cell count or CSF complement fixation antibody titer, however, is a sign of a relapse, and more intense antifungal therapy should be administered in this instance.[115]

BLASTOMYCES DERMATITIDIS

As discussed previously, infection with *Blastomyces dermatitidis* is primarily associated with outdoor activities including occupational exposure such as construction work, mining, and recreational activities. The AIDS epidemic has not affected the epidemiology of blastomycosis.[115] Initial infection with this fungus is essentially a pulmonary disease. The chest x-ray demonstrates nonspecific infiltrates, predominantly at the bases.[115] Dissemination to the CNS presents as single or multiple intracranial abscesses or granulomas, cranial and spinal extradural abscesses, and acute or chronic meningitis. Meningitis due to *B. dermatitidis* presents as a subacute infection with headache, anorexia, and weight loss. *B. dermatitidis* brain abscess or abscesses present with focal neurological deficits, seizures, and signs of increased ICP. Neuroimaging demonstrates evidence of a single or multiple homogeneously enhancing lesions. Chronic blastomycotic meningitis predominantly involves the basilar meninges and may be associated with hydrocephalus.[115] The one exception to the rule that fungal meningitis presents with a lymphocytic pleocytosis is *B. dermatitidis* meningitis, which may present with a polymorphonuclear leukocytic pleocytosis. A CSF cell count of greater than 5000 cells/mm^3 is not uncommon. The CSF glucose concentration may be markedly decreased, and the protein concentration is typically elevated. It is rare to identify *B. dermatitidis* from CSF obtained by lumbar puncture. Culture of cisternal or ventricular CSF has a better yield. There is no reliable *B. dermatitidis* antigen detection test available.[115] Treatment requires the administration of intravenous amphotericin B (0.5 to 0.8 mg/kg/d). Lifelong suppressive therapy with itraconazole in AIDS patients is recommended.

ASPERGILLUS FUMIGATUS

Aspergillus species are ubiquitous, and infection is acquired by inhaling conidia. CNS aspergillosis is rare in immunocompetent individuals. Isolated aspergilloma are unusual, except in intravenous drug abusers. Individuals who are granulocytopenic and those who have received organ transplantation are at risk for brain abscesses owing to aspergillosis. CNS aspergillosis typically occurs preferentially in major vascular territories and presents as isolated or multiple ischemic infarctions or subarachnoid hemorrhage from a ruptured mycotic aneurysm.[115] The majority of patients with aspergillosis will have an unremitting fever, despite broad-spectrum antibiotics, and pulmonary infiltrates on chest radiographs.[118] The diagnosis is made through sputum culture or lung tissue biopsy culture. CSF analysis is usually not helpful because meningitis is unusual.[115] Aspergillus is rarely, if ever, cultured from blood. Treatment should include intravenous amphotericin B (0.8 to 1.0 mg/kg/d) or preferably a lipid preparation of amphotericin B, either liposomal amphotericin B (Ambisome) 5 mg/kg/d or amphotericin B lipid complex (ABLC) 5 mg/kg/d.

CANDIDA

CNS candidiasis occurs in patients who have undergone organ transplantation, those receiving chronic corticosteroid therapy, those with a prolonged stay in the intensive care unit requiring invasive monitoring devices, and those who are treated with broad-spectrum antibiotics. CNS infections due to *Candida* present as either meningitis or cerebritis from multiple small parenchymal abscesses.[115] CNS infection due to *Candida* often occurs in conjunction with fungemia.[119] The majority of patients with CNS *Candida* infections have positive fungal blood cultures and are neutropenic.[119] Scattered, irregular ring-enhancing lesions surrounded by edema may be present on neuroimaging studies. A definitive diagnosis is made through CSF or tissue biopsy and culture. Standard therapy includes intravenous amphotericin B (0.5 to 0.7 mg/kg/d) plus flucytosine (100 mg/kg/d in four divided doses).

ZYGOMYCETES

The Mucoraceae are in the Zygomycetes class and cause the disease mucormycosis. This disorder is typically an acute fulminant CNS infection that occurs primarily in immunocompetent patients with ketoacidosis and in diabetic transplant recipients receiving immunosuppressive agents. The infection tends to originate in the palate or paranasal sinuses and spreads through the orbits and paranasal sinuses into the brain. The infection is often manifest by a black eschar on the palate or nasal mucosa with a blackish purulent discharge from the involved areas. Examination of the CSF demonstrates an elevated opening pressure, a pleocytosis with a predominance of polymorphonuclear cells, a normal glucose concentration, and an elevated protein concentration. Diagnosis is made by a biopsy of the black eschar.[120] The treatment of CNS mucormycosis involves debridement of all devitalized tissues and high-dose amphotericin B (1.0 mg/kg/d) or Ambisome (5 mg/kg/d) or ABLC (5 mg/kg/d).[115]

Amebic Infections

Naegleria and *Acanthamoeba* are free-living amebae that infect the CNS. *Naegleria fowleri* causes an acute fulminant meningoencephalitis, known as primary amebic meningoencephalitis, and is acquired by swimming or waterskiing in small, shallow freshwater lakes as a result of direct contamination through the nasal cavity. Infection with this organism has also been acquired from swimming in chlorinated pools; presumably, the organism gets into the pool through cracks in the pool. In Africa, cases have been reported during the dry and windy season by inhalation of dust containing amebic cysts.[109]

Acanthamoeba CNS infections are generally not water related and occur in immunosuppressed and debilitated individuals. This organism has been isolated from the nasopharynx of asymptomatic individuals. *Acanthamoeba* keratitis has been reported in healthy contact lens wearers.[109]

N. fowleri invades the nasal mucosa and ascends to the brain through the cribriform plate via the fila olfactoria, extensions of the olfactory nerves.[121] Amebae can then spread throughout the meninges. The temporal and frontal lobes are most severely affected. *Acanthamoeba* spp. reach the nervous system through the bloodstream from a distant site of infection or from a corneal infection of the eye and typically cause a subacute or chronic meningoencephalitis, or inflammatory lesions in multiple areas of the brain, particularly the white matter, the basal ganglia, the brain stem, and the cerebellum. A necrotizing vasculitis is common owing to invasion of arterial walls by trophozoites.[121]

The incubation period for infection by *N. fowleri* is usually 4 to 7 days. The patient presents with severe bifrontal headache, high fever, nausea, vomiting, and meningismus, a clinical presentation resembling bacterial meningitis. Twenty-four to forty-eight hours later, signs of encephalitis with focal neurological deficits, confusion, delirium, stupor, and finally coma occur. Meningoencephalitis due to *Naegleria* is typically a fatal disease with death occurring within 2 to 4 days. Because of involvement of the olfactory bulbs and tracts, early symptoms of abnormal smell or taste sensation have been reported. The incubation period of *Acanthamoeba* is longer than that of *Naegleria* infections and is typically weeks to months. The insidious onset of symptoms and signs of focal encephalitis or focal mass lesions follows. The presentation may include seizures, hemiparesis, visual disturbances, headache, low-grade fever, and ataxia.

A diagnosis of *N. fowleri* meningoencephalitis is rarely made while the patient is alive. Examination of the CSF demonstrates a leukocytosis with a neutrophilic predominance, an increased protein concentration, and a decreased glucose concentration. The ameboid movements of the trophozoites can be seen on fresh or wet unstained specimens of CSF. Trophozoites can also be demonstrated in the brain by light or electron microscopy. Serological tests for *Naegleria* are of limited value because patients usually die before the results are available. In contrast, serological tests for *Acanthamoeba* infections are helpful in diagnosis. Neuroimaging scans may demonstrate one or multiple abscesses of *Acanthamoeba*. Examination of the CSF shows a mild lymphocytic pleocytosis with a normal to decreased glucose concentration and a mild increase in protein concentration.[109]

The drug of choice for acute *N. fowleri* meningoencephalitis is intravenous amphotericin B (1 mg/kg/d) for at least 2 to 3 weeks. A few survivors of this infection have been documented, but one survivor required treatment with a combination of intravenous and intrathecal amphotericin B, intravenous and intrathecal miconazole, and rifampin, sulfisoxazole, and dexamethasone. The outcome may be improved by adding intrathecal amphotericin B (0.5 mg on alternate days) to parenteral amphotericin B.[109, 122, 123] *Acanthamoeba* abscesses are treated with surgical excision and amphotericin B. Although amphotericin B is amebicidal for *N. fowleri*, it is much less active against *Acanthamoeba*.[121] No effective vaccine for free-living amebae infections exist. Children should be prevented from swimming in contaminated fresh water, and *Acanthamoeba* keratitis can be prevented by using appropriate antimicrobial contact lens cleaning solutions.[121]

Neurocysticercosis

Epidemiology and Risk Factors. Neurocysticercosis is considered the most common parasitic disease of the CNS. In countries where this infection is endemic, it is the most common cause of late-onset epilepsy. Humans acquire cysticercosis by the ingestion of food contaminated with *Taenia solium* eggs, most often undercooked pork but also water and vegetables contaminated with human feces.[124]

Pathogenesis and Pathophysiology. After food contaminated with *T. solium* eggs is ingested, the eggs hatch into oncospheres in the stomach of the host. Oncospheres cross the intestinal wall, enter the bloodstream, and are carried to the eye, skeletal muscle, and the CNS. After 2 months, cysticerci develop in the brain parenchyma, subarachnoid space, ventricular space, or spinal cord. When the parasite invades the CNS, it may either stimulate an intense inflammatory response or an inflammatory response that develops so slowly that the cysticerci may live in the CNS for several years. When the parasite lodges in the brain parenchyma, the inflammatory response results in a thin capsule of fibrous tissue surrounding the cyst. With the passage of time, the capsule thickens. The parasite may be destroyed, and the site where the cyst was located is replaced by a granuloma composed of astroglial and fibrous tissue that subsequently becomes mineralized with deposits of calcium salts. The process of calcification of the granuloma takes several years after the disappearance of the parasite.[124] In any individual, one or several hundred cysticerci may exist. Cysts that develop in the subarachnoid space are associated with an inflammatory response in the subarachnoid space with subsequent fibrosis of the arachnoid membranes. Hydrocephalus is a complication of the inflammation and fibrosis in the subarachnoid space that interferes with the normal CSF resorption in the arachnoid granulations. Cysts that grow in the sylvian fissure and the subarachnoid space at the base of the skull may grow as large as 10 to 15 cm. A single cyst that is lodged inside the fourth ventricle can produce a valve mechanism on the outflow of CSF and can lead to subacute hydrocephalus with episodes of sudden increases in ICP related to movements of the head. This ventricular form of neurocysticercosis is the result of the arrival of the oncospheres at the choroid plexus of the lateral ventricles via the bloodstream with the parasites remaining in the ependyma of the choroid plexus. In meningeal and spinal cord cysticercosis, the oncospheres also enter the CNS at the choroid plexus, but the passage of the parasites along the CSF pathways is rapid, and the oncospheres hatch in the arachnoid membranes along the neural axis and evolve into cysticerci.[124]

Clinical Features. The diagnosis of neurocysticercosis should be considered in any patient who is a resident or immigrant from areas endemic for cysticercosis, or who has traveled to areas endemic for cysticercosis, and has new onset partial seizures, with or without secondary generalization, cognitive impairment, confusion, stupor, or signs of raised ICP. In the majority of patients, the clinical manifestation of parenchymal granulomas is partial seizures. Patients with meningeal cysticercosis may present with headache, vertigo, vomiting, papilledema, an altered level of consciousness, and gait disturbances due to the intense and widespread immune response in the subarachnoid space and the subsequent development of hydrocephalus. Cysticerci located in the spinal canal may manifest with signs and symptoms similar to an intraspinal tumor.[124]

Evaluation. The lesions of neurocysticercosis are readily visualized by CT and MRI. Granulomas are the most common finding in patients with neurocysticercosis. A very early sign of cyst death is hypointensity of the vesicular fluid on MRI T2-weighted images when compared with CSF. The ELISA and the complement fixation test can be performed on CSF and are highly specific and sensitive for the detection of anticysticercus antibodies. It is recommended that both tests be done on the CSF to increase the probability of diagnosis. These CSF immunodiagnostic tests are also useful to distinguish the inactive sequelae of neurocysticercosis, such as granulomas and calcifications, from the active forms. The test results are negative in the absence of active forms of the parasite. These tests remain positive for a few months in patients who are successfully treated with an anticysticercus drug after the disappearance of cysts. Serum immunodiagnostic tests lack reliability for the diagnosis of neurocysticercosis. About 30 percent of healthy individuals from endemic areas will have positive serology. In addition, patients with parenchymal or ventricular neurocysticercosis with positive immunodiagnostic tests on CSF may have negative serology.[124]

Management. Albendazole and praziquantel are cysticidal. Approximately 85 percent of parenchymal cysts are destroyed by a single course of albendazole, and approximately 75 percent are destroyed by a single course of praziquantel. The sequential use of two drugs increases the possibility of successful elimination of parasites to more than 95 percent of parenchymal cysticerci; therefore, a trial of cysticidal therapy is recommended before surgery is attempted. The dose of albendazole is 15 mg/kg/d in two doses for 8 days. Praziquantel is given in a single day in three doses of 25 to 30 mg/kg every 2 hours. Dexamethasone (16 mg/d) is also recommended to decrease the inflammatory reaction due to the destruction of the parasites. If the lesions persist unchanged on neuroimaging study 3 months after therapy is completed, praziquantel 50 mg/kg/d in three divided doses for 15 days is recommended. During the first few days of cysticidal therapy, headache, vomiting, or seizures may develop owing to an intense inflammatory response from the host to the acute death of the parasites. These symptoms are particularly intense in patients with many cysts. In the management of parenchymal cysticercosis, a differentiation must be made between active and inactive forms of the parasite, such as granulomas and calcification, because no response to cysticidal therapy will occur in inactive disease. Seizure activity secondary to parenchymal cysts should be managed with anticonvulsants. Parenchymal cysts that are destroyed by cysticidal therapy, without leaving granulomas, do not result in long-term seizure disorders. In these patients, the early withdrawal of antiepileptic drugs is recommended. A seizure disorder that is secondary to granulomas requires long-term anticonvulsant therapy.[124]

Malaria

Human malaria is caused by one of four species of *Plasmodium*. The majority of cases of malaria worldwide are caused by *P. falciparum*, and *P. falciparum* is the only species that causes cerebral malaria. Malaria is transmitted to healthy individuals through the bite of an infected mosquito.[125] The World Health Organization defines cerebral malaria as "unarousable coma not attributed to any other cause in a patient with *P. falciparum* malaria."[126] Malaria can be transmitted by the bite of an *Anopheles* mosquito, through blood transfusions, and by intravenous injections with blood-contaminated needles. The incidence of cerebral malaria in a population is determined by the population's immunity. In holoendemic areas, which are areas of the world where significant transmission of malaria occurs annually with little change from year to year, native adults rarely develop cerebral malaria. Persons at risk for severe malaria in these areas are children from 1 to 4 years of age, new residents from nonendemic areas, returning residents who have lived abroad for years, residents who were maintained on chemoprophylaxis but have stopped, and pregnant women. Travelers to endemic areas are at high risk for infection. Infected mosquitoes can be transported from endemic areas via airplane, and travelers may acquire malaria during brief stopovers without disembarking from the airplane. *P. falciparum* malaria requires a minimum of 8 days for incubation, and 95 percent of all infections present within 4 weeks of the last mosquito exposure.[125]

Systemic signs of malaria include jaundice, retinal hemorrhage, hepatosplenomegaly, fatigue, diarrhea, vomiting, abdominal pain, chest pain, cough, myalgia, and arthralgia. The majority of patients are febrile. Cerebral malaria presents with headache followed by an altered level of consciousness and convulsions. On neurological examination, upper motor neuron signs are common as is decerebrate or decorticate posturing, delirium, hallucinations, delusions, and disorders of dysconjugate gaze. Coma is often associated with shock, acidosis, noncardiogenic pulmonary edema, hemolysis, anemia, renal insufficiency, and hypoglycemia. These are all potentially treatable complications.[127] Diagnosis is made by examining a blood smear for parasites. Blood smear should be examined every 12 to 24 hours for a period of 2 to 3 days, and the number of intraerythrocytic parasites should be counted.

In the United States, parenteral quinidine is the drug of choice for the treatment of cerebral malaria. Cerebral malaria is treated with a loading dose of 10 mg/kg of intravenous quinidine gluconate over a period of 1 to 2 hours followed by continuous infusion of 0.02 mg/kg/min. Loading doses of quinidine are not recommended for patients who have received mefloquine, quinine, or quinidine in the 24 hours before initiation of therapy. When the patient is able to take oral medication, therapy can be changed to one of the oral antimalarial agents to complete a total of 7 days of treatment from the initiation of intravenous therapy.[125] Quinidine is cardiotoxic, and patients receiving parenteral forms of this agent should be monitored for arrhythmias, prolongation of the QT interval, and widening of the QRS complex.

Recommendations for malaria chemoprophylaxis depend on the area to which the individual plans to travel. In the few areas where the parasite remains sensitive to chloroquine, this antimalarial agent should be taken in a weekly dose of 300 mg base. Chemoprophylaxis should begin 2 weeks before departure and should continue for 6 weeks after return. In areas where the parasite is resistant to chloroquine, mefloquine is recommended at a once per week oral dose of 250 mg beginning 2 weeks before departure and continued for 4 weeks after return.[128]

Acknowledgment

The technical assistance of Mrs. Linda Hagan in the preparation of this chapter is greatly appreciated.

Reviews and Selected Updates

Aksamit AJ: Cerebrospinal fluid in the diagnosis of central nervous system infections. *In* Roos KL (ed): Central Nervous System Infectious Diseases and Therapy. New York, Marcel Dekker, 1997, pp 731–746.

American Academy of Neurology Therapeutics and Technology Assessment Subcommittee: Assessment: DTP vaccination. AAN Practice Handbook. Minneapolis, American Academy of Neurology Publications, 1991, p 143–144.

Halperin JJ, Logigian EL, Finkel MF, Pearl RA: Practice parameters for the diagnosis of patients with nervous system Lyme borreliosis (Lyme disease). Quality Standards Subcommittee of the American Academy of Neurology. Neurology 1996;46:619–627.

Lanska DJ: Anthrax meningoencephalitis. Neurology 2002;59:327–334.

Marra CM: Neurosyphilis. *In* Roos KL (ed): Central Nervous System Infectious Diseases and Therapy. New York, Marcel Dekker, 1997, pp 237–252.

Morris SM: Suggested dosing regimens and adverse effects of antimicrobials used in central nervous system infections. Semin Neurol 2000; 20:393–398.

Parola P, Raoult D: Ticks and tickborne bacterial diseases in humans: an emerging infectious threat. Clin Infect Dis 2001;32:897–928.

Roos KL: Meningitis: 100 Maxims in Neurology. London, Arnold, 1997, pp 1–208.

Smith RR: Neuroimaging of central nervous system infections. *In* Roos KL (ed): Central Nervous System Infectious Diseases and Therapy. New York, Marcel Dekker, 1997, pp 619–666.

Sotelo J: Neurocysticercosis. *In* Roos KL (ed): Central Nervous System Infectious Disease and Therapy. New York, Marcel Dekker, 1997, pp 545–572.

Trujillo M, McCracken GH: Neonatal meningitis. *In* Roos KL (ed): Central Nervous System Infectious Diseases and Therapy. New York, Marcel Dekker, 1997, pp 25–44.

Wormser GP, Nadelman RB, Dattwyler RJ, et al: Practice guidelines for the treatment of Lyme disease, The Infectious Disease Society of America. Clin Infect Dis 2000;31(Suppl 1):1–14.

References

1. Trujillo M, McCracken GH: Neonatal meningitis. *In* Roos KL (ed): Central Nervous System Infectious Diseases and Therapy. New York, Marcel Dekker, 1997, pp 25–44.
2. Roos KL, Tunkel AR, Scheld WM: Acute bacterial meningitis in children and adults. *In* Scheld WM, Whitley RJ, Durack DT (eds): Infections of the Central Nervous System, 2nd ed. Philadelphia, Lippincott-Raven, 1997, pp 335–401.
3. Roos KL: Etiologic organism. *In* Roos KL (ed): Meningitis: 100 Maxims in Neurology. London, Arnold, 1997, pp 53–68.
4. Rasmussen HH, Sorensen HT, Moller-Petersen J, et al: Bacterial meningitis in elderly patients: Clinical picture and course. Age Ageing 1992;21:216–220.
5. Gorse GJ, Thrupp LD, Nudleman KL, et al: Bacterial meningitis in the elderly. Arch Intern Med 1984;144:1603–1607.
6. Swartz M: Acute bacterial meningitis. *In* Gorbach SL, Bartlett JG, Blacklow NR (ed): Infectious Diseases. Philadelphia, WB Saunders, 1992, pp 1160–1177.
7. Roos KL: Bacterial meningitis. *In* Roos KL (ed): Central Nervous System Infectious Diseases and Therapy. New York, Marcel Dekker, 1997, pp 99–126.
8. Roos KL: Pathogenesis and pathophysiology of bacterial meningitis. *In* Roos KL (ed): Meningitis: 100 Maxims in Neurology. London, Arnold, 1997, pp 6–20.
9. Zwahlen A, Nydegger UE, Vaudaux P, et al: Complement-mediated opsonic activity in normal and infected human cerebrospinal fluid: early response during bacterial meningitis. J Infect Dis 1982;145:635–646.
10. Simberkoff MS, Moldover NH, Rahal J Jr: Absence of detectable bactericidal and opsonic activities in normal and infected human cerebrospinal fluids: A regional host defense deficiency. J Lab Clin Med 1980;95:362–372.
11. Dinarello CA: Interleukin-1. Rev Infect Dis 1984;6:51–95.
12. Dinarello CA: An update on human interleukin-1: From molecular biology to clinical relevance. J Clin Immunol 1985;5:287–296.
13. Kruger J, Dinarello C, Chedid L: Promotion of slow wave sleep by a purified interleukin-1 preparation. Fed Proc 1983;42:356.
14. Spellerberg B, Tuomanen EI: The pathophysiology of pneumococcal meningitis. Ann Med 1994;26:411–418.
15. Tureen JH, Dworkin RJ, Kennedy SL, et al: Loss of cerebrovascular autoregulation in experimental meningitis in rabbits. J Clin Invest 1990;85:577–581.
16. Roos KL: Clinical presentation of bacterial meningitis. *In* Roos KL (ed): Meningitis: 100 Maxims in Neurology. London, Arnold, 1997, pp 20–35.
17. Kernig VM: Ueber ein Krankheits Symptom der acuten Meningitis. St. Petersburg Medizinische Wochenschrift 1882;7:398.
18. Verghese A, Gallemore G: Kernig's and Brudzinski's signs revisited. Rev Infect Dis 1987;9:1187–1192.
19. Feigin RD, McCracken GH, Klein JO: Diagnosis and management of meningitis. Pediatr Infect Dis J 1992;11:785–814.
20. Cushing H: Concerning a definite regulatory mechanism of the vasomotor centre which controls blood pressure during cerebral compression. Johns Hopkins Hosp Bull 1901;12:290–292.
21. Roos KL: Cerebrospinal fluid. *In* Roos KL (ed): Meningitis: 100 Maxims in Neurology. London, Arnold, 1997, pp 36–52.
22. Dougherty JM, Roth RM: Cerebral spinal fluid. Emer Med Clin North Am 1986;4:281–297.
23. Bonadio WA: The cerebrospinal fluid: Physiologic aspects and alterations associated with bacterial meningitis. Pediatr Infect Dis J 1992;11:423–432.
24. Powers WJ: Cerebrospinal fluid lymphocytosis in acute bacterial meningitis. Amer J Med 1985;79:216–220.
25. Cherubin CE, Marr JS, Sierra MF, Becker S: Listeria and gram-negative bacillary meningitis in New York City, 1972–1979. Amer J Med 1981; 71:199–208.
26. Unhanand M, Mustafa MM, McCracken GH, Nelson JD: Gram-negative enteric bacillary meningitis: A twenty-one-year experience. J Pediatr 1993;122:15–21.
27. Bonadio WA: Bacterial meningitis in children whose cerebrospinal fluid contains polymorphonuclear leukocytes without pleocytosis. Clin Pediatr 1988;27:198–200.
28. Committee on Infectious Diseases: Dexamethasone therapy for bacterial meningitis in infants and children. Pediatrics 1990;86:130–133.
29. Girgis NI, Farid Z, Mikhail IA, et al: Dexamethasone treatment for bacterial meningitis in children and adults. Pediatr Infect Dis J 1989; 8:848–851.
30. Gaillard JL, Abadie V, Cheron G, et al: Concentrations of ceftriaxone in cerebrospinal fluid of children with meningitis receiving dexamethasone therapy. Antimicrob Agents Chemother 1994;38:1209–1210.
31. Prober CG: The role of steroids in the management of children with bacterial meningitis. Pediatr 1995;95:29–31.
32. Tureen JH, Tauber MG, Sande MA: Effect of hydration status on cerebral blood flow and cerebrospinal fluid lactic acidosis in rabbits with experimental meningitis. J Clin Invest 1992;89:947–953.
33. Kaplan SL, Fishman MA: Supportive therapy for bacterial meningitis. Pediatr Infect Dis J 1987;6:670–677.

34. Roos KL: Therapy of bacterial meningitis. *In* Roos KL (ed): Meningitis: 100 Maxims in Neurology. London, Arnold, 1997, pp 69–108.
35. Annegers JF, Hauser WA, Beghi E, et al: The risk of unprovoked seizures after encephalitis and meningitis. Neurology 1988;38:1477–1510.
36. Ropper AH: Treatment of intracranial hypertension. *In* Ropper AH (ed): Neurological and Neurosurgical Intensive Care. New York, Raven Press, 1993, pp 29–52.
37. Dacey RG: Monitoring and treating increased intracranial pressure. Pediatr Infect Dis J 1987;6:1161–1163.
38. Klein JO, Feigin RD, McCracken GH: Report of the task force on diagnosis and management of meningitis. Pediatrics 1986;78:S959–982.
39. Dodge PR, Swartz MN: Bacterial meningitis: A review of selected aspects: II. Special neurologic problems, postmeningitic complications and clinico-pathologic correlations. N Engl J Med 1965; 272:1003–1010.
40. Fritz DP, Nelson PB: Brain abscess. *In* Roos KL (ed): Central Nervous System Infectious Diseases and Therapy. New York, Marcel Dekker, 1997, pp 481–498.
41. Garvey G: Current concepts of bacterial infection of the central nervous system: Bacterial meningitis and bacterial brain abscess. J Neurosurg 1983;59:735–744.
42. Molinari GF, Smith L, Goldstein MN, Satran R: Brain abscess from septic cerebral embolism: An experimental model. Neurology 1973; 23:1205–1210.
43. Britt RH, Enzmann DR, Yeager AS: Neuropathological and computed tomographic findings in experimental brain abscess. J Neurosurg 1981;55:590–603.
44. Britt RH, Enzmann DR: Clinical stages of human brain abscesses on serial CT scans after contrast infusion: Computerized tomographic, neuropathological, and clinical correlations. J Neurosurg 1983;59:972–989.
45. Hirschberg H, Bosnes V: C-reactive protein levels in the differential diagnosis of brain abscesses. J Neurosurg 1987;67:358–360.
46. Shapiro S: Cranial epidural abscess and cranial subdural empyema. *In* Roos KL (ed): Central Nervous System Infectious Diseases and Therapy. New York, Marcel Dekker, 1977, pp 499–506.
47. Bleck TP, Greenlee JE: Subdural empyema. *In* Mandell GL, Douglas RG, Bennett JE (eds): Principles and Practice of Infectious Diseases, 5th ed.. New York, Churchill Livingstone, 2000, pp 1028–1031.
48. Silverberg AL, DiNubile MJ: Subdural empyema and cranial epidural abscess. Med Clin North Am 1985;69:361–374.
49. Farmer TW, Wise GR: Subdural empyema in infants, children and adults. Neurology 1973;23:254–261.
50. Jacobson PL, Farmer TW: Subdural empyema complicating meningitis in infants: Improved prognosis. Neurology 1981;31:190–193.
51. Roos KL, Scheld WM: Central nervous system infections. *In* Crossley KB, Archer GL (eds): The Staphylococci in Human Disease. New York, Churchill Livingstone, 1997, pp 413–439.
52. Kubik CS, Adams RD: Subdural empyema. Brain 1943;66:18–42.
53. Kaufman DM, Miller MH, Steigbigel NH: Subdural empyema: Analysis of 17 recent cases and review of the literature. Medicine 1975;54:485–498.
54. Lee SH: Infectious diseases. *In* Lee SH, Rao KC (eds): Cranial Computed Tomography. New York, McGraw-Hill, 1983, pp 506–546.
55. Shapiro S: Spinal epidural abscess and spinal subdural empyema. *In* Roos KL (ed): Central Nervous System Infectious Diseases and Therapy. New York, Marcel Dekker, 1997, pp 507–518.
56. Bleck TP, D'Angelo CM, Whisler WW: Bacterial infections of the spinal cord and its coverings. *In* Vinken PJ, Bruyn GW, Klawans HL (eds): Handbook of Clinical Neurology. Vol 52. Elsevier, Amsterdam, 1988, pp 185–194.
57. Dandy WE: Abscesses and inflammatory tumors in the spinal epidural space (so-called pachymeningitis externa). Arch Surg 1926;13:477–494.
58. Hulme A, Dott NM: Spinal epidural abscess. BMJ 1954;1:64–68.
59. Verner EF, Musher DM: Spinal epidural abscess. Med Clin North Am 1985;69:375–384.
60. Sharif HS, Ibrahim A: Intracranial epidural abscess. Br J Radiol 1982;55:81–84.
61. Feldenzer J, McKeever P, Schaberg D, et al: Experimental spinal epidural abscess: A pathophysiological model in the rabbit. Neurosurgery 1987;20:859–867.
62. Feldenzer J, McKeever P, Schaberg D, et al: The pathogenesis of spinal epidural abscess: Microangiographic studies in an experimental model. J Neurosurg 1988;69:110–114.
63. Heusner AP: Nontuberculous spinal epidural infections. N Engl J Med 1948;239:845–854.
64. Slater LN, Welch DF: *Bartonella* infections, including cat-scratch disease. *In* Scheld WM, Whitley RJ, Durack DT (eds): Infections of the Central Nervous System, 2nd ed. Philadelphia, Lippincott-Raven, 1997, pp 591–602.
65. Whipple GH: A hitherto undescribed disease characterized anatomically by deposits of fat and fatty acids in the intestinal and mesenteric lymphatic tissues. Johns Hopkins Hosp Bull 1907;18:382–391.
66. Relman DA: Whipple's disease. *In* Scheld WM, Whitley RJ, Durack DT (eds): Infections of the Central Nervous System, 2nd ed. Philadelphia, Lippincott-Raven, 1997, pp 579–589.
67. Aksamit AJ: Cerebrospinal fluid in the diagnosis of central nervous system infections. *In* Roos KL (ed): Central Nervous System Infectious Diseases and Therapy. New York, Marcel Dekker, 1997, pp 731–746.
68. Glander DA: Tuberculous meningitis. *In* Roos KL (ed): Central Nervous System Infectious Diseases and Therapy. New York, Marcel Dekker, 1997, pp 153–166.
69. Starke JR: Tuberculosis. *In* Jenson HB, Baltimore RS (eds): Pediatric Infectious Diseases. Principles and Practice. Philadelphia, WB Saunders, 2002, pp 517–545.
70. Plorde JJ: Mycobacteria. *In* Ryan KJ (ed): Sherris Medical Microbiology. An Introduction to Infectious Diseases, 3rd ed. Norwalk, CT, Appleton and Lange, 1994, pp 401–415.
71. Zuger A, Lowy FD: Tuberculosis. *In* Scheld WM, Whitley RJ, Durack DT (eds): Infections of the Central Nervous System, 2nd ed. Philadelphia, Lippincott-Raven, 1997, pp 417–443.
72. Roos KL: Tuberculous meningitis. *In* Roos KL (ed): Meningitis: 100 Maxims in Neurology. London, Arnold, 1997, pp 158–170.
73. Molavi A, LeFrock JL: Tuberculous meningitis. Med Clin North Amer 1985;69:315–331.
74. Leonard JM, Des Prez RM: Tuberculous meningitis. Infect Dis Clin North Amer 1990;4:769–797.
75. Udani PM, Dastur DK: Tuberculous encephalopathy with and without meningitis: Clinical features and pathologic correlations. J Neurol Sci 1970;10:541–561.
76. Ober WB: Ghon but not forgotten: Anton Ghon and his complex. Pathol Annual 1983;18:79–85.
77. Slavin RE, Walsh TJ, Pollack AD: Late generalized tuberculosis: Aclinical pathologic analysis and comparison of 100 cases in the preantibiotic and antibiotic eras. Medicine 1980;59:352–366.
78. Berenguer J, Moreno S, Laguna F, Vicente T: Tuberculous meningitis in patients infected with the human immunodeficiency virus. N Engl J Med 1992;326:668–672.
79. Wiggelinkhuizen J, Mann M: The radioactive bromide partition test in the diagnosis of meningitis in children. J Pediatr 1980;97:843–847.
80. Committee on Infectious Diseases: Chemotherapy for tuberculosis in infants and children. Pediatrics 1992;89:161–164.
81. Ad Hoc Committee of the Scientific Assembly on Microbiology, Tuberculosis, and Pulmonary Infections: Treatment of tuberculosis and tuberculosis infection in adults and children. Clin Infect Dis 1995; 21:9–27.
82. Cegielski JP, Wallace RJ: Infections due to nontuberculous *Mycobacteria*. *In* Scheld WM, Whitley RJ, Durack DT (eds): Infections of the Central Nervous System, 2nd ed. Philadelphia, Lippincott-Raven, 1997, pp 445–461.
83. Waivers LE: Did Columbus discover more than America? NC Med J 1989;50:687–690.
84. Johnson RA, White M: Syphilis in the 1990s: Cutaneous and neurologic manifestations. Semin Neurol 1992;12:287–298.
85. Roos KL: Syphilitic meningitis. *In* Roos KL (ed): Meningitis: 100 Maxims in Neurology. London, Arnold, 1997, pp 171–181.
86. Marra CM: Syphilis and human immunodeficiency virus infection. Semin Neurol 1992;12:43–50.
87. Johns DR, Tierney M, Felsenstein D: Alteration in the natural history of neurosyphilis by concurrent infection with the human immunodeficiency virus. N Engl J Med 1987;316:1569–1572.
88. Katz DA, Berger JR: Neurosyphilis in acquired immunodeficiency syndrome. Arch Neurol 1989;46:895–898.
89. Roos KL: Neurosyphilis. Semin Neurol 1992;12:209–212.
90. Hook EW: Syphilis. *In* Scheld WM, Whitley RJ, Durack DT (eds): Infections of the Central Nervous System, 2nd ed. Philadelphia, Lippincott-Raven, 1997, pp 669–684.
91. Marra CM: Neurosyphilis. *In* Roos KL (ed): Central Nervous System Infectious Diseases and Therapy. New York, Marcel Dekker, 1997, pp 237–252.
92. Merritt HH, Moore M: Acute syphilitic meningitis. Medicine 1935;14:119–183.
93. Afzelius A: Erythema chronicum migrans. Acta Derm Venereol 1921;2:120.

94. Coyle PK: Lyme disease. *In* Roos KL (ed): Central Nervous System Infectious Diseases and Therapy. New York, Marcel Dekker, 1997, pp 213–236.
95. Scrimenti RJ: Erythema chronicum migrans. Arch Dermatol 1970; 102:104–105.
96. Younger DS: Lyme disease: A historical perspective. Semin Neurol 1997;17:69–70.
97. Speilman AC, Clifford CM, Piseman J, et al: Human babesiosis on Nantucket Island, USA: Description of the vector, Ixodes (*Ixodes*) *dammini* sp. (*Acarina ixodidae*). J Med Entomol 1979;15:218–234.
98. Burgdorfer W, Barbour AG, Hayes SF, et al: Lyme disease—a tick borne spirochete? Science 1982;216:1317–1319.
99. Sterre AC, Grodzicki RL, Kornblatt AN, et al: The spirochetal etiology of Lyme disease. N Engl J Med 1983;308:733–740.
100. Benach JL, Bosler EM, Hanrahan JP, et al: Spirochetes isolated from the blood of two patients with Lyme disease. N Engl J Med 1983;308:740–742.
101. Logigian EL: Peripheral nervous system Lyme borreliosis. Semin Neurol 1997;17:25–30.
102. Halperin JJ: Neuroborreliosis: Central nervous system involvement. Semin Neurol 1997;17:19–24.
103. Kaplan RF, Jones-Woodward L: Lyme encephalopathy—a neuropsychological perspective. Semin Neurol 1997;17:31–37.
104. Dumler JS, Bakken JS: Ehrlichial diseases of humans: Emerging tick-borne infections. Clin Infect Dis 1995;20:1102–1110.
105. Bakken JS, Dumler JS, Sheng-Min C, et al: Human granulocytic ehrlichiosis in the upper Midwest states: A new species emerging? JAMA 1994;272(3):212–218.
106. Dumler JS: Is human granulocytic ehrlichiosis a new Lyme disease? Review and comparison of clinical, laboratory, epidemiological, and some biological features. Clin Infect Dis 1997;25(Suppl 1):S43–47.
107. Spach DH, Liles WC, Campbell GL, et al: Tick-borne diseases in the United States. N Engl J Med 1993;329:936–947.
108. Ratnasamy N, Everett ED, Roland WE, et al: Central nervous system manifestations of human ehrlichiosis. Clin Infect Dis 1996;23:314–319.
109. Pourmand R, Roos KL: Seasonal (spring-summer) encephalitides. *In* Roos KL (ed): Central Nervous System Infectious Diseases and Therapy. New York, Marcel Dekker, 1997, pp 193–211.
110. Saag MS, Powderly WG, Cloud GA, et al: Comparison of amphotericin B with fluconazole in the treatment of acute AIDS-associated cryptococcal meningitis. N Engl J Med 1992;326:83–89.
111. Pruitt AA: Central nervous system infections in cancer patients. Neurol Clin 1991;9:867–888.
112. Ampel NM, Wieden MA, Galgiani JN: Coccidioidomycosis: Clinical update. Rev Infect Dis 1989;11:897–911.
113. Treseler CB, Sugar AM: Fungal meningitis. Infect Dis Clin North Amer 1990;4:789–808.
114. Roos KL, Bryan JP, Maggio WW, et al: Intracranial blastomycoma. Medicine 1987;66:224–235.
115. Christin L, Sugar AM: Fungal infections. *In* Roos KL (ed): Central Nervous System Infectious Diseases and Therapy. New York, Marcel Dekker, 1997, pp 167–192.
116. Conti DJ, Rubin RH: Infection of the central nervous system in organ transplant patients. Neurol Clin 1988;6:241–260.
117. Wheat LJ, Batteiger BE, Sathapatayavongs B: *Histoplasma capsulatum* infections of the central nervous system. Medicine 1990;69:244–260.
118. Coleman JM, Hogg GG, Rosenfeld JV, Waters KD: Invasive central nervous system aspergillosis: Cure with liposomal amphotericin B, itraconazole, and radical surgery—case report and review of the literature. Neurosurgery 1995;36:848–863.
119. Hagensee ME, Bauwens JE, Kjos B, Bowden RA: Brain abscess following marrow transplantation: Experience at the Fred Hutchinson Cancer Research Center, 1984–92. Clin Infect Dis 1994;19:402–408.
120. Roos KL: Fungal meningitis. *In* Roos KL (ed): Meningitis: 100 Maxims in Neurology. London, Arnold, 1997, pp 141–158.
121. Durack DT: Amebic infections. *In* Scheld WM, Whitley RJ, Durack DT (eds): Infections of the Central Nervous System, 2nd ed. Philadelphia, Lippincott-Raven, 1997, pp 831–844.
122. Seidel JS, Harmatz P, Visvesvara GS, et al: Successful treatment of primary amebic meningoencephalitis. N Engl J Med 1982;306:346–348.
123. Anderson K, Jamieson A: Primary amoebic meningoencephalitis. Lancet 1972;i:902–903.
124. Sotelo J: Neurocysticercosis. *In* Roos KL (ed): Central Nervous System Infectious Diseases and Therapy. New York, Marcel Dekker, 1997, pp 545–572.
125. Wools KK: Cerebral malaria. *In* Roos KL (ed): Central Nervous System Infectious Diseases and Therapy. New York, Marcel Dekker, 1997, pp 601–617.
126. WHO: Severe and complicated malaria. Trans R Soc Trop Med Hyg 1990;84(Suppl 2):1–65.
127. White NJ: The treatment of malaria. N Engl J Med 1996;335:800–806.
128. Cegielski JP, Warrell DA: Cerebral malaria. *In* Scheld WM, Whitley RJ, Durack DT (eds): Infections of the Central Nervous System, 2nd ed. Philadelphia, Lippincott-Raven 1997, pp 765–784.

CHAPTER 43

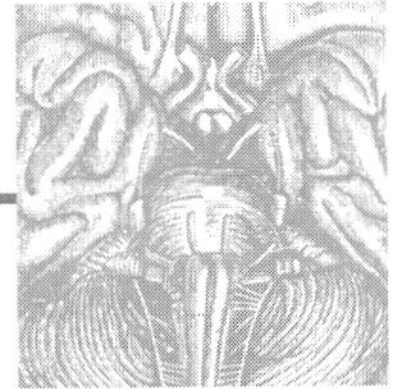

PAUL BROWN

Transmissible Spongiform Encephalopathy

History and Overview

The present widespread familiarity with the comparatively rare group of diseases called transmissible spongiform encephalopathies (TSEs) has come about through journalistic coinage of the term *mad cow disease* applied to its most recently identified member, bovine spongiform encephalopathy (BSE). That humans have proved susceptible to orally acquired infection by BSE has further fueled medical and public interest, and today TSEs are the focus of intensive campaigns of clinical, epidemiological, and experimental research that are considerably advancing knowledge of their behavior and fundamental nature.

In point of fact, the different diseases are merely variations on a theme and are more properly considered as a single disease taking different forms in humans and animals. Historically, these forms were given different names only because they were described before their shared properties were appreciated. As there is now good evidence that they all result from a "proteinaceous infectious particle," the TSEs are often referred to as *prion diseases*.

The first TSE to be described was scrapie, a disease of sheep that devastated the woolens industry in 18th century England. Scrapie remained the sole recognized example of TSE until the 20th century, when a number of additional animal and human diseases were identified that subsequently proved to be spontaneous or transmitted forms of TSE (Fig. 43–1). In animals, the disease has spread to mink (transmissible mink encephalopathy, or TME), deer and elk (chronic wasting disease or CWD), and most recently, to cattle (BSE). In humans, the prototypic disease was kuru, brought to epidemic proportions in an isolated population of New Guinea by endocannibalism. With cessation of this practice, the disease slowly disappeared. The other human varieties—Creutzfeldt-Jakob disease (CJD), Gerstmann-Sträussler-Scheinker disease (GSS), and fatal familial insomnia (FFI)—have a worldwide distribution and occur in sporadic, inherited, or environmentally acquired forms. The most important, numerically speaking, is the sporadic form of CJD, first described in the 1920s but not recognized as a TSE until the 1960s.

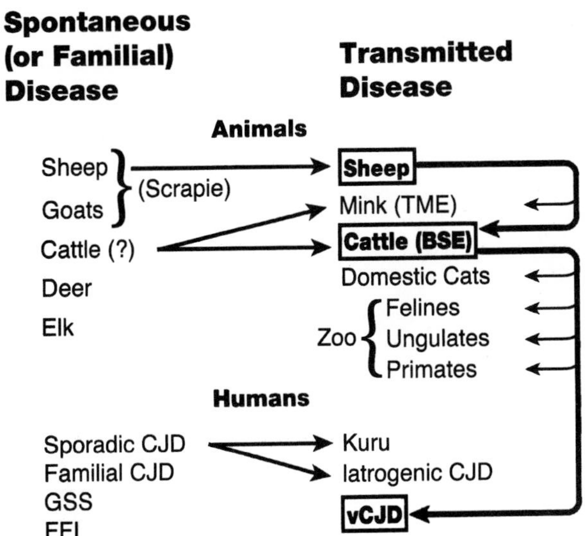

FIGURE 43–1. Inter-relationships between animal and human transmissible spongiform encephalopathies.

Sporadic Disease

Pathogenesis and Pathophysiology. A critical early observation by Alper and colleagues emphasized that infectivity of scrapie was not decreased by levels of ionizing irradiation sufficient to destroy the biological function of nucleic acid.[1] Subsequent research fostered a number of hypotheses about non-nucleic acid replication by membrane-complexed polysaccharides or proteins. Upon a background of repeated failures to detect any foreign disease-specific nucleic acid, the protein hypothesis was further bolstered in the 1980s by the demonstration that highly purified brain extracts from diseased subjects contained a host-encoded membrane-bound glycoprotein (PrP) that was inseparable from infectivity.[2]

The primary structure of the protein does not differ from that of the protein in healthy individuals. In consequence, the functional differences between the protein in normal and affected individuals—solubility, proteinase resistance, ease of separation from cell membranes and, most importantly, ability to replicate (infectivity)—must reside in post-translational secondary or tertiary alterations in protein folding. The normal form of the protein is rich in alpha-helical domains, whereas the abnormal isoform has fewer alpha-helices and a greatly increased amount of anti-parallel beta-sheet structure, the "signature" of amyloid protein[3] (Fig. 43–2). The mechanism by which such protein misfolding leads to replication is presumed to be either a process of polymerization akin to inorganic crystal formation[4] or a molecular constraint imposed by the misfolded protein upon normal molecules to assume its own abnormal configuration.[5]

The synaptic region appears to be the primary site of this pathological process, but extracellular aggregation can also produce microscopically visible amyloid plaques. The subsequent spread of infectious molecules is as puzzling as the original conversion event, but tissue sampling has demonstrated widespread infectivity not only within the brain (which contains by far the highest concentration of the infectious agent), but also in the spinal cord, cerebrospinal fluid, and (at much lower levels of infectivity) many peripheral organs. Infectivity has never been demonstrated in any external secretion or excretion (urine, feces, tears, sputum, or saliva).[6]

Epidemiology and Risk Factors. The sporadic form of the disease accounts for approximately 90 percent of all cases of spongiform encephalopathy, and occurs in a random distribution in all studied populations of the world at an annual frequency of about one case per million people.[7–9] There is no documented instance of the disease being "caught" from normal contact with other humans (whether in the preclinical or clinical stages of illness), nor is there any indication (by seasonality, geographical distribution, or disease clusters) of a nonhuman environmental source of infection. For the present, therefore, each such case must be considered a de novo event that has no antecedent cause or subsequent links to any chain of infection.

Clinical Features. The disease affects males and females equally and typically becomes manifest in late middle age. Peak incidence occurs in the 55- to 70-year-old age group, and the disease has a bell-shaped distribution curve that is skewed toward the younger age groups, including rare cases in adolescents (Fig. 43–3). The earliest symptoms usually appear gradually over a period of weeks but can occur suddenly. They are limited to mental deterioration in about a third of patients, physical disabilities in another third, and mixed mental and physical abnormalities in the remaining third (Table 43–1). The frequencies of various symptoms at the onset of illness, at medical presentation, and at an advanced stage of disease are shown in Table 43–2. Memory loss and either cerebellar or visual-oculomotor signs are comparatively frequent at the outset and, as the illness evolves, these are joined by pyramidal and extrapyramidal signs and a variety of involuntary movements, especially myoclonus. Progressive mental deterioration terminates in mutism and global dementia. Death commonly occurs within 6 months of the onset of illness, but a significant proportion of patients have more acute courses of a month or two, and about 10 percent have an extended course of 2 or more years (Fig. 43–4).

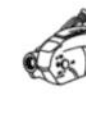

This description applies to the great majority of patients, but the literature is replete with case reports illustrating unusual variations on the theme. Among these are sudden or stuttering onsets that suggest a cerebrovascular accident or multiple sclerosis and syndromes that span a range of appearances from the Wernicke-Korsakoff syndrome or bulbar palsy to parkinsonism or amyotrophic lateral sclerosis. All represent the extremes in a continuum of multisystem disease based on the topographically unpredictable cerebral pathology of spongiform encephalopathy.

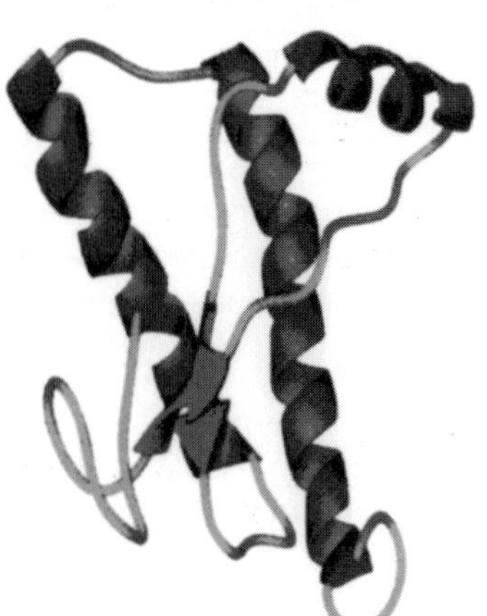

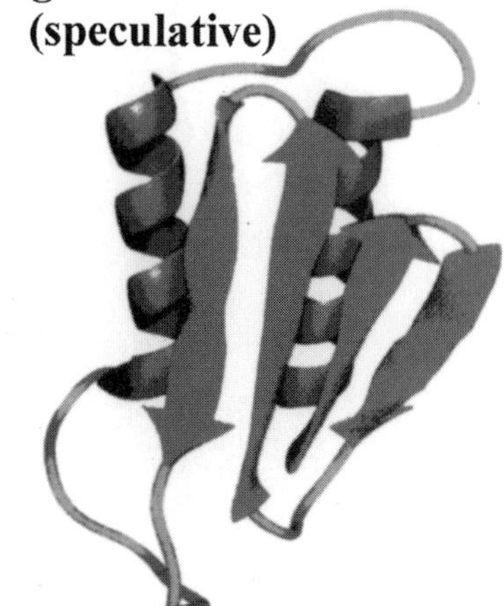

FIGURE 43–2. Proposed conversion of normal to pathological isoform of "prion" protein. Strings denote unstructured regions; coils denote alpha-helical structure; ribbons denote beta-sheet structure. Note the reduction in alpha-helical structure and corresponding increase in beta-sheet structure in the pathological isoform (the normal protein structure was determined by nuclear magnetic resonance analysis; the abnormal structure is hypothetical). Adapted from Prusiner SB: Shattuck Lecture—Neurodegenerative diseases and prions. N Engl J Med 2001;344: 1516–1526, Figure 1.

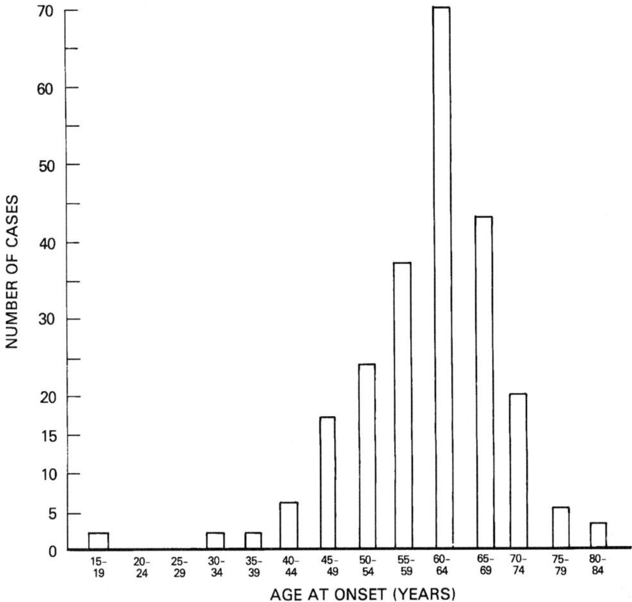

FIGURE 43–3. Age at onset of sporadic Creutzfeldt-Jakob disease (based on the NIH series of 232 experimentally transmitted cases).

Laboratory Evaluation. Three laboratory examinations are available as aids to diagnosis. The electroencephalogram (EEG) remains a valuable and easily performed examination.[10, 11] Early in the course of illness, the EEG may be normal or may show only some background slowing, and terminally it may simply reflect a dying brain. However, in the fully developed phase of disease, most patients show some form of periodic activity (Fig. 43–5). In its most pathognomonic form, the 1- to 2-cycle per second slow-wave triphasic spiking activity resembles an electrocardiogram; less specific but still suggestive is a "burst-suppression" pattern in which short runs of high voltage spikes alternate with periods of near electrical silence.

The second test is an immunological analysis of cerebrospinal fluid (CSF) to detect a protein kinase inhibitor called 14-3-3. This protein appears in CSF as a result of neuronal cell death, and although completely unrelated to the "prion" protein, its presence has nevertheless proved extremely useful as a surrogate marker of infection when used in an appropriate clinical setting and when routine examination of the CSF is normal.[11]

TABLE 43–1. **Sporadic Creutzfeldt-Jakob Disease: Overall Characteristics of the NIH Series of 232 Experimentally Transmitted Cases**

Male-to-female ratio	1.1
Median age at onset (range)	60 yr (16–82)
Neurological debut (%)	
Gradual (weeks to months)	86
Rapid (sudden to days)	14
Mental deterioration only	37
Mixed mental and neurological	34
Neurological signs only	29
Median duration of illness (range)	4.5 mo (1–130)

From Brown P, Gibbs C Jr, Rodgers-Johnson P, et al: Human spongiform encephalopathy: The National Institutes of Health series of 300 cases of experimentally transmitted disease. Ann Neurol 1994;35:513–529.

TABLE 43–2. **Sporadic Creutzfeldt-Jakob Disease: Symptomatology of the NIH Series of 232 Experimentally Transmitted Cases**

	Percentage of Patients with Symptoms or Signs		
Symptoms/Signs	**At Onset**	**On First Examination**	**During Course**
Mental deterioration	71	84	100
Memory loss	52	65	100
Behavioral abnormalities	29	38	55
Higher cortical function	16	36	73
Cerebellar	33	54	70
Visual/oculomotor	19	30	41
Vertigo/dizziness	12	14	19
Headache	11	12	20
Sensory	5	6	11
Involuntary movements	4	19	88
Myoclonus	0.5	9	80
Other (including tremor)	3	10	36
Pyramidal	1.5	16	62
Extrapyramidal	0.5	9	56
Lower motor neuron	0.5	2	11
Seizures	0	2	20
Pseudobulbar	0	0.5	7

From Brown P, Gibbs C Jr, Rodgers-Johnson P, et al: Human spongiform encephalopathy: The National Institutes of Health series of 300 cases of experimentally transmitted disease. Ann Neurol 1994;35:513–529.

The third test is magnetic resonance imaging (MRI), which has only recently been appreciated as a useful diagnostic procedure.[12] Many patients with sporadic disease at some point in the course of illness show a symmetrical or sometimes unilateral hyperintense signal in the basal ganglia (Fig. 43–6). Nonspecific abnormalities may be seen in other types of radiographic imaging procedures, such as computed tomography scans, which are primarily useful in exploring alternative diagnoses.

None of these tests is 100 percent sensitive or specific, especially on clinical presentation, but each can provide a highly useful clue either for or against the diagnosis of CJD during the course of illness (Table 43–3). Indeed, were all three tests positive, it would not even be necessary to see the patient before making the diagnosis of CJD, a far cry from the clinical situation confronting neurologists as recently as 10 years ago!

Brain biopsy was often used in the past to establish an antemortem diagnosis, revealing spongiform change in 95 percent of patients.[6] But the procedure was attended by significant morbidity and mortality (almost one quarter of patients died within 3 weeks of surgery); today, improved clinical skills together with EEG, CSF, and MRI examinations, have largely eliminated the need for biopsy. In fact, in most cases, the only current indication for biopsy is when there is reason to suspect an alternative treatable disease that cannot otherwise be diagnosed.

Differential Diagnosis. The spectrum of diseases with which spongiform encephalopathies can be mistaken is not

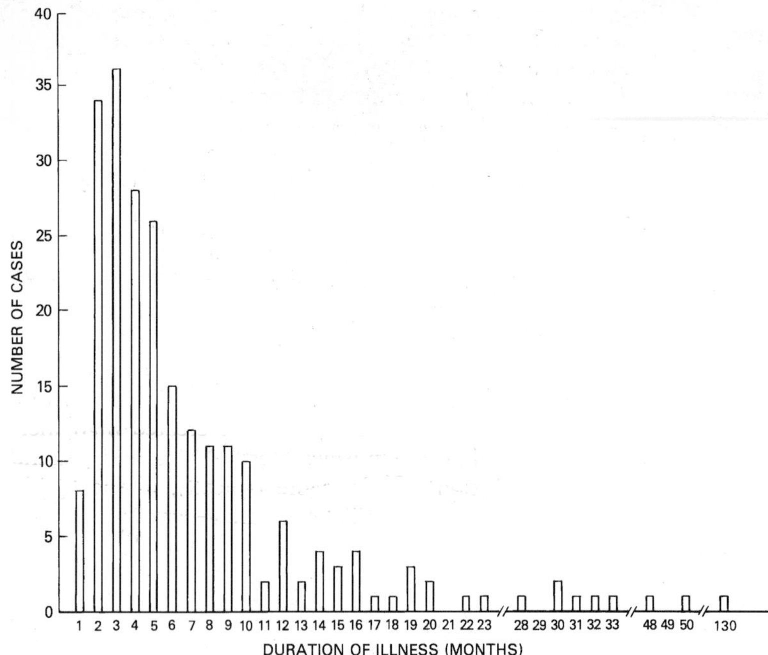

FIGURE 43–4. Duration of illness of sporadic Creutzfeldt-Jakob disease (based on the NIH series of 232 experimentally transmitted cases).

surprising in view of the variable distribution of neuropathological changes found at autopsy. As always, the guiding principle in differential diagnosis should be the investigation of all potentially treatable diseases before winnowing through untreatable neurodegenerative alternatives.

From a practical viewpoint, differential diagnosis can be separated into two categories: first and most important are diseases that can mimic the onset and early course of spongiform encephalopathy; the second category comprises diseases that can be confused with later stages of the illness. In the first cat-

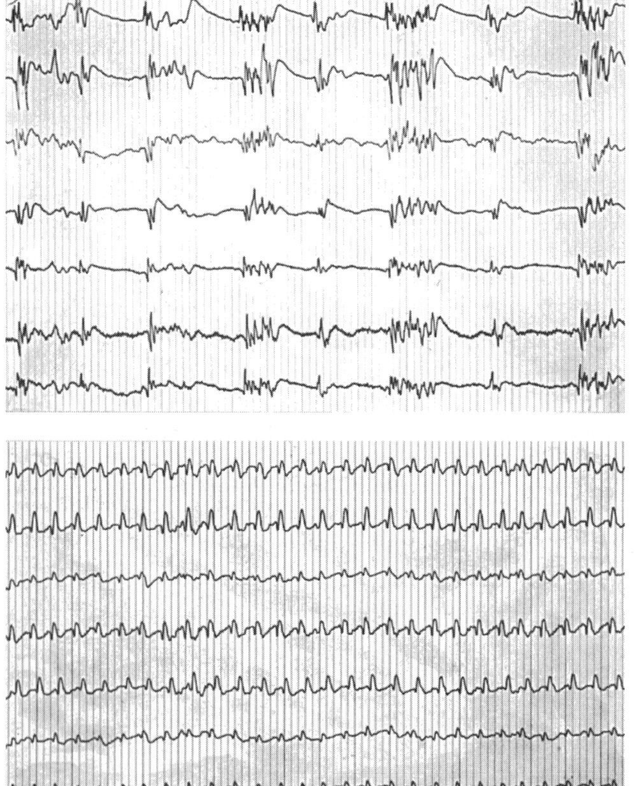

FIGURE 43–5. Periodic electroencephalographic recordings in sporadic Creutzfeldt-Jakob disease. Upper tracing shows a suggestive "burst-suppression" pattern, and lower tracing shows a virtually diagnostic 1- to 2-cycle/sec triphasic sharp wave pattern.

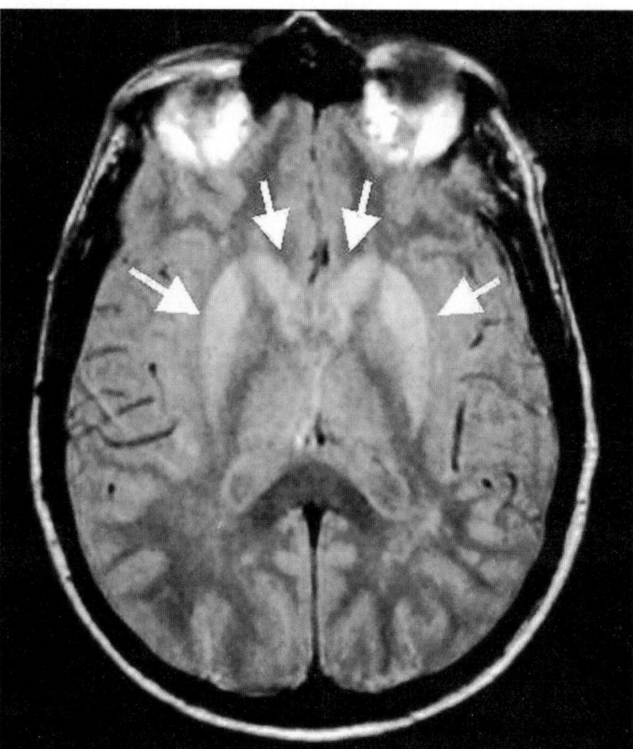

FIGURE 43–6. Magnetic resonance image (MRI) in sporadic Creutzfeldt-Jakob disease. Symmetrical hyperintense signal from the basal ganglia (in about 20 percent of cases, the signal is asymmetrical).

TABLE 43–3. **Sensitivity and Specificity of Laboratory Aids to Diagnosis**

Test	Sensitivity	Specificity
Electroencephalogram	67%	86%
Cerebrospinal fluid 14-3-3 protein	91%	91%
Magnetic resonance imaging	79%	(high)
Biopsy	95%	100%

egory are drug intoxications (bismuth, lithium, cyclical antidepressives), infections (herpes simplex encephalitis, cryptococcal meningoencephalitis, multiple cerebral abscesses), metabolic-endocrine disorders (hyperparathyroidism, Hashimoto's encephalitis, Wernicke-Korsakoff syndrome, and vitamin B_{12} deficiency), cerebrovascular accidents, neoplasms, and normal pressure hydrocephalus. In the second category are Parkinson's disease with dementia, diffuse Lewy body disease, amyotrophic lateral sclerosis with dementia, progressive supranuclear palsy, olivopontocerebellar atrophy, Huntington's disease, Ramsay Hunt syndrome, Pick's disease, and that most difficult of all differential diagnostic problems, Alzheimer's disease. Diagnostic uncertainty sometimes cannot be resolved prior to necropsy.

Management, Treatment, and Prevention. During hospitalization, "universal precautions" should be followed in managing the patient, including the handling and disposal of tissues, excretions, and other contaminated material.[13] Ordinary surface contact is not hazardous, but if blood or spinal fluid is involved, the exposed area of the worker's skin should be swabbed with bleach and then, after a minute or so, thoroughly washed with detergent and water. The golden rule is to avoid penetrating injury with anything that has penetrated the patient (e.g., needles), just as for patients with acquired immunodeficiency syndrome or hepatitis.

Despite early claims of clinical improvement in some patients with CJD who had been treated with the antiviral drugs amantadine or vidarabine, and more recently, with quinacrine, subsequent published and unpublished experience has failed to validate these successes. At best, only temporary pauses in the progression of disease occur.[14] Thus, management of the patient with CJD is still limited to good nursing care and the suppression of myoclonus or seizures, if they occur, with a benzodiazepine or anticonvulsant. Like all patients who become progressively helpless and bedridden, death is usually the result of sepsis from respiratory, skin, or urinary tract infections or, when swallowing becomes difficult, from aspiration.

Familial Disease

Pathogenesis and Pathophysiology. The molecular genetic basis for inherited disease remains to be defined, but it seems probable that mutation-induced alterations in the primary amino acid structure of PrP facilitate its transition from an alpha helix to a beta-pleated sheet configuration. If the magnitude of this facilitation were a million-fold, the one per million occurrence of sporadic disease would assume the appearance of a fully penetrant inherited disease linked to the mutation.[15] This explanation is unencumbered by any experimental evidence but is nonetheless consistent with the observed frequencies of the two forms of disease.

Epidemiology and Risk Factors. About 10 percent of cases of spongiform encephalopathy are familial and are associated with one of nearly 30 different insert and point mutations identified in the gene that encodes the amyloidogenic prion protein. All are inherited in an autosomal dominant genetic pattern, and all are experimentally transmissible.

Like sporadic disease, familial disease affects men and women equally, but its temporospatial distribution is determined by the origins and migrations of affected families. All case clusters of spongiform encephalopathy have a familial basis; for example, those in rural Slovakia and among Sephardic Jews, whose migrations have created high incidence pockets of disease in Israel, North Africa, and (via the Spanish Inquisition), Chile. More typically, in the highly mobile world of today, familial cases are geographically scattered, and individual patients may have lost all contact with and knowledge of their ancestors, leading to the mistaken appearance of sporadic mutation-positive cases.

Clinical Features. Familial disease can present as CJD, GSS, FFI, or as atypical Alzheimer-like syndromes, depending on which of the mutations is present in the family[15] (Table 43–4). For example, point mutations at codons 200 or 210 usually produce an illness that begins 5 to 10 years earlier but in other respects is indistinguishable from sporadic CJD, whereas repetitive octapeptide encoding insert mutations cause illnesses that may begin as early as the third or

TABLE 43–4. **Mutations of the Chromosome 20 "Prion" Gene Associated with Inherited Forms of Transmissible Spongiform Encephalopathy**

Mutation	Disease Phenotype
Octa-repeat insertions of 24, 48, 96, 120, 144, 168, 192, or 216 base pairs between codons 51 and 91	CJD, GSS, or atypical dementias
P102L (Pro Leu)	GSS: classical ataxic form
P105L (Pro Leu)	GSS: spastic paraparesis variant
A117V (Ala Val)	GSS: pseudobulbar variant
G131V (Gly Val)	GSS: classical ataxic form
Y145* (Tyr Stop)	Alzheimer-like dementia
D178N (Asp Asn)	CJD (129V on mutant allele)
D178N (Asp Asn)	FFI (129M on mutant allele)
V180I (Val Ile)	CJD
T183A (Thr Ala)	Alzheimer-like dementia
H187R (His Arg)	GSS: classical ataxic form
F198S (Phe Ser)	GSS with neurofibrillary tangles
E200K (Glu Lys)	CJD
D202N (Asp Asn)	GSS with neurofibrillary tangles
V2031 (Val Ile)	CJD
R208H (Arg His)	CJD
V2101 (Val Ile)	CJD
E211Q (Glu Gln)	CJD
Q212P (Gln Pro)	GSS with Lewy bodies
E217R (Glu Arg)	GSS with neurofibrillary tangles
M232R (Met Arg)	CJD
M232T (Met Thr)	GSS

CJD, Creutzfeldt-Jakob disease; GSS, Gerstmann-Sträussler-Scheinker Disease; FFI, fatal familial insomnia.[15]

fourth decade of life and produce a very slowly evolving dementia that ends in death after a period of 10 to 15 years with little or no brain pathology. Other mutations can produce a wide spectrum of intermediate disease syndromes.

GSS typically begins in members of affected families between ages 40 and 55 years as a slowly evolving ataxia, sometimes with associated mental deterioration, and progresses through a multisystem array of symptoms, including dementia and myoclonus, finally terminating fatally after an average duration of 5 to 10 years. It is characterized neuropathologically by a profusion of multifocal amyloid plaques in the cerebellum, with or without spongiform change. The classic syndrome (including Gerstmann's original case) is associated with a point mutation at codon 102, but more recently, variants of GSS have been described with mutations at other codons.[16, 17]

FFI is the most recently admitted member of the spongiform encephalopathy group and is unusual in that patients typically show early and pronounced autonomic and endocrine dysfunction, including intractable insomnia (often associated with daytime somnolence), and unexplained disorders of temperature, cardiovascular, and respiratory regulation.[18] Later in the course of the illness, more typical features of CJD supervene (pyramidal and extrapyramidal signs, cerebellar ataxia, and myoclonus), and death occurs after an average duration of 1 to 2 years. At autopsy, severe neuronal loss and astrogliosis are seen in the mediodorsal and anterior ventral thalamic nuclei, with variable pathology in the neocortex. The disease is caused by a mutation at codon 178, but curiously, it occurs only when the mutant allele specifies methionine at polymorphic codon 129; when valine is specified by codon 129, the pathogenic codon 178 mutation produces a CJD-like phenotype.[19]

From both diagnostic and genetic standpoints, it is important to remember that these clinical stereotypes have many exceptions, that significant phenotypic heterogeneity is the rule even among members of the same family, and that no matter what mutational phenotype is typical, at least one family member will have died from an illness that closely resembles sporadic CJD.

Laboratory Evaluation. In addition to the EEG, CSF, and MRI tests described for patients with sporadic disease, familial disease offers the possibility of identifying the specific causative mutation by molecular genetic analysis of DNA obtained from white blood cells in an anticoagulated blood specimen. Identification of the responsible mutation is not a mere academic exercise but has practical prognostic value for the patient's family: first, it permits a rough estimate of the likely age at onset and duration of illness, and second, it can have a crucial impact in counseling about the risk of disease inheritance because some mutations are not fully penetrant. For example, mutations at codons 200 and 210 have a penetrance of only 50 percent during a normal lifespan, so that although the mutation will be transmitted as an autosomal dominant trait, only half of the individuals who carry the mutation will become sick.[20, 21]

Management, Treatment, and Prevention. The care and outlook for patients with familial disease are no different from those for patients with sporadic disease; however, familial disease can be prevented in subsequent generations through the use of molecular genetic testing of amniotic fluid and elective therapeutic abortion of fetuses found to carry a lethal mutation.[22] This option should be carefully explained to family members for their ethical and medical consideration.

Iatrogenic Disease

Pathogenesis and Pathophysiology. Iatrogenic disease poses no difficulty in regard to pathogenesis; when the infectious agent is accidentally introduced into the body, whether directly into the nervous system or by peripheral routes, the seed is sown for its replication and spread, and the disease clinically appears when infectivity and neuropathology have reached a high enough level. The length of the incubation period between the infecting event and the onset of symptomatic disease ranges from about 2 years in cases in which infection is introduced directly into the brain, to an average of nearly 15 years in those who are inoculated subcutaneously (and some incubation periods are as long as 20 to 30 years).

Epidemiology. The first case of iatrogenic disease was recognized in the early 1970s in a U.S. recipient of a corneal graft from a patient who was later discovered to have died from CJD; soon afterward, two cases occurred in Swiss patients who had undergone stereotactic EEG with needles that had been previously used in a patient with CJD. A few years later, retrospective analysis of a series of British neurosurgical cases revealed that three of the patients had probably been infected by surgical instruments contaminated in an earlier operation on a CJD patient. These few reports constituted the totality of iatrogenic disease until the past decade, when separate outbreaks of disease were traced to contaminated batches of pituitary hormones and dura mater grafts obtained from human cadavers. There are currently over 300 recognized cases of iatrogenic disease, and a few cases in patients treated with growth hormone continue to appear each year, with increasingly longer incubation periods between the cessation of cadaveric hormone therapy in 1985 and the onset of CJD.

Clinical Features. Iatrogenic disease syndromes are significantly influenced by different routes of infection.[23] Introduction of the infectious agent into the brain parenchyma, directly or via the optic nerve, produces an illness that is in all respects similar to sporadic CJD[23] (Table 43–5). Introduction of the agent into the brain by a peripheral route of infection (hormone therapy) produces a distinctively different illness that begins with ataxia and even in its later stages may not include significant mental deterioration; this syndrome is strongly reminiscent of kuru, which was also acquired through peripheral routes of infection. Application of the agent to the brain surface through dura mater grafts produces an illness with intermediate characteristics, comprising either prominent cerebellar/visual or demential features. The duration of illness is unrelated to the route of infection, and the disease runs a course similar to that of sporadic CJD.

Laboratory Evaluation. Periodic EEG activity has been seen in about half of all patients, and the CSF 14-3-3 protein is present in most patients in whom it has been examined. MRI studies have not been reported, but would likely show the same features as sporadic CJD.

TABLE 43–5. **Iatrogenic Creutzfeldt-Jakob Disease**

Mode of Infection	Number of Patients	Agent Entry into Brain	Median Incubation Period (Range)	Clinical Presentation
Corneal transplant	3	Optic nerve	16, 18, 320 mos	Dementia/cerebellar
Stereotactic EEG	2	Intracerebral	16, 20 mos	Dementia/cerebellar
Neurosurgery	5	Intracerebral	17 mos (12–28)	Visual/dementia/cerebellar
Dura mater graft	136	Cerebral surface	9 yrs (1.5–18)	Cerebellar (visual, dementia)
Growth hormone	161	Hematogenous (?)	13 yrs (4–27)	Cerebellar
Gonadotrophin	4	Hematogenous (?)	13 yrs (12–16)	Cerebellar

Management, Treatment, and Prevention. Good nursing care and attention to symptomatic relief of movement disorders remain the only palliative measures available for these unfortunate victims of our own mistakes. The prevention of future episodes of iatrogenic disease is therefore an object of increasingly close scrutiny by physicians, research scientists, and government regulatory agencies alike.

In the past, neurosurgical instruments were subjected to the standard 15 to 20 minutes of steam autoclaving at 121°C; EEG needles were disinfected with benzene, ethanol, and formaldehyde vapor; cadaveric pituitary tissue extracts were sequentially passed through glacial acetic acid, acetone, and dilute NaOH; and dura mater grafts were irradiated. We know now that none of these procedures can be fully guaranteed to inactivate the infectious agent. Therefore, the temperature requirement for steam autoclaving of neurosurgical instruments has been raised to 134°C, stereotactic EEG needles are discarded after each use, and pituitary hormones are made with recombinant technology rather than from cadaveric sources.[13] Dura mater grafts are exposed to high (1N) concentrations of NaOH or avoided in favor of synthetic membrane patches. Renewed attention is being paid to other potential sources of infection from human-to-human transfers of tissue, tissue extracts, and blood or plasma derivatives[24]; donors at higher than usual risk of CJD such as growth hormone recipients or members of CJD families are deferred, and chemical or filtration processing steps are being devised to eliminate any potential contamination of biological products.

Variant Creutzfeldt-Jakob Disease (vCJD)

Epidemiology. vCJD was first recognized in the United Kingdom in 1996, approximately 10 years after the BSE epidemic had begun,[25] and the original cohort of 10 cases has since grown to more than 120, with six additional cases in France, one in Italy, and one in Ireland (countries in which BSE outbreaks have also occurred). New cases are being identified in the United Kingdom at the rate of about 20 per year, and predictive mathematical models that assume an average incubation period of 20 years or less—which is likely—estimate the eventual total tally to be several hundred cases.[26, 27] The most plausible explanation of vCJD is that humans became infected with the agent that causes BSE through the consumption of beef products containing central nervous system tissue (meat itself is not infectious, but mechanically recovered meat that is pressure-extracted from carcasses often contained spinal cord and paraspinal ganglia in addition to residual muscle shards).[28]

Clinical Features. The most distinctive feature of vCJD is the young age at onset of illness[29] (Fig. 43–7). The average age at onset is 27 years, with many adolescents, and only a single patient older than 50 years of age. The clinical presentation is also unusual in that the patient often has some form of psychiatric disturbance and complains of sensory symptoms, particularly limb pain (Table 43–6). However, symptoms more typical of early sporadic CJD (mental deterioration, incoordination, and visual complaints) may also be present at the outset, and as the illness progresses, the clinical distinction between the sporadic and variant forms of illness becomes progressively blurred. Nevertheless, the combination of psychiatric and sensory symptoms in an adolescent or young adult is enough to raise a suspicion of vCJD, at least in patients who have had extensive residence in the United Kingdom (and perhaps other European countries in which BSE occurs). The average duration of illness is 14 months, or about twice as long as that of sporadic CJD (Fig. 43–8).

Laboratory Evaluation. None of the vCJD patients has shown periodic EEG activity, nor has the CSF 14-3-3 protein test been as helpful as in sporadic cases of CJD. However, the MRI has become an extremely valuable examination,[12] as up to 80 percent of cases with vCJD show bilateral hyperintensity in the posterior thalamus (pulvinar), as opposed to the basal ganglia hyperintensity seen in sporadic disease (Fig. 43–9). One other interesting and so far unexplained feature

TABLE 43–6. **Variant Creutzfeldt-Jakob Disease: Symptomatology of the First 47 Cases in the United Kingdom**

	Percentage of Patients	
Symptom or Sign	Onset	Course
Mental	17	100
Psychiatric	66	98
Incoordination	9	98
Visual/oculomotor	0	34
Sensory	19	70
Pain	13	38
Involuntary movements	4	94
Myoclonus	0	70
Akinetic mutism	0	49

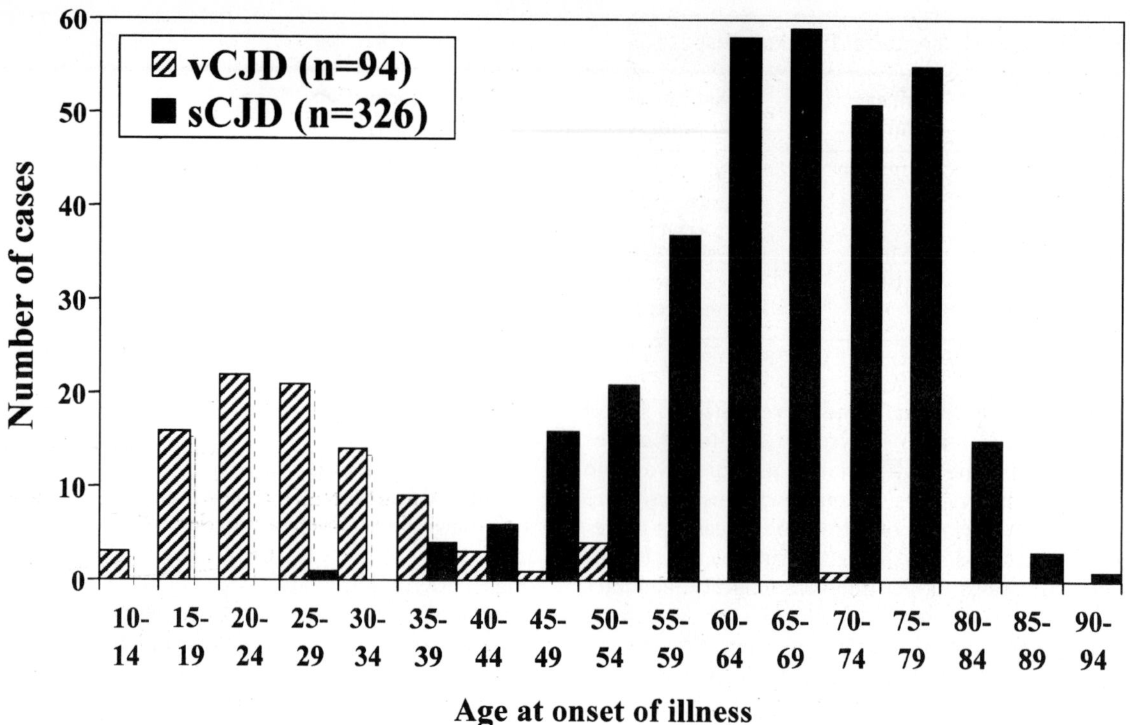

FIGURE 43–7. Comparison of age at onset of all cases of sporadic and variant Creutzfeldt-Jakob disease in the United Kingdom during the period 1994–2000. Data courtesy of Dr. Robert Will, National CJD Surveillance Unit, Edinburgh, UK.

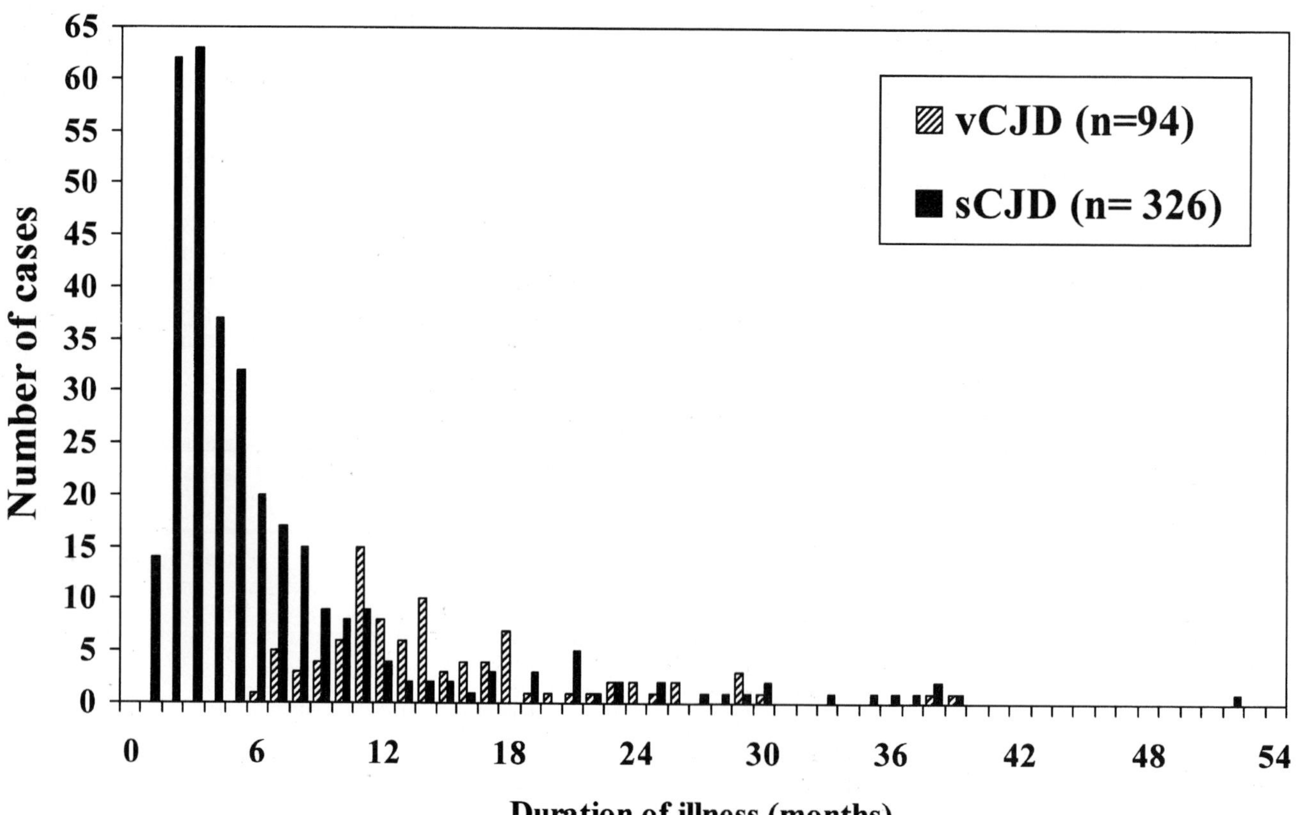

FIGURE 43–8. Comparison of duration of illness of all cases of sporadic and variant Creutzfeldt-Jakob disease in the United Kingdom during the period 1994–2000. Data courtesy of Dr. Robert Will, National CJD Surveillance Unit, Edinburgh, UK.

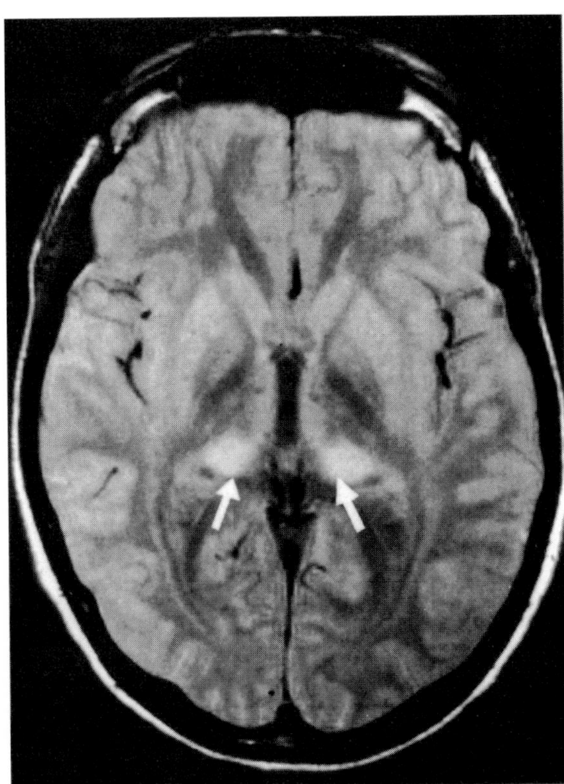

FIGURE 43–9. MRI in variant Creutzfeldt-Jakob disease. Symmetrical hyperintense signal from pulvinar.

of vCJD is its restriction to individuals with a homozygous methionine-coding genotype at polymorphic codon 129 of the prion protein gene. However, alternative genotypes could conceivably have longer incubation periods and only begin to appear in future cases. Neuropathological examination (without which a definitive diagnosis cannot be made) reveals diffuse spongiform changes that are especially severe in the basal ganglia, posterior thalamus, and cerebellum, and myriad amyloid plaques surrounded by halos of vacuolation—so-called "florid" or "daisy" plaques.[30]

Management, Treatment, and Prevention. The management, treatment, and prevention of vCJD are similar to other varieties of TSE. Neither BSE nor vCJD has occurred in the United States, and strict compliance with newly implemented importation and domestic animal feed bans should prevent any future occurrence.[28]

Reviews and Selected Updates

Brown P: 1755 and all that: A historical primer of transmissible spongiform encephalopathy. Brit Med J 1998;317:1688–1692.

Brown P, Gibbs CJ Jr, Rodgers-Johnson P, et al: Human spongiform encephalopathy: The National Institutes of Health series of 300 cases of experimentally transmitted disease. Ann Neurol 1994;35:513–529.

Brown P, Preece M, Brandel J-P, et al: Iatrogenic Creutzfeldt-Jakob disease at the millennium. Neurology 2000:55;1075–1081.

Brown P, Will RG, Bradley R, Asher DM, Detwiler L: Bovine spongiform encephalopathy and variant Creutzfeldt-Jakob disease: Background, evolution, and current concerns. Emerg Infect Dis 2001;7:6–16.

Caughey B, Chesebro B: Transmissible spongiform encephalopathies and prion protein interconversions. Adv Virus Res 2001;56:277–311.

Collie DA, Sellar RJ, Zeidler M, Colchester CF, Knight R, Will RG: MRI of Creutzfeldt-Jakob disease: Imaging features and recommended MRI protocol. Clin Radiol 2001;56:726–739.

Collinge J: Prion diseases of humans and animals: Their causes and molecular basis. Annu Rev Neurosci 2001;24:519–550.

Glatzel M, Aguzzi A: The shifting biology of prions. Brain Res Rev 2001; 36:241–248.

Prusiner SB: Neurodegenerative diseases and prions. New Engl J Med 2001;344:1516–1526.

Will RG, Zeidler M, Stewart GE, et al: Diagnosis of new variant Creutzfeldt-Jakob disease. Ann Neurol 2000;47:575–582.

References

1. Alper T, Cramp WA, Haig DA, Clarke MC: Does the agent of scrapie replicate without nucleic acid? Nature 1967;214:764–766.
2. Prusiner SB, Gabizon R, McKinley MP: On the biology of prions. Acta Neuropathol (Berl) 1987;72:299–314.
3. Zahn R, Liu A, Lührs T, et al: NMR solution structure of the human prion protein. Proc Natl Acad Sci (USA) 2000;97:145–150.
4. Gajdusek DC: Fantasy of a "virus" from the inorganic world: Pathogenesis of cerebral amyloidoses by polymer nucleating agents and/or "viruses." *In* Neth R, Gallo RC, Greaves MF, et al (eds): Modern Trends in Human Leukemia VIII. New York, Springer-Verlag, 1989, pp 481–499.
5. Kocisko DA, Come JH, Priola SA, et al: Cell-free formation of protease-resistant prion protein. Nature 1994;370:471–474.
6. Brown P, Gibbs C Jr, Rodgers-Johnson P, et al: Human spongiform encephalopathy: The National Institutes of Health series of 300 cases of experimentally transmitted disease. Ann Neurol 1994;35:513–529.
7. Brown P, Cathala F, Raubertas RF, et al: The epidemiology of Creutzfeldt-Jakob disease: Conclusion of a 15-year investigation in France and review of the world literature. Neurology 1987;37:895–904.
8. Will RG, Alperovitch A, Poser S, et al: Descriptive epidemiology of Creutzfeldt-Jakob disease in six European countries 1993–1995. Ann Neurol 1998;43:763–767.
9. Zerr I, Brandel J-P, Masullo C, et al: European surveillance on Creutzfeldt-Jakob disease: A case-control study for medical risk factors. J Clin Epidemiol 2000;53:747–754.
10. Steinhoff BJ, Racker S, Herrendorf G, et al: Accuracy and reliability of periodic sharp wave complexes in Creutzfeldt-Jakob disease. Arch Neurol 1996;53:162–166.
11. Zerr I, Pocchiari M, Collins S, et al: Analysis of EEG and CSF 14-3-3 proteins as aids to the diagnosis of Creutzfeldt-Jakob disease. Neurology 2000;55:811–815.
12. Collie DA, Sellar RJ, Zeidler M, Colchester CF, Knight R, Will RG: MRI of Creutzfeldt-Jakob disease: Imaging features and recommended MRI protocol. Clin Radiol 2001;56:726–739.
13. WHO Infection Control Guidelines for Transmissible Spongiform Encephalopathies: Report of a WHO Consultation. WHO/CDS/CSR/APH/2000.3. Geneva, Switzerland, 23–26 March 1999.
14. Brown P: Drug therapy in human and experimental transmissible spongiform encephalopathy. Neurology 2002, in press.
15. Brown P: BSE and transmission through blood. Lancet 2000;356:955–956.
16. Ghetti B, Piccardo P, Frangione B, et al: Prion protein amyloidosis. Brain Pathol 1996;6:127–145.
17. Collins S, McLean CA, Masters CL: Gerstmann-Sträussler-Scheinker syndrome, fatal familial insomnia, and kuru: A review of these less common human transmissible spongiform encephalopathies, J Chem Neurosci 2001;8:387–397.
18. Gambetti P, Parchi P, Petersen RB, et al: Fatal familial insomnia and familial Creutzfeldt-Jakob disease: Clinical pathological and molecular features. Brain Pathol 1995;5:43–51.
19. Goldfarb LG, Petersen RB, Tabaton M, et al: Fatal familial insomnia and familial Creutzfeldt-Jakob disease: Disease phenotype determined by a DNA polymorphism. Science 1992;258:806–808.
20. Goldfarb LG, Brown P, Cervenáková L, Gajdusek DC: Molecular genetic studies of Creutzfeldt-Jakob disease. Mol Neurobiol 1993;8:89–97.
21. Pocchiari M, Salvatore M, Cutruzzolá F, et al: A new point mutation of the prion protein gene in Creutzfeldt-Jakob disease. Ann Neurol 1993;34:802–807.
22. Brown P, Cervenáková L, Goldfarb LG, et al: Molecular genetic testing of a fetus at risk of Gerstmann-Sträussler-Scheinker syndrome. Lancet 1994;343:181–182.
23. Brown P, Preece M, Brandel J-P, et al: Iatrogenic Creutzfeldt-Jakob disease at the millennium. Neurology 2000;55:1075–1081.
24. Brown P: Transfusion medicine and spongiform encephalopathy. Transfusion 2001;41:433–436.

25. Will RG, Ironside JW, Zeidler M, et al: A new variant of Creutzfeldt-Jakob disease in the UK. Lancet 1996;347:921–925.
26. Ghani AC, Fergurson NM, Donnelly CA, Anderson RM: Predicted vCJD mortality in Great Britain. Nature 2000;406:583–584.
27. Valleron A-J, Boelle P-Y, Will R, Cesbron J-Y: Estimation of epidemic size and incubation time based on age characteristics of vCJD in the United Kingdom. Science 2001;294:1726–1728.
28. Brown P, Will RG, Bradley R, Asher DM, Detwiler L: Bovine spongiform encephalopathy and variant Creutzfeldt-Jakob disease: Background, evolution, and current concerns. Emerg Infect Dis 2001;7:6–16.
29. Will RG, Zeidler M, Stewart GE, et al: Diagnosis of new variant Creutzfeldt-Jakob disease. Ann Neurol 2000:47;575–582.
30. Ironside JW: Pathology of variant Creutzfeldt-Jakob disease. Arch Virol Suppl 2000;16:143–151.

CHAPTER 44

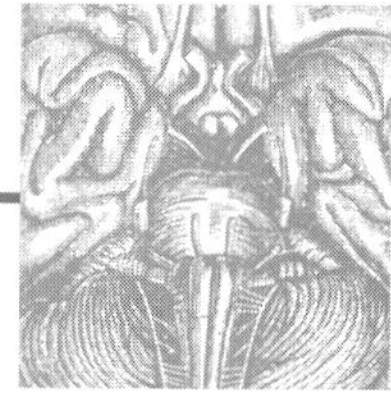

ANITA L. BELMAN and MIRJANA MALETIC-SAVATIC

Human Immunodeficiency Virus and Acquired Immunodeficiency Syndrome

Definitions and History

In 1981, the Centers for Disease Control and Prevention (CDC) reported the occurrence of *Pneumocystis carinii* pneumonia (PCP) in five Los Angeles homosexual men. Within months of this report, clusters of similar cases of young, previously healthy homosexual men, who had developed unusual neoplasms and unexplained opportunistic infections, were reported in New York and California. The disorder, which had the clinical and immunological hallmarks of a cell-mediated immunodeficiency (development of opportunistic infections, depressed numbers of circulating T-helper cells, with "reversed T4/T8 ratios"), was termed the *gay related immune deficiency (GRID) syndrome*. By the following year, the same syndrome complex was recognized in recipients of blood or blood products (mostly hemophiliacs) and in Haitians. Shortly thereafter, other high-risk groups were identified, namely men and women intravenous drug users and women whose only risk factor was sexual contact with men who were intravenous drug users, bisexuals, or both. These women's children were also a high-risk group. The disorder was renamed *the acquired immunodeficiency syndrome* (AIDS). Its epidemic nature was appreciated as increased numbers of cases were identified from specific geographic regions in the United States, Europe, and Africa. It was also appreciated that transmission of the disorder was from sexual contact, via mother to infant, or through blood-borne mechanisms. The agent, at that time, was thought to be most likely a virus that could survive the processing of blood factor VIII.

The etiological agent of AIDS, a retrovirus, was isolated in 1983[1–3] and named the human immunodeficiency virus (HIV) in 1986.[4] Once the agent was identified, studies confirmed the presence of HIV in sera that had been collected in central Africa in 1959 and the United States in 1968. It was not, however, until the early 1980s that HIV-1 infection began to reach epidemic proportions. Since then the epidemic has expanded relentlessly. From its beginning until December 2001, an estimated 66 million people worldwide have been infected with HIV-1.[5]

As a matter of definition, all individuals with AIDS are necessarily infected with HIV. However, patients with HIV infection do not qualify for classification as having AIDS unless certain criteria are fulfilled (Table 44–1, see later discussion). In certain settings (i.e., pediatric cases), the actual demonstration of HIV infection per CDC definition is not required for the diagnosis of AIDS (see Table 44–1).

Nervous system involvement complicating the course of AIDS was recognized in the very early years of the epidemic. In fact, the first reports of neurological complications appeared when the disorder was still termed GRID and thought to be restricted to homosexual males. Initially, in adults, neurological complications were believed to be caused strictly by central nervous system (CNS) opportunistic infections and neoplasms as a consequence of the immunodeficiency.[6] However, in 1985, distinct primary HIV-1–associated neurological disorders, unrelated to secondary infections or neoplasms, were described. In that same year, HIV-1 was isolated from brain, spinal cord, cerebrospinal fluid (CSF), and peripheral nerves.[7, 8] Between 1985 and 1988, further evidence from clinical, virological, and neuropathological studies indicated that neurological impairment in HIV-1–infected patients, referred to as *AIDS-dementia complex* in adults[9] and *AIDS encephalopathy/progressive encephalopathy* in children,[10] was associated with primary HIV-1 CNS infection. These studies included the following: (1) recovery of ribonucleic acid (RNA) and deoxyribonucleic acid (DNA) from the brain; (2) demonstration of intrathecal synthesis of anti-HIV

TABLE 44–1. **CDC Classification for HIV-1 Infection and Expanded Aids Surveillance Case Definition for Adolescents and Adults**

	Clinical Categories		
CD4+ Cell Categories	**(A) Asymptomatic or PGL**	**(B) Symptomatic Not (A) or (C) Conditions**	**(C) AIDS-Indicator Conditions**
(1) ≥500/mm^3	A1	B1	C1
(2) 200 to 499/mm^3	A2	B2	C2
(3) <200/mm^3 AIDS-indicator cell count	A3	B3	C3

PGL, persistent generalized lymphadenopathy.

Category A
Acute retroviral syndrome
Generalized lymphadenopathy
Asymptomatic disease
Pneumocystis carinii infection
Pneumonia, bacterial
Progressive multifocal leukoencephalopathy
Salmonellosis

Category B
Bacterial endocarditis, meningitis, pneumonia, or sepsis
Candidiasis, vulvovaginal: persisting (>1 month duration) or poorly responsive to therapy
Candidiasis, oropharyngeal (thrush)
Cervical dysplasia
Constitutional symptoms, such as fever (>38.5°C) or diarrhea lasting >1 month
Hairy leukoplakia, oral
Herpes zoster (shingles), involving at least two distinct episodes or more than one dermatome
Idiopathic thrombocytopenic purpura
Listeriosis
Nocardiosis
Pelvic inflammatory disease
Peripheral neuropathy

Category C
CD4 count <200/mm^3
Bacterial pneumonia, recurrent
Candidiasis of bronchi, trachea, or lungs
Candidiasis, esophageal
Cervical cancer, invasive
Coccidioidomycosis, disseminated or extrapulmonary
Cryptococcosis, extrapulmonary
Cryptosporidiosis, chronic intestinal (>1 month duration)
Cytomegalovirus disease (other than liver, spleen, or nodes)
Cytomegalovirus retinitis (with loss of vision)
HIV-1 encephalopathy
Herpes simplex: chronic ulcer(s) (>1 month duration) or bronchitis, pneumonitis, or esophagitis
Histoplasmosis, disseminated or extrapulmonary
Isosporiasis, chronic intestinal (>1 month duration)
Kaposi's sarcoma
Lymphoma, Burkitt's (or equivalent term)
Mycobacterial disease

antibodies; (3) localization of HIV-1 antigen in brain macrophages and monocytes by immunocytochemistry; (4) identification of viral particles within multinucleated giant cells and macrophages by electron microscopy; and (5) demonstration of increased levels of HIV-1 DNA in the brain compared with other organs by Southern blot analysis.[11–16] HIV-1 was also shown to belong to the lentivirus subfamily of retroviruses. In 1987, HIV/AIDS encephalopathy was recognized by the CDC as a major complication of HIV-1 infection and designated as one of the AIDS-defining conditions (i.e., a condition specific enough to diagnose AIDS in the context of documented HIV infection).[17]

It is now well-recognized that neurological disease at every anatomical level is a common complication of HIV-1 infection, and neurological symptoms and signs may be the initial manifestation of HIV/AIDS.[18, 19] Primary HIV-1–associated clinical syndromes are diverse and can occur not only at the onset, but also at other times during the course of infection. For example, a self-limited "aseptic meningitis"[20] may occur soon after initial infection, as may an acute encephalopathy,[21] myelopathy,[22] or neuropathy. During the next stage of HIV-1 disease (mild immune dysfunction), neurological complications such as "aseptic" meningitis, inflammatory demyelinating polyradiculopathy, myopathy, or zoster radiculitis may occur. With advancing HIV-1 disease (moderate to severe immunodeficiency), signs and symptoms of cognitive dysfunction, dementia, myelopathy, sensory neuropathy, and myopathy become more prevalent, as do nervous system opportunistic infections and neoplasms.[23]

In general, neurological involvement becomes increasingly more frequent with progression of HIV-1 disease; as the immunodeficiency worsens, the prevalence of associated neurological disorders increases. This chapter first presents a review of HIV, an overview of the virus' general role in disease, and the clinical criteria for AIDS. This is followed by a detailed account of HIV-1–related neurological disorders and a brief summary of the neurological malignancies and opportunistic infections that occur in the setting of AIDS.

Human Immunodeficiency Virus: Biology and General Medical Overview of Seroconversion and Early Infection

Pathogenesis and Pathophysiology. HIV-1, the etiological agent of AIDS, is a non-oncovirus RNA retrovirus that belongs to the *lentivirinae* genus of the Retroviridae family. Lentiviruses are species specific, contain RNA genome and reverse transcriptase, and have long periods of clinical latency and mechanisms to evade immune clearance. They target specific organs and cause persistent infection and multisystem disease in their natural hosts. Lentiviruses characteristically cause neurological disease. There are two distinct types of human AIDS viruses, HIV-1 and HIV-2, which are distinguished on the basis of their genome organizations and phylogenetic (i.e., evolutionary) relationships with other primate lentiviruses. Both have been further subclassified on the basis of phylogenetic criteria. Current data indicate that HIV-1 comprises three distinct virus groups (termed M, N, and O), with the predominant M group consisting of 11 classes, denoted subtypes A through K.[24] Similarly, HIV-2 strains infecting humans have been found to comprise six distinct virus groups (termed A through F).[24] Reconstruction of the phylogenetic relationships among the many strains of HIV-1 and HIV-2, as well as related viruses from African primates, has elucidated the simian origins of AIDS as well as factors that contributed to the beginning of the AIDS epidemic.

HIV-1, as other human retroviruses, is an enveloped virus containing RNA genomes of positive polarity. Structurally, HIV-1 is similar to other retroviruses (Fig. 44–1). There are two copies of the single-stranded RNA and reverse transcriptase (RNA-dependent DNA polymerase) in the central cylindrical core, which also contains four nucleocapsid proteins, p24, p17, p9, and p7. The nucleoprotein core is surrounded by a lipid bilayer membrane. The viral genome encodes for two classes of proteins: structural and regulatory. Three major segments code for the structural proteins: GAG

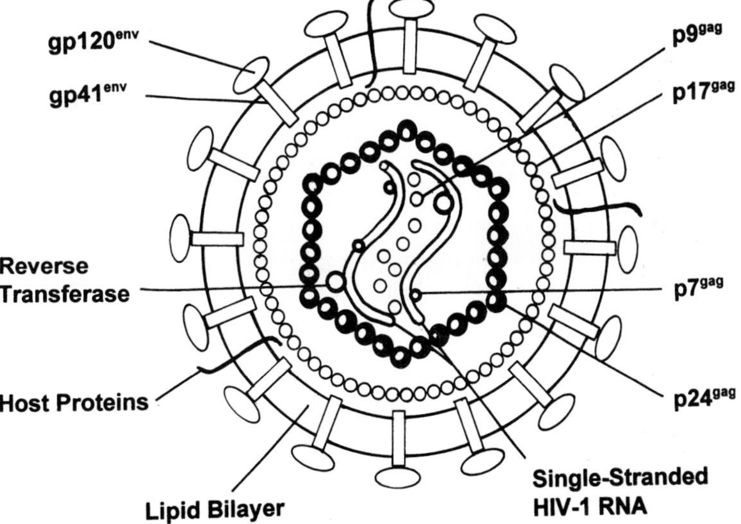

FIGURE 44–1. A schematic depiction of the HIV-1 virion. Virion protein components of the envelope and nucelocapsid are indicated. (Modified from Greene WC: The molecular biology of human immunodeficiency virus type 1 infection. N Engl J Med 1991;324:308–317.)

(the internal core protein), *POL* (the polymerase), and *ENV* (the envelope protein complex) (Fig. 44–2). These are situated in a left-to-right 5′-to-3′ order. The GAG gene encodes the internal core proteins of the virion particle (p24). The *POL* gene encodes the polymerase reverse transcriptase, a ribonuclease that copies the viral RNA into DNA, a ribonuclease (RNase H) that degrades the viral RNA once an initial DNA copy has been synthesized, and an endonuclease (integrase) that is responsible for integration of the DNA copy into the host cell genome. *POL* also encodes a protease that is required for the processing of the mature GAG and *POL* products from their polyprotein precursors during virion assembly. The *ENV* gene codes for the surface envelope glycoprotein gp160, which is cleaved into two major glycoproteins, gp120 and gp41. Gp120 forms surface spikes on the virion, and gp41 is a transmembrane glycoprotein. They mediate binding of the virus to the host target cell. Long terminal repeats are situated at each end of the retroviral genome and are involved in the regulation of viral expression and the initiation and termination of viral RNA transcription.

In general, retroviruses capable of replication contain only three genes (*GAG*, *POL*, and *ENV*). However, the viral genome of HIV-1 is more complex and contains additional genes for regulatory proteins. There are at least six genes (*TAT, REV, NEF, VIF, VPU*, and *VPR*) that regulate viral gene expression and are essential for virus replication. *TAT*, a transcriptional activator, stimulates the synthesis of HIV messenger RNAs early in the viral life cycle. *REV* modulates the pattern of viral RNAs expressed in infected cells, such as splicing and transport, and allows ordered production of viral proteins during the virus life cycle. The genes termed *VIF, VPU, VPR*, and *NEF* encode products that enhance the ability of the virus to productively infect host target cells and maximize the efficiency of viral replication. It is believed that the actions of these "additional" genes contribute to HIV-1's pathogenicity. Products of the *TAT, REV, VPR*, and *NEF* genes are neurotoxic.

The outer envelope of HIV-1 is derived from the host cell lipid bilayer during viral budding, when viral glycoproteins (coded by the *ENV* gene) are inserted. Electron microscopy has revealed that the HIV virion has an icosahedral structure containing 72 external spikes. These envelope spikes are responsible for binding to the receptor on the host cell and are important for cellular entry. They are composed of two components, gp120 and gp41. Gp120, the external protein, contains the receptor-binding determinants of the virus. The transmembrane protein, gp41, serves to anchor the envelope glycoprotein complex at the surface of the viral lipid bilayer and is responsible for cell entry through fusion with the cell membrane. The HIV-1 lipid bilayer also contains host proteins, including class I and class II histocompatibility antigens acquired during viral budding. Once within the cytoplasm of the host cell, the envelope of the virus is shed, its contents are released, and reverse transcription occurs. Reverse transcriptase enables the transcription of DNA from genomic RNA (contrary to the conventional informational flow from DNA to RNA to protein). The provirus DNA is then integrated into the host cell's DNA, where it may replicate, remain latent, or replicate at a restricted rate. When activated, the proviral DNA transcribes genomic and messenger RNA (Fig. 44–3). After the viral proteins are synthesized, new virions are assembled. Recently, two DNA microarray studies have illustrated a remarkably broad-based perturbation in host transcriptional responses, which is in part mediated by the HIV-encoded *NEF* protein. HIV therefore seems to function as a "master regulator" of cellular gene expression.[25] The virus matures by budding from the surface of cells or into vacuoles within the cells.[26]

HIV-1 targets, infects, and damages cells that have critically important functions in the host immune response. CD4 receptor is the principal target site for HIV. This target cell preference results from the high affinity binding of HIV-1 gp120 to the receptor molecule, CD4, which is used by HIV-1 during the initial stages of virus infection of host cells. Human CD4+ T-lymphocytes, monocytes/macrophages, and dendritic cells are the major cellular targets of HIV-1 infection in vivo.[27] Macrophages are an important reservoir of infection, including the microglia in the brain.[28] Dendritic cells bind HIV through DC-SIGN receptors and carry it from mucosal ports of entry to the lymph nodes, where they activate lymphocyte infection.[29] Based on the target cell preference, HIV-1 strains have been divided into T-tropic, which replicate in T lymphocytes, and M-tropic, which replicate in macrophages.

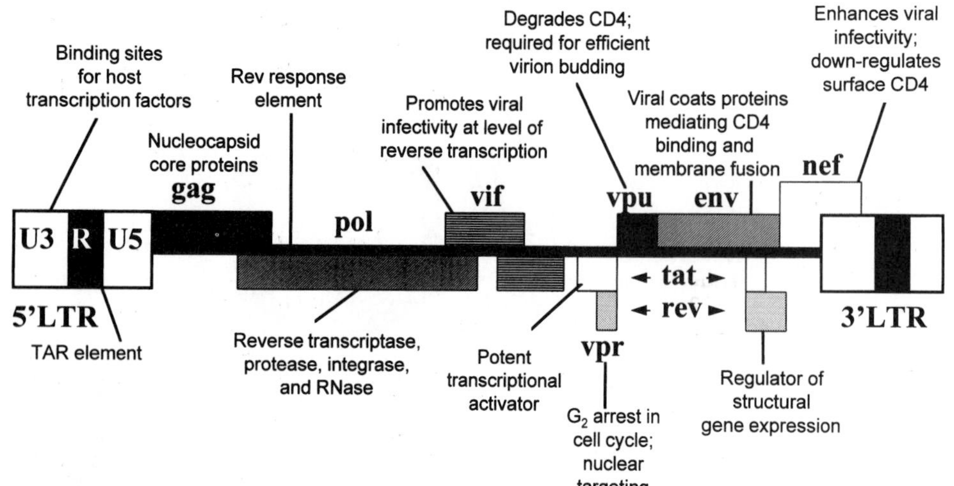

FIGURE 44–2. HIV-1 genomic structure. (Modified from Staprans SI, Feinberg MB: Natural history and immunopathogenesis of HIV-1 disease. *In* Sande MA, Volberding PA [eds]. The Medical Management of AIDS, 5th ed. Philadelphia, WB Saunders, 1997, pp 29–55.)

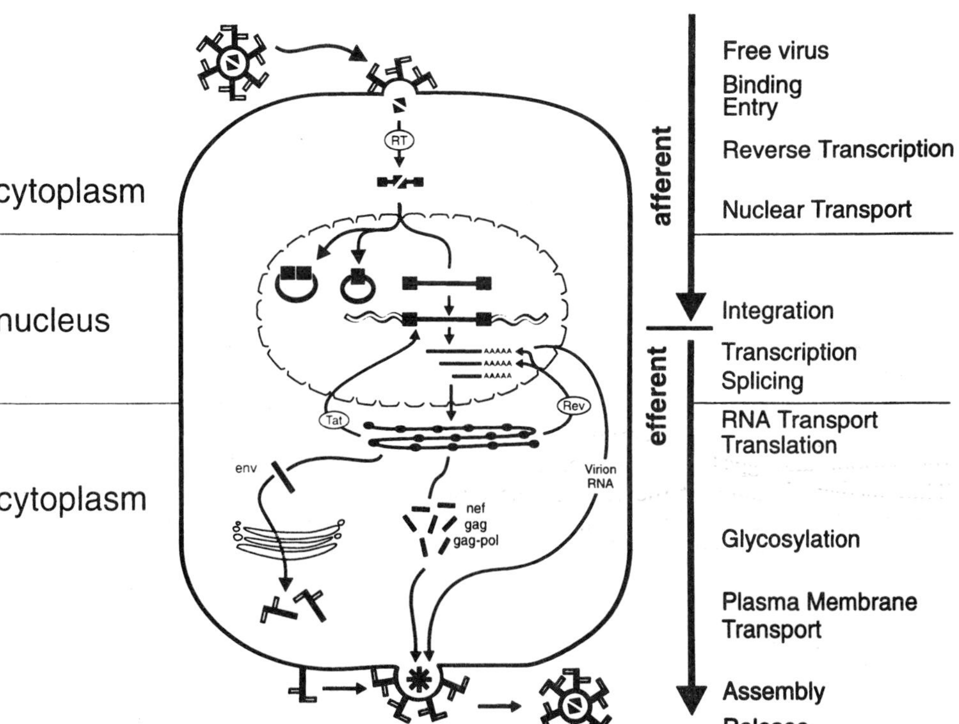

FIGURE 44–3. The human immunodeficiency virus life cycle (RNA-binding proteins: Tat, Rev; Retroviral genes: env, nef, gag, pol; RT, reverse transcriptase). (Reproduced with permission from Folks TM, Hart CE: The life cycle of human immunodeficiency virus type I. *In* DeVita VT, Hellman S, Rosenberg SA [eds]. AIDS: Biology, Diagnosis, Treatment and Prevention, 4th ed. Philadelphia, Lippincott-Raven, 1997, p 31.)

The CD4+ T-cell molecule is essential in interactions between helper-inducer T lymphocytes and antigen-presenting cells. It facilitates efficient recognition of antigens by CD4+ T cells, an obligate step in the generation of host immune responses. CD4+ lymphocytes serve as both essential regulators and effectors of the normal immune response. For example, they are involved in activation of macrophages, induction of cytotoxic T-lymphocyte function, natural killer and suppressor cell function, induction of B cells (dysfunction of which leads to impairment of the humoral arm of the immune system), growth and differentiation of lymphoid cells, regulation of hematopoietic colony stimulating factors, and other factors inducing nonlymphoid cell function. It is noteworthy that the CD4+ molecule is expressed at a very early stage of T-cell development, even on immature thymic T cells. Therefore, CD4+ T cells appear to be susceptible to HIV-1 infection and consequent destruction at essentially all stages of differentiation. The progressive loss of these critically important cells and basic components of the immune system ultimately leads to development of the profound immunodeficiency characteristic of advanced HIV-1 infection and eventually AIDS. In addition to the CD4 receptors, most recently, specific chemokine receptors have been shown to serve as important secondary cellular receptors, which guide the viral envelope glycoproteins into a specific conformation that allows membrane fusion and viral entry into the cell.[30, 31] T-tropic strains use CD4 receptor and chemokine CXR4 or fusin, while M-tropic strains use chemokine CCR5 receptor.[32] Interestingly, a genetic variant of CCR5, Delta32, has been found to be protective against HIV infection and to delay disease progression.

Even though most researchers agree that HIV induces both quantitative and qualitative defects in the CD4+ T-cell compartment, it is still not known how, in vivo, the virus destroys CD4+ T cells. In addition, it is not known whether cell loss is due to direct destruction by the virus or to some other, indirect factors.[33] Most researchers agree that HIV infection results in progressive loss of CD4+ T cells from the circulation as well as depletion of CD4+ T cells from total body stores. The normal young adult harbors about 2×10^{11} mature CD4+ T cells.[34] In the HIV-infected patient, the total number is halved by the time the peripheral blood CD4+ T-cell count falls to 200 cells/μL.[34, 35] In more advanced disease, destruction of parenchymal lymphoid spaces is so extensive that counting of CD4+ T cells has not even been attempted. With disease progression, there is also a decrease in the proportion of quiescent, naïve T cells and an increase in the proportion of activated, memory/effector T cells.[36] Among those cells that persist, many may be dysfunctional.[37] Hence, the circulating CD4+ T-cell count is very imprecise. However, it is still one of the best surrogate markers used to initiate treatment and to determine the prognosis late in infection.

Despite the enormous wealth of information accrued during the past decade concerning molecular properties and actions of the retrovirus, many fundamental questions remain concerning immunopathogenetic events. The following overview traces some of the major events once HIV-1 is transmitted to the host (Fig. 44–4). In-depth reviews that discuss postulated HIV's virological and immunological mechanisms have been published.[38–40] The virus, free or within cells, enters the blood or lymphatic vessels and is delivered to lymphoid tissue. It is suggested that macrophages may be the first target cell of HIV-1 early after invasion. Macrophages deliver HIV-1 to lymph nodes and other lymphoid tissue and may serve as a reservoir for HIV-1. A selection of HIV-1 strains may occur during this acute infection stage. Studies of HIV-1 isolates from donor-recipient transmission pairs show that donors have heterogeneous viral populations. In contrast, viral isolates from the newly infected

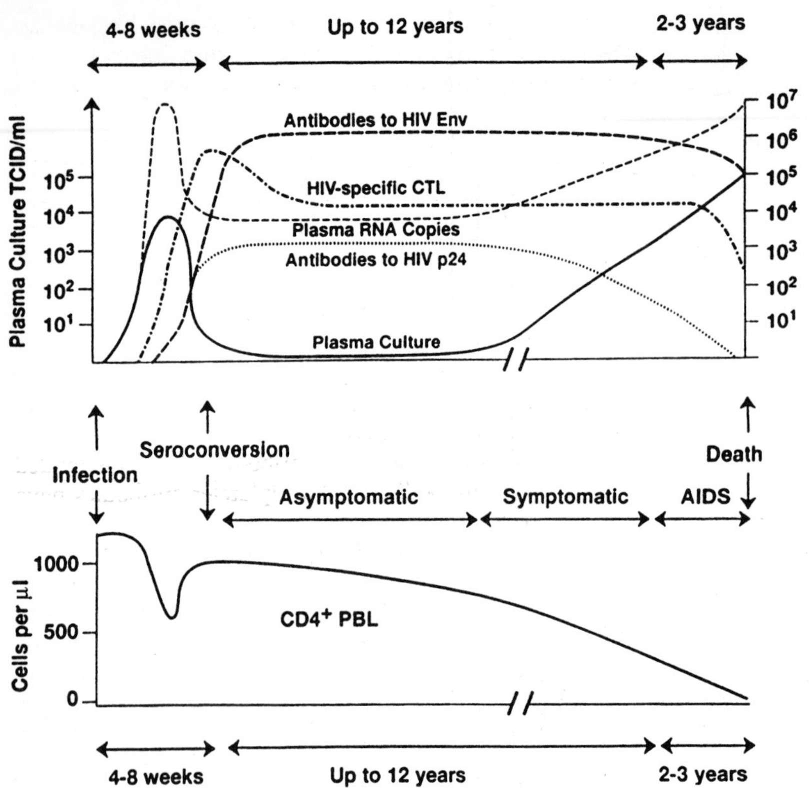

FIGURE 44–4. HIV-1 natural history. (Modified from Staprans SI, Feinberg MB: Natural history and immunopathogenesis of HIV-1 disease. *In* Sande MA, Volberding PA [eds]. The Medical Management of AIDS, 5th ed. Philadelphia, WB Saunders, 1997, pp 29–55.)

person are predominantly homogeneous in their envelope sequences and these viruses are mainly M-tropic.[41]

HIV-1 then enters the lymphoid tissue and an active immune response is mounted. A preferential infection of cells that are responding to or are proliferating in response to antigenic stimulation occurs. This leads to new cycles of HIV-1 replication and target cell infection.[42] Viral spread occurs to T cells and macrophages, and during the weeks after the initial infection, more cells are infected and more are lost. There is an increase in viral burden and an associated decline in the CD4+ lymphocyte counts. At this point, some individuals may develop symptomatic acute primary infection with both systemic and neurological signs (see later discussion). It is believed that a host immune response, cell-mediated and humoral, is mounted and controls the infection to some degree. Clinical symptoms of the acute illness resolve, and the amount of virus in peripheral blood falls. Monocytes, macrophages, and follicular dendritic cells are able to foster viral replication without cell death. These cells may serve as a reservoir for the retrovirus, allowing transport and dissemination (and possibly persistent infection) of the virus to nonlymphoid tissues such as the brain and other organ systems with subsequent development of organ-specific HIV-1–related disorders. For example, HIV-1 infection of gut epithelium may contribute to the diarrhea-wasting syndrome seen commonly in patients with more advanced HIV-1 infection, whereas infection of bone marrow progenitor cells may contribute to hematological abnormalities observed clinically in symptomatic HIV-1–infected patients. HIV-1 infection of these diverse organ cells may not be mediated by the CD4+ receptor but by others, such as the glycolipid galactosylceramide.

HIV seeds the meninges and CSF early during the course of infection.[43] Viral load is distributed unequally in the brain, mostly concentrating in the hippocampus and basal ganglia (caudate and globus pallidus), correlating with the clinical symptoms of HIV-associated dementia.[44] However, absolute brain viral load does not correlate well with the presence of HIV-associated dementia and the exact mechanisms by which HIV-1 infection leads to dementia are not understood. HIV-1 free viral particles, as well as infected monocytes, penetrate to the brain tissue through the disrupted blood-brain barrier, most likely due to the dysfunction of endothelial cells and changes in the basal lamina proteins, such as laminin, entactin, and collagen.[45] In addition, some viral proteins may be transported to the brain even through the intact blood-brain barrier, as was shown for *TAT*.[46] Both CD4 receptors and chemokine receptors CCR5 and CCR3 have been implicated in viral entry of HIV-1 M-strains into the brain microglial cells,[31] which then undergo a productive infection, syncytial formation, and cell death. In addition to the infection of microglia, HIV-1 infects astrocytes, mostly by T-tropic strains.[47] The mechanism is not known, as astrocytes lack both CD4 and cytokine receptors. The HIV-1 infection of astrocytes behaves differently than infection of microglial cells. Initially, the virus undergoes a productive infection, but then enters a latent phase and does not cause cell death.[47] It practically stays in astrocytes indefinitely, escaping all antiretroviral agents.

After the acute symptomatic or asymptomatic primary infection, there is a period of clinical latency. Patients enter a chronic clinically asymptomatic or minimally symptomatic period. Recent studies show that even during the clinically "latent" period of disease there is a high rate of viral expression and replication in lymphoid tissue.[48] In the stage of early and intermediate HIV-1 disease (Table 44–2), the greatest concentration of HIV-1–infected cells is still found in the lymphoid organs (lymph nodes, adenoids, tonsils, spleen).

TABLE 44–2. **Stages of HIV-1 Disease as Related to CD4+ Count**

Early HIV-1 infection	CD4+ ≥500 cells/μL
Intermediate HIV-1 infection	CD4+ 200–500 cells/μL
AIDS	CD4+ ≤200 cells/μL

There is, however, involvement of nonlymphoid tissues as well.[49] A very dynamic pattern of HIV-1 replication and turnover may occur. Ho and colleagues estimated that approximately 1 billion new virions are produced daily with replication occurring in lymphoid tissue.[48] At the same time, about 1 to 2 billion new CD4+ cells are produced. Persistence of virus in lymphoid tissue can cause chronic stimulation of the immune system.[50] This may lead to dysfunction and destruction of the responding T cells. Even before the occurrence of a marked decline in CD4+ cell numbers, specific defects in T-cell function can be noted. The effect on the immune system is widespread, affecting multiple aspects of lymphocytic function, the interaction of T cells with antigen-presenting cells, and disruption of lymphoid tissue architecture.

As CD4+ lymphocytes are lost as a result of virus-induced damage, the host's immune system attempts to compensate for depleted T cells by producing more cells, which become infected. It is hypothesized that homeostatic mechanisms exist to maintain a "normal" T-cell count. This hypothesis implies that the selective loss of CD4+ cells will induce production of both CD4+ and CD8+ cells in order to maintain homeostasis of T-cell number (referred to as "blind homeostasis"). CD4+ and CD8+ cells continue to be produced to maintain the total lymphocyte count as CD4+ cells are lost. This results in CD4+ cell lymphopenia and CD8+ lymphocytosis.[51] CD8+ lymphocytosis may in itself cause symptomatic complications. Approximately 18 months before the development of AIDS, this mechanism breaks down, resulting in lymphopenia. An increase in the rate of loss of CD4+ lymphocytes and perhaps in the appearance of more virulent viral phenotypes heralds the progression to AIDS.[52]

Regarding the pathophysiology of HIV-1 infection in children, a bimodal evolution of disease progression is noted (see later discussion). Infants with rapid disease progression (the first form) have high levels of detectable virus at birth and manifest severe clinical symptoms and immunological abnormalities within the first years of life. Some of these infants may lack anti–HIV-1 antibodies. This rapidly progressive course may reflect the effects of HIV-1 on the developing fetal thymus and immune system. In some cases, however, high levels of viral expression are found with normal CD4+ cell counts, suggesting that in this subset of children, early HIV-1 thymic infection may be impaired and resulted in immunological tolerance.

In children with slowly progressive disease (the second form), there is the occurrence of more frequent and severe infections with common childhood pathogens followed later by opportunistic infections. Although the principal target of HIV-1 is the human peripheral blood CD4+ T-lymphocyte, in children one of the first immunological abnormalities is impairment of B-cell function. This is manifested by polyclonal hypergammaglobulinemia, spontaneous B-cell proliferation, and increased in vitro spontaneous production of immunoglobulin. The development of polyclonal hypergammaglobulinemia may also be noted in adults.[53] Although the quantity of immunoglobulins is elevated, there are diminished in vivo vaccine responses to both T-cell dependent and T-cell independent antigens, as well as decreased responses to B-cell mitogens.[54] In vitro studies demonstrate diminished lymphocyte proliferation to B-cell mitogens. The decreased antibody responses predispose these infants and children to serious bacterial infections, which at times may be overwhelming. The B-cell activation may also result in polyclonal polymorphic B-cell lymphoproliferative disorders, such as lymphoid interstitial pneumonitis, parotitis, and unusual B-cell related complications such as B-cell lymphomas. Increased production of autoantibodies may also result from B-cell dysfunction. Circulating immune complexes, antinuclear antibodies, antibody to double-stranded DNA, red cell antibodies, and antiplatelet antibodies have been reported.

Epidemiology and Risk Factors. HIV-1 is transmitted by either sexual contact, parenteral exposure to blood, blood products, or body fluids; or from mother to infant. In the United States, western Europe, Australia, and in some Latin American countries, the majority of AIDS cases were initially among men infected through sexual contacts with other men. In the United States, the proportion that this group now represents has declined from approximately 72 percent in 1986 to 53 percent.[55] It is estimated that 75 percent of HIV-1 infection worldwide is the result of heterosexual transmission. Heterosexual transmission predominates in sub-Saharan Africa, the Caribbean, Southeast Asia (Thailand), and India. At present, in the United States, the number of women with heterosexually acquired infection continues to rise.

In the United States, western Europe, and Latin America, intravenous drug use (sharing of contaminated needles/equipment) was and remains a significant risk factor for transmission.[56] About 24 percent of AIDS cases in the United States were related to intravenous drug use. Iatrogenic spread of infection by the reuse of contaminated needles is also reported.[57] Since HIV-1 donor blood screening has been instituted, transfusion-acquired HIV-1 infection is rare in developed countries, but unfortunately it still occurs and accounts for a proportion of cases in undeveloped nations. Overall, in the United States, transfusion recipients and hemophiliacs represent less than 2 percent of cases.[58]

Maternal-to-infant transmission can occur in utero, during labor and delivery, or postnatally by breast-feeding.[59] Both the risk factors of mother-to-infant transmission and its timing are under active investigation. In utero transmission before 20 weeks' gestation is well documented. However, current evidence suggests that transmission during the third trimester and at parturition may be most common.[59–63] The rate of mother-to-infant infection is estimated at about 25 percent (range, 13 to 45 percent).[64] Maternal factors reported to be associated with increased risk of transmission include low CD4+ counts, high viral titers, advanced primary HIV-1 disease, AIDS, placental membrane inflammation, premature rupture of membranes, premature delivery, increased exposure of the infant to maternal blood, and low vitamin A.[57, 59, 60, 65, 66]

An estimated 40 million people worldwide are currently living with HIV, and at least 20 million people have already died, giving a cumulative total number of HIV infections of

66 million.[5] The worst of the epidemic is sub-Saharan Africa where, at the end of 2000, there were an estimated 25.3 million people living with HIV. Sub-Saharan Africa has accounted for around three quarters of the global death toll. There, HIV-1 transmission continues to be dominated by heterosexual sex, together with a significant level of mother-to-child transmission. Recent reports from UNAIDS show HIV spreading rapidly in other areas as well, including parts of China, eastern Europe, and central Asia. By the end of 2001, there were an estimated 2.7 million children under 15 living with HIV, over 90 percent of whom acquired infection from their mother.[67] Another tragic consequence of the epidemic is the increasing numbers of "AIDS orphans" (children under 15 years of age who have lost one or both parents to AIDS). By 2010, 25 million children are projected to be orphaned as a result of HIV/AIDS (*www.UNAIDS.org*).

In the developed countries, the epidemic changed due to initiation of the highly active antiretroviral therapy (HAART). In the course of 2000, an estimated 30,000 adults and children became infected with HIV in western Europe and 45,000 in North America, taking the total numbers living with HIV in these regions combined to 1.46 million. During 2001, 5 million people were newly infected with HIV-1 worldwide; 1.8 million were women and 800,000 were children; about 2000 HIV-1–infected infants were born per day![67] Persistent incidence at relatively low levels over the past decade has combined with longer survival.[58] Recently, UNAIDS provided a comprehensive review of the HIV/AIDS epidemic worldwide, with detailed distribution of the disease as well as predominant ways of transmission, which differ in different continents and countries.[67]

Although adolescents comprise only about 1 percent of total AIDS cases in the United States, approximately 20 percent of total AIDS cases are in the young adult age group (up to 29 years of age). Given that it may take about 10 years between infection with HIV-1 and the onset of symptoms, it can be assumed that many of these persons were infected as adolescents. In fact, it is estimated that at least 50 percent of the worldwide HIV-1 population were infected between ages 15 and 24 years.[68] In the United States and Europe, transfusion-acquired HIV-1 infection had been the most common cause of adolescent HIV-1 infection. However, since HIV donor blood screening has been instituted, the percentage of all cases that this group now represents has declined. At present, the most common risk factors for adolescents include sexual exposure and intravenous drug use.[57] It is estimated that approximately 65 percent of adolescents ages 13 to 19 years and 90 percent of 20- to 24-year-olds with AIDS were infected through these means.[68, 69] Because of improved medical management and the differential natural history of pediatric AIDS, an increasing number of vertically infected children are living into adolescence and even young adulthood. It is anticipated that the percentage that this group represents will continue to rise as more effective therapies for HIV-1 and its associated disorders lengthen survival.

Clinical Features and Associated Disorders. Within 2 to 6 weeks after HIV-1 infection, virus can be detected in the blood (see Fig. 44–4).[70] Primary HIV-1 infection may be associated with constitutional, dermatological, gastrointestinal, as well as neurological signs and symptoms (Table 44–3). A self-limiting acute viral syndrome (fever, myalgia, arthralgia, lymphadenopathy, maculopapular rash, and aseptic meningitis [see later discussion]) is described in a subset of patients a few weeks after primary infection and may last from 1 to 2 weeks.[71] The HIV-1 rash is characterized as an erythematous, nonpruritic, maculopapular rash that is symmetrical, may affect the face or trunk with or without involvement of the palms and soles, or may be generalized. Lesions may be 5 to 10 mm in diameter. Other patients are asymptomatic. Factors determining if a newly infected person will develop symptomatic primary infection are not clearly defined. Inoculum size, immunological state of the individual, transmission of HIV-1 from a person with late-stage disease, possibly viral strain differences, and other host factors may be important variables. It is suggested that those persons who are symptomatic with the acute retroviral syndrome (especially those with symptomatic disease lasting more than 2 weeks), those with neurological signs and symptoms, or those who acquired HIV-1 from a person with late-stage disease may be more likely to have more rapid disease progression than those without these early symptoms.[72] Clinical and laboratory features at the time of acute primary HIV-1 infection may also portend the subsequent course of disease.[72] Thrush, persistent fever, diarrhea, weight loss, oral hairy leukoplakia, cutaneous herpes zoster, and age greater than 35 years during this early phase of infection appear to be associated with more rapid disease progression.[73] Virological markers include infection with SI strain of virus, persistent p24 antigenemia, and high HIV RNA viremia after seroconversion. Immunological features that may have adverse prognostic significance include low p24 antibody titres, high gp120 antibody titres, presence of specific anti-HIV-1 IgM and IgA antibodies after infection, persistent low CD4+ lymphocyte count, high CD38 expression on CD8+ lymphocytes, and an oligoclonal T-cell response.

TABLE 44–3. **Clinical Manifestation of Primary HIV-1 Infection**

General	Fever
	Pharyngitis
	Lymphadenopathy
	Arthralgias/myalgias
	Headache, retro-orbital pain
	Lethargy, malaise
	Anorexia, weight loss
	Cough
Dermatological	Erythematous maculopapular rash
	Roseola-like rash
	Diffuse urticaria
	Desquamation
	Alopecia
	Palatal or gingival ulceration
Gastrointestinal	Nausea, vomiting
	Diarrhea
	Oral-pharyngeal candidiasis
Neurological	Headache
	Meningitis
	Encephalitis
	Peripheral neuropathy
	Radiculopathy
	Guillain-Barré syndrome
	Cognitive or affective impairment

Adapted from Hollander H: Primary HIV infection in management of HIV infections and their complications. *In* Sande MA, Volberding PA (eds): The Medical Management of AIDS, 5th ed. Philadelphia, WB Saunders, 1997.

Within 6 months of infection, most infected persons have detectable levels of anti-HIV antibodies.[74] A stage of clinical latency follows. Signs and symptoms of progressive immune dysfunction or of HIV-1 itself generally develop from 6 months to several years thereafter. Mild to moderate clinical manifestations during the intermediate stage of the disease (see Table 44–2) may include generalized lymphadenopathy, chronic diarrhea, night sweats, weight loss, fatigue, infections indicative of cell-mediated immunodeficiency (such as herpes zoster [see later discussion and Chapter 41], oral candidiasis, and oral hairy leukoplakia). These diverse clinical manifestations of HIV-1 infection may in part reflect the immunological response to the rapid and extensive dissemination of HIV-1.

The time to occurrence of AIDS is variable. A small percentage of patients may develop an AIDS-defining condition (see Table 44–1) during the first 2 years of infection, whereas some infected people remain healthy for more than 15 years. In the absence of treatment, about 50 percent of adults will develop AIDS within 10 years after infection.[75] As the CD4+ count declines, more serious opportunistic infections develop. The risk of developing an AIDS-defining condition increases as the duration of HIV-1 infection increases, and usually occurs in patients with less than 200 CD4+ cells/ μL. The natural history of vertically acquired HIV-1 infection in infants and children differs from that of adults. The adverse effects of HIV-1 on the developing immune system and nervous system often result in more rapid onset of clinical symptoms and progression to death. A bimodal evolution of symptomatic pediatric HIV-1 disease, with different rates of survival, is recognized from both clinical and data modeling studies. The first "hump" occurs in infancy, and the second (and larger "hump") later in childhood.[65, 69, 76] There is probably a trimodal evolution with the third "hump" (albeit smaller) occurring in the pre- and early adolescent years.[59, 69, 77] As in adults, latency to onset of symptoms in this group of children may be 10 years or more.

Infants in the first group develop symptomatic disease during the first years of life ("AIDS/HIV encephalopathy" [see later discussion], PCP, cytomegalovirus [CMV] infection, and/or wasting syndrome). The children in the second group have a more "benign" initial course (slower progression). Evidence of lymphoproliferative processes characteristic of pediatric HIV-1 infection is frequent and includes lymphadenopathy, hepatosplenomegaly, and parotid gland enlargement. Multiple or recurrent bacterial infections, ranging from otitis media, pneumonia, and bone and joint infection to sepsis and meningitis are common in both groups, as is failure to thrive, persistent oral candidiasis, and chronic or recurrent diarrhea.[54] Although these children have a form of HIV-1 disease that progresses more slowly, the disease may ultimately involve many organ systems, including the CNS, cardiovascular system (cardiomyopathy), and kidneys. A polyclonal, polymorphic B-cell lymphoproliferative disorder is commonly described with nodular lymphoid lesions in the lung as well as other organs and with lymphoid infiltrate in both nodal and extranodal sites. With HIV-1 disease progression, T-cell abnormalities develop, including lymphopenia, low absolute numbers of CD4+ cells, poor in vitro lymphocytic proliferation to T-cell mitogens, and cutaneous anergy. Infections indicative of cell-mediated immune dysfunction occur. PCP is the most common opportunistic infection, while disseminated candidiasis, *Mycobacterium avium–intracellulare* (MAI), and disseminated invasive CMV are the next most common. As in adults, CMV may produce colitis, pneumonitis, or retinitis. Other infections include disseminated ulcerative herpes simplex infections, cryptosporidiosis, and rarely, toxoplasmosis.

The 1993 revised CDC classification system for HIV-1 infection incorporates both clinical conditions and immunological parameters determined by CD4+ cell counts. There are three clinical categories: (A) asymptomatic infection, persistent generalized lymphadenopathy, acute primary HIV-1 infection; (B) symptomatic conditions occurring in an HIV-1–infected person, excluding those conditions specified in categories A and C; and (C) symptomatic conditions occurring in an HIV-1–infected person (AIDS-indicator diseases). Immunological categories are stratified according to CD4+ cell counts: (1) CD4+ cell greater than or equal to 500 cells/μL; (2) CD4+ cell 200 to 499 cells/μL; and (3) CD4+ cells less than 200 cells/μL (AIDS-indicator counts).

For the purpose of epidemiological surveillance, the CDC initially defined AIDS in children under age 13 years with the same restrictive clinical case definition as adults (i.e., required documentation of an opportunistic infections or an AIDS-related malignancy). Additionally, primary (congenital) or secondary immunodeficiency disorders and congenital infections had to be excluded. After HIV-1 was identified and with the advent of serological testing for the presence of anti-HIV-1 antibodies in 1985, only a small proportion of children with confirmed HIV-1 infection and HIV-1–related disease manifestations were found to fit the case definition criteria for AIDS. Subsequent revisions by the CDC broadened this definition. In 1985, biopsy-proven lymphoid interstitial pneumonitis was included as a pediatric AIDS indicator condition. In 1987, a major revision substantially expanded the criteria. This classification was based on laboratory evidence of HIV-1 infection, immunological function, and a spectrum of clinical manifestations (Table 44–4). In

TABLE 44–4. **CDC Classification System for HIV in Children (Revised 1994)**

Category N: Not Symptomatic

Children who have no signs or symptoms considered to be the result of HIV infection or who have only one of the conditions listed in category A

Category A: Mildly Symptomatic

Children with two or more of the conditions listed but none of the conditions listed in categories B and C:

- Lymphadenopathy (≥0.5 cm at more than two sites; bilateral equals one site)
- Hepatomegaly
- Splenomegaly
- Dermatitis
- Parotitis
- Recurrent or persistent upper respiratory infection, sinusitis, or otitis media

Category B: Moderately Symptomatic

Children who have symptomatic conditions other than those listed in category A or C that are attributed to HIV infection. Examples of conditions in clinical category B include but are not limited to the following:

- Anemia (<8 g/dL), neutropenia (<1000 cells/μL), or thrombocytopenia (<100,000/μL) persisting ≥30 d

Table continued on following page

TABLE 44–4. **CDC Classification System for HIV in Children (Revised 1994)** *Continued*

Bacterial meningitis, pneumonia, or sepsis
Candidiasis, oropharyngeal thrush
Cardiomyopathy
Cytomegalovirus infection
Diarrhea, recurrent or chronic
Hepatitis
Herpes simplex virus (HSV) stomatitis, recurrent
HSV bronchitis, pneumonitis, or esophagitis
Herpes zoster (at least two distinct episodes or more than one dermatome)
Leiomyosarcoma
Lymphoid interstitial pneumonia (LIP)
Nephropathy
Nocardiosis
Persistent fever (lasting >1 month)
Toxoplasmosis, onset before 1 month of age
Varicella

Category C: Severely Symptomatic

Children who have any condition listed in the 1987 surveillance case definition for acquired immunodeficiency syndrome (with the exception of LIP)

Serious bacterial infections
Candidiasis, esophageal or pulmonary
Coccidioidomycosis
Cryptococcosis
Cryptosporidiosis
Cytomegalovirus disease
Encephalopathy
HSV infection
Histoplasmosis
Kaposi's sarcoma
Lymphoma, primary, in brain
Lymphoma
Mycobacterium tuberculosis
Mycobacterium, other species or unidentified species
Mycobacterium avium complex or M. *kansasii*
Pneumocystis carinii pneumonia
Progressive multifocal leukoencephalopathy
Salmonella
Toxoplasmosis of the brain with onset >1 month of age
Wasting syndrome

Adapted from Centers for Disease Control and Prevention: Revised classification system for human immunodeficiency virus infection in children less than 13 years of age. MMWR 1994;43:1.

1994, revised CDC criteria based the diagnosis of AIDS in children on three indices: (A) infectious status, (B) clinical status, and (C) immunological status (Table 44–5).[78] The revised classification system reflects the child's disease and establishes mutually exclusive categories.

Differential Diagnosis. Serological testing for anti-HIV-1 antibody (enzyme-linked immunosorbent assay [ELISA]), with a confirmatory Western blot, usually provides the diagnosis. However, during the stage of acute HIV-1 infection before seroconversion, there may be a false-positive heterophil, which can confuse the diagnosis.[79] The clinical syndrome of acute HIV-1 infection in the adult is distinctive (see preceding discussion). It contrasts to the distribution of rubella rash, which is characterized as an erythematous fine and mild maculopapular rash that rapidly spreads in a cephalocaudal fashion from face to extremities, is usually generalized within 1 day, and clears within 72 hours to 4 days. A rash is also unusual in Epstein-Barr virus or CMV infection (less than 5 percent of patients) unless antibiotics have been given.

The infant or child with vertically acquired HIV-1 infection may present with several clinical manifestations. Differential diagnosis, therefore, is dependent on the presenting signs and symptoms and the age of the child. Later in infancy and in childhood, if the presenting symptoms are chronic or recurrent infections or opportunistic infections, the most important and likely diagnosis is an immunodeficiency disorder. An appropriate history, examination, and immunological analysis, including HIV-1 testing, can usually rule out these conditions.

Evaluation. The goal of the diagnostic workup is to establish the presence of HIV-1 infection and determine the stage of the disease, extent of immune dysfunction, and presence or absence of neurological involvement. Accurate staging helps to formulate a prognosis, plan prophylactic therapy for opportunistic infections, and determine antiretroviral therapeutic strategies for primary HIV-1 infection. Once HIV-1 infection is confirmed by anti-HIV-1 antibody testing (i.e., ELISA, with a confirmatory Western blot in adults), a complete history should be obtained, including a review of risk factors for HIV-1 exposure, drug and alcohol history, sexual history, travel history, and medical history. A complete baseline physical examination should be performed. Focused follow-up examinations are then recommended with attention directed to findings that indicate disease progression, such as general appearance and weight loss, dermatological conditions (seborrheic dermatitis, folliculitis, dermatophytosis, Kaposi's sarcoma, bacillary angiomatosis), oral lesions (candidiasis, hairy leukoplakia, aphthous ulcers, periodontal disease), localized lymphadenopathy, splenomegaly, and signs or symptoms of neurological/neuropsychiatric involvement (mood or affective disorders, psychomotor slowing, abnormal eye movements, hyper-reflexia, change of gait).

Initial laboratory studies should include CD4+/CD8+ counts (absolute cell counts and percentages) and, if possible, HIV-1 RNA levels. Complete blood count (CBC) with differential count, electrolyte and liver function panel, hepatitis

TABLE 44–5. **CDC Pediatric Human Immunodeficiency Virus Classification (1994)**

	Age of Child		
Immunological Categories	**<12 Months Cells/μL (percent)**	**1 to 5 Years Cells/μL (percent)**	**6 to 12 Years Cells/μL (percent)**
No evidence of suppression	≥1500 (≥25)	≥1000 (≥25)	>500 (≥25)
Evidence of moderate suppression	750 to 1499 (15 to 24)	500 to 999 (15 to 24)	200 to 499 (15 to 24)
Severe suppression	<750 (<15)	<500 (<15)	<200 (<15)

screen, reactive protein reagin or Venereal Disease Research Laboratory (VDRL) titer, anti-toxoplasma IgG antibodies, purified protein derivative with anergy panel, and chest x-ray should also be obtained. Ophthalmological, dental, and gynecological examinations (including a Papanicolau smear, chlamydia and gonorrhea studies) should be pursued. The stage of HIV-1 infection will then determine follow-up, prophylaxis, and therapeutic strategies.

In addition to declining CD4+ cell counts and CD4+/CD8+ lymphocyte ratios, other immunological markers of disease progression include elevated levels of serum beta-2 microglobulin, neopterin, serum acid labile interferon, and decreased or absent levels of anti-p24 antibody. Virological indicators of disease progression are p24 antigenemia, HIV culture, quantitative polymerase chain reaction (PCR) of proviral DNA in cells or RNA in serum, and the presence of syncytium-inducing strains of virus. Elevated erythrocyte sedimentation rate (ESR) and decreased hematocrit values serve as nonspecific markers.

HIV-1 infection in infants can be diagnosed by as early as 1 month and by 6 months in the vast majority of children.[80, 81] All children known to be at risk or exposed to HIV in utero need to be tested. HIV DNA PCR is the recommended test for infants. Neonates at risk should be tested before 48 hrs of age, and subsequently at 1 to 2 months, as well as between 3 and 6 months of age. Positive virological test at 48 hrs of age is indicative for in utero HIV infection. Negative virological test at 48 hrs of age but positive at the subsequent test times is indicative for the acquired infection during the intrapartum period. Two negative virological tests on separate blood samples, done at more than 1 month of age and at more than 4 months of age, tentatively exclude the diagnosis of HIV-1 infection in an exposed infant. If an infant is older than 6 months, two or more negative virologic tests or two negative HIV IgG antibody tests, performed at least 1 month apart, again tentatively exclude HIV infection if there is no evidence of clinical HIV symptomatology. Finally, at 18 months of age, if all virological tests are negative, HIV IgG antibody test is negative, there is no hypogammaglobulinemia, and there are no clinical signs of HIV infection, HIV infection can be definitely excluded.[80, 81]

The initial laboratory evaluations of children over age 18 months suspected of having HIV-1 infection should include HIV-1 serological testing (ELISA/Western blot), a CBC, and lymphocyte subsets (CD3, CD4, CD8 [and CD4:CD8 ratio]) enumeration. Other routine diagnostic tests, such as chest x-ray study, urinalysis, appropriate cultures for pathogens, a chemistry panel, and IgA, IgM, and IgG levels may also be warranted.

Management. Early recognition and diagnosis of HIV-1 infection is important to institute appropriate counseling, prevent further spread of the virus, limit the number of additional clinical and laboratory evaluations, and exclude possible other disorders. Thereafter, the mainstays of management of HIV-1 infection include antiretroviral therapy for primary HIV-1 infection and prophylaxis and treatment of opportunistic infections.[82] Drugs that treat HIV-1 infection attempt to interfere with the replication of HIV. Targeted points in the growth cycle of the virus include (1) blockage of viral entry (soluble CD4+ preparations); (2) prevention of transcription of RNA to DNA (reverse transcriptase inhibitors); (3) interference with translation (drugs acting on regulatory genes or their proteins); (4) inhibition of assembly (protease inhibitors); and (5) interruption of the release of virus (interferon) (see later discussion; Fig. 44–5). Guidelines for the evaluation and medical management of the HIV infected person and use of antiretroviral agents are available on the HIV/AIDS Treatment Information Service Website (*http://www.hivatis.org*) and should be consulted by the clinician, since this is a rapidly evolving field.

The 15 drugs currently approved for the treatment of HIV-1 infection fall into three therapeutic classes: the nucleoside (and nucleotide) analogue reverse transcriptase

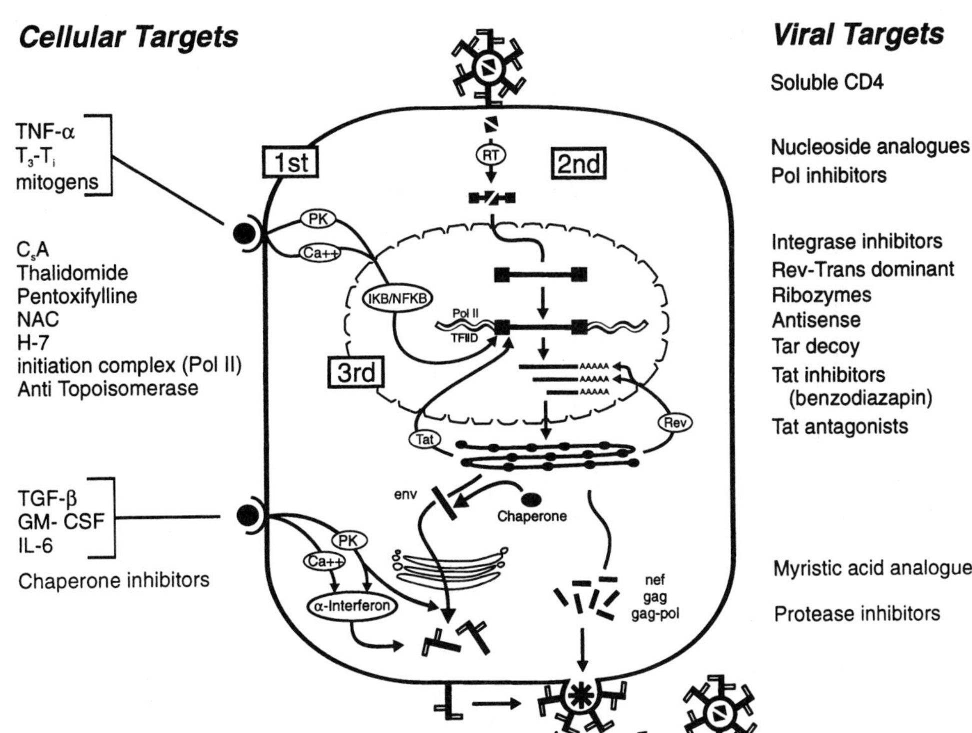

FIGURE 44–5. Potential locations for treatment intervention in the life cycle of the HIV. The boxes depict the cellular signaling pathways used for replication by HIV. The first box indicates the cellular surface receptors; the second depicts the intracellular signals that transmit the first signal; the third pathway is assembled in response to second messenger signaling and includes protein-DNA and protein-RNA interactions. (Reproduced with permission from Folks TM, Hart CE: The life cycle of human immunodeficiency virus type I. *In* DeVita VT, Hellman S, Rosenberg SA [eds]: AIDS: Biology, Diagnosis, Treatment and Prevention, 4th ed. Philadelphia, Lippincott-Raven, 1997, pp 29–43.)

inhibitors (NRTIs), the nonnucleoside reverse transcriptase inhibitors (NNRTIs), and the protease inhibitors (PIs). Retroviral drugs (NRTIs) include zidovudine (ZDV, AZT), didanosine (ddI), dideoxycytidine (ddC), stavudine (d4T), and lamivudine (3TC). These agents are nucleoside analogues that inhibit reverse transcriptase. NNRTIs inhibitors include delavirdine and nevirapine. Protease inhibitors include saquinavir, indinavir, ritonavir, and amprenavir. The primary goal of antiretroviral therapy is to maintain viral suppression as long as possible.[83] Effective treatment reduces plasma HIV RNA levels and increases CD4+ cell counts. Treatments offer the potential to delay onset of AIDS, prolong survival, and interrupt transmission.[83] Unfortunately, limitations have also been observed. Antiretrovirals do not completely inhibit viral replication, and HIV-1 disease progresses despite therapy. Studies show that treatment with antiretroviral drugs favors the fall of HIV RNA titers, the rise of CD4+ cell counts, the prolongation of time until HIV-1–related symptoms begin, and prolongation of survival. When to initiate primary HIV-1 therapy to an individual patient, however, remains unclear.

Recommendations for institution of antiretroviral therapy are guided by evaluation of the individual's clinical status and use of surrogate markers, such as CD4+ cell counts and plasma HIV-1 RNA levels.[83] Some investigators suggest treatment before the onset of HIV-related symptoms when the CD4+ cell count falls to or below 500/μL; HIV RNA titer is 30,000 to 50,000 copies/mL; or CD4+ cell count is rapidly declining. Treatment may also be considered if the HIV RNA titer is greater than 5000 copies/μL in those individuals whose CD4+ cell count is less than 500/μL.

It is not certain which initial antiretroviral agent or combination of agents should be used. The specific initial antiretroviral treatment should be based on an assessment of the potency, expected duration of benefit, resistance, toxicity, potential interactions with other medications, ease of use, and cost.[83] These medications are extraordinarily expensive and have certain common and distinct side effects (Table 44–6 and see Chapter 55). Because this information is rapidly changing, clinicians should review yearly updates on therapy recommendations (see later discussion). Clinical experience has shown that, over time, antiretroviral therapy has a diminished benefit. The optimum choice of secondary treatment is often a major dilemma. Many factors must be taken into consideration; for example, the patient's previous antiretroviral regimen, length of time the antiretroviral was taken, toxicities encountered, as well as side effects or toxicities of the new agent. Development of resistance to antiretroviral agents is a major problem, especially when protease inhibitors are administered as monotherapy or when not taken by the patient as directed.

The long-term clinical effectiveness of all available drugs is limited by the ability of patients to adhere to their complex dosing regimens and to tolerate their side effects. Over time, inadequate drug exposures due to limited drug efficacy or inadequate adherence may permit viral replication in the presence of the drug, leading to the emergence of drug-resistant viruses. In addition, because of their similar chemical structures and mechanisms of action, the emergence of viral resistance to one drug frequently results in cross-resistance to other, often all, members of the same therapeutic class. Therefore, there is an urgent need for new and effective drugs that will be convenient, well tolerated, and capable of suppressing viruses that are resistant to existing drugs.

Numerous clinical trials aimed to provide new treatment options for AIDS patients are currently ongoing. Among

TABLE 44–6. **Complications of Treatment with Specific Agents**

Agent	Complications
Nucleoside (and Nucleotide) Analog Reverse Transcriptase Inhibitors (NRTIs)	
Zidovudine	Anemia, neutropenia, nausea, anorexia, fatigue, insomnia, headache, myalgia, myopathy
Didanosine	Pancreatitis, peripheral neuropathy, hyperamylasemia, hyperuricemia, transaminase elevations
Dideoxycytidine	Peripheral neuropathy (dose-dependent), pancreatitis, rash, stomatitis, gastrointestinal disturbances
Stavudine	Peripheral neuropathy, arthralgia, myalgia, anemia, asthenia, gastrointestinal disturbances, headache, insomnia
Lamivudine	Pancreatitis, paresthesias, peripheral neuropathy, rash, cough, headache, dizziness, fatigue, hair loss, insomnia
Abacavir	Fatal hypersensitivity reactions, gastrointestinal disturbances, weight loss, sleep disorders
Zalcitabine	Peripheral neuropathy, pancreatitis, lactic acidosis, hepatic toxicity with steatosis, ulcers, cardiomyopathy
Nonnucleoside Reverse Transcriptase Inhibitors (NNRTIs)	
Delavirdine	Skin rash, multiple drug interactions, myalgias, gastrointestinal disturbances, encephalopathy
Nevirapine	Skin rash, hepatitis/hepatic failure, granulocytopenia, encephalopathy
Efavirenz	Psychiatric symptoms including depression and psychosis, dizziness, sleep alterations
Protease Inhibitors	
Saquinavir	Bleeding disorders, gastrointestinal disturbances, hepatic dysfunction, myalgias, arthralgias, skin rash
Indinavir	Nephrolithiasis/urolithiasis, hyperbilirubinemia, abdominal pains, nausea
Ritonavir	Diabetes, bleeding disorders, elevated cholesterol and plasma lipids, multiple drug interactions
Amprenavir	Bleeding disorders, fat redistribution, skin rash, multiple drug interactions, gastrointestinal disturbances
Nelfinavir	Diabetes, bleeding disorders, gastrointestinal disturbances, multiple drug interactions

NRTIs, the tenofovir prodrug, tenofovir disoproxil fumarate, has demonstrated antiviral activity in two phase III clinical trials and is currently under consideration for marketing approval for HIV-1 therapy. Two others, emtricitabine (FTC) and diaminopurine dioxolane/dioxolane guanosine (DAPD/DXG), show somewhat greater potency, the potential for once-daily dosing, good tolerability, and antiviral efficacy in phase I/II studies.[84, 85] In addition, several NNRTIs are in phase I/II trials,[86] and protease inhibitors tipranavir and BMS-232632 are in phase III clinical trials.[87, 88]

In addition, there are attempts to design new drugs that will have a novel mechanism of action compared to the existing drugs. The major classes of these new drugs are integrase inhibitors, viral entry inhibitors, and viral assembly inhibitors. Integrase is the third of the enzymatic proteins encoded by HIV-1, which catalyzes the insertion of the HIV-1 DNA into the genome of the host cell. Viral entry inhibitors are being designed to block HIV-1 entry by inhibiting gp120-CD4 binding, gp120-coreceptor binding, or gp41 function. In fact, each of these potential targets has been exploited by multiple inhibitors in cell culture systems. There is now at least one inhibitor in each class being tested in clinical trials. Assembly and release of HIV-1 are primarily governed by the viral GAG and *VPU* proteins. It might be possible to discover and develop drugs that block assembly or release by binding to one of these components. Indeed, there is one known example of a small molecule that has antiviral efficacy in vivo and is thought to inhibit assembly by binding to a GAG protein. This compound, a tripeptide with the sequence Gly-Pro-Gly-NH2 (GPG), is being developed by Tripep AB, who have presented unpublished results from a 2-week clinical trial.[89] All these attempts provide hope for future management and control of HIV-1 infection and AIDS.

Finally, there is now ongoing research to develop an HIV vaccine. Despite initial optimism and high expectations, there are many obstacles confonting the development of an effective vaccine.[90] HIV vaccines have been evaluated so far in over 70 phase I (dose-escalation safety and toxicity), five phase II (expanded safety and dose optimization), and two phase III (efficacy) clinical trials. These studies have evaluated safety and immunogenicity of preventive vaccines in more than 3,500 subjects.[91] These encouraging studies need to continue and expand in order to develop a safe and efficacious HIV vaccine.

HIV-Related Central Nervous System Disorders

ASEPTIC MENINGITIS

Retrospective studies have suggested that up to 10 percent of patients with HIV-1 infection and AIDS develop clinically apparent aseptic meningitis during the course of their illness. Additionally, HIV has been isolated in blood and CSF of patients with an acute self-limited aseptic meningitis at the time of HIV seroconversion. The clinical features in these cases are similar to those present in patients with aseptic meningitis owing to other viruses, outside the setting of HIV infection. Patients may have fever, meningeal signs, and headache that can be mild or severe with a dull or throbbing quality. These features may be accompanied by other constitutional signs that are characteristic of a viral syndrome including fatigue, malaise, myalgias, nausea, chills, and minor vomiting. Some individuals may have associated arthralgias, lymphadenopathy, and a maculopapular rash. This rash is erythematous, nonpruritic, and typically involves the face or trunk. At times, cranial neuropathies may be a concomitant finding, most often affecting the trigeminal, facial, or vestibulocochlear nerves.

The differential diagnosis of this clinical presentation includes other causes of aseptic meningitis (enteroviruses, varicella zoster), bacterial meningitis, intracranial mass (abscess), subarachnoid hemorrhage, and other causes of headache (migraine). In HIV-related aseptic meningitis, the CSF will reveal a mononuclear pleocytosis ranging from 20 to a few hundred cells/μL in the association of an elevated protein. The diagnosis will be made by the demonstration of HIV-1 infection, which may require repeat testing after the resolution of the acute presentation.

The treatment of aseptic meningitis is supportive in nature and includes symptomatic treatment. In association with fluids and bed rest, acetaminophen, aspirin, and nonsteroidal anti-inflammatory agents may be utilized to reduce fever and lessen headache.

HIV-ASSOCIATED COGNITIVE IMPAIRMENT—ADULTS

Over the past two decades, various terms have been used to describe the cognitive features, including mental slowness, diminished concentration, and a decline in memory in the setting of HIV infection. These cognitive changes are variably associated with changes in behavior (lethargy, apathy, and diminished emotional responses) and motor symptoms (clumsiness, gait abnormalities, tremor, and reduced motor control). The term *HIV-associated dementia* or *HIV dementia* incorporates the cognitive changes seen in HIV-1 infection as well as those occurring in the setting of AIDS. It is synonymous with the previously existing terms *AIDS dementia complex*[92] and *HIV encephalopathy*.[93] A separate term, *HIV-associated minor cognitive/motor disorder*, has been used to denote minor degrees of cognitive and motor impairment that are not sufficient for the diagnosis of dementia. According to the American Academy of Neurology AIDS Task Force,[64] this term is appropriate because it is unclear whether this degree of impairment uniformly progresses to overt dementia. The term *HIV-associated delirium* should be used in the setting of an alteration in consciousness with a rapid worsening of cognitive function in at least two domains (Table 44–7). The terms *HIV encephalitis*, *HIV-associated diffuse poliodystrophy*, and *HIV leukoencephalopathy* are pathological findings that may be seen at autopsy in patients with HIV dementia and should not be used to denote clinical syndromes.

Pathogenesis and Pathophysiology. Much has been learned about the biology of HIV-1, the cells it infects, and the mechanisms by which viral entry into cells occurs. However, just how HIV-1 exerts its effects on the CNS remains uncertain and continues to be the focus of ongoing research. Current knowledge indicates that HIV-1–infected macrophages/monocytes in blood are recruited to the brain by upregulation of chemoattractant-chemokines like MCP-1[94] and adhesion molecules on endothelial cells.

TABLE 44–7. **Classification of HIV-Associated Cognitive Dysfunction**

Category 1 (HIV-associated, minor)	0.5 SD below normal on standardized neuropsychological tests Decline in work or other activities of daily living (ADLs) Symptoms for 1 month Criteria for HIV-1–associated dementia or delirium is absent No other etiology
Category 2 (HIV-associated dementia)	Marked impairment in at least two ability domains Significant impairment in work and other ADLs Symptoms for 1 month No other etiology Free of delirium for a period sufficient to establish the presence of dementia
Category 3 (HIV-associated delirium)	Clouding of consciousness Marked, rapid worsening of cognitive function in ≥2 domains

SD, Standard deviation.

Upregulation enables transendothelial migration of activated macrophages/monocytes[95] and has been correlated with a high frequency of circulating activated monocytes expressing CD14/CD16 and CD14/CD9 in patients with HIV-associated dementia. Endothelial cells, oligodendrocytes, and neurons contain the virus only rarely, although a decrease in neuronal density and dendritic spines has been demonstrated.[96] Takahashi and coworkers have, however, demonstrated a latent HIV DNA provirus in some astrocytes.[97] Furthermore, development of HIV-associated dementia in advanced AIDS may correlate with the existence of neurotropic HIV-1 strains that have an increased propensity to invade CNS, rather than neurovirulent strains which have an increased propensity to cause CNS damage. In vitro studies of HIV-1 neurotoxicity indicate that changes in the envelope sequence might influence neuronal survival.[98] It has already been shown in in vitro models of simian immunodeficiency virus (SIV) and feline immunodeficiency virus that specific sequences of *ENV* or *NEF* genes confer neurovirulence.[99, 100]

Pathogenetic mechanisms of HIV-associated dementia are complex and most likely multifactorial. Activated macrophages release multiple proinflammatory cytokines, as well as other factors that might impair the function of virtually all neural cell types and interfere with the release of neurotransmitters and therefore synaptic transmission. This process would then correlate with the neuropsychological findings in HIV-associated dementia. Most recent studies have indicated the role of tumor necrosis factor (TNF)-alfa in HIV-induced neuronal apoptosis, and this finding promoted subsequent clinical trials with TNF-alfa antagonists.[101] However, little progress has been made. An initial trial with pentoxifylline was aborted due to the side effect profile of the drug.[102] A novel TNF-alfa antagonist, CPI–1189, is currently undergoing trials in the United States.

Studies of the viral load in HIV-associated dementia have indicated that plasma HIV RNA level is predictive of the development of dementia.[103] Similar data have been reported in SIV encephalitis.[104] However, HIV PCR analysis of the CSF viral load of patients with HIV-associated dementia has been controversial, because not all studies indicate a correlation between CSF HIV load and severity of dementia.[105–108] It is not clear how well the CSF viral load reflects brain parenchymal viral loads. It has been shown that CSF and parenchymal levels did not correlate when CSF levels were low (less than 10^5 copies/mL), but did correlate when CSF levels were high (more than 10^6 copies/mL). In addition, CSF HIV RNA levels sometimes correlated well with the treatment efficacy.[109, 110]

Macroscopic brain pathology from HIV-infected individuals with cognitive impairment shows cerebral atrophy of variable degrees. There is ventricular enlargement, particularly in the frontal and temporal lobes, widening of sulci, and attenuation of deep cerebral white matter with, at times, softening of the centrum semiovale.[111, 112] A spectrum of characteristic gross and microscopic changes has been described and categorized by an international working group consensus in 1991 as follows (Table 44–8). HIV-1 encephalitis is characterized by foci of inflammatory cells, microglia, and macrophages, called *microglial nodules*, as well as multinucleated giant cells (Fig. 44–6). Location tends to be perivascular with predominance in the basal ganglia and subcortical white matter, although to a lesser degree the cortical gray matter may also

TABLE 44–8. **CNS Neuropathological Findings in HIV**

Gross Examination
Cerebral atrophy of variable degrees
Ventricular enlargement
Widening of sulci
Attenuation of deep cerebral white matter
Microscopic Examination
HIV-1 encephalitis
Perivascular foci of inflammatory cells, microglia, macrophages, MGC involving the basal ganglia and subcortical white matter predominantly
HIV-1 leukoencephalopathy
Diffuse myelin pallor and white matter damage, reactive astrogliosis, macrophages
Calcific vasculopathy
Small vessel mineralization of basal ganglia, frontal white matter (children > adults)
Leukoencephalopathy and gliosis
Basal ganglia calcific vasculopathy (infants and children)
Diffuse poliodystrophy

MGC, Multinucleated giant cells.

Modified from Budka H, Wiley CA, Kleihues P, et al: HIV-1 associated disease of the nervous system: review of nomenclature and proposal for neuropathology-based terminology. Brain Pathol 1991;1:143–152.

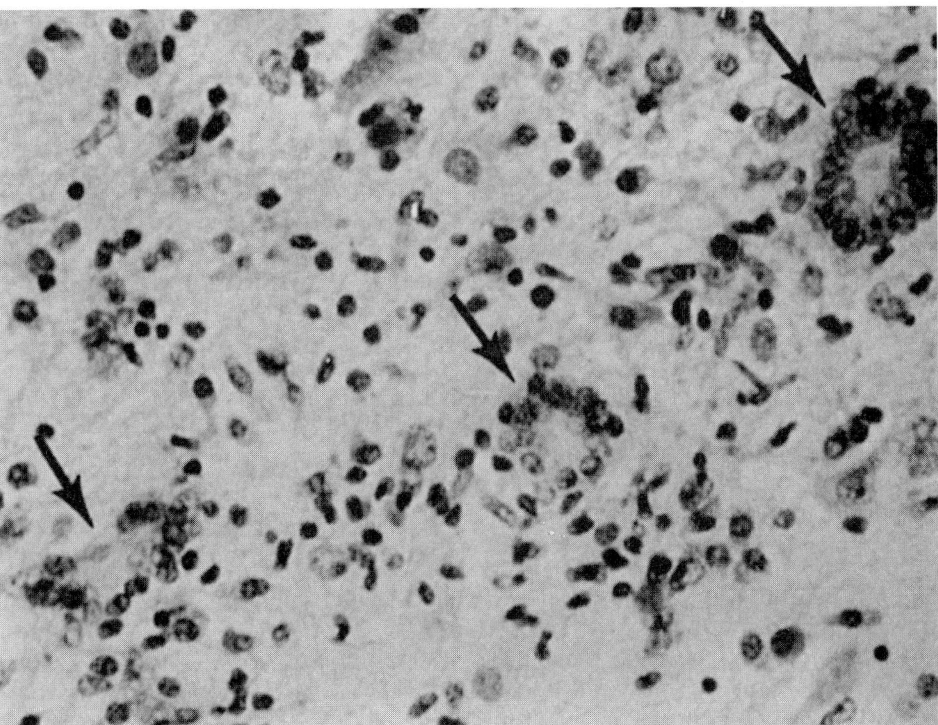

FIGURE 44–6. Multinucleated giant cells *(arrows)* obtained on biopsy from the brain of an AIDS patient. (Reproduced with permission from Belman AL, Diamond G, Dickson D, et al: Am J Dis Child 1988;142:29–35.)

be affected. In adult series, HIV encephalitis is reported in up to 90 percent (15 to 90 percent) of AIDS cases studied. The severity of pathological findings in HIV encephalitis is generally greater in adults than infants and young children.[113] HIV-1 leukoencephalopathy is characterized by diffuse myelin pallor and extensive damage to white matter with myelin loss. Associated findings such as reactive astrogliosis, the presence of macrophages, and multinucleated giant cells may also be present. Symmetrical white matter pallor can be seen in the hemispheres (Fig. 44–7) and less often in the cerebellum. Leukoencephalitis was reported in one third of patients clinically diagnosed with HIV dementia[114] and in 38 percent of autopsy series cases.[115] A diffuse poliodystrophy has also been described in approximately 50 percent of cases. More recently, neuronal loss, dendritic changes, and reduced levels of synaptophysin have also been demonstrated by quantitative methods with a frontal and parieto-occipital predominance.[116, 117]

Microscopic examinations reveal that HIV-1 is most frequently localized in cells of bone marrow lineage (blood-derived macrophages), intrinsic microglia (the resident mononuclear phagocytic system of the brain), and multinucleated giant cells (formed by the fusion of these cell types). It is these cells that support productive infection.[15, 16, 118] Their presence correlates both with the degree of dementia and the detection of HIV-1.[119] By immunocytochemistry, HIV-1 antigen is localized most often in the basal ganglia, subthalamic nucleus, substantia nigra, dentate nucleus, and white matter.[120] PCR studies, though, show HIV to be more abundant in subcortical white matter than basal ganglia, deep white matter, or cortex.[121] With more sensitive and specific techniques of viral detection, both a greater number of infected cells and cell types infected have recently been demonstrated. These include endothelial cells,[122] astrocytes,[123, 124] and neurons,[125] although this may be restricted infection.

The clinicopathological correlates of HIV-1–associated CNS disease are not clearly delineated, nor is the exact role of the virus defined. Although studies have confirmed direct HIV-1 CNS infection early in the disease, the development of clinical HIV-1–associated CNS disease does not occur until the late stage of HIV-1 infection when the patient is

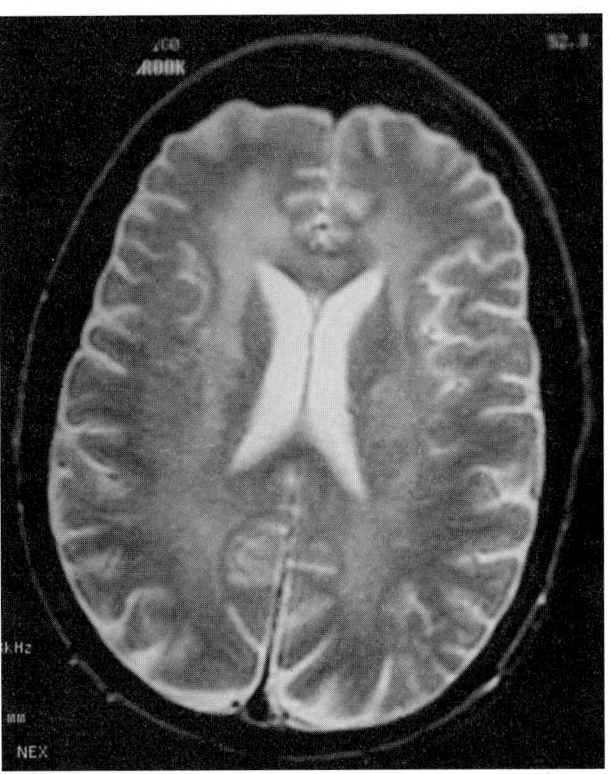

FIGURE 44–7. A 30-year-old male with AIDS. This T2-weighted magnetic resonance image demonstrates atrophy and diffuse white matter hyperintensity. (Courtesy of Clemente Roque, M.D.)

immunosuppressed. Moreover, the pathological changes seen at autopsy in some cases do not always correlate with the clinical course. Some patients with clinically severe neurological disease may have relatively mild neuropathological findings. Even in those cases with more marked pathological findings, there may be a relatively small proportion of infected cells and those actively replicating. Indeed, one prospective study found 50 percent of patients with clinically diagnosed dementia had neither the hallmark features of HIV encephalitis nor white matter pallor, and only 25 percent of dementia cases had multinucleated giant cells.[114] Brain levels of HIV RNA correlate with the pathological features of encephalitis, but do not clearly distinguish demented from nondemented subjects.[44, 108] These discrepancies have suggested that other factors besides direct cellular damage by HIV-1 may be important in pathogenesis.[126] Both virological and neuroimmunological processes have been implicated (Table 44–9). Many questions remain unanswered concerning the role of the virus, CNS viral load, evolution of neurotropic strains, mechanisms underlying viral protein and cytokine-mediated effects and toxicities, yet undefined host factors, and viral-host interactions.

Epidemiology and Risk Factors. Of the 1 to 1.5 million HIV-1–infected persons in North America,[127] up to 30 percent will manifest some form of cognitive impairment during the course of their infection. However, estimates vary as to the frequency and degree of neurocognitive deficits. Two major factors account for the differences in estimate. First, persons with HIV infection who came to medical attention in the early years of the epidemic were generally in more advanced stages of the disease. Early reports were thus probably biased toward a higher frequency rate of dementia. Second, terminology, study design, and methodology differed among studies, particularly with regard to the classification schemes used to categorize levels of HIV-1–related neurocognitive impairment. Thus, initial clinical reports described characteristics of a disorder with cognitive, motor, and behavioral manifestations, which was described in unitary terms as a single diagnostic entity, "AIDS dementia complex" (ADC).[9] Delineation of clinical stages and precise definitions of clinical characteristics were not uniformly used across different studies. This lack of precise definition led to considerable variation in estimates of dementia in HIV-infected persons.[128]

Current figures suggest that dementia develops in 10 to 20 percent of patients with AIDS, occurring at an annual incidence of approximately 7 percent after AIDS onset.[18] HIV dementia occurs as a late complication of HIV-1 infection when patients are immunosuppressed. It develops as the first AIDS-defining illness in only 3 percent of adults.[92] More generally, patients at risk for dementia are those who are farther along in the disease process and who have experienced moderate to severe immunosuppression, constitutional symptoms (e.g., anemia, weight loss, and poor nutrition), and systemic opportunistic processes.[129, 130] Higher plasma HIV RNA levels and lower CD4 counts are predictive of dementia, as well as of sensory neuropathy.[103] A recent study has suggested that presence of E4 isoform of apolipoprotein E indicates higher risk for development of dementia. Education and premorbid capacities are factors as well: individuals with lower levels of education and premorbid function show more frequent cognitive deficits; those with higher levels of education appear to benefit from the protective effects of "cognitive reserve" despite the impact of the virus on the CNS.[131] Concurrent with the widespread use of antiretrovirals, a decline in the frequency of HIV dementia was reported.[132–134]

Nonetheless, estimates of HIV dementia suggest its prevalence ranges from approximately 5 percent to approximately 14 percent.[135] Unfortunately, there are no clear estimates at present of the rates of either HIV-associated minor cognitive/motor disorder or HIV-associated delirium. Most investigators believe that symptomatic HIV-1 infection presents at least some risk of neurocognitive impairment, but estimates of the rate of impairment vary. Neurocognitive findings on asymptomatic individuals have varied considerably as well. An early report[136] suggested an increased incidence of impairment among asymptomatic patients. However, subsequent studies[137, 138] indicated no significant differences between asymptomatic HIV-positive patients and controls on selected cognitive measures. Still other concurrent efforts have again indicated mild deficits in asymptomatic individuals relative to control subjects.[139–141] Among studies that have shown impairment in HIV-infected asymptomatic individuals, estimates of rates of impairment range from 9.1 percent to 30.5 percent.

Clinical Features and Associated Disorders. Clinical features of HIV-associated dementia encompass changes in behavior, cognition, and neurological function. Initial clinical features of HIV-related cognitive impairment vary considerably in terms of time of presentation and severity.

TABLE 44–9. **Possible Factors in the Pathogenesis of HIV-Associated CNS Disease**

Viral Proteins
Blocking of transmitters
Possible interference with neurotrophic factors and cell function
Toxicity of viral polypeptides
Cytokines
Direct toxicity
Neuroimmune-mediated CNS dysfunction/injury
Stimulation of astrocytes
Excitotoxins
Toxic Effects of Other Soluble Factors
Blood-Brain Barrier Disruption
Exposure of parenchymal cells to circulating cytokines and systemic factors
Ingress of HIV-1-infected cells and free virus
Autoimmunity
Deregulation and T-cell activation
Molecular mimicry
Immune response to HIV antigens
Increased CNS HIV-1 Viral Load
Transactivation
Infectious agents
Cytokine induced
Emergence of neurovirulent strains
Host factors

Data from Johnson RT, McArthur JC, Narayon O, et al: The neurobiology of human immunodeficiency virus infections. FASEB J 1988;2:2970–2981.

Symptoms are often sufficiently subtle that they may be overlooked or mistaken for psychiatric problems. Neuropsychological findings have not been completely consistent across the literature, particularly with regard to asymptomatic individuals and persons with a mild disorder. In part, this is due to the varying measures that have been used with subjects, as well as the variety of parameters used to define subject groups. It is also likely due simply to the fact that presentation varies from individual to individual. There are indications that a subgroup of seropositive, asymptomatic individuals may show deficits, particularly in memory and executive functioning.[139, 141] These deficits may be related to declines in CD4+ lymphocyte counts and may precede clinical evidence of AIDS.

HIV dementia has been termed subcortical in nature, at least with respect to initial presentation, whereas subsequent deterioration is more global in nature. In early stages, typical symptoms of behavioral changes include apathy, inertia, and mild depressive symptoms. Change of personality and social withdrawal are very common. In some cases, however, behavioral changes are quite opposite, and agitation and mania may be the presenting manifestations.[142] Cognitive symptoms are intermixed and include forgetfulness, difficulty with sustained concentration, and psychomotor slowing. Manifestations of these problems in daily life may include problems in keeping track of appointments, telephone numbers, or medications; misplacement of personal items; difficulty following the direction of conversations or the plots of films or books. Other neurological features that occur early include primarily motor abnormalities, such as slow and clumsy handwriting, other fine-motor problems, insecure balance, and impaired gait.

On neuropsychological testing, these patients may have memory loss with particular difficulty in retrieval of newly learned information, impaired manipulation of known material, and slowed psychomotor and information processing speed. Simple attention and language skills are not typically affected during the initial stages of HIV-related cognitive impairment,[134] although these functions may also mildly deteriorate as the disease progresses.

HIV dementia in the setting of AIDS occurs along with increasing constitutional symptoms, immunosuppression, and opportunistic processes. With advancing dementia, the patient is likely to develop global behavioral deterioration. Mutism and abulia are typical but euphoria and denial of deficit, lack of insight/awareness, and hallucinations can be alternative syndromes. The most pronounced neurocognitive deficits remain in the areas of retrieval of new information and psychomotor function, although deficits in executive function, language, attention, and new learning become more pronounced as well. Neurological examination is notable for diffuse signs of CNS dysfunction, for example, slowed and erroneous motor programming, hyper-reflexia, hypertonia, and frontal release signs. Myelopathy and neuropathy might occur. Motor function and posture testing may be notable for marked psychomotor retardation, spasticity and weakness, ataxia and, ultimately, decorticate posturing. Although myoclonus is not consistently a feature of late dementia, generalized seizures may occur.[143]

Progression of the dementia varies widely from individual to individual. In some, it may occur rapidly over the course of 3 to 6 months, whereas others may show relatively mild and stable dementia up until death. The reason for this difference between rapid progressors and slow progressors is not known, but those with CD4+ cell counts <100/μL at the onset of HIV dementia tend to progress more quickly. It is interesting to note that despite the widespread use of antiretrovirals, survival after diagnosis of HIV dementia has not improved significantly in recent years.

Differential Diagnosis. The differential diagnosis of HIV dementia is often problematic, particularly in the early period. Initial symptoms overlap with and can be mistaken for adjustment and mood disorders, alcohol and other substance abuse, medication effects, metabolic encephalopathy, and other brain disorders.[144] It is important to pursue information from those close to the patient regarding the individual's history and current behavior, in order to rule out psychiatric or substance abuse complications as causes of an apparent dementia. Metabolic derangements (e.g., hypoxia and sepsis) must be considered. Other CNS processes, such as CMV encephalitis, toxoplasmosis, primary lymphoma, progressive multifocal leukoencephalopathy, and cryptococcus can complicate the diagnostic process and must be excluded as causes of cognitive deterioration. Time course, level of consciousness, presence of fever and headache, and focal signs and symptoms on neurological examination may help differentiate these conditions. Of these disorders, CMV encephalitis is probably the most frequent and problematic differential diagnosis. In approximately 10 percent of all patients with AIDS, it presents as a rapidly developing encephalopathy. CMV encephalitis can be distinguished from HIV dementia by the presence of co-existing CMV infection, electrolyte abnormalities, and periventricular abnormalities.

Depression frequently complicates cognitive function in HIV infection. HIV-infected individuals are known to have higher rates of major depression than those seen in the general population, and it is thought that in most cases depression predates HIV infection.[144] It appears that a substantial number of HIV-positive individuals can experience depression in concert with neurocognitive impairment, whereas others may show significant deficits without depressed mood, suggesting that although depression is a frequent concomitant of cognitive impairment in HIV infection, it does not play an etiological role in such impairment.[145] All of the preceding factors necessitate the need to screen individuals at high risk, who have unsuppressed plasma levels of HIV RNA and CD4+ cell counts <200/μL. In those individuals, a complete cognitive and behavioral evaluation and particularly neuropsychological testing is warranted.

Evaluation. A thorough neurological examination and history are essential. In the early stage, there may only be mild abnormalities of rapid eye and limb movements, as well as diffuse hyper-reflexia. Increased tone, especially in the lower extremities, hyper-reflexia, clonus, frontal release signs, and tremor are seen with disease progression. Focal neurological signs are suggestive of another CNS process (opportunistic infections, neoplasm, vascular events). In addition to mental changes, CNS-based motor complications are also frequently seen in association with HIV dementia, especially myelopathies, myopathies, and neuropathies (see later discussion).

Neuropsychological assessment is particularly useful for characterizing the dementia and for tracking its progress; it can also help in monitoring the patient's response to antiretrovirals and other medications. Critical domains and specific assessment tools are listed in Table 44–10 and are reviewed in Chapter 27. Particularly important are tests of both explicit and implicit learning and memory, complex attention, information processing speed, and psychomotor speed, such as Trailmaking, Grooved Pegboard, and Symbol-Digit tests. These areas are most likely to appear abnormal during early stages of HIV dementia and to demonstrate deterioration as the dementia progresses. On the other hand, calculation and language are usually not affected in initial stages of HIV-associated dementia.[134] Although neuropsychological assessment can be helpful with respect to the objective quantification of the nature and severity of cognitive impairment and the tracking of such impairment over time, it should be noted that neuropsychological testing in the case of HIV infection tends to be sensitive rather than specific. Clearly, numerous disease processes may present with a similar neurocognitive picture. Consideration of this issue is particularly important because HIV-infected individuals often present with histories that include other problems (e.g., alcohol/drug abuse, depression and other psychiatric disorders, learning disabilities, head injury). In addition, concurrent CNS processes such as metabolic encephalopathy and opportunistic infections can cause similar cognitive deficits, and some of these can be specifically treated.

TABLE 44–10. **Assessment Tools for Patients with HIV-Related Cognitive Deficits**

General Intellect
Wechsler Scales (WAIS-R, WAIS-III)
Stanford Binet IV
Kaufman Brief Intelligence Test

Attention—Simple and Complex
Continuous performance tests (simple and choice reaction time)
Auditory and visual span
Serial calculation tasks (Serial 3 addition, Serial 7 subtraction, Paced Auditory Serial Addition Test, etc.)
Stroop Test
Contingency Naming Test

Speech/Language/Academic Achievement
Confrontation naming
Praxis
Verbal fluency
Reading, spelling, arithmetic tests

Visuospatial/Vasoconstrictive
Block design and puzzle assembly tasks (WAIS-R, WAIS-III)
Rey-Osterrieth Complex Figure
Developmental Test of Visual-Motor Integration (VMI)
Bender Visual-Motor Gestalt Test

Learning/Memory
Wechsler Memory Scale (WMS-R, WMS-III)
Rey Auditory-Verbal Learning Test (RAVLT)
Selective Reminding Test
Hopkins Verbal Learning Test
California Verbal Learning Test
Rey-Osterrieth Complex Figure

Sensory-Perceptual/Psychomotor
Sensory-perceptual examination
Grooved or Purdue Pegboard
Finger tapping
Symbol Digit Modalities Test
Motor programming (limb movements, Luria-Christensen, Manual Imitation subtest from Test of Memory and Learning)
Motor learning (mirror writing, rotary pursuit)

Executive Functions/Reasoning
Trail Making Test
Wisconsin Card Sorting Test
Category Test
Tower Tasks (Tower of London, Tower of Hanoi, Tower of Texas, Tower of Toronto)
Contingency Naming Test

Emotional/Personality Functions
SDM IV Interview Schedules
Beck Scales
Symptom Checklist 90-Revised
Millon Clinical Multiaxial Inventory
Minnesota Multiphasic Personality Inventory-Second Edition (MMPI–2)

Cerebrospinal fluid in HIV dementia is abnormal, but similar abnormalities can be found in HIV-seropositive patients who are neurologically normal. CSF is usually acellular or shows mild lymphocytic pleocytosis. Total protein is elevated in about 65 percent of cases, with elevated beta-2 microglobulin and increased total IgG fraction. Elevated beta-2 microglobulin, an immune activation marker, has the greatest diagnostic value, particularly in cases of mild dementia in the absence of opportunistic infections. Beta-2 microglobulin level of >3.8 mg/dL has a positive predictive value of 88 percent.[146] Work by Martin and colleagues[140] has also suggested that elevated CSF quinolinic acid concentrations in HIV-infected individuals are associated with deficits in motor learning and reaction time. Even though the CSF HIV RNA levels are not diagnostic for HIV-associated dementia, they should be measured because they correlate with its severity.[147]

Imaging studies are essential for differentiation between HIV-associated dementia and opportunistic infections. Computed tomography (CT) and magnetic resonance imaging (MRI) may not show abnormalities in persons with HIV-associated minor cognitive and motor disorder, despite positive neuropsychological findings. In mild HIV dementia, neuroimaging suggests subcortical and cortical atrophy with MRI abnormalities seen in deep white matter. White matter abnormalities, which may represent disruptions of the blood-brain barrier, progress and are more diffuse with increasing severity of dementia.[148] The degree of atrophy also correlates with cognitive impairment.[149] Volumetric MRI indicates caudate atrophy as well as decreased gray matter.[150, 151] Proton MR spectroscopy is recently emerging as a tool to assess brain damage as well as treatment efficacy over time. N-acetylaspartate, a marker of neuronal viability, can be changed in cortical areas,[152] whereas myoinositol, a marker for glial turnover, may indicate tissue damage even earlier.[153] Positron-emission tomography (PET) studies have suggested that subcortical hypermetabolism occurs during early HIV dementia, particularly in the basal ganglia and thalamus. This hypermetabolism later appears to progress to subcortical and cortical hypometabolism.[154, 155] Single-photon emission computed tomography (SPECT) indicates abnormalities in cerebral blood flow in both neurologically normal HIV carriers and in demented patients. However, cocaine ingestion may also produce similar PET and SPECT patterns and should be ruled out. Neither PET nor SPECT scans are useful as diagnostic tools for HIV-associated dementia, and their patterns do not correlate with treatment efficacy.

Electroencephalographic (EEG) abnormalities have been reported in some asymptomatic seropositive patients,[156] but this is not the experience of all investigators.[157] Patients with early dementia may show EEG abnormalities, but up to 50 percent of subjects have normal recordings. As dementia becomes severe, diffuse slowing is frequently noted, consistent with widespread dysfunction.[9] In spite of the observations, EEG can be used only as an adjunct tool and has no specific diagnostic or predictive value.

Management. Over the past several years, major advances have been made in antiretroviral therapy and care for patients with HIV-associated dementia. There are now 15 FDA-approved antiretroviral agents in the United States, and many studies have monitored the response to therapy through regular measurement of CSF-to-plasma drug level ratios, CSF HIV RNA levels, and CD4+ counts, all currently part of standard clinical care for AIDS patients.

Initial studies reported a decline in the number of new cases with HIV dementia after the introduction of zidovudine therapy in 1987.[132] The dose was 1000 to 1200 mg/d, and other groups reported a decrease in the number of patients developing new HIV-1 dementia when treated with zidovudine 1200 mg/d compared with patients taking lower doses.[158] There were, however, only two placebo-controlled monotherapy antiretroviral trials showing that zidovudine improved neuropsychological performance.[159, 160] The response was dose-dependent, with recommended doses of 2000 mg/d.[161] Since 1992, as new antiretroviral drugs emerged, polytherapy has replaced monotherapy in the treatment of HIV-associated dementia. Although there have been only a few systematic studies, they indicate that the use of combination antiretroviral therapy without protease inhibitors can reduce risk of developing HIV dementia,[162] and can improve neuropsychological performance in patients with HIV dementia.[163] With the introduction of protease inhibitors in 1996, trials of combination of antiretrovirals and protease inhibitors showed improvement of neuropsychological performance compared to monotherapy or no treatment.[164, 165] In 1998, a new reverse transcriptase inhibitor, abacavir, was tested in a placebo-controlled, double-blinded fashion and showed that CSF viral load decreased and neuropsychological performance improved when the drug was used in combination with antiretrovirals. Most recently, two other drugs, stavudine and nevirapine, have been shown to be useful when combined with antiretrovirals, particularly due to their pharmacokinetic properties, tolerability, and dosing.

In addition to the antiretrovirals and protease inhibitors, several adjunctive therapies have been clinically tested in order to block macrophage activation and restricted release of neurotoxic factors. These include Lexipafant, an antagonist of platelet-activating factor;[166] memantine, an open-channel NMDA antagonist;[167] peptide T;[168] and selegiline.[169] As patients with HIV-associated dementia are very susceptible to adverse effects of psychoactive drugs, hypnotics and anxiolytics should be avoided. Risperidone in small doses may be useful in agitated and combative patients; stimulants such as methylphenidate may be tried for excessive inertia.

In summary, even though there are no specific guidelines for antiretroviral therapy in HIV-associated dementia, combination of antiretrovirals with or without protease inhibitors and adjunctive medications are generally recommended. These agents have complex side effects and are very expensive, making them inaccessible to the majority of HIV-infected patients worldwide.

HIV-ASSOCIATED CENTRAL NERVOUS SYSTEM DISORDERS—CHILDREN

Neurological involvement was reported as a frequent complication of pediatric AIDS in the early years of the epidemic. A devastating progressive encephalopathy (PE) was described,[170] as was more stable neurological impairment.[171] It was observed that by the time HIV-1 infection had advanced to full-blown AIDS, cognitive and motor impairment of varying duration, progression, and severity were extremely common. In the majority of cases, neuropathological studies revealed no evidence of CNS opportunistic infections or neoplasms.[14, 171, 172] The clinical syndrome of *progressive encephalopathy in children* (variously termed *AIDS encephalopathy, HIV-1 encephalopathy, PE, subacute PE, HIV-1–associated CNS disease, HIV-1–associated PE of childhood*) is now recognized to be similar to the adult counterpart, HIV dementia,[17] and is directly related to HIV-1 brain infection.

Pathogenesis and Pathophysiology. In adults, the pathophysiological mechanisms underlying HIV-1–associated CNS disease are not yet clearly defined. In infants and children, the study of neuropathophysiological mechanisms and their clinicopathological correlates is even more complex because developmental-maturational issues must also be considered. Adult, horizontally transmitted HIV-1 CNS infection and disease occur in mature, fully developed, and completely myelinated nervous system. The immune system and CNS elements of the mononuclear phagocyte system (intrinsic microglia) are also fully developed. Pediatric, vertically transmitted HIV-1 infection and disease occur in an immature, evolving organism. It is believed that HIV-1 invades the CNS early in the course of infection. Maternal-infant transmission may occur during gestation in some patients, whereas in others, the infection may occur during the perinatal period. The time of infection (gestational versus perinatal, and if gestational, in which trimester) is likely to be an important factor. The developmental stages of the nervous and immune system when exposed to the direct and indirect effects of the virus must be considered. Innumerable dynamic interactions occur between these two systems during development, and these undoubtedly interact in complex ways with HIV-1 variables. The maturational stage of CNS development when exposed to the effects of the virus is likely to manifest as different patterns of pediatric HIV-1 CNS disease.[173]

The nervous system may also be affected secondarily by complications related to the immunodeficiency, including CNS neoplasms, infections with pathogens other than HIV-1, and strokes. The nervous system may also be affected by systemic AIDS-related conditions (neurological complications of systemic illness), nutritional deficiencies, endocrinological and metabolic derangements, and by toxic/metabolic complications that arise as a consequence of therapy.

These conditions are not mutually exclusive, and co-existing conditions are common.[173, 174]

In addition, the developing nervous system in HIV-1-infected infants (as in non–HIV-1–infected infants) may be adversely affected by maternal conditions during pregnancy, such as substance abuse, inadequate nutrition, deficient prenatal care, and AIDS-associated illnesses (e.g., infections with pathogens other than HIV-1).[173] Premature delivery is associated with some of these high-risk maternal conditions. The prematurely born HIV-1–infected infant, like any premature infant, is, in turn, at risk for developing perinatal CNS complications—intraventricular hemorrhages, periventricular leukomalacia, hypoxic encephalopathy—that carry the risk of neurological sequelae.

Epidemiology and Risk Factors. The true incidence of pediatric HIV-1–associated CNS disease is not yet known. A review of the published literature is difficult to interpret because of differences in terminology, definitions, study populations, and study designs [65, 76, 174–177] Extrapolating from the experiences of many investigators, it appears that HIV-1–associated CNS disease in children generally parallels the progression and severity of immunodeficiency and systemic disease.

Over 1 million children are currently infected with HIV-1 worldwide, and over 1,000 new pediatric cases occur daily, as reported by Association Francois-Xavier Bagnoud.[178] This epidemic of pediatic HIV-1 infection and disease represents a major international health crisis. The pediatric HIV-1–associated CNS disease follows a bimodal distribution with an "early," very aggressive form that occurs within the first 2 years of life and a "late" form that occurs years after the perinatal infection. The latter corresponds in its course to the adult HIV-associated dementia. The incidence of the "early" form is much higher than the incidence of adult CNS infection 1 to 2 years after infection: approximately 10 percent in the first year and 4 percent in the second year, compared to 0.5 percent in adults. In these children, HIV-1–associated CNS disease is frequently the initial clinical manifestation: in up to 56 percent of infants less than 1 year old and 32 percent of older children, compared to 9 percent of adults.[65, 76, 179–182] The incidence of the "late" form is similar in children and adults: less than 1 percent.[181–183] Even though the initiation of zidovudine therapy in the second and third trimester in HIV-1–infected mothers significantly decreased the incidence of perinatally infected infants, the lack of resources in many third world countries limits treatment availability. Pediatric HIV-1 infection and disease remain significant worldwide problems.[182] Due to improving therapies over the years, there is a growing population of perinatally infected children who survive well into adulthood.[184]

Clinical Features and Associated Disorders. HIV-associated CNS disease is a clinical diagnosis, supported by neuroimmunological/virological testing, neuroimaging and psychometric evaluation.[183] HIV-1–infected newborns are usually well at birth, and clinically recognizable neurological features of HIV-1–associated CNS disease are exceedingly rare. However, some HIV-1–infected neonates do have neurological problems owing to co-morbid conditions. Observations in both clinical care settings and longitudinal research studies show that the rate and pattern of disease progression have considerable clinical diversity.[128, 173] In some infants and young children, neurological deterioration is rapidly progressive; in others it occurs over a period of weeks to months, followed by a relatively stable period and then further deterioration. Clinical deficits may not evolve uniformly, and some children develop progressive and disabling motor problems yet maintain relatively stable cognitive and socially adaptive skills. In contrast, others have more impaired cognitive than motor function. Finally, there is a subset of children who have relatively minor and stable motor and cognitive findings, defined as *HIV-1-associated static encephalopathies*.[171, 173, 177, 179, 183, 185] In an effort to delineate further the clinical characteristics of HIV-1–associated CNS disease syndromes in children, a classification scheme was adopted based on: (1) age of onset of clinically apparent disease; (2) rate and pattern of disease progression; and (3) domains of function most affected.[177]

The most severe, devastating, and clearly recognized syndrome is HIV-1–associated PE of childhood.[64] This entity corresponds to the HIV-associated dementia of adults.[186, 187] Age of onset is usually in the first year of life (3 to 8 months of age), but may begin later. It can develop in perinatally infected infants even though they are immunocompetent.[181, 182] There is some evidence that the development of PE during the first year of life correlates with the viral load and not strictly with the CD4+ lymphocyte markers.[188] Even in severe cases of PE, CSF and brain viral load can be significantly lower compared to plasma levels. Furthermore, there is no evidence that prenatal ZDV treatment prevents early development of PE.[182]

Neurological signs of PE of childhood consist of a well-defined triad, including impaired brain growth, progressive motor dysfunction, and loss, plateau, or inadequate acquisition rates of neurodevelopmental milestones.[80, 183] The clinical diagnosis of PE is made if one of the preceding clinical findings is present in a child who was neurologically normal at baseline or if two of the preceding clinical findings are present in a neurologically abnormal child at baseline.[80] Microcephaly at birth in an HIV-1–exposed neonate is suggestive of in utero HIV-1 infection, and indicates high risk for the development of PE in the first year of life.[182] Acquired microcephaly is easier to detect in children less than 3 years of age, due to the rapid head growth. In older children, head circumference velocity decreases, and a much longer interval is required in order to detect impaired brain growth. In these cases, serial neuroimaging studies are valuable, because progressive loss of brain parenchyma can be observed.[189] Progressive motor dysfunction results in fine and gross motor impairments, gait disturbance, and spasticity. Opisthotonic posturing and rigidity may develop and are usually superimposed on spasticity. Some children display extrapyramidal syndromes, with rigidity, dysarthria or oromotor dyspraxia, dysphagia with drooling, hypomimetic facies, and gait abnormalities.[190] Feeding difficulties due to pseudobulbar signs are frequent. Even though these children appear alert and wide-eyed, they have a paucity of spontaneous facial expressions. Despite these features, there is little facial weakness, and the lingual, buccal and forehead muscles show full and symmetrical movement when the child cries. Nonetheless, the child is hypophonic and has decreased spontaneous and responsive vocalizations. Play deteriorates and previously acquired language skills or adaptive skills are progressively lost. Psychometric measures document a decline in the composite cognitive score. At endstages, the child is apathetic, withdrawn, and quadriparetic with markedly impaired higher cortical function.[10, 191] Functions associated with cranial nerves and brain stem nuclei are usually spared, although autopsies often reveal HIV-1 within these structures.[192]

Cognitive decline, loss of interest in school performance, social withdrawal, emotional lability, decreased attention, and psychomotor slowing are reported as signs of HIV-1–associated PE in school-age children.[10, 171, 177, 193] With advancing disease, psychometric tests show a decline in the composite IQ score. No specific neuropsychometric marker has yet been developed to predict the appearance of PE in asymptomatic children.

Additional neurological and psychiatric manifestations are common. Among them, seizures are particularly frequent and develop not only because of focal pathology, [183] but also because there is a higher incidence of unprovoked seizures in PE compared to the general pediatric population.[187] Even though HIV-1 is well known to affect cerebrovascular tissue, infarcts are not common.[194] However, the syndrome of "reversible occipital parietal encephalopathy" has been described and relates directly to vascular pathology in HIV-1 infections.[195] Vacuolar myelopathies and neuropathies are very rare in children and often result as complications of intercurrent illnesses, such as measles or CMV, or due to drug-related adverse effects.[80, 194, 196] ZDV-associated myopathy has been reported and can be ameliorated with carnitine supplementation.[197, 198] In addition, cardiomyopathy is present in about 30 percent of children with PE and cardiac evaluation is important in all children with PE.[181]

Psychiatric and behavioral manifestations are numerous, and include acute psychoses, common at the endstage of disease,[199] depression, anxiety, adjustment disorders,[183, 200] attention-deficit hyperactivity disorder (ADHD),[201, 202] as well as language and communication impairments that lead to learning disabilities. [203]

A less severe neurological syndrome also occurs in the first 2 years of life.[179, 191] Most of these infants are hypotonic and have marked delays in attaining motor milestones. Cognitive impairment of a variable degree and expressive language problems are common.[177, 185] Poor brain growth as determined by serial head circumference measurements may be present.[13, 173, 179, 191] In early childhood, some of the children develop a diparesis-type syndrome,[177] whereas others fortunately remain stable and continue to acquire mental, motor, and adaptive skills. A change in gait is often the first sign of HIV-1 motor involvement in early childhood, as the child begins to toe walk. These individuals become hyper-reflexic and have increased tone in the lower extremities.[177] The rate of progression and the severity of deficits vary. Some children maintain independent ambulation for years, although they have a mildly spastic gait and are clumsy.[173, 179] Impairment of fine motor ability is frequent. Progression and severity in other children may be more rapid and marked. Some require orthotics for ambulation, whereas others become wheelchair-bound within months.[171, 177] Cognitive impairment is frequent but not invariable. In a subset of children, cognitive function is not affected, and composite IQ scores remain within the normal range. For most, the degree of impairment ranges from borderline intelligence to mild or moderate retardation.[10, 171]

A subset of the children, who had a prolonged stable course, ultimately developed further neurological deterioration, formerly referred to as "plateau followed by further deterioration." The course then becomes similar to that of subacute PE.[171] Progressive atrophy and white matter changes are invariably seen. In contrast, other children show improvement and steadily acquire additional developmental skills. Their rate of acquisition of new skills accelerates compared with their previous plateau performance.[171] Children, who in infancy and early childhood had marked delays in motor and mental development and were followed from birth in prospective studies, continued to acquire milestones and skills, although the rate and quality deviated from the norm.[177] This suggests that HIV-1 may compromise the normal developmental process and result in a stable or static encephalopathy.

It is as yet unknown whether HIV-1–associated CNS disease manifestations in adolescents differ in early signs and progression from that of adults or of children, although it is anticipated that manifestations will be similar to adults.

Differential Diagnosis. The differential diagnosis includes other neurodegenerative disorders, infectious etiologies, and psychiatric conditions. CNS opportunistic infections and primary CNS lymphoma are not common in HIV-infected infants and young children, except in cases of congenital opportunistic infections. They are more prevalent in older children and adolescents.[80] However, opportunistic infections should always be considered in a case of acute behavioral changes, headache, focal findings on neurological exam, or overall deterioration.[204] Fungal opportunistic infections (cryptococcal meningitis), *Toxoplasma gondii* abscess, primary CNS lymphoma (sometimes associated with Epstein-Barr virus [EBV]), and herpes simplex or CMV encephalitis, can all have the previously listed presentations.[80, 205, 206] Noncongenital CNS opportunistic infections are common in children older than 6 years of age, when CD4+ levels are less than 200, and particularly when less than 100 cells/μL.[206]

Evaluation. The evaluation of the HIV-1–infected child with neurological involvement requires the clinical skills and major diagnostic tools of the neurologist.[179] The approach to the diagnosis of HIV-1–associated CNS disease, including differential diagnosis (secondary complications, co-morbid complications), involves a careful medical and developmental history, HIV-1 systemic disease history, current immunological status, neurological examination, psychological assessment, and neuroimaging studies.[173, 179] The diagnosis of HIV-1–associated PE is relatively straightforward if the patient has been followed prospectively. Longitudinal assessments of the infant or child reveal progressive involvement. The diagnosis is also fairly straightforward if the child on initial examination is found to have motor deficits (e.g., spasticity, ataxia, weakness, abnormalities of tone, change in gait), and by a careful history, either the new onset or progression of motor impairment can be documented (again, when other causes for progressive motor dysfunction have been excluded). Confirmation of progression can at times be obtained by review of family photographs of the child.

However, diagnostic difficulties arise when an HIV-1–infected youngster who was not followed from birth or infancy by the examiner is found at the initial neurological evaluation to have deficits or delays. Because the frequency of neurological and developmental impairment in this population is high, it is often impossible for the clinician to ascribe these findings to HIV-1–associated CNS disease rather than to possible co-morbid conditions. A careful history is paramount. If there are no other risk factors, the diagnosis is likely. The child should have a formal psychological assessment and be re-evaluated by the neurologist and psychologist in 2 to 4 months.[207]

Head circumference measurements are very helpful, and because these measurements are commonly recorded in primary care settings, a careful review of medical records will usually document at least one or two past head circumference measurements. This comparison allows the examiner to plot serial measurements, and the pattern of downward deviation and "crossing percentiles" makes the diagnosis of HIV-1–associated CNS disease likely. Diagnostic probability is especially high if acquired microcephaly is documented.

Examination of CSF for HIV-1 in cases of suspected HIV-associated PE is not always helpful, as CSF quantitative HIV-1 microculture, p24 antigen, or HIV-1 PCR, as well as anti-HIV-1 IgG are not present in all cases.[80, 208] Perinatally infected infants may even have undetectable levels of CSF HIV RNA despite clinical PE.[182]

Neuroimaging studies are particularly helpful and in fact critical to proper diagnosis. If calcification of basal ganglia, with or without mineralization of the frontal white matter, is present, it is probable that the child has HIV-1–associated CNS disease. If cerebral atrophy is present in the absence of documented perinatal complications, steroid use, or other known causes of atrophy, the diagnosis likewise becomes extremely likely. Neuroimaging evidence of atrophy accompanied by acquired microcephaly clearly strengthens the diagnostic certainty. In addition, a recent study by Civitello and collaborators indicated correlation between quantitative cerebral atrophy on CT scans and CSF viral load. In recent years, magnetic resonance spectroscopy (MRS) is emerging as a possible tool for monitoring disease progression and treatment efficacy.[209, 210] Follow-up neuroimaging studies should be requested in addition to the previously mentioned serial neurological and psychological evaluations.

Treatment. As in HIV-associated dementia of adults, retroviral therapy revolutionized the treatment of HIV-1–infected children. In addition, emergence of NRTIs and NNRTIs and protease inhibitors further improved the approach to aggressive treatment of HIV-1 infection in children. Initial monotherapy with ZDV did not have a sustained benefit in all children,[211] and was replaced with monotherapy with NRTIs such as ddI, 3TC, and d4T.[212, 213] However, it was soon evident that polytherapy with ZDV and ddI was clearly better in preventing and treating HIV-associated PE, compared with monotherapy with each agent.[214, 215] In addition, a successful introduction of protease inhibitors in HIV-associated dementia of adults led to pediatric guidelines for treatment of HIV-associated PE. Currently, recommendations include an initial antiretroviral regimen consisting of two compatible NRTI agents and one highly active protease inhibitor.[81]

Adjunctive therapies of HIV-associated PE correspond to some agents tried in adults, such as methyl group donors (S-adenosylmethionine and gluthatione, baclofen for spasticity, NSAIDs for pain, stimulants for psychomotor slowing, and selective serotonin reuptake inhibitors for depression). Hypnotics and anxiolytics should be avoided, as HIV-1–infected individuals are highly susceptible to adverse effects. Good nutrition is essential, and some anecdotal reports indicate benefits of omega-3 and omega-6 polyunsaturated fatty acid supplements.

In addition, optimal treatment of HIV-associated PE in children is also directed to assist in neurodevelopment, and a battery of services, including not only physical and occupational therapists, but also speech pathologists for both language delays and feeding difficulties should be provided.

HIV-ASSOCIATED MYELOPATHIES

Spinal cord involvement associated with HIV-1 infection has diverse causes. As with other neurological disorders associated with HIV-1 infection, different conditions occur with increased prevalence during different stages of HIV-1 infection. Some conditions are related to HIV-1 itself, whereas others are associated with other infectious, neoplastic, vascular, or nutritional and metabolic etiologies.[22, 216–218] A self-limiting myelitis at the time of seroconversion and a vacuolar myelopathy (VM) that occurs during more advanced HIV-1 disease stages are related to primary HIV-1 infection.[22, 130] Other infectious agents reported include the herpesviruses (VZV, HSV-2, CMV); HTLV-1 or 2; *Treponema pallidum*, *Mycobacterium tuberculosis*, and other bacterial pathogens; as well as toxoplasmosis, cryptococcus, and aspergillosis. Epidural and paraspinal abscesses due to bacteria, fungi, or mycobacteria should also be considered. Intramedullary lesions due to infectious agents have also been described. Compressive lesions may be caused by neoplasms, of which lymphoma is most common.[6] In addition, direct involvement of the spinal cord, although rare, has been caused by lymphoma or multiple myeloma. Vascular causes of noninfectious spinal cord disease in AIDS include ischemic myelopathy due to disseminated intravascular coagulation. Finally, vitamin B_{12} and folate deficiency should always be investigated in HIV-1–infected patients who present with myelopathy.[219]

Pathogenesis. There is no evidence of the direct HIV-1 infection of the spinal cord in patients with VM. The virus can be identified within macrophages, which are abundant in areas of vacuolization, but not in neurons or microglia. It is possible that macrophage-derived factors, such as interferon, interleukin-1 (IL-1), and TNF-alfa, are directly toxic to myelin, or that these factors may be responsible for a metabolic abnormality that affects myelin.[220] These possibilities are supported by the notion that VM clinically and pathologically resembles myelopathy of vitamin B_{12} or folate deficiency. Cobalamin deficiency is common in AIDS patients, but there is no correlation between VM and vitamin B_{12} serum levels, nor between vitamin B_{12} supplementation and VM clinical course. However, the similarity between VM and vitamin B_{12} myelopathy suggests that the trans-methylation pathway using cobalamin as a cofactor may be involved in the white matter vacuolization. HIV-1 may ultimately lead to impairment of trans-methylation and myelin vacuolization through the activation of macrophages or other mechanisms.[221]

Pathology. VM is characterized by the presence of intramyelinic and periaxonal vacuoles in the lateral and posterior columns of the spinal cord. The axons are usually intact in areas of mild or moderate vacuolization, but in advanced cases with severe vacuolization, the axons are disrupted. Initially, the vacuolization is symmetrical, but with the progression of the disease, it often becomes asymmetrical. The myelopathy usually affects the mid-portion of the thoracic cord, but vacuolization can be present in other portions of the thoracic cord, the cervical cord, and lumbar cord.[222]

Clinical Course. VM complicates the clinical course of 5 to 27 percent of all HIV-1–infected patients. It is reported in up to 55 percent of autopsy series and, in one recent clinicopathological series examining adult AIDS patients, VM occurred in 47 percent.[57, 218, 223] VM usually appears late in the course of HIV infection, although there are occasional reports of AIDS initially presenting as VM.[224] The disease develops insidiously, and frequently it is not diagnosed until 3 to 16 weeks after onset. Initial symptoms include urinary urgency and increased frequency, sexual dysfunction, complaints of stiffness or heaviness of the legs, with initially no weakness or pain. As the disease progresses, walking becomes difficult, with painful spastic paraparesis, mild paresthesias, and urinary incontinence.

Neurological examination typically demonstrates spastic paraparesis with asymmetrical weakness, hyper-reflexia, clonus, extensor plantar responses, and mild or moderate loss of vibration and joint position sense in the lower extremities.[150] Sensory level is usually absent. Sensory ataxia may be present, due to the severe proprioceptive loss. If there is an associated sensory neuropathy, ankle reflexes may be hypoactive and hypesthesia to pain may be present in a stocking distribution.

Evaluation. The clinical examination confirming the preceding findings is essential for the diagnosis, since there are no confirmatory tests for VM. Spine MRI is usually normal, but may show atrophy of the affected thoracic or cervical region. In addition, increased signal on T2 images may be observed, whereas enhancement after gadolinium injection is very rare.[225] CSF studies may show a mild pleocytosis (<20 cells/mL) and increase in protein content. Somatosensory evoked potentials are an important diagnostic and prognostic tool to detect abnormal central conduction time even before the clinical manifestation of VM. When used sequentially, this test can monitor the progression of the disease or response to therapy.

Differential Diagnosis. VM is a diagnosis of exclusion that can be made only after other causes of myelopathy have been excluded. The differential diagnosis includes opportunistic infections (HTLV-1 or 2, CMV, herpes simplex 2, toxoplasmosis, tuberculosis, syphyllis, cryptococcus, or aspergillosis), metabolic disease (vitamin B_{12} and folate deficiency), neoplastic lesion (lymphoma, multiple myeloma), and toxic myelopathy induced by nitrous oxide.

Treatment. There have been very few clinical trials, and no specific treatment is available. Zidovudine and high doses of vitamin B_{12} given intramuscularly have failed. No clinical benefit has been shown with corticosteroids, intravenous immunoglobulin (IVIg), or protease inhibitors. A double-blinded controlled study with L-methionine is ongoing, based on the hypothesis that abnormal trans-methylation can cause VM.[226] Currently, therapy is primarily supportive and symptomatic.

HIV-Related Peripheral Nervous System Disorders

HIV-ASSOCIATED NEUROPATHIES

Peripheral neuropathies are a frequent complication of HIV-1 infection and AIDS. A wide range of disorders has been described, and their causes are diverse. Some neuropathies are related to HIV-1 itself, or HIV-induced immune-mediated mechanisms. In other cases, neuropathies may be related to toxic complications of therapy, complications of systemic HIV-1 illness, nutritional deficiencies, metabolic derangements, opportunistic infections, or neoplasms (Table 44–11). Drug-induced injury can also exacerbate HIV-associated neuropathic disease. "D" drugs (didanosine, stavudine, and zalcitabine) are most likely to induce such injury, particularly when used in combination with one another or with hydroxyurea.[227] Because these drugs have a primary affinity for mitochondrial gamma-DNA polymerase, drug-induced peripheral nerve injury has been added to the enlarging spectrum of antiretroviral-associated mitochondrial toxicity syndromes.

The major HIV-1–associated peripheral neuropathy syndromes have well-defined clinical characteristics (Table 44–12). Distinctive clinical features that aid in the diagnosis, management and, at times, prognosis of patients are stage of HIV-1 disease, CD4+ lymphocyte count, rate of symptom progression, degree of weakness relative to sensory loss, and characteristic electrophysiological findings.

Different neuropathic syndromes occur with increased prevalence at particular stages of HIV-1 disease. Some syndromes are encountered frequently whereas others are rare. In general, the overall incidence of peripheral neuropathies increases with advancing systemic disease, progressive immunodeficiency, and declining CD4+ counts.[228] By the time patients develop AIDS, clinical and electrophysiological evidence of neuropathy is present in up to one third of

TABLE 44–11. Peripheral Neuropathies Associated with HIV-1 Infection

Toxic Neuropathy
Vincristine, isoniazid, dapsone, choloramphenicol, metronidazole, pyridoxine, dideoxyinosine (didanosine), dideoxycytidine (zalcitabine), d4T (stavudine)
Nutritional Deficiencies
Vitamin B_1, B_{12} deficiency
HIV-1–Associated Peripheral Neuropathy Syndromes
Inflammatory polyneuropathy
Acute
Chronic
Distal symmetrical polyneuropathy
Progressive polyradiculopathy
Mononeuritis multiplex
Autonomic Neuropathy
Sensory Ganglionitis
Motor Neuron Disease

TABLE 44–12. **HIV-1–Associated Peripheral Neuropathies: Clinical Features**

Neuropathy	HIV Disease Stage ($CD4^+$ cells/μL)	Onset	Symptoms	Signs	Diagnostic Studies	Comments
Inflammatory Demyelinating Polyneuropathy (AIDP or CIDP)	AIDP: early (pre-AIDS) CIDP: early > late (variable)	Subacute	Progressive symmetrical weakness, paresthesias	Moderate to severe weakness ± mild sensory loss Areflexia	EMG: demyelination CSF: ↑ ↑ Protein ↑ WBC	Indistinguishable clinically from AIDP and CIDP in non-HIV-infected states
Distal Symmetrical Polyneuropathy	Late (variable <200–400)	Subacute	Pain is predominantly symmetrical distal dysesthesias/paresthesias, numbness, burning pain	Stocking-glove sensory loss (symmetrical length-dependent) ↓ ankle DTRs	EMG: distal axonopathy	Most common HIV-1–related form of neuropathy
Progressive Polyneuropathy	Late (<200)	Acute	Prominent lower extremity syndrome, back pain, radicular pain, paresthesias, lower extremity weakness, urinary incontinence	Bilateral lower extremity weakness → flaccid paraparesis, saddle anesthesia, bowel and bladder dysfunction ↓ ankle and knee DTRs	EMG polyradiculopathy CSF: ↑ ↑ WBC + CMV culture	Prominent lower extremity syndrome resembling spinal cord compression
Mononeuritis Multiplex	Early: limited Late: extensive progressive (variable)	Acute or subacute	Facial weakness, wrist drop, foot drop Focal deep aching pain	Asymmetrical multifocal cranial and peripheral neuropathy	EMG: multifocal axonal neuropathy Nerve Bx: inflammation vasculitis ± CMV inclusions	Laryngeal nerve involvement can occur and lead to hoarseness with vocal cord paralysis

AIDP, Acute inflammatory demyelinating polyneuropathy; CIDP, chronic inflammatory demyelinating polyneuropathy; Bx, biopsy.
Modified from So YT, Holtzman DM, Abrams DI, Olney RK: Peripheral neuropathy associated with acquired immunodeficiency syndrome; prevalence and clinical features from a population-based survey. Arch Neurol 1988;45:945–948.

patients.[228] Even higher rates of nerve pathology are reported in autopsy studies. Acute demyelinating polyneuropathy, brachial plexopathy, and mononeuritides may occur at the time of acute infection or seroconversion. Acute inflammatory demyelinating polyneuropathy (AIDP) and chronic inflammatory demyelinating neuropathy (CIDP), although rare, are the most common form of peripheral neuropathy during the latent, asymptomatic, or mildly symptomatic stage of HIV-1 disease when CD4+ cell counts are greater than or equal to 500 cells/μL. As immunodeficiency progresses and as CD4+ cell counts decline to the 200 to 500 cells/μL range, the most frequent neuropathies encountered are mononeuritis multiplex and herpes zoster neuropathy. With HIV-1 disease progression (CD4+ < 200 cells/μL), the occurrence of distal symmetrical polyneuropathy increases, as does the prevalence of other types of neuropathies such as autonomic neuropathy, mononeuritis multiplex, cranial mononeuropathies, mononeuropathies-radiculopathies associated with neoplasms, and toxic neuropathies. Progressive polyradiculopathy occurs in advanced HIV-1 disease when the patient is severely immunosuppressed (CD4+ < 50 cells/μL).

Inflammatory Demyelinating Polyneuropathies

Although they are relatively uncommon, both AIDP and CIDP are well-recognized complications of HIV-1 infection.[229] Unlike other HIV-associated neuropathies, the inflammatory neuropathies occur primarily in patients early in the course of the illness, before AIDS develops, and may be the initial manifestation of the disease. AIDP, in particular, may occur coincidentally with seroconversion.[230] Clinical and electrophysiological features of inflammatory demyelinating polyneuropathies are similar to those of patients without HIV-1 infection (see Chapter 41). Patients with AIDP present with progressive, ascending symmetrical weakness of the lower and upper extremities. Although sensory symptoms may be present, the examination commonly shows sensory deficits that are mild in comparison to the degree of weakness. Areflexia is a common finding. The CSF protein may be elevated, and a majority of patients have a mononuclear pleocytosis of up to 50 cells/μL, a helpful differentiating feature from AIDP in non-HIV-1–infected patients. Nerve conduction velocity (NCV) studies and sural nerve biopsy frequently demonstrate demyelination. As in non-HIV-1–infected patients with AIDP, the pathophysiological mechanism is thought to be due to autoimmune dysfunction. AIDP is a monophasic illness that responds well to the treatment, but can also remit without therapy. IVIg and plasmapheresis are the treatments of choice.

The natural history of HIV-1–associated CIDP is unknown. As in treatment of CIDP in non-HIV-1–infected patients, prednisone, IVIg, or plasmapheresis are reported to be efficacious (see Chapter 49).

Distal Symmetrical Polyneuropathies

Pathogenesis and Pathophysiology. Pathophysiological mechanisms of this form of HIV-associated polyneuropathy remain unclear. Several hypotheses have been proposed: (1) direct effects of HIV-1;[8, 231–233] (2) HIV-1–mediated effects of activated macrophages and the production of cytokines (TNF-alpha, IL-1, and IL-6);[234] (3) nutritional deficiencies; and (4) toxins. Further studies are needed to clarify the role of these agents in the pathogenesis of distal symmetrical polyneuropathy (DSPN) in AIDS. Infectious etiologies (mainly CMV) have also been implicated; however, some investigators believe that infection-related DSPN should be considered as a separate and distinct category.[57]

Pathological examination of nerve biopsies shows degeneration of first unmyelinated and then myelinated axons,[232, 235] with mild epineurial and endoneurial perivascular mononuclear inflammation. The inflammatory cells are characterized as T lymphocytes and activated macrophages. In the endoneurium, suppressor/cytotoxic cells (CD8+) predominate over helper/inducer (CD4+) cells. A more equal ratio is seen in the epineurium and perineurium. Immunoglobulin, complement, or fibrin are not seen. Associated demyelination may be present, but does not appear to be macrophage mediated or segmental.[232] Distal axonal degeneration is noted in both central and peripheral projections of dorsal root ganglion cells and is a frequent autopsy finding in AIDS patients. Gracile tract degeneration in the upper thoracic and cervical segments may also be seen.[233] Loss of dorsal root ganglion cells and mononuclear infiltration is usually mild in comparison with the degree of axonal degeneration and inflammation of distal nerves.

Epidemiology. DSPN is the most frequent type of HIV-associated neuropathy and an incidence of 2.81 percent is estimated in HIV-1-infected patients; however, it can be detected clinically in more than 35 percent of patients with AIDS.[229, 236, 237]

Clinical Features. Characteristically, sensory symptoms in the form of neuropathic pain far exceed motor dysfunction in DSPN.[238] Typical symptoms are burning pain, numbness, or tingling of the toes or over the soles. Some patients develop contact hyperalgesia. Upper extremity involvement occurs somewhat later in the course of the neuropathy. Muscle weakness is not a prominent symptom. The most common signs are those typical of a predominantly sensory length–dependent neuropathy with depressed or absent ankle tendon reflexes, elevated sensory threshold, increased vibratory thresholds, decreased pinprick and temperature, and stocking-and-glove distribution. Joint position sensation is relatively normal. If present, weakness is minimal and is generally restricted to intrinsic foot muscles.[218, 229]

Differential Diagnosis. HIV-1–associated DSPN should be differentiated from other neuropathic lesions,[239] including toxic neuropathies attributable to chemotherapeutic and retroviral (NRTI) agents (e.g., vincristine, isoniazid, ddC, ddI, d4T)[240, 241] and tarsal tunnel syndrome. Electrodiagnostic studies do not differentiate between toxic neuropathies and other causes of DSPN. The diagnosis of toxic neuropathy is based on the temporal association of the peripheral neuropathy with drug treatment and improvement after the suspected agent is removed. However, patients with severe immunosuppresion (CD4+ < 100/μL), anemia, and a prior history of DSPN are at highest risk to develop NRTI-associated DSPN. Co-morbid conditions, such as diabetes, vitamin B_{12} deficiency, or excessive alcohol intake, may exacerbate, unmask, or predispose HIV-1 patients to develop this neuropathy sooner than expected.

Evaluation. The electrodiagnostic features of DSPN in AIDS are consistent with distal and symmetrical degeneration of sensory and motor axons, in a pattern similar to other forms of DSPN. NCV studies usually demonstrate absent or low-amplitude sural nerve action potentials (SNAP).[229] Late responses are also delayed in a pattern consistent with axonal neuropathy. Reduction in the amplitudes of the peroneal or tibial compound muscle action potential (CMAP) is less common. Electromyography (EMG) may demonstrate signs of active or chronic partial denervation with re-innervation in distal leg muscles.[229, 238] Serum vitamin B_{12} levels, folate, ESR, antinuclear antibodies, fasting blood glucose, liver enzymes, creatinine, thyroid function tests, and serum protein electrophoresis are usually normal.[229] CSF examination is nonspecific and often shows mild abnormalities in cell count and protein level (as is common in HIV-1–infected patients).[242]

Management. DSPN is often a disabling condition owing to severe pain. The main treatment is symptomatic and includes those agents used in the treatment of painful non-AIDS peripheral neuropathies, ranging from analgesics and NSAIDs to anticonvulsants (see Chapter 20). Recent studies indicated beneficial effects of gabapentin[243] and lamotrigine[244] in the treatment of HIV-associated DSPN. A controlled study using recombinant human nerve growth factor in HIV neuropathy failed to show prominent evidence of nerve fiber regeneration, although significant reduction of pain occurred. Other treatments, such as antidepressants, mexiletine, and even acupuncture, have been tried in HIV-associated DSPN, but have proved ineffective.[245, 246]

Mononeuritis Multiplex

Two forms of mononeuritis multiplex (MM), both relatively rare, have been recognized as a complication of HIV-1 infection and AIDS. The first form affects patients in early stages of HIV-1 infection (CD4+ cell counts greater than 200 cell/μL), and the second affects those individuals with advanced disease.[235, 247] Patients in early HIV-1 stages have a more benign disease, the extent of nerve involvement is more restricted, and the course is self-limited. Motor and sensory deficits develop over the course of a few weeks in the distribution of discrete peripheral nerves. This form of MM is a self-limited disease and does not usually require specific treatment. As in non-AIDS MM, an autoimmune vasculitis is proposed (see Chapter 50).[248, 249] This form of mononeuritis neuropathy should be differentiated from compressive neuropathies of the ulnar or peroneal nerves, seen particularly in patients who are bed-bound with profound weight loss.

In contrast, more widespread, multifocal weakness is characteristic of the second type of MM, which occurs primarily in patients with low CD4+ counts. The clinical presentation is typically subacute with progression over several weeks or a few months. Asymmetrical, multifocal sensory and motor deficits in the distribution of several major peripheral nerves or spinal roots are characteristic of this neuropathy. Significant motor deficits are present, and deep tendon reflexes mediated by the affected nerves are diminished or absent. Cranial neuropathy is common, and some patients have hypophonia, hoarseness, and vocal cord paresis.[235] The asymmetrical weakness in discrete distributions of peripheral nerves and occasional laryngeal nerve involvement help distinguish these patients from those with the more frequently encountered CIDP. Before establishing the diagnosis, other causes of MM should be excluded, such as herpes zoster and lymphomatous nerve root infiltration.

Electrodiagnostic studies show multifocal neuropathy with mixed demyelination and axonal loss, reduced CMAP and SNAP amplitudes, and mild reduction in conduction velocities. Compressive or entrapment neuropathies are excluded by these studies. Pathological specimens from patients with advanced AIDS show polymorphonuclear infiltrates, with mixed axonal and demyelinative lesions, as well as evidence of CMV.[248, 249] The late form of MM requires specific anti-CMV therapy, including ganciclovir, foscarnet, or cidofovir, alone or in combination.

Progressive Polyneuropathy/Radiculitis

This syndrome develops primarily in patients with very low CD4+ counts and advanced HIV-1 disease. With the introduction of HAART, the incidence of progressive polyneuropathy significantly declined. It is generally considered to be due to secondary viral, infectious, or neoplastic processes in the immune-compromised host and not directly related to HIV infection. Presenting features of progressive lumbar polyneuropathy include an acute cauda equina syndrome with rapid progression of bilateral leg weakness and urinary/fecal incontinence. Back pain is a prominent feature in some patients. Initially, weakness is restricted to the lower extremities, as is areflexia. Paresthesias are common, but sensory deficits are rarely marked. Perineal or perianal sensory changes are characteristic but not always present. Areflexia and sensory disturbance (albeit mild) help differentiate this syndrome from weakness due to myopathy or the wasting syndrome (see later). Sphincteric disturbances and sparing of the upper extremities separate this disorder from AIDP, CIDP, and mononeuritis multiplex. EMG demonstrates denervation in lower extremity muscles as well as in lumbar paraspinal muscles. NCV abnormalities may be present in up to one third of patients and indicates a co-existing polyneuropathy. CSF examination is the most important confirmatory study. Elevated protein content and hypoglycorrhachia are common. About half of patients have a marked pleocytosis, with cell counts in excess of 500 cells/μL. The other half has a less striking mononuclear cell count.

CMV infection is the most important infectious cause of this syndrome[250] and may be detected by CSF culture and the use of CMV PCR testing. This disorder should be treated with ganciclovir and foscarnet (see Chapter 41), and early treatment may partially reverse the neurological deficits. Delayed diagnosis and treatment leads to poor prognosis.

A polyradiculopathy syndrome may also be caused by pathogens other than CMV (e.g., herpes zoster infections, *Treponema pallidum*, *Mycobacterium tuberculosis*, toxoplasmosis of the conus medullaris) and by leptomeningeal lymphoma.[251] Therefore, CSF studies should include viral cultures, VDRL titer, and cytological studies. A lumbosacral spine MRI excludes a compressive or mass lesion and may show enhancement of nerve roots. When herpes zoster radiculitis is present, lesions are improved and the incidence of neuralgia reduced by acyclovir. Parenteral acyclovir (30 mg/kg/d) should be used when cervical or lumbar dermatomes are involved, in an attempt to prevent severe myeloradiculitis. Amitriptyline, carbamazepine, and capsaicin can be used in the setting of postherpetic neuralgia.

Autonomic Neuropathy

Autonomic neuropathy has been reported in nearly 50 percent of HIV-1–infected patients. The severity of autonomic impairment is correlated with the degree of immunosuppression. Patients primarily experience dizziness, diarrhea, bladder and sexual dysfunction, and sometimes palpitations. Both sympathetic and parasympathetic systems are involved. Sometimes, autonomic neuropathy is caused by pentamidine, and this drug should be excluded in every patient. Treatment is symptomatic and may require cardiovascular monitoring.

HIV-1–RELATED MYOPATHIES

Muscle disorders related to HIV-1 infection include HIV-1–associated polymyositis, ZDV toxic myopathy, pyomyositis or infectious myopathy, cardiomyopathy, and the so-called wasting syndrome myopathy. Of these conditions, HIV-1–associated polymyositis and toxic myopathy related to ZDV are the most common. Distinguishing between these two forms of myopathy at times may be difficult.

Pathogenesis and Pathophysiology. The pathophysiological mechanisms underlying HIV-related myopathy are uncertain. A wide spectrum of histopathological findings has been described, including inflammatory infiltrates[252–254] noninflammatory myofiber degeneration,[253] nemaline rod bodies,[252, 253] cytoplasmic bodies, and mitochondrial abnormalities.[255] Muscle biopsy examination usually shows characteristic myopathic features such as variation in fiber size or degenerating muscle fibers. Features of polymyositis (necrotic fibers and lymphocytic infiltrates in the perimysium and perivascular space) are also noted in some patients, although the degree of these changes is variable.[256] In a subset of patients, Gomori trichrome-stained sections of muscle show prominent abnormalities of mitochondria giving the appearance of ragged-red fibers.[257–259] In other subsets of patients, electron microscopy examination shows granular material that appears as electron-dense rod bodies.[253] Variable amounts of inflammatory infiltrates have been described in both of these types.

Before the widespread use of ZDV, overt myopathy or a polymyositis-like syndrome was reported but not frequently. With increasing use of ZDV, and especially at the initially high 1200 mg/d dosage, reports of myopathy in ZDV-treated patients and those who improved following ZDV withdrawal appeared in the literature.[259–261] Studies showed ZDV to be an inhibitor of the gamma-polymerase of the mitochondrial matrix,[262] and ZDV toxicity in skeletal muscle mitochondria was demonstrated in some[255, 258, 260, 263–265] but not all studies.[264, 265]

Investigators have suggested that muscle changes may be due to the virus, the length of time of the patient's infection, and the length of time taking ZDV. Whether there are pathological features that distinguish between HIV-1– and ZDV-related myopathies remains uncertain.[257, 258, 260, 266] One clinical study of HIV-related myopathy conducted in unselected patients of all disease stages found that none of the patients taking ZDV had symptomatic myopathy thought to be related to ZDV. However, some patients had characteristic ZDV morphological changes on muscle biopsy.[266] The clinical relevance of the structural changes described earlier, the causal role of ZDV, and thus, the pathogenesis of HIV-related myopathy remain unclear and the subject of controversy.

HIV-1 has been localized in infiltrating monocyte/macrophage cells by immunocytochemistry.[267] Myofibers do not appear to be directly infected.[253] This suggests that it is unlikely that HIV-1 has a direct role in myopathy. As in other forms of polymyositis (see Chapter 50), immune-mediated mechanisms are proposed. It is postulated that activated macrophages secrete toxic factors (cytokine hypothesis) that mediate myofiber damage. TNF, which causes cachexia in laboratory animals and is produced mainly by monocytes, is also implicated as is IL–1 alpha (shown to accumulate in muscle fibers of HIV-infected patients).[268] HIV-1–infected CD8+ cells produce cytokines that expose muscle fiber antigens against which there is no self-tolerance. It has also been suggested that homology between viral GAG protein and muscle ribonucleoproteins triggers an autoimmune process leading to cellular infiltration and myofiber damage.[269]

Epidemiology and Risk Factors. Risk factors are not yet clearly defined. One study of 50 unselected patients in all stages of HIV-1 infection found that 26 percent of patients had myopathy. An autopsy series reported myopathic changes in 26 percent of AIDS cases.[254] A retrospective analysis of patients enrolled in an antiretroviral clinical trial showed a 0.4 percent incidence of myopathy in patients not treated with ZDV (placebo group), which rose to 3 percent in ZDV-treated patients (D. Simpson, personal communication). HIV-associated myopathy may develop in patients in all stages of HIV-1 infection and does not appear to be associated with degree of immunosuppression.[253]

Clinical Features and Associated Disorders. Muscle weakness is the predominant sign and symptom.[253, 257] Patients present with slowly progressive symmetrical and predominantly proximal weakness of the upper and lower limbs. Patients have difficulty arising from a chair or climbing stairs. Myalgia is present in 25 to 50 percent of affected patients. Neurological examinations reveal symmetrical weakness of proximal muscle groups with prominent involvement of neck and hip flexors. HIV-1–associated polymyositis can occur at any stage of HIV-1 infection. Presentation is similar to sporadic polymyositis with proximal muscle weakness, myalgias, and elevated CK.

There are no clinical features that differentiate HIV from ZDV myopathy. ZDV myopathy usually occurs after at least several months of therapy and there appears to be a dose and duration effect. Although some patients may improve after ZDV withdrawal (resolution of muscle pain and a slower recovery of strength),[259, 260] others do not.[257] To add further confusion, ZDV rechallenge in some patients does not cause a relapse.[261]

Differential Diagnosis. Other myopathic complications of HIV-1 infection include wasting syndrome and infectious myopathies. Patients with advanced HIV-1 disease frequently develop a wasting syndrome (Slim's disease) consisting of fatigue, profound involuntary weight loss, and diffuse weakness. Affected individuals are cachectic, weak, and have a general loss of muscle bulk. The frequent finding of the wasting syndrome in persons with severe HIV-1 infection makes it difficult to delineate a myopathic component. Although a myopathy can also cause a wasting syndrome characterized by involuntary weight loss and chronic muscle weakness,[270] at times it is difficult to distinguish between the two. HIV-1–associated myopathy can occur at any stage of HIV-1 infection. Thus, if myopathy develops in early HIV-1 infection before other AIDS-defining illnesses and immunosuppression, the diagnosis of HIV-related myopathy is likely if systemic or nutritional factors have been excluded and criteria for a diagnosis of myopathy are met. The importance of determining a specific diagnosis of myopathy in patients is evidenced by some patients' improvement with prednisone therapy.[270]

Infectious causes of myopathy in patients with AIDS, although infrequent, should be considered in the differential diagnosis. Pathogens reported in muscles of AIDS patients include *Toxoplasma gondii*,[271] CMV, *Microsporidia*, *Cryptococcus neoformans*, MAI, and *Staphylococcus aureus*.[254]

HIV-infected individuals may present with acute rhabdomyolysis characterized by a myopathic syndrome (myalagia, muscle weakness) associated with serum CK levels greater than 1,500 IU/L. The cause of acute rhabdomyolysis in HIV-1 disease is unknown, although investigators have suggested several etiologies, including HIV-1 itself, drug toxicity (e.g., ddI, sulfadiazine, pentamidine), and opportunistic infections.[272]

Evaluation. The diagnosis of myopathy is made by the presence of limb weakness with CK elevation, along with supportive electrodiagnostic and muscle biopsy studies. As in the diagnosis of polymyositis (non-HIV-1 related), if three of four features are present, the diagnosis is considered probable, and if two of four features are present, the diagnosis is possible (see Chapter 50). Electrophysiological studies show typical myopathic EMG features (small, brief, and polyphasic motor unit potentials that recruit with full interference patterns and fibrillation potentials).[257] Some patients also have NCV abnormalities indicative of coincident DSPN.[253]

In HIV myopathy, CK levels are usually elevated to a moderate degree, with a median level of approximately 500 IU/L.[253, 258–260] The CK elevation parallels the degree of myonecrosis observed in coincident muscle biopsies but does not seem to correlate with weakness and is not a specific marker of HIV myopathy (patients may have elevated CK without clinical features of myopathy).

Muscle biopsy is useful in the evaluation and management of patients. Some investigators propose that the histological finding of ragged-red fibers supports the diagnosis of ZDV myopathy.[258, 260] However, not all ZDV patients with myopathy have ragged-red fibers on biopsy; thus, the absence of the finding does not exclude a toxic myopathy.

Management. Because it is often difficult to distinguish patients with ZDV-related myopathy from those without, the initial management of patients with significant limb weakness and objective evidence of myopathy includes ZDV withdrawal. An 18 to 100 percent rate of improvement in muscle strength is reported from different series.[257, 259, 266] Some patients show further deterioration or no improvement after cessation of ZDV but do respond to treatment with corticosteroids. Thus, if signs and symptoms persist after ZDV withdrawal (about 1 month), a muscle biopsy should be considered. If there are signs of inflammation, a trial of steroids is warranted. Prednisone may be effective in treatment of polymyositis or rod-body myopathy.[252, 257]

HIV-Associated Neoplasms

Primary CNS lymphoma (PCNSL), non-Hodgkin's lymphoma metastatic to the CNS, and Kaposi's sarcoma are the principal brain neoplasms associated with HIV/AIDS. Of these neoplasms, PCNSL is the most common in both adults and children and is designated as an AIDS-defining condition. Neurological involvement associated with Kaposi's sarcoma is rare. Metastatic CNS lesions are found at the junction between gray and white matter, and on MRI scans, they enhance with contrast material. They are often highly vascular tumors and can hemorrhage.

PRIMARY CENTRAL NERVOUS SYSTEM LYMPHOMA

Primary CNS lymphoma (see Chapter 46) develops in approximately 5 percent of patients with AIDS and is found at autopsy in up to 10 percent of cases. It is the initial AIDS-defining illness in 0.6 percent of adults. In children, PCNSL is the most common mass lesion, and in adults, it is the second most common after toxoplasmosis. PCNSL develops in patients with advanced HIV-1 disease who are severely immunosuppressed. The incidence of PCNSL in the AIDS population may be increasing as longevity is extended by medical management and antiretroviral agents. Lymphomas are usually of the diffuse immunoblastic, diffuse large cell, or small-cell noncleaved B-cell type[273] with a predilection for the deep cerebral gray matter, corpus callosum, periventricular white matter, and cerebellar vermis. Strong evidence links PCNSL to EBV. EBV is frequently detected in the tumor tissue, and detection of EBV DNA by PCR in CSF is a sensitive and specific test for establishing a diagnosis in the appropriate clinical setting.[274] It is suspected that in HIV-1–infected patients, destruction of T cells enables a subpopulation of immortalized and latently infected B cells to persist in the CNS, leading to the development of non-Hodgkin's lymphoma, particularly PCNSL. Clinical presentation includes headache, mental status changes (confusion, lethargy, memory problems), seizures, cranial nerve palsies, and focal neurological deficits, such as hemiparesis or aphasia.[13, 273] In children, neurological deterioration at times may be rapidly progressive and fulminant.[14] As this clinical presentation is nonspecific, neuroimaging is recommended, with MRI as the procedure of choice.

Neuroimaging characteristics of lymphoma include: (1) hyperdense or isodense multiple mass lesions with variable ring enhancement; (2) diffusely infiltrating contrast-enhancing lesions; (3) periventricular contrasting lesions; (4) thallium-avid on SPECT; and (5) hypermetabolic area on PET scan.[274–276] Surrounding edema is variable, and a large solitary mass may be seen as well as multiple lesions. Diffusion-weighted MRI and MRS have been used to distinguish abscess, *Toxoplasma* encephalitis, and primary lymphoma, although with limited success.[277, 278] In addition to brain MRI, spinal MRI is indicated on the basis of clinical examination, as well as CSF studies for EBV DNA, ocular slit lamp exam, bone marrow, chest x-ray, and abdominopelvic CT scan.

The differential diagnosis of intracranial lesions in AIDS patients includes a variety of infectious, neoplastic, and cerebrovascular processes. In adults, the most common mass lesion is toxoplasmosis. Unlike *Toxoplasma* encephalitis, PCNSL lesions may cross the midline in the corpus callosum and be associated with patchy nodular ventricular enhancement.

Recommendations for the management of intracranial mass lesions in AIDS patients have recently been published. Large lesions with mass effect and threatening impending herniation require open biopsy with decompression. SPECT should be performed when available, because it appears to be highly specific for PCNSL. A combination of SPECT, PET scan, and CSF EBV analysis, if all positive, establish the diagnosis in virtually 100 percent of patients, eliminating the necessity for brain biopsy.[279] Biopsy in AIDS patients is generally avoided, not only because of the possibility for HIV-1 contamination, but also because of a high risk for significant hemorrhage after biopsy in AIDS patients.[280] In adults, empirical treatment for toxoplasmosis should be instituted in all other cases except when a single intracranial mass lesion accompanies negative serology for toxoplasmosis, when all the preceding diagnostic approaches should be initiated.

Primary CNS lymphoma are radiosensitive tumors, but prognosis is extremely poor.[281, 282] Reduction in tumor size has been noted in patients following whole brain radiation therapy and steroids (300 cGy in 10 fractions for a total of 3000 cGy).[282, 283] A 2- to 4-month survival after diagnosis is reported. In general, chemotherapy regimens have not significantly altered long-term survival rates. Prognosis for long-term survival is grim, with death resulting from concurrent illness and opportunistic infections rather than lymphoma. Absence of opportunistic infections at the time of diagnosis is associated with a longer median survival. Selected patients may be candidates for combined chemotherapy and radiation therapy.[284]

METASTATIC NON-HODGKIN'S LYMPHOMA

Non-Hodgkin's lymphoma occurs in 5 percent of AIDS patients. This malignancy develops in patients who are severely immunosuppressed, and, like PCNSL, it is linked etiopathologically to EBV. Non-Hodgkin's lymphoma often presents as an aggressive tumor, and there is a propensity for CNS metastasis. Approximately one third to one half of patients with non-Hodgkin's lymphoma develop metastatic CNS disease. Leptomeningeal involvement is common, with extension along the Virchow-Robins spaces, the cranial and spinal nerve sheaths, and the CSF pathways. Clinical features include mental status changes, seizures, cranial neuropathies and radiculopathies, and paraspinal masses.[285] Neuroimaging studies often reveal hydrocephalus with basilar meningeal enhancement. Diffuse leptomeningeal and cortical enhancement may also occur. CSF studies show depressed glucose levels. Lymphoma cells may be seen on cytological studies. Combination chemotherapy regimens have not been as successful in prolonging life in patients with AIDS-associated non-Hodgkin's lymphoma as they have in non-AIDS–non-Hodgkin's lymphoma patients. The poor response and short survival may be due to severe immunosuppression and the occurrence of opportunistic infections.

TABLE 44–13. **HIV-1–Associated Opportunistic Infections of the Central Nervous System**

Bacterial
Mycobacterium tuberculosis
Mycobacterium avium-intracellulare
Treponema pallidum
Nocardia
Salmonella
Listeria monocytogenes

Viral
Cytomegalovirus
Herpes simplex viruses 1 and 2
Varicella zoster virus
JC virus
Epstein-Barr virus

Fungi
Cryptococcus neoformans
Candida
Coccidioides immitis
Aspergillus
Histoplasma capsulatum

Protozoa
Toxoplasma gondii
Trypanosoma cruzi
Acanthamoeba

Modified from Marra CM: Opportunistic infections in AIDS, Infections of the Nervous System II. Minneapolis, MN, American Academy of Neurology, 1997, pp 234–259.

Opportunistic Infections in AIDS

A variety of opportunistic infections occur in the setting of AIDS and may affect the CNS (Table 44–13). The susceptibility of individuals with HIV to opportunistic infections is related to the degree of immunosuppression and correlates to the peripheral blood CD4+ lymphocyte count (Table 44–14). A full discussion of the clinical features,

TABLE 44–14. **Correlation Between Central Nervous System Disease Susceptibility and Peripheral Blood CD4 Count**

	CD4+ Count (Cells/μl)			
	>500	**500–200**	**<200**	**<100**
Toxoplasma encephalitis			X	X
Cryptococcal meningitis			X	X
Syphilitic meningitis	X	X	X	X
Tuberculous meningitis		X	X	X
Coccidioidal meningitis			X	X
Cytomegalovirus encephalitis or polyradiculopathy				X
Progressive multifocal leukoencephalopathy				X

Modified from Marra CM: Opportunistic infections in AIDS, Infections of the Nervous System II. Minneapolis, MN, American Academy of Neurology, 1997, pp 234–260.

evaluation, and management of infection with these organisms is detailed in the preceding chapters on viral (see Chapter 41) and nonviral (see Chapter 42) infections.

Reviews and Selected Updates

Note: Because of the rapidity of scientific advances in the field of HIV/AIDS, the authors recommend the following Internet resources for up-to-date information: *http://www.hivatis.org*; *http://www.unaids.org*; *http://www.nih.gov/medlineplus/aids.html.*

American Academy of Neurology: Human immunodeficiency virus (HIV) infection and the nervous system. Neurology 1989;39:119–122.

American Academy of Neurology: Report of the American Academy of Neurology on the ethical role of neurologists in the AIDS epidemic. Neurology 1992;42:1116–1117.

Berger JR, Levy RM: AIDS and the Nervous System, 2nd ed. New York, Lippincott-Raven, 1996, pp 223–254.

Carr A, Cooper DA: Primary HIV infection. *In* Sande MA, Volberding PA (eds): The Medical Management of AIDS, 5th ed. Philadelphia, WB Saunders, 1997, pp 89–106.

Condra JH, Miller MD, Hazuda DJ, Emini EI: Potential new therapies for the treatment of HIV-1 infection. Annu Rev Med 2002;53:541–555.

Feinberg MB: Virologic aspects of HIV infection. *In* Cotton D, Watts DH (eds): The Medical Management of AIDS in Women. New York, Wiley-Liss, 1997, pp 67–95.

Graham BS, Karzon DT: AIDS vaccine development. *In* Merigan TC Jr, Bartlett JG, Bolognesi D (eds): Textbook of AIDS Medicine. Baltimore, Lippincott, Williams, and Wilkins, 1998, pp 689–724.

Hahn BH, Shaw GM, De Cock KM, Sharp PM: AIDS as a zoonosis: Scientific and public health implications. Science 2000;287:607–614.

Janssen RS: Epidemiology and neuroepidemiology of human immunodeficiency virus infection. *In* Berger JR, Levy R (eds): AIDS and the Nervous System, 2nd ed. Philadelphia, Lippincott-Raven,1992, pp 13–37.

Kahn JO, Walker BD: Acute human immunodeficiency virus type 1 infection. N Engl J Med 1998;339:33–39.

McCune JM: The dynamics of CD4+ T-cell depletion in HIV disease. Nature 2001;410:974–979.

Tagliati H, Simpson D, Mogello S, et al: Cerebellar degeneration associated with human immunodeficiency virus infection. Neurology 1998; 50:244–251.

References

1. Barre-Sinoussi F, Chermann JC, Rey F, et al: Isolation of a T-lymphotrophic retrovirus from a patient at risk for acquired immunodeficiency syndrome. Science 1983;220:868–871.
2. Gallo RC, Salahuddin SZ, Popovic M, et al: Frequent detection and isolation of cytopathic retroviruses (HTLV–11) from patients with AIDS. Science 1984;224:500–503.
3. Levy JA, Hoffman AD, Kramer SM, et al: Isolation of lymphotrophic retroviruses from San Francisco patients with AIDS. Science 1984;225:840–842.
4. Coffin J, Haase A, Levy JA, et al: Human immunodeficiency viruses. Science 1986;232:697.
5. Joint United Nations Programme on HIV/AIDS and World Health Organization. AIDS Epidemic Update: December 2001. Geneva, UNAIDS, 2000.
6. Snider WD, Simpson DM, Nielsen S, et al: Neurological complications of acquired immune deficiency syndrome: Analysis of 50 patients. Ann Neurol 1983;14:403–418.
7. Levy JA, Shimabukuro J, Hollander H, et al: Isolation of AIDS associated retrovirus from cerebrospinal fluid and brain of patients with neurological symptoms. Lancet 1985;2:586–588.
8. Ho DD, Rota TR, Schooley RT, et al: Isolation of HTLV-III from CSF and neural tissues of patients with AIDS-related neurologic syndromes. N Engl J Med 1985;313:1493–1497.
9. Navia BA, Jordan BD, Price RW: The AIDS demential complex: 1. Clinical features. Ann Neurol 1986;19:517–524.
10. Belman AL, Ultmann MH, Horoupian D, et al: Neurologic complications in infants and children with acquired immune deficiency syndrome. Ann Neurol 1985;18:560–566.
11. Goudsmit J, Wolters EC, Bakker M, et al: Intrathecal synthesis of antibodies to HTLV-III in patients without AIDS or AIDS related complex. Br Med J 1986;292:1231–1234.
12. Epstein LG, Goudsmit J, Paul DA, et al: Expression of human immunodeficiency virus in cerebrospinal fluid of children with progressive encephalopathy. Ann Neurol 1987;21:397–401.
13. Epstein LG, Sharer LR, Oleske JM, et al: Neurologic manifestations of human immunodeficiency virus infection in children. Pediatrics 1986;78:678–687.
14. Sharer LR, Epstein LG, Cho ES, et al: Pathologic features of AIDS encephalopathy in children: Evidence for LAV/HTLV-III infection of the brain. Hum Pathol 1986;17:271–284.
15. Gabuzda DH, Ho DD, de la Monte SM, et al: Immunohistochemical identification of HTLV-III antigen in brain of patients with AIDS. Ann Neurol 1986;20:289–295.
16. Pumarola-Sune T, Navia BA, Cordon-Cardo D, et al: HIV antigen in the brains of patients with the AIDS dementia complex. Ann Neurol 1987;21:490–496.
17. CDC: Revision of the CDC surveillance case definition for acquired immunodeficiency syndrome. MMWR 1987;36(Suppl 1S):1–15.
18. Levy RM, Bredesen DE, Rosenblum ML: Neurological manifestations of the acquired immunodeficiency syndrome (AIDS): Experience at UCSF and review of the literature. J Neurosurg 1985;62:475–495.
19. Levy RM, Janssen RS, Bush TJ, Rosenblum ML: Neuroepidemiology of acquired immunodeficiency syndrome. J AIDS 1988;1:31–41.
20. Ho DD, Sarngadharan MG, Resnick L, et al: Primary human T-lymphotropic virus type III infection. Ann Intern Med 1985;103:880–883.
21. Carne CA, Tedder RS, Smith A, et al: Acute encephalopathy coincident with seroconversion for anti-HTLV III. Lancet 1985;2: 1206–1208.
22. Denning DW, Anderson J, Rudge P, Smith H: Acute myelopathy associated with primary infection with human immunodeficiency virus. Br Med J 1987;294:143–144.
23. Jannsen RS, Cornblath DR, Epstein LG, McArthur J, Price R: HIV infection and the nervous system: Report from the American Academy of Neurology Task Force. Neurology 1989;39:111–122.
24. Human Retroviruses and AIDS: A compilation and analysis of nucleic acid and amino acid sequences. Los Alamos National Laboratory, 1998. http://hiv-web.lanl.gov.
25. Arendt CW, Littman DR: HIV: Master of the host cell. Genome Biol 2001;2(11):Reviews 1030.
26. Perez OD, Nolan GP: Resistance is futile: Assimilation of cellular machinery by HIV-1 Immunity. Immunology 2001;15:687–690.
27. Levy JA: Pathogenesis of human immunodeficiency virus infection. Microbiol Rev 1993;57:183–289.
28. Kaul M, Garden GA, Lipton SA: Pathways to neuronal injury and apoptosis in HIV-associated dementia. Nature 2001;410:988–994.
29. Geijtenbeek TB, et al: DC-SIGN, a dendritic cell-specific HIV-1-binding protein that enhances trans-infection of T cells. Cell 2000; 100:587–597.
30. He J, Chen Y, Farzan M, et al: CCR3 and CCR5 are co-receptors for HIV-1 infection of microglia. Nature 1997;385:645–649.
31. Albright AV, Shieh JTC, Itoh T, et al: Microglia express CCR5, CXCR4, and CCR3, but of these, CCR5 is the principal barrier is enhanced by lipopolysaccharide. J Virol 1999;73:205–213.
32. O'Brien SJ, Moore JP: The effect of genetic variation in chemokines and their receptors on HIV transmission and progression to AIDS. Immunol Rev 2000;177:99–111.
33. Zinkernagel RM: Are HIV-specific CTL responses salutary or pathogenic? Curr Opin Immunol 1995;7:462–470.
34. Haase AT: Population biology of HIV-1 infection: Viral and CD4+ T cell demographics and dynamics in lymphatic tissues. Annu Rev Immunol 1999;17:625–656.
35. Rosok BI, et al: Reduced CD4 cell counts in blood do not reflect CD4 cell depletion in tonsillar tissue in asymptomatic HIV-1 infection. AIDS 1996;10:F35–F38.
36. Gorochov G, et al: Perturbation of CD4+ and CD8+ T-cell repertoires during progression to AIDS and regulation of the CD4+ repertoire during antiviral therapy. Nature Med 1998;4:215–221.
37. Clerici M, Shearer G: A Th1 to Th2 switch is a critical step in the aetiology of HIV infection. Immunol Today 1993;14:107–111.
38. Levy JA: HIV and the Pathogenesis of AIDS. Washington, DC, ASM Press, 1994.
39. Weiss RA: Gulliver's travels in HIV land. Nature 2001;410:963–967.
40. Wyatt R, Sodroski J: The HIV-1 envelope glycoproteins: Fusogens, antigens and immunogens. Science 1998;280:1884–1888.
41. Wolfs TF, Zwart G, Bakker M, Goudsmit J: HIV-I genomic RNA diversification following sexual and parenteral virus transmission. Virology 1992;189:103–110.

42. Dear ES, Moudgil T, Meyer Rd, Ho DD: Transient high levels of viremia in patients with primary human immunodeficiency virus type I infection. N Engl J Med 1991;324:961–964.
43. Di Stefano M, Gray F, Leitner T, Chiodi F: Analysis of ENV V3 sequences from HIV-1–infected brain indicates restrained virus expression throughout the disease. J Med Virol 1996;49:41–48.
44. Wiley CA, Soontornniyomkij V, Radhakrishnan L, et al: Distribution of brain HIV load in AIDS. Brain Pathol 1998;8:277–284.
45. Buttner A, Mehraein RB, Weis S: Vascular changes in the cerebral cortex in HIV-1 infection. II. An immunohistochemical and lectinhistochemical investigation. Acta Neuropathol (Berl) 1996;92:35–41.
46. Schwarze SR, Ho A, Vocero-Akbani A, Dowdy SF: In vivo protein transduction: Delivery of a biologically active protein into the mouse. Science 1999;285:1569–1572.
47. McCarthy M, He J, Wood C: HIV-1 strain-associated variability in infection of primary neuroglia. J Neurovirol 1998;4:80–89.
48. Ho DD, Neumann AU, Perelson AS, et al: Rapid turnover of plasma virions and CD4 lymphocytes in HIV-I infection. Nature 1995; 373:123–126.
49. Pantaleo G, Graziosi C, Demarest JF, et al: HIV infection is active and progressive in lymphoid tissue during the clinically latent stage of disease. Nature 1993;362:355–358.
50. Pantaleo G, Fauci A: New concepts in the immunopathogenesis of HIV infection. Ann Rev Immunol 1995;13:487–512.
51. Adleman LM, Wolfsy D: T-cell homeostasis: Implications in HIV infection. J AIDS 1993;6:144–152.
52. Kleet IP, Vos AH, deGoede RE, et al: Prognostic value of HIV-1 syncytium-inducing phenotype for rate of CD4+ cell depletion and progression to AIDS. Ann Intern Med 1993;118:681–688.
53. Amandari A, Gallo P, Zamarchi R, et al: IgG oligoclonal bands in sera of HIV-I infected patients are mainly directed against HIV-I determinant retroviruses. AIDS Res Hum 1990;6:581–586.
54. Andiman WA, Mezger J, Shapiro E: Invasive bacterial infections in children born to women infected with human immunodeficiency virus type-1. J Pediatr 1994;124:846–852.
55. CDC: Recommendations of the U.S. Public Health Service Task Force on the use of zidovudine to reduce perinatal transmission of human immunodeficiency virus. MMWR 1994;43(No RR-11).
56. Centers for Disease Control and Prevention: HIV/AIDS Surveillance Report. Mid-year edition 1994. New York Oxford University Press, 1996, pp 1–27.
57. Jannsen RS: Epidemiology and neuroepidemiology of human immunodeficiency virus infection. *In* Berger JR, Levy RM (eds): AIDS and the Nervous System, 2nd ed. Philadelphia-New York, Lippincott-Raven, 1996, pp 13–38.
58. Centers for Disease Control and Prevention: HIV/AIDS Surveillance Rep. 2000;12:35.
59. Mofenson LM, Wolinsky SM: Current insights regarding vertical transmission. *In* Pizzo PA, Wilfert CM (eds): Pediatric AIDS: The Challenge of HIV Infection in Infants, Children and Adolescents, 2nd ed. Baltimore, Williams & Wilkins, 1994, pp 179–203.
60. Boyer PJ, Dillon M, Navaie M, et al: Factors predictive of maternal-fetal transmission of HIV-1: Preliminary analysis of zidovudine given during pregnancy and/or delivery. JAMA 1994;271:1925–1930.
61. Mayaux MJ, Burgard M, Teglas JP, et al: Neonatal characteristics in rapidly progressive perinatally acquired HIV-1 disease. JAMA 1996; 275:606–610.
62. St. Louis ME, Kamenga M, Brown C, et al: Risk for perinatal HIV-1 transmission according to maternal immunologic, virologic, and placental factors. JAMA 1993;269:2853–2859.
63. Vigano A, Principi N, Villa ML, et al: Immunologic characterization of children vertically infected with human immunodeficiency virus, with slow or rapid disease progression. J Pediatr 1995;126(3): 368–374.
64. American Academy of Neurology AIDS Task Force: Nomenclature and research case definitions for neurologic manifestations of human immunodeficiency virus type 1. Neurology 1991;41:778–785.
65. Blanche S, Mayaux MJ, Rouzioux C, et al: Relation of the course of HIV infection in children to the severity of the disease in their mothers at delivery. N Engl J Med 1994;330:308–312.
66. Landesman SH, Kalish LA, Burns DN, et al: Obstetrical factors and the transmission of human immunodeficiency virus type 1 from mother to child. The Women and Infants Transmission Study. N Engl J Med 1996;334:1617–1623.
67. Piot P, Bartos M, Ghys PG, Walker N, Schwartlander B: The global impact of HIV/AIDS Nature 2001;410:968–973.
68. Hein K, Dell R, Futterman D, et al: Comparison of HIV+ and HIV– adolescents: Risk factors and psychosocial determinants. Pediatrics 1995;95:96–104.
69. Grubman S, Gross E, Learner-Weiss N, et al: Older children and adolescents living with perinatally acquired human immunodeficiency virus infection. Pediatrics 1995;95:657–663.
70. Allain JP, Paul DA, Laurian Y, Senn D: Serologic markers in early stages of human immunodeficiency virus infection in heomophiliacs. Lancet 1986;2:1233–1236.
71. Cumming PD, Wallace EL, Schorr JB, Dodd RY: Exposure of patients to human immunodeficiency virus through the transfusion of blood components that test antibody-negative. N Engl J Med 1990;321: 941–946.
72. Penderson C, Londhardt BO, Jensen BL, et al: Clinical course of primary HIV infection consequences for subsequent course of infection. Br Med J 1989;299:154–157.
73. Lifson AR, Rutherford GW, Jaffe HW: The natural history of human immunodeficiency virus infection. J Infect Dis 1988;158: 1360–1367.
74. Horsburgh CR, Ou CY, Jason J, et al: Duration of human immunodeficiency virus infection before detection of antibody. Lancet 1989; 2:637–640.
75. Hendriks JCM, Medley GF, van Griensven GJP, et al: Treatment-free incubation period of AIDS in a cohort of homosexual men. AIDS 1993;7(2):231–239.
76. Barnhart HX, Caldwell MB, Thomas P, et al: Natural history of human immunodeficiency virus disease in perinatally infected children: An analysis from the Pediatric Spectrum of Disease Project. Pediatrics 1996;97:710–716.
77. Persaud D, Chadwani S, Rigaud M, et al: Delayed recognition of human immunodeficiency virus infection in preadolescent children. Pediatrics 1992;90:688–669.
78. CDC: 1994 revised classification system for human immunodeficiency virus infection in children less than 13 years of age: Official authorized addenda—human immunodeficiency virus infection codes and official guidelines for coding and reporting ICD-9-CM. MMWR 1994;43 (No RR-12).
79. Gaines H, van Sydow M, Pehrson PO, Lundbergh P: Clinical picture of primary HIV infection presenting as a glandular fever-like illness. Br Med J 1988;297:1363–1368.
80. Working Group on Antiretroviral Therapy and Medical Management of Infants, Children and Adolescents with HIV Infection: Antiretroviral therapy and medical management of pediatric HIV infection. Pediatrics 1998;102(Suppl):1005–1062.
81. Working Group on Antiretroviral Therapy and Medical Management of HIV-Infected Children: Guidelines for the use of antiretroviral agents in pediatric HIV infection. J Int Assoc Phys AIDS Care 1999;5 (Suppl):4–20. *http://www.iapac.org.*
82. U.S. Department of Health and Human Services Clinical Practice Guidelines: 1. Managing early HIV infection, Number 7. 2. Evaluation and management of early HIV infection. AHCPR Publication No. 94-057-2 January, 1994.
83. Volberding PA: Antiretroviral therapy. Management of HIV infections and their complications. *In* Sande MA, Volberding PA (eds): Medical Management of AIDS, 5th ed. Philadelphia, WB Saunders, 1997, pp 113–124.
84. Van Der Horst C, Sanne I, Wakeford C, et al: Two randomized, controlled equivalence trials of emtricitibine (FTC) to lamivudine (3TC). 8th Conference on Retroviruses and Opportunistic Infections, 2001, p 48.
85. Richman DD, Kessler H, Eron J, et al: Anti-HIV activity and tolerability of DAPD, a novel dioxolane guanosine RT inhibitor: initial results of a phase I/II 14-day monotherapy clinical trial. 7th Conference on Retroviruses and Opportunistic Infections, 2000, p 200.
86. Gruzdev B, Horban A, Boron-Kaczmarska A, et al: TMC120, a new non-nucleoside reverse transcriptase inhibitor, is a potent antiretroviral in treatment naive, HIV-1 infected subjects. 8th Conference on Retroviruses and Opportunistic Infections, 2001.
87. Wang Y, Daenzer C, Wood R, et al: The safety, efficacy and viral dynamics analysis of tipranavir, a new-generation protease inhibitor, in a phase II study in antiretroviral-naive HIV-1-infected patients. 7th Conference on Retroviruses and Opportunistic Infections, 2000, p 201.
88. Squires K, Gatell J, Piliero P, et al: AI424–007: 48-week safety and efficacy results from a Phase II study of a once-daily HIV-1 protease inhibitor (PI), BMS–232632. 8th Conference on Retroviruses and Opportunistic Infections, 2001, p 47.

89. Vahlne A: Tripeptides that inhibit HIV-1: Discovery and mode of action. HIV Therapeutics: Searching for the Next Generation. San Diego, CA, Abstract T1, 2001.
90. Nabel GJ: Challenges and opportunities for development of an AIDS vaccine. Nature 2001;410:1002–1007.
91. Dolin R: Human studies in the development of human immunodeficiency virus vaccines. J Infect Dis 1995;172:1175–1183.
92. Navia BA, Price RW: The aquired immunodeficiency syndrome dementia complex as the presenting or sole manifestation of human immunodeficiency virus infection. Arch Neurol 1987;44:65–69.
93. Centers for Disease Control: Revision of the CDC surveillance case definition for aquired immunodeficiency syndrome. MMWR 1987; 36(Suppl 1S):3S–15S.
94. Conant K, Garzinodemo A, Nath A, et al: Induction of monocyte chemoattractant protein-1 in HIV-1 tat-stimulated astrocytes and elevation in AIDS dementia. Proc Natl Acad Sci USA 1998;95: 3117–3121.
95. Persidsky Y, Stins M, Way D, et al: A model for monocyte migration through the blood-brain barrier during HIV-1 encephalitis. J Immunol 1997;158:3499–3510.
96. Wiley CA, Masliah E, Morey M, et al: Neocortical damage during HIV infection. Ann Neurol 1991;29:651–657.
97. Takahashi K, Wesselingh SL, Griffin DE, et al: Localization of HIV-1 in human brain using polymerase chain reaction/in situ hybridization and immunocytochemistry. Ann Neurol 1996;39:705–711.
98. Bratanich AC, Liu C, McArthur JC, et al: Brain-derived HIV-1 tat sequences from AIDS patients with dementia show increased molecular heterogeneity. J Neurovirol 1998;4:387–393.
99. Flaherty MT, Hauer DA, Mankowski JL, et al: Molecular and biological characterization of a neurovirulent molecular clone of simian immunodeficiency virus. J Virol 1997;71:5790–5798.
100. Mankowski JL, Flaherty MT, Spelman JP, et al: Pathogenesis of simian immunodeficiency virus encephalitis: Viral determinants of neurovirulence. J Virol 1997;71:6055–6060.
101. Shi B, Raina J, Lorenzo A, et al: Neuronal apoptosis induced by HIV-1 Tat protein and TNF-alfa: Potentiation of neurotoxicity mediated by oxidative stress and implications for HIV-1 dementia. J Neurovirol 1998;4:281–290.
102. McArthur JC, Selnes OA, DalGan GJ, et al: Phase I/II trial of pentoxifylline in HIV-associated dementia and myelopathy. Neuroscience of HIV infection: Basic and Clinical Frontiers. Vancouver, BC, 1994. Abstract B8.
103. Childs EA, Lyles RH, Selnes OA, et al: Plasma viral load and CD4 lymphocytes predict HIV-associated dementia and sensory neuropathy. Neurology 1998;52:607–613.
104. Westmoreland SV, Halpern E, Lackner AA: Simian immunodeficiency virus encephalitis in rhesus macaques is associated with rapid disease progression. J Neurovirol 1998;4:260–268.
105. Conrad AJ, Schmid P, Syndulko K, et al: Quantifying HIV-1 RNA using the polymerase chain reaction on cerebrospinal fluid and serum of seropositive individuals with and without neurologic abnormalities. J AIDS 1995; 10:425–435.
106. Bossi P, Dupin N, Coutellier A, et al: Absence of any clinical interest of HIV-1 RNA in CSF for diagnosis of HIV encephalitis (abstract). Interscience Conference of Antimicrobial Agents and Chemotherapy, Toronto, 1997.
107. Ellis RJ, Hsia K, Spector SA, et al: Cerebrospinal fluid human immunodeficiency virus type 1 RNA levels are elevated in neurocognitively impaired individuals with acquired immunodeficiency syndrome. Ann Neurol 1997;42:679–688.
108. McArthur JC, McClernon DR, Cronin MF, et al: Relationship between human immunodeficiency virus-associated dementia and viral load in cerebrospinal fluid and brain. Ann Neurol 1997;42:689–698.
109. Letendre SL, Caparelli E, Ellis RJ: Levels of serum and cerebrospinal fluid (CSF) indinavir (IDV) and HIV RNA in HIV-infected individuals (abstract 407). 6th Conference on Retroviruses and Opportunistic Infections, 1999.
110. Marra CM, Coombs RW, Collier AC: Changes in CSF and plasma HIV-1 RNA and in neuropsychological test performance after starting HAART (abstract 408). 6th Conference on Retroviruses and Opportunistic Infections, 1999.
111. Gelman BB, Guinto FC: Morphometry, histopathology, and tomography of cerebral atrophy in the acquired immunodeficiency syndrome. Ann Neurol 1992;32:31–40.
112. Kozlowski PB, Sher JH, Rao, et al: Central nervous system in pediatric AIDS registry. *In* Lyman WD, Rubinstein A (eds): Pediatric AIDS, Clinical, Pathologic and Basic Science Perspectives. Ann NY Acad Sci 1993;693:295–296.
113. Vazeux R, Lacroix-Ciaudo C, Blanche S, et al: Low levels of human immunodeficiency virus replication in the brain tissue of children with severe acquired immunodeficiency syndrome encephalopathy. Am J Pathol 1992;140:137–144.
114. Glass JD, Wesselingh SL, Selnes OA, McArthur JC: Clinical-neuropathologic correlation in HIV-associated dementia. Neurology 1993;43:2230–2237.
115. Budka H: Neuropathology of human immunodeficiency virus infection. Brain Pathol 1991;1:163–175.
116. Wiley CA, Masliah E, Morey, et al: Neocortical damage during HIV infection. Ann Neurol 1991;29:651–657.
117. Masliah E, Achim CL, Ge N, et al: Spectrum of human immunodeficiency virus–associated neocortical damage. Ann Neurol 1992;32: 321–329.
118. Dickson DW, Lee SC, Hatch W, et al: Macrophages and microglia in HIV-related CNS neuropathology. *In* Price RW, Perry S (eds): HIV, AIDS and the Brain. New York, Raven Press, 1993, pp 99–118.
119. Harrison MJG, McArthur JC: AIDS and Neurology. Edinburgh, Churchill Livingstone, 1995.
120. Kure K, Weidenheim KM, Lyman WD, Dickson DW: Morphology and distribution of HIV-1 qp 41-positive microglia in subacute AIDS encephalitis. ACTA Neuropathol (Berl) 1990;80:393–400.
121. Wesselingh SL, Power C, Glass J, et al: Intracerebral cytokine messenger RNA expression in acquired immunodeficiency syndrome dementia. Ann Neurol 1993;33:576–582.
122. Moses AV, Bloom FE, Pauza CD, Nelson JA: Human immunodeficiency virus infection of human brain capillary endothelial cells occurs via a CD4/galactosylceramide-independent mechanism. Proc Natl Acad Sci USA 1993;90:10474–10478.
123. Blumberg BM, Gelbard HA, Epstein LE: HIV-1 infection of the developing nervous system central role of atrocytes in pathogenesis. Virus Res 1994;32:253–267.
124. Tornatore C, Chandra R, Berger JR, Major EO: HIV infection of subcortical astrocytes in the pediatric central nervous system. Neurology 1994;44:482–487.
125. Nuovo GJ, Gallery F, MacConnell P, Braun A: In situ detection of polymerase chain reaction-amplified HIV-1 nucleic acids and tumor necrosis factor-RNA in the central nervous system. Am J Pathol 1994;144:659–666.
126. Johnson RT, McArthur JC, Narayan O: The neurobiology of human immunodeficiency virus infections. FASEB J 1988;2:2970–2981.
127. Centers for Disease Control and Prevention: HIV/AIDS Surveillance Report 1995;7:1–39.
128. Price RW, Brew BJ: The AIDS dementia complex. J Infect Dis 1988;158:1079–1083.
129. Janssen RS, Nwanyanwu OC, Selik RM, Stehr-Green JK: Epidemiology of human immunodeficiency virus encephalopathy in the United States. Neurology 1992;14:289–297.
130. Navia BA, Price RW: The AIDS dementia complex is the presenting or sole manifestation of HIV infection. Arch Neurol 1987;44:65–69.
131. Satz P, Morgenstern H, Miller EN, et al: Low education as a possible risk factor for cognitive abnormalities in HIV 1: Findings from the Multicenter AIDS Cohort study (MACS). J AIDS 1993;6: 503–511.
132. Portegies P, de Gans J, Lange JM, et al: Declining incidence of AIDS dementia complex after introduction of zidovudine treatment [erratum in Br Med J 1989;299:1141] Br Med J 1989;299:819–821.
133. Brodt HR, Kamps BS, Gute P, et al: Changing incidence of AIDS-defining illnesses in the era of antiretroviral combination therapy. AIDS 1997;11:1731–1738.
134. McArthur JC, Sacktor N, Selnes OA: Human immunodeficiency virus-associated dementia. Semin Neurol 1999;19:129–150.
135. McArthur JC, Hoover DR, Bacellar H, et al: Dementia in AIDS patients: Incidence and risk factors. Neurology 1993;43:2245–2252.
136. Grant I, Atkinson JH, Hesselink JR, et al: Evidence for early central nervous system involvement in the acquired immunodeficiency syndrome (AIDS) and other human immunodeficiency virus (HIV) infections: Studies with neuropsychologic testing and magnetic resonance imaging [Erratum: Ann Intern Med 1988;108:496]. Ann Intern Med 1987;107:828–836.
137. McArthur JC, Cohen BA, Selnes OA, et al: Low prevalence of neurological and neuropsychological abnormalities in otherwise healthy HIV-1-infected individuals: Results from the Multicenter AIDS Cohort Study. Ann Neurol 1989;26:601–611.

138. Miller EN, Selnes OA, McArthur JC, et al: Neuropsychological performance in HIV-1-infected homosexual men: Multicenter AIDS Cohort Study (MACS). Neurology 1990;40:197–203.
139. Bornstein RA, Nasrallah HA, Para MF, et al: Neuropsychological performance in symptomatic and asymptomatic HIV infection. AIDS 1993;7:519–524.
140. Martin A, Heyes MP, Salazar AM, et al: Impaired motor skill learning, slowed reaction time, and elevated cerebrospinal fluid quinolinic acid in a subgroup of HIV-infected individuals. Neuropsychology 1993;7:149–157.
141. Stern Y, Marder K, Bell K, et al: Multidisciplinary baseline assessment of homosexual men with and without human immunodeficiency virus infection: Neurological and neuropsychological findings. Arch Gen Psychiatry 1991;48:131.
142. Navia BA, Jordan BD, Price RW: The AIDS dementia complex: I. Clinical features. Ann Neurol 1986;19:517–524.
143. So YT, Engstrom JW, Olney RK, et al: The spectrum of electrodiagnostic abnormalities in patients with human immunodeficiency virus infection. Muscle Nerve 1990;13:855.
144. Atkinson JH, Grant I: Neuropsychiatry of human immunodeficiency virus infection. *In* Berger JR, Levy RM (eds): AIDS and the Nervous System, 2nd ed. Philadelphia, Lippincott-Raven, 1996.
145. Marsh NV, McCall DW: Early neuropsychological change in HIV infection. Neuropsychology 1994;8:44–48.
146. McArthur JC, Nance-Sproson TE, Griffin DE, et al: The diagnostic utility of elevation in cerebrospinal fluid beta 2-microglobulin in HIV-1 dementia. Neurology 1992;42:1707–1712.
147. McArthur JC, Grant I: HIV neurocognitive disorders. *In* Gendelman HE, Lipton SA, Epstein L, Swindells S (eds: The Neurology of AIDS. New York, Chapman and Hall, 1998, pp 499–523.
148. Levy RM, Rosenbloom ML, Perrett LV: Neuroradiologic findings in AIDS: A review of 200 cases. Am J Roentgenol 1986;147:977–983.
149. DiSclafani V, Mackay RD, Meyerhoff DJ, et al: Brain atrophy in HIV infection is more strongly associated with CDC clinical stage than with cognitive impairment. J Int Neuropsychol Soc 1997;3:276–287.
150. Dal Pan GJ, McArthur JH, Aylward E, et al: Patterns of cerebral atrophy in HIV-1 infected individuals: Results of a quantitative MRI analysis. Neurology 1992;42:2125–2130.
151. Aylward EH, Henderer JD, McArthur JC, et al: Reduced basal ganglia volume in HIV 1 associated dementia: Results from quantitative neuroimaging. Neurology 1993;43:2099–2104.
152. Masliah E, Achim CL, Ge N, et al: Spectrum of human immunodeficiency virus-associated neocortical damage. Ann Neurol 1992; 32:321–329.
153. Chang L, Ernst T, Leonido-Yee M, et al: Cerebral metabolic abnormalities correlates with clinical severity of HIV-1 cognitive motor complex. Neurology 1999;52:100–108.
154. Rottenberg DA, Moeller JR, Strother SC, et al: The metabolic pathology of the AIDS dementia complex. Ann Neurol 1987;22:700–706.
155. van Gorp WG, Mandelkern MA, Gee M, et al: Cerebral metabolic dysfunction in AIDS: Findings in a sample with and without dementia. J Neuropsychiatry 1992;4:280–287.
156. Koralnik IJ, Beaumanoir A, Hausler R, et al: A controlled study of early neurologic abnormalities in men with asymptomatic human immunodeficiency virus infection. N Engl J Med 1990;323:864–870.
157. Nuwer MR, Miller EN, Visscher BR, et al: Asymptomatic HIV infection does not cause EEG abnormalities: Results from the Multicenter AIDS Cohort Study (MACS). Neurology 1992;42:1214–1219.
158. Hamilton JD, Hartigan PM, Simberkoff MS, et al: A controlled trial of early versus late treatment with zidovudine in symptomatic HIV-I infection. N Engl J Med 1992;326:437–443.
159. Fischl MA, Richman DD, Grieco MH, et al: The efficacy of AZT in the treatment of patients with AIDS and AIDS-related complex. N Engl J Med 1987;317:185–191.
160. Schmitt FA, Bigley JW, McKinnis R, et al: Neuropsychological outcome of AZT treatment of patients with AIDS and AIDS-related complex. N Engl J Med 1988;319:1573–1578.
161. Sidtis JJ, Gatsonis C, Price RW, et al: Zidovudine treatment of the AIDS dementia complex: Results of a placebo-controlled trial. Ann Neurol 1993;33:343–349.
162. Graham NMH, Hoover DR, Park LP, et al: Survival in HIV-infected patients who have received zidovudine: Comparison of combination therapy with sequential monotherapy and continued zidovudine monotherapy. Ann Intern Med 1996;124:1031–1038.
163. Price RW, Yiannoutsos C, Zaborski L, et al: Neurological substudies of ACTG protocol 193A: Quantitative neurological performance measures and treatment outcomes. 5th Conference on Retroviruses and Opportunistic Infections, 1998.
164. Sacktor N, Skolasky R, Esposito D, et al: Combination antiretroviral therapy including protease inhibitors improves psychomotor speed performance in HIV infection. Neurology 1998a;50(Suppl 4):A248.
165. Ferrando S, van Gorp W, McElhiney M, et al: Highly active antiretroviral treatment in HIV infection: benefits for neuropsychological function. AIDS 1998;12:F65–F70.
166. Jain KK: Evaluation of memantine for neuroprotection in dementia. Expert Opin Investig Drugs 2000;9:1397–1406.
167. Schifitto G, Sacktor N, Marder K, et al: Randomized trial of the platelet-activating factor antagonist lexipafant in HIV-associated cognitive impairment. Neurological AIDS Research Consortium. Neurology 1999;53:391–396.
168. Heseltine PNR, Goodkin K, Atkinson JH, et al: Randomized double-blind placebo-controlled trial of peptide T for HIV-associated cognitive impairment. Arch Neurol 1997;55:41–51.
169. The Dana Consortium on the Therapy of HIV Dementia and Related Cognitive Disorders: Safety and efficacy of the antioxidant OPC–14117 in HIV associated cognitive impairment. Neurology 1997;49:142–146.
170. Epstein LG, Sharer LR, Joshi VV, et al: Progressive encephalopathy in children with acquired immune deficiency syndrome. Ann Neurol 1985;17:488–496.
171. Belman AL, Diamond G, Dickson D, et al: Pediatric AIDS: Neurologic syndromes. Am J Dis Child 1988;142:29–35.
172. Dickson DW, Belman AL, Kim TS, et al: Spinal cord pathology in pediatric acquired immunodeficiency syndrome. Neurology 1989;39: 227–235.
173. Belman AL: AIDS and the child's central nervous system. Pediatr Clin North Am 1992;39:691–714.
174. Tovo PA, Demartino M, Gabiano C, et al: Prognostic factors and survival in children with perinatal HIV-I infection. Italian register for HIV infection in children. Lancet 1992;39:1249–1253.
175. Cogo P, Laverda AM, Ades AE, et al for the European Collaborative Study: Neurologic signs in young children with human immunodeficiency virus infection. Pediatr Infect Dis J 1990;9:402–406.
176. Lobato MN, Caldwell MB, Ng P, Oxtoby MJ: Encephalopathy in children with perinatally acquired immunodeficiency syndrome virus infection. Pediatric Spectrum of Disease Clinical Consortium. J Pediatr 1995;126:170–175.
177. Belman AL: Infants, children and adolescents. *In* Berger JR, Levy RM (eds): AIDS and the Nervous System, 2nd ed. Lippincott-Raven, New York, 1996, pp 223–254.
178. Association Francois-Xavier Bagnoud, 1999. *http://www.fxb.org.*
179. Belman AL, Calvelli T, Nozyce M, et al: Neurologic and immunologic correlates in infants with vertically transmitted HIV infection. Neurology 1990;[Suppl]40(1):409.
180. Davis SL, Halsted C, Levy N, Ellis W: Acquired immunodeficiency virus syndrome presenting as progressive infantile encephalopathy. J Pediatr 1987;110:884–888.
181. Cooper ER, Hanson C, Diaz C, et al: Encephalopathy and progression of human immunodeficiency virus disease in a cohort of children with perinatally acquired human immunodeficiency virus infection. Women and Infants Transmission Study Group. J Pediatr 1998;132: 808–812.
182. Tardieu M, Le Chenadec J, Persoz A, et al: HIV-1-related encephalopathy in infants compared to children and adults. French Pediatric HIV Infection Study and The SEROCO Group. Neurology 2000;54: 1089–1095.
183. Mintz M: Clinical features and treatment interventions for human immunodeficiency virus-associated neurological disease in children. Semin Neurol 1999;19:165–176.
184. Grubman S, Gross E, Lerner-Weiss N, et al: Older children and adolescents living with perinatally acquired human immunodeficiency virus infection. Pediatrics 1995;95:657–663.
185. Ultmann MH, Belman AL, Ruff HA, et al: Developmental abnormalities in infants and children with acquired immune deficiency syndrome (AIDS) and AIDS-related complex. Dev Med Child Neurol 1985;27:563–571.
186. Working Group of the American Academy of Neurology AIDS Task Force: Nomenclature and research case definitions for neurologic manifestations of human immunodeficiency virus type 1 infection. Neurology 1991;41:778–785.
187. Mintz M: Clinical comparison of adult and pediatric NeuroAIDS. Adv Neuroimmunol 1994;4:207–221.

188. Pratt RD, Nichols S, McKinney N, et al: Virologic markers of human immunodeficiency virus type 1 in cerebrospinal fluid of infected children. J Infect Dis 1996;174:288–293.
189. Scarmato V, Frank Y, Rozenstein A, et al: Central brain atrophy in childhood AIDS encephalopathy. AIDS 1996;10:1227–1231.
190. Mintz M: Neurological and developmental problems in pediatric HIV infection. J Nutr 1996;126:S2663–S2673.
191. Belman AL, Diamond G, Park Y, et al: Perinatal HIV infection: A prospective longitudinal study of the initial CNS signs. Neurology 1989;39[Suppl]:278–279.
192. Raphael SA, De Leon G, Sapin J: Symptomatic primary human immunodeficiency virus infection of the brain stem in a child. Pediatr Infect Dis J 1989;8:654–656.
193. Belman AL, Lantos G, Horoupian D, et al: AIDS: Calcification of the basal ganglia in infants and children. Neurology 1986;36:1192–1199.
194. Sharer LR, Mintz M: Neuropathology of AIDS in children. *In* Scaravilli F (ed): AIDS: The Pathology of the Nervous System. Berlin, Springer Verlag, 1993, pp 201–214.
195. Frank Y, Pavlakis S, Black K, Bakshi S: Reversible occipital parietal encephalopathy syndrome in AIDS. Neurology 1998;51:915–916.
196. Floeter MK, Civitello LA, Everett CR, et al: Peripheral neuropathy in children with HIV infection. Neurology 1997;49:207–212.
197. Walter EB, Drucker RP, McKinney RE, Wilfert CM: Myopathy in human immunodeficiency virus-infected children receiving long-term zidovudine therapy. J Pediatr 1991;119:152–155.
198. Semino-Mora MC, Leon-Monzon ME, Dalakas MC: Effect of L-carnitine on the zidovudine-induced destruction of human myotubes. Part I: L-carnitine prevents the myotoxicity of ZDV in vitro. Lab Invest 1994;71:102–112.
199. Hernandez M, Barros J: A new challenge in children with HIV: Psychosis. 7th Annual Conference of the Association of Nurses in AIDS Care, 1994.
200. Mintz M: Clinical features of HIV infection in children. *In* Gendelman HE, Lipton S, Epstein L, Swindells SY (eds): The Neurology of AIDS. New York, Chapman and Hall, 1998, pp 385–407.
201. Brouwers P, Moss H, Wolters P, et al: Neurobehavioral typology of school-aged children with symptomatic HIV disease. J Clin Exp Neuropshychol 1992;14:113.
202. Brouwers P, van der Vlugt H, Moss H, et al: White matter changes on CT brain scan are associated with neurobehavioral dysfunction in children with symptomatic HIV disease. Child Neuropsychol 1995;1:93–105.
203. Wolters PL, Brouwers P: Evaluation of neurodevelopmental deficits in children with HIV infection. *In* Gendelman HE, Lipton S, Epstein L, Swindells SY (eds): The Neurology of AIDS. New York, Chapman and Hall, 1998. pp 425–442.
204. Report of the Quality Standards Subcommittee of the American Academy of Neurology: Evaluation and management of intracranial mass lesions in AIDS. Neurology 1998;50:21–26.
205. Kingma DW, Mueller BU, Frekko K, et al: Low-grade monoclonal Epstein-Barr virus-associated lymphoproliferative disorder of the brain presenting as human immunodeficiency virus-associated encephalopathy in a child with acquired immunodeficiency syndrome. Arch Pathol Lab Med 1999;123:83–87.
206. Kovacs A, Schluchter M, Easley K, et al: Cytomegalovirus infection and HIV-1 disease progression in infants born to HIV-1 infected women. N Engl J Med 1999;341:77–84.
207. USPHS/IDSA: 1997 report on the prevention of opportunistic infections in persons infected with human immunodeficiency virus. MMWR 1997;46:RR–12.
208. Zaknun D, Orav J, Kornegay J, et al: Correlation of RNA PCR, acid dissociated p24 antigen, and neopterin with progression of disease: A retrospective, longitudinal study of vertically acquired human immunodeficiency virus type 1 infection in children. J Pediatr 1997;130:898–905.
209. Civitello L, Brouwers P, DeCarli C, et al: Relation between neuroimaging abnormalities and cerebrospinal fluid viral load in children with human immunodeficiency viral disease. Ann Neurol 1999;46:521.
210. Pavlakis SG, Lu D, Frank Y, et al: Brain lactate and N-acetylaspartate in pediatric AIDS encephalopathy. Am J Neuroradiol 1998;19:383–385.
211. Sei S, Stewart SK, Farley M, et al: Evaluation of HIV type 1 RNA levels in cerebrospinal fluid and viral resistance to zidovudine in children with HIV encephalopathy. J Infect Dis 1996;174:1200–1206.
212. Lewis LL, Venzon D, Church JA, et al: Lamivudine in children with human immunodeficiency virus infection: A phase I/II study. J Infect Dis 1996;174:16–25.
213. Kline MW, Van Dyke RB, Lindsey JC, et al: A randomized comparative trial of stavudine (d4T) versus zidovudine (ZDV) in children with human immunodeficiency virus infection. Pediatrics 1998;101:214–220.
214. Englund JA, Baker CJ, Raskino C, et al: Zidovudine, didanosine, or both as the initial treatment for symptomatic HIV-infected children. AIDS Clinic Trials Group (ACTG) Study 152 Team. N Engl J Med 1997; 336:1704–1712.
215. Raskino C, Pearson DA, Baker CJ, et al: Neurologic, neurocognitive, and brain growth outcomes in HIV-infected children receiving different nucleoside antiretroviral regimens. Pediatrics 1999; 104:E32.
216. Berger JR: Spinal cord syphilis associated with human immunodeficiency virus infection: A treatable myelopathy. Am J Med 1992;92:101–103.
217. Britton DB, Mesa-Tejada R, Fenoglio CM, et al: A new complication of AIDS: Thoracic myelitis caused by herpes simplex virus. Neurology 1985;35:1071–1074.
218. Dal Pan G, Glass J, McArthur J: Clinicopathologic correlations of HIV-1 associated myelopathy. Neurology 1994;44:2159–2164.
219. Di Rocco A: Diseases of the spinal cord in human immunodeficiency virus infection. Semin Neurol 1999; 19:151–155.
220. Tan SV, Guiloff RJ, Henderson DC, et al: AIDS-associated vacuolar myelopathy and tumor necrosis factor-alfa. J Neurol Sci 1996; 138:134–144.
221. Tan SV, Guiloff RJ: Hypothesis on the pathogenesis of vacuolar myelopathy dementia, and peripheral neuropathy in AIDS. J Neurol Neurosurg Psychiatry 1998;65:23–28.
222. Tan SV, Guiloff R, Scaravalli F : AIDS-associated vacuolar myelopathy: a morphometric study. Brain 1995;118:1247–1261.
223. Petito CK, Navia BA, Cho ES, et al: Vacuolar myelopathy pathologically resembling subacute combined degeneration in patients with acquired immune deficiency syndrome. N Engl J Med 1985; 312:874–879.
224. Jerez P, Palao A, Leiva C: HIV myelopathy as the presenting symptom of acquired immunodeficiency syndrome. Rev Neurol 1998; 26:1008–1010.
225. Chong J, Di Rocco A, Danisis F, et al: MR abnormalities in AIDS-associated vacuolar myelopathy. Am J Neuroradio 1999;20:1412–1416.
226. Di Rocco A, Tagliati M, Danisi F, et al: L-methionine for AIDS-associated vacuolar myelopathy. Neurology 1998;51:266–268.
227. McArthur J: HIV-related peripheral neuropathies and their treatment. 8th Conference on Retroviruses and Opportunistic Infections, Chicago, 2001. Abstract L8.
228. Hall CD, Snyder CR, Messenheimer JA, et al: Peripheral neuropathy in a cohort of human immunodeficiency virus-infected patients. Incidence and relationship to other nervous system dysfunction. Arch Neurol 1991;48:1273–1274.
229. Cornblath DR, McArthur JC: Predominantly sensory neuropathy in patients with AIDS and AIDS-related complex. Neurology 1988;38:794–796.
230. Vendrell J, Heredia C, Pujol M, et al: Guillain-Barré syndrome associated with seroconversion for anti-HTLV-III. Neurology 1987;37:544.
231. Apostolski S, McAlarney J, Quattrini A, et al: The gp 120 glycoprotein of human immunodeficiency virus type 1 binds to sensory ganglion neurons. Ann Neurol 1993;34:855–863.
232. Bailey RO, Baltch AL, Benkatesh R, et al: Sensory motor neuropathy associated with AIDS. Neurology 1988;38:886–891.
233. Rance NE, McArthur JC, Cornblath D, et al: Gracile tract degeneration in patients with sensory neuropathy and AIDS. Neurology 1988;38:265–271.
234. Yoshioka M, Shapshak P, Srivasta AK, et al: Expression of HIV-1 and interleukin–6 in lumbosacral dorsal root ganglia of patients with AIDS. Neurology 1994;44:1120–1130.
235. Lipkin WI, Parry G, Kiprov D, et al: Inflammatory neuropathy in homosexual men with lymphadenopathy. Neurology 1985;35:1479–1483.
236. Fuller GN, Jacobs JM, Guiloff RJ: Nature and incidence of peripheral nervous syndromes in HIV infections. J Neurol Neurosurg Psychiatry 1993;56:372–381.
237. Barohn RJ, Gronseth GS, LeForce BR, et al: Peripheral nervous system involvement in a large cohort of human immunodeficiency virus-infected individuals. Arch Neurol 1993;50:167–171.
238. Leger JM, Bouche P, Bolgert F, et al: The spectrum of polyneuropathies in patients infected with HIV. J Neurol Neurosurg Psychiatry 1989;52:1369–1374.

239. Leger JM, Henin D, Belic L, et al: Lymphoma-induced polyradiculopathy in AIDS: Two cases. J Neurol 1992;239:132–134.
240. Kieburtz KD, Seidlin M, Lambert JS, et al: Extended follow-up of peripheral neuropathy in patients with AIDS and AIDS-related complex treated with dideoxyinosine. J AIDS 1992;5:60–64.
241. Kieburtz KD, Ciang DW, Schiffer RB, et al: Abnormal vitamin B_{12} metabolism in human immunodeficiency virus infection: Association with neurological dysfunction. Arch Neurol 1991;48:312–314.
242. Hollander H: Cerebrospinal fluid normalities and abnormalities in individuals infected with human immunodeficiency virus. J Infec Dis 1988;158:855–858.
243. Newsahn G: HIV neuropathy reated with gabapentin. AIDS 1998;12:219–221.
244. Simpson DM, Olney R, McArthur JC, Khan A, Goldbold J, Ebel-Frommer K: A placebo-controlled trial of lamotrigine for painful HIV-associated neuropathy. Neurology 2000;54:2115–2119.
245. Kieburtz K, Simpson DM, Cohen B, et al: A randomized trial of amitriptyline and mexiletine for painful neuropathy in HIV infection. Neurology 1998;51:1682–1688.
246. Shlay JC, Chaloner K, Cohen D, et al: Acupuncture and amitriptyline for pain due to HIV-related peripheral neuropathy: A randomized controlled trial. JAMA 1998;280:1590–1595.
247. So YT, Olney RK: The natural history of mononeuritis multiplex and simplex in HIV infection. Neurology 1991;41(Suppl 1):375.
248. Said G, Lacroix-Ciando C, Fujimura H, et al: The peripheral neuropathy of necrotizing arteritis: A clinicopathological study. Ann Neurol 1988;23:461–465.
249. Said G, Lacroix C, Chemouilli P, et al: Cytomegalovirus neuropathy in acquired immunodeficiency syndrome: A clinical and pathological study. Ann Neurol 1991;29:139–146.
250. Eidelberg D, Sotrel A, Vogel H, et al: Progressive polyradiculopathy in acquired immune deficiency syndrome. Neurology 1986; 36:912–916.
251. Lanska MJ, Lanska DJ, Shmidley JW: Syphilitic polyradiculopathy in an HIV-positive man. Neurology 1988;38:1297–1301.
252. Dalakas MC, Pezeshkpour GH, Gravell M, Sever JL: Polymyositis associated with AIDS retrovirus. JAMA 1986;256:2381–2383.
253. Simpson DM, Bender AN: Human immunodeficiency virus–associated myopathy: Analysis of 11 patients. Ann Neurol 1988;24:79–84.
254. Wrzolek MA, Sher JH, Kozlowski PB, Rao C: Skeletal muscle pathology in AIDS: An autopsy study. Muscle Nerve 1990;13:508–515.
255. Arnaudo E, Dalakas M, Shanske S, et al: Depletion of muscle mitochondrial DNA in AIDS patients with zidovudine-induced myopathy. Lancet 1991;337:508–510.
256. Gabbai A, Schmidt B, Castelo A, et al: Muscle biopsy in AIDS and ARC: Analysis of 50 patients. Muscle Nerve 1990;13:541–544.
257. Simpson DM, Citak KA, Godfrey E, et al: Myopathies associated with human immunodeficiency virus and zidovudine: Can their effects be distinguished? Neurology 1993;43:971–976.
258. Mhiri C, Baudrimont M, Bonne G, et al: Zidovudine myopathy: A distinctive disorder associated with mitochondrial dysfunction. Ann Neurol 1991;29:606–614.
259. Bessen LJ, Greene JB, Louie E, et al: Severe polymyositis-like syndrome associated with zidovudine therapy of AIDS and ARC. N Engl J Med 1988;318:708.
260. Dalakas MC, Illa I, Pezeshkpour GH, et al: Mitochondrial myopathy caused by long-term zidovudine therapy. N Engl J Med 1990; 322:1098–1105.
261. Panegyres PK, Tan M, Kakulas BA, et al: Necrotising myopathy and zidovudine. Lancet 1988;I:1050–1051.
262. Simpson MV, Chin CD, Keilbough SA, et al: Studies on the inhibition of mitochondrial DNA replication of 3′-azido–3′-deoxythymidine and other deoxynucleoside analog which inhibit HIV-1 replication. Biochem Pharmacol 1989;38:1033–1036.
263. Chariot P, Monnet I, Gherardi R: Cytochrome c reaction improves histopathological assessment of zidovudine myopathy. Ann Neurol 1993;34:561–565.
264. Herzbert NH, Zorn I, Zwart R, et al: Major growth reduction and minor decrease in mitochondrial enzyme activity in culture human muscle cells after exposure to zidovudine. Muscle Nerve 1992;15:706–710.
265. Miller RG, Carson PJ, Moussavi RS, et al: Fatigue and myalgia in AIDS patients. Neurology 1991;41:1603–1607.
266. Grau JM, Masanes F, Pedro E, et al: Human immunodeficiency virus type infection and myopathy: Clinical relevance of zidovudine therapy. Ann Neurol 1993;34:206–211.
267. Chad DA, Smith TW, Blumenfeld DA, et al: HIV-associated myopathy: Immunocytochemical identification of an HIV antigen (gp 41) in muscle macrophages. Ann Neurol 1990;28:579–582.
268. Gherardi R, Florea-Strat A, Fromont G, et al: Cytokine expression in the muscle of HIV-infected patients: Evidence for interleukin-1 alpha accumulation in mitochondria of AZT fibers. Ann Neurol 1994;36:752–758.
269. Illa I, Nath A, Dalakas M: Immunocytochemical and virological characteristics of HIV-associated inflammatory myopathies/similarities with seronegative polymyositis. Ann Neurol 1991;29:474–481.
270. Simpson DM, Bender AN, Farraye J, et al: Human immunodeficiency virus wasting syndrome may represent a treatable myopathy. Neurology 1990;40:535–538.
271. Gherardi R, Baudrimont M, Lionnet F, et al: Skeletal muscle toxoplasmosis in patients with acquired immunodeficiency syndrome: A clinical and pathological study. Ann Neurol 1992;32:535–542.
272. Mahe A, Bruet A, Chabin E, Fendler J-P: Acute rhabdomyolysis coincident with primary HIV-1 infection. Lancet 1989;2:1454–1455.
273. Rosenblum MK, Levy RM, Bredesen DE, et al: Primary central nervous system lymphoma in patients with AIDS. Ann Neurol 1988;23(Suppl):S13–S16.
274. Brink NS, Sharvell Y, Howard MR, et al: Detection of Epstein-Barr virus and Kaposi's sarcoma-associated herpes virus DNA in CSF from persons infected with HIV who had neurological disease. J Neurol Neurosurg Psychiatry 1998;65:191–195.
275. Castagna A, Cinque P, D'Amico A, et al: Evaluation of contrast-enhancing brain lesions in AIDS patients by means of Epstein-Barr virus detection in CSF and ^{201}thallium single photon emission tomography. AIDS 1997;11:1522–1523.
276. Johnson BA, Fram EK, Johnson PC, et al: The variable MR appearance of primary lymphoma of the central nervous system: comparison with histopathologic features. AJNR 1997;18:563–572.
277. Chinn RJS, Wilkinson ID, Hall-Craggs MA, et al: Toxoplasmosis and primary central nervous system lymphoma in HIV infection: Diagnosis with MR spectroscopy. Radiology 1995;197:649–654.
278. Chang L, Miller B, McBride D, et al: Brain lesions in patients with AIDS: H-1 MR spectroscopy. Radiology 1995;197:527.
279. Antinori A, De Rossi G, Ammassari A, et al: Value of combined approach with thallium-201 single-photon emission computed tomography and Epstein-Barr virus DNA polymerase chain reaction in CSF for the diagnosis of AIDS-related primary CNS lymphoma. J Clin Oncol 1999;17:554–560.
280. Skolasky RL, Dal Pan GJ, Olivi A, et al: HIV-associated primary CNS lymphoma morbidity and utility of brain biopsy. J Neurol Sci 1999;1:32–38.
281. DeAngelis L, Yaholom J, Heineman M: Primary CNS lymphoma: Combined treatment with chemotherapy and radiotherapy. Neurology 1990;40:80.
282. Baumgartner JE, Rachlin JR, Beckstead JH, et al: Primary central nervous system lymphomas: Natural history and response to radiation therapy in 55 patients with acquired immunodeficiency syndrome. J Neurosurg 1990;73:206–211.
283. Goldstein J, Dickson DW, Rubinstein A, et al: Primary CNS lymphoma in a pediatric patient with acquired immunodeficiency syndrome treatment with radiation. Cancer 1990;66:2503–2508.
284. Chamberlin MC: Pediatric AIDS: A longitudinal comparative MRI and CT brain imaging study. J Child Neurol 1993;8(2):175.
285. Zeigler JL, Beckstead JA, Volberding PA, et al: Non-Hodgkin lymphoma in 90 homosexual men. N Engl J Med 1984;311:565–570.

CHAPTER 45

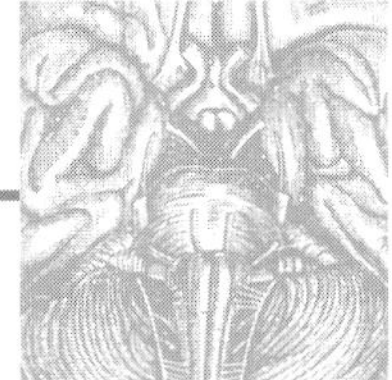

CHIN-SANG CHUNG and LOUIS R. CAPLAN

Neurovascular Disorders

Historical Background

During the 17th and 18th centuries, physicians and morphologists recognized that the brains of patients who died of apoplexy often contained hemorrhages and softenings and that brain damage could result from either bleeding or deprivation of the vital blood supply. During the 19th and early 20th centuries, physicians became interested in correlating the neurological symptoms and signs found in stroke patients during life with the anatomical region of damage in the brain found after death. Anatomical-clinical correlations defined the territories of supply of the various vessels within the anterior and posterior brain circulations and noted the findings in patients with infarcts in the territories of the various arteries. During the middle years of the 20th century, clinicians focused increasingly on the clinical findings in patients with brain hemorrhages and infarcts. In 1935, Aring and Merritt analyzed the clinical findings in patients who died at the Boston City Hospital from large strokes and tried to separate the signs of embolism, thrombosis, and brain hemorrhage. Kubik and Adams, in 1946, reported the first detailed clinicopathological analysis of a stroke syndrome—occlusion of the basilar artery (BA). In 1951, Miller Fisher described the clinical findings in patients who had internal carotid artery (ICA) occlusions in the neck. Fisher emphasized that warning spells, which he dubbed transient ischemic attacks (TIAs), often preceded strokes in his patients and that the causative vascular disease was located in the neck, where it could theoretically be repaired by surgeons, rather than intracranially in the middle cerebral arteries (MCAs), where most of the prior literature had indicated that the usual vascular lesions were located. Shortly thereafter, Hutchinson and Yates showed that patients with posterior circulation infarcts and TIAs also often had occlusive disease in the neck, at the origins of the extracranial vertebral arteries (VAs), rather than in the head. Wallenberg and Kubik and Adams had identified the vascular pathology. In 1961, Miller Fisher described the clinical findings in patients with large fatal brain hemorrhages located in the putamen, thalamus, pons, and cerebellum.[1] Stimulated by these seminal reports and their own clinical experiences, physicians became more interested in the clinical features of stroke, brain ischemia, and cerebrovascular disease.

During the third quarter of the 20th century, most neurologists had only modest interest in stroke, and most patients were cared for by non-neurologists. Furthermore, few investigations were available that could be performed safely during life to clarify the nature, location, and extent of stroke-related brain damage or the causative cardiac and cerebrovascular lesions. Physicians during this era turned to classifications based solely on the temporal features of symptoms. The terms TIAs, reversible ischemic neurological deficit, stroke-in-evolution, progressing stroke, and completed stroke became popular and were used as a basis for treatment. These terms were arbitrarily and variously defined, however, and proved unpredictive of the presence of brain infarction, prognosis, and stroke mechanism; they are now obsolete and of historical interest only. TIA is the only term that remains useful, mainly for ease in communication but not as a guide to diagnosis or treatment.[2]

During the last quarter of the 20th century, an explosion of technical advances in brain imaging (computed tomography [CT] and later magnetic resonance imaging [MRI]) and technology occurred that could give information about the cervicocranial arteries (subtraction angiography, magnetic resonance angiography [MRA], computed tomographic angiography [CTA], and extracranial and transcranial ultrasound). Knowledge of the role of blood cells and coagulation factors in causing or contributing to thromboembolism also advanced. During this time, potential treatments proliferated: agents that modify platelet functions; standard anticoagulants including heparin, heparinoids, low-molecular-weight heparins, and warfarin; endarterectomy and surgical bypass of stenotic or occluded arteries; thrombolytic treatment using intravenous injection of recombinant tissue plasminogen activator (rtPA); angioplasty and stenting; and neuroprotective drugs aimed at increasing the brain's tolerance of ischemia. Treatment now is based mainly on three considerations: first, nature, location, and severity of the causative cardiac, vascular, and hematological disorders; second, the pathogenesis of the stroke; and third, the state of the brain (normal, stunned, infarcted, or containing a hematoma). The newer available diagnostic technologies now make it possible to collect these data safely and quickly in most stroke patients.

Overview of Strokes

CLASSIFICATION OF STROKES

Ischemia

Brain ischemia results from the occlusion of cervicocranial vessels or hypoperfusion to the brain caused by various processes: atherothrombosis, embolism, or hemodynamic abnormalities. Atherothrombosis occurs in the large cervicocranial arteries in the neck and head and in the small penetrating arteries. A localized thrombus is formed in situ on an atherosclerotic arterial narrowing; it impedes distal blood flow and causes ischemia and ensuing infarction of the brain tissue supplied by the artery. The neurological symptoms and signs depend on the location of the brain vessel affected. In brain embolism, a brain artery is suddenly blocked by embolic material thrombus that has developed more proximally in the heart (cardiogenic), aorta, proximal arteries (intra-arterial), or venous system (paradoxical). These donor sites give rise to various types of particulate matter (white platelet-fibrin and red erythrocyte-fibrin thrombi, cholesterol crystals, fragments of atherosclerotic plaques, calcific fragments of valves and plaques, air, fat, myxomatous tumor fragments, bacterial vegetations), which then travel within the cervicocranial arteries to reach a recipient site. If the embolic material lodges at a recipient site, the resulting hypoperfusion causes an infarct that often becomes hemorrhagic when the embolus moves distally or fragments and reperfusion occurs. The clinical findings depend on the location of the recipient brain artery affected.

Critically lowered global blood flow to the brain (too severe to be compensated by cerebral autoregulation mechanisms) is caused by cardiac pump failure or hypovolemia. During such episodes, most patients are hypotensive. This condition causes infarction in the border zones between the major cerebral arteries (so-called watershed infarction) as well as widespread bilateral cerebral dysfunction. The major zones of damage are between the anterior cerebral arteries and MCAs, and between the MCAs and posterior cerebral arteries (PCAs) in the parieto-occipital regions of the cerebral hemispheres (Fig. 45–1). Loss of vision, decreased alertness, and weakness affecting predominantly the shoulder, hand, and thigh result.

Hemorrhage

Rupture of a brain vessel causes leakage of blood into the brain parenchyma, cerebrospinal fluid (CSF) spaces around the brain, or both. Bleeding injures the neighboring tissues by interrupting and cutting vital brain pathways, by exerting local pressure on the surrounding brain structures, and by causing ischemia of tissues adjacent to the hematoma. Further increase in intracranial pressure (ICP) causes shifts and herniations of brain tissues and may compress the brain stem. There are two large subcategories of spontaneous intracranial hemorrhages. Intracerebral hemorrhage (ICH)

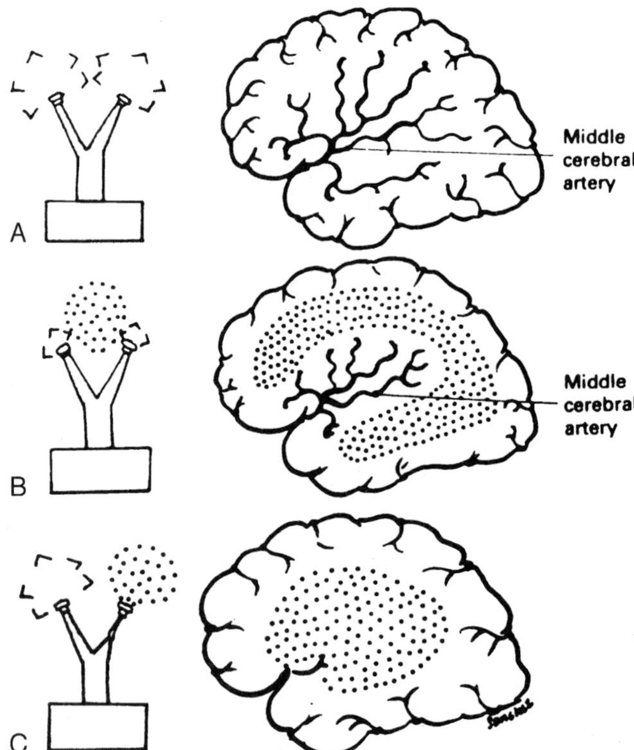

FIGURE 45–1. In heart (pump) failure and watershed infarction, normal pump and arterial circulation do not occur *(A)*; instead, due to low pump pressure and border zone ischemia *(B)*, water goes to the center of hoses (arteries) and stippled areas show poor flow. In contrast, with "blocked hose" and middle cerebral artery infarction *(C)*, water flow is deficient in the center of supply *(stippled area)*. (Adapted from Caplan LR: Stroke: Clinical Approach. Boston, Butterworth-Heinemann, 1993.)

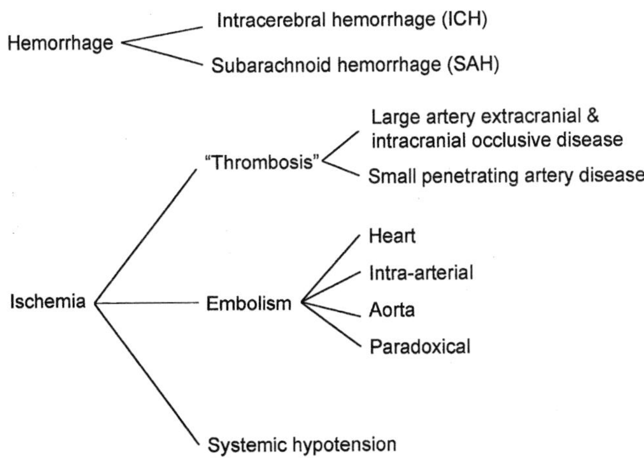

FIGURE 45–2. Differential diagnosis of stroke.

is bleeding in the brain parenchyma itself, and subarachnoid hemorrhage (SAH) refers to bleeding around the brain into the subarachnoid spaces and CSF. These two types of hemorrhages have different etiologies, clinical courses, and outcomes and thus require different management strategies.

The differential diagnosis of stroke is depicted in Figure 45–2.

STROKE INCIDENCE AND PREVALENCE

Stroke is a major public health problem, ranking among the top three causes of death in most countries. It affects the brains of almost a half million people every year, causing 150,000 deaths, and there are now approximately 3 million stroke survivors in the United States. Overall, age-adjusted incidence rates range between 100 and 300 per 100,000 population per year. Stroke is the major cause of serious disability in adults and is responsible for $20 billion per year in lost wages in the United States. Stroke incidence rates declined during the 1950s and 1960s but increased during the 1980s. This increase may be due to increased diagnostic recognition related to advances in neuroimaging technology, increased survival of patients with ischemic heart disease, better detection of milder cases of stroke, and other undefined factors during the past 10 years.[3]

Stroke accounts for about 10 percent of all deaths in most industrialized countries, and the great majority of deaths are among persons over age 65. The average age-adjusted mortality rate is 50 to 100 per 100,000 population per year in the United States. Stroke mortality rises exponentially with age, virtually doubling every 5 years. Stroke death rates are higher among African-Americans. The stroke mortality rate has steadily declined in the United States since 1915; the decline in black mortality rates has exceeded that of whites and spans all age groups. Improved survival after stroke contributes to this trend most significantly.

Ischemic stroke accounts for more than 80 percent of all strokes. ICH usually accounts for 10 to 30 percent of cases depending on the origin of the patient, with greater relative frequencies reported in Asians and blacks. Frequency of SAH is usually a third to a half that of ICH. Among patients with brain ischemia, cardioembolism accounts for 20 to 30 percent of cases, atherothrombotic infarction accounts for 14 to 40 percent, and small deep infarcts due to penetrating artery disease (lacunes) account for 15 to 30 percent of cases.[4]

There are major sex and racial differences in the distribution of occlusive cerebrovascular lesions. Extracranial occlusive diseases usually affect white men, are located at the origins of the internal carotid and VAs in the neck, occur twice as often in men, and are strongly associated with coronary and peripheral vascular occlusive disease, systolic hypertension, and hyperlipidemia. Compared with white men, blacks, persons of Asian origin, and women have more severe diseases of the intracranial arteries and their perforating branches. Intracranial stenosis is usually less frequently associated with coronary and peripheral vascular disease.

RISK FACTORS FOR STROKE

Knowledge of stroke risk factors has advanced substantially during the past several decades and exceeds that of many other major neurological diseases. Improved detection and modification of risk factors has reduced the impact of stroke. Important nonmodifiable stroke risk factors include advanced age, gender, ethnicity, and genetic determinants. Although there is little that can be done to control these factors, they identify people who may be at increased risk for going on to future strokes. Modifiable risk factors include hypertension, cardiac disease (particularly atrial fibrillation [AF], diabetes mellitus, cigarette smoking, alcohol consumption, hyperlipidemia, sedentary lifestyle, and asymptomatic carotid stenosis. Each of these risk factors carries a different relative risk, and prevalence varies among different groups of people. Although the risk from a specific factor may be only moderate, if its prevalence rate is high, it may be responsible for a significant number of strokes.[5]

Based on epidemiological data from the Framingham study, a risk profile table can be used to estimate a person's 10-year probability of stroke occurrence. Stroke rates increase dramatically with age. About two thirds of all strokes occur after age 65. In the Framingham study the mean age of stroke patients was 65.4 years for men and 66.1 years for women. As the population ages, the burden of stroke becomes greater.[6] In terms of gender, the stroke incidence rate is greater in men than in women.

Hypertension is the most significant modifiable risk factor for stroke, and stroke incidence is proportional to the level of the blood pressure. This is particularly true in blacks because of higher prevalence, earlier onset, greater severity, and poorer control of hypertension in this population. Decreasing systolic blood pressure by about 10 mm Hg reduces the relative risk of stroke by 35 to 40 percent.[7] Improved control of hypertension has resulted in a recent dramatic decline in stroke frequency, most notably in black women. The combination of hypertension, diabetes, and cigarette smoking is particularly risky and requires aggressive interventions. Diabetes mellitus is also a significant risk factor and is present in about 10 percent of stroke patients.[6] It is common among blacks and particularly contributes to the development of intracranial atherosclerosis.

Cigarette smoking is a very important preventable cause of stroke, and about 30 percent of stroke patients smoke. Heavy cigarette smoking (more than a pack per day) carries 11 times the ischemic stroke risk and 4 times the SAH risk of people who do not smoke.[8] Smoking has an especially toxic effect on women taking oral contraceptives, in whom it carries 22 times the risk of developing stroke than occurs in nonsmoking women who use other forms of birth control. With cessation of cigarette smoking, the risk of stroke declines after 2 to 5 years.

A J-shaped relationship exists between alcohol and stroke. Those who keep to 1 to 2 units per day have a lower ischemic stroke risk than those who do not drink at all. On the whole, the relative risk for ischemic stroke increases significantly with heavy alcohol consumption of 5 or more units of alcohol per day.[9]

Heart diseases are clearly associated with increased risk of ischemic stroke, particularly AF, valvular heart disease, myocardial infarction, coronary artery disease, congestive heart failure, left ventricular hypertrophy on electrocardiogram (ECG), and mitral valve prolapse. AF, which alone carries a fivefold increased risk of stroke, is particularly important in the elderly and among those with coronary artery disease or heart failure or valvular heart disease. Ischemic stroke associated with AF is nearly twice as likely to be fatal as non-AF stroke. Recurrence is more frequent, and functional deficits are more likely to be severe among survivors. Because stroke is usually the initial manifestation of embolism in AF, prevention is critical to reducing disability and mortality.[10] Abnormal serum lipid levels are regarded as risk factors. High-density lipoprotein (HDL) is protective against stroke whereas apolipoprotein (a) increases the risk. Higher HDL levels are more protective against atherosclerotic disease (extracranial carotid artery disease and intracranial atherosclerotic disease). Apolipoprotein (a) has both atherogenic and coagulation effects. Apolipoprotein a1 (Apo a-1) and apolipoprotein-b (Apo b) are major protein components of lipoproteins HDL and low-density lipoprotein (LDL), respectively. Recent studies have shown that carotid atheroma is linked with increased LDL (Apo b) and may be inversely related to HDL (Apo a-1).[5] Lipid-lowering agents, particularly HMG-CoA reductase inhibitors or statins, which lower LDL and triglyceride levels and increase HDL, have been shown to reduce the risk for stroke in patients with a history of coronary artery disease or myocardial infarction in recent trials.[11] Physical activity lowers the risk of stroke even in the elderly.[5, 12]

Recently factors causing blood vessel endothelial injury (homocysteine and chronic infections such as *Chlamydia pneumoniae* and periodontal disease) have been found to increase the risk of stroke. Homocysteine is both genetically and environmentally controlled. A genetic defect in the enzyme cystathionine ß synthetase is associated with hyperhomocysteinemia. An environmental deficiency of vitamin B_{12}, folic acid, or vitamin B_6 affects homocysteine metabolism and increases circulating plasma levels. Dietary supplementation with these vitamins reduces homocysteine levels, thus possibly preventing risk for endothelial injury that can lead to stroke. Excessive alcohol consumption and physical inactivity are also associated with elevated homocysteine levels.[13] *C. pneumoniae* is a common cause of community-acquired pneumonia, pharyngitis, and sinusitis. It can infect and injure the endothelium, thus increasing the likelihood of platelet aggregation.[14]

TRANSIENT ISCHEMIC ATTACKS AND STROKES

Miller Fisher first described the phenomenology of TIAs as "prodromal fleeting attacks of paralysis, numbness, tingling, speechlessness, unilateral blindness or dizziness," which nearly always preceded cerebral infarction in patients with occlusion of the ICA.[15] TIA is a strong indicator of a subsequent stroke. The first year after a TIA carries the greatest stroke risk (5%).[4] TIA is arbitrarily defined as a focal neurological deficit lasting less than 24 hours, but attacks are usually much shorter, most episodes clearing within 1 hour. If neurological deficits last 4 hours or longer, patients often have infarcts in the locations corresponding to the transient symptoms. The clinical features of TIAs are usually similar to those of infarctions located in the arteries affected except for the transient nature of the clinical episodes. Because TIAs are a manifestation of underlying cardiovascular or blood diseases, the underlying cardiac, hematological, and cerebrovascular diseases that potentially cause TIAs should be thoroughly investigated to manage the patients optimally. For accurate diagnosis and management, detailed clinical information is essential and helps to predict the underlying cause. Data should include the duration of the neurological deficit, heterogeneity or stereotypy, time from first TIA and from last TIA, number of spells, and nature of symptoms (motor, sensory, visual, motor and sensory, distribution on the body). There are many laboratory tests that are helpful in defining the most probable causative mechanisms of TIAs, but they should be selected and ordered on the basis of judicious interpretation of clinical data. Management of patients with TIAs should be directed toward specific vascular lesions and underlying causative diseases.[2, 16] Further details are discussed later in relation to the individual disease entities.

DIAGNOSIS

To determine the stroke mechanism or mechanisms, the following clinical bedside data should be obtained through careful history taking: (1) ecology—past and present personal and family illnesses; (2) the presence and nature of past strokes and TIAs; (3) the time of onset of the symptoms; (4) activity at stroke onset; (5) the temporal course and progression of the findings; and (6) accompanying symptoms. A general physical examination should then be done to add more data that can be used for diagnosis of the stroke mechanism. Elevated blood pressure, cardiac enlargement or murmurs, bruits in the carotid and supraclavicular region, and symmetry of blood pressure and pulses in the arms are important check points during physical examination of stroke patients (see Chapter 22).[1]

The presence of some findings, such as headache, vomiting, loss of consciousness, and seizures, is helpful in diagnosing subtypes of strokes. Headache at onset is an invariable feature of SAH and is also common in patients with large ICHs and large cerebral infarcts due to large artery occlusive disease and brain embolism. Headache is rare in patients with lacunar infarction due to penetrating artery disease. Vomiting is very common in patients with SAH and ICH and in those with brain stem and cerebellar infarcts. Vomiting is very rare in patients with cerebral hemispheric infarction due to large artery occlusive disease or embolism. Seizures at or shortly after the onset of the stroke are relatively common in patients with lobar hemorrhages and those with brain embolism but do not occur in patients with lacunar infarcts. Loss of consciousness at onset is common in patients with large SAHs and in those with embolism to the BA but is rare in strokes due to other mechanisms. Patients with large ICHs often have headache, vomiting, and progressive loss of alertness as the hematoma enlarges and ICP rises.

Neuroimaging studies include CT scan, MRI, diffusion and perfusion-weighted MRI, single photon emission computed tomography (SPECT), and positron-emission tomography (PET). CT scans are best for differentiating ischemic stroke from hemorrhagic stroke. MRI can detect an acute ischemic stroke earlier than CT and is the preferred technique for identifying brain stem and cerebellar infarcts. Diffusion-weighted MRI can often identify acute brain infarcts within minutes of ischemia onset. SPECT and PET scans image the perfusion and metabolic state of the brain and can quantify cerebrovascular reserve capacity. Vascular imaging can be divided into noninvasive and invasive studies. Four commonly used noninvasive tests are Duplex scans (B-mode and Doppler combined), transcranial Doppler ultrasonography (TCD), MRA, and CTA. Duplex scans show an accurate image of the extracranial carotid and vertebral arteries. TCD is useful for the evaluation of the intracranial cerebral arteries by measuring flow velocities and directions. MRA and CTA are useful for the evaluation of intracranial and extracranial large arteries. Combined use of these noninvasive tests is usually adequate for evaluation of most stroke patients. MR venography is now a very useful diagnostic tool for showing cerebral venous sinus thrombosis and has largely replaced invasive conventional cerebral angiography. When there is any suspicion of significant vascular lesions such as severe intra- or extracranial stenosis, aneurysm, arteriovenous malformation (AVM), or vasculitides, standard transfemoral artery catheterization and angiography are usually done to further define and characterize the lesions and, when possible, to intervene to treat vascular lesions at the same time. Important laboratory tests for stroke patients are listed in Table 45–1.

TABLE 45–1. **Laboratory Studies for Stroke Patients**

Neuroimaging
Structural imaging
Computed tomography (CT)
Magnetic resonance imaging (MRI)
Functional imaging
Single photon emission tomography (SPECT)
Positron-emission tomography (PET)
Magnetic resonance spectroscopy (MRS)
Diffusion and perfusion MRI
Vascular Imaging
Noninvasive
B-mode ultrasound
Continuous wave and pulsed Doppler (Duplex)
Transcranial Doppler ultrasound (TCD)
Magnetic resonance angiography (MRA)
Invasive
Digital subtraction angiography (DSA)
Conventional angiography
Heart Studies
Echocardiography: transthoracic, transesophageal
24-Hour ambulatory cardiac monitoring
Cardiac nuclear scanning
Blood Tests
Coagulation and platelet function tests

Diseases That Cause Brain Ischemia

ATHEROTHROMBOTIC DISEASE

Pathogenesis and Pathophysiology. Atherothrombosis implies a reduction or occlusion of blood flow caused by a localized thrombotic process in one or more atherosclerotic cervicocranial arteries. Branching points of arteries are the predilection sites of development of atherosclerosis (Fig. 45–3). In atherosclerosis, fibrous and muscular tissues of the vessel wall overgrow in the subintima, and fatty materials form plaques that can encroach on the lumen. Platelets adhere to the crevices in the plaques and form clumps that serve as nidi for the deposition of fibrin, thrombin, and clot.

Plaques and ulcers are associated with denudation of the endothelium and decreased release of endothelium-relaxing factors including nitric oxide. Endothelins can promote platelet activation and thrombus formation. Intraluminal thrombi are of different types: so-called "white clots," which are mainly composed of platelets and fibrin, and "red thrombi," which are red blood cells enmeshed in fibrin. White platelet clumps form most often in fast-moving streams, adhering to crevices and irregularities along the intimal surface. Fibrin-dependent red thrombi develop in slow-moving streams, for example, arteries with severe luminal narrowing. Narrowing of arteries decreases blood flow, leading to stagnation of the blood column and activation of clotting factors. Clot and fibrin-platelet clumps form and

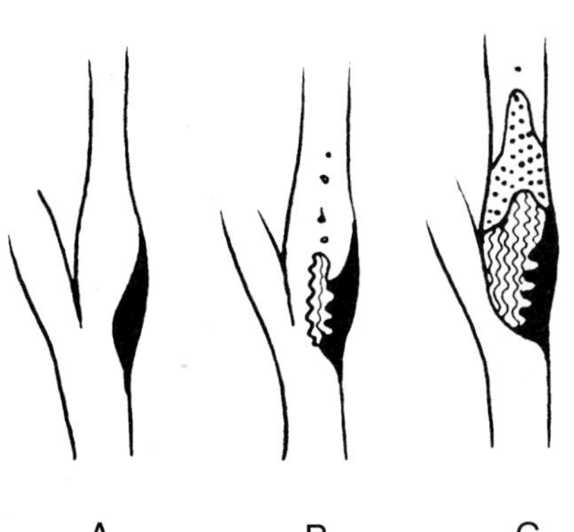

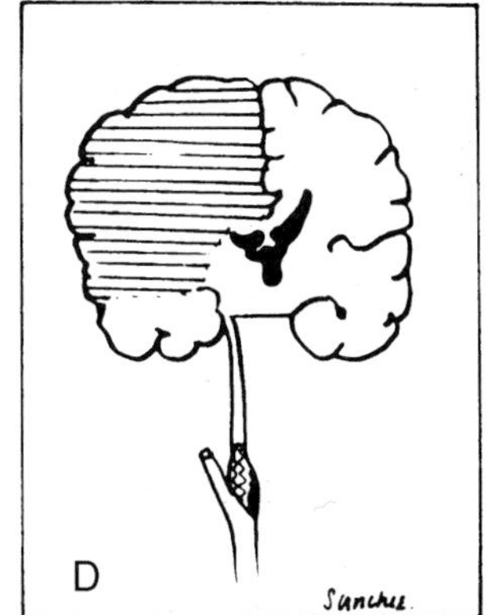

FIGURE 45–3. Internal carotid artery atherosclerotic lesions: *A,* plaque; *B,* plaque with platelet-fibrin emboli; *C,* plaque with occlusive thrombus; *D,* recent ischemic cerebral infarct due to internal carotid artery occlusion. (Adapted from Caplan LR: Stroke: Clinical Approach. Boston, Butterworth-Heinemann, 1993.)

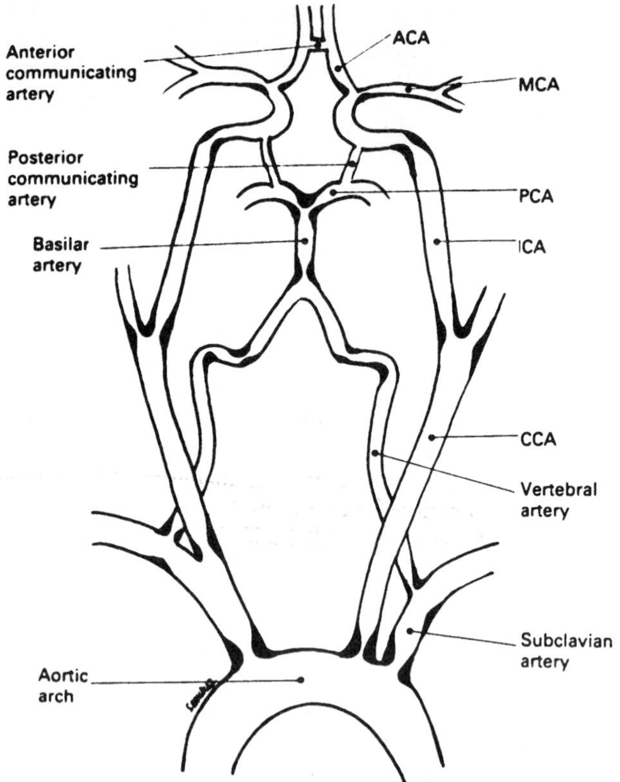

FIGURE 45–4. Sites of predilection for atherosclerotic narrowing; black areas represent plaques. (Adapted from Caplan LR: Stroke: Clinical Approach. Boston, Butterworth-Heinemann, 1993.)

break off, blocking distal arteries and further impeding flow in the affected parent artery (see Fig. 45–3).[1]

Epidemiology and Risk Factors. Atherosclerosis affects chiefly the large extracranial and intracranial arteries (Fig. 45–4), but there are important sex and racial differences in the distribution and incidence of lesions at these sites. White men have more severe disease of the extracranial arteries, whereas in blacks, persons of Asian origin, and women, there is a predilection for narrowing of the intracranial arteries.[4]

Patients with extracranial large artery disease have a high incidence of coronary artery disease (angina pectoris and myocardial infarction), peripheral vascular occlusive disease (claudication), hypertension, and hypercholesterolemia. Death is more often due to fatal coronary artery disease than stroke.

Clinical Features and Associated Disorders. Development of neurological deficits preceded by brief, frequent shotgun-like TIAs in the same vascular territory usually suggests atherothrombosis as the vascular mechanism. Stroke caused by a thrombotic process often develops during or just after sleep. Atherothrombotic infarctions are usually characterized by postural sensitivity of symptoms, occlusion or severe stenosis of a large artery, absence of distal embolus by angiography, infarct on CT or MRI near the border zone territory of the affected artery, and the presence of risk factors for atherosclerosis such as hypertension, diabetes mellitus, and smoking. The neurological symptoms and signs depend on the vessels involved and the regions of brain ischemia.

Differential Diagnosis and Evaluation. The diagnosis of large artery occlusive disease is based on the demographic and epidemiological situation of the patient, analysis of the time course of the brain ischemia, physical examination of the heart and neck vessels, and tests that define the anatomy and function of the cervicocranial arteries. Brain imaging (by CT or MRI) is usually important to define the presence, location, and size of any infarction and may show unexpected ("silent") infarcts not predicted from the history and physical examination. Ultrasound has now become the cornerstone of noninvasive vascular diagnosis. Duplex scans of the origins of the carotid and vertebral arteries combined with color-flow Doppler ultrasound can define and quantify most extracranial ICAs and VA lesions. TCD can detect many intracranial occlusive lesions, especially those involving the MCAs, intracranial VAs, and the PCAs. TCD also yields information about the impact of occlusive extracranial lesions on intracranial blood flow. MRA and CTA are also helpful in imaging the large extracranial and intracranial arteries. When ultrasound and MRA or CTA are concordant and define the occlusive vascular lesions, catheter angiography is usually not necessary.

Management. The very basic goal of management of ischemic stroke patients in the acute phase is protection of the so-called penumbra zone. This zone comprises the brain tissues at risk of irreversible ischemic damage. Brain tissues adjacent to the ischemic core are often impaired functionally ("stunned"), but ischemia is potentially reversible if the circulation is restored soon enough. To achieve this goal, several therapies can be used: (1) occluded vessels can be recanalized (thrombolytic therapy) if possible, (2) blood volume and cerebral blood flow can be maximized and blood viscosity can be reduced, (3) perfusion pressure must be maintained sufficiently (by careful control of blood pressure, reduction of cerebral edema, and lowering of ICP), and (4) the progression of occlusive processes should be blocked using anticoagulants and agents that alter platelet function in some instances. All these measures should be guided by the severity and reversibility of the lesion; the nature, location, and severity of the underlying stroke mechanism; and the viscosity and coagulability of the blood. Recanalization is usually performed by thrombolysis and will be discussed later in this chapter. Hemodilution therapy decreases blood viscosity by lowering the hematocrit level. Blood pressure should not be aggressively lowered during the acute phase because this decreases pressure in the collateral channels and may extend the infarct.

For prevention of recurrence of ischemia in the future, prophylactic treatment should be guided by the mechanism of the stroke. Theoretically, red clots would respond more to anticoagulants like warfarin and heparin, and white clots would be better prevented with platelet antiaggregants, such as aspirin. Surgery (endarterectomy), angioplasty, or warfarin may be indicated for patients with tight stenotic lesions perfusing clinically important tissues at risk for further ischemia. The choice of warfarin versus surgery or angioplasty depends on the accessibility of the lesions to treatment, the risk of surgery and angioplasty, the patient's wishes, the likelihood of the patient's compliance with anticoagulant usage, and any contraindication to the use of anticoagulants. Anticoagulation using intravenous heparin or subcutaneous low-molecular-weight heparin may be used for as long as 2 to 3 weeks to prevent propagation and embolization of clot. Long-term warfarin use is usually not needed after the clot organizes and adheres to the vessel wall in atherothrombotic stroke (usually 3 to 4 weeks). Because platelet adhesion, activation, and aggregation are fundamental components of thrombus formation during vascular occlusion, antiplatelet agents are effective in the prevention of ischemic stroke. Antiplatelet agents are given regularly to reduce the risk of recurrent stroke and other vascular events following a noncardioembolic (atherothrombotic, lacunar, or cryptogenic) stroke or TIA if there is no contraindication.[17] Aspirin, 50 to 325 mg daily, can prevent platelet-fibrin emboli in patients with minor or moderate stenosis. An increase in the dose of aspirin (especially if an in vitro aspirin effect is not shown at the lower dose) or use of ticlopidine should be tried if symptoms recur. The combination of aspirin, 25 mg, and extended-release dipyridamole, 200 mg bid, is more effective than aspirin alone for the prevention of stroke and has a similarly favorable serious adverse effect profile based on indirect comparisons. The thienopyridine derivatives, ticlopidine hydrochloride and clopidogrel, are also antiplatelet agents. They produce significantly less gastrointestinal hemorrhage and upper gastrointestinal upset than aspirin. Compared with aspirin, the thienopyridines produced a proportional reduction of 9 percent in the odds of a vascular event, corresponding to an absolute reduction of 11 events prevented per 1000 patients treated for about 2 years in a large randomized trial. Ticlopidine hydrochloride, 250 mg twice a day, is effective for prevention. The side effects include diarrhea, skin rash, leukopenia, thrombocytopenia, and thrombotic thrombocytopenic purpura (TTP), which require careful monitoring of clinical findings and blood tests during the first 3 months.[18] Clopidogrel is a newer antiplatelet agent that inhibits ADP-induced platelet aggregation and is at least as effective as aspirin.[19] The safety and tolerability seems to be superior to that of ticlopidine, although a few cases of TTP have been reported. For patients who are allergic to aspirin, clopidogrel is preferred to ticlopidine.

The uncertain magnitude of additional benefit and the considerable extra cost of these alternative regimens make their routine use in stroke prevention difficult to justify. It is reasonable to consider the addition of modified-release dipyridamole to aspirin in patients who continue to have ischemic cerebrovascular events on aspirin and to use clopidogrel among patients for whom aspirin is contraindicated or poorly tolerated. If the patient has a primary coagulopathy, polycythemia, or thrombocytosis, these disorders should be treated more specifically.

Prognosis and Future Perspectives. In patients with large artery occlusions, the risk of infarction is maximal in the days after occlusion. After the first week, the likelihood of further infarction is much less. Prognosis depends on whether the initial thrombus propagates distally or embolizes to intracranial arteries and the extent of collateral circulation that develops. Optimization of blood pressure and blood volume during the time when the collateral circulation is developing helps to augment blood flow to the penumbral zones and thus limits the extent of infarction. Of course, patients with large artery atherostenosis are at risk during the subsequent months and years of narrowing and occlusion of other arteries, so preventive measures instituted at the time of the initial symptoms may help in preventing or delaying further strokes. The effectiveness of surgery and angioplasty for various occlusive lesions is now under study in large trials. At times, thrombolysis and angioplasty may be used together because patients with thrombi superimposed on severe atherosclerotic occlusive disease often experience reocclusion of the artery after thrombolysis unless the atherostenosis is repaired. The optimal thrombolytic agent, portal of delivery, dose, timing, and target population for thrombolysis are now being studied.

OCCLUSIVE DISEASE OF SMALL PENETRATING ARTERIES

The small penetrating arteries deep within the brain parenchyma are the sites of various occlusive processes that are different from those of the larger arteries.

Pathogenesis and Pathophysiology. Lipohyalinosis, a destructive vasculopathy linked to severe hypertension, affects arteries 40 to 200 μm in diameter. The arterial lumen is compromised not by an intimal process but by thickening of the vessel wall itself. Subintimal lipid-laden foam cells and pink-staining fibrinoid material thicken the arterial walls, sometimes compressing the lumen. In places, the arteries are replaced by tangles and wisps of connective tissue that obliterate the usual vascular layers. The small, deep infarcts that result from occlusion of these arteries are usually called lacunes.[20] Small, deep infarcts can also result from microatheromas that form at the origin of penetrating arteries, as well as by plaques within the parent arteries that obstruct or extend into the branches (junctional plaques). Rarely, they are occluded by microemboli (Fig. 45–5). Vascular lesions involving the mouths of penetrating arteries are called intracranial branch atheromatous disease.[21]

A recently recognized entity named CADASIL (cerebral autosomal dominant arteriopathy with subcortical infarcts and leukoencephalopathy) is a familial arterial disease of the brain that begins in early adult life. Its gene is mapped to

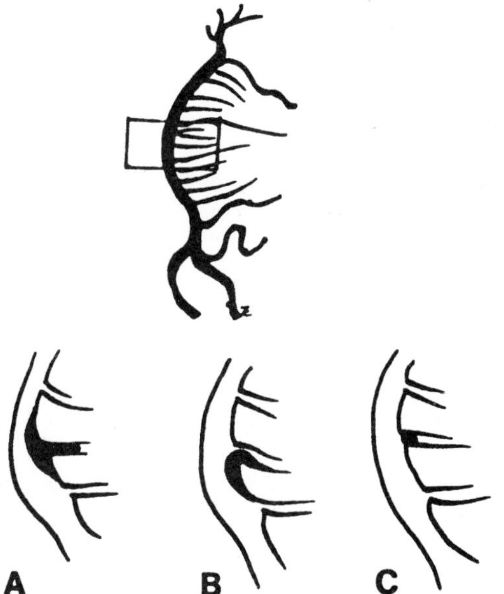

FIGURE 45–5. Branch atheromatous diseases of the basilar artery. *A,* Plaque within parent artery blocking the branch artery orifice. *B,* Plaque extends into the branch from the parent artery (junctional plaque). *C,* Microatheroma originating in orifice of branch. (Adapted from Caplan LR: Intracranial branch atheromatous disease: A neglected, understudied, and underused concept. Neurology 1989;39:1246–1250; with permission.)

chromosome 19. The CADASIL vasculopathy affects the media of leptomeningeal and perforating arteries of the brain. The media is thickened by an eosinophilic granular material of unknown origin. Clinically, patients present with recurrent subcortical infarcts, progressive or stepwise dementia, migraine with aura, and depression. Usually, there is no hypertension or other vascular risk factors. Prominent subcortical white matter and basal ganglia hyperintensities are noted on T2-weighted MRI. Vascular studies are usually not helpful diagnostically.[22]

Epidemiology and Risk Factors. Hypertension is the most significant risk factor for small vessel occlusive diseases and is responsible for about 80 to 90 percent of lacunar infarctions. In addition to hypertension, diabetes mellitus and smoking are also significantly associated with small vessel occlusive disease, particularly with branch atheromatous disease. Blacks and Asians, races with a predilection for hypertension, also have a higher frequency of penetrating artery disease and lacunar infarction than whites.

Clinical Features and Associated Disorders. The arteries commonly affected are the lenticulostriate branches of the MCAs, the thalamogeniculate and thalamoperforant branches of the PCAs, and midline and paramedian penetrating branches of the vertebral and basilar arteries (Fig. 45–6). Infarcts do not involve the cerebral cortex but usually affect the subcortical structures such as the basal ganglia, thalamus, internal capsule, subcortical white matter, and brain stem. Clinical findings are characteristically less severe, neurological dysfunctions are restricted within a few systems, and cognitive and behavioral abnormalities are less common. Lacunar infarcts present diverse clinical syndromes.[20]

Deep infarcts in some regions such as the caudate nucleus, anterior thalamus, and genu of the internal capsule can produce apathy, inertia, and reduced interest in the environment. Bilateral extensive lacunar infarcts are often associated with white matter damage and clinical dementia. Neurological deficits in patients with lacunar infarction can progress gradually or stepwise for 1 to 7 days.

Differential Diagnosis and Evaluation. The major differential diagnostic considerations are restricted cortical and brain stem infarcts due to large artery occlusive disease or embolism and small ICHs. The diagnosis of penetrating artery disease is based on (1) the presence of risk factors, especially present or past hypertension, and diabetes; (2) clinical neurological symptoms and signs typical for or compatible with occlusion of a single perforating artery; and (3) CT or MRI showing a lacunar cerebral infarct or a brain stem infarct in the territory of a single penetrator, or at least no cortical infarct. In uncertain cases, vascular and cardiac imaging may be needed to clarify the diagnosis of penetrating versus large artery occlusive disease.[1]

Management. Treatment consists primarily of controlling the underlying causative process—hypertension. Antiplatelet agents have not been shown to be effective in this condition but are frequently prescribed. Heparin and warfarin anticoagulants are probably ineffective. But if a patient with a small artery territory infarct has an embolic source, anticoagulation may be indicated to prevent future recurrence. No specific treatment is currently available for CADASIL.

Prognosis and Future Perspectives. Recovery from lacunar infarctions or branch atheromatous diseases is usually better than that from cortical infarctions. However, many patients develop recurrent lacunar infarcts and white matter ischemia. The syndrome of vascular dementia, pseudobulbar dysarthria and dysphagia, gait abnormalities, and parkinsonian-like signs are common features in patients with extensive brain damage caused by penetrating artery disease. To date, there have been no controlled trials of patients with acute lacunar infarcts, but these are badly needed in the future. Also badly needed are studies of prevention of further brain damage in patients who already have lacunar infarcts and white matter damage.

BRAIN EMBOLISM

Pathogenesis and Pathophysiology. There are three major sources of embolism—cardiogenic, intra-arterial, and paradoxical (Fig. 45–7). Emboli from any source tend to be arrested in a recipient artery, depending on the location of branch points and the size of the embolic material. Once

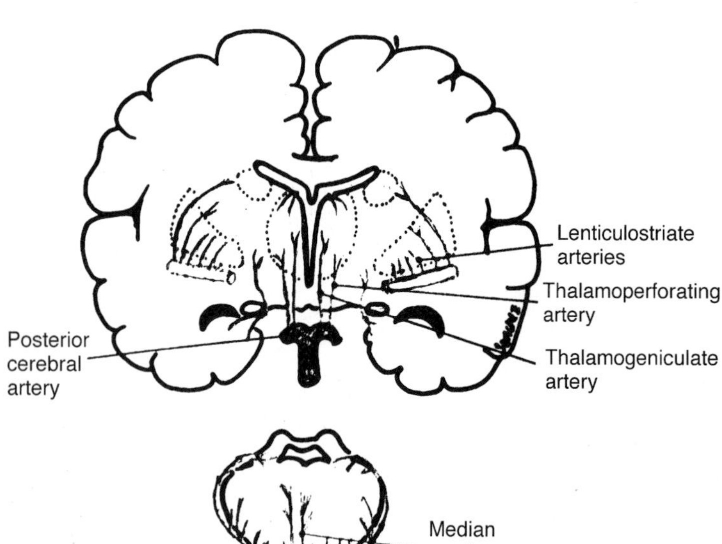

FIGURE 45–6. Penetrating arteries prone to lipohyalinosis and microaneurysms; the thalamogeniculate and lenticulostriate vessels and arteries to the pons. (Adapted from Caplan LR: Caplan's Stroke: A Clinical Approach, 3rd ed. Boston, Butterworth-Heinemann, 2000.)

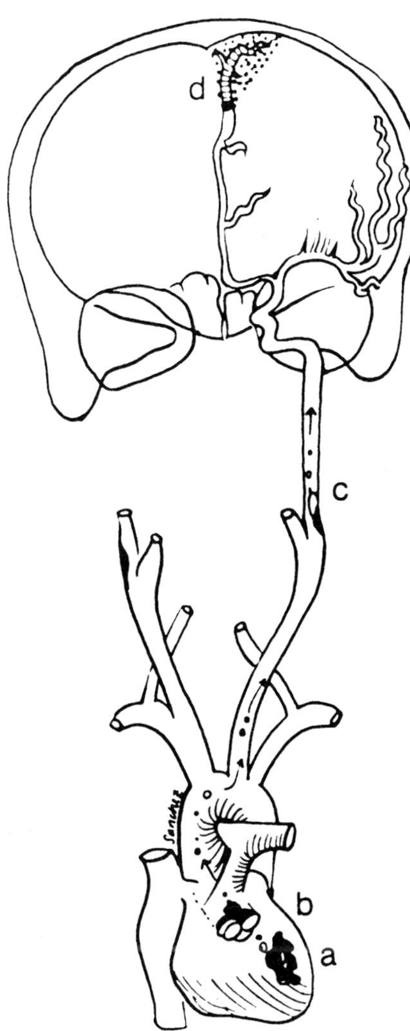

FIGURE 45–7. Examples of potential sources of embolism: cardiac mural thrombus (*a*); vegetation on heart valve (*b*); emboli from carotid plaque (*c*). Also shown: infarcted cortex in area supplied by terminal anterior cerebral artery due to embolism (*d*). (Adapted from Caplan LR: Caplan's Stroke: A Clinical Approach, 3rd ed. Boston, Butterworth-Heinemann, 2000.)

lodged, embolic matter often migrates distally within 48 hours, allowing reperfusion of the previously ischemic zone. This reperfusion frequently causes extravasation of blood through the disintegrated endothelial linings and hemorrhagic conversion of the ischemic lesions, so-called hemorrhagic infarction.

Recent advances in technology have improved the identification of previously unrecognized potential cardiogenic embolic sources and have documented the fact that a higher proportion of ischemic strokes than previously suspected are embolic in origin. Arrhythmias, especially AF and sick sinus syndrome, are important causes of brain embolism. Valvular disease—rheumatic, congenital, calcific, and bacterial and nonbacterial vegetations—is another very important donor source for embolism. Thrombi also form within the heart in patients with myocardial infarcts, myocardiopathies, ventricular aneurysms, and other diseases that cause endocardial and myocardial damage.

Atherosclerotic stenosis of the ICA or VA causes intra-arterial thromboembolism when the thrombus formed on the ulcerative plaque dislodges and travels up to a distal intracranial cerebral artery. Usually emboli are composed of clot, platelet clumps, or fragments of plaques. Embolism is especially apt to occur just after a clot is formed, before it becomes organized and adheres to the arterial wall. Cholesterol crystals, fat, tumor, and foreign body material, particularly talc and cornstarch injected by drug abusers, are less frequent intra-arterial embolic materials. Another important source of intra-arterial embolism is atheromatous aortic plaques. Transesophageal echocardiographic studies have shown that protruding, often mobile and pedunculated, atheromas and clots can be found in the thoracic aorta and are a relatively common source of embolism.[23] Angiography and cardiac surgery with clamping of the aorta promote embolism from aortic lesions.

A less common form of embolism, paradoxical embolism, occurs when the heart serves as a conduit for emboli arising from blood clots in the peripheral veins; these clots pass through septal defects, a patent foramen ovale (PFO), or pulmonary arteriovenous fistulas to reach the brain and systemic circulation (Fig. 45–8). Because PFOs usually open during exertion, stroke frequently occurs during Valsalva maneuvers, exertion, and sexual intercourse.

Epidemiology and Risk Factors. At least 30 percent of ischemic strokes are caused by cardiogenic embolism. The

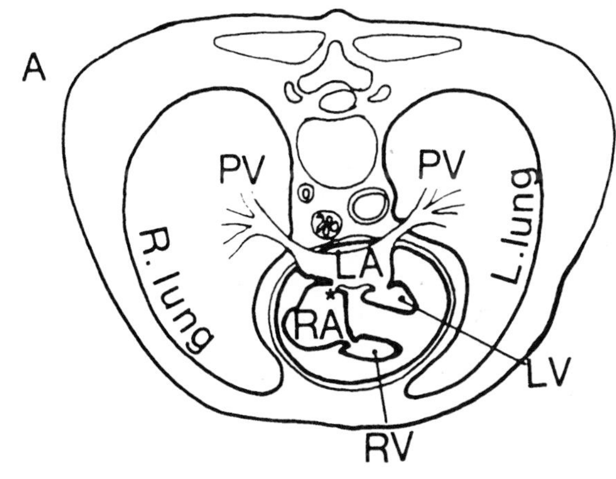

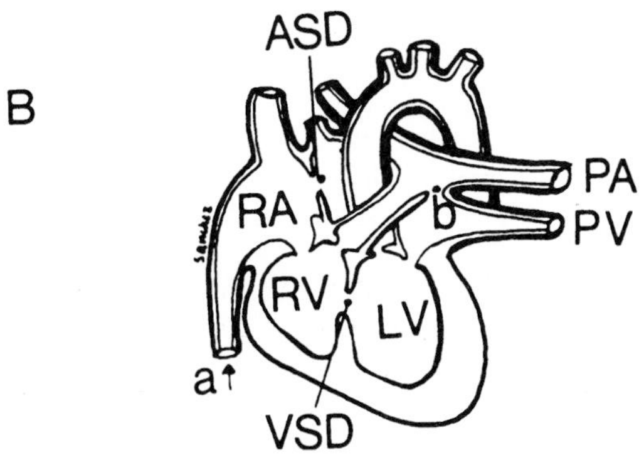

FIGURE 45–8. Common routes of paradoxical embolism. *A,* Cross section through the thorax showing patent foramen ovale (*asterisk*). *B,* Right-to-left shunts; atrial septal defect (ASD), ventricular septal defect (VSD), and fistula between the pulmonary artery and pulmonary vein. Clot from the leg vein ascends via the inferior vena cava. RA = right atrium; LA = left atrium; LV = left ventricle; PA = pulmonary artery; PV = pulmonary vein. (Adapted from Caplan LR: Caplan's Stroke: A Clinical Approach, 3rd ed. Boston, Butterworth-Heinemann, 2000.)

lesions with the highest risk are probably AF, acute myocardial infarction with mural thrombosis, ventricular aneurysms, prosthetic heart valves, rheumatic heart disease with atrial enlargement, myocardiopathies, and bacterial and marantic endocarditis. Cardiac surgery now also poses an important risk of embolism from the heart and aorta.

Clinical Features and Associated Disorders. Brain embolism usually presents abruptly with clinical abnormalities. Fluctuations or worsening symptoms and sudden improvements are common during the first 24 to 48 hours, probably because of emboli passing distally. Usually embolic infarcts are large, and deficits are more severe in patients with emboli than with in situ occlusions. Single or infrequent but longer-lasting TIAs may precede embolic infarctions. Embolic events often occur during activity or sudden straining, coughing, or sneezing. Infarcts may involve multiple vascular territories and are mixed in age. Early angiographic or TCD studies may show the presence of distal intra-arterial emboli. Hemorrhagic conversion of infarcted areas is commonly noted on CT and MRI scans. Infarcts are often wedge-shaped and involve the cerebral cortical surface.

Intra-arterial sources of cerebral embolism are usually atheromatous plaques at the carotid bifurcation, but occasionally responsible proximal vascular lesions are detected at the originating sites of the common carotid arteries or VAs from the subclavian arteries or aorta. Cardiac sources of emboli are listed in Table 45–2.

Differential Diagnosis and Evaluation. Embolic strokes are often difficult to separate from in situ thrombosis engrafted on stenotic lesions and ICH. Patients with brain hematomas more often develop signs gradually, whereas embolic strokes often begin instantly and in about 80 percent of patients reach their maximum intensity at or near onset. Decreased consciousness, headache, and vomiting are more common acutely in patients with hematomas than in those with embolic infarction. Still, CT is most often needed to differentiate hematomas from ischemia. In patients with preexisting arterial stenotic lesions and superimposed acute thrombosis, preceding TIAs are common and may occur several times over a period of weeks or months. The region of ischemia is also smaller than it is in patients with embolism, and the signs tend to accumulate over a longer period of time, producing frequent fluctuations and stepwise changes in neurological signs.

Angiography performed in the first 12 hours shows emboli in a high percentage of cases, but after 48 hours most emboli are no longer detectable. The most common recipient arteries are the MCAs and ACAs in the anterior circulation and the VAs, distal BA, and PCAs in the posterior circulation. The clinical signs and imaging findings are the same as those described in the discussion of these vessels in the section on thrombotic stroke. In patients in whom brain embolism is suspected, the possible embolic sources should be evaluated to prevent further strokes. Evaluation of cardiac and aortic sources usually involves TEE and sometimes cardiac rhythm monitoring. Noninvasive vascular tests (ultrasound, MRA, CTA) can be used to evaluate arterial sources. TCD monitoring for embolic signals can help identify the presence of embolism and may suggest the source.

Management. Treatment of cerebral embolism consists of two major strategies: acute thrombolytic therapy to lyse the embolus and prevention of recurrence of embolic stroke using long-term prophylactic therapy, removal of embolic source(s), or both. Thrombolytic therapy has usually been tried in patients with acute embolic stroke to recanalize the occluded artery, restore cerebral blood flow, reduce ischemia, and limit neurological disability. Recanalization may assist the recovery of reversibly ischemic tissue. So far, there have been several large trials of intravenous thrombolysis in acute stroke and it has been shown that thrombolytic therapy is unequivocally effective when it is started within 3 hours of clearly defined symptom onset.[17, 23] Intravenous rtPA is given in a dose of 0.9 mg/kg (maximum of 90 mg), with 10 percent of the total dose given as an initial bolus and the remainder infused over 60 minutes for eligible patients. So far, strict adherence to eligibility criteria and protocol of the NINDS trial is recommended.[17, 24]

TABLE 45–2. **Common Cardiac Sources of Emboli**

Coronary Artery Diseases
Myocardial infarcts
Ventricular aneurysms
Mural thrombi
Hypokinetic segments (focal and global)
Cardiomyopathies and Endocardiopathies
Endocardial fibroelastosis
Alcoholic cardiomyopathy
Cocaine cardiomyopathy
Myocarditis
Sarcoidosis
Amyloidosis
Valvular Diseases
Mitral stenosis, rheumatic
Aortic stenosis, rheumatic
Bicuspid aortic valve
Mitral annulus calcification (MAC)
Calcific aortic stenosis
Mitral valve prolapse (MVP)
Bacterial endocarditis
Nonbacterial thrombotic (marantic) endocarditis—systemic lupus erythematosus (SLE)
Prosthetic valves
Arrhythmias
Atrial fibrillation and flutter
Sick sinus syndrome
Intracardiac Lesions, Defects, and Shunts
Myxomas
Fibroelastomas
Malignant cardiac tumors
Metastatic tumors
Ball-valve thrombi
Cardiac Chamber Abnormalities
Atrial and ventricular thrombi
Spontaneous contrast on echocardiography
Septal Abnormalities for Paradoxical Embolism
Atrial septal defects
Patent foramen ovale
Atrial septal aneurysms
Pulmonary arteriovenous fistulas

Modified from Caplan LR: Stroke: A Clinical Approach, 2nd ed. Boston, Butterworth-Heinemann, 1993.

Several prognostic factors must be considered for selecting candidates for intravenous thrombolysis. Younger age, absence of cardiac disease or diabetes, lower blood pressure on admission, lower neurological score, absence of early ischemic parenchymal changes and large artery thrombus visible on baseline brain CT, and a developed collateral circulation are all factors associated with a more favorable outcome.[25] The most feared complication of thrombolytic therapy is intracranial hemorrhage, mainly into the evolving infarction. Risk factors for developing brain hemorrhage include time to treatment, dose of thrombolytics, blood pressure level, severity of neurological deficit, and severity of ischemia. Besides hemorrhage, potential complications of thrombolysis include reperfusion injury, arterial reocclusion, and secondary embolization due to thrombus fragmentation. Thus, adequate hospital facilities and personnel are required for administration of thrombolytic therapy as well as for monitoring and managing potential complications. Following tPA administration, BP should be closely monitored and kept <180/105 mm Hg and antithrombotic agents should be avoided for 24 hours.[17, 26]

Local intra-arterial thrombolysis has the advantage of a higher local drug concentration and a lower systemic concentration. Another advantage is its administration in better selected patients with demonstration of an occluded brain artery, because angiographic proof is a diagnostic requirement and a catheter is in place for local delivery of treatment. The Prolyse in Acute Cerebral Thromboembolism Trial (PROACT I) tested the effects of recombinant pro-urokinase and showed no difference in outcome between drug and placebo treatment. On repeat angiography 1 hour after treatment, however, partial or complete recanalization was significantly higher in treated versus control patients. Hemorrhagic transformation causing neurological deterioration within 24 hours of treatment occurred in 15.4 percent of the recombinant pro-urokinase-treated patients and 7.1 percent of the placebo-treated patients.[27] The PROACT II study, as reported by Furlan and colleagues, showed convincing effectiveness of intra-arterial pro-urokinase in patients with MCA thromboemboli.

If a patient arrives later than 3 hours after symptom onset, thrombolysis is usually not recommended. In such instances, anticoagulation seems to be beneficial for those who are at high risk for early recurrent embolism (i.e., patients with mechanical heart valves, an established intracardiac thrombus, AF associated with significant valvular disease, or severe congestive heart failure). But when potential contraindications to anticoagulation are present, such as a large infarction (based on clinical syndrome or brain imaging findings), uncontrolled hypertension, or other bleeding conditions, early anticoagulation should be avoided. For patients with ischemic stroke who are not receiving thrombolysis or anticoagulation, early aspirin therapy (160 to 325 mg/d) should be started within 48 hours of stroke onset and may be used safely in combination with low doses of subcutaneous heparin or low-molecular-weight heparins or the heparinoid danaparoid for deep vein thrombosis prophylaxis.[17] For long-term prevention of recurrent embolic stroke, long-term anticoagulation (target INR of 2.5; range, 2.0 to 3.0) is recommended for patients with AF or other high-risk cardiac sources who have had a recent stroke or TIA. Usually intravenous heparin is started, followed by oral warfarin. Antiplatelet agents are used for these patients with minor-risk cardiac sources.[17]

Cardiac sources of embolism must be corrected surgically if indicated. Recently transcatheter closure of PFO is done for patients with paradoxical embolic stroke.[28] If a tightly stenotic carotid artery is present, either surgery (if feasible) or longer-term warfarin is indicated. When stenosis is not severe, antiplatelet agents such as aspirin or clopidogrel may be used. Warfarin is effective in preventing embolism in patients with nonrheumatic AF. Warfarin also decreases the incidence of embolism in patients with rheumatic mitral stenosis and in those with mechanical heart valves. When warfarin anticoagulation is used, it is advisable to keep the INR at around 3.[29] In older patients, long-term anticoagulation poses important risks and problems. Aspirin may be useful for prophylaxis in some patients with cardiac lesions of low embolic potential and in patients with absolute or relative contraindications to warfarin use.

Carotid artery stenosis is a very common source of intra-arterial embolism. Carotid endarterectomy (CEA) has been used as a method of stroke prophylaxis, but there has been controversy about its safety and efficacy.[30] Two large randomized trials showed that, among such patients, immediate CEA produced a relative reduction of over one half in the risk of major stroke or death over the next 2 to 3 years.[31, 32] Symptomatic carotid stenosis of 70 percent or more is a surgical indication. Reduction in stroke risk after CEA is evident within 6 months of surgery and peaks by 2 years.[32] A CEA in patients with symptomatic moderate carotid stenosis of 50 to 69 percent yields only a moderate reduction in the risk of stroke; patients with less than 50 percent do not benefit from surgery.[33] Asymptomatic carotid stenosis of 60 to 99 percent may be indications for CEA,[34] but a recent analysis has shown that the risk of stroke among such patients is relatively low and that 45 percent of strokes are lacunes or cardioembolism rather than carotid artery–related stroke. Thus absolute benefit of CEA may be low.[35] In elderly patients the benefit of CEA has been uncertain and physicians have been reluctant to recommend CEA to them. Advanced age is associated with an increased risk of stroke in the medically treated group. Therefore, elderly patients benefit more from CEA than younger patients in each category of symptomatic ICA stenosis.[36]

Carotid angioplasty and stenting is a potential alternative to endarterectomy. It has similar major risks and effectiveness at prevention of stroke compared with carotid surgery. Endovascular treatment has the advantage of avoiding minor local complications such as damage to the lower cranial nerves or local hematoma formation.[37]

Prognosis and Future Perspectives. Prognosis depends on the nature of the potential embolic sources and the effectiveness of prophylaxis. The advent of monitoring for emboli with TCD technology has opened new diagnostic possibilities. Further advances in this technology with the use of multiple concurrent channels (such as EEG) will allow better recognition of the source and of the nature and frequency of release of embolic material.

SYSTEMIC HYPOTENSION (BORDER ZONE INFARCTION)

Pathogenesis and Pathophysiology. Inadequate pumping of the heart results in a global lack of blood flow to the brain. This occurs when there is too little blood in the system (shock, hypovolemia), when the pump itself fails (myocardial failure or severe arrhythmia), or when systemic hypotension is present. Collateral blood flow is affected first by a generalized lowering of blood pressure. In contrast to thromboembolic stroke, hypoperfusion is global and causes so-called border zone or watershed infarcts in the areas between the major regions of vascular supply (see Fig. 45–1). Infarcts are usually bilateral but may also occur unilaterally when there is severe stenosis of the ipsilateral proximal carotid or other large arteries. The most common area of border zone ischemia is in the temporoparietal region between the MCA and PCA supply regions.[38]

Epidemiology and Risk Factors. Causes of stroke due to cerebral hypoperfusion include orthostatic hypotension (due to diabetic dysautonomia or antihypertensive therapy), orthostatic brain ischemia (without hypotension), perioperative complications (especially cardiac surgery), myocardial ischemia, cardiac arrhythmias, severe carotid stenosis or occlusion, or combinations of these.

Clinical Features and Associated Features. Faintness, pallor, dim vision, dim hearing and lightheadedness, dizziness, and lack of thought clarity are commonly noticed. The patient's symptoms increase with sitting or standing, and the blood pressure is low. Profuse sweating is common. Temporoparietal border zone ischemia most often causes visual abnormalities. Balint's syndrome is common and consists of asimultagnosia (difficulty in seeing multiple objects at one time), optic ataxia (abnormal hand-eye coordination in one or both visual hemifields), and apraxia of gaze (difficulty in directing the eyes where willed). Ischemia in the anterior border zone between the ACA and MCA affects mostly the convexal surface of the precentral and postcentral gyri and causes arm and thigh weakness, usually with sparing of the face, feet, and often the hands. Occasionally patients have ischemia in the cerebellar border zones between the posteroinferior, anterior, and superior cerebellar arteries and have some gait and limb ataxia.[1]

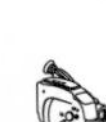

Differential Diagnosis and Evaluation. Frequently watershed infarction is diagnosed on the basis of one or more of the following: documented hypotension, a history of syncope or near-syncope preceding the event, and characteristic patterns of infarction on CT or MRI.

Orthostatic hypotension is defined as a persistent decline of greater than 20 mm Hg in systolic pressure from the supine to the standing position.[39] Hypotension due to other causes is defined as systolic blood pressure of 90 mm Hg or less or at least a 25 percent drop from pre-existing levels. Symptoms of syncope, near-syncope, or cardiac arrhythmia should be sought. Laboratory tests include (1) systemic blood tests including complete blood count (CBC), blood urea nitrogen, and electrolytes; (2) cardiac studies—ECG, echocardiography, and Holter monitoring; and (3) neuroimaging—CT, MRI, and SPECT.

Management. Correction of underlying disorders is essential. Care should be taken when performing interventional procedures such as CEA or cardiac surgery. Excessive use of antihypertensive drugs should be avoided. Recurrences are common, and, if they are not treated early, the outlook is poor. The mortality rate is around 10 percent, and there is a high association with myocardial infarction.

SELECTED NONATHEROSCLEROTIC OCCLUSIVE DISEASES

Noninflammatory Vascular Diseases

Fibromuscular dysplasia (FMD) is a rare condition that affects any or all of the three layers in the arterial walls of both extracranial and intracranial arteries, particularly those of the bilateral ICAs. FMD causes fibrous dysplastic tissue and proliferating smooth muscle cells in the media, presenting as constricting bands and a string-of-beads appearance on arteriography.[1] FMD is commonly found in middle-aged women and is most often asymptomatic. Because of its frequent association with cerebral aneurysms, FMD is often found during the evaluation of SAH.[40] FMD also causes arterial dissections, producing ischemic stroke syndromes, but it may present as a TIA or stroke without any evident compromise of the vascular lumen, possibly due to functional constriction. The stroke recurrence rate is quite low, even with no therapy. If the patient is hypertensive, the renal arteries should be studied.[1, 40]

Moyamoya disease is defined as progressive occlusion of the intracranial ICAs at their intracranial bifurcations and formation of collateral channels through the basal penetrating branches of the cerebral arteries. Pathologically, this condition is characterized by endothelial hyperplasia and fibrosis with intimal thickening and abnormalities of the internal elastic laminas and arterial walls of the perforating arteries, probably due to greatly increased flow through these small vessels. Inflammatory changes are absent. Moyamoya vessels are also found in patients with sickle cell disease, neurofibromatosis, and FMD, and in young women (especially those who smoke cigarettes and take oral contraceptives).[1] Although the disease was first described in young Asians, it has subsequently been found to be widespread and is not limited to Asians. Clinically, children under age 15 years usually present with transient episodes of hemiparesis, headache, seizures, or other focal neurological deficits, often precipitated by physical exercise or hyperventilation. In contrast, adults usually present with brain hemorrhages—usually in the thalamus, basal ganglia, or deep white matter. Occasionally the hemorrhages are SAH. Cerebral angiography, the standard method of diagnosis, shows progressive abnormalities in the intracranial ICAs bilaterally. MCA and ACA branches are also frequently involved. Collateral vessels appear as a cloud of smoke.[41] Recently, MRA has been used as a noninvasive alternative to conventional angiography in typical moyamoya disease. Some patients with moyamoya disease stabilize clinically, often after they have developed disabilities. The best treatment is not known. A variety of surgical revascularization procedures called encephaloduroarteriosynangiosis have been used, but whether they improve the outcome is uncertain.

Cerebrovascular Diseases Especially Related to Pregnancy

There is no increased risk of stroke associated with oral contraceptive use in healthy, nonsmoking, normotensive women. Although there is a three to fourfold increased risk of venous thromboembolism with current oral contraceptive use, the absolute risk is very small and is half that associated with pregnancy.[42, 43]

Although the incidence of ischemic stroke is not much increased during pregnancy and the early puerperium, pregnancy does increase the risk of cerebral hemorrhage. The incidence rates for ischemic stroke associated with pregnancy vary from 5 to 210 per 100,000 deliveries. Ischemic strokes seem to be most common in the puerperal period and third trimester, with few cases occurring in the first trimester. Hypertension contributes independently to the risk of pregnancy-related stroke, especially in older women with chronic hypertension.[44]

Eclampsia is the main cause of both ischemic and hemorrhagic stroke. Eclampsia accounts for about half of ischemic strokes, and eclampsia-related ICH carries a poor prognosis. Stroke is responsible for 4.3 percent of maternal deaths. Up to one third of pregnancy-related brain infarcts may be due to intracranial venous thrombosis, which is most frequent in the third trimester and in the early postpartum period. Dehydration, infection, and sepsis may contribute to venous thrombosis. Patients with eclampsia present with focal neurological deficits of sudden onset in addition to headaches, seizures, or altered consciousness, which usually resolve in several days. The precise pathogenesis is still poorly understood.

Other causes of ischemic stroke during pregnancy include premature atheroma, amniotic embolism, choriocarcinoma, reversible postpartum cerebral angiopathy, arterial dissection, postpartum cardiomyopathy, paradoxical embolism, border zone infarction, use of ergot, pregnancy-related cardiac diseases, hematological disorders, antiphospholipid antibody syndrome, and homocystinuria. Prognosis is worse than in nonpregnant women or men of the same age.[45, 46]

Cerebral venous thrombosis (CVT) is an uncommon condition that develops in association with venous stasis, increased clotting tendency, and traumatic or infective changes in the venous walls. More than 100 causes have been reported, including endocrine, hematological, immunological, vasculitic, infective, and neoplastic diseases. In neonates and children, regional infections (otitis media and mastoiditis), neonatal asphyxia, severe dehydrations, and congenital heart diseases are common associated diseases. In young women, pregnancy, puerperium, oral contraceptive pills, and various connective tissue diseases such as systemic lupus erythematosus are the major causes. Risk of CVT is increased in carriers of prothrombin and factor V gene mutations, which may be enhanced in women receiving oral contraceptives. Other causes include malignancies, antithrombin III protein C and protein S deficiencies, and Behçet's disease.[47]

Thrombi in CVT are rich in red blood cells and fibrin but poor in platelets ("red thrombus") and are then replaced by fibrous tissue over time. Occlusion of a dural sinus often results in severe brain edema, venous infarction in the cortex and adjacent white matter, while deep cerebral vein thrombosis causes venous infarcts in the basal ganglia, thalamus, or both. The venous hypertension caused by blockage of blood draining from the skull can also lead to brain hemorrhages. Brain edema, ischemia, and hemorrhages result from extensive thromboses. The sagittal sinus is involved most often, followed by the lateral sinuses and the cavernous sinus.

CVT has a variable mode of onset and usually has a favorable outcome. The most common symptom is headache, which can be severe and persistent and is often due to increased ICP. Others include vomiting, seizures, and focal neurological symptoms and signs that result from brain ischemia, edema, or hemorrhage. Clinical patterns include (1) isolated intracranial hypertension mimicking pseudotumor cerebri and presenting with headache, papilledema, and cranial nerve VI palsy; (2) focal neurological signs simulating arterial strokes or seizure attacks; and (3) a cavernous sinus syndrome.

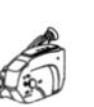

Differential diagnoses include benign intracranial hypertension ("pseudotumor cerebri"), migraine, meningitis, encephalitis, cerebral arterial infarction, ICH, brain abscess, brain tumor, and eclampsia. Diagnosis is based on clinical data, CT or MRI, and MR venographic findings. Conventional angiography is rarely needed when MRI is available. Venous infarcts appear as unilateral or bilateral or single or multifocal. Hemorrhagic infarction and small hematoma are common because of the increased pressure in draining veins.[48]

Management of patients with CVT includes reducing ICP and administering anticoagulant therapy, thrombolytic therapy, and antibiotics in case of an infected thrombus. Steroids and osmotic diuretics are used in patients with brain edema or increased ICP. Anticonvulsants are given for seizures. Patients show a clear and definite improvement in outcome when treated with anticoagulation using intravenous heparin followed by warfarin. Unfractionated or low-molecular-weight heparin can be used safely during the acute phase, followed by oral anticoagulation for 3 to 6 months (target INR of 2.5; range, 2.0 to 3.0) even in the presence of hemorrhagic infarction before treatment. In patients who demonstrate progressive neurologic deterioration despite adequate anticoagulation, other options, such as superselective local intrathrombus infusion of a thrombolytic agent together with IV heparin, are under investigation.[17, 49–51]

CVT usually resolves spontaneously, and the prognosis is generally better than previously thought but remains largely unpredictable. If left untreated, CVT is potentially life threatening, particularly in deep cerebral vein thrombosis. Recent reports attributed better outcomes to greater awareness of CVT, noninvasive imaging techniques, and a relative decline of infective etiologies. Among survivors only a minority develop a permanent deficit such as focal limb weakness, epilepsy, or optic atrophy. Poor prognostic factors include rapid evolution of thrombosis, coma, infancy or old age, involvement of deep cerebral and cerebellar veins, and septic thrombi.[17, 48]

Arterial dissection, especially spontaneous dissection of the cervicocranial arteries, is an important cause of ischemic strokes, especially in young people under 50 years of age. Congenital changes in the media or elastic layer of the arteries or edema of the arterial wall following mechanical stress promote cervicocranial arterial dissection. They include Marfan's disease, Ehlers-Danlos syndrome, pseudoxanthoma elasticum, or fibromuscular dysplasia, migraine, chiropractic manipulation of the neck, sports and other activities involving sudden neck stretching, or prolonged holding of the neck in an eccentric position. The pharyngeal portion of the extracranial ICA and the first and third segments of the VA are more mobile and thus most vulnerable to dissection.[52, 53]

A tear within the arterial wall leads to bleeding, which dissects along the longitudinal course of the artery. When the dissection develops between the intima and the media, the expanded arterial wall can compromise the lumen and may cause hemodynamic strokes such as TIAs or infarcts. But more freqeuntly the dissection causes thromboembolism. Because clots formed in the lumen of the dissected artery are usually loosely adherent to the intima, they may readily embolize distally, causing embolic infarction. Strokes usually develop within the first few days after the dissection, and late strokes are unusual.[52] The intraluminal clot is absorbed within several weeks, and the lumen usually returns to its normal size. When dissections extend between the media and the adventitia, tears through the adventitia may lead to SAH. If the adventitia is not torn, fusiform aneurysmal masses or pouches may develop.

Cervicocranial arterial dissection causes ipsilateral throbbing headache; local sharp pain in the neck, jaw, pharynx, or face; an ipsilateral Horner's syndrome; or cranial nerve palsies.[54] Pain in the neck and head is an important symptom that helps to separate the dissection from other causes of brain ischemia. At times, both carotid arteries and even the VAs are dissected at the same time.

CT and MRI can directly visualize the intramural bleeding and expansion, confirming the diagnosis. MRA and ultrasound testing are reliable noninvasive tools for diagnosis and follow-up of extracranial ICA dissections, but conventional angiography is more useful for VA dissections.[53] Angiography

TABLE 45–3. **Some Important Vasculitides**

Condition	Demography	Pathology Vessel Type	Clinical Environment	Other Features
Polyarteritis nodosa	1:25 f/m ratio; 30 to 50 years old	Necrotizing, small-medium muscular arteries	Strokes; kidney, peripheral nerves	Fever, hypertension, circulating immune complexes
Churg-Strauss syndrome	1:1.4 f/m ratio; 10 to 50 years old	Fibrinoid necrosis with eosinophils; small-medium arteries, veins, capillaries	Asthma; skin, kidney, encephalopathy, peripheral nerves	Eosinophilia, fever, rhematoid factor
Hypersensitivity vasculitis	Any age and sex	Leukocytoclastic vasculitis, postcapillary venules	Peripheral nerves and plexus, encephalopathy, palpable purpura	Drug-induced cryoglobulins, circulating immune complexes
Wegener's granulomatosis	1:1.2 f/m ratio; any age	Granulomas in organs, necrotizing arteritis	Sinuses, respiratory tract, kidneys, cranial and peripheral nerves	cANCA-positive; upper and lower respiratory tract involvement
Sarcoidosis	20 to 30 years old; no sex predilection, blacks > whites	Perivenous, granulomas	Peripheral nerves, muscle, eyes, lungs, skin, lymph nodes, brain granulomas	Granulomas in skin, muscle, liver, nodes
Temporal arteritis	1:2 to 1:3 f/m ratio; >50 years	Segmental granulomatous, external carotid, and aortic branches	Eyes, peripheral nerves, occasional strokes	High ESR, jaw claudication, scalp tender
Isolated CNS angiitis	1:2 f/m ratio; any age	Mononuclear perivascular cell, granulomas	Brain only, seizures, confusion	High CSF protein, no systemic symptoms
Takayasu's arteritis	9:1 f/m ratio; Asians; age range 15–40 yr	Acute inflammatory giant cell; large arteries of aortic arch	Syncope, lightheadedness, headache, absent arm pulses (strokes rare)	Systemic symptoms, hypertension
Behçet's disease	1:9 f/m ratio; Japan and Mediterranean heritage	Perivascular cell loss and demyelinization, perivascular plasma cells and lymphocytes	Aphthous oral ulcers, genital ulcers, eye inflammation, meningitis, brain stem lesions	Strokes and meningoencephalitis with focal brain stem lesions
Cogan's disease	Young adults	Arteritis of small and medium-sized arteries	Interstitial keratitis of eye, uveitis, ear involvement	Vertigo, tinnitus, decreased hearing, cornea opacification
Eales' disease	Mostly young men, aged 20 to 30 years old; middle East and Indian heritage	Inflammation of retinal arteries and veins	Retinal and vitreous hemorrhages, meningitis, occasional brain and spinal cord infarcts	Characteristic sheathing of retinal arteries and veins and vitreous hemorrhages
Microangiopathy of the brain, retina, ear	Almost always women, 15 to 30 years old	Obliterative, noninflammatory arteries and arterioles	Retina, ear, brain	High CSF protein
Kohlmeier-Degos syndrome	Young adults 15 to 30 years old	Fibrous vascular proliferation, rare inflammation	Small, yellow, aised skin lesions; GI tract; brain infarcts	Skin, GI, and brain infarcts
Sneddon's disease	Females > males; age 30 to 50	Proliferative thrombo-occlusive disease of skin and brain and small arteries and arterioles	Livedo reticularis of skin and brain infarcts	Antiphospholipid antibodies common

cANCA, Classic antineutrophil cytoplasmic antibody; CSF, cerebrospinal fluid; ESR, erythrocyte sedimentation rate; f/m, female-to-male; GI, gastrointestinal.

may show regions of severe narrowing ("string sign"), or the ICA may be totally occluded, beginning more than 2 cm distal to the ICA origin, sparing the siphon, and having a gradually tapering segment. Localized aneurysmal sacs or outpouchings may be seen. Duplex scans can show increased arterial diameter, decreased pulsatility, intravascular abnormal echoes, and hemodynamic evidence of decreased flow. TCD can demonstrate diminished intracranial velocities in the ICA siphon and the MCAs or the intracranial VAs and also show the post-dissection collateral blood flow.

Although there have been no controlled trials of medical therapy, prevention of embolization of clots at or shortly after the dissection is critically important because the risk of thromboembolic strokes is particularly high during the acute period. Unless there are contraindications, anticoagulation with intravenous administration of heparin followed by oral warfarin with a target INR of 2.0 to 3.0 is generally used for 3 to 6 months.[52]

Most extracranial dissections heal spontaneously with time. Arteries retaining some residual lumen invariably heal and become normal, but, when complete occlusion has occurred, the arteries often do not recanalize and remain occluded. In patients with SAH intracranial dissections can be repaired surgically. Recurrence is uncommon, occurring in 3 to 8 percent of patients with dissection.[55]

Inflammatory Vascular Disorders

This subject is discussed in depth in Chapter 50. Table 45–3 outlines some of the important vasculitides and their key features.

Drug-Related Vasculopathies

Illicit drug use and abuse has unfortunately become an important cause of stroke, especially in young individuals. This topic is discussed in Chapter 39. Table 45–4 outlines the common drugs implicated and some features of the strokes that they cause.

Migraine-related Stroke

Stroke is a rare but potentially devastating complication of migraine. Infarction is thought to be due to prolonged intense vasospasm associated with migraines. Intense vasospasm can impede flow, promoting thrombosis. Platelets are activated during migraine and the vasoconstrictive process itself may stimulate the endothelium to release factors that promote thrombosis. Severe vasoconstriction and thrombi have been demonstrated in patients with migraine who have PCA and BA territory infarcts.[56] To complicate matters, atherosclerotic lesions in the coronary arteries of humans—and in the extracranial and retinal arteries of experimental animals—seem to predispose them to superimposed vasoconstriction. Thus, vasoconstriction can complicate atherostenosis. TCD shows promise of identifying vasoconstriction by showing high velocities that change with time and with various pharmacological treatments.

Hemorrhage can occasionally complicate a severe migraine attack. Intense vasoconstriction leads to ischemia of a local brain region, accompanied by edema and ischemia of the small vessels perfused by the constricted artery. Then, when vasoconstriction abates, blood flow to the region is augmented, and the reperfusion can cause hemorrhage from the damaged arteries and arterioles. The mechanism is the same as that found in hemorrhage after CEA and in reperfusion after brain embolization. Prophylactic agents (most often calcium channel blockers, cyproheptadine, or methysergide) should be maintained as well as agents that modify platelet function and coagulation. Aspirin may be prescribed, but warfarin can be used in patients with prior infarcts.[57]

Stroke in Coagulation Disorders

Brain ischemia and hemorrhage often result from hematological disorders. Changes in the formed cellular constituents of the blood may be quantitative or qualitative. Polycythemia increases blood viscosity, decreases cerebral blood flow, and increases the risk of thrombosis. Sickle cell disease and sickle cell hemoglobin-C disease are examples of qualitative red blood cell abnormalities that affect blood flow. Sickle cell disease causes occlusive changes in large intracranial arteries and small penetrating vessels. Subcortical, cortical, and border zone infarcts are often found on CT and MRI.

Increased platelet counts, especially those over 1 million, are associated with hypercoagulability. Thrombocytosis can be primary (so-called essential thrombocythemia), associated with other myeloproliferation or, less often, secondary to systemic disease. Essential thrombocythemia is associated with strokes and digital arterial occlusions. There are also qualita-

TABLE 45–4. **Drug Abuse and Strokes**

Drug	Route	Ischemia	Hemorrhage	Other Features
Heroin	IV	Strokes—brain and spinal cord	No	Increased gamma globulins
Amphetamines	Oral, IV	No ischemic strokes	SAH, ICH; aneurysms and AVMs rare	Hypertension
Cocaine HCl	Nasal, IV	Ischemic strokes	SAH and ICH; aneurysms and AVMs common	Hypertension
Crack cocaine	Nasal, IV	Ischemic strokes very common	SAH and ICH; aneurysms and AVMs common	Hypertension
Mashed pills	IV	Ischemic strokes	No	Talc particles in eyes and lungs

SAH, Subarachnoid hemorrhage; ICH, intracerebral hemorrhage; AVM, arteriovenous malformation.

tive abnormalities of platelet function. In some patients, increased coagulability has been attributed to increased adhesion and aggregation of platelets (so-called sticky platelets) in the absence of thrombocytosis.

Leukemia is complicated occasionally by brain hemorrhages and microinfarcts. When the white blood cell count is very high (increased leukocrit), the white blood cells can pack capillaries, leading to microinfarcts and vascular rupture with small hemorrhages in the brain. Larger intraparenchymatous hemorrhages and SAHs are most often related to thrombocytopenia, due to replacement of the bone marrow with leukocyte precursors.

Abnormalities of the coagulation cascade can also cause hypercoagulability and lead to venous and arterial occlusions and brain infarction. Table 45–5 lists some of the most common abnormalities.

Stroke in Immunological Abnormalities

Circulating antibodies, like lupus anticoagulant (LA) and anticardiolipin antibodies, may be related to stroke. The LA is a phospholipid antibody that interferes with the formation of the prothrombin activator. In the laboratory, there is a prolonged activated partial thromboplastin time (PTT). Some patients with LA have systemic lupus erythematosus, but most do not. When antiphospholipids of the IgG, IgM, or IgA classes are found in the absence of a known systemic illness, and patients present with an increased incidence of spontaneous abortions, thrombophlebitis, pulmonary embolism, and large- and small-artery occlusions, the disorder is now referred to as primary antiphospholipid lupus anticoagulant syndrome. The APLA-associated stroke syndrome is characterized by its younger age at onset, predominance in women, and high risk of recurrent thrombo-occlusive events. Some patients have mitral and aortic valve vegetations and ocular ischemia. In addition to the presence of LA or anticardiolipins, or both, laboratory abnormalities include false-positive Venereal Disease Research Laboratory, thrombocytopenia, antinuclear antibodies, and prolonged activated PTT. The risk of recurrent thrombosis in patients with the antiphospholipid-antibody syndrome is high. More than one half of the patients have at least one recurrent thrombo-occlusive stroke, most occurring within the first year. Long-term anticoagulation therapy is recommended, maintaining the INR at or above 3.[58, 59]

TABLE 45–5. Some Common Coagulation Disorders Causing Hypercoagulability

1. Deficiencies of natural coagulation inhibitors
   Antithrombin III
   Protein C
   Protein S
2. Resistance to activated protein C
3. Increased levels of serine protein coagulation factors (can occur in patients with inflammatory diseases), factors V, VII, and VIII
4. Cancer, especially mucinous adenocarcinomas
5. Abnormalities of the normal fibrinolytic system
   Tissue plasminogen activator (t-PA)
   Plasminogen activator inhibitor (PAI)
6. Dysfibrinogenemias, including increased levels of fibrinogen

Disseminated intravascular coagulation occurs when a primary disorder leads to local or diffuse clotting and the coagulation cascade is activated, with generation of excess intravascular thrombin. The coagulation system then is activated further, fibrin is deposited into the microcirculation, hemostatic elements have a shortened survival, and the fibrinolytic system is activated. The most common disorders inciting disseminated intravascular coagulation are infections, obstetric and vascular emergencies, cancer, nonbacterial thrombotic endocarditis, head trauma, SAH, brain tumors, and vascular malformations. The laboratory findings usually include thrombocytopenia, reduced fibrinogen levels, prolongation of prothrombin time (PT) and PTT, and increased levels of fibrin split products. Neurological findings are frequent and include an encephalopathy with multifocal signs and frank thrombotic and embolic infarcts. Bleeding can also occur.

Whole blood viscosity is one of the major determinants of cerebral blood flow, especially in the microcirculation. Whole blood viscosity is very dependent on the hematocrit and fibrinogen levels, and these are often elevated in patients with stroke.[60] Hyperviscosity also is probably pathogenetically related to Binswanger's disease (subcortical arteriosclerotic encephalopathy).[61] Less often, viscosity is increased by high levels of globulins as in Waldenström's macroglobulinemia or in other disorders with abnormal proteins or cryoglobulins, such as multiple myeloma, or by very high levels of serum lipids, especially chylomicra.

TTP is characterized clinically by fever, renal failure, thrombocytopenia, and microangiopathic hemolytic anemia. Transient focal neurological signs and a more diffuse encephalopathy are common, but occasionally, persistent neurological deficits due to occlusion of medium-sized arteries or brain hemorrhages occur. Plasma exchange can be an effective treatment.

Hemorrhagic Cerebrovascular Diseases

PRIMARY INTRACEREBRAL HEMORRHAGE

Pathogenesis and Pathophysiology. Chronic hypertension causes fibrinoid necrosis in the penetrating and subcortical arteries, weakening of the arterial walls, and formation of small aneurysmal outpouchings, so-called Charcot-Bouchard microaneurysms, that predispose the patient to spontaneous ICH. Bleeding usually arises from the deep penetrating arteries of the circle of Willis, including the lenticulostriate, thalamogeniculate, and thalamoperforating arteries and perforators of the BA. Acute rises in blood pressure and blood flow can also precipitate ICH even in the absence of pre-existing severe hypertension. A ruptured vascular malformation is the second most common cause of ICH.

Bleeding is limited by the resistance of tissue pressure in the surrounding brain structures. If a hematoma is large, distortion of structures and increased ICP cause headache, vomiting, and decreased alertness. Because the cranial cavity is a closed system, enlargement of a hematoma or development of severe edema may shift brain tissues into another compartment, so-called herniation, and cause deterioration in the clinical condition.

Epidemiology and Risk Factors. ICH is a major cause of morbidity and death and accounts for 10 to 15 percent of all strokes in whites and about 30 percent in blacks and individuals of Asian origin. Pregnancy may increase the risk of ICH. Eclampsia accounts for more than 40 percent of ICHs in pregnancy and is a common cause of death from eclampsia. Locations of hypertensive ICHs are putamen (40%), lobar (22%), thalamus (15%), pons (8%), cerebellum (8%), and caudate (7%) (Fig. 45–9).

Spontaneous ICH can also occur in association with bleeding diatheses, especially the prescription of anticoagulants, primary or metastatic brain tumors or granulomas, and use of sympathomimetic drugs. Aneurysms rarely bleed only into the brain, but when they do, they cause a local hematoma near the brain surface.

Clinical Features and Associated Disorders. Hematomas are often classified as putaminal, thalamic, caudate, lobar, pontine, or cerebellar, and each has its specific neurological features in addition to the symptoms and signs of sudden increased ICP. Even hematomas arising in the same anatomical location may develop different clinical features and have varied prognoses because they differ in size, intraregional location, direction of intraparenchymal extensions, and presence of ventricular hemorrhage.[62, 63]

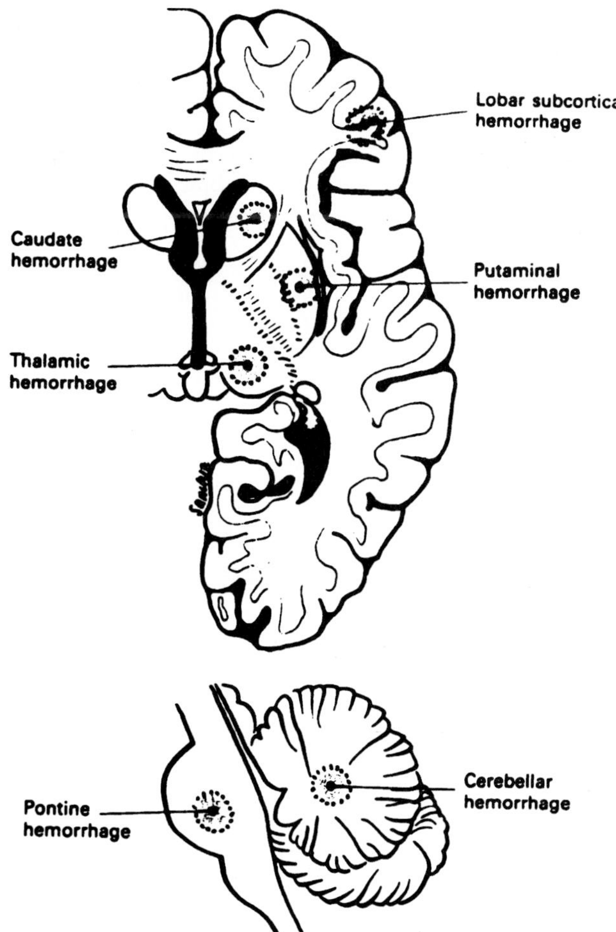

FIGURE 45–9. Horizontal cerebral section *(top)* and sagittal brain stem section *(bottom)*, showing most common sites of intracerebral hemorrhage. (Adapted from Caplan LR: Caplan's Stroke: A Clinical Approach, 3rd ed. Boston, Butterworth-Heinemann, 2000.)

The earliest signs relate to blood issuing into parenchymatous structures. For example, a hematoma in the left putamen and internal capsule would first cause weakness of the right limbs; a cerebellar hematoma would cause gait ataxia. As the hematomas enlarge, the focal symptoms increase. If the hematoma becomes large enough to raise ICP, then headache, vomiting, and decreased alertness develop. Some hematomas remain small and the only symptoms relate to the focal collection of blood. Table 45–6 notes the most important features of hematomas at the most common sites (see Chapter 21).

Differential Diagnosis and Evaluation. Diagnostic considerations include infarcts in similar regions and subdural and epidural hematomas. Rarely, brain tumors and abscesses can have a rapid onset mimicking ICH. It is very important to identify the cause of the hemorrhage. Hypertension, bleeding diatheses (especially as a result of iatrogenic prescription of coumadin), trauma, and amyloid angiopathy are the most frequent causes. In young, normotensive patients, especially those with lobar and intraventricular hemorrhages, vascular malformations are the most likely source of bleeding. Aneurysms can also rarely bleed directly into brain parenchyma. Some primary and metastatic brain tumors, especially renal carcinoma and choriocarcinoma, have a propensity to develop hemorrhages within the tumor, thus causing an abrupt onset or worsening of neurological symptoms. During the initial evaluation, blood samples for basic laboratory studies, including CBC, chemistries, coagulation studies (PT, PTT, bleeding time, and platelet count), arterial blood gas analysis, and toxicology screen, are obtained.

The CT scan is an essential tool for diagnosis, management, and follow-up of ICH. It accurately documents the size and location of the hematoma, the presence and extent of any mass effect, and the presence of hydrocephalus and intraventricular hemorrhage. CT scans should be performed immediately in patients suspected of having an ICH. Follow-up CT scans are requested when there is a change in clinical signs or state of alertness in order to monitor changes in the size of the lesion and ventricular system and to detect important pressure shifts. If the clinical syndrome and CT findings are typical of hypertensive hemorrhage in the basal ganglia, caudate nucleus, thalamus, pons, or cerebellum, angiography is usually not necessary. If the hemorrhage is in an atypical location or the patient is young and not hypertensive, angiography is indicated to exclude an AVM, aneurysm, vasculitis, or tumor. Patients who have ICH after cocaine use have a high likelihood of vascular malformations and aneurysms and need angiography.

Management. Prompt and careful management of patients with ICH may be life saving and is important even in those who will later undergo surgical intervention. Adequate airway and respiratory support should be established. Blood gases should be measured in patients with reduced alertness. Endotracheal intubation is performed for patients presenting in coma, for those who are unable to protect their airway, and for those who have respiratory failure. Wide swings in blood

TABLE 45–6. **Signs in Patients with Intracerebral Hemorrhages at Various Sites**

Location	Motor/Sensory	Eye Movements	Pupils	Other Signs
Putamen or internal capsule	Contralateral hemiparesis and hemisensory loss	Ipsilateral conjugate deviation	Normal	Left: aphasia Right: left-sided neglect
Thalamus	Contralateral hemisensory loss	Down and in upgaze palsy	Small; react poorly	Somnolence, decreased alertness; left: aphasia
Lobar				
Frontal	Contralateral limb weakness	Ipsilateral conjugate gaze	Normal	Abulia
Temporal	None	None		Hemianopia Left: aphasia
Occipital	None	None		Hemianopia
Parietal	Slight contralateral hemiparesis and hemisensory loss			Hemianopia; left: aphasia; right: left neglect; poor drawing and copying
Caudate	None or slight contralateral hemiparesis	None	Normal	Abulia, agitation, poor memory
Pons	Quadriparesis	Bilateral horizontal gaze paresis, ocular bobbing	Small; reactive	Coma
Cerebellar	Gait ataxia, ipsilateral limb hypotonia	Ipsilateral gaze or cranial nerve VI paresis	Small	Vomiting, inability to walk, tilt when sitting

pressure, especially hypertension, are common in the initial period following hemorrhage. Intravenous labetalol or sodium nitroprusside with concomitant intra-arterial pressure monitoring is an effective method of controlling such elevations. Continuous cardiac monitoring for arrhythmias is important. Hypotension, however, from cardiac or other etiologies can be devastating due to the impact on cerebral perfusion pressure. Control of local tissue pressure and ICP is also important to guarantee adequate cerebral perfusion pressure. The available medical and surgical treatment modalities are outlined in Table 45–7. They are not competitive, but a combined approach utilizing both medical and surgical modalities will often yield satisfactory results.[64, 65]

Emergency surgical treatments have been tried for several decades. Early studies showed that there was no value in surgical removal of hematomas over standard medical management. More recent studies of hematoma removal have shown promise for open surgical decompression, but only if it is accomplished early after the onset of symptoms. The best candidates for surgery may be patients with moderate to large hematomas who are still awake. Recent advances in neuroimaging techniques have made it possible to drain hematomas percutaneously, using stereotactic surgery. A burr hole is made, and the drainage instrument is guided stereotactically, using CT, to the core of the hematoma, which is then evacuated. Fibrinolytic agents also can be instilled to soften and lyse coagulated hematomas. As yet, there is too little experience to allow comparison of open versus stereotactic drainage of hematomas, although stereotactic surgical aspiration of ICH is probably safe and is promising.[66]

Prognosis and Future Perspectives. Survival depends on the location, size, and rapidity of development of the hematoma. ICHs are at first soft and dissect along white matter fiber tracts. If the patient survives the initial changes in ICP, blood is absorbed and a cavity or slit forms that may disconnect brain pathways. Patients with small hematomas located deep and near midline structures often develop secondary herniation and mass effect, and these patients have a high mortality rate. Survivors invariably have severe neurological deficits. In patients with medium-sized hematomas, the deficit varies with the location and size of the hematomas. Most patients survive with some residual

TABLE 45–7. **Treatment of Intracerebral Hemorrhage**

Medical

Medical decompression for increased intracranial pressure
- Intubation and mechanical hyperventilation
- Dexamethasone (Decadron), 4 mg every 6 hours
- Mannitol, 0.5 to 1 g/kg every 4 hours intravenously (IV)
- Glycerol, 1 to 1.5 ounces orally every 6 hours
- Furosemide (Lasix), 40 mg (4 mg/min) IV*

Control of hypertension
- Labetalol, 10 mg IV, followed by 10-mg doses as needed
- Trimethaphan camsylate (Arfonad), 0.5 to 1 mg/min IV by drip
- Nitroprusside sodium, 15 to 200 μg/min
- Hydralazine hydrochloride (Apresoline), 50 to 100 mg twice daily orally

Reversal of bleeding diathesis
- Fresh frozen plasma
- Antihemophilic factor
- Phytonadione (vitamin K, AquaMEPHYTON), 20 to 40 mg IV
- Platelet transfusion
- Fresh blood transfusion

Surgical

Drainage of hematoma—stereotactic drainage or surgical evacuation
Ventricular drainage or shunt
Removal of bleeding arteriovenous malformation or tumor
Repair of aneurysm

*FDA approved for this indication.
Modified from Chung C-S, Caplan LR: Parenchymatous brain hemorrhage. *In* Rakel RE (ed): Conn's Current Therapy. Philadelphia, WB Saunders, 1995, p 794.

neurological signs. Further experience with the procedure will help define its place in ICH management.[67]

SUBARACHNOID HEMORRHAGE

SAH is a common and often devastating condition. Despite considerable advances in diagnostic, surgical, and anesthetic techniques as well as perioperative management, the outcome for patients with SAH remains poor.[68]

Pathogenesis and Pathophysiology. The cause of SAH is a ruptured aneurysm in 85 percent of cases, nonaneurysmal perimesencephalic hemorrhage (with excellent prognosis) in 10 percent, and a variety of rare conditions such as vascular malformations in 5 percent. Aneurysms, often referred to as berry or congenital, are outpouchings on arteries, probably caused by a combination of congenital defects in the vascular wall and degenerative changes. Aneurysms usually occur at branching sites on the large arteries of the circle of Willis at the base of the brain (Fig. 45–10). When an aneurysm ruptures, blood is released under arterial pressure into the subarachnoid space and quickly spreads through the cerebrospinal fluid (CSF) around the brain and spinal cord. Aneurysms are less often caused by arterial dissection through the adventitia of arterial walls, embolism of infected or myxomatous material to the vasa vasorum of distal cerebral arteries (mycotic aneurysms), and degenerative elongation and tortuosity of arteries (dolichoectasia). Patients with fibromuscular dysplasia, polycystic kidney disease, and connective tissue diseases have a higher incidence of aneurysms. Embolization of bacteria, fungi, and tumor tissue to the adventitia of cranial arteries can cause mycotic aneurysms. Endocarditis and cardiac myxomas are the usual causes. About one fifth of patients with aneurysms have more than one vascular anomaly or other aneurysms.

AVMs are the second most common identifiable cause of nontraumatic SAH, accounting for approximately 10 percent of SAHs. Rupture of AVMs often causes ICH and SAH. Bleeding of AVMs is usually less vigorous and under less pressure than aneurysmal bleeding. Other less frequent causes of SAH include bleeding diatheses, trauma, bleeding into meningeal tumors, and the use of sympathomimetic drugs such as methamphetamine and cocaine. Amyloid angiopathy is an important cause of SAH during the geriatric years.

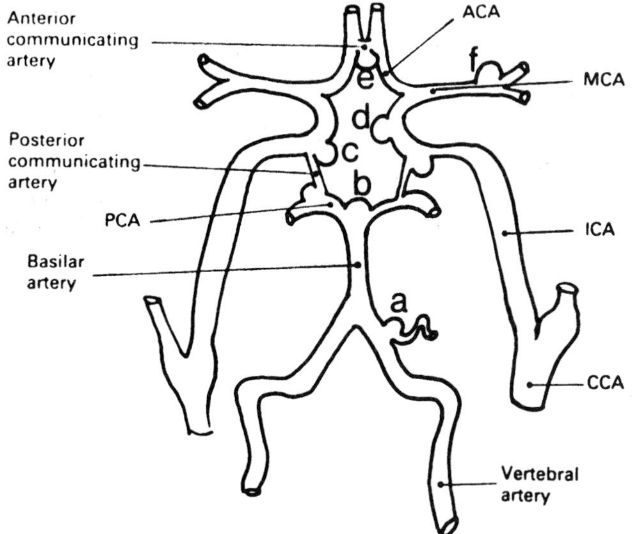

FIGURE 45–10. Most common sites of intracranial aneurysms: posterior inferior cerebellar artery (*a*), basilar artery (*b*), posterior communicating artery (PCA) (*c*), internal carotid artery (ICA) (*d*), anterior communicating artery (ACA) (*e*), and bifurcation of the middle cerebral artery (MCA) (*f*). (Adapted from Caplan LR: Caplan's Stroke: A Clinical Approach, 3rd ed. Boston, Butterworth-Heinemann, 2000.)

Epidemiology and Risk Factors. SAH is a significant cause of worldwide morbidity and mortality, predominantly among young adults of both genders. Most patients are under 60 years of age. Population-based incidence rates for SAH vary from 6 to 16 per 100,000, with the highest rates reported in Finland and Japan. The annual prevalence of aneurysmal SAH in the United States probably exceeds 30,000 persons. Unlike other stroke types, the incidence of SAH has not declined over time. Any apparent decrease is attributable to a higher rate of CT scanning, by which other hemorrhagic conditions are excluded. The incidence of SAH increases with age (mean age of approximately 50 years) and is higher in women than in men. Blacks are at higher risk than whites. Case fatality is approximately 50 percent overall (including pre-hospital deaths) and one third of survivors remain dependent. Population-based mortality rates for SAH have progressively declined, and the survival rate after SAH has improved since the 1970s. Risk factors are the same as for stroke in general; genetic factors operate in only a minority. They include smoking, hypertension, and heavy alcohol use. Use of oral contraceptives, hormone replacement therapy, hypercholesterolemia, and physical activity are not significantly related. During pregnancy, there is also a greater risk of AVM rupture.[45] The risk of SAH is increased during the third trimester of pregnancy. SAH due to aneurysm rupture is a leading cause of maternal mortality, contributing to between 6 and 25 percent of maternal deaths.[68, 69]

Clinical Features and Associated Disorders. A sudden increase in ICP and meningeal irritation cause sudden severe, explosive headache; cessation of physical and intellectual activity; vomiting; and alteration of consciousness. Drowsiness, restlessness, and agitation are especially common. Severe focal neurological signs such as hemiplegia and hemianopia are absent at onset unless the aneurysm also bleeds into the brain. Expanding aneurysms or focal surrounding collections of blood within the cisterns and subarachnoid space can affect the cranial nerves and adjacent brain structures, causing characteristic focal features that depend on the location of the aneurysm. Table 45–8 lists these common focal signs. SAH commonly causes various complications, which are discussed later in association with the management of patients with SAH. A poor clinical condition on admission may be caused by a remediable complication of the initial bleed or a recurrent hemorrhage in the form of intracranial hematoma, acute hydrocephalus, or global brain ischemia.

Diagnosis and Evaluation. The patient's history and neurological examination form the essential cores of SAH diagnosis and grading of clinical status. A CT scan performed within the first 24 hours detects approximately 95 percent of all SAH cases and is also useful in identifying large AVMs. When the clinical signs strongly suggest the diagnosis of SAH but the CT scan is normal, a lumbar puncture to detect blood in the CSF is necessary. After the diagnosis of SAH has been made, cerebral angiography is performed to define and

TABLE 45-8. **Focal Signs in Patients with Aneurysms at Various Sites**

Site of Aneurysms	Clinical Finding
Internal carotid—post communicating	Cranial nerve III palsy
Middle cerebral artery	Contralateral face or hand paresis Aphasia (left side) Contralateral visual neglect (right side)
Anterior communicating	Bilateral leg paresis Bilateral Babinski's signs
Basilar artery apex	Vertical gaze paresis Coma
Intracranial vertebral artery/posterior inferior cerebellar artery	Vertigo Elements of lateral medullary syndrome

localize aneurysm(s).[69] Catheter angiography for detecting aneurysms is gradually being replaced by CT angiography.[68] Severe migraine and meningitis are the major differential diagnostic considerations.

Management. The treatment of patients with SAH involves the prevention and management of the relatively common secondary complications of SAH, rebleeding, vasospasm, hydrocephalus, hyponatremia, and seizures. Rebleeding may be related to variations or changes in blood pressure rather than to absolute blood pressure. Bed rest, analgesics to relieve headache, and stable maintenance of blood pressure using antihypertensive medications in hypertensive patients are generally recommended. Surgical clipping of the aneurysm effectively prevents rebleeding, but there is a dearth of controlled trials assessing the relative benefit of early operation (within 3 days) versus late operation (day 10 to 12), or that of endovascular treatment versus any operation. Interventional endovascular occlusive procedures are often used for aneurysms that cannot be surgically clipped. Because antifibrinolytic therapy has been found to be associated with a higher risk of brain ischemia and no benefits in overall outcome, use of antifibrinolytic agents is usually recommended only in certain clinical situations, for example, patients with low risk of vasospasm or a beneficial effect of delaying surgery.

Cerebral vasospasm is the delayed narrowing of large capacitance arteries at the base of the brain after SAH, which is often associated with radiographic or cerebral blood flow evidence of diminished brain perfusion in the territory of the constricted arteries. About one half of patients with SAH have vasospasm, and this problem may resolve or progress to cerebral infarction. Fifteen to 20 percent of patients with vasospasm die despite maximal therapy. Angiographic vasospasm has a typical temporal course: onset between 3 to 5 days after hemorrhage, maximal narrowing at 5 to 14 days, and gradual resolution over 2 to 4 weeks. Measures of proven value in decreasing the risk of delayed cerebral ischemia are a liberal supply of fluids, avoidance of antihypertensive drugs, and administration of the calcium antagonist nimodipine. Patients should be closely monitored in an intensive care setting for hemodynamic function using TCD. Once ischemia has occurred, so-called "triple H therapy" composed of hypertension, hypervolemia, and hemodilution is recommended. Transluminal angioplasty can be tried.[68]

Acute obstructive hydrocephalus after SAH complicates about 20 percent of cases. Ventriculostomy is recommended in severe cases, although this intervention may be associated with increased rebleeding and infection. Chronic communicating hydrocephalus also occurs frequently. Temporary or permanent CSF diversion is recommended in symptomatic patients. In many patients, hydrocephalus and increased subarachnoid fluid can be managed by repeated lumbar punctures.

Hyponatremia occurs in 10 to 34 percent of cases after SAH. Hypotonic fluids should be avoided, and fluid restriction should not be instituted to treat hyponatremia. Volume should be maintained using isotonic solutions.

Seizure-like episodes occur in 25 percent of patients after SAH. Because of the potential risk of rebleeding, some recommend the administration of prophylactic anticonvulsants. The long-term use of anticonvulsants is not routinely recommended for patients with no seizure episodes and should be considered only for patients with risk factors such as prior seizure, hematoma, infarcts, or MCA aneurysms.

During pregnancy, the management options after SAH are early clipping or early delivery (spontaneous or by cesarean section), with a possible risk of rebleeding during delivery when aneurysms are unclipped. Cesarean section may be appropriate for patients with an acute hemorrhage who are near term, but management is otherwise similar to nonpregnant patients. Craniotomy and clipping have been successfully performed in women at early, mid-, and late stages of pregnancy. No difference is present in prognosis between pregnant and nonpregnant patients with SAH.

Reduction of exposure to the risk factors for SAH might result in a decreased incidence of SAH. Treatment of hypertension with antihypertensive medication, cessation of smoking, and moderation of alcohol use reduces the risk of SAH. Screening of certain high-risk populations for unruptured aneurysms is of uncertain value. Advances in MRA may facilitate screening in the future. In patients with acceptable surgical risk, clipping of unruptured aneurysms larger than 5 to 7 mm is often recommended.[68, 69]

Prognosis and Future Perspectives. At times, the initial bleeding is so severe that death or irreversible brain damage occurs. If the bleeding is limited, the patient survives but is at risk for rebleeding in the days and weeks after the initial SAH. For untreated, ruptured aneurysms, there is a 3 to 4 percent risk of rebleeding in the first 24 hours, 1 to 2 percent risk per day in the first month, and a long-term risk of 3 percent per year after 3 months. Urgent evaluation and treatment of patients with suspected SAH is strongly recommended. Many recent advances in endovascular treatment of aneurysms and AVMs may improve the outcome in patients with lesions that are inaccessible to surgery. The major problem is early recognition and referral to neurological centers for early definitive treatment.[68, 69]

ARTERIOVENOUS MALFORMATIONS

Pathogenesis and Pathophysiology. Vascular malformations are congenital in origin. They are classified into several subtypes according to the predominant vasculature. The most common type is venous angiomas, which are composed of anomalous veins without any direct feeding artery. The next most common is telangiectasia, usually found deep within the brain, particularly in the brain stem. It is composed of vessels morphologically resembling capillaries but slightly larger and is often found at necropsy. Another less common vascular abnormality, which also rarely causes symptoms, is the venous varix. Two other common symptomatic angiomas are AVMs and cavernous angiomas. AVMs are composed of clusters of abnormal arteries and veins of varying size, without intervening capillaries.[70]

Epidemiology and Risk Factors. Vascular malformations are the second most common cause of nontraumatic SAH and ICH. Vascular malformations are one tenth as common as aneurysms; an estimated 1000 new cases are identified in the United States each year. They rupture most commonly during the second and third decades of life. Hemorrhage from malformation is most common during early pregnancy or delivery.

Clinical Features and Associated Disorders. As AVMs enlarge, symptoms are related to a number of mechanisms. They can cause bleeding, seizures, vascular headache, and chronic ischemia. Bleeding is most likely due to fragility of the abnormal vessels. The angiomas that most frequently rupture are of the AVM type. Symptoms and signs depend on the location of hemorrhage. There are usually signs of meningeal irritation due to bleeding into the CSF. Not all ruptures are symptomatic, but evidence of previous bleeding is often observed at necropsy. About one half of the patients present with epilepsy. Progressive neurological signs may develop secondary to a mechanism called intracerebral steal or compression of adjacent brain tissue by the pulsating blood vessels. Chronic migrainous headaches are also a frequent complaint in patients with vascular malformations. Patients with unruptured AVMs may present with increased ICP and papilledema. Angiomas in the brain stem may cause serious bleeding or progressive neurological deficits, which may be fluctuating in clinical course and may simulate multiple sclerosis. Rarely, angiomas, particularly aneurysms of the vein of Galen, present with hydrocephalus by disrupting the normal flow of CSF. Bruits may be audible either to the patient or to the examiner. If there is enough shunting through a large AVM, high-output congestive heart failure may develop, especially in children. In spinal AVMs, the patients may present with back pain, myelopathic symptoms, and root dysfunction. However, headache often accompanies spinal AVM rupture, mimicking aneurysmal SAH. A number of patients with spinal AVMs have intracranial symptoms, including headache, mental status changes, loss of consciousness, papilledema, decreased vision, nystagmus, diplopia, seizures, cranial nerve VI palsy, and oculomotor paresis. Some cavernous angiomas are familial. Patients with hereditary hemorrhagic telangiectasias (Osler-Weber-Rendu syndrome) have a higher than normal incidence of vascular malformations.[1]

Differential Diagnosis and Evaluation. Diagnostic considerations include aneurysms and brain infarcts and tumors. Diagnosis of AVMs can be suspected clinically when young patients present with ICH, seizures, or frequent unilateral headaches. CT scan, MRI, MRA, and TCD are helpful noninvasive tests. However, a confirmative diagnosis is made using angiography, through which therapeutic embolization can sometimes be performed at the same time. On angiography, a typical AVM shows large feeding arteries; a central tangle of vessels; enlarged, tortuous draining veins; and rapid arterial-to-venous shunting of blood.

Management. Direct surgical excision of AVMs has been improved with the use of the operating microscope and often can be carried out with low rates of morbidity and mortality. The major complications of surgical excision are loss of normal brain tissue, with additional loss of neurological function, and the so-called breakthrough phenomenon. This term describes massive brain swelling and ICH occurring postoperatively, which is caused by redirection of the large volume of blood into small vessels that are unable to handle the large volume of blood that previously flowed into the AVM. Endovascular treatment of AVMs using embolization techniques can be used alone, before surgery, or at the time of surgery. It is particularly useful in treating lesions that are not surgically accessible and as an adjunct to surgical removal. Complications include hemorrhage, ischemic stroke, and angionecrosis due to toxicity of the embolic materials.[71] Radiotherapy of AVMs with high-energy x-rays, gamma rays, and protons induces subendothelial deposition of collagen and hyaline substances, which narrow the lumen of small vessels and shrink the nidus of the malformations by progressive occlusion of vessels during the months after treatment. Recent techniques focus the radiation beam on small regions. An example is the so-called gamma knife, a system that uses a cobalt source to generate highly collimated gamma rays that converge on a focal point. Modified linear accelerators can now deliver radiation to a defined volume of tissue with very good accuracy. Complications include radionecrosis of normal brain, bleeding, hydrocephalus, immediate post-therapy seizures, loss of body temperature regulation, and possibly long-term cognitive function deficits.[72] Forms of medical management include strict control of blood pressure and avoidance of anticoagulants and antiplatelet drugs. Because pregnancy increases risk of bleeding, appropriate contraception may be recommended in fertile women with an AVM.

Prognosis and Future Perspectives. In the short term, the prognosis of ruptured AVMs and cavernous angiomas is better than that of aneurysms. The rebleeding rate is low during the first few months. Only 6 percent of patients rebleed during the first year, and vasospasm occurs only rarely. Mortality from the first hemorrhage is low, only about 10 percent. However, in the long term, the prognosis of AVMs is not as good. With subsequent hemorrhages, the mortality rate is higher, about 20 percent. With each recurrence, the chances of additional bleeding increase. Improved noninvasive diagnosis using MRI and MRA and improved methods of treatment (endovascular and radiotherapy) promise to help reduce the rates of morbidity and mortality of this serious vascular condition.

Traumatic Neurovascular Diseases

CAROTID–CAVERNOUS SINUS FISTULAS

A carotid–cavernous sinus fistula (CCF) is an abnormal communication between the cavernous sinus and the carotid arterial system. CCFs usually develop after head trauma but can occur spontaneously. CCFs are classified into direct and dural types. The most common type is the direct type (70 to 90 percent) in which there is a direct connection between the intracavernous portion of the ICA and the cavernous sinus. This is a high-flow type often caused by a traumatic tear of the arterial wall. The dural types are communications between the cavernous sinus and meningeal arterial branches of the ICA, of the external carotid artery, or of both. They develop spontaneously or in the setting of atherosclerosis, systemic hypertension, or collagen vascular disease and during and after childbirth. These fistulas usually are of the low-flow type and almost always produce symptoms and signs spontaneously without antecedent trauma.

Patients with a direct CCF may develop monocular visual loss and abnormalities of the oculomotor nerves (III, IV, VI) ipsilaterally or bilaterally. Ocular manifestations include diplopia, proptosis, ocular bruit, chemosis, ocular pulsation, dilatation of retinal veins, optic disc swelling, visual loss, and, potentially, glaucoma. There are often signs of intracranial hypertension. Trigeminal nerve dysfunction is the most common cranial nerve abnormality. Dural types usually occur in middle-aged or elderly women. They present similar clinical symptoms and signs but are less severe than those of the direct type.

If a CCF is suspected, CT or MRI and ocular ultrasonography are performed and often show enlarged extraocular muscles, dilated superior ophthalmic veins, and an enlarged affected cavernous sinus. The ultimate diagnostic test is cerebral arteriography of both the bilateral internal and external carotid arteries. Recently CT angiography has been used for diagnosis.[73]

Urgent treatment is indicated in patients who have rapidly deteriorating vision, hemorrhage, and intracranial hypertension. Surgical repair of the damaged portion of the intracavernous ICA is only rarely used these days. Endovascular occlusion using detachable balloons has a success rate of 90 to 100 percent with low complication rates (2 to 5 percent).[74] The recurrence rate is 1 to 3.9 percent, and recurrence often responds to second balloon treatment. Early complications include migration of balloons and thromboembolism resulting in stroke; delayed complications are pseudoaneurysm formation and persistent ophthalmoplegias. If the condition is left untreated, almost all patients have progressive ocular problems, including increasing proptosis, chemosis, and visual loss. The most feared complications are central retinal vein occlusion and secondary glaucoma. Endovascular techniques have greatly improved the prognosis of CCFs. Most symptoms and signs usually disappear within days after treatment or at least improve with this procedure, but complete resolution may take weeks to months.[75,76]

SUBDURAL HEMATOMAS

A subdural hematoma (SDH) results from venous bleeding after blunt head trauma, which causes brain motion within the skull, shearing off the bridging veins between the surface of the brain and adjacent dural venous sinuses. The blood leaks and collects slowly in the subdural space. A chronic SDH usually develops after minor trauma, typically in an elderly person under anticoagulation or in an alcoholic individual with some degree of brain atrophy. Bleeding may continue around the atrophic brain, causing headaches, behavioral changes, altered level of consciousness, or a focal neurological deficit such as hemiparesis. Patients under anticoagulation and those with bleeding disorders may develop spontaneous SDH. Occasionally, subdural collections develop after lumbar puncture. Head trauma is often forgotten or considered too inconsequential to mention. A fall frequently causes retrograde amnesia and the patient may not have been fully aware of the injury. An SDH may be absorbed spontaneously or may form an encapsulated and liquefied hematoma. After about 2 weeks, membranes form around the hematoma. The outer membrane is thicker and more vascular than the inner membrane. The center of the encapsulated SDH liquefies and may enlarge due to repeated bleeding from the vascular outer membrane, assuming a progressively larger biconvex lens shape. Acute SDHs develop after severe head trauma and carry a poor prognosis, with a mortality rate of 50 percent even if treated.

The most common presentations of SDHs are headache, decreased level of alertness, and abnormalities of cortical function. Headache is usually ipsilateral to the hematoma and may be worse at night. Drowsiness and decreased alertness reflect an increase in ICP. There is often slight weakness, hyper-reflexia, and Babinski sign contralateral to the hematoma. Slight aphasia may develop in patients with left-sided hematomas, and neglect of the right side of space occurs in patients with right subdural hematomas. Usually, the neurological abnormalities are soft and seldom are as profound as those deficits that occur in patients with large hemisphere infarcts or intracerebral hematomas. Seizures may occur and probably indicate some contusion of the underlying brain tissue as the hematoma enlarges, headache worsens, and the level of consciousness often decreases. An ipsilateral Babinski sign or elements of an ipsilateral cranial nerve III palsy, or both, may develop and indicate midbrain compression. The diagnosis is usually obvious in patients with head injury. The insidious development of symptoms, especially in patients who provide no history of trauma, can readily mimic brain tumor or abscess. Cerebral infarcts and hematomas usually present with more acute-onset symptoms and signs and more severe focal deficits. On a CT scan, an acute SDH appears as a sickle-shaped, hyperdense lesion over the outer surface of the brain lying against the inner surface of the skull and dura. A chronic SDH appears hypodense on CT scans. MRI clearly demonstrates the extra-axial hematoma and particularly is useful when a subacute hematoma appears isodense on CT.

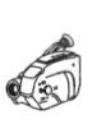

If an SDH is left untreated, it may cause a severe neurological deficit or death. SDHs should be surgically evacuated. The prognosis is primarily related to the degree of associated brain injury. In older patients and in those with brain atrophy, re-expansion of the compressed brain may be delayed. Because subdural bleeding may recur, a drain must be left in for days and the patient must be watched carefully for continued bleeding. Recovery is usually excellent in patients in whom SDHs are recognized and treated. Small SDHs are common and may heal spontaneously without surgical treatment. Because SDHs represent a very treatable cause of cognitive dysfunctions and neurological signs in the elderly prone to falls, improved screening of these patients would be an important public health advance.[77]

EPIDURAL HEMATOMAS

An epidural hematoma (EDH) develops when blood collects between the skull and the dura mater as the result of a severe head injury causing a fracture of the squamous portion of the temporal bone and producing a tear in the middle meningeal artery. Rarely, an EDH may be venous in origin due to laceration of the middle meningeal vein or a dural venous sinus. Blood escaping under arterial pressure dissects the dura inward away from the bone and forms a hematoma. The most common location of EDH is along the lateral wall of the middle cranial fossa. The underlying brain is displaced inward, and brain herniation may follow. Epidural hematomas are less common when compared with subdural hematomas. They may be an important cause of death in patients with severe head injury. Subdural, intracerebral, and subarachnoid hemorrhages often co-exist. Classically, the patient often has a lucid interval just after head trauma and then often has a progressive reduction in the level of consciousness as the hematoma enlarges. The initial injury causes brain concussion and loss of consciousness from which the patient awakens; the patient may have some degree of headache but seems to have otherwise recovered. The acute development of epidural bleeding causes pressure on the ipsilateral cerebral hemisphere and headache, reduction in consciousness, and abnormalities of function of the ipsilateral hemisphere. Downward transtentorial herniation may develop rapidly, causing dilatation of the ipsilateral pupil due to cranial nerve III compression and an ipsilateral hemiparesis due to compression of the contralateral cerebral peduncle of the midbrain against the contralateral tentorial edge. Altered mental status and hemiparesis develop before signs of brain herniation. Diagnosis is made by CT. The hematoma typically appears as a biconvex lens–shaped hyperdense lesion. There is an underlying skull fracture. Epidural hematomas should be surgically evacuated as soon as possible. There is no place for conservative management. Rapid drainage can be life saving, and the outcome is usually excellent when the hematomas are rapidly removed. Death usually results from unrecognized EDH.[78]

SPINAL CORD STROKES

Pathogenesis and Pathophysiology. Spinal cord strokes are very rare in comparison to strokes in the brain. Spinal cord infarcts are most often caused by interruption of the blood flow in one or more of the arteries that feed into the anterior spinal arterial system, which runs in the ventral midline from the medullospinal junction rostrally to the conus medullaris and the filum terminale caudally. This system is supplied by 5 to 10 single radicular arteries. The cervical region is supplied by the branches of the intracranial VA and inferiorly by branches of the thyrocervical and costocervical branches of the subclavian arteries. The thoracic and lumbar spinal cord segments are fed by radicular arterial branches of the deep cervical and intercostal arteries and branches of the aorta. The lower thoracic cord is supplied by direct branches from the aorta, the largest of which is the artery of Adamkiewicz, which most often enters between T12 and L2. The sacral cord and cauda equina are supplied by branches of the hypogastric and obturator arteries. This system is vulnerable to interruption of flow through any one of the feeding arteries. Resulting infarcts usually affect the anterior horns and the lateral and ventral white matter columns. In contrast to the anterior spinal artery system, there are paired posterior spinal arteries, which are fed by small posterior radicular arteries. The posterior spinal arteries supply the posterior columns and posterior gray horns of the spinal cord. Because of the multiple feeding channels, this system is very resistant to interruption of its blood supply. Interruption of blood flow in anterior spinal branches is probably most often due to diseases within the aorta, including aortic aneurysms, surgery on the aorta, aortic dissections, and emboli from atheromatous aortic plaques. Disc cartilage can also fragment and enter spinal arteries and veins and lead to infarction. Arteriovenous fistulas are an important cause of spinal cord infarction in older men. Direct communications developing between radicular arteries and veins outside the dura mater greatly increase pressure in the venous system, and large drainage veins develop on the surface of the spinal cord. At the same time, shunting of blood decreases flow to the spinal cord from the feeding artery. In order to maintain adequate spinal perfusion, the pressure of blood in the arterial system must exceed venous pressure. The spinal-dural AV fistula often creates a situation in which venous pressure exceeds arterial pressure intermittently, and ischemia develops. At first, ischemia can be intermittent, and spinal cord TIAs can result. Adhesive arachnoiditis following infection of the meninges (syphilis, tuberculosis, and Lyme borreliosis) and parasitic invasion of the spinal arteries (schistosomiasis) can cause obliteration of spinal arteries and lead to cord ischemia. Hypoxic-ischemic injury to the spinal cord also develops in patients with severe systemic hypotension and shock. Spinal cord hemorrhage most often results from trauma. Bleeding diathesis, especially anticoagulation, is another important cause. Aneurysms of intradural arteries and intradural AVMs and cavernous angiomas are other causes of spinal cord hemorrhages.

Clinical Features and Diagnosis. Spinal cord infarcts usually develop abruptly. Most spinal strokes are thoracic or lumbar, so that the lower extremities are selectively involved. The most common signs are motor and include both lower motor neuron and upper motor neuron abnormalities within the lower limbs. Paraplegia is usually symmetrical. There may be a pain and temperature level along the thorax. Sphincter function is most often lost. Posterior column functions (vibration and position sense) are usually spared. The findings are most often roughly symmetrical. When the lesion is asymmetrical or unilateral, sensory dissociation occurs, producing a Brown-Séquard–like pattern. In patients with spinal-dural AV fistulas, TIAs and steplike development of deficits are common.

Almost always, the symptoms and signs allow recognition that the lesion is spinal. Occasionally, medullary and pontine infarction can be a consideration. Tumors, abscesses, and syrinxes usually cause symptoms that develop gradually, but hemorrhage into a spinal cord tumor, most often an ependymoma, can be an important consideration. Spinal cord compression caused by cancer, epidural and subdural infections, and hematomas are other considerations. Almost all compressive spinal cord lesions involve the vertebral column. Plain bone x-ray studies and CT, MRI, and bone scans can yield information about osseous lesions that could compress the spinal cord. MRI is the best method to visualize the spinal cord, dura mater, and overlying bony structures. MRI can show spinal hemorrhages and infarcts and can identify the presence of spinal cord compression. MRI is not very sensitive for the detection of spinal-dural AV fistulas. Myelography may be needed to show the characteristic dilated veins that course on the surface of the spinal cord. Lumbar puncture is helpful in identifying spinal hemorrhage and infection. Spinal angiography is often necessary to characterize spinal vascular malformations and fistulas.

Management and Prognosis. There is little information about treatment of patients with spinal cord infarcts. Definitive treatment depends, as it does in the brain, on identification of the etiology in the individual patient. Hemorrhage, infection, and infarction can be separated by MRI and lumbar puncture. Identification of spinal-dural AV fistulas is very important because obliteration of the abnormalities can prevent further spinal cord damage. Rehabilitation and management of sphincter functions is similar to that pursued in other diseases of the spinal cord. Outcome depends almost entirely on the cause of the spinal cord vascular damage. In the future, we need to develop more accurate ways to study the aortic blood supply to the spinal cord. Intravascular ultrasound is promising. Perhaps further development of MRA and venography will be helpful and obviate the need for spinal angiography, which can be hazardous. Basic research on spinal cord protection may help limit damage in patients with vascular spinal cord insults.[1]

Strokes in the Young

Strokes in children younger than age 15 are often different from those found in adults. Brain infarcts tend to be limited more to the deeper regions of the cerebral hemispheres, especially the striatocapsular areas. Vascular occlusive lesions are more often intracranial and affect mostly the intracranial carotid and the middle cerebral and basilar arteries. Extracranial lesions are less common; when they occur, they usually involve the pharyngeal portions of the carotid and vertebral arteries rather than the arterial origins that are involved more commonly in adults. Vasoconstriction, dissection, fibromuscular dysplasia, trauma, and contiguous infection are the major conditions that affect the extracranial arteries of children. When the vascular occlusive process or embolism involves the MCA, vascular compromise is maximal in the territory of the lenticulostriate branches. Because of the invariable absence of severe occlusive disease, collateral circulation over the convexities is abundant. This explains the striatocapsular localization of infarcts. Because atherosclerosis is very rare in youth, the types of vasculopathies that cause brain ischemia in children are much more diverse than in adults, and the differential diagnosis is very broad. Congenital cardiac disease is an important cause of stroke in children. Table 45–9 lists the most important causes of brain ischemia in children younger than age 15 years.

ICH and SAH, especially from aneurysms and vascular malformations, comprise a much higher percentage of strokes in children than they do in adults.[79]

In young adults, premature atherosclerosis and stroke risk factors are much more important than in youths. Cardiac disease and hematological diseases and cancer provide a higher proportion of infarcts in young adults than during the geriatric years. Table 45–10 lists the major differential considerations of brain ischemia in persons 15 to 40 years of age.[1]

TABLE 45–9. Differential Diagnosis of Pediatric Brain Ischemia (1–15 Years)

Migraine
Trauma: Dissection and other vascular injuries; abuse including whiplash-shake injuries; oral foreign body trauma to the internal carotid artery
Cardiac: Congenital heart disease with right-to-left shunts; tetralogy of Fallot; transposition of great vessels; tricuspid atresia; atrial and ventricular septal defects; cardiomyopathies; endocarditis; pulmonary arteriovenous fistula
Drugs: Especially cocaine and heroin
Infections: Bacterial meningitis, especially *Hemophilus influenzae*, pneumococci, and streptococci; facial, otitic, and sinus infections; AIDS; dural sinus occlusion and infection; tuberculous meningitis
Genetic and metabolic: Neurofibromatosis; hereditary disorders of connective tissue (Marfan's and Ehlers-Danlos syndromes, pseudoxanthoma elasticum); homocystinuria; Menkes' kinky hair syndrome; hypoalphalipoproteinemia; familial hyperlipidemias; methylmalonicaciduria; MELAS syndrome (mitochondrial myopathy, encephalopathy, lactic acidosis, strokes)
Hematological and neoplastic: Sickle cell anemia; purpuras; leukemia; L-asparaginase and aminocaproic acid (Amicar) treatment; radiation vasculopathy; hypercoagulable states (e.g., caused by decrease in natural inhibitors such as antithrombin III)
Arteritis: Collagen vascular disease; local infections; Takayasu's disease; Behçet's disease
Venous sinus thrombosis: Head and neck infections; dehydration; coagulopathy; paroxysmal nocturnal hemoglobinuria; puerperal or pregnancy-related
Systemic disease: Rheumatic; gastrointestinal; renal; hepatic; pulmonary
Moyamoya disease

From Caplan LR, Estol CE: Strokes in youths. *In* Adams HP (ed): Cerebrovascular Disease. New York, Marcel Dekker, 1993, pp 233–254.

TABLE 45–10. **Differential Diagnosis of Ischemia in Young Adults (15–40 Years)**

Migraine
Arterial dissection
Drugs, especially cocaine and heroine
Premature atherosclerosis, hyperlipidemias, hypertension, diabetes, smoking, homocystinuria
Female hormone–related (oral contraceptives, pregnancy, puerperium): eclampsia; dural sinus occlusion; arterial and venous infarcts; peripartum cardiomyopathy
Hematological: Deficiency of antithrombin III, protein C, protein S; fibrinolytic system disorders; deficiency of plasminogen activator; antiphospholipid antibody syndrome; increased factor VIII; cancer; thrombocytosis; polycythemia; thrombotic thrombocytopenic purpura; disseminated intravascular coagulation
Rheumatic and inflammatory: Systemic lupus erythematosus; rheumatoid arthritis; sarcoidosis; Sjögren's syndrome; scleroderma; polyarteritis nodosa; cryoglobulinemia; Crohn's disease; ulcerative colitis
Cardiac: Interatrial septal defect; patent foramen ovale; mitral valve prolapse; mitral annulus calcification; myocardiopathies; arrhythmias; endocarditis
Penetrating artery disease (lacunes); hypertension, diabetes
Others: Moyamoya disease; Behçet's disease; neurosyphilis; Takayasu's disease; Sneddon's disease; fibromuscular dysplasia; Fabry's disease; Cogan's disease

From Caplan LR, Estol CE: Strokes in youths. *In* Adams HP (ed): Cerebrovascular Disease. New York, Marcel Dekker, 1993, pp 233–254.

Reviews and Selected Updates

American Academy of Neurology: Assessment: Carotid endarterectomy. Neurology 1990;40:682–683.

Barnett HJ, Mohr JP, Stein BM, Yatsu FM (eds): Stroke: Pathophysiology, Diagnosis, and Management, 3rd ed. New York, Churchill Livingstone, 1997.

Batjer HH, Caplan LR, Friberg L, Greenlee RG Jr, Kopitnik TA Jr, Young WL (eds): Cerebrovascular Disease. Philadelphia, Lippincott-Raven, 1997.

Bogosslavsky J, Caplan LR (eds): Stroke Syndrome, 2nd ed. Cambridge, Cambridge University Press, 2001.

Caplan LR: Brain Ischemia: Basic Concepts and Clinical Relevance. New York, Springer-Verlag, 1995.

Caplan LR, Hurst JW, Chimowitz MI: Clinical Neurocardiology. New York, Marcel Dekker, 1999.

Caplan LR, Reis D, Siesjo B, et al (eds): Primer of Cerebrovascular Disease. San Diego, Academic Press, 1996.

Donnan G, Norrving B, Bamford J, Bogousslavsky J (eds): Lacunar and Other Subcortical Infarctions. Oxford, Oxford University Press, 1995.

Furlan A, Higashida R, Wechsler L, et al: Intra-arterial prourokinase for acute ischemic stroke. The PROACT II study: a randomized controlled trial. Prolyse in acute cerebral thromboembolism. JAMA 1999;282:2003–2011.

Quality Standards Subcommittee of the American Academy of Neurology: Practice Advisory: Thrombolytic therapy for acute ischemic stroke—summary statement. Neurology 1996;47:835–839.

References

1. Caplan LR: Caplan's Stroke: A Clinical Approach, 3rd ed. Boston, Butterworth-Heinemann, 2000.
2. Caplan LR: TIAs: We need to reurn to the question, "What is wrong with Mr. Jones?" Neurology 1988;38:791–793.
3. Brown RD, Whisnant JP, Sicks JD, et al: Stroke incidence, prevalence, and survival. Secular trends in Rochester, Minnesota, through 1989. Stroke 1996;27:370–372.
4. Sacco RL: Current epidemiology of stroke. *In* Fisher M, Bogousslavsky J (eds): Current Review of Cerebrovascular Disease. Philadelphia, Current Medicine, 1993, pp 3–14.
5. Sacco RL: Newer risk factors for stroke. Neurology 2001;57(Suppl 2):S31–S34.
6. D'Agostino RB, Wolf PA, Belanger AJ, et al: Stroke risk profile: Adjustment for antihypertensive medication. The Framingham Study. Stroke 1994;25:40–43.
7. Whisnant JP: Effectiveness versus efficacy of treatment of hypertension for stroke prevention. Neurology 1996;46:301–307.
8. Caplan LR, Dyken ML, Easton JD: American Heart Association Family Guide to Stroke. New York, Random House, 1994, p 63.
9. Sacco RL, Elkind M, Boden-Albala B, et al: The protective effect of moderate alcohol consumption on ischemic stroke. JAMA 1999;281:53–60.
10. Lin HJ, Wolf PA, Kelly-Hayes M, et al: Stroke severity in atrial fibrillation. The Framingham Study. Stroke 1996;27:1760–1764.
11. Amarenco P: Hypercholesterolemia, lipid lowering agents, and the risk for brain infarction. Neurology 2001;57(Suppl 2):S35–S44.
12. Sacco RL, Boden-Albala B, Gan R, et al: Stroke incidence among whites, blacks and Hispanic residents of an urban community: The Northern Manhattan Stroke Study. Am J Epidemiol 1998;147:259–268.
13. Yoo JH, Chung CS, Kang SS: Relation of plasma homocyst(e)ine to cerebral infarction and cerebral atherosclerosis. Stroke 1998;29: 2478–2483.
14. Elkind MS, Lin IF, Grayston JT, Sacco RL: *Chlamydia pneumoniae* and the risk of first ischemic stroke. The Northern Manhattan Stroke Study. Stroke 2000;31:1521–1525.
15. Fisher CM: Occlusion of the internal carotid artery. Arch Neurol 1951;65:346–377.
16. Feinberg WM, Albers GW, Barnett HJM, et al: Guidelines for management of transient ischemic attacks. From the Ad Hoc committee on guidelines for the management of transient ischemic attacks of the Stroke Council of the American Heart Association. Circulation 1994;89:2950–2965.
17. Albers GW, Amarenco P, Easton JD, Sacco RL, Teal P: Antithrombotic and thrombolytic therapy for ischemic stroke. Chest 2001;119: 300S–320S.
18. Bennett CL, Davidson CJ, Raisch DW, et al: Thrombotic thrombocytopenic purpura associated with ticlopidine in the setting of coronary artery stents and stroke prevention. Arch Intern Med 1999;159:2524–2528.
19. CAPRIE Steering Committee: A randomised, blinded trial of clopidogrel versus aspirin in patients at risk of ischaemic events. Lancet 1996;348:1329–1339.
20. Fisher CM: Lacunar infarcts—a review. Cerebrovasc Dis 1991;1:311–320.
21. Caplan LR: Intracranial branch atheromatous disease: A neglected, understudied, and underused concept. Neurology 1989;39:1246–1250.
22. Chabriat H, Tounier-Lasserue F, Vahedi K: Autosomal dominant migraine with MRI white-matter abnormalities mapping to the CADASIL locus. Neurology 1995;45:1086–1091.
23. Heinzlef O, Cohen A, Amarenco P: Aortic arch atheroma. In Fisher M, Bogousslavsky J (eds): Current Review of Cerebrovascular Disease, 3rd ed. Philadelphia, Butterworth-Heinemann, 1999, pp 107–116.
24. The National Institute of Neurological Disorders and Stroke rt-PA Stroke Study Group: Tissue plasminogen activator for acute ischemic stroke. N Engl J Med 1995;333:1581–1587.
25. von Kummer R, Holle R, Rosin L, et al: Does arterial recanalization improve outcome in carotid territory stroke? Stroke 1995;26: 581–587.
26. Lyden PD, Grotta JC, Levin SR: Intravenous thrombolysis for acute stroke. Neurology 1997;49:14–29.
27. Del Zoppo GJ, Higashida RT, Furlan AJ, et al: PROACT: A phase II randomized trial of recombinant pro-urokinase by direct arterial delivery in acute middle cerebral artery stroke. Prolyse in acute cerebral thromboembolism. Stroke 1998;29:4–11.

28. Wahl A, Meier B, Haxel B, et al: Prognosis after percutaneous closure of patent foramen ovale for paradoxical embolism. Neurology 2001;57:1330–1332.
29. The European Atrial Fibrillation Trial Study Group: Optimal oral anticoagulant therapy in patients with nonrheumatic atrial fibrillation and recent cerebral ischemia. N Engl J Med 1995;333:5–10.
30. Moore WS, Barnett HJM, Beebe HG, et al: Guidelines for carotid endarterectomy. A multidisciplinary consensus statement from the Ad Hoc committee, American Heart Association. Circulation 1995;91:566–579.
31. North American Symptomatic Carotid Endarterectomy Trial Collaborators: Beneficial effect of carotid endarterectomy in symptomatic patients with high-grade stenosis. N Engl J Med 1991;325:445–453.
32. European Carotid Surgery Trialists' Collaborative Group: Randomised trial of endarterectomy for recently symptomatic carotid stenosis: Final results of the MRC European Carotid Surgery Trial (ECST). Lancet 1998;351:1379–1387.
33. Barnett HJM, Taylor DW, Eliasziw M, et al: Benefit of carotid endarterectomy in patients with symptomatic moderate or severe stenosis. N Engl J Med 1998;339:1415–1425.
34. Executive Committee for the Asymptomatic Carotid Atherosclerosis Study. Endarterectomy for asymptomatic carotid artery stenosis. JAMA 1995;273:1421–1428.
35. Inzitari D, Elisziw M, Gates P, et al: The causes and risk of stroke in patients with asymptomatic internal-carotid artery stenosis. N Engl J Med 2000;342:1693–1700.
36. Alamowitch S, Eliasziw M, Algra A, et al, for The North American Symptomatic Carotid Endarterectomy Trial (NASCET) Group: Risk, causes, and prevention of ischemic stroke in elderly patients with symptomatic internal carotid artery stenosis. Lancet 2001;357:1154–1160.
37. CAVATAS investigators: Endovascular versus surgical treatment in patients with carotid stenosis in the Carotid and Vertebral Artery Transluminal Angioplasty Study (CAVATAS): A randomised trial. Lancet 2001;357:1729–1737.
38. Bogousslavsky J, Regli F: Unilateral watershed cerebral infarcts. Neurology 1986;36:373–377.
39. Dobkin BH: Orthostatic hypotension as a risk factor for symptomatic occlusive cerebrovascular disease. Neurology 1989;39:30–34.
40. Mettinger KL, Ericson K: Fibromuscular dysplasia and the brain. Stroke 1982;13:46–52.
41. Suzuki J: Moyamoya Disease. Berlin, Springer-Verlag, 1986.
42. Bousser MG, Kittner SJ: Oral contraceptives and stroke. Cephalalgia 2000;20:183–189.
43. Burkman RT, Collins JA, Shulman LP, Williams JK: Current perspectives on oral contraceptive use. Am J Obstet Gynecol 2001;185(Suppl 2): S4–S12.
44. Grosset DG, Ebrahim S, Bone I, et al: Stroke in pregnancy and the puerperium: What magnitude of risk? J Neurol Neurosurg Psychiatry 1995;58:129–131.
45. Sharshar T, Lamy C, Mas JL: Incidence and causes of strokes associated with pregnancy and puerperium. A study in public hospitals of Ile de France. Stroke in Pregnancy Study Group. Stroke 1995;26:930–936.
46. Simolke GA, Cox SM, Cunningham FG: Cerebrovascular accidents complicating pregnancy and the puerperium. Obstet Gynecol 1991;78:37–42.
47. Martinelli I, Sacchi E, Landi G, et al: High risk of cerebral-vein thrombosis in carriers of a prothrombin-gene mutation and in users of oral contraceptives. N Engl J Med 1998;338:1793–1797.
48. Bousser MG: Cerebral venous thrombosis: Nothing, heparin, or local thrombolysis? Stroke 1999;30:481–483.
49. Fink JN, McAuley DL: Safety of anticoagulation for cerebral venous thrombosis associated with intracerebral hematoma. Neurology 2001;57:1138–1139.
50. Frey JL, Muro GJ, McDougall CG, et al: Cerebral venous thrombosis: Combined intrathrombus rtPA and intravenous heparin. Stroke 1999;30:489–494.
51. de Bruijn SFTM, Stam J, for the Cerebral Venous Sinus Thrombosis Study Group: Randomized, placebo-controlled trial of anticoagulant treatment with low-molecular-weight heparin for cerebral sinus thrombosis. Stroke 1999;30:484–488.
52. Schievink WI: Spontaneous dissection of the carotid and vertebral arteries. N Eng J Med 2001;344:899–906.
53. Caplan LR, Tettenborn B: Vertebrobasilar occlusive disease: Review of selected aspects. 1. Spontaneous dissection of extracranial and intracranial posterior circulation arteries. Cerebrovasc Dis 1992;2:256–265.
54. Baumgartner RW, Arnold M, Baumgartner I, et al: Carotid dissection with and without ischemic events. Local symptoms and cerebral artery findings. Neurology 2001;57:827–832.
55. Bassetti C, Carruzzo A, Sturzenegger M, et al: Recurrence of cervical artery dissection. A prospective study of 81 patients. Stroke 1996;27:1804–1807.
56. Caplan LR: Migraine and vertebrobasilar ischemia. Neurology 1991;41:55–61.
57. Tzourio C, Kittner SJ, Bousser MG, Alperovitch A: Migraine and stroke in young women. Cephalalgia 2000;20:190–199.
58. Levine SR, Brey RL, Sawaya KL, et al: Recurrent stroke and thrombo-occlusive events in the antiphospholipid syndrome. Ann Neurol 1995;38:119–124.
59. Khamashta MA, Cuadrado MJ, Mujic F, et al: The management of thrombosis in the antiphospholipid-antibody syndrome. N Engl J Med 1995;332:993–997.
60. Coull BM, Beamer N, de Garmo P, et al: Chronic blood hyperviscosity in subjects with acute stroke, transient ischemic attack, and risk factors for stroke. Stroke 1991;22:162–168.
61. Caplan LR: Binswanger's disease—revisited. Neurology 1995;45:626–633.
62. Chung CS, Caplan LR, Han W, et al: Thalamic haemorrhage. Brain 1996;119:1873–1886.
63. Chung CS, Caplan LR, Yamamoto Y, et al: Striatocapsular haemorrhage. Brain 2000;123:1850–1862.
64. Chung CS, Caplan LR: Parenchymatous brain hemorrhage. *In* Rakel RE (ed): Conn's Current Therapy. Philadelphia, WB Saunders, 1995, pp 794–798.
65. Broderick JP, Adams HP, Barsan W, et al: Guidelines for the manangement of spontaneous intracerebral hemorrhage. A statement of healthcare professionals from a special writing group of the stroke council, American Heart Association. Stroke 1999;30:905–915.
66. Gebel JM, Borderick JP: Intracerebral hemorrhage. Neurol Clin 2000;19:419–438.
67. Heros RC, Morcos JJ: Cerebrovascular surgery: Past, present, and future. Neurosurgery 2000;47:1007–1033.
68. van Gijn J, Rinkel GJ: Subarachnoid haemorrhage: Diagnosis, causes and management. Brain 2001;124:249–278.
69. Mayberg MR, Batjer HH, Dacey R, et al: Guidelines for the management of aneurysmal subarachnoid hemorrhage. A statement for healthcare professionals from a special writing group of the Stroke Council, American Heart Association. Circulation 1994;90:2592–2605.
70. McCormick WF: The pathology of vascular ("arteriovenous") malformations. J Neurosurg 1966;27:807–816.
71. Fournier D, TerBrugge KG, Willinsky R, et al: Endovascular treatment of intracerebral arteriovenous malformations: Experience in 49 cases. J Neurosurg 1991;75:228–233.
72. Heros R, Korosue K: Radiation treatment of cerebral arteriovenous malformations. N Engl J Med 1990;323:127–129.
73. Anderson K, Collie DA, Capewell A: CT angiographic appearances of carotico-cavernous fistula. Clin Radiol 2001;56:514–516.
74. Kwan E, Hieshima GB, Higashida RT, et al: Interventional neuroradiology in neuro-ophthalmology. J Clin Neuro-Ophthalmol 1989;9:83–97.
75. Redekop G, Marotta T, Weill A: Treatment of traumatic aneurysms and arteriovenous fistulas of the skull base by using endovascular stents. J Neurosurg 2001;95:412–419.
76. Annesley-Williams DJ, Goddard AJ, Brennan RP, et al: Endovascular approach to treatment of indirect carotico-cavernous fistulae. Br J Neurosurg 2001;15:228–233.
77. El-Kadi H, Kaufman HH (eds): Chronic subdural hematoma. Neurosurgery Clinics of North America 2000;11(3).
78. Samudrala S, Cooper PR: Traumatic intracranial hematomas. *In* Wilkins RH, Rengachary SS (eds): Principles of Neurosurgery, 2nd ed. Vol. 3. London, Wolfe, 1994, pp 2797–2807.
79. Caplan LR, Estol CE: Strokes in youths. *In* Adams HP (ed): Cerebrovascular Disease. New York, Marcel Dekker, 1993, pp 233–254.

CHAPTER 46

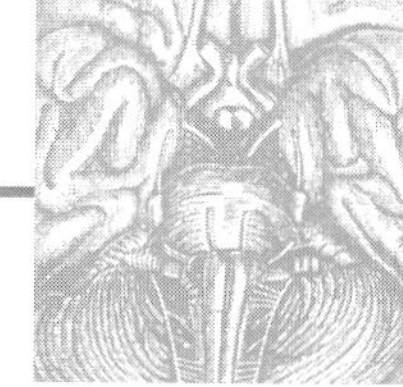

TODD J. JANUS and W. K. ALFRED YUNG

Primary Neurological Tumors

History

Primary malignant brain tumors have been a cause of increasing concern in the last several years. There has been a steady rise in the incidence of primary brain tumors, with an almost 25 percent increase during the past two decades, perhaps due to improved detection with neuroradiological imaging.[1, 2] Although the incidence of some tumors such as lung cancer has declined, and improvements in therapy have increased survival for other tumors such as breast cancer, the incidence of brain tumors continues to increase. Just as important as the rise in incidence is the fact that the need for treatment of these neoplasms is urgent because they afflict the young in disproportionate numbers, significantly affecting their chances of living productive lives.

According to statistics gathered by the American Cancer Society for 2002, the annual incidence of brain and other nervous system cancers is 17,000 involving 9600 men and 7400 women (Table 46–1). More than half of these cases are malignant gliomas. The annual death rate for brain and other nervous system tumors remains high. For comparison, the estimated annual incidence of breast cancer is 205,000 and 30,800 for leukemia. In children, brain tumors are the most common solid tumor and are second only to leukemias in overall incidence.

Early studies date back centuries to descriptions or drawings of lethal brain tumors discovered at autopsy. In 1828, John Ambercrombie published the first pathological descriptions of brain tumors in his monograph *Pathological and Practical Research on Disease of the Brain and Spinal Cord.* The first acknowledged resection of a brain tumor was performed in London in 1884, after Hughes Bennett provided sufficient clinical localization to permit Rickham Godlee to perform a craniotomy. Even then, doctors were quick to announce their findings in the lay press, and a report documenting the operation was published in *The London Times* a mere 21 days following the procedure. Formal reports of the operation were later published in the medical literature. The first monograph

TABLE 46–1. **Frequency of Primary CNS Tumors**

Children (0–14 Years)		Adults (≥15 Years)	
Type	**Percentage**	**Type**	**Percentage**
Glioblastoma	20	Glioblastoma	50
Astrocytoma	21	Astrocytoma	10
Ependymoma	7	Ependymoma	2
Oligodendroglioma	1	Oligodendroglioma	3
Medulloblastoma	24	Medulloblastoma	2
Neuroblastoma	3	Neurilemmoma	2
Neurilemmoma	1	Pituitary adenoma	4
Craniopharyngioma	5	Craniopharyngioma	1
Meningioma	5	Meningioma	17
Teratoma	2	Pinealoma	1
Pinealoma	2	Hemangioma	2
Hemangioma	3	Sarcoma	1
Sarcoma	1		
Others	5	Others	5
Total	100	Total	100

on brain tumors was prepared 4 years later by Sir Byron Bramwell.

Pathological criteria for the diagnosis of primary brain tumors remained under study and were controversial for almost a century. Even at the turn of the century, surgeons complained bitterly that a lack of precise pathological criteria hindered diagnosis. Fedor Krause, in his three-volume *Surgery of the Brain and Spinal Cord* (1912), described several successful tumor surgical procedures in which the neuropathologist was either unable or unwilling to venture a diagnosis. Bailey and Cushing published the first modern treatise on brain tumors and pathological description in 1932. Previously, they had histologically defined and coined the term *medulloblastoma*.[3] Use of this term to refer to a blue cell tumor of the posterior fossa continues to spark debate.[4]

In the first half of this century, Cushing continued to develop and refine the techniques of neurosurgical removal and localization, including angiography and pneumoencephalography. Greg Walter described the first use of electroencephalography for tumor localization in 1936. Improvements in radiotherapy and chemotherapy[5] during the second half of this century marked the emergence of neuro-oncology as a multidisciplinary field. In the 21st century, analysis of the biological markers and genetic behavior of these tumors is expected to advance the ability of clinicians to treat effectively this class of cancers.

Neuroectodermal Tumors

LOW-GRADE GLIOMA, ASTROCYTOMA, AND PILOCYTIC ASTROCYTOMA

Pathogenesis and Pathophysiology. The diagnosis of glioma remains one of the most difficult areas of neuro-oncology. As advances occur in the understanding of biological behaviors and cellular markers of these tumors, the diagnostic criteria continue to change. The popularity of stereotactic biopsy has resulted in problems of firm diagnosis because small tissue samples may not be representative of the entire tumor. Furthermore, previously determined diagnostic criteria have been found to be inconsistent; therefore, comparing results of clinical trials of radiotherapy and chemotherapy have often been unreliable because the patient populations for individual studies were not homogeneous. Finally, histological interpretation does not necessarily predict biological behavior in the individual patient.

Recent attempts to devise a grading system that provides ease of interpretation and interobserver consistency have had limited success. For example, the St. Anne-Mayo (Daumas-Duport) system proposed a modification of previous grading schemes that relied on histological criteria, including nuclear atypia, mitosis, vascular endothelial proliferation, and necrosis as differentiating features. A point system was assigned to these histological variables, as follows: grade 1 tumors had none of these features, grade 2 tumors had one feature, grade 3 had two features, and grade 4 had three or more features. In the initial evaluation, these groups led to distinct median survival curves, but a subsequent review of 251 cases at the Massachusetts General Hospital found no statistical difference in survival between patients with grade 2 and 3 tumors.[6] Even when the histological criteria are consistent, clinical features such as age or extent of resection alter the survival characteristics. For example, a patient with an astrocytoma at age 20 has a median survival of 5 to 10 years, whereas a patient at age 60 may have a survival similar to that characteristic of a malignant astrocytoma.

The modified Ringertz system remains the most reasonable grading scheme for astrocytic gliomas. It separates these tumors into three categories (Table 46–2): astrocytoma, anaplastic astrocytoma, and glioblastoma multiforme. This grading system appears to correlate best with survival. The recent World Health Organization classification incorporates the Ringertz system, assigning grades II to IV, respectively, to these histological categories and including a fourth category, pilocytic astrocytoma, as grade I (Fig. 46–1). Even with current research, necrosis remains the only significant histological predictor of survival.

Astrocytomas can infiltrate and invade vital neural systems and may prohibit complete surgical removal. They

TABLE 46–2. **Histological Criteria for Cerebral Gliomas**

Astrocytomas
1. Uniform cells closely resembling mature resting or reactive, nonanaplastic astrocytes
2. Moderate cell density
3. Mitoses absent or very rare

Anaplastic astrocytoma
1. Increased cellular and/or nuclear pleomorphism
2. Increased cell density
3. Increased mitoses
4. Vascular endothelial proliferation

Glioblastoma multiforme
1. All of above
2. Foci of coagulative necrosis

eventually lead to death because of this disruption of neural systems or because of increased intracranial pressure due to volume expansion. Histologically, they appear to be characterized by increased cell number and nuclear pleomorphism without necrosis. Mitotic figures should not be present. Microcystic changes separate these tumors from a glial reaction.

Pilocytic astrocytomas are commonly found in the cerebellum, brain stem, thalamus, and optic nerve tracts of preteenage youths, but they can occur in individuals up to 30 or 40 years of age. They have a gelatinous appearance, are often well circumscribed, and, if in a favorable location, can be totally excised. Histologically, they have a highly recognizable pattern marked by fibrillary astrocytes and stellate cells. Rosenthal fibers and microcystic changes are often evident. Pleomorphic xanthoastrocytomas are cerebral tumors with lipid-filled cytoplasm found in teens and young adults. Subependymal giant cell astrocytomas are common in the initial decades of life of patients with tuberous sclerosis and arise from the lateral ventricles. Brain stem gliomas are seen in younger individuals and usually are present in the pons or medulla. They rarely undergo biopsy. Magnetic resonance imaging (MRI) usually demonstrates a "fat" pons without gadolinium enhancement. Cervicomedullary gliomas carry a more favorable prognosis than pontine gliomas because brain stem gliomas in the medulla tend to be lower-grade tumors.

Epidemiology and Risk Factors. Gliomas are the most common tumors of the brain and spinal cord.[7] Astrocytomas occur most commonly in the 20- to 40-year-old age group and represent about 15 percent of all primary CNS tumors (see Table 46–1). The incidence of low-grade gliomas appears to be on the rise, perhaps because they are often diagnosed incidentally when patients undergo neuroradiological imaging for other reasons such as trauma.[8] Patients with astrocytomas

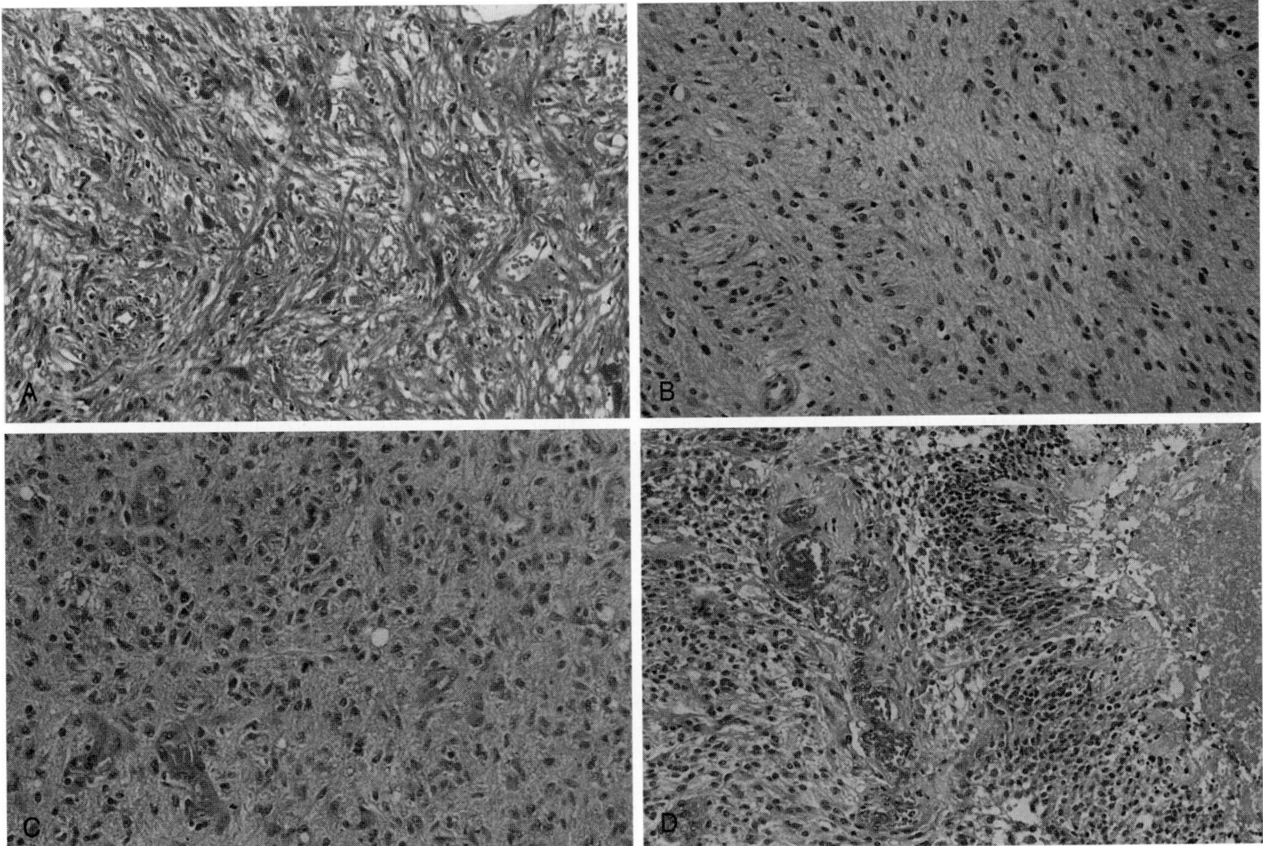

FIGURE 46–1. Histopathological picture of four types of astrocytomas. *A,* Pilocytic astrocytoma, elongated bipolar tumor cells forming a dense fibrillary matrix with numerous Rosenthal fibers. *B,* Astrocytoma, elongated hyperchromatic nuclei with diffused infiltration of the white matter (note lack of nuclear pleomorphism). *C,* Anaplastic astrocytoma, demonstrating nuclear pleomorphism, frequent mitosis, and vascular proliferation. *D,* Glioblastoma, small, anaplastic tumor cells, vascular proliferation, and areas of necrosis with pseudopalisading of tumor cells.

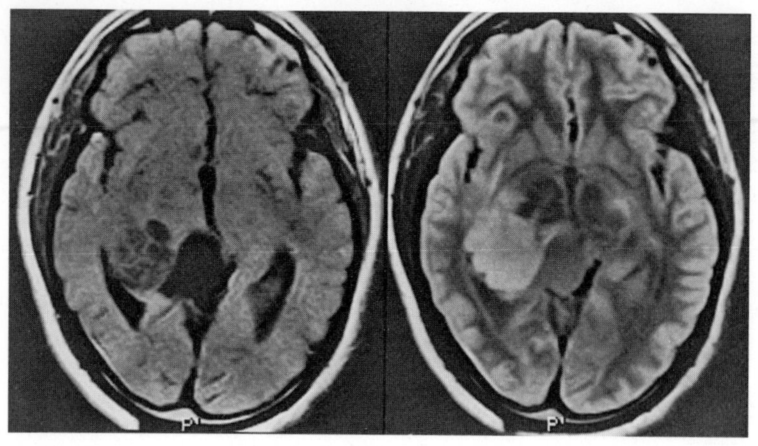

FIGURE 46–2. MRI of a low-grade astrocytoma, demonstrating a hypointense right temporal lesion without contrast enhancement on T1 and hyperintense signal on T2.

have a more favorable median survival than those with glioblastomas. But because astrocytomas are usually found in young people, even a survival time of 5 to 10 years appears unfavorable to the patient and the family. As a rule of thumb, gliomas in children are more often found in the posterior fossa, whereas gliomas in adults are most often located in the cerebral hemispheres. So far, there are no known risk factors associated with the development of astrocytomas.

Clinical Features and Associated Disorders. Patients presenting with low-grade gliomas may have a very gradual onset of symptoms, including headache or subtle neurobehavioral changes. Slowly evolving neurological deficits also raise suspicion of a malignant lesion. These tumors can grow very slowly, and diagnosis may be difficult on initial presentation. For example, increased difficulty with schoolwork or other cognitive tasks is easily blamed on social problems but may indicate a neurological malignancy. Patients with brain stem gliomas present with oculomotor problems or symptoms that may be confused with spinal cord involvement.

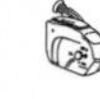

Seizures can also occur and may be either focal or generalized; if subtle, they may be mistakenly associated with psychological problems such as anxiety or panic attacks. Among patients with a new onset of seizures, about 5 percent are found to harbor a tumor, although approximately 25 percent of patients with gliomas have seizures. If patients who have previously had seizures experience an alteration in seizure characteristics or frequency, or if the seizures become refractory to medication, a re-evaluation with MRI scanning with gadolinium may be warranted. Occasionally, patients with new-onset seizures have normal MRI scans. In these patients, the seizures may be increasingly difficult to control. Repeat neuroradiological imaging after 3 to 6 months may uncover an astrocytoma or other mass lesion.

Differential Diagnosis. The differential diagnosis of astrocytomas includes other malignant gliomas (anaplastic astrocytoma, oligodendroglioma, and glioblastoma multiforme) or primary CNS lymphoma and metastatic lesions. Nonmalignant diagnoses such as abscesses and viral infections including herpes encephalitis or demyelinating processes should also be considered. In most patients the symptoms evolve slowly over a period of weeks. Occasionally, in older patients a stroke may be diagnosed because a low-attenuation lesion vaguely following a vascular pattern is discovered after a sudden onset of new symptoms. Later, with deterioration of the patient's condition, which is occasionally diagnosed as a progressive stroke in evolution, repeat imaging shows an expanding mass, later diagnosed as a tumor and most likely responsible for the initial symptoms. One must always beware of attempts to diagnose lesions histopathologically based on radiological imaging.

Evaluation. Low-grade gliomas are often seen as diffusely hypodense or isodense lesions with some flattening of the cortical gyral areas on computed tomography (CT) or significant changes on T2-weighted images on MRI (Figs. 46–2 and 46–3). There is correspondingly less edema formation. Often low-grade tumors are not enhanced or there may be

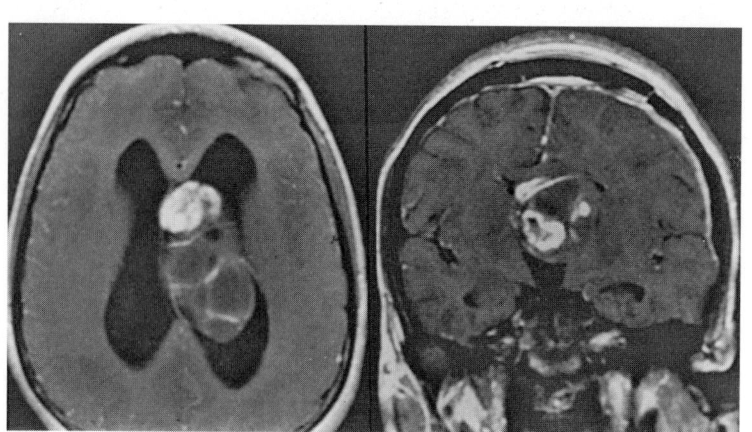

FIGURE 46–3. MRI of a juvenile pilocytic astrocytoma (JPA) of the thalamus, demonstrating contrast enhancement among a hypointense lesion budding into the lateral ventricle.

very small areas of enhancement that become more evident on triple-dose gadolinium injection. The presence or absence of enhancement does not predict the pathological diagnosis in an individual patient.

Surgical evaluation is usually needed to establish the diagnosis. Although a pilocytic astrocytoma of the cerebellum can often be fully resected, hemispheric astrocytomas are diffuse, and occasionally only a biopsy can be performed. Attempts should be made to perform a biopsy of any small enhancing areas to increase the likelihood of obtaining a representative sample for pathological examination. Surgical intervention for brain stem gliomas was previously thought to be impossible except in some cystic tumors that were amenable to decompression. Recent reports suggest that CT-guided biopsy may be feasible. The morbidity rate was found to be around 5 percent, and, surprisingly, 12 percent of the patients who underwent biopsy were found to have a benign pathology, usually infectious in nature.[9] Nonmalignant causes were seen more often in patients with focal enhancing lesions. Therefore, biopsy may be reasonable in selected patients at centers qualified to perform such procedures.

Management. Although surgery can be curative in patients with pilocytic astrocytomas, it is rarely an option or successful in those with low-grade gliomas. Previous therapeutic interventions were designed to treat symptomatic patients. With an increase in the number of patients diagnosed incidentally and presymptomatically, specific treatment regimens for these patients remain highly controversial. Further, the small number of patients diagnosed with these tumors has led to limited enrollment in clinical trials. The evolution of histological criteria, variable patient clinical status, and prolonged patient accrual periods have all led to more heterogeneous criteria for patient inclusion in treatment studies. Thus, there are no large randomized studies available by which to evaluate the results of postsurgery radiotherapy or chemotherapy in these patients. Recently, questions have been raised about whether purported tumors found on radiological imaging even need to undergo biopsy, let alone treatment with radiation.[10] Because histological criteria cannot predict biological behavior, some clinicians advocate the use of serial neuroradiological imaging to establish the growth characteristics of these tumors without intervention that might distort the natural history. One recent study examines the neurocognitive effects of radiation therapy as compared to watchful waiting and found a significant risk of neurocognitive dysfunction with the radiotherapy. The majority patients in this study, however, were not biopsied, and thus the true number of patients with a low-grade glioma is not known.[11]

Most studies favor maximal surgical removal and radiotherapy, although certain subgroups of patients may benefit more from this combined treatment than others. Concern has been raised that because these tumors are so slow growing, standard radiation therapy with 60 to 66 Gy for 6 weeks may not provide treatment when the tumor is less radiation sensitive. Delaying radiotherapy would also delay the neurotoxic effects of radiation that are found many years after treatment, thereby perhaps improving the patient's quality of life. There are incidental reports of successful treatment with chemotherapy following radiotherapy; however, no data are available to support these treatments. Chemotherapy is useful if recurrence is documented and surgical biopsy confirms that the tumor has undergone malignant degeneration.

Pilocytic astrocytomas can be treated with surgical removal alone. Radiotherapy should be reserved for patients in whom resection has been incomplete and evidence of tumor progression is found on clinical evaluation and neuroradiological imaging. Tumors in patients over age 20 can behave more aggressively and should be closely monitored. Cranial irradiation and chemotherapy should be considered following surgery in older patients.

Previous studies have not systematically evaluated the neurobehavioral impact of radiotherapy on long-term survivors. A decline in neurocognitive status 3 to 4 years following radiotherapy has been found in children.[12] Patients must be made aware of the risk of late-onset cognitive decline. Astrocytomas in older patients, especially those over age 45, are most likely to represent a poor sampling of heterogeneous tumors. Survival data indicate that these tumors behave like the more malignant gliomas and should be treated aggressively with radiation and chemotherapy as for anaplastic astrocytoma or glioblastoma multiforme.

The primary treatment for brain stem gliomas is radiotherapy to the area of tumor. Recent work has suggested that the brain stem may tolerate higher doses of radiation of up to 72 Gy. Early transient clinical deterioration may result from radiation to the brain stem, but patients thereafter usually improve.[13] Chemotherapy has no consistent benefit, although in anecdotal cases, treatment with nitrosoureas alone has been reported to prolong survival. Prolonged survival in some patients may be the result of misdiagnosis. Patients should be followed closely during the first years after diagnosis to establish the biological behavior of the tumor. To facilitate comparison, radiological scanning should be performed in a standardized manner using exclusively MRI or CT. Neuroradiological imaging may demonstrate a change in the original resection area consistent with either tumor regrowth and malignant degeneration or radiation necrosis. Pathological confirmation is required to resolve this diagnostic ambiguity and to exclude other possible explanations. No reliable predictor is available except histological examination. Radiation necrosis is becoming more common as newer radiotherapy techniques and higher-dosage radiation therapy protocols are developed. Radiation damage is related to total dose, and there has been a shift toward directing the radiation beam more closely to the tumor areas and less to the surrounding normal brain. Higher local doses in excess of 66 Gy to the tumor bed may lead to increased risk of necrosis. Studies have shown that the tumor can extend outside radiographically abnormal areas, leading to concern that as radiotherapy protocols attempt to spare the normal areas, the patient may have an increased risk of far-site recurrence. Presently, far-site recurrences are usually present with local-site regrowth of tumor.

People who undergo cranial radiation while taking phenytoin have an increased risk of developing Stevens-Johnson syndrome.[14] Patients have a higher risk of recurrent seizures with gliomas and a higher incidence of side effects with the use of anticonvulsants, especially if seizures were present at the time of discovery of the tumor.[15] Complications of the tumor and its treatment include neurobehavioral decline, an increased risk of cerebrovascular events, and seizures. Seizures should be treated with the appropriate medical therapy. Any sudden change in the frequency of seizures or the occurrence of new neurological findings should prompt re-evaluation with MRI. Occasionally, seizures can become refractory to medication, although the tumor does not progress. In this instance, surgical intervention may be required. Serial examinations should be conducted to determine whether neurobehavioral sequelae of the tumor and its treatment are present. Careful early testing may uncover problems that can be addressed with counseling, training, and an alteration in lifestyle or work environments to enhance the patient's quality of life. Complications resulting from the tumor and the treatment may indicate a need for prolonged rehabilitation or assisted care.

Prognosis and Future Perspectives. Patients with low-grade astrocytomas may have prolonged survival with surgery and radiotherapy. Five-year survival occurs in about 25 percent of patients with surgery alone and in 50 percent when radiation is added.[16] Patients with pilocytic astrocytomas can be cured with complete surgical resection; 5-year survival in these patients approaches 90 percent. A similar length of survival can be expected in patients with xanthoastrocytomas, whereas those with brain stem gliomas have a poor prognosis with a survival of only months.

Further examination of these tumors with molecular or genetic markers may provide clinicians with information that will allow them to predict which of these tumors will become more aggressive forms and which treatment strategies can best prevent this progression. Large randomized trials are needed to study the effects of observation versus radiotherapy or even surgery for low-grade gliomas.

ANAPLASTIC ASTROCYTOMA AND GLIOBLASTOMA MULTIFORME

Pathogenesis and Pathophysiology. Malignant tumors are thought to evolve from lower-grade tumors, although they can evolve spontaneously, perhaps as the result of abnormalities of certain gene functions. Alteration of one gene may lead to transformation to a low-grade glioma; subsequent cell divisions can lead to the accumulation of multiple genetic alterations that ultimately result in a tumor with the histological characteristics of a glioblastoma multiforme. Alternatively, a putative glioblastoma multiforme "gene" may be affected immediately, resulting in a high-grade malignancy. A low-grade astrocytoma that is first diagnosed in a young patient may, many years later, recur as an anaplastic astrocytoma and then subsequently as a glioblastoma multiforme. In another situation, a glioblastoma may occur in a patient with only a short history of neurological symptoms and a radiographically small tumor.

In recent years, multiple genetic alterations have been associated with malignant gliomas in different stages of malignant progression. These changes involve chromosomal changes in terms of deletion, addition, duplication, mutation, or amplification of specific genes, as illustrated in Table 46–3. The most frequently observed alterations include deletions in chromosomes 17p, 9p, and 10q as well as multiple copies of chromosome 7. Some changes are specific to certain types of tumor; for example, losses of genetic materials from chromosomes 1p, 9p, 10p, 10q, 11p, 13q, and 17p are often found in astrocytic tumors, whereas deletions in 19q are seen more often in oligodendrogliomas, and those of 22q occur in meningiomas. Mutations of the *p53* gene are found in low-grade as well as high-grade gliomas, indicating that they may

TABLE 46–3. **Molecular Phenotypes in Gliomas**

Oncogenes	Suppressor Genes	Growth Factors/ Growth Factor Receptors
erb-B	p16 (MTS1)	FGF/FGFR
mdm-2	p53	EGF/EGFR
ras	Retinoblastoma (Rb)	PDGF/PDGFR
c-fos	Chromosome 10q and 10p	TGF-α
ros	Chromosome 1p, 11p, 19q, 22q	TGF-β
gli		IGF-I, IGF-II, VEGF

FGF, Fibroblast growth factor; FGFR, fibroblast growth factor receptor; EGF, epidermal growth factor; EGFR, epidermal growth factor receptor; PDGF, platelet-derived growth factor; PDGFR, platelet-derived growth factor receptor; TGF, transforming growth factor; IGF, insulin-like growth factors; VEGF, vascular endothelial growth factor.

represent early events in the malignant transformation of normal astrocytes to astrocytic tumors. Alterations of the *p16* and *Rb* (retinoblastoma) genes as well as the loss of chromosome 10 and amplification of the epidermal growth factor receptor (EGFR) *ERBB* gene are found mostly in glioblastomas, suggesting that these changes are associated with late-stage tumor progression. Other, less frequently observed genetic abnormalities in malignant gliomas include overexpression of the platelet-derived growth factor (PDGF), transforming growth factor (TGF)-α and TGF-β, basic fibroblast growth factor (bFGF), vascular endothelial growth factor (VEGF), insulin-like growth factors I and II, and the *MYC*, *GLI*, *RES*, *FOS*, and *ROS* oncogenes.[17]

The *p53* gene encodes a 53-kD protein that functions as a transcriptional factor and is mapped to the short arm of chromosome 17. The wide-type (WT) p53 protein has been shown to have tumor suppression activity, and mutation of the *WT* gene has resulted in loss of this tumor suppressive function, thus increasing the transformation risk of the normal cells. Deletion of the short arm of chromosome 17 (17p13) on which the *p53* gene resides has been observed in over 60 percent of malignant astrocytomas. Mutations of *p53* are rare in low-grade astrocytomas but are equally common in anaplastic astrocytomas and glioblastomas, suggesting that this *p53* mutation may represent an early event in the genesis of glioma. However, other studies have demonstrated a higher frequency of *p53* mutations in glioblastomas than in anaplastic astrocytomas. The fact that *p53* mutations are detectable in small numbers of cells in a group of low-grade astrocytomas and are more frequently seen in the recurrent high-grade astrocytomas may indicate that the histological progression of low-grade astrocytoma to high-grade anaplastic astrocytoma is associated with clonal expansion of the transformed astrocytes carrying the same *p53* mutations. The p53 protein is also a nuclear protein involved in the regulation of cell cycle proliferation. It mediates its growth effect through two major mechanisms: induction of apoptosis and transient cell cycle arrest at G1 by induction of the p21 WAF1 (Cip1) protein. Furthermore, *p53* gene function is inhibited by the oncogene mdm-2. Thus amplification of the mdm-2 protein may result in an alternative pathway for apoptosis independent of *p53*.

Loss of or deletions associated with chromosome 10 have been observed in high-grade malignant astrocytomas examined by cytogenetic and molecular techniques. Loss of an entire copy of chromosome 10 occurs in 80 to 90 percent of glioblastomas, and approximately 40 percent of these tumors also show amplification of the *EGFR* gene. Such a high frequency of loss of genetic material involving an entire copy or a large segment of chromosome 10 strongly suggests the presence of one or more tumor suppressor genes (*TSG*) on chromosome 10. This conclusion is partially substantiated by experiments in which a copy of normal chromosome 10 was reinserted into a glioblastoma cell; the resulting hybrid cells showed reversal of the malignant phenotype in vitro and in vivo. The hybrid cells were not able to form colonies in soft agar nor tumors in nude mice.

Epidermal growth factor receptor *ERBB*, a 170-kD glycoprotein, is amplified and overexpressed in 40 to 60 percent of gliomas. About 40 percent of gliomas show increased autophosphorylation activity of EGFR. However, no apparent relationship between amplification of EGFR and tumor grading can be established except that amplification of EGFR occurs almost exclusively in glioblastomas. Several structurally and functionally altered EGFRs have also been found in approximately 40 percent of gliomas that show amplification of the *EGFR* gene. One class of mutant EGFR resembles the ERBB oncoprotein and is unable to bind EGF, but its intrinsic tyrosine kinase activity is not fully activated. A second mutant has an 83-amino acid deletion in domain 4, high-affinity EGF binding, enhanced tyrosine kinase activity, and the ability to transduce EGF-mediated glioma cell proliferation. The third mutant, which is seen in about 30 percent of glioblastoma with amplified EGFR, has an in-frame deletion of 267 amino acids in domains 1 and 2 and exhibits low-affinity binding for EGF, which then activates the intrinsic kinase activity. This mutant has been shown to have transformation activity. The fourth mutant is a larger (190-kD) protein that has autoactivated tyrosine kinase activity.

The *TGF-α* gene, which encodes for the 6-kD TGF-α peptide, has increased expression in many glioblastomas and anaplastic astrocytomas. TGF-α protein can be detected in all tumor specimens tested, and the higher-grade tumors show stronger staining with anti-TGF-α monoclonal antibodies. In several glioma cell lines, TGF-α is cell associated and is not secreted into the medium. Together with EGFR, TGF-α forms an autocrine growth mechanism. Moreover, TGF-α also has been shown to have angiogenesis activity that is capable of stimulating endothelial cell growth, thus forming small capillaries feeding the tumor.

Vascular endothelial growth factor, a 34- to 43-kD dimeric glycoprotein, induces endothelial cell proliferation, angiogenesis, and capillary permeability. Three mRNA forms are produced by alternative splicing and code for three protein products, $VEGF_{189}$, $VEGF_{165}$, and $VEGF_{121}$. VEGF, as opposed to EGF, is mitogenic specifically for tumor endothelial cells that display increased expression of VEGF receptors, suggesting that VEGF acts as the mediator for tumor angiogenesis. VEGF has also been shown to increase capillary permeability, suggesting that it may play an important role in tumor-induced edema. Because increased tumor vascularity and peritumoral edema are key features of high-grade astrocytomas, and because VEGF plays a unique role in angiogenesis and edema, it is especially important to understand VEGF's role in glioma transformation and progression.

Fibroblast growth factors are a family of heparin-binding proteins that express both mitogenic and angiogenic properties. Elevated levels of aFGF and bFGF are expressed in human glioma cells. More recently, elevated levels of bFGF and bFGF receptor have been described in a human glioma cell line in which the influence of endogenously excreted bFGF on cellular proliferation is downregulated by antisense oligonucleotide primers. Immunostaining experiments have also demonstrated elevated levels of bFGF in glioma cells as well as endothelial cells in all glioma specimens tested.

The *p16* gene, also known as the *MTS1* gene, is localized to the 9p21 region. It is a potent inhibitor of the cyclin-dependent kinases 4 and 6 (cdk4 and cdk6) and is often mutated and deleted in a variety of human cancers including gliomas. The p16 protein functions by forming a complex with D1 cyclin and prevents D1 cyclin and cdk4 from forming a phosphoprotein complex, thus paralyzing the activation of the *Rb* gene and resulting in a G1 blockade. A mutation or deletion of the *p16* gene allows formation of an active Rb protein, thus allowing cells to proceed through the normal cell cycle and maintain continued proliferation.

Mutations of the *Rb* gene, a well-characterized tumor suppressor gene, have been reported in 20 to 30 percent of malignant gliomas. They usually are associated with glioblastomas, suggesting that alteration of the *Rb* gene represents a late event. Hypophosphorylated Rb protein is essential to allow cells to remain in G1 without entering mitosis and proceeding to the G2 to M phases. Mutation and deletion of the *Rb* gene renders this critical step inactive and allows cells to continue to go through proliferation.

Epidemiology and Risk Factors. Malignant astrocytomas, including anaplastic astrocytoma and glioblastoma multiforme, are seen more often in adults and are characterized by a shorter survival time than low-grade astrocytomas. They constitute over 50 percent of all malignant tumors diagnosed and are the third most frequent type of cancer in the 15- to 34-year-old age group and the fourth most frequent in the 35- to 54-year-old age group. Incidence increases with age, especially after 50 years, and a higher frequency of glioblastoma multiforme than anaplastic astrocytoma is seen in successive decades. Malignant astrocytomas arise primarily in the frontal lobes and cerebral hemispheres. Anaplastic astrocytomas are differentiated from astrocytomas by histological evidence of increasing cellular atypia and nuclear pleomorphism. The addition of necrosis labels the tumor as glioblastoma multiforme. There are increasing numbers of reports of glioblastoma multiforme found outside the CNS.[18]

Clinical Features and Associated Disorders. Symptoms of these high-grade tumors can arise gradually, reflecting the manner of evolution of astrocytomas. More often, immediate symptoms are found, such as seizures (either focal or generalized), speech disturbances, a change in or increasingly severe headache, vomiting, nausea, visual disturbances, and weakness or sensory disturbances. Careful interviews with the patient or family members may lead to the unappreciated discovery of neurobehavioral symptoms. Elderly patients may have memory loss, suggesting dementia. Occasionally, older patients present with a sudden onset of focal neurological findings that are believed to be a vascular event. Neuroradiographic imaging abnormalities (often CT

performed without contrast dye) are consistent with a vascular distribution, leading to a mistaken diagnosis of stroke. However, instead of improving, these patients often continue to deteriorate. Such patients should be re-evaluated with MRI performed with gadolinium. Malignant gliomas are considered to have no definite hereditary association. There are case reports of family members who have had similar tumors in an autosomal dominant fashion, and studies have found a familial association in 7 percent of cases.[19] Turcot's syndrome is a genetic disease in which gastrointestinal adenomatous polyps and primary brain tumors, including gliomas and medulloblastoma, are combined. It is dominantly inherited and has been associated with the gene for familial adenomatous polyposis and should be considered a variant. Gliomas are also associated with neurofibromatosis (see subsequent discussion) and tuberous sclerosis.

Differential Diagnosis. Patients with malignant astrocytomas have a differential diagnosis similar to that listed for astrocytomas. Practitioners must be aware that a definitive diagnosis cannot be made on the basis of the neuroradiological evaluation alone. It is essential to obtain tissue diagnosis by surgical resection or biopsy when feasible. The main differential is between an abscess and a malignant tumor (either a primary brain tumor, lymphoma, or metastasis). Because of the increasing number of multifocal gliomas, the presence of multiple lesions does not always indicate metastatic disease from a systemic cancer.

Evaluation. Patients often present with a single lesion. Physicians may be tempted to undertake an extensive search for a primary cancer elsewhere that is often unfruitful, ultimately requiring resection of the lesion. Patients with large lesions that are amenable to resection should undergo a complete neurological and physical examination with rectal examination and stool guaiac analysis, a pelvic examination in women and a testicular examination in men, complete blood count, serum chemistries, coagulation profile, chest x-ray, and MRI of the brain with high-dose gadolinium (Fig. 46–4). If no other lesions are seen, biopsy and surgical resection are indicated to determine the pathological diagnosis. Even if the tumor is found to be metastatic, resection of a single metastasis has been shown to prolong survival.[20]

Comprehensive neurobehavioral studies should be performed prior to surgery to determine pretreatment deficits. After surgery, re-evaluation may be indicated to define areas of improvement and provide a baseline before further therapy is undertaken. These studies can help patients and their families define those areas that may be a problem for the patient and a focus for rehabilitation. Such studies can help as the patient begins to adjust to daily living at home, and they can also increase the ease of patient care. Recent data documenting the risk of cognitive impairment after surgery have not shown that significant worsening occurs. Indeed, in some patients, surgical debulking may improve cognitive status as well as other neurological symptoms and signs of disease.[20]

Management. Patients are often treated with steroids, usually dexamethasone, immediately on discovery of a lesion in the brain. Unless the patient is in danger of herniation or has another serious problem that specifically requires steroids, however, such treatment is not indicated. Cases of primary CNS lymphoma in patients without acquired immunodeficiency syndrome (AIDS) have increased in frequency (see later discussion). Dexamethasone can be

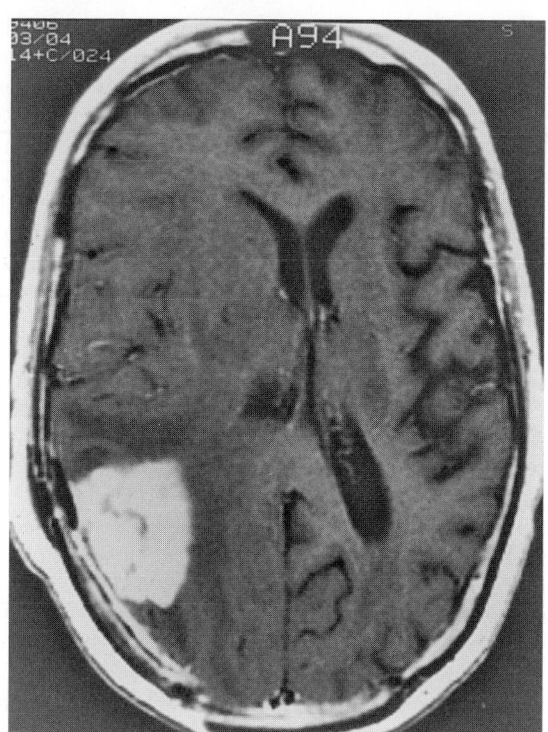

FIGURE 46–4. MRI picture of a glioblastoma multiforme demonstrating a large contrast-enhancing left temporal lesion with irregular border, as well as a central lucency suggesting an area of necrosis.

oncolytic to some tumors, especially leukemias and lymphomas, leading to resolution of lesions and causing diagnostic confusion. Therefore, the authors favor delaying the use of steroids until after the tumor has been evaluated but before surgery. Dexamethasone is the steroid of choice because it is a glucocorticoid with no mineralocorticoid activity and has better CNS penetration than other steroid preparations. Occasionally, patients with large lesions may require dexamethasone for several days before surgery. After surgical debulking has been performed, steroids can be rapidly tapered. Radiation oncologists often maintain patients on low doses of dexamethasone throughout radiotherapy, usually 2 to 4 mg a day. Medications with H_2 blockade activity are routinely given with steroids to prevent ulcers, although some believe the risk of ulceration is not sufficiently high to warrant its use. After radiotherapy is complete, steroids can usually be stopped by gradually tapering the dose.

All patients in whom the tumor is suspected require surgical intervention for pathological confirmation. Recently, there has been an increase in the use of limited surgery with stereotactic biopsy. In patients in whom mass lesions can be safely removed, however, maximum surgery is indicated. Small biopsies may not provide sufficient tissue to allow accurate neuropathological interpretation, leading to incorrect therapeutic interventions. All patients should be offered treatment in clinical trials whenever possible. The advent of computer listings of available studies on the Internet may facilitate enrollment in these studies.

The use of anticonvulsant medications prophylactically in patients with newly discovered mass lesions remains controversial. There are no studies that allow a direct answer to the question of whether patients are at increased risk of seizures. This question is complicated by the fact that virtually all patients undergo surgical decompression or biopsy and are given anticonvulsants at that time. The authors do not routinely administer anticonvulsants until a patient has sustained a seizure. Certainly, any patient presenting with seizures should be treated with anticonvulsants.

Cranial radiation following surgery remains the mainstay of treatment. Maximum radiation dose of 6000 to 6500 cGy is recommended. Recent radiotherapy techniques involve the application of approximately 4600 cGy to a larger field with a 2- to 3-cm margin encompassing the contrast-enhancing tumor and an additional 2000 cGy delivered to a reduced field encompassing only the contrast-enhancing abnormality. Irradiation to the brain during pregnancy has been shown to be feasible with minimal risk to the fetus.[21] Brachytherapy, in which radioactive seeds are applied into the tumor area, has been shown to be beneficial in some patients with glioblastoma multiforme. This technique, however, is associated with substantial morbidity; the high risk of radiation necrosis necessitates reoperation in approximately 50 percent of patients undergoing interstitial brachytherapy. It is therefore useful only in a limited number of patients with polar tumors. Stereotactic radiation may increase survival in those patients with radiosensitive tumors[22]; however, neither the neurobehavioral effects of this treatment nor randomized studies have been reported. Effects of radiation include hypersomnolence during treatment and cognitive dysfunction. These effects are more commonly seen in patients with prolonged survival after radiotherapy.

Chemotherapy regimens continue to evolve and have produced improvement in the overall time of tumor progression and patient survival. It appears that anticonvulsant use may affect efficacy by altering metabolic clearance of the chemotherapy agent.[23] The standard treatment includes the use of nitrosourea-based regimens such as carmustine (BCNU) alone or the triple drug regimen of lomustine (CCNU), procarbazine, and vincristine (PCV).[24] Recently temozolomide monotherapy has been approved for the treatment of recurrent anaplastic astrocytoma, and for glioblastoma multiforme in Europe. The role of this agent in combination with other chemotherapeutic and biologic agents and in different schedules is under study. Salvage chemotherapy regimens with agents such as carboplatin, etoposide, procarbazine, interferons, and diaziquone (AZQ) produce mixed results, but some responses occur. Newer agents under study alone and in combination regimens include thalidomide and metalloproteinase inhibitors. The efficacy of chemotherapy declines with patient age.[25] Blood-brain barrier disruption agents, carotid artery infusion, gene therapy, and combination therapy with multiple agents have not demonstrated overall survival benefit. An analysis of the changes in normal biological function or chromosomal aberrations occurring in tumor cells and their response to chemotherapy is under way.[26, 27]

Prognosis and Future Perspectives. Overall, prognosis is related to histological diagnosis, age, performance status, and treatment. Patients who receive more complete surgical resection tend to survive longer. Follow-up resection after tumor regrowth also prolongs survival and increases overall well-being in many patients. Median survival for patients with a glioblastoma multiforme, without accounting for age, is approximately 1 year. Patients with anaplastic astrocytoma have a life expectancy of 3 to 5 years. Prolonged survival with diagnosis of a malignant glioma can occur but may suggest incorrect pathological diagnosis of tissue type. In a review of patients entered in Radiation Therapy Oncology Group (RTOG) studies, histology was the most important determinant of survival for patients younger than 50 years of age, whereas performance status was the most important variable for patients over age 50.[28]

Clinical trials have to be conducted to better define the effects of treatment, including surgery, radiotherapy, and chemotherapy. Accrual of all brain tumor patients into clinical studies stands at 10 percent. Careful analysis and evaluation of all patients with these tumors is needed. Recent concerns have been raised about possible enrollment bias.[29] Newer imaging techniques may enhance the ability to evaluate both the disease and the treatment response. Positron-emission tomography has not been demonstrated to separate reliably the tumor from the treatment effects. Recent studies of gene therapy for these tumors have demonstrated infrequent short-term responses. Overall utility of this approach using newer viral vectors remains under investigation and is highly experimental. The combination of gene therapy with other modalities, including concomitant chemotherapy, remains to be studied.

OLIGODENDROGLIOMA AND OLIGOASTROCYTOMA

Pathogenesis and Pathophysiology. Because these tumors arise from oligodendrocytes, they usually occur in the white matter of the cerebrum, and because there are relatively more oligodendrocytes in the frontotemporal area, oligodendrogliomas have a predilection for these areas. Usually surgical specimens contain areas that are identifiable as astrocytoma. Increasing difficulty in the diagnosis of these tumors centers on the percentage of oligodendroglioma cells needed to categorize these tumors as pure oligodendrogliomas rather than mixed oligodendroglioma-astrocytoma (oligoastrocytoma). The grading system of Smith[30] has been used by most neuropathologists for the histological categorization of oligodendroglioma. Only necrosis has been found to be a predictor of biological behavior; mitotic activity apparently becomes more important with advancing age.[31] On microscopic examination most tumors show tumor cell infiltration into the cortex, and many tumor cells show an artifactual halo around the nucleus (the so-called fried-egg appearance). A delicate vascular pattern is also a prominent feature (Fig. 46–5).

Epidemiology and Risk Factors. Oligodendrogliomas occur most commonly in young adults. The peak incidence occurs in the third to fifth decade, and the tumor occurs predominantly among men. There are no known established risk factors. Recent epidemiological work has suggested that gliomas may be associated with repeated exposure to high-voltage electrical lines. These tumors have a poorer prognosis with age. Although typically considered to represent about 2 percent of intracranial primary tumors, recently the incidence has been increasing owing to changes in neuropathological diagnostic criteria. For example, at the University of Iowa, 25 patients were diagnosed with oligodendroglioma from 1961 to 1991, whereas from 1992 to 1995, 48 such diagnoses were made.

Clinical Features and Associated Disorders. Because of their infiltrative nature, oligodendrogliomas commonly cause

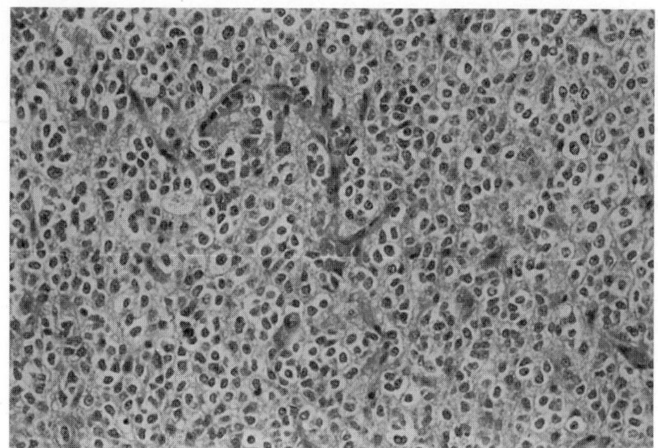

FIGURE 46–5. Histopathological picture of an oligodendroglioma. Nuclei are surrounded by swollen, clear cytoplasm, demonstrating a "fried-egg" appearance, and fine vascular channels.

seizures. Occasionally, patients with medically refractory seizures who undergo surgical abolition of the seizure focus are found to have an oligodendroglioma. These tumors can infiltrate and surround the neuronal networks without causing loss of function until they achieve a rather large volume. Retrospectively, subtle neurobehavioral changes can be detected long before the tumor is discovered. As with other gliomas, patients may also present with symptoms of hydrocephalus, headache, and sudden focal neurological findings consistent with acute hemorrhage into the tumor. There is also a higher risk of dissemination through the cerebrospinal pathways, resulting in spinal cord or patchy symptoms within the neuroaxis, which are sometimes confused with metastatic disease.[32] Rarely, oligodendrogliomas can metastasize outside the CNS.

Differential Diagnosis and Evaluation. Evaluation of oligodendrogliomas is the same as that discussed earlier for astrocytomas and glioblastoma multiforme. The differential diagnosis for oligodendroglioma and oligoastrocytoma is similar to that for astrocytomas. Because oligodendrogliomas are more often non-contrast enhancing on MRI scans, they may be confused with low-grade gliomas. With CT imaging, hypodense areas may also cause confusion with stroke or gliosis. Oligodendrogliomas are commonly found to have calcium deposits, and in many cases, contrast-enhancing areas are also found in the lesions on CT imaging. However, patients should undergo MRI to better define the areas of tumor involvement. Surgical diagnosis and attempts to achieve maximum cytoreduction are mandatory. Small stereotactic or open biopsies may lead to a misdiagnosis of astrocytomas, thereby affecting subsequent radiotherapy and chemotherapy treatment of these tumors.

Management. Neurological problems such as seizures should be treated with appropriate medications as discussed earlier for astrocytomas. Patients should be monitored closely for tumor regrowth or dissemination within the neuroaxis. The treatment of these tumors has become increasingly controversial. Some believe that these tumors are biologically less aggressive and can be observed with serial imaging until tumor growth is apparent either clinically or radiographically. Others believe that all oligodendrogliomas should be treated with radiation after histological confirmation. A large study at Duke University has suggested that radiotherapy may not benefit patients with oligodendrogliomas.[33] Recent studies have also suggested that anaplastic oligodendrogliomas are more responsive to chemotherapy and should be treated with PCV in addition to radiation, especially for Smith grade B, C, and D lesions.[34–37] Others have suggested that although chemotherapy for these oligodendrogliomas before radiotherapy may be harmful, this combination of chemotherapeutic agents is beneficial for patients with oligoastrocytomas.[38] Finally, some reports have appeared of treatment with chemotherapy alone for patients who have a more benign-appearing histological diagnosis.[39] An ongoing RTOG study of anaplastic oligodendrogliomas randomized between radiotherapy alone and chemotherapy with PCV followed by radiotherapy may shed further light on this discussion. Until better information is available, every effort should be made to enroll all patients in clinical studies.

Prognosis and Future Perspectives. Patients with oligodendrogliomas presenting with seizures seem to survive longer, possibly due to earlier discovery of the tumor. Reported overall median survival ranges from 5 to 10 years depending on the study, the reporting period, and the treatment regimen. Survival statistics will probably change as the diagnostic criteria continue to evolve. Survival for patients with oligoastrocytomas is similar to that for patients with anaplastic astrocytomas. Better neuropathological criteria for diagnosis of these tumors and higher enrollment of patients into clinical trials will provide better and timelier data on the optimal treatment for these tumors. As molecular definitions of these tumors are further refined, we may begin to base treatment of these tumors less on histological criteria and more on the presence of genetic abnormalities.

EPENDYMOMA

Pathogenesis and Pathophysiology. There are no known risk factors for these tumors. Ependymomas arise from ependymal cells lining the ventricles and the spinal cord central canal. Histologically, ependymomas are well demarcated from the surrounding structures and are marked by pseudorosettes, often located in the perivascular region. Blepharoplasts, intracellular structures associated with cilia formation, are also present. Anaplastic ependymomas have increasing features of nuclear atypia, necrosis, and mitotic figures. Myxopapillary ependymomas are usually confined to the filum terminale and have a distinctive fibrillary pattern with mucin secretion.[40]

Epidemiology and Risk Factors. Ependymomas represent less than 5 percent of all intracranial tumors. They occur in younger patients, usually in children, with a slight predominance among young men, although they can present in adults up to 30 years of age. An infratentorial location is more common in children, whereas supratentorial ependymomas are more common in adults. Cerebrospinal fluid (CSF) dissemination and systemic metastasis can occur.

Clinical Features and Associated Disorders. Patients with ependymomas have symptoms corresponding to the part of the neuroaxis affected by the tumor. For example, tumors arising in the spinal cord can lead to localized back pain, sensory disturbances with a demonstrated dermatomal line, weakness of both legs, or disturbances of bowel or bladder control. Ependymomas arising in the fourth ventricle, brain stem, or lateral ventricles can present with evidence of headaches or other symptoms of hydrocephalus (especially nausea and vomiting), ataxia, and increasing head circumference. Neck pain and behavioral changes also are common presenting complaints in children. Because ependymomas may be present for as long as 3 to 6 months before they come to clinical attention, symptoms may sometimes be labeled chronic.

Differential Diagnosis and Evaluation. The differential diagnosis of these tumors includes other CNS tumors such as medulloblastoma and low-grade glioma. Other more benign lesions such as meningioma do not have similar characteristics on MRI. Patients require surgical intervention when this tumor is diagnosed pathologically. Prior to surgery, the entire neuroaxis should be imaged with gadolinium MRI to determine involvement of other sites such as "dropped" metastasis. The resection attempt should be as extensive as possible, but occasionally this is not feasible. At least 2 weeks following surgery and before radiotherapy, the CSF should be evaluated for seeding of the cerebrospinal pathways with tumor cells.

Management. After surgery radiotherapy is the mainstay of treatment for patients with residual tumor.[41] Craniospinal irradiation is often given to treat clinically undetected seeding of cerebrospinal spaces. In patients with negative CSF examination after surgery, this is not indicated because it may hamper future treatment of localized recurrence. Myxopapillary ependymomas can often be cured with complete surgical resection. Chemotherapy has been shown to be of minimal benefit in patients with anaplastic ependymoma, although chemotherapy regimens including carboplatin and etoposide have been shown to prolong survival in several small series.[42] The use of craniospinal irradiation results in extensive treatment of the vertebral bone marrow, leaving little reserve for the cytotoxic chemotherapy. With newer cytokines such as the colony-stimulating factors that stimulate bone marrow function, patients may be able to tolerate more chemotherapy, allowing better appraisal of its use in these patients. Recurrence is usually local, although patients can develop distant metastasis. An increased risk of recurrence is associated with incomplete resection. Surgical resection, if feasible, should be strongly considered when the tumor recurs, followed by conventional radiotherapy to previously nonirradiated areas. Salvage chemotherapy also remains an option at recurrence.

Prognosis and Future Perspectives. Survival may be increased in patients who undergo resection of tumor and radiotherapy. Overall survival is similar to that for low-grade gliomas or oligodendrogliomas. Patient age of less than 5 years and a posterior fossa location of the tumor can have a worse outcome. No histological predictors of survival are available at this time. Future improvements in therapy can be expected with better understanding of the histological variants, application of radiotherapy and chemotherapy to more malignant subtypes of these tumors, and a better understanding of the molecular basis of tumor pathogenicity.

MEDULLOBLASTOMA

Pathogenesis and Pathophysiology. Almost two thirds of these tumors are located in the midline cerebellum, and over 90 percent are located in the vermis with encroachment on the cisterna magna. Laterally placed tumors are more common in adults. The macroscopic appearance is that of a soft friable tumor with central necrosis. In adults, these tumors are highly demarcated, but in children, they are less so. Microscopically, neuropathological analysis has attempted to define these tumors as a subset in a larger category termed *primitive neuroectodermal tumors*.[43] This classification stems from the belief that these tumors result from the germinal neuroepithelium during embryogenesis and thus can differentiate into tumor cells with neuronal, glial, or ependymal characteristics. Medulloblastomas are often classified as small blue cell tumors with little cytoplasm and pseudorosettes, which may signify neuronal differentiation (Fig. 46–6). A desmoplastic variant has been proposed for tumors in adults and may signify a different cell of origin.

Epidemiology and Risk Factors. Medulloblastomas are usually located infratentorially, accounting for approximately 2 percent of all CNS tumors in adults and 25 percent of intracranial tumors in children, second only to cerebellar astrocytomas. Although 50 percent of medulloblastomas are seen in children in the first decade of life, approximately 25 percent occur in patients over the age of 18. Tumors diagnosed in the seventh decade of life have been reported. There is a small second peak in incidence in patients 20 to 25 years of age. Interestingly, there seems to be a seasonal variation, with higher incidences in children born during the winter months and in those with congenital cerebral defects, possibly suggesting that these tumors are a remnant of embryonic dysfunction. Familial cases are known, including four cases in monozygotic twins, although there is no proven familial association. An association with leukemias and other CNS tumors, such as glioblastoma multiforme in first-degree relatives, has been noted.

Clinical Features and Associated Disorders. Patients often present with subtle problems that evolve over extended periods of time. In some patients, symptoms can exist for over 3 months before the tumor is diagnosed. The most common complaints include symptoms of increased intracranial pressure such as headache (especially in the morning) and vomiting. In younger children, behavioral changes such as decreases in activity or appetite may exist. Examination may demonstrate papilledema, truncal or limb ataxia, or nystagmus.

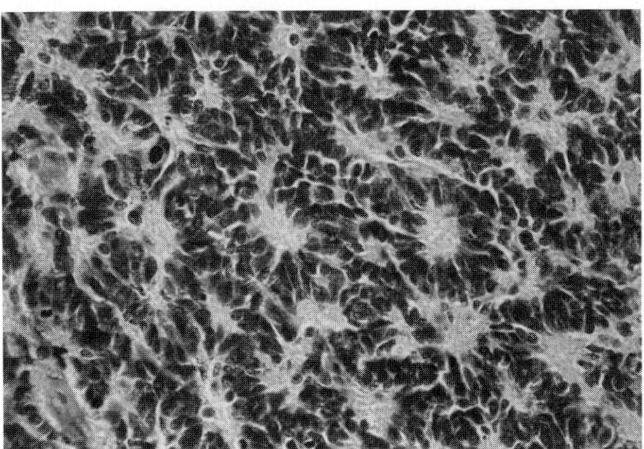

FIGURE 46–6. Histopathological picture of a medulloblastoma, showing primitive, undifferentiated tumor cells with numerous neuroblastic (Homer-Wright) rosettes.

A few patients have an increased head circumference or symptoms of leptomeningeal seeding similar to that seen in metastatic meningitis. There is a higher incidence of medulloblastoma in patients with nevoid basal cell syndrome, Turcot's syndrome, ataxia telangiectasia, and xeroderma pigmentosa.

Differential Diagnosis and Evaluation. The differential diagnosis for these tumors includes other primary CNS tumors such as ependymomas or gliomas, as discussed earlier, or metastatic tumors. Although CT scans are more readily available and may reveal evidence of hydrocephalus, all patients should undergo MRI with gadolinium. Occasionally, subarachnoid seeding is evident on initial imaging. CT or MRI scans usually demonstrate a hypodense mass with variable heterogeneous enhancement. Patients often present with evidence of obstructive hydrocephalus that requires immediate neurosurgical intervention such as shunting. Often conservative management with corticosteroids allows surgical planning, and some reports suggest that shunting should not be performed if at all possible. Some believe that midline lesions are more commonly medulloblastomas whereas hemispheric lesions are more often astrocytomas, but histological confirmation is mandatory. Gross total resection of tumor should always be the goal.

Management. Once the diagnosis has been established, patients should receive craniospinal MRI with gadolinium enhancement to study the entire neuroaxis for tumor dissemination. This also allows examination of the resection bed without worry about postoperative enhancement caused by the surgery. If MRI of the spine is contraindicated, myelography can be performed. Patients should undergo cytological evaluation of CSF at least 2 weeks after surgery. Although medulloblastomas have been known to spread outside the nervous system, especially to the bone and lungs, staging with bone marrow biopsy and imaging of the chest or radioactive bone scan should be performed only when such spread is clinically suggested. Reoperation should be considered at the time of tumor regrowth.

Patients have an increased risk of recurrence if gross total resection was not possible, if they are less than 4 years old, or if the tumor has a lateral location, evidence of CSF dissemination, or a differentiated cellular histological appearance. Those patients younger than 18 months should undergo chemotherapy alone, whereas older patients should receive both radiotherapy and chemotherapy. Patients without the features just mentioned are considered to have a decreased risk of recurrence and can receive craniospinal irradiation and observation, with chemotherapy given only with evidence of recurrence.

Radiotherapy remains the mainstay of postsurgical treatment. Typically, craniospinal irradiation with increased doses to the tumor bed is performed because undetected tumor may be disseminated in the spinal cord. Recent advances in chemotherapy include the use of CCNU, carboplatin, and vincristine.[44] Treatment failure is usually evident at the original site alone; cerebrospinal dissemination may occur, or systemic involvement may be seen in a later stage. Almost half the patients show evidence of cerebral hemispheric involvement at recurrence. Refinements in radiotherapy may increase the incidence of systemic dissemination at relapse.[45]

Neurobehavioral abnormalities such as mutism, pseudobulbar affect, or derangements of eyelid opening have been documented in children undergoing posterior fossa tumor resection.[46] These usually resolve within months of surgery. Patients may have problems with CSF drainage, requiring shunting. Children are at risk of decline in intellectual performance related to radiotherapy and possibly chemotherapy, especially if they are younger than 7 years old. Recent work has detailed the effects of radiotherapy and chemotherapy on progressive neurocognitive decline in these patients.[47] Endocrinological problems resulting from pituitary failure, including delay of puberty, may be seen. Children who survive for a long time display decreases in perceptual motor tasks, manual dexterity, learning, and physical growth and development.[48]

Prognosis and Future Perspectives. Medulloblastoma seems to follow Collin's law that the risk of recurrence of tumor is highest during the period equal to the patient's age at diagnosis plus 9 months.[49] Survival is correlated with the extent of surgical resection for those over the age of 3 in whom dissemination is absent.[50] Five-year survival can occur in nearly 75 percent of patients who undergo high-dose craniospinal irradiation after gross total resection. Survival is poorer in patients younger than 5 years of age. Adults seem to have the same survival duration as children.[51]

PRIMARY CNS LYMPHOMA

Pathogenesis and Pathophysiology. The reason for the increase in primary CNS lymphoma (PCNSL) in the immunocompetent and immunocompromised population is unclear. Because there are no lymphatics in the CNS, the mechanism for neoplastic transformation remains unknown. Viral causes have been suggested. In studies of AIDS-related PCNSL, the Epstein-Barr virus was found in a majority of cases,[52] but this was not found in samples analyzed from immunocompetent patients. Herpes virus type 6 has also been proposed as a causative agent. PCNSL is considered a non-Hodgkin's lymphoma, usually of B-cell origin, with a high-grade diffuse large cell, immunoblastic, or lymphoblastic type. T-cell PCNSL has been reported but is rare. Microscopically, the tumors aggregate near blood vessels and may provoke a normal reactive immune response. The tumor cells stain positive for appropriate immunohistological B-cell or T-cell markers. In the older literature, PCNSL was described as a reticulum cell sarcoma because the tumor stroma stained positive for reticulum.

Epidemiology and Risk Factors. The incidence of PCNSL has shown a three- to fivefold rise during the past 20 years.[53] Because the treatment for PCNSL is vastly different from that for malignant gliomas, clinicians should always keep the diagnosis of PCNSL in mind during the evaluation of a patient with a new cerebral lesion, The peak incidence occurs in the fifth and sixth decades, there is a slight predominance in men, and the tumor is commonly associated with immunodeficiency states including AIDS, drug-induced causes like immunosuppressive therapy for organ transplants, and other genetic immune deficiency states.

Clinical Features and Associated Disorders. Patients with PCNSL commonly present with focal findings or evidence of elevated intracranial pressure. Those patients with frontal lesions or the elderly may have neurocognitive changes that are sometimes confused with a dementing process. Seizures are common, especially in immunocompromised patients, and, although ocular involvement is also frequent, only occasionally do patients have ocular complaints such as blurred vision.

Differential Diagnosis. The differential diagnosis for PCNSL includes primary gliomas, demyelinating processes such as multiple sclerosis, and acute encephalomyelitis. In the immunocompromised population toxoplasmosis, progressive multifocal leukoencephalopathy, and other infectious causes should also be considered.

Evaluation. Neuroradiologically, PCNSL may be missed on CT; hence, MRI is the imaging modality of choice. Because PCNSL is often densely cellular and highly vascular, lesions usually enhance brightly on MRI with gadolinium, although exceptions have been reported in the literature. In the non-AIDS population, lesions are usually multifocal and periventricular in location. Immunocompromised patients are more likely to have single lesions, which are often confused with those of toxoplasmosis, and radiographically they have a higher incidence of necrosis with the appearance of ring enhancement. Edema is usually minimal. Leptomeningeal spread of PCNSL is present in more than a quarter of patients. Cytological examination of CSF in patients in whom lumbar puncture can be performed is mandatory. CSF should be evaluated for the concentration of beta-2-microglobulin and compared to serum levels as a marker of disease. Slit-lamp evaluation can sometimes provide diagnosis of vitreous or choroid involvement.

Because steroids can be oncolytic and can change the appearance of PCNSL on CT or MRI scans, whenever possible patients should not be given steroids before diagnostic studies have been completed. A marked reduction in tumor size and contrast-enhancing pattern occurs shortly after steroid therapy is initiated. All immunocompetent patients should undergo biopsy for pathological confirmation of disease. Although neurosurgical intervention with maximum cytoreduction is favored in patients with malignant gliomas, in those with PCNSL, which is very sensitive to radiotherapy and chemotherapy, stereotactic biopsy for tissue confirmation is a reasonable option. However, because of concern about the disease and the lack of identifying markers to separate PCNSL from malignant gliomas, open biopsy and tumor resection is usually performed. Once the diagnosis of PCNSL has been established, further resection is not warranted.

In the AIDS population, stereotactic biopsy is the rule. In AIDS patients in whom a single lesion is seen on MRI, treatment is often first performed with antitoxoplasmosis agents. Patients who are unresponsive to treatment, as evidenced by clinical or radiographic deterioration, then receive biopsy. Patients with multifocal disease and negative toxoplasmosis antibody titers should undergo biopsy. Occasionally, some patients may harbor both toxoplasmosis and lymphoma.

Management. After the diagnosis has been confirmed, patients should have a complete neuroradiological evaluation of the spinal cord with gadolinium-enhanced MRI. If not performed previously, a full ophthalmological evaluation and cytological examination of CSF are also required. Because systemic lymphomas spread into the CNS in approximately 10 percent of patients, the initial evaluation should include a complete physical examination, chest x-ray, abdominal CT, routine serum chemistries, and CBC to rule out systemic lymphoma. Further evaluation such as bone marrow biopsy or lymphangiograms is usually not necessary because the diagnostic yield is low.

Treatment of PCNSL includes the use of steroids, which may produce a significant decrease in tumor burden.[54] Radiotherapy alone has produced little overall increased survival beyond 12 months[55] and is no longer appropriate except in patients with AIDS or other immunocompromised states who cannot receive steroids or chemotherapy. Routine treatment now includes chemotherapy, both intrathecally and systemically, followed by radiotherapy. Chemotherapy has been shown to markedly improve survival, especially when methotrexate is included (Fig. 46–7). In 1992, DeAngelis and colleagues reported that a regimen that included intrathecal and systemic methotrexate, procarbazine, vincristine, and dexamethasone followed by radiation therapy and subsequent treatment with systemic ara-C yielded an increase in median survival of 41 months compared with 10 months for patients receiving radiotherapy alone.[56] Other reports of preradiation treatment with high-dose methotrexate have provided similar results.[57] There have been reports that radiotherapy followed by the PCV chemotherapy typically used for malignant gliomas may also induce remission.[58] Methotrexate following radiotherapy should be avoided because it is associated with an increased risk of treatment-related encephalopathy. Occasionally, ocular recurrence requires directed radiotherapy to the orbit. Immunocompromised patients with AIDS should receive whole brain radiotherapy. Craniospinal radiotherapy should be avoided in patients with localized disease.

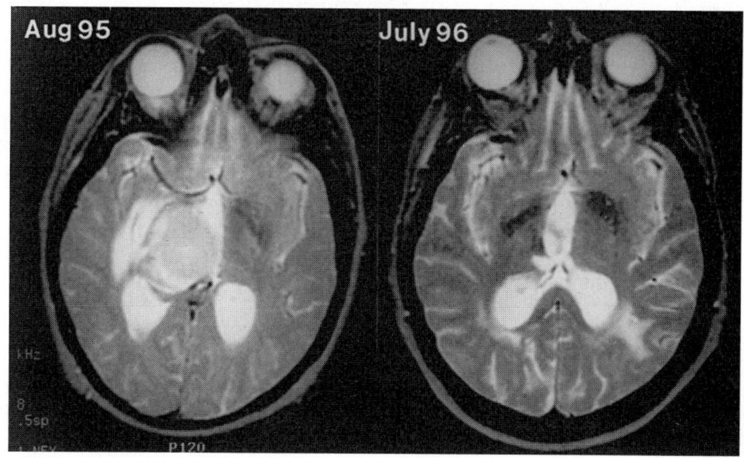

FIGURE 46–7. MRI of a patient with primary CNS lymphoma (HIV negative). *Left,* Before therapy; *right,* after 6 months of therapy with preradiotherapy methotrexate, procarbazine, vincristine, and dexamethasone, followed by radiotherapy and postradiation Ara-C.

Prognosis and Future Perspectives. Survival of patients with PCNSL who receive no treatment except surgery is poor, usually only several months. Radiotherapy alone can extend survival to about 1 year. Chemotherapy combined with radiation therapy can extend survival to about 3 to 4 years. Future work should examine the response of this tumor to various combinations of chemotherapy. An interesting issue is the study of whether radiotherapy should be performed only at relapse or at the failure of chemotherapy. There is evidence that radiotherapy may be afforded to patients of a younger age (<60) because radiotherapy in older patients may increase the risk of postradiation dementia.[59] Further examination of the origins of this tumor and a study of the pathological parameters related to treatment response may offer more information that can be used to direct management.

Nerve Sheath Tumors

ACOUSTIC SCHWANNOMA AND TRIGEMINAL NEURILEMMOMA

Pathogenesis and Pathophysiology. Acoustic neuromas, found incidentally on imaging performed for other reasons or due to new symptoms as described following, have a variable course. Less than 10 percent have a familial association. There appears to be no association with unilateral acoustic neuromas or with either form of neurofibromatosis. Some investigators have tried to examine the growth rates of these tumors by performing serial neuroimaging of the tumors to gauge their growth. Some suggest that the female predominance of these tumors indicates a sex hormonal influence.

Epidemiology and Risk Factors. Neuromas (schwannoma and neurilemmoma) are benign tumors that usually involve the sensory and motor cranial nerves, most commonly cranial nerves VIII, V, and VII. Neuromas represent about 10 percent of all intracranial tumors, the majority being acoustic neuromas. They present most frequently in the fourth and fifth decades of life, predominantly among women. Except for bilateral acoustic neuromas, which occur in neurofibromatosis II (see subsequent discussion), they are unilateral.

Clinical Features and Associated Disorders. Acoustic neuromas are considered slow growing, but they grow in a physiologically important area, the cerebellopontine angle, thus leading to multiple subtle complaints that may evolve slowly over many years. Symptoms may progress slowly, although sudden presentations can be seen. Patients usually present with hearing loss (especially sound discrimination), tinnitus, loss of balance, nystagmus, loss of facial sensation, or loss of function of the facial muscles or the muscles of mastication. Pain is uncommon but may sometimes mimic trigeminal neuralgia. Cerebellar findings such as ipsilateral limb can occur; ataxia and gait abnormalities may be noted when extremely large tumors have extended into the cerebellum. In patients with trigeminal pain, multiple sclerosis may be diagnosed initially; only with further hearing loss and a lack of involvement of intracranial areas of the nervous system will re-evaluation be conducted. Meningiomas are occasionally confused with neuromas, and, rarely, cholesteatomas or choroid plexus papillomas are identified at surgery.

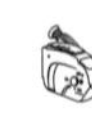

Evaluation. Sometimes early neuroradiological examination may fail to detect these tumors. Patients with increasing symptoms that are not amenable to medical treatment may require repeat studies. MRI with gadolinium enhancement remains the imaging modality of choice because it permits better definition of soft tissue involvement and identification of alternative diagnoses. Neuromas most often demonstrate bright enhancement with contrast agents. CT is performed to evaluate bony erosion of the skull. All patients should undergo audiometry and brain stem auditory evoked potentials at presentation to define pretreatment abnormalities.

Management. Surgical removal remains the mainstay of treatment. Recent reports have focused on the use of stereotactic irradiation or gamma knife surgery. No large series are available to compare their efficacy with that of surgery alone. After surgery patients are at risk of hearing loss and facial nerve paralysis. In patients with smaller tumors, hearing can sometimes be preserved. Radiotherapy has been shown to delay tumor regrowth after subtotal resection but carries a risk of radiation damage to other cranial nerves and brain stem vascular events. Chemotherapy has so far not been sufficiently explored.

NEUROFIBROMA

Pathogenesis and Pathophysiology. Both types of neurofibroma are associated with a gene localized to chromosome 17q11.2 for neurofibromatosis type I (NFI)[60] and to chromosome 22 for neurofibromatosis type II (NFII). The *NFI* gene encodes a protein termed *neurofibromin* that is involved in regulation of the RAS protein.

Epidemiology and Risk Factors. NFI, also known as von Recklinghausen's disease, comprises a constellation of tumors of the CNS. NFII is defined by bilateral acoustic neuromas. Patients with NFI have an increased risk of astrocytic tumors, including optic pathway glioma and brain stem gliomas.[61] Patients with NFII are at risk of ocular abnormalities, other cranial nerve schwannomas, and meningiomas. Spinal cord gliomas are seen more commonly in patients with NFII. NFI has a frequency of about 1 in 4000, and the frequency of NFII is 1 in 40,000. Both are inherited as autosomal dominant traits, with NFI having incomplete penetrance (see Chapter 32).

Clinical Features and Associated Disorders. In NFII, the bilateral acoustic neuromas usually become evident at the same time. Presenting complaints include tinnitus or hearing loss. Most patients have a first-degree relative who is similarly afflicted. Patients with NFII are also at risk of meningioma, gliomas, ependymoma, and schwannoma. Symptoms are the same as those discussed under the respective tumors.

Differential Diagnosis and Evaluation. Patients with NFI must be closely examined for any history consistent with visual disturbances or other visual abnormalities or signs of nerve root impingement, including bowel and bladder dysfunction or constipation. Patients may show evidence of peripheral nerve dysfunction caused by impingement by a neurofibroma. Patients may also have a plethora of other complications.[62] Only when the clinical findings suggest changes requiring intervention should tests be performed. Yearly MRI scans of the brain and spinal cord looking for tumor are not indicated. Some clinicians advocate yearly screening of children with visual evoked potentials for early detection of optic gliomas.[61] Patients and their spouses need genetic counseling for family planning purposes[63] and extensive social work intervention to help with issues related to the disease and the possibility of tumor generation.

Patients with NFII should be closely observed for any changes in auditory function, including hearing loss and tinnitus. During the neurological examination, particular attention should be focused on other cranial nerve abnormalities. Physicians should monitor the patient for any evidence of vertigo or difficulty with balance, possibly with yearly brain stem auditory evoked potentials. Formal audiometry on a yearly basis is a reasonable alternative as well; yearly MRI scanning is not generally indicated but may be repeated serially to allow a gauge of tumor enlargement.

Management. Patients with NFI should be monitored closely for development of treatable abnormalities, as previously described. Optic gliomas can be treated with surgical removal when feasible or with radiotherapy.[64] Malignant degeneration of a schwannoma or a neurofibroma (neurofibrosarcoma) occurs in 5 percent of patients. Patients with NFII require intervention to remove the acoustic neuromas, as described previously. In these patients, referral to a center that has facilities to perform a cochlear implant should be considered because these patients are at great risk of bilateral hearing loss. Patients receiving radiotherapy, especially children, are at risk for further neurobehavioral deterioration and endocrine abnormalities.

Prognosis and Future Perspectives. Further investigation into the genotype and how it relates to the variable phenotypic expression and manifestation of tumors remains to be conducted. A better understanding of the mechanism of action of the genes responsible for these diseases and the way in which malignant degeneration occurs may advance treatment of patients not only with NF, but with gliomas as well. In utero diagnosis remains a possibility. Genetic analysis of families and in family planning should be thoroughly explored.

OTHER PERIPHERAL NERVE TUMORS

Benign tumors of the peripheral nerves are often localized to single sites and are related to pressure or trauma. For example, Morton's neuroma is commonly associated with increased pressure or tight fitting shoes and represents fibrotic swelling of the nerve in response to repeated insult. Located on the plantar surface of the foot, it is treated with excision or observation. Symptoms include localized pain, tenderness, and weakness of the distally affected muscles innervated by the nerve. Ganglion cysts may result from repeated trauma, leading to undue inflammation and cystic degeneration. In other cases, transected stump nerves undergo unorganized sprouting, leading to a large clump of disorganized cells and their processes.

Spinal Cord Tumors

Although rare, spinal cord tumors continue to carry a grave prognosis for patients. They are difficult to resect and treat. Both the tumor itself and the treatment often lead to profound physical and neurological disability due to spinal cord damage. Spinal cord tumors represent about 7 percent of all primary tumors of the CNS and are seen more commonly in children, in whom they represent up to a fourth of all intra-axial tumors by location. The most common histological type is that of the glioma histology, especially astrocytomas and ependymomas. Their frequency is undoubtedly related to the percentage of total tissue of the spinal cord involved.

Often patients are brought to medical attention because of weakness of the legs, loss of bowel or bladder control, back pain, or, rarely, loss of sensation. In children, these symptoms may be confused with "regression" of the child's development, "growth pains," or muscle disease. Often a child's lesion is discovered incidentally during evaluation for a minor injury such as a sledding accident, when studies are performed to calm the fears of worried parents. Cervical or foramen magnum lesions may present with torticollis or nuchal rigidity.

Most patients are evaluated by MRI, which demonstrates an enlarged or thickened cord. Frequently, the spinal canal may be enlarged around the area of the slowly expanding tumor. Once the tumor has been identified, the entire neuroaxis should be studied for any other areas of involvement. Although a tissue diagnosis may be suggested by the tumor's location and radiographic pattern, pathological confirmation is essential prior to treatment. All patients should be evaluated by a neurosurgeon for consideration of biopsy or evacuation of the lesion. Preoperative and postoperative testing with evoked potentials can be performed to monitor disease evolution. Because of the location, patients are at a significant risk of morbidity from the tumor and any treatment for it.

Treatment of these tumors includes surgical evacuation when possible, followed by radiotherapy to a malignant lesion and the surrounding cord. Low-grade tumors may be monitored closely for evidence of recurrence or malignant degeneration. In children, consideration of a delay in radiotherapy will allow the treating physician to weigh risk-benefit options and consider the possibility of unwanted side effects due to the treatment. Although chemotherapy has not been systematically studied in these patients, one would intuitively expect that agents with known effects on supratentorial tumors would also be effective on spinal tumors with a similar histology. Patients with spinal column defects, such as scoliosis, that are related to the tumor or treatment can be treated appropriately with surgery (if necessary) and physical therapy.

Pituitary Tumors

ADENOMAS

Pathogenesis and Pathophysiology. Pituitary adenomas are neuroepithelial tumors of the adenohypophysis. They are generated in a stepwise fashion from initiation to growth evolution, probably in a fashion similar to that characteristic of other CNS tumors. This growth may be caused by derangements in the metabolic processing of cells of the adenohypophysis due to mutations of as yet undetermined gene alterations. Several putative gene alterations have been proposed, including the retinoblastoma gene and, because of its association with pituitary adenomas, the multiple endocrine neoplasia type I (*MEN-I*) tumor suppressor gene. Approximately 3 to 4 percent of adenomas of the pituitary are associated with *MEN-I*. Certainly other gene elements will also be found to play a role as laboratory investigations continue. An alternative hypothesis suggests that overstimulation or deranged signaling from the hypothalamus leads to pituitary cell dysfunction and inappropriate growth.

Pituitary adenomas can be classified by size, hormonal secretion, or histological appearance. Tumors less than 1 cm in diameter are considered microadenomas, and those larger than 1 cm are considered macroadenomas. Alternatively, pituitary adenomas can be classified as hormone secretors or nonsecretors. Approximately 15 to 20 percent of these tumors do not secrete hormones under current detection techniques. Of those that do, the majority secrete prolactin, followed by growth hormone (GH), adrenocorticotropic hormone (ACTH), gonadotropins, and thyrotropic hormone. Some tumors secrete multiple hormones and are termed *null tumors*. Null tumors that contain a buildup of mitochondria are termed *oncocytomas*, but this fact has no clinical relevance. Histologically, cells can appear acidophilic, basophilic, or chromophobic on routine staining techniques. By histological analysis, the tumor can be difficult to differentiate from normal tissue or metastatic disease. Immunohistochemical staining and evaluation by a neuropathologist is essential.

Epidemiology and Risk Factors. Aside from craniopharyngiomas in childhood, pituitary adenomas are the most common tumor in the region of the sella, comprising about 6 percent of all CNS tumors. Although pituitary adenomas are clinically evident more often in young women, autopsy series suggest that they appear equally in men and women. Recently, in a survey of clinically normal asymptomatic men and women, a 10 percent incidence of focally abnormal areas within the pituitary was found on MRI scans with contrast agent.[65]

Clinical Features and Associated Disorders. The reason most pituitary adenomas can be detected while they are relatively small is because they are located in a clinically sensitive area that controls hormonal function, just below the hypothalamus, and in close proximity to the optic chiasm (Table 46–4). If hormonal derangements do not bring the patient to medical attention, the tumor may be discovered during ophthalmological examination for a visual disturbance. Early pressure on the optic chiasm may result in a superior bitemporal quadrantanopia and can lead to a full bitemporal hemianopia. Alternatively, pressure symptoms such as headache may lead the patient to seek medical advice. The headaches can be diffuse and nonpulsatile and may be mistaken for daily headaches. As the adenoma enlarges, the patient may note hypothalamic dysfunction, basal forebrain abnormalities, anosmia, and seizures.

Symptoms of pituitary dysregulation are common. Prolactin-secreting tumors may lead to clinical presentation in women because of menstrual irregularities (usually amenorrhea), galactorrhea, and an inability to conceive. Men have a decrease in potency and libido. Abnormal prolactin function may also result from other pituitary tumors due to obstruction of the dopaminergic pathways between the hypothalamus and the pituitary. GH-secreting pituitary adenomas usually present at a younger age with evidence of acromegaly. Gonadotropin-secreting tumors cause precocious puberty, infertility, or impotence. ACTH alterations cause the typical features of Cushing's syndrome including hypertension, diabetes mellitus, fat deposition around the neck and shoulders (buffalo hump), acne, myopathy, and purple striae. Occasionally, patients present with psychiatric disturbances such as psychosis, mood alterations, or sleep disturbances, especially when the regulation of cortisol or prolactin is altered.

Differential Diagnosis. The differential diagnosis of a pituitary adenoma includes other space-occupying lesions in this area such as meningioma, metastatic tumors, craniopharyngioma, glioma, or, rarely, pituitary carcinoma. These alternatives can in most cases be resolved by surgical intervention performed with histological diagnosis. Confusion about compression of the sella area due to hemorrhage, a carotid aneurysm, or an empty sella caused by herniation of the meninges into the sella can often be resolved by appropriate neuroradiological imaging. An appropriate history will resolve questions about possible trauma to the area from a skull base fracture, previous surgery in an area near the sella, or a history of irradiation. Autoimmune or infectious causes of problems, including sarcoidosis, histiocytosis X, bacterial meningitis, tuberculosis, or abscess, are typically resolved by

TABLE 46–4. **Clinical Features of Derangement of Pituitary Hormone Function**

Hormone		Clinical Features
Prolactin	Excess	Hypogonadism, galactorrhea, amenorrhea, infertility, sexual activity dysfunction, impotence
	Deficiency	Infertility, ? impotence
Growth hormone	Excess	Acromegaly—hypertension, diabetes mellitus, coarse facial features, increased height, gigantism, nerve entrapment, visceromegaly, headaches, visual impairment, myopathy
	Deficiency	Growth failure, dwarfism
Thyroid-stimulating hormone	Excess	Weight loss, personality changes, psychosis, cardiac dysfunction, myopathy
	Deficiency	Cold intolerance, headache, constipation, paresthesias, infertility
Follicle-stimulating hormone, luteinizing hormone	Excess	Precocious puberty, amenorrhea, infertility
	Deficiency	Delayed puberty, impotence, amenorrhea
Adrenocorticotropic hormone	Excess	Cushing's syndrome—easy bruising, amenorrhea, hirsutism, hypertension, diabetes mellitus, acne, moon facies, truncal obesity, purple striae, psychiatric disturbance
	Deficiency	Nausea, malaise, weakness, hypotension

the presence of other findings of these diseases. Lymphocytic hypophysitis and Sheehan's syndrome often occur in the peripartum. Finally, one must always be vigilant to detect prescription or recreational drugs that interfere with normal pituitary function.

Evaluation. X-ray examination of the skull is of limited use in the evaluation of the patient with a suspected pituitary adenoma. CT scanning with bone windows is usually selected first, but this may miss a very small adenoma. MRI with contrast enhancement defines the soft tissue characteristics and is more sensitive to tumor identification in patients with large tumors. Angiography may be necessary to define the arterial supply for surgical planning and to exclude the presence of aneurysm. Neuro-ophthalmological evaluation for accurate mapping of visual disturbances is important prior to surgery. Evaluation of pituitary function is needed in all patients (Table 46–5). All patients require evaluation for cortisol insufficiency, especially to guard against cortisol insufficiency postoperatively.

Management. Prolactin-secreting tumors can be managed with the use of dopamine agonists such as bromocriptine (0.5 to 2.5 mg/d). These drugs interfere with the dopaminergic pathways between the hypothalamus and the pituitary. Ketoconazole has been proposed to stop the effects of ACTH hypersecretion. Use of somatostatin for GH-secreting tumors is still under investigation. Surgery remains the best way to produce a definitive diagnosis. The typical surgical pathway is a transsphenoidal approach and is usually curative. Use of radiotherapy (including stereotactic radiation) remains effective for patients with evidence of recurrence and for those who are not surgical candidates or who have not benefited from postsurgical medical intervention. After surgery, patients remain at risk for visual field defects or pituitary insufficiency, including panhypopituitarism requiring hormonal supplementation.

Prognosis and Future Perspectives. Because of the success of surgical intervention, these tumors have a very favorable prognosis. Recurrence is usually confined to patients in whom resection is incomplete. Further refinements in the medical treatment for microadenomas may allow nonsurgical treatment throughout life in some patients.

TABLE 46–5. **Tests for Anterior Pituitary Function***

Pituitary Function	Hormone	Laboratory Test
Thyrotropin (TSH)	Thyroxine	TSH, free thyroxine (free T_4)
Gonadotropins (LH/FSH)	Testosterone Estrogen Progesterone	Male: testosterone Female†: estradiol, progesterone
Corticotropin (ACTH)	Cortisol	Morning ACTH Fasting AM cortisol 24-Hour urine free cortisol Dexamethasone suppression test
Somatotropin	Somatomedin	Morning growth hormone Somatomedin-C
Lactotropin	Prolactin	Prolactin

*Test results may be altered by pharmacological agents.
†Tests should be performed and related to normal values for timing of menstrual cycle.

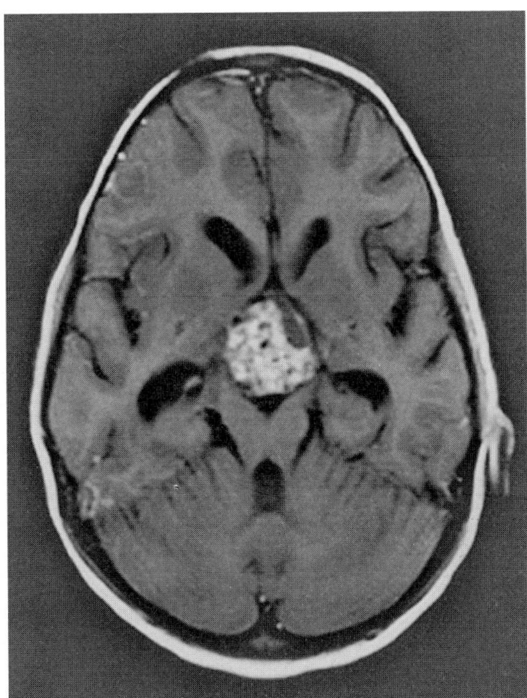

FIGURE 46–8. MRI of a craniopharyngioma, demonstrating a cystic contrast-enhancing mass in the suprasellar area extending upward, compressing the hypothalamus.

CRANIOPHARYNGIOMA

Pathogenesis and Pathophysiology. Craniopharyngiomas are thought to be congenitally derived and to arise from remnants of Rathke's pouch. Embryonic collections of epithelial cells remain after absorption of the hypophyseal-pharyngeal duct, from which the infundibulum/tuber cinereum is derived (Fig. 46–8). The squamous cells are found to be metaplastic and may be present for a significant period before transformation occurs. Alternative proposals suggest that these tumors are derived from a malformation of the embryonic cells that can linger in the area and are not absorbed during fetal life for a significant period of time, leading to abnormal growth. There are two main histological types, one seen in children and the other in adults, suggesting the possibility of two different explanations for their origin.

These tumors range in size from very small round nodules to large loculated cysts. Two main histological types are found. In the majority of children, an adamantinomatous form that appears to resemble tooth-forming material is composed of interspersed fibrous and necrotic tissue as well as many multiloculated cysts. Cholesterol and an oily, thick cystic fluid may also be present, and this fluid can spill from the sack into the subarachnoid space, causing a chemical meningitis. These types of craniopharyngiomas are more often found to have calcium deposits that can be visualized on plain skull radiographs. In adults, a squamous papillary form occurs; although it has no adamantinomatous features, a less cystic stratified squamous epithelium is found histologically. Keratin deposition may also occur. In many cases, it may be difficult to differentiate these two main forms, leading some to propose the presence of a third mixed form.

Epidemiology and Risk Factors. Craniopharyngioma is an epithelial tumor arising from the region of the sella and represents 3 percent of all primary intracranial neoplasms. It is the most common childhood tumor involving the sella area. Although it is the third most common tumor in childhood, about 50 percent of all cases occur in adults. There are no known risk factors.

Clinical Features and Associated Findings. Because this tumor is located near the pituitary, the resulting syndromes resemble those characteristics of pituitary adenomas. Symptoms can arise slowly over many months. The most common presenting complaints are compression of the chiasm, causing visual disturbances in the form of bitemporal visual field loss or obstruction of the CSF pathways, yielding papilledema, headache, nausea, or vomiting. Involvement of the hypothalamus or pituitary may lead to endocrinological disorders. With enlargement, pressure on the third ventricle in children can lead to a failure to attain developmental milestones or, in adults, a dementing process. In 90 percent of cases, endocrinological abnormalities are present, usually involving the anterior pituitary, yet most patients do not seek initial evaluation for problems related to endocrinological dysfunction. Notwithstanding, almost half of affected children are of short stature, and a quarter are obese at presentation. The primary endocrinological disturbance found is related to GH production; next in frequency are disturbances in luteinizing hormone/follicle-stimulating hormone, ACTH, and thyroid-stimulating hormone. In contrast to pituitary adenomas, abnormalities of prolactin are seen in only about a fifth of cases.

Differential Diagnosis. Craniopharyngiomas usually have a characteristic radiographic appearance that generally excludes other pathological processes. The differential diagnosis of these tumors includes pituitary adenomas, which have no calcifications, and separation of these two possibilities without surgery may be difficult in adults. Rathke's pouch cysts are usually single cysts and lack a solid component. Meningiomas often possess a "dural tag," and a cleavage plane can be visualized on imaging studies. In adults, metastatic tumors such as melanoma should also be considered.

Evaluation. Neuroradiographic studies should be designed to aid in surgical planning. Plain skull radiographs may show enlargement of the sella or calcium deposits, thereby giving a hint of potential diagnoses, especially in children. CT scans with and without contrast agent and paying attention to the sella in the coronal section may show bony alterations, whereas MRI with and without gadolinium can define the soft tissue extension of the tumor and the presence of cysts. Craniopharyngiomas tend to extend downward into the sella, whereas pituitary adenomas, in contrast, extend upward from the sella. Occasionally, angiography is required to define lateral displacement that can interfere with arterial blood supply, especially the internal carotid artery. Full endocrinological evaluation is mandatory before and after surgery (see Table 46–5).

Management. Surgical resection remains the mainstay of treatment to establish diagnosis and to relieve pressure from the surrounding structures.[66] Patients need corticosteroids at the time of surgery regardless of their preoperative status. All patients require assessment of fluid and electrolyte balance, which should be monitored closely in the operative period. Derangements in water and electrolyte balance caused by diabetes insipidus, the syndrome of inappropriate antidiuretic hormone secretion, or cerebral salt wasting[67] are common in the postoperative period. Following total removal of the tumor, further treatment is usually not required. With subtotal removal, patients can be evaluated with serial neuroradiological imaging, and reoperation at regrowth of the tumor can be considered. Alternatively, depending on the amount of residual tumor, radiotherapy is also an option. There is increasing controversy about the role of stereotactic radiation or gamma knife as the sole treatment modality. Follow-up periods for patients treated with radiosurgery have been relatively short, and further research in this area is required. Instillation of radioactive phosphorus may be considered in some patients with cystic lesions.[68] Endocrinological evaluation and postoperative treatment are similar to the regimen followed for patients with pituitary adenomas. Children require close observation with careful monitoring of neurocognitive and hormonal status.

Prognosis and Future Perspectives. Even when these tumors are detected before any neurological deficits become apparent, the prognosis remains guarded. Recurrence approaches 30 percent within 5 years and is higher in children and in those who have undergone incomplete resection. A significant number of patients continue to require hormonal supplementation. Further work is needed to determine ways to identify more aggressive tumors for which the use of radiotherapy and chemotherapy at initial tumor diagnosis may prevent recurrence.

Meningiomas

Pathogenesis and Pathophysiology. Many classification schemes are used for meningiomas, usually based on the histological appearance (Table 46–6). Meningiomas have a firm off-white appearance, and because they are extra-axial, they are usually well demarcated from the surrounding brain. Microscopically, they display a characteristic whorled pattern with calcifications (psammoma bodies). Discussion abounds about the classifications and subtypes and the histological characteristics of these tumors and their clinical course. For

TABLE 46–6. **Classifications of Meningiomas**

Histological Label	Features
Fibroblastic	Narrow, long cells in sheets; less commonly, whorls, psammoma bodies
Syncytial	Meningothelial cells, whorls, psammoma bodies
Transitional	Features of both syncytial and fibroblastic
Angioblastic	Intertwined, complex, thickened blood vessels, reticulin background, seldom contain whorls, psammoma bodies

example, proposed papillary and clear cell forms appear to be found more commonly in younger people and children and seem to behave more aggressively. Various cell-labeling tests and analysis of estrogen and progesterone receptor concentrations have been proposed to predict biological growth. However, the pathological features of brain invasion and mitotic activity are the most important pathological determinants of aggressive behavior. Hemangiopericytomas are highly vascular tumors that are seen equally often in usually younger men and women. Histologically similar tumors can be found in non-CNS regions. They are more prone to malignant behavior.

Epidemiology and Risk Factors. Meningiomas are extra-axial tumors that arise from dural elements within the cranial and spinal spaces. Although considered benign, they can enlarge and cause compression of neural elements and can behave aggressively, invading the bone or brain and threatening life. They comprise about 15 percent of all intracranial tumors and increase in incidence with age. Meningiomas have estrogen and progesterone receptors, possibly explaining why they occur in women almost a third more often than in men. Because of these receptors, meningiomas show increased growth during pregnancy. Further, meningiomas in the spine are almost always found in women. However, in blacks, men are more often affected. Several risk factors have been proposed for their occurrence, including trauma, infections, electrical exposure, and exposure to radiotherapy. Meningiomas are common in patients with NFII, in whom multiple tumors are commonly found.

Clinical Features and Associated Findings. Meningiomas can arise in virtually any extra-axial location in the CNS, although certain locations predominate (Table 46–7). Patients can present with epilepsy or subtle symptoms such as progressive headache, memory loss, or cognitive changes, which occur over an extended period of time. Slow progressive dementia and chronic depression in an older patient are also common presentations. Location of the tumor along the motor strip may present, possibly suddenly, with hemiparesis. Sagittal tumors along the falx may cause the development of bilateral leg weakness. Sphenoid area tumors may cause ophthalmological or cavernous sinus symptoms, and olfactory groove meningiomas may lead to anosmia. Because these tumors grow slowly, they may be identified incidentally in asymptomatic patients. Although hydrocephalus is extremely rare, children are more likely to present with symptoms of this entity.

TABLE 46–7. **Locations and Presentations of Meningiomas**

Location	Presenting Manifestation
Parasagittal	Urinary incontinence, dementia, gradual paraparesis, seizures
Lateral convexity	Variable depending on structures compressed, including slow hemiparesis, speech abnormalities
Olfactory groove	Anosmia, visual disturbance, dementia, Foster-Kennedy syndrome
Suprasellar	Hormonal failure, bitemporal hemianopia, optic atrophy
Sphenoid ridge	Extraocular nerve paresis, exostoses, proptosis, seizures

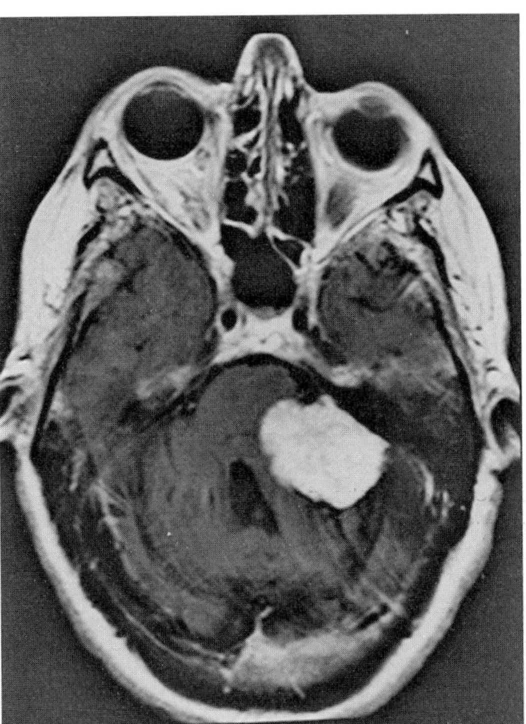

FIGURE 46–9. MRI of a posterior fossa meningioma, demonstrating an extra-axial, homogeneously contrast-enhancing mass arising from the tentorium and compressing the cerebellar hemisphere.

Differential Diagnosis. Meningiomas are often "diagnosed" from neuroradiological scans. The typical features and location do offer a reasonable amount of certainty in this diagnosis, yet clinicians must always be vigilant for unexpected possibilities. The ability to characterize these tumors radiographically still does not allow differentiation of a benign from a malignant meningioma. Malignant forms are more commonly seen in men, and unexpected metastatic deposits may be discovered. Suprasellar lesions may be confused with pituitary adenoma or craniopharyngioma. Extremely vascular lesions may be hemangiopericytomas.

Evaluation. MRI with gadolinium remains the diagnostic method of choice. Contrast agents demonstrate significant homogeneous enhancement (Fig. 46–9) and may highlight a dural "tail." CT may complement MRI findings and should include bone windows to show evidence of hyperostosis, calcifications within the tumor, and bone invasion. MRI angiography or routine angiography may reveal a tumor blush and can help with presurgical planning. In elderly patients preoperative and postoperative neuropsychological testing can be performed to evaluate patient response to and recovery from surgical resection.

Management. Meningiomas can be cured surgically. The location and size of the tumor and its involvement with close vital structures partially determine the extent of resection that is feasible. For example, sphenoid ridge meningiomas are rarely fully removed. The main decision is whether surgery is required. In patients in whom the tumor is an incidental finding or who are poor surgical risks, observation with serial scanning may be appropriate.[69] In those with large meningiomas, angiography and embolization are frequently used to aid in surgical removal. Extremely vascular lesions may be hemangiopericytomas. Following surgery, whether complete or near-complete, patients should be observed with serial MRI or CT scans for evidence of regrowth. Recurrence is related to extent of resection and location because the site of resection may preclude complete removal. Radiotherapy can be given for relapse following a second surgery or for anaplastic meningiomas.[70] Stereotactic radiotherapy and brachytherapy are under evaluation, with early results promising, although observation times have been short. Patients must be watched closely for evidence of cognitive decline from these intensive radiation doses. Chemotherapy with cytotoxic agents has met with limited success. Because meningiomas do possess estrogen and progesterone receptors, endocrine manipulation of the tumor residua with hormonal or biological agents such as tamoxifen or beta-interferon is under study and at this point remains investigational. Study of RU-486 has shown no benefit.

Prognosis and Future Perspectives. As the population continues to age, the frequency of meningiomas can only increase. Techniques for neurosurgical removal in the elderly must be further refined.[71] Histological variations and groups must be standardized to allow more timely and thorough evaluation of therapeutic treatments designed for a homogeneous population of tumors. Because meningiomas are amenable to resection but can remain to invade and disrupt vital neurological structures, future work must include detailed studies of their nonsurgical management, in relation to both timing and type of therapy. Attempts to predict biological behavior through histological and cell kinetic studies can help in management by identifying which patients are at increased risk of tumor regrowth and which have the potential to respond to medical management.

Congenital Tumors

DERMOID, EPIDERMOID, AND TERATOMA

These rare embryonic remnant tumors may present anywhere in the CNS but most commonly occur in the posterior fossa and the cauda equina. They are congenital tumors and may be seen at any age; however, they are more likely to occur in children or young adults of either sex. They are slow growing and present with symptomatology specific for compressive syndromes at their location within the CNS. These symptoms can be insidious, and blockage of CSF flow occurs rarely. Seizures or headaches are not common. Skin lesions are commonly associated with these tumors, and any infant with a dermal sinus tract should undergo neuroradiological evaluation to exclude these growths. Communication with a dermal tract may lead to recurrent meningitis, and any patient with repeated meningitis, whether associated with a bacterial cause or not, should undergo evaluation for an unnoticed dermal sinus. Prenatal diagnosis with ultrasound and resection shortly after birth are now possible.[72]

Epidermoid tumors, or cholesteatomas, are composed of ectodermal remnants and present as cystic structures in lateral positions within the CNS, especially around the brain stem or thoracic cord. Neuroradiological imaging usually demonstrates a hyperdense structure with poor enhancement characteristics. MRI scans demonstrate low but variable signals on T1-weighted images and high but variable signals on T2-weighted images. CT scans may demonstrate bone destruction and calcium within the lesion. These tumors have a thick ring that may be calcified and can appear "pearl-like." Epidermoids can interdigitate around vital neuronal structures, complicating surgical removal. Care should be taken during removal to prevent spilling the contents to avoid a chemical meningitis. Complete surgical removal is curative.

Dermoid tumors, composed of ectoderm and mesoderm, are more likely to be found in the midline, especially in the lumbar area and in the brain stem. Neuroradiological imaging usually shows an appearance similar to that of epidermoids with poor enhancement characteristics. These tumors are round multilobulated lesions containing fluid that also leads to a risk of chemical meningitis if the cysts are ruptured. Dermoids should be considered whenever lumbar puncture yields fat in the CSF.[73] Surgical removal is usually curative.

Teratomas are composed of ectoderm, mesoderm, and endoderm and are most often seen in infants and children, especially in the pineal region or the spinal canal. Because these tumors are composed of cells of all embryonic layers, they can generate hair, teeth, or other elements. Surgical removal, often not complete, is curative. Observation and an attempt at more complete re-resection may be feasible.

PINEAL AND GERM CELL TUMORS

Pineal region tumors account for about 1 percent of all brain tumors. They can be extremely difficult to diagnose and treat because of their location. Tissue confirmation is important because of the varied histologies found in this region as well as the implications of these differences in influencing treatment options. Occasionally, small samples of benign lesions may be confused with more malignant processes.

Patients with pineal region tumors often present with symptoms of hydrocephalus caused by compression of the cerebral aqueduct that result in elevated intracranial pressure (Table 46–8). Patients may present acutely with nausea, vomiting, lethargy, headaches, or changes in sensorium and mentation. Enlargement and infiltration of the nearby structures, including the midbrain, may lead to a kinetic mutism. Further expansion to involve the superior colliculus can lead to Parinaud's syndrome, characterized by paralysis of upgaze, near-light dissociation, and convergence-retraction nystagmus. Further compression may result in paralysis of downgaze. In patients with germ cell tumors, precocious puberty, especially in boys, may be observed.

The primary differentiation of lesions in this location can be separated into tumors and cysts or, in infants, a vein of Galen aneurysm. Tumors can be divided into germ cell tumors (germinomas, teratomas, or choriocarcinomas), intrinsic pineal tumors (pinealcytomas or pinealblastomas), metastatic lesions, or other tumors including ependymomas, astrocytomas, or meningiomas. Patients should undergo MRI with gadolinium or, if this is unavailable, CT with a suitable contrast agent. This will help to localize the tumor and define the involvement of local structures. Occasionally, angiography is required for surgical planning or to exclude an aneurysm of the vein of Galen.

TABLE 46–8. **Presentation and Evaluation of Pineal Region Lesions**

Type	Clinical Presentation	Evaluation	Treatment
Germ cell tumor	Headache, Parinaud's syndrome, endocrine dysfunction, nausea, vomiting, diabetes insipidus	MRI with gadolinium, hormone evaluation; when feasible, CSF evaluation including beta-hCG	Biopsy radiotherapy
Pineoblastoma	Headache, Parinaud's syndrome, endocrine dysfunction, nausea, vomiting	MRI with gadolinium	Resection radiotherapy
Glial neoplasms (astrocytomas, ependymomas, etc)	Slowly progressive, headache, nausea, vomiting	MRI with gadolinium	Resection, chemotherapy, radiotherapy
Meningioma	Slowly progressive, headache, late nausea, vomiting	MRI with gadolinium	Resection, radiotherapy with incomplete resection
Lymphoma	Headache, Parinaud's syndrome, endocrine dysfunction, nausea, vomiting, diabetes insipidus	MRI of craniospinal contents; when feasible, CSF evaluation including beta-2-microglobulin	Biopsy, chemotherapy, (?) radiotherapy
Metastatic tumors	Often history of cancer	MRI with gadolinium, evaluation for other metastatic deposits	Resection, radiotherapy, (?) chemotherapy
Pineal cysts	Slowly progressive, headache, late nausea, vomiting, or incidental finding	MRI with gadolinium	Observation, reduction
Vein of Galen	Most commonly male, high cardiac output, cranial bruit, enlarging head	CT with contrast	Surgery, (?) embolization

CSF, Cerebrospinal fluid; CT, computed tomography; hCG, human chorionic gonadotropin; MRI, magnetic resonance imaging.

MRI can help in differentiating possible pathological causes. For example, teratomas usually contain fat and calcium, whereas meningiomas may reveal a dural tag. All patients should undergo CSF analysis including cytological examination when feasible. Measurement of alpha-fetoprotein and beta-human chorionic gonadotropin (hCG) in the CSF should be compared with serum levels. Any clinical evidence of pituitary dysfunction should prompt thorough endocrinological studies.

Pineal region tumors require histological confirmation. Total resection is curative for benign lesions, whereas maximum resection may improve the overall survival of patients with malignant lesions. Hydrocephalus requiring shunting is common. Pineal or germ cell tumors require postoperative MRI for evaluation of seeding of the cerebrospinal pathway. Patients with germ cell tumors should undergo CSF evaluation when feasible. Testing should include a comparison of serum with CSF beta-hCG and alpha-fetoprotein, which can be used as markers for disease. Radiotherapy can be curative for localized lesions. Patients with evidence of cerebrospinal dissemination require craniospinal radiation. Because these tumors are so radiation sensitive, the use of chemotherapy with cisplatin and etoposide has often been reserved for patients with recurrent disease or those with more malignant tumors such as yoke-sac tumors or malignant choriocarcinoma. Although systemic germ cell tumors are very sensitive to chemotherapy, CNS germ cell tumors appear to be less responsive. Use of chemotherapy before or after primary treatment with radiotherapy remains to be studied. Relapse most commonly occurs locally or with CSF dissemination. Overall, survival approaches 75 percent at 5 years, and survival of patients with germinomatous germ cell tumors is over 90 percent.

Other Tumors

HEMANGIOBLASTOMA

Hemangioblastoma, a benign vascular tumor, is seen primarily in middle-aged adults but often presents at a younger age in patients with von Hippel-Lindau disease. These tumors are primarily located in the posterior fossa, although they can occur anywhere within the neuroaxis. They are usually cystic and are sometimes classified as a variant of meningiomas (angioblastic variant). Histologically, they are characterized by distinctive vascular channels with fat-laden cells. Occasionally they can be mistaken for xanthochromic astrocytomas.[74]

The clinical presentation is similar to that of other posterior fossa lesions. The neuroradiological appearance is that of a well-demarcated, cystic lesion with a distinctly enhanced tumor nodule on administration of contrast material. Identification should prompt a search for other lesions, including lesions of the cervical spine, especially in those with von Hippel-Lindau disease; retinal examination and evaluation for intra-abdominal neoplasms such as renal cell carcinoma or pheochromocytoma should also be done. Angiography is performed to help in this search for radiographically silent lesions and to aid in preoperative planning. Surgery is usually curative, although the use of stereotactic radiation is being explored. Because these tumors are known to express an erythropoietin-like factor, the accompanying erythrocytosis may be a marker for the extent of resection or for occult lesions in patients with known hemangioblastoma or von Hippel-Lindau disease.

CHORDOMA

Chordomas are often considered "benign" tumors that are amenable to surgical resection alone. However, they can be invasive and can metastasize, and, without complete resection, they can produce local regrowth. They are considered embryonal tumors and are remnants of the notochord. The primary histological feature is the presence of large mucin-containing physaliferous cells. Areas of hemorrhage and calcification may also be seen. Chordomas may degenerate to a more malignant histological appearance, the chondrosarcoma. Chordomas originate in essentially two locations, the clivus or sphenoid region and the sacrococcygeal region, although they can arise in other areas as well, including infiltration into the facial structures. They are relatively rare and account for less than 1 percent of primary CNS tumors. They usually occur at midlife and predominate in men. Men who have smaller non-necrotic tumors seem to have a better overall outcome.[75]

Clinical presentations of patients with clivus or cervical region tumors include headache, oculomotor nerve abnormalities, or other cranial nerve dysfunction, especially in the lower motor nerves. Tumors in the sacrococcygeal region present with symptoms similar to those typical of cauda equina or conus medullaris disruption. Radiological evaluation should include both CT for examination of bone abnormalities and MRI to evaluate soft tissue destruction. These tumors are extra-axial, and displacement of brain stem or other structures may be seen. Nerves exiting from the nervous system may become entrapped in the tumor. Chordomas can be confused with craniopharyngiomas, meningiomas, metastatic carcinoma, or possibly adenoma. They show variable enhancement with contrast dye. Angiography may be necessary to define the arterial structures prior to surgery. The differential diagnosis for these tumors includes the malignant variant, chondrosarcoma, and other lesions known to occur in this region such as meningiomas or schwannomas, metastatic tumors such as carcinomas, or, remotely, craniopharyngiomas.

Definitive surgery for diagnosis and maximum tumor removal is imperative. Patients should be referred to large centers staffed by neurosurgeons who are adept at skull-base surgery. Tumors usually exhibit regrowth at the site of the previous resection. Radiotherapy, including directed stereotactic radiotherapy, is improving overall survival; however, radiotherapy should be reserved for patients who show evidence of tumor after surgery.

In a recent report of 60 patients with chordoma or chondrosarcoma, overall regrowth-free survival at 5 years was found in 84 percent of patients with near-total resection and in 64 percent of patients with partial resection.[76] Extent of surgical resection was the greatest predictor of overall survival. Importantly, extent of surgical resection did lead to some decrease in patient performance postoperatively, but with rehabilitation, most patients regained their level of preoperative performance in about 6 months.

GLOMUS JUGULARE (CAROTID BODY) TUMORS

Glomus jugulare tumors arise from the paraganglionic tissue surrounding the jugular vein in the area of the middle ear. These tumors most often present late in life, in the sixth or seventh decade, and may have a genetic predisposition. They are locally invasive and highly vascular. Although presenting symptoms include complaints similar to those typical of acoustic neuromas, with tinnitus or hearing loss, the key differentiating features of these tumors are pain and the presence of loud pulsations in the ear. Occasionally, blood may drain from the ear. On examination, the patient may have tumor visible in the ear canal and, with larger lesions, evidence of cranial nerve or cerebellar dysfunction. The differential diagnosis includes neuromas, cholesteatomas, meningiomas, vascular malformations, or metastatic disease.

MRI with gadolinium enhancement demonstrates a brightly enhancing lesion and defines the spread and involvement of the local structures. Angiography is important to define the presence of vascular involvement before any attempts are made to remove the tumor surgically. Often, preoperative embolization of the involved vascular territories and intraoperative electrophysiological monitoring will help in surgical removal, which can be curative. Radiotherapy, including the use of stereotactic radiation or gamma knife, is an option for patients who are poor risks for surgery or who have residual disease that appears to be growing on serial MRI examinations. Prognosis is excellent.

COLLOID CYSTS

Colloid cysts are benign tumors that are amenable to curative neurosurgical resection. They must be diagnosed promptly before symptoms develop that can lead to acute conditions and sudden death. They are rare tumors but, with the advent of neuroradiological imaging, can be identified incidentally when imaging is performed for other reasons. They typically present in midlife, although pediatric diagnoses are known. They are located most frequently in the third ventricle and can cause variable symptoms due to intermittent obstruction of CSF pathways.

Patients may have weakness in the legs not associated with loss of consciousness, headache that is progressive, or paradoxical lightning headache that is relieved by positional changes of the head. Papilledema may be present on examination. Occasionally, patients with colloid cysts present with symptoms consistent with normal pressure hydrocephalus. Imaging with noncontrast CT demonstrates ventricular obstruction and dilatation with a hyperdense mass in the third ventricle. Coronal MRI usually demonstrates the mass in the anterior third ventricle. These tumors can be confused with basilar aneurysms or choroid plexus papilloma, although these lesions are not as hyperdense on noncontrast neuroradiological studies. Management includes immediate attention to hydrocephalus, often with ventricular drainage. Early surgical intervention is recommended to prevent neurological deterioration.[77]

CHOROID PLEXUS PAPILLOMA

Choroid plexus papillomas are extremely rare vascular tumors that are often located in the ventricular areas of infants and children of both sexes. Although the lateral ventricles are the most common location, these tumors can present in the third or fourth ventricles, especially in adults. Although some believe the childhood predilection suggests that these tumors are congenitally derived, no risk factors are known.

Patients commonly present with symptoms of increased intracranial pressure. In infants and small children these manifestations can include changes in behavior and decreased feeding. Seizures are not uncommon, and hemorrhages are known to occur. The main differential factor is that of malignant degeneration to a choroid carcinoma or an ependymoma. Choroid plexus carcinomas are more common in children, whereas in adults the differentiation of a choroid plexus carcinoma from a metastatic carcinoma may be difficult.[78] Occasionally, these tumors can be confused with colloid cysts, although the latter lesions have much different imaging characteristics, as discussed previously.

Evaluation usually begins with CT or MRI. CT scan reveals hydrocephalus with a brightly enhancing rounded mass located within or near the ventricular system. MRI usually establishes the intraventricular location and may identify leptomeningeal seeding of malignant forms. Calcifications may be present. These tumors can be extremely vascular, necessitating angiography prior to surgery.

Shunting may be required prior to surgery to allow time for thorough surgical preparation. Because papillomas are usually well-demarcated lobules that shell out easily, these tumors can be cured with surgical resection. Those that are more adherent suggest a more malignant type. Choroid plexus papillomas require no further treatment beyond serial neuroradiographical studies to survey for early asymptomatic regrowth. In patients with choroid plexus carcinomas, further treatment is important. Patients require evaluation of the neuroaxis of any evidence of seeding by craniospinal MRI and CSF evaluation. Because radiotherapy is not favored in young children, chemotherapy is the mainstay of treatment for choroid plexus carcinomas that are not completely resected, those that show evidence of regrowth, and those that have malignant potential. No large series exist in regard to the choice of optimal chemotherapeutic agents, although carboplatin and etoposide are commonly used. Some advocate presurgical chemotherapy in patients who require reoperation.

Reviews and Selected Updates

American Cancer Society: Cancer Facts and Figures 2002. Atlanta, American Cancer Society, 2002.

Brat DJ, Castellano-Sanchez A, Kaur B, Van Meir EG: Genetic and biologic progression in astrocytomas and their relation to angiogenic dysregulation. Adv Anat Pathol 2002;9:24–36

Chinot O: Chemotherapy for the treatment of oligodendroglial tumors. Semin Oncol 2001;28(4 Suppl 13):13–18.

Glantz MJ, Cole BF, Forsyth PA, et al: Practice parameter: Anticonvulsant prophylaxis in patients with newly diagnosed brain tumors. Report of the Quality Standards Subcommittee of the American Academy of Neurology. Neurology 2000;54:1886–1893.

Keles GE, Lamborn KR, Berger MS. Low-grade hemispheric gliomas in adults: A critical review of extent of resection as a factor influencing outcome. J Neurosurg 2001;95:735–745.

Kleihues P, Louis DN, Scheithauer BW, et al: The WHO Classification of Tumors of the Nervous System. J Neuropathol Exper Neurol 2002;61:215–225.

Kurpad SN, Zhao XG, Wikstrand CJ, et al: Tumor antigens in astrocytic gliomas. Glia 1995;15:244–256.

Levin VA: Chemotherapy for brain tumors of astrocytic and oligodendroglial lineage: The past decade and where we are heading. Neuro-oncol 1999;1:69–80.

Ligon AH, Perhouse MA, Jasser SA, Yung WKA: Identification of a novel gene product, RIG, that is down-regulated in human glioblastoma. Oncogene 1997;14:1075–1081.

Obbens EA, Schneider AG, Shapiro WR: Brain tumors. Cancer Chemother Biol Response Modif 1996;16:625–643.

Piepmeir JM, Christopher S: Low-grade gliomas. J Neuro-oncol 1997;34:1–3.

Rich JN, Guo C, McLendon RE, Bigner DD, Wang XF, Counter CM: A genetically tractable model of human glioma formation. Cancer Res 2001;61:3556–3560.

Wefel JS, Janus TJ: Neurology and neuropsychology in oncology. *In* Principles and Practice of Behavioral Neurology and Neuropsychology. Rizzo M, Eslinger P (eds): Philadelphia, Saunders, Churchill Livingstone & Mosby 2003 (in press).

References

1. Haapasalo HK, Sallinen PK, Helén PT, et al: Comparison of three quantitation methods for PCNA immunostaining: Applicability and relation to survival in 83 astrocytic neoplasms. J Pathol 1993;171:207–214.
2. Helseth A: Increasing incidence of primary central nervous system tumors in the elderly: Real increase or improved detection? J Natl Cancer Inst 1993;85:1871–1872.
3. Bailey P, Cushing H: Medulloblastoma cerebelli: A common type of midcerebellar glioma of childhood. Arch Neurol Psychiatry 1925;14: 192–213.
4. Fields WS: Primary Brain Tumors: A Review of Histologic Classification. New York, Springer-Verlag, 1989.
5. Fewer D, Wilson CB, Boldrey EB, et al: The chemotherapy of brain tumors. JAMA 1972;22:549–552.
6. Kim TS, Halliday AL, Hedley-White ET, Convery K: Correlates of survival and the Daumas-Duport grading system for astrocytomas. J Neurosurg 1991;74:27–37.
7. Radhakrishnan K, Mokri B, Parisi JE, et al: The trends in incidence of primary brain tumors in the population of Rochester, Minnesota. Ann Neurol 1995;37:67–73.
8. Desmeules M, Mikkelsen T, Mao Y: Increasing incidence of primary malignant brain tumors: Influence of diagnostic methods. J Natl Cancer Inst 1992;84:442–445.
9. Rajshekhar V, Chandy MJ: Computerized tomography-guided stereotactic surgery for brainstem masses: A risk-benefit analysis in 71 patients. J Neurosurg 1995;82:976–981.
10. Recht LD, Lew D, Smith TW: Suspected low-grade glioma: Is deferring treatment safe? Ann Neurol 1992;31:431–436.
11. Surma-aho O, Niemela M, Vilkki J, et al: Adverse long-term effects of brain radiotherapy in adult low-grade glioma patients. Neurology 2001;56:1285–1290.
12. Radcliffe J, Packer RJ, Atkins TE, et al: Three- and four-year cognitive outcome in children with noncortical brain tumors treated with whole-brain radiotherapy. Ann Neurol 1992;32:551–554.
13. Packer RJ, Zimmerman RA, Kaplan A, et al: Early cystic/necrotic changes after hyperfractionated radiation therapy in children with brainstem gliomas. Cancer 1993;71:2666–2674.
14. Delattre J-Y, Safai B, Posner JB: Erythema multiforme and Stevens-Johnson syndrome in patients receiving cranial irradiation and phenytoin. Neurology 1988;38:194–198.
15. Moots PL, Maciunas RJ, Eisert DR, et al: The course of seizure disorders in patients with malignant gliomas. Arch Neurol 1995;52:717–724.
16. Shaw EG, Scheithauer BW: Management of supratentorial low-grade gliomas. Oncology 1993;7:97–107.
17. Kyritsis AP, Yung WKA: Molecular genetics and tumor suppressor genes in gliomas. Bailliere's Clin Neurol 1996;5:295–305.
18. Park CC, Hartmann C, Folkerth R, et al: Systemic metastasis in glioblastoma may represent the emergence of neoplastic subclones. J Neuropathol Exp Neurol 2000;59:1044–1050.
19. Ikizler Y, van Meyel DJ, Ramsay DA, et al: Gliomas in families. Can J Neurol Sci 1992;19:492–497.
20. Patchell RA, Tibbs PA, Walsh JW, et al: A randomized trial of surgery in the treatment of single metastasis to the brain. N Engl J Med 1990;322:494–500.
21. Sneed PK, Albright NW, Wara WM, et al: Fetal dose estimates for radiotherapy of brain tumors during pregnancy. Int J Radiat Oncol Biol Phys 1995;32:823–830.
22. Gannett D, Stea B, Lulu B, et al: Stereotactic radiosurgery as an adjunct to surgery and external beam radiotherapy in the treatment of patients with malignant gliomas. Int J Radiat Oncol Biol Phys 1995;33:461–468.
23. Chang SM, Kuhn JG, Robins HI, et al: A Phase II study of paclitaxel in patients with recurrent malignant glioma using different doses depending upon the concomitant use of anticonvulsants: A North American Brain Tumor Consortium report. Cancer 2001;91:417–422.

24. Levin VA, Silver P, Hannigan J, et al: Superiority of post-radiotherapy adjuvant chemotherapy with CCNU, procarbazine and vincristine (PCV) over BCNU for anaplastic gliomas: NCOG 6G61 final report. Int J Rad Oncol Biol Phys 1990;8:321–324.
25. Grant R, Liang BC, Page MA, et al: Age influences chemotherapy response in astrocytomas. Neurology 1995;45:929–933.
26. Belanich M, Pastor M, Randall T, et al: Retrospective study of the correlation between the DNA repair protein alkyltransferase and survival of brain tumor patients treated with carmustine. Cancer Res 1996;56:783–788.
27. Shapiro JR, Pu PY, Mohamed AN, et al: Chromosome number and carmustine sensitivity in human gliomas. Cancer 1993;71:4007–4012.
28. Curran P, Scott CB, Horton J, et al: Recursive partitioning analysis of prognostic factors in three Radiation Therapy Oncology group malignant gliomas trials. J Natl Cancer Inst 1993;85:704–710.
29. Kirby S, Brothers M, Irish W, et al: Evaluating glioma therapies: Modeling treatments and predicting outcomes. J Natl Cancer Inst 1995;87:1884–1888.
30. Smith MT, Ludwig CL, Godfrey AD, Armbrustmacher VW: Grading of oligodendrogliomas. Cancer 1983;52:2107–2114.
31. Burger PC, Rawlings CE, Cox EB, et al: Clinicopathologic correlations in the oligodendroglioma. Cancer 1987;59:1345–1352.
32. Chen R, MacDonald DR, Ramsay DA: Primary diffuse leptomeningeal oligodendroglioma—case report. J Neurosurg 1995;83:724–728.
33. Bullard DE, Rawlings CE, Phillip SB, et al: Oligodendroglioma. An analysis of the value of radiation therapy. Cancer 1987;60:2179–2188.
34. Glass J, Hochberg FH, Gruber ML, et al: The treatment of oligodendrogliomas and mixed oligodendroglioma-astrocytomas with PCV chemotherapy. J Neurosurg 1992;76:741–745.
35. Cairncross JG, MacDonald DR, Ramsay DA: Aggressive oligodendroglioma: A chemosensitive tumor. Neurosurgery 1992;31:78–82.
36. Cairncross G: Chemotherapy for anaplastic oligodendroglioma. J Clin Oncol 1994;12:2013–2021.
37. Streffer J, Schabet M, Bamberg M, et al: A role for preirradiation PCV chemotherapy for oligodendroglial brain tumors. J Neurol 2000;247:297–302.
38. Kyritsis AP, Yung WKA, Bruner J, et al: The treatment of anaplastic oligodendrogliomas and mixed gliomas. Neurosurgery 1993;32:365–371.
39. Mason WP, Krol GS, DeAngelis LM: Low grade oligodendroglioma responds to chemotherapy. Neurology 1996;46:203–207.
40. Sonneland PRL, Scheithauer BW, Onofrio BM: Myxopapillary ependymoma. A clinicopathologic and immunocytochemical study of 77 cases. Cancer 1985;56:883–893.
41. Waldron JN, Laperriere NJ, Jaakkimainen L, et al: Spinal cord ependymoma: A retrospective analysis of 69 cases. Int J Radiat Oncol Biol Phys 1993;27:223–229.
42. Goldwein JW, Glauser TA, Packer RJ, et al: Recurrent intracranial ependymomas in children. Survival, patterns of failure, and prognostic factors. Cancer 1990;66:557–563.
43. Rorke LB: The cerebellar medulloblastoma and its relationship to primitive neuroectodermal tumors. J Neuropathol Exp Neurol 1983;142:1–15.
44. Packer RJ, Sutton LN, Elterman R, et al: Outcome for children with medulloblastoma treated with radiation and cisplatin, CCNU, and vincristine chemotherapy. J Neurosurg 1994;81:690–698.
45. Tarbell NJ, Loeffler JS, Silver B, et al: The change in patterns of relapse in medulloblastoma. Cancer 1991;68:1600–1604.
46. Pollack IF, Polinko P, Albright AL, et al: Mutism and pseudobulbar symptoms after resection of posterior fossa tumors in children: Incidence and pathophysiology. Neurosurgery 1995;37:885–893.
47. Ris MD, Packer R, Goldwein J, Jones-Wallace D, Boyett JM: Intellectual outcome after reduced-dose radiation therapy plus adjuvant chemotherapy for medulloblastoma: A Children's Cancer Group study. J Clin Oncol 2001;19:3470–3476.
48. Johnson DL, McCabe MA, Nicholson HS, et al: Quality of long-term survival in young children with medulloblastoma. J Neurosurg 1994;80:1004–1010.
49. Brown WD, Tavar CJ, Sobel EL, Gilles FH: Medulloblastoma and Collins' law: A critical review of the concept of a period of risk for tumor recurrence and patient survival. Neurosurgery 1995;36:691–697.
50. Albright AL, Wisoff JH, Zeltzer PM, et al: Effects of medulloblastoma resections on outcome in children: A report from the Children's Cancer Group. Neurosurgery 1996;38:265–270.
51. Frost PJ, Laperriere NJ, Wong CS, et al: Medulloblastoma in adults. Int J Radiat Oncol Biol Phys 1995;32:951–957.
52. DeAngelis LM, Wong E, Rosenblum M, Furneaux H: Epstein-Barr virus in acquired immune deficiency syndrome (AIDS) and non-AIDS primary central nervous system lymphoma. Cancer 1992;70:1607–1611.
53. Fine HA, Mayer RJ: Primary central nervous system lymphoma. Ann Intern Med 1993;119:11.
54. Singh A, Strobos RJ, Singh BM, et al: Steroid-induced remission in CNS lymphoma. Neurology 1982;32:1267–1271.
55. Loeffler JS, Ervin TJ, Mauch P, et al: Primary lymphomas of the central nervous system: Patterns of failure and factors that influence survival. J Clin Oncol 1985;3:490–494.
56. DeAngelis LM, Yahalom J, Thaler HT, Kher U: Combined modality therapy for primary CNS lymphoma. J Clin Oncol 1992;10:635–643.
57. Glass J, Gruber ML, Cher L, Hochberg FH: Preirradiation methotrexate chemotherapy of primary central nervous system lymphoma. Long-term outcome. J Neurosurg 1994;81:188–195.
58. Chamberlain MC, Levin VA: Adjuvant chemotherapy for primary lymphoma of the central nervous system. Arch Neurol 1990;447:1113–1116.
59. Bessell EM, Lopez-Guillermo A, Villa S, et al: Importance of radiotherapy in the outcome of patients with primary CNS lymphoma: An analysis of the CHOD/BVAM regimen followed by two different radiotherapy treatments. J Clin Oncol 2002;20:231–236.
60. Wallace MR: Type 1 neurofibromatosis gene: Identification of a large transcript disrupted in three NF1 patients. Science 1990;249:181–186.
61. North K, Cochineas C, Tang E, Fagan E: Optic gliomas in neurofibromatosis type 1: Role of visual evoked potentials. Pediatr Neurol 1994;10:117–123.
62. Creange A, Zeller J, Rostaing-Rigattieri S, et al: Neurological complications of neurofibromatosis type 1 in adulthood. Brain 1999;122: 473–481.
63. Rosenberg RN, Iannaccone ST: The prevention of neurogenetic disease. Arch Neurol 1995;52:356–362.
64. Janss AJ, Grundy R, Cnaan A, et al: Optic pathway and hypothalamic/chiasmatic gliomas in children younger than age 5 years with a 6 year follow-up. Cancer 1995;75:1051–1059.
65. Hall WA, Luciano MG, Doppman JL, et al: Pituitary magnetic resonance imaging in normal human volunteers. Ann Intern Med 1994;120:817–820.
66. Maira G, Anile C, Rossi GF, Colosimo C: Surgical treatment of craniopharyngiomas: An evaluation of the transsphenoidal and pterional approaches. Neurosurgery 1995;36:715–724.
67. Harrigan MR: Cerebral salt wasting syndrome: A review. Neurosurgery 1996;38:152–160.
68. Pollock BE, Lunsford LD, Kondziolka D, et al: Phosphorus-32 intracavitary irradiation of cystic craniopharyngiomas: Current technique and long-term results. Int J Radiat Oncol Biol Phys 1995;33:437–446.
69. Olivero WC, Lister JR, Elwood PW: The natural history and growth rate of asymptomatic meningiomas: A review of 60 patients. J Neurosurg 1996;83:222–224.
70. Younis GA, Sawaya R, DeMonte F, et al: Aggressive meningeal tumors: Review of a series. J Neurosurg 1995;82:17–27.
71. Buhl R, Hasan A, Behnke A, Mehdorn HM: Results in the operative treatment of elderly patients with intracranial meningioma. Neurosurg Rev 2000;23:25–29.
72. Ferreira J, Eviatar L, Schneider S, Grossman R: Prenatal diagnosis of intracranial teratoma. Prolonged survival after resection of a malignant teratoma diagnosed prenatally by ultrasound: A case report and literature review. Pediatr Neurosurg 1993;9:84–88.
73. Roeder MB, Bazan C, Jinkins JR: Ruptured spinal dermoid cyst with chemical arachnoiditis and disseminated intracranial lipid droplets. Neuroradiology 1995;37:146–147.
74. Chandler J, Friedman WA: Radiosurgical treatment of a hemangioblastoma: Case report. Neurosurgery 1994;34:353–355.
75. O'Connell JX, Renard LG, Liebsch NJ, et al: Base of skull chordoma: A correlative study of histologic and clinical features of 62 cases. Cancer 1994;74:2261–2267.
76. Gay E, Sekhar LN, Rubinstein E, et al: Chordomas and chondrosarcomas of the cranial base: Results and follow-up of 60 patients. Neurosurgery 1995;36:887–897.
77. Cabbell KL, Rodd DA: Stereotactic microsurgical craniotomy for the treatment of third ventricular colloid cystsainage. Neurosurgery 1996;38:301–307.
78. Kohno M, Matsutani M, Sasaki T, Takakura K: Solitary metastasis to the choroid plexus of the lateral ventricle—report of three cases and a review of the literature. J Neuro-oncol 1996;27:47–52.

CHAPTER 47

RAMSIS K. BENJAMIN, ASHA DAS,
and FRED H. HOCHBERG

Metastatic Neoplasms and Paraneoplastic Syndromes

Neurological complications occur in as many as 40 percent of patients with systemic cancer. These conditions are feared and devastating with uniform morbidity. An estimated 170,000 patients annually experience brain or spinal cord difficulties either from direct or remote effects of a systemic neoplasm.[1] One fifth of the yearly cost of cancer in the United States is relegated to therapy for patients who harbor systemic malignancies metastatic to the nervous system or those with primary tumors commencing in the brain. From first symptoms, patients experience an uninterrupted cycle of repetitive hospitalizations, neurological morbidity, complicated surgical, radiation, or medical therapies, followed by extended periods of rehabilitation care. The costs commonly exceed $100,000 per patient.[2] Both the prevalence and associated costs of these disorders will invariably rise as patients with cancer live longer and have the benefit of sophisticated blood and imaging diagnostic procedures. Also, the nonmetastatic effects of cancer, including the complications of radiation therapy and chemotherapy, are becoming better understood, more apparent, and more disabling. This chapter provides both the primary caregiver and neurological specialist with the bases for the recognition of these disorders and focuses on neurological issues in day-to-day management as well as those problems handled best at specialized neurooncological centers. The neurological complications of cancer are outlined in Table 47–1. This chapter concentrates on metastatic effects of cancer and the paraneoplastic syndromes. The primary tumors of the nervous system are discussed in Chapter 46.

Direct Metastatic Disease

INTRAPARENCHYMAL METASTASES

Pathogenesis and Pathophysiology. To establish a metastasis in brain, cancers enter a cascade of events. First, tumor cells from the primary site of malignancy must reach a critical volume in proximity to a blood vessel. The cells then dislodge from the primary tumor and enter vessels through their basement membrane, stroma, and subendothelial membrane. In the vessel lumen, the cancer cells embolize to the microvasculature of other organs, extravasate, and grow within the parenchyma. To enter this cascade tumor cells utilize proteolytic enzymes, particularly metalloproteinases[3] and cathepsins, and tend not to retain fibronectin, collagen, or laminin, possibly as the result of a change in their specific integrin receptors. Metastases have the propensity to adhere to the vascular *addressins* on endothelial cells. Tumor growth is stimulated by trophic factors that stimulate growth of cells and their blood vessels. These factors are produced by the

TABLE 47–1. Classification of Neurological Complications of Cancer

I. Metastasis of Cancer to the Nervous System (Direct/Metastatic)
   A. Intracranial (intraparenchymal and dural)
   B. Leptomeningeal and ventricular
   C. Bony (calvarium and skull base)
   D. Spinal (vertebral, epidural, and intramedullary)
   E. Nerves (cranial nerves, peripheral nerves, nerve plexus, or nerve roots)
II. Nonmetastatic Neurological Complications of Cancer
   A. Vascular disorders
      1. Cerebral hemorrhage in cancer patients
      2. Intracerebral hematoma (intratumoral, coagulopathy, hypertension)
      3. Subdural hematoma
      4. Subarachnoid hemorrhage
      5. Cerebral infarction
      6. Atherosclerosis
      7. Intravascular coagulation
      8. Nonbacterial thrombotic endocarditis
      9. Septic occlusion
      10. Tumor embolus
      11. Venous occlusion
   B. Infections
      1. Bacteria (*Listeria, Nocardia*)
      2. Fungi (*Cryptococcus, Coccidioides, Histoplasma*)
      3. Parasites (*Toxoplasma, Strongyloides*)
      4. Viruses (varicella-zoster, papovavirus, cytomegalovirus, herpes simplex)
   C. Metabolic and nutritional encephalopathy
      1. Drugs
      2. Sepsis
      3. Oxygen deprivation (hypoxia, ischemia)
      4. Hypercapnia
      5. Fluid and electrolyte imbalance
      6. Hepatic failure
      7. Vitamin deficiencies
      8. Endocrine disorders
   D. Side effects of chemotherapy, radiation therapy, surgery, or other diagnostic procedures
   E. Paraneoplastic syndromes

Data from Posner JB: Neurologic Complications of Cancer. Philadelphia, F.A. Davis, 1995.

tumor cells themselves as well as by the target organs.[4] As the cells grow, they survive by avoiding the killing effects of macrophages, natural killer cells, and cells of the reticuloendothelial system.

Epidemiology and Risk Factors. Virtually all systemic cancers have the capacity to disseminate to the brain or spinal cord. In adults, melanoma has the highest predilection, followed by cancers of the lung, breast, and kidneys. However, lung and breast cancers are more common than melanoma, and therefore produce more cases of intracranial metastasis (Fig. 47–1).[5] If patients survive for years, metastases emerge from sarcoma and tumors of the gastrointestinal tract, thyroid, uterus, ovary, pancreas, and prostate. Hematological malignancies such as chronic leukemia and Hodgkin's disease are uncommon causes of brain metastases, and caution should be exercised when diagnosing cerebral metastases in patients with these neoplasms. In the pediatric population, osteogenic sarcoma, rhabdomyosarcoma, and testicular germ cell tumors are the most frequent solid brain metastases.

The interval between the appearance of the primary cancer and that of the cerebral metastasis varies widely. The delay reflects the speed of tumor growth and the time required to pass through intermediate organs such as the lung. The pulmonary circulation accounts for the usual passage of tumor cells to the cranial vault.[6] When tumors present first in the brain, they are usually of covert lung, melanoma, or breast origin, whereas those presenting decades after systemic cancer tend to be of breast, ovarian, or uterine origin. These latter cases may also reflect a covert lung cancer or melanoma. The average interval between the diagnosis of the primary carcinoma and the development of brain metastasis is 4 months for lung carcinoma and 3 years for breast cancer.

Two thirds of brain metastases are to the parenchyma of the brain. The remaining one third involve tumors overlying the brain in the subdural or extradural spaces and usually compress the brain. Brain involvement is in proportion to both tissue volume and blood flow. The cerebral hemispheres receive the majority of blood flow and are the site of nearly 75 percent of metastases, whereas the smaller and less vascular cerebellum, thalamus, and brain stem account for 15, 5, and 3 percent, respectively.[7] Most commonly invaded are the frontal lobes followed by parietal, occipital and temporal lobes, in descending order.[8] Highly vascularized areas, including the leptomeninges, ventricles, and pituitary gland, receive a disproportionately large number of cancers.

Hemispheric metastases lodge in regions where arterioles rapidly diminish in size to small capillaries. This caliber reduction occurs at the cortical gray-white junction and the "watershed" zones, those areas along the margins of arteriolar supply from major intracranial arteries. The latter zone covers 29 percent of the total brain volume, but harbors 62 percent of all brain metastases.[8]

In general, tumors of the pelvis or retroperitoneal space have proclivity for the infratentorial locations of the posterior fossa: the cerebellum, pons, and their coverings. These cancers spread through the paravertebral venous plexus, known as Batson's plexus, draining the primary locations. From other organs, systemic tumors drain into the pulmonary circulation and then to supratentorial locations.[9] Forty-four percent of cerebellar metastases are single and solitary; the rest are multiple. Less common than these parenchymal brain metastases are those tumors compressing dura from sites in bone of the calvarium (plasmacytoma or myeloma), or those surrounding cranial sinuses (carcinomas of the sinus epithelium or parotid, submandibular, or maxillary glands), and the cranial lymphoid epithelial tumors (lymphoma or plasmacytoma of the sinuses, lacrimal glands, and orbit) that spread directly through the bone and periosteum to the dura. In addition cancers of breast and prostate origin also produce these dural masses, often confused with subdural hematoma. Certain tumors of the skull base, often of lymphoma or sinus origin, have the potential of invading the neural foramina and the cranial nerves without damaging the bone.[10]

Rarely metastases develop in another tumor, such as breast cancer metastasizing to meningioma or to a vascular malformation.[11] When two different primary tumors exist (such as glioma and gastrointestinal cancer or meningioma in a

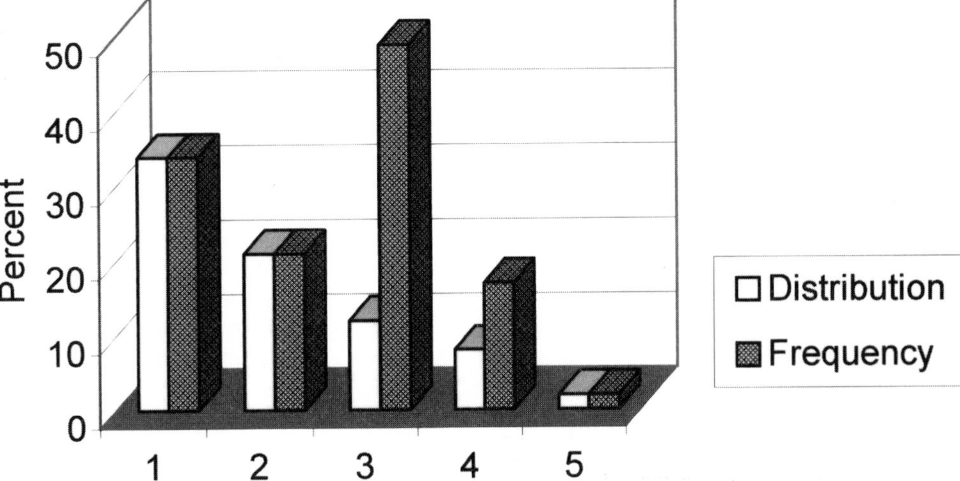

FIGURE 47–1. Primary tumors in patients with intracranial metastases: Distribution versus frequency. Tumor type: 1=lung; 2=breast; 3=melanoma; 4=urogenital tract; 5=prostate.

patient with breast cancer), the suspicion is raised of shared risk factors and treatment effects. Certainly, primary brain tumors have been reported in the setting of systemic malignancy and likely reflect common cancer-causing exposures, the effects of radiation therapy, or shared genetic predisposition. Those brain tumors occurring after bladder cancer may reflect the carcinogenic effects on the bladder and brain of occupational chemical exposure. If brain tumor risk is increased in patients with breast, endometrial, and colorectal cancer, this linkage may reflect the common exposure to reproductive hormones. The occurrence of sporadic cases of brain tumors after acute leukemia, sinus cancer, or pituitary tumors is probably due to tumor induction after cranial irradiation. Additionally, shared genetic predispositions can explain associations between brain tumors and sarcoma (Li-Fraumeni syndrome on chromosome 17), colorectal cancer[12] and familial polyposis (Turcot's and Gardner's syndromes, respectively; both on chromosome 5), nevoid basal cell carcinoma in association with medulloblastoma (chromosome 9), neurofibromatosis, von-Hippel Lindau, and a few others.

Clinical Features. Cognitive deficits, weakness, and headaches are the typical symptoms of intracranial metastases and are similar to those of other brain masses. These difficulties reflect the edema surrounding tumor, hydrocephalus, or compression of the dura (Table 47–2) much more than the actual mass of the tumor itself. Frequently the tumor volume accounts for less than 10 percent of mass volume. After steroid therapy, symptoms disappear in many metastatic lesions. Headache, the presenting complaint in one half of patients, is mild, not particularly disabling, and seldom migrainous. When visual or auditory features suggest migraine, these symptoms should raise concern for seizure activity. Headache may be worse in the morning as a result of increased edema from CO_2 retention during sleep. Headache is ominous when associated with emesis, hiccoughs, yawning, transient visual loss or altered awareness. Seizures are commonly associated with tumors that metastasize to the gray matter of the brain and can be the presenting complaint in up to one third of patients with new or previously treated intracranial metastasis. Seizure frequency among cancer patients, however, is not sufficiently high enough to support the use of prophylactic anticonvulsants. Careful examination discloses weakness in two thirds of patients, but less than half complain of focal weakness. Similarly, although only one third of patients note behavioral or mental status changes, when careful mental status testing is done, impaired cognitive function is apparent in three fourths of patients.[13] Small metastases in the frontal, temporal, and occipital lobes may be missed when not associated with focal weakness. Thus, the apathy, inattention, and abulia that accompany frontal lobe lesions are commonly attributed to exogenous depression. Psychotic thought disorders, unusually querulous and "viscous" personality changes, food intolerance, or hallucinations of smell and tingling may accompany lesions of the temporal lobe. Right parietal lobe lesions alter the ability to attend to one side of space, and may produce apraxia of dressing. Multiple metastases, often of breast or lung origin, can produce a confusional state. Cerebellar metastases, likely the most symptom-inducing lesions of all intracranial tumors, are heralded by headache or gaze-evoked nystagmus, associated rarely with dizziness. Often walking appears wide-based and staggering. If the lesion is close to the fourth ventricle there may be vomiting or hiccups, but dysarthria and tremor are uncommon.[14]

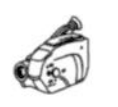
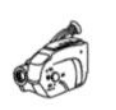

Hemorrhage within a metastatic brain tumor occurs in one tenth of patients who develop acute symptoms. Metastases of choriocarcinoma, melanoma, and bronchogenic, thyroid, and renal cell carcinomas are most prone to bleeding.[15, 16] These

TABLE 47–2. **Presenting Symptoms and Signs of Brain Metastasis**

Symptom	Common Signs
Headache	Focal weakness or unexplained falls
Mental status change	Focal sensory deficits
Altered level of consciousness	Speech difficulty
Seizures occurring when older than 35 years of age	Aphasia, focal weakness
Papilledema or visual obscurations	Ataxia
Visual complaints or unexplained motor vehicle accidents	Visual field defect

hemorrhages occur within the metastatic deposit, may be confluent, and often must be treated with emergency craniectomy and decompression. Subdural hematomas in cancer patients are less common and usually occur in the context of head trauma or anticoagulant medication use.

Differential Diagnosis. Mass lesions in the brain are not necessarily metastatic. Indeed, one out of 10 presumed metastases are actually of other origin, including primary central nervous system (CNS) tumors, abscess, granuloma, acute demyelinating disease, resolving cerebral hematoma, stroke, and radiation necrosis. Many nontumor masses have characteristic magnetic resonance (MR) diffusion signals and spectroscopy (MRS) patterns. Brain abscesses occur with frequencies of less than 2 percent of those for intracranial tumors but are on the rise in immunodeficient populations. Granulomas in the brain result from infection with *Mycobacterium*, *Candida*, *Aspergillus*, *Cryptococcus*, and *Histoplasma* species. Sarcoidosis masses and meningeal infiltrates are similar to infiltrates of Whipple's disease. Demyelinating lesions of acute disseminated encephalomyelitis present as focal neurological dysfunction with seizures and edematous mass(es). These masses occur as large ring-enhancing lesions in a setting of recent respiratory infection or immunization.[17]

Nonbacterial thrombotic endocarditis (NBTE) produces embolization of cardiac vegetations to the arteries of the brain or occludes these vessels as a result of intravascular thrombosis from an associated coagulation disorder. Tumors of hematopoietic origin and of the lung, gastrointestinal tract, breast, and genitourinary tract most commonly result in NBTE. Although most patients with NBTE have disseminated cancer, the brain vascular syndromes seldom are seen when tumor is not present. Stroke, metabolic encephalopathy, or complicated migraine is observed. Coagulopathy, with arterial or venous brain infarcts, in the presence of anticardiolipin antibodies (Hughes syndrome) or abnormalities of Russell viper venom coagulation studies, may involve patients with breast cancer and leukemia. Intravascular coagulation usually produces multiple small vessel occlusions as a diffuse encephalopathy, frequently with focal signs.[18]

Evaluation. No test other than magnetic resonance imaging (MRI) with contrast medium is required to exclude or confirm brain metastasis, especially at the gray-white junction (Fig. 47–2).[19] Computed tomography (CT) with contrast, often the first study obtained in an emergency setting, detects multiple metastases in 50 percent of patients,[7] 20 percent fewer than those detected on enhanced MRI.[20] Metastases as small as 3 mm can be identified using MRI at gapless 3-mm sections accompanying single-dose and then triple-dose administrations of gadolinium, often with delayed imaging times (Fig. 47–3).[21] The characteristic features of metastases include increased signal on T1-weighted images. Edema appears as T2-weighted hyperintensity surrounding the hypointense tumor. The latter may exhibit irregular rim enhancement. Several newer techniques, including magnetization transfer imaging, proton MRS (with elevated ratios of choline to creatine), and diffusion-weighted MRI (reflecting increased flow of water into cells as a result of deficient membrane pumps), can further delineate brain tumors from infections, abscesses, and strokes.[22–26] Diffusion-weighted imaging (DWI) is sensitive to the diffusion of water protons and can be quantified by a measure known as the apparent diffusion coefficient (ADC). Restricted diffusion due to cytotoxic edema appears dark on ADC maps. On the other hand, vasogenic edema appears hyperintense owing to increased extracellular water content in the edematous region. In cases of abscess, the DWI is bright, whereas lobulated or cystic metastases are hypointense.

In the absence of a known malignancy the physician should obtain a history, breast and prostate exam, CT of the chest and abdomen, blood chemistry and differential cell counts, liver enzyme studies, tumor marker studies including prostate-specific antigen, carcinoembryonic antigen (CEA), CA-125, and mammography where appropriate. Without a known systemic cancer, as occurs in 5 to 10 percent of patients, the surgeon is obligated to provide surgical material from the brain for diagnosis of the primary tumor. The histological evaluation of these specimens includes use of antibodies that are tumor and/or organ specific (Table 47–3).

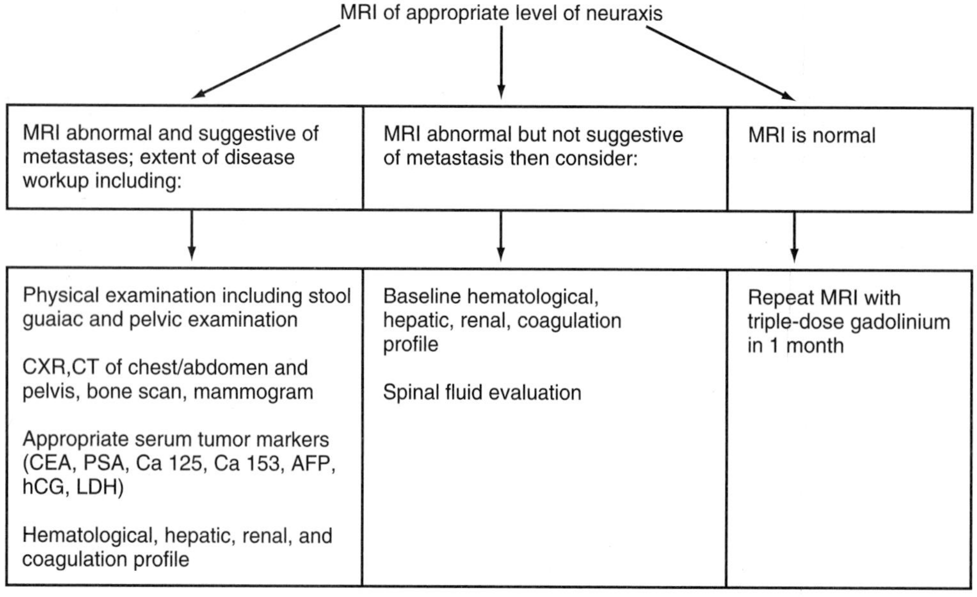

FIGURE 47–2. Evaluation of patients with suspected metastatic cancer to the central nervous system. AFP, alpha-fetoprotein; CEA, carcinoembryonic antigen; CT, computed tomography; CXR, chest x-ray; hCG, human chorionic gonadotropin; LDH, lactate dehydrogenase; LEMS, Lambert-Eaton myasthenic syndrome; MRI, magnetic resonance imaging; PSA, prostate-specific antigen.

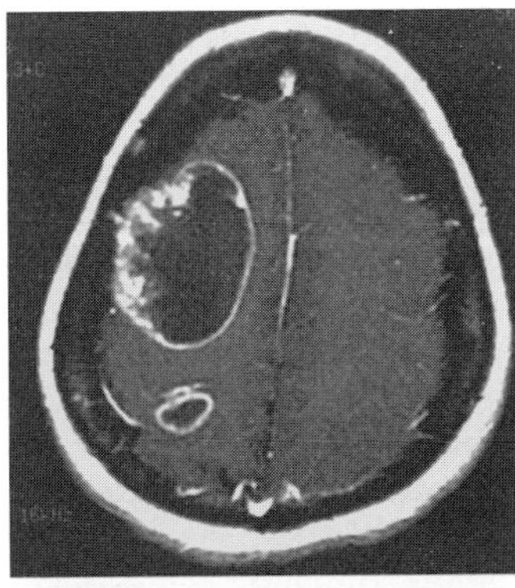

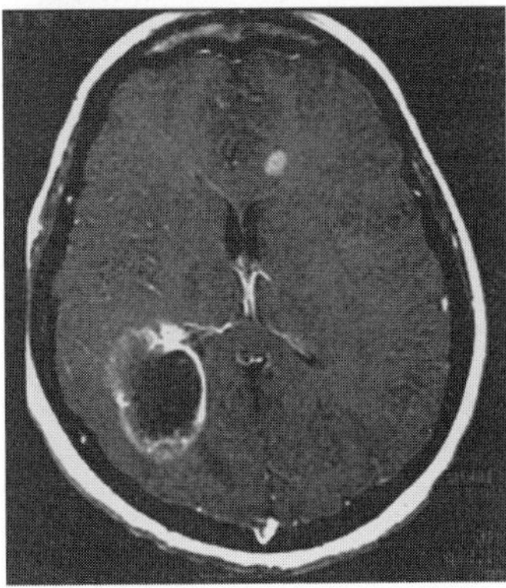

FIGURE 47–3. Multiple metastases on MRI scan are associated with lung carcinoma. (Courtesy of Todd Brack, DO.)

Management. The optimal treatment of patients with brain metastasis continues to evolve. Untreated, brain metastases are fatal within 1.5 months of diagnosis. These patients succumb from neurological, not systemic, causes. Corticosteroids produce a clinical response in 70 percent of these patients, but extend the median survival to only 2 months. The palliative addition of whole-brain radiotherapy (WBRT), 30 Gy in 10 fractions, has extended median survival to 3 to 6 months.[27] With palliative radiotherapy the rates of neurological deaths are reduced to the level of those seen from systemic disease.[28] Radiosurgery utilizes single fractions provided by "gamma knife" or similar photon devices or linear accelerators, proton beams of cyclotron derivation, or interstitial x-ray generators. These treatments are optimized for symptomatic lesions less than 3 cm in size (volume <12 cm^3), which are spherical and located in noneloquent brain areas.[29] In general, technologies with rapid "fall-off" of radiation penumbra are best offered to sites close to the optic chiasm or the brain stem. Adjunctive whole-brain irradiation is often added after radiosurgery to prevent recurrence in local or distant sites.

Conventionally fractionated photon radiotherapy is successfully given to "radiosensitive" tumors (lung, breast, or germ cell origin), whereas "radioresistant" lesions (melanoma, renal cell carcinoma, colon cancer, or sarcoma origin) are best treated with single or multiple radiosurgical fractions. Prophylactic cranial irradiation provided in the setting of small-cell lung cancer reduces the likelihood of CNS relapse by 20 percent, although it does not provide long-term survival benefit.[30]

Surgical excision is indicated in solitary lesions, cases of impending morbidity or death from edema, or in those with an unknown malignancy for whom operation will provide the diagnosis. Usually areas of sizable tumor with attendant edema, impending hydrocephalus, or compression of the fourth ventricle are targets of operative intervention. Finally, new chemotherapeutic agents as single or combination treatments—temozolomide,[31, 32] topotecan,[33] capecitabine,[34] liposomal doxorubicin, and weekly paclitaxel,[35] cisplatin, and etoposide[36]—have shown some promise and may play a greater role in the management of brain metastasis in the future.

Prognosis and Future Perspectives. Brain metastasis from breast cancer carry a better prognosis than spread from lung cancer, melanoma, or colorectal cancer.[37] Therapy is often based on the prognosis of the systemic cancer. With surgical resection and WBRT, patients with solitary brain metastases survive longer and remain functionally independent in comparison to recipients of radiation alone.[38, 39] In a retrospective study by Lentzsch et al,[40] women with breast cancer and brain metastasis had a median survival of 1 month, 6.5 months, and 21 months when rendered corticosteroids only, WBRT, and surgery alone, respectively. Although stereotactic radiosurgery and WBRT show comparable results,[41–43] this finding is counterintuitive and is the subject of a large clinical trial that is ongoing. In a recent randomized prospective trial[39] adjuvant WBRT with 50.4 Gy in surgically resected solitary metastasis yielded a dramatic reduction in both local and distant tumor recurrence relative to surgery alone (18 percent vs 70 percent), but without an overall change in survival rate. In general these studies do not take into account the quality of life of radiation recipients, a subject of great concern to older individuals likely at

TABLE 47–3. **Histological Stains with Tumor Specificity***

Histological Stain	Tumor Specificity
Keratin	Carcinomas
Mucicarmine (chromogranin)	Neuroendocrine tumors
HMB-45	Melanoma
S-100	Melanoma, sarcoma
CEA	Adenocarcinomas of colon, stomach, lung, breast, pancreas, uterus, ovary; medullary carcinoma of thyroid, squamous carcinoma
Estrogen and progesterone receptors	Breast and uterus
Muscle-specific actin	Rhabdomyosarcomas
Alpha-fetoprotein, human chorionic gonadotropin	Genitourinary tumor
Placental alkaline phosphatase	Germ cell tumors
Prostatic acid phosphatase or prostate-specific antigen	Prostate carcinomas
Leukocytic common antigen, immunoglobulins, L26, UCHL 1, Leu-M1, and CD30	Lymphoma

*The approach suggested in the evaluation of patients with suspected brain metastases is identified in Figure 47–1.

TABLE 47–4. Common Primary Sites of Cancer in Patients with Leptomeningeal Metastases

Breast
Lung
Lymphoma
Melanoma
Adenocarcinoma of unknown origin

Data from Olsen ME, Chernik NL, Posner JB: Leptomeningeal metastases from systemic cancer: A report of 47 cases. Trans Am Neurol Assoc 1971;96:291–293; and Wasserstrom WR, Glass JP, Posner JB: Diagnosis and treatment of leptomeningeal metastases from solid tumors: Experience with 90 patients. Cancer 1982;49:759–772.

risk of memory and intellectual alterations. Multiple brain metastases of breast origin or absent systemic primary lesions may benefit from surgical removal of all lesions,[44] or of radiosurgery if operation is impossible. Similarly, reoperation for recurrent hemorrhagic, edematous, or posterior fossa brain metastases can prolong survival and improve quality of life. For most patients, poor prognosis is associated with extensive systemic disease, multiple lesions, Karnofsky performance score below 70, recurrence within 4 months, and age older than 40 years.[28, 45] Patients with breast metastasis younger than 40 years, however, carry a poorer prognosis than older subjects.[40] Future trends are likely to focus on the role of improved chemotherapy, expanded use of radiosurgery to include larger and more numerous lesions, the concomitant use of oxygen-enhancing radiosensitizers, and improvements in automated MRI-based radiotherapy techniques.

MENINGEAL AND VENTRICULAR METASTASES

Pathogenesis and Pathophysiology. Leptomeningeal metastases (meningeal carcinomatosis) can develop when malignant cells reach the cerebrospinal fluid (CSF). Tumor cells may enter through the leptomeningeal veins, the choroid plexus, veins draining the bone marrow, of the skull or as a result of inadvertent shedding during neurosurgical procedures. Malignant cells may grow along cranial or peripheral nerve roots. Rarely, metastases to the parenchyma of brain or spinal cord seed into the CSF, usually when there is involvement of the cerebellum in proximity to the subarachnoid space or fourth ventricle.[46]

Epidemiology and Risk Factors. At least 5 percent of patients with disseminated cancer develop leptomeningeal metastases.[47, 48] Unlike the multiplicity of cell types responsible for intracerebral metastases, metastases to the subarachnoid space, ventricular system, and choroid plexus are frequently adenocarcinoma (usually of breast, lung, or prostate origin), melanoma, or lymphoma (Table 47–4). Although days to years may pass before the meninges are invaded, the diagnosis of leptomeningeal involvement is most commonly made 6 months to 3 years after the primary tumor is discovered.

Clinical Features and Associated Findings. Leptomeningeal metastases are usually clinically silent, and when present are seldom separable from those of parenchymal brain involvement. The physician who awaits the appearance of nuchal rigidity, pain with straight leg raising, or headache likely has waited too long. The telltale clinical sign is the appearance of subtle but multiple clinical deficits.[49] Commonly combined are cranial nerve deficits with dulled sensorium and obstipation or urinary hesitancy. Infiltrates of the pia and Virchow-Robin spaces affect the cerebrum, cranial nerves, and spinal roots. A subtle abducens paresis may be combined with reduced pin sensation over the legs or asymmetry of deep tendon reflexes. Communicating hydrocephalus, with associated diminished attention, gait apraxia, urinary incontinence, and hyperactivity of ankle reflexes and Babinski responses, results from obstruction of the arachnoid granulations by layers of tumor cells. As the intracranial pressure rises and there is stretching of the dura and trigeminal innervation, bifrontal, diffuse, or radiating skull-based headache may develop. Nausea, vomiting, or lightheadedness ensues, often with confusion and memory loss. Episodes of altered consciousness, seizures, nausea and vomiting, dizziness or lightheadedness, and gait ataxia reflect changes in cranial pressure or localized nonatheromatous changes in arterial or venous perfusion (Table 47–5). The cranial nerves are either compressed by infiltrates of tumor cells or rendered ischemic when tumor invades the feeding vessels. Diplopia from subtle cranial nerve VI compression, facial numbness, central hearing alteration, and impaired visual acuity are common but frequently overlooked. The compromised spinal nerve roots induce diffuse back pain, radicular pain, and paresthesias. Involvement of the cauda equina produces obstipation, constipation, and urinary hesitancy.

Differential Diagnosis. Multifocal neurological symptoms are common to many metastatic sites. Cranial and spinal nerve dysfunction may be mimicked by cranial or spinal epidural foci of cancer; multiple infiltrates of intra-axial lymphoma; infections with *Borrelia*, parasitic organisms, or fungi in the immunosuppresssed patient; or coagulation abnormalities during chemotherapy. Paraneoplastic radiculopathy (see later), aseptic or bacterial meningitides (see Chapter 42), and hydrocephalus all should be part of the physician's concern.

Evaluation. The diagnosis of meningeal cancer is generally difficult. A single CSF examination reveals tumor cells in 50 percent of patients, rising to 98 percent after two procedures with 10 mL aliquots of fluid drawn in the vicinity of the disease.[50] It is recommended that fluid from both ventricular and lumbar areas be sampled if possible, especially when assessing response to treatment.[47] CSF from the first cervical interspace is much closer than lumbar CSF to cranial nerve tumors and the resulting specimens are more reflective of the underlying disease. CSF cytology may remain persistently negative on repeated fluid examinations in 10 percent of patients with leptomeningeal disease.[48] Although tumor markers such as CEA and beta-2 microglobulin in the spinal

TABLE 47–5. Cerebral Symptoms and Signs in Patients with Leptomeningeal Metastases from Solid Tumors

Symptoms	Common Signs
Headache	Papilledema
Mental status changes	Dysarthria/dysphasia
Nausea/vomiting	Extensor plantar
Vertigo/lightheadedness	Hemiparesis
Seizures	Diabetes insipidus

fluid provide useful information, their assessment is not a common practice because the results are neither specific nor sensitive. For example, CEA may indicate leptomeningeal carcinoma, especially metastatic lung cancer, and beta-2 microglobulin corresponds with hematological neoplasm. Certain tumors, such as sarcomas or malignant gliomas, are seldom detected in CSF as their cells strongly adhere to the leptomeninges or occur as focal nodules rather than widespread leptomeningeal disease.[51] MRI is a valuable tool in the investigation of leptomeningeal metastasis. Often gadolinium-enhanced MRI is definitive in the absence of CSF cytological abnormalities or provides equal sensitivity to CSF cytology[52] (Fig. 47–4). Typically, MRI delineates leptomeningeal or subependymal enhancement, dural enhancement, superficial cerebral lesions, enhancement of cranial nerves, or communicating hydrocephalus, the latter occurring most often in patients with solid, rather than hematological, tumors.[53] The single most characteristic finding is the appearance of thickened, often nodular, lumbar nerve roots within the subarachnoid space. An adjunct to CSF studies will be the increasing use of polymerase chain reaction–based analyses for infectious agents (including those of herpetic, toxoplasmosis, or cysticercal origin), rearrangements of immunoglobulin genes (lymphoma), and tumor-specific marker proteins.

Management. Therapy is based on irradiation and chemotherapy. As a general rule, symptomatic or nodular foci of tumor require irradiation, whereas chemotherapy is provided to patients without these findings. Chemotherapy can be administered either systemically or intrathecally, but in most instances intrathecal chemotherapy via an Ommaya device is the preferable route of administration. The device, a small Silastic membrane in communication with either the ventricle or subarachnoid space, serves as a painless delivery port. Complications from its use occur in fewer than 5 percent of patients and include the risk of infection, failure, bleeding, or drug toxicities to white matter. Commonly used chemotherapeutic agents include methotrexate (12 mg twice a week with an oral leucovorin rescue), cytarabine (50 mg twice a week or liposomal cytarabine bimonthly), and thiotepa (10 mg twice a week) until CSF is cleared of malignant cells. Liposomal cytarabine, recently approved for meningeal lymphoma, commonly produces an aseptic meningeal reaction necessitating the use of corticosteroids. Radiation therapy of tumor nodules larger than 5 mm is provided as local boosts designed to spare the bone marrow of the iliac crests and vertebrae. If chemotherapy fails, radiation to the entire neuraxis at doses of 30 Gy in 10 fractions can be recommended. Intrathecal radiolabeled I^{131} monoclonal antibodies,[54] lymphokine-activated killer cells, and oral etoposide are other therapeutic alternatives. Many tumors of lymphoma or breast origin are sensitive to methotrexate therapy. This drug, given intravenously in gram equivalent doses (3.5 to –8 g/m^2), is a suitable alternative to intrathecal approaches and produces therapeutic concentrations throughout the ventricular and lumbar CSF as well as the brain parenchyma.[55]

Prognosis and Future Perspectives. Although a percentage of patients with leukemia, lymphoma, and breast cancer respond to some treatment, the prognosis for patients with non–small-cell lung cancer, melanoma, and other adenocarcinomas is extremely poor. Patients with leptomeningeal spread from breast cancer survive a median period of 7 months. The survival is reduced for other solid tumors. Without treatment, the patients succumb within 6 weeks. The survival extends to 3 to 6 months with radiation therapy to symptomatic sites and intrathecal chemotherapy.[48] Treatment with experimental radiolabeled monoclonal antibodies increases the mean survival to 24 months in 50 percent of patients, with a few long-term survivors.[54] Future trends are likely to concentrate on treatments utilizing slow-release chemotherapy agents or those with high penetrance of the CSF after parenchymal administration.

SKULL-BASE METASTASES

Metastases to the skull base usually fall within the province of the otolaryngological surgeon or oncologist. Cancers of the breast, lung, and prostate have a propensity to produce skull-base metastases, which can entrap the cranial nerves and vessels at their exit foramina (Table 47–6). Greenberg has identified five clinical syndromes: orbital, parasellar, middle fossa, jugular foramen, and occipital condyle.[56] Skull-base metastases most commonly involve the 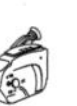 middle cranial fossa, in the area of Gasserian ganglion. Other sites include the jugular foramen, affecting cranial nerves IX, X, and XI to produce posterior auricular pain; occipital condyle, causing ipsilateral hypoglossal palsy and occipital pain; parasellar region, exhibiting as unilateral frontal sensory loss, headaches, and ophthalmoplegia; and orbit,

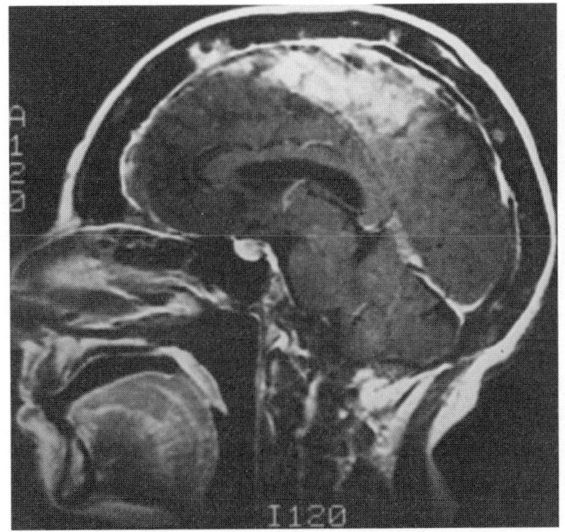

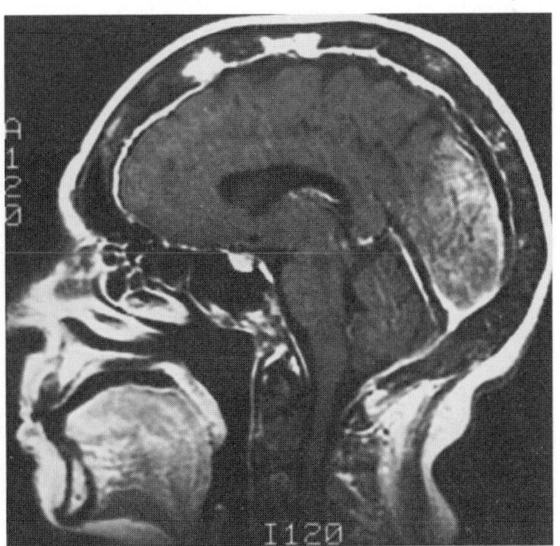

FIGURE 47–4. Meningeal carcinomatosis. Sagittal MRI scans showing deposition of tumor. (Courtesy of M. Huckman, MD.)

presenting as proptosis and external ophthalmoplegia. Often the cancer appears as a thin skin of tumor cells, termed *en plaque*.

Owing to their insidious subacute onset, skull-based metastases are difficult to identify on MRI or CT where masses may coalesce with changes of prior irradiation or surgical extirpation. Often the T2-weighted changes in contiguous bone after radiotherapy may be confused with tumor. Radionucleotide bone scans with careful evaluation of the skull may improve diagnosis. Treatment depends on the nature of the underlying tumor and is typically confined to irradiation as previously described.

SPINAL METASTASES

Pathogenesis and Pathophysiology. The vertebral column is the most common site of skeletal metastases, which may be due to the rich concentration of growth factors in its bone marrow stroma. Spread from the primary site to the spine occurs through the arterial system, retrograde spread of malignant cells through Batson's plexus particularly during Valsalva maneuvers,[57] and direct invasion of the tumor through the intervertebral foramina from a paraspinal mass. An epidural mass lesion can produce damage to the spinal cord either by mass effect, resulting in mechanical distortion with demyelination or axonal destruction, or from vascular compromise, producing venous congestion and vasogenic edema of the spinal cord with resultant venous hemorrhage and loss of myelin and ischemia.

Epidemiology and Risk Factors. Seventy-five percent of patients with breast cancer and one third of patients with solid tumors have spinal metastases at autopsy, though only 5 to 10 percent of patients with solid tumors ever develop epidural spinal cord compression. The most commonly identified cancers causing epidural spinal cord compression are cancers of breast, lung, prostate, and renal systems, lymphoma, sarcoma, and melanoma (Table 47–7). Eighty-five percent of cases of epidural spinal cord compression arise from metastases to the vertebral column. The vertebral body is the portion most frequently involved. The pedicle or posterior arch is less frequently involved. In 10 to 15 percent of cases, epidural spinal cord compression arises from lymphoma or renal cell cancer spreading through the intervertebral foramina (Fig. 47–5).[58, 59]

TABLE 47–6. **Syndromes of Base of Skull Metastases and Their Associated Symptoms**

Syndrome	Signs and Symptoms
Orbital and parasellar	Progressive, dull, continuous pain in the supraorbital area over the affected eye, diplopia, proptosis of the involved eye, external ophthalmoplegia, first-division trigeminal sensory loss
Parasellar	Ipsilateral frontal headache, oculomotor or abducens palsies without associated proptosis or visual loss
Middle fossa	Facial pain or numbness referable to the second or third divisions of trigeminal nerve
Jugular foramen	Paralysis of cranial nerves IX through XI
Occipital condyle	Unilateral occipital pain and unilateral tongue paralysis

Data from Greenberg HS, Deck MDF, Vikram B, et al: Metastasis to the base of the skull: Clinical findings in 43 patients. Neurology 1981;31:530–537.

TABLE 47–7. **Common Primary Malignancies in Patients with Symptomatic Spinal Cord Compression**

Breast
Lung
Prostate
Lymphoreticular system
Sarcomas
Kidney
Unknown primary

Several studies have shown that metastatic epidural spinal cord compression occurs at multiple noncontiguous sites in 10 to 38 percent of cases. Multifocal involvement is particularly high in patients with breast and prostate cancer. Usually the tumor occupies the anterior or anterolateral spinal cord. This has significance for clinicians as posterior decompression will not address the main mass of tumor. The overall sites of spinal involvement are 70 percent thoracic, 20 percent lumbosacral, and 10 percent cervical,[58] although lumbar spine involvement is three times more likely than cervical spine involvement in patients with prostate cancer.[60]

Clinical Features and Associated Findings. Back pain and leg weakness are the major findings, and MRI is the diagnostic procedure of choice. Local, radicular, or referred pain is the most common initial symptom, preceding any objective neurologic deficit (Table 47–8). The pain is localized, reflecting stretching of the pain-sensitive bony periosteum, and is constant, progressive, and worsened by coughing, sneezing, or straining. As the pain increases in the prone position, some patients adopt postures of sleep in a sitting position to obtain relief. Movements such as turning over in bed or rising from a lying position may be excruciating. Tenderness is found to percussion over the involved vertebral body. Patients without pain or neurological deficit probably do not have epidural spinal cord compression or intradural metastasis.

In general, the clinical symptoms correlate closely with the site of compression. For example, laterally placed masses that compress the lateral corticospinal and spinothalamic fibers cause a Brown-Séquard syndrome consisting of ipsilateral hemiparesis and loss of vibration and position sense along with contralateral loss of pain and temperature sensation below the lesion. Compression of the posterior tracts of the spinal cord affects dorsal fibers for position and vibratory sensations but does not alter pain and temperature sensations or strength. The corticospinal tracts and the posterior columns are most vulnerable to compression, and therefore leg weakness and gait disturbances are common presentations. Spinothalamic and descending autonomic fibers are less vulnerable. Although neurological findings often reflect direct compressive effects of tumor, clinicians should always consider spinal cord ischemia from compression of radicular arteries or venous drainage. In this case, neurological signs

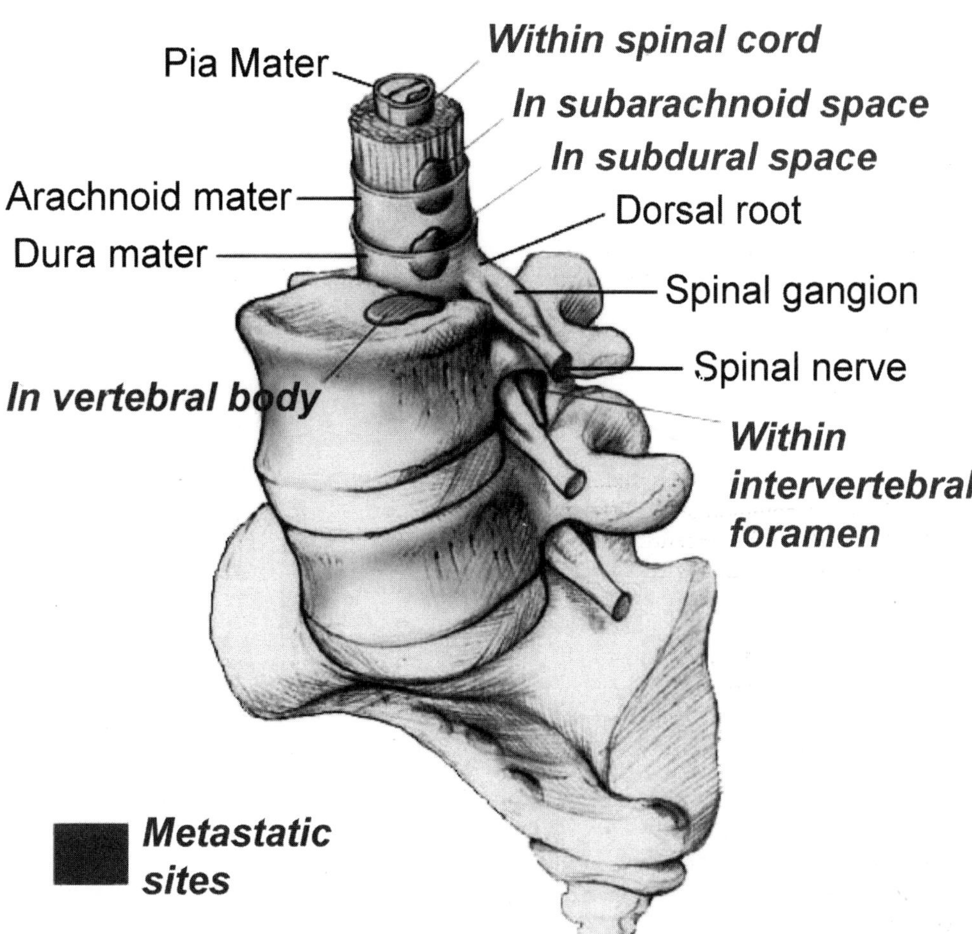

FIGURE 47–5. Sites of metastases to the spine. Adapted from Benjamin R: Neurologic complications of prostate cancer. (Am Fam Physician 2002;65: 1834–1840.)

may suggest a wider area of spinal cord damage than apparent from the site of metastasis. Weakness, spasticity, and hyperreflexia are the earliest signs of epidural spinal cord compression. Loss of pain and temperature sensation and bowel and bladder dysfunction occur late in the disease. Gait ataxia due to spinocerebellar tract compression or altered position sense may be the only sign of epidural cord compromise.

The longitudinal location of the lesion is clinically important as it is the major determinant of morbidity as well as the most significant clinical indicator for the surgeon and radiation therapist. The most reliable clinical sign is the level of sensory loss to pin testing. Other approaches may also be fruitful, including identification of the level of altered "wheal and flare" reaction to skin scratch, reduction of vibration sense over the posterior vertebrae, or loss of perception of the directional movement (toward or away from the head) of the skin of the back. Cervical lesions cause quadriplegia, and thoracic lesions cause paraplegia. The conus medullaris syndrome behaves like an acute intramedullary lesion. It is due to upper lumbar lesions and results in normal or near normal motor function, early bowel and bladder dysfunction, and extensor plantar responses with bilateral Achilles tendon stretch loss. Lesions below the first lumbar vertebral body compromise the cauda equina, causing radicular pain, early lower motor neuron weakness, asymmetrical hyporeflexia (especially of Achilles and patellae), plantarflexion of the toes, and possibly bowel and bladder incontinence.

TABLE 47–8. **Signs and Symptoms of Spinal Cord Compression**
Pain
Weakness
Autonomic dysfunction
Sensory loss
Ataxia

Differential Diagnosis. Other spinal diseases occur in cancer patients. Disc herniation or steroid-related compression fracture can be painful, as can ischemic or hemorrhagic lesions of the spinal cord and epidural space. Painful involvement of the brachial or lumbar plexus by tumor (lung, breast, ovarian, or uterine) or the painless effects of localized prior radiotherapy or chemotherapy must be considered. Other conditions include leptomeningeal cancer, demyelinating disease, paraneoplastic myelitis or motor neuropathy, necrotizing myelopathy, and epidural fat deposition associated with chronic corticosteroid use.

Evaluation. Visualization of the epidural space can be accomplished with MRI and should be provided to cancer patients with back pain. The MRI study, which should include the entire spinal axis, has largely replaced CT myelography. Imaging of the entire spinal axis discloses multiple epidural deposits in 15 percent of cases and sets the stage for the simulation of radiation portals and the design of surgical decompression. Clinicians reviewing MRI studies should address the issue of spine stability, the extent of spondylolisthesis, the presence of T2-weighted or FLAIR signal abnormalities within the spinal cord, and the extent of preservation of the three columns supporting the vertebrae. The treatment plan is based on the extent and evolution of neurological difficulties as well as the MRI-defined cord damage and spinal stability.

Routine radiography or bone scintigraphy should not be used to evaluate epidural disease but can provide clues to metastatic disease. Epidural metastasis is found in 87 percent of patients with more than 50 percent collapse of the vertebra on radiographs, 31 percent of those with pedicle erosion without major vertebral collapse, and 7 percent of those with tumor limited to the vertebral body without collapse.[61] Vertebral body collapse is, therefore, a highly specific indicator of epidural disease. Normal spine radiographs do not exclude epidural disease. For example, in patients with lymphoma, more than 60 percent of patients with epidural disease showed no demonstrable spinal abnormality.[62] Bone scintigraphy is generally more sensitive, but less specific, than plain radiography. A positive bone scintigram with a normal radiograph is associated with epidural disease in 17 percent of patients with back pain and no neurological findings.[63] Therefore, clinicians should obtain early MRI studies, even in the setting of normal bone scintigraphy and plain radiographs.

Management. The management of metastatic epidural compression is evolving and involves the provision of either radiation therapy or surgical decompression. For most patients, early management includes obtaining MRI scans and alleviating pain with opioids, corticosteroids, and radiation therapy. The treatment of pain should follow the analgesic ladder as developed by the World Health Organization, with rescue doses for breakthrough pain.[64, 65] Clinical and laboratory studies demonstrate that corticosteroids improve neurological function and relieve pain in the short term, but their contribution to ultimate recovery is unknown. Corticosteroids should be administered by vein immediately, often prior to definitive scanning. The benefit of dexamethasone is dose-related. In most centers, the immediate intravenous dose is 10 to 100 mg followed by 4 to 24 mg either intravenously or orally four times a day. Larger doses are used in patients with profound or rapidly progressive neurological injury, with lower doses in those with mild or equivocal signs. The administration of corticosteroids is usually continued in a tapering dose throughout radiation therapy, the latter consisting of 30 Gy in 10 fractions.[66, 67] Rarely does mannitol diuresis provide any benefit.

Excellent results follow anterior[68, 69] and posterior decompression[70] with appropriate stabilization. There is no consensus concerning the treatment of neoplastic spinal cord compression. Traditionally, surgery is provided to patients with controlled systemic disease (> 6 months life expectancy) whose instability of spine and spinal cord damage cannot be reversed with radiation therapy. To this group can be added those patients with paraplegia or quadriplegia at diagnosis, or patients whose condition deteriorates during or relapses after radiation therapy. Although surgical morbidity occurs in one third of these patients, chiefly from wound breakdown and sepsis,[71] surgery may be the only hope at regaining ambulation. Older literature identified no difference between radiation and surgical treatment of epidural disease, reflecting the indiscriminate use of posterior laminectomy regardless of the anatomy of the compression. However, it is likely that ongoing randomized trials will define a new role for surgery that maximizes tumor resection, stabilizes the spine, and returns a minority of patients to independent walking. Several reports have demonstrated the value of the anterior approach in patients who fail radiation therapy, with short-term improvement rates ranging from 60 to 80 percent. Recompression at the operative site occurs in more than one third of previously irradiated patients, whereas a high proportion of patients undergoing surgery as their first intervention maintain their ambulatory status until death.[72, 73]

Prognosis and Future Perspectives. The major determinant of treatment outcome is the patient's pretreatment neurological status. Patients who walk at the onset of radiation are likely to maintain ambulation, even after surgical intervention.[70, 74, 75] The rate of progression of neurological symptoms is also important, as slow progression predicts a better recovery. Future trials will undoubtedly stratify patients by tumor histology and the extent of T2 or FLAIR abnormalities within the spinal cord.

PERIPHERAL NERVE METASTASES

Cancer can affect peripheral nerves either by compression or direct invasion. Direct invasion occurs from hematogenous spread of tumor to peripheral nerves or dorsal root ganglia, or by direct extension from surrounding structures. Typically, head and neck malignancies, melanoma, lung and breast cancer, and abdominal and pelvic tumors cause either cranial or peripheral nerve dysfunction. In general, this involvement is late in the disease, with the possible exception of head and neck cancer, neurotropic skin cancers, and lymphoma. Frequently pain, sensory symptoms, or weakness reflect involvement of single or multiple cranial nerves, spinal roots, nerve plexi, or peripheral nerves. However, these painful syndromes can be mimicked by neurotoxicities of chemotherapy, radiation, or paraneoplastic mononeuropathies. Pain characterizes metastatic plexopathy, whereas painless lesions tend to be radiation-induced. Myokymia exists on the electromyogram in approximately two thirds of patients with radiation fibrosis, but rarely in tumor involvement.[76]

Acute ischemic or inflammatory neuropathies and complications of paraneoplastic neurological syndromes should also be considered. These can include the vasculitis that accompanies disseminated zoster infections; the neuropathic effects of vinca alkaloids, paclitaxel (Taxol), suramin, and platinum compounds; and the painful inflammations of the dorsal root ganglia and nerves that accompany a variety of tumors. Definitive diagnosis often requires neuroimaging studies of the appropriate area. Cranial neuropathies mandate both CT and MRI studies of the foramina of the skull base whereas lesions of the brachial and lumbar plexus obligate fat-suppressed MRI studies performed in coronal planes. If imaging studies fail to reveal the presence of tumor, exploration of the affected area is recommended depending on the extent of the underlying malignancy, degree of patient's disability, and surgical accessibility and morbidity. Control of pain, frequently severe and unrelenting, is a priority. This control may be achieved with systemic chemotherapy or focal radiation. Additionally, pain control with analgesics or anesthetic blocks may be successful. Prognosis is often good for both pain control and functional improvement after treatment of lymphoma, breast cancer, and some head and neck malignancies.

Paraneoplastic Syndromes

The neurological paraneoplastic syndromes represent nonmetastatic complications of cancer and constitute disorders affecting multiple levels of the nervous system (Table 47–9). These are rare, with an incidence below 1 percent. In descending occurrence, syndromes include sensory neuropathy (34 percent), Lambert-Eaton myasthenic syndrome (25 percent),[77] paraneoplastic cerebellar degeneration (< 25 percent), and limbic encephalitis (5 percent).[78] In 60 to 80 percent of patients, the neurological syndrome precedes the diagnosis of neoplasm.[78,79] Months to years may pass between symptom onset and identification of the causative malignancy. Often multiple "staging" examinations are needed to identify the indolent and small focus of tumor. On occasion, a paraneoplastic syndrome develops in the setting of prior cancer that can no longer be identified. The syndromes reflect an antibody or neurochemically mediated effect rather than the direct target of malignant spread, the compressive effects of metastatic disease, or alterations from metabolic or nutritional disorders, infection, stroke, or therapy.

TABLE 47–9. Paraneoplastic Syndromes Affecting the Nervous System

Brain and Cranial Nerves
Cerebellar degeneration
Opsoclonus-myoclonus
Limbic encephalitis and other dementias and brain stem encephalitis as part of encephalitis, encephalomyelitis
Optic neuritis
Retinopathy/photoreceptor degeneration

Spinal Cord and Dorsal Root Ganglia
Necrotizing myelopathy; myelitis, as part of encephalomyelitis
Subacute motor neuronopathy
Motor neuron disease
Myelitis
Sensory neuronopathy

Peripheral Nerves
Subacute or chronic sensorimotor peripheral neuropathy
Acute polyradiculoneuropathy (Guillain-Barré syndrome)
Mononeuritis multiplex and microvasculitis of peripheral nerve
Brachial neuritis
Autonomic neuropathy
Peripheral neuropathy with islet-cell tumors
Peripheral neuropathy associated with paraproteinemia

Neuromuscular Junction and Muscle
Lambert-Eaton myasthenic syndrome
Myasthenia gravis
Dermatomyositis, polymyositis
Acute necrotizing myopathy
Carcinoid myopathies
Myotonia
Cachectic myopathy
Stiff-person syndrome

Data from Rusciano D, Burger MM: Mechanisms of metastases. *In* Levine AJ, Schmidek HH (eds): Molecular Genetics of Nervous System Tumors. New York, John Wiley & Sons, 1993.

TABLE 47–10. Neoplasms and Antigens Associated with Specific Paraneoplastic Syndromes

Syndrome	Tumor Type	Antigen
PEM/SSN	SCLC	Hu, CV2 Amphiphysin
Limbic encephalitis	SCLC Testicular Breast	Hu, CV2 Ta (Ma2)
PCD	Breast/ovary SCLC Hodgkin's Breast	Yo Hu, CV2, VGCC Tr, metabotropic Glu receptor Ri
POM	Breast Non-SCLC, SCLC Neuroblastoma	Ri Hu Hu
CAR, MAR	SCLC, renal Melanoma	Recoverin Retinal bipolar cell
LEMS	SCLC	P/Q-type VGCC Synaptotagmin CV2
Stiff-person syndrome	Breast, colon	Amphiphysin
Paraneoplastic chorea syndrome	SCLC, lymphoma	Hu, CRMP-5

PEM/SSN, Paraneoplastic encephalomyelopathy/subacute sensory neuronopathy; PCD, paraneoplastic cerebellar degeneration; POM, paraneoplastic opsoclonus-myoclonus; CAR, cancer-associated retinopathy, MAR, melanoma-associated retinopathy; LEMS, Lambert-Eaton myasthenic syndrome; SCLC, small-cell lung cancer; VGCC, voltage-gated calcium channel; Glu, glutamate; CRMP-5, collapsin response-mediator protein 5.

Patients with these syndromes harbor antibodies in their serum and CSF that recognize antigens shared by neurons and tumor cells. About 15 percent of these antibodies can be detected with commercial assays, but specialized laboratories exist to identify novel antibodies in the remainder. Paraneoplastic syndromes result when an appropriate immune response against a tumor antigen (onconeural or oncofetal antigen) cross-reacts with similar antigens expressed by the nervous system.[80,81] For example, oat cell lung cancer expresses various nicotinic acetylcholine receptors.[82] Finding a tumor-specific antionconeural autoantibody (anti-Yo, -Hu, -Ri, -Ma, etc) in a patient with a neurological syndrome predicts the identification of an underlying carcinoma of a specific histological type (Table 47–10). Thus far, immunoglobulin G (IgG) accounts for the only class of antibody responsible for paraneoplastic syndrome, and IgG1 being the major subclass.[83] The role of these antibodies in disease causation has been proven in only Lambert-Eaton myasthenic syndrome (LEMS).[77,84,85] Interestingly, tumor growth suppression has been suggested by these antibodies.[86,87] Experimental approaches exist by which to harness these antibodies for both cancer imaging and therapy using "chimeric" molecules.

Traditionally, paraneoplastic syndromes are classified according to the affected anatomical level. The clinical features of only a few of the major syndromes are highlighted.

Management and prognosis are discussed for the entire group of disorders at the end of the chapter.

CENTRAL NERVOUS SYSTEM

Encephalomyelopathies

Pathogenesis and Pathophysiology. Strong evidence exists that paraneoplastic encephalomyelitis results from attacks by humoral and cellular arms of the immune system.[88] Tumor cells must invade regional lymph nodes to trigger the immune response that leads to a paraneoplastic syndrome.[89, 90]

Some patients with small-cell lung cancer (SCLC) harbor high titers of IgG antibodies (G1 subclass far greater than G2, G3, and G4) against a set of 35-40 kD antigens that are selectively expressed in the nuclei of neurons throughout the human nervous system. These antibodies, designated as anti-Hu, constitute a family of RNA binding proteins characterized by an RNA recognition motif of 80 amino acids.[91] They are present in higher concentrations in the CSF than in the serum, suggesting that their synthesis likely occurs within the CNS.[92] They can be detected within the neuronal nuclei of patients with paraneoplastic encephalomyelitis, and the sites of antibody accumulation correlate closely with those areas most affected by the paraneoplastic syndrome.[93] Although there exists a strong relationship between the presence of high titers of anti-Hu antibody and the development of paraneoplastic encephalomyelitis and sensory neuronopathy, the exact role of these antibodies in the pathogenesis of this disease is unclear. These proteins are likely to promote neuronal differentiation and maintenance of the neuronal phenotype. The mechanism for the inflammatory infiltrates, which consist of B cells, CD4+ and CD8+ lymphocytes, and macrophages within the dorsal root ganglion and the CNS, remains to be elucidated.

Epidemiology and Risk Factors. In a study by Graus and colleagues[94] the median age of patients with paraneoplastic encephalomyelitis was 63 years, three quarters being men. Tumor, confirmed by radiographic or pathological study, was evident in 83 percent, the majority of small cell lung origin. Testicular tumors were discovered in 20 percent of patients who elaborated anti-Ta (anti-Ma2) antibodies. Hypothalamic and brain stem involvement occurred in nearly three fourths of the patients with these antibodies.[95]

All sSCLC with or without paraneoplastic symptoms express the Hu antigen, and anti-Hu antibodies have been detected in 90 percent of these patients. Sixteen percent of patients with SCLC without neurological dysfunction develop low titers of anti-Hu antibody. There is no overlap between the titers of anti-Hu antibodies in small cell lung cancer with paraneoplastic encephalomyelitis and sensory neuronopathy (average titer, 4592 U/mL) and those without neurological symptoms (average titer, 76 U/mL). Titer levels provide information of SCLC aggression. All patients with low titers of anti-Hu antibody have the tumor confined to the thorax at diagnosis, whereas in those lacking anti-Hu antibody, more than 50 percent have systemic metastases at diagnosis.[96] These findings, and the common localized nature of tumors that underlie paraneoplastic encephalomyelitis and sensory neuronopathy, suggest that antibody status contributes to indolent disease.

A novel neuronal autoantibody, CRMP-5, has been described in the setting of SCLC and rarely with thymoma. These patients have varied neurological presentations with subacute dementia and peripheral neuropathies occurring most commonly. Chorea, abnormalities of olfaction and taste, and optic neuropathy have also been observed.[97]

Clinical Features and Associated Findings. Paraneoplastic encephalomyelopathy (PEM) afflicts multiple sites of the nerveous system to produce "limbic encephalitis," "encephalomyelitis," "cerebellitis/cerebellar degeneration," "brain stem encephalitis," "subacute sensory neuronopathy," and "autonomic neuropathy." Some of these patients have "anti-Hu syndrome" as they possess high titers of the antibody. In general, the syndromes are never purely confined to one anatomical location. Sensory neuronopathy produces asymmetrical burning or electrical dysesthesias of the limbs. Symptoms emerge over weeks to affect all elementary and discriminative sensations and to produce loss of deep tendon reflexes (see later discussion). Limbic encephalitis causes depression and memory loss, with progressive confusion, hallucinations, hypersomnia, and seizures, a pattern often wrongly identified as dementia.[98, 99] Brainstem encephalitis may involve the medulla to produce vomiting, vertigo, nystagmus, ataxia, and bulbar palsy. With more rostral midbrain disease, eye movements become restricted and movement disorders predominate, with possible mixtures of parkinsonian tremor and rigidity, dystonic contraction of agonist and antagonist musculature, and myoclonus.[100] Autonomic neuropathy can lead to gastroparesis, orthostatic hypotension, dryness of secretions, bladder dysfunction, and has a risk of sudden death. When cerebellar degeneration develops in patients with SCLC, it is usually a minor component of a more widespread paraneoplastic encephalomyelitis and sensory neuronopathy.

Evaluation and Differential Diagnosis. MRI has aided in establishing the diagnosis, but remains limited because many syndromes affect gray rather than white matter. The MRI of limbic encephalitis can be normal or reveal subtle T2-weighted alterations of the amygdala and hippocampus where prominent neuronal loss and gliosis occur. Electroencephalograms may show epileptic discharges in the temporal lobes.

A variety of encephalitides resemble PEM. Infections from herpes simplex and zoster, toxoplasmosis and other viral agents, Wernicke's encephalopathy, Leigh's disease, and leptomeningeal carcinomatosis can all mimic the syndrome. The peripheral manifestations are hard to distinguish from the dorsal root ganglion effects of vitamin B_{12} deficiency, cytomegalovirus ganglionitis, Sjögren's syndrome and autoimmune disorders, tabes dorsalis, diabetes, chemotherapy-related neuropathy, and direct tumor infiltration.

Paraneoplastic Cerebellar Degeneration

Pathogenesis and Pathophysiology. Cytotoxic T-cell lymphocytes may play a role in the autoimmune destruction of Purkinje neurons. In this disorder, cells present in the CSF are directed against Purkinje cell structures including cytoplasmic Yo proteins of the Golgi apparatus, ribosomes, and endoplasmic reticulum.[101–103] The antibody generated against the Yo antigen, is uniquely IgG1 subclass,[104] and accurately predicts an underlying neoplasm.[89] Subcategories of anti-Yo include autoantibody cdr34, cdr62-1, and cdr62-2 (breast cancer, ovarian, and other gynecological malignancies) with rare contributions of adenocarcinoma of the lung.[105] The major epitope for anti-Yo antibody appears to be a leucine zipper motif, leading to the supposition of its interference with DNA transcription.[106] Also, HLA class I A24 has been observed in patients with paraneoplastic cerebellar degeneration (PCD) and anti-Yo antibody.[107]

Another antibody, designated as anti-Ri antibody, binds neuron-specific RNA nucleic protein of 55-80 kD, and is seen in patients with breast, gynecological, and lung cancers.[105] Unlike the anti-Yo paraneoplastic cerebellar degeneration in patients who are older women, some anti-Ri patients are young men with Hodgkin's disease. Sera of patients with Hodgkin's disease react with the Tr protein, a new onconeural antigen in Purkinje cells.[108] A further subgroup of cerebellar degeneration is associated with SCLC and LEMS and antibodies against the presynaptic voltage-gated calcium channel,[109] antimetabotropic glutamate receptor,[110] and CV2.[111] Anti-CV2 antibody is not an antionconeural antibody, but rather it stains the cytoplasmic antigen of oligodendrocytes.

Epidemiology and Risk Factors. Cerebellar degeneration is most commonly associated with breast and lung cancer, particularly SCLC; gynecological cancers; and lymphoma. Anti-Yo antibody patients are commonly women with breast cancer. When men have PCD, lung cancer is commonly the cause. Patients with Hodgkin's disease usually elaborate anti-Tr antibody after the tumor has been detected. The median survival for patients with breast cancer and PCD approximates 8 years, five times longer than patients with gynecologic malignancies.[89]

Clinical Features and Associated Findings. Neurological manifestations can precede detection of the associated cancer in more than one half of patients by months, occasionally up to 4 years, or develop up to 2 years after the diagnosis of cancer. Neurological signs generally develop over weeks to months but rarely, anti-Ri-positive patients develop symptoms within one day's time. Gait ataxia progresses to truncal and appendicular ataxia, dysarthria, and nystagmus. Although the symptoms eventually plateau when Purkinje cells disappear, disability is usually persistent.

Evaluation and Differential Diagnosis. In the acute setting the MRI is normal, but cerebellar atrophy is soon noted and folia become more visible. The cerebellum becomes atrophic and scarred by glia when Purkinje cells are virtually lost. The CSF may contain oligoclonal bands with or without an elevated IgG synthesis index. Clinicians must exclude direct metastatic invasion of the cerebellum or its meningeal coverings, the effects of medication such as cytarabine, strokes, disseminated encephalomyelitis, multiple sclerosis, and cerebellitis.

Paraneoplastic Opsoclonus-Myoclonus

Paraneoplastic opsoclonus-myoclonus (POM) can occur in the context of Purkinje cell loss, changes in the dentate nucleus, or demyelination of cerebellar white matter. Less certain are examples without neuronal loss and scattered perivascular lymphocytes.[112] Most patients lack specific antineuronal antibodies, but some with POM produce high titers of anti-Ri antibody that cross-reacts with an antigen in the nuclei of all CNS neurons and in tumor cells of affected patients. Anti-Ri antibody recognizes proteins of 55 to 80 kD in molecular weight. The distribution of these proteins is widespread, but anti-Ri–associated immunological responses appear to target the basis pontis and optic tectum.[113]

This syndrome occurs in association with childhood neuroblastoma. About 50 percent of adult cases with POM are idiopathic, and paraneoplastic causes represent 20 percent of cases.[114] Breast and lung cancers account for 80 percent of all tumors.[115, 116] The disorder produces chaotic saccades of the eye that increase with eye closure and fixation, in combination with myoclonus involving facial muscles, limbs, or trunk. Sleep does not ablate the eye movements. The majority of patients die within a few months. Sporadically, opsoclonus-myoclonus may occur after viral infections, with medication use such as intravenous phenytoin or diazepam, or in cases of amitriptyline overdose.

Cancer-Associated Retinopathy (CAR)

Sera from patients with cancer-associated retinopathy (CAR, or paraneoplastic retinal degeneration) contain antibodies against antigens that are both a photoreceptor cell–specific protein and a protein expressed by SCLC.[117] Pathologically, widespread degeneration of the outer retinal layers occurs with relative preservation of the other layers. This syndrome is usually associated with SCLC and melanoma, the latter condition called melanoma-associated retinopathy (MAR). In CAR, an antibody to a calcium-binding protein named recoverin is frequently found. Recoverin regulates rhodopsin kinase in a calcium-dependent fashion.[118] Patients with MAR produce an antibody to the retinal bipolar cells.[117, 119] The distinctive clinical triad consists of photosensitivity, ring scotomatous visual field loss, and attenuated caliber of retinal arterioles.[120] Nocturnal blindness and painless visual loss may also develop. Some chemotherapeutic agents such as platinum, nitrosoureas, procarbazine, tamoxifen, radiation fields inclusive of the optic nerves and chiasm, and the infiltrative effects of lymphoma may cause retinopathy with similar clinical features and should be considered as part of the differential diagnosis. Characteristic features of CAR and MAR exist on electroretinographic studies, and serological markers can be performed in research laboratories.

PERIPHERAL NERVOUS SYSTEM

Peripheral Neuropathies

Approximately 5 percent of cancer patients have symptomatic neuropathy, 12 percent have abnormalities on quantitative sensory testing, and 40 percent have electrophysiological abnormalities.[121] Typically, women with SCLC or breast carcinoma present with asymmetrical upper limb pain, paresthesia, and sensory loss preceding the diagnosis of cancer by months to 2 years. When proprioception is lost, the extremities may appear tremulous; patients position their extremities poorly in space and adopt athetoid postures. Subacute sensory neuronopathy is an inflammatory process that selectively involves the cells of the dorsal root ganglia. The acute lymphocytic response gives way to scar tissue.[122] With lost dorsal root cells, secondary demyelinative changes occur in the dorsal columns and peripheral sensory nerves. Paresthetic pain and sensory loss ensue.

The sensory symptoms may be acute, subacute, or relapsing. A simple mnemonic, the 2-3-4 rule, may aid the clinician to remember its time course and associations. Generally, two thirds of patients with subacute sensory neuronopathy develop symptoms before the discovery of tumor, three fourths have concomitant paraneoplastic encephalomyelitis, and four fifths have small cell lung cancer.

An acute neuropathy often indistinguishable from acute inflammatory demyelinating polyneuropathy has been described with Hodgkin's disease. Clearly "double-crush" syndromes occur by which these neuropathies have superimposed nerve damage of compressive (e.g., carpal tunnel syndrome, tardy ulnar palsy), neurotoxic (vincristine, paclitaxel), metabolic, and atrophic origins.

Stiff-person syndrome, characterized by painful muscle spasms and rigidity, has been described in association with breast cancer and autoantibodies against amphiphysin, a 128-kD neuronal antigen concentrated at synapses.[123]

Neuromuscular Junction and Muscle Disorders

In LEMS, autoantibodies develop to the neuronal voltage-gated calcium channels, especially the P/Q type,[124] or to synaptotagmin, a synaptic vesicle protein acting as a calcium sensor.[125, 126] The former occurs far more frequently than the latter (85 to 90 percent versus 10 to 30 percent). Calcium channel function is disrupted by the antibody, leading to reduced acetylcholine release at the neuromuscular junction and at synapses of autonomic nerves. Changes in membrane voltage and depolarization of the neuronal membrane by influx of potassium ions leads to the opening of calcium channels. Calcium ions flow into the nerve terminal, and neurotransmitter vesicles fuse with the neuronal membrane. When muscle biopsy specimens from LEMS patients receive a single supramaximal stimulus, miniature end-plate potentials are normal in amplitude but reduced in number, suggesting a reduction in the number of quanta of acetylcholine being released into the neuromuscular junction.

Fifty percent of LEMS cases have an associated malignancy, usually of small-cell lung origin. Less commonly, LEMS occurs in association with autoimmune disorders, including thyroid disease, pernicious anemia, vitiligo, and type I diabetes mellitus. Fatigue commonly precedes weakness, and gait difficulties occur when the patient moves from a sitting to a standing posture. The combination of proximal muscle weakness and hyporeflexia are hallmarks of this disease. Autonomic difficulties are commonly present but often not specifically recognized. Cholinergic alterations at both nicotinic and muscarinic synapses produce dry eyes and mouth and erectile failure. Although symptomatic orthostatic hypotension is seldom clinically significant, it can usually be demonstrated with a tilt-table study. Ocular symptoms are rare, but sluggish pupillary responses can often be elicited. When the examiner requests that the patient perform repetitive or sustained muscle contraction, there is obvious improvement in strength of the lower extremity proximal muscles as the patient continues the task. This pattern is in distinct contrast to myasthenia gravis where fatigability is the hallmark. Neurophysiological studies are confirmatory, and the weakened muscles exhibit resting and volitional reduced amplitude compound motor action potential (CMAP), not improved by low frequencies of stimulation. With rapid stimulation at 20 to 50 Hz, electrical facilitation occurs, characterized by a twofold increase in CMAP. When the repetitive stimulation ("rep-stim") at rates of 2 Hz is associated with no facilitation and a decremental response, these LEMS patients also have some element of myasthenia gravis.

Motor Neuron Diseases

Rarely, cancer patients experience a disorder of the spinal cord that is similar to motor neuron disease (amyotrophic lateral sclerosis, ALS). Motor neuronopathy with possible conduction block and loss of anterior horn cells in association with cancer should always suggest a paraneoplastic syndrome. Patients with the predominant motor neuron syndrome may have the anti-Hu antibody. Following successful treatment of the cancer, neurological symptoms may remit as long as anterior horn cells are still present. The appearance of motor neuron disease and encephalomyelitis should raise the suspicion of anti-Hu syndrome in association with SCLC. On the other hand, the appearance of motor neuron disease and conduction block abnormalities, with or without paraproteinemia, should raise the suspicion of non-Hodgkin's lymphoma.[127] With Hodgkin's disease there appears a subacute motor neuronopathy with progressive painless, asymmetrical lower motor neuron weakness. The tendon reflexes are decreased. Unlike ALS, the bulbar muscles are usually spared, fasciculations are rare, and the course is benign. Lower motor neuron syndromes should raise the suspicion of lymphoma,[128] and upper motor neuron syndromes, SCLC or breast cancer. Several reports exist of a rapidly developing necrotizing myelopathy that mimics an acute transverse myelitis in patients with lung cancer. This involves the spinal cord at the thoracic level, which produces CSF protein elevation. The MRI can show patchy gadolinium enhancement and T2-weighted signal abnormality.[129] Pathologically, widespread spinal cord necrosis is seen with little inflammatory response or evidence of vasculitis.[130]

MANAGEMENT AND PROGNOSIS OF PARANEOPLASTIC SYNDROMES AS A GROUP

Paraneoplastic syndromes may be separated into those that are responsive and those that are unresponsive to therapy. In general the inflammatory syndromes or those with circulating antibodies respond to therapy. These include LEMS with antibodies to gated sodium channels, stiff-person syndrome with antibodies to glutamic acid dehydrogenase, and opsoclonus-myoclonus. Less responsive are inflammatory processes, including limbic encephalitis and microvasculitis of nerve and muscle. Refractory to therapy are cell degenerative processes, including Purkinje cell cerebellar degeneration, retinopathy with ganglion cell loss, and motor neuronopathy with reduction of anterior horn cells.

Releantless progression is seen in the three fourths of patients with paraneoplastic syndromes that involve neuronal or myelin loss. Control of the underlying tumor may halt the progression after the passage of several months, but commonly physicians are unaware of the halt in progression. Broad therapeutic guidelines are difficult to outline but the physician is guided by several rules. Expedient procedures are warranted (see Fig. 47–6) and should include the exclusion of alternative diagnoses, the provision of appropriate scanning,

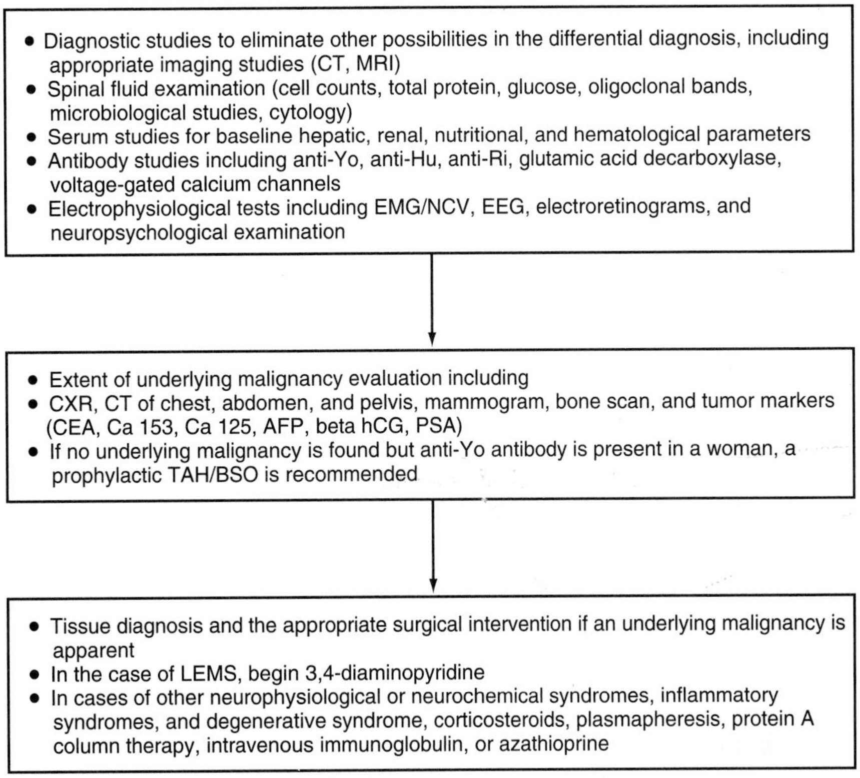

- Diagnostic studies to eliminate other possibilities in the differential diagnosis, including appropriate imaging studies (CT, MRI)
- Spinal fluid examination (cell counts, total protein, glucose, oligoclonal bands, microbiological studies, cytology)
- Serum studies for baseline hepatic, renal, nutritional, and hematological parameters
- Antibody studies including anti-Yo, anti-Hu, anti-Ri, glutamic acid decarboxylase, voltage-gated calcium channels
- Electrophysiological tests including EMG/NCV, EEG, electroretinograms, and neuropsychological examination

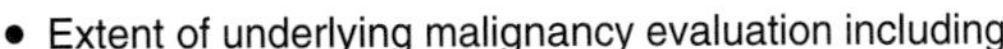

- Extent of underlying malignancy evaluation including
- CXR, CT of chest, abdomen, and pelvis, mammogram, bone scan, and tumor markers (CEA, Ca 153, Ca 125, AFP, beta hCG, PSA)
- If no underlying malignancy is found but anti-Yo antibody is present in a woman, a prophylactic TAH/BSO is recommended

- Tissue diagnosis and the appropriate surgical intervention if an underlying malignancy is apparent
- In the case of LEMS, begin 3,4-diaminopyridine
- In cases of other neurophysiological or neurochemical syndromes, inflammatory syndromes, and degenerative syndrome, corticosteroids, plasmapheresis, protein A column therapy, intravenous immunoglobulin, or azathioprine

FIGURE 47–6. Evaluation of paraneoplastic syndromes. AFP, alpha-fetoprotein; CEA, carcinoembryonic antigen; CT, computed tomography; CXR, chest x-ray study; EEG, electroencephalogram; EMG/NCV, electromyography/nerve conduction velocities; hCG, human chorionic gonadotropin; LEMS, Lambert-Eaton myasthenic syndrome; MRI, magnetic resonance imaging; PSA, prostate-specific antigen; TAH/BSO, total abdominal hysterectomy/bilateral salpingo-oophorectomy.

and serological marker studies. Certain syndromes justify a thorough search for an underlying cancer and the provision of appropriate treatment with surgery, chemotherapy, or radiation therapy. Concomitant treatment of the paraneoplastic syndrome should be provided rather than awaiting tumor response. Immunosuppressive therapy is necessary but may be difficult to coordinate with concurrent chemotherapy. LEMS should be treated with 3,4-diaminopyridine. Because of the renal toxicity of guanidine, use of this drug should probably be avoided in a patient who may be undergoing chemotherapy with agents that require renal clearance. The remaining neurophysiological or neurochemical and inflammatory and degenerative paraneoplastic syndromes should be managed with immunosuppressive therapy. The vasculitides respond to corticosteroids and azathioprine. The antibody-mediated syndromes appear to benefit equally from intravenous immunoglobulin or plasmapheresis. For the former, a 2-day course is preferred but hematological complications may obligate slower administration.[131]

Reviews and Selected Updates

Byrne TN: Spinal cord compression from epidural metastases. N Engl J Med 1992;327:614–619.

Forsyth PA, Dalmau J, Graus F: Motor neuron syndromes in cancer patients. Ann Neurol 1997;41:722–730.

Glantz MJ, Cole BF, Forsyth PA, et al: Practice parameter: Anticonvulsant prophylaxis in patients with newly diagnosed brain tumors. Neurology 2000;54:1886–1893.

Inuzuka T: Autoantibodies in paraneoplastic neurological syndrome. Am J Med Sciences 2000;319:217–226.

Posner JB: Neurologic Complications of Cancer. Philadelphia, F.A. Davis, 1995.

Posner JB: Paraneoplastic syndromes. Curr Opin Neurol 1997;10:471–476.

Rusciano D, Burger MM: Mechanisms of metastases. *In* Levine AJ, Schmidek HH (eds): Molecular Genetics of Nervous System Tumors. New York, John Wiley & Sons, 1993.

References

1. Davey P: Brain metastases. Curr Probl Cancer 1999;233:59–98.
2. Posner JB: Neurologic Complications of Cancer. Philadelphia, F.A. Davis, 1995.
3. Stetler-Stevenson WG: The role of matrix metalloproteinase in tumor invasion, metastasis, and angiogenesis. Surg Oncol Clin N Am 2001;10:383–392.
4. Rusciano D, Burger MM: Mechanisms of metastases. *In* Levine AJ, Schmidek HH (eds): Molecular Genetics of Nervous System Tumors. New York, John Wiley & Sons, 1993.
5. Chidel MA, Suh JH, Barnett GH: Brain metastases: Presentation, evaluation, and management. Cleve Clin J Med 2000;67:120–127.
6. Sze G, Milano E, Johnson C, Heier L: Detection of brain metastases: Comparison of contrast enhanced MR with unenhanced MR and enhanced CT. Am J Neuroradiol 1990;11:785–791.
7. Delattre JY, Krol G, Thaler HT, et al: Distribution of brain metastases. Arch Neurol 1988;45:741–744.
8. Hwang TL, Close TP, Grego JM, et al: Predilection of brain metastasis in the gray and white matter junction and vascular border zones. Cancer 1996;77:1551–1555.
9. LeChevalier T, Smith FP, Caille P, et al: Sites of primary malignancies in patients presenting with cerebral metastases: A review of 120 cases. Cancer 1985;56:880–882.
10. Zimm S, Wampler GL, Stablein D, et al: Intracerebral metastases in solid tumor patients: Natural history and results of treatment. Cancer 1981;48:384–394.
11. Zon LI, Johns WD, Stomper PC, et al: Breast carcinoma metastatic to a meningioma: Case report and review of the literature. Arch Intern Med 1989;149:959–962.
12. Ahsan H, Neugent AI, Bruce JN: Association of malignant brain tumors and cancers of other sites. J Clin Oncol 1995;13:2931–2935.
13. Posner JB: Management of central nervous system metastases. Semin Oncol 1977;4:81–91.
14. Fadul C, Misulis KE, Wiley RG: Cerebellar metastases: Diagnostic and management considerations. J Clin Oncol 1987;5:1107–1115.
15. Mandybur TI: Intracranial hemorrhage caused by metastatic tumors. Neurology 1977;27:650–655.
16. Rogers LR: Cerebrovascular complications in cancer patients. Neurol Clin 1991;9:889–899.
17. Bakshi R: Solitary inflammatory demyelination in the brain or spinal cord with tumor-like MRI presentation. Arch Neurol 2001;58:677.

18. Rogers LR, Cho ES, Kempin S, et al: Cerebral infarction from nonbacterial thrombotic endocarditis. Am J Med 1987;83:746–756.
19. DeAngelis LM: Metastatic disease of the nervous system. Curr Treat Options Neurol 1999;1:409–416.
20. Akeson P, Larsson EM, Kristofferson DT, et al: Brain metastases: Comparison of gadolinium injection-enhanced MR imaging at standard and high dose, contrast-enhanced CT, and non–contrast-enhanced MR imaging. Acta Radiologica 1995;36:300–306.
21. Yuh WTC, Tali ET, Nguyen HD: The effect of contrast dose, imaging time, and lesion size in the MR detection of intracerebral metastasis. Am J Neuroradiol 1995;16:373–380.
22. Pui MH: Magnetization transfer analysis of brain tumor, infection, and infarction. J Magn Reson Imaging 2000;12:395–399.
23. Shukla-Dave A, Gupta RK, Roy R, et al: Prospective evaluation of in vivo proton MR spectroscopy in differentiation of similar appearing intracranial cystic lesions. Magn Reson Imaging 2001;19:103–110.
24. Grand S, Passaro G, Ziegler A, et al: Necrotic tumor versus brain abscess: Importance of amino acids detected at 1H MR spectroscopy—initial results. Radiology 1999;213;785–793.
25. Park SH, Chang KH, Song IC, et al: Diffusion-weighted MRI in cystic or necrotic intracranial lesions. Neurorad 2000;42:716–721.
26. Holtas S, Geijer B, Stromblad LG, et al: A ring-enhancing metastasis with central high signal on diffusion-weighted imaging and low apparent diffusion coefficients. Neurorad 2000;42:824–827.
27. Coia LR: The role of radiation in the treatment of brain metastases. Int J Radiat Oncol Biol Phys 1992;23:229–238.
28. Gaspar L, Scott C, Rotman M, et al: Recursive partitioning analysis (RPA) of prognostic factors in three Radiation Therapy Oncology Group (RTOG) brain metastases trials. Int J Radiat Oncol Biol Phys 1997;37:745–751.
29. Patchell RA: The treatment of brain metastases. Cancer Invest 1996;14:169–177.
30. Rubenstein JH, Dosoretz DE, Katin MJ, et al: Low doses of prophylactic cranial irradiation effective in limited stage small-cell carcinoma of the lung. Int J Radiat Oncol Biol Phys 1995;33:329–337.
31. Abrey LE, Olson JD, Boutros DY, et al: A phase II study of temozolomide for recurrent brain metastases. Proc Am Soc Clin Oncol 2000;19:166 (abstract 643).
32. Christodoulou C, Bafaloukos D, Kosmidis P, et al: Phase II study of temozolomide in heavily pretreated cancer patients with brain metastases. Ann Oncol 2001;12:249–254.
33. Oberhoff C, Kieback DG, Wurstlein R, et al: Topotecan chemotherapy in patients with breast cancer and brain metastases: results of a pilot study. Onkologie 2001;24:256–260.
34. Wang ML, Yung WK, Royce ME, et al: Capecitabine for 5-fluorouracil–resistant brain metastases from breast cancer. Am J Clin Oncology 2001;24:421–424.
35. Schwonzen M, Kurbacher CM, Mallmann P: Liposomal doxorubicin and weekly paclitaxel in the treatment of metastatic breast cancer. Anti-Cancer Drugs 2000;11:681–685.
36. Franciosi V, Cocconi G, Michiara M, et al: Front-line chemotherapy with cisplatin and etoposide for patients with brain metastases from breast carcinoma, nonsmall cell lung carcinoma, or malignant melanoma: A prospective study. Cancer 1999;85:1599–1605.
37. Cappuzzo F, Mazzoni F, Maestri A, et al: Medical treatment of brain metastases from solid tumors. Forum 2000;10:137–147.
38. Vecht CJ, Haaxma-Reiche H, Noordijk EM, et al: Treatment of single brain metastasis: Radiotherapy alone or combined with neurosurgery? Ann Neurol 1993;33:583–590.
39. Patchell RA, Tibbs PA, Regine WF, et al: Postoperative radiotherapy in the treatment of single metastases: A randomized trial. JAMA 1998;280: 1485–1489.
40. Lentzsch S, Reichardt P, Weber F, et al: Brain metastases in breast cancer: Prognostic factors and management. European J Cancer 1999;35:580–585.
41. Fernandez-Vicioso E, Suh JH, Kupelian PA, et al: Analysis of prognostic factors for patients with solitary brain metastasis treated by stereotactic radiosurgery. Radiat Oncol Invest 1997;5:31–37.
42. Auchter RM, Lamond JP, Alexander E, et al: A multiinstitutional outcome and prognostic factor analysis of radiosurgery for resectable single brain metastasis. Int J Radiat Oncol Biol Phys 1996;35:27–35.
43. Cho Kh, Hall WA, Lee AK, et al: Stereoradiosurgery for patients with single brain metastasis. J Radiosurg 1998;1:79–85.
44. Bindal RK, Sawaya R, Leavens ME, et al: Surgical treatment of multiple brain metastases. J Neurosurg 1993;79:210–216.
45. Bindal RK, Sawaya R, Leavens ME, et al: Reoperation for recurrent metastatic brain tumors. J Neurosurg 1995;83:600–604.
46. Olson ME, Chernik NL, Posner JB: Leptomeningeal metastases from systemic cancer: A report of 47 cases. Trans Am Neurol Assoc 1971;96:291–293.
47. Chamberlain MC, Kormanik PA, Glantz MJ: A comparison between ventricular and lumbar cerebrospinal fluid cytology in adult patients with leptomeningeal metastases. Neuro-Oncol 2001;3:42–45.
48. Grossman SA, Krabak MJ: Leptomeningeal carcinomatosis. Cancer Treat Rev 1999;25:103–119.
49. Balm M, Hammack J: Leptomeningeal carcinomatosis. Presenting features and prognostic factors. Arch Neurol 1996;53:626–632.
50. Glantz MJ, Cole BF, Glantz LK, et al: Cerebrospinal fluid cytology in patients with cancer. Minimizing false negative results. Cancer 1998;82:733–739.
51. Glass JP, Melamed M, Chernik NL, et al: Malignant cells in cerebrospinal fluid (CSF): The meaning of a positive CSF cytology. Neurology 1979;29:1369–1375.
52. Straathof CS, de Bruin HG, Dippel DW, et al: The diagnostic accuracy of magnetic resonance imaging and cerebrospinal fluid cytology in leptomeningeal metastasis. J Neurology 1999;246:810–814.
53. Freilich RJ, Krol G, DeAngelis LM: Neuroimaging and cerebrospinal fluid cytology in the diagnosis of leptomeningeal metastasis. Ann Neurol 1995;38:51–57.
54. Coakham HB, Kemshead JT: Treatment of neoplastic meningitis by targeted radiation using (131)I-radiolabelled monoclonal antibodies. Results of responses and long term follow-up in 40 patients. J Neuro-Oncol 1998;38:225–232.
55. Balis FM, Blaney SM, McCully CL, et al: Methotrexate distribution within the subarachnoid space after intraventricular and intravenous administration. Cancer Chemother Pharmacol 2000;45:259–264.
56. Greenberg HS, Deck MDF, Vikram B, et al: Metastasis to the base of the skull: Clinical findings in 43 patients. Neurology 1981;31:530–537.
57. Geldof AA: Models for cancer skeletal metastasis: A reappraisal of Batson's plexus. Anticancer Res 1997;17:1535–1539.
58. Posner JB: Back pain and epidural spinal cord compression. Med Clin North Am 1987;71:185–205.
59. Byrne TN: Spinal cord compression from epidural metastases. N Engl J Med 1992;327:614–619.
60. Bubendorf L, Schopfer A, Wagner U, et al: Metastatic patterns of prostate cancer: An autopsy study of 1589 patients. Hum Pathol 2000;31:578–583.
61. Graus F, Krol G, Foley KM: Early diagnosis of spinal epidural metastasis (SEM): Correlation with clinical and radiological findings (abstr). Proc Am Soc Clin Oncol 1985;4:269.
62. Haddad P, Thaell JF, Kiely JM: Lymphoma of the spinal extradural space. Cancer 1976;38:1862–1866.
63. Portenoy RK, Galer BS, Salamon O, et al: Identification of epidural neoplasm: Radiography and bone scintigraphy in the symptomatic and asymptomatic spine. Cancer 1989;64:2207–2213.
64. Abrahm JL: Management of pain and spinal cord compression in patients with advanced cancer. ACP-AIM End of Life Care Consensus Panel. American College of Physicians—American Society of International Medicine. Ann Intern Med 1999;131:37–46.
65. Foley KM: Management of cancer pain. *In* DeVita VT, Helman S, Rosenberg SA (eds): Cancer: Principles & Practice of Oncology, 5th ed. Philadelphia, Lippincott-Raven, 1997, pp 2807–2814.
66. Loblaw DA, Laperriere NJ: Emergency treatment of malignant extradural spinal cord compression: An evidence-based guideline. J Clin Oncol 1998;16:1613–1624.
67. Maranzano E, Latini P: Effectiveness of radiation therapy without surgery in metastatic spinal cord compression: Final results from a prospective trial. Int J Radiat Oncol Biol Phys 1995;32:959–967.
68. Gokaslan Z: Spine surgery for cancer. Cur Opin Oncol 1996 8:178–181.
69. Grant R, Papadopoulos S, Sandler H, et al: Metastatic epidural spinal cord compression: Current concepts and treatment. J Neurooncol 1994;19:79–92.
70. Bilsky MH, Boland P, Lis E, et al: Single-stage posterolateral transpedicle approach for spondylectomy, epidural decompression, and circumferential fusion of spinal metastases. Spine 2000;25:2240–2249.
71. Ghogawala Z, Mansfield FL, Borges LF: Spinal radiation before surgical decompression adversely affects outcomes of surgery for symptomatic metastatic spinal cord compression. Spine 2001;26:818–824.
72. Sundaresan N, Galicich JH, Lane JM, et al: Treatment of neoplastic epidural cord compression by vertebral body resection and stabilization. J Neurosurg 1985;63:676–684.
73. Sundaresan N, DiGiacinto GV, Hughes JE, et al: Treatment of neoplastic spinal cord compression: Results of a prospective study. Neurosurgery 1991;29:645–650.

74. Bridwell K, Jenny A, Saul T, et al: Posterior segmental spinal instrumentation (PSSI) with posterolateral decompression and debulking for metastatic thoracic and lumbar spine disease: Limitations and technique. Spine 1998;13:1383–1394.
75. Cahill DW, Kumar R: Palliative subtotal vertebrectomy with anterior and posterior reconstruction via single posterior approach. J Neurosurg (Spine 1) 1999;90:42–47.
76. Kori SH, Foley KM, Posner JB: Brachial plexus lesions in patients with cancer: 100 cases. Neurology 1981;31:45–50.
77. Inuzuka T: Autoantibodies in paraneoplastic neurological syndrome. Am J Med Sciences 2000;319:217–226.
78. A nationwide survey on paraneoplastic neurological syndromes. Project group on paraneoplastic neurological syndromes, Neuroimmunological Disease Research Committee, the Ministry of Health and Welfare, Japan. Rinsho Shinkeigaku 1997;37:93–98.
79. Moll JW, Vecht CJ: Immune diagnosis of paraneoplastic neurological disease. Clin Neurol Neurosurg 1995;97:71–81.
80. Dalmau JO, Posner JB: Paraneoplastic syndromes affecting the nervous system. Semin Oncol 1997;24:318–328.
81. Posner JB, Dalmau JO: Paraneoplastic syndromes of the nervous system. Clin Chem Lab Med 2000;38:117–122.
82. Sciamanna MA, Griesmann GE, Williams CL, et al: Nicotinic acetylcholine receptors of muscle and neuronal ([alpha]7) types co-expressed in a small-cell lung carcinoma. J Neurochem 1997;69:2302–2311.
83. Greeenlee JE, Boyden JW, Pingree M, et al: Antibody types and IgG subclasses in paraneoplastic neurological syndromes. J Neurol Sci 2001;184:131–137.
84. Fukuoka T, Engel AG, Lang B, et al: Lambert-Eaton myasthenic syndrome: II. Immunoelectron microscopy localization of IgG at the mouse motor end-plate. Ann Neurol 1987;22:200–211.
85. Lang B, Newsom-Davis J, Wray A, et al: Autoimmune aetiology for myasthenic (Eaton-Lambert) syndrome. Lancet 1981;2:224–226.
86. Darnell RB, DeAngelis LM: Regression of small-cell lung carcinoma in patients with paraneoplastic neuronal antibodies. Lancet 1993; 341:21–22.
87. Peterson K, Rosenblum MK, Kotanides H, et al: Paraneoplastic cerebellar degeneration. I. A clinical analysis of 55 anti-Yo antibody–positive patients. Neurology 1992;42:1931–1937.
88. Benyahia B, Liblau R, Merle-Beral H, et al: Cell mediated autoimmunity in paraneoplastic neurological syndromes with anti-Hu antibodies. Ann Neurol 1999;45:162–167.
89. Rojas I, Graus F, Keime-Guilbert F, et al: Long-term clinical outcome of paraneoplastic cerebellar degeneration and anti-Yo antibodies. Neurology 2000;55:713–715.
90. Chartrand-Lefebvre C, Howarth N, Grenier P, et al: Association of small cell lung cancer and anti-Hu paraneoplastic syndrome: Radiographic and CT findings. Am J Radiol 1998;170:1513–1517.
91. Marusich M, Furneaux H, Henion P, Weston J: Hu neuronal proteins are expressed in proliferating neurogenic cells. J Neurobiol 1994;25:143–155.
92. Vega F, Graus F, Chen QN, et al: Intrathecal synthesis of the anti-Hu antibody in patients with paraneoplastic encephalomyelitis or sensory neuropathy. Neurology 1994;44:2145–2147.
93. Jean WC, Dalmau J, Ho A, Posner JB: Analysis of the IgG subclass distribution and inflammatory infiltrates in patients with anti-Hu associated paraneoplastic encephalomyelitis. Neurology 1994;44:140–147.
94. Graus F, Keime-Guibert F, Rene R, et al: Anti-Hu-associated paraneoplastic encephalomyelitis: Analysis of 200 patients. Brain 2001; 124:1138–1148.
95. Rosenfeld MR, Eichen JG, Wade DF, et al: Molecular and clinical diversity in paraneoplastic immunity to Ma proteins. Ann Neurol 2001;50:339–348.
96. Manley GT, Smitt PAES, Dalmau J: Hu antigens: Reactivity with Hu antibodies, tumor expression, and major immunogenic sites. Ann Neurol 1995;102–110.
97. Yu Z, Kryzer TJ, Griesmann GE, et al: CRMP–5 neuronal autoantibody: Marker of lung cancer and thymoma-related autoimmunity. Ann Neurol 2001;49:146–154.
98. Alamowitch S, Graus F, Uchuya M, et al: Limbic encephalitis and small cell lung cancer. Clinical and immunological features. Brain 1997;120:923–938.
99. Boylan LS: Limbic encephalitis and late-onset psychosis. Am J Psychiatry 2000;157:1343–1344.
100. Posner JB: Paraneoplastic syndromes. Neurol Clin 1991;9:919–936.
101. Hida C, Tsukamoto T, Awano H, et al: Ultrastructural localization of anti-Purkinje cell antibody-binding sites in paraneoplastic cerebellar degeneration. Arch Neurol 1994;51:555–558.
102. Albert ML, Austin LM, Darnell RB: Detection and treatment of activated T cells in the cerebrospinal fluid of patients with paraneoplastic cerebellar degeneration. Ann Neurol 2000;47:9–17.
103. Tanaka M, Tanaka K: A candidate peptide reacting with cytotoxic T cell in paraneoplastic cerebellar degeneration with anti-Yo antibody. Clin Neurol 1999;39:603–605.
104. Amyes E, Curnow J, Stark Z, et al: Restricted IgG1 subclass of anti-Yo antibodies in paraneoplastic cerebellar degeneration. J Neuroimmunol 2001;114:259–264.
105. Drlicek M, Bianchi G, Bogliun G, et al: Antibodies of the anti-Yo and anti-Ri type in the absence of paraneoplastic neurological syndromes: A long-term survey of ovarian cancer patients. J Neurol 1997;244:85–89.
106. Sakai K, Ogasawara T, Hirose G, et al: Analysis of autoantibody binding to 52-kd paraneoplastic cerebellar degeneration–associated antigen expressed in recombinant proteins. Ann Neurol 1993;33:373–380.
107. Tanaka M, Tanaka K: HLA A24 in paraneoplastic cerebellar degeneration with anti-Yo antibody. Neurology 1996;47:606–607.
108. Graus F, Dalmau J, Valldeoriola F, et al: Immunological characterization of a neuronal antibody (anti-Tr) associated with paraneoplastic cerebellar degeneration and Hodgkin's disease. J Neuroimmunol 1997;74:55–61.
109. Clouston PD, Saper CB, Arbizu T, et al: Paraneoplastic cerebellar degeneration: III. Cerebellar degeneration, cancer, and the Lambert-Eaton myasthenic syndrome. Neurology 1992;42:1944–1950.
110. Kinoshita A, Shigemoto R, Nakashini S, et al: Autoantibodies to metabotropic glutamate receptor 1 (mGluR1) in paraneoplastic cerebellar ataxia. Proceedings of the 39th Annual Meeting of the Societas Neurologica Japonica. Tokyo, Oshita. 1998, p 74.
111. Honnorat J, Antoine JC, Derrington D, et al: Antibodies to a subpopulation of glial cells and a 66kDa development protein in patients with paraneoplastic neurological syndromes. J Neurol Neurosurg Psychiatry 1996;61:270–278.
112. Young CA, MacKenzie JM, Chadwick DW, Williams IR: Opsoclonus myoclonus syndrome: An autopsy study of three cases. Eur J Med 1993;2:239–241.
113. Hormigo A, Dalmau J, Rosenblum MK, et al: Immunological and pathological study of anti-Ri–associated encephalopathy. Ann Neurol 1994;36:896–902.
114. Vigliani MC, Palmucci L, Polp P, et al: Paraneoplastic opsoclonus-myoclonus associated with renal cell carcinoma and responsive to tumor ablation. J Neurol Neurosurg Psychiatry 2001;70:814–815.
115. Bataller L, Graus F, Saiz A, Vilchez JJ: Spanish Opsoclonus-Myoclonus Study Group. Clinical outcome in adult onset idiopathic or paraneoplastic opsoclonus-myoclonus. Brain 2001;125:437–443.
116. Antunes NL, Matthay KK, et al: Antineuronal antibodies in patients with neuroblastoma and paraneoplastic opsoclonus-myoclonus. J Ped Hem Oncol 2000;22:315–320.
117. Thirkill CE, Keltner JL, Tyler NK, Roth AM: Antibody reactions with retina and cancer associated antigens in 10 patients with cancer-associated retinopathy. Arch Ophthalmol 1993;111:931–937.
118. Ohguro H, Rudnicka-Nawrot M, Buczylko J, et al: Structural and enzymatic aspects of rhodopsin phosphorylation. J Biol Chem 1996; 271:5215–5224.
119. Milam AH, Saari JC, Jacobson SG: Autoantibodies against retinal bipolar cells in cutaneous melanoma-associated retinopathy. Invest Ophthalmol Vis Sci 1993;34:91–100.
120. Jacobson MD, Thirkill CE, Tipping SJ: A clinical triad to diagnose paraneoplastic retinopathy. Ann Neurol 1990;28:162–167.
121. McLeod JG: Paraneoplastic neuropathies. *In* Dyck PJ, Thomas PK (eds): Peripheral Neuropathy, 3rd ed. Philadelphia, WB Saunders, 1993, pp 1583–1590.
122. Tanaka K, Tanaka M, Inuzuka T, et al: Cytotoxic T lymphocyte mediated cell death in paraneoplastic sensory neuropathy with anti-Hu antibody. J Neurol Sci 1999;163:159–162.
123. DeCamilli P, Thomas A, Cofiell R, et al: The synaptic vesicle-associated protein amphiphysin is the 128 kD autoanigen of stiff-man syndeom with breast cancer. J Exp Med 1993;178:2219–2223.
124. Motomura M, Johnson I, Lang B, et al: An improved diagnostic assay for Lambert-Eaton myasthenic syndrome. J Neurol Neurosurg Psychiatry 1995;58:85–87.
125. Takamori M, Takahishi M, Yasukawa Y, et al: Antibodies to recombinant synaptotagmin and calcium channel subtypes in Lambert-Eaton myasythenic syndrome. J Neurol Sci 1995;133:95–101.
126. Kelly RB: Synaptotagmin is just a calcium sensor. Curr Biol 1995;5:257–259.

127. Younger DS, Rowland LP, Latov N, et al: Lyphoma, motor neuron disease, and amyotrophic lateral sclerosis. Ann Neurol 1991;29:78–96.
128. Forsyth PA, Dalmau J, Graus G, et al: Paranoplastic motor neuron disease. Ann Neurol 1993;34:277.
129. Glantz MJ, Biran H, Myers Me, et al: the radiographic diagnosis and treatment of paraneoplastic central nervous system disease. Cancer 1994;73:168–175.
130. Ojeda VJ: Necrotizing myelopathy associated with malignancy: A clinicopathologic study of two cases and literature review. Cancer 1984;53:1115–1123.
131. Das A, Hochberg FH, McNeils S: A review of the therapy of paraneoplastic neurologic syndromes. J Neuro-Oncol 1999;41:181–194.

CHAPTER 48

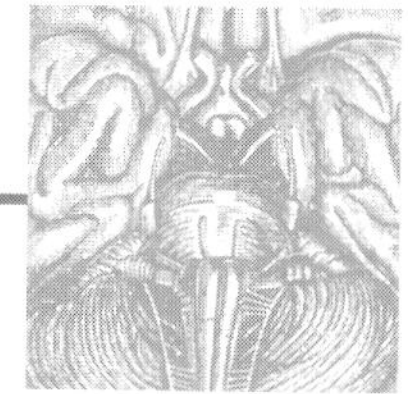

ISTVAN PIRKO and JOHN H. NOSEWORTHY

Demyelinating Disorders of the Central Nervous System

History

Multiple sclerosis (MS) is now known to be a common malady even though it was first recognized as a distinct clinicopathological entity less than 150 years ago.[1] The lack of clear medical reports before the early 1800s is sometimes interpreted as evidence that MS is a relatively new disease. However, it is more likely that the evolution of medicine into science, led to more precise observation and description of human diseases, including MS. Saint Lidwina of Schiedam (1380–1433) developed a relapsing neurological disorder at the age of 18 and may be the first case of clinically described MS.[2] Ollivier was the first to report a clinical case in the medical literature in 1824.[1] Shortly thereafter, Carswell illustrated a case of what is now clearly recognizable as MS in his atlas of anatomical pathology. Cruveilhier published gross pathological and clinical descriptions of MS. Vulpian first suggested the rubric of "sclerose en plaque" in 1866. Charcot was primarily responsible for establishing MS as a unique and recognizable syndrome.[3] He also described the clinical spectrum and the histological appearance. Pierre Marie was the first to suggest an infectious cause of MS in 1884, a hypothesis that is still debated. Toxins were also considered to be responsible in the early 1900s. A major advance toward the understanding of demyelinating diseases was the discovery of experimental allergic encephalomyelitis (EAE) by Rivers in 1935.[4] A variety of different demyelinating diseases have subsequently been described (Table 48–1).

Role of Myelin

Myelin provides insulation for axons and is necessary for saltatory conduction. It is composed of tightly wrapped lipid bilayers with specialized protein constituents. Peripheral nervous system (PNS) myelin is formed by the extension of Schwann cells, and central nervous system (CNS) myelin is produced by oligodendrocytes. The myelin coating is interrupted at regular intervals (nodes of Ranvier) where the axon membrane with its concentration of voltage-gated sodium channels is exposed to the extracellular environment

TABLE 48–1. **Primary (Idiopathic) Inflammatory Demyelinating Disorders of the Central Nervous System**

Acute disseminated encephalomyelitis
Monophasic
Multiphasic
Relapsing (controversial)
Monosymptomatic syndromes
Optic neuritis
Acute transverse myelitis (partial and complete)
Brain stem demyelination
Multiple sclerosis
Neuromyelitis optica
Marburg's disease
Schilder's myeloclastic diffuse sclerosis (controversial)
Balo's concentric sclerosis

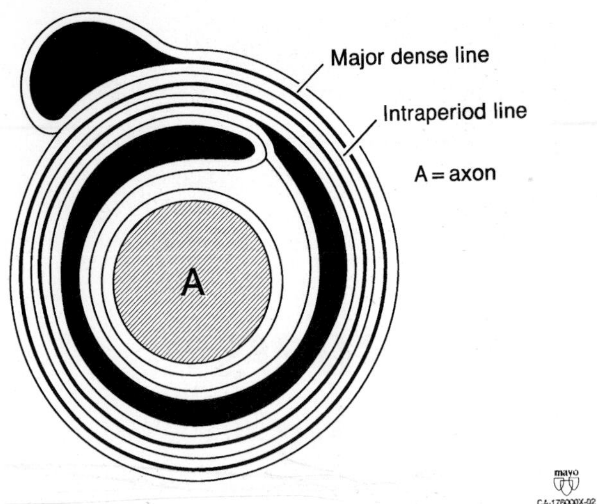

FIGURE 48–1. Major constituent components of CNS myelin. (Modified from Raine CS: Morphological aspects of myelin and myelination. *In* Morrell P [ed]: Myelin. New York, Plenum Press, 1984, p 26.)

(Fig. 48–1).[5] The presence of myelin is essential to maintain conduction velocity; its loss or damage can lead to significantly slower conduction or conduction block. Other factors affect conduction velocity including certain antibodies and chemicals like nitric oxide. In certain cases, blockade may be the initial event in the cascade of events leading to demyelination.

CNS and PNS myelin differ in a number of important ways. Schwann cells myelinate only one internodal segment from a single PNS axon, whereas oligodendrocytes myelinate multiple CNS axons. The proteins also differ. Proteolipid protein accounts for approximately 50 percent of the CNS myelin proteins. Mutations in this highly conserved protein cause Pelizaeus-Merzbacher disease. Protein zero is the major PNS myelin protein and performs a function similar to PLP in compacting the intraperiod line. Myelin basic protein (MBP) makes up 30 percent of CNS and 10 percent of PNS myelin proteins. MBP is not an integral protein but binds to the cytoplasmic surface and is responsible for compaction at the major dense line. Myelin associate glycoprotein accounts for about 1 percent of both peripheral and central myelin. Myelin oligodendrocyte glycoprotein and cyclic nucleotide phosphodiesterase are minor constituents of CNS myelin and are not found in the PNS. Peripheral myelin protein 22 is a minor component of PNS myelin.

Multiple Sclerosis

MS is an inflammatory relapsing or progressive disorder of CNS white matter and is a major cause of disability in young adults. Pathologically, it is characterized by multifocal areas of demyelination, loss of oligodendrocytes, and astrogliosis but with relative preservation of axons. Although certain clinical features are characteristic of MS, investigative studies are often needed to confirm the clinical suspicion and exclude other possibilities. Recently, there have been advances in understanding the etiology, mechanisms of myelin injury, and potential for repair, and several partially effective agents are now approved for use in relapsing-remitting and secondary progressive MS.

Pathogenesis and Pathophysiology. (Fig. 48–2). The pathogenesis and pathophysiology of MS remains incompletely understood. Several mechanisms may be important to MS plaque formation: autoimmunity, infection, bystander demyelination, and heredity. Although convincing proof is lacking, dietary factors and toxin exposure have been hypothesized to contribute as well. These mechanisms are not mutually exclusive, and the true pathophysiology is likely to depend on more than one of them.

AUTOIMMUNITY. During ontogenesis, autoreactive lymphocytes normally undergo clonal depletion, but some escape and are merely suppressed, becoming tolerant to their antigens. Low levels of autoreactive T and B cells persist even in normal individuals. Autoimmune disorders occur when the tolerance of these cells toward their antigen is broken. The decreased suppressor activity of circulating lymphocytes from patients with MS and other presumed autoimmune diseases may reflect loss of tolerance.[6] One potential mechanism that may break tolerance is molecular mimicry between self and foreign antigens. Autoreactive T4 lymphocytes may become activated on exposure to structurally similar foreign antigens. Some evidence suggests that molecular mimicry is relevant in MS. Not only do several viral and bacterial peptides share structural similarities with MBP, but it has also been demonstrated that these antigens may activate MBP-specific T-cell clones derived from MS patients.[7] Blood-brain barrier leakage alone may break tolerance because it gives CNS-reactive lymphocytes easy access to otherwise inaccessible antigens. Alternatively, a primary event such as an infection or injury may release CNS antigens into the periphery, where they may activate corresponding autoreactive cells.[8] The major support for autoimmunity in the pathogenesis and pathophysiology of MS is by analogy to EAE, the major animal model for MS. EAE is, however, an artificial situation and there is no spontaneous autoimmune animal model of MS.

INFECTION. The role of viral infections in the initiation and maintenance of MS has been debated for some time. Several viral infections are known to cause demyelination in animals, including visna virus of goats and sheep, canine distemper virus, and Theiler's murine encephalomyelitis virus. Viral infections in humans can also cause demyelination (progressive multifocal leukoencephalopathy [JC papilloma virus], subacute sclerosing panencephalitis [measles virus], and human T-cell lymphotropic or leukemia virus type 1 [HTLV-1]-associated myelopathy). The epidemiology of MS suggests that environmental factors may promote the disease state, possibly due to one or more viruses. A virus may be involved in the pathogenesis of MS in several ways:

1. Transient or persistent infection outside the CNS may activate autoreactive T cells by means of molecular mimicry or by other nonspecific means (as superantigens do).
2. Transient CNS infection may initiate a cascade of events that fosters autoimmunity (breach the blood-brain barrier, release CNS antigens).
3. Recurrent CNS infections may precipitate repeated inflammation and demyelination.
4. Persistent CNS viral infection could either incite inflammatory reactions detrimental to oligodendrocytes or directly injure them.

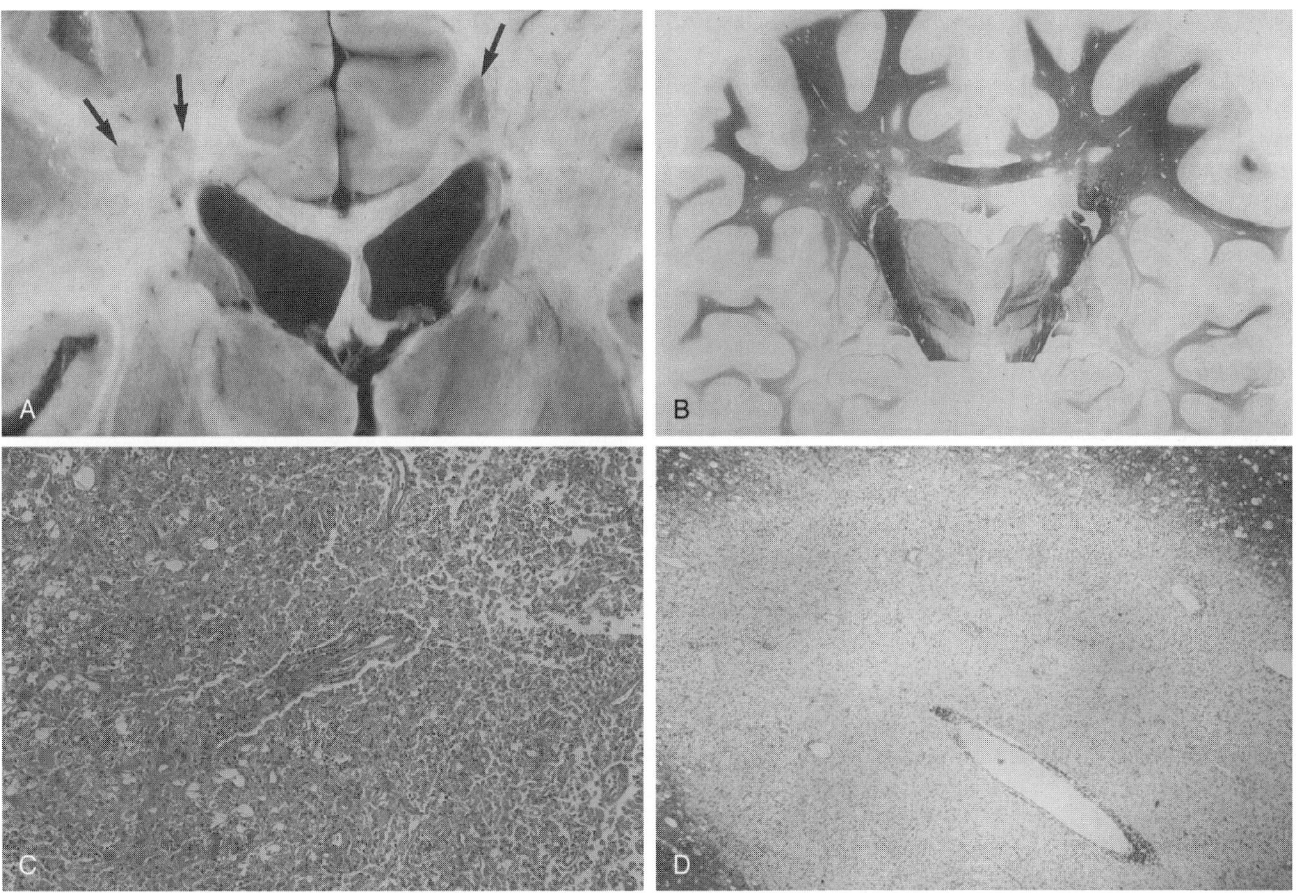

FIGURE 48–2. Pathology of MS. *A*, Coronal brain slice showing several focal areas of sclerosis *(arrows)*. *B*, Luxol fast blue stain of a coronal brain section showing numerous discrete areas of myelin loss. *C*, Hematoxylin and eosin stain of a chronic lesion showing perivascular mononuclear cells and prominent gliosis. *D*, Luxol fast blue/periodic acid–Schiff stain showing perivascular inflammation and loss of myelin.

Beyond speculation and epidemiological observations, there is slim evidence for a viral infection in MS. Early serological studies are difficult to interpret because of nonspecific immune activation and resulting elevation of titers to many different viruses. Many MS patients have elevated cerebrospinal fluid (CSF) titers to measles and herpes simplex (HSV) viruses, but this appears nonspecific. Virus has rarely been cultured from CSF of MS patients, but a new strain of HSV (the MS strain) and a new virus (Inoue-Melnick virus) were first isolated from the CSF of MS patients.[9, 10] Newer molecular techniques to search for a viral genome in CSF and brain have rejected the claim that HTLV-1 is associated with MS. The finding that human herpesvirus 6 (HHV6), although present in 70 percent of brains from both controls and MS patients, is localized to the oligodendrocyte nuclei near plaques of MS patients and to oligodendrocyte cytoplasm in controls indicates that persistent CNS viral infection is common.[11] This raises the possibility that MS may depend on an aberrant host response to this normal condition or that a defective virus that lacks the ability to evade immune detection may be to blame.

More recently, measles and canine distemper virus antibodies were found elevated in blood and CSF samples of MS patients, although their relationship is not clear to the disease process. In a study from Denmark, patients with serological markers for late-stage Epstein-Barr virus (EBV) infection had a threefold increase in the likelihood of developing MS. A follow-up study from Sweden failed to reach this conclusion. In general, serum samples of MS patients may contain higher titers of antibodies to the following infectious organisms: adenovirus, canine distemper virus, HSV, HHV6, influenza, measles, mumps, parainfluenza, rubella, vaccinia, and varicella zoster virus (VZV). Similarly, CSF samples from MS patients may show higher titers of adenovirus, *Chlamydia pneumoniae*, cytomegalovirus (CMV), EBV, HHV6, corona, influenza A&B, measles, mumps, *Mycoplasma pneumoniae*, parainfluenza 1, 2, and 3; respiratory syncytial virus, rubella, vaccinia, and VZV. There has been an interest recently in a potential link between *C. pneumoniae* infection and the development of MS. No direct cause-effect relationship has been observed between any of these infections and MS.

"BYSTANDER" DEMYELINATION. Immune actions may mediate myelin injury in a nonspecific manner. Many soluble products of the immune response other than immunoglobulins are known or suspected to be toxic to myelin and oligodendrocytes. Activated complement is capable of lysing oligodendrocytes in an antibody-independent fashion.[12] The proinflammatory cytokine tumor necrosis factor-alpha causes myelin disruption and oligodendrocyte apoptosis in vitro.[13] Arachidonic acid metabolites may also participate in myelinolysis, and reactive oxygen species released by macrophages cause lipid peroxidation that can damage myelin. Other soluble substances that are potentially toxic to myelin include nitric oxide and vasoactive amines.

HEREDITY. Epidemiological findings support a polygenic hereditary predisposition to MS. A number of candidate genes have been investigated, often with conflicting results. The only definitive genetic association in MS is with the serologically defined human leukocyte antigen (HLA) DR15, DQ6. This is one of the DR2 haplotypes and also known as Dw2 in cellular terminology and DRB1*1501,DQA1*0102, DQB1*0602 in molecular nomenclature. Though its link to MS is well established, the risk conferred by this haplotype is small (relative risk of 3 to 4), and it is neither necessary nor sufficient for the development of MS. Linkage to this locus has not been proven, indicating that it plays only a minor role in familial susceptibility. Other susceptibility genes likely contribute, possibly the T-cell receptor variable beta region and the IgG heavy-chain variable region (especially the VH2-5 gene). But their specific roles have not been established. Other genes under study have been the MBP coding gene, the CTLA-4 gene on chromosome 2q33, and the interleukin-1ra associated gene, in concurrence with the HLA-DR15 haplotype. Mitochondrial mutations are also under investigation, and an LHON-associated mtDNA mutation may be an important cofactor in developing MS in some patients. The ApoE4 gene, as in Alzheimer's disease, has been associated with a higher incidence of MS. On the other hand, ApoE3 is considered to have neurotropic, immunomodulatory, and antioxidant properties. These findings are yet to be confirmed by larger studies.

Twenty percent of MS patients have at least one affected relative. Only about 4 percent of first-degree relatives of patients develop MS, but this represents a 20- to 40-fold increase in risk compared with the general population. Unaffected family members sometimes have abnormal findings on cranial magnetic resonance imaging (MRI), implying that this risk is even higher. One study of MS rates in adopted relatives of MS patients verified that the familial distribution is due to genetic factors rather than shared environment.[14] Twin studies lend support to both genetic and environmental influences on MS development. Genetically identical monozygotic twins are more often concordant for MS than dizygotic twins (26 percent and 2.4 percent, respectively), indicating a genetic component;[15] however, even after following monozygotic twins past age 50 or using MRI data, less than 50 percent are concordant, suggesting a role for environmental factors.

Epidemiology and Risk Factors. MS is not a rare disease. It affects millions worldwide and approximately 250,000 to 350,000 in the United States alone. Symptoms usually begin during young adulthood, with the peak onset at age 24. Approximately 0.3 percent of MS cases are diagnosed before age 15. Women are affected nearly twice as often as men. MS has a predilection for Caucasians, especially those of northern European heritage. Other races and ethnic populations are resistant to a variable extent. MS is virtually unknown among black Africans but occurs in African-Americans at half the rate of whites, possibly due to racial admixture or environmental factors. MS is rare in tropical areas, and the prevalence increases proportional to the distance from the equator, excluding polar regions. The prevalence is less than 5 cases per 100,000 in tropical areas; in high prevalence areas it can be higher than 30 per 100,000,[16] reaching up to 100/100,000 in selected areas. Although usually interpreted as the effect of environmental factors, the prevalence gradient is at least partially due to racial susceptibility.[17]

Perhaps the most incriminating evidence for the role of environmental factors in the development of MS is the changing risk with migration and the occurrence of MS clusters and epidemics. Immigrant populations tend to acquire the MS risk inherent to their new place of residence. Migration from high to low prevalence before the age of 15 lowers the MS risk, whereas migration after this age does not affect risk.[18] Migration from low to high prevalence areas increases the risk of MS, but the effect of age is less clear. Many clusters of MS have been reported.[19, 20] The occurrences of MS epidemics in Iceland and the Faroe Islands have been proposed to be the result of exposure to a pathogen brought by British troops during their occupation in World War II.

Epidemiological data support the view that MS is caused or triggered by an environmental factor in persons who are genetically susceptible. The familial frequency and distribution implies that several genes contribute to susceptibility, and this is consistent with the low relative risk conferred by the genetic loci studied so far. Data from clusters, migration studies, and family studies reveal that there is a latent period of some 20 years between exposure to the environmental factor and the development of clinical symptoms and that the age at exposure is around 15, the putative age at acquisition.

The precise environmental events that lead to CNS demyelination are uncertain. Viral infection is the most plausible, but because of the nonspecific elevation of viral titers and long latent period, there is little direct evidence. Minor respiratory infections precede 27 percent of relapses in patients with established MS. Measles infection was found to have occurred at a later age in MS patients than controls, although the incidence of MS has not been reduced by immunization against measles. Head injury and trauma have received attention as putative triggering events, but cohort studies have not verified any link. Pregnancy does not alter the risk of developing MS, but it does seem to influence disease activity. The relapse rate drops by about one third during the last two trimesters, but this is offset by an increase in relapse rate in the postpartum period. Most studies have found no long-term effects of pregnancy on the prognosis for progression or disability, although one did report a favorable effect.[21] A multitude of other environmental factors have been suspected to alter the risk for MS (cold climate, precipitation, amount of peat in the soil, exposure to dogs, and consumption of meat, processed meat, and dairy products), but none has been verified to be an independent risk factor.

Clinical Features and Associated Findings. MS can cause a wide variety of clinical features. Many signs and symptoms are characteristic, and a few are virtually pathognomonic for the disorder. Conversely, some symptoms are atypical and some are so rare as to suggest a different diagnosis (Table 48–2). The course of the illness is also variable, but it remains a critical consideration in the diagnosis of MS.

Sensory symptoms are the most common presenting manifestation in MS (21 to 55 percent) and ultimately develop in nearly all patients.[22] Loss of sensation (numbness), paresthesias (tingling), dysesthesias (burning), and hyperesthesias are common. These may occur in practically any distribution:

TABLE 48–2. **Diagnosis of Multiple Sclerosis**

Clinical Features Suggestive of MS	Clinical Features Not Suggestive of MS*
Onset between ages 15 and 50	Onset before age 10 or after 55
Relapsing-remitting course	Continued progression from onset without relapses
Optic neuritis	Early dementia
Lhermitte's sign	Seizures
Partial transverse myelitis	Aphasia
Internuclear ophthalmoplegia	Agnosia
Sensory useless hand	Apraxia
Acute urinary retention (especially in young men)	Homonymous or bitemporal hemianopia
Paroxysmal symptoms	Encephalopathy
Diurnal fatigue pattern	Extrapyramidal symptoms
Worsening symptoms with heat or exercise	Uveitis
	Peripheral neuropathy

*Whereas features listed in the right column may be seen in MS, they are atypical and should prompt consideration of alternate explanations.

one or more limbs, part of a limb, trunk, face, or combinations. The more distinctive sensory relapses of MS consist of the sensory cord syndrome and the useless hand syndrome. A common scenario is that of numbness or tingling beginning in one foot, ascending first ipsilaterally and then contralaterally. The sensory symptoms may ascend to the trunk, producing a sensory level, or may involve the upper extremities. Associated symptoms commonly include poor balance, weakness, urinary urgency, constipation, and Lhermitte's sign (see later). Brown-Séquard syndrome may occur with sensory disassociation and hemiparesis. The sensory cord syndrome reflects an evolving demyelinating lesion that begins in the medial posterior column ipsilateral to the first symptoms. Sensory cord syndromes are common in MS and suggest the diagnosis when they occur in young persons and remit spontaneously or in response to corticosteroids. Patients with the sensory useless hand may note subjective numbness and lose discriminatory and proprioceptive function, resulting in difficulty writing, typing, buttoning clothes, and holding onto objects, especially when not looking at their hand. This can occur bilaterally even without lower extremity symptoms. The responsible lesion is in the lemniscal pathways either in the cervical spinal cord or in the brain stem. This syndrome usually remits over several months. The useless hand syndrome is a very specific symptom and is only rarely caused by other disorders.

A large portion of MS patients have persistent sensory loss, usually consisting of diminished vibratory and position sensation in distal extremities. Itching may occur in a dermatomal distribution with relapse or in paroxysms. Pain is not a major manifestation of MS, but distressing lower extremity dysesthetic pain associated with spinal cord involvement, radicular pain from lesions at the root entry zone, paroxysms (see later), and an uncomfortable sensation of pressure or tightness surrounding a leg or the trunk may be present.

Pyramidal tract dysfunction is common in MS and causes weakness, spasticity, loss of dexterity, and hyper-reflexia. Motor deficits can occur acutely or in a chronic progression with weakness of one or more limbs and facial weakness, leg stiffness that impairs gait and balance, or extensor and flexor spasms. Exercise or heat frequently worsens subtle deficits. Muscle atrophy is usually due to disuse, but lesions of lower motor neuron fibers or of the anterior horn itself can cause a pseudoradiculopathy with segmental weakness, atrophy, and diminished reflexes. Motor symptoms are presenting manifestations of MS in 32 to 41 percent of all cases; their prevalence is higher than 60 percent in longstanding MS.

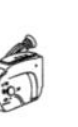

The initial symptom of MS is optic neuritis (ON) in 14 to 23 percent of patients and more than 50 percent experience a clinical episode of ON during their lifetime. The most common manifestation is visual loss in one eye that evolves over a few days. Periocular pain, especially with eye movement, usually accompanies and may precede the visual symptoms. Bilateral simultaneous ON is uncommon in adults, but formal visual field testing reveals unexpected defects in the clinically normal eye in a substantial number of patients. Children and Asian patients are more likely to have bilateral simultaneous ON. Examination shows an afferent pupillary defect, diminished visual acuity, subdued color perception, and often a central scotoma. Funduscopic examination is usually normal but occasionally will reveal papillitis (more common in children) or venous sheathing. Most patients begin to recover within 2 weeks, and significant visual recovery is common. There may be persistent visual blurring, altered color perception, or Uhtoff's sign (see later). MS patients without a clinical history of ON often have evidence of optic nerve involvement on funduscopic examination or visual evoked potentials.

Cerebellar pathways are frequently involved during the course of MS, but a predominately cerebellar syndrome is uncommon at onset. The manifestations include dysmetria, dysdiadochokinesia, action tremor with terminal accentuation, dysrhythmia, breakdown of complex motor movements, and loss of balance. Patients with longstanding MS may develop a "jiggling" gait and an ataxic dysarthria with imprecise articulation, scanning speech, or varying inflection, giving it an explosive character.

Urinary urgency, frequency, and urge incontinence (due to detrusor hyper-reflexia or detrusor-sphincter dyssynergia) result from spinal cord lesions and are frequently encountered in MS patients. The combined incidence of bowel and bladder dysfunction in MS is thought to be higher than 70 percent. Symptoms of bladder dysfunction may be transient and occur with an exacerbation but are commonly persistent. Impaired vesicular sensation causes a high capacity bladder and may lead to bladder atonia with thinning and disruption of the detrusor muscle. Incontinence results in constant dribbling of urine in this irreversible condition. Interruption of brain stem micturition center input sometimes leads to cocontracture of the urinary sphincter and detrusor muscles (detrusor-sphincter dyssynergia). The resulting high pressure may lead to hydronephrosis and chronic renal failure if untreated.

Constipation is a common problem, occurring in 39 to 53 percent of MS patients, especially with limited activity and spinal cord involvement. Fecal incontinence is a socially devastating symptom that is often associated with perineal sensory loss in MS patients.

Sexual dysfunction is seldom mentioned, even though it is a frequent problem in MS. Nearly two thirds of patients report diminished libido. One third of men have some degree of erectile dysfunction, and a similar percentage of women have deficient vaginal lubrication. Besides direct neurological impairment, sensory loss, physical limitations, depression, and fatigue additionally contribute to sexual difficulties in MS patients. In addition, the partner's attitude and psychological factors dealing with self-image, self-esteem, and fear of rejection may also lead to impotence or loss of libido.

Intense vertigo associated with nausea and emesis is an occasional manifestation of MS relapse. In the absence of a clear diagnosis of MS, these symptoms are often attributed to vestibular neuronitis. Patients may also develop a persistent but mild vertigo that is precipitated by movement, or this may be a residual finding after an acute relapse. Internuclear ophthalmoplegia, caused by a lesion in the medial longitudinal fasciculus, is the most common cause of diplopia in MS patients. When symptomatic, it produces horizontal diplopia on lateral gaze that usually remits. Examination discloses incomplete or slow adduction of the eye ipsilateral to the lesion and nystagmus of the contralateral eye during abduction (see Chapter 9). Dissociated nystagmus may be the only finding of an old or subtle internuclear ophthalmoplegia. Bilateral internuclear ophthalmoplegia is strongly suggestive of MS, although this rarely may occur with tumor, infarct, mitochondrial cytopathy, Wernicke's encephalitis, and Chiari malformation. Vertical and diagonal diplopia usually results from skew deviation. Nystagmus, slow saccadic movements, broken ocular pursuits, and ocular dysmetria are other eye findings produced by lesions of cerebellar and vestibular pathways (see Chapter 12). Abducens paresis occurs on occasion, but oculomotor and trochlear nerve impairment is rare.

Corticospinal, spinothalamic, lemniscal, vestibular, and cerebellar pathways can all be affected. Cranial nerve impairment may be seen with lesions that affect brain stem nuclei or exiting and entering fibers. Usually this occurs in association with other symptoms. Because of the long spinal tract and nucleus, the trigeminal nerve is frequently involved. Facial nerve paresis does occasionally occur, but MS is an extremely rare cause of Bell's palsy in patients without previous symptoms. Acute unilateral hearing loss is an uncommon manifestation. Dysphagia is often due to impairment of cranial nerves IX, X, and XII and generally appears late in the course of some patients.

Once thought uncommon, cognitive disorders are now known to be present in 40 to 70 percent of MS patients.[23] Age, duration of MS, and physical disability do not predict the presence of cognitive dysfunction, but the total lesion load seen on MRI does seem to correlate with the degree of cognitive decline. Brain atrophy, enlarged ventricles, and thinning of the corpus callosum also portend symptoms of cognitive dysfunction. The problems are often subtle and may not be detected on standard mental status evaluation. The pattern of cognitive decline is typified by decrease of episodic memory, processing speed, verbal fluency, and difficulty with abstract concepts and complex reasoning. To a lesser extent, executive functioning and visual perception, semantic memory, and attention span may also be also decreased. General intelligence is not typically affected. As expected, cortical symptoms such as aphasia, apraxia, and agnosia are unusual. Homonymous hemianopia, which can be caused by cortical or subcortical lesions, is also uncommon. Despite prominent cerebral white matter involvement, many of the disconnection syndromes such as alexia without agraphia, conduction aphasia, and pure word deafness have not been reported in MS patients.

Affective disorders are more frequent in MS patients than in the general population. These include both anxiety and depression. In long-term studies, the incidence of depression in MS patients is close to 75 percent. Neither depression nor anxiety are related to physical or cognitive disability or MRI lesion load. Patients sometimes experience uncontrollable weeping or less commonly laughter incongruent with their mood. Interruption of inhibitory corticobulbar fibers is responsible for these symptoms (pseudobulbar affect).

Fatigue is a pervasive symptom among MS patients that is not related to disability or depression. Over 75 percent of MS patients experience fatigue during their disease course. A diurnal pattern is characteristic and follows the normal circadian pattern of body temperature fluctuations, with the worse symptoms occurring in afternoon hours (peak core body temperature) often giving way to improvement in the late evening.

MS symptoms may fluctuate in a predictable fashion. Transient worsening of symptoms frequently follows exercise or elevation of body temperature. One example is Uhtoff's phenomenon, in which visual blurring occurs during strenuous activity or with passive exposure to heat. These episodes resolve when the body temperature cools to normal or after a period of rest. An intercurrent infection with fever can induce worsening of symptoms and may be confused with a relapse. Heat sensitivity is presumably related to conduction block, as demyelinated axons are more prone to failed conduction than normal, myelinated fibers.[24]

Paroxysmal symptoms are characteristic of MS and are believed to be due to the lateral spread of excitation (ephaptic transmission) between denuded axons in areas of demyelination. Symptoms are typically brief (seconds to 2 minutes) and recur frequently, occasionally dozens of times per day. They may be precipitated by hyperventilation, certain sensory input, or particular postures. Tonic spasms (paroxysmal dystonia) most often affect the arm and leg on one side, but the face, one limb, or bilateral limbs are sometimes involved. These spasms may result from lesions anywhere along the corticospinal tract. They often begin during the recovery phase after an acute relapse and remit after a few months. Intense pain and ipsilateral or crossed sensory symptoms may accompany them. Paroxysmal weakness occurs, but it is uncommon. A wide variety of paroxysmal sensory symptoms may occur with MS, including tingling, prickling, burning, or itching, and sharp neuralgic pain is common. Trigeminal neuralgia may appear in patients with MS. The occurrence of trigeminal neuralgia in a person younger than age 40 is suggestive of MS. Lhermitte's sign (transient sensory symptoms usually precipitated by neck flexion) is usually described as an electrical or tingling sensation that travels down the spine or into the extremities. Although quite common in MS, Lhermitte's sign can also occur with a wide variety of other disorders, such as vitamin B_{12} deficiency, spondylosis, Chiari malformation, and tumors, and after cisplatin chemotherapy. Several other paroxysmal symptoms are occasionally encountered, including paroxysmal dysarthria and ataxia, paroxysmal diplopia, and combinations of these symptoms. Facial myokymia and hemifacial spasm are additional transient (lasting months) phenomena sometimes due to brain stem demyelination. Trismus, kinesigenic dystonia, paroxysmal kinesigenic choreoathetosis, and segmental myoclonus have also been described in case reports of MS patients as rare and unusual examination findings.

Seizures occur in about 10 percent of MS patients. Focal motor seizures, possibly with secondary generalization, are the most frequent. The occurrence of seizures usually follows one of two patterns. On occasion, focal onset seizures begin early in the course of MS and later remit. The start of seizures late in the course of MS more often poses a chronic problem and may be difficult to control.

The eye is the only organ outside the nervous system that is sometimes involved in MS. Uveitis and retinal periphlebitis each occur in at least 10 percent of MS patients. Uveitis can involve the posterior, intermediate (pars planitis), or rarely anterior portion and resembles that seen in other inflammatory (e.g., sarcoid, Reiter's syndrome, Behçet's syndrome, inflammatory bowel disease, systemic lupus erythematosus) and infectious (e.g., syphilis, tuberculosis, Lyme disease) conditions. Periphlebitis is seen as venous sheathing on funduscopic examination and is histologically identical to the perivascular inflammation present in brain white matter. It is interesting that inflammation commonly occurs in the retina, which has a peripheral type of myelin produced by Schwann cells.

There are occasional reports of peripheral nerve or nerve root demyelination in MS patients as well as central demyelination in acute inflammatory demyelinating polyradiculoneuropathy and chronic inflammatory demyelinating polyradiculoneuropathy (see Chapter 49). Some of these cases may be due to the incidental occurrence of two unrelated disease processes. However, because the PNS and CNS share many antigens, including MBP, it is possible that an autoimmune reaction or a viral infection could involve both the CNS and PNS.

Persons with one autoimmune disorder generally have an increased risk of others. Even though there are several reports of systemic and organ-specific autoimmune diseases in MS patients, population-based studies have not confirmed any increase in prevalence of these disorders among MS patients.[25] In fact, there appears to be a negative association between MS and rheumatoid arthritis.

Multifocal CNS involvement and acute relapses, remissions, and/or slow progression of neurological deficits typify MS. A single episode of neurological dysfunction can be suggestive of MS if it follows the typical time course of a relapse: progression over less than 2 weeks (usually days), with or without a period of stabilization, and improvement or resolution (often over months). Insidious progression of deficits localized to a single site in the CNS can also be due to MS, but other causes must be excluded. The temporal course of MS can be described by one of four categories: relapsing-remitting (RR), secondary progressive (SP), primary progressive (PP), and progressive relapsing (PR).[24] Many physicians use the term *relapsing progressive*, which encompassed patients with SP, PR, and even those with RR MS who have stepwise relapse-related worsening disability. This term has recently been abandoned. Other terms that relate to the course of MS but have no consensus regarding their definition are sometimes encountered. *Benign* MS generally refers to patients who have had MS for a long time but have little or no disability. *Malignant* MS is sometimes used to describe patients with frequent relapses and incomplete recovery but is also used in reference to patients with acute fulminant demyelinating syndromes (see later). The term *"clinically isolated syndrome"* (*CIS*) refers to patients presenting with their first episode of region-restricted episodes of CNS inflammatory demyelination. This may remain an isolated syndrome (no recurrence), it may remain a forme fruste of acute disseminated encephalomyelitis (ADEM) (see later) or may be the harbinger for one of the relapsing forms of MS. The probability of recurrent demyelinating episodes (e.g., clinically definite MS) has been the subject of several important investigations, and several clinical features and test results are of predictive value. Optic nerve, spinal cord, and brain stem are the most common sites of these recurrent monosymptomatic events, and the time profile follows that of MS relapses. The pathogenesis, pathophysiology, epidemiology, clinical features, associated disorders, differential diagnosis, evaluation, and management are the same as in MS.

The prognosis for visual recovery after each episode of ON is good, and most patients regain normal visual acuity. Profound visual loss, recurrent ON, and age older than 35 are associated with a higher risk for poor recovery. Investigators have concluded that recurrent multifocal demyelinating episodes, fulfilling the diagnostic requirements of clinically definite MS, develop in 50 percent or more of patients after isolated ON when follow-up is extended beyond 20 years.[26] Most of this risk is incurred within the first few years, although significant risk may continue into the fourth decade after the event. Children much more often develop simultaneous bilateral ON and have a lower risk for subsequent MS than adults. Factors that are associated with an increased risk of *developing* MS as a disseminated illness are the presence of venous sheathing, recurrent ON, family history of MS, white race, previous vague or nonspecific neurological symptoms, and the presence of OCB-s, elevated IgG index, or IgG synthesis rate in CSF. The severity of acute transverse myelitis is inversely related to the risk of acquiring further symptomatic demyelinating lesions. Complete transverse myelitis with profound loss of motor, sensory, and sphincter function imparts a relatively low risk of 3 to 14 for the later diagnosis of MS. Partial transverse myelitis with preservation of significant motor function at peak is associated with a much higher incidence of MS. Although monosymptomatic brain stem demyelination is not as common as either ON or acute transverse myelitis, similar conclusions have been reached. In the only study available, two thirds of these patients with cerebral white matter lesions detected on MRI developed MS within 5 years, compared with none of 5 patients with normal head MRI.[27,28]

A recently published 10-year follow-up of the original Queen Square series continues to demonstrate the value of the baseline cranial MRI study in determining risk of recurrence (MS risk). In this cohort study of 81 CIS patients, approximately two thirds had at least one asymptomatic lesion (54 of 81, 67 percent) at baseline. After 5 years of follow-up, slightly more than half with one to three asymptomatic baseline cerebral lesions had developed MS (13 of 24) compared with the majority of cases presenting with at least four baseline lesions (28 of 33, 85 percent). After 10 years of follow-up, the majority of patients with any asymptomatic cerebral lesions had developed definite MS (45 of 54, 83 percent).[29] This information is helpful for treating patients in the setting of CIS (see treatment implications, later).

Differential Diagnosis. Only a few diseases cause neurological deficits that regress spontaneously and relapse in different areas of the CNS over the course of many years. However, because of the remarkable heterogeneity of MS, many disorders may resemble MS (Table 48–3), especially in the first years of active disease.

Other primary idiopathic inflammatory demyelinating CNS disorders may be mistaken for MS. ADEM usually causes monophasic CNS demyelination. Although it frequently involves multifocal areas of white matter simultaneously, ADEM cannot be reliably differentiated from the initial clinical episode of MS. Fulminant brain demyelination in persons without previous symptoms of MS is more likely due to ADEM or other conditions (Schilder's myelinoclastic diffuse sclerosis, Balo's concentric sclerosis, Marburg's variant of MS). Neuromyelitis optica differs from MS primarily in the topography and intensity of the lesions (see later discussion).

Several systemic or organ-specific inflammatory conditions can involve the CNS white matter. ON, myelitis, and other syndromes sometimes occur with systemic lupus erythematosus. Whether this autoimmune disease increases the risk of developing MS or causes similar syndromes by a different pathological process is unknown. Sarcoidosis can affect the nervous system in several ways, including multifocal, corticosteroid-responsive white matter lesions. Sjögren's syndrome sometimes occurs with MS, but this may only represent a chance association. Neuro-Behçet's disease has a predilection for the brain stem. Occasionally, isolated demyelinating syndromes are associated with inflammatory bowel disease.

A wide variety of vasculitic syndromes (e.g., primary angiitis of the CNS, periarteritis nodosa, Wegener's granulomatous angiitis, vasculitis associated with rheumatoid arthritis, Susac's syndrome, Eales' disease) may mimic MS. However, these syndromes can usually be distinguished by involvement of the cortex, seizures, early dementia, personality changes, psychosis, infarcts involving large vessel territories on MRI, and lack of improvement. Findings characteristic to the particular vasculitis (uveitis and vitreal hemorrhage in Eales' disease, retinal and cochlear involvement in Susac's syndrome, upper and lower respiratory tract involvement in Wegener's granulomatosis) also aid in the correct diagnosis.

A few infections must also be considered in the differential diagnosis of MS. Both Lyme disease and syphilis may cause multifocal white matter lesions. HTLV-1 causes a chronic progressive myelopathy (HTLV-1–associated myelopathy/tropical spastic paraparesis). Acute or recurrent myelitis can be caused by VZV. Progressive multifocal leukoencephalopathy and *Toxoplasma* abscesses should be considered in immunocompromised patients with progressive neurological decline. Bacterial endocarditis with brain abscess formation, subacute sclerosing panencephalitis, or chronic rubella encephalomyelitis may need to be considered in the appropriate circumstances.

Cerebrovascular disease is only rarely mistaken for MS. Occasionally, an MS relapse has an abrupt onset that may mimic an infarct, especially in those not previously diagnosed with MS. The usual circumstance is that of a hemisensory or hemimotor deficit imitating a lacunar infarct. Disorders with multiple cerebral infarcts (emboli, hypercoagulable states, Sneddon's syndrome, CADASIL, vasculitis) may produce an MRI appearance and course resembling MS. Vascular malformations may also produce symptoms similar to MS.

Additional neurological illnesses capable of producing multifocal lesions rarely mimic MS. Metastatic tumors and multifocal gliomas are often cited examples but rarely is this distinction difficult for an experienced clinician. Lymphoma more commonly masquerades as MS because the lesions may involve the white matter, may be multifocal, and are corticosteroid responsive. In addition, demyelination sometimes presents as one (or a few) mass lesion(s). In this situation, biopsy may be needed for diagnosis. Neoplasms can cause paraneoplastic syndromes that may be confused with MS. A high index of suspicion must be kept for older age at presentation, subacute ataxia, early dementia, and personality changes. A few metabolic disorders may resemble MS, such as vitamin B_{12} deficiency, vitamin E deficiency (seen in Bassen-Kornzweig syndrome, hypobetalipoproteinemia, and Refsum's disease), and central pontine or extrapontine myelinolysis. Leukodystrophies are usually not difficult to distinguish from MS. Krabbe's disease (galactocerebroside-beta-galactosidase deficiency), metachromatic leukodystrophy (MLD; arylsulfatase A deficiency), and the usual adult form of adrenoleukodystrophy (ALD) and adrenomyeloneuropa-

TABLE 48–3. Differential Diagnosis of Multiple Sclerosis

Other inflammatory demyelinating CNS conditions	Cerebrovascular disorders
Acute disseminated encephalomyelitis	Multiple emboli
Neuromyelitis optica	Hypercoagulable states
Systemic or organ-specific inflammatory diseases	Sneddon's syndrome
Systemic lupus erythematosus	Neoplasms
Sjögren's syndrome	Metastasis
Behçet's disease	Lymphoma
Inflammatory bowel disease	Paraneoplastic syndromes
Vasculitis	Metabolic disorders
Periarteritis nodosa	Vitamin B_{12} deficiency
Primary CNS angiitis	Vitamin E deficiency
Susac's syndrome	Central (or extra) pontine myelinolysis
Eales' disease	Leukodystrophies (especially adrenomyeloneuropathy)
Granulomatous diseases	Leber's hereditary optic neuropathy
Sarcoidosis	Structural lesions
Wegener's granulomatosis	Spinal cord compression
Infectious disorders	Chiari malformation
Lyme neuroborreliosis	Syringomyelia/syringobulbia
Syphilis	Foramen magnum lesions
HTLV-1 associated myelopathy	Spinal arteriovenous malformation/dural fistula
Viral myelitis (HSV, VZV)	Degenerative diseases
Progressive multifocal leukoencephalitis	Hereditary spastic paraparesis
Subacute sclerosing panencephalitis	Spinocerebellar degeneration
	Olivopontocerebellar atrophy
	Psychiatric disorders
	Conversion reactions
	Malingering

HTLV-1, Human T-cell lymphotropic virus type 1; HSV, herpes simplex virus; VZV, varicella-zoster virus; CNS, central nervous system.

thy (AMN) exhibit both central and peripheral dysmyelination. Blood leukocyte or fibroblast culture enzyme activity levels will confirm the diagnosis of Krabbe's disease and MLD, and elevated levels of very long-chain fatty acids occur in ALD/AMN. Mitochondrial disorders should also be given consideration because symptoms and MRI appearance may be similar to MS. A relapsing remitting disorder identical to MS is sometimes seen in patients with the mutations responsible for Leber's hereditary optic neuritis.[30] This usually occurs in female patients, and there may not be a family history of visual loss. A number of rare biochemically defined illnesses and other genetic disorders may occasionally merit consideration (including cobalamin and folate dysmetabolism, adult polyglucosan body disease, hereditary spastic paraparesis, spinocerebellar degeneration, and hereditary cerebroretinal vasculopathy).[31]

Several additional disorders must be excluded before diagnosing primary progressive MS (PP MS). Spinal cord compression from spondylosis or tumor may produce chronic progressive myelopathy. Chiari malformations, syringomyelia, syringobulbia, other foramen magnum lesions, spinal arteriovenous malformations, and dural fistulas may also need consideration. Careful imaging readily identifies these structural abnormalities. Degenerative diseases such as olivopontocerebellar atrophy may mimic PP MS. MRI and CSF examination will help distinguish between the two.

Conversion reactions and somatization disorders are commonly encountered in a busy referral practice and must be accurately diagnosed to afford optimal patient management.

Evaluation. The diagnosis of MS is based on the demonstration of white matter lesions disseminated in time and space in the absence of another identifiable explanation. MS remains a clinical diagnosis, although MRI, evoked potentials, and CSF examination can help clarify less certain cases. For research purposes, various categories of MS have been defined based on the certainty of the diagnosis.[32] At least two attacks and evidence of two separate CNS lesions (clinical or paraclinical) are required for the designation of *clinically definite* MS (CD MS). Two attacks and evidence of one CNS lesion or one attack and evidence of two CNS lesions (clinical or paraclinical) is considered *clinically probable* MS. Cases that fulfill the criteria for clinically probable MS and have supportive CSF findings are labeled as *laboratory-supported definite* MS. Patients with a clear history of at least two attacks and supportive CSF but a normal neurological examination and no paraclinical evidence of CNS lesions are categorized as having *laboratory-supported probable* MS. Suspected cases that do not fit any of these criteria may be regarded as *possible* MS. Paraclinical evidence generally refers to abnormalities on evoked potential studies or imaging procedures.

As a result of increasing availability of refined paraclinical diagnostic modalities (especially MRI) and an overall better understanding of the disease process, new diagnostic criteria for MS were proposed by an international expert panel in 2001.[33] Three out of four of the following findings should be present on MRI: (1) one gadolinium enhancing lesion, or nine T2 hyperintense lesions; (2) at least one infratentorial lesion; (3) at least one juxtacortical lesion; and (4) at least three periventricular lesions.

According to the clinical diagnostic criteria, if a patient had two or more attacks with objective evidence on examination of two or more anatomical areas involved, no additional data is required to make the definite diagnosis. However, if such diagnostic studies were done and are not supportive of a diagnosis of MS, then the diagnosis should be reconsidered.

If a patient presents with a history of two or more attacks, but objective clinical evidence only suggests one lesion, the following additional data is needed to confirm the diagnosis: the disease process has to be disseminated in space as demonstrated by MRI; alternatively, two or more MRI-detected lesions consistent with MS plus positive CSF would suffice to meet the newly defined criteria. The clinician also may elect to await a further attack implicating a different anatomical site.

In case a patient had one attack, with objective clinical evidence of two or more lesions, dissemination in time as demonstrated by serial MRIs separated by at least 3 months or a second clinical attack would clarify the diagnosis. If a patient has a clinically isolated syndrome, or "monosymptomatic" presentation, the following criteria should be met: dissemination in space as demonstrated by MRI (again separated by at least 3 months), or two or more MRI-detected lesions consistent with MS plus positive CSF and dissemination in time on serial MRI scans, or a second clinical attack.

In case the patient presents with a progressive course, the presence of positive CSF is required, and dissemination in space should be present, as suggested by nine or more T2-weighted brain lesions, or two or more cord lesions, or four to eight brain lesions plus one cord lesion on MRI. Alternatively, abnormal visual evoked potentials (VEP) with four to eight brain lesions, or fewer than four brain lesions plus one cord lesion, and dissemination in time on serial MRI scans, or continued progression for a year would meet the diagnostic criteria.

"Positive CSF" according to this set of criteria is defined by either the presence of oligoclonal bands detected by established methods (preferably isoelectric focusing) different from any such bands in serum, or by a raised IgG index. The presence of both enhancing and nonenhancing white matter lesions on a single MR image must not be used as evidence of dissemination in time as well as space, because these can also be seen in ADEM. Oligoclonal bands (OCBs) and an elevated IgG index provide supportive CSF findings.

Ancillary tests are frequently required to confirm the diagnosis of MS and to exclude other possibilities in uncertain cases. Laboratory tests on peripheral blood can help to exclude many of the infectious and other inflammatory disorders. A chest x-ray is generally needed to assess for sarcoid or paraneoplastic disorders if these are under consideration. An ophthalmological examination may be needed to search for alternative causes of visual loss. Imaging studies, CSF examination, and evoked potentials are often helpful because characteristic abnormalities are frequently present.

MRI of the head is the most sensitive study for MS and is far more useful than computed tomography. Eighty-five to 95 percent of CD MS patients have abnormalities on head MRI (Fig. 48–3). Focal areas of increased T2-weighted and decreased T1-weighted signal reflect the increased water content associated with demyelinated plaques. The MRI appearance of MS lesions, however, is not specific and similar abnormalities may be seen in normal aging, small penetrating vessel infarcts, Lyme disease, tropical spastic paraparesis/HTLV-1–associated myelopathy, sarcoid, systemic

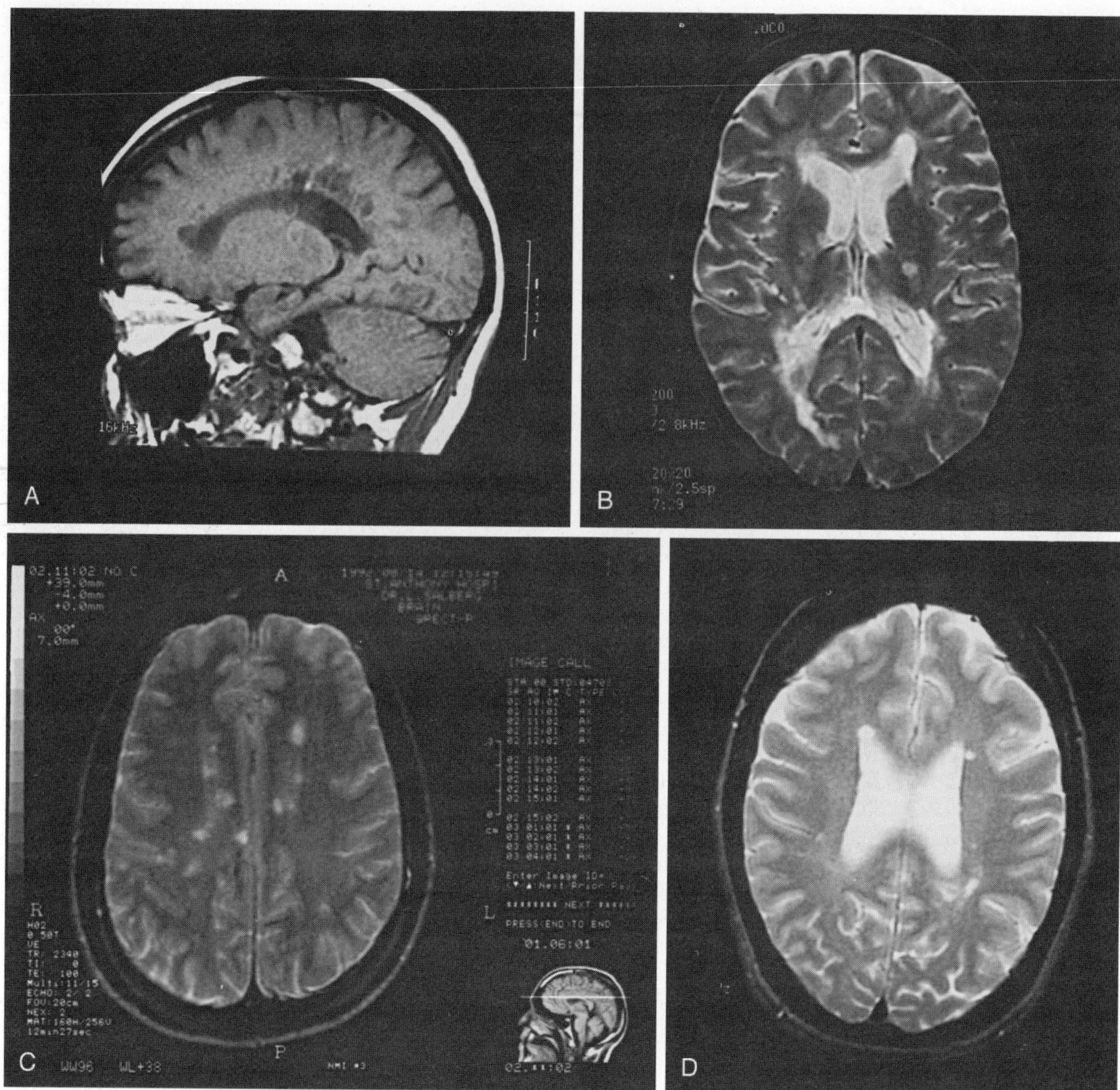

FIGURE 48–3. Head MRI of patients with MS. *A,* T1-weighted sagittal image showing multiple hypointense periventricular lesions. *B,* Axial T2-weighted image showing confluent periventricular high-intensity lesions most prominent at the frontal and occipital horns. A focal lesion is also present in the posterior limb of the left internal capsule. *C* and *D,* Periventricular lesions suggestive of MS.

lupus erythematosus, Sjögren's syndrome, mitochondrial cytopathies, vasculitis, and ADEM. The specificity for MS can be increased by consideration of lesion number, size, location, and shape.[34] This is especially important in persons older than age 50. MRI characteristics, other than the ones suggested by the international criteria outlined previously, are size larger than 6 mm, oval shape (often with the long axis directed perpendicular to lateral ventricles), and locations in the periventricular area, corpus callosum, and posterior fossa.

Longitudinal MRI studies have shown the evolution of MS lesions.[35] Gadolinium enhancement, indicating blood-brain barrier disruption, sometimes precedes the development of T2-weighted lesions and typically lasts for 4 weeks in the brain (occasionally longer, especially in large hemisphere lesions), and perhaps somewhat longer in the spinal cord. FLAIR imaging is especially helpful for evaluating periventricular lesions that may go unnoticed on regular T2-weighted scans. The disadvantage of the technique is its relative insensitivity to posterior fossa lesions. Proton density weighted images are also part of the usual sets of images used in the MR diagnostics of MS. These images can be evaluated similarly to T2-weighted images. Technically they are usually acquired together with the T2-weighted datasets, as a first echo in conventional fast spin echo sequences, where the subsequent echoes can be used for generating the T2-weighted images. New T2-weighted lesions have a fuzzy border and enlarge over a few weeks. After a period of stabilization, the T2-weighted lesion regresses and becomes more sharply delineated from the surrounding white matter as edema resolves. Most of the time, a residual abnormality with increased T2 weighting and decreased T1-weighted signal remains, reflecting demyelination and gliosis. The low attenuation T1 signal, or "T1 black hole," is more often seen in secondary progressive MS and is thought to represent actual tissue loss. In several well-documented cases, hypointense

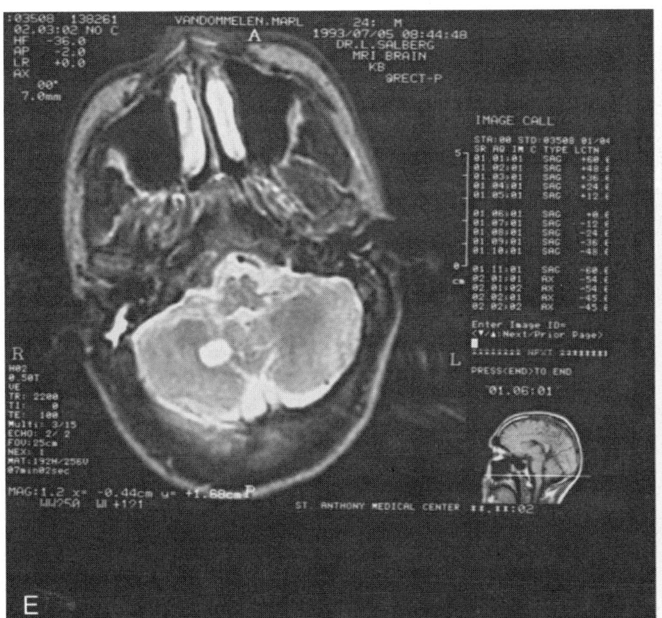

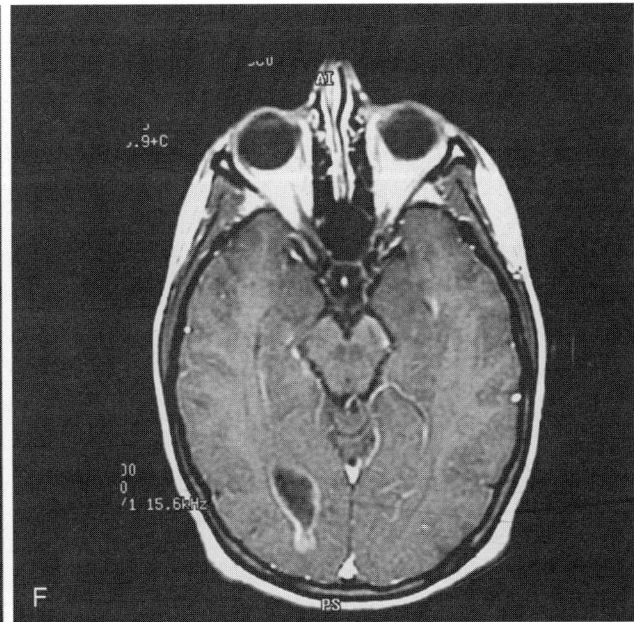

FIGURE 48–3 *Continued. E,* A single large right cerebellar hemisphere lesion seen on T2-weighted MRI. *F,* Peripherally gadolinium-enhanced large right occipital white matter lesion. Enhancement can also be seen along the temporal horn of the lateral ventricles.

lesions on T2-weighted scans were described in subcortical gray matter structures in MS patients. On a molecular level these areas are thought to represent iron deposition; their significance in MS is not fully understood. The MRI activity of disease, defined as either the number of new, recurrent, and enlarging lesions or the number of gadolinium-enhancing lesions, is usually higher than the clinical activity. This may be either because of the involvement of asymptomatic areas of the CNS or because of a pathophysiological difference between symptomatic and nonsymptomatic lesions based on the presence or absence of axonal dysfunction.

There is only poor correlation between disability and lesion load (volume of white matter abnormalities) determined by head MRI. Sometimes individuals have severe impairment and few MRI abnormalities, and the converse may occur. This disparity is partially explained by variable spinal cord involvement, but a pathophysiological difference may account for some of the discrepancy. There is a better correlation between "T1 black holes" and disability.

MR spectroscopy is rapidly becoming an accepted diagnostic modality, where information can be obtained about the biochemical constituents of the imaged substance. With this technique, a cubic volume of interest is defined based on a regular MR image set. Simultaneous acquisition of multiple volume units is possible. With long echo time (TE) studies, NAA (N-acetyl aspartate), choline, creatinine, and lactate peaks can be identified on the MR spectrum. With short TE studies, myoinositol, lipids, and some neurotransmitters may be identified. The resolution of the MR spectrum (the "number of lines" in the spectrum) is proportionate to the magnetic field strength used. NAA is the second most abundant amino acid constituent in the brain after glutamate. It is localized almost exclusively in neurons. Creatinine is used as the "constant" peak in a MR spectrum, since it is the least likely to be altered by CNS-specific processes. Therefore, numeric MRS data are usually presented as ratios related to creatinine. The NAA/creatinine ratio is decreased in areas of axonal or neuronal loss. It correlates well with disability. It can be decreased in normal appearing white matter, also in early stages of lesion formation, thus representing a challenge to the usual dogma of axonal loss being secondary to myelin damage. This decrease of the NAA/creatinine ratio may return to normal following the resolution of the acute phase. This process may be related either to reversibility of neuronal injury or to disappearance of edema in the involved areas. In general, more reduced NAA peaks are seen in progressive forms of MS with more profound tissue loss. If a relatively large hemispheric lesion shows decreased NAA content, similar findings may be seen in the other hemisphere in a "mirror" location. The lactate peak can be elevated in a variety of acute processes, and as such, carries relatively low specificity. The short TE spectrum is used less frequently; the "mobile lipid" peak (which is also though to represent macromolecular protein fragments) is increased in areas of acute demyelination.

Another innovative MRI technique is magnetization transfer imaging. The principle behind this imaging modality is relatively simple. In complex macromolecular systems, there is a baseline magnetization exchange in equilibrium between macromolecular protons and mobile protons. If the macromolecular protons are saturated before each excitation (and subsequent data acquisition) with a prolonged off-resonance broadband pulse, then the signal intensity of the image will be reduced due to magnetization transfer exchange between the saturated ("bound") and free ("mobile") protons. By obtaining duplicate sets of images (with and without magnetization transfer pulse), a magnetization transfer ratio can be calculated. The ratio reflects the integrity of the macromolecular environment. It is reduced by approximately 3 to 5 percent in areas of edema, but it is more significantly reduced in areas of demyelination or axonal loss. If the ratio "normalizes" in a lesion, no subsequent tissue loss is usually seen on other imaging modalities. Despite these advantages, the magnetization transfer imaging is technically difficult because it produces variable findings depending on the technical environment and is not universally available. It has not been accepted as a standard technique for evaluation of MS patients.

Diffusion-weighted imaging is well known from its widespread use in the diagnosis of ischemic stroke. This technique can show early stages of MS plaque formation, according to some studies. The increase in apparent diffusion coefficient correlates with acute plaques, and seems to best correspond with T1-enhancing lesions; this technique may show the lesions at an even earlier stage.

MRI has become an important component of recent clinical trials. Because of the high sensitivity of MRI for disease activity, it is reasoned that periodic MRI may determine treatment efficacy more quickly than monitoring relapse rate or disability level. Many studies have used MRI as a secondary outcome, but clinical outcomes are still used as the primary outcome for definitive trials. Additional MRI techniques have also proven useful in the diagnosis of MS. MRI of the spinal cord shows discrete lesions in about 80 percent of CD MS patients. Several semiautomatic methods exist to determine lesion volume, ventricle volume, or hemispheric volume. These are generally applied for research purposes only, and are not part of the usual workup of MS.

CSF evaluation remains a valuable diagnostic tool for MS. A lymphocytic pleocytosis occurs during acute exacerbations in about one third of patients, but this seldom exceeds 50 cells. Eighty percent of the lymphocytes are CD3 positive. The ratio of CD4 to CD8 cells is 2:1. Less than 20 percent of the cells are B cells. CSF protein is normal in up to 60 percent; levels above 100 mg/dL are unusual and may suggest a different disorder. The proportion of gamma globulin is high owing to the synthesis of immunoglobulins within the blood-brain barrier. The majority of CSF immunoglobulin is IgG, although IgM and IgA may also be elevated. Measures of intrathecal IgG production have been devised that are more useful than simple gamma-globulin levels. The IgG index and synthesis rate are elevated in 70 to 90 percent of CD MS patients and occasionally in other disorders (see later). Agarose gel electrophoresis, or the more sensitive isoelectric focusing of CSF proteins, often reveals discrete bands of immunoglobulin, each a monoclonal antibody. It is pertinent to compare serum and CSF banding patterns because peripheral monoclonal gammopathies may produce CSF bands. To reduce false-positive results, only unique CSF OCBs should be reported. Between 85 and 95 percent of CD MS patients have OCBs; however, early in the course they are not as prevalent. Once present, OCBs persist and the pattern does not vary, although new bands occasionally appear. Unlike subacute sclerosing panencephalitis, in which the majority of OCBs are antibodies specific for measles virus, the antigenic specificity of OCBs in MS is unknown. Five to 10 percent of noninflammatory CNS samples and 30 percent of inflammatory samples are also positive for OCBs.[36] In other inflammatory or infectious illnesses OCBs are often transient features. Their persistence is more suggestive of MS. The presence of myelin components, antimyelin antibodies, and kappa light chains in CSF has also been used in the diagnosis of MS. However, the sensitivity and specificity of these products is less than that of OCBs.

Evoked potentials are summed cortical electrical responses to peripheral sensory stimulation that can be used to localize sites of pathology and measure conduction velocity along sensory pathways. VEP and somatosensory evoked potentials (SSEP) may detect subclinical sites of demyelination, thus providing evidence of multifocality. Brain stem auditory evoked potentials (BAEP) are occasionally informative. More than 90 percent of persons with a history of ON have an abnormal VEP, and 85 percent of CD MS patients have abnormalities on VEP-s even when the history of ON is absent. Slowed conduction is present on SSEP in nearly three fourths of patients with CD MS. BAE-s are the least sensitive, with abnormalities in less than 50 percent. MRI has largely supplanted the use of evoked potentials in MS because of the greater sensitivity in the diagnosis and the detailed anatomical information it provides. In 2001, the American Academy of Neurology released practice parameters regarding the usefulness of evoked potential studies in MS. According to these recommendations, VEPs are considered probably useful (Class II evidence) to identify patients at increased risk for developing clinically definite MS. SSEPs are possibly useful, whereas the evidence for BAEPs supporting the diagnosis of CD MS is insufficient.

Management. There is no available prevention or cure for MS. Treatments focus on three areas: treating acute exacerbations and hastening their recovery; altering the natural history of MS; and providing symptomatic relief of current symptoms by enhancing physical abilities and preventing or treating complications. A fourth management topic concerns special treatment issues related to pregnancy.

ACUTE EXACERBATIONS. Corticosteroids are the most commonly used treatment for MS, although there have been few studies to address their efficacy. Adrenocorticotropic hormone (ACTH) was shown to speed recovery from an exacerbation but had no effect on the ultimate degree of recovery. Because of the unpredictable cortisone response to ACTH, oral prednisone and later intravenous methylprednisolone became the preferred treatments. The Optic Neuritis Treatment Trial verified that intravenous methylprednisolone but not prednisone increased the recovery rate and unexpectedly increased the time to the next relapse, thus delaying the diagnosis of CD MS.[37] Moreover, the prednisone-treated group had twice as many recurrences. The finding was not replicated in a second study but it has affected the practice of treating acute MS exacerbations. The current recommendation is to treat disabling attacks with 500 to 1000 mg of intravenous methylprednisolone per day for 3 to 5 days with or without a short tapering dose of oral corticosteroids. According to the practice parameters for steroid treatment of acute ON attacks released by the American Academy of Neurology in 2001, oral prednisone in doses of 1mg/kg/d has no proven value. Higher dose of oral or parenteral methylprednisolone may result in quicker and more thorough recovery of visual function. There is no evidence of long-term benefit for visual function.

A recent study suggested that intravenous steroids may also have long-term effects on disease progression when given regularly.[38] In this study, RR MS patients randomized to receive regularly scheduled pulses of IV methylprednisolone (every 4 months for 3 years, then every 6 months for 2 years) demonstrated stability or improvement in disability measures, fewer "T1 black holes," and less brain atrophy than did control patients randomized to receive steroids only with relapses. These findings suggest a possible long-term benefit of pulsed IV methylprednisolone therapy on brain atrophy and disability. This as yet unconfirmed approach to long-term therapy might be considered a reasonable "control arm" in future Phase III trials of experimental therapies.

Up to one third of patients do not have an adequate recovery after a relapse despite the use of corticosteroids. Plasma exchange (PLEX) alone was found beneficial in a substantial proportion of patients with severe inflammatory demyelinating episodes who had failed to improve following treatment with high-dose IV methylprednisolone.[39, 40] A randomized, sham-controlled, double-blind trial in 22 patients (seven exchanges over 14 days) without concomitant use of immunosuppressants in acute demyelinating events confirmed these findings.[41] Moderate or greater clinical improvement was observed in over 42 percent of participants. A trial of seven PLEX treatments (alternate days) is a reasonable option for patients who fail to respond to conventional IV methylprednisolone therapy in acute, severe episodes of demyelinating diseases.

ALTERATION OF THE NATURAL COURSE. The primary goal of drug treatment is to alter the natural course of the disease (e.g., reducing the frequency and severity of relapses, preventing the chronic progressive phase, and slowing the progression of disability). The disease activity seen on MRI is often used as a secondary outcome, although MRI measures currently correlate imperfectly with clinical outcome. Knowledge on altering the course of MS is largely restricted to three patient groups, those with RR MS, those with clinically isolated syndromes, and those with secondary progressive MS.

Altering the Course of Relapsing-Remitting Multiple Sclerosis

BETA-INTERFERONS. Interferons are a class of peptides that have antiviral and immunoregulatory functions. Both interferon alpha and interferon-beta are part of the anti-inflammatory TH2 response. Interferon-beta 1b (Betaseron) was the first drug approved by the U.S. Food and Drug Administration (FDA) specifically for the treatment of MS. A large clinical study in RR MS patients demonstrated a reduction in the frequency of relapses by about one third with subcutaneous injection every other day.[42] The severity of relapses was also lessened. Interferon-beta 1b had a striking effect on MRI measures of disease activity. The placebo-control group continued to accumulate white matter lesions, whereas patients in the high-dose arm (8 million IU) had stabilization of their MRI lesion load. No difference was found in the disability levels, however. Side effects include injection site reactions, flulike symptoms (low-grade fever, myalgias, headache; these lessen in frequency after treatment for a few months), mild liver enzyme elevation, and lymphopenia. Depression and attempted suicide were more common in the treated groups. One particularly disturbing result was the production of neutralizing autoantibodies (NAbs) in 38 percent of patients after 3 years of treatment. Not only do patients with these antibodies thereafter fail to respond to this drug, but there is also a concern that NAbs may cross-react with natural interferon-beta and interfere with its function. All positive sera for NAbs seem to cross-react with both interferon-beta 1a and 1b. Switching from one preparation to the other does not change the pattern of antibody response.[43] The long-term effects of NAbs are unknown. Recent studies seem to support that NAb formation reduces clinical and MRI effects although often NAb formation subsides with time. There are no firm guidelines for monitoring NAb formation. Most physicians do not measure NAbs but rather change therapies empirically when patients appear to be failing treatment.

Interferon-beta 1a (Avonex) has the same amino acid sequence as natural interferon-beta and differs from interferon-beta 1b by one amino acid as well as by the presence of carbohydrate moieties. Once-weekly intramuscular interferon-beta 1a has been found to have effects similar to that of interferon-beta 1b in reducing the frequency of MS relapses. In addition, a favorable effect on disability was also demonstrated and side effects were less common. NAbs occurred half as often as with interferon-beta 1b. Interferon-beta 1a has been approved for "relapsing MS" by the FDA.[44]

The "correct" dose of interferon continues to be debated. In a recent placebo-controlled trial, patients randomized to a high dose of interferon-beta 1a (44 mcg three times/week) seemed overall to do better than those receiving half this weekly dose. Both groups outperformed placebo and the high dose seemed to have more effect on relapse severity, hospitalizations, MRI activity and lesion volume accumulation, and possibly on delaying disability in the most severely disabled patients. At the end of the 2 years of follow-up, placebo-treated patients were randomized to 22 or 44 mcg sc three times weekly; patients on active treatment were continued on their original dose.[45] The authors reported a benefit for the higher dose and for those treated for the full 4 years, again suggesting that early treatment and perhaps higher doses of interferons may be beneficial. The primary outcome, however, was relapse count per patient per 4 years and, as such, patients treated early had a significant advantage using this outcome measure. There were trends favoring the higher dose (relapse rate, MRI volumes; not for time to first confirmed progression, however). The authors did not make statistical adjustments for multiple comparisons and there were many dropouts in the high-dose groups, making it difficult to draw firm conclusions. Again, the answer to the question about the benefit of early treatment can best come from long-term (perhaps 8 to 10 years) studies using "hard outcomes" (e.g., time to progression, major milestones in disability). Relative treatment advantages of interferon-beta 1a and 1b have not been clearly established but are under study.[46, 47] A pilot study in RR MS patients suggests that interferon-alpha may also have a therapeutic effect.[48]

GLATIRAMER ACETATE. Glatiramer acetate is a synthetic mixture of polypeptides produced by the random combinations of four amino acids that are frequent in MBP. After a preliminary study suggested efficacy,[49] a Phase III randomized, double-blind, placebo-controlled, multicenter trial showed a 29 percent reduction in relapse rate.[50] The FDA has approved this medication for use in RR MS. Even though this disease-modifying therapy requires daily subcutaneous administration, the side effects are relatively minor compared to the interferons, and patients do not need regular laboratory monitoring (Table 48–4). Glatiramer acetate reduces new lesion formation, the number of T2 enhancing lesions, lesion volumes, and the percentage of new lesions that will evolve into T1 "black holes," although the MRI effect is not apparent until the agent has been used for at least 6 months.[51–53]

TABLE 48–4. **Therapeutic Options in MS**

MS Type	Agent	Dosage	Proven Benefits	Adverse Effects	Monitoring
Acute Episodes	Methylprednisolone (Solu-Medrol)	500–1000 mg IV for 3–7 days	Hastens recovery Effects on blood-brain barrier (transient restoration) Long-term effects (as of yet uncertain)	Usual steroid-related side effects	As usually with short-term steroid therapy
	Plasma exchange	7 exchanges every other day	Promotes recovery in patients not responding to high-dose IV steroids	Problems with venous access site (hematoma, bleeding, pneumothorax); Anemia (usually asymptomatic); Risk of infection and sepsis Fatigue, thrombosis, hypotension Citrate toxicity (perioral numbness) Heparin-associated thrombocytopenia	CBC before therapy and at regular intervals
Relapsing-Remitting	Interferon beta-1b (Betaseron, Betaferon)	8 million IU subcutaneously every other day	Relapse rate reduction MRI benefits: reduces development of new lesions, delays increase in volume of lesions	Flulike symptoms Hepatotoxicity Leukopenia, anemia, thrombocytopenia Myalgias, depression, anorexia Menstrual disorders Hypocalcemia, injection site reaction, necrosis, neutralizing antibodies, pregnancy category C	CBC and LFT before therapy, every week in the first month, every month in the first 3 months, then every 3 months
	Interferon beta-1a (Avonex)	30 mcg IM once weekly	Relapse rate reduction May delay progression of disability MRI benefits: reduces development of new lesions, delays increase in volume of lesions	Flulike symptoms Hepatotoxicity Anemia, eosinophilia Syncope Depression Nausea, dyspepsia, anorexia Neutralizing antibodies Injection site reaction, necrosis Pregnancy category C	CBC and LFT before therapy, every week in the first month, every month in the first 3 months, then every 3 months

	Glatiramer acetate (Copaxone)	20 mcg SC daily	Relapse rate reduction Moderate, delayed MRI effects	Pain/edema at injection site Flushing Transient chest pain Transient dyspnea Transient eosinophilia Facial edema Palpitations Nausea, anorexia Anxiety Vasodilation Lymphadenopathy Pregnancy category B	None
	Interferon beta-1a (Rebif)	22 mcg or 44 mcg SC every other day	Relapse rate reduction MRI benefits: reduces development of new lesions, delays increase in volume of lesions Possible dose-related benefit in patients with more severe disease	Flulike symptoms Hepatotoxicity Anemia, granulocytopenia, lymphopenia Blocking antibodies Injection site reaction Pregnancy category C	CBC and LFT before therapy, every week in the first month, every month in the first 3 months, then every 3 months
	Intravenous immunoglobulin (IVIG)	0.15–0.2 g/kg IV every 2 months for 2 years	Relapse rate reduction One phase III trial to date	Hyperviscosity syndrome Aseptic meningitis Headaches Neutropenia Anemia Pseudohyponatremia Renal failure	IgA level before therapy Renal function tests before therapy and at regular intervals
Secondary Progressive	Interferon beta-1b (Betaseron, Betaferon)	8 million IU subcutaneously every other day	Reduces disability regardless of relapse rate Relapse rate reduction MRI benefits	See above	See above
	Mitoxantrone (Novantrone)	5 or 12 mg/m^2 every 3 months Not to exceed 100–140 mg/m^2 cumulative lifetime dose (cardiac toxicity)	Relapse rate reduction* Delays progression of disability MRI benefits	Cardiomyopathy Menstrual disorders Leukopenia Nausea, vomiting Urticaria, skin rash Acute leukemia Pregnancy category D	Echocardiogram to determine EF before initiating therapy and every 6 months, more frequently if cumulative dose to exceed 100 mg/m^2 ECG LFTs before each infusion CBC before each infusion

*At the time of submission, this phase III trial has not been published in a peer-reviewed journal.
CBC, Complete blood count; ECG, electrocardiogram; LFT, liver function tests; MRI, magnetic resonance imaging.

IVIG. Monthly treatment with low-dose (0.15 to 0.2 g/kg) intravenous immunoglobulin in RR MS patients resulted in fewer and less severe relapses in addition to slowing the accumulation of disability in a single randomized trial. The outcome was very similar to that of injectable interferons, suggesting an alternative treatment option for RR MS patients.[54] This therapy is less accepted in the United States. More studies with larger number of patients and extended follow-up are needed to confirm these observations. Recent studies have failed to demonstrate that IVIg administration reverses longstanding deficits from MS and ON.[55–57]

Altering the Course of a Clinically Isolated Syndrome. When should treatment be initiated in patients with demyelinating disease? Two recently published multicenter studies have addressed this issue in persons at high risk of developing MS. In the CHAMPS study,[58] 383 patients with their first episode of presumed demyelinating disease ("clinically isolated syndrome") in the setting of an abnormal, asymptomatic baseline cranial MRI scan, were randomized to receive either weekly interferon-beta 1a 30 mcg IM or placebo after an initial course of steroid therapy. This study was terminated early when the primary outcome measure of conversion to "clinically definite MS"status was reached in a greater number of placebo-treated patients. These findings were not unexpected given the known effect of interferons on reducing relapse rate but do provide some support for early treatment. The duration of follow-up in this study (71 percent 1 year, 34 percent 2 years) is insufficient to determine long-term benefit from early intervention, however. In a second placebo-controlled study of 309 patients with either monosymptomatic (61 percent) or multifocal onset (39 percent) early demyelinating disease, early treatment with low dose interferon-beta 1a (22 mcg sc once weekly), reduced conversion to CD MS (34 percent versus 45 percent) at 2 years.[59] Again, there is no data on whether these treatments offer long-term benefit. These two studies provide support for considering early treatment in patients presenting with first attack, presumed MS (e.g., in the presence of multiple asymptomatic MRI lesions), but further studies are needed in order to determine whether this approach will provide a prolonged benefit on disease course.

Altering the Course of Secondary Progressive MS. Within 15 years of onset, almost 60 percent of RR MS patients will enter the secondary progressive phase of the disease. Treatment approaches aimed to affect the natural course of disease are available for these patients.

INTERFERONS. Interferon-beta 1b may have a beneficial effect on the overall outcome of SP MS and may also alter MR lesions,[60, 61] but this question remains incompletely answered. In the placebo-controlled European study[62] of inteferon-beta 1b in SP MS, the time to worsening was extended for treated patients. Treated patients were less likely to be wheelchair-bound and had fewer hospitalizations. Another analysis[63] of this study confirmed the benefits, though the dropout rate in this study was relatively high. The patients who responded best to interferon therapy were those who experienced relapses during their disease course. MRI monitoring suggested that the benefit on T2 lesion activity was seen early and persisted into the second half of the second year of treatment. T2 lesion load increased in placebo- but not interferon-treated patients in the first 2 years of treatment.[64]

Contrasting with these results, in another trial involving patients with SP MS,[65] both high dose (44 mcg) and lower dose (22 mcg) inteferon-beta 1a failed to change the primary outcome of time to disability worsening. Positive effects were seen on relapse rate and reduction of MRI activity but the effect on disability did not replicate the European interferon-beta 1b report.

MITOXANTRONE. In a European Phase III study of the anthracenedione chemotherapeutic agent mitoxantrone,[66] significant benefits were observed in a group of SP MS patients. Several clinical and functional outcome measures were reported to stabilize or improve with every 3 month administration of this intravenous medication. Secondary MRI outcome measures, including enhancing lesion formation and overall T2 lesion load, were also better in the treated patients. The greatest concern regarding this medication is its cardiac toxicity: the cumulative lifetime maximum dose was established at 140 mg/m^2. Besides the cardiac side effects, mitoxantrone may cause menstrual irregularities or overall ablation of the menstrual cycle. A case of treatment-induced acute promyelocytic leukemia was also reported in the literature. This therapy has been approved by the FDA treatment of SP MS, but no peer-reviewed full report has been published. It has also been used with methylprednisolone.[67]

OTHER IMMUNOMODULATOR THERAPIES. Cyclophosphamide is an alkylating agent that has indiscriminate cytotoxic effects on rapidly dividing cells, including lymphocytes, making it a potent immunosuppressant. Several studies have claimed a beneficial effect in both relapsing and progressive patients. Because one of the major studies included ACTH, IV methylprednisolone is sometimes given with the cyclophosphamide. Other trials have not found a favorable effect. Because of the inconsistent results, high potential for serious side effects, and adverse reactions, including hemorrhagic cystitis and malignancy, cyclophosphamide is not widely used. Some centers, however, use cyclophosphamide in patients with aggressive disease in whom more conventional treatments have failed.

Azathioprine, a purine analog antimetabolite, has marginal efficacy in the treatment of MS. A meta-analysis of all blinded, placebo-controlled studies confirmed a slight benefit of slowed progression and less frequent relapses.[68] The toxicity of azathioprine and its slow onset of action have prevented its widespread use. Besides the liver toxicity and hematological effects, the induction of malignancies has been a concern. One retrospective study did not find an increased incidence of cancer in MS patients treated with azathioprine, but this remains a potential risk.

Methotrexate is a folate antagonist that is effective in rheumatoid arthritis. Weekly low-dose oral methotrexate was found to delay upper extremity dysfunction in SP MS patients, although it had no effect on the more traditional measures of disability, including the Expanded Disability Status Scale (EDSS).[69]

The use of cyclosporine in the treatment of MS has been evaluated in three clinical trials, none of which have demonstrated a convincing benefit. In addition, side effects such as hypertension and elevation of creatinine were common.

Numerous additional therapies have been tested, and many others are undergoing evaluation. The antiherpesvirus drug acyclovir has been shown to reduce relapse frequency in a small prospective trial. Total lymphoid irradiation was found to slow the chronic progression of MS, but because this approach precludes the later initiation of immunosuppressant drugs and may be associated with a higher mortality rate, it is not widely used. Cladribine is a nucleoside derivative that was found to decrease relapse rate and slow the progression in patients with SP MS in an initial investigation.[70] The drug is better tolerated than other parenteral immunosuppressants, although bone marrow suppression is a risk. In a more extensive clinical trial,[71] cladribine therapy did not change disability scores, but significant reduction in enhancing lesions and overall T2 lesion burden was observed with higher dose treatment. A study of a small number of patients treated with autologous stem cell transplantation[72] suggested possible clinical stabilization or minor improvement over a 15-month period of follow-up in both secondary and primary progressive MS. The induction chemotherapy (BEAM regimen) resulted in one fatality in this trial; similar incidences are known in patients undergoing this procedure. The small number of patients and the different methods used (some patients received CD34+ selected graft) makes the interpretation of this data very difficult. Trials with higher number of patients under standardized circumstances are needed to verify the validity of these observations.

SYMPTOMATIC TREATMENT OF EXISTING DISABILITIES. Spasticity is common even in patients with only minimal weakness. It is usually prudent to begin treatment of mild spasticity with a stretching program. A randomized controlled crossover trial[73] of physical therapy (8-week blocks of therapy twice a week, for 45 minutes/session) showed significant benefit on several outcome measures related to improved mobility. No apparent differences were observed between home-based or hospital-based therapy. The addition of an evening dose of benzodiazepine may help relieve extensor spasms and clonus that may interfere with sleep. As spasticity worsens it becomes necessary to use baclofen. Doses should be escalated slowly to prevent the occurrence of overt side effects, and up to 120 mg/day may be required. Although baclofen is well tolerated in most patients, limiting side effects such as sedation and increased muscle weakness may occur, and rarely a paradoxical increase in spasticity is noted. Liver enzyme elevation and nonconvulsive status epilepticus presenting as encephalopathy have also been reported in association with baclofen. Abrupt withdrawal of baclofen may result in hallucinations or seizures, making it necessary to taper doses. Despite symptomatic improvement, antispasticity measures may not increase function or independence. In paraplegic patients with severe spasticity and intolerance to the required oral dose, intrathecal baclofen delivered by a subcutaneously implanted pump allows a much smaller dose and is often effective in alleviating intractable spasticity and may lessen urinary urgency. Tizanidine seems to be as effective as baclofen. Dantrolene has been used for spasticity, although the therapeutic window is small.

For treating fatigue, medications are only partially effective. Amantadine at 100 mg bid is the standard initial treatment, although pemoline 37.5 mg daily is also superior to placebo. The stimulating effects of the selective serotonin reuptake inhibitors may also be somewhat effective in combating MS-related fatigue. Modafinil, a medication approved for the treatment of narcolepsy, has also been used with good success. Often, however, patients need to limit activities and schedule rest periods. Paroxysmal symptoms are highly responsive to medical treatment. A small dose of carbamazepine is often very effective. If not tolerated, several alternative medications may be tried, including phenytoin, acetazolamide, baclofen, and gabapentin. In addition, misoprostol has been claimed to be effective in MS-related trigeminal neuralgia. After about 1 month of treatment, a periodic attempt at tapering off these medications is a reasonable approach because these symptoms usually remit. Seizures are treated no differently than in non-MS conditions. Heat sensitivity may require avoidance of precipitating activities, but this depends on the nature of symptoms and the situation in which they occur. If the precipitating activity cannot be avoided, a cooling jacket may be an option. A potassium channel blocker, 4-aminopyridine improves temperature sensitivity in some patients but occasionally causes seizures or disturbing paresthesias. Action tremor is a common disabling symptom. Unfortunately, it is often only marginally amenable to medical therapy. Clonazepam may offer some relief, but tolerance frequently develops, necessitating increasing doses. Isoniazid and carbamazepine have also been found marginally beneficial. One clinical trial showed ondansetron to reduce tremor-related disability. Anecdotal reports suggest that gabapentin may be partially effective. Improvements in stereotactic neurosurgery have made thalamotomy a legitimate option in those whose disability is mainly due to tremor and not ataxia.

Dysesthetic pains are difficult to control but sometimes respond to tricyclic antidepressants, carbamazepine, or baclofen. Gabapentin and tramadol may also be effective. Standard analgesics are not often useful in MS-associated pain, and narcotics should be avoided in the treatment of chronic pain.

Emotional incontinence may be amenable to a low dose of a tricyclic antidepressant.

Symptoms of a hyper-reflexic bladder (urgency, frequency, and urge incontinence) are often manageable with anticholinergics such as oxybutynin, propantheline, or imipramine. A flaccid bladder can sometimes be aided by bethanechol, although intermittent self-catheterization is more often needed. Symptoms that suggest urinary retention (a feeling of incomplete emptying, frequency, hesitancy, or a need to apply pressure to the lower abdomen to urinate) should prompt evaluation with urinalysis and a post-void residual urine measurement. Residuals in excess of 15 mL are abnormal; and if they are above 50 mL, consideration should be given to urological consultation for more thorough investigation and to blood chemistries to determine urea and creatinine levels. Detrusor-sphincter dyssynergia, diagnosed by cystometrography, is treated with anticholinergics, sometimes with the addition of an alpha-1 blocking agent (terazosin) or intermittent catheterization. It is important to reassess bladder function periodically, and residual urine volumes should be monitored if there are any persistent changes in function or symptoms. Intermittent catheterization should be considered when post-void residuals reach 100 mL. A chronic indwelling urinary catheter should be avoided if reasonably possible. It is usually not necessary to use antibiotics prophylactically in the prevention of urinary tract infections. Urinary calculi may be prevented by acidification of the urine with cranberry juice. Constipation can usually be managed with bulk laxatives and stool softeners. More severe cases may require osmotic agents, bowel stimulants, anal stimulation, suppositories, or enemas. Bedridden patients may develop fecal impaction unresponsive to these measures and require manual disimpaction. Fecal incontinence can be minimized by adherence to a schedule for bowel movements.

The clinician should determine the precise nature of any sexual dysfunction in patients with MS. Physical difficulty from spasticity may be alleviated by premedication with baclofen, and a fast-acting anticholinergic such as oxybutynin may calm urinary urgency. Sexual dysfunction should not be automatically attributed to MS. It may be necessary to investigate hormonal levels and to obtain urological or gynecological consultation. Manual lubrication with gel is a ready solution to vaginal dryness. Erectile dysfunction responds very well to sildenafil. Less frequently, vacuum devices, intracavernous injections of papaverine (or combinations of papaverine, prostaglandins, and epinephrine; triple agent), or penile implant are also used in the treatment of erectile dysfunction. Thalamotomy or thalamic stimulation may provide some short-term clinical benefit to patients disabled by appendicular cerebellar tremor and ataxia. The benefits on disability and quality of life are much less clear, however, and the early benefits may wain within 1 to 3 years.[74, 75] Further studies are needed to clarify how best to select patients for these ablative and stimulation treatment interventions.

It is advisable for MS patients to attain good health habits, including proper diet and fitness. Smoking, excess alcohol intake, and obesity should be avoided. Exercise can help maximize function by increasing and maintaining joint mobility, strength, and stamina; may promote improved sleep hygiene; and may reduce the severity of fatigue. Physical and occupational therapy can play an important role in regaining independence. Canes, walkers, and wheelchairs or scooters may be needed to maintain safe mobility. Hand controls can be installed in automobiles for patients with lower extremity dysfunction. In debilitated, immobilized patients, periodic shifts in posture to change weight-bearing regions and air or water mattresses prevent bedsores. Passive range of motion exercises prevent contractures. When ventilatory dysfunction occurs, it should be evaluated and activity schedules should be appropriately modified.[76]

Two recently completed randomized trials failed to demonstrate benefit from IVIg administration in patients with longstanding weakness or visual loss from MS and ON.[55, 56]

SPECIAL CONSIDERATIONS DURING PREGNANCY. Before initiation of any drug in a woman of reproductive age, the potential for teratogenicity must be discussed. In general, immunomodulator therapy should be avoided if one is planning a pregnancy. The treatment of acute exacerbations is unchanged during pregnancy, although one might have a higher threshold for treatment. Both corticosteroids and plasma exchange are relatively safe during pregnancy. None of the drugs used to alter the disease course, however, should be used during pregnancy, and they should be stopped if pregnancy occurs. The cytotoxic immunosuppressants have teratogenic effects, and interferon-beta induces spontaneous abortion in animals. The effects of many of the other drugs are unknown. It is best if these drugs are stopped several months before a planned pregnancy.

Prognosis and Future Perspectives. Because most information on the prognosis of MS is reported in terms of the EDSS, it is important to have some understanding of this scale. The EDSS is a 10-point scale, with each increase representing worsening symptoms of function. The score is derived from severity scores in each of six systems as well as ambulation and work ability. A score of 0 means no signs or symptoms; 1 to 3 represent mild disability with no or minimal impairment of ambulation; 3.5 to 5.5 refer to moderate disability and impairment of gait; the need for a cane to walk one-half block (100 m) receives a score of 6; an EDSS of 8 refers to the need for a wheelchair and effective upper extremity function; an EDSS of 10 refers to death related to MS.

MS has a highly variable outcome, ranging from asymptomatic to fulminant with death ensuing in a matter of months. Autopsy series have estimated that unsuspected MS may occur in as many as 0.2 percent of the population. Even when symptomatic, MS may cause only nuisance symptoms. Benign MS, when defined as unrestricted ambulation or EDSS of 3 or less 10 years after onset, accounts for about one third of cases. However, many of these patients acquire more disability at a later time. When considering all patients with MS, Weinshenker found that 15 years after onset, 80 percent had EDSS worse than 3, 50 percent had reached EDSS of 6 or more, 10 percent were at EDSS 8, and 2 percent had died. The percentage of patients with initially RR MS who develop SP MS increases steadily with disease duration.[77] At 10 years, 40 to 50 percent have continual deterioration; after 25 years, approximately 80 percent have slow progression.

Natural history studies have identified several prognostic indicators that predict outcome to a limited extent. Factors associated with a better prognosis (slower accumulation of disability, longer time before chronic progression) include young age at onset, female gender, RR course (as opposed to PP MS), initial symptoms of sensory impairment or ON, first manifestations affecting only one CNS region, high degree of recovery from initial bout, longer interval between first and second relapse, low number of relapses in the first 2 years, and less disability at 5 years after onset (both EDSS and number of systems affected—sensory, motor, sphincter, brain stem, vision, cerebral). Despite the indolent nature, a PP course is the worst prognostic factor, with the median time to reach EDSS 6 of only 6 years, compared with approximately 20 years in RR patients. Men and patients with an older age at onset are more likely to have PP MS.

The survival of MS patients is only slightly below expected. Seventy-six percent of patients are alive 25 years after onset, which is 85 percent of that seen in age- and sex-matched controls.[25] MS is rarely the direct cause of death, although respiratory failure from cervical myelopathy or extensive cerebral and brain stem demyelination and death occasionally occurs with acute or subacute exacerbations.[78] Complications of MS such as pneumonia, pulmonary emboli, aspiration, urosepsis, and decubiti are responsible for 50 percent of deaths. Most of the other deaths are from heart disease, cancer, cerebrovascular disease, and trauma. Suicide is the only cause of death that is overrepresented among these cases. The suicide rate among MS patients may be as high as two to seven times that of non-MS persons.

Neuromyelitis Optica

Neuromyelitis optica (NMO) is an uncommon neurological illness characterized by the occurrence of optic neuropathy and myelopathy in close temporal relationship. The separation from MS has come under question, owing to the frequent dissemination of lesions outside the optic nerves and spinal cord. Part of the difficulty lies with the broad, imprecise, and inconsistent definition. The names Devic's syndrome, Devic's disease, and NMO are often used interchangeably, although the first name encompasses all patients who fit the preceding definition and the second and third should only be used to refer to those patients presumed to have a distinct disorder. The term *opticospinal* MS is often used in the Far East to denote patients with exclusive or predominant involvement of optic nerves and spinal cord, encompassing most patients with Devic's syndrome.

Pathogenesis and Pathophysiology. Devic's syndrome may occur with ADEM, autoimmune disorders (e.g., systemic lupus erythematosus), MS, and possibly viral infections. Not surprisingly, the pathological descriptions are quite varied because these patients are invariably a heterogeneous group. Classically, acute spinal cord lesions demonstrate diffuse swelling and softening that extend over several levels or involve nearly the entire cord in a continuous or patchy distribution. Acutely, there is destruction with dense macrophage infiltration involving white and gray matter, loss of myelin and axons, and lymphocytic cuffing of vessels. In chronic lesions, the cord is atrophic and necrotic, with cystic degeneration and gliosis. In the absence of perivascular cuffing, these extensive lesions resemble infarctions. The prominent spinal cord swelling in the confines of the restrictive pia presumably may raise intramedullary pressure, leading to the collapse of small parenchymal vessels, further propagating tissue injury. Proliferation of vessels with thickened and hyalinized walls similar to that seen after infarction or other extensive injury may occur.[78] Less fulminant lesions commonly coexist and are much more typical of inflammatory demyelination. The optic nerves, chiasm, and occasionally cerebral hemispheres are involved in a similar fashion with either demyelinating lesions, necrotizing lesions, or both.

Epidemiology and Risk Factors. Devic's syndrome occurs in patients of varied ages (range, 1 to 73). The mean age at onset of monophasic Devic's syndrome is 27, whereas relapsing NMO (see later) tends to occur in an older age group (mean age at onset of 43). Monophasic Devic's syndrome affects males and females equally, whereas relapsing NMO affects females predominantly (F:M, 3.8:1). One third of patients have a preceding infection within a few weeks of neurological symptom onset. Most commonly this is a nonspecific upper respiratory tract infection, flu, or gastroenteritis. The most common specific infections preceding the development of Devic's syndrome are chickenpox and pulmonary tuberculosis. Devic's syndrome has also followed vaccination for swine flu and mumps. Only a few instances of a possible familial occurrence of Devic's syndrome have been reported, and in one of these families, a unique mitochondrial mutation was found. Devic's syndrome is said to be more common in Japan and East Asia, although even there it is uncommon (less than 5 per 100,000). There are 3 cases described in the literature with familial occurrence of Devic's disease in the Far East. In a genetic study, HLA-DPB1*0501 was more frequently associated with "opticospinal MS,", whereas HLA-DPB1*0301 is the most strongly associated allele with conventional MS in the Japanese.

Clinical Features and Associated Findings. Symptoms of ON and myelitis develop over hours to days and are often preceded or accompanied by headache, nausea, somnolence, fever, or myalgias. Continued progression of symptoms over weeks or months occasionally occurs. Most patients (greater than 80 percent) develop bilateral optic neuritis. Bitemporal or junctional field deficits, indicating chiasm involvement, are sometimes present early in the course of the ON. Visual loss is often accompanied by periocular pain, and myelitis onset is sometimes heralded by localized back or radicular pain. Lhermitte's sign is common. Severe degrees of neurological deficits are usual, and the degree of recovery is variable.

Patients who present with Devic's syndrome can follow one of several possible courses. Approximately 35 percent have a monophasic illness, 55 percent develop relapses nearly limited to the optic nerves and spinal cord (relapsing NMO or opticospinal MS), and rarely patients have a fulminantly progressive course without relapses or a course typical of MS.[79] According to a study conducted at the Mayo Clinic,[80] patients with a monophasic course usually presented with rapidly sequential events (median, 5 days) with only moderate recovery. Patients showing characteristics of the relapsing form of Devic's had a median interval of 166 days between index events, followed within 3 years by clusters of severe relapses isolated to the optic nerves and spinal cord. Most relapsing patients developed severe disability in a stepwise manner. Approximately one third died from respiratory failure. Features of NMO distinct from "typical" MS included normal initial brain MRI, > 50 cells/μfL in CSF with polymorphonuclear predominance, and lesions extending over three or more vertebral segments on spinal cord MRI. Relapsing NMO is often associated with autoimmune disorders, most commonly systemic lupus erythematosus. These patients also frequently have an elevated erythrocyte sedimentation rate and nonspecific elevation of autoantibodies, including antinuclear antibodies, anti-ds-DNA, and antiphospholipid antibodies. Tonic spasms and neuropathic lower extremity pain are common sequelae to the spinal cord damage. Symptoms referable to brain stem lesions (nystagmus, ophthalmoparesis, and vertigo) can occur in these patients as well.

Differential Diagnosis. The differential diagnoses for Devic's syndrome includes MS, ADEM, pulmonary tuberculosis, and viral infection (especially in the immunocompromised patient). In patients with an apparent affected family member, consideration should be given to mitochondrial disease. Relapsing NMO should raise the suspicion for associated autoimmune disorders. Because Devic's syndrome can occur in persons older than age 60, when an unrelated ischemic optic neuropathy could occur, and because isolated or recurrent myelopathy may precede the ON, additional consideration must be given to spinal cord compression, spinal cord tumor, and spinal arteriovascular malformation (AVM) or dural fistula.

Evaluation. Imaging is needed to exclude structural lesions and provide information on the pathological process.

Optic nerve or chiasm enlargement, T2-weighted signal changes, and enhancement may be seen on head MRI during the acute phase. Increased T2-weighted signal in the medulla is not uncommon and usually represents extension of high cervical lesions. Spine MRI characteristically shows cord swelling, signal changes, and enhancement extending over at least three levels (Fig. 48–4). This appearance may resemble a spinal cord tumor, prompting consideration for biopsy.

On magnetization transfer (MT) MRI, no significant difference was found on normal-appearing white matter of Devic's patients and controls, whereas MS patients had a significantly lower MT ratio peak and histogram average.[81] T1 hypointense lesions and linear lesions that cross over more than two segments are more suggestive of Devic's disease.

An occasional patient may need prone and supine myelography to exclude a spinal dural-based AVM. Laboratory investigations reveal an elevated erythrocyte sedimentation rate in one third, positive antinuclear antibodies in nearly one half, and occasionally other autoantibodies (e.g., thyroperoxidase antibodies).[82] It is reasonable to exclude syphilis, Lyme disease, and human immunodeficiency virus by laboratory testing. In a few patients with the Far East variety of Devic's disease, hyperprolactinemia was described predominantly with optic nerve involvement. A chest x-ray helps to exclude pulmonary tuberculosis and sarcoidosis. CSF examination is an essential part of the evaluation for Devic's syndrome, and repeated studies are sometimes necessary to ensure that there is no infection in that the CSF findings are sometimes atypical for inflammatory demyelination.

A marked pleocytosis is often present, sometimes exceeding 100 cells. Moreover, neutrophils are commonly seen in CSF and may predominate, a situation virtually unknown in MS.[79, 82] The protein concentration is often very high and in 41 percent exceeds 100 mg/dL. Anti-MOG antibodies are the predominant autoantibody detected in CSF; anti-MBP or anti-S100beta antibodies are less frequently seen. In addition, matrix metalloproteinase-9 levels are higher in CSF samples of MS patients compared to Devic's disease. Despite the intense inflammatory response, OCBs are conspicuously absent in the majority, being present in fewer than 20 percent of patients. CSF serology for the herpesvirus family (HSV types 1 and 2, VZV, EBV, and CMV) is important, and poly-

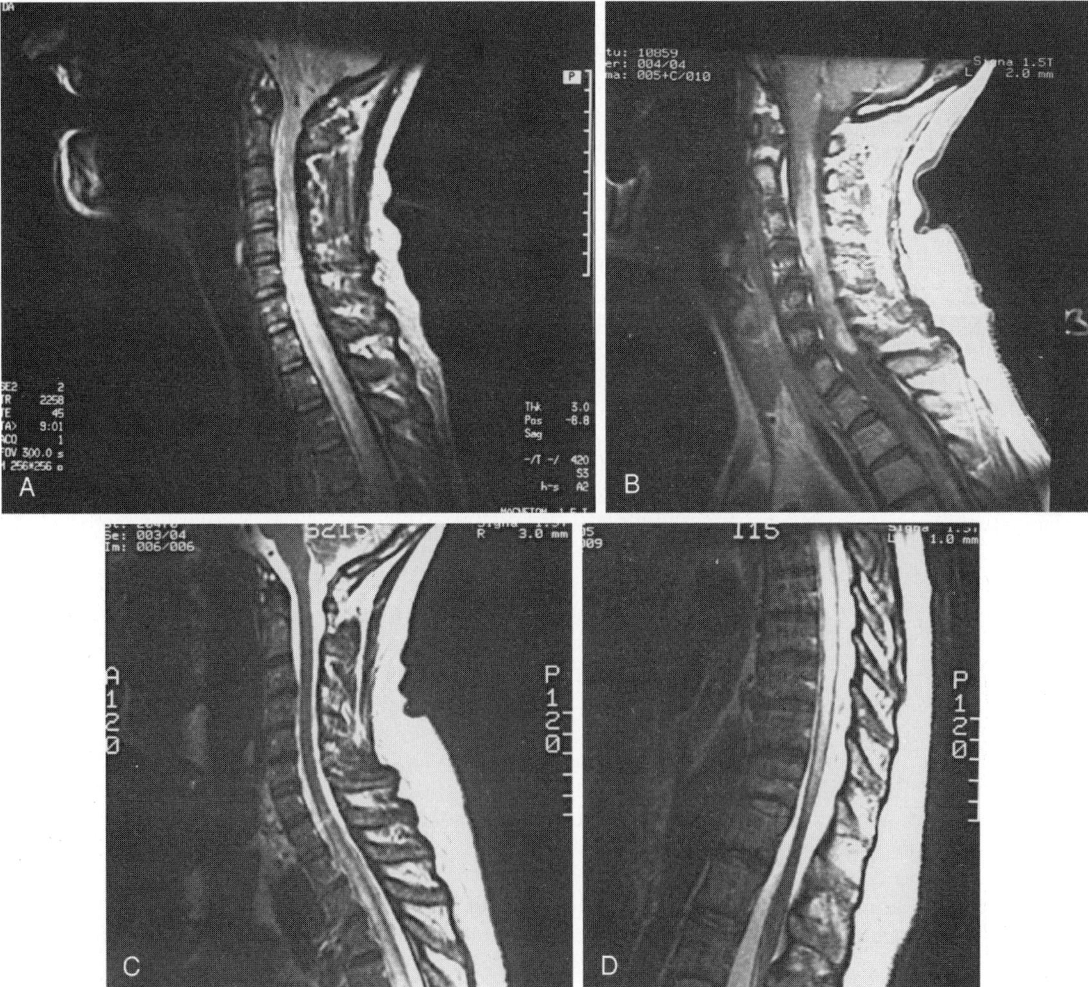

FIGURE 48–4. Spine MRI of patients with relapsing NMO. *A*, Sagittal T2-weighted image of the cervical spine showing cord expansion and signal abnormalities extending through the cervical and upper thoracic cord. *B*, T1-weighted sagittal MRI showing cord swelling and extensive gadolinium enhancement from C1 to C7. Further enhancement is seen in the upper thoracic area. *C* and *D*, Sagittal T2-weighted spine MRI showing a diffuse hyperintense lesion extending from T1 to the conus.

merase chain reaction testing should be done in cases suggestive of viral infection (immunocompromised patients).

Management. Patients with acute or subacute Devic's syndrome may respond to corticosteroids (e.g., intravenous methylprednisolone). Limited experience suggests that they may respond to plasma exchange even when intravenous methylprednisolone does not produce significant improvement. Attempts at preventing relapses and the subsequent disability are often disappointing even with the use of immunosuppressive agents (e.g., azathioprine, cyclophosphamide). IVIG and mitoxantrone are other considerations, although there have been no controlled studies to assess these agents.

Supportive care is important in the management of NMO. These patients are prone to many complications and require measures to prevent deep venous thrombosis and pulmonary embolism, urinary tract infection, decubiti, and contractures. Mechanical ventilation may be needed either temporarily or permanently. Patients with monophasic Devic's syndrome generally have simultaneous or rapid onset of the ON and myelitis (interval usually less than 1 month). Although some have significant residual disability, many recover remarkably and have little or no permanent deficits. A history of previous vague neurological symptoms or definite demyelinating events is predictive of future relapses, either typical of MS or relapsing NMO. Those patients destined for recurrent myelitis and ON have a longer interval between the onsets of myelitis and ON. The vast majority of patients with relapsing NMO have very aggressive disease with frequent and severe exacerbations and a poor prognosis.

Acute Disseminated Encephalomyelitis

ADEM is a monophasic inflammatory demyelinating disorder that characteristically begins within 6 weeks of an antigenic challenge such as infection or immunization. It occurs more often in the young and causes the rapid development of multifocal or focal neurological deficits. Perivenous inflammation, edema, and demyelination are the pathological hallmarks of ADEM, although these lesions commonly enlarge and coalesce, forming lesions pathologically indistinguishable from MS. Moreover, perivascular changes typical of ADEM are common in patients with MS. There is considerable overlap in the epidemiological, clinical, CSF, imaging, and pathological features between ADEM and MS, often making it difficult to distinguish between the two with reasonable confidence when encountering patients with a single demyelinating event.

Pathogenesis and Pathophysiology. ADEM closely resembles the experimental allergic encephalomyelitis animal model of MS (EAE) both clinically and pathologically, and is most likely due to a transient autoimmune response toward myelin. The occurrence of ADEM after vaccination with the rabbit spinal cord preparation of rabies virus led to the discovery of EAE. Infections and non–CNS-containing vaccinations may induce ADEM by molecular mimicry or by activating autoreactive T-cell clones in a nonspecific manner. Lymphocyte reactivity toward MBP has been identified in blood and CSF from patients with ADEM, but its absence in others indicates a role for other antigens. Increased peripheral blood gamma interferon–producing T-cells have been described in ADEM.

Epidemiology and Risk Factors. ADEM can occur at any age but perhaps because of the higher frequency of immunization and exposure to new antigens, it is most common during childhood. Unlike MS, both sexes are affected with equal frequency. No association has been noted with pregnancy.

ADEM has been reported to follow a number of different immunizations, usually within 6 weeks, including those for pertussis, diphtheria, measles, mumps, rubella, influenza (postvaccination ADEM), tetanus, and yellow fever. In addition, there are case reports of ADEM following hepatitis B vaccination. However, the only epidemiologically and pathologically proven association is with rabies vaccination, which also causes demyelinating peripheral neuropathies. The original Pasteur rabies vaccine, prepared in rabbit spinal cord, was associated with an incidence of ADEM of approximately 1 per 3,000 to 35,000 vaccinations and is no longer in use. A later vaccine, made in duck embryo, which contains little neural tissue, carries a risk for ADEM of 1 per 25,000 vaccines. The use of human diploid cell lines, which contain no nervous system tissue, for the production of rabies vaccine has virtually eliminated the risk of ADEM. The association of bee stings with ADEM has also been reported.

Parainfectious ADEM usually follows onset of the infectious illness, often during the recovery phase, but because of the latency between pathogen exposure and illness it may precede clinical symptoms of infection or the two may occur simultaneously. The most commonly reported associated illness is a nonspecific upper respiratory tract infection. There have been a vast number of specific infections associated with ADEM, such as virus infections (including rubella, mumps, VZV, EBV, CMV influenza, coxsackievirus, and hepatitis-C) and infection with *Mycoplasma, Borrelia burgdorferi*, and *Leptospira*. Measles carries the highest risk for ADEM of any infection, occurring in 1 per 400 to 1,000 cases. Although ADEM has been reported in association with measles immunization, the risk is far lower than the risk of acquiring measles and its neurological complications.

Clinical Features and Associated Disorders. A prodrome of headache, low-grade fever, myalgias, and malaise often precedes the onset of ADEM by a few days. In a German study of 40 cases,[83] the most frequent clinical signs were motor deficit (80 percent), followed by sensory deficits, brain stem signs, and cerebellar signs. CSF findings were variable; normal results were present in up to 20 percent of patients. Oligoclonal bands were positive in over 60 percent. Almost all patients improved during the acute phase of the disease. Of the 26 patients with the final diagnosis of ADEM, 21 had minor or no symptoms, 2 died, the rest had moderate symptoms. Compared to MS patients, the ADEM patients were older, and more often had a preceding infection, clinical signs of brain stem involvement, a higher CSF albumin fraction, and infratentorial lesions. Neurological symptoms develop rapidly in the acute phase and are commonly associated with encephalopathy, stupor, coma, meningismus, and seizures. Peak severity occurs within several days, and recovery may begin soon afterward. Occasionally, ADEM may evolve over a few months and there may be a second clinical deterioration or subacute progression for a time. In these unusual cases, the distinction from MS is difficult. Three recent large retrospective series and an accompanying editorial have highlighted that there remain no clinical or laboratory features that accurately allow one to predict which adult or pediatric ADEM patients will develop.[83–86]

Differential Diagnosis. One of the primary concerns after a single demyelinating episode is whether other bouts can be expected (e.g., MS). Several features may tip the balance toward one or the other, but the proper diagnosis becomes apparent only with time. Classically, ADEM is characterized by the multifocal involvement at onset whereas MS often presents with monosymptomatic deficits such as ON. However, ADEM may cause unifocal symptoms and MS may present with multifocal CNS involvement, especially in children. The monosymptomatic deficits caused by ADEM are more commonly severe, such as bilateral ON and complete transverse myelitis. Although OCBs occur transiently in about one third of ADEM cases, their persistence implies a diagnosis of MS. The subsequent disappearance of OCBs, when performed by consistent techniques, is evidence against MS. The MRI appearance of these two disorders is often identical,[86] but the presence of basal ganglia or cortical lesions, or large globular white matter lesions, is more frequent in ADEM.

The fulminant development of ADEM is distinctive but not pathognomonic, because a rare form of MS known as Marburg's MS is also rapid in onset and often deadly. The appearance of brain stem, periventricular, and multiple, large cerebral white matter lesions and the presence of OCBs may distinguish Marburg's variant from ADEM.

On rare occasions, inflammatory demyelinating lesions may reach a large size and resemble tumors (especially lymphoma) on MRI, necessitating biopsy for clarification. There is usually one dominant lesion, but smaller separate lesions may be identifiable. These have been referred to as both ADEM and MS in the literature. The prognosis for recovery is often quite good, although approximately one third suffer subsequent attacks. Some develop typical MS, whereas others have recurring tumor-like lesions. The term *multiphasic ADEM* has been used when patients have large recurrences in the same location, and *relapsing ADEM* refers to recurrences at different sites. The relationship of these entities with MS is unclear.

Balo's concentric sclerosis refers to the pathological finding of alternating bands of demyelination and remyelination. These patients typically have large lesions and subacute deficits similar to those described earlier. Typical demyelinating lesions commonly coexist, and rarely CD MS patients are noted to have similar-appearing lesions. The reason for this peculiar alternating pattern is unknown.

Schilder's myelinoclastic diffuse sclerosis is another rare condition that may be confused with ADEM or other demyelinating conditions. This is a progressive demyelinating disorder that usually begins in childhood. The features are often atypical and include dementia, aphasia, homonymous hemianopia, seizures, psychosis, elevated intracranial pressure, and the absence of OCBs. The most characteristic finding is the presence of two large, roughly symmetrical lesions on MRI, one in each hemisphere. The diagnosis is made by excluding the known inherited leukodystrophies, especially adrenoleukodystrophy.

Management. Treatment with intravenous methylprednisolone seems to halt progression and allow recovery to begin sooner, just as with MS. Plasma exchange can be tried in those with severe deficits and little response to corticosteroids. IVIG has also been used successfully according to case reports in the literature. One fulminant case responded to hypothermia only.

Reviews and Selected Updates

American Academy of Neurology: Practice advisory on selection of patients with multiple sclerosis for treatment with betaseron. Neurology 1994; 44:1537–1540.

Gronseth GS, Ashman EJ: Practice parameter: The usefulness of evoked potentials in identifying clinically silent lesions in patients with suspected MS. Neurology 2000;54:1720–1725.

Hemmer B, Cepok S, Nessler S, Sommer N: Pathogenesis of multiple sclerosis: an update on immunology. Curr Opin Neurol 2002;15:227–231.

Hogancamp WE, Rodriguez M, Weinshenker BG: The epidemiology of multiple sclerosis. Mayo Clin Proc 1997;72:871–878.

Hogancamp WE, Rodriguez M, Weinshenker BG: Identification of multiple sclerosis–associated genes. Mayo Clin Proc 1997;72:965–976.

Kaufman DI, Trobe JD, Eggenberger ER, Whitaker JN: Practice parameter: The role of corticosteroids in the management of acute monosymptomatic optic neuritis. Neurology 2000;54:2039–2044.

Kurtzke JF: Rating neurological impairment in multiple sclerosis: Expanded Disability Status Scale (EDSS). Neurology 1983;33:1444–1452.

Noseworthy JH, Lucchinetti C, Rodriguez M, Weinshenker BG: Medical progress: Multiple sclerosis. N Engl J Med 2000;343:938–952.

Raine CS: The Dale E. McFarlin Memorial Lecture: The immunology of the multiple sclerosis lesion. Ann Neurol 1994;36(Suppl):S61–S72.

References

1. Ebers GC: MS—an historical overview. *In* Paty DW, Ebers GC (eds): Multiple Sclerosis: Contemporary Neurology Series. Philadelphia, F.A. Davis (in press).
2. Medaer R: Does the history of multiple sclerosis go back as far as the 14th century? Acta Neurol Scand 1979;60:189–192.
3. Fredrikson S, Kam-Hansen S: The 150-year anniversary of multiple sclerosis: Does its early history give an etiological clue? Perspect Biol Med 1989;32:237–243.
4. Rivers TM, Schwentker F: Encephalomyelitis accompanied by myelin destruction experimentally produced in monkeys. J Exp Med 1935;61: 698–702.
5. Raine CS: Morphological aspects of myelin and myelination. *In* Morell P (ed): Myelin. New York, Plenum Press, 1997.
6. Tjernlund U, Cesaro P, Tournier E, et al: T-cell subsets in multiple sclerosis: A comparative study between cell surface antigens and function. Clin Immun Immunopathol 1984;32:185–197.
7. Wucherpfennig KW, Strominger JL: Molecular mimicry in T cell-mediated autoimmunity: Viral peptides activate human T cell clones specific for myelin basic protein. Cell 1995;80:695–705.
8. Allegretta M, Nicklas JA, Sriram S, et al: T cells responsive to myelin basic protein in patients with multiple sclerosis. Science 1990;247:718–721.
9. Bergstrom T, Andersen O, Vahlne A: Isolation of herpes simplex virus type 1 during first attack of multiple slerosis. Ann Neurol 1989; 26:283–285.
10. Melnick JL, Seidel E, Inoue YK, et al: Isolation of virus from the spinal fluid of three patients with multiple sclerosis and one with amyotrophic lateral sclerosis. Lancet 1982;1:830–833.
11. Challoner PB, Smith KT, Parker JD, et al: Plaque-associated expression of human herpesvirus 6 in multiple sclerosis. Proc Natl Acad Sci USA 1995;92:7440–7444.
12. Wren DR, Noble M: Oligodendrocytes and oligodendrocyte/type-2 astrocyte progenitor cells of adult rats are specifically susceptible to the lytic effects of complement in absence of antibody. Proc Natl Acad Sci USA 1989;86:9025–9029.
13. Selmaj KW, Raine CS: Experimental autoimmune encephalomyelitis: Immunotherapy with anti-tumor necrosis factor antibodies and soluble tumor necrosis factor receptors. Neurology 1995;45(Suppl 6):S44–S49.
14. Ebers GC, Sadovnick AD, Risch NJ: A genetic basis for familial aggregation in multiple sclerosis. Nature 1995;377:150–151.

15. Sadovnick AD, Ebers GC: Genetics of multiple sclerosis. Neurol Clin 1995;13:99–118.
16. Kurtzke JF: MS: changing times. Neuroepidemiology 1991;10:1–8.
17. Page WF, Kurtzke JF, Murphy FM, et al: Epidemiology of multiple sclerosis in U.S. veterans: V. Ancestry and the risk of multiple sclerosis. Ann Neurol 1993;33:632–639.
18. Dean G, Kurtzke JF: On the risk of multiple sclerosis according to age at immigration to South Africa. BMJ 1971;3:725–729.
19. Sheremata WA, Poskanzer DC, Withum DG, et al: Unusual occurrence on a tropical island of multiple sclerosis. Lancet 1985;2:618.
20. Armon C, Daube JR, O'Brien PC, et al: When is an apparent excess of neurologic cases epidemiologically significant? Neurology 1991;41: 1713–1718.
21. Runmarker B, Andersen O: Pregnancy is associated with a lower risk of onset and a better prognosis in multiple sclerosis. Brain 1995;118: 253–261.
22. Paty D, Noseworthy J, Ebers G: Diagnosis of MS. *In* Paty DW, Ebers GC (eds): Multiple Sclerosis: Contemporary Neurology Series. Philadelphia, F.A. Davis (in press).
23. McIntosh-Michaelis SA, Roberts MH, Wilkinson SM, et al: The prevalence of cognitive impairment in a community survey of multiple sclerosis. Br J Clin Psychol 1991;30:333–348.
24. Lublin FD, Reingold SC: Defining the clinical course of multiple sclerosis: Results of an international survey. Neurology 1996;46:907–911.
25. Wynn DR, Rodriguez M, O'Fallon WM, et al: A reappraisal of the epidemiology of multiple sclerosis in Olmsted County, Minnesota. Neurology 1990;40:780–786.
26. Rodriguez M, Siva A, Cross SA, et al: Optic neuritis: A population-based study in Olmsted County, Minnesota. Neurology 1995;45:244–250.
27. Morrissey SP, Miller DH, Kendall BE, et al: The significance of brain magnetic resonance imaging abnormalities at presentation with clinically isolated syndromes suggestive of multiple sclerosis: A 5-year follow-up study. Brain 1993;116:135–146.
28. Filippi M, van Waesberghe JH, Horsfield MA, et al: Interscanner variation in brain MRI lesion load measurements in MS: Implications for clinical trials. Neurology 1997;49:371–377.
29. O'Riordan JI, Thompson AJ, Kingsley DP, et al: The prognostic value of brain MRI in clinically isolated syndromes of the CNS. A 10-year follow-up. Brain 1998;121:495–503.
30. Harding AE, Sweeney MG, Miller DH, et al: Occurrence of a multiple sclerosis-like illness in women who have a Leber's hereditary optic neuropathy mitochondrial DNA mutation. Brain 1992;115: 979–989.
31. Natowicz MR, Bejjani B: Genetic disorders that masquerade as multiple sclerosis. Am J Med Genet 1994;49:149–169.
32. Poser CM, Paty DW, Scheinberg L, et al: New diagnostic criteria for multiple sclerosis: Guidelines for research protocols. Ann Neurol 1983;13:227–231.
33. McDonald WI, Compston A, Edan G, et al: Recommended diagnostic criteria for MS: Guidelines from the International panel on the diagnosis for multiple sclerosis Ann Neurol 2001;50:121–127.
34. Offenbacher H, Fazekas F, Schmidt R, et al: Assessment of MRI criteria for a diagnosis of MS. Neurology 1993;43:905–909.
35. Francis GS, Evans AC, Arnold DL: Neuroimaging in multiple sclerosis. Neurol Clin 1995;13:147–171.
36. Ebers GC, Paty DW: CSF electrophoresis in one thousand patients. Can J Neurol Sci 1980;7:275–280.
37. Beck RW: The optic neuritis treatment trial: Three-year follow-up results. Arch Ophthalmol 1995;113:136–137.
38. Zivadinov R, Rudick RA, De Masi R, et al: Effects of IV methylprednisolone on brain atrophy in relapsing-remitting MS. Neurology 2001;57:1239–1247.
39. Weiner HL, Dau PC, Khatri BO, et al: Double-blind study of true vs. sham plasma exchange in patients treated with immunosuppression for acute attacks of multiple sclerosis. Neurology 1989;39:1143–1149.
40. Rodriguez M, Karnes WE, Bartleson JD, et al: Plasmapheresis in acute episodes of fulminant CNS inflammatory demyelination. Neurology 1993;43:1100–1104.
41. Weinshenker BG, O'Brien PC, Petterson TM, Noseworthy JH, et al: A randomized trial of plasma exchange in acute central nervous system inflammatory demyelinating disease. Ann Neurol 1999;46: 878–886.
42. The IFNB Multiple Sclerosis Study Group: Interferon-beta 1b is effective in relapsing-remitting multiple sclerosis. I. Clinical results of a multicenter, randomized, double-blind, placebo-controlled trial. Neurology 1993;43:655–661.
43. Antonelli G, Simeoni E, Bagnato F, et al: Further study on the specificity and incidence of neutralizing antibodies to interferon (IFN) in relapsing remitting multiple sclerosis patients treated with IFN beta 1-a or IFN beta-1b. J Neurol Sci 1999;168:131–136.
44. Jacobs LD, Cookfair DL, Rudick RA, et al: Intramuscular interferon beta-1a for disease progression in relapsing multiple sclerosis. Ann Neurol 1996;39:285–294.
45. PRISMS Study Group: PRISMS-4: Long term efficacy of interferon beta-1a in relapsing MS. Neurology 2001;56:1628–1636.
46. PRISMS (Prevention of Relapses and Disability by Interferon-1a Subcutaneously in Multiple Sclerosis) Study Group: Randomised double-blind placebo-controlled study of interferon-1a in relapsing/remitting multiple sclerosis. Lancet 1998;352:1498–1504.
47. David K, Li B, Paty DW: Magnetic resonance imaging results of the PRISMS trial: A randomized, double-blind, placebo-controlled study of interferon-1a in relapsing-remitting multiple sclerosis. Ann Neurol 1999;46:197–206.
48. Brod SA, Lindsey JW, Vriesendorp FS, et al: Ingested IFN-alpha: Results of a pilot study in relapsing-remitting MS. Neurology 2001; 57:845–852.
49. Bornstein M, Miller A, Slagle S, et al: A pilot trial of Cop 1 in exacerbating-remitting multiple sclerosis. N Engl J Med 1987;317: 408–414.
50. Johnson KP, Brooks BR, Cohen JA, et al: Copolymer 1 reduces relapse rate and improves disability in relapsing-remitting multiple sclerosis: Results of a phase III multicenter, double-blind placebo-controlled trial: The Copolymer 1 Multiple Sclerosis Study Group. Neurology 1995; 45:1268–1276.
51. Filippi M, Rovaris M, Rocca MA, et al: Glatiramer acetate reduces proportion of new MS lesions evolving into black holes. Neurology 2001;57:731–733.
52. Wolinsky JS, Narayana PA, Johnson KP: United States open-label glatiramer acetate extension trial for relapsing multiple sclerosis: MRI and clinical correlates. Multiple Sclerosis Study Group and the MRI Analysis Center. Mult Scler 2001;7:33–41.
53. Comi G, Filippi M, Wolinsky JS, et al: European/Canadian multicenter, double-blind, randomized, placebo-controlled study of the effects of glatiramer acetate on magnetic resonance imaging—measured disease activity and burden in patients with relapsing multiple sclerosis. European/Canadian Glatiramer Acetate Study Group. Ann Neurol 2001; 49:290–297.
54. Strasser-Fuchs S, Fazekas F, Deisenhammer F, et al: The Austrian Immunoglobulin in MS (AIMS) study: Final analysis, Mult Scler 2000;6:9–13.
55. Noseworthy JH, O'Brien PC, Petterson TM, et al: A randomized trial of intravenous immunoglobulin in inflammatory demyelinating optic neuritis. Neurology 2001;56:1514–1522.
56. Noseworthy JH, O'Brien PC, Weinshenker BG, et al: IV immunoglobulin does not reverse established weakness in MS: A double-blind, placebo-controlled trial. Neurology 2000;55:1135–1143.
57. Stangel M, Boegner F, Klatt CH, et al: Placebo controlled pilot trial to study the remyelinating potential of intravenous immunoglobulins in multiple sclerosis. J Neurol Neurosurg Psychiatry 2000;68:89–92.
58. Jacobs LD, Beck RW, Simon JH, et al: Intramuscular interferon beta 1a therapy initiated during a first demyelinating event in MS. N Engl J Med 2000;343:898–904.
59. Comi G, Filippi M, Barkhof F, et al: Effect of early interferon treatment on conversion to definite multiple sclerosis: a randomised study. Lancet 2001;357:1576–1582.
60. Barkhof F, Van Waesberghe JT, Filippi M, et al: T1 hypointense lesions in secondary progressive MS: Effect of interferon beta 1-b treatment. Brain 2001;124:1396–1402.
61. European Study Group on Interferon 1b in Secondary Progressive MS: Placebo-controlled multicentre randomised trial of interferon 1b in treatment of secondary progressive multiple sclerosis,. Lancet 1998;352:1491–1497.
62. Miller DH, Molyneux PD, Barker GJ, et al: Effect of interferon-1b on magnetic resonance imaging outcomes in secondary progressive multiple sclerosis: Results of a European multicenter, randomized, double-blind, placebo-controlled trial. Ann Neurol 1999;46:850–859.
63. Kappos L, Polman C, Pozzilli C, et al: Final analysis of the European multicenter trial on IFNß-1b in secondary-progressive MS. Neurology 2001;57:1969–1975.
64. Molyneux PD, Kappos L, Polman C, et al: The effect of interferon beta-1b treatment on MRI measures of cerebral atrophy in secondary progressive multiple sclerosis. Brain 2000;123:2256–2263.

65. Li DK, Zhao GJ, Paty DW: Randomized controlled trial of interferon beta 1a in SPMS (SPECTRIMS), MRI results. Neurology 2001;56: 1505–1513.
66. Hartung HG, Gonsette R: Mitoxantrone in progressive MS a placebo controlled, randomized, observer blinded phase III multi-center study—clinical results. Mult Scler 1998;4:325.
67. Edan G, Miller D, Clanet M, et al: Therapeutic effect of mitoxantrone combined with methylprednisolone in MS. J Neurol Neurosurg Psychiatry, 1997;62:112–118.
68. Yudkin PL, Ellison GW, Ghezzi A, et al: Overview of azathioprine treatment in multiple sclerosis. Lancet 1991;338:1051–1055.
69. Goodkin DE, Rudick RA, VanderBrug Medendorp S, et al: Low-dose (7.5 mg) oral methotrexate reduces the rate of progression in chronic progressive multiple sclerosis. Ann Neurol 1995;37:30–40.
70. Sipe JC, Romine JS, Koziol JA, et al: Cladribine in treatment of chronic progressive multiple sclerosis. Lancet 1994;344:9–13.
71. Rice GP, Filippi M, Comi G: Cladribine and progressive MS. Neurology 2000;54:1145–1155.
72. Fassas A, Anagnostopulos A, Kazis A, et al: Autologous stem cell transplantation in progressive MS—an interim analysis of efficacy. J Clin Immunol 2000;20:24–30.
73. Wiles CM, Newcombe RJ, Fuller KJ, et al: Controlled randomized crossover trial of the effects of physiotherapy on mobility in chronic MS. J Neurol Neurosurg Psych 2001;70:174–179.
74. Alusi SH, Aziz TZ, Glickman S, et al: Stereotactic lesional surgery for the treatment of tremor in multiple sclerosis: A prospective case-controlled study. Brain 2001;124:1576–1589.
75. Alusi SH, Worthington J, Glickman S, Bain PG: A study of tremor in multiple sclerosis. Brain 2001;124:720–730.
76. Carter JL, Noseworthy JH: Ventilatory dysfunction in multiple sclerosis. Clin Chest Med 1994;15:693–703.
77. Weinshenker BG, Bass B, Rice GP, et al: The natural history of multiple sclerosis: A geographically based study. I. Clinical course and disability. Brain 1989;112:133–146.
78. Mandler RN, Davis LE, Jeffery DR, et al: Devic's neuromyelitis optica: A clinicopathological study of 8 patients. Ann Neurol 1993;34:162–168.
79. Hogancamp WE, Weinshenker BG: The spectrum of Devic's syndrome. Neurology 1996;46(Suppl):254.
80. Wingerchuk DM, Hogancamp WF, O'Brien PC, Weinshenker BG: The clinical course of neuromyelitis optica (Devic's syndrome). Neurology 1999; 53:1107–1114.
81. Filippi M, Rocca MA, Moiola L, et al: MRI and magnetization transfer imaging changes in the brain and cervical cord of patients with Devic's neuromyelitis optica. Neurology 1999;53:1705–1710.
82. O'Riordan JI, Gallagher HL, Thompson AJ, et al: Clinical, CSF, and MRI findings in Devic's neuromyelitis optica. J Neurol Neurosurg Psychiatry 1996;60:382–387.
83. Schwarz S, Mohr A, Knauth M, et al: Acute disseminated encephalomyelitis: A follow-up study of 40 adult patients. Neurology 2001;56:1313–1318.
84. Hynson JL, Kornberg AJ, Coleman LT, et al: Clinical and neuroradiologic features of acute disseminated encephalomyelitis in children. Neurology 2001;56:1308–1312.
85. Hartung HP, Grossman RI: ADEM: Distinct disease or part of the MS spectrum? Neurology 2001;56:1257–1260.
86. Kesselring J, Miller DH, Robb SA, et al: Acute disseminated encephalomyelitis: MRI findings and the distinction from multiple sclerosis. Brain 1990;113:291–302.

CHAPTER 49

ROBERT W. SHIELDS, JR., and ASA J. WILBOURN

Demyelinating Disorders of the Peripheral Nervous System

History and Definitions

Waldrop, in 1834, reported a single patient who probably had acute inflammatory demyelinating polyradiculoneuropathy (AIDP), thereby providing the first clinical description of a demyelinating polyneuropathy. Landry, in 1859, described 10 patients who very likely had the same disorder; he recounted most of the clinical features now considered typical for AIDP. Guillain, Barré, and Strohl, in 1916, reported two soldiers who were recovering from rapidly evolving, principally motor polyneuropathies. They emphasized the loss of the deep tendon reflexes (DTRs) and the presence, on cerebrospinal fluid (CSF) examination, of an elevated protein level with a normal cell count (albuminocytological dissociation). Their paper probably has been the most influential of all the articles concerned with demyelinating neuropathies; from it, the commonly used eponymic title for AIDP derives (i.e., Guillain-Barré syndrome, or GBS). Haymaker and Kernohan, in 1949, reviewed the pathology they had found in 50 fatal cases of AIDP. Their paper confirmed, both on a clinical and a pathological basis, that Landry's ascending paralysis and GBS were, in fact, the same disorder. In 1955, Waksman and Adams first produced experimental autoimmune neuritis (EAN) by injecting peripheral nerve tissue, with adjuvants, into rabbits. In 1969, Asbury, Arnason, and Adams observed lymphocytic infiltration and segmental demyelination on pathological examination of spinal roots and nerves in all 19 patients they studied who had died of GBS, thus establishing a pathological link between GBS and EAN.[1–4]

The first diagnostic criteria for AIDP were proposed in 1935. Several others have been proposed since then. Formulated in 1978 by Asbury, Arnason, Karp, and McFarlin, the most widely used set resulted from a colloquium sponsored by the National Institute of Neurological and Communicative Disorders and Stroke; it was triggered by claims against the United States government for AIDP resulting from the 1976 swine influenza vaccination program. The electrodiagnostic (EDX) features of AIDP were first described in detail by Lambert and Mulder in 1964.[1–4]

Osler and Targowla reported chronic progressive and relapsing forms of polyradiculoneuropathy in the 1890s. But in 1958 Austin first catalogued many of the clinical features of what is now termed chronic inflammatory demyelinating polyradiculoneuropathy (CIDP). Austin's report triggered the widespread use of corticosteroids in patients thought to have this disorder.[2–4] Nonetheless, there was no generally accepted clinical presentation for CIDP until 1975, when Dyck and co-workers established it as a distinct clinical entity, based on their review of 53 patients.[5] Because the features of CIDP are relatively nonspecific, a number of polyneuropathies and polyradiculoneuropathies associated with specific diseases resemble, and may represent instances of, it.

Overview of Peripheral Nervous System Myelination and Electrophysiology

The peripheral nervous system (PNS) comprises less than 0.1 percent of all nerve tissue. The somatic PNS, when defined anatomically by the presence of Schwann cells, includes the primary roots, dorsal root ganglia, mixed spinal nerves, plexuses, nerve trunks, autonomic nervous system, and cranial nerves III to XII. Peripheral nerve trunks are composed of a great number of axons, which are grouped into individual bundles or fascicles. These structures vary in number, depending on the nerve, its size, and the site at which it is studied. Schwann cells ensheath every PNS axon nearly throughout their extent. Peripheral nerve fibers are divided into two groups, either myelinated or unmyelinated, depending on whether they have one or several axons per Schwann cell. In the human sural nerve, the ratio of unmyelinated to myelinated axons is approximately 3.7 to 1.[6]

A myelinated peripheral nerve fiber consists of an axon and a series of Schwann cells located sequentially on its external surface. Each Schwann cell encircles the axon segment adjacent to it with a multilayered cell membrane structure, the myelin sheath. The short, constricted, myelin-free axon segment where consecutive Schwann cells abut each other is called the node of Ranvier. This region contains voltage-gated Na^+ channels. The myelin-coated axon segment between two nodes of Ranvier is an internode. Saltatory conduction is the characteristic means of impulse transmission along myelinated fibers. The myelinated axon is depolarized only at the nodes of Ranvier, thereby permitting it to conduct much faster than an unmyelinated fiber. Approximate linear correlations have been noted between myelin thickness and conduction velocity (CV).[6] Myelinated motor axons conduct impulses centrifugally to the extrafusal muscle fibers, whereas myelinated sensory axons transmit impulses centripetally from the muscle spindles and Golgi tendon organs; they subserve the sensations of touch, pressure, and vibration.[7, 8]

Segmental demyelination (SD), or damage to the myelin sheath, can be either primary or secondary. With primary SD, only the myelin portion of the nerve fiber is affected; the axon is spared. Through several different mechanisms, numerous disorders can cause primary SD, including diphtheria toxin, lead salts, acute and chronic compression, and GBS. Nonetheless, both clinically and electrophysiologically, the demyelination that results is quantitatively the same. With secondary SD, damage to the myelin results from initial changes in the axon, typically consisting of chronic shrinking and atrophy. Axon atrophy with secondary SD occurs in some chronic polyneuropathies (e.g., uremia).[9] Pathophysiologically, whether it is primary or secondary, SD produces conduction abnormalities—slowing or block—as well as abnormal (ectopic) impulse generation. Clinically, these abnormalities can result in muscle weakness, impairment of large fiber sensory modalities, fasciculations, myokymia, cramps, and paresthesias.[8]

The underlying pathology of a specific peripheral polyneuropathy frequently can be predicted by its EDX features. Based on these patterns, most peripheral polyneuropathies can be divided into two types: (1) axonal degeneration or axon loss (frequently referred to as axonal) and (2) SD. Both familial and acquired polyneuropathies can be found in each group. For example, axon loss polyneuropathies include familial Charcot-Marie-Tooth type II (Dyck classification) and acquired arsenic polyneuropathy, whereas SD polyneuropathies include familial Charcot-Marie-Tooth type I, as well as acquired AIDP and CIDP. Most classifications make no distinctions between peripheral polyneuropathies and peripheral polyradiculoneuropathies, although often their clinical and EDX presentations differ. All of the acquired disorders discussed in this section actually are polyradiculoneuropathies, regardless of the terminology used.

With axon loss polyneuropathies and polyradiculoneuropathies, the main EDX features include the following: On nerve conduction studies, there is uniform reduction of amplitudes, ultimately culminating in unelicitable responses at all stimulation points. This change is not accompanied by any significant alterations in latencies or CV, because they are being measured along surviving, unaffected axons. On NEE, fibrillation potentials occur, accompanied by reduced motor unit potential (MUP) recruitment, if the motor nerve involvement is severe, and chronic neurogenic MUP changes, if the disorder is chronic and rather severe.

With generalized SD disorders, the underlying pathophysiology may be conduction slowing, conduction block, or both, depending on the severity of involvement of the individual fibers. Whenever SD conduction slowing affects all, or nearly all, of the large myelinated fibers to the same degree, then only the latencies and CVs are affected on NCS. In these cases, the amplitudes and durations of the responses are unaltered. Alternatively, if conduction is slowed along different fibers to different degrees, then the NCS responses become dispersed, and as they do so, the amplitudes decrease (Fig. 49–1). With SD conduction block lesions, the NCS responses decrease in amplitude but are not dispersed

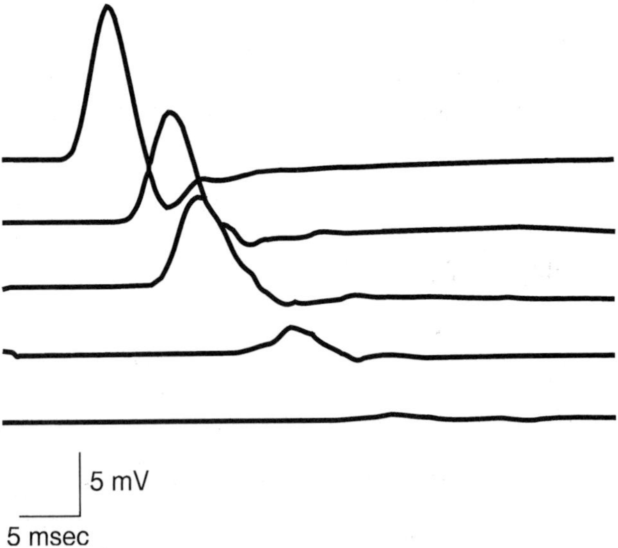

FIGURE 49–1. Motor nerve conduction studies of the ulnar nerve in a patient with CIDP, recording from the hypothenar eminence with stimulation at wrist (*top trace*), distal to the elbow (*second trace*), above the elbow (*third trace*), axilla (*fourth trace*), and at supraclavicular notch (*bottom trace*). With stimulation at more proximal sites, there is a cumulative effect of segmental demyelinating lesions, resulting in dispersion of the responses with conduction block.

(Fig. 49–2). Importantly, all types of SD lesions affect only a focal area of nerve, so the CVs, durations, and amplitudes on stimulating distal to that area (while recording still more distally) are unaffected, because conduction is being determined along a normal segment of nerve. On NEE, conduction slowing produces no changes, whereas conduction block, if severe, causes reduced MUP recruitment.[7]

Some confusion exists regarding the pathophysiological and clinical correlations found with these two basic types of peripheral nerve lesions. Unelicitable responses and low-amplitude nondispersed responses are the NCS counterpart of weakness and of fixed sensory deficits, due to involvement of large myelinated fibers. They indicate that, regardless of cause, impulses are not able to traverse the nerve segments between the stimulating and recording sites. The only two pathophysiological processes that produce such NCS amplitude changes are axon degeneration and SD conduction block. In contrast, SD conduction slowing has very few clinical counterparts. If differential slowing is present, certain neurological examination techniques that require transmission of highly synchronized nerve volleys may be altered (e.g., DTRs and vibratory sensation). However, SD conduction slowing generally does not produce clinical weakness when it affects motor axons. The fact that nerve impulses are reaching the muscle fibers a few milliseconds later than normal is of no clinical significance.[7]

Based on various EDX features, familial and acquired demyelinating disorders often can be differentiated from one another, and the acquired disorders can be subdivided into acute and chronic types. Familial SD polyneuropathies are length-dependent polyneuropathies and have predictable presentations that vary principally with the severity of the process. Some of their features are (1) NCS of the same type (i.e., motor or sensory) are affected earlier and more severely in the lower extremity than in the upper extremity; (2) in a given limb, the sensory NCS, compared with the motor NCS, tend to be involved earlier and more severely; (3) NCS of the same type, assessing nerve segments at approximately the same limb level, are affected to approximately the same degree; (4) NCS performed on corresponding nerves in contralateral limbs are affected equally; (5) along any specific nerve, conduction rate abnormalities are uniform; (6) late responses, H-responses and F waves, usually are unelicitable; (7) NEE abnormalities appear first and ultimately are most severe in the more distal lower extremity muscles.[10]

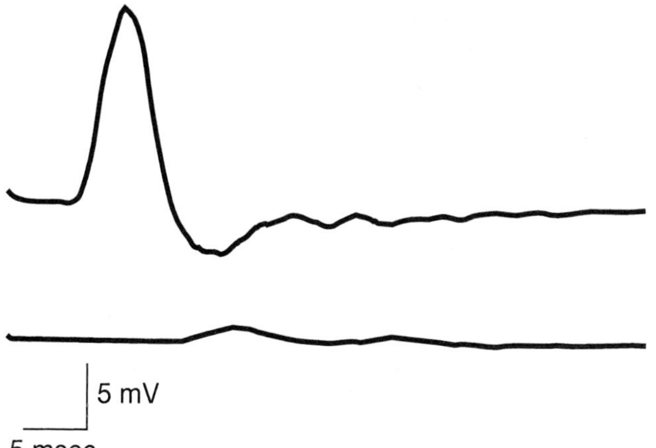

FIGURE 49–2. Motor nerve conduction studies of the median nerve in a patient with motor neuropathy with multifocal conduction block, recording from the thenar eminence with stimulation at wrist (*top trace*) and above the elbow (*bottom trace*). A severe conduction block is noted in the segment of nerve between the two stimulating sites.

In contrast to the familial demyelinating polyneuropathies, the acquired demyelinating disorders are all polyradiculoneuropathies. Nonetheless, at times they have an EDX presentation identical to that seen with the familial polyneuropathies, and in those instances, they cannot be distinguished from the familial types in the EDX laboratory. This most frequently occurs in patients with CIDP and with AIDP in the recovery stages. More often, however, the EDX findings with the acquired disorders deviate sufficiently from those listed earlier so that they can be recognized. This is particularly the case with AIDP relatively early in its course. There are several such variations: (1) nerves of the same type may show abnormalities that are more severe in the upper extremities than in the lower extremities—for example, the sural NCS may be normal, whereas the median sensory NCS may be grossly abnormal; this combination of changes virtually is never seen with a familial demyelinating polyneuropathy; (2) abnormalities may be focal or multifocal, rather than generalized, along a specific peripheral nerve; thus, a conduction block or focal slowing may be found only between the elbow and wrist segment of the median nerve, whereas it may be absent from more distal and more proximal segments or, conversely, progressive conduction blocks or progressive differential slowing may be found along a nerve; (3) nerves of the same type, in the same limb, at the same level, often show very dissimilar findings; (4) homologous nerves in contralateral limbs may be affected differently; (5) in a given limb, motor NCS may be more abnormal than sensory NCS; (6) H-responses and F waves may be variably affected; with acute disorders they may be abnormal when the standard NCS are normal, if the SD conduction changes are restricted to the proximal segments of the PNS; (7) on NEE, abnormalities may be found in any muscle, or they may be generalized, rather than manifesting a distal-proximal gradient.[2–4, 10–12]

With acute SD polyradiculoneuropathies, conduction blocks often dominate the NCS, whereas with chronic SD polyradiculoneuropathies, conduction slowing typically is prominent. This chapter focuses on several acquired forms of neuropathies, most of which are characterized by SD.

Acute Inflammatory Demyelinating Polyradiculoneuropathy (Guillain-Barré Syndrome)

Until approximately a decade ago, GBS was considered to be a single clinical entity, a rapidly evolving sensorimotor polyradiculoneuropathy resulting from widespread demyelination in the PNS, due to inflammation. Consequently, GBS was viewed as synonymous with AIDP. However, it is now obvious that demyelination is only one of the causes for the combination of clinical features labeled GBS; different pathological processes can lead to the same clinical presentation (Table 49–1).[13, 14] In 1986, Feasby and coworkers reported that some patients who were considered to

TABLE 49–1. **Acquired Demyelinating Disorders of the Peripheral Nervous System**

Acute
Guillain-Barré syndrome
  Acute inflammatory demyelinating polyradiculoneuropathy (AIDP)
  Acute axon loss ("axonal") polyradiculopathy
    Acute motor axonal neuropathy
    Acute motor-sensory axonal neuropathy

Chronic
Chronic inflammatory demyelinating polyradiculopathy (CIDP)
Monoclonal gammopathies of undetermined significance (MGUS)
  MGUS IgM neuropathy with anti-MAG antibody
  MGUS IgG, IgA, IgM neuropathy without anti-MAG antibody
CIDP with multiple myeloma
CIDP with osteosclerotic myeloma
CIDP with Waldenström's macroglobulinemia
Motor neuropathy with multifocal conduction block

have GBS had axon loss rather than SD as their underlying pathophysiology; these cases have been labeled the acute axonal form of GBS.[15] More recently, it has been appreciated that this subdivision must be further separated into two groups: the first with both motor and sensory fibers affected, labeled AMSAN or the acute motor-sensory axonal neuropathy pattern,[16] and the second with only motor fibers affected, particularly at the root level, labeled AMAN or the acute motor axonal neuropathy pattern or acute motor neuropathy.[16, 17] The following discussion reflects the prototype of GBS and these variations.

Pathogenesis and Pathophysiology. All subdivisions of GBS appear to be autoimmune diseases resulting from aberrant immune responses against various components of peripheral nerve fibers. Antibodies to ganglioside GM_1 appear to play an important role, as do T cells.[18] With AIDP, both humoral and cell-mediated factors are operative. Although the specific mechanisms of injury are unclear, the pathology that results is well documented, its hallmarks being inflammatory lesions, consisting of circumscribed areas containing lymphocytes, macrophages, and localized demyelination scattered throughout the PNS. The roots, plexuses, proximal nerve trunks, some cranial nerves, and autonomic fibers may be involved, often with a predilection, at least soon after onset, for the roots and distal peripheral nerve fibers. The myelin sheath is the specific target structure. Macrophages penetrate the basal lamina surrounding the axon, displace the Schwann cell from the myelin sheath, and then phagocytose the myelin lamellae.[19] Pathophysiologically, these focal areas of demyelination result in conduction slowing or conduction block, depending on the severity of the process. Almost invariably, some axon loss also occurs, but it is much less marked.[11, 12] With the acute axonal form of GBS, the roots are far more extensively affected than the peripheral nerves. Wallerian degeneration is prominent in the ventral roots alone with the AMAN form, and in both the ventral and dorsal roots with the AMSAN pattern. In those axons that have not undergone wallerian degeneration, macrophages are present within the periaxonal spaces, surrounding compressed but otherwise normal-appearing axons. Just as AIDP has some minor associated axon loss, the acute axonal forms of GBS have some sparse SD present along surviving myelinated fibers; thus, the lesions are "predominately" rather than "purely" axon loss in type.[16] Pathophysiologically, the so-called acute axonal forms present as axon loss polyradiculoneuropathies affecting motor, or motor and sensory, fibers, depending on the particular subgroup.[15–17]

Epidemiology and Risk Factors. AIDP is a relatively rare disorder, having an average yearly incidence rate of 1 to 2 cases per 100,000 population. It occurs worldwide, affects all races, and attacks more males than females. Persons of any age are at risk, although the incidence is higher in the elderly. Most cases are sporadic, but clusters have been reported. Actual common-origin clusters typically derive from an obvious trigger factor, such as antirabies vaccination. Most studies have not reported a seasonal variation. Unlike the situation with CIDP, no clear relationship has been demonstrated between AIDP and human leukocyte antigen.[2, 3] AIDP is responsible for more than 90 percent of the GBS cases that occur in North America, Europe, and Australia.[20] The acute motor axonal form of GBS, at least in Northern China, has many epidemiological features that differ from those described earlier. It occurs principally in epidemics and during the summer months, has a very strong association with preceding *Campylocbacter jejuni* infections,[20] and typically affects children and young adults.[15, 16] It is also occurring, or at least being recognized more frequently, in North American, Japan, and especially Latin America. The AMSAN form affects mainly adults, regardless of the region where they live.[20]

Antecedent events (so-called triggers) are associated with GBS in approximately 70 percent of cases. These usually occur 1 to 3 weeks before the onset of clinical symptoms, rarely as much as 6 weeks earlier. The one most often reported is a mundane upper respiratory infection. However, a great number of others have been described, although the linkage often has been inconclusive. Nonetheless, the evidence is rather convincing connecting a few vaccines (especially rabies), a few viral infections (particularly human immunodeficiency virus [HIV], Epstein-Barr virus, and cytomegalic inclusion virus), a few bacterial infections (especially *C. jejuni*), and even surgery with bouts of GBS (Table 49–2). None of these infections is uniquely linked to any particular subgroup of GBS. However, severe axon loss often follows *C. jejuni* infections, just as severe sensory involvement often is preceded by cytomegalovirus infections.[18] Increasing attention is being focused on *C. jejuni* infection, which clinically is manifested as a gastroenteritis.[2–4] This particular bacterium appears to play a major role in the acute axonal form of GBS that occurs in epidemics in China.[15, 16] Fewer than 40 cases of GBS occurring during pregnancy have been reported. Apparently, this is an incidental co-existence, which can develop during any particular trimester. Nonetheless, a few women have experienced GBS with successive pregnancies.[2, 4]

Clinical Features and Associated Disorders. The cardinal features of GBS are weakness, paresthesias, and diminished or absent DTRs.[4] Most patients are essentially well and lack systemic symptoms, including fever, when their PNS symptoms begin. Often they have recently experienced one

TABLE 49–2. Antecedent Events Associated with Guillain-Barré Syndrome

Viral
Influenza
Herpes
Cytomegalovirus*
Epstein-Barr virus*
Hepatitis
Human immunodeficiency virus*
Surgery
Bacterial
*Campylobacter jejuni**
*Mycoplasma pneumoniae**
Spirochetal
Borrelia burgdorferi
Vaccination
Rabies (some strains)
Vaccinia

*Stronger association.

of the many antecedent events already described. The initial neurological symptoms vary from patient to patient. Distal, usually symmetrical paresthesias (so-called pins and needles) involving the toes, fingers, or both herald the onset of the disorder in at least 50 percent of patients. As the disease progresses, these paresthesias typically spread proximally but seldom extend beyond the ankles and wrists. Facial paresthesias, which are usually perioral, are less common. Weakness can be the presenting feature, but more often it is first noted a few days after the paresthesias begin. Typically, it begins in the lower extremities, especially in the proximal muscles so that patients may experience difficulty climbing stairs and rising from chairs for a day or two before they realize that they are ill. Weakness soon spreads (ascends) to the upper extremities. Less often, weakness begins simultaneously in the upper and lower extremities, with the lower extremities usually more severely affected. The progressive phase of the illness lasts from a few days to 3 to 4 weeks. Approximately 50 percent of patients reach the nadir of clinical function by 2 weeks and 80 percent by 3 weeks. The flaccid weakness that is ultimately present varies considerably in severity and distribution from one patient to another. However, it often is profound, involving all four limbs, the respiratory muscles, and the face. Facial diplegia, or bilateral facial weakness, is seen in approximately 50 percent of patients. Occasionally, fasciculations are noted. Although the prominent features are motor in nature, pain that is deep, poorly localized, and sometimes accompanied by muscle cramping commonly occurs. Usually, it is most severe in the shoulder girdle, back, and posterior thighs and is notoriously more severe at night.[2–4]

On clinical examination, one of the earliest findings is decreased or unelicitable DTRs. This finding may either precede or follow by a few days the demonstration of weakness on formal examination. Substantial sensory abnormalities are found infrequently and contrast with the high incidence of sensory symptoms. Typically, vibration and proprioception, the sensory modalities mediated over large myelinated fibers, are the most severely affected. In some cases, profound proprioceptive loss results in sensory ataxia and pseudoathetosis. Generally, once symptoms have peaked, they persist unchanged for approximately 2 to 4 weeks (the so-called plateau phase) and then begin to recede in an extremely variable fashion from patient to patient.[2–4]

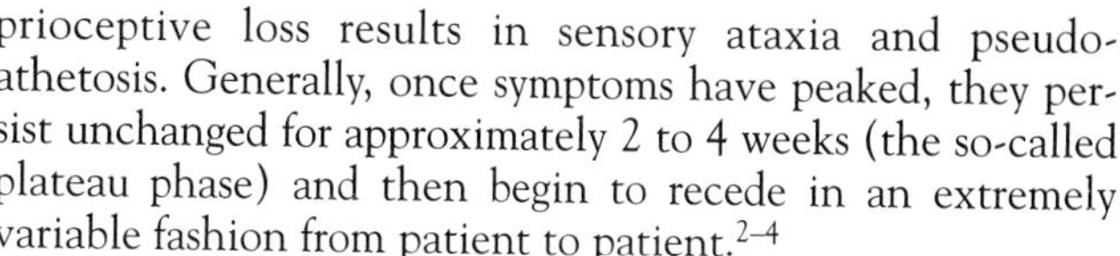

Several atypical presentations or clinical variants of GBS have been described. The acute axonal form is more rapid in onset and more severe, and ultimate recovery is often poor. As noted earlier, this GBS subgroup is mainly responsible for the summer epidemics in China and is linked to a preceding *C. jejuni* infection. The pure motor form, in which no sensory symptoms occur, is now known to be one of the presentations of the acute axonal variant. The Miller-Fisher syndrome consists principally of a triad of ophthalmoplegia, ataxia, and areflexia essentially occurring in isolation. The CSF protein usually is elevated, but the EDX findings are more suggestive of axon loss than SD. Miller-Fisher syndrome generally is a benign disorder and does not require specific immune therapy. Finally, a pure sensory form has been reported, although the diagnostic criteria for GBS proposed in 1978 exclude this variant.[2–4] Nonetheless, some convincing cases have been described and suggest that the spectrum of GBS may need to be expanded to include a predominantly sensory AIDP.[21, 22]

With GBS, there is some overlap between antecedent events and associated conditions. GBS has been linked, often through single case reports, to a number of systemic diseases. However, for most of these cases, the relationship is more probably a chance association. There are a few exceptions. So many cases of GBS have occurred in patients with HIV infection that some type of cause-and-effect relationship seems very likely. Similarly, although the data are not as compelling, a link between Hodgkin's disease and GBS also appears to exist.[2–4]

Differential Diagnosis. GBS is the most common type of rapidly evolving, generalized PNS disorder. Nonetheless, a great number of other disorders can be mistaken for it, particularly early in its course (Table 49–3). Ropper and coworkers, for example, list 50 entities that must be considered in the differential diagnosis of typical GBS.[4] Certain preconditions must be met for many of these entities to be included. Thus, generally the patient must have recently traveled to various tropical regions for fish and snake poisonings to be considered; traveled to underdeveloped countries for rabies, polio, and diphtheria to be included; recently been in the woods in certain areas for tick paralysis or Lyme disease to be viable diagnostic possibilities; or been receiving parenteral hyperalimentation for hypophosphatemia to occur. Obtaining a detailed history and performing a careful physical examination will allow the correct initial diagnosis of GBS in most instances.

Transverse myelitis may superficially resemble GBS, particularly if spinal shock has occurred and the lower extremity DTRs are not able to be elicited. However, asymmetrical involvement, a definite sensory level, complete absence of upper extremity weakness, urinary incontinence, and CSF pleocytosis all speak against GBS. Heavy metal intoxication, principally subacute arsenic or acute thallium poisoning, can mimic GBS clinically; moreover, in the initial phase of arsenic poisoning, both the CSF and EDX findings may be identical to typical GBS. However, these disorders should be included in the differential diagnosis of GBS only if there were preceding bouts of gastroenteritis. Associated central

TABLE 49-3. **Differential Diagnosis of Guillain-Barré Syndrome**

Hysteria/conversion reaction
Malingering
Brain stem infarction (Locked-in syndrome)
Acute myelopathies
Poliomyelitis
Rabies
Enteroviruses
Necrotic
Transverse
Focal compression
Cauda equina lesions
Peripheral neuropathies
Heavy metals; arsenic, thallium, gold
Alcohol
Organophosphates
Hexacarbons
Diphtheria
Drugs
Lyme disease
Critical illness
Vasculitis
Neuromuscular transmission disorders
Botulism
Tick-bite paralysis
Myasthenic syndrome
Myasthenia gravis
Snake venom
Sea urchin venom
Hypermagnesemia
Muscle disorders
Hypokalemia
Hyperkalemia

nervous system involvement is also common, particularly with thallium poisoning, and sometimes more than one person is affected simultaneously, strongly suggesting a common source.

Vasculitic neuropathies occasionally are mistaken for GBS. However, systemic signs, including fever, are common; the sensory and motor involvement in the limbs usually is both distal in location and asymmetrical; cranial nerve involvement, respiratory complications, and sphincter dysfunction are uncommon. Moreover, the CSF typically is normal (except with systemic lupus erythematosus), and EDX studies reveal changes suggestive of axon loss, rather than SD.

Acute intermittent porphyria can produce a PNS disorder that can be mistaken for GBS. However, its evolution is usually longer, and abdominal pain, constipation, and altered mental status are almost constant findings. The motor deficits often begin in the upper extremities; the Achilles DTRs may be preserved; sensory loss often is proximal; and seizures may occur. Moreover, the CSF protein typically is normal, and the EDX studies demonstrate axon loss rather than SD. Finally, both porphobilinogen and alpha-aminolevulinic acid are excreted in the urine in increased amounts during attacks of acute intermittent porphyria.

Botulism in adults, nearly always foodborne, has a clinical presentation that resembles that of GBS. However, frequently several cases occur simultaneously, excluding sporadic GBS from consideration. Even with single cases, immediately preceding gastrointestinal symptoms are prerequisite, and constipation often is prominent throughout the course. Blurred vision, dry mouth, ptosis, and dilated pupils that poorly respond to both light and accommodation are very common. Weakness descends from the bulbar region, so that neck weakness and respiratory muscle weakness may be far more prominent than limb weakness. Other features include rare sensory loss and a normal CSF. EDX changes include motor unit disintegration, affecting the motor amplitudes on NCS and highly polyphasic, disintegrated MUPs, usually with fibrillation potentials, on NEE. Finally, early in its course GBS can be mistaken for a functional disorder (e.g., hysteria). Most neurologists can recount situations in which patients were released from emergency rooms with hysterical symptoms, only to be admitted to an intensive care unit (ICU) a few days later to receive treatment for GBS. This most often occurs when the patient has a history of psychiatric illness; the sensory complaints can be mistaken for those caused by hyperventilation, and weakness is at an early stage, so that gait disturbances are present but limb strength seems intact on formal testing; and before the DTRs are lost.[2–4]

Evaluation. Routine hematology studies usually are normal. The two critical laboratory studies are CSF analysis and EDX examination. CSF that contains increased protein concentration with a normal cell count—albuminocytological dissociation—has been considered one of the diagnostic findings in the GBS since Guillain, Barré, and Strohl's original 1916 report. Elevated CSF protein, typically ranging from 46 to 300 mg/dL, is seen in most patients, particularly after the first week of illness. Conversely, the CSF cell count usually remains normal, although it may be elevated (greater than 10 mononuclear leukocytes per microliter) in patients whose GBS is superimposed on acquired immunodeficiency syndrome (AIDS) or Lyme disease. The CSF protein, however, is often not elevated very early after symptom onset. Moreover, in approximately 10 percent of patients with GBS, usually those with mild cases, elevated CSF protein cannot be found, even with repeated sampling, during the entire course of the illness. On EDX examination, very often changes strongly suggestive of SD, particularly conduction block, less often differential slowing or focal slowing, are seen on assessment of one or more often several nerves; generally, these changes are much more apparent on motor NCS than sensory NCS. Moreover, patterns of abnormalities suggestive of an acquired SD polyradiculoneuropathy, such as upper extremity sensory NCS responses that are unelicitable or of low amplitude while normal in the lower extremity, often are found. Similar to the CSF analysis, EDX is generally least helpful for diagnosis during the very initial phase of the illness, precisely the period when a definite diagnosis is being sought so that specific treatment can be rapidly initiated. Thus, during the first several days of the illness, in many patients the CSF protein is not elevated and the EDX studies are normal or, if abnormal, nondiagnostic.[11, 12] Among 31 patients who had EDX examinations within the first week of onset of motor symptoms (i.e., weakness), a definite diagnosis of GBS was possible in just 55 percent, and usually not until the fifth day.[23] One very common misconception regarding the EDX studies is that substantial slowing of motor CV is a typical finding with early GBS. In fact, such NCS slowing seldom is seen during that stage of GBS and it is far more commonly found in the late plateau or recovery stages.

Management. There is no known prevention for sporadic GBS, although those persons who previously had a bout after immunization should avoid future immunizations if at all possible.[3] In contrast, whenever GBS occurs in epidemic form, as it does in China and other underdeveloped countries, its incidence may be reduced by improved public health measures.

The treatment of GBS has two components: supportive care and specific therapy. Supportive care remains the cornerstone of therapy, because most patients recover function if they advance past the acute phase of the illness. The major reduction in deaths from GBS over the past few decades has been due to advances in supportive care, particularly in mechanical ventilation.[2–4]

Most authorities recommend that patients with suspected GBS be hospitalized, regardless of how mild their disorder appears initially. This advice is based on instances of rapid deterioration occurring over a brief period of time, leading to respiratory failure. Once they are hospitalized, patients must be assessed and monitored to avoid the major life-threatening complications of GBS, including respiratory failure, dysautonomia, and venous thromboembolism. Respiratory compromise is the most common serious complication and underlies the reason that approximately 30 percent of GBS patients who are hospitalized require treatment in an ICU. Weakness of the respiratory muscles, particularly the diaphragm, is most often responsible for respiratory failure. Other factors include weakness of various bulbar-innervated muscles and pulmonary complications, including atelectasis, pneumonia, and pulmonary embolism.[2–4, 24] Respiratory function can be assessed with arterial blood gas analysis and peak expiratory flow pressure measurements. Vital capacity measurements provide the most useful information regarding the degree of respiratory compromise.[2, 25] Respiratory function must be monitored closely. Generally, intubation is required whenever the vital capacity falls to 15 mL/kg. Intratracheal intubation is complicated in patients with GBS because of dysautonomia, which can result in marked hypotension, arrhythmias, and sudden death due to various drugs and to airway manipulation and because of hyperkalemia, induced by succinylcholine, which can cause arrhythmias and cardiac arrest. Tracheotomies usually are not performed unless airway assistance is still needed at the end of the second week of the illness.[25]

Dysautonomia occurs to some extent in the majority of GBS patients but more frequently and more severely in those with respiratory failure and severe motor deficits. Severe paroxysmal hypertension, orthostatic hypotension, and various cardiac arrhythmias are all complications that may prove difficult to manage.[24] Pulmonary embolism occurs in about 5 percent of patients immobilized with GBS, typically after the second week of immobilization. In one series, it was responsible for approximately 28 percent of deaths. Preventive measures include subcutaneous heparin—switched to warfarin if patients are long term—and intermittent calf pneumatic compression devices.[2–4, 24] Other complications are urinary tract infections and gastrointestinal disorders, including bleeding secondary to stress ulcers and erosive gastritis, ileus, and fecal impaction. Hyponatremia can develop, usually in ventilated patients and due to inappropriate release of antidiuretic hormone. This electrolyte imbalance responds to fluid restriction.[4, 24, 26]

Two non–life-threatening complications of GBS that require attention are pain and psychological trauma. To treat pain, a number of medications have been used with varying success. These include analgesics such as aspirin and narcotics. However, narcotics must be given with caution because they tend to exacerbate respiratory failure and to produce ileus. Antidepressants and anticonvulsants generally have not been effective. A few reports have described sustained pain relief for a few days following a single IM injection of 40 to 60 mg of methylprednisolone. Simple physical measures, such as the application of cold or hot packs, gentle massage, or repositioning with the limbs in slight flexion, may bring pain relief.[24] The psychological stress on essentially paralyzed GBS patients must also be appreciated. Their fears and concerns, particularly regarding recovery potential, must be addressed throughout all phases of the illness.[24, 26]

The specific treatment of choice for GBS since 1978 has been plasmapheresis. It can be beneficial in patients of all ages, although there are only anecdotal reports, rather than large-scale studies, to support its value in children with GBS. Also, pregnancy is not a contraindication to plasmapheresis; at least two pregnant women have been treated with this method without incident.[4] Although plasmapheresis has no effect on either mortality or relapse rates, measurable objective improvement occurs in nearly every other aspect of the disorder in at least 50 percent of treated patients. Thus, compared with nontreated patients, improvement begins earlier in the course and is appreciably better at 1 month after onset. With plasmapheresis, less mechanical ventilation is required, and both ICU and hospitalization time is decreased. To be effective, plasmapheresis must be instituted early in the course of the disorder, preferably within the first week. The precise regimen has not been established, although most investigators have used 150 to 250 mL/kg over 7 to 10 days of treatment.[2–4] The drawbacks of plasmapheresis include its expense and rare complications such as hypotension and sepsis. There is a risk of acquiring viral infections, such as hepatitis and possibly AIDS, if fresh frozen plasma is used as the replacement fluid. (Plasma appears to offer no benefit over albumin with saline.[4])

Some preliminary studies using intravenous immunoglobulin (IVIg) treatment for GBS have produced encouraging results. This mode of treatment has advantages over plasmapheresis in regard to its being simpler to administer and costing slightly less. However, the transmission of viral infections, including AIDS, is a significant concern, because IVIg is made from plasma pooled from thousands of donors.[4] Both corticosteroids, in conventional doses, and adrenocorticotropic hormone (ACTH) have proved to be ineffective in the treatment of GBS. In fact, a few studies have suggested that ACTH is actually detrimental.[2, 4] High-dose corticosteroids could conceivably be of benefit, but there are potential complications, particularly bowel perforations and serious infections. Nonetheless, if they are shown to be effective, they will be very appealing treatment options compared with plasmapheresis because of their being relatively inexpensive and easy to administer.[4]

During the first two trimesters of pregnancy, the management of women with GBS is identical to that of nonpregnant patients in regard to both supportive care and specific therapy. During the third trimester, owing to increased respiratory demand, supportive care becomes crucial, because the risk of respiratory failure increases, culminating during delivery. Adequate ventilation must be ensured during this period. Due to an increase in premature labor and delivery, a perinatal infant mortality rate of approximately 10 percent mars late pregnancy complicated by GBS.[4] GBS is not considered an indication for cesarean section, and infants do not acquire GBS, even transiently, from their affected mothers.[2, 4]

Prognosis and Future Perspectives. Even as late as 1953, Guillain always contended that GBS was an inherently nonfatal disorder, a benign disease that left little, if any, residual effects. Such optimism is not supported by many series published over the past 30 years. Excluding those with mild disease, most patients are hospitalized for at least 1 month and often considerably longer, particularly if mechanical ventilation is required. Overall, approximately 5 percent of patients die; mortality rates of 15 to 20 percent have occurred in ICUs, most often from adult respiratory distress syndrome. Approximately 75 percent of patients recover without serious neurological residuals, and recovery typically ensues over the 6 to 12 months after onset and is usually maximal by 18 months after onset. Some patients may be left with persistent minor weakness, paresthesias, or sensory loss.[4] Approximately 7 to 15 percent of patients have permanent, substantial neurological sequelae (e.g., bilateral footdrop, intrinsic hand muscle weakness and wasting, sensory ataxia, burning dysesthesias). Only a very few, however, are permanently bedridden by the disorder.[2–4] Several factors during the acute phase of the illness have been linked to subsequent poor recovery. These include older patient age (particularly age 60 or older); rapid, early evolution, leading to quadriparesis within a week; and very low motor NCS amplitudes on distal stimulations early in the course of the disease (suggesting severe axon loss, but equally consistent, at least theoretically, with severe distal SD conduction blocks). The latter has proved to be the single most reliable outcome predictor.[12] Not surprisingly, most of the prognostic factors listed merely indicate that a poor long-term prognosis is directly related to the severity of the acute episode.

As the past decade has illustrated, much is yet to be learned about GBS. What is the exact initiating mechanism for demyelination with AIDP?[19] How frequently does C. *jejuni* infection serve as the antecedent event with GBS, and exactly how does it cause the disorder? Unlike certain other known triggers (e.g., cytomegalovirus), C. *jejuni* rarely invades PNS tissue directly, so the possibility that GBS results from various PNS structures being injured as a bystander when the immune system attacks a virus within the PNS is untenable.[14] Is the acute axonal form of GBS seen in North America and Europe typically caused by C. *jejuni* infection? These questions are of much more than academic interest, because the answers to them can influence treatment and possibly prevention of this disorder.

Chronic Inflammatory Demyelinating Polyradiculoneuropathy (CIDP)

Pathogenesis and Pathophysiology. CIDP is an apparent immune-mediated disorder of the PNS. The term CIDP was coined to emphasize that the disorder is a chronic process that results in demyelination as well as an inflammatory cell response in peripheral nerves and spinal nerve roots; typically, there is a mononuclear cell infiltration involving the endoneurium and epineurium of peripheral nerve fibers.[27] The predominant pathological feature is SD, although usually there is some degree of axon loss as well (Figs. 49–3 and 49–4). These pathological changes have been found to involve roots, plexuses, proximal nerve trunks, and, occasionally, cranial nerves and sympathetic trunks, as well as some autonomic nerves.[28] The predilection for CIDP to involve roots and proximal nerve trunks is responsible for the prominent proximal weakness that may be encountered in this disorder and helps distinguish it from most other generalized polyneuropathies. The predominant involvement of myelin in CIDP results in a characteristic pattern of findings on EDX

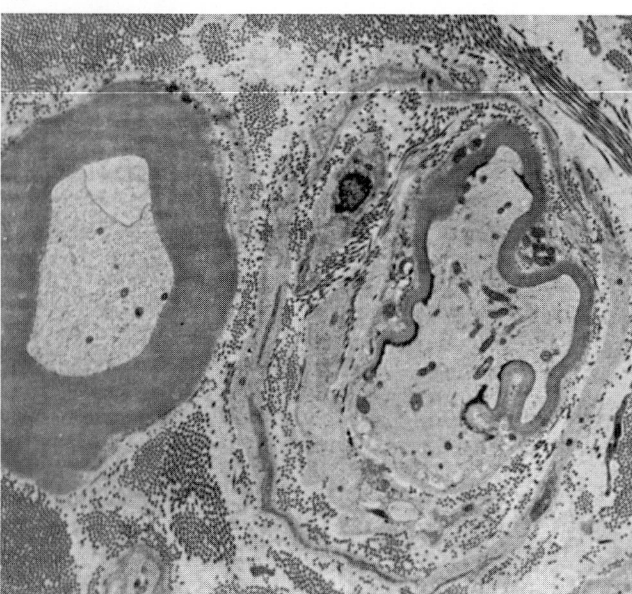

FIGURE 49–3. Electron microscopy of sural nerve in CIDP. A normal myelinated fiber (*left*) adjacent to a myelinated fiber that has thin and partially absent myelin (*right*).

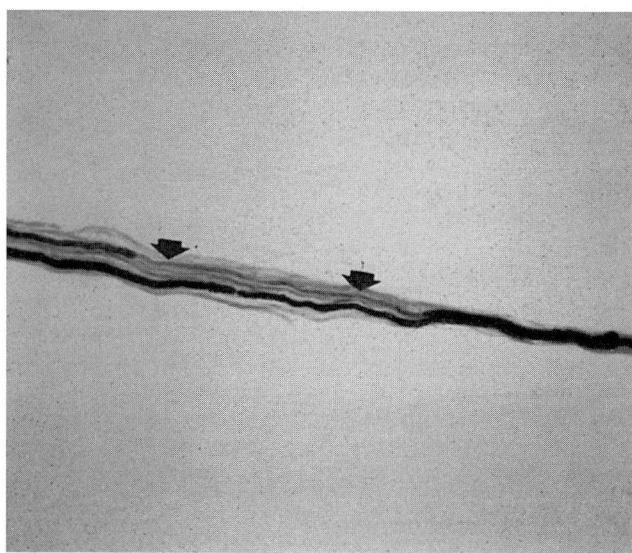

FIGURE 49–4. Teased nerve fiber preparation showing segmental demyelination in a sural nerve in CIDP.

testing, including slowed nerve CV and conduction block; the latter process correlates with the clinical deficits. Also, the distinctive distribution of NCS abnormalities that may occur with acquired SD polyradiculopathies (already described) is often seen.[10]

The evidence that CIDP is immune-mediated is compelling although still somewhat inconclusive. In many respects, it is similar to the evidence advanced for AIDP being an immune-mediated disorder. The onset or relapses of CIDP on occasion seem to be triggered by a preceding event, such as an infection or vaccination that could initiate an immune-mediated response. In addition, most patients with CIDP respond to corticosteroids and other immunosuppressants, plasma exchange, and IVIg, therapies designed to treat immune-mediated disorders. Furthermore, CIDP shares many clinical and pathological features with experimental models of immune-mediated peripheral neuropathy, particularly EAN. This has led to speculation that the pathogenesis of CIDP is similar to that of AIDP and EAN. Lastly, the presence of immune-effector cells and the deposition of antibody and complement on myelinated fibers is impressive but indirect evidence of an immune-mediated process in which both cellular and humoral immune systems are operative.[29]

More recent studies have provided additional evidence of an immune-mediated mechanism for CIDP. Passive transfer of sera and IgG from CIDP patients to experimental animals has resulted in histological and electrodiagnostic evidence of demyelination of peripheral nerve fibers.[30] In addition, IgG antibodies directed at protein zero (P0), the major integral membrane protein of peripheral myelin, have been found in 28 percent of CIDP patients, and in two thirds of these patients, the sera caused conduction block and demyelination when injected into experimental animals.[31]

A disorder clinically similar to CIDP but with pathological and EDX features, indicating an axon loss process, has been reported.[28] Whether this actually represents a so-called axonal form of CIDP similar to the axonal form of GBS remains to be established.[32]

Epidemiology and Risk Factors. The age of onset of CIDP has been reported to range from 1 year through the eighth decade or later, with a mean in the fourth decade. Both sexes are affected, although there is a slight male predominance. With the mean age of onset being in the fourth decade, women of childbearing age may develop CIDP. Furthermore, there is evidence that the disorder may relapse or worsen during pregnancy and in the postpartum period.[33] Patients with certain histocompatibility antigens have an increased risk of developing CIDP. In particular, there is an increased incidence of histocompatibility locus antigens AW30, AW31, A1, B8, and DR w3. Furthermore, CIDP, GBS, and multiple sclerosis have all been associated with the presence of the M3 allele of the alpha-1 antitrypsin system located on chromosome 14.[3]

Clinical Features and Associated Disorders. By definition, CIDP is a chronic disorder that typically evolves slowly, almost always requiring a period of 8 weeks or longer for symptoms to reach their peak, and they typically do so over many months. CIDP can follow either a slowly progressive monophasic course, which occurs in approximately two thirds of patients, or a cyclical relapsing course seen in the remainder.[5, 33]

The symptoms of CIDP can be variable, but usually weakness tends to predominate over sensory symptoms.[5, 27] The distribution of weakness often conforms to a typical peripheral neuropathy pattern of symmetrical involvement, with the lower extremities being affected more than the upper extremities and distal muscles being affected more than proximal muscles. However, in many patients, the weakness is asymmetrical, and in others, it is more prominent proximally. The degree of weakness varies markedly from patient to patient. In the majority of patients, it is mild to moderate in degree, but rarely, the weakness can be severe and generalized, sometimes associated with respiratory failure necessitating ventilatory support. Muscle cramping and fasciculations are infrequent symptoms.[5, 27, 28]

Sensory symptoms are usually confined to mild paresthesia or modest sensory loss. However, in those patients with chronic progressive courses, sensory symptoms may become more prominent. In addition to numbness and paresthesia, pain sometimes is reported, although this occurs in less than 20 percent of patients. Very infrequently, CIDP may present with predominantly sensory symptoms, including numbness, paresthesia, and sensory ataxia. In a subset of these patients, this PNS disorder appears essentially confined to sensory fibers, prompting speculation that the apparent immune-mediated response is directed at a unique antigen in the myelin of sensory fibers. However, in most instances in which the disorder begins as a sensory neuropathy, it later evolves to a more typical pattern of sensory and motor involvement. On occasion, the cranial nerves may be affected, causing symptoms of diplopia, facial weakness or numbness, dysarthria, and dysphagia. Autonomic symptoms are uncommon, although incontinence and erectile impotence have been reported.[5, 27, 28]

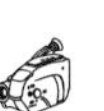

The physical signs noted in CIDP reflect the clinical symptoms. Distal symmetrical weakness, with the lower extremities more severely affected than the upper extremities, is the rule. However, asymmetrical involvement and more prominent proximal involvement can occur, and they serve as important clinical clues to the diagnosis of CIDP. Generalized hyporeflexia or areflexia is characteristic. Sensory loss often conforms to a distal to proximal gradient, in the so-called stocking-glove pattern, with all modalities affected to a nearly equal extent. Occasionally, sensory ataxia may be observed. Cranial nerve findings may include signs of facial, bulbar, and neck weakness. Papilledema is an unusual clinical feature, and its precise pathophysiology is unclear. It has been attributed to altered resorption of CSF over the arachnoid villi due to elevations of CSF protein or to increased intracranial pressure.[3] Rather rare clinical features include pupil abnormalities consistent with parasympathetically denervated pupil, Horner's syndrome, and postural or cerebellar-type tremors.[34] Occasionally, hypertrophied nerves may be palpated in patients with very chronic CIDP. Rarely, the spinal nerve roots may be hypertrophied to such an extent that they act as masses, compressing the spinal cord, and may produce a syndrome of spinal cord compression.[34]

More recently, additional terminologies have been proposed to define special variants of CIDP.[35] Idiopathic distal acquired demyelinating symmetric (DADS-I) neuropathy has been suggested as a term to describe a variant of CIDP with clinical features of a sensorimotor polyneuropathy that is often predominantly sensory and strictly respects a distal to proximal gradient of involvement. In addition, DADS-I may be less responsive to the standard therapies for typical CIDP. When this phenotype occurs in the setting of a monoclonal gammopathy of uncertain significance (MGUS), it is referred to as DADS-M (see later discussion).[35] This entity will be discussed in the section dealing with MGUS. Multifocal acquired demyelinating sensory and motor (MADSAM) neuropathy, or Lewis-Sumner syndrome, has been proposed as a term to describe a multifocal or mononeuritis multiplex variant of CIDP.[36] In this syndrome, sensory and motor symptoms and signs may conform to the distribution of individual peripheral nerves. Onset is often in the upper extremities, sensory symptoms may be prominent, and progression tends to be slow and insidious. CSF findings are similar to those seen in typical CIDP, and EDX findings are indicative of multifocal SD. These patients tend to respond to the standard therapies used for typical CIDP. MADSAM neuropathy may occasionally resemble multifocal motor neuropathy with conduction block, a disorder with different clinical, CSF, and EDX features as well as very different therapeutic implications.

Some patients with CIDP have abnormalities on MRI scans of the head consistent with multiple sclerosis.[37] Whether these isolated patients represent the coincidental occurrence of two disorders or an immune-mediated disorder of both central and peripheral myelin remains unclear.

There is no conclusive evidence that CIDP patients have a higher incidence of other medical conditions, including autoimmune disorders. However, associated disorders, including systemic lupus erythematosus, Hashimoto's thyroiditis, thyrotoxicosis, chronic active hepatitis, inflammatory bowel disease, urticaria, eczema, and psoriasis, do occur in some CIDP patients.[3] A CIDP-like disorder may occur in the setting of MGUS, as well as with multiple myeloma, osteosclerotic myeloma, and other lymphoproliferative disorders. These disorders are discussed as distinct entities in the following sections.

Differential Diagnosis. On purely clinical grounds, CIDP may be confused with a wide variety of chronic sensorimotor polyneuropathies, including those related to diabetes, uremia, hypothyroidism, acromegaly, toxins, and alcoholic-nutritional mechanisms. Although CIDP may produce distinguishing clinical features, such as predominant motor symptoms and signs, asymmetrical involvement, proximal motor involvement, and cranial nerve symptoms and signs, the paramount factor in separating CIDP and related disorders from the rather large group of nonspecific, chronic axon loss sensorimotor polyneuropathies is the presence of acquired SD features on EDX testing. Thus, EDX evaluation is the key step in identifying the acquired SD polyneuropathies, including CIDP. The differential diagnosis of this category includes not only CIDP, but also the CIDP-like disorders that may be associated with multiple myeloma, osteosclerotic myeloma (including the POEMS syndrome, an acronym that stands for *p*olyneuropathy, *o*rganomegaly, *e*ndocrinopathy, *M*-protein, and *s*kin changes), MGUS, and Waldenström's macroglobulinemia. These disorders may be distinguished from CIDP by the presence of an M-protein in the serum or urine, the presence of lytic or sclerotic lesions on skeletal bone survey, or both. A disorder essentially identical to CIDP can result from HIV infection. Consequently, testing for HIV is indicated in patients at risk. CIDP may be a presenting feature of HIV infection, preceding seroconversion for up to 6 months. For this reason, repeating HIV testing 6 months after the onset of a CIDP-like disorder is appropriate in patients at risk.

Familial hypertrophic polyneuropathies that produce EDX features of SD along with axon loss may sometimes be confused with CIDP. With the familial disorders, a positive family history typically is recorded, but in some instances, it is not. CIDP can usually be distinguished on clinical grounds by its more rapid tempo of evolution and a cyclical or relapsing course. The EDX findings may also be helpful in differentiating CIDP from these disorders. In the familial disorders, the SD features on NCS tend to be symmetrical, with uniform involvement of all nerves. Focal conduction block and focal conduction slowing usually are not observed. Despite these numerous distinguishing features, occasionally it still may be difficult to distinguish a long-duration CIDP from a familial hypertrophic SD polyneuropathy. In such circumstances, a trial of therapy is usually indicated.

On occasion, CIDP may be difficult to differentiate from AIDP. Patients with more subacute courses of CIDP have been described, and sometimes CIDP may begin with a relatively acute onset. Over time, CIDP usually declares itself by a typical chronic relapsing course or a more slowly progressive monophasic course. The distinction between AIDP and CIDP is significant because the ultimate course, prognosis, and treatment are different.[28, 29]

Evaluation. As noted earlier, the performance of a comprehensive EDX evaluation to uncover findings consistent with acquired SD is key in the evaluation and diagnosis of CIDP and related disorders. These EDX findings clearly distinguish CIDP and related disorders from the vastly more common group of clinically similar axon loss sensorimotor polyneuropathies. The general laboratory features of CIDP are relatively nonspecific and are not particularly useful in confirming the diagnosis. Routine laboratory tests typically are normal. The CSF protein, however, is frequently elevated to a moderate degree; in one series, it ranged from 23 to 600 mg/dL with a mean of 138 mg/dL. Nonetheless, it should be emphasized that in 10 percent of patients with CIDP, the CSF protein may be normal.[5] Even sural nerve biopsies generally do not provide specific or diagnostic features, although in the majority of patients they will document the presence of inflammation and demyelination, two features that characterize CIDP. However, these findings are not pathognomonic. Furthermore, the sural nerve biopsy may be normal in nearly 25 percent of patients.[27] It is important to appreciate that a normal CSF protein and sural nerve biopsy are not necessarily inconsistent with the diagnosis of CIDP. On the other hand, a normal EDX examination essentially excludes this diagnosis.

The critical component in the evaluation of a patient with suspected CIDP is to exclude the CIDP-like disorders. This requires careful screening of the serum and urine for the presence of M-proteins. Because a small amount of M-protein may still be undetected by routine serum protein electrophoresis testing, the search for M-protein should include an assessment incorporating immunoelectrophoresis or immunofixation techniques. The presence of an M-protein in the setting of a CIDP-like disorder may signify a polyneuropathy associated with multiple myeloma, osteosclerotic myeloma, MGUS, Waldenström's macroglobulinemia, or another lymphoproliferative disorder. Also, a skeletal x-ray study is indicated, because a significant percentage of patients with osteosclerotic myeloma may not disclose an M-protein on immunofixation. HIV testing should also be performed in all patients at risk with a CIDP-like disorder.

Management. CIDP is a very treatable disorder, with most patients showing favorable responses to one of the many therapeutic modalities available. Some of the earliest reports of CIDP indicated that it was often steroid responsive.[28] Subsequently, a controlled clinical trial clearly established the value of corticosteroids in the treatment of CIDP, regardless of whether the course was monophasic and progressive or cyclical and relapsing.[38] Controlled trials have also established the efficacy of IVIg and plasma exchange in CIDP.[39, 40]

When constructing a treatment plan for patients with CIDP, it is important to balance clinical symptoms against the risks and potential benefits of the therapy. Clearly, patients with rather modest or minimal symptoms may not require treatment. Instead, they should be followed and observed closely. However, in those with a progressive course or with substantial clinical symptoms, treatment may begin with IVIg, plasma exchange therapy, or corticosteroids. Although both IVIg and plasma exchange are relatively expensive therapeutic modalities, either is justified as an initial treatment. Their advantage is that they obviate the need for chronic corticosteroid or other immunosuppressant treatment and thus avoid the associated side effects and complications of these therapies. Both IVIg and plasma exchange are comparable in efficacy and expense. Nonetheless, IVIg may have certain advantages over plasma exchange. It may require fewer treatments, is somewhat less invasive, and may be administered at home. It is imperative, however, that patients considered for IVIg therapy be assessed for IgA deficiency, because anaphylactic reactions have occurred following the administration of IVIg in patients with IgA deficiency. Furthermore, caution should be exercised in administering IVIg to patients who have underlying renal dysfunction, because the risk of renal failure is increased following IVIg treatment. Traditionally, IVIg therapy is administered at a dose of 400 mg/kg/d over 5 consecutive days.[29] An alternative recommendation is to use IVIg at 400 mg/kg/d once per week over 6 to 8 consecutive weeks.[34] Follow-up doses, typically single doses of 400 mg/kg, are administered at intervals needed to maintain the clinical response. Plasma exchange therapy requires expertise in its use and is clearly more technically demanding than is IVIg treatment. Plasma exchange usually is administered twice weekly for the first 3 weeks and then once or twice weekly for an additional 3 weeks.[28] Patients typically respond to IVIg or plasma exchange within the first several weeks of treatment and may demonstrate sustained improvement for many weeks or months. Relapses may require periodic isolated treatments with a single dose of IVIg or single plasma exchange. If a patient responds successfully to infrequent booster treatments of either IVIg or plasma exchange, it is reasonable to maintain this form of treatment rather than adding corticosteroids or other immunosuppressants.

In patients who are not candidates for either IVIg or plasma exchange, or in whom responses are not satisfactory, chronic immunosuppressive therapy must be considered. Corticosteroids typically are used at relatively high doses initially and then slowly tapered while monitoring the clinical response. Most patients who respond will do so during their first few months of treatment. In those patients who cannot tolerate corticosteroids and in those who do not obtain a satisfactory clinical response to them, a trial of other immunosuppressants may be a reasonable alternative.[28] Anecdotal evidence suggests that azathioprine, cyclophosphamide, cyclosporine, total lymphoid irradiation, alpha- and beta-interferon, and mycophenolate may be of value in treating some patients with CIDP.[41]

In addition to these various immunosuppressive therapies, patients should undergo a thorough physical therapy assessment to determine if they require aids to ambulation, including orthotic devices such as ankle-foot orthosis for footdrop. Other physical therapy modalities, including stretching and range-of-motion exercises, may be helpful while a patient is responding to medical therapy.

Prognosis and Future Perspectives. The prognosis is favorable for most patients with CIDP who are properly diagnosed and treated. In one large group of patients whose disease duration averaged 5.7 years and who were followed for a minimum of 24 months, nearly 40 percent were asymptomatic and nearly 50 percent had either minor symptoms that did not have any impact on their level of function or had only very modest restrictions in lifestyle.[42] Future research objectives will focus on the specific immune-mediated mechanisms and pathophysiology of CIDP. From a purely clinical perspective, further trials are needed to better define optimal therapeutic protocols using the modalities that have already proved effective, including IVIg, plasma exchange, and corticosteroids.

Monoclonal Gammopathies of Undetermined Significance

Pathogenesis and Pathophysiology. A heterogenous group of peripheral neuropathies has been associated with the presence of an MGUS. However, the precise relationship of the monoclonal (M) protein to the peripheral nerve disorder remains unclear. By definition, MGUS indicates the presence of an M-protein of less than 3 g/dL in concentration, with less than 5 percent plasma cells in bone marrow, none or only a very small amount of M-protein in the urine, and the absence of other abnormalities, including lytic or sclerotic bone lesions, anemia, hypercalcemia, and renal insufficiency. Furthermore, the M-protein should remain at stable and low concentrations over time.[43] The natural history of MGUS indicates that with advancing time-specific hematological and lymphoproliferative disorders, such as multiple myeloma, Waldenström's macroglobulinemia, amyloidosis, and lymphoma, may develop. Nevertheless, most patients who undergo a comprehensive evaluation for an M-protein in their serum ultimately will have it attributed to MGUS. MGUS is rather common, occurring in up to 1.7 percent of patients older than age 50 and in 3 percent of patients older than age 70.[43]

Acquired SD polyneuropathies with features similar to that of CIDP have been observed in MGUS with IgG, IgA, and IgM M-proteins. These observations, coupled with the response of these disorders to the typical therapeutic interventions used for CIDP, have fostered the belief that these disorders are also immune-mediated. However, the only strong evidence to support this theory is found in the MGUS neuropathy associated with IgM M-protein. In this disorder, the M-protein binds and reacts to myelin and to an oligosaccharide determinant that is shared by the myelin glycoproteins myelin-associated glycoprotein (MAG) and P0 and the glycolipids sulfated glucuronyl paragloboside (SGPG) and sulfated glucuronyl lactosaminyl paragloboside (SGLPG).[44] Approximately 50 percent of patients with IgM MGUS neuropathy have anti-MAG antibodies. The finding of deposits of anti-MAG M-protein and complement on affected myelin sheaths, the presence of widening of myelin lamellae at the sites of antibody deposition, and the experiments that document the development of polyneuropathy in animals following passive transfer of patients' serum support the concept that the IgM M-protein with anti-MAG activity plays an important pathogenetic role in the development of the polyneuropathy.[44] Other observations, however, have detracted from this theory, including the fact that the concentration of the IgM M-protein may not always correlate with the severity of the polyneuropathy nor with the clinical response after treatment.[45]

Similar to CIDP, the demyelinating polyneuropathy associated with MGUS typically produces physiological alterations suggestive of an acquired SD polyradiculoneuropathy, often accompanied by a modest degree of axon loss. MGUS can also produce a pure axonal sensorimotor polyneuropathy.[44, 45]

Epidemiology and Risk Factors. MGUS polyneuropathy tends to occur later in life than CIDP, with the mean age of onset in the mid- to late sixth decade. In most large series, a distinct male predominance is noted. There are no other particular risk factors, and MGUS neuropathy seldom occurs in women of childbearing age.[44, 45]

Clinical Features and Associated Disorders. In general, the MGUS polyneuropathies associated with IgG and IgA conform to a sensorimotor polyneuropathy that shares many clinical features with CIDP, including predominant proximal weakness. Nonetheless, there may be some differences. Sensory symptoms usually are more prominent than in CIDP. In addition, the initial phase of the disorder often progresses much slower than it does in CIDP, and the course is less likely to be cyclical or relapsing. Also, cranial nerve involvement and autonomic involvement are rare. Nevertheless, clinical syndromes indistinguishable from CIDP may be seen with MGUS polyneuropathy.

The clinical syndrome seen with MGUS IgM polyneuropathy appears to differ from that seen both with CIDP and with MGUS polyneuropathy associated with IgG and IgA. This disorder typically conforms to a distal and symmetrical polyneuropathy and has been termed DADS-M (i.e., distal acquired demyelinating symmetrical neuropathy associated with an M-protein).[35] With this disorder, sensory symptoms may be even more prominent and can be the initial presenting feature. Typically, progressive sensory impairment is followed later by motor involvement. Sensory ataxia, particularly affecting the gait, is a common finding, as are tremors of the upper extremities that resemble essential tremor.[46] Similar to the other MGUS polyneuropathies, the clinical features tend to progress more slowly and are less severe than the initial symptoms associated with CIDP. Moreover, relapsing and cyclical courses are not seen, and cranial nerve or autonomic involvement rarely is encountered.

There is no definitive evidence that other disorders, particularly other immune-mediated disorders, are present to a greater extent in patients with MGUS polyneuropathy. It should be emphasized, however, that the diagnosis of MGUS depends on the stability of the M-protein concentration. Because a significant number of patients with MGUS will later develop malignant forms of monoclonal gammopathy, these patients require repeated evaluations and monitoring of the M-protein over time.

Differential Diagnosis. The differential diagnosis of MGUS polyneuropathy producing acquired SD changes on EDX examination is identical to that of CIDP. It is key to exclude the other causes for monoclonal gammopathy, including multiple myeloma, isolated plasmacytoma, Waldenström's macroglobulinemia, osteosclerotic myeloma (including the POEMS syndrome), heavy chain diseases, malignant lymphoma, and amyloidosis. It should also be noted that MGUS polyneuropathy may manifest as an axon loss polyneuropathy and, consequently, should be included in the differential diagnosis of axon loss sensorimotor polyneuropathy discussed elsewhere.[43–45]

Evaluation. In IgG and IgA MGUS demyelinating polyneuropathy, the EDX examination typically shows changes suggestive of a chronic, acquired SD polyradiculoneuropathy similar to that seen in CIDP. In patients with IgM MGUS, the EDX examination may disclose a distinctive pattern of distal, symmetrical demyelinating change.[35, 47] Searching for an M-protein is an important component in the evaluation of any patient with a significant sensorimotor polyneuropathy. As noted earlier, if the serum protein electrophoresis is negative or unrevealing, additional testing should be performed using immunoelectrophoresis or immunofixation techniques. These methods are more sensitive in detecting small amounts of M-protein that may be important in the identification of MGUS polyneuropathy.[43] Once an M-protein is detected in the setting of a sensorimotor polyneuropathy, a careful evaluation must follow to assess for a lymphoproliferative disorder. This evaluation typically entails routine laboratory studies to assess for anemia, hypercalcemia, and renal insufficiency. In addition, M-protein should be sought in the urine, and a skeletal bone survey should be obtained to assess for multiple myeloma, isolated plasmacytomas, or osteosclerotic changes typical of osteosclerotic myeloma. Although radionuclide bone scans may be valuable in this assessment, the skeletal plain x-ray study is more sensitive for the detection of osteosclerotic lesions. A bone marrow aspirate should also be performed. HIV testing also should be performed in patients at risk, with guidelines similar to those noted for CIDP.

Routine laboratory studies in MGUS polyneuropathy typically are unremarkable. The CSF protein is consistently increased in a fashion similar to that seen with CIDP. Sural nerve biopsy may also disclose features of inflammation and SD with some axon loss, which are very similar to the pathological changes noted in CIDP. None of these findings, however, is specific for MGUS polyneuropathy, and none serves to differentiate it from CIDP and other related disorders.

Although it is unclear whether the presence of antibodies has any definite clinical implication regarding the management, prognosis, or pathophysiology of IgM MGUS polyneuropathy,[35] patients with IgM MGUS are usually assessed for anti-MAG antibodies, often in conjunction with anti-SGPG and anti-SGLPG antibodies.

Management. The data regarding benefits of therapeutic intervention with steroids, immunosuppressants, plasma exchange, and IVIg are largely anecdotal but tend to indicate that MGUS polyneuropathy responds in a fashion similar to CIDP.[45] A controlled trial of plasma exchange did disclose efficacy in MGUS polyneuropathy but appeared to demonstrate greater improvement in polyneuropathies associated with IgG and IgA M-proteins compared with those associated with IgM M-proteins.[48] It appears that IgM MGUS polyneuropathy, especially in the setting of a distal sensory polyneuropathy phenotype (i.e., DADS-M), is the least responsive to therapy, with only 30 percent of patients demonstrating improvement following immunomodulating treatments.[35] Although convincing data are lacking, there is general agreement that these patients should be treated following the same guidelines used for CIDP. However, because MGUS polyneuropathy tends to be a more slowly progressive disorder than CIDP, it may be more difficult to define a precise threshold when treatment is indicated. Furthermore, treatment must be aggressive and sustained to provide ample time to observe a clinical response.

Prognosis and Future Perspectives. In comparison to CIDP, the prognosis in patients with MGUS polyneuropathy as a group may be less favorable. Despite the fact that the initial severity of weakness and sensory impairment is considerably less in MGUS polyneuropathy compared with cyclical relapses of CIDP or to the peak of a monophasic course of CIDP, MGUS polyneuropathy tends to be slowly progressive and ultimately, if the condition is left untreated, may result in more severe clinical deficits and disability.[42] Also, MGUS polyneuropathy, overall, is somewhat less responsive to therapy than CIDP. Patients with MGUS polyneuropathy who have prominent features of acquired SD on EDX testing appear to have the greatest chance for significant improvement following therapeutic intervention. Those patients with DADS-M may be less responsive to plasma exchange and other interventions. In a study of 25 treated patients with MGUS polyneuropathy who had a mean duration of illness of 6.6 years and were followed for a minimum of 24 months, 12 percent were asymptomatic and another 60 percent had either minimal, nondisabling symptoms or minor symptoms that caused only modest restrictions in their lifestyle.[42]

Very fundamental nosological issues regarding MGUS polyneuropathies need to be clarified. Does the presence of an M-protein in the setting of a SD polyneuropathy mimicking CIDP indicate a separate and distinct clinical entity? What is the pathogenetic role of the M-protein in MGUS polyneuropathy? Is the subset of MGUS polyneuropathy associated with IgG and IgA M-proteins distinct clinically and pathogenetically from that associated with an IgM M-protein? More specifically, does the presence of anti-MAG antibodies in IgM MGUS polyneuropathy signify a distinct clinical and pathogenetic disorder that can be separated from CIDP and the other MGUS polyneuropathies? And finally, what are the natural histories of these disorders and what represents optimal therapies for the various types of MGUS polyneuropathy?

Multiple Myeloma

Pathogenesis and Pathophysiology. Multiple myeloma is a hematological disorder characterized by a proliferation of a single clone of plasma cells that produces a specific immunoglobulin. This disorder may affect patients between the ages of 40 and 70, but the peak incidence is in the seventh decade. Multiple myeloma typically causes bone pain, general fatigue, and weakness and is often accompanied by anemia, chronic renal failure, and hypercalcemia. Over 99 percent of patients will have an M-protein detected in the serum or urine on immunoelectrophoresis or immunofixation.[43] Skeletal bone surveys reveal osteolytic or rarely osteoblastic lesions in approximately two thirds of patients. The diagnosis can be established by bone marrow aspiration, which documents prominent collections of immature plasma cells.

Peripheral neuropathy is a rare complication of multiple myeloma, and when present, it is more likely due to associated amyloidosis than a remote effect of the multiple myeloma. However, an axon loss polyneuropathy as well as an acquired SD polyneuropathy may occur as a remote effect. The precise pathogenesis of the polyneuropathy is unknown, but mechanisms similar to those proposed for MGUS polyneuropathy may be operative.

Epidemiology and Risk Factors. Patients with polyneuropathy secondary to multiple myeloma tend to present at a younger age than patients with multiple myeloma without polyneuropathy.[49] Most reports document a prominent male predominance in the patients with neuropathy. In the majority of patients, polyneuropathy is the presenting sign of the multiple myeloma and, in fact, may predate the diagnosis of multiple myeloma for many months or years. It is extremely rare for multiple myeloma to affect women of childbearing age, and thus there is no known influence or risk associated with pregnancy.

Clinical Features and Associated Disorders. Multiple myeloma typically produces a chronic, slowly progressive, symmetrical, sensorimotor polyneuropathy. However, in some patients, a more rapid evolution may occur with prominent motor weakness that can evolve to quadriparesis with respiratory involvement. Rarely, cranial nerve involvement, characterized by facial weakness or ophthalmoplegia, may be observed. Generalized hyporeflexia or areflexia is a common finding. Autonomic involvement seldom occurs, and when present in a patient with multiple myeloma, it raises the more likely possibility of an underlying amyloid neuropathy.

There are no additional disorders that are directly associated with the polyneuropathy secondary to multiple myeloma. However, the clinical disorders that often accompany multiple myeloma may be present. These include metabolic abnormalities such as anemia, leukocytosis, thrombocytosis, hypercalcemia, hyperuricemia, and chronic renal failure. Amyloidosis is also a common associated disorder that may itself produce a polyneuropathy with prominent small fiber involvement characterized by burning dysesthesia and pain as well as by generalized dysautonomia. Direct involvement of bone marrow by multiple myeloma may result in compression fractures of the spine, which, in turn, may cause compressive myelopathy, compressive radiculopathies, or both.

Differential Diagnosis. The differential diagnosis of an acquired SD polyneuropathy occurring in the setting of multiple myeloma is identical to that already described for CIDP. In particular, the presence of an M-protein and an acquired SD polyneuropathy requires a careful, methodical evaluation for multiple myeloma, osteosclerotic myeloma, lymphoma, macroglobulinemia, and MGUS. HIV testing should be performed in patients at risk.

Evaluation. The EDX examination shows evidence of a chronic, acquired SD polyradiculoneuropathy. The presence of an M-protein in the serum or urine occurs in nearly all patients. General laboratory studies in multiple myeloma may sometimes disclose evidence of anemia, chronic renal failure, hypercalcemia, and occasionally hyperuricemia, leukocytosis, and thrombocytosis. Skeletal survey may disclose osteolytic or occasionally osteoblastic lesions in approximately two thirds of patients. However, the diagnosis of multiple myeloma is made on bone marrow aspiration, which demonstrates increased numbers of immature plasma cells in the bone marrow. As noted earlier, the presence of a polyneuropathy in a patient with multiple myeloma is more likely to be due to amyloidosis. Confirmation of systemic amyloidosis with appropriate biopsy of such tissues as the rectal mucosa or abdominal fat pad may be helpful; however, sural nerve biopsy for amyloid may provide definitive evidence of amyloidosis as the mechanism of the underlying polyneuropathy. Amyloid neuropathy can be distinguished from polyneuropathy associated with multiple myeloma by EDX testing, which typically discloses changes of axon loss rather than demyelination.

Management. The treatment of acquired SD polyneuropathy caused by multiple myeloma consists of optimal treatment of the myeloma. This usually involves chemotherapy, typically with steroids and melphalan. In some patients, as the multiple myeloma clinically improves with treatment, the polyneuropathy does also. In others, however, the polyneuropathy may persist or worsen despite successful treatment of the multiple myeloma. In patients with isolated plasmacytoma, local surgery or radiation therapy may result in satisfactory improvement in the polyneuropathy.[49]

Prognosis and Future Perspectives. The published data are insufficient to define clearly the specific prognosis of acquired SD polyneuropathy occurring in the setting of multiple myeloma. Obviously, patients with associated systemic amyloidosis have a poorer prognosis than patients with polyneuropathy due solely to the remote effect of multiple myeloma.[45]

Much is yet to be learned regarding the pathogenesis of the polyneuropathies associated with multiple myeloma. In particular, the role of the M-protein in their pathogenesis and the possibility of an immune-mediated pathophysiology needs to be carefully explored. However, owing to their rare occurrence, it has been difficult to amass enough clinical experience to define properly the clinical and pathogenetic mechanisms of these heterogeneous disorders.

Osteosclerotic Myeloma

Pathogenesis and Pathophysiology. Osteosclerotic myeloma may be considered a rare variant of multiple myeloma, comprising only 3 percent of all patients with myeloma. Many of the typical features of multiple myeloma, including anemia, hypercalcemia, chronic renal failure, fatigue, weakness, and bone pain, are rare or at least uncommon in osteosclerotic myeloma. Furthermore, the level of M-protein is lower, and there are fewer plasma cells in the bone marrow. In contrast to multiple myeloma, however, an associated polyneuropathy is relatively common in osteosclerotic myeloma, occurring in over 50 percent of patients.[45] Furthermore, the polyneuropathy associated with osteosclerotic myeloma may frequently be a component of the so-called POEMS syndrome.[50]

The precise pathophysiology of the polyneuropathy associated with osteosclerotic myeloma and the multi-organ features of POEMS syndrome is unknown. It is likely that the plasma cells secrete an immunoglobulin or some other substance that may cause both the polyneuropathy and the other systemic features of POEMS syndrome.[50]

Epidemiology and Risk Factors. Patients with polyneuropathies secondary to osteosclerotic myeloma typically range in age from the late fourth decade through the seventh decade with a mean age in the late fifth decade. There is a rather prominent predilection for the disorder to occur in males. For the preceding reasons, it would be exceedingly rare for this disorder to occur in women of childbearing age.

Clinical Features and Associated Disorders. The clinical features of polyneuropathy associated with osteosclerotic myeloma typically conform to those of a rather chronic, progressive sensorimotor polyneuropathy. In the majority of patients, the polyneuropathy progresses to the point of rather remarkable weakness involving proximal as well as distal muscles and may result in significant disability. Typically, weakness is a more prominent symptom than sensory impairment. Autonomic symptoms are rare, and cranial nerve involvement is absent except for instances of papilledema. General systemic symptoms of bone pain, fatigue, and weakness typical of multiple myeloma usually are not seen.[50]

The neurological examination typically discloses prominent weakness that is worse distally but with occasional proximal involvement. Sensory loss is less prominent and tends to affect the large fiber modalities of touch pressure, joint position sense, and vibratory sensation more so than smaller fiber modalities of pain and temperature. Papilledema may be seen in up to 50 percent of patients.[50]

One or more additional features of the POEMS syndrome often are observed, but in many cases, these are not prominent and must be carefully sought. Hepatomegaly may be found in up to 50 percent of patients, whereas lymphadenopathy and splenomegaly are less common. Manifestations of endocrinopathy include diabetes mellitus, hypothyroidism, impotence, gynecomastia, testicular atrophy, amenorrhea, hyperprolactinemia, and hyperestrogenemia. Skin changes include hyperpigmentation, thickening of the skin, hypertrichosis, skin angiomas, clubbing, and white nails. Some skin changes are suggestive of scleroderma. Peripheral edema, ascites, and pleural effusions may also be seen. POEMS syndrome, sometimes referred to as Crow-Fukase syndrome, is not unique to osteosclerotic myeloma. It has been observed in multiple myeloma, Waldenström's macroglobulinemia, and angiofollicular lymph node hyperplasia, also referred to as Castleman's disease.[50]

Differential Diagnosis. In nearly all patients with polyneuropathy associated with osteosclerotic myeloma, the diagnosis is made during a comprehensive evaluation for a cryptogenic polyneuropathy. The findings on EDX examination of features consistent with an acquired SD polyneuropathy provide the differential diagnosis of CIDP and the related disorders, as noted earlier. Furthermore, the presence of an M-protein necessitates a hematological evaluation, which encompasses skeletal bone study and bone marrow aspirate. Careful attention to the possibility of the systemic features of the POEMS syndrome can yield important clues to the diagnosis of polyneuropathy associated with osteosclerotic myeloma.

Evaluation. Typically, the fact that there are EDX changes suggestive of an acquired SD polyradiculoneuropathy will already have been determined. The M-protein associated with osteosclerotic myeloma is usually IgG or IgA and is almost always of the lambda light chain type.[45] The concentration is typically low and rarely more than 3 g/dL, the usual range seen in multiple myeloma. An important point is that approximately 25 percent of patients with osteosclerotic myeloma may not have an M-protein detected in the serum or urine.[45] Thus, to evaluate a patient properly for this disorder, a skeletal survey is essential to uncover osteosclerotic lesions, the hallmark of the syndrome. These lesions typically involve the spine, pelvis, ribs, and proximal long bones of the limbs; occasionally they are not prominent and may be misinterpreted as benign bone sclerosis. Usually, the bony lesions show both osteosclerotic and lytic changes—sometimes they have the appearance of an osteosclerotic rim around a lytic lesion. The CSF usually is normal, except for an elevation of protein comparable to that noted in CIDP. EDX studies show features of an acquired SD polyneuropathy, although in some patients, axonal degeneration may be prominent. Sural nerve biopsies typically show combinations of both axon loss and segmental demyelination with occasional small foci of inflammatory cell infiltrates in the perivascular epineurium. Bone marrow aspirate usually discloses less than 5 percent of plasma cells. Routine laboratory studies most often are unrevealing, although thrombocytosis may be observed in nearly half of patients, with other features, including leukocytosis and polycythemia, present in a smaller number of patients.

Management. Patients with solitary osteosclerotic lesions appear to have the very best response to therapy. Local radiation of single or multiple lesions may result in substantial improvement in the polyneuropathy in the majority of patients. In patients with multiple osteosclerotic lesions, chemotherapy may result in improvement and stabilization of the polyneuropathy, although the responses appear to be less satisfactory than in those with isolated osteosclerotic lesions.

Prognosis and Future Perspectives. The polyneuropathy associated with osteosclerotic myeloma tends to be slowly progressive and may produce rather prominent generalized weakness and considerable disability, including wheelchair or bed confinement. The majority of patients with isolated osteosclerotic lesions respond to treatment, demonstrating stabilization, if not improvement, of their polyneuropathies. Patients with multiple osteosclerotic lesions do not respond as well.

Future research into this entity must provide a unifying pathophysiology that can explain the multisystem involvement of the POEMS syndrome. The pathogenetic role of the M-protein lambda light chain is a likely candidate for further study. From a clinical viewpoint, a more systematic study of the optimal mode of therapy is needed. However, the relatively rare occurrence of this entity will make it difficult to perform controlled therapeutic trials.

Waldenström's Macroglobulinemia

Waldenström's macroglobulinemia is a chronic lymphoproliferative disorder characterized by a clonal proliferation of B lymphocytes or lymphoplasmacytic cells in bone marrow or in lymph nodes, or both, and a high concentration of monoclonal IgM M-protein, typically exceeding 3 g/dL. In addition to the clinical features caused by the circulating macroglobulin, including hyperviscosity syndrome and cryoglobulinemic features, a polyneuropathy occurs in approximately one third of patients.[51] Half of all those with polyneuropathy are positive for anti-MAG antibodies.[45] In this latter group of patients, the pathophysiology of the polyneuropathy may be similar to that seen with MGUS IgM anti-MAG–positive polyneuropathy. However, a more heterogenous group of polyneuropathies, predominantly axon loss in type but occasionally demyelinating, may be encountered in those patients who are anti-MAG negative, similar to what is observed in the other IgM MGUS polyneuropathies. The pathophysiology of these polyneuropathies also is similar to that noted for the MGUS polyneuropathies without anti-MAG activity. Waldenström's macroglobulinemia tends to occur in the middle to older age groups, with a mean age of onset in the early seventh decade, and there is a slight male predominance. The late age of onset essentially precludes it occurring in pregnant women.

The clinical features of the demyelinating polyneuropathy associated with macroglobulinemia and anti-MAG activity is essentially identical to that noted in MGUS IgM anti-MAG–positive patients.[45] The disorder typically is a chronic sensorimotor polyneuropathy with prominent sensory involvement, including sensory ataxia. Other peripheral nerve syndromes may occur in macroglobulinemia, however, including asymmetrical mononeuropathy associated with cryoglobulinemia and a rather typical amyloid polyneuropathy. A hyperviscosity syndrome may occur in 15 percent of patients with macroglobulinemia, usually in the setting of an underlying lymphoma.[51] This syndrome produces a wide spectrum of symptoms, including general fatigue, blurred vision, and dizziness. Blurred vision may be secondary to distended retinal veins, retinal hemorrhages, and papilledema. Easy bleeding of mucous membranes is also observed and usually is due to abnormal platelet function induced by the IgM M-protein. In addition, the IgM M-protein may function as a cryoglobulin and contribute to other systemic symptoms, including renal disease, altered liver function studies, arthralgia, Raynaud's syndrome, and cryoglobulinemic neuropathy.[51] Moreover, a chronic hemolytic anemia occurs in approximately 10 percent of patients. Nearly one third of patients have lymphadenopathy or splenomegaly.

The presence of a high concentration of IgM M-protein in the context of an acquired SD polyneuropathy requires a careful evaluation for lymphoproliferative disorders. This usually necessitates skeletal bone survey to assess for multiple myeloma and osteosclerotic myeloma as well as bone marrow aspiration. The presence of lymphadenopathy and organomegaly coupled with the other systemic features of macroglobulinemia provide the key clinical clues to the diagnosis.

Evidence of an acquired SD polyradiculoneuropathy should be found on EDX studies. The evaluation of patients with IgM M-protein and acquired SD polyneuropathy is identical to that described for MGUS polyneuropathy. Testing for anti-MAG activity is essential to identify the subset of patients with macroglobulinemia who may have a more specific immune-mediated disorder. Results of nerve biopsies and CSF analysis are similar to those seen in MGUS IgM anti-MAG polyneuropathy. Routine laboratory studies in patients with macroglobulinemia often disclose anemia, monoclonal blood lymphocytosis, and Bence Jones proteinuria as well as elevated serum beta-microglobulin in nearly half of patients. Also, the presence of cryoglobulins is not an uncommon finding. Diagnosis is confirmed by the presence of a high concentration of IgM M-protein in the setting of underlying lymphoma characterized by infiltration of bone marrow, lymph nodes, and spleen.

Waldenström's macroglobulinemia typically is treated with combinations of chemotherapy and plasmapheresis. Chemotherapy for underlying lymphoma often incorporates a combination of an alkylating agent and a glucocorticoid. Plasma exchange often is recommended for patients who develop polyneuropathy and in those with clinical features of hyperviscosity syndrome and cryoglobulinemia.[51] Waldenström's macroglobulinemia is a serious disease with a median survival time of approximately 4 years. Therapeutic intervention with chemotherapy and plasmapheresis may be helpful in stabilizing or improving the associated polyneuropathy.

Multifocal Motor Neuropathy with Conduction Block

Pathogenesis and Pathophysiology. Multifocal motor neuropathy (MMN) with conduction block, sometimes referred to as motor neuropathy with multifocal conduction block, is a rare disorder that is characterized by asymmetrical motor weakness and EDX features of acquired SD lesions affecting one or more localized segments of motor nerve fibers. Its pathogenesis is unknown, but an immune-mediated mechanism is supported by pathological features of inflammatory demyelinating changes, favorable clinical response to immunosuppressant and immune-modulating therapies, and many striking similarities with CIDP.[52] Pathological features include demyelination, occasionally with evidence of remyelination in the form of onion bulb formation, and perivascular inflammatory infiltrates, primarily of lymphocytes. These changes have been observed in cranial nerves as well as in proximal and distal segments of peripheral nerves examined at autopsy.[53] Although motor fiber involvement is responsible for most of the clinical and EDX features, similar pathological changes of demyelination with inflammation also have been reported in sensory nerves, including sural nerve specimens examined at nerve biopsy. Reflecting this, occasionally sensory NCS abnormalities are seen.

Antibodies to the GM_1 ganglioside have been reported in a high percentage of patients with MMN.[52] This factor has led to the concept that these antibodies are playing a pathogenetic role in this disorder. However, direct evidence in support of this proposal is lacking.[54] Furthermore, the presence of anti-GM_1 antibodies is relatively nonspecific, because they can be found in a wide range of other neuromuscular disorders. Very high titers of GM_1 antibody appear to have greater specificity for lower motor neuron syndromes, including MMN.[55] Nonetheless, patients with MMN who do not have antibodies to GM_1 still respond to immune-modulating therapies. This field is rapidly evolving. It is possible that the presence of antibodies to GM_1 and other antigens may eventually prove more useful in the diagnosis of lower motor neuron syndromes, including MMN.[55]

Epidemiology and Risk Factors. MMN is a rare disorder. The age of onset spans many decades, from the teenage years through late adult life, but the condition tends to begin in young adults. There is a slight male predominance. There is no known predilection for this disorder to affect women during pregnancy or to worsen during pregnancy or in the postpartum period.

Clinical Features and Associated Disorders. MMN characteristically is a progressive disorder that causes multifocal and asymmetrical weakness and occasionally muscular atrophy accompanied by cramps and sometimes fasciculations.[52] This disorder often begins in the upper extremities, and although it may spread to involve the lower extremities, it may remain localized to or more prominent in the upper extremities throughout its course. Whereas some weakened muscles may be atrophic, other involved muscles may be of normal bulk despite chronic weakness, a clinical sign suggesting that SD conduction block is the mechanism of weakness rather than axon loss. Cranial nerve involvement is uncommon, although atrophy and weakness of the tongue and other bulbar symptoms and signs have been noted. Even though the condition predominately affects motor function, most patients will eventually experience sensory symptoms, including a sense of numbness or tingling, often in the absence of objective sensory loss. Sensory symptoms and signs are most common in patients with long-standing MMN. The DTRs frequently are absent or depressed in the distribution of the affected nerves, but surprisingly, they are sometimes preserved.

MMN typically follows a very chronic indolent course that may span many years. On occasion, the disease appears episodic, with patients having a stable nonprogressive course lasting many months or years before another episode develops. Alternatively, some patients have a more subacute course that may lead to rather prominent widespread weakness and disability over several months. Rare instances of CNS involvement have been reported in patients with typical MMN. However, these clinical features are usually modest and seldom resemble the combined features of upper and lower motor neuron disease noted in amyotrophic lateral sclerosis (ALS).[52]

Differential Diagnosis. Many of the clinical and EDX features of MMN bear a close similarity to CIDP and related disorders. In fact, MMN has been regarded by some as a variant of CIDP.[52] Thus, patients presenting with predominately motor weakness accompanied by EDX features of acquired SD need to be assessed for the same conditions included in the differential diagnosis of CIDP. As noted earlier, MMN may on occasion resemble MADSAM. However, it is important to differentiate MMN from MADSAM, as the latter condition more closely resembles typical CIDP. Unlike MMN, in MADSAM sensory symptoms and signs may be noted early in its course, the CSF protein is often elevated, anti-GM_1 antibodies are absent, and patients may respond to all of the typical therapies known to be effective in CIDP.[35] In addition, some patients with MMN may superficially resemble patients with motor neuron disease or ALS. Usually, MMN can be differentiated from these disorders by its more chronic and indolent course, the absence of upper motor neuron symptoms and signs, and most important, the presence of acquired SD features on EDX testing.

Evaluation. Because MMN may represent a variant of CIDP, it is important to evaluate patients with MMN in the same fashion as patients with possible CIDP. A careful search for an M-protein, skeletal bone survey for osteosclerotic or osteolytic lesions, and HIV testing in patients at risk should be considered in patients with clinical features suggesting MMN. The CSF is usually normal in all aspects, including its protein content, thereby signifying the predilection of MMN to involve peripheral nerves rather than spinal nerve roots. The majority of patients with MMN will have high titers of anti-GM_1 antibodies. As noted earlier, the presence of the anti-GM_1 antibody is not specific to MMN and is not required for the diagnosis. The EDX features of this disorder provide its laboratory confirmation: They disclose evidence of multifocal conduction block, generally confined to motor fibers (see Fig. 49–2). Typically, the lesion sites are not common locations for entrapment or compressive neuropathies; for example, a focal conduction block may be found along the ulnar nerve in the forearm, rather than at the elbow.

Management. Because MMN is a rare disorder, the data are limited regarding the efficacy of the various available treatment modalities. Anecdotal reports suggest that prednisone, azathioprine, and plasmapheresis rarely are effective. However, both IVIg and high-dose intravenous cyclophosphamide may be of benefit.[52, 56] Randomized, double-blinded, placebo-controlled trial data have confirmed the efficacy of IVIg in MMN.[57, 58] Clearly, IVIg is the preferred treatment over IV cyclophosphamide, owing to the greater risks and complications of the latter drug. In a fashion similar to CIDP, IVIg may be administered periodically to maintain clinical improvement. It should be emphasized that the treatment of MMN must be individualized. Many patients with MMN, for example, have very modest clinical symptoms that persist unchanged for many years. The appropriate management of such patients may be observation alone rather than have them undergo the risk and expense of IVIg or cyclophosphamide treatments.

Prognosis and Future Perspectives. The rarity of this disease and its relatively recent initial description in 1982 are factors that limit experience with its natural history. Nevertheless, most patients with MMN seem to display a chronic, slowly progressive or stable course over many years. With the advent of IVIg treatment as well as intravenous cyclophosphamide, it is likely that in many patients the disorder can be stabilized, resulting in modest, if any, disability.

Key fundamental issues to be resolved regarding MMN include its precise pathophysiology, including the role of anti-GM_1 antibodies and its relationship to CIDP. From a clinical perspective, more experience is required to better formulate optimal therapeutic interventions.

Reviews and Selected Updates

Arnason BGW, Soliven B: Acute inflammatory demyelinating polyradiculoneuropathy. *In* Dyck PJ, Thomas PK, Griffin JW, et al (eds): Peripheral Neuropathy, 3rd ed. Philadelphia, WB Saunders, 1993, p 1437.

Cornblath DR, Sumner AJ, Daube J, et al: Conduction block in clinical practice. Muscle Nerve 1991;14:869–871.

Hahn AF: Guillain-Barré syndrome: An evolving concept: Editorial review. Curr Opin Neurol 1997;10:363–365.

Hartung H-P, van der Meché FGA, Pollard JD: Guillain-Barré syndrome, CIDP and other chronic immune-mediated neuropathies. Curr Opin Neurol 1998;11:497–513.

O'Leary CP, Willison HJ: Autoimmune ataxic neuropathies (sensory ganglionopathies). Curr Opin Neurol 1997;10:366–370.

Pollard JM: Chronic inflammatory demyelinating polyradiculoneuropathy. Curr Opin Neurol 2002;15:279–283.

Van der Meché FGA, Vermeulen M, Busch HFM: Chronic inflammatory demyelinating polyneuropathy. Brain 1989;112:1563–1571.

References

1. Asbury AK: Guillain-Barré syndrome: Historical concepts. Ann Neurol 1990;27:S2–S6.
2. Hughes RAC: Guillain-Barré Syndrome. London, Springer-Verlag, 1990.
3. Parry GJ: Guillain-Barré Syndrome. New York, Thieme Medical Publishers, 1993.
4. Ropper AH, Wijdicks EPM, Truax BT: Guillain-Barré Syndrome. Philadelphia, F.A. Davis, 1991.
5. Dyck PJ, Lais AC, Ohta M, et al: Chronic inflammatory polyradiculoneuropathy. Mayo Clin Proc 1975;50:621–637.
6. Mitsumoto H, Bradley WG: Structure and development of nerves. *In* Vinkin PJ, Bruyn GW, Klawans HL, Matthews WB (eds): Neuropathies: Handbook of Clinical Neurology, Vol. 51. Amsterdam, Elsevier Science, 1987, pp 1–22.
7. Wilbourn AJ: The electromyographic examination. *In* Rothman RH, Simeone FA (eds): The Spine, 3rd ed. Philadelphia, WB Saunders, 1992, pp 155–172.
8. Sivak M, Ochoa J, Fernadez JM: Positive manifestations of nerve fiber dysfunction: Clinical, electrophysiologic, and pathologic correlates. *In* Brown WF, Bolton CF (eds): Clinical Electromyography, 2nd ed. Boston, Butterworth-Heinemann, 1993, pp 117–147.
9. Asbury AK, Thomas PK: The clinical approach to neuropathy. *In* Asbury AK, Thomas PK (eds): Peripheral Nerve Disorders, 2nd ed. Boston, Butterworth-Heinemann, 1995, pp 1–28.
10. Wilbourn AJ: Nerve conduction studies in axonopathies and demyelinating neuropathies. Syllabus: 1989 AAEE Course A: Fundamentals of Electrodiagnosis. Rochester, MN, American Association of Electromyography and Electrodiagnosis, 1989, pp 7–20.
11. Albers JW, Donofrio PD, McGonagle TK: Sequential electrodiagnostic abnormalities in acute inflammatory demyelinating polyradiculoneuropathy. Muscle Nerve 1985;8:528–539.
12. Cornblath DR: Electrophysiology in Guillain-Barré syndrome. Ann Neurol 1990;27(Suppl):S17–S20.
13. Thomas PK: The Guillain-Barré syndrome: No longer a simple concept. J Neurol 1992;239:361–362.
14. Griffin JW, Ho TW: The Guillain-Barré syndrome at 75: The *Campylobacter* connection. (Editorial.) Ann Neurol 1993;34:125–127.
15. Feasby TE, Gilbert JJ, Brown WF, et al: An acute axonal form of Guillain-Barré polyneuropathy. Brain 1986;109:1115–1126.
16. Griffin JW, Li CY, Ho TW, et al: Guillain-Barré syndrome in northern China. Brain 1995;118:577–595.
17. Visser LH, Van der Meché FGA, Van Doorn PA, et al: Guillain-Barré syndrome without sensory loss (acute motor neuropathy). Brain 1995;118:841–847.
18. Hughes RAC, Hadden RDM, Gregson NA, Smith KJ: Pathogenesis of Guillain-Barré syndrome. J Neuroimmunol 1999;100:74–97.
19. Hartung H-P, Pollard JD, Harvey GK, Toyka KV: Immunopathogenesis and treatment of the Guillain-Barré syndrome—Parts 1 & 2. Muscle Nerve 1995;18:137–153, 154–164.
20. Asbury AK: New concepts of Guillain-Barré syndrome. J Child Neurol 2000;15:183–191.

21. Oh SJ, Laganke C, Claussen GC: Sensory Guillain-Barré syndrome. Neurology 2001;56:82–86.
22. Hughes RAC: Sensory form of Guillain-Barré syndrome. Lancet 2001;357:1465.
23. Gordon PH, Wilbourn AJ: Early electrodiagnostic findings in Guillain-Barré syndrome. Arch Neurol 2001;58:913–917.
24. Ropper AH: Intensive care of acute Guillain-Barré syndrome. Can J Neurol Sci 1994;21:S23–S27.
25. Teitelbaum JS, Borel CO: Respiratory dysfunction in Guillain-Barré syndrome. Clin Chest Med 1994;15:705–714.
26. Hund EF, Borel CO, Cornblath DR, et al: Intensive management and treatment of severe Guillain-Barré syndrome. Crit Care Med 1993;21:433–446.
27. Prineas JW, McLeod JG: Chronic relapsing polyneuritis. J Neurol Sci 1976;27:427–458.
28. Dyck PJ, Prineas J, Pollard J: Chronic inflammatory demyelinating polyradiculoneuropathy. *In* Dyck PJ, Thomas PK (eds): Peripheral Neuropathy. Philadelphia, WB Saunders, 1993, pp 1498–1517.
29. Koski CL: Guillain-Barré syndrome and chronic inflammatory demyelinating polyneuropathy: Pathogenesis and treatment. Semin Neurol 1994;14:123–130.
30. Yan WX, Taylor J, Andrias-Kauba S, et al: Passive transfer of demyelination by serum or IgG from chronic inflammatory demyelinating polyneuropathy patients. Ann Neurol 2000;47:765–775.
31. Yan WX, Archelos JJ, Hartung H-P, et al: P0 protein is a target antigen in chronic inflammatory demyelinating polyradiculoneuropathy. Ann Neurol 2001;50:286–292.
32. Feasby TE: Axonal CIDP: A premature concept? Muscle Nerve 1996;19:372–374.
33. McCombe PA, McManis PE, Frith JA, et al: Chronic inflammatory demyelinating polyradiculoneuropathy associated with pregnancy. Ann Neurol 1987;21:102–104.
34. Midroni G, Dyck PJ: Chronic inflammatory demyelinating polyradiculoneuropathy: Unusual clinical features and therapeutic responses. Neurology 1996;46:1206–1212.
35. Saperstein DS, Katz JS, Amato AA, et al: Clinical spectrum of chronic acquired demyelinating polyneuropoathies. Muscle Nerve 2001;24: 311–324.
36. Saperstein DS, Amato AA, Wolfe GI, et al: Multifocal acquired demyelinating sensory and motor neuropathy: The Lewis-Sumner syndrome. Muscle Nerve 1999;22:560–566.
37. Mendell JR, Kolkin S, Kissel JT, et al: Evidence for central nervous system demyelination in chronic inflammatory demyelinating polyradiculoneuropathy. Neurology 1987;37:1291–1294.
38. Dyck PJ, O'Brien PC, Oviatt KF, et al: Prednisone improves chronic inflammatory demyelinating polyradiculoneuropathy more than no treatment. Ann Neurol 1982;11:136–141.
39. Dyck PJ, Daube J, O'Brien P, et al: Plasma exchange in chronic inflammatory demyelinating polyradiculoneuropathy. N Engl J Med 1986;314:461–465.
40. Dyck PJ, Litchy WJ, Kratz KM, et al: A plasma exchange versus immune globulin infusion trial in chronic inflammatory demyelinating polyradiculoneuropathy. Ann Neurol 1994;36:838–845.
41. Lindenbaum Y, Kissel JT, Mendell JR: Treatment approaches for Guillain-Barré syndrome and chronic inflammatory demyelinating polyradiculoneuropathy. Neurol Clin 2001;19:187–204.
42. Simmons Z, Albers JW, Bromberg MB, Feldman EL: Long-term follow-up of patients with chronic inflammatory polyradiculoneuropathy, without and with monoclonal gammopathy. Brain 1995;118:359–368.
43. Kyle RA: Monoclonal proteins in neuropathy. Neurol Clin 1992;10:713–735.
44. Latov N: Evaluation and treatment of patients with neuropathy and monoclonal gammopathy. Semin Neurol 1994;14:118–122.
45. Bosch EP, Smith BE: Peripheral neuropathies associated with monoclonal proteins. Med Clin North Am 1993;77:125–139.
46. Smith IS: The natural history of chronic demyelinating neuropathy associated with benign IgM paraproteinemia. A clinical and neurophysiological study. Brain 1994;117:949–957.
47. Kaku DA, England JD, Sumner AJ: Distal accentuation of conduction slowing in polyneuropathy associated with antibodies to myelin-associated glycoprotein and sulphated glucuronyl paragloboside. Brain 1994;117:941–947.
48. Dyck PJ, Low PA, Windebank AJ, et al: Plasma exchange in polyneuropathy associated with monoclonal gammopathy of undetermined significance. N Engl J Med 1991;325:1482–1486.
49. Delauche MC, Clauvel JP, Seligmann M: Peripheral neuropathy and plasma cell neoplasias: A report of 10 cases. Br J Haematol 1981;48:383–392.
50. Soubrier MJ, Dubost J-J, Sauvezie BJM: French Study Group on POEMS Syndrome: A study of 25 cases and a review of the literature. Am J Med 1994;97:543–553.
51. Diniopoulos MA, Alexanian R: Waldenström's macroglobulinemia. Blood 1994;83:1452–1459.
52. Parry GJ, Sumner AJ: Multifocal motor neuropathy. Neurol Clin 1992;10:671–684.
53. Oh SJ, Claussen GC, Odabasi Z, Palmer CP: Multifocal demyelinating motor neuropathy: Pathologic evidence of "inflammatory demyelinating polyradiculoneuropathy." Neurology 1995;45:1828–1832.
54. Parry GJ: Anti-ganglioside antibodies do not necessarily play a role in multifocal motor neuropathy. Muscle Nerve 1994;17:97–99.
55. Kornberg AJ, Pestronk A: The clinical and diagnostic role of anti-GM_1 antibody testing. Muscle Nerve 1994;17:100–104.
56. Nobile-Orazio E, Meucci N, Barbieri S, et al: High-dose intravenous immunoglobulin therapy in multifocal motor neuropathy. Neurology 1993;43:537–544.
57. Federico P, Zochodne DW, Hahn AF, et al: Multifocal motor neuropathy improved by IVIg: Randomized, double-blind, placebo-controlled study. Neurology 2000;55:1256–1262.
58. Leger JM, Chassande B, Musset L, et al: Intravenous immunoglobulin therapy in multifocal motor neuropoathy: A double-blind, placebo-controlled study. Brain 2001;124:145–153.

CHAPTER 50

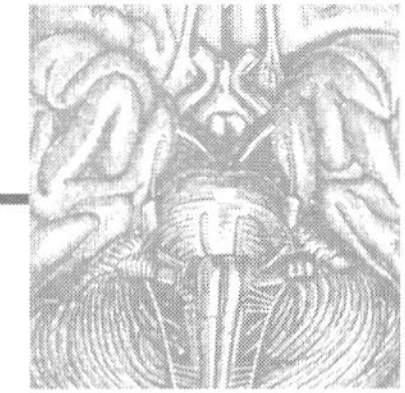

RUSSELL BARTT and KATHLEEN M. SHANNON

Autoimmune and Inflammatory Disorders

History and Definitions

Pathological disorders mediated by immune processes directed against autologous tissues were first recognized in the early 1900s by Erlich, who used the term "horror autotoxicus" to describe this phenomenon. The first descriptions of necrotizing arteritis appeared in an 1852 treatise on aneurysms by Karl Rokitansky.[1] In 1866, the term periarteritis nodosa was used to describe a single patient with a typical histological appearance of necrotizing arteritis.[1] Most of the descriptions evolved in the 1940s and 1950s by people such as Jacob Churg and Friedreich Wegener. With few exceptions, these syndromes continue to be defined by the classic pathological appearance.

The ability of the immune system to differentiate between one's body and a wide variety of potential pathogens and toxins is remarkable. Under normal circumstances, the immune system may react against certain of its own tissues such as neoplasms and senescent red blood cells. While extensive growth in immunology has led to a better understanding of the pathophysiology of these diseases, often the etiology remains obscure.

Lymphocytes recognize foreign antigens through receptors on their surface, and the differentiation between self and nonself is essential to normal function. Several factors may account for this ability to avoid self-reactivity: self-directed T-lymphocytes may be deleted from the repertoire at an early age; self-antigens may not be presented to the lymphocytes in such a way as to induce an immune response; self-antigens may be in "immunologically privileged" tissues, which are not routinely exposed sufficiently to the circulating lymphocytes; or self-response may be downregulated by other components of the immune system.[2] It is believed that evasion of these mechanisms leads to autoimmune disease by one of the following pathways: (1) normal regulatory control to a given self-antigen may be lost or bypassed; (2) self-antigens may express major histocompatibility complexes II (MHC-II), normally present only on immunologically competent cells; these self-tissues may then present antigens to lymphocytes; or (3) a foreign antigen with a similar molecular structure may mimic a self-antigen and result in cross-reactivity.[2]

The autoimmune response may be directed at a relatively specific tissue antigen such as the acetylcholine receptor in myasthenia gravis (organ-specific response). Alternatively, the self-antigen may be in many tissues and be relatively nonorgan specific, causing diseases such as systemic lupus erythematosus.

Vasculitis is a common manifestation of a diverse group of diseases. Though they may result from etiologically and pathogenetically different diseases, all share the pathological finding of inflammation of the vessel wall. Tissue injury results from the occlusion of inflamed vessels. Vasculitides can be organized by the size of the vessels involved (e.g., large, medium, or small vessel vasculitis shown in Fig. 50–1) or by the predominant cell type involved, as discussed later.[1]

For *neutrophil-predominant vasculitis* to occur, an inflammatory stimulus must perturb the homeostasis of circulating leukocytes and endothelial cells. Adhesion to certain areas of the vasculature is induced by cytokine-stimulated expression of adhesion molecules (e.g., ICA-1, VCAM-1). In severe inflammation, there is mural necrosis with rupture and hemorrhage or leakage of plasma factors into tissues where soluble coagulation factors contact inflammatory debris causing fibrinoid necrosis.

Mononuclear-predominant vasculitis (lymphocytes, monocytes, macrophages) can occur as a discrete entity or can evolve from neutrophil-predominant vasculitis. Unlike neutrophils, monocytes have a regulatory role as well as an effector role in inflammation. Therefore, the histological demonstration of T-lymphocytes does not prove that the process is mediated by a T-lymphocyte immune response. Mononuclear-predominant vasculitis is seen in giant cell arteritis, Takayasu's arteritis, and primary angiitis of the central nervous system.

Immune complex vasculitis results from deposition of heterologous or autoantigen immune complexes in vessel walls either from the circulation or by in situ formation. Most circulating immune complexes are cleared from the circulation without causing vascular inflammation. Molecular size and electrical charge influence the ability to survive in the circulation and deposit in vessel walls. Medium-sized cationic particles are the most pathogenic.

Antineutrophil cytoplasmic antibodies (ANCA) are associated with some vasculitides that involve small vessels including epineural vessels. It is not known if ANCA cause the vasculitis or are an epiphenomenon. Peripheral neuropathies are frequently encountered in ANCA vasculitides, but it is unclear how many neuropathies are ANCA associated.

Infections can cause vasculitis by direct effects of the agents themselves and by the immune-mediated response. Infectious vasculitides will not be covered in this chapter.

Connective tissue diseases as a whole are syndromes with immunological reactivity to various tissue components. Clinically, however, there may be overlap with other autoimmune conditions. Tissue components of the vasculature may be involved, and a vasculitis may dominate the clinical picture. This is demonstrated by the frequent occurrence of mononeuritis multiplex in the connective tissue diseases, as a result of peripheral nerve ischemia secondary to inflammation of the vasa nervorum.

Other autoimmune conditions are not targeted at the vessels but are part of a connective tissue syndrome. Those disorders affecting the neurological system are discussed in the last section of this chapter.

Inflammatory Vasculopathies; Arteritis

EXTRACRANIAL GRANULOMATOUS ARTERITIS (GIANT CELL "TEMPORAL" ARTERITIS)

Pathogenesis and Pathophysiology. Giant cells are the pathological hallmark of this large vessel, T-cell–mediated vasculitis. CD4 cells aggregate with a response centered on the internal elastic lamina. These cells may contain elastic fiber fragments. Giant cell arteritis (GCA) affects the aorta and its branches, including the cervicocephalic arteries (carotid and vertebral), reflecting its predilection for the internal elastic lamina. Intracranial arteries are usually not involved, although proximal branches of the internal carotid artery have been lesioned. The superficial temporal artery

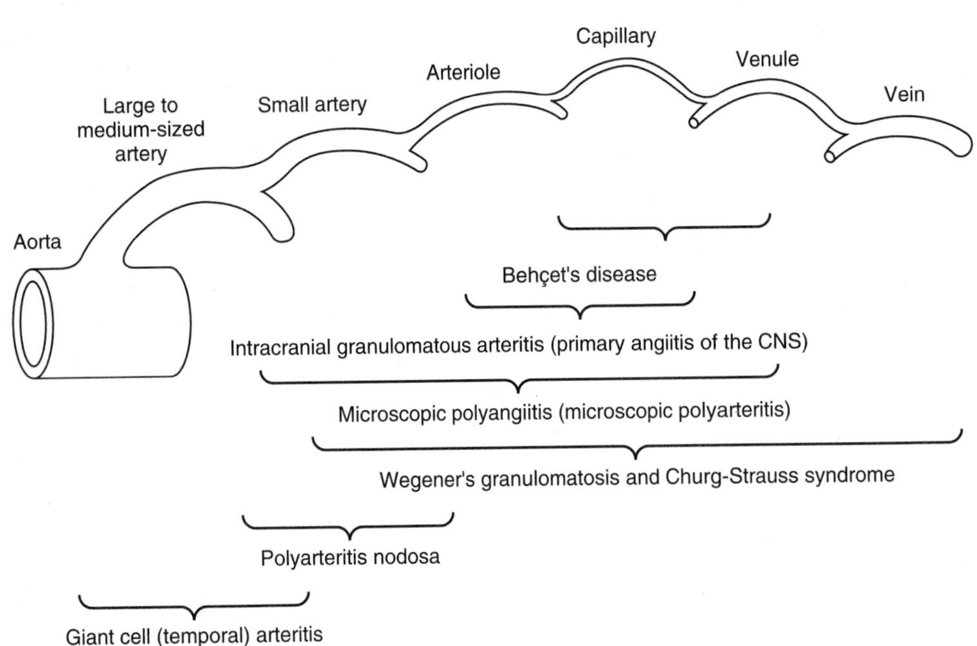

FIGURE 50–1. Classification of the vasculitides by vessel size. (Adapted from Jennette JC, Falk RJ: Clinical and pathological classification of ANCA-associated vasculitis: What are the controversies? Clin Exp Immunol 1995;101[Suppl 1]:18–22.)

and intraorbital branches of the carotid artery are involved in many cases. Vertebral arteries may be affected in very severe cases, though basilar artery involvement is rare. Aortic rupture can also occur. There is an overlap between GCA and polymyalgia rheumatica (PMR).

Epidemiology and Risk Factors. Age is a strong risk factor for disease. Maximum incidence is in the 70s with the median age of onset being 75,[3] and virtually no cases in the population less than 50 years of age. Overall, women have a higher age-adjusted incidence than men, 16.5 versus 5.7 per 100,000 per year of the U.S. population aged 50 and older.[3] The incidence rate reported has increased each decade from the 1950s into the 1970s. Additionally, the number of negative biopsies in cases suspected of having GCA has also increased. As opposed to an actual increase in the disease, an explanation for these findings may represent better identification of potential cases as a result of heightened awareness of the disease.[3] There has been a tendency to reclassify cases of PMR to GCA when the disease has been more aggressive, was accompanied by visual symptoms or headache, or was relatively resistant to low-dose corticosteroid therapy.

Clinical Features and Associated Disorders. GCA was first described in 1890, but was best described in 1932 as giant cell inflammation of the temporal artery with a systemic syndrome of fever, anorexia, weight loss, fatigue, and anemia. PMR was described as an illness of the elderly with proximal muscle pain and stiffness along with a systemic syndrome. PMR was felt to be a variant of rheumatoid arthritis, with synovitis but without rheumatoid factor. In time it became clear that there was overlap between GCA and PMR. However, the greater sensitivity of PMR to steroids contributed to continued separation of the two syndromes.[4] Most likely, both are part of a spectrum of disease characterized by variable degrees of synovitis and arteritis related to a common yet unknown etiopathogenic agent.[4] PMR occurs in 58 percent of patients with GCA and is the initial symptom in 25 percent. Criteria for the diagnosis of GCA and PMR are listed in Table 50–1.[5]

Pain is commonly experienced by patients with GCA. Headache, sometimes with scalp tenderness, occurs in 72 percent of patients and is present in 33 percent at the time of diagnosis.[6] Jaw claudication is an occasional feature. Neck or back pain is present in 25 percent of patients with GCA who do not have PMR.[6]

Vascular disease may manifest in several ways. Bruits may be audible over involved arteries. Carotid bruits occur in 10 to 20 percent and are frequently bilateral. Claudication or upper limb bruits occur in approximately 60 percent of patients, and about 40 percent of patients with carotid bruits will have some ischemic brain or eye complication. However, permanent visual loss and stroke occur with about the same frequency regardless of the presence of bruits.[6] About 4 percent of patients with GCA will experience a transient ischemic attack (TIA) or stroke (Chapters 22 and 45). The proportion of such events occurring in the vertebrobasilar circulation is greater in GCA patients than that seen in the general stroke population. Within the vertebrobasilar system, these events may not respect distinct vascular territories.[6] There are some reports of myelopathy in GCA, presumably from vertebral or anterior spinal artery involvement.[6]

The risk of blindness remains poorly defined in GCA and PMR. Overall, eye findings occur in 8 to 23 percent of people with GCA. Amaurosis fugax occurs in 10 to 12 percent. Anterior ischemic optic neuropathy results from posterior ciliary and, less frequently, retinal arteritis. Occasionally, the findings are entirely retrobulbar. However, acute optic disc edema followed by the development of optic pallor over 2 to 4 weeks may be seen.[6] Diplopia is seen in 2 to 14 percent of patients, usually related to extraocular muscle dysfunction, but rarely as a result of brain stem disease. Clinical findings may fluctuate daily as a characteristic feature.[6] When permanent visual loss occurs, the onset is typically abrupt, and within 2 weeks, contralateral involvement occurs in 25 to 50 percent of cases.[7]

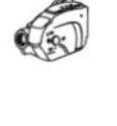

Vertigo or unilateral hearing loss may rarely be the result of an infarct of the vestibulocochlear nerve. Other cranial nerves, such as V, VII, or XII, have been affected in isolation or as part of a mononeuritis multiplex. Occasionally, other cranial neuropathies have occurred, causing facial pain, hemianesthesia of the tongue, or lingual paralysis.

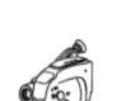

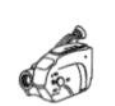

Peripheral nerve disorders are common in many of the vasculitides. Involvement of the vasa nervorum may result in a mononeuritis multiplex. Many areas of involvement of peripheral nerves may overlap, suggesting a distal symmetrical polyneuropathy.[6]

Although myalgia is a common symptom and localized inflammation has been described in patients with GCA, inflammatory myositis is not a recognized feature of the illness. Myopathy in GCA usually results from corticosteroid use (see Management).

Differential Diagnosis. Numerous symptoms occur in GCA that are not specific for the condition. Certainly, the

TABLE 50–1. **Criteria for the Diagnoses of Giant Cell Arteritis and Polymyalgia Rheumatica**

Giant Cell Arteritis (Must Meet All Five Criteria)	Polymyalgia Rheumatica (Must Meet All Seven Criteria)
1. Confirmatory biopsy	1. Shoulder/pelvic girdle muscle pain
2. Tenderness to palpation ± pulselessness in temporal artery	2. Morning stiffness
3. Any or all of:	3. Duration of symptoms for at least 2 weeks
visual disturbance	4. Absence of true arthritis
temporal or occipital headache	5. Absence of objective signs of muscle disease
jaw claudication	6. Westergren ESR >30 mm/hr OR C-reactive protein >6 μg/mL
4. Westergren ESR >30 mm/hr OR C-reactive protein >6 μg/mL	7. Prompt response to steroid therapy
5. Prompt response to steroid therapy	
Duration of symptoms for at least 2 weeks	

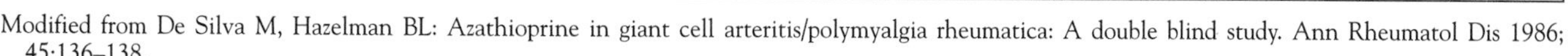

Modified from De Silva M, Hazelman BL: Azathioprine in giant cell arteritis/polymyalgia rheumatica: A double blind study. Ann Rheumatol Dis 1986; 45:136–138.

population that is at the greatest risk for the development of GCA is also at risk for atherosclerotic vascular disease. This situation presents problems in evaluating individual patients as well as interpreting the literature. The presence of constitutional symptoms such as weight loss and fevers and an elevated erythrocyte sedimentation rate (ESR), with or without a pain syndrome, should raise GCA as a serious consideration.

Evaluation. The examination in suspected GCA should include inspection, auscultation, and palpation of extracranial arteries. Blood pressure in both arms should be assessed for asymmetry. Routine blood work commonly shows anemia. Serological evaluation, including ESR, and C-reactive protein assessment are necessary.[3] Abnormalities of the temporal artery may be apparent on color duplex ultrasonography. Characteristic signs include a dark halo around the arterial lumen and stenoses or occlusions of temporal artery segments.[7] Angiography may demonstrate segmental stenosis or occlusion of the temporal artery. Superior temporal artery angiography is less reliable than biopsy.[6] Biopsy of the superficial temporal artery may show giant cells, but several sections usually need to be examined.[3]

Management. Early studies evaluating steroid efficacy were flawed and some do not reach statistical significance by today's standards. Overall, however, there appears to be a modest beneficial effect of high-dose steroids consistent with the understanding of the effect of steroids on other vasculitic syndromes.[4] The prevention of blindness is considered worth the approximately 50 percent risk of adverse effects (symptomatic vertebral collapse in 26%, myopathy in 17%) from steroid therapy.[4] Prednisone remains the mainstay of treatment with initial dose of 40 to 60 mg/d and treatment over the next few years. Tapering should be done slowly. In the rapidly deteriorating patient or one with a neurological syndrome, IV methylprednisolone can be used, typically 1 g/d divided into two to four doses. No well-controlled trials have examined differences in dosing regimens. If relapse occurs while tapering, then the target dose to taper to should be higher than the dose at the time of relapse. ESR monitoring is very helpful in determining relapses and responses to dose changes.[6]

A number of other immunosuppressives have been used, including azathioprine, methotrexate, dapsone, and cyclophosphamide, with inconsistent results. Cyclophosphamide may be the most consistently effective.[6] Azathioprine was compared in a double-blind fashion to placebo in GCA patients already taking prednisone. Because the immunosuppressive effect of azathioprine is delayed, a statistically significant difference in prednisone dose was reached only after 1 year of therapy.[5]

Prognosis and Future Perspectives. Although GCA can cause death, stroke, or myocardial infarction, the survival of GCA patients does not significantly differ from that of age-matched controls.[3] In a series of 21 GCA patients who died, in only one case was the cause of death attributed to GCA.[3] Catastrophic neurological sequelae such as blindness and stroke are uncommon and have been lessened in frequency by the use of steroids.

INTRACRANIAL GRANULOMATOUS ARTERITIS OR PRIMARY ANGIITIS OF THE CENTRAL NERVOUS SYSTEM

Pathogenesis and Pathophysiology. This disorder has carried a number of names, including noninfectious granulomatous angiitis with a predilection for the central nervous system (CNS), granulomatous angiitis of the CNS, primary angiitis of the CNS (PACNS), and vasculitis confined to the CNS. First described in 1959, very few cases were described antemortem until the widespread availability of angiography in the 1960s. The term PACNS is most appropriate because it requires the absence of a systemic disease but does not require the presence of granulomatous lesions.[8,9] Pathologically there are monocytes/histiocytes, lymphocytes, and plasma cells infiltrating the walls of small arteries, particularly in the leptomeninges.[10] In 85 percent of cases, multinucleated giant cells are seen among the inflammatory cells.[11] Small leptomeningeal arteries are preferentially affected, although occasional involvement of the internal carotid and vertebral arteries is seen. Numerous small foci of infarction are common, but there may be large areas of ischemia, sometimes with superimposed hemorrhage.[9] Unlike polyarteritis nodosa, there is no predilection for the branching points of arteries.[10] The etiology is unknown, but there is growing speculation of a viral cause. There is no evidence that the disease is mediated by immune complexes, although there may be a direct immune interaction at the level of the vessel wall.[9]

Epidemiology and Risk Factors. Most patients are young or middle aged (range, 3 to 74 years). In the literature, early cases suggested a female predominance of 2:1; however, currently there does not appear to be a gender difference.[12] The majority of cases do not have any identifiable pre-existing condition.

Clinical Features and Associated Disorders. Typically, the patient has a headache of gradual onset and a diffuse encephalopathy or dementia. Later, focal neurological signs develop. In one large review of 108 cases (including 99 from the literature), 53 percent of cases presented with both focal and diffuse findings, 32 percent with focal findings only, and 11.1 percent with diffuse findings only (Table 50–2).[13] Headache is the most common presenting symptom and is often associated with nausea and vomiting. Occasionally, cranial neuropathies, cerebellar dysfunction, and cauda equina syndromes have been the initial symptoms. Isolated cord involvement has been noted in a few patients. The syndrome may be acute or insidious and may fluctuate with periods of apparent remission. Systemic symptoms like fever, weight loss, arthralgias, and myalgias are typically absent and when present suggest an alternative diagnosis.[11]

It has been proposed that PACNS may fall into subgroups by clinical criteria.[11] According to these criteria, "true" PACNS lasts longer than 3 months, is characterized by focal and diffuse neurological dysfunction, and is associated with typical biopsy findings. The cerebrospinal fluid (CSF) is abnormal with a picture suggesting chronic meningitis. The outcome is poor if untreated. A more "benign angiopathy" of the CNS has an acute onset, normal CSF analyses, primary diagnosis by angiography, and a benign clinical course. Postpartum cerebral angiopathy has been described in women in the immediate postgravid state. There are eight well-documented cases in which headaches, nausea, vomiting, focal CNS signs, and abnormal CSF developed in women who showed no signs of toxemia or hypertension.[11] Cerebral angiography showed alternating areas of stenosis and ectasia with "sausaging" of multiple vessels. Normalization of angiography changes demonstrated by serial studies over 4 weeks suggests that the basis of the arteritis is

TABLE 50–2. **Clinical Features of Primary Angiitis of the Central Nervous System**

	Literature Cases N = 40	Cleveland Clinic Cases N = 8	Combined Cases N = 48
Mean age in years (range)	45 (3–74)	33 (10–73)	43 (3–74)
Sex ratio, M:F	21:18	4:4	25:23
Abrupt onset (%)	22 (56)	5 (62)	29 (60)
Signs and symptoms			
Focal	4 (10)	0	4 (8)
Diffuse	6 (15)	1 (12)	7 (14)
Both	29 (74)	7 (88)	38 (78)

Modified from Calabrese LH, Mallek JA: Primary angitis of the central nervous system. Medicine (Baltimore) 1987;67:20–39.

at least in part vasospastic.[11] The strength of the relationship between this condition and PACNS remains unclear.

PACNS associated with immunosuppressive illness represents a small subset of these cases, which include lymphomas, leukemias, myeloproliferative disorders, immunosuppressive therapy for inflammatory bowel disease or following renal transplant, and human immunodeficiency virus.[11] These are unique cases in which the immunosuppressed state may appear crucial to susceptibility to the condition.

Differential Diagnosis. Other small vessel vasculitides such as Wegener's granulomatosis have presented as temporal or CNS vasculitis. Pulmonary lesions should be helpful in this differential.[12] GCA occurs in an older population than PACNS. Those patients with PACNS affecting large and small arteries are older than those with small vessel involvement alone. Immunological or epitope changes may be related to age.[12] Infections and more systemic forms of vasculitis need to be considered in the differential diagnosis of PACNS. Tuberculosis and other mycobacteria, meningovascular syphilis, fungal infections, hepatitis B, and herpes ophthalmicus are other possibilities.[11] Drugs, particularly stimulants, can cause a vasculitis. Noninflammatory vasculopathies such as fibromuscular dysplasia and moyamoya may be considered, and these diagnoses are best addressed by angiography.[9]

Evaluation. Most important in the diagnosis of PACNS is appropriate clinical suspicion. The ESR is elevated in 66 percent of the patients, on average 44 mm/hr, ranging up to 116 mm/hr. The ESR may be more helpful to exclude a systemic vasculitis than to include a CNS vasculitis.[10]

CSF should be examined if the diagnosis of PACNS is considered. The CSF is abnormal in 81 percent of those examined. Mixed or lymphocytic pleocytosis is present in 68 percent, ranging up to 330 cells/hpf.[9] Seventy percent have elevations of CSF protein averaging 118 mg/dL, but ranging up to 825 mg/dL.[9] Serial lumbar punctures in the same patient may show spontaneous fluctuations in pleocytosis and protein. An abnormal electroencephalogram is 81 percent sensitive, and diffuse slowing is the most common finding. Focal slowing or sharp wave discharges are noted on occasion.[9] Computed tomography (CT) brain scans have disparate findings, showing infarcts, low-density lesions, or gyriform enhancement.[9] Magnetic resonance imaging (MRI) may show focal areas of infarction in multiple vascular territories. Normal MRI scans are rare but have been seen in some biopsy-proven cases.[11] The combination of anormal MRI and normal CSF is a powerful negative predictor of CNS vasculitis, although rare exceptions may occur.

In patients with angiograms, "classic arteritis" is seen in 65 percent, and less specific abnormalities in 19 percent. Thirteen percent of angiograms are normal. High-resolution film magnification is preferred to digital subtraction angiography in its ability to resolve changes in small-caliber vessels. The "arteritic" appearance of vasculitis is not completely specific and has been seen in vasculopathies due to other causes such as atherosclerosis, infection, and drugs and toxins. Considered in the context of the patient's age, clinical syndrome, laboratory studies, and CSF studies, angiography remains very helpful in establishing the diagnosis short of biopsy.

If the angiogram is normal or atypical, leptomeningeal and cortical biopsy should be performed.[9] Owing to the focal nature of the lesions, there is significant risk for sampling error. In a series of 108 cases (including 99 from the literature), the yield of leptomeningeal and cortical tissue was 87 percent and 57.9 percent, respectively. In 43 pathologically confirmed cases, 11 premortem biopsies were false negatives (diagnostic sensitivity, 74.4%). The morbidity of biopsy in patients with suspected vasculitis is 3.3 percent, but up to 50 percent of cases referred for biopsy in whom PACNS is suspected have an alternative diagnosis discovered. These statistics emphasize the necessity for biopsy and the potential harm of empirical immunosuppressive therapy in lieu of biopsy.

Because of the false-negative rates in biopsy and angiography, decisions about diagnosis and monitoring of treatment must be tailored to the individual case and incorporate as much clinical and laboratory information as possible. However, highly toxic therapy should not be considered unless cerebral and leptomeningeal biopsy has been performed.[10]

Management. There are no controlled treatment trials to date. High-dose (60 to 80 mg/d) prednisone combined with a calcium channel blocker is recommended. With good clinical response, tapering in a few months' time is reasonable. If lack of response or recurrence develops, oral cyclophosphamide (1 to 2 mg/kg/d) should be added and continued for 6 to 12 months until all signs of disease have disappeared. Angiography can be used to reassess disease activity, and repeated biopsies may be needed in some cases.[11] The rationale for treatment of PACNS is summarized in Table 50–3. Postpartum cerebral angiitis should be treated with a short course of high-dose steroids and calcium channel blocker.[11]

TABLE 50–3. **Treatment Outcome in Primary Angiitis of the Central Nervous System**

Treatment	N	Deaths	Poor Outcome	Complete Recovery
None	20	19	0	1
Steroids alone	13	6	3	4
Steroids + cytotoxic agent	13	1	2	10

Patients treated with steroids alone have a rate of relapse as high as 90 percent. Treatment with cyclophosphamide and low-dose prednisone for up to 6 months is associated with a relapse in 30 percent, and if treatment is continued for 12 months, a relapse is seen in only 10 percent.

Prognosis and Future Perspectives. The prognosis in PACNS is guarded; outcome depends on the severity of the disease and the response to the treatments described previously. The prognosis is favorable in young women with "benign angiopathy" or "postpartum angiopathy," and poorer in those with "true" PACNS. Considerable work remains to be done to further the understanding of the etiology, pathogenesis and pathophysiology, clinical subtypes, optimal treatment, and the long-term outlook of the disorder.

TAKAYASU'S ARTERITIS

Pathogenesis and Pathophysiology. Takayasu's arteritis (TA), first described by Takayasu and Onishi in Asian patients with absent limb pulses and retinopathy,[14] is now well recognized in Western countries as well. The burden of disease is in the aorta and its main branches with symptoms attributable to vascular compromise or a systemic immune response. In tissue specimens, giant cells are seen invading the media and adventitia of affected vessels.

There are a number of changes that suggest an immunopathogenesis, including hypergammaglobulinemia, increased ratio of CD4 to CD8 cells in the periphery, circulating immune complexes, antiaortic antibodies, and a positive rheumatoid factor. Nearly half of Japanese patients have statistically significant associations with Bw52 or DR12. The immunogenetics of TA are less well defined in Western patients.[15] It is currently believed that in a genetically predisposed individual and in a conducive hormonal milieu, exposure to an unknown antigen precipitates an uncontrolled, inflammatory immune response that primarily targets large vessels.[16] Because of descriptions occurring in India where tuberculosis is endemic, a relationship between TA and tuberculosis infection was briefly considered but later abandoned.[14, 16]

Epidemiology and Risk Factors. Despite increased ascertainment, TA remains rare in the Western Hemisphere (2.6 cases/million). The ratio of women to men is about 8.5:1, and TA is more common in lower socioeconomic classes.[14] In a prospective study of 60 patients, in which 45 were followed for 6 months to 20 years (median, 5.3 years), mean age of onset was 21 years.[15] If only Western cases are considered, the mean age of onset is 41 years.[16] Within the United States, the racial makeup of cases largely reflects the relative proportions of ethnic groups among U.S. residents, except that Asians account for an unusually large number of cases (10% of casess vs. 2.9% of the U.S. population).[15] There are occasional reports among family members suggesting a possible genetic component. Associations between TA and various other autoimmune diseases have been reported.[16]

Clinical Features and Associated Disorders. Although early descriptions suggested that TA had a triphasic course. with early systemic complaints followed by symptoms related to vascular inflammation and finally sequelae of vascular stenoses, this pattern is not universal. In addition, the clinical manifestations of TA may differ depending on geographic region. Aortic arch disease predominates in Japanese patients, and thoracic and abdominal aortic disease predominates in Thailand, Mexico, and India. Within a given vascular territory, the presence of symptoms depends largely on the extent of collateral circulation to involved organs. For example, gastrointestinal symptoms are rare even though stenoses and mesenteric vessel occlusions are common.[16]

In the preceding 60-patient series, all had vascular symptoms or signs.[16] Eighty percent of patients had bruits, most in the carotid arteries. Carotodynia was present in 32 percent of the series. Elevated blood pressure occurred in 33 percent, mostly owing to lesions of the renal arteries or descending aorta. Asymmetrical blood pressures were present in 50 percent of the patients, a finding suggesting that four extremity blood pressures can be used in diagnosis and in clinical follow-up. Diminished or absent extremity pulses occur in over half of the patients with TA. HLA-Bw52 has been associated with an increased risk of aortic valve insufficiency and a worse prognosis in Japanese patients.[15]

Among the 60 patients cited previously, nervous system symptoms occurred in over half. Fifty-seven percent of those with vertebral artery involvement and 23 percent of those without vertebral artery involvement experienced lightheadedness or dizziness. TIA and stroke each occurred in 5 of the 60 patients. These events are presumably related to artery-to-artery or cardiogenic emboli. Visual disturbances affected one third of the patients, most of whom had carotid or vertebral artery involvement. These visual disturbances are almost always bilateral; however, monocular blindness did occur in one patient.[15] Pregnancy does not appear to potentiate disease activity, and there is no difference in fertility rates, cesarean section rates, or neonatal death among TA patients when compared with the general population.[14] It is recommended that those who wish to become pregnant do so during an inactive disease phase. Because of increased cardiovascular demands, the third trimester may be most difficult for these patients. Aortic regurgitation or heart failure may develop, and hypertension may be a problem even in the absence of pre-eclampsia. Typically, these problems abate after delivery.[14] Moderate doses of corticosteroids have not had significant effects on the fetus.[16]

Differential Diagnosis. Diagnostic criteria for TA are shown in Table 50–4.[16] Other causes of large vessel disease should be entertained. Possible causes of inflammatory aortitis include syphilis, tuberculosis, systemic lupus erythematosus, and giant cell arteritis. Developmental abnormalities such as Ehlers-Danlos syndrome and Marfan's syndrome can give an abnormal appearance to the aorta and be misleading. Aortic abnormalities can also occur as the result of radiation fibrosis, neurofibromatosis, and ergotism.

TABLE 50–4. **Criteria for the Diagnosis of Takayasu's Arteritis**

Onset or Worsening of Two of the Following:
Unexplained systemic illness (fever or musculoskeletal complaints)
Increased sedimentation rate
Features of vascular ischemia or inflammation
Claudication
Diminished or absent pulse
Asymmetrical blood pressure (arms or legs)
Bruit
Vascular pain
Typical angiographic features

Modified from Kerr GS: Takayasu's arteritis. Curr Opin Rheumatol 1994; 6:32–38.

Evaluation. ESR >20 mm/hr (>40 mm/hr during pregnancy) is considered by most to be an indicator of active disease.[14] In one series, ESR was elevated in 72 percent during active disease and 44 percent during clinical remission.[15] The correlation between ESR and biopsy evidence of disease activity is poor. As many as 42 percent of patients with normal ESR have active lesions on biopsy.[17] Repeated ESR evaluations over time may be most useful as an indicator of relative disease activity in a given patient. Other markers of disease activity, including endothelin-1, von Willebrand's factor, and factor VIII antigen, have not been well evaluated.[17] The disease is presumed to be inactive when there is an absence of clinical features, the ESR is normal, and the angiogram is unchanged. Unfortunately, the correlation between ESR and biopsy evidence of disease activity is poor.[17]

Noninvasive tests have been used as diagnostic aids. Ultrasonography and MRI have been used with varying results, but nothing yet has the sensitivity and specificity of an angiogram.[16] Angiography is considered the diagnostic gold standard but carries the risks of an invasive procedure and the risk of rupture of diseased vessels (Fig. 50–2). An angiogram does not differentiate between acute and chronic lesions, however, and cannot assess disease activity. In one series, the disease burden was distributed as follows: aortic lesions 65 percent, carotid 58 percent, renal 38 percent, and vertebral 35 percent. Long stenotic lesions were seen in 98 percent of patients. Aneurysms were seen in 27 percent of patients and were present in 5 percent of carotid and 2 percent of vertebral arteries.[15]

Management. Glucocorticoids are the mainstay of therapy. Other immunosuppressive therapies are used for patients who fail to respond to steroid therapy or who relapse during steroid withdrawal. Azathioprine is frequently used, and cyclophosphamide has been used with some success. Methotrexate appears to be relatively well tolerated and is beneficial in helping patients successfully taper steroids or avoid relapse.[16] Beta-adrenergic blockers and angiotensin-converting enzyme (ACE) inhibitors can be used to treat hypertension due to vascular stenosis that is not surgically correctable. ACE inhibitors must be used with caution in patients with bilateral renal artery stenosis. Although effective for heart failure, vasodilators are not helpful in patients with renal artery stenosis.[16] Antiplatelet therapy is probably not indicated to prevent thrombotic events, because native-vessel thrombosis is not a common feature.

Surgical treatment has an auxiliary role, because renal artery stenosis with severe hypertension is common. Percutaneous coronary transluminal angioplasty (PCTA) successfully restores patency in as many as 80 percent of these patients. Bypass surgery can be done for repeated PCTA failure. Bypass of carotid arteries from the ascending aorta can be done as well. In general, success of bypass surgery is improved during disease inactivity (88% vs. 53%).

Prognosis and Future Perspectives. Most patients experience morbidity from TA or the treatment of the disease. Five- to 10-year survival rates are in the range of 80 to 97 percent. Myocardial infarction, stroke, cardiac failure, aneurysmal rupture, and renal failure are causes of death.[5]

In the future, more accurate noninvasive diagnostic tools, including vascular imaging and serum markers for disease activity, will likely improve the accuracy of TA diagnosis. Safer and more efficacious immune-modulating therapies are also needed based on a better elucidation of the etiopathogenesis of the disorder.

POLYARTERITIS NODOSA, CHURG-STRAUSS SYNDROME, AND OVERLAP SYNDROMES

Pathogenesis and Pathophysiology. Classic polyarteritis nodosa (PAN) is a necrotizing, nodular vasculitis that preferentially affects medium and small arteries, and sometimes arterioles. The pathophysiology is believed to be a deposition of immune complexes in the involved arteries. PAN is associated with a number of infections, particularly hepatitis B, tuberculosis, and *Streptococcus*. In those cases associated with hepatitis B, hepatitis B surface antigen, IgM, and complement can be demonstrated in the vasculitic lesions. In most

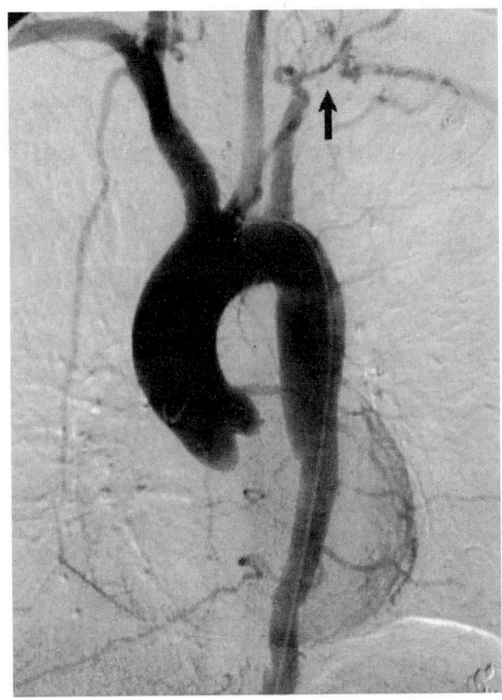

FIGURE 50–2. Angiogram of a 46-year-old Hispanic woman with intercostal angina and pulseless left radial artery. Note the stenosis of the descending aorta (40%) and of the left subclavian artery indicated by the arrow (95%).

cases, however, no association with an infectious agent can be demonstrated.[18]

Churg-Strauss syndrome (CSS), also known as allergic angiitis and granulomatosis, is a systemic vasculitis marked by systemic hypereosinophilia and multiple organ involvement, which usually includes asthma. These signs and symptoms are somewhat distinctive and serve to reduce confusion with the other vasculitides. Pathological features include a necrotizing vasculitis affecting small or occasionally medium-sized arteries and veins, eosinophilic infiltration, and extravascular granulomata.[19]

Microscopic polyangiitis (MPA) is similar to PAN but is characterized histologically by involvement of arterioles, capillaries, venules, and rarely medium-sized arteries.[18] PAN and MPA overlap considerably, and the American College of Rheumatology criteria for diagnosis do not distinguish between the two entities.[18]

Epidemiology and Risk Factors. PAN occurs from infancy to old age, with peak incidence in the fifth and sixth decades of life and an estimated male-to-female ratio of 2.5:1. In a series of patients with CSS, the mean age of diagnosis was 49.7 years (range, 17 to 75 years), and women were affected more often than men.[19] MPA, considered an overlap syndrome, shares the epidemiology of PAN, and an incidence separate from that of PAN is difficult to discern.

Clinical Features and Associated Disorders. Patients with PAN typically present with systemic signs and symptoms, including weakness, leg and abdominal pain, and fever. Arthralgias and hypertension are often present. Maculopapular or nodular skin rash is common, as is livedo reticularis. Cardiac symptoms result from hypertension, pericarditis, or coronary vasculitis, and pulmonary involvement is atypical. The CNS is rarely involved, but stroke, delirium, seizures, and myelopathy have been reported.[20, 21] Disease affecting the peripheral nervous system (PNS) is common in PAN and usually appears in the pattern of mononeuritis multiplex or asymmetrical polyneuropathy.[22]

CSS usually begins with upper respiratory symptoms such as sinusitis and rhinitis. Symptoms of systemic vasculitis involving skin, heart, and peripheral nerves follow. In a series of 42 patients with CSS, 62 percent had nervous system involvement, almost entirely restricted to the PNS. Mononeuropathy multiplex (58.6%), distal symmetrical polyneuropathy (24.1%), asymmetrical polyneuropathy (3.5%), and one patient with a lumbar radiculopathy (3.5%) were included. Three of the patients in the series (10.3%) had cerebral infarctions.[19] Inflammatory myopathy has also been described in other series.

Little information is available on pregnancy and vasculitis. One woman with CSS worsened with two pregnancies, then died of cardiac disease during her third. Another woman had symptom remission during pregnancy.

Rapidly progressive glomerular nephritis is one of the major characteristics of MPA. The clinical outcome can be poor with chronic renal failure. Relapses may be more common than in PAN.[18] In MPA, peripheral neuropathy occurs in only 10 to 20 percent of patients.[18]

Differential Diagnosis. Nonspecific systemic symptoms at presentation may lead to consideration of infection, neoplasm, or connective tissue disease.[23] The presence of mononeuritis multiplex strongly suggests vasculitis. In the absence of organ system involvement other than the CNS, the differential diagnosis rapidly expands to include virtually any vasculopathy, inflammation, or infectious disease. In the appropriate clinical setting, particularly with perinuclear antineutrophil cytoplasmic antibody (pANCA) positivity, the diagnosis may be made clinically without need for tissue diagnosis.[19]

Evaluation. The ESR is typically elevated in PAN patients, averaging 60 mm/hr.[22] Other laboratory studies may show leukocytosis, anemia, thrombocytosis, and abnormal urinary sediments. Hepatitis B surface antibody is seen in a subset of patients. pANCA is detected in almost 20 percent of PAN patients, and it has been suggested that these pANCA-positive PAN patients may actually have MPA.[1]

Electromyography (EMG) and nerve conduction velocity studies demonstrate chronic partial denervation, impaired motor and sensory nerve conduction, and sometimes conduction block due to focal ischemic lesions.[22] Sural nerve biopsies in patients with peripheral neuropathy demonstrated pathological findings in 30 of 34 patients, showing vasculitis of epineural arterioles, resulting in a central fascicular pattern of nerve damage.[22] In suspected cases of PAN-associated myopathy, muscle enzymes, EMG, and biopsy are diagnostic.[24] Biopsy of symptomatic tissues such as peripheral nerve and skin may also be diagnostic. CSF may also be helpful in detecting CNS involvement with lymphocytosis and elevated protein. MRI is nonspecific but helpful in localizing involvement in the CNS. Angiography establishes the diagnosis in about 80 percent of patients, demonstrating aneurysms and changes in blood vessel caliber or stenotic lesions.[18]

In CSS, eosinophilia in the peripheral blood (defined as greater than 1.5×10^9/L) is very helpful in leading toward a correct diagnosis.[19] In the clinical setting of peripheral eosinophilia, asthma, and findings typical of vasculitis or multiple necrotizing cutaneous lesions, the diagnosis can be made without biopsy,[19] although other hypereosinophilic syndromes discussed later in this chapter must also be considered. Approximately 70 percent of CSS patients are pANCA positive.[1]

MPA may cause mononeuritis multiplex without other defining disease features, and evaluation of the PNS as described previously is essential.[22] Skin lesions, when present, provide a convenient means of tissue diagnosis with minimal risk. Even in the presence of CNS vasculitis, visualization of arteritis by angiography is usually impossible because the involved vessels are smaller than 700 μm in diameter.[25] MPA is the vasculitis most closely associated with pANCA, and 50 to 90 percent of patients are pANCA positive.[1]

Management. Glucocorticosteroids are the mainstay of immunosuppressive therapy for all of the vasculitides. In PAN and MPA, prednisone 1 mg/kg daily (possibly higher), in divided doses, should be given until inflammatory features are controlled. Prolonged treatment may be required, and the lowest effective dose should be sought on an alternate-day regimen.[26] Retrospective trials of cytotoxic agents have suggested efficacy, but other studies report no added benefit.[26] Nonetheless, if steroids are not effective or organ system damage is progressive, cyclophosphamide, at doses of 2.5 to 3.5 mg/kg/d, or another cytotoxic agent should be used.[26] Antiviral agents, such as vidarabine, have been reported to be successful in cases of hepatitis B–associated PAN.[26]

Antiplatelet agents such as aspirin should be used throughout the course of treatment, due to a potential platelet aggregating effect of steroids in vasculitis patients.[26]

CSS is managed in the same fashion as PAN and MPA, but CSS patients are more responsive to initial treatment with steroids and less often require cytotoxic treatment.[26] In a series of 29 CSS patients, only 2 required cytotoxic therapy in addition to steroids.[19]

Prognosis and Future Perspectives. Prior to immunosuppressive therapy, patients with systemic vasculitides had a 5-year survival rate of about 13 percent.[22] Most deaths were attributed to renal or pulmonary failure with vascular events in the gastrointestinal tract or CNS comprising the rest. Since the use of steroids, the 5-year survival has improved to about 47 to 57 percent, although older patients have a worse outcome.[22]

With PNS involvement, if inflammatory features respond to treatment, there is often an improvement in the neuropathy.[22]

All the 29 patients with CSS in the Mayo Clinic series received steroid therapy and 10 patients had improvement of their neurological syndrome. In the mean follow-up of 3.9 years, four patients died, one from a cerebral infarct.[18] With MPA, the clinical outcome can be poor with chronic renal failure. Relapses may be more common than in PAN.[18]

WEGENER'S GRANULOMATOSIS

Pathogenesis and Pathophysiology. The almost universal involvement of the upper or lower airway in Wegener's granulomatosis (WG) has led to a theory that the condition results from exposure to an inhaled antigen with resultant granulomatous inflammation and altered immunoreactivity.[27] Cell-mediated immunity and immune complexes are felt to play significant roles. There may be genetic or other predisposing host factors. A strong association with cytoplasmic antineutrophil cytoplasmic antibodies (cANCA) suggests a pathogenic role. It has been shown in vitro that cANCA causes neutrophils to undergo a respiratory burst and degranulation, releasing toxic superoxides.[28] However, there is no direct evidence to confirm that it is an etiological factor in WG.

Epidemiology and Risk Factors. The incidence of WG in the United States is about 1 in 30,000. Among 180 patients referred to the National Institute of Allergy and Infectious Diseases, 97 percent with WG were white with equal numbers of men and women. The mean age was 41 years (range, 9 to 79 years), and 15 percent were less than 19 years of age.[29] The ease of identification of the disorder with cANCA has increased disease ascertainment.

Clinical Features and Associated Disorders. Criteria for the diagnosis of WG are listed in Table 50–5.[30] Ninety percent of patients with WG have upper and/or lower airway symptoms. Median duration of these symptoms at the time of diagnosis is 4.7 months. Nasal, sinus, and ear abnormalities are seen at presentation in 73 percent and during the illness in 92 percent. Lung disease develops in 85 percent of cases over the course of the illness, although it is asymptomatic in one third of cases. Eighteen percent of patients present with asymptomatic glomerulonephritis, and 77 percent develop glomerulonephritis, usually within the first 2 years of disease onset.[29]

TABLE 50–5. Criteria for the Diagnosis of Wegener's Granulomatosis

Two or More of the Following:
Purulent or bloody nasal discharge or oral ulcers
Radiographic evidence of nodules, fixed infiltrates, or cavities
Microscopic hematuria
Biopsy evidence of granulomatous inflammation

Modified from Nishino H, DeRemee RA, Rubino FA, Parisi JE: Wegener's granulomatosis associated with vasculitis of the temporal artery: Report of five cases [see comments]. Mayo Clin Proc 1993;68:115–121.

In a prospective series, peripheral nervous system involvement occurred in 24 percent of patients at the time of diagnosis of WG.[31] CNS involvement occurs in 8 percent of patients and includes stroke, cranial nerve abnormalities, and diabetes insipidus.[29] In literature series, neurological involvement with WG occurs in 22 to 54 percent of patients. Virtually any portion of the neuraxis can be affected, but the most common manifestation is peripheral neuropathy, particularly mononeuropathy multiplex.[32]

Headache in WG is due to sinusitis, pachymeningitis, or cerebral vasculitis. Multiple forms of cranial nerve problems occur. Exophthalmos, ophthalmoplegia, and optic nerve involvement due to granulomatous involvement may be a presenting symptom of WG.[27] Ocular symptoms are present in 15 percent of patients at onset and 52 percent of patients during the disease course. The most helpful diagnostic finding is proptosis (2% at onset, 15% overall), because it is highly suggestive of WG when associated with upper or lower airway disease. Proptosis is usually painful and leads to visual loss owing to anterior ischemic optic neuropathy in about half of affected patients. Extraocular muscle entrapment can cause diplopia.[29] Recurrent serous or suppurative otitis media may cause partial (33%) or total unilateral (1%) or bilateral (1%) hearing loss.[29] Multiple cranial neuropathies rarely occur as a result of pachymeningitis.[27]

Intracranial vasculitis, cerebritis, and meningitis are uncommon.[27, 33] Because the small vessels are typically involved in WG, angiography is usually normal.[27]

PNS involvement can take several forms. Mononeuritis multiplex is a frequent neurological complication (as in PAN and MPA) and is highly suggestive of vasculitis as an etiology.[27] Forty-four percent of peripheral nerve syndromes present in this manner with the common peroneal nerve typically involved along with one or more other nerves.[31]

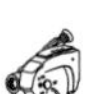

Polyneuropathy, either symmetrical or asymmetrical, occurs with slightly greater frequency.[22] Axonal features predominate on electrodiagnostic studies, and demyelinating features are uncommon.[31] Although myalgias and arthralgias are frequent complaints in WG, myopathy is a relatively uncommon manifestation.[27] In general, pregnancy adversely affects clinical signs.[34]

Differential Diagnosis. Constitutional symptoms such as fever and weight loss occur to varying degrees and may initially lead the diagnostic evaluation toward chronic infection or malignancy. In those patients with clinical involvement of the orbit or retro-orbital space, malignancy and endocrinopathies are likely considerations. When symptoms are isolated to the respiratory tract, diagnoses of recurrent infection or allergy are common. In patients with milder disease, diagnosis may be delayed up to 5 to 15 years after the initial symptoms.[29]

Evaluation. Routine blood studies show leukocytosis and normochromic normocytic anemia in most and thrombocytosis in many patients. ESR averages 71 mm/hr (range, 17 to 140) and correlates well with disease activity before treatment in 80 percent of patients.[29]

The high specificity of cANCA for Wegener's and its limited variants has been confirmed in large studies. In the appropriate clinical setting, a positive cANCA may obviate the need for tissue diagnosis. A negative cANCA, however, does not exclude the possibility of WG. The sensitivity depends on extent and activity of the disease process. There is greater than 90 percent sensitivity in the systemic vasculitic phase of disease, but only 65 percent in patients with predominantly granulomatous disease limited to the upper and lower respiratory tract. In patients with no active disease, the sensitivity is about 30 percent.[35]

In patients with CNS manifestations of the disease, MRI is a valuable initial step in evaluation. T2-weighted sequences and gadolinium-enhanced images are most sensitive to ischemic changes secondary to vasculitis.[25] When clinical suspicion of CNS vasculitis is high, angiography and biopsy should be pursued despite a normal MRI.[25] Because the size of vessels involved in CNS WG is small, the greatest utility of angiography may be the exclusion of other vasculitides or nonvasculitic vascular disease.[25, 27]

Open lung biopsy is positive greater than 90 percent of the time, whereas bronchoscopy-directed biopsy shows vasculitis in only 7 percent. The typical appearance is that of a granulomatous vasculitis with necrosis, giant cells, and microabscesses.[29]

Management. Treatment includes prednisone (1 mg/kg/d) and oral cyclophosphamide (2 mg/kg/d). Fulminant disease is treated with more aggressive cyclophosphamide (up to 5 mg/kg/d) with subsequent doses based on white cell counts. According to response, doses are adjusted to eliminate prednisone and maintain patients on cyclophosphamide alone. Then cyclophosphamide is tapered until disease recurrence or discontinuation. Using this regimen, 75 percent remit completely, and an additional 16 percent have marked improvement. Eight percent of patients have seemingly intractable disease, but achieve remission in up to 4 to 6 years. Remission is achieved at least once in 96 percent of patients. However, 46 percent of patients have at least one relapse, and 44 percent have relapses of more than 5 consecutive years' duration.[29] Methotrexate may be of some value in patients with milder disease or cyclophosphamide intolerance.[30]

The role of serial cANCA titers in determining the risk of relapse in treated patients is unknown, and it is premature to recommend altering immunosuppressive therapy in response to a changing titer.[35]

Prognosis and Future Perspectives. The disease and its treatment carry significant morbidity. Cushingoid features are universal among steroid-treated patients. With cyclophosphamide, there is a 2.4-fold overall increase in the rate of malignancies, including a 33-fold increase in bladder and 11-fold increase in lymphoma, compared with rates of the National Cancer Registry for a similar cohort. Serious infections occur in half of the patients, with a rate of 0.11 infections per patient year. The mortality rate is 20 percent; more than 50 percent of the deaths are attributed to active disease or treatment-related complications. Renal disease, coronary disease, infection, malignancy, and combined renal and pulmonary disease are contributory.[29]

VASCULITIS ASSOCIATED WITH ANTIPHOSPHOLIPID ANTIBODIES

Pathogenesis and Pathophysiology. Antiphospholipid antibodies (aPL) are a heterogenous family of antibodies of the IgG, IgM, or mixed classes with varying cross-reactivities. Antibodies within this family include anticardiolipin antibodies, antibodies responsible for the false-positive Venereal Disease Research Laboratory serology, and the lupus anticoagulant. Antiphospholipid antibodies may be detected in a number of clinical settings. Normal elderly may have aPL of unclear significance. They may be seen in patients treated with phenothiazines, antiarrhythmics, and anticonvulsants, or in the context of infections or malignancy. Antiphospholipid antibodies are commonly seen in patients with systemic autoimmune disorders such as systemic lupus erythematosus (SLE). The primary aPL syndrome comprises recurrent venous or arterial thrombosis, fetal loss, thrombocytopenia, and positive results on serological tests for lupus anticoagulant or anticardiolipid antibodies.[36]

The nervous system antigen targeted by aPL has not been identified. All cell membranes contain phospholipids, though they are generally protected from the immune system by the bilayer membrane structure. The ability to form aPL may depend on an induced conformational change in membrane structure and interaction with cofactors. Certain known vascular risk factors such as diabetes, hypertension, cigarette smoking, and lipid disorders may trigger the conformational change, exposing the vascular endothelium to the immune system. Old age, smoking, and diabetes mellitus may elevate glycoprotein cofactors such as beta-2 glycoprotein I. This cofactor normally inhibits the intrinsic coagulation pathway and adenosine diphosphate–mediated platelet aggregation; interference with its action may promote thrombosis and platelet aggregation.[37] In addition, aPL may interact with natural anticoagulants such as placental anticoagulant proteins, plasminogen activators, and proteins C and S. These antibodies may also provoke complement activation or may interfere with the function of prostaglandin I2. Although the exact mechanism or mechanisms remain ill-defined, the preponderance of evidence is that aPL cause an autoimmune-mediated prothrombotic state.[36]

Pathological examination of affected cerebral and carotid arteries shows a noninflammatory vasculopathy with fibromuscular dysplasia, fibrin thrombi, and widespread obstruction by a proliferation of intimal fibrous tissue or myointimal cells. In later stages, fibrous webs may form across arterial lumens.[38, 39]

Epidemiology and Risk Factors. The frequency of aPL depends heavily on the population being studied. A review of a number of studies suggests that aPL can be detected in 2 to 12 percent of the normal population, 10 to 26 percent of patients with first stroke, 10 to 40 percent of women with recurrent fetal loss, and 40 to 50 percent of patients with SLE.[36] In a prospective study of 147 people with aPL and thromboses within or outside the nervous system, a number of concomitant risk factors for thrombosis were identified in

76 percent. These included pregnancy, hypertension, hyperlipidemia, and diabetes.[40]

Clinical Features and Associated Disorders. The complications of aPL fall into four classes: peripheral venous thrombosis and pulmonary embolism (type I), coronary or peripheral artery thrombosis (type II), cerebrovascular or retinal vessel thrombosis (type III), and mixtures (type IV).[41] Nervous system abnormalities associated with aPL include cerebral or spinal arterial or venous infarction, chorea, hemidystonia, seizures, migraine, Guillain-Barré syndrome, transient global amnesia, motor neuron disease, myasthenia gravis, and behavioral abnormalities such as affective disorder or dementia.[36, 42–46] Several clinical features of transient focal neurological events in aPL-positive patients distinguish these individuals from their aPL-negative cohort. Amaurosis fugax and episodes of unilateral paresthesias without headache and without a family history of migraine suggest aPL positivity in young persons.[47]

The risks associated with aPL in otherwise healthy persons are ill-defined. Clearly, patients with aPL and a single thrombotic event are at greater risk of subsequent thrombotic events. However, the risk of primary thrombotic events in otherwise healthy persons with aPL remains poorly understood.

Differential Diagnosis. The primary aPL syndrome must be distinguished from other causes of atherosclerotic and nonatherosclerotic vascular disease. Other connective tissue diseases such as SLE or aPL associated with exposure to inciting drugs can be discerned using history, physical examination, and laboratory tests. An analysis of 1000 patients with SLE from the medical literature yielded an average frequency of 34 percent for the lupus anticoagulant and 44 percent for anticardiolipin antibody.[48] Within the context of SLE, the presence of aPL is highly correlated with a history of thrombosis, neurological disorders, and thrombocytopenia.

Evaluation. The diagnosis of primary antiphospholipid syndrome rests on the demonstration of aPL (anticardiolipin antibodies, lupus anticoagulant, or false-positive serological test for syphilis) in a person with a characteristic syndrome. Associated connective tissue diseases such as SLE and Sjögren's syndrome should be excluded with appropriate clinical investigation and autoantibody studies. Patients with CNS focal events should be evaluated using MRI, and scans may demonstrate large infarcts or hyperintense white matter abnormalities.[49]

Management. The management of aPL employs antithrombotic agents and immunosuppression. However, there are no prospective controlled data that support a given course of therapy. Young patients with thrombotic events and aPL are generally treated with antithrombotics (warfarin, subcutaneous heparin, low-molecular-weight heparin, and antiplatelet therapy). In a prospective study of 147 patients with aPL and an index nervous system lesion or evidence of thrombosis, anticoagulation using warfarin to an International Normalized Ratio of greater than 3 (with or without aspirin) was superior to less aggressive warfarin therapy (with or without aspirin), aspirin alone, and no therapy.[40] The highest risk of recurrent thrombosis in this study was within 6 months of discontinuation of warfarin, suggesting the need for chronic therapy.[40] There remains no consensus, however, on the nature and duration of optimal anticoagulation. Corticosteroid and other immunotherapies in the aPL syndrome are also controversial. The titers of aPL may be reduced with effective doses of immunosuppressants or with plasmapheresis, but the clinical efficacy of these modalities in the prevention of recurrent thrombosis is unknown.[50] Intravenous immune globulin (IVIg) infusions, usually with concomitant corticosteroids and antithrombotic therapy, have successfully prevented fetal loss in women with aPL and recurrent fetal loss. However, there are no reliable data in women with nervous system thrombosis, and the association of IVIg therapy and thrombotic events in other nervous system conditions warrant caution in the use of this technique. More definitive recommendations are likely to result from prospective trials of various therapies in aPL-positive patients with stroke.[36, 51]

Prognosis and Future Perspectives. Patients with the highest titers of IgG aPL have a relatively high risk of recurrent thrombotic events, especially stroke, deep venous thrombosis, and spontaneous abortion. Patients with aPL and cerebral thrombosis face a recurrence risk up to 20 percent per year for TIA or stroke and 56 percent per year for noncerebral thrombosis.[36] While the risks associated with aPL seem well defined among patients with SLE or those who have had thrombotic events, the prognostic import of a finding of isolated aPL remains obscure.

THROMBOANGIITIS OBLITERANS (BUERGER'S SYNDROME)

Pathogenesis and Pathophysiology. Discovered in 1879 and described in 1908, Buerger's disease, or thromboangiitis obliterans (TO), is an uncommon vasculitis of the small and medium-sized distal arteries and veins and almost exclusively affects cigarette smokers. There was confusion about the existence of TO for many years. The better classification of other vasculitides and the development of angiography have led to the identification of TO as a separate condition.

Almost all cases of TO have occurred in tobacco users, suggesting that the inflammatory response may be allergic. Smokers with and without TO demonstrate a similar cellular immune response to a purified tobacco glycoprotein.[52] Anticollagen antibodies and cellular immune reactions to type I and III collagen are present in patients with TO. Other potential mechanisms involved include a derangement of the endothelial cell, which could be the result of decreased plasminogen activator inhibitor 1 release.[52] There are reported familial occurrences that raise the question of a genetic susceptibility, and an increased association with HLA-A9 and HLA-B5 has been demonstrated in some with the disease. Some cases have occurred in association with other disorders such as IgA nephropathy and hypereosinophilia and with positive serological tests for rickettsial organisms. It has also been proposed that the abnormality may be a hypercoagulable state with secondary inflammation. However, the exact pathogenesis remains somewhat elusive.

Pathological findings are not routinely reported because most of the surgeries are performed on limbs with severe ischemia.[52] Three stages of pathological changes have been identified. Initially, non-necrotizing panarteritis occurs with preservation of vascular wall architecture. The media and internal elastic lamina remain intact, a finding that differentiates TO from other vasculitides where there is destruction of the elastic lamina. Infiltrates of inflammatory cells and granulomas in the thrombus differentiate the occlusive lesions of TO from atherosclerosis where thrombi are composed of only fibrin, red blood cells, and platelets. Intrathrombotic granulomas are a distinctive hallmark of TO. Following this development, there is organization of the thrombus, with the type of inflammatory cells involved changing from neutrophils to lymphocytes and occasionally with eosinophils. Lastly, recanalization occurs with evidence of perivascular fibrosis. Aneurysms are an uncommon finding because the vascular wall remains intact.

Epidemiology and Risk Factors. TO typically occurs in young smokers. The incidence is approximately 8 to 12 per 100,000 in the general population, thereby representing less than 1 percent of all patients with vascular disease. According to a report from the Mayo Clinic, there has been a tenfold decline in U.S. case incidence from 1947 to 1986. Japan, Eastern Europe, Southeastern Asia, and Israel have not shown similar declines.[52] The median age of onset is 34.5 years of age. All are tobacco users. Men are affected about three times as often as women, but this ratio varies in different countries in relation to the gender predominance of smokers.[52]

Clinical Features and Associated Disorders. Clinically, intermittent claudication begins in the feet and involves the legs more proximally as the disease progresses. The arms become affected in 90 percent of cases. Large arteries are rarely involved. Symptoms include ischemic pain at rest in 80 percent, claudication in 60 percent, and Raynaud's phenomenon in 35 percent of patients. Common signs are ischemic ulcers in 75 percent and distal gangrene in 80 percent.[52, 53] The neurological consequences of TO are sensory symptoms, which occur in 69 percent of patients.[52] Sensory polyneuropathy may be secondary to severe ischemic changes or to fibrous encasement of distal neurovascular bundles.[52]

Differential Diagnosis. Differential diagnoses include other vasculopathies and autoimmune diseases such as SLE, scleroderma, polyarteritis nodosa, antiphospholipid antibody syndrome, GCA, or TA. Other conditions such as pseudoxanthoma elasticum and Ehlers-Danlos syndrome may be considered as well. It is important to exclude proximal sources of emboli and atherosclerosis.[52]

Evaluation. The ESR is abnormal in only 15 percent of patients. Angiography demonstrates involvement of small and medium-sized vessels with segmental occlusions and collateral vessels in the distal vessels of the feet and hands.[52] The absence of lesions proximally strongly favors the diagnosis of TO.

Management. It is imperative that the patient discontinues tobacco exposure. Forty-two percent of patients who continued smoking after the diagnosis required amputation, whereas only 5 percent of those who ceased smoking underwent amputation. The use of anticoagulants and antiplatelet agents may be beneficial on occasion, although the results of medical therapy have been generally poor. Ilprost, a prostacyclin analogue, improves leg pain in 35 percent and heals ulcers in 22 percent of patients. Despite clear evidence of inflammation, corticosteroids have not been of benefit.

Prognosis and Future Perspectives. Twenty percent of patients require limited resection of the toes or feet, and another 20 percent have a proximal, below-the-knee amputation. Only 6 percent of patients require finger or upper extremity amputation. The sensory changes parallel the course of the vascular disease and stabilize if the ischemic changes are controlled. Survival rates at 5 and 10 years approach that of the normal population.

Connective Tissue Diseases

RHEUMATOID ARTHRITIS

Pathogenesis and Pathophysiology. Rheumatoid arthritis (RA) is an immune complex disease. The most important autoantibody in RA is the rheumatoid factor (RF), an antibody, usually of the IgM or IgG class, which reacts with immunoglobulins. The original triggering mechanism may be exposure to a microbial antigen. Autoantibodies to other cellular antigens such as histones, single-stranded DNA, filaments, collagen, and nuclear antigens have been described. Immune complexes composed of IgG combined with IgM or IgG anti-IgG antibodies cause inflammation of the synovium in the joints. Although the largest and most pathogenic immune complexes are found in the joints, others can be detected in the blood of patients with extra-articular manifestations such as vasculitis.

Epidemiology and Risk Factors. RA is a chronic multisystem disease that affects 1 to 2 percent of the population. Disease onset is between 35 and 50 years of age in 80 percent of cases. Women account for 75 percent of cases. An increased risk in nulliparous women and a putative protective effect of oral contraception suggest a hormonal role in disease expression. Although there is a genetic predisposition to developing the disorder, genetic factors probably account for only about 30 percent of the risk of developing RA.[54]

Clinical Features and Associated Disorders. The onset of RA is typically insidious, with prodromal malaise, fatigue, and generalized weakness. Characteristic symmetrical polyarthritis develops within weeks to months. Articular signs and symptoms preferentially affect the cervical spine and the metacarpophalangeal, proximal interphalangeal, wrist, elbow, knee, ankle, forefoot, and subtalar joints. Progression of joint disease leads to bony erosion and joint deformity. Extra-articular manifestations, including rheumatoid nodules in subcutaneous, cutaneous, connective, and pulmonary tissues; pleuritis; interstitial fibrosis; pneumonitis; and pericardial effusions tend to occur in patients with high levels of circulating RF. Felty's syndrome (RA, splenomegaly, neutropenia, anemia, and thrombocytopenia) is seen in some patients with long-standing disease.

A few patients develop systemic vasculitis, heralded by the development of ischemic skin lesions, mononeuritis multiplex, or documented visceral vasculitis. Although this syndrome is usually seen in men who have had RA for more than 10 years, it may be seen in women at disease presentation.[55]

Neurological manifestations occur in patients with moderate to severe RA. They may be caused by direct effects of the disease process or secondary effects from bone or joint involvement. Rheumatoid nodules frequently form in the dura mater, where they tend to be asymptomatic except in cases of extensive involvement with pachymeningitis.[56] The occurrence of symptomatic CNS vasculitis is rare, even in the setting of active systemic vasculitis.[57, 58] Clinical signs of rheumatoid CNS vasculitis include seizures, dementia, hemiparesis, cranial nerve palsy, blindness, hemispheral dysfunction, cerebellar ataxia, and dysphasia. Pathological examination reveals chronic perivasculitis, transmural chronic inflammatory cell infiltration, intimal collagen proliferation with luminal narrowing, and fibrinoid necrosis of the media of small arteries.[57] Changes in the articular architecture of the cervical spine may produce CNS dysfunction at the cervicomedullary junction or spinal cord level. Significant disease of the cervical spine is present in up to 70 percent of patients with advanced disease. The major changes in the cervical spine include vertebral body erosion and collapse,[59] rheumatoid discitis, dural thickening and fibrosis with spinal cord compression, and most commonly atlantoaxial subluxation. Subluxation of C1 on C2 may be in the anterior, posterior, or vertical directions, or there may be multiple cervical subluxations resulting in a "staircase appearance" of the cervical spine.[60] Cervical subluxation is often asymptomatic. In patients who are symptomatic, the most striking features are myelopathic. However, other symptoms have been reported, including occipital headache[61] and obstructive hydrocephalus.[62] Brain stem syndromes result from pseudoaneurysm of the vertebral artery,[63] direct compression of the medulla by eroded, displaced odontoid fragments, and rheumatoid granulomata. Neurological manifestations more commonly result from intermittent or sustained anterior cord compression, sometimes complicated by compression-induced ischemia in the distribution of branches of the anterior spinal artery. Most patients with radiographical evidence of subluxation are asymptomatic. Common symptoms and signs include neck pain, weakness affecting arms before legs, flexor spasms, sphincter disturbances, paresthesias, hyperreflexia, and sensory changes.[60]

Peripheral nerve disease in RA results from nerve entrapment, segmental demyelination, or vasculitic involvement of the vasa nervorum. Entrapment or compression of peripheral nerves occurs in 45 percent of patients and affects the median, ulnar, posterior interosseous, tibial, common peroneal, or posterior tibial nerves.[64] Other patterns of neuropathy seen in RA are distal sensorimotor or sensory polyneuropathy and mononeuritis multiplex. Vasculitic changes underlie all types of noncompressive neuropathies in RA.[65] Myositis may be seen but is not usually a prominent feature of the disorder.

Differential Diagnosis and Evaluation. RA must be distinguished from degenerative osteoarthritis and from deforming inflammatory arthritis associated with other connective tissue disorders. The diagnosis of RA is based on a clinical picture of symmetrical polyarthritis, radiological confirmation of joint erosion, and the demonstration of antibodies including RF by immunological tests. CNS signs should be explored using MRI studies of the brain and spinal cord as clinically indicated. EMG is useful in the differentiation of various peripheral nerve syndromes.

Management. The treatment of RA is generally divided into first-, second-, and third-line therapies. First-line therapy for joint disease employs nonsteroidal anti-inflammatory drugs. Second-line therapies include gold, D-penicillamine, sulfasalazine, and hydrochloroquine. Third-line agents include corticosteroids and cytotoxic agents. Rheumatoid vasculitis with central or peripheral nervous system manifestations should be treated as any other systemic vasculitis using immunosuppression with corticosteroids and cytotoxic agents. The role of other immunotherapies such as plasmapheresis or IVIg is not known.[66] The prognosis is similar to that of systemic necrotizing vasculitis. Cervical subluxation should be treated conservatively with analgesics, muscle relaxants, and neck immobilization. Protection from inadvertent and iatrogenic trauma is essential. Patients with severe vertebral displacement and marked or progressive myelopathy should be considered for surgical fixation.[67]

Prognosis and Future Perspectives. RA is a chronic disease, and the remission rate over 10 years is less than 10 percent.[68] RA is associated with excess mortality, with a threefold increase in the risk of death. Causes of death attributable to the disease process include infection and renal disease, whereas those likely related to treatment are gastrointestinal disorders.[69] Vasculitic peripheral neuropathy often improves, but the survival of patients with systemic rheumatoid vasculitis is poorer than others with RA.[22] Atlantoaxial subluxation is most often clinically static, and surgical fixation is not necessary in the majority of cases.[67]

SYSTEMIC LUPUS ERYTHEMATOSUS

Pathogenesis and Pathophysiology. SLE is defined by its clinical features and the almost invariable presence of autoantibodies directed against certain components of cell nuclei.[70] The immunological features of SLE are the lupus erythematosus cell, antinuclear antibodies, immune complexes, complement activation, tissue deposition of immunoglobulins and complement, and other autoantibodies. A nonspecific B-cell polyclonal activation may be responsible for the initiation of the disease; however, evidence of antigen-specific activation of antibody production also exists. Both of these mechanisms likely operate simultaneously to bring about manifestations of the disease.[70] Additionally, the linkage of certain antibodies with particular human leukocyte antigen loci and a 30 to 50 percent coincidence of SLE in monozygotic twins suggest a genetic factor in the pathogenesis of the disease.[70]

Tissue damage results from both immune complex–mediated vasculopathy and direct effects of antibodies reacting with cell-surface or serum components.[70] The clinical manifestations of SLE include those that result from immune responses as well as those that result from organ damage (e.g., uremia).

A number of drugs including procainamide, hydralazine, chlorpromazine, methyldopa, antibiotics, and anticonvulsants can produce a lupus-like syndrome. Some of these drugs induce the formation of histone-dependent antinuclear antibodies (ANA), and the syndromes usually abate with cessation of the drug. Drug-induced lupus is milder than idiopathic SLE and does not cause renal or CNS disease.

Epidemiology and Risk Factors. SLE is prevalent but varies throughout the world. In North America and northern Europe, the incidence is about 1 in 2500. There appears to be a higher incidence in Hispanics and African-Americans and a tendency toward more severe disease; however, based in part on socioeconomic factors, a potential ascertainment bias exists. There is a predominance of disease in women, with an incidence of 1 in 700, particularly among African-Americans, with an incidence of 1 in 245. The incidence in children and older adults is about 1 per 100,000.[70] Environmental risk factors have been implicated, including exposure to ultraviolet light, viral infection, and physical or emotional stress.

Neurological events are common in SLE. In one series, 91 patients were followed for 599 patient years. In 25 percent of the 288 hospital admissions, neurological problems were primary or secondary reasons for admission. Only 14 percent had no symptoms or signs attributable to nervous system disease.[71]

Clinical Features and Associated Disorders. SLE has diverse clinical manifestations that can affect virtually every organ system. A number of the common manifestations are not specific to SLE. Criteria for the diagnosis of SLE are listed in Table 50–6.[72]

The criteria for the diagnosis of neurological SLE are the presence of psychosis or seizures in the absence of offending drugs or known metabolic disturbance such as uremia or severe electrolyte imbalance. The term CNS-SLE or neuropsychiatric lupus has been used to describe collectively the neurological or behavioral events in patients with SLE. The neurological complications of SLE extend beyond this oversimplification, and there are often multiple factors related and unrelated to the disease that contribute to neurological dysfunction.

A few studies have looked specifically at the neurological and behavioral events in SLE.[71, 73] Seizures represent approximately 25 percent of the neurological problems in patients with SLE and may occur at times of disease inactivity.[74] In most cases, the genesis of seizures was multifactorial and included pre-existing epilepsy, trauma, azotemia, systemic infection, meningitis, or stroke. About 30 percent of patients with SLE and seizures have no other predisposing features.[71] Seizures are positively associated with coagulopathy and stroke, and negatively associated with cardiac disease.[71]

Stroke accounts for 15 to 20 percent of neurological events in SLE and is a significant cause of morbidity.[71] Although stroke was as likely to occur during disease inactivity in the study by Kaell, 86 percent of another series of patients with large vessel occlusive disease stroke had active SLE at the time of the stroke.[73, 74] In more than half the cases, strokes are multiple, although earlier strokes may have been asymptomatic.[74] Headache heralded ischemic stroke in 60 percent of cases in one series.[73] Strokes may result from emboli, coagulopathy, atherosclerotic disease, or arterial dissection.[74] Libman-Sacks valvular disease or ventricular dysfunction may be identified in some patients. Valvular

TABLE 50–6. **Criteria for the Diagnosis of Systemic Lupus Erythematosus**

Criterion	Definition
Malar rash	Fixed erythema, flat or raised, over the malar eminences, tending to spare the nasolabial folds
Discoid rash	Erythematous raised patches with adherent keratotic scaling and follicular plugging; atrophic scarring may occur in older lesions
Photosensitivity	Skin rash occurring as a result of exposure to sunlight, by patient history or physician observation
Oral ulcers	Oral or nasopharyngeal ulceration, usually painless, observed by a physician
Arthritis	Nonerosive arthritis involving two or more peripheral joints, characterized by tenderness, swelling, or effusion
Serositis	Pleuritis—convincing history of pleuritic pain or rub heard by a physician or pleural effusion *or* Pericarditis—documented by electrocardiogram or rub or evidence of pericardial effusion
Renal disorder	Persistent proteinuria >0.5 g per day or greater than 3+ if quantitation not performed *or* Cellular casts—may be red cell, hemoglobin, granular, tubular, or mixed
Neurological disorder	Seizures—in the absence of offending drugs or metabolic derangements *or* Psychosis—in the absence of offending drugs or known metabolic derangements
Hematological disorder	Hemolytic anemia—with reticulocytosis *or* Leukopenia—less than 4000/μL on two or more occasions *or* Lymphopenia—less than 1500/μL on two or more occasions *or* Thrombocytopenia—less than 100,000/μL in the absence of offending drugs
Immunological disorder	Positive LE cell preparation *or* Anti-DNA: antibody to native DNA in abnormal titer *or* Anti-Sm: presence of antibody to Smith nuclear antigen *or* False-positive serological test for syphilis known to be positive for 6 months and confirmed by *Treponema pallidum* immobilization or fluorescent treponemal antibody absorption test
Antinuclear antibody	An abnormal titer of antinuclear antibody by immunofluorescence or equivalent assay at any point in time and in the absence of drugs known to be associated with drug-induced lupus syndrome

Modified from Tan EM, Cohen AS, Fries JF, et al: The 1982 revised criteria for the classification of systemic lupus erythematosus. Arthritis Rheum 1982; 25:1271–1277.

vegetations on postmortem examination can be found despite a normal echocardiogram.[73]

Antiphospholipid antibodies such as anticardiolipin antibody and lupus anticoagulant may play a significant role in many of the thrombotic events in SLE.[73] Statistically, the presence of these antibodies significantly raises the incidence of primary stroke; the recurrence rate among aPL-positive SLE patients with prior stroke exceeds 50 percent.[71] Antiphospholipid antibodies in patients with SLE are more likely to be associated with valvular and other cardiac disease.[73] Vasculitis is a rare cause of CNS dysfunction in SLE.[71, 73] Long-term corticosteroid treatment may play a role in premature cerebral and coronary atherosclerotic disease, which may contribute to stroke risk.[73] Hemorrhagic stroke occurs less commonly but frequently results in coma or death.[71]

Behavioral changes occur for a variety of reasons and represent at least one third or more of the neurological complications seen with SLE. Psychosis, delirium, altered alertness, disorientation, suicide attempts, and behavioral outbursts account for most cases.[71] Steroids are rarely implicated as a cause of behavioral change. Systemic or CNS infections are involved in many cases and may be fatal.[71] Opportunistic infections, including cytomegalovirus, aspergillus, *Listeria*, and *Strongyloides stercoralis* are common, and the CSF may not show inflammatory changes in the presence of infection.[71, 74]

Chorea has been described in patients with SLE and may be associated with the presence of aPL in the absence of a radiographic lesion in the basal ganglia.[71] PNS abnormalities are less common than in other collagen vascular disorders, occurring in 2 to 21 percent of cases.[75] A predominantly distal, axonal sensorimotor polyneuropathy is more common than mononeuritis multiplex.[75]

Pregnancy in patients with active disease, particularly with nephritis and hypertension, is associated with a substantial risk of disease exacerbation and injury to the fetus. The presence of aPL has been associated with both stroke and second-trimester abortion.[70, 73] For patients in remission, however, the risks during pregnancy are similar to those of unaffected patients.[70]

Differential Diagnosis. The diagnosis of SLE is largely dependent on demonstrating a constellation of relatively specific findings to differentiate it from other systemic diseases. In approaching a patient with a given neurological syndrome, the differential diagnosis is generated by the predominant clinical picture, but SLE should always be kept in mind in a patient with CNS or PNS problems and dermatological or renal disease.

Evaluation. Various techniques can detect serum immune complexes, but the presence or quantity of the complexes is not specific to SLE. The most common antibody in SLE is the ANA that stains homogeneously on immunofluorescence and is directed against nucleosomal DNA histone complexes. Over 95 percent of SLE patients have ANA in significant titers. Normal ANA titers are strong evidence against the diagnosis. Antibodies to native or double-stranded DNA and Sm, a ribonuclear protein antigen, are more specific than other ANA for the diagnosis of SLE.[70]

Depressed serum complement levels are useful though not specific in recognizing disease activity and risk for renal and CNS involvement in SLE. Levels should be assessed during disease inactivity for comparison, and routine levels can serve as a guide for treatment. The aPL anticardiolipin antibody and lupus anticoagulant can be directly assessed in the serum.[73]

CSF studies in SLE are nonspecific. Pleocytosis, elevated protein, and oligoclonal bands do not consistently correlate with the clinical syndrome or its severity.[71] CSF may be helpful in identifying the responsible pathogen in CNS infection but is not entirely sensitive.[71] Electroencephalography (EEG) may be useful in a certain number of cases. The most common finding is generalized or focal slowing, and focal epileptiform discharges are seen in patients with seizures. The demonstration of a normal EEG may be useful in differentiation of psychosis and delirium.[71]

MRI and CT scans are valuable in detecting strokes in this population. MRI has also demonstrated reversible changes suggesting breakdown of the blood-brain barrier in association with seizures or headaches.[71]

There are no accepted criteria for the diagnosis of CNS-SLE.[71] Of the diagnostic tests such as antineuronal antibodies, CSF-guanine levels, nuclear imaging, CT or MRI, or CSF oligoclonal bands, none has proven to be a single index of nervous system involvement.[74]

Management. Many patients with mild symptoms such as myalgias, arthralgias, low-grade fevers, or arthritis can be managed with nonsteroidal anti-inflammatory medications. Some patients with skin rash and mucositis are effectively managed with antimalarial medications.[70] When end organs are jeopardized, glucocorticoid therapy is indicated, and prednisone at an initial dose of 60 mg/d is usually sufficient.[70] Treatment response can be followed clinically and serologically. Because there are no clear guidelines for the steroid management of SLE, the risks of steroid therapy should be weighed against the more immediate risks of the disease activity.

Treatment of the CNS complications of SLE depends on the pathogenic factors involved. Antithrombotic therapy with antiplatelet agents or anticoagulants is probably required for patients with aPL-associated vascular events, but this treatment has not been proven.[71, 73] Increased doses of corticosteroid may be of benefit if there are significant levels of aPL.[73] Diffuse CNS involvement, mononeuritis multiplex, or findings suggestive of a vasculitis are best treated with corticosteroids; cytotoxic agents may be of additional benefit, although this has not been well demonstrated.[70] There are no specific guidelines for therapy during pregnancy. However, anticoagulation is probably indicated for pregnant SLE patients with aPL.[70]

Prognosis and Future Perspectives. Although the natural history is highly variable, the 10-year survival rate approaches 90 percent. Patients with nephritis and systolic hypertension have a significantly worse prognosis.[70] Although acutely dangerous, seizures and psychosis are generally associated with good long-term recovery.[74] Patients with neurological episodes with more than one potential etiological factor such as hypertension, uremia, infection, drug abuse, and electrolyte abnormalities are more likely to recover significant function than those experiencing primary SLE-related events.[74] Stroke and systemic infection carry a relatively poor short-term outcome.[71, 73]

Additional investigation of mechanisms involved in the generation of SLE-induced organ damage will serve to direct future therapies. Of relevance to SLE and other autoimmune diseases are therapies that may eliminate specific autoantibodies involved in the pathogenesis of the disease such as anti-idiotype antibodies and sensitization of T cells against specific autoantibodies.

PROGRESSIVE SYSTEMIC SCLEROSIS

Pathogenesis and Pathophysiology. Progressive systemic sclerosis (PSS) is a condition associated with thickening of the skin and tethering to subcutaneous tissues as well as smooth muscle atrophy and fibrosis of internal organs such as the gastrointestinal tract, lungs, heart, and kidneys. The disorder is characterized pathologically by increased collagen deposition and perivascular inflammation in the skin, subcutaneous tissues, and internal organs.

Antinuclear antibodies are typically found, usually in a nucleolar pattern; antibodies to Scl-70, a soluble nuclear antigen, are specific, though insensitive. The demonstration of antibodies to smooth muscle and cytotoxicity to cultured endothelial cells suggests that autoimmunity plays a role in pathogenesis. The etiology of PSS is unknown, but glandular inflammatory processes appear to be related to cell-mediated immunity or to antibody-mediated cytotoxicity rather than to immune complex deposition.[66] Immune complex disease appears to be responsible for rare cases of associated vasculitis.

Epidemiology and Risk Factors. The incidence of PSS ranges from 0.6 to 2.3 per million.[76] Women, usually between the ages of 40 and 60 years, are affected three times as often as men. The association with certain HLA class II antigens suggests a hereditary predisposition.

Clinical Features and Associated Disorders. Some patients have a relatively benign form of the disorder limited to cutaneous changes in the distal extremities. In the generalized form of the illness, cutaneous abnormalities may predominate, but systemic symptoms, including generalized malaise, are common. Vascular changes in the hands progress from Raynaud's phenomenon to frank necrosis and induration and fibrosis of the skin (sclerodactyly) with atrophy of the underlying muscle. Rigidity of ligamentous tissue in the inner ear leads to conductive hearing loss. There may be fibrotic changes in the myocardium, pericardium, pleura, or lung. Glomerulonephritis with renal crisis is a frequent cause of morbidity and mortality. Mucosal gastrointestinal lesions occur, preferentially in the distal esophagus. Keratoconjunctivitis, lens subluxation, and cataracts are typical ocular signs, and musculoskeletal changes, including atrophy and osteolytic lesions, joint symptoms, and myopathy, occur in 50 percent of patients.[77]

The frequency of nervous system involvement varies; in one series of 727 patients, 6 had nervous system changes.[77] In a more recent report of 48 patients, 56 percent had neurological disturbances.[75] Electrophysiological studies suggest subclinical nervous system dysfunction in many asymptomatic patients.[78]

Although rare, CNS disease has been reported. It may present as global cognitive decline or as a focal lesion. Encephalopathy, migraine, psychiatric changes, seizures, and focal neurological deficits have been reported.[75, 79] Three cases with presumed cerebral arteritis have been reported, one a reversible encephalopathy with angiographic evidence of vasculitis, one with hemiplegia and aphasia with angiographic evidence of vasculitis, and one with right thalamic hemorrhage.

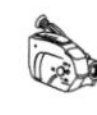

Trigeminal neuropathy is a frequent presenting feature of PSS and is the most common cranial neuropathy found in the disorder. It develops insidiously or acutely and affects primarily the central part of the face. Pain is common and may resemble that of tic douloureux.[78] Median and ulnar entrapment neuropathies have been reported in up to 20 percent and distal polyneuropathy in up to 15 percent of patients.[80] Most peripheral neuropathies can be ascribed to metabolic and nutritional factors. However, some cases of sensorimotor neuropathy occurring before the onset of other symptoms or very early in the disease course suggest that PSS may be etiological. In addition, a prospective evaluation of 29 patients with limited or widespread systemic sclerosis demonstrated raised tactile thresholds in 28, suggesting that subclinical peripheral nerve dysfunction is common in the disorder.[81] Autonomic neuropathy is common,[82] and recent evidence suggests that gastrointestinal dysmotility may be related to a neuropathic process.[83]

EMG in most cases of sensorimotor neuropathy reveals axonopathy, and histological features include collagenous infiltration of the peripheral nerves and the adventitia of vasa nervorum. Low-grade distal nerve trunk ischemia may contribute to neuropathy.[84] Biopsy of the sural nerve reveals segmental demyelination, axonal degeneration, loss of large myelinated fibers, and an increase of collagen fibers, without evidence of vasculitis.[85]

Differential Diagnosis. Chronic graft-versus-host disease following bone marrow transplant can mimic the picture of PSS, though esophageal and renal involvement are usually not seen. Sclerodermatous skin changes can be seen in response to certain chemotherapeutic agents.

Evaluation. The diagnosis of PSS is generally made clinically. Evidence of disturbed gastrointestinal motility and vasculopathy on nailfold capillary microscopy are confirmatory. Generalized or focal CNS abnormalities can be investigated using MRI. Nerve conduction velocities (NCV) and EMG are useful in the elucidation of neuropathy syndromes, and NCV can be used to detect subclinical neuropathy.

Management. Symptomatic treatments include nonsteroidal anti-inflammatory drugs for arthritis and vasoactive drugs for Raynaud's phenomenon. Neuropathic pain, especially that associated with trigeminal neuropathy, can be treated with carbamazepine or tricyclic antidepressants. Penicillamine, colchicine, prednisone, and immunosuppressants have been used for more severe disease manifestations, but their relative effectiveness has not been determined.[66]

Prognosis and Future Perspectives. The 10-year survival rate in PSS approximates 50 percent.[86] In some cases the disease is rapidly progressive, and death occurs within 1 year. The most common causes of death are renal failure and cardiac complications. Individual survival is largely dependent on the extent of involvement. Digital sclerodactyly alone carries a very benign prognosis. Prognosis is worse with diffuse disease, older onset age, and early involvement of internal organs.[87]

MIXED CONNECTIVE TISSUE DISEASE

Pathogenesis and Pathophysiology. In 1971, Sharp described patients in whom a new type of antibody to ribonuclease-sensitive extractable nuclear antigen was accompanied by clinical features of more than one connective tissue disease. He called the syndrome mixed connective tissue disease (MCTD) and described several serologic characteristics: (1) high titers of hemagglutinating antibody to saline-extractable nuclear antigen; (2) marked sensitivity of this antibody to ribonuclease with moderate sensitivity to trypsin and resistance to deoxyribonuclease; (3) high titers of speckled pattern on fluorescent ANA testing; and (4) absence of Smith antibody. Saline-extractable nuclear antigen appears to represent two moieties: ribonucleoprotein (RNP) and the Smith (Sm) antigen, a glycoprotein. Whereas high titers of anti-RNP antibodies appear to be associated with MCTD, the presence of anti-Sm correlates highly with the diagnosis of SLE. The etiopathogenesis of MCTD is poorly understood but is felt to relate to formation of autoreactive T cells in response to exposure to microbial antigens, which are similar to an autoantigen.[88] Patients with MCTD may have ANA in a speckled pattern, RF, and cold-reactive lymphocytotoxic and anticardiolipin antibodies.[89]

Epidemiology and Risk Factors. The prevalence of MCTD is unknown. It is intermediate in frequency between SLE and systemic sclerosis.[90] Women are more frequently affected than men by a factor of 4 to 79:1.[91] Although most frequently seen in the second and third decades of life, it has been reported in children and the elderly as well.[89] There is an association between the 68-kd-U1 snRNP and the DR4 haplotype in both SLE and MCTD.[92] The existence of MCTD as a discrete syndrome is not universally accepted, because the serological markers are not specific for the diagnosis[90] and the disorder frequently evolves over a number of years into SLE or PSS.[90, 93] Nevertheless, the term is still considered helpful to describe a number of patients with a mixed clinical picture.

Clinical Features and Associated Disorders. Patients with MCTD have clinical features of at least two connective tissue disorders, among them SLE, PSS, and polymyositis. Nearly all have arthralgia, nondeforming arthritis, inflammatory myositis, Raynaud's phenomenon, sclerodactyly, and a tapered or sausage-like appearance of the digits, sometimes with digital ischemia and ulceration. Pitting edema of the forehead and erythematous malar or violaceous eyelid rash may be present. Disorders of esophageal motility affect more than 75 percent of patients. Lymphadenopathy is common and sometimes marked, suggesting lymphoma. Fever, hepatosplenomegaly, pleuritis, pericarditis, and cardiac and hair changes are seen in 20 to 40 percent of cases. Pulmonary disease is very common, and although it may be asymptomatic, pulmonary hypertension is the most common cause of death.[94, 95] Frequent laboratory abnormalities include leukopenia, anemia, and hypergammaglobulinemia.[95] Renal disease is evident in some patients with MCTD. Proteinuria, sometimes with nephrotic syndrome, hematuria, glomerulonephritis, or proliferative vascular lesions, may be seen.

Neurological sequelae of MCTD occur in 10 to 55 percent of cases.[96–98] The CNS complications of MCTD resemble those seen in SLE, whereas the PNS complications resemble those seen in PSS. CNS effects occur in the context of active systemic disease and are largely steroid responsive, whereas PSS effects occur irrespective of systemic disease activity and are largely steroid resistant. The most common disorders are vascular-type headache, aseptic meningitis, psychosis, and convulsions.[98, 99] Ischemic and hemorrhagic cerebrovascular disorders, optic neuritis, cerebellar ataxia, chorea, and transverse myelitis occur less commonly.[97, 98, 100–102]

The PNS is a more frequent target of MCTD than the CNS. In published series, unilateral or bilateral trigeminal neuropathy occurs in about 10 percent of MCTD patients.[96, 98, 103] The maxillary and mandibular branches are usually involved.[104] Some patients may have involvement of the motor root with masseter atrophy.[98, 104] Although dysfunction of regional cranial nerves is rare, associations with facial neuropathy have been reported.[104, 105] Vasculitic polyneuropathy has been reported in up to 10 percent of patients with MCTD.[98] There have been rare reports of carpal tunnel syndrome[106] and neuromuscular junction dysfunction.[107] The importance of myositis in MCTD is underscored by its inclusion as a diagnostic criterion in virtually all series of patients.[89] Concurrent changes of overlying skin mimic dermatomyositis in some patients.[97]

Differential Diagnosis. The most important distinction is between MCTD and other connective tissue disorders such as PSS, SLE, and polymyositis. This distinction is blurred over time as the disease generally comes to resemble one of these connective tissue diseases.

Evaluation. The diagnosis of MCTD is made in patients with symptoms and signs of more than one connective tissue disease and the characteristic serological markers. CNS manifestations are evaluated with MRI, which may demonstrate signs of vascular disease. In patients with seizures, EEG shows focal or generalized slowing and often epileptiform activity.[98] CSF in patients with headaches or aseptic meningitis may be normal or show a lymphocytic pleocytosis or increased protein. Elevations of serum creatine kinase occur in about half of those with myopathic symptoms. EMG changes may confirm the presence of myopathy, and biopsy may show inflammatory myositis.[97]

Management. The treatment of nervous system involvement in MCTD is based on anecdotal data rather than controlled clinical trials. CNS disorders such as headache, aseptic meningitis, psychosis, convulsions, optic neuritis, and transverse myelitis have been reported by various authors to be responsive to corticosteroids,[97, 98] plasmapheresis, or immunosuppressive drugs.[101] Disorders of the PNS, including trigeminal and peripheral neuropathy, are relatively steroid resistant.[98, 104, 106] Myositis is believed to mirror the systemic signs of MCTD and be quite sensitive to corticosteroid therapy.

Prognosis and Future Perspectives. The majority of patients with MCTD evolve clinical features typical of another connective tissue disease within 5 years of diagnosis.[88] Long-term follow-up of 194 patients in several series revealed that 13 to 28.2 percent had died by 13 years' follow-up.[90, 107] More benign prognosis appears to be associated with the presence of Raynaud's phenomenon, less widespread and severe organ system involvement, and HLA-DR2 or DR4.[107, 108]

The most compelling research questions are whether MCTD is a discrete diagnostic entity and what factors predict its evolution into other connective tissue diseases. Better elucidation of environmental triggering antigens and the autoantigen immune target may lead to more effective therapies, particularly for steroid-resistant symptoms.

SJÖGREN'S SYNDROME

Pathogenesis and Pathophysiology. Sjögren's syndrome (SS) is a chronic inflammatory disease of unknown cause characterized by inflammation of the salivary and lacrimal glands and synovial tissues. Involved tissues have infiltrates of lymphocytes and plasma cells. Autoantibodies include RF, ANA (SS-A and SS-B type), and antibodies directed against salivary duct antigens.

Epidemiology and Risk Factors. SS is seen in 0.5 to 2.0 percent of the population; among the collagen vascular diseases, it is second in prevalence only to RA.[109] Ninety percent of patients are women. Onset usually occurs during middle age.[109] Genetic susceptibility is suggested by an association with HLA-B8, HLA-DR3, HLA-DR2, and HLA-DRw52. SS occurs in isolation in 50 percent of cases and in the context of RA, SLE, scleroderma, or another connective tissue disease in the remaining patients.[109]

Clinical Features and Associated Disorders. Primary SS predominantly affects exocrine glands, with lymphocytic infiltration and fibrosis of lacrimal and salivary glands. Ocular, oral, and dental complications occur as a result of decreased tear and saliva production.[109] Extraglandular manifestations occur in at least 25 percent of patients. Lymphadenopathy and hepatosplenomegaly are common. Cutaneous vasculitis may present with a picture of nonthrombocytopenic purpura or urticaria. Symmetrical, nondeforming arthritis of the small joints occurs in more than 80 percent of patients. Renal disease, usually interstitial nephritis, is seen in up to 40 percent of cases. Less commonly, the lungs may be involved, with interstitial pneumonitis and restrictive or obstructive abnormalities of pulmonary function. Vasculitis, usually localized to the skin, PNS, and muscle, occurs in up to 20 percent. Lymphoproliferative disorders occur, and there is an increased risk of lymphoma in these patients.

Although neurological disorders have been thought to be rare manifestations of SS, as many as 25 to 80 percent of patients have nervous system dysfunction, sometimes in advance of other symptoms.[110–112] CNS complications include mild aseptic meningitis; cognitive, affective, or personality disorders; focal cerebral deficits; and seizure.[110, 111] 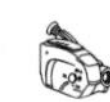 Optic neuropathy, nystagmus, ataxia, internuclear ophthalmoplegia, and parkinsonism or other movement disorders have occasionally been reported.[113] Spinal cord involvement may take one of three forms: progressive myelopathy, acute transverse myelitis, or intraspinal hemorrhage.[110]

PNS signs and symptoms occur in 10 to 32 percent of cases.[114] Most commonly, there is a sensory or mixed motor-sensory polyneuropathy or entrapment neuropathy. The polyneuropathy may be abrupt or insidious in onset, is often asymmetrical, affects proprioceptive and kinesthetic senses, and causes mild distal motor weakness in the legs.[115] Mononeuritis multiplex occurs somewhat less commonly, and cranial nerve involvement, specifically trigeminal, oculomotor, and abducens nerves, can occur.[115]

Differential Diagnosis. The diagnosis of primary SS is made in the presence of two of the typical manifestations of xerostomia, xerophthalmia, and arthritis. Illnesses that should be considered in the differential diagnosis are all causes of parotitis, including malignancy, nutritional and endocrine disorders, sarcoidosis, infections, and amyloidosis.

Evaluation. Xerophthalmia can be demonstrated by Schirmer's test, staining of the corneal and conjunctival epithelium by Rose Bengal dye, or demonstration of epithelial strands by slit-lamp examination. Xerostomia can be assessed by nuclear scanning of the salivary glands, radiological sialography, or calculation of salivary flow rate. Biopsy of minor salivary glands, found on the inner aspect of the lower lip, is well tolerated and diagnostic when lymphocytic aggregation is demonstrated. Anemia, leukopenia, and elevated ESR are common. Hypergammaglobulinemia and positive RF are common but not specific for the diagnosis. SS-B antibodies are relatively specific for primary SS. SS-A antibodies are seen in primary SS and SS associated with SLE. Half of SS patients have antibodies against salivary duct antigens.

The EEG is abnormal in nearly 50 percent of patients with CNS dysfunction, but the findings are nonspecific. CT and MRI scans usually show focal regions of abnormality in patients with clinical evidence of focal pathology.[110] Electrophysiological studies are consistent with demyelination, denervation, or both. CSF may be normal or may show pleocytosis and elevated protein. CSF is characterized by protein elevation and evidence of intrathecal immunoglobulin synthesis, with increased IgG and oligoclonal bands.[110] Pathological studies are limited, but perivascular inflammation and diffuse vasculitis involving the cerebral blood vessels, as well as acute necrotizing arteritis of the spinal cord, have been described.[114] Peripheral nerve tissue shows demyelination and acute or chronic vasculitis or perivasculitis.[115] Dorsal root ganglionitis, with lymphocytic infiltration and degeneration of ganglion cells, has also been reported to accompany subacute sensory neuronopathy, which is a rare complication of SS.[116]

Management. Ocular and oral symptoms are managed conservatively, with artificial tears and saliva and good oral hygiene. Corticosteroids may be needed to control arthritis and symptoms related to vasculitis.

Prognosis and Future Perspectives. Primary SS is generally compatible with prolonged survival. A small number of patients develop more serious disease manifestations, including primary biliary cirrhosis, renal disease, chronic active hepatitis, pancreatitis, visceral lymphocytic infiltration, lymphoma, immunoblastic sarcoma, or Waldenström's macroglobulinemia. Future research should focus on the etiopathogenesis of the disorder in order to increase understanding of the cause and potential treatments.

Other Autoimmune Conditions

MYASTHENIA GRAVIS

Pathogenesis and Pathophysiology. Myasthenia gravis (MG), although described for many years, was first associated with decreased numbers of muscle acetylcholine receptors about 25 years ago.[117] Since then, the identification of anti-acetylcholine receptor antibodies (AChR-ab), the development of an animal model of the disease, and an overall improved knowledge of immune mechanisms have led to a very precise understanding of the pathophysiology of MG.[117]

The immune effector cells in MG are both T and B cells. Although the key to acetylcholine receptor damage is through the AChR-ab, sensitized T cells and complement play a role in the continued stimulation of B cells and in cell-mediated postsynaptic destruction at the neuromuscular junction.[118] The histological hallmarks of MG include decreased numbers of acetylcholine receptors, simplification of the postsynaptic clefts, and widening of the synaptic space with a normal presynaptic nerve terminal.[117]

The thymus is unequivocally involved in the pathogenesis of the disease, and its surgical removal often is associated with improvement in disease severity.[118] Thymic abnormalities are either hyperplastic or neoplastic. Hyperplasia is associated with areas of germinal centers that may enlarge the gland beyond the normal size for age. Neoplasms occur in about 12 percent of patients and are usually locally invasive epithelial cell tumors (thymomas or rarely carcinomas).[117, 118]

In addition to immune activation against acetylcholine receptors, there is functional blockade of postsynaptic receptors, which can in part explain the response to acetylcholinesterase inhibitors and the relatively quick response to therapies that reduce the number of AChR-ab.[117]

Epidemiology and Risk Factors. MG can occur throughout life, with a bimodal peak of incidence in younger women (second and third decades) and older men (fifth and sixth decades).[118] Overall, MG has a prevalence of 1 in 25,000 in the United States.[117] There are cases of overlap of MG with other autoimmune diseases and case reports of families with various autoimmune conditions including MG. This suggests a partial genetic predisposition.[117]

Clinical Features and Associated Disorders. The typical features of MG are fatigability and weakness of skeletal muscles without reflex, sensory, or coordination abnormalities. Many cases begin with involvement of ocular muscles such as diplopia and ptosis. Weakness may remain confined to ocular muscles for long periods or involve bulbar muscles, which control chewing, swallowing, and articulation. The disorder remains confined to ocular muscles in up to 15 percent of patients but becomes generalized in the majority.[117] Examination of neck extensors and flexors is often more sensitive in demonstrating generalized disease than the motor examination of other muscle groups.[117] Under periods of physical stress, such as infection or surgery, a precipitous worsening may occur, and failure of respiratory muscles can be life threatening. Classification of disease severity is usually assessed according to a scale devised by Osserman, where grade I is ocular disease only, grade II is generalized weakness of mild (IIa) or moderate (IIb) intensity, grade III is severe generalized disease, and grade IV is myasthenic "crisis" with respiratory failure.[117]

Transient neonatal MG can occur from passive transfer of maternal AChR-ab causing a myasthenic syndrome that may require ventilatory assistance.[117] These symptoms typically resolve in under 2 weeks, with routine clearance of antibodies from the neonate's circulation.

Differential Diagnosis. A number of disorders may mimic MG and include other disorders of neuromuscular transmission, metabolic or toxic syndromes, and neurogenic weakness.[117] Botulism and Lambert-Eaton myasthenic syndrome (LEMS) can cause ophthalmoplegia and fatigue. Botulism affects cranial nerves early, affects the pupillary light response, and shows an incremental response on repetitive nerve stimulation. Botulinum toxin may be detectable in the stools. LEMS is often associated with an oat-cell carcinoma of the lung, dry mouth and eyes, and more distal weakness that may improve with exercise. The presence of voltage-gated calcium channel antibodies in the serum and a dramatic increase in compound motor potentials on postexercise repetitive nerve stimulation are confirmatory objective signs.[117] The congenital myasthenic syndromes appear as MG but are not autoimmune in nature.[118]

Certain drugs, including penicillamine, curare, aminoglycosides, quinine, procainamide, and calcium channel blockers, may cause a myasthenia-like syndrome or exacerbate weakness in MG patients. Hyperthyroidism, or Graves' disease, may cause generalized fatigue or worsen MG and is detectable by abnormal thyroid function tests.[117] Cranial nerve abnormalities may cause symptoms that mimic MG.[117]

Evaluation. Timed endurance tasks such as prolonged upgaze, holding outstretched arms in abduction, or vital capacities at every visit are often helpful in providing objective information about fatigability.[117] Laboratory tests useful in excluding other diagnoses include thyroid function tests, antithyroid antibody, ANA, voltage-gated calcium channel antibodies, and chest x-ray.

Improvement of weakness after edrophonium chloride (Tensilon) injection is a useful sign, although false-negative and false-positive tests do occur.[119] The test is performed by first fatiguing the patient with a task that includes signs that can be easily clinically assessed (ptosis, vital capacity, slurred speech). The diagnostic test is then performed by injection of 1 mg as a test dose, then injecting 9 mg intravenously with attention to the fatigued muscles. A rapid improvement or recovery of the fatigued muscles (resolved ptosis, normalized vital capacity, clear and strong voice) over the subsequent 2 minutes is a positive test. If ptosis is present, the "ice pack test" may be diagnostic. Local cooling improves the safety factor of neuromuscular junctions, possibly by slowing the kinetics of acetylcholinesterase. In a prospective series, 80 percent of MG patients responded after 2 minutes of ice pack application to the affected eye, and the nonresponders with MG had complete ptosis. Ptosis due to other etiologies did not respond.[120] This test is easier to administer in a clinic setting than edrophonium chloride and does not require cardiac monitoring.

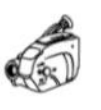

In recent years, the detection of AChR-ab in the serum, using a commercially available immunoprecipitation test, has significantly changed the evaluation of MG patients.[119] The sensitivity of AChR-ab in ocular myasthenia is 70 percent and in generalized disease is 80 percent.[119]

Repetitive nerve stimulation may demonstrate a reduction of the compound muscle action potential, potentiated after 1 minute of exercise, consistent with a postsynaptic transmission defect. For patient comfort, the test should first be performed on a distal muscle; negative studies on distal muscles should prompt more extensive study of proximal muscles. Clinically weak muscles are more likely to demonstrate the decremental response.[119] The sensitivity of repetitive nerve stimulation is about 75 percent. It may be normal in ocular MG but is virtually always abnormal in generalized MG.[119]

The demonstration of increased "jitter" by single-fiber EMG is the most sensitive test for MG. The sensitivity ranges from 80 percent in ocular MG to virtually 100 percent in moderate generalized MG. In 9 percent of MG cases, this is the only abnormal test.[119] Using AChR-ab, repetitive stimulation and single-fiber EMG identifies all MG cases.[119, 121]

CT scanning or MRI of the chest should be done in all patients to screen for the presence of thymoma or thymic hyperplasia. Thymic enlargement or detectable thymic tissue in a patient over age 40 raises the suspicion of thymoma.[117]

Chest imaging is also indicated in patients who have had thymectomy but are experiencing unexplained worsening of MG symptoms. Residual thymic tissue may be found in some of these patients.

Management. Acetylcholinesterase inhibitors (mainly pyridostigmine) inhibit the enzymatic elimination of acetylcholine, increasing its concentration at the postsynaptic membrane. They play a supporting role in the management of symptoms throughout the disease course but do not affect the primary immune mechanism of the disease.[118] Cholinergic toxicity causing transient weakness can result from overuse of pyridostigmine and can be difficult to distinguish from the weakness of MG. MG is rarely controlled by symptomatic treatment alone, and immunomodulating therapy is often required.

There is general consensus that thymectomy is helpful in the treatment of MG; however, a randomized controlled study has never been done.[117] With thymoma, there is a clear role for thymectomy. For nonthymomatous MG, thymectomy may increase the likelihood of disease remission or improvement.[122] Typically, patients with generalized MG (Osserman stage 2b or worse) are selected for thymectomy. Thymectomy for ocular MG (Osserman stage 1) has been supported by nonrandomized, uncontrolled data but remains a controversial issue.[123] The beneficial effects of thymectomy usually occur in the first year but may be seen as late as 5 years from the time of surgery.[118] Thymectomy is never an urgent procedure but can be done on optimally stabilized patients and in centers with experience in managing the perioperative course of MG patients. The trans-sternal approach is preferred because it allows for direct visualization and complete removal of the thymus and adipose tissue of the anterior mediastinum. In contrast, the transcervical approach by indirect mediastinoscopy is associated with a higher occurrence of residual thymus tissue, although this method is cosmetically more appealing.[117, 118] Controlled comparison of these two approaches has not demonstrated superiority of one over the other.[122]

Corticosteroids have been the mainstay of immunotherapy for MG. Seventy to 80 percent of patients have complete remission of their disease within weeks to months of adequate doses of prednisone.[118] The starting dose is dependent upon the severity of symptoms, but most patients require 40 to 60 mg/d. Alternate-day dosing is encouraged to lessen adverse side effects and should be tapered to the lowest effective dose.[117]

Cytotoxic therapies are useful in MG and should be considered in patients who are not able to achieve sufficiently low doses of prednisone or who are having significant steroid side effects. Azathioprine 2 to 3 mg/kg/d is effective in a number of patients as an adjunct to prednisone, and its use allows lowering of the total dose of the prednisone to more tolerable levels. Some patients respond well enough to discontinue the prednisone.[118] Cyclosporine is a more effective and more toxic immunosuppressive agent.[117] The typical dose is 5 mg/kg/d. Improvement occurs in the first several months of therapy.[117] Nephrotoxicity, hypertension, neutropenia, and remote risk of leukemia are potential complications of therapy, and blood levels need to be monitored to reduce the incidence of these toxic side effects.[118] Mycophenolate mofetil is a novel immunosuppressant that blocks purine synthesis in T- and B-cell lymphocytes, selectively inhibiting proliferation. It is relatively well tolerated with less frequent but similar side effects as other cytotoxic therapies. Dosing is 1 gram given twice daily. Initial studies have shown efficacy in MG with a relatively short time to therapeutic benefit (2 weeks to 2 months), and larger studies are ongoing.[124, 125]

Plasma exchange and intravenous pooled immune globulin are effective short-term treatments for MG. For the treatment of MG crisis or before thymectomy, five courses of plasma exchange, given on alternate days, cause rapid improvement that lasts for several weeks. Venous access, a mild increased risk of infection, hypotension during exchanges, deep venous thrombosis, and cost are drawbacks to this treatment.[117] There is preliminary evidence to support the use of pooled IVIg in the treatment of MG. Like plasma exchange, the treatment is given over a few days (0.4 g/kg/d times 5 days) and the effect is relatively short-lived, lasting a few weeks.[118]

Prognosis and Future Perspectives. Before 1958, approximately one third of MG patients died, one third failed to improve, and one third improved spontaneously.[117] Currently, the mortality rate is essentially zero, and most patients lead normal lives. Lifelong immunomodulating therapy is often required.[117]

Novel approaches for potential treatment of MG are increasing with advancing knowledge of the immune system. Targeting specific T cells and B cells, which are "programmed" to mediate anti-acetylcholine receptor activity, is the focus of recent experimental work.[117] Such therapy would tightly target the effector arm of the immune system. This strategy is limited by evidence that T cells have a number of targets and lack of knowledge of which T cells are relevant to the pathogenesis of MG. Animal models suggest that the nonselective removal of the T helper cells may also be beneficial.[117] Lastly, there is renewed interest in inducing tolerance to self-antigens by ingesting them. Oral ingestion of anti-acetylcholine receptor antibodies has been found to prevent the disease in rat models of MG.[117] New insights generated by this work will lead to safer and more effective therapies.

DERMATOMYOSITIS AND POLYMYOSITIS

Pathogenesis and Pathophysiology. Dermatomyositis (DM) and polymyositis (PM) have been thought to have an autoimmune origin for many years. This concept is based on indirect associations with other autoimmune disorders, mononuclear inflammatory cells in affected muscles, and responsiveness to immunosuppressive agents. Genetic factors play a role, as evidenced by reports of identical twins with DM, families with other connective tissue diseases and DM or PM, and increased associations with HLA-DR3. Without convincing evidence of support, it has been hypothesized that these inflammatory myositides are the result of a viral infection.

In DM, several observations suggest that circulating immune complexes or antibodies induce vascular injury. Intramuscular blood vessels show endothelial hyperplasia with tubuloreticular profiles, fibrin thrombi, and obliteration of capillaries. Even in cases where light microscopy is normal, electron microscopy reveals microtubular inclusions and vacuoles in the lining of endomesial capillaries, suggesting that the capillary lining may be the target of the immune response. Perifascicular atrophy results from ischemic changes secondary to the endomesial vasculopathy. Similar changes occur in skin vasculature leading to the rash, which is often part of the DM syndrome.

In PM, there is strong histochemical evidence for cell-mediated immune mechanisms in the pathogenesis. The inflammatory exudate is predominantly CD8$^+$ T cells within the endomysium. These exudates are seen in muscle cells undergoing necrosis and phagocytosis. Further evidence suggests that these T cells (and monocytes) are a few distinct clones (i.e., oligoclonal) and are not simply nonspecific inflammatory effectors.

Epidemiology and Risk Factors. Both of these syndromes affect women slightly more than men. PM typically occurs after age 20 years and rarely in childhood, whereas DM affects both children and adults. The incidence of the inflammatory myopathies is less than 1 in 100,000 population. Although the adult cases of PM and DM present in the fifth and sixth decades of life, the majority of cases of DM are childhood onset with typical age of 5 to 14 years.

The risk of cancer in association with adult PM or DM ranges from 6 to 45 percent in DM and 0 to 28 percent in PM. A population-based retrospective study in 788 DM patients and 396 PM patients over 20 years reported the rate of cancer occurrence to be 9 percent in the PM group and 15 percent in the DM group. The majority of these cancers were within 5 years of the diagnosis of the myopathy. In PM, the relative risk of malignancy was 1.7 for women and 1.8 for men, with the most common site of malignancy in men being the lung (relative risk, 5.6). In DM, the relative risk for malignancy was 2.4 in men and 3.4 in women, with the ovary most often affected (relative risk, 16.7).[126] Patients with associated malignancy have a higher than average age of DM or PM onset.

Clinical Features and Associated Disorders. Childhood DM is a relatively uniform disorder usually characterized by erythematous rash and skin lesions and coincidental muscle weakness. This photosensitive rash usually begins as periorbital heliotrope (blue-purple) discoloration with subsequent erythematous involvement of extensor surfaces of the limbs and joints. The anterior neck and chest rash may form a "V" sign or rash over the shoulders in a "shawl" sign. The proximal muscles of the limbs are more affected than distal ones, the abductors of the leg affected more than the adductors, and the extensors more than the flexors. Ectopic calcifications are present in subcutaneous tissues and muscle in about half of the cases. Associated complications include hemorrhagic gastrointestinal vasculitis and pulmonary fibrosis.

Adult DM shares the same skin features with childhood DM and often helps secure a clinical diagnosis. On occasion the skin manifestations are subtle or absent and the diagnosis of DM over PM relies on the muscle biopsy appearance.

The clinical features of muscle involvement are similar in DM and PM. Muscle pain and tenderness are common and usually more prominent in the arms. Onset of symptoms is subacute or insidious. As the disease progresses, dysphagia and neck flexor weakness begin. Respiratory muscles are impaired in severe cases and result in a restrictive pulmonary defect. In addition, pulmonary interstitial fibrosis may appear as a complication of the disease and may even precede the muscle weakness. There is an increased frequency of electrocardiographic abnormalities (dysrythmias, heart block, etc.), and occasionally patients may have pericarditis as part of their syndrome.

A number of other related conditions may have myositis as a feature and are considered to be "overlap" syndromes when the diagnostic criteria for both conditions are fulfilled. These are other autoimmune diseases such as PSS, SS, SLE, RA, and MCTD.

Differential Diagnosis. The main clinical differentiation to be made is between DM/PM and other acquired myopathies or inflammatory diseases. The rash of DM limits the potential diagnoses to the overlap syndromes. The diagnosis of PM is one of exclusion. Inclusion body myositis may appear similar to PM, and the serum creatinine phosphokinase (CK) is elevated although typically not to the same extent. Endocrinopathies such as hyperthyroidism and Cushing's syndrome can behave similarly. Toxic exposures and drugs that induce myopathy should be sought as potential etiologies. Additionally, inherited neuromuscular or metabolic disease may have a similar appearance. Serological testing and muscle biopsy should resolve the differences in most cases.

Evaluation. In a patient with a possible inflammatory myopathy, the diagnosis is strengthened or confirmed by serum CK, EMG, and most important, muscle biopsy to help exclude overlap syndromes. ESR is neither a sensitive nor a specific indicator of PM or DM but does correlate in general with inflammatory diseases. Testing for autoantibodies such as ANA and anti-Sm (SLE), SS-A and SS-B (Sjögren's), PM-Scl and anti-Ku (scleroderma), anticentromere (CREST syndrome), and anti-U1 snRNP (MCTD and SLE) may be useful in considering the overlap syndromes.

Serum CK is the most sensitive muscle enzyme for the detection of destruction of muscle cells. Typically, tenfold elevations can be seen; however, it is possible to have normal levels even during active disease. There are elevations of both muscle and brain isoenzyme forms of CK, reflecting both necrosis and new fiber regeneration. The CK is often used for a marker of disease activity.

Certain autoantibodies are associated with the inflammatory myopathies. Of these autoantibodies (such as anti-nRNP, PM-Scl, and antisynthetases), the anti-Jo-1 is the most useful because 75 percent of patients with anti-Jo-1 have interstitial lung disease.

Electrodiagnostic studies are helpful to evaluate clinically weak muscles for evidence of a myopathic pattern of activity and to exclude a neurogenic component. Muscle biopsy is the gold standard in the diagnosis of inflammatory myopathies and to exclude other neuromuscular diseases. Histopathological evaluation is the mainstay of diagnosis of these conditions. Treatment of the condition, however, should not be delayed while awaiting the histopathology results.

Management. Immunosuppressive therapy is the mainstay of treatment. Prednisone is the agent of choice for DM and PM, and treatment should begin with 80 to 100 mg/d (or 1 mg/kg/d) given in a single morning dose. This dose should be maintained for 3 to 4 weeks. If a clinical response has occurred, then tapering of the dose on every other day (by 5 to 10 mg every 3 to 4 weeks) should take place with an eventual goal of 80 to 100 mg every other day. This dose can then be tapered slowly over a period of months. The inability to taper the prednisone without disease reactivation or a lack of clinical response suggests the need for another agent. Corticosteroids may cause a clinical worsening secondary to steroid myopathy. Worsening in the absence of CK elevation and absence of neck flexor weakness may point to steroid myopathy in treated patients with inflammatory myopathy.

Azathioprine is most helpful in combination with corticosteroids and has a steroid-sparing effect. The recommended dose is approximately 2 mg/kg/d, and side effects may include gastrointestinal upset, a flulike syndrome, hepatotoxicity, and bone marrow suppression. A several-month delay in effectiveness is common and should be expected. Azathioprine can be used alone but is probably not as effective.

Methotrexate, cyclophosphamide, and cyclosporine A are agents that also may be useful in the treatment of DM or PM. These agents have associated potential toxicities to bone marrow, to liver, and during pregnancy. The effectiveness of these agents is not well studied, but they may be promising, particularly in patients who are not responding to prednisone, azathioprine, or both.[127] A randomized evaluation of methotrexate versus cyclosporine A in steroid nonresponders demonstrated clinical improvement in both groups without superiority of one therapy.[128] Mycophenolate mofetil may also be useful but has not been well studied at this time. In a small series, clinical response occurred in patients who had not responded to the combination of prednisone and methotrexate or prednisone and IVIg.[129]

IVIg is an expensive, relatively safe, and promising treatment for DM and PM. The dose is 2 g/kg, divided over 2 to 5 days initially, then 0.4 g/kg given at intervals based upon the clinical response. The exact mechanism of action is not clear but is felt to affect circulating autoantibodies, the autoimmune target, or complement activation. Side effects include increased serum viscosity with potentiation of thromboembolic events, aseptic meningitis, rash, anaphylaxis in IgA-deficient individuals, and a low risk of transmissible diseases such as hepatitis C. Many patients who have failed other treatments may respond to IVIg. Plasmapheresis has been shown ineffective in a controlled clinical trial.

Prognosis and Future Perspectives. Childhood DM has a variable prognosis. Some cases may have complete reversal of signs and symptoms after months, but 7 percent of cases have a fatal condition. The disease may recur, even after prolonged remission. Overall, the prognosis for DM and PM is relatively favorable with 10-year survival rates as high as 90 percent. Patients with interstitial lung disease have a mortality that approaches 40 percent at 3 years. Other factors that adversely affect prognosis include advanced age at onset, acute onset, involvement of respiratory muscles, dysphagia, fever, and inadequate therapy.

Potential avenues for treatment include more specific immunotherapies. Proteins that could bind the antigenic targets and interfere with recognition by auto-directed T cells or products that mimic the antigenic target are possible new avenues of treatment.

EOSINOPHILIC MYOSITIS AND RELATED SYNDROMES

Pathogenesis and Pathophysiology. True eosinophilic myositis occurs in the setting of a subacute or chronic unexplained peripheral blood eosinophilia. Patients with hypereosinophilia may be asymptomatic or may have end-organ damage, including myositis. The skeletal muscle in such patients resembles polymyositis with an eosinophil-predominant infiltrate.[130]

Eosinophilic fasciitis is likely a separate condition with eosinophilia, elevated ESR, and hypergammaglobulinemia. Clinically, these patients present with taut skin and flexion contractures secondary to intense diffuse fasciitis. Pathologically eosinophilic inflammation of the fascia extends into adjacent muscle, but there is no primary muscle involvement.[130]

Eosinophilia-myalgia syndrome (EMS) is a more recently described condition. A number of patients developed peripheral eosinophilia, fatigue, and myalgia associated with the chronic ingestion of L-tryptophan. Biopsies demonstrate inflammatory infiltrates of small and medium-sized vessels and connective tissues consisting of various cell types (histiocytes, $CD4^+$ and $CD8^+$ lymphocytes, and mast cells) but few if any eosinophils.[130] An autoimmune disorder or idiosyncratic response is suspected.[130] Since the withdrawal of L-tryptophan from the market, the number of cases reported has dramatically dropped.[131] It is likely that the vehicle, not L-tryptophan, was the responsible agent. The toxic oil syndrome, which was the result of a toxic contaminant in the production of rapeseed oil in Spain, is nearly an identical syndrome with identical pathology as EMS.[130]

Epidemiology and Risk Factors. The number of cases of eosinophilic myositis is small. The syndrome is associated with the systemic hypereosinophilic syndromes almost as a rule. With eosinophilic fasciitis, men 30 to 60 years of age are more often affected, and about half have a history of intense exertion prior to the onset.

In a study of 205 patients with EMS associated with L-tryptophan ingestion, 79 percent were women and almost all were Caucasian.[132] The EMS from L-tryptophan ingestion was associated with contamination by 1,1′-ethyldenebis tryptophan and 3-phenylamino alanine. The doses taken in the EMS patients were generally higher than the at-risk patients who did not develop the syndrome. One of the toxic contaminants in rapeseed oil was 3-phenylamino-1,2-propanediol, an alanine derivative similar to the 3-phenylamino alanine in the EMS outbreak.[130]

Clinical Features and Associated Disorders. The systemic syndrome associated with eosinophilic myositis involves other organs such as lungs, heart, and skin. There may be heart block, dysrythmias, and pulmonary infiltrates, resulting in death. Esophageal motility can be affected in some patients. Proximal muscle weakness and elevated CK, suggestive of myositis, may be accompanied by signs of neuropathy.[130]

Diffuse fasciitis presents acutely, usually after a short prodromal period with low-grade fever, myalgias, and fatigue. Thickening of the subcutaneous tissues ensues, sparing the face, with pitting edema of involved areas. Over the next weeks there may be limitations of movement of the small joints and to a lesser degree of large joints. Proximal and distal muscle weakness has been described in a few patients. Spontaneous remissions are common, and a rapid response to treatment is a rule.[130]

EMS begins insidiously, with severe fatigue and myalgias. Low-grade fever, transient maculopapular rash, muscle pains, and cramps and weakness of the extremities with or without paresthesias may all be part of the syndrome. The features of the syndrome in a given patient will vary depending on whether fasciitis, myositis, peripheral neuropathy, or mixed features predominate.[130] There are some vague reports of an acute encephalopathy at presentation.[131] Cognitive changes have been described 1 to 23 months after the acute syndrome. Objective neurocognitive changes were present in almost two thirds of those with subjective complaints of mental difficulties. Affected were verbal and visual memory, conceptual reasoning, and motor speed. No risk factors for the development of cognitive changes have been identified, and the pathogenesis of these changes remains unknown.[131] Proposed mechanisms include a direct toxic effect, eosinophil-derived neurotoxin or major basic protein, and effects of cytokines.[131]

Differential Diagnosis. Other conditions usually considered with this group of diseases are other autoimmune or inflammatory states such as polyarteritis nodosa, RA, allergic granulomatosis, hypersensitivity vasculitis, scleroderma, or parasitic infections. History, organ involvement, serological studies, and tissue biopsy may be necessary to distinguish among these conditions.

Evaluation. In eosinophilic myositis, the severity of peripheral blood eosinophilia is helpful in terms of diagnosis and reflects the severity of tissue eosinophilic inflammation. RF may be present, a feature that does not occur with eosinophilic fasciitis or EMS. ESR is often moderately elevated in all of these states. Serum CK, EMG, and muscle biopsy aid in the diagnosis of eosinophilic myositis. The serum CK is often elevated with true myositis, but may be normal in eosinophilic fasciitis. In EMS and in toxic oil syndrome, the CK is normal or only slightly elevated.[130]

The EMG reveals a myopathic pattern with eosinophilic myositis. There have been reports of myopathic changes in EMS and eosinophilic fasciitis, but this is less common. When peripheral neuropathy is associated with eosinophilic myositis, EMG may demonstrate axonal or demyelinative lesions.[130]

In EMS, one should be aware of potential signs of cognitive dysfunction and differentiate them from fatigue or depression. If there is a question of an encephalopathy, neuropsychological testing is recommended with follow-up assessments. The cognitive changes in EMS may begin or progress while other symptoms and signs of the syndrome are improving.[131]

Management. Treatment of eosinophilic myositis is initiated with high-dose prednisone at 1 mg/kg/d. With control of the symptoms and peripheral blood eosinophilia, gradual reduction of dose on an alternate-day regimen can be initiated. Cytotoxic agents may be of benefit if steroid doses remain high or if it is mandatory to reduce the steroid dose because of side effects. Improvement of survival has resulted.[130]

Eosinophilic fasciitis often will improve spontaneously, but resolution is faster with corticosteroid treatment. Relapses are infrequent. Although the treatment and resolution are in most cases good, the acute phase of the illness can be complicated by aplastic anemia, and either a megakaryocytic or idiopathic thrombocytopenia. Delayed lymphoproliferative disorders have also occurred.[130]

There are no specific recommendations on the treatment of EMS other than cessation of the inducing agent. Corticosteroids may induce clinical improvement and remission of eosinophilia. The drugs should be tapered after clinical benefit is maintained.[132] Beneficial responses to other medications have been reported, but the number of patients is too small to draw significant conclusions.[132]

Prognosis and Future Perspectives. In a 1982 study of 57 patients with hypereosinophilic syndromes, the average survival was 9 months, with 12 percent of patients surviving 3 years.[130] Eosinophilic fasciitis has a good prognosis with spontaneous recovery or response to corticosteroids in most patients. Occasional patients develop recurrence of fasciitis or secondary myeloproliferative disorder.[130] In a follow-up of over 200 patients with EMS, at 18 to 24 months, almost all of the symptoms and signs of the syndrome had improved or resolved completely.[132] Neurocognitive deficits and peripheral neuropathy are less likely to respond to therapy.[132]

With the exception of EMS, the pathogenesis of these syndromes is unclear, and directing more specific therapies is difficult. The hypereosinophilic syndromes in particular are associated with a high morbidity and mortality despite treatment with nonspecific immunosuppression. The identification of the driving force behind these inflammatory states will likely lead to novel approaches to influence the effects of these diseases, probably at the level of the cytokines and their regulatory effects.

INCLUSION BODY MYOSITIS

Pathogenesis and Pathophysiology. The specific hallmarks of inclusion body myositis (IBM) are inflammation, vacuolated muscle fibers, intracellular amyloid deposits, and 15- to 18-nm tubulofilamentous inclusions. Although there are familial forms of this disease, either autosomal dominant or recessive, inflammation is only rarely seen in those cases,[133] and, therefore, the familial forms are best referred to as inclusion body myopathies.

The inflammatory cells that are present in affected muscle are mostly $CD8^+$ lymphocytes or macrophages expressing MHC II surface markers. These findings suggest a directed response against specific antigens and a role of immune-mediated cytotoxicity. In addition, there are changes in the mitochondria and the nuclei of the myofibers, amyloid protein, and abnormally present filaments that suggest a possible "neurodegenerative" pathogenic mechanism. It is also suggested that the expression of an abnormal gene product may lead to a cytodestructive process and help explain the inflammatory and neurodegenerative evidence.[133]

Epidemiology and Risk Factors. IBM is the most common inflammatory muscle disease occurring over the age of 50.[134] Patients are greater than 30 years of age and usually greater than 50 at the time of onset of symptoms. Men are more often affected than women, in contrast with other autoimmune and inflammatory diseases.[135] There are no known risk factors other than genetic risk in those families with a history of IBM.

Clinical Features and Associated Disorders. The clinical weakness of IBM may resemble that of PM or DM but more typically evolves over years and resembles a limb-girdle dystrophy. Distal weakness is common, and dysphagia occurs in as many as 60 percent of patients. The weakness and atrophy may be asymmetrical and involve solitary muscles such as the quadriceps, iliopsoas, biceps, or triceps. Over years, there is more symmetry and weakness of the involved muscles. IBM is suspected when a patient with the diagnosis of PM does not respond to corticosteroid therapy, has early involvement of distal muscles such as long-finger flexors of the hand and wrist and extensors of the foot, or has dysphagia.[134] Unlike other inflammatory myopathies, patients with IBM do not have an increased risk of malignancy.

Differential Diagnosis. As alluded to previously, the other diagnoses to consider in these patients are PM, DM, or a myositis as the result of another systemic illness. With an earlier and gradually progressive onset, there may be features in common with limb-girdle muscular dystrophy. If there is focal atrophy or weakness, the possibility of a mononeuropathy or plexopathy should be considered. These can be differentiated with electrodiagnostic testing. The lack of respiratory involvement, EMG features, and slow course differentiate IBM from motor neuron disease. However, atypical presentations without the classical features can lead to diagnostic uncertainty. Muscle biopsy and quantitative EMG can often clarify these cases.[136]

Evaluation. As in DM and PM, the diagnosis of IBM relies on the assessment of CK, EMG, and most important, muscle biopsy. Suggested diagnostic criteria are listed in Table 50–7.[133] CK levels are often mildly elevated but should be less than 12 times normal.[133] EMG may show fibrillation potentials, positive sharp waves, complex repetitive discharges, and a mixture of myopathic, normal, and neurogenic motor units. These findings are not specific to the diagnosis of IBM, though short- and long-duration polyphasic potentials may be more prominent in IBM than other myopathies. Conventional EMG may not demonstrate myopathic motor units and can lead to misdiagnosis, especially if "neurogenic" spontaneous activity is seen. Quantitative EMG, particularly of single motor unit potentials, can be useful in identifying the motor units as myopathic in these circumstances.[136]

Muscle biopsy alone can make the diagnosis of IBM but may not always show the typical pathological features of the disease, even in patients with clinically typical presentations. Additional sections, additional stains (i.e., Congo red to assess for amyloid deposits), or another biopsy may increase this yield.[133]

Management. IBM is generally resistant to all therapies, but a trial of corticosteroids and one aggressive immunosuppressive agent is probably reasonable. Although initial reports suggested IVIg was useful in IBM, subsequent studies, including one with placebo control, have shown response in only about one third of patients.[133, 134] A controlled study of IVIg plus prednisone versus IVIg plus placebo demonstrated no difference between the groups and no improvement in strength.[137] A randomized pilot study of beta-interferon-1a did not show benefit after 6 months of therapy.[138]

Prognosis and Future Perspectives. IBM is typically a slowly progressive disease. Further studies with currently available or novel therapies may require larger numbers of patients and a longer duration of treatment to demonstrate a pattern of benefit or predict which subset of patients may respond. A better understanding of the etiological mechanisms of the unusual constellation of pathological findings will likely tailor new approaches to treatment.

TABLE 50–7. Characteristic Features and Diagnostic Criteria for Inclusion Body Myositis

Characteristic Features

Clinical

Duration of illness >6 months
Age of onset >30 years old
Weakness of proximal and distal arm and leg muscles; must include at least one of the following features:
- Finger flexor weakness
- Wrist flexor > wrist extensor weakness
- Quadriceps muscle weakness (≤ grade 4 MRC)

Laboratory

Serum creatine kinase <12 times normal
Muscle biopsy:
- Inflammatory myopathy characterized by mononuclear cell invasion of non-necrotic muscle fibers
- Vacuolated muscle fibers
- Intracellular amyloid deposits or 15- to 18-nm tubulofilaments by electron microscopy

Electromyography consistent with inflammatory myopathy

Diagnostic Criteria

Definite *inclusion body myositis*

Patients must exhibit all of the muscle biopsy features including invasion of non-necrotic fibers by mononuclear cells, vacuolated muscle fibers, and intracellular (within muscle fibers) amyloid deposits or 15- to 18-nm tubulofilaments
None of the other clinical or laboratory features are mandatory if the muscle biopsy features are diagnostic

Possible *inclusion body myositis*

If the muscle shows only inflammation (invasion of non-necrotic muscle fibers by mononuclear cells) *without* other pathological features of inclusion body myositis, *then* a diagnosis of possible inclusion body myositis can be given if the patient exhibits the characteristic clinical and laboratory features

Modified from Griggs RC, Askanas V, DiMauro S, et al: Inclusion body myositis with IVIg: A double-blind, placebo-controlled study [see comments]. Neurology 1997;48:712–716.

BEHÇET'S DISEASE

Pathogenesis and Pathophysiology. In 1937, Hulusi Behçet (1889–1948), a Turkish dermatologist, described the syndrome that bears his name. Behçet's disease (BD) is a relapsing inflammatory disorder without a defined cause. It may be a viral or autoimmune disorder, although familial cases and an association with HLA-B5 and HLA-B1 support a genetic role.[139, 140] Although it was previously thought to be a hypercoagulable state, elevation of procoagulant factors such as aPL are now known to be a secondary feature of the syndrome.[140] Pathologically, there is infiltration of smaller venules with lymphocytes and plasma cells, disrupted architecture of vessels, and occlusion with fibrin to fibrotic replacement, depending on the age of the lesion. There may be involvement of larger arteries or veins, resulting in thrombosis, aneurysm formation, or hemorrhage.[140]

Epidemiology and Risk Factors. The syndrome occurs with a prevalence rate as high as 37 per 100,000 in rural Turkey but only 0.4 per 100,000 in the United Kingdom.[141] Although children may be affected, mean age of onset is in the third decade. Neurological signs may occur at presentation but more typically occur several years later.[142] It is unclear if there are risk factors independent of genetic predisposition. In an autopsy series, 20 percent of 170 patients with BD had neurological involvement.[141]

Clinical Features and Associated Disorders. Criteria established by an international study group include recurrent major or minor aphthous or herpetiform ulceration of the mouth (mandatory) and involvement of at least one of the organ systems discussed later. Ocular signs include uveitis and vitritis, which are often present bilaterally, hypopyon, and vasculitis of the retinal vessels, sometimes with permanent visual loss.[140] Skin lesions include small, oval to round buccal and genital aphthous ulcerations, erythema nodosum, and pustules. Patients may have pathergy, the delayed development of a pustular or nodular skin reaction at the site of needle puncture.[140] A polyarteritis may occur, and larger arteries or veins may be affected, producing superior or inferior vena cava syndrome, intermittent claudication, edema, pulmonary infarct or fistula, or myocardial infarction.[140]

Although nervous system involvement occurs in up to 33 percent of patients with BD, it is not a defining criterion for the disease.[143] The nervous system is affected in one of a few ways, and often these syndromes may overlap. Brain stem involvement with meningoencephalitis is the most common location of parenchymal disease in two of the larger series reported.[141, 144] Usually the syndrome presents subacutely over days, with headache, oculomotor abnormalities, and ataxia. Only a few patients have respiratory insufficiency resulting in ventilatory support. Isolated cranial nerve dysfunction has also been seen with the facial nerve most often affected. Intramedullary spinal cord lesions, including complete transverse myelitis, are seen less often.[141] Meningoencephalitis or aseptic meningitis may present with chronic headache and typically mild pleocytosis.[129, 144] Vasculitis of venules or veins may cause significant thrombosis. In a prospective study of 31 patients with BD and neurological involvement, 10 patients had intracranial venous thrombosis. All had intracranial hypertension, but only two had focal neurological deficits due to cortical vein thrombosis.[143] Angiography may confirm a suspected thrombosis that is not visualized by MRI or may be performed in the appropriate setting if MRI is not available. CSF studies are typically abnormal with pleocytosis, elevated protein, and normal glucose but may be normal despite grossly abnormal MRI studies.[143] Serial CSF studies may be intermittently abnormal regardless of CNS disease activity.[142] In contrasting the CSF profiles of these presentations, the opening pressure was abnormal in the cases of meningitis and venous thrombosis. Pleocytosis was predominantly neutrophilic in the meningitis cases and lymphocytic/monocytic in cases of venous thrombosis or parenchymal lesions of the hemisphere, brain stem, or spinal cord.[141, 144] Glucose is typically normal.[144]

Differential Diagnosis. Other diagnostic considerations include inflammatory conditions or systemic infections such as SLE, polyarteritis nodosa, and bacterial endocarditis. The presence of arthritis may lead to the diagnosis of RA or postviral polyarthritis. Prominent neurological signs suggest other conditions including meningitis, encephalitis, stroke, and multiple sclerosis. Meningitis can be caused by bacterial or viral infection or drugs (i.e., ibuprofen, trimethoprim) or can be recurrent Mollaret's meningitis. Focal brain lesions may resemble those of multiple sclerosis or be radiologically identical to other vasculitic syndromes.[143]

Evaluation. Since there is no definite test to confirm the diagnosis of BD, the constellation of symptoms and signs over time allows the diagnosis to be made. A thorough history, physical examination, and review of previous symptoms are required. ESR is likely to be elevated if there is large vessel vasculitis but may be normal if the only evidence of disease is uveitis. Fibrin split products and platelet count may be elevated. Antiphospholipid antibodies are present in 15 to 35 percent of patients.[140] These changes are felt to be secondary effects of the inflammatory process.

Skin manifestations may lead to a diagnostic skin biopsy in patients with accessible lesions. Only occasionally is vasculitis proven, however. There is often infiltration of the dermis with lymphocytes and plasma cells, and deposits of IgM and C3 sometimes occur in cutaneous vessels.[140] A test for pathergy can be done by making a few sterile puncture sites in the forearm. Formation of nodule or pustule supports the diagnosis of BD; however, the absence of pathergy does not exclude BD as a potential diagnosis.[140] Visual complaints should be evaluated by an ophthalmologist to prevent morbidity owing to visual loss. Neurological evaluation is guided by the clinical presentation of the patient. MRI is superior to CT in detection of BD-related lesions.[143] T2-weighted MRI images may show multiple high-intensity lesions. Lesions occur in the cerebral white matter (70 percent), brain stem (60 percent), and deep gray matter (40 percent). They may be confluent and more extensive than suspected clinically. They do not have a predilection for the periventricular white matter. A lumbar puncture with assessment of opening pressure will identify those cases of intracranial hypertension secondary to venous thrombosis and confirm the presence of meningitis or meningoencephalitis.[143] CSF pleocytosis may range from 0 to 850 cells/mL (mean, 82), with the percentage of lymphocytes ranging from 25 to 100 (mean, 63), protein ranging from 16 to 101 mg/dL (mean, 43), and glucose ranging from 40 to 89 mg/dL (mean, 59).[142] Blood-brain barrier function may be abnormal as measured by the albumin ratio of CSF to serum; oligoclonal bands may be demonstrated.[145]

Management. Corticosteroids palliate inflammation at any disease stage by reducing the current vascular inflammation.[140] Therefore, their use is justified during disease activation. However, corticosteroids are not effective in the prevention of blindness or the morbidity and mortality that can be associated with neurological sequelae.[140] Other agents (e.g., alkylating agents) are needed in the long-term management of the disease to prevent or reduce significant morbidity.

Chlorambucil is helpful in controlling uveitis or meningoencephalitis. The dose is 0.1 mg/kg/d with gradual reduction in the dose if the disease remains controlled. Prolonged treatment at doses of 2 to 4 mg/d may be required to keep control. Routine blood counts should be followed, and the risk of sterility is a factor if treatment continues longer than 1 year.[140] Cyclosporine at 6 mg/kg/d is tried if chlorambucil is ineffective or not tolerated. Monitoring of routine blood counts, blood urea nitrogen, creatinine, and cyclosporine levels is necessary owing to the renal disease that can result from cyclosporine.[140] Azathioprine, methotrexate, and colchicine (which is widely used in Japan) may also be effective.

The treatment of major vessel occlusion is not clearly agreed upon. Treatment with prednisone and an alkylating agent should be initiated. Anticoagulation has been shown useful in patients with intracranial venous infarction,[143] although this treatment should be avoided in patients with pulmonary vasculitis.[140] Low-dose aspirin may reduce secondary thrombosis without significantly increasing the bleeding risk.[140]

Prognosis and Future Perspectives. Mucocutaneous lesions can exist for years without substantial morbidity or mortality. Ocular and neurological involvement, however, can lead to significant disability or mortality. The patients who experience intracranial hypertension and vein occlusions have a generally good prognosis if satisfactory treatment is provided at presentation. Patients with parenchymal disease often have sequelae felt to be related to the degree of axonal damage. A relapsing course of disease is seen in about 30 to 40 percent of neuro-BD patients, and patients with brain stem involvement and younger age of disease onset tend to have a worse prognosis.[141] Appropriate evaluation and prompt treatment reduce this morbidity.[140] After several years, most patients enter a period of relative disease inactivity and are less prone to complications as a result.[140]

Reviews and Selected Updates

Condemi JJ: The autoimmune diseases. JAMA 1992;268:2882–2892.

Dalakas MC: How to diagnose and treat the inflammatory myopathies. Semin Neurol 1994;14:137–145.

Engel AG, Hohlfeld R, Banker BQ: The polymyositis and dermatomyositis syndromes. *In* Engel AB, Franzini-Armstrong C (eds): Myology. New York, McGraw-Hill, 1994, pp 1335–1383.

Jennette JC, Falk RJ: Small vessel vasculitis. N Engl J Med 1997; 337(21):1523.

Jennette JC, Falk RJ, Milling DM: Pathogenesis of vasculitis. Semin Neurol 1994;14:291–299.

Moore PM, Richardson B: Neurology of the vasculitides and connective tissue diseases. J Neurol Neurosurg Psychiatry 1998;65:10–22.

Rosenwasser LJ: The vasculitic syndromes. *In* Bennett JC, Plum F (eds): Cecil Textbook of Internal Medicine. Philadelphia, WB Saunders, 1996, pp 1490–1498.

Siva A: Vasculitis of the nervous system. J Neurol 2001;248:451–468.

References

1. Jennette JC, Falk RJ: Clinical and pathological classification of ANCA-associated vasculitis: What are the controversies? Clin Exp Immunol 1995;101(Suppl 1):18–22.
2. Roitt IM: Principles of autoimmunity. *In* Brostoff J, Scadding GK, Male DK, Roitt IM (eds): Clinical Immunology. London, Gower Medical Publishing, 1991, pp 401–412.
3. Huston KA, Hunder GG, Lie JT: Temporal arteritis. A 25-year epidemiologic, clinical, and pathologic study. Ann Intern Med 1978;88: 162–167.
4. Turnbull J: Temporal arteritis and polymyalgia rheumatica: Nosographic and nosologic considerations. Neurology 1996;46:901–906.
5. De Silva M, Hazelman BL: Azathioprine in giant cell arteritis/polymyalgia rheumatica: A double blind study. Ann Rheumatol Dis 1986;45: 136–138.
6. Caselli RJ, Hunder GG: Neurologic complications of giant cell (temporal) arteritis. Semin Neurol 1994;14:349–353.
7. Movsas TZ, Liu GT, Galetta SL, Balcer LJ, Volpe NJ: Current neuro-ophthalmic therapies. Neurol Clin 2001;19:145–172.
8. Schmidt WA, Kraft HE, Vorpahl K, et al: Color duplex ultrasonography in the diagnosis of temporal arteritis. N Engl J Med 1997;337:1336–1342.
9. Calabrese LH, Mallek JA: Primary angiitis of the central nervous system. Medicine (Baltimore) 1987;67:20–39.
10. Schmidley JW: Central nervous system vasculitis. *In* Bradley WG, Daroff RB, Fenichel GM, Marsden CD (eds): Neurology in Clinical Practice: Principles of Diagnosis and Management. Boston, Butterworth-Heinemann, 1995, pp 1086–1088.
11. Calabrese LH, Furlan AJ, Gragg LA, Ropos TJ: Primary angiitis of the central nervous system: Diagnostic criteria and clinical approach. Cleve Clin J Med 1992;59:293–306.
12. Rhodes RH, Madelaire NC, Petrelli M, et al: Primary angiitis and angiopathy of the central nervous system and their relationship to systemic giant cell arteritis. Arch Pathol Lab Med 1995;119: 334–349.
13. Calabrese LH, Mallek JA: Primary angiitis of the central nervous system. Medicine (Baltimore) 1988;67:20–39.
14. Bassa A, Desai DK, Moodley J: Takayasu's disease and pregnancy. S Afr Med J 1995;85:107–112.
15. Kerr GS, Hallahan CW, Giordano J, et al: Takayasu arteritis. Ann Intern Med 1994;120:919–929.
16. Kerr GS: Takayasu's arteritis. Curr Opin Rheumatol 1994;6:32–38.
17. Lagneau P, Michel JB, Vuong PN: Surgical treatment of Takayasu's disease. Ann Surg 1987;205:157–166.
18. Guillevin L, Lhote F: Polyarteritis nodosa and microscopic polyangiitis. Clin Exp Immunol 1995;101:22–23.
19. Sehgal M, Swanson JW, DeRemee RA, Colby TV: Neurologic manifestations of Churg-Strauss syndrome. Mayo Clin Proc 1995;70:337–341.
20. Smith DL, Kim JA, Wang B: Polyarteritis nodosa-induced quadriplegia [letter]. Ann Intern Med 1995;122:731–732.
21. Carr J, Bryer A: An isolated myelopathy as a presentation of polyarteritis nodosa [letter]. Br J Rheumatol 1993;32:644.
22. Hawke SH, Davies L, Pamphlett R, et al: Vasculitic neuropathy. A clinical and pathological study. Brain 1991;114:2175–2190.
23. Kattah JC, Chrousos GA, Katz PA, et al: Anterior ischemic optic neuropathy in Churg-Strauss syndrome. Neurology 1994;44:2200–2202.
24. Fort JG, Griffin R, Tahmoush A, Abruzzo JL: Muscle involvement in polyarteritis nodosa: Report of a patient presenting clinically as polymyositis and review of the literature. J Rheumatol 1994;21: 945–948.
25. Hurst RW, Grossman RI: Neuroradiology of central nervous system vasculitis. Semin Neurol 1994;14:320–340.
26. Valente RM, Conn DL: Current therapies for systemic vasculitis. Semin Neurol 1994;14:380–386.
27. Nishino H, Rubino FA, Parisi JE: The spectrum of neurologic involvement in Wegener's granulomatosis. Neurology 1993;43:1334–1337.
28. Kafka SP, Condemi JJ, Marsh DO, Leddy JP: Mononeuritis multiplex and vasculitis. Association with anti-neutrophil cytoplasmic autoantibody [see comments]. Arch Neurol 1994;51:565–568.
29. Hoffman GS, Kerr GS, Leavitt RY, et al: Wegener granulomatosis: An analysis of 158 patients [see comments]. Ann Intern Med 1992;116:488–498.
30. Sneller MC, Hoffman GS, Talar-Williams C, et al: An analysis of forty-two Wegener's granulomatosis patients treated with methotrexate and prednisone. Arthritis Rheum 1995;38:608–613.
31. de Groot K, Schmidt DK, Arlt AC, et al: Standardized neurologic evaluations of 128 patients with Wegener granulomatosis. Arch Neurol 2001;58:1215–1221.
32. Nishino H, DeRemee RA, Rubino FA, Parisi JE: Wegener's granulomatosis associated with vasculitis of the temporal artery: Report of five cases [see comments]. Mayo Clin Proc 1993;68:115–121.
33. Weinberger LM, Cohen ML, Remler BF, et al: Intracranial Wegener's granulomatosis [see comments]. Neurology 1993;43:1831–1834.
34. Connolly JO, Lanham JG, Partridge MR: Fulminant pregnancy-related Churg-Strauss syndrome. Br J Rheumatol 1994;33:776–777.
35. Specks U, Homburger HA: Anti-neutrophil cytoplasmic antibodies. Mayo Clin Proc 1994;69:1197–1198.
36. Feldmann E, Levine SR: Cerebrovascular disease with antiphospholipid antibodies: Immune mechanisms, significance, and therapeutic options. Ann Neurol 1995;37(Suppl 1):S114–S130.
37. Gharavi AE, Sammaritano LR, Bovastro JL Jr, Wilson WA: Specificities and characteristics of beta 2 glycoprotein I–induced antiphospholipid antibodies. J Lab Clin Med 1995;125:775–778.
38. Szpak GM, Kuczynska-Zardzewialy A, Popow J: Brain vascular changes in the case of primary antiphospholipid syndrome. Folia Neuropathol 1996;34:92–96.
39. Hughson MD, McCarty GA, Sholer CM, Brumback RA: Thrombotic cerebral arteriopathy in patients with the antiphospholipid syndrome. Mod Pathol 1993;6:644–653.
40. Khamashta MA, Cuadrado MJ, Mujic F, et al: The management of thrombosis in the antiphospholipid-antibody syndrome [see comments]. N Engl J Med 1995;332:993–997.
41. Bick RL, Baker WF Jr: The antiphospholipid and thrombosis syndromes. Med Clin North Am 1994;78:667–684.
42. Levine SR, Welch KM: The spectrum of neurologic disease associated with antiphospholipid antibodies. Lupus anticoagulants and anticardiolipin antibodies. Arch Neurol 1987;44:876–883.

43. Gorman DG, Cummings JL: Neurobehavioral presentations of the antiphospholipid antibody syndrome. J Neuropsych Clin Neurosci 1993;5:37–42.
44. Brey RL, Gharavi AE, Lockshin MD: Neurologic complications of antiphospholipid antibodies. Rheum Dis Clin North Am 1993;19: 833–850.
45. Levine SR, Brey RL: Neurological aspects of antiphospholipid antibody syndrome. Lupus 1996;5:347–353.
46. Hasegawa M, Yamashita J, Yamashima T, et al: Spinal cord infarction associated with primary antiphospholipid syndrome in a young child. Case report. J Neurosurg 1993;79:446–450.
47. Tietjen GE, Levine SR, Brown E, et al: Factors that predict antiphospholipid immunoreactivity in young people with transient focal neurological events [published erratum appears in Arch Neurol 1994 Jan;51(1):12]. Arch Neurol 1993;50:833–836.
48. Love PE, Santoro SA: Antiphospholipid antibodies: Anticardiolipin and the lupus anticoagulant in systemic lupus erythematosus (SLE) and in non-SLE disorders. Prevalence and clinical significance. Ann Intern Med 1990;112:682–698.
49. Provenzale JM, Heinz ER, Ortel TL, et al: Antiphospholipid antibodies in patients without systemic lupus erythematosus: Neuroradiologic findings. Radiology 1994;192:531–537.
50. Neuwelt CM, Daikh DI, Linfoot JA, et al: Catastrophic antiphospholipid syndrome: Response to repeated plasmapheresis over three years. Arthritis Rheum 1997;40:1534–1539.
51. Brey RL, Levine SR: Treatment of neurologic complications of antiphospholipid antibody syndrome. Lupus 1996;5:473–476.
52. Olin JW: Thromboangiitis obliterans. Curr Opin Rheumatol 1994; 6:44–49.
53. Colburn MD, Moore WS: Buerger's disease. Heart Dis Stroke 1993;2:424–432.
54. Alarcon GS: Epidemiology of rheumatoid arthritis. Rheum Dis Clin North Am 1995;21:589–604.
55. Vollertsen RS, Conn DL: Vasculitis associated with rheumatoid arthritis. Rheum Dis Clin North Am 1990;16:445–461.
56. Bathon JM, Moreland LW, DiBartolomeo AG: Inflammatory central nervous system involvement in rheumatoid arthritis. Semin Arthritis Rheum 1989;18:258–266.
57. Ramos M, Mandybur TI: Cerebral vasculitis in rheumatoid arthritis. Arch Neurol 1975;32:271.
58. Beck DO, Corbett JJ: Seizures due to central nervous system rheumatoid meningovasculitis. Neurology 1983;33:1058–1061.
59. Lorber A, Pearson CM, Rene RM: Osteolytic vertebral lesions as a manifestation of rheumatoid arthritis and related disorders. Arthritis Rheum 1961;4:514.
60. Castro S, Verstraete K, Mielants H, et al: Cervical spine involvement in rheumatoid arthritis: A clinical, neurological and radiological evaluation. Clin Exp Rheumatol 1994;12:369–374.
61. Santavirta S, Konttinen YT, Lindqvist C, Sandelin J: Occipital headache in rheumatoid cervical facet joint arthritis. Lancet 1986;2:695.
62. Collee G, Breedveld RC, Algra PR, Padberg GW: Rheumatoid arthritis with vertical atlanto-axial subluxation complicated by hydrocephalus. Br J Rheumatol 1987;26:56.
63. Fedele FA, Ho G, Dorman BA: Pseudoaneurysm of the vertebral artery: A complication of rheumatoid cervical spine disease. Arthritis Rheum 1986;29:136.
64. Nakano KK: The entrapment neuropathies of rheumatoid arthritis. Orthop Clin North Am 1975;6:837.
65. Puechal X, Said G, Hilliquin P, et al: Peripheral neuropathy with necrotizing vasculitis in rheumatoid arthritis. A clinicopathologic and prognostic study of thirty-two patients. Arthritis Rheum 1995; 38:1618–1629.
66. Nadeau SE, Watson RT: Neurologic manifestations of vasculitis and collagen vascular syndromes. *In* Baker AB, Joynt RJ (eds): Clinical Neurology. Philadelphia, Harper & Row, 1985.
67. Rana NA: Natural history of atlanto-axial subluxation in rheumatoid arthritis. Spine 1989;14:1054–1056.
68. Wolfe F, Ross K, Hawley DJ, et al: The prognosis of rheumatoid arthritis and undifferentiated polyarthritis syndrome in the clinic: A study of 1141 patients [see comments]. J Rheumatol 1993;20:2005–2009.
69. Myllykangas-Luosujarvi RA, Aho K, Isomaki HA: Mortality in rheumatoid arthritis. Semin Arthritis Rheum 1995;25:193–202.
70. Mills JA: Systemic lupus erythematosus [see comments]. N Engl J Med 1994;330:1871–1879.
71. Futrell N, Schultz LR, Millikan C: Central nervous system disease in patients with systemic lupus erythematosus. Neurology 1992;42: 1649–1657.
72. Tan EM, Cohen AS, Fries JF, et al: The 1982 revised criteria for the classification of systemic lupus erythematosus. Arthritis Rheum 1982;25:1271–1277.
73. Mitsias P, Levine SR: Large cerebral vessel occlusive disease in systemic lupus erythematosus. Neurology 1994;44:385–393.
74. Kaell AT, Shetty M, Lee BC, Lockshin MD: The diversity of neurologic events in systemic lupus erythematosus. Prospective clinical and computed tomographic classification of 82 events in 71 patients. Arch Neurol 1986;43:273–276.
75. Hietaharju A, Jantti V, Korpela M, Frey H: Nervous system involvement in systemic lupus erythematosus, Sjögren syndrome and scleroderma. Acta Neurol Scand 1993;88:299–308.
76. Steen VD, Medsger TA: Epidemiology and natural history of systemic sclerosis. Rheum Dis Clin North Am 1990;16:1–10.
77. Tuffanelli DL, Winkelmann RK: Systemic scleroderma: A clinical study of 727 cases. Arch Dermatol 1961;84:359.
78. Hietaharju A, Jaaskelainen S, Kalimo H, Hietarinta M: Peripheral neuromuscular manifestations in systemic sclerosis (scleroderma). Muscle Nerve 1993;16:1204–1212.
79. Escudero D, Latorre P, Codina M, et al: Central nervous system disease in Sjögren's syndrome. Ann Med Interne (Paris) 1995;146:239–242.
80. Hietaharju A, Yli-Kerttula U, Hakkinen V, Frey H: Nervous system manifestations in Sjögren's syndrome. Acta Neurol Scand 1990;81: 144–152.
81. Schady W, Sheard A, Hassell A, et al: Peripheral nerve dysfunction in scleroderma. Q J Med 1991;80:661–675.
82. Dessein PH, Joffe BI, Metz RM, et al: Autonomic dysfunction in systemic sclerosis: Sympathetic overactivity and instability. Am J Med 1992;93:143–150.
83. Howe S, Eaker EY, Sallustio JE, et al: Antimyenteric neuronal antibodies in scleroderma. J Clin Invest 1994;94:761–770.
84. Corbo M, Nemni R, Iannaccone S, et al: Peripheral neuropathy in scleroderma. Clin Neuropathol 1993;12:63–67.
85. Nitta Y, Sobue G: Progressive systemic sclerosis associated with multiple mononeuropathy. Dermatology 1996;193:22–26.
86. Silman AJ: Scleroderma. Baillieres Clin Rheumatol 1995;9:471–482.
87. Mayes MD: Scleroderma epidemiology. Rheum Dis Clin North Am 1996;22:751–764.
88. Kallenberg CG: Overlapping syndromes, undifferentiated connective tissue disease, and other fibrosing conditions. Curr Opin Rheumatol 1993;5:809–815.
89. Alarcon-Segovia D: Clinical manifestations of the antiphospholipid syndrome. J Rheumatol 1992;19:1778–1781.
90. Black C, Isenberg DA: Mixed connective tissue disease—goodbye to all that. Br J Rheumatol 1992;31:695–700.
91. Nakae K, Furusawa F, Kasukawa R, et al: A nationwide epidemiological survey on diffuse collagen diseases: Estimation of prevalence rate in Japan. *In* Kasukawa R, Sharp GC (eds): Mixed Connective Tissue Disease and Anti-Nuclear Antibodies. Amsterdam, Excerpta Medica, 1987, pp 9–13.
92. Hietarinta M, Ilonen J, Lassila O, Hietaharju A: Association of HLA antigens with anti-SCL-70-antibodies and clinical manifestations of systemic sclerosis (scleroderma). Br J Rheumatol 1994;33:323–326.
93. van den Hoogen FH, Spronk PE, Boerbooms AM, et al: Long-term follow-up of 46 patients with anti-(U1)snRNP antibodies. Br J Rheumatol 1994;33:1117–1120.
94. Sullivan WE, Hurst DJ, Harmon CE, et al: A prospective evaluation emphasizing pulmonary involvement in patients with mixed connective tissue disease. Medicine (Baltimore) 1986;63:92–107.
95. Mukerji B, Hardin JG: Undifferentiated, overlapping, and mixed connective tissue diseases. Am J Med Sci 1993;305:114–119.
96. Nimelstein SJ, Brody S, McShane D, Holman HR: Mixed connective tissue disease: A subsequent evaluation of the original 25 patients. Medicine (Baltimore) 1980;59:239.
97. Lazaro MA, Maldonado Cocco JA, Catoggio LJ, et al: Clinical and serologic characteristics of patients with overlap syndrome: Is mixed connective tissue disease a distinct clinical entity? Medicine (Baltimore) 1989;68:58–65.
98. Bennett RM, Bong DM, Spargo BH: Neuropsychiatric problems in mixed connective tissue disease. Am J Med 1978;65:955.
99. Fujimoto M, Kira J, Murai H, et al: Hypertrophic cranial pachymeningitis associated with mixed connective tissue disease: A comparison with idiopathic and infectious pachymeningitis. Intern Med 1993;32:510–512.
100. Graf WD, Milstein JM, Sherry DD: Stroke and mixed connective tissue disease. J Child Neurol 1993;8:256–259.

101. Flechtner KM, Baum K: Mixed connective tissue disease: Recurrent episodes of optic neuropathy and transverse myelopathy. Successful treatment with plasmapheresis. J Neurol Sci 1994;126:146–148.
102. McKenna F, Eccles H, Neumann VC: Neuropsychiatric disorders in mixed connective tissue disease. Br J Rheumatol 1986;25:225–226.
103. Farrell DA, Medsger TA: Trigeminal neuropathy in progressive systemic sclerosis. Am J Med 1982;73:57–62.
104. Hagen NA, Stevens JC, Michet CJ: Trigeminal sensory neuropathy associated with connective tissue diseases. Neurology 1990;40:891–896.
105. Alfaro-Giner A, Penarrocha-Diago M, Bagan-Sebastian JV: Orofacial manifestations of mixed connective tissue disease with an uncommon serologic evolution. Oral Surg Oral Med Oral Pathol 1992;73:441–444.
106. Vincent FM, Van Houzen RN: Trigeminal sensory neuropathy and bilateral carpal tunnel syndrome: The initial manifestation of mixed connective tissue disease. J Neurol Neurosurg Psychiatr 1980; 43:458–460.
107. Yasuda M, Loo M, Shiokawa S, et al: Mixed connective tissue disease presenting myasthenia gravis. Intern Med 1993;32:633–637.
108. Gendi NS, Welsh KI, Van Venrooij WJ, et al: HLA type as a predictor of mixed connective tissue disease differentiation. Ten-year clinical and immunogenetic follow-up of 46 patients. Arthritis Rheum 1995;38:259–266.
109. Talal N: Sjögren's syndrome: Historical overview and clinical spectrum of disease. Rheum Dis Clin North Am 1990;18:507–515.
110. Alexander E: Central nervous system disease in Sjögren's syndrome. New insights into immunopathogenesis. Rheum Dis Clin North Am 1992;18:637–672.
111. Spezialetti R, Bluestein HG, Peter JB, Alexander EL: Neuropsychiatric disease in Sjögren's syndrome: Antiribosomal P and anti-neuronal antibodies. Am J Med 1993;95:153–160.
112. Font J, Valls J, Cervera R, et al: Pure sensory neuropathy in patients with primary Sjögren's syndrome: Clinical, immunological, and electromyographic findings. Ann Rheum Dis 1990;49:775–778.
113. Tesar JT, McMillan V, Molina R, Armstrong J: Optic neuropathy and central nervous system disease associated with primary Sjögren's syndrome. Am J Med 1992;92:686–692.
114. Alexander GE, Provost TT, Stevens MB, Alexander EL: Sjögren's syndrome: Central nervous system manifestations. Neurology 1981;31:1391–1396.
115. Kaltreider HB, Talal N: The neuropathy of Sjögren's syndrome: Trigeminal nerve involvement. Ann Intern Med 1969;70:751.
116. Malinow K, Yannakakis GD, Glusman SM, et al: Subacute sensory neuronopathy secondary to dorsal root ganglionitis in primary Sjögren's syndrome. Ann Neurol 1986;20:535.
117. Drachman DB: Myasthenia gravis. N Engl J Med 1994;330:1797–1810.
118. Richman DP, Agius MA: Myasthenia gravis: Pathogenesis and treatment. Semin Neurol 1994;14:106–110.
119. Oh SJ, Kim DE, Kuruoglu R, et al: Diagnostic sensitivity of the laboratory tests in myasthenia gravis. Muscle Nerve 1992;15:720–724.
120. Golnik KC, Pena R, Lee AG, Eggenberger ER: An ice test for the diagnosis of myasthenia gravis. Ophthalmology 1999;106:1282–1286.
121. Somnier FE, Trojaborg W: Neurophysiological evaluation in myasthenia gravis. A comprehensive study of a complete patient population. Electroencephalogr Clin Neurophysiol 1993;89:73–87.
122. Gronseth GS, Barohn RJ: Thymectomy for autoimmune myasthenia gravis (an evidenced based review): Report of the quality standards subcommittee of the American Academy of Neurology. Neurology 2000;55:7–15.
123. Roberts PF, Venuta F, Rendina E, et al: Thymectomy in the treatment of ocular myasthenia gravis. J Thor Cardiovasc Surg 2001;122:562–567.
124. Ciafaloni E, Massey JM, Tucker-Lipscomb B, Sanders DB: Mycophenolate mofetil for myasthenia gravis: An open-label pilot study. Neurology 2001;56:97–99.
125. Mowzoon N, Sussman A, Bradley WG: Mycophenolate (CellCept) treatment of myasthenia gravis, chronic inflammatory polyneuropathy and inclusion body myositis: J Neurol Sci 2001;185:119–122.
126. Sigurgeirsson B, Lindelof B, Edhag O, Allander E: Risk of cancer in patients with dermatomyositis or polymyositis. A population-based study. N Engl J Med 1992;326:363–367.
127. Tietjen GE: Migraine and antiphospholipid antibodies [see comments]. Cephalalgia 1992;12:69–74.
128. Vencovsky J, Jarosova K, Machacek S, et al: Cyclosporine A versus methotrexate in the treatment of polymyositis and dermatomyositis. Scand J Rhematol 2000;29:95–102.
129. Tausche AK, Meurer M: Mycophenolate mofetil for dermatomyositis. Dermatology 2001;202:341–343.
130. Banker BQ: Other inflammatory myopathies. *In* Engel AG, Franzini-Armstrong C (eds): Myology. New York, McGraw-Hill, 1994, pp 1461–1486.
131. Krupp LB, Masur DM, Kaufman LD: Neurocognitive dysfunction in the eosinophilia-myalgia syndrome. Neurology 1993;43:931–936.
132. Hertzman PA, Clauw DJ, Kaufman LD, et al: The eosinophilia-myalgia syndrome: Status of 205 patients and results of treatment 2 years after onset. Ann Intern Med 1995;122:851–855.
133. Griggs RC, Askanas V, DiMauro S, et al: Inclusion body myositis and myopathies. Ann Neurol 1995;38:705–713.
134. Dalakas MC, Sonies B, Dambrosia J, et al: Treatment of inclusion-body myositis with IVIg: A double-blind, placebo-controlled study [see comments]. Neurology 1997;48:712–716.
135. Barohn RJ: The therapeutic dilemma of inclusion body myositis. Neurology 1997;48:567–568.
136. Dabby R, Lange DJ, Trojaborg W, et al: Inclusion body myositis mimicking motor neuron disease. Arch Neurol 2001;58:1253–1256.
137. Dalakas MC, Koffman B, Fujii M, et al: A controlled study of intravenous immunoglobulin combined with prednisone in the treatment of IBM. Neurology 2001;56:323–327.
138. The Muscle Study Group: Randomized pilot trial of βINF1a (Avonex) in patients with inclusion body myositis. Neurology 2001;57: 1566–1570.
139. Moore PM, Calabrese LH: Neurologic manifestations of systemic vasculitides. Semin Neurol 1994;14:300–306.
140. O'Duffy JD: Vasculitis in Behçet's disease. Rheum Dis Clin North Am 1990;16:423–431.
141. Kidd D, Steuer A, Denman AM, Rudge P: Neurologic complications in Behçet's syndrome. Brain 1999;122:2183–2194.
142. Devlin T, Gray L, Allen NB, et al: Neuro-Behçet's disease: factors hampering proper diagnosis. Neurology 1995;45:1754–1757.
143. Wechsler B, Dell'Isola B, Vidailhet M, et al: MRI in 31 patients with Behçet's disease and neurological involvement: Prospective study with clinical correlation. J Neurol Neurosurg Psychiatry 1993;56:793–798.
144. Al-Fahad SA, Al-Araji AH: Neuro-Behçet's disease in Iraq: A study of 40 patients. J Neurol Sci 1999;170:105–111.
145. McLean BN, Miller D, Thompson EJ: Oligoclonal banding of IgG in CSF, blood-brain barrier function, and MRI findings in patients with sarcoidosis, systemic lupus erythematosus, and Behçet's disease involving the nervous system. J Neurol Neurosurg Psychiatry 1995;58:548–554.

CHAPTER 51

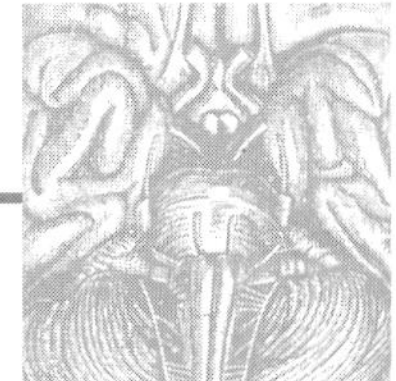

RANDOLPH W. EVANS and JACK E. WILBERGER

Traumatic Disorders

Disorders due to head, spine, and peripheral nerve injuries are among the most commonly seen by neurologists. The impact of these injuries can be devastating for individuals and society, because injuries occurring in a fraction of time can result in death or lifelong impairments associated with chronic pain syndromes. Motor vehicle accidents continue to be a leading cause of neurological trauma despite efforts at primary prevention. Although some neurological injuries such as those due to gunshot and stab wounds reflect a violent society, others, like a lightning strike, are random and capricious. Basic and clinical neuroscience research is directed toward prevention and better treatment of traumatic neurological injury.

Acute Head Injury

Pathogenesis and Pathophysiology. Head injury (HI) accounts for a disproportionate share of morbidity and mortality in traumatized patients. The past two decades have witnessed a significant decline, however, in overall HI mortality from the mid-30 percent range in the 1970s to less than 20 percent in the 1990s. This improvement has paralleled an understanding of the secondary injury process and an appreciation that all neurological damage does not occur at the moment of insult but evolves over the ensuing hours and days from various biochemical and molecular derangements. This understanding has led to the development of aggressive treatment strategies to prevent intracranial pressure (ICP) elevations and ischemia. This understanding has led also to extensive clinical therapeutic trials to identify pharmacological neuroprotective agents. The structural injury to the brain at the time of impact is rarely the sole determinant of outcome. Hypoxia, hypotension, mass lesions, increased ICP, ischemia, free radical production, excitotoxicity, and loss of calcium homeostasis are also important.

The frequent occurrence and deleterious effects of the secondary insults of hypoxia and hypotension have long been known.[1, 2] Mortality is doubled when these insults are superimposed on severe HI (Fig. 51–1), and, similarly, concomitant elevated ICP increases morbidity.[3] Considerable research has focused on the biochemical and molecular mechanisms of secondary injury. Although these events are multifactorial and interrelated, their timing sequence justifies consideration of each component (Fig. 51–2).

The contribution of oxygen free radicals to secondary injury following HI is a subject of active research.[4, 5] Free radicals generated by HI, including superoxide, hydroxyl, hydrogen peroxide, singlet oxygen, and nitrous oxide, have the potential to damage proteins and the phospholipid components of cells and organelle membranes. Additionally, extensive membrane depolarization, induced by trauma, allows for a nonselective opening of the voltage-sensitive calcium channels and an abnormal accumulation of calcium within neurons and glia. Such calcium shifts are associated with activation of lipolytic and proteolytic enzymes, protein kinases, protein phosphatases, dissolution of microtubules, and altered gene expression.[6] Another method of abnormal calcium influx is via activation of excitatory amino acid receptors such as glutamate and aspartate. Excitotoxicity occurs in a widespread fashion after trauma, resulting in cell swelling, vacuolization, and death.[7]

Head injury can result in various types of primary injury occurring at the moment of impact, including lacerations of

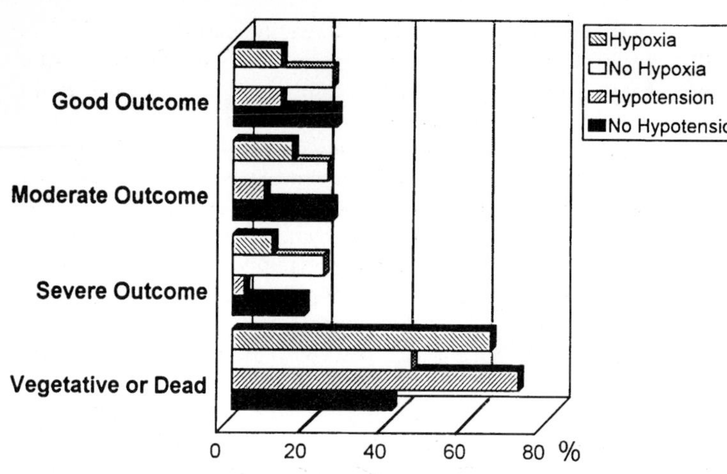

FIGURE 51–1. Influence of hypoxia and hypotension on mortality after head injury.

the scalp, skull fractures, cortical contusions and lacerations, diffuse axonal injury, and intracranial hemorrhage. A coup contusion occurs at the site of impact in the absence of a fracture. A contrecoup contusion occurs in the brain diametrically opposite the point of impact. Acceleration/deceleration forces may cause tearing of nerve fibers at the moment of impact, which is called *shearing injury* or *diffuse axonal injury*. Types of intracranial hematomas include extradural, subarachnoid, subdural, and intracerebral hematomas.

Epidemiology and Risk Factors. Closed HI leads to 500,000 hospitalizations per year resulting in over 175,000 deaths and significant disability. Although the statistics are somewhat variable, it is estimated that the incidence of HI currently approaches 222 in 100,000 population per year.[8] The peak incidence occurs in men 15 to 24 years of age. Whereas motor vehicle accidents still account for the majority of injuries, the increasing mandate for seat belt use and availability of air bags appear to be reducing injuries. The incidence of penetrating HI from gunshot wounds is ever increasing, and in some urban communities it is now the most common type of injury seen.

A number of classification schemes have been developed for assessment of neurological damage after HI. The most reliable scheme, from a clinical and prognostic standpoint, is based on the Glasgow Coma Scale (GCS):

GCS 3–7 Severe
GCS 8–12 Moderate
GCS 13–15 Mild

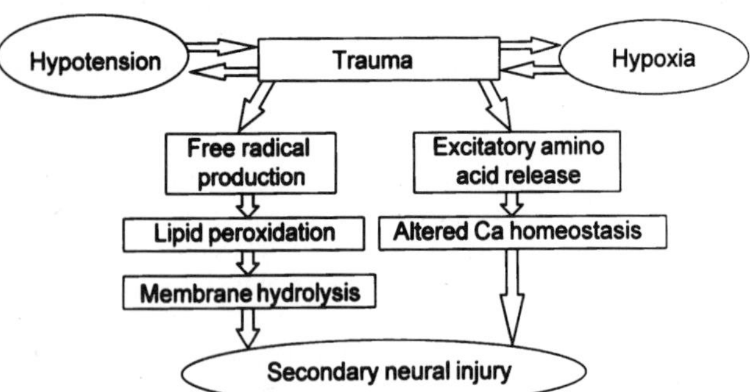

FIGURE 51–2. Biochemical/molecular substrates of the secondary injury cascade. (From Salaman M: Current Techniques in Neurosurgery, 2nd ed. Philadelphia, Current Medicine, 1993.)

Mild HI is termed a *concussion*. Concussions are infrequently associated with structural brain injury and rarely lead to significant long-term sequelae. The postconcussion syndrome is distinct. Attention to neuropsychological testing has shown the possibility of significant cognitive disability following a concussion.[9] Moderate HI may be associated with significant structural injury such as hemorrhage or contusion, but death is uncommon. Severe HI generally results in some form of cognitive and/or physical disability or in death, especially with very low GCS scores.

The accurate classification of HI is critical in both triage and management. Severe HI should be treated at facilities with appropriate neurotrauma resources, whereas moderate HI requires close clinical observation for possible neurological deterioration. In the setting of mild HI, the most important management issues are related to the need for computed tomographic (CT) scanning, possible inpatient observation, and appropriate follow-up.

Clinical Features and Associated Disorders. HI is frequently associated with skull fracture, and the significance of the fracture depends on the type of head injury. When associated with severe HI, linear fractures have little practical significance, whereas with mild HI, the presence of a skull fracture increases the risk of an intracranial abnormality by as much as fourfold.[10] Basilar skull fractures may be complicated by cerebrospinal fluid (CSF) leak, infection, and/or cranial nerve palsies. Patients with basilar skull fractures generally deserve closer clinical monitoring than those with linear skull fracture. In infants and young children, however, linear fractures may be complicated by leptomeningeal cysts or "growing" skull fractures. When such lesions occur, a mass may develop over the fracture site as CSF collects from a disruption of arachnoid intregrity underlying the injury. Cysts always require surgical correction; it is important to follow young children for several months for this possible occurrence.

Infrequently, blunt trauma to the head can tear the middle meningeal artery, diploic veins, or the dural sinuses, resulting in a collection of blood in the epidural space, which is an epidural hematoma. Epidural hematomas are associated with a skull fracture in 85 percent of cases. They most commonly occur in the temporal region, although they can also occur in other locations such as the frontal or parietal regions or within the posterior fossa. The classically described lucid interval associated with this entity is rarely seen because most patients are unconscious from the time of injury. Examination of the head may reveal a laceration and skull fracture over the region of the hematoma. If uncal herniation (i.e, herniation of the mesial temporal lobe) occurs from mass effect, findings may include an ipsilateral cranial nerve III palsy and contralateral hemiparesis. An ipsilateral hemiparesis can occur as a result of compression of the contralateral cerebral peduncle against the edge of the tentorium. Most epidural hematomas require immediate surgical intervention; however, there are exceptions, particularly in alert pediatric patients.[11]

Acute subdural hematomas occur in approximately 20 percent of patients with severe HI. Impact injury to the brain can rupture the parasagittal bridging veins (which drain blood from the surface of the hemisphere into the dural venous sinuses) leading to hematoma formation within the subdural space. Subdural hematomas can also occur without head injury in patients with a coagulopathy or on anticoagulants. Subdural hematomas can also be due to rupture of cerebral aneurysms. Subdural hematomas are usually located over the hemispheres, although other locations, such as between the occipital lobe and tentorium cerebelli or between the temporal lobe and base of the skull, can occur. About 50 percent of patients with acute subdural hematomas are unconscious from the time of injury. Focal findings can occur because of herniation, as described for epidural hematomas. Surgery within the first 4 hours from injury is generally associated with improved outcome; however, this basic tenet of HI management has been challenged.[12, 13]

A subdural hematoma becomes subacute between 2 and 14 days after the injury when there is a mixture of clotted and fluid blood. A subdural hematoma becomes chronic when the hematoma is filled with fluid more than 14 days after the injury. Most patients with chronic subdural hematomas are late middle age or elderly. Up to 50 percent of those with chronic subdural hematomas, however, have no history of head injury. Patients with chronic subdural hematomas may have multiple types of presentations such as the following: headache and nausea without focal findings; a slow progression of focal signs; altered mental status, apathy, and unsteady gait; an acute focal neurological deficit; fluctuating neurological deficits that may clear; and seizures. Thus, it is easy to see how the various presentations of chronic subdural hematoma can lead to misdiagnoses such as stroke, transient ischemic attack, brain tumor, depression, and dementia. Although occasionally chronic subdural hematomas can be treated with diuretics and corticosteroids, symptomatic patients generally require surgery.

Cerebral contusions are frequently associated with intracranial mass lesions, although they may occur as a result of the coup-contrecoup phenomenon, especially in the temporal and inferior frontal regions. The clinical presentation depends upon the location and severity of the contusion and whether other lesions are present. Patients with small focal contusions can present with speech or motor deficits, whereas larger contusions can act as a mass lesion. Contusions themselves rarely require surgical intervention; however, they necessitate careful clinical and CT follow-up because they may evolve into delayed post-traumatic intracerebral hematomas.[14]

Diffuse axonal injury (DAI) is a frequent CT and pathological correlate of severe head injury, accounting for about 50 percent of primary brain injuries. DAI is usually associated with a poor outcome.[15] DAI is readily identifiable on CT as multiple punctate hemorrhages, typically in the deep white matter and corpus callosum and occasionally in the brain stem. DAI may also occur as a result of mild head injury and may culminate in subtle types of cognitive deficits.

Approximately 10 to 15 percent of patients with clinically severe HI have a normal CT scan. In such situations, the possibility of extracranial or intracranial vascular disruptions must be considered, and angiography should be considered. Occasionally, magnetic resonance imaging (MRI) may demonstrate lesions not appreciated on CT in this setting.

Approximately 5 to 10 percent of patients with severe HI have an associated spine and/or spinal cord injury. Initial HI evaluation and management thus require simultaneous evaluation and management for potential spinal injuries. The majority of patients with severe HI have multisystem injury. Possibility of other significant and potentially life-threatening injuries should be evaluated and the proper treatment priorities accordingly established.

Multiple medical complications can also occur after HI.[16] Cardiovascular effects of head injury include neurogenic hypertension and cardiac dysrhythmias. Respiratory complications such as neurogenic pulmonary edema, aspiration pneumonia, and pulmonary emboli usually caused by deep venous thrombosis are rather common. Other complications include disseminated intravascular coagulation, hyponatremia due to the syndrome of inappropriate antidiuretic hormone secretion, diabetes insipidus, and stress gastritis.

Differential Diagnosis. Many nontraumatic disorders may mimic HI, including drug or alcohol intoxication, metabolic disturbances, and subarachnoid or other types of intracranial hemorrhages. When an intoxicated person falls or becomes involved in a fight and sustains a head injury, the emergency evaluation can be further complicated. Often, a patient presents after an apparent traumatic event that itself was precipitated by primary underlying intracranial pathology. Examples include the following: a stroke that causes loss of control while driving; a generalized seizure resulting in a head injury; a gait disturbance (due, for example, to Parkinson's disease, diabetes with a sensory ataxia, or cervical spondylitic myelopathy) causing a fall and an HI; and delirium or dementia as a cause of the fall. The physician should not only treat the injury, but should also try to find out if there is an underlying cause.

Evaluation. The primary evaluation of a patient with HI necessitates a careful neurological evaluation. Because a significant number of these patients have multiple types of trauma, however, systemic evaluation and stabilization take precedence. The ABCs of trauma resuscitation must be followed. As noted previously, correction of hypoxia and hypotension has a significant impact on outcome from HI.

The neurological evaluation of these patients is often complicated by many physical and iatrogenic factors. In comatose patients, a cervical spine series should be performed to exclude fractures before checking the oculocephalic reflex. Severe ocular trauma may obviate examination of pupillary reflexes. Alcohol intoxication and the use of sedatives or muscle relaxants to facilitate patient transport adversely affect the trauma-related neurological findings. Extremity fractures limit the extent of the neurological examination.

The GCS score has been the most reliable indicator of the severity of injury and deterioration or improvement. The initial GCS score often influences early treatment decisions. Thus, an intimate familiarity with the examination essentials to establish the GCS score is important: eye opening, verbal response, and motor response (Table 51–1).[17]

Once the GCS score has been established, a more detailed head and neurological examination can be pursued. A careful examination of the head is essential for findings such as scalp lacerations, skull fractures, blood in the external auditory canal, a hemotympanum, or Battle's sign (ecchymosis of the scalp overlying the mastoid bone). Any laterality to the neurological findings (i.e., a dilated pupil, hemiparesis) suggests a focal mass lesion. The higher the GCS score, the more important a detailed mental status examination becomes in determining management. For penetrating HI and especially gunshot wounds, there must also be a full and careful documentation of entry and exit wounds, powder burns, and foreign bodies.

In pediatric patients, the possibility of child abuse must be borne in mind, especially when the primary structural brain injury is subdural hematoma. The *shaken baby syndrome* refers to violent shaking of an infant or small child resulting in retinal hemorrhages and subarachnoid or subdural hemorrhage, but with minimal or no external evidence of severe trauma.[18] When such concerns arise, there must be a careful systemic survey for evidence of other injuries—retinal hemorrhages, skin bruising, new and old long bone fractures.

The more severe the HI, the greater the urgency for CT scanning as an integral part of initial evaluation to exclude lesions that require neurosurgical intervention. The only exception is when other life-threatening injuries take precedence. With minor HI, CT is not routinely indicated. Similarly, if CT is to be obtained, plain skull radiographs are unnecessary. Additional diagnostic evaluations such as MRI, cerebral angiography, and transcranial Doppler examination may be appropriate depending on clinical and/or CT findings.

Management. The management of minor HI is primarily directed toward a determination of which patients require CT scanning and/or in-hospital observation. Considerable effort has been expended to determine the risk of deterioration in this group of patients so that appropriate triage protocols may be established. A meta-analysis of a large number of series indicates that approximately 2.5 percent of patients presenting to an emergency room with minor HI require neurosurgical intervention.[19] This observation has led to current recommendations that only patients with GCS scores of 15 be discharged without prior CT scanning. Risk factors that must be taken into consideration when making this determination include palpable depressed skull fracture, seizures, extremes of age, persistent headache or vomiting, therapeutic anticoagulation, and suspected abuse. Unless there are significant associated extracranial injuries, it is rare for a minor HI to necessitate more than 24 hours of hospital observation.

Moderate HI is generally associated with significant symptoms and/or findings and necessitates CT scanning and hospitalization for serial neurological monitoring. Repeat CT scanning is indicated if there is any deterioration in neurological functioning. Delayed hematomas are occasionally seen after moderate HI. These usually represent bleeding into areas of contusion not well visualized initially, and patients typically present 24 to 48 hours after injury.[20]

The management of severe HI requires intensive support and monitoring. Because all patients are comatose, intubation and artificial ventilation are mandatory. Blood pressure monitoring and support are crucial to prevent hypotension. Monitoring via Swan-Ganz catheterization may be helpful to maximize perfusion. The first priority is complete and rapid physiological resuscitation. Hypotension (systolic blood pressures less than 90 mm Hg) and hypoxia (PaO_2 less than 60 mm Hg) should be avoided if possible and corrected if present.

The institution of ICP monitoring remains somewhat controversial; however, ICP monitors are appropriate in this setting and provide the most reliable guide to treatment of the underlying brain injury. Because elevation of ICP more than 20 mm Hg is a significant predictor of a poor outcome, an appropriate threshold to begin aggressive ICP treatment appears to be 20 to 25 mm Hg.[3, 21]

Considerable interest has been focused on cerebral perfusion pressure (CPP) in treating severe HI.[22] CPP is determined by subtracting the ICP value from mean arterial blood pressure and represents the pressure driving cerebral blood flow. Thus, CPP and cerebral blood flow can be positively affected by either lowering ICP or elevating systemic blood pressure. It is generally believed that active attempts to maintain CPP above 70 mm Hg improves outcome; however, there are no systematic scientific studies to validate this.

The primary treatments for elevated ICP have traditionally included hyperventilation, diuretics, and, in extreme circumstances, barbiturates. If an ICP monitor is in place, the drainage of CSF may have significant therapeutic benefits. Care must be taken if hyperventilation is implemented, because the cerebral vasoconstriction induced may produce ischemia. Thus, $PaCO_2$ levels lower than 25 mm Hg are rarely indicated unless ICP is totally refractory to all other therapeutic interventions. When extreme hyperventilation is required, methods of monitoring for cerebral ischemia, such as jugular venous oxygen saturation ($SJVO_2$), may provide useful clinical information.[23, 24] Recently attempts have been made to correlate cerebral perfusion with noninvasive cere-

TABLE 51–1. **Glasgow Coma Scale**

Eye opening	
Spontaneous	4
To Voice	3
To Pain	2
None	1
Verbal response	
Oriented	5
Confused	4
Inappropriate	3
Incomprehensible	2
None	1
Motor response	
Obeys commands	6
Localizes pain	5
Withdraws	4
Flexion	3
Extension	2
Flaccid	1
Total 3–15	

bral oximetry.[25] Mannitol is the primary diuretic used to control ICP. Effective doses range from 0.25 to 1.0 g/kg, which are typically given as intermittent boluses. Care must be taken to prevent hypernatremia and hyperosmolarity when giving frequent boluses.

High-dose barbiturate therapy is generally reserved for those situations in which ICP becomes refractory to other available therapies.[26] Many potential complications, including cardiovascular instability, are associated with barbiturate use, however, and extremely careful monitoring is necessary. Although steroids have been often used to treat severe HI, there are no data to support their use to either control ICP or to affect its long-term outcome.[27] Their current use in this setting is thus usually discouraged.

Decompressive craniectomy for intractable brain swelling is an older treatment that has recently received renewed attention. A number of operations have been developed for or applied to decompression of the brain at risk for the sequelae of uncontrollable intracranial hypertension. These include Cushing's subtemporal decompression, temporal lobectomy, and the more widely utilized hemispheric and bifrontal decompressive craniectomies. Recent literature suggests, but does not prove, that decompressive procedures, in the appropriate setting, may decrease mortality and improve outcome.

Research has focused on attempting to identify neuroprotective agents to ameliorate secondary injury and thus improve outcome from severe HI. Two large-scale prospective randomized trials of the free radical scavengers tirilazad mesylate and polyethylene glycol-superoxide dismutase (PEG-SOD) have been reported to show no significant reduction in mortality or outcome.[28] Recently completed trials with *N*-methyl-D-aspartate (NMDA)–receptor antagonists in an attempt to limit excitotoxicity have not shown any benefit in the clinical setting; however, final results have yet to be published. A small randomized controlled trial reported by Marion and colleagues demonstrated that moderate hypothermia for 24 hours in patients with severe traumatic brain injury and GCS of 5 to 7 on admission hastened neurological recovery and may have improved the outcome. However, a large, multicenter clinical trial did not bear out these positive findings, actually demonstrating a nonstatistically significant increase in mortality in GCS 3–4 patients treated with hypothermia.

Prognosis and Future Perspectives. Minor HI is rarely associated with significant long-term sequelae. It is well established, however, that a significant minority of patients suffer chronic disability attributable to neurobehavioral sequelae.[29] The exception to this is sports-related minor HI in which death from the second impact syndrome or cognitive disability from cumulative concussions may occur.

Second impact syndrome refers to malignant cerebral edema resulting from relatively mild head trauma occurring after a recent concussion. The syndrome is believed to be due to impaired cerebral autoregulation. It has been well documented that fatal brain swelling may occur in the setting of one minor HI followed in short order by a second minor HI in athletes who are still symptomatic from the first injury.[30] The cumulative effects of multiple minor HIs is recognized in boxing as the *punch drunk syndrome* (see later); however, the occurrence of this syndrome in association with other sports is controversial.

TABLE 51–2. **When to Return to Play After Removal from Contest**

Grade of Concussion	Time Until Return to Play*
Multiple Grade 1 concussions	1 week
Grade 2 concussion	1 week
Multiple Grade 2 concussions	2 weeks
Grade 3—brief loss of consciousness (seconds)	1 week
Grade 3—prolonged loss of consciousness (minutes)	2 weeks
Multiple Grade 3 concussions	1 month or longer, based on clinical decision of evaluating physician

*Only after being asymptomatic with normal neurological assessment at rest and with exercise.

From Practice parameter: The management of concussion in sports (summary statement). Report of the Quality Standards Subcommittee. Neurology 1997;48:584.

For sports-related minor HI, the American Academy of Neurology has defined three grades of concussion and recommended guidelines for return to play.[31] For Grades 1 and 2, there is transient confusion and no loss of consciousness. Resolution of concussion symptoms or mental status abnormalities occurs in less than 15 minutes in Grade 1 and more than 15 minutes in Grade 2. Grade 3 concussion is any loss of consciousness. Players with Grade 1 concussion may return to play the same day if they have a normal sideline neurological assessment including a detailed mental status examination. Players with Grade 2 and 3 concussions should not return to play the same day. Guidelines for return to play after removal from the contest (Table 51–2) are necessary because of concern over the cumulative effects of even mild HI and the rare occurrence of second impact syndrome.[32]

Dementia, long recognized as a sequela of multiple head injuries in boxing, was termed *punch drunk* by Martland in 1928 and *dementia pugilistica* by Millspauch in 1937. Neuropathological study of brains of boxers with dementia pugilistica demonstrate β-amyloid protein–containing diffuse plaques and neurofibrillary tangles, which are pathological features of Alzheimer's disease. Increased expression of β-amyloid precursor protein is part of an acute-phase response to neuronal injury, which can lead to deposition of β-amyloid protein.[33]

Patients with moderate HI usually experience both cognitive and physical disabilities and typically require rehabilitation services after acute hospitalization. Nevertheless, the incidence of severe long-term disability is small.

In contrast, few patients with severe HI recover completely to their preinjury state. The most common system to rate recovery is the Glasgow Outcome Scale: Good Recovery (GR), Moderate Disability (MD), Severe Disability (SD), Vegetative (V), and Death (D).[34] The tirilazad mesylate and PEG-SOD trials provide excellent information on current severe HI outcomes (Table 51–3).

The most active area of research in head injury today is in the field of molecular genetics. It has been noted that certain genes are upregulated, whereas others are downregulated, after both trauma and ischemia. Particular attention has been focused on the apolipoprotein E gene and its various alleles.

TABLE 51–3. **Current Prognosis from Severe Head Injury**

	Outcomes				
Study	**Good Recovery (%)**	**Moderate Disability (%)**	**Severe Disability (%)**	**Vegetative (%)**	**Death (%)**
Tirilazad (n = 557)	44.8	19.6	14.4	21.4	—
PEG-SOD (n = 162)	27	19	20	9	25

Data from Young B, Runge JW, Waxman KJ, et al: Effects of pegorgotein on neurologic outcome of patients with severe head injury. JAMA 1996;276:538–543.

Certain alleles have been associated with an increased susceptibility and severity of head injury, and others have been linked to improved recoveries after head injury.[35, 36] Considerably more research will be required to more completely define and ultimately understand and possibly clinically manipulate these "head injury" genes.

Postconcussion Syndrome

Sequelae of mild HI have been recognized for the past few hundred years.[37] In 1866, Erichsen initiated the controversy with his description of patients with persistent complaints after mild head and neck injury due to "molecular disarrangement" of the spinal cord. This condition was known as *railway spine* because many cases were the result of railway accidents. Rigler introduced the concept of compensation neurosis in 1879, because he believed that many persons with persistent symptoms were trying to obtain financial compensation for the injuries. Charcot believed that the impairment was actually the result of hysteria and neurasthenia. Similar debates about the organicity of persistent complaints after mild head injury are still common today, especially in medicolegal cases. The use of the term *postconcussion syndrome* dates back to 1934.

Pathogenesis and Pathophysiology. Mild head injury may result in cortical contusions due to coup and contrecoup injuries and diffuse axonal injury resulting from sheer and tensile strain damage. Subdural and epidural hematomas can also occasionally result. Release of excitatory neurotransmitters, including acetylcholine, glutamate, and aspartate may be a neurochemical substrate for mild HI.

Epidemiology and Risk Factors. Mild HI accounts for 75 percent or more of all brain injuries. The annual incidence of mild HI in the United States is about 140 in 100,000 population, with the relative causes as follows: motor vehicle accidents, 45 percent; falls, 30 percent; occupational accidents, 10 percent; recreational accidents, 10 percent; and assaults, 5 percent. Falls are the more likely cause in the elderly, whereas motor vehicle accidents are more common in the young. Men are more commonly injured, with a 2:1 ratio, and about one half of all patients are between the ages of 15 and 34 years. Between 20 and 40 percent of persons with mild HI in the United States do not seek treatment. Approximately 50 percent of patients with mild HI develop the postconcussion syndrome.[38]

Clinical Features and Associated Disorders. The postconcussion syndrome, which is usually the result of mild head trauma, comprises one or more of a large array of symptoms and signs (Table 51–4).[39, 40] The most common complaints are headaches, dizziness, fatigue, irritability, anxiety, insomnia, loss of concentration and memory, and noise sensitivity. Loss of consciousness does not have to occur for the postconcussion syndrome to develop. Headaches have been estimated to occur in 30 to 90 percent of patients who are symptomatic after mild injury. Headaches may occur more often and with longer duration in patients with mild rather than severe HI. Tension-type headaches account for about 85 percent of all post-traumatic headaches. Neck injuries, which often occur at the time of the HI, may cause referred headaches due to myofascial, intervertebral disc, and facet joint injury. Greater occipital neuralgia may occur from a direct blow to the nerve or may be associated with muscle spasm of the superior trapezius and semispinalis capitis muscles in the suboccipital region. Similar headaches may arise from the C2–C3 facet joint, which are known as *third occipital headaches*. Temporomandibular joint injury may also cause tension-type headaches.

Migraine headaches with and without aura can develop in the hours to weeks after a mild HI. Immediately after mild HI in sports such as soccer, football, rugby, and boxing, children, adolescents, and young adults may have a first-time migraine with aura. This syndrome may be triggered multiple times after additional mild HI and has been termed *footballer's migraine*. Cluster headaches can rarely develop after mild HI. Various other less common causes of post-traumatic headaches are found, including supraorbital and infraorbital neuralgia, dysesthesias over scalp lacerations, carotid or vertebral artery dissections, and subdural and epidural hematomas (see Table 51–1). Subdural hematomas can result in headaches that are nonspecific and that can be mild to severe, paroxysmal or constant, and bilateral or unilateral.

Cranial nerve symptoms and signs also occur. About one half of patients after mild HI report dizziness, which can be caused by various types of central and peripheral pathology, including labyrinthine concussion, benign positional vertigo, and brain stem injury. Blurred vision, reported by 14 percent of patients, is usually caused by convergence insufficiency. Blurred vision is occasionally the result of cranial nerve III, IV, and VI palsies. Decreased smell and taste are reported by 5 percent of patients after mild HI; the symptoms can be due to damage to the olfactory filaments. Approximately 10 percent of patients describe light and noise sensitivity after mild HI.

Nonspecific psychological symptoms such as personality change, irritability, anxiety, and depression are reported by over one half of patients within 3 months of mild HI. Fatigue and disruption of sleep patterns are also often reported. Post-traumatic stress disorder, which has many symptoms similar to those of the postconcussion syndrome, may occur after mild HI.

Four weeks after a mild HI, 20 percent of patients complain of impaired memory and concentration. Neuropsychological

TABLE 51–4. **Sequelae of Mild Head Injury**

Headache types and causes
- Muscle contraction or tension type
  - Cranial myofascial injury
  - Secondary to neck injury (cervicogenic)
    - Myofascial injury
    - Intervertebral discs
    - Cervical spondylosis
    - C2–C3 facet joint (third occipital headache)
  - Secondary to temporomandibular joint injury
- Migraine
  - Without and with aura
  - Footballer's migraine
- Greater and lesser occipital neuralgia
- Mixed
- Cluster
- Supraorbital and infraorbital neuralgia
- Due to scalp lacerations or local trauma
- Dysautonomic cephalgia
- Orgasmic cephalgia
- Carotid or vertebral artery dissection
- Subdural or epidural hematomas
- Hemorrhagic cortical contusions

Cranial nerve symptoms and signs
- Dizziness
- Vertigo
- Tinnitus
- Hearing loss
- Blurred vision
- Diplopia
- Convergence insufficiency
- Light and noise sensitivity
- Diminished taste and smell

Psychological and somatic complaints
- Irritability
- Anxiety
- Depression
- Personality change
- Fatigue
- Sleep disturbance
- Decreased libido
- Decreased appetite

Cognitive impairment
- Memory dysfunction
- Impaired concentration and attention
- Slowing of reaction time
- Slowing of information processing speed

Rare sequelae
- Subdural and epidural hematomas
- Seizures
- Transient global amnesia
- Tremor
- Dystonia

Modified from Evans RW: Post-concussion syndrome. *In* Evans RW, Baskin DS, Yatsu FM (eds): Prognosis of Neurological Disorders. New York. Oxford University Press, 1992.

testing has documented cognitive impairments, including a reduction in information processing speed, attention, reaction time, and memory for new information.

Differential Diagnosis. The incidence of complications that require neurosurgical consultation after mild HI has been estimated to be between 1 and 3 percent. For adults with mild HI and an initial GCS score of 13 to 15, the incidence of subdural hematomas is approximately 1 percent and epidural hematomas about 0.5 percent.

Evaluation. Single photon emission computed tomography and positron-emission tomography (PET) scans, brain stem auditory evoked potential studies, and brain mapping currently lack adequate sensitivity and specificity to justify use in the evaluation of the postconcussion syndrome. Electroencephalogram (EEG) studies are usually not indicated except for evaluating post-traumatic seizure disorders. Neuropsychological testing can be quite useful for the evaluation of patients with persistent cognitive complaints.

Management. Treatment should be individualized after the patient's particular problems are diagnosed. Tension- and migraine-type headaches can be treated with the usual prophylactic and symptomatic medications. Greater occipital neuralgia may improve with local anesthetic nerve blocks, which can be combined with an injectable corticosteroid. Physical therapy and transcutaneous electrical nerve stimulators (TENS units) may also help tension-type headaches. For patients with cognitive difficulties, the efficacy of cognitive retraining has not yet been established by prospective studies. Patients with prominent psychological symptoms may benefit from supportive psychotherapy and use of antidepressant and antianxiety-type medications. Simple reassurance is often the major treatment because most patients improve after 3 months. One of the most important roles for the physician is education of the patient and family members, other physicians, and, when appropriate, employers, attorneys, and representatives of insurance companies.

Prognosis and Future Perspectives. The probability of having persistent symptoms and neuropsychological deficits is the same whether a patient is only dazed or loses consciousness for less than 1 hour.[41] Persistent symptoms occur more often in women than men, in patients over the age of 40 years, and in those with a prior history of head trauma. Two years after the injury, about 20 percent of patients still complain of headaches. Cognitive deficits usually resolve within 3 months after the injury, although a small minority of patients report persistent problems for months or years. When patients have unusual or persistent complaints, the possible contributions of personality disorders, psychosocial problems, or secondary gain should be considered.

A compensation case or lawsuit is often filed in circumstances in which another party may be responsible for the HI, such as a motor vehicle accident or on-the-job injury. In this circumstance, when patients have persistent complaints, many physicians are appropriately concerned about compensation neurosis or malingering being the cause. Patients with claims, however, have similar symptoms that improve with time and similar cognitive test results as those without claims. For many claimants, the end of litigation does not mean the end of symptoms or return to work. They are not cured by a verdict.

Cranial Neuropathies

Blunt trauma can result in a stretching injury of cranial nerves, which, when severe, can result in nerves being torn loose from the brain stem. Stretching injuries often occur at points of attachment or at points of angulation. Skull fractures and penetrating trauma such as gunshot wounds can cause nerve lacerations.

Blunt trauma most often damages cranial nerves I, VII, and VIII; less often II, III, IV, and VI; and least often V, IX, X, XI, and XII. The incidence of cranial neuropathies increases with more severe HI. For example, the overall incidence of anosmia is about 7 percent but increases to 30 percent in patients with anterior fossa fractures or severe HI. Even trivial HI can result in anosmia. Injury to the optic nerves and chiasm has been reported in up to 5 percent of patients with HI. Ocular motility disorders occur in up to one third of patients sustaining closed HI; the abducens nerve is the most commonly injured. Trigeminal nerve and branch injuries often occur as a result of facial trauma. Facial nerve injuries frequently occur with temporal bone fractures.

The site of likely trauma, clinical features, evaluation, management, and prognosis are summarized in Table 51–5.

Post-traumatic Epilepsy

Pathogenesis and Pathophysiology. Post-traumatic seizures may be associated with the typical pathological changes that may be seen in brain injuries, including reactive gliosis, axon retraction balls, wallerian degeneration, microglial scar formation, and cystic white matter lesions.[42] When a contusion or cortical laceration is present, the breakdown of hemoglobin releases iron. Based on animal and cell culture studies, iron may increase intracellular calcium oscillation and may increase free radical formation through activation of the arachidonic acid cascade, producing increased intracellular calcium resulting in excitotoxic damage, neuronal death, and glial scarring, which lead to epileptiform activity.[43] These findings suggest a possible role for neuroprotective treatment in the future. There is also evidence suggesting that post-traumatic seizures may be a result of alterations of intrinsic membrane properties of pyramidal neurons together with enhanced NMDA synaptic conductances.[44]

Epidemiology and Risk Factors. Head injury is the cause of about 4 percent of all cases of epilepsy. In teenagers and young adults, HI is the most common cause of symptomatic epilepsy. Post-traumatic seizures can be divided into different types based on the time of onset after the injury. Immediate seizures occur within minutes of the injury. Early seizures occur within 1 week, whereas late seizures occur after 1 week.

The incidence of early post-traumatic seizures is about 4 percent. Early seizure rates are higher in patients with more severe HI, intracranial and subdural hematomas, depressed skull fractures, focal neurological signs, loss of consciousness, or post-traumatic amnesia present for more than 24 hours, and in children under the age of 5 years.

Late seizures have an incidence of about 2 percent.[43] Risk factors for late seizures include penetrating missile wounds; an early seizure; intracerebral, epidural, and subdural hematomas; GCS score of 10 or less; depressed and linear skull fractures; and cortical contusions.

Clinical Features and Associated Disorders. About one third of early seizures occur during each of the following times: within the first hour, between 1 and 24 hours, and between 1 and 7 days. Over 60 percent of early seizures are partial, whereas the others are generalized tonic-clonic. About 10 percent of patients develop status epilepticus. Immediate concussive convulsions are not an epileptic phenomenon but instead are due to a brief traumatic functional decerebration resulting from loss of cortical inhibition.[45] Antiepileptic medication is not indicated for concussive convulsions.

About 50 percent of patients with late seizures have their first seizure within 1 year of the injury and about 80 percent within 2 years. Over 60 percent of the seizures are generalized tonic-clonic with or without focal onset, whereas the others are simple or complex partial seizures.

Differential Diagnosis. In some cases, post-traumatic seizures must be distinguished from disorders that can result in psychogenic nonepileptic events including conversion, factitious behavior, malingering, reinforced behavior pattern, somatization, post-traumatic stress disorder, hypochondriasis, panic disorder, depersonalization, dissociative disorder, and hyperventilation syndrome. Because mild HI uncommonly result in seizures, nonepileptiform events should be considered when these patients have "funny spells," or episodes that are atypical for epilepsy.[46]

Evaluation. A detailed history from the patient and witnesses, if any, of the event; review of pertinent medical records; and general and neurological examination are often the bases for diagnosing post-traumatic seizures. Although an EEG study is certainly important, epileptiform activity is seen in only 50 percent of patients. Video or ambulatory EEG may be worthwhile in occasional cases when the diagnosis is unclear. A CT or MRI scan of the brain may also be indicated.

Management. In patients with risk factors for early seizures, prophylactic treatment with phenytoin reduces the incidence of early seizures. Within the first few weeks, however, phenytoin can be gradually withdrawn because the incidence of late seizures is not reduced by continuing treatment.[47] Instituting long-term anticonvulsant treatment is beneficial for patients after an initial late seizure.

Prognosis and Future Perspectives. The remission rate for post-traumatic epilepsy is about 50 percent. An EEG is of no specific value in predicting either the development or remission of post-traumatic epilepsy. A greater number of seizures and abnormal findings on neurological examination decrease the chance of remission.

Post-traumatic Movement Disorders

An association between injuries and involuntary movements has been suggested since the 19th century speculation of Parkinson, Charcot, and Gowers. When a movement disorder begins shortly after a brain injury, a cause-and-effect relationship is apparent. An association is less obvious with longer latencies after the injury and after peripheral trauma where there may be a temporal but not causal relationship.[48] In some cases, the patient may not have noticed or reported a mild movement disorder that was present before the injury.[49, 50]

Pathogenesis and Pathophysiology. Direct trauma to subcortical and substantia nigral neurons can result in move-

TABLE 51–5. **A Summary of Traumatic Cranial Neuropathies**

Cranial Nerve	Site of Likely Trauma	Clinical Features	Evaluation	Management	Prognosis
I	Any part of head. More common with occipital than frontal trauma	Decreased or absent sense of smell	Check for possible ethmoid fractures, CSF rhinorrhea, and injury to orbital surface of frontal lobes	Educate patient	Reso in up to 50% of cases, usually during first 3 months but up to 5 years after injury
II	Intracanalicular often associated with a skull base fracture	Decreased or loss of vision. Scotomas, sector, and altitudinal defects can occur	Check visual acuity, fields, and for afferent pupillary defect. CT scan and ultrasound A and B are useful to assess for possible compressive lesions	Controversial for indirect optic neuropathy: include observation, high-dose steroids, and surgery. Surgical decompression often recommended in cases of delayed onset of visual loss	Extremely variable; from 0–100% depending upon the study
III	Where the nerve enters the dura at the posterior end of the cavernous sinus. Uncal herniation much less common	Dilated pupil and turned out eye present in complete palsy. Anisocoria and diplopia in partial lesions	CT and/or MRI scans to look for a compressive lesion	Symptomatic such as eyepatch, semitransparent tape to glasses and prisms for diplopia. Muscle shortening procedures may be helpful for permanent diplopia	Recovery begins within 2–3 months when nerve in continuity. Aberrant regeneration often occurs with findings such as lid elevation or pupillary constriction with attempted adduction or depression
IV	Stretching or contusion of the nerve as it exits the dorsal midbrain near the anterior medullary velum	Trauma is the most common cause of trochlear palsies. Bilateral palsies are rather common	Same as above	Same as above	Only 50% recover because of frequent avulsion of the trochlear nerve
V	Trigeminal nerves and branches are commonly injured with facial trauma, especially supraorbital and supratrochlear nerves. The infraorbital nerve is often injured in orbital floor blowout fractures	Injury to the gasserian ganglion and trigeminal trunk is rare after closed head trauma	Imaging studies to exclude underlying fractures	Decompression of the infraorbital nerve in orbital floor fractures. Symptomatic for hyperpathia due to supra- and infraorbital neuropathies with medications such as carbamazepine, tricyclics, and baclofen	Hyperpathia in the distribution of the nerve may be permanent
VI	As the nerve ascends the clivus, in fractures of the petrous bone along with VII and VIII, in the superior orbital fissure along with III and IV, and in its subarachnoid course due to raised intracranial pressure	Bilateral palsies are rather common	Same as above	Same as above	Recovery often occurs after 4 months

Table continued on following page

TABLE 51–5. **A Summary of Traumatic Cranial Neuropathies** *Continued*

Cranial Nerve	Site of Likely Trauma	Clinical Features	Evaluation	Management	Prognosis
VII	Most commonly within the petrous bone but can be injured anywhere along its course	Injured in 50% with a transverse temporal bone fracture. Facial palsy in 25% with a longitudinal fracture, often with a delayed onset	CT scan to evaluate temporal bone trauma. A nerve conduction study 5 or more days after the injury is helpful to assess the degree of nerve injury	Facial nerve decompression is usually indicated for transverse fractures. Artificial tears and eye patch at night to prevent exposure keratitis	Spontaneous recovery usual after longitudinal fractures. When due to transverse fractures, 50% recovery after decompression
VIII	Labyrinthine concussion without a skull fracture is the most common site. Conductive hearing loss follows longitudinal temporal bone fractures in over 50% of cases. Transverse fractures result in vestibular and cochlear nerve laceration in over 80%	Findings associated with a fracture of the petrous portion of the temporal bone include hemotympanum or tympanic membrane perforation with blood in the external canal, hearing loss, vestibular dysfunction, peripheral facial nerve palsy, CSF otorrhea, and ecchymosis of the scalp over the mastoid bone (Battle's sign). Benign positional vertigo occurs in about 25% of patients following head trauma	Examine the external canals and tympanic membranes. An audiogram including pure-tone and speech audiometry, acoustic reflexes, and middle ear function is used to assess hearing loss. An electronystagmogram (ENG) is used to assess vestibular function. CT scan to evaluate temporal bone trauma	A hearing aid may help those with sensorineural hearing loss. Surgical correction is indicated for conductive hearing loss due to ossicular chain disruption. Positioning maneuvers, such as Epley's or Semont's, which move the debris out of the semicircular canal and into the utricle, can be curative for benign positional vertigo	Following temporal bone fractures, patients with low- or high-frequency hearing loss may have some recovery, but those with low- and high-frequency loss usually do not recover. Vertigo due to a labyrinth concussion usually resolves within a year
IX, X, XI, XII	Gunshot or stab wounds occasionally cause injury. A fracture of the occipital condyle, Collet-Sicard syndrome, can injure all four nerves. The peripheral portion of XI can be injured in surgical procedures such as posterior cervical lymph node biopsies. The hypoglossal and recurrent laryngeal nerves can be traumatized in anterior neck operations such as carotid endarterectomy	Lower cranial nerve findings associated with signs of brain stem compression are consistent with an intracranial lesion, whereas the presence of a Horner's syndrome is consistent with an extracranial lesion	A careful clinical examination is mandatory. CT and MRI are both useful, depending upon the case	Treatment of Collet-Sicard syndrome is supportive with elevation of the head for drainage of excess saliva and IV or nasogastric nutrition until normal swallowing returns. Accessory nerve injuries in the neck may require exploration with neurolysis or resection and repair or grafting, depending on the degree of injury	Collet-Sicard syndrome may show slow partial recovery. Patients with vagal, spinal accessory, and hypoglossal nerve injuries associated with carotid endarterectomy often recover

ment disorders occurring shortly after an injury. Movement disorders occurring months following the injury have been hypothesized to be related to sprouting, remyelination, ephaptic transmission, inflammatory changes, oxidative reactions, and central synaptic reorganization. Peripheral trauma that precedes the development of a movement disorder may alter sensory input, leading to central cortical and subcortical reorganization.[51, 52]

Epidemiology and Risk Factors. Movement disorders due to trauma are rare, and specific epidemiological and risk factor studies have not been performed.

Clinical Features and Associated Findings. Although HI does not result in Parkinson's disease with pathological findings of Lewy bodies, HI may result in a temporary exacerbation of motor function in patients with pre-existing Parkinson's disease.[49] Parkinsonism is a rare complication of single closed HI and may also occur after penetrating bullet and knife injuries of the brain stem. Repeated HI as in the case of boxers with dementia pugilistica may result in parkinsonism in association with many other neurological signs. Parkinsonian tremor may rarely be associated with peripheral body trauma, although a direct causal relationship cannot be established.[53]

Postural and kinetic tremor can be due to direct traumatic lesions of the dentatothalamic circuit. Benedikt's syndrome (unilateral cranial nerve III palsy and contralateral ataxic hemiparesis) can be associated with rest and postural and kinetic tremor. Postural-kinetic tremors of the arms, legs, or head may occur within weeks of mild HI even without loss of consciousness. Peripheral trauma can induce tremor, which can occur along with reflex sympathetic dystrophy, dystonia, and myoclonus.[52, 53] Myoclonus, dystonia, and athetosis may be present in patients with post-traumatic tremors.

Contralateral dystonia can be due to a lesion in the striatum, particularly the putamen. Causes include perinatal trauma, closed HI (severe much more often than mild), and thalamotomy. The onset of dystonia may have a latency period from 1 month to 9 years. Spastic dystonia due to pyramidal and extrapyramidal injury and paroxysmal nocturnal dystonia are variants of post-traumatic dystonia. Often patients develop post-traumatic dystonia as a delayed sequela of severe HI, initially characterized by coma and quadriplegia. After the patient awakens and the plegia improves, severe action dystonia develops. Minor or moderate local peripheral trauma can be associated with focal dystonia, sometimes in patients with reflex sympathetic dystrophy. Examples of peripherally induced dystonia include the following: blepharospasm after surgery on the eyelids; oromandibular dystonia after dental procedures; spasmodic dysphonia after facial injuries; cervical dystonia after neck injuries such as whiplash; and foot dystonia after stubbing a toe.

A recent report by Kraus and colleagues studied survivors of severe HI, admitted to the hospital with GCS of 8 or less. Of the 264 survivors, follow-up was obtained on 221, and 22 percent reported or showed evidence of movement disorders, half transient and half persistent. Tremor, usually kinetic, and dystonia were the most common disorders and usually developed with a post-trauma latency of 2 to 24 months.

Chorea, choreoathetosis, and ballismus can follow blunt head trauma with injury to the striatum, subthalamic nucleus, and anterior thalamus. The onset is usually days to months following the trauma.

Action myoclonus, palatal myoclonus, and segmental myoclonus may result from head injury not associated with anoxia or epilepsy. Segmental myoclonus may also occur after spinal cord injury.

A deep, burning pain followed by persistent, involuntary, and irregular movements of the toes and feet, termed *painful legs and moving toes*, can be associated with minor foot and ankle injuries. Hemifacial spasm has been rarely associated with trauma. Additionally, after amputation, the remaining stump can involuntarily jerk.

Differential Diagnosis. Because the relationship between many injuries and the movement disorder may be circumstantial and retrospective, an idiopathic movement disorder is always a diagnostic consideration. The possibility of psychogenic movement disorders, which may be more common in women, should also be considered. Because movement disorders often develop several weeks or months after trauma and because patients often receive neuroleptic medications after acute injuries, drug-induced movement disorders are another possible cause.

Evaluation. Neuroimaging such as MRI and occasionally PET can demonstrate responsible brain lesions. Depending on the case, testing to exclude other potential causes of the movement disorder such as Wilson's disease may also be appropriate.

Management and Prognosis. Post-traumatic parkinsonism may respond to dopaminergic and cholinergic medications. Post-traumatic action tremors only occasionally respond to standard medical treatment. Selected cases may benefit from botulinum toxin injections into involved muscles and ventrolateral thalamotomy. Medications are usually not helpful for dystonia associated with central and peripheral trauma, although botulinum toxin injections can produce temporary relief.[51] Post-traumatic chorea and choreoathetosis may respond to valproic acid and haloperidol, whereas trauma-induced cortical myoclonus can be treated with clonazepam.

Spinal Cord Injury

Over the past decade there have been significant advances in transport, emergency management, pharmacological resuscitation, comprehensive acute care, and rehabilitation. Nevertheless, spinal cord injury (SCI) remains a physically and emotionally devastating problem. The neurologist may thus be confronted with the need for recognition of a potential spinal injury or SCI and institute appropriate stabilization procedures.

Pathogenesis and Pathophysiology. The pathophysiology of SCI may be divided into two distinct phases—primary and secondary injury. Primary injury refers to the structural damage occurring instantly after the traumatic event. Further primary injury may occur, however, if an injured spine is not adequately immobilized. Secondary injury refers to a pathophysiological cascade initiated shortly after injury, including such insults as ischemia, hypoxia, edema, and various harmful biochemical events. Because it is extremely rare for the primary injury to cause transection of the spinal cord, and it has been shown that less than 10 percent of the cross-sectional area of the spinal cord supports locomotion, it is very important to focus clinical attention of the secondary injury process.[54]

Ischemia is a very prominent feature of post-SCI events. Within 2 hours of injury there is a significant reduction in spinal cord blood flow. This ischemia may be confounded by loss of the normal autoregulatory response of the spinal cord vasculature. When autoregulation is lost, blood flow becomes dependent on systemic pressures. Thus, in the multitraumatized patient or the patient with vasogenic spinal shock complicating the SCI, severe systemic hypotension may exacerbate the spinal cord ischemia.

Edema formation is another feature of the secondary injury process. Edema develops first at the injury site and subsequently spreads into adjacent and sometimes distant segments of the cord. The relationship between this edema and worsening of neurological function is not well understood.

Many biochemical mechanisms have been implicated in the evolution of the pathological changes and physiological derangements occurring after SCI. Electrolyte disturbances have been well documented, including increased intracellular calcium level, increased extracellular potassium level, and increased sodium permeability. Other events such as excitatory neurotransmitter accumulation, arachidonic acid release, endogenous opiate activation, and prostaglandin production have all been implicated as damaging elements of the postinjury cascade. Other events, free radical production and lipid peroxidation, are believed to play a central role in this process. Ultimately, however, all of these events cumulatively result in ischemia, edema formation, membrane destruction, cell death, and eventually permanent neurological deficits.

Epidemiology and Risk Factors. Spinal cord injury occurs at a rate of 30 to 40 per million population per year, resulting in approximately 10,000 new cases each year. The prevalence of SCI is over 200,000.[55] SCI occurs primarily in young males 18 to 25 years of age. The primary precipitant of injury is motor vehicle accidents, although in some areas of the country, swimming and diving-related accidents may take precedence. Sports-related injuries account for less than 5 percent of the total. In some urban areas the incidence of gunshot-related SCI is increasing (Fig. 51–3). SCI rarely occurs in isolation, and over 75 percent of these patients has some other systemic injury. In 10 to 15 percent, there is an associated head injury. This concern has led to the widely quoted clinical maxim that all multitraumatized patients or any patient with a severe head injury should be presumed to have a spine injury or SCI until proven otherwise.

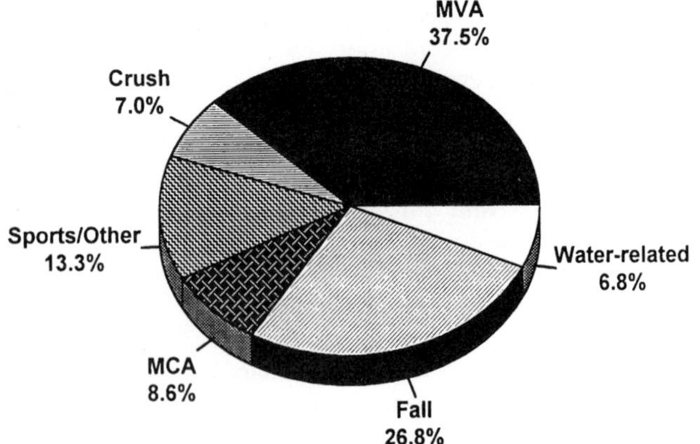

FIGURE 51–3. Epidemiology of spinal cord injury. MCA, motor cycle accident; MVA, motor vehicle accident.

Clinical Features and Associated Disorders. Although general physical assessment of the patient may raise concerns over a possible SCI, a detailed neurological assessment is the only reliable means to rule out this diagnosis. A standardized means of performing and recording the neurological examination has been advocated by the American Spinal Injury Association (ASIA) and has been accepted internationally by both clinicians and researchers (Fig. 51–4). With a complete transverse myelopathy, all motor and sensory function below the level of injury is absent. The neurological level of injury is the most caudal or lowest spinal cord segment with normal sensation and a muscle strength of 3/5 or better. An incomplete injury is present when there is preservation of any motor or sensory function below the zone of injury, including sacral sparing.

Acute SCI can result in spinal shock with a total flaccid paralysis below the level of the lesion. Basic knowledge of myotomes, dermatomes, and deep tendon reflexes is essential for localization. Injury to the upper cervical cord can also damage brain stem structures either because of direct trauma or because of vascular injury of the vertebral arteries. This cervicomedullary syndrome is characterized by respiratory dysfunction, hypotension, variable tetraparesis, hyperesthesia from C1 to C4, and sensory loss of the face with an onionskin pattern.

Partial or incomplete lesions of the spinal cord can result in four patterns of deficit. In the central cervical cord syndrome, the paresis involves the upper extremities, especially the hands, more than the lower extremities. The mechanism of injury is acute cord compression between bony bars or spurs anteriorly and thickened ligamentum flavum posteriorly, resulting in relatively more injury to the medial segments of the corticospinal tracts, which control arm function. The anterior cord syndrome, complete paralysis and hyperesthesia at the level of the lesion but intact light touch and vibration sense, is due to a large disc herniation compressing the anterior cord but without compression of the dorsal columns. The posterior cord syndrome is posterior column damage with impaired light touch and proprioception resulting from hyperextension injuries with fractures of the vertebral arch. The Brown-Séquard syndrome, caused by a lesion of half of the spinal cord, is defined by ipsilateral motor and proprioceptive loss and contralateral pain and temperature loss with the upper level one or two segments below the level of the lesion. This syndrome can occur after various injuries, including penetrating trauma, hyperextension and flexion injuries, locked facets, and compression fractures.

The conus medullaris syndrome is due to a compression injury at T12 that can occur from a disc herniation or a burst fracture of the body of T12. Because almost all the lumbar cord segments are opposite the T12 vertebral body, a severe compression can produce dysfunction in any or all of the lumbar as well as the sacral segments. Flaccid paralysis of the legs and anal sphincter with variable sensory deficits can be present. Because the spinal cord usually terminates at the L1–L2 disc space, trauma below this level injures the nerve roots. The cauda equina syndrome, which is compression of nerve roots below the L1 level, can be caused by frac-

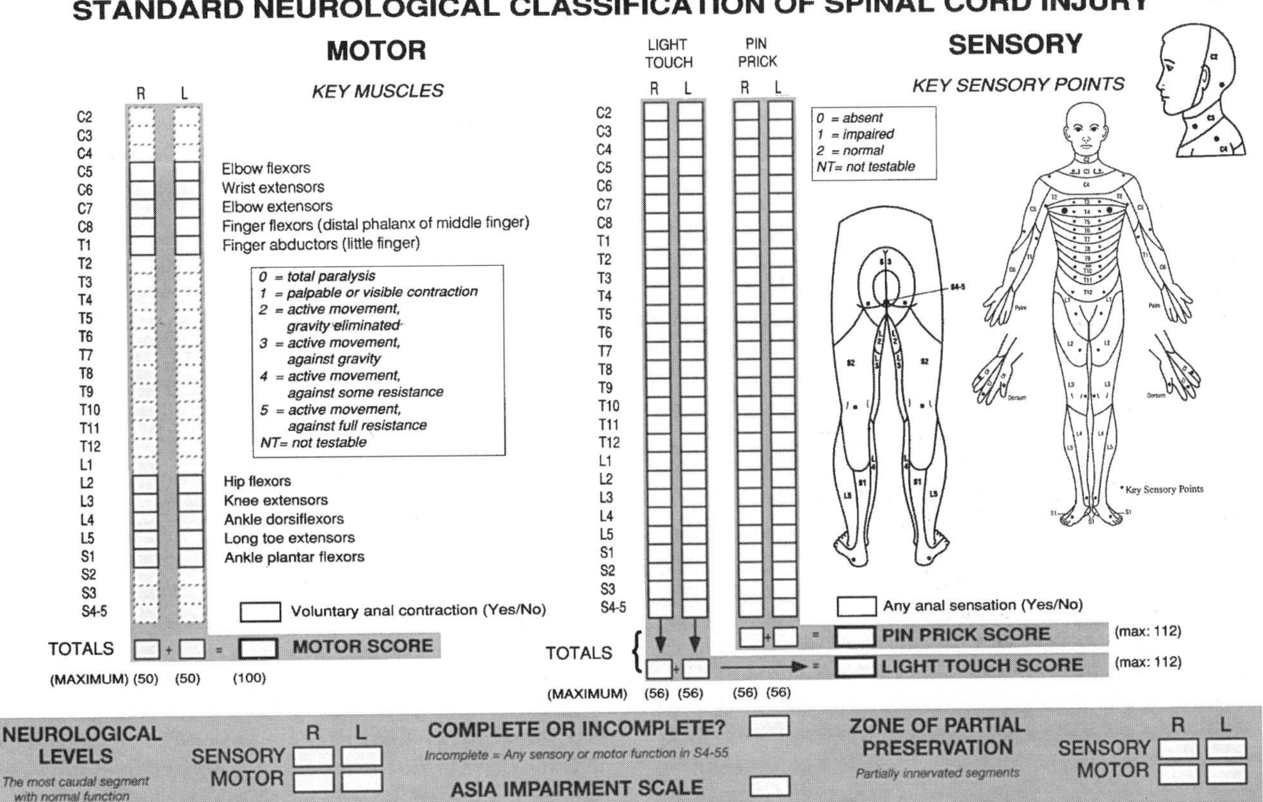

FIGURE 51–4. The ASIA system for examination and classification of spinal cord injury. (From American Spinal Injury Association: Standards for Neurological and Functional Classification of Spinal Cord Injury, Revised 1992, p 278.)

tures and dislocations of the spine or large posterocentral intervertebral disc herniations. Lower motor neuron deficits result with variable sensorimotor, reflex, bladder, bowel, and sexual dysfunction.

In the unconscious patient, neurological evaluation for SCI is very difficult. The only clues to the presence of a significant SCI may be a lack of facial grimacing to peripherally applied painful stimuli, indicating a sensory loss over the trunk, or a lack of withdrawal behavior in the arms or legs in response to painful stimulation applied to the head or face.

The biomechanics of the pediatric spine are fundamentally different from that of the adult. These differences—ligamentous laxity, wedge-shaped vertebrae, horizontally oriented facets—account for distinct clinical presentations. The clinical differences between adult and pediatric SCI include the following: disproportionate involvement of the upper cervical spine in pediatric patients, high frequency of spinal cord injury without radiographic abnormality, high susceptibility to the delayed onset of neurological deficits in children, and a higher proportion of complete neurological injuries in children (Table 51–6).[56, 57]

A unique SCI syndrome—the burning hands syndrome—was first described in sports injury.[58] This syndrome appears to be a variation of central cord syndrome associated with severe burning paresthesias and dysesthesias in the hands and/or the feet. Other signs of neurological dysfunction are minimal or absent. Over 50 percent of the time there is an underlying spine fracture-dislocation. It is important to differentiate this syndrome from the much more common and usually innocuous "burner" or "stinger" of brachial plexus origin.

The syndrome of neurapraxia is also of special concern after athletic injury. Affected individuals experience dramatic, although transient, neurological deficits including quadriplegia. Frequently this syndrome is associated structurally with degenerative or congenital spinal canal stenosis. Many attempts have been made to quantitate the level of risk

TABLE 51–6. **Spine and Spinal Cord Injuries**

Characteristics	Adult	Pediatric
Mechanism of Injury	Motor vehicle accidents	Pedestrian/falls
Level of Injury		
C1–C3	1–2%	60%
C3–C7	85%	30–40%
Thoracolumbar	10–15%	5%
Type of Injury		
Fracture-dislocation	>70%	25%
Subluxation alone	<20%	>50%
SCIWORA	Rare	Up to 50%
Delayed Neurological Deficits	Rare	Up to 50%

SCIWORA, Spinal cord injury without radiological abnormalities.

to these individuals from continued athletic participation; however, considerable controversy still exists.[59, 60]

The majority of spinal cord–injured patients have at least one other system injury. Occasionally these injuries take precedence in evaluation and treatment. If one level of bony injury has been identified, it is necessary to survey the entire spine because there is a 10 to 15 percent incidence of spine injury at other levels.

Various problems may occur with chronic SCIs. Within a few weeks of the injury, hyperactive reflexes develop, which are associated with hypertonicity of the extremities. Although moderate spasticity is not a problem for the patient, severe spasticity may lead to flexor spasms and contractures. Central deafferentation pain, dysesthesias described as burning, stinging, or freezing, may be present. Autonomic dysfunction can occur as early as 2 to 3 weeks after complete or incomplete lesions of the cervical or thoracic cord. Orthostatic hypotension is frequent when the patient is first allowed to sit. Autonomic hyper-reflexia or "mass reflex" may be triggered by noxious stimuli such as fecal impaction, urinary tract infections, distention of the bladder, uterine contraction, and decubiti. Manifestations include nausea, throbbing headache, skin blanching and diaphoresis below the level of the cord lesion, and paroxysmal hypertension.

When patients develop progressive neurological deficits any time from several months to many years after SCI, posttraumatic syringomyelia may be responsible. Present in up to 3 percent of patients, four kinds of trauma may be responsible: repeated microtrauma, arachnoiditis, severe single trauma, and minor single trauma.[61] One mechanism of syrinx formation is an initial hematomyelia with subsequent resorption and formation of a cyst cavity.

Differential Diagnosis. Very few disorders mimic acute SCI. Occasionally a patient with hysterical paralysis presents a diagnostic and therapeutic dilemma. It should be borne in mind that true SCI is almost always associated with obvious physiological disturbances such as bradycardia, hypotension, and respiratory compromise.

Evaluation. The injured spine may become a radiological diagnostic dilemma, and one must constantly bear in mind the normal radiological appearance of the spine. The initial evaluation should always include plain radiographs of the cervical or thoracolumbar spine, depending on the neurological findings.[62–64] If an abnormality is identified, complete spine films must be obtained because there is a 10 to 15 percent incidence of multiple fractures following trauma.

Additional useful information can often be obtained by performing flexion-extension views. Extreme caution must be taken if instability is suspected, however. To better interpret plain films or to better define a definite abnormality, CT is extremely helpful. MRI is sometimes necessary for the complete evaluation of SCI. MRI is the only diagnostic modality that allows direct visualization of the injured cord.[65]

A number of guidelines have been developed to aid the clinician in clearing the potentially injured spine. The most widely quoted of these are the Eastern Association for the Surgery of Trauma guidelines.[66]

The first principle in evaluating the cervical spine is a clear visualization of all seven cervical vertebrae. At times, a swimmer's view is necessary to visualize this region. If the C7–T1 junction cannot be imaged on plain films, a CT should be performed.

All films should be reviewed for alignment of the vertebral bodies and the facet joints, vertebral body height, and interpedicular distance and normal soft tissue configuration. When evaluating the C1–C2 region, careful attention must be given to the distance separating the anterior arch of C1 and the odontoid process. In an adult, this distance is normally less than 2 mm; in children up to 5 mm distance is acceptable. If any questions arise over possible pathological separation, flexion-extension films may be helpful. Alternatively, MRI may be employed to evaluate the competency of the transverse axial ligament.[67]

Another important consideration when evaluating cervical spine films is the entity of pseudosubluxation. Pseudosubluxation of up to 3 to 4 mm of C2 on C3 may appear in up to 40 percent of normal radiographs in children younger than 8 years old. A similar abnormality can occur at C3–C4 in up to 20 percent. If there is any question about this entity, flexion-extension views should be helpful. A true subluxation cannot be reduced, as contrasted with a pseudosubluxation.

The usual mechanism for atlas fractures involves axial compression of the head with downward displacement of the occipital condyles into the lateral masses of C1. The most important radiographical view is the open-mouth odontoid. With a C1 fracture, the lateral masses of C1 are offset laterally with respect to C2. CT scanning clearly demonstrates the associated C1 ring fractures (Fig. 51–5).

Dens fractures occur as a consequence of either forced hyperextension or hyperflexion of the head. With hyperflexion injuries and associated transverse axial ligament damage, the dens is displaced anteriorly with forward subluxation of C1 on C2. With hyperextension injuries the dens is displaced posteriorly with associated posterior subluxation of C1 on C2. Three type of dens fractures may be seen—type 1, fracture line across tip of dens; type 2, at the base of the dens; and type 3, with a fracture extending into the body of C2. CT scanning may not demonstrate a dens injury if the fracture line is axially oriented.

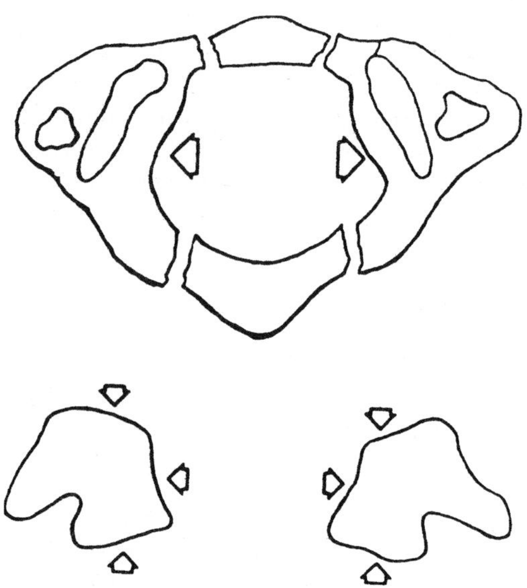

FIGURE 51–5. A C1 burst or Jefferson's fracture.

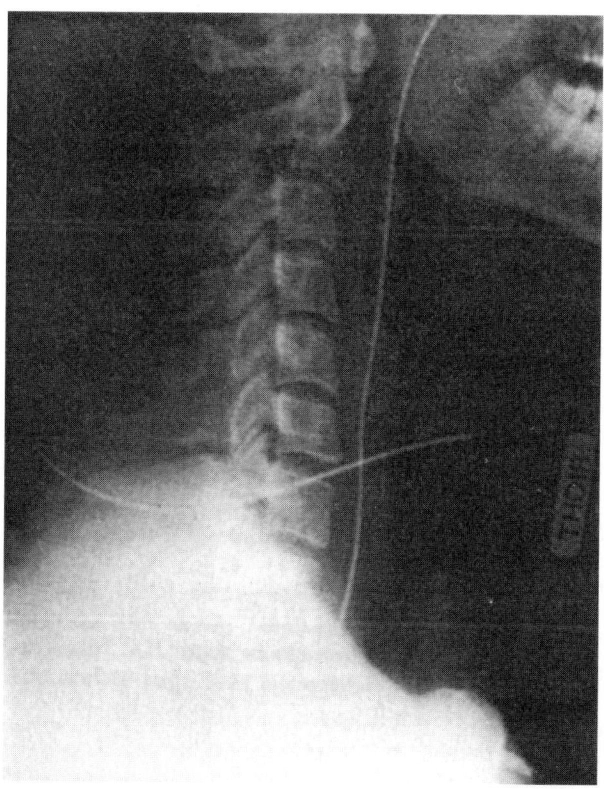

FIGURE 51–6. Plain radiograph of a typical C2-hangman's fracture.

Another type of axis fracture is the hangman's fracture, usually resulting from hyperextension. Typically there are fractures through both pedicles of C2 with associated forward subluxation of C2 on C3 (Fig. 51–6).

Except in infants and young children, over 85 percent of cervical fractures occur below C3. Locked facets, either unilateral or bilateral, and compression fractures are the most common lesions. These types of injuries are characteristically produced by flexion complicated by axial loading.

Compression fractures are characterized radiographically by loss of vertebral height, retropulsion of bone into the spinal canal, and kyphotic angulation. The hallmark of facet dislocation is subluxation (Fig. 51–7).

The most common fracture of the thoracolumbar spine is the compression or burst fracture brought about by flexion and axial loading. The T12–L1 level is the one most frequently affected. Typical radiographical features are loss of vertebral height, retropulsion of bone fragments, and kyphotic angulation. The degree of bony disruption and spinal canal compromise is well demonstrated on CT (Fig. 51–8).

A small but definite subtype of SCI occurs without any demonstrable radiographical abnormality, including the appearance on MRI. This type is more likely to occur in children rather than adults; it is often associated with a delayed onset of symptoms after injury, and there is a very poor prognosis for neurological recovery.[68]

MRI is becoming increasingly useful in the evaluation of SCI. MRI is adequate for demonstrating most bony injury and is superior to all other modalities for exposing the soft tissue and ligaments. Additionally, MRI is the only modality that allows direct visualization of the injured cord (Fig. 51–9).

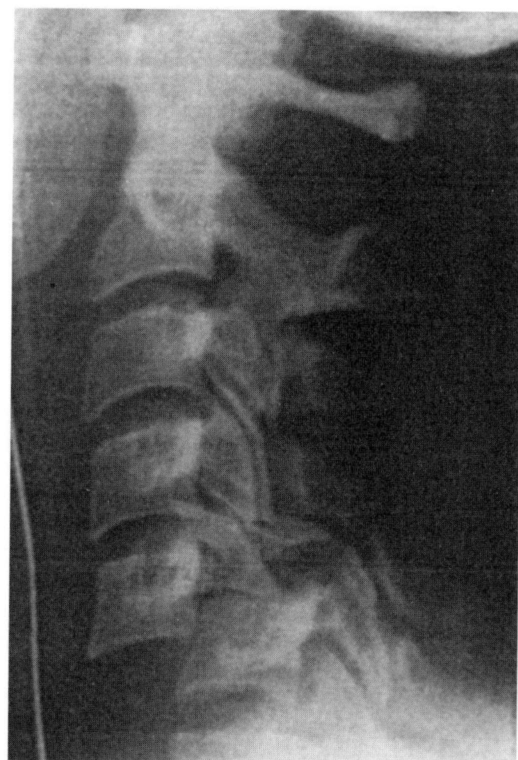

FIGURE 51–7. Plain lateral radiograph demonstrating C5–C6 subluxation secondary to bilateral facet dislocation. (From Wilberger JE: Spinal Cord Injuries in Children. Mount Kisco, NY, Futura Publishing, 1986, p 29.)

Several patterns of cord injury have been identified on MRI—transection, contusion, hemorrhage, edema—and preliminary studies suggest a correlation between initial and follow-up MRI findings and neurological prognosis.[69] When MRI is not available, not feasible, or contraindicated, intrathecally enhanced CT scan is the best alternative. Myelography can also be performed initially when movement of the patient is feasible.

Management. Resuscitation and stabilization of the patient's condition must be accomplished simultaneously

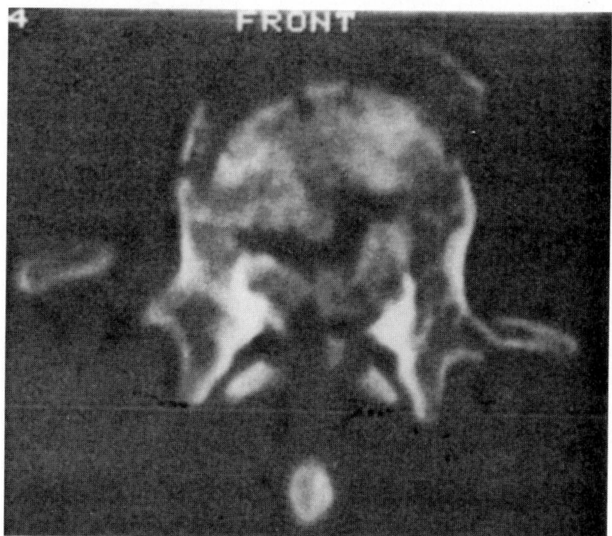

FIGURE 51–8. CT scan slice of an L1 compression-burst fracture with significant spinal canal compromise.

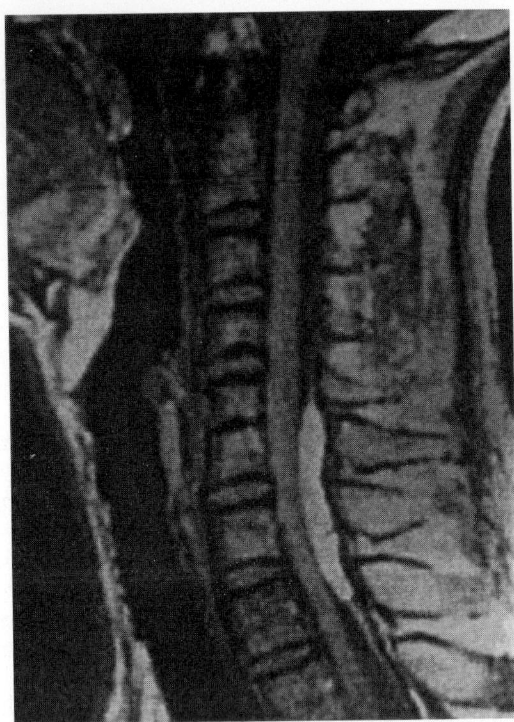

FIGURE 51–9. Sagittal MRI image showing a large dorsal epidural hematoma after posterior element fracture.

with immobilization and stabilization of the spine in the patient with SCI. Because of the frequent occurrence of multisystem injury, the principles of advanced trauma life support must be methodically applied. If significant chest or abdominal injuries co-exist, immediate treatment should be directed to those injuries considered most life-threatening.

In the initial management, establishment and maintenance of the airway takes precedence. With known or suspected SCI, neck manipulation should be minimized. Appropriate large-bore intravenous lines should be placed and fluid resuscitation provided. If possible, both a Foley catheter and a nasogastric tube should be placed. When SCI is related to sports injury, the sensational nature of these cases often generates considerable interest. When these injuries do occur it is important to immobilize the athlete on the field and to leave intact any protective headgear, unless airway maintenance is threatened.

During the process of general stabilization, the clinician must remain constantly aware of the principles of spine stabilization. As noted earlier, intubation when necessary should be accomplished with the neck in as neutral position as possible. Adequate stabilization of the cervical spine requires both a hard cervical collar to prevent flexion or extension and side supports to prevent rotation. This immobilization can be accomplished by using sandbags or bolsters on the sides of the head or by taping the head to a rigid backboard. Thoracolumbar injuries are stabilized on a backboard. It is important to remember, however, that insensate patients with SCI left on hard backboards rapidly develop decubiti.

Once the patient's condition is stabilized and appropriate diagnostic studies have been accomplished, more definitive spine stabilization can be undertaken. For cervical injuries, this involves immobilization and reduction of any dislocations, usually by skeletal traction. Many devices are currently available for this purpose; the most commonly used are Gardner-Wells tongs and halo rings. Once a traction device has been placed, weights can be added to aid in spinal realignment. It has been generally recommended that no more that 5 pounds of weight be applied for each cervical level involved (i.e., for a C5 level dislocation no more than 30 pounds should be applied). In routine clinical practice, however, especially for injuries such as bilateral facet dislocations, weights in excess of 50 pounds may be necessary to achieve reduction. Some controversy exists over how rapidly reduction should be undertaken; however, most agree that with incomplete SCI, rapid intervention is most appropriate.

When traction is applied, the patient must be continually monitored both radiographically and clinically. Overtension of the spine may cause cranial nerve deficits or neurological worsening. Muscle relaxants such as diazepam are often helpful adjuncts in reducing spasm, which may inhibit efforts at reduction. Fluoroscopy may be useful for frequent radiographical monitoring during active attempts at reduction through traction. If closed reduction through traction fails, a decision must be made about open reduction and surgical stabilization. Although there are no good scientific data to indicate any definite advantages with respect to neurological improvement from rapid aggressive surgical intervention in these cases, there is a growing tendency to advocate such an approach.[70–73]

Generally, realignment of the thoracolumbar spine cannot be accomplished with external traction. Affected patients are immobilized on rotating beds until a decision is made regarding surgical intervention.

The best current initial medical and pharmacological therapy of SCI is based on the potentially reversible pathophysiological changes that occur in relation to spinal cord blood flow and the beneficial effects that have been demonstrated with high-dose methylprednisolone treatment.

Because of the known tendency for spinal cord perfusion to fall abruptly after SCI, systemic blood pressure should be vigorously supported and on occasion mild hypertension induced to ensure adequate perfusion for at least the first 24 hours after injury.[74] Fluid resuscitation should consist of an appropriate combination of crystalloid and colloid or blood replacement, if necessary. In most instances, lactated Ringer's solution or normal saline is the best initial fluid. If, despite adequate fluid replacement, the blood pressure cannot be normalized, pressors such as dopamine or phenylephrine hydrochloride (NeoSynephrine) may be instituted. An additional temporary measure to improve peripheral vascular resistance may be a pneumatic antishock garment.

Because spinal cord blood flow is dependent not only on perfusion pressure, but also on blood rheology, it is important to consider measures to reduce blood viscosity, thereby increasing perfusion. Optimal viscosity for this purpose is achieved with a blood hematocrit in the range of 33 to 37 percent.

A wide variety of hemodynamic derangements is seen in association with SCI, and there is some indication that their correction improves the chances for neurological recovery. Thus placement of a Swan-Ganz catheter is appropriate after SCI to better detect and treat these problems.

If treatment is initiated within 8 hours of injury, methylprednisolone can be given as an intravenous bolus of 30 mg/kg followed by continuous infusion of 5.4 mg/kg/hr. If treatment is initiated within 3 hours of injury, the continuous infusion should be continued for 24 hours. Patients initiating treatment 3 to 8 hours after injury should have the continuous infusion for 48 hours. The odds of a methylprednisolone-treated patient improving motor function is greater than 2:1 when compared with other pharmacological therapies, whereas the odds of improving sensory function is 3:1.[75, 76] Methlyprednisolone should not be given if more than 8 hours have elapsed since the SCI, because patients treated in this manner have a slightly worse outcome. Recently, considerable controversy has arisen over the scientific validity of the studies showing the benefits of methlyprednisolone, and the clinician should weigh the potential benefits versus the possible risks of this treatment.

The only other pharmacological treatment of SCI that has demonstrated potential benefit is GM-1 ganglioside (SYGEN). When given after methylprednisolone on a daily basis for up to 2 months following injury, this therapy increases the rate of neurological recovery. Ultimately, however, the final degree of functional improvement was no different than the level attained by placebo treatment.[77]

Once the immediate problems attendant on the SCI have been stabilized, attention must be directed to preventing the many complications—pulmonary, cardiovascular, urinary tract, gastrointestinal, skin—that typically threaten in the first week to 10 days after SCI (Fig. 51–10).

Pulmonary problems are the single most common cause of morbidity and mortality following SCI. The higher the anatomical level of injury, the greater the risk of neurological problems. Impaired deep breathing and coughing, on the basis of either pain or neurological compromise, increase the risks of atelectasis and pneumonia. Additionally, the need for maintaining recumbency to allow for immobilization of the spinal injury further compromises respiratory status.[78] Careful serial observation must be maintained to guard against the insidious development of respiratory insufficiency. Measurements of arterial blood gases or pulse oximetry should be supplemented by measurements of vital capacity at regular intervals. Pulmonary toilet is enhanced by regular nasotracheal suctioning, frequent chest physiotherapy, and the use of rotating beds or frames.[79]

Several cardiovascular problems may complicate acute management—vasogenic spinal shock, paroxysmal hypertension, arrhythmias, and thermoregulatory dysfunction. Vasogenic spinal shock results from peripheral pooling of blood from loss of sympathetic vasomotor control; it generally requires treatment with vasopressors. The most common arrhythmia is bradycardia, which may be so pronounced as to produce hypotension. On occasion, temporary pacing may be required. Thus, all patients with SCI should be monitored hemodynamically for the first several days after injury.

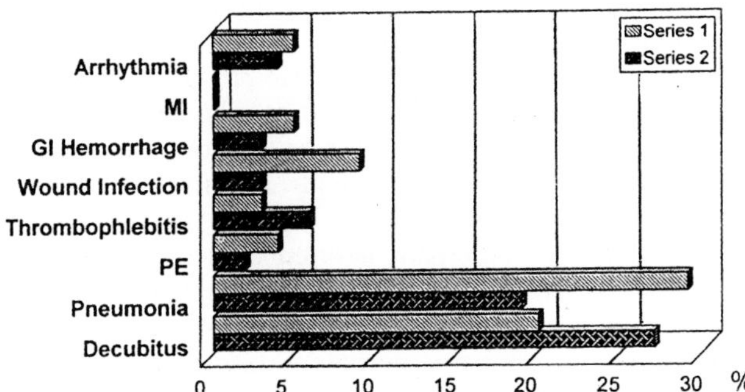

FIGURE 51–10. Frequency of acute complications after spinal cord injury. MI, myocardial infarction; PE, pulmonary embolus. (From American Spinal Injury Association: Standards for Neurological and Functional Classification of Spinal Cord Injury, Revised 1992, p 278.)

The gastrointestinal (GI) tract must be monitored for the development of paralytic ileus, which almost universally occurs. Associated abdominal distention may adversely affect respiratory function. Judicious use of nasogastric suctioning should prevent these problems. Once the ileus has resolved, it is important to initiate and maintain regimens of bowel regulation and retraining to prevent constipation and impaction and their undesirable effects.

The primary source of infection after SCI is the genitourinary tract. The bladder can also account for significant long-term disabilities consequent to associated renal damage if appropriate care is not taken early on. Because reflex micturition almost always begins within several days of injury, long-term Foley catheterization is discouraged in favor of intermittent catheterization. Prophylactic antibiotics are not indicated, and bladder re-education should begin promptly.

Attention to skin care is vitally important. Immobility and lack of sensation predispose to skin breakdown. Prolonged pressure over bony prominences must be avoided. Pressure reduction can only be accomplished by frequent turning.[80]

Considerable disagreement exists regarding the place of surgery after SCI and, should surgical treatment be decided upon, what should be done and when.

General agreement exists as to the necessity for immediate immobilization and early stabilization of fractures and dislocations of the spine. Immobilization and early stabilization can be accomplished without surgical intervention (i.e., with external orthoses such as the halo) in over 60 percent of SCI cases. The timing and method of internal surgical stabilization are points of controversy. The single widely accepted indication for acute surgical intervention is documented neurological deterioration in association with ongoing spinal cord compression from bone and disc fragments, hematoma, or unreduced subluxation. Nevertheless, the presence of an incomplete SCI with persistent spinal cord deformity and presence of complete SCI when the perceived possibility exists for recovering some neurological function have been advocated as rationales for early aggressive surgical intervention.[11–13]

Oral and injectable diazepam, baclofen, dantrolene, and clonidine are helpful for the treatment of spasticity. When these medications are inadequate, other treatments include motor point blocks with phenol, botulinum toxin injections, and intrathecal perfusion with baclofen or morphine. Central deafferentation pain may respond to treatment with tricyclic antidepressants, valproic acid, carbamazepine, mexiletine, and intrathecal morphine. Occasional patients may be helped by surgical approaches such as dorsal root entry zone lesions and implantation of a dorsal column stimulator.

Prognosis and Future Perspectives. It is important to attempt to quantify the natural history of the degree and extent and time course of neurological recovery after SCI to prognosticate function, determine the effectiveness of various interventions, and develop a comprehensive rehabilitation plan.

Waters and co-workers[81] reported a study of 148 patients with complete SCI followed for 5 years with annual examinations using the ASIA scoring system. Very little, if any, significant recovery was documented after 1 year of follow-up. In these patients, however, 18 percent had at least one level of improvement at 1 year in their neurological level of injury and 7 percent had two levels of improvement. Ditunno and co-workers[82] undertook a study to determine the recovery of key muscles of the upper extremities in motor-complete quadriplegics. One hundred fifty patients were followed for 24 months. Recovery persisted in muscles with no initial motor power from the ninth to twenty-fourth month, with ultimately 64 percent achieving some increased function. The recent National Acute Spinal Cord Injury Study found a plateauing of recovery between 6 and 12 months after injury.[79, 80] If an athlete suffers an SCI, return to any level of competition is medically precluded. Risks to the individual from other less severe spinal injuries are debated, however. In general, any injury that necessitates internal surgical spinal stabilization probably obviates return to contact sports. More minor injuries that heal correctly with bracing may not limit athletic involvement.[83]

Whiplash Injuries

The term *whiplash* refers to the mechanism of the neck injury, which can result from hyperextension followed by flexion that occurs when an occupant of a motor vehicle is hit from behind by another vehicle. Some clinicians use the term to also describe other types of collisions wherein the neck is subjected to different sequences and combinations of flexion, extension, and lateral motion. The term was first used in 1928. Other terms used include cervical sprain, cervical myofascial pain syndrome, acceleration-deceleration injury, and hyperextension injury.[84, 85]

Pathogenesis and Pathophysiology. Animal and human studies have demonstrated structural damage, including muscle tears, rupture of ligaments, avulsions and herniations of intervertebral discs, retropharyngeal hematoma, nerve root damage, cervical sympathetic chain injury, and hemarthrosis of facet joints.

Epidemiology and Risk Factors. In 1999, there were 11,900,000 motor vehicle accidents, including 3,555,000 rear-end collisions, in the United States. Although neck injuries can commonly occur after side or front impact collisions, rear-end collisions are responsible for about 85 percent of all whiplash injuries. More than 1 million people sustain whiplash-type injuries per year in the United States. Women have persistent neck pain more often than men, especially women in the 20- to 40-year age group, by a ratio of 7:3. The greater susceptibility of women to whiplash injuries may be due to a narrower neck with less muscle mass supporting a head of roughly the same volume compared with men.

Clinical Features and Associated Disorders. Following a motor vehicle accident with a whiplash-type mechanism of injury, 62 percent of patients presenting to the emergency room complain of pain. The onset of pain is within 24 hours in 93 percent of the injured. The most common cause of the neck pain is myofascial injury. Cervical disc herniations, cervical spine fractures, and dislocations are uncommon. Cervical facet joint injury can also be a source of pain.[86]

Eighty percent of patients with whiplash-type injuries complain of headaches during the first 4 weeks after the accident. The headaches are usually of the muscle contraction type and are often associated with greater occipital neuralgia. Whiplash trauma can also injure the temporomandibular joint and can cause jaw pain often associated with headache. Headache may be referred from the C2–C3 facet joint that is innervated by the third occipital nerve. Occasionally, whiplash injuries can precipitate new migraine with recurring episodes including classic migraine with aura, migraine attacks without aura, and basilar migraine.

Dizziness is a common complaint and can be due to dysfunction of the vestibular apparatus, cervical proprioceptive system, brain stem, and cervical sympathetic nerves.

Paresthesias of the upper extremities can be referred from trigger points, brachial plexopathy, facet joint disease, entrapment neuropathies, cervical radiculopathy, and spinal cord compression. Thoracic outlet syndrome, which occurs four times more often in women than men, is a common cause of paresthesias, which often radiate down the ulnar arm and forearm into the fourth and fifth fingers. Eighty-five percent of these cases are of the non-neurogenic type with subjective complaints but no objective findings.

Cognitive impairment due to a whiplash injury without direct head trauma is a controversial topic with evidence for and against. [87]

Interscapular pain and low back pain are frequent complaints after whiplash injuries and are reported in 20 percent and 35 percent of patients, respectively, after the injury. Visual symptoms, especially blurred vision, are often reported by patients and are usually due to convergence insufficiency, although oculomotor palsies can occasionally occur. Rare sequelae include cervical dystonia or torticollis, transient global amnesia, esophageal perforation and descending mediastinitis, hypoglossal nerve palsy, cervical epidural hematoma, superior laryngeal nerve palsy, and internal carotid and vertebral artery dissections.

Differential Diagnosis. Whenever patients have pain complaints without objective findings, nonorganic explanations should be considered. Other possible causes of pain complaints after whiplash injuries include psychological problems, secondary gain and malingering in cases in which litigation is pending, and social and peer copying.[88, 89]

Evaluation. A cervical spine MRI study is helpful to evaluate patients with persistent complaints of neck pain and paresthesias or those with abnormal results on examination. When radiographical abnormalities are present, the possibility that they are pre-existent should be considered. Cervical spondylosis, degenerative disc disease, and cervical disc protrusions occur with increasing frequency with older age and are often asymptomatic.

Management. Neck pain is often treated initially with ice, then with heat, nonsteroidal anti-inflammatory drugs, muscle relaxants, and pain medications. Use of soft cervical collars should be kept to a minimum during the first 2 to 3 weeks and then avoided. Range-of-motion exercises, physical therapy, trigger point injections, and TENS units may be helpful for patients with persistent complaints. Percutaneous radiofrequency neurotomy may be beneficial for the treatment of chronic facet joint pain documented by anesthetic blocks.[90]

Prognosis and Future Perspectives. Neck pain and headaches can persist for months and sometimes years in a minority of patients. According to various studies, neck pain and headache, respectively, have been reported as persisting for the following intervals after the accident[91, 92]: 1 month, 64 percent and 82 percent; 3 months, 38 percent and 35 percent; 1 year, 19 percent and 21 percent; and 2 years, 16 percent and 15 percent. Psychosocial factors and personality traits are not predictive of the duration of symptoms. Risk factors for more severe symptoms include older age, female gender, a rear-end collision, and a rotated or inclined head position at the moment of impact. Despite the common belief that pending litigation is responsible for persistent symptoms, litigants and nonlitigants have similar psychological profiles and similar recovery rates. Most patients who are still symptomatic at the time when litigation is settled are not cured by a verdict.

Brachial and Lumbosacral Plexopathies

Pathogenesis and Pathophysiology. Trauma can result in variable injury to the myelin, axon, and connective tissue covering of plexus elements. Mild injuries may result in focal demyelination with conduction slowing. More severe injuries may cause demyelinating conduction block (neurapraxia), which can occur alone or in association with axon degeneration. Axonotmesis, which is loss of the relative continuity of the axon and myelin but preservation of the connective tissue framework, leads to wallerian degeneration. *Neurotmesis* refers to an injury in which the axons and investing connective tissues lose their continuity. A combination of different grades of injury can occur. An axonal nerve injury in continuity may heal as a neuroma that consists of axons growing in all directions surrounded by connective tissue. Root avulsion is the traumatic separation of a nerve root from the spinal cord.[93]

Epidemiology and Risk Factors. Closed lesions usually resulting from traction are the most common causes of traumatic brachial plexopathy. Stretch injuries are responsible for about 70 percent of serious brachial plexus injuries. High-velocity closed injuries, which usually involve the supraclavicular plexus, are primarily due to motor vehicle accidents, occupational injuries, and falls. Falls, which result in scapular and proximal humeral fractures and humeral head dislocations, are the most common causes of infraclavicular injuries. Brachial plexus injury, usually involving the lower trunk or medial cord, occurs in 5 percent of patients undergoing coronary artery bypass surgery. Brachial plexus injury is probably due to traction associated with sternal retraction.[94] Most brachial plexus avulsion injuries are due to motor vehicle accidents, especially motorcycle accidents; industrial accidents; obstetrical injury; falls; objects falling on the shoulder; and sports injuries (most commonly football, bicycling, skiing, and equestrian activities). Root avulsions more commonly involve the C7, C8, and T1 roots, whereas extraforaminal ruptures more commonly affect the C5 and C6 roots.

The less common open lesions, which most often affect the infraclavicular plexus, are often associated with injuries to major limb vessels and the lung. Gunshot wounds, which account for 25 percent of the cases of surgical repair of the brachial plexus in the United States, usually involve the infraclavicular or retroclavicular plexus and less often the supraclavicular plexus. Laceration injuries of the brachial plexus are usually the result of broken glass and knives.

Injury to the lumbosacral plexus is uncommon because it is protected by the pelvic bony ring. Pelvic fractures, which are usually due to motor vehicle accidents, crush injuries, and falls from a height, result in lumbosacral plexus injury in about 7 percent of cases.

Clinical Features and Associated Disorders. Plexus injuries can result in sensory loss, paresthesias, motor loss, and pain, which can be particularly severe after root avulsions. A detailed knowledge of the anatomy of the brachial and lumbosacral plexus is essential to localizing lesions (see Chapters 15, 19, and 20).

Burners and *stingers* are synonymous terms that refer to the radicular and plexus symptoms following sudden depression of the shoulder in contact sports, usually football. The player experiences burning dysesthesias going down the ipsilateral upper extremity, often into the thumb, and sometimes weakness of the biceps and shoulder girdle muscles. The symptoms usually resolve within a few minutes, although occasional cases last for weeks.

Other causes of acute compression of the brachial plexus include the following: prolonged compression in someone inebriated or comatose; compression of the plexus against the first rib due to heavy backpacks carried by students or soldiers; prolonged firing of shotguns or rifles; and shoulder restraints in motor vehicles. In addition to coronary artery bypass surgery, other intraoperative causes of plexus injury include malpositioning of the arm, often affecting the upper plexus; damage during other procedures such as radical mastectomies, transaxillary arterial bypasses, and biopsies; orthopedic procedures on the humerus or shoulder; and, ironically, first rib resections and scalenotomies performed to treat thoracic outlet syndrome.[94] False aneurysms of the axillary artery due to trauma and hematomas from transaxillary percutaneous angiograms can also injure elements of the plexus. Stretch injuries of the plexus in neonates, often resulting from shoulder dystocia, most commonly involve the upper trunk (Erb's palsy) and only occasionally the lower trunk (Klumpke's palsy).

Repetitive activity such as working at a keyboard or playing a musical instrument and single injuries such as a fall or whiplash-type injury commonly result in the non-neurogenic type of thoracic outlet syndrome. Patients may complain of aching of the shoulder and arm with paresthesias going down the arm into the fourth and fifth fingers. The symptoms may be worse at night, with repetitive activity, and/or with use of the arm overhead. Although they are nonspecific causes, medial supraclavicular palpation and the exaggerated military posture may reproduce the symptoms. Most of the patients are women; long necks, droopy shoulders, and pendulous breasts may be contributing factors. No objective findings appear on examination or electrodiagnostic studies.[93]

In addition to pelvic fractures and gunshot wounds, there are other important causes of lumbosacral plexus injury. During labor and delivery, pressure on the lumbosacral trunk by the fetal head or forceps may result in a postpartum footdrop. Ischemic injury of the plexus can result from inadvertent injection of drugs into the gluteal arteries, leading to a propagating thrombus to the iliac arteries. Blunt trauma to the abdomen can rarely result in a retroperitoneal hemorrhage into the psoas muscle, which compresses the lumbar plexus, causing pain and extremity weakness. Neuromas may form after partial or complete injuries to peripheral nerves. The only neuromas that are symptomatic are those that contain sensory nerve fibers. Sensory nerves of the hands and feet are especially likely to form painful neuromas. Symptomatic neuromas produce a burning or aching pain that may radiate proximally or distally. Tinel's sign may be present. The diagnosis can be confirmed by temporary relief of symptoms after injection of local anesthetic. Injection of a corticosteroid may significantly improve or cure symptoms in some cases. Various surgical approaches such as nerve grafting, decompression and translocation, excisional neurectomy, and transposition may be appropriate, depending on the case.[95]

Differential Diagnosis and Evaluation. Cervical and lumbosacral disc herniations and peripheral nerve injuries should be considered. The clinical examination can often localize the lesion as pre- or postganglionic or to various elements of the plexus. For example, the presence of a Horner's syndrome indicates lesions of the roots of C8 and T1 proximal to the site where the white rami communican exits to enter the sympathetic chain. Depending on the specific injury, various imaging techniques including plain radiographs, CT and MRI scans, arteriography, venography, and myelography may be indicated.[96] Pseudomeningoceles, which are formed when a nerve root is avulsed and the meninges are pulled through the neural foramina, may be detected on myelography, followed by CT scan as well as MRI. Electromyogram (EMG) and nerve conduction studies can be helpful in localizing and determining the extent of the lesion.

Management. Management depends on the location of the lesions, the grade of nerve injury, and the presence of root avulsions. Patients with acute transections of the brachial plexus due to lacerations with a knife or glass should undergo relatively rapid primary repair. For closed stretch injuries with severe axonal degeneration present on electrophysiological studies 3 to 5 months after the injury, surgical exploration and repair are indicated.[97] Because missile wounds usually leave the nerve in continuity, initial management is often conservative. Although avulsion of nerve roots has been regarded as an untreatable injury, animal and human studies suggest that implantation of ventral roots into the spinal cord may lead to recovery of motor function especially with use of neurotrophic factors.[98–100]

Up to 80 percent of patients with obstetrical palsy have no paresis or mild paresis by the age of 1 year. Surgery for infants with obstetrical palsy not improving is controversial, with recommendations for the time of surgery ranging from 3 to 9 months of age. Non-neurogenic thoracic outlet syndrome may respond to Peet's exercises, which strengthen the muscles of the pectoral girdle and improve posture. In very occasional cases, scalenotomy or first rib resection may be indicated. Physical and surgical rehabilitation may help to improve function after brachial plexus injuries.

Pain following brachial plexus injuries may be difficult to manage with various treatments depending upon the type and severity of the pain. Treatments range from pain pills, anticonvulsants, and TENS units to stellate ganglion blocks and sympathectomy, dorsal column stimulators, and dorsal root entry zone lesions. Similar considerations apply to lumbosacral plexus injuries. When indicated, surgery may be helpful in some cases of pelvic fractures, gunshot wounds, stab wounds or lacerations, and iatrogenic injuries.

Prognosis and Future Perspectives. In cases of neurapraxia, spontaneous recovery may occur within 3 to 4 months of the injury. Because of the long regeneration distances and lack of collateral sprouting, the intrinsic hand muscles with lower trunk lesions and the muscles below the knee with sacral plexopathies reinnervate poorly after severe axon loss lesions. For severe brachial plexus lesions, satisfactory results may occur postoperatively in up to 70 percent of patients after primary repair and up to 48 percent after a nerve graft. Fifty to 85 percent of patients with non-neurogenic thoracic outlet syndrome may improve with exercises.[99]

Reflex Sympathetic Dystrophy and Causalgia

In 1864, the Philadelphia neurologist S. Wier Mitchell and colleagues reported the cases of Union soldiers who sustained gunshot wounds at the battle of Gettysburg resulting in partial nerve lesions of the brachial plexus and peripheral nerves followed by a severe burning pain of the hand or foot associated with trophic changes.[101] Mitchell coined the term *causalgia*, which is from the Greek for "burning pain," to describe this syndrome.

Pathogenesis and Pathophysiology. The pathophysiology of reflex sympathetic dystrophy (RSD) and causalgia is poorly understood. Various mechanisms proposed include the following: sympathetic hyperactivity, ephaptic transmission between sympathetic and primary afferents, a reverberating circuit in the spinal internuncial pool, sensitization of wide dynamic range neurons in the dorsal horn, and neurogenic inflammation. Despite common perception and nomenclature, some researchers strongly argue that the sympathetic nervous system is not involved.[102]

Epidemiology and Risk Factors. Causalgia may occur in up to 5 percent of patients after partial peripheral nerve injury, but it does not occur when a nerve is completely severed. The incidence of RSD is 1 to 2 percent after various fractures but is particularly common following Colles' fracture, occurring in about 30 percent. RSD may occur after various other injuries, including minor soft tissue trauma, operations such as carpal tunnel release and arthroscopic knee surgery, myocardial and cerebral infarction, and frostbite and burns. In up to 25 percent of RSD cases, a precipitant cause is not identified. RSD occurs in all ages with a median of 40 years. Females account for about 70 percent of cases.

Clinical Features and Associated Disorders. RSD is a syndrome with variable major components of burning pain, autonomic dysfunction, edema, dystrophy and atrophy, and sometimes a movement disorder.[103] When this pain syndrome follows peripheral nerve injury, the term *causalgia* is used. Various other terms for reflex sympathetic dystrophy are used including Sudeck's atrophy, algodystrophy, post-traumatic dystrophy, reflex neurovascular dystrophy, shoulder-hand syndrome, sympathetic maintained pain syndrome, and complex regional pain syndrome.

The symptoms of RSD and causalgia may develop within days to months after injury. The pain, which begins in the area of the injury or event, may then spread throughout the extremity and, in perhaps 5 percent of cases, involves the contralateral extremity (rarely, three and four extremities may become involved). The burning, aching, or constant pain is associated with hyperalgesia (lower pain threshold with enhanced pain perception), allodynia (pain induced by innocuous mechanical and thermal stimuli, especially cold), and hyperpathia (an exaggerated response to a stimulus, which may be delayed and may persist after cessation of the stimulus). Spontaneous paroxysmal shooting, sharp, or electrical sensations may be described. Decreased sensation may be present in affected areas. Proprioception may be limited. As in other pain disorders, RSD patients are often depressed and anxious.

Edema over the site of injury and distally may be present. At first, the involved extremity is usually warm, red, and dry but occasionally may be cold. Over time, the extremity usually becomes cool, pale, cyanotic, and hyperhydrotic. Early on, the nails may become thickened and the hair darker. Later, the hair may be lost in the affected areas, the skin may become shiny, and the nails may break. Dystrophy and atrophy of subcutaneous tissue, muscles, and bone may be present. Nodular fasciitis of the palmar or plantar skin may be present. RSD affecting the hand may be associated with a frozen shoulder.[104] Motor manifestations variably present include weakness, an enhanced physiological tremor, spasm and increased reflexes, focal dystonia, and an inability to initiate movement. Exercise or use may aggravate RSD complaints.

Differential Diagnosis. Other disorders that may have some features of RSD include chronic arterial insufficiency, thrombophlebitis, infection, collagen vascular disorders, postherpetic neuralgia, entrapment neuropathies (which can co-exist with RSD), painful neuromas, plexopathies and radiculopathies, phantom limb pain, and central pain syndromes. When pain complaints are the major problem, psychological causes such as depression, factitious disorders, conversion, and malingering should be considered.

After amputation of an extremity, up to 85 percent of patients describe phantom limb pain, which may still be present in about 30 percent 1 year later. The patients describe pain, which may be a continuous numbing or an intermittent sharp, stabbing, shooting, cramping, or burning sensation, as being present either in the stump or in the absent limb. Both peripheral and central mechanisms for the pain have been suggested, with one study showing evidence of plastic changes in the primary somatosensory cortex.[105] Despite various medical and surgical treatments, the pain is often intractable.

Evaluation and Management. The diagnosis of RSD and causalgia is based on the symptoms and signs. Laboratory testing sometimes used includes thermography and a triple-phase bone scan (which may reveal abnormal uptake and increased periarticular uptake in 30 percent of patients); abnormal findings are not specific. Pain relief following sympathetic blockade or an intravenous phentolamine test is supportive of the diagnosis. The possibility of a placebo response should be considered.

The inciting disorder should be appropriately diagnosed and treated. Although many treatments have been proposed, there is a lack of prospective and controlled studies with controversy over inclusion criteria. Medications reported as useful include the following: narcotic and nonsteroidal anti-inflammatory drugs; adrenergic blockers such as clonidine and prazosin; tricyclic antidepressants; anticonvulsants such as carbamazepine and gabapentin; corticosteroids; and intranasal calcitonin. Physical therapy modalities, rehabilitation, TENS units, and psychological treatment are often worthwhile. A series of five sympathetic anesthetic blocks of the stellate ganglion for upper extremity or lumbar chain for lower extremity cases can be beneficial. If the blocks improve the pain but only temporarily, many clinicians recommend sympathectomy. Dorsal column stimulators and morphine intrathecal pumps are sometimes recommended for refractory cases. Some patients with dystonia associated with reflex sympathetic dystrophy may respond to treatment with intrathecal baclofen.

Prognosis and Future Perspectives. Prognostic information is quite limited. Many clinicians believe that recovery occurs more frequently when treatment is begun early in the course. Pain may still be present in 25 percent of cases with RSD after 1 year and in 60 percent of patients with causalgia after 3 years. Reported response rates for surgical sympathectomy range from 12 to 97 percent. RSD may resolve early in the clinical course only to return weeks or months later.

Mountain Sickness

Pathogenesis and Pathophysiology. As the partial pressure of oxygen decreases with increasing altitude, ventilation rises, leading to respiratory alkalosis. Although hypocapnia alone results in cerebral vasoconstriction, hypoxia produces a net decline of cerebral vascular resistance and increased cerebral blood flow. Hypoxia can result in cerebral edema, which may be due to cerebral vasodilatation and elevated cerebral capillary hydrostatic pressure. An increase in sympathetic activity follows, causing an elevated heart rate, pulmonary vasoconstriction, and an initial increase and later decrease of cerebral blood flow.[106]

Epidemiology and Risk Factors. Acute mountain sickness (AMS) develops in about 25 percent of visitors to moderate altitudes (6300 to 9700 feet). About 100 million tourists visit altitudes above 2000 meters worldwide per year. Symptoms usually occur within the first 12 hours of arrival but may be delayed 24 hours or more. Risk factors for AMS include those who are younger than 60 years, are less physically fit, live at sea level, have a history of AMS, are obese or female, or have underlying lung problems.[107] AMS develops into high-altitude cerebral edema (HACE) in perhaps 1.5 percent of cases. Alcohol use inhibits acute ventilatory adaptation to mild hypoxia at moderate altitude and may be a risk factor.

Clinical Features and Associated Disorders. AMS, which usually occurs above 8200 feet, is defined by the presence of a headache and at least one of the following symptoms: gastrointestinal (anorexia, nausea, or vomiting), fatigue or weakness, dizziness or lightheadedness, and difficulty sleeping.[108] The headache is usually bilateral but may be unilateral. HACE, which is uncommon below 12,000 feet, is defined by the presence of a change in mental status and/or ataxia in a person with AMS or the presence of both mental status change and ataxia in a person without AMS. HACE, which can lead to coma and death, may be associated with urinary incontinence, papilledema, cranial nerve palsies, tremor, and abnormalities in limb tone.

High-altitude pulmonary edema (HAPE), which can occur along with HACE, usually occurs above 9840 feet. High-altitude retinal hemorrhage is common in people who go above 15,0000 feet.

Evaluation and Management. The diagnosis is usually a clinical one that is made in the setting of a recent altitude ascent. Altitude sickness may be prevented in those planning higher ascents by starting below 8000 feet, resting the first day, and then ascending about 1000 feet per day. Sleeping at a lower altitude at night may be helpful because hypoxia is worse with sleep. It is also important for climbers to keep well hydrated and avoid alcohol. Acetazolamide, at a dose of 125 to 250 mg twice daily starting 24 hours before ascent and continuing for 2 days, may prevent AMS and improve sleep. Other medications which may reduce the risk and symptoms of AMS include the following: aspirin 320 mg 1 hour before arrival at high altitude and then one every 4 hours for two doses (for a total of three doses)[109]; dexamethasone 2 mg every 6 hours or 4 mg every 12 hours orally starting 24 to 48 hours before arrival at high altitude and continuing for several days; and perhaps Gingko biloba 120 mg a day orally.

AMS may be treated symptomatically with rest, mild analgesics, alcohol avoidance, and adequate hydration. Depending upon the severity of symptoms, avoiding going any higher or slowing the rate of ascent or descent may be necessary. Acetazolamide 250 mg po bid may also help acute symptoms. For HACE, immediate descent should be initiated if possible, and, if not, HACE may be treated with the use of a portable hyperbaric bag (2 to 4 psi for a minimum of 2 hours), administration of oxygen (2 to 4 L/min), and dexamethasone (8 mg orally, IM, or IV initially and then 4 mg q 6 hr). Acetazolamide should be given in instances where descent or evacuation is delayed.

Prognosis and Future Perspectives. AMS usually resolves after 16 to 72 hours at altitude. When descent is impossible and treatment is unavailable, HACE and HAPE have a mortality up to 50 percent.

Decompression Sickness

Pathogenesis and Pathophysiology. With descent, the partial pressure of the gases breathed by the diver increases proportionately, according to Dalton's law. Although oxygen is metabolized, tissues soak up inert nitrogen and become saturated. With ascent, the nitrogen moves from the tissues to the blood and is exhaled by the lungs, which is a process termed *decompression*. When ascent is too rapid and the tissues are supersaturated, dissolved gas changes to free gas, which creates bubbles. When the filtering capacity of the pulmonary capillaries is exceeded, the bubbles enter the arterial circulation. Symptoms depend on those tissues in which the bubbles accumulate. Bubbles in the paravertebral veins, Batson's plexus, can result in stasis and venous infarction in the spinal cord. Cerebral injury can develop from bubbles occluding vessels or directly disrupting tissue. Symptoms may also result from secondary effects such as activation of complement, platelet aggregation, and release of vasoactive mediators.

Epidemiology and Risk Factors. Decompression sickness (DCS), also referred to as *the bends* or *caisson disease*, usually affects divers and caisson workers but can also occur in pilots during rapid ascent in a nonpressurized cabin. About 900 cases of DCS are reported yearly in the United States among recreational scuba divers. Most accidents occur in inexperienced divers. The incidence of DCS for recreational divers is one per 5000 to 10,000 dives, and for commercial divers, one incident per 500 to 1000 dives. Up to 50 percent of cases of DCS occur in divers who claimed to have been diving within the limits set by a standard table or decompression computer. Divers with a patent foramen ovale are five times more likely to sustain serious decompression problems because bubbles can go directly from the right to left atrium without being filtered by the lungs.[110] Right-to-left shunts are more common in those with migraine with aura who are more likely to suffer DCS.[111]

Clinical Features and Associated Disorders. DCS, which can occur after diving to a depth of more than 25 feet, usually appears within a few minutes to a few hours after the end of a dive. Mild DCS (type I) is defined by pain usually in the joints (bends) and/or itching of the skin. Serious DCS (type II) is characterized by neurological problems. Involvement of the thoracic spinal cord, the most commonly affected area, leads to low back or pelvic pain and dysesthesias, which may be accompanied by sensory loss, weakness, and incontinence. Less often, the brain may be involved, resulting in various symptoms and signs such as headache, confusion, lethargy, vertigo, speech disturbance, hemiparesis, visual impairment, and seizures, depending upon the site of the insult.[112]

Rupture of alveoli, which may occur when a diver ascends without venting air from the lungs or from blockage of part of the bronchial tree, can result in additional arterial gas embolism. During ascent or shortly after surfacing, divers may develop various problems ranging from acute respiratory distress and headache to cardiorespiratory arrest and seizures. Depending on the site of embolism to the brain, cortical blindness, dysphasia, and hemiplegia may occur. Arterial gas embolism and DCS may co-exist.

Evaluation and Management. DCS is typically diagnosed based on the findings on history and physical examination. The results of MRI studies of the brain and spinal cord may often be normal or may show only nonspecific abnormalities in cases of DCS.[112] Initially, high concentrations of oxygen should be administered by face mask to increase the resorption of gas bubbles. Fluid administration, ideally a hyperosmolar drink, may result in more rapid elimination of gases and treat dehydration. As soon as possible, the patient should undergo recompression in a hyperbaric chamber while breathing oxygen.[113]

Prognosis and Future Perspectives. Prompt treatment usually results in a complete recovery. Neurological deficits may persist in cases where recompression is delayed or not done.[114]

Lightning and Electrical Injuries

Pathogenesis and Pathophysiology. Although incompletely understood, the two major causes of tissue damage are thermal injury and electroporation, which is the production and expansion of transient aqueous pores in the lipid bilayer component of the cell membrane.[115]

Epidemiology and Risk Factors. About 100 lightning- and 1500 technical electricity-related deaths per year occur in the United States. The following routes can produce lightning injury. A direct strike is the most damaging, which is more common if the person is carrying a metal conductor such as an umbrella or golf club above shoulder level. A side flash or splash injury occurs when lightning first strikes a tall object such as a tree and then arcs to the person standing next to the object or when lightning first strikes a person or animal and then the second victim. A ground or stride current occurs when lightning strikes the ground first and then travels along the surface before reaching the person. Occasionally, people can sustain injury indoors while on the telephone from current conducted through the lines or in the bath or shower from ground current traveling along the water pipes.

Technical electrical injuries can occur from exposure to high-voltage electricity (1000 volts or more) and low-voltage electricity. High voltage electricity injuries, which are almost always work related, account for about 70 percent of electrical injuries and deaths. Low-voltage injuries typically happen in the home with the following common circumstances: the use of electrical appliances while standing on a wet floor or while in the bathtub, children playing with outlets or wires, or use of faulty electrical equipment. When the energized conductor is held in the hand, alternating current exposure in the range of 8 to 22 mA at 60 Hz may result in long exposure due to a state of tetanic contraction of flexor muscles of the forearm and hand, which is paradoxically termed *let go current*.[116]

Clinical Features, and Associated Disorders. Lightning and electrical injuries may result in sudden death or cerebral hypoxia from inducing ventricular fibrillation. Transient loss of consciousness, confusion, and amnesia may also occur.[117] Lightning injury may result in keraunoparalysis, which is a transient paralysis usually of the lower extremities associated with sensory loss and pale skin. Lightning and electrical injuries may also cause acute spinal cord, focal brain, and peripheral nerve damage and rhabdomyolysis. Deep burns are more common with electrical than with lightning injuries. Delayed neurological disorders associated with lightning and electrical injuries include cognitive deficits, motor neuron disease, parkinsonism, choreoathetosis, dystonia, myoclonus, basilar artery thrombosis, seizures, myelopathy, generalized polyneuropathy, and reflex sympathetic dystrophy.[118–120] An additional type of injury is secondary trauma, such as from falls.

Management, Prognosis, and Future Perspectives. Evaluation and management depend on the sites, types, and extent of injury.[121] About one third of lightning strikes are fatal. The symptoms and signs of keraunoparalysis typically resolve within a few hours. Victims of lightning and electrical injuries who are comatose due to a hypoxic encephalopathy as a result of cardiac arrest usually have a poor prognosis. Most patients with spinal cord injuries due to lightning and electrical injuries have permanent disability.

Reviews and Selected Updates

Bethea JR, Dalton Dietrich W: Targeting the host inflammatory response in traumatic spinal cord injury. Curr Opin Neurol 2002;15:355–360.

Bracken M, Shepard MJ, Holford TR, et al: Treatment of acute spinal cord injury. JAMA 1997;277:1597–1604.

Cooper PR, Golfinos JG (eds): Head Injury, 4th ed. New York, McGraw-Hill, 2000.

Evans RW: Neurology and Trauma. Philadelphia, WB Saunders, 1996.

Harris OA, Colford JM, Good MC, Matz PG: The role of hypothermia in the management of severe brain injury. Arch Neurol 2002;59:1077–1083.

Kelly JP, Rosenberg JH: Diagnosis and management of concussion in sports. Neurology 1997;48:575–580.

Kline DG: Atlas of Peripheral Nerve Surgery, revised ed. Philadelphia, WB Saunders, 2001.

Krauss JK, Tränkle R, Kopp KH: Post-traumatic movement disorders in survivors of severe head injury. Neurology 1996;47:1488–1492.

Levin HS, Hanten G, Chang C-C, et al: Working memory after traumatic brain injury in children. Ann Neurol 2002;52:82–88.

Marion DW, Penrod LE, Kelsey SF, et al: Treatment of traumatic brain injury with moderate hypothermia. N Engl J Med 1997;336:540–546.

Narayan RK, Wilberger JE, Povlishock JT (eds): Neurotrauma. New York, McGraw-Hill, 1996.

References

1. Miller JD, Becker DP: Secondary insults to the injured brain. J R Coll Surg Edinb 1982;27:292–298.
2. Chesnut RM, Marshall LF, Klauber MR, et al: The role of secondary brain injury in determining outcome from severe head injury. J Trauma 1993;34:216–222.
3. Marmarou A, Anderson RL, Ward JD, et al: Impact of ICP instability and hypotension on outcome in patients with severe head trauma. J Neurosurg 1991;75:S59–S66.
4. Hall ED, Yonkers PA, Andrus JK, et al: Biochemistry and pharmacology of lipid antioxidants in acute brain and spinal cord injury. J Neurotrauma 1992;19:S425–S442.
5. Braughler JM, Hall ED: CNS trauma and stroke. Biochemical considerations for oxygen radical formation and lipid peroxidation. Free Radic Biol Med 1989;6:289–301.
6. Siesjo B: The role of calcium in cell death. *In* Price D, Aguayo A, Thoenen H (eds): Neurodegenerative Disorders: Mechanisms and Prospects for Therapy. London, Wiley & Sons, 1991, pp 35–59.
7. Bullock R, Fujisawa H: The role of glutamate antagonists for the treatment of CNS injury. J Neurotrauma 19:S443–S446.
8. Lobosky JF: Epidemiology of head injury. *In* Narayan RK, Wilberger JE, Povlishok JT (eds): Neurotrauma. New York, McGraw-Hill, 1996.
9. Rimel RW, Giordani B, Barth JT: Disability caused by minor head injury. Neurosurgery 1981;9:221–229.
10. Masters SJ, McClean PM, Arcarese JS, et al: Skull x-ray examination after head trauma: Recommendations by a mulitidisciplinary panel and validation study. N Engl J Med 1987;316:84–91.
11. Pang DA, Horton JA, Herron JM: Nonsurgical management of extradural hematomas in children. J Neurosurg 1983;59:958–971.
12. Seelig JM, Becker DP, Miller JD, et al: Traumatic acute subdural hematoma. Major mortality reduction in comatose patients treated within four hours. N Engl J Med 1981;304:1511–1518.
13. Wilberger JE, Harris M, Diamond DL: Acute subdural hematoma: Morbidity, mortality and operative timing. J Neurosurg 1991;74:212–218.
14. Sprick C, Bettag M, Bock WJ: Delayed traumatic intracranial hematomas—clinical study of seven years. Neurosurg Rev 1989;12:228–230.
15. Wilberger JE, Rothfus W, Tabas J, et al: Tissue tear hemorrhages: CT and clinicopathologic correlations. Neurosurgery 1990;27:160–165.
16. Kaufman HH, Timberlake GA, Voelker J: Medical complications of head injury. *In* Evans RW (ed): Neurology and Trauma. Philadelphia, WB Saunders, 1996.
17. Teasdale G, Jennet B: Assessment of coma and impaired consciousness: A practical scale. Lancet 1974;2:81–84.
18. Duhaime AC, Gennarelli TA, Thibault LE, et al: The shaken baby syndrome. A clinical, pathological, and biomechanical study. J Neurosurg 1987;66:409–415.

19. Stein SC, Ross SE: Mild head injury: A plea for routine early CT scanning. J Trauma 1992;33:11–13.
20. Gudeman SK, Kishore PRS, Miller JD, et al: The genesis and significance of delayed traumatic intracerebral hematoma. Neurosurgery 1979;5:309–312.
21. Marshall LF, Gautile T, Klauber MR, et al: The outcome of severe closed head injury. J Neurosurg 1991;75:S28–S36.
22. Rosner MJ, Rosner SD, Johnson AH: Cerebral perfusion pressure: Management protocol and clinical results. J Neurosurg 1995;83: 949–962.
23. Diringer MN, Videen TO, Yundt K, et al: Regional cerebrovascular and metabolic effects of hyperventilation after severe traumatic brain injury. J Neurosurg 2002;96:103–108.
24. Imberti R, Bellinzona G, Langer M: Cerebral tissue PO_2 and $SJVO_2$ changes during moderate hyperventilation in patients with severe traumatic brain injury. J Neurosurg 2002;96:97–102.
25. Dunham CM, Sosnowski C, Porter J, et al: Correlation of noninvasive cerebral oximetry with cerebral perfusion in the severe head injured patient. J Trauma 2002;52:40–46.
26. Eisenberg H, Frankowski R, Contant C, et al: High-dose barbiturate control of elevated intracranial pressure in patients with severe head injury. J Neurosurg 1988;69:15–23.
27. Braakman R, Schouten HJA, Blaauw-Van Dishoeck M, Minderhoud JM: Megadose steroids in severe head injury. J Neurosurg 1983;58: 326–330.
28. Young BF, Runge JM, Waxman KS: Effects of pegorgotein on neurologic outcome of patients with severe head injury. JAMA 1996;276:538–543.
29. Levin HS, Gary HE, Eisenberg HM, et al: Neurobehavioral outcome one year after severe head injury: Experience of the traumatic coma data bank. J Neurosurg 1990;73:699–709.
30. Saunders RL, Harbaugh RE: The second impact in catastrophic contact sports head trauma. JAMA 1984;252:538–539.
31. Practice Parameter: The management of concussion in sports (summary statement). Report of the Quality Standards Subcommittee. Neurology 1997;48:581–585.
32. Kelly JP, Rosenberg JH: Diagnosis and management of concussion in sports. Neurology 1997;48:575–580.
33. Roberts GW, Gentleman SM, Lynch A, et al: β-amyloid protein deposition in the brain after severe head injury. Implications for the pathogenesis of Alzheimer's disease. J Neurol Neurosurg Psychiatry 1994;57:419–425.
34. Jennett B, Snoek J, Bond MR, et al: Disability after severe head injury: Observations on the use of the Glasgow outcome scale. J Neurol Neurosurg Psychiatry 1981;44:285–293.
35. Liaquat I, Dunn LT, Nicoll JAR, et al: Effect of apolipoprotein E genotype on hematoma volume after trauma. J Neurosurg 2002;96:90–96.
36. Friedman G, Froom P, Sazbon L, et al: Apolipoprotein E-e4 genotype predicts a poor outcome in survivors of traumatic brain injury. Neurology 1999;52:244–248.
37. Evans RW: The postconcussion syndrome: 130 years of controversy. Semin Neurol 1994;14:32–39.
38. Bazarian JJ, Atabaki S: Predicting postconcussion syndrome after minor traumatic brain injury. Acad Emerg Med 2001;8:788–795.
39. Evans RW: The postconcussion syndrome and the sequelae of mild head injury. *In* Evans RW (ed): Neurology and Trauma. Philadelphia, WB Saunders, 1996.
40. Evans RW: The postconcussion syndrome. *In* Aminoff MJ (ed): Neurology and General Medicine, 3rd ed. Philadelphia, WB Saunders, 2001.
41. Evans RW: The post-concussion syndrome. *In* Evans RW, Baskin DS, Yatsu FM (eds): Prognosis of Neurological Disorders, 2nd ed. New York, Oxford, 2000.
42. Willmore LJ: Posttraumatic epilepsy: Cellular mechanisms and implications for treatment. Epilepsia 1990;31[Suppl 3]:S67–S73.
43. Annegers JF, Grabow JD, Groover RV, et al: Seizures after head trauma: A population study. Neurology 1980;30:683–689.
44. Bush PC, Prince DA, Miller KD: Increased pyramidal excitability and NMDA conductance can explain posttraumatic epileptogenesis without disinhibition: A model. J Neurophysiol 1999;82:1748–1758.
45. Perron AD, Brady WJ, Huff JS: Concussive convulsions: Emergency department assessment and management of a frequently misunderstood entity. Acad Emerg Med 2001;8:296–298.
46. Evans RW: Funny spells. Semin Neurol 1995;15:115–225.
47. Temkin NR, Dismen SS, Wilensky AJ, et al: A randomized double-blind study of phenytoin for prevention of post-traumatic seizures. N Engl J Med 1990;323:497–502.
48. Weiner WJ: Controversy. Can peripheral trauma induce dystonia? No! Mov Dis 2001;16:13–22.
49. Goetz CG, Pappert EJ: Trauma and movement disorders. Neurol Clin 1992;4:907–919.
50. Goetz CG, Pappert EJ: Movement disorders: Post-traumatic syndromes. *In* Evans RW (ed): Neurology and Trauma. Philadelphia, WB Saunders, 1996, pp 569–580.
51. Jankovic J: Post-traumatic movement disorders: Central and peripheral mechanisms. Neurology 1994;44:2006–2014.
52. Jankovic J: Controversy. Can peripheral trauma induce dystonia and other movement disorders? Yes! Mov Dis 2001;16:7–12.
53. Cardoso F, Jankovic J: Peripherally induced tremor and parkinsonism. Arch Neurol 1995;52:263–270.
54. Blight AR, Decrescito V: Morphometric analysis of experimental spinal cord injury in the cat: The relation of injury intensity to survival of myelinated axons. Neuroscience 1986;19:321–341.
55. Lobosky J: The epidemiology of spinal cord injury. *In* Narayan RK, Wilberger JE, Povlishok JT (eds): Neurotrauma. New York, McGraw-Hill, 1996.
56. Hadley MN, Zabramski JM, Browner CM, et al: Pediatric spinal trauma: Review of 122 cases of spinal cord and vertebral column injuries. J Neurosurg 1988;68:18–24.
57. Ruge JR, Sinson GP, McLone DG, et al: Pediatric spinal injury: The very young. J Neurosurg 1988;68:25–30.
58. Wilberger JE, Maroon JC: Burning hands syndrome revisited. Neurosurgery 1987;20:599–605.
59. Torg JS, Yu A, Pavlov H, et al: Neuroapraxia of the cervical spinal cord with transient quadriplegia. J Bone Joint Surg 1986;68A:1354–1370.
60. Cantu RC: Functional cervical spinal stenosis: A contraindication to participation in contact sports. Med Sci Sports Exerc 1993;25:51–61.
61. Van den Bergh R: Pathogenesis and treatment of delayed post-traumatic syringomyelia. Acta Neurochir 1991;110:82–86.
62. Bachulis BL, Long WB, Hynes GD, Johnson MC: Clinical indications for cervical spine radiographs in the traumatized patient. Am J Surg 1987;153:473–478.
63. Woodring JH, Lee C: Limitations of cervical radiography in the evaluation of acute cervical trauma. J Trauma 1993;34:32–39.
64. Samuels LE, Kerstein MD: Routine radiographic evaluation of the thoracolumbar spine in blunt trauma patients: A reappraisal. J Trauma 1993;34:85–89.
65. Kalfas I, Wilberger JE, Goldberg A, et al: MRI in acute spinal cord trauma. Neurosurgery 1988;23:295–299.
66. Pasquale M, Fabian TC: Practice management guidelines for trauma from the Eastern Association for the Surgery of Trauma. J Trauma 1998; 44:941–956.
67. Dickman CA, Greene KA, Sonntag VKH: Injuries involving the transverse atlantal ligament: Classification and treatment guidelines based upon experience with 39 injuries. Neurosurgery 1996;38:44–50.
68. Pang D, Wilberger JE: Spinal cord injury without radiographic abnormality in children. J Neurosurg 1982;57:114–129.
69. Goldberg AL, Rothfus WE, Deeb Z, et al: The impact of magnetic resonance imaging in the diagnostic evaluation of acute cervicothoracic spinal trauma. Skeletal Radiol 1992;17:89–95.
70. Wilberger JE: Diagnosis and management of spinal cord trauma. J Neurotrauma 1991;8:75–86.
71. Duh MS, Bracken MD, Shepard MJ, Wilberger JE: Surgical treatment of spinal cord injury—the National Acute Spinal Cord Injury Study II experience. Neurosurgery 1994;35:240–249.
72. Levi L, Wolf A, Rigamonti D, et al: Anterior decompression in cervical spine trauma. Does the timing of surgery affect the outcome? Neurosurgery 1991;29:216–222.
73. Weinshel SS, Maiman DJ, Beok P, Scales L: Neurologic recovery in quadriplegia following operative treatment. J Spinal Disord 1990;3:244–249.
74. Guha A, Tator CH, Smith CR, Piper I: Improvement in post-traumatic spinal cord blood flow with the combination of a calcium channel blocker and a vasopressor. J Trauma 1989;29:1440–1447.
75. Bracken MB, Shepard MJ, Collins WF, et al: A randomized, controlled trial of methylprednisolone or naloxone in the treatment of acute spinal cord injury. Results of the Second National Acute Spinal Cord Injury Study. N Engl J Med 1990;322:1405–1411.
76. Bracken MB, Shepard MJ, Collins WF, et al: Methylprednisolone or naloxone in the treatment of acute spinal cord injury: One year follow-up results of the National Acute Spinal Cord Injury Study. J Neurosurg 1992;76:23–32.
77. Geisler FH, Coleman WP, Grieco G, et al: The Sygen Multi-Center Acute Spinal Cord Injury Study. Spine 2001;26(Suppl 24):S87–S98.

78. Cameron GS, Scott JW, Jousse AT, et al: Diaphragmatic respiration in the quadriplegic patient and the effect of position on vital capacity. Ann Surg 1955;141:451–456.
79. Harris R, Reines HD: Prevention of pulmonary complications in spinal cord injury with the Roto Rest bed. *In* Green BA, Summer WR (eds): Continuous Oscillation Therapy: Research and Practical Applications. Miami, University of Miami Press, 1986, pp 115–132.
80. Curry K, Casady L: The relationship between extended periods of immobility and decubitus ulcer formation in the acutely spinal cord injured individual. J Neurosci Nurs 1992;24:185–189.
81. Waters RL, Adkins RH, Yakura JS: Definition of complete spinal cord injury. Paraplegia 1991;29:573–581.
82. Ditunno JF, Sipski ML, Posuniak EA, et al: Wrist extensor recovery in traumatic quadriplegia. Arch Phys Med Rehab 1987;68:287–290.
83. Wilberger JE, Maroon JC: Cervical spine injuries in athletes. Phys Sports Med 1990;18:27–47.
84. Evans RW: Some observations on whiplash injuries. Neurol Clin 1992;10:975–997.
85. Evans RW: Whiplash injuries. *In* Gilman S (ed): MedLink Neurobase. San Diego, MedLink Corporation, 2002.
86. Lord S, Barnsley L, Bogduk N: Cervical zygapophyseal joint pain in whiplash. Spine: State Art Rev 1993;7:355–372.
87. Di Stefano G, Radanov BP: Course of attention and memory after common whiplash: A two-year prospective study with age, education and gender pair-matched patients. Acta Neurol Scand 1995;91:346–352.
88. Pearce JMS: The polemics of chronic whiplash injury. Neurology 1994;44:1993–1997.
89. Cassidy JD, Carroll LJ, Cotye P, et al: Effect of eliminating compensation for pain and suffering on the outcome of insurance claims for whiplash injury. N Engl J Med 2000;342:1179–1186.
90. Lord SM, Barnsley L, Wallis BJ, et al: Percutaneous radio-frequency neurotomy for chronic cervical zygapophyseal-joint pain. N Engl J Med 1996;335:1721–1726.
91. Radanov BP, Sturzenegger M, De Stefano G, Schnidrig A: Relationship between early somatic, radiological, cognitive and psychosocial findings and outcome during a one-year follow-up in 117 patients suffering from common whiplash. Br J Rheumatol 1994;33:442–448.
92. Radanov BP, Sturzenegger M, Di Stefano G: Long-term outcome after whiplash injury. A 2-year follow-up considering features of injury mechanism and somatic, radiologic, and psychosocial findings. Medicine (Baltimore) 1995;74:281–297.
93. Wilbourn AJ: Plexus injuries. *In* Evans RW (ed): Neurology and Trauma. Philadelphia, WB Saunders, 1996, pp 375–400.
94. Wilbourn AJ: Iatrogenic nerve injuries. Neurol Clin 1998;16:55–82.
95. Stewart JD: Focal Peripheral Neuropathies, 3rd ed. Philadelphia, Lippincott, Williams & Wilkins, 2000.
96. Tavakkolizadeh A, Saifuddin A, Birch R: Imaging of adult brachial plexus traction injuries. J Hand Surg [Br] 2001;26:183–191.
97. Burchiel KM, Johans TJ, Ochoa J: The surgical treatment of painful traumatic neuromas. J Neurosurg 1993;78:714–719.
98. Kline DG, Hudson AR: Nerve injuries. Philadelphia, WB Saunders, 1995.
99. Carlstedt T, Grane P, Hallin RG, Noren G: Return of function after spinal cord implantation of avulsed spinal nerve roots. Lancet 1995;346: 1323–1325.
100. Ramer MS, Priestley JV, McMahon SB: Functional regeneration of sensory axons into the adult spinal cord. Nature 2000;403:312–316.
101. Mitchell SW, Morehouse GR, Keen WW: Gunshot Wounds and Other Injuries of Nerves. Philadelphia, JB Lippincott, 1864.
102. Schott GD: Reflex sympathetic dystrophy. J Neurol Neurosurg Psychiatr 2001;71:291–295.
103. Schwartzman RJ: New treatments for reflex sympathetic dystrophy. New Engl J Med 2000;343:654–656.
104. Veldman PHJM, Reynen HM, Arntz IE, Goris RJA: Signs and symptoms of reflex sympathetic dystrophy: Prospective study of 829 patients. Lancet 1993;342:1012–1015.
105. Flor H, Elbert T, Knecht S, et al: Phantom-limb pain as a perceptual correlate of cortical reorganization following arm amputation. Nature 1995;375:482–484.
106. Krasney JA: A neurogenic basis for acute altitude illness. Med Sci Sports Exerc 1994;26:195–208.
107. Honigman B, Theis MK, Koziol-McLain J, et al: Acute mountain sickness in a general tourist population at moderate altitudes. Ann Intern Med 1993;118:587–592.
108. Hackett PH, Roach RC: High-altitude illness. New Engl J Med 2001;345:107–114.
109. Burtscher M, Likar R, Nachbauer W, Philadelphy M: Aspirin for prophylaxis against headache at high altitudes: Randomised, double blind, placebo controlled trial. BMJ 1998;316:1057–1058.
110. Moon RE, Vann RD, Bennett PB: The physiology of decompression illness. Sci Am 1995;273:70–77.
111. Wilmshurst PT, Nightingale S, Walsh KP, Morrison WL: Effect of migraine of closure of cardiac right-to-left shunts to prevent recurrence of decompression illness or stroke or for haemodynamic reasons. Lancet 2000;356:1648–1651.
112. Greer HD, Massey EW: Neurological injury from undersea diving. *In* Evans RW (ed): Neurology and Trauma. Philadelphia, WB Saunders, 1996, pp 529–539.
113. Moon RE: Treatment of diving emergencies. Crit Care Clin 1999;15:429–455.
114. Broome JR: Aspects of neurologic decompression illness: A view from Bethesda. J R Nav Med Serv 1995;81:120–126.
115. Lee RC, Gaylor DC, Bhatt D, et al: Role of cell membrane rupture in the pathogenesis of electrical trauma. J Surg Res 1988;44:709–719.
116. Cherington M: Central nervous system complications of lightning and electrical injuries. Semin Neurol 1995;15:233–240.
117. Primeau M, Engelstatter GH, Bares KK: Behavioral consequences of lightning and electrical injury. Semin Neurol 1995;15:279–285.
118. Jafari H, Couratier P, Camu W: Motor neuron disease after electrical injury. J Neurol Neurosurg Psychiatry 2001;71:265–267.
119. Wilbourn AJ: Peripheral nerve disorders in electrical and lightning injuries. Semin Neurol 1995;15:241–255.
120. O'Brien CF: Involuntary movement disorders following lightning and electrical injuries. Semin Neurol 1995;15:263–267.
121. Jain S, Bandi V: Electrical and lightning injuries. Crit Care Clin 1999;15:319–331.

CHAPTER 52

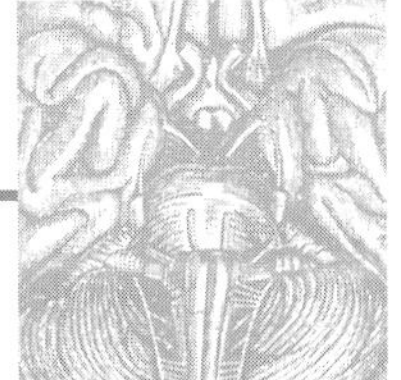

NANCY FOLDVARY-SCHAEFER and ELAINE WYLLIE

Epilepsy

History and Definitions

Epilepsy, from the Greek *epilepsia* (a taking hold of or seizing), is a chronic disorder characterized by a spontaneous tendency for recurrent seizures. Seizures are the clinical manifestation of abnormally hyperexcitable cortical neurons. Whereas all patients with epilepsy have seizures, many more patients have a single seizure during life and are not considered to have epilepsy.

The earliest descriptions of epilepsy appear in Mesopotamian writings from the fifth millennium BC. Persons with epileptic seizures were believed to be possessed by demons or evil spirits, and as a result, the disorder became known as the *sacred disease*. In the book *On the Sacred Disease*, a collection of Hippocratic writings from around 400 BC, the notion that epilepsy was caused by the gods and should be treated by the invocation of supernatural powers was challenged. In these writings, epilepsy was described as a hereditary disease caused by an overflow of phlegm in the brain. Treatment interventions, including proper diet and hygiene, were suggested in lieu of superstitious remedies. Nevertheless, during the middle ages, the drinking of human blood, trephination, skull cauterization, and sterilization were routinely practiced to cleanse the body of evil spirits and reduce the likelihood of transmission.[1]

By the eighteenth century, epilepsy became recognized as a chronic disorder of cerebral function. In the latter half of the nineteenth century, the British neurologist John Hughlings Jackson hypothesized that epilepsy was due to hyperexcitable cerebral gray matter. By correlating focal motor seizure semiology with postmortem pathological examinations, Jackson was the first to localize epileptogenic lesions. In 1886, the first surgery for epilepsy was performed by Sir Victor Horsley, who resected a traumatic cortical scar in a patient with focal motor seizures, rendering him seizure-free.

The invention of the electroencephalogram in 1929 had a profound impact on the diagnosis and classification of the epilepsies. During the 1930s and 1940s, Wilbur Penfield and colleagues mapped the primary sensory and motor cortices in human subjects, advancing the concept of functional localization. In the past several decades, a universally accepted classification of epileptic seizures and syndromes emerged through advancements in electrophysiology, neuroimaging, and molecular biology.

Epilepsy affects 6 to 7 per 1000 population in the United States, and 40 to 50 new cases per 100,000 develop annually.[2] The risk of epilepsy increases from approximately 1 percent at birth through early adulthood to 3 percent by age 75 years. In two thirds of cases, the etiology is not identified.

Basic Mechanisms of Epileptogenesis

To understand the mechanisms related to the development of epilepsy, some basic principles of normal neurophysiology must be reviewed. Electrical signals in neurons take two forms: the action potential, which propagates down the axon of the neuron from the soma to the axon terminal, translocating information within a neuron; and transmission of information between neurons, which is accomplished primarily by chemical synapses.

A complex series of events underlie these electrical signals. Central to the understanding of these events is that the neuronal membrane is semipermeable to different ions carrying electrical current. The neuronal membrane's permeability exhibits rapid changes that can dramatically alter the voltage across it. At the resting membrane potential, sodium ions (Na^+), which are concentrated in the extracellular space, flow into the cell, and intracellular potassium ions (K^+) flow out. A Na^+-K^+ pump, utilizing adenosine triphosphate (ATP), replaces the displaced ions. Influx of positively charged ions (Na^+ and calcium ions [Ca^{2+}]) raises the membrane potential in the direction of depolarization, whereas chloride ion (Cl^-) influx and K^+ efflux hyperpolarizes the membrane. When a cell membrane is depolarized to threshold, Na^+ channels open, allowing the ions to flow intracellularly, which produces an action potential. Potassium efflux from the cell leads to repolarization of the membrane. The propagation of action potentials along axons transmits information throughout the nervous system. When the presynaptic axon terminal is stimulated by an action potential, there is an influx of Ca^{2+}, triggering the release of neurotransmitters that bind to postsynaptic membrane receptors. This process produces excitatory and inhibitory postsynaptic potentials (EPSPs and IPSPs) whose summation and synchronization comprise the electrical activity recorded from the surface electroencephalogram (EEG). Glutamate and aspartate are the primary excitatory neurotransmitters in the central nervous system. Gamma-aminobutyric acid (GABA) is the major inhibitory neurotransmitter in the brain.

A number of cortical cytoarchitectural and anatomical factors influence the propagation of electrical activity. The cerebral cortex is subdivided into neocortex, paleocortex, and archicortex. The archicortex includes the hippocampus and dentate gyrus, and the paleocortex consists of the piriform and olfactory cortices. The neocortex constitutes the remaining cortical regions characterized by the infolding of gyri and sulci. Epilepsy is a disorder that affects neocortical and archicortical neurons and their interconnections with brain stem and diencephalic structures.

The gray matter of the neocortex contains six types of neurons: pyramidal, stellate, horizontal, fusiform, basket, and Martinotti's cells (Fig. 52–1). The vertically aligned pyramidal cells are the main output neurons; they have extensive dendritic arborizations and excitatory synaptic endings that facilitate propagation of electrical activity. The granule, or stellate, cells are the major interneuronal pool. They are the second most numerous cells in the neocortex and are responsible for the propagation of both excitatory and inhibitory information. Axons of the horizontal and granule cells and collaterals of pyramidal and fusiform cells traverse parallel to the surface of the cortex. Pyramidal, fusiform, stellate, and Martinotti's cell axons form radial networks that travel vertically as projection or association fibers.

Projection fibers are afferent and efferent fibers conveying impulses to and from the cortex. Efferent fibers arise from the cortex and descend through the corona radiata and internal capsule. Afferent fibers arise primarily from the thalamus and project via the internal capsule to all regions of the cortex. Fibers interconnecting various cortical regions within the same hemisphere are known as *association fibers*. These

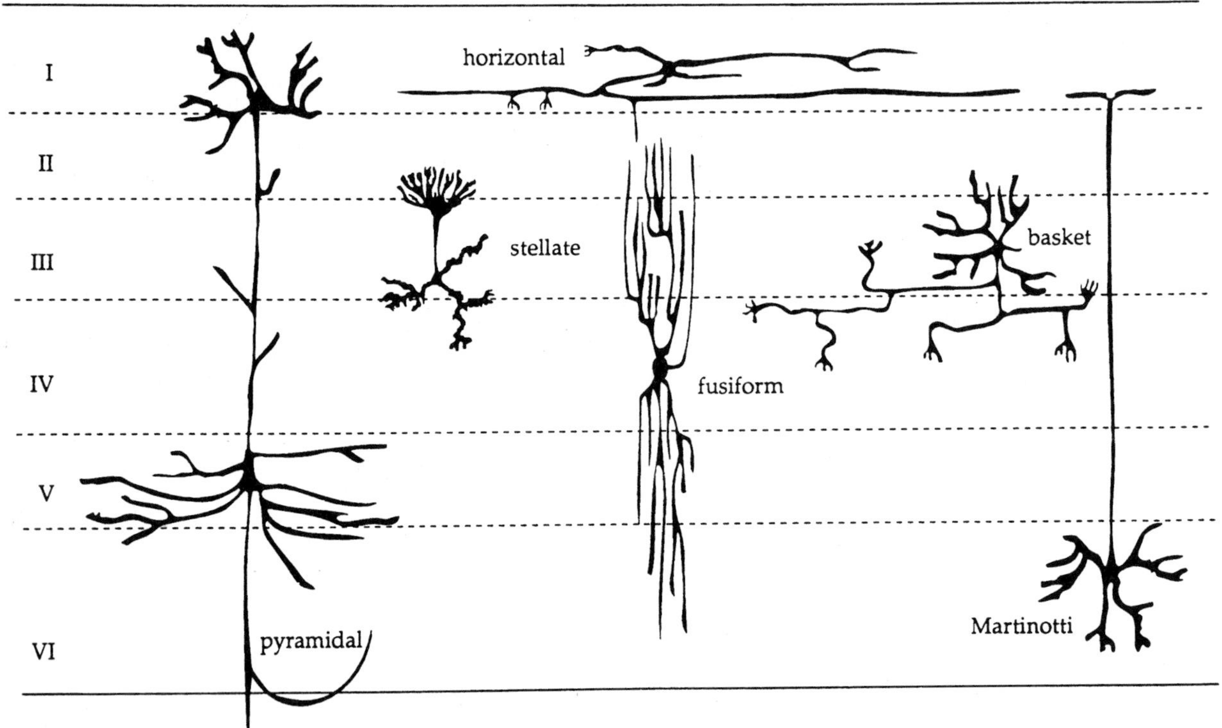

FIGURE 52–1. Types and orientation of neurons within the six-layer neocortex. (From Pansky B, Allen DJ: Review of Neuroscience. New York, Macmillan, 1980, p 287.)

include three main bundles: the uncinate fasciculus, connecting the orbital frontal gyri with anterior portions of the temporal lobe; the arcuate fasciculus, connecting the superior and middle frontal gyri with parts of the temporal lobe; and the cingulum, connecting medial regions of the frontal and parietal lobes with parahippocampal and adjacent temporal cortical regions. Commissural fibers interconnect corresponding cortical regions of the two hemispheres and are represented by the corpus callosum and the anterior commissure. These pathways are important in the relay of information between hemispheres.

The pathophysiology of epilepsy involves alterations of normal physiological processes. An epileptic seizure is produced by synchronous and sustained firing of a population of neurons in the brain. The behavioral manifestations of a seizure reflect the function of the cortical neurons involved in the generation and spread of abnormal electrical activity. Epileptogenicity refers to the excitability and synchronization of neuronal networks that produce epileptiform activity in the brain. Both excitatory and inhibitory influences may be altered, creating a predisposition to excessive synchrony within neuronal populations.

Differences exist between patients who experience a single seizure and those with a tendency for recurrent seizures. Single seizures have various causes, including electrolyte disturbances, drugs, and toxins. Increased extracellular K^+ leading to regenerative hyperexcitability underscores seizures that accompany metabolic aberrations. In hyponatremia, the extracellular space shrinks, leading to an increased concentration of extracellular K^+ and increased nonsynaptic or ephaptic coupling. This rise in K^+ facilitates neuronal firing. Similarly, because membrane excitability varies inversely with the extracellular concentration of Ca^{2+}, hypocalcemia can contribute to the synchronization and spread of abnormal electrical activity. Other metabolic disturbances such as hypomagnesemia, hyperglycemia, hypoxia, and ischemia can also produce seizures.

Alterations of neurotransmission, the ionic milieu, neuronal morphology, and neuronal networks are instrumental in the production of recurrent unprovoked seizures. Animal models using maximal electroshock and chemoconvulsants such as pentylenetetrazol have been used for decades to investigate the pathophysiology of generalized and focal seizures.

Experimentally induced focal epilepsies have been produced by the application of topical metals, such as cobalt, aluminum, and iron, to the sensorimotor cortex. Pathological examination of these lesions reveals gliosis and neuronal loss. Neurons in the surrounding area may demonstrate abnormal dendritic morphology, including denuded spines and reduced branching. Iron salts applied or injected into the cortex of experimental animals have been used in the investigation of post-traumatic epilepsy. Although the precise mechanisms of iron-induced epilepsy are unclear, iron is known to bind strongly with ATP and inhibit Na^+-K^+-ATPase activity, leading to neuronal hyperexcitability. Additionally, iron reacts with the neuronal cell lipid membrane, producing free radicals and resulting in lipid peroxidation.

The kindling model is currently used in the study of partial epilepsy, particularly that involving the mesial temporal structures. *Kindling* refers to the processes that mediate long-lasting changes in brain function in response to repeated, gradually augmented stimulation of the brain. In the kindled animal, there is a permanent state of enhanced seizure susceptibility. These models are important not only in the understanding of the pathophysiological basis of epilepsy, but also in the screening of new compounds that may have anticonvulsant activity.

The structures most susceptible to the development of recurrent seizures include the motor cortex and the hippocampal formation and amygdaloid complex of the limbic system. The motor cortex is comprised of three areas: primary motor cortex, premotor cortex, and supplementary motor area. The motor cortex exerts its control by way of descending corticospinal and corticobulbar tracts and pathways originating in the brain stem. The motor cortex receives input from the thalamus, parietal lobe, and prefrontal cortex. These afferents allow seizures arising in restricted areas to propagate diffusely.

The amygdaloid complex (see Chapter 3) is an aggregate of subcortical nuclei within the rostral pole of the mesial temporal lobe having reciprocal interconnections with the septal area, hypothalamus, and brain stem nuclei. The hippocampal formation extends along the floor of the temporal horn of the lateral ventricle and is comprised of the dentate gyrus, hippocampus proper (CA fields), and the subicular complex (see Chapter 4). Hippocampal or mesial temporal sclerosis is characterized by variable degrees of pyramidal cell loss and gliosis in the hippocampal subfields and dentate gyrus. This condition represents the most common pathological substrate of partial epilepsy in adolescents and adults.

The notion that epilepsy is an inherited disorder was suggested more than 2000 years ago. The prevalence of epilepsy in relatives of affected individuals ranges from 0.5 to 15 percent.[3] Rates are higher in idiopathic than symptomatic epilepsies. Studies of twins have demonstrated concordance rates as high as 70 percent in monozygotic and 10 percent in dizygotic pairs,[3] implying that factors other than genetics play a role in the occurrence of seizures in these groups. Thus far, three syndromes have been mapped to a single gene locus: juvenile myoclonic epilepsy to chromosome 6q, benign familial neonatal convulsions to 20p, and progressive myoclonic epilepsy of the Unverricht-Lundborg type to 21q. Several other epilepsies, including childhood/juvenile absence epilepsy, benign childhood epilepsy with centrotemporal spikes, childhood epilepsy with occipital paroxysms, and epilepsy with grand mal seizures on awakening appear to exhibit mendelian inheritance patterns and are likely to be mapped in the future. Additionally, as the result of various metabolic abnormalities, tumor formation, or impairment of normal brain growth or differentiation, seizures may occur in a large group of inherited neurological disorders. The investigation of these disorders may further elucidate the processes involved in epileptogenesis.

Epileptic Seizures

Efforts to classify epileptic seizures date back to the earliest of medical literature. In 1964, the Commission on Classification and Terminology of the International League Against Epilepsy proposed the first official classification of epileptic seizures, which was revised in 1981.[4, 5] Based on this classification, seizures are divided into *focal*, those in which the first clinical and/or electrographical manifestations indicate initial activation of a limited population of neurons in part of one hemisphere, and *generalized*, those in which the initial manifestations suggest initial activation of neurons throughout both hemispheres. Focal seizures are further subdivided into *simple* and *complex*, based on level of consciousness. Seizures in which consciousness is preserved are referred to as *simple partial seizures*. Those in which consciousness is impaired are classified as *complex partial seizures*. Secondarily generalized seizures are generalized seizures preceded by focal clinical and/or electrographical manifestations that occur in patients with focal epilepsy. The revised classification uses seizure semiology and EEG features to establish whether seizures are focal or generalized. For example, a seizure characterized by staring and loss of awareness is classified as *absence* when generalized spike-wave complexes are noted on the EEG, and as *complex partial* when associated with focal epileptiform discharges. This classification is currently under revision. Debate continues regarding terminology and the classification of seizures in infants and neonates.

The following discussion describes the clinical semiology of the various types of seizures. A later section describes epilepsy syndromes, which are characterized by combinations of seizure types and clinical, historical, and electrographical manifestations.

GENERALIZED SEIZURES

Tonic-Clonic Seizures

Tonic-clonic seizures (TCS) are the most common type of seizure encountered in childhood, adolescence, and adulthood. The manifestations of generalized TCS can be divided into several phases beginning with vague prodromal symptoms that may occur hours to days before the actual convulsion. Common premonitory symptoms include headache, mood change, anxiety, irritability, lethargy, changes in appetite, dizziness, and lightheadedness. The tonic phase may be preceded by a series of brief, bilateral muscle contractions lasting a few seconds. The tonic phase begins with brief flexion of the trunk, accompanied by upward deviation of the eyes, mydriasis, and a characteristic vocalization as contraction of abdominal muscles produces forced expiration across a spasmodic glottis. This process is followed by a period of generalized extension lasting 10 to 15 seconds. With evolution of the clonic phase, tonic contractions alternate with periods of muscle atonia of gradually increasing duration until contractions cease. The seizure terminates with a final generalized tonic spasm. Loss of consciousness and autonomic alterations occur during the tonic and clonic phases. Secondarily, generalized seizures may be preceded by focal or lateralized clinical behaviors such as involuntary jerking of an extremity or head version before the onset of bilateral motor manifestations. Similarly, focal weakness of an extremity during the postictal state (Todd's paralysis) indicates seizure origin from the contralateral hemisphere. TCS commonly produce hypocarbia, owing to a combined respiratory alkalosis and lactic acidosis, transient hyperglycemia, mild cerebrospinal fluid (CSF) pleocytosis, and elevated serum prolactin. The immediate postictal state is characterized by coma that is gradually replaced by a confusional state. Once consciousness is regained, lethargy, myalgia, and headache are often reported. Most TCS are less than 1 minute in duration. Potential complications include oral and head trauma, vertebral body stress fractures, aspiration pneumonia, pulmonary edema, and sudden death.

Generalized TCS occurring in patients with idiopathic generalized epilepsies are associated with normal background activity and bilaterally synchronous and symmetrical spikes, polyspikes, or spike-wave complexes in the interictal EEG. Secondarily generalized TCS are usually associated with background abnormalities and focal or lateralized slowing and epileptiform activity. During the tonic phase of a TCS, generalized low-amplitude 20- to 40-Hz activity evolves into a bilaterally synchronous and symmetric 10-Hz rhythm, which is referred to as the *epileptic recruiting rhythm*. Generalized polyspikes interrupted by slow waves characterize the clonic phase. The postictal period is characterized by generalized suppression or low-amplitude slow activity.

Experimental animal models using systemic chemoconvulsants and maximal electroshock provide some insight into the neuronal structures involved in the production of TCS. Lesions involving the pontine reticular formation produce the tonic phase in several animal models. Involvement of forebrain structures is required for the production of clonus, suggesting that an interaction of brain stem and neocortical structures takes place. These findings, however, have not been confirmed in humans.

TCS are observed in patients with idiopathic and symptomatic epilepsies and in association with systemic disease.[6] 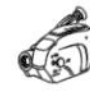 Hyponatremia, hypoglycemia, alcohol withdrawal, and drugs are common causes of isolated seizures particularly in hospitalized patients. Drugs that may precipitate TCS include tricyclic antidepressants, antipsychotics, anticholinergics, antihistamines, methylxanthines, antibiotics, and withdrawal from barbiturates and benzodiazepines. The prognosis for patients with idiopathic generalized TCS is better than that for those with focal or secondary generalized seizures, which tend to persist if untreated. The remission rate is greatest in patients who develop TCS in childhood in the absence of other seizure types.

Tonic, Atonic, and Clonic Seizures

Tonic and atonic seizures are clinically distinct, although they are often present in the same patient. 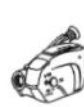 Tonic seizures are characterized by sustained, nonvibratory contractions of axial musculature, usually involving flexion of the upper extremities and flexion or extension of the lower extremities. Impairment of consciousness and autonomic alterations occur, but to a lesser extent than in TCS. Seizures last typically less than 10 seconds, but they may be as long as 1 minute in duration. Tonic seizures are typically abrupt in onset and are followed by a rapid return to baseline. Seizures commonly occur in clusters during drowsiness and nonrapid eye movement (non-REM) sleep, frequently occurring dozens of times per day. Tonic seizures during wakefulness commonly produce injuries owing to sudden, unexpected falls. The interictal EEG typically shows a poorly organized background with generalized spike-wave discharges of less than 3.0 Hz (slow spike-wave complexes) or focal or multifocal spikes and sharp waves. Ictal patterns include generalized attenuation, known as an *electrodecremental response*, low-voltage fast activity (15 to 25 Hz), high-amplitude 10-Hz rhythms, and generalized theta or delta activity.

The pathophysiology of tonic seizures is poorly understood. Lesions of brain stem nuclei produce the tonic phase of TCS and are implicated in the generation of tonic seizures as well. Other animal studies have suggested that discharges in the reticular gray matter caudal to the thalamus may produce EEG desynchronization, autonomic phenomena, and tonic seizures. Tonic seizures are typically observed in children with symptomatic generalized epilepsy, such as Lennox-Gastaut syndrome. Prolonged tonic seizures may be mistaken for generalized TCS, decerebration, paroxysmal dystonia, convulsive syncope, and the tonic spasms seen in patients with neurodegenerative disorders such as multiple sclerosis. Tonic seizures arising from the supplementary motor area are characterized by bilateral electrographical manifestations on surface EEG, although motor activity is asymmetrical and consciousness is usually preserved.

Atonic seizures, or drop attacks, are characterized by abrupt loss of postural tone lasting 1 to 2 seconds. Consciousness is usually impaired, although recovery is rapid. Seizures may be limited to head and neck musculature producing a head drop, or they may involve all postural musculature resulting in sudden unexpected falls and injuries. The loss of tone may be preceded by a series of myoclonic jerks. The terms *atonic* and *astatic* are not synonymous. The latter refers to loss of erect posture resulting in a fall, which may occur with atonic, tonic, and myoclonic seizures. Like tonic seizures, atonic seizures are observed in neurologically abnormal children with symptomatic generalized epilepsy syndromes. Atonic seizures may be mistaken for breath-holding spells, syncope, and cataplexy. The ictal EEG demonstrates polyspike-wave or spike-wave discharges. More prolonged seizures may be accompanied by generalized spike-wave discharges followed by diffuse generalized slowing that is maximal at the vertex and central regions. This slow wave activity can be accompanied by severe, generalized hypotonia. Postictal changes are not prominent. With no experimental animal models available, the pathophysiology of atonic seizures is poorly understood. Because corpus callosotomy is effective in some patients with atonic seizures, interhemispheric mechanisms are suspected.

Generalized clonic seizures are rare and are usually seen in children with febrile illnesses. These seizures are characterized by an abrupt loss of consciousness with hypotonia or a generalized tonic spasm, followed by a series of myoclonic jerks. Motor involvement may be asymmetrical, migratory, or focal. Significant autonomic changes and postictal confusion do not occur. Clonic seizures may be mistaken for TCS, when the onset is not observed, and myoclonic seizures when the phenomenology of the movement is more arrhythmical and random. In addition, nonepileptic clonic jerks may be seen in syncope and breath-holding spells and during the recovery phase of cataplexy. The interictal EEG in patients with clonic seizures reveals generalized spike- or polyspike-wave discharges. Seizures are accompanied by a generalized 10-Hz rhythm intermixed with slow waves of variable frequency. As in TCS, neocortical structures are implicated in the generation of clonic seizures.

Absence Seizures

Absence seizures (AS) are subdivided into typical and atypical forms. Typical AS are characterized by sudden behavioral arrest and unresponsiveness that may be accompanied by eyelid or facial clonus; automatisms; and autonomic, tonic, or atonic features. The duration rarely exceeds 10 seconds, and no aura or postictal state is observed. Atypical AS generally exceed 10 seconds in duration, begin and end more gradually, and produce less marked alteration of consciousness. Tonic, atonic, and myoclonic features are commonly observed.

Brief AS without automatisms or motor features may be mistaken for daydreaming or inattention. Absences with automatisms must be differentiated from temporal lobe complex partial seizures because treatment and natural history differ. Temporal lobe complex partial seizures usually exceed 30 seconds in duration and are characterized by prominent oral and hand automatisms, auras, and postictal confusion. Frontal lobe complex partial seizures may be more difficult to differentiate owing to their brevity, tendency to cluster, and higher incidence of bilateral EEG changes.

The interictal EEG in patients with typical AS reveals generalized 3.0-Hz spike-wave complexes superimposed on normal background activity. Bursts of generalized 3.0- to 4.0-Hz spike-wave complexes slowing to 2.5- to 3.0-Hz are observed during seizures (Fig. 52–2). Typical AS are commonly precipitated by hyperventilation and infrequently by photic stimulation. Behavioral changes are usually observed during bursts exceeding 3 seconds. Atypical AS are associated with 0.5- to 2.5-Hz slow spike-wave complexes superimposed on abnormal background activity. Unlike typical AS, atypical absences are rarely provoked by hyperventilation or photic stimulation.

Animal models of generalized absence seizures and in vitro electrophysiological techniques have shed light on the pathogenesis of AS.[7] The corticoreticular theory postulates that typical AS involve the generation of abnormal oscillations within thalamocortical circuitry. Thalamic neurons have the ability to shift between oscillatory and tonic firing modes. During normal wakefulness, EEG desynchronization and tonic thalamocortical neuronal firing take place. With oscillatory rhythmical firing, the thalamic EPSP threshold is raised, which produces dampening of signal transmission to the cortex, resulting in impairment of consciousness. Oscillatory behavior relies on the nucleus reticularis thalami, which is composed of GABAergic neurons that project to thalamic relay nuclei and to one another. The nucleus reticularis thalami receive excitatory glutaminergic inputs as well. Biochemically, a phase-locked $GABA_A/GABA_B$–mediated inhibition followed by glutamate-mediated excitation appears to be operative within the thalamocortical circuitry. The $GABA_A/GABA_B$-mediated inhibition triggers the key event, a low-threshold Ca^{2+} current in the nucleus reticularis thalami neurons, leading to recurrent depolarization and repetition of the cycle. Neurons of the reticular nucleus of the thalamus and voltage-dependent Ca^{2+} channels (T-channels) of thalamic relay neurons are required to sustain the series of oscillatory burst firings between thalamic relay neurons and neocortical pyramidal cells. Generalized AS represent a potentiation of the rhythmicity so that the rhythmical firing mode predominates. The anti-absence agents ethosuximide

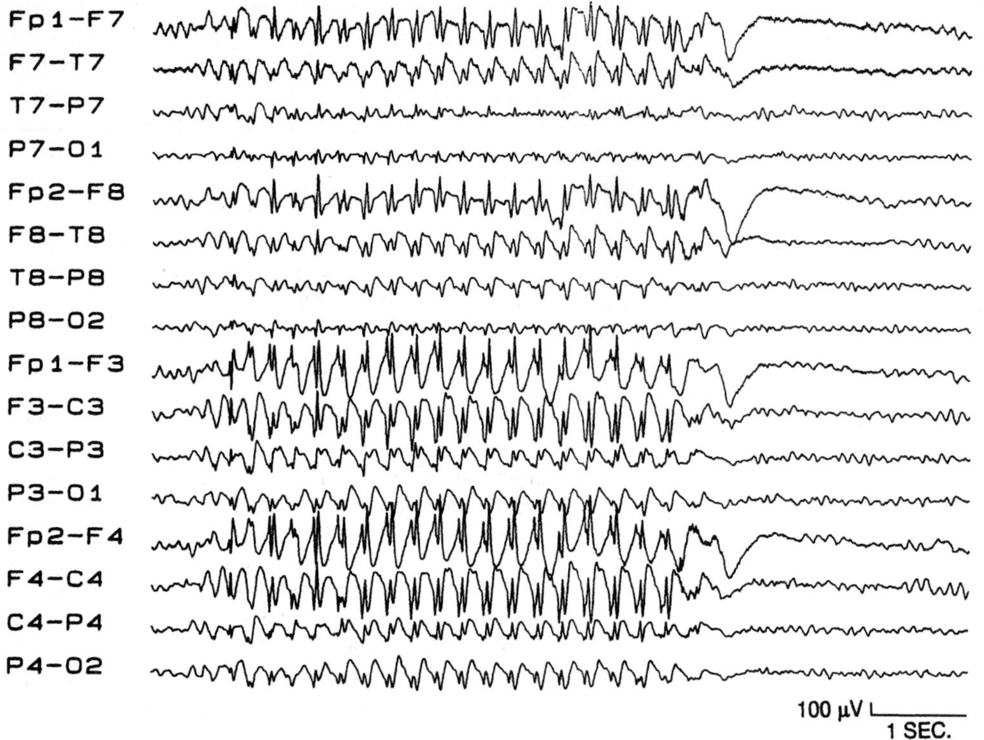

FIGURE 52–2. 3.0-Hz spike-wave complexes during a seizure in a child with absence epilepsy.

and valproic acid suppress T-channel currents, whereas other anticonvulsant agents do not.

The high concordance for seizures and the 3.0-Hz spike-wave trait in monozygotic twins supports a genetic basis for AS. Typical AS occur in neurologically normal children with idiopathic generalized epilepsy. Atypical absences are observed in patients with diffuse or multifocal cerebral dysfunction resulting from acquired or inherited neurological disorders such as Lennox-Gastaut Syndrome (see later).

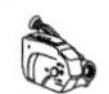

Myoclonic Seizures

Myoclonic seizures are single or repetitive, bilaterally synchronous and symmetrical, rapid muscular contractions. Jerks are often restricted to facial and shoulder girdle muscles, although involvement of the trunk and limbs may occur. Consciousness is usually preserved. The EEG reveals generalized polyspikes or spike-wave complexes, which may or may not be time-locked to the muscular contraction. Interictal findings vary from normal background rhythms with generalized epileptiform discharges to severe background abnormalities with multifocal spike discharges, depending on the etiology.

Myoclonic seizures are commonly observed in neonates and children with idiopathic or symptomatic epilepsy. These seizures should be differentiated from nonepileptic events, including movement disorders, hypnic jerks, nocturnal myoclonus, and segmental myoclonus of spinal cord or brain stem origin. Nonepileptic reticular and cortical reflex forms of myoclonus may occur in the setting of anoxia, trauma, stroke, or degenerative or neoplastic disorders.

The pathophysiology of myoclonic seizures is poorly understood, partly because of the diversity of syndromes in which they appear and the difficulty in differentiating nonepileptic from epileptic myoclonus. Three subgroups of epileptic myoclonus have been described based on etiology, distribution, and the back-averaged EEG.[8] In idiopathic generalized epileptic myoclonus, generalized myoclonic jerks preceded by spike discharges are thought to be produced by abnormal subcortical influences on a diffusely hyperexcitable neocortex. Reticular reflex myoclonus consists of generalized, synchronous muscle contractions that precede the electrographical correlate and originate in brain stem structures. Cortical reflex myoclonus is characterized by unilateral or asynchronous jerks restricted to a few contiguous muscles preceded by spike discharges in the contralateral sensorimotor cortex. This form of myoclonus is thought to represent a form of focal epilepsy.

PARTIAL (FOCAL) SEIZURES

Simple Partial Seizures

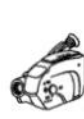

Simple partial seizures are epileptic seizures characterized by motor, sensory, autonomic, or psychic symptomatology during which consciousness is preserved. The term *aura* is reserved for subjective symptoms of epileptic origin reported by the patient in the absence of objective signs. Simple partial seizures can occur in isolation or preceding complex partial or tonic-clonic seizures. Multiple symptoms or signs may occur during a single seizure. Simple partial seizures with motor features include focal tonic and clonic activity, vocalizations, speech arrest, and version, defined as sustained, forced, involuntary turning of the eyes or head. The epileptic focus is usually in the hemisphere contralateral to the motor manifestations. The classic "Jacksonian march" in which focal clonus in distal muscles gradually spreads proximally along the motor homunculus occurs only rarely. Simple partial seizures with sensory symptoms include somatosensory, visual, auditory, vertiginous, gustatory, and olfactory disturbances. Autonomic phenomena include epigastric sensation, pallor, sweating, flushing, piloerection, and pupillary dilatation. Seizures with psychic symptoms include affective and cognitive disturbances and illusions or hallucinations of memory (déjà vu, jamais vu), visions, sounds, self-image, and time.

Simple partial seizures should be differentiated from the prodromal symptoms that precede complex partial seizures and TCS. Movement disorders, including paroxysmal dyskinesias and tonic spasms, transient ischemic attacks, migraine, and psychiatric disease, should be considered in patients with transient symptoms without impairment of consciousness.

Less than one third of simple partial seizures are associated with changes on surface EEG recordings. EEG changes are more common when the epileptic focus is close to the recording electrodes, such as in seizures arising from the perirolandic area. Neurons within an epileptogenic focus produce a synchronized burst of action potentials known as the *paroxysmal depolarization shift*, which is responsible for the generation of partial seizures. This paroxysmal depolarization shift is believed to produce focal interictal epileptic discharges.

The signs and symptoms of simple partial seizures reflect the function of the cortex involved in the generation and propagation of the abnormal electrical activity. A strong association exists between semiology and site of seizure origin.[9] Seizures with motor manifestations usually arise from the frontal lobes, although tonic activity and version may be seen in parietal and occipital lobe epilepsy. Autonomic, affective, and psychic phenomena are produced by activation of temporal lobe and, less commonly, frontal lobe structures. Activation of epileptogenic foci in the insula and parietal operculum produces gustatory symptoms. Olfactory disturbances occur with orbitofrontal and mesial temporal lobe seizures. Elementary visual or auditory phenomena indicate activation of primary visual and auditory cortices in the occipital and superior temporal lobes, respectively. Complex illusions and hallucinations occur with activation of association areas. Whereas the first sign or symptom of a focal seizure aids in the localization of the epileptogenic focus, postictal focal motor, sensory, or visual field deficits can reliably identify the hemisphere of seizure origin. Consequently, whenever possible, a careful neurological examination should be performed immediately following a seizure.

Common pathological substrates of partial seizures include mesial temporal sclerosis, congenital malformation, neoplasm, CNS infection, head trauma, and cerebrovascular disease. With modern neuroimaging techniques, the ability to detect neuronal migration disorders, mesial temporal sclerosis, and low-grade gliomas has improved dramatically. The most common etiologies for partial seizures in children are congenital malformations and low-grade gliomas. Mesial temporal sclerosis predominates in young adults, and cerebrovascular disease is the most common cause of new-onset partial epilepsy in older adults.

Complex Partial Seizures

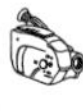

Complex partial seizures are partial seizures that are associated with an alteration of consciousness. The term *psychomotor* describes a particular semiology characterized by automatisms and impairment of consciousness, usually of temporal lobe origin. Complex partial seizures are also observed in frontal, parietal, and occipital lobe epilepsies. As in simple partial seizures, the clinical manifestations reflect the origin and propagation pattern of the epileptic focus. Seizures often begin with a motionless stare or arrest of activity followed by oroalimentary, hand, or gestural automatisms; eye movements; speech disturbances; and automatic behavior.

Complex partial seizures must be differentiated from typical and atypical AS. Psychogenic seizures, fugue states, panic attacks, inattention, sleep disorders, syncope, transient global amnesia, metabolic derangements, drug and alcohol ingestion, migraine, transient ischemic attacks, and fluctuations in mental status in patients with dementia should also be considered in the evaluation of patients with transient alterations in consciousness.

The interictal EEG in patients with complex partial seizures demonstrates focal or lateralized sharp waves, spikes, and slow waves. Several ictal patterns are observed. Rhythmical sinusoidal activity or repetitive spike discharges maximal over one region or hemisphere is most common. Nearly one third of complex partial seizures are not accompanied by EEG changes. A lack of EEG correlate is more likely to occur with brief seizures arising from deep regions such as orbitofrontal cortex or mesial temporal structures. The neuronal substrates of complex partial seizures are the same as in simple partial seizures except that alteration of consciousness implicates more extensive spread, usually involving both cerebral hemispheres.

General Approach to the Initial Seizure

Approximately 6 percent of the population experiences an afebrile seizure at least once in their lifetime.[10] The decision to initiate antiepileptic drug (AED) therapy after a single seizure is based on the risk of recurrence versus that of treatment. Nearly 30 percent of treated patients experience unacceptable side effects requiring discontinuation of anticonvulsant medication.[11] In addition, although the initiation of AED therapy significantly reduces the risk of recurrence, it does not guarantee remission. Recurrence rates after single unprovoked seizures range from 27 to 71 percent.[10] The most reliable predictors of recurrence are (1) evidence of a neurological abnormality based on known etiology, neurological examination, or neuroimaging studies; (2) epileptiform abnormalities on EEG; and (3) partial versus generalized seizures. The risk of recurrence increases with the number of abnormalities identified.

Patients who experience their first seizure should be evaluated with an EEG and a magnetic resonance imaging (MRI) study. The need for laboratory studies, toxicological screens, and CSF analysis should be determined on an individual basis. Seizures due to drugs, alcohol, and metabolic disturbances require treatment of the underlying cause instead of AED therapy. Patients with evidence of neurological abnormalities that are likely to persist should be treated with anticonvulsants after discussing the potential risks and benefits. Treatment is generally continued for a period of 1 to 2 years, after which medication is gradually withdrawn if seizures have not recurred. Approximately 80 percent of recurrences appear within 2 years, and the majority do so within 6 months.[10] As a result, most states have laws requiring that driving be restricted for periods ranging from 3 to 12 months after a single unprovoked seizure. Individual state laws vary, as do the requirements for the reporting of patients to state authorities by physicians.

Epilepsies and Epilepsy Syndromes

Certain epileptic disorders are characterized by specific clusters of signs and symptoms that are considered epileptic syndromes. Because most of these syndromes have numerous etiologies, few have been defined as specific diseases. Proposed in 1989, the current classification of the epilepsies subdivides epilepsies and epileptic syndromes into three categories based on clinical history, EEG manifestations, and etiology.[12] *Localization-related epilepsies and syndromes* are typified by seizures that originate from a localized cortical region. The *generalized epilepsies and epilepsy syndromes* are characterized by seizures with initial activation of neurons within both cerebral hemispheres.

The syndromes are further divided into idiopathic and symptomatic types. *Idiopathic* refers to syndromes that arise spontaneously without a known cause, presumably having a genetic basis. Most affected patients are of normal intelligence and have normal results on neurological examinations. *Symptomatic* denotes epilepsies with an identified cause such as mesial temporal sclerosis. The term *cryptogenic* describes syndromes that are presumed to be symptomatic but have no known etiology and that occur in patients with or without abnormalities on neurological examination. Epilepsies that are characterized by both partial and generalized seizures and focal and generalized epileptiform discharges, but without a clear predominance of one over the other, are classified as *undetermined*. The term *lesional* epilepsy refers to focal epilepsy in which a lesion is identified on neuroimaging studies that is the probable cause of seizures. Lesions include mesial temporal sclerosis, congenital malformations, neoplasms, vascular malformations, and ischemic insults. The distinction between lesional and nonlesional focal epilepsy is particularly important in patients being considered for epilepsy surgery. In this population, surgical outcome is dependent upon the completeness of resection of epileptogenic lesion, which is accomplished more readily when a well-defined structural abnormality is present. In addition to the classic dichotomy between localization-related and generalized epilepsies, a number of special syndromes are also highlighted.

LOCALIZATION-RELATED (FOCAL) EPILEPSIES AND EPILEPTIC SYNDROMES

Benign Focal Epilepsies of Childhood

Benign focal epilepsies of childhood are idiopathic localization-related epilepsies characterized by partial seizures, focal EEG abnormalities, and absence of a known etiology. These are age-related syndromes occurring in neurologically normal children that have a tendency for spontaneous remission. Benign childhood epilepsy with centrotemporal spikes (BCECT) is the most common, comprising 15 to 20 percent of all childhood epilepsies.[13] In comparison, benign childhood epilepsy with occipital paroxysms (BCEOP), benign frontal epilepsy of childhood, and benign epilepsy with affective symptoms are rare.

Age of onset of BCECT ranges from 2 to 13 years, with peak incidence of 9 years. Simple partial seizures with sensorimotor symptoms of the face and oropharynx, hemiconvulsions, and TCS followed by Todd's paralysis occur typically during non-REM sleep. Nearly 80 percent of patients experience isolated or infrequent seizures. A family history of epilepsy is reported in 15 to 30 percent of patients. Centrotemporal sharp waves are observed in the EEGs of 15 to 30 percent of first-degree relatives. An autosomal dominant mode of inheritance with age-dependent penetrance is suspected. In BCEOP, seizures consist of visual symptoms with frequent evolution to hemiclonic, complex partial, and TCS. Tonic eye deviation and vomiting with alteration of consciousness are also observed. Headache, nausea, and vomiting occur postictally in 20 to 30 percent of patients.

BCECT can be distinguished from the symptomatic epilepsies by seizure semiology, EEG manifestations, response to AEDs, and absence of abnormalities on neurological examination and neuroimaging studies. Similar seizure patterns and electrographical features may be seen in patients with lesions of the operculum and perirolandic cortex, however. Migraine, lesional occipital lobe epilepsy, MELAS (mitochondrial myopathy, lactic acidosis, and stroke-like episodes), and bilateral occipital cortico-subcortical calcifications with focal motor seizures should be considered in patients presenting with symptoms of BCEOP.

The interictal EEG in BCECT shows stereotypical unilateral or bilateral high-voltage diphasic centrotemporal sharp waves superimposed on normal background activity. Epileptiform activity tends to be markedly enhanced during non-REM sleep. The results of neuroimaging studies are normal. In BCEOP, high-amplitude, rhythmical, unilateral or bilateral occipital or posterior temporal spikes or sharp waves appear with eye closure and attenuate with eye opening.

Children with benign focal epilepsy who experience isolated or rare nocturnal seizures do not necessarily require treatment with AEDs. Treatment should be considered in patients with frequent TCS or seizures during wakefulness, however. Phenytoin, carbamazepine, phenobarbital, valproic acid, and gabapentin are effective; however, carbamazepine and gabapentin are often preferred for their lower incidence of adverse reactions. Medication withdrawal should be considered after 1 to 2 years of seizure control or by age 16 years, when spontaneous remission usually occurs. Spontaneous remission by 16 to 18 years occurs in all patients with BCECT, although 1 to 2 percent experience rare TCS in adulthood. Satisfactory seizure control is achieved in only 60 percent of patients with BCEOP, 5 percent of whom develop new seizure types in adulthood.

Temporal Lobe Epilepsy

Temporal lobe epilepsy (TLE) constitutes nearly two thirds of localization-related epilepsies that appear during adolescence and adulthood.[14] Mesial temporal lobe epilepsy (MTLE), in which seizures arise from the hippocampus or amygdala, is most common, although neocortical onset occurs. The natural history is variable, and as many as 30 to 40 percent of patients continue to have seizures despite appropriate medical management.[14] Seizure onset ranges from the latter half of the first decade of life to early adulthood. In many cases, seizures begin several years after febrile seizures, head trauma, or CNS infection. Complicated febrile seizures are reported in 40 percent of patients with refractory TLE.

Visceral sensations, fear, anxiety, olfactory disturbances, and psychic phenomena are commonly reported by patients with seizures arising from the mesial temporal lobe. Auditory hallucinations or complex visual phenomena usually indicate neocortical temporal origin. Complex partial seizures are characterized by behavioral arrest, staring, automatisms and occasionally, dystonic posturing of an extremity contralateral to the seizure focus. Seizure duration typically ranges from 30 to 120 seconds. Postictal confusion usually occurs, and language disturbances may follow seizures arising from the dominant hemisphere. Approximately 50 percent of patients also experience secondarily generalized TCS. Stress, sleep deprivation, and menstruation are common provoking factors. Status epilepticus is rare, and the results of the neurological examination are usually normal.

Mesial temporal sclerosis is the most common pathological substrate of TLE. Marked neuronal loss in the CA1, CA3, CA4, and the dentate granule cells is observed. The pyramidal cells in CA2, subiculum, entorhinal cortex, and temporal neocortex are relatively spared. Loss of granule cell innervation leads to reactive synaptogenesis, which results in an excitatory process capable of initiating and propagating seizures. The coexistence of mesial temporal sclerosis and extralimbic lesions is observed in 30 percent of surgical specimens. Seizure semiology may be indistinguishable in epilepsy arising from the orbitofrontal cortex, cingulate gyrus, and temporal lobe. Temporal lobe seizures should be differentiated from fugue states, syncope, psychogenic seizures, transient global amnesia, and absences.

The interictal EEG reveals slowing and spikes or sharp waves in the temporal region that are accentuated during non-REM sleep. The yield of EEG abnormalities is increased with sphenoidal or additional inferior temporal electrodes (Fig. 52–3). Bitemporal independent discharges are observed in 30 percent of cases. The ictal EEG commonly begins with a regionalized or generalized attenuation followed by a gradual buildup of rhythmical theta or alpha frequencies intermixed with epileptic discharges (Fig. 52–4). EEG manifestations are typically maximal in the anterior or mesial temporal region in patients with MTLE and lateral or posterior temporal area in neocortical TLE.

High-resolution MRI demonstrates hippocampal atrophy and abnormal signal intensities that are highly correlated with mesial temporal sclerosis in many patients with MTLE. Fluorodeoxyglucose DG (^{18}FDG) positron-emission tomography (PET) demonstrates temporal lobe hypometabolism in over 80 percent of cases. Both ictal and interictal single-photon emission computed tomography (SPECT) show unilateral abnormalities, although the spatial resolution is inferior to that of PET, and technical factors, such as time of injection in relation to seizure onset, dramatically influence results.

Carbamazepine, phenytoin, oxcarbazepine, and lamotrigine are first-line agents for the treatment of complex partial seizures with or without secondarily generalized TCS.[15] Outcome is poorer and the incidence of adverse effects is higher with phenobarbital or primidone monotherapy.[15] A comparison study of carbamazepine and valproic acid revealed similar efficacy against TCS, although carbamazepine was superior for the control of complex partial seizures and produced fewer adverse effects.[16] The newer anticonvulsant medications gabapentin, topiramate, tiagabine, levetiracetam, and zonisamide are effective as adjunctive therapy. Sixty to 70 percent of patients achieve good control or remission with appropriate medical management. Factors predictive of less favorable outcome include onset before 2 years of age, frequent complex partial and tonic-clonic seizures, known etiology, status epilepticus, and history of febrile convulsions. Those who fail to respond to medical management after 1 to 2 years and those with structural lesions in the temporal lobe should be referred to an epilepsy center for surgical evaluation.

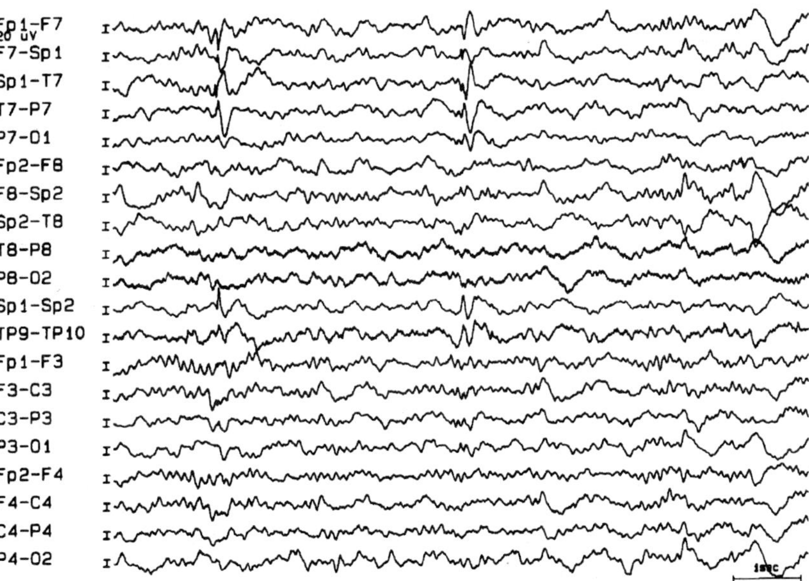

FIGURE 52–3. Interictal EEG on an adult woman with left mesial temporal lobe epilepsy due to mesial temporal sclerosis. Spike discharges are present in the left mesial temporal region maximal at the left sphenoidal (SP1) electrode.

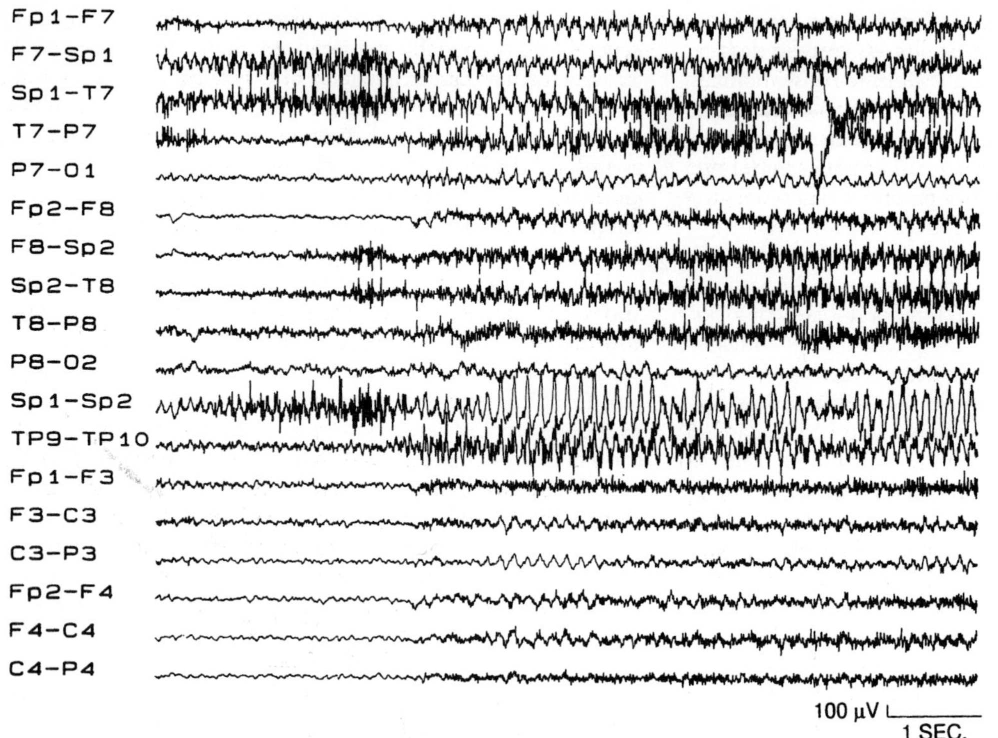

FIGURE 52–4. Rhythmic theta activity maximal at the left sphenoidal electrode during a seizure in a patient with mesial temporal lobe epilepsy.

Extratemporal Neocortical Epilepsy

The incidence of neocortical epilepsy is derived from surgical series of medically refractory patients. Consequently, the incidence and natural history of extratemporal epilepsy are unknown. Frontal lobe epilepsy is most common after TLE, followed by parietal and occipital lobe epilepsies.[17]

Various seizure patterns are observed in frontal lobe epilepsy. Frontal lobe complex partial seizures are differentiated from those of temporal lobe origin by their abrupt onset, shorter duration, absence of prolonged postictal state, and tendency for status epilepticus and seizure clusters. Generalized motor activity, sexual automatisms, vocalizations, version, and focal clonic and tonic activity are observed. Seizures arising from the orbitofrontal cortex and cingulate gyrus produce staring, automatisms, and autonomic and affective manifestations. Brief, recurrent, nocturnal seizures characterized by asymmetrical tonic posturing and vocalizations with preserved consciousness are observed in supplementary motor area epilepsy. Opercular area seizures are associated with salivation, mastication, speech arrest, laryngeal symptoms, autonomic signs, and gustatory or epigastric disturbances. Seizures originating in the dorsolateral frontal convexity are characterized by focal tonic and clonic activity, version, and speech arrest. Koshewnikow's syndrome, characterized by repetitive focal motor seizures, myoclonus, and focal motor status epilepticus, is observed in seizures originating in the perirolandic region.

In parietal lobe epilepsy, auras consist of lateralized somatosensory symptoms, vertigo, and epigastric or cephalic sensations. Automatisms and asymmetrical tonic posturing are observed with ictal propagation to the temporal or frontal lobes, respectively. Occipital lobe seizures are characterized by elementary visual hallucinations that may be limited to the contralateral hemifield, sensations of eye movement, eye blinking, and ictal blindness.

With the exception of head trauma, which commonly produces contusions of the frontal and temporal polar regions and orbitofrontal cortex, the location of the epileptic focus does not predict etiology. The various etiologies of neocortical epilepsies include neoplasm, head injury, CNS infection, vascular malformation, and neuronal migration disorder.[18] No cause is identified in 25 percent of cases.

Neocortical epilepsy should be differentiated from MTLE, which has a more favorable response to surgical intervention. Movement disorders, parasomnias, and psychogenic seizures may mimic frontal lobe seizures. Parietal and occipital lobe seizures may be mistaken for transient ischemic events. The differentiation of migraine and occipital lobe epilepsy may be difficult because both commonly produce transient visual phenomena followed by nausea, vomiting, and headache.

The yield of EEG abnormalities is dependent on the size of the epileptogenic focus and its distance from the recording electrodes. The EEG recording may be normal when seizures arise from deep, midline, or basal locations unless special recording techniques or montages are employed. Abnormalities consist of nonspecific slowing, focal or bilateral epileptiform discharges, and low-voltage fast activity. Secondary bilateral synchrony, in which a unilateral deep or midline focus produces bilaterally synchronous and symmetrical epileptiform activity, may be mistaken for generalized epileptic discharges found in idiopathic generalized epilepsy. In comparison with MTLE, a higher incidence of nonlocalized and nonlateralized ictal EEG patterns is observed. Consequently, intracranial monitoring is usually required in medically refractory cases when MRI fails to reveal focal pathology.

The management of neocortical epilepsy is similar to that for patients with TLE. No studies comparing the response to AEDs and remission rate in neocortical epilepsy and TLE are available. Patients with structural abnormalities on MRI and those who prove to be medically resistant after 1 to 2 years of treatment should be referred to an epilepsy center for surgical consideration. The outcome of surgical treatment depends on the extent of resection of the epileptogenic zone, which may be limited by involvement of cortical regions subserving motor or language functions. Following complete resection of an epileptogenic lesion, 40 to 70 percent of patients become seizure-free.[17,18] The prognosis is less favorable when imaging studies fail to reveal a focal abnormality.

GENERALIZED EPILEPSIES AND EPILEPTIC SYNDROMES

Idiopathic, Age-Related Forms

Benign Neonatal Familial and Nonfamilial Convulsions. Benign idiopathic neonatal convulsions (BINNC) and benign familial neonatal convulsions (BFNNC) are rare neonatal syndromes, characterized by seizures beginning in the first week of life. Most infants are neurologically normal, and spontaneous remission usually occurs. BINNC account for 2 to 7 percent of neonatal convulsions.[19] BFNNC is less common, with only 150 cases having been reported in the literature.[19]

Seizures in BINNC have been referred to as *fifth-day fits* because of their presentation between the fourth and sixth days of life. Recurrent focal or generalized clonic seizures, apneic events, and status epilepticus are observed. A family history of epilepsy may be present. In BFNNC, seizures begin on the second or third day of life and tend to recur for several months. Although most infants have no other abnormalities on examination, minor neurological findings have been reported. The etiology and pathophysiology of BINNC are unknown; BFNNC is an inherited disorder characterized by autosomal dominant transmission with a genetic defect located on chromosome 20q.

A diagnosis of BFNNC can be made only when other causes of convulsions are excluded and a family history of neonatal seizures with spontaneous remission is present. The diagnosis of both syndromes is usually made retrospectively after neurological deterioration and other seizure disorders fail to emerge. Laboratory and neuroimaging study results are unrevealing, although the EEG commonly shows "theta pointu alternant," which is a discontinuous, unreactive theta rhythm associated with neonatal seizures of various etiologies. In other cases, the EEG recording is normal or shows focal or multifocal abnormalities.

Anticonvulsant therapy has not had a consistent effect on the duration of seizures. Neonates with infrequent seizures and those in whom a family history of BFNNC is present do not require AED therapy. Prognostically, both syndromes are considered benign, although follow-up beyond early childhood has not been reported. Febrile and afebrile seizures during childhood have been described in 11 percent of patients with BFNNC and in 0.5 percent of patients with BINNC.[19]

Myoclonic Epilepsies of Infancy and Childhood. Myoclonus and myoclonic seizures are observed in various disorders affecting infants and children. Myoclonic seizures may be overshadowed by more striking seizure patterns and neurological abnormalities. As a result, the classification of these disorders is imprecise. Several syndromes demonstrating consistent etiological, clinical, and electrophysiological features have been described, however.[20]

Early myoclonic encephalopathy is a disorder affecting severely neurologically impaired infants shortly after birth. Erratic fragmentary myoclonus and generalized myoclonic, tonic, and focal motor seizures are observed. The EEG shows a suppression-burst pattern that evolves to hypsarrhythmia or multifocal spike discharges within months. Antiepileptic medications are ineffective, and 50 percent of patients do not survive beyond the first year of life. Inborn errors of metabolism and congenital malformations are present in some cases.

Early infantile epileptic encephalopathy, or Ohtahara's syndrome, is characterized by tonic spasms beginning in the first few months of life, a suppression-burst pattern on EEG, and rapid progression from normal to severe neurological disability. Only 50 percent of infants survive beyond the first year of life. Hypsarrhythmia, slow spike-wave complexes, or multifocal spikes are observed beyond the neonatal period. Ohtahara's syndrome represents the first in the spectrum of age-related epileptic encephalopathies, frequently evolving to West's syndrome, followed by Lennox-Gastaut syndrome. Congenital malformations are commonly found. Anticonvulsant treatment is usually ineffective, and the prognosis is poor.

Benign myoclonic epilepsy of infancy is characterized by myoclonic seizures in neurologically normal children in the first or second years of life. TCS may develop in adolescence. A history of febrile seizures is common, and a family history of seizures is reported in 30 percent of cases. The interictal EEG is usually normal, and seizures are readily controlled with valproic acid.

Severe myoclonic epilepsy in infancy appears in the first year of life as prolonged, recurrent febrile seizures. Other seizure patterns including atypical absences, myoclonic seizures, and myoclonic status epilepticus appear in early childhood. Affected children are initially normal but develop psychomotor retardation by the second year of life, which is often accompanied by ataxia, pyramidal signs, and myoclonus. The EEG reveals generalized epileptiform discharges. Medical treatment is generally ineffective, and prognosis is poor.

Epilepsy with myoclonic absences is characterized by rhythmical myoclonic seizures with impairment of consciousness beginning in childhood. Seizures are provoked by hyperventilation, and the EEG reveals 3.0-Hz spike-wave complexes. Nearly 50 percent of patients are cognitively impaired before seizure onset. Valproic acid and ethosuximide may be effective, but seizures are often medically refractory.

Absence Epilepsy. Previously referred to as "petit mal," absence epilepsy (AE) accounts for 3 to 4 percent of all seizure disorders.[21] Childhood AE, which appears in children between the ages of 4 and 8 years, comprises 80 percent of cases. Juvenile AE constitutes the remainder, in which seizures begin around the age of 12 years. Typical AS occur several to hundreds of times per day. TCS occur in approximately 30 percent of childhood-onset AE (CAE) and 80 percent of juvenile-onset AE (JAE) patients. Absence status, consisting of prolonged periods of mental clouding associated with repetitive spike-wave complexes, occurs in 10 to 20 percent of CAE and 40 percent of JAE cases. Myoclonic seizures, which are not routinely seen in CAE, occur in 15 percent of JAE. Neurological examination results and intelligence are normal. AE is presumed to be an inherited disorder, although the gene responsible for its expression has not been identified. A family history of epilepsy is present in approximately

30 percent of patients. In one study, the concordance rate for seizures and the spike-wave trait in monozygotic twins was found to be 64 percent and 82 percent, respectively, suggesting that a combination of genetic and nongenetic factors is operative.[22]

AE should be distinguished from daydreaming, inattention, and temporal or frontal lobe seizures. In general, the diagnosis is readily confirmed by EEG, which demonstrates 3.0-Hz spike-wave complexes in CAE. Irregular 3.5- to 6.0-Hz polyspike-wave complexes are more commonly observed in juvenile-onset cases. Background activity is otherwise normal. Hyperventilation accentuates spike-wave complexes in nearly 80 percent of cases. Additionally, nearly 30 percent of patients are photosensitive. Neuroimaging, including MRI and CT scans, is usually unrevealing and is not required unless atypical features are present.

Ethosuximide or valproic acid controls absence seizures in 80 percent of cases. Because ethosuximide is not effective against TCS, valproic acid is the drug of choice in patients with both seizure types. The disease in 5 to 20 percent of patients is not satisfactorily controlled with monotherapy, and patients may benefit from a combination of agents, benzodiazepines, or acetazolamide. Lamotrigine and topiramate may also be effective.

AS typically go into remission by early adulthood, although TCS are more likely to persist. Rhythmical occipital delta activity on EEG is associated with a more favorable course and lower incidence of TCS. Subnormal intellect, resistance to antiepileptic medication, and presence of myoclonic seizures portend a worse prognosis. A meta-analysis showed remission rates ranging from 21 to 89 percent with differences relating to inclusion criteria, follow-up lengths, and outcome definitions.[23] Seventy-eight percent of patients with AS alone were seizure-free compared with 35 percent when TCS were also present.[23]

Juvenile Myoclonic Epilepsy. Juvenile myoclonic epilepsy (JME) accounts for 4 to 10 percent of all epileptic syndromes.[24] JME appears in neurologically normal adolescents between the ages of 12 and 18 years. Myoclonic seizures consist of bilaterally synchronous and symmetrical jerks of the neck, shoulders, and arms that may be single or repetitive. Consciousness is usually preserved. TCS preceded by a series of myoclonic jerks occur in over 90 percent of patients. One third have absences as well. Myoclonic seizures and TCS occur predominantly in the early morning hours shortly after awakening and are provoked by sleep deprivation, alcohol ingestion, fatigue, and menstruation.

Juvenile myoclonic epilepsy is a genetically determined syndrome with a gene locus on the short arm of chromosome 6 (6p). Nearly 50 percent of JME patients have relatives with seizures and 30 percent have asymptomatic family members with generalized epileptiform abnormalities on EEG. JME should be differentiated from the progressive myoclonic epilepsies (PMEs) and other idiopathic epilepsies in which absence, myoclonic, and tonic-clonic seizures are observed. The PMEs are characterized by progressive neurological deterioration, myoclonus, and seizures, and may be mistaken for JME early on before severe neurological disabilities develop (see later).

The interictal EEG reveals bilaterally synchronous 4.0- to 6.0-Hz polyspike-wave complexes superimposed on normal background activity (Fig. 52–5). A photoparoxysmal response is elicited in 30 percent of patients. Myoclonic seizures are accompanied by bursts of generalized, synchronous, and symmetrical 10- to 24-Hz polyspikes followed by irregular slowing. AS are associated with 3.0-Hz spike-wave or 4.0- to 6.0-Hz polyspike-wave complexes. MRI and CT studies generally yield normal results and need not be routinely performed unless atypical features are present.

Patients should be advised to avoid precipitating factors. Photosensitive patients should also limit their exposure to

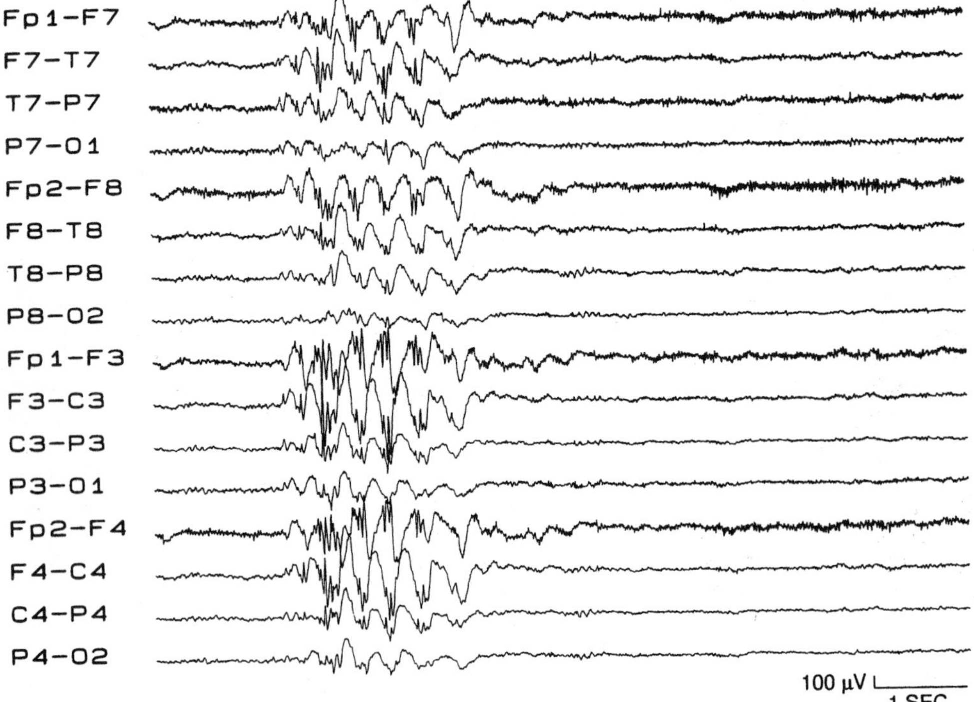

FIGURE 52–5. Generalized polyspike-wave complexes in a patient with juvenile myoclonic epilepsy.

flashing lights. Valproic acid has long been considered the drug of choice and is effective in 85 to 90 percent of patients. Lamotrigine is being used as first-line therapy with increasing frequency due to a lower incidence of adverse effects. Ethosuximide may be used for refractory absences. Uncontrolled myoclonic seizures may respond to benzodiazepines. Phenytoin, carbamazepine, primidone, phenobarbital, topiramate, zonisamide, and acetazolamide may be effective against refractory TCS. Women of childbearing age should be counseled of the teratogenic potential of the AEDs, in particular, the association of valproic acid with neural tube defects. The prognosis of JME is excellent, and seizures are well controlled in most patients if precipitating factors are avoided. Because over 90 percent of patients relapse after medication withdrawal, AED therapy should be maintained even in patients with long seizure-free intervals.

Epilepsy with Generalized Tonic-Clonic Seizures. Generalized TCS are observed in six idiopathic generalized epilepsy syndromes, which include CAE, JAE, JME, epilepsy with generalized TCS on awakening, epilepsies precipitated by specific modes of activation, and generalized idiopathic epilepsies not included in the other syndromes. A significant degree of overlap exists between these syndromes. Rarely, more than one has been present in the same patient at different periods in life.

By definition, idiopathic generalized TCS are not preceded by auras, although vague prodromal symptoms such as headache and malaise have been described hours or days before seizures. Seizures are usually infrequent; they tend to occur at the same time in the sleep-wake cycle of a given patient. Sleep deprivation, photic stimulation, alcohol consumption, menstruation, and stress are potent activators. The age of onset ranges from 6 to 20 years, usually peaking in puberty. Neurological examination results and intelligence are normal.

The family history of epilepsy exceeds that of the general population, suggesting a genetic etiology. Linkage to the gene locus of JME was demonstrated in a group of adolescents with generalized TCS on awakening, but such a phenomenon was not seen in patients with randomly occurring generalized TCS.[25] A higher incidence of microdysgenesis exists in patients with idiopathic generalized epilepsy compared with controls, but the significance of this finding is unknown. The differential diagnosis includes generalized TCS due to drugs, alcohol intoxication and withdrawal, and medical disorders, including metabolic derangements and electrolyte imbalance.

The EEG reveals diffuse, bilaterally synchronous 3.0-Hz or 4.0- to 6.0-Hz spike-wave or polyspike-wave complexes, similar to that seen in the other idiopathic generalized epilepsies. Background activity and neuroimaging study results are normal. Phenytoin, carbamazepine, valproic acid, and phenobarbital are effective, and newer antiepileptic medications such as lamotrigine, topiramate, and zonisamide may be beneficial. Patients should be instructed to avoid sleep deprivation and other precipitating factors. Eighty to 95 percent of patients experience prolonged seizure-free periods. Relapses after medication withdrawal are variable, tending to be lower in children than adults.

Cryptogenic or Symptomatic Forms

West's Syndrome. West's syndrome is an age-dependent epilepsy consisting of the triad of infantile spasms, psychomotor retardation, and a characteristic EEG pattern known as *hypsarrhythmia*. The syndrome is named for WJ West, the nineteenth century neurologist who described the features he observed in his own son. Infantile spasms occur in 24 to 42 of 100,000 births.[26] Spasms and psychomotor retardation appear in the first year of life in 85 percent of cases, the majority between 3 and 7 months. Infantile spasms are sudden, brief, usually bilaterally symmetrical flexor contractions of the neck, trunk, or limbs. Eye movements, autonomic signs, and brief lapses of consciousness may be observed. Less commonly, extension of the head, trunk, and limbs may be seen. Spasms are commonly repetitive, occurring in clusters on awakening, or during drowsiness, handling, feeding, or fever. Initially, the movements can be so slight that they may go unnoticed. Neurodevelopmental abnormalities may precede the onset of spasms. Moderate to severe cognitive disability occurs in 76 to 95 percent of patients. Associated abnormalities include generalized hypotonicity, microcephaly, paralysis, ataxia, blindness, and deafness. Because one third of patients lack the characteristic EEG features and 5 percent do not develop psychomotor retardation, the distinction between West's syndrome and the myoclonic epilepsies of infancy may be difficult. In addition, infantile spasms may be mistaken for nonepileptic phenomena that occur in infants with diffuse cerebral dysfunction, such as head-banging, colic, and decerebration.

West's syndrome is classified as symptomatic or cryptogenic based on the presence or absence of a known etiology. The proportion of symptomatic cases has increased in the years paralleling advances in neuroimaging. Tuberous sclerosis is one of the most common etiologies, comprising nearly 25 percent of symptomatic cases. Congenital malformations, including midline defects, neurocutaneous disorders, and neuronal migration disorders, comprise 30 percent of cases in neuropathological series.[27] Another 30 percent occur in the setting of perinatal complications such as trauma or hypoxic ischemic injury. Tumors, CNS infections, metabolic disorders, and inherited diseases such as Aicardi's syndrome are less common. A family history of epilepsy or febrile seizures is present in 10 to 15 percent of cases.

Although the underlying pathophysiology of infantile spasms is unknown, the age-dependency and diffuse EEG abnormalities imply widespread cortical dysfunction. Increased synthesis and activity of corticotrophin-releasing hormone (CRH) has been postulated as a mechanism that might predispose to the development of spasms. Increased CRH may follow an abnormal stress during early life or an errant response to common stressors, resulting in growth or hyperfunction of certain CRH-containing neuronal pathways. Supporting this theory are various animal studies demonstrating the excitatory effects of CRH on neurons, including those in the hippocampus, and the beneficial effects of adrenocorticotropin (ACTH) and glucocorticoids in the treatment of spasms. Although ACTH and glucocorticoids may have intrinsic anticonvulsant activity, they may also suppress CRH production via the hypothalamic-pituitary-adrenal axis and thereby alleviate the excitatory effects of CRH on certain neuronal networks.

The typical EEG reveals hypsarrhythmia, a chaotic pattern of high-amplitude slow waves with multifocal epileptiform discharges and poor interhemispheric synchrony (Fig. 52–6). Sleep is markedly disrupted and REM sleep is reduced.

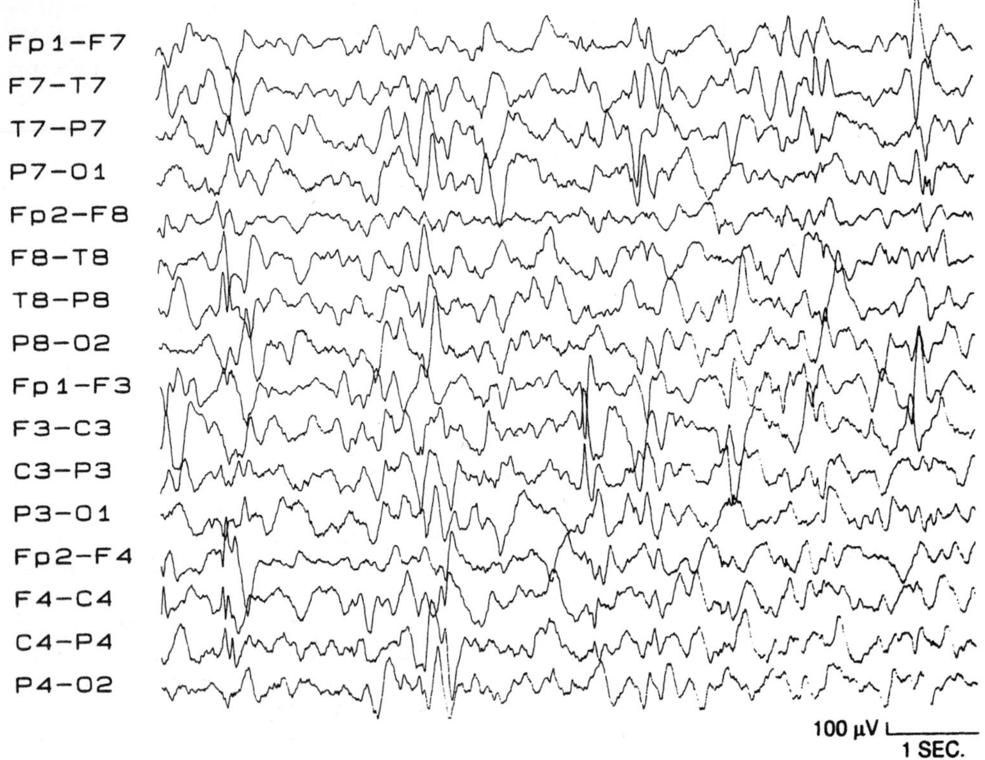

FIGURE 52–6. Hypsarrhythmia in an infant with West's syndrome.

An electrodecremental response consisting of generalized low-voltage fast activity accompanies spasms. By 3 years of age, hypsarrhythmia typically evolves to slow spike-wave complexes or multifocal spikes and sharp waves. Abnormalities on neuroimaging studies are found in over 60 percent of infants. These abnormalities include generalized atrophy, white matter hyperintensities, and focal or multifocal lesions. Regional hypometabolism on PET studies has been demonstrated in some patients with focal cortical lesions.

The dose and duration of steroid therapy has not been standardized. The most common treatment is ACTH 40 IU/d administered intramuscularly. Approximately 75 percent of patients achieve initial seizure control using this regimen. The response rate tends to increase with duration of therapy. Within 2 months of remission, however, approximately 30 to 50 percent of patients suffer relapse after the first course of steroids. The relapse rate may be somewhat lower in cryptogenic than symptomatic cases. No differences in long-term response rates are observed with low- and high-dose therapy. Although there have been few reports using oral steroids, a noncontrolled study comparing hydrocortisone with ACTH found no difference in the rate of response.[28] Others have achieved better results early on with high-dose ACTH as compared with prednisone or prednisolone therapy.[28] Side effects are common and include electrolyte disturbances and cardiac, infectious, and neuropsychiatric complications. Valproic acid, pyridoxine, vigabatrin, lamotrigine, topiramate, and immune globulin have shown some efficacy, as has nitrazepam, which is not currently commercially available in the United States. Favorable results have been reported following lesionectomy or hemispherectomy in patients with focal abnormalities on MRI or PET scans.[27]

Infantile spasm and the hypsarrhythmia tend to diminish with increasing age. Complete resolution is achieved in 50 percent of patients by 2 years and 72 to 99 percent by 5 years of age.[27] Over 50 percent of patients develop Lennox-Gastaut syndrome, multifocal or secondarily generalized epilepsy, or other forms of epilepsy during childhood. Only 5 percent of patients experience spontaneous remission without neurological sequelae. Mental retardation is observed in 50 to 60 percent of cases. The condition ultimately leads to death in 5 to 20 percent of patients. Factors associated with a poor prognosis include delay in treatment, unilateral spasms, neurological deficits, abnormal neuroimaging study results, atypical EEG manifestations, and known etiology.

Lennox-Gastaut Syndrome. Lennox-Gastaut syndrome is responsible for 2 to 3 percent of childhood epilepsies.[29] The syndrome is characterized by multiple seizure types, slow spike-wave complexes, and diffuse cognitive dysfunction. Seizure onset ranges from 1 to 8 years of age, with a peak incidence between 3 and 5 years of age. Tonic seizures during sleep or on awakening occur in virtually all cases. Atonic, atypical absence, and myoclonic seizures are commonly observed. Status epilepticus, consisting of repetitive tonic seizures or clouding of consciousness lasting hours to weeks, is seen in nearly two thirds of patients. Severe mental retardation is found in 50 percent of cases, preceding the onset of seizures in 20 to 60 percent. In addition, disturbances of behavior and personality are common.

Approximately 70 percent of cases occur in children with acquired or genetic disorders affecting the nervous system. Congenital malformations, hypoxic-ischemic encephalopathy, CNS infections, and neurocutaneous disorders, particularly tuberous sclerosis, are frequent causes. Thirty percent of patients have a history of West's syndrome. A family history of epilepsy may be found in cryptogenic cases; however, familial Lennox-Gastaut syndrome has not been reported. This syndrome should be differentiated from epilepsy with myoclonic astatic seizures. In the latter, multiple seizure types occur in previously normal children, 50 percent of whom develop mental retardation. A genetic etiology is suspected for myoclonic astatic seizures.

The EEG reveals 2.0- to 2.5-Hz slow spike-wave complexes and multifocal spikes superimposed on abnormal background activity. Runs of generalized paroxysmal fast activity and rhythmical 10-Hz spikes are observed during sleep. Atypical AS are associated with runs of slow spike-wave complexes. Tonic seizures are accompanied by an electrodecremental response or generalized 10- to 25-Hz spikes. Neuroimaging studies commonly demonstrate generalized cerebral atrophy and focal or multifocal abnormalities.

In general, seizures respond poorly to anticonvulsant treatment, and polytherapy is usually required. Benzodiazepines, valproic acid, and lamotrigine are the most effective agents, although the former may precipitate tonic status. Topiramate may also be effective. Sedation should be minimized because of the tendency for seizures to increase in sleep. Phenytoin and rectal diazepam are effective for serial tonic seizures and status epilepticus. Refractory cases may benefit from a trial of felbamate, the ketogenic diet, or corpus callosotomy, which reduces tonic and atonic seizures in some cases.

The prognosis for seizure control and mental development is poor. Daily seizures occur in most patients. Factors that portend a poor prognosis include known etiology, onset before 3 years of age, prior West's syndrome, refractory tonic seizures, and severe mental retardation. Seizures usually persist into adulthood, and fatal injuries related to seizures occur in 5 percent of cases.

SPECIAL EPILEPSY SYNDROMES

Progressive Myoclonic Epilepsies (PMEs)

The PMEs represent a group of disorders of various etiology that collectively account for 1 percent of all epilepsy syndromes.[30] The natural history varies with the specific disorder from mild neurological impairment to severe disability progressing to death in early childhood. Onset is typically during childhood or adolescence, although some of the disorders may appear at any age. Clinically, the PMEs are characterized by progressive myoclonus, seizures, variable degrees of cognitive impairment, and other neurological deficits. Myoclonus is commonly precipitated by action, sustained posture, or sensory stimulation including touch, cold, or light. Fragmentary and asynchronous myoclonic jerks primarily involving the limbs occur without associated alteration of consciousness. Myoclonus varies from mild to debilitating, depending on the specific disorder. Dementia is a characteristic sign of many of the PMEs but is not a universal feature. The severity of intellectual deterioration is related to the degree of cortical loss and varies among individuals affected with the same disorder. Other neurological findings include ataxia, spasticity, visual impairment, hearing loss, peripheral neuropathy, and extrapyramidal signs such as choreoathetosis. TCS represent the most common seizure type, although atypical absence and focal seizures are observed in some patients.

The disorders comprising the PMEs may be classified into the following categories: (1) those with well-defined biochemical defects; (2) those with a known pathological or biochemical marker yet poorly defined mechanism; and (3) the "degenerative" PMEs, in which there are no known pathological or biochemical markers (Table 52–1). The PMEs with known biochemical defects include the sialidoses, sphingolipidoses, and myoclonic epilepsy with ragged red fibers (MERRF) (see Chapter 31).

Of the PMEs with a known pathological or biochemical marker but imprecisely defined mechanism, Lafora's disease and neuronal ceroid lipofuscinosis (see Chapter 30) are most common. *Lafora's disease* is a rapidly progressive autosomal recessive disorder affecting individuals in late childhood or adolescence, although adult onset rarely occurs. Generalized TCS or partial seizures of occipital lobe origin are usually the initial manifestation. Progressive cognitive decline is a universal feature. Severe resting and action myoclonus develops early in the course of illness. Ataxia, decreased vision, and spasticity are variably present. Death occurs within 2 to 10 years of symptom onset. Skin, liver, and muscle biopsies demonstrate periodic acid–Schiff stain polyglucosan inclusions, or Lafora's bodies, which are a hallmark of the disease.

Other rare PMEs having known biological or pathological markers but poorly defined mechanisms include the *childhood form of Huntington's chorea, juvenile neuroaxonal dystrophy*, and *action myoclonus–renal insufficiency syndrome*.

Unverricht-Lundborg's disease, or Baltic myoclonus, and *dentatorubropallidoluysian atrophy* (see Chapters 34 and 35) represent the degenerative PMEs in which no pathological or biochemical markers are known to exist. Baltic myoclonus has long been shrouded in controversy, and its existence as a separate entity has only recently been confirmed. This disorder occurs predominantly in Finland, Estonia, and Sweden. The disease is autosomal recessive, and the responsible gene has been linked to the long arm of chromosome 21. The syndrome is characterized by myoclonus and TCS beginning between the ages of 8 and 13 years in individuals with no prior neurological abnormalities. The myoclonus is severe and can be precipitated by movement, stress, light, noise, or tactile stimulation. Repetitive myoclonic jerks in the morning may culminate in generalized TCS later in the day. Ataxia, intention tremor, and dysarthria usually develop in the later stages of illness. Gradual intellectual decline is observed, although severe dementia does not occur. Depression is a common feature and death typically occurs within 14 years of onset.

Dyssynergia cerebellaris myoclonica, or the Ramsay Hunt syndrome, describes a nonspecific disorder characterized by a gradually progressive cerebellar syndrome followed by myoclonus and infrequent TCS beginning in childhood or adolescence. The disorder does not represent a specific disease. Seizures and epileptiform electrographical findings are rare. Consequently, Ramsay Hunt syndrome is generally not considered a manifestation of PME, but rather it is better considered to be a presentation of various progressive ataxias.

In general, treatment of the PMEs is difficult. Myoclonus responds best to valproic acid and benzodiazepines, particularly clonazepam. L-tryptophan, 5-hydroxytryptophan with carbidopa, and piracetam may also be useful. Mechanical techniques may be useful in lessening the incapacitating effects of action myoclonus. Valproate, clonazepam, and phenobarbital alone or in combination may be used to control seizures. Phenytoin typically exacerbates ataxia and myoclonus and should be avoided.

TABLE 52–1. **Etiologies of the Progressive Myoclonic Encephalopathies**

Disorders	Age at Onset	Clinical Features	Prognosis	Laboratory/Diagnosis	Inheritance/Deficiency
With Well-Defined Biochemical Defects					
Sialidoses					
Type I	8–15	Myoclonus, visual deficit, CRS, TCS, ataxia, spasticity, burning sensation in extremities	Poor	↑ urinary sialyloligosaccharides Demonstration of enzymatic deficiency	AR, Chromosome 20q α-N-acetyl-neuramidase
Type II	Adolescence or adulthood	Myoclonus, visual deficit, CRS, TCS, ataxia, coarse facies, dysostosis multiplex, ↓ hearing, corneal opacities, dementia	Poor	↑ urinary sialyloligosaccharides Demonstration of enzymatic deficiency	AR, Chromosome 20q β-galactosidase α-N-acetyl-neuramidase
Sphingolipidoses					
Gaucher's type III	Childhood to adulthood	Myoclonus, SNGP, impaired saccades, dementia, seizures, ataxia	Poor	β-glucocerebroside storage in lymphocytes Demonstration of enzymatic deficiency	AR β-glucocerebrosidase
GM_2 gangliosidosis	Childhood to adolescence	Myoclonus, ataxia, spasticity, dystonia, tremor, seizures, optic atrophy, dementia	Poor	Demonstration of enzymatic deficiency	AR β-N-acetylhexosaminidase
MERRF	Any age	Myoclonus, TCS, dementia, ataxia, lipomas, myopathy, neuropathy, deafness, optic atrophy	Variable	Ragged-red fibers in skeletal muscle; ↑ lactate; respiratory chain defect	Substitution at pair 8344-mitochondrial DNA, sporadic
With Biological or Pathological Markers					
Ceroid lipofuscinosis					
Late infantile	1–4	Myoclonus, visual failure, optic atrophy, ataxia, speech alterations, dementia, TCS	Death by 10 years	↑ urinary dolichol phosphates; lipopigment inclusions (skin, rectal, brain) on EM	AR
Juvenile	4–10	Myoclonus, ↓ vision, optic atrophy, dementia, ataxia, EPS, seizures, dysarthria, psychosis	Death by 20 years		AR, Chromosome 16
Adult	>10	Myoclonus, ataxia, seizures, dementia, vision not impaired	Death 10 years after onset		AR
Lafora's disease	6–18	Myoclonus, occipital/TCS, ataxia, dementia, ↓ vision, depression	Death 2–10 years after onset	Polyglycan inclusions in sweat glands	AR
Degenerative					
Unverricht-Lundborg	6–15	Myoclonus, TCS, ataxia, dysarthria, depression, dementia absent	Variable, usually mild impairment	None	AR, Chromosome 21q

AR, Autosomal recessive; CRS, cherry-red spot; DNA, deoxyribonucleic acid; EM, electron microscopy; EPS, extrapyramidal signs; SNPG, supranuclear gaze palsy; TCS, tonic-clonic seizures.
Adapted from Berkovic et al[30].

Neonatal Seizures

Seizures are a common manifestation of cerebral dysfunction in the first 4 weeks of life. The incidence of neonatal seizures is unknown owing to the lack of consensus on which behaviors constitute epileptic seizures in this population.[31, 32] Neonatal seizures are paroxysmal events associated with alteration in neurological function that may or may not have an electrographical correlate. Brief, recurrent, focal or multifocal clonic, focal or generalized tonic, and myoclonic seizures are observed. Although these seizure types have already been discussed, brief mention as to their clinical appearance in neonates is appropriate.

Focal clonic seizures consist of rhythmical twitching of a limb or one side of the face that may be sustained for long periods without apparent spread. Multifocal clonic seizures are characterized by random, migratory clonic movements involving limb and facial muscles bilaterally. Tonic seizures may be focal or generalized. Generalized tonic seizures are characterized by bilaterally symmetrical extension of the trunk and limbs often associated with apnea and upward deviation of the eyes. Focal tonic seizures include asymmetrical flexion of the trunk and eye deviation. Myoclonic seizures consisting of focal or generalized brief muscle jerks occur rarely. The term *subtle seizures* includes behaviors that are not clearly epileptic, including oral-buccal-lingual movements, eye movements, pedaling, swimming, and autonomic phenomena. These signs are commonly observed in premature infants. Because of incomplete CNS myelination, which prevents synchronous and symmetrical propagation patterns, generalized TCS are not observed in the neonatal period.

Neonatal seizures are caused by a wide variety of disorders affecting the brains of neonates. Clinically, the etiologies of neonatal seizures may be classified based on age of seizure onset (Table 52–2).[33] Hypoxic-ischemic encephalopathy is the most common etiology of neonatal seizures overall and the most common etiology encountered within the first 24 hours of life. Other causes of seizures within the first day of life include bacterial meningitis, sepsis, subarachnoid hemorrhage, intrauterine infection, laceration of the tentorium or falx, drug effects, and pyridoxine dependency. From 24 to 72 hours of life, additional etiologies include cerebral contusion with subdural hemorrhage, drug withdrawal, congenital malformations, and metabolic disorders. When seizures appear beyond the third day of life, inborn errors of metabolism, herpes simplex infection, kernicterus, and neonatal adrenoleukodystrophy should be considered. Neonatal seizures should be differentiated from tremor, clonus, decerebration, and jitteriness, which commonly occur in neonates with diffuse cerebral dysfunction. Unlike epileptic events, these nonepileptic phenomena can often be elicited by limb repositioning or tactile stimulation and suppressed by physical restraint.

The EEG is important in determining adequacy of therapy and in predicting neurological outcome. Prolonged or serial recordings should be performed in pharmacologically paralyzed infants at risk for developing seizures. The severity of background abnormalities is correlated with the extent of neurological impairment. Infants with suppressed, undifferentiated, or suppression-burst patterns have a high incidence of neurological and developmental sequelae. In contrast, isolated sharp waves are commonly seen in neurologically normal neonates without seizures and are not predictive of seizures or the future development of epilepsy. Ictal patterns are more variable in neonates than in older patients; typically, they consist of runs of focal paroxysmal activity of varying frequency and polarity. Clonic, focal tonic, and generalized myoclonic seizures are consistently accompanied by EEG changes, whereas generalized tonic, focal or multifocal myoclonic, and subtle seizures are not.

Cranial ultrasound or CT studies should be performed to rule out structural lesions. CSF analysis and metabolic screens are indicated when infection or inborn errors of metabolism are suspected.

Severely impaired neonates with clinical seizures unaccompanied by EEG changes should not be treated with anticonvulsant medication. In this setting, AEDs are not likely to reduce the clinical manifestations, and affected patients have a high incidence of adverse reactions. Antiepileptic drug therapy is recommended when recurrent clinical events are accompanied by EEG seizure patterns. Phenobarbital is the most widely used agent, although phenytoin and benzodiazepines are also effective. Because protein binding is altered in sick infants, monitoring of total and free drug levels is advised. Pyridoxine, 50 to 100 mg, should be administered intravenously with simultaneous EEG recording when seizures are refractory to conventional agents. In the absence of CNS pathology and significant EEG abnormalities, neurologically normal infants do not require prolonged therapy and should be withdrawn from medication before hospital discharge. Neonates with abnormal findings on neurological examinations and focal cerebral pathology have a high risk of recurrence and should be treated for longer periods.

The mortality rate for neonates with seizures is 40 percent for full-term and 50 percent for premature infants. Subsequent epilepsy develops in nearly 25 percent of patients. Aside from etiology and findings on neurological examination, the presence and severity of background abnormalities on EEG are the most reliable predictors of outcome. Most infants with normal background features on EEG have normal development, whereas severe background abnormalities, independent of electrographical seizures, portend a poor prognosis.

Febrile Convulsions

Febrile seizures occur in 2 to 5 percent of children, representing the most common seizure disorder in this age group.[34] Approximately 30 percent of patients experience a single recurrence, and of this group, half will experience multiple seizures.[35] The age of onset ranges from 3 months to 5 years with a peak incidence from 18 to 24 months. Seizures occur during a sudden rise in temperature early in the course of an illness in the absence of intracranial infection or a defined etiology. Simple febrile seizures, which are single, generalized convulsions less than 15 minutes in duration, comprise 80 to 90 percent of cases. Seizures that exceed 15 minutes in duration, occur more than once in a 24-hour period, or show focal motor manifestations are classified as complex or complicated febrile seizures. Patients with complex febrile seizures have a higher rate of subsequent epilepsy.

The risk of seizures in family members of patients with febrile seizures is two to three times that of the general population. Generalized epileptiform activity and photosensitivity

TABLE 52–2. **Etiologies of Neonatal Seizures by Peak Time of Onset**

Disorder	24 Hours	24–72 Hours	3–7 Days	7–28 Days
Cerebrovascular	Hypoxic ischemic encephalopathy Subarachnoid hemorrhage Intraventricular hemorrhage	Intraventricular hemorrhage (preemies) Cerebral infarction Intraventricular hemorrhage Subdural hemorrhage Subarachnoid hemorrhage	Cerebral infarction Intracerebral hemorrhage	
Traumatic	Laceration of tentorium or falx	Cerebral contusion		
Infectious	Bacterial meningitis Sepsis Intrauterine infection	Bacterial meningitis Sepsis		Herpes simplex encephalitis
Iatrogenic	Anesthetic toxicity	Drug withdrawal		
Nutritional	Pyridoxine dependency Hypoglycemia	Pyridoxine dependency Hypoglycemia	Hypocalcemia	
Developmental		Congential malformations Neurocutaneous disorders	Congenital malformations Neurocutaneous disorders	Congenital malformations
Metabolic		Hypoparathyroidism Hypocalcemia Glycine encephalopathy Glycogen synthase deficiency Urea cycle disorders Nonketotic hyperglycinemia	Hypoparathyroidism Kernicterus Ketotic hyperglycinemia Urea cycle disorders	Adrenoleukodystrophy Fructose dysmetabolism Gaucher's disease type II GM_1 gangliosidosis Ketotic hyperglycinemia Maple syrup urine disease Urea cycle disorders

Adapted from Fenichel[33].

have been reported in asymptomatic relatives of affected patients. These findings support a genetic etiology, although the mode of inheritance is unknown. Similarly, the relationship between febrile seizures and MTLE is poorly understood. Prolonged febrile convulsions are associated with various physiological alterations capable of producing ischemic changes in hippocampal neurons. Whether these changes are operative in the development of epilepsy or whether they simply represent the effect of recurrent seizures remains a matter of debate.

Febrile seizures should be distinguished from seizures due to intracranial infection, electrolyte disturbance, inborn errors of metabolism, and nonepileptic events such as breath-holding spells. The extent of laboratory and radiological evaluation depends on results of the clinical history and examination. Because the condition of most children with simple febrile seizures has returned to baseline by the time of evaluation, laboratory testing, EEG, and neuroimaging studies are generally unrevealing. Patients with complex febrile seizures, especially those with focal motor manifestations, should undergo a neuroimaging study to rule out structural lesions. CSF analysis is indicated in cases of suspected CNS infection. Patients presenting with their first febrile seizure before 6 months and after 5 years of age should be thoroughly evaluated because secondary causes are more likely.

Single seizures do not necessarily require treatment with AEDs. Repetitive seizures and status epilepticus should be terminated with intravenous benzodiazepines or phenobarbital. Prophylactic anticonvulsants are usually not recommended because of the high incidence of behavioral and cognitive adverse reactions and their failure to reduce the risk of subsequent epilepsy. Parents should be assured of the benign nature of the disorder and instructed in the administration of antipyretics, tepid sponge bathing, and emergency first aid. Rectal diazepam should be considered in children with frequent febrile illnesses. The risk of recurrent febrile seizures is highest in children younger than 1 year of age and those with complicated seizures. Two to 9 percent of affected children develop afebrile seizures. Patients with abnormal findings on neurological examinations or abnormal development, family history of afebrile seizures, and complicated seizures have a higher risk of subsequent epilepsy.

Acquired Epileptic Aphasia

Approximately 200 cases of acquired epileptic aphasia, or Landau-Kleffner syndrome, are reported in the literature.[36] This syndrome is characterized by an acquired aphasia with epileptiform activity over the temporal or temporo-parieto-occipital regions and psychomotor and behavioral difficulities. An auditory verbal agnosia and reduction of spontaneous speech typically begin before 6 years of age, after the initial acquisition of verbal language. Consequently, many patients are misdiagnosed as deaf or autistic. Infrequent tonic-clonic, focal motor, and atonic seizures are observed in 75 percent of cases. Psychomotor disturbances or personality disorders occur in 70 percent of patients. Seizures persisting into adolescence tend to be infrequent and nocturnal. Males are affected twice as often as females. Interruption of subcortical fibers resulting in the deafferentation of language cortex has been hypothesized as the underlying pathogenesis; however, no etiological factors have been identified. In cases in which brain biopsies were performed, no specific abnormalities have been identified.[36]

The waking EEG in Landau-Kleffner syndrome is characterized by multifocal spikes in the temporal and parieto-occipital regions superimposed on normal background activity and markedly enhanced sleep. Audiography, auditory evoked potentials, and neuroimaging study results are normal. Landau-Kleffner syndrome bears striking resemblance to epilepsy with continuous spike waves during slow-wave sleep (CSWS). In both disorders, EEG abnormalities are markedly accentuated, and at times continuous, during sleep. Seizures are more frequent and global neurological deterioration emerges rather than aphasia in CSWS, however.

Administration of intravenous diazepam may produce dramatic but transient improvements in language and EEG abnormalities. The benefit of long-term anticonvulsant therapy has not been demonstrated, however. In most cases, seizures and EEG abnormalities undergo remission spontaneously by 15 years of age, and speech typically recovers by adulthood. Onset after 6 years of age and early speech therapy are associated with a more favorable prognosis.

Epilepsy and Pregnancy

Epilepsy is the most common neurological disorder encountered by obstetricians. Approximately 0.3 to 0.5 percent of all pregnancies and over 1 million women of child-bearing age are affected.[37] Seizure frequency during pregnancy typically parallels preconception seizure control, and 50 to 75 percent of women experience no significant change. Breakthrough seizures are usually due to noncompliance, stress, or sleep deprivation. The incidence of status epilepticus is similar to nonpregnant epileptic controls. The risk of spontaneous abortion, bleeding diatheses, premature labor, pre-eclampsia, eclampsia, and placental defects in women with epilepsy is two to four times higher than in nonepileptic women. In most cases, labor and delivery progress without complications. Elective cesarean section should be performed when there is poor seizure control during the third trimester, in cases of severe stress-induced seizures, and in patients with neurological deficits interfering with labor. Emergency cesarean section is indicated in women with recurrent seizures during labor and delivery and when seizures result in fetal distress.

Most seizures during pregnancy occur in association with subtherapeutic anticonvulsant levels. The serum concentration of AEDs gradually declines during pregnancy, reaching a nadir near term and returning to preconception levels by 8 to 12 weeks postpartum. During pregnancy, a reduction in protein binding leads to a higher percentage of unbound, free drug that is more rapidly excreted by the kidneys. The dilutional effects of water retention and increased hepatic microsomal activity, which enhances drug metabolism, are additional factors that contribute to subtherapeutic drug concentrations and breakthrough seizures.

Seizures may be the initial manifestation of a host of diseases that present during pregnancy. Ischemic stroke, paradoxical embolus, vasculitis, and metastatic choriocarcinoma may appear at any time during pregnancy with seizures and focal neurological deficits. Vascular anomalies should be considered when seizures develop in pregnancy because the risk of bleeding due to arteriovenous malformations and aneurysms tends to increase as pregnancy progresses. Eclampsia, oxytocin-induced water intoxication, toxicity of local anesthetics, amniotic fluid embolus, thrombotic thrombocytopenic purpura, cerebral venous thrombosis, pheochromocytoma, and subarachnoid hemorrhage may produce seizures in the peripartum period. These disorders should be considered in the differential diagnosis of patients with new onset of seizures during pregnancy.

The evaluation and treatment of pregnant women with epilepsy are summarized in Table 52–3.[38] Patients should be treated with monotherapy when possible, because the incidence of fetal malformations increases with the number of AEDs administered. Total and free antiepileptic drug levels should be monitored regularly. Serum drug concentrations should be maintained in the therapeutic range near term to prevent seizures during labor. Dosage adjustments should be made when seizures occur that pose a significant risk to the mother and fetus.

Several anticonvulsants may lead to folate deficiency, which is associated with an increased incidence of neural tube defects in offspring of epileptic women. Women with epilepsy of childbearing age should take multivitamins containing folate 1 mg/d. Folate therapy should be instituted in those not already taking the preparation as soon as pregnancy is recognized. Fetal ultrasound and maternal alpha-fetoprotein testing should be performed during the second trimester to assess for fetal malformations. In women taking carbamazepine or valproic acid, the risk of fetal neural tube defects is 1 percent and 2 percent, respectively. These drugs should be avoided in women with a family history or prior pregnancy complicated by such defects.

Obstetrical and neonatal outcome is normal in over 90 percent of pregnant patients with epilepsy. Proper nutrition, regular prenatal care, folate supplementation, and optimal seizure control improve the chance of a favorable outcome. Women with new onset of seizures should be carefully evaluated for medical and neurological etiologies, drugs, and alcohol use. If nonepileptic events are suspected, ambulatory EEG or video EEG monitoring should be considered before empirical institution of anticonvulsant therapy.

Epileptic women of childbearing age taking hepatic enzyme–inducing AEDs and oral contraceptive agents should be advised of the risk of contraceptive failure due to the accelerated metabolism of steroids. To prevent pregnancy, moderate- or high-dose estradiol preparations or barrier methods are recommended. In women planning pregnancy, anticonvulsant regimens should be reassessed before conception, and the agent most likely to control seizures should be maintained at the lowest effective serum concentration. Drug withdrawal may be considered in patients with prolonged seizure-free periods and seizures not impairing consciousness.

TABLE 52–3. **Guidelines for the Management of Epilepsy During Pregnancy**

- Baseline antiepileptic drug (AED) levels (total/free) and folate (serum/RBC)
- Folate supplementation 0.5 to 1.0 mg/d
- Maternal alpha-fetoprotein at week 15 to 16
- AED levels and fetal ultrasound at 18 to 19 weeks
- Repeat fetal ultrasound at 22 to 24 weeks
- AED levels at 34 to 36 weeks; make adjustments to assure therapeutic drug levels at term
- Vitamin K 20 mg/d during eighth month or 10 mg IV 4 hours before birth *and* 1 mg IM to newborn at birth
- Monthly AED levels postpartum for 12 weeks

Status Epilepticus

Status epilepticus (SE) is a medical emergency that demands prompt diagnosis and treatment if severe neurological sequelae and death are to be minimized. An estimated 125,000 to 195,000 episodes of SE occur in the United States annually, resulting in 22,000 to 42,000 deaths.[39] Despite improvements in medical management, the incidence of significant morbidity and mortality remains high. SE is defined as continuous clinical or electrical seizure activity or repetitive seizures with incomplete neurological recovery interictally for a period of at least 30 minutes. Patients having continuous seizure activity for 10 minutes or longer should be treated as if in SE, because most seizures terminate spontaneously within 1 to 2 minutes. In addition, impending SE should be suspected in patients experiencing three or more TCS within a 24-hour period, particularly when this represents an increase from the typical frequency.

Status epilepticus is classified as generalized or partial (focal), and convulsive or nonconvulsive. Generalized convulsive status includes tonic-clonic, tonic, clonic, or myoclonic SE, although the majority of cases consist of recurrent TCS. Nonconvulsive SE includes absence and complex partial SE, both of which are characterized by clouding of consciousness with or without minor motor manifestations. EEG is usually required to distinguish the two. Any type of simple partial seizure, including seizures with sensory, motor, language, autonomic, or psychic manifestations, can evolve into SE. Partial SE characterized by focal clonic activity is referred to as *epilepsia partialis continua*. This condition is seen in patients with lesions involving the perirolandic region such as in children with Rasmussen's encephalitis.

In adult patients, the most common type of SE is secondary generalized convulsive SE (GCSE), characterized by intermittent or continuous overt convulsive activity accompanied by coma and epileptiform activity on EEG. The manifestations change over time such that discrete convulsions give way to increasingly subtle clinical manifestations, which is a condition known as *subtle SE*. Eventually, electrical status without clinical manifestations is all that remains. Occasionally, subtle SE occurs without prior convulsive activity in patients with severe diffuse cerebral dysfunction. Generalized convulsive activity produces various systemic effects, including hypoxia, hyperpyrexia, blood pressure instability, and cerebral dysautoregulation. Metabolic derangements, including respiratory and metabolic acidosis, hyperazotemia, hypokalemia, hyponatremia, hyperglycemia followed by hypoglycemia, and marked elevations of plasma prolactin, glucagon, growth hormone, and corticotropin may be observed. Rhabdomyolysis may produce myoglobinuria and renal failure.

Acute CNS insults, including anoxia, head injury, stroke, neoplasm, and infection, account for 50 percent of cases. In children, the most common precipitants are fever and infection, whereas cerebrovascular disease predominates in older adults. Approximately 20 percent of all SE cases occur in epileptic patients during medication adjustment or as a result of noncompliance. In one third of patients, the cause for SE is undetermined. SE should be suspected in patients with unexplained coma with or without motor manifestations. Nonepileptic phenomena, including tremor, myoclonus, eye movements, and oral-buccal movements that frequently occur following anoxia, brain stem or bilateral cerebral ischemia, drug overdose, and severe metabolic and electrolyte disturbances may be difficult to differentiate clinically from nonconvulsive SE. Occasionally, prolonged psychogenic seizures are misinterpreted and treated as SE.

A protocol for the treatment of GCSE is provided in Table 52–4. Treatment should begin with assessment of cardiorespiratory function. An oral airway should be secured and oxygen administered when needed. Blood should be drawn for AED, glucose, blood urea nitrogen, electrolytes, calcium, magnesium, and drug screens. An intravenous infusion with isotonic saline solution should be placed and glucose 25 g and thiamine 100 mg administered. A history and neurological examination should be performed once the patient's condition is stabilized. When an acute CNS insult or infection is suspected, further investigations, including neuroimaging (cranial CT) and lumbar puncture, should be performed once treatment is initiated. EEG is useful when the diagnosis of GCSE is in doubt, during pharmacological coma, or when assessing the adequacy of treatment.

Generalized convulsive seizures and electrical seizures in patients with subtle SE should be terminated as rapidly as possible, because the duration of SE is a major determinant of morbidity and mortality. Absence, complex partial, and focal motor SE may be treated less aggressively, because the risk of neurological sequelae is significantly lower. GCSE should be treated with medications administered intravenously until seizures are aborted. The most common cause of treatment failure is when the appropriate medication is administered in inadequate dosages via an inappropriate route.

Once an intravenous line has been secured, lorazepam (0.1 mg/kg (no faster than 2 mg/min) should be administered. Because of its high lipid solubility and rapid CNS entry, diazepam frequently abolishes seizure activity within minutes, only for seizures to recur within 30 minutes as the drug redistributes to other fatty tissues. Consequently, lorazepam is preferred for its longer duration of action.

In most circumstances, following treatment with a benzodiazepine, fosphenytoin should be administered. Fosphenytoin, a phosphate ester of phenytoin, was released by the Food and Drug Administration (FDA) in 1996 for use in the treatment of escalating seizures requiring parenteral treatment and SE. Its advantages over phenytoin include a more rapid rate of infusion (150 mg/min) and lower incidence of hypotension and cardiac arrhythmias. If seizure activity continues after fosphenytoin loading, additional boluses should be given to achieve a serum concentration of 25 to 30 mcg/mL. This regimen is effective in terminating over 90 percent of cases. Anticonvulsant medications should be administered in a setting equipped to provide advanced cardiac life support. Patients should be continuously monitored during parenteral administration of AEDs for signs of respiratory depression, hypotension, and cardiac arrhythmias.

If seizures persist, elective intubation should be performed before further treatment is administered, particularly if other CNS depressants have been previously administered. Only 6 percent of cases prove refractory to this approach and require anesthetic doses of barbiturates titrated to achieve burst-suppression. With the availability of agents with shorter half-lives, phenobarbital is used less frequently. Pentobarbital is the most commonly used agent for refractory SE. A loading dose of 5 mg/kg followed by a maintenance infusion of 1 to 3 mg/kg/hr titrated to burst-suppression is recommended. Treatment is continued for 6 to 48 hours, after which the drug is withdrawn and the EEG observed for recurrence of seizure activity. Midazolam, lidocaine, and propofol have

TABLE 52–4. **Management of Status Epilepticus**

Step 1

Assess Airway, Breathing, Circulation

1. Administer O_2, monitor cardiac rhythm, oxygen saturation, and vital signs
2. Establish intravenous line with normal saline
3. Bedside glucose test
4. Draw blood for AED levels, CBC, electrolytes, calcium and magnesium, glucose and toxicology screen
5. Administer thiamine 100 mg and dextrose 50% 50 mL IV (D_{25} 2 mL/kg in children)
6. Obtain history and perform examination

Step 2

1. Administer intravenous lorazepam 0.1 mg/kg in adults, 0.05 to 0.5 mg/kg in children (up to 2 mg/min) or diazepam 0.25 mg/kg in adults, 0.1 to 1.0 mg/kg in children (up to 5 mg/min). Repeat after 10 minutes if seizures persist
2. Administer fosphenytoin 20 PE (phenytoin equivalents)/kg load (up to 150 PE/min)
3. If seizures persist, give additional fosphenytoin 5–10 PE/kg to a total dose of 30 PE mg/kg or serum concentration of 30 μg/mL

Step 3

1. Intubate, place arterial line, and draw arterial blood gas and phenytoin level
2. Consider intravenous phenobarbital 20 mg/kg (100 mg/min or 3 mg/kg/min in children)

Step 4

1. Consider pharmacological coma with pentobarbital 5–8 mg/kg load, followed by continuous infusion of 2–4 mg/kg/hr titrated to burst-suppression for 6 to 48 hrs

   or

2. Midazolam 0.2 mg/kg load followed by continuous infusion beginning at 1 μg/kg/min increasing by 1 μg/kg/min every 15–30 minutes as needed to a maximum rate of 10 μg/kg/min

been used for refractory SE; however, no controlled studies using these agents are available, and experience with them is limited. For the treatment of absence SE, intravenous benzodiazepines followed by ethosuximide or valproic acid are usually effective. Depending on the situation, simple and complex partial SE may be treated with oral anticonvulsants, fosphenytoin (IM or IV), or intravenous benzodiazepines. The use of phenobarbital or pharmacological coma is rarely indicated.

Morbidity and mortality in SE are largely dependent on the speed of intervention, age of the patient, and etiology. Although mortality in adults ranges from 1 to 32 percent, subtle SE and GCSE exceeding 1 hour in duration carry a poor prognosis. A favorable outcome is observed in children, patients with pre-existing epilepsy, and individuals with drug-induced SE.

Nonepileptic Seizures

Nonepileptic seizures, also referred to as *psychogenic* or *pseudo* seizures, constitute 15 to 20 percent of admissions to epilepsy units.[40] Affected women outnumber men by a factor of 3.5:1. Psychogenic seizures are infrequent before 12 years of age but have been observed in children as young as 5 years old. Peak incidence is in the third to fourth decades, although onset may occur later in life. The incidence of epilepsy in patients with psychogenic seizures ranges from 10 to 60 percent.[40]

Psychogenic seizures are episodes involving affective, autonomic, or sensorimotor manifestations that are precipitated by emotional distress. Palpitations, choking sensations, dizziness, malaise, acral paresthesias, sensory disturbances, crying, and alterations in consciousness with or without motor manifestations are observed. Unlike epileptic seizures, motor activity generally consists of side-to-side head movements, opisthotonus, pelvis thrusting, trembling, and random asynchronous movements. Micturition, injuries, amnesia, and postictal somnolence may occur. Psychogenic seizures tend to be less stereotyped, more gradual in evolution, and longer in duration than epileptic seizures.

Psychogenic seizures are believed to represent subconsciously mediated behavior resulting from emotional distress. Unlike malingerers, affected individuals do not feign illness for obvious secondary gain. Psychogenic seizures occur in patients with conversion disorders, anxiety and panic disorder, depression, post-traumatic stress disorder, schizophrenia, and personality disorders. Additionally, over two thirds of patients have a history of sexual or physical abuse in childhood.

Patients with psychogenic seizures frequently present to neurologists or epilepsy monitoring units having been diagnosed with epilepsy and treated with anticonvulsants. Seizures may be difficult to differentiate from frontal lobe seizures characterized by violent motor activity and sexual automatisms. Malingering and physiological nonepileptic events such as cerebral hypoperfusion, hypoxia, hypoglycemia, electrolyte disturbances, alcohol and drugs effects, migraine, gastroesophageal reflux, parasomnias, and movement disorders including paroxysmal dyskinesias may produce similar symptoms.

The EEG is the most valuable diagnostic tool. The persistence of normal background activity in a comatose patient essentially rules out epilepsy as a cause of that spell. Because 30 percent of complex partial seizures and 70 percent of simple partial seizures are not accompanied by EEG changes, however, events characterized by subtle behavior without complete loss of consciousness should be interpreted with caution. Induction procedures are commonly employed to provoke seizures in the EEG laboratory. Serum prolactin is elevated following 60 percent of complex partial seizures and 90 percent of TCS, provided that the serum sample is obtained within 10 minutes of the seizure. Normal values do not reliably predict a nonepileptic event, however.

The patient should be informed of the diagnosis of psychogenic seizures, and consideration should be made for AED withdrawal. A psychiatric evaluation should be obtained and underlying psychological disorders addressed. Psychotherapy and pharmacological treatment of psychiatric disease is indicated in most cases. Typically, a team approach involving neurologist, psychiatrist, and therapist is most effective.

Neuropharmacology of the Antiepileptic Drugs

PHARMACOLOGICAL PRINCIPLES

Pharmacokinetics refers to drug concentrations and their variability over time based on absorption, distribution, and elimination (Table 52–5). Absorption is defined as the passage of a drug from the site of administration to the vascular space. Absorption is measured in terms of rate and bioavailability, which is the amount of drug that reaches the systemic circulation. Both vary with route of administration and drug formulation. Bioavailability is 100 percent following intravenous administration, the route against which others are measured. With oral administration, absorption is influenced by gastric pH, bowel motility, splanchnic blood flow, and concomitant medications and food intake. Large variations in absorption occur with intramuscular administration, making this an undesirable route if high drug concentrations are required rapidly.

Following absorption, drugs are distributed into other compartments. The extent of distribution is expressed as the volume of distribution (V_d), a hypothetical volume of total body fluid within which a drug is evenly distributed. Distribution depends on extent of protein binding, solubility, and blood flow. Most AEDs are partially protein bound, and only the free, or unbound, fraction penetrates the blood-brain barrier to produce an effect. The V_d required to dissolve an amount of drug (D) to achieve a given concentration (ΔC = desired minus actual concentration) can be calculated by using the equation

$V_d = D \div \Delta C$
By solving for
$D = V_d \times \Delta C$
the dose of drug required to achieve a particular serum concentration can be determined.

Elimination of anticonvulsant medications occurs through hepatic metabolism and renal excretion. The major metabolic pathway in humans is the hepatocyte endoplasmic

TABLE 52-5. **Pharmacokinetic Parameters of Antiepileptic Drugs***

Drug	V_d (L/kg)	Protein Binding (%)	$t_{1/2}$ (hr)	Elimination Route (%)		Maintenance Dose (mg/kg/d)	Dosing Interval	Loading Dose (mg/kg)	Range (μg/mL)
				Renal	Liver				
Carbamazepine	0.8	75	9–15	1	99	10–25	BID–TID	—	4–12
Clonazepam	3.0	85	20–60	<5	>90	0.03–0.3	BID	—	5–70†
Clorazepate	1.2	97	50–100	<5	>90	0.5–1.0	BID	—	0.5–1.9†
Ethosuximide	0.7	0	30–60	<20	>80	15–40	q D	—	40–100
Felbamate	0.8	25	13–22	50	50	15–60	BID–TID	—	30–100
Gabapentin	0.7	0	5–7	100	0	1800–3600 mg/d	TID	—	4–8
Lamotrigine	1.0	55	12–62	10	90	300–500 mg/d	BID	—	2–4
Levetiracetam	0.5–0.7	<10	6–8	100	0	1000–3000 mg/d	BID	—	20–60
Oxcarbazepine	0.8	40	9	1	99	1200–2400 mg/d	BID	—	5–50
Phenobarbital	0.6	45	75–110	25	75	1–4	q D	18–20	10–40
Phenytoin	0.8	90	9–36	5	95	4–7	q D, BID	15–20	10–20
Primidone	0.7	0–20	10–15	40	60	10–20	TID	—	5–15
Tiagabine	1.4	96	7–9	2	98	32–56 mg/d	BID–QID	—	5–70
Topiramate	0.7	15	12–24	65	35	200–800 mg/d	BID	—	2–25
Valproate	0.2	90	6–18	2	98	10–60	BID–TID	—	50–150
Zonisamide	1.5	40	63	35	65	100–600 mg/d	q D	—	10–40

*Normal values for adults on monotherapy; pediatric dosages may vary.
†ng/mL.
Range, Therapeutic range of serum concentration; qD, once daily; BID, twice daily; TID, three times daily; V_d, volume of distribution; $t_{1/2}$, elimination half-life.

reticulum P-450 mixed oxidase system. Phenobarbital, primidone, phenytoin, carbamazepine, and topiramate induce this enzyme system, thereby facilitating metabolism of other hepatically metabolized drugs, including oral contraceptives, folic acid, warfarin, quinidine, and steroids. Conversely, valproic acid is an enzyme inhibitor which, when combined with other hepatically metabolized agents, impairs their metabolism, potentially leading to toxicity. Analgesics, cardiac drugs, antimicrobials, antiulcer agents, and psychotropics may also interfere with the metabolism of AEDs and produce toxic reactions. Carbamazepine, valproic acid, primidone, oxcarbazepine, and diazepam are converted to active metabolites having additional anticonvulsant properties.

Half-life ($t_{1/2}$) is the time required for the serum concentration of a drug to decrease by 50 percent following complete absorption and distribution of a single dose. A drug's half-life determines the dosing frequency and, as a rule, the dosing interval should not exceed one half-life. Drugs with short half-lives should be administered multiple times per day to prevent large fluctuations in serum concentration that may produce adverse effects or breakthrough seizures. Those with longer half-lives may be administered once daily, which generally improves compliance.

A drug's half-life may be altered by hepatic enzyme induction or inhibition and impaired renal function. With the exception of phenytoin, metabolism of anticonvulsant medications follows linear, or first-order, kinetics, in which the rate of metabolism is directly proportional to serum concentration. Phenytoin is metabolized through nonlinear, or zero-order, kinetics. The enzymes responsible for the elimination of phenytoin become saturated at levels within the therapeutic range. Once enzyme systems are saturated, the rate of metabolism fails to increase proportionately with further dosage increments, and modest increases in dosage result in marked increases in serum concentration. To avoid toxicity, the daily dosage of phenytoin should be increased by no more than 50 mg when serum concentration exceeds 10 to 12 μg/mL.

PRINCIPLES OF ANTIEPILEPTIC DRUG TREATMENT

The selection of an AED is based on efficacy against specific seizure types and the potential for producing adverse reactions. First-line agents against TCS include phenytoin, carbamazepine, valproic acid, oxcarbazepine, and lamotrigine. Ethosuximide, valproic acid, and lamotrigine are effective against AS. Valproic acid and lamotrigine are the drugs effective against tonic-clonic, absence, and myoclonic seizures. Myoclonic seizures are responsive to valproic acid, lamotrigine, and benzodiazepines. Carbamazepine and phenytoin, oxcarbazepine, lamotrigine, and valproic acid are effective in the treatment of partial seizures. Although primidone and phenobarbital are effective against tonic-clonic and partial seizures, they are not considered first-line agents because of their sedative properties. In controlled trials, most of the newer AEDs have been shown to produce a 30 to 50 percent reduction in seizures in approximately one third of patients with partial epilepsy.[41–47] Lamotrigine is also effective in the treatment of seizures in patients with Lennox-Gastaut syndrome. Topiramate is effective as adjunctive treatment of generalized seizures.[48] Felbamate has a broad spectrum of action but is no longer indicated for routine use because of hematological and hepatic toxicity. The potential for long-term complications has not been established for newer AEDs, and their cost is significantly greater than the older agents.

Dose-related adverse effects commonly occur in patients taking anticonvulsant medication and usually resolve spontaneously or with reduction in dosage or discontinuation of the drug. Gastrointestinal distress, dizziness, dysarthria, diplopia, and ataxia are commonly reported with the use of all of the AEDs. The benzodiazepines, phenobarbital, primidone, and phenytoin may produce sedation and cognitive impairment. Skin eruptions represent the most commonly encountered idiosyncratic reaction associated with AEDs. Generally appearing within the first 3 months of treatment, rashes are usual benign, and they resolve with dosage reduction or discontinuation. Severe reactions, including Stevens-Johnson syndrome, exfoliative dermatitis, and toxic epidermal neurolysis, occur rarely. AEDs can produce megaloblastic anemia, leukopenia, thrombocytopenia, aplastic anemia, asymptomatic elevations of hepatic transaminases, and life-threatening hepatotoxicity. Chronic idiosyncratic reactions include disorders of connective tissue and nervous system, endocrinopathies, and autoimmune disease.

DRUG INTERACTIONS

The goal of treatment is to control seizures using a single agent maintained at serum concentrations that do not produce adverse effects. If seizures persist, the dosage should be gradually increased until seizure control is achieved or intolerable side effects appear. Trough blood levels should be obtained during steady-state conditions, generally no sooner than five half-lives after a dosage adjustment. A second agent is introduced only after an adequate trial of the first drug has failed. If polytherapy is required, drugs should be chosen with different mechanisms of action and side effect profiles to maximize anticonvulsant benefit and minimize toxicity. Interactions among the various AEDs must also be kept in mind in the selection of drug combinations (Table 52–6). Patients whose seizures continue despite adequate trials of several AEDs should be referred to an epilepsy center for further evaluation.

Clinical and laboratory monitoring is routinely performed in patients taking the older AEDs. The utility of routine laboratory monitoring in patients treated with the newer agents is unclear. Blood levels help to achieve maximal medication effect and identify patients who are noncompliant. The older agents have an established therapeutic range within which most patients experience an improvement in seizure control and few or no adverse reactions. The therapeutic range should serve as a general guide only. Some patients become seizure-free with subtherapeutic serum concentrations, whereas others require levels in the "toxic" range to achieve satisfactory seizure control.

No standard recommendations exist for the timing of laboratory monitoring. Hematological parameters should be assessed periodically during carbamazepine, ethosuximide, and valproic acid therapy. Hepatic transaminases should be monitored in patients taking carbamazepine, valproic acid, phenytoin, primidone, and phenobarbital. Hematological and hepatic status must be monitored regularly in patients treated with felbamate. Laboratory monitoring is particularly important in the setting of hepatic or renal dysfunction and during pregnancy. Free levels are useful when protein binding is altered, such as in pregnancy, uremia, and hypoalbuminemia, and with highly protein-bound drugs such as phenytoin and valproic acid.

CLINICAL USE AND ADVERSE EFFECTS OF SPECIFIC ANTIEPILEPTIC DRUGS

Phenobarbital, first marketed in the United States in 1912, is the oldest of the currently available AEDs. It is effective against partial, tonic-clonic, tonic, and clonic seizures and is the most commonly prescribed agent for neonatal seizures. Phenobarbital enhances GABA transmission by interacting with the $GABA_A$ receptor-chloride channel complex, and it acts at glutamate receptors to decrease excitatory synaptic transmission. Long-term use is associated with chronic connective tissue disorders. Safety, affordability, and a broad spectrum of action contribute to its continued use in the United States and worldwide. Common neurological side effects include sedation, nystagmus, ataxia, and irritability and hyperactivity in children. Phenobarbital is available in 16 mg capsules, 8-, 15-, 16-, 30-, 32-, 60-, 65-, and 100-mg tablets, elixir (15 mg/ 5 mL and 20 mg/5 mL), and injectable formulations.

Primidone has been available in the United States since 1954 for the treatment of partial and generalized seizures. Primidone is metabolized to phenobarbital and phenylethymalonamide, both of which possess anticonvulsant properties. The adverse effects are similar to phenobarbital, although initiation of primidone is associated with a higher incidence of GI distress, dizziness, ataxia, and diplopia. Primidone is available in 50- and 250-mg scored tablets and elixir (250 mg/5 mL).

Phenytoin became available in 1938 and remains a first-line agent in the treatment of tonic-clonic and partial seizures and status epilepticus. Its primary mechanism of action is inhibition of sustained high-frequency firing through blockade of voltage-gated Na^+ channels. Phenytoin precipitates in muscle and can cause tissue necrosis if administered intramuscularly. Long-term complications include gingival hyperplasia, hirsutism, coarsening of facial features, hyperpigmentation, acne, pseudolymphoma, cerebellar degeneration, movement disorders including chorea and dystonia, and disorders of vitamin D metabolism. Phenytoin is available in 30- and 100-mg extended release capsules, 30- and 100-mg prompt release capsules, 50-mg chewable tablets, suspension (125 mg/5 mL), and injectable forms. *Fosphenytoin sodium*, a phosphate ester prodrug of phenytoin, has essentially replaced the injectable formulation of phenytoin. Because of its higher water solubility, fosphenytoin can be safely administered intramuscularly and intravenously at a rate of 150 mg phenytoin equivalent per minute.

Ethosuximide has been marketed in the United States since 1960 for the treatment of AS. It is the drug of choice in AE without TCS, against which it is ineffective. Ethosuximide blocks T-type Ca^{2+} channels that trigger and sustain rhythmical burst discharges in thalamic neurons. Trimethadione, which is no longer available in the United States, is the only other agent with a similar mechanism of action. Ethosuximide does not induce hepatic microsomal enzymes and is not protein-bound. Idiosyncratic reactions include headache, hiccups, blood dyscrasias, lupus-like syndromes, behavioral disturbances, and parkinsonism. Ethosuximide is available in 250-mg capsules and syrup (250 mg/5 mL).

Carbamazepine, available in the United States since 1974, has a similar mechanism and spectrum of action as phenytoin. The carbamazepine–10, 11-epoxide metabolite also pos-

TABLE 52–6. **Expected Antiepileptic Drug Interactions*,†**

Drug	Pheno-barbital	Primi-done	Pheny-toin	Carba-maze-pine	Valproate	Ethosuxi-mide	Gabapen-tin	Lamotri-gine	Felba-mate	Topira-mate	Tiagab-ine	Oxcar-baze-pine	Leveti-racetam	Zonisa-mide
Phenobarbital			V	9	9	9	0	9	9	NA	9	9	0	9
Primidone			V	9	9	9	0	9	0	NA	9	9	0	9
Phenytoin	0	0		9	9	9	0	9	9	9	9	9	0	9
Carbamazepine	0	0	9	A	9	9	0	9	9	9	9	9	9	9
Valproate	8	8	V	0‡		V	0	8	V	9	8	9	0	0
Ethosuximide	0	0	V	0	0		0	0	0	0	0	0	0	0
Gabapentin	0	0	0	0	0	0		0	0	0	0	0	0	0
Lamotrigine	0	0	0	0	9	0	0		NA	NA	NA	0	0	NA
Felbamate	0	8	8	9?	8	NA	0	NA		NA	NA	NA	0	NA
Topiramate	0	0	V	0	9	0	0	0	NA		NA	NA	0	NA
Tiagabine	0	0	0	8	9	0	0	0	NA	0		NA	0	NA
Oxcarbazepine	8	8	8	0	0	0	0	NA	NA	NA	NA		0	NA
Levetiracetam	0	0	0	0	0	0	0	0	0	0	0	0		0
Zonisamide	0	0	0	0	0	0	0	0	NA	NA	NA	NA	0	

*The effect on serum concentrations of concomitant AEDs (*top*) by the addition of the AEDs in the first column.
†Possible interactions of felbamate, gabapentin, lamotrigine, and topiramate may not yet be available.
‡Increases CBZ 10,11-epoxide concentration.
V, Variable; NA, not available; A, autoinduction.

sesses anticonvulsant properties. Autoinduction occurs during the first several weeks of therapy, necessitating gradual titration. Concomitant use of propoxyphene, erythromycin, and cimetidine results in significant accumulation of carbamazepine. Despite its association with aplastic anemia, serious hematological complications are rare. A mild, dose-related leukopenia may occur, which does not require discontinuation of the drug unless the total white blood cell count falls below 2500/μL or the total granulocyte count is less than 750/μL. Neurological side effects include drowsiness, vertigo, ataxia, and diplopia. Idiosyncratic reactions include hyponatremia due to inappropriate antidiuretic effect; disturbances of thyroid, adrenal, and sex hormones; cardiac conduction disturbances; impaired renal function; movement disorders; and a lupus-like syndrome. Carbamazepine is available in 200-mg tablets; 100-mg chewable tablets; 100-, 200-, and 400-mg extended-release capsules (Tegretal XR), 200- and 300-mg extended-release capsules (Carbatrol), and suspension (100 mg/5 mL).

Valproic acid is a branched-chain fatty acid that was approved for use in the United States in 1978. The enteric-coated preparation, divalproex sodium, became available in 1983. Multiple mechanisms likely contribute to its broad spectrum of action, including inhibition of sustained repetitive firing through blockade of voltage-gated Na^+ channels. Valproic acid is effective against generalized and partial seizures. including absence, myoclonic, and tonic-clonic seizures. High protein binding and hepatic enzyme inhibition contribute to the high incidence of drug interactions. Adverse reactions include tremor, weight gain, alopecia, hyperammonemia, carnitine deficiency, and thrombocytopenia. Fulminant hepatic failure and fatal pancreatitis have been reported. Valproate is available in 250-mg tablets and syrup (250 mg/5 mL), and divalproex sodium in 125-, 250-, and 500-mg tablets and 125-mg sprinkles for mixture with food. An intravenous formulation (Depakon) is available for use in patients who are unable to take oral formulations.

For the past 30 years, benzodiazepines have been used in the treatment of nearly every type of seizure disorder. As a class, benzodiazepines bind to their receptor on the $GABA_A$ receptor–chloride ionophore complex, increasing the frequency of Cl^- channel opening and potentiating GABA transmission. Long-term usage is limited by their sedative properties and development of tolerance to the anticonvulsant effect. Only *clonazepam* and *clorazepate* are used for the long-term treatment of seizures. *Lorazepam* and *diazepam* have a major role in the treatment of status epilepticus. Clonazepam is available as 0.5-, 1-, and 2-mg tablets. Clorazepate is available as 3.75-, 7.5-, and 15-mg capsules and 3.75-, 7.5-, 11.25-, 15-, and 22.5-mg tablets.

Felbamate was approved in the United States in 1993 for the treatment of partial seizures in adults and as adjunctive therapy in patients over 2 years of age with Lennox Gastaut syndrome. Just over 1 year later, the FDA recommended limiting its use due to its association with aplastic anemia. Currently, the FDA recommends that felbamate be used only in situations in which the risk of seizures exceeds the risks of the drug. As of December 1995, there have been 32 cases of aplastic anemia reported, including 10 fatalities, and numerous cases of hepatitis. The mechanism of action of felbamate is unknown, although it likely has multiple actions, including blockade of voltage-gated Na^+ channels, potentiation of GABA transmission, and inhibition of excitatory neurotransmission through interaction with the NMDA receptor. Felbamate is effective against partial and generalized seizures, including AS. Common adverse effects include insomnia, weight loss, nausea, anorexia, dizziness, and lethargy. Although there is no evidence that laboratory monitoring will prevent serious complications, the manufacturer currently recommends monitoring liver function studies, complete blood count, and reticulocyte count monthly. Felbamate is available in 400-mg capsules, 600-mg tablets, and suspension (600 mg/5 mL). To avoid drug interactions, concomitant AEDs should be reduced by 20 to 30 percent when felbamate therapy is initiated.

Gabapentin was approved in the United States in 1993 and is currently indicated as adjunctive therapy of partial and secondary generalized seizures in patients over 3 years of age.[41] Despite being an amino acid derivative of GABA, gabapentin does not interact with GABA receptors or potentiate gabaminergic transmission. Absorption is dose-dependent, and doses exceeding 1200 mg produce only modest increases in bioavailability. Lack of protein binding and hepatic metabolism contribute to the absence of significant drug interactions. Gabapentin is eliminated by the kidneys unchanged, which necessitates dosage adjustments in renally compromised patients. The most common adverse effects include somnolence, dizziness, ataxia, fatigue, and nystagmus. Gabapentin is available in 100-, 300-, and 400-mg capsules, 600- and 800-mg tablets, and syrup (250 mg/mL).

Lamotrigine received FDA approval in the United States in 1994 for the adjunctive treatment of partial seizures in patients older than 12 years of age.[42] Since then, it has also been approved in conversion to monotherapy in adults with partial seizures and as adjunctive treatment of generalized seizures in patients with Lennox Gastaut syndrome over the age of 2 years. Its mechanism of action and spectrum of activity are similar to those of phenytoin and carbamazepine. Lamotrigine does not induce hepatic microsomal enzymes and does not significantly affect the metabolism of other drugs. The half-life of lamotrigine, however, is significantly prolonged by the concomitant use of valproic acid and shortened by agents that induce hepatic microsomal enzymes. The most common adverse effects are dizziness, headache, diplopia, ataxia, somnolence, and vomiting. Hepatic or hematological abnormalities have not been reported, and routine laboratory monitoring is not required. Lamotrigine is associated with skin rash in approximately 10 percent of patients. Severe hypersensitivity reactions may also occur, particularly in very young patients receiving valproic acid, and in the setting of rapid initiation or high initial doses. Lamotrigine is available in 100-, 150-, and 200-mg tablets and 2-, 5-, and 25-mg chewable tablets.

Topiramate received FDA approval in December 1996 for use as an adjunctive agent in adults with partial seizures with and without secondary generalized TCS.[43] The drug is also indicated for the treatment of partial seizures in children and as adjunctive treatment of generalized seizures in patients over the age of 2 years.[48] Topiramate has several mechanisms of action, including effects at voltage-gated Na^+ channels, enhancement of GABA activity at $GABA_A$ receptors, and antagonism of glutamate receptors. The drug does not affect the metabolism of concomitant AEDs. Adverse effects include cognitive dysfunction, visual disturbance, weight loss, and nervousness. Topiramate is not associated with organ toxicity, although renal stones develop in 1.5 percent of patients. It is available in 25-, 100-, and 200-mg tablets and 15- and 25-mg sprinkles.

Tiagabine was FDA approved in 1997 and is indicated as adjunctive treatment of partial seizures in patients over 12 years of age.[44] Tiagabine is a potent inhibitor of GABA uptake, the primary inhibitory neurotransmitter in the CNS. By blocking uptake, the drug increases the extracellular concentration of GABA and prolongs its inhibitory effect. Common adverse effects include dizziness, asthenia, somnolence, and nervousness. Tiagabine is available in 4, 12, 16, and 20 mg tablets.

Levetiracetam received FDA approval in 1999 for use as an adjunctive agent in adults with partial and secondary generalized seizures.[45] Its mechanism of action is unknown, however, levetiracetam is effective in a broad range of animal models of partial and generalized epilepsy. There are no significant drug interactions, as this agent is excreted in the urine largely unchanged. Adverse effects include somnolence, dizziness, headache, asthenia, and agitation. Levetiracetam is available in 250-, 500-, and 750-mg tablets.

Oxcarbazepine received approval for use in the United States in 2000 as monotherapy or adjunctive treatment of partial seizures in adults and adjunctive treatment of partial seizures in children 4 years of age and older.[46] The 10-monohydroxy metabolite (MHD) of the drug is responsible for its anticonvulant effect. Unlike carbamazepine, oxcarbazepine does not induce its own metabolism. The major advantage of this drug over carbamazepine is the lower incidence of adverse effects. Severe hyponatremia (sodium <125 mmol/L) is reported in 2 to 3 percent of patients. Oxcarbazepine is available in 150-, 300-, and 600-mg tablets and suspension (300 mg/5 mL).

Zonisamide was approved in the United States in 2000 as an adjunctive agent in adults with partial seizures.[47] It may also be effective against generalized seizures and infantile spasms. The precise mechanism of action is unknown. However, zonisamide appears to block sodium and calcium channels, binds to the GABA/benzodiazepine receptor complex, and weakly inhibits carbonic anhydrase. Zonisamide is chemically classified as a sulfonamide and is therefore relatively contraindicated in patients with sulfonamide hypersensitivity. Common adverse effects include dizziness, somnolence, headache, agitation, and weight loss. Nephrolithiasis is reported in 2 to 3 percent of patients. Zonisamide has a long half-life and may be administered once per day. It is available in 100-mg capsules.

Surgical Treatment

GENERAL PRINCIPLES

Candidates for epilepsy surgery are those patients with seizures refractory to appropriate medical management and a well-defined epileptogenic focus not involving eloquent cortex. Surgery is contraindicated in patients with generalized epilepsy, benign childhood epilepsy, progressive diseases, and significant noncompliance. Mental retardation, psychiatric disease, and the coexistence of epileptic and nonepileptic seizures are not absolute contraindications. Dominant hemisphere seizure origin, bilateral or multifocal epileptic discharges on EEG, and neurological deficits on examination should not preclude surgical consideration. Rarely, surgery is considered in patients with seizures arising from more than one epileptogenic focus. Surgery should be performed as early as possible, because intractable seizures portend a poor prognosis for seizure remission and psychosocial outcome. Once adequate trials of several first-line AEDs prove ineffective, the likelihood of improvement with adjunctive agents is low.

SURFACE AND INTRACRANIAL ELECTROENCEPHALOGRAPHY

The goal of the presurgical evaluation is to define the epileptogenic zone, which is the region of cortex capable of generating seizures. Complete removal of the epileptogenic zone is necessary to produce a seizure-free state.[49] The clinical history and EEG are used to identify patients who may be candidates for surgery. The yield of surface EEG, however, is limited by the attenuating effects of the skull and intervening tissue, distance of the recording electrodes from the generator of ictal activity, and variable orientation of generator. Cerebral activity from mesial or basal cortical areas is particularly apt to escape detection. Modified electrode placements and semi-invasive techniques such as sphenoidal electrodes increase the yield of surface recordings. In general, the distribution of interictal abnormalities extends beyond the epileptogenic zone. Nevertheless, interictal epileptiform discharges generally provide more reliable localizing information than ictal recordings because of the tendency for seizures to spread rapidly to contiguous regions.

Intracranial EEG may be required when surface EEG and neuroimaging studies fail to delineate the epileptogenic zone adequately. Although more sensitive than surface EEG, intracranial EEG provides a limited view of cerebral activity, because recordings are obtained only from areas where electrodes are placed.

The successful use of intracranial EEG requires that noninvasive studies provide enough information to ensure appropriate electrode placement. Intracranial monitoring is performed with depth and subdural electrodes. Depth electrodes are multiple-contact wires placed stereotactically into the brain. Their primary indication is for the identification of the epileptogenic zone in patients with TLE and bitemporal abnormalities on surface EEG or MRI. Electrodes embedded in thin Silastic plates arranged in strips or grids can be placed through burr holes or craniotomy within the subdural space over cortical areas of interest. This technique allows for the recording of multiple regions over one or both hemispheres and mapping of eloquent cortex. Complications of depth and subdural electrodes include intraparenchymal hemorrhage, infection, and cerebral edema in 1 to 2 percent of patients.

NEUROIMAGING

Advances in neuroimaging have revolutionized the approach to patients with partial epilepsy. MRI has replaced CT as the study of choice, although CT remains superior in the detection of calcified lesions. SPECT and PET scans measure functional changes produced by seizures. All patients with partial epilepsy should undergo an MRI during the course of their illness to rule out structural lesions. The use of special imaging sequences and thin cuts increases the

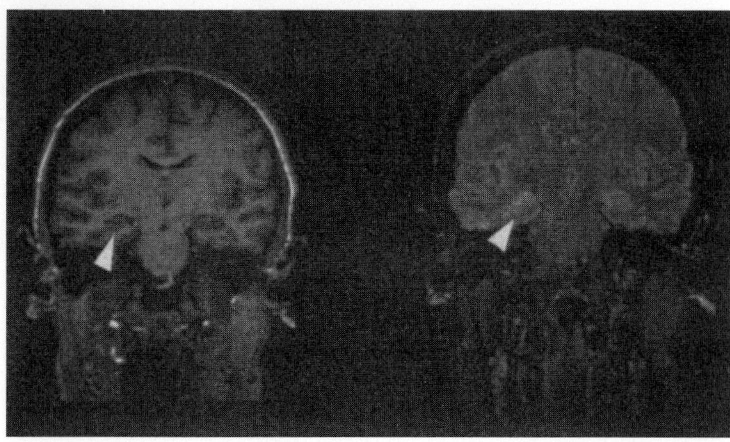

FIGURE 52–7. MRI showing atrophy (T1-weighted image on left) and increased signal (fluid-attenuated inversion-recovery sequence on right) in the right hippocampus in a patient with right mesial temporal lobe epilepsy.

detection of small neoplasms, developmental abnormalities, and mesial temporal sclerosis. In most cases, mesial temporal sclerosis is associated with unilateral hippocampal atrophy on T1-weighted images and increased signal in the mesial temporal structures on T2-weighted sequences (Fig. 52–7). These findings are highly predictive of seizure remission and lack of material-specific memory deficits following mesial temporal resection. Magnetic resonance spectroscopy is a new tool that demonstrates regional metabolic alterations in epileptogenic tissue.

Cerebral glucose metabolism measured with ^{18}FDG PET is reduced in some patients with partial epilepsy. Temporal lobe hypometabolism is seen in 60 to 90 percent of patients with intractable TLE (Fig. 52–8).[50] The extent of abnormality is usually larger than the epileptogenic zone, frequently extending into the ipsilateral basal ganglia, thalamus, and frontoparietal cortices. The yield of PET in nonlesional extratemporal epilepsy is significantly lower. The short half-life of the isotope precludes its use for ictal studies.

SPECT is more readily available than PET because it utilizes commercially available isotopes and does not require an on-site cyclotron. Technetium 99m-hexamethylene-propylene-amine-oxime SPECT reveals hypoperfusion in the epileptogenic temporal lobe during the interictal state in over 50 percent of patients with TLE.[51] False lateralization has been reported in 15 to 20 percent of cases. The resolution of SPECT is inferior to that of PET, and quantitative analysis is not available. The long half-lives of the isotopes make

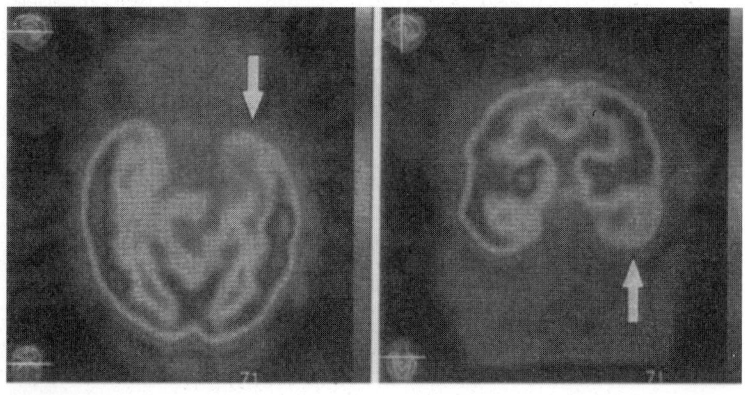

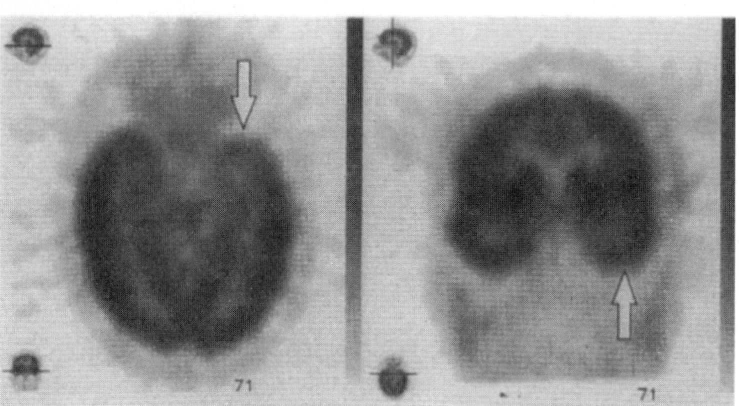

FIGURE 52–8. ^{18}FDG PET demonstrating significant hypometabolism involving the left temporal lobe in a patient with left mesial temporal lobe epilepsy. The darkness scale is divided into 10 equal intervals, each representing a 10-percent change in hypometabolism. The level of darkness at the top of the scale represents an increase in metabolism as compared to the normal state, with glucose metabolism decreasing as one progresses down the darkness scheme. (See CD-ROM for color version.) (Photo courtesy of C. Oliver Wong, MD, PhD, FACP.)

ictal and immediate postictal SPECT a useful noninvasive localizing tool. The results of ictal SPECT depend on the time of injection of the isotope from seizure onset. Under optimal circumstances, 65 to 90 percent of studies demonstrate hyperperfusion ipsilateral to seizure origin (Fig. 52–9).[51] Delayed injections produce widespread hyperperfusion and a higher incidence of false lateralization.

SPECIFIC SURGERIES

Temporal Lobectomy

Anterior temporal lobectomy is the most common surgical procedure for the treatment of intractable epilepsy in adolescents and adults. The resection typically includes the anterior 3.0 to 3.5 cm of the inferior and middle temporal gyri, uncus, part of the amygdala, and the anterior 2.0 to 3.0 cm of the hippocampus and adjacent parahippocampal gyrus. In patients with mesial temporal sclerosis, selective amygdalohippocampectomy may suffice. Lesionectomy with preservation of the mesial temporal structures may be indicated in patients with discrete temporal lobe lesions without evidence of mesial involvement. Language mapping is required when lesions are located near the language cortex. The use of tailored resections based on intraoperative electrocorticography remains controversial. A seizure-free state is achieved in 60 to 70 percent of patients, although auras may persist.[52] A risk of verbal memory impairment exists in patients with normal preoperative memory scores undergoing dominant hemisphere anterior temporal lobectomy. Transient dysnomia after dominant anterior temporal lobectomy occurs in approximately 30 percent of patients.

Extratemporal Lesion Resection, Hemisperectomy, Corpus Callosotomy

The procedure of choice for patients with extratemporal epilepsy due to a structural brain lesion is complete resection of the lesion and surrounding epileptogenic cortex. Lesionectomy is the most common type of epilepsy surgery performed in infants and children. Subtotal removal of a structural lesion is associated with a lower likelihood of seizure remission. Patients with nonlesional extratemporal epilepsy generally require intracranial monitoring to delineate the epileptogenic zone, and cortical mapping if the proposed resection is located in or around eloquent cortex. Surgical outcome in these cases depends on the certainty with which the epileptogenic zone is defined and the completeness of the resection. Only 25 to 35 percent of patients become seizure-free, and another 20 to 30 percent has a significant reduction in seizures.[53]

Hemispherectomy is indicated in patients with intractable partial and secondarily generalized seizures in whom an entire

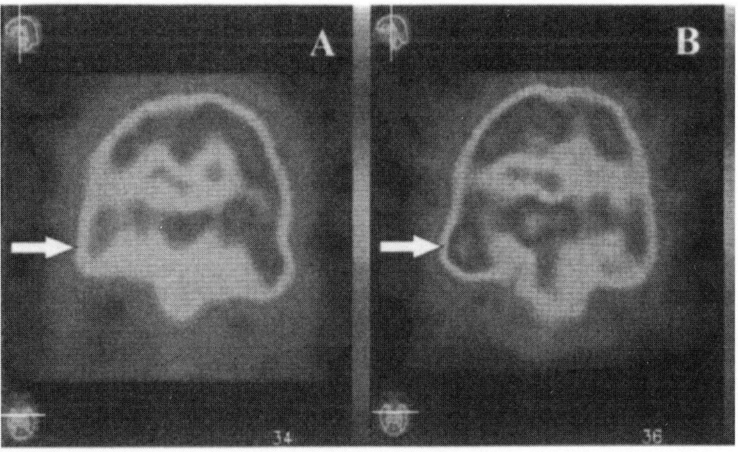

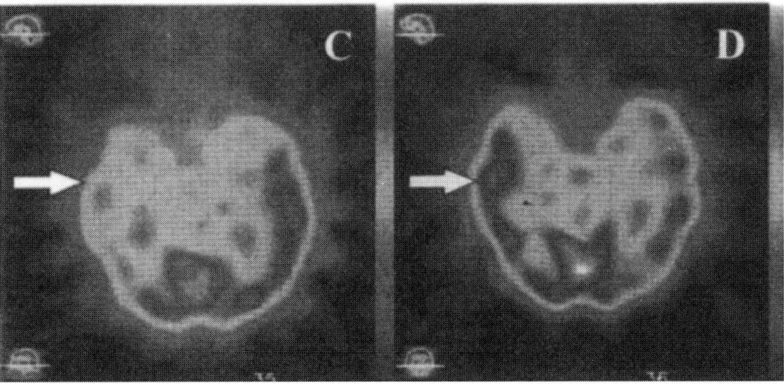

FIGURE 52–9. Interictal and ictal Tc-99m SPECT in coronal and transverse planes in a patient with right mesial temporal lobe epilepsy. There is a reduction in blood flow in the right temporal lobe interictally and hyperperfusion in the same region during a typical partial seizure. (See CD-ROM for color version.) (Photo courtesy of C. Oliver Wong, MD, PhD, FACP.)

hemisphere is considered epileptogenic with little or no remaining functional cortex. The procedure is usually performed in patients with Rasmussen's encephalitis, Sturge-Weber syndrome, hemimegancephaly, or large hemispheric infarctions. Functional hemispherectomy consists of the removal of the frontal and temporal lobes and complete disconnection of the remaining cortex and corpus callosum. This procedure is an alternative to total hemispherectomy, which is associated with a high rate of cerebral hemosiderosis and hydrocephalus. Seizures are completely abolished in nearly 80 percent of patients.[54]

Corpus callosotomy should be considered in patients with frequent secondary generalized tonic-clonic, tonic, and atonic seizures that lead to falls and injuries. The goal of the procedure is to disrupt the major central pathways necessary for the propagation of generalized seizures. Complete callosal section may result in mutism, apraxia, or frontal lobe dysfunction. For this reason, the procedure is often performed in two stages beginning with sectioning of the anterior two thirds followed by section of the remainder of the corpus callosum, if necessary. Nearly two thirds of patients experience a significant reduction in seizures, although few are rendered seizure-free.[55]

Reviews and Selected Updates

American Academy of Neurology: Assessment: Generic substitution for antiepileptic medication. Neurology 1990;40:1641–1643.

Engel J Jr, Pedley TA (eds): Epilepsy: A Comprehensive Textbook. Philadelphia, Lippincott-Raven, 1998.

Gastaut H, Broughton R (eds): Epileptic Seizures. Springfield, IL: Charles C Thomas, 1972.

Helmstaedter C, Reuber M, Elger CCE: Interaction of cognitive aging and memory deficits related to epilepsy surgery. Ann Neurol 2002;52:89–94.

Hirtz D, Ashwal S, Berg A, et al: Practice parameter: Evaluating a first non-febrile seizure in children: Report of the Quality Standards Subcommittee of the American Academy of Neurology. Neurology 2000;55:616–623.

Levy RH, Mattson RH, Meldrum BS (eds): Antiepileptic Drugs. New York, Raven Press, 1995.

Quality Standards Subcommittee of the American Academy of Neurology: Practice parameter: a guideline for dicontinuing antiepileptic drugs in seizure-free patients—summary statement. Neurology 1996;47:600–602.

Quality Standards Subcommittee of the American Academy of Neurology: Practice parameter: management issues for women with epilepsy (summary statement). Neurology 1998;51:944–948.

Roger J, Bureau M, Dravet C, et al (eds): Epileptic Syndromes in Infancy, Childhood and Adolescence. London, John Libbey & Company, 1992.

Wyllie E (ed): The Treatment of Epilepsy: Principles and Practice, 3rd ed. Philadelphia, Lippincott, Williams & Wilkins, 2001.

References

1. Temkin O: The Falling Sickness, 2nd ed. Baltimore, Johns Hopkins University Press, 1971.
2. Annegers JF: The epidemiology of epilepsy. *In* Wyllie E (ed): The Treatment of Epilepsy: Principles and Practice. Philadelphia, Lea & Febiger, 1993, pp 157–164.
3. Treiman LJ, Treiman DM: Genetic aspects of epilepsy. *In* Wyllie E (ed): The Treatment of Epilepsy: Principles and Practice. Philadelphia, Lea & Febiger, 1993, pp 145–156.
4. Commission on Classification and Terminology of the International League Against Epilepsy: A proposed international classification of epileptic seizures. Epilepsia 1964;5:297–306.
5. Commission on Classification and Terminology of the International League Against Epilepsy: Proposal for revised clinical and electrographic classification of epileptic seizures. Epilepsia 1981;22:489–501.
6. Messing RO: Seizures as a manifestation of systemic disease. Neurol Clin 1986;4:563–584.
7. Snead OC: Basic mechanisms of generalized absence seizures. Ann Neurol 1995;37:146–157.
8. Hallett M: Myoclonus: Relation to epilepsy. Epilepsia 1985;26(Suppl 1):S67–S74.
9. Palmini A, Gloor P: The localizing value of auras in partial seizures: A prospective and retrospective study. Neurology 1992;42:801–808.
10. So NK: Recurrence, remission, and relapse of seizures. Cleve Clin J Med 1993;60:439–444.
11. Hauser WA: Should people be treated after a first seizure? Arch Neurol 1986;43:1287–1288.
12. Commission on Classification and Terminology of the International League Against Epilepsy: Proposal for revised classification of epilepsies and epileptic syndromes. Epilepsia 1989;30:389–399.
13. Loiseau P: Benign focal epilepsies of childhood. *In* Wyllie E (ed): The Treatment of Epilepsy: Principles and Practice. Philadelphia, Lea & Febiger, 1993, pp 503–512.
14. Hauser WA: The natural history of temporal lobe epilepsy. *In* Lüders H (ed): Epilepsy Surgery. New York, Raven Press, 1991, pp 133–141.
15. Mattson RH, Cramer JA, Collins JF, et al: Comparison of carbamazepine, phenobarbital, phenytoin, and primidone in partial and secondarily generalized tonic-clonic seizures. N Engl J Med 1985;313:145–151.
16. Mattson RH, Cramer JA, Collins JF, et al: A comparison of valproate with carbamazepine for the treatment of complex partial seizures and secondarily generalized tonic-clonic seizures in adults. N Engl J Med 1992;327:765–771.
17. Van Ness PC: Frontal and parietal lobe epilepsy. *In* Wyllie E (ed): The Treatment of Epilepsy: Principles and Practice. Philadelphia, Lea & Febiger, 1993, pp 525–532.
18. Sveinbjornsdottir S, Duncan JS: Parietal and occipital lobe epilepsy: A review. Epilepsia 1993;34(3):493–521.
19. Plouin P: Benign idiopathic neonatal convulsions (familial and non-familial). *In* Roger J, Bureau M, Dravet C, et al (eds): Epileptic Syndromes in Infancy, Childhood, and Adolescence, 2nd ed. London, John Libbey & Company, 1992, pp 3–12.
20. Lombroso CT: Early myoclonic encephalopathy, early infantile epileptic encephalopathy, and benign and severe infantile myoclonic epilepsies: A critical review and personal contributions. J Clin Neurophysiol 1990;7(3):380–408.
21. Delgado-Escueta AV, Treiman DM, Walsh GO: The treatable epilepsies. N Engl J Med 1983;308:1508–1514.
22. Berkovic SF: Childhood absence epilepsy and juvenile absence epilepsy. *In* Wyllie E (ed): The Treatment of Epilepsy: Principles and Practice. Philadelphia, Lea & Febiger, 1993, pp 547–551.
23. Bouma PAD, Westendrop RGJ, van Dijk JG, et al: The outcome of absence epilepsy: A meta-analysis. Neurology 1996;47;802–808.
24. Serratosa JM, Delgado-Escueta AV: Juvenile myoclonic epilepsy. *In* Wyllie E (ed): The Treatment of Epilepsy: Principles and Practice. Philadelphia, Lea & Febiger, 1993, pp 552–570.
25. Greenberg DA, Durner M, Resor S, et al: The genetics of idiopathic generalized epilepsies of adolescent onset: Differences between juvenile myoclonic epilepsy and epilepsy with random grand mal and with awakening grand mal. Neurology 1995;45:942–946.
26. Jeavons PM, Livet MO: West syndrome: Infantile spasms. *In* Roger J, Bureau M, Dravet C, et al (eds): Epileptic Syndromes in Infancy, Childhood, and Adolescence, 2nd ed. London, John Libbey & Company, 1992, pp 53–65.
27. Dulac O, Plouin P: Infantile spasms and West syndrome. *In* Wyllie E (ed): The Treatment of Epilepsy: Principles and Practice. Philadelphia, Lea & Febiger, 1993, pp 464–491.
28. Dulac O, Schlumberger E: Treatment of West syndrome. *In* Wyllie E (ed): The Treatment of Epilepsy: Principles and Practice. Philadelphia, Lea & Febiger, 1993, pp 595–603.
29. Beaumanoir A, Dravet C: The Lennox-Gastaut syndrome. *In* Roger J, Bureau M, Dravet C, et al (eds): Epileptic Syndromes in Infancy, Childhood, and Adolescence, 2nd ed. London, John Libbey & Company, 1992, pp 115–132.
30. Berkovic SF, Cochius J, Andermann E, Andermann F: Progressive myoclonus epilepsies: Clinical and genetic aspects. Epilepsia 1993;34(Suppl 3):S19–S30.
31. Volpe JJ: Neonatal seizures: Current concepts and revised classification. Pediatrics 1989;84:422–428.
32. Mizrahi EM, Kellaway P: Characterization and classification of neonatal seizures. Neurology 1987;37:1837–1844.
33. Fenechel G: Paroxysmal disorders. *In* Fenichel GM (ed): Clinical Pediatric Neurology: A Signs and Symptoms Approach. Philadelphia, WB Saunders, 1988, pp 1–41.
34. Nelson KF, Ellenberg JH: Predictors of epilepsy in children who have experienced febrile seizures. N Engl J Med 1976;295:1029–1033.

35. Freeman JM: Febrile seizures: A consensus of their significance, evaluation, and treatment. Pediatrics 1980;66:1009–1012.
36. Beaumanoir A: The Landau-Kleffner syndrome. *In* Roger J, Bureau M, Dravet C, et al (eds): Epileptic Syndromes in Infancy, Childhood, and Adolescence, 2nd ed. London, John Libbey & Company, 1992, pp 231–243.
37. Yerby M: Pregnancy and epilepsy. Epilepsia 1991;32(Suppl 6):S51–S59.
38. Delgado-Escueta AV, Janz D: Consensus guidelines: Preconception counseling, management, and care of the pregnant woman with epilepsy. Neurology 1992;42(Suppl 5):149–160.
39. DeLorenzo RJ, Hauser WA, Towne AR, et al: A prospective, population-based epidemiologic study of status epilepticus in Richmond, Virginia. Neurology 1996;46:1029–1035.
40. Lesser R: Psychogenic seizures. Neurology 1996;46:1499–1507.
41. McLean MJ: Gabapentin. Epilepsia 1995;36(Suppl 2):S73–S86.
42. Messenheimer JA: Lamotrigine. Epilepsia 1995;36(Suppl 2):S87–S94.
43. Privitera M, Fincham R, Penry J, et al: Topiramate placebo-controlled dose-ranging trial in refractory partial epilepsy using 600, 800, and 1,000 mg daily dosages. Neurology 1996;46:1678–1683.
44. Uthman BM, Rowan AJ, Ahmann PA, et al: Tiagabine for complex partial seizures. Arch Neurol 1998;55:56–62.
45. Cereghino JJ, Biton V, Abou-Khalil B, et al: Levetiracetam for partial seizures: results of a double-blind, randomized clinical trial. Neurology 2000;55:236–242.
46. Sachedo R, Beydoun A, Schachter S, et al: Oxcarbazepine (Trileptal) as monotherapy in patients with partial seizures. Neurology 2001;57: 864–871.
47. Leppik IE: Zonisamide. Epilepsia 1999;40(Suppl 5):S23–S29.
48. Biton V, Montouris GD, Ritter F, et al: A randomized, placebo-controlled study of topiramate in primary generalized tonic-clonic seizures. Neurology 1999;52:1330–1337.
49. Lüders HO, Awad I: Conceptual considerations. *In* Lüders H (ed): Epilepsy Surgery. New York, Raven Press, 1991, pp 51–62.
50. Henry TR, Mazziotta JC, Engel J Jr: Interictal metabolic anatomy of mesial temporal lobe epilepsy. Arch Neurol 1993;50:582–588.
51. Gaillard WD: Metabolic and functional neuroimaging. *In* Wyllie E (ed): The Treatment of Epilepsy: Principles and Practice, 3rd ed. Philadelphia, Lippincott, Williams & Wilkins, 2001, pp 1053–1066.
52. Doyle WK, Spencer DD: Anterior temporal resections. *In* Engel J Jr, Pedley TA (eds): Epilepsy: A Comprehensive Textbook. Philadelphia, Lippincott-Raven, 1998, pp 1807–1817.
53. Comair YG, Young Choi H, Van Ness PC: Neocortical resections. *In* Engel J Jr, Pedley TA (eds): Epilepsy: A Comprehensive Textbook. Philadelphia, Lippincott-Raven, 1998, pp 1819–1828.
54. Villemure JG, Peacock W: Multilobar resections and hemispherectomy. *In* Engel J Jr, Pedley TA (eds): Epilepsy: A Comprehensive Textbook. Philadelphia, Lippincott-Raven, 1998, pp 1829–1839.
55. Smith MC, Byrne R, Kanner AM: Corpus callosotomy and multiple subpial transection. *In* Wyllie E (ed): The Treatment of Epilepsy: Principles and Practice, 3rd ed. Philadelphia, Lippincott, Williams & Wilkins, 2001, pp 1175–1184.

CHAPTER 53

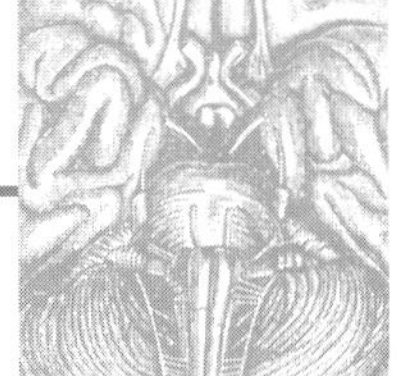

STEPHEN D. SILBERSTEIN and WILLIAM B. YOUNG

Headache and Facial Pain

History and Definitions

Headache is a problem that has plagued humans since the beginning of recorded time. The earliest written reference to migraine is found in an epic poem written in Sumeria around 3000 BC[1]: "The sick-eyed says not I am sick-eyed. The sick-headed not I am sick-headed." From Mesopotamia comes a description of a headache sufferer with an associated visual disturbance, in which "the head is bent with pain gripping his temples . . . and his eyes are afflicted with dimness and cloudiness." Hippocrates described the visual aura that can precede the migraine headache and the relief that can be induced by vomiting.[2] Aretaeus of Cappadocia is credited as the discoverer of migraine because of his classic description of the symptoms in the 2nd century AD.[2] Migraine clearly was well known in the ancient world.

In 1778, Fothergill introduced the term fortification spectra to describe the visual aura of migraine. A hundred years later, Airy gave a vivid description of the same phenomenon, which he called teichopsia, quoting Tennyson[1]: " . . . as yonder walls rose slowly to a music slowly breathed, a cloud that gathered shape." In 1783, Tisso distinguished migraine from common headache and ascribed it to a supraorbital neuralgia "provoked by reflexes from the stomach, gallbladder, or uterus."[3] Over the next century, DuBois, Reymond, Mollendorf, and later Eulenburg proposed different vascular theories for migraine.

Liveing wrote the first monograph on migraine entitled *On Megrim, Sick-headache, and Some Allied Disorders: A Contribution to the Pathology of Nerve-Storms*[4] and was the originator of the neural theory of migraine, ascribing the problem to "disturbances of the autonomic nervous system," which he called "nerve storms." In 1900, Dey[1] suggested that migraine resulted from intermittent swelling of the hypophysis with compression of the trigeminal nerve. Later in the 20th century (1950), Harold Wolff developed the experimental approach to the study of headache[1] and elaborated the vascular theory of migraine, which has come under attack as the pendulum again swings to the neurogenic theory.[1]

In 1962, an Ad Hoc Committee established descriptive definitions of migraine, tension-type headache (TTH), and other headache disorders. In 1988, the International Headache Society (IHS) published a formal classification system for the diagnosis of headache disorders.[5] This system is being re-evaluated, modified, and improved. The IHS classification system (Table 53–1) divides headache into primary and secondary disorders. In a primary headache disorder, headache itself is the illness and no other etiology is diagnosed. In a secondary headache disorder, headache is the symptom of an identifiable structural or metabolic abnormality.

Headache

MIGRAINE HEADACHE

Pathogenesis and Pathophysiology. Although the exact pathophysiology of migraine is unknown, several theories

TABLE 53–1. **International Headache Society Criteria**

Migraine
Migraine with aura
Migraine without aura

Tension-Type Headache
Episodic tension-type headache
Chronic tension-type headache

Cluster Headache and Chronic Paroxysmal Hemicrania
Cluster headache
Chronic paroxysmal hemicrania

Miscellaneous Headaches Unassociated with Structural Lesion
Idiopathic stabbing headache
Cold stimulus headache
Benign cough headache
Benign exertional headache
Headache associated with sexual activity

Headache Associated with Head Trauma

Headache Associated with Vascular Disorders

Headache Associated with Nonvascular Intracranial Disorders

Headache Associated with Substances or Their Withdrawal

Headache Associated with Noncephalic Iinfections

Headache Associated with Metabolic Disorders

Headache or Facial Pain Associated with Disorders of Cranium, Neck, Eyes, Ears, Nose, Sinuses, Teeth, Mouth, or Other Facial or Cranial Structures

Cranial Neuralgias, Nerve Trunk Pain, and Deafferentation Pain

exist. Any migraine theory must explain the prodrome, the aura, the headache with its associated symptoms, and the postdrome. The traditional vascular theory proposed that the migraine aura was caused by intracerebral vasoconstriction and the headache by painful reactive vasodilation. This theory cannot explain the prodromal features of migraine or the reason some antimigraine drugs have no effect on the cerebral vasculature.[6] Furthermore, this theory has not been substantiated by cerebral blood flow (CBF) studies.

The comprehensive neurovascular theory, which has replaced the vascular theory, is based on CBF studies, magnetic resonance spectroscopy, and magnetoencephalography research. It suggests that hypothalamic and limbic system disturbances may produce the prodromal symptoms of migraine, and that neuronal dysfunction with secondary vascular changes is responsible for the aura and headache of migraine. During the aura of classic migraine, a wave of decreased CBF spreads forward from the occipital cortex, preceding the aura symptoms and persisting into the headache phase. This change in CBF may be caused by cortical spreading depression (a short-lasting wave of neuronal activation, followed by inhibition), which may also produce the aura symptoms and activate trigeminal nerve endings. In the headache of migraine with aura (classic migraine), increased CBF occurs after the headache begins, and this change continues until the headache subsides. There is no change in CBF in migraine without aura (common migraine).[6]

It is unclear how the brain stem nucleus for facial pain (the nucleus caudalis trigeminalis) is activated, but it may be that cortical spreading depression or biochemical dysfunction, or both, stimulates its peripheral nerve terminals. Activation of the central midbrain region during migraine has been demonstrated and has resulted in the speculation that this region may be the generator of migraine.[7] An imbalance between facilitation and inhibition to the nucleus caudalis trigeminalis may render it more sensitive to nonpainful stimuli that are misinterpreted as painful. This theory may explain why migraine sufferers have an increased propensity to head pain (such as so-called ice-pick headache) even during migraine-free periods.

Peripheral mechanisms may also play a role in migraine. Stimulation of the trigeminal nerve results in release of substance P, calcitonin gene–related peptide, and neurokinin A.[8] These chemicals cause neurogenic inflammation and may further enhance neuronal sensitivity and altered blood flow in the microcirculation. Neurogenic inflammation–induced meningeal inflammation may produce some of the pain of migraine.

Serotonin (5-HT) also appears to play a role in migraine pathogenesis.[9] Stimulation of the midbrain serotonergic cells results in increased CBF, and reserpine, a central nervous system (CNS) 5-HT–depleting agent, can precipitate migraine headaches. Similarly, sleep reduces CNS 5-HT neuronal firing and is a well-established method of aborting migraine attacks. Biochemical studies demonstrate that plasma 5-HT concentrations decrease during a migraine attack, and urinary excretion of 5-hydroxyindoleacetic acid, the main 5-HT metabolite, may increase. 5-HT receptor distribution and function, however, are not uniform in the brain. Some receptors modulate CBF, whereas others modulate pain, sleep, thermoregulation, motor activity, emotional behavior, and sensory responsiveness. Activation of inhibitory $5\text{-HT}_{1B/1D}$ receptors decreases the release of 5-HT, norepinephrine, acetylcholine, and substance P. When activated, the inhibitory $5\text{-HT}_{1B/1D}$ heteroreceptor, located on trigeminal nerve terminals, blocks neurogenic inflammation. Antimigraine drugs that are 5-HT agonists, such as dihydroergotamine (DHE) and sumatriptan, have high affinity for this receptor. Additionally, many drugs used to prevent migraine headaches are 5-HT_2 antagonists. 5-HT_3 receptor stimulation causes nausea, vomiting, and autonomic reflex activation.[9] Other neurotransmitters and mediators, such as catecholamines, histamine, vasoactive peptides, endogenous opiates, prostaglandins, free fatty acids, and steroid hormones, are also implicated in the pathogenesis of migraine, but their specific effects are less clearly established.

Epidemiology and Risk Factors. Migraine occurs in 18 percent of women, 6 percent of men, and 4 percent of children in the United States.[10] This disorder usually begins in the first three decades of life, with prevalence peaking in the fifth decade (Fig. 53–1). Most migraineurs have a family history of migraine. At least 60 percent of women with migraine experience clear improvement during later pregnancy, yet in some women, migraine worsens during the first trimester. Additionally, many women experience improvement of their migraine with natural, but not surgical, menopause.

Lance and Anthony found improvement in 58 percent of 120 women migraineurs who had borne children.[11] Bousser found that migraine was improved or disappeared in 69.4 per-

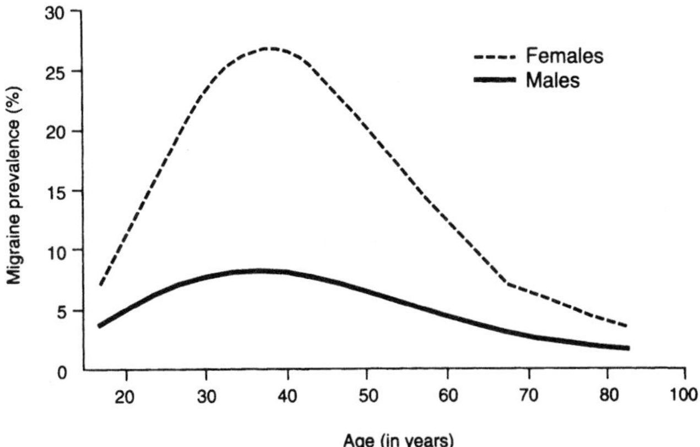

FIGURE 53–1. Migraine prevalence by age. (From Silberstein SD, Lipton RB: Epidemiology of migraine. Neuroepidemiology 1993;12:179–194. Reproduced with permission of S. Karger AG, Basel.)

cent of pregnancies, worsened in 6.8 percent, was unchanged in 11 (7.9 percent), was variable in 5.4 percent, and appeared for the first time in 10.9 percent.[12] Although disappearance or improvement did not differ significantly in migraine with or without aura, worsening was much more common in migraine with aura. Headache occurs frequently in the postpartum period, particularly in known migraineurs. Migraineurs do not have an increased risk of complications during pregnancy, and the children of migraineurs do not have an increased incidence of birth defects.[13]

Migraine is a risk factor (that is, comorbid) for affective disorders. Compared with nonmigraineurs, migraineurs have a 4.5-fold increased risk of major depression, a six-fold risk of manic episodes, a three-fold increase in anxiety disorder, and a six-fold prevalence in panic disorder. Migraineurs without depression develop depression at follow-up at three times the rate of nonmigraineurs. Furthermore, depressed patients without migraine develop migraine at three times the rate of nondepressed patients.[14] The prospective data indicates that the cross-sectional or lifetime association between migraine and major depression could result from a bidirectional influence. These recent epidemiological studies support the association between migraine and major depression previously reported in clinic-based studies.

It has been proposed that major depression in migraineurs might represent a psychological reaction to repeated, disabling migraine attacks. Migraine has an earlier average age of onset than major depression in the population and in persons with comorbid disease. Nonetheless, the bidirectional influence of each condition on the risk for the other is incompatible with the simple causal model.[14] Specifically, persons with depression but not migraine have an increased risk for migraine before painful attacks ever develop.[14] Furthermore, Breslau and Davis[15] reported that the risk for new episodes of major depression (or panic disorder) did not vary by the proximity of migraine attacks. Migraineurs may have affective spectrum disorders with associated irritable bowel syndrome, fibromyalgia, and chronic fatigue syndrome. Epilepsy, stroke, and mitral valve prolapse are also more common in migraineurs.

Contrary to the findings of clinic-based studies, population-based studies have shown migraine to be more prevalent in families of lower socioeconomic class. In addition, the economic impact of migraine and other headaches is enormous; the annual cost of headaches in terms of absenteeism, decreased productivity, and the cost of diagnostic tests and treatment ranges from 5 to 17 billion dollars. Despite 10 million physician visits each year, migraine is still underdiagnosed and undertreated.[10]

Clinical Features and Associated Disorders. The migraine attack can be divided into four phases: (1) the prodrome, which occurs hours or days before the headache; (2) the aura, which immediately precedes the headache; (3) the headache itself; and, (4) the postdrome.[16] Although most migraineurs experience more than one phase, no phase is obligatory for diagnosis. Migraine with aura may occur with or without the headache, but migraine without aura requires the headache for its diagnosis (Table 53–2). Premonitory phenomena occur hours to days before the onset of headache in about 60 percent of migraineurs (Table 53–3). They include psychological, neurological, constitutional, and autonomic features. The migraine aura is a complex of focal neurological symptoms (positive or negative phenomena) that precedes or accompanies an attack. Most aura symptoms develop over 5 to 20 minutes and usually last less than 60 minutes. The aura can be characterized by visual, sensory, or motor phenomena and may also involve language or brain stem disturbances. If the aura is prolonged, it may meet the criteria of what was formerly termed a complicated migraine. Headache, when present, usually occurs within 60 minutes of

TABLE 53–2. **Diagnostic Criteria for Migraine**

Migraine with Aura (Classic Migraine)

Diagnostic Criteria

At least two attacks fulfilling the following:

At least three of the following four characteristics:

1. One or more fully reversible aura symptoms
2. At least one aura symptom over more than 4 minutes or two or more symptoms occurring in succession
3. No single aura symptom lasts more than 60 minutes
4. Headache follows aura with a free interval of less than 60 minutes (it may also begin before or simultaneously with the aura)

Migraine Without Aura

Diagnostic Criteria

At least five attacks fulfilling the following:

Headache lasting 4 to 72 hours (untreated or unsuccessfully treated)

Headache has at least two of the following characteristics:

1. Unilateral location
2. Pulsating quality
3. Moderate or severe intensity (inhibits or prohibits daily activities)
4. Aggravation by walking stairs or similar routine physical activity

During headache at least one of the following:

1. Nausea and/or vomiting
2. Photophobia and phonophobia

For Both Disorders

History, physical and neurological examinations, and appropriate investigations must adequately exclude secondary disorders. If a secondary condition co-exists, the migraine is considered primary only if the original migraine onset did not occur in close temporal relation with the other disorder.

TABLE 53-3. **Migraine Prodrome Symptoms**

Psychological	Constitutional and Autonomic
Depression	Stiff neck
Hyperactivity	Food cravings
Euphoria	Cold feelings
Talkativeness	Anorexia
Irritability	Sluggishness
Drowsiness	Diarrhea or constipation
Restlessness	Thirst
Neurological	Urination
Photophobia	Fluid retention
Difficulty concentrating	
Phonophobia	
Dysphasia	
Hyperosmia	
Yawning	

the end of the aura, and most patients do not feel well during the period from the end of the aura to the beginning of the headache. Many patients experience a variety of cognitive or emotional symptoms during this time.[17]

The most frequently occurring aura is visual in nature. Elementary visual disturbances, including scotomata, photopsia, phosphenes (simple flashes), specks, geometrical forms, shimmering, or undulations are the most common and may occur singly or number in the hundreds. Interestingly, these elementary visual disturbances are more likely to occur during than before the headache. An occipital lobe origin is presumed based on their presence in both eyes and often in a hemifield distribution. More complicated hallucinations include teichopsia or fortification spectrum, which is the most characteristic visual aura and nearly diagnostic of migraine. An arc of scintillating lights, usually but not always beginning near the point of fixation, may form into a herringbone-like pattern that expands to encompass an increasing portion of a visual hemifield. It migrates across the visual field with a scintillating edge of often zigzag, flashing, or occasionally colored phenomena.[17, 18] Visual distortions and hallucinations, speculated to represent some of Lewis Carroll's descriptions in *Alice's Adventures in Wonderland*, occur more commonly in children. They are characterized by a complex disorder of visual perception that may include metamorphopsia, micropsia, macropsia, zoom vision (opening up or closing down in the size of objects), or mosaic vision (fracture of image into facets).[18]

Paresthesias are the second most common aura and typically start in the hand, migrate up the arm, and then extend to involve the face, lips, and tongue. Paresthesias can become bilateral and may be followed by numbness and loss of positional sense.[17, 18] They typically progress over a period of more than 5 minutes and are often associated with a visual aura. More complex symptoms include difficulties in the perception and use of the body; speech and language disturbances; states of double or multiple consciousness associated with déja vu or jamais vu; and elaborate, dreamy, nightmarish, trancelike, or delirious states. Motor symptoms, when they occur, are usually associated with sensory symptoms, but true weakness is rare and usually unilateral.

The typical migraine headache is unilateral, throbbing, moderate to marked in severity, and aggravated by physical activity. Not all of these features are required. The pain may be bilateral at the onset or start on one side and become generalized.[17, 19] The onset is usually gradual. The pain peaks and then subsides, and usually lasts between 4 and 72 hours in adults and 2 and 48 hours in children. The frequency of attacks is extremely variable, from a few in a lifetime to several a week, and the average migraineur experiences from one to three headaches a month. The head pain varies greatly in intensity, although most migraineurs report pain ratings of five or greater on a 0 to 10 pain scale. Pain is throbbing in 85 percent of cases,[17, 19] although throbbing pain is not diagnostic of migraine because it is often described in other headache types.

The pain of migraine is invariably accompanied by other features. Anorexia is common, and nausea occurs in almost 90 percent of patients, while vomiting occurs in about one third of patients.[20] Many patients experience sensory hyperexcitability manifested by photophobia, phonophobia, and osmophobia, and seek a dark, quiet room. Blurred vision, nasal stuffiness, diarrhea, polyuria, pallor, or sweating may be noted during the headache phase. There may be localized edema of the scalp or face, scalp tenderness, prominence of a vein or artery in the temple, or stiffness and tenderness of the neck. Impairment of concentration and mood are common. Lightheadedness, rather than true vertigo, and a feeling of faintness may occur. The extremities tend to be cold and moist. Following the headache, during the postdrome phase, the patient may feel tired, "washed out," irritable, and listless, and may have impaired concentration, scalp tenderness, or mood changes. Some people feel unusually refreshed or euphoric after an attack, whereas others note depression and malaise.

A variety of migraine clinical subtypes have been described. Attacks of migraine lasting longer than 72 hours define *status migrainosus*. It is often associated with pernicious nausea, vomiting, dehydration, and despair.[17] *Basilar migraine*, previously called "basilar artery migraine," was originally believed to be a disorder of adolescent girls, and although there is a clear female predominance, it is now known to affect all age groups. Severe headache is preceded by a visual aura, then brain stem signs of ataxia, vertigo, tinnitus, diplopia, nausea and vomiting, nystagmus, dysarthria, bilateral paresthesia, and a change in level of consciousness and cognition. Confusional migraine, which occurs more commonly in boys than in girls, is characterized by headache accompanied by inattention, distractibility, and difficulty maintaining speech and other motor activities. Spells of basilar and confusional migraine can present a confusing picture and should be considered in patients with paroxysmal brain stem disturbances.[5, 17]

Hemiplegic migraine occurs in two forms, sporadic and familial, both of which typically begin in childhood and cease with adulthood.[21] The age of onset of hemiplegic migraine may be earlier than that of common migraine. The attacks are frequently precipitated by minor head injury. Accompanying changes in consciousness ranging from confusion to coma are a feature of hemiplegic migraine, especially in childhood, and occur in 23 percent of patients. The hemiplegia may be part of the aura and last less than 1 hour, or it may continue through the headache phase and last for days or weeks. Familial hemiplegic migraine has an autosomal dominant mode of inheritance with variable penetrance.

In 20 percent of unselected familial hemiplegic migraine families, patients can have fixed cerebellar symptoms and signs such as nystagmus and progressive ataxia. All of these families have been shown to be linked to chromosome 19.[22] Mutations within CACNA1A, a gene encoding for the α1A subunit of a neuronal P/Q type calcium channel, cause both familial hemiplegic migraine and episodic ataxia type 2 (EA2). Another gene has been mapped to chromosome 1, CACNA1A.[23] All EA2 families have been linked to chromosome 19.[24]

Periodic focal neurological dysfunction, which may be part of the migraine aura, can occur in isolation without the headache.[17, 18] These phenomena can be part of migraine, but they are accepted as migraine only after a full investigation and prolonged follow-up. Occasional headaches occurring in association with the same symptoms as an aura help confirm the migraine diagnosis for the episodes without headache, because patients who have migraine with aura often experience aura without headache.

Late-life migrainous accompaniments are transient neurological phenomena that frequently are not associated with headache.[25] Attacks of episodic focal neurological dysfunction, which last from 1 minute to 72 hours, can occur with variable recurrence. Fisher considered scintillating scotoma to be diagnostic of migraine, even when it occurred in isolation, whereas other episodic neurological symptoms (paresthesias, aphasia, and sensory and motor symptoms) needed more careful evaluation (Table 53–4). Transient migrainous accompaniments may occur for the first time after the age of 45 and can easily be confused with transient ischemic attacks of cerebrovascular origin.

Ophthalmoplegic migraine[5] is associated with acute attacks of cranial nerve III palsy associated with a dilated pupil and migrainous unilateral eye pain. Cranial nerves IV and VI may rarely be involved. The duration of ophthalmoplegia varies from hours to months. The differential diagnosis includes intracranial aneurysms and chronic sinusitis with a mucocele. Some cases of ophthalmoplegic migraine fit the criteria for the Tolosa-Hunt syndrome of painful ophthalmoplegia:[26] (1) steady, gnawing, boring eye pain; (2) involvement of nerves of the cavernous sinus; (3) symptoms lasting days or weeks; (4) spontaneous remission, with recurrent attacks occurring after months or years; (5) computed tomography (CT) or magnetic resonance imaging (MRI) limiting disorder to the cavernous sinus; and (6) steroid responsiveness. Using contrast-enhanced MRI, Mark et al.[27] recently reported six patients with typical clinical features of ophthalmoplegic migraine who had enhancement of the cisternal segment of the oculomotor nerve during the acute phase of headache. This was followed by resolution of the enhancement over several weeks as the symptoms resolved. Enhancement can occur in a variety of conditions.[28–31] A lumber puncture is needed to rule out infectious and neoplastic causes. This disorder may be due to a viral infection of the oculomotor nerve similar to Bell's palsy (a viral neuritis with nerve enhancement).[32] Contrast-enhanced MRI and MR angiography (MRA) is the procedure of choice in evaluating patients with oculomotor palsy. If MR shows enhancement of the cisternal portion of the oculomotor nerve and lumbar puncture is negative, a presumptuous diagnosis of ophthalmoplegic migraine can be made, but follow-up is necessary to be sure the symptoms resolve.[27]

TABLE 53–4. Main Criteria for the Diagnosis of Late-Life Migrainous Accompaniments

- Scintillations (or other visual display), paresthesias, aphasia, dysarthria, and paralysis
- Build-up of scintillations
- March of paresthesias
- Progression from one accompaniment to another, often with a delay
- Two or more similar attacks
- Headache in 50 percent of attacks
- Episodes last 15 to 25 minutes
- Characteristic mid-life "flurry" of attacks
- Generally benign course
- Normal angiography
- Rule out cerebral thrombosis, embolism and dissection, epilepsy, thrombocythemia, polycythemia, and thrombotic thrombocytopenia

Various pain patterns have been described in migraine. Patients who have daily headaches that persist for months often have transformed migraine, with a past history of episodic migraine typically beginning in their teens or twenties.[33] Most of these patients are women, 90 percent of whom have a history of migraine without aura. The headaches grow more frequent, and the associated symptoms of photophobia, phonophobia, and nausea become less severe and less frequent than during typical migraine. Patients often develop a pattern of daily, or nearly daily, headaches that phenomenologically resemble chronic TTH, with mild to moderate pain but with photophobia, phonophobia, or gastrointestinal features. Other features of migraine, including unilaterality and aggravation by menstruation and other trigger factors, may persist. Attacks of full-blown migraine superimposed on a background of less severe headaches often occur. In the past, this was called mixed tension-vascular headache. Most patients with transformed migraine overuse symptomatic medication. Stopping the overused medication frequently results in distinct headache improvement. Eighty percent of patients with transformed migraine have depression. The depression often lifts when the pattern of medication overuse and daily headache is interrupted.

Because of the limitations of patient recall, a past history of migraine and an escalation of symptoms over 3 months may be impossible to obtain. Three alternative diagnostic links to migraine have been proposed: (1) a prior history of IHS migraine; (2) a clear period of escalating headache frequency with decreasing severity of migrainous features; or (3) current superimposed attacks of headaches that meet all of the IHS criteria for migraine except duration.

There are a number of disorders that may present with migraine symptoms. Cerebral autosomal dominant arteriopathy with subcortical infarcts and leukoencephalopathy (CADASIL) is an inherited arterial disease of the brain that has been mapped to chromosome 19.[34] The complete CADASIL syndrome consists of recurrent episodes of focal brain deficits (recurrent strokes) that start in midadult life and often lead to dementia, residual motor disability, and pseudobulbar palsy. Even before clinical symptoms or signs have developed, at-risk individuals may demonstrate an abnormal MRI, with extensive areas of increased T2 signals in the white matter. Many cases of FHM (all with associated cerebellar features) map to chromosome 19, close to the gene locus for CADASIL. The main clinical presentation of CADASIL is recurrent subcortical events, either transient or (more often) permanent. The arteriopathy underlying CADASIL is neither atherosclerotic nor amyloid and involves the media of small cerebral arteries and to a lesser extent extracerebral arteries, including skin arterioles. Skin biopsy can be diagnostic. Ultrastructural examination reveals abnormal patches of agranular osmophilic material within the basal membranes of vascular smooth-muscle cells.[35]

In 1996, Joutel et al identified Notch3 as the defective gene in CADASIL.[36] Members of the Notch gene family encode evolutionarily conserved transmembrane receptors and are involved in cell fate specification during embryonic development. The Notch3 gene includes 33 exons encoding a protein of 2321 amino acids. Its extracellular domain contains 34 epidermal growth factor-like repeats that are involved in ligand-binding, whereas the intracellular domain carries the intrinsic signal-transducing activity. CADASIL gene identification has provided the information needed to set up a direct genotypic diagnostic test.[35]

Mitochondrial encephalopathy with lactic acidosis and stroke-like spells (MELAS) syndrome may present with otherwise typical migraine or migraine with neurological deficits. Ornithine transcarbamylase deficiency, a urea cycle enzyme abnormality, may resemble confusional migraine in children and young adults, with migraine-like headaches, cyclic vomiting, confusion, hallucinations, visual disturbances, and ataxia.

Differential Diagnosis. Migraine-like headaches with or without aura may occur as a result of a wide variety of structural abnormalities of the brain, including tumors, infections, and vascular malformations. Such headaches may be thought of as secondary migraine. Cerebrovascular disorders such as infarction, transient ischemic attack, venous thrombosis, vasculitis, and carotid or vertebral dissection should be included in the differentiation of migraine. Idiopathic intracranial hypertension (IIH), low pressure headache, and intracranial neoplasms may also mimic migraine, as may metabolic abnormalities, hypoxia, hypoglycemia, dialysis, pheochromocytoma, and various chemicals and medications. Raeder's syndrome, with carotid artery abnormalities along the base of the skull, may also resemble migraine. Sinusitis or glaucoma may occasionally resemble migraine, and sometimes epilepsy produces intermittent headaches. Although rare, the aura of migraine may lead directly to a partial or complex partial seizure, termed migralepsy.[37] Other primary headache disorders such as TTH, cluster headache, and hypnic headache should be considered (see Table 53–1).[17]

Evaluation. Patients who have normal neurological examinations and benign recurrent headaches that fit the IHS criteria of migraine do not require brain imaging.[38] Patients who have abnormal neurological examinations, atypical histories, or a sudden unexplained change in the frequency or major characteristics of their headaches should be imaged. There is no consensus whether all patients with chronic daily headaches should be imaged with CT or MRI, even if they fulfill the criteria for typical migraine. Unless a metabolic abnormality is suspected, blood tests for diagnostic purposes are rarely indicated. However, routine blood tests and an electrocardiogram are often valuable before initiating therapy for migraine.

Management. The US headache consortium guidelines helped organize and prioritize treatment options.[39, 40]

ACUTE TREATMENT. For acute management, the choice depends on the severity and frequency of the headaches, the pattern of the associated symptoms, the presence of comorbid illnesses, and the patient's treatment response profile. Most migraineurs describe headache-provoking (trigger) factors (Table 53–5), with alcohol, stress, menstruation, and diet being the most common. Patients should attempt to avoid these triggers and keep regular exercise, meal, and sleep patterns.[17] In the pharmacological treatment of migraine, there are two strategies: (1) acute medications (Table 53–6), which are used to terminate attacks, and (2) preventive medications (Table 53–7), which are used to prevent future ones. Some drugs, such as metoclopramide, can prevent a headache attack when they are administered during the prodrome. Acute headache treatment medication can be specific or nonspecific. Nonspecific medications (analgesics, antiemetics, anxiolytics, nonsteroidal anti-inflammatory drugs [NSAIDs], steroids, neuroleptics, opioids) are used to control the pain and associated symptoms of migraine or other pain disorders, while specific medications (ergots and selective 5-HT1 agonists [triptans]) control the migraine attack but are not useful for nonheadache pain disorders. Headaches are stratified by severity and disability and treated with the medications most likely to be effective for that attack, taking into account the drug's efficacy, safety, and side effects. When there is significant early nausea or vomiting, patients will need to be treated with antiemetics or with nonoral drugs for migraine control.[41] The sooner treatment is begun, the more effective it will be. Caffeine, butalbital, isometheptene, and dichloralphenazone are adjunctive medications included in combination preparations to improve efficacy.[17]

For patients with mild-to-moderate headaches, analgesics, NSAIDs, or a caffeine adjuvant compound can be useful. The authors use a triptan or DHE as a first-line drug for severe attacks and as a backup for less severe attacks that do not adequately respond to simple or combination analgesics. The subcutaneous injection is useful for patients who need rapid relief. Oral triptans may be used for gradual-onset headache, when rapid pain relief is not required. In given patients, more than one treatment plan can be used; for example, patients may successfully use naproxen sodium for mild-to-moderate headaches, but require a triptan for more severe headaches.[42, 43]

TABLE 53–5. **Trigger Factors of Migraine**

Psychological	**Physical**
Stress	Exercise
Tension	Fatigue
Anxiety	Sexual activity
Letdown	High altitude
Neurological and Medical	**Dietary**
Bright lights or glare	Missed or delayed meals
Odors	Certain foods
Changes in sleep patterns	Alcohol
Hormonal changes (menstruation)	
Changes in weather or temperature	

TABLE 53–6. **Abortive Pharmacotherapy for Various Headache Types**

Agent	Starting Dose	Maximum Daily Dose	Use
Ergot Alkaloids			
Dihydroergotamine	0.25–1 mg IM/IV	2 mg IV	M,C
	1 mg SC	3 mg SC/IM	
	2–3 mg IN	6 mg IN	
Ergotamine	1–2 mg PO/SL/PR	6 mg PO/SL/PR	M,C
Serotonin Agonists			
Sumatriptan	6 mg SC	12 mg SC	M,C
	25–100 mg PO	300 mg PO	
Rizatriptan	5–10 mg PO	30 mg PO	M
Naratriptan	2.5 mg PO	5 mg PO	M
Zolmitriptan	2.5–5 mg PO	10 mg PO	M,C
Frovatriptan	2.5 mg	7.5 mg	M
Almotriptan	6.25–12.5 mg PO	25 mg PO	M
Opioid Analgesics			
Butorphanol	1 mg IN	8 mg IN	M,C
	2 mg IM	4 mg IM	
Hydromorphone	2–4 mg PO	16 mg PO	M
Meperidine	50–150 mg PO/PR/IM/IV	400 mg PO/IM/IV	M
Morphine	5–10 mg PO/PR/IM/IV	60 mg PO/IM/IV	M
Nonopioid Analgesics			
Ketolorac	10 mg PO	40 mg PO	M,T
	30–60 mg IM	120 mg IM	
Naproxen sodium	275–825 mg PO	1650 mg PO	M,T
Neuroleptics			
Chlorpromazine	25–50 mg IV/IM	400 mg IV/IM	M,T
	25–100 mg PR	400 mg PR	
Prochlorperazine	5–10 mg IV/IM	40 mg IV/IM	M,T
	25 mg PR	75 mg PR	
Thiothixene	5 mg PO	20 mg PO	M
	5 mg IM	20 mg IM	
Corticosteroids			
Dexamethasone	4–8 mg PO	32 mg PO	M,C
Prednisone	40–100 mg PO	200 mg PO	M,C
Miscellaneous Agents			
Oxygen	7–10 L/min for 15 min via face mask		C

M, Migraine; C, cluster headache; T, tension-type headache; IN, intranasal; SC, subcutaneous; IM, intramuscular; PO, per mouth; IV, intravenous; SL, sublingual; PR, per rectum.

A self-administered rescue medication is needed when other treatments fail. Rescue medications include potent opioids, neuroleptics, and corticosteroids. The triptans are effective but expensive, and about one third of patients have recurrent headaches with this drug. Patient-administered triptans and DHE have the best efficacy-to-adverse-effect ratio of all the acute treatment medications and are the most cost-effective because their use results in fewer emergency room visits. Because nausea and vomiting are symptoms that are commonly associated with migraine headaches, oral medications may be unsuitable, and alternative formulations, as well as antiemetics, are often needed. Intravenous (IV) neuroleptics, corticosteroids, and DHE are highly effective. Patients with severe rebound headache, significant psychiatric or medical comorbidity, or a severe intractable headache that has failed to respond to outpatient treatment may require inpatient treatment with IV medication.[17] Before deciding that a drug is ineffective, the clinician should test its effects on at least two different attacks. One must be sure that the dose is adequate and no other factors interfere with its effect. It may be necessary to change formulation or route of administration or add an adjuvant. Changing the drug should be considered when the response is incomplete or too slow, the headache recurs, the results are inconsistent after an adequate trial at an adequate dose, or the side effects are bothersome. Medication-overuse headache is a serious clinical problem and, in general, treatment with acute headache medication should be limited to 2 to 3 days per week. Medication-overuse headache results from the too-frequent use of acute headache medications, often resulting in more frequent headaches that are refractory to treatment.[42]

PREVENTIVE TREATMENT. Preventive medications (see Table 53–7) are usually taken, whether or not headache is present, to reduce attack frequency, duration, or severity.[44] Preventive drug treatments include antidepressants, beta-blockers, calcium channel blockers, NSAIDs, serotonin antagonists (methysergide, cyproheptadine), and anticonvulsants. Preventive treatment is used when there is:

TABLE 53–7. **Preventive Pharmacotherapy for Various Headache Types**

Agent	Starting Daily Dose*	Maximum Daily Dose*	Use
Beta Blockers			
Atenolol	50 mg	200 mg	M,T
Metoprolol	50 mg	450 mg	M,T
Nadolol	20 mg	240 mg	M,T
Propranolol	40 mg	320 mg	M,T
Timolol	10 mg	60 mg	M,T
Calcium Channel Blockers			
Diltiazem	120 mg	360 mg	M,C
Nifedipine	30 mg	180 mg	M,C
Verapamil	120 mg	720 mg	M,T,C
Serotonin Antagonists-Agonists			
Cyproheptadine	4 mg	36 mg	M
Methysergide	2 mg	14 mg	M,T,C
Antidepressants			
Amitriptyline	10 mg	150 mg	M,T
Doxepin	10 mg	150 mg	M,T
Fluoxetine	10 mg	80 mg	M,T
Imipramine	10 mg	200 mg	M,T
Nortriptyline	10 mg	125 mg	M,T
Phenelzine	30 mg	90 mg	M,T
Anticonvulsants			
Divalproex	250 mg	3000 mg	M,T,C
Topiramate	15–25 mg	1000 mg	M,T,C
Gabapentin	300 mg	3600 mg	M,T
Miscellaneous Agents			
Lithium	300 mg	1800 mg	C

*All doses are oral.
M, migraine; T, tension-type headache; C, cluster headache.

(1) recurring migraine that significantly interferes with the patient's daily routine despite acute treatment; (2) failure of, contraindication to, overuse of, or troublesome side effects from acute medications; (3) special circumstances, such as hemiplegic migraine or attacks with a risk of permanent neurological injury; (4) very frequent headaches (more than two per week) with the risk of developing rebound headache; and (5) patient preference; that is, the desire to have as few acute attacks as possible.

If preventive medication is indicated, the agent should be chosen from one of the major categories, based on documented efficacy, side effect profiles, ease of use, and coexistent comorbid conditions. Medications used to treat migraine can be divided into five major categories: (1) drugs with documented high efficacy and mild-to-moderate adverse effects (AEs), which include beta-blockers, amitriptyline, and divalproex; (2) drugs with documented high efficacy but with significant AEs or complex management limitation, which include methysergide and monoamine oxidase inhibitors; (3) drugs with lower documented efficacy and mild to moderate AEs, which include selective serotonin reuptake inhibitors, calcium channel antagonists, gabapentin, riboflavin, and NSAIDs; (4) drugs without trial-document data on efficacy and used because of open-label observations with mild-to-moderate AEs or major AEs or complex management limitation; and (5) drugs with limited or no efficacy, which include cyproheptadine, lithium, and phenytoin. Treatment selection is based on the best risk-to-benefit ratio for the individual patient. Medication should be started at a low dose and increased slowly until headache severity or frequency decreases, the maximum recommended dose is reached, or adverse effects develop. Dose titrations may take several months. When the headaches have been controlled for 6 months, attempts can be made to taper and discontinue therapy. Patients should be monitored for acute medication overuse, which may result in chronic refractory headaches and withdrawal symptoms when the medication is discontinued.[17] Recently, botulinum toxin type A injection has been reported to be effective in migraine prevention.[45]

The pregnant headache patient should be treated conservatively, with nonpharmacological treatments the first choice. If the patient does not respond to this form of therapy, acetaminophen (alone or with prochlorperazine or narcotics) can be used, and NSAIDs may be used in the first two trimesters. Very severe attacks should be treated with IV fluids, prochlorperazine, or narcotics. Prednisone has occasionally been used, but aspirin, barbiturate, and benzodiazepine use should be limited. Ergotamine and sumatriptan should be avoided completely. In the breast-feeding migraineur, ergotamine and lithium should not be used, because these drugs readily transfer to the baby via breast milk and can cause significant toxicity. Benzodiazepines, antidepressants, and neuroleptics may be used cautiously. Acetaminophen is preferable to aspirin.[17]

Prognosis and Future Perspectives. The prognosis of migraine is generally good. It usually improves and may disappear in the sixth or seventh decade of life. The natural history of transformed migraine is less certain. With aggressive treatment, most patients improve, although many continue to have lower intensity chronic daily headache or frequent episodic migraine. Future research will involve the search for the migraine gene. Gene-directed therapy may be a therapeutic option in the next decade. The gene for CADASIL has been cloned, and familial hemiplegic migraine has been linked to chromosomes 19 and 1. The gene on chromosome 19 is the α_1 subunit of a neuronal P/Q calcium channel.

TENSION-TYPE HEADACHE

Pathogenesis and Pathophysiology. Although many patients with TTHs have muscle tenderness, TTH is not the result of sustained contraction of the pericranial muscles with subsequent ischemic pain in response to emotion or stress. Muscle ischemia is not present during headache. Electromyographic activity is increased in some muscles, independent of tenderness and pain. Reduced CNS 5-HT levels may be responsible for abnormal pain modulation, producing the decreased pain thresholds that are observed in patients with chronic TTH. A "myofascial-supraspinal-vascular" model has been proposed for TTH.[46] When pain facilitation is present, normal subthreshold stimuli may produce significant pain even if myofascial nociceptor hypersensitivity is not present. The cranial muscle ache of a TTH attack may, therefore, be due to increased neuronal sensitivity and pain facilitation due to chronic or intermittent dysfunction of the monoaminergic or serotonergic function in the hypothalamus, brain stem, and spinal cord.[47] Chronic TTH may be associated with a perceived increase in stressful life events. Depression is common in patients with chronic TTH, and neurotransmitter abnormalities in 5-HT, norepinephrine, dopamine, and enkephalins have been proposed as the etiology.

Epidemiology and Risk Factors. TTH is the most common headache type, with a lifetime prevalence of 69 percent in men and 88 percent in women.[19] TTHs can begin at any age, but onset during adolescence or young adulthood is most common. About 40 percent of patients evaluated in headache clinics suffer from daily headache, whereas only 3 percent of the population has daily headache.[48] Headache prevalence declines with increasing age, and severity decreases in the women who continue to report headaches but does not change in men. Only patients with more severe frequent headaches that are unresponsive to over-the-counter preparations seek medical attention.

Clinical Features and Associated Disorders. The IHS criteria for a TTH require that patients experience at least 10 previous headaches, each lasting 30 minutes to 7 days (median, 12 hours), with at least two of the following characteristics: a pressing/tightening (nonpulsating) quality, mild to moderate intensity, bilateral location, and no aggravation with physical activity. In addition, the patient should not have nausea or vomiting or a combination of photophobia and phonophobia. Episodic TTH occurs less than 15 days a month, whereas chronic TTH occurs 15 or more days a month.[47]

The onset of TTH is gradual, often occurring after or during stress, and is typically worse late in the day. There is no prodrome. The pain is usually a nagging, tight, or viselike bilateral pressure that is located in the forehead, the temples, or the back of the head. It may radiate to the neck and shoulders. There are no associated autonomic or gastrointestinal symptoms except for occasional anorexia. The frequency of episodic TTH ranges from 2 to 12 days a month, with a median of 6 days a month. The headaches may be associated with menstruation.[47, 48]

Twenty-five percent of TTH patients also have migraine. Patients with episodic TTH are no different from controls in terms of stress, depression, anxiety, emotional conflicts, sleeping problems, and fatigue. Patients with chronic TTH are often depressed.[47]

Differential Diagnosis. Migraine is the primary headache disorder that may be confused with TTH. Both can be bilateral, nonthrobbing, and associated with anorexia. Migraine is more severe, often unilateral, and frequently associated with nausea. IIH, brain tumor headache, chronic sphenoid sinusitis, and cervical, ocular, and temporomandibular disorders need to be considered.[47, 48]

Evaluation. Most patients with a long history of unchanged episodic TTHs do not require extensive evaluation if they have normal neurological examinations and are otherwise healthy. Patients with chronic TTHs should be imaged with CT or MRI, even if their general and neurological examinations are normal. A metabolic screen, complete blood count, electrolytes, and kidney and thyroid function studies are also appropriate.[47]

Management. TTH patients usually self-medicate with over-the-counter analgesics (aspirin, acetaminophen, NSAIDs), with or without caffeine. If these medications are not effective, prescription NSAIDs or combination analgesic preparations can be used. Narcotics and combination analgesics that contain sedatives or caffeine should be limited, because overuse may cause dependence. Symptomatic medication overuse can cause episodic TTHs to convert to chronic TTHs Patients with both migraine and TTHs benefit from specific migraine medication such as sumatriptan or DHE (see Tables 53–6 and 53–7).[47, 48]

Preventive therapy should be administered when a patient has frequent headaches that produce disability or may lead to symptomatic medication overuse. Medications used for TTH prevention include antidepressants, beta blockers, and anticonvulsants. Antidepressants, the medication of first choice, should be started at a low dose and increased slowly every three to seven days. An adequate trial period of at least one to two months must be allowed. The addition of biofeedback therapy or beta-blocking agents may improve the therapeutic benefit derived from antidepressants.[47, 48]

Prognosis and Future Perspectives. Episodic TTH is a benign recurrent condition that usually improves with time. Some patients may, however, progress to chronic TTH, especially when analgesic overuse is present. The prognosis of chronic TTH is controversial, because many studies include patients with more severe headaches and co-existing conditions, such as migraine and psychiatric disorders.

CLUSTER HEADACHE

Pathogenesis and Pathophysiology. The pathogenesis of cluster headaches is increasingly clear. Trigeminovascular system involvement has been demonstrated by a marked increase in the level of calcitonin gene-related peptide in the cranial venous circulation during attacks.[49] Parasympathetic system activation in cluster headache has been corroborated by the finding of dramatically elevated levels of vasoactive intestinal polypeptide during attacks[49] with robust ipsilateral autonomic features. This finding provides an anatomical basis for the expression of first division trigeminal pain and ipsilateral autonomic symptoms that occur during cluster attacks. Cluster events are probably related to alterations in the circadian pacemaker, which may be due to hypothalamic dysfunction. Attacks increase following the beginning and end of daylight savings time, and there is a loss of circadian rhythm for blood pressure, temperature, and hormones, including prolactin, melatonin, cortisol, and beta endorphins. Evidence for the role of the hypothalamus in cluster headache pathogenesis has come from functional and morphometric neuroimaging. Using positron-emission tomography imaging, May and colleagues demonstrated marked activation in the ipsilateral ventral hypothalamic gray matter during nitroglycerin-induced acute cluster headache attacks.[50] Neurogenic inflammation, carotid body chemoreceptor dysfunction, central parasympathetic and sympathetic tone imbalance, and increased responsiveness to histamine have been proposed as the cause of cluster pain.[51]

Epidemiology and Risk Factors. With an incidence of 0.01 to 1.5 percent in various populations, cluster headache prevalence is lower than that of migraine or TTH. Prevalence is higher in men than in women and in black patients compared with white patients. The male-to-female ratio is about 6:1. However, recent evidence suggests a progressively decreasing male preponderance. The male-to-female ratio based on the year of onset in Manzoni's study[52] decreased from 6.2:1 in the 1960s to 2.1:1 in the 1990s.[53] A family history of cluster headache is rare. The most common form of cluster headache is episodic cluster. The rarest form is chronic cluster headache without remissions, with only about 10 percent of patients suffering from this variety of cluster. Cluster headache can begin at any age, but it generally begins in the late twenties. Cluster headache rarely begins in childhood, and only about 10 percent of patients develop cluster when they are in their sixties.[51, 54]

Clinical Features and Associated Disorders. Patients with cluster headache have multiple episodes of short-lived but severe, unilateral, orbital, supraorbital, or temporal pain. At least one of the following associated symptoms must occur: conjunctival injection, lacrimation, nasal congestion, rhinorrhea, facial sweating, miosis, ptosis, or eyelid edema. Episodic cluster consists of headache periods of 1 week to 1 year, with remission periods lasting at least 14 days, whereas chronic cluster headache has either no remission periods or remissions that last less than 14 days.[51, 54]

The pain of a cluster attack rapidly increases (within 15 minutes) to excruciating levels. The attacks often occur at the same time each day and frequently awaken patients from sleep. If the condition is left untreated, the attacks usually last from 30 to 90 minutes, but may last up to 180 minutes. The pain is deep, constant, boring, piercing, or burning in nature, located in, behind, or around the eye. It may radiate to the forehead, temples, jaws, nostrils, ears, neck, or shoulder. During an attack, patients often feel agitated or restless and feel the need to isolate themselves and move around. Gastrointestinal symptoms are uncommon. The attack frequency varies from one every other day to eight a day, occurring in cluster periods that last a week to a year. Remissions between cluster periods generally lasts 6 months to 2 years. Most patients have one or two cluster periods a year that last 2 to 3 months, with one to two attacks a day.[51]

Peptic ulcer disease is the only known associated medical disorder. Secondary cluster-like headache may occur due to structural lesions near the cavernous sinuses.[51, 54]

Differential Diagnosis. The differential diagnosis of cluster headache includes chronic paroxysmal hemicrania, migraine, trigeminal neuralgia, temporal arteritis, pheochromocytoma, Raeder's paratrigeminal syndrome, Tolosa-Hunt syndrome, sinusitis, and glaucoma.[51] Raeder's syndrome has characteristics similar to cluster headaches. It may be associated with severe pain, unilateral and supraorbital distribution, and an associated partial Horner's syndrome. It is distinct from cluster headache in that there are no distinct attacks and the pain is constant.

Evaluation. There are no studies that address the need for testing in cluster-like headache. In most cases, a careful history is all that is needed to make the diagnosis. MRI of the head is justified only in atypical cases or cases with an abnormal neurological examination (except when the abnormality is a Horner's syndrome).

Management. Patients with cluster headaches should avoid alcohol and nitroglycerin, yet other dietary and drug restrictions have little effect. Pharmacological treatment for cluster headaches is divided into abortive and preventive therapy, and recommendations are mainly based on uncontrolled trials (Table 53–8).[51, 54] Oral preparations are absorbed slowly and are not recommended for the treatment of acute attacks. Effective abortive treatments that provide

TABLE 53–8. **Cluster Headache Prophylaxis**

Drug	Dosage	Adverse Effects
Episodic Cluster Headache*		
Divalproex	500–3000 mg/d	Nausea, lethargy, tremor, bodyweight gain, hair loss; rarely abnormal liver function, pancreatitis
Ergotamine	Up to 4 mg/d	Nausea, paresthesia, intermittent claudication, ergotism
Lithium	300 mg bid or tid (0.4–0.8 mmol/L)	Weakness, nausea, thirst, tremor, lethargy, slurred speech, blurred vision
Methysergide	2–14 mg/d	Muscle cramps, nausea, diarrhea, abdominal discomfort
Prednisone	40–100 mg/d, taper over 1 to 2 weeks	Insomnia, restlessness, personality changes, hyponatremia, edema, hyperglycemia, osteoporosis, myopathy, gastric ulcers, hip necrosis
Topiramate	50–200 mg/d	Weight loss, paresthesia, renal stones, cognitive dysfunction
Verapamil	120–720 mg/d	Constipation, edema, dizziness, nausea, hypotension, fatigue
Chronic Cluster Headache†		
Divalproex	500–3000 mg/d	Same as episodic
Lithium	300 mg bid or tid (0.4 to 0.8 mmol/L)	Hypothyroidism and polyuria
Methysergide	2–14 mg/d	Fibrotic reactions
Topiramate	50–200 mg/d	Weight loss, paresthesia, renal stones, cognitive dysfunction
Verapamil	120–720 mg/d	Same as episodic

*Begin early in the cluster period and continue until the patient has been headache-free for at least 2 weeks.
†Combinations are often required.
bid, Twice daily; tid, three times daily.

rapid onset of action include oxygen, sumatriptan, DHE, and (perhaps) topical local anesthetics. Inhaled oxygen, 7 to 10 L/min for 10 minutes following headache onset, is 70 percent effective and is often the treatment of first choice. Parenteral injections of sumatriptan or DHE mesylate provide significant relief for about 80 percent of patients. An intranasal local anesthetic may provide relief for some patients.[51, 54]

Most patients with cluster headache require preventive treatment because each attack is too short in duration and too severe in intensity to treat with only abortive medication. In addition, ergotamine, DHE, sumatriptan, and oxygen may just postpone rather than abort the attack. Preventive therapy for cluster includes ergotamine, calcium channel blockers, methysergide, lithium, corticosteroids, divalproex, topiramate, melatonin, and capsaicin. Occasionally, indomethacin is effective. If medical therapy fails completely, surgical intervention may be beneficial for the psychologically stable patient with strictly unilateral chronic cluster. The surgery consists of neuronal ablation procedures directed toward the sensory input of the trigeminal nerve and autonomic pathways, and is generally effective in 75 percent of patients.[51] A new procedure, gamma knife radiosurgery, was reported to be effective in 6 medically recalcitrant cluster headache patients.[55] The prognosis of cluster headaches is guarded; it is a chronic headache that may last for the patient's life. Drug therapy may help convert some patients from chronic to episodic cluster.[51]

CHRONIC PAROXYSMAL HEMICRANIA

Chronic paroxysmal hemicrania resembles cluster headache in character but distinguishes itself by its dramatic responsiveness to indomethacin therapy. The pathophysiology of chronic paroxysmal hemicrania is unknown. Changes in intraocular pressure that occur during attacks suggest autonomic dysfunction, and the periodicity of this disorder suggests a central generator.[56] Chronic paroxysmal hemicrania is a rare disorder that affects women more than men (ratio approximately 7:1), in contrast to cluster headache. It appears to have approximately 2 percent the prevalence of cluster headache.[56]

Like cluster headache patients, chronic paroxysmal hemicrania patients have severe unilateral headaches associated with unilateral nasal stuffiness, lacrimation, conjunctival eye tearing, ptosis, and eyelid edema. Headaches average 13 minutes in duration and occur an average of 11 times a day. Occasionally, there is a continuous dull ache between attacks. In 10 percent of patients, attacks may be triggered by flexing, rotating, or pressing the upper portion of the neck.[56] Typically, there are no remissions. Rarely, a patient may present with episodic paroxysmal hemicrania with remissions that last weeks or months. Patients may evolve from the episodic to the chronic form of the illness. By definition, chronic and episodic hemicrania are responsive to indomethacin. No other medical or psychiatric disorders have been associated with chronic paroxysmal hemicrania.[56]

The differential diagnosis of chronic paroxysmal hemicrania is similar to that of cluster headache. In addition, patients with "jabs and jolts syndrome" might occasionally resemble chronic paroxysmal hemicrania patients. A rare headache disorder called short unilateral neuralgiform headache with conjunctival injection and tearing should be considered, although the headaches are much shorter in duration (15 to 30 seconds) and occur much more frequently (many times per hour) than those of chronic paroxysmal hemicrania.

In the evaluation of chronic paroxysmal hemicrania, a trial of indomethacin is necessary to establish the diagnosis. Brain imaging with MRI or CT should be undertaken to exclude symptomatic causes of apparent chronic paroxysmal hemicrania. The treatment of choice is indomethacin (in a dose up to 200 mg/d). Aspirin may also be beneficial, but the relief afforded is usually not complete. Chronic paroxysmal hemicrania may last indefinitely, but over time, there may be a reduced indomethacin requirement. Temporary remissions and spontaneous cures have been described. Selective prostaglandin synthesis inhibitors, indomethacin-like drugs without the gastrointestinal side effects of the current NSAIDs, are in development and may be beneficial.

IDIOPATHIC INTRACRANIAL HYPERTENSION

Pathogenesis and Pathophysiology. The pathophysiology of IIH is unknown. Postulated mechanisms include increased cerebrospinal fluid (CSF) production, decreased CSF absorption, and increased venous sinus pressure. Some studies suggest that interstitial brain edema and a decreased rate of absorption at the arachnoid villi are the major contributors. The disturbances of CSF hydrodynamics in IIH persist for years.[57] Increased CSF pressure in IIH may result from a rise in venous sagittal sinus pressure secondary to extracellular edema causing venous obstruction or from low conductance for CSF reabsorption producing a compensatory increase in CSF pressure. Patients were evaluated with cerebral venography and manometry, and they demonstrated elevated venous pressure in the superior sagittal and proximal transverse sinuses. This elevated pressure dropped at the level of the lateral third of the transverse sinus, resembling a mural thrombosis on venography. Two patients with intracranial hypertension due to minocycline did not have venous hypertension. The authors suggested that most patients with IIH may have partial venous outflow obstructions, blurring the distinction between idiopathic and symptomatic causes.[58, 59] In another study, the authors suggested that IIH was due to either venous obstruction or elevated central venous pressure, despite the absence of signs or symptoms of heart failure. The pathophysiology of IIH without papilledema is presumably similar to that with papilledema.

Epidemiology and Risk Factors. IIH with papilledema occurs with a frequency of about 1 case per 100,000 per year in the general population and 19.3 cases per 100,000 per year in obese women aged 20 to 44.[58] The patient with IIH is commonly a young, obese woman with chronic daily headaches, normal laboratory studies, an empty sella, and a normal neurological examination (except for papilledema) (Fig. 53–2).[58]

Clinical Features and Associated Disorders. The symptoms of IIH consist of generalized increased intracranial pressure, with headache occurring in most, but not all, patients. Bifrontotemporal headache is most common. Unilateral headache with increased CSF pressure due to IIH may be an exacerbation of migraine or a new local phenomenon. Transient visual obscuration (an episode of visual clouding in one or both eyes usually lasting seconds) occurs with all forms of increased intracranial pressure with papilledema but is not

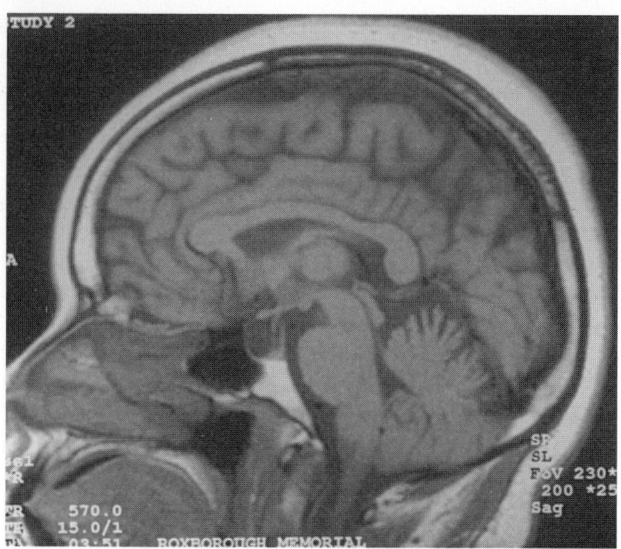

FIGURE 53–2. An empty sella is shown.

a specific symptom. Transient visual obscurations can occur in patients without increased intracranial pressure who have elevated optic discs from other causes. Persons without papilledema do not have transient visual obscurations. Pulsatile tinnitus, diplopia, and visual loss can occur. Some patients report shoulder and arm pain (perhaps secondary to nerve root dilatation) and retro-orbital pain.[58]

Idiopathic intracranial hypertension without papilledema has been described in some patients. The headache and demographic characteristics are identical to those of patients with papilledema except for (1) possible association with prior head trauma or meningitis; (2) extended delay in diagnosis, which requires lumbar puncture in the absence of papilledema; and (3) no evidence of the visual loss seen in patients with IIH with papilledema.[58] There are no disorders associated with IIH other than obesity.

Differential Diagnosis. IIH may be either truly *idiopathic*, with no clear identifiable cause, or *symptomatic*, a result of venous sinus occlusion, radical neck dissection, hypoparathyroidism, vitamin A intoxication, systemic lupus erythematosus, renal disease, or drug side effects (nalidixic acid, danocrine, steroid withdrawal).

Evaluation. The diagnosis of IIH (with or without papilledema) is based on lumbar puncture following neuroimaging (paying attention to empty sella and sinus thrombosis). If CSF biochemical and cytological analyses are unremarkable and intracranial pressure is elevated to greater than 200 mm H_2O (in nonobese subjects), IIH is the likely diagnosis. Secondary causes should also be considered in the evaluation. Over 50 diseases, conditions, toxins, or pharmaceuticals have been associated with IIH. Patients, particularly obese women, with chronic daily headaches and symptoms of increased intracranial pressure—for example, pulsatile tinnitus, a history of head trauma or meningitis, an empty sella on neuroimaging studies, or a headache that is unrelieved by standard therapy—should have a diagnostic lumbar puncture.[58]

Management. The treatment of IIH is multidimensional (Table 53–9). Obese patients should be encouraged to lose weight. If patients are asymptomatic and do not have visual loss, treatment is not indicated. In these cases, careful ophthalmological follow-up is necessary. If there is headache with visual loss or papilledema, aggressive treatment should be instituted.

Headache associated with IIH and papilledema frequently responds to the same treatments used for migraine and TTH. If rigorous headache therapy is unsuccessful, or if there is visual loss, then a 4- to 6-week trial of furosemide or a potent carbonic anhydrase inhibitor (acetazolamide) should be given. High-dose steroids may be effective, but headache commonly recurs when the drugs are withdrawn. Lumbar puncture typically relieves headache in patients with IIH and papilledema. Some intractable headache patients have a dissociation between the CSF pressure and the headache. In some patients, lumbar puncture reduces the pressure and relieves the headache; in others, there is no improvement. Surgical treatment of IIH has been directed toward preventing visual loss secondary to papilledema, and headache improvement occurs in many patients when optic nerve sheath fenestration is performed.[58]

Prognosis and Future Perspectives. Most patients with IIH and papilledema can be managed successfully. The prognosis for headache control of IIH without papilledema is more guarded, although there appears to be no risk of visual deterioration. The development of drugs to control CSF production, perhaps acting via 5-HT_{2C} receptors, may revolutionize the treatment of IIH in the near future.

LOW PRESSURE HEADACHE

Pathogenesis and Pathophysiology. The most common cause of low pressure headache is a lumbar puncture. Head or back trauma, craniotomy, and spinal surgery can produce CSF hypotension as a result of a dural tear or traumatic avulsion of a nerve root resulting in a CSF leak. In addition, craniotomy and trauma can produce intracranial hypotension not associated with a CSF leak. This may be a result of decreased CSF formation, decreased CBF, or both. Low pressure syndromes can occur secondary to CSF rhinorrhea, either spontaneous, post-traumatic, or due to a pituitary tumor. Spontaneous dural tears must be ruled out in all cases of spontaneous intracranial hypotension. Infusion of hypertonic solution or a systemic medical illness, including severe dehydration, hyperpnea, meningoencephalitis, uremia, and severe systemic infection, can cause CSF hypotension. Postural headache can also occur in patients who have had CSF shunts, and this can be one of the complications of treating IIH (see Table 53–9).[58] Intracranial hypotension may also respond to caffeine and an epidural blood patch

TABLE 53–9. **Possible Treatments of Idiopathic Intracranial Hypertension**

Eliminate symptomatic causes
Weight loss if obese
Standard headache treatment
Carbonic anhydrase inhibitors and loop diuretics
Short course of high-dose corticosteroids
Serial lumbar punctures
Lumboperitoneal or ventriculoperitoneal shunt
Optic nerve sheath fenestration

even without correction of an underlying leak, suggesting that the CSF pressure indicator of some patients may be set too low.

Cases of spontaneous intracranial hypotension have been reported in which the radionuclide cisternogram showed rapid uptake in the bladder and kidneys and rapid transport of isotope with no evidence of a CSF leak. This finding is believed to be abnormal and consistent with CSF hyperabsorption. Many researchers believe that this abnormality is solely due to an occult CSF leak. Slowing of isotope flow, which is evidence for decreased CSF production, has also been reported. This could lead to brain sagging with compression of the pituitary-hypothalamic axis and further reduction in CSF production. Slit-like ventricles and tight basilar cisterns have been reported on CT scans of patients with spontaneous intracranial hypotension, leading to speculation that this contributed to decreased CSF production. However, small ventricles (due to a compensatory increase in brain volume) is most likely a result, rather than a cause, of decreased CSF production.[58]

Occult CSF leakage may also be a major cause of IIH, according to some studies. A history of minor trauma is often elicited. In one report, approximately half the patients had a history of minor trauma or an inciting event. Traumatic rupture of spinal epidural cysts (formed during development), perineural cysts, or a nerve sheath tear could then produce a cryptic CSF leak. CSF can also leak into the petrous or ethmoidal regions or through the cribriform plate, and the patient may swallow the fluid and be unaware of the leak.

Epidemiology and Risk Factors. The incidence of spontaneous intracranial hypotension or secondary intracranial hypotension is unknown. Postlumbar puncture headache is more common in women, who are affected twice as often as men, and in younger patients. The incidence depends on the type of procedure: surgical lumbar puncture, 13 percent; obstetrical, 18 percent; and diagnostic, 32 percent.[60]

Clinical Features and Associated Disorders. Low pressure headache is the most common complication of lumbar puncture, occurring in 15 to 30 percent of patients. Onset varies from 15 minutes to 4 days following lumbar puncture, but it can take as long as 12 days. If it is left untreated, the headache can last 2 to 14 days (most commonly 4 to 8 days) or even months.[58] The headache of intracranial hypotension may be frontal, occipital, or diffuse. It is accentuated by the erect position and relieved with recumbency. The pain is severe, dull, or throbbing in nature and is usually not relieved with analgesics. It is aggravated by head-shaking, coughing, straining, sneezing, and jugular compression. The more severe the headache, the more frequently it is associated with dizziness, nausea, vomiting, and tinnitus, and the longer the patient is upright, the longer it takes the headache to subside with recumbency. Physical examination is usually normal; however, there may be mild neck stiffness and a slow pulse rate (so-called vagus pulse).[58, 60] Spinal fluid pressure usually ranges from 0 to 65 mm. The CSF composition is usually normal, but there may be a slight protein elevation and a few red blood cells in the fluid. Reversible Arnold-Chiari type malformation has been reported in association with a low CSF pressure headache.[60, 61]

Differential Diagnosis. The differential diagnosis of a spontaneous positional headache is limited, but other disorders, such as a colloid cyst of the third ventricle, need to be considered.

Evaluation. The diagnosis of low CSF pressure headache is easily made in the presence of orthostatic headache, particularly if there is an obvious etiology, such as head or back trauma, a recent lumbar puncture or craniotomy, or an associated medical illness. If no obvious cause is apparent or the diagnosis is uncertain, lumbar puncture (perhaps at the time of cisternography) is indicated, following a neuroimaging procedure (CT or MRI). The opening pressure usually ranges from 0 to 70 mm H_2O. However, in the Mayo Clinic series of spontaneous intracranial hypotension, the opening pressure was, at times, in the normal range, especially if the measurement was made after a period of recumbency.[60]

Diffuse pachymeningeal enhancement is the most common head MRI abnormality in CSF leaks and CSF volume depletion. This enhancement is limited to the pachymeninges without any evidence of leptomeningeal involvement. Descent of the brain "sagging" or "sinking" is also a common finding and is manifested by descent of the cerebellar tonsils (which may sometimes mimic type 1 Arnold-Chiari malformation),[62] decrease in the size of the pre-pontine cistern, inferior displacement of the optic chiasm, effacement of perichiasmatic cisterns, and crowding of the posterior fossa.

Subdural fluid collections are usually but not always bilateral. Decrease in the size of the ventricles, or "ventricular collapse," is sometimes obvious, though often subtle, and is best noted by comparing a head MRI obtained after recovery with a previous MRI taken during the symptomatic phase. Other abnormalities include pituitary enlargement;[63] engorged venous sinuses;[64] and elongation of the brain stem in the anteroposterior plane.[65] Spine MRI may reveal extra-arachnoid or extradural fluid.[66, 67] Dural enhancement[68] and engorgement or prominence of the epidural venous plexus can occur.

If the cause of the low pressure is known, one should proceed with the appropriate treatment modalities. If, however, treatment is unsuccessful, one should re-evaluate with the radioisotope cisternography or ionic myelography to identify CSF leaks, which can be caused by very small dural tears or nerve avulsions.[58]

Management. The treatment of low CSF pressure headache begins with noninvasive therapeutic modalities. If these modalities fail, a brief trial of steroids with a quick taper is recommended. Intravenous or oral caffeine therapy may also be highly effective. If the patient continues to be symptomatic after noninvasive therapies, a blood patch should be used. If the headache of intracranial hypotension recurs, a repeat blood patch can be performed or a continuous intrathecal saline infusion can be attempted. In the latter procedure, an epidural catheter is placed at the L2–L3 level and a saline infusion begun at a rate of 20 mL/hour and continued for as long as 72 hours.[58, 69]

Prognosis. Most patients with intracranial hypotension can be cured once a diagnosis is made. Occasionally, none of the treatments provides relief for a patient with a refractory CSF leak or a refractory low pressure headache without apparent cause.[58, 60] The development of atraumatic lumbar puncture needles has resulted in a decreased incidence of postlumbar puncture headache.[60]

OTHER HEADACHE SYNDROMES

Headache of Intracranial Neoplasms

Headache occurs at presentation in up to half of patients with brain tumors and develops in the course of the disease in 60 percent. Headache is partly dependent on the location of the tumor, and it is a rare initial symptom in patients with pituitary tumors, craniopharyngiomas, or cerebellopontine angle tumors.[58] In a modern series, 111 consecutive patients with primary (34 percent) or metastatic (66 percent) brain tumor were diagnosed using neuroimaging. In this series, headache was present in 48 percent of patients with primary and metastatic tumor and was similar in quality to TTH in 77 percent and migraine in 9 percent of patients. Unlike primary TTH, brain tumor headaches were worsened by bending in 32 percent of patients, and nausea or vomiting was present in 40 percent.[70] Increased intracranial pressure was defined by the presence of papilledema, obstructive hydrocephalus, communicating hydrocephalus from leptomeningeal metastasis, or a lumbar puncture opening pressure greater than 250 mm of CSF.

Eighty-six percent of patients with increased intracranial pressure had headache that was typically constant, bilateral, and frontal in location with a pressure-like or aching character. Only 1 percent had unilateral headache. The pain was severe in intensity, associated with nausea and vomiting, and resistant to common analgesics. Ataxia occurred in 61 percent. In contrast, only 36 percent of patients with a supratentorial tumor without increased intracranial pressure had headache. These headaches were milder and more likely to be intermittent, yet they were constant in 20 percent of patients. Nausea, vomiting, and ataxia were much less common.[70]

Patients with a history of prior headache were more likely to have a brain tumor headache. In many cases, this headache was similar in character to the prior headache, but it was more severe or frequent, or associated with neurological signs or symptoms.[70] There is a significant overlap between brain tumor headache and migraine or TTH. Morning or nocturnal headache associated with vomiting and increased headache frequency can be seen with both migraine and brain tumors. Brain tumor headache is more common in patients with a history of prior headache, increased intracranial pressure, and large tumors with a midline shift.[58] Headache of recent onset or a headache that has changed in character requires a thorough evaluation, particularly if the headache is severe or is accompanied by nausea or vomiting. Any neurological sign or symptom that is accompanied by a headache and cannot be easily explained by the aura of migraine must be carefully evaluated, as well.

Headache Due to Vascular Anomalies

Thunderclap headache is defined as the sudden onset of a severe headache that reaches maximum intensity within 1 minute. Benign thunderclap headache can be further defined by the absence of a subarachnoid hemorrhage and other intracranial pathology. This can be due to acute onset migraine and is very difficult to differentiate from a subarachnoid hemorrhage.[71, 72] An extensive neurological evaluation, including CT and lumbar puncture, is indicated in patients presenting with their first or worst headache, particularly one associated with focal neurological signs, stiff neck, or changes in cognition. CT can miss subarachnoid blood in as many as 25 percent of cases, particularly if it is not performed until days after the onset of headache.[71] MRI is unreliable in detecting an acute subarachnoid hemorrhage. Only with a lumbar puncture can one unerringly diagnose subarachnoid hemorrhage. Day and Raskin[72] have stated that all patients presenting with severe, sudden-onset headache should be evaluated for an aneurysm, even if CT, MRI, and lumbar puncture do not show evidence of subarachnoid hemorrhage, based on reports of unruptured aneurysms presenting as thunderclap headaches.[73]

Raps and associates[74] looked at the clinical spectrum of unruptured intracranial aneurysms. Acute, severe thunderclap headache, comparable to subarachnoid hemorrhage but without nuchal rigidity, was seen in 7 of 111 patients (6.3 percent) with unruptured aneurysms, most of which were located in the anterior circle of Willis. Because the true frequency of unruptured aneurysm among patients with thunderclap headache is unknown, all patients in whom unruptured aneurysm is a possibility should undergo at least an MRA. The routine use of cerebral angiography is proscribed by the risk of permanent (0.1 percent) and transient (1.2 percent) deficits in this low-yield population.[74]

Cough and Exercise Headache

Although coughing and exertion rarely provoke headache, these maneuvers can aggravate any type of headache. However, transient, severe head pain on coughing, sneezing, weight-lifting, bending, straining at stool, or stooping defines exertional headache.[75] Exertional headache mainly affects middle-aged men, and it runs its course over a few years. It is uncommon, and only 93 diagnoses were made at the Mayo Clinic over a 14-year period by Rooke,[76] who proposed the term benign exertional headache. In a population-based study,[77] benign cough headache and benign exertional headache each occurred with a prevalence of about 1 percent.

The IHS distinguishes between benign cough headache and benign exertional headache, entities that do not have identical clinical features, diagnostic evaluations, and treatment responses.[5] Benign cough headache is defined as a bilateral, throbbing headache of sudden onset lasting less than 1 minute and precipitated by coughing in the absence of any intracranial disorder. Benign exertional headache lasts from 5 minutes to 24 hours and is produced by physical exercise without any associated systemic or intracranial disorder. In general, benign exertional headache starts at a much younger age than benign cough headache. Benign cough headache has been infrequently reported, and the mean age of onset is 55, with a range of 19 to 73 years. Benign cough headache is twice as common in patients older than 40 years of age and is four times more common in men than in women.[78] The pain begins immediately[78, 79] or within seconds after muscular effort, coughing, sneezing, lifting, straining at stool, blowing, crying, or singing. The pain is severe in intensity with a bursting, explosive, or splitting or stabbing quality that lasts a few seconds or minutes. The headache can be unilateral 35 percent of the time and may be maximal at the vertex or in the occipital, frontal, or temporal region. Bending the head or lying down may be impossible.[78, 79] Benign cough headache is not generally associated with nausea or vomiting, and the neurological examination is usually normal. Vomiting, if present, suggests an organic basis for the headache.[78, 79] As many as 25 percent of patients with benign cough headache have an antecedent respiratory infection.

Benign exertional headache and benign cough headache can be confused with other mechanically precipitated disorders, such as effort migraine and coital headaches. In fact, 40 percent of patients with coital headache of the vascular type had benign exertional headache, suggesting a relationship between these entities. Most patients are free of pain between attacks of head pain, but in some cases, the paroxysms are followed by dull, aching pain that may persist for hours. Benign exertional headache lasts longer than benign cough headache and is bilateral and throbbing.[78, 79] Five of the 21 patients reported by Symonds had such additional headaches.[75] Because these patients often describe the problem as a continuous headache, they should be asked directly about the role of exertion as a trigger factor for their headaches. Autonomic symptoms are unusual in this disorder.

If a patient presents with cough or exertional headache, MRI must be performed to rule out posterior fossa abnormalities, which can cause this headache syndrome. These abnormalities include brain tumors, such as posterior fossa meningiomas, acoustic neurinomas, and other tumors; midbrain cysts; basilar impression; and Chiari malformations.[78, 79]

Of the 219 cases of exertional and cough headache reviewed by Sands and colleagues,[78] 48 had an identifiable organic etiology. Pascual and co-workers[79] have suggested that symptomatic cough headache is more likely to be associated with a Chiari malformation and begin at an earlier age in life than benign cough headache. Symptomatic exertional headaches began later in life and lasted longer than benign exertional headaches. Most acute cases of exertional headaches were due to subarachnoid hemorrhage.

The long-term outlook for these patients is favorable. If the headaches are frequent or severe, prophylactic therapy is required, because the short duration of the headaches usually renders abortive therapy impractical. Patients with benign cough headache often respond dramatically to indomethacin in doses ranging from 25 to 150 mg daily.[80] If there is gastrointestinal intolerance to indomethacin, concomitant treatment with misoprostol, sulcralfate, proton-pump inhibitors, or antacids may be helpful. When indomethacin fails, Raskin[80] reports that naproxen, ergonovine, and phenelzine are useful, but propranolol is not. Patients with benign exertional headaches often respond to ergotamine or propranolol. Symonds[75] performed four lumbar punctures or pneumoencephalograms on 21 patients with benign cough headache syndrome. One patient, a 38-year-old woman, developed a typical postlumbar puncture headache; her cough headache syndrome remitted for 3 weeks but then recurred. On the basis of this observation, some specialists recommend lumbar puncture to treat this disorder.[80, 81]

Coital Headache

Headache associated with sexual activity may be precipitated by masturbation or coitus, in the absence of any intracranial disorder. Three types of sexual headaches are recognized in the IHS classification.[5] The first, the dull type, is described as a dull ache in the head and neck that intensifies as sexual excitement increases. Type 2, also known as vascular or explosive, is a sudden, severe, explosive headache occurring at orgasm. Type 3 is a postural headache, resembling that of low CSF pressure, developing after coitus.[79, 82] Following the IHS criteria, Rasmussen and Olesen[83] have shown that the lifetime prevalences of these headaches are 1 percent in each case (95 percent confidence interval [CI], 0 to 2 percent).

The coital type 2 headache, which usually begins at or shortly before orgasm, is of high intensity, frontal or occipital in location, explosive or throbbing in nature, and persists for a few minutes to 48 hours. Type 1, a less ominous type of headache, begins earlier in intercourse, is occipital or diffuse in location, is characterized as dull and aching, and is most severe at orgasm. For a new type 2 coital headache of sudden onset, a CT scan should be performed, and even if this is negative, a lumbar puncture should be obtained. Aneurysm without rupture has presented as coital headache. Again, MRA may be a reasonable alternative. Coital headache is often associated with benign exertional headache.[79, 84]

Sinus Headache

Sinus infections are much less common today than they were in the preantibiotic era. The diagnosis of sinusitis is usually based on symptoms indicating maxillary or frontal sinus involvement. This may occur secondary to, and is frequently a result of, ethmoid disease. The ultimate cause is usually obstruction of the sinus ostia. Acute sinusitis lasts from 1 day to 3 weeks. Subacute sinusitis lasts from 3 weeks to 3 months, whereas chronic sinusitis lasts for more than 3 months. The IHS criteria for acute sinus headache includes a purulent discharge, abnormal neuroimaging, and the simultaneous onset of headache and sinusitis. These criteria may not be valid for sphenoid sinusitis, because purulent discharge is often lacking and headache may precede sinus drainage. Once drainage begins, obstruction is relieved and the headache may begin to abate.

Maxillary sinusitis pain is typically located in the cheek, the gums, and the teeth of the upper jaw; ethmoid sinusitis pain is located between the eyes; and frontal sinusitis pain is located in the forehead. Ethmoid and maxillary sinusitis are usually associated with rhinitis. Sphenoid sinusitis is an uncommon infection that accounts for approximately 3 percent of all cases of acute sinusitis. It is usually accompanied by pansinusitis; less commonly, it occurs alone. Although sphenoid sinusitis is an uncommon cause of headache, it is potentially associated with significant morbidity and mortality, and requires early identification and aggressive management. The physical examination may not be helpful, because not all patients are febrile and sinus tenderness is not always present.

Standard radiography is inadequate for the evaluation of sinusitis, because it does not evaluate the anterior ethmoid air cells, the upper two thirds of the nasal cavity, or the infundibular, middle meatus, and frontal recess air passages. Neuroimaging (CT or MRI) is necessary to definitively diagnose sphenoid sinusitis, because plain x-ray studies are nondiagnostic in about 26 percent of cases. Diagnostic endoscopy with the flexible fiberoptic rhinoscopy allows direct visualization of the nasal passages and sinus drainage areas (osteomeatal complex), and is complementary to CT or MRI.

Management goals for the treatment of sinusitis include (1) treatment of bacterial infection, (2) reduction of ostial swelling, (3) sinus drainage, and (4) maintenance of sinus ostia patency. Uncomplicated sinusitis, other than sphenoid sinusitis, should be treated with a broad spectrum oral antibiotic for 10 to 14 days. Treatment failure and recurrent infections are indications for neuroimaging and endoscopy to search for a source of obstruction. Treatment of complications consists of high doses of intravenous antibiotics and surgical drainage, if appropriate, of any enclosed space.[85]

Neck and Facial Pain

TRIGEMINAL NEURALGIA

Trigeminal neuralgia (TN) probably results from the focal demyelination of the trigeminal nerve or ganglia.[86,87] Symptomatic causes include intrinsic and extrinsic tumors near the gasserian ganglia and multiple sclerosis (MS) plaques located around the root entry zone of the trigeminal nerve. In the past, dental disease or dental procedures were thought to occasionally cause TN. However, the delineation of the syndrome of pretrigeminal neuralgia, which mimics dental illness, casts doubt on whether dental procedures can ever cause TN.[88] Most cases of so-called idiopathic TN may be due to pulsations of an aberrant vascular loop on the trigeminal nerve.[86] These pulsations induce a series of neural events that result in changes in wide dynamic range neurons in the trigeminal nucleus caudalis.

The annual prevalence of TN is approximately 6 per 100,000 persons. Women are affected more than men. TN usually affects the elderly, with onset in the sixth or seventh decade in over 50 percent of patients. MS is the disease most clearly linked with TN, and 2 to 8 percent of patients with TN also have MS.[87] The second and third division of the trigeminal nerve are most frequently affected by the brief, repetitive, lightning-like pains of TN. In over 90 percent of cases, there is a trigger zone that, when stimulated, induces a train of painful sensations. Eating, talking, a light touch, or even a draft of air may induce an attack. During a severe attack, the face may contort; in some patients, it remains in that position until the pain eases—hence, the term tic. After a paroxysm, there is a relatively refractory phase during which is it difficult to trigger an attack.[87]

There are no known associated disorders except for the known or suspected causes of secondary TN. Psychological problems may occur secondary to chronic pain. Secondary causes of idiopathic TN other than MS include syringomyelia, postmedullary infarction, aneurysm, basilar impression, and tumors, which include acoustic neuromas, epidermoids, meningiomas, schwannomas, and cholesteatomas. In the evaluation of suspected TN, an MRI of the brain is indicated, even if there is no loss of sensation or other abnormality on neurological examination. The value of a dental evaluation is uncertain.

Medical therapy should be tried first. Carbamazepine, gabapentin, baclofen, and IV phenytoin are the most effective treatments. Oral phenytoin, valproic acid, clonazepam, topiramate, lamotrigine, and pimozide are alternatives. Distal nerve blocks or ablative procedures generally are not recommended owing to a high incidence of early recurrence. More proximal procedures include retrogasserian glycerol injections and radiofrequency gangliolysis, which have acceptable recurrence rates and minor complications. The Jannetta procedure involves intracranial exploration of the trigeminal nerve root and removal of aberrant blood vessels. It is the most successful surgical procedure, but it also has the most complications.[87] Most patients with TN can be successfully treated with medical therapy; many will require lifelong medication, and some will require surgical intervention.

CERVICOGENIC HEADACHE AND OCCIPITAL NEURALGIA

This is a controversial entity whose existence has been questioned. Pain from cervical structures is referred to the head through the C1 to C4 cervical roots. Accepted causes of head pain from the neck include developmental abnormalities, tumors, ankylosing spondylitis, rheumatoid arthritis, and osteomyelitis. Controversial causes include cervical disc herniations, degenerative disc disease, and whiplash injuries.[89] Occipital neuralgia is thought by some to occur as a result of an injury to the occipital nerve, which may be vulnerable to compression as it passes through the semispinalis capitis muscle. Referred pain of cervical origin has often been referred to as occipital neuralgia, modifying the definition of this disorder. The prevalence of cervicogenic headache and occipital neuralgia is unknown. Risk factors include whiplash injury.

Some patients who are said to have cervicogenic headache have a pattern of unilateral pain that originates in the neck and spreads to the oculofrontal area. The headache is of moderate severity. The upper cervical region is often tender; palpation often results in radiation of pain to the head. Relief may occur after anesthetizing the occipital nerve or C2 cervical root. Some authors believe that nausea, vomiting, photophobia or phonophobia, and eye changes may accompany this headache, thus confusing its diagnosis with migraine. The situation is further complicated by the ability of occipital nerve blocks to relieve migraine headaches.[89] Occipital neuralgia is an even more controversial entity. The pain, which is in the distribution of the occipital nerve, is aching or burning in quality.

Even if a structural abnormality of the neck is identified, migraine and TTH should be considered in the differential diagnosis of cervicogenic headache. Abnormal cervical x-ray studies and MRI are common and cannot be used by themselves to establish the diagnosis. A positive response to neuroblockade should *not* be considered diagnostic. Physical therapy, muscle relaxants, low doses of tricyclic antidepressants, and nerve blocks or trigger point injections are appropriate for most cases of so-called cervicogenic headache. Correction of anatomical abnormalities has been advocated, although surgery is often useless or harmful. Occipital neurectomy is usually unsuccessful and may cause anesthesia dolorosa. Most patients respond slowly to conservative management. There are no valid outcome studies. The results of ablative procedures are uncertain; with longer term follow-up, the initial benefit was lost.

GLOSSOPHARYNGEAL NEURALGIA

The pathophysiology of glossopharyngeal neuralgia (GN) is similar to that of TN because the pain characteristics are so remarkably similar. Most cases are idiopathic, although vascular compression has been described.[90] Secondary GN may be due to oropharyngeal malignancies, peritonsillar infection, an osteophytic stylohyoid ligament, and carotid aneurysm. The incidence of GN is reported to be between 1/70 and 1/100 the incidence of TN.[91] The pain of GN is similar to that of TN, although a few patients experience a dull pain that persists for minutes or hours. The pain is located in the ear, tonsil, larynx, tongue, or combinations of these areas. Triggers include swallowing, chewing, or talking. Coughing may accompany the pain. Anesthetizing the throat may temporarily relieve the pain. Unlike TN, MS has not been associated with GN. The differential diagnosis of GN includes TN, geniculate neuralgia, and neck/tongue syndrome. MRI of the brain, x-ray studies to visualize the stylohyoid ligament and styloid process, and careful examination of the pharynx are indicated when evaluating the patient with a present diagnosis of GN. Medical management is identical to the treatment of GN. Surgical options include ablation of the glossopharyngeal nerve and microvascular decompression.

CAROTIDYNIA

The existence of carotidynia as a single pathological entity has been appropriately questioned.[92,93] Acute monophasic carotidynia may have a viral etiology. Carotidynia often means nonspecific neck pain with carotid artery tenderness. Many cases of recurring carotidynia, however, are due to migraine. At present, the epidemiology and risk factors are not known. The clinical features of carotidynia generally include neck pain and carotid artery tenderness, particularly near the bifurcation. Occasionally, there is face pain rather than neck pain. A number of temporal patterns have been reported, with pain lasting seconds, minutes, hours, days, weeks, or months. Some cases of carotidynia may be associated with migraine. Symptomatic causes of carotidynia include carotid dissection, stenosis or occlusion with or without intraplaque hemorrhage, aneurysm, fibromuscular dysplasia, giant cell arteritis, and post–carotid endarterectomy. If the temporal profile suggests a monophasic illness rather than a recurrent condition, anatomical investigation, including ultrasound, MRI, MRA, or angiography, may be necessary. Indomethacin is often effective in treating the pain of carotidynia and migraine treatment may also be effective.[92, 93] Because carotidynia does not represent a single illness, the prognosis depends on the cause.

Reviews and Selected Updates

Dahlöf C: Integrating the triptans into clinical practice. Curr Opin Neurol 2002;15:317–322.

Lance JW, Goadsby PJ (eds): Mechanism and Management of Headache, 6th edition. Butterworth-Heinemann Ltd, Oxford, 1998.

Lipton RB, Silberstein SD: Comorbidity of migraine. Neurology 1994;44(Suppl 7):S4–S5.

Olesen J, Tfelt-Hansen P, Welch KMA (eds): The Headaches, 2nd ed. New York, Raven Press, 2001.

Quality Standards Subcommittee: Appropriate use of ergotamine and dihydroergotamine (DHE) in the treatment of migraine and status migrainosus. AAN Practice Handbook, 1994, pp 225–228.

Silberstein SD: Practice parameter: Evidence-based guidelines for migraine headache (an evidence-based review). Report of the Quality Standards Subcommittee of the American Academy of Neurology. Neurology 2000;55:754–763.

Silberstein SD, Goadsby PJ (eds): Headache. Newton, MA, Butterworth-Heinemann, 1997.

Silberstein SD, Lipton RB, Dalessio D (eds): Wolff's Headache and Other Head Pain, 7th ed. New York, Oxford University Press, 2001.

References

1. Silberstein SD, Silberstein MM: Clinical symptomatology and differential diagnosis of migraine. *In* Tollison CD, Kunkel RS (eds): Headache: Diagnosis and Treatment. Baltimore, Urban and Schwarzenberg, 1993, pp 59–75.
2. Critchley M: Migraine: From Cappadocia to Queen Square. *In* Smith R (ed): Background to Migraine, Vol 1. London, Heinemann, 1967.
3. Sachs O: Migraine: Understanding a common disorder. Berkeley, University of California Press, 1985.
4. Liveing E: On Megrim, Sick Headache, and Some Allied Disorders: A Contribution to the Pathology of Nerve-Storms. London, Churchill, 1873.
5. International Headache Society: Classification and diagnostic criteria for headache disorders, cranial neuralgias, and facial pain. Cephalalgia 1988;8(Suppl 7):1–96.
6. Goadsby PJ: Pathophysiology of headache (Chapter 5). *In* Silberstein SD, Lipton RB, Dalessio D (eds): Wolff's Headache and Other Head Pain, 7th ed. New York, Oxford University Press, 2001, pp 57–72.
7. Weiller C, May A, Limmroth V, et al: Brain stem activation in spontaneous human migraine attacks. Nat Med 1995;1:858–860.
8. Moskowitz MA: The neurobiology of vascular head pain. Ann Neurol 1984;16:157–168.
9. Silberstein SD: Review: Serotonin (5HT) and migraine. Headache 1994;34:408–417.
10. Lipton RB, Hamelsky SW, Stewart WF: Epidemiology and impact of headache (Chapter 7). *In* Silberstein SD, Lipton RB, Dalessio D (eds): Wolff's Headache and Other Head Pain, 7th ed. New York, Oxford University Press, 2001, pp 85–107.
11. Lance JW, Anthony M: Some clinical aspects of migraine. Arch Neurol 1996;15:356–361.
12. Silberstein SD: Headaches, pregnancy, and lactation. *In* Yankowitz J, Niebyl JR, eds: Drug Therapy in Pregnancy, 3rd ed.. Philadelphia, Lippincott Williams & Wilkins, 2001, pp 231–246.
13. Uknis A, Silberstein SD: Review article: Migraine and pregnancy. Headache 1991;31:372–374.
14. Silberstein SD, Lipton RB, Breslau N: Migraine: Association with personality characteristics and psychopathology. Cephalalgia 1995; 15:337–369.
15. Breslau N, Davis GC: Migraine, major depression and panic disorder: A prospective epidemiologic study of young adults. Cephalalgia 1992;12:85–89.
16. Blau JN: Migraine prodromes separated from the aura: Complete migraine. BMJ 1980;281:658–660.
17. Silberstein SD, Lipton RB: Overview of diagnosis and treatment of migraine. Neurology 1994;44(Suppl 7):S6–S16.
18. Silberstein SD, Young WB: Migraine aura and prodrome. Semin Neurol 1995;45:175–182.
19. Selby G, Lance JW: Observations on 500 cases of migraine and allied vascular headache. J Neurol Neurosurg Psychiatry 1960;23:23–32.
20. Silberstein SD: Migraine symptoms: Results of a survey of self-reported migraineurs. Headache 1995;35:387–396.
21. Bradshaw P, Parsons M: Hemiplegic migraine, a clinical study. Q J Med 1965;133:65–85.
22. Ducros A, Deiner C, Joutel A, et al: The clinical spectrum of familial hemiplegic migraine associated with mutations in a neuronal calcium channel. N Eng J Med 2001;345:17–24.
23. Gardner K, Barmada MM, Ptacek LJ, Hoffman EP: A new locus for hemiplegic migraine maps to chromosome 1q31. Neurology 1997; 49:1231–1238.
24 Ducros A, Joutel A, Vahedi K: Mapping of a second locus for familial hemiplegic migraine to 1q21-q23 and evidence of further heterogeneity. Ann Neurol 1997;42:885–890.
25. Fisher CM: Late-life migraine accompaniments as a cause of unexplained transient ischemic attacks. Can J Neurol Sci 1980;7:9–17.

26. Hansen SL, Borelli-Miller L, Strange P, et al: Ophthalmoplegic migraine: Diagnostic criteria, incidence of hospitalization and possible etiology. Acta Neurol Scand 1990;81:54–60.
27. Mark AS, Casselman J, Brown D, et al: Ophthalmoplegic migraine: Reversible enhancement and thickening of the cisternal segment of the oculomotor nerve on contrast-enhanced MR images. Am J Neuroradiol 1998;19:1887–1891.
28. Nelson JA, Wolfe MD, Yuh WT, Peeples ME: Cranial nerve involvement with Lyme borreliosis demonstrated by magnetic resonance imaging. 1992;42:673.
29. Pachner AR, Duray P, Steere AC: Central nervous system manifestations of Lyme disease. Arch Neurol 1989;46:790–795.
30. Blake PY, Mark AS, Kattah J, Kolsky M: MR of oculomotor nerve palsy. Am J Neuroradiol 1995;16:241–251.
31. Schmitt T, Erbguth F, Taghavy A: Oculomotor paralysis as the leading symptom of meningovascular syphilis: Report of two patients and review of the literature. Nervemarzt 1993;64:668–672.
32. May M: Idiopathic (Bell's) palsy, herpes zoster and other facial nerve disorders of viral origin. *In* May M (ed): The Facial Nerve. New York, Thieme Medical, 1986, pp 365–399.
33. Silberstein SD, Lipton R, Solomon S, Mathew N: Classification of daily and near daily headaches: Proposed revision to the IHS classification. Headache 1994;34:1–7.
34. Tournier-Lasserve E, Joutel A, Melki J, et al: Cerebral autosomal arteriopathy with subcortical infarcts and leukoencephalopathy maps to chromosome 19q12. Nat Genet 1993;3:256–259.
35. Joutel A, Vahedi K, Corpechot C, et al: Strong clustering and stereotyped nature of Notch3 mutations in CADASIL patients. Lancet 1997;350:1511–1515.
36. Joutel A, Corpechot C, Ducros A, et al: Notch3 mutations in CADASIL, a hereditary adult-onset condition causing stroke and dementia. Nature 1996;383:707–710.
37. Marks DA, Ehrenberg BL: Migraine-related seizures in adults with epilepsy with EEG correlation. Neurology 1993;43:2476–2483.
38. Frishberg BM: The utility of neuroimaging in the evaluation of headache in patients with normal neurologic examinations. Neurology 1994;44:1191–1197.
39. Ramadan NM, Silberstein SD, Freitag FG, Gilbert TT, Frishberg B: Evidence-based guidelines of the pharmacological management for prevention of migraine for the primary care provider. Unpublished manuscript, 1999.
40. Matchar DB, Young WB, Rosenberg JA, et al: Evidence-based guidelines for migraine headache in the primary care setting: Pharmacological management of acute attacks. http://www aan com 2000.
41. Silberstein SD: Preventive treatment of migraine: an overview. Cephalalgia 1997;17:67–72.
42. Silberstein SD, Saper JR, Freitag, FG: Migraine: Diagnosis and treatment (Chapter 9). *In* Dalessio DJ, Silberstein SD (eds): Wolff's Headache and Other Head Pain, 7th ed. New York, Oxford University Press, 2001, pp 121–237.
43. Silberstein SD, Lipton RB: Overview of diagnosis and treatment of migraine. Neurology 1994;44:6–16.
44. Silberstein SD: Preventive headache treatment. Cephalalgia 1997; 17:67–72.
45. Silberstein SD, Mathew N, Saper J, Jenkins S: Botulinum toxin type A as a migraine preventive treatment. Headache 2000;40:445–450.
46. Olesen J: Clinical and pathophysiological observations in migraine and tension-type headache explained by integration of vascular, supraspinal and myofascial inputs. Pain 1991;46:125–132.
47. Silberstein SD: Chronic daily headache and tension-type headache. Neurology 1993;43:1644–1649.
48. Silberstein SD, Lipton RB: Chronic daily headache. *In* Silberstein SD, Goadsby P (eds): Headache. Newton, MA, Butterworth-Heinemann, 1997, pp 201–225.
49. Goadsby PJ, Edvinsson L: Human in vivo evidence for trigeminovascular activation in cluster headache. Brain 1994;117:427–434.
50. May A, Bahra A, Buchel C, Frackowiak RS, Goadsby PJ: Hypothalamic activation in cluster headache attacks. Lancet 1998;352:275–278.
51. Silberstein SD: Pharmacological management of cluster headache. CNS Drugs 1994;2:199–207.
52. Manzoni GC: Male preponderance of cluster headache is progressively decreasing over the years. Headache 1997;37:588–589.
53. Manzoni GC: Cluster headache and lifestyle: Remarks on a population of 374 male patients. Cephalalgia 1999;19:88–94.
54. Manzoni GC, Prusinski A: Cluster headache: Introduction (Chapter 89). *In* Olesen J, Tfelt-Hansen P, Welch KMA (eds): The Headaches, 2nd ed. Philadelphia, Lippincott, Williams & Wilkins, 2000, pp 675–678.
55. Ford RG, Ford KT, Swaid S, et al: Gamma knife treatment of refractory cluster headache. Headache 1998;38:1–9.
56. Russell D, Vincent M: Chronic paroxysmal hemicrania. *In* Olesen J, Tfelt-Hansen P, Welch KMA (eds): The Headaches, 2nd ed. Philadelphia, Lippincott, Williams & Wilkins, 2000, pp 741–750.
57. King JO, Mitchell PJ, Thomson KR, Tress BM: Cerebral venography and manometry in idiopathic intracranial hypertension. Neurology 1995;5:2224–2228.
58. Mokri B: Headache associated with abnormalities in intracranial structure or function: Low cerebrospinal fluid pressure headache (Chapter 17). *In* Silberstein SD, Lipton RB, Dalessio D (eds): Wolff's Headache and Other Head Pain, 7th ed. New York, Oxford University Press, 2001 pp 417–433.
59. Malm J, Kristensen B, Markgren P, Ekstedt J: CSF hydrodynamics in idiopathic intracranial hypertension: A long-term study. Neurology 1992;42:851–858.
60. Lay CL, Campbell JK, Mokri B: Low cerebrospinal fluid pressure headache. *In* Silberstein SD, Goadsby P (eds): Headache. Newton, MA, Butterworth-Heinemann, 1997, pp 355–368.
61. Kasner SE, Rosenfeld J, Farber RE: Spontaneous intracranial hypotension: Headache with a reversible Arnold-Chiari malformation. Headache 1995;35:557–559.
62. Atkinson JL, Weinshenker BG, Miller GM, Piepgras DG, Mokri B: Acquired Chiari I malformation secondary to spontaneous cerebrospinal fluid leakage and chronic intracranial hypotension syndrome in seven cases. J Neurosurg 1998;88:237–242.
63. Mokri B, Atkinson JL, Dodick DW, et al: Absence pachymeningeal gadolinium enhancement on cranial MRI despite symptomatic CSF leak. Neurology 1999;53:402–404.
64. Bakshi R, Mechtler LL, Kamran S, et al: MRI findings in lumbar puncture headache syndrome: Abnormal dural-meningeal and dural venous sinus enhancement. Clin Imaging 1999;23:73–76.
65. Pakiam AS, Lee C, Lang AE: Intracranial hypotension with Parkinsonism, ataxia, and bulbar weakness. Arch Neurol 1999;56:869–872.
66. Mokri B, Piepgras DG, Miller GM: Syndrome of orthostatic headaches and diffuse pachymeningeal gadolinium enhancement. Mayo Clin Proc 1997;72:400–413.
67. Rabin BM, Roychowdhury S, Meyer JR, et al: Spontaneous intracranial hypotension: Spinal MR findings. Am J Neuroradiol 1998;19:1034–1039.
68. Moayeri NN, Henson JW, Schaefer PW, et al: Spinal dural enhancement on magnetic resonance imaging associated with spontaneous intracranial hypotension. Report of three cases and review of the literature. J Neurosurg 1998;88:912–918.
69. Bart AJ, Wheeler AS: Comparison of epidural saline infusion and epidural blood placement in the treatment of post lumbar puncture headache. Anesthesiology 1978;48:221–223.
70. Forsyth PA, Posner JB: Headaches in patients with brain tumors. A study of 111 patients. Neurology 1993;43:1678–1683.
71. Adams HP, Kassell NF, Torner JC, Sahs AL: CT and clinical correlations in recent aneurysmal subarachnoid hemorrhage: A preliminary report of the cooperative aneurysm study. Neurology 1983;33:981–988.
72. Day JW, Raskin NH: Thunderclap headache: Symptom of unruptured cerebral aneurysm. Lancet 1986;2:1247–1248.
73. Ng PK, Pulst S-M: Not so benign "thunderclap headache." Neurology 1992;260:42.
74. Raps EC, Rogers JD, Galetta SL, et al: The clinical spectrum of unruptured intracranial aneurysms. Arch Neurol 1993;50:265–268.
75. Symonds C: Cough headache. Brain 1956;79:557–568.
76. Rooke ED: Benign exertional headache. Med Clin North Am 1968; 52:801–808.
77. Rassmussen BK, Jensen R, Schroll M, Olesen J: Epidemiology of headache in a general population—a prevalence study. J Clin Epidemiol 1991;44:1147–1157.
78. Sands GH, Newman L, Lipton R: Cough, exertional, and other miscellaneous headaches. Med Clin North Am 1991;75:733–743.
79. Pascual J, Iglesias F, Oterno A, et al: Cough, exertional, and sexual headaches: An analysis of 72 benign and symptomatic cases. Neurology 1996;46:1520–1524.
80. Raskin NH: The indomethacin-responsive syndromes. *In* Headache. New York, Churchill-Livingstone, 1988, pp 255–268.
81. Raskin NH: The cough headache syndrome: Treatment. Neurology 1995;45:1784.
82. Silbert PL, Edis RH, Stewart-Wynne EG, Gubbay SS: Benign vascular sexual headache and exertional headache: Interrelationships and long term prognosis. J Neurol Neurosurg Psychiatry 1991;54:417–421.

83. Rasmussen BK, Olesen J: Symptomatic and nonsymptomatic headaches in a general population. Neurology 1992;42:1225–1231.
84. Johns DR: Benign sexual headache within a family. Arch Neurol 1986;43:1158–1160.
85. Silberstein SD: Nose and sinus-related headaches. *In* Gilman S, Goldstein GW, Waxman SG (eds): Neurobase, La Jolla, CA, Arbor, 1995.
86. Jannetta PJ: Arterial compression of the trigeminal nerve at the pons in patients with trigeminal neuralgia. J Neurosurg 1967; 26(Suppl):159–162.
87. Zakrzewska JM: Trigeminal neuralgia. *In* Major Problems in Neurology. London, WB Saunders Company, Ltd., 1995, pp 5–20.
88. Fromm GH, Graff-Radford SB, Terrence CF, Sweet WH: Pretrigeminal neuralgia. Neurology 1990;40:1493–1495.
89. Edmeads J: Disorders of the neck: cervicogenic headache (Chapter 19) *In* Silberstein SD, Lipton RB, Dalessio D (eds): Wolff's Headache and Other Head Pain, 7th ed. New York, Oxford University Press, 2001, pp 447–458.
90. Rushton JG, Stevens JC, Miller RH: Glossopharyngeal (vagoglossopharyngeal) neuralgia: A study of 217 cases. Arch Neurol 1981;38:201–205.
91. Young WB, Silberstein SD: Headache in the elderly. *In* Pathy MSJ (ed): Principles and Practice of Geriatric Medicine, 3rd ed. London, John Wiley & Sons, Ltd. 1998.
92. Bousser MG, Good J, Kittner SJ, Silberstein SD: Headache associated with vascular disorders (Chapter 15). *In* Silberstein SD, Lipton RB, Dalessio D (eds): Wolff's Headache and Other Head Pain, 7th ed. New York, Oxford University Press, 2001, pp 349–392.
93. Chabriat H, Tournier-Lasserve E, Vahedi K, et al: Autosomal dominant migraine with MRI white matter abnormalities mapping to the CADASIL locus. Neurology 1995;45:1086–1091.

CHAPTER 54

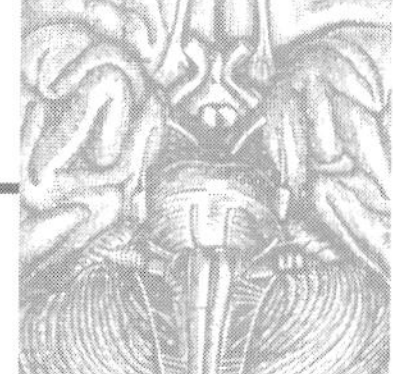

FLAVIA B. CONSENS and RONALD D. CHERVIN

Sleep Disorders

History

Sleep disorders are common age-old problems that can lead to distress and discomfort, impaired daytime functioning, and serious complications. In ancient Greece, Democritus believed that physical illness was the cause of daytime sleepiness and that poor nutrition was the main cause of insomnia. Effects of sleep on epilepsy and asthma were recognized in the Middle Ages, and Thomas Willis, a British physician of the 17th century, described nightmares and restless legs. For most of recorded history, however, sleep problems were considered a result of medical or psychiatric illnesses rather than primary disorders. Sleep was viewed as a passive process, akin to death, and the idea that disordered sleep physiology could lead to specific syndromes was unknown.

With the discovery of rapid-eye-movement (REM) sleep in 1953, the concept of sleep as a passive shutting down of cortical activity began to change to a view of sleep as an active process initiated by specific events of the nervous system and with two distinct states: REM and non-REM (NREM). The discovery of the association of narcolepsy with sleep-onset REM periods, as opposed to the usual onset of sleep in the NREM state, led to the idea that narcolepsy was a primary disorder of the sleep process and to the corollary that clinical syndromes could be caused by such disruption of sleep processes.

Forty years ago, the only sleep disorder of interest to most neurologists was narcolepsy; all other sleep problems generally were considered manifestations of psychiatric problems. The discoveries of sleep apnea and periodic leg movements, the use of sleep laboratories to study sleep patterns, the discovery of effective treatments for sleep apnea, and the recognition that untreated sleep apnea is associated with increased cardiovascular morbidity and mortality have dramatically changed the approach to sleep disorders. At present, most sleep medicine specialists have primary training in neurology or pulmonary medicine, and the practicing neurologist is often expected by colleagues to be familiar with the major sleep disorders.[1]

Insomnia

Insomnia refers to the subjective sense that sleep is inadequate, insufficient, or interrupted. It is subjective because sleep requirements vary among individuals and because the restorative aspect of sleep is difficult to measure. Insomnia has many causes, and effective treatment requires an understanding of the basis for the symptoms.

Pathogenesis and Pathophysiology. Causes of insomnia include emotions and thoughts that interfere with sleep; medications and use of illicit drugs or alcohol; external stimuli, such as noise, excessive heat or cold, or bright light; alterations in the central nervous system (CNS) that initiate and maintain sleep; and bodily dysfunctions such as pain, decreased mobility, arousals, and disturbing sensations or movements. Mental activity during sleep may contribute to the impression that sleep is not restorative. In most patients, several elements contribute to insomnia, and it is useful to identify the predisposing, precipitating, and perpetuating factors.[2]

Personality and age affect the predisposition to insomnia. Tense, nervous, worried persons who internalize problems and have somatic responses to stress are at higher risk for insomnia than relaxed, phlegmatic types. Medical illnesses, deterioration of CNS functions responsible for sleep initiation and maintenance, and increased sensitivity to the sleep-disrupting effects of medications and other drugs contribute to the increase in insomnia with age.

Stress often precipitates insomnia. Medical or psychiatric illness and the medications used to treat them, death or illness of a loved one, divorce or separation, a move to a new location, and a change in occupational status are common precipitants. A change in sleep-wake schedule or a change in the sleeping environment may also bring on insomnia.

Once insomnia begins, anxiety about sleep, conditioned negative associations, poor sleep habits, or secondary gain often perpetuate insomnia. Performance anxiety associated with the belief that good sleep is a requirement for effective functioning the next day makes falling asleep difficult. As sleep fails to occur, the patient becomes increasingly anxious. Soon the entire process of preparing for sleep becomes tied to anxiety and fear of insomnia. Some patients respond to insomnia by increasing the amount of time spent in bed with the hope that they will then obtain enough sleep. The usual result is increased time awake in bed rather than increased time asleep, which increases the negative conditioning associated with sleeplessness. The secondary gain associated with nighttime snacks and alcohol use, television use, time off from work, and the role of sickly child or dependent adult also may perpetuate insomnia.

Some insomniacs have the impression that they sleep very little, even when laboratory recordings reveal normal or near-normal sleep. The cause of this faulty impression, referred to as *sleep state misperception*, is unknown. Ruminative thoughts that recur with each awakening during the night may give the impression of uninterrupted consciousness and thereby contribute to the failure to perceive sleep. A subtle disturbance of sleep undetected by standard polysomnography could also be a factor.

Epidemiology and Risk Factors. About 10 percent of adults in the United States have chronic insomnia, and another 15 percent have short-term insomnia. The prevalence is higher in women and in older persons. Community residents older than 50 years have a prevalence of insomnia of 23 percent.[3] Depression, anxiety disorders, and substance abuse disorders are substantially more common in insomniacs than in the general population.[4] Although insomnia is distressing to many individuals, less than one third of insomniacs complain about the problem to physicians, perhaps because they believe that physicians are not interested in the problem or are unable to treat it effectively.

Clinical Features and Associated Disorders. Patients with insomnia complain of difficulty falling asleep, difficulty staying asleep, early morning awakening, or a sense that sleep is nonrestorative. During nocturnal sleeplessness, some patients toss and turn in bed. Others watch television, read, eat, drink, or use the bathroom. Persons who do not like to waste time often do housework or homework. Common daytime symptoms include poor concentration, fatigue, irritability, mood changes, anxiety, and muscle aching. Fatigue is sometimes accompanied by sleepiness, but most insomniacs are unable to nap even if they lie down.

As insomnia continues, many patients become preoccupied with sleep. Evening rituals designed to promote relaxation may last for an hour or more. Many patients ruminate at night and during the day about the ill effects of poor sleep and its effects on daytime function. For some patients, insomnia is less severe on weekend nights and during vacations, when concerns about the effects on daytime function are less.

Although most insomniacs have significant sleep disruption, patients with sleep state misperception describe severe chronic insomnia even though they have relatively normal sleep. Such patients often report that they obtain as little as 2 hours of sleep per night and frequently have no sleep at all. Some describe long periods of resting in bed without sleeping.

Insomnia can occur with virtually any sleep disorder as well as with a host of medical and psychiatric disorders (Table 54–1). A psychiatric disturbance is present in about 40 percent of insomniacs.[4] Overuse and abuse of alcohol and sedative medications is common. Several community-based studies have found that sleep disturbances are powerful risk factors for the development of new episodes of major depression in the following year.[5]

Differential Diagnosis. The differential diagnosis of insomnia is extensive (Table 54–2), and a given patient may have several contributing factors, such as poor sleep hygiene, environmental factors, maladaptive conditioning, hypnotic dependence, and a predisposition to poor sleep. It is critical to determine whether the insomnia is secondary to a psychiatric or medical disorder; in such cases, the insomnia is best treated by optimal management of the underlying disorder.

It is sometimes difficult to determine whether insomnia is due to depression, especially a masked depression in which the patient denies sadness or hopelessness, because dysphoria is a common feature of all types of insomnia. A history of depressive episodes before insomnia began, a history of episodic insomnia at times of mood disturbance, and the occurrence of other depressive symptoms favor a primary diagnosis of an affective disorder. Although most insomniacs are anxious, the anxiety is usually focused on sleep, and generalized anxiety disorder as a cause of insomnia should be suspected only if anxiety affects many aspects of life.

When insomnia is caused by learned sleep-preventing associations, the diagnosis is *psychophysiological insomnia*, the most common form of primary insomnia.[1] Patients with psychophysiological insomnia tend to prefer regular routines and view good sleep as a necessity. For such patients, an awakening that would ordinarily be just long enough for a change in body position is instead followed by anxiety that sleep will not return or will not be restful. The anxiety about the consequences of not sleeping induces full alertness, and a rapid return to sleep becomes impossible.

Poor sleep hygiene as the cause of insomnia should be suspected in patients who have never had good sleep habits, perhaps because they were not required to sleep at regular times as children or because their internal sleep systems were initially so robust that they were able to sleep well despite poor habits. Insomnia due to caffeine or medication is common. With increasing age or because of other factors, some people may become less able to tolerate the effects of poor sleep habits. Sleep state misperception should be suspected in

TABLE 54–1. **Medical and Psychiatric Disorders Associated with Sleep Disturbances**

Infectious diseases	Sleeping sickness, febrile illnesses
Cardiac diseases	Congestive heart failure, nocturnal angina
Pulmonary diseases	Chronic obstructive pulmonary disease, asthma
Gastrointestinal diseases	Gastroesophageal reflux, peptic ulcer disease, inflammatory bowel disease
Neurological disorders	Degenerative disorders of the CNS, neuromuscular disorders
Rheumatological disorders	Rheumatoid arthritis
Renal disorders	Chronic renal failure
Psychiatric disorders	Acute psychosis, depression, anxiety disorders, panic disorder, alcoholism
Endocrine disorders	Cushing's disease, hyperthyroidism, hypothyroidism, diabetes, menopause
Skeletal and soft tissue disorders	Achondroplasia, craniofacial malformations, Down syndrome, mucopolysaccharidoses
Miscellaneous	Cancer, pruritus, Prader-Willi syndrome

CNS, Central nervous system.

patients who do not toss and turn or get out of bed despite complaints of severe insomnia.

Loud snoring, witnessed apneas, or frequent kicking movements suggest that insomnia may be due to sleep apnea or periodic leg movements. Patients with periodic breathing patterns with central apneas, such as Cheyne-Stokes pattern, frequently complain of insomnia. If the main problem is difficulty falling asleep, an anxiety disorder or a delayed sleep phase syndrome (DSPS) may be responsible. Early morning awakening with excessive rumination suggests depression or obsessive-compulsive disorder.

Evaluation. The history is the most crucial part of the evaluation. Circumstances at the onset of insomnia should be assessed, and the course of the insomnia should be determined, along with any factors the patient has identified that make insomnia better or worse. Times of going to bed, falling asleep, nighttime awakenings, and getting out of bed for good nights and bad nights should be determined, along with associated behaviors, thoughts, and emotions. Information about the patient's weekday and weekend schedule of work, alcohol use, caffeine intake, meals, and medication use is also essential. Sleep logs that contain this information are very useful.

Psychiatric evaluation is helpful if a psychiatric etiology is a consideration. Polysomnography is useful if there is a suspicion that apnea or periodic leg movements are the cause of the symptoms, if there is a failure to respond to treatment, or if sleep state misperception is suspected.

Management. Treatment of insomnia is based on the underlying causes. From a therapeutic perspective, the factors that perpetuate insomnia are often the most important because they may be most amenable to change. Improved sleep hygiene can lead to marked improvement (Table 54–3), but poor sleep hygiene is sometimes a result of other problems, particularly psychiatric problems.

Behavioral treatments are a major part of treatment for patients with psychophysiological insomnia.[2] Between 70 and 80 percent of patients treated with nonpharmacological interventions benefit from treatment.[6] With sleep restriction therapy, mild sleep deprivation produced by eliminating naps and temporarily restricting time in bed to 1 to 2 hours less than the nightly reported amount of sleep tends to make sleep more continuous. Once sleep is consolidated, the time in bed can be gradually increased. With stimulus control therapy, the principle is to associate the bed and sleep environment only with sleep and intimacy; no reading, eating, or watching TV in bed is permitted. Patients are encouraged to get out of bed and to do something relaxing if unable to sleep after 15 to 20 minutes.

TABLE 54–2. **Causes of Insomnia in Adults**

Disorder	Key Diagnostic Feature
Intrinsic Disorders	Insomnia related to processes within the body
Psychophysiological insomnia	Conditioned negative associations
Sleep state misperception	Marked discrepancy between subjective and objective sleep
Idiopathic insomnia	Insomnia caused by constitutional factors
Restless legs syndrome	Leg discomfort relieved by movement
Periodic limb movement disorder	Kicking movements during sleep
Sleep apnea and related disorders	Snoring, witnessed apnea
Extrinsic Disorders	Insomnia due to processes outside the body
Inadequate sleep hygiene	Poor sleep habits
Environmental sleep disorder	Unsuitable sleeping environment
Adjustment sleep disorder	Insomnia related to specific stresses
Hypnotic dependent sleep disorder	Inability to obtain restful sleep without hypnotics
Drug- and medication-related insomnia	Insomnia caused by medications
Altitude insomnia	Insomnia only at high altitude
Circadian Rhythm Sleep Disorders	Schedule-dependent insomnia
Sleep Disorders Due to Medical or Psychiatric Illness	Insomnia fluctuates with severity of the underlying illness

TABLE 54–3. **Principles of Sleep Hygiene**

Go to bed and arise from bed at the same time each day
Avoid daytime naps or limit them to one midafternoon nap
Avoid evening alcohol use
Avoid caffeinated drinks late in the day
Reduce or eliminate tobacco use, especially at night or in the evening
Exercise in moderation; avoid evening exercise
Use the bed only for sleep and sexual activity
Keep the bedroom dark, quiet, and cool
Avoid stress and worrisome thoughts in the evening before sleep

Hypnotics are often helpful in patients with acute situational insomnia and in some patients with chronic insomnia. In a recent randomized trial among patients with late-life insomnia, both behavioral and pharmacological approaches were effective for the short-term management of insomnia, but improvement in sleep was better sustained over time with behavioral treatment.[7] Some chronic insomniacs do well using hypnotics 1 to 2 nights per week when they feel they simply must have a good night's sleep. Others find it reassuring to have a hypnotic available in the medicine cabinet; the knowledge reduces anxiety, and actual use may be minimal. Others use a hypnotic nightly for years with good response and no dose escalation. Still others obtain no benefit from hypnotics, become dependent, or both. Other problems with hypnotics include nocturnal confusion, next-day memory impairment, and sedation. Low doses of sedating tricyclic antidepressants are sometimes useful as alternatives to standard hypnotics (Table 54–4). As a sedative, melatonin is much less effective than conventional hypnotics.

Patients with sleep state misperception should be educated about the distinction between subjective insomnia and objective sleep disruption; they may be reassured to know that restorative sleep-related processes are occurring even though they do not sense it. Behavioral treatment and hypnotics are helpful for some, perhaps because the amnestic effects interrupt the subjective impression that consciousness has been maintained during sleep.

TABLE 54–4. **Medications Used for Insomnia**

Short-acting benzodiazepines	Triazolam 0.125 to 0.25 mg Midazolam 7.5 to 15 mg
Intermediate-acting benzodiazepines	Temazepam 15 to 30 mg Oxazepam 15 to 30 mg Lorazepam 1 to 2 mg Alprazolam 0.25 to 0.5 mg
Long-acting benzodiazepines	Flurazepam 15 to 30 mg Diazepam 2.5 to 10 mg Clorazepate 7.5 to 15 mg Clonazepam 0.5 to 2 mg Prazepam 10 mg Halazepam 20 mg Chlordiazepoxide 10 to 20 mg
Imidazopyridines	Zaleplon 5 to 10 mg Zolpidem 10 to 20 mg
Cyclopyrrolones	Zopiclone 7.5 to 15 mg
Antihistamines	Diphenhydramine 25 to 50 mg
Sedating antidepressants	Amitriptyline 10 to 75 mg Doxepin 10 to 75 mg Trazodone 25 to 100 mg Imipramine 25 to 100 mg

Prognosis and Future Perspectives. The course of insomnia is variable; many patients have a lifetime of sleep problems, whereas others have episodic bouts of poor sleep separated by years of tranquil nights. Insomniacs who continue with symptoms after 12 months have an increased risk for depression, anxiety disorders, and alcohol abuse.[4] Other complications include benzodiazepine dependence, decreased job performance and self-esteem, and an increased risk of motor vehicle accidents.

Primary Disorders of Daytime Somnolence

NARCOLEPSY

Narcolepsy is a genetically based neurological disorder associated with abnormalities of REM sleep and of sleep-wake control. Although the disorder has been recognized for more than 100 years, the discoveries of sleep apnea, other syndromes of excessive sleepiness, and the association of narcolepsy with REM sleep abnormalities and specific human leukocyte antigen (HLA) markers helped delineate narcolepsy as a distinct syndrome. Clinically, the usual hallmarks are excessive sleepiness and cataplexy.

Pathogenesis and Pathophysiology. Animal models of narcolepsy show either loss of dorsolateral hypothalamic neurons that produce hypocretin (also called orexin) or lack of receptors for this neurotransmitter.[8] Hypocretin levels in cerebrospinal fluid were undetectable in seven of nine narcoleptic patients,[9] and brains of such patients also showed reduced numbers of hypocretin neurons.[10] One human hypocretin mutation has been identified, in a patient with atypical early-onset and severe narcolepsy[11] (Fig. 54–1).

More than 90 percent of narcoleptics have a specific HLA haplotype that includes HLA-DQB1-0602, which is present in less than one third of the general population.[12] The penetrance of the HLA-associated gene is low, and the risk for narcolepsy in first-degree relatives, although 40 times greater than in the general population, is only about 1 percent.[13]

The low penetrance of the HLA-associated gene and discordance for narcolepsy in identical twins indicates that unknown environmental factors play an important role in the pathogenesis of narcolepsy.[14] Canine narcolepsy, which is clinically similar to the human disease, is associated with monoaminergic abnormalities, and the gene that causes one form of canine narcolepsy has been isolated.[15] The gene for canine narcolepsy is tightly linked to a DNA region involved in immune regulation.[16] Despite the association of human narcolepsy with an HLA-associated gene, there is no direct evidence to indicate that narcolepsy is an autoimmune disease.

Abnormalities of REM sleep control probably contribute to narcoleptic symptoms. The muscle atonia that occurs with sleep paralysis and cataplexy is similar to the muscle atonia of REM sleep, and hypnagogic hallucinations probably represent an intrusion of REM sleep imagery into consciousness

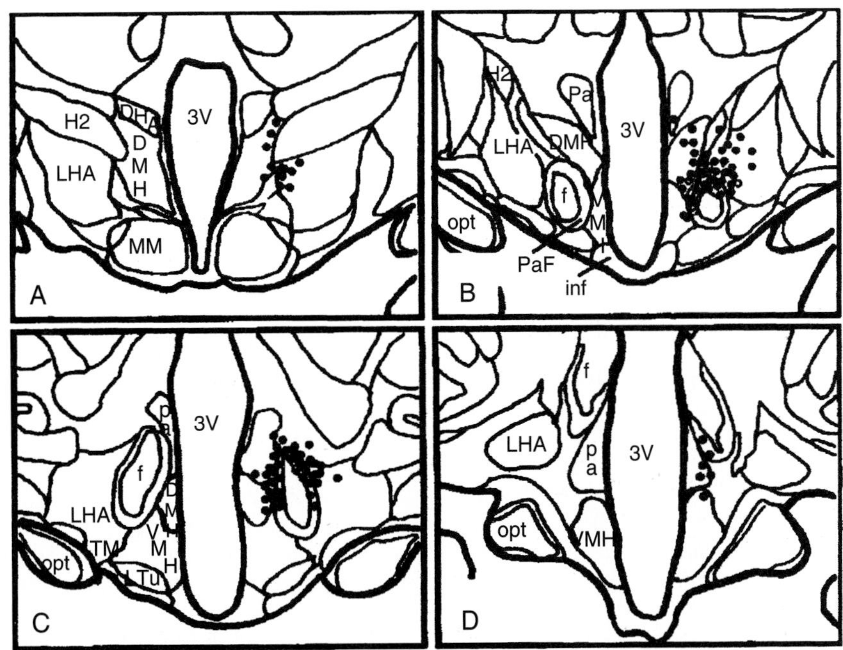

FIGURE 54–1. Distribution of hypocretin-containing cells in the human hypothalamus. The *preprohypocretin* mRNA expressing neurons are localized discretely in the perifornical area. Their distribution is illustrated on schematic diagrams of representative coronal planes through the human hypothalamus. Each *black circle* represents three to five cells detected in emulsion-coated sections. DHA, dorsal hypothalamic area; DMH, dorsal hypothalamic nucleus; f, fornix; H2, lenticular fasciculus; Inf, infundibular nucleus; LHA, lateral hypothalamic area; MM, mammillary nucleus; opt, optic tract; Pa, paraventricular hypothalamic nucleus; PaF, parafornical nucleus; TM, tuberomammillary nucleus; VMH, ventromedial hypothalamic nucleus. (Reprinted with permission from Peyron C, Faraco J, Rogers W, et al: A mutation in a case of early onset narcolepsy and a generalized absence of hypocretin peptides in human narcoleptic brains. Nature Medicine 2000;6:991–997.)

during transitions between wakefulness and sleep. However, the REM sleep abnormalities appear to be part of a broader problem of impaired sleep-wake regulation that includes an inability to sustain sleep, along with the daytime inability to remain awake.[17]

Epidemiology and Risk Factors. The prevalence of narcolepsy with cataplexy in a white population is about 1 in 4000.[18] Estimates for other populations range from 1 in 600 to less than 1 in 10,000. Narcolepsy affects men and women equally.

Clinical Features and Associated Disorders. Most patients report symptoms beginning gradually in the second decade of life. The appearance of symptoms before age 5 is rare; occasional patients develop narcolepsy after age 50. The primary symptoms include sleepiness and sleep episodes, cataplexy, sleep paralysis, hypnagogic and hypnopompic hallucinations, and nocturnal sleep disruption. Sleepiness and cataplexy may develop simultaneously, or cataplexy can begin years or decades later. Excessive sleepiness is present most of the time, although the severity fluctuates during the day and is variable among individuals. Boring sedentary situations and warm afternoons following lunch are especially difficult settings. Work performance is most often affected in sedentary jobs requiring sustained vigilance. Physical activity usually provides relief, but sleepiness returns as soon as the patient sits down. Brief daytime sleep episodes, often called sleep attacks, are common.

Cataplexy is a brief episode of bilateral weakness, without altered consciousness, that is brought on by strong emotion. Laughter, anger, embarrassment, excitement, elation, surprise, shock, and humor without actual laughter can induce the attacks. These events last a few seconds and are associated with buckling of the knees, sagging of the jaw or face, drooping eyelids, and mild dysarthria. Twitching around the face or eyelids may accompany the weakness. Severe attacks produce almost complete paralysis, and prolonged episodes may be associated with auditory, visual, or tactile hallucinations. Cataplexy can be dangerous if it occurs during driving. Unlike sleepiness, definite cataplexy—defined as brief bilateral loss of strength without altered consciousness that responds to tricyclic antidepressants—is virtually pathognomonic for narcolepsy.

Sleep paralysis refers to episodes of partial or total paralysis that last a few seconds or minutes and occur at the beginning or at the end of a sleep period. The paralysis, which occurs in about 60 percent of narcoleptics, may be accompanied by a struggle to move, to speak, or to wake up. Patients often feel awake or half-awake and are usually aware of being in bed. Frightening hallucinations and a sense of suffocation may accompany the paralysis. Despite the intense psychic experience, patients appear to be asleep with eyes closed and with occasional twitches, slight moans, or irregular respirations.

Hallucinations are referred to as hypnagogic when they occur at the onset of sleep, and they are termed hypnopompic when they occur at the end of sleep. The hallucinations, which almost always include visual imagery, differ from dreams in that a thematic story is lacking and some awareness of the surroundings is preserved. Sometimes the hallucinations are so vivid and realistic that the subject may have difficulty believing that they are not real and may take actions to escape from the images.

Daytime drowsiness may also lead to complaints of memory difficulties, blurred vision, and amnestic episodes of automatic behavior lasting seconds to an hour or more during which patients drift in and out of sleep while engaging in aimless or semipurposeful activity. Disrupted nighttime sleep with frequent awakenings may be a prominent complaint. Other sleep disorders, such as obstructive sleep apnea, periodic limb movement disorder, and REM behavioral disorder, are more common than in the general population.

Differential Diagnosis. Sleepiness should be distinguished from tiredness, fatigue, apathy, and weakness. Sleepiness is more likely to occur in boring sedentary situations, is relieved to some extent by movement or stimulation, and is associated with a feeling of impending sleep or a need to fight against sleep onset. Descriptions of daytime sleep episodes as periods of loss of awareness may suggest a diagnosis of syncope, partial complex seizures, or absence seizures. Premonitory drowsiness, sleeplike appearance with absence of pallor, ease of arousability, and the association with sedentary situations are useful differentiating features. There are several causes of excessive sleepiness (Table 54–5). Unplanned daytime sleep episodes, or so-called sleep attacks, are an indication of severity of sleepiness rather than a marker of a qualitatively different process. They can occur with any disorder that causes severe sleepiness and are not specific for narcolepsy.

The association with emotion, the duration of episodes, and the preservation of consciousness help differentiate cataplexy from atonic seizures, myasthenia gravis, periodic paralysis, or drop attacks associated with vertebrobasilar insufficiency. Because cataplexy is not invariably present in narcoleptics, its absence does not exclude the diagnosis.

Sleep paralysis and hypnagogic hallucinations are less useful for diagnosis because they can occur as isolated symptoms in otherwise normal persons, often precipitated by sleep deprivation or a change in sleep schedule, as well as in other sleep disorders.[19]

Evaluation. Because a variety of conditions can cause excessive sleepiness, sleep studies are generally required for accurate diagnosis. Nocturnal polysomnography can determine the presence and severity of sleep apnea, periodic limb movements, and nocturnal sleep disturbance. A multiple sleep latency test (MSLT), usually performed the following day, provides a measure of the severity of sleepiness and an indication of the presence or absence of early onset of REM sleep.[20]

TABLE 54–5. **Causes of Daytime Sleepiness**

- Narcolepsy
- Sleep apnea and other breathing disorders of sleep
- Insufficient sleep syndrome
- Medication effects
- Periodic limb movement disorder
- Idiopathic hypersomnia
- Brain lesions that compromise pathways involved in sleep-wake regulation
- Circadian rhythm sleep disorders
- Nocturnal sleep disruption caused by medical, neurological, or psychiatric illness

TABLE 54–6. **Medication Dosages for Treatment of Narcolepsy and Idiopathic Hypersomnia**

Amphetamines	Dextroamphetamine 5 to 60 mg/day
	Methamphetamine 5 to 40 mg/day
Nonamphetamines	Methylphenidate 5 to 80 mg/day
	Pemoline 18.75 to 112.5 mg/day
	Mazindol 2 to 8 mg/day
Wake-promoting agent	Modafinil 100 to 400 mg/day

Early onset of REM sleep occurs with about 50 percent of sleep episodes, and the presence of two or more sleep-onset REM periods during the four to five nap opportunities provided by the MSLT is the usual diagnostic criterion for narcolepsy. However, this finding is not specific. Other potential causes of early-onset REM sleep include circadian rhythm disturbances, REM sleep deprivation, sleep apnea, and drug or alcohol withdrawal.[19, 21, 22] Some patients with brain pathology in areas concerned with sleep-wake regulation also may have early onset of REM sleep.

HLA typing has limited value for diagnosis. As the HLA haplotype associated with narcolepsy is present in about 20 to 35 percent of the general population, more than 99 percent of persons with the haplotype do not have narcolepsy.

Management. Medications and behavioral measures should be designed to enhance alertness during critical times of the day such as at work, during school, and while driving. The importance of good sleep hygiene and the risks associated with sleepiness while driving must be emphasized. Naps during lunch or other breaks are often helpful.

STIMULANTS. Medications such as modafinil, methylphenidate, dextroamphetamine, and pemoline improve alertness in most narcoleptics (Table 54–6).[23] Stimulants should be initiated at low doses and increased gradually until symptoms are controlled or side effects appear. In general, the lowest effective dose should be used, but some patients may not recognize the severity of their sleepiness, and reports from family members should also be obtained to assess the effectiveness of treatment.

Although chronic use of stimulants can lead to irritability, insomnia, habituation, addiction, and psychosis, the risk for amphetamine abuse is no higher among narcoleptics than in other population groups. With appropriate management, most narcoleptics are able to take stimulants regularly for decades without harmful side effects. When sleepiness fails to respond to medications after a period of good control, the possibility of sleep apnea or chronically insufficient sleep should be considered.

Nonsedating tricyclic antidepressants and serotonin reuptake inhibitors are effective treatments for cataplexy and sleep paralysis, probably by blockade of norepinephrine and serotonin reuptake (see Table 54–6). Patients with severe cataplexy may develop tolerance to the effects of tricyclics, and abrupt withdrawal can lead to a temporary rebound increase in cataplexy. Gamma-hydroxybutyrate (GHB) reduces cataplexy, increases slow-wave sleep, and probably improves daytime sleepiness in narcoleptics. This medication is now available in the United States, with special regulations to prevent abuse.

Prognosis and Future Perspectives. Sleepiness is a lifelong problem for most narcoleptics, whereas cataplexy, hypnagogic hallucinations, and sleep paralysis improve with age in about one third of patients. Sleepiness is often adequately but not completely controlled by current therapeutic strategies. In the future, new agents such as GHB and new strategies based on better understanding of hypocretin functions should improve the lives of many affected patients.

IDIOPATHIC HYPERSOMNIA

Idiopathic hypersomnia is clinically similar to narcolepsy in that daytime sleepiness occurs despite adequate amounts of apparently normal sleep at night, but cataplexy does not occur and there is no association with specific HLAs. The pathogenesis is unknown. Circulating somnogenic factors or focal lesions that affect systems involved in sleep-wake regulation may play a role in some cases. Idiopathic hypersomnia is less common than narcolepsy by a ratio of about 1:10. Recent viral illness may be a risk factor.

Symptoms often develop gradually during adolescence or young adulthood. There appear to be at least two types of idiopathic hypersomnia, but many patients have mixed features. With the classic type, patients complain of an increased need for sleep, difficulty awakening in the morning, and sleep drunkenness with disorientation and confusion in the morning.[24] Daytime naps are long and unrefreshing, and patients may sleep as much as 14 to 18 hours during the day and night. With the second type, daytime sleepiness is sometimes irresistible, similar to narcolepsy, but short naps are usually refreshing.

Other diagnostic considerations in patients who complain of long periods of unrefreshing sleep include atypical depression and chronic fatigue syndrome. In both of these disorders, patients often spend many hours in bed, but actual sleep time is increased only mildly or not at all. Idiopathic hypersomnia is usually considered in a patient who complains of sleepiness and has no apparent cause for sleepiness based on the clinical history and a nocturnal polysomnogram. For such patients, the differential diagnosis includes narcolepsy, upper airway resistance syndrome, insufficient sleep syndrome, and obstructive sleep apnea that occurs during some nights but not others. The diagnosis of idiopathic hypersomnia is not easy because it requires ruling out all other causes to the extent possible. Post-traumatic hypersomnia should be considered when sleepiness develops after head trauma.

Evaluation should include one or more nights of polysomnography, MSLT, psychiatric assessment, and a trial of increased sleep. The upper airway resistance syndrome may be difficult to detect on polysomnography unless airway resistance is assessed with monitoring of endoesophageal pressure during polysomnography.[25] Patients with narcolepsy may not have REM sleep abnormalities on an initial MSLT. Atypical depression or other psychiatric conditions may be associated with complaints of sleepiness, although the MSLT is usually not abnormal. Sleepiness caused by chronically insufficient sleep should improve after a trial of 1 to 2 hours of additional sleep each night. After these diagnoses have been excluded, one is left with the diagnosis of idiopathic hypersomnia.

Management is similar to the approach used for narcolepsy. Patients with the narcoleptic type of sleepiness often respond to stimulants, whereas those with long sleep periods and difficult awakening may not. For most patients, the disorder is chronic. A minority of patients improve with time, and in some, the disorder resolves completely.

OBSTRUCTIVE SLEEP APNEA

Obstructive sleep apnea syndrome (OSA) is characterized by airway narrowing during sleep that leads to nighttime sleep disruption and associated daytime symptoms. The recognition that OSA is a common and treatable disorder with serious complications has been the most important factor in the growth of sleep medicine over the past 20 years.

Pathogenesis and Pathophysiology. Narrowing and occlusion of the upper airway during sleep is the basis for OSA. Obstruction usually occurs in the pharynx, which lacks supporting cartilage and bone, and is therefore more collapsible than other portions of the upper airway. Upper airway size is determined by the anatomy of the bones and soft tissues of the neck and face, by the pressures acting on the pharyngeal tissues, and by their compliance. During wakefulness, contraction of pharyngeal muscles occurs just before the onset of inspiration and increases the outward pressure on the pharyngeal wall by pulling the soft palate, tongue, mandible, and hyoid bone forward. This outward pressure balances the inward pressure produced by negative pressure developed within the thorax and helps maintain airway patency.[26] Activity of upper airway dilator muscle is affected by arterial blood gas concentration; by proprioceptive input to respiratory neurons from the jaw, mouth, and thorax; and by receptors sensitive to changes in upper airway transmural pressure. For example, increased negative upper airway pressure leads to increased activity of the genioglossus, which pulls the tongue forward and tends to open the airway.

Pharyngeal muscles relax during sleep, which leads to narrowing of the pharyngeal airway and increased resistance to airflow. The relaxation alone may be sufficient to close the airway in some persons. In others, inspiratory muscle activity increases to compensate for the increased airway resistance, and the increased negative pressure generated by the extra effort leads to airway collapse. Ultimately, the airway opens only after an arousal, or brief awakening leads to increased activity of pharyngeal dilators. The patient then takes a few deep breaths and returns to sleep, whereupon the cycle repeats itself. Pharyngeal narrowing without complete occlusion may cause decreased ventilation. These episodes, referred to as hypopneas, lead to arousals, sleep fragmentation, daytime sleepiness, and hypoxemia and thus have the same functional effect as apneas.

Pharyngeal narrowing with high resistance to airflow is sometimes associated with compensatory increased respiratory effort that minimizes changes in tidal volume, ventilation, and oxygenation but still leads to arousals and sleep fragmentation. The functional effect is similar to OSA but without the associated hypoxemia. When such episodes are the predominant type of respiratory event, the disorder is referred to as the *upper airway resistance syndrome*.[25] The body weight of patients with this disorder is often normal or near-normal, and there appears to be a higher proportion of women and children with the syndrome than occurs with OSA, perhaps because their upper airways tend to be less compliant.

Airway narrowing may be due to a variety of causes (Table 54–7), including craniofacial malformations (high arched palate, a long low-placed soft palate, dental malocclusion, or retrognathia), neurological diseases with incoordination of preinspiratory activation of upper airway dilators,

TABLE 54–7. **Causes of Upper Airway Narrowing**

Genetic and developmental factors that influence craniofacial development
Anatomical malformations that affect craniofacial structures such as Crouzon's syndrome, Treacher Collins syndrome, Pierre Robin syndrome, Arnold-Chiari malformation, achondroplasia, rheumatoid arthritis, and Klippel-Feil syndrome
Enlarged tongue, soft palate, or uvula associated with obesity, Down syndrome, hypothyroidism, and acromegaly
Pharyngeal dilator weakness associated with neuromuscular diseases and medullary lesions
Infiltration of pharyngeal tissue associated with obesity, mucopolysaccharidoses, and mucosal edema and inflammation
Structural lesions such as enlarged tonsils and adenoids and pharyngeal tumors
Dyscoordinated breathing from abnormal respiratory control associated with Arnold-Chiari malformation, dysautonomias, and degenerative CNS disorders
Abnormally compliant airway associated with Marfan's syndrome

CNS, Central nervous system.

mouth breathing with posterior displacement of the mandible, or weakness from neuromuscular diseases. The site of airway occlusion may be at the level of the velopharynx, the oropharynx, the hypopharynx, the epiglottis, or the larynx. In some patients, the occlusion may be at more than one level or at different sites during different stages of sleep owing to differential activity of muscles involved in maintenance of airway patency.

The reason for the more frequent occurrence of OSA in men than in women is not known. Men tend to have longer, narrower upper airways, which may predispose them to airway collapse. The airway may be more compliant in men and may close at lower pressures for a given airway diameter. Women also show a greater augmentation of genioglossus activity in response to inspiratory loading, which may indicate a less collapsible airway. Testosterone may lead to increased bulk of neck muscles and may lead to a preferential deposition of fat in upper airway structures. For poorly understood reasons, the frequency and severity of OSA syndrome in women after menopause is higher than in premenopausal women.[27]

In susceptible persons, OSA may be precipitated or made worse by sleep deprivation, evening alcohol use, sedative medications, and the supine sleeping position. Even small doses of alcohol enhance upper airway muscle relaxation that occurs during sleep, thereby exacerbating OSA. Alcohol also blunts chemoreceptor responses to blood gases and raises the arousal threshold, which increases the duration of apneas.

Arterial oxyhemoglobin saturation (SaO_2) falls during apneas and hypopneas at a rate of 0.1 to 1.6 percent per second. The severity of hypoxemia is a function of baseline oxygenation, lung oxygen stores, the degree of airway narrowing, and apnea duration. Drops in SaO_2 to below 70 percent are common in severe OSA. Apneas during REM sleep tend to produce greater decreases in SaO_2 owing to decreased lung oxygen reserves and increased duration of apneas.

Arteriolar constriction as a result of hypoxemia, acidosis, and increased sympathetic tone contribute to increases in blood pressure during apneas that may reach 190 mm Hg systolic and 110 mm Hg diastolic. Right-to-left shifts of the cardiac interventricular septum and decreased cardiac output may occur as a result of increased negative intrathoracic pressure associated with attempts to breathe. Increased vagal tone associated with fluctuations in intrathoracic pressure, stimulation of the carotid body by hypoxemia, and increased sympathetic tone that accompanies the arousals at the end of apneas contribute to bradycardia, periods of asystole, atrioventricular block, premature ventricular contractions, and ventricular tachyarrhythmias. Sleep-disordered breathing is associated strongly with systemic hypertension.[28]

The repeated arousals to resume breathing, along with reduced amounts of REM sleep and slow-wave sleep, appear to be the major causes of daytime sleepiness in patients with OSA.

Epidemiology and Risk Factors. Habitual snoring, which is more common in males than in females, occurs in 6 to 12 percent of children and 5 to 20 percent of adults. OSA has a prevalence of about 1 percent in children, 2 percent in adult women, and 4 percent in adult men.[29, 30]

Clinical Features and Associated Disorders. The usual presenting symptoms are snoring, excessive sleepiness, daytime sleep episodes, and a sense that sleep is not restful. Morning headaches, frequent nocturnal urination, and nocturnal restlessness are also common. Some patients have no complaints and present only because the bed partner has noted periods of apnea. Others are referred because of a suspicion that OSA contributes to headaches, pulmonary or systemic hypertension, cardiac arrhythmias, or impotence.

Loud snoring, sometimes exceeding 90 dB, occurs in more than 80 percent of patients and usually begins years before the onset of sleep apnea. Some patients report that they cannot go on camping trips and must have separate hotel rooms on business trips because of their obnoxious snoring. Increasing volume of snoring, snoring that has changed in character, and loud rhythmical snoring punctuated by snorts and choking noises are suggestive of OSA. Snoring is produced by vibration of the soft tissues of the upper airway. The intensity and quality vary depending on the stage of sleep, the position of the body, the rate of airflow, the anatomical structure of the individual's nose and throat, and the amount of floppy airway tissue with potential to vibrate. Although snoring is common in patients with OSA, it is not universal. Snoring will not occur even with a very narrow pharynx if floppy tissue is absent.

Restless sleep is caused by the arousals at the end of apneas, which may be accompanied by jerks, twitches, and gross body movements. Changes in body position may occur several times per hour as patients attempt to find a sleeping position compatible with airway patency. With severe apnea, patients may sleep in a chair, on the couch, sitting up on the side of the bed, or leaning against a wall. Despite the restlessness, patients usually have the impression that sleep has been continuous or interrupted only by a few trips to the bathroom. A few patients describe repeated awakenings and complain mainly of insomnia.

Tiredness, sleepiness, and a sense that sleep is not refreshing are characteristic symptoms of sleep apnea, often accompanied by impaired memory and concentration. The sleepiness often increases gradually over several years as patients gain weight. Some patients feel mentally dull or disoriented each morning. Daytime sleepiness is usually most apparent after lunch, while driving or reading, or in other boring sedentary situations. Patients often minimize difficulties with sleepiness and describe it as no worse than in colleagues or peers. With more severe apnea, patients may fall asleep on the telephone or during sexual intercourse and may have episodes of "automatic behavior" during which complex activities are performed such as driving for miles with no recollection. Although daytime sleepiness is common, its absence does not rule out OSA.

Other common symptoms include irritability, impotence or reduced libido, excessive sweating at night, and dry mouth. Symptoms of gastroesophageal reflux may be present if the repeated episodes of negative intrathoracic pressure associated with apneas lead to passage of gastric contents through the lower esophageal sphincter.

In children, snoring and restless sleep are common complaints, along with poor attention, decreased school performance, enuresis, and hyperactivity. Daytime sleepiness is often less pronounced than in adults unless apnea is severe.

On physical examination, patients are often obese and have thick necks. Long narrow facies, high arched palate, retrognathia, an enlarged edematous uvula, prominent tonsils, and redundant pharyngeal tissue are other common findings. Patients with severe OSA may have findings consistent with right-sided heart failure.

Obstructive sleep apnea occurs in 10 to 40 percent of obese persons and in at least 25 percent of patients with hypertension. In untreated severe OSA, the prevalence of hypertension may be as high as 50 percent. A number of other disorders contribute to the development of OSA (see Table 54–7).

Central sleep apnea, which is much less common than OSA, is a disorder in which apneas occur but there is no associated attempt to breathe. The disorder may be idiopathic, or it may be caused by congestive heart failure or brain stem pathology. Many patients have both central sleep apnea and OSA, presumably because activation of upper airway afferents during airway occlusion leads to inhibition of attempts to breathe.

Differential Diagnosis. Loud snoring with gasping or choking sounds, witnessed apneas, restless sleep, hypertension, and neck circumference greater than 16.5 inches are useful predictors of OSA, but a definitive diagnosis usually requires polysomnography. Among children, snoring or noisy breathing, daytime mouth breathing, and parental observation of apneas and struggles to breathe are suggestive symptoms. The absence of snoring and obesity does not rule out OSA in either adults or children. In patients with excessive daytime sleepiness, other diagnostic considerations include narcolepsy, idiopathic hypersomnia, periodic limb movement disorder (PLMD), central sleep apnea, and the insufficient sleep syndrome. The differential diagnosis of nocturnal choking and gasping includes gastroesophageal reflux, nocturnal asthma, congestive heart failure, nocturnal panic attacks, and sleep-related laryngospasm.

Evaluation. A nocturnal polysomnogram with monitoring of sleep stage, airflow, respiratory effort, electrocardiogram, leg movements, and body position is the most commonly used tool for diagnosis. If upper airway resistance syndrome is suspected, intraesophageal pressure measurements should be obtained as part of the polysomnogram. The polysomnogram helps determine the presence and type of apnea, assess the relation of breathing disturbance to sleep stage and body position, determine the severity of hypoxemia and sleep disturbance, and identify cardiac arrhythmias. Apneas and hypopneas usually last 10 to 30 seconds and typically are followed by transient arousals. During REM sleep, apneas and hypopneas are usually longer, sometimes as long as 2 to 3 minutes, and are more likely to be associated with hypoxemia and cardiac arrhythmias. There are usually reduced amounts of stages 3 and 4 sleep and REM sleep. With mild OSA, apneas may occur only after alcohol ingestion or only when the patient is supine. With severe OSA, apneas occur continuously throughout the night and in all body positions.

In patients with high pretest probability of moderate or severe OSA, a home-monitoring study may be sufficient for diagnosis. A variety of home-monitoring devices are available; the simplest types measure only a single variable, such as oxygen saturation, whereas more complex devices may record as many channels as a typical laboratory polysomnogram. Home-monitoring studies cost less than laboratory studies, but they do not allow for visual observation, correction of artifacts or faulty sensors, or therapeutic interventions. It is also more difficult to assess mild sleep apnea. Finally, current models suggest that even inexpensive home studies with excellent sensitivity and specificity still may not be cost-effective in comparison to laboratory polysomnography.[31]

Additional studies may be indicated in some patients. An MSLT helps assess the presence and severity of excessive sleepiness. Although fiberoptic endoscopy of the upper airway, cephalometric radiographs, and magnetic resonance imaging (MRI) can be used to assess airway anatomy, such studies during wakefulness are of limited value in determining the site of obstruction because airway dynamics differ in sleep and wakefulness. Arterial blood gases and pulmonary function tests are indicated if obesity-hypoventilation syndrome or other causes of hypoventilation are suspected but they are not needed for routine evaluation of suspected OSA. In selected cases, evaluation for hypothyroidism may be indicated.

Some patients described as loud snorers do not snore during sleep studies. In such cases, snoring may be intermittent and related to alcohol use, body position, or allergies. Loud snoring that cannot be verified with objective assessment is sometimes an indication of marital problems.

Management. The goal of treatment is to keep the airway open during sleep, which should lead to improved sleep, better oxygenation, and enhanced daytime alertness. Treatment for OSA depends on the severity of the disorder. There is little doubt that treatment is needed for severe OSA because it is associated with increased risks of motor vehicle accidents, hypertension, stroke, myocardial infarction, cardiovascular death, and death while sleeping, if left untreated or treated ineffectively.[32–37] For patients with a mild case of the disorder—those with fewer than 20 apneas plus hypopneas per hour of sleep, little or no nocturnal hypoxemia, mild or absent daytime sleepiness, and no hypertension or serious cardiac arrhythmias—the health benefits of treatment are less certain, and it is unknown at present whether asymptomatic patients with mild sleep apnea need to be treated.

The introduction in the 1980s of continuous positive airway pressure (CPAP) administered via a nasal mask revolutionized the management of OSA.[38] Nasal CPAP functions as an air splint to maintain positive intraluminal pressure in the upper airway. Although nasal CPAP can be used by children as well as by adults and is effective in 80 to 90 percent of patients, the proportion who use CPAP on a regular basis is substantially less. If nasal obstruction prevents the use of nasal CPAP, treatment with decongestants, steroid inhalers, septoplasty, or other forms of nasal surgery may be required. Other factors that may prevent the use of CPAP or reduce its benefit include a poorly fitting or uncomfortable mask, sinus infections, claustrophobia, chronic mouth breathing, incomplete efficacy, and lack of motivation. The more expensive bilevel positive airway pressure (BPAP) devices provide different pressures during inspiration and expiration and are sometimes better tolerated, particularly by patients with claustrophobia. Other problems associated with nasal CPAP include noise from the machine, air swallowing, allergic rhinitis, and discomfort from misdirection of airflow into the eyes. Barotrauma to the lungs is extremely rare.

For patients who cannot tolerate CPAP or prefer not to use it, a number of other treatments may be used. Removal of enlarged tonsils and adenoids is often successful in children and sometimes in adults. Uvulopalatopharyngoplasty (UPP) with removal of the uvula, portions of the soft palate, and redundant pharyngeal tissue eliminates snoring in more than 80 percent and produces improvement of OSA in about 50 percent of patients, but complete resolution of sleep apnea is uncommon. Laser-assisted UPP is a staged outpatient procedure that eliminates snoring in about 60 percent of patients but is probably less effective for OSA than standard UPP. Maxillofacial surgery, with advancement of the mandible, the maxilla, or both, appears to be beneficial for selected patients. Orthodontic appliances that advance the tongue or mandible can improve airway patency during sleep, reduce snoring, and decrease the frequency of respiratory events during sleep, but they rarely eliminate sleep apnea completely. Weight reduction is often helpful, but it may be difficult to achieve. Protriptyline at doses of 5 mg at bedtime may provide some benefit in mild cases. For some patients with mild OSA, avoidance of precipitating factors such as sleep deprivation, evening alcohol use, sedative medications, and the supine sleeping position is the only treatment needed. Whatever treatment is used, the outcome should be assessed with a sleep study because many patients experience more subjective than objective improvement.

Prognosis and Future Perspectives. Some patients develop increasingly severe apnea with age, but worsening of the condition may be due to weight gain. The natural history of sleep apnea in the absence of weight gain is unknown. Habitual snoring remits in as many as 35 percent.

RESTLESS LEGS SYNDROME AND PERIODIC LIMB MOVEMENT DISORDER

Restless legs syndrome (RLS) is characterized by unpleasant sensations of the legs that are worse in the evening and at night and that are relieved by movement.[1] Most patients with RLS also have movements of the legs that occur periodically at 20- to 30-second intervals for minutes to hours during sleep. Although the term nocturnal myoclonus sometimes is used to describe these movements, they usually are not sudden lightning-like movements. Rather, they typically last for about 1 second and consist of extension of the great toe with variable degrees of ankle extension, knee extension, and hip extension or flexion. With PLMD, periodic movements occur during sleep, but the unpleasant evening and nighttime sensations are absent. Arousals associated with the PLMs may lead to complaints of insomnia or daytime sleepiness, or the disorder may be asymptomatic.

Pathogenesis and Pathophysiology. Although the pathophysiological basis for RLS and PLMD is unknown, disinhibition of a CNS pacemaker that affects reticular excitability may contribute. The similarity of PLMs to the extensor response to plantar stimulation (Babinski's sign) or to a triple flexion response suggests that pyramidal or dorsal reticulospinal tract dysfunction is involved.[39] Functional dopamine or opiate insufficiency, perhaps related to abnormal iron metabolism, may also play a role. Abnormal sensory input may be a factor in some patients.

Epidemiology and Risk Factors. The prevalence of RLS is about 2 to 5 percent for the adult population and increases with age. Men and women are affected equally, and symptoms begin after age 40 in most patients. About one third to one half of patients report that other family members are affected, and in some families, the syndrome occurs in a pattern consistent with an autosomal dominant inheritance. PLMD without waking symptoms of RLS occurs in about 5 percent of persons between ages 30 and 50 years and in 30 to 45 percent or more of persons older than 65 years of age.[40]

Clinical Features and Associated Disorders. Patients with RLS complain of a gradual buildup of a subcutaneous crawling, pulling, itching, aching, or pins-and-needles sensation that affects the muscles or bones of the calves and thighs. As the sensation builds, the associated urge to move gradually becomes irresistible and movement provides temporary relief. Most patients have insomnia with difficulty getting to sleep and frequent awakenings during which they may flex and extend the legs, repeatedly turn over in bed, or get out of bed and walk. About 80 to 90 percent of patients with RLS have PLMs, usually during light NREM sleep, that contribute to awakenings and arousals.

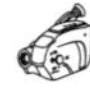

During the day and especially during attempts to remain still, many patients fidget, swing their legs, or have movements that are similar to the extensor movements during sleep. Apart from the movements, neurological examination is usually normal.

In PLMD, the condition is associated with arousals that lead to sleep disruption and complaints of insomnia or daytime sleepiness, but the sensory symptoms and waking dyskinesias that accompany RLS do not occur. Although severely affected patients may produce movements throughout sleep, PLMD may also be entirely asymptomatic, causing no disruption of sleep patterns, and is sometimes brought to medical attention either as an incidental finding on a polysomnogram or because the spouse is unable to sleep owing to the leg jerks and kicks.

RLS and PLMD may be induced or aggravated by a variety of conditions, including iron deficiency, anemia, and chronic renal failure. Peripheral neuropathy may be a factor in some cases, although peripheral nerve function is clinically normal in most affected patients. Symptoms occur in 10 to 20 percent of pregnant women and usually resolve postpartum. Other disorders that may be associated with PLMD or RLS include venous disease, degenerative CNS disorders, and vitamin deficiency.

Differential Diagnosis. The diagnosis of RLS is based on the history. The essential elements are the urge to move associated with sensory phenomena in the legs, motor restlessness, and exacerbation at rest and in the evening and night.[41] The differential diagnosis may include akathisia, peripheral neuropathy, claudication, and leg cramps. With akathisia caused by phenothiazines, there is restlessness of the body and a compulsion to move, but the sensory component is less than with RLS and it is usually not exacerbated at night. Neuropathic dysesthesias are usually more distal than proximal, are felt more on the surface than in deeper structures, and are not relieved by movement. Claudication is brought on by exercise and relieved by rest, which is the reverse of the pattern with RLS. Leg cramps are associated with palpable tightness of muscles that does not occur with RLS.

Differential diagnosis of PLMD includes sleep starts and a variety of other movements during sleep. Sleep starts are vigorous myoclonic jerks of the extremities or trunk that occur at sleep onset but do not recur periodically. Most other types of movements and behaviors during sleep are not periodic.

Evaluation. Evaluation of patients with suspected RLS should include complete blood count and serum iron and ferritin levels. Renal function tests and electromyography and nerve conduction studies are indicated only in selected patients. Polysomnography is useful for suspected PLMD.

Management. Evening and bedtime doses of dopaminergic agonists or levodopa-carbidopa provide considerable benefit in RLS and PLMD.[42] Some patients require additional doses during the night or controlled-release formulations. Unfortunately, some patients treated with levodopa develop tolerance and require increasing doses, whereas others develop increased daytime symptoms of restless legs. If necessary, levodopa-carbidopa can be given around the clock to such patients. Temporary withdrawal and reinstitution of therapy a few weeks later may improve efficacy. Fortunately, most patients treated with dopamine agonists such as pramipexole do not develop these complications. Pramipexole is generally a good first-line agent for RLS.

Benzodiazepines, particularly clonazepam, can be used either alone or in combination with dopaminergic agents for RLS and for PLMD. Daytime sedation, tolerance, and loss of efficacy are the major problems encountered with these drugs. Opiates such as propoxyphene, codeine, and hydrocodone also reduce the unpleasant sensations and can be used alone or in combination with dopaminergic agents and benzodiazepines.[43] Clonidine, baclofen, carbamazepine, and gabapentin are sometimes helpful.

For patients with PLMD without RLS, it may be difficult to determine the extent to which PLMD contributes to daytime symptoms. The decision to treat PLMD depends on the frequency of movements and associated arousals and on the clinical assessment of the degree to which other sleep disorders contribute to symptoms.

Prognosis and Future Perspectives. RLS has a variable course. Some patients have long periods of relative stability, whereas others worsen with age. Permanent remissions are rare.

Chronobiological Disorders

People who sleep at the wrong time of day or who cannot sleep at the right time of night often have one of the six major chronobiological disorders: jet lag syndrome, shift work sleep disorder, DSPS, advanced sleep phase syndrome, non–24-hour sleep-wake disorder, and irregular sleep-wake pattern disorder.[1]

Pathogenesis and Pathophysiology. Circadian rhythm disturbances are caused by a shift in the usual phase relation between the internal biological clock and the desired sleep-wake schedule. The suprachiasmatic nucleus of the hypothalamus functions as the biological clock. In the absence of entraining influences, the output of the nucleus has a period slightly longer than 24 hours. Thus, persons living in temporal isolation adopt a 24.5- to 25-hour sleep-wake schedule and cycle in and out of phase with the external environment. The phase of the biological clock can be shifted by only a few stimuli, of which the most potent is bright light.[44] Bright light exposure helps maintain synchronization between the internal clock and the external world, but the phase-shifting effects of light are limited in most circumstances to no more than 2 hours each day. The retinohypothalamic pathway, the primary afferent tract to the suprachiasmatic nucleus, mediates the effects of light on circadian rhythms. Intensity, duration, and timing of light exposure determine its effect on the phase of the circadian system. Light pulses just before or during the first half of the dark phase produce phase delays, whereas light pulses during the second half of the dark phase or just after the end of the dark phase produce phase advances. Melatonin, a pineal hormone that is secreted mainly at night in humans, appears to have phase-shifting properties that are opposite to the effects of bright light: Melatonin administered in the afternoon produces phase advances, whereas melatonin given in the morning produces phase delays.

With east-west jet travel or with changing work schedules, most persons attempt to shift their schedule of sleep and wakefulness quickly to meet the social demands of the new schedule, but the internal clock cannot adjust and sleep-wake patterns are disrupted. Night workers also sleep about 1 to 1.5 hours less than day workers, and their attempts to sleep at night when they are not working often prevent them from synchronizing the internal clock to the night shift schedule. As the internal clock shifts by about 1 hour per day after a phase advance—such as an eastbound flight—and by 1.5 hours per day after a phase delay—such as a westbound flight— it may be several days before sleep-wake patterns and the internal clock shift to the new schedule.[45, 46]

Phase shifts also may occur during weekends if bedtimes and rise times are delayed, at least in part because of altered timing of light exposure. In patients with DSPS,[47] phase delays induced by sleeping later are not corrected during the week. Adolescence, the usual time of appearance of DSPS, is associated with increased sleep needs, but social factors and greater independence usually prevent earlier bedtimes. As a result, many adolescents sleep later on weekends and develop DSPS. Leaving home for college may exacerbate DSPS because parents can no longer act as backups to the alarm clock. In advanced sleep phase syndrome, the pattern is the opposite, with excessively early bedtimes and early awakenings due to phase advance of the biological clock.

Degeneration or destruction of the suprachiasmatic nucleus or its effector pathways is the usual cause of irregular sleep-wake pattern disorder. Non–24-hour sleep-wake disorder is usually caused by retinal, prechiasmal, or chiasmal lesions that interrupt the retinohypothalamic tract. Although most affected persons are blind, chiasmal lesions that interrupt the retinohypothalamic tract may cause the syndrome even when visual loss is incomplete. Without retinal input, the internal clock moves in and out of phase with the environmental clock. When the phase difference is small, patients may be able to maintain sleep hours close to the societal norm, but when the phase difference is large, synchronization cannot be maintained and sleep times become highly irregular. Prolonged periods of wakefulness lasting up to 40 to 50 hours may be followed by sleep periods of 12 to 20 hours and then resumption for a few days of a relatively normal schedule.

The first mammalian circadian clock gene was cloned recently, and its mutation causes altered behavior, affecting the free-running rhythm period and causing loss of persistence of circadian rhythms. Additional circadian clock genes have already been described.[48]

Epidemiology and Risk Factors. Circadian rhythm sleep disorders are common. Jet lag symptoms affect the majority of persons who fly across five or more time zones. Sleep disruption is a problem for a large proportion of the more than 20 million shift workers, particularly for older workers during the days and nights following a shift change. DSPS may affect as many as 7 percent of urban adolescents. The other disorders are less common. The irregular sleep-wake pattern disorder occurs mainly in institutionalized persons with severe static or progressive encephalopathies. The non–24-hour sleep-wake disorder appears to be a major cause of sleep-wake complaints in blind persons.

Clinical Features and Associated Disorders. Symptoms of jet lag, which may last as long as 7 to 10 days after trips across five or more time zones, include difficulty falling asleep or remaining asleep in the new environment, along with sleepiness during the new daytime. Symptoms, which are usually worse with eastward flight than with westward flight, may be exacerbated by sleep loss and alcohol use during the flight. Chronic jet lag with sleepiness, sleep disruption, malaise, irritability, and reduced performance may occur in airline personnel and in other frequent jet travelers. Night workers and those who work rotating shifts often develop sleep problems similar to jet lag because an 8-hour shift in the sleep schedule produces effects similar to flight across eight time zones. Nighttime sleep on weekends may prevent shifts in phase to match the new schedule and may exacerbate sleep problems during the week. Adolescent patients with DSPS have difficulty falling asleep at night and difficulty waking up on time when they try to maintain a conventional sleep-wake schedule. Patients with advanced sleep phase syndrome complain of evening sleepiness and early morning awakening. Sleep onset between 6 and 9 PM and awakening between 1 and 3 AM are typical.

With the irregular sleep-wake pattern disorder, sleep episodes of varying length occur at irregular intervals. Patients or caretakers complain of difficulty falling asleep, difficulty remaining asleep, and daytime somnolence. The picture is often complicated by nocturnal agitation and by the use of sedatives or antipsychotic medications to control the agitation.

Patients with the non–24-hour sleep-wake disorder may complain of difficulty falling asleep in the evening, difficulty waking up in the morning, or difficulty staying awake during the day. Cyclical fluctuation in severity of the complaints is typical because sleep problems are much greater when the phase difference between the temperature rhythm and the desired sleep-wake schedule is high.

DSPS may be the initial manifestation of depression in adolescents. In adults with poor social adaptation, the syndrome may provide secondary gain as a means to reduce or avoid social interaction. Irregular sleep-wake syndrome is often associated with encephalopathy and non–24-hour sleep-wake syndrome with blindness.

Differential Diagnosis. The differential diagnosis of chronobiological disorders includes most of the other disorders that cause insomnia or sleepiness. Inadequate sleep hygiene and chronically insufficient sleep often contribute to sleep disturbance in shift workers and night workers; temporal association of sleep disturbance with night or rotating shift work and remission during vacations is suggestive of shift work sleep disorder. Depression, marital or family problems, job dissatisfaction, or other psychosocial factors should be considered in a permanent shift worker who develops sleep problems after years of stable functioning.

DSPS that presents in adolescence is sometimes misdiagnosed as narcolepsy, depression, chronic fatigue, or a learning disorder. Knowledge that sleepiness occurs mainly in the morning and continuous restful sleep occurs when patients go to bed late and arise late helps the clinician arrive at the correct diagnosis.

Evaluation. The history and sleep logs provide the most useful information for diagnosing circadian rhythm sleep disorders. Maintenance of a sleep log for 2 to 4 weeks is usually sufficient except for patients with the non–24-hour sleep-wake pattern, whose cyclical sleep patterns may only be revealed after several weeks of maintaining sleep logs. In DSPS, sleep logs show sleep onset and awakening from sleep that are much later than the social norm. Bedtimes and wakeup times are often even later on weekends. Sleep logs in patients with irregular sleep-wake patterns show no consistent sleep times: There may be several 2- to 4-hour sleep periods scattered over the 24-hour period, with marked variability in the timing and duration of sleep from one day to the next.

If sleep apnea or narcolepsy is suspected, polysomnography and MSLT may be helpful, but MSLT interpretation is difficult if the patient has not been on a regular schedule. Psychiatric assessment is indicated if depression appears to be a contributing factor.

Management. Appropriate scheduling of sleep and of exposure to bright light are the keys to management of circadian rhythm sleep disorders. To minimize jet lag, the pretravel sleep schedule should be shifted 1 to 2 hours closer to the destination schedule. Although hypnotic use during the trip may minimize in-flight sleep loss, the potential for effects on memory and cognition must be considered, especially in the elderly. After travel, correctly timed exposure to bright light and immediate adoption of the new time zone schedule help reduce symptoms. At present, melatonin, which may be beneficial for jet lag, is not available in the United States except as an unregulated health food supplement.

Treatment of shift work sleep disorder depends on the frequency of shift changes, the direction of shift rotation, the desired schedule during nights of work, and the daytime obligations of the shift worker.[49] Shift rotations from days to evenings to nights tend to be better tolerated than rotations in the opposite direction. Although sleep is usually best for night workers who sleep during the day 7 days per week, most persons are unwilling to spend days off asleep. A biphasic sleep schedule with a 2- to 3-hour nap in the afternoon and 4 to 6 hours of sleep in the morning after work is sometimes the best option. Bright light at night and dark bedrooms in the daytime are beneficial, but daytime sedative use is usually of no value.

For DSPS, the patient should be instructed to advance the times of going to bed and arising from bed by about 15 minutes each day or two beginning with the usual weekend sleep times. Alternative approaches with more rapid phase shifts are quicker, but they are more socially disruptive and require strong motivation. Once the desired schedule is achieved, it must be rigorously maintained 7 days per week. Morning bright light is helpful, but patients should understand that the schedule is the most critical element.

Although DSPS almost always can be treated effectively with strict scheduling, psychosocial factors often interfere with the planned treatment. Awakening in time to get to school often has become a focus for conflict between the parents and the patient, and many patients, particularly those with depression, lack the motivation to maintain the schedule. Failure to attempt even a minimal shift in schedule is usually an indication of major family discord, depression, or poor motivation.

Advanced sleep phase syndrome can be treated with daily 15-minute delays in bedtime and evening exposure to bright light. Treatment of the irregular sleep-wake pattern disorder is difficult, although morning exposure to bright light, increased daytime activity, and prohibition of morning and evening naps may be helpful. Management of the non–24-hour sleep-wake syndrome is also difficult, but blind patients who retain some retinal input to the suprachiasmatic nucleus benefit from appropriately timed exposure to high-intensity bright light.[50]

Parasomnias

Parasomnias are disorders in which the chief complaint is related to undesirable physical and mental phenomena that occur mainly or exclusively during sleep.[1] Twenty-three parasomnias are recognized (Table 54–8).[25] This section reviews some parasomnias that are of particular interest to neurologists.

TABLE 54–8. **Parasomnias**

Disorder	Key Features
Confusional arousals	Sudden arousals, usually from slow- wave sleep, associated with confusion and disorientation
Sleepwalking	Arousal with complex motor behavior, usually from slow-wave sleep; walking, running, talking, and eating may occur
Sleep terrors	Sudden arousal, usually from slow-wave sleep, with fearful agitated behavior, often with screaming or crying and inconsolability
Rhythmic movement disorder	Stereotyped repetitive rhythmical movements—such as head-banging, head-rocking, and body-rolling—during light sleep and transitions between sleep and wakefulness
Sleep starts	Sudden myoclonic jerks at sleep onset of the trunk, head, or extremities
Sleep talking	Talking during sleep, usually during arousals
Nocturnal leg cramps	Painful cramps of the foot or calf that produce awakenings
Nightmares	Frightening dreams
Sleep paralysis	Paralysis occurring at the onset or end of sleep or during nocturnal awakenings
Impaired sleep-related penile erections	Impaired or absent penile erections during REM sleep
Sleep-related painful erections	Painful erections occurring during REM sleep
REM sleep–related sinus arrest	Periods of cardiac asystole during REM sleep
REM sleep behavior disorder	Dream-enacting behavior with loss of the normal muscle atonia during REM sleep
Sleep bruxism	Stereotyped repetitive grinding of the teeth during sleep or arousals from sleep
Sleep enuresis	Incomplete bladder control during sleep beyond the expected age for bladder control
Sleep-related abnormal swallowing syndrome	Impaired swallowing of saliva during sleep
Nocturnal paroxysmal dystonia	Brief stereotyped episodes of sudden dystonic posturing and ballistic movements, arising from NREM sleep
Sudden unexplained nocturnal death syndrome	Sudden death during sleep in healthy young adults
Primary snoring	Snoring without sleep apnea
Infant sleep apnea	Sleep apnea in infants
Congenital central hypoventilation syndrome	Hypoventilation during sleep that is not due to primary lung disease or respiratory muscle weakness
Sudden infant death syndrome	Sudden unexplained death in infancy
Benign neonatal sleep myoclonus	Irregular myoclonic jerks of the trunk and extremities during NREM sleep in neonates

REM, Rapid eye movement; NREM, nonrapid eye movement.

AROUSAL DISORDERS

Pathogenesis and Pathophysiology. The arousal disorders—confusional arousals, sleepwalking, and sleep terrors—are grouped together based on the hypothesis that impaired ability to arouse fully from slow-wave sleep is responsible for the phenomena.[51] The disorders, which are most common during childhood when the amount of slow-wave sleep is at its peak, probably exist on a continuum. Confusional arousals are associated with low levels of motoric and autonomic activation; sleepwalking with motoric activation but little autonomic activation; and sleep terrors with pronounced autonomic, emotional, and motoric activation. The variable activation patterns lead to considerable overlap between the three syndromes.

Epidemiology and Risk Factors. Children are affected more than adults with a peak incidence between ages 4 and 10 years; however, onset in adulthood can occur. About 1 to 6 percent of children have recurrent sleep terrors. An increased prevalence in first-degree relatives suggests that genetic factors may play a role. In susceptible persons, sleepwalking and sleep terrors may be precipitated or aggravated by stress, sleep deprivation, fever, sleep apnea, and noise.

Clinical Features and Associated Disorders. Sleep terrors are episodes of fearful agitation with decreased responsiveness and inconsolability that begin abruptly, usually from slow-wave sleep in the first third of the night. Severe episodes are often accompanied by screaming and attempts to leave the bed or the room. Patients may fall down stairs and may react violently to attempts to restrain them. After several minutes the patient calms down and returns to sleep. Morning recall is usually absent, although some patients have a vague recollection of a terrifying situation such as suffocation and occasional patients recall more elaborate dreamlike experiences.

Sleepwalking is characterized by complex automatisms during sleep typified by getting out of bed and walking. Some subjects eat;[52] others attempt to leave the home through a door or window. Patients sometimes sit or stand in bed without getting out of bed. Although sleepwalkers often respond inappropriately, they sometimes follow instructions to return to bed.

Confusional arousals are brief episodes associated with talking, moaning, or agitation that rarely require treatment.

Although sleep terrors and sleepwalking may be precipitated by stress in susceptible individuals, most affected children do not have severe psychopathology. Arousal disorders appear to be increased in Tourette's syndrome, post-traumatic stress disorder, and children with violent, abusive families.

Differential Diagnosis. The differential diagnosis of arousal disorders includes sleep-related epilepsy, REM sleep behavior disorder (RBD),[53] nightmares, confusional states, and nocturnal delirium. Although the patient's history is often sufficient for diagnosis, symptoms of screaming, walking, running, and vague, frightening perceptions may accompany nocturnal complex partial seizures. Atypical presentations that suggest the possibility of seizures include onset in adulthood; multiple nightly episodes; stereotyped behaviors with chewing, swallowing, and salivation; and poor or no response to medications.[54] RBD occurs mainly in adults and is usually associated with dream recall; the vague recollections that accompany some episodes of sleep terrors are usually fragmentary without the plot or story that characterizes dream mentation. Behavior may, however, be similar to that observed with sleep terrors, and some patients have a so-called overlap syndrome with elements of sleep terrors and RBD.

In hysterical dissociative phenomena, such as fugue states and multiple personalities, the patient is not asleep and behavior is purposeful, more complex, and longer lasting. The electroencephalogram (EEG) is consistent with waking state.

Evaluation. For otherwise normal children with typical behaviors of sleepwalking or sleep terrors that occur during the first third of the night, the diagnosis can usually be made based on clinical criteria. When the diagnosis is uncertain, polygraphic monitoring with simultaneous video monitoring is indicated for 1 or 2 nights, particularly if the events are occurring several times per week. If nocturnal seizures are a consideration, several additional EEG channels should be included in the recording montage, along with a video recording of the patient and the capability to record or play back activity at a sufficient paper speed to identify interictal and ictal epileptiform activity.[54] Standard polysomnographic recording techniques used for identifying sleep apnea are generally insufficient for a definitive diagnosis.

Polysomnographic monitoring usually demonstrates the onset of sleep terror episodes during stage 3 or 4 sleep. The EEG during the episode may show rhythmical delta activity or other nonwaking patterns, whereas the EEG shows waking activity during psychogenic dissociative episodes and REM sleep activity during RBD. Psychiatric evaluation is indicated if a dissociative disorder is suspected, because many patients have severe psychopathology.

Management. Sleep terrors and sleepwalking usually improve with age and resolve before adolescence. Treatment may be required if the associated behaviors are potentially injurious or if the behavior is excessively disruptive to the family. Good sleep hygiene with regular sleep hours and adequate amounts of nocturnal sleep are important initial recommendations. Ground-floor bedrooms, window locks, and absence of sharp objects or toys on the bedroom floor are other useful measures. If injuries have occurred or appear likely to occur, treatment of the patient at bedtime with imipramine, diazepam, or clonazepam is usually effective. Hypnosis or other behavioral treatments may be helpful for some patients, and psychiatric treatment is indicated when the disorder is linked to significant psychopathology.

Prognosis and Future Perspectives. Episodes tend to decrease in frequency and severity during adolescence. The natural history of adult-onset arousal disorders is unknown.

REM SLEEP BEHAVIORAL DISORDER

Normal REM sleep is associated with skeletal muscle atonia interrupted by irregular muscle twitches. With the RBD, the muscle atonia that accompanies REM sleep is incomplete, and patients have motor automatisms in which they appear to act out their dreams.[53]

RBD occurs mainly in older persons and is more common in men than in women. Patients with Parkinson's disease, Alzheimer's disease, dementia with Lewy bodies, multi-infarct dementia, multiple system atrophy, olivopontocerebellar degeneration, narcolepsy, and focal brain stem lesions are at increased risk for RBD, but over half of patients have no major abnormality on neurological examination or MRI. Some studies have suggested that the disorder may be an early marker or risk factor for parkinsonian syndromes.

The disorder may begin fairly abruptly, or it may be preceded by months of progressively increasing nocturnal movements, vocalizations, and disturbing dreams. Presenting complaints include nocturnal shouting, violent behavior with "acting out" of dreams, and injuries during sleep to the patient or bed partner.[55] During the episodes, which usually last a few minutes, behavior may be limited to talking, laughing, and waving of the arms or it may include punching, kicking, or jumping out of bed. Some patients have a so-called Jekyll and Hyde syndrome with quiet peaceable behavior during the day that contrasts with the swearing and violence that accompanies REM sleep.

The timing and duration of episodes parallel the distribution of REM sleep across the night. Some patients have complex behaviors with virtually every REM period, whereas others have the behaviors less than once per week. Episodes usually do not occur during naps or during the first hour of sleep because REM sleep is uncommon at these times. Patients can usually be awakened from an episode without the confusion or difficulty arousing that characterizes sleep terrors.

Dream mentation and dream-enacting behaviors are uncommon with other disorders associated with complex motor activity during sleep (Table 54–9). The recurrence of episodes at approximately 90-minute intervals and the rapid return to full alertness on awakening are also useful distinguishing features.

Polysomnography with simultaneous audio and video monitoring and additional channels for limb movement monitoring is indicated when RBD is suspected. On polysomnography, the atonia that normally accompanies REM sleep is disrupted by periods of increased tone and increased phasic muscle activity, even during REM periods that are not associated with disruptive behavior. One night of recording is usually sufficient, but sometimes two nights are required. Brain imaging, daytime EEG, or neuropsychological tests may be indicated in patients with abnormal neurological examinations, but they are not needed in patients with idiopathic RBD.

In 80 to 90 percent of patients, behavior is eliminated or reduced to minor movements and vocalizations with bedtime doses of clonazepam, which appears to be more effective than other benzodiazepines. Incomplete atonia persists during REM sleep even with treatment. If clonazepam is ineffective or not tolerated, imipramine, levodopa-carbidopa, diazepam, temazepam, clonidine, or carbamazepine are occasionally useful.

Idiopathic RBD is a chronic disorder with few if any remissions. A substantial proportion of patients who are otherwise neurologically normal at the time of presentation develop Parkinson's disease over the next several years.

TABLE 54–9. **Causes of Episodic Nocturnal Complex Motor Activity**

Disorder	Stage of Sleep or Wakefulness in Which Episodes Arise
Sleepwalking	NREM sleep, usually slow-wave sleep
Sleep terrors	NREM sleep, usually slow-wave sleep
Partial complex seizures of temporal lobe origin	Usually NREM sleep
Partial complex seizures of frontal lobe origin	Usually NREM sleep
Hypnogenic paroxysmal dystonia	Usually NREM sleep
Panic disorder	NREM sleep
REM sleep behavior disorder	REM sleep
Nightmares	REM sleep
Nocturnal delirium	Wakefulness
Dissociative episodes	Wakefulness
Malingering	Wakefulness

REM, Rapid eye movement; NREM, nonrapid eye movement.

HYPNOGENIC PAROXYSMAL DYSTONIA

The clinical characteristics of hypnogenic paroxysmal dystonia (also called nocturnal paroxysmal dystonia) closely resemble partial seizures originating in the supplementary motor area, and in most patients, the attacks are epileptic.[56, 57] Unusual cases with long-lasting attacks are presumed to be caused by a basal ganglia disturbance.

The disorder is rare. Lesions of the supplementary motor area or of mediobasal regions of the frontal lobe appear to be the major risk factors.

Patients with this disorder have brief spells of ballistic choreoathetoid movements and dystonic postures that arise abruptly from NREM sleep. The violent movements are usually bilateral, but they may predominate on one side and the patient usually is awake with eyes open during the episode.

Differential diagnosis includes partial seizures of temporal lobe origin, sleep terrors, nocturnal dissociative disorder, and RBD. Although the bizarre behaviors may suggest a psychiatric disorder, the abrupt onset from sleep, the highly stereotyped behaviors, and the absence of dream mentation and dream-enacting behaviors are helpful distinguishing features. Sleep terrors rarely occur more than 3 to 4 times per night, whereas episodes of hypnogenic paroxysmal dystonia often occur 10 to 40 times per night.

Polysomnography with video-EEG monitoring is the most useful diagnostic test.[54] The documentation of abrupt onset from sleep with stereotyped behavior is usually sufficient to exclude psychiatric causes, but definitive determination of whether the episodes are epileptic is often difficult. In some cases, ictal discharges may be recorded from frontal regions, but it may be necessary to record dozens of episodes over the course of several nights before a focal ictal discharge is revealed. In some cases, intracranial electrode placement is required.

Epileptic and nonepileptic forms may respond to carbamazepine and other antiepileptic agents, but as in other patients with seizures of frontal lobe origin, some patients show no response to any anticonvulsant.

The course is variable. Spontaneous remissions may occur that last for years, even when the disorder is epileptic. Other patients have numerous nightly episodes that are refractory to all treatments. Daytime seizures sometimes develop.

Sleep Abnormalities in Neurological Disorders

SLEEP DISORDERED BREATHING AND NEUROMUSCULAR DISEASES

Breathing disturbances in neuromuscular diseases are due to weakness of respiratory muscles, upper airway muscles, or both. Respiratory muscle weakness is usually severe in Duchenne muscular dystrophy and also occurs in myotonic dystrophy, limb-girdle dystrophy, polymyositis, poliomyelitis, amyotrophic lateral sclerosis, myasthenia gravis, and congenital myopathies.

Weakness of the diaphragm is the most important cause of respiratory disturbance during sleep. Diaphragmatic workload increases in NREM sleep owing in part to airway narrowing caused by decreased tone in upper airway muscles, in part to sleep-related changes in lung mechanics and respiratory muscle activation, and in part to the increased load associated with the horizontal position. With neuromuscular disorders, weakness of upper airway muscles may further reduce airway diameter, leading to increased respiratory load. Diaphragm workload increases even further during REM sleep, because accessory muscles of respiration are inhibited and the diaphragm must perform almost all of the work of breathing. The increased workload during sleep may lead to diaphragm fatigue with hypoxia, hypercapnia, acidosis-induced muscle dysfunction, and progressively worsening hypoventilation during the latter portion of the night.

Weakness of upper airway muscles may also lead to obstructive apneas and hypopneas, but weakness of inspiratory muscles may prevent generation of sufficient force to produce snoring.

Obesity, kyphoscoliosis, and other factors that increase work of breathing may precipitate sleep-related hypoventilation in patients with diaphragm weakness. Patients with bulbar symptoms are at increased risk for upper airway obstruction during sleep. Although patients with daytime respiratory symptoms are at greatest risk, many patients without daytime complaints have significant sleep-related hypoventilation.

Patients may complain of frequent awakenings, nocturnal dyspnea or restlessness, inability to sleep supine, or morning headaches. Patients with marked diaphragm weakness may be unable to sleep in a bed and may sleep in a chair or on the couch. Daytime sleepiness is usually not a prominent complaint until sleep disturbance is severe. In occasional patients with motor neuron disease or myopathy, sleep complaints caused by nocturnal hypoventilation are the initial manifestation of the neuromuscular disease.

Other causes of sleep disturbance, including PLMD and the effects of medications, must be considered. Patients with progressive disorders may have sleep disturbance caused by depression.

Evaluation should include spirometry obtained in the sitting and supine positions because patients with diaphragm weakness may have a pronounced reduction in vital capacity when they are supine. Arterial blood gases, assessment of diaphragm motion with fluoroscopy, and complete pulmonary function testing are helpful in selected patients. Polysomnography allows assessment of breathing in REM and NREM sleep in various body positions and sleep stages. Measurement of end-tidal pCO_2, which can be performed as part of the recording, provides a quantitative assessment of ventilation.

Weight reduction may produce marked benefits if obesity has led to decompensation of marginal pulmonary function during sleep. Nocturnal oxygen may be beneficial if hypoventilation is not severe, but it must be administered cautiously in patients with daytime hypercapnia because of the risk of precipitating respiratory failure in patients whose breathing is dependent on hypoxic drive. For patients with upper airway obstruction, nasal CPAP is excellent treatment, and if hypoventilation is not reversed with CPAP, BPAP devices that provide a higher pressure during inspiration than during expiration can be used, especially for patients with expiratory muscle weakness. Negative-pressure cuirass ventilators and intermittent positive-pressure ventilation can be used if additional ventilatory support is needed. Tracheostomy combined with positive-pressure ventilation may be needed for some patients. The prognosis depends on the underlying neuromuscular disorder.

SLEEP DISORDERS ASSOCIATED WITH DEGENERATIVE DISORDERS OF THE CENTRAL NERVOUS SYSTEM

Degenerative neurological diseases can lead to sleep disturbance through effects of the disease on neuronal systems involved in sleep-wake regulation, on systems involved with regulation of breathing during sleep, or on systems involved with motor control during sleep. Degenerative processes that affect the suprachiasmatic nucleus or the retina may produce circadian rhythm disturbances. OSA may occur if weakness, spasticity, or rigidity affect bulbar muscles, and central or obstructive apneas may occur if respiratory control systems of the lower brain stem are involved. Patients who have degenerative processes that affect motor systems are at increased risk for PLMD, RLS, and RBD.

Degenerative disorders may also cause sleep disturbance due to the effects on sleep continuity of immobility, discomfort, and nocturnal disorientation. Depression and the effects of psychoactive medications also contribute to sleep problems in many patients, but sleep disturbance is also common in unmedicated nondepressed patients.

Frequent awakenings scattered throughout the night represent the most common pattern of sleep disturbance in these patients. Awakenings combined with disorientation in demented persons often lead to the so-called sundown syndrome with nocturnal wandering, confusion, and agitation. This problem is highly stressful to family members and is a major cause of institutionalization of the demented elderly.[58, 59] Daytime somnolence, often caused by nocturnal sleep disruption, may exacerbate difficulties with memory and attention.

Obstructive and central sleep apneas and irregular respiratory patterns during sleep are common in patients with autonomic disturbances, in those with bulbar symptoms, and in those with degeneration of pontomedullary systems involved in the coordination of breathing.[60, 61]

For the patient with a degenerative neurological disorder and sleep complaints, the differential diagnosis may include direct and indirect effects of the disease, medication effects, poor sleep hygiene with excessive time in bed, circadian rhythm sleep disorders, RLS and PLMD, sleep-related breathing disorders, sundowning, and RBD.

The history is the most important element for diagnosis. The relation of the onset of sleep disturbance to the onset of the degenerative disorder helps determine whether the two are related. For patients with insomnia or disruptive nocturnal behavior, the frequency and duration of awakenings should be noted, along with the times of naps and medications. Mood should be assessed because depression is a common contributor to sleep disturbance in this population. A sleep log may provide evidence of a circadian rhythm disorder and also helps quantify the sleep disturbance and its effect on the caregiver. Sleep laboratory evaluation may be required in some cases, particularly if sleep apnea, PLMD, or RBD are suspected.

The management of disturbed sleep in patients with degenerative disorders requires a determination of the severity of sleep disturbance and its probable causes, an assessment of the impact of disrupted sleep on the patient and family, and a consideration of the benefits and drawbacks associated with particular treatments. Although the underlying pathology usually cannot be halted or reversed, there may be elements contributing to disordered sleep that can be ameliorated or removed. Good sleep hygiene with a regular sleep-wake schedule, exposure to bright light in the morning, and minimal amounts of time spent in bed during the day are important first steps. Morning and evening naps should be avoided in most patients, but afternoon naps may help some patients obtain more total sleep. Caffeine and alcohol should be eliminated, and psychoactive medications should be minimized.

Sleep-related breathing disturbances should be treated to the greatest extent possible, particularly in patients with autonomic disturbances because they appear to be at high risk for death during sleep.[62] OSA may respond to treatment with nasal CPAP. Although the CPAP apparatus may be manageable initially, its use may become impossible as the degenerative disorder progresses, particularly if dementia is a prominent symptom. In most patients with advanced disease, the complications associated with tracheostomy outweigh its benefits.

Disruptive nocturnal behavior that is due to RBD usually responds to treatment with clonazepam in patients who can tolerate the medication, but it is a difficult symptom to manage when the condition is due to other causes. Benzodiazepines exacerbate nocturnal confusion and impair memory in the demented. Some patients benefit from low doses of thioridazine, butyrophenone, or sedating tricyclic antidepressants, but their anticholinergic properties may worsen cognitive disturbance.

Reviews and Selected Updates

Aldrich MS: Sleep disorders. Curr Opin Neurol Neurosurg 1992;5:240–246.

Benca RM: Consequences of insomnia and its therapies. J Clin Psychiatry 2001;62(Suppl 10):33–38.

Billiard M: Narcolepsy: Clinical features and aetiology. Ann Clin Res 1985;17:220–226.

Guilleminault C: Narcolepsy syndrome. *In* Kryger MH, Roth T, Dement WC (eds): Principles and Practice of Sleep Medicine. Philadelphia, WB Saunders, 1994, pp 549–561.

Krahn LE, Black JL, Silber MH: Narcolepsy: New understanding of irresistible sleep. Mayo Clin Proc 2001;76:185–194.

Rosen R, Zozula R: Education and training in the field of sleep medicine. Curr Opin Pulm Med 2000;6:512–518.

Wu H, Yan-Go F: Self-reported automobile accidents involving patients with obstructive sleep apnea. Neurology 1996;46:1254–1257.

References

1. ICSD—International Classification of Sleep Disorders: Diagnostic and Coding Manual. Diagnostic Classification Steering Committee, Thorpy MJ, Chairman. Rochester, Minnesota, American Sleep Disorders Association, 1990.
2. Spielman AJ, Nunes J, Glovinsky PB: Insomnia. Neurol Clin North America 1996;14:513–543.
3. Roberts RE, Shema SJ, Kaplan GA, Strawbridge WJ: Sleep complaints and depression in an aging cohort: A prospective perspective. Am J Psychiatry 2000;157:81–88.
4. Ford DE, Kamerow DB: Epidemiologic study of sleep disturbances and psychiatric disorders: An opportunity for prevention. JAMA 1989;262: 1479–1484.
5. Ford DE, Cooper-Patrick L: Sleep disturbances and mood disorders: An epidemiologic perspective. Depress Anxiety 2001;14:3–6.
6. Morin CM, Hauri PJ, Espie CA, Spielman AJ, Buysse DJ, Bootzin RR: Nonpharmacologic treatment of chronic insomnia. An American Academy of Sleep Medicine review. Sleep 1999;22:1134–1156.
7. Morin CM, Colecchi C, Stone J, Sood R, Brink D: Behavioral and pharmacological therapies for late-life insomnia: A randomized controlled trial. JAMA 1999;281:991–999.
8. Overeem S, Mignot E, Gert van Dijk J, Lammers GJ: Narcolepsy: Clinical features, new pathophysiologic insights, and future perspectives. J Clin Neurophysiol 2001;18:78–105.
9. Nishino S, Ripley B, Overeem S, Lammers GJ, Mignot E: Hypocretin (orexin) deficiency in human narcolepsy. Lancet 2000;355:39–40.
10. Thannickal TC, Moore RY, Nienhuis R, et al: Reduced number of hypocretin neurons in human narcolepsy. Neuron 2000;27: 469–474.
11. Peyron C, Faraco J, Rogers W, et al: A mutation in a case of early onset narcolepsy and a generalized absence of hypocretin peptides in human narcoleptic brains. Nat Med 2000;6:991–997.
12. Mignot E, Lin X, Arrigoni J, et al: DQB1*0602 and DQA1*0102 (DQ1) are better markers than DR2 for narcolepsy in Caucasian and black Americans. Sleep 1994;17(Suppl 8):S60–S67.
13. Guilleminault C, Mignot E, Grumet FC: Familial patterns of narcolepsy. Lancet 1989;2:1376–1379.
14. Aldrich MS, Hollingsworth Z, Penney JB: Dopamine receptor autoradiography of human narcoleptic brain. Neurology 1992;42:410–415.
15. Lin L, Faraco J, Li R, et al: The sleep disorder canine narcolepsy is caused by a mutation in the hypocretin (orexin) receptor 2 gene. Cell 1999;98:409–412.
16. Mignot E, Wang C, Rattazzi C, et al: Genetic linkage of autosomal recessive canine narcolepsy with a mu immunoglobulin heavy-chain switch-like segment. Proc Natl Acad Sci USA 1991;88:3475–3478.
17. Broughton R, Valley V, Aguirre M, et al: Excessive daytime sleepiness and the pathophysiology of narcolepsy-cataplexy: A laboratory perspective. Sleep 1986;9:205–215.
18. Hublin C, Kaprio J, Partinen M, et al: The prevalence of narcolepsy: An epidemiologic study of the Finnish twin cohort. Ann Neurol 1994;35:709–716.
19. Aldrich MS: The clinical spectrum of narcolepsy and idiopathic hypersomnia. Neurology 1996;46:393–401.
20. Carskadon MA, Dement WC, Mitler MM, et al: Guidelines for the multiple sleep latency test (MSLT): A standard measure of sleepiness. Sleep 1986;9:519–524.
21. Chervin RD, Aldrich MS: Sleep onset REM periods during multiple sleep latency tests in patients evaluated for sleep apnea. Am J Respir Crit Care Med 2000;161:426–431.
22. Moscovitch A, Partinen M, Guilleminault C: The positive diagnosis of narcolepsy and narcolepsy's borderland. Neurology 1993;43:55–60.

23. Mitler MM, Aldrich MS, Koob GF, Zarcone VP: ASDA standards of practice: Narcolepsy and its treatment with stimulants. Sleep 1994;17:352–371.
24. Roth B: Functional hypersomnia. *In* Guilleminault C, Dement WC, Passouant P (eds): Narcolepsy. New York, Spectrum, 1976, pp 333–349.
25. Guilleminault C, Stoohs R, Clerk A, et al: A cause of excessive daytime sleepiness. The upper airway resistance syndrome. Chest 1993;104:781–787.
26. Isono S, Remmers JE: Anatomy and physiology of upper airway obstruction. *In* Kryger MH, Roth T, Dement WC (eds): Principles and Practice of Sleep Medicine, 2nd ed. Philadelphia, WB Saunders, 1994, pp 642–656.
27. Dancey DR, Hanly PJ, Soong C, Lee B, Hoffstein V: Impact of menopause on the prevalence and severity of sleep apnea. Chest 2001;120:151–155.
28. Nieto FJ, Young TB, Lind BK, et al: Association of sleep-disordered breathing, sleep apnea, and hypertension in a large community-based study. Sleep Heart Health Study. JAMA 2000;283:1880–1881.
29. Ali NJ, Pitson DJ, Stradling JR: Snoring, sleep disturbance and behaviour in 4–5 year olds. Arch Dis Child 1993;68:360–366.
30. Young T, Palta M, Dempsey J, et al: The occurrence of sleep disordered breathing among middle-aged adults. N Engl J Med 1993;328:1230–1235.
31. Chervin RD, Murman DL, Malow BA, Totten V: Cost-utility of three approaches to the diagnosis of sleep apnea: Polysomnography, home testing, and empirical therapy. Ann Intern Med 1999;130:496–505.
32. Findley L, Unverzagt ME, Suratt PM: Automobile accidents involving patients with obstructive sleep apnea. Am Rev Respir Dis 1988;138:337–340.
33. Seppala T, Partinen M, Penttila A, et al: Sudden death and sleeping history among Finnish men. J Intern Med 1991;229:23–28.
34. He J, Kryger MH, Zorick FJ, et al: Mortality and apnea index in obstructive sleep apnea. Experience in 385 male patients. Chest 1988;94:9–14.
35. Partinen M, Guilleminault C: Daytime sleepiness and vascular morbidity at seven-year follow-up in obstructive sleep apnea patients. Chest 1990;97:27–32.
36. Koskenvuo M, Kaprio J, Telakivi T, et al: Snoring as a risk factor for ischemic heart disease and stroke in men. BMJ 1987;294:16–19.
37. Hung J, Whitford EG, Parsons RW, Hillman DR: Association of sleep apnoea with myocardial infarction in men. Lancet 1990;336:261–264.
38. Sullivan CE, Issa FG, Berthon-Jones M, Eves L: Reversal of obstructive sleep apnoea by continuous positive airway pressure applied through the nares. Lancet 1981;1:862–865.
39. Smith RC: Relationship of periodic movements in sleep (nocturnal myoclonus) and the Babinski sign. Sleep 1985;8:239–243.
40. Ancoli-Israel S, Kripke DF, Klauber MR, et al: Periodic limb movements in sleep in community-dwelling elderly. Sleep 1991;14:496–500.
41. Walters AS, Aldrich MS, Allen R, et al (The International Restless Legs Syndrome Study Group): Towards a better definition of the restless legs syndrome. Mov Disord 1995;10:634–642.
42. Brodeur C, Montplaisir J, Godbout R, Marinier R: Treatment of restless legs syndrome and periodic movements during sleep with L-dopa: A double-blind, controlled study. Neurology 1988;38:1845–1848.
43. Hening WA, Walters A, Kavey N, et al: Dyskinesias while awake and periodic movements in sleep in restless legs syndrome: Treatment with opioids. Neurology 1986;36:1363–1366.
44. Czeisler CA, Kronauer RE, Allan JS, et al: Bright light induction of strong (type 0) resetting of the human circadian pacemaker. Science 1989;244:1328–1333.
45. Aschoff J, Hoffman K, Pohl H, Wever R: Re-entrainment of circadian rhythms after phase shifts of the zeitgeber. Chronobiologia 1975;2:23–78.
46. Moore-Ede MC, Sulzman FM, Fuller CA: The Clocks That Time Us. Cambridge, MA, Harvard University Press, 1982.
47. Weitzman ED, Czeisler CA, Coleman RM, et al: Delayed sleep phase syndrome. A chronobiological disorder with sleep-onset insomnia. Arch Gen Psychiatry 1981;38:737–746.
48. King DP, Takahashi JS: Molecular genetics of circadian rhythms in mammals. Ann Rev Neurosci 2000;23:713–742.
49. Czeisler CA, Johnson MP, Duffy JF, et al: Exposure to bright light and darkness to treat physiologic maladaptation to night work. N Engl J Med 1990;322:1253–1259.
50. Czeisler CA, Shanahan TL, Klerman EB, et al: Suppression of melatonin secretion in some blind patients by exposure to bright light. N Engl J Med 1995;332:6–11.
51. Broughton RJ: Sleep disorders: Disorders of arousal? Science 1968;159:1070–1078.
52. Schenck CH, Hurwitz TD, Bundlie SR, Mahowald MW: Sleep-related eating disorders: Polysomnographic correlates of a heterogeneous syndrome distinct from daytime eating disorders. Sleep 1991;14:419–431.
53. Schenk CH, Bundlie SR, Patterson AL, Mahowald MW: Rapid eye movement sleep behavior disorder. JAMA 1987;257:1786–1789.
54. Aldrich MS, Jahnke B: Diagnostic value of video-EEG polysomnography. Neurology 1991;41:1060–1066.
55. Schenck CH, Milner DM, Hurwitz TD, et al: A polysomnographic and clinical report on sleep-related injury in 100 adult patients. Am J Psychiatry 1989;146:1166–1173.
56. Lugaresi E, Cirignotta F, Montagna P: Nocturnal paroxysmal dystonia. J Neurol Neurosurg Psychiatry 1986;49:375–380.
57. Meierkord H, Fish DR, Smith SJ, et al: Is nocturnal paroxysmal dystonia a form of frontal lobe epilepsy? Mov Disord 1992;7:38–42.
58. Bliwise DL: Sleep in normal aging and dementia. Sleep 1993;16:40–81.
59. Evans LK: Sundown syndrome in institutionalized elderly. J Am Geriatr Soc 1987;35:101–108.
60. Chokroverty S, Sachdeo R, Masdeu J: Autonomic dysfunction and sleep apnea in olivopontocerebellar degeneration. Arch Neurol 1984;41:926–931.
61. Guilleminault C, Briskin JG, Greenfield MS, Silvestri R: The impact of autonomic nervous system dysfunction on breathing during sleep. Sleep 1981;4:263–278.
62. Munschauer FE, Loh L, Bannister R, Newsom-Davis J: Abnormal respiration and sudden death during sleep in multiple system atrophy with autonomic failure. Neurology 1990;40:677–679.

CHAPTER 55

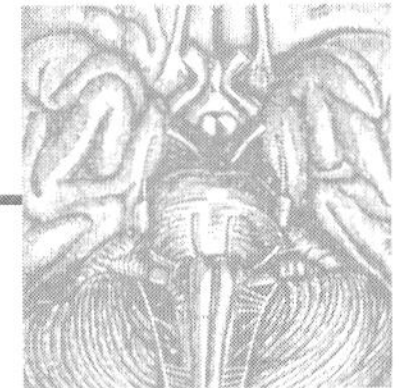

KATIE KOMPOLITI and STACY S. HORN

Drug-Induced and Iatrogenic Neurological Disorders

History and Definitions

Adverse reactions to prescription or over-the-counter medications are a frequent cause of neurological morbidity and patient hospitalization. Therefore, it is essential that the

TABLE 55–1. **Selected Neuroleptics**

Nonproprietary/Trade Name	Sedative Effects	Extrapyramidal Effects	Hypotensive Effects
Phenothiazines			
Chlorpromazine hydrochloride (Thorazine)	+++	++	+++
Mesoridazine besylate (Serentil)	+++	+	++
Thioridazine hydrochloride (Mellaril)	+++	+	+++
Fluphenazine hydrochloride (Prolixin)	+	+++	+
Perphenazine (Trilafon)	++	++	+
Trifluoperazine hydrochloride (Stelazine, Suprazine)	+	+++	+
Thioxanthenes			
Thiothixene hydrochloride (Navane)	++	+++	++
Other Heterocyclic Compounds			
Haloperidol (Haldol)	+	+++	+
Loxapine succinate (Loxitane)	+	++	+
Molindone hydrochloride (Moban)	++	++	+
Pimozide (Orap)	+	+++	+
Atypical Neuroleptics			
Clozapine (Clozaril)	+++	0	+++
Quetiapine (Seroquel)	+++	+	+++
Olanzapine (Zyprexa)	+++	++	+++
Risperidone (Risperdal)	+++	++	+++

+, Rare; ++, moderately common; +++, very common.

possibility of an iatrogenic condition be considered in any patient presenting with acute, subacute, or chronic neurological symptoms. Identification of the responsible agent is simple when neurological symptoms are highly characteristic of the offending agent. However, in most cases, symptoms of intoxication are nonspecific and mimic neurological entities, or they exacerbate pre-existing neurological disease. Some effects relate directly to neurotoxicity, and others are secondary to damage of other organ systems such as renal or hepatic.

The nervous system may be adversely affected by several mechanisms. There may be interference with energy production necessary to maintain normal neural structure and function; exposure to foreign material may result in allergic or other immunological phenomena; drugs may affect the nervous system through their effects on neurotransmitters; the offending agent may interfere with nerve nutrition through involvement of the nutrient vessels; and alterations in acid-base balance or in ionic concentrations may occur. Advances in molecular biology research techniques are being applied to understanding the biochemical foundations of toxic reactions and to identifying subjects at risk of intoxication.

Tranquilizers, Antidepressants, and Anxiolytics

NEUROLEPTICS

The neuroleptic agents or major tranquilizers (Table 55–1) exert their antipsychotic activity by blocking dopaminergic receptors at the level of the limbic system, forebrain, and basal ganglia. They also have antihistaminergic, anticholinergic, and anti–alpha$_1$ adrenergic properties. The newer so-called atypical agents include clozapine, olanzepine, quetiapine, and risperidone. Many newer agents have some affinity for 5-HT$_2$ serotonin receptors as well (clozapine, risperidone). The atypical neuroleptics have become favored due to their lower side effect profile. Many newer agents have some affinity for 5-HT$_2$ serotonin receptors as well (clozapine, risperidone). Neuroleptics, as a class, are associated with a variety of important neurological complications. These can be classified as acute, subacute, and chronic side effects (Table 55–2).

Encephalopathy

Neuroleptics may cause a toxic confusional state, especially in the elderly, and confusion occurs more frequently with the low-potency, high-anticholinergic activity subclass (chlorpromazine, thioridazine, mesoridazine). These drugs

TABLE 55–2. **Neuroleptic Neurotoxicity**

- Acute
  - Akathisia
  - Dystonia
  - Encephalopathy
  - Lowering of seizure threshold
  - Neuroleptic malignant syndrome*
- Subacute
  - Neuroleptic malignant syndrome*
  - Parkinsonism
- Tardive
  - Akathisia
  - Chorea (classical tardive dyskinesia)
  - Dystonia
  - Myoclonus
  - Tics

*Neuroleptic malignant syndrome can occur as an acute, subacute. or chronic side effect of neuroleptics.

can also produce profound sedation, especially with initiation of therapy.[1]

Seizures

Neuroleptics also lower the seizure threshold and have been associated with exacerbation of pre-existing epilepsy as well as the de novo appearance of seizures. Clozapine use has been associated with generalized and myoclonic seizures that may develop during the titration phase at low dosages (<300 mg/d) and at high dosages during maintenance therapy (>600 mg/d).[2]

Neuroleptic Malignant Syndrome

The pathogenesis of neuroleptic malignant syndrome (NMS) is not completely understood. Alterations in dopaminergic transmission, changes in sympathetic outflow, alterations in central serotonin metabolism, and abnormalities in muscle membrane function have been implicated. NMS has been associated with all groups of neuroleptics, although high-potency agents, specifically haloperidol and fluphenazine, have been most frequently cited. Neuroleptic malignant syndrome has been described with the atypical neuroleptic medications clozapine, risperidone, and olanzapine.[3–5]

Neuroleptic malignant syndrome tends to occur with the initiation of treatment or increases in dose and is more common with depot forms of neuroleptics. Affective disorder, concomitant lithium carbonate administration, psychomotor agitation, dehydration, exhaustion, and mild hyperthermia seem to increase susceptibility toward this condition.[6]

The principal features of NMS are hyperthermia, muscle rigidity, autonomic dysfunction, and mental status changes. Laboratory findings include elevated creatine kinase (CK), polymorphonuclear leukocytosis, elevated aldolase, alkaline phosphatase, lactic dehydrogenase, alanine aminotransferase and aspartate aminotransferase, hypocalcemia, hypomagnesemia, low iron, proteinuria, and myoglobinuria.[6] Approximately 40 percent of patients with NMS develop medical complications that may be life threatening. NMS is a clinical diagnosis based on the presence of the proper historical setting and the characteristic constellation of signs. Disorders with similar features include malignant hyperthermia, heat stroke induced by neuroleptics, lethal catatonia, other drug reactions, and vascular, infectious, or postinfectious brain damage.

Neuroleptic malignant syndrome is a potentially fatal disease, and a high index of suspicion is required for early recognition and intervention. Treatment includes discontinuing the offending agent, providing supportive measures, and administering dantrolene or bromocriptine or a combination of the two.

Acute Dystonia

Acute neuroleptic-induced dystonia can be seen early in the course of neuroleptic therapy or with dosage increases. It is often seen following a single parenteral dose of neuroleptics. The manifestations can be diverse, although the most typical clinical signs involve oculogyric crises and opisthotonic posturing. Risk factors include young age, male gender, and use of high-potency neuroleptics.[7] Acute dystonic reactions are self-limited and, if left untreated, usually subside within 24 hours. Parenteral administration of anticholinergics, such as benztropine or diphenhydramine, offers immediate relief in the majority of cases, but oral anticholinergics should be continued for a few days until the causative neuroleptic is cleared.

Acute Akathisia

Akathisia is a severe form of restlessness associated with the need to move. Typically the patient paces incessantly in place and cannot sit down without continual volitional movement of the legs or feet. The pathophysiology of the syndrome is not well understood but may relate to the development of acute imbalance between the dopaminergic and cholinergic systems. This neuroleptic side effect usually occurs within the first days of therapy or with dosage increases, and it resolves with withdrawal of the neuroleptic agent. Anticholinergics, amantadine, beta-blockers, clonidine, and benzodiazepines have also been used with variable success.[1, 6] Late-onset akathisia may be a form of tardive dyskinesia (TD; see later) and may be more difficult to treat.

Parkinsonism

Neuroleptic-induced parkinsonism is the result of striatal dopaminergic underactivity due to dopaminergic D_2 receptor blockade. Clinically, it cannot be distinguished from idiopathic Parkinson's disease, although its development occurs as a subacute syndrome within the first weeks of drug introduction or dosage increase. Parkinsonian symptoms resolve over a few weeks to 6 months after stopping the causative agent or with the use of antiparkinsonian drugs. Proposed risk factors for development of neuroleptic-induced parkinsonism are female gender, older age, and the use of high-potency agents.[1, 7] Treatment consists of discontinuing or reducing the dosage of the offending agent. A lower-potency neuroleptic or one of several novel neuroleptics that lack prominent striatal receptor blockade, such as clozapine, can be substituted. Anticholinergics, amantadine, and electroconvulsive therapy are also possible treatments.

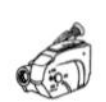

Tardive Dyskinesia

Tardive dyskinesia usually appears after several months or years of treatment with antipsychotic medications and almost never before 3 months. No consistent neuropathological changes have been seen in patients with TD, and the predominant hypothesis for its genesis is denervation supersensitivity of the striatal dopamine receptors following chronic blockade.[6] Risk factors for the development of TD include old age, female gender, presence of affective disorders, history of neuroleptic-induced parkinsonism, presence of organic brain disease, high-potency neuroleptics, sufficient duration of treatment with neuroleptics, and possibly the use of anticholinergic medications, previous electroconvulsive treatment, and drug holidays.

In addition to the well-known oral-buccal-lingual masticatory movements and generalized chorea, dystonia, akathisia, tics, and myoclonus have been described. Once TD has appeared, its peak severity is reached rapidly and is often maintained. Following neuroleptic withdrawal, TD may transiently worsen, but this exacerbation is short lived. TD resolves in up to 33 percent of patients within 2 years after discontinuation of the offending agent.[8] A recent prospective study comparing risperidone and haloperidol in 350 patients who had not been exposed to neuroleptics before showed that each drug had a similar incidence of dystonia, parkinsonism, akithisia, and dyskinesia.[9]

At present, prevention is the treatment of choice for TD. Therefore, neuroleptics should be used only when specifically needed and at the lowest possible doses. Once TD develops, the causative agent should be discontinued, if possible. Alternatively, the patient should be switched to an atypical neuroleptic like clozapine, which not only does not regularly cause TD but may even improve its symptoms.[6] If neurological impairment, disfigurement, or discomfort exists, treatment with the dopamine depleters reserpine or tetrabenazine should be considered. Noradrenergic antagonists (propranolol, clonidine), gamma-aminobutyric acid (GABA) agonists (clonazepam, diazepam, valproate, baclofen), botulinum toxin injections, and, to a lesser degree, vitamin E, buspirone, and calcium channel blockers have been used with variable success.[1, 6]

ANTIDEPRESSANTS

Tricyclic Antidepressants

Tricyclic antidepressants (TCAs) act by blocking primarily norepinephrine or serotonin reuptake and also affect the cholinergic and histaminergic systems (Table 55–3). They have a narrow therapeutic index and can be associated with significant central nervous system (CNS) toxicity. Risk factors for CNS toxicity include plasma level, type of TCA, and concomitant administration of other psychotropic drugs.[10]

Sedation is a very common side effect of TCAs and is most prominent when drug therapy is initiated or when the dosage is increased. Sleep in TCA-treated patients is associated with a decrease in rapid-eye-movement (REM) sleep and may result in a hangover.[11] Confusional states and delirium occur particularly in the elderly or in those treated with high doses, concomitant administration of neuroleptics, or antiparkinsonian medications. Confusion also occurs especially with the use of TCAs with high anticholinergic activity (amitriptyline, imipramine).[11, 12] Anticholinergic effects of TCAs are also responsible for memory impairment, especially in the elderly. TCAs can exacerbate the naturally occurring tendency for depressed patients to become manic and are responsible for a rare but unusual difficulty in articulation that resembles stammer and has been called speech blockade.[10]

Tricyclic antidepressants lower the seizure threshold and may be associated with an increased risk of seizures in individuals who have a history of epilepsy or who are predisposed to have seizures. For imipramine, the most frequently studied TCA, the literature indicates a seizure rate of between 0.3 and 0.6 percent at effective doses. In general, seizures are observed after long-term treatment with high doses of TCAs or after a rapid increase in dose.[10]

A high-frequency postural and kinetic tremor may be present in as many as 10 percent of patients treated with imipramine. Myoclonus, akathisia, and choreoathetoid movements are additional rare side effects seen with TCAs.[1, 10]

Tricyclic antidepressants are a serious cause of drug-related death in the United States. The signs and symptoms of TCA overdose are cardiovascular instability, CNS depression, and anticholinergic toxicity. TCA-induced drowsiness and coma can be reversed by the cholinergic agonist physostigmine.[11]

Selective Serotonin Reuptake Inhibitors

The selective serotonin reuptake inhibitors (SSRIs) are potent and selective inhibitors of serotonin reuptake at the presynaptic terminal. They are considered first-line therapy for depression because of their prescribing ease and superior side effect and safety profile. SSRI-induced side effects are usually transient and rarely result in discontinuation of the medication. In addition, they appear to be safer than TCAs when an overdose occurs.

The major side effects of the SSRIs referring to the CNS include nausea, headache, dry mouth, insomnia and somnolence, agitation, nervousness, sweating, dizziness, tremor, and sexual dysfunction.[13] Fluoxetine is often associated with anxiety, nervousness, insomnia, and anorexia. Paroxetine, fluvoxamine, and nefazodone are associated with sedation. Sexual dysfunction manifests itself as ejaculatory delay in men and anorgasmia in women. There have been reports suggesting that fluoxetine can induce or exacerbate suicidal tendencies, and several mechanisms have been proposed. However, because suicide is an important feature of depression, it is difficult to draw conclusions, whereas on the other

TABLE 55–3. **Action of Tricyclic Antidepressants**

Drug	Anticholinergic Action	Serotonin Reuptake Inhibition	Norepinephrine Reuptake Inhibition
Imipramine	+ +	+	+ +
Desipramine	+	+ / –	+ + +
Amitriptyline	+ + +	+ +	+ +
Nortriptyline	+	+	+ +
Protriptyline	+ + +	+ / –	+ + +
Trimipramine	+ +	+ / –	+
Doxepin	+ +	+	+
Clomipramine	+ +	+ + +	+

+ + +, Significant; + +, moderate; +, low, +/–, inconsistent.

hand, it is difficult to exclude the possibility that suicidal ideation occurs as a rare adverse reaction with some drugs.[12]

SSRIs have been shown to inhibit the cytochrome P-450 system both in vitro and in vivo and, therefore, to result in increased levels of drugs that are substrates of cytochrome P-450 as well (i.e., TCAs). There has been debate over whether the combination of SSRIs and monoamine oxidase inhibitors (MAOIs) or TCAs can lead to the serotonin syndrome, characterized by hyperpyrexia, myoclonus, rigidity, hyper-reflexia, shivering, confusion, agitation, restlessness, coma, autonomic instability, low-grade fever, nausea, diarrhea, diaphoresis, flushing, and, rarely, rhabdomyolysis and death.[13, 14] This occurrence is probably uncommon but should be watched for and immediately handled with supportive care and drug withdrawal if it occurs. Several case reports in the literature suggest that SSRIs can produce extrapyramidal symptoms in the form of akathisia, dyskinesia, acute dystonia, and deterioration in Parkinson's disease, but controlled clinical studies are needed to determine the validity of these observations.

Monoamine Oxidase Inhibitors

Monoamine oxidase is an intramitochondrial enzyme responsible for the breakdown of intracellular dopamine, norepinephrine, and serotonin. MAOIs inhibit monoamine oxidase, resulting in an increase in the concentration of monoamines in the synapse. Therefore, when patients taking MAOIs ingest vasoactive amines in foods and beverages (e.g., cheese, chocolate, pickled herring, chicken livers, caviar, broad beans, wine, beer), or take certain medications (e.g., amphetamines, ephedrine, reserpine, L-dopa, tryptophan), the vasoactive amines are not catabolized but enter the bloodstream and are taken up by the nerve terminals (Table 55–4). The result is a cataclysmic syndrome consisting of sudden severe headache, stiff neck, profuse sweating, mydriasis, neuromuscular irritability, extreme hypertension, and cardiac arrhythmias. The most effective treatment is phentolamine, or sodium nitroprusside, and for less severe cases, chlorpromazine.[1, 10, 12, 13] When MAOIs are taken in combination with TCAs in high doses or in overdose, or when MAOIs are taken with the narcotic analgesic meperidine, a severe condition of hyperpyrexia can occur.[13]

TABLE 55–4. Potential Interactions with MAOIs

Drug-Food Interactions
Cheese
Smoked fish, pickled fish, caviar
Prepared or nonfresh meat, fermented and dry sausage
Chianti, vermouth, beer
Broad pea pods
Ripe banana pulp and banana peel
Yeast extract and brewer's yeast
Hydrolyzed protein extracts (used as a base for soup, gravy, and sauces)
Sauerkraut
Drug-Drug Interactions
Sympathomimetics
L-Dopa
Meperidine
Hypoglycemics
Tricyclic antidepressants
L-Tryptophan
Selective serotonin reuptake inhibitors
Reserpine

MAOIs, Monoamine oxidase inhibitors.

The MAOIs cause odd mixtures of sedation and stimulation. All three available drugs—tranylcypromine, phenelzine, and isocarboxazid—can cause insomnia, daytime sedation, aberrant changes in the sleep-wake cycle, and suppression of rapid-eye-movement sleep. In some patients, tranylcypromine can have amphetamine-like effects such as tremor and heightened locomotion activity about 1 hour after each dose, but it also causes sedation. This and other drugs in the group can produce mild euphoria as a prolonged effect.[12] Other side effects include myoclonic jerks, paresthesias of the extremities, and sexual dysfunction.

Lithium Carbonate

Lithium carbonate is indicated for the treatment of mania and for maintenance therapy in patients with a history of bipolar disorder. The majority of patients suffer side effects at therapeutic doses, although most patients classify them as mild. A fine postural or intentional tremor occurs in up to 80 percent of patients on lithium therapy. This side effect may resolve spontaneously, respond to a decrease in dose, or be treated with beta-adrenergic blockers.[15] Case reports have described choreiform movements or parkinsonism associated with lithium treatment.

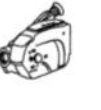

Poor memory, loss of concentration, fatigue, muscle weakness, slowed reaction time, and lack of spontaneity are common during the course of treatment. These side effects cannot be consistently related to drug serum levels, duration of treatment, dose, age, or other variables. A toxic confusional state may occur in the absence of signs of toxicity and at relatively low serum lithium levels. This is characterized by disorientation, confusion, lack of continuity of thought, memory loss, lability of mood, and reduced comprehension. The symptoms are preceded by a steady or precipitous rise in oral lithium dose, often within the first weeks of treatment, but may occur at serum lithium levels as low as 1.0 mEq/L. The condition usually remits within a few days following reduction or withdrawal of the dose.[1]

Lithium intoxication manifests itself with nausea, vomiting, diarrhea, tremor, drowsiness, ataxia, muscle twitching, and slurred speech. As intoxication advances, ataxia, alteration of the level of consciousness, and, eventually, seizures and coma occur. Until recently, it was thought that patients who survived severe lithium intoxication suffered no permanent neurological damage. However, reports indicate that the basal ganglia and the cerebellum can be permanently damaged following lithium intoxication.[1]

Finally, lithium has been associated with syndromes similar to myasthenia gravis, NMS, lowering of the seizure threshold, pseudotumor cerebri, headaches, polyneuropathy, and downbeating nystagmus. A case report with neuropathological evaluation of a patient who expired due to lithium toxicity showed severe cerebellar atrophy of the internal granule and Purkinje cell layers with attendant Bergmann gliosis.[16]

Benzodiazepines

Benzodiazepines potentiate GABA action in the nervous system and act on the spinal cord as well as in many areas within the brain, including the cerebellum, the limbic system, and the cerebral cortex. Although the therapeutic index of benzodiazepines is 10 to 30 times that of the barbiturates and hence their absolute toxicity is less, adverse reactions are 7 times more frequent with benzodiazepines.[1] This statistic apparently relates to the vast number of patients consuming these agents.

The most frequent toxic symptoms are increased drowsiness or paradoxical excitation. After large doses, exacerbation of depression and antisocial behavior have been reported. Withdrawal seizures can occur as well. Encompassing the range from subtle cognitive impairments to frank delirium, toxicity due to benzodiazepines is associated with impairment of immediate and delayed memory, psychomotor performance, and rebound insomnia.

Physiological dependence on benzodiazepines is accompanied by a withdrawal syndrome that is typically characterized by sleep disturbance, irritability, increased tension and anxiety, panic attacks, hand tremor, sweating, difficulty in concentration, nausea, weight loss, palpitations, headache, muscular pain, and stiffness. Factors that contribute to the development of withdrawal symptoms are primarily dose, duration, concurrent medication, and pharmacokinetics of individual drugs. The shorter-acting drugs can produce a more intense withdrawal syndrome following chronic administration.[17] No specific treatment exists for the withdrawal syndrome, which commonly lasts for up to 6 weeks, although tapering the benzodiazepine dose, sedative antidepressants, or the substitution of a longer-acting benzodiazepine may help.

Even short-term benzodiazepine use can lead to the development of tolerance, necessitating larger doses of drug to be administered.

Anesthetics

INHALATIONAL GENERAL ANESTHETICS

Halothane, Enflurane, Isoflurane, and Sevoflurane

Halothane, a halogenated hydrocarbon, was first synthesized in 1951. It was introduced into clinical practice in 1956 in the United Kingdom and in 1958 in the United States. It quickly replaced the other volatile agents because it was nonflammable, easy to administer, and relatively safe. Halothane, enflurane, isoflurane, and sevoflurane depress cerebral metabolism, with isoflurane having the greatest effect.[18] Electrical activity of the cerebral cortex recorded by a fronto-occipital electroencephalogram (EEG) shows progressive replacement of fast, low-voltage activity by slow, high-amplitude waves as anesthesia gets deeper.[19] Since cerebral blood flow generally increases during halothane anesthesia, cerebrospinal fluid (CSF) pressure increases. After several hours of anesthesia with halothane, the changes in cerebral blood flow and metabolism return to normal. Recovery of mental function after anesthesia with halothane is not complete for several hours.[19]

Tonic-clonic activity and spike and wave EEG complexes have been reported with enflurane anesthesia. Deepening anesthesia and hyperventilation may exacerbate these phenomena. This excitatory action of enflurane does not appear to be associated with aggravation of seizures in epileptic patients; nevertheless, enflurane is best avoided in such patients.[18, 19]

Rarely, the induction of anesthesia with halothane or any of the other halogenated inhalational anesthetics triggers an uncontrolled hypermetabolic reaction in the skeletal muscle of susceptible patients. There is defective uptake of Ca^{2+} by the sarcoplasmic reticulum, resulting in elevation of intracellular free Ca^{2+} levels. The resultant syndrome of malignant hyperthermia has an incidence of 1 in 12,000 and a mortality rate of 24 percent.[18] It is more common in men and children, in association with various myopathies, and in genetically susceptible individuals. Mutations in the gene encoding the skeletal muscle ryanodine receptor (*RYR1*) are considered a common cause of the disorder, and to date, more than 20 *RYR1* mutations have been reported in European and Canadian families.[20] Malignant hyperthermia is produced most often by halothane, which is more common than enflurane, which, in turn, is more common than isoflurane. The concomitant use of suxamethonium and gallamine, neuroleptics, infection, stress, heat, and alcohol tend to increase the risk of malignant hyperthermia. Larach and colleagues demonstrated that generalized muscle rigidity that occurs as a result of an anesthetic is a valuable, but not absolute, predictor of a patient's susceptibility to malignant hyperthermia, its presence being associated with an eighteenfold increase in risk of being susceptible, as determined by subsequent muscle biopsy testing.[21]

Clinically, there is a rapid rise in body temperature, generalized muscular rigidity, high metabolic rate with increased oxygen consumption and carbon dioxide production, tachycardia, tachyarrythmias, metabolic acidosis, and hyperkalemia. The most reliable method of diagnosis is by muscle biopsy and in vitro contracture tests with halothane and caffeine.[19] Treatment consists of cessation of known triggering agents, supportive measures, and the administration of dantrolene.

Nitrous Oxide

Nitrous oxide (N_2O), or so-called laughing gas, was first used as a dental anesthetic. When used by itself, it produces a light level of anesthesia; when used to supplement more potent anesthetics, it reduces the dose requirements for those agents. However, its euphorogenic properties, ready availability, and low cost have contributed to its popularity as a recreational gas. Human nitrous oxide toxicity is associated with its occupational, iatrogenic, and recreational use.

Nitrous oxide toxicity is due to inactivation of methionine synthase, a vitamin B_{12}–dependent enzyme, resulting in defective biosynthesis of DNA and myelin in nervous tissue. Monkeys exposed to 15 percent nitrous oxide develop the biochemical changes and neurological signs of vitamin B_{12} deficiency very rapidly. Morphologically, their spinal cords show degeneration of both the myelin sheaths and axis cylinders in the posterior columns and in the lateral and anterior corticospinal and spinocerebellar tracts.[22]

Nitrous oxide is more likely to produce megaloblastosis or subacute combined degeneration-like clinical presentation when it is used repetitively or for periods longer than 3 hours or in individuals with vitamin B_{12} deficiency. Occupational exposure of medical and dental personnel during its use as an analgesic is not likely to produce adverse neurological effects except in vitamin B_{12}–deficient individuals or in those routinely exposed to high nitrous oxide levels.[23] An epidemiological survey of over 30,000 dental personnel occupationally exposed to nitrous oxide found an incidence of neurological complaints of less than 2 percent in the population at risk.[22] In the elderly, in whom subclinical vitamin B_{12} deficiency reportedly ranges from 7.3 to 21 percent, the frequency of neuropathic symptoms after anesthesia due to nitrous oxide may be under-recognized.[24]

Clinically, nitrous oxide neuropathy presents with numbness, paresthesias, ataxia, and clumsiness in the extremities. Many but not all of the symptoms resolve with time if exposure is discontinued. With further exposure, weakness, gait disturbance, impotence, and loss of sphincter control can occur.[22] Administration of folinic acid or methionine have been shown to protect against megaloblastosis and neurotoxicity occurring following nitrous oxide administration.[23]

Tension pneumoencephalus can follow any intracranial neurosurgical procedure if nitrous oxide has been used. Following dural closure, the increase in volume due to nitrous oxide can result in pressure changes that may lead to seizures, brain stem herniation, and death. Discontinuing nitrous oxide at the time of dural closure can prevent tension pneumoencephalus. Nitrous oxide can expand air emboli in the bloodstream. In patients undergoing posterior fossae exploration in the sitting position, nitrous oxide increases the risk of air emboli and should be avoided.[22]

LOCAL ANESTHETICS

When applied locally, local anesthetics reversibly block the action potentials responsible for nerve conduction. The most commonly used local anesthetics are cocaine, lidocaine, bupivacaine, chloroprocaine, etidocaine, mepivacaine, prilocaine, ropivacaine, procaine, and tetracaine. Local anesthetics entering the systemic circulation produce adverse effects primarily on the CNS. Usually, when they are administered locally, they cannot reach sufficient systemic concentrations to interfere with the function of organs where conduction or transmission of impulses occurs.[25] Nevertheless, when systemic absorption occurs after topical use of local anesthetics, as is the case in children when tetracaine, adrenaline, and cocaine is applied to mucous membranes, CNS toxicity has been described.[26, 27]

The first sign of systemic toxicity following administration of local anesthetics is drowsiness, followed by tremor, restlessness, convulsions, and, ultimately, CNS depression with respiratory failure.[28] Lidocaine and cocaine can produce changes in mood and behavior. Finally, local anesthetics can affect neuromuscular transmission. This effect is due to blockade of the ion channel of the acetylcholine receptor.[25]

EPIDURAL AND SPINAL ANESTHESIA

Epidural anesthesia is administered by injecting local anesthetic into the epidural space and can be performed in the sacral hiatus or in the lumbar, thoracic, or cervical regions of the spine. Spinal anesthesia follows the injection of local anesthetic into the CSF in the lumbar space. Significant differences between epidural and spinal anesthesia are that the dose of local anesthetic used in epidural anesthesia can produce high concentrations in blood following absorption from the epidural space and that there is no zone of differential sympathetic blockade with epidural anesthesia; thus the level of sympathetic block is close to the level of sensory block.[25]

Probable causes of neurological complications following epidural and spinal anesthesia include trauma, the nature of the injected material, infection, vascular lesions, or pre-existing pathology. The incidence of transient paralysis following epidural anesthesia is 0.1 percent, and the incidence of permanent paralysis is 0.02 percent.[29] Neurological sequelae after spinal anesthesia are rare as well. Neurological complications of spinal or epidural anesthesia tend to be more severe in the presence of spinal stenosis.

During the administration of epidural anesthesia, damage to a single nerve can occur and is the most frequent complication. Paresthesia, with or without motor weakness, is the presenting symptom, and the majority of patients recover completely. Paraplegia, resulting from myelopathy or cauda equina syndrome, can occur secondary to epidural hematoma or abscess, adhesive arachnoiditis, or anterior spinal artery occlusion. An epidural hematoma or abscess should be suspected if severe backache appears in combination with weakness and hypoalgesia of the lower extremities. Signs and symptoms of extradural abscess may be delayed for several days until the abscess has developed. Adhesive arachnoiditis may result from inadvertent subarachnoid administration of toxic chemicals or chemical contamination of anesthetic solutions. Chemical contaminants such as detergents or antiseptics act as irritants and induce a meningeal reaction that may progress to constrictive adhesive arachnoiditis. Clinically, gradual progressive weakness and sensory loss of the lower extremities occurs beginning several weeks to months after the procedure. Precontrast and postcontrast magnetic resonance imaging (MRI) scans are usually sufficient to diagnose arachnoiditis. Spinal cord infarction is usually associated with prolonged arterial hypotension and can occur whether or not epinephrine was added to the local anesthetic.[29–31] Finally, dural puncture may cause severe and prolonged headache because of leakage of CSF into the extradural space. The incidence of dural puncture is about 1 percent.[30] Fortunately, most patients never develop a spinal headache or the problem resolves spontaneously in a few days. The use of an extradural injection of autologous blood (a so-called blood patch) is usually effective in treating spinal headaches.

The neurological syndromes that appear after spinal anesthesia are similar to the ones described following epidural anesthesia. The most benign is aseptic meningitis, characterized by high fever, headache, nuchal rigidity, and photophobia. Symptoms usually appear within 24 hours of spinal anesthesia, and recovery occurs spontaneously within several days to a week.[29] Cauda equina syndrome is characterized by urinary and fecal incontinence, localized sensory loss in the perineal area, and varying degrees of leg weakness. These symptoms are evident after the effect of anesthesia has worn off and may be permanent or may show gradual regression over weeks or months. Single nerve injury, lumbosacral polyradiculopathy, adhesive arachnoiditis, spinal cord ischemia, and postural headache can occur under circumstances similar to the ones described for epidural anesthesia.

Spinal anesthesia is sometimes regarded as contraindicated in patients with pre-existing disease of the spinal cord. Although there is no experimental evidence to support this hypothesis, it is prudent to avoid spinal anesthesia in patients with progressive diseases of the spinal cord.[25]

Drugs Used to Treat Myasthenia Gravis

CHOLINESTERASE INHIBITORS

Cholinesterase inhibitors interfere with the hydrolysis of acetylcholine at the cholinergic synapses. Peripherally active agents have been the mainstay of myasthenic treatment until the advent of immunosuppressive therapy in the 1960s. Pyridostigmine bromide and neostigmine bromide are the most commonly used cholinesterase inhibitors. Pyridostigmine bromide is preferred because it has fewer gastrointestinal side effects and a longer duration of action.

Side effects of cholinesterase inhibitors result from overstimulation of the cholinergic system at the level of the muscarinic receptors of the smooth muscle, the nicotinic receptors of the skeletal muscle, the autonomic glands, and the CNS. Signs of cholinergic excess include nausea, abdominal cramps, excessive secretions, and bronchospasm. This syndrome is distinct from myasthenia gravis and is usually diagnosed accurately. However, because overstimulation can lead to subsequent depolarization blockade and enhanced weakness, exacerbation of myasthenia and cholinergic crisis can be dangerously confused. In situations in which there is a question of too much or too little cholinesterase inhibition, edrophonium (Tensilon) given in 1-mg increments may be helpful. More likely, however, admission to an intensive care unit (ICU) for transient cessation of cholinesterase inhibition is needed to elucidate whether the dose should be raised or lowered.

It has been suggested that chronic administration of cholinesterase inhibitors may damage the neuromuscular junction. This concern is based in part on the chronic effects on the neuromuscular junction known to occur in animals after large doses of prostigmine and reported decrease in improvement after thymectomy when the use of cholinesterase inhibitors increased. Nevertheless, the latter was a retrospective review, and therefore, there is no evidence that would discourage the use of cholinesterase inhibitors to treat myasthenia gravis when needed.[32]

GLUCOCORTICOSTEROIDS

Neurological side effects of glucocorticosteroids are well described and may be as serious as the diseases being treated. Neuropsychiatric disorders and myopathy are common. Most of the neurological sequelae are often related to dosage and duration of therapy and may be reversible by modification of the drug regimen.[33] Glucocorticosteroid use can be associated with a broad spectrum of neuropsychiatric disorders, ranging from emotional lability and anxiety to confusion, mood disorders, and psychosis. Behavioral symptoms usually begin within 5 to 14 days of starting steroids, but they may also occur during withdrawal of therapy. With the exception of multiple sclerosis, pre-existing neurological disease does not appear to increase the risk of steroid-induced mental status abnormalities. Alternate-day steroid therapy may decrease the overall incidence of behavioral changes, although it may rarely induce a cyclic behavior, with mania occurring on high-dose days and depression occurring on low-dose days.

Steroid myopathy is probably the most common drug-related disorder of muscle. There are two forms of myopathy: a common, well-known, chronic form involving type II fiber atrophy and a rare acute form that occurs during treatment for status asthmaticus and may be associated with rhabdomyolysis. The exact incidence of the more typical chronic myopathy is uncertain, but in one series of patients with rheumatic disease, it was reported to be 7 percent.[33] The syndrome consists of insidious onset of painless, symmetrical proximal muscle weakness and atrophy, with the lower extremities involved first. Bulbar muscles are spared, but the diaphragm may be involved. The time of onset is variable, and the symptoms may begin from several weeks to several months after beginning treatment. The serum CK is normal and electromyography (EMG) reveals short-duration, low-amplitude motor unit action potentials. Muscle biopsy shows type II atrophy, and electron microscopy reveals glycogen accumulation and enlarged mitochondria. Treatment consists of tapering and discontinuing the offending agent or substituting another steroid. The uncommon acute myopathy has been reported mainly in asthmatic patients who are receiving IV steroids, paralytic agents, and mechanical ventilation. The pathogenesis is unclear.[33]

Steroid-induced deposition of fat in the epidural space occurs in patients taking more than 40 mg of prednisone for at least 4 months. Most of these patients are already cushingoid when consequent neurological symptoms occur. The earliest and most common feature is low back pain, and depending on the level of the lipomatosis, signs of myelopathy, cauda equina syndrome, or radiculopathy may develop. MRI can be a very useful diagnostic tool. Fat appears to be hyperintense on T1-weighted images and less intense on T2-weighted images, in contrast with inflammatory processes, which are brighter on T2-weighted images. Unless it is contraindicated, laminectomy has been the treatment of choice. Further studies are needed to clarify the response to steroid tapering without surgical decompression before the onset of significant myelopathy. There have been isolated reports of corticosteroid-induced lipomatosis in the perineural spaces of peripheral nerves, leading to entrapment neuropathies.[33]

Increased intracranial pressure (ICP) has been associated with steroid use, and the vast majority of cases involve male children. No particular dose has been implicated, but the duration of treatment is usually prolonged. Symptom onset generally occurs after discontinuation, tapering, or change in the type of steroid. Signs and symptoms are consistent with elevated ICP: headache, nausea, vomiting, papilledema, and diplopia with abducens nerve palsy. The disorder is usually self-limited. Patients have improved after changing the type or dose of steroids (using lower or higher dose) or lumbar puncture.[33]

Glucocorticosteroids have been reported to enhance physiological tremor. Propranolol can be useful in controlling this movement disorder if steroid withdrawal is not possible. Intrathecal administration of glucocorticosteroids can be associated with sterile meningitis, arachnoiditis, and pachymeningitis. Epidural steroids can have the same complications because the epidural and subarachnoid spaces are not totally separate but communicate via arachnoid villi and epidural veins. Additionally, inadvertent subarachnoid injections occur during about 2.5 percent of epidural attempts.[33]

AZATHIOPRINE

Side effects due to azathioprine (the nitroimidazole derivative of 6-mercaptopurine) can be classified as toxic (myelosuppression, hepatotoxicity) and idiosyncratic (fever, rigors, arthralgias, pneumonitis, and gastrointestinal symptoms). Although the toxic effects are due to 6-mercaptopurine, the hypersensitivity reactions are believed to be caused by the nitroimidazole moiety.

Azathioprine toxicity can occur during long-term treatment of myasthenia gravis.[34, 35] Among 104 treated patients with myasthenia gravis, side effects occurred in 35 percent and included, in decreasing frequency, hematological, 18 percent; gastrointestinal, 13 percent; infectious, 13 percent; and elevation of liver enzymes, 6 percent. The medicine was discontinued temporarily in 11 percent of the patients. In five patients, a malignant tumor was diagnosed, but a causal relationship seemed likely in only one.[34] Neurological toxicity is rare with azathioprine. Two patients with recurrent meningitic reactions following azathioprine ingestion have been presented in the literature; they were being treated for lupus of the CNS.[36]

CYCLOSPORINE

Cyclosporine is reviewed under Transplant Drugs.

Antibiotics (Tables 55–5 and 55–6)

ANTIBACTERIAL AGENTS

Penicillins, Cephalosporins, and Imipenem

Historically, radiculitis, paraplegia, hemiplegia, and convulsions occurred after penicillin was administered into the CSF, but because this route of administration has been abandoned, such reactions are exceedingly rare. The neurotoxic clinical manifestations of penicillins, cephalosporins, and imipenem include myoclonus, seizures, confusion, hallucinations, encephalopathy, nystagmus, and agitation.[37, 38] Imipenem, cefazolin, and benzyl penicillin are the most epileptogenic.[39] These drugs antagonize the inhibitory neurotransmitter GABA. Status epilepticus occurred in two patients treated with cefapime; seizures did not respond to anticonvulsant therapy but subsequently resolved with discontinuation of this fourth-generation cephalosporin.[40]

Risk factors for neurotoxicity are high-dose intravenous use (e.g., >30 to 40 million units of benzyl penicillin per day), decreased renal function, abnormal blood-brain barrier, cardiopulmonary bypass, age more than 50 years, pre-existing CNS disease, concurrent use of drugs that may lower the seizure threshold (such as theophylline or ciprofloxacin), and concomitant use of nephrotoxic drugs. Blockade of a system for transporting the beta-lactams out of the CSF in diseases causing meningeal inflammation adds to the risk of increased meningeal antibiotic penetration during inflammation.

Penicillin gluteal injection may cause sudden and irreversible paraplegia. The actual incidence of such a complication is not known, but there have been eight cases reported in the literature. The proposed mechanism is accidental

TABLE 55–5. **Central Neurotoxicity of Antibiotics**

Syndrome	Drug
Seizures/encephalopathy	Amphotericin B
	Bismuth
	Cephalosporins
	Cycloserine
	Erythromycin
	Imipenem-cilastatin
	Isoniazid
	Metronidazole
	Penicillins
	Quinolones
	Rifampin
Aseptic meningitis	Cephalosporins
	Penicillins
	Trimethoprim-sulfamethoxazole
Benign intracranial hypertension	Amphotericin B
	Nalidixic acid
	Nitrofurantoin
	Tetracyclines
	Trimethoprim-sulfamethoxazole
Cerebellar ataxia	Metronidazole
Optic neuritis	Chloramphenicol
	Ethambutol
	Isoniazid
Cochlear/vestibular damage	Aminoglycosides
	Erythromycin
	Minocycline
	Vancomycin

TABLE 55–6. **Peripheral Neurotoxicity of Antibiotics**

Syndrome	Drug	Relative Toxicity
Peripheral neuropathy	Chloramphenicol	S > M
	Chloroquine	S
	Colistin	S
	Dapsone	M
	Ethionamide	S
	Isoniazid	S > M
	Metronidazole	S
	Nitrofurantoin	SM
Neuromuscular blockade	Aminoglycosides	
	Ampicillin?	
	Clindamycin	
	Erythromycin	
	Polymyxins	
	Tetracyclines	

S, Sensory; M, motor.

intra-arterial injection, causing distal spasm and the upstream ascent of penicillin with ensuing embolic or spastic occlusion, or both, of the anterior spinal artery. Treatment of this complication is unsatisfactory, but it can be prevented by giving injections in the lateral thigh.[41]

Penicillins and cephalosporins have also been reported to cause recurrent aseptic meningitis.[42] Ampicillin has been reported to aggravate weakness in myasthenia gravis. Intrathecal beta-lactams have the potential to cause adhesive arachnoiditis.[39]

Aminoglycosides

The toxicity of all aminoglycosides is similar—mainly ototoxicity and neuromuscular blockade (Table 55–7). Acute ototoxicity is based on calcium antagonism and blockade of ion channels, and chronic mechanisms are related to tissue-specific toxicity of a noxious metabolite. Genetic analyses suggest that ototoxicity to aminoglycosides may be related to genetic mutations in mitochondrial ribosomal RNA in susceptible individuals.[43] Excitotoxicity has also been implicated as the mechanism for ototoxicity with aminoglycoside use. A recent animal study showed that spiral ganglion neuronal loss can be prevented by neurotrophin 3, and protection against hair cell damage occurs with *N*-methyl-D-aspartate receptor antagonists.[44, 45]

The frequency of ototoxicity ranges from 2 to 4 percent in retrospective studies and up to 25 percent in studies with specialized testing. The incidence and severity of damage appear to increase with patient age, total drug dose, and concomitant use of other ototoxic drugs.[46] Auditory toxicity is more common with the use of amikacin and kanamycin, whereas vestibular toxicity predominates following gentamicin and streptomycin therapy. Tobramycin is associated equally with vestibular and auditory damage. Cochlear toxicity is more often silent, as the hearing loss first affects the high frequencies (>4000 Hz) before involving the speech frequencies. Cochlear toxicity presents clinically as deafness, tinnitus, and ear pain, whereas vestibular toxicity presents as ataxia, dizziness, vertigo, chronic sense of imbalance, nystagmus, or oscillopsia.[39] Routine audiometry or studies of auditory brain stem evoked responses can be used to monitor ototoxicity. Monitoring vestibular toxicity is complex and needs even more specialized testing.[39] Aminoglycoside hearing loss is usually irreversible and may even progress following discontinuation of drug therapy.[46] Careful monitoring of peak and trough levels, especially in high-risk groups, helps prevent toxicity.

A potentially fatal neurotoxic effect of all aminoglycosides is neuromuscular blockade, due in part to a curare-like effect of the aminoglycosides and also to a competition with calcium by these antibiotics. This side effect is related to dose and serum level. Aminoglycosides are relatively contraindicated in both presynaptic (e.g., botulism) and postsynaptic (e.g., myasthenia gravis) disorders of neuromuscular transmission.[39] They may further potentiate ether and other drugs used to induce muscular relaxation during anesthesia. Neomycin and netilmicin are the most toxic, and tobramycin and kanamycin are the least toxic. Sudden or prolonged respiratory paralysis due to aminoglycosides may be reversed by calcium infusion, cholinesterase inhibitors, and aminopyridines.[39]

TABLE 55–7. **Aminoglycoside Neurotoxicity**

Drug	Cochlear Toxicity	Vestibular Toxicity	Neuromuscular Toxicity
Neomycin	+	++	+++
Kanamycin	++	+	+
Streptomycin	+	++	++
Gentamicin	+	++	++
Tobramycin	+	+	+
Amikacin	++	+	++
Netilmicin	++	+	+++

+++, Very common; ++, moderately common; +, rare.

Sulfonamides

Sulfonamides inhibit the synthesis of tetrahydrofolic acid, the one-carbon donor needed for the synthesis of methionine, serine, and purines. Although sulfonamides are associated with low incidence of neurotoxicity, a variety of adverse reactions can occur during therapy.[1] Recurrent aseptic meningitis is a well-recognized side effect of sulfonamide therapy, more specifically trimethoprim-sulfamethoxazole, and presents clinically with episodes of headache, nuchal rigidity, confusion, and myalgias. CSF analysis may show low glucose levels with or without pleocytosis; however, this study is not a reliable method to differentiate antibiotic-induced meningitis from partially treated bacterial meningitis.[42]

In addition, headache, fatigue, tinnitus, generalized convulsions, optic neuritis, agraphia, aphasia, stammering, teleopsia, macropsia, polyneuritis, and myelopathy can occur with sulfonamides. Euphoria, nausea, vomiting, somnolence, poor concentration, and impairment of judgment may be observed on the second or third day of treatment. The pathophysiology of the neurotoxic signs may relate to a drug-induced hypersensitivity reaction, because they often occur in the context of serum sickness or drug-induced vasculitis. Pathologically, a variety of lesions have been reported in fatal cases, including focal necrosis and demyelination of the cerebral white matter, hypothalamus, and pons, as well as hemorrhages in the fourth ventricle, brain stem, cerebral gray matter, and nuclear structures.[1, 39]

Quinolones

Seizures have been reported with ciprofloxacin as well as other quinolones, and the use of nalidixic acid, the first clinically useful quinolone, is contraindicated in patients with a history of epilepsy. In vitro studies suggest that the epileptogenic effect of the quinolones may be due to inhibition of GABA binding to its receptor site in the brain. This effect seems to be related to quinolone concentrations at the receptor site (dose related) and to particular substituents in quinolone structure. Simultaneous use of theophylline or nonsteroidal anti-inflammatory drugs may increase the risk for quinolone-associated toxic effects on the CNS, as the combination has an additive inhibitory effect on GABA sites.[47]

CNS side effects are seen in 1 to 4 percent of patients but are usually minor, including dizziness or mild headache. Quinolones have been reported to cause tremor, restlessness, hallucinations, delirium, psychosis, and benign intracranial hypertension, especially in high-dose therapy.[47] Especially in cases of renal impairment, the dose should be carefully monitored to avoid CNS toxicity.

Metronidazole

Metronidazole, a nitroimidazole derivative, is used for anaerobic and protozoal infections, as well as for the treatment of Crohn's disease. It is generally well tolerated, but it is associated with minor, transient adverse side effects. However, peripheral neuropathy is a potentially serious effect associated with the use of metronidazole. The mechanism of metronidazole peripheral neuropathy is undetermined, but the drug binds to the RNA of rat nerve cells, which may diminish protein synthesis and lead to subsequent nerve degeneration.

Neuropathy is particularly prevalent in patients who receive more than 2 g/day, a total dose of 50 g or more, and a treatment duration of at least 30 days. In long-term administration, 10 to 50 percent of patients develop a sensory neuropathy that is predominantly distal and symmetrical. Sensory deficits are prominent, with the sural and peroneal nerves most often affected. The paresthesias and discomfort associated with metronidazole neuropathy usually improve when metronidazole is discontinued or the dose is decreased. Symptoms gradually subside within 4 to 48 months following drug cessation. Rarely, neuropathic symptoms persist for an extended duration, worsen, or are irreversible. These atypical clinical courses may be related to metronidazole-induced nerve degeneration.

Metronidazole has rarely been associated with seizures in humans. It is believed that the total cumulative dose of metronidazole is more closely associated with seizure potential than the serum level.[48] Confusion, irritability, depression, headache, optic neuropathy, and aseptic meningitis have been reported as drug complications. These rare complications can be associated with large doses or prolonged administration, and they disappear rapidly with cessation of the drug.

Erythromycin and Newer Macrolides

Macrolides are among the safest anti-infective drugs in clinical use. An uncommon neurological side effect is temporary hearing loss. Whereas erythromycin-induced hypoacusis is a dose-dependent effect, its occurrence in patients otherwise free from predisposing factors suggests that it is idiosyncratic.[49] Usually, this reaction has occurred during treatment with 4 g or more of the lactonate derivative of oral erythromycin. Because erythromycin is metabolized by the liver, patients with hepatic abnormalities may be at higher risk for this ototoxic reaction. Tinnitus rather than a distinct difficulty hearing is the usual complaint.[1] This adverse reaction is reversible with dose reduction or discontinuation, and in patients with impaired renal or liver function, a lower prescribed daily dose may prevent or reduce its development. Azithromycin, a new macrolide antibiotic, has also been reported to cause sensorineural hearing loss.[50, 51] Erythromycin interacts with carbamazepine, causing carbamazepine levels to increase rapidly when erythromycin is introduced. Careful monitoring of the carbamazepine blood level and clinical symptoms of toxicity should be performed in patients receiving both drugs. Worsening of weakness in patients with myasthenia gravis, through a possible presynaptic mechanism, is generally mild, although respiratory failure may be precipitated.[39] Clarithromycin treatment has been associated with acute psychotic episodes.[52]

Tetracyclines

Vestibular toxicity has been reported in approximately 50 percent of patients receiving minocycline, a tetracycline derivative. Toxicity is more common in women, and the incidence is estimated to be at 70 percent. Although vestibular toxicity is more likely in patients with pre-existing vestibular disease, many patients have no such history. The symptoms begin a few days after the initiation of treatment and consist of lightheadedness, dizziness, loss of balance, nausea, and extreme vertigo. The reaction is transient, and even in the most severe cases, it resolves within a few days.[53]

Pseudotumor cerebri occurs in both adults and infants taking tetracyclines, but infants are more susceptible. The syndrome is characterized by headache, papilledema, elevated CSF pressure, and bulging fontanelles in infants. Signs and symptoms disappear within a few days after drug discontinuation, although papilledema may persist for weeks.[53] The intravenous administration of tetracyclines has rarely been reported to exacerbate myasthenia. This may be the result of magnesium in the diluent, binding of calcium by non–protein-bound tetracycline, or direct action at the neuromuscular junction.[39]

Nitrofurantoin

Nitrofurantoin therapy has been associated with polyneuropathy. Generally seen with prolonged therapy, neuropathy can occur as early as the first week of treatment. It is usually subacute, begins in the distal extremities with paresthesias, and tends to ascend progressively to involve the motor system with weakness and areflexia. Although this polyneuropathy clinically resembles Guillain-Barré syndrome, the spinal fluid is usually normal, except for 25 percent of patients, in whom there is a slight increase in protein without pleocytosis. When neuropathy is recognized, drug withdrawal is essential, although 10 to 15 percent of patients do not improve, and 15 percent have only partial recovery. The prognosis appears to relate to the extent of the neuropathy at the time of drug withdrawal but not to the total dose exposure or the duration of therapy.[1]

ANTITUBERCULOUS DRUGS

Isoniazid (INH)

Isoniazid inhibits the phosphorylation of pyridoxine and chelates whatever pyridoxal phosphate remains. Because pyridoxal phosphate is a cofactor that is important to the GABA system, it has been hypothesized that the centrally diminished GABA activity may relate to the pathophysiology of isoniazid-induced seizures. In chronic toxicity, isoniazid predominantly inhibits the phosphorylation of pyridoxine to induce a peripheral neuropathy.[1] INH has a narrow therapeutic window making drug intoxication easily possible. The usual dosage of INH is 5 mg/kg/d for adults and 10 to 15 mg/kg/d for children.

Seizures have been reported with dosages as low as 20 mg/d and severe neurotoxicity with dosages of 80 mg/d.[54]

The incidence of pyridoxine-associated polyneuropathy is 0.2 to 2 percent, and the clinical features include numbness and tingling of the feet with diminished or absent deep tendon reflexes and occasional optic neuropathy. Isoniazid-associated neuropathy can be prevented by concomitant administration of pyridoxine, 50 mg/d.[39] In patients not receiving pyridoxine, high-risk groups for neuropathy include slow acetylators, adults, alcoholics, malnourished individuals, and those receiving more than 5 mg/kg/d.

Acute isoniazid intoxication due to overdosage is associated with generalized seizures, ataxia, psychosis, and coma. Metabolic acidosis, hyperglycemia, and aciduria may accompany the acute neurological syndrome. Pyridoxine should be administered immediately, along with standard anticonvulsant and supportive measures. Because seizures are a complication of isoniazid therapy, the drug is not recommended for patients with pre-existing seizure disorder if another drug can be chosen. When isoniazid is required in patients who are already receiving phenytoin, the phenytoin dose has to be adjusted because isoniazid decreases its clearance.[1, 39]

More unusual isoniazid-related neurotoxic syndromes include drug-induced lupus with meningitis, psychosis, obsessive-compulsive disorder, and acute mania.

Rifampin

Rifampin may induce an encephalopathy with features suggestive of a psychosis. Other rare adverse reactions are dizziness, headache, drowsiness, confusion, inability to concentrate, and ataxia.[39] Rarely, paresthesias and pain suggestive of peripheral neuropathy are reported.

Ethambutol

Optic neuropathy has been associated with ethambutol treatment. This appears to be a demyelinating process, and the reason for the optic nerve's sensitivity to this drug is unknown. Symptoms are seen in as many as one third of patients taking doses of 35 mg/kg/d for 6 months. Doses of 25 mg/kg/d are safe for not more than 2 months, and the safe maintenance dose is 15 mg/kg/d. Toxicity is manifested by impairment of visual acuity, loss of color discrimination, constricted visual fields, and central and peripheral scotomata. The drug should be stopped at the first sign of visual change, and recovery can be anticipated, although it may take weeks to months.[55] Ten patients with ocular toxicity due to ethambutol were followed for up to 3 years. Only 50 percent of these patients experienced visual recovery, and permanent ocular toxicity was highest in patients over 60 years of age.[56] Animal studies suggest that the visual loss from ethambutol may be mediated through excitotoxic mechanisms on the retinal ganglion cells by decreased ATPase activity and perturbed mitochondrial function.[57] Other side effects include mild peripheral neuropathy and a metallic taste in the oral cavity.

ANTIFUNGAL DRUGS

Amphotericin B

Encephalopathy, occasionally with parkinsonian features, can be associated with intravenous administration of amphotericin B. Autopsy examination of afflicted patients discloses diffuse noninflammatory degeneration of the white matter, characterized by demyelination and infiltration by foamy macrophages. The leukotoxic effect of amphotericin B is related to its binding to myelin and an increase in membrane permeability, resulting in leakage of intracellular components.[58] Clinically, the patients develop a subacutely evolving neurological disorder characterized by personality change and confusion, rapidly progressing to akinetic mutism. Neuroimaging studies disclose diffuse nonenhancing lesions of the cerebral white matter that include hypodensity on computed tomography and increased signal on T2-weighted MRI. Amphotericin-associated leukoencephalopathy can be fatal, although there have been cases of slow recovery after discontinuation of the drug.

Polymyxin B

The incidence of neurotoxicity from parenteral polymyxin B averages 7 percent. Polymyxin has both presynaptic and postsynaptic effects, and it can worsen neuromuscular weakness, leading to respiratory failure, particularly in patients with renal failure or in combination with other drugs known to block neuromuscular transmission.[39] The various adverse effects of polymyxins include paresthesias, peripheral neuropathy, diplopia, dysphagia, ototoxicity, muscle weakness, dizziness, ataxia, seizures, and confusion.[1, 39]

ANTIMALARIALS

Chloroquine

Chloroquine, once considered too toxic for humans, has been the antimalarial of choice for 40 years. Although a range of serious CNS effects has been documented during chloroquine therapy, the incidence is unclear.[59] Abnormal involuntary movements, including torticollis, blepharospasm, and dystonic tongue protrusion, have been reported during chloroquine therapy, especially in patients younger than 30 years of age.[1] Headache, nausea, and tinnitus with progressive hearing loss, optic nerve dysfunction, seizures, psychosis, mania, and myasthenic syndrome have also been reported.

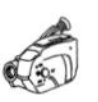

When used chronically, as in rheumatoid arthritis, chloroquine has been implicated in the development of peripheral neuropathy, cranial nerve palsies, and myopathy. The peripheral neuropathy is a distal sensorimotor polyneuropathy that is reversible after drug withdrawal.[1]

Antiretroviral Medications

Patients infected with the human immunodeficiency virus (HIV) are living longer than before due to a better understanding of the disease process and newer pharmacological agents often used in combination to control viral loads. Their use, however, comes with a price of toxic side effects. The currently available classes of antiretrovirals for HIV infection include protease inhibitors, nucleoside reverse transcriptase inhibitors (NRTI), and non-nucleoside reverse transcrip-

TABLE 55–8. **Antiretroviral Medications**

Protease Inhibitors
Amprenavir (Agenerase)
Indinavir (Crixivan)
Nelfinavir (Viracept)
Ritonavir (Norvir)
Saquinavir (Fortovase, Invirase)

Nucleoside Reverse Transcriptase Inhibitors
Abacavir (Ziagen)
Combivir (Lamivudine + Zidovudine)
Didanosine (Videx, DDI)
Lamivudine (Epivir, Epivir-HBV, 3TC, Heptovir)
Stavudine (Zerit, d4T)
Zalcitabine (Hivid, ddC)
Zidovudine (Retrovir, AZT, Azidothymidine, ZDV)

Non-Nucleoside Reverse Transcriptase Inhibitors
Delavirdine (Rescriptor)
Efavirenz (Sustiva)
Nevirapine (Viramune)

tase inhibitors (NNRTI). New drug regimens support the use of concomitant medications from each class in HIV-positive individuals to prevent the complications of acquired immunodeficiency syndrome. Table 55–8 contains a list of available HIV medications.[60]

PROTEASE INHIBITORS

The major side effects of protease inhibitors are metabolic in nature and include diabetes, hyperlipidemia, and fat redistribution.[60] These effects are not directly neurological.

NUCLEOSIDE REVERSE TRANSCRIPTASE INHIBITORS

The most frequent neurological side effect of NRTI is peripheral neuropathy. This problem is typically a distal, symmetrical, predominantly sensory neuropathy and has been described with zalcitabine, didanosine, and stavudine.[61] EMG demonstrates an axonal neuropathy. It may be difficult to determine the origin of the neuropathy, because HIV infection can also cause a distal sensory neuropathy. The treatment includes removal of the offending agent.[60, 62, 63] Myopathy of mitochondrial origin has been reported with both NNRTI and NRTI. This proximal and symmetrical myopathy is associated with a mitochondrial pattern of ragged-red fibers on histological examination. Removal of the offending agent is the best treatment. The onset of this syndrome in association with NRTI and NNRTI likely occurs preferentially in subjects who already have a genetic predisposition to mitochondrial disorders.[64]

NON-NUCLEOSIDE REVERSE TRANSCRIPTASE INHIBITORS

The major neurological side effects of the NNRTI include dizziness, somnolence, diminished concentration, and confusion. The patient may also experience psychiatric disturbances, including agitation, depersonalization, hallucinations, insomnia, vivid dreams, depression, and euphoria. These symptoms are most severe at initiation of therapy and typically resolve with elimination of the offending medication.[60]

Antineoplastic Chemotherapy

(Table 55–9)

ALKYLATING AGENTS

Nitrogen Mustard (Mechlorethamine)

Nitrogen mustard (NM) administered intravenously in a dose of 0.4 mg/kg is not usually associated with neurotoxicity. Hemiplegia, coma, chills, and fever, with increased ICP and CSF pleocytosis, however, were reported in one patient 7 days after each of two standard intravenous doses of NM (0.4 mg/kg).[65] On both occasions the signs and symptoms subsided after therapeutic measures to decrease ICP. When the patient died 4 years later from unrelated reasons, a gross and microscopical examination of the brain revealed focal areas of gliosis with loss of neurons. Massive intravenous injections of NM have caused hearing loss and vertigo, presumably from damage to cranial nerve VIII, seizures, somnolence, and confusion.[66] Intracarotid NM injection has been associated with hemiplegia, seizures, coma, and death.[65] One pathological study showed diffuse cerebral edema, which was greater on the side of the injection, and extensive gliosis and demyelination, presumably from a previous injection.[1]

Cyclophosphamide

One of the most widely used alkylating agents, cyclophosphamide is associated with very little neurological toxicity. Rapid intravenous infusion of cyclophosphamide has been associated with facial or scalp burning, oropharyngeal tingling, nasal congestion, rhinorrhea, sneezing, and lacrimation. These uncomfortable sensations of the skin and mucous

TABLE 55–9. **Anticancer Drugs and Neurotoxins**

Encephalopathy
BCNU
Cisplatin
Cytosine arabinoside
5-Fluorouracil
Ifosfamide
L-Asparaginase
Methotrexate
Procarbazine
Interferon
Interleukin-2

Cerebellar Syndromes
Cytosine arabinoside
5-Fluorouracil
Procarbazine

Myelopathy
Adriamycin (intrathecal)
Methotrexate (intrathecal)
Cytosine arabinoside
Thiotepa
Vincristine (intrathecal)

Parkinsonism
Cyclophosphamide
Cytosine arabinoside
Methotrexate
5-Fluorouracil

Peripheral Neuropathy
Cisplatin
Cytosine arabinoside
Hexamethylmelamine
Procarbazine
Vincristine

Strokelike Syndromes
Cytosine arabinoside
BCNU
L-Asparaginase
Methotrexate
5-Fluorouracil

membranes occur more frequently than was previously noted, and changing infusion duration or the concentration of cyclophosphamide, or administering anticholinergics intranasally, can result in variable degrees of improvement.[67]

Inappropriate secretion of antidiuretic hormone has occurred rarely and is exacerbated by the high fluid loading required in high-dose cyclophosphamide therapy to prevent renal toxicity. Biopsy-proven progressive multifocal leukoencephalopathy (PML) has been described in a man treated with cyclophosphamide and prednisone for Wegener's granulomatosis. On discontinuation of immunosuppression, dramatic recovery took place.[68]

Ifosfamide

Ifosfamide, an analogue of cyclophosphamide, is derived from nitrogen mustard and is used to treat a wide variety of pediatric and adult tumors. CNS effects of ifosfamide are frequent, are often severe, and can limit drug use.[69] Neurotoxic effects include changes in mental status ranging from drowsiness to coma, ataxia, tremor, myoclonus, seizures, facial spasms, and focal neurological signs.[69–72] Symptoms are usually self-limited, clearing 48 to 72 hours after cessation of therapy, but persistent neuropsychological abnormalities and even fatalities can occur. The encephalopathy and accompanying seizures that can manifest as nonconvulsive status epilepticus may respond to intravenous diazepam.[72, 73] Predisposing factors for CNS toxicity include dehydration, decreased renal function, previous cerebrovascular events or brain metastases, pelvic tumors, and decreased serum albumin.[74]

Chlorambucil

Seizures have rarely been reported with chlorambucil administration. They occur almost exclusively in children, in the setting of overdosage or nephrotic syndrome. They consist of myoclonic seizures followed by generalized tonic-clonic seizures. The EEG can show paroxysmal discharges that continue for several days after seizure activity.[1] Although the drug is generally considered to be non-neurotoxic, acute CNS abnormalities consisting of lethargy, ataxia, seizures, and coma have been reported with overdose.[66] PML has occurred in a patient with rheumatoid arthritis after treatment with chlorambucil. Of interest is that PML can develop as a late complication, even after the medicine is stopped.[75]

Thiotepa

Owing to its low neurotoxicity, thiotepa, an intravenously administered alkylating agent, is one of the few anticancer drugs that can be injected into the CSF. In one series of 10 patients with meningeal leukemia and carcinomatosis treated with multiple courses of intrathecal thiotepa, clinical neurotoxicity developed in only 2.[1] This neurotoxicity consisted of progressive myelopathy, manifested as progressive lower extremity weakness, back and leg pain, areflexia, and sensory deficits. EMG revealed diffuse lower motor neuron abnormalities. The histopathological changes in the spinal cord were localized to the white matter and consisted of demyelination and gliosis of the posterior columns and the nerve roots of the cauda equina.[76]

Busulfan

Generalized seizures are a frequent side effect of high-dose busulfan (total dose 16 mg/kg) as part of a preparative regimen for allogeneic bone marrow transplantation. No neurological deficits are found after the episodes, and there are no recurrences. Maintenance of therapeutic blood concentrations of anticonvulsant prophylactic regimens is recommended.[77] There has been one case of busulfan administration associated with the development of myasthenia gravis, although the relationship among the myasthenia, the busulfan, and the leukemia was not clarified.[1]

ANTIMETABOLITES

Methotrexate

Methotrexate is a competitive inhibitor of dihydrofolate reductase, acting primarily during DNA synthesis (S-phase) as an antifolate antineoplastic drug. It prevents two primary reactions, the conversion of folic acid to tetrahydrofolic acid and the conversion of tetrahydrofolic acid to folinic acid, thereby blocking DNA, RNA, and protein synthesis by limiting the availability of reduced folates.[1, 66, 78] As an oral or intravenous drug in the usual prescribed doses, methotrexate is a neurologically safe agent. It has limited ability to cross the blood-brain barrier, and the CSF concentration is less than 10 percent of that in plasma after oral or parenteral administration. When given intrathecally or in higher doses, however, methotrexate is associated with a number of neurological syndromes. Proposed mechanisms of methotrexate neurotoxicity include depletion of cerebral reduced folates, reduced cerebral protein, altered blood-brain barrier permeability, and impaired neurotransmitter synthesis.[66] The risk of neurotoxicity is increased with increasing total intrathecal methotrexate dose, prolonged elevated CSF methotrexate levels, concurrent radiation therapy, or systemic high-dose methotrexate therapy. Toxicity is also more frequent and severe in younger patients and when methotrexate is used as treatment for meningeal tumor rather than for prophylaxis.[66]

Acute methotrexate neurotoxicity includes an acute chemical meningitis with fever, headache, nuchal rigidity, and CSF leukocytosis. This condition is usually mild to moderate; begins within hours of intrathecal administration; lasts for 1 to 3 days, although it may persist for 2 weeks; resolves spontaneously; and does not recur with subsequent therapy.[1, 66, 78] An acute strokelike encephalopathy with seizures, confusion, hemiparesis, and coma may complicate high-dose methotrexate (more than 1 g/m^2) in as many as 15 percent of patients.[66] Other acute complications that occur within hours of intrathecal administration are acute transverse myelopathy with paraplegia, which may be permanent, and transient radiculopathies, possibly related to epidural or subdural injection, or the development of hematomas.[66, 78] Accidental intrathecal methotrexate overdose may produce an ascending myelopathy and necrotizing leukoencephalopathy.[66] Doses of 50 mg or less probably produce few serious sequelae. A moderate overdose (50 to 100 mg) without early CSF drainage may produce an acute chemical meningitis. Massive overdose (more than 500 mg) causes myelopathy and encephalopathy, which may be fatal. Intensive systemic support, high-dose leucovorin, and alkaline diuresis, plus rapid CSF drainage and ventriculolumbar perfusion, may permit survival and recovery of neurological function.

Delayed neurotoxicity from repeated intrathecal or intraventricular methotrexate is more frequent than acute intoxication, and encephalopathy is the most important late effect. Pathologically, this is a leukoencephalopathy, with areas of coagulative necrosis, demyelination, and mineralizing microangiopathy. Clinically, it is characterized by progressive personality and intellectual decline, dementia, hemiparesis, and sometimes seizures. MRI and CT usually show extensive, patchy white matter lesions. The long-term effects of the treatment (or prophylaxis) of childhood leukemia and brain tumor include behavioral changes, poor school performance, memory loss, intellectual decline, growth retardation, hormonal disturbances, and abnormal CT scans. Although radiotherapy may account for many of these complications, intrathecal methotrexate alone may produce intellectual and behavioral problems or exacerbate those produced by radiotherapy.[66]

5-Fluorouracil

5-Fluorouracil is a fluorine-substituted analogue of the pyrimidine uracil. It inhibits the enzyme thymidylate synthetase, blocking DNA synthesis by reducing thymidine monophosphate formation. It is associated with a characteristic cerebellar syndrome in 1 percent of patients when the recommended doses are used. When doses exceed the usual recommendations, the incidence of this cerebellar syndrome may be as high as 3 to 7 percent. The mechanism of 5-fluorouracil neurotoxicity is unknown, but its conversion to fluocitrate and fluoacetate in the CNS with subsequent inhibition of the Krebs cycle has been postulated.[66, 78, 79] Concomitant administration of alpha-interferon, cisplatin, leucovorin, or thymidine potentiates the toxic effects.[66]

Clinically, 5-fluorouracil induces pancerebeller dysfunction, characterized by the acute or subacute onset of gait ataxia, limb incoordination, dysarthria, nystagmus, and, sometimes, diplopia. The symptoms are usually controlled by dose reduction or increase in intervals between treatments. Although the syndrome is reversible, cases of re-emergence after subsequent treatment have been reported.[66, 78, 79]

Other neurotoxic reactions associated with 5-fluorouracil include encephalopathy, as well as a parkinsonian syndrome in 40 percent of patients.[79] The encephalopathy is usually mild to moderate but can range from lethargy to coma with high-dose infusions. All of the neurological symptoms associated with 5-fluorouracil are usually reversible on cessation of the drug, and no pathological changes have been noted in the brain at postmortem examination.[79]

Cerebral demyelination has been described with 5-fluorouracil monotherapy. In a patient who completed chemotherapy with 5-fluorouracil, an MRI showed areas of demyelination that enhanced with contrast. A repeat MRI of the brain was completed in 2 months and showed a decreased number of demyelinating lesions. The demyelination was felt to be causally related to partial dihydropyrimidine dehydrogenase deficiency in combination with 5-fluorouracil administration.[80] Ischemic strokes following administration of 5-fluorouracil and cisplatin have occurred in five patients. In each, no other cause for stroke could be identified in spite of an extensive workup. Each patient developed ischemic stroke in the second or third treatment cycle with development of symptoms in close relation to medication administration.[81]

Cytosine Arabinoside (Cytarabine)

Cytosine arabinoside is an analogue of pyrimidine nucleosides and readily crosses the blood-brain barrier. The drug destroys proliferating cells as an S-phase–specific cytotoxic agent. In many animals, in which cellular proliferation is active in the external granular layer of the cerebellum, cytosine arabinoside selectively destroys this layer and causes disarrangement and abnormal arborization of the Purkinje cells.[82]

Although the drug has little neurotoxicity following usual intravenous doses, in high doses it can cause an acute cerebellar syndrome in up to 14 percent and less commonly seizures and encephalopathy. When given intrathecally, it may result in myelopathy or cauda equina syndrome that is incompletely reversible. Combined intrathecal cytarabine and cranial irradiation may lead to necrotizing encephalopathy. Intravenous therapy may cause a peripheral neuropathy.[82] The incidence and severity of neurotoxicity increases with increasing dose (more than 18 g/m^2/course), increasing age (rare in patients younger than age 20, occurring in 3 percent of those from age 20 to 50, and in 19 percent of those older than age 50), and following subsequent rather than initial courses.[66] Symptoms of neurotoxicity typically begin 6 to 8 days after the initiation of cytosine arabinoside with nystagmus and ataxia, peak over the following 2 to 3 days (confusion, somnolence, ataxia, dysarthria, and sometimes seizures or coma), start to improve within 1 week, and resolve completely within 2 weeks in most patients.[66] Cerebellar atrophy may be seen on CT or MRI, and pathological changes are remarkable for Purkinje cell loss, reactive Bergmann's gliosis, and, occasionally, demyelination.

NATURAL PRODUCTS

Vinca Alkaloids

Vincristine and vinblastine are alkaloid derivatives of the periwinkle plant, whose major and dose-limiting toxicity is neurological. The mechanism of action of these agents is probably related to inhibition of microtubule formation in the mitotic spindle, resulting in an arrest of dividing cells at the metaphase stage. Peripheral neuropathy is almost universal in patients receiving these drugs, and neurotoxicity is attributed to the inhibition of axoplasmic transport by their effect on axonal microtubules.[65, 66] Patients with pre-existing neuropathy (diabetic, familial, compressive, or nutritional) may have more severe neuropathy. Generally, the longer the exposure, the more numerous and severe the neuropathic side effects.

The earliest and most consistent objective manifestation of vincristine neurotoxicity is suppression of the Achilles tendon reflex. This is followed rapidly by losses of other reflexes, distal symmetrical sensory loss (pin and temperature more than vibration and proprioception), weakness, footdrop, and muscle atrophy. Autonomic neuropathy with constipation, ileus, urinary retention, impotence, or postural hypotension may occur. Cranial neuropathy occurs, usually

involving the oculomotor nerve, often causing bilateral ptosis. Affected nerves include the abducens, trigeminal, facial, and recurrent laryngeal nerves, the latter resulting in hoarseness or stridor. Nerve conduction velocities are normal, because the process is an axonopathy.[1, 65, 66, 79] Cases of life-threatening vincristine neuropathy have been described in patients with an underlying neuropathic disorder such as hereditary sensory motor neuropathy. To avoid vincristine exposure to subjects with pre-existing neuropathy, a pretreatment neurological examination and careful family history are useful.[83] A proximal myopathy can occur with prolonged vincristine therapy even in the absence of neuropathy and is distinguishable because of its proximal distribution of weakness.[84, 85] A painful myopathy may occur in children. Vincristine does not cross the blood-brain barrier, so CNS toxicity is rare, although seizures may develop as a result of inappropriate secretion of antidiuretic hormone.[79] Vinblastine has similar neurotoxic reactions but only at doses that are usually not prescribed because of concomitant severe hematological reactions.[79]

L-Asparaginase

L-Asparaginase is an enzyme that hydrolyzes asparagine to aspartic acid and ammonia, depleting asparagine and inhibiting protein synthesis. When it was first introduced, the drug was used at high doses that produced an acute encephalopathy that proved to be dose limiting. At usually prescribed doses, the encephalopathy is not seen.[79]

Because L-asparaginase inhibits protein synthesis, plasma protein deficits occur, including those involved in coagulation and fibrinolysis. Decreased levels of fibrinogen, factor IX, factor XI, plasminogen, antithrombin III, protein C, protein S, alpha$_2$-antiplasmin, histidine-rich glycoprotein, and alpha$_2$-macroglobulin also occur.[86] L-Asparaginase has been linked to hemorrhagic and thrombotic cerebrovascular complications, including cortical infarction, capsular infarction, intracerebral hemorrhage, hemorrhagic infarction, and cerebral venous and dural sinus thrombosis. During treatment, progressive prolongations in prothrombin time, partial thromboplastin time, and thrombin time are seen. In patients who have had complications resulting from L-asparaginase and who require further treatment, therapy to prevent subsequent complications is controversial. Fresh frozen plasma alone or with low-dose heparin or antithrombin III has been proposed.[86] Because fresh frozen plasma lessens the decrease in coagulation proteins normally seen with L-asparaginase, it is a reasonable treatment for patients with thromboembolic complications from the medicine.

ANTIBIOTIC ANTINEOPLASTIC AGENTS

Bleomycin

The existence of pure bleomycin toxicity has not been established, because the drug is ordinarily used in conjunction with other chemotherapeutic agents. Mental status changes and peripheral neuropathy have been reported with bleomycin therapy, although no pathological changes have been associated in brain or peripheral nerves in such patients. In animals, cochlear damage has been demonstrated, although there is no comparable clinical evidence in humans.[1]

Adriamycin and Actinomycin D

Adriamycin and actinomycin D produce no neurological side effects in humans in the usually prescribed doses, and when administered systemically, the drugs do not enter the CSF. Adriamycin can produce a severe form of myelopathy and encephalopathy after accidental intrathecal injection. Experimentally, it can produce cerebral damage after intracarotid injection and anterior horn cell loss after direct injection into a peripheral nerve.[66]

Actinomycin D causes tremors, myoclonus, seizure, ascending myelopathy, and encephalopathy when it is injected into the CSF in animal models. In pathological studies, demyelination and necrosis have been found in the brain.[1]

OTHER CHEMOTHERAPEUTIC AGENTS

Nitrosoureas

The nitrosoureas include BCNU (carmustine), CCNU (lomustine), methyl-CCNU (semustine), PCNU, and ACNU. As alkylating agents, they bind DNA and produce interstrand and intrastrand cross-links and carbamoylated proteins. They readily cross the blood-brain barrier and have little or no neurotoxicity at the usual dose regimens used (BCNU IV 200 mg/m^2 or 80 mg/m^2/day for 3 days). Encephalopathy with confusion and seizures may follow high doses of the drug (BCNU IV 600 to 800 mg/m^2 or more).[66] Several patients developed multifocal neurological abnormalities 3 to 12 weeks following high doses of BCNU (1500 to 3000 mg) followed by autologous bone marrow transplantation to rescue the bone marrow from the drug toxicity. Postmortem examination revealed foci of coagulative necrosis.[79] Intracarotid BCNU (usually 100 to 200 mg/m^2) can produce severe local pain in the ipsilateral face, eye, and head during infusion and, sometimes, retinopathy, blindness, or ocular necrosis. Intracarotid infusions above the ophthalmic artery may prevent ocular toxicity. A severe ipsilateral encephalopathy with seizures, hemiparesis, progressive neurological deficits, and cerebral necrosis (pathologically similar to radiation necrosis) has been described following intracarotid BCNU administration.[66] Concurrent cranial radiotherapy and intracarotid BCNU may increase the risk of neurotoxicity.

Cisplatin

Cisplatin most likely acts by binding to DNA, forming intrastrand and interstrand cross-links. Cisplatin neurotoxicity is common and dose limiting. Ototoxicity is a dose-limiting complication, occurring most commonly at doses of 120 mg/m^2 or more. Direct toxicity of the drug on the organ of Corti appears to be the cause of the induced deafness, because nystagmus and vertigo have rarely been reported. Deafness is more common in elderly patients and is exacerbated by radiation therapy to the head. The patient cannot hear high-frequency sounds; the hearing loss is bilateral and largely reversible, but it can be permanent. Deafness often begins within 3 to 4 days of the initial treatment and slowly improves over the succeeding weeks after treatment is stopped. The combination of slow infusion and pretreatment with intravenous hydration and often mannitol to enhance renal excretion has reduced the problem of ototoxicity.[66, 79]

Peripheral neuropathy is a second prominent complication and involves predominantly large fibers. It is dose related and cumulative (with a total dose usually more than 300 to 600 mg/m^2). Symptoms may begin or progress even after cisplatin has been stopped.[66] Encephalopathy with confusion and seizures can occur, especially with high doses, but may be due to fluid or electrolyte disturbances that accompany cisplatin therapy, such as hyponatremia, hypocalcemia, and hypomagnesemia. Cerebral herniation with severe headache, increasing hemiparesis, seizures, coma, and death has been reported in patients with large intracranial tumors receiving cisplatin, possibly due to overhydration and electrolyte disturbances producing cerebral edema and seizures.[1, 66] Finally, retinopathy and cranial neuropathy occasionally follow cisplatin therapy.

Procarbazine

Procarbazine is a weak MAOI that acts primarily as an alkylating agent. High-dose intravenous or intracarotid procarbazine can produce severe encephalopathy. At usual oral doses (60 to 150 mg/m^2/d), a mild reversible encephalopathy (drowsiness, confusion, agitation) or peripheral neuropathy (paresthesias, reduced deep tendon reflexes, and muscle aches) develop in as many as 20 percent of patients.[66]

Because of its monoamine oxidase inhibition, procarbazine can predispose the patients receiving it to a variety of drug interactions, including synergistic sedative effects with phenothiazines, barbiturates, and narcotics, as well as alcohol intolerance. The caution advised with other MAOIs regarding the tyramine effect with cheese or wine has not been a clinical problem with procarbazine.[1, 65, 66]

Hexamethylmelamine

Hexamethylmelamine can act as an alkylating agent or as an antimetabolite. It has both central and peripheral neurotoxic effects. In the usual doses administered (8 mg/kg/d), neurological problems are seen in up to 20 percent of patients. The clinical manifestations include encephalopathy (confusion, agitation, hallucinations, parkinsonism) and peripheral neuropathy (distal sensory loss, weakness). In the case of the peripheral neuropathy, pyridoxine may be beneficial.[1, 66]

Transplant Drugs

CYCLOSPORINE

Neurotoxicity is a well-recognized sequela of cyclosporine, and the most common complications are tremor and altered mental status. Cyclosporine neurotoxicity can occur in 1 in 10 patients after liver transplantation. Behavioral signs

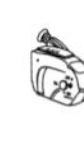

include acute psychosis, restlessness, wide mood swings with inappropriate crying and laughing, cortical blindness, visual hallucinations, stupor, and akinetic mutism. Additionally, seizures, extrapyramidal symptoms, action myoclonus, and quadriparesis have been reported. In patients with neurological signs, cyclosporine levels are usually outside the normal range, and after lowering the dose or withholding administration, neurotoxicity clears in most cases. MRI abnormalities are consistent with cortical or white matter high-signal changes with a predilection for the occipital lobes.[87–91] One autopsy case of a patient who died from cyclosporine toxicity revealed diffuse patchy white matter edema and astrocytic injury without infectious/inflammatory process.[89] Although the mechanism of cyclosporine neurotoxicity has not been fully elucidated, one theory suggests that hypocholesterolemia may result in upregulation of the low-density lipoprotein receptors, which increases intracellular transport of cyclosporine. Access may be particularly high in the white matter with a relatively high density of low-density lipoprotein receptors. Another theory implicates endothelin, a potent vasoconstrictive neuropeptide, in combination with breakdown of the blood-brain barrier, resulting in local ischemia. Other possible etiological mechanisms of cyclosporine neurotoxicity include hypomagnesemia, hypertension, aluminum overload, and high-dose methylprednisolone administration.[87, 92] One study used in vitro multinuclear magnetic resonance to study the effects of cyclosporine on high-energy phosphate metabolism in brain cells and perfused rat brain slices.[93] Both the clinical manifestations and the neuroimaging abnormalities of cyclosporine neurotoxicity usually resolve with a reduction or discontinuation of cyclosporine.[87, 92]

NEW TRANSPLANT IMMUNOSUPPRESSIVES

These are relatively new drugs, so more extensive use will be needed to determine the entire realm of neurological side effects. Among the new transplant immunosuppressives are basiliximab, daclizumab, mycophenolate mofetil, sirolimus, and tacrolimus. Typical neurological effects of long-term immunosuppression, including infections such as meningitis, encephalitis, and abscess formation, are similar with the newer agents.[94] Direct neurological toxicity is more common with tacrolimus, a calcineurin inhibitor like cyclosporine, while the others exhibit toxicity that spares the nervous system.

Although tacrolimus may be a better immunosuppressant than cyclosporine, it may have worse neurological effects.[95, 96] In a multicenter, randomized, parallel-group study of 545 patients undergoing primary liver transplantation, tacrolimus was associated with a higher incidence of neurological symptoms than cyclosporine.[97] The risk of tacrolimus-treated patients developing tremor was related to the initial intravenous dose, the rate of administration, and the total daily dose. Headache was significantly correlated with dose while insomnia was not.[97] Factors that may promote the development of serious complications include advanced liver failure, hypertension, hypocholesterolemia, elevated serum levels, hypomagnesemia, and methylprednisone.[98] Calcineurin inhibition by tacrolimus and cyclosporine alters sympathetic outflow, which may play a role in the mediation of neurotoxic and hypertensive adverse events. The symptoms may be reversed by reducing the dose of immunosuppressant or by discontinuation. However, some patients have experienced permanent or even fatal neurological damage even after discontinuation of tacrolimus.[98, 99] Occipital white matter appears to be uniquely susceptible to the neurotoxic effects of tacrolimus as is the case with cyclosporine. The encephalopathy associated with tacrolimus has been reported to involve the cortex as well.[95] MRI has been reported to reveal bilateral symmetrical regions of signal abnormality with abnormal contrast enhancement. The abnormal signal was more evident in FLAIR (fluid-attenuated-inversion-recovery) sequences.[100] Epilepsy[101] and cerebral hemorrhage[102] have been reported with tacrolimus-induced neurotoxicity.

In contrast to CNS toxicity, peripheral nervous system involvement is uncommon. Nevertheless, both demyelinating[103] and axonal polyneuropathy[104] have been described.

Cardiac Drugs (Table 55–10)

DIGITALIS

Adverse effects on the CNS occur in 40 to 50 percent of patients with clinical digitalis toxicity and may develop before, with, or after signs of cardiac toxicity. Neurological complications include nausea, vomiting, visual disturbances, seizures, confusion, delirium, mania, hallucinosis, and syncope. Explanations for the high frequency of neurotoxicity with digitalis have been inadequate, and the few pathological studies compiled have not demonstrated consistent lesions.[1]

The most frequent and often the first neurotoxic reaction is nausea due to direct stimulation of the medullary chemoreceptor trigger zone. Nausea associated with digitalis toxicity is often accompanied by vomiting, and when vomiting is chronic, it may lead to malnourishment and cachexia. The incidence of digitalis-related visual disturbances has been estimated at 40 percent. Clinically, it presents with blurred vision, scotomas, diplopia, defects of color vision, and amaurosis. Electrodiagnostic and labeled tracer studies have implicated retinal dysfunction in the pathogenesis.[105]

Seizures are most commonly seen in the pediatric population. The mechanism by which digitalis induces seizures has been postulated to involve inhibition of membrane ATPase and subsequent neuronal irritability. Confusion, delirium, mania, and hallucinosis have been reported in as many as 15 percent of patients with digitalis toxicity.[1] Although the mechanism for the symptoms is unknown, they are not the result of altered cardiac function. On the other hand, transient cognitive changes that are believed to be due to intermittent cerebral hypoperfusion can resemble transient global amnesia or be manifested as syncope.

TABLE 55–10. **Neurological Complications of Cardiac Medications**

Complication	Drugs
Ataxia	Amiodarone
Encephalopathy/Delirium	Digoxin Beta-blockers Lidocaine
Extrapyramidal	Amiodarone Calcium channel blockers
Hallucinations	Beta-blockers Digoxin
Headaches	Lidocaine Quinidine
Insomnia	Beta-blockers
Sedation	ACE inhibitors
Seizures	Digoxin Lidocaine
Visual disturbances	Digoxin Quinidine

BETA-BLOCKERS

Neuropsychiatric symptoms occur frequently during treatment with beta-blockers. The pharmacology of CNS side effects is unclear, although presynaptic and postsynaptic adrenergic inhibition has been implicated, as has serotonergic antagonism.[1] Nonselective beta-blockers seem to cause CNS-related side effects to a greater extent than $beta_1$-selective blockers.[106] It is unclear to what degree lipophilicity is responsible for this kind of side effect. Lassitude or insomnia and depression are the most common reactions, although vivid dreams, nightmares, hypnagogic hallucinations, and psychotic behavior have been reported with high doses (more than 500 mg/day of propranolol). Pre-existing major psychiatric illness and hyperthyroidism may predispose to the preceding symptoms.

CALCIUM CHANNEL BLOCKERS

Calcium channel blockers, particularly flunarizine and cinnarizine, have been associated with dystonia, parkinsonism, akathisia, and TD. Theoretical explanations for these events include the inhibition of calcium influx into striatal cells and direct dopaminergic antagonistic properties. Recent evidence also suggests that inhibition of proton pumping and catecholamine uptake are possible mechanisms.[107] In addition, the chemical structures of flunarizine and cinnarizine, which are related to neuroleptics, may explain the greater incidence of such side effects with these agents compared with those of calcium channel blockers available in the United States. Suggested risk factors appear to be advanced age and a family history of tremors or Parkinson's disease, or both.[108] The onset and type of presentation is unpredictable. The long-term evolution was assessed in a prospective follow-up study of 32 patients with diagnoses of calcium channel blocker–induced parkinsonism. Eighteen months following discontinuation of the offending agent, 44 percent of the patients had depression, 88 percent had tremor, and 33 percent still had criteria for diagnosis of parkinsonism.[109] 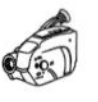

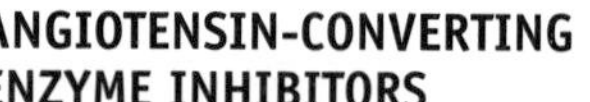

ANGIOTENSIN-CONVERTING ENZYME INHIBITORS

The incidence of CNS effects with angiotensin-converting enzyme (ACE) inhibitors is similar to that of beta-blockers. The precise role of ACE in the CNS is not well defined. Mild lethargy, sedation, and fatigue are the most common complaints.[110] As opposed to beta-blockers, ACE inhibitors appear to have the lowest association with depression and, therefore, are the drugs of choice when depression is a risk.

Approximately 2 to 4 percent (depending on renal function and dose) of 100 patients on captopril develop diminution or loss of taste perception. This sign is reversible and usually resolves within 2 to 3 months, even with continued drug administration.

NITRATES

The major problem with nitrate therapy is headache. According to proposed mechanisms, nitric oxide is the common mediator in experimental vascular headaches possibly resulting in headache through vasodilatation of extracerebral arteries.[111] Nitroglycerin produces a throbbing or pulsating sensation in many patients and an overt headache in many others. Often, the headaches attenuate or disappear with time, but 15 to 20 percent of patients are not able to tolerate long-acting nitrates because of headache. Patients should be encouraged to use analgesics during the initial days or weeks of nitrate therapy and should be educated as to the nature of this problem and its probable resolution with time.[112]

Nitroglycerin therapy can cause dose-related increases in ICP, which, in rare cases, can result in a clinically overt syndrome. Finally, the hypotensive effects of nitroglycerin can result in dizziness and lightheadedness or even syncope.

ANTIARRHYTHMIC AGENTS

Amiodarone

Amiodarone is a di-ionated benzofurane derivative used primarily in the treatment of refractory ventricular and atrial arrhythmias. Amiodarone can be toxic for almost every organ in the body, including the central and peripheral nervous systems, especially when taken at high doses for long periods of time. The most common neurotoxic findings include tremor, ataxia, proximal muscle weakness, and wasting. Tremor usually appears early in the course of therapy and is usually a bilateral 6- to 10-Hz action tremor of the arms, which is indistinguishable from essential tremor. It can involve all limbs and may be asymmetrical, although to date it has not been reported to be unilateral. Rarely, the tremor is associated with parkinsonian features. Other manifestations of basal ganglia dysfunction that have been reported in association with amiodarone include myoclonus, hemiballismus, and dyskinesias of the extremities and orofacial area. Basal ganglia dysfunction associated with amiodarone is dose related, and reversibility is inversely related to duration of therapy.[113]

Lidocaine

Lidocaine is widely administered parenterally and topically. It is oxidized to active and inactive metabolites by hepatic enzymes in the cytochrome P-450 mixed oxidase system. Toxic effects of lidocaine occur frequently and involve the cardiovascular system and CNS. Although lidocaine-associated CNS effects can be seen with other local anesthetics, lidocaine is far more common as the causative drug, and this relates to its rapid absorption across the blood-brain barrier. The high frequency of toxicity is probably due to a diffuse excitation of neuronal systems and begins as altered behavior.[1] At concentrations less than 6 μg/mL, dizziness, drowsiness, paresthesias, and visual disturbances predominate; confusion, dysarthria, coma, convulsions, cardiac arrhythmias, and respiratory arrest are more often seen at concentrations greater than 6 μg/mL. The toxicity of lidocaine can be viewed as a self-enhancing phenomenon: If administration is not terminated immediately, a marked respiratory acidosis results, which creates more of the active, ionized form of the drug.[114] Treatment focuses on adequate oxygenation and support because the half-life of bolus lidocaine given immediately is 6 to 8 minutes. However, because repeated injections change the kinetics of lidocaine and prolong its half-life to approximately 90 minutes, more long-lasting effects can be seen.[114] Although most reports of adverse reactions involve intravenous lidocaine, toxic signs have also been reported with topical or oral use.

Quinidine

Quinidine is present in the cinchona bark, along with quinine and other alkaloids. Nervous system manifestations are usually not significant, but with overdosage or in susceptible individuals, quinidine causes a type of intoxication similar to that of quinine. The corresponding clinical syndrome, namely cinchonism, is manifested as headache, nausea, vomiting, blurring of vision, transient visual obscurations, and ringing of the ears.[1] The visual symptoms are short lived but can be confused with visual transient ischemic attacks or the visual accompaniments of migraine. More persistent quinidine amblyopia is the result of direct damage to the retinal ganglion cells.[115] Finally, there have been two case reports of dementia associated with chronic quinidine use, which reversed after drug discontinuation.[116]

Dietary Compounds and Miscellaneous Drugs

CAFFEINE

Caffeine and other xanthine derivatives, including aminophylline, are CNS stimulants that excite all levels of the CNS, with the cortex being the most sensitive. Caffeine increases energy metabolism throughout the brain but decreases cerebral blood flow, inducing a relative brain hypoperfusion. The drug activates noradrenaline neurons and may act as a second messenger at dopamine receptors to affect the local release of dopamine.[117] Mobilization of intracellular calcium and inhibition of specific phosphodiesterases occurs at high, nonphysiological concentrations of caffeine. The most likely mechanism of action of methylxanthine is the antagonism at the level of adenosine receptors.

Caffeine's psychostimulant action on humans is often subtle and difficult to detect. Its effects on learning, memory, performance, and coordination are related to methylxanthine-induced arousal, vigilance, and fatigue. An increased awareness of the environment or hyperesthesia may be an unpleasant experience to some patients. The patient becomes loquacious and restless and often complains of ringing in the ears and giddiness. In high doses, xanthines affect the spinal cord, resulting in increased reflex excitability, tremulous extremities, and tense muscles.[1] Caffeine clearly alters sleep patterns, and if taken within 1 hour of attempted sleep, it increases sleep latency, decreases total sleep time, and worsens the subject's estimate of sleep quality. Less time is spent in stage 3 and 4 sleep and more in stage 2 sleep. Xanthine-associated seizures are seen as a complication of aminophylline therapy, especially when the drug is administered intravenously. They are usually generalized but can be focal. Cessation of the use of products containing caffeine can cause a withdrawal syndrome that includes headaches, drowsiness, fatigue, decreased performance, and, in some instances, nausea and vomiting. These symptoms begin within 12 to 24 hours after the last use of caffeine, peak at 20 to 48 hours, and last approximately 1 week.[118] Excessive caffeine ingestion can cause low serum potassium levels. Caffeine-induced hypokalemia resulted in paralysis in a pregnant woman, which resolved after potassium supplementation and decrease in caffeine intake.[119]

NICOTINE

Nicotine increases circulating levels of norepinephrine and epinephrine, and it stimulates the release of striatal dopamine. It exerts stimulant effects through specific nicotinic receptors, whose activation may facilitate dopaminergic transmission centrally.[120] Nicotine has been reported to affect a number of neurological diseases, such as spinocerebellar degeneration, multiple system atrophy, multiple sclerosis, tic disorders, parkinsonism, and myoclonic epilepsy.[121]

Nicotine, despite being a powerful stimulant, has no major therapeutic application. Unaccustomed smoking may elicit transient nystagmus, dizziness, unsteadiness, and nausea. Nystagmography and posturography performed in nonsmokers or occasional smokers has found multidirectional nystagmus (mainly horizontal or upbeat), associated with significant increase in postural sway.[122] Its high toxicity and presence in tobacco smoke give nicotine a considerable medical importance. Clinically, tremors and convulsions are major neurological signs of nicotine intoxication. Respiration is stimulated, and vomiting is induced. Nicotine also has marked antidiuretic activity resulting from direct hypothalamic stimulation. If nicotine is acutely ingested, it can be fatal at approximately 60 mg of the base product. Autonomic overactivity with dilated pupils, irregular pulse, sweating, and muscle twitching are characteristic signs of nicotine toxicity. Coma may supervene rapidly, although convulsions are usually not present. If death occurs, it is due to paralysis of respiratory muscles. Cardiac arrhythmias are significant and are another potential cause of demise.[1] Chronic intoxication due to nicotine, consisting of nausea, vomiting, dizziness, and prostration, occurs among tobacco pickers or croppers. The illness lasts intermittently between 12 and 14 hours and clears, only to recur when workers return to work. There are no mortalities or long-term sequelae, however. During the 1973 harvesting season, an estimated 9 percent of the 60,000 tobacco growers in North Carolina reported illnesses. Ingestion of leaves from the tree tobacco plant (*Nicotiana glauca*) has been reported to result in severe muscle weakness, bulbar palsies, flexor muscle spasms, hypertension, nausea, vomiting, and respiratory compromise.[123]

VITAMINS

These vital trace substances are generally associated with vitamin deficiency syndromes, but because health enthusiasm has reached passionate proportions for many individuals, physicians are encountering neurotoxic syndromes from overdosage. The first recognized toxicity of vitamins was related to the fat-soluble vitamins, but water-soluble vitamins have been found to be harmful at times when they are ingested in large quantities.

Vitamin A

Vitamin A toxicity results in a syndrome of increased ICP, headaches, blurred vision, and cranial nerve VI palsy. On funduscopic examination, gradual papilledema develops.[124, 125] The mechanism whereby increased ICP develops is not known, although biochemically, the vitamin stimulates the synthesis of glycoproteins and mucopolysaccharides, which may alter fluid balance centrally. The generally recommended daily vitamin A allowance is 5000 IU, and toxicity occurs with intake as little as four times that dose.[125] Similar toxicity has been noted with one of the vitamin A–like substances, *cis*-retinoic acid, when used for acne in a person taking recommended intakes of vitamin A.[125] In addition there is considerable evidence of the teratogenic effects of vitamin A in the mouse, rat, hamster, and guinea pig. Malformations include cleft palate, fused ribs, spina bifida, meningocele, hydronephrosis, and heart and genitourinary abnormalities.[124]

Vitamin D

Massive amounts of vitamin D mobilize bone calcium and phosphorus. Where there is bone demineralization and degeneration, nerve root and spinal cord compression can occur. Meningeal symptoms and trigeminal neuralgia are two additional reported findings without clear pathogenesis. Trigeminal neuralgia may relate to bony foraminal changes. Alterations in the calcium balance in the form of hypercalcemia can produce metastatic calcifications in the brain with resultant mental retardation or a clinical picture of generalized weakness, muscle aches, cramps, and mild metabolic encephalopathy.[125] When renal impairment occurs, progressive secondary encephalopathy, not directly related to the vitamin, develops. Vitamin D, like vitamin A, is a teratogen, and when the vitamin is consumed in large amounts by pregnant women, it can produce specific abnormalities of the facies, brain, heart, and kidney of the fetus.[125]

Vitamin E

Excessive vitamin E ingestion may produce subtle signs and symptoms of toxicity, such as easy fatigability, muscle weakness, headache, and delayed wound healing. Symptoms usually disappear with cessation of excessive intake. Increased bleeding tendencies have also been reported with large amounts of vitamin E, but no intracranial bleeding has been reported as resulting from it. No toxic effects have been reported at doses of 800 IU daily.[125] Even with supraclinical doses, associated with high levels of plasma tocopherol, ventricular CSF levels are exceedingly low.[126]

Thiamine

Effects of excess thiamine on the CNS include nervousness, convulsions, headache, weakness, trembling, and neuromuscular paralysis.[124] The decreased use of thiamine, especially parenterally for various functional disorders, appears to have resulted in a reduction of toxic reactions.

Thiamine deficiency results in Wernicke's encephalopathy, manifesting with ophthalmoplegia or nystagmus, ataxia and confusion, or mild memory impairment (see Chapter 40). It can therefore mimic brain stem stroke.[127] Thiamine deficiency has also been reported to manifest as polyneuropathy[128] or chorea.[129] Iatrogenic causes include total parenteral nutrition, drastic weight-reducing diet, hemodialysis, colonic surgery, or gastrectomy.[130–132] MRI can demonstrate high-signal lesions on T2 in the diencephalon, mesencephalon, as well as enhancing lesions of the floor of the hypothalamus.[133]

Pyridoxine

Pyridoxine, previously considered benign, has been found to have direct toxic effects on the peripheral nervous system. Animals treated with high doses of pyridoxine develop vacuolation and degeneration of dorsal root and ganglion cells, along with a widespread degeneration of sensory nerve fibers. When consumed in daily doses of 2 g or more, it has been reported to produce a syndrome consisting of difficulty walking with lightning-like dysesthesias in the back. Numbness of the extremities occurs, and most important, facial dysesthesias, so uncommon with most toxic neuropathies other than trichloroethane, quickly develop. Areflexia, stocking-and-glove sensory loss, and profound sensory ataxia with preserved strength are typical. On EMG, marked slowing of the sensory nerve conduction is seen with normal motor conduction.[1, 125] Treatment consists of cessation of pyridoxine, and in some cases there is a dramatic, although often slow, recovery.

When low to moderate doses of pyridoxine are added to the diet of a parkinsonian patient receiving levodopa without carbidopa supplementation (e.g., Sinemet), it will precipitiously cause an exacerbation of the disease. Pyridoxine is a cofactor for dopa decarboxylase and enhances the systemic conversion of dopa to dopamine: Because dopamine cannot cross the blood-brain barrier, this enhanced peripheral synthesis of dopamine in fact diminishes central delivery of dopa for effective antiparkinsonian therapy. When sufficient carbidopa is added to levodopa (usually at least 100 mg/d), this pyridoxine toxicity is probably insignificant.

MONOSODIUM GLUTAMATE

In 1968, Kowk, a Chinese physician, described a transient neurological syndrome that occurred when he ate at American-Chinese restaurants. He suggested that monosodium glutamate could be the provoking agent because this product is used widely in Chinese restaurants to enhance the flavor of food. The pathophysiology of the syndrome has been suggested to relate to glutamate. As an excitatory agent, glutamate may alter synaptic transmission. Some authors suggest that the symptoms of monosodium glutamate syndrome may relate to cholinergic overstimulation or non-neurological vascular mechanisms. The syndrome has three major symptoms, occurring within 15 minutes after ingestion of Chinese food and lasting approximately 1 hour: a dysesthetic facial pressure, burning dysesthesias over the trunk, and chest pain. Headache, which may be migrainous in quality, is more frequently seen in patients with a prior history of headaches. Other vague symptoms such as malaise and light-headedness may accompany the triad. It is not fully established that monosodium glutamate is, in fact, the causative agent. Therefore, important contributing influences may also be the vehicle, whether the subject has been fasting, and whether a load of carbohydrate accompanies the ingestion of monosodium glutamate.[1]

SEX HORMONES AND CONTRACEPTIVE AGENTS

Female hormones in the form of oral contraceptives or postmenopausal replacement therapy have become widely prescribed. It is clear that oral contraceptives increase by three to eight times the risk of stroke in women taking them. Oral contraceptive–associated strokes can occur in any vascular distribution. Factors predisposing to cerebrovascular disease in women on birth control pills include the use of compounds containing high levels of estrogen, multiparity, and a change in migraine headache pattern. Of probable but less certain importance are previous thrombotic or embolic disease and hypertension. Inherited resistance to activated protein C, which is caused by a single factor V gene mutation, is a frequent risk factor for thrombosis. Activated protein C resistance was found to be highly prevalent in women with a history of thromboembolic complications during pregnancy or use of oral contraceptives. The gene defect is common in the general population, and the question is raised as to whether it would be reasonable to perform general screening for activated protein C resistance early during pregnancy or before prescription of oral contraceptives.[134]

Chorea is another serious problem related to oral contraceptives. The involuntary movements appear days or weeks after starting birth control pills and may be more frequent in patients with a prior history of Syndenham's chorea. The chorea starts abruptly and may involve only one side of the body.[135] A similar phenomenon occasionally occurs during pregnancy when a woman develops severe involuntary movements that spontaneously resolve when the pregnancy ends (chorea gravidarum). Birth control chorea may disappear within 48 hours of cessation of the medication, although the abatement can take longer.

Whereas pseudotumor cerebri can occur in patients taking oral contraceptives, other conditions that may cause blurring of the optic disc are papilledema related to venous sinus obstruction or retrobulbar optic neuritis, which also occurs in patients on birth control pills. Vascular headaches may also appear for the first time or suddenly change in pattern when oral contraceptives are started. Common migraine may become classic migraine, with patients experiencing symptoms or signs of focal cerebral dysfunction at the onset of the headache. In cases in which migraines either appear for the first time, increase in frequency, or become focal, cessation of oral conraceptives is suggested. On the other hand, a subgroup of headache patients find relief of headache pain while taking oral contraceptives. These headaches may have a close relationship to menstruation, and while on the oral contraceptives, the patient has minimal pain.

CHELATING AGENTS

2,3,Dimercaptol-1-propranol

2,3,Dimercaptol (British antilewisite [BAL]) was synthesized during World War II as an antidote for arsenic-containing lewisite gas. This compound has also been found to be effective against the toxic manifestations of arsenic, mercury, gold, antimony, and other heavy metals. With doses of 2.5 mg/kg of body weight, toxic symptoms develop in less than 1 percent of individuals; with twice that dose, there is a 50 to 60 percent increase in the occurrence of intoxication. Symptoms appear within 10 to 20 minutes after injection of the drug and subside within 50 to 90 minutes. The usual reaction consists of headache, burning sensations in the mouth and eyes, muscular aches, paresthesias, pain in the teeth, lacrimation, salivation, rhinorrhea, and profuse sweating. Restlessness, anxiety, and general agitation may also develop, with progression in some instances to generalized convulsions and stupor. Abdominal pain, apprehension, blepharospasm, piloerection, tachycardia, and palpitations may also occur. Because of the transient nature of the toxic symptoms, no treatment is needed in BAL poisoning. Twenty-five milligrams of ephedrine sulfate given before the injection of BAL may lessen the incidence of toxic reactions.[1]

Penicillamine

The most commonly encountered neurotoxic effect of penicillamine is loss or abnormality of taste, which has been correlated with high doses and long duration of therapy.[1] Hypogeusia occurs in 25 to 30 percent of patients at doses of 1 g daily within 6 weeks. It may be reversible by decreasing the dosage or discontinuing the drug and may not occur at all in dosages of 500 mg or less. Zinc infiltration of taste receptors has been postulated as causing the hypogeusia induced by penicillamine.

Dermatomyositis and polymyositis characterized by typical tender proximal muscle weakness with elevation of muscle enzymes may occur during penicillamine therapy. Another neurological side effect of penicillamine therapy, especially in rheumatoid arthritis patients, is a myasthenic syndrome. This can start as ptosis, diplopia, or dysphagia but progresses to generalized weakness if early signs go undetected. The edrophonium test usually confirms the clinical suspicion, and laboratory studies demonstrate autoantibodies to acetylcholine receptors. Withdrawal of the drug and treatment with cholinesterase inhibitors reverse the weakness over several months.[136]

CHOLESTEROL-LOWERING AGENTS

Clofibrate

Clofibrate, an aromatic monocarboxylic acid, is capable of inducing myotonia in humans and experimental animals, and this is clinically significant because it is widely used to reduce serum triglyceride levels. The mechanism by which it induces myotonia is believed to be through a decrease in chloride conductance.

Lovastatin and Pravastatin

Lovastatin and pravastatin are HMG-CoA reductase inhibitors that are effective cholesterol-lowering agents used in the treatment of hypercholesterolemia. They can induce myotonia by blocking chloride channels on the muscle membrane.[137] Lipid-lowering agents can also cause a myopathy.

TABLE 55–11. Lipid-Lowering Agents Associated with Myopathy

3-Hydroxy-3-Methylglutaryl Coenzyme A (HMG-CoA) Reductase Inhibitors
Lovastatin (Mevacor)
Pravastatin (Pravachol)
Simvastatin (Zocor)
Atorvastatin (Lipitor)

Fibric Acid Derivatives
Benzafibrate
Clofibrate
Fenofibrate
Gemfibrozil (Lopid)

Niacin

The risk of myopathy is highest when multiple lipid-lowering agents are used together and can be as high as 5 percent. Clinically, patients have myalgias, elevated CK levels, and proximal weakness. Recovery is typical after discontinuation of the offending medications. Table 55–11 lists the lipid-lowering agents associated with myopathy.[138, 139]

Neurological Sequelae of Diagnostic and Therapeutic Procedures

CORONARY ARTERY BYPASS GRAFT SURGERY

Coronary artery bypass graft (CABG) surgery is the most frequently performed cardiac surgery in North America, with nearly 400,000 procedures performed annually in the United States and Canada.[140] Early retrospective studies of open heart surgery found that stroke and anoxic encephalopathy were common postoperative neurological complications, occurring in more than 20 percent of patients. Improvement in surgery and extracorporeal circulation may have initially reduced the frequency of permanent, disabling neurological sequelae. Nevertheless, subsequent prospective studies have shown that neurological complications account for the major adverse sequelae of this procedure. Because these problems can be severe, they must be taken into account when decisions are weighed as to whether medical or surgical therapy would be more appropriate in a given case.

Central Nervous System Complications

Stroke as a complication of CABG procedures occurs in 0.9 to 5.9 percent of cases.[140] Off-pump CABG has been reported to carry a smaller risk for stroke.[141] Most territorial infarcts result from macroemboli from diseased valves, left ventricular thrombus, or atheromatous emboli from a rigid ascending aorta. Stroke occurs more frequently with valvular heart surgery than with CABG operations. A permanent neurological disability after valve replacement occurs in 5 to 10 percent of patients. In contrast, the risk of a severe disability complicating CABG surgery is less than 2 to 5 percent.[142, 143] The difference is due to the greater risk of cardiac macroemboli with operations that require opening of the heart chambers. Removal or repair of diseased, calcified mitral or aortic valves is associated with the dispersion of tissue and surgical debris in the cardiac chambers. Extracranial carotid artery disease is often suggested as an important cause of stroke during CABG surgery. This theory proposes that severe carotid occlusive disease, combined with intraoperative hypotension, results in cerebral ischemia. However, most perioperative strokes occur in the absence of carotid occlusive disease or have their onset in the postoperative period. Most studies have failed to demonstrate a correlation between perioperative stroke and asymptomatic carotid artery stenosis. Nevertheless, it is common practice in some hospitals to perform a prophylactic staged or combined carotid endarterectomy in asymptomatic patients discovered to have carotid stenosis.[142] Because the majority of patients undergoing combined carotid endarterectomy and CABG have asymptomatic carotid stenosis, one has to take into consideration the added stroke risk from carotid stenosis.[144] Additional intracranial carotid artery disease may be an independent factor for stroke after CABG, and, therefore, a comprehensive evaluation of the arterial tree to delineate the risk assessment for CABG surgery is warranted.[145] Although CABG surgery frequently results in a tendency for bleeding (as a result of heparin administration, low fibrinogen levels, and thrombocytopenia induced by hemodilution and sequestration) and occasional disseminated intravascular coagulation, intracranial hemorrhage is an infrequent cause of stroke.[142]

Attempts to prevent neurological sequelae after cardiac surgery have focused on improved surgical and cardiopulmonary bypass techniques, as well as identifying the high-risk patient. Age, preoperative stroke (within 3 months), severe aortic atheroma, opening of cardiac chambers, and sustained mean arterial pressure of less than 30 to 40 mm Hg are probable risk factors for postoperative neurological sequelae. Less proven but still possible risk factors are prolonged cardiopulmonary bypass, severe carotid or cerebrovascular disease, postoperative atrial fibrillation, congestive heart failure, and diabetes mellitus.[140, 142]

Minor cognitive impairment following CABG procedures occurs in as many as 75 percent of patients tested 8 days postoperatively and may be present in up to a third of patients, even 1 year after surgery. These patients show a reduction of one standard deviation in neurocognitive testing postoperatively.[140] In a prospective longitudinal cognitive assessment of 261 patients who underwent CABG, the incidence of cognitive decline was 53 percent at discharge, 24 percent at 6 months, and 42 percent in 5 years.[146] The pathogenesis of the cognitive decline following CABG is believed to be secondary to disseminated brain microemboli occurring during cardiac surgery. An alkaline phosphatase map of the afferent cerebral microvasculature has revealed thousands to millions of focal, small capillary and arteriolar dilatations in patients and dogs who have recently undergone CABG. These capillary and arteriolar dilatations are usually empty, suggesting that gas bubbles or fat emboli are a prime cause. Some authors believe that membrane oxygenators and 40-μ arterial line filters are an essential part of protecting the brain against microembolic events, although this remains to be proved in practice.[140]

The global encephalopathy that can follow heart surgery varies from confusion to coma or a psychotic delirium. Nonmetabolic coma is a rare complication of open heart surgery, occurring in less than 1 percent of patients. It may be due to global anoxia-ischemia, massive stroke, or multiple strokes. On the other hand, the incidence of clinically detectable diffuse encephalopathy varies from 3 to 12 percent.[140] Post-CABG encephalopathy is often multifactorial and can be related to medications, hypoxia, fever, sepsis, metabolic derangements, hemodynamic instability, and ICU psychosis. These patients may be slow to emerge from anesthesia, are often agitated or restless, and have poor visual fixation, small reactive pupils, and, occasionally, Babinski's sign. Improvement usually occurs during the first postoperative week. In otherwise uncomplicated cardiac surgery, disseminated microemboli during extracorporeal circulation may be the cause of this encephalopathy.[142] Seizures occur in less than 1 percent of patients and can accompany coma, encephalopathy, or delirium, or they may occur independently. The vast majority occur within the first 24 hours after surgery.

Peripheral Nervous System Complications

In a prospective analysis of 412 consecutive patients undergoing coronary bypass surgery, 55 (13 percent) developed new peripheral nervous system complications postoperatively.[147] The most common complication was brachial plexopathy, occurring in 23 patients. Most frequently the lower trunk or the medial cord of the brachial plexus was involved. The plexus injuries may be due to torsional traction, compression, or cannulation of the jugular vein. Male gender and hypothermia during surgery were associated with an increased risk. The usual clinical presentation involves intrinsic hand weakness and a decreased or absent triceps reflex. Sensory loss is sometimes present in the affected hand; some patients have prominent pain, and a minority of them have Horner's syndrome. Most brachial plexus injuries are reversible within 1 to 3 months, implicating conduction block as the primary pathophysiological mechanism. Such injuries may be prevented by minimizing the opening of the sternal retractor, placing the retractor in the most caudal location, and avoiding asymmetrical traction. Unilateral phrenic nerve injuries with hemidiaphragmatic paralysis occur in at least 10 percent of patients during open heart surgery and can be manifested as atelectasis or persistent singultus. Finally, mononeuropathies resulting from compression or trauma during surgery may involve the accessory, facial, lateral femoral cutaneous, peroneal, radial, recurrent laryngeal, saphenous, and ulnar nerves.[147]

CARDIAC CATHETERIZATION

CNS complications of cardiac catheterization are rare and occur in 0.1 to 1.0 percent of patients. The majority of these complications are focal neurological deficits, which are believed to result secondary to embolism from either manipulation of the guidewire or catheter flushing in the ascending aorta when the brachial route is chosen.[142] Resolution of the focal deficits within 48 hours occurs in approximately half of the patients. In one big series, the carotid circulation accounted for 30 to 40 percent of focal deficits and consisted of hemiparesis, hemisensory deficits, and dysphasia. The vertebrobasilar circulation accounted for 60 percent of the deficits, with combinations of cortical blindness, hemianopic visual field defects, and intrinsic brain stem signs.[142]

TABLE 55–12. Neurological Complications of Cardiac Transplantation

Early Onset (First 2 Weeks)
Anoxic-ischemic encephalopathy
Brachial plexopathy/mononeuropathy
Cerebrovascular disease
Metabolic encephalopathy/sepsis
Psychosis
Seizures
Vascular headache

Late Onset
Cerebrovascular disorders
Cyclosporine/prednisone toxicity
Lymphoma
Metabolic encephalopathy/sepsis
Opportunistic infections
Psychosis
Seizures

PERCUTANEOUS TRANSLUMINAL CORONARY ANGIOPLASTY

Focal neurological complications following percutaneous transluminal coronary angioplasty occur in 0.2 to 0.3 percent of patients and are similar to those seen in catheterization patients.[142]

CARDIAC TRANSPLANTATION

Neurological complications recognized in the first weeks after cardiac transplantation are similar to those seen after routine CABG surgery or heart valve repair (Table 55–12). They include cerebrovascular disease, anoxic-ischemic encephalopathy, seizures, and peripheral nerve disorders.[148] Vascular headaches accompanied by nausea and vomiting may occur the first week after transplantation and are felt to be associated with a rapid shift from low preoperative to high postoperative mean arterial pressures. Psychotic behavior with hallucinations, delusional thought process, and disorganized behavior can occur during the first 2 weeks after transplantation or as a late complication. When it occurs in the first 48 hours and is accompanied by disorientation and impaired memory, it probably represents a behavioral response to intraoperative cerebral ischemia-hypoxia. If it begins 2 to 5 days after surgery, memory is preserved, and there is rapid resolution with environmental reorientation, then a multifactorial ICU psychosis may be present. If psychotic behavior presents 2 to 4 weeks following transplantation, then a full evaluation for an opportunistic infection is indicated.[148]

Immunosuppression remains the major cause of late neurological complications after cardiac transplantation. Opportunistic infections can occur as early as 2 weeks after surgery and immunosuppression, but usually there is an interval of at least a month. Focal meningoencephalitis or brain abscess, meningitis, and encephalitis are three common presentations of infections in cardiac transplant recipients. *Aspergillus*, *Toxoplasma gondii*, *Cryptococcus*, *Listeria*, *Candida*, and *Nocardia* are the most frequent nonviral organisms. The most frequent viral infections are caused by the herpesviruses, with cytomegalovirus being the most common.[142, 148] Aseptic meningitis has been reported in 5 percent of patients receiving OKT3 and presents as mental status and behavioral changes.[142]

The use of cyclosporine since the early 1980s has allowed significant lowering of corticosteroid requirements and has reduced the frequency of its side effects. There have been a number of neurological effects ascribed to cyclosporine, however, including tremor, lowered seizure threshold, confusion, muscle weakness, ataxia, paresthesias, visual hallucinations, and a leukoencephalopathy with cortical blindness.[142, 148] These neurotoxic side effects rapidly remit with reduction of the dose of cyclosporine. When seizures occur and anticonvulsants are indicated, selection of the best agent may be difficult because phenytoin, phenobarbital, and carbamazepine can decrease the blood levels of cyclosporine. Finally, immunosuppression predisposes the patient to the development of primary or secondary lymphoma of the brain.

RADIATION DAMAGE

Therapeutic radiation may affect the nervous system in two settings: (1) damage to neural structures or blood vessels when they are included in the radiation port, whether the cancer undergoing radiation therapy is within or outside the nervous system (Table 55–13); (2) secondary nervous system involvement when radiation causes new tumors to develop or when radiation damages endocrine organs that are necessary

TABLE 55–13. Radiation-Induced Injury: Direct Damage to the CNS

Time after Radiation	Clinical Findings	Mechanisms
Acute (minutes to days)	Brain Increased intracranial pressure	Vasogenic edema
Early delayed (weeks to months)	Brain Diffuse: somnolence/lethargy Focal: simulates recurrent tumor Spinal cord Lhermitte's sign	Demyelination
Late delayed (months to years)	Brain Diffuse: dementia Focal: simulates recurrent tumor Spinal cord Transverse myelopathy Motor neuron syndrome	Glial and vascular damage

for nervous system function. The presence and severity of these reactions are governed by a number of factors, including the total radiation dose, the radiation fraction size, and the volume of tissue irradiated. The age of the patient, the presence of pre-existing brain injury by tumor or surgery, infection, vascular disease due to hypertension or diabetes mellitus, and chemotherapy may influence the susceptibility of the patient to injury as well.[149]

Primary Brain Damage

Injury to the brain resulting from the radiosensitivity of normal brain tissue encompassed in the treatment volume can be classified as acute, early delayed, and late delayed reactions. Acute reactions occur during or immediately after the course of radiation therapy and typically develop in patients with increased ICP from primary or secondary brain tumors, particularly in the absence of corticosteroid coverage. Clinically, patients present with symptoms suggesting increased ICP or exacerbation of pre-existing neurological symptoms or signs.[150] The pathogenesis of the disorder is unknown, although it is thought to be due to radiation-induced edema secondary to blood-brain barrier breakdown. Acute symptoms are uncommon with dose-fractionation schedules consisting of 180 to 200 rad/d, given 5 days per week to a total dose of 6000 rad. Daily doses of up to 600 rad are well tolerated, but higher daily dose fractions should be administered with caution. Acute reactions, when they occur, are usually mild and transient. The preceding situations have two implications for the clinician: First, patients with large brain tumors and signs of increased ICP should not receive more than 200 rad per fraction. Second, all patients undergoing brain radiation should be given dexamethasone, preferably at least 24 hours before starting radiation therapy.

Early delayed reactions occur a few weeks to a few months after radiation. The symptoms often simulate tumor progression, with accentuation of pre-existing signs and symptoms, or may present as somnolence and lethargy without lateralizing signs. The early delayed reaction is transient and usually associated with an uneventful recovery. Rarely, however, it can be fatal. This is more likely to occur following radiation of the posterior fossa resulting in brain stem encephalopathy.[149, 150] Pathologically, there is extensive demyelination with central necrosis, absence of oligodendroglia, and gliosis accompanied by minimal vascular change and preservation of neurons and axons. The pathogenesis of the early delayed reaction is thought to be a temporary inhibition of myelin synthesis due to radiation-induced effects on the oligodendroglial cells. The turnover time of myelin is 5 weeks to 2 months, which corresponds to the latency and recovery time of the syndrome. The main significance of early delayed radiation injury lies in the need to differentiate this condition, which is transient and requires no therapy, from late radiation injury and tumor progression.

Late delayed reactions occur several months to years after treatment. Late delayed injury constitutes the major hazard of CNS exposure to therapeutic radiation. There are several theories as to the pathogenesis of late delayed brain injury. These theories include vascular injury, direct effect on glial cells, or autoimmune demyelination. It is probable that several mechanisms are involved, and the importance of each depends on the radiation dose and the latent interval. Evidence suggests that demyelination is important in the early delayed reaction and that the effect on the small and medium arterioles becomes progressively more important with time. Histologically, the typical lesion is an area of coagulative necrosis in the white matter, with relative sparing of the overlying cortex. Microscopically, the most striking abnormalities are found in blood vessels, with hyalinized thickening and fibrinoid necrosis of the walls often associated with vascular thrombosis, vascular hemorrhages, and accumulation of perivascular fibrinoid material.

There is little information on the incidence of late radiation injury, because there is a paucity of prospective, well-controlled studies. The available data suggest that the risk of injury increases with doses in excess of 6000 rad delivered in 30 fractions over 6 weeks.[150] The daily fraction size in addition to total dose has a substantial effect on the risk of inducing damage to the CNS. Concomitant administration of chemotherapeutic agents may potentiate radiation injury.

In patients who were treated for primary or metastatic brain tumors, symptoms of radiation damage usually recapitulate those of the brain tumor, leading the physician to suspect tumor recurrence. In patients irradiated for head and neck tumors, whose brains were included in the radiation portal, new focal neurological signs are the rule. When injury occurs at the site of an intracerebral tumor, it is not possible to differentiate the effects of radiation from those of residual or recurrent tumor on the basis of CT or angiographic findings. MRI provides no additional information that can be used to differentiate between lesions. In both conditions, an increase in tissue water content causes an increase in mobile proton density and prolongation of T1 and T2 relaxation times. These changes result in decreased signal in T1-weighted images and increased signal in T2-weighted and proton density images. Contrast enhancement, resulting from blood-brain barrier breakdown, can be seen as well. Diffuse white matter injury is seen as periventricular white matter lesions, appearing as high-signal areas on proton density and T2-weighted images. These abnormalities are usually symmetrical and indistinguishable from the deep white matter changes seen in older people with risk factors for cerebral vascular disease.[150, 151] The CT, MRI, and angiographic picture of radiation necrosis cannot be differentiated from tumor recurrence. This differentiation is reliably achieved by fluorodeoxyglucose (FDG [^{18}F]) positron-emission tomography examination, based on the decreased FDG accumulation in an area of necrosis.[152]

Surgical resection of favorably situated focal lesions may result in considerable improvement or in complete recovery from the secondary effects of brain injury. After surgery, improvement most commonly occurs in patients with focal necrosis who have been irradiated for primary extracranial lesions. Resection is of little value in patients with diffuse lesions or brain stem involvement. Corticosteroids may result in improvement or stability of neurological deficit by reducing brain edema, although they cannot reverse the ongoing process.[150] Other agents that have been used in the treatment of radiation necrosis include heparin, coumadin, pentoxyfylline, low-iron diet, desferioxamine, pentobarbital, and hyperbaric oxygen therapy. New agents that are still in different stages of study include cytokine inhibitors, antiapoptotic agents, and drugs preventing radiation-induced loss of endothelial cells when given prior to radiation.[153]

Primary Spinal Cord Damage

Although there are no acute effects of radiation on the spinal cord, early delayed radiation myelopathy is common, especially after radiation of the neck. The patient develops Lhermitte's sign, which persists for weeks and months with spontaneous resolution; the sign is believed to be caused by demyelination of the posterior columns of the spinal cord.

Late delayed radiation myelopathy appears either as progressive myelopathy or a motor neuron syndrome. Radiation myelopathy usually presents as Brown-Séquard syndrome, which progresses to cause paraparesis or quadraparesis over weeks to months. Pathologically, there are areas of necrosis with a predilection for the white matter. Vascular changes are similar to those of the brain and sometimes can result in hemorrhage.[154] The myelogram and MRI are usually normal, although in the acute phase, spinal cord swelling or contrast enhancement of focal lesions may be seen. Motor neuron syndrome characteristically follows pelvic radiation for testicular tumors. This is characterized by muscle weakness, accompanied by atrophy, fasciculations, and areflexia. There are no sensory, sphincter, or sexual changes. The symptoms progress over months to years and eventually stabilize.[150]

Cranial and Peripheral Nerve Damage

Radiation injuries to the cranial and peripheral nervous systems are rare. The risk of brachial plexus injury increases with total dose in excess of 6000 rad, with daily fraction sizes of 200 rad, and with the use of large daily fraction sizes. Optic nerve and chiasmal injury are major risks in patients with pituitary or parapituitary tumors who are treated with high daily dose fractions. In patients with pituitary tumors, the use of fraction sizes of 180 to 200 rad, with the total dose limited to 4500 rad, minimizes the risk of such injury. The retina is sensitive as well, and clinically evident injury may occur with doses as low as 4600 rad when the whole retina is included in the radiation field.[150]

Secondary Involvement of the Nervous System

Secondary involvement of the nervous system following head and neck radiation for tumors not involving the nervous system can result in the development of radiation-induced tumors years to decades later. These radiation-induced tumors can be meningiomas, sarcomas, gliomas, thyroid cancer, and malignant schwannomas. The development of vascular malformations as a complication of radiotherapy is well described in the literature. Lesions of large intracranial or extracranial blood vessels may also follow radiation therapy by years. The supraclinoid portion of the internal carotid artery is particularly vulnerable to the occlusive effects of radiation.

Finally, radiation of the head and neck can result in primary hypothyroidism, hypercalcemic hyperparathyroidism, and hypothalamic-pituitary dysfunction. Radiation-induced hypothyroidism can present as encephalopathy, ataxia, and peripheral neuropathy. Thyroid function should be part of the evaluation of every patient with neurological dysfunction who has undergone prior radiation to the head and neck.

VACCINATIONS

Worldwide vaccination programs have had unparalleled success during this century in reducing the incidence of serious infectious diseases. Neurological sequelae of vaccinations have been reported, although assigning a causative relationship for vaccine injuries is difficult because randomized double-blind placebo-controlled studies have not been systematically conducted. There are five types of vaccines available: whole-killed organisms, live-attenuated viruses, toxoids or components, conjugated vaccines, and recombinant vaccines (Table 55–14).

Whole-Killed Organisms

Vaccines composed of whole-killed organisms include the influenza, poliomyelitis (IPV), pertussis, and rabies vaccines. Administration of the inactive antigens provokes an immune response that creates immunity without causing the disease. Vaccines made from whole-killed organisms may cause a variety of immune-mediated reactions.

Pertussis. Standard pertussis vaccine prepared from killed whole cell *Bordetella pertussis* organisms has been in widespread use since the early 1950s.[155] It has been effective in reducing the incidence of pertussis in the United States to low levels. Despite marked reduction in disease, the use of the vaccine has caused concern because of questions of encephalopathy resulting in permanent brain damage or death. Pertussis vaccine is ordinarily combined with diphtheria and tetanus toxoids (DPT), and all reported side effects are based on DPT and not pertussis vaccine alone. The Child Neurology Society, after reviewing the reports linking the whole-cell pertussis vaccine and neurological illness, has issued a consensus statement concluding that the pertussis vaccine is associated with a short-term increased risk of seizures, most of which are febrile seizures, and complete recovery is expected. The risk for febrile seizures is elevated on the day of receipt of DPT vaccine and 8 to 14 days after the receipt of measles-mumps-rubella vaccine, but these risks do not appear to be associated with any long-term adverse consequences.[156] In regard to encephalopathy, the report concluded: "At present, there is no means by which a diagnosis of pertussis vaccine–encephalopathy can be established in an individual basis."

Influenza. Annual vaccination against influenza is constituted depending on the prevalent strains that are expected to appear in the United States the following year. A small

TABLE 55–14. **Types of Vaccines**

Killed organisms	Toxoids (Components)
Influenza	Acellular pertussis
Japanese encephalitis	Diphtheria
Pertussis	Tetanus
Poliomyelitis (IPV)	Conjugated
	Haemophilus influenza type B
Live-attenuated viruses	Recombinant
Measles	Hepatitis B
Mumps	Smallpox
Poliomyelitis (OPV)	
Rubella	
Varicella	

increase in the incidence of Guillain-Barré syndrome has been reported after the 1976 vaccination against the so-called swine flu. The significance of this association was initially questioned but later confirmed.[157]

Inactivated Poliomyelitis Vaccine. IPV was introduced in 1955, is still preferred in most European countries, and is devoid of neurological complications. In spite of this safety, the vaccine was not used in the United States until recently. Since the risk of contracting poliomyelitis is extremely low in the United States and all of the new cases are associated with the oral poliomyelitis vaccine, IPV has again become the vaccination of choice.

Rabies. The rabies vaccine used in the United States is both safe and efficacious. It is prepared by inactivated rabies virus grown on human diploid cells. Unfortunately, many underdeveloped countries prepare the vaccine by growing inactivated virus in the brains or spinal cords of mature animals. The myelin basic protein present in this vaccine (Semple) is responsible for encephalomyelitis and polyneuritis.

Live-Attenuated Viruses

Vaccines composed of live-attenuated viruses include the measles, mumps, rubella, oral poliomyelitis, and varicella vaccines. They are intended to cause an asymptomatic infection. The immunity provided by these vaccines is lifelong, but they can occasionally cause symptomatic infection, sometimes with associated neurological involvement.

Measles-Mumps-Rubella (MMR). MMR vaccine may cause fever, rash, conjunctivitis, or other measle-like symptoms in the second week after immunization. A double-blind placebo-controlled crossover study of the MMR vaccine performed in twins living in the same household found that statistically significant differences between placebo and vaccine occur during the second week and can be attributed to the development of measles infection.[158] Seizures can also occur during the second week following immunization and are almost always simple febrile seizures.[156] The evidence is inadequate to accept or reject a causal relationship between encephalopathy, subacute sclerosing panencephalitis, residual seizure disorder, sensorineural deafness, optic neuritis, transverse myelitis, multiple sclerosis, Guillain-Barré syndrome, inflammatory bowel disease, type 1 diabetes mellitus, idiopathic thrombocytopenic purpura, rheumatoid arthritis, or other autoimmunce disease and MMR.[159–162]

Reports have suggested an association with mumps vaccines and aseptic meningitis and sensorineural deafness. This is probably associated with the Urabe mumps strain, which is not used in the United States. Finally, with regard to the rubella vaccine, the Institute of Medicine concluded that there is insufficient evidence to indicate a causal relationship between the rubella vaccine and radiculoneuritis and other neuropathies.[163]

There has been an attempt to associate a recent increase in the incidence of autism to MMR vaccination. Nevertheless, there is no evidence that any correlation exists between the prevalence of MMR vaccination and the rapid increase in the risk of autism over time.[164–167]

Oral Poliomyelitis Vaccine. The oral poliomyelitis vaccine (OPV) consists of live-attenuated virus, and after its introduction in 1961, it replaced IPV in the United States because of ease of administration, combined intestinal as well as serum immunity, and spread from immunized to nonimmunized persons. The main disadvantage of OPV is that it can cause paralytic disease in 1 of 2.5 million doses distributed. At present, all cases of poliomyelitis in the United States are vaccine related.[159] High-risk groups are infants receiving their first dose and immunocompromised individuals who either receive the vaccine or are in contact with vaccine recipients. Finally, evidence favors acceptance of a causal relationship between OPV and Guillain-Barré syndrome.[159]

Toxoids

Toxoid vaccines include tetanus and diphtheria and acellular pertussis. They are denatured bacterial toxins that prevent disease but not infection.

Tetanus and Diphtheria. Adverse reactions to diphtheria and tetanus immunizations cannot be assessed separately because they are always given together. Several reports have implicated DT in causing polyradiculoneuritis, brachial plexus neuritis, and acute transverse myelitis. The Institute of Medicine has reported that current evidence favors acceptance of a causal relationship between diphtheria and tetanus toxoid and Guillain-Barré syndrome and brachial neuritis.[159] It has also concluded that evidence rejects a causal relationship between diphtheria and tetanus toxoid and encephalopathy and infantile spasms.[159]

Acellular Pertussis. Acellular pertussis vaccines contain two or more denatured elements of *Bordetella pertussis* required for immunity but do not contain endotoxin. In a recent study, the five-component acellular pertussis vaccine has been found to have a favorable safety profile with sustained protection against pertussis. The two-component acellular vaccine and the whole-cell vaccine were less efficacious.[168]

OBSTETRICAL AND GYNECOLOGICAL PROCEDURES AND SURGERY

The peripheral nervous system can be injured in a variety of ways during pregnancy and delivery. Injury can occur at the level of the nerve roots, lumbosacral plexus, or individual peripheral nerves (Table 55–15).

The risk of injury to spinal cord or nerve roots from spinal or epidural anesthesia used for delivery is 0.1 percent or less. Various types of injury that have been described include epidural hematomas, chemical radiculitis or arachnoiditis, direct needle injury to the root, or spinal infarction secondary to hypotension.[169]

Lumbosacral plexus injuries occur during labor or delivery and can be easily confused with a herniated disc. They occur in fetal-pelvic disproportion or in primiparous patients with large babies that necessitate midforceps delivery. The anterior division of the lumbosacral trunk (L4 or L5) is compressed by the fetal head or the obstetric forceps against the pelvic brim. These patients often complain of buttock or leg pain, which intensifies with uterine contractions. A footdrop or weakness of the tibialis anterior is the most common finding.[170]

A number of isolated nerve lesions may occur as a complication of obstetrical maneuvers. The obturator nerve may be injured when the patient is in the lithotomy position,

TABLE 55–15. **Neurological Complications of Obstetrical and Gynecological Procedures and Surgery**

Site of Injury	Mechanism	Symptoms
Spinal cord and nerve roots	Spinal or epidural anesthesia (hematoma, chemical injury, infarction)	Myelopathy/radiculopathy
Lumbosacral plexus	Disporportion, large babies, midforceps use	Buttock/leg pain weakness: footdrop
Genitofemoral nerve	Pelvic surgery	Sensory loss: labia, femoral triangle
Ilioinguinal and iliohypogastric nerves	Surgery with low transverse abdominal incision	Sensory loss: suprapubic area, upper-medial thigh, anterior labial majus
Lateral femoral cutaneous	Inguinal lymphadenectomy	Sensory loss: anterior-lateral thigh
Pudendal nerve	Radical pelvic surgery	Sensory loss: clitoris, perineum, anus, incontinence
Obturator nerve	Lithotomy position, at the obturator foramen, pelvic surgery	Sensory loss: medial thigh, weakness: thigh adduction
Femoral nerve	Stirrups with thighs flexed and abducted and hip flexed and externally rotated, retractors	Sensory loss: anterior thigh, weakness: thigh flexion, reflex loss: patellar
Sciatic nerve	Stirrups, intramuscular injections, sacroiliac fossa bleeding	Sensory loss: lateral leg, foot weakness: foot flexion or extension, knee flexion, reflex loss: ankle
Common peroneal nerve	Lithotomy position, at the head of the fibula	Sensory loss: lateral and dorsum of the foot, weakness: footdrop and inversion

because of angulation as the nerve leaves the obturator foramen. Clinically, the patient has weakness of adduction of the thigh and sensory loss over the medial thigh.

The femoral nerve is injured when the thighs are markedly flexed and abducted or the hips are abducted and externally rotated. Results of the injury include impaired extension of the knee, impaired flexion of the thigh, sensory loss over the anterior thigh, and loss of the patellar reflex.

The saphenous nerve can be injured by pressure from leg braces when the patient is in the lithotomy position. The sciatic nerve can be injured when the patient is placed in stirrups on the obstetrical table or with a misplaced deep intramuscular injection. Clinically, the patient experiences sensory loss over the lateral leg and the whole foot, weakness of both dorsal and plantar flexion of the foot and of the extension of the knee, and loss of the ankle jerk. Isolated tibial injury is uncommon. The common peroneal is usually compressed at the head of the fibula from the leg braces with the patient in the lithotomy position.[170] Clinically, the patient has footdrop and inversion and sensory loss on the lateral aspect and the dorsum of the foot.

Nerve injury is an infrequent complication of gynecological surgery (see Table 55–15). The most frequently reported injury has been to the femoral nerve, followed by the sciatic and the obturator nerves.[171] Stretch, compression, ligation, and transection are the most commonly reported intraoperative precipitators of symptoms, and postoperative scar formation may lead to entrapment symptoms at anatomical locations remote from the procedure.

Mechanisms of femoral neuropathy include self-retaining retractors, especially in thin patients with low transverse incisions and deep retractor blades; hyperflexion of the thigh; and control of bleeding deep in the pelvis and in the region of the psoas muscle. The clinical presentation is as described earlier.

Sciatic nerve injury can occur as a result of sacroiliac fossa bleeding, intramuscular injections, and the sacrospinus vaginal vault suspension procedure. Obturator nerve injury has been associated with pelvic surgery and specifically with pelvic lymphadenectomy.

Other less commonly encountered nerve injuries that may occur in association with gynecological surgery include the genitofemoral nerve, which may be injured during pelvic lymphadenectomy, and can result in numbness or tingling over the labia and the skin over the femoral triangle. The ilioinguinal and iliohypogastric nerves may be severed during an operation using a low transverse abdominal incision. The clinical syndrome consists of numbness or tingling over the suprapubic region, the upper medial thigh, and the anterior part of the labium majus. Finally, the lateral femoral cutaneous nerve may be injured during an inguinal lymphadenectomy, and the pudendal nerve may be injured during radical pelvic surgery or during the performance of the sacrospinous vaginal vault suspension. Damage of the lateral femoral cutaneous nerve results in paresthesias over the lateral aspect of the front of the thigh as far as the knee, and damage of the pudendal nerve results in urinary and fecal incontinence and paresthesias of the clitoris, labia, perineum, and anus.

In contrast to brachial plexopathy, radiation-induced neural damage to the lumbosacral plexus is a rare complication. Although a few permanent lumbosacral lesions have been reported in patients treated with conventionally fractionated external beam, this syndrome is more often seen in patients treated with intracavitary irradiation for cervical or endometrial carcinoma.[172]

Careful surgical technique is probably the most important factor in prevention of the preceding complications. In addition, careful placement of the self-retaining retractor and careful positioning of the patient in stirrups is of paramount importance. With mild injuries, the prognosis for recovery is excellent, but recovery may be prolonged and incomplete if axonal degeneration has occurred. Recovery usually takes 4 weeks for the sensory function and 1 to 4 months for the motor function. Physical therapy, splinting or bracing to prevent contractures, and electrical stimulation are the usual treatment modalities used.

CRITICAL ILLNESS POLYNEUROPATHY

The occurrence of muscle weakness in patients with sepsis and multiple organ failure managed in the ICU has been recognized with increasing frequency in the past 15 years. This weakness is due to an axonal polyneuropathy, otherwise called critical illness polyneuropathy. It must be differentiated from myopathy or disturbance of the neuromuscular junction that can also occur in the intensive care setting.[173] Neither the cause nor the exact mechanism of critical illness polyneuropathy has been elucidated. Nutritional, toxic, metabolic, and vascular factors have all been proposed as likely causes, but none has been proved so far.[173]

The difficulty in examining critically ill patients may explain why this complication has only recently been recognized. The presence of encephalopathy or generalized edema can make the clinical diagnosis difficult to obtain. Predominantly proximal weakness can lead to quadriparesis. The facial muscles can be mildly weak, but the muscles of the eyes, tongue, and jaw are relatively spared.[174] Deep tendon reflexes are partially preserved. Nevertheless, the signs of limb weakness and loss of previously elicited tendon reflexes are not present in all patients, even those who are subsequently shown by electrophysiological studies to have a moderately severe polyneuropathy.[174]

Electrophysiological studies demonstrate acute axonal damage to the peripheral nerves. Signs of primary demyelination, such as marked slowing of nerve conduction velocities, prolongation of distal latencies, dispersion of compound muscle action potentials, conduction block, and increased F-wave latencies, are absent even in severe cases of polyneuropathy.[173] Parenchymatous axonal damage and marked neurogenic atrophy are constant features of nerve biopsy.

Before the recognition of critical illness polyneuropathy, these cases were usually misdiagnosed as acute demyelinating Guillain-Barré syndrome. The essentials for diagnosis of Guillain-Barré syndrome (e.g., absent reflexes, albuminocytological dissociation in the CSF, and evidence of demyelination in the electrophysiological studies), however, are not present in most critically ill patients with neuromuscular weaning failure. Furthermore, prolonged neuromuscular blockade following long-term treatment with muscle relaxant drugs, aminoglycoside antibiotics, neuromuscular blocking agents in combination with high-dose corticosteroids for treatment of life-threatening status asthmaticus, and infectious, metabolic, or toxic myopathies or neuropathies should be included in the differential diagnosis of weakness and prolonged dependence on the ventilator.[173, 174]

Sepsis and multiple organ failure still has a high mortality rate, even in fully equipped ICUs. Clinical recovery from the neuropathy is rapid and nearly complete in those patients who survive, although it may appear to be incomplete on electrodiagnostic studies. Thus, neuropathy acquired during critical illness, although causing a delay in weaning from ventilatory support and hospital discharge, does not worsen long-term prognosis.[173]

Reviews and Selected Updates

Armstrong CL, Hunter JV, Ledakis GE, et al: Late Cognitive and radiographic changes related to radiotherapy. Initial perspective findings. Neurology 2002;59:40–48.

Batchelor TT, Taylor LP, Thaler HT, Posner JB: Steroid myopathy in cancer patients. Neurology 1997;48:1234–1238.

Child Neurology Society Consensus Report: Pertussis immunization and the central nervous system. Ann Neurol 1991;29:458–460.

Dashe JF, Pessin MS, Murphy RE, Payne DD: Carotid occlusive disease and the risk of stroke in coronary artery bypass graft surgery. Neurology 1997;49:678–686.

Goetz CG, Kompoliti K, Horn S: Neurotoxic agents. *In* Joynt RJ, Griggs RC (eds): Baker's Clinical Neurology. Philadelphia, Lippincott-Raven, 2002.

Hardman JG, Limbird LE: Goodman and Gilman's The Pharmacological Basis of Therapeutics, 10th ed. New York, McGraw-Hill, 2001.

Piyasirisilp S, Hemachudha T: Neurological adverse events associated with vaccination. Curr Opin Neurol 2002;15:333–338.

References

1. Goetz CG: Neurotoxins in Clinical Practice. New York, Spectrum, 1985.
2. Pacia SV, Devinsky O: Clozapine-related seizures: Experience with 5,629 patients. Neurology 1994;44:2247–2249.
3. Stanfield SC, Privett T: Neuroleptic malignant syndrome associated with olanzapine therapy: A case report. J Emerg Med 2000;19:355–357.
4. Karagianis JL, Phillips LC, Hogan KP, et al: Clozapine-associated neuroleptic malignant syndrome: Two new cases and a review of the literature. Ann Pharmacother 1999;33:623–630.
5. Bajjoka I, Patel T, O'Sullivan T: Risperdone-induced neuroleptic malignant syndrome. Ann Emerg Med 1997;30:698–700.
6. Lang AE, Weiner WJ: Drug-Induced Movement Disorders. Mount Kisco, NY, Futura, 1992.
7. Pappert EJ: Neuroleptic-induced movement disorders: Acute and subacute syndromes. *In* de Wolff FA (ed): Intoxication of the Nervous System, Part II. Amsterdam, Elsevier Science B V, 1994.
8. Kane JM, Woerner M, Borenstein M, et al: Integrating incidence and prevalence of tardive dyskinesia. Psychopharmacol Bull 1986;22:254–258.
9. Rosebush PI, Mazurek MF: Neurologic side effects in neuroleptic-naïve patients treated with haloperidol or risperdone. Neurology 1999;52:782–785.
10. Blackwell B: Adverse effects of antidepressant drugs. Part 1: Monoamine oxidase inhibitors and tricyclics. Drugs 1981;21:201–219.
11. Krishel S, Jackimczyk K: Cyclic antidepressants, lithium, and neuroleptic agents. Pharmacology and toxicology. Emerg Med Clin North Am 1991;9:53–86.
12. Cole JO, Bodkin JA: Antidepressant drug side effects. J Clin Psychiatry 1990;51:21–26.
13. Andrews JM, Nemeroff CB: Contemporary management of depression. Am J Med 1994;97:24S–32S.
14. Carbone JR: The neuroleptic malignant and serotonin syndromes. Emerg Med Clin North Am 2000;18:317–325.
15. Groleau G: Lithium toxicity. Emerg Med Clin North Am 1994;12:511–531.
16. Mangano WE, Montine TJ, Hulette CM: Pathologic assessment of cerebellar atrophy following acute lithium intoxication. Clin Neuropathol 1997;16:30–33.
17. Gudex C: Adverse effects of benzodiazepines. Soc Sci Med 1991;33:587–596.
18. Berthoud MC, Reilly CS: Adverse effects of general anaesthetics. Drug Saf 1992;7:434–459.
19. Marshall BE, Longnecker DE: General anesthetics. *In* Hardman JG, Limbird LE (eds): Goodman and Gilman's The Pharmacological Basis of Therapeutics, 9th ed. New York, McGraw-Hill, 1996, pp 307–330.
20. Sambuughin N, Sei Y, Gallagher KL, et al: North American malignant hyperthermia population: Screening of the ryanodine receptor gene and identification of novel mutations. Anesthesiology 2001;95:594–599.
21. Larach MG, Rosenberg H, Larach DR, Broennle AM: Prediction of malignant hyperthermia susceptibility by clinical signs. Anesthesiology 1987;66:547–550.
22. Brodsky JB, Cohen EN: Adverse effects of nitrous oxide. Med Toxicol 1986;1:362–374.
23. Louis-Ferdinand RT: Myelotoxic, neurotoxic and reproductive adverse effects of nitrous oxide. Adverse Drug React Toxicol Rev 1994;13: 193–206.
24. Kinsella LJ, Green R: "Anesthesia paresthetica": Nitrous oxide–induced cobalamin deficiency. Neurology 1995;45:1608–1610.
25. Catterall W, Mackie K: Local anesthetics. *In* Hardman JG, Limbird LE (eds): Goodman and Gillman's The Pharmacological Basis of Therapeutics, 10th ed. New York, McGraw-Hill, 2001, pp 367–384.

26. Terndrup TE, Walls HC, Mariani PJ, et al: Plasma cocaine and tetracaine levels following application of topical anesthesia in children. Ann Emerg Med 1992;21:162–166.
27. Tipton GA, DeWitt GW, Eisenstein SJ: Topical TAC (tetracaine, adrenaline, cocaine) solution for local anesthesia in children: Prescribing inconsistency and acute toxicity [see comments]. South Med J 1989;82:1344–1346.
28. Reynolds F: Adverse effects of local anaesthetics. Br J Anaesth 1987;59:78–95.
29. Kane RE: Neurologic deficits following epidural or spinal anesthesia. Anesth Analg 1981;60:150–161.
30. Scott DB, Hibbard BM: Serious nonfatal complications associated with extradural block in obstetric practice. Br J Anaesth 1990;64:537–541.
31. Yuen EC, Layzer RB, Weitz SR, Olney RK: Neurologic complications of lumbar epidural anesthesia and analgesia. Neurology 1995;45:1795–1801.
32. Sanders DB, Scoppetta C: The treatment of patients with myasthenia gravis. Neurol Clin 1994;12:343–368.
33. Lacomis D, Samuels MA: Adverse neurologic effects of glucocorticosteroids. J Gen Intern Med 1991;6:367–377.
34. Hohlfeld R, Michels M, Heininger K, et al: Azathioprine toxicity during long-term immunosuppression of generalized myasthenia gravis. Neurology 1988;38:258–261.
35. Kissel JT, Levy RJ, Mendell JR, Griggs RC: Azathioprine toxicity in neuromuscular disease. Neurology 1986;36:35–39.
36. Lockshin MD, Kagen LJ: Meningitic reactions after azathioprine. N Engl J Med 1972;286:1321–1322.
37. Fishbain JT, Monahan TP, Canonico MM: Cerebral manifestations of cefepime toxicity in a dialysis patient. Neurology 2000;55:1756–1757.
38. Herishanu YO, Zlotnik M, Mostoslavsky M, et al: Cefuroxime-induced encephalopathy. Neurology 1998;50:1873–1875.
39. Thomas RJ: Neurotoxicity of antibacterial therapy. South Med J 1994;87:869–874.
40. Dixit S, Kurle P, Buyan-Dent L, et al: Status epilepticus associated with cefepime. Neurology 2000;54:2153–2155.
41. Tesio L, Bassi L, Strada L: Spinal cord lesion after penicillin gluteal injection. Paraplegia 1992;30:442–444.
42. River Y, Averbuch-Heller L, Weinberger M, et al: Antibiotic induced meningitis. J Neurol Neurosurg Psychiatry 1994;57:705–708.
43. Fischel-Ghodsian N: Genetic factors in aminoglycoside toxicity. Ann NY Acad Sci 1999;884:99–109.
44. Duan M, Agerman K, Ernfors P, et al: Complementary roles of neurotrophin 3 and a *N*-methyl-D-aspartate antagonist in the protection of noise and aminoglycoside-induced ototoxicity. Proc Natl Acad Sci USA 2000;97:7597–7602.
45. Sha SH, Schacht J: Are aminoglycoside antibiotics excitotoxic? Neuroreport 1998;9:3893–3895.
46. Lortholary O, Tod M, Cohen Y, Petitjean O: Aminoglycosides. Med Clin North Am 1995;79:761–787.
47. Halkin H: Adverse effects of the fluoroquinolones. Rev Infect Dis 1988;10:S258–S261.
48. Semel JD, Allen N: Seizures in patients simultaneously receiving theophylline and imipenem or ciprofloxacin or metronidazole. South Med J 1991;84:465–468.
49. Sacristan JA, Soto JA, de Cos MA: Erythromycin-induced hypoacusis: 11 new cases and literature review. Ann Pharmacother 1993;27:950–955.
50. Mamikoglu B, Mamikoglu O: Irreversible sensorineural hearing loss as a result of azithromycin ototoxicity. A case report. Ann Otol Rhinol Laryngol 2001;110:102.
51. Lo SH, Kotabe S, Mitsunaga L: Azithromycin-induced hearing loss. Am J Health Syst Pharm 1999;56:380–383.
52. Warner A: Clarithromycin—a precipitant for acute psychotic stress. Psychosomatics 2000;41:539.
53. Klein NC, Cunha BA: Tetracyclines. Med Clin North Am 1995;79: 789–801.
54. Wallace KL: Antibiotic-induced convulsions. Crit Care Clin 1997;13:741–762.
55. Holdiness MR: Neurological manifestations and toxicities of the antituberculosis drugs. A review. Med Toxicol 1987;2:33–51.
56. Tsai RK, Lee YH: Reversibility of ethambutol optic neuropathy. J Ocular PharmTher 1997;13(5):473–477.
57. Heng JE, Vorwerk CK, Lessell E, et al: Ethambutol is toxic to retinal ganglion cells via an excitotoxic pathway. Invest Ophthalmol Visual Sci 1999;40:190–196.
58. Walker RW, Rosenblum MK: Amphotericin B–associated leukoencephalopathy. Neurology 1992;42:2005–2010.
59. Phillips-Howard PA, ter Kuile FO: CNS adverse events associated with antimalarial agents. Fact or fiction? Drug Saf 1995;12:370–383.
60. Stenzel MS, Carpenter CC: The management of the clinical complications of antiretroviral therapy. Infect Dis Clin North Am 2000; 14:851–878.
61. Manji H: Neuropathy in HIV infection. Curr Opin Neurol 2000;13: 589–592.
62. Verma A, Schein RM, Jayaweera DT, et al: Fulminant neuropathy and lactic acidosis associated with nucleoside analog therapy. Neurology 1999;53:1365–1367.
63. Raffi R, Musini JM, Reliquet V, et al: Peripheral neuropathy during stavudine-didanosine combination therapy (QUINTET Trial). Meeting Abstracts 1998;12:93.
64. Shaikh S, Ta C, Basham AA, et al: Leber hereditary optic neuropathy associated with antiretroviral therapy for human immunodeficiency virus infection. Am J Ophthalmol 2001;131:143–145.
65. Weiss HD, Walker MD, Wiernik PH: Neurotoxicity of commonly used antineoplastic agents (second of two parts). N Engl J Med 1974;291:127–133.
66. Macdonald DR: Neurologic complications of chemotherapy. Neurol Clin 1991;9:955–967.
67. Kosirog-Glowacki JL, Bressler LR: Cyclophosphamide-induced facial discomfort. Ann Pharmacother 1994;28:197–199.
68. Morgenstern LB, Pardo CA: Progressive multifocal leukoencephalopathy complicating treatment for Wegener's granulomatosis. J Rheumatol 1995;22:1593–1595.
69. Miller LJ, Eaton VE: Ifosfamide-induced neurotoxicity: A case report and review of the literature. Ann Pharmacother 1992;26:183–187.
70. Merimsky O, Reider-Groswasser I, Wigler N, Chaitchik S: Encephalopathy in ifosfamide-treated patients. Acta Neurol Scand 1992;86: 521–525.
71. Meanwell CA, Blake AE, Latief TN, et al: Encephalopathy associated with ifosphamide/mesna therapy. Lancet 1985;1:406–407.
72. Simonian NA, Gilliam FG, Chiappa KH: Ifosfamide causes a diazepam-sensitive encephalopathy. Neurology 1993;43:2700–2702.
73. Wengs WJ, Talwar D, Bernard J: Ifosfamide-induced nonconvulsive status epilepticus. Arch Neurol 1993;50:1104–1105.
74. Davies SM, Pearson AD, Craft AW: Toxicity of high-dose ifosfamide in children. Cancer Chemother Pharmacol 1989;24(Suppl 1):S8–S10.
75. Sponzilli EE, Smith JK, Malamud N, McCulloch JR: Progressive multifocal leukoencephalopathy: A complication of immunosuppressive treatment. Neurology 1975;25:664–668.
76. Gutin PH, Levi JA, Wiernik PH, Walker MD: Treatment of malignant meningeal disease with intrathecal thioTEPA: A phase II study. Cancer Treat Rep 1977;61:885–887.
77. Murphy CP, Harden EA, Thompson JM: Generalized seizures secondary to high-dose busulfan therapy. Ann Pharmacother 1992;26:30–31.
78. Weiss HD, Walker MD, Wiernik PH: Neurotoxicity of commonly used antineoplastic agents (first of two parts). N Engl J Med 1974;291:75–81.
79. Shapiro WR, Young DF: Neurological complications of antineoplastic therapy. Acta Neurol Scand Suppl 1984;100:125–132.
80. Franco DA, Greenburg HS: 5-FU multifocal inflammatory leukoencephalopathy and dihydropyrimidine dehydrogenase deficiency. Neurology 2001;56:110–112.
81. El Amrani M, Heinzlef O, Debroucker T, et al: Brain infarction following 5-fluorouracil and cisplatin therapy. Neurology 1998;51:899–901.
82. Baker WJ, Royer GL Jr, Weiss RB: Cytarabine and neurologic toxicity. J Clin Oncol 1991;9:679–693.
83. ldebrandt G, Holler E, Woenkhaus M, et al: Acute deterioration of Charcot-Marie-Tooth disease 1A (CMT 1A) following 2 mg of vincristine chemotherapy. Ann Oncol 2000;11:743–747.
84. Wald JJ: The effects of toxins on muscle. Neurol Clin 2000;18:695–718.
85. George KK, Pourmand R: Toxic myopathies. Neurol Clin 1997;15:711–730.
86. Feinberg WM, Swenson MR: Cerebrovascular complications of L-asparaginase therapy. Neurology 1988;38:127–133.
87. Pace MT, Slovis TL, Kelly JK, Abella SD: Cyclosporin A toxicity: MRI appearance of the brain. Pediatr Radiol 1995;25:180–183.
88. Chen YC, Chao TY, Chen CY, Ho CL: Cyclosporine-induced encephalopathy in a patient with relapsed acute myeloid leukemia treated with unrelated allogeneic bone marrow transplantation. J Formos Med Assoc 2000;99:248–251.
89. Gopal AK, Thorning DR, Back AL: Fatal outcome due to cyclosporine neurotoxicity with associated pathological findings. Bone Marrow Transplant 1999;23:191–193.

90. Shah AK: Cyclosporine A neurotoxicity among bone marrow transplant recipients. Clin Neuropharmacol 1999;22:67–73.
91. Shbarou RM, Chao NJ, Morgenlander JC: Cyclosporin A-related cerebral vasculopathy. Bone Marrow Transplant 2000;26:801–804.
92. Wijdicks EF, Wiesner RH, Krom RA: Neurotoxicity in liver transplant recipients with cyclosporine immunosuppression. Neurology 1995;45:1962–1964.
93. Breil M, Chariot P: Muscle disorders associated with cyclosporine treatment. Muscle Nerve 1999;22:1631–1636.
94. Hong JC, Kahan BD: Immunosuppressive agents in organ transplantation: Past, present, and future. Sem Nephrol 2000;20:108–125.
95. Parvex P, Pinsk M, Bell LE, et al: Reversible encephalopathy associated with tacrolimus in pediatric renal transplants. Pediatr Nephrol 2001;16:537–542.
96. Mueller AR, Platz KP, Schattenfroh N, Bechstein WO, Christe W, Neuhaus P: Neurotoxicity after orthotopic liver transplantation in cyclosporin A- and FK 506-treated patients. Transpl Int 1994;7(Suppl 1):S37–S42.
97. Neuhaus P, McMaster P, Calne R, et al: Neurological complications in the European multicentre study of FK 506 and cyclosporin in primary liver transplantation. Transpl Int 1994;7(Suppl 1):S27–S31.
98. Bechstein WO: Neurotoxicity of calcineurin inhibitors: Impact and clinical management. Transpl Int 2000;13:313–326.
99. Misawa A, Takeuchi Y, Hibi S, Todo S, Imashuku S, Sawada T: FK506-induced intractable leukoencephalopathy following allogeneic bone marrow transplantation. Bone Marrow Transplant 2000;25:331–334.
100. Furukawa M, Terae S, Chu BC, Kaneko K, Kamada H, Miyasaka K: MRI in seven cases of tacrolimus (FK-506) encephalopathy: Utility of FLAIR and diffusion-weighted imaging. Neuroradiology 2001;43:615–621.
101. Suzuki Y, Ueda H, Toribe Y, Ida S: Mesial temporal lobe epilepsy in a patient with Wilson's disease receiving FK506 (tacrolimus) after liver transplantation. No To Hattatsu 2001;33:342–346.
102. Mori A, Tanaka J, Kobayashi S, et al: Fatal cerebral hemorrhage associated with cyclosporin-A/FK506-related encephalopathy after allogeneic bone marrow transplantation. Ann Hematol 2000;79:588–592.
103. Laham G, Vilches A, Jost L, Nogues M: Acute peripheral demyelinating polyneuropathy and acute renal failure after administration of FK506. Medicina (B Aires) 2001;61:445–446.
104. Boukriche Y, Brugiere O, Castier Y, Stocco J, Mal H, Fournier M: Severe axonal polyneuropathy after a FK506 overdosage in a lung transplant recipient. Transplantation 2001;72:1849–1850.
105. Piltz JR, Wertenbaker C, Lance SE, et al: Digoxin toxicity. Recognizing the varied visual presentations. J Clin Neuroophthalmol 1993;13:275–280.
106. Dahlof C, Dimenas E: Side effects of beta-blocker treatments as related to the central nervous system. Am J Med Sci 1990;299:236–244.
107. Terland O, Flatmark T: Drug-induced parkinsonism: Cinnarizine and flunarizine are potent uncouplers of the vaculoar h+-ATPase in catecholamine storage vesicles. Neuropharmacol 1999;38:879–882.
108. Daniel JR, Mauro VF: Extrapyramidal symptoms associated with calcium-channel blockers. Ann Pharmacother 1995;29:73–75.
109. Garcia-Ruiz PJ, Garcia de Yebenes J, Jimenez-Jimenez FJ, et al: Parkinsonism associated with calcium channel blockers: A prospective follow-up study. Clin Neuropharmacol 1992;15:19–26.
110. Gengo FM, Gabos C: Central nervous system considerations in the use of beta-blockers, angiotensin-converting enzyme inhibitors, and thiazide diuretics in managing essential hypertension. Am Heart J 1988;116:305–310.
111. Christiansen I, Iversen HK, Olesen J: Headache characteristics during the development of tolerance to nitrates: Pathophysiological implications. Cephalalgia 2000;20:437–444.
112. Abrams J: Nitrates. Med Clin North Am 1988;72:1–35.
113. Werner EG, Olanow CW: Parkinsonism and amiodarone therapy. Ann Neurol 1989;25:630–632.
114. Greenblatt DJ, Bolognini V, Koch-Weser J, Harmatz JS: Pharmacokinetic approach to the clinical use of lidocaine intravenously. JAMA 1976;236:273–277.
115. Fisher CM: Visual disturbances associated with quinidine and quinine. Neurology 1981;31:1569–1571.
116. Gilbert GJ: Quinidine dementia. JAMA 1977;237:2093–2094.
117. Nehlig A, Daval JL, Debry G: Caffeine and the central nervous system: Mechanisms of action, biochemical, metabolic and psychostimulant effects. Brain Res Brain Res Rev 1992;17:139–170.
118. Hughes JR: Clinical importance of caffeine withdrawal. N Engl J Med 1992;327:1160–1161.
119. Appel CC, Myles TD: Caffeine-induced hypokalemic paralysis in pregnancy. Obstet Gynecol 2001;97:805–807.
120. Pomerleau OF: Nicotine and the central nervous system: Biobehavioral effects of cigarette smoking. Am J Med 1992;93:2S–7S.
121. Yokota T, Kagamihara Y, Hayashi H, et al: Nicotine-sensitive paresis. Neurology 1992;42:382–388.
122. Pereira CB, Strupp M, Holzleitner T, Brandt T: Smoking and balance: Correlation of nicotine-induced nystagmus and postural body sway. Neuroreport 2001;12:1223–1226.
123. Mellick LB, Makowski T, Mellick GA, Borger R: Neuromuscular blockade after ingestion of tree tobacco (*Nicotiana glauca*). Ann Emerg Med 1999;34:101–104.
124. Diploma JR, Ritchie DM: Vitamin toxicity. Annu Rev Pharmacol Toxicol 1977;17:133–148.
125. Barness LA: Adverse effects of overdosage of vitamins and minerals. Pediatr Rev 1986;8:20–24.
126. Pappert EJ, Tangney CC, Goetz CG, et al: Alpha-tocopherol in the ventricular cerebrospinal fluid of Parkinson's disease patients: Dose response study and correlation with plasma levels. Neurology 1996;47:1037–1042.
127. Chang GY: Acute Wernicke's syndrome mimicking brainstem stroke. Eur Neurol 2000;43:246–247.
128. Koike H, Misu K, Hattori N, et al: Postgastrectomy polyneuropathy with thiamine deficiency. J Neurol Neurosurg Psychiatry 2001;71:357–362.
129. Hung SC, Hung SH, Tarng DC, Yang WC, Huang TP: Chorea induced by thiamine deficiency in hemodialysis patients. Am J Kidney Dis 2001;37:427–430.
130. Merkin-Zaborsky H, Ifergane G, Frisher S, Valdman S, Herishanu Y, Wirguin I: Thiamine-responsive acute neurological disorders in nonalcoholic patients. Eur Neurol 2001;45:34–37.
131. Toth C, Voll C: Wernicke's encephalopathy following gastroplasty for morbid obesity. Can J Neurol Sci 2001;28:89–92.
132. D'Aprile P, Tarantino A, Santoro N, Carella A: Wernicke's encephalopathy induced by total parenteral nutrition in patient with acute leukaemia: Unusual involvement of caudate nuclei and cerebral cortex on MRI. Neuroradiol 2000;42:781–783.
133. Sparacia G, Banco A, Lagalla R: Reversible MRI abnormalities in an unusual paediatric presentation of Wernicke's encephalopathy. Pediatr Radiol 1999;29:581–584.
134. Hellgren M, Svensson PJ, Dahlback B: Resistance to activated protein C as a basis for venous thromboembolism associated with pregnancy and oral contraceptives. Am J Obstet Gynecol 1995;173:210–213.
135. Nausieda PA, Koller WC, Weiner WJ, Klawans HL: Chorea induced by oral contraceptives. Neurology 1979;29:1605–1609.
136. Andonopoulos AP, Terzis E, Tsibri E, et al: D-Penicillamine induced myasthenia gravis in rheumatoid arthritis: An unpredictable common occurrence? Clin Rheumatol 1994;13:586–588.
137. Sonoda Y, Gotow T, Kuriyama M, et al: Electrical myotonia of rabbit skeletal muscles by HMG-CoA reductase inhibitors. Muscle Nerve 1994;17:891–897.
138. Wald JJ: The effects of toxins on muscle. Neurol Clin 2000;18:695–718.
139. George KK, Pourmand R: Toxic myopathies. Neurol Clin 1997;15: 711–730.
140. Brillman J: Central nervous system complications in coronary artery bypass graft surgery. Neurol Clin 1993;11:475–495.
141. Trehan N, Mishra M, Sharma OP, Mishra A, Kasliwal RR: Further reduction in stroke after off-pump coronary artery bypass grafting: A 10-year experience. Ann Thorac Surg 2001;72:S1026–S1032.
142. Furlan AJ, Sila CA, Chimowitz MI, Jones SC: Neurologic complications related to cardiac surgery. Neurol Clin 1992;10:145–166.
143. Shaw PJ, Bates D, Cartlidge NE, et al: An analysis of factors predisposing to neurological injury in patients undergoing coronary bypass operations. Q J Med 1989;72:633–646.
144. Farooq MM, Reil TD, Gelabert HA, et al: Combined carotid endarterectomy and coronary bypass: Adecade experience at UCLA. Cardiovasc Surg 2001;9:339–344.
145. Yoon BW, Bae HJ, Kang DW, et al: Intracranial cerebral artery disease as a risk factor for central nervous system complications of coronary artery bypass graft surgery. Stroke 2001;32:94–99.
146. Newman MF, Kirchner JL, Phillips-Bute B, et al: Longitudinal assessment of neurocognitive function after coronary-artery bypass surgery. N Engl J Med 2001;344:395–402.
147. Lederman RJ, Breuer AC, Hanson MR, et al: Peripheral nervous system complications of coronary artery bypass graft surgery. Ann Neurol 1982;12:297–301.

148. Hotson JR, Enzmann DR: Neurologic complications of cardiac transplantation. Neurol Clin 1988;6:349–365.
149. Sheline GE, Wara WM, Smith V: Therapeutic irradiation and brain injury. Int J Radiat Oncol Biol Phys 1980;6:1215–1228.
150. Gutin PH, Leibel SA, Sheline GE: Radiation Injury to the Nervous System. New York, Raven Press, 1991.
151. Tsuruda JS, Kortman KE, Bradley WG, et al: Radiation effects on cerebral white matter: MR evaluation. Am J Roentgenol 1987; 149:165–171.
152. Doyle WK, Budinger TF, Valk PE, et al: Differentiation of cerebral radiation necrosis from tumor recurrence by [18F]FDG and 82Rb positron emission tomography. J Comput Assist Tomogr 1987;11:563–570.
153. New P: Radiation injury to the nervous system. Curr Opin Neurol 2001;14:725–734.
154. Allen JC, Miller DC, Budzilovich GN, Epstein FJ: Brain and spinal cord hemorrhage in long-term survivors of malignant pediatric brain tumors: A possible late effect of therapy. Neurology 1991;41:148–150.
155. Edwards KM, Karzon DT: Pertussis vaccines. Pediatr Clin North Am 1990;37:549–566.
156. Barlow WE, Davis RL, Glasser JW, et al: The risk of seizures after receipt of whole-cell pertussis or measles, mumps, and rubella vaccine. N Engl J Med 2001;345:656–661.
157. Safranek TJ, Lawrence DN, Kurland LT, et al: Reassessment of the association between Guillain-Barré syndrome and receipt of swine influenza vaccine in 1976–1977: Results of a two-state study. Expert Neurology Group. Am J Epidemiol 1991;133:940–951.
158. Peltola H, Heinonen OP: Frequency of true adverse reactions to measles-mumps-rubella vaccine. A double-blind placebo-controlled trial in twins. Lancet 1986;1:939–942.
159. Stratton KR, Howe CJ, Johnston RB Jr: Adverse events associated with childhood vaccines other than pertussis and rubella. Summary of a report from the Institute of Medicine. JAMA 1994;271:1602–1605.
160. Miller E, Waight P, Farrington CP, Andrews N, Stowe J, Taylor B: Idiopathic thrombocytopenic purpura and MMR vaccine. Arch Dis Child 2001;84:227–229.
161. Patja A, Paunio M, Kinnunen E, Junttila O, Hovi T, Peltola H: Risk of Guillain-Barré syndrome after measles-mumps-rubella vaccination. J Pediatr 2001;138:250–254.
162. Shoenfeld Y, Aron-Maor A: Vaccination and autoimmunity—"vaccinosis": A dangerous liaison? J Autoimmun 2000;14:1–10.
163. Howson CP, Fineberg HV: Adverse events following pertussis and rubella vaccines. Summary of a report of the Institute of Medicine. JAMA 1992;267:392–396.
164. Edwardes M, Baltzan M: MMR immunization and autism. JAMA 2001;285:2852–2853.
165. Kaye JA, del Mar Melero-Montes M, Jick H: Mumps, measles, and rubella vaccine and the incidence of autism recorded by general practitioners: A time trend analysis. BMJ 2001;322:460–463.
166. Fombonne E, Chakrabarti S: No evidence for a new variant of measles-mumps-rubella-induced autism. Pediatrics 2001;108:E58.
167. Farrington CP, Miller E, Taylor B: MMR and autism: Further evidence against a causal association. Vaccine 2001;19:3632–3635.
168. Gustafsson L, Hallander HO, Olin P, Reizenstein E, Storsaeter J: A controlled trial of a two-component acellular, a five-component acellular, and a whole-cell pertussis vaccine. N Engl J Med 1996;334: 349–355.
169. Rosenbaum RB, Donaldson JO: Peripheral nerve and neuromuscular disorders. Neurol Clin 1994;12:461–478.
170. Fox MW, Harms RW, Davis DH: Selected neurologic complications of pregnancy. Mayo Clin Proc 1990;65:1595–1618.
171. Hoffman MS, Roberts WS, Cavanagh D: Neuropathies associated with radical pelvic surgery for gynecologic cancer. Gynecol Oncol 1988;31:462–466.
172. Georgiou A, Grigsby PW, Perez CA: Radiation induced lumbosacral plexopathy in gynecologic tumors: Clinical findings and dosimetric analysis. Int J Radiat Oncol Biol Phys 1993;26:479–482.
173. Hund EF, Fogel W, Krieger D, et al: Critical illness polyneuropathy: Clinical findings and outcomes of a frequent cause of neuromuscular weaning failure. Crit Care Med 1996;24:1328–1333.
174. Zochodne DW, Bolton CF, Wells GA, et al: Critical illness polyneuropathy. A complication of sepsis and multiple organ failure. Brain 1987;110:819–841.

Index

Note: Page numbers followed by the letter f refer to figures; page numbers followed by the letter t refer to tables.

C

H

M

T

U

V

W

X

systematized or fragmentary, and the content may be variable, but persecutory delusions are most common.

Schizophrenia is the most common psychotic illness, and in the United States there is a 1 to 1.5 percent lifetime prevalence of this disorder. The disorder is equally prevalent in men and women and tends to occur more frequently in urban populations and in lower socioeconomic groups. The peak age of onset in men is 15 to 25, while in women the peak occurs at 25 to 35 years of age. Numerous studies suggest that the inheritance of schizophrenia has a genetic component, which is most likely polygenetic. Certain genetic abnormalities have been found that cause specific schizophrenic syndromes. Fifty percent of monozygotic twins of schizophrenics develop the disorder compared with 10 percent of dizygotic twins. The diagnosis of schizophrenia is a clinical diagnosis because there are no pathognomonic findings. At present, two or more of the following features must be present for a significant period of time during a 1-month period: delusions, hallucinations, disorganized speech, grossly disorganized or catatonic behavior, and negative symptoms. Only one of these is required if delusions are bizarre, if hallucinations consist of a voice keeping up a running commentary, or if two or more voices are conversing with each other. There are five subtypes of schizophrenia including paranoid, disorganized, catatonic, undifferentiated, and residual types.[1, 26]

Schizophrenia is a chronic disorder, but many of the dramatic and acute symptoms subside over time. Most patients have low-level delusions and hallucinations and end up in psychiatric hospitals or supervised shelters. There is an improved prognosis when the onset occurs after age 30 and the active psychotic symptoms have a rapid onset. Additionally, good premorbid social and occupational function, the presence of a probable precipitant, and the absence of a family history are associated with an improved outcome. Although genetic abnormalities have been clearly implicated, the neurobiology of schizophrenia has not been categorized. Unlike neurodegenerative disorders such as Parkinson's disease and Alzheimer's disease, schizophrenia appears to reach a plateau. Many researchers believe that schizophrenia represents a neurodevelopmental disorder rather than a neuronal degeneration. It is associated with mild but consistent MRI changes. Until recently schizophrenia has been hypothesized to be largely a dopaminergic disorder, but recent focus has shifted to a broader pharmacologic theory including glutamate, serotonin, and norepinephrine. No convincing evidence of primary abnormalities in any of these neurochemical systems has been developed.

Schizophrenia should be differentiated from other primary psychiatric disorders that may have psychosis as a feature, including schizoaffective disorder, the major affective disorders, autism, malingering, and obsessive-compulsive disorder. Symptoms of psychosis can be caused by a large number of medical and neurological conditions and may be precipitated by legal and illicit drugs (Table 3–3). Psychosis and other psychiatric symptoms may present early in the course of medical or neurological disorders, and the clinician must consider this in the differential diagnosis. Of note, a significant link has been established between temporal lobe tumors and psychosis, even if patients with epilepsy are not considered. Tumors of the limbic system, particularly the cingulate gyrus, amygdala-hippocampal region, and the area around the third ventricle, are also commonly associated with psychotic behaviors. Typically, patients with organic causes of psychosis have a higher amount of insight into the illness and are distressed by their symptoms. Clinicians should be aggressive in pursuing a medical or neurological cause of psychosis in patients with no diagnosed psychiatric disease, particularly if there are unusual symptoms, altered consciousness, or concomitant medical or neurological signs. Additionally, a concomitant medical or neurological condition may cause an exacerbation or recrudescence of psychosis in patients with an established psychiatric disease. Neither infarcts nor hemorrhages cause psychosis, so acute-onset psychotic syndromes in the elderly should not be blamed on vascular events.

TABLE 3–3. **Differential Diagnosis of Psychosis**

Infections
Acquired immunodeficiency syndrome (AIDS)
Creutzfeldt-Jakob disease
Herpes encephalitis
Neurosyphilis

Structural
Neoplasm
Trauma
Normal pressure hydrocephalus

Toxins
Heavy metals
Carbon monoxide

Nutritional
Vitamin B_{12} deficiency
Pellagra

Hereditodegenerative
Cerebral lipidoses
Fabry's disease
Fahr's disease
Hallervorden-Spatz disease
Homocystinuria
Huntington's disease
Diffuse Lewy body disease
Metachromatic leukodystrophy
Lafora's disease
Wilson's disease

Drugs
Amphetamines
Anticholinergics
Levodopa
Dopaminergics
Deprenyl
Alcohol
Barbiturate withdrawal
Cocaine
Phencyclidine

Other
Epilepsy

APATHY SYNDROMES

Patients with apathy demonstrate a lack of interest not only in their usual interests and hobbies but also in routine daily activities. Apathy may arise from unilateral or bilateral lesions of the caudate nuclei, bilateral lesions in the lenticular nuclei, or frontal lobe lesions. Apathy is a common aspect